To access your Student Resources, visit the Web address below:

http://evolve.elsevier.com/Nagelhout/anesthesia/

Evolve Learning Resources for Nagelhout/Zaglaniczny: Nurse Anesthesia, 3rd edition offers the following features:

- **WebLinks**
  An exciting resource that lets you link to hundreds of websites carefully chosen to supplement the content of the textbook. The WebLinks are regularly updated, with new ones added as they develop.

- **Case Studies**
  Actual case scenarios designed to apply knowledge and stimulate critical thinking.

Nurse Anesthesia

Nurse Anesthesia

Third Edition

John J. Nagelhout, PhD, CRNA
Director, School of Anesthesia
Kaiser Permanente/California State University, Fullerton
Southern California Permanente Medical Group
Pasadena, California

Karen L. Zaglaniczny, PhD, CRNA, FAAN
Director, Perioperative Services Education and Research
Director, Graduate Program of Nurse Anesthesia
William Beaumont Hospital
Royal Oak, Michigan

With 493 Illustrations

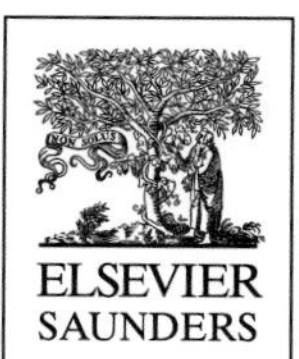

ELSEVIER
SAUNDERS

11830 Westline Industrial Drive
St. Louis, Missouri 63146

NURSE ANESTHESIA 0-7216-0363-7

Notice

Anesthesia is an ever-changing field. Standard safety precautions must be followed, but as new research and clinical experience broaden our knowledge, changes in treatment and drug therapy may become necessary or appropriate. Readers are advised to check the most current product information provided by the manufacturer of each drug to be administered to verify the recommended dose, the method and duration of administration, and contraindications. It is the responsibility of the licensed prescriber, relying on experience and knowledge of the patient, to determine dosages and the best treatment for each individual patient. Neither the publisher nor the author assumes any liability for any injury and/or damage to persons or property arising from this publication.

Previous editions copyrighted 2001, 1997

International Standard Book Number 0-7216-0363-7

Executive Editor: Michael Ledbetter
Senior Developmental Editor: Lisa P. Newton
Publishing Services Manager: Catherine Albright Jackson
Senior Project Manager: Celeste Clingan
Design Project Manager: Bill Drone

Printed in United States of America

Last digit is the print number: 9 8 7 6 5 4 3 2

Contributors

John Aker, CRNA, MS
Co-Chief Nurse Anesthetist
Department of Anesthesia
University of Iowa
Iowa City, Iowa

Charles R. Barton, MSN, MEd, CRNA
Director, Graduate Anesthesia Program
College of Nursing
University of Akron
Akron, Ohio;
Chairman, CRNA Liaison Committee
International Trauma Anesthesia and Critical Care Society
Baltimore, Maryland

Donald M. Bell, CRNA, DNSc
Assistant Professor of Nurse Anesthesia
Associate Director for Didactic Education
Nurse Anesthesia Concentration
The University of Tennessee – College of Nursing
Knoxville, Tennessee

Chuck Biddle, CRNA, PhD
Professor
Department of Nurse Anesthesia
Virginia Commonwealth University
Richmond, Virginia

Michael Boytim, CRNA, MN
Assistant Director
Kaiser Permanente School of Anesthesia
California State University, Fullerton
Pasadena, California

Charlene V. Brouillette, CRNA, MS, APRN
Instructor, Nurse Anesthesia Program
Louisiana State University Health Sciences Center
New Orleans, Louisiana

Richard J. Brown, CRNA, PhD
Assistant Professor and Program Director
Nurse Anesthesia Specialization
University of North Dakota
Grand Forks, North Dakota

Joseph F. Burkard, DNSc, CRNA
Clinical Research Coordinator
Navy Nurse Corps Anesthesia Program
San Diego, California

Anthony Chipas, CRNA, PhD
Program Director and Associate Professor
Medical University of South Carolina
Charleston, South Carolina

Gary D. Clark, CRNA, EdD
Associate Professor and Coordinator of Special Projects
Department of Biological Sciences
Associate Program Director
MS in Nurse Anesthesia Program
Webster University
St. Louis, Missouri

Angela Darsey, MN, CRNA
Medical College of Georgia
Augusta, Georgia

Lyle C. Dorman, MSN, CRNA
Certified Registered Nurse Anesthetist
Anesthesia and Pain Medicine Associates of Augusta, Georgia
Augusta, Georgia

Michael P. Dosch, CRNA, MS
Program Director
University of Detroit Mercy Graduate Program in Nurse Anesthesiology
Detroit, Michigan

Sass Elisha, CRNA, MSN
Assistant Professor
Kaiser Permanente School of Anesthesia
California State University, Fullerton
Pasadena, California

Wayne E. Ellis, PhD, CRNA
Director, Program in Anesthesia
Trover Foundation – Murray State University
Madisonville, Kentucky

Ladan Eshkevari, CRNA, MS, Dipl Ac
Assistant Professor of Nurse Anesthesia
School of Nursing and Health Studies
Georgetown University
Washington, DC

Michael D. Fallacaro, DNSc, CRNA
Professor and Chairman
Department of Nurse Anesthesia
Virginia Commonwealth University
Richmond, Virginia

Nadine A. Fallacaro, MS, CRNA
Clinical Assistant Professor
Department of Nurse Anesthesia
Virginia Commonwealth University
Richmond, Virginia

Margaret Faut-Callahan, CRNA, DNSc, FAAN
Professor and Chair, Adult Health Nursing
Director, Nurse Anesthesia Program
Rush University, College of Nursing
Chicago, Illinois

Michael A. Fiedler, PhD, CRNA
Associate Professor and Chair
Department of Nurse Anesthesia
Ida V. Moffett School of Nursing
Samford University
Birmingham, Alabama

Francis Gerbasi, CRNA, PhD
Director of Accreditation and Education
American Association of Nurse Anesthetists
Park Ridge, Illinois

Silas N. Glisson, PhD
Professor
Department of Anesthesiology
Northwestern University
Feinberg School of Medicine
Chicago, Illinois

Ira P. Gunn, MLN, CRNA, FAAN
LTC, United States Army—Retired
Consultant
Nurse Anesthesia Affairs
El Paso, Texas

Richard E. Haas, EdM, MS, CRNA
Assistant Professor
Nursing Anesthesia Program
Medical College of Georgia
Augusta, Georgia

Walter R. Hand, Jr., CRNA, DNSc
Contact Nurse Anesthetist
Womack Army Medical Center
Fayetteville, North Carolina

Don R. Hill, MN, CRNA
Staff CRNA
The Medical Center of Central Georgia
Macon, Georgia

Betty J. Horton, CRNA, DNSc
Director of Accreditation and Education (Retired)
American Association of Nurse Anesthetists
Council on Accreditation of Nurse Anesthesia Educational Programs
Park Ridge, Illinois

Donna M. Jasinski, DNSc, CRNA
Associate Professor and Program Director
School of Nursing and Health Studies
Georgetown University
Washington, DC

Joseph Anthony Joyce, CRNA
Staff Nurse Anesthetist
Wesley Long Community Hospital
Moses Cone Health System
Greensboro, North Carolina

Mary Karlet, CRNA, PhD
Director, Nurse Anesthesia Program
Duke University
Durham, North Carolina

Mark A. Kossick, DNSc, CRNA
Director, Nurse Anesthesia Program
Associate Professor
University of Maryland School of Nursing
Baltimore, Maryland

Jeanne B. Learman, CRNA, MS
Anesthesia Department Manager
Eaton Rapids Medical Center
Eaton Rapids, Michigan;
Anesthesia Department Manager
Clinton Memorial Hospital
St. Johns, Michigan

Julie Ann Lowery, CRNA, MS
Department of Anesthesia
University of North Carolina
Chapel Hill,
North Carolina

Rex Marley, MS, CRNA, RRT
Staff Nurse Anesthetist
Northern Colorado Anesthesia Professional Consultants
Fort Collins, Colorado

Denise Martin-Sheridan, CRNA, PhD
Professor and Associate Graduate Director
Center for Nurse Anesthesiology
Albany Medical College
Albany, New York

John P. McDonough, CRNA, EdD, ARNP
Professor and Director,
Anesthesiology Nursing
Florida International University
Miami, Florida

Elizabeth Monti-Seibert, MSN, CRNA
Director of Clinical Education
Department of Nurse Anesthesia
Virginia Commonwealth University
Richmond, Virginia

Sonja J. Myers, CRNA, MS
Clinical Preceptor
Nurse Anesthesiology Program
Center for Nurse Anesthesiology
Albany Medical College;
Staff Anesthetist
Department of Anesthesiology
Albany Medical Center
Albany, New York

John J. Nagelhout, PhD, CRNA
Director, School of Anesthesia
Kaiser Permanente/California State University, Fullerton
Southern California Permanente Medical Group
Pasadena, California

R. Lee Olson, MS, CRNS
Deputy Director
Navy Nurse Corps Anesthesia Program
Bethesda, Maryland

Sandra M. Ouellette, CRNA, MEd, FAAN
Director, Nurse Anesthesia Program
Wake Forest University Baptist Medical Center
University of North Carolina – Greensboro
Winston-Salem, North Carolina

Sherry H. Owens, CRNA, MSN
Assistant Director,
Nurse Anesthesia Program
Wake Forest University Baptist Medical Center
Winston-Salem, North Carolina

Timothy J. Palmer, CRNA, MS
Anesthesia Education Coordinator
Clinical and Didactic Faculty
Oakland University Graduate Program of Nurse Anesthesia
William Beaumont Hospital
Royal Oak, Michigan

DeAnna Powell, MN, CRNA
Medical College of Georgia
Augusta, Georgia

Bernadette T. Roche, CRNA, EdD
Administrative Director
Evanston Northwestern Healthcare
School of Anesthesia
Evanston, Illinois;
Assistant Professor
DePaul University, Department
of Nursing
Chicago, Illinois

Allan J. Schwartz, CRNA, DDS
Independent Certified Registered Nurse Anesthetist
CRNA Services, P.C.
Columbia, Missouri

Brent Sommer, CRNA, MPHA
Assistant Professor and
Clinical Coordinator
Program of Nurse Anesthesia
Samuel Merritt College
Oakland, California;
Senior Anesthetist
The Permanente Medical Group, Inc.
Oakland, California

Julie A. Stone, EdD, CRNA
Assistant Professor
Director, MS in Nurse Anesthesia Program
Webster University
St. Louis, Missouri

Charles A. Vacchiano, PhD, CRNA
Specialty Advisor for Research,
Navy Nurse Corps
Director, Biomedical Sciences
Naval Aerospace Medical Research Laboratory
NAS Pensacola, Florida

Edward Waters, CRNA, MN
Instructor
Kaiser Permanente School of Anesthesia
California State University, Fullerton
Pasadena, California

Joe R. Williams, CRNA, MS
Director, Nurse Anesthesia Program
University of Alabama at Birmingham
Birmingham, Alabama

Wanda O. Wilson, CRNA, PhD
Associate Professor and Program Director
University of Cincinnati College of Nursing
Master's Program – Nurse Anesthesia Major;
Assistant Director – Anesthesia Services
Department of Anesthesia
University of Cincinnati Medical Center
Cincinnati, Ohio

E. Laura Wright, MNA, CRNA
Assistant Professor – Critical Care
Nurse Anesthesia Program
University of Alabama at Birmingham
Birmingham, Alabama

Karen L. Zaglaniczny, PhD, CRNA, FAAN
Director, Perioperative Services Education and
Research
Director, Graduate Program of Nurse Anesthesia
William Beaumont Hospital
Royal Oak, Michigan

Foreword

As a new century dawns, nurse anesthetists continue to provide the highest quality anesthesia services to their patients. To put this into perspective, consider that nurse anesthetists safely and compassionately administered anesthesia throughout the entire last century and even prior to that. The writings of Alice Magaw, published between 1899 and 1906, provide a noteworthy benchmark. Magaw detailed the use of chloroform and other anesthesia with the open-drop technique in more than 14,000 surgical cases without a single fatality attributable to anesthesia. She was the first nurse anesthetist to publish articles on the practice of anesthesia and was considered "the mother of anesthesia" during a time when surgeons selected nurses to specialize in anesthesia to provide greater safety for patients requiring anesthesia.

Many pharmacologic and technologic changes in anesthesia have occurred, however, since those noble beginnings. The chapter titles of this textbook serve as an atlas to this expanded knowledge base: "Clinical Monitoring in Anesthesia;" "Anesthesia Equipment;" "Pharmacokinetics;" "Inhalation Anesthetics;" "Intravenous Induction Agents;" "Local Anesthetics;" "Opioid Agonists and Antagonists;" and "Neuromuscular Blocking Agents, Reversal Agents, and Their Monitoring;" to name a few. Look at the specialty components of anesthesia contained in this book: "Cardiac Anesthesia," "Respiratory Anesthesia," "Thermal Injury and Anesthesia;" "Trauma Anesthesia;" "Outpatient Anesthesia;" "Regional Anesthesia;" "Anesthesia for Ophthalmic Procedures;" "Anesthesia and Orthopedics;" "Anesthesia for Ear, Nose, Throat, and Maxillofacial Surgery;" "Anesthesia and Laser Surgery;" and the list goes on. The continuum for practice in the 21st century is that of professionals learning anew how to ensure the best possible care for their patients.

When Agatha Hodgins and other nurse anesthetist pioneers gathered in a classroom in the anesthesia department of the University Hospital of Cleveland on June 17, 1931, they established what was to become the American Association of Nurse Anesthetists (AANA). This group sought to place better qualified people in the field, to keep those already in nurse anesthesia abreast of modern developments, and to give protection and recognition to this group of professionals.

When the AANA values statement was adopted in 1995, it was not surprising that it reflected this earlier philosophy. The AANA values the following:

- Its members and the advancement of the profession of nurse anesthesia
- Quality service to the public through diverse practice settings based on collaboration and personal choice
- Integrity, accountability, competence, and professional commitment
- Scientific inquiry and contributions to the fields of anesthesiology, nursing, and related disciplines
- Participation in the formation of health care policy.

These value statements are supported by knowledgeable practitioners ever in pursuit of their craft.

Nurse Anesthesia is a textbook that builds on a formidable knowledge base and draws on the expertise of CRNAs and other professionals practicing in today's fast-paced, ever-changing environment. I look upon this volume as a means to demonstrate the profession's growth and encourage CRNAs and student nurse anesthetists to read it and reflect upon the dynamic field they have chosen.

I would like to close with one of my favorite quotations from Ralph Waldo Emerson, which I believe reflects all professionals on their prospective journeys:

To laugh often and much, to win the respect of intelligent people . . .
To earn the appreciation of honest critics . . . , to find the best in
Others . . . , to leave the world a bit better. . . .

Bon voyage.

John F. Garde, CRNA, MS, FAAN

Preface to the Third Edition

The publication of this third edition of our textbook *Nurse Anesthesia* symbolizes several advances in the profession of nurse anesthesia and the practice of clinical anesthesia. As advance practice professionals, Nurse Anesthetists continue to lead nursing in their clinical expertise and contributions to the advancement of nursing research and education. Nurse Anesthetists maintain their tireless efforts at improving patient safety and satisfaction in light of the increasing complexity and demands of modern medical and surgical interventions.

This edition of our text reflects the advances and scope of modern anesthesia practice. In the few short years since the second edition was produced, several new areas required further discussion as well as extensive revisions to existing materials. New chapters on Chemistry and Physics and Anesthesia for Therapeutic and Diagnostic Procedures have been added. Anesthesia is no longer exclusively confined to the operating room. Increasingly, nurse anesthetists are providing anesthesia care in radiologic suites, various office-based settings, and non-hospital clinics. Changes in our approach to preoperative assessment, anesthesia management, and post-anesthesia recovery are consistently evolving as these new practice settings become more common. In addition, every chapter has undergone extensive revision to reflect the most recent scientific and clinical information available.

We are grateful to the returning and new authors and anesthesia experts who have joined us in producing this edition. They bring a wealth of experience and expertise in their particular areas. The broad range of knowledge enjoyed by nurse anesthetists is reflected in the diversity of subject matter and the in-depth coverage of the many facets of anesthesia. This text will be useful to both students and experienced practitioners. Basic factual material is included for nurses who are new to anesthesia as well as extensive discussions of the current approaches to anesthesia management and their scientific foundations for practicing nurse anesthetists.

As always, we have totally revised our companion handbook that accompanies this text. We have produced the handbook in three sections to include basic pathophysiology, surgical procedures, and drugs. Our intent is not to reproduce the material in this textbook but rather to provide complementary useful clinical information for the practicing clinician. We are very excited that there will also be a PDA version to accompany the textbook and handbook that will include useful calculators and clinical information, which can be accessed electronically in the operating room at a moment's notice.

Production of an educational resource of this size and complexity would not be possible without the efforts of many experts. First, we thank the authors for their expert contributions and the many hours they have spent researching, writing, and revising their chapters. We would like to express our sincere gratitude to Retta Smith who assisted in every aspect of the production and editing of the textbook. Special gratitude is expressed to the staff at Elsevier, including Michael Ledbetter, Lisa Newton, Catherine Jackson, and Celeste Clingan.

In the ten years since we have produced the first edition of this text we are consistently amazed and grateful for the professional contributions that Nurse Anesthetists make to academic medicine and nursing, clinical practice, and society as a whole. We are proud that this textbook has played a part in the continuous evolution of our specialty.

John J. Nagelhout
Karen L. Zaglaniczny

Preface to the Second Edition

The publication of the first edition of this text was a significant event in the professional evolution of certified registered nurse anesthetists. An array of nurse anesthetists pooled their knowledge and expertise to produce the first compendium of nurse anesthesia practice. The many diverse areas that influence our profession—including physiology, pharmacology, biochemistry, clinical and basic research, and clinical practice—are woven together into a comprehensive guide to modern clinical anesthesia. We are gratified by how the book has been received by the anesthesia community.

The second edition builds on previous strengths and includes extensive revisions that reflect the rapid changes occurring in anesthesia patient care. We increased the focus on clinically related issues to make the book even more useful to practitioners in their everyday practice. Chapters have been completely revamped and updated. Several chapters have been combined to allow for easier access to related information. The chapter on preoperative evaluation has been expanded to reflect the importance of this area to perioperative care. We have added new chapters on non–operating room and office anesthesia to reflect the broadening demands on anesthesia providers.

The production of a textbook of this magnitude is not possible without the dedication and hard work of many people. First, we would like to thank the authors, without whose thoughtful and expert contributions and dedication this book would not be possible. A special thanks to William Loechel, our illustrator. The hundreds of original medical drawings he produced for the first and second editions are a tribute to more than 50 years of study and experience in the field. As computers become the norm, the artistry of his hand drawings remains a testament to a lifetime of accomplishment and excellence. Special gratitude is expressed to the staff at Harcourt Health Sciences and W.B. Saunders, including Michael Ledbetter, Lisa Newton, Victoria Legnini, Thomas Eoyoung, Maura Conner, Catherine Jackson, and Jodi Everding. We would also like to thank Retta Smith and Emily Maclean for the hundreds of hours they spent helping prepare, edit, and proofread this text. Finally, we would like to thank our families and friends for their support throughout our careers, which has made production of this textbook possible.

John J. Nagelhout
Karen L. Zaglaniczny

Preface to the First Edition

Clinical anesthesia practice has evolved over the past 100 years into a specialty founded on scientific principles and focused on patient care. With the advancement of scientific technology and the ongoing application of innovative techniques, there is a continuing need for instructional materials to enhance clinical nurse anesthesia practice. This textbook is a tribute to the profession of nurse anesthesia and will serve as a resource guide in the daily provision of anesthesia care.

Nurse anesthesia is a comprehensive textbook that serves as a resource of knowledge and information for current anesthesia students and practitioners. Its focus is the application of sound scientific principles to modern clinical anesthesia practice for all types of surgical procedures and patient populations encountered daily by anesthesia providers.

The textbook is organized in seven sections: "Introduction and Overview," "Scientific Foundations," "Technology Related to Anesthesia Practice," "Preoperative Preparation," "Intraoperative Management," "Postoperative Considerations," and "Current Topics," which addresses issues related to clinical anesthesia practice. The chapters in each section detail the necessary and current information requisite for that area. The content and organization of the clinical practice chapters provide a functional learning overview of the topic.

The introduction and overview relate the history and specialty practice of nurse anesthesia and the guidelines for management of an anesthesia department. The section on scientific foundations includes a discussion of chemistry and physics, organ and system physiology, pathophysiology, and pharmacologic principles as they relate to anesthesia practice. The technology section describes the concepts associated with anesthesia equipment and invasive and noninvasive patient monitoring. The preoperative preparation section reviews the necessary concepts related to the preoperative assessment, interpretation of diagnostic data, and preoperative medication of patients. The intraoperative management section comprehensively covers the major principles and specialties related to clinical anesthesia. These chapters include a discussion of both the basic principles and the advanced practice principles related to the clinical management of patients undergoing transplantation, as well as cardiac, thoracic, and ophthalmic procedures. The section on postoperative considerations details postoperative care and pain management. The current topics section provides the practitioner with knowledge about legal aspects, statistics, computers, and research as they relate to clinical anesthesia practice.

We recognize that many topics discussed in this textbook will undergo change as advances in the anesthesia profession are realized. The challenge for students and practitioners will be to integrate new knowledge from a variety of sources and to be receptive and sufficiently skilled to incorporate the dynamic changes as they occur in clinical anesthesia practice.

John J. Nagelhout
Karen L. Zaglaniczny

Acknowledgments

We would like to thank the following authors for their contributions to the first and second editions of this textbook.

Roy Alisoglu
Steve L. Alves
Anne E. Aprile
Victoria Base-Smith
Colleen M. Beauchamp
Baher Boctor
Danny R. Bowman
Joanne M. Cafarelli
Cynthia Cappello
Marge Chick
Diane Bleak Dayton
George G. DeVane
Ronda L. Erway
Jan L. Frandsen
Donna J. Funke
Vance G. Gainer Jr.
Stanley M. Hall
Celestine Harrigan
Shelly Harthrong-Lethiot
Randolf R. Harvey
Bernadette Henrichs
Frederick C. Hill, Jr.
Holly E. Holman
Maria Iacopelli
Jeanne M. Kachnij
Kenneth M. Kirsner
Jeffrey F. Kopecky
Michael J. Kremer
Gail LaPointe
Kim Litwack
Janet Maroney
Michael P. Mitton
Ann Misterovich
Diane Moniz
Ralph O. Morgan, Jr.
Howard J. Normile
Richard S. Purdham
Julie A. Rigoni Neville
Janet Rojo
Linda Saber McIntosh
Susanna Sands
Elaine Sartain-Spivak
James Scarsella
Lisa A. Sebastian
Jeffrey P. Serwin
Barry Shaw
Jeffrey A. Sinkovich
Kathy Swender
Michael Troop
John Weisbrod
Hilary V. Wong

Contents

CHAPTER 1

NURSE ANESTHESIA: A HISTORY OF CHALLENGE

IRA P. GUNN

The anesthetic properties of nitrous oxide and diethyl ether have been known since the late 1700s. Priestley, Davy, and later Faraday remarked on these properties and their possible use for anesthesia during surgical operations. It was not until these two drugs had become popular through their recreational use in "laughing gas and ether frolics," however, that their application as possible adjuncts to surgery was attempted. Before this time, alcohol, ice, tourniquets, and even unconsciousness brought about by blows to the head or strangulation were tried in the effort to relieve the pain of surgical amputations and the drainage of abscesses. For most lifesaving surgeries, however, strong men were placed around patients to hold them down for the surgeon.[1]

Crawford Long, a Georgia physician, first used diethyl ether for the removal of a small cyst in 1842. Unfortunately he did not report his findings. It was William T. G. Morton, a dentist, who in 1846 first demonstrated the use of ether for surgical anesthesia in an operating room (now known as the "ether dome") at Massachusetts General Hospital in Boston. After the procedure, Dr. Warren, the surgeon, reportedly exclaimed, "Gentlemen, this is no humbug."[1] An observer who was an eminent surgeon stated, "I have seen something today that will go around the world."[1]

Over the grave of Dr. Morton, the citizens of Boston erected a monument with the following inscription[1]:

Inventor and Revealer of Anaesthetic Inhalation
Before Whom, in All Time, Surgery was Agony
By Whom Pain in Surgery was Averted and Annulled
Since Whom Science Has Control of Pain

From the vantage point of the physician who wrote the inscription, optimism seemed justified; however, another century and a half would pass before the last line would be substantially fulfilled. For approximately the first 100 years after this demonstration, in many areas anesthesia was a mixed blessing.

THE PERIOD OF THE FAILED PROMISE

In the early years the discovery and application of anesthesia to surgical procedures did not yield the promising results expected for several reasons—principally the morbidity and mortality associated with both anesthesia and surgery. With surgery, the main culprit was infection; with anesthesia, it was the "occasional anesthetists."

The Problem of Infection

Justifying the greater use of surgery necessitated adequate resolution of the problem of infection. Achievement of this goal required Florence Nightingale during the Crimean War (1854 through 1856) and others to demonstrate that hospitals did not have to be "pest houses." With cleanliness, good ventilation, adequate nutrition, and care provided by a qualified staff, patients could go into hospitals to get well rather than merely to die. Oliver Wendell Holmes, a U.S. attorney who became a physician, and Ignaz Philipp Semmelweis, a Viennese physician, hypothesized that infection spread by the medical provider was the major cause of the puerperal fever that resulted in so many maternal deaths and that merely washing one's hands between patients could reduce this morbidity and mortality. Semmelweis developed his hypothesis while observing midwives, noting that their deliveries were associated with a lower incidence of infection and death than those assisted by medical students. The primary difference he observed was that the midwives washed their hands between patients; in contrast, the medical students often went from the autopsy rooms to the delivery wards without washing their hands or changing their clothes. Both Holmes and Semmelweis were severely criticized by their colleagues for their hypothesis.[2] At the time, the germ theory had been alluded to but had not been confirmed.

Before the medical establishment would accept the germ theory and the means of prevention of infection in the mid 1880s, Koch and Pasteur had to confirm the theory and Lister and several German physicians had to advocate the concept of antisepsis through the use of germ-killing chemicals. Furthermore, it was up to Pasteur to introduce the heating of milk to eliminate the "germs" that it contained and, finally, to Koch and another German, von Bergmann, to demonstrate asepsis through physical and steam sterilization, respectively.[2,3] With the problem of infection greatly reduced (but not completely resolved), the problem of the occasional anesthetists became more apparent as a cause of surgical morbidity and mortality.

The Problem of the Occasional Anesthetists

Many have attributed the problem of the occasional anesthetists in part to the limited prestige and the low pay that they received for their work. For these reasons, physicians did not choose to specialize in anesthesia practice. Most physicians chose either medicine or surgery as their principal specialty, and if they did perform anesthesia, it was, for the most part, in an effort to gain a front-row seat to surgery.[3] Often the patient was not afforded the continuous vigilance needed for balancing the two basic needs of every anesthetic procedure: patient safety and appropriate surgical conditions.

The 1890s were ushered in with scathing debates over the morbidity and mortality associated with anesthesia. Many surgeons and physicians began to understand the need for anesthesia providers who devoted their practice to the administration of anesthetics. These debates took place in Europe and the United States. In England, a physician model of anesthesia was chosen; in the United States, no particular model gained acceptance. However, history has shown that at the time of the debates some surgeons took the problems associated with the "anesthetizer or narcotizer" to heart and were determined to develop an anesthesia specialty.[3] Furthermore, they seemed to recognize the apparent need for anesthetists who, as Thatcher defined later, would "(1) be satisfied with the subordinate role that the work required, (2) make anesthesia their one absorbing interest, (3) not look on the situation of anesthetist as one that put them in a position to watch and learn from the surgeon's technic [sic], (4) accept the comparatively low pay, and (5) have the natural aptitude and intelligence to develop a high level of skill in providing the smooth anesthesia and relaxation that the surgeon demanded."[3]

As a result, as long ago as the mid 1870s many surgeons began to encourage the Catholic Hospital Sisters and the new professional nurses who graduated from nursing schools patterned after the Nightingale plan to train as anesthetists.

HISTORICAL BEGINNINGS OF THE NURSE ANESTHETIST

In the United States the first evidence that "nurses" may have been involved in administering anesthesia is found in accounts of the Civil War. At that time it was reported that a woman, Mrs. Harris, used chloroform and stimulants at the Battle of Gettysburg. It is not known whether Mrs. Harris was a nurse. However, in the military annals chronicling the war, one passage does connect a nurse with the use of chloroform. In a report of the care of a Private Budlinger of the 76th Ohio Unit, it was recorded that "after breathing it for a few minutes without any apparent effect, more chloroform was added and reapplied by a nurse in attendance."[4]

Thatcher[3] reported that both male and female nurses were taught to induce anesthesia and were used as anesthetists in the Franco-Prussian War (1870 to 1871). She also reported that during this period patients were turned over to nurses who would drop more anesthetic agents onto patients' masks while anesthetizers went to start another anesthetic, a practice that was severely criticized in the 1890s. Therefore, the practice of using nurses for administering a part or all of an anesthetic was employed on both sides of the Atlantic in the latter half of the nineteenth century, setting the stage for greater use of nurses for this purpose in times of peace and war. Health-care needs created by wars have often led to progress for medical therapeutics and health-care delivery modalities; this has been particularly true with regard to the historical confirmation of the use of nurses as anesthetists in the United States.

The First Nurse Anesthetists

Although early evidence of the use of nurses as anesthetists is somewhat fragmentary, reports of anesthesia provided by nurses became more and more frequent beginning in the 1880s. Sister Mary Bernard founded the Sisters of St. Joseph of Wichita, Kansas, and in 1877 entered St. Vincent's Hospital in Erie, Pennsylvania, to train as a nurse. A year later, she took over the anesthesia duties of the hospital and therefore has been credited with being the first nurse anesthetist in the United States.[3] Evidence abounds that this success was rapidly repeated in the Midwest. The Franciscan Sisters, who were active in the building and staffing of St. John's Hospital in Springfield, Illinois, were particularly successful in preparing Hospital Sisters as nurse anesthetists and sending them out to other Midwestern hospitals for practice. Having been prepared by another community of the Sisters of St. Francis (Syracuse, New York), Sister Mary Erhard went to Hawaii in 1886, where she administered anesthesia and performed other nursing duties on the island of Maui for approximately 42 years.[3]

The St. Mary's Experience

Another community of the Sisters of St. Francis in Rochester, Minnesota, also made a significant contribution to the historical evolution of lay nurse anesthetists. The mother superior of this order went to Dr. William W. Mayo (who, along with his sons William and Charles, as well as other physicians, was destined to achieve international fame for his surgery after the advent of asepsis) and offered to build a hospital if Mayo would take charge of it. Mayo agreed, and St. Mary's Hospital was built and opened in 1889. It was planned that Edith and Dinah Graham, two hometown graduates of the School of Nursing at Woman's Hospital in Chicago, would direct and supervise the new hospital's nursing service and administer anesthesia.[3]

Within a few weeks, the Catholic Sisters took on the nursing service positions and gave the jobs of anesthetist, office nurse, general bookkeeper, and secretary to the two trained nurses. Mayo, believing that there was no reason why intelligent nurses would not make good anesthetists, instructed both of these nurses in their anesthesia duties.[3,5] Dinah Graham administered anesthesia for only a short period of time, but Edith was active in its administration until she married Dr. Charles H. Mayo. Her successor and friend Alice Magaw, who also was a graduate of the School of Nursing at Women's Hospital in Chicago, took over the anesthesia administration. Magaw's achievements, along with those of another nurse, Florence Henderson, contributed significantly to the international fame enjoyed by the Mayos and St. Mary's Hospital for excellence in surgery and anesthesia. It was Dr. Charles H. Mayo who gave "Magaw the title Mother of Anesthesia"[5] (Box 1-1).

BOX 1-1 Alice Magaw

A scientist at heart, Alice Magaw saw the importance of observing, recording, analyzing, and publishing her findings concerning anesthesia practice at St. Mary's Hospital in Rochester, Minnesota. Her findings were published in various medical journals, including *Northwestern, The Lancet, St. Paul Medical Journal, Transactions of the Minnesota State Medical Association,* and *Surgery, Gynecology, and Obstetrics* in 1899, 1900, 1901, 1904, and 1906, respectively. In 1906 she reported the results of more than 14,000 anesthetic cases in which not a single death was attributed to anesthesia. In reporting her experiences and findings, Magaw advocated selected techniques and cited their advantages.[3,5]

Having heard of the success of using nurses in anesthesia in Rochester or having observed it firsthand, many surgeons invited nurses to specialize in the field and to become their anesthetists. In many places the nurse anesthetist was employed by the hospital administrator and was not placed under the authority of the nursing superintendent, so that the nurse's availability for providing anesthesia would be ensured. The pay of the nurse anesthetist often was equivalent to that of the nursing superintendent.

In the South, another practice pattern became prevalent: the nurse anesthetist was employed by the surgeon to serve as anesthetist and office nurse. This mode of practice was still in use in some parts of the United States in the early 1950s.

The Lakeside Experience

Agatha Hodgins, a Canadian nurse, went to Cleveland, Ohio, to work at Lakeside Hospital. Dr. George Crile chose her to become his anesthetist in 1908, and as such she became perhaps even more renowned than Alice Magaw. She is the founder of the American Association of Nurse Anesthetists (AANA). Like St. Mary's Hospital, Lakeside Hospital became an international showcase for its success in surgery and anesthesia and was the recipient of many requests for anesthetist training from both physicians and nurses. Its reputation grew from the work of the American Ambulance, a Lakeside Hospital surgical unit established in France before the United States' entry into World War I. This unit's staff included both Crile and Hodgins, who traveled to France in 1914 to conduct research. While in France, they took on the additional mission of training some English and French physicians and nurses in the art and science of anesthesia. It was after this experience that Crile, in working with the General Medical Board of the Council for National Defense and the Red Cross to develop base hospitals for use in France during the war, ensured the placement of nurse anesthetists in these units, as well as their involvement (and that of some physicians) in the teaching and training of other physicians and nurses in the specialty.[5]

The Great War, a Small Battlefield

Anne Penland was a nurse anesthetist with the Presbyterian Hospital of New York unit, Base Hospital Number 2. She had the honor of being the first U.S. nurse anesthetist to go officially to the British front, where she so won the confidence of British medical officers that the British decided to train their own nurses in anesthesia, ultimately relieving more than 100 physicians for medical and surgical work. Several hospitals were selected for this training of British nurses, including the American Base Hospital Number 2, with Penland as the instructor.[6]

One of the very poignant stories involving nurse anesthetists in World War I comes from Penland's diary. She was serving in a casualty clearing station, a small surgical unit usually made up of a surgeon, an anesthetist, an operating room nurse, and an orderly, situated close to the front in the Flanders section of Belgium. The casualties were heavy, and she was working the night shift and went on duty at 7 PM. Shortly after Penland arrived on duty, Lieutenant Osler, son of the distinguished Professor of Medicine Sir William Osler, was brought in with penetrating wounds of the chest, abdomen, and leg. Penland's surgeon, Major Darrasch, sent for Major Brewer, Chief of Surgery at Columbia College of Physicians and Surgeons; Major Crile from Lakeside Hospital in Cleveland; and Major Harvey Cushing, neurosurgeon from the Harvard Unit, all serving in casualty clearing stations within close proximity of one another.[6] Penland writes the following:

> *All of them knew his father well. Major Crile brought his blood transfusion apparatus and Major Darrach operated, assisted by Major Brewer, Major Cushing kept his finger on the boy's pulse, and I gave a few drops of ether. It isn't often that in a small country-side, so many famous surgeons could be brought together in such a short span of time. The transfusion went beautifully, his pulse became perceptible, then gradually stronger, and his color became quite pink. The operation lasted thirty minutes; the abdomen was opened and found to have several perforations in the gut which were sutured. The chest and leg wounds were only dressed.*
>
> *Thursday, August 20 [sic 30]. We were still operating at seven this morning when Major Darrach was sent for to see Lieut. Osler; his breathing had suddenly become embarrassed, and he died in a few minutes. It is a glorious thing to give one's life for one's country, but how unutterably sad; such numbers of lives being sacrificed in a strange land with no loved ones there. What grief and agony to those waiting at home!"*[6]

The Proliferation of Nurse Anesthetists

Before World War I, surgeons and hospitals sought nurse anesthetists so enthusiastically that four formalized postgraduate programs were developed and implemented before the United States entered the war: at St. Vincent's Hospital in Portland, Oregon (1909); at St. John's Hospital in Springfield, Illinois (1912); at New York Postgraduate Hospital in New York City (1912); and at Long Island College Hospital, Brooklyn, New York (1914).[3] Other nurse anesthesia programs were developed as a part of the undergraduate nursing curriculum as a specialty option. Isabel Adams Hampton Robb, a pioneer nursing leader and the first superintendent of the Johns Hopkins School of Nursing, which had opened in 1889, had in 1893 published a nursing textbook entitled *Nursing: Its Principles and Practices for Hospital and Private Use*; this textbook included a chapter entitled "The Administration of Anaesthetics."[5]

Many institutions in which anesthesia was taught to both physicians and nurses aimed solely at covering the anesthesia services in a particular hospital setting. The reputation gained by U.S. nurse anesthetists in World War I generated the climate for a great expansion of nurse anesthesia educational programs and an even greater demand for their graduates. A challenge to the program at Lakeside Hospital, however, brought this educational program to a halt until potential regulatory problems could be resolved.[3,5]

ANESTHESIA: MEDICINE, NURSING, DENTISTRY, OR WHAT?

Although few physicians chose to specialize in anesthesia before World War II, one such physician, Francis Hoeffer McMechan—a Cincinnati native—began a crusade to claim the field solely for physicians in approximately 1911. Although McMechan had become disabled shortly after entering the field of medicine and was no longer able to practice, he and his wife undertook his mission through writing, publishing, and speaking on the issue. To what extent professional nurse anesthetists owe the Lakeside challenge in 1915 and the concomitant Kentucky challenge of nurse anesthetists to McMechan is unknown, but there can be little doubt that McMechan bore some responsibility for them.[5] These legal challenges were based on allegations that anesthesia was the practice of medicine and that the administration of anesthesia by nurses was illegal because it constituted the practice of medicine. The two challenges, however, took separate forms.

The Lakeside challenge went to the Ohio Board of Medicine, which sent a letter to Crile in 1916. The board notified Crile of its position that no one other than a registered physician was permitted to administer anesthesia and that the state attorney general concurred with its position. Essentially, the board of medicine issued an order that Lakeside Hospital's School of Nursing was to cease its anesthesia program or lose its accreditation. Not wanting to be responsible for the loss of the school's accreditation, Crile obeyed the order pending the outcome of a hearing conducted in 1917. At the hearing Crile took the position that Lakeside Hospital was only following the lead of many of the major clinics in the country. Crile managed to persuade the board of medicine to lift its order, and he was able to reinstitute his nurse anesthesia educational program and his use of nurse anesthetists. Crile and supporting physicians took the additional step of petitioning the Ohio legislature to amend the state Medical Practice Act so that it ensured the legality of the nurse anesthetist's profession and activities by exception. The 1919 amendment essentially stated that nothing in the bill could be construed to prevent a registered nurse from administering anesthesia under the supervision and in the immediate presence of a physician, provided that such a nurse had taken a prescribed course in anesthesia at a hospital in good standing.[3]

In the Kentucky challenge, the Louisville Society of Anesthetists passed a resolution proclaiming that only physicians should administer anesthesia, and it received a concurring opinion from the state attorney general in 1916. The Kentucky State Medical Association followed with a resolution stating that it was unethical for a physician to use a nonphysician anesthetist or to use a hospital that permitted nurses to administer anesthesia. This resolution led surgeon Louis Frank and his nurse anesthetist, Margaret Hatfield, to ask the state board of health to join them in a suit against the Kentucky State Medical Association.[3]

The attorney charged with representing the state board of health was the same attorney general who had issued the opinion in 1916 that prompted the medical association's actions. Frank and Hatfield lost at the lower court level but won on appeal.[3] In 1917 Judge Hurt of the Kentucky Court of Appeals, writing the opinion for the court, not only confirmed the right of nurses to administer anesthesia under the conditions that were in vogue at the time, but also enunciated the following clear opinion with regard to the purpose and limits of state licensure of professionals:

> *[These] laws have not been enacted for the peculiar benefit of the members of such professions, further, than they are members of the general community, but they have been enacted for the benefit of the people.*
>
> *While the practice of medicine is one of the most noble and learned professions, it is apparent that such a construction ought not to be given to the statute, which regulates the profession, that the effect of it would be to invade the province of the professions of pharmacy, dentistry or trained nursing, all of which are professions, which relate to the alleviation of the human family of sickness and bodily afflictions, and to make duties belonging to these professions, also "the practice of medicine" within the meaning of the statute.*
>
> *Nor should such a construction be given to it as to deprive the people from all services, which could be rendered to them in sickness and affliction, except gratuitous services, or else by licensed physicians, unless the legislature intended that such should be the result of the enactment of the statute. We are of the opinion that, in the performance of the service by appellate Hatfield, in the way, and under the circumstances as agreed upon, as being the facts of this case, that she is not engaged in the practice of medicine within the meaning of the statute laws*[3] *(Box 1-2).*

The results of these two challenges were not enough to deter the small group of physician anesthetists from other challenges. A California court case (1933 through 1936) in which Dagmar Nelson, a nurse anesthetist, was charged with the practice of medicine has been considered as the defining test case of whether nurse anesthetists are practicing medicine or nursing when they administer anesthesia. This case was decided in favor of Dagmar Nelson at each level of the California civil court system. The California Supreme Court ruled again that the functioning of the nurse anesthetist under the supervision and in the direct presence of the surgeon or the surgeon's assistants was the common practice in operating rooms; therefore the nurse anesthetist was not diagnosing and treating within the meaning of the medical practice act[3,5] (Box 1-3).

BOX 1-2 Alice Maude Hunt

Alice Maude Hunt was the first nurse anesthetist to be appointed to a university medical school faculty. In 1922 she became an instructor in anesthesia at the Yale University School of Medicine, and later she was promoted to assistant professor. As an instructor, Hunt taught both nurses and physicians. Hunt also pioneered the use of nitrous oxide and oxygen as an anesthetic modality.[3]

BOX 1-3

Nurse Anesthetists Involved in Anesthesia Machine Development

Between 1912 and 1916 Agatha Hodgen and Graham Clark, a gas manufacturer, developed and perfected the Ohio mooncalf anesthesia machine at Lakeside Hospital in Cleveland.[3] Between 1913 and 1922 Margaret Boise and Hugh Young, a urologist, developed the Boise-Young machine. It was first used at Johns Hopkins Hospital in Baltimore, where Boise and Young were both on staff. In the early 1930s Helen Lamb worked with Richard von Foregger in developing anesthesia machines for use at Barnes Hospital in St. Louis. The Foregger machine was very popular and outlived most of its predecessors.[3]

ORGANIZATIONAL AND PROFESSIONAL SURVIVAL

Thatcher stated, "In times of prosperity, professional people give little thought to the principles of group survival and are satisfied with the most tenuous of bonds with their fellow workers. It is only when common problems become too big for individual solutions that the average professional person becomes conscious of the protection that can be found in organization."[3] Certainly, nurse anesthetists across the country were experiencing challenges. The hostility of physician anesthetists in California led to the development of a local organization of nurse anesthetists there in 1929. Other groups of nurse anesthetists often held meetings and in some instances met at the American Nurses Association (ANA) meetings. Some schools of anesthesia formed alumni associations, which served as the early model for nursing organizations[3] (Box 1-4).

In 1926 Agatha Hodgins called together the Lakeside Hospital alumni group to form a national organization, with 133 names being submitted for membership, and tentative bylaws were drawn up. Hodgins' concept of a national organization, however, did not take hold until 1931, after the Great Depression led physician anesthetists to exacerbate their challenges to nurse anesthetists in the interest of protecting their own incomes.[3] At approximately the same time the ANA undertook an effort to consolidate the fields of office nursing and nurse anesthesia within the construct of organized nursing.

Hodgins maintained that nurse anesthetists were a highly specialized group of nurses: they were not exactly nurses, but they were not physicians either; rather, professionally they fell between the two. The concept of advanced practice nursing, although not by that title, was taking root in the forms of both the public health nurse and the nurse-midwife.[2] Nurse-midwifery was emerging at the time that the nurse anesthetists were seeking affiliation with the ANA.[7] Diers describes midwives (not nurse-midwives) as the "oldest of women healers, having been referred to in biblical times in the book of Genesis."[7] They were well established in Europe, and with the influx of immigrants into the United States and the urbanization of this country, midwives worked with public health nurses, caring for indigent populations that lived and worked in appalling conditions.[2]

The Sheppard-Towner Act of 1921 provided federal monies to public health nursing programs for the preparation and use of midwives. Midwives rapidly demonstrated their competence by lowering infant and maternal mortality rates and by reducing the incidence of infant neonatal ophthalmia. As with the nurse anesthetists, physicians began to perceive midwives as threats to their livelihoods. They withdrew support for the Sheppard-Towner Act because public health nurses, along with midwives, were not under the direction of physicians. The legislation was permitted to lapse, and the funding was lost. Nurse-midwifery did not begin in the United States until 1925, when Mary Breckenridge, a British nurse and midwife, established the Frontier Nursing Service in Kentucky.[2,7]

Although the evolution of the nurse anesthesia profession and that of nurse-midwifery shared some common problems, as nursing specialties both were somewhat ahead of their time and were a not looked on with great favor by organized nursing as whole. To what extent they may have brought some of these intranursing problems on themselves will perhaps never be known. When organizing their specialty associations, neither group was able to work out agreeable conditions for merging with the ANA.[5,7]

As a result the National Association of Nurse Anesthetists was established in 1931, and in 1933 the name was changed to the American Association of Nurse Anesthetists. The AANA developed a loose affiliation with the American Hospital Association, which furnished the AANA with its first office space. The AANA also held its national meetings in conjunction with the American Hospital Association. The AANA set as its first priority the establishment of standards for educating nurse anesthetists. It also filed its first amicus curiae brief in support of Dagmar Nelson of California. In establishing its educational standards the AANA also recognized the need to certify nurse anesthetists on the basis of an examination after graduation from accredited educational programs. Unfortunately, World War II delayed these plans.[3]

BOX 1-4 Agatha Hodgen

In addition to her practice, pedagogy, and organizational work, Agatha Hodgen was involved in the testing of some of the early anesthesia machines designed to administer a combination of nitrous oxide and oxygen. Working with surgeon George Crile, she pioneered the use of nitrous oxide–oxygen techniques for patients undergoing thyroid surgery for Graves' disease.[3,5]

WORLD WAR II AND NURSE ANESTHETISTS

Once again, nurse anesthetists distinguished themselves in time of war. According to Adriani,[8] when World War II broke out there were only seven anesthesiology residencies involving at least 1 year of training. Rosemary Stevens, a noted hospital historian, reports that in 1940 there were only 285 physicians in the full-time practice of anesthesiology, of whom only 30.2% were certified.[9] In another of her books, Stevens states that in 1942 nurse anesthetists outnumbered anesthesiologists by 17 to 1.[10] The military had to prepare both physicians and nurses in the specialty to meet its needs for anesthesia providers. By the end of World War II the Army Nurse Corps had educated more than 2000 nurse anesthetists, using a 4- to 6-month curriculum patterned after that required by the AANA.[11] The shortage of nurse anesthetists could have been alleviated somewhat if U.S. law had not precluded male nurses from being commissioned and appointed in the Army and Navy Nurse Corps. A growing number of male nurses were specializing in anesthesia before World War II. They were also precluded from membership in the AANA at that time.[5]

Nurse anesthetists served at home and in all theaters of operation of World War II. They were serving in Hawaii when Pearl Harbor was attacked. Mildred Irene Clark, who was originally from North Carolina and later retired in Michigan, joined the United States Army in 1938. Under Army auspices she became a student of and graduated from Hilda Salomon's nurse anesthesia educational program. Using her own military leave time, Clark went to the Mayo Clinic to observe and learn intravenous anesthesia techniques under Dr. John Lundy and Florence McQuillen, nurse anesthetist (Woodson MIC: personal oral communication, Oct. 1994).

Clark was on assignment as a nurse anesthetist at the Schofield Barracks Hospital in Hawaii at the time of the attack on Pearl Harbor. Clark was among other nurse anesthetists on active duty who set up educational programs for preparing additional nurse anesthetists. Clark completed her illustrious career in 1967 as the Chief of the Army Nurse Corps, the first and only nurse anesthetist to hold this position.

Ann Mealor, another Army nurse anesthetist, was sent from Walter Reed Army Medical Center to the Philippines in 1941. She was assigned as Chief Nurse and Chief Nurse Anesthetist of the hospital on Corregidor in September, just 3 months before the attack on Pearl Harbor. In addition to providing anesthesia services, she was responsible for a staff of 12 nurses.[5] Denny Williams, another Army nurse anesthetist, was assigned to the Philippines in 1936. She subsequently met and married a U.S. engineer and terminated her Army career. (At that time and for some years to come, Army nurses could not be married and remain within the Army.) At the beginning of the war, Williams' husband was called up to join a U.S. Army battalion. Captain Maude Davidson, chief nurse of the Sternberg Army Hospital, Manila, requested that Williams be available for assisting the hospital in the provision of anesthesia services to the large number of casualties expected; she gladly agreed. When the Army nurses were ordered to Bataan and subsequently to Corregidor, Williams went with them. It was on Corregidor that Denny Williams, Ann Mealor, and two other Army nurse anesthetists, Doris Kehoe and Phyllis Arnold Iacobucci, were taken prisoner by the Japanese, along with some 62 other Army nurses. These nurses were interned at the Santo Tomas Internment Camp in Manila in May 1942. The prisoners of Santo Tomas were liberated by U.S. forces on February 3, 1945. All of the Army and Navy nurses who had been prisoners of war in the Philippines survived their ordeal despite starvation diets, deprivation, and tropical diseases. Throughout their imprisonment they provided nursing and anesthesia services for their fellow prisoners at the prison hospital, although access to drugs and equipment was severely limited. After Williams learned of her husband's death almost 3 years after his capture, she returned to the Army Nurse Corps and served on active duty as a nurse anesthetist until her retirement in the early 1960s.[12,13] Kehoe stayed in the Army, transferred later to the Air Force, and subsequently retired. Military nurse anesthetists served in U.S. hospitals wherever they went in support of U.S. troops, both on land and at sea on hospital ships. (The Air Force was established as a separate service of the military forces in 1949.)

Although male nurses were precluded from serving as nurses, they could and did serve in both enlisted and commissioned status, based on their educational qualifications. Some served as military medics and corpsmen. Ahead of many organizations, the AANA first accepted black female nurse anesthetists as members in 1944, and male nurses in 1947. Hilda Salomon, the AANA's fourth president, had wanted to open up the membership to these groups during her presidency in the mid 1930s. However, at that time the recommendations were considered too radical.[5]

As World War II drew to a close, the AANA's plans for instituting a certification examination for membership were realized, and the first examination was given in June 1945. The examination was taken by 92 candidates. Provisions had been made for many nurse anesthetists to be grandmothered into the AANA on the basis of their education and experience before 1939. Of note, the title "Certified Registered Nurse Anesthetist" (CRNA) was not accepted for the identification of nurse anesthetist members of the AANA until 1957 (Box 1-5).[5]

BOX 1-5

Anesthesia for Specialty Surgery

Anesthesia for pulmonary surgery was pioneered by Helen Lamb (the AANA's fifth president), working in conjunction with surgeon Evart Graham of Barnes Hospital in St. Louis, who pioneered pulmonary surgery.[3] Anesthesia for cardiac surgery, particularly pericardectomy, was pioneered by Gertrude Fife (the AANA's second president), working with pioneer cardiac surgeon Claude Beck in Cleveland.[3] Anesthesia for the correction of tetralogy of Fallot and the repair of other congenital heart defects was pioneered by Olive Berger (the AANA's fourteenth president), working with surgeon Alfred Blalock at Johns Hopkins University Hospital in Baltimore.[15] Anesthesia for pediatric cardiothoracic procedures was pioneered by Betty Lank, head nurse anesthetist at Boston's Children's Hospital, working with Dr. R. E. Gross. In 1938 Lank (AANA Trustee, 1949 to 1950) devised a miniature to-and-fro system, along with a handmade miniature mask and head strap, successfully demonstrating the efficacy of the use of closed-system cyclopropane for infants and children for the first patent ductus arteriosus ligation performed by Gross, and initiating the evolution of congenital cardiac surgery.[16-18]

A SHORT-LIVED PEACE FOR NURSE ANESTHETISTS AND THE NATION

Physicians and nurse anesthetists often worked in harmony to achieve their mission of providing high-quality anesthesia care to U.S. and Allied troops. World War II may be noted for alerting physicians to the potential of anesthesia as a specialty. The number of anesthesiology residencies greatly increased. The impact of World War II, as reported by Stevens,[9] resulted in an increase in the number of anesthesiologists from the 285 full-time anesthesiologists in 1940, with 30.2% certified, to 1231 in 1949, with 38.3% certified. Beginning in early 1947, challenges once again faced nurse anesthetists.[3]

The American Society of Anesthesiologists (ASA) was founded in 1936* and declared its intention to make anesthesia an all-physician specialty. It changed the title "physician anesthetist" to "anesthesiologist" in an attempt to eliminate the confusion that occurred when people referred to anesthesia providers simply as "anesthetists." The ASA also promulgated ethical guidelines for its members that made working with and

*The ASA has changed the date of its founding in recent years. Some small groups of physician anesthetists were formed earlier, as were some nurse anesthetist alumni associations. Earlier literature from the ASA, including its amicus curiae to the U.S. Supreme Court in the Hyde Case (October Term, 1982), gives the 1936 date.

teaching nurse anesthetists unethical. Despite the ethical code of the ASA, many anesthesiologists, recognizing that the number of qualified anesthesia providers was insufficient to meet the nation's need, continued to participate in educating nurse anesthetists to work with them. John Adriani, chairman of the Anesthesiology Department at Charity Hospital in New Orleans, was among the more prominent of these.[5]

The historical problems between nurse anesthetists and physician anesthetists have been detailed in books by Thatcher[3] and Bankert[5] on the history of nurse anesthesia, as well as in Rosemary Stevens' history of hospitals and history of medical specialization.[9,10] Stevens[10] wrote the following:

> *Since hospitals needed doctors in private practice to bring in hospital patients, the doctors had a strong power base of their own. Nevertheless, the traditional relationship between private practitioners and hospitals as the private doctor's workshop was difficult to justify and sustain by the late 1930s, for hospitals had obvious technologies of their own. Laboratories, x-ray, and anesthesia equipment could be operated by technicians and/or nurses, with or without the direct supervision of medical specialists.*
>
> *Anesthesia, often bitterly contested in a three-way tussle for control among surgeons, nurse anesthetists, and medical anesthesiologists, was the most dramatic case in point.... The employment of hospital based [medical] specialists became a major battleground for hospitals and doctors in the 1930s.... A leading anesthesiologist pressed for a propaganda campaign in the media in 1940 because he was tired, he said, of watching movies where dramatic operating scenes focused on the heroism and authority of the surgeon and represented anesthesiologists only in images of filling rubber bags and jiggling valves.*

Even with the number of physician and nurse anesthetists prepared during World War II, particularly by the military, and the increasing number of anesthesiology residencies after the war, an acute and serious shortage of qualified anesthesia providers remained. Despite this shortage, some physician anesthetists, including some leaders among their specialty associations, set out to make anesthesia an all-physician specialty and initiated a public relations campaign not directly aimed at surgeons, but rather aimed at destroying the confidence of the U.S. public in nurse anesthetists. This onslaught consisted of a series of articles, published principally in women's magazines, questioning the competence of nurse anesthetists and advocating the use of physician anesthetists. Surgeons and hospital administrators who had long experienced the achievements of nurse anesthetists came to the nurses' support. The American Medical Association, the American College of Surgeons, the Southern Surgical Association, and the American Hospital Association passed resolutions decrying the actions of these physicians and affirming their support of both physician and nurse anesthetists.[3]

The effort to make anesthesiology an all-physician specialty began before Beecher and Todd[14] completed and reported their findings in the first anesthesia outcome study in the United States. Beecher had been an anesthesiology consultant to the Army Surgeon General during World War II and had also worked previously with nurse anesthetists. After the war, Beecher and Todd performed a 5-year (1948 through 1952) prospective study of anesthesia outcomes in 10 university hospital settings. They reported the results in 1954.[14] The results shocked and dismayed many anesthesiologists. After studying approximately 600,000 anesthetic procedures, they found that the mortality rates based on the providers were as follows: anesthesiologists, having done 62,200 cases, had a rate of 1:890; anesthesia residents, a category that included some medical and surgical residents on their anesthesia rotation, having done a total of 287,800 cases, had a rate of 1:1200; and nurse anesthetists, having done twice the number of cases as anesthesiologists, or 128,100 cases, had one half the mortality rate of anesthesiologists, or 1:1800. Furthermore, using a 7-point score for assessing patient physical status, Beecher and Todd found that there was no difference in this assessment across groups of providers. The findings were so surprising to physicians that they made assumptions that anesthesiologists were performing more complex surgical cases.[14] Perhaps this was true in some institutions, but the evidence in the literature demonstrates that, in the time frame of this study, nurse anesthetists in university-type hospitals were pioneering anesthesia for specialty surgery. One such example was Olive Berger, Chief Nurse Anesthetist at Johns Hopkins Medical Center, who in 1948 reported on a series of 480 anesthetics administered to 475 patients who underwent surgery for cyanotic congenital heart disease, including procedures for tetralogy of Fallot. Of that series, physicians administered anesthesia in 41 cases, and in the remainder anesthesia was administered by nurse anesthetists. Berger herself administered anesthesia in 289 of those cases. The patients ranged from 4 months to 45 years of age, with only 54 patients over age 20.[15] The pioneering work of Betty Lank, Chief Nurse Anesthetist at Boston's Children's Hospital, with regard to designing equipment and using cyclopropane for infants undergoing congenital heart repairs,[16] has been acknowledged by noted anesthesiologists Hamel and Lamont[17] and Smith.[18] Beecher and Todd's study had little or no effect on those anesthesiology leaders who were trying to claim the specialty solely for medicine. (Note that one must recognize the vast difference in the state of the art at the time of the study and that existing today to understand the magnitude and importance of these findings. Change in the health-care field as a result of advancing knowledge and technology, particularly in anesthesiology, has been logarithmic rather than linear.)

The national peace had been short-lived when North Korea invaded South Korea in June 1950. The United States committed its troops in support of South Korea. South Korea had been liberated from the Japanese after World War II, and the United States had troops there to help it rebuild. Again, nurse anesthetists lived up to their reputation as highly qualified and competent anesthesia professionals. The National Women's Press Club named the Army nurse as its Woman of the Year in 1953. An Army nurse anesthetist, Lieutenant Mildred Rush from Massachusetts, was designated to accept the award on behalf of all Army nurses.[5]

In 1951 U.S. Representative Frances Payne Bolton, from Ohio, introduced legislation to authorize the commissioning of male nurses as officers in the military nurse corps. It was not passed. However, in 1955, Public Law 294, also introduced by Representative Bolton, did pass, authorizing male nurses for reserve commissions. President Dwight D. Eisenhower signed it into law. Of note, the first male nurse commissioned in the

Army Nurse Corps was a nurse anesthetist, Edward L. T. Lyon of New York. Representative Bolton attempted to correct the inequity of the 1955 law that restricted male nurses to reserve commissions by introducing legislation in 1961, 1963, and 1965. Representative Stratton of New York introduced a bill that was identical to Bolton's in 1965. The first and only male nurse draft in U.S. history was accomplished in April 1966; a bill authorizing male nurses for regular commissions in the Army, Navy, and Air Force was passed and signed into law in September 1966.[19]

ACCREDITATION OF NURSE ANESTHESIA EDUCATIONAL PROGRAMS

During the Korean War in 1952, the AANA began its accreditation program for nurse anesthetist education. The Korean GI Bill—federal legislation that made Korean War veterans eligible for federal funds for education—prompted the AANA to seek recognition of its accreditation program from the United States Office of Education (USOE), then a part of the U.S. Department of Health, Education, and Welfare. Such a bill had been passed for the veterans of World War II, but because of abuses of that legislation the Korean War legislation mandated that to receive the educational benefits, veterans had to attend schools or programs that were accredited by an accrediting agency recognized by the USOE. Therefore, to make it possible for nurse veterans who wanted to enter nurse anesthesia programs and acquire the federal benefits, the AANA became recognized as the accreditor of nurse anesthesia education by the USOE in 1955.[5]

Unfortunately, challenges to the nurse anesthesia profession over the years have continued and have taken many forms. Although the public relations campaign of 1947 did not do away with nurse anesthetists, the campaign, in combination with the anesthesiologists' attempts to make this field into an all-physician specialty, significantly decreased the number of nurses who entered the field. In the 1960s, when only approximately 3% of medical school graduates chose to enter anesthesiology residencies, shortages of anesthesia providers became more pronounced. A general shortage of physicians in the country prompted the U.S. government to open up educational visas to graduates of foreign medical schools, permitting them to enter the United States to obtain residency training. Many stayed in the country to practice. By the late 1960s, approximately 55% of anesthesiology medical residencies were filled by foreign medical school graduates (Box 1-6).[20]

BOX **1-6**

Mechanical Control of Respirations for Intrathoracic Surgery

Developed by Dr. Claude Beck, Dr. F. Mautz, and Gertrude Fife (the AANA's second president), the technique of mechanical control of respirations during intrathoracic surgery was perfected at Lakeside Hospital in Cleveland by Dr. Beck and Miriam Shupp (the AANA's fourth president), with the technical and commercial assistance of K. Wolfe and H. J. Rand III.[3]

THE NEW AGE OF NURSE ANESTHESIA: THE 1960s

The decade of the 1960s was a transitional period in health care in general, as well as in anesthesiology. Passage of the Medicare and Medicaid legislation, with projections for a greater need for health services in the latter half of the decade, culminated in many meetings of various health-care professionals and specialists. The new legislation prompted the expansion of educational programs and the development of new programs for health professionals, such as nurse practitioners and physician assistants, as well as the resurgence of nurse-midwifery. The increased federal funding for educating health professionals, for establishing additional academic health centers, and for research led to an escalation of new knowledge and new technology that pushed health-care delivery toward an ever-increasing degree of specialization.

Health care became even more hospital based and concentrated on acute care to the detriment of preventive and health-maintenance services. Public health services received less attention and, in many instances, fewer resources. The Medicaid program (designed to provide health-care services for the poor) was intended to supplant, in some instances, public health services, which had often been associated with indigent care. Unfortunately, the concomitant pursuit of new knowledge and new technology and the concentration on acute care were often funded at the expense of Medicaid and other public health programs. It was at this time that serious work in organ transplantation was beginning; this work would lead to the development of artificial anatomic parts designed to replace worn out or destroyed body parts. As knowledge grew, so did specialization, with a spurt of subspecialization occurring in many medical fields. Subspecialization began to be seen in anesthesiology, which was to hit subspecialization peak in the 1980s and 1990s.

Anesthesiologists held meetings to define the future needs of anesthesiology. The meetings clearly delineated the philosophic differences among anesthesiologists concerning the ASA's goal to have an all-physician specialty and the practical reality that confronted many anesthesiologists in the 1960s, which made such a goal seem impossible. No consideration was given to calling a meeting with the AANA to jointly plan for the future.

Two schools of thought gained prominence in anesthesiologic circles during the 1960s. Adherents of the first advocated rapprochement with nurse anesthesia and support of nurse anesthesia educational programs,[20] and adherents of the second supported the identification of another type of anesthesia practitioner based on a physician assistant model and whom the anesthesiologist could control.[21,22] In 1962 Robert D. Dripps,[21] a highly respected pioneer anesthesiologist from the University of Pennsylvania, wrote, "There are not now enough physician-specialists to administer all anesthetics in the country. It is unlikely that there ever will be. Who then will be available, how will they be trained, how *supervised and controlled* [emphasis added]? The terms *nurse anesthetist* and *nurse technician* arouse strong emotional reaction in some quarters. Perhaps it is well to recognize this and to try to solve the problem of additional personnel in another way."[21] Dripps also suggested the preparation of persons in associate degree programs in community college settings.[21]

At a 1967 meeting designed for debate of the manpower issue (and after which a number of the papers were published in an issue of the quarterly *Clinical Anesthesia*), H. H. Bendixon, a renowned academician and research anesthesiologist, stated the following:

> *The total national anesthetic case load cannot possibly at present or within the foreseeable future, be administered by trained physician anesthetists. We could not at present take the responsibility for the total anesthetic case load, working with nurse anesthetists, because trained nurses are not available in sufficient numbers.... We need to increase the number of U.S. graduates in our residencies.... We should reduce sharply the recruitment of foreign physicians into technician service. This trend has been a mistake and a waste of valuable training.... I do not have the facilities or the time to predict our manpower needs for the next decade or two, but I offer the general observation that the shortage of nurses and technicians is far more serious than the physician shortage. We need to train more nurses* and to assume responsibility for the work *[emphasis added].*[20]

In 1972, when proposing and justifying his proposal to prepare anesthesiology assistants (a specialist type of physician assistant), John Steinhaus, chairman of the Department of Anesthesiology at Emory University, wrote the following:

> *There was general agreement at this conference [Crisis in Anesthesia Manpower, 1965 Conference] that physician manpower should be increased and that programs in anesthesia research should be expanded. Although it was recognized that nurse anesthetists contribute a large portion of anesthesia service, there was no agreement as to the role this group should play in the future. The definition of the relationship between the physician and the nurse in general medicine has been difficult, [and] that between the anesthesiologists and the nurse anesthetist is even more so.*[22]

This emphasis on "control," "supervision," and "assumption of responsibility for nurse anesthetist practice" was of no surprise to nurse anesthetists nor to those who knew and understood the history of health care in the United States. Barbara Safreit, Associate Dean, Yale Law School, wrote the following in her 1992 monograph, *Health Care Dollars and Regulatory Sense: the Role of Advanced Practice Nursing*:

> *As Eliot Friedson has noted, in the mid-to-late 1800s, physicians rose from the ranks of previously undifferentiated occupations devoted to healing, and claimed preeminence through their highly organized effort to obtain the "exclusive right to practice." Having obtained that right, however, physicians also recognized their need for the services of other practitioners of healing, who were "useful to the physician and necessary to his practice, even if dangerous to his monopoly." Friedson concludes that, to solve this dilemma, physicians obtained from "the state control over those occupations' activities" so as to limit what they could do and to supervise or direct their activities.*[23]

Having been the principal providers of anesthesia services since the late 1880s and often the anesthesia experts in operating rooms, nurse anesthetists had developed a strong sense of autonomy in their practice and were not inclined to give this up. Many had developed a conviction that was subsequently enunciated by the Ohio Supreme Court in a malpractice case. The court's legal opinion was that a physician's legal obligation to direct or supervise a nurse anesthetist's practice is not the same thing as control, and only when a physician actually exerts control over a nurse anesthetist's practice could he or she be held responsible for that practice.[24]

In fact, in the 1960s nursing as a profession was coming of age. Nursing moved its education from hospital-based programs to institutions of higher education and was exerting efforts toward identification of its unique professional role. It also focused on determining its independent and collaborative roles with medicine and with other professionals. Some nurse educators perceived nursing that involved physicians at all as a dependent role, as did many physicians. Other nurses, particularly those moving into so-called "expanded" roles—roles that had similarities to those of nurse anesthetists—asserted that they were engaged in collaborative practice with physicians and other types of health professionals, as opposed to dependent roles. With the women's movement also becoming more prominent, occupations that were predominantly held by women were attempting to remove the barriers that restricted earnings, as well as women's roles and rightful positions in the hierarchies of professions, industry, government, and universities. Although the number of men in nurse anesthesia was much greater than that in general nursing—probably because the former offered a higher degree of autonomy and greater remuneration—it was still held back by the same constraints that had been exerted on other traditionally "female" occupations and specialties.

The shortage of anesthesia personnel in the 1960s, within the confines of the forces that were shaping history itself, produced and sowed several seeds that exhibited varying degrees of growth. More nurse anesthesia educational programs were developed, and the number of nurse anesthetists being prepared increased. Many of the programs were small training programs, which were not able, subsequently, to comply with accreditation requirements that were changed in 1975 as a result of new criteria placed on accrediting agencies by the USOE.

In 1964 the ASA and AANA established a liaison committee that met twice a year. C. R. Stephens, a noted anesthesiologist who had worked with nurse anesthetists for many years, wrote in a 1969 report to the ASA, "Progress has not been rapid, but the dialogue has enhanced understanding."[25]

The AANA and ASA developed and adopted a joint statement on anesthesia providers. It was published by both organizations in January 1972. This statement first recognized that both anesthesiologists and nurse anesthetists were needed in the field, and that only those who were first prepared in total patient care should be prepared as anesthetists. It went on to recognize that "the ideal circumstances of qualified anesthesiologists and nurse anesthetists working together as an anesthesia care team may not be totally possible in the future."[26] By 1975, because of some substantive differences between the ASA and AANA, the ASA had withdrawn its support of the statement. Some within nurse anesthesia also were happy to see its demise. The compromises made by both groups to achieve the statement had been too much for the purists and traditionalists of both professional groups. Among anesthesiologists were those of the traditional paradigm to which medicine was and is devoted. Nurse anesthetists were of two schools: the true traditionalists, who had worked exceedingly hard to overcome challenge after challenge, maintaining for the profession a relatively high degree of autonomy for those days; and the newer nurse anesthetists, who had somewhat broader views regarding the happenings of the 1960s, who saw the potential for change of the traditional health-care paradigm, and who wanted to bring this change about sooner rather than later.

Some nurse anesthetists saw the need for nurse anesthesia to upgrade its educational programs and to move into universities and colleges while retaining the hospital base for clinical education. I was instrumental in convincing the U.S. Army to develop and implement a graduate nurse anesthesia program in cooperation with the University of Hawaii's School of Nursing in the fall of 1969. This was the first prototype of a university-based nurse anesthesia program that led to a graduate degree. Although this program did not survive military reductions at the end of the Vietnam War, it served as an impetus for future change.

John Garde and Sister Mary Arthur Schramm pioneered programs in the baccalaureate framework in the early 1970s. From these beginnings, nurse anesthesia education has moved swiftly to include academically qualified faculty; a baccalaureate requirement for admission to accredited programs; and, in 1988, a mandated requirement for all programs to offer a graduate degree.[27]

A little-known seed of the 1960s was the attempt by some state nurse anesthetist organizations to gain recognition by their states, either within the state nurse practice act or as a separate act. Codification in state practice acts was perceived not only as a matter of governmental recognition; more important, it provided a legal framework for public protection of patients who received nurse anesthesia services. Arizona was the first state to gain such inclusion in the nurse practice act in the mid 1960s. State codification has, in fact, become more of a necessity for advanced practice nurses (APNs) over the years. This has not been a problem for medicine because it claimed the whole of health care in its initial practice acts. Ever since, nurses and other health professionals have had to carve out their practices in state statutes to protect against charges of "practicing medicine" as the practice evolved. This expanded scope of practice, resulting from both evolutionary and revolutionary changes in health care and its delivery, made state codification of nurse anesthetists' roles even more important. California found codification necessary for its nurse anesthetists to reverse an attorney general's opinion that rendered it unlawful for nurses to provide regional anesthesia. The attorney general maintained that the California statute did not distinguish among types of nurses, and therefore opinions had to apply to all nurses.[28] To date, nurse anesthetists are addressed in one or more places within state statutes or regulations in all 50 states. Tobin[29] states, "Although it is clear that legitimacy of nurse anesthesia as a profession is widely accepted, the manner, type, and frequency of statutory and regulatory recognition of CRNA practice varies considerably." Historically and to the present day, state and federal regulations regarding nurse anesthetists and their practice have been battle sites where anesthesiologist–nurse anesthetist differences are publicly fought.

AMERICAN ASSOCIATION OF NURSE ANESTHETISTS' INCREASING FEDERAL INVOLVEMENT IN THE 1970s

The recognition of the AANA as the accreditor of nurse anesthesia programs by the U.S. Commissioner of Education in 1955 marked the AANA's first formalized relationship with federal agencies other than the military services and the Veterans Administration (VA). With the passage of federal Medicare and Medicaid legislation and of subsequent legislation that provided for the funding of the education of additional health professionals, many nurse anesthetists saw the need for a federal presence for the AANA. In the late 1960s a resolution was passed at an AANA business meeting that mandated the AANA to monitor federal legislation and to acquire a lobbyist. The signers of the resolution did not dream that the profession's governmental activities would grow sufficiently in the subsequent 20 years to require establishment of an AANA federal affairs office in Washington, D.C.

In 1970 the ASA procured a grant from the Bureau of Health Manpower of the U.S. Department of Health, Education, and Welfare (the forerunner of the current Department of Health and Human Services and the Department of Education) to perform a demographic study of anesthesia providers, both CRNAs and anesthesiologists. The Bureau of Health Manpower requested that the AANA furnish a listing of its membership with members' home or practice locations to use in the study. This was the extent to which the AANA was asked to participate in the study. When the study was completed and sent to the funding agency in 1972, it carried a notation that it had been conducted in cooperation with the AANA. As a result, governmental reviewers, in addressing its recommendations, did not think anything was amiss when one of the recommendations was for anesthesiologists to become more involved in the education and credentialing of nurse anesthetists.

This study was also made available by the ASA to the U.S. Office of Education's Department of Eligibility and Agency Evaluation, the group that reviewed accrediting agencies. John Profitt, director of this department, began communicating with the AANA on how this recommendation could best be implemented without knowing that the AANA had never been a party to the recommendation. This set the stage for a major confrontation between the ASA and AANA in the mid 1970s concerning which organization was going to control nurse anesthesia educational programs and credential their graduates. This very public challenge came at a time when major change was taking place in the criteria by which the Office of Education recognized accrediting agencies. These new criteria reflected many of the trends of the 1960s, including requirements defined in the civil rights legislation of that decade, such as public accountability, nondiscrimination, the involvement of the community of interests in decision-making, students as the consumers of educational programs, requirements for due process, and grievance procedures to ensure fair and equitable treatment of students and faculty, as well as the typical educational standards concerning curriculum, instruction, and evaluation.

When these criteria were published in the *Federal Register* in August 1974, it became apparent that a great deal of change would have to be made in the AANA's educational standards, particularly as they related to the administration of accredited programs. It would also be necessary to change the organizational structure of the AANA to ensure that the accrediting groups' degree of autonomy would be maintained. It was decided that the body and mechanism for certification would be patterned after that planned for accreditation, in the belief that greater autonomy in private credentialing was the wave of the future. I was designated as project manager to spearhead this process, with Ruth P. Satterfield and Mary Cavagnaro (both AANA educational consultants) serving as principal advisors and assistants. Edward Kaleita was the newly appointed AANA educational director at that time.

After consultation with various educational and association leaders within the AANA, it became apparent that the time was right to implement new standards that incorporated not only the Office of Education's criteria but also those that set the stage for moving nurse anesthesia educational programs into university frameworks. Furthermore, with its accrediting mechanism under constant challenge by anesthesiologists, the AANA considered it necessary to demonstrate more definitive compliance with the Office of Education's criteria than did other accrediting agencies. These efforts resulted in the development of the credentialing council structure of the AANA.

The councils were first established as ad hoc structures in January 1975 because the AANA was one of the first accrediting agencies to be reviewed by Office of Education under the new criteria in March 1975. The new organizational structure was confirmed with bylaw changes at the annual meeting in August 1975. Separate councils for accreditation (Council on Accreditation for Nurse Anesthesia Educational Programs and Schools) and certification (Council on Certification of Nurse Anesthetists) were established as multidisciplinary bodies composed of members of the community of interests, including CRNAs, anesthesiologists, a hospital administrator, a student, and potential consumers of anesthesia services (i.e., the general public). These councils were given full autonomy in decision-making concerning the credential that each council was authorized to confer. The Council on Practice was established to serve as an appeal body for the two councils, as well as to attend to matters that might be of public concern. (Some younger CRNAs have questioned why the Council on Practice was established to serve as an appellate body for the credentialing councils. The AANA did not have a standing committee on practice at the time; the AANA Board of Directors served that function, as needed. I believed that all credentialing, public or private, exists primarily to protect the public and that practice is the interface between the public and the educational program and practitioner. Therefore, I recommended "Council on Nurse Anesthesia Practice" as the name for this appellate body; this name was subsequently accepted by the AANA Board of Directors and the members. The implementation within the AANA structure a few years later of a standing committee on practice necessitated a name change so that confusion would be avoided. The name was changed to the "Council for Public Interest in Nurse Anesthesia" in 1987.)

In 1979 the AANA membership established the Council on Recertification, which was responsible for the recertification program mandated in 1976 and implemented in 1978. Recertification has been and continues to be based primarily on continuing educational requirements and is required every 2 years. This program evolved from an AANA voluntary program implemented in 1968 for procuring certificates of excellence; the program was based on the acquisition of 100 contact hours of continuing education over a 5-year period. There is an evolving trend that could lead in the near future to a multifaceted approach for recertification, including the possibility of retesting.

The very public challenge leveled by the ASA against the AANA was answered, and recognition by the Office of Education was continued. It was this challenge that brought about the rapprochement between nurse anesthesia and the mainstream of nursing, a schism that had existed since the AANA's organization. Nursing believed that allowing physicians to take over the professional credentialing process of a long-standing nursing specialty could lead to other attempts by medicine to gain control over other nursing groups. Therefore, support for the AANA with regard to this challenge was forthcoming from the major players within the nursing community. The involvement of many CRNA practitioners, program directors, and students in acquiring letters of support for the AANA's credentialing mechanisms and their presence at Office of Education hearings also served as a training ground for subsequent lobbying of the federal government and of Congress. The Council on Accreditation has been recognized by the Council on Post-Secondary Accreditation (COPA), a private counterpart to governmental recognition since 1985. COPA has now evolved into the Council for Higher Education Accreditation.

The anesthesiologists' challenge of the AANA's credentialing prerogatives was a major one, disrupting many good relationships between individual CRNAs and anesthesiologists. This situation was further exacerbated by the AANA's first venture to seek legislation for direct reimbursement for CRNAs within the Medicare program in 1976. Medicine had long believed that physicians should be the only health-care professionals directly reimbursed for patient services and had been exceptionally active at the federal level in attempting to enforce this view in Medicare and Medicaid. The AANA was somewhat politically naive at this time, and the effort failed. However, the challenge before the Office of Education served to educate many CRNA leaders in the federal political and regulatory process, and these lessons were successfully drawn on when direct reimbursement was again on the AANA's legislative agenda in the 1980s.

Another change affecting nurse anesthetists and all professionals was the 1976 Supreme Court decision in the case of *Goldfarb v. Virginia State Bar*, 421 US 773 (1976), which ruled that members of learned professions were not exempt from federal antitrust laws. This decision was subsequently confirmed in the case of *National Society of Professional Engineers v. United States*, 435 US 679 (1978).

In both these cases, the U.S. Supreme Court indicated that in some circumstances the attempts by professional groups to self-regulate the quality of their services or the ethics of their profession might be treated differently from other economic activities. However, the court in these and later decisions left little doubt that it would view these efforts with considerable suspicion and that exemption of the "learned professions," if extant at all, would be very narrowly defined.[30] Therefore, nurse anesthetists and other professionals are subject to antitrust laws. However, they also can use them when they are victims of a conspiracy to restrict their practices or another antitrust violation.

Although there have been many incidents in the education and practice of nurse anesthetists in which suspicion of antitrust violations has arisen, antitrust violations are often difficult to prove and are exceedingly lengthy and costly to pursue. The cases filed by two CRNAs, Tafford Oltz (*Oltz v. St. Peters Community Hospital*, 861 F2d 1440, 1450 [9th Cir 1988]) and Vinnie Bhan (*Bhan v. NME Hospitals, Inc.*, 84-2256, DC No. CV-S-83-295 LKK [October 2, 1985]), demonstrated these facts. Oltz had held clinical privileges and had worked as a private practitioner at St. Peters Community Hospital in Helena, Montana. His clinical privileges were terminated when the hospital gave an exclusive contract to a group of anesthesiologists. Oltz alleged, and the court agreed, that the hospital and the anesthesiologists had conspired to terminate his privileges so that the anesthesiologists would have access to his cases. Another factor involved in this case was that Oltz offered regional anesthesia as a part of his practice, and the anesthesiologists at St. Peters were not as interested in providing this type of anesthesia. Also, there were cost savings to the public when Oltz administered anesthesia compared with when the anesthesiologists did. The court found that St. Peters Community Hospital had a significant market share of health-care services within its service area, and as a result, the awarding of an exclusive contract to the anesthesiologists and the termination of Oltz's privileges damaged competition. The verdict in favor of Oltz and the damages awarded were appealed by the hospital. (Oltz had previously settled with the anesthesiologists.) On appeal, the Ninth Circuit Court upheld the decision of the lower court with regard to the antitrust violation but remanded the case back to the lower court for retrial on the damages. Oltz again won in the retrial on damages, but the hospital once again appealed on a liability issue. Once again, Oltz won at the appellate court level, and the case was finally settled in August 1994, more than 12 years after it had been filed. Although nondisclosure was a condition of the final settlement of monetary damages in this case, the court awarded Oltz (the plaintiff) $1.6 million in attorney fees.[31]

The Bhan case was filed for similar reasons. However, the defendants challenged Bhan's standing—that is, his legal right to file an anticompetitive suit against NME, Inc. The anesthesiologists involved asserted that Bhan, who was licensed as a nurse and nurse anesthetist, could not legally compete with licensed physicians because of the differences in their legal scopes of practice. The defendant's argument prevailed at the lower court; however, the decision was reversed on appeal.

The Circuit Court reasoned that "the issue is not whether the two groups perform identical services, but whether there is reasonable interchangeability of use or . . . cross-elasticity of demand between the services provided by nurse anesthetists and by MD anesthesiologists."[32]

The Circuit Court concluded, "*No doubt the legal restrictions upon nurse anesthetists create a functional distinction between nurses and MD anesthesiologists. They do not, however, necessarily preclude the existence of a reasonable interchangeability of use or cross-elasticity of demand sufficient to constrain the market power of MD anesthesiologists and thereby to affect competition*" (emphasis added).[32] The court continued, stating that "as a matter of law, Bhan's allegations are sufficient to establish that he is a proper party to bring this antitrust action."[32]

Bhan lost his case because the hospital that terminated his privileges was ruled not to have sufficient market share in the community for the action to serve as a constraint on competition. The sine qua non of antitrust laws is the fact that they exist to protect competition, not competitors, and therefore the proof must be that competition within a defined economic market is adversely affected. However, the appellate court ruling that gave Bhan and CRNAs standing to sue anesthesiologists under antitrust laws sets a significant legal precedent for the profession.

FEDERAL LEGISLATIVE INITIATIVES IN THE 1980s

After the turbulent 1970s it was hoped that a somewhat more peaceful environment would prevail in the 1980s. CRNAs were actively sought health-care professionals and practiced principally in three types of settings. The majority of civilian CRNAs worked as employees of hospitals or of anesthesiologists. In addition, a small but growing number of CRNAs were private practitioners. Their major problem at the time was an inability to gain direct reimbursement from many governmental programs, as well as from many private payers.

The private practitioners wanted the AANA to become more involved in assisting CRNAs to obtain direct reimbursement from both governmental and private payers for the anesthesia services that the CRNAs provided. Many of the contracts between CRNA private practitioners and hospitals for the provision of anesthesia services stipulated that the hospital serve as a billing service for them; this allowed the hospital to take a small percentage of the income generated from their services. These CRNAs believed that this arrangement was not to their advantage for a variety of reasons. First, some hospital administrators did not want the hospital to act as the billing agent and preferred the CRNA to be employed if they had to be the billing agent. Second, it was not always in the best interest of CRNAs for the hospital administrator to know the amount of income that the CRNAs were generating.

During 1980 and 1981, some AANA leaders were somewhat intimidated by the reaction of the anesthesiologists when the AANA first sought direct reimbursement for CRNAs. Therefore, direct reimbursement was not one of their priorities. Furthermore, the efforts and expenditures necessary to fight the challenges of the 1970s had depleted the AANA's treasury, and the leaders believed that the AANA needed time for retrenchment.

Every profession must attend to certain activities through its professional association; for CRNAs these include monitoring and ensuring appropriate and timely standards of practice and education; establishing and enforcing ethical codes; issuing practice policies; ensuring the availability of malpractice insurance for its members; monitoring governmental regulations and those of private credentialing agencies, such as the Joint Commission on Accreditation of Healthcare Organizations; and intervening, whenever possible, in the interest of its members. Many of these areas also needed attention.

Although all professions have an inherent conflict of interest in terms of their obligations to the public versus those to their members, the implementation of the AANA's council structure freed the AANA to take a more vigorous stance with regard to protection of its members' interests. This was made possible by the AANA's provision of autonomy to the Councils on Accreditation, Certification, and Recertification and their appellate body, the Council on Public Interest, which eliminated the AANA's overt conflict of interest in credentialing for the public welfare while pursuing efforts aimed at members' benefit.

The AANA, as a professional association with more than 18,000 members in the early 1980s, was somewhat different from most other such associations. Although authority for policy making was vested within its board of directors, the power within the AANA shifted from time to time from the executive director to the board of directors. Florence McQuillen was executive director of the AANA from 1948 to 1970, and as Bankert reports, "No single Association leader before or after 'Mac' would exercise comparable control over all facets of [the AANA's] business."[5] However, AANA members, holding dearly to their rights as members, have repeatedly turned down suggestions that it might be time to adopt a house-of-delegates governing mechanism. CRNAs have expressed their desire to maintain their right to speak about issues at the annual meeting, to offer resolutions and bylaw changes to the membership if they can obtain sufficient cosigners, and to vote directly for their officers and directors. The voting body for appointments other than those of AANA officials has consisted and continues to consist of the members who attend the annual meeting.

Because these prerogatives have been maintained, the AANA's annual business meetings, despite having a skilled parliamentarian, have been lively and characterized by member debates. The members have been known on limited occasions to vote down recommendations of their board of directors; at the 1993 annual meeting, against the recommendations of their board of directors, members even voted themselves a dues increase that they believed was warranted. As a result of this modus operandi, members, having access to the floor at business meetings, have presented issues that might otherwise not have been brought to the floor or that might have been acted on much later. The members' ability to vote and elect their leadership also gives them the opportunity to change leaders and to put in leaders who are sympathetic to their interests.

Such was the case in the early 1980s. Although many CRNAs were tired of the challenges of the 1970s and wanted nothing better than a few peaceful years, others recognized that many things were happening that would have direct impact on CRNAs and their practice and that the work ahead did not allow for rest. Among these issues were the federal and state governments' concerns regarding the cost of governmental health programs such as Medicare and Medicaid, the adequacy of the national health-care manpower mix, and the impact of the cost of health insurance on businesses and industry. Hospital costs had been singled out as a major problem, and studies were ongoing with regard to control of these costs. Because almost 50% of CRNAs were employed by hospitals at that time, anything aimed at controlling hospital costs could affect CRNAs. Many of the flaws in the system that related to cost escalation were based on incentives within health insurance or reimbursement mechanisms that actually promoted higher costs. Despite the AANA's many successes over the years, those AANA members who saw the increasing pressures building in society to address the emerging health-care problems believed that the AANA must change its operations to have a more proactive stance if CRNAs were to continue to meet future challenges successfully. In the election of AANA officers and board members in 1981 and 1982, CRNAs saw an opportunity to put into power a group of CRNAs willing and able to make every effort to move the AANA forward with regard to affairs of government, even if this action meant taking unpopular positions with physician colleagues.

Pat Fleming assumed the office of AANA president in August 1982. Although she had run for president in 1981 on the platform of "A Choice for Change," she did not realize the extent to which political events would influence her actions as president and set into motion a series of legislative initiatives that demanded the AANA's attention on a continuing basis throughout the subsequent years. The principal events during her presidency that necessitated priority action by the AANA were the Tax Equity and Fiscal Responsibility Act of 1982 (TEFRA), the decision to file an amicus curiae brief with the United States Supreme Court concerning the case of *Jefferson Parish Hospital District v. Hyde*, 104 SCt 1551 (1984), and the federal enactment into law of the Medicare Prospective Payment System (PPS) for Hospitals.

Tax Equity and Fiscal Responsibility Act of 1982

When the AANA first approached the Senate Finance Committee in 1976 and 1977 regarding direct reimbursement for CRNAs, the committee expressed concerns over the escalating Medicare costs for what formerly had been called "hospital-based services," including anesthesiology, pathology, and radiology. At the time the committee was exploring means for containing these costs. Despite the actions taken, by 1982 additional efforts were being made to constrain these costs. This effort took the form of the TEFRA legislation.

Before the passage of TEFRA in 1982, hospitals could bill Medicare under Part A for anesthesia services rendered by nurse anesthetists in hospitals and under Part B for anesthesia services rendered by nurse anesthetists in outpatient settings. The reimbursement was based on "a reasonable charge." The hospital also derived profits from the use of anesthesia drugs, supplies, and capital equipment.

Anesthesiologists could not bill for hospital-employed CRNAs' services, but they could bill for their own services in conjunction with medical direction of such CRNAs. This, however, was at a rate different from what they could bill for their own employed CRNAs. Although Medicare did not require anesthesiologists to actually be in the operating room with CRNAs to be reimbursed, its manual (4-76, 2050.2, Rev. 3-512, 2.21) did require that "the physician be close by and available to provide immediate and personal assistance and direction." The manual stated that availability by telephone would not constitute direct, personal, and continuous service.

However, in many instances during this period, anesthesiologists were billing for services when they were not present in the hospital or even in town. Some chose not to come out at night or on weekends to supervise care provided in emergencies, yet they billed as if they had been present. Anesthesiologist supervision or billing capability for concurrent cases was not limited to any specific fixed numbers, permitting abuse. During this time some surgeons were openly critical of the number of fees being paid to anesthesiologists for concurrent services, particularly when the anesthesiologists were not available. Some of these surgeons and other providers complained to both private insurers and Medicare. As a result, some private payers began limiting reimbursement to not more than two concurrent procedures, and Medicare's Inspector General focused on anesthesia reimbursement in the search for potential fraud. Around this time Richard Veruille, the AANA's Washington counsel, stated that a source in the Inspector General's office of what was then the U.S. Department of Health, Education, and Welfare had told him that approximately 25% of Medicare fraud and abuse investigations concerned anesthesia services.

Among other things, TEFRA addressed anesthesia, radiology, and laboratory payments. The legislation indicated a need to ensure that anesthesiologists demonstrate that they provided certain services as a part of a given anesthetic procedure to qualify for payment. (These services have been referred to as the seven conditions for anesthesiologist payment when medically directing CRNAs. These seven conditions initially were those conditions specified by the ASA in its *Guidelines to the Ethical Practice of Anesthesiology*, adopted October 25, 1978, effective February 12, 1979, for anesthesiologists when medically directing nonphysicians in an anesthesia care team (ACT) configuration. Therefore, the ASA has considered them standards of practice. Although changes have been made in the ASA's ethical guidelines, the last of which was in 2003, according to the online copy of the ethical code [http://www.asahq.org/publicationsAndServices/Standards/10.pdf] these components of it have not been changed.)

Subsequent to the enactment of the law, the Health Care Financing Administration (HCFA) proposed rules for implementation of TEFRA. The proposed rules separated reimbursement for anesthesiologists based on supervision or direction.

Essentially the proposed rules called for anesthesiologist payments on the basis of direction to be limited to not more than two concurrent procedures administered by CRNAs. Such a payment took two forms, depending on the CRNA's employer. When the CRNAs were employed by the anesthesiologist, each service was billed as though the anesthesiologist had administered each case. When the CRNAs were hospital employees, the time units for the anesthesiologist were cut in half. When the anesthesiologist's service was supervision and not direction (i.e., supervising three or more CRNAs), the payment was to be made under Part A on the basis of reasonable charge. The hospital could still bill for the CRNA services of their own employees under Part A if the services were provided within the hospital and under Part B if the services were provided in a surgical center.

The AANA opposed the 2:1 ratio for the following reasons:

1. No research indicated differences in anesthesia outcomes based on fixed supervision or direction ratios in the provision of anesthesia services.
2. Because such ratios did not take into consideration the characteristics of the anesthesia workload or the population served within a given hospital, they were inappropriate for determining cost-effective personnel resources for a given facility.
3. Implementation of such ratios would significantly increase the cost of anesthesia services to individual Medicare beneficiaries and decrease the acceptance of Medicare assignment by anesthesiologists (which did not have a high assignment acceptance rate).
4. If the HCFA considered it necessary to differentiate between supervision and direction on the basis of an anesthesiologist's involvement, a 4:1 ratio would be more cost-effective in the long run, at least to beneficiaries, because anesthesiologists could derive greater income and would be more inclined to accept Medicare assignment. The AANA further stated that, although the use of a ratio might be appropriate with regard to reimbursement, a ratio should never be used to imply a quality standard.

The HCFA published final rules implementing TEFRA.[20] The HCFA chose the 4:1 ratio rather than the originally proposed 2:1 ratio. They also imposed the seven conditions that an anesthesiologist must satisfy with regard to an anesthetic procedure if he or she is to obtain reimbursement for the medical direction of CRNAs:[33]

1. Perform a preanesthesia evaluation
2. Prescribe the anesthesia plan
3. Personally participate in induction and emergence and other demanding procedures in the plan
4. Monitor the course of anesthesia administration at frequent intervals
5. Remain physically available for the immediate diagnosis and treatment of emergencies
6. Provide needed postanesthesia care
7. Refrain from personally performing an anesthesia procedure when purporting to be engaged in medical direction

Over the years, various interpretations have somewhat loosened these conditions; for example, in an emergency, an anesthesiologist engaged in medically directing CRNAs may go to the obstetrics area and administer a regional anesthetic.

The HCFA also stated the following in the *Federal Register*:

> The distinction we are making is between physician services to providers and individuals, not between good and bad anesthesia services. . . . Therefore the criteria for "medical direction" should not be interpreted as standards of practice or standards of quality, but rather as a description of those elements of common medical practice that are expected to be present when a physician has significant involvement with an individual patient *[emphasis added]*.[34]

Hyde v. Jefferson Parish Hospital District No. 2

The case of *Hyde v. Jefferson Parish Hospital District No. 2* centered on whether an exclusive contract by a group of anesthesiologists was, per se, a violation of the Sherman antitrust laws, because such a contract was the basis for denying Dr. Hyde clinical privileges in the East Jefferson Hospital, which was part of the larger Jefferson Parish Hospital District No. 2. At this hospital, a group of anesthesiologists who had an exclusive contract worked with hospital-employed CRNAs to cover anesthesia services. It was a fairly large hospital with a sizable workload. Dr. Hyde, who had clinical privileges at other hospitals in the area, decided he also wanted clinical privileges at East Jefferson Hospital. His request was denied solely on the basis of the exclusive contract. The legal question raised by the case was whether a patient who was admitted by his or her surgeon to East Jefferson Hospital for surgery in effect had any choice but to buy anesthesia from the hospital's exclusive group of anesthesiologists. It was alleged that this situation represented a tying arrangement, such as those previously found to be per se violations of the antitrust laws. (A tying arrangement would be similar to going to a store to buy bread but being unable to buy it by itself. Rather, one would be required to buy butter to get the bread, whether or not the purchaser used butter on bread.)

The Jefferson Parish Hospital District won the case at the lower court level. Dr. Hyde appealed to the U.S. Court of Appeals, which ruled in his favor. Jefferson Parish Hospital District then filed an appeal to the U.S. Supreme Court. This would ordinarily not be a case in which the AANA would consider filing an amicus curiae brief; however, in both the lower court and appellate court opinions, the judges cited some rather derogatory conclusions regarding nurse anesthetists that had been presented by anesthesiologists testifying for Dr. Hyde in an attempt to discredit the quality of anesthesia service provided by East Jefferson Parish Hospital. The AANA, in submitting its amicus curiae brief, chose not to take a position for or against exclusive contracts. It only wanted to "set the record straight" about the misrepresentation of nurse anesthetists and ensure that the Supreme Court in its decision did not perpetuate some of the myths cited by the other judges and was not swayed in its decision by such myths.

The AANA Board of Directors requested that the AANA legal counsel acquire permission to file such an amicus curiae brief and then to prepare it. Problems getting the AANA's legal counsel and law firm to follow the AANA's purpose for filing the amicus, identified only approximately 7 days before the due date of the brief, led President Fleming to turn the project over to Gene Blumenreich of the Fine and Ambrogne law firm in Boston. Blumenreich was legal counsel for the Massachusetts Association of Nurse Anesthetists at the time. Blumenreich was to be assisted by Richard Verville of Fine and Verville, the AANA's Washington, D.C. attorney, and by Susan Jenkins of Lyon and Kurz, also in the District of Columbia.

In the AANA amicus curiae brief the Supreme Court was asked to decide the issue on very narrow grounds, ignoring the previous courts' opinions as they related to nurse anesthetists.

It stated that nurse anesthetists were not a party to the suit, had not had representation during any of the proceedings, and had certainly had no opportunity to counter erroneous testimony. The amicus masterfully corrected the record on nurse anesthetists.[34]

The ASA also filed an amicus curiae brief, but in support of Dr. Hyde. The ASA concluded their brief as follows:

> *ASA submits that this is hardly the case in which to reverse thirty-five years of consistent Supreme Court precedent applying the per se rule in tying cases. In the circumstances of this case, which involves the administration of lethal drugs to human beings under carefully controlled conditions, the elimination of competition through a classic tying arrangement is not simply a matter of dollars and cents. It can adversely affect the quality of medical care. ASA believes that in this setting it is particularly important that competition be allowed to reward superior performance and innovation, while exposing the indifference to quality that may too often be the hallmark of a monopoly.*[35]

The Supreme Court, during its hearing on this case, gave evidence of noting the AANA's brief in its questioning of attorneys who argued the case. When the ruling came down, the Supreme Court had decided unanimously in favor of the hospital, not Dr. Hyde. The justices differed (five to four) as to why they decided in favor of the hospital. The majority opinion stated that the decision was based on the finding that "every refusal to sell two products separately cannot be said to restrain competition" and that no evidence had been presented to support the contention that the hospital had forced unwilling patients to buy this service. Because they found that this arrangement did not violate the per se rule, they applied the "rule of reason" and found no evidence of adverse effect on competition. East Jefferson Hospital did not have market power. The concurring opinion, written by Justice O'Connor and supported by three other justices, stated that it was time to abandon the per se rule and to focus on the adverse economic effects and the potential economic benefits of the exclusive contract. Finding no adverse competitive effects, and even citing a potential benefit from the exclusive contract in increasing a hospital's efficiency, these justices concurred that this exclusive contract was not a violation of the antitrust laws.[35]

The Hyde case is important, not only for clarifying the law, but for its opportunity to correct the legal records concerning CRNAs. Case transcripts represent sworn testimony. Although some testimony, and indeed judges' decisions, may represent opinion, some testimony is considered fact. Furthermore, within the court's jurisdictional area, judges' opinions become "common law" if not appealed or if upheld on appeal. Case records and opinions are filed and are used repeatedly by other attorneys and scholars in developing briefs or legal theories or in illustrating legal theory in textbooks. Decisions in court cases and judges' opinions can be overturned by appellate courts; grossly erroneous information in court transcripts can be corrected through briefs, such as amicus curiae, and legal rulings. Without refutation, erroneous information may be passed along and assumed to be fact by the unknowing. What happened in the Louisiana courts in this case is similar to what the anesthesiologists did to discredit CRNAs after World War II. The Hyde case alerted the AANA to the need to revitalize its public relations program, continue its watch for attempts to discredit CRNAs or the profession, and take action either to correct or to prevent further damage.

Medicare Prospective Payment System for Hospital Services

The AANA was still dealing with TEFRA when, in early 1983, without much fanfare and with less media exposure than usually accompanies such legislation, the PPS legislation was passed in an effort to control the hospital costs of the Medicare program. Until that time, hospitals were allowed to submit their bills on a cost-plus basis to Medicare and therefore had no incentives for controlling their costs. The PPS was scheduled to be phased in over a 4-year period. Hospitals would be reimbursed for their services on the basis of prospective pricing for various diagnosis-related groups. Thus, if the hospital services did not cost as much as the hospital was paid, the hospital reaped a profit; if the services' actual costs were greater than the amount paid, the hospital had to absorb the loss.

Verville, the AANA's Washington attorney, and the AANA's Government Relations Committee and consultants analyzed the legislation and found that CRNAs had inadvertently been put at a decided disadvantage in the workplace. The law actually was placing pressure on Medicare Part A (the hospital component) without constraint on Medicare Part B (the physician services component). The law provided that all services by providers, other than those with authorized payment under Medicare Part B, would be bundled in the hospital diagnosis-related group payment. First, the manner in which the diagnosis-related group payment had been calculated made it impossible for the anesthesia component of the payment to fully cover the cost of hospital-employed CRNAs and provided a partial payment for CRNAs to hospitals that did not employ them. Second, unbundling of services and payments was prohibited. Third, anesthesiologists who employed CRNAs and who had been billing for CRNA services under Part B by considering them as a physician service were impeded from acquiring payment for those services. These three problems served as a strong disincentive to the use of CRNAs. Although the full impact of these changes would not be felt for 4 years, it became obvious that immediate action had to be initiated to correct the disincentives.

The AANA developed an option paper that demonstrated the impact of the PPS legislation on nurse anesthetists, including its potential to result in higher costs for anesthesia services. AANA leaders believed that the only alternative for preventing the disincentives to using CRNA services found in the legislation was the acquisition of direct reimbursement rights for CRNAs under Medicare Part B or the placement of reimbursement for all anesthesia services (those provided by both anesthesiologists and CRNAs) under Medicare Part A. Based on its analysis and conclusions, the AANA's plans for resolving the problems that the PPS had created for CRNAs also took into consideration the fact that making anesthesia a hospital-based service was not politically feasible at that time. The AANA proposed and eventually acquired the following provisions:

1. A temporary pass-through of hospitals' CRNA costs for a 3-year period, which would assure hospitals that they would not lose money on CRNA services for Medicare patients
2. A single exception to the unbundling provisions of the law for anesthesiologist-employed CRNAs, because it was questionable whether anesthesiologists could be reimbursed for CRNA services without such a provision
3. Direct reimbursement for all CRNAs under Medicare, because provisions 1 and 2 were temporary, and CRNAs needed a mechanism under Medicare that would pay for CRNA services

The AANA and CRNAs agreed to accept assignment as a condition for passage of the direct reimbursement legislation. As a part of the Omnibus Budget Reconciliation Act of 1986, direct reimbursement for CRNAs was enacted into law to become effective January 1, 1989, with the two temporary provisions being extended to the effective date of the legislation. The various practice configurations of CRNAs required the development of two payment schedules—one for CRNAs not medically directed by anesthesiologists and the other for CRNAs working under an anesthesiologist's direction. This latter payment schedule resulted in significantly higher Medicare prices for anesthesia services compared with prices for services provided either by anesthesiologists who administered their own anesthesia or by non–medically directed CRNAs. Furthermore, as a part of this legislation, Congress mandated a study of reimbursement mechanisms that would not serve as disincentives to the use of CRNAs.[37]

The success that the AANA achieved with respect to Medicare during this period must be attributed to the commitment of the profession and its leaders to goals set during the Fleming administration. This required the commitment and concerted actions of the leaders of the succeeding AANA administrations—Patrick Downey, Barbara Adams, Richard Ouellette, Peggy McFadden, and Jan Mannino. Furthermore, AANA members owe much to Richard Verville, AANA's Washington attorney; Debbie Hardy, AANA lobbyist of Capitol Associates; and Jay Constantine, another lobbyist, who formerly had been the chief staff member of the Senate Finance Committee when the AANA first attempted to gain reimbursement, for expertise and expended untiring effort toward achieving these goals. Their commitment to this cause made them part of the AANA family, not merely retained experts.

Furthermore, these activities gave AANA members the opportunity to make certain that their legislators knew who CRNAs were; how much they contributed to the provision of anesthesia services in this country, along with its quality; and why such legislation was important to the nation, as well as to CRNAs—and they indeed met the challenge. Some of the legislators whom they were able to persuade to introduce and cosponsor AANA's direct reimbursement bills were Matsunaga (Democrat, Hawaii), Inouye (Democrat, Hawaii), Sasser (Democrat, Tennessee), Pell (Democrat, Rhode Island), Pressler (Republican, South Dakota), Humphrey (Republican, New Hampshire), Sarbanes (Democrat, Maryland), Melcher (Democrat, Montana), Burdick (Democrat, North Dakota), and Leahy (Democrat, Vermont) in the U.S. Senate and Barney Franks (Democrat, Massachusetts) and other cosponsors in the U.S. House of Representatives. Many of these legislators were fully aware that without nurse anesthetists, rural health care would have been nonexistent in many of their states. Nurse anesthetists, serving as the sole anesthesia providers in many of these areas, were also believed to be a key in retaining physicians in rural areas and in keeping hospitals in these areas open.

However, it is not enough to ensure that legislation is passed. Monitoring and intervention during the period of rulemaking must and did occur. Permanent rules were not in place until 1991.[36]

The activism of the AANA at this time was thought to have been partially responsible for the ASA's issuance of practice policies that if adhered to would have restricted CRNA practice and severely limited obstetric patients' access to regional anesthesia. The ASA's policy that "only physicians should perform regional anesthesia" was the basis for the action of a Maine attorney general when anesthesiologists in Portland, Maine, revoked the right of CRNAs to perform regional blocks and to teach them to their students. The Maine attorney general obtained a consent decree from the anesthesiologists that reversed their decision regarding CRNAs' performance and teaching of regional blocks.[5]

Quality-of-Care Studies

Despite the frequent challenges by the ASA, neither the AANA nor its members had given much time to considering the performance of quality-of-care studies relative to patient outcomes by CRNAs. There had been a constant market for nurse anesthesia services, and surgeons had provided them support and acclaim. There were no major indicators of any significant problems, although little question existed that studies demonstrating accountability in terms of patient outcomes were on the horizon. What was then called the "expanded role nurse" and now the "advanced practice nurse" essentially came on the health-care scene in the 1960s and 1970s. The nurse practitioner was the major new provider, along with the physician assistant, newly introduced by medicine. Certified nurse-midwives, who had existed in limited numbers before that time, began to expand their ranks and set up nurse-midwifery services. It was anticipated that these providers would offer many services previously restricted to physicians, and their practice and outcomes would be subjected to multiple studies. Because at that time nurse anesthetists quantitatively performed the greatest number of anesthetic procedures in the United States and few complaints were being heard, not much thought was given to studying their outcomes, except by a few physicians. Beecher and Todd's study, reported in 1954, had shown that nurse anesthetist mortality statistics were less than half those of anesthesiologists, even though the sample size for nurse anesthetists was twice that for anesthesiologists. Furthermore, the physical status of the patients in both groups was studied and was found to be similar.[14]

In a North Carolina retrospective study of anesthesia-related mortality during the period from 1969 to 1976, performed by a committee from the North Carolina Society of Anesthesiologists, the authors reported in 1981 that the findings based on providers (e.g., CRNAs, anesthesiologists, and CRNAs and anesthesiologists) were similar. No test of significance was made in this study because adequate data had not been collected to assess the likelihood that a variety of variables were factors in these cases.[37]

In the mid 1970s, amid major complaints about the VA health-care system, the U.S. House of Representatives mandated a study by the National Science Foundation regarding the care given to veterans. As a part of that study, physicians and surgeons reviewed a sample of VA medical facilities regarding the care being given. Most of the larger facilities were being used by medical schools both for medical student and graduate medical education. However, because of the shortfall of anesthesia residencies at that time, many nurse anesthetists were employed by the VA and worked in these facilities. The reviewers included surgery and anesthesia in their assessment and reported back to Congress in 1977 that there was no significant difference in the outcomes of anesthesia based on the provider of that care.[38]

In 1980 W. H. Forrest, an anesthesiologist, reported and published a portion of an institutional differences study conducted by the Stanford Center for Health Care Research. In looking at hospitals and anesthesia outcomes, dividing the hospitals between those predominantly served by nurse anesthetists and those predominantly served by anesthesiologists, he also came to the conclusion, using conservative statistical methods, that there were no significant differences in anesthesia outcomes between the two hospital groups defined by their anesthesia provider.[39] (I had opportunity to talk with Dr. Forrest regarding his study, and he mentioned that he had been castigated by his colleagues for reporting these results.)

It was apparent that the physicians and anesthesiologists were conducting the studies and demonstrating that CRNAs were doing a commendable job. Furthermore, the fact that many anesthesiologists would not believe the studies performed by their own colleagues gave little reason to think that these anesthesiologists would believe studies conducted by the AANA, if the AANA chose to do some, or even if the AANA paid to have someone else perform such studies.

Educational Funding for Nurse Anesthesia

In 1979 the AANA had been successful in acquiring passage of legislation that would have permitted funding for nurse anesthesia students. However, because the legislation was out of synchronization with the congressional appropriations cycle and because it ran up against some of the Reagan administration's policies, the funding was not available until 1983.[40]

By 1983 the AANA began to notice an increasing number of announcements concerning the closure of long-standing university-affiliated nurse anesthesia educational programs that had coexisted with anesthesiology residency programs. To be sure, the number of graduates of medical schools in the United States had more than doubled since the 1960s, and there was serious recruitment of graduates for anesthesiology residencies. The coming overall surplus of physicians, as identified by the Graduate Medical Education National Advisory Committee, along with its evidence that the field of anesthesiology demonstrated a shortage, added to the rapid influx of medical school graduates and physicians already certified in lower-paying specialty areas into anesthesiology residencies.[40]

The displeasure of many ASA leaders with the AANA's federal initiatives, along with concerns by some anesthesiologists that they were, in fact, participating in preparing their future competitors, led a sizable number of academic chairs to convert nurse anesthesia training slots into medical residency training spaces and to close the nurse anesthesia programs.[41,42] At this time, some anesthesiologist leaders expressed the belief that, once again, the reality of an all-physician specialty might be possible. Strangely, the more that anesthesiologists were prepared, the more that nurse anesthetists were being sought for employment by hospitals, surgical centers, and even anesthesiologists. It has been hypothesized that the decentralization of surgical facilities and the increasing specialization of health care, along with the aging of the population, are reflected in the increasing need for health professionals. Anesthesiology has been no exception.

The shortage of nurse anesthetists prompted salaries to rise to heights that our forebears never imagined. It also increased the workload of practically all CRNAs. The CRNA shortage prompted Congress to mandate a CRNA manpower study, which was reported in February 1990. It also prompted Richard Ouellette, a CRNA who was then serving a second term as association president, to appoint a National Commission on Nurse Anesthesia Education. Sandra Mare, a former AANA president and program director, was appointed to serve as its chairperson. The commission was multidisciplinary in nature, made up of leaders from nursing education, CRNA education, anesthesiology, hospital administration, managed care groups, health policy analysts, and health economists. Their charge was to study the problems concerning nurse anesthesia education and to advise and work with the association to increase its educational programs and the number of graduates from those programs. This study was reported in December 1990. The AANA implemented many of the commission's recommendations, with the consequence being a significant increase in the number of graduates from accredited programs.

Concomitant with the growing shortage of CRNAs were prevailing conditions favoring the possibility of some increases in federal funding for nurse anesthesia educational programs. These increases were tempered by the growing federal deficit, but funds were made available not only for student stipends but also for program development or for expansion and faculty development.

It was also in 1990 that the AANA's federal affairs department was moved to Washington, D.C., with the establishment of an AANA Washington office. A new team of lobbyists came on board to staff the Washington office.

THE CALL FOR HEALTH-CARE REFORM IN THE 1990s

Efforts Toward Cost Containment in Health Care

Health-care reform and cost containment in the delivery of care are important parts of nurse anesthesia history, because many issues involving nurse anesthetists have either evolved or been exacerbated as a result of this movement in which all health-care providers have a major interest. Understanding of these issues within the context of nurse anesthesia history requires some explanation.

The escalating costs of health care precipitated by the passage and implementation of the Medicare and Medicaid programs; the increased federal and state support of health-care professional education in response to the anticipated increase in the number of patients seeking health care, particularly among the elderly and the poor; and the rapid advance of science and technology had led many national leaders to discuss the need for health-care reforms as early as 1972.[43] The 1992 election of Bill Clinton as president of the United States on a platform that promised health-care reform brought both hope and concern to the public and to health-care providers with regard to what actual reforms would be enacted as legislation and how those reforms would affect health professionals. More specifically to anesthesia providers, what would be the role of anesthesiologists and nurse anesthetists in such reform? The president's health-care reform package was aimed at universal coverage and reflected a major shift in health-care delivery toward managed care. A component of the legislation would have preempted state laws and thereby removed legal barriers to the practice of APNs, permitting them to more directly compete with their physician counterparts in efforts to reduce costs. This provision would also have provided the necessary legal authority for APNs to render services for which they were educationally qualified to all segments within the population without physician supervision (in some instances collaborating with or referring patients to physicians).

For a variety of reasons, Clinton's health-care plan was defeated, but in general it was believed to involve too much change in too short a time; too much governmental involvement and control and too many mandates; and too high a cost, although spending caps were a part of its design. Large corporations, the health insurance industry, and in large measure the American Medical Association (AMA) were able to influence enough legislators and the public via major television advertising to kill the plan. As soon as the plan was pronounced dead, the health insurance industry, in conjunction with the major businesses that provided health insurance to their employees, forced a "managed care" system on a large portion of the insured population. This managed care system did not have some of the patient or physician protections that were built into Clinton's proposed plan. However, because of the cost savings projected for a managed care system, the U.S. government offered Medicare beneficiaries certain incentives to move to managed care plans. Subsequently, some states begin to pattern their Medicaid programs after the managed care concept, permitting, in some instances, managed care groups to bid to cover Medicaid patients.

Managed care, in theory and in its pure form, was supposed to (1) move the health-care system from its acute care orientation to a health maintenance, disease prevention system of care; (2) do away with some of the economic incentives found in the fee-for-service system—that is, the more services provided, the more money made—and thereby reduce unnecessary or minimally indicated health services (and concomitant procedures) that had been provided as a major component of the fee-for-service system that had been the major component of the health delivery system[44,45]; (3) promote a more ideal and less costly workforce mix, that is, more primary care providers and fewer specialists, fewer physicians and more nonphysician health professionals such as APNs; and (4) promote a shift from independent practice patterns to greater use of salaried personnel. In fact, in some of the incentives provided to physicians, particularly under capitation arrangements, it was also designed to encourage physicians to treat patients with less costly modalities, to reduce the number of screening and diagnostic tests performed, and to increasingly shorten the time patients spent in hospitals. Hospitals experimented with staffing patterns, in many instances reducing the number of nurses and employing more assistive personnel. Some anesthesiologist groups found their workload reduced by 40%.[46] Health providers tried to find ways to cope with all the changes, and in some instances they were successful.

Managed care, as implemented, took many forms as physicians scrambled to protect their autonomy and their income and patients sought to preserve some of their former health-care rights relative to the choice of provider. The traditional health maintenance organization (HMO) was considered a "one-stop shopping mall" for health-care needs. Kaiser Permanente's HMO was the classic example of a not-for-profit HMO model. It was designed principally to reduce costs by keeping people healthy or by picking up health problems early when they were less costly to correct. However, the following two elements caused the traditional HMO organization to be modified:

1. In efforts to maintain more autonomy and to avoid being placed on salaries, physicians designed physician provider organizations (PPOs), independent practice associations (IPAs), and other, similar entities to contract with insurers and HMOs and other provider service groups and be paid a contracted price per service in many instances, maintaining a fee-for-service practice although at reduced rates in the private sector. Thus, many avoided becoming employees or moving into a capitation environment.
2. Health-care delivery moved even more rapidly under these circumstances to a for-profit enterprise in which investors expected good returns for their investment. This movement also led to corporations with vast numbers of hospitals, followed by mergers, which reduced the alternatives available to the public and payers. Furthermore, groups of physicians began to form, contracting within and across states for the provision of services to specific institutions or chains of institutions. The environment was constantly changing, and security for most health-care professionals relative to their position was lost. For CRNAs there was often a shifting from hospital employment to anesthesiologist group employment, and some CRNAs were left without a position.

The shift from the not-for-profit health-care organizations to for-profit organizations has also affected where health-care dollars are being spent. It has been reported that in for-profit managed care organizations, 30.9% of income on average is spent for administration, payment of merger debt, executive salaries, and stockholders' dividends. In Kaiser Permanente's not-for-profit HMO operation, administrative costs are reported to be approximately 3.5%, while excellent patient services and outcomes are maintained.[47] Data have consistently shown that the cost of health-care services has been higher in the for-profit sector. Data in 1999 showed that higher costs in for-profit facilities had persisted. Although managed care, overall, was thought to be responsible for slowing the escalating cost increases in the mid 1990s, it became obvious that in some organizations much of that slowing was related to a reduction in services to patients, some of which were necessary and lifesaving; as a result, tragic stories hit the media. In some instances costs were shifted to patients when they developed a need for emergency care and had to have health care away from their point of contact for health services. A cry went across the land for a patient's bill of rights, but partisan differences as to just what those rights should be has stalled development of a consensus and passage of such legislation.

Regardless of the modus operandi for delivering health care, the large amount of money involved has also attracted a large amount of fraud, not only associated with the Medicare and Medicaid programs but involving private payers as well. The fraud has taken a variety of forms, including setting up dummy health services providers and billing for services never rendered; up-coding patient diagnoses by hospitals to increase their reimbursement rate; double billing by physicians and hospitals; fraudulent billing practices by individual providers; and fraud on the part of Medicare intermediaries, which are Medicare-designated payers who are supposed to be watchdogs for fraud. When caught, some claim ignorance as the basis for what happened, although it is evident that most fraud has been purposeful and intentional. Even with the increasing surveillance for fraud and personnel devoted to its discovery, it is recognized that much has gone undetected. The result of such fraud can only be higher health-care premiums or a reduction in services provided to beneficiaries. In trying to come to grips with fraud, whistle-blower laws now permit private individuals or groups to pursue cases in court and receive a portion of the award should the case be won. Such was the case in one of the suits brought by the Minnesota Association of Nurse Anesthetists and a group of CRNAs against the Allina Health Systems and some anesthesiology groups after the transfer of hospital-employed CRNAs to anesthesiologist group employment, which resulted in some adverse effects for some of the CRNAs.

For approximately 5 years, cost increases for health-care services slowed. However, in 1998 and 1999 health insurance premiums for managed care entities increased significantly, wiping out many of these cost savings. Furthermore, Medicare patients are being forced out of many managed care plans. Many managed care plans have gone bankrupt, and unrest within the health-care industry and among health professionals and consumers of health services is on the rise.

In summer 1999 two significant studies published in major journals indicated significant problems with the for-profit segment of the health-care industry, prompting some calls for another look at options for health-care reform. In one study the quality of care in for-profit HMOs, as measured by 14 quality-of-care measures using the Health Plan Employer Data and Information Set (HEDIS) from the National Committee for Quality Assurance's Quality Compass, 1997, demonstrated that "investor-owned HMOs deliver lower quality of care than not-for-profit plans."[48] In the other study the authors found that governmental spending "in for-profit areas was greater than in not-for-profit areas in each category of service examined . . . [but] the greatest increase in per capita spending between 1989 and 1995 [was] for hospital services . . . and home health care in areas where for-profit corporations dominated the scene."[49,50] Therefore, questions are beginning to be raised regarding efficacy of the current reforms wrought by the industrial giants and other health payers.[48-50]

Exacerbation of Tension and Conflict between CRNAs and Anesthesiologists

The health-care reform environment has fostered insecurity among health providers and a realization that many advocate the greater use of lower-cost, highly qualified nonphysician health-care providers. This has led to exacerbation of tensions and open conflicts between groups of providers whose scopes of practice permit a significant degree of competition. State legislative agendas have been swamped by legislative proposals to either expand or restrict scopes of practices of various health providers, to gain direct reimbursement rights, to acquire nondiscriminatory language in the use or credentialing of health professionals based on one licensure, to codify the practice of groups, to gain prescriptive rights, and a multiplicity of other types of legislation affecting various players in health-care delivery, including the consumers of care.

These shifts in delivery and payment systems significantly affect CRNAs and anesthesiologists. Theoretically, they can have an even greater impact on anesthesiologists than on CRNAs, because the use of CRNAs has some definite cost advantages without compromise in the quality of care.[14,37-39] This impact is greatly affected by excess training of anesthesiologists since the early 1980s, when they began to convert the training slots of nurse anesthesia programs to medical residency training slots, causing many of the nurse anesthesia programs to close. Although the AANA has worked to recoup the clinical training slots for CRNAs that had previously been lost, it has needed a dozen years to do so. In the meantime, the ratio of anesthesiologists to CRNAs, which in 1986 was 1:1.2,[51] in 1995 was 1.2:1.[54] In the mid 1990s, an excess of anesthesiologists resulted in the inability of a fair number of graduating residents to find positions. When publicized, this phenomenon elicited a response that included a significant drop in the number of graduates of U.S. medical schools who chose to enter the field of anesthesia and the transfer of some anesthesiology residents out of the specialty. Many anesthesiology residencies cut some of their training spaces, but others resorted to accepting increasing numbers of international medical graduates. As a result, 55% of the current anesthesiology residents are international medical graduates, approaching the 58% that was the peak for such residencies in the early 1970s.[53]

It should be noted that nonphysician health providers capable of competing with physicians within the area of their overlapping scopes of practice require removal of at least two legal barriers to do so with relative ease: (1) they need a legal status with regard to autonomy that is sufficient to allow them to engage in such competition, and (2) they must have the capability to be reimbursed for their services. Efforts by these professionals to achieve these legal conditions and others that facilitate their practice have presented significant threats to their physician counterparts. Such is the case between CRNAs and anesthesiologists.

Reimbursement Initiatives

Relationships between the AANA and the ASA have not improved significantly since the AANA sought direct reimbursement for CRNAs. Both organizations bear a responsibility to their individual memberships for their economic and professional welfare, and the welfare of CRNAs and that of anesthesiologists are not necessarily congruent. Therefore, early in the 1990s the two groups found themselves on opposing sides. When CRNAs won direct reimbursement rights in the mid 1980s, they had agreed to accept Medicare assignment, and the legislation called for a budget-neutral reimbursement methodology. Payment schedules were devised for anesthesiologists working alone, CRNAs working alone, and anesthesiologists medically directing CRNAs in the ACT practice setting. In the early 1990s the "single-payment-for-anesthesia" issue arose as a result of a Government Accounting Office (GAO) study.[54] This study demonstrated that payments for anesthesia services under the medical direction model of delivery were 120% to 140% greater than those when CRNAs or anesthesiologists were administering their anesthetics alone. Although this greater cost to Medicare was not consistent with the legislative intent of Congress, it did serve as an economic incentive for anesthesiologists to employ or use more CRNAs. The GAO recommended that the payment model be changed and that only a single anesthesia fee, not more than what would be charged when an anesthesiologist performed the service alone, be reimbursed for each anesthetic procedure.[54] Furthermore, the payment for anesthetic procedures under the medical direction model was suggested to be reimbursed at 50% for the CRNA service and 50% for the anesthesiologist service, which significantly reduced both the anesthesiologist's and the CRNA's portion of the fee. (Payment for additional anesthesia providers would continue to be allowed if adequate justification based on patient-specific factors such as physical status and surgical complexity was submitted along with the bill.) The AANA chose to support the single-payment concept. Efforts to contain health-care costs were already being made by the federal government, and the AANA believed this change was consistent with the legislation it had initiated in gaining direct reimbursement for CRNAs. The ASA opposed it. The single-payment reimbursement plan was implemented, and tension between the two groups again was exacerbated.

ASA Anesthesia Care Team Statement

At the heart of many of the AANA-ASA differences has been the ASA's definition of the ACT concept, which has often reflected what appears to be a lingering desire to make anesthesia an all-physician specialty, albeit today with technical assistants. In the mid 1970s the ASA appointed an Ad Hoc Anesthesia Care Team Committee, which fronted the effort by the ASA to take over the education and credentialing of CRNAs. In 1977 the ASA adopted a policy statement, *Suggestions to ASA Members for Delineation of Anesthesia Functions for Non-Physician Personnel.* This statement started with these words: "The provision of anesthesia by non-physician personnel should be under the direction of the physician responsible for the anesthesia."[55] It stated that the delineation of functions and local credentials should be based on the non-physician's education, training, and experience. It ended as follows: "Qualified personnel under the direction of a physician should be competent to: (1) induce anesthesia; (2) maintain anesthesia at the required levels; (3) support life functions during the perioperative period; (4) recognize and take appropriate action for abnormal patient responses during anesthesia; and (5) provide professional observation and resuscitation until the patient has regained control of his vital functions."[55] (These guidelines were published before significant numbers of graduates of U.S. medical schools were choosing anesthesiology as their specialty.)

In 1982 the ASA unilaterally defined the ACT and announced its control by anesthesiologists. Although it did not call CRNAs technicians in its statement, it essentially assigned CRNAs a technician's role, and ASA leadership did not hesitate to verbally distinguish anesthesiologists and CRNAs by using the professional-technician categorization in public pronouncements. Furthermore, in the 1982 edition of the statement, such a team was to be in existence only until the ASA's goal of one-on-one anesthesia could be accomplished, that is, when enough anesthesiologists were available to personally provide each anesthesia service.[56]

In 1987 the ASA modified its ACT statement, removing the offensive paragraph cited previously.[57] In 1995 the ASA made another modification to its ACT statement, stating that "the Society believes that the involvement of an anesthesiologist in the care of every patient undergoing anesthesia is essential. This may be accomplished through personal provision of anesthesia care or by medical direction of the anesthesia care team."[58] This was impractical, because in 1990 it had been estimated by the U.S. Office of Technology Assessment that approximately 25% of the U.S. population lived in rural areas. Further estimations indicated that up to 80% of the rural population received anesthesia services solely from CRNAs.[59] Furthermore, the majority of office anesthetic procedures in urban areas were also provided by CRNAs. Many health consumers needed CRNAs who were professionals, not merely technicians, and who were competent in a broad range of anesthesia and anesthesia-related modalities, including regional anesthesia techniques and resuscitation and stabilization. Their education prepared them as professionals, and their practice of anesthesia was the practice of professional nursing, not the practice of delegated medicine.

The AANA has recognized and continues to recognize the three basic practice patterns of CRNAs, including CRNAs working with anesthesiologists. Until the early 1980s, it was not unusual for CRNAs and anesthesiologists to work in the same institutions, yet not work together. CRNAs sometimes consulted these anesthesiologists or other medical specialists, but they did not work as a team in many settings. Furthermore, the AANA has always recognized that if CRNAs were required to work solely with or under the supervision or direction of anesthesiologists, millions of people would lose their access to anesthesia services. Rural America and in some instances other underserved populations have not drawn anesthesiologists to their location of health-care need, and for that matter many other medical specialists have not been drawn to those areas. CRNAs, working with primary care physicians and some surgeons, have been able to provide anesthesia for these populations because no state has required them to practice solely with anesthesiologists or under their supervision or direction.

Fruitful dialogue between the ASA and AANA has essentially been nonexistent since the mid 1980s because of stipulations placed on AANA-ASA dialogue by the ASA that the AANA must accept its ACT statement as a condition for such discussions. The AANA has not agreed with such stipulations for a variety of reasons, including the fact that it was never a party to the development of the statement. The ramifications should the AANA adopt the ASA statement as a national position on anesthesia delivery are unthinkable, primarily because this position would deny access to anesthesia services near the homes of some 20% to 25% of U.S. residents. Although the ASA and its leadership may sincerely believe in its position, it is also no less true that research data are inadequate to support such a position. Furthermore, the economic benefits that would be derived by anesthesiologists should such a proposal be implemented present them with a serious conflict of interest that would be difficult to explain.

The AANA's position not to adopt the ASA's ACT statement has been long-standing. According to AANA data, in 1998 approximately 37% of CRNAs were employed by anesthesiologists and approximately the same percentage were employed by hospitals. Many hospital-employed CRNAs work with anesthesiologists who have privileges in those hospitals. The practice pattern of CRNAs working with anesthesiologists has long been one of those approved by the AANA. The question has never been whether the two groups of providers will work together in hospitals in which both groups practice, but rather how and under what conditions? Many CRNAs believe that the ASA's medical direction model, as defined, demeans CRNAs, is restrictive of their practice, inhibits productivity of both providers, and is wasteful of anesthesia personnel. It is more costly than other models that recognize the full range of competencies of both providers and maximize these capabilities in practice, fostering a true collegial partnership.

In an article published November 8, 1999, the *AMA News* announced that the ASA's House of Delegates had approved an "educational affiliate membership" category for CRNAs and anesthesiologist associates. These providers would have to have their applications endorsed by two anesthesiologists, and "they would be required to sign on to the association's statements on ethics and the ACT, which advocates that anesthesiologists be in charge of the medical direction of all in providing anesthesia care."[60] To what extent anesthesiologist-employed CRNAs will be pressured or mandated by their employers to endorse these statements as a condition of employment will have to be evaluated with regard to potential for violation of antitrust or employment laws, both state and federal. The ACT statement has never been one on which the ASA has been willing to seek consensus, and this effort appears to attempt an end run around the AANA by declaring it a "nonissue." Such membership became available in 2001 and constitutes an issue to watch in the new millennium.[60]

State and Federal Regulations

Although the expanded-role movement for nurses got a major boost in the 1960s with the development of primary care nurse practitioners, it was not until the late 1980s that significant progress was made in removing some of the barriers to advanced nursing practice. States vary in their legal requirements concerning CRNA practice. If state laws or regulations mention any relationship with a physician, they specify it with phrases ranging from "under the supervision and/or direction of a physician" to "in collaboration with" or "with the consent of" a physician. Some 20 states now have no requirement for physician supervision of CRNAs in their Medical Practice Acts, their Nurse Practice Acts, or their hospital licensing regulations. Nine others have included a supervisory requirement only in their hospital licensing regulations.[61] Some attorneys believe that regulating professionals through hospital licensing regulations may be unlawful if it conflicts with other legislation (e.g., giving authority to boards of nursing for regulating nurses and nursing practice), but to my knowledge this has not been tested in the courts or by attorney general rulings.

In all states, it is a physician, usually the patient's attending physician or surgeon, who determines the patient's need for anesthesia or anesthesia-related services; therefore, anesthesiology has always been a referral service to anesthesiologists or CRNAs. It must be noted that the idiosyncratic language between doctors and nurses has reflected that referral over the years in the terminology of "ordering," for example, "an anesthetic." For the most part, such ordering has not been technique, drug, or device specific. It may have been as simple as posting a patient for anesthesia and surgery within the operating room. Historically, it has been accepted that each anesthesia provider knows what techniques, drugs, and devices are safest in his or her hands for a particular patient.

The states' changing regulatory scene regarding physician supervision and the continual complaints of CRNAs regarding the TEFRA regulations, which are believed by many CRNAs to adversely affect their ability to practice, came to a head in two additional initiatives pursued by the AANA in the 1990s. The HCFA requirement for physician supervision of CRNAs preempts state laws that permit them to practice without medical supervision. Furthermore, ASA leaders had started a campaign in the 1980s to convince surgeons who worked with CRNAs that the surgeons were legally liable for the CRNAs' practice. Many CRNAs thought this was an effort to discourage surgeons' use of CRNAs without anesthesiologist supervision. Physicians who employ CRNAs are legally liable for their employees under the master-servant legal doctrine, just as any other employer is liable for his or her employees. However, surgeons, who solely fulfill the legal requirement for supervision in states that require such supervision, are not automatically liable for the acts of CRNAs.[24] A surgeon may become liable under the following two conditions: (1) in cases in which the surgeon decides to control what the CRNA does, such as mandating a general anesthetic when the CRNA believes a regional anesthetic would be better; and (2) in instances in which hospital policies mandate a degree of supervision tantamount to control. (The early "captain of the ship" doctrine that made the surgeon responsible for everyone in the operating room has long since been nullified in the vast majority of states.) The inherent medical culture, including the emphasis that the ASA's leaders have placed on CRNA supervision, has led many anesthesiologists to believe that there are legal requirements for CRNAs to be supervised by a physician, even in states in which there are no such requirements. Many CRNAs believe anesthesiologists use this argument with hospital administrators and medical staff to create barriers for CRNAs who seek independent clinical privileges. Some CRNAs have expended tremendous time and effort to untangle the web the ASA and some of its members have been spinning. The HCFA regulations that mandate physician supervision of CRNAs under Medicare policy has presented a serious barrier to progress, and many CRNAs believe the federal regulation needs changing. Therefore, the AANA began to work with the HCFA to propose elimination of the federal requirement for physician supervision and to defer to state laws, recognizing that even if the state permitted independent practice for CRNAs and other APNs, institutional credentialing policy could require physician supervision if the medical staff believed strongly that it was needed.

In December 1997 the HCFA published its proposal for major change in its *Hospital Conditions of Participation*, and it included the elimination of the supervisory requirement for CRNAs.[61,62] The immediate response by the ASA has led to a major political fight involving both organizations, the HCFA, and both houses of the U.S. Congress. As of the closing months of 1999, the matter had not been resolved, and the proposed HCFA rules were pending until 2001 when the issue was resolved. Again, the conflict is characterized by quality-of-care rhetoric on the part of the ASA and its leaders and charges of economic motivations on the part of the AANA and many of its members. Little question exists that the loss the ASA suffered to the AANA in the 1970s in its effort to take over CRNA education and credentialing fostered an intent not to lose again. Two unfortunate tactics on the part of the ASA and its leaders in this confrontation have been the attempt by ASA to frighten the elderly about the anesthesia care they would receive from unsupervised CRNAs and their use of research in inappropriate and misleading ways.

Of interest, within the medical literature in the 1990s, with the *British Medical Journal* and the American College of Physicians Journal Club taking the lead, serious questions have been raised regarding the quality and relevance of research being published, the peer review system, and the selection of articles for publication.[63] One report in 1993 concluded that 95% of the medical research being published in journals was either flawed or irrelevant.[64] This has been demonstrated in the misuse of research, not just within anesthesia over the CRNA supervision issue, but in the public media as well.[39,65-74]

In 1997 the AANA, ASA, and HCFA came to an agreement to revise the TEFRA rules and make them less onerous and less prone to fraud by anesthesiologists. Whether it was the change in ASA presidents or the hostilities over the supervision issue is unclear, but the ASA withdrew its support for the changes before the HCFA proposed and finalized them, negating the chance for change that both CRNAs and many anesthesiologists would have preferred.

In this age of cost containment in health-care services, the TEFRA rules preclude cost-effective use of both CRNAs and anesthesiologists without the anesthesiologists' risking a crossing of the line into fraudulent practice. Some anesthesia groups consisting of both types of providers have decided to eliminate TEFRA as a concern by billing for each provider's services as though the provider were practicing alone. This permits the group to configure its practice to be more productive while basing assignments on individual patient needs. These groups have, in effect, formed the collegial partnership arrangement that the AANA has fostered.

In all organizational and interprofessional affairs, it is easier for individual professionals to accommodate one another than it is for organizations to do the same when vital differences separate them. Such has been the case with nurse anesthetists and anesthesiologists throughout their history in the United States.

ENDING THE TWENTIETH CENTURY

Nurse anesthetists were few in number but were making strong headway in this "new" nursing specialty as the nineteenth century closed and the twentieth century began. They made great strides in that time, achieving what surgeons had requested of them when asked to become anesthetists and make it their career (i.e., making anesthesia safer for patients). In fact, although some physicians devoted their practice to anesthesia, it was not until after World War II that physicians in any significant numbers made it a full-time practice. The strides made in anesthesia practice at the end of the twentieth century were attributable to all those who made it a life's work and contributed to its practice, research, and development. This includes CRNAs, surgeons, anesthesiologists, basic scientists, and engineers. As the twentieth century closed, nurse anesthesia education had moved from hospital-based certificate programs (of which there were four before World War I) to graduate school programs in university settings offering master's or higher degrees to their graduates.

At the close of the millennium, the shifts in delivery and payment systems under managed care significantly affected both CRNAs and anesthesiologists. The use of CRNAs had some definite advantages with regard to cost, without a compromise in the quality of anesthesia care. Many teaching hospitals, whose anesthesia services were primarily provided by medical residents and the anesthesiologist teaching staff, were affected by the lingering decline in numbers of U.S. graduates who enter anesthesiology residencies, caused in part by some decline in graduate medical educational funding. Where the residencies were reduced in number, many such hospitals replaced residents with significant numbers of CRNAs. Some academic health centers that had had no CRNAs for 20 to 25 years are now employing them. Although in the early 1990s there was some displacement of CRNAs in the workforce, at the time of this writing there is a shortage of CRNAs, and once again they are in high demand.

The efforts of proponents of managed care to reduce services that were not medically indicated did not reduce the need for anesthesia providers, as was expected. This resulted from the following:

1. The decentralization of services has invariably led to greater requirements for personnel resources. Anesthesia services are now required in hospitals, ambulatory surgicenters, and physician's offices (the fastest growing site for surgical procedures).
2. Subspecialization among anesthesiologists and even some CRNAs has decreased the flexibility of these providers for use in a variety of settings, which also has resulted in the need for additional anesthesia providers.
3. In large hospitals there has been a significant increase (22% to 66%) over the past 15 years in the number of women who seek pain management during labor.[75] In larger hospitals this has led to the staffing of obstetric services with anesthesia providers around the clock. Hawkins, without stating where or how she collected her data, states that anesthesiologists are for the first time the principal providers of obstetric anesthesia; however, there is a growing market for CRNAs in this field. Many CRNAs devote their practice to obstetric anesthesia, working with and without anesthesiologists. Furthermore, a significant proportion of a rural CRNA practice consists of obstetric anesthesia services.
4. The changing philosophy; advances in knowledge, methodologies, and technology; and greater recognition of the physical, emotional, social, economic, and personal benefits of pain management have led a large variety of professionals, including CRNAs and anesthesiologists, into acute and chronic pain management.

In addition, whereas the locum tenens business was seriously curtailed during the move into the managed care environment, such businesses are now booming for both CRNAs and anesthesiologists. Given the environment of uncertainty, some facilities seem to prefer to use locum tenens personnel rather than employing additional professionals. Some locum tenens CRNAs have been in the same facility for longer than a year and feel more secure being on contract than they would as employees.

Not all CRNAs have benefited from these changes. Some have reported staying in their positions without wage increases for 4 to 6 years, after having their salaries and benefits reduced because of declining hospital revenues within their areas. Although some of these CRNAs could remedy their situation if they believed they were in a position to move, many have not done so. In addition, anesthesia has been severely affected by the reduction of reimbursement rates for services by both governmental and private payers. Often CRNAs are unaware of the income they generate for their employers, and fear or misinformation may well be the greater culprit in keeping their incomes down. However, the variations in managed care penetration and other factors may also be at play in the differences in CRNA income during the 1990s.

Many groups and individuals have advocated greater use of nurses, particularly APNs, as alternatives to physicians where their scopes of practice overlap and their practices have demonstrated quality.[23,59,76-80] It appears that organizational medicine may be fearing decline in its power, authority, and income with the many changes occurring in health-care delivery. Although it recognizes the value of APNs, the AMA is making efforts to increase the barriers to independent APN practice rather than removing them.[81,82] The AMA's passage of an ASA-submitted resolution declaring that anesthesiology is the practice of medicine, and a public relations campaign and initiative to work with state medical boards to prevent any additional legislation and regulation that permits APNs and other nonphysician professionals more independence in practice, are only the latest AMA efforts to avert increased competition.[82,83] They have moved back from a position they took in 1970—a position that has been confirmed by state courts and legislators—that recognizes functional or task overlaps in scopes of practice among health professionals; that is, when a task is performed by a physician, it is the practice of medicine, but when it is performed by another health professional, it is the practice of that professional (e.g., when performed by a nurse, it is nursing).[84] The Texas Attorney General, in an opinion issued September 28, 1999, confirmed the concept of overlapping scopes of practice among health professionals and affirmed that state law does not require that CRNAs be supervised by physicians.[85]

A variety of reasons may explain why medicine is trying to reverse this well-accepted principle and fact; if what these professionals do is categorized as medicine, then the field of medicine can legally control them and their practice, and in an environment in which reimbursement for health professionals is declining, physicians can adjust payment to their employees for their own economic benefit. Much of the confusion over "delegation and ordering" stems from the late nineteenth century, when medicine claimed the whole of health care, necessitating other health professionals to legally carve their practices from that claimed by medicine.[20] However, it has become more recognized over time that although the purpose for which a profession is legally identified may be unique, state laws seldom give that profession a monopoly on practice modalities that are useful and included within the scope of practice of other professions.[86]

At the close of the previous century, several problems worked against resolution of the health-care–cost dilemma in the United States. Significant differences of opinion existed as to whether health care and its delivery could appropriately be subsumed under the market system of capitalism. With an excess of physician specialists, it became obvious that the laws of supply and demand had not worked to maintain health-care costs in an affordable range under the old fee-for-service delivery system. One of the major problems was that health-care needs of individuals and across populations are not as simple as those for food for sustenance or transportation for mobility. Another was that the greater the number of physicians, the greater the number of services provided, some of which may not be medically necessary.[43,44] Because health-care providers are legislatively regulated by the states, and on occasion by the federal government, using funding and reimbursement as a basis, lower-cost providers were not allowed to compete significantly with physicians. The Pew Foundation's Health Professions Commission studied the health-care system and its delivery extensively during the 1990s. Some of the Commission's findings and conclusions are detailed in its 1998 report, *Strengthening Consumer Protection: Priorities for Health Care Workforce Regulation*.[77] These findings include the following vision as a basis for better serving of the public interest: (1) "a move from state standards to national standards"; (2) provision for "significant overlap of practice authority among the health professions"; (3) "new venues and participants for regulatory policy making" predicated on the concept that "legislatures may not be the best venue to decide technical professional matters as lobbying, campaign contributions and allegiance to constituents often distort rational policy development"; (4) "integration of regulatory systems that protect health care consumers"; and (5) "increased regulatory focus on quality of care and competence assurance."[79] The report also recommended that Congress establish "a national policy advisory body that will research, develop and publish national scopes of practice and continuing competency for state legislatures to implement."[77] The question remains as to whether there is sufficient legislative will to move beyond rhetoric, unrestrained campaign financing, and special interest influence to devise a health-care delivery system based on an appropriate, cost-effective health workforce mix that would have the potential to provide affordable health care to all.

THE NEW MILLENNIUM BEGINS

The old saying, "the more things change, the more they remain the same" is fully illustrated in the first few years of the new millennium. For instance, the use of U.S. military forces increased in the 1990s, including campaigns such as Desert Storm (to drive the Iraqis out of Kuwait) and smaller engagements in Somalia, Bosnia, and Kosovo (to stop internal ethnic and religious killings). Terrorists attacked the World Trade Center in New York in 1995. This was followed in 2001 by a major terrorist attack and the full destruction of the World Trade Center in New York and a section of the Pentagon in Washington, D.C. The result was a continuing war in Afghanistan, where many of these terrorists were trained. Additional terrorist bombings in Saudi Arabia and in the port waters of Yemen with U.S. losses eventually led to a preemptive repeat of the Iraq war of 1991 in 2003. The initiative was led by the United States and Great Britain and was based on stated concerns about nuclear, biologic, and chemical weapons and their potential to fall into the hands of terrorists. The United States did not have the degree of backing and support from the United Nations that it did in 1991 and therefore had to rely more on its own troops and support personnel. A sizable number of CRNAs have been called up, along with many reserve and national guard units, to supplement the active military force in caring for military and civilian casualties at home and abroad. The U.S. Army and Air Force use more CRNAs than anesthesiologists; these "call-ups," therefore, create additional CRNA shortages in many civilian and stateside military hospitals at a time when the surgical workload continues to escalate. To increase the total number of CRNAs available, many nurse anesthesia educational programs have increased the number of students they enroll, and a few new programs have been opened or are obtaining initial accreditation status, which allows them to accept students.

Further, the anesthesiologist's challenges to CRNAs and their professional association continued unabated. The HCFA passed new Medicare regulations that eliminated its requirement for physician supervision of nurse anesthetists on January 18, 2001 (66 *FR* No. 12. 4674-4686, 1/18/2001)[87] to take effect March 19, 2001. The unfortunate aspect of the issuance of these regulations was its occurrence late in President Clinton's terms of office, which allowed incoming president George W. Bush time to act on them before they went into effect. Bush did not single out the CRNA Supervision regulation, but on the day he was sworn into office as President of the United States, he announced a 60-day moratorium on all regulations on which Clinton had signed off in his final days in office. The lobbying of the new President and his appointees began early and in earnest.

Bush's action was disappointing to CRNAs, although not surprising. Before taking further action on these regulations, Bush and Secretary Thompson of the U.S. Department of Health and Human Services changed the name of the HCFA to the Centers for Medicare and Medicaid Services (CMS). On July 5, 2001, Bush and the CMS proposed a new regulation that contained a provision allowing governors in those states in which no laws or regulations required physician supervision of CRNAs to opt out of the Medicare physician supervision requirement after discussions with the Boards of Medicine and Nursing. This moved the battle back to those states in which CRNAs had previously fought and won the supervision battle, requiring them to fight it again. Despite the ASA's fight to keep the original regulation that required physician supervision and the AANA's efforts to keep the Clinton regulation, the regulation proposed by Bush (66 *FR* 35395, 7/5/2001)[88] was adopted as the final regulation on November 13, 2001 (66 *FR* 56762, 11/13/2001).[89] The public relations and lobbying battle had been fierce and financially costly to both organizations. In reality, neither side got all that it wanted. Michael Scott, ASA's Director of Governmental and Legal Affairs, wrote the following: "What emerged from the Bush administration on the supervision issue was a compromise. . . . A more accurate characterization of what happened is that [the ASA's] ability to receive a fair hearing at [the Department of Health and Human Services] and the White House was enhanced by our relatively stronger support than AANA for [Republican] candidates in the 2000 and prior elections and by our early support in 2001 for the White House views on patient protection liability issues. We also were measurably aided by urgings of key Senators and Representatives, on both sides of the aisle, who believed that a real anesthesia patient safety issue was at stake and were willing to stand up and be counted."[90] Scott's last sentence is of questionable accuracy, although the early part of his statement demonstrates that when dealing in governmental affairs, AANA members must know how and must be willing to be involved in and to pay the costs associated with public relations and lobbying.

It appeared to many that in the 20 states in which no legal provisions existed for physician supervision of CRNAs, the governors would be inclined to provide "opt-outs" in their states; however, this has not been the case, for political reasons. To date only 10 state governors out of 20 have chosen to go this route. These include Iowa, Nebraska, Idaho, Minnesota, New Hampshire, New Mexico, Kansas, North Dakota, Washington, and Alaska.[91] Other state nurse anesthesia associations that have no state legal regulations requiring supervision of CRNA practice continue their efforts to get their governors to act on the "opt-out" provision.

Medicine developed its coalition to fight perceived incursions of its "turf" by nonphysician professionals in the late 1990s and has become better aligned to combat such initiatives at both the state and federal levels.[83] As a result, medicine has been more effective in blocking such initiatives,[92] which necessitates greater effort on the part of all nonphysician providers to strength their coalitions and get their own individual initiatives enacted into law.

During this period the ASA pursued other activities, perhaps in an attempt to intimidate CRNAs into discontinuing their efforts to eliminate physician supervision from their practice. The ASA announced a plan to consider opening an affiliate membership category—the Educational Member—to CRNAs and anesthesiologist assistants (AAs) within its organization and also to support efforts to increase the number of AA programs.[93] However, the ASA House of Delegates chose to open affiliate educational membership only to anesthesiologist assistants and anesthesiologist assistant students. The ASA has now opened educational membership status to AAs and CRNAs.[94]

After 30 years, in 2002 the ASA's Committee on the Anesthesia Care Team recommended to the ASA Board of Directors that the old statement on regional anesthesia be rescinded and a new one be adopted. The ASA's 1983 policy statement restricted the administration of regional anesthesia to anesthesiologists and other physicians. The ASA Board of Directors disapproved the recommendation pending action by the House of Delegates, which, after consideration, changed the statement to read that it was preferable for such techniques to be administered by anesthesiologists.[95] Despite the previous ASA regional anesthesia policy statement, many nurse anesthetists have been highly successful in incorporating regional techniques in their practice for years, dating back to World War II. Such techniques are preferable for some patients and some surgical procedures. Regional techniques are very frequently used for selected aspects of the management of pain, both acute and chronic. Experience with regional techniques also has become required in accredited nurse anesthesia educational programs.

The ASA has continued to claim that selected research shows that mortality is higher when CRNAs function without anesthesiologist supervision.[96] No such definitive research is available. The most recently published study, performed by Pine, Holt, and Yu using Medicare data from over 400,000 patients from 22 states, found that patients were equally safe when undergoing anesthesia provided by CRNAs, anesthesiologists, or an ACT composed of a CRNA and an anesthesiologist.[97]

Despite the differences in supervision philosophy between CRNAs and anesthesiologists, these two groups of providers have functioned and continue to function collaboratively in many settings with a high degree of success; hospital administrators, surgeons, and patients who have access only to CRNAs are equally satisfied and have the same degree of anesthesia success as those who receive anesthesia service from other providers.

Two programs for training anesthesiologist assistants were established in 1974. One was developed as a master's program, primarily for premedical graduates who were not accepted into medical schools. This program has been in continuous existence. The other was developed as a baccalaureate program and closed after a few years. After its curriculum was revised into a graduate course of study, it was reactivated. CMS and state laws or regulations, where they exist, require that the graduates of these programs function under the supervision of anesthesiologists. They cannot practice where there are no anesthesiologists on duty in the operating room suite to supervise their practice. There are only approximately 700 active practicing AAs. Although more have been graduated from these two schools in the past 30 years of their existence, approximately half of them have gone on to other pursuits, some to medical schools.

THOUGHTS FOR THE FUTURE

Nurse anesthesia has grown from humble beginnings to a fully mature professional specialty that, over the whole of its history, has been committed to the provision of high-quality services to patients and to excellence in education for its members. As more historians delve into its beginnings, they will find and report more of the many accomplishments of early nurse anesthetists in the development of anesthesia equipment and the pioneering of anesthesia techniques for specialty surgery. After physicians entered the field of anesthesiology in significant numbers, it was nurse anesthetists who assisted them and, even more so, covered the service commitment to allow physician investigators time to conduct needed research. The growing number of doctorate nurse anesthetists will increase the number of CRNA researchers and the research contributions they will make to this field of practice.

In the early 1960s ASA leaders stated that economics is the force that shapes the anesthesiology specialty the most.[98] Since that time, this has become even more apparent. Dr. Forrest Leffinwell, the ASA's president in 1961, warned the membership, "We often find ourselves in monopolistic positions, and the temptation is great to indulge in sharp practices. In such situations, the heaviest loser is apt to be the patient."[99] The ability of anesthesiologists to monopolize the training spaces in academic health-care centers in the 1980s not only increased the cost of the education of anesthesia providers significantly but also increased the cost of anesthesia services and contributed to the escalating cost of health care. Some 10 to 15 years later it is contributing to yet another shortage of CRNAs.

In the past, many anesthesiologists blamed nurse anesthetists for their lack of prestige within the medical community and for their difficulty in acquiring acceptance from their surgical colleagues.[8] Anesthesiologists failed to recognize that, as the providers of anesthesia services who spend long hours at the head of the operating table or within the operating room, they were limiting themselves to a process that is, in most instances, more in the nature of nursing than medicine. Although Collins[100] has called the anesthesiologist "the medical internist of surgery," few anesthesiology residencies have provided adequate time in their programs for residents to master the field of internal medicine and apply it to patients during their anesthesia experience. Anesthesiologists often are as likely as nurse anesthetists to consult with medical specialists regarding their patients.

The historical problems that have existed between physician anesthetists and nurse anesthetists are in part the result of the fact that anesthesia is neither solely medicine nor wholly nursing, as is the case in such specialties as pediatrics, obstetrics, and psychiatry. They are in part the result of the historical interprofessional "transactional neurosis" that exists between physicians and nurses, as reported by Stein.[101] Furthermore, the area of overlap between medicine and nursing in the field of anesthesia is far greater than that in other areas of specialization.

The traditional paradigm of medicine, in which physicians are in control of the whole of health care, is totally inconsistent with the legal requirements imposed by the state licenses of other health professionals, which make individuals responsible for their own professional actions. Furthermore, resolving the many challenges that nurse anesthetists have faced has led to the development of a whole body of common law based on legal decisions concerning common practices, and this law further confirms the legal appropriateness of their practice.

The field of nursing, including that of nurse anesthesia, has long believed that true collaboration—not control—is the best means for achieving greater productivity and for attaining better qualitative outcomes in the delivery of health-care services in any health-care system. No health professional is truly independent. The increased use of APNs can contain health costs for two reasons: the cost of an APN's preparation is only one tenth that of a physician's preparation,[102] and APNs generally practice a more conservative brand of health care, offering additional nursing services aimed at health promotion and making patients more responsible for their own health.[78]

Although no data are available comparing the conservatism in practice of CRNAs versus anesthesiologists, those of us who have been in the field for some time have observed it among our colleagues. APNs in all specialties refer patients to physicians when the patients require the services of physicians. An abundance of research demonstrates that, in the areas of practice, APNs' care outcomes are equal to and sometimes better than those of their physician colleagues.[14,23,37-39,76-78]

The socialization of physicians in medical schools makes it exceedingly difficult for them to believe the research concerning APN outcomes of care. Most physicians hesitate to move with the shifting paradigm under which cost-effective health-care services must be delivered in the future if universal coverage is to be achieved.

The future of nurse anesthetists will continue to be filled with challenges. Despite the need for better relationships between organizational anesthesiology and nurse anesthesia, society has benefited from both groups of providers. Anesthesiologists as a group are better off because of the existence of nurse anesthetists. The corollary to this statement is equally true. The fact that these two groups of providers are from different disciplines in health care has been beneficial to patients because the skills and attributes of both nursing and medicine can be brought to patients who need anesthesia services.

There are those who question how nurse anesthetists have survived so long, considering the many challenges that have confronted them. The reason for their professional longevity stems from many factors, including the following:

1. The practice of anesthesia is predominantly nursing in its essence, and the basic nursing programs of nurse anesthetists have served them well; furthermore, they have been well prepared for their work as anesthetists.
2. The work is such that it has attracted the best and the brightest among nurses.
3. Nurse anesthetists have historically had a commitment to excellence and to the provision of their services where and when needed at a reasonable cost, thereby making themselves available and accessible.
4. They have also had a commitment to their professional association, lending adequate support to make it strong and capable in its representation of their interests.
5. They have often weighed their interests against those of the public and, in so doing, have sought to make them congruent. If nurse anesthetists had not done so, their demise would have long since been reported.

CRNAs have been a vital health-care resource in the United States for over 100 years and have been the principal anesthesia providers in times of war and peace. Furthermore, they are the major "hands-on" anesthesia providers in this country, working with or without anesthesiologists. The first decade of the twenty-first century will be one of turbulence for all health-care professionals as they continue to jockey for advantage and their desired place in the coming health-care reform. However, the real question in health-care reform is one that to date has been almost too political to discuss—the impact of physician overages, their costs, and the costs they generate as the basic force driving the escalating expense of health care.

Greater use of expanded role nurses, now APNs, to meet the health needs of the U.S. public has been advocated since the 1960s. However, problems related to access, quality, and cost of care are worldwide, and many countries have been trying to deal with similar problems for just as long, even though the state of development among the nations varies significantly.

In 1986 the World Health Organization, the Pan American Health Organization, the World Federation of Medical Education, and the Secretariat of Health in Mexico collaborated on a conference in Acapulco on "Health Manpower out of Balance: Conflicts and Prospects." The meeting was reported in the United States in the *Journal of Public Health Policy* in 1988.[103] It also had been reported in *World Health*, the magazine of the World Health Organization, in April 1987. The organizations' conclusions were that nurses are the key to making health care more accessible and reducing the costs of health care in all countries. It was found that most countries in 1986, regardless of the level of development, were experiencing health manpower mixes that were out of balance. Worldwide, there were current and projected overages of physicians and shortages of nurses and other types of health workers, including community health aides. Little has changed since 1986 except that the disparity in the need for physicians and nurses has widened. The organizations also found that in countries that concentrated on the preparation of physicians and the delivery of physician care, national health-care budgets were expended, leaving many citizens without even rudimentary health services. Thus, either the costs of health care were overwhelming governments or a significant number of people within these countries were going without health care—or both.[103]

At the Acapulco conference, B. Abel-Smith reported on an analysis that had been performed regarding health workers and their salaries. In any given country studied, a rural health aide who had a primary school education plus 6 months of training was paid 2 currency units; nurses, medical assistants (similar to our physician assistants), and a sanitarian who all had completed a secondary education plus 3 additional years of education were paid 6 currency units; and a physician or dentist who had completed secondary education plus 5 to 8 years of additional education was being paid 20 currency units. Thus, pay was also considered to be somewhat out of balance.[103] Abel-Smith stated that "to reduce physician's earning to a more reasonable level vis-a-vis nurses and rural health workers might tax all the courage and political will of any government."[103]

In addition, at this meeting the consensus was growing among public health officials worldwide that to improve cost effectiveness in the delivery of health services, countries should work to limit physician numbers and services (i.e., limit their work to those services that only they can provide) and expand nurses' scope of practice to include much of the primary care provided by physicians. The participants at the meeting believed that nurses did a better job with regard to illness prevention and health maintenance. They estimated that nurses could pick up as much as 80% of the primary care services of physicians, thereby reducing the cost of these services below that paid to physicians. Although it might sound inconsistent to promote the greater use of nurses in the midst of nursing shortages, Gillian Briscoe pointed out that the dropout rate from nursing was (and continues to be) high, resulting from issues such as low wages, physician dominance, lack of respect or credit for one's work, and lack of control over one's own practice. It was believed that giving nurses more responsibility, more authority, and higher wages would improve retention within the profession of nursing.[103]

Although recognizing that a better health workforce mix had to be combined with better geographic distribution if health services were to be made maximally accessible, Briscoe stated, "An effective nursing work-force, which makes the best possible use of nursing skills, is essential if countries are to offer equal access for all to quality health care at a reasonable cost."[103]

We in the United States have experienced the difficulties of trying to optimize the use of APNs in health-care delivery since at least the mid 1960s. The proliferation of government-funded and government-supported medical schools has increased the numbers of physicians so significantly that APNs are now perceived by many physicians to be economic threats to physician incomes unless they are controlled by physicians, although they usually express this in terms of quality of care. Furthermore, immigration of international medical graduates into the United States continues, and U.S. citizens pay for their postgraduate medical education. A few of them specialize in primary care and go to underserved portions of the United States. However, a large portion of them go into the more narrow medical specialties and stay in America's urban areas, compounding the cost of health care directly attributable to physicians at physician payment rates.[104] (This assumption is backed by studies that have shown that a significant number of medical procedures rendered in areas in which the density of physicians is high are either not medically indicated or minimally medically indicated.[44,45]) With the ever-burgeoning growth of physicians, neither the distribution nor practice of APNs has contributed significantly to reductions in health-care costs, and their potential for cost containment has been imperiled.

The future for CRNAs, for all APNs, and indeed for all nurses will be what we make it. Nurse anesthetists can no longer live in the isolation of the specialty as we did in the first half of the twentieth century. The quality of U.S. nurses, the health needs of the U.S. public, and the high cost of health care in the United States today offer nurses their greatest opportunity and the national economy its greatest hope with regard to containment of health-care costs. Although many decision-makers know this, little is being done about it. There are major social, cultural, and political problems with which we must contend. Nurses, more than 2 million strong, must recognize that it is time that they be seen and heard in the halls and at the tables of health policy deliberations and decision-making. The only way that can happen is if we speak with one voice regarding health-care reform. Various groups of nurses may have different problems within their practice arenas, but we must recognize that at the top we all have the same problems, although to varying degrees: inadequate power and autonomy, too little authority, poor public and professional recognition relative to the value of our work, and in many instances inadequate remuneration for our services. The fact is, however, that the interests of nurses and of consumers of health services are congruent. We are capable of providing a major portion of health-care services at a cost that consumers and society can afford. Certainly, physicians are needed, but as was decided at the meeting in Acapulco, they should be more limited in number and in the services they provide. In the United States one way that this can be accomplished is by opening up the legal scopes of practice of nonphysician health professionals so that they can compete for services that fall into the overlap in their scopes of practice.

It is unclear whether regulated managed care entities can accomplish the job without having a more balanced health workforce mix that has a better capability of providing high-quality, cost-effective services. Many ascribe to a greater role for nurses in the delivery of health services and the education of the U.S. public regarding self-care and health maintenance. The Pew Health Professions Commission, through its Taskforce on Health Care Regulation, has identified the United States' Achilles' heel in making change: the political system itself and the degree to which campaign contributions and special interest groups have coopted politicians.[79] Successful change will not occur unless we make it happen, and unless it happens, the promise of nursing and of APNs, including CRNAs, and the hope for health care for all, will remain unrealized. If nursing is denied a major role in health-care reform, it not only will adversely affect health consumers, it also will adversely affect the pool from which nursing students are recruited. The best and the brightest will not likely pursue nursing as a career.

CRNAs can look to the past for courage to face the future. Because they have been capable of providing a quality service at prices society can afford and because they have been uniquely qualified for the work they perform, CRNAs have successfully met the challenges of the past with aplomb and vigor. The challenges of today are no less intense than those of the past, but they are made even more complex as they coincide with efforts to change the health-care system. Unrest and insecurity have intensified, and the positions taken by various health professional groups have hardened. I am sure that at the beginning of the twentieth century a small group of nurse anesthetists anticipated with great hope, yet also with great trepidation, what the new century would bring. Few could have predicted how far anesthesia and nurse anesthetists would advance in that century. The nurse anesthetists of the past, though, built a strong professional foundation. They achieved a great reputation for excellence and service for current CRNAs to live up to. Throughout the twentieth century nurse anesthetist leaders furthered our progress and upgraded our educational programs so that we are prepared for whatever the twenty-first century brings. They broadened our practice opportunities and in so doing presented us with new challenges. With the same courage and vigor as our nurse anesthesia ancestors had, we must rise to the occasion and advance our profession in the twenty-first century, not solely for our benefit or for that of those who follow in our footsteps, but primarily for the good of the people we serve.

As long as nurse anesthetists maintain and act in a manner consistent with their historical attributes, they will continue to be a vital health resource in preventing and relieving pain and in making anesthesia safe for people in need. In concert with our physician and other health-care colleagues, through collaboration and cooperation, we can reach the goal of health care for all at reasonable costs. Health care is not an independent operation; it requires a community of providers and educated consumers. CRNAs must be among those who lead the way in the twenty-first century.

REFERENCES

1. Smith TC, Wollman H. History and principles of anesthesiology. In: Goodman LS, Rall TW, and Murad F, eds. *Goodman and Gillman's the Pharmacological Basis of Therapeutics*. 7th ed. New York: Macmillan; 1985:260-275.
2. Donahue MP. *Nursing: The Finest Art. An Illustrated History*. St Louis: Mosby; 1985.
3. Thatcher V. *History of Anesthesia with Emphasis on the Nurse Specialist*. Philadelphia: Lippincott; 1953.
4. Otis GA, Huntington, DL. *The Medical and Surgical History of the War of the Rebellion*. Part III (vol. II), "Surgical History," Washington, DC: US Government Printing Office; 1883:905.
5. Bankert M. *Watchful Care: A History of America's Nurse Anesthetists*. New York: Continuum; 1989.
6. Lee E. *History of the School of Nursing of the Presbyterian Hospital New York, 1892-1942*. New York: Putnam; 1942:105-108.
7. Diers D. Nurse-midwives and nurse anesthetists: the cutting edge in specialist practice. In: Aiken L, Fagin C, eds. *Charting Nursing's Future: Agenda for the 1990s*. Philadelphia: Lippincott; 1992:159.
8. Adriani J. Four decades of association with the pioneers of anesthesiology. *Anesth Analg*. 1972;51:665-667.
9. Stevens R. *American Medicine and the Public Interest*. Berkeley: University of California Press; 1998:195, 543-544.
10. Stevens R. *In Sickness and in Wealth: American Hospitals in the Twentieth Century*. New York: Basic Books; 1989:181.
11. Bellafaire J. *The Army Nurse Corps, a Commemoration of World War II Service*. Washington, DC: US Army Center of Military History; 1991:6-7. CMH publication 72-14. Available at: http://www2.army.mil/cmh/books/wwii/72-14/72-14.htm. Accessed July 17, 1999.
12. Williams D. *To the Angels*. San Francisco: Denson Press; 1985.
13. Norman E. *We Band of Angels: The Untold Story of American Nurses Trapped on Bataan by the Japanese*. New York: Random House; 1999.
14. Beecher HK, Todd DP. A study of deaths associated with anesthesia and surgery. *Ann Surg*. 1954;140:2-34.
15. Berger OL. Anesthesia for the surgical treatment of cyanotic congenital heart disease. *J Am Assoc Nurse Anesthetists*. 1948;16: 79-90.
16. Lank BE. Cyclopropane anesthesia in infant surgery. *J Am Assoc Nurse Anesthetists*. 1947;15:3-11.
17. Hamel MH, Lamont A. Anesthesia in the surgical treatment of congenital pulmonary stenosis. *Anesthesiology*. 1946;7:477-498.
18. Smith RM. Progress in paediatric anaesthesia in the United States. *Anesth Hist Assoc Newsletter*. 1993;11:2.
19. Moore C, Feller C, eds. *Highlights in the History of the Army Nurse Corps*. Washington, DC: US Army Center of Military History; 1995:27-28, 40. CMH publication 85-1.
20. Bendixon HH. Debate: Anesthesia manpower shortage—fact or fiction? Fact. *Clin Anesth*. 1967;2:16-21.
21. Dripps RD. Decisions for the specialty. *Bull N Y Acad Med*. 1962;38:264-270.
22. Steinhaus JE, Evans JA, Frazier WT. The physician assistant in anesthesiology. *Anesth Analg*. 1973;52:794-798.
23. Safreit BJ. Health care dollars and regulatory sense: the role of advanced practice nursing. *Yale J Reg*. 1992;9:417-487.
24. Blumenreich GA. The irrelevant issue of surgeon's liability. In: *AANA Journal Legal Briefs: 1984-86*. Park Ridge, Ill: American Association of Nurse Anesthetists; 1987:16-17. Reprinted from *AANA J*. 1985;53:5.
25. Stephens CR. Nurses in anesthesia. In: *ASA Manpower Report*. Park Ridge, Ill: American Society of Anesthesiologists; 1969.
26. American Society of Anesthesiologists, American Association of Nurse Anesthetists. Joint statement of the ASA and AANA concerning qualifications of individuals administering anesthetics. *AANA News Bull*. 1972;26:3.
27. Gunn IP. The history of nurse anesthesia education: highlights and influences. In: *Report of the National Commission on Nurse Anesthesia Education*. Park Ridge, Ill: American Association of Nurse Anesthetists; 1990:33-41.
28. Wiseman E. Legislation: the California experience. *CRNA Forum* 1986;2:3-10.
29. Tobin MH. Governmental regulation of nurse anesthesia practice. In: Foster SD, Jordan LM, eds: *Professional Aspects of Nurse Anesthesia Practice*. Philadelphia: FA Davis; 1994.
30. Wing KR. Government enforcement of competition: the antitrust laws. In: Wing KR, ed. *The Law and the Public's Health*. 2nd ed. Ann Arbor, Mich: Health Administration Press; 1985.
31. Blumenreich GA, Markham JW Jr. Bhan vs NME Hospital, Inc: antitrust standing of CRNAs sustained. In: *AANA Journal Legal Briefs: 1984-86*. Park Ridge, Ill: American Association of Nurse Anesthetists; 1987:14-15. Reprinted from *AANA J*. 1985;53:6.)

32. US Department of Health and Human Services, Health Care Financing Administration. Final Rules for the Tax Equity and Fiscal Responsibility Act, 1982. *Federal Register.* 1983;48:8901-8951.
33. Brief of amicus curiae, the American Association of Nurse Anesthetists. No. 82-1031. In the Supreme Court of the United States, October Term, 1982, *Jefferson Parish Hospital District No. 2 and East Jefferson Hospital Board, Petitioners, v Edwin G. Hyde.* Respondent, Counsel of Record: Phil David Fine.
34. American Society of Anesthesiologists, Inc. Brief of Amicus Curiae in Support of Respondent No. 82-1031. In the Supreme Court of the United States, October Term, 1982, 3. Respondent, Counsel of Record: John Lansdale, Jr.
35. Blumenreich GA. *Jefferson Parish Hospital v. Hyde*—the last chapter. In: *AANA Journal Legal Briefs: 1984-86.* Park Ridge, Ill: American Association of Nurse Anesthetists; 1987:33-34. Reprinted from *AANA J.* 1984;52:4.)
36. Garde JF. The case study involving the prospective payment system legislation, diagnostic related groups and CRNAs. *Nurs Clin North Am.* 1988;23:521-553.
37. Bechtold AA. Committee on anesthesia study of anesthesia-related deaths—1969-1976. *N C Med J.* 1981;42:253.
38. National Academy of Sciences, National Research Council. *Health Care for American Veterans.* House Committee Print No. 36, Health Care for American Veterans, 1977:156.
39. Forrest WH. Outcome—the effect of the provider. In: Wolman H, ed. *Health Care Delivery in Anesthesia.* Philadelphia: George F. Stickley; 1980.
40. Hardy-Havens D. Federal legislative and regulatory impact on funding of nurse anesthesia education. In: *Report of the National Commission on Nurse Anesthesia Education.* Park Ridge, Ill: American Association of Nurse Anesthetists; 1990:123-129.
41. Zambricki C, Ouellette RG. On matters of concern about nurse anesthesia education. *AANA J.* 1987;55:499-505.
42. DePaolis-Lutzo MV. Factors influencing nurse anesthesia educational programs: 1982-1987. In: *Report of the National Commission on Nurse Anesthesia Education.* Park Ridge, Ill: American Association of Nurse Anesthetists; 1990:46-51.
43. Ribicoff A, Danaceau P. *The American Medical Machine.* New York: Harrow Books, Harper & Row; 1972.
44. Anders G. *Health against Wealth: HMOs and the Breakdown of Medical Trust.* New York: Houghton Mifflin; 1996:23-24.
45. Blustein J, Marmor TR. Cutting waste by making rules: promises, pitfalls, and realistic prospects. In: Lee PR, Estes CL, eds: *The Nation's Health.* 4th ed. Boston: Jones & Bartlett; 1994:333.
46. American Society of Anesthesiologists. *Practice Management: Managed Care* [videotape]. Park Ridge, Ill: American Society of Anesthesiologists; 1994.
47. Christensen KT. Ethically important distinctions among managed care organizations. *J Law Med Ethics.* 1995;23:223-229.
48. Himmelstein DU, Woolhandler S, Hellander I, Wolfe SM. Quality of care in investor-owned vs. not-for-profit HMOs. *JAMA.* 1999;282:159-163.
49. Silverman EM, Skinner JS, Fisher ES. The association between for-profit hospital ownership and increased Medicare spending. *N Engl J Med.* 1999;341:420-426.
50. Himmelstein DU, Woolhandler S. When money is the mission—the high costs of investor-owned care [editorial]. *N Engl J Med.* 1999;341:444-446.
51. Cromwell J, Rosenbach ML. Reforming anesthesia payment under Medicare. *Health Aff (Millwood).* 1988;7:5-19.
52. Reves JG. Anesthesiologist workforce projections. Paper presented at: American Association of Nurse Anesthetists' Assembly of States Meeting; November 11, 1995; St Louis, Mo.
53. Grogono AW. December 1998 update on residency composition 1960-1998. *ASA Newsletter.* 1998. Available at: http://www.asahq.org/Newsletters/1998/12_98/Update_1298.html. Accessed March 8, 1999.
54. US General Accounting Office, Human Resources Division, *Report to Congressional Committees. Medicare: Payments for Medically Directed Anesthesia Services Should Be Reduced.* Washington, DC: US General Accounting Office; 1992. Publication RRD-92-25.
55. American Society of Anesthesiologists. *American Society of Anesthesiologists' Guidelines: Suggestions to ASA Members for Delineation of Anesthesia Functions for Non-physician personnel.* Park Ridge, Ill: American Society of Anesthesiologists; 1977.
56. American Society of Anesthesiologists. *American Society of Anesthesiologists' Guidelines: The Anesthesia Care Team.* Park Ridge, Ill: American Society of Anesthesiologists; 1982.
57. American Society of Anesthesiologists. *American Society of Anesthesiologists' Guidelines: The Anesthesia Care Team.* 1987 rev ed. Park Ridge, Ill: American Society of Anesthesiologists; 1987.
58. American Society of Anesthesiologists. *American Society of Anesthesiologists' Guidelines: The Anesthesia Care Team.* 1995 rev ed. Park Ridge, Ill: American Society of Anesthesiologists; 1995.
59. US Congress, Office of Technology Assessment. *Health Care in Rural America.* Washington, DC: US Government Printing Office; 1990. Publication OTA-H-434.
60. Prager LO. Anesthesiologists decide to lay out the welcome mat. The American Society of Anesthesiologists proposed to create an educational arm for nurse anesthetists and others. But will the new affiliates attract any takers? *AMA News.* November 8, 1999. Available at: http://www.ama-assn.org/amednews/1999/pick_99/orga1108.htm.
61. Foster S. Comments of the American Association of Nurse Anesthetists on the Proposed Rule Regarding the Medicare and Medicaid Programs: Hospital Conditions of Participation; Provider and Supplier Approval. Park Ridge, Ill., AANA, Vol 1. 1998.
62. Proposed rules, the Medicare and Medicaid programs: hospital conditions of participation. *Federal Register.* 1997;62: 66725-66763.
63. Godlee F. Getting evidence into practice [editorial]. *BMJ.* 1998;317:6.
64. Haynes RB. Where's the meat in clinical journals? *ACP J Club.* 1993;119:A22-A23.
65. Abenstein JD, Warner MA. Anesthesia providers, patient outcomes, and costs. *Anesth Analg.* 1996;82:1273-1278.
66. Miller R. Perspective from the editor-in-chief: anesthesia providers, patient outcomes, and costs. *Anesth Analg.* 1996;82: 1117-1278.
67. Zambricki CS. Anesthesia providers, patient outcomes, and costs. The AANA responds to the Abenstein and Warner article in the June 1996 *Anesthesia and Analgesia* [editorial]. *AANA J.* 1996;64:413-416.
68. Stoelting RK. Letters to the editor: anesthesia providers, patient outcomes and costs, *Anesth Analg.* 83:1347, 1996.
69. Gaba DM: Anesthesia providers, patient outcomes and costs [letter]. *Anesth Analg.* 1996;83:1348.
70. Hanna K. Anesthesia providers, patient outcomes and costs [letter]. *Anesth Analg.* 1996;83:1348.
71. Kremer M. Anesthesia providers, patient outcomes and costs [letter]. *Anesth Analg.* 1996;83:1348-1349.
72. Abenstein JP, Warner MA. Anesthesia providers, patient outcomes and costs [letter]. *Anesth Analg.* 1996;83:1349-1350.
73. Martin-Sheridan D, Wing P. Anesthesia providers, patient outcomes, and costs: a critique. *AANA J.* 1996;64:528-534.
74. Boodman SG. Turf battle in the operating room. Does it matter who puts you to sleep—anesthesiologist or nurse anesthetists? *Washington Post.* May 5, 1998; Health section:12-16.
75. Hawkins J. *More women opt for pain relief during labor* [press release]. American Society of Anesthesiologists; October 12, 1999; Dallas.
76. The Pew Foundation Health Professions Commission, Taskforce on Health Care Workforce Regulation. *Critical Challenges: Revitalizing the Health Professions for the 21st Century.* San Francisco: Pew Health Professions Commission; 1995.

77. Finnocchio LJ, Dower CM, Blick NT, Gragnola CM, Taskforce on Health Care Workforce Regulation. *Strengthening Consumer Protection: Priorities for Health Care Workforce Regulation*. San Francisco: Pew Health Professions Commission; 1998.
78. US Congress, Office of Technology Assessment. *Nurse Practitioners, Physician Assistants, and Certified Nurse Midwives: A Policy Analysis (Health Technology Case Study 37*. Washington, DC: US Government Printing Office; 1986. Publication OTA-HCS-47.
79. Bauer JC. *Not What the Doctor Ordered: How to End the Medical Monopoly in Pursuit of Managed Care*. New York: McGraw-Hill (Health Care Financial Management Association); 1998.
80. Califano JA Jr. *America's Health Care Revolution. Who Lives? Who Dies? Who Pays?* New York: Random House; 1986.
81. American Medical Association House of Delegates. *Report 20 of the Board of Trustees: Supervision of Medical Care Delivered by Advanced Practice Nurses (Resolution 305, A-95)*. Adopted at the December 1995 meeting of the House of Delegates.
82. AMA declares "Anesthesiology is the practice of medicine." *Am Soc Anesthesiol Newsletter. February 1999*. Available at: http://www.asahq-org/Newsletters/1999/02_99/AMA_0299.html. Accessed April 25, 1999.
83. Greene J. The threat of the domino effect. The AMA plans to launch a Web-based advocacy campaign to help inform Federation members on efforts by nonphysician practitioners to expand scope of practice. *Amed News. June 21*, 1999. Available at: http://www.ama-assn.org/amednews/1999/pick_99/prfa0621.htm. Accessed June 23, 1999.
84. AMA Committee on Nursing: Medicine and nursing in the 1970s: a position statement. *JAMA*. 1970;213:1882.
85. Texas Attorney General Opinion No. JC-0117, September 28, 1999. Available at: http://intranet1.oag.state.tx.us/opinions/jc/JC0117.pdf. Accessed September 29, 1999.
86. Blumenreich GA. The overlap between the practice of medicine and the practice of nursing. *AANA J*. 1998;66:11-15.
87. It's official! HCFA removes physician supervision requirement for nurse anesthetists: editorial. *AANA Newsletter*. January 2001. Available at: http://www.aana.com/members/newsbulletin/2001_01/cover.asp. Accessed August 31, 2003.
88. Supervision rule published: what does it mean? What's next: editorial. *AANA Newsletter*. December 2001. Available at: http://www.aana.com/members/newsbulletin/2001_12/cover.asp. Accessed August 31, 2003.
89. Administration puts politics before patients; implements cumbersome anesthesia care rule: editorial. *AANA Capitol Corner*. November 13, 2001. Available at: http://www.aana.com/capcorner/finalrule_111301.asp. Accessed August 31, 2003.
90. Scott M. 2001: not shoes, nor ships, nor sealing wax. *ASA Newsletter*. December 2001. Available at: http://www.asahq.org/Newsletters/2001/12_01/scott.htm. Accessed August 31, 2003.
91. Kansas Governor Sebelius removes physician supervision for nurse anesthetists [AANA press release]. Available at: http://www.aana.com/press/2003/040103.asp. Accessed August 31, 2003.
92. Green J. Professional issues: physicians win big in states over scopes of practice. *Am Med News. July 2*, 2001. Available at: http://www.ama-assn.org/sci-pub/amnews/pick_01/prl10702.htm. Accessed July 7, 2001.
93. American Society of Anesthesiologists. Board of Directors annual meeting summary, membership for anesthetists. *ASA Newsletter*. October 1999. Available at: http://www.asahq.org/Newsletters/1999/10_99/board1099.html. Accessed August 31, 2003.
94. American Society of Anesthesiologists. Board of Directors annual meeting summary, educational affiliate membership. *ASA Newsletter*. October 2001. Available at: http://www.asahq.org/Newsletters/2001/10_01/bodsumm.htm. Accessed August 31, 2003.
95. American Society of Anesthesiologists. Board of Directors annual meeting summary, statement of regional anesthesia. *ASA Newsletter*. October 2002. Available at: http://www.asahq.org/Newsletters/2002/10_02/article1.htm. Accessed August 31, 2003.
96. Silber JH, Kennedy SK, Even-Shoshan O, et al. Anesthesiologist direction and patient outcomes. *Anesthesiology* 2000;93:152-163.
97. Pine M, Holt KD, Lou Y. Surgical mortality and type of anesthesia provider. *AANA J*. 2003;71:109-116.
98. Beecher HK. Trends in anesthesia. *JAMA*. 1962;180:44.
99. Leffingwell FE. Hallmarks of maturity [editorial]. *Anesthesiology*. 1961;22:830-831.
100. Collins V. *Principles of Anesthesiology*. 2nd ed. Philadelphia: Lea & Febiger; 1976:27-28.
101. Stein LI. The doctor-nurse game. *Am J Nurs*. 1968;68:101-105.
102. Gunn IP. Health educational costs, provider mix, and health care reform: a case in point—nurse anesthetists and anesthesiologists. *AANA J*. 1996;64:48-52.
103. Terris M. Meeting the needs for health workers: proportions, prerogatives, and priorities [editorial]. *J Public Health Policy*. 1988;3:309-318.
104. Pasko T, Seidman B. Physician Characteristics and Distribution in the US, 1999 ed. Chicago: American Medical Association; 1999.

CHAPTER 2

Specialty Practice of Nurse Anesthesia

Betty J. Horton

In existence for more than 100 years, the specialty practice of nurse anesthesia has become one of the most challenging and rewarding areas of advanced nursing practice. Nurse anesthetists, in association with their professional association, the American Association of Nurse Anesthetists (AANA), have been role models for members of other nursing groups and allied health organizations. The roles of the certified registered nurse anesthetist (CRNA) and the AANA are described in this chapter.

THE CERTIFIED REGISTERED NURSE ANESTHETIST

Definition

Founded in 1931, the AANA is a professional association that represents more than 30,000 CRNAs nationwide. More than 90% of CRNAs in the United States are members of the AANA.[1] CRNAs are anesthesia specialists who administer more than 65% of all anesthetics delivered annually to patients in the United States. As advanced practice nurses, CRNAs can serve in a variety of capacities in daily practice, such as clinician, educator, administrator, manager, and researcher. CRNAs administer anesthesia for all types of surgical cases, using all anesthetic techniques, and practice in every type of setting in which anesthesia is delivered, from university-based medical centers to freestanding surgical facilities. CRNAs are the sole anesthesia providers in more than two thirds of all rural hospitals and enable these medical facilities to provide obstetric, surgical, diagnostic, and trauma stabilization services.[2]

Qualifications and Capabilities

The following are required for an individual to become a CRNA:

1. Current and unrestricted state licensure as a registered professional nurse
2. Graduation from a nurse anesthesia educational program accredited by the Council on Accreditation of Nurse Anesthesia Educational Programs or its predecessor
3. Successful completion of the certification examination administered by the Council on Certification of Nurse Anesthetists or its predecessor[2,3]

Education

Nurse anesthesia educational programs range from 24 to 36 months of full-time study or the part-time equivalent.[4,5] All programs are required to award master's degrees to graduates who are entering nurse anesthesia practice. Courses of study leading to doctoral degrees also are available. Each accredited program provides an educationally sound curriculum that builds on prior nursing education and experience.

The curriculum incorporates studies in the sciences, basic and advanced principles of anesthesia, research, and professional aspects of nurse anesthesia. Students acquire knowledge, skills, and competencies in patient safety, perianesthetic management, critical thinking, communication, and the professional role. Students learn to integrate classroom content with direct application of state-of-the-art techniques in the provision of anesthesia care to all patient populations in all risk categories.

Clinical Curriculum Requirements. The clinical component of the nurse anesthesia curriculum focuses on preparing students for the full scope of current practice in a variety of work settings.[4] Each student must administer a minimum number of anesthetics involving a variety of procedures, techniques, and specialty cases. To meet this requirement, students provide anesthesia care under the supervision of qualified clinical instructors who are CRNAs or anesthesiologists. In most programs the minimum requirements for clinical experience are far exceeded before graduation.[5]

Admission Prerequisites. Admission to nurse anesthesia educational programs is highly competitive. Applicants must meet specific admission criteria that include possession of a baccalaureate degree and current licensure as a registered nurse (RN) in the United States or its territories or protectorates. At least 1 year of experience as an RN in an acute care setting is also a prerequisite for admission.[4]

Most applicants have acquired extensive clinical experience in such settings as coronary, respiratory, postanesthesia, and surgical intensive care units and emergency departments or as members of a trauma or cardiac surgical team.[5] Such experiences attest to the high level of clinical skills possessed by licensed professional nurses who apply to nurse anesthesia programs.

Clinical Practice

Professional certification indicates that an individual has met predetermined criteria that measure the knowledge, skills, and abilities necessary for entry level practice in a specialty area. Credentialing affords the public an awareness of the qualifications and capabilities of its health care providers. The title of CRNA signifies that the individual who holds it has fulfilled prescribed criteria and is qualified to provide in a competent and compassionate manner the services described within a CRNA's scope of practice. The standards for nurse anesthesia practice are listed in Box 2-1.

The AANA publishes a scope of practice for CRNAs[6] that includes but is not limited to the following tasks*:

1. Performing and documenting a preanesthetic assessment and evaluation of the patient, including requesting consultations and diagnostic studies; selecting, obtaining, ordering, and administering preanesthetic medications and fluids; and obtaining informed consent for anesthesia
2. Developing and implementing an anesthetic plan
3. Initiating the anesthetic technique, which may include general, regional, and local anesthesia and sedation
4. Selecting, applying, and inserting appropriate noninvasive and invasive monitoring modalities for continuous evaluation of the patient's physical status
5. Selecting, obtaining, and administering the anesthetics, adjuvant drugs, and accessory drugs and fluids necessary to manage the anesthetic
6. Managing a patient's airway and pulmonary status using current practice modalities
7. Facilitating emergence and recovery from anesthesia by selecting, obtaining, ordering, and administering medications, fluids, and ventilatory support
8. Discharging the patient from a postanesthesia care area and providing postanesthesia follow-up evaluation and care
9. Implementing acute and chronic pain management modalities
10. Responding to emergency situations by providing airway management, administering emergency fluids and drugs, and using basic or advanced cardiac life support techniques

Other functions included in a CRNA's scope of practice are administrative and management-related activities; quality assessment; education; research; committee work; and interdepartmental liaison activities.[6]

*Reprinted with permission from AANA, May 13, 2003.

BOX **2-1**

Standards for Nurse Anesthesia Practice

I. Perform a thorough and complete preanesthesia assessment.
II. Obtain informed consent for the planned anesthetic intervention from the patient or legal guardian.
III. Formulate a patient-specific plan for anesthesia care.
IV. Implement and adjust the anesthesia care plan based on the patient's physiologic response.
V. Monitor the patient's physiologic condition as appropriate for the type of anesthesia and specific patient needs.
   1. Monitor ventilation continuously.
   2. Monitor oxygenation continuously.
   3. Monitor cardiovascular status continuously.
   4. Monitor body temperature continuously.
   5. Monitor neuromuscular function and status.
   6. Monitor and assess patient's positioning.
VI. Document pertinent information on the patient's medical record completely, accurately, and in a timely manner.
VII. Transfer the responsibility for care of the patient to other qualified providers in a manner that assures continuity of care and patient safety.
VIII. Adhere to appropriate safety precautions, as established within the institution, to minimize the risks of fire, explosion, electrical shock, and equipment malfunction. Document on the patient's medical record that the anesthesia machine and equipment were checked.
IX. Take precautions to minimize the risk of infection to the patient, the CRNA, and other health care providers.
X. Assess anesthesia care to assure its quality and contribution to positive patient outcomes.
XI. Respect and maintain the basic rights of patients.

Adopted by the American Association of Nurse Anesthetists, June 1989. Revised 1992, 1996. © 1997, 2002 American Association of Nurse Anesthetists. Used with permission.

Activities outside the Operating Room

CRNAs are consulted on a 24-hour basis and are an integral part of the health care team, lending their experience in airway management, respiratory care, the management of fluid and electrolyte problems, pain management, resuscitative efforts, and other related clinical activities.[2] Many CRNAs are recognized by the American Heart Association as providers and instructors of advanced cardiac life support (ACLS), pediatric advanced life support (PALS), and neonatal advanced life support (NALS).

Nurse anesthesia education provides CRNAs with the theoretic basis necessary for participating in pain management. Many CRNAs are involved in the administration of regional nerve blocks and assist physicians in the diagnosis of neurologic deficits or in the modification of pain. Pain management is an expanding area of nurse anesthesia practice and research. CRNAs serve on a variety of institutional committees and participate as instructors in staff development and continuing educational programs for both professional and nonprofessional staff members. Accreditation standards require that each nurse anesthesia program includes CRNAs with graduate degrees as program director and assistant director.[5] As teachers, CRNAs instruct student nurse anesthetists and mentor junior faculty members.

CRNAs hold staff and committee appointments with state and federal governmental agencies, such as state boards of nursing and the U.S. Food and Drug Administration. CRNAs also are actively involved in standard-setting organizations, including the American National Standards Institute, the National Fire Protection Association, the American Society of Testing and Materials International, and the Association of Professionals in Infection Control and Epidemiology (S. Tunajek, personal oral communication, May 15, 2003).

Administrative Role. Current data indicate that hundreds of CRNAs perform administrative functions for departments of anesthesia.[7] The services provided by these administrators are extremely important to the overall functioning of an anesthesia department and correlate directly with the efficiency and quality of service provided. These functions include department management, quality assurance, risk management, continuing education, and data and fiscal management.[6]

Research. Conducting and participating in departmental, hospital-wide, and university- sponsored research projects fall within the CRNA's scope of practice.[6] Historically, nurse anesthetists have been involved in research since the beginning of the twentieth century. Early studies were generally descriptive in nature, whereas more recent investigations are scientifically designed quantitative and qualitative studies. Research findings have been published as theses and dissertations and in medical and nursing journals. CRNAs with doctoral degrees have qualified to be project directors or consultants for research projects including those conducted in universities.[2]

Involvement in research activities is encouraged by the profession through the AANA Foundation and at AANA meetings. The Foundation sponsors a doctoral mentorship program as a support group for CRNAs involved in research. Educational sessions on scientific inquiry, poster presentations, and communication of research findings are frequently part of the agenda of AANA meetings.

Both CRNA and student researchers are eligible to apply for grants that are awarded by the Foundation. CRNAs have also competed successfully for private and governmental grants. Their research findings have been presented at national and international meetings sponsored by other nurses, physicians, physiologists, pharmacologists, and the government.[2]

Nurse Anesthesia Programs

In mid 2003, 90 nurse anesthesia programs were available in the United States, including two in Puerto Rico. All of them offered master's degrees, reflecting a decision by the Council on Accreditation of Nurse Anesthesia Educational Programs to approve only graduate degree programs after January 1, 1998. In addition, all nurse anesthesia programs must meet specific accreditation standards to prepare students to take the national certification examination. On successful completion of the examination, the nurse anesthetist becomes a CRNA.

Practice Settings

The AANA has established professional standards of anesthesia care, as well as guidelines for nurse anesthesia practice. These standards are published in the *AANA Professional Practice Manual*, which is available from the AANA's national office. The standards and guidelines direct professional nurse anesthesia practice.[6]

CRNAs practice in traditional and critical access hospitals, ambulatory surgical centers, and U.S. military, public health services, and Veterans Administration health care facilities. CRNAs also practice in the offices of dentists, podiatrists, ophthalmologists, and plastic surgeons. Most CRNAs are hospital employees, although others are self-employed or work for anesthesiologist groups, military installations, universities, or clinics or in locum tenens situations.[8] Because CRNAs are licensed as nurses, they provide anesthesia services in collaboration with physicians—for example, surgeons, anesthesiologists, dentists, podiatrists, or other qualified practitioners.

ROLE OF THE PROFESSIONAL ORGANIZATION

Historical Background

In 1926, at the first meeting of the Lakeside Hospital alumni group of nurse anesthetists, Agatha Hodgins announced her vision of a national association of nurse anesthetists. Although Hodgins maintained the philosophy that nurse anesthesia should not be considered a part of nursing service but rather a part of general hospital service, on several occasions she approached the American Nurses Association (ANA) to propose the recognition of nurse anesthetists within that group. However, the ANA did not approve the proposal and requested more study on the matter. Determined to form a group of nurse anesthetists, Hodgins called on CRNAs around the country to convene at Western Reserve University–Lakeside Hospital in Cleveland, Ohio, to try to organize their own group. In 1931, 53 CRNAs from 12 states agreed to form the National Association of Nurse Anesthetists (NANA) and to continue their efforts to affiliate with the ANA.[9]

In 1933 the American Hospital Association invited the NANA to present its first national meeting in conjunction with the older, more established organization. After this meeting the NANA was confronted with one of the most important issues facing nurse anesthetists: education. NANA president Gertrude Fife called for the creation of a committee to investigate all schools of nurse anesthesia with the objective of creating a list of accredited schools. In addition she called for the establishment of a national board examination for nurse anesthetists. With this agenda set for the NANA in 1933, the members continued to move forward. In 1939 the organization's name was changed to the American Association of Nurse Anesthetists.[9]

Organizational Structure and Function

The AANA (at that time, the NANA) was first incorporated in Ohio on March 12, 1932. It was reincorporated in the state of Illinois on October 17, 1939 and was designated as a tax-exempt organization in accordance with subsection 501(c) of the Internal Revenue Code. The AANA's Education and Research Foundation was incorporated on July 15, 1981 and was designated as a tax-exempt organization in accordance with the same subsection of the Internal Revenue Code. The name was changed to the AANA Foundation in 1994 (K. Koch, personal oral communication, April 28, 2003).

The AANA's bylaws are essentially the AANA's working constitution, and they dictate how the association functions. The bylaws address areas such as the different classes of membership, decision-making procedures, the responsibilities of the AANA's elected officials, and the configuration of committees as well as the functions of their members.[5] AANA bylaws also define the national organization's relationship with state nurse anesthesia associations.

National Headquarters

In 1937 the AANA executive office moved from Cleveland to Chicago.[6] After having been situated in downtown Chicago, in 1980 the AANA purchased and moved into its first building on Higgins Road in Park Ridge, Illinois, a northwestern suburb of Chicago. A satellite office for federal affairs was opened in Washington, D.C. in 1990; lobbyists there advocated for nurse anesthesia education and practice. By early 1990 the AANA had outgrown the executive office in Park Ridge because of an expanding staff and increase in services. A 43,000–square-foot building was purchased in 1992 on South Prospect Avenue in the downtown area of Park Ridge. This building nearly tripled the size of the AANA's national headquarters, allowing the housing of all member services and subsidiaries at one site. The site is also large enough to house a learning center in which educational seminars are conducted for members on a variety of clinical and professional topics.

Departmental Organization

The AANA executive office consists of approximately 83 professional and support staff members. The organizational structure of the AANA comprises numerous departments, each with its own director, who reports to the executive director of the AANA. These departments include the executive unit, as well as departments for education, research, continuing education, information services and membership, finance, practice, state governmental affairs, federal governmental affairs, public relations and publications, and programs and meeting services. Member services are provided by each of these departments. The executive staff provides staff support to each standing and ad hoc committee of the AANA.[6]

The executive director is responsible for the administrative functions of the national office and reports directly to the elected AANA board of directors. As outlined in AANA bylaws, the executive director is responsible for keeping minutes on file of all AANA board meetings, for attending meetings of the board of directors and the executive committee, and for participating in other activities designated by the president. The executive director has no voting privileges but provides advice and guidance on policy formulation to the AANA board of directors. Other duties are to maintain professional AANA staff, negotiate and renew necessary service contracts for the AANA, oversee all financial decisions for the national office with direction from the board, and provide leadership to educational, legal, and legislative entities of the AANA. The executive director also represents the AANA to external organizations.[10]

Council Configurations and Relationships

Provisions within the AANA's bylaws have allowed the establishment of four separate autonomous councils that reside at the AANA's national office: the Council on Accreditation of Nurse Anesthesia Educational Programs, the Council on Certification of Nurse Anesthetists, the Council on Recertification of Nurse Anesthetists, and the Council for Public Interest in Anesthesia. These councils are solely responsible for their own internal affairs, including the election of officers and the direction of financial activities. In accordance with the bylaws, membership on these councils includes CRNAs, students, physicians, hospital administrators, and members of the public.[10]

The councils have been established with the intention of informing and assuring the public that accreditation, certification, recertification, and public interest activities are within the discipline of nurse anesthesia and are separate from and not unduly influenced by the national professional association. Communication between the AANA and the councils takes place through a formal liaison committee of council chairs and association officers that facilitates discussion of issues of mutual concern. An executive staff director serves each of the councils.

The Council on Accreditation of Nurse Anesthesia Educational Programs consists of individuals who are involved in the accreditation process of educational programs and the promulgation of educational standards. The purpose of the council is to formulate and adopt standards, guidelines, procedures, and criteria for the accreditation of nurse anesthesia educational programs. This process is subject to review and comment from the AANA board of directors and from the larger community interested in nurse anesthesia.[10]

The Council on Certification of Nurse Anesthetists consists of individuals who are involved in the process of certification of nurse anesthetists. The purpose of this council is to formulate and adopt the requirements, guidelines, and prerequisites for certification and eligibility for the certification examination.[10] The council is also responsible for administering the certification examination and for evaluating candidates' performance. The council grants initial certification to those candidates who successfully pass the examination and meet the other criteria for certification.

The Council on Recertification of Nurse Anesthetists consists of individuals who are involved in the evaluation and recertification of CRNAs (S. Caulk, personal oral communication, April 28, 2003). Its purpose is to formulate, adopt, and continuously evaluate the eligibility criteria for recertification. CRNAs are recertified on the basis of their participation in approved continuing educational activities, documentation of practice, and Registered Nurse/Advanced Registered Nurse Practitioner (RN/ARNP) licensure. Certification is also required that no condition exists that might adversely affect the ability of a CRNA to administer anesthesia or provide safe care to patients.[10]

The Council for Public Interest in Anesthesia is a multidisciplinary body composed of representatives of the public concerned with issues that involve public safety in anesthesia care. It acts as an autonomous appellate body in the credentialing of nurse anesthetists and their educational programs. Its major activities are the monitoring of social and health care trends and issues from the viewpoint of the public; the provision of recommendations to the AANA board of directors, committees, and councils on matters pertaining to accreditation, certification, and recertification; and the application of a public perspective in the review of practice issues as requested by the AANA.[10]

International Federation of Nurse Anesthetists

The International Federation of Nurse Anesthetists (IFNA) is a federation of national associations of nurse anesthetists. It is an affiliate member of the International Council of Nurses and a Nursing Partner of the World Health Organization. The IFNA represents more than 45,000 nurse anesthetists worldwide and is a growing organization with members in both developed and developing countries (R. Caulk, personal oral communication, April 23, 2002). The first organizational meeting was held in September 1988, and 11 countries were admitted as charter members in 1989. To date there are 32 member countries. In 1995 the executive office of the IFNA was established at the AANA headquarters. The IFNA has developed international standards for education, standards of practice, standards for patient monitoring, and a code of ethics for nurse anesthetists.[11] A World Congress is held every 4 years and is hosted by a member country.

Subsidiary

The AANA owns one subsidiary, the AANA Association Management Services (AAMS), which provides non–dues-related sources of revenue, as well as services for the general membership. There are currently three divisions within the AAMS. These divisions provide insurance-, management-, and publishing-related services to both internal and external clients (R. Rupp, personal oral communication, April 24, 2003).

Elected Leadership

The elected board of directors is responsible for managing the affairs of the AANA.[10] The board members include the president, the president-elect, the vice president, the treasurer, and seven regional directors. The officers are elected for 1-year terms and the regional directors for 2-year terms. Eligibility requirements for serving on the board include active involvement in state association activities, as well as proved leadership and interpersonal skills. A nominating committee oversees the recruitment and selection of individuals for the slate of candidates. All CRNAs are mailed a written ballot and are eligible to vote for candidates for all 11 positions.

The board of directors is the administrative authority for the AANA. It receives and considers the reports of the various committees and councils and makes recommendations as needed. Other responsibilities of the board include developing policy, overseeing the budget and related financial affairs, promulgating clinical standards and guidelines, participating in legislative activities, and serving as a liaison with external governmental and professional agencies.

Other Activities

In addition to maintaining the national office, the AANA conducts business largely through meetings of its membership segments. These meetings include the Assembly of School Faculty, the Fall and Mid-Year Assemblies of States, and the annual meeting. All AANA members are invited to attend and fully participate in these activities.

SUMMARY

The nurse anesthesia profession continues to grow from its strong foundation with the ongoing dedication of its members, volunteer leaders, and staff. As they encounter the challenges of health care reform, all CRNAs must take an active role in securing their future, because a profession is merely the sum of its members. As we look to the future, we can be guided by the AANA's vision statement:

> *The goal of the AANA is to] be the preeminent association of anesthesia providers by putting patients first and taking a leadership role in policy making, nurse anesthesia education, and research to ensure high-quality, safe anesthesia practice by CRNAs worldwide.*[12]

REFERENCES

1. Beutler, J. Report of the AANA Executive Director. *AANA News Bull.* 2002;12(special supplement):7-11.
2. American Association of Nurse Anesthetists. *Qualifications and Capabilities of the Certified Registered Nurse Anesthetist.* Park Ridge, Ill: American Association of Nurse Anesthetists; 1999.
3. Council on Certification of Nurse Anesthetists. *Candidate Handbook.* Park Ridge, Ill: Council on Certification of Nurse Anesthetists; 2003.
4. Council on Accreditation of Nurse Anesthesia Educational Programs. *Trial Standards for Accreditation of Nurse Anesthesia Educational Programs.* Park Ridge, Ill: Council on Accreditation of Nurse Anesthesia Educational Programs; 2003.
5. American Association of Nurse Anesthetists. *Education of Nurse Anesthetists in the United States.* Park Ridge, Ill: American Association of Nurse Anesthetists; 2002.
6. American Association of Nurse Anesthetists. *Scope and Standards for Nurse Anesthesia Practice.* Park Ridge, Ill: American Association of Nurse Anesthetists; 2002.
7. American Association of Nurse Anesthetists. AANA 2000 Manpower Survey details. *AANA News Bull.* 2000;54:8.
8. American Association of Nurse Anesthetists. *Nurse Anesthetists at a Glance.* Park Ridge, Ill: American Association of Nurse Anesthetists; 2002.
9. Garde JF. *The Nurse Anesthesia Profession: A Past, Present, and Future Perspective.* Park Ridge, Ill: American Association of Nurse Anesthetists; 1996.
10. American Association of Nurse Anesthetists. *Bylaws and Standing Rules of the American Association of Nurse Anesthetists.* Park Ridge, Ill: American Association of Nurse Anesthetists; 2002.
11. International Federation of Nurse Anesthetists. *Educational Standards for Preparing Nurse Anesthetists, Standards of Practice, Code of Ethics, and Monitoring Guidelines.* Helsinki, Finland: International Federation of Nurse Anesthetists; 2002.
12. American Association of Nurse Anesthetists. *Strategic Plan Highlights: Fiscal Years 2001-2003.* Park Ridge, Ill: American Association of Nurse Anesthetists, 2000.

CHAPTER 3

Nurse Anesthesia Research: Science of an Orderly, Purposeful, and Systematic Nature

Chuck Biddle

The certified registered nurse anesthetist (CRNA) brings a wealth of knowledge to the clinical arena. Although this knowledge comes from a variety of disciplines, including physiology, pharmacology, physics, nursing, medicine, and psychology, it should be appreciated that research and critical thinking first and foremost make this knowledge possible.

Research represents a rational approach to the making of practice choices among initially plausible alternatives and provides direction and a means for validating these choices. Whether selecting one intravenous opioid over another or choosing one particular pediatric induction technique instead of another, CRNAs rely on research to provide a solid foundation for clinical decision-making, thereby avoiding fads and inferior alternatives.

Without question, the dissemination of research findings to anesthesia practitioners is occurring at a higher rate than has ever before been seen. Not only are the results of research being presented with greater frequency at anesthesia symposia of all kinds, but research is also conspicuous in the literature previously devoted entirely to clinical anesthesia.

The impact of research on the day-to-day activities of the CRNA has become an especially relevant topic. Before the mid 1970s the vast majority of nurses functioned without much consideration of research or publication of their ideas. In the late 1970s we experienced a period of punctuated evolution. Major driving forces behind this evolution included movement into a graduate educational framework, a more sophisticated appreciation of the scientific underpinnings of our specialty, recognition of the importance of evidence-based practice (EBP; see the discussion of this topic later in this chapter), national attention to issues of patient outcome and patient safety, and a growing self-awareness of nurse anesthetists not only as providers of excellent clinical care but also as active participants as scholars in the field.

Because CRNAs primarily function with a practice-oriented perspective, the recommendations of Brown and colleagues[1] seem especially relevant. These scholars suggested that four characteristics of research are essential for the development of a scientific knowledge base for a discipline such as nurse anesthesia. First, research should be actively conducted by the members of the discipline. Second, research should be focused on clinical problems encountered by members of the discipline. Third, the approach to these problems must be grounded in a conceptual framework—that is, it must be scientifically based, emphasizing selection, arrangement, and clarification of existing relationships. Finally, the methods employed in studying the problems must be fundamentally sound.

WAYS OF KNOWING

The term *research* can be broadly defined as the application of a systematic approach to the study of a problem or question. However, we do not know all of the things that we claim to know on the basis of systematic inquiry. For example, tradition and custom are important sources of human knowledge. Those who live in the United States are raised in a democratic society and are taught that democracy is the best and most advanced form of government. This is a powerful and efficient route for communication of knowledge because it excuses individuals from initiating an independent effort to come to grips with the concept of democracy. In the absence of evaluation for validity, however, such a route may lead to blind acceptance.

Another source of our knowledge is authority. We know something to be true because an authoritative person such as a parent, policeman, clergyman, physician, or teacher tells us that it is true. Yet, despite the fact that authorities are fallible, the knowledge they pass on often remains unchallenged. Should we not ask the basis for what we are being told?

Personal experience (the trial-and-error method) represents a powerful source of knowledge. We make observations (e.g., that placing a hand on a hot stove causes a burn) and on their basis make predictions (e.g., that a stove may be hot) and future behavioral decisions (e.g., to avoid touching a stove). However, a risk remains: not only are certain events perceived differently by different people, but one person's experience may be too narrow to serve as the basis for the development of a reasonable and unbiased understanding of a given phenomenon. Although this mechanism is a practical way of knowing, it is highly fallible and represents a coarse and inefficient way to gain knowledge.

Logical reasoning is yet another way of knowing. The reasoning method has two components: inductive reasoning and deductive reasoning. Inductive reasoning results in generalizations that are derived from specific observations. Consider the following line of reasoning using James Bond, the character in several action and adventure movies, as an example: we observe that James Bond is mortal; we observe that a number of other people are mortal as well; on this basis, we conclude that all people are mortal. Deductive reasoning is the development of specific predictions from generalities. In this case, we see the following line of reasoning: we know that all men are mortal; we know that James Bond is a man; therefore we conclude that James Bond is mortal. Both methods are useful, but the former offers no mechanism for evaluation or self-correction, and the latter is not in itself a source of new information.

Perhaps the most advanced way of knowing is reflected in the scientific method. Although it too is fallible, the scientific method is more reliable and valid than other methods. It provides for self-evaluation with a system of checks and balances that minimizes bias and faulty reasoning. In essence, it is a systematic approach to solving problems and enhancing our understanding of phenomena. It has, at its foundation, the gathering and interpretation of information without prejudice.

THE NATURE OF RESEARCH

Research is by definition a dynamic phenomenon. Whether it is directed purely at the acquisition of knowledge for knowledge's sake (basic research) or at the specific solution of problems (applied research), it is a process that can be conceptualized in terms of at least four characteristics.

First, research can assume many different forms. Second, research must be valid, both internally and externally (Box 3-1). Internal validity is necessary but not sufficient for ensuring external validity. Third, research must be reliable. Reliability refers to the extent to which data collection, analysis, and interpretation are consistent and to which the research can be replicated. Fourth, research must be systematic. The elements of a systematic approach include the identification of the problem or problems, the gathering and critical review of relevant information, the collection of data in a highly orchestrated manner, an analysis of the data appropriate to the problem or problems faced, and the development of conclusions within the study's framework.

Science is not a routine, cut-and-dried process. Rather, scientific knowledge emerges from an enterprise that is intensely human, and, as a consequence, it is subject to the full spectrum of human strengths and limitations. The scientific discovery and understanding that attend participation in research and its results can be professionally exhilarating and satisfying.

EVIDENCE-BASED PRACTICE IN NURSE ANESTHESIA

EBP is an approach to patient care that is founded on the belief that clinical decisions must be based on results obtained from rigorously controlled investigations. It cautions against using studies with low external validity (e.g., animal studies) or those based on uncontrolled observations (e.g., case reports, retrospective studies) in rendering decisions that influence or dictate patient care interventions.

Although many recipes for and approaches to EBP exist, the essential ingredients common to all include the following:

1. Defining the patient's problem
2. Proficiently searching the relevant literature
3. Critically appraising the discovered literature
4. Rationally applying the relevant literature in the context unique to the patient

At the core of EBP is the notion of critical thinking (appraisal) of the applicable literature. Here, intellectual rigor is balanced with clinical experience as the clinician determines whether the evidence is applicable to a particular patient's situation.

The dizzying array of studies in our field coupled with the complexities and vagaries of our patient population produce an informational blitzkrieg that is both frustrating and daunting to clinicians who endeavor to remain on the cutting edge with respect to patient care decisions. We all rely, to one extent or another, on reviews of primary research to assist us in coming to understand and apply clinical research findings. Whenever possible, we should endeavor to use systematic reviews. Systematic reviews are those than incorporate a comprehensive study retrieval process that minimizes publication bias; selection criteria that identify only relevant studies; a critical appraisal of the emergent literature accomplished by knowledgeable and sophisticated clinicians and researchers; and reproducible decisions regarding the relevance and methodologic rigor of the selected primary research.

Recently the metaanalysis has begun to appear in the anesthesia literature. A metaanalysis is a systematic review that includes a quantitative statistical analysis of the findings that

BOX 3-1

Research Scenario: Internal versus External Validity

Internal Validity

The extent to which results can be accurately interpreted and the degree to which the independent variable (that which is manipulated) is responsible for a change in the dependent variable (that which is measured). For example, the patient's blood pressure is measured. A combination of thiopental, midazolam, isoflurane, and a new muscle relaxant is used for induction of anesthesia. A postinduction blood pressure is recorded, and the researcher concludes that the new muscle relaxant lowers blood pressure.

Questions

Has the researcher isolated the effect of the muscle relaxant from those of the other agents? Are there plausible or competing alternative explanations?

Analysis

Internal validity is low because the results cannot be interpreted with any degree of certainty.

External Validity

The extent to which the results can be generalized; this issue relates to the question "to whom can the results be applied?" For example, 35 obese men who are nonsurgical volunteers are anesthetized with a standard dose of a new induction drug. The clinical half-life of the drug is determined with plasma drug sampling and brain wave activity monitoring. The researcher concludes that future patients receiving the standard dose of the new drug will experience a clinical half-life of 11 minutes.

Questions

Is it reasonable to assume that obese patients might respond differently than their nonobese counterparts? Might women respond differently than men? Could surgical manipulation or other drug therapy have an impact on the pharmacokinetics of the new drug?

Analysis

External validity is low because the results cannot be generalized to any other individuals except those similar to the subjects in the study.

have emerged from several (or many) discrete studies examining a similar phenomenon. Examples of anesthesia-based metaanalyses include those by Tramer, who examined ondansetron as an antiemetic; Ballantyne and colleagues, who studied pulmonary outcomes in patients who had epidural analgesia; Lee and colleagues, who looked at acupuncture and acupressure as alternative approaches in the management of postoperative emetic symptoms; and Biddle, who evaluated the use of nonsteroidal antiinflammatory drugs in the treatment of acute postoperative pain.[2-5]

EBP helps us to avoid confusing (or even unsound) opinion with scientific evidence. EBP complements other foundational approaches to patient care and teaching. When solid evidence evolves into sound clinical decision-making, patients receive the best possible care. Some researchers argue that there is a crucial final step in the EBP model—namely, that clinicians self-evaluate their own EBP. In doing so clinicians provide an ongoing process of evaluation and sensitivity testing for practice-based decisions.

THE EIGHT CRITICAL STAGES IN THE RESEARCH PROCESS

Research accords several personal freedoms to those who engage in it: the freedom to pursue those opportunities in which one is interested, the freedom to exchange ideas with other interested colleagues, and the freedom to be a *deconstructionist*—that is, one who challenges existing knowledge. Yet, despite these freedoms, research must be logical, must progress in an orderly manner, and ultimately must be grounded within the framework of the scientific method. If research is a way of searching for truths, uncovering solutions to problems, and generating principles that result in theories, we must come to understand the process of research.

The research process can be described in many different ways; for purposes of simplicity, this process is defined as consisting of the following eight distinct stages:

1. Identification of the problem
2. Review of the relevant knowledge and literature
3. Formulation of the hypothesis or research question
4. Development of an approach for testing the hypothesis
5. Execution of the research plan
6. Analysis and interpretation of the data
7. Dissemination of the findings to interested colleagues
8. Evaluation of the research report

Stage 1: Identification of the Problem

The selection and formulation of the problem constitute an essential first step in the research process. The researcher decides the general subject of the investigation, guided principally by personal experience and by inductions and deductions based on existing sources of knowledge. The researcher makes the general subject manageable by narrowing of the focus of the problem. The following criteria must be met at this phase of the research process:

1. The problem area should be of sufficient importance to merit study.
2. The problem must be one that is practical to investigate.
3. The researcher should be knowledgeable and experienced in the area from which the problem has emerged.
4. The researcher should be sincerely motivated and interested in studying the problem.

We constantly encounter problems and situations that can be studied. At clinical anesthesia conferences, one hears remarks such as the following:

"It seems to me that a tiny dose of thiopental given just before propofol alleviates virtually any pain on injection."

"Do you think there is less nausea and vomiting in outpatients who are deliberately overhydrated?"

"I find that the use of the waveform generated by my pulse oximeter gives me valuable information about depth of anesthesia."

"I believe that the inspiratory pause mechanism on the Ohmeda 7810 ventilator significantly improves arterial oxygen tension in my patients with chronic obstructive pulmonary disease."

"I am convinced that sleepiness is a major cause of anesthesia accidents."

A study could emerge from each of these situations, built on ideas, hunches, or curiosity. A problem that lends itself to research often materializes from personal observations and in the sharing of ideas and experiences among those who are familiar with the phenomenon in question.

Once identified, the problem should be stated in terms that clarify the subject and restrict the scope of the study. Defining the terms involved in the problem statement also is critical, as demonstrated in Box 3-2.

The wording of the problem statement sets the stage for the type of study design used. Each step in the research process subsequently influences later steps, and this should be kept in mind at all times. A mistake made early inevitably creates difficulties at some later stage in the process. The novice researcher may be surprised to find that this first stage in the research process often consumes a large portion of the total time invested in the research effort. Yet the time is well spent, because research should not commence until a problem has been identified and formulated in a thoughtful and useful manner.

Common Mistakes

At this stage of the process, pitfalls can include an overly ready acceptance of the first research idea that comes to mind and selection of a problem that is too broad or vague to allow effective study.

BOX **3-2**

Research Scenario: Stating the Problem

Poor

I am unsure of the effectiveness of etomidate in patients.

Better

I am unsure at what dose etomidate induces unconsciousness in patients undergoing hysterectomy and what impact it has on heart rate, blood pressure, and vascular resistance.

Comments

- The problem should be focused.
- The terms should be clarified.
- The relationships should be understood.
- The problem should not be so narrow as to be trivial.

Stage 2: Review of the Relevant Knowledge and Literature

Once the problem has been identified, information is needed for putting the problem into proper context so that the research can proceed effectively. A well-conducted literature review provides the researcher with the following:

1. An understanding of what has already been accomplished in the area of interest
2. A theoretic framework within which the problem can be optimally stated, understood, and studied
3. An appreciation for gaps in current understanding of the phenomenon
4. Information for avoiding unanticipated difficulties
5. Examples of potentially useful or poorly constructed research designs and procedures
6. A background for interpreting the results of the proposed investigation

The knowledge that influences the problem originates from three general sources: personal files and experience, personal contacts with experts, and the library and Internet. Both manual indexes and computerized databases should provide the researcher with immediate and full access to the world's published literature. Additional literature searches may be required at different times throughout the research process.

Common Mistakes

At this stage in the research process, mistakes include hasty review of the literature, overly heavy reliance on secondary (book) rather than primary (journal) sources, lack of critical examination of the methods by which conclusions were reached, and incorrect copying of references so that they cannot be located again with ease.

Stage 3: Formulation of the Hypothesis or Research Question

In its most elemental form, a hypothesis is either a proposition of the solution to a problem or a stated relationship among variables. It establishes and defines the independent variable (the variable that is to be manipulated or is presumed to influence the outcome) and the dependent variable (the outcome that is dependent on the independent variable). The hypothesis is declarative in nature and assumes one of the following three forms:

1. A *directional hypothesis:* Patients premedicated with midazolam have less anxiety on arrival in the operating room than do those who were not premedicated.
2. A *nondirectional hypothesis:* Patients premedicated with midazolam experience a difference in anxiety on arrival in the operating room when compared with those who were not premedicated.
3. A *null hypothesis:* Patients premedicated with midazolam experience no difference in anxiety on arrival in the operating room compared with those who were not premedicated.

Research questions are generally reserved for investigations that are descriptive or exploratory in nature or for when the relationships among the variables are unclear. A research question might be more appropriate than a hypothesis in a study that proposes to determine the beliefs of anesthesia providers who interact with patients under specific circumstances. For example, consider the following research question: What are the attitudes of CRNAs in the northeastern United States who care for patients with acquired immunodeficiency syndrome (AIDS)?

Common Mistakes

At this point in the process, mistakes include use of a vague or unmanageable hypothesis and development of a research question that cannot be answered reasonably.

Stage 4: Development of an Approach for Testing the Hypothesis

After the research idea has taken shape in the form of a formal hypothesis or research question, a plan of attack is developed. The research proposal represents the stage at which the ideas of the project crystallize into a substantive form. The proposal includes the following:

1. A problem statement and clarification of the significance of the proposed study
2. The hypothesis or research question
3. A sufficient review of the literature for justification of the study
4. A description of the research design
5. A careful explanation of the sample to be studied
6. The type of statistical analysis to be applied

A research proposal is a useful and efficient way for the researcher to determine the completeness of the plan and is usually required if the researcher is to obtain departmental or institutional approval or is applying for financial support.

Research Methods

The research method is the way the truth of a phenomenon is coaxed from the world in which it resides and freed of the biases of the human condition. A variety of research methods are at our disposal, and researchers are not inflexibly wedded to any particular approach. Researchers do not follow a single scientific method but rather use a body of methods that are amenable to their fields of study.

Some of the methods available are highly recognizable, permanent components of the researcher's armamentarium, whereas others have evolved not only with respect to time, but also in response to the specific needs of a particular problem or discipline. The research method can be influenced by the way a researcher views a problem. For example, a researcher can test a hypothesis, search for a correlation, ask "why" or "how" questions, or probe a phenomenon on the basis of "what would happen if" suppositions.

The researcher can view the method on the basis of the fundamental task that it will accomplish. For example, two broad categories into which research efforts can be divided are basic research and applied research. Basic research adds to the existing body of knowledge and may not have immediate, practical use. Applied research is oriented toward solving an immediate, specific, and practical problem.

The research method can be characterized in terms of its temporal relationship to the problem. A retrospective study is the process of surveying the past; the thing in which we are interested has already occurred, and we are simply looking to see what did occur. In contrast, a prospective study looks forward to see what will happen in a given situation; here, the collection of data proceeds forward in time.

It is important to understand several terms fundamental to the research process. As mentioned previously, the dependent variable is the object of the study, or the variable that is being measured. The independent variable is the one that affects the dependent variable and is presumed to cause or influence it. Another way of looking at this relationship is that variables that are a consequence of or are dependent on antecedent variables are considered dependent variables.

Another set of variables consists of control variables, also known as "organismic," "background," or "attribute" variables. Control variables are not actively manipulated by the researcher, but because they might influence the relationships under study, they must be controlled, held constant, or randomized so that their effects are neutralized, canceled out, or at least considered by the researcher (Box 3-3).

The term *blinding* refers to the process of controlling for obvious and occult bias arising from subjects' or researchers' reactions to what is going on. In a single-blind design the researchers are unaware of which treatment or manipulation is actually being given to the subjects. In the double-blind design, neither the researcher nor the subject is aware of which treatment or manipulation the subject is receiving. Whereas randomization attempts to equalize the groups at the start of the study, blinding equalizes the groups by controlling for psychologic biases that might arise apart from any effect of the treatment. Many factors influence the decision to use a single-blind or a double-blind design. For example, in some situations, it may not be feasible to disguise a particular treatment or intervention.

Operationalization is the process of making the characteristics inherent in a given variable, condition, or process familiar or clear to others. If researchers do not operationalize the terms, phrases, and manipulations in the study, the net effect could be an ambiguous study. For example, in a study examining the effects of epidural anesthesia in critically ill patients, it would be essential to operationalize the terms *effects* and *critically ill patients*. Similarly, in a study comparing the quality of inhalation induction with isoflurane and halothane in pediatric patients, it is essential that the researcher operationalize the terms *inhalation induction* and *quality*. Operationalization of terms clearly designates performable and observable acts or procedures in such a way that they can be replicated immutably.

BOX **3-3**

Research Scenario: Understanding the Types of Variables

Study Group

A new intravenous drug that may be associated with fewer cardiovascular effects than thiopental during induction in pediatric patients is being studied. Fifty children ages 3 to 6 years undergoing intravenous inductions for hernia repair or eye muscle surgery are randomized to either the thiopental group or the new drug group. Blood pressure, heart rate, and rhythm are measured by a dedicated observer who is unaware of which drug the patients are receiving.

Analysis

The dependent variables are blood pressure, heart rate, and heart rhythm. The independent variable is the drug that the child receives—either the thiopental or the new drug. A number of control variables are present, including sex, fluid status, time of day, underlying medical history, and concurrent drug therapy. With randomization, such control variables should be equated or neutralized for the two groups, but even randomization is not an absolute guarantee.

Classifying Research on the Basis of Methodology

Although different authors use a variety of classification schemes, the following example provides a simple way for the researcher to select and classify a design. This scheme attends to the study's purpose and scope and to the nature of the problem at hand. Table 3-1 offers a simplified approach to classifying research design.

Quasi-experimental research differs from experimental research in that it is missing one or more of the key elements

TABLE **3-1** Classifying Research by Method

Type	Qualities and Purpose	Example
Experimental	At least one variable manipulated Random assignment to groups Dependent variable is measured Good for determining cause and effect Prospective in nature	Is there more or less pain on injection of one or the other drug? What did the manipulation do?
Ex post facto	Independent variable has already occurred Examines relationships by observing a consequence and looking back for associations Retrospective in nature (Latin for "from a thing done after")	Looking back over 5 years, did a relationship exist between the rate of myocardial infarction and the inhaled anesthetic that was administered?
Descriptive	Describes something as it occurred Incidence, relationships, and distributions are studied Deals more with "what is?" than "why is it so?" questions	What are the attitudes of CRNAs regarding the care of patients who have AIDS?
Historical	Describes "what was" rather than what effect variables had on others Events are described as accurately as possible through a process of critical inquiry	A test of the hypothesis is that Sister M. Bernard was the first nurse anesthetist
Qualitative Phenomenology Grounded theory Ethnography	Experiences lived by people Perception is viewed as our access to that experience Discovers and conceptualizes the essence of complex processes	What is the nature of the relationship of CRNAs and surgeons in private and in academic settings?

AIDS, *Acquired immunodeficiency syndrome*.

required for the experimental design. Either a control group or a randomization procedure may be absent from the design. For example, at an institution, outpatients may routinely receive ondansetron from a particular practitioner, whereas they routinely do not receive the drug from another practitioner. A prospective trial in which both practitioners use a standard anesthetic technique could be initiated. For example, isoflurane, an opioid, and atracurium could be administered; this would allow the two practitioners to use or not use ondansetron as they normally would. Outcome, measured in terms of the incidence of nausea and vomiting in the first 6 postoperative hours, is quantified, and the groups are compared. Although randomization is not achieved, a study that may not otherwise have been possible because of the inflexibility of the clinicians involved is successfully accomplished. Quasi-experiments, by yielding to one or more of the rigid criteria of the experimental design, offer an attractive alternative in certain circumstances.

Qualitative Research: an Alternative Paradigm

Up to this point, the traditional approach to a problem has been characterized by deductive reasoning, objectivity, manipulation, and control. An alternative approach involves a group of methods characterized by inductive reasoning, subjectivity, exploration, and process orientation. These methods fall under the rubric of qualitative research techniques.

Qualitative techniques include philosophic inquiry, histography, phenomenology, grounded theory, and ethnography. Generally speaking, qualitative research refers to systematic modes of inquiry directed principally at observing, describing, analyzing, interpreting, and understanding the patterns, themes, qualities, and meanings of specific contextual phenomena. Qualitative research seeks to gain insight by discovering the meanings associated with a given phenomenon and exploring the depth, richness, and complexity inherent in it.

For example, exploring how male and female CRNAs differ in the manner in which they deal with parental and child separation discomfort when a child is readied for induction of anesthesia might best be achieved through the use of a qualitative design. The actual experiences might be observed or videotaped. Those involved—anesthetists, parents, and children—might be interviewed immediately and at some time after the procedure. This study would be artificially constrained and disjointed if it were conducted in any setting other than the original one or if too many controls were brought to bear on the experiment.

The qualitative paradigm seems especially apropos when the researcher does not want to artificially distance a study from its contextual richness or when there is not enough information available on a particular subject for the adequate development of sound and testable hypotheses. The treatise on qualitative approaches by Marshall and Rossman[6] is recommended to interested readers.

Sampling

Under most circumstances, studying everyone who might be affected by a particular study is impractical, if not impossible. For example, if we want to know how effective intravenous nitroglycerin is in minimizing the rise in blood pressure associated with laryngoscopy in hypertensive patients, we cannot realistically study all hypertensive patients who undergo laryngoscopy. Rather, we would hope to find a smaller group of subjects who are representative of the relevant population at large. By accessing certain information in the sample, we can credibly make inferences or generalizations regarding the population at large.

Similarly, if we want to know how often anesthesia machines in small community hospitals receive preventive maintenance, we cannot visit all the community hospitals in the nation. Rather, we might randomly select a number of hospitals in a number of different states, visit those locations, and inspect the maintenance records. By studying this representative sample, we can make some reasonable and safe generalizations regarding the phenomenon of preventive maintenance at large.

Consider the anecdote about the four blind people who encountered an elephant during one of their daily walks (Figure 3-1). Each person felt a different part of the elephant. When asked to describe what they had encountered, the first person replied, "a tree trunk" (the elephant's leg). The second reported feeling "a large snake" (the elephant's trunk). The third reported that it was "most definitely a wall" (the elephant's torso). The last person reported that it was "a large, frayed rope" (the elephant's tail). This analogy illustrates that

Four blind people encounter an object and discuss what they found.
"A frayed rope"
"A wall"
"A tree trunk"
"A large snake"

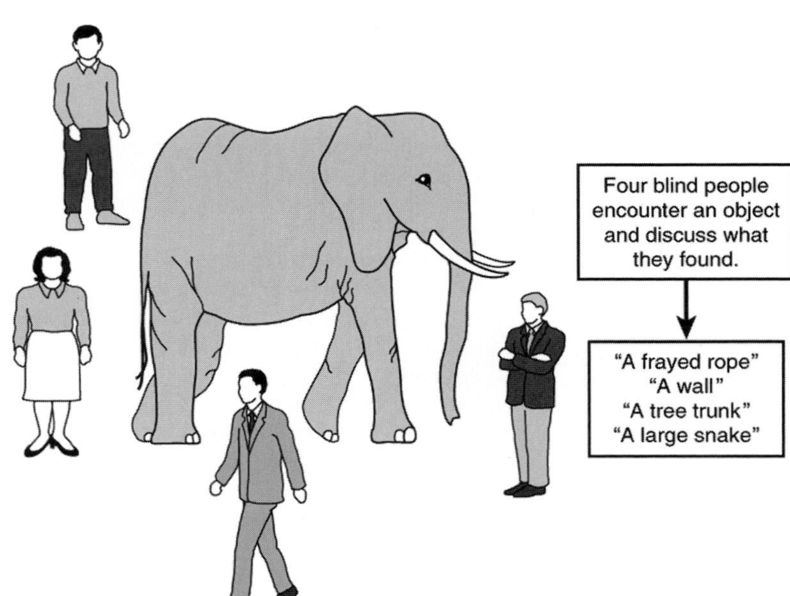

FIGURE **3-1**
The importance of sampling. A few discrete sampling points may not be adequate for describing a complex phenomenon.

a few discrete sampling points may not be adequate for describing a complex phenomenon. Not only is a random sample best, it also should be large enough and should sample a sufficient number of points in the population that a truly representative perspective is gained.

Different sampling techniques can be used, depending on the research design employed. In a true random sample (also known as "probability sampling"), all members of the population at large have a similar chance of being included in the study. This is rarely the case in clinical research, in which we are confined to dealing with those individuals who present themselves. In this situation, the sample is called a *convenience sample*. When a convenience sample is used in an experimental study, it is important to ensure that the subjects selected for the study are at least randomized when assigned to treatments or groups. In the ideal situation the researcher aims for both random selection (from the population at large) and random assignment (to the different groups in the study).

For example, in a study designed to quantify the rate of arterial desaturation in pediatric patients who are transported to the postanesthesia care unit with and without supplemental oxygen, the researcher is limited to those patients who are undergoing surgery. It is difficult to obtain a sample from the pediatric population at large and subject them to anesthesia and surgery. Rather, a convenience sample of patients who are having an operation is used. However, the researcher should randomly assign the study participants to one of the two treatment groups—those who receive supplemental oxygen or those who do not receive supplemental oxygen.

Obtaining a random sample, especially in clinical research, is often a complicated process. Most important is the realization that the concept of randomness is essential to minimizing human biases associated with both selection and assignment.

Instrumentation and Measurement

Two important concepts essential to measurement are validity and reliability. Instrument validity is the degree to which an instrument, such as a blood pressure cuff or a personality inventory, measures what one believes it is measuring. Instrument reliability refers to the degree of consistency with which an instrument measures whatever it is measuring—that is, whether the same result is obtained on repeated trials.

Validity and reliability are often easily established for measures of certain physiologic phenomena but may be troublesome in behavioral or psychologic evaluations. Imagine trying to determine reliability and validity for a thermometer. Contrast this to trying to establish validity and reliability for a psychologic tool that professes to measure a CRNA's attitude toward euthanasia; obviously, the latter is a much more difficult undertaking. Although a measure must be reliable to be valid, it can be reliable without being valid. For example, a skin temperature probe might reliably (consistently) measure temperature even in a variety of extreme settings, although it would not be viewed as a valid indicator of core temperature. Both reliability and validity are discussed in degrees rather than in "all-or-nothing" terms.

Many published instruments have reliability and validity testing reported. When choosing an instrument for a study, it is critical to consider whether the instrument's reliability and validity have been established. For example, if an instrument measures evoked responses in the esophagus as an indicator of depth of anesthesia, it must be determined whether the reliability and validity of the instrument have been established under the conditions of the anesthetic protocol being used in the proposed study. Coefficients of reliability and validity are presented on a scale of 0 to 1, with 1 being perfect.

Occasionally the researcher may encounter no reasonable measures to use for a study. For example, instruments for measuring such phenomena as arterial oxygen tension, end-tidal anesthetic concentration, and opioid metabolic by-products are well established. A researcher may need to develop a totally new instrument (questionnaire) to determine perceptions regarding the propriety of a given manufacturer's high-pressure promotional campaigns for newly released pharmaceutical products. In developing such a tool, it is helpful to have an expert in the discipline look over the instrument and provide feedback to ensure that the instrument is appropriate.

Researchers have a variety of instruments for measuring phenomena. These include the following:

- Written tests
- Rating scales
- Questionnaires
- Chemical tests
- Physical tests
- Electrical tests
- Visual observation
- Auditory observation
- Psychologic inventories

Levels of Measurement. In designing a study, the researcher must decide how to measure a phenomenon such as anxiety level, blood pressure, attitude toward health care, or rate of complications. There are four levels or degrees of measurement: nominal, ordinal, interval, and ratio. The type of data measured determines the kind of statistical analysis that can be done. Table 3-2 characterizes the four levels of measurement.

Nominal level measurement allows categorization of data, but the only numeric data that are obtained are frequencies. For example, in a study assessing the educational level of CRNAs in the profession, only the frequency of each category (certificates, bachelor's degrees, master's degrees, doctorates) can be reported. No statement can be made concerning the amount of the characteristic.

Ordinal level measurement allows for data to be ordered or ranked. In a sense, numbers are used to indicate the magnitude

TABLE 3-2 Characteristics of the Four Categories of Measurement

Category	Characteristics	Examples
Nominal	Identifies	Male or female Diagnosis
Ordinal	Identifies Orders	American Society of Anesthesiologists (ASA) class Order of race finish
Interval	Identifies Orders Equal intervals	Intelligence Calendar years Degrees Fahrenheit or Celsius
Ratio	Identifies Orders Equal intervals Has a true zero	Blood pressure Reaction time Weight Distance Degrees Kelvin

of the observations. For instance, the American Society of Anesthesiologists' Physical Status system provides for a relative ranking system for patients on the basis of their pathophysiologic status.

Interval level measurement uses numeric data that are ordered and spaced equally, such as temperature on the Fahrenheit or centigrade scale, calendar years, or intelligence quotients derived from an intelligence performance test. Here, the distance between adjacent scores is highly meaningful.

Ratio level measurement uses numeric data that can be ordered and equally spaced. It is based on a scale with an absolute zero point, such as temperature on the Kelvin scale, reaction time, height, and blood pressure. Both interval and ratio level measures can be referred to as "continuous" in nature.

Measurement can also be defined in terms of four broad categories: cognitive, affective, psychomotor, and physiologic. Each can manifest as one of the levels noted earlier. Cognitive measurement addresses the test subjects' knowledge or achievement. For example, what actions should be taken in the face of unexplained bradycardia? Affective measurements determine interests, values, and attitudes, thereby providing behavioral insights. For example, how do CRNAs in different locations feel about anesthetizing patients with AIDS? Psychomotor measurements test the subjects' ability or skill in performing specific tasks, such as evaluating performance with a new laryngoscopic design. Physiologic measurements look at the biologic functioning of the organism—for example, heart rate differences in men and women at basal conditions.

Although researchers sometimes develop unique instruments, which must be tested for reliability and validity, many published and acceptable instruments can be located in any number of sources.[7,8]

The Pilot Study

A pilot study is the implementation of a study on a small scale. It includes only a few subjects, who generally will not be included in the formal study. Its purpose is to troubleshoot the methodology for any anticipated design problems. The pilot study allows the researcher the opportunity to perform a dry run, ultimately facilitating the progression of the study.

Common Mistakes

At this point in the process, mistakes include failure to adequately operationalize definitions, failure to define the population or sample adequately, unrealistic expectations for subject recruitment and participation, underestimation of the difficulty of design execution, failure to establish instrument reliability and validity, and failure to appreciate the ethical dimensions of the investigation.

Stage 5: Execution of the Research Plan

Up to this point, the research process has involved the acquisition of knowledge regarding the subject, planning the project, and critical thinking about what is to occur. The next stage of the process involves actual data collection and the organization of the data into a format that allows data analysis.

The data collection must precisely follow the procedure that the researcher specified previously. The real payoff in research comes with the drawing of useful and bona fide conclusions once the data have been collected and precisely analyzed within the framework of the research design. The goal of the previous step—namely, maximization of both internal and external validity—would not be achieved if the researcher were to deviate from the plan.

Maintaining careful records of what was done and what results were recorded is essential. The labeling and sorting of data into the respective categories or chronologies should be extremely precise. No data should be discarded until the researcher knows that they are absolutely unnecessary. Many researchers "stockpile" raw data and their notes, because additional uses for the information may not manifest for months or even years after the initial project's completion and publication.

Common Mistakes

The mistakes associated with this stage include drifting from the stated methodology for convenience or administrative purposes, placing excessive demands on subjects, allowing personal bias to creep into the research plan, using observers or research assistants who are improperly trained, failing to obtain a sufficient sample size, and improperly using measurement instruments.

Stage 6: Analysis and Interpretation of the Data

A few words on statistics are in order. Not only is proper analysis essential to the design, analysis, and interpretation of the investigation, it also is necessary for understanding and evaluating research studies conducted by other investigators. Analysis has three general phases: the initial mechanical manipulation of the data, the analysis itself, and the thoughtful formulation of conclusions on the basis of the analysis.

For the purposes of this discussion, the following two questions are posed:

1. What is the rationale for the use of statistical analysis in research?
2. What are the more common statistical procedures used, and under what circumstances are they appropriate?

Descriptive Statistical Techniques

Once the data on the phenomenon under study have been collected, they often are categorized and described. For example, if the goal of a study is the determination of the incidence of headache and the change noted in blood pressure in 50 patients undergoing spinal anesthesia, the researcher would describe the demographics of the sample of patients in terms of sex, height, weight, or any other relevant variable.

The group or set of all the observations of the variable is called a *distribution*. The distribution yields information about the overall dispersion of the phenomenon within the sample, as well as the exact location of a given measure relative to the group as a whole. In the case of an interval- or ratio-level measurement, such as blood pressure, the distribution of values is probably Gaussian or bell shaped in nature (i.e., some pressures are low, most are intermediate, and some are high). By studying the distribution, the researcher can compare a particular measured value with all the values obtained for the phenomenon.

Alternatively, the researcher might use a technique that clusters data into rational blocks or intervals. For example, in the spinal anesthesia study, instead of listing all 50 initial blood pressures individually, the researcher could tabulate them according to frequency relative to a given interval. In this case, each measured blood pressure falls within a range, and the frequency of presentation in the sample is tabulated as shown in

Table 3-3. Instead of using the tabular form, the researcher could arrange the same data in graphic form, indicating the frequency of the phenomenon on the vertical *(y)* axis and the blood pressure values on the horizontal *(x)* axis. In histograms and bar graphs, the width of each bar corresponds to the limits of the interval, and the height of the bar corresponds to the frequency or percent of the cases occurring in a specific interval. A frequency polygram also is a commonly used tool for displaying data. Points are plotted directly over the midpoint of each of the intervals. The data given in Table 3-3 are presented in Figure 3-2 as a frequency polygram.

Other descriptive statistics include the mean (the arithmetic mean of the sample); the median (the point below which one half of the measurements lie); and the mode (the value occurring most frequently). The range shows the dispersion data from the highest to the lowest value. Variance and standard deviation (SD) must be computed and are based on the concept of deviation (the difference between an observed score and the mean value in the distribution). Variance is the square of the sum of all of the deviations divided by the number of scores, and the SD is the positive square root of the variance. Because of variation, investigators describe the data not only in terms of the typical or average value but also in terms of the amount of variation that is present. With respect to quantitative data such as blood pressure, number of attempts at intubation, or amount of blood loss, this task is generally a matter of characterizing the distribution of the attribute in terms of its central tendency and dispersion. This is achieved by providing the mean and the SD. The SD is a tool for describing the variation of individual observations around the mean. Standard error of the mean (SEM) is linked to the SD by the following simple mathematical formula:

$$\text{SEM} = \text{SD}/n$$

where *n* is the number of observations in the sample.

The SEM describes the variation of the sample mean (that for the actual data collected) around the true, but unknown, population mean (that for all possible observations). The difficulty with using the SEM is that as the number of subjects or observations increases, the standard error of the mean decreases. In theoretic terms, as *n* approaches infinity, SEM approaches 0. Researchers are urged to consult with a biostatistician and to develop a rationale before deciding to use the SEM or SD.

In general, the higher the level of measurement used (i.e., ratio > interval > ordinal > nominal), the greater the flexibility in selecting a descriptive statistic. Using the data from the spinal anesthesia study noted earlier, it would be appropriate to compute the SD for initial systolic blood pressure (ratio-level data). However, such a computation would be meaningless for nominal-level information, such as whether subjects are male or female.

TABLE 3-3 Frequency Distribution for Initial Systolic Blood Pressure

Interval (mm Hg)*	Frequency†
0-60	1
60-90	8
91-120	15
121-150	15
151-180	8
>180	3

**Interval equals the range or band into which a given measure is placed.*
†Frequency equals the number of observations falling into that interval.

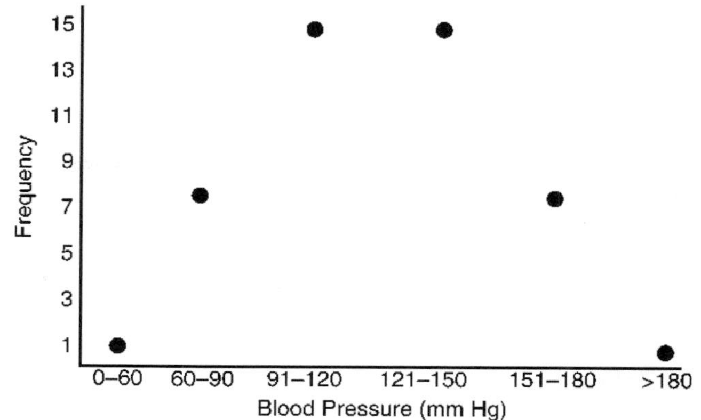

FIGURE **3-2**
The frequency polygram. Note the bell-shaped configuration that plotted data have assumed; this typically is the "normal" distribution of biologic data (e.g., weight, heart rate, minimum alveolar concentration, intelligence).

Correlational Statistical Techniques

The correlation coefficient is generally used for describing the extent to which two variables are related to each other or for quantifying the degree of that relationship. For example, it would be useful if one were studying the extent to which the level of carbon monoxide in the blood is related to cigarette smoking. Calculated correlations vary from +1.0 (a perfect direct correlation) to −1.0 (a perfect inverse correlation). A correlation of 0 indicates no relationship. Researchers often display the correlations visually in the form of a scattergram, which shows the shape of a relationship between two variables. There are many types of correlational techniques (Table 3-4).

In the hypothetic study of carbon monoxide level and cigarette smoking, a researcher might decide to use the product-moment correlation technique. The numeric value for carbon monoxide in the blood has a true 0 (ratio-level data) and a numeric value (ratio-level data) for daily cigarette smoking. The correlation between these variables would probably be positive and very high (e.g., 0.8 or even higher), which suggests that heavy use of cigarettes is associated with a high carbon monoxide level in the blood.

Conversely, assume that a study examines the relationship between gender (a nominal-level variable) and anesthetic

TABLE 3-4 Correlation Techniques Appropriate to Data Type

Correlation	Variable No. 1	Variable No. 2
Product-moment	Interval or ratio	Interval or ratio
Spearman's rank	Ordinal	Ordinal
Point biserial	Nominal or ordinal	Interval or ratio
Phi	Dichotomy	Dichotomy
Contingency	Nominal	Nominal

minimum alveolar concentration (a ratio-level variable). In this example, the researcher using the point biserial correlation technique would expect to see a very low correlation, because gender probably is not associated in any meaningful way with anesthetic requirements.

Inferential Statistical Techniques

Inferential statistical procedures provide a set of techniques that allow the researcher to infer that the events observed in the sample will also occur in the larger unobserved population from which the sample was obtained. There are two basic reasons for using inferential techniques. First, they can assist the researcher who is testing a hypothesis and must decide whether to accept or reject it. For example, a researcher, having a particular value in mind, poses the question, "Is this value reasonable in light of the evidence from the sample?" Second, inferential techniques can be used for estimation. For example, a researcher may have no particular value in mind but wants to know what the population value is. The researcher draws a sample, studies it, and makes an inference about the population characteristic (Figure 3-3). These two classic situations as addressed by inferential techniques are as follows:

- *Testing a hypothesis* (Table 3-5). Is there a significant difference in the incidence of nausea between those patients given thiopental and those who receive propofol?
- *Making an estimation*. What percentage of CRNAs perform a thorough machine check at the start of each day?

Researchers are seemingly preoccupied with the concept of significance. The level of significance (also designated as *alpha level* or P *value*) is a criterion used in making decisions regarding a hypothesis. For example, if P is less than 0.05, the probability that the difference observed between the samples was the result of chance alone is less than 5%. Accordingly, if P is less than 0.05, the probability that the difference between the samples was real (i.e., it resulted from the treatment), and not just the result of chance, is greater than 95%. It is conventional to establish the alpha level before the data analysis is begun; however, there seems to be an increasing trend toward reporting calculated P values after hypotheses have been tested. Commonly used levels in research are $P < 0.05$ and $P < 0.01$; $P < 0.10$ is sometimes used in preliminary or descriptive studies.

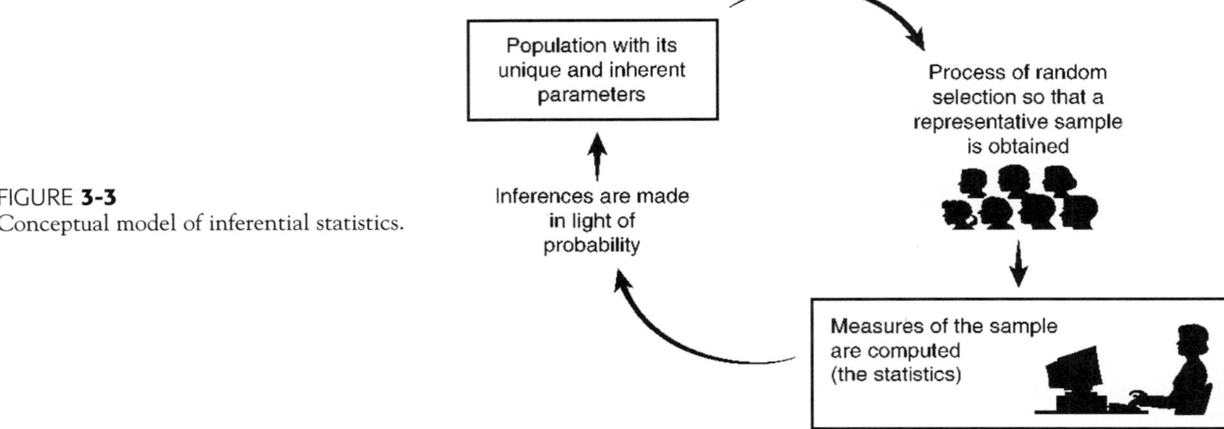

FIGURE **3-3**
Conceptual model of inferential statistics.

TABLE 3-5 Statistical Methods Used for Testing Hypotheses

Scale of Measurement	TYPE OF EXPERIMENT: Two Treatment Groups Consisting of Different Individuals	Three or More Treatment Groups Consisting of Different Individuals	Before and After a Single Treatment in the Same Individual	Multiple Treatments in the Same Individual	Association between Two Variables
Interval (and drawn from normally distributed populations*)	Unpaired *t*-test	Analysis of variance	Paired *t*-test	Repeated-measures analysis of variance	Linear regression and Pearson product-moment correlation
Nominal	Chi-squared analysis of contingency table	Chi-squared analysis of contingency table	McNemar's test	Cochrane Q	Contingency coefficient
Ordinal	Mann-Whitney rank sum test	Kruskal-Wallis statistic	Wilcoxon signed rank test	Friedman's statistic	Spearman's rank correlation

**If the assumption of normally distributed populations is not met, the observations should be ranked, and the methods for data measured on the ordinal scale should be used.*

Adapted with permission from Glantz SA. Primer of Biostatistics. *3rd ed. New York: McGraw-Hill; 1992.*

There is also a trend to simply report the calculated *P* value and leave the interpretations up to the reader.

Selecting the Appropriate Statistical Procedure

There are two major categories of inferential procedures: parametric analyses and nonparametric analyses. The major factors that dictate which category should be selected involve the assumptions that the investigator makes regarding the data. Tables 3-6 and 3-7 provide some guidelines for selecting a statistical procedure.

Power

The sensitivity of the planned experiment and analysis is known as its power. The concept of power is important to anyone planning a research project or evaluating a published paper. The estimate of an experiment's ability to accurately test the hypothesis under question should be computed before the research is begun. A researcher should ask the following two critical questions:

1. What is the chance that I will incorrectly determine that my treatment had an effect when it really did not (type I error)?
2. What is the chance that I will miss an effect that is actually present (type II error)?

Power estimates obtained during a study's design stage encourage investigators to thoughtfully enhance the study's sensitivity. Making such estimates forces the posing of questions regarding effect size (e.g., how potent is the effect of the independent variable on the dependent variable?) and sample size, both of which are essential in a study. Many adverse outcomes that occur as a result of anesthetic management are rare (e.g., death, postspinal hematoma, blindness, stroke), and studies proposing to measure such outcomes as a function of a particular interventional approach must be "powered" by a large sample size and other methodologic controls.

Established procedures and techniques can assist the researcher in determining what sample size must be used if a study is to have an acceptable chance of achieving its purpose (the testing of a given hypothesis). What is at stake is the issue of a trial's having sufficient rigor to detect whether a true difference between treatment groups exists. Other issues should be considered as well, and the reader is referred to the definitive text by Cohen[9] for further treatment of these issues. Careful attention to these issues may help prevent the commission of a type III error (conducting the wrong experiment). Most human subject committees and scientific journals require that study reports contain some discussion of power before they are seriously considered.

TABLE 3-6 Choice of Statistical Test Based on Assumptions

	Parametric Procedures	Nonparametric Procedures
Nature of the assumptions	Data are interval or ratio level; Each value is independent of the other values Value is normally distributed Groups have similar variance; Usually work best with large population	Data are nominal or ordinal level Not necessarily distributed "normally" (i.e., data do not "fit" a bell-shaped curve)
Examples of tests	*t*-Test for independent groups*; *t*-Test for dependent samples†; Analysis of variance	Chi-squared test Mann-Whitney test Kruskal-Wallis test

**For example, two totally unrelated groups are compared.*
†*For example, a pretest and posttest comparison on one group of people.*

TABLE 3-7 Choice of Statistical Test Based on Purpose

Test	Goal
t-Test, independent groups	To test the difference between the means of two independent groups
t-Test, dependent samples	To test for the difference between dependent, paired samples (e.g., pretreatment and posttreatment) outcome
Analysis of variance	To test the difference among the means of more than two independent groups or more than one independent variable
Chi-squared test	To evaluate the difference between observed and expected frequencies
Correlation coefficient (e.g., product-moment)	To test whether a relationship exists between two variables
Simple linear regression	Used when one independent variable *(x)* is used to predict a dependent variable *(y)*
Multiple linear regression	To understand the effects of two or more independent variables on a dependent measure
Analysis of covariance	To test for differences between group means after adjustment of the scores on the dependent variable in order to eliminate the effects of the covariate
Factor analysis	To reduce a large set of variables into a smaller, more manageable set of measures
Canonical correlation	To analyze the relationship between two or more independent variables and two or more dependent variables
Discriminant analysis	To make predictions regarding membership in categories or groups, in contrast to using interval- or ratio-level measures

Data analysis allows the researcher to organize this information in a focused manner so that the research question can be answered. Selecting the appropriate method of data analysis is essential to the proper execution of the research plan. Experienced and beginning researchers alike may need assistance when choosing an appropriate method for data analysis. Expert researchers, statisticians, and clinical nurse specialists may prove to be valuable resources for the beginning researcher.

Once the data collection and analysis have been completed, the researcher must interpret the results. These results are directly related to and should answer the research question or hypotheses. Researchers may find that the answers are different from those they were expecting. The answers, results, and outcomes should be interpreted and their implication for clinical practice described. The researcher also should discuss how the findings relate to other research studies and should present ideas for future practice.

Common Mistakes

At this step in the research process, mistakes include selecting an inappropriate statistical procedure, using only one statistical procedure when several should be used, overstating the importance of small differences that are statistically significant but of little clinical importance, interpreting correlational research as evidence of cause-and-effect relationships, and overgeneralizing the findings of the investigation. Some common errors in statistical usage are noted in Box 3-4.

Stage 7: Dissemination of the Findings to Interested Colleagues

The research process is not complete until the results, conclusions, and implications have been adequately communicated to those likely to be interested in the study. Clearly, a study that has been completed but whose results have not been disseminated is of little value. Communication of the research findings can be done through a variety of routes, including publication in journals or newsletters, oral and poster presentations at formal symposia, or even discussion with others interested in the phenomenon.

Researchers fail to publish the results of their work for many reasons. These include such claims as "my findings were not significant," "my results were negative," and "the sample size was small." Negative or insignificant results can be as valuable as positive ones. For example, it has been found that in most circumstances, the by-product of atracurium breakdown, laudanosine, is unlikely to have significant clinical effects.[10] This is an important negative finding that has contributed substantively to clinical understanding.

Similarly, small sample sizes may provide an element of control over variables not present in larger studies or may indicate some preliminary direction as to how to approach a problem. An example is the finding that epidural anesthesia or analgesia in conjunction with light general anesthesia may be preferable to a purely general anesthesia technique and may be associated with lower mortality rates in critically ill patients.[11] Although the sample size in this particular investigation is relatively small, the overall design is acceptable and contributes to our understanding of the issue by stimulating other investigators to pursue answers to the questions raised.

Because the goal of nurse anesthesia research is the improvement of practice, the dissemination of research findings to clinicians is a major challenge faced by nurse anesthesia researchers. In a report directed at a highly research-oriented audience, the introduction is usually somewhat detailed, emphasizing the theoretic basis for the research. The introduction is followed by an extensive methodologic section that focuses on establishing the reliability and validity of the instruments used. The findings of the study are presented next, with emphasis on the statistical procedures employed. Finally, the conclusion focuses on the limitations and implications of the study's results.

Writing for a Clinically Oriented Audience

Generally, clinicians find research literature difficult to understand and its clinical application cumbersome. Both authors and journal editors can do much to make research more palatable to the clinical reader, thereby improving the chance that the research findings will be broadly disseminated and integrated in clinical situations. A recipe for successful clinical writing follows.

Clinical readers of research want to extract information applicable to clinical practice as quickly as possible. Therefore, the introduction of the research report should be brief, should establish the practical importance of the study, and should present a clear statement of the study's purpose. A deliberate

BOX 3-4

Top 10 Common Errors in Statistical Usage

1. No justification for reporting statistical results
   - No control group (when one is possible)
   - Random sampling or random group assignment not performed (or reported)
   - Statistical test not specified
   - Obvious biases or threats to validity
   - No documentation of consent or institutional review board approval
2. Errors in use of the *t*-test
   - Multiple application without correction
   - Use of independent groups form for paired data and vice versa
   - Use for ordinal data
3. Negative conclusions when statistical test results are not significant
4. Use of a test for independent samples for paired data or repeated measures
5. Inappropriate or no follow-up to analysis of variance
6. Hypotheses generated by the data
7. Use of one-sided tests without justification (or disclosure)
8. Inadequate number for chi-squared analysis
9. Standard error of the mean used for specifying variability
10. Misinterpretation or misrepresentation of P value
    - Small P value called "highly significant"
    - No confidence intervals stated
    - Different interpretation of $P = 0.04$ and $P = 0.06$

effort should be made to connect the study with the realities of clinical practice.

With respect to the methods section, writing that "a quasiexperimental, Solomon three-group crossover design yielded data that were subjected to canonical and discriminant analysis" does little to satisfy the needs of the average clinical reader. Instead, stating how the subjects were obtained, what manipulations were made, how the measurements were taken, and how the statistical analysis was performed provides the reader with some straightforward information, allowing him or her to put the study into a clinical context. The methods section should completely describe both the research design and the statistical procedures used, and it should indicate why this approach was selected.

The results of the study should focus on the relevant findings and should describe them clearly and fully. Tables or figures, explicitly labeled and simple in design, should be used for representing the findings visually. Admittedly, the more complex the findings, the more difficult it is to avoid a statistical or technical focus.

In the discussion section the implications of the investigation for theory and future research are somewhat less important to the clinical reader than are the implications for practice. For example, assume that a study demonstrates that the proposed intervention is not ready to be implemented in practice. In this situation, the discussion section should emphasize why this is so and what can be done about it. Encyclopedic comparisons of the results with those of other investigators at this point probably will not contribute materially to the report and may, paradoxically, deter the reader. Alternatively, if a researcher finds that a particular intervention, strategy, or assessment is ready to be introduced into clinical practice, the discussion section should emphasize how and for whom it should be used. It should include considerations such as efficiency and cost, as well as suggestions for clinical implementation.

This recipe for making research reports more palatable to primarily clinically oriented readers is not meant to diminish the importance of highly theoretic research-oriented writing. Many CRNAs continue to generate and publish valuable theoretic papers that contribute materially to a scientific basis for practice. Researchers and writers must keep the CRNA audience in mind as they develop and disseminate their findings.

All researchers must understand that the results of their studies, once published, become part of the general knowledge of the scientific community at large. However, the use of this knowledge requires acknowledgment of the original researchers; also, published results may be subject to copyright protection laws (i.e., their use may require permission from the publisher). It is not until the information becomes common knowledge that others may use it freely without acknowledgment.

Common Mistakes

At this stage of the research process, common mistakes include not keeping the study focused on the original problem, overwriting, generalizing the findings too broadly, and failing to address the clinical significance of the study.

Stage 8: Evaluation of the Research Report

Both clinicians (in their reading for application) and researchers (in their writing and analysis) are called on to evaluate research reports despite the fact that many may not have received formal training in reading and interpreting professional literature. Evaluation is the process of appraising the quality of a phenomenon—in this case, the findings of research as they bear on the art and science of nurse anesthesia. Outside of the practice settings, humans evaluate hundreds of things every day: Are the apples on the grocery shelves to our liking? Does the description of the program in the television guide entice us to tune in? Is the weather too warm to wear a jacket? Have we cooked the eggs sufficiently? These seem trivial and informal compared with the clinical evaluations that the CRNA must perform daily: Is the patient's anesthesia too deep, too light, or about right? Should I administer more opioid? Is the patient dehydrated, or is the hematocrit level misleading me? Should I perform a rapid-sequence induction? What dose of thiopental do I use in this 80-year-old with a fractured hip? Both sets of questions, nonprofessional and professional, are highly evaluative and parallel the evaluative decision-making that occurs when anesthesia research literature is read.

Systematic evaluation of the research, which influences the practice of nurse anesthesia, consists of a formal appraisal of the quality and value of the research. This essential step in the research process is multidimensional and can be approached in many ways. The approach outlined in the following subsections involves asking carefully orchestrated, critical questions. The answers to the suggested questions are not necessarily a dichotomous yes or no, but rather are qualitative in nature. An overview of this approach is detailed in Box 3-5.

Gaining Experience at Evaluation: the Journal Club

Most clinicians and researchers are familiar with the concept of the journal club, a common curricular component of many programs in nurse anesthesia. A journal club offers a planned, periodic, and critical reading of anesthesia-oriented research and clinical articles pertaining directly to practice. Participants in a journal club are assigned to read selected articles; later, a discussion of the articles can proceed under the direction of an informed leader. Questions that should be asked during discussion and critique include the following:

1. What are the purposes and the research questions or hypotheses, and how does the related literature review bear on the purpose or problem?
2. What methods did the authors use to study or evaluate the problem?
3. How are the data presented, and in what manner are they analyzed?
4. What are the conclusions of the study, and what are the implications for practice?

Participation in a journal club can be a rewarding and intellectually stimulating activity that can be used for keeping one's knowledge of the field current and for gaining experience in evaluating the anesthesia-related literature.

Evaluating a Study: the Bottom Line

Ultimately, the nurse anesthetist evaluating a study is faced with the following three questions:

1. Do I disregard the study and its findings entirely, not applying them to either clinical practice or future analysis in any fashion?
2. Do I apply the study only in the sense of expanding my cognitive approach to anesthetic management? (In this scenario, although one may not materially or directly apply the study or its findings to practice, some intellectual growth or understanding is gained from the study, which subsequently is incorporated into one's repertoire.)
3. Do I make a direct application of the study to my practice?

Some questions to ask when one reads a study are listed in Box 3-6.

BOX 3-5

Research Scenario: A Guide for Researchers* and Clinicians† in Evaluating Research for Completeness and Clinical Application

Problem
Is it lucid, researchable, justified, and practical?

Hypothesis
Is it clear, with the variables under consideration identified?

Definitions
Are terms adequately defined and put into context?

Literature
Is it relevant, current, and organized?

Review
Is it logical, and does it justify the study?

Methods
Is the sample representative of the population being considered? Is the sample large enough? If human subjects were used, was institutional approval granted? Is the instrumentation described and valid? Is the design compatible with the problem and the hypothesis or research question? Is there any evidence of drift from established procedure? Are the data-gathering procedures defined? Is there enough information for replication of the study, if desired? Are the statistical procedures described, and are they appropriate?

Results
Are they presented clearly, concisely, and without bias? Are they organized and displayed logically in tables or figures? Are they relevant to the problem or hypothesis?

Discussion
Is it logically based on the results? Is it intimately grounded in the original problem or hypothesis? Is there overgeneralization of the findings? Is the writing impartial and scientific? How can this study be used in the practice setting? How similar is the study's environment to the real world? What are the risks associated with implementation of the recommendations?

**Researchers should benefit from this by critically asking themselves whether they have included answers to these questions in their report.*
†Clinicians should benefit from this by judging the report on the basis of completeness and utility and by finding out whether it contains answers to these questions.

BOX 3-6

Questions to Ask in the Reading of a Study

Object or Hypothesis
What are the objectives of the study or the questions to be answered?
What is the population to which the investigators intend to refer their findings?

Design of the Investigation
Was the study an experiment, planned observations, or an analysis of records?
How was the sample selected? Do possible sources of selection exist that would make the sample atypical or nonrepresentative? If so, what provision was made for dealing with this bias?
What is the nature of the control group or standard of comparison?

Observations
Are there clear definitions of the terms used, including diagnostic criteria, measurements made, and criteria of outcome?
Was the method of classification or of measurement consistent for all the subjects and relevant to the objectives of the investigation? Do possible biases in measurement exist, and, if so, what provisions were made to deal with them?
Are the observations reliable and reproducible?

Presentation of Findings
Are the findings presented clearly, objectively, and in sufficient detail to enable the reader to judge them for herself or himself?
Are the findings internally consistent? That is, do the numbers add up properly, can different tables be reconciled, and so on?

Analysis
Are the data worthy of statistical analysis? If so, are the methods of statistical analysis appropriate to the source and nature of the data, and is the analysis correctly performed and interpreted?
Is analysis sufficient for determining whether "significant difference" may be the result of lack of comparability of the group in gender or age distribution, in clinical characteristics, or in other relevant variables?

Conclusions
Which conclusions are justified by the findings? Which are not?
Are the conclusions relevant to the questions posed by the investigators?

Constructive Suggestions
Assume you are planning an investigation to answer the questions put forth in this study. If they have not been clearly asked by the authors, frame them in an appropriate manner. Suggest a practical design, criteria for observations, and type of analysis that would provide reliable and valid information relevant to the questions under study.

Adapted from Colton T. Statistics in Medicine. *Boston: Little, Brown; 1974. With permission from Little, Brown & Co., copyright 1974.*

Common Mistakes

At this stage of the research process, mistakes include failing to adequately evaluate a study's methods and findings and, in the process, uncritically accepting into practice information that may be misleading or incorrect. Although articles in professional journals should undergo critical review by peers who can detect mistakes, omissions, and alternative explanations, the ultimate responsibility for evaluating a study and determining the pros and cons of the implementation of its recommendations rests with the clinical reader.

FRAUD, DECEIT, AND HUMAN ERROR IN SCIENTIFIC RESEARCH

Scientists are human and suffer from the inherent frailties of the human condition. Even the most scrupulous and compulsive scientist can make an honest mistake, and such mistakes are tolerated by the community at large. Errors are costly in a variety of ways. Not only might an error result in months or years of wasted effort if it is not identified and rectified, but it also can mislead others who attempt to use or build on the original, flawed work.

Unfortunately, not all errors are honest. Scientific and academic misconduct occurs in a variety of forms. Although the motives of the involved parties are not always identifiable, some researchers feel pressure to publish, whereas others simply are intent on gaining attention by compiling a long list of publications or presentations. The bottom line is that scientific misconduct ultimately erodes the foundation on which science is built and may result in the administration of inappropriate therapy to those in need of treatment. Common examples of scientific and academic misconduct include the following:

- Plagiarism
- Alteration of data so that they conform to expectations
- Outright fabrication of data
- Intentional sloppiness in scientific work
- Selective publication of data in order to support one's beliefs
- Coercing subordinates to acknowledge oneself unreasonably
- Unapproved use or misuse of human or animal subjects
- Not giving appropriate credit in collaborative research

Guidelines for Dealing with Errors or Suspected Misconduct

The nurse anesthetist who is personally involved with or suspects scientific or academic misconduct on the part of a colleague is morally and professionally compelled to take action as soon as possible. Box 3-7 lists guidelines to adhere to if such a situation occurs.

STUDIES INVOLVING HUMAN SUBJECTS

The process of making a research project a reality involves coordination between patients' needs and rights and the study's parameters and goals. This process is controlled in some respects by criteria set up by various governing agencies. The 1947 Nuremberg Code, the 1964 Helsinki Declaration, and the 1971 guidelines of the U.S. Department of Health, Education, and Welfare were drafted to reflect the concern for individuals participating in research. In 1979 the National Commission for the Protection of Human Subjects of Biomedical and Behavioral Research was established to continue work in this area. The culmination of that work, the Belmont report, defines the limits between research and practice and outlines the ethical guidelines to be considered for patient participation in research projects. According to the report, the difference between standard practice and research is defined in terms of design and outcomes. The phrase *medical practice* refers to diagnosis, treatment, and preventive health care whose purpose is the enhancement of the well-being of an individual. The term *research* refers to procedures whose purpose is the examination of a question or the testing of a hypothesis in order to expand the existing body of knowledge.

Institutional Review of Research That Involves Humans and Animals

All protocols involving the living must be submitted to a local institutional review board (IRB). The IRB is charged with the protection of each subject participating in the study. It is the responsibility of the IRB to ensure that informed consent is adequate, that no coercion is used in the recruitment of subjects, and that the risks to the subjects are minimal or no greater than necessary. To accomplish this, the IRB carefully reviews the study's protocol and consent forms, considering the study's design and patient selection.

A number of factors must be considered when a study calls for the involvement of human participants. The risk-benefit assessment compares the benefits of participating in a study with the potential risks generated by the study. Risks can involve the patient, the family, or the community. The risk-benefit balance

BOX 3-7

Dealing with Errors and Misconduct

If the Situation Has Resulted from Your Own Actions

Immediately acknowledge the error to your colleagues and, if the error is in print, write to the journal editor or source in which the mistaken information was published.

If You Discover an Error in a Publication

Write a letter to the editor of the publication stating your case and supply any supportive materials you have.

If You Believe That a Colleague Has Engaged in Misconduct

1. Discuss the situation with a trusted and experienced colleague, maintaining the anonymity of the accused. This will help you to judge the motives of your own suspicions and to establish the veracity of your charges.
2. Once the facts have been established, contact the colleague privately to determine whether the concern can be satisfactorily explained or rectified.
3. If resolution is not at hand, discuss the situation with the department director, chairperson, or dean, as indicated by the hierarchic administrative arrangement. Many institutions and universities have written procedures that carefully outline the process to be followed in such situations.
4. In situations in which resolution is still not achieved or if a definable administrative structure is not in place, consider contacting the National Academy of Sciences, Sigma Xi, the American Association for the Advancement of Science, the American Association of University Professors, or other scientific or professional organizations.

Adapted from Colton T. Statistics in Medicine. *Boston: Little, Brown; 1974. With permission from Little, Brown & Co., copyright 1974.*

should be justified by an analysis of information to be gained from the research, a description of the available treatment alternatives, and the measures to be taken to minimize risks and discomfort.

Vulnerable populations (e.g., children, prisoners) require special considerations.

Providing a patient with the information necessary for him or her to make an informed decision about participation is fundamental. Informed consent should be easy to understand and should include a description of the research and plan of treatment, the risks and benefits, the alternatives to participation in the study, confidentiality, costs, and compensation. Informed consent also must include an assertion of the voluntary nature of the study, a statement that the patient may withdraw at any time without penalty, and a commitment to disclose any new findings that are discovered during the course of the study that may affect the subject's participation. In most instances, a signed consent form from a participant is necessary; ultimately, however, the IRB decides whether such a form is necessary.

Virtually all institutions and funding agencies have model consent forms whose format researchers must follow when developing a study. Consent forms (written in lay terminology) should include a brief description of the study, a summary of the anticipated risks and benefits of participation in the study, a statement regarding the maintenance of the participant's confidentiality, a disclaimer obviating the host institution of financial responsibility for damages that might occur, and the names and telephone numbers of the researchers. Under most circumstances, the individual who has agreed to participate in the study signs the consent form in the presence of the researcher and a witness who cosigns the consent. A copy of the consent form is given to the participant for his or her records.

CONTROVERSIES IN ANIMAL RESEARCH

Biomedical institutions now operate under guidelines that mandate the humane treatment of animals that are used in research. The use of animals for research is a subject of controversy fueled by disagreements among people who are highly supportive of the use of animals and those who strongly oppose it, such as supporters of the People for the Ethical Treatment of Animals (PETA) and the Animal Liberation Front (ALF). Researchers contemplating the use of animals in their research should carefully consult with their local IRB for guidance in this area.

SUMMARY

Although CRNAs are only now becoming prepared to assume the role of primary researchers, all CRNAs are in a position to read about the latest advances in nurse anesthesia practice and incorporate validated interventions into their clinical practice. Nurse anesthesia research is grounded fundamentally in solving patient care problems during the preoperative, intraoperative, and postoperative periods. Although much behavioral, educational, and product evaluation–oriented research has been conducted by nurse anesthesia researchers, all nurse anesthesia research is wedded inextricably to patient care. Research is essential to the professional evolution of nurse anesthesia as CRNAs become increasingly accountable for their own independent basis for practice.

A number of antiscience movements are operative in the world today (Figure 3-4). At the heart of all of these movements is the sophisticated use of the concept of proof by proclamation, rather than proof by experimentation. As active consumers and producers of scientific knowledge, nurse anesthetists can do their part by resisting the integration of aberrant and ill-founded thinking into their discipline. This can be achieved if each CRNA understands the need to maintain a critical dialogue regarding what can be incorporated into nurse anesthesia practice.

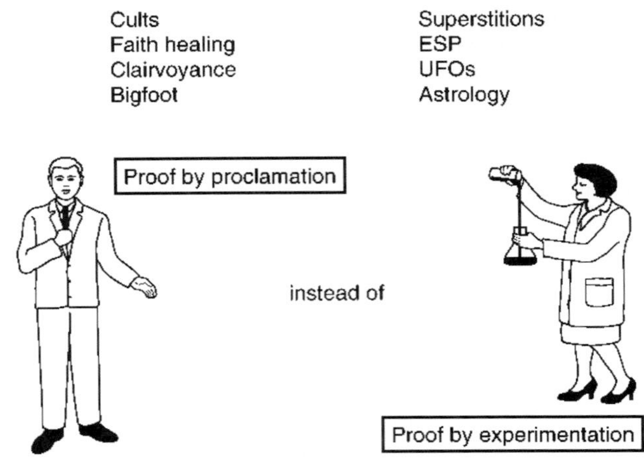

FIGURE **3-4**
Antiscience trends in the world today.

All CRNAs are mandated to understand and use research in their practices. The American Nurses Association strongly urges even undergraduate nursing students to learn how to read, interpret, and evaluate published research for applicability to nursing practice. Although the evolution of nursing research—and that of nurse anesthesia research in particular—has lagged behind that of many other disciplines, tremendous strides are being made as greater numbers of nurse anesthetists are prepared at both the master's and doctoral levels. It is essential that nurse anesthetists recognize the need to promote nurse anesthesia as a science-based profession. There is no better way to achieve this end than continuing to emphasize the importance of the research process.

REFERENCES

1. Brown J, Tanner C, Padrick K. Nursing's search for scientific knowledge. *Nurs Res.* 1984;33:26-32.
2. Tramer MR. Does meta-analysis increase our knowledge in the management of postoperative nausea and vomiting? *Int Anesthesiol Clin.* 2003;41(4):33-39.
3. Ballantyne JC, Carr DB, deFerranti S, Suarez T, Lau T, et al. The comparative effects of postoperative analgesic therapies on pulmonary outcome: cumulative meta-analysis of randomized, controlled trials. *Anesth Analg.* 1998;86(3):1460.
4. Lee A, Done ML. The use of nonpharmacologic techniques to prevent postoperative nausea and vomiting: a meta-analysis. *Anesth Analg.* 1999;88(6):1200-1202.
5. Biddle C. Meta-analysis of the effectiveness of nonsteroidal anti-inflammatory drugs in a standardized pain model. *AANA J.* 2002; 70(2):111-114.
6. Marshall C, Rossman GB. *Designing Qualitative Research.* Newbury Park, Calif: Sage; 1989.
7. Buros O. *Tests in Print.* Princeton, NJ: Gryphon Press, 1961.
8. Ward MJ, Lindeman C. *Instruments for Measuring Nursing Practice and Other Health Care Variables.* Denver: Western Interstate Commission for Higher Education; 1978.

9. Cohen J. *Statistical Power Analysis for the Behavioral Sciences*. 2nd ed. Hillsdale, NJ: Lawrence Erlbaum Associates; 1988.
10. Standaert FG. Magic bullets, science, and medicine. *Anesthesiology*. 1985;63:577-578.
11. Yeager MP. Epidural anesthesia and analgesia in high-risk surgical patients. *Anesthesiology*. 1987;67:729-736.

SUGGESTED READING

Introductory Texts

Isaac S, Michael WB. *Handbook in Research and Evaluation*. San Diego: Edits; 1990.

Knapp RG. *Basic Statistics for Nurses*. 2nd ed. New York: Wiley; 1985.

Treece RW, Treece JR Jr. *Elements of Research in Nursing*. St Louis: Mosby; 1986.

Wilson HS. *Research in Nursing*. Redwood City, Calif: Addison-Wesley; 1989.

Advanced Texts

Kerlinger F. *Foundations of Behavioral Research*. New York: Holt, Rinehart & Winston; 1986.

Polit DF, Hungler BP. *Nursing Research: Principles and Methods*. Philadelphia: Lippincott; 1987.

Waltz CF, Strickland OL, Lenz ER. *Measurement in Nursing Research*. Philadelphia: FA Davis; 1984.

CHAPTER 4

General Principles, Pharmacodynamics, and Drug Receptor Concepts

Silas N. Glisson

The practice of anesthesia requires a full spectrum of drugs from which an anesthetic plan can be implemented to achieve the desired level of surgical analgesia, hypnosis, and muscle relaxation. In addition to surgical anesthesia, pain medicine has evolved as a significant practice component. The identification of the active receptor site of cyclooxygenase (COX) and the subsequent genetic coding of COX-1 and COX-2 receptor proteins have ushered in an entirely new class of antiinflammatory and analgesic drugs for pain management.[1,2] Now that the human genome has been mapped and the field of molecular and cellular proteomics is exploring new concepts, specific receptor-targeted drugs are envisioned, as is a revolution in the way health care is delivered. Likewise, the methods employed to provide anesthesia care will undergo a profound change based on this new knowledge. Already studies are challenging long-held concepts of pharmacodynamics and pharmacokinetics that guide the clinical use of anesthetic agents. The primary site of anesthetic action is now considered to be membrane receptors and not the lipid bilayer surrounding the receptor.[3] Spinal cord receptors are being differentiated from receptors in the brain and targeted with specific drugs. Receptor superfamilies with definable amino acid subunits are the targets of new classes of anesthetic drugs such as α_2-agonists and analgesics such as COX-1 and COX-2 inhibitors.[2] The potentiation of the inhibitory γ-aminobutyric acid (GABA) receptors is considered a primary mechanism of action of inhalation and intravenous anesthetics. The recovery from intravenous anesthesia is described in terms of context-sensitive half-time, which is modified by the duration of anesthetic administration rather than drug redistribution and elimination profiles and is directly influenced by age.[4-7] The importance of the individual, with his or her unique genetic profile, is resurfacing as a major determinant of anesthesia outcome.[8] The number of patients who now make up the portion of the population classified as elderly—those aged 60 to 90 years—is ever increasing. Clinical experience has shown that the response to anesthetic drugs in elderly patients differs from that in younger patients. Age-related change in drug pharmacokinetics (e.g., decreased total clearance) has been shown not to be responsible for the decrease in drug dose necessary to achieve anesthetic endpoints in elderly patients. Studies to date in elderly patients, although limited, demonstrate an age-related decline in most receptor populations and an overall decrease in pharmacodynamic responses.[9-12] Preoperative assessment by the anesthetist may soon take on an entirely different meaning as patient information becomes more genetically oriented. The choice of anesthetic agents will be based on age-related receptor profiles and the patient's genetic ability to rapidly clear and recover from anesthetic drugs once their administration has been terminated. Until that time, anesthetists will continue to administer anesthesia based on age-indexed population drug profiles adjusted for individual pathologies (i.e., general principles of pharmacology).

The current medical economic climate necessitates the optimum selection and use of anesthetic drugs based on their pharmacologic profiles. The term *pharmacology* refers to the processes by which a drug produces one or more measured physiologic responses. The concept of a drug-induced tissue response has changed little since Ehrlich first proposed it (circa 1905). What has changed, and continues to change, is our understanding of the processes involved in a drug response.[13-16] Recent attention has focused on the biosphere, or the protein receptor site, as not only the locus of drug binding but also a primary regulator of the measured pharmacologic response. Secondary processes, including drug absorption, distribution, biotransformation, and excretion, also influence the pharmacologic response.[17]

DRUG RESPONSE EQUATION

The drug response equation is fundamental to pharmacologic principles.[15] As shown in the following equation, drug (D) combines with receptor (R) to form a drug receptor complex (DRC) that elicits a tissue response (TR).

Equation 4-1

$$D + R \leftrightharpoons (DRC) \leftrightharpoons TR$$

What remains unique about this equation is that, in most cases, the drug receptor complex represents a highly selective process. Yet the resultant tissue response tends to vary from individual to individual, reflecting each individual's receptor and genetic profile.

POPULATION VARIABILITY

Because the objective of pharmacologic intervention is to achieve a desired therapeutic response, anesthetists must recognize that a range of responses to a given drug and dosage is possible within a patient population. Therapeutic drug doses reflect average doses of a "normal" population of individuals. Specific therapeutic doses for population subsets (e.g., pediatric, neonatal, geriatric, patients with cardiac disease) are available, thereby narrowing the degree of response variability for a given drug and clinical population. The age, sex, body weight, body surface area, basal metabolic rate, pathologic state, and genetic profile of an individual directly influence the pharmacologic response.[18]

Given the increasing median age of the population in the United States, studies of the influence of age on the responses to anesthetic drugs have increased. Steady-state plasma concentrations of hypnotic drugs such as midazolam and propofol and minimum alveolar concentrations (MAC) for inhaled anesthetics (e.g., halothane, isoflurane, or sevoflurane) required to achieve desired anesthetic end-points decrease as age increases, independent of any age effect on drug pharmacokinetics.[7,9,12,19] Studies using positron emission tomography (PET) have demonstrated an age-related decrease in striatal and extrastriatal dopamine D2 receptors in humans and decreased muscarinic cholinergic receptor binding in monkeys.[10,11] The effective plasma concentration 50 (EC_{50}) needed to achieve sedation with midazolam infusion is reported to be decreased by 50% in elderly volunteers.[12] Unfortunately the specifics responsible for the observed age-related decrease in effective dose of anesthetic drugs is not presently known. Receptor hypersensitivity and decreased receptor protein both have been investigated as explanations for the response. Until a better understanding of the age-related changes exists, empirical dose reduction or the use of dosing algorithms for the elderly patient population is indicated.

Mean, Median, and Mode

A graphic description of the dose-response relationship is displayed in Figure 4-1. The theoretic normal distribution of quantal (desired) responses to increasing drug dose takes the shape of a Gaussian curve. Theoretically, the numbers of respondents on both sides of the mean (average dose) are equal, with the greatest percentage of individuals responding near the center of the curve. In a Gaussian distribution curve, the mean, median, and mode are equidistant from the two extremes.[17] Atypical responders fall at each end of the curve.

On the curve, the mean dose is the arithmetic average of the range of doses that produce a given response. The median dose is that dose on either side of which half of the responses occur.

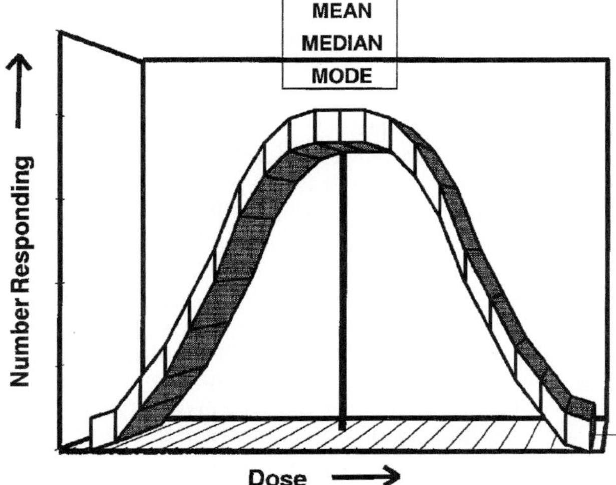

FIGURE **4-1**
The theoretic normal frequency distribution of a drug response in a normal population.

The mode dose is the dose representing the greatest percentage of responses. The mean, median, and mode doses are often close but are rarely the same in actual dose-response curves.

Standard Deviation

The terms *standard deviation* (SD) and *standard error of the mean* (SEM) describe population response variability.[18] The SD provides information regarding the actual responses measured and their difference from the calculated mean. In Figure 4-2, the SD makes up 68% of the responses (34% to the left and 34% to the right of the mean value); 2 and 3 SDs constitute 95% and 99.7% of the responses, respectively. The greater the SD, the less the mean reflects the central tendency of responses.

Standard Error of the Mean

The SEM describes the variance of the mean. It is equivalent to the SD of the mean. By repeating the dose-response measurements on different, normally distributed populations, a slightly different mean dose value is obtained each time, because the mean value is only an arithmetic average of the responses obtained. In Figure 4-3, 1 SEM represents the range

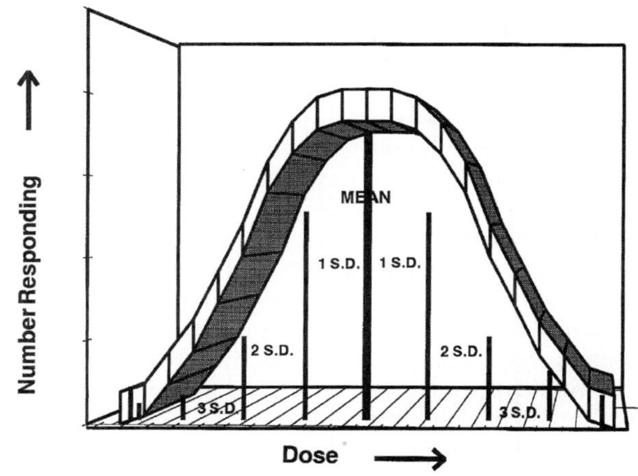

FIGURE **4-2**
A normal distribution curve showing the standard deviation (SD) in relation to the mean (average) dose value.

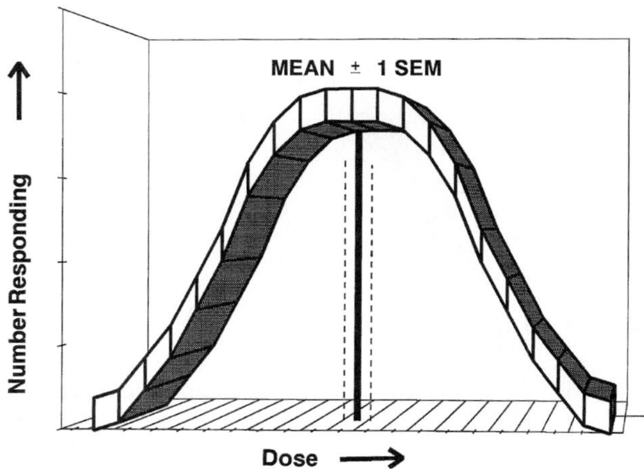

FIGURE **4-3**
A normal distribution curve showing the relationship of the standard error of the mean (SEM) to the mean (average) value.

within which the mean value would occur on repeat testing 68% of the time, and 2 and 3 SEMs represent the range within which the mean value would occur 95% and 99.7% of the time, respectively. Both the SD and the SEM are important statistical descriptors of observed drug responses in patient care and in research and reflect pharmacologic principles of population variance.[17,20]

DRUG DOSE RESPONSE

The administration of drugs is largely determined by a calculated mean therapeutic dose per kilogram of body weight or body surface area from a previously determined average dose for the normal population. This approach is responsible for underdosing and overdosing of patients, because population variability is not considered in the calculation. The individual therapeutic response to a fixed mean dose is frequently less than optimal.

Studies that employed sensitive quantitative measurement techniques have identified a response variability to given drug doses in the normal population that was far greater than previously demonstrated.[14] Clearly, the optimal dosing approach for patients when drugs are administered by the intravenous route is by titration until the desired therapeutic response is attained. This is particularly true in critical care and anesthesia patients, in whom drug onset and offset responses are relatively rapid.

Two types of dose-response curves—graded and quantal—describe average drug response and subject variability within a given population.

Graded Dose Response

The graded dose-response curve, which is plotted in linear fashion, characterizes the change in measured response as an administered dose is increased (Figure 4-4). The response curve has a hyperbolic shape, with the greatest change in response occurring to the left on a small portion of the x-axis. When plotted on a logarithmic scale, the graded dose-response curve takes an **S** shape: at the lowest dose, the measured response (e.g., vascular response to norepinephrine) is small or even nonexistent. At the highest doses, the response is maximal and approaches a plateau (Figure 4-5). Typically, at between 20% and 80% of the maximal response the curve approaches a straight line, because changes in dose and response reflect a proportional relationship.

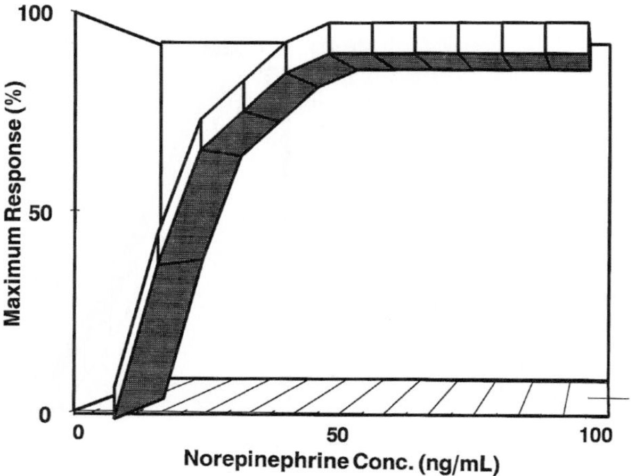

FIGURE **4-4**
A linear arithmetic-graded response curve showing blood vessel constriction to increasing norepinephrine concentrations.

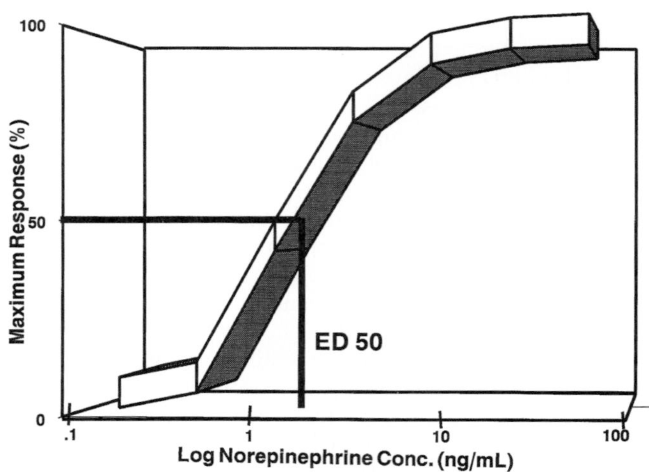

FIGURE **4-5**
A logarithmic plot of the data from Figure 4-4 showing blood vessel constriction to increasing concentrations of norepinephrine. The median effective dose (ED_{50}) is identified.

Plotting on a semilogarithmic scale, with the dose in log units, provides a more detailed representation of the entire graded dose-response curve, especially at the two extremes.[13,14] From a semilogarithmic plot of graded dose responses, the potency of different agonist drugs with similar mechanisms of action (i.e., action through the same receptor) can be compared, or the ability of an antagonist drug to reduce the response to an agonist (e.g., in phenoxybenzamine antagonism of norepinephrine-induced vasoconstriction) can be observed. It should be noted that "antagonist" drugs that do not bind to the agonist receptor are actually not antagonists. For example, neostigmine is not an antagonist of vecuronium because it does not compete with vecuromium for the muscle end-plate receptor site. Neostigmine inhibits acetylcholinesterase, which allows acetylcholine to compete effectively with vecuronium for the receptor, leading to a recovery of muscle tone as measured using train-of-four (a common diagnostic test for muscle strength used in the operating room). Therefore, its effect is at least a partial form of indirect antagonism.

Quantal Dose Response

Clinically, a quantal dose-response curve provides information on the frequency with which a given drug dose produces a desired therapeutic response in a patient population. The response is measured in an all-or-nothing fashion. The quantal response curve describes the variation in response to the threshold dose within a population of seemingly similar individuals (Figure 4-6). For example, with thiopental induction of anesthesia, a small number of patients become unconscious after administration of 2 mg/kg, more after administration of 3 mg/kg, and virtually all after administration of 4 to 6 mg/kg. Plotting the cumulative number of patients with all-or-nothing responses over a range of doses produces an **S**-shaped response curve. However, the quantal dose **S**-shaped curve differs from the graded dose-response **S**-shaped curve because it reflects population variation for the threshold dose needed to produce a given all-or-nothing desired response.

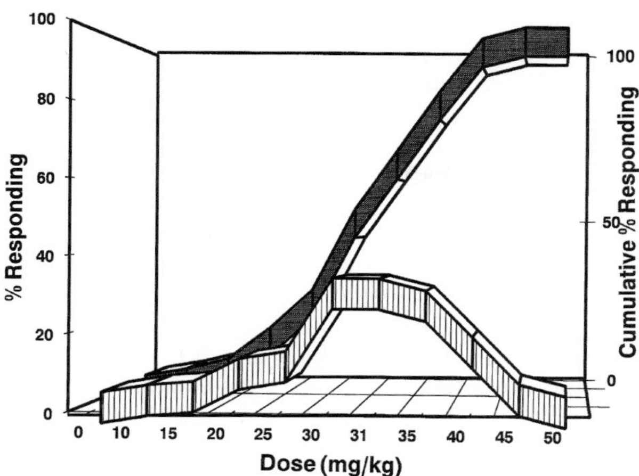

FIGURE **4-6**
A quantal dose-response curve indicating the frequency of all-or-nothing dose responses. The hashed line represents a histogram of the number of responses measured at each dose. The solid line represents the cumulative response curve of the total number of responses up to and including each dose.

Descriptive information about population dose-response characteristics can be obtained from quantal dose-response curves.[17,21] Two descriptors—effective dose 99% (ED_{99}) and lethal dose 1% (LD_1)—identify the therapeutic safety margin of a drug, as shown in the following equation.

Equation 4-2

$$\text{Safety margin} = LD_1 - ED_{99}/ED_{99} \times 100$$

When the therapeutic safety margin is great, the risk of drug-induced death is small and the margin of therapeutic safety is wide. The opposite is true when the therapeutic safety margin is small.

The term *therapeutic index* (LD_{50}/ED_{50}) describes a drug's median therapeutic safety margin for a particular therapeutic effect.[14] For example, chemotherapeutic drugs have a very narrow margin of safety. Drugs that produce surgical depths of anesthesia, such as sevoflurane and other halogenated anesthetics, also have a relatively narrow margin of safety. Sevoflurane is administered clinically in an amount that is 1.3- to 1.4-fold the MAC, or the dose at which 50% of the patients do not move on surgical stimulation. The MAC can be lethal if the volume percentage delivered is increased to 1.7- to 2.0-fold and this percentage is maintained for a prolonged period of time.

Another descriptor obtained from the quantal dose-response curve is the median effective dose (ED_{50})—the dose at which 50% of a population responds as desired. The ED_{50} is often used for comparing the potency of drugs within a class. Because the ED_{50} dose is derived from the linear portion of the quantal dose-response curve (20% to 80% of the responders), relatively accurate comparisons of drugs that cause similar responses can be made (see Figure 4-5). Important in each of these descriptions is the word *median*. Median ED_{50} dose values are derived average response doses from a population of patients.[17,18] Each individual within the population responds, more or less, to a median dose on the basis of his or her biologic variation or, specifically, genetic variations in drug receptor protein. Confidence limits for a given median dose and its therapeutic response can be calculated. Typically, the proportion of subjects responding to an ED_{50} dose ranges from 45% to 55%. Derived median population dose values provide a point of reference for achieving an individual's optimum therapeutic dose.

For intravenously administered drugs used in anesthesia, the trend is toward drugs that have brief onset-offset times and can be administered by infusion, often with the use of a computer-controlled pump.[16,22] For example, the desired anesthetic response to alfentanil and remifentanil can be effectively titrated after an initial loading dose.

Future developments related to drugs will include the availability of indwelling drug-analyzing probes similar to the continuous mass spectrometers currently used for analysis of end-tidal anesthetic gas concentrations. Real-time analysis of drug concentration can incorporate feedback control to drug infusion devices. Once the desired patient response is attained by titration, the dose can be set and automatically maintained with minimal fluctuations in blood and effect site drug concentrations and the tissue response. Currently, computer-controlled infusion pumps employ programs based on pharmacokinetic modeling studies in an attempt to approximate the required effect site drug concentration to achieve and maintain a desired level of anesthesia in patients. The continuing development of ultrafast onset-offset anesthetic drugs such as remifentanil and rocuronium will simplify titration of the anesthetic endpoint by the anesthetist and minimize undesired overdose effects.

DRUG RECEPTOR INTERACTIONS

Advances in molecular receptor pharmacology have provided a new understanding of patient drug responses.[13,15,23,24] The drug receptor interaction describes the formation of a single drug receptor complex, which leads to a fractional tissue response (FRT):

Equation 4-3

$$D + R \underset{k_2}{\overset{k_1}{\leftrightharpoons}} DR \xrightarrow{k_3} FTR$$

The desired tissue response is observed when sufficient receptors have been occupied and activated by free drug. This process obeys the law of mass action: at steady state, equilibrium exists between bound and unbound drug receptors and the concentration of free unbound drug at the site. Specific characteristics of the drug and the receptor determine the association and dissociation of a drug with regard to its receptor and the kinetic, *k*, rates, which are constants.[8]

Drug Affinity and Efficacy

The terms *affinity* and *efficacy* (intrinsic activity) describe the degree of drug receptor interaction for a given drug and receptor protein population (e.g., $GABA_A$, α_2 , and propofol). The observed tissue response reflects the quantity of drug receptor complexes intact at any given moment. Each drug receptor interaction elicits a quantum of excitation, and the summation of many individual quanta produces the tissue response.[15,23,25]

The time constant that describes the fractional tissue response after the drug receptor complex formation typically has been considered to be near zero or instantaneous. Until recently, the primary time constant thought to influence the onset of tissue response was the duration of the delay in the delivery of drug to the receptor sites. The phrase *pharmacokinetic analysis* of drug absorption and distribution describes onset time and magnitude of drug response. *Drug elimination kinetic analysis* describes the duration of the tissue response.

Drug-Receptor-Response Triad

Current understanding of receptor dynamics has added an additional and possibly the most descriptive component of the drug-receptor-response triad. When a drug combines with its receptor, a conformational change occurs in the receptor protein itself. Without the structural shift, no tissue response can occur. Evidence has not fully described the specifics of the drug-induced protein conformational change coupled with tissue response dynamics (nor have the time constants been determined). Evidence does suggest that events within the biosphere after drug association with the receptor are the principal regulatory variables of the response onset-offset time course.[13,16,25]

Until recently, the terms *drug absorption*, *distribution*, and *elimination* were used solely to describe the tissue response time course.[18,26] However, the response may be more complex than was originally thought. It is now known that drug delivery sufficient to occupy 1% of the receptors is, in many instances, all that is required for a maximum tissue response to occur.[15] Furthermore, the synthesis and destruction of receptor proteins occur at a much more rapid rate than was previously believed—within minutes rather than days. Receptor up-regulation and down-regulation can occur during drug infusion, with new receptor protein being synthesized in response to availability of free unbound drug.[13,14,27]

Drug Receptors

Drug receptor proteins are now considered to be located within the luminal membrane and at the surface of the ionic channel. A few are known to occupy intracellular sites. The drug lidocaine and other amide and ester local anesthetics act at intracellular receptor sites near the sodium channel. Studies of acetylcholine and its receptor at the neuromuscular junction indicate that less than 1% of the cell surface binds drug to receptor protein to achieve the tissue response.[8] Complete saturation of available receptors with drug molecules is not necessary for a desired tissue response to be elicited.

For intravenously administered drugs, sufficient drug for a maximal tissue response is delivered to the receptor site within the time required for a single complete circulation (approximately 1 minute), provided an adequate drug dose was administered initially. Current understanding of molecular pharmacology suggests that the delay recorded from initial drug administration to the onset of the tissue response reflects the time required for molecular orientation and attachment to the receptor—that is, the time course of the receptor protein conformational change and the tissue response time.[15,17] As long as both the drug and the receptor are hydrophobic, bonding occurs.[23] Intravenous anesthetics act by binding to membrane receptor channel proteins. The $GABA_A$ inhibitory receptor has been implicated and suggested as a primary site of intravenous anesthetic action, except in the case of ketamine.[28] Inhalation anesthetics have long been thought to produce their anesthetic action by dissolving in the lipid bilayer surrounding membrane ion channels and interfering with their ability to open and close. Recent electrophysiologic evidence, however, indicates that inhalation anesthetics, like intravenous anesthetics, bind to $GABA_A$ receptor proteins and cause inhibition of signal transduction by increasing the influx of chloride ions through membrane channels.[3,29,30]

Individual agonist drugs have at least three configuration points for attachment to their receptors. With more points of attachment, a more perfect drug-receptor fit occurs.[15] Agonist drugs can induce receptor proteins to alter their topography to achieve a more exacting fit with the drug. The alignment of a drug with its receptor is aided by various bonding forces, of which van der Waals forces and ionic bonding are prominent. Volatile anesthetics (e.g., halothane, desflurane, sevoflurane, isoflurane and nitrous oxide) bond to cell receptors by means of a nonspecific hydrophobic bonding mechanism.

Some protein receptors provide "silent bonding" sites.[15] The silent bonding sites are more correctly termed *acceptors*; the acceptor reduces the amount of unbound drug available for receptor complexing. Circulating albumin contains numerous acceptor sites.

DRUG ANTAGONISM

Pure Antagonists

Pure antagonist drugs are similar in molecular structure to their corresponding agonist drugs. However, owing to the addition or subtraction of one or more chemical moieties, they are unable to initiate the receptor protein conformational shift necessary for eliciting a tissue response. Such antagonist drugs have receptor affinity but lack intrinsic activity.

Antagonists that possess the property of weak affinity for the same receptor protein (e.g., atropine, esmolol) are competitive and are easily displaced by an agonist. Noncompetitive antagonists, such as phenoxybenzamine, have a strong affinity for the receptor protein and cannot be displaced by the agonist.[13,18] New receptor protein must be synthesized if agonist receptor complexing is to occur.[31] As with agonist drugs, not all receptors are bound by antagonists. Antagonists cause a rightward shift in the drug dose-response curve. The extent of rightward shift reflects the number of available receptors occupied by the antagonist drug (Figure 4-7). Comparison of the ED_{50} doses in Figure 4-7 shows a reduced affinity of the agonist for its receptor when the antagonist is present.

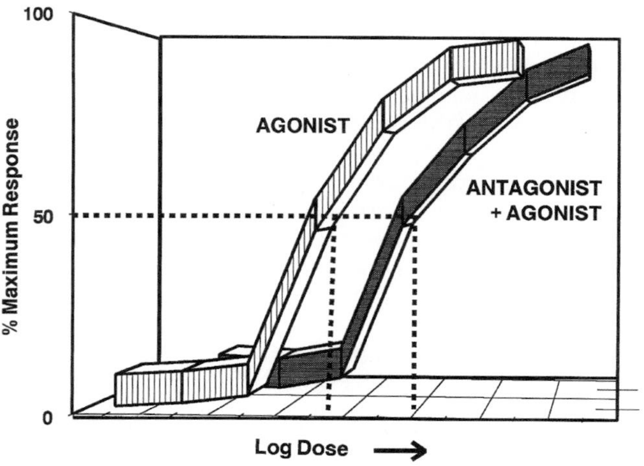

FIGURE **4-7**
A logarithmic dose-response curve that shows an agonist drug response alone and in the presence of an antagonist drug.

Agonist-Antagonists

Agonist-antagonists are the second major type of antagonist drugs.[14,23] As the name implies, agonist-antagonist drugs have receptor protein affinity and intrinsic activity, but often only one tenth to one fiftieth the potency of the pure agonist. Narcotic antagonists often are of the nonpure, agonist-antagonist type, such as nalbuphine. The mechanism by which agonist-antagonist drugs elicit less of a tissue response is not fully understood. An incomplete receptor protein conformational shift has been suggested.

Physiologic Antagonism

Physiologic antagonism, another form of antagonism, involves two agonist drugs that bind to different receptors.[14] For competitive antagonism, the agonist and antagonist have affinity for the same receptor protein; in contrast, in physiologic antagonism, both drugs bind to specific unrelated receptor proteins, initiate a protein conformational shift, and elicit individual tissue responses. The responses, however, generate opposing forces such as are observed with isoproterenol-induced vasodilation and norepinephrine-induced vasoconstriction. The net effect on blood pressure is less than it would be if either drug were used by itself. The drug response that predominates depends on the intrinsic activity of each and on the extent of the tissue response that can be elicited.

Chemical Antagonism

Chemical antagonism occurs when a drug or chemical is present in the local receptor environment. It does not take part in the drug-receptor complex formation, yet the measured agonist drug response is less than expected. When local pH is altered or when the oxygen concentration is outside the physiologic range, the drug tissue response is altered. For example, contraction of isolated blood vessels induced by norepinephrine is decreased by low oxygen concentrations and normal pH and is augmented by high oxygen concentrations (Figure 4-8).[14] Chemical antagonism is thought to alter the chemistry of receptor proteins such that the protein conformational shift caused by the drug's bonding is rendered incomplete; this results in the tissue response being less than maximum for the drug dose administered.[7] Occasionally, as shown in Figure 4-8, the presence of other drugs unrelated to the agonist, in this case halothane and sufentanil, potentiates rather than antagonizes the agonist's response.

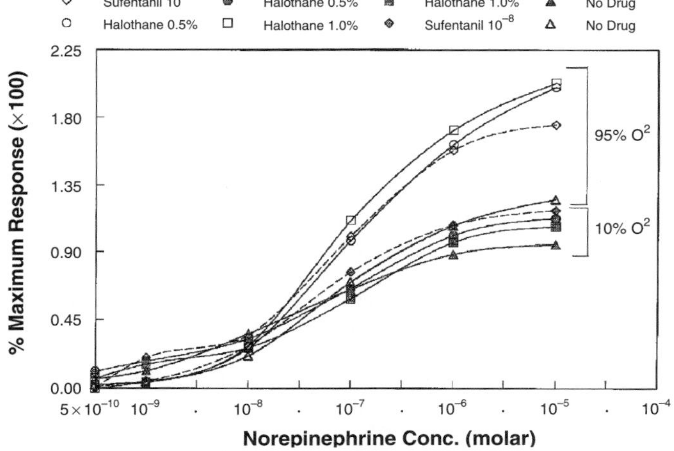

FIGURE **4-8**
A semilogarithmic plot of the responses of isolated rat aorta to norepinephrine with varying concentrations of oxygen, halothane, and the narcotic sufentanil.

Antagonist Dose Response

Tissue physiology also can be modified, particularly when energy-producing enzymes are involved in the response. Enzymes are particularly sensitive to changes in the local environment. Decreased enzymatic activity modifies tissue responsiveness, even when drug and receptor have perfect binding alignment. Chemical antagonism is more prevalent in critically ill individuals whose physiologic homeostasis is only marginal and is easily disturbed.[32] Drug responses in these individuals can be unpredictable, falling mostly to the right of the normal response curve. Occasionally, however, a greater than expected response occurs to an administered dose (potentiation).

RECEPTOR STRUCTURE

The historic concept of a drug receptor complex considered the receptor to be a single protein to which the drug aligned and attached itself. The transduction of signal to tissue (the increased ion movement into or out of the cell) occurred at a site near the receptor. Current evidence identifies the receptor and transduction site as being the same.

Types of Receptors

A variety of receptor types have been isolated and investigated, including GABA, opioid, α_2, acetylcholine, benzodiazepine, histaminic types, and the pain-related capsaicin receptor, as well as numerous others.[33-37] The nicotinic and muscarinic cholinergic receptors that bind acetylcholine have been extensively studied.[15,34,38,39] The acetylcholine receptor protein is a pentamer of five peptide subunits conceptually forming a five-sided ring, with the central portion serving as the transduction ion channel. Only two of the five subunits are involved in acetylcholine binding. The remaining three peptide subunits participate in the signal transduction process that involves a protein conformational shift, allowing inward movement of sodium ions through the opened ion channel. It is interesting to note that the $GABA_A$ receptor also has been shown to be composed of five peptide subunits arranged to form a pentameric ring.[27,33,39,40]

Signal Transduction

Signal transduction for the $GABA_A$ receptor involves inward chloride ion movement through the opened central channel. The protein compositions of acetylcholine and GABA receptors are remarkably similar, despite their functional differences—specifically, acetylcholine and sodium ion transduce an excitatory signal, and GABA and chloride ion transduce an inhibitory signal.[3,28,41,42]

For many drugs, the composition of the receptor protein and the signal transduction process may be identical, even though the drug-induced tissue response is not. The primary difference among drug receptor proteins may be only the selective binding subunits and the ion species moving through the channel.[27,33,34] The specific peptide subunits are ultimately responsible for the pharmacologic properties of specificity, affinity, and potency.

Drug Receptor Dynamics

The process by which the receptor protein undergoes a conformational shift to allow inward, and sometimes outward, ion movement is poorly understood. It may be more than mere chance that the pentameric ring structure of the receptor containing drug-specific peptide subunits is frequently met. Conceptually, when a drug binds to selective receptor peptide components, the outermost portion of the peptide ring may function as a backbone toward which the inner flexible surface is pulled.

By analogy, this "pulling" is similar to what occurs when a starfish opens its central mouth. The drug-induced conformational shift primarily involves a structural shortening of the protein filaments between the outer and inner surfaces. Such a process provides an open inner channel that allows the passage of ions through the receptor protein to achieve the intracellular response, thus initiating the dynamics of tissue response. Molecular pharmacology is rapidly identifying large numbers of specific cell binding sites involving etomidate, propofol, desflurane, and other anesthetics.[43,44] Drugs designed to bind only with selective sites to achieve a specific response are now available for clinical use (e.g., dexmedetomidine, S-ropivacaine).[37,45]

SUMMARY

The pharmacologic principles described in this chapter are essential to understanding drug responses in patients. The drug receptor subunit site now appears to be the primary regulator of onset-offset drug response. More and more evidence suggests that individual genetic variation in receptor proteins accounts for drug response variation within seemingly normal populations. In clinical anesthesia, the range of patient responses to a given drug dose reflects this genetic variation. The trend toward dosing by titration with rapid onset and offset anesthetic drugs minimizes the response variability factor by optimizing the use of available receptor proteins. The age-related decline in anesthetic drug dose needed to achieve a desired anesthetic end-point is related to a change in pharmacodynamics, not pharmacokinetics.

The anesthetist employs pharmacologic intervention to elicit a desired patient response. The site of the intervention is the biosphere, or the protein drug receptor, which is the primary regulator of the therapeutic response. Observed variation in patient drug response reflects the functionality of the biosphere and genetic variability.

The mean, median, and mode typically describe the dose-response relationship of a "normally distributed" population. In anesthesia, the patient population is rarely "normal." The drug response of population subsets can be expected to vary around the mean dosage. The trend toward dose titration by infusion allows individualization of the desired drug response, with fewer resultant overresponses and underresponses. The SD, SEM, and median effective dose provide a description of a population's response to a drug. Such descriptors provide only an approximate dosage; the anesthetist must adjust this dosage for each patient to achieve the desired physiologic response. Viewed at the molecular level, the observed response to a drug represents countless individual drug responses at the biosphere. Each drug-receptor interaction at the protein receptor elicits a fractional tissue response, and the sum of the fractional responses provides the observed response. In accordance with the law of mass action, when free drug binds to a receptor, a conformational shift occurs in the receptor protein. This shift causes a central space or channel to open, allowing specific ions to enter or leave the cell. The resultant tissue response continues until the drug dissociates from the receptor. Antagonist drugs also bind to the receptor but lack the ability to initiate the required protein conformational shift. The sum of fractional tissue responses elicited when an antagonist is present is inadequate for maintaining the desired tissue response.

Molecular pharmacology is identifying site-specific and age-related causes for the observed variation in patient drug response. Further investigation of the biosphere, genetics, and receptor protein subunits will provide a new understanding of pharmacodynamics for the anesthetist.

REFERENCES

1. Kurumbail RG, Stevens AM, Gierse JK, et al. Structural basis for selective inhibition of cyclooxygenase-2 by anti-inflammatory agents. *Nature*. 1996;348:644-648.
2. McMurry RW, Hardy KJ. Cox-2 inhibitors: today and tomorrow. *Am J Med Sci*. 2002;323:181-189.
3. Jenkins A, Franks NP, Lieb WR. Effects of temperature and volatile anesthetics on $GABA_A$ receptors. *Anesthesiology*. 1999;90:484-491.
4. Shafer SL, Varvel JR. Pharmacokinetics, pharmacodynamics, and rational opioid selection. *Anesthesiology*. 1991;74:53-63.
5. Hughes MA, Glass PSA, Jacobs JR. Context-sensitive half-time in multicompartment pharmacokinetic models for intravenous anesthetic drugs. *Anesthesiology*. 1992;76:334-341.
6. Bailey JM. Technique for quantifying the duration of intravenous anesthetic effect. *Anesthesiology*. 1995;83:1095-1103.
7. Schuttler J, Ihmsen HM. Population pharmacokinetics of propofol: a multicenter study. *Anesthesiology*. 2000;92:727-738.
8. Wakeling HG, Zimmerman JB, Howell S, Glass PS. Targeting effect compartment or central compartment concentration of propofol: what predicts loss of consciousness? *Anesthesiology*. 1999;90:92-97.
9. Jacobs JR, Reves JG, Marty J, et al. Aging increases pharmacodynamic sensitivity to the hypnotic effects of midazolam. *Anesth Analg*. 1995;80:143-148.
10. Inoue M, Suhara T, Sudo Y, et al. Age-related reduction of extrastriatal dopamine D2 receptor measured by PET. *Life Sci* 2001;69:1079-1084.
11. Kakiuchi T, Ohba H, Nishiyama S, et al. Age-related changes in muscarinic cholinergic receptors in the living brain: a PET study using N-[11C]methyl-4-piperidyl benzilate combined with cerebral blood flow measurement in conscious monkeys. *Brain Res*. 2001;916:22-31.
12. Albrecht S, Ihmsen H, Hering W, et al. The effect of age on the pharmacokinetics and pharmacodynamics of midazolam. *Clin Pharmacol Ther*. 1999;65:630-639.
13. Richards WG. *Quantum Pharmacology*. Boston: Butterworth; 1983:19-31.
14. Bourne HR, Roberts JM. Drug receptors and pharmacodynamics. In: Katzung BG, ed. *Basic and Clinical Pharmacology*. Los Altos, Calif: Lange Medical; 1984:9-22.
15. Csaky TZ. *Introduction to General Pharmacology*. New York: Appleton-Century-Croft; 1979:13-28.
16. Law Min JC. Iontophoretic study of speed of action of various muscle relaxants. *Anesthesiology*. 1992;77:351-356.
17. Levine RR. *Pharmacology: Drug Actions and Reactions*. Boston: Little, Brown; 1978:169-203.
18. DiPalma JR. *Basic Pharmacology in Medicine*. New York: McGraw-Hill; 1982:3-18.

19. Eger EI. Age, minimum alveolar anesthetic concentration, and minimum alveolar anesthetic concentration-awake. *Anesth Analg.* 2001;93:947-953.
20. Glantz SA. *Primer of Biostatistics.* New York: McGraw-Hill; 1981:10-29.
21. Gibaldi M. *Biopharmaceutics and Clinical Pharmacokinetics.* Philadelphia: Lea & Febiger; 1984:156-167.
22. Jacobs JR, Reves JG. Effect site equilibrium time is a determinant of induction dose requirement. *Anesth Analg.* 1993;76:1-6.
23. Gudzinowicz BJ, Younkin BK Jr, Gudzinowicz MJ. *Drug Dynamics for Analytical, Clinical, and Biological Chemists.* New York: Marcel Dekker; 1984:103-137.
24. Jenkinson DH. An introduction to receptors and their actions. In: Feldman SA, ed: *Drugs in Anesthesia: Mechanisms of Action.* London: Edward Arnold; 1987:3-31.
25. Greenblatt DJ, Shader RI. *Pharmacokinetics in Clinical Practice.* Philadelphia: Saunders; 1985:95-103.
26. Nierenberg DW, Melmon KL. Introduction to clinical pharmacology. In: Melmon KL, ed: *Clinical Pharmacology: Basic Principles in Therapeutics.* 4th ed. New York: McGraw-Hill; 2000;1-62.
27. Burt DR, Kamatchi GL. $GABA_A$ receptor subtypes: from pharmacology to molecular biology. *FASEB J.* 1991;5:2916-2923.
28. Franks NP, Lieb WR. Molecular and cellular mechanisms of general anesthesia. *Nature.* 1994;367:607-614.
29. Cheng G, Kendig JJ. Enflurane decreases glutamate neurotransmission to spinal cord motor neurons by both pre- and postsynaptic actions. *Anesth Analg.* 2003;96:1354-1359.
30. Campana JA, Miller KW, Forman SA. Mechanisms of actions of inhaled anesthetics. *N Engl J Med.* 2003;348:2110-2124.
31. El-Etr AA, Glisson SN. Alpha-adrenergic blocking agents. In: Ivankovich AD, ed: *Nitroprusside and Other Short-Acting Hypotensive Agents.* Boston: Little, Brown; 1978:239-259.
32. Power BM, Forbes AM, van Heerden PV, et al. Pharmacokinetics of drugs used in critically ill adults, *Clin Pharmacokinet.* 1998;34:25-56.
33. Olsen RW. Drug interactions at the GABA receptor-ionophore complex. *Annu Rev Pharmacol Toxicol.* 1982;22:245-277.
34. Pocock G, Richards CD. Cellular mechanisms in general anaesthesia. *Br J Anaesth.* 1991;66:116-128.
35. Wiklund RA, Rosenbaum SH. Medical progress: anesthesiology: first of two par. *N Engl J Med.* 1997;337:1132-1141.
36. Caterina MJ, Schumacher MA, Tominaga M, et al. The capsaicin receptor: a heat-activated ion channel in the pain pathway. *Nature.* 1997;389:816-824.
37. Pekka T. Receptor-specific reversible sedation. *Anesthesiology.* 1998;89:560-561.
38. Durieux ME. Muscarinic signaling in the central nervous system: recent developments and anesthetic implications. *Anesthesiology.* 1996;84:173-189.
39. Tassonyi E, Charpantier E, Muller D, et al. The role of nicotinic acetylcholine receptors in the mechanisms of anesthesia. *Brain Res Bull.* 2002;57:133-150.
40. Hucho F, Tsetlin VI, Machold J. The emerging three-dimensional structure of a receptor: the nicotinic acetylcholine receptor. *Eur J Biochem.* 1996;239:539-557.
41. Tanelian DL, Kosek P, Mody I, et al. The role of the $GABA_A$ receptor/chloride channel complex in anesthesia. *Anesthesiology.* 1993;78:757-776.
42. Rabow LE, Russek SJ, Farb DH. From ion currents to genomic analysis: recent advances in $GABA_A$ receptor research. *Synapse.* 1998;21:189-274.
43. Hara M, Kai Y, Ikemoto Y. Enhancement by propofol of the gamma-aminobutyric $acid_A$ response in dissociated hippocampal pyramidal neurons of the rat. *Anesthesiology.* 1994;81:988-994.
44. Tomlin SL, et al. Stereoselective effects of etomidate optical isomers on gamma-aminobutyric acid type A receptors and animals. *Anesthesiology.* 1998;88:708-717.
45. Wulf H. Do "lefthanders" make better local anesthetics? The relevance of stereoisomerism in clinical practice as shown by new local anesthetics. *Der Anaesthesist.* 1997;46:622-626.

UNIT II SCIENTIFIC FOUNDATIONS

CHAPTER 5

PHARMACOKINETICS

LADAN ESHKEVARI, DONNA JASINSKI

Pharmacokinetics is a term used to describe the study of the changes in the concentration of a drug during the processes of absorption, distribution, metabolism or biotransformation, and elimination from the body. Essentially, it is the study of what the body does to a drug once the agent has been introduced into the system. The knowledge of this discipline is important to the anesthetist, because the pharmacokinetics of drugs are a major factor in their onset, time course, offset, and variability of responses from patient to patient, as well as in the determination of the amount of drug available to act at the effect site. Pharmacokinetic concepts also play a vital role in the delivery of serum concentrations that will result in desired effects without untoward side effects.

Regardless of the route of administration, the vascular system delivers the drug to various tissues. Therefore most kinetic concepts revolve around assessment of blood level over time, even if the correlation with the amount of drug at the effector site is poor. Once in the blood the drug can either remain within the vascular system and body water, bound to proteins, or cross membranes to enter tissues. The unbound drug enters organs, muscles, fat, and, of greatest importance, the site of activity—the receptors. This transfer of drug to various sites depends on several intrinsic properties of the agent, such as molecular size, degree of ionization, lipid solubility, and protein binding. In addition to these drug properties, uptake also depends on the amount of blood flow to the tissue and the concentration gradient of the drug across membranes.

PROPERTIES THAT INFLUENCE PHARMACOKINETIC ACTIVITY

Molecular Size

The smaller the molecular size of an agent, the better it crosses the lipid barriers and membranes of tissues. When a drug is administered, it must be absorbed across biologic membranes that have very small openings or pores. Generally speaking, molecules with molecular weights greater than 100 to 200 do not cross the cell membranes. Transport across the membranes can occur passively or actively. Passive transport does not require energy and involves transfer of a drug from an area of high concentration to an area of lower concentration. Active transport mechanisms are generally faster and require energy. This transport system uses carriers that form complexes with drug molecules on the membrane surface and can involve movement of the drug molecule against a concentration gradient from an area of low concentration to an area of high concentration.[1] Figure 5-1 depicts the movement of a drug across cell membranes.

Degree of Ionization and Lipid Solubility

Most drugs are salts of either weak acids or weak bases. When introduced into the body they behave as a chemical in solution. As acids or bases they exist in solutions in both ionized and unionized forms. The charged (ionized) form is water soluble, and the uncharged (nonionized) form is lipophilic. Because the nonionized molecules are lipid soluble, they can diffuse across cell membranes such as the blood-brain, gastric, and placental barriers to reach the effect site. On the other hand, the ionized molecules are usually unable to penetrate lipid cell membranes easily because of their low lipid solubility. This results from the electrical charges exerted by the ionized drug molecules. These charged drugs are repelled by those sections of the cell membranes with similar charges, which prevents their diffusion across the membrane.[1] The higher the degree of ionization, the less access the drug has across tissues such as the gastrointestinal tract, the blood-brain and placental barriers, and liver hepatocytes. This is important in that ionized drugs are not absorbed well when taken orally and may not be metabolized by the liver to any significant extent. Instead, they commonly are excreted via the renal system.[2]

The degree of ionization of an agent, whether acidic or basic, at a particular site is determined by the dissociation constant (pK_a) of the agent and its pH gradient across the membrane. The pK_a is the negative log of the equilibrium constant for the dissociation of the acid or base. The relationship between the pK_a of the drug and the pH of the solution may be expressed by two equations. The first equation applies to drugs that are basic in nature:

Equation 5-1

$$pK_a = pH = \log\frac{(HA^+)}{(A^-)}$$

The second equation applies to acidic drugs:

Equation 5-2

$$pK_a = pH = \log\frac{(A^-)}{(HA^+)}$$

From these equations an estimate of the degree of drug absorption can be developed.[2,3] Acids are usually defined as proton donors, whereas bases are made up of molecules that can accept a proton. When the pH is equal to the pK_a, the two species exist in equal amounts; for example, because phenobarbital has a pK_a of 7.4 and blood has a pH of 7.4, in the bloodstream the drug is present in equal proportions of charged and uncharged forms.

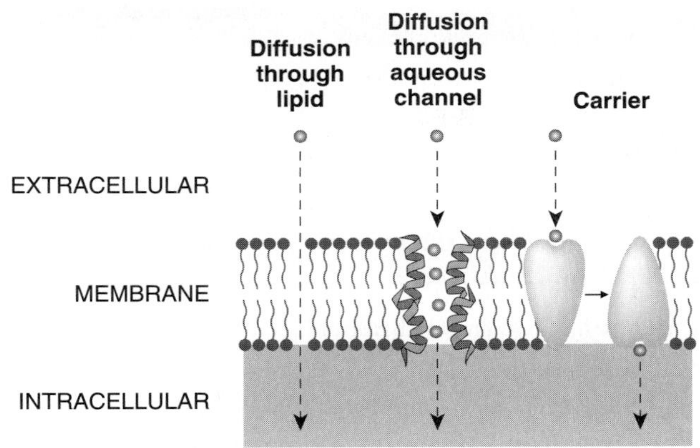

FIGURE **5-1**
Routes by which solutes can transverse cell membranes. (From Rang HP, Dale MM, Ritter JM, et al. Absorption and distribution of drugs. In: *Pharmacology*. 5th ed. Edinburgh: Churchill Livingstone; 2003:92.)

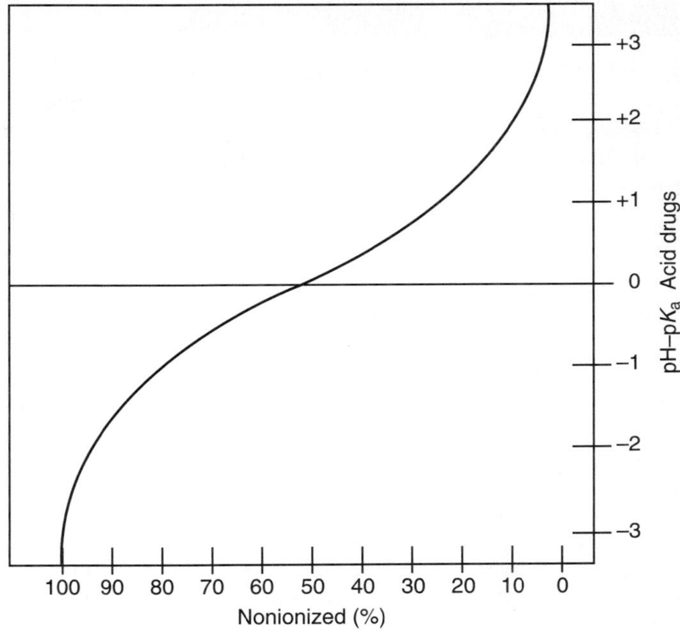

FIGURE **5-2**
When acidic drugs are placed in physiologic solutions, the degree of nonionization is greater if the pH of the solution minus the pK_a of the drug ($pH - pK_a$) is less than zero. Conversely, when the $pH - pK_a$ is greater than zero, more of the drug exists in an ionized, less absorbable, form.

It is of importance to note that relatively modest changes in the pH of the environment, when it is close to the pK, are more significant in changing the ratio of charged to uncharged forms than the same change in pH at some value far removed from the pK. For example, phenobarbital, with a pK of 7.4, is for the most part nondissociated and therefore is nonionized at a pH of 1.4. This results from the fact that the pH is well below the pK, and when phenobarbital is in a relatively strongly acidic environment with an abundance of protons, it does not give up its protons readily. If a drug is a weak acid and if the pH of the fluid environment is below the pK, most of the drug's protons are associated with the drug molecule, and the predominant species is uncharged and therefore lipid soluble. See Figure 5-2. Conversely, if the pH is below the pK for a drug that is a weak base, an abundance of protons exists, and most of the drug tends to ionize as the proton is donated by the drug molecule, which results in a species that is highly charged and therefore lipid insoluble.[2] See Figure 5-3. The effects of pK_a and pH on ionization are summarized in Box 5-1.

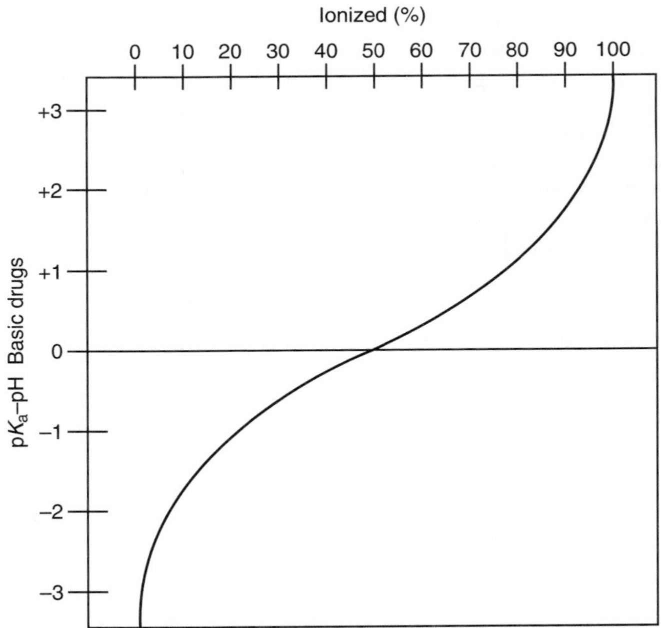

FIGURE **5-3**
$pK_a - pH$ versus the percent ionized. The degree to which a basic drug remains in its nonionized state depends on the medium in which it is placed. pK_a is the dissociation constant (see text for further explanation).

Ion Trapping

Ion trapping has several anesthesia-related applications. Influences on oral absorption of drugs, maternal-fetal transfer, and central nervous system toxicity of local anesthetics are commonly cited. The degree of ionization for a specific agent can vary across a membrane that separates fluids with different pH values. For example, morphine sulfate, a base, with a pK of 7.9 when present in the blood (which has a pH of 7.4) exists in appreciable amounts in both ionized and nonionized forms. The uncharged drug fraction moves freely across tissue membranes, and the charged fraction does not. As the drug enters the stomach, a very acidic environment with a pH of 1.9, morphine accepts protons and becomes ionized, and ion trapping occurs.[2] (Figure 5-4 illustrates this phenomenon using diazepam as an example.) The drug, however, will be absorbed later, as stomach contents move farther down the gastrointestinal tract to the more basic and favorable environment of the small intestine.

A similar scenario occurs when agents are transferred between a mother and a fetus, where the placenta is the membrane separating fluids with varying pH values—that of the fetus is more acidic than that of the mother. Again, the lipid-soluble fraction of basic agents such as lidocaine (pK 7.9) crosses the placenta easily. However, once there, because of the lower pH of the fetus the drug becomes more ionized and cannot easily cross the lipid bilayer of placenta, which results in

BOX 5-1

Relationship between pH, pK_a, and Ionization for Weak Acids and Weak Bases

Weak Base		*Weak Acid*	
$pH > pK_a$	Unionized form predominates	$pH > pK_a$	Ionized form predominates
$pH = pK_a$	Unionized equal to ionized	$pH = pK_a$	Unionized equal to ionized
$pH < pK_a$	Ionized form predominates	$pH < pK_a$	Unionized form predominates

Modified with permission from White M. Principles of pharmacokinetics. In: Bovill JG, Howie MB. Clinical Pharmacology for Anaesthetists. *London: Saunders; 1999:23.*

accumulation of drug in the fetus. Finally, in a local anesthetic overdose situation in which high concentrations of a basic local anesthetic agent have entered the central nervous system and caused toxicity, ion trapping may occur. If the patient experiences respiratory arrest and hypoxia, the resulting acidosis may trap the drug in the brain, resulting in prolonged and possibly more intense toxicity. Ion trapping also plays a role in the use of bicarbonate solutions and carbonated local anesthetics. A discussion of the effects of ion trapping on local anesthetics can be found in Box 9-2.

Protein Binding

Changes in protein binding have long been theorized to influence a drug's clinical effect. Two situations are commonly cited. The first involves a patient with a reduction in proteins such as occurs with severe liver or kidney disease, with protein deficiencies caused by poor nutrition, and during the last trimester of pregnancy, when fluid shifts alter distribution volume. The second situation involves a drug interaction between two or more highly protein-bound drugs.

Potential clinical changes are conceptualized by the following phenomena. Some drugs are bound extensively to proteins in the plasma because of their innate affinity for the circulating plasma proteins. The drug-protein molecule is too large to diffuse through blood vessel membranes and is therefore trapped within the circulatory system. Albumin is quantitatively the most abundant plasma protein, and although it is capable of binding basic, neutral, or acidic drugs, it favors acidic compounds. α_1-Acid glycoprotein (AAG) and β-globulin bind, for the most part, basic drugs.[4] Lipoproteins bind cyclosporine, and transcortin binds corticosteroids. Protein binding influences how a drug is distributed, because protein-bound drug is not free to act on receptors. High protein binding prevents the drug from leaving the blood to enter into tissue, which results in high plasma concentrations. The degree of protein binding for a drug is proportional to its lipid solubility such that the more lipid soluble an agent, the more highly protein bound it tends to be.[5] See Box 5-2.

The number of potential binding sites on plasma proteins for drugs is finite; therefore the kinetics for binding behaves like any saturable process in that protein binding can be overcome by adding more agent.[2] The bond between drug and protein is usually weak, and they can dissociate when the plasma concentration of the drug declines or a second drug that binds to the same protein is introduced. For example, when a drug has been in chronic use and is at steady state, an equilibrium will be reached between free and protein-bound drug. If a new drug with a high affinity for the same protein sites is introduced, the new drug competes with the chronic drug for binding sites. This leads to displacement of the first drug with an increase in free fraction of that agent. It is important to note that the displaced free drug does become available

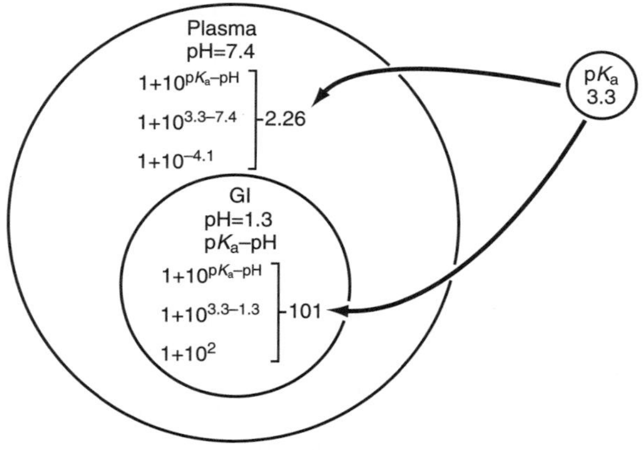

FIGURE **5-4**
For both weak acids and weak bases the total concentration of a drug is greater on the side of the membrane on which it is more highly ionized. Diazepam, a basic drug with a pK_a of 3.3, is more ionized at gastric pH than it is in plasma. Consequently it has a greater total concentration in the gastrointestinal compartment than it does in the plasma.

BOX 5-2

Binding of Drugs to Plasma Proteins

- Plasma albumin is most important; β-globulin and α_1-acid glycoprotein also bind some drugs.
- Plasma albumin binds, for the most part, acidic drugs (approximately two molecules per albumin molecule). Basic drugs may be bound by β-globulin and α_1-acid glycoprotein.
- Saturable binding sometimes leads to a nonlinear relationship between dose and free (active) drug concentration.
- Extensive protein binding slows drug elimination (metabolism and excretion by glomerular filtration).
- Competition between drugs for protein binding rarely leads to clinically important drug interactions.

Modified with permission from Rang HP, Dale MM, Ritter JM, et al. Absorption and distribution of drugs. In: Pharmacology. *5th ed. Edinburgh: Churchill Livingstone; 2003.*

for biotransformation and elimination, so unless these clearance mechanisms are at capacity, a rise in free fraction will lead to a small change in free plasma concentrations.

Protein binding is expressed in terms of the percentage of total drug bound. Drugs with protein binding greater than 90%, such as warfarin, phenytoin, propranolol, propofol, fentanyl and its analogues, and diazepam, are conceptualized to have an unexpected intensification of their effect if they are displaced from plasma proteins.[6] Drugs that exhibit less than 90% binding have so little change in free active fractions that they are not a concern. The example that is commonly used is the anticoagulant warfarin. Because warfarin is approximately 98% bound to plasma proteins, a reduction in bound fraction to 96% causes an increase in the free active fraction of the drug. Furthermore, when hypoalbuminemia exists, decreased albumin levels result in the availability of a greater amount of free drug. These theoretic concerns are rarely clinically relevant, as explained subsequently.

No clinically relevant examples of changes in drug disposition or effects can be clearly ascribed to changes in plasma protein binding. The idea that a drug displaced from plasma proteins increases the unbound drug concentration, increases the drug effect, and perhaps produces toxicity seems a simple and obvious mechanism. Unfortunately this simple theory, which is appropriate for a test tube, does not work in the body, which is an open system capable of eliminating unbound drug.

First, a seemingly dramatic change in the unbound fraction from 1% to 10% releases less than 5% of the total amount of drug in the body into the unbound pool, because less than one third of the drug in the body is bound to plasma proteins even in the most extreme cases (e.g., when warfarin is used). Drug displaced from plasma protein, of course, distributes throughout the volume of distribution, so that a 5% increase in the amount of unbound drug in the body produces at most a 5% increase in pharmacologically active unbound drug at the site of action.

Second, when the amount of unbound drug in plasma increases, the rate of elimination increases (if unbound clearance is unchanged), and after four half-lives the unbound concentration returns to its previous steady-state value. When drug interactions associated with protein binding displacement and clinically important effects have been studied, it has been found that the displacing drug is also an inhibitor of clearance, and it is the change in *clearance* of the *unbound* drug that is the relevant mechanism explaining the interaction.

The clinical application of plasma protein binding is only to help interpretation of measured drug concentrations. When plasma proteins are lower than normal, then total drug concentrations are lowered but unbound concentrations are not affected.[1]

Absorption

Routes of Drug Administration

An important variable in the bioavailability of drug at its effect site is the route by which the agent is administered. The route of administration determines how much of the drug is delivered to the systemic circulation. When the entire amount of drug given is delivered, the drug is said to have *100% bioavailability*. Many routes of drug administration are used; each has advantages and disadvantages (Table 5-1). The routes of drug administration are enteral (involves the gastrointestinal tract); parenteral (injected subcutaneously, intramuscularly, intravenously, intrathecally, or epidermally); pulmonary; and topical.[7] Absorption mechanisms of relevance to anesthesia are discussed in the following sections.

Enteral Administration. The oral route is the most common and convenient method for administration of drugs. It is relatively inexpensive, does not require sterile technique, and can be carried out with little skill. Several disadvantages, however, exist, because many conditions—such as emotions, physical activity, and food intake—change the gastrointestinal environment. Therefore orally administered drugs tend to have a lower bioavailability. The stomach has a large surface area, and the length of time a drug remains there is a significant factor in absorption. Because of the low pH in the stomach (1.5 to 2.5), drugs that are highly acidic, such as barbiturates, tend to remain nonionized and are highly absorbed. Basic drugs that remain intact in the stomach acids can pass through and are more readily absorbed in the intestine. The small intestine is highly vascular and has an alkaline environment (pH 7 to 8).[7]

The enteral route often results in failure of the drug to be absorbed into the systemic circulation. Alternatively, chemical alteration may occur before entry from the intestines. *Presystemic elimination* refers to the elimination of drug by the

TABLE 5-1 Routes of Administration

Route	Bioavailability (%)	Comments
Intravenous	100 (by definition)	Most rapid onset; allows for titration of doses; suitable for large volumes
Intramuscular	75 to 100	Moderate volumes feasible; may be painful
Subcutaneous	75 to 100	Smaller volumes than intramuscular; may be painful; suitable for implantation of pellets
Oral	5 to 100	Most convenient and economical; first-pass effect may be significant; requires patient cooperation
Rectal	30 to 100	Less first-pass effect than oral; useful in pediatric patients
Inhalation	5 to 100	Common anesthetic use for inhalation drugs, steroids, bronchodilators, and occasionally resuscitative drugs; very rapid onset (parallels intravenous administration)
Sublingual	60 to 100	Lack of first-pass effect; absorbed directly into systemic circulation
Intrathecal	Low (intentionally)	Specialized application, as with local anesthetics and analgesics, chemotherapy, and antibiotic administration; circumvents blood-brain barrier
Topical	80 to 100	Includes skin, cornea, buccal, vagina, and nasal mucosa; dermal application results in slow absorption; used for lack of first-pass effect; prolonged duration of action

gastrointestinal system before the drug reaches the systemic circulation. This occurs by means of three mechanisms: the stomach acids hydrolyze the drug (e.g., penicillin); enzymes in the gastrointestinal wall deactivate the drug; or the liver biotransforms ingested drug before it reaches the effect site.[2] This liver activity is called *first-pass* hepatic effect. Drugs absorbed from the gastrointestinal tract after oral ingestion enter the portal venous blood and pass through the liver first, with subsequent delivery to the tissue receptors. At the liver they may undergo extensive hepatic extraction and metabolism before they have a chance to enter the systemic circulation (Box 5-3). Agents such as these exhibit large differences between oral and intravenous dosages. To have the desired effect, oral dosages must be exaggerated to compensate for the initial metabolism that occurs before the drug reaches the effect site.

The sublingual and buccal routes of administration of drugs bypass the presystemic, portal system first-pass effect and are delivered rapidly to the superior vena cava for transport to the effect site.[1] Nitroglycerin is an example of a sublingual drug that is put under the tongue and absorbed by the rich blood supply there. If ingested the drug would be hydrolyzed by the stomach; therefore, sublingual administration is the ideal route for this agent. Protein hormones that would also be digested by the stomach are instead placed between the gum and cheek (buccal administration) and enter venous drainage without undergoing hepatic, presystemic elimination.[8,9]

Occasionally the rectal route of drug administration is the ideal route for prevention of emesis caused by irritation of the gastrointestinal mucosa by the drug. It is also a preferred method of drug delivery for patients in whom oral ingestion poses difficulty. For example, rectal acetaminophen is administered to infants and young children undergoing general anesthesia for postoperative pain control. Drugs placed in the proximal rectum are absorbed into the portal system via the superior hemorrhoidal vein. They will therefore undergo significant first-pass effect in the liver before entering the systemic circulation, leading to unpredictable responses.[1] Conversely, agents placed in the distal rectum do not undergo presystemic elimination and therefore have more predictable circulatory levels. The disadvantage historically associated with this route was the unpredictability of drug retention and absorption because of rectal contents.

BOX **5-3**

Examples of Drugs That Undergo Substantial First-Pass Elimination

Aspirin
Glyceryl trinitrate
Isosorbide dinitrate
Levodopa
Lidocaine
Metoprolol
Morphine
Propranolol
Salbutamol
Verapamil

Modified with permission from Rang HP, Dale MM, Ritter JM, et al. Drug elimination and pharmacokinetics. In: Pharmacology. *5th ed. Edinburgh: Churchill Livingstone; 2003.*

However, more recent studies have demonstrated that regardless of enema volume, agents are absorbed with consistent plasma concentrations within subjects.[10]

Parenteral Administration. *Parenteral administration* refers to administration by injection. The most rapid and predictable route to the systemic circulation is the parenteral route. With intramuscular injections the drug is instilled deep into the muscle, among the muscle fascicles.[2] Subcutaneous agents are placed under the skin. With both intramuscular and subcutaneous injections the systemic absorption of the drug is dependent on the capillary blood flow to the area and the lipid solubility of the agent.[1] Conversely, intravenous injections allow for rapid and accurate delivery of drug into the systemic circulation. Parenteral administration is the route of choice for anesthetists, as it is an exact method of achieving the desired effect from agents delivered.

Pulmonary Administration. The lungs provide a large surface area for drugs administered by inhalation. Bronchodilators and antibiotics are administered via devices such as nebulizers, used to propel aerosols into the alveolar sacs.[10] Anesthetic gases are also effectively administered through the lungs, as described in detail in Chapter 6.

Transdermal (Topical) Administration. The transdermal route is usually chosen for administration of a sustained release agent in order to provide the patient with a steady therapeutic plasma concentration. Drugs that are administered via this route must possess several characteristics. They usually exist in a combined form—both water soluble and lipid soluble. The water solubility is necessary so that the drug can penetrate the hair follicles and sweat ducts. The drug must be lipid soluble in order to exert effect at the receptors once in the system. These agents must have a molecular weight of less than 1000, dose requirements less than 10 mg in a 24-hour period, and a pH of 5 to 9.[1] The area to which the drug is applied must have a relatively thin epidermis with a sufficient blood supply (Figure 5-5).

Bioavailability

Bioavailability is the extent to which a drug reaches its effect site after its introduction into the circulatory system. The rate at which systemic absorption occurs establishes a drug's duration of action and intensity. Many factors play a role in the bioavailability of agents, including lipid solubility, solubility in aqueous and organic solvents, molecular weight, pH, pK_a, and blood flow. For example, drugs given in aqueous solution are more rapidly absorbed than those given in oily solution or solid form, because they mix more readily with the aqueous phase at the absorptive site.[11,12] A recent study demonstrated that propofol in the form of a water-soluble prodrug is metabolized to propofol which has a longer half-life, an increased volume of distribution, a delayed onset, and a greater potency.[13]

The environment into which the drug is introduced also has an impact on its bioavailability. The patient's age, sex, pathology, pH, blood flow, and temperature are all factors to consider. For example, pH plays a role when local anesthetic (a weak base) is injected into an infected wound (an acidic environment). In this instance the local anesthetic is highly ionized (basic agent in acidic environment) and therefore cannot enter the lipid nerve membrane to reach the site of action. Some important concepts influencing absorption are listed in Box 5-4.

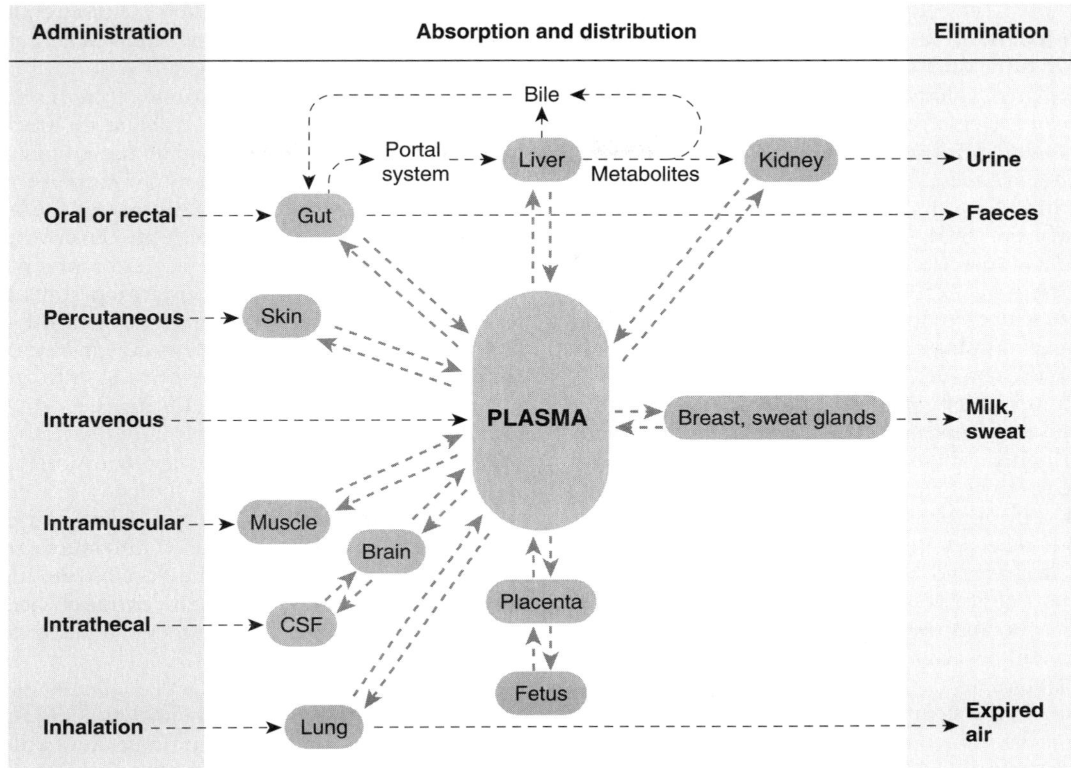

FIGURE **5-5**
The main routes of drug administration and elimination. (From Rang HP, Dale MM, Ritter JM, et al. Absorption and distribution of drugs. In: *Pharmacology*. 5th ed. Edinburgh: Churchill Livingstone; 2003:97.)

BOX **5-4**

Movement of Drugs across Cellular Barriers

- To traverse cellular barriers (e.g., gastrointestinal mucosa, renal tubule, blood-brain barrier, placenta), drugs must cross lipid membranes.
- Drugs cross lipid membranes mainly by passive diffusional transfer or by carrier-mediated transfer.
- The main factors that determine the rate of passive diffusional transfer across membranes are a drug's lipid solubility and the concentration gradient. Molecular weight is a less important factor.
- Drugs are weak acids or weak bases; their state of ionization varies with pH according to the Henderson-Hasselbalch equation.
- With weak acids or bases only the uncharged species (the protonated form for a weak acid; the unprotonated form for a weak base) can diffuse across lipid membranes; this gives rise to pH partition or ion trapping.
- The term *pH partition* refers to the fact that weak acids tend to accumulate in compartments of relatively high pH, whereas weak bases tend to leave compartments of high pH.
- Carrier-mediated transport (e.g., in the renal tubule, blood-brain barrier, gastrointestinal epithelium) is important for some drugs that are chemically related to endogenous substances.
- Drugs of very low lipid solubility, including those that are strong acids or bases, are generally poorly absorbed from the gut.
- A few drugs (e.g., levodopa) are absorbed by carrier-mediated transfer.
- Absorption from the gut depends on many factors, including the following:
  - Gastrointestinal motility
  - Gastrointestinal pH
  - Particle size
  - Physicochemical interaction with gut contents (e.g., chemical interaction between calcium and tetracycline antibiotics)
- Bioavailability is the fraction of an ingested dose of a drug that gains access to the systemic circulation. It may be low because absorption is incomplete or because the drug is metabolized in the gut wall or liver before reaching the systemic circulation.
- Bioequivalence implies that if one formulation of a drug is substituted for another, no clinically untoward consequences will ensue.

Modified with permission from Rang HP, Dale MM, Ritter JM, et al. Absorption and distribution of drugs. In: Pharmacology. *5th ed. Edinburgh: Churchill Livingstone; 2003.*

Distribution

Compartment Models. Compartment models depict the body as composed of distinct sections that represent theoretic spaces with calculated volumes and are used to describe the pharmacokinetics of agents. These models are useful for prediction of serum concentrations and changes in drug concentrations in other tissues. A single-compartment model represents the entire body, through which homogeneous distribution occurs (Figure 5-6). Although a one-compartment model is sufficient to describe the action of many drugs, it is generally insufficient to explain the kinetics of lipid-soluble anesthetic drugs. A two-compartment model is typically used to simplify and explain pharmacokinetic concepts that can be extrapolated to more complex models.[14]

In the two-compartment model, the first compartment is termed the *central compartment* and is composed of intravascular fluid and the highly perfused tissues such as the heart, lungs, brain, liver, and kidneys (Figure 5-7). The central compartment represents only approximately 10% of body mass in an adult, however, it receives approximately 75% of the cardiac output and is also referred to as the *vessel-rich group*. The peripheral compartment (vessel-poor group) is composed of muscle, fat, and bone and represents 90% of body mass. This second compartment receives approximately 25% of the cardiac output.[14] The terms *central* and *peripheral compartments* refer to differences in the size of the compartments and the rate at which a drug is distributed to them. In reality the compartments are not true anatomic areas but conceptual representation of two separate volumes in which a quantitative change in drug concentration occurs.[15]

Drugs leave the central compartment in two phases. Drugs leave by distribution into the tissues or via metabolism and excretion. In the initial phase, after an intravenous bolus dose, those organs with the highest blood flow have the largest amount of drug delivered to them. These highly perfused tissues equilibrate with the initial high serum concentration and attain a high concentration of drug (Table 5-2). As blood flows through the less perfused organs, the drug begins to be deposited in those tissues as well.[11] However, the tissue levels rise more slowly and do not reach as high a concentration as in the vessel-rich group or central compartment, with extraction occurring to a lesser degree. As blood flows through the tissues, serum concentrations drop because of this distribution, and the fall in plasma concentration is described mathematically via the alpha half-life.[16] When the plasma concentration falls below the tissue concentration, the drug reemerges from the highly perfused tissue, enters the plasma serum, and is again redistributed. The drug enters the central compartment for clearance from the body. The degree to which drugs distribute and redistribute from the central compartment to the peripheral compartment, and the resultant concentration of the drug established before elimination occurs, allows for the calculation of the volume of distribution.

Volume of Distribution

The volume of distribution is a proportional expression that relates the amount of drug in the body to the serum concentration. It is the apparent volume in which the drug is distributed after it has been introduced into the system.[1] Essentially it is calculated by dividing the dose of the drug administered intravenously by the plasma concentration before elimination occurs. The volume of distribution is used to calculate the loading dose of a drug that will achieve a steady-state concentration.[14] In practice a patient's volume of distribution is unknown, and an average volume of distribution is assumed and used to calculate a loading dose that will attain a therapeutic concentration rather than a steady-state concentration.

Equation 5-3

$$\text{Volume of distribution} = \frac{\text{Dose of drug}}{\text{Plasma concentration of drug}}$$

The volume of distribution is an independent variable and enables calculation of a loading dose if the desired plasma concentration is known. The volume of distribution is also of relevance in the drug's elimination from the body, because drugs can be eliminated only by the body's organs of elimination, such as the kidneys and liver. Therefore a drug with a large volume of

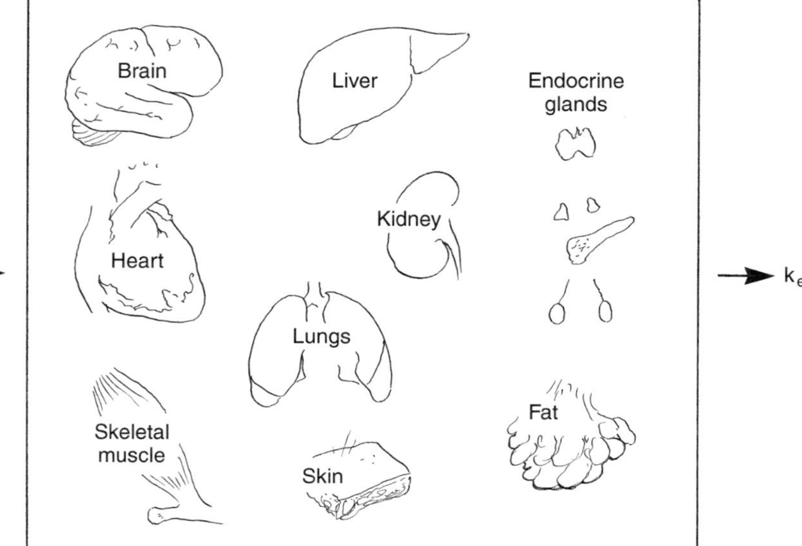

FIGURE **5-6**
In the one-compartment model, a drug instantaneously and homogeneously is distributed throughout the fluids and tissues that constitute the compartment. When changes in drug concentration occur in any of these tissues, a corresponding quantitative change occurs in drug concentration in all the other tissues.

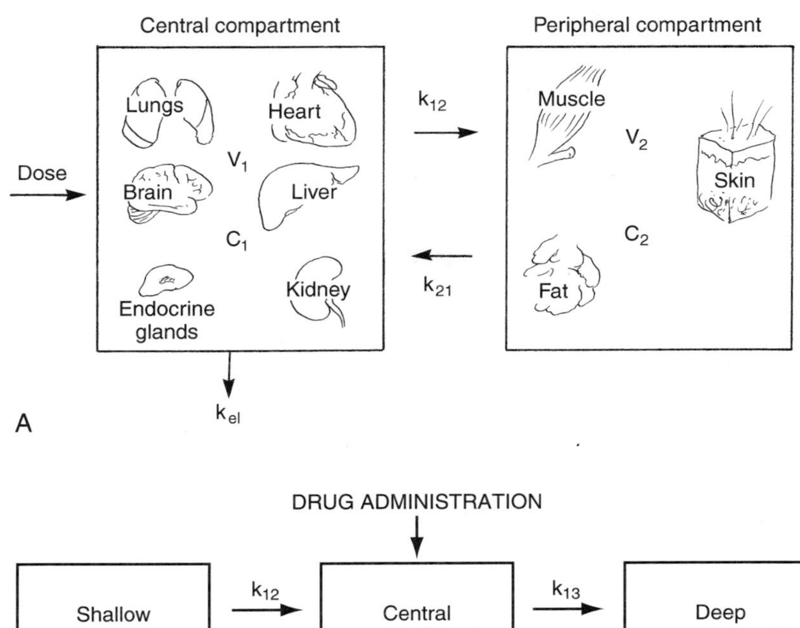

FIGURE **5-7**
A, In the two-compartment model the body is assumed to be made up of two compartments: a central compartment (C_1) made up of a small apparent volume (V_1), and a peripheral compartment (C_2) made up of a larger apparent volume (V_2). **B,** The three-compartment model is depicted as having a central compartment into which the drug is administered and two peripheral compartments to which reversible drug distribution occurs. k_{12}, Rate of distribution of drugs to the peripheral compartment; k_{21}, rate of redistribution of drugs back to the central compartment; k_{el}, rate of drug removal or elimination from the body; k_{13}, rate of distribution of drugs from the central compartment to a shallow peripheral compartment; k_{31}, rate of distribution of drugs from the shallow peripheral compartment back to the central compartment (see text for further explanation).

distribution has very low concentrations in the plasma, and very little drug would be available to the organs for elimination.[1]

The volume of distribution of a drug is affected by the physiochemical properties of that drug, such as lipid solubility, plasma protein binding, and molecular size.[2] Drugs that are free, unbound to plasma proteins, and lipid soluble easily cross membranes to tissues and therefore have large calculated volumes of distribution with low plasma concentrations. An example of a drug with a large volume of distribution is thiopental.[1] On injection of an induction dose this highly lipid-soluble drug is distributed quickly to peripheral tissue, thereby ending its action much more rapidly than its elimination half-life would predict. The patient wakes up in just a few minutes because of redistribution from the brain (central compartment) to the peripheral compartment; however, the patient may feel sleepy for hours because of the long elimination half-life of the drug from the whole body (11.6 hours).[2]

TABLE **5-2** Tissue Groups Based on Perfusion*

Characteristic	Vessel-Rich	Muscle	Fat	Vessel-Poor
Percentage of body weight	10	50	20	20
Percentage of cardiac output	75	19	6	0
Perfusion (ml/min/100 g)	75	3	3	0

**The vessel-rich group represents the central compartment, and the muscle, fat, and vessel-poor groups are peripheral compartments.*

The volume of distribution of a drug administered by bolus is also calculated by dividing the total dose administered by the area under the plasma concentration curve. The greater the area under the curve, the longer the drug acts and the drug intensity increases.[2] However, if the drug is infused or given in multiple doses and the amount given equals the amount eliminated, the central and peripheral compartments are in equilibrium. Therefore the volume of distribution at this steady state would differ if the agent were given as a bolus injection.[3]

Plasma Concentration Curve

A schematic depiction of the decline in plasma concentration of drug with time after rapid intravenous injection into the central compartment is plotted on a logarithmic graph. The y-axis of the graph represents the plasma concentration, and the x-axis reflects the time after the dose is injected. The first phase of the curve is the α phase, or the distribution phase, which represents the initial dispersal of drug into the tissue compartments from the central compartment. This slope is usually steep with drugs that are highly lipid soluble, which demonstrates the ability of these agents to cross membrane lipid bilayers and be distributed to the peripheral compartment rapidly, leading to a rapid fall in plasma levels.[1]

The second phase of the curve is a logarithmic plot of the slower elimination, or β, phase of the plasma concentration curve. Once equilibrium has been reached, the concentration

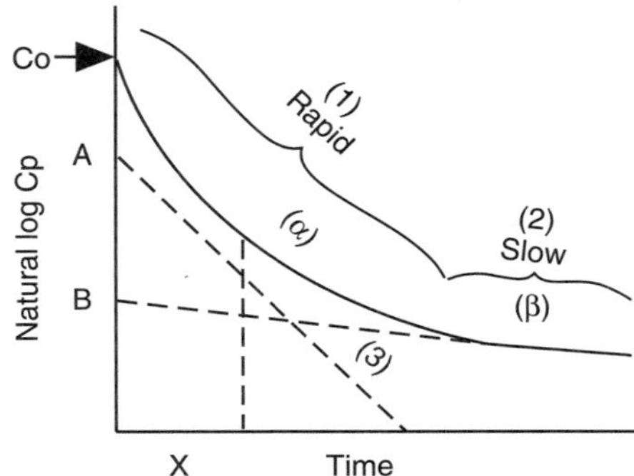

FIGURE **5-8**
The plot of the natural log of drug concentration. For drugs that conform to the two-compartment model, the plot of the natural log of the drug concentration is not linear along its entire length. Rather, it is curvilinear. The initial segment *(1)*, which represents the decline in drug concentration, is parabolic, then linear *(2)*. This decline in the drug concentration is also described as *biphasic*—a rapid phase, representing distribution, and a slow phase, representing elimination. The slope of the slow phase *(2)* is determined in a manner similar to that used for the elimination rate constant, k_{el}, in the one-compartment model.

falls exponentially because of elimination. This portion of the graph is much less steep and has a plateau shape, illustrating the more gradual decline in the drug's plasma concentration. The slope is flatter because it reflects the elimination of the drug from the circulation by the hepatic, renal, and other systems, which is a more gradual process. The plasma concentration curve is an example of a biexponential decay curve, because two distinct components of decay exist—a steep slope that describes distribution and a second, less steep slope that depicts the elimination phase (Figure 5-8).[2]

The elimination phase of the plot is used to determine the elimination half-life of drugs, which becomes important with regard to dosing intervals.

Steady State

A steady state occurs when, theoretically, a stable plasma concentration of a drug is achieved. In this instance all body compartments will have had ample opportunity to equilibrate with the circulating agent, and although tissue concentrations of the drug vary from organ to organ, they are not changing. At this point drug elimination is equal to the rate at which drug is made available, so the amount being eliminated in a given time equals the amount being added to the system at the same time.[17] This state is typically reached with chronic administration of a drug or by continuous intravenous administration. Some important distribution concepts are listed in Box 5-5.

Metabolism

Drug *metabolism* is synonymous with drug *biotransformation*. Metabolism is an enzyme-catalyzed change in the chemical structure of agents, and it usually involves more than one pathway. The main organ for drug metabolism is the liver, although metabolism can occur in the plasma, lungs, gastrointestinal tract, kidneys, heart, brain, and skin. The goal of metabolism is to change lipid-soluble agents into more water-soluble forms so that the kidneys can then eliminate them from the body. Metabolism usually leads to transformation of active drugs into inactive metabolites; however, numerous consequences can occur. For example, a drug can be metabolized to an active drug with the same or new activity, or an agent can be converted from an inactive prodrug to its active form, as occurs with the metabolism of inactive enalapril to active enalaprilat.

For most drugs administered in therapeutic doses, metabolism occurs as a first-order process, in that the drug is cleared at a rate proportional to the amount of drug present in the plasma. Thus a constant fraction of total drug is metabolized in a set time period. The greatest amount of drug eliminated per unit time occurs when the concentration is highest.[18]

Drugs such as alcohol undergo zero-order kinetics at therapeutic doses. This means that even at therapeutic levels they exceed the body's ability to excrete or metabolize them. In

BOX **5-5**

Drug Distribution

- The major compartments are as follows:
  - Plasma (5% of body weight)
  - Interstitial fluid (16%)
  - Intracellular fluid (35%)
  - Transcellular fluid (2%)
  - Fat (20%)
- Volume of distribution (V_d) is defined as the volume of plasma that would contain the total body content of the drug at a concentration equal to that in the plasma.
- Water-soluble drugs are mainly confined to plasma and interstitial fluids; most do not enter the brain after acute dosing.
- Lipid-soluble drugs reach all compartments and may accumulate in fat.
- For drugs that accumulate outside the plasma compartment (e.g., in fat, or by being bound to tissues) V_d may exceed total body volume.
- For many drugs, disappearance from the plasma follows an exponential time course characterized by the plasma half-life.
- Plasma half-life, in the simple case, is directly proportional to the volume of distribution and inversely proportional to the overall rate of clearance.
- With repeated dosage or sustained delivery of a drug, the plasma concentration approaches a steady value within 4 to 5 plasma half-lives. Elimination of a drug also takes 4 to 5 half-lives.
- A two-compartment model is often needed. In this case the kinetics are biexponential. The two components roughly represent the processes of transfer between plasma and tissues or distribution (α phase) and elimination from the plasma (β phase).
- Some drugs show nonexponential "saturation" kinetics, with important clinical consequences, especially a disproportionate increase in steady-state plasma concentration when the dose is increased.

Modified with permission from Rang HP, Dale MM, Ritter JM, et al: Absorption and distribution of drugs. In: Pharmacology. *5th ed. Edinburgh: Churchill Livingstone; 2003:42.*

zero-order kinetics the available enzyme systems for elimination of drugs are saturated. For these agents a constant amount of drug is cleared regardless of the plasma concentration, as opposed to a constant percentage as occurs with first-order kinetics. The amount of agent cleared per unit time during zero-order kinetics is the same amount, independent of its plasma concentration. The least common type is Michaelis-Menton models (e.g., phenytoin), which are dose dependent and follow zero order at high doses and first order after drug levels have fallen.

Drug metabolism occurs in two phases. Phase I reactions are oxidation, reduction, and hydrolysis reactions and generally result in increased polarity of the molecule, transforming a lipid-soluble compound to a water-soluble one. Phase II reactions involve conjugation reactions, in which a drug or metabolite is conjugated with endogenous substrate such as glucuronic, sulfonic, or acetic acid.

Phase I Reactions

Oxidation reactions generally are reactions in which oxygen is introduced into the molecule or the oxidative state of a molecule is changed so that its relative oxygen content is increased. The molecule of oxygen is split; one atom oxidizes each molecule of drug, and the other is incorporated into a molecule of water. The loss of electrons results in oxidation. Oxidative metabolism reactions are catalyzed by the enzymes of the cytochrome P-450 system.[19] Reduction pathways of metabolism also use the cytochrome P-450 system. When insufficient amounts of oxygen are present to compete for electrons, these enzymes transfer electrons directly to a substrate rather than to oxygen. Reduction involves the gain of electrons.[20]

Hydrolysis is the addition of water to an ester or amide to break the bond and form two smaller molecules. The addition of water to these compounds leads to an acid and alcohol in the case of esters and to an acid and an amine in the case of amides. Amide drugs rarely undergo hydrolysis even though they are formed by removing water. Steric hindrance limits the ability to add water to a drug (hydrolyze it) once the water has been removed. Examples of drugs that are hydrolyzed are listed in Table 5-3.

The end result of phase I reactions is typically a more polar compound that is easily excreted by the kidneys. It is also important to note that phase I reactions, by placing hydroxy or carboxy groups on drug molecules, enable Phase II reactions to occur.[1]

TABLE 5-3 Common Anesthesia-Related Drugs That Undergo Phase 1 Hydrolysis

Cholinesterase Catalyzed	Non–Esterase Dependent
Succinylcholine	Remifentanil
Mivacurium	Atracurium (partial pathway)
Cocaine	Cisatracurium (partial pathway)
Procaine	Esmolol
Chloroprocaine	
Tetracaine	
Neostigmine (partial pathway)	
Pyridostigmine (partial pathway)	
Edrophonium (partial pathway)	

Phase II Reactions

Phase II reactions are also referred to as *synthetic reactions*, because the body actually synthesizes a new compound by donating a functional group usually derived from an endogenous acid. The new compound is the conjugate of the drug or the drug product of the phase I reaction with either glucuronic acid, sulfuric acid, glycine, acetic acid, or a methyl group.[17]

The products of phase II reactions almost always have little or no biologic activity. Conjugation always leads to a more polar compound that is more highly ionized at physiologic pH and therefore more easily extractable by the kidney via glomerular filtration. The conjugation proceeds by joining the body's donated group (during phase I reactions) with an OH, COOH, or NH group to form an ester or amide bond. However, many drugs already possess an appropriate functional group for conjugation and therefore do not need to be modified by a prior phase I reaction in order to be conjugated.

Many intracellular sites exist for drug metabolizing enzymes, such as the endoplasmic reticulum, mitochondria, cytosol, lysosomes, and plasma membrane. Hepatic microsomal enzymes, responsible for biotransformation of numerous agents, reside mainly in the smooth hepatic endoplasmic reticulum. They are termed *microsomal enzymes* because microsomes are fragments of the endoplasmic reticulum that are obtained in vitro by physical disruption of the tissue and differential centrifugation. This microsomal fraction includes a protein called *cytochrome* (iron-containing hemoprotein) *P-450*, indicating its peak absorption at 450 nm, when it reacts with carbon monoxide. The cytochrome P-450 is also called the *mixed-function oxidase system*, as it includes both oxidation and reduction steps and has low substrate specificty.[2] Some extrahepatic sites of the P-450 system exist, such as the kidneys, lungs, skin, and intestinal mucosa.

Six well-characterized forms, or isozymes, of the cytochrome P-450 system are involved in drug metabolism in humans: CYP1A2, CYP2D6, CYP2C19, CYP2E1, CYP2C9, and CYP3A.[21] The letters *CYP* stand for cytochrome P-450; the first number denotes genetic family; the second letter describes the genetic subfamily; and, finally, the second number stands for the specific gene or isozyme.

It is important to note some characteristics of these isozymes. It should be appreciated that small differences in amino acid sequences of the different isozymes lead to differences in drug metabolism and account for genetic variability among individuals' abilities to metabolize agents.[21] Therefore hepatic enzyme activity varies among individuals and is determined genetically. Genetic variability exists in the expression of CYP2C19, CYP2C9, and CYP2D6. It is possible to increase enzyme activity by stimulating the enzymes over a period of time. This is called *enzyme induction* and is usually produced by exposure to certain drug or chemical compounds. Alcohol is one such compound; when ingested chronically it induces enzymatic activity. The system can more quickly break down agents that use the same enzymatic system for biotransformation. Other drugs capable of enzyme induction include phenobarbital, phenytoin, rifampin, and carbamazepine. This increased capacity to clear drugs leads to reduction in half-lives of agents and is important with regard to dosing intervals.[22,23]

Microsomal enzymes also can be inhibited. This usually occurs through exposure to certain drugs and chemicals, which leads to accumulation of the substrate agent. This can cause elevated plasma levels and potentially greater activity and toxicity. For example, erythromycin inhibits the metabolism of theophylline, and cimetidine inhibits metabolism of many drugs.[21] Box 5-6 contains a summary of important metabolic concepts. A list of cytochrome enzymes, metabolites, inducers, and inhibitors is given in Table 5-4.

Drug Elimination

Elimination Half-life

The elimination half-life ($t\frac{1}{2}$) is the time necessary for the plasma content of a drug to drop to half of its prevailing concentration after a rapid bolus injection. It takes the same amount of time to reduce a drug's concentration from 100 mg/L to 50 mg/L as to decrease the concentration from 10 mg/L to 5 mg/L. The amount of drug remaining in the body is related to the number of elimination half-lives that have elapsed (Table 5-5). For practical purposes, a drug is regarded as being fully eliminated when approximately 95% has been eliminated from the body. This usually occurs when four or five half-times have elapsed and is important with regard to dosing intervals, in that drug accumulation occurs if dosing intervals are shorter than this. The body has not been able to rid itself of the initial dose, and subsequent doses will lead to overdose and potential adverse effects. Instances can occur in which, although only 5% of the drug amount remains, it is still somewhat active; however, for the majority of agents four half-times is considered sufficient time for the drug's action to be terminated and the agent eliminated from the body. As noted earlier, most drugs leave the body at a constant rate or percentage over time. This is referred to as *first-order kinetics* or *dosage independence* and is the reason why half-life is constant. Other elimination rate kinetic models include zero-order (e.g., alcohol) elimination, in which a constant amount (not a percentage) is eliminated over time, and Michaelis-Menton models (e.g., phenytoin), which are dose dependent and follow zero order at high doses and first order once drug levels have fallen.[2]

BOX 5-6

Drug Metabolism

- Phase I reactions involve oxidation, reduction, and hydrolysis—usually form more chemically reactive products; sometimes pharmacologically active, as with thiopental; toxic or carcinogenic
- Phase II reactions are conjugation (e.g., glucuronidation) of a reactive group (often inserted during phase I reaction) and usually form inactive and readily excretable products
- Some conjugated products are excreted via bile, are reactivated in the intestine and then reabsorbed
- Induction of enzymes by other drugs and chemicals can greatly accelerate hepatic drug metabolism
- Some drugs show rapid "first-pass" hepatic metabolism and therefore poor oral bioavailability

Modified with permission from Rang HP, Dale MM, Ritter JM, et al. Drug elimination and pharmacokinetics. In: Pharmacology. *5th ed. Edinburgh: Churchill Livingstone; 2003:110.*

Context-Sensitive Half-Time

Deficiencies in the use of standard pharmacokinetic parameters such as half-life when describing anesthetic drug administration have led to the proposal for the introduction of a new model that accounts for continuous infusion or repeated dosing-induced changes in drug behavior.[24] Context-sensitive half-time was developed through use of computer simulations of typical anesthetic dosing practices to provide a more clinically relevant measure of drug concentrations, taking into consideration the method and duration of administration.[25] It is defined as the time to halving of the blood concentration after termination of drug administration by an infusion designed to maintain a constant concentration. It is believed that through incorporation of the effect compartment the context-sensitive half-time of the pharmacodynamic effect can be modelled.[26] A flaw in the concept is that it describes only the time to a 50% decrease in central compartment concentration, which may not be the decrement in drug level required to achieve recovery.[27] Whether context-sensitive half-time is a useful secondary kinetic descriptor may await its more widespread application.

Clearance

The clearance of a drug is an independent value and is governed by the properties of the drug and the body's capacity to eliminate it. It is defined as the volume of plasma completely cleared of drug by metabolism and excretion per unit of time. Clearance is directly proportional to the dose and inversely related to the agent's half-life as well as its concentration in the central compartment. Clearance is a very important pharmacokinetic concept, because it influences the steady-state concentration for a given drug given at repeated intervals or by infusion.

The two main organs for clearance are the liver and the kidneys. The rate of clearance is determined by the blood flow to these organs as well as by their ability to extract the drug from the bloodstream. Mathematically, clearance is equal to the product of the blood flow (Q) and extraction ratio (E):

Equation 5-4

$$\text{Clearance} = Q \times E$$

Total clearance is the sum of all organs' clearance values. The changes in clearance occur when blood flow to the liver or kidney is altered or when their extraction ratios are changed.

Hepatic Clearance. Drugs typically go through perfusion-dependent elimination or capacity-dependent elimination in the liver. Drugs that have a high extraction ratio of 0.7 or greater rely heavily on the perfusion of the liver to be cleared. These drugs are referred to as *high-clearance drugs*. Examples of high-clearance drugs are verapamil, morphine, and lidocaine. Hepatic blood flow for these agents far outweighs enzymatic activity in clearing the body of them, so a decrease in hepatic blood flow decreases the rate of clearance, and a high perfusion state leads to faster clearance. This is termed *perfusion-dependent* elimination.[1]

Capacity-dependent elimination occurs with agents that possess a low extraction ratio of 0.3 or lower. When a low extraction rate exists, only a small fraction of the agent is removed per unit time, and changes in hepatic perfusion do not have significant effect on hepatic clearance. Clearance of

TABLE 5-4 List of Cytochrome Enzymes, Metabolites, Inducers, and Inhibitors

Isozyme	Metabolic Substrates	Inducers	Inhibitors
CYP1A2	Theophylline—has a narrow therapeutic range, so inhibition of its metabolism can lead to toxic levels Imipramine Propanolol Clozapine	Tobacco smoke—smokers may require higher doses of these drugs because their metabolism is increased	Ciprofloxacin Erythromycin
CYP2C19—absent in 20%-30% of Asians, who therefore need a reduced dose when these drugs are administered	Diazepam Phenytoin Omeprazole (proton pump inhibitor for ulcers)		Omeprazole Ketoconazole (antifungal agent) Isoniazid
CYP2C9—absent in approximately 1% of whites	NSAIDs COX II inhibitors Warfarin Phenytoin		Fluconazole
CYP2D6—absent in approximately 7% of whites; hyperactive in approximately 30% of East Africans (Ethiopians) because they have multiple copies of the gene	Codeine → Morphine Some β-blockers Some tricyclic antidepressants		Fluoxetine Haloperidol Paroxetine Quinidine
CYP2E1	Acetaminophen Ethanol Some halogenated hydrocarbons such as halothane	Chronic ethanol Isoniazid	Disulfiram
CYP3A—present in GI tract and liver; responsible for a large amount of first-pass metabolism	Calcium channel blockers Most benzodiazepines HIV protease inhibitors HMG-CoA reductase inhibitors (lipid lowering agents) Cyclosporine (immunosuppressant) Most nonsedating antihistamines Cisapride (gastric motility agent)	Carbamazepine Rifampin Rifabutin (to treat TB) Ritonavir (to treat HIV) St. John's wort (herbal product used for depression and menopause)	Azole antifungal agents such as itraconazole Ketoconazole Fluconazole Cimetidine (broad range P450 inhibitor) Macrolide Antibiotics (but *not* azithromycin) Grapefruit juice

COX, *Cyclooxygenase;* GI, *gastrointestinal;* HIV, *human immunodeficiency virus;* HMG-CoA, *3-hydroxy-3-methylglutaryl coenzyme* A; NSAIDs, *nonsteroidal antiinflammatory drugs;* TB, *tuberculosis.*

TABLE 5-5 Relationship between Half-Life and Drug Remaining in the Body

Half-Life	Drug Eliminated (%)	Drug Remaining (%)
0	0	100
1	50	50
2	75	25
3	87.5	12.5
4	93.75	6.25
5	96.875	3.125

these drugs depends on hepatic enzymes and the degree of protein binding. Therefore alterations such as enzyme induction or suppression cause a change in the elimination of these drugs from the body. An increase in enzyme activity causes faster elimination from the body, and enzyme suppression has the opposite outcome. A decrease in protein binding (increase in availability of drug at hepatocytes) also leads to a greater rate of clearance. Examples of drugs with a low hepatic extraction ratio are thiopental, diazepam, and theophylline.[1]

Renal Clearance. The kidneys excrete water-soluble molecules with great ease. The excretion of drugs involves passive glomerular filtration, active tubular secretion, and some reabsorption. Selected substances that are actively secreted are noted in Table 5-6. The amount of drug made available to the renal tubule for elimination depends on the amount of free, unbound drug and the glomerular filtration rate. Water-soluble metabolites are filtered by the glomeruli and eliminated. The kidneys do not excrete lipid-soluble agents as efficiently as water-soluble compounds. For these agents elimination depends on the liver for metabolism into water-soluble molecules. Indeed, increased water solubility reduces the volume of

TABLE 5-6 Important Drugs and Related Substances Actively Secreted into the Proximal Renal Tubule

Acids	Bases
ρ-Aminohippuric acid	Amiloride
Furosemide	Dopamine
Glucuronic acid conjugates	Histamine
Glycine conjugates	Mepacrine
Indomethacin	Morphine
Methotrexate	Meperidine
Penicillin	Quaternary ammonium compounds
Probenecid	Quinine
Sulphate conjugates	5-Hydroxytryptamine (serotonin)
Thiazide diuretics	Triamterene
Uric acid	

Modified with permission from Rang HP, Dale MM, Ritter JM, et al. Drug elimination and pharmacokinetics. In: Pharmacology. *5th ed. Edinburgh: Churchill Livingstone; 2003.*

distribution of agents, leading to their excretion by the kidneys. Conversely, lipid-soluble molecules are reabsorbed from the renal tubules back into the systemic circulation. An example of a lipid-soluble drug that is almost completely reabsorbed (such that little or none of it is excreted unchanged) is thiopental.

The pH of the urine can also affect the elimination of drugs. Weak acids are better excreted in alkaline urine, and, conversely, weak bases are readily excreted in acid urine. The kidneys can use glomerular filtration for elimination of drugs that are highly polar (e.g., aminoglycoside antibiotics). Certain agents (e.g., penicillin) are eliminated via secretion. Some important clearance concepts are noted in Box 5-7.

BOX 5-7

Elimination of Drugs by the Kidney

- Most drugs, unless highly bound to plasma protein, cross the glomerular filter freely.
- Many drugs, especially weak acids and weak bases, are actively secreted into the renal tubule and therefore are more rapidly excreted.
- Lipid-soluble drugs are passively reabsorbed by diffusion across the tubule and are not efficiently excreted in the urine.
- Because of pH partition, weak acids are more rapidly excreted in alkaline urine, and vice versa.
- Several important drugs are removed predominately by renal excretion and are liable to cause toxicity in elderly persons and patients with renal disease.

Modified with permission from Rang HP, Dale MM, Ritter JM, et al. Drug elimination and pharmacokinetics. In: Pharmacology. *5th ed. Edinburgh: Churchill Livingstone; 2003:112.*

OTHER FACTORS THAT INFLUENCE PHARMACOKINETICS

Age

Age plays an important role in the manner in which drug disposition occurs. Elderly patients have a decrease in renal function, resulting in impaired excretion of agents that are eliminated in the urine.[6] Creatinine clearance, as an indicator of renal function, parallels the kidney's ability to excrete drugs and is a useful test in predicting renal pharmacokinetics in the elderly.[2] Liver blood flow decreases with age as well, decreasing the metabolism of agents with moderate to high extraction ratios. The elderly also have an increase in the fat compartment, leading to an increased volume of distribution, which can lead to accumulation of lipid-soluble agents.[9] Liver and renal function are also important in neonates. Elimination of drugs via the kidneys is altered in neonates because of poor renal function in the first year of life. Neonates and premature infants lack the ability to metabolize certain agents because of immature liver enzyme systems.[2] It is therefore important to consider extremes of age when administering any agent that may be highly lipid soluble with a high hepatic extraction ratio or that relies primarily on the kidneys for elimination.

Gender

Gender differences account for some variability in the pharmacokinetics of many agents. In a recent review of the literature, it was found that female patients had a 20% to 30% greater sensitivity to the muscle relaxant effects of vecuronium, pancuronium, and rocuronium.[13] It was also found that male patients were more sensitive to propofol than female patients and that it may be necessary to reduce propofol doses in male patients.[28] In 1999 Gan and co-workers studied emergence from general anesthesia with propofol, alfentanil, and nitrous oxide. Female patients emerged significantly more quickly than male patients. In fact, female patients were three times more likely than male patients to experience recall under general anesthesia.[29] Conversely, female patients were shown to be more sensitive to opioid receptor agonists, with their male counterparts requiring 30% to 40% more narcotics for management of pain.[28]

Temperature

Because temperature affects tissue metabolism and blood flow, it follows that the pharmacokinetics of agents are also affected by varying temperatures. In a 2002 study, Knibbe and colleagues examined the pharmacokinetics of long-term propofol sedation in critically ill patients. Temperature was a significant covariate for clearance of propofol. Warmer temperatures led to faster elimination of propofol regardless of the concentration of the drug in solution.[30]

Disease States

Comorbidity accounts for some of the variability observed in drug pharmacokinetics. The pharmacokinetics of ropivacaine in patients with and without uremia after axillary brachial plexus block was examined. An enhanced absorption and larger total plasma concentrations of ropivacaine and its main metabolite were noted in the patients with uremia.[31] Conversely, Goyal and colleagues found a negative correlation of propofol dose with preoperative hemoglobin concentration in patients with renal failure. They concluded that the hyperdynamic state caused by anemia in these patients was responsible for their higher propofol dose requirement.[32]

BOX 5-8

Summary of Pharmacokinetic Principles

- Clinical pharmacokinetics is the discipline that describes the absorption, distribution, metabolism, and elimination of drugs in patients who require drug therapy.
- Clearance is the most important pharmacokinetic parameter, because it determines the steady-state concentration for a given dosage rate. Physiologically, clearance is determined by blood flow to the organ that metabolizes or eliminates the drug and the efficiency of the organ in extracting the drug from the bloodstream.
- The dosage and clearance determine the steady-state concentration.
- The fraction of drug absorbed into the systemic circulation after extravascular administration is defined as its bioavailability.
- Pharmacokinetic models are useful for description of data sets, prediction of serum concentrations after several doses or different routes of administration, and calculation of pharmacokinetic constants such as clearance, volume of distribution, and half-life. The simplest case uses a single compartment to represent the entire body.
- The volume of distribution determines the loading dose.
- Half-life is the time required for serum concentration to decrease by one half after absorption and distribution are complete. Half-life is important because it determines the time required to reach steady state and the dosage interval. Half-life is a dependent kinetic variable, because its value depends on the values of clearance and volume of distribution.
- The half-life determines the time to reach steady state and the time for "all" drug to be eliminated from the body.
- If a drug obeys first-order pharmacokinetics, then a simple ratio of dosage to steady-state concentration can be used to estimate a new dosage as long as the clearance has not changed.
- Phenytoin is an example of a drug that obeys Michaelis-Menton rather than first-order pharmacokinetics. In this case, as plasma concentration increases, the clearance decreases and the half-life becomes longer.
- *Cytochrome P450* is a generic term for the group of enzymes that are responsible for most drug metabolism oxidation reactions. Several P450 isozymes have been identified, including CYP1A2, CYP2C9, CYP2C19, CYP2D6, CYP2E1, and CYP3A4.
- Factors to be taken into consideration when deciding on the best drug dose for a patient include age, gender, weight, ethnic background, other concurrent disease states, and other drug therapy.
- The importance of transport proteins in drug bioavailability and elimination is now better understood. The principal transport protein involved in the movement of drugs across biologic membranes is P-glycoprotein. P-glycoprotein is present in many organs, including the gastrointestinal tract, liver, and kidney.

Modified from Bauer LA: Clinical pharmacokinetics and pharmacodynamics. In: Dipiro JT, Talbert RL, Yee GC et al, eds. Pharmacotherapy: A Pathophysiological Approach. *5th ed. New York: McGraw-Hill; 2002:52-53; and Laizure SC, Yanishevsi Y, Evans WE. Clinical pharmacodynamics. In: Herfindal ET, Gourley DR, eds.* Textbook of Therapeutics: Drug and Disease Management. *7th ed. Philadelphia: Lippincott Williams & Wilkins; 2000:19-20.*

Other disease states can cause variability, as illustrated by a recent study that found an increase in the volume distribution of ketamine disproportional to increases in clearance in spinal cord injury inpatients in the intensive care unit, leading to a longer than expected half-life for the drug, again placing the patients at risk for overdose.[33]

A summary of some pharmacokinetic principles is given in Box 5-8.

REFERENCES

1. Katsung BG. Basic Principles. In: Katsung BG, ed. *Basic and Clinical Pharmacology*. 9th ed. New York: McGraw Hill; 2004:1- 64.
2. Wilkinson GR. Pharmacokinetics: the dynamics of drug absorption, distribution and elimination. In: Hardman JG, Limbird LE, eds. *Goodman and Gilman's the Pharmacological Basis of Therapeutics*. 10th ed. New York: McGraw-Hill; 2001:3-30.
3. Troop, M. Pharmacokinetics. In: Nagelhout JJ, Zaglaniczny KL, eds. *Nurse Anesthesia*. Philadelphia: Saunders; 2001:60-87.
4. du Souich P, Verges J, Eril S. Plasma protein binding and pharmacological response. *Clin Pharmacokinet*. 1993;24:435-440.
5. Shargel L, Yu AB. *Applied Biopharmaceutics and Pharmacokinetics*. Stanford, Conn: McGraw-Hill/Appleton and Lange; 1999:29-45.
6. Schywalsky M, Ihmsen H, Tzabazis A, et al. Pharmacokinetics and pharmacodynamics of the new propofol prodrug GPI 15715 in rats. *Eur J Anaesthesiol*. 2003;20:82-90.
7. Gibaldi M, Perrier D. Pharmacokinetics. In: *Drugs and the Pharmaceutical Sciences*. Vol 15. New York: Marcel Dekker; 1982:54-109, 451-457.
8. Gibaldi M, Boyes RN, Feldman S. Influence of first pass effect on availability of drugs on oral administration. *J Pharm Sci*. 1971;60:1338-1340.
9. Wu C-Y, Benet LZ, Hebert MF, et al. Differentiation of absorption and first pass gut and hepatic metabolism in humans: studies with cyclosporine. *Clin Pharmacol Ther*. 1995;58:492-497.
10. Wingard A. *Human Pharmacology*. St Louis: Mosby; 1994:12-32.
11. Hudson RJ. Basic principles of clinical pharmacology. In: Barash PG, Cullen BF, Stoelting RK, eds. *Clinical Anesthesia*. Philadelphia: Lippincott Williams & Wilkins; 1999:221-235.
12. Koup JR, Gibaldi M. Some comments on the evaluation of bioavailability data. *Drug Intell Clin Pharm*. 1980;14:327-330.
13. Kazama T, Morita K, Ikeda T, et al. Comparison of predicted induction dose with predetermined physiologic characteristics of patients and with pharmacokinetic models incorporating those characteristics as covariates. *Anesthesiology*. 2003:98:229-305.
14. Guyton AC, Hall JE. *Textbook of Medical Physiology*. Philadelphia: Saunders; 2000:797-800.
15. Fechner J, Ihmsen H, Hatterscheid D, et al. Pharmacokinetics and clinical pharmacodynamics of the new propofol prodrug GPI 15715 in volunteers. *Anesthesiology*. 2003:99(2), 303-313.
16. Wagner JG. *Fundamentals of Clinical Pharmacokinetics*. Hamilton, Ill: American Pharmaceutical Association; 1980:57-116.
17. Ortiz de Montellano P. *Cytochrome P-450: Structure, Mechanism, and Biochemistry*. New York: Plenum; 1986:45-67.

18. Rowland M, Tozer TN. *Clinical Pharmacokinetics: Concepts and Applications*. 3rd ed. Baltimore: Williams & Wilkins; 1995:33-62.
19. Smith CM, Reynard AM. *Textbook of Pharmacology*. Philadelphia: Saunders; 1992:57-86.
20. Boobis AR, Edwards RJ, Adams DA, et al. Dissecting the function of P450. *BR J Clin Pharmacol*. 1996;42:81-89.
21. Gonzalez FJ, Korzekwa KR. Cytochromes P450 expression systems. *Annu Rev Pharmacol Toxicol*. 1995;35:269-390.
22. Lin JH, Lu AY. Interindividual variability in inhibition and induction of cytochrome P450 enzymes. *Annu Rev Pharmacol Toxicol*. 2001:41:535-567.
23. Raunio H, Hakkola J, Hukkanen J, et al. Expression of xenobiotic-metabolizing cytochrome P450s in human pulmonary tissues. *Arch Toxicol Suppl* 1998:20:465-469.
24. Hughes MA, Glass PSA, Jacobs JR. Context-sensitive half-life in multi-compartment pharmacokinetic models for intravenous anesthetic drugs. *Anesthesiology*. 1992;76:334-341.
25. Kapila A, Glass PSA, Jacobs JR, et al. Measured context-sensitive half-times of remifentanil and alfentanil. *Anesthesiology*. 1995:83:968-975.
26. Fisher DM. (Almost) everything you learned about pharmacokinetics was (somewhat) wrong! *Anesth Analg*. 1996;8:901-903.
27. Recovery from anaesthesia: which is the best kinetic descriptor of a drug's recovery profile? [editorial] *Anaesthesia*. 1996;51, 997-999.
28. Pleym H, Spigset O, Kharasch ED, Dale O. Gender differences in drug effects: implications for anesthesiologists. *Acta Anaesthesiol Scand*. 2003:47:241-259.
29. Gan TJ, Glass PS, Sigl J, et al. Women emerge from general anesthesia with propofol/alfentanil/nitrous oxide faster than men. *Anesthesiology*. 1999:90:1283-1287.
30. Knibbe CA, Zuideveld KP, DeJongh J, et al. Population pharmacokinetics and pharmacodynamic modeling of propofol for long-term sedation in critically ill patients: a comparison between propofol 6% and propofol 1%. *Clinic Pharmacol Ther*. 2002:72:670-684.
31. Pere P, Salonen M, Jokinen M, et al. Pharmacokinetics of ropivacaine in uremic and nonuremic patients after axillary brachial plexus block. *Anesth Analg*. 2003:96:563-569.
32. Goyal P, Puri GD, Pandey CK, Srivastva S. Evaluation of induction doses of propofol: comparison between endstage renal disease and normal renal function patients. *Anaesth Intensive Care*. 2002:30:584-587.
33. Hijazi Y, Bodonian C, Bolon M, et al. Pharmacokinetics and haemodynamics of ketamine in intensive care patients with brain or spinal cord injury. *Br J Anaesth*. 2003:90:155-160.

CHAPTER 6

Pharmacokinetics of Inhalation Anesthetics

John J. Nagelhout

As with any drug, the basic action of an anesthetic in the body is largely a function of the drug's chemical structure and the resulting interaction with a cellular receptor complex (Figure 6-1). A number of heterogenous compounds exhibit anesthetic properties. The inorganic molecule nitrous oxide; hydrocarbons such as halothane; and halogenated ethers such as isoflurane, desflurane, and sevoflurane are all capable of binding to central nervous system and spinal cord neuronal membranes to produce reversible depression. A single specific anesthetic receptor has yet to be found, and in fact multiple sites of action probably exist; however, once a critical concentration of drug has entered the brain and spinal cord, loss of consciousness ensues.[1]

The administration of inhalation anesthetic gases plays a primary role in modern clinical anesthesia. In the early years of anesthesia, administration of a gas such as diethyl ether constituted the entire anesthetic regimen. Now, one or two gas anesthetics are combined with a variety of intravenous drugs to produce an anesthetic state. These intravenous drugs include sedative induction agents, analgesics, neuromuscular blocking drugs, and local anesthetics. The use of such a combination allows the anesthetist to use smaller and more easily manipulated doses of specific receptor agonists and antagonists. Used in the proper combination, the desired amount of anesthesia, analgesia, amnesia, and muscle relaxation can be achieved. Current anesthetic and surgical practice dictates that the anesthetic technique allow for a quick and pleasant induction and recovery with maximum patient safety and efficient caseload management. A sound understanding of the pharmacokinetics of the anesthetic gases is essential to such safe practice.

PRIMARY FACTORS CONTROLLING UPTAKE, DISTRIBUTION, AND ELIMINATION OF ANESTHETICS

The basic task of anesthetic administration involves taking a drug supplied as a liquid, vaporizing it in an anesthesia machine, and delivering it to the patient's brain and other tissues via the lungs. Therefore the main factors that influence the ability to anesthetize a patient are technical or machine specific, drug related, respiratory, circulatory, and tissue related. This process is shown conceptually in Figure 6-2.

A few assumptions usually are made. The level of anesthesia is related to the alveolar concentrations of anesthetic agents, which can be readily and continuously measured or inferred. The concentration or partial pressure of anesthetic in the lungs is assumed to be the same as that in the brain, because the drugs are highly lipid soluble and diffusible, and they quickly and easily reach equilibrium between the body compartments. For this reason, the dose of an individual drug is expressed in terms of the minimum alveolar concentration (MAC) necessary to produce anesthesia (lack of movement) on surgical stimulation.[2,3] The faster the lung (and therefore brain) concentration rises, the faster anesthesia is achieved. Conversely, the faster the lung (brain) concentration falls after discontinuation of the drug, the more quickly the patient emerges.[4]

Machine-Related Factors

Concepts regarding the anesthesia machine and its function are described in detail in Chapter 15. Two factors that may affect uptake early in anesthetic administration are drug solubility in the rubber and plastic machine parts and total machine liter flow of the gases chosen.

The rubber and plastic components of the machine as well as the ventilator and absorbent can retain small quantities of anesthetic gases. Theoretically, this could slow administration to the patient at the start of anesthetic delivery. The effect on uptake is minimal in actual clinical practice and essentially ceases after approximately 15 minutes of administration.[5] Nonetheless, sequestration of small amounts of gas in the machine apparatus has other implications, such as when anesthetizing patients with malignant hyperthermia. All gases except nitrous oxide are potent triggering agents for a hyperthermic episode. To avoid exposure resulting from residual trace amounts of gases, a thorough flush with 100% oxygen for at least 10 minutes, replacement of breathing circuits and the carbon dioxide canister, and draining, inactivation, or removal of vaporizers are advised when preparing for a patient who is susceptible to malignant hyperthermia.[6]

Low liter flows of oxygen and nitrous oxide carrier gas, although economical, deliver the anesthetic more slowly at the start of induction. Increasing liter flows for the first few minutes of the anesthetic minimizes this effect without unduly adding to cost.[7]

Drug-Related Factors

Blood-Gas Solubility

The blood-gas solubility coefficient of an anesthetic is an indicator of the speed of uptake and elimination.[8,9] It reflects the proportion of the anesthetic that will be soluble in the blood, "bind" to blood components, and not readily enter the tissues (blood phase), versus the fraction of the drug that *will* leave the blood and quickly diffuse into tissues (gas phase). The more soluble the drug (high blood-gas coefficient), the slower the brain and spinal cord uptake and therefore the

Isoflurane

N≡N=O

Nitrous oxide

Halothane

Desflurane

Sevoflurane

FIGURE **6-1**
Chemical structure of anesthetic agents. Nitrous oxide is inorganic, halothane is a halogenated hydrocarbon, and the rest are halogenated ethers.

slower the anesthesia achieved by the patient. Highly soluble drugs stay in the blood in greater proportion than less-soluble agents; therefore, less of the drug is released to the tissues during the early, rapid-uptake phase of induction. For example, halothane has a blood-gas solubility coefficient of 2.3 or, expressed as a ratio, 2.3:1. Therefore 2.3 times as much stays in the blood as a nonreleasable fraction for every molecule that enters the tissues and produces anesthesia. Conversely, agents with low solubility properties (low blood-gas coefficient) leave the blood quickly and enter the tissues, producing a rapid anesthetic state. Desflurane, for example, has a low blood-gas coefficient of 0.47 or, expressed as a ratio, 0.47:1. Only 0.47 molecule stays in the blood for every 1 (greater than twice as much) that enters the brain. Anesthesia is achieved quickly. Blood-gas solubility coefficients for the inhalation anesthetic agents are listed in Table 6-1.[10] The rate of rise of an anesthetic in the alveoli relative to the concentration administered is graphically depicted by plotting the fraction in the alveoli over the fraction inspired, as shown in Figure 6-3. As noted previously, the lower the blood-gas solubility, the faster the rise in lung concentration. The rate of rise of low solubility agents such as nitrous oxide and desflurane is greater than moderately soluble drugs such as halothane. Note that nitrous oxide exhibits a slightly faster rate of rise compared with desflurane despite a higher blood-gas coefficient. This variation in the usual trend is a result of the concentration effect—that is, nitrous oxide is given at much higher concentrations (50% to 70%) than desflurane (3% to 9%).

TABLE **6-1** General Anesthetic Properties of Inhalation Agents

Anesthetic	MAC (%)	Blood-Gas Partition Coefficient (at 37° C)	Oil-Gas Partition Coefficient (at 37° C)
Sevoflurane (Ultane)	2	0.6	50
Halothane (Fluothane)	0.75	2.3	224
Isoflurane (Forane)	1.15	1.4	99
Nitrous oxide	105	0.47	1.4
Desflurane (Suprane)	5.8	0.42	18.7

VENTILATION FACTORS

As with all diffusible drugs, anesthetics move down a concentration gradient. Continuous inhalation administration of the agent into the lungs promotes subsequent diffusion into the blood and tissues as the anesthetic progresses. Anesthetic uptake slows throughout the surgical procedure.[11] The anesthetic is delivered, along with the necessary amount of oxygen or an oxygen mix appropriate for the patient's condition. Supplemental nitrous oxide is commonly used. Basically, the faster and more deeply a patient breathes or is ventilated, the faster the patient loses consciousness at the start of anesthesia and emerges at the end.[9] This is often referred to as the *ventilation effect.*

Ventilation-perfusion deficits or poor lung function hinders inhalation drug administration.[12] Rapid-acting (low blood-gas solubility) agents are affected by these deficits to a greater extent than are slower-acting (high blood-gas solubility) drugs.[13] These decreases in speed can be partially compensated for by increasing the concentration of insoluble (fast) agents or increasing ventilation with soluble (slow) drugs.

Concentration or Dose

During the first few minutes of gas administration, a higher concentration of the drug than necessary for maintenance, or a loading dose, is delivered to speed initial uptake. This is commonly referred to as *overpressuring* or the *concentration effect.*[14] Overpressuring during initial administration is a common clinical practice and is more effective the more soluble the anesthetic. In other words, overpressuring can speed the effect of

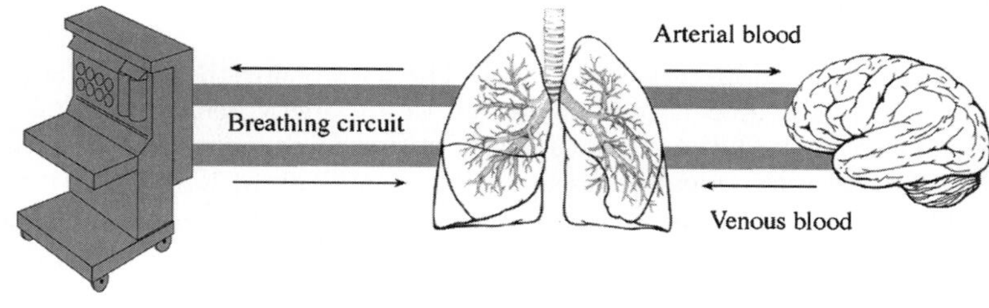

FIGURE **6-2**
The transfer of an anesthetic gas from the machine through the lungs into the blood and tissues.

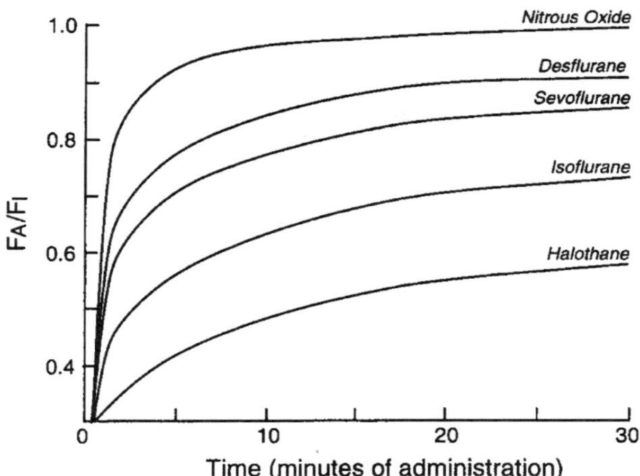

FIGURE **6-3**
The rate of rise (F_A/F_I) of the alveolar concentration of the inhalation anesthetics over time. The low blood gas anesthetics such as nitrous oxide and desflurane achieve a lung concentration much faster than the high solubility gases such as halothane. Note that nitrous oxide rises in the lungs more quickly than desflurane in spite of a slightly higher blood gas solubility. This is due to the concentration effect.

slow agents but has less of an effect on relatively fast agents. This practice follows the kinetic standard of using a loading dose to speed onset. After the first few minutes, the dose is decreased to normal maintenance levels.[15-17]

As noted previously, the dose of an anesthetic is expressed in terms of MAC—the relative concentration when the anesthetic is combined with all the other gases in the lungs. Induction and maintenance doses are given in Table 6-2.

Second-Gas Effect

Simultaneous administration of a relatively slow agent such as halothane and a faster drug such as nitrous oxide (in high concentrations) can speed the onset of the slower agent. This is known as the *second-gas effect*.[18] The uptake of the slower agent is increased by administering it with a high concentration of the faster anesthetic nitrous oxide. The faster the inherent speed of the second slower gas on its own, however, the less prominent the augmentation when given with nitrous oxide. For example, sevoflurane, which has a low blood solubility (blood-gas solubility coefficient 0.6) is rapidly taken up into tissues. Coadministration of sevoflurane with the slightly faster nitrous oxide produces only small and brief increases in sevoflurane uptake as compared with sevoflurane administration alone.[15-17] Others have questioned the validity of this concept.[19]

Tissue-Related Factors

Oil-Gas Solubility

The oil-gas solubility coefficient is an indicator of potency. The higher the solubility, the more potent the drug.[20,21] Oil-gas solubility coefficients are listed in Table 6-1. A high solubility coefficient reflects high lipid solubility. Because the anesthetic must traverse the blood-brain barrier and penetrate lipid cell membranes to produce its action, highly lipid-soluble drugs tend to be the most potent. Of the currently used agents, halothane (oil-gas partition coefficient 224) is the most potent, and nitrous oxide (oil-gas partition coefficient 1.4) is the least potent. Remember that two factors are at play: how fast the drug is delivered to the tissues (blood-gas solubility) and how efficiently it can access and affect the sites of action (oil-gas solubility). Recent investigations suggest that polarity along with lipophilicity plays an important yet not fully understood role in the mechanism of inhalation anesthetics.[22,23]

Circulatory Factors

The cardiovascular system exerts two major influences on anesthetic uptake and distribution.[24] First, the majority of the blood leaving the lungs with anesthetic is normally distributed to the vital organs or high–blood-flow areas, commonly referred to as the *vessel-rich group* or *central compartment*. Organs such as the heart, liver, kidneys, and brain receive proportionately more anesthetic sooner than the muscle and fat areas (Table 6-3). The longer the anesthetic is given, the greater the saturation of all body compartments.

Second, during induction, increases in increased cardiac output slow onset. All anesthetics are affected; however, the more soluble the agent (higher blood-gas coefficient, and therefore slower), the greater the effect. An increased cardiac output removes more anesthetic from the lungs, which slows the rise in lung and brain concentration.[25-27] This effect dissipates as the anesthetic proceeds.

Metabolism

Anesthetics are metabolized in the body to varying degrees.[28] The effect on uptake, distribution and elimination with the modern anesthetics other than halothane is minimal. Possible toxic metabolite formation also remains an important clinical issue.[29] Drug metabolism is associated with hepatotoxicity from halothane[30] and other agents and theoretically nephrotoxicity

TABLE **6-2** Inhalation Anesthetic Doses*

Anesthetic	Induction	Maintenance
Nitrous oxide	50%-70%	Same
Halothane (Fluothane)	0.5%-4%	0.5%-1.5%
Isoflurane (Forane)	1%-4%	0.5%-2%
Desflurane (Suprane)	3%-9%	2%-6%
Sevoflurane (Ultane)	4%-8%	1%-4%

**Doses vary according to patient status, procedure, and types of medications coadministered.*

TABLE **6-3** Tissue Compartments and Perfusion Comparisons

Characteristic	Vessel-Rich	Muscle	Fat	Vessel-Poor
Percentage of body weight	10	50	20	20
Percentage of cardiac output	75	19	6	0
Perfusion (ml/min/100 g)	75	3	3	0

TABLE 6-4 Anesthetic Metabolism

Agent	Average Metabolism (%)
Halothane	12-25
Sevoflurane	3-6
Nitrous oxide	<1
Isoflurane	<1
Desflurane	<0.1

from sevoflurane, although these incidents are rare.[31-34] Metabolism data for the anesthetics are given in Table 6-4. Nitrous oxide, desflurane, and isoflurane are the least metabolized and do not result in degradation-related toxicity.

Emergence

After surgery, when the anesthetic is discontinued, the same principles that influence onset apply. The anesthetic leaves the tissues via the blood and exits the lungs with ventilation. Routine practice is to administer 100% oxygen to assist recovery. If nitrous oxide was given, 100% oxygen prevents diffusion hypoxia as described subsequently. Anesthetics redistribute out of the tissues in a more uniform manner compared with the way they distribute into tissue during onset. An equilibrium is approached among tissues during the anesthetic period, so recovery tends to be smoother than induction with respect to the excitatory stage responses. The longer an anesthetic is administered, the slower the patient emerges. Differences among anesthetics are small but significant and are seen during the final 20% of the elimination process.[35]

Diffusion Hypoxia

During emergence, when high concentrations of a rapid (insoluble) anesthetic such as nitrous oxide has been given, the drug exits the body quickly through the lungs and is replaced by less-soluble nitrogen in air. This may result in a transient dilution of normal respiratory gases such as oxygen and carbon dioxide. This phenomenon is referred to as *diffusion hypoxia.* As mentioned, administration of 100% oxygen for several minutes when anesthesia is terminated avoids entirely this potential problem.

Diffusion of Nitrous Oxide into Closed Spaces

Nitrous oxide diffuses into air-containing cavities in the body during an anesthetic procedure. These air-containing spaces are normally rich in nitrogen, which is 34 times less soluble than nitrous oxide. If the space is expandable, it increases in volume. Examples of expandable air cavities include air embolism, pneumothorax, acute intestinal obstruction, intraocular air bubbles produced by sulfur hexafluoride gas injection, and pneumoperitoneum. Rigid air-containing spaces will undergo an increase in pressure. This includes tympanic membrane grafting after tympanomastoid procedures and intracranial air during diagnostic or surgical intracranial procedures. Nitrous oxide should be avoided in these situations. The endotracheal tube cuff, laryngeal mask airway, and balloon-tipped pulmonary artery catheters may expand during nitrous oxide anesthesia, and appropriate precautions and adjustments should be considered.[36,37]

Other Factors

The interaction of two agents with the carbon dioxide absorber in the breathing circuit should be noted, although this does not directly affect anesthetic kinetics.

Sevoflurane reacts with the carbon dioxide–absorbing granules in the anesthesia machine.[38-40] The reaction increases with heat and total gas flows less than 2 L/min.[41,42] Duration of the anesthetic administration naturally plays a role. The by-product, compound A, exhibits toxicity in animals.[43,44] To date, no clinical morbidity has been reported.

Carbon monoxide production has been reported after use of the inhalation anesthetics and carbon dioxide granules such as sodalime and baralyme.[45,46] Toxin production is increased with dehydrated granules.[47] Proper machine maintenance decreases the likelihood of problems. A new type of granule, Amsorb, is available and is less reactive with inhalation anesthetics.[48,49]

PEDIATRICS

The uptake of anesthetic drugs is faster in children than in adults.[50,51] In other words, a child goes to sleep faster than an adult patient.[52] The child's higher alveolar ventilation per weight accounts for this effect.

Infants and children have a higher cardiac output per weight than adults. As noted previously, the higher the cardiac output, the slower the onset. This effect is minimized, however, by the increased cardiac output distributed to the vessel-rich group in children. The infant's lower muscle mass allows more of the agent to concentrate in the vital organs. This overall effect is to promote uptake to the brain.

Finally, anesthetics appear to be less blood soluble (i.e., they work faster) in children than in adults. This effect varies with age and the agent.[53-55] The MAC or required dose of the anesthetics is higher in children and decreases with increasing age.[3]

Recent data suggest that during recovery from anesthesia with some inhalation agents, especially sevoflurane and desflurane, emergence reactions and agitation may occur in infants, children, and young adults.[56,57] Recent evidence suggests that this phenomenon is not pharmacokinetic or related to rapidity of emergence.[58] Coadministration of fentanyl reduces the incidence of emergence agitation.[59] Propofol and midazolam have no reducing effect.[60]

A glossary of pharmacokinetic concepts is given in Table 6-5.

SUMMARY

A thorough understanding of the basic kinetic principles involved in administering anesthetic gases and the development of clinical skills in their use are the cornerstones of modern anesthesia practice. Adults are generally induced with one of the several available intravenous agents and maintained with a combination of inhalation and intravenous drugs. The traditional inhalation or mask induction is still commonly performed with children, because it may not be possible to insert the intravenous needle until the child is anesthetized.

Better anesthesia machines and more sophisticated monitoring have greatly facilitated the quantification of clinical anesthetic levels and depth, contributing to the remarkable safety of modern anesthesia practice.

TABLE 6-5 **Inhalational Anesthetic Pharmacokinetic Concepts**

Concept	Comments
Ventilation effect	The greater the alveolar ventilation, the faster the patient achieves anesthesia.
Concentration effect	The higher the concentration of anesthetic delivered, the faster anesthesia is achieved. This is also referred to as *overpressuring*. As with any drug, the larger the initial dose administered, the faster the onset of action.
Blood-gas solubility coefficient	The blood-gas solubility coefficient is the indicator of an anesthetic's speed of onset and emergence. The higher the coefficient, the slower the anesthetic. Conversely, the lower the coefficient, the faster the anesthetic.
Oil-gas solubility coefficient	The oil-gas solubility coefficient is the indicator of an anesthetic's potency. The higher the coefficient the more potent the agent.
Second-gas effect	The second-gas effect is a phenomenon in which two anesthetics of varying onset speeds are administered together. A high concentration of a fast anesthetic such as nitrous oxide is administered with a slower second anesthetic gas. The slower gas achieves anesthetic levels more quickly than if it had been given alone.
Diffusion hypoxia	Diffusion hypoxia occurs when high concentrations of nitrous oxide are administered. At the end of the procedure, when nitrous oxide is discontinued, it leaves the body very rapidly, causing a transient dilution of the oxygen and carbon dioxide in the lungs. Hypocarbia and hypoxia may occur. Administration of 100% oxygen for approximately 3-5 min when nitrous oxide is discontinued alleviates this problem.
Cardiac output effect	Increases in cardiac output decrease the speed of onset of all anesthetics. The more soluble anesthetics are affected to a much greater extent than the insoluble anesthetics.
Ventilation-perfusion abnormalities	Ventilation-perfusion abnormalities reduce the speed of onset of all anesthetics and affect the insoluble agents to a much greater degree than the soluble agents.
Pediatrics	Children achieve anesthesia more rapidly than adults because of a higher ventilatory rate. This occurs despite the fact that the required dose and cardiac output is higher in children.
Obesity	Obesity has minimal clinical effects on anesthetic induction; however, emergence may be slower because of deposition of anesthetics in fat.

REFERENCES

1. Campagna JA, Miller KW, Forman SA. Mechanisms of action of inhaled anesthetics. *N Engl J Med*. 2003;348:2110-2124.
2. Ranipil IJ, Lockhart SH, Zwass Ms, et al. Clinical characteristics of desflurane in surgical patients: minimum alveolar concentration. *Anesthesiology*. 1991;74:429-433.
3. Quasha AL, Eger EI II, Tinker JH. Determinations and application of MAC. *Anesthesiology*. 1980;53:314-334.
4. Yasuda N, Lockhart SH, Eger EI II. Comparison of kinetics of sevoflurane and isoflurane in humans. *Anesth Analg*. 1991; 72:316-324.
5. Eger EI II, Ionescu P, Gong D. Circuit absorption of halothane, isoflurane, and sevoflurane. *Anesth Analg*. 1998;86:1070-1074.
6. The Malignant Hyperthermia Association of The United States. 11 East State Street, PO Box 1069, Sherbane, NY 13460. Available at: www.mhaus.org/index.cfm/fuseaction/Content.Display/PagePK/MedicalFAQs.cfm. Accessed Oct. 25, 2003.
7. Dole O, Brown BR. Clinical pharmacokinetics of the inhalation anesthetics. *Clin Pharmacokinet*. 1987;12:145-167.
8. Yasuda N, Lockhart SG, Eger EI, et al. Kinetics of desflurane, isoflurane and halothane in humans. *Anesthesiology*. 1991;74:489-498.
9. Carpenter RL, Eger EI, Johnson BH, et al. Pharmacokinetics of inhaled anesthetics in humans: measurements during and after simultaneous administration of enflurane, halothane, isoflurane, methoxyflurane and nitrous oxide. *Anesth Analg*. 1986;65:575-582.
10. Halsey JM. Physicochemical properties of inhalation anesthetics. In: Gray TC, Nunn JF, Utting JE, eds. *General Anesthesia*. London: Butterworth; 1980:45.
11. Pal SK, Lockwood GG, White DC. Uptake of isoflurane during prolonged clinical anaesthesia. *Br J Anaesth*. 2001;86:645-649.
12. Eger EI II, Severinghause JW. Effect of uneven pulmonary distribution of blood and gas on induction with inhalation anesthetics. *Anesthesiology*. 1964;25:620-626.
13. Peyton PH, Robinson GJB, Thompson B. Effect of ventilation-perfusion in homogeneity and N_2O on oxygenation: physiological modeling of gas exchange. *J Appl Physiol*. 2001:91(1): 17-25.
14. Eger EI II. The effect of inspired anesthetic concentration on the rate of rise of alveolar concentration. *Anesthesiology*. 1963; 24:153-157.
15. Korman B, Maples WW. Concentration and second gas effects: can the accepted explanation be improved. *Br J Anaesth*. 1997; 78:618-625.
16. Taheri S, Eger EI II. A demonstration of the concentration of second gas effects in humans anesthetized with nitrous oxide and desflurane. *Anesth Analg*. 1999;89:774-780.
17. Goldman LJ. Anesthetic uptake of sevoflurane and nitrous oxide during an inhaled induction in children. *Anesth Analg*. 2003;96:400-406.
18. Epstein RM, Rachow H, Salanitre E, et al. Influence of the concentration effect on the uptake of anesthetic mixtures: the second gas effect. *Anesthesiology*. 1964;25:364-371.
19. Sun X, Su F, Shi Y-Q, et al. The "second gas effect" is not a valid concept. *Anesth Analg*. 1999;88:188-192.
20. Strum DP, Eger EI II. Partition coefficient of sevoflurane in human blood, saline and olive oil. *Anesth Analg*. 1987;66:654-666.
21. Eger EI II. Partition coefficient of I-653 in human blood, saline and olive oil. *Anesth Analg*. 1987;66:971-973.
22. Zhang Y, Trudell JR, Masica MP, et al. The anesthetic potencies of alkanethiols for rats: relevance to theories of narcosis. *Anesth Analg*. 2000;91:1294-1299.

23. Koblin DD, Laster MJ, Ionescu P, et al. Polyhalogenated methy ethyl ethers: solubilities and anesthetic properties. *Anesth Analg.* 1999;88:1161-1167.
24. Eger EI II. Uptake of inhaled anesthetics: the alveolar to inspired anesthetic difference. In: *Anesthetic Uptake and Action*. Baltimore: Williams & Wilkins; 1974:77.
25. Watt SJ, Cook LB, Ohri S, et al. The relationship between anaesthetic uptake and cardiac output. *Anaesthesia.* 1996;51:24-28.
26. Kennedy RR, Baker AB. The effect of cardiac output changes on end-expired volatile anaesthetic concentrations—a theoretical study. *Anaesthesia.* 2001;56:11,1034.
27. Hendrickx JF, Van Zundert AA, De Wolf AM. Sevoflurane pharmacokinetics: effects of cardiac output. *Br J Anaesth.* 1998; 81:495-501.
28. Carpenter RL, Eger EI, Johnson BH, et al. The extent of metabolism of inhaled anesthetics in humans. *Anesthesiology.* 1986;65:201-205.
29. Reichle FM, Conzen PF. Halogenated inhalational anaesthetics. *Best Pract Res Clin Anaesthesiol.* 2003;17:29-46.
30. Splinter W. Halothane: the end of an era? *Anesth Analg.* 2002;95:1471.
31. Kharasch ED, Karol MD, Lanni C, et al. Clinical sevoflurane metabolism and disposition. *Anesthesiology.* 1995;82:1369-1377.
32. Kharash ED, Hankins DC, Thummel K. Human kidney methoxyflurane and sevoflurane metabolism. *Anesthesiology.* 1995;82:689-699.
33. Brown BR. Shibboleths and jigsaw puzzles: the fluoride nephrotoxicity enigma [editorial]. *Anesthesiology.* 1995;82:607-608.
34. Malan GBA. Renal toxicity with sevoflurane: a storm in a teacup? *Drugs.* 2001;61:2155-2162.
35. Bailey JM. Context-sensitive half-times and other decrements times of inhaled anesthetics. *Anesth Analg.* 1997;85:681-686.
36. Ouellette RG. The effect of nitrous oxide on laryngeal mask cuff pressure. *AANA J.* 2000;68:411-414.
37. Algren JT, Gursoy F, Johnson TD, et al. The effect of nitrous oxide diffusion on laryngeal mask airway cuff inflation in children. *Paediatr Anesth.* 1998;8(1):31-36.
38. Hanaki C, Fujii K, Morio M, et al. Decomposition of sevoflurane by soda lime. *Hiroshima J Med Sci.* 1987;36:61-67.
39. Frink EJ, Isner RJ, Malan TP, et al. Sevoflurane degradation product concentrations with soda lime during prolonged anesthesia. *J Clin Anesth.* 1994;6:239-242.
40. Goldberg ME, Cantillo J, Gratz I, et al. Dose of compound A, not sevoflurane, determines changes in the biochemical markers of renal injury in healthy volunteers. *Anesth Analg.* 1999;88:437-445.
41. Bito H, Ikeuchi Y, Ikeda K. Effects of low-flow sevoflurane anesthesia on renal function. *Anesthesiology.* 1999;86:1231-1237.
42. Mazze RI, Jamison RI. Low-flow (1 L/min) sevoflurane: is it safe? *Anesthesiology.* 1997;86:1225-1227.
43. Stabernack CR, Eger Ei II, Warnken UH, et al. Sevoflurane degradation by carbon dioxide absorbents may produce more than one nephrotoxic compound in rats. *Can J Anaesth.* 2003; 50:249-252.
44. Eger Ei II. Compound A: does it matter? *Can J Anaesth.* 2001; 48:427-430.
45. Baum J, Sachs G, vd Driesch C, et al. Carbon monoxide generation in carbon dioxide absorbents. *Anesth Analg.* 1995;81: 144-146.
46. Eger EI II. Stability of I-653 in soda lime. *Anesth Analg.* 1987; 66:983-985.
47. Kharasch E, Powers KM, Artru AA. Comparison of Amsorb, sodalime, and Baralyme degradation of volatile anesthetics and formation of carbon monoxide and compound a in swine in vivo. *Anesthesiology.* 2002;96:173-182.
48. Mchaourab A, Arain Sr, Ebert TJ. Lack of degradation of sevoflurane by a new carbon dioxide absorbent in humans. *Anesthesiology.* 2001;94:1007-1009.
49. Stabernack CR, Brown R, Laster MJ, et al. Absorbents differ enormously in their capacity to produce compound A and carbon monoxide. *Anesth Analg.* 2000;90:1428-1435.
50. Salanitre E, Rackow H: The pulmonary exchange of nitrous oxide and halothane in infants and children. *Anesthesiology.* 1969;30:388-394.
51. Brondom BW, Brondom RB, Cook DR. Uptake and distribution of halothane in infants: in vivo measurements and computer simulations. *Anesth Analg.* 1983;62:404-410.
52. Sarner JB, Levine M, Davis PJ, et al. Clinical characteristics of sevoflurane in children: a comparison with halothane. *Anesthesiology.* 1995;82:38-46.
53. Eger EI II, Bakham SH, Munson ES. The effect of age on the rate of increase of alveolar anesthetic concentration. *Anesthesiology.* 1971;35:365-372.
54. Lerman J, Schmitt-Bantel B, Gregory GA, et al. Effect of age on the solubility of volatile anesthetics in human tissues. *Anesthesiology.* 1986;65:307-311.
55. Malviya S, Lerman J. The blood-gas solubilities of sevoflurane, isoflurane, halothane, and serum constituent concentrations in neonates and adults. *Anesthesiology.* 1990;72;793-796.
56. Uezono Sl, Goto T, Terui K, et al. Emergence agitation after sevoflurane versus propofol in pediatric patients. *Anesth Analg.* 2000;91:563-566.
57. Beskow A, Westrin P. Sevoflurane causes more postoperative agitation in children than does halothane. *Acta Anaesthesiol Scand.* 1999;43:536-541.
58. Cohen IT, Fikel JC, Hannallah RS, et al. Rapid emergence does not explain agitation following sevoflurane anaesthesia in infants and children: a comparison with propofol. *Paediatr Anaesth.* 2003;1391:63-67.
59. Cohen IT, Finkel JC, Hannallah RS, et al. The effect of fentanyl on the emergence characteristics after desflurane or sevoflurane anesthesia in children. *Anesth Analg.* 2002;94: 1178-1181.
60. Cohen IT, Drewsen S, Hannallah RS. Propofol or midazolam does not reduce the incidence of emergence agitation associated with desflurane anaesthesia in children undergoing adenotonsillectomy. *Paediatr Anaesth.* 2002;12:604-609.

CHAPTER 7

INHALATION ANESTHETICS

MARK A. KOSSICK

Historically, major advances have been made in the development of inhalation anesthetics (Table 7-1). In 1800 the anesthetic property of nitrous oxide (N_2O) was first recognized by Humphry Davy. He achieved pain relief from a toothache while inhaling N_2O and later described the experience as one of merriment and exhilaration. Davy also predicted that N_2O could be used to advantage during surgical operations.[1] It is surprising to note that his nineteenth-century prediction not only came to pass but also remains true today. The predominant reason for this is the pharmacokinetic profile that N_2O possesses.

The present-day use of N_2O can be credited to Edmund Andrews, a professor of surgery in Chicago. In 1868 he declared that a safer anesthetic could result from combining oxygen (O_2) with N_2O.[2] Before that time N_2O was administered through a mouthpiece with a nose clamp to prevent the rebreathing of air.

One of the earliest "complete" anesthetic agents used was diethyl ether (C_2H_5—O—C_2H_5). The first ether anesthetic was administered in Georgia in March 1842 when C. W. Long anesthetized a patient for a minor operation.[3] However, the recognition of numerous unfavorable characteristics (excessive secretions with inhalation induction, laryngospasm, excessive depths of anesthesia) promoted its disappearance from clinical practice as newer agents were subsequently developed.

In the 1930s research into potential anesthetic agents was based on the principle of a structure-activity relationship.[4] One of the earliest inhalation anesthetics developed in this manner was divinyl ether. Halothane was introduced into clinical practice in 1956 by Bryce-Smith and O'Brien in Oxford[5] and Johnstone in Manchester[6] and represented a significant advancement in inhalation anesthesia. Its sweet odor, nonflammability, and high potency offered clinical characteristics that were absent from the previous inhaled anesthetics. The search for newer and improved inhalation anesthetics persisted as concerns with hepatotoxicity and arrhythmogenicity of this alkane derivative began to be documented.

With the recent start of a new millennium, researchers will no doubt continue to work toward the development of the "ultimate" inhalation anesthetic—one that is associated with no organ toxicity, allows for prompt adjustment of anesthetic depth, and permits a smooth, rapid emergence from anesthesia. Isoflurane (a methyl ethyl ether derivative), although not an "ideal" agent, represents a substantial improvement over the older agents with regard to these characteristics.

TABLE 7-1 History of the Introduction of Inhalational Anesthetics

Anesthetic	Year(s) Introduced
N_2O	1840s
Ether	
Chloroform	
Cyclopropane	1930s
Fluroxene	1951
Halothane	1956
Methoxyflurane	1960
Enflurane	1973
Isoflurane	1981
Desflurane	1993
Sevoflurane	1995

The two most recently released inhalation agents, sevoflurane (synthesized by Regan in the late 1960s) and desflurane (the 653rd compound of over 700 synthesized by Terrell and colleagues between 1959 and 1966), have become accepted by many anesthesia providers as viable anesthetics for a diverse surgical population based on their pharmacokinetic profiles. What remains as a significant variable in determining the use of sevoflurane and desflurane among anesthesia providers is the cost (relative to isoflurane) versus clinical benefit to the patient. Some properties of an ideal anesthetic agent are listed in Box 7-1.

RELATIONSHIP BETWEEN CHEMICAL STRUCTURE AND AGENT CHARACTERISTICS

An understanding of the chemical structure of inhalation agents provides insight into their physical properties (e.g., flammability). However, the relationship between the pharmacologic characteristics (e.g., arrhythmogenic properties) and chemical structure of agents is not as predictable. This section reviews the structure-activity relationships of anesthetic vapors and their clinical relevance. Some selected physical and chemical properties are listed in Table 7-2.

All commonly used inhalation agents are ethers (R—O—R) or aliphatic hydrocarbons (straight-chained or branched nonaromatic hydrocarbons) with no more than four carbon atoms (Figure 7-1). The length of the anesthetic molecule is significant in that immobility (anesthetic effect)

BOX 7-1

Properties of the Ideal Inhalation Anesthetic Agent*

- It should have a pleasant odor, be nonirritating to the respiratory tract, and result in pleasant and rapid induction of anesthesia.
- It should possess a low blood-gas solubility, which permits rapid induction of and rapid recovery from anesthesia.
- It should be chemically stable in storage and should not interact with the material of the anesthetic machine and circuits or with soda lime.
- It should be neither flammable nor explosive.
- It should be capable of producing unconsciousness with analgesia and preferably some degree of muscle relaxation.
- It should be sufficiently potent to allow the use of high inspired oxygen concentrations when necessary.
- It should not be metabolized in the body, should exert no systemic toxicity, and should not provoke allergic reactions.
- It should produce minimal and predictable depression of the cardiovascular and respiratory systems and should not interact with other drugs used commonly during anesthesia, e.g., pressor agents or catecholamines.
- It should be completely inert and eliminated completely and rapidly in an unchanged form via the lungs.
- It should be easy to administer using standard vaporizers.
- It should have a reasonable cost.
- It should not be epileptogenic or raise intracranial pressure.

**None of the inhalation anesthetic agents approaches the standards required of the ideal agent.*

Modified from Aitkenhead AR, Rowbotham DF, Smith G. Inhalation anaesthetic agents. In: Textbook of Anaesthesia. *4th ed. Edinburgh: Churchill Livingstone; 2001; and Bovill JG, Howie MB. Inhalational anaesthetics. In:* Clinical Pharmacology for Anaesthetics. *London: Saunders; 1999.*

TABLE 7-2 **Select Properties of Volatile Anesthetics**

Property	Halothane	Isoflurane	Desflurane	Sevoflurane	Nitrous oxide
MAC (EC_{50}; % atmosphere)	0.77	1.15	6	2	110
Blood-gas partition coefficient	2.3	1.43	0.42	0.60	0.47
Oil-gas partition coefficient	234	91	19	53	1.4
Specific gravity (g/ml)	1.87	1.50	1.47	1.50	NA
Boiling point (°C)	50	48.5	22.8	58.5	−88.5
Vapor pressure (mm Hg, 20° C)	243	238	669	120	Gas
Molecular weight (daltons)	197.4	184.5	168	200.1	44
Preservative	Thymol	None	None	None	None
Stability in CO_2 absorbers	Stable	Stable	Stable	Unstable	Stable
Extent metabolized (%)	12-25	0.2	0.02	3-5	Trace

EC_{50}, *effective concentration in 50% of the population;* MAC, *minimum alveolar concentration.*

Modified from Aitkenhead AR, Rowbotham DF, Smith G. Inhalation anaesthetic agents. In: Textbook of Anaesthesia. *4th ed. Edinburgh: Churchill Livingstone; 2001; and Lerman J. Pharmacokinetics of inhalation anesthetics. In Hemmings H, Hopkins P:* Foundation of Anesthesia Basic and Clinical Sciences. *London: Mosby; 2000.*

is attenuated or lost if carbon atom chain length exceeds a distance of four of five carbon atoms (5 angstroms [Å]).[7] The molecular shape of the agents is spherical or cylindric, with a length less than 1.5 times the diameter.[8]

Of primary importance to the development of volatile agents was the discovery of the impact of halogenation of organic compounds. Halogenation of hydrocarbons and ethers (the addition of fluorine [F], chlorine [Cl], bromine [Br], or iodine [I]) influences anesthetic potency, arrhythmogenic properties, flammability, and chemical stability (e.g., oxidation during storage and reactions with bases).

Anesthetic potency has been shown to increase when a halogen with a lower atomic mass unit (amu) is replaced by a heavier halogen (e.g., Br at 80 amu substituted for F at 19 amu). This relationship has been confirmed with previous research by Robbins,[9] Larsen,[10] and most recently Targ and colleagues.[11] Nonetheless, a ceiling effect exists with halogenation of anesthetic compounds. For example, adding F atoms to ether results in a continuum in which the ether becomes more potent, then acts as a strong convulsant, and finally changes to an inert compound with full fluorination.[12]

In general the potency of volatile agents has also been found to correlate with the physical property of lipid solubility. A decline in potency (meaning an *increase* in the minimum alveolar concentration [MAC] of volatile agents) is associated with a proportional decrease in oil-gas partition coefficient values. Exceptions to this principle exist and demonstrate that the correlation between potency and lipid solubility is not perfect.

With regard to arrhythmogenic properties, increasing the number of halogen atoms within a volatile agent favors the genesis of cardiac dysrhythmias.[12] Nevertheless, alkanes that contain five halogens (e.g., halothane) are more prone to induce arrhythmias than ethers with six halogen atoms (e.g., isoflurane).[13] Ether molecules also contain oxygen, which reduces arrythmogenic effects.

Flammability is reduced and chemical stability enhanced by substituting hydrogen atoms with halogens. The epitome

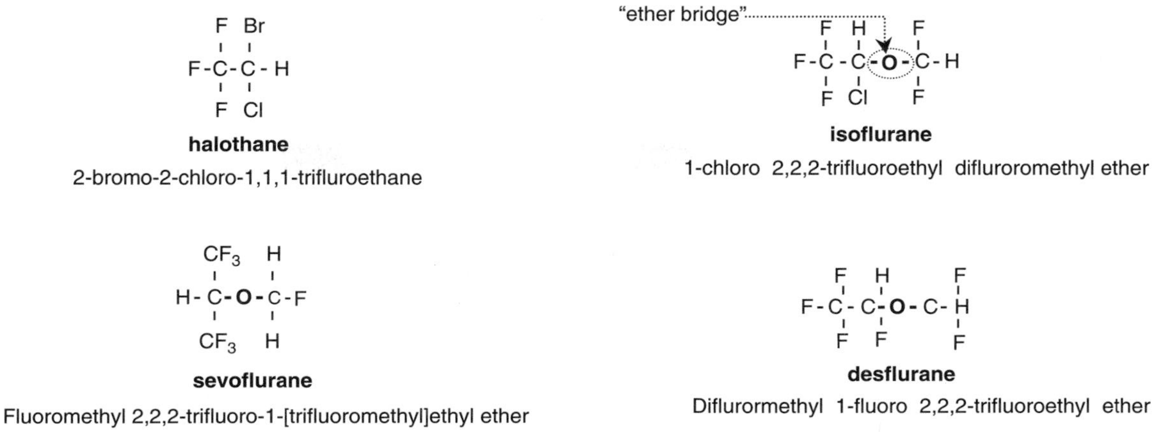

FIGURE **7-1**
Structural formulas of inhalational agents. The "ether bridges" (R—O—R) are seen with enflurane, sevoflurane, desflurane, and isoflurane. *R* refers to alkyl group.

of this relationship is demonstrated with desflurane, a compound that contains fluorine as its only halogen and therefore strongly resists biodegradation; desflurane is metabolized one tenth as much as isoflurane (less than 0.02% versus 0.2%).[14,15]

METABOLISM

As stated previously, the chemical structure of each inhalation agent determines the extent to which each volatile agent is metabolized. In general, increasing the number of fluorine atoms to an anesthetic molecule retards biodegradation (halothane has 3, and desflurane has 6). Table 7-3 depicts the degree to which each of the modern fluorinated inhalation agents is biodegraded. The two ends of the spectrum are represented by halothane (12% to 25% metabolized) and desflurane (0.02% metabolized).[14,16-18] The latter anesthetic has been shown to resist biodegradation even after 7.35 MAC-hours; volunteers were found to have a peak mean urinary excretion rate of trifluoroacetic acid (TFA) of 0.169 ± 0.107 μmol/hr. By comparison, isoflurane administered in lower doses has been found to yield a maximum TFA excretion rate of approximately 50 μmol/hr (approximately 300-fold greater than seen with desflurane).[19] The significance of these findings relates to the fact that TFA provides definitive and quantifiable evidence of the biodegradation of desflurane and is a sensitive marker of desflurane metabolism.[20]

TABLE **7-3** **Metabolism of Inhalational Agents as Determined by Percent Taken up That Is Biodegraded**

Anesthetic	Percent of Uptake That Is Biodegraded
Desflurane	0-0.02
Isoflurane	0-0.2
Sevoflurane	5-8
Halothane	12-25
Nitrous Oxide	Trace

The biodegradation of all currently used volatile anesthetics is predominantly by way of hepatic metabolism through oxidation (phase I).[21] Halothane is unique in that it can also be metabolized by an alternative reductive pathway.[22] Sevoflurane, introduced into clinical practice in the United States in 1995, continues to attract the interest of researchers, in large part because of concern for sevoflurane's olefin metabolite, which may impair renal function. In humans sevoflurane is metabolized from 5% to 8% of a given dose.[23] Sevoflurane's biotransformation is reviewed later in this chapter.

PHARMACODYNAMICS

Mechanisms of Action

The following properties of anesthetics must be taken into account when developing a theory that attempts to explain their mechanism of action:

1. Lipid solubility is directly proportional to potency (Meyer-Overton rule).[24,25]
2. Reversal of anesthetic effect can be achieved with the application of pressure, with some exceptions (species variation).[26]
3. No common chemical structure exists for the variety of compounds capable of producing anesthesia.
4. The molecular and structural changes responsible for producing anesthesia must occur within seconds and be reversible.
5. A reduction in body temperature lowers anesthetic requirements.

In keeping with most of these prerequisites is the unitary hypothesis. This theory proposes that all inhalation anesthetics work via a similar (undefined) mechanism of action but not necessarily at the same site of action. One factor that supports this hypothesis is the Meyer-Overton correlation, which recognizes that the more lipid soluble the agent, the greater its potency (the lower its MAC value). This correlation suggests that anesthesia is produced by the volume of anesthetic molecules present (dissolved) at the site, not by the type of volatile agent present. The additive effect observed among different anesthetics also supports the unitary hypothesis by suggesting independent sites of action.[27] Nonetheless, most investigators disagree with this theory.[28]

Recent investigations of the mechanism of action of volatile anesthetics have led to the redefining of the term *anesthesia*. From a parsimonious point of view, inhalation anesthesia involves use of compounds that produce amnesia and immobility in response to noxious stimuli. *Amnesia* in this context is defined as being unaware of the environment or unable to recall a previous episode of awareness. Any agent that produces both characteristics is termed a *full anesthetic*, and drugs that cause amnesia alone are termed *nonimmobilizers and nonanesthetics*.[29] The other traditional characteristics of an anesthetic state (analgesia, skeletal muscle relaxation) are viewed as "side effects" that are not essential to what defines anesthesia.[30] For clarification, this does not mean these side effects are of no concern to the anesthesia provider. Quite the contrary; adequate modulation of a patient's sympathetic response to painful stimuli can determine the success or failure of some anesthetics.

Research has shown that inhaled anesthetics are capable of producing their desired clinical endpoint at two primary sites (anatomic and molecular).[31] The first is within the spinal cord (inhibiting the motor response to a painful stimulus),[32] and the second is supraspinal.[33-35] The mechanisms of action associated with each of these effects (immobility and amnesia) are understood to be different. Investigators have also demonstrated that nonimmobilizers with lipophilic characteristics are able to produce amnesia but not immobility to noxious stimuli, which suggests two separate sites and mechanisms of anesthetic action.[31] In other research, spinal and cerebral receptors (γ-aminobutyric acid type A [$GABA_A$]) were shown to contribute to isoflurane's ability to produce immobility; therefore the anesthetic effect of immobility is modulated at the spinal cord and supraspinal level.[36] Other specific anatomic sites at which volatile anesthetics produce an effect include the reticular formation within the brain stem, cerebral cortex, and hippocampus.[37-40] Evidence of changes in cortical activity by volatile agents includes the alteration in electroencephalogram (EEG) activity. All inhalation agents cause a dose-dependent change in the EEG—an initial increase in voltage (and decrease in frequency), then a peak, followed by a decline.[37,41,42] Deeper levels of anesthesia produce burst suppression and eventually a flat EEG.[43] Nonspecific generalized EEG changes may also persist for several days postoperatively; as evidenced by one investigator who documented generalized EEG slowing for 6 to 8 days after 13.83 MAC-hours of halothane anesthesia.[44]

Increased or decreased neuronal excitability and enhanced or depressed inhibitory postsynaptic currents can occur, depending on which anesthetic agent or specific area within the central nervous system (CNS) is manipulated. In addition to supraspinal effects, modulation of afferent and efferent impulses within the spinal cord has also occurred with volatile anesthetics.[45-47]

On a molecular level, researchers have found that the most likely site of action for volatile anesthetics involves interactions with membrane proteins in specific receptors (stereoselective) and not perturbation of lipid bilayers.[48-50] Evidence is mounting that the primary receptor within the CNS that modulates anesthetic effects is the GABA receptor, specifically the subtype A.[46,49,51] This receptor is located abundantly in the CNS and is a ligand-gated Cl^- ion channel.[52] Agonism of this receptor by full anesthetics (volatile agents) results in enhanced Cl^- conductance,[53] which leads to inhibitory actions on local neurons.[52] Ultimately what is expressed is an extension of the amount of time the Cl^- channel remains open.[43] In contrast to full anesthetics, nonimmobilizers do not enhance the effect of GABA on these receptors.

An investigation by Kaech and colleagues revealed a new anesthetic site of action within the CNS; chloroform, diethyl ether, methoxyflurane, halothane, and isoflurane were each shown (in clinically relevant concentrations) to block the morphologic plasticity of dendritic spines.[54] Prior research demonstrated that dendritic spines can change shape in seconds.[55] This phenomenon occurs secondarily to motile actin, which is abundant in the spines.[56] These volatile agents were found to strongly inhibit actin motility, which blocked changes in dendritic spine shape (Figure 7-2); the inhibition was fully reversed after removal of the agents. The dendritic spines serve as excitatory postsynaptic contact sites.[57] They are extremely abundant in the cerebral cortex (greater than 10^{13}) and are also located in large numbers in the cerebellum, basal ganglia, and olfactory bulb.[58] The details of how these

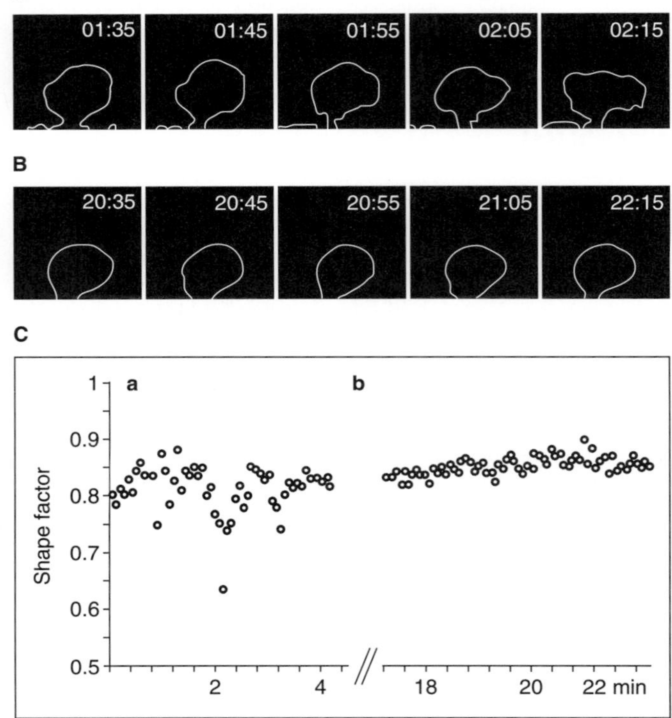

FIGURE **7-2**
Volatile anesthetics block dendritic spine motility. Outline profiles show changes in the shape of a dendritic spine visualized in a time-lapse recording of green fluorescent protein–actin tagged in the spine head. Selected images taken 10 seconds apart over a period of 5 minutes show changes in shape that occurred in control conditions, **(A)** compared with relative lack of shape change in the presence of clinically relevant concentrations of isoflurane **(B).** Data from all the frames recorded in this experiment are shown in the shape factor plot **(C)**, in which the variation in spine shape **(a,** *left***)** is blocked after medium containing isoflurane was perfused into the observation chamber **(b,** *right***)**. (Reprinted with permission from Kaech S, Brinkhaus H, Matus A. Volatile anesthetics block actin-based motility in dendritic spines. *Proc Natl Acad Sci U S A*. 1999;96:10433-10437.)[54]

rapid morphologic changes in dendritic spines contribute to an anesthetic state are unclear and merit further research. The CNS effects of amnesia and loss of consciousness likely are produced separately from the immobility conceptualized in the theory of MAC.[59] The concept of MAC refers to the concentration required to prevent movement in response to a surgical situation. This is the result of an effect at the spinal cord level via glycine, 5-hydroxytriptamine$_{2A}$, sodium, and N-methyl-D-asparate receptor action. Potassium, α-amino-3-hydroxy-5-methyl-4-isoxazolepropionic (AMPA) and kainate, GABA, opioid, α_2-, 5HT$_3$, and acetylcholine receptors are likely not involved in producing immobility. They may be involved in varying degrees in the amnestic and anesthetic effects in the CNS.

MINIMUM ALVEOLAR CONCENTRATION

A useful means of comparing the potencies of inhalation agents is to use the concept of MAC, defined as the minimum alveolar concentration at equilibrium (expressed as a percentage of 1 atmosphere) in which 50% of subjects do not respond to a painful stimuli (i.e., initial surgical skin incision).[60] The response is defined as gross, *purposeful* movement of the head or extremities. The MAC values for the modern inhalation agents are listed in Table 7-4.[61]

The MAC of volatile agents can be affected by numerous factors (Box 7-2). For example, with increasing age, MAC of all volatile anesthetics is reduced. As an illustration, the MAC of desflurane in humans aged 18 to 30 years is 7.25%, whereas the MAC value in humans 30 to 55 years of age is 6%.[60] A similar study with sevoflurane determined that elderly patients (mean age 71.4 years) had a MAC value of 1.48 compared with 1.71 for adults with a mean age of 47.5 years.[62]

Two other areas related to MAC are MAC-awake and MAC-BAR (block adrenergic response). MAC-awake is defined as the MAC at which 50% of subjects respond to the command, "Open your eyes." It has also been described as the anesthetic concentration that is between the end-tidal values that allow and prevent response to a command.[63] This end-tidal concentration is usually associated with a loss of recall and encompasses approximately one third of MAC values. MAC-awake can also be used in combination with MAC values to evaluate the potency of each agent with regard to amnestic properties. This is done by dividing MAC-awake by MAC (MAC-awake/MAC ratio). This parameter indicates that agents with ratios between 0.3 and 0.4 (e.g., desflurane, sevoflurane, isoflurane) are considered potent anesthetics. In contrast, N_2O, which has a ratio of 0.64, is considered a weak amnestic agent.

The MAC-BAR parameter represents the MAC necessary to block the adrenergic response (e.g., changes in plasma norepinephrine concentration, heart rate [HR], rate-pressure product, and mean arterial pressure) to skin incision. It can be expressed as a MAC-BAR$_{50}$ or MAC-BAR$_{95}$. The former is similar to AD$_{95}$ values, which represent the anesthetic dose that inhibits somatic evidence of light anesthesia in 95% of subjects in response to skin incision. Established MAC-BAR$_{50}$ values for volatile agents include (in 60% N_2O) 1.45 MAC ($0.75\% \times 1.5 = 1.125\%$) for halothane and 1.3 MAC for both isoflurane and desflurane.[64,65] The MAC-BAR$_{50}$ for sevoflurane in 66% N_2O is 2.2.[61] The MAC-BAR$_{95}$ of halothane is 2.1 and of enflurane is 2.6.[64] It should be emphasized that MAC-BAR values exceed the requirements for ablation of skeletal muscle movement with surgical stimulation; therefore the blocking of an adrenergic response requires a greater depth of anesthesia than does the prevention of skeletal muscle movement.[66] From a clinical standpoint patients usually require anesthetic concentrations that exceed MAC by 10% to 30%. At this alveolar concentration somatic evidence of light anesthesia is commonly abated, and fewer patients respond adrenergically to the stresses of surgery.

The concept of MAC has limitations when applied clinically to determine adequacy of anesthesia. It should be viewed as a general guide to the overall depth of anesthesia. One variable that restricts its application is the frequency at which surgical patients receive muscle relaxants, which attenuates the recognition of skeletal muscle movement in response to light planes of anesthesia. This results in the dependence of anesthesia providers on other traditional signs of anesthetic depth, such as changes in HR, blood pressure, pupillary size, and sweating. Unfortunately, a light plane of anesthesia can exist even with a decreased blood pressure and a normal HR (e.g., in patients with limited cardiac reserve). Pupillary changes can also be affected by opioids (miosis) and volatile agents (mydriasis) over time, even in the absence of surgical stimuli.[67] Also, the usefulness of a traditional clinical endpoint as a guide to depth of anesthesia can change over time. For example, one investigator found that decreases in blood pressure served as an estimate of anesthetic depth during the first hour of an anesthetic, but after 5 hours they were unreliable; additional declines in blood pressure did not occur even with increasing concentrations of halothane.[68] The challenge to the anesthesia provider is to estimate anesthetic depth based on a collation of variables (HR, blood pressure, synergistic and additive effects of anesthetic adjuvants, volume status, physiologic reserve, MAC, MAC-BAR, and MAC intubation values). The last variable (MAC intubation) is similar to MAC-BAR in that its values exceed the anesthetic requirements for surgical skin incision. Clearly, different stimuli require different end-tidal concentrations (brain anesthetic partial pressures) of volatile anesthetics.[69]

TABLE 7-4 Potencies of Volatile Anesthetics in Humans with and without N_2O Expressed in MAC and MAPP Values*

Anesthetic	MAC (MAPP)	In 60% N_2O MAC (MAPP)
Nitrous oxide	104 (798)	—
Desflurane	6† (45.60)	2.83‡ (21.51)
Sevoflurane	1.58-2.05† (12.01-15.58)	0.87-0.97‡ (6.61-7.37)
Isoflurane	1.15† (8.74)	0.50 (3.80)
Halothane	0.74-0.77† (5.62-5.85)	0.29 (2.20)

FiO_2, *Fraction of inspired oxygen;* MAC, *minimum alveolar concentration;* MAPP, *minimum alveolar partial pressure;* N_2O, *nitrous oxide.*
**MAC is expressed as volume percent of end-tidal gas at standard pressure. MAPP is calculated as MAC value times 760 mm Hg ÷ 100 (expressed in mm Hg).*
†Age 31 to 65 years.
‡Age 36 to 49 years.

BOX 7-2

Relationship of Physiologic and Pharmacologic Factors to the MAC of Inhaled Anesthetics

Factors That Reduce MAC
- Increase in age*
- Hypothermia
- Administration of depressant medications (e.g., opioids, opioid agonist-antagonist analgesics, benzodiazepines, barbiturates, chlorpromazine, hydroxazine)
- α_2 Agonists
- Acute ethanol consumption
- Metabolic acidosis
- Hypoxemia
- Hypotension
- Hyponatremia
- Pregnancy
- N_2O, ketamine, verapamil, intravenous local anesthetics, clonidine, alpha-methyl dopa, reserpine, chronic dextroamphetamine use, lithium
- Cholinesterase inhibitors

Factors That Increase MAC
- Decrease in age*
- Hyperthermia
- Hyperthyroidism
- Hypernatremia
- Chronic alcohol consumption
- Acute administration of dextroamphetamine
- Monoamine oxidase inhibitors
- Cocaine, levodopa

Factors with No Effect on MAC
- Duration of anesthesia
- Gender
- Hypocarbia and hypercarbia
- Metabolic alkalosis
- Hypertension
- Administration of propranolol, isoproterenol, promethazine, naloxone, aminophylline, and neuromuscular blocking agents.

MAC, *Minimum alveolar concentration;* N_2O, *nitrous oxide.*
**Exception: infants have a greater anesthetic requirement than neonates.*

INFLUENCE OF INHALATION AGENTS ON ORGANS AND SYSTEMS

Central Nervous System

The volatile agents can adversely affect the care provided to patients with CNS pathology. Such effects include areas related to intracranial compliance, autoregulation of cerebral blood flow (CBF; e.g., cerebrovascular reactivity to carbon dioxide [CO_2]), cerebral metabolic rate, cerebrospinal fluid pressure (CSFP), and neurologic assessment.

Cerebral Metabolic Rate and Cerebral Blood Flow

In general, volatile agents decrease cerebral metabolic rate of O_2 consumption ($CMRO_2$) in a dose-dependent manner, whereas their effect on CBF is variable; the latter has been reported by various researchers to be unchanged,[70,71] increased,[72,73] and decreased.[74,75] When vascular resistance is decreased, CBF, cerebral blood volume (CBV), and CSFP increase. The order of potency for increasing CBF varies; it is affected by the dose of volatile anesthetic,[1] the administration of other drugs (e.g., propofol, N_2O), the rate of change in end-tidal concentration of agent,[72] and the animal model used.[76] In other cases, differences in research findings lack a plausible explanation.

A distinct picture of a homogeneous versus heterogeneous change in CBF and $CMRO_2$ has developed for halothane and isoflurane. Halothane globally increases CBF, whereas isoflurane's sphere of influence predominates in the subcortical regions and hindbrain structures[77] (Figure 7-3).

Uncoupling of Cerebral Blood Flow and Metabolism

When decreases in $CMRO_2$ are accompanied by increases in CBF, *uncoupling* is said to occur. As noted above, volatile anesthetics are capable of producing this effect. This paradoxic response (decreased $CMRO_2$ in conjunction with increased CBF) seems not to occur with a MAC of 1 or less of halothane and isoflurane[78]; the magnitude of change is variable and dose dependent, meaning some flow-metabolism coupling mechanism is preserved.[70,74,78,79]

N_2O reduces cerebrovascular tone significantly. This effect is unmasked and enhanced when N_2O is combined with a volatile anesthetic (decreased autoregulation).[71,80,81] The mechanism for increased CBF may be related to a sympathoadrenal-stimulating effect of N_2O. The changes produced by N_2O in the $CMRO_2$ are the reverse of what takes place with volatile

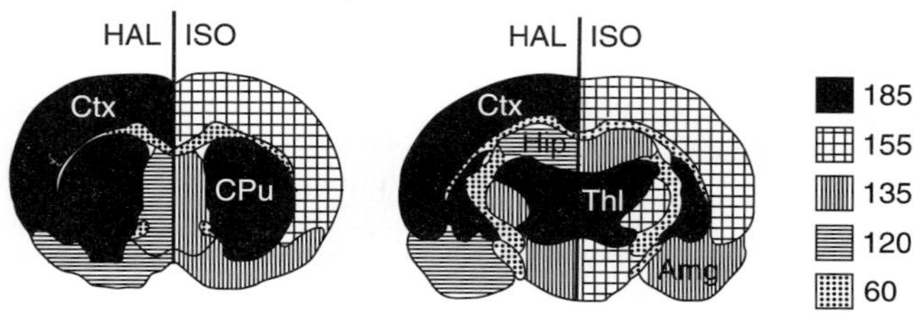

FIGURE **7-3**
Regional differences in the cerebral blood flow (CBF) effect of isoflurane and halothane. The figure is a schematic representation of CBF in a coronal autoradiographic image of rat brain. The key indicates the approximate CBF (ml/100 g/min). In the cortex CBF is less during anesthesia with isoflurane than with halothane. In the subcortex CBF is similar during anesthesia with the two agents in some structures, and in others it is greater with isoflurane. The average hemispheric CBF with the two agents is very similar. Similar CBF distribution differences occur in humans, although the mean global CBF is greater for halothane than for isoflurane.[23] (*Amg,* Amygdala; *CPu,* caudate-putamen; *Ctx,* cortex; *HAL,* halothane; *Hip,* hippocampus; *ISO,* isoflurane; *Thl,* thalamus.) (Reprinted with permission from Hansen TD, Warner DS, Todd MM, et al. Distribution of cerebral blood flow during halothane versus isoflurane anesthesia in rats. *Anesthesiology.* 1988;69:332-337.)

agents (i.e., increased $CMRO_2$),[82] although other investigators have reported no effect.[83] Nevertheless, a general impression is that N_2O probably increases $CMRO_2$ and CBF. The combination of elevated CBF and $CMRO_2$ still results in an uncoupling between flow and metabolism, because in goats the increase in $CMRO_2$ exceeds, albeit slightly, the elevation in CBF. In summary, the use of N_2O during neurosurgical procedures is acceptable as long as the anesthesia provider recognizes that its vasodilatory effects might adversely affect surgical outcome in patients with reduced intracranial compliance. Hyperventilation helps attenuate the increase in CBF that accompanies the use of N_2O.[84]

Cerebral Vasculature Responsiveness to Carbon Dioxide

The normal physiologic response of the cerebral vasculature to CO_2 is to vasoconstrict in the presence of hypocapnia and vasodilate with hypercarbia. This reflex is effective in the acute setting when used during neurosurgical procedures to counteract drug-induced vasodilation and to reduce brain bulk within a closed compartment (cranial vault).[85,86]

Differences exist among the volatile agents in their ability to interfere with the cerebral vasculature's responsiveness to CO_2. For example, halothane and sevoflurane (in 67% N_2O)[87] interfere with hypocapnia-induced vasoconstriction to a greater extent than does isoflurane. In contrast, dynamic cerebral autoregulation (the body's response to an acute acidic load assessed via middle cerebral artery blood velocity) is better preserved with sevoflurane than isoflurane when each is delivered at 1.5 MAC in combination with 100% O_2.[88] In patients undergoing craniotomy for tumor resection, desflurane with an air-O_2 mixture at 1 and 1.5 MAC has been shown to act similarly to isoflurane and maintain cerebrovascular reactivity to CO_2. The research findings previously reviewed suggest that increases in CBF produced by isoflurane, desflurane, and sevoflurane can be effectively prevented by hyperventilation and using concentrations less than 1 to 1.5 MAC. Researchers have also found desflurane to be without appreciable effects on neurologic parameters (e.g., intracranial pressure).[89]

Electroencephalogram and Evoked Potentials

The volatile agents produce a dose-related suppression of EEG activity (initial increase [later a decline] in amplitude and decreased frequency) and at high concentrations produce electrical quiescence.[43,90,91] At deeper levels of anesthesia the EEG may temporarily stop recording; at such times, *burst suppression* is said to have occurred. The effect of anesthetic agents on evoked potential is given in Box 26-4.

For procedures that require monitoring of the integrity of the spinal cord or mapping of cortical regions of the brain, the anesthetist should be aware that inhalation agents can skew somatosenory, motor, brain-stem auditory, and visual evoked potentials. Isoflurane, desflurane, sevoflurane, and N_2O produce a dose-dependent reduction in these evoked potentials.[37,92-94] The two evoked potential variables commonly assessed are latency and amplitude. An increase in latency or decrease in amplitude of evoked potentials can reflect ischemia or be secondary to the volatile agent. Latency is the time between the initiation of a peripheral stimulus (e.g., electrical stimulation of the median nerve at the wrist) and onset of the evoked potential (e.g., cortical) recorded by scalp electrodes.

Desflurane, sevoflurane, and isoflurane (without N_2O) have been shown to interfere with the recording of somatosensory evoked potentials (SSEPs) at light planes of anesthesia (<0.7 MAC)[92] and when MAC exceeds 1[93-95] to 1.3.[92] Of these three agents, isoflurane produces the greatest reduction in SSEP amplitude, whereas no difference exists among the effects of volatile anesthetics on latency. The addition of N_2O to isoflurane, desflurane, and sevoflurane can also produce a significant reduction in the amplitude of SSEPs.[93,95] It may be prudent to avoid the use of this agent in patients who have baseline low-amplitude evoked potentials.

Sevoflurane,[96,97] unlike desflurane and isoflurane,[41] can predispose pediatric and adult patients to epileptic activity, even though sevoflurane[98] can suppress drug-induced convulsive activity in a manner similar to desflurane[99] and isoflurane.[98] Sevoflurane combined with N_2O has produced epileptiform EEG activity during inhalation induction with adults in a single-breath technique. A hyperdynamic response can accompany the EEG changes if concurrent hyperventilation occurs. The incidence of epileptiform EEG changes has been shown to more than double in the presence of hypocapnia (100% versus 47%). Similar results have been observed in children aged 2 to 12 years.[100] In contrast, intravenous induction with thiopental followed by anesthetic maintenance with 2% end-tidal sevoflurane in air does not produce seizurelike changes in EEGs in children.[97] Epileptiform activity has also been reported to occur during the emergence from sevoflurane.[101]

Emergence and Neurologic Assessment

Although the objective of a smooth and rapid emergence from a general anesthetic is desirable for all surgical patients, it is especially meaningful for neurosurgical candidates. Delayed emergence in this specialty of anesthesia can have devastating consequences. A slow return of consciousness makes it difficult to perform the initial postoperative neurologic examination. It can also add to unnecessary therapeutic or diagnostic intervention and can predispose the patient to respiratory complications.[102]

Because of this, a large number of neurosurgical procedures are performed with a primary opioid-N_2O anesthetic technique supplemented with low concentrations of an inhalation agent. With the introduction of desflurane and sevoflurane, an acceptable alternative may now exist for the management of neuroanesthesia cases. The primary reason for this is the attractive pharmacokinetic profile of these volatile agents. Recovery profiles for both agents indicate they are superior to isoflurane. In side-by-side comparisons of desflurane and sevoflurane, desflurane permits a more rapid awakening than sevoflurane. It also has a lower incidence of nausea and vomiting, a variable that could be significant in the neurosurgical patient population.[103] In contrast, sevoflurane allows for acute changes in vaporizer settings without evoking neurocirculatory excitation (significant increases in sympathetic nerve activity, norepinephrine concentrations, HR, and mean arterial blood pressure); of particular interest was the finding that desflurane's sympathomimetic response occurred in response to a controlled adjustment in vaporizer settings (i.e., changing from 6% to 9%)—that is, in the absence of overpressurization.[104] Sevoflurane may be preferred over desflurane if concentrations equal to or in excess of 1 MAC are used during neurologic surgery.[72] Additional research is necessary to clarify whether the use of one volatile agent over another influences neurosurgical outcome.

Cardiovascular System

All inhalation agents are capable of altering hemodynamics, the extent being related to various preoperative and intraoperative factors (e.g., American Society of Anesthesiologists physical status; coadministration of vasoactive drugs, opioids, barbiturates). This section reviews the influence of volatile agents on the cardiovascular system.

Systemic Hemodynamics

Halothane, isoflurane, desflurane, and sevoflurane all reduce mean arterial pressure (MAP) (Figure 7-4), cardiac output (CO), and cardiac index (CI) in a dose-dependent fashion.[104,105] The mechanism by which each accomplishes this varies. For example, desflurane, sevoflurane, and isoflurane predominantly reduce MAP via a reduction in systemic vascular resistance (SVR), with the dose-response relationship being least with sevoflurane (Figure 7-5).[104,106] Halothane, by comparison, causes less disruption in inherent vascular tone and therefore predominantly reduces MAP by direct myocardial depression versus a reduction in preload.[107] N_2O activates the sympathetic nervous system and increases SVR,[108] which can also lead to an increase in central venous pressure (CVP).

In general, N_2O used in combination with inhalation agents increases SVR and helps support arterial blood pressure.[109] In contrast, with opioids the addition of N_2O augments cardiac depression instead of supporting it,[110] because N_2O also produces a direct negative inotropic effect. This property can be unmasked in patients with decreased left ventricular function secondary to coronary artery disease or valvular heart defects.[111] Criteria for selecting a volatile anesthetic should at times be based on the capacity of the agent to depress the normal and failing myocardium: halothane > isoflurane = sevoflurane = desflurane > N_2O (although research in a canine model showed that 70% N_2O was equipotent to 1 MAC isoflurane).[112,113]

Desflurane supports CI better than halothane at both low and high MAC levels (i.e., 1.66 MAC; Figure 7-6). With light levels of anesthesia, desflurane maintains the CI without an accompanied elevation in HR. For deeper levels of anesthesia, the CI is probably supported by the associated rise in HR. Some investigators believe the favorable circulatory profile of desflurane, isoflurane, and sevoflurane results from their ability to attenuate the body's circulatory compensatory mechanisms

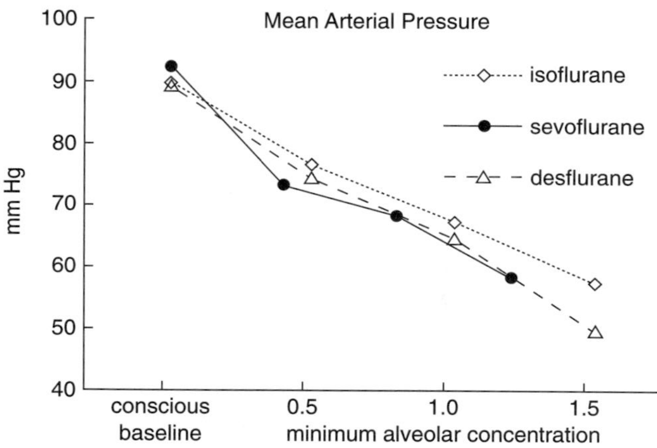

FIGURE **7-4**
Mean arterial pressure response to the administration of isoflurane, sevoflurane, and desflurane in healthy volunteers. With increasing minimum alveolar anesthetic concentration, progressive decreases in blood pressure occurred with each of the volatile anesthetics. (Data from Ebert TJ, Muzi M. Sympathetic hyperactivity during desflurane anesthesia in healthy volunteers: a comparison with isoflurane. *Anesthesiology*. 1993;79:444-453; and Ebert TJ, Muzi M, Lopatka CW. The neurocirculatory responses to sevoflurane anesthesia in humans: a comparison to desflurane. *Anesthesiology*. 1995;83:88-95. Reprinted with permission from Ebert TJ, Harkin C, Muzi M. Cardiovascular responses to sevoflurane: a review. *Anesth Analg*. 1995;81:S11-S22.)

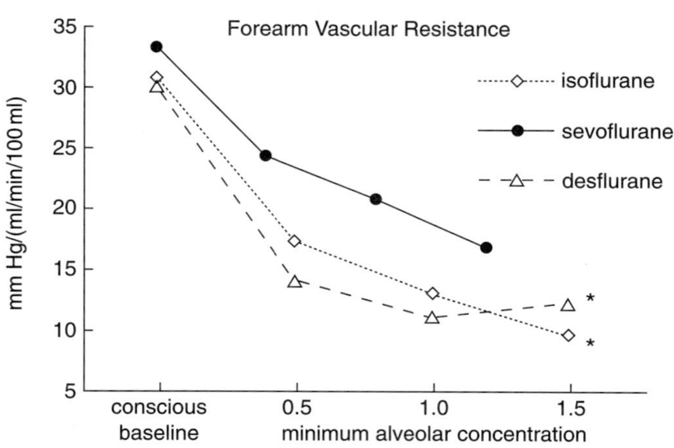

FIGURE **7-5**
Forearm vascular resistance response to the administration of isoflurane, sevoflurane, and desflurane in healthy volunteers. Forearm vascular resistance was, in general, progressively decreased with increasing minimum alveolar anesthetic concentrations of each of the volatile anesthetics; however, this decline was less in the group receiving sevoflurane. (Data from Ebert TJ, Muzi M. Sympathetic hyperactivity during desflurane anesthesia in healthy volunteers: a comparison with isoflurane. *Anesthesiology*. 1993;79:444-453; and Ebert TJ, Muzi M, Lopatka CW. The neurocirculatory responses to sevoflurane anesthesia in humans: a comparison to desflurane. *Anesthesiology*. 1995;83:88-95. Reprinted with permission from Ebert TJ, Harkin C, Muzi M. Cardiovascular responses to sevoflurane: a review. *Anesth Analg*. 1995;81:S11-S22.)

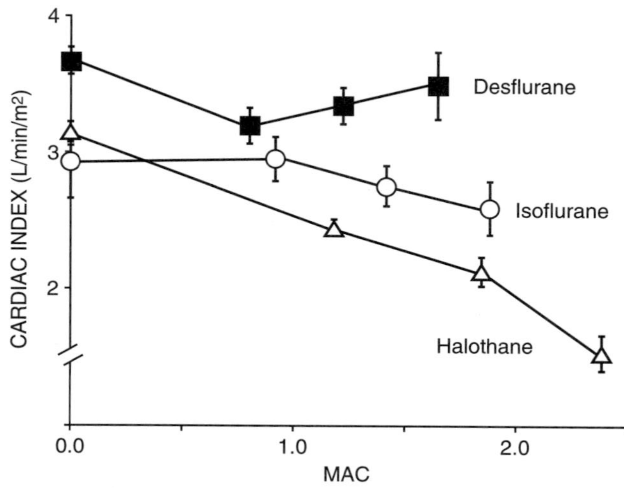

FIGURE **7-6**
Cardiac index measured in healthy normocarbic volunteers during conscious state (0) MAC and during various steady-state MAC levels of halothane, isoflurane,[90] and desflurane. (Reprinted with permission from Warltier DC, as modified from Weiskopf et al. Cardiovascular and respiratory actions of desflurane: Is desflurane different from isoflurane? *Anesth Analg*. 1992;75:S23.)

in a dose-related manner.[104,114] For example, halothane and isoflurane (but not sevoflurane) at 2 MAC abate the positive chronotropic response to head-up tilt.[115] Full recovery of baroreflex function after 2 hours of 1.3% end-tidal isoflurane and 2% end-tidal sevoflurane has been shown to occur in 2 hours.[116]

Regarding the impact of the duration of anesthesia on hemodynamics, desflurane is similar to halothane and isoflurane. As MAC-hours of anesthesia increase, each agent exerts less of a myocardial depressant effect, as evidenced by an increase in CO or CI over time.[107,117] This effect may be secondary to a continued reduction in SVR and increase in HR (with desflurane and halothane) after prolonged exposure to each of the agents.[117] Protracted anesthesia (8 hours) in healthy volunteers anesthetized with desflurane and sevoflurane leads to an increase in pupil size and HR independent of surgery.[67] These changes are not associated with increases in plasma catecholamines, blood pressure, or CO_2 production; therefore mydriasis and tachycardia as signs of anesthetic depth could be misleading at times.

Although anesthetic changes produced at the cellular level have already been discussed, it is sensible to briefly review the cellular effects of inhaled anesthetics on the aforementioned areas of the cardiovascular system. In vitro studies have revealed that halothane and isoflurane can reduce intracellular free Ca^{+2} concentrations in cardiac and vascular smooth muscle.[118] The mechanism for this is believed to be a reduction in Ca^{+2} influx through the sarcolemma along with a decreased release (a transient increase also occurs that results in decreased accumulation[119]) of Ca^{+2} from the sarcoplasmic reticulum.[113,118,120] The end result is a depression in the contractile state of the myocardium along with dilation of the peripheral vasculature. Other reported cellular effects of volatile agents include augmentation and attenuation of endothelium-derived relaxation factor, inhibition of acetylcholine-induced vascular relaxation,[121] and attenuation of Na^+-Ca^{2+} exchange that leads to a reduction in the quantity of intracellular Ca^{2+}.[122]

Heart Rate

Volatile agents and N_2O induce changes in HR relative to the concentration of the anesthetic being used. Alterations in HR are a result of several variables: antagonism of SA node automaticity,[123] modulation of baroreceptor reflex activity, and sympathetic nervous system activation via activation of tracheopulmonary and systemic receptors.[124]

Halothane and sevoflurane produce only minor alterations in HR, even when used in excess of 1 MAC,[125] although a rapid and large increase in the inspired concentration (e.g., from 0.5 MAC to 2.9 MAC) of sevoflurane (and isoflurane) may produce an increase in plasma epinephrine concentrations.[126] Isoflurane and desflurane can cause an increase in HR,[127] and when more than 1 MAC of desflurane is used (even without overpressurization), the dose-response relationship becomes more prominent, particularly when compared with sevoflurane (Figure 7-7).[104] Desflurane's steep dose-response to HR can potentially cause problems by diminishing the reliability of HR as a guide to anesthetic depth and by predisposing patients at risk for coronary artery disease to myocardial ischemia secondary to an increase myocardial O_2 demand.

Research has shown that pretreatment with fentanyl (1.5 mcg/kg or 4.5 mcg/kg) 5 minutes before an increase in end-tidal desflurane concentration from 4% to 8% modulates (but does not abolish) an increase in HR by 61% and 70%,

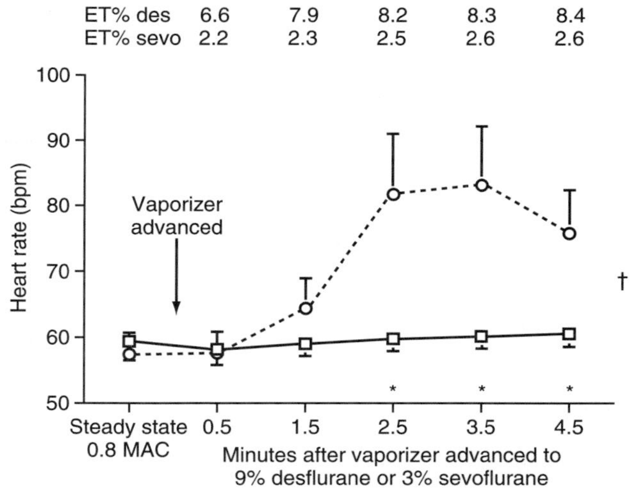

FIGURE **7-7**
The effects of sevoflurane *(solid line with squares)* and desflurane *(dashed line with circles)* on heart rate in healthy young volunteers when the inspiratory concentration is rapidly increased from a steady-state value of 0.83 minimum alveolar concentration (MAC) to 1.25 MAC. (Reprinted with permission from Ebert TJ. Neurocirculatory responses to sevoflurane in humans. *Anesthesiology*. 1995;83:88.)

respectively.[128] In the same study the increase in MAP was attenuated by 31% and 46%. Another group of investigators found that 5 mcg/kg of fentanyl followed by a continuous infusion of 2 mcg/kg/hr initiated 12 minutes before induction significantly blunted the HR and MAP response to a rapid increase in end-tidal desflurane concentration (5.4% to 11%).[129] The acute change in desflurane concentration occurred 20 minutes after intubation. The efficacy of fentanyl was also assessed 2 minutes after induction when desflurane was given in three incremental 1-minute steps (3.6%, 7.2%, 11%). Of interest was the finding that fentanyl was ineffective in diminishing the desflurane stimulatory effect during this induction period. Therefore the optimal use of fentanyl may be during steady-state periods of anesthesia when acute adjustments of desflurane are desired.

Esmolol (0.75 mg/kg) has been shown to attenuate HR response but not MAP and therefore may be less desirable than fentanyl.[128] Prior administration of intravenous lidocaine (1.5 mg/kg) has not been shown to be effective in modulating the sympathetic response associated with an acute change in desflurane end-tidal MAC value of 0.7 to 1.5.[130]

Coronary Blood Flow

The term *coronary steal* refers to a reduction in perfusion of ischemic myocardium with simultaneous improvement of blood flow to nonischemic tissue. Simply stated, blood has been taken from the "poor" and given to the "rich" (a "reverse Robin Hood" syndrome). In addition, this phenomenon has been demonstrated to occur more easily with "coronary steal–prone anatomy" (i.e., multivessel disease models).[131] Several articles have suggested that isoflurane and perhaps desflurane are capable of producing a coronary steal with clinically relevant concentrations,[132] but other researchers have not found this to occur.[133,134] One investigator's results suggest that the use of 0.5% isoflurane in combination with 50% N_2O might be protective to the myocardium (i.e., might improve the tolerance to pacing-induced myocardial ischemia).[135] Recent data suggest that the inhalation anesthetics exert a protective effect against ischemia and reperfusion injury referred to as *anesthetic preconditioning* (APC),[136] which is similar in concept to ischemic preconditioning. Inhalation anesthetics have a varying ability to protect against ischemia and reperfusion injury via effects on potassium-sensitive adenosine triphosphate (ATP) channels, nuclear synthesis of new growth factors, and other protective proteins and possibly up-regulation of G proteins coupled to adenosine, muscarinic, and opioid receptors.

An important qualifier to isoflurane's ability to maldistribute coronary blood flow is the presence of hypotension; when normotension is maintained, a steal phenomenon is abated.[135,137] Reduced blood flow to ischemic myocardium can also be reversed if normotension is reestablished with phenylephrine administration.[138] To summarize the effects of isoflurane, desflurane, and sevoflurane on the coronary circulation, it can be stated that each produces vasodilation, with sevoflurane doing so the least.[132,139] In the presence of hypotension a steal phenomenon can occur (as it can with inappropriate use of intravenous nitroglycerin or sodium nitroprusside), and this effect is reversible if normotension is reestablished. The magnitude of coronary vasodilation also is markedly less with isoflurane than with dipyridamole[140] and the endogenous nucleoside adenosine,[141] both of which produce coronary vasodilation even in the presence of normotension. Any of these three volatile anesthetics can be used in patients with a history of ischemic heart disease. If ECG monitoring demonstrates ST-segment or T-wave changes suggestive of myocardial ischemia (in the absence of abnormal hemodynamics), a change in primary anesthetic techniques may be warranted (e.g., substitution of isoflurane for sevoflurane).[132,134]

Dysrhythmias

The dysrhythmic potential of inhalation agents has long been recognized. All of the agents, with the exception of isoflurane and probably desflurane, are conducive to the development of bradycardias and disturbances in atrioventricular (AV) nodal conduction (excluding second- or third-degree AV block). The mechanism for this is the ability of inhalation agents to depress slow-response (sinoatrial and AV nodal tissue) and fast-response (atrial or ventricular musculature, Purkinje fibers) action potentials. When fibers become ischemic or injured, the volatile agents (particularly halothane) are prone to produce reentrant excitation.[142]

The ability of the volatile agents to reduce the quantity of catecholamines necessary to evoke dysrhythmias is commonly but inaccurately called "sensitization." It is more accurate to describe this phenomenon as an adverse drug interaction.[142] Researchers have determined the nasal and oral submucosal effective dose (ED_{50}) dosage of epinephrine for volatile agents to be 2.11 ± 0.15 mcg/kg for halothane and 6.72 ± 0.66 mcg/kg for isoflurane.[143] With these dosages, 50% of subjects developed three or more premature ventricular contractions or ventricular tachycardia during or immediately after a single injection of epinephrine (which required 3.5 to 11 minutes to complete). Variables that may influence epinephrine ED_{50} values are differences in systemic absorption, route of administration, existing plasma catecholamine levels, preexisting atrial or ventricular dysrhythmias, and the previous administration of induction agents (e.g., thiopental,[144] ketamine,[145] each of which increases the incidence of epinephrine-induced dysrhythmias). When these variables are taken into consideration it is not surprising that data regarding volatile agent "sensitization" are conflicting.[146] Regarding the two newest volatile agents, desflurane and sevoflurane, both appear to be similar to isoflurane in their epinephrine-arrhythmogenic potential.[147]

In general, it is reasonable to anticipate the fewest difficulties with dysrhythmias if the epinephrine dose remains 7 mcg/kg or less when isoflurane, desflurane, or sevoflurane is used[147] and 1 mcg/kg or less during the administration of halothane, the ED_{50} value of which is half that of epinephrine. In children anesthetized with halothane who are normocarbic and do not have congenital heart disease, the dose is 10 mcg/kg.[148] Additional protection can be achieved by combining 0.5% lidocaine with epinephrine; the net effect is an increase in the minimum threshold dose of epinephrine.[143]

N_2O in combination with halothane in canine studies appears to promote epinephrine dysrhythmias.[149] The mechanism by which this occurs is unknown, because no studies have examined the electrophysiologic effects of N_2O on the heart. Also, prolonged desflurane administration in combination with low-dose dopamine or dobutamine (5 mcg/kg/min) in patients undergoing advanced head and neck reconstructive surgery has been associated with increased postoperative mortality. The critical events that were associated with each death were acute bradycardia or tachycardia accompanied by ST-segment changes.[150]

One other point is worth mentioning in relation to rhythm disturbances and inhalation agents: patients who are given a general anesthetic (primary opioid supplemented with a volatile anesthetic) who are on amiodarone can have significant dysrhythmias intraoperatively or postoperatively (e.g., atropine-resistant bradycardia requiring isoproterenol infusions, AV sequential pacing). These significant rhythm disturbances can also result in death.[151] For clarification and emphasis it should be understood that amiodarone and its major metabolite are detectable in plasma for up to 9 months after discontinuation of therapy.[152]

Pulmonary Circulation

Pulmonary vascular resistance (PVR) is also affected by the volatile agents and N_2O. The effects of N_2O on PVR vary with age and preexisting levels of PVR. In adults with normal PVR the addition of N_2O results in a small increase in PVR,[153] presumably because of an increase in sympathetic nervous system tone.[108] If a subject has preexisting pulmonary hypertension, the addition of N_2O results in larger increases in PVR,[153] which may become clinically significant. Volatile agents (including 0.8 or 1.2 MAC desflurane) decrease pulmonary artery pressure; the opposite effect occurs when desflurane is administered at 1.6 MAC.[105]

The pulmonary vasculature also minimizes changes in alveolar-arterial O_2 tension gradient via hypoxic pulmonary vasoconstriction (HPV). This normal physiologic response to atelectasis or hypoxia is attenuated in vivo by halothane and isoflurane and markedly by N_2O.[154] All of the currently used volatile agents only marginally affect HPV. Consistent with this finding, one group of researchers noted only minimal impairment in oxygenation (approximately 20% reduction in HPV at 1 MAC) in patients having one-lung ventilation performed during thoracotomy procedures. Desflurane and sevoflurane delivered at 1 MAC without N_2O have also been shown to only slightly affect arterial oxygenation in patients placed in a lateral position while undergoing esophagogastrectomy.[155,156]

Respiratory System

As seen with other systems of the body, the volatile agents exert a dose-response effect on the respiratory system, primarily tidal volume (TV). Responsiveness to CO_2 is depressed and the TV reduced as concentrations of the agents are increased. The compensatory mechanism for the diminished TV with halothane, sevoflurane, and desflurane is an increase in respiratory rate (RR).[157,158] However, the increase in RR is not sufficient to prevent elevations in arterial CO_2 tension. In addition, isoflurane is unique in that it generally does not support minute volume (MV) as well, because it does not increase RR[157] unless it is combined with N_2O.[159] Surgical stimulation is another variable that helps overcome the respiratory depressant effects of isoflurane.[160]

Studies in humans have determined that the dose-response effect on $PaCO_2$ with anesthetic concentrations less than 1.24 MAC is of the following order: desflurane = isoflurane = sevoflurane ≥ halothane (at 1.1 MAC the effect of sevoflurane was similar to that of halothane, and at 1.4 MAC sevoflurane was a greater respiratory depressant). Emergence from an anesthetic can be associated with hypercarbia if MV is not adequately supported, because of the capacity of a volatile agent to depress the ventilatory response to $PaCO_2$ and PaO_2.[161,162] Hypercarbia also represents an increase in the apneic threshold (higher $PaCO_2$ values are required for spontaneous ventilation to occur). Patients should be closely monitored during emergence from an anesthetic and after adequate reversal of muscle relaxants to avoid acidemia or hypercarbia. During this phase of the anesthetic, significant end-tidal values of residual volatile anesthetic may persist, particularly if an opioid was recently administered (synergistic effect). It is important to recognize that impairment of the hypoxic ventilatory response by volatile agents is not abated with CNS arousal or acute pain.[163] Specifically, arousal of subjects to a level of wakefulness via a noxious stimulus does not reverse the depressed hypoxic ventilatory response (peripheral arterial chemoreceptors) seen with 0.1 MAC sevoflurane. These research findings have implications for patients whose MVs are maintained via a hypoxic drive (e.g., emphysematous patients with depressed central chemoreceptors).

The smoothness of an inhalation induction is directly related to the ability of an inhalation agent to avoid provoking an irritant response. Halothane, N_2O, and sevoflurane are considered the standards by which other agents are measured because of the low incidence of breath holding, coughing, secretions, and laryngospasm encountered during inhalational induction. In contrast, desflurane is considered a respiratory irritant when used for mask induction in concentrations greater than 6%[164]; therefore it is generally not used to induce anesthesia in pediatric[165] and adult patients. One alternative method for incorporation of desflurane in the pediatric population is to induce the child with halothane or sevoflurane, then change to desflurane for maintenance. For example, there is no significant difference in the incidence of respiratory complications (e.g., coughing, laryngospasm) when desflurane has been compared with other anesthetic maintenance techniques (the use of 67% N_2O combined with 1.4% to 6% desflurane, 0.25% to 1% isoflurane, or 50 to 200 mcg/kg/min propofol).[166] The induction method used for these three groups of patients included intravenous propofol followed by insertion of a laryngeal mask airway. The following techniques have been shown to lessen the incidence of the airway irritant properties of desflurane: administration of fentanyl 1.5 mcg/kg or morphine 0.1 mg/kg as a premedicant before an inhalational induction; a more gradual increase in the concentration of desflurane (1% increments after every 6 breaths)[167]; and performance of intravenous inductions with propofol.[168]

Kidneys

In general, autoregulation of the renal circulation remains intact during the administration of inhalation agents. Reductions in systolic blood pressure are accompanied by decreases in renal vascular resistance.[169] Nevertheless, compensatory reductions in renal vascular resistance can still lead to a decline in the glomerular filtration rate. This may contribute to the commonly observed intraoperative reduction in urinary output.

The potential for a volatile agent to produce renal damage is commonly assessed by the extent to which it elevates creatinine, blood urea nitrogen (BUN), and serum inorganic fluoride (F^-) concentrations.[170] With the older volatile agent methoxyflurane, a "toxic threshold" for peak serum concentration of F^- was established (50 μmol)[171]; at this value vasopressin-resistant polyuric renal insufficiency occurs.[172]

Of the currently used inhalation agents, desflurane has been shown in both healthy and chronic renal disease patients[173] to alter these indices of renal integrity the least. One group of researchers found that 3.1 MAC-hours of desflurane anesthesia produced only negligible changes in serum F^- levels.[14] Another study documented no change in serum creatinine and BUN in young, healthy volunteers after 7.4 MAC-hours of anesthesia.[174] These subjects were induced with desflurane and received no other drugs (with the exception of 60% N_2O in some volunteers). In another clinical investigation involving 10 healthy male volunteers, it was shown that after 1 MAC-hour of desflurane no change had occurred in the renal function tests of urinary retinol-binding protein and *N*-acetyl-β-glucosaminidase (NAG).[175] The significance of this is that NAG is considered a sensitive indicator of drug-induced proximal tubular necrosis,[176,177] and retinol-binding protein has been shown to be a specific marker for indicating the presence of tubular damage of any cause.[178] Recent advancements in clinical markers for renal integrity have shown two new, perhaps better, biomarkers of tubular injury. Isoforms of glutathione-*S*-transferase (GST) include alpha GST, which is located exclusively in the proximal tubules, and pi GST, found only in the distal tubules.[179] In humans the urinary levels of each of these enzymes have been shown to increase after acute tubular necrosis and renal infarction.[180]

In contrast to studies involving desflurane (and isoflurane),[181] research with sevoflurane has generated concerns regarding compromised renal function. However, the current debate has settled on the degradation of sevoflurane by CO_2 absorbents. Most researchers now accept that serum inorganic fluoride (F^-) levels associated with sevoflurane administration do not represent a significant risk to patients; including those with compromised renal function.[182-184] Millions of sevoflurane anesthetic procedures worldwide have failed to demonstrate any significant untoward renal outcomes in the general surgical population.

Previous research has shown that sevoflurane yields higher peak serum F^- levels than isoflurane.[185] In one study that compared isoflurane with sevoflurane, no patients had any evidence of renal dysfunction after 1 MAC-hour to more than 7 MAC-hours of surgical anesthesia. The mean peak plasma

F^- concentrations did not significantly increase with the isoflurane group but were elevated to a mean peak value of 29.3 ± 1.8 μmol/L 2 hours after sevoflurane anesthesia. This value decreased to 18 μmol/L by 8 hours after anesthesia. A peak plasma F^- level of 100 μmol/L was not reached by any patients[186] (this value has been associated with obvious defects in urine-concentrating ability[171]). A study investigating plasma inorganic F^- levels with sevoflurane anesthesia in morbidly obese versus nonobese patients also failed to detect any difference in sevoflurane's biotransformation and subsequent fluoride levels.[186]

A concern still exists on the part of some researchers regarding sevoflurane's degradation within anesthesia circuits by barium hydroxide lime and soda lime.[187,188] Sevoflurane, like isoflurane, is absorbed in appreciable volumes by soda lime and barium hydroxide lime.[187] In contrast, isoflurane is not broken down, even with the addition of CO_2, which causes an increase in temperature.[189]

The two by-products of sevoflurane's degradation that have been measured in a closed circuit are fluoromethyl-2,2-difluoro-1 (trifluoromethyl)-vinyl ether (also known as compound A, an olefin) and fluoromethyl-2-methoxy-2,2-difluoro-1-(trifluoromethyl) ethyl ether (compound B).[190] The former is known to produce proximal corticomedullary tubular necrosis in rats.[191,192] Clinical studies involving low-flow (1 L/min) sevoflurane anesthesia have found maximum compound A in concentrations that averaged 13.6 to 41.3 ppm with soda lime.[193,194] In these studies no evidence was found of depressed renal function, which was assessed via serum creatine, BUN, and osmolarity. Unfortunately, these tests are less sensitive than glucosuria, proteinuria, and increased alpha GST excretion in detection of nephrotoxicity induced by compound A.

Kharasch and colleagues[195] compared the effects of low-flow (1 L/min) sevoflurane versus isoflurane on renal function in patients with normal renal function. To further maximize the quantity of compound A produced, barium hydroxide lime was used as the CO_2 absorbent.[196] The average anesthetic duration was 3.7 hours for sevoflurane and 3.9 hours for isoflurane. The results showed that no difference existed between sevoflurane and isoflurane in serum creatinine, BUN, NAG, alpha GST excretion, or pi GST excretion. Each parameter was measured the morning of surgery, then 24 and 72 hours after anesthesia (inspired compound A concentrations were less than or equal to 67 ppm). The patients who received sevoflurane did have significantly greater inorganic fluoride concentrations (10 of 36 patients exceeded 50 μmol). This study demonstrates that low-flow sevoflurane anesthesia of moderate duration is as safe as low-flow isoflurane anesthesia in patients with normal kidney function.[195] Other investigators have reported similar results[183,184,197,198]—one with sevoflurane administered over 8 hours at 1.25 MAC with a fresh gas flow of 2 L/min and another with 3.1 MAC-hours of sevoflurane given with a fresh gas flow of 1 L/min or less. Noteworthy for the latter study was the use of Baralyme to increase the exposure of patients (who had stable renal insufficiency) to compound A. No statistically significant differences were found in serum creatinine, blood urea nitrogen, creatinine clearance, urine protein, and glucose between the low-flow isoflurane and low-flow sevoflurane groups.[198] Two other studies also found the effect of sevoflurane on renal tubules in patients with moderately impaired renal function to be similar to that of isoflurane.[183]

Despite the lack of change in tests results in the studies listed previously, Eger and co-workers found significant changes in alpha GST and pi GST values measured 1, 2, 3, and 5 to 7 days after 8 hours of 1.25 MAC sevoflurane. They worked with healthy volunteers who received their anesthetic through a standard circle absorber system with a fresh gas flow of 2 L/min. The change in the volunteers' GST values equated with an established threshold for renal injury—a threshold applicable to rats and humans with normal kidney function,[199] although the latter (a threshold applicable to humans) is debatable when other variables are taken into consideration.[200] To the researchers' credit, they did acknowledge the fact that despite the changes in alpha GST and pi GST, other measures of renal integrity failed to show a diminution in kidney function (serum creatinine, BUN, and a vasopressin stress test).[201]

In summary, continued research will aid anesthetists in determining the clinical significance of compound A and how its production might or should affect their anesthetic practices. It is widely recognized that the following variables increase the content of compound A low fresh gas flows, high concentrations of sevoflurane, drying of soda lime or Baralyme, and the use of Baralyme as the CO_2 absorbent.[202] One way to eliminate compound A is to replace soda lime or Baralyme with Amsorb. This new CO_2 absorbent does not contain strong bases (sodium hydroxide [NaOH] or potassium hydroxide [KOH]), which are responsible for the degradation of sevoflurane to compound A as well as the production of carbon monoxide from the breakdown of desflurane or isoflurane.[203] It is anticipated that the availability of Amsorb will bring about a revision of the current U.S. Food and Drug Administration (FDA)–approved package insert dosage guidelines for sevoflurane, which state that a minimum of 1 L/min of fresh gas flow should be used and that 2 MAC-hours at this flow rate should not be exceeded.

Liver

"Halothane hepatitis" has been investigated for nearly 40 years, since the first appearance in the literature of case reports of hepatic damage.[204] A better understanding of the pathophysiology of this phenomenon has improved diagnostic capabilities for volatile-agent hepatitis (e.g., with halothane, isoflurane).[205]

Halothane-associated hepatitis is most common in the adult population (children are not immune to the response[206]) and is expressed in one of two clinical forms. The first is a mild hepatic reaction that occurs secondarily to a direct hepatic effect or after reductive metabolism of halothane.[207] It is associated with low morbidity and moderately increased concentrations of elevated serum GST levels[208] or transient jaundice. It can occur shortly after the first exposure to a volatile agent, and the incidence may be as high as 20% to 50%.[209]

The second syndrome is characterized by fulminant hepatic failure with a high mortality rate. Multiple anesthetic exposures precede its onset, which has led researchers to theorize that an immune response evokes this syndrome. Oxidative metabolism of halothane by hepatic cytochrome P-450 releases an unstable intermediate, trifluoroacetyl chloride (CF_3COCl). This substance binds to liver proteins to form TFA-protein neoantigens.[209] Unfortunately, some patients form antibodies to TFA-protein neoantigens and on reexposure to halothane develop an immune response that is expressed as hepatic necrosis.[209,210] TFA-protein antibodies occur in up to 70% of patients with fulminant hepatic failure.[210] These antibodies do not appear in patients with normal liver function, in patients with hepatic injury resulting from other causes, or in subjects who previously received halothane but have not developed fulminant hepatic failure.

The predominant P-450 isoform responsible for the oxidation of halothane is cytochrome P-450 2E1. This may help explain why morbidly obese patients are prone to halothane hepatitis, in that the enzymatic activity of P-450 2E1 increases in this patient population.[211] In addition, the fatty liver infiltration observed in obese patients is associated with a greater quantity of P-450 2E1. These findings have led some researchers to propose that pretreatment with disulfiram to inhibit P-450 2E1 synthesis may be protective by shunting halothane metabolism to a reductive pathway.[211] The clinical applications for this finding are limited, given that halothane is not advocated for use in adult patients—particularly those with risk factors for development of halothane hepatitis (e.g., fatty liver infiltration, having multiple anesthetics, isoniazid and ethanol use).[212]

The overall incidence of the fulminant form of halothane hepatitis is reported to be 1:35,000 anesthetic administrations.[213] In a Swedish study the incidence was found to be much lower, at 1:110,000 anesthetic procedures.[214] In addition to the laboratory changes noted previously, the development of more specific serologic markers (i.e., hepatitis C, D, and E[215]) for detecting the presence of viral hepatitis has led to fewer false-positive diagnoses of halothane-associated hepatitis.

Isoflurane and desflurane are similar to halothane in that each possesses a common metabolic pathway via cytochrome P-450 that eventually yields TFA-protein molecules.[205,209] However, because of differences in the rate of biodegradation, these volatile agents are probably less likely to produce hepatic injury than halothane. For example, isoflurane is metabolized 100-fold less than halothane, and therefore it is estimated that fulminant hepatic failure caused by isoflurane may occur in 1:3,500,000 anesthetic procedures.[205] Several case reports and clinical studies suggest that a potential immunologic mechanism (including cross-sensitization) may exist for the development of "hepatitis," "isoflurane hepatitis," "sevoflurane hepatitis," and "desflurane hepatitis."[216-218] The literature contains several case reports linking each of these agents to liver damage. In one of these cases the patient developed fulminant hepatic failure that led to death.[217]

Although desflurane is metabolized the least of all volatile anesthetics, it has also been associated with hepatotoxicity.[218] In one case report a 65-year-old woman without a history of liver disease developed desflurane hepatitis 12 days postoperatively. The patient had a rash, nausea, polyarthralgias, marked elevations in liver transaminases, and jaundice. Serologic markers for hepatitis A, B, and C were negative. It was significant that the patient had undergone two prior halothane anesthetic procedures that lasted approximately 45 minutes each (death from a halothane anesthetic given 28 years after primary exposure has been documented[219]). The patient was discharged from the hospital 27 days after surgery, with continued improvement in liver function.

Sevoflurane is unique among the volatile anesthetics in that it is the only one that appears not to be biodegraded to TFA-protein molecules.[220] This step is a prerequisite to the formation of TFA-protein antibodies, so it is unlikely that sevoflurane will produce fulminate hepatic failure via an immunoallergic mechanism.[221] Nonetheless, there have been several case reports of hepatic injury associated with sevoflurane use,[222] including one that involved a child.[223]

In spite of the case reports listed above, it is extremely rare for isoflurane, sevoflurane, and desflurane to produce clinically significant liver damage. Their molecular structure (increased fluorination) resists hepatic degradation, and their pharmacodynamic profile is associated with no changes or a slight reductions in hepatic blood flow.

Current in vitro research suggests that N_2O is metabolized minimally (0.004%) by intestinal microflora, yielding molecular nitrogen (N_2).[224] The limited metabolism does not necessarily mean that N_2O is an inert substance within the body. On the contrary, studies have demonstrated that chronic exposure to N_2O can lead to inactivation of the vitamin B_{12} component of methionine synthetase,[225] which can disrupt deoxyribonucleic acid synthesis. Nevertheless, for routine surgical cases this is generally not an issue. Caution should be exercised with patients who are pregnant, patients who receive a general anesthetic more than once a week, and patients who are debilitated and have problems with wound healing.[226]

In summary, current research indicates that TFA-protein formation occurs regularly during halothane anesthesia. Why only a small percentage of patients produce TFA-protein antibodies is unknown. Risks of the development of depressed liver function or failure may be enhanced with frequent repeated exposure (possibly within a 4- to 8-week period) to halothane or another volatile agent (cross-sensitization). This is especially true for obese middle-aged women.[212]

Neuromuscular System

All volatile agents produce a dose-dependent relaxation of skeletal muscle, as well as potentiation of the effects of depolarizing and nondepolarizing muscle relaxants.[227] The mechanism by which this occurs is multifactorial, involving reduced neural activity within the CNS and a presynaptic or postsynaptic effect at the neuromuscular junction. Of the synaptic changes produced, the volatile agents predominantly affect the postjunctional membrane.

With the exception of halothane, it is variable as to which volatile agent potentiates neuromuscular blocking agents the most. Studies incorporating a broader methodology indicate that the greatest degree of potentiation of neuromuscular blockade occurs with sevoflurane, then isoflurane, and finally halothane.[228] Desflurane has been found by some investigators to potentiate the effects of neuromuscular blockers to the same extent as isoflurane[229] and sevoflurane.[230] Similarly, other studies have shown that sevoflurane and isoflurane equally augment and prolong[231] neuromuscular blockade produced by nondepolarizing muscle relaxants. In contrast, one investigation found that desflurane and sevoflurane enhanced the intensity of neuromuscular blockade with rocuronium, whereas the effect of isoflurane was no different from that observed with a total intravenous anesthetic (TIVA).[232]

The discrepancies reported with interactions between volatile agents and muscle relaxants may be the result of differences in research methodology (e.g., the type of muscle relaxant used in the study). For example, recovery of neuromuscular blockade after the use of cisatracurium and rocuronium is prolonged with sevoflurane but not isoflurane.[228,230] In contrast, the recovery profile for both volatile agents is the same after the use of vecuronium.[231]

Isoflurane and N_2O have been shown to potentiate the effects of succinylcholine. The former can accelerate the transition from a phase I to phase II block during an infusion of succinylcholine. In general, nondepolarizing muscle relaxant dosages are decreased by approximately 25%[232,233] (sometimes as much as 50%) of that required with TIVA when they are used in combination with a volatile agent. Of interest are two studies that found no difference in potentiation of nondepolarizing muscle relaxants and neuromuscular recovery profiles[228,230] between an isoflurane with N_2O and TIVA technique.

The volatile agents have also been shown to produce a time-dependent potentiation of (beginning in 5 to 10 minutes) and delayed recovery from nondepolarizing muscle relaxants. For example, after 30 minutes of exposure to sevoflurane, recovery from vecuronium to 25% of baseline neuromuscular function is prolonged by 89%, and after 60 minutes, recovery exceeds 100%.[234] The inhalation agents have also been implicated in impairing reversal of nondepolarizing neuromuscular block.[235] For the reasons listed above, anesthetists should carefully titrate muscle relaxants used in combination with inhalation anesthetics. Also, in select cases, a volatile anesthetic alone may produce adequate skeletal muscle relaxation without concurrent use of muscle relaxants. A summary of the systemic effects of the major inhalation anesthetics is given in Table 7-5. Some advantages and disadvantages are given in Box 7-3.

Malignant Hyperthermia

All of the volatile agents are capable of triggering malignant hyperthermia, including desflurane and sevoflurane.[236,237] These agents should not be used in malignant hyperthermia–susceptible patients, but if a reaction occurs it can generally be successfully treated with intravenous dantrolene. The use of nondepolarizing muscle relaxants has also been shown to delay a malignant hyperthermia response provoked by inhalation agents.

In research done with swine susceptible to malignant hyperthermia, the administration of succinylcholine with desflurane resulted in the development in two animals of profound hypotension and death despite administration of dantrolene and supportive therapy.[201] The clinical relevance of this response remains to be determined.

N_2O is considered at most a weak trigger of malignant hyperthermia in susceptible patients. The premise for this is a report of a case in which N_2O was responsible for a hyperthermic response in an 11-year-old girl who required dental care.[238] Overall, the clinical use of N_2O, in combination with many other agents (e.g., barbiturates, propofol, ketamine, etomidate, opiates, amide and ester anesthetics), is considered acceptable in patients susceptible to malignant hyperthermia.[239]

SUMMARY

Inhalation agents remain the most common class of drugs used to maintain a general anesthetic. With the introduction of desflurane and sevoflurane, the ability to titrate a volatile anesthetic has improved (less hysteresis in pharmacodynamic responses). The limited metabolism of these agents also offers an advantage over many of the older agents. The net effect has been enhanced safety for the patient in these

TABLE 7-5 Effects of the Inhalation Anesthetics

	Halothane	Isoflurane	Desflurane	Sevoflurane
Alveolar equilibration	Slow	Moderate	Fast	Fast
Recovery	Slow	Moderate	Very fast	Fast
Liver				
Hepatotoxicity	Yes	No	No	No
Metabolism (%)	12-25	0.2	0.02	3-5
Musculoskeletal relaxation	Moderate	Significant	Significant	Significant
Cardiovascular System				
Heart rate	Reduced	Increased	Increased	Stable
Cardiac output	Reduced	Slightly reduced	Stable	Slightly reduced
SVR	Stable	Reduced	Reduced	Reduced
MAP	Reduced	Reduced	Reduced	Reduced
Coronary vasodilation	Minimal	Marked	Minimal	Moderate
Sensitization of myocardium	Yes	No	No	No
Respiratory System				
Respiratory irritation	No	Significant	Significant	No
Respiratory depression	Yes	Yes	Marked	Yes
Central Nervous System				
Seizure activity on EEG	No	No	No	No
Renal System				
Renal toxic metabolites	No	No	No	No

EEG, *Electroencephalogram;* SVR, *systemic vascular resistance;* MAP, *mean arterial pressure.*
Modified from Mushambi MC, Smith G. Inhalation anaesthetic agents. In: Aitkenhead AR, Rowbotham DF, Smith G, eds. Textbook of Anaesthesia. *4th ed. Edinburgh: Churchill Livingstone; 2001:152-168.*

BOX 7-3

Clinical Advantages and Disadvantages of Selected Inhalation Anesthetics

Anesthetic	Advantages	Disadvantages
Nitrous oxide	Analgesia Rapid uptake and elimination Little cardiac or respiratory depression Nonpungent Allows less potent anesthetic to be administered	Expansion of closed air spaces Requires high concentrations Diffusion hypoxia Suppression of methionine synthetase that affects vitamin B_{12} utilization Teratogenic?
Halothane	Inexpensive Effective in low concentrations Excellent bronchodilator	Slow uptake and elimination Susceptible to biotransformation Idiosyncratic hepatic necrosis Catecholamine-induced ventricular ectopy Use is rapidly declining Impairs pulmonary macrophage activity and bronchial ciliary mucous transport Trigger for malignant hyperpyrexia
Isoflurane	Moderate muscle relaxation Decreases cerebral metabolic rate Minimal biotransformation No significant systemic toxicity Maintains cardiac output because of vasodilation Inexpensive	Pungent odor Airway irritant Fewer negative inotropic effects than halothane Trigger for malignant hyperpyrexia
Desflurane	Rapid uptake and elimination Stable molecules Minimal biotransformation No significant systemic toxicity	Airway irritant Low boiling point Sympathetic stimulation Expensive Low boiling point and high saturation vapor pressure Needs special, electrically heated vaporizer Rapid increases in inspired concentration can lead to reflex tachycardia and hypertension Trigger for malignant hyperthermia
Sevoflurane	Rapid uptake and elimination Nonpungent Excellent for inhalation induction Cardiovascular effects broadly comparable to those of isoflurane	Susceptible to biotransformation Reacts with soda lime and baralyme Increases serum fluoride concentration Expensive 3%-5% metabolized, but current evidence is that it causes neither hepatic nor renal toxicity

aspects of anesthesia care. Ultimately, the total cost of anesthesia care may also be reduced; continued research, which influences practice guidelines, will eventually determine to what extent.

REFERENCES

1. Frost EAM. A history of nitrous oxide. In: Eger EI, ed. *Nitrous Oxide*. New York: Elsevier; 1985:1-22.
2. Andrews E. The oxygen mixture, a new anaesthetic combination. *Chicago Med Exam*. 1868;9:656-661.
3. Keys TE. *The History of Surgical Anesthesia*. New York: Krieger; 1978.
4. Calverley RK. Fluorinated anesthetics. 1. The early years, 1932-1946. *Surv Anesthesiol*. 1986;30:170-173.
5. Bryce-Smith R, O'Brien HD. Fluothane: a non-explosive anaesthetic agent. *Br Med J*. 1956;2:969-972.
6. Johnstone M. The human cardiovascular response to Fluothane anesthesia. *Br Med J*. 1956;28:392-410.
7. Eger EI, Halsey MJ, Harris RA, et al. Hypothesis: volatile anesthetics produce immobility by acting on two sites approximately five carbon atoms apart. *Anesth Analg*. 1999;88:1395-1400.
8. Halsey MJ. A reassessment of the molecular structure-functional relationships of the inhaled general anaesthetics. *Br J Anaesth*. 1984;56(suppl 1):9S-25S.
9. Robbins JH. Preliminary studies of the anaesthetic activity of fluorinated hydrocarbons. *J Pharmacol Exp Ther*. 1946; 86:197-204.
10. Larsen ER. Fluorine compounds in anesthesiology. In: Tarrant P, ed. *Fluorine Chemistry Reviews*. New York: Marcel Dekker; 1946:3.
11. Targ AG, Yasuda N, Eger EI, et al. Halogenation and anesthetic potency. *Anesth Analg*. 1989;68:599-602.
12. Rudo FG, Krantz JC Jr. Anaesthetic molecules. *Br J Anaesth*. 1974;46:181-189.

13. Terrell RC. Physical and chemical properties of anaesthetic agents (with an appendix on the manufacture of isoflurane). *Br J Anaesth.* 1984;56(suppl 1):3S-7S.
14. Sutton TS, Koblin DD, Gruenke LD, et al. Fluoride metabolites after prolonged exposure of volunteers and patients to desflurane. *Anesth Analg.* 1991;73:180-185.
15. Holaday DA, Fiserova-Bergerova V, Latto IP, Zumbiel MA. Resistance of isoflurane to biotransformation in man. *Anesthesiology.* 1975;43:325-332.
16. Carpenter RL, Eger EI, Johnson BH, Unadkat JD, Sheiner LB. The extent of metabolism of inhaled anesthetics in humans. *Anesthesiology.* 1986;65:201-205.
17. Carpenter RL, Eger EI, Johnson BH, Unadkat JD, Sheiner LB. Pharmacokinetics of inhaled anesthetics in humans: measurements during and after the simultaneous administration of enflurane, halothane, isoflurane, methoxyflurane, and nitrous oxide. *Anesth Analg.* 1986;65:575-582.
18. Yasuda N, Lockhart SH, Eger EI, et al. Kinetics of desflurane, isoflurane, and halothane in humans. *Anesthesiology.* 1991;74: 489-498.
19. Mazze RI, Cousins MJ, Barr GA. Renal effects and metabolism of isoflurane in man. *Anesthesiology.* 1974;40:536-542.
20. Koblin DD. Characteristics and implications of desflurane metabolism and toxicity. *Anesth Analg.* 1992;75(suppl 4): S10-S16.
21. Baden JM, Rice SA. Metabolism and toxicity of inhaled anesthetics. In: Miller RD, ed. *Anesthesia.* Vol 1. 5th ed. Philadelphia: Churchill Livingstone; 2000:147-173.
22. Spracklin DK, Thummel KE, Kharasch ED. Human reductive halothane metabolism in vitro is catalyzed by cytochrome P450 2A6 and 3A4. *Drug Metab Dispos.* 1996;24:976-983.
23. Kharasch ED, Karol MD, Lanni C, Sawchuk R. Clinical sevoflurane metabolism and disposition. I. Sevoflurane and metabolite pharmacokinetics. *Anesthesiology.* 1995;82:1369-1378.
24. Meyer HH. Theorie der alkoholnarkose. *Arch Exp Pathol Pharmakol.* 1899;42:109-118.
25. Overton CE. *Studien uber die Narkose, zugleich ein Beitrag zur allgemeinen Pharmakologie.* Jena, Germany: G Fischer; 1901.
26. Wann KT, Macdonald AG. Actions and interactions of high pressure and general anaesthetics. *Prog Neurobiol.* 1988;30: 271-307.
27. DiFazio CA, Brown RE, Ball CG, Heckel CG, Kennedy SS. Additive effects of anesthetics and theories of anesthesia. *Anesthesiology.* 1972;36:57-63.
28. Gelman S. A step toward consensus on general anesthesia. *Anesth Analg.* 1998;86:446.
29. Eger EI, Koblin DD, Harris RA, et al. Hypothesis: inhaled anesthetics produce immobility and amnesia by different mechanisms at different sites. *Anesth Analg.* 1997;84:915-918.
30. Eger EI, Koblin DD. A step toward consensus on general anesthesia [letter; comment]. *Anesth Analg.* 1998;86:446.
31. Kandel L, Chortkoff BS, Sonner J, Laster MJ, Eger EI. Nonanesthetics can suppress learning. *Anesth Analg.* 1996;82: 321-326.
32. Kendig JJ. In vitro networks: subcortical mechanisms of anaesthetic action. *Br J Anaesth.* 2002;89:91-101.
33. Sonner J, Li J, Eger EI. Desflurane and nitrous oxide, but not nonimmobilizers, affect nociceptive responses. *Anesth Analg.* 1998;86:629-634.
34. Dutton RC, Maurer AJ, Sonner JM, Fanselow MS, Laster MJ, Eger EI. Short-term memory resists the depressant effect of the nonimmobilizer 1-2-dichlorohexafluorocyclobutane (2N) more than long-term memory. *Anesth Analg.* 2002;94:631-639.
35. Eger EI, Xing Y, Pearce R, et al. Isoflurane antagonizes the capacity of flurothyl or 1,2-dichlorohexafluorocyclobutane to impair fear conditioning to context and tone. *Anesth Analg.* 2003;96:1010-1018.
36. Zhang Y, Stabernack C, Sonner J, Dutton R, Eger EI. Both cerebral GABA(A) receptors and spinal GABA(A) receptors modulate the capacity of isoflurane to produce immobility. *Anesth Analg.* 2001;92:1585-1589.
37. Clark DL, Rosner BS. Neurophysiologic effects of general anesthetics. I. The electroencephalogram and sensory evoked responses in man. *Anesthesiology.* 1973;38:564-582.
38. Berg-Johnsen J, Langmoen IA. Mechanisms concerned in the direct effect of isoflurane on rat hippocampal and human neocortical neurons. *Brain Res.* 1990;507:28-34.
39. Angel A. Central neuronal pathways and the process of anaesthesia. *Br J Anaesth.* 1993;71:148-163.
40. Pearce RA. Volatile anaesthetic enhancement of paired-pulse depression investigated in the rat hippocampus in vitro. *J Physiol.* 1996;492(part 3):823-840.
41. Rampil IJ, Lockhart SH, Eger EI, Yasuda N, Weiskopf RB, Cahalan MK. The electroencephalographic effects of desflurane in humans. *Anesthesiology.* 1991;74:434-439.
42. Watts AD, Herrick IA, McLachlan RS, Craen RA, Gelb AW. The effect of sevoflurane and isoflurane anesthesia on interictal spike activity among patients with refractory epilepsy. *Anesth Analg.* 1999;89:1275-1281.
43. Osawa M, Shingu K, Murakawa M, et al. Effects of sevoflurane on central nervous system electrical activity in cats. *Anesth Analg.* 1994;79:52-57.
44. Bruchiel KJ, Stockard JJ, Calverley RK, Smith NT, Scholl ML, Mazze RI. Electroencephalographic abnormalities following halothane anesthesia. *Anesth Analg.* 1978;57:244-251.
45. Borges M, Antognini JF. Does the brain influence somatic responses to noxious stimuli during isoflurane anesthesia? *Anesthesiology.* 1994;81:1511-1515.
46. Collins JG, Kendig JJ, Mason P. Anesthetic actions within the spinal cord: contributions to the state of general anesthesia. *Trends Neurosci.* 1995;18:549-553.
47. Zhou HH, Mehta M, Leis AA. Spinal cord motoneuron excitability during isoflurane and nitrous oxide anesthesia. *Anesthesiology.* 1997;86:302-307.
48. Franks NP, Lieb WR. Molecular and cellular mechanisms of general anaesthesia. *Nature.* 1994;367:607-614.
49. Jenkins A, Franks NP, Lieb WR. Effects of temperature and volatile anesthetics on GABA(A) receptors. *Anesthesiology.* 1999;90:484-491.
50. Franks NP, Jenkins A, Conti E, Lieb WR, Brick P. Structural basis for the inhibition of firefly luciferase by a general anesthetic. *Biophys J.* 1998;75:2205-2211.
51. Mihic SJ, McQuilkin SJ, Eger EI, Ionescu P, Harris RA. Potentiation of gamma-aminobutyric acid type A receptor-mediated chloride currents by novel halogenated compounds correlates with their abilities to induce general anesthesia. *Mol Pharmacol.* 1994;46:851-857.
52. Bloom FE. Neurotransmission and the central nervous system. In: Hardman JG, Limbird LE, eds. *Goodman & Gilman's the Pharmacological Basis of Therapeutics.* 9th ed. New York: McGraw-Hill; 1996:267-293.
53. Lin LH, Chen LL, Zirrolli JA, Harris RA. General anesthetics potentiate gamma-aminobutyric acid actions on gamma-aminobutyric acidA receptors expressed by *Xenopus* oocytes: lack of involvement of intracellular calcium. *J Pharmacol Exp Ther.* 1992;263:569-578.
54. Kaech S, Brinkhaus H, Matus A. Volatile anesthetics block actin-based motility in dendritic spines. *Proc Natl Acad Sci U S A.* 1999;96:10433-10437.
55. Fischer M, Kaech S, Knutti D, Matus A. Rapid actin-based plasticity in dendritic spines. *Neuron.* 1998;20:847-854.
56. Kaech S, Fischer M, Doll T, Matus A. Isoform specificity in the relationship of actin to dendritic spines. *J Neurosci.* 1997;17:9565-9572.
57. Shepherd GM. The dendritic spine: a multifunctional integrative unit. *J Neurophysiol.* 1996;75:2197-2210.
58. Shepherd GM, Koch C. *The Synaptic Organization of the Brain.* Oxford, UK: Oxford University Press; 1998.

59. Sonner JM, Antognini JF, Dutton RC, et al. Inhaled anesthetics and immobility: mechanisms, mysteries, and minimum alveolar anesthetic concentration. *Anesth Analg*. 2003;97:718-40.
60. Eger EI, Saidman LJ, Brandstater B. Minimum alveolar anesthetic concentration: a standard of anesthetic potency. *Anesthesiology*. 1965;26:756-763.
61. Rampil IJ, Lockhart SH, Zwass MS, et al. Clinical characteristics of desflurane in surgical patients: minimum alveolar concentration. *Anesthesiology*. 1991;74:429-433.
62. Nakajima R, Nakajima Y, Ikeda K. Minimum alveolar concentration of sevoflurane in elderly patients. *Br J Anaesth*. 1993;70:273-275.
63. Stoelting RK, Longnecker DE, Eger EI. Minimum alveolar concentrations in man on awakening from methoxyflurane, halothane, ether and fluroxene anesthesia: MAC awake. *Anesthesiology*. 1970;33:5-9.
64. Roizen MF, Horrigan RW, Frazer BM. Anesthetic doses blocking adrenergic (stress) and cardiovascular responses to incision—MAC BAR. *Anesthesiology*. 1981;54:390-398.
65. Daniel M, Weiskopf RB, Noorani M, Eger EI. Fentanyl augments the blockade of the sympathetic response to incision (MAC-BAR) produced by desflurane and isoflurane: desflurane and isoflurane MAC-BAR without and with fentanyl. *Anesthesiology*. 1998;88:43-49.
66. de Jong RH, Eger EI. MAC expanded: AD50 and AD95 values of common inhalation anesthetics in man. *Anesthesiology*. 1975;42:384-389.
67. Tayefeh F, Larson MD, Sessler DI, Eger EI, Bowland T. Time-dependent changes in heart rate and pupil size during desflurane or sevoflurane anesthesia. *Anesth Analg*. 1997;85:1362-1366.
68. Cullen DJ, Eger EI, Stevens WC, et al. Clinical signs of anesthesia. *Anesthesiology*. 1972;36:21-36.
69. Zbinden AM, Petersen-Felix S, Thomson DA. Anesthetic depth defined using multiple noxious stimuli during isoflurane/oxygen anesthesia. II. Hemodynamic responses. *Anesthesiology*. 1994;80:261-267.
70. Heath KJ, Gupta S, Matta BF. The effects of sevoflurane on cerebral hemodynamics during propofol anesthesia. *Anesth Analg*. 1997;85:1284-1287.
71. Bedforth NM, Girling KJ, Harrison JM, Mahajan RP. The effects of sevoflurane and nitrous oxide on middle cerebral artery blood flow velocity and transient hyperemic response. *Anesth Analg*. 1999;89:170-174.
72. Bedforth NM, Hardman JG, Nathanson MH. Cerebral hemodynamic response to the introduction of desflurane: a comparison with sevoflurane [comment]. *Anesth Analg*. 2000;91:152-155.
73. Kolbitsch C, Lorenz IH, Hormann C, et al. A subanesthetic concentration of sevoflurane increases regional cerebral blood flow and regional cerebral blood volume and decreases regional mean transit time and regional cerebrovascular resistance in volunteers. *Anesth Analg*. 2000;91:156-162.
74. Mielck F, Stephan H, Buhre W, Weyland A, Sonntag H. Effects of 1 MAC desflurane on cerebral metabolism, blood flow and carbon dioxide reactivity in humans. *Br J Anaesth*. 1998;81:155-160.
75. Mielck F, Stephan H, Weyland A, Sonntag H. Effects of one minimum alveolar anesthetic concentration sevoflurane on cerebral metabolism, blood flow, and CO_2 reactivity in cardiac patients. *Anesth Analg*. 1999;89:364-369.
76. Manohar M, Parks CM. Porcine systemic and regional organ blood flow during 1.0 and 1.5 minimum alveolar concentrations of sevoflurane anesthesia without and with 50% nitrous oxide. *J Pharmacol Exp Ther*. 1984;231:640-648.
77. Hansen TD, Warner DS, Todd MM, Vust LJ, Trawick DC. Distribution of cerebral blood flow during halothane versus isoflurane anesthesia in rats. *Anesthesiology*. 1988;69:332-337.
78. Hansen TD, Warner DS, Todd MM, Vust LJ. The role of cerebral metabolism in determining the local cerebral blood flow effects of volatile anesthetics: evidence for persistent flow-metabolism coupling. *J Cereb Blood Flow Metab*. 1989;9:323-328.
79. Lam AM, Matta BF, Mayberg TS, Strebel S. Change in cerebral blood flow velocity with onset of EEG silence during inhalation anesthesia in humans: evidence of flow-metabolism coupling? *J Cereb Blood Flow Metab*. 1995;15:714-717.
80. Strebel S, Kaufmann M, Anselmi L, Schaefer HG. Nitrous oxide is a potent cerebrovasodilator in humans when added to isoflurane. A transcranial Doppler study. *Acta Anaesthesiol Scand*. 1995;39:653-658.
81. Reinstrup P, Ryding E, Algotsson L, Berntman L, Uski T. Regional cerebral blood flow (SPECT) during anaesthesia with isoflurane and nitrous oxide in humans. *Br J Anaesth*. 1997;78:407-411.
82. Nakanishi O, Ishikawa T, Imamura Y, Hirakawa T. Inhibition of cerebral metabolic and circulatory responses to nitrous oxide by 6-hydroxydopamine in dogs. *Can J Anaesth*. 1997;44:1008-1013.
83. Petersen-Felix S, Zbinden AM, Fischer M, Thomson DA. Isoflurane minimum alveolar concentration decreases during anesthesia and surgery. *Anesthesiology*. 1993;79:959-965.
84. Wollman H, Alexander SC, Cohen PJ. Cerebral circulation during general anesthesia and hyperventilation in man. *Anesthesiology*. 1965;26:329.
85. Smith AL, Wollman H. Cerebral blood flow and metabolism: effects of anesthetic drugs and techniques. *Anesthesiology*. 1972;36:378-400.
86. Cho S, Fujigaki T, Uchiyama Y, Fukusaki M, Shibata O, Sumikawa K. Effects of sevoflurane with and without nitrous oxide on human cerebral circulation. Transcranial Doppler study. *Anesthesiology*. 1996;85:755-760.
87. Nishiyama T, Matsukawa T, Yokoyama T, Hanaoka K. Cerebrovascular carbon dioxide reactivity during general anesthesia: a comparison between sevoflurane and isoflurane. *Anesth Analg*. 1999;89:1437-1441.
88. Summors AC, Gupta AK, Matta BF. Dynamic cerebral autoregulation during sevoflurane anesthesia: a comparison with isoflurane. *Anesth Analg*. 1999;88:341-345.
89. Muzzi DA, Losasso TJ, Dietz NM, Faust RJ, Cucchiara RF, Milde LN. The effect of desflurane and isoflurane on cerebrospinal fluid pressure in humans with supratentorial mass lesions. *Anesthesiology*. 1992;76:720-724.
90. Hoffman WE, Edelman G. Comparison of isoflurane and desflurane anesthetic depth using burst suppression of the electroencephalogram in neurosurgical patients. *Anesth Analg*. 1995;81:811-816.
91. Schwender D, Daunderer M, Klasing S, Finsterer U, Peter K. Power spectral analysis of the electroencephalogram during increasing end-expiratory concentrations of isoflurane, desflurane and sevoflurane. *Anaesthesia*. 1998;53:335-342.
92. Rehberg B, Ruschner R, Fischer M, Ebeling BJ, Hoeft A. Concentration-dependent changes in the latency and amplitude of somatosensory-evoked potentials by desflurane, isoflurane and sevoflurane. *Anasthesiol Intensivmed Notfallmed Schmerzther*. 1998;33:425-429.
93. Schindler E, Muller M, Zickmann B, Osmer C, Wozniak G, Hempelmann G. Modulation of somatosensory evoked potentials under various concentrations of desflurane with and without nitrous oxide. *J NeurosurgAnesthesiol*. 1998;10:218-223.
94. Vaugha DJ, Thornton C, Wright DR, et al. Effects of different concentrations of sevoflurane and desflurane on subcortical somatosensory evoked responses in anaesthetized, non-stimulated patients. *Br J Anaesth*. 2001;86:59-62.
95. Schindler E, Thiel A, Muller M, Milosevic M, Langer C, Hempelmann G. Changes in somatosensory evoked potentials after sevoflurane and isoflurane. A randomized phase III study. *Anaesthetist*. 1996;45(suppl 1):S52-S56.
96. Iijima T, Nakamura Z, Iwao Y, Sankawa H. The epileptogenic properties of the volatile anesthetics sevoflurane and isoflurane in patients with epilepsy. *Anesth Analg*. 2000;91:989-995.
97. Nieminen K, Westeren-Punnonen S, Kokki H, Ypparila H, Hyvarinen A, Partanen J. Sevoflurane anaesthesia in children

after induction of anaesthesia with midazolam and thiopental does not cause epileptiform EEG. *Br J Anaesth.* 2002;89:853-856.
98. Murao K, Shingu K, Tsushima K, Takahira K, Ikeda S, Nakao S. The anticonvulsant effects of volatile anesthetics on lidocaine-induced seizures in cats. *Anesth Analg.* 2000;90:148-155.
99. Fang Z, Laster MJ, Gong D, et al. Convulsant activity of nonanesthetic gas combinations. *Anesth Analg.* 1997;84: 634-640.
100. Vakkuri A, Yli-Hankala A, Sarkela M, et al. Sevoflurane mask induction of anaesthesia is associated with epileptiform EEG in children. *Acta Anaesthesiol Scand.* 2001;45:805-811.
101. Hilty CA, Drummond JC. Seizure-like activity on emergence from sevoflurane anesthesia. *Anesthesiology.* 2000;93: 1357-1359.
102. Parr SM, Robinson BJ, Glover PW, Galletly DC. Level of consciousness on arrival in the recovery room and the development of early respiratory morbidity. *Anaesth Intensive Care.* 1991;19: 369-372.
103. Eger EI, Bowland T, Ionescu P, et al. Recovery and kinetic characteristics of desflurane and sevoflurane in volunteers after 8-h exposure, including kinetics of degradation products. *Anesthesiology.* 1997;87:517-526.
104. Ebert TJ, Muzi M, Lopatka CW. Neurocirculatory responses to sevoflurane in humans. A comparison to desflurane. *Anesthesiology.* 1995;83:88-95.
105. Malan TP Jr, DiNardo JA, Isner RJ, et al. Cardiovascular effects of sevoflurane compared with those of isoflurane in volunteers. *Anesthesiology.* 1995;83:918-928.
106. Lowe D, Hettrick DA, Pagel PS, Warltier DC. Influence of volatile anesthetics on left ventricular afterload in vivo. Differences between desflurane and sevoflurane. *Anesthesiology.* 1996;85:112-120.
107. Bahlman SH, Eger EI, Halsey MJ, et al. The cardiovascular effects of halothane in man during spontaneous ventilation. *Anesthesiology.* 1972;36:494-502.
108. Ebert TJ. Differential effects of nitrous oxide on baroreflex control of heart rate and peripheral sympathetic nerve activity in humans. *Anesthesiology.* 1990;72:16-22.
109. Dolan WM, Stevens WC, Eger EI, et al. The cardiovascular and respiratory effects of isoflurane-nitrous oxide anaesthesia. *Can Anaesth Soc J.* 1974;21:557-568.
110. Eisele JH, Reitan JA, Massumi RA, Zelis RF, Miller RR. Myocardial performance and N_2O analgesia in coronary-artery disease. *Anesthesiology.* 1976;44:16-20.
111. Houltz E, Caidahl K, Hellstrom A, Gustavsson T, Milocco I, Ricksten SE. The effects of nitrous oxide on left ventricular systolic and diastolic performance before and after cardiopulmonary bypass: evaluation by computer-assisted two-dimensional and Doppler echocardiography in patients undergoing coronary artery surgery. *Anesth Analg.* 1995;81:243-248.
112. Pagel PS, Kampine JP, Schmeling WT, Warltier DC. Effects of nitrous oxide on myocardial contractility as evaluated by the preload recruitable stroke work relationship in chronically instrumented dogs. *Anesthesiology.* 1990;73:1148-1157.
113. Schotten U, Greiser M, Braun V, Karlein C, Schoendube F, Hanrath P. Effect of volatile anesthetics on the force-frequency relation in human ventricular myocardium: the role of the sarcoplasmic reticulum calcium-release channel. *Anesthesiology.* 2001;95:1160-1168.
114. Ebert TJ, Perez F, Uhrich TD, Deshur MA. Desflurane-mediated sympathetic activation occurs in humans despite preventing hypotension and baroreceptor unloading. *Anesthesiology.* 1998;88:1227-1232.
115. Adachi H. Sevoflurane anesthesia maintains reflex tachycardia on position change from supine recumbent to head-up tilt. *J Anesth.* 1996;10:129-132.
116. Nagasaki G, Tanaka M, Nishikawa T. The recovery profile of baroreflex control of heart rate after isoflurane or sevoflurane anesthesia in humans. *Anesth Analg.* 2001;93:1127-1131.
117. Price HL, Skovsted P, Pauca AL, Cooperman LH. Evidence for beta-receptor activation produced by halothane in normal man. *Anesthesiology.* 1970;32:389-395.
118. Rusy BF, Komai H. Anesthetic depression of myocardial contractility: a review of possible mechanisms. *Anesthesiology.* 1987;67:745-766.
119. Wheeler DM, Katz A, Rice RT, Hansford RG. Volatile anesthetic effects on sarcoplasmic reticulum Ca content and sarcolemmal Ca flux in isolated rat cardiac cell suspensions. *Anesthesiology.* 1994;80:372-382.
120. Bosnjak ZJ, Aggarwal A, Turner LA, Kampine JM, Kampine JP. Differential effects of halothane, enflurane, and isoflurane on Ca^{2+} transients and papillary muscle tension in guinea pigs. *Anesthesiology.* 1992;76:123-131.
121. Muldoon SM, Hart JL, Bowen KA, Freas W. Attenuation of endothelium-mediated vasodilation by halothane. *Anesthesiology.* 1988;68:31-37.
122. Haworth RA, Goknur AB. Inhibition of sodium/calcium exchange and calcium channels of heart cells by volatile anesthetics. *Anesthesiology.* 1995;82:1255-1265.
123. Bosnjak ZJ, Kampine JP. Effects of halothane, enflurane, and isoflurane on the SA node. *Anesthesiology.* 1983;58:314-321.
124. Weiskopf RB, Eger EI, Daniel M, Noorani M. Cardiovascular stimulation induced by rapid increases in desflurane concentration in humans results from activation of tracheopulmonary and systemic receptors. *Anesthesiology.* 1995;83:1173-1178.
125. Eger EI, Smith NT, Cullen DJ, Cullen BF, Gregory GA. A comparison of the cardiovascular effects of halothane, fluroxene, ether and cyclopropane in man: a resume. *Anesthesiology.* 1971; 34:25-41.
126. Wajima Z, Inoue T, Yoshikawa T, Imanaga K, Ogawa R. Changes in hemodynamic variables and catecholamine levels after rapid increase in sevoflurane or isoflurane concentration with or without nitrous oxide under endotracheal intubation. *J Anesth.* 2000;14:175-179.
127. Weiskopf RB, Moore MA, Eger EI, et al. Rapid increase in desflurane concentration is associated with greater transient cardiovascular stimulation than with rapid increase in isoflurane concentration in humans. *Anesthesiology.* 1994;80:1035-1045.
128. Weiskopf RB, Eger EI, Noorani M, Daniel M. Fentanyl, esmolol, and clonidine blunt the transient cardiovascular stimulation induced by desflurane in humans. *Anesthesiology.* 1994;81:1350-1355.
129. Pacentine GG, Muzi M, Ebert TJ. Effects of fentanyl on sympa thetic activation associated with the administration of desflurane. *Anesthesiology.* 1995;82:823-831.
130. Gormley WP, Murray JM, Trinick TR. Intravenous lidocaine does not attenuate the cardiovascular and catecholamine response to a rapid increase in desflurane concentration. *Anesth Analg.* 1996;82:358-361.
131. Gross GJ, Warltier DC. Coronary steal in four models of single or multiple vessel obstruction in dogs. *Am J Cardiol.* 1981;48:84-92.
132. Hirano M, Fujigaki T, Shibata O, Sumikawa K. A comparison of coronary hemodynamics during isoflurane and sevoflurane anesthesia in dogs. *Anesth Analg.* 1995;80:651-656.
133. Cason BA, Verrier ED, London MJ, Mangano DT, Hickey RF. Effects of isoflurane and halothane on coronary vascular resistance and collateral myocardial blood flow: their capacity to induce coronary steal. *Anesthesiology.* 1987;67:665-675.
134. Kersten JR, Schmeling T, Tessmer J, Hettrick DA, Pagel PS, Warltier DC. Sevoflurane selectively increases coronary collateral blood flow independent of KATP channels in vivo. *Anesthesiology.* 1999;90:246-256.
135. Priebe HJ, Foex P. Isoflurane causes regional myocardial dysfunction in dogs with critical coronary artery stenoses. *Anesthesiology.* 1987;66:293-300.
136. Katz KLG, Camara AK, Novalija E, et al. Anesthetic preconditioning: effects on latency to ischemic injury in isolated hearts. *Anesthesiology.* 2003;99:385-391.

137. Priebe HJ. Isoflurane causes more severe regional myocardial dysfunction than halothane in dogs with a critical coronary artery stenosis. *Anesthesiology*. 1988;69:72-83.
138. Wilton NC, Knight PR, Ullrich K, Martin B, Gallagher KP. Transmural redistribution of myocardial blood flow during isoflurane anesthesia and its effects on regional myocardial function in a canine model of fixed coronary stenosis. *Anesthesiology*. 1993;78:510-523.
139. Mignella R, Buffington CW. Inhaled anesthetics alter the determinants of coronary collateral blood flow in the dog. *Anesthesiology*. 1995;83:799-808.
140. Habazettl H, Conzen PF, Hobbhahn J, et al. Left ventricular oxygen tensions in dogs during coronary vasodilation by enflurane, isoflurane and dipyridamole. *Anesth Analg*. 1989;68:286-294.
141. Conzen PF, Habazettl H, Vollmar B, Christ M, Baier H, Peter K. Coronary microcirculation during halothane, enflurane, isoflurane, and adenosine in dogs. *Anesthesiology*. 1992;76:261-270.
142. Atlee JL, Bosnjak ZJ. Mechanisms for cardiac dysrhythmias during anesthesia. *Anesthesiology*. 1990;72:347-374.
143. Johnston RR, Eger EI, Wilson C. A comparative interaction of epinephrine with enflurane, isoflurane, and halothane in man. *Anesth Analg*. 1976;55:709-712.
144. Atlee JL, Malkinson CE. Potentiation by thiopental of halothane—epinephrine-induced arrhythmias in dogs. *Anesthesiology*. 1982;57:285-288.
145. Roberts FL, Burstrom RE, Atlee JL. Effects of ketamine and etomidate on epinephrine-induced ventricular dysrhythmias in dogs anesthetized with halothane. *Anesthesiology*. 1984;61:A36.
146. Atlee JL, Roberts FL. Thiopental and epinephrine-induced dysrhythmias in dogs anesthetized with enflurane or isoflurane. *Anesth Analg*. 1986;65:437-443.
147. Moore MA, Weiskopf RB, Eger EI, Wilson C, Lu G. Arrhythmogenic doses of epinephrine are similar during desflurane or isoflurane anesthesia in humans. *Anesthesiology*. 1993;79:943-947.
148. Karl HW, Swedlow DB, Lee KW, Downes JJ. Epinephrine-halothane interactions in children. *Anesthesiology*. 1983;58:142-145.
149. Liu WS, Wong KC, Port JD, Andriano KP. Epinephrine-induced arrhythmias during halothane anesthesia with the addition of nitrous oxide, nitrogen, or helium in dogs. *Anesth Analg*. 1982;61:414-417.
150. Murray JM, Luney SR. Fatal cardiac ischaemia associated with prolonged desflurane anaesthesia and administration of exogenous catecholamines[comment]. *Can J Anaesth*. 1998;45:1200-1202.
151. Liberman BA, Teasdale SJ. Anaesthesia and amiodarone. *Can Anaesth Soc J*. 1985;32:629-638.
152. Holt DW, Tucker GT, Jackson PR, Storey GC. Amiodarone pharmacokinetics. *Am Heart J*. 1983;106(part 2):840-847.
153. Schulte-Sasse U, Hess W, Tarnow J. Pulmonary vascular responses to nitrous oxide in patients with normal and high pulmonary vascular resistance. *Anesthesiology*. 1982;57:9-13.
154. Lennon PF, Murray PA. Attenuated hypoxic pulmonary vasoconstriction during isoflurane anesthesia is abolished by cyclooxygenase inhibition in chronically instrumented dogs. *Anesthesiology*. 1996;84:404-414.
155. Wang JY, Russell GN, Page RD, Jackson M, Pennefather SH. Comparison of the effects of sevoflurane and isoflurane on arterial oxygenation during one lung ventilation. *Br J Anaesth*. 1998;81:850-853.
156. Wang JY, Russell GN, Page RD, Oo A, Pennefather SH. A comparison of the effects of desflurane and isoflurane on arterial oxygenation during one-lung ventilation. *Anaesthesia*. 2000;55:167-173.
157. Fourcade HE, Stevens WC, Larson CP Jr, et al. The ventilatory effects of Forane, a new inhaled anesthetic. *Anesthesiology*. 1971;35:26-31.
158. Green WB Jr. The ventilatory effects of sevoflurane. *Anesth Analg*. 1995;81(suppl):S23-S26.
159. Murat I, Saint-Maurice JP, Beydon L, MacGee K. Respiratory effects of nitrous oxide during isoflurane anaesthesia in children. *Br J Anaesth*. 1986;58:1122-1129.
160. Eger EI, Dolan WM, Stevens WC, Miller RD, Way WL. Surgical stimulation antagonizes the respiratory depression produced by Forane. *Anesthesiology*. 1972;36:544-549.
161. Hirshman CA, McCullough RE, Cohen PJ, Weil JV. Depression of hypoxic ventilatory response by halothane, enflurane and isoflurane in dogs. *Br J Anaesth*. 1977;49:957-963.
162. Knill RL, Gelb AW. Ventilatory responses to hypoxia and hypercapnia during halothane sedation and anesthesia in man. *Anesthesiology*. 1978;49:244-251.
163. Sarton E, Dahan A, Teppema L, et al. Acute pain and central nervous system arousal do not restore impaired hypoxic ventilatory response during sevoflurane sedation. *Anesthesiology*. 1996;85:295-303.
164. Jones RM, Cashman JN, Mant TG. Clinical impressions and cardiorespiratory effects of a new fluorinated inhalation anaesthetic, desflurane (I-653), in volunteers. *Br J Anaesth*. 1990;64:11-15.
165. Zwass MS, Fisher DM, Welborn LG, et al. Induction and maintenance characteristics of anesthesia with desflurane and nitrous oxide in infants and children. *Anesthesiology*. 1992;76:373-378.
166. Ashworth J, Smith I. Comparison of desflurane with isoflurane or propofol in spontaneously breathing ambulatory patients. *Anesth Analg*. 1998;87:312-318.
167. Kong CF, Chew ST, Ip-Yam PC. Intravenous opioids reduce airway irritation during induction of anaesthesia with desflurane in adults [comment]. *Br J Anaesth*. 2000;85:364-367.
168. Van Hemelrijck J, Smith I, White PF. Use of desflurane for outpatient anesthesia. A comparison with propofol and nitrous oxide. *Anesthesiology*. 1991;75:197-203.
169. Bernard JM, Doursout MF, Wouters P, et al. Effects of enflurane and isoflurane on hepatic and renal circulations in chronically instrumented dogs. *Anesthesiology*. 1991;74:298-302.
170. Cousins MJ, Mazze RI, Kosek JC, Hitt BA, Love FV. The etiology of methoxyflurane nephrotoxicity. *J Pharmacol Exp Ther*. 1974;190:530-541.
171. Cousins MJ, Mazze RI. Methoxyflurane nephrotoxicity. A study of dose response in man. *JAMA*. 1973;225:1611-1616.
172. Crandell WB, Pappas SG, Macdonald A. Nephrotoxicity associated with methoxyflurane anesthesia. *Anesthesiology*. 1966;27:591-607.
173. Zaleski L, Abello D, Gold MI. Desflurane versus isoflurane in patients with chronic hepatic and renal disease. *Anesth Analg*. 1993;76:353-356.
174. Weiskopf RB, Eger EI, Ionescu P, et al. Desflurane does not produce hepatic or renal injury in human volunteers. *Anesth Analg*. 1992;74:570-574.
175. Jones RM, Koblin DD, Cashman JN, Eger EI, Johnson BH, Damask MC. Biotransformation and hepato-renal function in volunteers after exposure to desflurane (I-653). *Br J Anaesth*. 1990;64:482-487.
176. Price RG. Urinary enzymes, nephrotoxicity and renal disease. *Toxicology*. 1982;23:99-134.
177. Price RG. Measurement of N-acetyl-beta-glucosaminidase and its isoenzymes in urine methods and clinical applications. *Eur J Clin Chem Clin Biochem*. 1992;30:693-705.
178. Bernard AM, Vyskocil AA, Mahieu P, Lauwerys RR. Assessment of urinary retinol-binding protein as an index of proximal tubular injury. *Clin Chem*. 1987;33:775-779.
179. Beckett GJ, Hayes JD. Glutathione S-transferases: biomedical applications. *Adv Clin Chem*. 1993;30:281-380.
180. Sundberg A, Appelkvist EL, Dallner G, Nilsson R. Glutathione transferases in the urine: sensitive methods for detection of kidney damage induced by nephrotoxic agents in humans. *Environ Health Perspect*. 1994;102(suppl 3):293-296.

181. Stevens WC, Eger EI, Joas TA, Cromwell TH, White A, Dolan WM. Comparative toxicity of isoflurane, halothane, fluroxene and diethyl ether in human volunteers. *Can Anaesth Soc J*. 1973;20:357-368.
182. Frink EJ Jr, Ghantous H, Malan TP, et al. Plasma inorganic fluoride with sevoflurane anesthesia: correlation with indices of hepatic and renal function. *Anesth Analg*. 1992;74:231-235.
183. Higuchi H, Adachi Y, Wada H, Kanno M, Satoh T. The effects of low-flow sevoflurane and isoflurane anesthesia on renal function in patients with stable moderate renal insufficiency. *Anesth Analg*. 2001;92:650-655.
184. Story DA, Poustie S, Liu G, McNicol PL. Changes in plasma creatinine concentration after cardiac anesthesia with isoflurane, propofol, or sevoflurane: a randomized clinical trial. *Anesthesiology*. 2001;95:842-848.
185. Oikkonen M. Isoflurane and enflurane in long anaesthesias for plastic microsurgery. *Acta Anaesthesiol Scand*. 1984;28:412-418.
186. Frink EJ Jr, Malan TP, Atlas M, Dominguez LM, DiNardo JA, Brown BR Jr. Clinical comparison of sevoflurane and isoflurane in healthy patients. *Anesth Analg*. 1992;74:241-245.
187. Liu J, Laster MJ, Eger EI, Taheri S. Absorption and degradation of sevoflurane and isoflurane in a conventional anesthetic circuit. *Anesth Analg*. 1991;72:785-789.
188. Steffey EP, Laster MJ, Ionescu P, Eger EI, Gong D, Weiskopf RB. Dehydration of Baralyme increases compound A resulting from sevoflurane degradation in a standard anesthetic circuit used to anesthetize swine. *Anesth Analg*. 1997;85:1382-1386.
189. Strum DP, Johnson BH, Eger EI. Stability of sevoflurane in soda lime. *Anesthesiology*. 1987;67:779-781.
190. Hanaki C, Fujii K, Morio M, Tashima T. Decomposition of sevoflurane by sodalime. *Hiroshima J Med Sci*. 1987;36:61-67.
191. Gonsowski CT, Laster MJ, Eger EI, Ferrell LD, Kerschmann RL. Toxicity of compound A in rats. Effect of increasing duration of administration. *Anesthesiology*. 1994;80:566-573.
192. Keller KA, Callan C, Prokocimer P, et al. Inhalation toxicity study of a haloalkene degradant of sevoflurane, Compound A (PIFE), in Sprague-Dawley rats. *Anesthesiology*. 1995;83:1220-1232.
193. Bito H, Ikeda K. Plasma inorganic fluoride and intracircuit degradation product concentrations in long-duration, low-flow sevoflurane anesthesia. *Anesth Analg*. 1994;79:946-951.
194. Bito H, Ikeda K. Renal and hepatic function in surgical patients after low-flow sevoflurane or isoflurane anesthesia. *Anesth Analg*. 1996;82:173-176.
195. Kharasch ED, Frink EJ Jr, Zager R, Bowdle TA, Artru A, Nogami WM. Assessment of low-flow sevoflurane and isoflurane effects on renal function using sensitive markers of tubular toxicity. *Anesthesiology*. 1997;86:1238-1253.
196. Eger EI, Ionescu P, Laster MJ, Weiskopf RB. Baralyme dehydration increases and soda lime dehydration decreases the concentration of compound A resulting from sevoflurane degradation in a standard anesthetic circuit. *Anesth Analg*. 1997;85:892-898.
197. Ebert TJ, Arain SR. Renal responses to low-flow desflurane, sevoflurane, and propofol in patients. *Anesthesiology*. 2000;93:1401-1406.
198. Conzen PF, Kharasch ED, Czerner SF, et al. Low-flow sevoflurane compared with low-flow isoflurane anesthesia in patients with stable renal insufficiency. *Anesthesiology*. 2002;97:578-584.
199. Eger EI, Gong D, Koblin DD, et al. Dose-related biochemical markers of renal injury after sevoflurane versus desflurane anesthesia in volunteers. *Anesth Analg*. 1997;85:1154-1163.
200. Kharasch ED, Hankins DC. P450-dependent and nonenzymatic human liver microsomal defluorination of fluoromethyl-2,2-difluoro-1-(trifluoromethyl)vinyl ether (compound A), a sevoflurane degradation product. *Drug Metab Dispos*. 1996;24:649-654.
201. Eger EI, Koblin DD, Bowland T, et al. Nephrotoxicity of sevoflurane versus desflurane anesthesia in volunteers. *Anesth Analg*. 1997;84:160-168.
202. Fang ZX, Kandel L, Laster MJ, Ionescu P, Eger EI. Factors affecting production of compound A from the interaction of sevoflurane with Baralyme and soda lime. *Anesth Analg*. 1996;82:775-781.
203. Versichelen LF, Bouche MP, Rolly G, et al. Only carbon dioxide absorbents free of both NaOH and KOH do not generate compound A during in vitro closed-system sevoflurane: evaluation of five absorbents. *Anesthesiology*. 2001;95:750-755.
204. Brody GL, Sweet RB. Halothane anesthesia as a possible cause of massive hepatic necrosis. *Anesthesiology*. 1963;24:29.
205. Elliott RH, Strunin L. Hepatotoxicity of volatile anaesthetics. *Br J Anaesth*. 1993;70:339-348.
206. Walton B. Halothane hepatitis in children. *Anaesthesia*. 1986;41:575-578.
207. Brown BR Jr, Gandolfi AJ. Adverse effects of volatile anaesthetics. *Br J Anaesth*. 1987;59:14-23.
208. Hussey AJ, Aldridge LM, Paul D, Ray DC, Beckett GJ, Allan LG. Plasma glutathione S-transferase concentration as a measure of hepatocellular integrity following a single general anaesthetic with halothane, enflurane or isoflurane. *Br J Anaesth*. 1988;60:130-135.
209. Ray DC, Drummond GB. Halothane hepatitis. *Br J Anaesth*. 1991;67:84-99.
210. Kenna JG, Neuberger J, Williams R. Specific antibodies to halothane-induced liver antigens in halothane-associated hepatitis. *Br J Anaesth*. 1987;59:1286-1290.
211. O'Shea D, Davis SN, Kim RB, Wilkinson GR. Effect of fasting and obesity in humans on the 6-hydroxylation of chlorzoxazone: a putative probe of CYP2E1 activity. *Clin Pharmacol Ther*. 1994;56:359-367.
212. Cousins MJ, Plummer JL, Hall PD. Risk factors for halothane hepatitis. *Aust N Z J Surg*. 1989;59:5-14.
213. Bunker JP, Forrest WH, Mosteller F, Vandam LD. *A Study of the Possible Association between Halothane Anaesthesia and Post Operative Hepatic Necrosis*. Washington, DC: US Government Printing Office; 1969.
214. Bottiger LE, Dalen E, Hallen B. Halothane-induced liver damage: an analysis of the material reported to the Swedish Adverse Drug Reaction Committee, 1966-1973. *Acta Anaesthesiol Scand*. 1976;20:40-46.
215. Kuo G, Choo QL, Alter HJ, et al. An assay for circulating antibodies to a major etiologic virus of human non-A, non-B hepatitis. *Science*. 1989;244:362-364.
216. Lewis JH, Zimmerman HJ, Ishak KG, Mullick FG. Enflurane hepatotoxicity. A clinicopathologic study of 24 cases. *Ann Intern Med*. 1983;98:984-992.
217. Carrigan TW, Straughen WJ. A report of hepatic necrosis and death following isoflurane anesthesia. *Anesthesiology*. 1987;67:581-583.
218. Martin JL, Plevak DJ, Flannery KD, et al. Hepatotoxicity after desflurane anesthesia. *Anesthesiology*. 1995;83:1125-1129.
219. Martin JL, Dubbink DA, Plevak DJ, et al. Halothane hepatitis 28 years after primary exposure. *Anesth Analg*. 1992;74:605-608.
220. Green WB, Eckerson ML, Depa R, Brown BR. Covalent binding of oxidative metabolites to hepatic protein not detectable after exposure to sevoflurane or desflurane. *Anesthesiology*. 1994;81:A437.
221. Kenna JG, Jones RM. The organ toxicity of inhaled anesthetics. *Anesth Analg*. 1995;81(suppl):S51-S66.
222. Watanabe K, Hatakenaka S, Ikemune K, Chigyo Y, Kubozono T, Arai T. A case of suspected liver dysfunction induced by sevoflurane anesthesia. *Masui*. 1993;42:902-905.
223. Ogawa M, Doi K, Mitsufuji T, Satoh K, Takatori T. [Drug induced hepatitis following sevoflurane anesthesia in a child]. *Masui*. 1991;40:1542-1545.
224. Hong K, Trudell JR, O'Neil JR, Cohen EN. Metabolism of nitrous oxide by human and rat intestinal contents. *Anesthesiology*. 1980;52:16-19.
225. Deacon R, Lumb M, Perry J, et al. Inactivation of methionine synthase by nitrous oxide. *Eur J Biochem*. 1980;104:419-423.

226. Nunn JF, O'Morain C. Nitrous oxide decreases motility of human neutrophils in vitro. *Anesthesiology*. 1982;56:45-48.
227. Bevan JC, Reimer EJ, Smith MF, et al. Decreased mivacurium requirements and delayed neuromuscular recovery during sevoflurane anesthesia in children and adults. *Anesth Analg*. 1998;87:772-778.
228. Lowry DW, Mirakhur RK, McCarthy GJ, Carroll MT, McCourt KC. Neuromuscular effects of rocuronium during sevoflurane, isoflurane, and intravenous anesthesia. *Anesth Analg*. 1998;87:936-940.
229. Kumar N, Mirakhur RK, Symington MJ, Loan PB, Connolly FM. A comparison of the effects of isoflurane and desflurane on the neuromuscular effects of mivacurium. *Anaesthesia*. 1996;51:547-550.
230. Wulf H, Kahl M, Ledowski T. Augmentation of the neuromuscular blocking effects of cisatracurium during desflurane, sevoflurane, isoflurane or total IV anaesthesia. *Br J Anaesth*. 1998;80:308-312.
231. Saitoh Y, Tanaka H, Fujii Y, Makita K, Amaha K. Post-tetanic burst count and train-of-four during recovery from vecuronium-induced intense neuromuscular block under different types of anaesthesia. *Eur J Anaesthesiol*. 1998;15:524-528.
232. Wulf H, Ledowski T, Linstedt U, Proppe D, Sitzlack D. Neuromuscular blocking effects of rocuronium during desflurane, isoflurane, and sevoflurane anaesthesia. *Can J Anaesth*. 1998;45:526-532.
233. Bock M, Klippel K, Nitsche B, Bach A, Martin E, Motsch J. Rocuronium potency and recovery characteristics during steady-state desflurane, sevoflurane, isoflurane or propofol anaesthesia. *Br J Anaesth*. 2000;84:43-47.
234. Ahmed AA, Kumagai M, Otake T, Kurata Y, Amaki Y. Sevoflurane exposure time and the neuromuscular blocking effect of vecuronium. *Can J Anaesth*. 1999;46(part 1):429-432.
235. Morita T, Kurosaki D, Tsukagoshi H, Shimada H, Sato H, Goto F. Factors affecting neostigmine reversal of vecuronium block during sevoflurane anaesthesia. *Anaesthesia*. 1997;52:538-543.
236. Gronert GA, Theye RA. Halothane-induced porcine malignant hyperthermia: metabolic and hemodynamic changes. *Anesthesiology*. 1976;44:36-43.
237. Ducart A, Adnet P, Renaud B, Riou B, Krivosic-Horber R. Malignant hyperthermia during sevoflurane administration. *Anesth Analg*. 1995;80:609-611.
238. Ellis FR, Clarke IM, Appleyard TN, Dinsdale RC. Malignant hyperpyrexia induced by nitrous oxide and treated with dexamethasone. *Br Med J*. 1974;4:270-271.
239. Gronert GA, Antognini JF, Pessah IN. Malignant hyperthermia. In: Miller RD, ed. *Anesthesia*. Vol 1. 5th ed. Philadelphia,: Churchill Livingstone; 2000:1033-1052.

CHAPTER 8

INTRAVENOUS INDUCTION AGENTS

NADINE A. FALLACARO, MICHAEL D. FALLACARO

BARBITURATES

The first intravenous agents used for general anesthesia were the opioids, which were widely accepted for relief of the suffering patient. However, not until barbiturates were introduced in the 1930s was intravenous anesthesia taken seriously. Waters and Lundy introduced the thiobarbiturate thiopental in 1935. Despite the discovery of more than 2000 barbiturate agents since then, thiopental remains the barbiturate of choice for general anesthesia.

Chemical Structure

Structural Activity Relationships

Barbituric acid is a cyclic compound formed from the condensation of urea and malonic acid. This compound has no intrinsic central nervous system (CNS) depressant activity by itself. Drugs that are derivatives of barbituric acid are categorized as barbiturates (Figure 8-1).

Various substitutions to the barbituric acid compound can create different pharmacologic actions. By replacing both hydrogen atoms at position 5 with *alkyl-* or *aryl-* groups, the pharmacologic action is as a sedative hypnotic.

These derivatives of barbituric acid are known as *oxybarbiturates* or as the *true barbiturates*. Although insoluble in water, these compounds are soluble in nonpolar solvents, such as chloroform and oil; this solubility is a common feature of organic CNS depressants. These drugs have a relatively slower onset of action and a prolonged duration. Alterations in molecular side-chain lengths affect potency; longer chains result in a higher potency. The structures of the barbiturates used in anesthesia are shown in Figure 8-2.

The replacement of the number 2 carbon atom of the barbituric acid molecule with a sulfur atom produces the thiobarbiturates (thiopental and thiamylal). These compounds have a more rapid onset and a shorter duration of action than the oxybarbiturates.

The sulfurization of oxybarbiturates increases lipid solubility. Any structural change that increases the lipid solubility of barbiturates decreases the duration of action and the latency to onset of action. It also accelerates metabolic degradation, often increasing hypnotic potency.[1]

The ultra–short-acting barbiturate methohexital is produced by the methylation of the active barbiturate phenobarbital at C-1.

Methylation produces an agent that has a more rapid onset and a shorter duration but increased excitatory side effects. The addition of a methyl radical at C-5 confers some convulsant activity, such as involuntary muscular movement (Table 8-1).

Barbiturates are weak acids (the dissociation constant [pK_a] of thiopental is 7.6, and of methohexital is 7.9) and are prepared as sodium salts. They are usually combined with 6% anhydrous sodium carbonate, which is used for preventing precipitation of the insoluble free acid form of the barbiturate by atmospheric carbon dioxide.[2] The solution produced has an alkalinity of 10.5 to 11. Barbiturates must be reconstituted before administration using aseptic technique with sterile water for injection, U.S. Pharmacopeia (USP) 0.09% sodium chloride injection, USP; or 5% dextrose injection, USP. If lactated Ringer's solution or acidic solutions of drugs are used for reconstitution, the barbiturate precipitates out in the form of free acids. This moderate alkalinity also makes this solution incompatible with opioids, catecholamines, and muscle relaxants, all of which are acidic in solution. Intraarterial or extravascular infusion of this alkaline solution can cause severe tissue injury. One advantage of the alkalinity of barbiturates is the bacteriostatic property it confers. If properly reconstituted and refrigerated, it is stable at room temperature for 2 weeks.[2] Wong and associates[3] studied the risk of contamination in vials left out at room temperature for up to 25 days and found neither significant change in pH nor positive bacteriologic growth. Abbott Laboratories advises that thiopental be at room temperature for no longer than 24 hours after it is reconstituted. When reconstituted with sterile water, methohexital remains stable

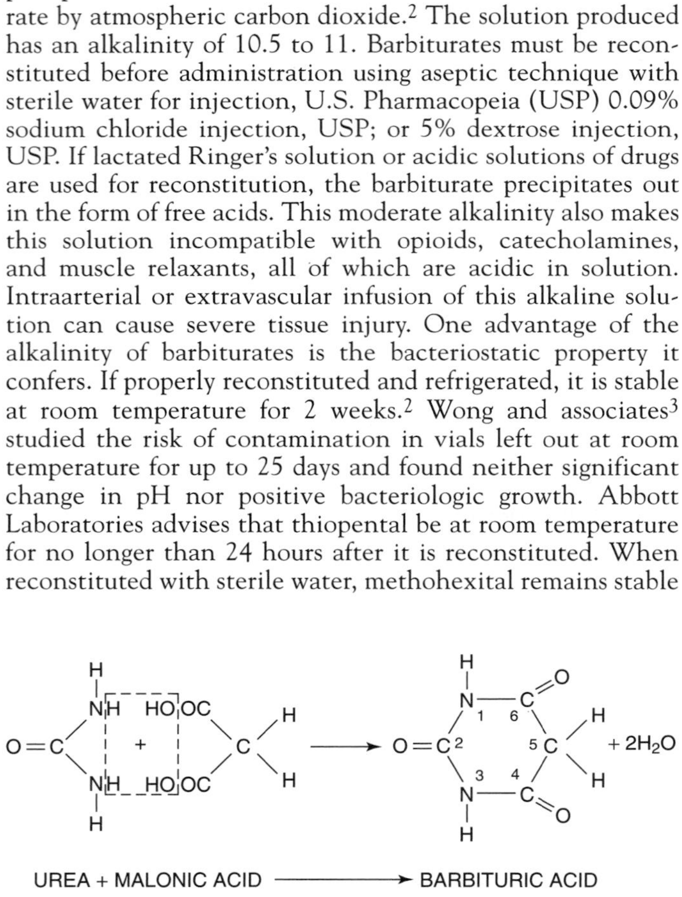

FIGURE **8-1**
Formation of barbituric acid.

BENZODIAZEPINES

Diazepam

Midazolam

Flumazenil

BARBITURATES

Methohexital

Thiopental

MISCELLANEOUS

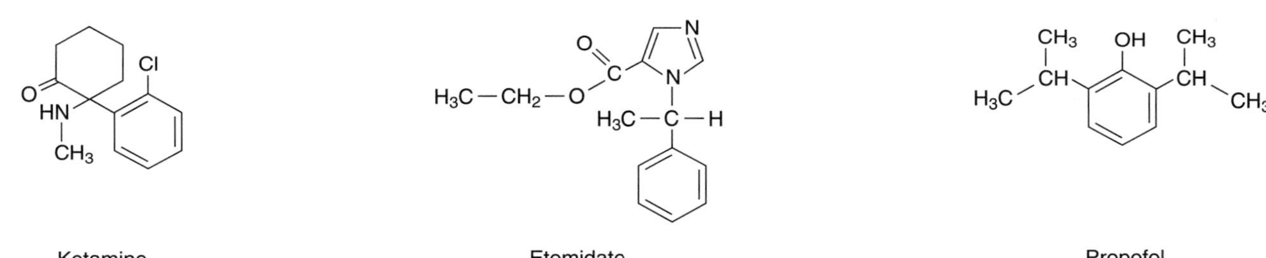

FIGURE **8-2**
Agents used for the induction of general anesthesia.

for 6 weeks.[4] The preparations of the induction drugs are listed in Table 8-2.

Pharmacokinetics

Stereoisomers

Barbiturates are enantiomeric. Many barbiturates have asymmetric side chains attached to the number 5–carbon atom of the barbiturate ring. They contain equal amounts of stereoisomers and are marketed as racemic compounds. In thiopental, thiamylal, pentobarbital, and secobarbital, the L-isomers are the most potent. Methohexital has four stereoisomers that have varying degrees of activity. The β-L-stereoisomers are the most potent, but they create excessive motor activity. Methohexital is therefore a racemic mixture of the α-L-stereoisomers, which are the least potent and do not cause excessive motor activity.[5]

Protein Binding

Barbiturates are reversibly bound to plasma proteins, most commonly to plasma albumin.[4] This binding has a significant effect on the pharmacologic actions of these drugs, because bound

TABLE **8-1** **Chemical Modification of Barbiturates**

	Placement	**Substitute**	**Example**
Oxybarbiturates	C-2	Oxygen	Pentobarbital, secobarbital
Thiobarbiturates	C-2	Sulfur	Thiopental, thiamylal
Methylated oxybarbiturates	C-1	Methyl	Methohexital, hexobarbital

- Thiomethylated and n-methylated drugs are ultra short acting.
- Synthesized by condensation of urea and malonic acid to form barbituric acid ring (barbital).
- Metabolized via liver cytochrome enzymes by desulfuration (thiopental) producing the clinically active oxy-analogue pentobarbital, which contributes to the hangover effect. Oxidation of carbon-5 radicals and to a lesser extent ring hydrolysis also occur.
- Methohexital undergoes demethylation. Oxidation at carbon-5 and ring hydrolysis occur.

TABLE 8-2 Pharmaceutic Preparation of Intravenous Anesthetic Agents

Class	Drug Name	Available Solution	Pain on Injection*
Thiobarbiturates	Thiopental (Pentothal)	pK_a 7.5; sodium salts mixed with anhydrous sodium bicarbonate; pH 10.5-11	+++
N-methylated oxybarbiturate	Methohexital (Brevital)	pK_a 7.9; same as thiopental; pH 10-11	+
Benzodiazepines	Diazepam (Valium)	0.5% in 40% propylene glycol and 10% alcohol	+++
		0.5% emulsion formula; intralipid	+/−
	Lorazepam (Ativan)	0.4% in propylene glycol	+
	Midazolam (Versed)	0.5% buffered aqueous solution (pH 3.5)	O
Imidazoles	Etomidate (Amidate)	Water soluble at acidic pH, lipophilic at physiologic pH (pK_a 4.24); 0.2% solution in 30% propylene glycol (pH 5)	+++
Alkylphenol	Propofol (Diprivan)	1% solution in an aqueous emulsion containing 10% soy bean oil, 2.25% glycerol, and 1.2% egg phosphatide, EDTA (pK_a 11); AstraZeneca	++
	Generic	Generic formulation from Baxter contains metabisulfate and a lower pH of 4.5-6.4 (use with caution in patients with allergies and asthma)	
Arylcyclohexylamines	Ketamine (Ketalar)	White crystalline salt 1% or 10% aqueous solution (pH 3.3-5.5; pK_a 7.5)	O

EDTA, *disodium ethylenediaminetetraacetate*.
*O, *None*; +, *mild*; ++, *moderate*; +++, *marked*.

drugs are unable to cross biologic membranes. The greater the amount of free drug available, the greater the pharmacologic effect caused. Thiopental is approximately 80% protein bound, making it more highly protein bound than the oxybarbiturates.[1] The sulfur substitution may be responsible for the change in the affinity of the thiobarbiturate compound for protein.[6] Factors that change protein binding are listed in Table 8-3.

When competition with other drugs for protein binding sites occurs, the unbound fraction of thiopental is increased. Such competitive drugs include aspirin, indomethacin, naproxen, and coumadin. The greater the unbound fraction, or amount of free drug available, the shorter the duration of action as more rapid redistribution occurs.[7] Decreased plasma protein concentrations that occur in some patients (e.g., those with uremia or hepatic disease and those in the third trimester of pregnancy) also cause an increase in circulating free drug levels.

Physiologic pH favors the un-ionized fraction of thiopental. Its high lipid solubility accounts for its rapid movement across the blood-brain barrier and the quick onset of anesthesia it provides. Phenobarbital has much lower lipid solubility, a characteristic that accounts for its slower onset of action.

Distribution of the barbiturates out of blood to the various tissue compartments continues until equilibrium occurs. This phenomenon is expressed as a tissue-blood partition coefficient. The tissue-blood partition coefficient for the brain is 1.4, that for muscle is 1.5, and that for fat is 11. The net transfer of molecules stops when the partial pressures in each phase are equal.[5]

TABLE 8-3 Factors That Alter Protein Binding

Factors	Percent Bound
Decreased lipid solubility	Decreases binding
Increased pH (≤8.0)	Increases binding
Increased drug concentration	Decreases binding
Increased protein concentration	Increases binding
Increased competition for binding sites with other drugs	Decreases binding

Barbiturate distribution depends on lipid solubility, protein binding, and degree of ionization. Of these, lipid solubility is the most important. Drugs that are highly lipid soluble cross cell membranes rapidly. There is a more rapid transfer into the CNS when the drug is more soluble. Solubility also accounts for transplacental drug transfer. Thiopental, being highly soluble, easily crosses the placental barrier.

Ionization

In order to cross cellular membranes, agents must be nonionized and non–protein bound. Ionized or protein-bound drugs are unable to cross physiologic membranes and remain in high concentrations within the circulation. The pK_a of the drug and the pH determine the proportion of the compound that is ionized and the proportion that is nonionized. Once sodium thiopental is in the extracellular fluid, the base combines with hydrogen (H^+) ions to form the nonionized thiopental. It is this nonionized thiopental that is able to cross the blood-brain barrier. The 7.5 pK_a of thiopental is close to the physiologic pH of 7.4. Because formation of the nonionized pharmacologically active thiopental compound depends on the H^+ concentration, tissue pH exerts some control over the amount of active compound formed. Because the pK_a of thiopental is so close to physiologic pH, 61% of the compound exists in the nonionized state at a pH of 7.4. The pH is not uniform throughout the body; intracellular pH is more acidic than extracellular fluid pH, creating a difference in concentration of ionized and nonionized thiopental at either side of the membrane. Acidosis increases the amount of nonionized thiopental in the extracellular fluid and allows greater diffusion across membranes into tissues.

The distribution, redistribution, and elimination of thiopental have been studied extensively in various physiologic and pharmacologic models. In the first decade of clinical use of thiopental, its short duration was attributed to rapid metabolism and elimination.[1] Brodie and associates[8] changed that theory by introducing the idea of redistribution into fat stores to account for the short duration of action. Price and colleagues,[9] however, not convinced that adipose tissue uptake was rapid enough to account for this effect, looked to other tissue groups for an explanation of uptake that would terminate thiopental's drug action. These investigators found that the fat uptake of thiopental was too slow and that the relatively poorly perfused tissues, muscle, connective tissue, bone, and skin, in full, were responsible for depleting the brain of thiopental in the time considered.[9]

The role of metabolism in the short duration of effect of thiopental was reexamined with consideration given to the rapid decrease in plasma levels of barbiturates. After an intravenous injection of thiopental, its presence is restricted to the central blood volume, where its concentration is high. Distribution to the tissues is dependent on drug concentration in blood and cardiac output, which perfuses tissues and organs. The vessel-rich group of organs receives a major percentage of the cardiac output. The brain receives 20% of the cardiac output and achieves a peak plasma concentration of thiopental in one circulation time, accounting for the rapid onset of anesthesia after a bolus injection. In a three-compartment pharmacokinetic model, the brain is placed within, or in immediate proximity to, the central compartment.[10] After an intravenous injection, the first phase of distribution transports most of the injected drug to the vessel-rich group. Two phases begin shortly thereafter in which the drug is distributed to all other tissues, causing the drug blood levels to fall. A rapid phase of distribution begins with a redistribution of blood to the vessel-poor group, which is composed primarily of muscle tissues. This phase lasts 2 to 4 minutes, during which a patient would awaken from an initial bolus dose of thiopental. The second distribution phase is slow because of the equilibration of the drug concentration into peripheral compartments.[7] Although the capacity to store thiopental in fat is high, limited blood flow delays equilibration. The slow phase becomes predominant after four to five rapid distribution half-lives, or 12 to 17 minutes.

Distribution and redistribution of thiopental are largely dependent on cardiac output. Alterations in cardiac function and circulating blood volume may change some pharmacologic characteristics, including duration and therapeutic effect. Impaired cardiac function or hypovolemia decreases tissue perfusion to peripheral compartments; this phenomenon does not change the initial concentration of circulating drug in the central compartment after injection. Less hemodilution of the drug results in higher drug concentrations to the vessel-rich groups, such as the CNS (causing anesthesia) and the heart (causing cardiac depression).[5] Sympathetic stimulation from pain or increased anxiety increases cardiac output and speeds distribution to peripheral compartments from the brain, thereby decreasing the duration of the anesthesia.[11]

As tissue saturation of thiopental approaches equilibrium with the blood, termination of the drug action depends on the slow uptake of the drug into the vessel-poor group and on elimination.

Metabolism

Investigators have looked for the rationale behind the rapid termination of the anesthetic effects of thiopental and methohexital. The role of hepatic metabolism has been extensively examined. The pharmacokinetics of the induction drugs is given in Table 8-4.

By use of a pharmacokinetic model with the brain concentration of thiopental as an approximation of the central compartment concentration, measurements were made 1 minute after intravenous bolus administration. Only 14% of the injected dose was lost through metabolism. This percentage correlated very well with a hepatic extraction ratio of 0.15. After 15 minutes, the amount of drug lost to metabolism was 18%, only a 4% change from the previous measurement. However, the CNS effects were greatly diminished, indicating that the redistribution of the central compartment, and not hepatic metabolism, was responsible for awakening.[12] The pharmacokinetic movement of thiopental is given in Figure 8-3. Note that thiopental rapidly enters the brain and other vital organs with peak effects at 1 minute after bolus injection. The brain concentration then falls rapidly over the next 10 to 15 minutes as the drug redistributes more evenly throughout the body to muscle and fat.

In comparisons of methohexital and thiobarbiturates the distribution kinetics are very similar, but the clearance-elimination half-times are different.[9] The hepatic extraction ratio for methohexital is three times greater than that for thiopental. Although hepatic metabolism has a much greater role in the termination of action of methohexital than of thiopental, the total difference in hepatic extraction after 30 minutes was not great enough to account for the much larger difference in clearance between the two agents.[13-14] Redistribution again is proved to be of much greater importance than hepatic metabolism in awakening from thiobarbiturate anesthesia.

TABLE 8-4 Select Pharmacokinetic Values for Intravenous Anesthetic Agents

Drug Name	Distribution Half-Life (min)	Elimination Half-Life (hr)	Clearance (ml/kg/min)	Volume of Distribution (L/kg)	Protein Binding (%)
Thiopental	2-4	10-12	3.5	2.5	80
Methohexital	5-6	2-4	10	2.3	85
Diazepam	10-15	20-50	0.3	0.8-1.3	98
Lorazepam	3-10	10-20	1.4	0.7-1.5	98
Midazolam	7-15	2-4	7-11	1-1.7	94
Etomidate	2-4	2-5	22.5	2.5-4.5	75
Propofol	2-4	1-5	25	2-8	98
Ketamine	11-17	2-3	14.5	2.5-3.5	12

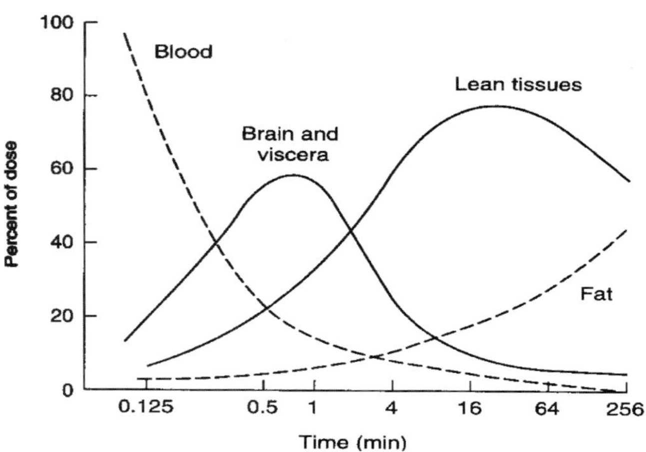

FIGURE **8-3**
Pentothal kinetics. Note that thiopental rapidly enters the brain and other vital organs with peak effects at 1 minute after bolus injection. The brain concentration then falls rapidly over the next 10 to 15 minutes as the drug redistributes more evenly throughout the body to muscle and fat.

The metabolism and elimination of barbiturates are almost entirely the result of hepatic biotransformation by microsomal enzymes and renal excretion. The role of the kidney in metabolism is small, because thiobarbiturates are highly protein bound and thus are not freely filtered at the glomerulus. The lipid solubility of barbiturates allows them to be easily reabsorbed into the circulation via the renal tubules. Whereas oxybarbiturates are metabolized by hepatocytes alone, other tissues (brain and kidney) are capable of metabolizing thiobarbiturates to a small extent.[12]

The most significant metabolic pathway involves the oxidation of the side-chain radicals at the C-5 position.[1,2] Omega oxidation produces thiopental carboxylic acid, which is not pharmacologically active. Thiobarbiturates can undergo desulfurization to the corresponding oxybarbiturate (pentobarbital) and further breakdown to inactive metabolites. The amount of pentobarbital produced has been studied in low- and high-dose administration techniques. After a 450- to 1275-mg intravenous bolus injection of thiopental, serum levels of pentobarbital at 15 minutes were found to be too low to produce pharmacologic effects.[14] Doses of thiopental for cerebral resuscitation (300 to 500 mg/kg given over 2 to 3 days) produced concentrations of pentobarbital that were pharmacologically active at approximately 10% of thiopental concentration.[15] In dosages used for achieving anesthesia for induction, the amount of pentobarbital produced is not significant.

Methohexital undergoes *N*-demethylation in addition to C-5 oxidation. Only minute amounts of active metabolites are generated.[1]

Barbiturates combine with cytochrome P-450 enzymes and compete for biotransformation with other substrates. In addition, they are responsible for the increased microsomal activity of these enzymes, probably by increasing their numbers rather than by altering their properties.[1]

In a study of the effect of hepatic cirrhosis on thiopental metabolism, Pandele and colleagues[16] found that the pharmacokinetics were only slightly modified. Besides altered protein binding, hepatic blood flow and hepatic intrinsic clearance are decreased in the cirrhotic patient.[17] The decrease in hepatic blood flow is not a key factor because of thiopental's low hepatic extraction ratio. The liver's intrinsic abilities to metabolize drugs and influence protein binding are linked because only unbound drug is available for biotransformation. With the increase in free drug that occurs in hypoalbuminemic states, the rate of clearance should increase, but it remains unchanged. Although the findings of Pandele and co-workers[16] were statistically insignificant, the impairment of intrinsic metabolism of hepatocytes was decreased in liver disease. Redistribution still has a major influence on the duration of therapeutic effect.

Burch and Stanski[18] studied the effects of renal failure on thiopental pharmacokinetics. They determined that in chronic renal disease the intrinsic hepatic metabolism and thiopental distribution remain essentially unchanged. Additionally, they found an increase in unbound drug that was caused by altered protein binding and therefore an increase in hepatic drug clearance. This increase in hepatic drug clearance was offset, however, by an increase in the volume of distribution attributed to increases in unbound drug available for distribution to the tissues. As a result, the elimination half-life is unchanged because differences in altered clearance and volume of distribution were approximately equal.[18] Injection of thiopental into an acidemic patient results in a higher proportion of un-ionized, unbound drug and therefore a more profound pharmacologic effect. Alterations in the blood-brain barrier that accompany uremia increase sensitivity to CNS depressants as well. A shorter titrated administration of thiopental and methohexital avoids the transient high concentration of these drugs that could cause CNS and cardiovascular depression.

Mechanism of Action

γ-Aminobutyric acid (GABA) is a major inhibitory transmitter in the CNS. The barbiturate mechanism of action is linked to postsynaptic enhancement of GABA-mediated inhibition.[19] The $GABA_A$ receptor, which is a ligand gated ion channel receptor, is activated by the binding of the neurotransmitter GABA. This binding of GABA to the $GABA_A$ receptor initiates the movement of chloride (Cl^-) through ion channels into the cell. This results in hyperpolarization of postsynaptic cell membrane and the inhibition of neuronal cell excitation. A model has been developed that includes sites of action for GABA on the postsynaptic membrane, as well as sites of action for barbiturates and benzodiazepines. Propofol, etomidate, ethanol, and volatile anesthetics may also have binding sites on this receptor.[20] The GABA receptor and its function are described in Figure 8-4. The intravenous anesthetics mentioned earlier achieve hypnotic activity by binding to their distinctive sites on the $GABA_A$ receptor. They may also have GABA-mimetic effects, allowing the influx of Cl^- in the absence of GABA. Barbiturates increase the mean open time of GABA receptor channels by increasing the frequency with which longer openings occur, not by changing the duration of these channel openings.[21]

Pharmacodynamics

Central Nervous System Effects

Thiopental has a firmly rooted place as an anesthetic induction agent because of its ability to promptly (within 15 to 30 seconds) and predictably induce a loss of consciousness. In recent years, however, propofol has become as popular an induction agent because it is associated with less postanesthesia drowsiness. Its spectrum of CNS depression effects ranges from sedation to

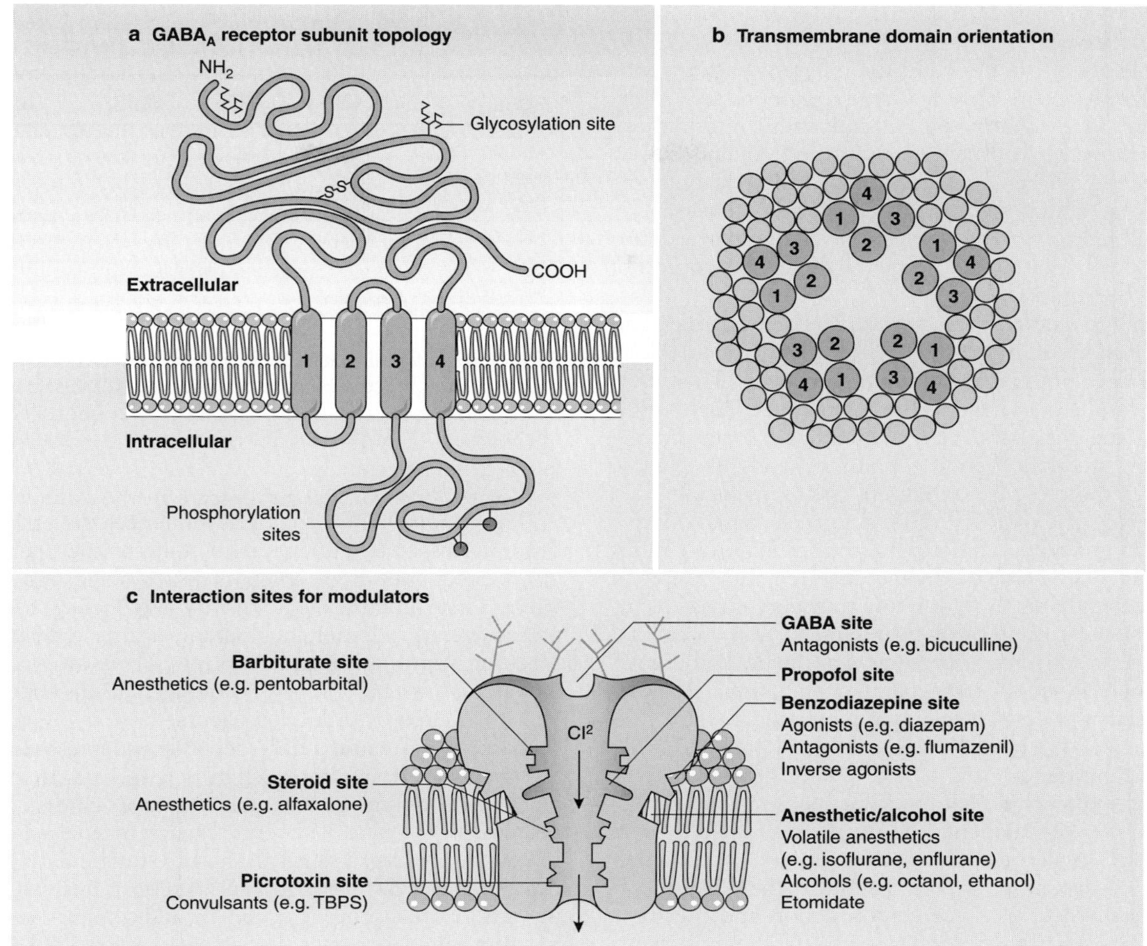

FIGURE **8-4**
The GABA$_A$ receptor. (a) The generic GABA$_A$ receptor subunit has four hydrophobic transmembrane segments that are thought to form amphipathic α-helices. The N-terminal domain contains *N*-glycosylation sites and a conserved cystine bridge; it forms the agonist-binding site. The large intracellular loop undergoes phosphorylation in several isoforms. (b) Plane view of the transmembrane hydrophobic segments showing interactions to form a central ion-conducting pore lined by the second transmembrane domains. The hetero-oligomeric structure consists of five subunits, with each subunit contributing to the ion channel pore. (c) The GABA$_A$ receptor gates an anion channel permeable to Cl^- and HCO_3^-. The general anesthetics are distinguished from the benzodiazepines (which allosterically modulate GABA binding to potentiate GABA responses) by their ability to activate/gate the GABA$_A$ receptor channel directly. A separate site at the interface between the third and fourth transmembrane segments appears to interact with volatile anesthetics, alcohols and etomidate, as demonstrated by site-directed mutagenesis studies. (From Hopkis PM, Winlow W. Mechanisms of anesthesia. In: Hemmings HC, Hopkins PM, eds. *Foundations of Anesthesia Basic and Clinical Sciences*. St Louis: Mosby; 2000;244.)

dose-dependent unconsciousness. It is not useful in the maintenance of anesthesia, however, because it does not possess any intrinsic analgesic properties. On the contrary, it has been found to be antianalgesic or hyperalgesic, especially at low blood levels. Patients may exhibit a heightened response to pain at low doses (sedation) or at emergence.[22] In studies of somatic pain the pain threshold to deep pain stimulus (tibial pressure) was decreased with thiopental.

Loss of consciousness occurs when the bolus of thiopental enters the cerebral circulation and crosses the blood-brain barrier. Factors that alter the onset of anesthesia are lipid solubility, protein binding, degree of ionization, plasma drug concentration, and cardiac output.

With regard to the evaluation of the effect of thiopental on the brain, the electroencephalograph (EEG) produces characteristic changes associated with dose-dependent stages of anesthesia.[23] Stage 1 occurs as the patient loses consciousness and the EEG waveform displays a slight increase in amplitude and a slowing in frequency. Stage II EEG patterns show a marked slowing of the frequency of delta and theta waves and correspond to the loss of the corneal reflex and to amnesia. Stage III is marked by burst suppression, in which bursts of electrical activity are interspersed with periods of isoelectric waveforms. There is a lack of awareness to pain in stage III, and, as does stage II, stage III corresponds to surgical anesthesia. The isoelectric periods are more prolonged in stage IV, and a flat

EEG is produced in stage V. Stages IV and V are induced for barbiturate coma.[23]

The complexity of the EEG and the different patterns produced by different agents have led investigators to seek alternative measures for evaluating pharmacodynamic information. The term *spectral-edge frequency* refers to the frequency below which 95% of the EEG energy or power is located or the highest frequency at which significant EEG energy exists. The spectral-edge tracing for the thiopental effect on the brain would theoretically imitate the curve for the concentration of thiopental in the brain.[24]

Hudson and co-workers[25] used spectral-edge frequency and continuous infusions of thiopental to show that acute tolerance to thiopental does not exist as originally believed. The difference in study results was explained by thiopental concentration differences in the peripheral venous blood and brain circulation.[26] Energy production in the brain depends on glucose metabolism. In the presence of oxygen, glucose is metabolized through the glycolytic pathway, citric acid cycle, and oxidative phosphorylation to produce adenosine triphosphate (ATP) for the maintenance of cerebral energy requirements. Cerebral metabolism depends on ATP for ion transport across membranes, on molecular transport within neurons, and on cellular metabolism of carbohydrates, proteins, and lipids. Barbiturates have a pronounced effect on cerebral metabolism. A dose-dependent decrease occurs in cerebral metabolic oxygen consumption rate ($CMRO_2$) and cerebral blood flow.[27] Under pentobarbital anesthesia, the $CMRO_2$ was decreased 30% when the reaction to painful stimuli was blocked.[28] In studies using large doses of thiopental in dogs, the $CMRO_2$ was decreased by 50% when the EEG was isoelectric. Any further increase in dosage was unable to alter the $CMRO_2$.[27] Pharmacologically decreasing cerebral function and causing a resultant decrease in $CMRO_2$ diminish the ATP requirements of the brain, thereby maintaining a supply-and-demand state that is favorable for electrophysiologic and cellular mechanics of brain cells. A parallel decrease in cerebral blood flow occurs with barbiturates. When $CMRO_2$ is decreased, cerebral blood flow and intracranial pressure are decreased. Barbiturates are used as a mechanism for brain protection before potential ischemic events. Collateral circulation to the ischemic areas is promoted by decreasing brain function and metabolic needs. The decreased cerebral blood flow in well-perfused tissue allows collateral circulation to the ischemic areas to increase, because the acidemic milieu favors vasodilation. Normal systemic blood pressure and cerebral perfusion pressure must be maintained.[29] The effects on cerebral metabolism and blood flow are useful in inducing anesthesia, especially in patients undergoing intraoperative somatosensory evoked potential (SEP) recording. Thiopental causes only minor alterations in SEP; wave amplitude is maintained, allowing for SEP monitoring.[30]

Thiopental administration decreases intraocular pressure.[31] Mechanisms thought to be responsible for this decrease include an increase in the outflow of aqueous humor, relaxation of extraocular muscles, and peripheral vasodilation.[32] Additionally, in doses used for anesthesia, thiopental has anticonvulsant properties and can abruptly stop seizures. CNS effects of the intravenous induction drugs are given in Table 8-5.

TABLE 8-5 Central Nervous System Effects of Intravenous Anesthetics*

Agent	CBF	CPP	$CMRO_2$	ICP	IOP
Thiopental	↓↓	↓↓	↓↓	↓↓	↓
Methohexital	↓↓	↓↓	↓↓	↓↓	↓
Etomidate	↓↓	0	↓↓	↓↓	↓
Propofol	↓↓	↓↓	↓↓	↓↓	↓↓
Ketamine	↓↓	↑	↑	↑	↑
Midazolam	↑↓	↓	↓	↓	↓

CBF, *Cerebral blood flow*; $CMRO_2$, *cerebral metabolic rate of oxygen consumption*; CPP, *cerebral perfusion pressure*; ICP, *intracranial pressure*; IOP, *intraocular pressure*.
*↓, *Decreases*; ↑, *increases*; 0, *no effect*.

Cardiovascular Effects

Among the many factors that influence the cardiovascular effects seen with barbiturates are rate of administration and dose. Lower doses are associated with fewer cardiovascular effects.

The condition of the patient influences the patient's hemodynamic response. Patients who come to the operating room often experience high levels of psychologic and physiologic stress. Their pharmacologic history may include use of antihypertensives, β-adrenergic blocking agents, calcium channel blocking agents, and antidepressants. These drugs alter the cardiovascular system compensatory mechanisms that respond to changes caused by induction agents.[33]

Barbiturates cause a dose-dependent depression of the cardiovascular system, resulting in a reduction in cardiac output.[34] One of the factors that decreases cardiac output is a decrease in the tone of systemic capacitance vessels that results in venous pooling.[35] With an increase in circulating volume in the periphery, decreases in venous return, left ventricular filling, and cardiac output occur. In addition, a direct negative inotropic effect occurs, with decreased myocardial contractility and sympathetic nervous system outflow that result in decreased sympathetic tone and vasodilation.[36] The systemic vascular resistance is either unchanged or increased.[34] The increased systemic vascular resistance is probably a compensatory mechanism that occurs in response to the decreased cardiac output. Baroreceptor reflexes are minimally depressed and respond to the change in cardiac output with an increase in heart rate. Barbiturates do not sensitize the myocardium to catecholamines and are not arrhythmogenic in the presence of normal oxygen and carbon dioxide balance.

The anesthetist should use caution when using barbiturate induction agents in medically compromised patients. The hypovolemic patient may have a 69% reduction in cardiac output and a significant decrease in systemic blood pressure.[37] Patients who are unable to tolerate the tachycardia and associated increase in myocardial oxygen demand (e.g., those with coronary artery disease, pericardial tamponade, or congestive heart failure) should receive an alternative induction agent that has fewer cardiovascular depressant properties. The cardiac effects are compared in Table 8-6.

Respiratory Effects

Barbiturates can cause a dose-related, centrally mediated respiratory system depression. Dose, speed of injection, premedication, and concomitant use of other CNS depressants increase the degree of respiratory depression. The central origin of the respiratory effects has been determined from the inverse relationship between EEG depth and minute ventilation.[38] Peak respiratory depression occurs and dissipates rapidly, probably

TABLE 8-6 Cardiac and Respiratory Effects of Intravenous Anesthetic Agents

Drug Name	Mean Arterial Pressure	Heart Rate	Cardiac Output	Venous Dilation	Systemic Vascular Resistance	Respiratory Depression	Bronchodilation
Thiopental	−	+	−	++	−/+	−	0
Methohexital	−	++	−	+	−/+	−	0
Etomidate	0	0	0	0	0	0/−	0
Propofol	− −	−	−	++	− −	− −	0/+
Ketamine	++	++	+	0	+/−	0	++
Diazepam	0/−	−/+	0	+	−/0	0	0
Midazolam	0/−	−/+	0	+	−/0	0	0

−, *Mild decrease;* − −, *moderate decrease;* +, *mild increase;* ++, *moderate increase;* 0, *no effect.*

because of the pharmacokinetics of distribution and redistribution. Originally, thiopental was considered to be spasmogenic, and its use was thought to increase the risk for laryngospasm and bronchospasm. Actually, airway and laryngeal reflexes remain intact unless large doses are used. Stimulation of the airway at light levels of anesthesia would therefore explain the occurrence of laryngospasm. Comparative respiratory effects of the intravenous induction drugs are given in Table 8-6.

Age

Various studies have examined the effects of barbiturates on the elderly and the requirements of this population for a decreased dose for induction of anesthesia.[39] Using the EEG spectral-edge frequency effect versus time curve for each patient, investigators found that with increasing age the dose of thiopental necessary to achieve anesthesia decreased 50% to 67%, the initial volume of distribution was decreased, and brain sensitivity was not a factor. A reevaluation by Stanski and Maitre showed that the initial volume of distribution was not age related and that EEG pharmacodynamics did not change with increased age. The rapid distribution phase is altered in the elderly population, resulting in a longer period of higher plasma concentrations of thiopental before redistribution. This longer time period allows an increased amount of thiopental to be available to the brain, often causing dramatic pharmacologic effects.[11]

Other

Thiobarbiturates cause a dose-dependent histamine release. Anaphylactic and anaphylactoid reactions have been reported. Extravascular injection of thiopental in subcutaneous tissue can cause chemical irritation ranging from tenderness to venospasm and tissue necrosis.[22,40]

Intraarterial injection of thiopental causes immediate arteriospasm, vasoconstriction, and intense pain along the course of the artery. Blanching of the arms, hand, and fingers occurs and may result in gangrene if not immediately treated. Interventions include the following: (1) dilution of drug by injection of normal saline; (2) treatment of vasospasm with papaverine 40 to 80 mcg, procaine 1% 10 ml, or lidocaine injection into the artery; (3) administration of stellate ganglion or brachial plexus block to increase circulation; (4) heparinization (if not contraindicated); and (5) local infiltration of the area with phentolamine. Treatments for extravascular injections of thiopental are given in Box 8-1.

All barbiturates are able to rapidly cross the placenta into the fetal circulation. Rapid redistribution of thiopental in the mother during the time between dosing and delivery may account for the difference in the level of consciousness between the neonate and the mother.[41] Higher doses (8 mg/kg) were associated with higher maternal and fetal blood levels.[42]

Thiopental

The two commonly used barbiturates in anesthesia are thiopental and methohexital. Thiopental is prepared as a 2.5% solution. The usual induction dose of these agents is 3 to 4 mg/kg. It produces few excitatory symptoms, has a rapid onset and a short duration, and is associated with some pain on injection. Patient age, size, physical condition, and current disease must be taken into consideration when a dose is chosen.

Contraindications

Absolute contraindications to thiopental include a history of allergic reaction to barbiturates and acute intermittent porphyria or variegate porphyria. Acute exacerbations of this

BOX 8-1

Precautions for Use of Intravenous Barbiturates

- Reduce dose and rate of injection in cardiovascularly compromised and hypovolemic patients.
- Solution has high pH (>10).
  - Avoid eye splash
  - Extravascular injection is painful and can cause tissue damage
  - Intraarterial thiopental—causes arterial spasm thrombosis and distal limb ischemia:
    - Stop the injection but leave the needle in the artery
    - Arterial injection of lidocaine (10 ml of 1%) provides analgesia and vasodilatation
    - A brachial plexus block has the same action for a more prolonged period
    - Papaverine (70-80 mg in 20 ml of saline) is an effective vasodilator
    - Anticoagulate with a heparin
  - Methohexital does not result in thrombosis although it may be painful
- Porphyria is an absolute contraindication to the use of barbiturates.

Modified from Windsor A, Bowen P, Sebel P. Intravenous anaesthetics. In: Bovill JG, Howie MB, eds. Clinical Pharmacology for Anaesthetists. *London: Saunders; 1999:65.*

phenomenon do not occur with every exposure to a drug, but when they do occur, the mortality rate is as high as 10%. All symptoms are related to neurologic disturbances, especially the autonomic nervous system, and may include abdominal pain, nausea and vomiting, hypertension, tachycardia, seizures, and mood disturbances.[17] Other induction agents (ketamine and propofol) are available for use in affected patients.

Methohexital

An ultra–short-acting barbiturate, methohexital is also primarily used for procedures outside of the operating room such as electroconvulsive therapy (ECT), dental procedures, and cardioversion.[43] Its popularity is not as great as that of the thiobarbiturates because of actions such as excitatory movements (myoclonia) on induction, pain on injection, hiccough, and seizures.[43,44] Spontaneous muscle movements may be influenced by the total amount of drug given and the rapid rate of injection. The hepatic extraction ratio of methohexital is 0.5 (three times greater than that of thiopental). Therefore, hepatic blood flow is a major factor in methohexital clearance. The pharmacokinetics (distribution, redistribution, protein bonding, lipid solubility) of thiopental and methohexital are similar. Although the hepatic clearance of methohexital is greater than that of thiopental, the difference is not as great as would be expected. Hence, redistribution is the most important determinant in the termination of effects for both drugs.[13]

Simulated driving tests showed mental impairment 8 hours after methohexital administration, even though clinical recovery with methohexital was more rapid than with thiopental.[45] The cardiovascular and respiratory effects of methohexital are also similar to those of thiopental.

Methohexital is 2.5 times more potent than the thiobarbiturates, and the incidence of pain on injection is 5%, compared with 1% to 2% with the thiobarbiturates.[43] Key points of barbiturate pharmacology are noted in Box 8-2.

NONBARBITURATE INTRAVENOUS ANESTHETICS

Etomidate

Etomidate (1-[1-phenylethyl]-1*H*-imidazole-5-carboxylic acid ethyl ester) is an intravenous induction agent whose CNS effects result in hypnosis. No intrinsic analgesic properties are associated with the use of this drug.[46] Extensively studied in Europe, etomidate has a cardiovascular stability and a wider margin of safety that appeared to challenge the long-standing role of thiopental as the induction agent of choice in intravenous anesthesia. Side effects such as pain on injection and myoclonia, however, have limited a wider acceptance of the drug. Etomidate is a carboxylated imidazole derivative that was synthesized in 1965 and introduced to European anesthesia practice in 1972.[47] Etomidate has two isomers, but the (+) isomer is the only one with hypnotic properties[37] (see Figure 8-2 for the chemical structure of etomidate).

Etomidate is currently supplied as a 2-mg/ml preparation; each milliliter contains 35% propylene glycol as a solvent and has a pH of 8.1. This formulation has been changed over the years in an effort to decrease the incidence of pain on injection and spontaneous muscle movements. Previously used preparations included polyethylene glycol, aqueous ethanol, Cremophor EL, and an aqueous solution.[48]

BOX 8-2

Key Points of Barbiturate Pharmacology

- Barbiturates bind to a specific site on the $GABA_A$ receptor, depressing neuronal excitability.
- Barbiturates reduce cerebral blood flow (CBF), cerebral metabolic rate ($CMRO_2$), and intracranial pressure. The reduction in $CMRO_2$ is brought about by decreased electrical activity in neurons. CBF decreases with decreased $CMRO_2$, because flow-metabolism coupling is preserved.
- Cerebral protective efforts of barbiturates are controversial.
- Barbiturates cause CNS and myocardial depression and vasodilation, leading to hypotension and decreased cardiac output.
- Respiratory effects include transient hyperventilation followed by prolonged hypoventilation, chiefly through reduction in tidal volume. The slope of the ventilatory response to hypercarbia is decreased.

GABA, *γ-Aminobutyric acid.*

Pharmacokinetics

Etomidate is rapidly metabolized in the liver by hepatic microsomal enzymes and plasma esterases. Ester hydrolysis is the primary mode of metabolism in the liver and plasma. Etomidate is hydrolyzed to form inactive carboxylic acid metabolites. Approximately 10% of the administered dose can be recovered in bile, 13% can be recovered in feces, and the remainder is eliminated by the kidney.[49]

The rapid distribution half-life of etomidate accounts for its extremely short duration of action (see Table 8-4). The drug is lipid soluble and has a volume of distribution that is several times greater than its body weight. Shortly after intravenous injection (within 1 minute) the brain concentration rises rapidly because of the drug's lipid solubility, and extensive redistribution to organs and tissues occurs.

The total body clearance of etomidate is rapid—five times greater than that of thiopental. The hepatic extraction ratio is 67%. The rapid distribution and clearance of etomidate make it especially useful in repeated doses and continuous infusions. Studies examining dose-response relationships have found a lack of accumulation with this compound.[46]

Awakening occurs 7 to 14 minutes after bolus administration. This attribute, combined with the cardiovascular stability of the drug, has led to extensive use of etomidate as a hypnotic-sedative infusion agent in critical care units. Etomidate is 76% protein bound, mostly to albumin. As with other intravenous anesthetics, variations in the amount of available plasma protein alter the amount of free drug available to exert pharmacologic actions. Disease states that produce alterations in plasma protein content should alert the anesthetist to decrease the administered dose.

The mechanism of action of etomidate involves GABA modulation. GABA antagonists can antagonize the effects of etomidate.[4] In clinical investigations of 2500 cases, Doenicke and co-workers[50] confirmed that no histamine is released by etomidate (see Figure 8-4).

Pharmacodynamics

Central Nervous System Effects. Etomidate produces a dose-dependent CNS depression within one arm-brain circulation. Its duration of action is also dose dependent,[46] with awakening occurring 5 to 10 minutes after a 0.2- to 0.4-mg/kg dose. The drug is devoid of analgesic properties because it is unable to block afferent pain stimulus to the thalamus.

Cerebral blood flow and cerebral metabolic rate of oxygen consumption are both decreased by etomidate.[51,52] In a study of fully alert patients without neurologic deficit or impaired consciousness, an etomidate induction was followed by an infusion of 2 to 3 mg/min. Cerebral blood flow decreased 34%, and cerebral metabolism was also reduced (mean decrease of 45%). Decreased oxygen consumption and the associated decrease in carbon dioxide production can cause cerebrovascular vasoconstriction, decreased cerebral blood flow, and decreased intracranial pressure. Also noted during this trial was the maintenance of cerebral blood vessel responsiveness to changes in carbon dioxide levels.[51]

In a study of patients with intracranial pathology, etomidate (0.2 mg/kg given intravenously) was shown to decrease intracranial pressure while maintaining cerebral perfusion pressure. Because of the cardiovascular stability of this drug, mean arterial pressure did not decrease below cerebral autoregulation values, at which cerebral blood flow would become pressure dependent. Cerebral perfusion pressure was maintained adequately in all study subjects.[52]

The electroencephalographic changes that follow administration of etomidate are similar to those that follow administration of other intravenous induction anesthetics. When compared with thiopental, a lack of beta-wave activity was present during induction, along with a longer duration of stages III and IV.[53]

One negative characteristic of etomidate is its excitatory phenomenon of muscle movements and tremors.[53,54] Referred to as *myoclonia*, this phenomenon is defined as sudden, generalized, asynchronous muscle contractions.[55] Myoclonia can affect many muscle groups or a single muscle. The movements can be so severe that they resemble, and are often mistaken for, seizures. In EEG patterns monitored during etomidate anesthesia, no specific EEG disturbances occurred during or after myoclonic episodes.[53] The origin of these muscle movements is thought to be related to uneven drug distribution into brainstem or deep cerebral structures and not to CNS stimulation.[33,53] Etomidate has been associated with epileptic seizures.[56] The incidence of myoclonia ranges between 10% and 60% and varies with the type and the amount of premedication given. Investigators associated the 35% incidence of myoclonic movement with painful stimuli (e.g., drug injection, mandibular lifting). Horrigan and colleagues[54] reported that premedication with fentanyl (100 mg) given intravenously 2 minutes before induction did not significantly decrease motor activity. However, other studies reported better outcomes with fentanyl and diazepam given before induction.[50,57] Etomidate is shown to decrease intraocular pressure. The use of etomidate in sensory-evoked potential (SEP) recording is avoided, because the drug increases wave amplitudes recorded on the scalp. This alteration makes assessing neurologic function with SEP difficult.[33]

Cardiovascular Effects. A major advantage of etomidate over thiopental and other intravenous induction agents is the hemodynamic stability of etomidate. Originally documented in animal studies,[58,59] these findings were later confirmed in humans. In studies of subjects who did not have cardiac disease but had compensated heart disease, changes in heart rate, pulmonary artery pressure, cardiac index, systemic vascular resistance, and arterial blood were not significant.[60] In one study of high-risk patients with significant cardiac disease, hemodynamic stability was maintained with induction doses of 0.3 mg/kg. Also, minimal changes in heart rate, blood pressure, central venous pressure, and intrapulmonary shunting have been demonstrated after etomidate administration.[61] Patients with aortic and mitral valve disease, however, are noted to have significant decreases in systemic blood pressure (17% to 19%), pulmonary artery pressure (11%), and pulmonary capillary wedge pressure (17%).[62] Slight decreases in blood pressure are thought to be caused by decreases in systemic vascular resistance. Myocardial oxygen supply and demand are kept constant by a balance of decreased myocardial blood flow and decreased oxygen consumption.[63] No reports have been made of cardiac dysrhythmias associated with etomidate administration. Both renal and hepatic blood flow are maintained by the stability of cardiac output (see Table 8-6). In summary, at equivalent anesthetic doses, propofol depresses cardiorespiratory function to the greatest degree, followed by thiopental; etomidate depresses it the least.

Respiratory Effects. Etomidate affects the respiratory system in a dose-dependent manner. Minute volume decreases, but respiratory rate increases. The respiratory depression seen with thiopental use is significantly greater than that seen with etomidate use.[63] The ventilatory response to carbon dioxide is decreased, and etomidate administration may cause brief periods of apnea followed by a period of hyperventilation (see Table 8-6).[64]

Adrenocortical Effects. The pharmacokinetics of etomidate (rapid onset, short duration, lack of cumulative response, hemodynamic stability, lack of histamine release, and hypnosis) made it the agent of choice for sedation in critically ill patients. After 10 years of use in Europe, a study reported an increased mortality rate in critically ill patients who received etomidate infusions. This phenomenon was attributed to adrenocortical hypofunction, demonstrated by decreased levels of plasma cortisol.[65] After infusions of etomidate were discontinued, this decrease in adrenal hormone level lasted for 4 days.[66]

Multiple studies have shown adrenal hormone levels to be decreased for 5 to 8 hours after infusion or an induction dose (0.4 mg/kg).[66,67] These effects are caused by a reversible dose-dependent inhibition of adrenocortical enzymes. These enzymes are the cytochrome P-450–dependent mitochondrial enzymes and 11β-hydroxylase. To a lesser degree, 17α-hydroxylase is also affected. The result yields an increase in cortisol precursors but a decrease in cortisol, aldosterone, and corticosterone levels. This enzyme inhibition results in decreased ascorbic acid synthesis, which is necessary for steroid production.[68] These effects are caused by a reversible dose-dependent inhibition of the adrenal cortical enzyme 11β-hydroxylase.

The adrenocortical hypofunction that results from the administration of etomidate administered for the induction of anesthesia is reversible. See Figure 8-5.

Other Effects. Etomidate has been formulated in various solvents in an effort to decrease pain on injection and myoclonia. When etomidate was in a saline base, the incidence of burning and pain was 33% to 80%. After etomidate was reformulated with propylene glycol, no significant difference existed in painful sensations between thiopental and etomidate (18% for both agents).[54] The effects of this reformulation on the incidence of myoclonia, however, have been negligible. Different studies have produced conflicting reports on patients' perception of pain on injection. Some of the variables identified as contributing to pain on injection include site and speed of injection, size of vessel used, and premedication (opioids, benzodiazepines, lidocaine).

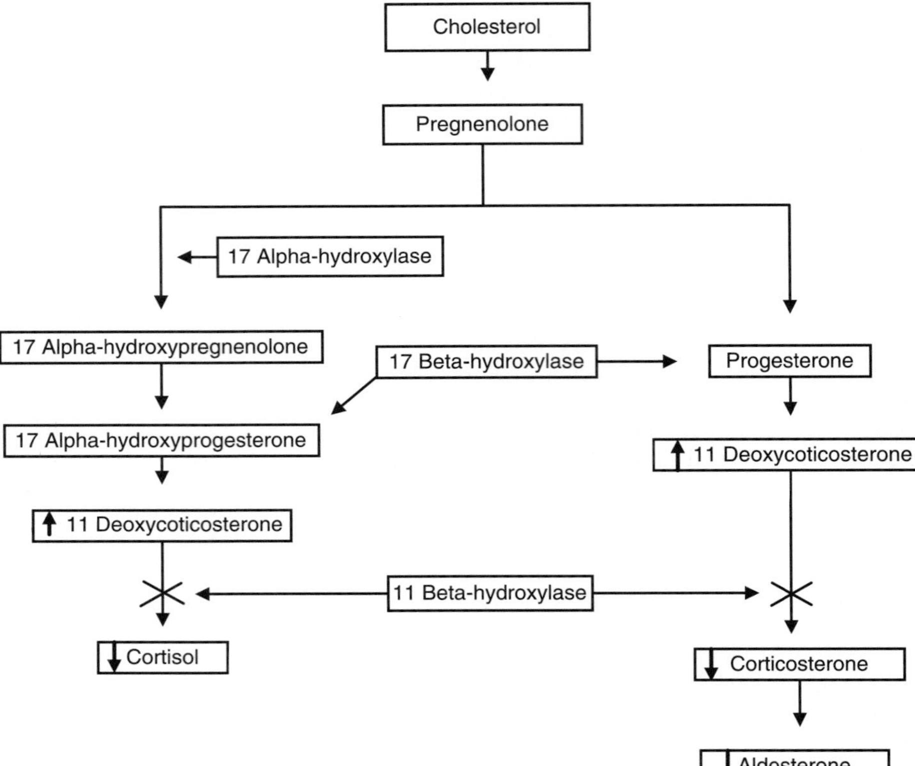

FIGURE **8-5**
Adrenocorticoid suppression by etomidate. Etomidate produces prolonged inhibition of 11β-hydroxylase, which leads to reductions in cortisol and aldosterone.

BOX **8-3**

Key Points of Etomidate Pharmacology

- Etomidate reduces intracranial pressure, cerebral blood flow, and $CMRO_2$.
- The involuntary movements (myoclonia), tremor, and that may occur during induction and recovery are not associated with an epileptiform EEG pattern.
- Etomidate causes myocardial depression and hypotension to a lesser degree than other induction agents do.
- Etomidate depresses the slope of the ventilatory response to carbon dioxide in a manner similar to that of barbiturates and propofol. However, minute ventilation increases, chiefly through an increase in respiratory rate.
- Etomidate inhibits the hepatic enzyme 11β-hydroxylase, which is essential in the production of both corticosteroids and mineralocorticoids. However, clinically significant reductions in steroid production occur only with prolonged infusions or repeated dosing.
- Etomidate increases postoperative nausea and vomiting.

$CMRO_2$, *Cerebral metabolic rate of oxygen consumption;* EEG, *electroencephalogram.*
Modified from Windsor A, Bowen P, Sebel P. Intravenous anaesthetics. In: Bovill JG, Howie MB, eds. Clinical Pharmacology for Anaesthetists. *London: Saunders; 1999:70.*

One study showed that the use of propylene glycol slightly increased thrombophlebitis. Unlike thiopental, no vascular injury occurs after intraarterial injection of etomidate. Nausea and vomiting are more common with etomidate (30% to 40%) than with thiopental (19% to 20%).[69,70] Opioids also increase the susceptibility to nausea and vomiting. Key points of etomidate pharmacology are given in Box 8-3.

KETAMINE

In the search for the ideal induction agent, phencyclidine and its congeners were introduced into clinical practice. However, they were deemed to be unacceptable because they caused serious psychic disturbances, including hallucinations and delirium.[71,72] These agents produced a dissociative state of anesthesia, a concept described by Corssen and Domino,[73] in which the patient is in a catatonic state, feels separated from the environment, and has analgesia and amnesia. Continued research into the congeners of phencyclidine produced ketamine (Ketaject, Ketalar), which was found to be an acceptable drug for anesthesia. Ketamine produced profound analgesia and less-severe psychic reactions when it was first introduced in clinical studies.[74]

The structural formula for ketamine is given in Figure 8-2. The chemical structure of ketamine is 2-(O-chlorophenyl)-2-(methylamino)cyclohexanone. It has a pK_a of 7.5, is partially water soluble, and is slightly acidic (pH 3.5 to 5.5). Pharmacologic preparations contain a preservative, Phemerol (benzethonium chloride), at a ratio of 1:10,000.

Structural Activity

Ketamine is an optically active drug with a chiral center that exists as two optical isomers. A racemic mixture is available for use at this time, although investigators have looked at the different pharmacologic properties of the two stereoisomers. In studies of the S(+) isomer, the R(−) isomer, and the racemic mixture, many pharmacologic differences were found. The S(+) isomer was found to have less spontaneous motor activity; patients were calm and cooperative in the recovery room and had fewer complaints of pain and much lower levels of postoperative anxiety than with either the R(−) isomer or the racemic mixture. The R(−) isomer caused more instances of combativeness and delirium on emergence from anesthesia.[75]

Mechanisms of Action

The primary site of the analgesic action of ketamine is the thalamoneocortical system. Ketamine causes antagonism at *N*-methyl-D-aspartate amino acid (NMDA) receptors in the brain, resulting in a selective depressant effect on the medial thalamic nuclei that is responsible for blocking afferent signals of pain perception to the thalamus and cortex. The NMDA receptor is a ligand gated ion channel where anions Ca^{2+} and Na^{+} are voltage dependent. L-glutamate, an amino acid, is probably the most important excitatory neurotransmitter in the CNS. At the NMDA receptor it causes the opening of the ion channel. A rapid influx of Na^{+}, Ca^{2+}, and K^{+} results in the depolarization of the normally negative postsynaptic membrane that initiates the action potential. Ketamine is a noncompetitive antagonist at this receptor.[76,77] Afferent impulses are transmitted to cortical regions of the brain but are not interpreted, so responses to visual, auditory, and pain stimuli are inappropriate.[74] Although cortical association areas are depressed, the limbic system, which is thought to cause excitatory behavior, is simultaneously activated. The NMDA receptor is shown and described in Figure 8-6.

The analgesia produced by ketamine has a spinal cord component. By injecting bradykinin intraarterially as a noxious stimuli, Nagasaka and co-workers[78] were able to demonstrate that ketamine blocked the stimulated excitatory activity of wide dynamic range neurons in the dorsal horn, thereby preventing transmission of noxious stimuli to the brain. Ketamine may also act as an agonist at opiate receptors.[79]

Neurotransmitter systems have been implicated in ketamine's mechanism of action. The use of acetylcholine was reduced in the caudate nucleus and hippocampus in rats during ketamine anesthesia, a finding that indicates that ketamine may induce electrophysiologic changes that reduce acetylcholine turnover. Physostigmine has been shown to reverse the sedative effect of ketamine but not its analgesic effect.[80]

Metabolism

Hepatic microsomal enzyme systems are responsible for the biotransformation of ketamine. The primary pathway for ketamine metabolism by the cytochrome P-450 system is demethylation to form the metabolite I, norketamine. Hydroxylation of norketamine occurs at one of two positions in the cyclohexone ring to form hydronorketamine metabolites I, II, and III. These metabolites form a glucuronide derivation via conjugation to produce a more water-soluble compound that is eliminated primarily via renal excretion. Thermal dehydration forms dehydroxynorketamine, a cyclohexene derivative (metabolite II).[37,81]

The pharmacologic activity of the metabolite norketamine is approximately 20% to 30% of ketamine's activity. The activity of the other metabolites is unknown.[82]

Pharmacokinetics

The distribution kinetics of ketamine follows a two-compartment model. Ketamine is able to cross the blood-brain barrier quickly to achieve a rapid pharmacologic effect.[83] Peak plasma concentrations are reached within 5 minutes of intravenous injection, and termination of action occurs within 10 to 15 minutes. Ketamine is less protein bound than thiopental (12%), so more drug is immediately available for distribution to the CNS. Brain concentrations decrease rapidly as ketamine is redistributed from the central compartment to peripheral tissue compartments. Redistribution to low–blood-flow tissue compartments accounts for the termination of drug effect and return to consciousness. The slow elimination half-life of the drug is the result of hepatic metabolism and excretion. A large amount of ketamine remains in peripheral tissues as active drug and may be responsible for prolonged or cumulative effects.[84] Hepatic extraction of ketamine is high, because the mean total body clearance is approximately the same as the hepatic blood flow.[85] Ketamine elimination is therefore dependent on hepatic blood flow. Halothane alters the distribution kinetics of ketamine and its metabolite I by decreasing hepatic blood flow, thereby prolonging the duration of action. Pharmacokinetic values remain consistent with analgesic and anesthetic doses of ketamine, which implies that distribution of ketamine is not dose dependent (see Table 8-4).

Intramuscular Route

Given intramuscularly, ketamine reaches peak plasma concentrations within 22 minutes.[86] Dosages range from 4 to 6 mg/kg[76] to 5 to 10 mg/kg. The onset of anesthetic effects is seen within 2 to 3 minutes. Analgesic doses of ketamine (0.44 mg/kg) can be used for painful procedures without causing loss of consciousness and psychic disturbances.[37] After intramuscular administration, approximately 93% of the drug is bioavailable.[87] A consideration with the intramuscular route is the delayed onset of anesthesia. See Table 8-7 for complete dosing information.

Placental Transfer

Ketamine is highly lipid soluble and readily crosses the placenta into fetal tissue. When standard induction doses of 2 to 2.5 mg/kg were given to mothers, neonates were depressed on delivery.[88] Decreasing this dose to 0.2 to 1 mg/kg spared the newborn this CNS depression because of the rapid redistribution of the drug in the mother and the shunting of the drug past the fetal circulation.

Pharmacodynamics

Central Nervous System Effects

Ketamine produces a dissociative state of anesthesia, so called because the patient appears to be dissociated from the environment. The onset of anesthesia is slower than with thiopental or methohexital and may make judgments regarding the onset of sleep and analgesia difficult. In the dissociative state, as originally described by Corssen,[37] the patient is cataleptic: the eyes remain open, the pupils are reactive to light, the corneal reflexes are intact, and horizontal nystagmus is present. Lacrimation and eye blinking continue, and salivary gland secretions are increased. Airway reflexes also remain intact (e.g., laryngeal reflex, pharyngeal reflex, coughing, sneezing, and swallowing). Skeletal muscle tone is increased, and occasional, purposeless movements occur that are unrelated to painful stimuli.

Movement in response to painful stimuli is often required for judgments of adequate anesthesia. After administration of

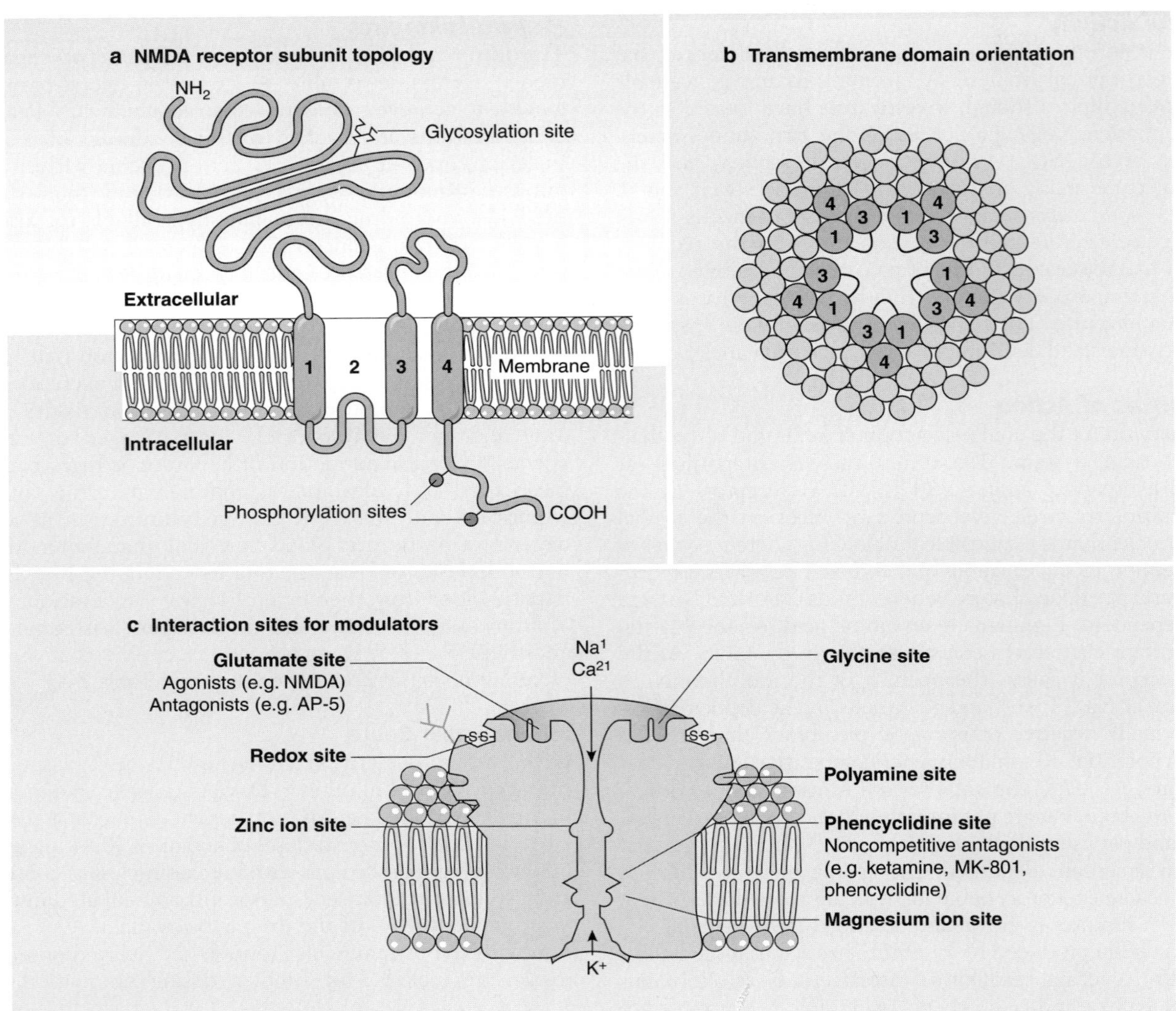

FIGURE **8-6**
The *N*-methyl-D-aspartate amino acid (NMDA) receptor. (a) The NMDA NRI receptor has three transmembrane segments and a fourth hydrophobic segment (designated 2) that loops into the membrane without traversing it. Mutation studies suggest that this loop is the putative channel-lining segment and that blockade by dizocilpine (MK-801), phencyclidine, and ketamine occurs through binding to a site that overlaps the Mg^{2+} site in the pore. The C-terminal domain undergoes phosphorylation, which regulates channel activity and mediates interactions with intracellular anchoring proteins. (b) Transmembrane hydrophobic segments interact to form a central ion-conducting pore lined by the second hydrophobic segments. The stoichiometry of the hetero-oligomer is not known but may be four or five (as shown), by analogy with the homologous nicotinic cholinergic receptor. (c) The NMDA receptor gates a cation channel that is permeable to Na^+, Ca^{2+}, and K^+ and is gated by Mg^{2+} in a voltage-dependent fashion. Agonists (glutamate, NMDA) and the coagonist glycine, required for full activation, bind to the extracellular domain. (From Hopkis PM, Winlow W. Mechanisms of anesthesia. In: Hemmings HC, Hopkins PM, eds. *Foundations of Anesthesia Basic and Clinical Sciences*. St Louis: Mosby; 2000:250.)

a single dose, full reorientation to person, place, and time takes place in 15 to 30 minutes.[89] Ketamine is a profound analgesic that has a preference for skin, bones, and joints. Analgesia occurs with subdissociative doses[85] of ketamine, and this agent may be used for painful procedures without inducing a loss of consciousness. Analgesia is present after the anesthetic effects are terminated and correlates well with plasma levels of ketamine. Anesthetic levels are present with plasma levels of 640 to 1000 μg/ml, and analgesic levels are present with plasma ketamine concentrations of 100 to 150 μg/ml.[81]

Cerebral blood flow is increased 60% to 80% by ketamine and returns to normal within 20 to 30 minutes of administration. This increase in blood flow is attributed to the excitatory effects of ketamine; these effects increase the cerebral metabolic rate of oxygen consumption, which in turn increases central blood flow and cerebrospinal fluid pressure. This indirect effect of ketamine can be attenuated with hyperventilation; this finding indicates that the response of cerebral vessels to carbon dioxide is left intact with ketamine anesthesia.

TABLE 8-7 Recommendations for Using Ketamine as a Sedative, Analgesic, or Anesthetic during the Perioperative Period

Premedication

- A benzodiazepine administered either orally (e.g., 15-30 mg of diazepam or 2-5 mg of lorazepam) 60-90 min before surgery or IV (e.g., midazolam 0.05-0.1 mg/kg) immediately before induction of anesthesia as an adjunctive agent
- If preoperative sedation is contraindicated, a benzodiazepine can be administered IV after induction of anesthesia but before termination of surgery; an antisialagogue (e.g., glycopyrrolate, 0.005 mg/kg IV) can effectively decrease secretions if administered 5-10 min before induction

Induction of Anesthesia

- Ketamine 0.5-1.5 mg/kg IV, or 4-6 mg/kg IM; lower doses of ketamine are used if thiopental (1-2 mg/kg IV), midazolam (0.075-0.15 mg/kg), or propofol (0.75-1.5 mg/kg IV) is used as a co-induction agent in place of the premedicant or if the patient is elderly or critically ill

Maintenance of Anesthesia

- Ketamine 15-45 mcg/kg/min (1-3 mg/min) by continuous IV infusion with supplemental nitrous oxide, 70%; after a barbiturate (or propofol) induction a higher initial maintenance infusion rate is required (e.g., 30-90 mcg/kg/min)

Sedation and Analgesia

Ketamine 0.2-0.8 mg/kg IV (over 2-3 min) or 2-4 mg/kg IM, followed by a continuous ketamine infusion (5-120 mcg/kg/min) with or without supplemental oxygen

IM, *Intramuscular;* IV, *intravenous.*
From Gajraj N, White PF. Clinical pharmacology and applications of ketamine. In: Bowdle T, Horita A, Kharasch ED, eds. The pharmacologic Basis of Anesthesiology. *New York: Churchill Livingstone; 1994:375-392.*

On loss of consciousness and onset of analgesia, ketamine induces a transition from alpha to theta waves (slow waves with moderate-to-high amplitude) on the EEG. Alpha waves do not reappear until after consciousness returns and analgesia is lost.[74]

Ketamine anesthesia emergence is associated with psychic disturbances immediately on return of consciousness.[90] These emergence reactions are the result of visual, auditory, proprioceptive, and confusional illusions.[91] Descriptions of this phenomenon include vivid illusions, sensations of drunkenness, delirium, restlessness, altered states of consciousness, extracorporeal sensations, and combativeness.[75,91] The onset occurs with the first verbal contact and usually resolves with full return of orientation to person, place, and time.[37] Recurrent dreams have been reported to occur weeks after a ketamine anesthetic.[92] The benzodiazepines diazepam and midazalam were found to significantly decrease the incidence of these reactions.

Cardiovascular Effects

Ketamine, unlike other intravenous anesthetics, acts as a circulatory stimulant, producing increases in systemic blood pressure, heart rate, cardiac output, and central venous pressure.[73,75,90] Systemic vascular resistance responded differently among patients undergoing cardiac catheterization and angiography (±25%), possibly because of patient variability in autonomic tone and disease states. Other studies have failed to show significant effects in systemic vascular resistance but have found evidence of an increase in pulmonary vascular resistance (42%), pulmonary artery pressure (47%), and right ventricular stroke work. These values persisted throughout the 12-minute measurement period, although they were somewhat decreased (pulmonary vascular resistance, 42% at 3 to 5 minutes and 25% at 12 minutes; mean pulmonary arterial pressure, 47% at 3 to 5 minutes and 23% at 12 minutes). In patients with congenital heart disease and increased pulmonary pressure and resistance, ketamine administration did not adversely affect myocardial function (ejection fractions remained constant).[93]

Ketamine administration causes an increase in myocardial contractility, thereby affecting the myocardial oxygen balance. This increase in myocardial oxygen consumption has not been shown to cause inadequate myocardial perfusion, because a concomitant rise in coronary artery perfusion occurs that is produced by a decrease in coronary artery vasodilation.[93]

Ketamine-induced activation of the sympathetic nervous system that results in endogenous catecholamine release is believed to be the mechanism for the cardiostimulatory properties experienced after administration of the drug. Injection of ketamine directly into the CNS via the carotid artery causes an immediate increase in blood pressure, heart rate, and cardiac output.[94] The positive inotropic effect of ketamine in vitro results from an inhibition of neuronal and extraneuronal uptake of norepinephrine. This norepinephrine then activates β-adrenergic receptors.[95] Studies have indicated that the negative inotropic effects of ketamine are the result of a decrease in the available calcium ions (Ca^{2+}) intracellularly, caused by an interference with Ca^{2+} delivery mechanisms (net transsarcolemma Ca^{2+} influx).[96] When the positive inotropic effects of ketamine are blocked, the negative inotropic effects predominate and may result in decreased blood pressure and cardiac output. This phenomenon may be seen clinically in the critically ill patient who, as a result of protracted illness, has decreased available catecholamine stores and limited ability to compensate. With an intact sympathetic nervous system, the positive inotropic effects dominate and counteract the negative inotropic effects. By decreasing sympathetic responses, some inhalation anesthetics are able to block the cardiovascular effects of ketamine to produce a decrease in systemic blood pressure and cardiac output.[97] The cardiovascular stimulation produced by ketamine may be deliberately decreased by the prior administration of benzodiazepines in patients in whom that response should be avoided.[90]

Ketamine has been used successfully in patients who are hemodynamically compromised because of shock, trauma, debilitation, or hypovolemia.

Changes in systemic blood pressure are dose related; systolic and diastolic blood pressures increase when larger doses of ketamine are administered (0.5 to 2.0 mg/kg). However, the heart rate response to different dosages reaches a plateau, with no significant change in rate occurring between doses of 0.5 and 2 mg/kg.

Ketamine has been used successfully for both pediatric and adult cardiac surgery patients with congenital and acquired disease processes.[93,98] See Table 8-6.

Respiratory Effects

The effects of ketamine on the respiratory system are minor and of short duration. Respiratory depression, which is reflected in a decrease in tidal volume over respiratory rate, begins 2 to 3 minutes after parenteral administration.[74]

Significant respiratory depression, demonstrated by decreased oxygen constant and increased partial pressure of arterial carbon dioxide, follows rapid bolus intravenous injection and may last 5 to 10 minutes. The addition of other CNS depressants augments the respiratory depression produced by ketamine. With slow administration or infusion methods, arterial blood gases remain within normal limits, and the central response to carbon dioxide is maintained.[75]

Ketamine increases pulmonary compliance and decreases pulmonary resistance in patients with bronchospastic disease. In case reports the effects of ketamine on resolving bronchospasm coincide with peak blood levels toward the end of the drug's distribution half-life, with recurrence of bronchospasm. Increased circulation catecholamine levels stimulated by ketamine, along with bronchial smooth muscle relaxation and vagolytic actions, are thought to be the reason for the bronchodilating effects of the drug. Tracheal, bronchial, and salivary muscle gland secretions are increased with ketamine, requiring the use of an antisialagogue. The muscle tone of the tongue and jaw is retained, and protective pharyngeal and laryngeal reflexes are left intact. Coughing, gagging, and swallowing remain in response to airway stimulation, although silent pulmonary aspiration has occurred in some patients.[75] See Table 8-6.

Intraocular Effects

Research into the effects of ketamine administration on intraocular pressure has yielded varied results. Some investigators have reported marked increases in intraocular pressure with ketamine administration, whereas others have concluded that no change in intraocular pressure occurs.[99] Measurement techniques and adjunctive anesthetics may have affected these results. Ketamine causes nystagmus, increased muscle tone, and muscle spasms, which may not be appropriate for ophthalmic procedures.[100] The common clinical effects of ketamine are given in Box 8-4.

Obstetric Use

Ketamine can be used in obstetrics for analgesia or anesthesia. As an induction agent, ketamine in doses of 0.5 to 1 mg/kg produces rapid anesthesia without compromising uterine tone, uterine blood flow, or neonatal status at delivery. For analgesia, 0.25 mg/kg of ketamine provides pain-related relief, airway stability, and a sustained maternal blood pressure and uninhibited uterine contractions. Use of doses reserved for surgical procedures (2 to 2.2 mg/kg) results, however, in a depressed neonate on delivery.[101,102] Clinical uses of ketamine are given in Box 8-5. Recommendations for using ketamine as a sedative, analgesic, or anesthetic during the postoperative period are listed in Table 8-7. Key points of ketamine pharmacology are given in Box 8-6.

BOX 8-4

Primary Clinical Characteristics and Effects of Ketamine

- Phencyclidine derivative
- Causes unconsciousness, amnesia referred to as *dissociative anesthesia*
- Increases cerebral metabolic rate, cerebral blood flow, intracranial pressure
- Causes nystagmus, increased intraocular pressure
- Is an analgesic
- Increases blood pressure and pulse
- Potent bronchodilator
- Maintains respirations and airway reflexes (note: a period of initial apnea may occur, especially with high doses and rapid administration)
- Increases salivation and respiratory secretions
- Increases muscle tone
- Increases postoperative nausea and vomiting
- Associated with emergence delirium, nightmares, and hallucinations
- Requires caution in patients with hypertension, angina, congestive heart failure, increased intracranial pressure, increased intraocular pressure, psychiatric disease, airway problems

BENZODIAZEPINES

Benzodiazepines are used in many clinical situations because of their multiple pharmacologic properties, including sedation, hypnosis, muscle relaxation, antianxiety effects, anticonvulsant effects, and amnesia. They also are noted to have a low incidence of side effects. Benzodiazepines used clinically in the United States are listed in Table 8-8.

Although similar compounds were first synthesized in 1933, the first benzodiazepine synthesized was chlordiazepoxide (Librium) in 1955. It was not introduced into clinical practice until 1960, when it was found to have antianxiety and hypnotic effects. Diazepam was synthesized in 1959, and its metabolite, oxazepam (Serax), was synthesized in 1961. Lorazepam (Ativan) was derived from oxazepam in 1971.[103] The last benzodiazepine to be developed was midazolam (in 1976, by Fryer and Walser), which was the first of the benzodiazepine group to be formulated with anesthesia as its target clinical use.[4] The benzodiazepines available for clinical use have different potencies, pharmacokinetics, and intensities of clinical properties.

Chemical Structure

The chemical structure of the benzodiazepines shares some common features: (1) the benzodiazepine ring system; (2) the presence at positions 1 and 4 (except in clobazam) of two nitrogen atoms; (3) a phenyl group at position 5; and (4) an electronegative group at position 7 (see Figure 8-2).[103]

BOX 8-5

Clinical Uses of Ketamine

Induction of Anesthesia in High-Risk Patients
- Shock or cardiovascular instability
- Severe dehydration
- Bronchospasm
- Severe anemia
- One-lung anesthesia

Obstetric Patients
Induction of General Anesthesia
- Severe hypovolemia
- Acute hemorrhage
- Acute bronchospasm

Low Dose for Analgesia
- To supplement regional anesthetic techniques at the time of delivery or during the postpartum period

Adjunct to Local and Regional Anesthetic Techniques
- For sedation and analgesia during performance of nerve block procedures
- To supplement an inadequate block

Outpatient Surgery
- For brief diagnostic and therapeutic procedures
- To supplement local and regional block techniques

Use outside the Operating Room
- In burn units (e.g., débridement, dressing changes)
- In emergency rooms (e.g., closed reduction)
- In intensive care units (e.g., sedation, painful procedures)
- In recovery rooms (e.g., postoperative sedation and analgesia)
- During x-ray examinations

Modified from Gajraj N, White PF. Clinical pharmacology and applications of ketamine. In: Bowdle TA, Horita A, Kharasch ED, eds. The Pharmacological Basis of Anesthesiology. *New York: Churchill Livingstone; 1994:375-392.*

BOX 8-6

Key Points of Ketamine Pharmacology

- Site of action appears to be primarily in the thalamus and limbic systems; ketamine acts via the NMDA receptor as a noncompetitive antagonist.
- Onset of effect is relatively slow (2-5 min).
- Ketamine produces a rise in cerebral perfusion pressure by increased sympathetic outflow, which causes a rise in mean arterial pressure.
- Ketamine is a bronchodilator, preserves airway reflexes, and increases tracheobronchial and salivary secretions.
- Emergence phenomena, including vivid dreams, floating sensations, and delirium, can occur after ketamine administration. They are more common in adults than children and are reduced by benzodiazepine or barbiturate administration.

NMDA, *N-methyl-D-aspartate.*
Modified from Windsor A, Bowen P, Sebel P. Intravenous anaesthetics. In Bovill JG, Howie MB, eds. Clinical Pharmacology for Anaesthetists. *London: Saunders; 1999:68.*

Midazolam has a unique chemical structure in comparison with the other benzodiazepines. The imidazole ring is responsible for its basic formulation, which permits the preparation of salts that are water soluble at a pH of 4.0. In a chemical reaction that depends on the environmental pH, the diazepine ring opens reversibly between positions 4 and 5. Midazolam is water soluble and does not require a lipoidal vehicle (such as propylene glycol) for parenteral use.[103] Minimal, if any, side effects of venous irritation or phlebitis occur. Once in physiologic solution with a pH greater than 4.0, the diazepine ring closes, and midazolam becomes lipophilic, an effect that accounts for its rapid onset of action and the acceptance it has received as an alternative intravenous induction agent.[103]

Diazepam, lorazepam, and midazolam are the most commonly used benzodiazepines in anesthesia practice.

In each milliliter of solution of diazepam, 0.4 ml of propylene glycol and 0.1 ml of ethyl alcohol are present as solvents, 0.015 ml of benzyl alcohol is present as a preservative, and sodium benzoate or benzoic acid in water is present as a buffer. Each milliliter contains 5 mg of diazepine, and the pH is 6.2 to 6.9.[102]

Each milliliter of lorazepam solution contains 0.18 ml of polyethylene glycol and 2% benzyl alcohol, a preservative. Lorazepam is available in solutions of 2 or 4 mg/ml.[102]

Injectable midazolam is compounded with 0.8% sodium chloride and 0.01% disodium edetate and 1% benzyl alcohol as a preservative. A pH of 3 is adjusted with hydrochloric acid and, if necessary, sodium hydroxide. Each milliliter of preparation contains 1 or 5 mg of midazolam.

Mechanisms of Action

In 1977 specific benzodiazepine receptors were identified in vivo.[104] Benzodiazepine binding sites were found in great density in the olfactory bulb, cerebral cortex, cerebellum, and substantia nigra, with lesser concentrations in the lower brain stem and spinal cord. The clinical effects of benzodiazepines are a result of their occupation of the benzodiazepine receptors within a complex of receptors on the synaptic membrane of the effector neuron. This complex is a GABA-α-receptor complex that modulates GABA, the major inhibitory neurotransmitter in the CNS. This complex is composed of protein subunits that contain binding sites for benzodiazepines, GABA, the barbiturates, ethanol, and a chloride ion channel. When these sites are occupied, GABA receptor modulation increases the frequency of chloride channel opening, which results in postsynaptic membrane hyperpolarization, and neuronal transmission is inhibited.[104] A ceiling effect exists on the CNS depression produced by benzodiazepines and is a result of a limitation of the extent of modulation of GABA. Different receptor subtypes and concentration dependent receptor occupancy may have a role in whether anxiolysis, sedation, or hypnosis occurs when a benzodiazepine is administered.

Three classes of ligands that bind to the benzodiazepine receptors have been identified: agonists, antagonists, and inverse agonists. Midazolam is a receptor agonist that has an increased binding affinity for GABA, resulting in the opening of the chloride channels. Antagonists (e.g., flumazenil) form reversible bonds with the agonist receptor but produce no agonist activity.[152] Inverse agonists cause CNS stimulation by interfering with GABA transmission, which is inhibitory.[105]

The pharmacologic effects of agents depend on which receptors in the CNS are occupied. The brain stem or cortical receptors mediate sedation, the forebrain and hippocampus mediate amnesia, and the benzodiazepine receptors in the amygdala, hippocampus, and other limbic areas mediate anxiolytic properties. See Figure 8-4.

Diazepam

Pharmacokinetics

The elimination pharmacokinetics of benzodiazepines can be examined in both two- and three-compartment models (Table 8-8). Benzodiazepines have been classified according to their elimination half-lives. These classifications take into account the elimination half-lives of both the parent drug and the active metabolites it produces. Diazepam is long lasting, lorazepam has an intermediate duration, and midazolam is short lasting.[106]

Diazepam has a very slow distribution half-life, which limits its usefulness as an acceptable induction agent. Its inability to cause unconsciousness rapidly may be the result of its ability to produce profound CNS depression and renders it unacceptable.[106] Diazepam is extremely lipid soluble, a characteristic that promotes extensive distribution to the tissues. The volume of distribution is large, a characteristic of all benzodiazepines. Also characteristic is extensive protein binding, which can be affected by disease states that decrease plasma protein levels. The total body clearance of diazepam is only 0.24 to 0.53 ml/min/kg and is totally dependent on hepatic metabolism.

The hepatic extraction ratio of diazepam is very low, making it dependent on hepatic blood flow, protein binding, and hepatic metabolism. Cimetidine, a hepatic enzyme inhibitor, decreases the hepatic biotransformation of diazepam and prolongs its effects.[107] The pharmacologic effects seen with benzodiazepines are terminated primarily by redistribution of the drug out of the CNS. Oral diazepam has a 100% bioavailability, which reflects no first-pass removal of the drug by the liver. Intramuscular administration of similar doses, however, results in a plasma blood level of only 50% to 60% of that administered. Diazepam does not stay in solution after intramuscular injection. After the solvent dissolves, the diazepam precipitates, leaving less drug available for absorption. The preparation with propylene glycol also causes pain and irritation at the injection site.

Diazepam exhibits a near-linear relationship between elimination half-life and patient age.[108] Pharmacokinetics in the elderly are altered as a result of slowed drug absorption; increased percentage of adipose tissue in body mass; decreased plasma proteins, hepatic blood flow, and metabolism; and decreased cardiac output and circulation time. A prolonged circulation time allows for a slower onset and a higher plasma drug level that remains in the CNS longer before it redistributes; this phenomenon exaggerates the effects of the drug.[109]

Hepatic microsomal enzymes are responsible for the metabolism of diazepam. Diazepam is demethylated to dimethyl diazepam (nordiazepam), which is an active metabolite that, although less potent, is responsible for prolonged drug effect as a result of its slower metabolism. Diazepam can also be hydroxylated to 3-hydroxydiazepam, which is then demethylated to oxazepam, which is also pharmacologically active and commercially marketed. The termination of action of diazepam is caused by redistribution, and the distribution half-life is 30 to 66 minutes, much longer than that of other induction agents.

Pharmacodynamics

Central Nervous System Effects. Diazepam produces all the characteristic CNS depressant effects of the benzodiazepines from sedation to anxiolysis and sleep. Diazepam produces anterograde but not retrograde amnesia; the amnesia is dose related. Benzodiazepines also possess anticonvulsant activity, and diazepam has been shown to be effective in the treatment of status epilepticus and sedative-hypnotic withdrawal syndromes. In vitro studies in animals have shown it to be effective in the prevention of seizures induced by local anesthetics. EEG changes include disappearance of the alpha rhythm and the onset of higher-frequency beta-rhythm activity.[110] See Table 8-5.

Respiratory Effects. Some respiratory depression occurs with diazepam, as evidenced by a decrease in minute ventilation and slope of the carbon dioxide response curve.[107] This response curve is not shifted to the right, as occurs with some other CNS depressants. Increased respiratory depression and apnea are possible when benzodiazepines are combined with other CNS depressants, such as opioids.

TABLE 8-8 Benzodiazepines Used Clinically in the United States

Generic Name	Trade Name	Half Life (hr)	Clinical Application
Alprazolam	Xanax	12-15	Anxiolysis
Chlordiazepoxide	Librium	8-18	Treatment of alcohol withdrawal, etc.
Clonazepam	Klonopin	18.7-39	Treatment of epilepsy
Clorazepate	Tranxene	2.4	Treatment of epilepsy and alcohol withdrawal
Diazepam	Valium	36-50	Sedation; induction and maintenance of anesthesia
Estazolam	ProSom	14	Treatment of insomnia
Flurazepam	Dalmane	2-3	Treatment of insomnia
Lorazepam	Ativan	10-22	Anxiolysis and sedation
Midazolam	Versed	1.7-2.6	Sedation; induction and maintenance of anesthesia
Oxazepam	Serax	3-21	Anxiolysis
Prazepam	Centrax	63-70	Anxiolysis
Quazepam	Doral	25-41	Treatment of insomnia
Temazepam	Restoril	10-21	Treatment of insomnia
Triazolam	Halcion	2-3	Treatment of insomnia
Flumazenil	Romazicon	0.7-1.3	Reversal of benzodiazepine agonists

Uses

Diazepam has been used successfully for preanesthesia medication and sedation during therapeutic or diagnostic procedures. Three main concerns with its use are pain on injection, thrombophlebitis, and duration of action. Dosages should be adjusted in elderly patients and in patients with hepatic or renal disease. Intravenous diazepam has been associated with patient dissatisfaction regarding pain and postoperative thrombophlebitis. The use of small veins and a rapid rate of injection can increase the high rate of these complications. The longer duration of action compared with that of midazolam explains the currently limited anesthetic use of diazepam.

Midazolam

Midazolam is an imidazobenzodiazepine that is similar to diazepam in potency but is shorter acting. Its chemical structure differs from that of the classic benzodiazepines in that it has an imidazole ring that gives the drug basicity, which allows the preparation of the drug as a salt. This quality makes the drug soluble and stable in aqueous solutions. No solvents are necessary as a vehicle for injection, and the venous irritation produced by other benzodiazepines is therefore omitted. A methyl group exists at position 1; this group produces a very short duration of action, because it is rapidly metabolized by hepatic oxidizing enzymes. The imidazole ring structure is altered by physiologic pH, and at a pH of less than 4 the ring is 80% to 85% in the closed ring form and 15% to 20% in the open form. When the pH is greater than 4, the ring structures are totally closed, and the drug becomes highly lipophilic, which results in a rapid onset of action.[103] The closed ring form has an increased affinity for hydrolysis by hepatic microsomal oxidative mechanisms, which contributes to the drug's short duration of action.

Absorption

Oral midazolam is rapidly absorbed and subject to first-pass hepatic extraction, which results in a systemic availability of less than 50% of the administered dose. The greater the dose, the larger the percent of active drug available.[111]

Intramuscular injection produces a bioavailability of between 80% and 100%. Peak plasma concentrations are reached within 45 minutes of intramuscular injection.[112]

Mechanisms of Action

The pharmacologic effects of midazolam include all actions common to benzodiazepines, such as anticonvulsant effects, hypnosis, amnesia, muscle relaxant effects, and anxiolysis. Midazolam has a higher affinity for benzodiazepine receptors in the CNS than diazepam. In animal studies, the anticonvulsant effects of midazolam were found to be equivalent to diazepam, although of shorter duration. Midazolam was also found to be a more effective sedative than diazepam but for a shorter duration.[113]

Pharmacokinetics

The rapid onset of this drug is a result of its high lipid solubility at physiologic pH and its ability to rapidly cross the blood-brain barrier. Midazolam is extensively protein bound (95% to 96%), which may contribute to clinically evident alterations in the effects of the drugs in patients with alterations in protein states.[114] Termination of action is dependent on a rapid redistribution of the drug. Midazolam may be described in a three-compartment model, with elimination occurring from the central compartment.

Metabolism of midazolam is via hydroxylation in the liver. It has a high hepatic extraction ratio (7 to 9 ml/min/kg) and a high clearance, resulting in the shortest elimination half-life of the benzodiazepines. The metabolites of midazolam are alpha-hydroxymidazolam (which has minimal potency), 4-hydroxymidazolam (which is similar in potency to alpha-hydroxymidazolam but is produced in very small amounts), and alpha-4-hydroxymidazolam (which is also produced in small amounts but is practically inactive). Combined, the metabolites do not contribute significantly to the pharmacologic effects of midazolam or its duration of action. All metabolites are excreted in the urine as glucuronide conjugates.[115]

In animal studies, three metabolites of midazolam were evaluated for pharmacologic activity. Alpha-hydroxymidazolam levels measured 30 minutes after administration in mice were one tenth to one fortieth as potent than those of midazolam. The metabolite 4-hydroxymidazolam had similar levels of potency, and alpha-4-hydroxymidazolam was practically inactive.

Pharmacodynamics

Cardiovascular Effects. Blood pressure was not significantly changed and heart rate was only slightly increased in conscious dogs. Under barbiturate anesthesia, midazolam caused slight dose-related decreases in systolic and diastolic blood pressure. In humans the use of midazolam is associated with a relatively stable cardiac profile.[114] When the drug was used for induction of anesthesia in healthy humans (0.15 mg/kg given intravenously over 15 seconds), systolic blood pressure was decreased 5%, diastolic blood pressure was decreased 10%, and heart rate was increased 18% (significance $P < 0.05$).[116] The decrease in arterial blood pressure is the result of a reduction in systemic vascular resistance.

Respiratory Effects. Midazolam, as well as all the other benzodiazepines, produces less respiratory depression in usual doses than older sedatives, such as the barbiturates or phenothiazines. As expected with any CNS depressant drug, however, respiratory depression may occur in the very young, elderly, or debilitated, as well as in patients receiving other respiratory depressant agents.[116]

Central Nervous System Effects. Amnesia is an important pharmacologic effect of midazolam. Intravenous administration produces anterograde amnesia in low doses. Amnesia occurs within 2 to 5 minutes of administration and remains for 20 to 30 minutes.[117] In one study partial amnesia remained for 90 minutes in 40% of the patients studied.

Previous studies have shown that midazolam produces a decrease in cerebral blood flow and cerebral metabolic oxygen consumption without significant cardiovascular depression.[118]

Knudsen and co-workers[118] studied 30 patients with different serum concentrations of midazolam and the presence of nitrous oxide. They concluded that no drug response relationship existed between midazolam and cerebral blood flow or oxygen consumption. In this study, mean arterial pressure and arterial partial pressure of CO_2 were maintained at constant levels.

Uses

The popularity of midazolam in modern anesthesia is widespread. Its rapid onset and short duration and half-life make it ideal for use as a preoperative anxiolytic and a perioperative sedative drug.

FLUMAZENIL

Flumazenil is the sole benzodiazepine antagonist available in the United States (see Figure 8-2). It is a competitive antagonist with a high affinity for the receptor site. It produces prompt and effective specific reversal of benzodiazepine agonist effects after anesthesia and overdose.[119,120] Actual available receptors for occupancy by flumazenil effect its pharmacologic action. Benzodiazepine affinity for the receptors and concentration of free benzodiazepines at the sites determine receptor occupancy of flumazenil. Its relatively short duration and half-life make the possibility of resedation clinically relevant, especially in overdose situations. A slow titration of 0.2-mg doses (2 ml) is given intravenously (up to 1 mg) until the desired level of consciousness is achieved. Doses rarely exceed 1 mg for the reversal of midazolam-induced sedation and 3 mg for suspected benzodiazepine overdose. Withdrawal reactions are possible in patients who are benzodiazepine dependent, and its use in these patients is contraindicated. Flumazenil does not reverse the actions of ethanol or barbiturates.[121] Side effects are rare, although mild anxiogenic effects have been reported.[122] Seizures have been reported in patients with suspected tricyclic and antidepressant overdose, and the use of flumazenil in these situations and in patients with a known history of seizures should be avoided.[123]

PROPOFOL

Chemistry

Propofol is a 2,6-diisopropyl phenol (see Figure 8-2). It is prepared in a milky-white emulsion of 10% soybean oil, 2.25% glycerol, and 1.2% purified egg lecithin. This unique vehicle has been reported to be especially favorable to bacterial contamination. The pH of Diprivan (propofol) is 7 to 8.5, and the pK_a is 11. The pH of the generic form of propofol is 4.5 to 6.4, and the pK_a is 11. Diprivan contains 0.005% disodium edetate, and the generic propofol contains 0.025% sodium metabisulfite to retard the growth of organisms. These preservatives may be effective in decreasing the risk of bacterial contamination. However, these formulations may still support bacterial growth. It is recommended that aseptic conditions be maintained and disinfection of the vial with 70% isopropyl alcohol be employed when syringes are prepared for use. Opened vials and syringes should be discarded if they are not used within 6 hours of preparation.[124]

Pharmacokinetics

Propofol exhibits a generally favorable kinetic profile, which is one of its main clinical benefits in comparison with other induction drugs.[125,126] See Table 8-4.

Rapid redistribution from the central to the peripheral compartments produces a quick initial decline in blood levels. This effect leads to a rapid reawakening after sedative and anesthetic doses. The characteristic of propofol that differentiates it from thiopental is its rapid metabolic clearance, which actually exceeds hepatic blood flow.[126] It was concluded by Veroli and colleagues[127] that extrahepatic routes of metabolism exist, because metabolites of propofol were found in the urine during the anhepatic phase of a liver transplantation. Residual drug undergoes hepatic elimination, and effects can be prolonged in patients with liver disease. The drug's kinetics are also influenced by age, with the elderly requiring lower doses.[128] Children require higher doses because they have an increased volume of distribution based on body weight. Their rate of clearance is also higher.[129] Accumulation can occur with prolonged infusion because of extensive tissue saturation.[130]

Mechanism of Action

Like other intravenous induction agents, propofol appears to exert its effect via an interaction with the inhibitory neurotransmitter GABA and the $GABA_A$ glycoprotein receptor complex.[131] Recent studies are also implicating the excitatory amino acid neurotransmitter glutamate and NMDA receptors in the anesthetic action of propofol but to a lesser extent. Other actions include a rapid, pleasant recovery and antiemetic and antipruritic effects.[132]

Other Pharmacologic Actions

It is recognized that propofol possesses mild antiemetic effects that are most prominent when given by continuous infusion.[133,134]

Patients experience varying degrees of pain on injection of propofol.[135] Different formulations have not changed this spontaneous complaint, and various techniques of administration have been employed to minimize this problem. The addition of lidocaine to the emulsion has been employed with good results. Lidocaine (1% or 2%) 0.1 or 0.2 mg/kg reduces the pain on injection.[136,137] A study using chilled propofol failed to reduce the incidence of pain.[136] The lidocaine may also be given before the administration of propofol. The use of larger veins for intravenous access in the antecubital fossa or forearm can decrease the incidence of pain on injection. The pain on infusion is not associated with an increased incidence of phlebitis. Intraarterial injection of propofol does not cause vascular injury.

PHARMACODYNAMICS

Central Nervous System Effects

The use of propofol in neuroanesthesia, as well as in prolonged sedation, in neurologic intensive care unit settings has increased steadily since its introduction. Significant reductions in cerebral blood flow, $CMRO_2$, intracranial pressure, and cerebral perfusion pressure have been reported with the use of numerous administration techniques.[138] These effects result in part from the decreased mean arterial pressure and cerebral vasoconstriction produced by standard doses in a manner comparable to the effects of barbiturates and etomidate.[139] Craen and co-workers[140] have found that cerebral autoregulation and reactivity to changes in CO_2 were preserved with propofol.

EEG data produced a delta rhythm without evidence of epileptiform activity and burst suppression with higher doses.[141] Even with these findings, controversy exists over the use of propofol in the epileptic patient.[142] Three epileptic patients were reported to experience increased epileptiform activity on EEG after the administration of propofol 2 mg/kg.[143] Studies in epileptic patients showed a different response in that the EEG showed no increase in epileptogenic activity at any of the sites monitored.[144] It was also found that activation of or extension of EEG activity was greater with thiopental than with propofol (although not statistically significant).[145] Propofol has been used successfully to manage status epilepticus.[146] Seizures induced by propofol may be spontaneous excitatory movements secondary to selective disinhibition of subcortical centers. Adequate dosage may prevent the occurrence of these movements. Myoclonia may occur on induction, but the incidence appears to be lower than that with etomidate, thiopental, and methohexital. Opisthotonos has also been associated with propofol. Intraocular pressure is decreased by propofol.[147]

The use of propofol for ECT has been somewhat controversial as a result of this drug's effects on seizure duration. Several studies have shown that propofol reduces the duration of the ECT-induced seizure when compared with barbiturates.[148,149] The efficacy of ECT as an antidepressant is based on the duration of the seizure; a shortened seizure implies a less effective therapy. Researchers have found that a reduction in seizure duration does not decrease the efficacy of the ECT and that propofol is an appropriate agent for use in this procedure.[149,150] Some patients with a prolonged seizure response would benefit from the shorter seizure time caused by propofol. ECT is associated with cardiovascular changes (elevated blood pressure and heart rate) that may be prevented or modified with the use of propofol.[151]

Cardiovascular Effects

Propofol produces significant cardiac depression in the usual induction doses. The effects are more pronounced than those seen with equivalent doses of thiopental, midazolam, or etomidate. As with most cardiac-depressing sedatives, the effect is the result of a combination of CNS, cardiac, and baroreceptor depression and systemic vasodilation. Decreased cardiac contractility and negative inotropy have been identified in animal studies on isolated papillary muscle. A decrease in dose or alternative agents should be considered in the elderly or cardiac-compromised patients. Propofol has been used successfully for cardiac anesthesia when combined with fentanyl in low-dose or infusion regimens.[152] See Table 8-6.

Respiratory Effects

Respiratory depression, more prominent than that seen with thiopental, has been reported with induction doses of propofol. Decreases in tidal volume are more prominent than decreases in respiratory rate, although apnea is common on initial administration of induction doses.[153]

Studies have shown propofol to have a relative bronchodilating effect in asthmatic patients, nonasthmatic patients, and patients who smoke. Respiratory resistance was lower and the incidence of wheezing was decreased after tracheal intubation, compared with the effects of etomidate, thiopental, and methohexital.[154,155]

The effect on airway reflexes by propofol is controversial. McKeating and co-workers[156] compared propofol with thiopental and found more satisfactory conditions for intubation with propofol than with thiopental. In a study of 90 patients, Kallar[157] confirmed that intubation without muscle relaxants could be done more successfully with propofol compared with thiopental and methohexital.

Uses

Propofol is widely used for the induction of anesthesia in doses of 0.5 to 2.5 mg/kg. Infusion rates of 25 to 200 mg/min are common for intraoperative sedation for a wide variety of surgical and diagnostic procedures. Higher rates of 100 to 200 mcg/kg/hr are required for hypnosis. Induction doses for children are higher (2.5 to 3.5 mg/kg) as a result of their larger central volume of distribution and more rapid rate of clearance. Use of propofol is especially popular in shorter procedures in an ambulatory setting and in monitored anesthesia care. Other uses include sedation for cardioversion, electroconvulsive therapy, malignant hyperthermia, facilitation of laryngeal mask airway insertion, and obstetric anesthesia.[158]

Contraindications

Few absolute contraindications exist for propofol other than cases in which a known hypersensitivity exists to propofol or its components. The new generic formulation of propofol, which contains sodium metabisulfite, does issue a precaution to its use. The sulfite may cause allergic-type reactions such as anaphylactic symptoms and life-threatening or less-severe asthmatic episodes in certain susceptible people. Sulfite sensitivity is more common in patients with asthma than in patients without asthma.[40] As noted, caution is advised in elderly, debilitated, and cardiac-compromised patients. Although propofol has been used successfully in pediatric intensive care units for prolonged sedation, a fatal syndrome occurs with long-term high-dose infusions of propofol. The majority of patients have been children, but several cases in adults have been identified. The syndrome has occurred in patients with acute inflammatory disease with infection or sepsis or acute neurologic disease. Propofol is a triggering agent when catecholamines and corticosteroids are also administered. Fatty acid metabolism and mitochondrial activity are impaired, creating a supply-and-demand situation that results in cardiac and peripheral muscle necrosis. Symptoms include cardiac failure, rhabdomyolysis, severe metabolic acidosis, and renal failure. Caution is advised for infusion doses of over 5 mg/hr for longer than 48 hours.[159] Key points are listed in Box 8-7. Induction doses of the intravenous anesthetic are given in Table 8-9.

Recent Reformulations of Propofol

Propofol was initially manufactured as a preservative-free product. However, after initial introduction, reports of bacterial contamination of propofol emulsion started to appear, suggesting that some cases of postoperative infection might have been the result of the injection of contaminated product. The concern that the preservative-free product could easily be contaminated through handling led the original patent holder, AstraZeneca, to reformulate the preparation. Antimicrobial studies demonstrated that disodium ethylenediaminetetraacetate (EDTA) at a

BOX **8-7**

Key Points of Propofol Pharmacology

- The high clearance rate of propofol permits rapid emergence after continuous infusions of drug.
- Central nervous system effects include reduction in cerebral blood flow, $CMRO_2$ and ICP. Cerebral perfusion pressure may be lowered, despite the reduction in ICP, because of the reduction in mean arterial pressure.
- Propofol decreases blood pressure, cardiac output, and systemic vascular resistance to a greater extent than thiopental or etomidate at equipotent doses.
- Respiratory effects include an initial brief increase followed by a decrease in minute ventilation, very similar to thiopental. The reduction in minute ventilation is chiefly through reduction in tidal volume.

$CMRO_2$, *Cerebral metabolic rate of oxygen consumption;* ICP, *intracranial pressure.*
Modified from Windsor A, Bowen P, Sebel P. Intravenous anaesthetics. In: Bovill JG, Howie MB, eds. Clinical Pharmacology for Anaesthetists. *London: Saunders; 1999:66.*

TABLE 8-9 Induction Doses of the Intravenous Anesthetics

Agent	Dose (mg/kg)
Thiopental	2-4
Methohexital	1-2
Etomidate	0.2-0.3
Propofol	1-2.5
Ketamine	0.1-0.2 (see Table 8-7)
Midazolam	0.1-0.2

concentration of 0.005% successfully retards microbial growth and has no adverse effects on the physicochemical stability of the product.

At approximately the same time that the EDTA preparation of propofol was being formulated, another manufacturer was marketing a sulfite-containing product. This product, generic propofol injectable emulsion 1%, (Baxter Pharmaceutical Products) contains sodium metabisulfite 0.25 mg/ml and is formulated in a slightly more acidic medium (pH 4.5 to 6.4) than the AstraZeneca product (pH 7 to 8.5). The release of these products has initiated a number of studies examining whether the new additives might have any effect on the stability of the emulsion product. It has been determined that both EDTA- and sulfite-containing propofol products promote the formation of a propofol dimer. Although the propofol dimer was found in only trace amounts in the propofol-EDTA product (<0.015%), its concentration in the sulfite-propofol product was significantly higher (0.18%). In addition, reports have been made of yellow discoloration in sulfite-propofol products, which could result from increased dimer production. Of interest, both products are promoted by their respective manufacturers as being "preservative free," because the concentrations of both EDTA and sodium metabisulfite are below the USP minimum standard that would require other labeling.[160] See Table 8-2.

Allergy

Lecithin (from the Greek *lekithos*, meaning "egg yolk") is a phospholipid compound composed of a range of phosphatidyl esters such as phosphatidyl choline, ethanolamine, and serine. These are combined with varying amounts of triglycerides and fatty acids. Lecithin was originally obtained from eggs, although now soya beans and other vegetables with a high lecithin content are also useful sources. Apart from its use as an antioxidant synergist, lecithin has important surfactant properties and is used as an emulsifying agent.

It is questionable whether propofol injection, because of its lecithin content, should be avoided in patients with egg allergy. No adverse effects have been reported to date, and, although hypersensitivity reactions to both soya bean extract and lecithin have been demonstrated, they have been reported only when the allergens have been inhaled or ingested. Furthermore, patients who are designated as having a so-called "egg allergy" generally demonstrate an IgE-mediated hypersensitivity to allergenic proteins found in egg whites. The derivation and chemical structure of egg lecithin suggest that the risk associated with its administration to such individuals is very low. Current evidence suggests that egg-allergic patients are not more likely to develop anaphylaxis when exposed to propofol.[40,160]

SUMMARY

The availability of a variety of unique intravenous drugs that contain the necessary properties for use in induction has allowed the clinician to tailor the induction to fit the needs of the patient and surgeon. This characteristic has made it much easier to care for an increasingly diverse and complex patient population. The intravenous anesthetics can be chosen with consideration for the health status of the patient, the type of procedure to be performed, and the patient's susceptibility to possible adverse effects to produce the remarkably safe techniques and excellent outcomes achieved today.

REFERENCES

1. Goodman LS, Gilman A. *The Pharmacologic Basis of Therapeutics*. New York: Macmillan; 1942.
2. Stoelting RK. *Pharmacology and Physiology in Anesthetic Practice*. 3rd ed. Philadelphia: Lippincott; 1999:113-120.
3. Wong CL, Wariner CB, McCormack JP, et al. Reconstituted thiopentone retains its alkalinity without bacterial contamination for up to four weeks. *Can J Anaesth*. 1992;39:504-508.
4. Ghoneim MM, et al. Binding of thiopental to plasma proteins. *Anesthesiology*. 1976;45:635-639.
5. Miller RD. *Anesthesia*. 5th ed. New York: Churchill Livingstone; 2000:209-214.
6. Eger EI II. *Anesthetic Uptake and Action*. Baltimore: Williams & Wilkins; 1974.
7. Stanski DR. Pharmacokinetics of barbiturates. In: Prys-Roberts C, Hug CC Jr, eds: *Pharmacokinetics of Anaesthesia*. Oxford: Blackwell Scientific; 1984:86-93.
8. Brodie BB, Bernstein E, Mark LC. The role of body fat in limiting the duration of thiopental. *J Pharmacol Exp Ther*. 1952;105:421-426.
9. Price HL, Kornat PH, Safer JN. The uptake of thiopental by body tissues and its relation to the duration of narcosis. *Clin Pharmacol Ther*. 1960;1:16-22.
10. Nguyen KT, Stephens DP, McLeish MJ, et al. Pharmacokinetics of thiopental and pentobarbital enantiomers after intravenous administration of racemic thiopental. *Anesth Analg*. 1996; 83:552-558.
11. Stanski DR, Maitre PO. Pharmacokinetics and pharmacodynamics of thiopental: the effect of age revisited. *Anesthesiology*. 1990;72:412-422.
12. Shanks CA, Avram MJ, Krejcie TC, et al. A pharmacokinetic-pharmacodynamic model for quantal responses with thiopental. *J Pharmacokinet Biopharm* 1993;21:309-321.
13. Hudson RJ, Stanski DR, Burch PG. Pharmacokinetics of methohexital and thiopental in surgical patients. *Anesthesiology*. 1983;59:215-219.
14. Jones DJ, Nguyen KT, McLeish MJ, et al. Determination of (R)-(+)- and (S)-(−)-isomers of thiopentone in plasma by chiral high-performance liquid chromatography. *J Chromatogr* 1996; 675:174-179.
15. Abramson NS. Randomized clinical study of thiopental loading in comatose survivors of cardiac arrest. *N Engl J Med*. 1986; 314:397-399.
16. Pandele G, et al. Thiopental pharmacokinetics in patients with cirrhosis. *Anesthesiology*. 1983;59:123-126.
17. Diasio RB. Principles of drug therapy. In: Goldman L, Avsiello D, eds: *Cecil Textbook of Medicine*. Philadelphia: Saunders; 2004: 124-134.
18. Burch PG, Stanski DR. Thiopental pharmacokinetics in renal failure. *Anesthesiology*. 1981;55:A176.
19. Olsen RW, et al. Barbiturate and benzodiazepine modulation of GABA receptor binding and function. *Life Sci*. 1986;39: 1969-1976.

20. Hemmings HC, Hopkins PM. *Foundations of Anesthesia, Basic and Clinical Sciences*. Philadelphia: Mosby; 2000:241-245.
21. MacDonald RL, Rogers CJ, Twyman RE. Barbiturates regulation of kinetic properties of the $GABA_A$ receptor channel of mouse spinal neurons in culture. *J Physiol.* 1989;417:483-500.
22. Gentry WB, Henthorn TK. Barbiturates. In: White PF, ed. *Textbook of Intravenous Anesthesia.* Baltimore: Williams & Wilkins; 1997:65-76.
23. Ross AK, Glass PSA. Pharmacology and physiology of intravenous anesthesia. In: Miller RD, ed. *Atlas of Anesthesia.* Philadelphia: Churchill Livingstone; 1998.
24. Rampil ID, et al. Spectral edge frequency: a correlate of anesthesia depth. *Anesthesiology.* 1980;53:S12.
25. Hudson RJ, et al. A model for studying depth of anesthesia and acute tolerance to thiopental. *Anesthesiology.* 1980;59:301-308.
26. Barratt R, Granans GG, Torda TA. The influence of sampling site in the distribution phase kinetics of thiopentone. *Anaesth Intensive Care* 1984;56:1385-1391.
27. Michenfelder JG. The interdependency of cerebral function and metabolic effects following massive dose of thiopental in the dog. *Anesthesiology.* 1974;41:231-236.
28. Albrecht RF, et al. Cerebral blood flow and metabolic changes from induction to onset of anesthesia with halothane or pentobarbital. *Anesthesiology.* 1977;47:252-256.
29. Asrup J, et al. Minimal cerebral blood flow and metabolism during craniotomy: effect of thiopental loading. *Acta Anaesthesiol Scand.* 1984;28:478-481.
30. McPherson RW, Sell B, Traystman RJ. Effects of thiopental, fentanyl and etomidate on upper extremity somatosensory evoked potentials in humans. *Anesthesiology.* 1986;65:584-589.
31. Joshi C, Bruce DL. Thiopental and succinylcholine: action in intraocular pressure. *Anesth Analg.* 1975;54:471-475.
32. Calla S, et al. Comparison of the effects of etomidate and thiopental on intraocular pressure. *Br J Anaesth.* 1987;59:437-439.
33. Prys-Roberts C, Meloche R, Foex P. Studies of anaesthesia in relation to hypertension. I. Cardiovascular responses of treated and untreated patients. *Br J Anaesth.* 1971;43:122-137.
34. Flickenger H, et al. Effect of thiopental induction on cardiac output in man. *Anesth Analg.* 1961;40:693-700.
35. Eckstein JW, Hamilton WK, Mcammond JM. The effect of thiopental on peripheral venous tone. *Anesthesiology.* 1961;22: 525-528.
36. Skorsted P, Price ML, Price HL. The effects of short acting barbiturates on arterial pressure, preganglionic sympathetic activity and barostatic reflexes. *Anesthesiology.* 1970;33:10.
37. Corssen G. *Intravenous Anesthesia and Analgesia.* Philadelphia: Lea & Febiger; 1988.
38. Patrick RT, Faulconer A. Respiratory studies during anesthesia with ether and with Pentothal sodium. *Anaesthesiology.* 1952;13:252.
39. Sedik H. Use of intravenous methohexital as a sedative in pediatric emergency departments. *Arch Pediatr Adolesc Med.* 2001;155:665-668.
40. Hepner DL, Castell MC. Anaphylaxis during the perioperative period. *Anesth Analg.* 2003;97:1381-1395.
41. Morgan DJ, et al. Pharmacokinetics and plasma binding of thiopental. II. Studies at cesarean section. *Anesthesiology.* 1981; 54:474-480.
42. Kosaka Y, Takahashi T, Mark LC. Intravenous thiobarbiturate anesthesia for cesarean section. *Anesthesiology.* 1969;31: 489-506.
43. Chernin EL, Smiler B. The cost-effectiveness of methohexital versus propofol: the stability of reconstituted methohexital should eliminate waste. *Anesth Analg.* 1999;89:1064.
44. Todd MM, Drummond JL, Sang H. The hemodynamic consequences of high dose methohexital anesthesia in humans. *Anesthesiology.* 1984;61:495-501.
45. Korttila K, et al. Recovery and simulated driving after intravenous anesthesia with thiopental, methohexital, propanidid, or alphadione. *Anesthesiology.* 1975;43:291-299.
46. Kay B. A dose response relationship for etomidate with some observations on cumulation. *Br J Anaesth.* 1976;48:213-215.
47. Doenicke A. Etomidate: a new intravenous hypnotic. *Acta Anaesthesiol Belg.* 1974;25:307-315.
48. Giese JL, Stanley TH. Etomidate: a new intravenous anesthetic induction agent. *Pharmacotherapy.* 1983;3:251-258.
49. Thoheim MM, VanHamme MJ. Hydrolysis of etomidate. *Anesthesiology.* 1979;50:242-244.
50. Doenicke A, et al. Histamine release with intravenous application of short acting hypnotics. *Br J Anaesth.* 1973;45: 1097-1104.
51. Renou AM, et al. Cerebral blood flow and metabolism during etomidate anaesthesia in man. *Br J Anaesth.* 1978;50: 1047-1050.
52. Moss E, et al. Effect of etomidate on intracranial pressure and cerebral perfusion pressure. *Br J Anaesth.* 1979;51:347-352.
53. Ghoneim MM, Yamada T. Etomidate: a clinical and electroencephalographic comparison with thiopental. *Anesth Analg.* 1977;56:479-485.
54. Horrigan RW, et al. Etomidate vs. thiopental with and without fentanyl: a comparative study of awakening in man. *Anesthesiology.* 1980;52:362-364.
55. Jankovic J. Tics, myoclonus and stereotypes. In: Goldman L, Bennett JC, eds: *Cecil Textbook of Medicine.* 21st ed. Philadelphia: Saunders; 2000:2086.
56. Gancher S, Laer KO, Krieger W. Activation of epileptogenic activity by etomidate. *Anesthesia.* 1984;61:616-621.
57. Korttila K, Tammisto T, Uromaa U. Comparison of etomidate in combination with fentanyl or diazepam, with thiopentone as an induction agent for general anesthesia. *Br J Anaesth.* 1979; 51:1151-1156.
58. Prakash O, et al. Cardiovascular effects of etomidate with emphasis on regional myocardial blood flow and performance. *Br J Anaesth.* 1981;53:591-599.
59. Skovsted P, Sapthavichaikul S. The effects of etomidate on arterial pressure, pulse rate and preganglionic sympathetic activity in cats. *Can J Anaesth.* 1977;24:565-570.
60. Gooding JM, Corssen G. Effect of etomidate on the cardiovascular system. *Anesth Analg.* 1977;56:717-719.
61. Gooding JM, et al. Cardiovascular and pulmonary responses following etomidate induction of anesthesia in patients with demonstrated cardiac disease. *Anesth Analg.* 1979;58:40-41.
62. Colvin MP, et al. Cardiorespiratory change following induction of anaesthesia with etomidate in patients with demonstrated cardiovascular disease. *Br J Anaesth.* 1979;51:551-556.
63. Daehlin L, Gran L. Etomidate and thiopentone: a comparative study of their respiratory effects. *Curr Ther Res* 1980;27:5.
64. Morgan M, Lumley J, Whitwan JG. Respiratory effects of etomidate. *Br J Anaesth.* 1977;49:233-236.
65. Ledingham IM, Watt I. Influence of sedation on mortality in critically ill multiple trauma patients. *Lancet.* 1983;1:1270.
66. Fragen RJ, et al. Effects of etomidate on hormonal response to surgical stress. *Anesthesiology.* 1984;61:652-656.
67. Absalom A, Pledger D, Kong A. Adrenocortical function in critically ill patients 24 h after a single dose of etomidate. *Anaesthesia.* 1999;54:861-867.
68. Boidin MP, Erdman WE, Faithfull NS. The role of ascorbic acid in etomidate toxicity. *Eur J Anaesthesiol.* 1986;37:417-422.
69. Fragen RJ, Caldwell N. Comparison of the new formulation of etomidate with thiopental: side effects and awaking times. *Anesthesiology.* 1979;50:242-244.
70. Giese JL, et al. Etomidate versus thiopental for induction of anesthesia. *Anesth Analg.* 1985;64:871-876.
71. Lear E, et al. Cyclohexamine (CI-400): a new intravenous agent. *Anesthesiology.* 1961;20:525.
72. Maddox VH. The historical development of phencyclidine. In: Domino EF, ed. *PCP (Phencyclidine). Historical and Current Perspectives.* Ann Arbor, Mich: NPP Books; 1981:46-54.
73. Corssen G, Domino EF. Dissociated anesthesia: further pharmacologic studies and first clinical experience with the phencyclidine derivative. *Anesth Analg.* 1966;45:26-40.

74. Domino EF, Chodoff P, Corssen G. Pharmacologic effects of CI-581, a new dissociated anesthetic in man. *Clin Pharmacol Ther*. 1965;6:279-291.
75. Schuttler J, Zsigmond EK, White PF. Ketamine and its isomers. In: White PF, ed. *Textbook of Intravenous Anesthesia*. Baltimore: Williams & Wilkins; 1997:171-190.
76. Franks NP, Lieb WR. Molecular and cellular mechanisms of general anesthesia. *Nature*. 1994;367:607-614.
77. Leeson PD, Iverson LL. Perspective: the glycine site on the NMDA receptor—structure-activity relationships and therapeutic potential. *J Med Chem* 1994;37:4053-4060.
78. Nagasaka H, et al. The effect of ketamine on the excitation and inhibition of dorsal horn WDR neuronal activity induced by bradykinin injection into the femoral artery in cats after spinal cord transection. *Anesthesiology*. 1993;78:722-732.
79. Smith DJ, Westfall DF, Adams JD. Ketamine interacts with opioid receptors as an agonist. *Anesthesiology*. 1980;53:55.
80. Toro-Matos A, et al. Physostigmine antagonizes ketamine. *Anesth Analg*. 1980;59:764-767.
81. Kharasch ED, Labroo R. Metabolism of ketamine stereoisomers by human liver microsomes. *Anesthesiology*. 1992:77:1201-1207.
82. Ihmsen H, Geisslinger G, Schuttler J. Stereoselective pharmacokinetics of ketamine: R(−)-ketamine inhibits the elimination of S(+)-ketamine. *Clinical Pharmacology & Therapeutics*. 2001; 70:431-438.
83. Henthorn TK, Krejcie TC, Niemann CU, et al. Ketamine distribution described by a recirculatory pharmacokinetic model is not stereoselective. *Anesthesiology*. 1999;91:1733-1743.
84. Nimmo WS, Clements JA. Ketamine. In: Prys-Roberts C, Hug CC, eds. *Pharmacokinetics of Anaesthesia*. Oxford: Blackwell Scientific; 1984:235.
85. Roytblat L, Korotkoruchko A, Katz J, et al. Postoperative pain: the effect of low-dose ketamine in addition to general anesthesia. *Anesth Analg*. 1993;77:1161-1165.
86. Grant IS, Nimmo WS, Clements JA. Pharmacokinetics and analgesic effects of IM and oral ketamine. *Br J Anaesth*. 1981; 53:805-810.
87. Stanski DR, Watkins DW, eds. *Drug Disposition in Anesthesia*. New York: Grune & Stratton; 1982.
88. Woolf CJ, Chong MS. Preemptive analgesia: treating postoperative pain by preventing the establishment of central sensitization. *Anesth Analg*. 1993;77:362-379.
89. Corssen G, Bjarnesen W. Recent advances in intravenous anesthesia, *AANA J*. 1966;34:416-427.
90. Zsigmond EK, Domino EF. Clinical pharmacology of ketamine. In: Domino EF, ed. *Status of Ketamine in Anesthesiology*. Ann Arbor, Mich: NPP Books; 1990:27-76.
91. Engelhardt W. Recovery and psychomimetic reactions following S-(+)-ketamine. *Anaesthetist*. 1997;46(suppl 1):38-42.
92. Gray C, Swinhoe CF, Myint Y, et al. Target controlled infusion of ketamine as analgesia for TIVA with propofol. *Can J Anaesth* 1999;46:957-961.
93. Pedersen T, et al. Effects of low dose ketamine and thiopentone on cardiac performance and myocardial oxygen balance in high risk patients. *Acta Anaesthesiol Scand*. 1982;26:235-239.
94. Ivankovick AD, et al. Cardiovascular effects of centrally administered ketamine in spats. *Anesth Analg*. 1974;53:924-933.
95. Cook DJ, Carron EG, Housemans PR. Mechanisms of the positive inotropic effect of ketamine in isolated ferret ventricular papillary muscle. *Anesthesiology*. 1991;74:880-888.
96. Kongsayreepong S, Cook DJ, Housmans PR. Mechanisms of direct, negative inotropic effect of ketamine in isolated ferret and frog ventricular myocardium. *Anesthesiology*. 1993;80:313-322.
97. Bidwal AV, et al. The effects of ketamine on cardiovascular dynamics during halothane and enflurane anesthesia. *Anesth Analg*. 1975;54:588-592.
98. Corssen G. Ketamine for high risk cardiac patients. *Anesthesiology*. 1972;36:413.
99. Yoshikawa K, Marai Y. The effect of ketamine on intraocular pressure in children. *Anesth Analg*. 1971;50:199-202.
100. Ausinsch B, et al. Ketamine and intraocular pressure in children. *Anesth Analg*. 1976;55:773-775.
101. Little B, et al. Study of ketamine as an obstetrical agent. *Am J Obstet Gynecol*. 1972;113:247-260.
102. Galloon S. Ketamine for obstetrical delivery. *Anesthesiology*. 1976;44:522-544.
103. Walser A, et al. Quinazolines and 1,4 benzodiazepines. Synthesis and reactions of imidazo(1,5-a)(1,4)-benzodiazepines. *J Org Chem*. 43:936, 1978.
104. Goodchild CS. GABA receptors and benzodiazepines. *Br J Anaesth*. 1993;71:127-133.
105. Mohler H, Richards JG. The benzodiazepine receptor: a pharmacologic control element of brain function. *Eur J Anaesthesiol*. 1988;2(suppl):15-24.
106. Greenblat DJ, Shader RI, Harmatz JS. Benzodiazepines: a summary of pharmacokinetic properties. *Br J Clin Pharmacol*. 1981;11:11-16.
107. Stanski DR, Watkins DW, eds. *Drug Disposition in Anesthesia*. New York: Grune & Stratton; 1982.
108. Roy-Bryne P, Crowley D, eds. *Benzodiazepines in Clinical Practice: Risk and Benefits*. Washington, DC: American Psychiatric Press; 1991.
109. Cote P, Gueret P, Bourassa MG. Systemic and coronary hemodynamic effects of diazepam in patients with normal and diseased coronary arteries. *Circulation*. 1974;50:1210-1216.
110. Tomichek RL, et al. Cardiovascular effects of diazepam-fentanyl anesthesia in patients with coronary artery disease. *Anesth Analg*. 1982;61:217-218.
111. Allonen H, Ziegler G, Klotz U. Midazolam kinetics. *Clin Pharmacol Ther*. 1981;30:653-661.
112. Versed [product information]. Nutley, NJ: Hoffmann-LaRoche; 1991.
113. Dundee JW, et al. Midazolam: a review of its pharmacological properties and therapeutic use. *Drugs*. 1984;28:519-543.
114. Dundee JW, Halliday NJ, Loughran PG. Variations in response to midazolam. *Br J Clin Pharmacol*. 1984;17:645-646.
115. Heizmann P, Eckert M, Ziegler WH. Pharmacokinetics and bioavailability of midazolam in man. *Br J Clin Pharmacol*. 1983;16:435-495.
116. Greenblatt DJ, et al. Effect of age, gender, and obesity on midazolam kinetics. *Anesthesiology*. 1984;61:27-35.
117. Dundee JW, Wilson DB. Amnesia action of midazolam. *Anaesthesia*. 1980;35:459-461.
118. Knudsen L, et al. The effects of midazolam on cerebral blood flow and oxygen consumption. *Anaesthesia*. 1990;45:1016-1019.
119. Nagelhout J, Gerbasi F, Zaglaniczny KL, et al. The effect of flumazenil on patient recovery and discharge following ambulatory surgery. *AANA J*. 1999;67:229-236.
120. Klotz V, Kanto J. Pharmacokinetics and clinical use of flumazenil. *Clin Pharmacokinet*. 1988;14:1-12.
121. Martens F, et al. Clinical experience with the benzodiazepine antagonist flumazenil: suspected benzodiazepine or ethanol poisoning. *Clin Toxicol*. 1990;28:341-356.
122. Brogen RN, Goa KL. Flumazenil: a preliminary review of its benzodiazepine antagonist properties, intrinsic activity and therapeutic use. *Drugs*. 1988;35:448-467.
123. Spivey WH. Flumazenil and seizures: analysis of 43 cases. *Clin Ther*. 1992;14:292-305.
124. Propofol. St Louis: Mosby Drug Consult, 2003.
125. Schuttler J, Ihmsen H. Population pharmacokinetics of propofol: a multicenter study. *Anesthesiology*. 2000;92:727-738.
126. Fechner J, Ihmsen H, Hatterscheid D, et al. Pharmacokinetics and clinical pharmacodynamics of the new propofol prodrug GPI 15715 in volunteers. *Anesthesiology*. 2003;99:303-313.
127. Veroli P, et al. Extrahepatic metabolism of propofol in man during the anhepatic phase of orthotopic liver transplantation. *Br J Anaesth*. 1992;68:183-186.

128. Dindee JW, et al. Sensitivity to propofol in the elderly. *Anesthesia.* 1986;41:482-485.
129. Hannollah RS. Induction dose of propofol in children. *Semin Anesth.* 1992;11(suppl 1):48-49.
130. Abanese J, et al. Pharmacokinetics of long term propofol infusion used for sedation in ICU patients. *Anesthesiology.* 1990;73: 214-217.
131. Perduto VA, Concas AS, et al. Biochemical and electrophysiologic evidence that propofol enhances GABA-ergic transmission in rat brain. *Anesthesiology.* 1991;75:1000-1009.
132. Irifune M, Takarada T, Shimizu Y, et al. Propofol induced anesthesia in mice is mediated by γ-aminobutyric acid-A and excitatory amino acid receptors. *Anesth Analg.* 2003;97:424-429.
133. Mukherjee K, Seavell C, Rawlings E, et al. A comparison of total intravenous with balanced anaesthesia for middle ear surgery: effects on postoperative nausea and vomiting, pain, and conditions of surgery. *Anaesthesia.* 2003;58:176-180.
134. Pollard BJ, Elliott RA, Moore EW. Anaesthetic agents in adult day case surgery. *Eur J Anaesthesiol.* 2003;20:1-9.
135. Cork RC, Scipione P. Appendix: patient perceptions of propofol versus thiopental-isoflurane for outpatient anesthesia *Semin Anesth.* 1992;11(suppl 1):50-54.
136. Parmar AK, Koay CK. Pain on injection of propofol. A comparison of cold propofol with propofol mixed with lignocaine. *Anaesthesiology.* 1998;53:79-83.
137. Gehan G, et al. Optimal dose of lignocaine for preventing pain on injection of propofol. *Br J Anaesth.* 1991;66:324-326.
138. Herregods L, et al. Effect of propofol on elevated intracranial pressure: preliminary results. *Anesthesia.* 1988;43:107-109.
139. Aikire MT, et al. Cerebral metabolism during propofol anesthesia in humans studied with positron emission tomography. *Anesthesiology.* 1995;82:393-403.
140. Craen RA, et al. Human cerebral autoregulation is maintained during propofol air/O_2 [abstract]. *Anesthesiology.* 1992;77: A220.
141. Mahla ME, et al. Prolonged anesthesia with propofol or isoflurane: intraoperative electroencephalographic patterns and postoperative recovery, *Semin Anesth.* 1992;11(suppl 1):31-32.
142. Collier C, Kelly K. Propofol and convulsions: the evidence mounts. *Anesth Intensive Care.* 1991;19:573-575.
143. Hodkinson BP, Firth RW, Mee EW. Propofol and the electroencephalogram. *Lancet.* 1987;2:1518.
144. Samra SK, et al. The effects of propofol sedation on seizures and intracranially recorded epileptiform activity in patients with partial epilepsy. *Anesthesiology.* 1995;82:843-851.
145. Hewitt PB, et al. Effects of propofol on the electrocorticogram in epileptic patients undergoing cortical resection. *Br J Anaesth.* 1999;82:199-202.
146. MacKensie SJ, Kapadia F, Grant IS. Propofol infusion for control of status epilepticus. *Anaesthesia.* 1990;45:1043-1045.
147. DeFriez CB, Wond HC. Seizures and opisthotonos after propofol anaesthesia. *Anesth Analg.* 1992;75:630-632.
148. Boey WK, Lai FO. Comparison of propofol and thiopentone as anaesthetic agents for electroconvulsive therapy. *Anaesthesia.* 1990;45:623-628.
149. Mcartensson B, et al. A comparison of propofol and methohexital as anesthetic agents for ECT: effects on seizure duration, therapeutic outcome, and memory. *Biolog Psychiatry* 1994; 35:179-189.
150. Malsch E, Gratz I, Mani S. Efficacy of electroconvulsive therapy (ECT) after propofol (P) or methohexital (M) anesthesia [abstract]. *Anesth Analg.* 1992;74:S192.
151. Malsch E, Mani S, Gratz I. The effect of antihypertensive medication on the cardiovascular (CV) response to electroconvulsive therapy (ECT) after methohexital (M) or propofol (P) anesthesia [abstract]. *Anesthesiology.* 1992;77:A76.
152. Patrick MR, et al. A comparison of the hemodynamic effects of propofol (Diprivan) and thiopentone in patients with coronary artery disease. *Postgrad Med J.* 1985;61(suppl 3):23-27.
153. Goodman NW, Black AMS, Carter JA. Some ventilatory effects of propofol as a sole anesthetic agent. *Br J Anaesth.* 1987; 59:1497-1503.
154. Eames WO, et al. Comparison of effects of etomidate, propofol, and thiopental on respiratory resistance after tracheal intubation. *Anesthesiology.* 1996;84:1307-1311.
155. Pizov R, et al. Wheezing during induction of general anesthesia in patients with and without asthma: a randomized, blinded trial. *Anesthesiology.* 1995;82:1111-1116.
156. McKeating K, Bali IM, Dundee JW. The effects of thiopentone and propofol on upper airway integrity. *Anaesthesia.* 1988; 43:638-640.
157. Kallar SK. Propofol allows intubation without relaxants [abstract]. *Anesthesiology.* 1992;73(A22):3A.
158. Smith I, et al. Propofol: an update on its clinical use. *Anesthesiology.* 1994;81:1005-1043.
159. Vasite B, Rasulo F, Candiani A, et al. The pathophysiology of propofol infusion syndrome: a simple name for a complex syndrome. *Intensive Care Med.* 2003;9:1417-1425.
160. MacPherson RD. Pharmaceutics for the anaesthetist. *Anaesthesia.* 2001;56:965-979.

CHAPTER 9

Local Anesthetics

Joe R. Williams

Local anesthetics are drugs that reversibly block the conduction of electrical impulses along nerve fibers. Their ability to perform this function depends on various factors, including the microscopic and gross anatomy of the nerve being blocked and the physicochemical properties of the local anesthetics used. Anesthesia providers are primarily interested in the neural blocking effect that this group of drugs has on the spinal cord, spinal nerve roots, and peripheral nerves.

Equally important in considering the local anesthetics is the knowledge that absorption of these drugs into the circulation can produce significant systemic effects. The intrinsic potency and the fate of the drugs after absorption influence their ability to produce systemic effects and possible toxicity. Symptoms of toxicity can occur whether the drug is administered by local infiltration, intravenously, or regionally.

ANATOMY OF THE PERIPHERAL NERVE

The *axon*, an extension of a centrally located neuron, is the functional unit of peripheral nerves. A cell membrane, or *axolemma*, and intracellular contents, or *axoplasm*, are the major components of the axon. *Schwann cells*, whose functions are support and insulation, surround each axon. In unmyelinated nerves, single Schwann cells cover several axons. Conversely, in larger nerves the Schwann cell sheath covers only one axon and has several concentric layers of a liquid substance known as *myelin*.

Between Schwann cells are small segments of nerve that do not contain myelin. These areas, known as *nodes of Ranvier*, have limited diffusion barriers for drugs to penetrate and therefore may be the primary sites at which local anesthetics exert their action. In addition, these uncovered areas contain a large number of sodium (Na^+) channels; these channels are able to generate an action potential so intense that it can jump from node to node.[1] This phenomenon, known as *saltatory conduction*, significantly facilitates conduction speed along the axon.[2] Because of their better insulation, myelinated nerves are larger, conduct impulses faster, and are more difficult to block with local anesthetics than are unmyelinated nerves[3,4] (Figure 9-1).

Peripheral nerves have structures containing bundles of axons called *fasciculi*. Three layers of connective tissue—the *endoneurium*, *perineurium*, and *epineurium*—also are components of the peripheral nerve.[4,5] The endoneurium, which is a delicate connective tissue composed of longitudinally arranged collagen, surrounds and embeds the axons in the fasciculi. The *perineurium*, which consists of layers of flattened, overlapping cells, binds a group of fascicles together. The *epineurium*, which surrounds the perineurium, is composed of areolar connective tissue that functionally holds the fascicles together to form the peripheral nerve.[5] These layers of connective tissue are important because they serve as barriers through which local anesthetics must diffuse if they are to exert their pharmacologic action (Figure 9-2).

NEURON ELECTROPHYSIOLOGY AND THE ACTION MECHANISM OF LOCAL ANESTHETICS

Electrophysiology

Measurement with an electrode placed in the axoplasm of a resting peripheral nerve demonstrates a negative membrane potential of −70 to −90 mV.[5,6] This voltage difference across the neuronal membrane at steady state is called the *resting membrane potential* (Figure 9-3). An ionic imbalance between the axoplasm and the extracellular fluid causes the electrical potential.[7,8] Several physiologic mechanisms create the ionic gradient; the primary one is an active, energy-dependent process executed by a sodium-potassium pump (Na^+-K^+pump) located in the axolemma.[7,8]

Although the membrane is relatively permeable to the outward diffusion of K^+, an intracellular-to-extracellular K^+ ratio of 150 to 5 mmol, or 30 to 1, exists. An important contributor to this concentration difference is the impermeability of the membrane to other cotransported ions, such as Na^+.[8] In addition, the movement of K^+ out of the neuron leaves an excess of intracellular negatively charged organic ions. The negative charge results in an electrostatic counterforce that limits K^+ movement out of the neuron.

Two opposing forces influence K^+ movement into and out of the neuron. First, a concentration gradient pushes K^+ outward. Second, an electrostatic gradient, created by the impermeability of the membrane to cations, tends to keep the K^+ in the cell. The net effect of these counterforces is modest movement of K^+ out of the cell, and this movement creates an intracellular negative charge. The Nernst equation expresses the charge created by the K^+ concentration gradient:[9]

The Nernst equation follows:

Equation 9-1

$$\text{Membrane potential} = -58 \log \frac{(K^+ \text{ 30 inside})}{(K^+ \text{ outside})}$$

Determination of the resting membrane potential is not as simple as the Nernst equation for K^+ indicates, because Na^+ and

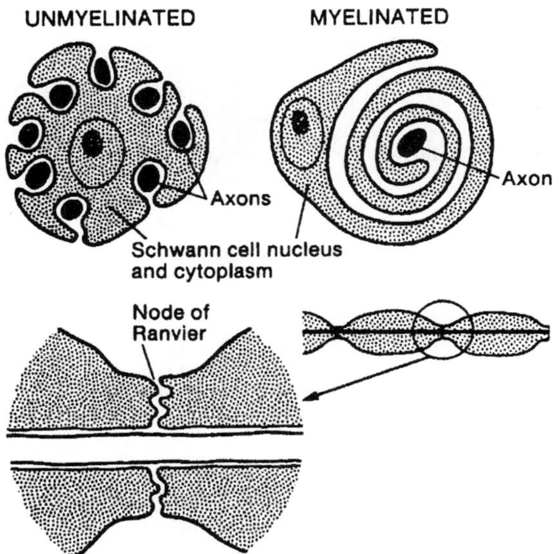

FIGURE **9-1**
Upper aspect, Transverse sections of myelinated and unmyelinated nerves. Note the concentric configuration of myelin around the axon of the myelinated nerve. *Lower aspect*, Break in the myelin sheath known as the node of Ranvier. Local anesthetics have better access to the axon at this site. (From Carpenter RL, Mackey DC. Local anesthetics. In: Barash GP, Cullen, BF, Stoelting RK, eds. *Clinical Anesthesia*. 2nd ed. Philadelphia: Lippincott, Williams & Wilkins; 1989:514. Reprinted with permission.)

chloride ions have a minor role in establishing the intracellular resting potential.[6]

When an electrical impulse is applied to a resting nerve, the membrane potential is reversed because of the intracellular movement of Na^+. This occurs because of the higher concentration of Na^+ outside the cell and the stimulation-induced increase in membrane permeability to this ion. The sudden influx of Na^+ that occurs in response to stimulation overrides the efflux of K^+ directed at maintaining the resting membrane potential. Once the process has reversed the membrane potential to 20 mV, an outward electrochemical gradient develops; this gradient resists the concentration-dependent, inward diffusion of Na^+.[5] This state of equilibrium causes the Na^+ channels to close. Shortly after Na^+ enters the cell, K^+ channels begin to open, and the ion rapidly diffuses out of the neuron, according to its concentration gradient. The active removal of intracellular Na^+ by the Na^+-K^+ pump and the passive diffusion of K^+ outward restore the resting membrane potential. During repolarization, three Na^+ ions leave the cell for each two K^+ ions that enter[10] (Figure 9-4).

The sequence of events that results in an action potential results from the passage of ions through pores, or "channels," located in the axolemma. These channels, which are composed of globular proteins, have transmural orientation to the phospholipid molecules that constitute the axolemma.[11] Although K^+ and calcium channels are important, the Na^+ channels are the most significant and best understood with respect to the initiation and propagation of the action potential.[12-14]

Mechanism of Action

Sodium channels have three functional states: closed (resting), open, and inactive. The resting state exists when the membrane polarizes to its resting potential.[12] When a nerve is stimulated, reversal of the membrane potential occurs until the threshold potential is reached. When this happens, a conformational change in the proteins that compose the channel occurs; this results in the open state. An inactive state, characterized by the return of the Na^+ channel to an impermeable state, follows the open state. This state, which prevents initiation of an action potential, lasts until the restoration of the resting membrane potential[12] (Figure 9-5).

Local anesthetics produce their effects by blocking Na^+ channels. The following four possible mechanisms of action have been suggested:

1. One theory postulates that local anesthetics produce their effect by displacing calcium from the axolemma. According to this theory, calcium controls sodium permeability in the axolemma.
2. Investigators have suggested that local anesthetics produce their effects by altering the membrane surface charge. Such changes in charge could hyperpolarize the membrane or influence the process of repolarization.
3. Because local anesthetics are relatively lipophilic molecules, they could "dissolve" into the axolemma, resulting in membrane expansion. Such conformational changes in the membrane could result in distortion and closure of the sodium channel.
4. Although all of the aforementioned effects may influence the mechanism of action of local anesthetics, at present these theories do not have as much support in the literature as the specific receptor theory. The specific receptor theory states that

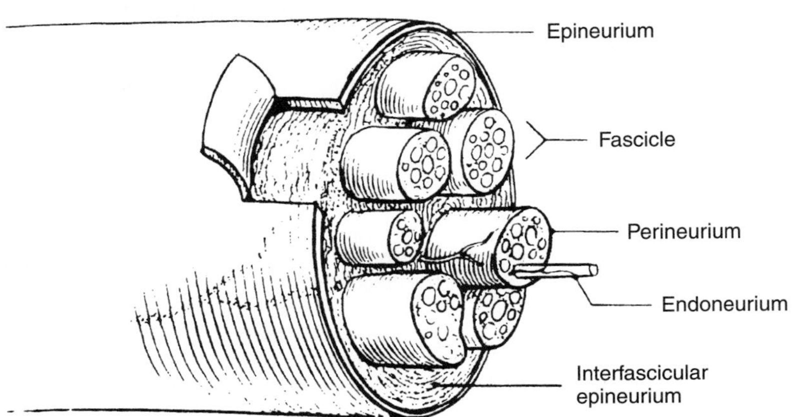

FIGURE **9-2**
Drawing showing the principal connective tissue layers of nerve, including epineurium, interfascicular epineurium, perineurium, and endoneurium. These structures serve as diffusion barriers for local anesthetics. (From Kline DG, Hudson AR. Acute injuries of peripheral nerves. In: Youmans JR, ed. *Youman's Neurological Surgery*. 4th ed. Vol 3. Philadelphia: Saunders; 1995:2104. Reprinted with permission.)

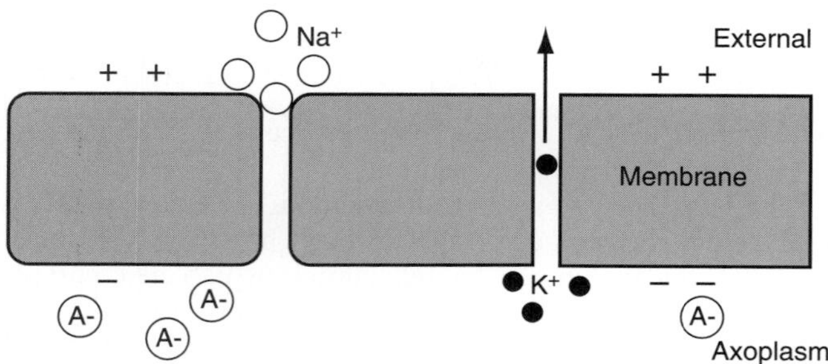

FIGURE **9-3**
In the polarized, resting state, the membrane is permeable to the movement of potassium (K^+) out of the axon (*closed circles*) and impermeable to the influx of sodium (Na^+) into the cell (*open circles*). The selective movement of the positively charged cation K^+ out of the cell results in an intracellular negative charge. (From de Jong RH. *Local Anesthesia*. St Louis: Mosby; 1994:29. Reprinted with permission.)

local anesthetics block the propagation of the action potential by binding reversibly to specific receptors within or adjacent to the internal opening of the Na^+ channel.[2] Studies have indicated that these receptors, located on the intracellular side of the cell membrane, have a greater affinity for the charged or protonated form of the local anesthetics.[12,15] Consequently, local anesthetics must first penetrate the cell membrane before they produce their effects. This penetration is greatly facilitated if the drug is in the uncharged or un-ionized state. See Figure 9-6.

Studies indicate that local anesthetics have a greater tendency to bind to receptors in the open or inactive state (*phasic* or *frequency-dependent block*). The open or inactive state may increase the affinity for binding, the physical access of the drug to the receptor, or both.[13,16] Because of this preference, local anesthetics are more likely to block rapidly firing nerves than nerves in which action potentials are less frequent. Compared with motor fibers, sensory fibers often fire at greater frequencies; hence, sensory blockade occurs before motor blockade with a given concentration of a local anesthetic.[7] This may be one of the factors that influence the "margin of safety," as

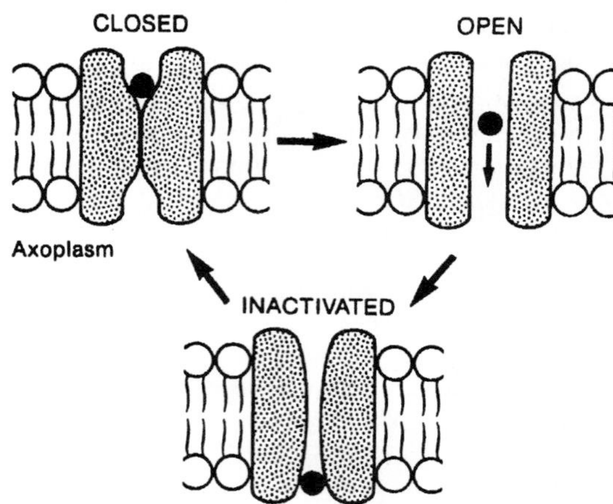

FIGURE **9-5**
The Na^+ channel in the closed, open, and inactive state. The channel remains in the inactive state until the resting membrane potential is reestablished. Once this has occurred, it returns to the closed position and can reopen. Local anesthetics bind to Na^+ channel receptors best when the channels are in the open or inactive state. (From Carpenter RL, Mackey DC. Local anesthetics. In: Barash GP, Cullen BF, Stoelting RK, eds. *Clinical Anesthesia*. 2nd ed. Philadelphia: Lippincott, Williams & Wilkins; 1989:514. Reprinted with permission.)

discussed under the topic of differential block in the next section. The following is a summary of possible events that lead to neural blockade with the use of local anesthetics:

1. Local anesthetics gain access to the interior of the neuron. This occurs by the diffusion of neutral, uncharged molecules across the cell membrane.
2. Both charged and neutral molecules bind to the receptor located on the cytoplasm side of the Na^+ channel (however, the protonated moiety has a greater binding affinity than the neutral molecule).
3. Local anesthetics bind more readily to open or inactive channels than to resting channels. This type of binding prevents the channels from returning to the resting or repolarized state, which results in blockade.[11]

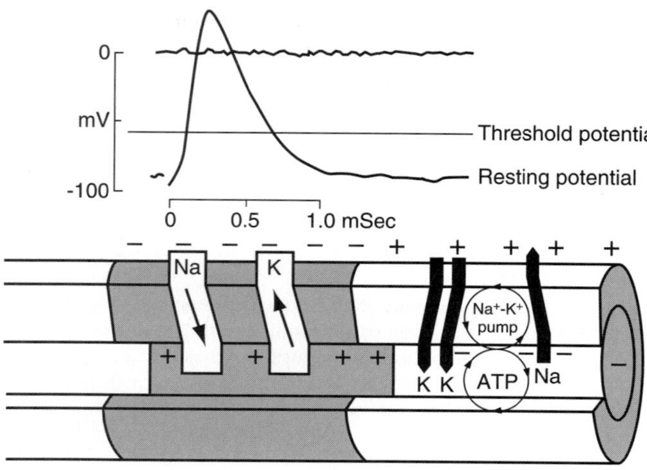

FIGURE **9-4**
Local anesthetic mechanism of action and clinical use. (From Covino BG, Vassallo HG. *Local Anesthetics: Mechanism of Action and Clinical Use*. New York: Grune & Stratton; 1976:20.)

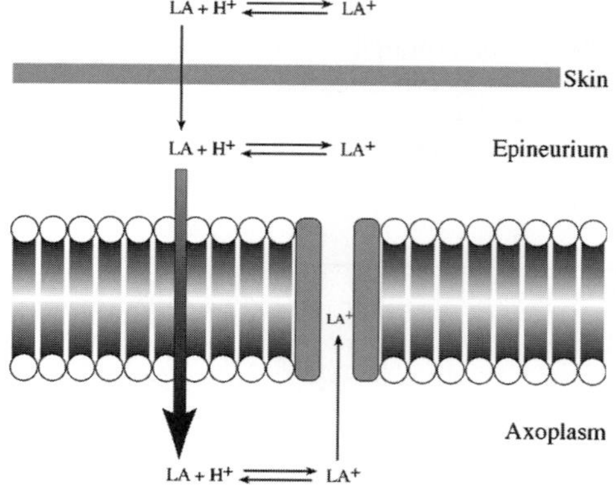

FIGURE **9-6**
Schematic conceptualization of local anesthetics action. *LA*, Nonionized form of the local anesthetic; *LA+*, ionized form. Equilibrium forms outside the nerve between the ionized and nonionized portions. The nonionized portion (*LA*), which is lipid soluble, enters the nerve. Once inside the axoplasm the drug reequilibrates, and the ionized fraction (*LA+*) attaches to the local anesthetic receptor on the inside of the sodium channel.

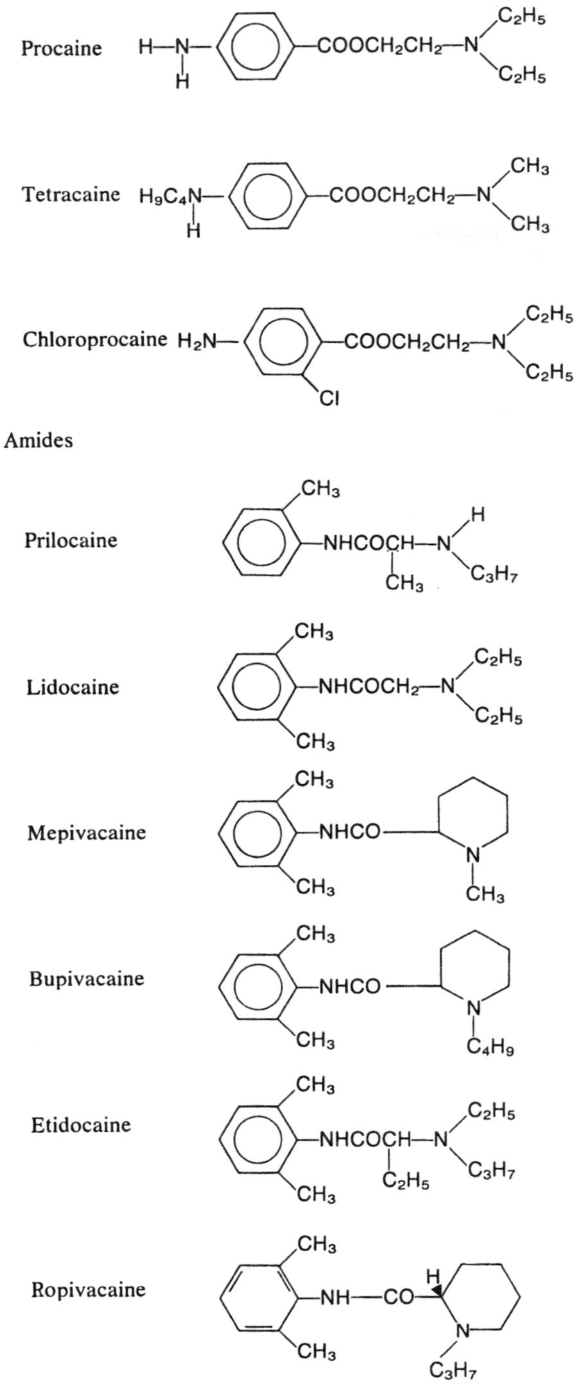

Procaine $H_2N-C_6H_4-COOCH_2CH_2-N(C_2H_5)_2$

Tetracaine $H_9C_4NH-C_6H_4-COOCH_2CH_2-N(CH_3)_2$

Chloroprocaine $H_2N-C_6H_3(Cl)-COOCH_2CH_2-N(C_2H_5)_2$

Amides

Prilocaine $C_6H_4(CH_3)-NHCOCH(CH_3)-N(H)(C_3H_7)$

Lidocaine $C_6H_3(CH_3)_2-NHCOCH_2-N(C_2H_5)_2$

Mepivacaine $C_6H_3(CH_3)_2-NHCO-$ (piperidine ring, $N-CH_3$)

Bupivacaine $C_6H_3(CH_3)_2-NHCO-$ (piperidine ring, $N-C_4H_9$)

Etidocaine $C_6H_3(CH_3)_2-NHCOCH(C_2H_5)-N(C_2H_5)(C_3H_7)$

Ropivacaine $C_6H_3(CH_3)_2-NH-CO-$ (piperidine ring, H, $N-C_3H_7$)

FIGURE **9-9**
Chemical structure of the most commonly used local anesthetics. Note the chemical substitutions on the benzene ring and the amine end of the molecules. (Modified with permission from Longnecker DE, Murphy FL. *Introduction to Anesthesia*. 9th ed. Philadelphia: Saunders; 1997:204.)

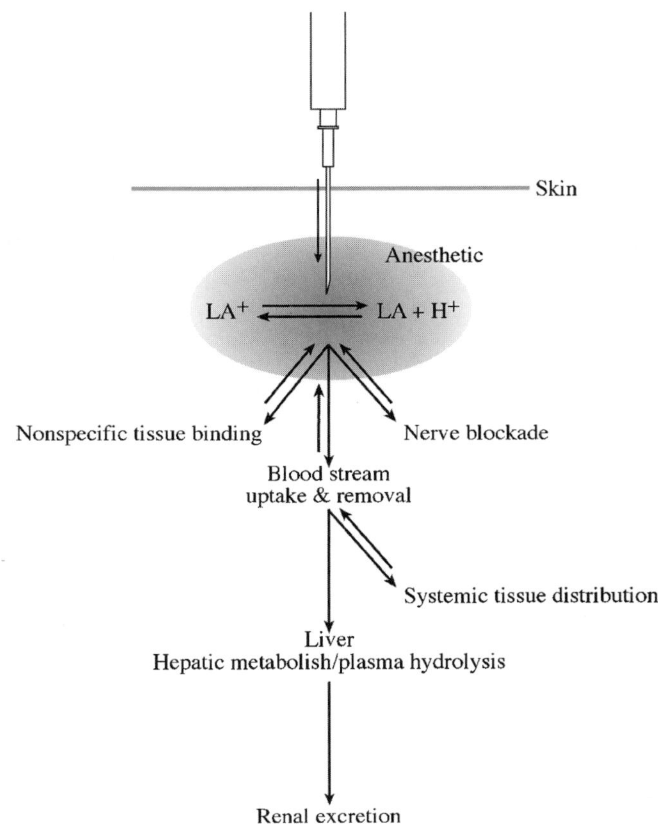

FIGURE **9-10**
Representation of the fate of a local anesthetic injected into tissue.

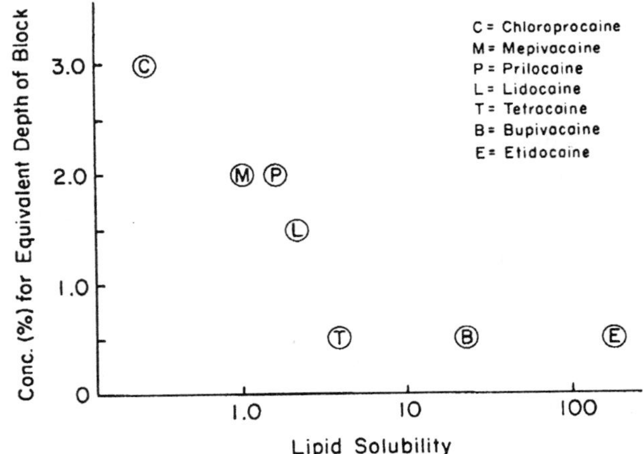

FIGURE **9-11**
The relationship between lipid solubility and the potency of local anesthetics. (From Covino BG. Clinical pharmacology of local anesthetic agents. In: Cousins MJ, Bridenbaugh PO, eds. *Neural Blockade*. Philadelphia: Lippincott, Williams & Wilkins; 1988:114. Reprinted with permission.)

that lidocaine has greater vasodilating properties than prilocaine and therefore may be absorbed away more rapidly; this means that less drug is available for interaction with the neuron.[31]

Duration of Action

The duration of action of local anesthetics demonstrates a relationship to protein binding and lipid solubility.[9,27,32] In theory, drugs that have a high affinity for protein and lipids attach more firmly to these substances in the vicinity of the Na^+ channel receptor. This means that the drug remains in the channel for a longer time, producing prolonged conduction blockade[27] (Figure 9-12).

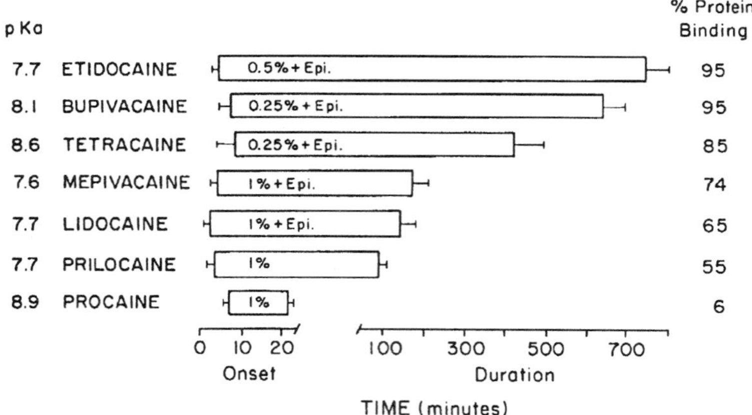

FIGURE **9-12**
The relationship between pK_a and onset of action and protein binding and duration of action. (From Covino BG. Clinical pharmacology of local anesthetic agents. In: Cousins MJ, Bridenbaugh PO, eds. *Neural Blockade*. Philadelphia: Lippincott, Williams & Wilkins; 1988:115. Reprinted with permission.)

The addition of larger chemical radicals to the amide or aromatic end of the drugs results in greater protein binding. The duration is directly proportional to plasma protein binding, presumably because the local anesthetic receptor on the neural membrane is also composed of protein.[5,6,33] It has been posited that local anesthetics that have increased protein-binding properties (e.g., etidocaine 90%, ropivacaine 94%, bupivacaine 97%, levobupivacaine 97%) produce longer-duration anesthesia as a consequence of more efficient binding of the anesthetic to the Na^+ ion channel.[34] For example, bupivacaine and etidocaine are more than 90% bound to plasma protein; however, their homologues, mepivacaine and lidocaine, are only 65% to 75% bound, respectively.[32] The duration of action of bupivacaine and etidocaine is significantly longer than for mepivacaine or lidocaine. The lipid solubility of these drugs was discussed earlier in this chapter.

As in the case of potency, the effect that local anesthetics have on the vasculature at the injection site influences the duration of action. This is discussed in detail in the section on vasomotor action and absorption.

Onset of Action

As stated previously, local anesthetics must diffuse through the axolemma before they can interact with receptors. How readily they diffuse through the nerve membrane depends on their chemical structure, lipid solubility, and state of ionization. Of these, ionization is the most important, because the charged form of a drug does not penetrate membranes well.[28,30,33]

Local anesthetics are bases and therefore proton acceptors. As with all bases, a drug's pK_a is the pH at which 50% of the drug is in the charged form while the remaining half is uncharged. A basic drug becomes predominantly ionized if it is placed in an environment with a pH that is significantly less than its pK_a. Therefore drugs that have a greater pK_a are ionized to a greater extent at body pH than those with a lower pK_a. For example, if lidocaine (pK_a 7.74) is placed in plasma (pH 7.4), 65% of the drug is ionized and 35% remains un-ionized. Similarly, if tetracaine (pK_a 8.6) is placed in plasma, 95% of the drug becomes ionized and 5% remains un-ionized.[27]

Because their ionization is less, local anesthetics with lower pK_a (7.6 to 7.8), such as lidocaine, mepivacaine, prilocaine, and etidocaine, tend to have a more rapid onset of action than drugs with a greater pK_a (8.1 to 8.6), such as bupivacaine, tetracaine, and procaine. Chloroprocaine is one exception; it has a high pK_a and a rapid onset, probably because the clinical use of high concentrations of the drug attenuates the ionization effect.[27] These properties are beneficial in the classification of local anesthetics. The classification presented in Table 9-1 assists in the selection of the appropriate drug with respect to pharmacokinetic properties and toxicity.[35]

TABLE **9-1** **Classification of Local Anesthetics Based on Onset, Duration of Action, and Potency**

Characteristics	Drug	Common Name	Relative Potency*	Onset	Duration of Action (min)
Low potency and short duration of action	Procaine	Novocaine	1	Slow	60-90
	Chloroprocaine	Nesacaine	1	Fast	30-60
Intermediate potency and duration	Mepivacaine	Carbocaine	2	Fast	120-240
	Prilocaine	Citanest	2	Fast	120-240
	Lidocaine	Xylocaine	2	Fast	90-200
High potency and long duration	Tetracaine	Pontocaine	8	Slow	180-600
	Bupivacaine	Marcaine, Sensorcaine	9	Intermediate	180-600
	Etidocaine	Duranest	6	Fast	180-600
	Ropivacaine	Naropin	10	Slow	180-600
	Levobupivacaine	Chirocaine	9	Slow	180-600

**On a milligram-for-milligram basis with procaine, 1 mg.*
Modified from Covino BG. Pharmacology of local anesthetics. Res Staff Physician, *June 1982. Modified with permission from* Resident and Staff Physician *(June 1982) by Romaine Pierson Publishers, Inc.; and* Mosby's Drug Consult; *St Louis: Mosby; 2003; vol 4 (online).*

Vasomotor Action and Absorption

All local anesthetics except cocaine and ropivacaine produce relaxation of vascular smooth muscle.[31] The resultant vasodilation increases blood flow to the tissue, where the drug is deposited. This results in an increase in the drug's absorption, which limits its duration of action and increases the probability of toxic effects. It is interesting to note that ropivacaine is the only parenterally administered local anesthetic that has vasoconstrictive properties.[2] This factor is related to its longer duration of action and lower toxicity when compared with other local anesthetics.[36] Cocaine also has vasoconstrictive properties because of its ability to block reuptake of norepinephrine. It is used only topically.

As indicated previously, not all local anesthetics have the same ability to produce vasodilation. For example, lidocaine is a more potent vasodilator than mepivacaine or prilocaine.[31] This may explain why lidocaine has a slightly shorter duration of action when compared with other drugs with an intermediate duration of action. Bupivacaine, etidocaine, and levobupivacaine have equal vasodilating properties and produce a longer duration of vasodilation when compared with intermediate-acting drugs.[31]

The speed of absorption and entry into the systemic circulation obviously has significant implications for toxicity. Absorption of drugs occurs most rapidly after intercostal blocks, followed by caudal-lumbar epidural, brachial plexus, sciatic-femoral, and subcutaneous blocks. Table 9-2 shows the approximate peak plasma levels after lidocaine injection (400 mg) for intercostal versus brachial block[8] (Figure 9-13). These data indicate that toxicity probably occurs more frequently after intercostal block than after brachial plexus block if the dose administered is the same.

The total dose of local anesthetic, rather than the volume or concentration, linearly determines the peak plasma concentration.[37] For example, 400 mg of lidocaine yields the same peak plasma concentration regardless of whether 40 ml of a 1% or 80 ml of a 0.5% solution is administered (Figure 9-14).

The addition of a vasoconstrictor, such as epinephrine, to local anesthetics can reduce the rate of vascular absorption. The availability of the drug is increased for neuronal uptake, resulting in a longer and more profound block. Of importance, the slower rate of absorption also attenuates the peak plasma concentration of the drug, thereby reducing systemic toxicity. The magnitude of this effect depends on the drug, the dose, and the concentration of both the local anesthetic and the vasoconstrictor, as well as the site of injection.[8] For example, addition of epinephrine to mepivacaine prolongs the time to maximum arterial plasma drug concentration in all situations; however, a 2% solution used for an intercostal block has the greatest effect.[38]

Epinephrine does not prolong the duration of blockade to the same extent with all local anesthetics. For example, it prolongs the duration for local infiltration, peripheral nerve block, and epidural anesthesia with procaine, mepivacaine, and lidocaine.[28,39-42] In the case of prilocaine, bupivacaine, and etidocaine, infiltration and peripheral nerve blocks are prolonged with epinephrine, whereas no significant effect occurs with epidural anesthesia.[42,43] The rationale for this discrepancy

TABLE 9-2 Peak Plasma Concentration of Lidocaine (400 mg) with Intercostal versus Brachial Plexus Block

Site of Injection	Peak Plasma Level
Intercostal	7 g/ml
Brachial plexus	3 g/ml

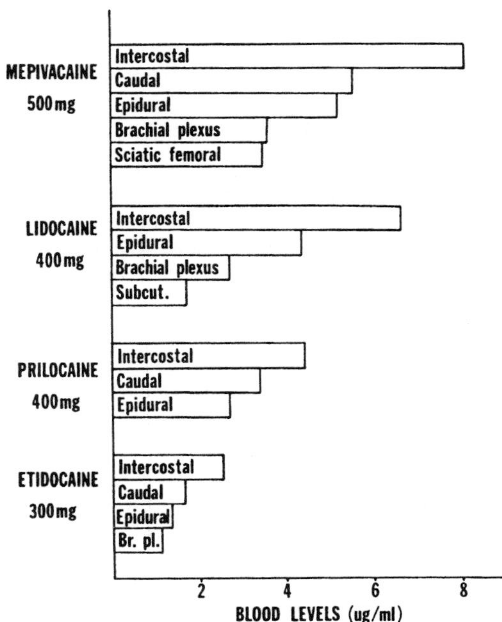

FIGURE **9-13**
Peak plasma levels of local anesthetics after injection at various anatomic sites. (From Covino BG, Vassallo HG. *Local Anesthetics: Mechanism of Action and Clinical Use*. New York: Grune & Stratton; 1976:97.)

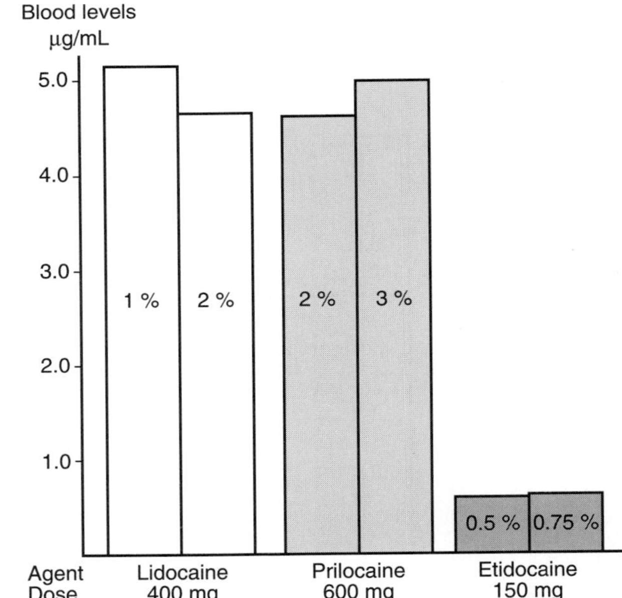

FIGURE **9-14**
Peak plasma concentrations after the epidural injection of fixed doses of lidocaine, prilocaine, and etidocaine administered at varying concentrations. (From Covino BG, Vassallo HG. *Local Anesthetics: Mechanism of Action and Clinical Use*. New York: Grune & Stratton; 1976:107. Reprinted with permission.)

might be that epidural fat significantly absorbs ropivacaine, bupivacaine, and etidocaine, owing to their lipid solubility. These drugs are released slowly from the fat depot, which could prolong the block.[41,43-45] This process overrides the effects of epinephrine on duration of action. In addition, the drug concentration can contribute to the differential effect seen with epinephrine. For example, epinephrine can prolong epidural blocks with 0.125% or 0.25% bupivacaine when used in patients in labor.[44,45] Conversely, epinephrine has little effect with the epidural administration of 0.5% or 0.75% bupivacaine.[46]

The addition of epinephrine does not attenuate the peak plasma level of all local anesthetics; for example, epinephrine significantly reduces the peak plasma concentration of lidocaine and mepivacaine, regardless of the site of administration. On the other hand, epinephrine does not significantly affect the peak plasma level of prilocaine, bupivacaine, or etidocaine after epidural anesthesia. The lack of effect seen with prilocaine may be explained by its slower absorption and rapid tissue redistribution. In the case of bupivacaine and etidocaine, it may be explained by the significant lipid solubility and uptake of these drugs in epidural adipose tissue[26] (Figure 9-15).

Studies that have compared vasoconstrictors conclude that epinephrine is superior to drugs such as phenylephrine and norepinephrine in producing vasoconstriction with local anesthetics.[47,48] The usual concentration of epinephrine that is used for this purpose is 1:200,000 or 5 mcg/ml.

Miscellaneous Factors That Influence Onset and Duration

Local anesthetics are basic drugs. As discussed previously, they have both water- and lipid-soluble properties. Factors that raise the pH of their environment increase their lipid solubility, and, conversely, lower pH environments result in increased water solubility. These changes to pH result in altered proportions of lipid-water soluble fractions of the drugs, which may have clinical consequences. At times the term used for this phenomenon is *ion trapping*. Ion trapping results from changes in pH in relationship to the agent's pK_a. Instances in which ion trapping may have clinical consequences are noted in Box 9-2.

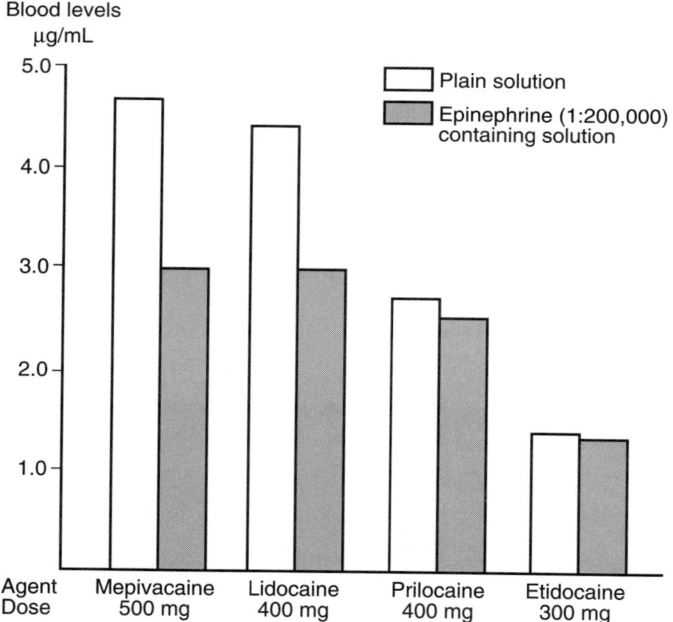

FIGURE **9-15**
Peak plasma level of local anesthetics injected into the epidural space with and without epinephrine. (From Covino BG, Vassallo HG. *Local Anesthetics: Mechanism of Action and Clinical Use*. New York: Grune & Stratton; 1976:104. Reprinted with permission.)

Local anesthetics have been carbonated to speed onset. In isolated nerve preparations, carbonation gives a more rapid onset and greater intensity of block.[49] Diffusion of carbon dioxide through the nerve membrane can lower the intracellular pH. When local anesthetics accompany this process, they become more ionized within the neuron; this results in an increase in the concentration of the drug in the protonated form at the intracellular binding site.

Controversy exists concerning whether carbonation improves onset time in the in vivo situation.[50] Separate double-blind studies of lidocaine and bupivacaine have failed to

BOX **9-2**

Ion Trapping: Clinical Situations in Which Differences between pK_a and pH May Affect Patient Response

- In the event of local anesthetic overdose, associated respiratory depression may occur, resulting in hypoxia and acidosis. The acidosis resulting from hypoxia may increase the ionized fraction of local anesthetic within the cerebral circulation, thereby decreasing the ability of the anesthetic to cross the blood-brain barrier, leave the brain, and reenter the systemic circulation. This phenomenon may prolong and enhance the central nervous system toxicity of local anesthetics.
- Local anesthetic accumulation in the fetal circulation is enhanced by the fact that fetal pH is lower than maternal pH, which may result in high fetal levels of local anesthetics.
- Local anesthetics injected into acidotic, infected tissues are rendered ineffective because of the loss of lipid solubility. The lipid solubility of local anesthetics is diminished in an acidotic environment because of an increased concentration of the ionized, water-soluble form of the drug. The loss of lipid solubility prevents absorption into the nerve, thereby preventing access to the site of action.
- Carbonation of local anesthetics speeds the onset and intensity of action of neural blockade. Carbon dioxide readily diffuses into the nerve, lowering the pH within the nerve. The lipid-soluble form of local anesthetic, after passing through the neuronal membrane, receives protons from the intraneuronal environment and ionizes. An increase in the ionized fraction within the neuron produces a higher concentration of the active form of the anesthetic available at the sodium channel, the site of action.
- Commercially available local anesthetics are prepared in a slightly acidic formulation that improves the stability of the drug by increasing the concentration of the ionized, water-soluble form of the drug. Addition of sodium bicarbonate to the local anesthetic mixture increases the pH of the solution, thereby increasing the concentration of the non-ionized, lipid soluble form of the drug. Improving the lipid solubility of the local anesthetic improves diffusion of the local anesthetic through the neuronal membrane, leading to a more rapid onset of action.

yield positive results.[51] This inconsistency may exist because the injected carbon dioxide is rapidly buffered in vivo, so intracellular pH is not greatly affected.[50,51]

The addition of sodium bicarbonate to local anesthetics may reduce the latency of onset and increase the duration of action.[52,53] In theory this would increase the pH of the local anesthetic solution, resulting in the presence of more drug in the non-ionized state. As stated previously, this form of the drug readily diffuses across the cell membranes and could decrease the latency of onset. Studies done with bupivacaine and lidocaine have indicated that this alteration does facilitate the onset and duration of action.[52,53]

The major limitation to the addition of bicarbonate is the precipitation that can occur in the local anesthetic solution. Table 9-3 indicates the propensity for precipitation, which depends significantly on the local anesthetic and whether the solution contains epinephrine. It also should be noted that the amount of bicarbonate that can be added without precipitation depends on whether the epinephrine is commercially or "freshly" mixed.[52] Manufacturers acidify local anesthetic solutions in order to increase solubility and stability (the free base is more susceptible to photodegradation and aldehyde formation), which results in a longer shelf-life. For example, the pH range of plain lidocaine is 6.5 to 6.8 and 3.5 to 4.5 for preparations that contain epinephrine. The lower pH is used with epinephrine because of the instability of this compound in alkaline solutions. Table 9-3 indicates proposed mixing regimens for bicarbonate and local anesthetics that prevent precipitation.[54]

Another benefit of alkalization is that it may result in less pain on injection.[55,56] The mechanism of action for this effect could be more complex than just an increase in pH. It may be that the nociceptive nerve fibers may not be as sensitive to the un-ionized form of the drug. It also is possible that the un-ionized drug diffuses so rapidly through the tissue and axolemma that a sensory block occurs almost instantaneously.[55,56]

The addition of dextran to local anesthetics may increase their duration of action.[57,58] Studies indicate that this alteration does not consistently prolong the block. Animal studies demonstrate that dextran is effective if the pH of the solution is high (pH 8).[59]

The addition of hyaluronidase to local anesthetics facilitates the spread of the drugs in the tissue. This additive accomplishes the effect via the hydrolysis of hyaluronic acid, which is a polysaccharide that inhibits the diffusion of foreign substances within the interstitial tissue. Also, it has been suggested that hyaluronidase reduces hematoma size if a needle that is used with the regional technique punctures a major blood vessel. The addition of hyaluronidase can result in certain undesirable effects, such as the initiation of allergic reactions, a shortening of the duration of anesthetic action, and an increase in drug toxicity.[60] Nevertheless, some clinicians still use the drug with local anesthetics for certain regional techniques in an attempt improve the success rate and onset of action.

Clinicians mix local anesthetics to obtain a more rapid onset and a longer duration of action. For example, a chloroprocaine and bupivacaine mixture might yield a rapid onset because of the former and a prolonged duration because of the latter. Studies exploring these combinations have yielded conflicting results.[61,62] This combination probably does yield a faster onset; however, the duration of action is shorter than that seen with only bupivacaine.[56]

TABLE 9-3 Sodium Bicarbonate and Local Anesthetic Mixtures

Local Anesthetic	Concentration (%)	HCO_3^- (ml/20 ml)*	pH after Addition of HCO_3^-
2-Chloroprocaine	2	4	7.51
	3	4	7.43
Mepivacaine	1	4	7.26
	1.5	2	7
Etidocaine	1	0.015	5.90
	1 + epi†	0.100	5.73
	1 + epi‡	0.015	5.85
	1.5 + epi†	0.100	5.76
Bupivacaine	0.25	0.10	6.97
	0.5	0.05	6.62
	0.5 + epi†	0.30	6.37
	0.5 + epi	0.05	6.78
	0.75	0.05	6.56
	0.75 + epi	0.30	6.32
	0.75 + epi‡	0.05	6.58
Lidocaine	1	4	7.43
	1 + epi†	4	7.21
	1 + epi‡	4	7.37
	1.5	4	7.31
	1.5 + epi†	4	7.16
	1.5 + epi‡	4	7.35
	2	4	7.24
	2 + epi†	4	7.08
	2 + epi‡	4	7.26

epi, *Epinephrine.*
**Data compiled for sodium bicarbonate 4% (weight/volume; 0.48 mEq/ml).*
†*Commercially added epinephrine, 1:200,000.*
‡*Freshly added epinephrine, 1:200,000.*
Modified from Peterfreund RA, Satta S, Ostheimer GW. Adjustment of local anesthetic solutions with sodium bicarbonate: laboratory evaluations of alkalization and precipitation. Reg Anesth. *1989;14:265-270.*

Distribution

The absorption or injection of local anesthetics into the systemic circulation results in rapid distribution throughout the body.[63] Distribution results in a rapid decrease in the plasma concentration, owing to the movement of drug into tissues that have the greatest perfusion. A secondary, slower disappearance follows; this reflects either distribution into tissues with a more limited blood supply, drug metabolism and excretion, or both of these processes. In a two-compartment model, distribution is known as the *alpha phase of plasma decay*, and the slower elimination component is referred to as the *beta phase of plasma decay*[63] (Figure 9-16). Some describe the pharmacokinetics of drugs, including local anesthetics, using a three-compartment model. In a three-compartment model, the distribution phase is subdivided into rapid (alpha) and slow (beta) phases. The elimination (gamma) phase remains conceptually similar to the usual two-compartment model.

Although local anesthetics are distributed throughout the body, their concentration varies in different tissues. Immediately after vascular uptake, more greatly perfused tissues, such as those of the lungs, receive more of these drugs than do less perfused tissues.[64] Once equilibration occurs, the local anesthetic leaves the highly perfused tissue and is deposited in tissue with less perfusion. Muscle tissue receives the greatest amount of local anesthetic from distribution. This is not

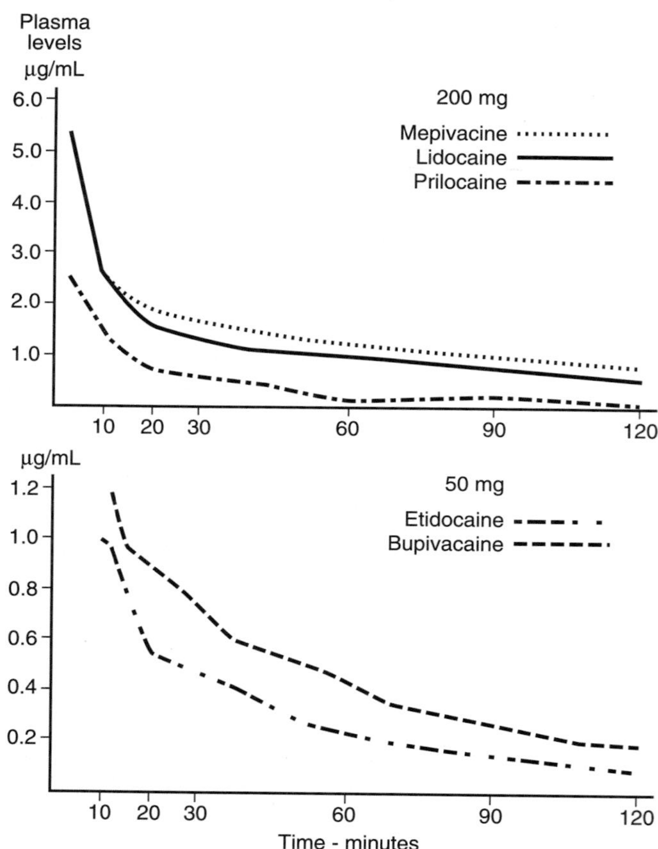

FIGURE **9-16**
Plasma concentration curves of three intermediate-acting (*top*) and two long-acting (*bottom*) local anesthetics. Note that prilocaine and etidocaine are cleared more rapidly than the other local anesthetics in their respective groups. (From Covino BG, Vassallo HG. *Local Anesthetics: Mechanism of Action and Clinical Use*. New York: Grune & Stratton; 1976:108.)

because it has a greater affinity for these drugs, but rather because muscle acts as a depot, owing to its greater tissue mass.[9]

The distribution process varies significantly with different local anesthetics. For example, the disappearance rate of prilocaine is more rapid than that of mepivacaine or lidocaine. Of the longer-acting amides, etidocaine has a shorter distribution half-life than bupivacaine.[63] Ropivacaine also has shorter half-life than bupivacaine. Levobupivacaine appears to have a half-life similar to that of bupivacaine.[64-66] Distribution of the ester local anesthetics occurs as it does with the amides; however, their site and rate of metabolism tend to result in distribution having a lesser effect on plasma concentration.[67]

Metabolism

The metabolism of local anesthetics differs according to their chemical classification as either amides or esters. Ester hydrolysis is the primary metabolic route of ester local anesthetics. The hydrolysis occurs through the action of esterase in plasma, red blood cells, and the liver.[63,68-70] Primarily, plasma cholinesterase rapidly metabolizes the ester local anesthetics. Enzymatic hydrolysis in the plasma is rapid (half-life is 1 minute). An outcome of rapid hydrolysis is that toxic effects are short lived. Table 9-4 shows the clearance rates for the ester local anesthetics.[71]

TABLE **9-4** Clearance Half-Life of Local Anesthetics

Drug	Clearance (L/min)	Half-Life (min)
Chloroprocaine	—	0.3
Procaine	—	0.75
Tetracaine	—	—
Prilocaine	2.84	5
Lidocaine	0.95	9.6
Mepivacaine	0.78	7.2
Bupivacaine	0.47	28
Levobupivacaine	0.35	120
Ropivacaine	7.2	112
Etidocaine	1.22	19

The plasma half-lives of procaine and chloroprocaine are shorter than 1 minute. The rapid rate of clearance of these drugs significantly reduces the incidence and severity of toxicity. Conversely, tetracaine is the most toxic ester and therefore is of limited clinical use. Saturated, inhibited, or genetically atypical plasma cholinesterase can significantly prolong the plasma half-life of ester local anesthetics.[70,72] For example, atypical plasma cholinesterase has been shown to significantly reduce the rate of procaine metabolism.[73] Drugs that are metabolized by plasma cholinesterase, such as succinylcholine or mivacurium, could also reduce the metabolism of ester local anesthetics.

In theory, patients who have liver disease severe enough to reduce plasma cholinesterase could be more prone to develop toxicity from ester local anesthetics. In fact, the plasma half-life of procaine is longer in patients with liver disease.[70] However, toxicity is unlikely in patients with liver disease who receive procaine and 2-chloroprocaine because of these drugs' intrinsic rate of metabolism and the esterase activity that is maintained in the erythrocytes.[68]

Metabolism of the amide local anesthetics occurs primarily in the liver. Metabolism is predominantly by microsomal cytochrome P-450.[74] The rate of hepatic metabolism—and therefore clearance—is slowest for bupivacaine, followed in order by mepivacaine, lidocaine, etidocaine, and prilocaine.[75] This suggests that prilocaine, with intermediate potency, and etidocaine, with high potency, would be the least toxic drugs in their respective potency-related groups. It is obvious that clearance functions are independent of such factors as potency, lipid solubility, protein binding, and chemical structure. Table 9-5 presents pharmacokinetic data for the amide local anesthetics.[76]

Hepatic enzyme activity and blood flow are the primary factors that determine the rate of elimination of amide local anesthetics.[77] The hepatic extraction ratio represents the activity level specific to the liver for metabolizing a drug. This ratio names the percentage of drug removed with each pass through the liver. The clearance of drugs that have higher hepatic extraction ratios, such as etidocaine, depends on adequate hepatic blood flow.[77] Hepatic enzyme activity is important when drugs with lower ratios, such as bupivacaine, are used[35,77] (see Figure 9-16). Table 9-6 indicates the extraction ratios for the amide local anesthetics.[71]

Consequently, pathologic conditions that influence hepatic function prolong the plasma half-life of these drugs by a reduction in hepatic blood flow, enzyme activity, or both. For example, lidocaine has a plasma half-life of 1.8 hours; however, in

TABLE **9-5** Pharmacokinetics of Amide Local Anesthetics

Agent	Half-Life Alpha (min)	Half-Life Beta (min)	Half-Life Gamma (min)	V_{dss} (L)	Clearance (L)
Prilocaine	0.5	5	2	261	2.84
Lidocaine	1	9.6	1.6	91	0.95
Mepivacaine	0.7	7.2	1.9	84	0.75
Bupivacaine	2.7	28	3.5	72	0.47
Etidocaine	2.2	19	2.6	133	1.22
Ropivacaine	2.7	1.9	—	66.9	0.73

V_{dss}, *volume of distribution at steady state.*
Modified from Longnecker DE, Murphy FL. Introduction to Anesthesia. *9th ed. Philadelphia: Saunders; 1997:204.*

severe hepatic disease, its half-life is 4.9 hours. This probably results from both an enzymatic and a perfusion effect. A second example is found in congestive heart failure, which significantly reduces the rate of elimination of lidocaine because of a concomitant reduction in hepatic blood flow[78] (Table 9-7). These data indicate that reduced doses of amide local anesthetics should be used for patients with hepatic or circulatory dysfunction. Both of these pathologic states are common in the geriatric patient, necessitating the use of lower doses of anesthesia.

Only 1% to 5% of the injected dose of local anesthetic is accounted for by unchanged renal and hepatic excretion. However, the inactive, more water-soluble metabolites of local anesthetics appear in the urine.[71] Although renal dysfunction affects the clearance far less than does hepatic failure, it can result in the accumulation of potentially toxic metabolites.[71]

The use of local anesthetics in pregnancy deserves some special pharmacokinetic and pharmacodynamic consideration. Clinical observations and studies both indicate that the spread and depth of spinal and epidural anesthesia are increased in pregnant women.[79] At first this was thought to be the result only of mechanical factors produced by a gravid uterus. For example, mechanical factors result in dilation of epidural veins, which leads to narrowing of the epidural and subarachnoid space, thereby reducing the dose requirement.[79] However, hormonal changes may explain some of this finding: there is a greater segmental spread of local anesthetics administered in the epidural during the first trimester of pregnancy.[80] A relationship appears to exist between the progesterone level in cerebrospinal fluid and the segmental spread of the drugs. Studies performed on isolated nerve taken from pregnant animals demonstrate more sensitivity to local anesthetic block than in nonpregnant animals.[81,82] Pregnancy appears to influence the potency of the local anesthetics.

TABLE **9-6** Hepatic Extraction of Amide Local Anesthetics

Drug	Hepatic Extraction Ratio
Lidocaine	0.68
Bupivacaine	0.37
Etidocaine	0.73

TABLE **9-7** Effect of Disease on Lidocaine Pharmacokinetics

	Half-Life (hr)	V_{dss} (L/kg)	Clearance (ml/kg/min)
Normal	1.8	1.32	10
Renal disease	1.3	1.2	13.7
Heart failure	1.9	0.88	6.3
Liver disease	4.9	2.31	6

V_{dss}, *volume of distribution at steady state.*
From Thompson PD, Melmon KL, Richardson JA, et al. Lidocaine pharmacokinetics in advanced heart failure, liver disease and renal failure in humans. Ann Intern Med. *1973;78:499.*

TOXICITY OF LOCAL ANESTHETICS

Local anesthetics exert their action by inhibiting the passage of Na^+ ions through nerve membranes. Stabilized excitable tissue in the application region prevents normal function of afferent neurons. If the plasma concentration of these drugs becomes significantly elevated, this "stabilizing" property can lead to toxicity of the cardiovascular system and CNS. Toxic reactions to local anesthetics may be either local or systemic. Local reactions include pain, hematoma, abscess, ecchymosis, tissue necrosis, and neurotoxicity.[83] (Because tissue necrosis is often associated with the concomitant administration of epinephrine, the local anesthetic may not be the primary cause.) The most common causes of systemic local anesthetic toxicity are inadvertent intravascular injection and administration of an excessive dose.

Central Nervous System Toxicity

In one study, local anesthetics were infused into volunteers until they demonstrated symptoms of CNS toxicity.[84] This study demonstrated that, although often similar, the patterns of CNS toxic effects varied among individuals. For example, some volunteers initially experienced tinnitus, whereas others became irrational. Despite individual variability, a sequence of symptoms was identified when all subjects were compared. Sequential symptoms are shown in Figure 9-17.

All of the symptoms noted in Figure 9-17 are the result of CNS effects, except for circumoral numbness, which is a result

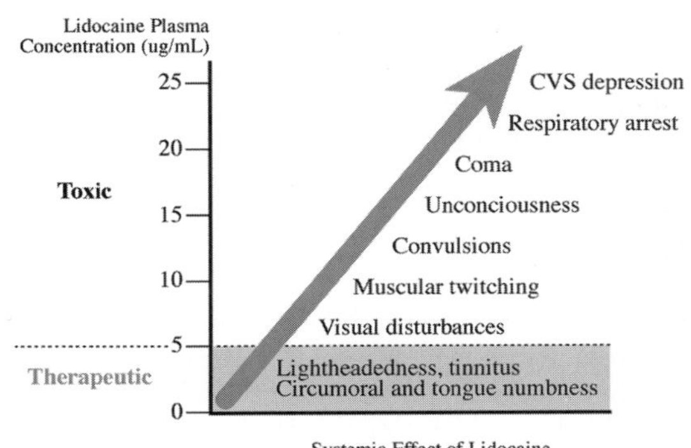

FIGURE **9-17**
Clinical signs after increased central nervous system concentration of lidocaine.

of extracellular extravasation of the drug in the tongue and mouth.[85] It has been noted that more of these symptoms are seen when plasma concentrations increase slowly. Conversely, a sudden increase in plasma concentration, as might occur with failure of an intravenous regional technique, may result in convulsion as the initial symptom.[84] Some patients manifest CNS depression as the initial symptom, especially if they have received a CNS depressant for sedation. For example, a CNS depressant, such as midazolam, administered for anxiety associated with a regional technique precludes the manifestation of the excitability component of the local anesthetic reaction.

The effect of local anesthetics on the brain is depression of neuronal function. At first this may appear paradoxic because many of the symptoms, such as muscle twitching and convulsion, indicate stimulation. The explanation lies in the fact that the local anesthetics selectively depress inhibitory functions in the cerebral cortex. Consequently, stimulatory activity results because facilitory neurons function are unopposed.[86] If plasma levels increase significantly, both inhibitory and facilitory pathways are depressed, and generalized CNS depression results.[86]

The potential for a local anesthetic to produce CNS toxicity relates to its potency. For example, animal studies have indicated that lidocaine 20 mg/kg results in convulsion. More potent drugs, such as etidocaine and bupivacaine, produced seizures at 8 mg/kg and 5 mg/kg, respectively.[87] This results in a CNS toxicity ratio of 4:2:1, which correlates with the relative potency of these agents in establishing epidural anesthesia. Studies in human subjects have also demonstrated a similar correlation between potency and CNS toxicity.[86]

The acid-base status of animals and humans is important in the determination of CNS toxicity. For example, studies in cats have indicated that the convulsive threshold decreases by approximately 50% when carbon dioxide tension increases from 25 to 40 mm Hg to 45 to 81 mm Hg.[88] Both respiratory and metabolic acidosis increase the propensity for toxicity, whereas alkalosis reduces it. Several factors may be responsible for this effect. An elevation in carbon dioxide tension leads to cerebral vasodilation, which results in the delivery of more drug to the brain. Also, diffusion of carbon dioxide across the neuronal membrane causes a reduction in intracellular pH. This results in ionic trapping of the local anesthetic within the neurons.[89] Finally, more free drug is available for diffusion into the CNS because of the reduction in plasma protein binding caused by acidosis.[89]

Some clinicians advocate having patients voluntarily hyperventilate while breathing oxygen when they first experience premonitory signs of CNS toxicity.[10] Acute lowering of the intracerebral carbon dioxide tension may prevent seizure by raising the local anesthetic seizure threshold. However, if seizure should occur, the patient is less likely to develop hypoxia because of the denitrogenation that occurs when a high concentration of oxygen is breathed.[10]

Cardiovascular Toxicity

Studies have indicated, with some notable exceptions, that the cardiovascular system, when compared with the CNS, is more resistant to toxicity of local anesthetics. For example, in animals the doses that cause significant cardiovascular depression are approximately threefold greater than those that produce convulsion.[90] Nevertheless, toxicity to the cardiovascular system does occur and is extremely important, because it can result in grave clinical outcomes. As with the CNS, cardiovascular toxicity appears to be related to the anesthetic potency of the drugs.

Local anesthetics produce toxicity by influencing the heart and peripheral vascular system. The peripheral vascular effects of these drugs appear to be biphasic.[91] At low concentrations, they produce vasoconstriction and an increase in systemic vascular resistance. As doses are increased, vasodilation occurs, resulting in significant hypotension.[91]

In the heart, these drugs influence electrophysiologic and contractile functions. An example of this is the prolongation of conduction time through the heart that occurs with the use of bupivacaine.[92] On electrocardiography, these effects result in an increase in the PR interval and in the duration of the QRS complex. As the dose of these drugs is increased, complete atrioventricular block, sinus bradycardia, or both can occur, possibly leading to cardiac arrest. Cardiac pacing, as indicated in the treatment of extreme bradycardia or cardiac arrest, may be difficult in this situation. By stabilizing nerve tissue, local anesthetics may elevate the pacing threshold.

In addition, because these drugs depress automaticity, extreme bradycardia is not well tolerated.[88] The effect of local anesthetics on conductivity, automaticity, and pacing potential is attributable to the blockade of Na^+ channels.[13,14]

Local anesthetics also depress contractility of the myocardium.[92] The mechanism for this depression is unknown; however, it is probably related to the blockade of Na^+ channels and the displacement of calcium from the cardiac muscle.[93] The negative inotropic effect results in a depression in V_{max} (maximum velocity of shortening of cardiac muscle fibers), a reduction of cardiac output, and an elevation in left ventricular end-diastolic pressure and volume. As stated previously, a relationship exists between myocardial depression and the potency of a drug.[94] For example, tetracaine is 8 to 10 times more potent than procaine as a local anesthetic and also as a myocardial depressant.[95,96]

The selectivity in the cardiovascular toxicity of local anesthetics is thought to be significant. For example, bupivacaine and etidocaine appear to produce toxicity at lower doses than a less potent drug such as lidocaine.[97,98] More important, the cardiovascular toxicity seen with the potent drugs is severe and recalcitrant to treatment and may occur prior to CNS toxicity.[99,100] Studies on isolated papillary muscles have demonstrated greater depression of Na^+ current by bupivacaine than by lidocaine. Also, the highly lipid-soluble bupivacaine dissociates from the channel more slowly than lidocaine.[101] Lastly, tachycardia, by a frequency-dependent effect, facilitates the binding of bupivacaine to Na^+ channels, thereby enhancing cardiac toxicity.[102]

This selectivity has special implications in the consideration of ventricular arrhythmias. Bupivacaine can produce severe and even fatal ventricular arrhythmias in patients; however, lidocaine, mepivacaine, and tetracaine rarely produce arrhythmias. The arrhythmogenic effect of bupivacaine is probably a result of the inhibition of both fast Na^+ and slow calcium channels. Because this drug dissociates slowly from Na^+ channels, it is possible that it produces a persistent, slow conduction velocity, reentry pathways, and ventricular tachycardia, which lead to ventricular fibrillation.[101,102] Studies on the cardiotoxicity of ropivacaine and levobupivacaine suggest that they are much safer in this regard.[103,104] On comparison, ropivacaine is less cardiotoxic than levobupivacaine, which is less cardiotoxic than bupivacaine. The number of reported cases of bupivacaine toxicity has declined significantly in recent years with increased vigilance in clinical practice.[105,106]

Several cases of cardiovascular toxicity in pregnant patients have been reported. These reports have led to the assumption that pregnancy possibly has a role in increasing sensitivity to the cardiovascular toxicity of local anesthetics. It has been noted that bupivacaine produces cardiovascular collapse at a lower plasma concentration in pregnant animals than in nonpregnant animals.[101,107] This difference possibly results from pregnancy-induced hormonal changes.[106] Neither pregnant animals nor humans have demonstrated this degree of toxicity in response to lidocaine or mepivacaine. It does not appear that this differential effect is the result of an increase in the myocardial uptake of bupivacaine.[108] Although the mechanism is unknown, case reports and animal studies have resulted in the recommendation that bupivacaine 0.75% not be used in obstetrics.

Hypercarbia, acidosis, and hypoxia potentiate the negative chronotropic and inotropic effects of lidocaine and bupivacaine in isolated myocardial tissue. This effect is most significant in the case of bupivacaine. Animal studies demonstrate that the use of bupivacaine in the presence of hypoxia and acidosis also increases the frequency of arrhythmias and death.[109] These facts emphasize the importance of good airway management during seizure activity resulting from the toxicity of local anesthetics.

Allergic Reactions

Local anesthetics can produce allergic, hypersensitive, and anaphylactic reactions, although the incidence of true allergy is very low. The use of ester local anesthetics is associated with a much greater incidence of these reactions than the use of amides. This is because the esters are derivatives of *para*-aminobenzoic acid, which is an allergenic compound.[110] Cross-reactivity among the ester-type local anesthetics is high and among the amide types is low but still possible. Although reports indicate that amide local anesthetics can produce allergic reactions, the incidence in this class is much lower. Skin testing is possible but at times difficult to interpret.[106,111,112]

Intradermal experiments demonstrate the difference between amides and esters.[113] Both amides and esters were injected intradermally in patients with no history of allergic response to local anesthetics. Of these patients, 30% had skin reactions to esters, but no reactions to the amides were observed. None of these patients had systemic anaphylactic reactions. True immunologic reactions to local anesthetics are rare, encompassing less than 1% of all adverse reactions.[114] Cross-allergy between ester and amide type local anesthetics is rare.

Some commercially available amide local anesthetics are in solution with the preservative methylparaben. This substance, which has a chemical structure similar to that of *para*-aminobenzoic acid, can increase the incidence of allergic reactions with the amide local anesthetics.[115] Patients who are allergic to ester local anesthetics, whether determined through the patient's history or through intradermal skin testing, should be treated with a preservative-free amide local anesthetic to avoid a possible allergic reaction to the *para*-aminobenzoic acid metabolite of methylparaben.[114]

In clinical practice, adverse reactions after injection of local anesthetics are frequently observed. In most cases, they can be attributed to (1) toxic events (both cardiovascular and neurotoxic) related to the dose of the local anesthetic or vasoconstrictor (epinephrine) or accidental intravascular injections; (2) psychomotor reactions; and (3) reactions caused by preservatives or hidden allergens (e.g., the latex in surgical gloves).[114]

Methemoglobinemia

The use of prilocaine can produce methemoglobinemia, because of the metabolite *o*-toluidine, which oxidizes hemoglobin to methemoglobin.[116] The tendency of prilocaine to produce methemoglobin is dose related. Significant methemoglobin does not result until the dose administered epidurally reaches 600 mg.[116] High concentrations of methemoglobin produce a brownish-gray cyanosis, tachypnea, and metabolic acidosis. Severe methemoglobinemia causes signs and symptoms related to tissue hypoxia, headache, and irritability. Loss of consciousness may occur in 50% to 60% of cases.[117] Spontaneous reversal of methemoglobin occurs in 2 to 3 hours; however, the administration of methylene blue can result in immediate reversal. The formation of the usual clinical levels of methemoglobin is of little consequence in healthy patients; however, patients with severe anemia or heart failure cannot tolerate the reduction in oxygen-carrying capacity. Prilocaine should not be used in obstetrics, because clinical doses can result in a 10% conversion of fetal hemoglobin to methemoglobin, leading to neonatal cyanosis.[118] Benzocaine and benzocaine-containing mixtures such as Cetacaine may also produce methemoglobinemia.[119]

Local Tissue Toxicity

Chloroprocaine is the only local anesthetic that has produced prolonged sensory and motor deficits after epidural and subarachnoid administration.[120] Because of this, animal experiments were conducted to determine the effect of chloroprocaine on neural function.[121,122] It appears that nerve damage is likely to result if chloroprocaine 3% is added to a solution of sodium bisulfite 0.2% at a pH of 3. However, chloroprocaine and sodium bisulfite at these concentrations did not produce damage if put into a solution with a pH of 7. Also, chloroprocaine 3% with a pH of 3 does not produce nerve damage if sodium bisulfite is omitted. Sodium bisulfite, without chloroprocaine and at a pH of 3, can produce nerve damage. These data indicate that the combination of low pH and sodium bisulfite causes neurotoxic effects.[120-122] It does not appear that chloroprocaine itself is neurotoxic. Clinically used preparations now omit sodium bisulfite because of this problem. A comparison of the common features of local anesthetic reactions are given in Box 9-3.

Prevention of Toxicity

Animal studies have demonstrated that pretreatment with benzodiazepines is effective in prevention of local anesthetic–induced CNS seizures.[123,124] Although this has been demonstrated in several species, the results are difficult to extrapolate to humans. Owing to ethical considerations, it is difficult to perform well-controlled clinical studies in humans, and without clinical studies it is impossible to determine the appropriate dose and timing for administration. Nevertheless, the results of the animal studies tend to indicate that benzodiazepines are the drugs of choice, especially if sedation is needed for a regional technique. Administration of midazolam 5 to 10 minutes before the injection of the local anesthetic seems prudent.

The dose administered is important in determination of toxicity. The dose of local anesthetics that produces toxicity is difficult to predict because, as previously discussed, the site of injection has a significant influence on the peak plasma level. Nevertheless, as shown in Table 9-8, manufacturers have issued recommended dose limits for single, nonvascular injections.[76]

BOX 9-3

Common Features of Local Anesthetic Reactions

Cause	Major Clinical Features	Comments
Local Anesthetic Toxicity		
Intravascular injection	Immediate convulsion or cardiac toxicity;	
Relative overdose	onset in 5 to 15 minutes of irritability, progressing to convulsions	
Reaction to vasoconstrictor	Tachycardia, hypertension, headache	
Vasovagal Reaction	Rapid onset, bradycardia, hypotension, pallor, faintness	Apprehension
Allergy		
Immediate	Anaphylaxis (hypotension, bronchospasm, edema)	Allergy to amides is extremely rare
Delayed	Urticaria	Cross-allergy possible, e.g., with preservatives in local anesthetics and food

Some techniques for the recognition, prevention, and treatment of an accidental overdose of a local anesthetic are listed in Boxes 9-4 and 9-5.

Treatment of Systemic Toxicity

The severity of toxic effects depends on the drug used and the amount administered. Drugs such as lidocaine, prilocaine, and chloroprocaine produce toxicity of limited duration because of short distribution times and elimination half-lives. A drug such as bupivacaine, ropivacaine, or levobupivacaine, which have longer half-lives, produces more protracted toxicity.

A primary concern when toxicity occurs is the treatment of CNS symptoms. During convulsions oxygen consumption increases and ventilation is significantly compromised; this situation can result in respiratory acidosis and hypoxemia. Therefore the assurance and maintenance of a patent airway and ventilation with oxygen are the initial actions taken.

If distribution allows the plasma concentration of the drug to rapidly fall below the convulsive threshold, airway management and ventilation with oxygen may be the only treatment needed. However, convulsions may be severe and protracted, making airway management difficult. The administration of ultra–short-acting barbiturates treats convulsions in this situation. Care is taken to use a minimal dose, because an excessive dose can potentiate cardiovascular and postconvulsive CNS depression. Thiopental, 50 to 100 mg, is usually satisfactory.

TABLE 9-8 Manufacturers' Recommended Single-Injection Dose

Drug	Concentration (%)	Dose* (mg/kg)
Chloroprocaine	3	11 (14)
Lidocaine	1	4 (7)
Lidocaine	2	4 (7)
Mepivacaine	2	4 (7)
Prilocaine	3	7 (8.5)
Bupivacaine	0.75	2.5 (3.2)
Etidocaine	1	6 (8)
Etidocaine	2	(8)
Ropivacaine	0.75	3 (3.5)
Levobupivacaine	0.75	2.5 (3.2)

**Values are drug alone (drug with epinephrine).*

BOX 9-4

Techniques to Prevent Regional Block Toxicity

Patient Evaluation
- Identification of significant systemic disease, age, and surgical requirements to permit individualization of local anesthetic dose

Premedication
- A moderate dose of midazolam or other appropriate central nervous system depressant

Preparation

Resuscitative Drugs
- Midazolam, propofol or thiopental, succinylcholine, atropine, cardiac support drugs

Equipment
- Oxygen administration and suction equipment
- Airway management supplies, including airway, laryngoscope, and endotracheal tube and laryngeal mask airway
- Ensure adequate intravenous access is available before beginning procedure
- Be aware of allergies to locals and preservatives
- Physically separate neural blockade tray from any other drugs

Prevention
- Personally check dose of local anesthetic and vasoconstrictor
- Administer a test dose of 5%-10% of total dose
- Aspirate frequently and discard bloody solutions
- Monitor for cardiovascular signs such as increase in heart rate if epinephrine is used

Maintain constant verbal contact with patient and vigilance for premonitory signs of toxicity after time of peak plasma concentration

BOX **9-5**

Treatment of Acute Local Anesthetic Toxic Response

Airway
- Secure clear airway

Breathing
- Administer oxygen with face mask
- Encourage adequate ventilation, which prevents acidosis and ion trapping
- Use artificial ventilation, intubation as required

Circulation
- Increase intravenous fluids to treat hypotension
- Administer cardiovascular support drugs as required to treat blood pressure and heart rate changes
- Administer antiarrhythmic agents as required

Drugs
- Administer incremental doses of benzodiazepine, thiopental, or propofol as needed to prevent or treat seizure
- Administer muscle relaxant to secure airway
- Use cardiovascular support and resuscitation agents as required

Outcomes
- Local anesthetic toxicity may result in convulsions or abrupt respiratory and cardiac changes; however, with rapid and appropriate treatment long-term sequelae are rare

Also, use of a rapid-onset and short-acting muscle relaxant, such as succinylcholine, helps control the convulsive state. It should be noted that if this mode of treatment is used, the patient should undergo endotracheal intubation.

If hypotension occurs, conservative treatment includes the correction of hypoxia and acidosis.[125] The patient's legs should be elevated and the intravenous infusion increased. Vasopressors are administered if hypotension is persistent and severe. Sympathomimetic drugs with alpha and beta effects can be used to treat hypotension resulting from local anesthetic–induced myocardial depression and vasodilatation. Ephedrine, 15 to 30 mg, is usually the agent of choice. Atropine, 0.4 mg, adequately treats bradycardia that may be present. Significant doses of atropine, dopamine, or epinephrine can be used to treat severe hypotension and bradycardia that might occur, especially in the case of bupivacaine toxicity.[126]

Widening of the QRS complex usually precedes cardiovascular collapse. Cardiopulmonary resuscitation and cardioversion are used for treating ventricular tachycardia and fibrillation. The electrical energy needed for cardioversion may be greater than normal. With bupivacaine-induced cardiovascular collapse, resuscitation can be difficult and may require large doses of epinephrine, atropine, or both.

ADVANCES IN LOCAL ANESTHESIA

Ropivacaine

Researchers have attempted to identify drugs that have a long duration of action but do not have the cardiovascular toxicity of bupivacaine. Ropivacaine was designed to meet these specifications. Chemically, ropivacaine differs from bupivacaine in that it has a propyl group in place of the butyl group on the nitrogen atom in the piperidine ring. In addition, local anesthetics that have asymmetric carbon atoms can exist in either sinister (S−) or rectus (R−) stereoisomers. Bupivacaine exists as a racemic compound in that it has both S− and R− isomers. Conversely, ropivacaine exists only in the S− stereoisomer form. This difference between ropivacaine and bupivacaine has resulted in less cardiotoxicity.[127]

Isolated in vitro studies of ropivacaine have indicated that it is less potent than bupivacaine in its ability to block Na^+ channels. More important, this compound has a more rapid rate of reversal of Na^+ channel blockade than bupivacaine.[128,129] This may result in less toxicity.[103,130] As stated earlier in the section on cardiovascular toxicity, the slow dissociation of local anesthetics from Na^+ channels can result in the development of recalcitrant ventricular arrhythmias.

Ropivacaine and bupivacaine have been administered intravenously at equal doses in dog studies. These studies have demonstrated that ropivacaine produces less slowing in cardiac conduction velocity, less cardiovascular collapse, and less ventricular fibrillation than bupivacaine.[131-133] Conversely, studies in sheep have indicated that the mortality rate from ventricular fibrillation is the same for the two drugs.[134] Also important, studies in animals have shown that cardiac resuscitation is more successful after ropivacaine use when toxic doses of both drugs were administered by intravenous bolus.[135]

Clinical studies have indicated that the therapeutic profiles of both ropivacaine and bupivacaine are similar, but differences do exist. Ropivacaine appears less potent than bupivacaine and produces less motor blockade at low concentrations.[136-138]

The elimination half-life of ropivacaine is less than that of bupivacaine.[127] A study in which two drugs were infused at a rate of 10 mg/min demonstrated that 25% more ropivacaine was needed to produce minor symptoms. When the infusions were stopped, the toxic symptoms disappeared more rapidly in the subjects who had received ropivacaine. These findings seem to indicate that ropivacaine has a pharmacokinetic advantage over bupivacaine.[139] In summary, the most important aspect of the overall clinical profile of ropivacaine is reduced CNS and cardiac toxicity and less motor blockade, most likely because of a lower potency.[140]

Levobupivacaine

Levobupivacaine, a new local anesthetic, is the S(−) enantiomer of bupivacaine.[141-143] Levobupivacaine is clinically similar to bupivacaine and has a long duration of action. The advantage of levobupivacaine is a reduced CNS and cardiac toxicity profile compared with that of bupivacaine.[144]

In a study in human volunteers, levobupivacaine and ropivacaine appear to have similar CNS toxicity profiles. Because levobupivacaine is more potent then ropivacaine, the conclusion can be reached that levobupivacaine also has a higher therapeutic index.[145-147] Cost is a major factor in the decision regarding which long-acting agent to use. The type of block, the dose and concentration of local anesthetic required, and the realistic risk of bupivacaine toxicity compared with that associated with the new agents must be considered.[148]

Eutectic Mixture of Local Anesthetics

For years, researchers have sought to develop techniques and drugs that produce anesthesia on application to intact skin. As a result of their work, the eutectic mixture of local anesthetics

(EMLA) was developed. EMLA is a mixture of lidocaine and prilocaine that, when applied to skin, accumulates at the site of dermal pain receptors and nerve endings.

The clinical effectiveness of EMLA has been studied in the performance of venipuncture in children. A study of 41 ill children revealed that the application of EMLA for 45 minutes before the procedure resulted in lower pain scores than if no pretreatment was used. The effectiveness was not seen in situations classified as "difficult venipunctures." As might be expected, EMLA also was not as effective in children under age 7 years than it was in older children.[149]

Pharmacokinetic studies indicate that satisfactory dermal analgesia is achieved 1 hour after application with an occlusive dressing; maximal analgesia occurs 2 to 3 hours after application.[150] When EMLA is applied to areas of abnormal skin (e.g., where psoriasis or eczema is present), absorption is faster, plasma levels are higher, and the duration of anesthesia is shorter. This results from an impairment of diffusion barriers and an increase in regional blood flow.[151] Systemic absorption of lidocaine and prilocaine is dependent on the duration and surface area of application. Blood levels of 5% and 2.8% of those needed to produce systemic toxicity are seen with use of lidocaine and prilocaine, respectively, when the drugs are applied in accordance with appropriate dosage recommendations.[152] Toxicity is more likely to occur in infants and small children than in adults. Also, toxicity can result if the emulsion is applied to broken or inflamed skin or to areas of 2000 cm^2 or greater or if it is left on for longer than recommended periods.[150]

The recommended dose of EMLA for minor dermal procedures, such as venipuncture, is 2.5 g; the dose is applied over a 20- to 25-cm^2 skin surface at least 60 minutes before the procedure. Analgesia does not occur until 15 minutes after application of the drug. For painful procedures, 2 g of EMLA per 10 cm^2 of skin surface area are applied and left in place for at least 2 hours.[151] EMLA should not be used in infants younger than age 12 months. The rationale for this limitation is that EMLA contains prilocaine. Prilocaine can cause a dose-related increase in oxidation of hemoglobin to methemoglobin, which is especially problematic in neonates.[153] Studies have indicated that simultaneous use of EMLA and drugs that cause oxidation of hemoglobin (e.g., sulfonamides, benzocaine, aniline drugs, nitrites) also increases this risk.[150] The use of EMLA for mucous membrane anesthesia is not recommended, because of the rapid rate of absorption.

A common use of local anesthetics is to produce analgesia for the irrigating, débridement, and suturing of traumatic dermal lacerations. An ideal local anesthetic for this use would be painless, produce minimal systemic toxicity, maintain tissue viability, and not distort the wound margins.[154] In an attempt to produce some of these characteristics, three previously available agents—tetracaine, epinephrine, and cocaine (TAC)—were combined for use on traumatic lacerations. The relative concentration of each component is as follows: tetracaine 0.5%, epinephrine 1:200, cocaine 10%.[155] This combination has been as effective as infiltration of local anesthetics for the closure of certain types of laceration. Tetracaine and cocaine can produce excellent topical anesthesia, and cocaine and epinephrine result in vasoconstriction at the site of application. The vasoconstriction that results from the combination should slow the absorption of the local anesthetics, which should reduce toxicity and facilitate the quality and duration of anesthesia produced.

The clinical use of TAC has not been without problems. TAC is more expensive to administer than lidocaine when the latter is used for local infiltration. Because the combination contains cocaine, TAC must be treated as a Schedule II controlled substance.[156] Therefore it must be kept in a locked cabinet and records of its use must be kept. This further increases the cost of administering the drug combination.

The drug combination in TAC can produce significant toxicity. Both cocaine and tetracaine can individually produce significant systemic toxicity. Cocaine can also increase the α-adrenergic response to epinephrine by blocking the reuptake of epinephrine into the peripheral adrenergic nerve terminal. The types of severe toxicity seen with TAC have been status epilepticus and death.[156] It appears that complications are more likely to occur when TAC is administered topically to mucous membrane. The maximum recommended safe dose is 3 to 4 ml in adults and 0.05 ml/kg in children.[155] Because of toxicity seen with TAC, other non–cocaine-containing drug combinations have been used and demonstrated similar effectiveness.[156]

An over-the-counter anesthetic cream (ELA-Max) and gel (Topicaine) are also available. ELA-Max contains 4% lidocaine in a liposomal delivery system and is more than twice as fast as compared with EMLA. Topicaine is a 4% microemulsion gel with an onset of approximately 1 hour and a duration of 1 hour after removal.

Sustained Release of Local Anesthetics

Pain can be easily alleviated with local anesthetics; however, their clinical usefulness is limited by their relatively short duration of action. Even long-acting local anesthetics, such as bupivacaine, etidocaine, ropivacaine, and levobupivacaine are of limited use in relieving pain that lasts longer than 2 to 12 hours.[157] In order to address this problem, indwelling catheters with continuous infusion of mixtures of local anesthetic and opiates are commonly used. The use of indwelling catheters is associated with problems such as blockage or breakage, migration subdurally (after epidural insertion), and infection.

Because of the problems associated with indwelling catheters, researchers are investigating the use of liposomal microspheres for the slow release of local anesthetics. Liposomal microspheres consist of a phospholipid bilayer that encapsulates an aqueous core. Pharmacokinetically the liposomes act as a depot for local anesthetics and allow for the slow clearance of the drugs into the injected tissue. Liposomal microspheres impregnated with lidocaine and bupivacaine and injected into the epidural space have resulted in a prolonged duration of neural blockade. In addition, it appears that the administration of local anesthetics by this method results in lower plasma concentrations than those seen when the drugs are administered as regular preparations.[157] The lower plasma concentrations should certainly result in an attenuation of CNS and cardiac toxicity. It will be interesting to see if this new technology will have a significant impact on the clinical use of local anesthetics.

CLINICAL USE OF LOCAL ANESTHETICS

Specific regional anesthetic techniques and blocks are discussed in detail in Chapter 42.

Topical Anesthesia

The application of local anesthetics to the mucous membranes of the nose, mouth, tracheobronchial tree, esophagus, and genitourinary tract can produce satisfactory anesthesia. Local anesthetics used for this purpose are tetracaine (2%), lidocaine (2% to 10%), and cocaine (1% to 5%). Cocaine and lidocaine yield their maximum anesthetic effect in 2 to 5 minutes; the onset of tetracaine is slightly slower, at 3 to 8 minutes. The duration of action of tetracaine (30 to 60 minutes) is longer than that of lidocaine or cocaine (30 to 45 minutes).[158]

Absorption of local anesthetics from the mucous membrane is significant and therefore can result in systemic toxicity. Tetracaine has the most rapid rate of absorption, followed by cocaine and lidocaine, respectively. Peak plasma levels occur 5 minutes after the application of tetracaine or cocaine to the pyriform fossae of the laryngopharynx.[158] The peak plasma level in this study was one third to one half that seen with intravenous bolus infusion. Lidocaine applied to the trachea manifests peak plasma levels in 15 to 20 minutes. However, high peak blood levels can occur after tracheal application of these drugs. This probably occurs because the drugs migrate to the distal airways and alveoli, where a large vascular surface is available for absorption. For example, absorption is faster if the drugs are instilled while the patient is in the erect position rather than in the supine position.[159]

Cocaine is a unique local anesthetic in that it produces vasoconstriction. This action facilitates nasal surgery because it results in shrinking of the mucosa. Cocaine produces vasoconstriction by blocking norepinephrine and epinephrine uptake into the adrenergic nerve ending. This uptake is responsible for the termination of the action of catecholamines. Epinephrine is usually injected shortly after the application of cocaine, setting the stage for a significant drug interaction. Because absorbed cocaine can block the uptake of epinephrine systemically, a toxic effect can result from the injection of epinephrine. This interaction can result in life-threatening ventricular arrhythmias. The possibility is even more significant if the patient is taking other adrenergic uptake blockers, such as tricyclic antidepressants, or catecholamine metabolism blockers, such as monoamine oxidase inhibitors.

Local Infiltration Anesthesia

Local infiltration involves the injection of local anesthetics into tissue in order to block diffuse nerve endings. Most local anesthetics are used for this purpose. The addition of epinephrine almost doubles the duration of action of all the local anesthetics; however, this effect is greater with the short- and intermediate-acing drugs. Also, epinephrine reduces the peak plasma concentration attained by the local anesthetics.

Epinephrine should not be injected around end-arteries, such as are present in the fingers, toes, ear, nose, and penis. A large volume of 1:200,000 solution can be absorbed and can result in significant adrenergic stimulation. Doses of 5 mcg/kg or less are usually safe. This could be harmful to certain patients, such as those with ischemic heart disease or hypertension.

The local anesthetics most often used for infiltration are lidocaine (0.5% to 1%), procaine (0.5% to 1%), and bupivacaine (0.125% to 0.25%). The selection of the drug depends on the duration of anesthesia needed and on the tissue area to be blocked. For example, procaine is used for short procedures, whereas bupivacaine provides anesthesia for longer surgeries. If significant volumes are needed to block large areas, lidocaine and procaine are less likely to result in toxicity than bupivacaine. When injected without epinephrine, 4.5 mg/kg of lidocaine, 7 mg/kg of procaine, or 2.5 mg/kg of bupivacaine is the recommended maximum dose.[160] With the addition of epinephrine, these doses can be increased by one third.

The main disadvantage of local infiltration is that a large volume of local anesthetic must be used for blocking relatively small areas. Also, patients often object to the pain of injection, which may be attenuated by a slow rate of injection and by the alkalization of the local anesthetic. A single-blind study of 42 adult volunteers compared the effect that rate of administration versus buffering has on the pain associated with subcutaneous infiltration of local anesthetics. The findings indicated that the rate of injection had a greater effect on pain than did buffering; even with buffered drugs, rapid injection rates increased pain.[160]

Tumescent liposuction and anesthesia require infiltration of large volumes of crystalloids or "wetting" solution subcutaneously. Wetting solutions are used to facilitate fat suctioning, for their local anesthesia effect and to decrease blood loss. These solutions commonly contain lidocaine 0.05% to 0.1% (0.5-1 mg/ml) and epinephrine 0.5 to 1.5 mg/L. Many surgeons also add sodium bicarbonate to increase absorption, speed onset, and decrease pain of infiltration. Steroids such as triamcinolone may also be added to decrease scarring and aid healing. Even though these are dilute solutions, large amounts of local may be absorbed. Fortunately the epinephrine slows absorption, and the peak plasma levels of lidocaine are within normal ranges. Intravenous fluid administration with these techniques should be limited. A reasonable goal is two times the volume of aspirate. Intravenous fluids and wetting solution are counted in the total fluids.[161,162]

Nerve Block Anesthesia

Injection of local anesthetics around peripheral nerves or plexuses can provide anesthesia for a large area, obviating the need for excessive doses or volumes.

Many clinicians classify nerve blocks as major or minor. *Minor nerve blocks* refer to anesthesia for individual nerves, such as the ulnar and median nerves at the elbow. Major nerve blocks produce anesthesia for two or more nerves that supply large areas. Analgesia of the brachial plexuses, which innervate the arms, is an excellent example of a major nerve block. This classification of nerve block is important, because it influences many local anesthetic parameters.

Most local anesthetics manifest a rapid onset of action in all minor nerve blocks. This occurs because minor nerves are single nerves that have limited diffusion barriers for local anesthetics. The duration of action with these blocks is similar to those seen with local infiltration. Also, the addition of epinephrine prolongs the duration of block provided by all the drugs to an extent similar to that of local infiltration. The duration of block with epinephrine varies from 30 to 60 minutes with chloroprocaine to 240 to 480 minutes with bupivacaine.[163] Toxicity is usually not a problem because of the small volumes (5 to 20 ml) and concentrations required for minor nerve blocks. Chloroprocaine, lidocaine, and bupivacaine, which represent the three potency or duration groups, are usually selected for these blocks. The selection is dependent on the duration of the anesthesia required.

Major nerve blocks differ from minor nerve blocks in that they usually require a higher concentration of local anesthetic and in that their time of onset can vary significantly. For example, the onset time for major blocks with lidocaine or mepivacaine is 7 minutes; in contrast, with bupivacaine, 23 minutes is required.[164] Differences most likely exist because of the greater diffusion barriers of the larger nerves. As a result, latency of onset becomes dependent on the factors that influence the diffusion of drug through tissues, such as the ionization state.

If an appropriate concentration is used, the duration of major nerve blocks is the same as or longer than that observed with minor nerve blocks. Epinephrine prolongs major blocks with all anesthetics; however, it has a smaller effect with local anesthetics that have a longer duration of action, such as bupivacaine, ropivacaine, etidocaine, and levobupivacaine. A significant variation exists in the duration of a brachial plexus block when compared with other conduction blocks. For example, bupivacaine can produce a brachial plexus block that lasts from 4 to 30 hours.[163]

Spinal Anesthesia

Spinal anesthesia is currently conducted with bupivacaine, lidocaine, or tetracaine combined with analgesics such as fentanyl or sufentanil. Tetracaine is usually administered as a hyperbaric solution obtained by mixing 2 ml of 1% solution with 2 ml of 10% dextrose. Hypobaric solutions can be obtained by mixing the tetracaine with sterile water to yield a 0.1% solution. Isobaric solutions are acquired by mixing 20 mg of tetracaine crystals with cerebrospinal fluid. The use of the latter two formulations is indicated for specific surgical procedures. Tetracaine provides approximately 75 to 150 minutes of anesthesia; the duration can be increased by 50% with the addition of 0.2 to 0.3 mg of epinephrine.

The mixture of bupivacaine (0.75%) and dextrose 8.25% results in a hyperbaric solution. Bupivacaine is similar to tetracaine in that it is indicated for surgical procedures lasting 2 to 2.5 hours. However, some clinicians believe that bupivacaine may produce less hypotension and may better obliterate tourniquet pain in orthopedic procedures of the lower extremities.[164] It has largely replaced tetracaine as the most widely used spinal anesthetic drug. Epinephrine prolongs the duration of action of bupivacaine as it does tetracaine.[165]

Lidocaine has the fastest onset and the shortest duration of action when compared with the other two drugs. The hyperbaric from of the drug usually is mixed as a 5% concentration in 7.5% dextrose. The duration of anesthesia usually is 30 to 90 minutes.[165] Epinephrine also significantly increases the duration of action of this drug. Lidocaine is generally indicated for short procedures.

Transient neurologic symptoms (TNSs) have been reported commonly after the use of lidocaine for spinal anesthesia.[166-168] Risk factors include lidocaine spinal anesthesia, lithotomy position, and outpatient procedures, especially knee arthroscopy. Avoidance of lidocaine in these situations is justified. Symptoms include a burning. aching, cramplike, and radiating pain in the anterior and posterior aspect of the thighs. Half of affected patients report that the pain radiates to the lower extremities, and lower back pain is common. Symptoms occur within 12 to 24 hours after surgery and resolve within several hours to 4 days. Treatment is supportive and should include nonsteroidal anti-inflammatory agents. This transient syndrome is completely sensory in nature and has no motor involvement and can therefore be differentiated from more serious abnormalities such as epidural hematoma, cauda equina syndrome, and nerve root damage.[169]

Epidural Anesthesia

Almost all local anesthetics can be used for epidural anesthesia. However, clinicians avoid tetracaine and procaine because of their long latency of onset. The intermediate-acting local anesthetics have a duration of 1 to 2 hours. The long-acting drugs produce anesthesia for 3 to 5 hours.[163] Epinephrine significantly prolongs the duration of the intermediate-acting agents but has little effect on the long-acting drugs. In addition, it has been postulated that clonidine might prolong the duration of action of local anesthetics by a mechanism similar to that observed with epinephrine. Studies show that clonidine reduces local blood flow, and the decrease in blood flow correlates with the injected dose. Higher doses were needed (300 mcg), and this reduction may be relevant only at the higher doses.[165] The onset is 5 to 15 minutes with all the drugs except bupivacaine, which has a longer onset of 10 to 20 minutes. Bupivacaine (0.25% and 0.5%) produces a good sensory block but has minimal effect on motor function. This makes it an ideal drug for obstetric anesthesia. Ropivacaine has been successfully used for epidural anesthesia; however, it is less potent than bupivacaine, which likely accounts for a reduced motor block.[103] Etidocaine (1% to 1.5%) produces adequate analgesia and a profound motor block; therefore this drug is not used in obstetric anesthesia.

Prolonged Administration

It is common in clinical practice to administer local anesthetics by continuous infusion for several days after surgery or for weeks during treatment of chronic pain. It has been noted that administration of local anesthetics by continuous infusion can result in the attenuation of effectiveness. Also, it has been demonstrated that allowing pain to return between bolus epidural injections results in attenuation of intensity and duration of the block. Animal studies have indicated that the mechanism for the tolerance associated with local anesthetics probably has both a pharmacokinetic and pharmacodynamic component. For example, repeated injections of the sciatic nerve in rats result in a lower intraneural lidocaine content and a shorter duration of block (pharmacokinetic). Tachyphylaxis in rats is associated with hyperalgesia, indicating a pharmacodynamic component.[170,171]

SUMMARY

Local anesthetic techniques are becoming more commonplace in outpatient procedures, obstetrics, and pain services. The nurse anesthetist must thoroughly understand the pharmacologic properties of local anesthetics in order to administer and manage local, topical, and regional anesthesia appropriately. For example, this knowledge is important in the selection of a drug with an appropriate dose, concentration, time to onset, and duration of action for a selected regional technique.

Local anesthetics are drugs used for blocking the conduction of nerve impulses. They accomplish this primarily by blocking Na^+ channels on the cytoplasmic side of the axolemma. To do this, they must diffuse through tissue barriers. These include the supportive structures within the nerve trunk, such as the endoneurium, perineurium, and epineurium.

Different local anesthetics have similar chemical structures: they have an aromatic ring, an intermediate carbon chain, and an amine moiety. However, the structures differ with respect to the type of boundary that connects the aromatic ring to the carbon chain and because of substitutions on the amine and aromatic ends of the molecules. These structural differences can make a significant difference in the time to onset, duration, and potency, as well as the site and rate of metabolism, of these drugs. Therefore, the chemical structure is a primary determinant of which drug is selected in a given clinical situation.

Local anesthetics can be inadvertently injected intravascularly or can be absorbed systemically in quantities large enough to produce significant effects on the CNS and the cardiovascular system. In the CNS they produce depression that can result in seizures and coma. Cardiovascular toxicity may also be problematic. Manifestations of cardiovascular toxicity are myocardial depression, cardiac conduction abnormalities, and vasodilation, which can result in cardiovascular collapse and cardiac arrest. Toxicity can be prevented through the avoidance of intravascular injection and the administration of appropriate doses. Less common forms of toxicity are allergic reactions, local tissue effects, and methemoglobinemia.

Local anesthetics can be used topically, as well as for local infiltration, nerve block, spinal anesthesia, and epidural anesthesia. Onset, duration, concentration, dose, and rate of absorption vary significantly with the site of anesthesia and with the local anesthetic administered.

REFERENCES

1. Koster J. Passive membrane properties of the neuron. In: Kandel ER, ed: *Principles of Neural Sciences*. Norwalk, Conn: Appleton & Lange; 1991:3.
2. Skidmore RA. Local anesthetics. *Dermatol Surg*. 1996;22:511-522.
3. Guyton AC, Hall JE. *Textbook of Medical Physiology*. 10th ed. Philadelphia: Saunders; 2000:62-65.
4. Jaffe RA, Rowe MA. Differential nerve block. Direct measurements on individual myelinated and unmyelinated dorsal root axons. *Anesthesiology*. 1996;84:1455-1464.
5. Wildsmith JAW. Peripheral nerve and local anesthetic drugs. *Br J Anaesth*. 1986;58:692-699.
6. Guyton AC, Hall JE. *Textbook of Medical Physiology*. 10th ed. Philadelphia: Saunders; 2000:52-59.
7. Stevens CE. The neuron. *Sci Am*. 1979;241:55.
8. Tetzlaff JE: *Clinical Pharmacology of Local Anesthetics*. Boston: Butterworth-Heinemann; 2000.
9. Guyton AC, Hall JE. *Textbook of Medical Physiology*. 10th ed. Philadelphia: Saunders; 2000:44-45.
10. de Jong RH. *Local Anesthesia*. Springfield, Ill: Charles C Thomas; 1994:65-66, 82-84.
11. Singer SJ, Nicolson GL. The fluid mosaic model of the structure of cell membranes. *Science*. 1972;175:723.
12. Ragsdale DS, McPhee JC, Scheuer T, Catterall WA. Common molecular determinants of local anesthetic, antiarrhythmic, and anticonvulsant block of voltage-gated Na^+ channels. *Proc Natl Acad Sci U S A*. 1996;93:9270-9275.
13. Butterworth JF, Strichartz GR. Molecular mechanisms of local anesthesia: a review. *Anesthesiology*. 1990;72:711.
14. Power I, Kam P. *Principles of Physiology for the Anaesthetist*. London: Arnold; 2001:1-15.
15. Ragsdale DS, McPhee JC, Scheuer T, Catterall WA. Molecular determinants of state-dependent block of Na^+ channels by local anesthetics. *Science*. 1997;265:1724-1728.
16. Starmer CF, Grant AO, Strauss HC. Mechanisms of use-dependent block of sodium channels in excitable membranes by local anesthetics. *Biophys J*. 1984;46:15.
17. Huang LYM, Elarenstein G. Local anesthetic QX-572 and benzocaine act at separate sites on the batrachotoxin-activated sodium channel. *J Physiol*. 1981;77:137-153.
18. Wynn RL. Recent research on mechanisms of local anesthetics. *Gen Dent*. 1995;4:316-318.
19. Franz DN, Perry RS. Mechanism for differential block among single myelinated and nonmyelinated axons by procaine. *J Physiol (Lond)*. 1973;236:193.
20. Rosenburg PH, Heavner JE. Temperature dependent nerve blocking action of lidocaine and halothane. *Acta Anaesthesiol Scand*. 1980;24:324.
21. Bromage PR. *Epidural Anesthesia*. Philadelphia: Saunders; 1978:525.
22. Truant AP. Differential physical-chemical and neuropharmacologic properties of local anesthetic agents. *Anesth Analg*. 1959;38:478-484.
23. Gasser HS, Erlanger J. The role of fiber size in the establishment of nerve block by pressure or cocaine. *Am J Physiol*. 1929;88:581-591.
24. Collins WF, Nulsen FE, Randt CT. Relation of peripheral nerve fiber size and sensation in man. *Arch Neurol*. 1960;3:381-385.
25. Raymond SA, Gissen AJ. Mechanisms of differential nerve block. In: Strichartz GR, ed. *Local Anesthetics*. Berlin: Springer-Verlag; 1987:95.
26. Gissen A, Covino B, Gregus J. Differential sensitivity of fast and slow fibers in mammalian nerve. II. Margin of safety for nerve transmission. *Anesth Analg*. 1982;61:7:561-569.
27. Given BG. Pharmacology of local anesthetic agents. *Br J Anaesth*. 1986;58:701.
28. Gissen AJ, Given BG, Groggiest JP. Differential sensitivity of mammalian nerves to local anesthetic drugs. *Anesthesiology*. 1980;53:467.
29. Wildsmith JAW, et al. Differential nerve blocking activity of amino-ester local anesthetics. *Br J Anaesth*. 1985;57:612.
30. Wildsmith JA, Gissen AJ, Gregus J, et al. Differential nerve blockade: esters v. amines and the influence of pK_a. *Br J Anaesth*. 1987;59:379-384.
31. Blair MR. Cardiovascular pharmacology of local anesthetics. *Br J Anaesth*. 1975;47(suppl):247-252.
32. Tucker GT, et al. Binding of amide-type local anesthetics in human plasma: relationships between binding, physiochemical properties, and anesthetic activity. *Anesthesiology*. 1970;33:287.
33. Ritchie JM, Ritchie B, Greengard P. The active structure of local anesthetics. *J Pharmacol Exp Ther*. 1965;150:152.
34. Covino BG, Wildsmith, JA. Clinical pharmacology of local anesthetic agents. In: Cousins MJ, Bridenbaugh PO, eds. *Neural Blockade in Clinical Anesthesia and Management of Pain*. Philadelphia: Lippincott–Raven; 1998:111-144.
35. Covino BG. Pharmacology of local anesthetic agents. *Br J Anaesth*. 1986;58:701-716.
36. Cederholm I, Akerman B, Evers H. Local analgesic and vascular effects of intradermal ropivacaine and bupivacaine in various concentrations with and without addition of adrenaline in man. *Acta Anaesthesiol Scand*. 1994;38:322-327.
37. Scott DB, et al. Factors affecting plasma level of lidocaine and prilocaine. *Br J Anaesth*. 1972;44:1040.
38. Cox B, Durieux ME, Marcus MA. Toxicity of local anaesthetics. *Best Pract Res Clin Anaesthesiol*. 2003;17:111-136.
39. Faccenda KA, Finucane BT. Complications of regional anaesthesia. Incidence and prevention. *Drug Saf*. 2001;24:413-442.
40. Tagariello V, Caporuscio A, De Tommaso O. Mepivacaine: update on an evergreen local anaesthetic. *Minerva Anestesiol*. 2001;67(suppl 1):5-8.
41. Naguib M, Magboul MM, Samarkandi AH, Attia M. Adverse effects and drug interactions associated with local and regional anaesthesia. *Drug Saf*. 1998;18:221-250.
42. Swerdlow M, Jones R. The duration of action of bupivacaine, prilocaine and lidocaine. *Br J Anaesth*. 1970;42:335.
43. Albert J, Tofstrom B. Bilateral ulnar blocks in the evaluation of local anaesthetic agents. *Acta Anesthesiol Scand*. 1965;9:203.
44. Eisennach JC, Grice SC, Dewan PM. Epinephrine enhanced analgesia produced by epidural bupivacaine during labor. *Anesth Analg*. 1987;66:467.
45. Sandler AN, Arlander E, Finucane BT, et al. Pharmacokinetics of three does of epidural ropivacaine during hysterectomy and comparison with bupivacaine. *Can J Anaesth*. 1998;45:843-849.
46. Sinclair CJ, Scott DB. Comparison of bupivacaine and etidocaine in extradural blockade. *Br J Anaesth*. 1984;56:147.
47. Neal JM. Effects of epinephrine in local anesthetics on the central and peripheral nervous systems: neurotoxicity and neural blood flow. *Reg Anesth Pain Med*. 2003;28:124-134.

48. Chen TY, Tseng CC, Wang LK, Tsai Ty, Chen BS, Chang CL. The clinical use of small-dose tetracaine spinal anesthesia for transurethral prostatectomy. *Anesth Analg.* 2001;92:1020-1023.
49. Bokesch PM, Raymond SA, Strichartz GR. Dependence of lidocaine potency on pH and PCO_2. *Anesth Analg.* 1987;66:9.
50. Gosteli P, van Gessel E, Gamulin Z. Effects of pH adjustment and carbonation of lidocaine during epidural anesthesia for foot or ankle surgery. *Anesth Analg.* 1995;81:104-149.
51. Nickel PM, Bromage PR, Sherrill DL. Comparison of hydrochloride and carbonated salts of lidocaine for epidural analgesia. *Reg Anesth.* 1986;11:66.
52. Chassard D, Berrada K, Bouletreau P. Alkalinization of local anesthetics: theoretically justified but clinically useless. *Can J Anaesth.* 1996;43:384-393.
53. Ramos G, Pereira E, Simonetti MP. Does alkalinization of 0.75% ropivacaine promote a lumbar peridural block of higher quality? *Reg Anesth Pain Med.* 2001;26:357-362.
54. Peterfreund RA, Datta S, Ostheimer GW. Adjustment of local anesthetic solutions with sodium bicarbonate: laboratory evaluations of alkalization and precipitation. *Reg Anesth.* 1989; 14:265, 270.
55. McKay W, Morris R, Mushlin P. Sodium bicarbonate attenuates pain on skin infiltration with lidocaine with or without epinephrine. *Anesth Analg.* 1987;66:572-574.
56. Christoph RA, et al. Pain reduction in local anesthetic administration through pH buffering. *Ann Emerg Med.* 1988;17:117-120.
57. Navaratnarajah M, Davenport HT. The prolongation of local anaesthetic action with dextran. The effect of molecular weight. *Anesthesia.* 1985;40:259-262.
58. Alkhawajah A, Farag H. The effect of dextran on the pharmacokinetics of lignocaine during epidural anaesthesia. *J Int Med Res.* 1992;20:127-135.
59. Rosenblatt RM, Fung DL. Optional ratio of bupivacaine and dextran for regional anesthesia. *Reg Anesth.* 1979;4:2.
60. Dempsey GA, Barrett PJ, Kirby IJ. Hyaluronidase and peribulbar block. *Br J Anaesth.* 1997;78:671-674.
61. Cunningham ML, Kaplan JA. A rapid onset long acting regional anesthesia technique. *Anesthesiology.* 1974;41:509.
62. Cohen SE, Thurlow A. Comparison of a chloroprocaine-bupivacaine mixture with chloroprocaine and bupivacaine used individually for obstetric epidural analgesia. *Anesthesiology.* 1979;51:288.
63. Reynolds F. Adverse effects of local anaesthetics. *Br J Anaesth.* 1987;59:78-95.
64. Sandler AN, et al. Pharmacokinetics of three doses of epidural ropivacaine during hysterectomy and comparison with bupivacaine. *Can J Anaesth.* 1998;45:843-849.
65. Johnson RF, et al. A comparison of the placental transfer of ropivacaine versus bupivacaine. *Anesth Analg.* 1999;89: 703-708.
66. Santos AC, Karpel B, Nobel G. The placental transfer and fetal effects of levobupivacaine, racemic bupivacaine, and ropivacaine. *Anesthesiology.* 1999;90:6.
67. Lofstrom JB, et al. Lung uptake of lidocaine. *Acta Anesthesiol Scand.* 1978;70:80.
68. Calvo R, Carlos R, Erell S. Effects of disease and acetazolamide on procaine hydrolysis by red cell enzymes. *Clin Pharmacol Ther.* 1980;27:175.
69. Bowill JG, Howie MB. *Clinical Pharmacology for Anaesthetists.* London: Saunders; 1999:157-172.
70. Aitkenhead AR, Rowbotham DJ, Smith G. *Textbook of Anaesthesia.* Edinburgh: Churchill Livingstone; 2001:184-191.
71. Arthur GR. Pharmacokinetics of local anesthetics. *Handbook Exp Pharmacol.* 1987;81:165-186.
72. Smith AR, Hot D, Resano F. Grand mal seizures after 2-chloroprocaine epidural anesthesia in a patient with plasma cholinesterase deficiency. *Anesth Analg.* 1987;66:677.
73. Davis L, Britten JJ, Morgan M. Cholinesterase. Its significance in anaesthetic practice. *Anaesthesia.* 1997;52:244-260.
74. Markham A, Faulds D. Ropivacaine: a review of its pharmacology and therapeutic use in regional anesthesia. *Drugs.* 1996;52: 429-449.
75. Tucker GT, et al. Hepatic clearance of local anesthetics in man. *J Pharmacokinet Biopharm.* 1977;5:111.
76. Longnecker DE, Murphy FL. *Introduction to Anesthesia.* Philadelphia: Saunders; 1992:204.
77. Tucker GT, et al. Hepatic clearance of local anesthetics in man. *J Pharmacokinet Biopharm.* 1977;5:111.
78. Thompson PD, et al. Lidocaine pharmacokinetics in advanced heart failure, liver disease and renal failure in humans. *Ann Intern Med.* 1973;78:499.
79. Nakayama M, Yamamoto J, Ichinose H, Yamamoto S, Kanaya N, Namiki A. Effects of volume and concentration of lidocaine on epidural anaesthesia in pregnant females. *Eur J Anaesthesiol.* 2002;19:808-811.
80. Fagraeus L, Urban BJ, Bromage PR. Spread of analgesia in early pregnancy. *Anesthesiology.* 1983;58:184.
81. Datta S, et al. The effect of pregnancy on bupivacaine induced conduction blockade in the rabbit vagus nerve. *Anesth Analg.* 1987;66:123.
82. Datta S, et al. Differential sensitivities of mammalian nerve fibers during pregnancy. *Anesth Analg.* 1983;62:1070.
83. McCaughey W. Adverse effects of local anesthetics. *Drug Saf.* 1992;77:74-78.
84. Scott DB. Evaluation of the toxicity of local anaesthetic agents in man. *Br J Anaesth.* 1975;47:56.
85. Scott DB. Toxic effects of local anaesthetic agents on central nervous system. *Br J Anaesth.* 1986;58:732.
86. Graf BM. The cardiotoxicity of local anesthetics: the place of ropivacaine. *Curr Top Med Chem.* 2001;1:207-214.
87. Liu PL, et al. Comparative CNS toxicity of lidocaine, endocaine, bupivacaine and tetracaine in awake dogs following rapid IV administration. *Anesth Analg.* 1973;62:375.
88. Englesson S. The influence of acid-base changes on central nervous system toxicity of local anesthetic agents: an experimental study in cats. *Acta Anaesthesiol Scand.* 1974;18:79.
89. Covino BG. Clinical pharmacology of local anesthetic agents. In: Cousins MJ, Bridenbaugh PO, eds. *Neural Blockade in Clinical Anesthesia and Management of Pain.* Philadelphia: Lippincott; 1998:100-105.
90. Covina BG. Toxicity of local anesthetics. *Adv Anesth.* 1986;3:37.
91. Johns RA, DiFazio CA, Longnecker DE. Lidocaine constricts or dilates rat arterioles in a dose-dependent manner. *Anesthesiology.* 1985;62:141.
92. Gristwood RW. Cardiac and CNS toxicity of levobupivacaine: strengths of evidence for advantage over bupivacaine. *Drug Saf.* 2002;25:153-163.
93. Feldman HS, Covino BM, Sage DJ. Direct chronotropic and inotropic effects of local anesthetic agents in isolated guinea pig atria. *Reg Anesth.* 1982;7:149.
94. Mather LE, Chang DH. Cardiotoxicity with modern local anaesthetics: is there a safer choice? *Drugs.* 2001;61:333-342.
95. Till R, et al. Acute cardiovascular toxicity of procaine, chloroprocaine and tetracaine anesthetized ventilated dogs. *Reg Anesth.* 1982;7:14.
96. Mulroy MF. Systemic toxicity and cardiotoxicity from local anesthetics: incidence and preventive measures. *Reg Anesth Pain Med.* 2002;27:556-561.
97. Morishima HO, et al. Is bupivacaine more cardiotoxic than lidocaine? *Anesthesiology.* 1983;59:A409.
98. Morishima HO, et al. Etidocaine toxicity in the adult, newborn, and fetal sheep. *Anesthesiology.* 1981;58:342.
99. Davis ML, de Jong RH. Successful resuscitation following massive bupivacaine overdose. *Anesth Analg.* 1982;61:62-64.
100. Albright GA. Cardiac arrest following regional anesthesia with etidocaine and bupivacaine. *Anesthesiology.* 1979;51: 285.

101. Heavner JE. Cardiac toxicity of local anesthetics in the intact isolated heart model: a review. *Reg Anesth Pain Med.* 2002;27: 545-555.
102. Graf BM. The cardiotoxicity of local anesthetics: the place of ropivacaine. *Curr Top Med Chem.* 2001;1:207-214.
103. Polley LS, et al. Relative analgesic potencies of ropivacaine and bupivacaine for epidural analgesia in labor. *Anesthesiology.* 1999;90:944-950.
104. Chan VWS, et al. Comparison of ropivacaine and lidocaine for intravenous regional anesthesia in volunteers. *Anesthesiology.* 1999;90:1602-1608.
105. Kopaz DJ, Allen HW. Accidental intravenous levobupivacaine. *Anesth Analg.* 1999;89:1027-1029.
106. Tetzlaff J. Local anesthesia: are the new agents any better? *Audio Digest Anesthesiol.* 2002;44:4.
107. Crandall JT, Kotelks DM. Cardiotoxicity of local anesthetics during pregnancy. *Anesth Analg.* 1985;61:60.
108. Morishima HO, et al. Bupivacaine toxicity in pregnant and non-pregnant ewes. *Anesthesiology.* 1985;63:134.
109. Sage DJ, et al. Influence of bupivacaine and lidocaine on isolated guinea pig atria in the presence of acidosis and hypoxia. *Anesth Analg.* 1984;63:1.
110. Malamed SF. Allergy and toxic reactions to local anesthetics. *Dent Today.* 2003;22:114-116, 118-121.
111. Finder RL, Moore PA. Adverse drug reactions to local anesthesia. *Dent Clin North Am.* 2002;46:747-757.
112. Tetzlaff JE. *Clinical Pharmacology of Local Anesthetics.* Boston: Butterworth-Heinemann; 2000:47-52.
113. Aldrete AJ, Johnson AA. Evaluation of ventracutaneous testing for investigation of allergy to local anesthetic agents. *Anesth Analg.* 1970;49:173.
114. Eggleston ST, Lush LW. Understanding allergic reactions to local anesthetic. *Ann Pharmacother.* 1996;30:851-857.
115. Nagel JE, Fuscaldo JT, Fireman R. Paraben allergy. *JAMA.* 1977;237:1594.
116. Climic CR, et al. Methaemoglobinemia in mothers and fetus following continuous epidural analgesia with prilocaine. *Br J Anesth.* 1967;30:195.
117. Law RMT, et al. Measurement of methemoglobin after EMLA analgesia for newborn circumcision. *Biol Neonate.* 1996;70: 213-217.
118. Frey B, Kehrer B. Toxic methaemoglobin concentrations in premature infants after application of a prilocaine-containing cream and peridural prilocaine. *Eur J Pediatr.* 1999;158:785-788.
119. Gupta PM, Deepa SL, Edwawrd LA. Benzocaine-induced methemoglobinemia. *South Med J.* 2000;93;1:83-86.
120. Gissen AJ, Datta S, Lambert D. The chloroprocaine controversy: is chloroprocaine neurotoxic? *Reg Anaesth.* 1984;9:135.
121. Wang DC, et al. Chronic neurological deficits and Nesacaine-C—an effect of the anesthetic, 2-chloroprocaine, or the antioxidant, sodium bisulfite? *Anesth Analg.* 1984;63:445-447.
122. Ford DJ, Raj DR. Peripheral neurotoxicity of 2-chloroprocaine and bisulfite in the cat. *Anesth Analg.* 1987;66:719.
123. Feinstein MB, Lenard W, Mathias J. The antagonism of local anesthetic induced convulsions by the benzodiazepine derivative diazepam. *Arch Intern Pharmacodyn Ther.* 1970;187: 144-154.
124. Wesseling H, Bovenhorst GH, Wier JW. Effects of diazepam and pentobarbitone on convulsions induced by local anesthetics in mice. *Eur J Pharmacol.* 1971;1:150-154.
125. Rosen M, et al. Bupivacaine-induced cardiotoxicity in hypoxic and acidotic sleep. *Anesth Analg.* 1985;64:491.
126. Kasten GW, Martin ST. Successful cardiovascular resuscitation after massive intravenous bupivacaine overdosage in anesthetized dogs. *Anesth Analg.* 1985;64:491.
127. Reynolds F. Ropivacaine. *Anesthesiology.* 1991;46:339.
128. Wang GK. Binding affinity and stereoselectivity of local anesthetics in single batrachotoxin-activated sodium channels. *J Gen Physiol.* 1990;96:105.
129. Bader AM, et al. Comparison of bupivacaine- and ropivacaine-induced conduction blockade in the isolated rabbit vagus nerve. *Anesth Analg.* 1989;68:724.
130. Polley LS, et al. Is ropivacaine less potent than bupivacaine? *Anesthesiology.* 1999;90:941-943.
131. Ritz S, Haggmark S, Johansson G. Cardiotoxicity of ropivacaine: a new amide local anesthetic. *Acta Anaesthesiol Scand.* 1989;33:93.
132. Hurley RJ, et al. The effects of epinephrine on the anesthetic and hemodynamic properties of ropivacaine and bupivacaine after epidural administration in the dog. *Reg Anesth.* 1991;16:303.
133. Feldman HS, Arthur GR, Covino BG. Comparative systemic toxicity of convulsant and supraconvulsant doses of ropivacaine, bupivacaine, and lidocaine in the conscious dog. *Anesth Analg.* 1989;69:794.
134. Rutten AJ, et al. Hemodynamic and central effects of intravenous bolus doses of lidocaine, bupivacaine, and ropivacaine in sheep. *Anesth Analg.* 1989;69:291.
135. Feldman HS, et al. Treatment of acute systemic toxicity after the rapid intravenous injection of ropivacaine and bupivacaine in the conscious dog. *Anesth Analg.* 1991;73:373.
136. Stienstra R. The place of ropivacaine in anesthesia. *Acta Anaesthesiol Belg.* 2003;54:141-148.
137. McClellan KJ, Faulds D. Ropivacaine: an update of its use in regional anaesthesia. *Drugs.* 2002;60:1065-1093.
138. Owen MD, Dean LS. Ropivacaine. *Expert Opin Pharmacother.* 2002;1:325-336.
139. Scott BD, et al. Acute toxicity of ropivacaine compared with that of bupivacaine. *Anesth Analg.* 1989;69:563.
140. Pollock JE. Local anesthetic toxicity. *Audio Digest Anesthesiol.* 2003;45:11.
141. Gunter JB, et al. Levobupivacaine for ilioinguinal/iliohypogastric nerve block in children. *Anesth Analg.* 1999;89:647-649.
142. McClellan KJ, Spencer CM. Levobupivacaine. *Drugs.* 1998;56: 355-362.
143. Markham A, Faulds D. Ropivacaine: a review of its pharmacology and therapeutic use in regional anaesthesia. *Drugs.* 1996;52:429-449.
144. Foster RH, Markham A. Levobupivacaine: a review of its pharmacology and use as a local anaesthetic. *Drug.* 2000;59;3:551-579.
145. Stewart J, Kellett N, Castro D. The central system and cardiovascular effects of levobupivacaine and ropivacaine in healthy volunteers. *Anesth Analg.* 2003;97;412-416.
146. Lacassie HJ, Columb MO, Laccie HP, Lantadilla RA. The relative motor blocking potencies of epidural bupivacaine and ropivacaine in labor. *Anesth Analg.* 2002;95:204-208.
147. Polley LS, Columb MO, Naughton NN, et al. Relative analgesic potencies of ropivacaine and bupivacaine for epidural analgesia in labor: implications for therapeutics indexes. *Anesthesiology.* 1999;90:944-950.
148. Panni M, Segal S. New local anesthetics. Are they worth the cost? *Anesthesiol Clin North Am.* 2003;21:19-38.
149. Robieux I, et al. Assessing pain and analgesia with a lidocaine/prilocaine emulsion in infants and toddlers during venipuncture. *J Pediatr.* 1991;118:970.
150. EMLA [package insert]. Westboro, Mass: Astra Pharmaceutical Products; 1993.
151. Goede IA, Betcher DL. EMLA. *J Pediatr Oncol Nurs.* 1994;11:38.
152. Ohlsen C, Englesson S, Evers H. An anesthetic lidocaine/prilocaine cream (EMLA) for epicutaneous applications tested for cutting split skin grafts. *Scand J Plast Reconstr Surg.* 1985;19:201.
153. Jokobson B, Nilsson A. Methemoglobinemia associated with a prilocaine/lidocaine cream and trimethoprim/sulfamethoxazole: a case report. *Acta Anaesthesiol Scand.* 1985;29:453.
154. Grant S, Hoffman RS. Use of tetracaine, epinephrine, and cocaine as a topical anesthetic in the emergency department. *Ann Emerg Med.* 1992;21:987.
155. Strichartz GR, Berde CB. Local anesthetics. In: Miller RD, ed. *Anesthesia.* 5th ed. New York: Churchill Livingstone; 2000: 508-509.

156. Smith G, et al. New non–cocaine-containing topical anesthetics compared with tetracaine-adrenaline-cocaine during repair of lacerations. *Pediatrics*. 1997;100:825.
157. Jeffrey JM, et al. Extended duration nerve blockade using large unilamellar vesicles that exhibit a proton gradient. *Anesthesiology*. 1996;85:635.
158. Astrom A, Persson NH. The toxicity of some local anesthetics after application on different mucous membranes and its relation to anesthetic action on the nasal mucosa of the rabbit. *J Pharmacol Exp Ther*. 1961;132:87.
159. Scarfone RJ, Jasani M, Gracely EJ. Pain of local anesthetics: rate of administration and buffering. *Ann Emerg Med*. 1998;31:36-40.
160. Campbell D, Adriani I. Absorption of local anesthetics. *JAMA*. 1958;168:873.
161. Strichartz GR, Berde CB. Local anesthetics. In: Miller RD, ed. *Anesthesia*. 5th ed. New York: Churchill Livingstone; 2000: 491-522.
162. Morell RC. What the anesthesiologist needs to know about tumescent anesthesia. *Audio Digest Anesthesiol*. 2002;44:10.
163. Bromage PR, Geriel M. An evaluation of two new local anesthetics for major conduction blockade. *Can J Anesth*. 1970;17:55.
164. Concepcion MA, et al. Tourniquet pain during spinal anesthesia: a comparison of plain solutions of tetracaine and bupivacaine. *Anesth Analg*. 1988;67:828.
165. Mazoit JX, et al. Clonidine and or adrenaline decrease lidocaine plasma peak concentration after epidural injection. *Br J Clin Pharmacol*. 1996;42:242-245.
166. Phillip J, Sharma SK, Gottumukkala VN, et al. Transient neurologic symptoms after spinal anesthesia with lidocaine in obstetric patients. *Anesth Analg*. 2001;92:405-409.
167. Freedman JM, Li DK, Drasner K, et al. Transient neurologic symptoms after spinal anesthesia: an epidemiologic study of 1863 patients. *Anesthesiology*. 1998;89;633-641.
168. Sime AC. AANA Journal course: transient neurologic symptoms and spinal anesthesia. *AANA J*. 2000;68:163-168.
169. Pollock JE. Transient neurologic symptoms: etiology, risk factors, and management. *Reg Anesth Pain Med*. 2002;27:581-586.
170. Lee KC, et al. Thermal hyperalgesia accelerates and MK-801 prevent the development of tachyphylaxis to rat sciatic nerve blockade. *Anesthesiology*. 1994;81:1284.
171. Choi R, et al. Pharmacokinetic nature of tachyphylaxis to lidocaine: peripheral nerve blocks and infiltration anesthesia in rats. *Life Sc*. 1997;61:177-184.

CHAPTER 10

Opioid Agonists and Antagonists

Wanda O. Wilson

HISTORY

In the past opium was used as a topical, an intravenous, and an inhaled analgesic. One of the earliest uses of opium is found in the Greek literature dating from 300 BCE. Opium sponges, referred to as *soporific sponges*, were used for the control of pain as early as the fourteenth century. An attempt to administer opioids by the intravenous route was attributed to Elscholtz in 1665, approximately 200 years before the invention of the syringe and needle. The first attempt to administer an opium vapor by inhalation was documented in 1778. It was not until 1853, when the syringe and needle were introduced into clinical practice by Wood, that an accurate dose of opioid could be administered intravenously.

In 1803 Sertürner reported the isolation of a pure substance from opium that he named morphine, after Morpheus, the Greek god of dreams. Abuse of opium and isolated alkaloids led to the synthetic production of potent analgesics. Other opium alkaloids were soon discovered—codeine by Robiquet in 1832 and papaverine by Merck in 1848. The goal of the synthetic manufacture of analgesics was the creation of potent analgesics that would have high specificity for receptors, were not addictive, and were free of side effects. Synthetic production led to the development of opioid agonists, partial agonists, agonists-antagonists, and antagonists.

Opioid is a term used to refer to a group of drugs, both naturally occurring and synthetically produced, that possess opium- or morphine-like properties. Opioids exert their effects by mimicking naturally occurring substances, endogenous opioid peptides or endorphins. The term *narcotic* is derived from the Greek word for stupor and refers to potent morphine-like analgesics with potential to produce dependence. The term *narcotic* is not useful in a pharmacologic or clinical discussion because of its legal connotations.

At least four systems of classification are used to describe opioids. The first divides the opioids into four categories: agonists, partial agonists, agonists-antagonists, and antagonists (Table 10-1). A second descriptive classification separates the opioids into classes according to their lipophilicity. Another system of categorization is based on the chemical derivation of the opioids and divides them into naturally occurring, semisynthetic, and synthetic compounds, with each group having subgroups (Box 10-1). A final simple classification system describes the drugs as either weak or strong.

The term *opioid* is derived from *opium* (*opos*, the Greek word for sap), an extract from the poppy plant, *Papaver somniferum*. The properties of opium are attributable to the 20 different isolated alkaloids, and the alkaloids are divided chemically into two types: phenanthrene (from which morphine and codeine are derived) and benzylisoquinoline (from which papaverine, a nonanalgesic drug, is derived). Modification of the morphine molecule with retention of the five-ring structure results in the semisynthetic drugs heroin and hydromorphone. When the furan ring is removed from morphine, the resulting four-ring synthetic opioid levorphanol is formed. The phenylpiperidines (e.g., meperidine, fentanyl) and the phenylheptylamines (e.g., methadone, propoxyphene) all have only two of the original five rings of the basic morphine molecular structure. A close relationship exists between the stereochemical structure and potency of opioids, with the *levo-* isomers being the most potent.[1] All opioids, despite the diverse molecular structures, share an *N*-methylpiperidine moiety, which seems to confer analgesic activity.[2] Figure 10-1 illustrates the structures of the commonly used opioids.

TABLE 10-1 Opioid Agonists, Partial Agonists, Agonists-Antagonists, and Antagonists at Sites of Activity

Opioid	Mu	Kappa	Delta
Morphine	Agonist	Agonist	Agonist
Meperidine	Agonist	Agonist	Agonist
Fentanyl	Agonist	Agonist	Agonist
Sufentanil	Agonist	Agonist	Agonist
Alfentanil	Agonist	Agonist	Agonist
Remifentanil	Agonist	Agonist	Agonist
Butorphanol	Antagonist	Partial agonist	Agonist
Nalbuphine	Antagonist	Partial agonist	Agonist
Naloxone	Antagonist	Antagonist	Antagonist
Naltrexone	Antagonist	Antagonist	Antagonist
Nalmefene	Antagonist	Antagonist	Antagonist

Opioid drugs produce pharmacologic activity by binding to opiate receptors primarily located in the central nervous system (CNS), supraspinal and spinal; however, evidence of sites outside the CNS, such as peripheral sites, has emerged.[3] Supraspinal analgesia occurs through activation of postsynaptic opioid receptors in the medulla and midbrain, which causes inhibition of neurons involved in pain pathways via increased flux of potassium ions. Spinal analgesia occurs by activation of presynaptic opioid receptors, which leads to decreased calcium influx and decreased release of neurotransmitters involved in nociception. Clinically, supraspinal and spinal opioid analgesic

BOX 10-1

Classification of Opioids Based on Derivation of Drug

Naturally Occurring Opium Alkaloids

Phenanthrene derivatives
- Morphine
- Codeine

Benzylisoquinoline derivatives

Papaverine

Semisynthetic Derivatives of Opium Alkaloids

Morphine derivatives
- Oxymorphone
- Hydromorphone
- Heroin

Thebain derivatives
- Buprenorphine
- Oxycodone

Synthetic Opioids

Morphinans
- Levorphanol
- Nalbuphine

Phenylheptylamines
- Methadone
- Propoxyphene

Phenylpiperidine
- Alfentanil
- Fentanyl
- Naloxone
- Naltrexone
- Meperidine
- Sufentanil
- Remifentanil

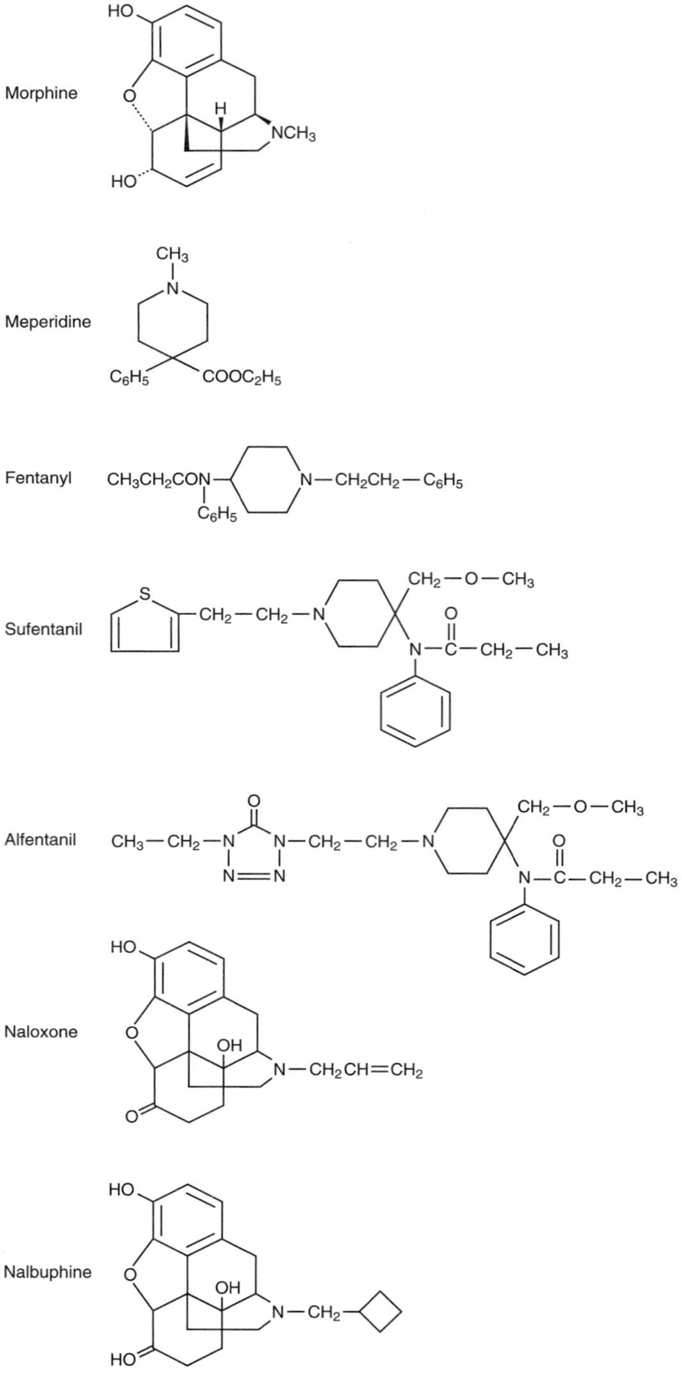

FIGURE **10-1**
Selected opioid agonists and antagonists used as anesthesia adjunct drugs.

mechanisms are synergistic.[4] This explains why opioids such as fentanyl and sufentanil produce more profound analgesia when delivered epidurally than when delivered systemically despite the similar blood concentrations measured with both routes of administration.[2,5]

Inflammatory hyperalgesic conditions appear to be especially amenable to peripheral opioid antinociceptive actions.[4] The mechanism of peripheral actions appears to be activation of opioid receptors located on primary afferent nerves.

Opiate Receptors

The discovery of opioid receptors can be traced back to the 1940s and 1950s, when pharmaceutical companies were involved in research in anticipation of the development of an effective nonaddictive analgesic. In 1973 the examination of vertebrate species led to the discovery of three opiate receptor classes that mediate analgesia.[3] Questions emerged as to why the receptors existed, and further research led to the hypothesis that the receptors possess endogenous functions.

After the discovery of opiate receptors in the early 1970s, the search began for endogenous substances that were their agonists. In 1975 three such agonists were identified: enkephalins, endorphins, and dynorphins.[3] Each group is derived from a distinct precursor polypeptide and has a characteristic anatomic distribution. By the early 1980s three precursor molecules to these agonists were identified and named after the active fragments: proenkephalin, pro–adrenocorticotropic hormone (ACTH)–endorphin (also called *proopiomelanocortin*), and prodynorphin.[2,3] Opioid peptides share the common amino-terminal sequence of Try-Gly-Gly-Phe-(Met or Leu), which has been labeled the *opioid motif* or *message* and is necessary for interaction at the receptor site.[2] The peptide selectivity resides in the carboxy-terminal extension, providing the *address*.[2] In 1975 Hughes and Kosterlitz identified the first endogenous substance with opioid activity.

Martin and co-workers[6] were the first to provide evidence for opiate receptor subtypes (Table 10-2). Their findings provided evidence for the existence of three opiate receptors: mu, kappa, and sigma, named after their respective agonists—morphine, ketocyclazocine, and SK&F 10047. Each major opioid receptor has a unique anatomic distribution in the brain, spinal cord, and periphery.[7]

Stimulation of the mu receptor produces supraspinal analgesia, euphoria, and a decrease in ventilation. Studies of mu receptor subtypes revealed that the mu-1 subtype mediates analgesia and the mu-2 subtype mediates ventilatory depression, bradycardia, and dependence. Kappa stimulation produces spinal analgesia, sedation, and miosis. Currently, kappa-opioid drugs are being investigated for antiinflammatory actions that reduce disease severity of arthritis in a dose-dependent manner.[8] Sigma stimulation is responsible for an increase in ventilation, motor movement, and hallucinations. The delta receptor, discovered later, is responsible for spinal analgesia, responds to enkephalins, and serves to modulate activity of the mu receptors.[9] Evidence supports the existence of three kappa and two delta receptor subtypes.[3] Because sigma receptor stimulation produces effects so different from that of the opiate receptors and its effects cannot be reversed by antagonists, the sigma receptor is no longer considered an opiate receptor.

At the cellular level, endogenous peptides and exogenous opioids produce effects by altering patterns of interneuronal communications. Receptor binding initiates a series of physiologic functions that result in cellular hyperpolarization and inhabitation of neurotransmitter release, effects that are mediated by second messengers.[9] All opioid receptors appear to be coupled to G-proteins,[1] which regulate the activity of adenylate cyclase as well as performing other functions. G-protein interactions affect ion channels. Mu opioid receptors are coupled to potassium conductance, and activation increases potassium conductance, which inhibits neurotransmitter release and hyperpolarizes the cell membrane. Delta receptor activation increases potassium conductance and affects voltage-dependent calcium current, whereas kappa opioids appear to inhibit calcium entry through voltage-dependent calcium channels.[4,10]

PHARMACOKINETICS AND PHARMACODYNAMICS

Effects of opioids result from the combination of opioids with one or more receptors at specific tissue sites. The relationship between opioid dose and effects varies with pharmacokinetic and pharmacodynamic characteristics. Pharmacokinetics determines the relationship between drug dose and its concentration at receptor sites and refers to the study of plasma drug concentration versus time. Pharmacodynamics relates to the concentration of the drug at its site of action and the intensity of its effects. Changes in drug concentration over time in the blood, at the effect site and other sites, are determined by physiochemical properties of the drug as well as biologic functions involved in the processes of absorption, redistribution, biotransformation, and elimination.

Clinically, opioids are administered parenterally, even though the drugs are well absorbed from the gastrointestinal (GI) tract. Some opioids undergo extensive first-pass metabolism in the liver, greatly reducing their bioavailability and therapeutic efficacy after oral dosing. The early rapid decline in plasma concentration after the peak is the distribution phase, and the slower decline is the elimination phase. Orally administered morphine has one third the potency of parenterally administered morphine.[11] Drugs with greater lipophilicity are better absorbed through nasal and buccal mucosa and dermis.

TABLE 10-2 Characteristics of Opioid Receptor Subtypes*

	MU RECEPTOR			
Effects	**Mu-1**	**Mu-2**	**Kappa Receptor**	**Delta Receptor**
Analgesia	Supraspinal	Spinal	Supraspinal, spinal	Supraspinal, spinal; modulates mu-receptor activity
Cardiovascular effects	Bradycardia	Bradycardia		
Respiratory effects		Depression	Possible depression	Depression
Central nervous system effects	Euphoria; sedation; prolactin release; hypothermia; catalepsy; indifference to environmental stimulus	Euphoria; dopamine turnover; possible growth hormone release	Sedation; dysphoria; psychotomimetic reactions (hallucinations, delirium)	
Pupil	Miosis	Miosis	Miosis	
Gastrointestinal effects		Inhibition of peristalsis; nausea, vomiting		
Genitourinary effects	Urinary retention	Urinary retention	Diuresis (inhibition of vasopressin release)	Urinary retention
Pruritus		Yes		Yes
Physical dependence	Low abuse potential	Yes	Low abuse potential	Yes

**Other opioid subtypes exist in animals, such as kappa-1, kappa-2, and kappa-3. Mu-1 and mu-2 agonists have not been developed for human use.*

Physiochemical properties of opioids influence both pharmacokinetics and pharmacodynamics. To reach effector sites in the CNS, opioids must cross biologic membranes from the blood to receptors on neural cell membranes. The ability of opioids to cross the blood-brain barrier depends on molecular size, ionization, lipid solubility, and protein binding. The physiochemical characteristics, pharmacokinetic variables, and partition coefficients (octanol and water as a measure of lipid solubility) for several of the commonly used opioid analgesics are summarized in Table 10-3. Pharmacokinetic parameters of opioids vary, in part, according to population and study differences. When the table is reviewed, it is most important to note how the opioids relate to one another. For example, the fact that fentanyl and morphine have similar elimination half-lives can explain how the drugs develop a similar duration of action when high doses of fentanyl are used.

Opioids are usually metabolized to more polar and less active or inactive compounds. Common mechanisms of metabolism include *N*-dealkylation, *O*-demethylation, glucuronidation, and hydrolysis. Some opioids, such as morphine, have active metabolites that can produce the therapeutic effects of the parent compound. Opioid metabolites and parent compounds are excreted primarily by the kidneys and secondarily by the biliary system and the GI tract.

Clinical Effects

Systemic Effects

Potency, speed of onset, and duration of action of the opioid analgesics are the most clinically relevant pharmacodynamic measures. The relative potencies of commonly used opioids, based on acute administration, and are listed in Table 10-4. However, apparent potencies can change over time and can be a function of the route of administration. For example, morphine administered over a long period of time may seem to become more potent as a result of the gradual accumulation of active metabolites.[5] Tolerance usually predominates with any opioid drug and results in a diminishing effect with multiple dosing.

Probably of greatest importance in determining the speed of onset of analgesia of systemically administered analgesics is the gradient between blood and brain tissue. Although other factors, such as percent of free, non-ionized drug in the blood and lipid solubility, appear to play a significant role in the drug entry rate into the CNS, empirically these factors do not correlate with drug onset. For example, alfentanil has a shorter time to onset of drug effect than either fentanyl or morphine. Fentanyl, however, is more than seven times more lipid soluble than alfentanil, and morphine has 16 times more non-ionized free drug available to the CNS for any given dose. Alfentanil's rapid onset is probably the result of its small volume of distribution, which allows a rapid effect-site equilibrium.[4]

TABLE 10-4 Potencies of Opioids

Drug	Relative Potency, IM	Relative Potency, Oral
Morphine	10	30
Meperidine	80	300
Methadone	10	12.5
Fentanyl	0.1	N/A
Butorphanol	2	N/A
Nalbuphine	12	N/A

IM, *intramuscular;* N/A, *not applicable.*

All the opioid agonists have similar clinical effects that vary in some degree from one drug to another. Sedation, respiratory depression, nausea, constipation, cough suppression, euphoria, dysphoria, and miosis are also known dose-dependent effects of the opioid agonists, in addition to analgesia. The commonly produced clinical effects of opioid agonists are given in Box 10-2. Morphine and related opioids affect the central nervous, renal, cardiovascular, GI, and endocrinologic systems.

CNS actions include analgesia, euphoria, respiratory depression, changes in temperature regulation and diuresis, miosis, and nausea. The effect of opioids on electroencephalographic and evoked potential activity is minimal; therefore neurophysiologic monitoring can be conducted during opioid anesthetic techniques. Analgesia results from the activity of morphine at several spinal and supraspinal sites within the CNS (Table 10-5). Nociceptive reflexes and neurotransmitter release are inhibited, and this inhibition produces analgesia.[12]

Most opioids produce miosis by stimulating the autonomic segment of the nucleus of the oculomotor nerve. The respiratory depression produced by opioids is the result of direct depression of the respiratory centers and activation of the mu-2 receptors in the brainstem. Respiratory rate, minute volume, and tidal volume are decreased.

TABLE 10-3 Physicochemical Characteristics and Pharmacokinetics

Opioids	pK_a	Percent Non-ionized	Protein Binding (%)	V_c (L/kg)	V_d (L/kg)	Clearance (ml/min/kg)	Elimination Half-Life (hr)	Partition Coefficient (octanol/water)
Morphine	7.9	23	35	0.23	2.8	15.5	1.7-3.3	1
Meperidine	8.5	7	70	0.6	2.6	22.7	3-5	21
Methadone	9.3	N/A	85	0.15	3.4	1.6	23	115
Fentanyl	8.4	8.5	84	0.85	4	13	2-4	820
Sufentanil	8	20	93	0.1	2	12	2-3	1750
Alfentanil	6.5	89	92	0.12	0.6	5	1-2	130
Remifentanil	7.26	58	93	0.1-0.2	0.39	41	0.1-0.3	N/A
Butorphanol	8.6	17	80	0.1	5	38.6	2.65	140
Nalbuphine	8.71	N/A	N/A	0.45	4.8	23.1	3.7	N/A

N/A, *not applicable;* V_c, *volume of distribution central compartment;* V_d, *volume of distribution.*

BOX **10-2**

Common Clinical Effects of Opioid Agonists

Acute	Chronic
Analgesia	Tolerance
Respiratory depression	Physical dependence
Sedation	Constipation
Euphoria	
Dysphoria	
Vasodilation	
Bradycardia	
Cough suppression	
Miosis	
Nausea and vomiting	
Skeletal muscle rigidity	
Smooth muscle spasm	
Constipation	
Urinary retention	
Biliary spasm	
Pruritus, rash	
Antishivering (meperidine only)	

Opioids can act either as diuretics or as antidiuretics, depending on the opioid receptors stimulated. Opioids that are agonists at kappa receptors cause diuresis, whereas those that are agonists at mu receptors produce an antidiuretic effect. The increase in smooth muscle tone from opioid administration can result in urinary retention because of action on the urinary sphincter. However, with systemic opioids the tone of the detrusor muscle may be enhanced, leading to a sensation of urgency and inability to void.[12] Urinary retention is a common side effect with intrathecal and epidural opioid administration.

Opioids have no major effects on nerve conduction at the neuromuscular junction or at the skeletal muscle membrane. A generalized hypertonus of skeletal muscle can be produced by large intravenous doses of most opioid agonists. Although morphine can produce rigidity, the problem is most often associated with fentanyl, alfentanil, sufentanil, and remifentanil.

TABLE **10-5** Opioid Mediated Analgesia in the Central Nervous System

Central Nervous System Location	Opioid Receptor
Supraspinal	
Periaqueductal gray area	Mu = kappa > delta
Raphe nuclei	
Caudal linear	Kappa
Dorsal	Kappa > mu
Median	Mu > kappa
Magnus	Mu > kappa
Pallidus	Delta
Gigantocellular reticular	Mu = kappa = delta
Spinal	
Spinal cord	Mu = delta = kappa
Dorsal root ganglia	Mu = delta = kappa

The difficulty is caused in part by loss of chest wall compliance and by constriction of pharyngeal and laryngeal muscles. It is commonly referred to as *tight chest* or *truncal rigidity*. Opioid-induced muscle rigidity is thought to be mediated by mu receptors at supraspinal sites, including the nucleus raphe pontis and sites lateral to it in the hindbrain.[9] These effects are reduced or eliminated by an antagonist and by muscle relaxants.

The degree to which opioids affect the cardiovascular system depends on the specific opioid agent used. All opioids induce some degree of peripheral vasodilation and diminish the responses of baroreceptor reflexes. Much of the hypotension produced by morphine is attributed to histamine release, which is absent with meperidine, fentanyl, sufentanil, alfentanil, and remifentanil.[4] $Histamine_1$ antagonists only partially block the vasodilation that results from the administration of morphine. The antagonist naloxone effectively reverses morphine-induced vasodilation. The vasoconstriction response initiated by an increase in the partial pressure of carbon dioxide also is inhibited by morphine.[2] At high doses most opioids produce significant bradycardia via medullary vagal stimulation.[2] An exception is meperidine, which often causes tachycardia as a result of its having a structure similar to that of atropine or via a reflex response to hypotension.[4] Morphine may also cause tachycardia as a reflex to the hypotension that results from the histamine release.[4]

Opioids have several effects on the GI tract in addition to the nausea produced via the CNS. The effects include constipation, nausea, and vomiting. Opioids decrease gastric motility, prolong gastric emptying, and potentially increase the incidence of esophageal reflux. Opioids directly stimulate the chemoreceptor trigger zone, causing nausea in some patients and both nausea and vomiting in others. The use of morphine decreases biliary, pancreatic, and intestinal secretions, leading to delayed digestion of food in the small intestines. Constipation is probably the result of decreased GI transit via mu-2 receptor action both within the brain and in the peripheral nerve plexus.[2]

Other GI effects from the administration of opioids include an increase in tone of smooth muscle sphincters, which results in increased pressure in the common bile duct and constriction of the sphincter of Oddi. Study results are conflicting. One study demonstrated that morphine produced greater biliary spasm than meperidine, whereas another demonstrated no significant differences between morphine and meperidine but found that fentanyl produced larger increases in intrabiliary pressure.[13] Pentazocine has shown less biliary sphincter spasm than any of the other opioids.

Endocrinologic effects of opioids include the release of vasopressin and inhibition of the stress-induced release of corticotropin and of gonadotropins from the pituitary. Release of thyrotropin from the adenohypophysis is also inhibited. Basal metabolic rate and temperature may also be decreased in patients receiving chronic opioids, although animal data indicate that acute administration either systemically or intrathecally can increase temperature.[2] Opioids slightly decrease body temperature by resetting the equilibrium point of temperature regulation in the hypothalamus.[2]

Neuraxial

Opioids delivered by epidural or subarachnoid routes behave differently in onset, duration, and side effects than the same drugs given systemically. Pain that is unresponsive to systemic opioids may respond to the same drugs given centrally, reducing some side effects while increasing the incidence of others. Systemic opioids suppress nociception in lamina II and V cells of the dorsal horn of the spinal cord, leaving lamina IV and VI cells, which mediate nonnociceptive information, relatively unaffected.[14]

Spinal administration of opioids is a selective and potent means of producing analgesia. Intrathecal administration allows injection of the opioids directly into the cerebrospinal fluid (CSF), a more efficient method of delivering the drug to the spinal cord opiate receptors. The analgesic response is the result of activity at spinal opiate receptors, especially kappa receptors in the substantia gelatinosa, lamina II of the dorsal horn.[14] Opioids can be given with local anesthetics intraoperatively at the initiation of spinal anesthesia or postoperatively for pain control.[15] Side effects with spinal administration are similar to those with systemic administration, except that pruritus and urinary retention occur with much greater frequency. Less lipid-soluble agents such as morphine and hydromorphone produce a delayed ventilatory depression, the result of migration of opioid via the CSF to the midbrain vestibular centers.

Respiratory depression is the most common serious complication associated with intrathecally and epidurally administered opioids. Two different levels of respiratory depression can occur after neuraxial morphine administration. An early phase observed soon after administration reflects rapid systemic absorption and is similar to parenteral dosing. A later, more insidious depression that occurs over a period of 8 to 12 hours has been related to rostral flow of CSF and delivery of morphine to the brain stem respiratory center.[16] Awareness of the delayed respiratory depression has resulted in increased monitoring of patients and dose reduction, thereby greatly reducing the incidence of serious respiratory depression to that seen with patient-controlled analgesia (PCA) opioids.

Generalized pruritus has been observed with neuraxial morphine and to a lesser extent with other opioids. Mild itching, usually involving the face or chest, is common; however, the intensity of itching can become so annoying that it interferes with sleep. Pruritus is commonly seen with opioids such as fentanyl and sufentanil that do not release histamine. Pruritus can be treated with antihistamines or with opiate receptor antagonists. The incidence of postoperative nausea and vomiting increases for patients treated with neuraxial opioids. Nausea may result either from the rostral spread of the drug in the spinal fluid to the brain stem or vascular uptake and delivery to the vomiting center and chemoreceptor trigger zone.[17]

Urinary retention after spinal opioid analgesia has been related to inhibition of sacral parasympathetic outflow, which results in relaxation of the bladder detrusor muscle and an inability to relax the sphincter.[4]

Opioids with higher lipid solubilities (see Table 10-3) tend to be rapidly absorbed into the spinal tissues after central administration, resulting in a faster onset of action. However, higher lipid solubility is associated with a small area of distribution of the drug along the length of the spinal cord and therefore a more limited area of analgesia.[5,7] Higher lipid solubility is also associated with faster clearance of the drug out of the epidural and intrathecal space, resulting in a shorter duration of action and higher blood concentrations of the opioid.[14,16] Intraspinal opioids are advantageous in selective analgesia, which occurs in the absence of motor and sympathetic blockade.

Epidural anesthesia and analgesia have been successfully used in obstetric patients and surgical patients. Epidural doses of opioids, however, are much higher than doses of opioids for intrathecal use. Small portions of epidural opioids cross the dura, enter the CSF, and penetrate spinal tissue in amounts proportional to their lipid solubility. The remaining drug is absorbed by the vasculature, producing plasma levels comparable to those after intramuscular injections and providing supraspinal analgesia.[16] In fact, the doses of the more lipid-soluble agents approach those of systemic doses.

Opioid Delivery

Initially, the most common method of administering opioids in the practice of anesthesia was intermittent bolus injection, which produces wide swings in drug plasma concentration. Intermittent periods of deep and light anesthesia are produced. Continuous opioid infusion is a more common method of administration, because the plasma concentration can be maintained more accurately and consistently with continuous infusion than with intermittent bolus injection. Continuous infusion of opioids is associated with hemodynamic stability, reduces the total necessary dose of opioids, and decreases the need for opioid reversal agents.

Continuous intravenous administration involves the infusion of a loading dose that "fills" the volume of distribution, followed by continuous drug replacement that keeps the volume of distribution "filled" as the drug is eliminated.[18]

Equation 10-1

$$\text{Loading dose (mcg/kg)} = V_d\ \text{(ml/kg)} \times C_p\ \text{(mcg/ml)}$$
$$\text{Maintenance infusion (mcg/kg/min)} = Cl\ \text{(ml/kg/min)} \times C_p\ \text{(mcg/ml)}$$

where V_d is volume of distribution, C_p is plasma concentration, and Cl is drug clearance. See Table 10-3 for the V_d and Cl of various opioids.

The rate of continuous infusion does not remain constant but rather is adjusted to meet the patient's needs and to control varying surgical stimuli. The volume of distribution is decreased for patients with hypovolemia and trauma and for geriatric patients. The anesthetist must exercise proper judgment when administering the maintenance dose, considering factors such as enzyme induction, hepatic failure, and adjunctive drug use. Table 10-6 provides dose ranges for continuous infusions.

Continuous intravenous infusion can be administered by gravity flow with a manual control device (e.g., Buretrol), an infusion pump, or a syringe pump. The least accurate method is the gravity flow device, the accuracy of which depends on counting the drops delivered. Most infusion pumps deliver medication in units of milliliters per hour. Syringe pumps are

TABLE 10-6 Infusion Rates*

Opioid	Induction (mcg/kg)	Maintenance (mcg/kg/min)
Fentanyl	5.75	0.01-0.05
Sufentanil	1-10	0.0025-0.15
Alfentanil	40-100	0.25-10
Remifentanil	5-20	0.05-0.10

**Lower dose range with nitrous oxide and benzodiazepines; higher dose range with oxygen only.*

advantageous because they are programmed to administer drug in units of micrograms per kilogram per minute. Some advantages of continuous infusion techniques are listed in Box 10-3.

Anesthesia practitioners are exploring nonparenteral routes of opioid delivery. Fentanyl is the prototypic opioid for transdermal application. Transdermal administration of fentanyl does not require cooperation from the patient; also, first-phase hepatic metabolism is not a factor, and the route does not produce discomfort. Currently available formulations permit delivery of 25 to 100 mcg per hour for 24 to 72 hours. Janssen Pharmaceutica has developed a fentanyl patch under the brand name Duragesic, which has been studied primarily in the cancer patient population.[13] The transdermal fentanyl patch provides a relatively constant plasma concentration for 72 hours. It is not currently recommended for use in managing postoperative pain.

Oral transmucosal fentanyl citrate is used for providing analgesia in children. Fentanyl is dissolved in a sucrose solution and shaped into a lozenge. The transmucosal route is effective, owing to the characteristics of the oral mucosa. The oral mucosa is thinner than the skin and is supplied by numerous blood and lymphatic vessels. The opioid administered transmucosally is also absorbed directly into the systemic circulation without passing through the liver. Pruritus is a common side effect with transmucosal administration.

Nasal administration of sufentanil preoperatively in the pediatric patient has been studied. The children remained calm, and some experienced somewhat decreased ventilatory compliance. Recovery room time was not increased, and the highest incidence of nausea and vomiting occurred in the group that received the highest dose of sufentanil. Nasal butorphanol is currently available and is widely used in the management of migraine headaches.

Spinal and epidural opioid administration has been successfully used in obstetric patients, surgical patients, and patients with postoperative pain. Neuraxial administration of opioids is a selective and potent means of producing analgesia. See Table 10-7 for neuraxial opioid dosages.[14,16]

Specific Opioids

Naturally Occurring Opioids

Morphine. Morphine, the prototype for opioid agonists, is the most abundant alkaloid in raw opium. The primary therapeutic use of morphine is the abatement of moderate to severe pain. Morphine can be administered via the intramuscular, intravenous, subcutaneous, oral, intrathecal, and epidural routes. Effects of intravenous morphine on the time course of sedation and analgesia occur with sedation first, followed by analgesia.[19] Morphine-induced sedation, therefore, should not be considered as an indicator of appropriate analgesia. When given intrathecally morphine has the longest duration of action of the specific opioids. Morphine is among the least lipophilic of the opioids, resulting in slow penetration of biologic membranes, less accumulation in lipid membranes or fatty tissues, and slower onset.

Morphine is glucoronidated in the liver at both the 3 position (which produces morphine-3-glucuronide, M3G) and the 6 position (which produces morphine-6-glucuronide, M6G), in a 2:1 ratio.[20,21] As a result of the active metabolite, M6G, morphine appears to produce a more prolonged effect, often excessive sedation, in the patient with renal failure. Within the CNS, M6G metabolite is 100 times more potent than the parent drug, whereas M3G metabolite is inactive.[20-22] The greater hydrophilicity of M6G than the parent drug normally impedes its passage into the CNS. However, after chronic administration or in patients with renal failure, M6G at a high blood level can enter the CNS by mass action.

Morphine produces a nonimmunologic release of histamine from tissue mast cells, resulting in local itching, redness, or hives near the site of intravenous injection or generalized flushing. When sufficient histamine is released, the patient may exhibit signs of decreased systemic vascular resistance, hypotension, and tachycardia. Localized histamine release after a morphine injection is not uncommon.

Codeine. Considered a weak opioid, codeine is generally not used for treatment of severe pain.[7] Approximately 10% of the administered dose of codeine is O-demethylated to morphine, which accounts for most of its analgesic activity.[7,11] It has good antitussive activity, but on a weight basis codeine is a less potent antitussive than morphine. Combinations of codeine with acetaminophen remain very popular as prescribed analgesics.

Semisynthetic Opioids

Hydromorphone. Derived from morphine in the 1920s, hydromorphone has a pharmacokinetic profile similar to that

TABLE 10-7 Doses of Neuraxial Opioids*

Opioid	Single Dose	Infusion Rate
Epidural		
Morphine	2-5 mg	0.1-1 mg/hr
Meperidine	25-50 mg	5-20 mg/hr
Methadone	5 mg	0.3-0.5 mg/hr
Fentanyl	50-100 mcg	25-100 mcg/hr
Sufentanil	25-50 mcg	10-50 mcg/hr
Butorphanol	2-4 mg	0.2-0.4 mg/hr
Subarachnoid		
Morphine	0.25-0.3 mg	
Meperidine	10 mg	
Fentanyl	10-20 mcg	
Sufentanil	5-10 mcg	

**Doses adjusted for age and level of regional injection.*

BOX 10-3

Advantages of Continuous Opioid Infusion

- Hemodynamic stability
- Decreased side effects
- Reduced need for opioid-reversal agents
- Reduced use for vasopressor drugs
- Suppression of cortisol and vasopressin response to cardiopulmonary bypass
- Reduced total dosage of opioids
- Decreased recovery time

of morphine. Hydromorphone is absorbed from the oral, rectal, and parenteral sites. Because of its lipid solubility, it is sometimes used instead of morphine for epidural or spinal administration when a wide area of analgesia is needed.[23] Studies performed on parenteral hydromorphone relative to morphine tend to demonstrate similar analgesia and side effect profiles. Because of the lack of any known active metabolites, it is often recommended for patients with renal failure.[2]

Oxycodone. Since its approval for use in the treatment of pain, oxycodone has been studied in the setting of various pain conditions. Its relative potency in oral form is similar to that of oral codeine. Intravenous and oral oxycodone has differing potency results compared with morphine.

Synthetic Opioids

Methadone. Introduced in the 1940s, methadone is used primarily for relief of chronic pain, treatment of opioid abstinence syndromes, and treatment of heroin addiction. Supplied as a racemic mixture of two optical isomers, most of methadone's activity comes from the *l*-isomer. Unlike most opioids, it has a long half-life, allowing less frequent dosing.[24] Because its prolonged effect is the result of extensive protein binding (90%) with slow release and a lower intrinsic ability of the liver to metabolize it, methadone does not require a specific formulation. It also has the advantage of a high bioavailability and no active metabolites. Disadvantages include accumulation and a longer time to reach steady state than other opioids.

Meperidine. Meperidine, a mu-receptor agonist, exerts its pharmacologic action on the CNS and the neural elements in the bowels. It is structurally similar to atropine and has an atropine-like antispasmodic effect. After demethylation in the liver, meperidine is partially metabolized to normeperidine, which is half as analgesic as meperidine but lowers the seizure threshold and induces CNS excitability. Normeperidine's elimination half-life is significantly longer than that of meperidine. With accumulation of normeperidine, subjects may experience a CNS excitation characterized by tremors, muscle twitches, and seizures. Because of accumulation of normeperidine, limitations on its use should be considered in patients with renal failure and those with cancer who are receiving high doses of meperidine. Side effects may include dry mouth and blurring of vision.

Meperidine is effective in reducing shivering from diverse causes, including general and epidural anesthesia. Intravenous doses of 25 to 50 mg reduce or eliminate visible shivering, as well as the accompanying increase in oxygen consumption.[9] It produces local anesthesia when applied locally or intrathecally, but it can also cause significant local tissue irritation.[2]

Alfentanil. After bolus injection, alfentanil has a more rapid onset of action and shorter duration than fentanyl, even though it is less lipid soluble. The high non-ionized fraction (90%) of alfentanil at physiologic pH and its small volume of distribution increase the amount of drug available for binding in the brain. Although alfentanil is effective epidurally, the duration of analgesia is short, and for this reason it has never achieved popularity. Alfentanil is metabolized in the liver by oxidative *N*-dealkylation and O-demethylation in the cytochrome P-450 system, and the inactive metabolites are excreted in the urine. Alfentanil has great patient-to-patient variability, as seen in the original studies, in which a high coefficient of variation was reported. Erythromycin has been shown to prolong the metabolism of alfentanil and interact with alfentanil to produce clinical symptoms of prolonged respiratory depression and sedation.

Fentanyl. A single administered dose of fentanyl has a short duration of action (approximately 20 to 40 minutes). It produces a profound dose-dependent analgesia, ventilatory depression, and sedation. The action of a single dose of fentanyl is terminated by redistribution. The high lipid solubility of fentanyl allows for rapid tissue uptake.[13] Fentanyl and its derivatives all undergo significant first-pass uptake in the lungs with temporary accumulation before release. When fentanyl is given in multiple doses or as a continuous infusion, the termination of action reflects elimination but not redistribution. Clearance of fentanyl is dependent on hepatic blood flow. Fentanyl is metabolized by *N*-dealkylation and hydroxylation to inactive metabolites that are eliminated in the urine and bile. The delayed postoperative respiratory depression that can occur has been attributed to sequestering of fentanyl in the gastric juice and muscles; the drug returns to the plasma and produces a secondary peak of action. Fentanyl elimination is prolonged in the elderly and the neonate.

Initially used intravenously during surgery, fentanyl later was administered for intrathecal, epidural, and postoperative PCA intravenous use. Fentanyl release from transdermal patches (Duragesic) is proportional to the surface area, with 25 mcg/hr being released per 10 cm^2 of patch.[13] It takes up to 24 hours after patch application for blood concentrations of fentanyl to stabilize, because a subcutaneous depot of drug must be saturated before the drug is consistently absorbed into the bloodstream. After removal, the decline in blood concentration follows an apparent 17-hour half-life; the true elimination half-life of fentanyl remains at approximately 3 hours, but continued absorption from the subcutaneous depot during elimination makes it appear longer.

Transmucosal fentanyl (Oralet) was initially developed in the form of a lollipop as an adjunct to pediatric anesthesia. A similar fentanyl product (ACTIQ) is available in higher strengths and is used for relief of breakthrough cancer pain.[13,25] The pharmacokinetics of this form are dose related, with an apparent elimination half-life of approximately 6 hours. Not all opioids are absorbed sublingually. Hydromorphone, oxycodone, and heroin are minimally absorbed, whereas absorption for morphine is 18%; fentanyl, 51%; and methadone, 34%.[26]

Remifentanil. Remifentanil is a moderately lipophilic, piperidine-derived opioid with an ester link. The addition of the ester group allows the drug to be easily and rapidly metabolized.[27] Kinetic studies indicate that the drug has a small volume of distribution (V_d 0.39 ± 0.25) and an elimination half-life of 8 to 20 minutes. It is metabolized by hydrolysis catalyzed by general esterase enzymes. It is not dependent on cholinesterase enzyme for metabolism and therefore is not influenced by quantitative or qualitative changes in cholinesterase. Succinylcholine metabolism does not influence remifentanil breakdown.

Because of the potential for respiratory depression and muscle rigidity, bolus dosing in the preoperative or postoperative care unit or during monitored anesthesia care is not recommended. Because of its unique metabolic pathway, remifentanil has brevity of action, a precise and rapid titratable effect because of rapid onset and offset, and noncumulative effects and results in rapid recovery after discontinuation of its administration. However, because of the rapidity of emergence from remifentanil anesthesia, it is important to develop and to start a plan for alternative analgesic therapy in the postoperative period.[28]

The commercial preparation of remifentanil is a water-soluble, lyophilized powder that contains a free base and glycine as a vehicle to buffer the solution. Because of potential glycine neurotoxicity, remifentanil should not be administered epidurally or intrathecally.[2]

Sufentanil. Sufentanil is more tightly bound to receptors than fentanyl and has minimal nonspecific brain-tissue binding. Despite its high lipophilicity and potency, sufentanil has a shorter elimination half-life and duration of effect than fentanyl because of its high degree of plasma protein binding, lower volume of distribution, tighter binding to receptors, and minimal binding to brain tissue. Hepatic clearance of sufentanil approaches liver blood flow. Sufentanil metabolism involves *O*-demethylation and *N*-dealkylation, with minimal amounts being excreted unchanged in the urine.

The effects of age on the distribution and elimination of sufentanil are reflected in a decrease in the initial volume of distribution for the elderly. The reduced volume of distribution of sufentanil in elderly patients is associated with increased respiratory depression.

Tramadol. Tramadol is a synthetic codeine analog that is a weak mu opioid receptor agonist, with analgesic effects produced by inhibition of norepinephrine and serotonin uptake.[29,30] Tramadol is a racemic mixture; the (+) enantiomer binds to the mu receptor and inhibits serotonin uptake, whereas the (−) enantiomer inhibits norepinephrine uptake and stimulates α_2-adrenergic receptors.[2] It has an elimination half-life of 5 to 6 hours and is an effective analgesic for the treatment of mild to moderate pain. Tramadol can cause seizures and possibly exacerbate them in patients with predisposing factors. Tramadol-induced analgesia is not entirely reversed by naloxone, but tramadol respiratory depression can be reversed. In overdose situations, most of the toxicity is related to monoamine uptake inhibition rather than to opioid effects.[2]

Partial Agonists and Agonists-Antagonists

Buprenorphine

Buprenorphine, a synthetic derivative, is a potent partial agonist opioid that binds mainly to the mu receptors.[31] Its slow dissociation from the receptor is a result of its long duration of action (approximately 8 hours). Its high affinity for the mu receptor accounts for the reduced ability of naloxone to reverse buprenorphine's effects. Clinically significant respiratory depression can occur with therapeutic doses. Buprenorphine exhibits a ceiling effect in which an increase in the dose does not increase respiratory depression; this is believed to result from the fact that the drug's antagonistic effects become more apparent at higher doses. It also has minimal effect on GI motility and smooth muscle sphincter tone. A transdermal system of buprenorphine was developed for treatment of moderate to severe cancer pain.[32] Administered transdermally, it provides analgesia and has a low incidence of adverse events.

Butorphanol

Butorphanol, a highly lipophilic opioid, acts as an agonist at the kappa and sigma receptors and as a weak antagonist at mu receptors. It is more potent than morphine in the production of analgesia. It produces respiratory depression, but its ceiling effect is below that of mu agonists. Butorphanol has been used as a nasal spray formulation without the restriction of being a controlled substance in the United States, but since its release in 1991 it has been shown to have significant abuse potential.[33] Butorphanol has also been studied for epidural use, although it tends to produce significant sedation. It has been shown to be effective in the treatment of postoperative shivering, but the mechanism of this effect is unknown.

Dezocine

Dezocine, an agonist-antagonist, demonstrates a greater anesthetic sparing effect than other agonist-antagonists. It demonstrates less affinity for sigma receptors, but it does have significant activity at kappa receptors and has a high affinity for mu receptors.[2]

Nalbuphine

Nalbuphine has the ability to reverse respiratory depression that results from opioid use and to maintain analgesia. Nalbuphine acts as both an agonist and an antagonist at the opioid receptors. Nalbuphine's analgesic response is equal to that of morphine. Nalbuphine provides an agonist effect at the kappa and sigma receptors and an antagonist effect at the mu receptor. A ceiling effect for respiratory depression and difficulty with reversal with naloxone has been demonstrated with both nalbuphine and butorphanol.[9,12] Nalbuphine has been used to antagonize pruritus induced by epidural and intrathecal morphine. Nalbuphine effectively antagonizes fentanyl-induced respiratory depression, maintains analgesia, and does not produce adverse endocrinologic and circulatory changes.

During laparoscopic cholecystectomy, opioid use can cause spasms of the sphincter of Oddi, which complicates the interpretation of intraoperative cholangiography. In one case study, nalbuphine was effectively used to reverse a spasm produced by morphine at the time of contrast medium injection. Nalbuphine, 10 mg intravenously, released an occluded common bile duct around the sphincter of Oddi within 3 minutes.[2]

Pentazocine

Pentazocine has analgesic and weak antagonistic effects. It is considered to be a competitive antagonist at the mu receptor and an agonist at the kappa and sigma receptors. Although it does not reverse morphine-induced respiratory depression, it can precipitate withdrawal in morphine-dependent patients.

Antagonists

Naloxone

Naloxone, an oxymorphone derivative, is a pure opioid antagonist. Naloxone blocks the opioid receptor sites and reverses respiratory depression and opioid analgesia. The reversal of respiratory depression and analgesia occurs as a result of competitive antagonism at the mu, kappa, and delta receptors. The duration of action of naloxone is less than that of most opioid agonists, allowing the return of respiratory depression in some patients treated with naloxone. Naloxone is effective only when it is administered intravenously or intramuscularly.

Naloxone may antagonize intrinsic analgesic systems, as evidenced by its ability to blunt the placebo effect and to inhibit the analgesia of electroacupuncture. Studies have demonstrated that naloxone's effect on reversing the effects of morphine is in fact titratable. Administration of low doses of naloxone can reverse the side effects of epidural opioids while preserving the analgesic effects. This effect is also seen in reversal of the side effects of intravenous morphine.[34]

The effects of naloxone use range from discomfort to pulmonary edema to sudden death. Pulmonary edema after naloxone administration has been observed in patients with a documented history of cardiovascular disease. Prough and coworkers[35] reported two cases of acute onset of pulmonary edema in young male patients who received either 100 or 200 mcg of naloxone. The report discusses the ability of naloxone to inhibit endogenous pain suppression pathways and to allow unopposed noradrenergic transmission from medullary centers that can produce neurogenic pulmonary edema. Neurogenic pulmonary edema results from an increase in catecholamine levels in healthy patients as well as in patients with a history of cardiovascular disease. Cautious titration of naloxone is of paramount importance in both cardiovascular patients and healthy patients. Andree[36] reported two cases of sudden death after naloxone administration. This study suggests that naloxone produces increases in blood catecholamine levels that predispose to ventricular fibrillation and subsequent cardiac arrest.

Nalmefene

Structurally similar to naloxone, nalmefene (Revex) is a long-acting parenteral opioid antagonist. It has an elimination half-life of approximately 10 hours (compared with naloxone's half-life of 1 hour) and a duration of action of 8 hours when it is given in the usual doses.[37] The clinical effects of nalmefene are similar to those of naloxone.

Reversal of postoperative respiratory depression is accomplished with the administration of nalmefene 0.1 to 0.5 mcg/kg titrated at 2- to 5-minute intervals. In acute opioid overdose, it is recommended that 0.5 to 1.6 mcg be given intravenously. Administration of doses higher than 1.6 mcg does not elicit additional effects and is not recommended. As with all antagonists, slow titration of small doses may minimize side effects. As with naloxone, nalmefene should not be administered to opioid-dependent patients.[38]

Naltrexone

As a synthetic cogener of oxymorphine, naltrexone has antagonist and receptor binding properties that are similar to those of naloxone but with a higher oral efficacy and longer duration of action. Its activity is the result of both the parent drug and its 6-beta metabolite. The parent and metabolite have half-lives of 6 and 13 hours, respectively.

Naltrexone has a duration of action of approximately 24 hours. Naltrexone is administered to patients addicted to opioids so that the euphoric effects of opioids can be prevented. When doses greater than 100 mg are administered to the opioid-addicted patient, plasma concentrations are reached within 2 hours, and the agent's half-life is approximately 10 hours. Naltrexone produces an active metabolite with a half-life even longer than that of naltrexone.[2] A major disadvantage associated with the use of naloxone and naltrexone is the potential for reversal of opioid analgesia.

Clinical Use

Cardiovascular Considerations

Opioids have been shown to produce greater cardiovascular stability when compared with inhalation agents. An advantage of the use of fentanyl and its analogs during cardiac surgery is their lack of cardiovascular depression.[39] Less depression of cardiac output and less decrease in systemic vascular resistance occur. A goal of management of the cardiac patient is providing continuous cardiac protection. Opioids can provide the cardiac patient with a stable heart rate and blood pressure. Opioids blunt sympathetic stimulation and maintain perfusion pressure without producing cardiac depressant effects. The degree of myocardial impairment influences patient responses. Critically ill patients or patients with significant myocardial dysfunction appear to require lower doses of an opioid for anesthesia. Patients with poor left ventricular function may develop higher plasma and brain concentrations for a given loading dose or infusion rate of opioids than patients with good left ventricular function.

Before the 1970s morphine was the drug of choice for patients who underwent open heart procedures. Side effects associated with morphine anesthesia included venodilation, tachycardia, hypotension, and a high incidence of awareness. These side effects promoted the search for a more predictable opioid for use in such patients. In the late 1970s fentanyl became the primary agent for patients who were to undergo open heart surgery. Patients given fentanyl had a greater degree of cardiovascular stability than patients given morphine.[40] The bradycardia that occasionally occurs with the use of fentanyl can be countered with the administration of pancuronium bromide or treated with anticholinergics or sympathomimetics. Fentanyl does not produce the hypotension that can be seen with the use of morphine. Fentanyl rarely produces histamine release and has little effect on peripheral vascular resistance except in massive doses. The combination of benzodiazepines and fentanyl produces decreases in blood pressure, cardiac output, and stroke volume and an increase in central venous pressure. For patients dependent on catecholamines for blood pressure maintenance, fentanyl must be titrated slowly and in small doses so that arterial blood pressure remains constant. High-dose fentanyl, 15 to 50 mcg/kg, is used in cardiac anesthesia for producing cardiac stability. Because of the prolonged respiratory depression, postoperative ventilation is necessary for cardiac patients who have received high-dose fentanyl.

In the late 1970s the opioid sufentanil was introduced into the practice of anesthesia. Sufentanil is 5 to 10 times more potent than fentanyl and has approximately the same or a slightly shorter duration of action. Sufentanil provides excellent cardiovascular stability for the cardiac patient. Sufentanil has a greater vasodilating effect than fentanyl does, and bradycardia and hypotension may occur when it is used as the induction agent. The vasodilating effects of sufentanil are not associated with histamine release. High-dose sufentanil for patients undergoing cardiac surgery is administered in the range of 8 to 30 mcg/kg. Considerations for postoperative ventilation are the same as for patients receiving high-dose fentanyl. Hemodilution, hypotension, altered regional blood flow, and hypothermia alter the pharmacokinetics of drugs during cardiac anesthesia.[40]

Remifentanil, with its fast decay in plasma concentration, even with high doses and long infusion times, ensures a rapid recovery from cardiac surgery.[39] It allows rapid and precise control of analgesia during surgery. However, because of its rapid offset, the requirement for postoperative analgesia needs to be considered before the remifentanil infusion is discontinued at the end of surgery.

Obstetrics

Concerns attendant with the use of opioids in obstetrics are the implications of respiratory depression in the mother, which results in acid-base imbalance in the fetus and possible hypoxia, and the transfer of opioids across the placenta to the fetus. The plasma concentration of opioids available for placental transfer depends on the distribution of the opioids, on the metabolism and excretion of opioids and metabolites, on protein binding, and on the acid-base status of the mother.

Many different opioids have been used successfully in the obstetric setting. Opioids, whether administered intravenously, intramuscularly, epidurally, or intraspinally, are effective in obstetric patients during and after labor and delivery. Meperidine, administered both systemically and epidurally, has been shown safe and effective, as have fentanyl, sufentanil, and morphine when used for epidural analgesia during labor.[41] However, use of opioids without local anesthetics is likely to be effective in only the very early stages of labor; local anesthetics will ultimately need to be added.[41]

Butorphanol and nalbuphine, synthetic agonist-antagonists, are used in obstetric practice for analgesia during labor. Because of its strong kappa-receptor activity, butorphanol can modulate visceral pain and be effective for the relief of labor pain. The major advantage attributed to these drugs is the ceiling effect for respiratory depression. Butorphanol systemically was found to be similar to intramuscular meperidine for labor analgesia.[42]

Nalbuphine is considered equipotent to morphine and is used in obstetric practice to reverse the itching associated with epidural morphine while maintaining the analgesia.[41] Major side effects associated with both nalbuphine and butorphanol are drowsiness and dizziness. They can cause psychomimetic effects in the obstetric patient and rarely cause a sinusoidal fetal heart pattern after administration.[42]

Pediatrics

Opioids have been widely used in recent years for infants and children as adjuncts to inhaled anesthetics, as the primary or major anesthetic component for balanced anesthesia techniques, and as analgesics for postoperative pain. Morphine, meperidine, methadone, fentanyl, sufentanil, alfentanil, and, more recently, remifentanil have been safely used in the pediatric population.[43,44] Dosage varies a great deal, depending on the age and size of the patient and the purpose and plan for anesthetic and postoperative management.

Pediatric patients are at increased risk for complications associated with anesthesia, and the younger the patient, the greater the risk. Failure to recognize and treat perioperative stress may account for the poor anesthesia outcomes in pediatric patients. Infants who undergo surgery experience stress as a result of catabolism and substrate mobilization. Critically ill neonates have a precarious metabolic balance and poor metabolic reserve, and they experience the metabolic cost of rapid growth. The added stress of surgery can be detrimental to the metabolic state of the neonate. Opioid-related suppression of the stress response in infants can improve these patients' postoperative course.

Fentanyl is the opioid most commonly used in the pediatric population. Its major advantage relates to its rapid onset and brief duration of action. It induces a very stable cardiovascular response. Excellent recovery characteristics and ventilatory function were provided when fentanyl, either 2 mcg/kg or 10 mcg/kg, was used for anesthesia in full-term infants who underwent hernia repair. It did not result in apnea and produced better pain control in comparison with other opioids; however, time to discharge was prolonged.

Effective analgesia can also be achieved in pediatric patients by injecting epidural (bolus or continuous infusion) and intrathecal opioids.[45] Control of respiratory depression, the major complication, requires careful dosing and monitoring. Other side effects, including pruritus, nausea, vomiting, and urinary retention, are often easily managed by administration of a small dose of naloxone.

Neurosurgery

Administration of opioids can increase CSF pressure if ventilation is not controlled and if the $PaCO_2$ is allowed to increase. Opioid premedication should therefore be used cautiously when elevated intracranial pressure is suspected. However, opioids are useful during induction of anesthesia in neurosurgical patients to blunt the stress of intubation. When ventilation is controlled, opioids have little effect on cerebral metabolic rate and blood flow.

Studies have been conducted on the use in neurosurgery of multiple opioids, including morphine, fentanyl, alfentanil, sufentanil, remifentanil, and meperidine. Results of these studies on opioids during intraoperative neurologic monitoring were similar for all types of evoked potentials. The effects of opioids on evoked responses are generally mild; effects are maximal when the drug is peaking and then remain rather stable.[46] Studies also found that spinal morphine and fentanyl produced minimal changes.[46]

Opioids, even in relatively high doses, can be used for patients who require intraoperative monitoring without compromising the ability to monitor neurologic function adequately.[47] Large intravenous bolus administration of opioids should be avoided at times of potential surgical compromise to neurologic function to prevent confusion regarding the interpretation of the measurements. Continuous infusions of opioids provide stable recordings, whereas bolus injections can affect both the evoked potentials and the wake-up test. Continuous infusions of remifentanil allow a rapid return to consciousness for neurologic examination if a wake-up test is needed during surgery.

Trauma

Opioids are commonly the agents of choice in the anesthetic management of trauma patients.[48] Opioid use provides cardiovascular stability for trauma patients, who are often in an unstable condition. Patients with major trauma have hypotension, hypovolemia, and hypothermia.

The selection of a specific opioid must be based on knowledge of its characteristics and the experience of the anesthesia provider. It is important to avoid the use of opioids that produce histamine release and hypotension. Histamine release after intravenous administration of equipotent doses of meperidine, morphine, fentanyl, and sufentanil for anesthesia induction must be considered. Morphine results in a great degree of histamine release. Patients receiving either meperidine, sufentanil, or fentanyl do not experience histamine release.

The hemodynamic instability of trauma patients decreases opioid anesthetic requirements. The decreased anesthetic requirements that are the result of hemodynamic instability can result in surgical recall. The most distressing component of recall was pain. Less distressing components were voices and awareness of the experience of surgery.

Ambulatory Surgery

Because of patient preferences, improved technology, and financial considerations, more and more surgical procedures are being performed in an ambulatory setting. Choosing the ideal anesthetic for ambulatory surgery patients is difficult because of the variation in duration and stimulation among procedures.

Fentanyl, alfentanil, and remifentanil have all been used in the ambulatory setting. Comparison of the pharmacokinetics of these three opioids has shown that fentanyl is more lipid soluble and has a larger volume distribution, a longer elimination half-life, and a more basic pK_a. Alfentanil has a more acidic pK_a; therefore the component of non-ionized drug is larger, and this allows a more rapid onset of action. Because alfentanil has a shorter elimination half-life, it is excreted more rapidly than fentanyl but not as rapidly as remifentanil. Fentanyl and alfentanil can be administered as a single bolus or intermittent infusion in the ambulatory setting, but remifentanil can be administered only as an infusion. Fentanyl is a better choice for ambulatory surgery patients than nalbuphine, because nalbuphine is associated with a greater incidence of nausea, vomiting, unpleasant dreams, and hospital admission.

Pharmacokinetic differences between adults and children can influence opioid effect in outpatient pediatric surgery. The use of opioids in both adults and children is an effective technique for inducing and maintaining analgesia in the ambulatory setting. Considerations with regard to opioid use in ambulatory surgical settings include drug ionization, elimination half-life, plasma clearance, and bolus versus infusion techniques.

POSTOPERATIVE PAIN CONTROL

In the 1980s several devices that enabled patients to control their postoperative pain were marketed. PCA requires that patients be taught preoperatively about the equipment. PCA programming requires selection of the opioid, dosage, and a lockout interval measured in minutes. To decrease postoperative discomfort, the patient triggers the device, which then delivers a dose of the chosen opioid.

The incidence of respiratory depression is low with the use of PCA devices. The potential for operator, patient, and mechanical errors during PCA exists but has been reduced with the improvement of devices. Continuous infusion can be used to supplement PCA dosages, but it can increase side effects without an increase in analgesia.

The role of intrathecal and epidural opioids has been evolving since their first use in 1979. From intermittent boluses of epidural morphine only to combinations of other opioids with bupivacaine in continuous infusions or patient-controlled epidural analgesia, the safety and efficacy of this form of analgesia have been defined. However, with the introduction of ketorolac and the use of less invasive surgical approaches, fewer cases require the effect and cost of epidural analgesia.

SUMMARY

Opioids are a group of drugs that bind to receptor sites in the CNS, supraspinal and spinal, and at peripheral sites, producing morphine-like effects. Opioid analgesia results from the inhibition of nociceptive reflexes and the release of neurotransmitters. Because of their multiplicity of sites and mechanisms of action, opioids are a uniquely valued means for analgesia and anesthesia. Opioids can be used for preoperative medication, as induction agents, as maintenance anesthetics, and for treatment of postoperative pain. The newer methods of opioid delivery have been growing in popularity. Opioids provide the anesthesia practitioner with a multitude of delivery modalities. The introduction of other forms of delivery (e.g., inhalation) will further expand their role in perioperative pain management.

REFERENCES

1. Bailey PL, Egan TD, Stanley TH. Intravenous opioid anesthetics. In: Miller RD, ed. *Anesthesia.* 5th ed. Philadelphia: Churchill Livingstone; 2000:273-376.
2. Gutstein HB, Akil H. Opioid analgesics. In: Hardman JG and Limbird LE, eds. *Goodman and Gilman's the Pharmacological Basis of Therapeutics.* 10th ed. New York: McGraw-Hill; 2001:569-620.
3. Synder SH, Pasternak GW. Historical review: opioid receptors. *Trends Pharmacol Sci.* 2003;24:198-205.
4. Stoelting RK. *Pharmacology and Physiology in Anesthesia Practice.* Philadelphia: Lippincott-Raven; 1999.
5. Klepstad P, Kaasa S, Borchgrevink PC. Start of oral morphine to cancer patients: effective serum morphine concentrations and contribution from morphine-6-glucuronide to the analgesia produced by morphine. *Eur J Clin Pharmacol.* 2000;55:713-719.
6. Martin WR, Eades CG, Thompson JA, et al. The effects of morphine and nalorphine-like drugs in nondependent and morphine dependent chronic spinal dogs. *J Pharmacol Exp Ther.* 1976;197:517-532.
7. Inturrisi CE. Clinical pharmacology of opioids and pain. *Clin J Pain.* 2002;18:S3-S13.
8. Walker JS. Anti-inflammatory effects of opioids. *Adv Exp Med Biol.* 2003;521:148-160.
9. Coda BA. Opioids. In: Barash PG, Cullen BF, Stoelting RK, eds *Clinical Anesthesia.* 4th ed. Philadelphia: Lippincott-Raven; 2001: 345-375.
10. McCleskey EW, Gold MS. Ion channels of nociception. *Annu Rev Physiol.* 1999;61:835-856.
11. Holtzman SG, Sung YF. Pain control with opioid analgesics. In: Brody TM, Larner J, Minneman KP, eds. *Human Pharmacology.* 4th ed. St Louis: Mosby; 1998:395-408.
12. Rosow CE, Dershwitz M. Pharmacology of opioid analgetic agents. In: Longnecker DE, Tinker JH, Morgan GE, eds. *Principles and Practice of Anesthesiology.* 2nd ed. St Louis: Mosby; 1998:1233-1259.
13. Peng P, Sandler A. A review of the use of fentanyl analgesia in the management of acute pain in adults. *Anesthesiology.* 1999;90:576-599.
14. Carr DB, Cousins MJ. Spinal route of analgesia: opioids and future options. In: Cousins M, Bridenbaugh P, eds. *Neural Blockade.* 3rd ed. Philadelphia: Lippincott-Raven; 1998:915-983.
15. Bernards CM. Understanding the physiology and pharmacology of epidural and intrathecal opioids. *Best Pract Res Clin Anaesthesiol.* 2002;16:489-505.
16. Sinatra RS, Ayoub CM. Postoperative analgesia: epidural and spinal techniques. In: Chestnut DH, ed. *Obstetric Anesthesia Principles and Practice.* St Louis: Mosby; 1999:521-555.
17. Sinatra R. Acute pain management and acute pain services. In: Cousins M, Bridenbaugh P, eds. *Neural Blockade.* 3rd ed. Philadelphia: Lippincott-Raven; 1998:803-815.

18. Glass P, Shafer SL, Reves JG. Intravenous drug delivery systems. In: Miller RD, ed. *Anesthesia*. 5th ed. Philadelphia: Churchill Livingstone; 2000:377-411.
19. Paqueron X et al. Is morphine-induced sedation synonymous with analgesia during intravenous morphine titration? *Br J Anaesth*. 2002;89:697-701.
20. Christup LL. Morphine metabolites. *Acta Anaesthesiol Scand*. 1997;41:116-122.
21. Smith MT. Neuroexcitatory effects of morphine and hydromorphone: evidence implicating the 3-glucuronide metabolites. *Clin Exp Pharmacol Physiol*. 2000;27:524-528.
22. Cann C, et al. Unwanted effects of morphine-6-glucoronide and morphine. *Anaesthesia*. 2002;57:1200-1203.
23. Quigley C. Hydromorphone for acute and chronic pain. *Cochrane Database Syst Rev*. 2002;10.
24. Bruera E, Sweeney C. Methadone use in cancer patients with pain: a review. *J Palliat Med*. 2002;5:127-138.
25. Farrar J, et al. Oral transmucosal fentanyl citrate: randomized, double-blinded, placebo-controlled trial for treatment of breakthrough pain in cancer patients. *Anesthesiology*. 1998;90:611-616.
26. Weinberg D, et al. Sublingual absorption of selected opioid analgesics. *Clin Pharmacol Ther*. 1988;44:335-342.
27. Gan TJ, Howell S. A review of pharmacokinetics and pharmacodynamics of remifentanil. *Anesth Analg*. 1999;89:S7-S14.
28. Munoz HR, et al. Effect of timing of morphine administration during remifentanil-based anaesthesia on early recovery from anaesthesia and postoperative pain. *Br J Anaesth*. 2002;88:814-818.
29. Lewis KS, Han NH. Tramadol: a new centrally acting analgesic. *Am J Health Syst Pharm*. 1997;54:643-652.
30. Duthe DJ. Remifentanil and Tramadol. *Br J Anaesth*. 1998;81:51-57.
31. Tzschentke TM. Behavioral pharmacology of buprenorphine, with a focus on preclinical models of reward and addiction. *Psychopharmacology*. 2002;161:1-16.
32. Budd K. Buprenorphine and the transdermal system: the ideal match in pain management. *Int J Clin Pract Suppl*. 2003;133:9-14.
33. Fisher M, Glass S. Butorphanol: a study in problems of current drug information and control. *Neurology*. 1997;48:1156-1160.
34. Gan T, et al. Opioid sparing effects of a low-dose infusion of naloxone in patient-administered morphine sulfate. *Anesthesiology*. 1997;87:1075-1081.
35. Prough DS, et al. Acute pulmonary edema in healthy teenagers following conservative doses of intravenous naloxone. *Anesthesiology*. 1984;60:485-486.
36. Andree R. Sudden death following naloxone administration. *Anesth Analg*. 1980;59:782-784.
37. Glass P, Jhaveri R, Smith LR. Comparison of potency and duration of action of nalmefene and naloxone. *Anesth Analg*. 1994;78:536-541.
38. Henderson CA, Reynolds JE. Acute pulmonary edema in a young male after intravenous nalmefene. *Anesth Analg*. 1997;84:218-219.
39. Bovill JG, Boer F. Opioids in cardiac anesthesia. In: Kaplan JA. *Cardiac Anesthesia*. 4th ed. Philadelphia: Saunders; 1999: 573-610.
40. Eaton MP, Bailey PC. Cardiovascular pharmacology of anesthetics. In: Estafanous FG, Barash PG, Reves JG, eds. *Cardiac Anesthesia Principles and Clinical Practice*. 2nd ed. Philadelphia: Lippincott; 2001:295-318.
41. Riley ET, Ross BK. Opioid techniques. In: Chestnut DH, ed. *Obstetric Anesthesia Principles and Practice*. St Louis: Mosby; 1999:386-408.
42. Wakefield ML. Systemic analgesia: parenteral and inhalational agents. In: Chestnut DH, ed. *Obstetric Anesthesia Principles and Practice*. St Louis: Mosby; 1999:346-358.
43. Davis PJ et al. A randomized multicenter study of remifentanil compared with alfentanil, isoflurane, or propofol in anesthetized pediatric patients undergoing elective strabismus surgery. *Anesth Analg*. 1997;84:982-989.
44. Ross AK, et al. Pharmacokinetics of remifentanil in anesthetized pediatric patients undergoing elective surgery or diagnostic procedures. *Anesth Analg*. 2001;93:1393-1401.
45. Cote CJ. Pediatric anesthesia. In: Miller RD, ed. *Anesthesia*. 5th ed. Philadelphia: Churchill Livingstone; 2000:2088-2117.
46. Sloan T. Evoked potentials. In: Albin MS, ed. *Textbook of Neuroanesthesia with Neurosurgical and Neuroscience Perspectives*. New York: McGraw-Hill; 1997:221-276.
47. Black S, Mahla ME, Cucchiara RF. Neurologic monitoring. In: Miller RD, ed. *Anesthesia*. 5th ed. New York: Churchill Livingstone; 2000:1324-1350.
48. Alpen MA, Morse C. Managing the pain of traumatic injury. *Crit Care Nurs Clin North Am*. 2001;13:243-257.

CHAPTER 11

Neuromuscular Blocking Agents, Reversal Agents, and Their Monitoring

Richard E. Haas, Angela Darsey, DeAnna Powell

HISTORY

In the nineteenth century, Claude Bernard, a famous French physiologist and philosopher, carried out experiments with curare, then in use by the Amazonian Indians of South America.[1] He noted that animals the Indians hunted for food were paralyzed by arrows poisoned with curare and subsequently died of asphyxiation.[2] Bernard's experiments with the poison with which the Indians tipped their arrows formed the basis for our ideas of the neuromuscular junction, neuromuscular transmission, and neuromuscular pharmacology.[3] Indeed, curare had been used since 1857 as an anticonvulsant treatment in tetany and other types of spastic disorders.[4]

Laewen also described the use of curare in anesthetized humans in a German report in 1912.[3] For readers who are interested in historical aspects of this topic, a fascinating and more complete report of the earliest work of these and other researchers, beginning as early as the year 1548, is available in an outstanding review article by Bisset.[5]

In 1936 Dale and colleagues[6] found that acetylcholine (ACh) was the chemical neurotransmitter that activated the postjunctional muscle membrane receptors after excitation of the nerve terminal. This finding contradicted the once widely held theory that direct electrical transmission from the nerve to the muscle occurs.[6] This discovery provided the impetus for further research concerning pharmacologic agents that could either enhance the action of ACh or prevent it, thereby causing a temporary and reversible state of therapeutic paralysis.

Griffith and Johnson[7] of Montreal, Canada, are universally acknowledged as the persons responsible for the introduction of neuromuscular blockers into anesthetic practice. Their groundbreaking report laid the foundations for other studies that followed. Within a year of their study, Cullen[4] reported on the use of curare in 131 general anesthetic procedures. His only report of an adverse reaction dealt with a 44-year-old woman who experienced "complete paralysis and severe salivation," accompanied by muscular twitching.[4]

Despite initial successes with the neuromuscular blockers, an early study nearly doomed their use before they became widely accepted. Henry Beecher and Donald Todd,[8] two physicians in the anesthesia department of Harvard Medical School, reviewed 599,548 anesthetic procedures administered at 10 institutions between 1948 and 1952. As part of this review they examined the death rate in patients receiving *curares* (the term by which they described any neuromuscular blocking agent, including tubocurarine chloride, decamethonium bromide, succinylcholine chloride, gallamine triethiodide, and dimethyltubocurarine [*d*-tubocurarine] iodide). Beecher and Todd found that the overall death rate for persons treated with neuromuscular blockers was 1:370, compared with a death rate of 1:2100 in patients who did not receive these agents.[8]

After reviewing the conditions of the patients; the educational background and training of the practitioners who administered the anesthetic (e.g., physician, nurse anesthetist, or physician-in-training); the size of the institution; the sexes, races, and ages of the patients; and numerous other combinations of these factors, the investigators reached the following conclusions.

> *[I]n our judgment the situation is one where neither experience of individual nor experience of institution appears to protect. This adds up to evidence that neither mistakes nor preventable error of any kind are involved in the main, but rather the inherent toxicity of the "curares" themselves.*[8]

In the litigious environment of modern anesthetic practice, such a statement may have ended the administration of these agents. Certainly, it would have slowed their development. The positive attributes of the agents, however, were discussed later in the same paper, as Beecher and Todd added this caveat:

> *Having presented the foregoing evidence and comment, one can ask what, then, is to be done about these agents? Are they to be banned as a practical solution of the problem? We believe not. These data strongly suggest that great caution in the use of muscle relaxants should be exercised, that the agents available at present be considered as on trial, and that they be employed only when there are clear advantages to be gained by their use, that they not be employed for trivial purposes or as a corrective for generally inadequate anesthesia.*[8]

Beecher and Todd's admonition still echoes through the halls of anesthetic practice today. Although the safety and efficiency of neuromuscular blocking agents have markedly increased, the sage advice is still germane for the practitioner: neuromuscular blocking agents, like all anesthetic agents, are best used where and when they are indicated. Nevertheless, as one leg of the anesthetic triad that includes analgesia, amnesia, and muscle relaxation, neuromuscular blockade has become an accepted, if not integral, part of most modern anesthetic techniques. A broad spectrum of these agents now exists, each a part of the armamentarium of anesthetic practice. Their individual pharmacokinetic and pharmacodynamic attributes enable the anesthetist to tailor the use of the agent to the physiologic needs of the patient and the requirements of the surgeon.

GENERAL PHARMACODYNAMICS OF NEUROMUSCULAR BLOCKERS

The following template and conventions are used in the subsequent discussions of the individual neuromuscular blocking agents. All doses, unless otherwise specified, are listed as a mean dose followed by the standard deviation of that mean dose in parentheses. An overview of the agent is presented first. Next, its pharmacodynamic profile, including onset, duration, and elimination, is discussed. The pharmacodynamic effects of the agent are subsequently examined. The effect of the agent on other systems, such as the central nervous system, cardiovascular system, and others, is then reviewed. Finally, the effects of the agent on special populations, such as children, the elderly, and the obese (among others) are discussed. In an effort to simplify learning for those still in training, we place these discussions in the context of each individual agent rather than looking at the special populations as a whole. For the practicing nurse anesthetist faced with an unfamiliar agent, this format should increase the ease and facility with which one can quickly find information regarding any neuromuscular blocking agent.

DEPOLARIZING AGENTS

Succinylcholine Chloride

Succinylcholine chloride (Anectine, Quelicin, Sucostrin) is familiar to every nurse anesthetist in practice. Research on this agent abounds, yet its use remains controversial. Although its continued use in clinical practice represents the standard of care for a variety of cases, opinions regarding its use remain divided because of some of its untoward effects.

In 1906 Hunt and de Taveau described succinylcholine as a valerylcholine whose physiologic action caused the heart to slow and the blood pressure to rise.[3] Boret and colleagues were the first to study its actual neuromuscular blocking effects in 1949.[3] The use of succinylcholine was considered to represent a tremendous breakthrough in neuromuscular blockade. The disadvantages of curare were being debated, and some thought succinylcholine was a drug that offered the benefits of curare without its drawbacks. The first use of succinylcholine in the United States occurred in 1952. Foldes and co-workers[9] described this agent in the following manner:

> *Compared to other muscle relaxants used in anesthesiology, succinylcholine possesses several advantages, the outstanding one, in our experience, being its easy controllability, which permitted almost instantaneous changes in degree of muscular relaxation. With succinylcholine, both increasing and decreasing muscular relaxation took less than a minute.*[9]

The disadvantages of succinylcholine have been well recorded through years of clinical experience. The antagonistic action by which skeletal muscle is depolarized can also stimulate cardiac cholinergic receptors.[10] This stimulation can result in a profound bradycardia. Prolonged neuromuscular blockade can result from excessive doses of succinylcholine in patients with atypical, inhibited, or deficient levels of plasma cholinesterases.[3,10]

Succinylcholine is the only existing depolarizing muscle relaxant licensed for use in the United States. Remembering the composition of the drug is helpful in better understanding its effects and side effects. Succinylcholine results from the joining of two ACh molecules and is represented by the chemical formula $C_{14}H_{30}N_2O_4$. Although succinylcholine mimics the action of ACh by depolarizing the motor end plate, its degradation is distinct.[11] In contrast to the degradation of ACh by acetylcholinesterase (AChE), succinylcholine is hydrolyzed by plasma cholinesterase (pseudocholinesterase).[11] The popularity of this muscle relaxant is rooted in its unique ability to provide a quick onset and short duration of effect.[11] A bolus of 0.5 to 1.5 mg/kg is the recommended dose for adequate adult paralysis and relaxation for intubation.[11] The dose of succinylcholine that provides the desired effect in 95% of the population (ED_{95}) is 0.5 mg/kg.[12]

Pharmacodynamics

Onset. Succinylcholine has an extremely rapid onset and remains the gold standard against which other agents are compared. A typical intubating dose of 1 to 1.5 mg/kg results in a maximum suppression of muscle twitch and good-to-excellent intubating conditions within 1 to 1.5 minutes of administration.[12,13] Onset of action of succinylcholine at the larynx with administration of 1 mg/kg is 34 seconds.[14] The onset as measured at peripheral sites such as the adductor pollicis is slightly longer at 1 minute.[15] The rapid onset of succinylcholine is based on its action as an agonist at the nicotinic receptor rather than as a competitive antagonist. This action results in the need for significantly less drug at the receptor site to produce neuromuscular block.[16] In contrast, most nondepolarizing neuromuscular blocking agents (NMBAs) require 75% or more receptor occupancy for paralysis to result. Variable onset must be considered in patients with altered physiology. Patients with atypical plasma cholinesterase may exhibit prolonged onset after succinylcholine administration.[16] A summary of the dose, onset, and duration of the neuromuscular blocking drugs is given in Table 11-1.

Duration. The plasma half-life of succinylcholine is 2 to 4 minutes.[17] The clinical duration of succinylcholine (i.e., the length of time during which its clinical effects can be recognized) is 5 to 10 minutes, with full recovery evident at 12 to 15 minutes.[14] Twitch recovery of 25% as measured by the laryngeal adductor pressure responses is 4.3 minutes, whereas 90% to 95% twitch recovery has been reported to occur in 8 minutes.[14] Other studies have yielded similar results, with researchers citing a range of duration of 7 to 12 minutes.[10,12]

Elimination. Succinylcholine is degraded via hydrolysis by plasma cholinesterases. These enzymes, although found in the plasma, are produced by the liver. Initially hydrolysis results in the transformation of succinylcholine into succinylmonocholine and choline (Figure 11-1). Succinylmonocholine is further degraded by plasma cholinesterase into succinic acid and choline. Succinylcholine metabolism is so rapid that only 10% of the injected dose ever reaches the neuromuscular junction.[11] A summary of the elimination routes for the neuromuscular blocking drugs is given in Table 11-2.

Pharmacodynamic Summary. The onset of succinylcholine given in a dose of 1 to 1.5 mg/kg is 30 to 90 seconds. The clinical duration of succinylcholine is 8 to 15 minutes. It is degraded via the plasma cholinesterase into succinic acid and choline.

TABLE 11-1 Neuromuscular Blocking Agents: Dose, Onset, and Duration*

Agent	ED_{95} (mg/kg)	Intubating Dose (mg/kg)	Time to Onset	Duration of Action (min)
Succinylcholine (Anectine)	1	1-1.5	30-60 sec	Ultrashort, 5-15
Mivacurium (Mivacron)	0.25	0.75	2-4 min	Short, 20-30
Atracurium (Tracrium)	0.15	0.5	2-4 min	Intermediate, 30-60
Cis-Atracurium (Nimbex)	0.05	0.1	2-4 min	Intermediate, 30-60
Rocuronium (Zemuron)	0.3	0.6-1	1-1.5 min	Intermediate, 30-60
Vecuronium (Norcuron)	0.05	0.1	2-4 min	Intermediate, 30-60
Pancuronium (Pavulon)	0.05	0.08-1.8	2-4 min	Long, 60-90
Pipecuronium (Arduan)	0.05	0.08-1	2-4 min	Long, 60-90
Doxacurium (Nuromax)	0.025	0.075	2-4 min	Long, 60-90

ED_{95}, *Effective dose for 95% paralysis.*
**All data for adult patients without significant disease.*

Central Nervous System. The use of succinylcholine is controversial because of its many side effects. One such concern is that it clearly has the potential to increase intracranial pressure (ICP).[14] Research conducted on animal subjects exhibited a 10- to 15-mm Hg rise in ICP for as much as 5 to 8 minutes after administration.[17] This precise mechanism of action is unknown; however, it is thought to be related to cerebral activation.[18]

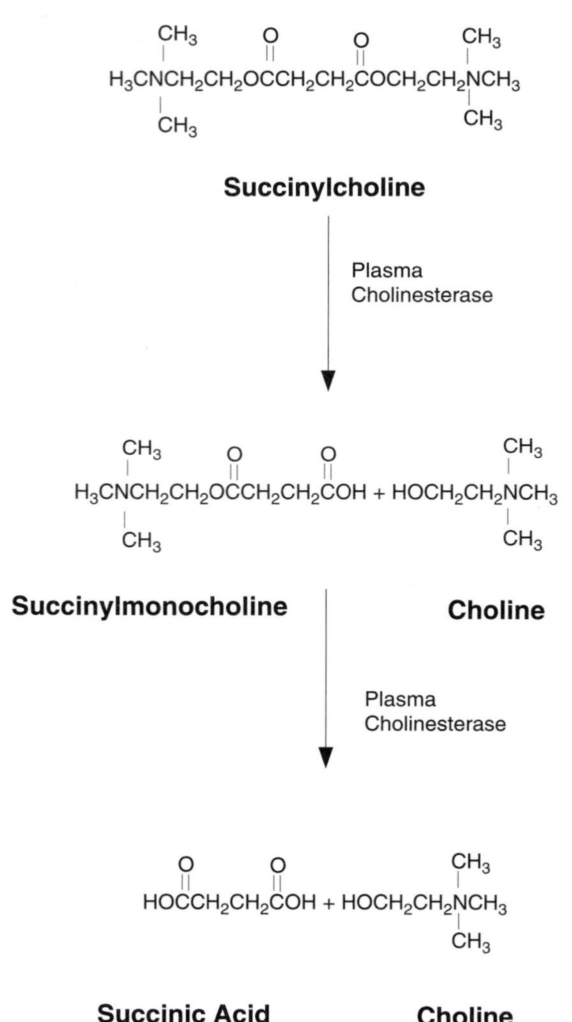

FIGURE **11-1**
Metabolism of succinylcholine.

Caution is warranted with administration of succinylcholine to patients undergoing anticonvulsant therapy.[19] Patients often experience an upregulation of ACh receptors with drugs such as phenytoin and carbamazepine.[20] The response-concentration curve is shifted to the left with these drugs and reduces the amount of succinylcholine needed by as much as 30%.[20] Therefore administration of succinylcholine to these patients results in prolonged paralysis.[19]

Cardiovascular System. Succinylcholine influences the nicotinic receptors in both the parasympathetic and sympathetic nervous systems, as well as muscarinic receptors in the heart.[11,17] The ability of succinylcholine to stimulate the heart may result in positive and negative inotropy, with higher doses resulting in the former.[17] Stimulation of the ACh receptors may result in additional hemodynamic alterations including both hypotension and hypertension.[21] The presence of bradycardia associated with succinylcholine administration is thought to be related to its metabolite, succinylmonocholine, which causes stimulation of cholinergic receptors in the sinoatrial node.[21] Stimulation of the sympathetic nervous system may result in various cardiac dysrhythmias including sinus arrest, premature ventricular contractions, and atrioventricular nodal blockade with junctional rhythm.[17,22,23] Additional cardiovascular problems, which may occur with the administration of succinylcholine, include peaked T waves; such problems are associated with a large potassium release that results in reported serum levels of 7.4 ± 2.8 mmol/L.[22]

An intubating dose of succinylcholine increases serum potassium levels by 0.5 to 1 mEq/L.[17] Although this may not be significant in the normokalemic patient, it may be life threatening in patients with preexisting hyperkalemia.[24] Gronert[23] presents a case that involved an 11-year-old girl who experienced cardiac arrest after receiving succinylcholine. Her cardiac arrest and eventual death were directly attributed to a high potassium release after the succinylcholine administration (10.2 mEq/L). The exaggerated potassium release after the succinylcholine administration in this case was determined to be related to a familial myopathy as evidenced by extremely high patient levels of creatine kinase.[23]

Some clinicians believe that a second dose of succinylcholine indicated by any event should be preceded by intravenous (IV)

TABLE 11-2 Neuromuscular Blockers: Elimination Mechanism

Agent	Elimination Mechanism	Comments
Mivacurium	Plasma cholinesterase	Prolonged in patients with cholinesterase deficiency
Atracurium	Hofmann elimination; non-specific esterases cholinesterase	Non–organ-dependent elimination produces consistent duration in patients with significant hepatic and renal disease, as well as the elderly
Cis-Atracurium	Hoffman elimination; non-specific esterases	Similar to atracurium but without the histamine release
Rocuronium	Renal; hepatic	May be prolonged with hepatic and renal disease
Vecuronium	Renal (20%-30%); hepatic (40%-80%)	May be prolonged with hepatic disease
Pancuronium	Renal	May be prolonged with renal disease
Pipecuronium	Renal	May be prolonged with renal disease
Doxacurium	Renal; possibly hepatic	May be prolonged with renal disease
Succinylcholine	Plasma cholinesterase	Prolonged in patients with cholinesterase deficiency

atropine 0.3 to 0.6 mg for its anticholinergic effects; however, others do not.[24,25]

Hepatic System. Both serum and liver pseudocholinesterase (PChE) degrade succinylcholine, suggesting that liver damage may prolong the effects of the drug.[17] Additional side effects of succinylcholine have been documented in patients with hepatic disease. Although limited information exists regarding the influence of the drug on the hepatic system, documentation exists on the development of severe hyperkalemia associated with liver disorders and concomitant succinylcholine administration. The discussion of hyperkalemia later in this chapter provides more information regarding this phenomenon.

Cholinesterase is a generic term used for a family of related enzymes that hydrolyze choline esters at a faster rate than other esters under optimal conditions. The major function of cholinesterase is to terminate the action of ACh at cholinergic nerve endings in synapses or in effector organs. Two types of cholinesterase exist in the human body, with several variations and a confusing set of names. One type of cholinesterase is AchE, also known as *true*, *specific*, *genuine*, and *type 1* cholinesterase. This enzyme is found in erythrocytes, nerve endings, the lungs, the spleen, and the gray matter of the brain. This enzyme is a membrane-bound glycoprotein and exists in several molecular forms. The other subgroup, pseudocholinesterase (PChE), also known as *plasma*, *serum*, *benzoyl*, *false*, *butyryl*, *nonspecific*, and *type II* cholinesterase, exists in plasma and has more than 11 isoenzyme variants. PChE is also present in the liver, smooth muscle, intestines, pancreas, heart, and white matter of brain.

Measurements of PChE activity can serve as a sensitive measure of the synthetic capacity of the liver. In the absence of known inhibitors, any decrease in activity reflects impaired synthesis of the enzyme. A moderate decrease (30% to 50%) is seen in acute hepatitis and long-standing chronic hepatitis, whereas a severe decrease (50% to 70%) is seen in advanced cirrhosis and in some carcinomas with metastases to the liver. Decreased levels of PChE are also found in patients with acute infections, pulmonary embolism, muscular dystrophy, myocardial infarction, or pregnancy and after surgical procedures. Essentially normal levels are noted in patients with chronic hepatitis, mild cirrhosis, or obstructive jaundice. Increased levels have been observed in cases of nephrotic syndrome, thyrotoxicosis, and hemochromatosis; in obese patients with diabetes; and in patients with anxiety and other psychiatric states. Patients generally develop neuromuscular symptoms at approximately 60% of normal activity, and serious neuromuscular effects are seen at approximately 20% of normal. Reference intervals are 2900 to 7100 U/L.

Genetic Variants and the Dibucaine Inhibition Test. Some patients exhibit genetic variations that cause a prolonged response and apnea when the patient is exposed to succinylcholine or mivacurium. The atypical variants of cholinesterase are not able to hydrolyze these drugs in the usual fashion. Low levels or even the absence of serum cholinesterase is indicative of atypical variants. By treating the patient's serum with dibucaine and measuring the residual PChE activity compared with the PChE of an untreated sample, the metabolic sensitivity to succinylcholine and mivacurium may be measured. However, patients with acute or chronic liver disease, organophosphate poisoning, or chronic renal disease, patients in the late stages of pregnancy, and patients undergoing estrogen therapy may have markedly decreased PChE activities. PChE phenotype interpretation is based on the total PChE activity and the percent of inhibition caused by dibucaine. Although over 25 different phenotypes exist, most are extremely rare (Table 11-3).

Renal System. Succinylcholine may be used in surgical patients with renal disease when preoperative potassium levels are normal. One author states that the use of succinylcholine in patients with elevated preoperative potassium levels is absolutely contraindicated.[26] This recommendation came in response to a report of a renal patient whose potassium level increased from 6.2 mEq/L preoperatively to 8.9 mEq/L after the administration of succinylcholine.[26] Researchers note that succinylcholine use in these patients may quickly lead to cardiovascular arrhythmias and even cardiac arrest.[22,23,26] Conversely, Bevan and Donati[27] state that the administration of succinylcholine to patients with a preexisting elevated potassium level does not result in higher levels.

Special Populations

Elderly Patients. The medical conditions associated with aging make the use of succinylcholine potentially dangerous in elderly patients.[28]

Osteoporosis is one such disease in the elderly that may contraindicate the use of succinylcholine. The fasciculations associated with succinylcholine administration may cause pathologic fractures and worsening of preexisting fractures that are commonly present in this patient population.[28]

TABLE 11-3 Select Inherited Variants of Plasma Cholinesterase

PChE Variant	Genetic Label*	Frequency (%)	Enzyme Activity	Duration of Succinylcholine or Mivacurium
Usual	Homozygote U	96	Normal	Normal; dibucaine number 70-80
—	Heterozygote U/A	3	Decreased	Slightly prolonged; dibucaine number 50-69
Atypical	Homozygote A	0.3	Decreased by 70% or more	Significantly prolonged; dibucaine # 16-30
Fluoride	Homozygote F	0.03	Decreased by 60%	Moderately prolonged
Silent	Homozygote S	0.04	No activity	Significantly prolonged

PChE, *Plasma cholinesterase.*
**The gene controlling the synthesis of PChE is known to exist in at least four allelic forms, though 25 other forms and another gene locus have been speculated. The allelic forms are designated EU, EA, EF, and ES. The phenotypes most susceptible to apnea after succinylcholine or mivacurium administration are AA, SS, FF, FS, AS, AF, and, to some extent, UA.*

In one case a 76-year-old man undergoing electroconvulsive therapy (ECT) therapy received succinylcholine with significant adverse effects.[28] Two different ECT sessions associated with the administration of succinylcholine resulted in the development of ventricular tachycardia, hypertension, and eventual asystole.[28] The substitution of mivacurium during subsequent ECT therapies resulted in mild hypertension with no arrythmias.[28] Furthermore, it is important to remember that reduced plasma cholinesterase levels in elderly men allow for a reduced dose of succinylcholine.[29]

Obese Patients. No contraindication to the use of succinylcholine exists in obese patients. For example, the potency of succinylcholine in obese adolescents and nonobese adolescents is similar, with an ED_{50} of 158 mcg/kg and 147 mcg/kg, respectively. It is noted, however, that PChE levels may be increased in obese adolescents, which leads to the possibility of higher dose requirements in these patients.[30] Succinylcholine use has been reported in 14 morbidly obese patients (body mass indices ranging from 35.8 to 58) who underwent laparoscopic gastric bypass surgery.[31] The authors administered doses ranging from 120 to 140 mg and successfully intubated all of the patients. Only two of the 14 patients complained of postoperative myalgia that was linked by the authors to the administration of the agent, which prompted the authors to recommend the use of succinylcholine as an integral part of the induction of general anesthesia in affected patients.[31]

Pediatrics. Few issues have caused more debate in anesthetic circles than the use of succinylcholine in children. Its ability to be administered intramuscularly or sublingually, as well as intravenously, has led to its use on a fairly large scale for many years.[32,33,34] Nevertheless, the drug is not without its drawbacks. With a structure so close to that of ACh, succinylcholine has resulted in cardiac arrhythmias, particularly bradycardia and sinus arrest, in children who are primarily vagal autonomically. These side effects, however, can usually be prevented with the administration of 0.1 mg of atropine before the initial dose of succinylcholine is given.[35]

Other side effects have proved more worrisome. The jaw-opening ability and the presence or absence of masseter spasm, often considered a precursor of malignant hyperpyrexia, was reported in a prospective study of 63 children anesthetized with halothane then relaxed with succinylcholine, pancuronium, or vecuronium. Although vecuronium and pancuronium did not cause problems with jaw opening, succinylcholine was associated with this problem, and some of the succinylcholine patients were difficult to intubate.[36] Masseter spasm was noted to be more frequent in children in whom succinylcholine was administered concomitantly with halothane when compared with children who received succinylcholine and thiopental.[22]

A random sample of 6500 anesthetic records (53% of 12,169 anesthetic procedures performed) was reviewed. Fifteen cases of masseter spasm were identified. In each case the patient underwent halothane induction and was then given succinylcholine intravenously.[37] Seven of the 15 cases of masseter spasm developed in children between ages 8 and 10 years.[37] An increased incidence of masseter spasm in children with strabismus who were anesthetized with halothane and received IV succinylcholine was noted. Of 1468 halothane anesthetic procedures, 15 cases of masseter spasm were discovered, and of these 15 cases, 6 occurred in the 211 patients with strabismus.[38]

There have also been reports of intractable cardiac arrest in children given succinylcholine. Rosenberg and Gronert[39] described the deaths of four boys younger than age 8 years after the administration of halothane or succinylcholine during 1991 and 1992. At least one case was linked to unrecognized Duchenne's muscular dystrophy. Earlier case reports were published of prolonged cardiac arrest in an apparently healthy child who was later diagnosed with Duchenne's muscular dystrophy.[40]

These concerns and others led to controversy in January 1994. Several authors noted that succinylcholine was contraindicated in children unless the situation warrants an emergency tracheal intubation.[41,42,43] Another group acknowledged that adverse reactions could occur but questioned whether the term *contraindicated* was too strong, in light of the low incidence of reported problems.[41,44] Still others stated that the wording was appropriate in light of the fact that these complications could occur in healthy-appearing individuals with occult neuromuscular disease, offering the clinician no warning and rendering it difficult to prepare for possible problems.[42,43] This debate continues. Cote states,

> *Succinylcholine remains the drug of choice when rapid onset of muscle relaxation is essential. Eventually, a rapid acting nondepolarizing muscle relaxant will replace succinylcholine; until such a drug is commercially available, succinylcholine must still be used for specific indications. Currently succinylcholine is used only for airway emergencies and not for routine intubation in pediatric patients.*[45]

Other Factors. Common side effects and contraindications of succinylcholine are noted in Table 11-4 and Box 11-1.

Intraocular Pressure. Intraocular pressure (IOP) is known to increase by 5 to 15 mm Hg for as much as 10 minutes

TABLE 11-4 Side Effects of Succinylcholine

Side Effect	Probable Cause
Hyperkalemia	Normally, serum K^+ increased by up to 0.5 mEq/L secondary to potassium leaking from the depolarized muscle; in patients with crush injuries, burns, denervating injuries, or malignant hyperthermia, K^+ levels may rise much higher
Dysrhythmias	Secondary to hyperkalemia or ganglionic effects of succinylcholine; wide electrocardiographic complexes leading to cardiac arrest have been seen in children with dystrophin-deficient muscular dystrophies, Duchenne muscular dystrophy, and Becker muscular dystrophy
Myalgia	Secondary to fasciculation, even though some patients complain of muscle pain without having shown evidence of fasciculation
Myoglobinemia	A rare complication after extensive fasciculation or in malignant hyperthermia
Elevated intragastric pressure	Secondary to contraction of abdominal muscles during fasciculation; however, the elevations of intragastric pressure seen after succinylcholine are less significant than occur with CO_2 insufflation during laparoscopic procedures
Elevated intracranial pressure	Postulated to be secondary to fasciculation and increased central venous pressure; doubt exists that succinylcholine has much of an effect; a traumatic intubation by itself may cause increased intracranial pressure; counteracted by the usual initial administration of an induction agent
Elevated intraocular pressure	Mechanism is not known; appears not to be related to the contraction of ocular muscles during succinylcholine-induced fasciculation
Malignant hyperthermia	Associated with a genetic predisposition; mechanism by which succinylcholine triggers the syndrome is not understood
Masseter spasm	Seen more often in children than in adults, perhaps more so when succinylcholine is used with halothane than with thiopental; sometimes followed by malignant hyperthermia

CO_2, *Carbon dioxide;* $K+$, *potassium.*
Modified from Nejman AM. Muscle relaxants. In: Kirby RR, Gravenstein N, Lobarto EB, et al, eds. Clinical Anesthesia Practice. *2nd ed. Philadelphia: Saunders; 2002:707-714.*

after succinylcholine administration.[17] This increase is related to both the dilation of choroidal vessels and the contraction of extraocular muscles.[22] One author, however, disputes the finding of extraocular muscle contraction as a mechanism for increased IOP, noting that patients with extraocular muscle disease undergoing elective enucleation still experienced increases in IOP.[46]

This rise in IOP with succinylcholine administration is significantly less than the IOP increase associated with coughing or bucking. Patients who receive succinylcholine and are intubated 1 minute after its administration had IOPs that were not significantly higher than baseline.[47] A Medline review of articles from 1966 to June 2003 revealed no documented reports of the extrusion of globe contents on concomitant administration of succinylcholine. A recent review has essentially refuted the issue of eye damage following succinylcholine administration in open globe injuries. It appears as a theoretical but not a clinical concern. Securing the airway remains the primary issue.[17]

BOX 11-1

Contraindications to the Use of Succinylcholine

- Hyperkalemia
- Burn patients with burns over 35% TBSA, third-degree burn
- Severe muscle trauma
- Neurologic injury (e.g., paraplegia, quadriplegia)
- Hyperkalemia resulting from renal failure
- Severe sepsis (e.g., abdominal)
- Muscle wasting, prolonged immobilization, extensive muscle denervation
- Malignant hyperthermia
- Duchenne muscular dystrophy
- Selected muscle disorders (see Table 11-5)
- Should be used in children under 8 years old only in emergency situations; not for routine intubation
- Genetic variants of pseudocholinesterase
- Allergy

TBSA, *Total body surface area.*

Hyperkalemia. Succinylcholine administration results in a short-lived hyperkalemia. A 0.5- to 1-mEq/ L increase in serum potassium levels within 3 minutes after administration is usual. The effects were reported as lasting less than 10 to 15 minutes.[26] At least two explanations exist with regard to potassium release with succinylcholine administration.[23,26]

A muscle receives signals to perform various functions from action potentials. As the action potential traverses the neuron, an influx of sodium and release of potassium occur.[26] This mechanism of potassium release during normal muscle signaling is the same mechanism by which serum potassium increases because of the depolarization associated with receiving succinylcholine.[26]

Hyperkalemia may be profound in certain patients. One particular case involved a 15-year-old girl who received succinylcholine after liver transplant and developed fatal hyperkalemia with a potassium of 9 mEq/L.[23] Other diseases and pathologic states associated with an exaggerated potassium release after succinylcholine administration include burns, spinal cord injuries, Parkinson's disease, tetanus, and muscular dystrophy. Thapa and Brull propose that this relates to a "proliferation of postsynaptic ACh receptors beyond the neuromuscular junction (extra junctional receptors) with the result that potassium flux is not restricted to the neuromuscular junction."[26] Patients with receptor upregulation are also noted to experience hyperkalemia. Two main factors are related to hyperkalemia associated with receptor upregulation. Not only is the number of receptors increased, but also the receptor subunits are altered and result in longer channel open time, resulting in a large efflux of potassium.[23]

Patients with musculoskeletal weakness or injury are at risk to develop hyperkalemia when exposed to succinylcholine. When curare is administered to rats in doses that resulted in weakening but not total paralysis, they developed increased numbers of ACh receptors. The administration of succinylcholine to these animals resulted in significantly higher serum potassium levels than were present in the precurarized state.[48] This study proved prescient, as three researchers subsequently reported succinylcholine-induced deaths in patients who had prolonged neuromuscular blockade.[49-51] The immobility does not have to be induced by physical illness or pharmacologic paralysis. In one unusual case, a catatonic schizophrenic undergoing an electroencephalographic study also experienced hyperkalemia.[52]

Finally, other severe illnesses not associated with immobility may also result in this syndrome. In one case a patient with severe mucositis after chemotherapy had a fatal response to the administration of succinylcholine.[53] In another case a patient with a botulism-infected wound was exposed to succinylcholine and subsequently experienced a cardiac arrest.[54] The use of various muscle relaxants in patients with muscle disorders is reviewed in Table 11-5.

Succinylcholine has been implicated in hyperkalemia after its administration to burn patients and is contraindicated in these patients.[55] Receptor upregulation resulting from thermal trauma has been associated with several documented cases of cardiac arrest involving succinylcholine administration.[23] Indeed, plasma potassium levels as high as 15 mEq/L have been reported after the administration of succinylcholine, with this effect occurring 4 to 10 days after the burn but lasting as long as 120 days after the burn.[56] It is generally reported that the administration of succinylcholine to a burn patient more than 24 hours after the burn is unsafe; however, others note that succinylcholine can be safely used with burn patients for up to 7 days after the burn, as receptor upregulation does not begin until 24 to 48 hours after the burn.[57,58] Clearly, succinylcholine should be used only after the greatest deliberation regarding risks versus benefits, especially in light of the development of the newer, quicker-onset nondepolarizing agents.[10]

Malignant Hyperthermia. Succinylcholine has been associated with a specific condition known as *malignant hyperthermia* (MH).[22] The occurrence of MH in patients who receive a combination of succinylcholine with volatile anesthetic agents ranges from 1:4000 to 1:40,000.[22] Patients who develop MH show signs such as muscle rigidity, convulsions, metabolic acidosis, and a rapid increase in temperature. One study showed evidence that the preservative used in succinylcholine, called *chlorocresol*, actually produced a response similar to that of MH in both rabbits and isolated human muscle samples.[59]

It is important to note, however, that not all signs and symptoms of MH in response to succinylcholine arise immediately, nor are they easily identified. One report focused on a

TABLE 11-5 Response of Neuromuscular Blocking Agents in Select Muscle Disorders

Neuromuscular Disorder	Succinylcholine	Nondepolarizing Neuromuscular Blocking Agents
Multiple sclerosis	Contraindicated	Increased sensitivity; anesthetic stress may increase the rate of relapse
Motor neuron disease (amyotrophic lateral sclerosis [ALS, Lou Gehrig's Disease])	Contraindicated	Increased sensitivity
Guillain-Barré syndrome	Contraindicated	Increased sensitivity; avoid agents with cardiac side effects
Charcot-Marie-Tooth disease	Contraindicated	Response to atracurium and mivacurium normal; all others, increased sensitivity
Muscular dystrophies	Contraindicated	Increased sensitivity
Myotonias	Contraindicated	Increased sensitivity; anticholinesterase agents may precipitate myotonia
Myasthenic syndromes	Resistant; prolonged duration of action may be present with plasmapheresis or anticholinesterase therapy	Extreme sensitivity
Mitochondrial myopathies	Contraindicated	Increased sensitivity
Hyperkalemic periodic paralysis	Contraindicated	Normal response
Hypokalemic periodic paralysis	Contraindicated	Normal response
Malignant hyperthermia	Contraindicated	Normal response
Myasthenia gravis	Resistant	Increased sensitivity
Huntington's chorea	Increased sensitivity	Increased sensitivity
Upregulation of acetylcholine receptors because of spinal cord trauma, stroke, or prolonged immobility	Contraindicated	Usually resistant, but depends on time since injury

Modified from Naguib M, Flood P, McArdle J, et al. Advances in neurobiology of the neuromuscular junction: implications for the anesthesiologist. Anesthesiology. 2002;96:202-231; and Malignant Hyperthermia Association of America, 11 East State Street, PO Box 1069, Sherburne, NY 13460.

27-year-old man who underwent two anesthetic procedures, both of which used succinylcholine, and who developed a low-grade fever but no masseter spasm or muscle rigidity.[60] His temperature rose 4 days after the second surgery; he developed sepsis-like symptoms and subsequently died. Postmortem examination of muscle tissue resulted in the diagnosis of MH despite the unusual presentation.[60] A second case of delayed response was reported during resuscitation from upper torso trauma, during which masseter spasm was encountered after the administration of succinylcholine.[61] In this instance the onset of MH did not occur until 2.5 hours after the administration of succinylcholine, and the patient was successfully treated with dantrolene.[61] One final case reported an MH-sensitive patient who did not disclose his history and received succinylcholine and isoflurane without any MH-like response to either agent.[62]

A family history of MH is an absolute contraindication to succinylcholine administration.[24,63] A complete discussion of the physiologic and treatment aspects of MH can be found in Chapter 30.

Myalgias and Fasciculations. Postoperative muscle pain, particularly in the subcostal region, trunk, neck, upper abdominal muscles, and shoulders, is a common occurrence after succinylcholine administration.[24,64] Such myalgias are attributed to the occurrence of fasciculations resulting from repetitive firing of the motor nerve terminals, which causes uncoordinated muscle contractions.[64] Patients who experience muscle pain most often are women and those persons who rarely participate in muscular activity.[24] Conversely, patients at extremes of age, as well as pregnant patients, are least affected. The average occurrence of these postoperative muscle pains is 50%, with a wide range of incidence from 1.5% to 89%.[65]

Prevention is the key to avoiding postoperative muscle pain. Postoperative myalgias associated with succinylcholine increase in severity with early ambulation, which may consequently delay postoperative healing.[64] Administration of a defasciculating dose of a nondepolarizing neuromuscular blocking agent helps decrease myalgias by as much as 10% to 50%.[64,65] Without this defasciculating dose of a nondepolarizing neuromuscular blocker, postoperative myalgias may last from 2 to 7 days.[64] Postulated mechanisms of action of various pretreatment agents are given in Table 11-6.

Phase II Block. Administration of large doses of succinylcholine results in an alteration of the block.[24] It changes to resemble more of a nondepolarizing block, as evidenced by fade in response to tetanic stimuli, posttetanic potentiation, and antagonism with drugs such as neostigmine.[66] This most commonly is referred to as a *desensitization* or *phase II block.* One case report of potentiation of a preexisting phase II block after vancomycin administration has been noted.[66] An 82-year-old man undergoing surgery on the larynx had received a total of 2.8 mg of succinylcholine per kilogram by the end of his case. A phase II block was noted, with fade of the fourth twitch in a train-of-four (TOF). The patient was successfully extubated, his airway was adequately supported, and he was transferred to the postanesthesia care unit (PACU). During transfer to the PACU a vancomycin drip was initiated. Shortly thereafter the patient was noted to be paralyzed and apneic. This was attributed to vancomycin potentiation of a previously noted phase II block. The interaction with vancomycin and other therapeutic drugs such as neomycin, tobramycin, gentamicin, and streptomycin is thought to be related to both inhibition of the presynaptic ACh release, changes in calcium modulation, and postsynaptic competition with the motor nerve end plate.[66]

To avoid a phase II block practitioners avoid succinylcholine infusions and doses exceeding 6 to 8 mg/kg. Phase II block occurs less frequently with high dose succinylcholine in addition to volatile agents but is more frequently seen during concomitant administration with nitrous opioid anesthesia.[24] It has been proposed that the cellular mechanism of action of a phase II block is attributed to both ionic and conformational changes of the cell that result after any prolonged depolarization.[21] More specifically, this is a late occurrence related to the prolonged exposure of the motor end plate to succinylcholine. This block is also noted as a "dual block" resulting from its transition from phase I with a depolarizing agent to phase II with a depolarizing agent and resembling a nondepolarizing block.[67]

TABLE 11-6 Postulated Mechanisms of Action of Pretreatment Agents

Component in Mechanism of Postoperative Myalgia	Pretreatment Agent	Postulated Mechanism of Action
Neuromuscular junction	Nondepolarizing neuromuscular blockers	Prejunctional
	Phenytoin	Prejunctional
	Self-taming	Neuromuscular desensitization
Muscle fibers, stretch receptors	Stretching exercises	Desensitization of stretch receptors
	Vitamin C	Prevents damage to muscle fibers
Cell membrane, intracellular calcium mechanisms	Lidocaine	Cell membrane stabilization
	Calcium gluconate	Cell membrane stabilization
	Dantrolene	Interferes with intracellular calcium transfer
Fasciculations	Dose of succinylcholine	Synchronicity of muscle contractions
	Magnesium	Abolishes fasciculations
Muscle damage	Aspirin or nonsteroidal antiinflammatory drugs	Interrupt prostaglandin-mediated destructive cycle
	Chlorpromazine	Inhibits cellular phospholipases

Modified from Wong SF, Chung F. Succinylcholine-associated postoperative myalgia. Anaesthesia. *2000;55:144-152.*

NONDEPOLARIZING AGENTS

Mivacurium Chloride

Mivacurium (Mivacron) was marketed as the first "short-acting" NMBA (see Figure 11-2). Its chemical formula is (*R*-(*R**, *R**-(*E*)))-2,2′-((1,8-dioxo-4-octene-1,8-diyl) bis(oxy-3,1-propenediyl) bis(1,2,3,4-tetrahydro-6,7-dimethoxy-2-methyl-1-(3,4,5-trimethoxyphenyl) methyl) isoquinolinium) chloride.[68] Mivacurium chloride is (*R*-(*R**, *R**-(*E*)))-2,2′-((1,8-dioxo-4-octene-1,8-diyl) bis(oxy-3,1-propenediyl)) bis(1,2,3,4-tetrahydro-6,7-dimethoxy-2-methyl-1-((3,4,5-trimethoxyphenyl) methyl) isoquinolinium) dichloride. Mivacurium is classified as a benzylisoquinolinium and consists of a mixture of three different isomers.[69,70] The *trans-trans* and *cis-trans* are the two most active stereoisomers, contributing 57% and 36%, respectively, to the composition of mivacurium. Animal studies show that the *cis-cis* isomer contributes only 6% of the composition, with one tenth the activity of the *trans-trans* and *cis-trans* isomers.[70] The intubating dose of mivacurium is 0.2 mg/kg.[11] Problems associated with histamine release may be avoided by administering the drug in two divided doses. The first dose is 0.15 mg/kg, followed by a second dose of 0.1 mg/kg after a 30-second interval.[71] Perioperative relaxation is achieved with a dose of 0.05 mg/kg.[11] The ED_{95} of mivacurium is 0.08 mg/kg.[63,72,73,74] Its degradation by plasma cholinesterase provides it with a short duration.[69] The structures of the nondepolarizing muscle relaxants are listed in Figure 11-2.

Pharmacodynamics

Onset. The times to 90% suppression of first twitch (T1) in American Society of Anesthesiologists Physical Classification I or II (ASA I or II) adults has been studied. Those receiving a dose of 0.20 mg/kg achieved this 90% reduction in 2.2 (0.8) minutes, whereas in those receiving a dose of 0.25 mg/kg, onset times decreased to 1.5 (0.8) minutes. The onset time of mivacurium in healthy adults receiving 0.18 mg/kg along with nitrous-oxide–opioid anesthesia was 3.7 minutes.[75] The onset of mivacurium using the adductor muscles of the larynx as well as the adductor pollicis was determined to be 2.5 (0.7) minutes at the vocal cords and 4 (1.3) minutes at the adductor pollicis with a dose of 0.07 mg/kg.[76]

Finally the use of mivacurium versus succinylcholine in laparoscopy patients was compared. Onset time to maximum depression of T1 was 6.1 minutes (0.6) in patients who received a dose of 0.015 mg/kg and opioid–nitrous oxide anesthesia (group II) and 5.7 (0.8) minutes in patients who received an identical dose with nitrous oxide–enflurane anesthesia (group III). Times to 70% blockade of T1 in groups II and III were 2.4 (1) minutes for group II and 2.4 (1.8) minutes for group III, whereas times to 90% blockade of T1 were 3.4 (0.3) minutes for group II and 3.8 (0.3) minutes for group III.[77]

Duration. Mivacurium chloride was developed specifically to fill the niche between the short-acting succinylcholine and intermediate-acting atracurium and vecuronium in the neuromuscular blockade armamentarium.[63] The duration of mivacurium is 15 to 20 minutes, approximately twice that of succinylcholine,[11] and is dose related. The time to 25%, 75%, and 95% spontaneous recovery of T1 was measured in patients who received nitrous oxide–opioid anesthesia after an infusion

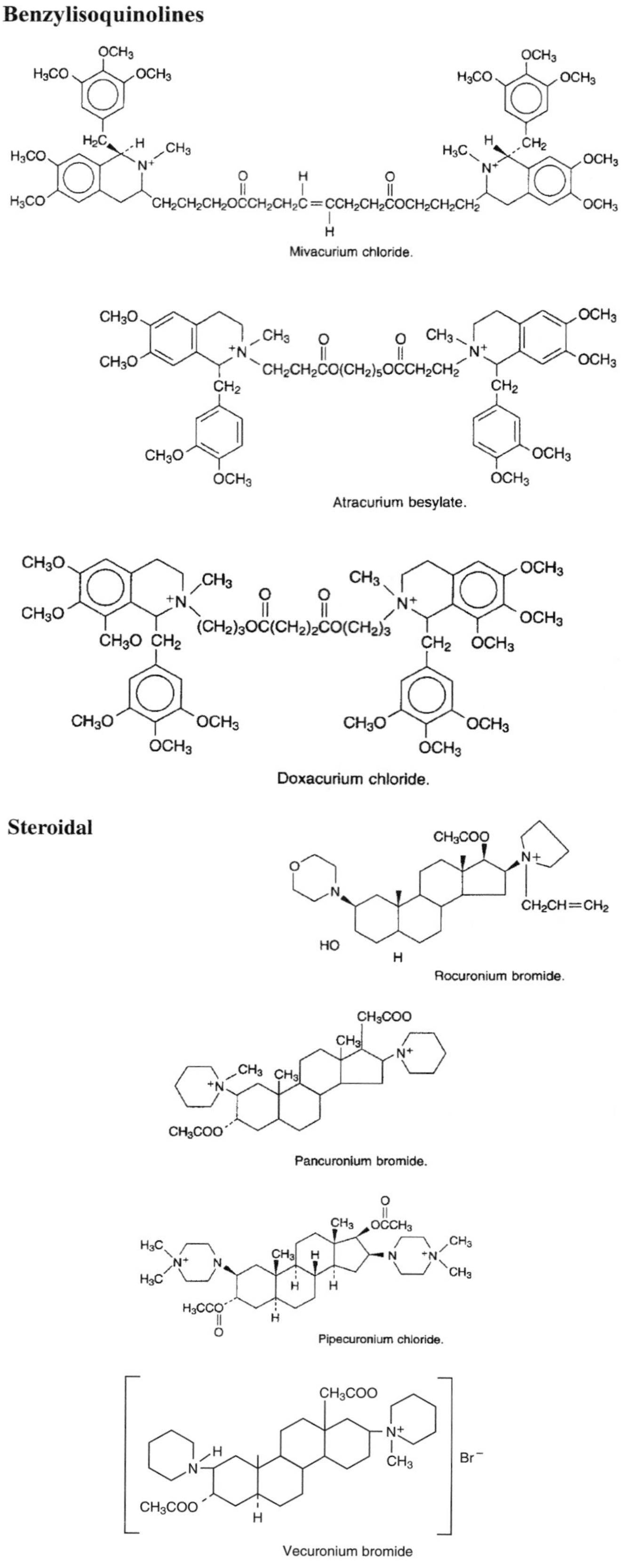

Benzylisoquinolines

Mivacurium chloride.

Atracurium besylate.

Doxacurium chloride.

Steroidal

Rocuronium bromide.

Pancuronium bromide.

Pipecuronium chloride.

Vecuronium bromide

FIGURE **11-2**
Structure of nondepolarizing muscle relaxants.

dose of 10 mcg/kg/min. These patients recovered in 6.9 (1.6), 11.5 (1.8), and 14.7 (2.8) minutes, respectively.[71]

Additionally, the time to 25% spontaneous recovery of twitch (among other times) was measured in patients who received 0.15 mg of mivacurium per kilogram, and it was found that patients who received opioid–nitrous oxide anesthesia recovered this value in 24 (8) minutes, whereas those who received enflurane–nitrous oxide anesthesia recovered to the same extent in 22 (10) minutes.[77] Others, however, using the same dose, reported a return to 95% of twitch height in 26 minutes in adult patients who received nitrous oxide, oxygen, and opioid anesthesia.[63] Initial bolus doses of mivacurium may result in varying recovery times.[72] Brandom and associates,[78] who administered mivacurium to adult patients who received nitrous oxide, oxygen, and opioid anesthesia, noted that the time for the first twitch in a TOF to return to 5% of the baseline height was 17.5 (1.8) minutes after an initial dose of 0.25 mg/kg was administered.

Elimination. Like that of succinylcholine, mivacurium's degradation by plasma cholinesterase results in its short action.[70] The rate of metabolism (measured in vitro) was found to be 88% that of succinylcholine.[72] In vivo, the rate of degradation has been found to be 50% to 90% that of succinylcholine.[68] Mivacurium is metabolized into two molecules of a quaternary alcohol and a dicarboxylic acid, and these metabolites are subsequently eliminated in the bile and urine.[63] Any disease process that interferes with the production of this enzyme results in the prolongation of action of this agent.[78]

Succinylcholine should not be administered to patients with atypical plasma cholinesterase. Patients with a deficiency of plasma cholinesterase exhibit prolonged blockade. Patients who are heterozygous for the atypical plasma cholinesterase gene experienced recovery times that were prolonged approximately 50% compared with those in patients without the gene.[79,80] Patients who had a homozygous occurrence of the atypical plasma cholinesterase gene experienced significantly prolonged recovery times as well.[80,81]

Renal excretion via the urine results in the elimination of up to 7% of mivacurium.[82]

Pharmacodynamic Summary. The onset time of mivacurium is dose dependent and ranges from 1.5 minutes with 0.25 mg/kg up to 4 minutes with 0.15 mg/kg. The duration of mivacurium is 15 to 20 minutes. The metabolites of mivacurium are excreted in the urine, after the agent itself has been broken down by plasma cholinesterases.[83]

Central Nervous System

AChE, the enzyme responsible for terminating cholinergic transmission at both the neuromuscular junction and the central nervous system, is a naturally occurring enzyme found in humans that hydrolyzes mivacurium.[84] Patients undergoing long-term anticonvulsant therapy have been reported to demonstrate a decreased duration of action with regard to NMBA.[85,86] Resistance to mivacurium in this patient population has not been established.[87]

Cardiovascular System

The arrival of mivacurium on the nondepolarizing neuromuscular blocker scene once again initiated research to determine whether this ultra–short-acting neuromuscular blocker would achieve the important goal of hemodynamic stability. Early researched showed that when the dose of this agent exceeded 0.15 mg/kg, decreases in arterial blood pressure lasting several minutes could occur.[69,85] Savarese and colleagues,[88] for example, found that rapid injections of mivacurium at a dose of 0.2 mg/kg resulted in a decrease in mean arterial pressure of 18%, whereas doses of 0.25 mg/kg and 0.3 mg/kg resulted in decreases of 13% and 32%, respectively. Other researchers echoed or amplified these results, warning against the use of the rapid injection of doses higher than 0.15 mg/kg.[85,89] The hypotension has been linked to histamine release, such as that occurring with higher doses of atracurium. In a study comparing the speed of onset of mivacurium with that of succinylcholine, Poler and associates[77] noted that patients in experimental groups who received mivacurium at a dose of 0.15 mg/kg experienced cutaneous flushing: 40% in the group anesthetized with alfentanil and nitrous oxide and 60% in the group anesthetized with enflurane and nitrous oxide. Of interest, this effect was not associated with hypotension.[77] The cardiovascular effects of mivacurium have been examined in 90 adult patients, ASA class I or II, undergoing elective surgery. Of these patients, 45 received a balanced anesthetic technique using nitrous oxide, oxygen, and narcotic, and the remaining 45 received nitrous oxide, oxygen, and isoflurane. In both groups and at doses ranging from 0.05 to 0.15 mg/kg, no statistically significant differences in mean arterial pressure or heart rate occurred.[90] The effects of stimulation of histamine receptors and cardiac effects are listed in Box 11-2.

Hepatic System

Patients with severe hepatic disease were noted to have an increased sensitivity to mivacurium that was inversely related to their plasma cholinesterase levels.[91] At a dose of 0.15 mg of mivacurium per kilogram, the effects of this agent in nine patients with hepatic disease were compared with the effects in nine healthy patients. No difference existed in the time of onset of the agent: 2.1 (0.9) minutes in patients with hepatic failure versus 1.9 (1) minutes in healthy control patients.[82] The times to 25% recovery of initial twitch and to 95% of initial twitch were prolonged in the patients with hepatic failure when compared with those in healthy patients. The time to 25% recovery of initial twitch was 15.7 (9.3) minutes in patients with hepatic failure, compared with 5.5 (2.2) minutes in healthy patients. The time to 95% recovery of initial twitch was 86.3 (44.2) minutes in patients with hepatic failure, compared with 27.4 (10.8) minutes in healthy control patients. The prolongation of action was attributable to the well-known decrease in plasma cholinesterase activity experienced by patients with severe hepatic insult.

Renal System

Mivacurium was also administered to patients with renal failure.[82] The onset time was 2.6 (0.9) minutes compared with 1.9 (1) minutes in normal control patients. The time to recovery of 95% of twitch was 51 (15.5) minutes in the experimental group, compared with 27.4 (10.8) minutes in the control group. These researchers found that in patients with renal failure, 7% of the administered dose of the agent was found unchanged in the urine within 6 hours of administration. The small amount that was excreted via this mechanism was attributed to the enzymatic breakdown pathway of the agent.[73,74,82] Patients with renal

BOX **11-2**

Effects of Stimulation of Histamine Receptors by Neuromuscular Blockers and Cardiac Effects

H_1 Receptors	*H_2 Receptors*
Increased capillary permeability	Increased gastric acid production
Bronchoconstriction	Systemic and cerebral vasodilation
Intestinal contraction	Positive inotropic effects
Negative dromotropic effects	Positive chronotropic effects

Mivacurium and atracurium release modest amounts of histamine. Slight histamine release may occur with succinylcholine. The amount of histamine release is dependent on dose and speed of injection.

With endogenous histamine release all receptor responses are elicited.

Prophylaxis against histamine release requires administration of both H_1- and H_2-receptor blockers.

Cardiac Effects

- Atracurium and mivacurium cause histamine release, therefore produce hypotension and tachycardia
- Pancuronium is vagolytic and causes slight catecholamine release (indirect sympathomimetic) producing tachycardia
- Succinylcholine usually results in slight tachycardia; however, sudden abrupt bradycardia may result from repeat dosing in adults and any dose in children. Many types of arrhythmias have been reported

H, *Histamine*.

disease who receive mivacurium may have a prolonged action of the drug when there is an alteration (decrease) in plasma cholinesterase activity.[14]

Special Populations

Elderly Patients. Mivacurium was administered to elderly patients and younger control patients at a dose of 0.10 mg/kg.[92] No significant differences were noted in degree of neuromuscular blockade or time to 25% recovery (19.9 [1.2] minutes in the elderly versus 18 [1.7] minutes in young control patients). The responses of 32 elderly patients were compared with those of an equal-sized group of young adults. The dose requirements were the same for both groups, and the agent had a slightly longer, but significantly different duration of action in the elderly. The mean time to the return of a 0.7 TOF ratio was 21 minutes in the older patients, versus 16.5 minutes in the younger patients.[93]

The choice of mivacurium over succinylcholine for elderly patients receiving ECT was endorsed by one author, who cited the problems experienced by older patients with the side-effects attributed to succinylcholines.[94] Although mivacurium has a small histamine release, it has no direct cardiovascular side effects, making it an acceptable agent in elderly patients with cardiovascular instability.[24]

Obese Patients. No adverse effects of mivacurium were discovered with regard to its administration in obese patients. When mivacurium was used for a laparoscopic cholecystectomy on an obese patient with myotonic dystrophy, no neuromuscular or pulmonary complications were reported.[95]

Pediatrics. The properties of mivacurium and those of succinylcholine were compared in children. Children aged 2 to 12 years were given an IV dose of 0.2 mg of mivacurium per kilogram, and the effects were compared with those in a group of children who received 1 mg of succinylcholine per kilogram. The time to onset of 75% of blockade suppression was 83 seconds (range 29 to 235 seconds) in the mivacurium group, compared with 32 seconds (range 14 to 73 seconds) in the succinylcholine group. Time to recovery to 25% of maximal twitch depression was 615 seconds (range, 308 to 1227 seconds) in the mivacurium group, compared with 196 seconds (range, 117 to 327 seconds) in the succinylcholine group.[96] Other researchers attempted to compare intramuscular mivacurium to intramuscular succinylcholine but were never able to achieve more than 80% twitch depression, even at a dose of 800 mg/kg, at which point the study was terminated.[97]

Other Factors

Thermal Injury. The resistance to neuromuscular relaxants in burn patients is mainly attributed to alterations in receptor sites.[98] In addition, thermal injury leads to decreases in plasma cholinesterase levels, which is especially noteworthy in drugs such as mivacurium in which breakdown is initiated and completed by plasma cholinesterase. The administration of a dose of 0.2 mg/kg resulted in good relaxation conditions in burn patients, and the onset of mivacurium was very similar to that in the control groups, indicating that it may be safely used in patients with thermal injury.[98]

Atypical Plasma Cholinesterase. Caution is warranted with mivacurium administration to patients with known alterations in plasma cholinesterase activity. Prolonged paralysis after a test dose of 30 mcg/kg in a patient with a previously known plasma cholinesterase deficit has been reported.[99] Conversely, patients with elevated plasma cholinesterase activity were difficult if not impossible to paralyze.[100] Therefore, it is essential to obtain a thorough history regarding the patient and family before the administration of mivacurium (see Table 11-3).

Rocuronium Bromide

The introduction of vecuronium and atracurium, both of which were marketed as intermediate-acting nondepolarizing muscle relaxants, improved the flexibility of the clinician in matching the agent to the expected duration of surgery.[101] Slow onset, solution stability, and histamine release remained problems to be overcome.[102] Rocuronium (Zemuron) has been developed to partially fill this void; it combines a duration and cardiovascular profile comparable to those of vecuronium with an onset that is only slightly longer than that of succinylcholine.[68,101-103] It exists in a solution that is stable at room temperature for up to 30 days.[104]

A derivative of vecuronium, rocuronium bromide is chemically designated as 1-[17β-(acetyloxy)-3α-hydroxy-2β-(4-morpholinyl)-5α-androstan-16β-yl]-1-(2-propenyl) pyrrolidinium bromide, and it has one seventh to one eighth the potency of its derivative.[13,24,103] It is a monoquaternary structure that also shares its aminosteroid structure with pancuronium.[105] It has a molecular weight of 609.7 and a molecular formula of $C_{32}H_{53}BrN_2O_4$ (Figure 11-2).[101] The pH of rocuronium is adjusted to 4, and the agent contains no preservative. Each 1 ml of solution contains 10 mg of rocuronium bromide and 2 mg of sodium acetate.[103]

Results of clinical studies of both healthy children and healthy adults suggest an ED_{95} of approximately 0.3 mg/kg.[12] Its steady-state volume of distribution in healthy adults is 207 (14) ml/kg and is slightly smaller for children age 4 to 8 years.[103] Rocuronium is approximately 30% bound to human plasma proteins, somewhat less than other neuromuscular blockers.[103] Other researchers dispute these data. For example, Chaudhry and associates[106] found the agent in vitro to be 72% bound to plasma proteins. Even so, with regard to this characteristic, rocuronium compares very favorably with similar agents, such as vecuronium, which is 91% bound.[103] This decreased plasma protein binding may lead to a more rapid onset, because more unbound drug is readily available at the neuronal binding sites.[85,103,107]

Pharmacodynamics

Onset. Rocuronium, a vecuronium derivative, was introduced in 1992.[13] It became a widely accepted alternative to succinylcholine during rapid sequence intubation (RSI) because of its quick onset of action and cardiovascular stability.[13,27] Rocuronium is the ideal NMBA for RSI when succinylcholine is contraindicated.[21] The disadvantages of use of rocuronium during RSI include its long duration of action.[21] Rocuronium has been shown to be safe for use during RSI in patients with increase IOP when succinylcholine cannot be used.[108,109]

Administration of rocuronium with doses ranging from 0.6 mg/kg to 1.2 mg/kg provides good to excellent intubating conditions within 45 to 90 seconds.[14,27,110] A 95% probability of successful intubation at 60 seconds was noted after a 1.04-mg/kg dose.[111] The onset of muscle relaxants is related to potency. The less potent an agent, the faster the onset. Rocuronium has an onset of action that is inversely proportional to its potency.[68] Rocuronium is less potent than other steroidal-based neuromuscular blockers.[85,112,113] This decrease in potency and the decrease in the amount of drug that is protein bound allow a larger mass of drug at the prejunctional and postjunctional cholinoreceptors.[14,85] This large drug mass at the receptor site yields a faster onset.[103,106]

Duration. With regard to length of action, rocuronium is classified as intermediate in duration.[16] Its duration of action is similar to that of vecuronium, and its duration depends, like that of many other agents, on the dose administered.[13] An intubating dose of 0.6 mg/kg to 1 mg/kg provides a clinical duration of 30 to 90 minutes.[13,14] The administration of 0.6 mg/kg resulted in 10% recovery of T1 within 27.2 (5.5) minutes, whereas 25%, 75%, and 90% recovery of T1 occurred in 31.1 (5.6) minutes, 39.3 (6.2) minutes, and 41.2 (6.1) minutes, respectively.[86] Recovery of the TOF ratio to 0.8 when rocuronium was administered with sevoflurane, isoflurane, and propofol occurred in 103 (30.7), 69(20.4), and 62(21.1) minutes, respectively.[114]

Elimination. The primary means of rocuronium elimination is deacetylation via the liver.[86,115] Renal excretion accounts for 35% of elimination.[24] Plasma levels of rocuronium follow a three-compartment open model. This results in extensive redistribution after IV injection. Therefore, before elimination occurs, serum levels of the drug are low enough to result in recovery.[12] The elimination half-life of rocuronium is 60 to 120 minutes. The elimination half-lives of the agent in children, normal adults, and elderly persons are 38.3 (11.7) minutes, 56 (20) minutes, and 137 (101) minutes, respectively.[85,116]

Pharmacodynamic Summary. The onset of rocuronium is 45 to 90 seconds. the duration of rocuronium is 30 to 90 minutes. Elimination of the agent is via the liver and kidneys.

Central Nervous System

Concurrent administration of anticonvulsants with drugs such as rocuronium may result in a shorter duration of action.[86] One explanation is that the formation of cytochrome P-450 in the liver may be induced, a phenomenon that increases the breakdown of the agents.[107] A combination of hepatomegaly and induced enzymes associated with long term anticonvulsant therapy explains the increased clearance of rocuronium.[86]

Cardiovascular System

Rocuronium bromide has undergone considerable scrutiny to determine whether its use ensures adequate cardiovascular stability. Rocuronium is practically devoid of cardiovascular side effects including histamine release.[12,27] Hemodynamic variables were measured in patients scheduled to undergo coronary artery bypass grafting. The patients received a dose of 0.6 mg of rocuronium per kilogram bromide on induction.[117] Heart rate and mean arterial pressure were not significantly changed in these patients, although small increases in cardiac index (11%) and stroke volume index (15%) and a reduction in pulmonary capillary wedge pressure (25%) occurred. No evidence of histamine release was found, nor was evidence of cardiac ischemia with doses up to 0.6 mg/kg.[117,118,119]

These results were reconfirmed in the adult population of patients (ASA class I, II, and III) who received varying doses of rocuronium for intubation.[120]

Hepatic System

The duration of action of rocuronium, as well as the onset, is typically prolonged in patients with hepatic disease such as cirrhosis.[14] Patients with hepatic dysfunction demonstrate an elimination half-life that is increased to 173 (111) minutes compared with the normal 60 to 120 minutes.[12,116] This supports the finding that the route of plasma clearance of rocuronium is predominantly by hepatic uptake, through which most of the drug is excreted unchanged in the bile.[82,85] Cautious dosing is warranted, with vigilant monitoring of neuromuscular function, in these patients.[14]

Earlier research showed that the elimination of rocuronium took place primarily via the bile.[82,85] However, patients with cirrhosis received 0.6 mg of rocuronium per kilogram for muscle relaxation while undergoing elective surgery. The onset time was somewhat prolonged. The times were 158 (56) seconds in patients with cirrhosis versus 108 (33) seconds in healthy controls, and the times to both 75% recovery of twitch (77 [25] minutes) and 90% recovery of twitch (88 [29] minutes) were significantly longer than in healthy control patients.[121] The report attributed this prolongation to the larger volume of distribution of the patients with cirrhosis rather than to liver parenchymal failure, although the authors noted that they were not able to demonstrate a significant increase in the apparent volume of distribution.[121]

Renal System

A small portion of rocuronium is excreted unchanged in the urine, resulting an elimination half-life of 112 (79) minutes in patients with renal dysfunction.[82,85,116] The onset time of rocuronium is not affected by renal failure. However, a prolonged duration of action of rocuronium results from a decrease in renal excretion.[122] In another study the NMBA rocuronium was administered to patients with chronic renal failure by Khunel-Brady and associates.[123] Because the hepatic route appeared to be primarily responsible for the elimination of rocuronium, patients received 0.15 mg of the agent per kilogram, resulting in an onset of 126 (54) seconds in normal control patients, compared with 182 (82) seconds in patients with renal failure.[82,85,124] The recovery times to 25% of twitch height were 28.0 (5.5) minutes for normal control patients and 25.6 (11.7) minutes for those with renal failure.[123] The researchers stated that the limited differences between duration times in these two groups suggest that in moderate doses, "the neuromuscular effects of rocuronium are little dependent on renal elimination."[123]

Special Populations

Elderly Patients. The pharmacokinetics and pharmacodynamics of rocuronium have been measured in elderly patients and compared with those in younger control patients.[92] A dose of 600 mcg/kg was administered to both groups, and onset times to 90% twitch suppression and to maximal twitch depression and recovery times were measured. The data showed no significant difference in time to onset of 90% blockade or in time to maximal block. The time until recovery of T1 was then measured. Recovery times in all categories (10%, 25%, 50%, 75%, 90%, 10% to 25%, and 25% to 75% twitch), however, were significantly prolonged in the elderly.[125] The prolongation of rocuronium in the elderly was the result of a decrease in clearance and an increase in the volume of distribution.

Obese Patients. Because of a decrease in elimination of rocuronium, obese patients have a prolonged duration of action with this drug.[14] The median duration (range) of blockade in patients with a body mass index (BMI) of >28 was 31.5 minutes (21 to 26), whereas in those with a BMI of 20 to 24, the effects of rocuronium lasted for 26 minutes (20 to 36).[126]

Pediatrics. The advent of rocuronium, with its rapid onset of action, provided an alternative to succinylcholine for rapid management of the airway. Rocuronium has a high margin of safety and is often one of the preferred NMBAs for intubation of children in emergency situations.[104] When administered in a dose of 0.6 mg/kg to children age 1 to 5 years, the onset to 90% depression of twitch is 0.8 (0.1) minute. Recovery time to 25% of maximal twitch depression is 26.7 (1.9) minutes.[119] A dose of 0.8 mg/kg results in a mean onset time that is somewhat shorter (28.2 [8.7]) seconds, with a clinical duration of 32.3 (12.4) minutes. No hemodynamic changes were associated with the administration of this agent.[119,127]

Atracurium Besylate

Atracurium (Tracrium) was developed as a result of a joint venture between the Department of Pharmaceutical Chemistry at the University of Strathclyde and the Wellcome Research Laboratories.[128] The objective of the investigators was to develop an agent with the following characteristics:

1. Competitive bis-quaternary neuromuscular blocker
2. Highly selective in action
3. Degradable without renal or hepatic intervention[128,129]

The resulting agent was a bis-quaternary competitive neuromuscular blocker in the form of a besylate salt.[128-130] Atracurium besylate is designated as 2,2′-[1,5-pentanediyl-bis[oxy(3-oxo-3,1-propanediyl)]] bis[1-[(3,4-dimethoxyphenyl) methyl]-1,2,3,4-tetrahydro-6,7-dimethoxy-2-methylisoquinolinium] dibenzenesulfonate.[131] It has a molecular weight of 1243.49 and a molecular formula of $C_{65}H_{82}N_2O_{18}S_2$ (see Figure 11-2).[131] The pH of atracurium is adjusted to 3.25 to 3.65, and the agent contains the preservative benzyl alcohol. Atracurium loses potency at the rate of 6% per year when it is refrigerated at 5° C. At room temperature the agent degrades approximately 5% per month, and its recommended unrefrigerated shelf life is 14 days.[131] It was developed with an intermediate duration in mind, and it spontaneously degrades to inactive products. It is well absorbed intravenously, with an ED_{95} of 0.10 to 0.25 mg/kg.[130,132]

Atracurium is rapidly distributed throughout the extracellular space after IV injection and has a volume of distribution of 153 (13) ml/kg.[68] It is approximately 82% protein bound and probably does not distribute into the fat, because it is ionized.[133] Obese patients who received atracurium demonstrated no difference in recovery indices or recovery times when compared with control patients of normal weight because of the agent's lack of organ dependency for elimination.[134,135,136]

Pharmacodynamics

Onset. As expected, atracurium has an onset time that is inversely proportional to dosage, in the range of 1.2 to 2.8 minutes. When various doses of atracurium were given to 70 patients anesthetized with fentanyl, thiopental, and nitrous oxide– oxygen anesthesia, clinical effects were seen at doses of 0.3 to 0.6 mg/kg.[112]

Other investigators, however, have found the onset to be longer, in the range of 2.31 to 3.55 minutes.[137-139]

Duration. The duration of atracurium increases as its dose increases. Duration of maximum effect and duration to 95% recovery of peak contraction are reported in the range of 5.6 to 69.5 minutes.[137,140,141]

Elimination. The development of atracurium arose from the discovery of the plant *Leontice leontopetalum* and one of its components, designated *petaline*.[132] This component was similar to tubocurarine and was observed to undergo an unexpectedly facile degradation in mild alkali by the well-known Hofmann elimination pathway with loss of water and formation of a tertiary base.[132] Stenlake's pursuit of this research led to the development of atracurium, which does not rely on any organ system for its breakdown and elimination. Study of the clinical pharmacology of atracurium reveals that its molecules decompose by Hofmann elimination as well as nonspecific ester hydrolysis.[128,132,134,142]

Atracurium degrades via Hofmann elimination: in mild alkaline states fission occurs at the quaternary nitrogen position, and laudanosine is subsequently released.[142,143] The agent then degrades further, after ester hydrolysis, into a quaternary alcohol and a quaternary acid.[105,112,128,142] These metabolites are excreted primarily in the bile and the urine.

Pharmacodynamic Summary. Onset time of atracurium is 1 to 3 minutes. The duration of atracurium is 20 to 60 minutes. It is degraded via Hofmann elimination, and its metabolites are subsequently excreted in bile and urine.

Central Nervous System

CNS stimulation has been noted in studies of animals after atracurium administration.[133] This CNS stimulation is primarily attributed to laudanosine, one of the metabolites produced from the breakdown of atracurium.[143] Two other metabolites produced from atracurium degradation include a quaternary alcohol and a quaternary acid, which have no CNS effects.[112,128,133,142] Studies in conscious dogs have shown that bolus doses sufficient to produce serum levels of 1.2 mcg/ml of laudanosine are associated with convulsions.[144] However, in a case report in which a patient received atracurium infusion for tetanus at a mean rate of 1.3 mg/kg/hr over a 71-day period, laudanosine concentrations were no more than 0.985 mcg/ml, and the patient incurred no CNS dysfunction.[144]

With renal failure laudanosine levels are roughly 3.5 times those of patients with normal renal function (1200 ng/ml versus 4300 ng/ml).[145] Despite this level, no adverse CNS reactions have been found.[146,147]

Cardiovascular System

Once the development of atracurium was completed, researchers attempted to determine whether it would provide a suitable and more stable neuromuscular blockade than that effected by agents already in use. Atracurium has been associated with increases in heart rate and decreases in blood pressure at doses of 0.5 mg/kg and greater because of histamine release.[148-151] Systolic and diastolic pressures significantly decrease, and cardiac output was significantly increased at 2, 5, and 10 minutes after a bolus dose. The increase in cardiac output is the result of a markedly decreased systemic vascular resistance. Nearly all of the hemodynamic changes associated with the administration of atracurium have been linked to the release of histamine.[152-154] In an effort to attenuate these changes the combined use of histamine$_1$-and histamine$_2$-receptor blockade after the use of high-dose atracurium has been attempted.[154] A dose of atracurium of 1.5 mg/kg, or roughly six times the ED_{95}, was administered. The patients were divided into four groups (a control group, a diphenhydramine group, a cimetidine group, and a diphenhydramine-cimetidine group), anesthesia was induced, and a dose of 1.5 mg of atracurium per kilogram was administered. Despite the antihistamine pretreatment, only the group receiving the combined histamine$_1$ and histamine$_2$ blockers had an attenuated cardiovascular response to the atracurium, and even this group underwent a modest decrease in mean arterial pressures (although the effect was not statistically significant).[154] The effects of histamine release on other organ systems are discussed later in this chapter.

Hepatic System

Atracurium has pharmacokinetic factors that are unaffected by hepatic diseases, specifically its breakdown pathway via Hofmann elimination.[130] The pharmacokinetics of atracurium in patients with hepatic and renal disease were compared with those in nonimpaired control subjects. No differences in plasma elimination half-lives were noted, although actual neuromuscular blockade parameters were not tested.[155,156]

The effect of atracurium infusions in patients with fulminant hepatic failure who were awaiting liver transplantation as well as during liver transplantation has been studied. Plasma clearances and half-lives were similar to those reported in healthy individuals, and no cumulative effects were noted.[147,157]

Renal System

Atracurium represented the first attempt to produce an NMBA that would not depend on the kidneys for its excretion.[158] Shortly after the introduction of the agent, its effects were assessed in patients with normal renal function and in patients in renal failure. At doses of 0.5 mg of atracurium per kilogram, no significant differences were noted in the onset time of 1.8 (0.1) minutes in normal patients and 2 (0.4) minutes in those with renal failure.[141] Furthermore, the duration of action was only slightly prolonged; 69.5 (5.2) minutes in normal patients versus 77.4 (3.2) minutes in those with renal failure.[141] Others have studied the effects of atracurium on patients with renal failure after the administration of a dose of 0.3 to 0.4 mg/kg. The recovery times from 25% twitch to 75% twitch in patients with renal failure (17.3 [2.6] minutes) were somewhat longer than those in normal control patients (10.3 [1.3] minutes).[140] The mean duration of the blockade for renal patients (time for recovery from 0% twitch to 25% twitch) was slightly but not significantly shorter than that of normal control patients (27 [5] minutes versus 30 [5] minutes).[140]

This reinforced an earlier study in which a slightly larger (0.5 mg/kg) dose of atracurium was administered to normal control patients and anephric patients. The researchers found a longer time to first depression of twitch response (32 $\pm$ 13.6 seconds versus 53 $\pm$ 8.1 seconds) in anephric patients, as well as a longer time to maximal depression of twitch response (109.7 $\pm$ 27.8 seconds versus 183.6 $\pm$ 58 seconds). In comparisons of the times to reappearance of twitch after complete ablation and return to 10% recovery of initial twitch, no significant difference existed between anephric patients and patients with normal renal function.[159]

Special Populations

Elderly Patients. Atracurium was administered to patients older than 60 years, and its effects were compared with those in two groups of younger control patients (those aged 40 to 60 years and those younger than 40 years old). A bolus of 0.3 mg/kg, followed by an infusion that was regulated by keeping twitch height within 10% of maximal twitch depression, was administered. No significant difference existed in the steady-state dose requirement, return from 10% to 25% twitch height, and return from 25% to 75% twitch height.[160] It appears that atracurium, with its unique Hofmann elimination, is age independent. Other researchers have suggested that recovery from comparable levels of blockade may be slightly prolonged in the elderly.[161] Shorten and colleagues[162] measured histamine release after the administration of atracurium in both elderly and younger control patients; they found that histamine release was greater in the elderly than in control patients.

Obese Patients. The effects of atracurium and vecuronium have been examined in obese patients. Doses of either 0.1 mg of vecuronium per kilogram or 0.5 mg of atracurium per kilogram were given to patients whose weight was at least 130% of ideal body weight. Recovery indexes (5% to 25% and 25% to 75% twitch) and recovery times (50%, 75%, and 100% twitch) were measured in these patients and in healthy control patients.[134] The atracurium group demonstrated no significant difference in any of the indices or recovery times.[134] The researchers stated that "the mechanism for the delayed recovery from vecuronium in the obese demonstrated by this study is likely to be impaired hepatic clearance and/or an overdose effect with recovery occurring in the redistribution phase."[134]

Pediatrics. The dose requirements of an atracurium infusion have been evaluated in neonates, infants, and children undergoing elective surgery, and these patients have been categorized into seven groups based on body weight. The researchers calculated dose on the basis of both weight (milligrams per kilogram per hour) and body surface area (milligram per square meter per hour) and found that with the exception of neonates, whose requirement is some 25% lower, atracurium dose by weight is consistent, regardless of patient age.[163] The doses to maintain first twitch height between 5% and 10% of control values were 0.52 (0.03) mg/kg/hr in infants and children and 0.40 (0.02) mg/kg/hr in neonates.[163]

Other Factors

Intraocular Pressure. The effects of atracurium on IOP were compared with those seen in a control group receiving succinylcholine. In 30 patients age 16 to 65 years who met criteria for ASA class I or II and who required surgery for nonophthalmic indications, IOP was measured before and after intubation. Patients who received succinylcholine and were then intubated 1 minute after its administration had IOPs that were not significantly higher than baseline. Patients who received atracurium and then were intubated 2 minutes after its administration had IOPs that were significantly lower than baseline. The authors found that clinicians would have to weigh the risks of waiting 2 minutes to intubate versus the benefits of decreased IOP in the emergency patient with both a full stomach and a nonintact globe.[47]

cis-Atracurium

The most notable of the 10 stereoisomers of atracurium, *cis*-atracurium besylate (Nimbex) has gained popularity in the clinical arena since the mid 1990s. It is a nondepolarizing muscle relaxant, three times more potent than atracurium but with a slower onset of action. The agent is available as a sterile, nonpyrogenic aqueous solution in 5-, 10-, and 20-ml vials.[164] The pH is 3.25 to 3.65, and the concentration is 2 mg/ml (except in the 20-ml vial, in which the concentration is 10 mg/ml for convenience in the intensive care unit setting).[164] Advantages of *cis*-atracurium include maintenance of cardiovascular stability and a lack of histamine release after injection.[165,166]

Pharmacodynamics

Onset. *cis*-Atracurium is regarded as intermediate in its onset and duration of action. In adults the ED_{95} is 0.05 mg/kg during N_2O-O_2 opioid anesthesia.[167] It has been noted to be five times more potent than rocuronium, with a slower onset of action, longer duration, and slower spontaneous recovery.[168,169] An IV bolus of 0.1 mg/kg (twice the ED_{95}) produces desired levels of relaxation within 3.1 (1) minutes.[170] Doses of three to four times the ED_{95} (0.15 mg/kg to 0.2 mg/kg) decrease the mean time of onset to 3.4 and 2.8 minutes, respectively.[171]

Duration. After doses of three to four times the ED_{95}, the average time for the first twitch in a TOF to recover to 25% of control is 65 minutes.[172] Further studies report that the duration of *cis*-atracurium with an intubating dose of 0.25 mg/kg is 55 to 75 minutes.[14] Full recovery at the aforementioned dose results in 75 to 100 minutes.[14] Additional sources report the duration as 55 to 61 minutes.[173]

Elimination. *cis*-Atracurium, like atracurium, undergoes Hofmann elimination (which is pH and temperature dependent) in the plasma and tissues.[174] Hofmann elimination accounts for 77% of total body clearance, and non-specific estenases is responsible for 23% of total body clearance. Of the organ-dependent clearance, 16% occurs through renal pathways.[174] Studies have demonstrated a half-life of approximately 26 to 36 minutes, with an increase in the rate of degradation as pH increases.[175] As with atracurium, one of *cis*-atracurium's metabolites is laudanosine. However, *cis*-atracurium liberates one fifth as much laudanosine as atracurium.[176]

Pharmacokinetic Summary. The onset of *cis*-Atracurium is 2 to 4 minutes. The duration of *cis*-atracurium is 40 to 75 minutes. The agent is degraded via Hofmann elimination, and its metabolites are partially excreted in the urine.

Central Nervous System

The increased potency of *cis*-atracurium results in laudanosine production that is four times less than that of its parent compound, atracurium.[14] *cis*-Atracurium, which is given in lower doses than atracurium because of its increased potency, is less likely to produce any significant change in metabolic levels and therefore has no significant CNS effects.[146]

Cardiovascular System

Administration of *cis*-atracurium to patients with cardiovascular instability is extremely safe. This is attributed to the lack of histamine release associated with the administration of the drug.[27] It has been noted to have a lack of both cardiovascular side effects and histamine release in doses up to eight times the ED_{95} (0.4 mg/kg).[166,172] A study involving 70 patients undergoing elective myocardial revascularization examined the hemodynamic consequences of *cis*-atracurium administration. There were no episodes of hypotension or cutaneous flushing after the *cis*-atracurium administration when measured 2, 5, and 10 minutes after injection at doses of twice the ED_{95} (0.10 mg/kg).[117] The cardiovascular effects of the neuromuscular blocking agents are summarized in Box 11-2.

Hepatic System

Although the major pathway of total body clearance for *cis*-atracurium is Hofmann elimination, the liver accounts for 7% of elimination.[174] Patients with liver disease have minimal adverse effects with *cis*-atracurium; in fact, clearance rate has been noted to be slightly increased in these patients.[14]

Renal System

cis-Atracurium is considered an acceptable and safe agent for use in patients with renal failure. Prolongation of onset and duration are statistically insignificant, based on a study comparing the effects of *cis*-atracurium when used in patients with renal failure versus those with normal renal function.[177] Doses of three times the ED_{95} (0.15 mg/kg) were given to 39 patients, who were all induced with fentanyl and thiopental. Onset time, mean arterial blood pressure, heart rate, and time to recovery of 25% T1 were assessed, and there was no significant variation between the two populations.[177]

Special Populations

Elderly Patients. Based on a study of young adults and geriatric patients (>65 years of age) who received *cis*-atracurium, pharmacokinetic differences are not dramatic. Onset of action of *cis*-atracurium is slightly delayed in the elderly patient (mean prolongation of 1 minute), and the duration of action is similar.[178] Plasma clearance of *cis*-atracurium was the same in the two groups.[178] Volume of distribution was measured as slightly higher in the elderly in comparison with the young group at 13.28 (9.9 to 16.7) L and 9.6 (7.6 to 11.7) L, respectively. These marginal differences between the two groups were attributed to biphasic equilibration.

Cis-atracurium has been noted to have a prolonged elimination because of an increased volume of distribution. Clearance, however, is not decreased.[14]

Obese Patients. No contraindications to *cis*-atracurium administration in obese populations were noted. As with most muscle relaxants, it is recommended to calculate the dosage to approximately 20% above lean body mass in obese patients.[14]

Pediatrics. In the pediatric population, the ED_{95} of *cis*-atracurium is 0.04 mg/kg.[179] A dose of 0.1 mg/kg in children provides an onset of 2 minutes with a duration of 30 minutes. It is further suggested that 0.2 mg/kg provides optimal intubating conditions for members of this population.[14] The stability of *cis*-atracurium makes it ideal for administration to children.

Vecuronium Bromide

Vecuronium bromide (Norcuron) is a potent nondepolarizing neuromuscular blocker. Studies comparing vecuronium with pancuronium, its predecessor, found vecuronium to be 1.5 times more potent than its parent compound.[88,180] Both agents were developed by manipulation of the steroid nucleus. The molecule was successfully altered from bis-quaternary pancuronium to a monoquaternary compound, creating an agent with a more rapid onset and a shorter duration. Vecuronium is more lipophilic than pancuronium, although it is still predominantly a hydrophilic compound. This change in its solubility is thought to be the cause of its differing pharmacokinetic profile.[130,181,182]

The chemical formula of vecuronium bromide is $C_{34}H_{57}BrN_2O_4$, and the drug has a molecular weight of 637.74 (Figure 11-2).[181] It is chemically designated as piperidinium, 1-[(2β, 3α, 5α, 16β, 17β)-3, 17-bis(acetyloxy)-2-(1-piperidinyl) androstan-16-yl]-1-methyl-, bromide.[181]

Vecuronium is available as a 10- or 20-mg sterile, nonpyrogenic powder for IV use only. Once reconstituted the solution has a pH of 4 and is stable for 24 hours at 25° C.[181] Researchers' determinations of ED_{90} to ED_{95} of vecuronium are variable. An ED_{90} of 0.044 to 0.056 mg/kg was reported when vecuronium was administered with nitrous oxide–oxygen and narcotic anesthesia.[128] Miller and associates constructed dose-response curves to derive the ED_{90}, which they found to be 0.023 to 0.044 mg/kg.[130] The agent has a steady-state volume of distribution of 0.21 to 0.27 L/kg.[182,183]

Pharmacodynamics

Onset. Vecuronium has an onset of action that is 1.5 times that of pancuronium, a proportion similar to that of its potency.[88,184] At a dose of twice the ED_{95}, 0.1 mg/kg, the maximum suppression of muscle twitch occurs within 3 minutes of administration.[138] The onset varies with the concurrent anesthetic administered and is inversely proportional to the dose.[116] With balanced anesthesia, a 0.1-mg/kg dose of vecuronium resulted in an onset of 3.1 minutes, whereas in patients receiving isoflurane, nitrous oxide, and oxygen anesthesia, the onset time decreased to 1.8 minutes.[137,182,185,186]

Duration. Duration of action varies with the type of anesthetic being administered and the dose of the agent. This phenomenon has been noted with other nondepolarizing agents as well as with vecuronium.[186] Haines[137] reported a duration of 36.2 ± 6.4 minutes after a dose of 0.1 mg of vecuronium per kilogram was given patients undergoing balanced anesthesia. Larijani and associates[88] reported a duration of 30 to 45 minutes. The time from 25% twitch recovery to 75% twitch recovery at a dose of 0.1 mg/kg was 11 to 12 minutes.[180]

Elimination. Vecuronium undergoes elimination via an orthodox three-compartment model. Because it is more lipophilic than other agents in its class, vecuronium does not depend solely on the kidneys for elimination. Only 20% to 30% of the administered dose is recovered unchanged in the urine within 24 hours.[88,116,130] A major portion of the dose, 40% to 80%, is taken up by the liver and excreted in the bile.[184] Small amounts of its metabolites (3-hydroxy, 17-hydroxy, and 3, 17-hydroxy) can be detected by thin-layer chromatography, but the amounts are minimal and have little if any neuromuscular blocking activity.[88,130] Reported elimination half-lives range from 51 to 90 minutes in healthy adults.[6,180,187,188] Total clearances have been reported from 3 to 5.6 ml/kg/min.[6,180,187,188]

Pharmacodynamic Summary. The onset of vecuronium is 2 to 3 minutes. The duration of vecuronium is 30 to 45 minutes. It is eliminated by the kidneys (20% to 30%) and liver (40% to 80%).

Central Nervous System

Two studies involving administration of vecuronium to patients on chronic anticonvulsive therapy were conducted. In the first a patient taking carbamazepine received vecuronium for muscle relaxation during bowel surgery. Recovery time to 15% of control value was nearly halved (18 minutes versus 34 minutes) when compared with a group of control subjects not taking anticonvulsants.[189] In the second a patient had two neurosurgical procedures, one before taking the anticonvulsant phenytoin and one after taking it.[190] A dose of 93 mcg of vecuronium per kilogram in the first surgery resulted in neuromuscular blockade of 40 minutes before three of four twitches in a TOF returned. In the second surgery a dose of 119 mcg/kg gave only 25 minutes of relaxation, a decrease of some 37%.[190]

Cardiovascular System

Another advantage of the modified steroid nucleus is that it provides a safer cardiovascular profile. The presence of the AChE-like fragment provides a high affinity for the nicotinic receptors of the neuromuscular junction and a lower affinity for the cardiac muscarinic receptors.[116,180]

Studies dealing with cardiovascular stability were the most prominent areas of research associated with vecuronium on its introduction, and vecuronium given at an ED_{90} dose of 0.050 mg/kg resulted in an increase in heart rate of less than 1%, an increase in mean arterial pressure of 2%, and an increase in cardiac output of 2.6%.[191] A comparison study that measured hemodynamic variables in elective cardiac surgical patients found that at a dose of 0.12 mg/kg, vecuronium did not result in any statistically significant changes in heart rate, systolic blood pressure, diastolic blood pressure, mean arterial blood pressure, or cardiac output.[151] In patients scheduled for elective cardiac surgery vecuronium was associated with a higher incidence of bradyarrhythmias than pancuronium was and, furthermore, the administration of an anticholinergic (glycopyrrolate) was sufficient therapy for these arrhythmias.[192]

Hepatic System

Vecuronium has also been administered to patients with hepatic disease. Early studies showed that no significant difference existed in pharmacokinetic parameters among animals and humans who had no renal function, leading investigators to believe that hepatic mechanisms might play a role in its clearance.[193-196] Lebrault for example, compared patients with cirrhosis who received 0.2 mg of vecuronium per kilogram with healthy control patients and found that elimination half-life was prolonged approximately 60%. This effect resulted in a time to return of 50% twitch height of 130 (52) minutes in the former group, compared with 62 (16) minutes in healthy patients. Differences in clearance among alcoholic patients with liver disease are dose dependent. Hepatic uptake may be a major determinant of vecuronium clearance, because animal data suggest that a relatively small fraction of a dose of vecuronium is metabolized. If higher doses of vecuronium saturate the hepatic uptake capacity of patients with alcoholic liver disease, clearance would decrease. The clinical implication of dose-dependent clearance would be that large or repeated doses may result in accumulation of vecuronium in the plasma of patients with liver disease.[196]

Renal System

Vecuronium was also carefully studied for its effects in patients with renal failure. Lynam administered vecuronium in a dose of 0.1 mg/kg to patients with renal failure and compared the effects with those in normal control patients. Onset times between the two groups were not significantly different: 1.9 (0.8) minutes in patients with absent renal function versus 1.8 (0.6) minutes in patients with normal renal function. Spontaneous recovery began at 40.4 (24.9) minutes in patients with normal renal function, versus 60.6 (20.4) minutes in patients with absent renal function. The clinical duration of action was 54.1 (25.2) minutes in patients with normal kidneys, whereas patients with absent renal function experienced a clinical duration of 98.6 (37.7) minutes.[124] The prolongation, according to the researchers, is the result of decreased clearance of vecuronium from patients with compromised renal function. Other authors, however, state they cannot attribute this prolongation of action to decreased elimination, decreased degradation of the agent, or decreased redistribution of the agent. However, they agree with the researchers' observations of prolonged action of the agent in patients with renal failure.[197]

Special Populations

Elderly Patients. Vecuronium has been found to have a prolonged duration of action in the elderly. A decreased dose of vecuronium in the elderly resulted in the same amount of neuromuscular blockade, as well as prolonged duration, when compared with the effects in younger control patients.[180] Other researchers, however, have found no significant difference in recovery index between younger adults and the elderly.[188] A "priming" dose of vecuronium (0.01 mg/kg) given to speed onset has been used in the elderly. A significant decrease in pulmonary parameters and a significant decrease in oxygen saturation were noted. The advantages of this technique in the elderly should be weighed against the risks.[198]

Obese Patients. Obesity is associated with a slower recovery with vecuronium administration because of a decrease in clearance in obese patients. Obese patients who received vecuronium exhibited prolonged time in recovery, significantly so in the 5% to 25% index, the 25% to 75% index, and the time to 75% recovery when compared with nonobese control patients.

Pediatrics. Vecuronium is commonly administered to children because of its intermediate duration of action.[14] It is also associated with minimal residual paralysis in the pediatric population.[14] However, the neonatal patient may experience increased duration in comparison with children. This is thought to be related to an increased volume of distribution in neonates.[14] Using identical milligram per kilogram doses, researchers have reported that onset times are shorter in both infants and children compared with adults.[116] Although children have a faster recovery time, infants and neonates have a somewhat prolonged recovery time from this agent.[68,116] Doses of vecuronium are 16.5 mcg/kg in infants (younger than 1 year), 19 mcg/kg in children (age 1 to 18 years), and 15 mcg/kg in adults (older than 18 years). They also exhibit a more rapid onset, presumably resulting from faster circulation times in infants and children.[180,199] Recovery times after a bolus dose of 0.07 mcg/kg are 70 minutes in infants, compared with 53 minutes in adults.[199,200]

Other Factors

Intraocular Pressure. The effect of vecuronium on IOP during normal-sequence induction, rapid-sequence induction, and steady-state anesthesia has been evaluated. During a normal-sequence induction, at a dose of 0.15 mg/kg, vecuronium reduced IOP from preoperative control values on intubation. This improvement was also noticed during rapid-sequence induction and intubation. During steady-state anesthesia, a dose of 0.1 mg of vecuronium per kilogram was associated with a significant reduction in IOP.[201]

Hypothermia. The importance of keeping the patient's core body temperature normothermic cannot be overstated. Hypothermic patients exhibit a prolonged duration of action to all muscle relaxants including vecuronium blockade. Hypothermia is thought to inhibit the means of elimination of vecuronium via carrier-mediated active transport, which is temperature dependent.[202]

Pancuronium Bromide

Pancuronium bromide (Pavulon) was first synthesized for Organon in England in 1966. Researchers, especially Lewis and co-workers, were searching for an agent that was nondepolarizing, had a rapid onset, had an intermediate duration of action, was easily reversed, and had no significant unwanted side effects.[6] After clinical use by Baird and Reid in 1967 in Europe, the agent was introduced into the United States in 1972.[154,203]

Pancuronium bromide's chemical designation is 2β, 16β-dipiperidine-5α-androstane-3α, 17-β-diol diacetate dimethobromide (see Figure 11-2). It has a volume of distribution of 0.18 to 0.26 L/kg; is an odorless, white, crystalline powder; and has a melting point of 215° C.[6,116] Extensive testing revealed an effective dose of 0.02 to 0.05 mg/kg in mice, rats, rabbits, cats, and dogs.[6] Further research determined the ED_{95} of pancuronium to be 0.075 mg/kg in human beings.[124,155]

Pharmacodynamics

Onset. The mean time to depression of twitch to 5% of control values after a dose of twice the ED_{95} (0.14 mg/kg) is

4.4 (0.5) minutes.[204] At a dose of 1.5 ED_{95}, which is estimated as 0.08 mg/kg, an onset time to 90% blockade was 2.3 ± 0.3 minutes.[205,206]

Duration. Pancuronium was produced as an intermediate- to long-acting nondepolarizer that would not have the histamine-releasing effects of metocurine or *d*-tubocurarine.[203] Numerous authors have reported the duration of action of pancuronium since the development of the agent. In a comparative study with vecuronium, *d*-tubocurarine, and metocurine at an ED_{90} dose of 0.062 mg/kg the mean duration of blockade was 109 (8) minutes.[191]

Elimination. Pancuronium theoretically undergoes triphasic elimination via the kidney through glomerular filtration, and a small amount of the drug is also released in the bile.[88,116] Up to 24 hours after the injection of pancuronium, anywhere from 43% to 67% of the unchanged drug may be found in the urine.[191]

Pharmacodynamic Summary. The onset of pancuronium is 2 to 3 minutes. The duration of pancuronium is 60 to 90 minutes. The majority of the agent undergoes renal elimination, but hepatic breakdown is also part of the degradation of this agent.

Central Nervous System

Patients who are using anticonvulsants may present anesthetic providers with a confounding pharmacodynamic variable that alters the effects of neuromuscular blocking agents. Patients who were receiving the oral anticonvulsants carbamazepine and phenytoin were given pancuronium for neuromuscular relaxation during surgery. Using this agent for relaxation in neurosurgical patients at doses of 0.084 mg/kg, the researchers measured the time to return of 15% of control values of T1 of a TOF. Patients who received pancuronium had a response time of 7.5 minutes if they were taking carbamazepine, 44 minutes if they were taking phenytoin, and 3.8 minutes if they were taking both, as compared with 68.5 minutes in control subjects.[207]

These findings were supported by studies conducted by other researchers. Patients taking carbamazepine and who received a dose of 37 mcg of pancuronium per kilogram needed only 35 minutes to achieve a return to three of four twitches in a TOF.[190] In the same patient's second surgery a dose of 47 mcg/kg yielded a duration of only 15 minutes to a return of four of four twitches (a decrease of over 40%).[190] Similar findings have been noted in patients undergoing long-term phenytoin therapy.[208]

Cardiovascular System

With the development of pancuronium and its use as an intermediate- to long-acting neuromuscular blocker, researchers again sought no adverse cardiovascular system effects. Significant increases in heart rate 3 minutes after the administration of the agent were noted in patients with coronary artery disease who were scheduled for coronary artery bypass graft and who received a dose of 0.1 mg of pancuronium per kilogram despite administration of narcotics.[152,209,210] Increases in heart rate are often accompanied by increases in mean arterial pressure. The tachycardia results from a vagolytic and possibly indirect sympathominetic action.

Hepatic System

The development of pancuronium also resulted in research to determine whether the agent might be safely administered to patients with hepatic disease. After the administration of 0.10 to 0.25 mg of pancuronium bromide per kilogram, 14 patients who had cirrhosis were compared with 12 patients who had no liver disorders. Distribution half-life was increased nearly 100% in the patients with cirrhosis, whereas the elimination half-life was nearly doubled in the same patients.[211] Pancuronium is acetylated to a limited extent in the liver, but in humans, only the 3-OH deacetylated metabolite has been found, and it is present in small fractions (5% to 10%).[211] The effect of the various alterations on the physiology of patients with cirrhosis was a prolonged action of pancuronium.[116,211]

Renal System

Pancuronium elimination is markedly decreased in patients with chronic renal failure, which therefore leads to the prolongation of neuromuscular blockade.[212]

Special Populations

Elderly Patients. The factors that affect the pharmacokinetics and pharmacodynamics of various neuromuscular blockers include decreased kidney function (secondary to decreased renal blood flow) and decreased glomerular filtration rate, as well as decreased hepatic blood flow.[68,213] These are the primary reasons for decreased clearance of pancuronium in the elderly.[14]

Of further concern is the presence of tachycardia associated with pancuronium administration.[209,210] The elderly frequently have problems with hypertension or cardiovascular disease. The presence of tachycardia in these patients, particularly those with marginal cardiovascular reserve, could be dangerous.[214]

Obese Patients. Pancuronium is one of the only neuromuscular blockers in which patient weight is independent of the drug's duration of action.[14]

Pediatrics. In children who received pancuronium at a dose of 0.13 mg/kg, the recovery time to 5% of twitch height was 65 (6) minutes.[215] The use of pancuronium in the neonate has been shown to result in hypertension. However, pancuronium may be the drug of choice for hypotensive neonates or those in shock.[216]

Other Factors

Intrauterine Surgery. The use of both pancuronium and pipecuronium for fetal blockade in utero for intrauterine surgery has been described. With the use of ultrasound guidance techniques an intramuscular injection of 0.2 mg of either pancuronium or pipecuronium per kilogram was administered, resulting in an onset of 4.5 minutes (no significant difference between agents) and allowing surgery to proceed. The duration of blockade was 54 (17) minutes in the pancuronium group and 48 (21) minutes in the pipecuronium group. Pancuronium was associated with four cases of fetal tachycardia (50% of the group) and two cases of beat-to-beat variability, whereas pipecuronium caused no cardiovascular changes.[217]

Pipecuronium Bromide

Molecular modifications to the pancuronium molecule, first observed before 1980 by chemists of the Gedeon Richter Company of Hungary, resulted in the formation of pipecuronium (Arduan). This change resulted in increased potency and decreased vagolytic side effects. Changing the 2,16-β-piperidino of pancuronium to the 2,16-β-piperizino, with the quaternization of the distal nitrogen, results in pipecuronium (see Figure 11-2).[68] The chemical name of the agent is 2β, 16-bis [4′-dimethyl-1-piperazinol] 3α, 17β-dia-cetoxy-5-androstane-dibromide.[212] Pipecuronium has a volume of distribution of 309 (103) ml/kg.

Pharmacodynamics

Onset. Onset and potency are inversely related in nondepolarizing neuromuscular blockers, and pipecuronium is no exception.[218] The onset of pipecuronium is 2.8 (0.5) minutes in normal patients after a dose of 100 mg/kg.[219] Onset time when one ED_{95} dose of pipecuronium (45 mcg/kg) was used was measured by two parameters: the maximum depression of a single twitch and the maximum depression of the first twitch (T1) of a TOF. With the use of the single-twitch method, onset was 5.7 (1.4) minutes in patients receiving fentanyl and nitrous oxide anesthesia and 4.3 (1.1) minutes for those receiving halothane anesthesia. When a TOF pattern was measured, the results for the fentanyl–nitrous oxide and halothane groups were 3.5 (0.6) minutes and 3.5 (0.5) minutes, respectively.[220]

Duration. The development of a nondepolarizer with a long course of action and none of the vagolytic effects of pancuronium was the *raison d'être* for pipecuronium, and its developers have been successful in achieving their goal of long duration. After one ED_{95} dose of pipecuronium (45 mcg/kg), the time to the return of 25% twitch height in patients anesthetized with either fentanyl nitrous oxide and oxygen anesthesia or halothane, nitrous oxide, and oxygen anesthesia was 41 (12.6) minutes or 51 (14.8) minutes, respectively. Return of twitch to 90% of control values was 83 (12.3) minutes in the fentanyl group and 87 (15.5) minutes in the halothane group.[220,221] At a dose of 50 mcg/kg, a return of twitch to 25% of control value was found at 24 (9) minutes after injection.[222]

Elimination. In a study of the use of pipecuronium in patients with renal failure compared with normal control subjects, researchers had several important findings. Each member of each group received 70 mg of pipecuronium per kilogram, and clinical and pharmacokinetic parameters were subsequently measured. The time to return to 25% of twitch height from control values was 98 (36) minutes in the normal control subjects, compared with 103 (60) minutes in the renal failure group. Using a three-compartment pharmacokinetic model, however, the investigators discovered a beta half-life of 131 minutes for the normal control subjects, compared with 236 minutes for the renal failure patients. The researchers attributed these differences to increased volumes of distribution in renal patients (secondary to fluid shifts), decreased clearance times, and possible altered protein binding. Despite the lack of statistical significance in the differences between clinical relaxation times, the researchers noted that the duration of the agent in the renal failure patient was "unpredictable."[223]

Pharmacokinetic Summary. The onset of pipecuronium is 3 to 6 minutes. The duration of pipecuronium is 30 to 100 minutes. Most of the agent is degraded and eliminated via the kidneys.

Central Nervous System

Pipecuronium is an acceptable NMBA for use in patients with intracranial hypertension, as it does not raise IOP.[224,225]

Cardiovascular System

Pipecuronium was developed primarily with the goal of cardiovascular stability in mind. This stability results from its lack of histamine release and the absence of vagolytic properties, as well as the absence of autonomic ganglionic blockade.

No significant changes occur in heart rate, systolic blood pressure, diastolic blood pressure, and cardiac output after administration of pipecuronium.[226] The cardiovascular stability of pipecuronium was evaluated in 20 patients undergoing elective coronary artery bypass surgery. Systolic systemic arterial pressure, diastolic systemic arterial pressure, central venous pressure, systolic pulmonary arterial pressure, and pulmonary capillary wedge pressure all decreased significantly after the injection of pipecuronium. Furthermore, the values for cardiac output, rate pressure product, left ventricular stroke work index, and left ventricular power decreased simultaneously. The investigators attributed this finding to the fact that, unlike pancuronium, pipecuronium fails to counteract the negative chronotropic effect of opiate anesthesia. Pipecuronium bromide at a bolus dose of 200 mcg/kg did not produce tachycardia. Although vagolytic drugs were absent, neither unacceptably low heart rates nor ventricular escape beats were registered. The improvement in oxygen delivery-demand ratio, associated with the use of pipecuronium in this particular anesthetic technique, may be of benefit in patients with ischemic heart disease.[223]

Hepatic System

The biliary excretion of pipecuronium is minimal with only approximately 2% of the agent excreted in the bile within 24 hours.

Renal System

Pipecuronium was also evaluated for its suitability in patients with renal failure. Pipecuronium is approximately 38% excreted via the urinary system.[227] When 0.07 mg of pipecuronium per kilogram was administered to 20 patients with end-stage renal disease, no significant difference in the time of onset was noted. Mean duration was nearly the same in both groups; however, a wide range of data was reported in the experimental group, with the reappearance of 25% twitch occurring anywhere from 30 to 267 minutes after the administration of the agent.[149]

Special Populations

Elderly Patients. Pipecuronium has been evaluated for its use in the elderly. No significant differences in volume of distribution, elimination half-life, drug clearance, and similar recovery indices in the elderly have been reported.[228]

Obese Patients. A review of the literature revealed no studies documenting the effects of pipecuronium in obese patients.

Pediatrics. Pipecuronium has been administered to children. It was given to children age 1.7 to 11.5 years in doses of 20 mcg/kg, followed by incremental 10-mcg/kg doses until twitch was 95% suppressed. The ED_{95} doses were 59.4 (5.4) mcg/kg in adults and 79.3 (9.8) mcg/kg in children when both groups underwent a nitrous oxide–narcotic technique. This dose decreased in both groups when they received isoflurane for their primary anesthesia Onset time in children ranged from

11 (0.4) minutes in a narcotic–nitrous oxide group to 13.3 (0.2) minutes in a halothane group. Whereas the clinical duration of blockade was 38.7 ± 5.9 minutes in the nitrous oxide–narcotic group, with no significant difference occurring in the isoflurane group, this value decreased to 25.7 ± 2 minutes in the halothane group.[229]

Doxacurium Chloride

By the mid 1970s clinicians were already searching for longer-acting neuromuscular blockers that would have better cardiovascular stability than that of existing agents.[230] By altering the structure of the older benzylisoquinoliniums, researchers were able to develop doxacurium (Nuromax), a potent, long-acting neuromuscular blocker that had no adverse cardiovascular side effects.[231] Early research with both dogs and rhesus monkeys demonstrated that in these models clinically efficacious doses of doxacurium were not associated with adverse side effects.[232,233]

Doxacurium chloride is a bis-quaternary benzylisoquinolinium diester. It is designated as *trans, trans*-2-2′[succinyl-bis (oxytrimethylene)] bis[1,2,3,4-tetra-hydro-6,7,8-trimethoxy-2-methyl-1-(3,4,5-tri-methoxybenzyl) isoquinolinium] dichloride. Its molecular formula is $C_{56}H_{78}Cl_2N_2O_{16}$, and it has a molecular weight of 1106.14.[233] The agent has a pH of 3.9 to 5 and contains 0.9% benzyl alcohol.[234] It is well absorbed intravenously and has an ED_{95} of 23 to 33 mcg/kg.[68,133,235] (See Figure 11-2.)

Pharmacodynamics

Onset. At its ED_{95} dose, the onset of doxacurium is 12 minutes.[236] Researchers who wished to take advantage of the agent's smooth cardiovascular profile but did not want to wait for its slow onset began to test varying doses of the agent in the hopes of speeding its time of onset. At twice the ED_{95} (50 mcg/kg) the time to 90% of blockade decreased to 5.4 (1.5) minutes, whereas at 80 mcg/kg (three times the ED_{95}) this number decreased still further, to 3.5 (1.2) minutes.[149]

Duration. Researchers were interested primarily in the duration of the agent when they set out to produce what became doxacurium.[150] What developed turned out to be the most potent of all neuromuscular blocking drugs.[68] The duration of doxacurium at an ED_{95} dose of 30 mcg/kg was 128 (26.4 minutes).[231] As with most other blockers, increasing the dose led to prolongation of the neuromuscular blockade. Furthermore, in the presence of inhalation agents, the dose-response curves were shifted significantly to the left.[150]

In normal patients, doxacurium has a volume of distribution of 220 ± 110 ml/kg, and this value is unchanged in patients with renal or hepatic failure.[237] It is approximately 42% protein bound in the plasma after IV injection.[238] The beta half-life of doxacurium is 76 to 99 minutes.[238] Although inhalation agents increase the potency of doxacurium, the duration and recovery are not affected by these agents.[239]

Elimination. It appears that little or no metabolism of doxacurium occurs in humans, despite a chemical structure that is related to that of atracurium and mivacurium.[68] Early in vitro studies showed that doxacurium was catalyzed by purified pooled human plasma cholinesterase at approximately 6% of the rate of succinylcholine.[231] Researchers have reported 30% to 50% of the agent being excreted unchanged in the urine 6 to 12 hours after administration.[149,232] Other researchers have suggested that an alternate pathway may exist for the elimination of doxacurium.[232,233,235]

Pharmacodynamic Summary. The onset of doxacurium is 3 to 6 minutes. The duration of doxacurium after an intubation dose ranges from 90 to 150 minutes.[14] The mechanism of elimination of doxacurium is unclear but probably involves redistribution, enzymatic hydrolysis, and renal and hepatobiliary components.

Central Nervous System

Nondepolarizing neuromuscular blockers administered in patients receiving long-term anticonvulsant therapy have shorter durations of actions.[240-242]

Cardiovascular System

Doxacurium is a long-acting nondepolarizing muscle relaxant that may be used in patients with cardiac instability. The preference for its use in these patients is related to the prolonged paralysis it causes without a significant elevation in heart rate—the result of minimal histamine release.[243] The increasing number of older and sicker patients undergoing complicated surgery resulted in the need for longer acting, yet cardiovascularly stable, neuromuscular blockers. Doxacurium was developed and formulated to meet this need. In doses ranging from 10 to 40 mcg/kg, doxacurium causes neither tachycardia nor hypotension.[244-246]

Hepatic System

The long-acting muscle relaxants pipecuronium and doxacurium were evaluated for use in patients with hepatic failure. Initial studies revealed that doxacurium was excreted primarily unchanged in the kidney, so investigation was begun to see if the agent could be used safely in patients with hepatic failure. A dose of 15 mg of doxacurium per kilogram was administered to nine patients undergoing cadaveric liver transplantation because of end-stage hepatocellular disease. The maximum neuromuscular blockade in this group was a mean of 70.4% (37%), with an onset of 10.6 (2.2) minutes and a clinical duration (return of twitch to 25% of maximum) of 51.6 (29.4) minutes. When compared with data from control patients without liver disease, these data revealed slower onset, less blockade, and prolonged clinical duration.[237]

Renal System

Doxacurium was also evaluated for its suitability in patients with renal disease because some researchers postulated a significant hepatobiliary excretion route of elimination.[233] Cashman and co-workers[233] evaluated the effects of this agent when they administered a dose of 25 mcg/kg to patients in end-stage renal failure and compared the results with those in normal control patients. When measuring the time (T1) to onset of various levels of blockade (25%, 50%, and 75%), the researchers found no significant difference between the onset times in patients with renal disease and those in healthy control patients.[234] The time to the reappearance of twitch was 35.5 (22.6) minutes in patients with renal failure and 37.8 (10.9) minutes in patients with no renal disease. The mean clinically useful duration was 120.8 minutes, compared with 66.7 minutes in patients without renal disease. As with other agents, the researchers noted that there was "wide variability" in the experimental group.[233] This wide range of responses serves as a reminder of the importance of monitoring neuromuscular blockade closely during the administration of this agent.

Special Populations

Elderly Patients. The increasing number of older and sicker patients undergoing complicated surgery resulted in a need for longer acting, yet cardiovascularly stable, neuromuscular blockers. Doxacurium and pipecuronium were developed at nearly the same time, and both were designed to meet this need. In studies in ASA class I and II men and women undergoing elective surgery, doxacurium in doses ranging from 10 to 40 mcg/kg caused neither tachycardia nor hypotension.[244] In a follow-up study in which doses of 10 to 80 mcg/kg were used, heart rate and mean arterial pressure varied little from control values. The largest differential occurred at a dose of 20 mcg/kg, at which heart rate dropped to 89% of control values and mean arterial pressure decreased to 89% of control values, whereas the rest of the data were within 8% of control values.[231,246]

Obese Patients. Doxacurium administration to obese patients results in a prolonged paralysis and recovery time. This is most likely related to the fact that obesity decreases both clearance and sensitivity of the neuromuscular junction.[247]

Pediatrics. Sarner and colleagues[248] administered doxacurium in varying doses to children age 2 to 12 years who were undergoing elective surgery. One group (A) received a bolus dose of 10 mcg/kg, followed by incremental doses of 2.5 to 10 mcg/kg, and the other two groups received bolus doses of either 27.5 mcg/kg (B) or 50 mcg/kg (C). Onset time to maximum blockade was 6.7 (1.9) minutes in the B group, compared with 5.3 (3.2) minutes in the C group.[248] The time to 25% recovery was 16.3 (8.8) minutes in the A group, 27.8 (10.3) minutes in the B group, and 50.6 (15.6) minutes in the C group.[248] These doses resulted in shorter times to onset and to 25% recovery from block, and the recovery index (25% twitch recovery to 75% twitch recovery) was roughly half of that of adults.[248]

ANTICHOLINERGICS

Anticholinergic, *antimuscarinic*, and *parasympatholytic* are three common terms used to describe compounds that originate from alkaloids of the belladonna plant. Each group name divides these compounds into subgroups that have a more similar mechanism of action. For the purposes of this section, all of the compounds are referred to as *antimuscarinics*. Atropine (*dl*-hyoscyamine) is the prototype of this group, and many of the currently available products are structural derivatives obtained both naturally and synthetically.[249,250] Atropine is found in the plant *Atropa belladonna*, or deadly nightshade, and in *Datura stramonium*, also known as *jimson weed*.[133] Preparations of these plants have been used by clinicians for centuries; belladonna was used as a poison during the time of the Roman Empire and in the Middle Ages. In 1867 Bezold and Bloebaun began to study the cardiac effects of belladonna's vagal inhibition, and in 1931 Mein isolated atropine in the pure form.[250]

Scopolamine (hyoscine) is also a naturally occurring compound and is isolated from the *Hyoscyamus niger*, or henbane, as the *l*(−)-stereoisomer. Atropine, in contrast, is isolated as *l*(−) hyoscine, but it rapidly racemizes, so the *d,l*-hyoscyamine racemic mixture is the commercially prepared product. The *l*(−) isomers of both compounds are at least 100 times more potent than the *d*.(+) isomers.[133]

Atropine and scopolamine are naturally occurring tertiary amines. Semisynthetic congeners of the belladonna alkaloids represented by glycopyrrolate are usually quaternary ammonium derivatives. These quaternary ammonium derivatives often have potent peripheral effects without CNS activity.[250]

Naturally occurring atropine and scopolamine, as well as semisynthetic glycopyrrolate, are amino-alcohol esters. Atropine and scopolamine are formed by combining tropic acid and a complex organic base, either tropine or scopine. Glycopyrrolate contains mandelic acid rather than tropic acid. Structurally the integrity of the ester must be maintained for antimuscarinic activity; neither the free acid nor the free base exhibits substantial antimuscarinic activity.[235,250] The presence of a free hydroxyl (-OH) group in the acid portion is also important. Both tropic acid and mandelic acid contain an asymmetric carbon, which results in the formation of optical isomers.[235] These isomers result in differing antimuscarinic potency and activity. Antimuscarinic compounds are well absorbed and distributed throughout the body, and the response by receptors is dose dependent because of varying sensitivities. The difference in structure between the tertiary and the quaternary compounds causes the presence or absence of CNS absorption. The highly charged quaternary compounds cannot diffuse through the lipid-soluble blood-brain barrier like their tertiary predecessors, which results in the fact that the former have little if any CNS effect.

Like ACh, these agents contain a cationic portion that can fit into muscarinic cholinergic receptors. This interaction allows antimuscarinics to reversibly combine with the receptors and thereby prevent the access of the neurotransmitter ACh to the same sites. Although ACh is also an active neurotransmitter at the postganglionic nicotinic receptors, usual doses of anticholinergics have little or no effect on these receptors.[250] This interaction is reversible and can be overcome by sufficiently increasing the concentration of ACh at the receptor sites of the effector organ.[249] In anesthesia these agents are used for treating the undesirable effects of surgical manipulation, cardiovascular dysfunctions, and side effects of other anesthetic agents.[234]

All the antimuscarinics are absorbed orally to some extent, although this route is often unpredictable. Intramuscular or IV administration is usually the route used. Scopolamine has the additional advantage of transdermal absorption.[250] Atropine is well absorbed from the gastrointestinal tract by inhalation via endotracheal administration and by IV and intramuscular routes. Given orally, 90% of the dose is absorbed and reaches peak plasma levels within 1 hour. Intramuscular and IV administration results in peak plasma levels within 30 minutes and 2 to 4 minutes, respectively. Atropine is well distributed throughout the body. It crosses both the blood-brain barrier and the placental barrier. Both the kidneys and liver aid in the elimination of atropine. Although elimination is biphasic, the terminal half-life is 2 to 3 hours. Metabolism by the liver results in several metabolites: tropic acid, tropine, and glucuronide conjugates. Approximately 30% to 50% of a dose is excreted unchanged in the urine. Small amounts of atropine may also be eliminated in expired air as carbon dioxide and in the feces.[235]

Glycopyrrolate is a quaternary ammonium compound whose ionization limits gastrointestinal absorption, blood-brain barrier penetration, and placental penetration. After IV administration, glycopyrrolate has an onset of 1 minute. Intramuscular and subcutaneous administration results in an onset of 15 to 30 minutes. Vagal blockade can persist for 2 to

3 hours. Serum levels of glycopyrrolate decline quickly, and less than 10% of the drug remains in the serum after 5 minutes. Glycopyrrolate is excreted in the feces and urine, primarily as unchanged drug. Small amounts are metabolized to inactive metabolites. Eighty-five percent of an IV dose is excreted in the urine within 48 hours.[133]

Scopolamine is readily absorbed after intramuscular and subcutaneous injection, as well as after oral and transdermal administration. Amnesia occurs within 10 minutes of IV administration and persists for up to 2 hours. Antiemetic effects are seen within 15 to 30 minutes of intramuscular administration and persist for up to 4 hours. Transdermal systems have an antiemetic onset of 4 hours and duration of 72 hours. Scopolamine reversibly binds to plasma proteins, although the extent to which this phenomenon occurs is controversial. Because it is a tertiary amine, scopolamine crosses both the blood-brain barrier and the placental barrier. Metabolism by the liver accounts for all but approximately 4% to 5% of the drug. All the metabolites and a small portion of unchanged drug are excreted in the urine.[235]

Atropine and glycopyrrolate are commonly administered for the prevention of the muscarinic effects of anticholinesterase inhibitors. Atropine induces its vagolytic effect more rapidly than glycopyrrolate. Atropine appears to be somewhat better suited for use with edrophonium, whereas the onset times of glycopyrrolate and either pyridostigmine or neostigmine are more closely matched. When administered with edrophonium, the usual recommended dose of atropine is 7 mcg/kg.[130,234] With 0.5 to 2.5 mg of neostigmine or 10 to 20 mg of pyridostigmine, the recommended dose of atropine is 0.6 to 1.2 mg and that of glycopyrrolate is 0.2 to 0.6 mg.[235,251,252] (See Table 12-2 for a comparison of the anticholinergics.)

CHOLINESTERASE INHIBITORS

Cholinesterase inhibitors are used for the reversal of the effects of nondepolarizing neuromuscular blockers. Physostigmine, or eserine, is the prototype of this group. It is obtained from the *Calabar* or ordeal bean, the dried ripe seed of *Physostigma venenosum*. This bean was once used by West African tribes as a poison in witchcraft trials.[253] In 1840 Daniell, a British medical officer, brought the Calabar bean to England for early pharmacologic study. The pure alkaloid was isolated in 1864 and named *physostigmine* by Jobst and Hesse, its discoverers.[253] Although discovered and used before World War II, physostigmine did not receive as much attention as it did shortly before and during the war. Physostigmine has the potential to be synthesized into a highly potent compound that could be used in chemical warfare. Organophosphates are descendants of physostigmine and have undergone extensive study and development. These compounds have become the insecticides and, regrettably, some of the "nerve gases" with which we are familiar today.[249]

Neostigmine was introduced into therapeutics in 1931, after Stedman and associates began substituting phenyl esters of alkyl carbamic acids into the chemical structure of physostigmine.[253] The original use of neostigmine was in the treatment of myasthenia gravis, a disease for which it is still used.

Edrophonium was developed later through a similar structural adjustment: the deletion of the carbamyl group.[14] This alteration made the compound extremely useful in the treatment of myasthenic crisis, as well as in anesthetic reversal, because of the difference in its pharmacokinetic profile compared with that of its precursors.

Three groups of indirect-acting cholinesterase inhibitors exist, and they are classified by their mechanism of action. The mechanism of each is primarily the result of its structural relationship and interaction with AChE, a protein with a molecular weight of approximately 320,000 and the capacity to hydrolyze an estimated 300,000 molecules of ACh per minute.[14,253,254] Reversible inhibitors and agents that form carbamyl esters can be used therapeutically.

Edrophonium, pyridostigmine, and neostigmine all contain an ionized center that actively combines either at the active center or at the site specifically removed from the active center of AChE . Edrophonium is a simple alcohol that contains a quaternary ammonium group.[254] It is considered a reversible inhibitor of cholinesterase, because it electrostatically attaches to the anionic site of AChE and is stabilized by hydrogen binding at the esteratic site of the enzyme. Because a true chemical bond is not formed, ACh competes with edrophonium for the binding site of AChE and therefore has a shorter duration of action than those of compounds that form a bond.[255]

Neostigmine and pyridostigmine are carbamic acid esters of alcohols and contain a quaternary or tertiary ammonium group.[254] These agents form a carbamyl-ester complex at the esteratic site of cholinesterase.[14] This drug-enzyme complex then degrades in the same manner as the ACh-cholinesterase complex. The carbamate group is transferred to acetylcholinesterase, leaving it unable to hydrolyze ACh.[14,253]

The indirect-acting cholinesterase inhibitors exert their effect by inhibiting AChE, thereby increasing the concentration of endogenous ACh around the cholinoreceptors.[254] This provides a twofold mechanism in the reversal of neuromuscular blockade. Increasing the concentration of ACh in the junctional cleft changes the agonist-antagonist ratio, thereby increasing the likelihood that the agonist will reoccupy the receptor site once occupied by the neuromuscular blocker, as well as occupying sites not previously engaged. Second, the life of the ACh within the cleft is increased. Because ACh is so rapidly hydrolyzed, it is seldom still available to occupy a receptor site when the antagonist spontaneously dissociates. The increased concentration of ACh prolongs the time it remains in the cleft, allowing time for the antagonist dissociation and the reactivation of the receptor site.[256] Evidence also suggests that these agents have direct influences on neuromuscular transmission independent of enzyme inhibition. These include at least three distinct although possibly interacting mechanisms, including a weak agonist action, the formation of desensitized receptor complex intermediates, and the alteration of the conductance properties of active channels.[257]

Although the result of inhibition of AChE is the same when edrophonium, neostigmine, or pyridostigmine is administered, the means by which these agents accomplish this task varies. Edrophonium binds reversibly with the negatively charged enzyme site by electrostatic attraction of its positively charged nitrogen. This effect prevents catalytic binding with ACh for the short time that edrophonium occupies the binding site. Although the duration of receptor site occupation is short for edrophonium, the duration of its effects is prolonged by the fact that once it leaves the receptor site, it finds another to occupy and continues with this process until eliminated.[256]

Enzymatic inactivation is accomplished by neostigmine and pyridostigmine. Electrostatic interaction between the ionized centers of drug and enzyme takes place initially, as with edrophonium. This phenomenon then leads to a hydrolytic chemical reaction in which a shift in covalent bonds occurs, resulting in the formation of a carbamylated enzyme.[256] This methy-carbamyl AChE is much more stable and resistant to hydrolysis than the acetyl enzyme, resulting in an enzyme that is incapable of inactivating ACh.[253]

These differences in chemical deactivation of AChE result in differing pharmacokinetic profiles. Edrophonium, neostigmine, and pyridostigmine are all quaternary ammonium compounds that are poorly lipid soluble. Penetration through lipid barriers (e.g., gastrointestinal tract, placenta, and blood-brain barrier) is minimal, if present at all, at moderate doses.[14]

Edrophonium is the most rapid acting of these agents, with an onset time after IV administration of 30 to 60 seconds and a duration of 5 to 10 minutes. Intramuscular administration results in an onset of 2 to 10 minutes.[258] Renal excretion accounts for approximately 75% of the edrophonium eliminated, although in the absence of renal function, hepatic metabolism accounts for the inactivation of 30% of the injected dose; this amount undergoes conjugation to inactive edrophonium glucuronide.[14] The elimination half-life of edrophonium is 110 minutes in the healthy patient and 304 minutes in the anephric patient.[14,256] The volume of distribution is 1.1 L/kg and 0.7 L/kg in normal and anephric patients, respectively.[14]

Although similar in structure and mechanism of AChE deactivation, neostigmine is more potent than pyridostigmine and has a more rapid onset of action. After IV administration of neostigmine, onset occurs within 4 to 8 minutes. Duration of action is 0.5 to 2 hours, although other sources suggest durations from 60 minutes to 4 hours. Renal excretion accounts for roughly 50% of the neostigmine eliminated, primarily by glomerular filtration.[14,256] The remaining 50% of the neostigmine dose is hydrolyzed by plasma esterases and hepatic metabolism to 3-hydroxyphenyltrimethyl ammonium (3-OH PPM) and conjugated 3-OH PPM. These metabolites have approximately one tenth the activity of the parent compounds and are renally eliminated. The elimination half-life of neostigmine is 70 to 80 minutes, increasing to 181 to 183 minutes in anephric patients.[255,259] The volume of distribution of 0.7 L/kg in healthy patients increases to 0.8 L/kg in those with renal failure.[256]

Pyridostigmine is the cholinesterase inhibitor with the longest onset and duration, primarily because of slower hydrolization of the pyridostigmine-enzyme complex. Onset of action after IV administration is from 2 to 5 minutes.[252] Duration of action has been reported to be from 90 minutes to 3 to 6 hours.[14,254] Pyridostigmine is 75% eliminated by the kidneys.[14,256] The remaining 25% is metabolized by the hepatic microsomal enzyme system to 3-hydroxy–methyl pyridinium, its major metabolite, and six other minor metabolites.[14,251] All of these metabolites are excreted in the urine.[251] The elimination half-life and volume of distribution are 113 minutes and 1.1 L/kg, respectively.[14,256] In patients with renal failure the elimination half-life dramatically rises to 379 minutes, whereas the volume of distribution decreases slightly to 1 L/kg.[14,256]

An exhaustive study by Kopman,[242] in which he compared neostigmine with edrophonium in the reversal of neuromuscular blockade of steady-state infusions of vecuronium, pancuronium, and atracurium, found the following:

1. Five minutes after a reversal dose of 0.75 mg of edrophonium per kilogram, neither the pancuronium group (0.05-mg/kg bolus dose plus 0.3 mcg/kg per minute steady-state infusion) nor the atracurium group (0.3-mg/kg bolus dose followed by 6 mcg/kg per minute steady-state infusion) experienced adequate reversal of neuromuscular blockade.
2. Neostigmine reversal (dose of 0.05 mg/kg) of atracurium blockade (same parameters as in number 1) was prompt and complete.
3. Patients receiving vecuronium (bolus dose of 0.05 mg/kg and steady-state infusion of 1 mcg/kg per minute) experienced adequate neuromuscular blockade reversal with either neostigmine or edrophonium.

Important evidence suggests that many patients are often inadequately reversed and exhibit clinically significant residual blockade in the postoperative period.[260,261] Qualitative assessment of the signs of recovery are frequently misinterpreted by even the most experienced clinicians. Debaene and colleagues[261] noted that 45% of patients arrived in the recovery room with residual muscular block after intermediate-duration relaxant administration. Residual paralysis was evident even up to 2 hours after relaxant administration. This can have several important consequences, such as interference with pulmonary function, recovery of protective reflexes, and protection of the airway and a reduction of the ventilatory response to hypoxia. They suggest that all patients should receive reversal agents regardless of the recovery status noted on clinical testing.

The pharmacology of the reversal agents is summarized in Table 11-7. The common clinical signs of muscle recovery after administration of a muscle relaxant are listed in Box 11-3. Some considerations that apply when reversal is incomplete are noted in Box 11-4. Factors that may prolong paralysis are listed in Table 11-8.

TABLE 11-7 Commonly Used Anticholinesterase and Anticholinergic Agents

Agent	Dose Range (mcg/kg)	Onset (min)	Duration (min)	Comments
Neostigmine	25-75	5-15	45-90	Most commonly used reversal agent; may increase incidence of postoperative nausea and vomiting
Pyridostigmine	100-300	10-20	60-120	Slow onset, long duration and slow reversal
Edrophonium	500-1000	5-10	30-60	Not recommended for deep block; rapid onset, short duration
Atropine	15	1-2	1-2 hr	Should be combined with edrophonium because of more rapid onset
Glycopyrrolate	10-20	2	2-4 hr	Less initial tachycardia than atropine

BOX **11-3**

Common Clinical Signs of Recovery from Neuromuscular Blockers

Adequate tidal volume and rate
Respirations are smooth and unlabored
Patient opens eyes widely on command with no diplopia
Sustained protrusion and purposeful movement of the tongue
Effective swallowing and sustained bite
A head or leg lift is sustained for at least 5 seconds
In small children a strong knee-to-chest movement is equivalent
Strong, constant hand grip
Effective cough
Adequate vital capacity of at least 15 ml/kg
Adequate inspiratory force of at least 25 to 30 cm H_2O negative pressure
Sustained tetanic response to 50 Hz for 5 seconds
Train-of-four ratio >0.90 with no fade
No fade to double burst stimulation

BOX **11-4**

Considerations When Return of Muscle Function is Incomplete

- As with any reversal agent, the ability to counteract a nondepolarizing blocking agent depends on the amount of spontaneous recovery before the administration of anticholinesterase drug.
- Has enough time been allowed for the anticholinesterase to antagonize the block (at least 15 to 30 minutes)?
- Is the neuromuscular blockade too intense to be antagonized?
- Has an adequate dose of antagonist been given?
- Are the other anesthetics and adjunctive agents contributing to patient weakness?
- Has metabolism or excretion of the relaxant been reduced by a possibly unrecognized process?
- Have acid-base and electrolyte status, temperature, age, drug interactions, and other factors that may prolong relaxant action been contemplated?
- The safest approach when any question as to successful reversal remains is to provide proper sedation and controlled ventilation until adequate recovery is ensured.

TABLE **11-8** Factors That May Prolong Paralysis

Pathophysiologic Causes	Pharmacologic Causes
Acid maltase deficiency	Aminoglycoside toxicity
Adrenocortical dysfunction	Penicillin toxicity
Acute intermittent porphyria	Steroid myopathy
Amyotrophic lateral sclerosis	
Anoxia and ischemia	***Antihypertensive***
Carcinomatous polyneuropathy	Ganglionic blockers
Cholinesterase deficiency or genetic variance	Calcium channel blockers
Compressive neuropathy	β-blockers
Critical illness polyneuropathy	Furosemide
Diphtheria	***Antidysrhythmics***
Eaton-Lambert syndrome	Quinidine
Guillain-Barré syndrome	Bretylium
Hypokalemia and hypocalcemia	Procainamide
Hypomagnesemia	Local anesthetics in large doses
Hypophosphatemia	
Hypothermia	
Motor neuron disease	***Antibiotics***
Multiple sclerosis	Aminoglycoside antibiotics
Muscular dystrophy	Polymyxin B
Myasthenia gravis	Clindamycin
Myotonic syndromes	Tetracycline
Neurofibromatosis	
Nonspecific nutritional deficiency	***Miscellaneous Drugs***
Poliomyelitis	Cyclosporine
Pyridoxine abuse	Steroids
Polymyositis	Volatile anesthetics
Renal failure (variable prolongation)	Dantrolene
	Magnesium
Respiratory acidosis	Lithium
Sepsis	Azathioprine
Thiamine deficiency	Organophosphate (poisoning)
Tick bite paralysis	
Trauma	
Vitamin E deficiency	
Wound botulism	

Modified from Nejman AM. Muscle relaxants. In: Kirby RR, Gravenstein N, Lobato EB, et al, eds. Clinical Anesthesia Practice. *2nd ed. Philadelphia: Saunders; 2002:707-714.*

MONITORING OF NEUROMUSCULAR BLOCKADE

Monitoring of neuromuscular blockade has been in widespread use for over 20 years.[2] The peripheral nerve stimulator (PNS) is the most commonly used method of monitoring neuromuscular blockade. It indirectly determines the relaxation of musculature.[262] The PNS is an electrical device that delivers a series of shocks to the patient through electrodes applied to the skin near a nerve.[262] On activation of the PNS, muscle contraction is visible in the absence of neuromuscular blockers.

Depolarization and contraction of a muscle are caused by the traveling of an action potential along the course of a nerve. As the impulse reaches the motor endplate, ACh is released across the synaptic cleft. It subsequently travels toward the receptor sites on the muscle membrane, resulting in depolarization and subsequent contraction of the muscle.[2] The PNS elicits the same activity, which makes it useful for the monitoring of neuromuscular blockade.

The administration of NMBAs places patients in a high-risk situation. Respiratory function is compromised. The monitoring of neuromuscular blockade is essential and provides the anesthetist a more accurate assessment of the patient. Inadequate doses of NMBAs may result in complications during surgical procedures because of unexpected patient movement. In contrast, overdosage may result in increased drug cost and labor-intensive intervention (e.g., mechanical ventilation).

Contraction of the adductor muscle of the thumb via stimulation of the ulnar nerve is the preferred method of determining the level of neuromuscular blockade.[262] Disposable

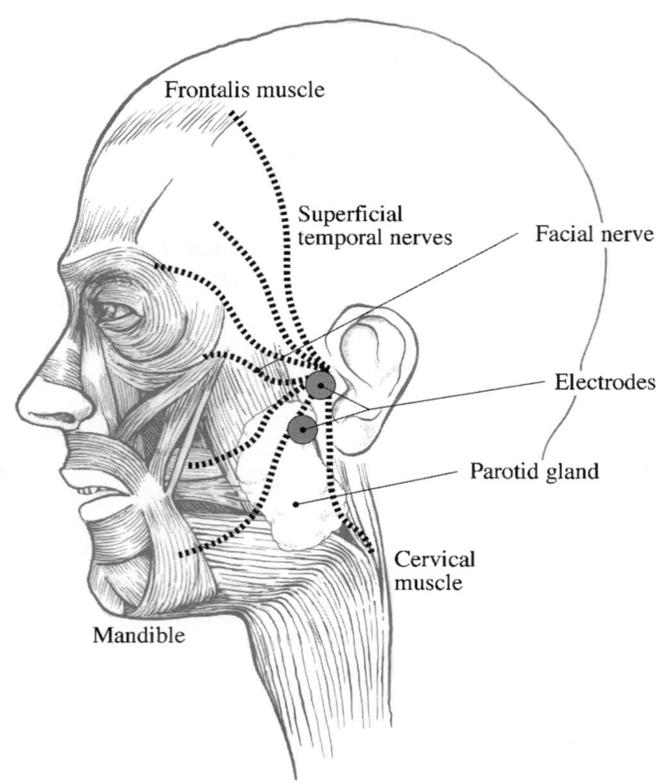

FIGURE **11-3**
Facial neuromuscular blockade.

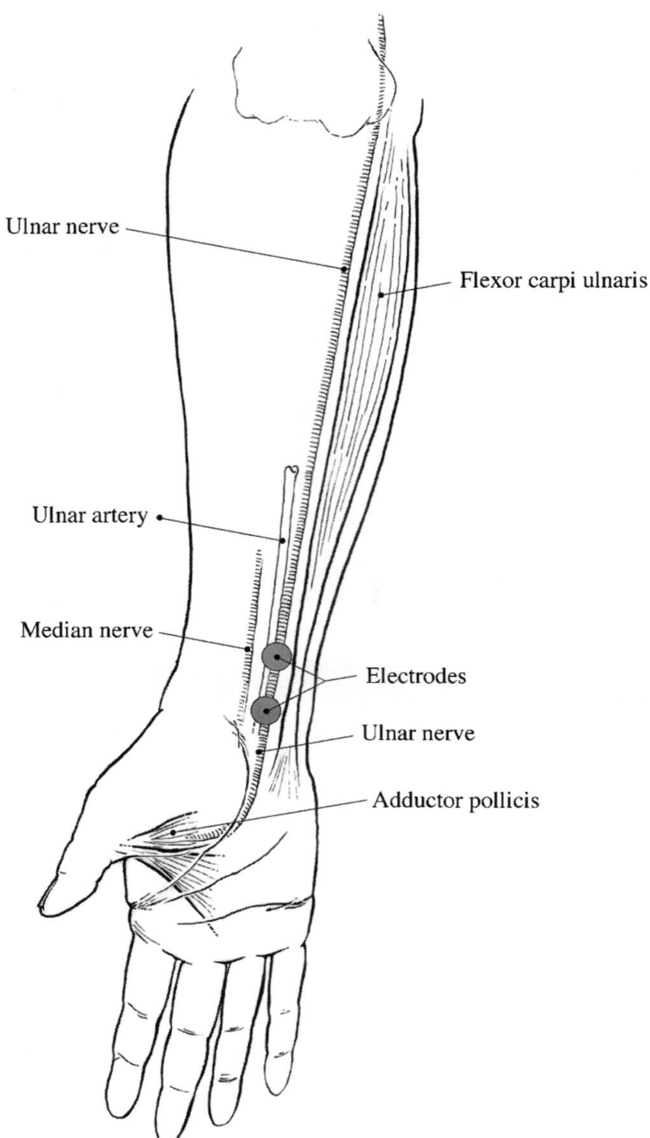

FIGURE **11-4**
Ulnar neuromuscular blockade.

electrodes are applied over the ulnar nerve.[262] The distal electrode is placed over the proximal flexor crease of the wrist, and the other electrode is placed over and parallel to the carpi ulnaris tendon.[262] On stimulation of these electrodes with the PNS, adduction of the thumb is visible.[262] Other monitoring sites include the first dorsal interosseous muscle in the hand, the abductor muscle of the little finger, the nerves of the foot, and the facial nerve, which stimulates the orbicular muscle around the eye or the orbicular muscle that contracts the lip.[263] The facial and ulnar nerves are the most commonly used sites (Figures 11-3 and 11-4).

The first (and simplest) type of stimulation is a single twitch at 0.1 to 1 Hz for 0.1 to 0.2 ms.[263] These impulses can be delivered automatically every 10 seconds, automatically every second, or manually, depending on the sophistication of the neurostimulating mechanism.[263] The most common means of stimulation is the TOF, which delivers four separate stimuli, each with a duration of less than 0.5 ms at a frequency of 2 Hz.[264] In the event that four twitches remain after NMBA administration, it is important to remember that the patient may be 0% to 50% blocked. As relaxation increases, the twitches in the TOF pattern progressively fade. The fourth twitch disappears first, which represents a block of less than 50%. Disappearance of the third and second twitches indicates a 75% and 90% block, respectively.[262] Assessment of the TOF test is noted in Figure 11-5.

Other types of stimulation that may be delivered are tetany, posttetanic count, and double-burst stimulation (DBS).[264] Tetany may be used to determine whether "fade" occurs after the administration of nondepolarizing neuromuscular blockers.[227,228] It consists of continuous electrical stimulation for 1 second at 50, 100, and as much as 200 Hz.[265] Posttetanic count and double-burst stimulation are somewhat newer techniques of monitoring the degree of neuromuscular block. The posttetanic count mode releases a 50-Hz tetanic stimulation for 5 seconds, followed in 3 seconds by a series of single 1-Hz twitch stimulations.[265] The number of twitches inversely correlates with the time necessary for the return of the first twitch of a TOF stimulation; however, these values vary and should be investigated for each individual agent.[27,266] DBS is a means of administering two brief bursts of three impulses at 50 Hz, separated by a time period of 750 ms.[264] This is proposed to be a more accurate means of assessing nondepolarizing blockade, in part because of its ability to be detected by tactile sensation.[264,265] Neuromuscular monitoring terminology and tests are summarized in Box 11-5 and Tables 11-9 and 11-10. Some key points related to tests of neuromuscular transmission are given in Boxes 11-6 and 11-7.[267]

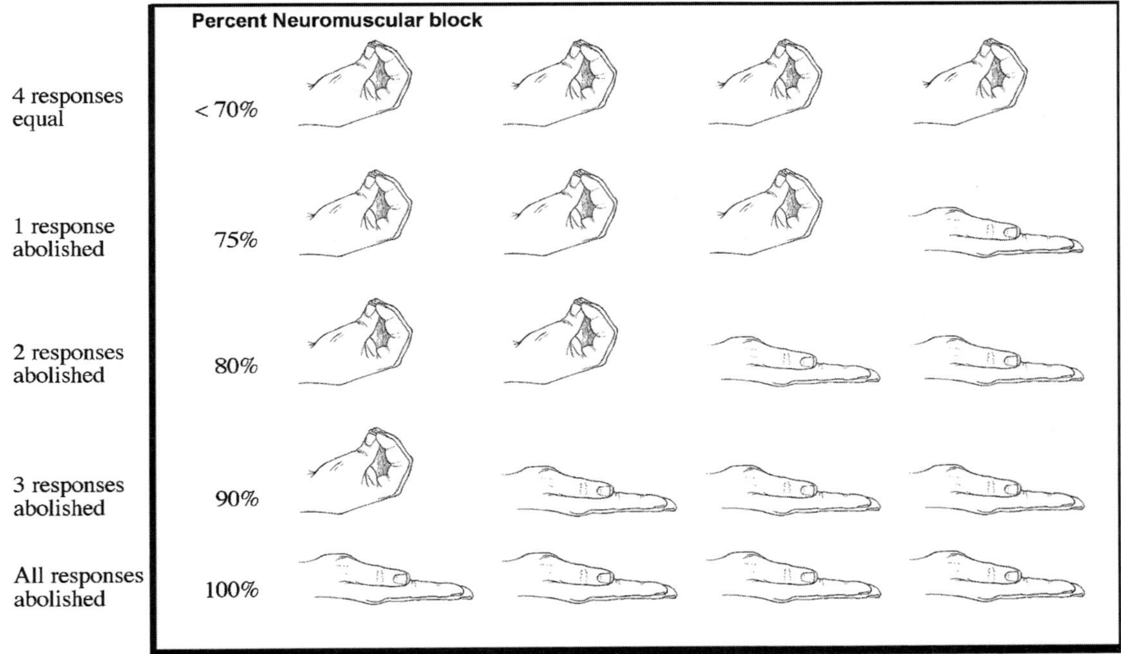

FIGURE **11-5**
Train-of-four test.

BOX **11-5**

Commonly Used Neuromuscular Terminology

- *Onset time*: time from drug administration to maximum effect
- *Clinical duration*: time from drug administration to 25% recovery of the twitch response
- *Total duration of action*: time from drug administration to 90% recovery of twitch response
- *Recovery index*: time from 25% to 75% recovery of the twitch response
- *Train-of-four ratio*: compares the fourth twitch of a train of four with the first twitch; when the fourth twitch is 90% of the first, recovery is indicated

TABLE **11-9** **Neuromuscular Monitoring Modalities**

Monitoring Test	Definition	Comments
Single twitch	A single supramaximal electrical stimulus ranging from 0.1-1 Hz	Requires baseline before drug administration; generally used as qualitative rather than quantitative assessment
Train-of-four	A series of four twitches at 2 Hz every half-second for 2 seconds	Reflects blockade from 70%-100%; useful during onset, maintenance, and emergence
Tetanus	Generally consists of rapid delivery of a 30-, 50-, or 100-Hz stimulus for 5 seconds	Should be used sparingly for deep block assessment; painful
Posttetanic count	50-Hz tetanus for 5 seconds, a 3-second pause, then single twitches of 1 Hz	Used only when train-of-four or double-burst stimulation response is absent; count less than eight indicates a deep block, and prolonged recovery is likely
Double-burst stimulation	Two short bursts of 50-Hz tetanus separated by 0.75 seconds	Similar to train-of-four; useful during onset, maintenance, and emergence; may be easier to detect fade than with train of four; tactile evaluation

TABLE 11-10 Key Points Related to Tests of Neuromuscular Transmission and Reversal

Test	Acceptable Clinical Result to Suggest Normal Function	Approximate Percent of Receptors Occupied When Response Returns to Normal Value	Comments, Advantages, and Disadvantages
Tidal volume	At least 5 ml/kg	80	Necessary but insensitive as an indicator of neuromuscular function
Single twitch strength	Qualitatively as strong as baseline	75-80	Uncomfortable; need to know twitch strength before relaxant administration; insensitive as an indicator of recovery, but useful as a gauge of deep neuromuscular blockade
Train-of-four (TOF)	No palpable fade	70-75	Uncomfortable, but more sensitive as indicator of recovery than single twitch; used as a gauge of depth of block by counting the number of responses perceptible
Sustained tetanus at 50 Hz for 5 seconds	At least 20 ml/kg	70	Very uncomfortable, but a reliable indictor of adequate recovery
Vital capacity	At least 20 ml/kg	70	Requires patient cooperation but is the goal for achievement of full clinical recovery
Double-burst stimulation	No palpable fade	60-70	Uncomfortable, but more sensitive than TOF as an indicator of peripheral function; no perceptible fade indicates TOF of at least recovery of 60%
Inspiratory force	At least −40 cm H_2O	50	Difficult to perform with endotracheal intubation but a reliable gauge of normal diaphragmatic function
Head lift	Must be performed unaided with patient supine and sustained for 5 seconds	50	Requires patient cooperation but remains the standard test of normal clinical function
Hand grip	Sustained at a level qualitatively similar to preinduction	50	Sustained strong grip, though also requires patient cooperation; is another good gauge of normal function
Sustained bite	Sustained jaw clench on tongue blade	50	Very reliable with patient cooperation; corresponds with TOF of 85%

Modified with permission from Savarese JJ, Caldwell JE, Lien CA, et al. Pharmacology of muscle relaxants and their antagonists. In: Miller RD, ed. Anesthesia. *5th ed. Philadelphia: Churchill Livingstone; 2000.*

BOX 11-6

General Guidelines for Successful Neuromuscular Monitoring

- During onset, paralysis begins with the eye muscles, followed by the extremities, trunk (from the neck muscles downward through the intercostals), abdominal muscles, and finally the diaphragm. Recovery returns in the opposite manner. Protective reflex muscles of the pharynx and upper esophagus recover later than the diaphragm, larynx, hands, or face.
- Monitoring of the facial nerve for determination of onset and readiness for intubation may be preferable to monitoring of the ulnar nerve.
- Monitoring of the offset and recovery from neuromuscular blockade is probably better at the ulnar nerve.
- Tactile evaluation of double-burst stimulation may be better to differentiate "fade" than train of four.
- When there is only one response to train-of-four (TOF) stimulation, successful reversal may take as long as 30 minutes.
- At a TOF count of two to three responses, recovery may take up to 10 to 12 minutes after administration of long-acting relaxants and 4 to 5 minutes after intermediate-acting drugs.
- When the fourth response to TOF stimulation appears, adequate recovery can be achieved within 5 minutes of reversal with neostigmine or 2 to 3 minutes after use of edrophonium.

BOX 11-7

Characteristics of Neuromuscular Blockade

Depolarizing (Phase I) Block

- Muscle fasciculation precedes the onset of neuromuscular blockade
- Sustained response to tetanic stimulation
- Absence of posttetanic potentiation, stimulation, or facilitation
- Lack of fade to train-of-four or double-burst stimulation
- Block antagonized by prior administration of nondepolarizer as pretreatment (approximately 20% more succinylcholine required)
- Block potentiated by anticholinesterase drugs

Nondepolarizing (Phase II) Block

- Absence of muscle fasciculation
- Appearance of tetanic fade and posttetanic potentiation, stimulation, or facilitation
- Train-of-four and double-burst fade
- Reversal with anticholinesterase drugs
- In rare cases may be produced by an overdose and desensitization with succinylcholine at doses >6 mg/kg

SUMMARY

Like every other agent used in the practice of anesthesia, neuromuscular blocking agents are useful tools in the hands of skilled clinicians. In the *Physicians' Desk Reference*, each neuromuscular blocking agent entry is accompanied by stern words of warning regarding the importance of immediate access to advanced airway support and a trained individual to provide that support. It should go without saying that these agents ought never be administered without first appropriately sedating the patient. The exception is if the patient's condition is so marginal that even the most careful use of sedation could increase the chance for morbidity or death. The decision to use neuromuscular blockers in the absence of sedation should be made only after the most careful and thorough consideration. The prevention of movement should provide the surgeon with the optimum field on which his life-saving skills can be practiced.

REFERENCES

1. Bloch H. Francois Magendie, Claude Bernard, and the interrelation of science, history, and philosophy. *South Med J*. 1989;82:1259-1261.
2. Rowlee SC. Monitoring neuromuscular blockade in the intensive care unit: the peripheral nerve stimulator. *Heart Lung*. 1999;28:352-362.
3. Lee C. Succinylcholine: its past, present and future. In: Katz RL, ed. *Muscle Relaxants: Basic and Clinical Aspects*. Orlando: Grune & Stratton; 1985:69-70.
4. Cullen SC. The use of curare for the improvement of abdominal muscle relaxation during inhalational anesthesia: a report on one hundred and thirty-one cases. *Surgery*. 1943;14:261-266.
5. Bisset NG. War and hunting poisons of the new world. I. Notes on the early history of curare. *J Ethnopharmacol*. 1992;36:1-26.
6. Karis JH, Gissen AJ. Evaluation of the new neuromuscular blockers. *Anesthesiology*. 1971;35:149-157.
7. Griffith HR, Johnson GE. The use of curare in general anesthesia. *Anesthesiology*. 1942;3:418-420.
8. Beecher HK, Todd DP. A study of the deaths associated with anesthesia and surgery. *Ann Surg*. 1954;140:2-34.
9. Foldes FF, McNall PG, Borrego-Hinojosa JM. Succinylcholine: a new approach to muscular relaxation in anesthesiology. *N Engl J Med*. 1952;247:596-600.
10. Flynn PB. Pharmacokinetics and pharmacodynamics of succinylcholine. *Anesthesiol Clin North Am*. 1993;11:309-324.
11. Leuwer M. Do we need muscular blockers in ambulatory anaesthesia? *Curr Opin Anaesthesiol*. 2000;13:625-629.
12. Donati F. Neuromuscular blocking drugs for the new millennium: current practice, future trends-comparative pharmacology of neuromuscular blocking drugs. *Anesth Analg*. 2000;90:S2-S6.
13. Mendez DR, Goto CS, Abramo TJ, Weibe RA. Safety and efficacy of rocuronium for controlled intubation with paralytics in the pediatric emergency department. *Pediatr Emerg Care*. 2001;17:233-236.
14. Savarese JJ, Caldwell JE, Lien CA, Miller RD. Pharmacology of muscle relaxants and their antagonists. In: Miller RD, ed. *Anesthesia*. Vol 1. 5th ed. Philadelphia: Churchill Livingstone; 2000:412-490.
15. Heier T, Feiner JR, Lin J, Brown R, Caldwell JE. Hemoglobin desaturation after succinylcholine-induced apnea: a study of the recovery of spontaneous ventilation in healthy volunteers. *Anesthesiology*. 2001;94:754-759.
16. Kopman AF, Klewicka MM, Neuman GG. Molar potency is not predictive of the speed of onset of atracurium. *Anesth Analg*. 1999;89:1046.
17. Vachon CA, Warner DO, Bacon DR. Succinylcholine and the open globe. Tracking the teaching. *Anesthesiology*. 2003;99:220-223.
18. Drummond JC, Patel PM. Cerebral physiology and the effects of anesthetics and techniques. In: Miller RD, ed. *Anesthesia*. Vol 1. 5th ed. Philadelphia: Churchill Livingstone; 2000:695-733.
19. Melton AT, Antognini JF. Prolonged duration of succinylcholine in patients receiving anticonvulsants: evidence for mild upregulation of acetylcholine receptors. *Can J of Anaesth*. 1993;40:939-942.
20. Nguyen A, Ramzan I. Acute in vitro neuromuscular effects of carbamazepine and carbamazepine-10,11-epoxide. *Anesth Analg*. 1997;84:886-890.
21. Morgan JE, Mikhail MS, Murray MJ. *Clinical Anesthesiology*. 3rd ed. New York: Lange Medical Books/McGraw-Hill; 2001.
22. Cook DR. Can succinylcholine be abandoned? *Anesth Analg*. 2000;90:S24-S28.
23. Gronert GA. Cardiac arrest after succinylcholine. *Anesthesiology*. 2001;94:523-529.
24. Calvey TN, Williams NE. Drugs acting on the neuromuscular junction. *Principles and Practice of Pharmacology for Anaesthetists*. Cambridge: Blackwell Science; 1997:317-361.
25. Calvey TN, Williams NE. *Principle and Practice of Pharmacology for Anaesthetists*. 3rd ed. Cambridge: Blackwell Science; 1997.
26. Thapa S, Brull SJ. Succinylcholine-induced hyperkalemia in patients with renal failure: an old question revisited. *Anesth Analg*. 2000;91:237-241.
27. Bevan DR, Donati F. Muscle relaxants. In: Barash PG, Cullen BF, Stoelting RK, eds. *Clinical Anesthesia*. 3rd ed. Philadelphia: Lippincott-Raven; 1997:385-412.
28. Janis K, Hess J, Fabian JA, Gillis M. Substitution of mivacurium for succinylcholine for ECT in elderly patients. *Can J Anaesth*. 1995;42:612-613.
29. Muravchick S. Anesthesia for the elderly. In: Miller RD, ed. *Anesthesia*. Vol 2. 5th ed. Philadelphia: Churchill Livingstone; 2000:2140-2156.
30. Rose J, Theroux MC, Katz MS. The potency of succinylcholine in obese adolescents. *Anesth Analg*. 2000;90:576-578.
31. Brodsky JB, Foster PE. Succinylcholine and morbid obesity. *Obes Surg*. 2003;13:138-139.
32. Liu LM, DeCook TH, Goudsouzian NG, et al. Dose response to intramuscular succinylcholine in children. *Anesthesiology*. 1981;55:599.

33. Sutherland GA, Bevan JC, Bevan DR. Neuromuscular blockade in infants following intramuscular succinylcholine in two or five percent concentration. *Can J Anesth.* 1983;30:342-346.
34. Mazze RI, Dunbar RW. Intralingual succinylcholine administration in children: an alternative to intravenous and intramuscular routes? *Anesth Analg.* 1968;47:605-615.
35. Brandom BW, Cook DR. Muscle relaxants in children. In: Katz RL, ed. *Muscle Relaxants: Basic and Clinical Aspects.* Orlando: Grune & Stratton; 1985:215-232.
36. Van Der Speck AFL, Fang WB, Ashton-Miller JA, Stohler CS, et al. The effects of succinylcholine on mouth opening. *Anesthesiology.* 1987;67:459-465.
37. Schwartz L, Rockoff MA, Koka BV. Masseter spasm with anesthesia: incidence and implications. *Anesthesiology.* 1984;61:772-775.
38. Carroll JB. Increased incidence of masseter spasm in children with strabismus anesthetized with halothane and succinylcholine. *Anesthesiology.* 1987;67:559-561.
39. Rosenberg H, Gronert G. Intractable cardiac arrest in children given succinylcholine. [letter]. *Anesthesiology.* 1992;77:1054.
40. Delphin E, Jackson D, Rothstein P. Use of succinylcholine during elective pediatric anesthesia should be reevaluated. *Anesth Analg.* 1987;66:1190-1192.
41. Morell RC, Berman JM, Royster RI, et al. Revised labeling regarding the use of succinylcholine in children and adolescents (part I) [letter]. *Anesthesiology.* 1994;80:242.
42. Katz R, Wright C. Revised labeling regarding the use of succinylcholine in children and adolescents (parts I and II) [reply to letter]. *Anesthesiology.* 1994;80:243-244.
43. Kent RS. Revised labeling regarding the use of succinylcholine in children and adolescents (part II) [letter]. *Anesthesiology.* 1994;80:244-245.
44. Facts and Comparisons Staff: Cholinergic muscle stimulants. In: *Drug Facts and Comparisons.* 48th ed. St Louis: Wolters Kluwer; 1994:2860-2867.
45. Cote CJ. Pediatric anesthesia. In: Miller RD, ed. *Anesthesia.* 3rd ed. New York: Churchill Livingstone; 2000:2088-2117.
46. Kelly RE, Dinner M, Turner LS, Haik B, Abramson DH, Daines P. Succinylcholine increases intraocular pressure in the human eye with the extraocular muscles detached. *Anesthesiology.* 1993;79:948-952.
47. Edmondson L, Lindsay SL, Lanigan LP, et al. Intra-ocular pressure changes during rapid sequence induction of anesthesia. *Anaesthesia.* 1988;43:1005-1010.
48. Yanez P, Martyn JA. Prolonged *d*-tubocurarine infusion and/or immobilization cause upregulation of acetylcholine receptors and hyperkalemia to succinylcholine in rats. *Anesthesiology.* 1996;84:384-391.
49. Berkahn JM, Sleigh JW. Hyperkalemic cardiac arrest following succinylcholine in a long-term intensive care patient. *Anaesth Intensive Care.* 1997;25:588-589.
50. Markewitz BA, Elstad MR. Succinylcholine-induced hyperkalemia following prolonged pharmacologic neuromuscular blockade. *Chest.* 1997;111:248-250.
51. Sato K, Nishiwaki K, Kuno N, et al. Unexpected hyperkalemia following succinylcholine administration in prolonged immobilized parturients treated with magnesium and ritodrine. *Anesthesiology.* 2000;93:1539-1541.
52. Cooper RC, Baumann PL, McDonald WM. An unexpected hyperkalemic response to succinylcholine during electroconvulsive therapy for catatonic schizophrenia. *Anesthesiology.* 1999;91:574-575.
53. Al-Khafaji AH, Dewhirst WE, Cornell CJ Jr, Quill TJ. Succinylcholine-induced hyperkalemia in a patient with mucositis secondary to chemotherapy. *Crit Care Med.* 2001;29:1274-1276.
54. Chakravarty EF, Kirsch CM, Jensen WA, Kagawa FT. Cardiac arrest due to succinylcholine-induced hyperkalemia in a patient with wound botulism. *J Clin Anesth.* 2000;12:80-82.
55. Stene JK, Grande CM. Anesthesia for trauma. In: Miller RD, ed. *Anesthesia.* 3rd ed. New York: Churchill Livingstone; 2000:2137-2172.
56. Gronert GA, Theye RA. Pathophysiology of hyperkalemia induced by succinylcholine. *Anesthesiology.* 1975;43:89-99.
57. MacLennan N, Heimbach DM, Cullen BF. Anesthesia for major thermal injury. *Anesthesiology.* 1998;89:749-770.
58. Gronert GA. Succinylcholine hyperkalemia after burns. *Anesthesiology.* 1999;91:320-322.
59. Tegazzin V, Scutari E, Treves S, Zorzato F. Chlorocresol, an additive to commercial succinylcholine, induces contracture of human malignant hyperthermia-susceptible muscles via activation of the ryanodine receptor Ca^{2+} channel. *Anesthesiology.* 1996;84:1380-1385.
60. Karger B, Teige K. Fatal malignant hyperthermia—delayed onset and atypical course. *Forensic Sci Int.* 2002;129:187-190.
61. Ramirez JA, Cheetham ED, Laurence AS, Hopkins PM. Suxamethonium, masseter spasm and later malignant hyperthermia. *Anaesthesia.* 1998;53:1111-1116.
62. Claxton BA, Cross MH, Hopkins PM. No response to trigger agents in a malignant hyperthermia-susceptible patient. *Br J Anaesth.* 2002;88:870-873.
63. Basta SJ. Clinical pharmacology of mivacurium chloride: a review. *J Clin Anesth.* 1992;4:153-162.
64. Wong SF, Chung F. Succinylcholine-associated postoperative myalgia. *Anaesthesia.* 2000;55:144-152.
65. Collins L, Prentice J, Vaghadia H. Tracheal intubation of outpatients with and without muscle relaxants. *Canadian Journal of Anaesthesia.* 2000;47(5):427-432.
66. Albrecht RF, Lanier WL. Potentiation of succinylcholine-induced phase II block by vancomycin. *Anesth Analg.* 1997;77:1300-1302.
67. Baraka A, Baroody M, Yazbeck V. Repeated doses of suxamethonium in the myasthenic patient. *Anaesthesia.* 1993;48:782-784.
68. Lien CA. What is really new about the new relaxants? *Anesthesiol Clin North Am.* 1993;11:729-778.
69. Plaud B, Marty G, Debaene B, et al. Cardiovascular effects of mivacurium in hypertensive patients. *Anesth Analg.* 2002;95:379-384.
70. Lacroix M, Donati F, Varin F. Pharmacokinetics of mivacurium isomers and their metabolites in healthy volunteers after bolus administration. *Anesthesiology.* 1997;86:322-330.
71. Lien CA, Belmont MR, Roth DL, Okamoto M, Abalos A, Savarese JJ. Pharmacodynamics and the plasma concentration of mivacurium during spontaneous recovery and neostigmine-facilitated recovery. *Anesthesiology.* 1999;91:119-126.
72. Ali HH, Savarese JJ, Embree PB, et al. Clinical pharmacology of mivacurium chloride (BW B1090U) infusion: comparison with vecuronium and atracurium. *Br J Anaesth.* 1988;61:541-546.
73. Maddineni VR, Mirakhur RK, McCoy EP, et al. Neuromuscular effects and intubating conditions following mivacurium: a comparison with suxamethonium. *Anaesthesia.* 1993;48:940-945.
74. Goldberg ME, Larijani GE, Azad SS, et al. Comparison of tracheal intubating conditions and neuromuscular blocking profiles after intubating doses of mivacurium chloride or succinylcholine in surgical outpatients. *Anesth Analg.* 1989;69:93-99.
75. Kim KS, Jeon JW, Koh MS, Shim JH, Cho SY, Suh JK. The duration of immobilization causes the changing pharmacodynamics of mivacurium and rocuronium in rabbits. *Anesth Analg.* 2003;96:438-442.
76. Plaud B, Debaene B, Lequeau F, Meistelman C, Donati F. Mivacurium neuromuscular block at the adductor muscles of the larynx and adductor pollicis in humans. *Anesthesiology.* 1996;85:77-81.
77. Poler SM, Watcha MF, White PF. Mivacurium as an alternative to succinylcholine during outpatient laparoscopy. *J Clin Anesth.* 1992;4:127-133.

78. Brandom BW, Woelfel SK, Cook DR, et al. Comparison of mivacurium and suxamethonium administered by bolus and infusion. *Br J Anaesth*. 1989;62:488-543.
79. Ostergaard D, Jensen FS, Jensen E, et al. Mivacurium-induced neuromuscular blockade in patients heterozygous for the atypical gene for plasma cholinesterase [abstract]. *Anesthesiology*. 1989;71:A782.
80. Apfelbaum JL. Muscle relaxants for outpatient surgery: old and new. *J Clin Anesth*. 1992;4:2S-8S.
81. Ostergaard D, Jensen E, Jensen FS, et al. The duration of action of mivacurium-induced neuromuscular block in patients homozygous for the atypical plasma cholinesterase gene. *Anesthesiology*. 1991;75:A774.
82. Cook DR, Freeman JA, Lai AA, et al. Pharmacokinetics of mivacurium in normal patients and in those with hepatic or renal failure. *Br J Anaesthesia*. 1992;69:580-585.
83. Puhringer FK, Khuenl-Brady KS, Koller J, et al. Evaluation of endotracheal intubating conditions of rocuronium and succinylcholine in outpatient surgery. *Anesth Analgesia*. 1992;75:37-40.
84. McGehee DS, Krasowski MD, Fung DL, Wilson B, Gronert GA, Moss J. Cholinesterase inhibition by potato glycoalkaloids slows mivacurium metabolism. *Anesthesiology*. 2000;93:510-519.
85. Mirakhur RJ. Newer neuromuscular blocking drugs. *Drugs*. 1992;44:182-199.
86. Wicks TC. The pharmacology of rocuronium bromide. *AANA*. 1994;62:33-38.
87. Hernandez-Palazon J, Tortosa JA, Martinez-Lage JF, Perez-Ayala M. Rocuronium-induced neuromuscular blockade is affected by chronic phenytoin therapy. *J Neurosurg Anesthesiol*. 2001;13:79-82.
88. Savarese JJ, Ali HH, Basta SJ, et al. The cardiovascular effects of mivacurium chloride in patients receiving nitrous oxide-opiate-barbiturate anesthesia. *Anesthesiology*. 1989;70:386-394.
89. Larijani GE, Gratz I, Silverberg M, et al. Clinical pharmacology of the neuromuscular blocking agents. *Ann Pharmacol*. 1991;25: 54-64.
90. Weber S, Brandom BW, Powers DM, et al. Mivacurium chloride (BW B1090U) induced neuromuscular blockade during nitrous oxide-isoflurane and nitrous oxide-narcotic anesthesia in adult surgical patients. *Anesth Analg*. 1988;67:495-499.
91. Green DW, Fisher M, Sockalingham I. Mivacurium compared with succinycholine in children with liver disease. *Br J Anaesth*. 1998;81:463-465.
92. Basta SJ, Dresner DL, Shaff LP, et al. Neuromuscular effects and pharmacokinetics of mivacurium in elderly patients under isoflurane anesthesia. *Anesth Analg*. 1989;68:S18.
93. Ostergaard D, Viby-Mogensen J, Pedersen NA, Holm H, Skovgaard LT. Pharmacokinetics and pharmacodynamics of mivacurium in young adult and elderly patients. *Acta Anaesthesiol Scand*. 2002;46:684-691.
94. Janis K, Hess J, Fabian JA, Gillis M. Substitution of mivacurium for succinylcholine for ECT in elderly patients.[comment]. *Can J Anaesth*. 1995;42:612-613.
95. Yazigi A, el Hage C, Richa F, Antakly MC. Mivacurium in an obese patient with myotonic dystrophy—a case report. *Middle East J Anesthesiol*. 1997;14:77-82.
96. Mangat PS, Evans DE, Harmer M, et al. A comparison between mivacurium and suxamethonium in children. *Anaesthesia*. 1993;48:866-869.
97. Cauldwell CB, Lau M, Fisher DM. Is intramuscular mivacurium an alternative to intramuscular succinylcholine? *Anesthesiology*. 1994;80:320-325.
98. Martyn JA, Goudsouzian NG, Chang Y, Szyfelbein SK, Schwartz AE, Patel SS. Neuromuscular effects of mivacurium in 2- to 12-year old children with burn injury. *Anesthesiology*. 2000;92:31.
99. Vanlinthout LE, Bartels CF, Lockridge O, Callens K, Booij LH. Prolonged paralysis after a test dose of mivacurium in a patient with atypical serum cholinesterase. *Anesth Analg*. 1998;87: 1199-1202.
100. Naguib M, Gomaa M, Samarkandi AH, et al. Increased plasma cholinesterase activity and mivacurium resistance: report of a family. *Anesth Analg*. 1999;89:1579.
101. Foldes FF, Nagashima H, Nguyen HD, et al. The neuromuscular effects of ORG9426 in patients receiving balanced anesthesia. *Anesthesiology*. 1991;75:191-196.
102. Booij LH, Knape HT. The neuromuscular blocking effects of ORG 9426. *Anaesthesia*. 1991;46:341-343.
103. Rocuronium bromide for injection [package insert]. West Orange, NJ: Organon; 2004.
104. Doobinin KA, Nakagawa TA. Emergency department use of neuromuscular blocking agents in children. *Pediatr Emerg Care*. 2000;16:441-447.
105. Rose M, Fischer M. Rocuronium: high risk for anaphylaxis? *Br J Anaesth*. 2001;86:678-682.
106. Chaudrhy I, Foldes FF, Ohta Y, et al. The protein binding effect of ORG9426 and its inhibitory effect on human cholinesterases. *Anesthesiology*. 1991;75:A786.
107. Szenohradszky J, Caldwell JE, Sharma ML, et al. Interaction of rocuronium (ORG 9426) and phenytoin in a patient undergoing cadaver renal transplantation: a possible pharmacokinetic mechanism? *Anesthesiology*. 1994;80:1167-1170.
108. Chiu CL, Jaais F, Wang CY. Effect of rocuronium compared with succinylcholine on intraocular pressure during rapid sequence induction of anaesthesia. *Br J Anaesth*. 1999;82:757-760.
109. Meistelman C. Update on neuromuscular pharmacology. *Curr Opin Anesthesiol*. 2001;14:399-404.
110. Sieber TJ, Zbinden AM, Curatolo M, Shorten GD. Tracheal intubation with rocuronium using the "timing principle." *Anesth Analg*. 1998;86:1137-1140.
111. Kirkegaard-Nielsen H, Caldwell JE, Berry PD. Rapid tracheal intubation with rocuronium. *Anesthesiology*. 1999;91: 131-136.
112. Basta SJ, Ali HH, Savarese JJ, et al. Clinical pharmacology of atracurium besylate (BW 33A): a new non-depolarizing muscle relaxant. *Anesth Analg*. 1982;61:723-729.
113. Bartkowski RR, Witkowski TA, Azad S, et al. Rocuronium onset of action: a comparison with atracurium and vecuronium. *Anesth Analg*. 1993;77:574-578.
114. Lowry DW, Mirakhur RK, McCarthy G, Carroll MT, McCourt KC. Neuromuscular effects of rocuronium during sevoflurane, isoflurane, and intravenous anesthesia. *Anesth Analg*. 1998;87: 936-940.
115. Adejumo SW, Hunter JM. Muscle relaxants in the critically ill. *Curr Opin Crit Care*. 1999;5:263.
116. Ducharme J, Donati F. Pharmacokinetics and pharmacodynamics of steroidal muscle relaxants. *Anesthesiol Clin North Am*. 1993;11:283-307.
117. McCoy EP, Maddineni VR, Elliott P, et al. Haemodynamic effects of rocuronium during fentanyl anaesthesia: comparison with vecuronium. *Can J Anesth*. 1993;40:703-708.
118. Hudson ME, Rothfield KP, Tullock WC, et al. Haemodynamic effects of rocuronium bromide in adult cardiac surgical patients. *Can J Anesth*. 1998;45:139-143.
119. Woelfel SK, Brandom BW, Cook DR, et al. Effects of bolus administration of ORG-9426 in children during nitrous oxide halothane anesthesia. *Anesthesiology*. 1992;76:939-942.
120. Dubois MY, Lapeyre G, Lea D, et al. Pharmacodynamic effects of three doses of ORG 9426 used for endotracheal intubation in humans. *J Clin Anesth*. 1992;4:472-475.
121. Khalil M, D'Honneur G, Duvaldestin P, et al. Pharmacodynamics and pharmacokinetics of rocuronium in patients with cirrhosis. *Anesthesiology*. 1994;80:1241-1247.
122. Robertson E, Bunschoten P, Driessen J, Booij L. A comparison of the pharmacodynamics of rocuronium in patients with and without renal failure. *Anesthesiology*. 1998;89(suppl):987A.
123. Khunel-Brady KS, Pomaroli A, Puhringer F, et al. The use of rocuronium (ORG 9426) in patients with chronic renal failure. *Anaesthesia*. 1993;48:873-875.

124. Lynam DP, Cronnelly R, Castagnoli KP, et al. The pharmacodynamics and pharmacokinetics of vecuronium in patients anesthetized with isoflurane with normal renal function or with renal failure. *Anesthesiology*. 1988;69:227-231.
125. Matteo RS, Ornstein E, Schwartz AE, et al. Pharmacokinetics and pharmacodynamics of rocuronium (ORG9426) in elderly surgical patients. *Anesth Analgesia*. 1993;77:1193-1197.
126. Gin T, Chan MT, Lai Chan K, Mo Yuen P. Prolonged neuromuscular block after rocuronium in postpartum patients. *Anesth Analg*. 2002;94:686-689.
127. O'Kelly B, Farcsi F, Frossard J, et al. Neuromuscular blockade following ORG 9426 in children during N_2O-halothane anesthesia. *Anesthesiology*. 1991;75:A787.
128. Torda TA. The "new" relaxants: a review of the clinical pharmacology of atracurium and vecuronium. *Anaesth Intensive Care*. 1987;15:72-82.
129. Payne JP. Atracurium. In: Katz RL, ed. *Muscle Relaxants: Basic and Clinical Aspects*. Orlando: Grune & Stratton; 1985:87-101.
130. Miller RD, Rupp SM, Fisher DM, et al. Clinical pharmacology of vecuronium and atracurium. *Anesthesiology*. 1984;61:444-453.
131. Atracurium [package insert]. Research Triangle Park, NC: Burroughs Wellcome; 1992.
132. Stenlake JB, Waigh RD, Urwin J, et al. Atracurium: conception and inception. *Anaesthesia*. 1983;55:3S-10S.
133. Service AHF. Skeletal muscle relaxants. In: McEvoy GK, ed. *AHFS*. Bethesda, Md: American Society of Hospital Pharmacists; 1994:817.
134. Weinstein JA, Matteo RS, Ornstein E, et al. Pharmacodynamics of vecuronium and atracurium in the obese surgical patient. *Anesth Analg*. 1988;67:1149-1153.
135. Papadimitriou L, Foustanos A. Continuous intravenous infusion of atracurium in idiopathic obesity [letter]. *Anaesthesia*. 1988;43:900.
136. Payne JP, Hughes R. Evaluation of atracurium in anaesthetized man. *Br J Anaesth*. 1981;53:45-54.
137. Haines M. A comparison of the onset time, duration of action, and fade characteristics of atracurium and vecuronium. *AANA J*. 1993;61:592-596.
138. Healy TE, Pugh ND, Kay B, et al. Atracurium and vecuronium: effect of dose on the time of onset. *Br J Anaesth*. 1986;58:620-624.
139. Gramstad L, Lilleaasen P, Minsaas B. Comparative study of atracurium, vecuronium (ORG NC 45) and pancuronium. *Br J Anaesth*. 1982;54:827-829.
140. Ward S, Boheimer N, Weatherley BC, et al. Pharmacokinetics of atracurium and its metabolites in patients with normal renal function and in patients in renal failure. *Br J Anaesth*. 1987;59:697-706.
141. Fahey MR, Rupp SM, Fisher DM, et al. The pharmacokinetics and pharmacodynamics of atracurium in patients with and without renal failure. *Anesthesiology*. 1984;61:699-702.
142. Shea JHA. Atracurium: a review of a new non-depolarizing muscle relaxant. *AANA J*. 1984;52:299-302.
143. Hughes R, Chapple DJ. The pharmacology of atracurium: a new competitive neuromuscular blocking agent. *Br J Anaesth*. 1981;53:31-44.
144. Peat SJ, Potter DR, Hunter JM. The prolonged use of atracurium in a patient with tetanus. *Anaesthesia*. 1988;43:962-963.
145. Parker CJR, Jones JE, Hunter JM. Disposition of infusions of atracurium and its metabolite, laudanosine, in patients in renal and respiratory failure in an ITU. *Br J Anaesth*. 1994;61:531-540.
146. Buck ML, Reed MD. Use of nondepolarizing neuromuscular blocking agents in mechanically ventilated patients. *Clin Pharmacokin*. 1991;10:32-48.
147. Bion JF, Bowden MI, Chow B, et al. Atracurium infusions in patients with fulminant hepatic failure awaiting liver transplantation. *Intensive Care Med*. 1993;19:S94-S98.
148. Schramm W, Papousek A, Michalek-Sauberer A, Czech T, Illievich U. The cerebral and cardiovascular effects of cisatracurium and atracurium in neurosurgical patients. *Anesth Analg*. 1998;86:123-127.
149. Modica P, Templehoff R. Effect of chronic anticonvulsant therapy on recovery from atracurium. *Anesth Analg*. 1989; 68:S198.
150. Caldwell JE, Canfell PC, Castagnoli KP, et al. The influence of renal failure on the pharmacokinetics and duration of action of pipecuronium bromide in patients anesthetized with halothane and nitrous oxide. *Anesthesiology*. 1989;70:7-12.
151. Savarese JJ, Kitz RJ. Does clinical anesthesia need new neuromuscular blockers? *Anesthesiology*. 1975;42:236-239.
152. Ferres CJ, Carson IW, Lyons SM, et al. Haemodynamic effects of vecuronium, pancuronium, and atracurium in patients with coronary artery disease. *Br J Anaesth*. 1987;59:305-311.
153. Gallo JA, Cork RC, Puchi P. Comparison of effects of atracurium and vecuronium in cardiac surgical patients. *Anesth Analg*. 1988;67:161-165.
154. Hoskings MP, Lennon RL, Gronert GA. Combined H_1 and H_2 receptor blockade attenuates the cardiovascular effects of high dose atracurium for rapid sequence endotracheal intubation. *Anesth Analg*. 1988;67:1089-1092.
155. Estafanous FG. Anesthetics and muscle relaxants in patients with heart disease: historical perspective. *J Cardiovasc Anesth*. 1990;6(suppl 4):3-13.
156. Ward S, Neill EAM. Pharmacokinetics of atracurium in acute hepatic failure (with acute renal failure). *Br J Anaesth*. 1987;55:1169-1172.
157. Farman JV, Turner JM, Blanloeil Y. Atracurium infusion in liver transplantation. *Br J Anaesth*. 1986;58:96S-102S.
158. Hughes R. Atracurium: an overview. *Br J Anaesth*. 1986;58:2S-5S.
159. Hunter JM, Jones RS, Utting JE. Comparison of vecuronium, atracurium and tubocurarine in normal patients and in patients with no renal function. *Br J Anaesth*. 1984;56:941-951.
160. d'Hollander AA, Luyckx C, Barvais L, et al. Clinical evaluation of atracurium besylate requirement for a stable muscle relaxation during surgery: lack of age related effects. *Anesthesiology*. 1983;59:237-240.
161. Kitts JB, Fisher DM, Canfell PC, et al. Pharmacokinetics and pharmacodynamics of atracurium in the elderly. *Anesthesiology*. 1990;72:272-275.
162. Shorten GD, Goudsouzian NG, Ali HH. Histamine release following atracurium in the elderly. *Anaesthesia*. 1993;48:568-571.
163. Kalli I, Meretoja OA. Infusion of atracurium in neonates, infants and children: a study of dose requirements. *Br J Anaesth*. 1988;60:651-654.
164. Nimbex Injection [package insert]. Research Triangle Park, NC: Glaxo Wellcome; 1995.
165. Doenicke AW, Czeslick E, Moss J, Hoernecke R. Onset time, endotracheal intubating conditions, and plasma histamine after cisatracurium and vecuronium administration. *Anesth Analg*. 1998;87:434-438.
166. Konstadt SN, Reich DL, Stanley TE, et al. A two-center comparison of the cardiovascular effects of cis-atracurium (Nimbex) and vecuronium in patients with coronary artery disease. *Anesth Analg*. 1995;81:1010-1014.
167. Bryson HM, Faulds D. cis-Atracurium besylate. A review of its pharmacology and clinical potential in anaesthetic practice. *Drugs*. 1997;53:848-866.
168. Naguib M, Samarkandi AH, Ammar A, et al. Comparative clinical pharmacology of rocuronium, cis-atracurium, and their combination. *Anesthesiology*. 1998;98:1116-1124.
169. Tran T, Fiset P, Varin F. Pharmacokinetics and pharmacodynamics of cis-atracurium after a short infusion in patients under propofol anesthesia. *Anesth Analg*. 1998;87:1158-1163.
170. Mellinghoff H, Radbruch L, Diefenbach C, et al. A comparison of cis-atracurium and atracurium: onset of neuromuscular block after bolus injection and recovery after subsequent infusion. *Anesth Analg*. 1996;83:1072-1075.
171. Bluestein LS, Stinson LW, Lennon RL, et al. Evaluation of cis-atracurium, a new neuromuscular blocking agent, for tracheal intubation. *Can J Anaesth*. 1996;43:925-931.

172. Savarese JJ, Lien CA, Belmont MR, et al. The clinical pharmacology of new benzylisoquinoline-diester compounds, with special consideration of cis-atracurium and mivacurium. *Anaesthetist.* 1997;46:840-849.
173. Donnelly AJ, Cunningham FE, Baughman VL. *Anesthesiology and Critical Care Drug Handbook.* 4th ed. Hudson, Ohio: Lexi-Comp Corporation; 2001.
174. Kisor DF, Schmith VD, Wargin WA, et al. Importance of the organ-independent elimination of cis-atracurium. *Anesth Analg.* 1996;83:1065-1071.
175. Welch RM, Brown A, Ravitch J, et al. The in vitro degradation of cis-atracurium, the R, cis-R'-isomer of atracurium, in human and rat plasma. *Clin Pharmacol Ther.* 1995;58:132-142.
176. Smith CE, van Miert MM, Parker CJ, et al. A comparison of the infusion pharmacokinetics and pharmacodynamics of cis-atracurium, the 1R-cis1'R-cis isomer of atracurium, with atracurium besylate in healthy patients. *Anaesthesia.* 1997;52: 833-841.
177. Soukup J, Czeslick E, Bunk S. *cis*-Atracurium in patients with compromised kidney function. Pharmacodynamic and intubation conditions under isoflurane-nitrous oxide anesthesia. *Anaesthetist.* 1998;47:669-676.
178. Sorooshian SS, Stafford MA, Eastwood NB, Boyd AH, Hull CJ, Wright PM. Pharmacokinetics and pharmacodynamics of cisatracurium in young and elderly adult patients. *Anesthesiology.* 1996;84:1083-1091.
179. Mellinghoff H, Diefenbach C. The clinical pharmacology of *cis*-atracurium. *Anaesthetist.* 1997;46:481-485.
180. Fahey MR, Morris RB, Miller RD, et al. Clinical pharmacology of ORG NC45 (Norcuron): a new nondepolarizing muscle relaxant. 1981;55:6-11.
181. Baird WLM, Savage DS. Vecuronium—the early years. *Anesthesiol Clin North Am.* 1985;3:347-360.
182. Shanks CA, Avram MJ, Fragen RJ, et al. Pharmacokinetics and pharmacodynamics of vecuronium administered by bolus and infusion during halothane or balanced anesthesia. *Clin Pharmacol Ther.* 1987;42:459-464.
183. Belmont MR. Pharmacodynamics and pharmacokinetics of benzylisoquinolinium (curare-like) neuromuscular blocking drugs. *Anesthesiol Clin North Am.* 1993;11:251-281.
184. Cronnelly R, Fisher DM, Miller RD, et al. Pharmacokinetics and pharmacodynamics of vecuronium (ORG NC45) and pancuronium in anesthetized humans. *Anesthesiology.* 1983;58: 405-408.
185. Gramstad L, Lilleaasen P, Minsaas B. Onset time and duration of action for atracurium, ORG NC 45 and pancuronium. *Br J Anaesth.* 1982;54:827-830.
186. Rorvik K, Husby P, Gramstad L, et al. Comparison of large dose of vecuronium with pancuronium for prolonged neuromuscular blockade. *Br J Anaesth.* 1988;61:180-185.
187. Fisher DM, Rosen JI. A pharmacokinetic explanation for increasing recovery time following larger or repeated doses of nondepolarizing muscle relaxants. *Anesthesiology.* 1986;65: 286-291.
188. Sohn YJ, Bencini A, Scaf AHJ, et al. Pharmacokinetics of vecuronium in man. *Anesthesiology.* 1982;57:A256.
189. Ornstein E, Matteo RS, Halevy JD, et al. Accelerated recovery from doxacurium in carbamazepine treated patients. *Anesthesiology.* 1989;71:A785.
190. Norman J. Resistance to vecuronium. *Anaesthesia.* 1993;48: 1068-1069.
191. Booij LHDJ, Edwards RP, Sohn YJ, et al. Comparative cardiovascular and neuromuscular effects of ORG NC 45, d-tubocurarine and metocurine. *Anesthesiology.* 1979;51:S280.
192. Cozantis DA, Pouttu J, Rosenberg PH. Bradycardia associated with the use of vecuronium. *Anaesthesia.* 1987;42:192-194.
193. Lebrault C, Berger JL, D'Hollander AA, et al. Pharmacokinetics and pharmacodynamics of vecuronium (ORG NC 45) in patients with cirrhosis. *Anesthesiology.* 1985;62:601-605.
194. Fahey MR, Morris RB, Miller RD, et al. Pharmacokinetics of ORG-NC45 (Norcuron) in patients with and without renal failure. *Br J Anaesth.* 1981;53:1049-1052.
195. Durant NN, Marshall IG, Savage DS, et al. The neuromuscular and autonomic blocking activities of pancuronium, Org NC 45, and other pancuronium analogues, in the cat. *J Pharm Pharmacol.* 1979;31:831-836.
196. Arden JR, et al. Vecuronium in alcohol liver disease: a pharmacokinetic and pharmacodynamic analysis. *Anesthesiology.* 1988;68: 771-776.
197. Lepage JY, Malinge M, Cozian A, et al. Vecuronium and atracurium in patients with end-stage renal failure. *Br J Anaesth.* 1987;59:1004-1010.
198. Mahajan RP, Hennessy N. Effect of priming dose of vecuronium on lung function in elderly patients. *Anesth Analg.* 1993;77: 1198-1202.
199. Fisher DM, Miller RD. Neuromuscular effects of vecuronium (ORG NC45) in infants and children during N_2O, halothane anesthesia. *Anesthesiology.* 1983;58:519-523.
200. Goudsouzian NG, Martyn JJ, Liu LM, et al. Safety and efficacy of vecuronium in adolescents and children. *Anesth Analg.* 1983;62:1083-1088.
201. Mirakhur RK, Shepher WF, Lavery GG, et al. The effects of vecuronium on intraocular pressure. *Anaesthesia.* 1987;42:944-949.
202. Caldwell JE, Heier T, Wright PM, et al. Temperature-dependent pharmacokinetics and pharmacodynamics of vecuronium. *Anesthesiology.* 2000;92:84.
203. Rupp SM, Fisher DM, Miller RD, et al. Pharmacokinetics and pharmacodynamics of vecuronium in the elderly. *Anesthesiology.* 1983;59:A270.
204. Rathmell JP, Brooker RF, Prielipp RC, et al. Hemodynamic and pharmacodynamic comparison of doxacurium and pipecuronium with pancuronium during induction of cardiac anesthesia: does the benefit justify the cost? *Anesth Analg.* 1993;76:513-519.
205. Murray DJ, Mehta MP, Forbes R, et al. Cardiovascular and neuromuscular effects of bwa938u: comparison with pancuronium. *Anesthesiology.* 1987;67:A367.
206. Lebowitz PW, Ramsey FM, Savarese JJ, et al. Combination of pancuronium and metocurine: neuromuscular and hemodynamic advantages over pancuronium alone. *Anesth Analg.* 1981;60:12-17.
207. Desai P, Hewitt PB, Jones RM. Influence of anticonvulsant therapy on doxacurium and pancuronium induced paralysis. *Anesthesiology.* 1989;71:A784.
208. Haas R, Masters J. Comparative recovery from three nondepolarizing neuromuscular blockers in a patient before and after chronic anticonvulsant therapy: a case report. *AANA J.* 1997;65:475-478.
209. Gravlee GP, Ramsey FM, Roy RC, et al. Rapid administration of a narcotic and neuromuscular blocker: a hemodynamic comparison of fentanyl, sufentanil, pancuronium, and vecuronium. *Anesth Analg.* 1988;67:39-47.
210. Emmott RS, Bracey BJ, Goldhill DR, et al. Cardiovascular effects of doxacurium, pancuronium, and vecuronium in anaesthetized patients presenting for coronary artery bypass surgery. *Br J Anaesth.* 1990;65:480-486.
211. Duvaldestine P, Agoston S, Henzel D, et al. Pancuronium pharmacokinetics in patients with liver cirrhosis. *Br J Anaesth.* 1978;50:1131-1136.
212. McLeod K, Watson MJ, Rawlins MD. Pharmacokinetics of pancuronium in patients with normal and impaired renal function. *Br J Anaesth.* 1976;48:341-345.
213. Matteo RS, Backus WW, McDaniel DD, et al. Pharmacokinetics and pharmacodynamics of d-tubocurarine and metocurine in the elderly. *Anesth Analg.* 1985;64:23-29.
214. Martin-Sheridan D. Geriatrics and anesthesia practice. In: Nagelhout J, Zaglaniczny K, eds. *Nurse Anesthesia.* Philadelphia: Saunders; 2001;1169-1176.
215. Goudsouzian NG, Liu LMP, Cote CJ. Comparison of equipotent doses of non-depolarizing muscle relaxants in children. *Anesth Analg.* 1981;60:862-866.

216. Berry FA. Neonatal anesthesia. In: Stoelting RK, ed. *Clinical Anesthesia.* 3rd ed. Philadelphia: Lippincott-Raven; 1997: 1091-1114.
217. Fan SZ, Susetio L, Tsai MC. Neuromuscular blockade of the fetus with pancuronium or pipecuronium for intrauterine procedures. *Anaesthesia.* 1994;54:284-286.
218. Tassonyi E, Neidhart P, Tatti B, et al. Hemodynamic effects of pipecuronium bromide during fentanyl-midazolam anesthesia induction for coronary artery bypass grafting. *Anesthesiology.* 1986;65:A284.
219. D'honneur G, Khalil M, Dominique C, et al. Pharmacokinetics and pharmacodynamics of pipecuronium in patients with cirrhosis. *Anesth Analg.* 1993;77:1203-1206.
220. Stanley JC, Mirakhur RD, Sampaio MM, et al. Onset and duration of action of pipecuronium bromide. *Anesthesiology.* 1989; 71:A776.
221. Foldes FF, Nagashima H, Nguyen HD, et al. Neuromuscular and cardiovascular effects of pipecuronium. *Can J Anesth.* 1990;37: 554-555.
222. deGouw NE, Crul JF, Vandermeersch E, Mulier JP, van Egmond J, van Aken H. Interaction of antibiotics on pipcuronium-induced neuromuscular blockade. *J Clin Anesth.* 1993;5:212-215.
223. Wierda JM, Karliczek GF, Vandenbrom RH, et al. Pharmacokinetics and cardiovascular dynamics of pipecuronium bromide during coronary artery surgery. *Can J Anesth.* 1990;37: 183-191.
224. Thiel A, Wyderka T, Wagner RM, Ebel H, Hempelmann G. Effects of pipecuronium and pancuronium on cerebrospinal fluid pressure in neurosurgical patients. *Acta Anaesthesiol Belg.* 1996; 47:59-65.
225. Shaheen B, Wig J, Grewal S, Tewari MK. Effect of pipecuronium and pancuronium on intracranial pressure and cardiovascular parameters in patients with supratentorial tumours. *Neurol India.* 2000;48:37-42.
226. Larijani GE, Bartkowski RR, Azad SS, et al. Clinical pharmacology of pipecuronium bromide. *Anesth Analg.* 1989;68:734-739.
227. Wierda JM, Szenohradszky J, DeWit AP, et al. The pharmacokinetics, urinary, and biliary excretion of pipecuronium bromide. *Eur J Anaesthesiol.* 1991;8:451-457.
228. Ornstein E, Matteo RS, Schwartz AE, et al. Pharmacokinetics and pharmacodynamics of pipecuronium bromide in elderly surgical patients. *Anesth Analg.* 1992;74:841-844.
229. Pittet JF, Tassonyi E, Morel DR, et al. Pipecuronium-induced neuromuscular blockade during nitrous-oxide fentanyl, isoflurane, and halothane anesthesia in adults and children. *Anesthesiology.* 1989;71:210-213.
230. Glass PSA, Ginsberg B, Quill T, et al. Onset, duration and reversal following doxacurium chloride (BW A938U) when combined with isoflurane. *Anesth Analg.* 1988;67:S73.
231. Lennon RL, Hosking MP, Houck PC, et al. Doxacurium chloride for neuromuscular blockade before tracheal intubation and surgery during nitrous oxide-oxygen-narcotic-enflurane anesthesia. *Anesth Analg.* 1988;68:255-260.
232. Cook DR, Freeman JA, Lai AA, et al. Pharmacokinetics and pharmacodynamics of doxacurium in normal patients and in those with hepatic or renal failure. *Anesth Analg.* 1991;72:145-150.
233. Cashman JN, Luke JJ, Jones RM. Neuromuscular block with doxacurium (BW A938U) in patients with normal or absent renal function. *Br J Anaesth.* 1990;64:186-192.
234. Stoelting RK. Anticholinesterase drugs and cholinergic agonists. *Pharmacology and Physiology in Anesthetic Practice.* Philadelphia: Lippincott; 1999:224-237.
235. Dresner DL, Basta SJ, Ali HH. Pharmacokinetics and pharmacodynamics of doxacurium in young and elderly patients during isoflurane anesthesia. *Anesth Analg.* 1990;71:498-502.
236. Maddineni VR, Cooper R, Stanley JC, et al. Clinical evaluation of doxacurium chloride. *Anaesthesia.* 1992;47:554-557.
237. Basta SJ, Savarese JJ, Ali HH, et al. Clinical pharmacology of doxacurium chloride. *Anesthesiology.* 1988;69:478-486.
238. Atherton DP, Hunter JM. Clinical pharmacokinetics of the newer neuromuscular blocking drugs. *Clin Pharmacokinet.* 1999;36: 169-189.
239. Kern C, Tassonyi E, Rouge JC, Wilder-Smith OH, Pittet JF. Doxacurium pharmacodynamics in children during volatile and opioid-based anaesthesia. *Anaesthesia.* 1996;51:361-364.
240. Lieberman BA, Norman P, Hardy BG. Pancuronium-phenytoin interaction: a case of decreased duration of neuromuscular blockade. *Int J Clin Pharmacol Ther Toxicolol.* 1988;26:371-374.
241. Ornstein E, Matteo RS, Weinstein JA, Halevy JD, et al. Accelerated recovery from doxacurium induced neuromuscular blockade in patients receiving chronic anticonvulsant therapy. *J Clin Anesth.* 1991;3:108-111.
242. Kopman AF. Recovery times following edrophonium and neostigmine reversal of pancuronium, atracurium, and vecuronium steady state infusions. *Anesth Analg.* 1986;65:572-578.
243. Roth DL, Rothstein P, Thomas SJ. Anesthesia for cardiac surgery. In: Stoelting RK, ed. *Clinical Anesthesia.* Vol 1. Philadelphia: Lippincott-Raven; 1997:835-869.
244. Basta SJ, Savarese JJ, Ali HH, et al. Neuromuscular and cardiovascular effects in patients of BW A938U: a new long-acting neuromuscular blocking agent. *Anesthesiology.* 1986;65:A281.
245. Embree PB. Long-acting nondepolarizing neuromuscular blocking agents. *AANA J.* 1993;61:382-387.
246. Mehta MP, Murray D, Forbes R, et al. The neuromuscular pharmacology of BW A938U in anesthetized patients. *Anesthesiology.* 1986;65:A280.
247. Fisher DM, Reynolds KS, Schmith VD, et al. The influence of renal function of the pharmacokinetics and pharmacodynamics and simulated time course of doxacurium. *Anesth Analg.* 1999;89:786.
248. Sarner JB, Brandom BW, Cook DR, et al. Clinical pharmacology of doxacurium chloride (BW A938U) in children. *Anesth Analg.* 1988;67:303-306.
249. Katzung BG. Acetylcholine receptor antagonists. In: Katzung BG, ed. *Basic and Clinical Pharmacology.* 3rd ed. Norwalk, Conn: Appleton & Lange; 1987:75-83.
250. Brown JH, Taylor P. Muscarinic receptor agonists and antagonists. In: Gilman A, ed. *Goodman and Gilman's Pharmacological Basis of Therapeutics.* 9th ed. New York: McGraw-Hill; 1995:141-160.
251. Facts and Comparisons. Cholinergic muscle stimulants. In: *Drug Facts and Comparisons.* 48th ed. St Louis: Wolters Kluwer; 1994: 2860-2867.
252. Fragen RJ. Role of reversal agents. *J Clin Anesth.* 1992;4(suppl 1): 9S-15S.
253. Service AHF. Parasympathomimetic agents. In: McEvoy GK, ed. *AHFS 94 drug information.* Bethesda, Md: American Society of Hospital Pharmacists; 1994:721-728.
254. Taylor P. Anticholinesterase agents. In: Gilman A, ed. *Goodman and Gilman's Pharmacological Basis of Therapeutics.* 9th ed. New York: McGraw-Hill; 1995:161-176.
255. Sparr HJ, Mellinghoff H, Blobner M, et al. Comparison of intubating conditions after rapacuronium (ORG 9487) and succinylcholine following rapid sequence induction in adult patients. *Br J Anaesth.* 1999;82:537-541.
256. Haas RE, Johnson TW, Werlinger DJ. Cardiovascular effects of atropine and glycopyrrolate on anesthetized children. *AANA J.* 1987;55:529-538.
257. Naguib M, Flood PM, McArdle JJ, et al. Advances in neurobiology of the neuromuscular junction: implications for the anesthesiologist. *Anesthesiology.* 2002;96:202-231.
258. Service AHF. Myasthenia gravis. In: McEvoy GK, ed. *AHFS 94 drug information.* Bethesda, Md: American Society of Hospital Pharmacists; 1994:1565-1567.
259. Goulden MR, Hunter JM. Rapacuronium (ORG 9487): do we have a replacement for succinylcholine? *Br J Anaesth.* 1999;82: 489-492.
260. Eriksson LI. Evidence-based practice and neuromuscular monitoring. *Anesthesiology.* 2003;98:1037.

261. Debaene B, Plaud B, Pierre Dilly M, et al. Residual paralysis in the PACU after a single intubating dose of nondepolarizing muscle relaxant with an intermediate duration of action. *Anesthesiology*. 2003;98:1042.
262. Pena O, Prestjohn S, Guzzetta CE. Agreement between muscle movement and peripheral nerve stimulation in critically ill pediatric patients receiving neuromuscular blocking agents. *Heart Lung*. 2000;29:309-318.
263. Silverman DG, Brull SJ. Monitoring neuromuscular block. *Anesthesiology*. 1994;12:237-260.
264. Bevan DR. Recovery from neuromuscular block and its assessment. *Anesth Analg*. 2000;90:S7-S13.
265. Viby-Mogensen J. Neuromuscular monitoring. In: Miller RD, ed. *Anesthesia*. Vol 1. 5th ed. Philadelphia: Churchill Livingstone; 2000:1351-1366.
266. Rupp SM. Monitoring neuromuscular blockade: twitch monitoring. *Anesthesiol Clin North Am*. 1993;11:361-378.
267. Kervin MW. Residual neuromuscular blockade in the immediate postoperative period. *J Perianesth Nurs*. 2002;17: 152-158.

CHAPTER 12

Cardiac Pharmacology

John J. Nagelhout, John P. McDonough

The provision of high-quality anesthetic care obviously requires that the anesthetist understand autonomic and cardiovascular physiology as well as the pharmacology of drugs that affect the autonomic and cardiovascular systems. With the population of the nation aging, it is not unreasonable to expect that the age of patients coming to surgery will also increase. With advancing age, patients will require operative intervention for treatment of increased levels of cardiac disease and autonomic dysfunction. When these patients undergo surgical intervention, they have the chronic disorders of the cardiovascular system that are associated with advancing age. In addition to the performance of the usually expected procedures associated with anesthesia management, it is the duty of the anesthetist to manage the patient's cardiovascular diseases during the period the patient is under anesthesia care. Many patients require attentive monitoring and interventional management of preload, afterload, peripheral resistance, cardiac contractility, and coronary perfusion and the maintenance of balance between myocardial oxygen supply and demand. Failure to accomplish these tasks may well result in increased frequencies of both perioperative morbidity and mortality. Many patients who are taking drugs that affect the autonomic and cardiovascular systems will likely need to continue taking them through the morning of surgery. In addition, different drugs affecting the autonomic and cardiovascular systems, such as α- and β-agonists or antagonists and nitrates, may have to be added to the management plan during the administration of the anesthetic.

AUTONOMIC DRUGS–SYMPATHOMIMETIC AMINES

The sympathomimetic amines include the three naturally occurring catecholamines epinephrine, norepinephrine, and dopamine and a number of synthetic agents such as phenylephrine and dobutamine. These drugs are used in a variety of situations, including the treatment of anesthesia-induced hypotension, bradycardia, anaphylaxis, shock, heart failure, and cardiac resuscitation.

The basic structure of the sympathomimetic amines is β-(3,4-dihydroxyphenyl)-ethylamine (Figure 12-1); this structure consists of a substituted benzene ring and an ethylamine side chain.[1] The effects elicited by this pharmacologic class are the result of the stimulation of β-adrenergic, α-adrenergic, and dopamine adrenergic receptors. The efficacy of a particular sympathomimetic amine depends on its concentration at the receptor site, its affinity for specific receptors, and the population of receptors available for binding. The population of receptors available is influenced not only by absolute numbers of receptors, but also by the percentage of receptors that are present and have not been pharmacologically antagonized.

Epinephrine

Epinephrine, one of the naturally occurring catecholamines, is the final product in the chain of catecholamine synthesis. Although both epinephrine and norepinephrine have agonistic activity at both α- and β-receptors, norepinephrine has minimal β_1 activity in low doses, whereas epinephrine strongly stimulates both β_1- and β_2-receptors.

Epinephrine is useful not only in the treatment of anaphylaxis and cardiopulmonary resuscitation; its combination of α and β effects also makes it an appropriate choice for the treatment of some shock states in which poor tissue oxygen delivery and hypotension are combined. In small doses epinephrine may well be useful as a sympathomimetic agent in patients who are not responsive to indirect acting agents and in those in whom simultaneous β_1- and β_2-receptor stimulation may be helpful. With epinephrine, the dominance of α or β effects is dose related.

Epinephrine's β_1 effect produces marked positive inotropic, chronotropic, and dromotropic actions. It should be noted that as heart rate, left ventricular stroke work, stroke volume, and cardiac output increase, so does myocardial oxygen consumption. In addition, the corresponding increased automaticity of all foci, including those that are ectopic, may lead to arrhythmia. Marked vigilance must be maintained in an effort to ensure that an imbalance of myocardial oxygen supply and demand does not occur. It should be recalled that the effects resulting from epinephrine administration are capable of both increasing myocardial demand and decreasing supply.

Beneficial effects of β_2 stimulation include bronchodilation, vasodilation, and stabilization of mast cells, with a resultant diminution of histamine release. Concurrently, α stimulation promotes a decrease in bronchial secretion. The net effect is a decrease in airway resistance with an improvement in oxygenation.

With low doses of epinephrine, β_2 stimulation in the peripheral vasculature promotes the redistribution of blood flow to skeletal muscle, thereby producing a decrease in systemic vascular resistance. As the dose of epinephrine is increased, the α effect predominates, with resultant vasoconstriction and an increase in systemic pressures. The systolic pressure is increased, whereas the diastolic pressure remains relatively unchanged, with a resultant increase in pulse pressure. It should be noted that if the coronary arteries are not obstructed, autoregulation increases oxygen delivery to meet the increased demand.[2] However, in the presence of a coronary

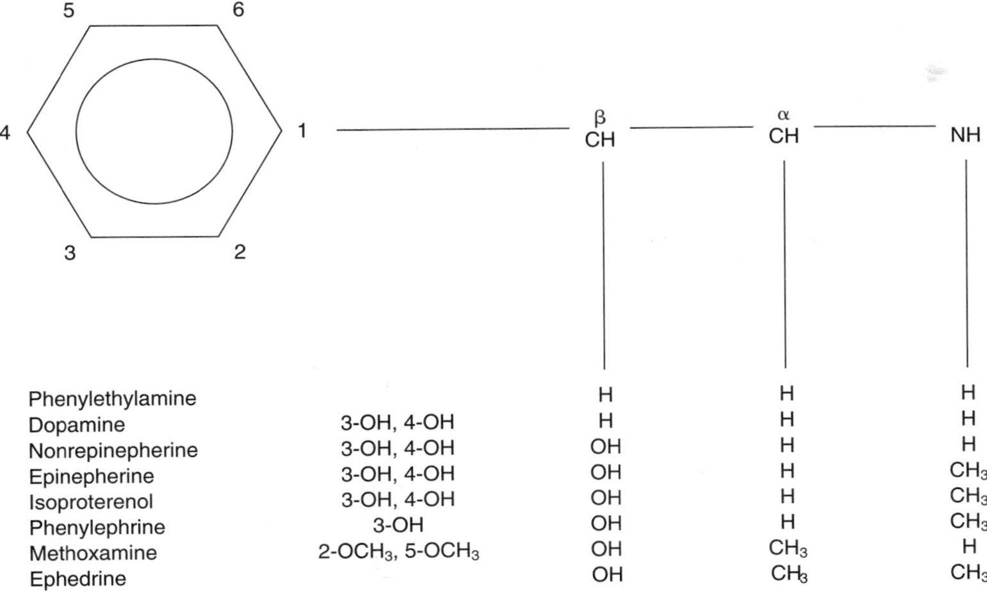

FIGURE **12-1**
Phenylethylanoleamine derivatives. Basic chemical structure of the sympathomimetic amines with drug-specific substitutions. (Modified from Hoffman BB. Catecholamines, sympathomimetic drugs and adrenergic receptor antagonists. In: Hardman JG, Limbird LE, Goodman Gilman A, et al, eds. *Goodman and Gilman's the Pharmacological Basis of Therapeutics*. 10th ed. New York: McGraw-Hill; 2001:218.)

artery lesion, oxygen delivery may not be able to meet demand, and myocardial ischemia results.[3]

The increased α effect that occurs with greater doses of epinephrine also results in renal and splanchnic vasoconstriction. Renal vascular resistance and ultimately renal blood flow are decreased. β Stimulation leads to activation of the renin-angiotensin system and also to an increase in lipolysis, glycogenolysis, gluconeogenesis, ketone production, and lactate release by skeletal muscle.[4] Insulin secretion is inhibited by an overriding β_2 stimulation. Epinephrine-induced β_2 stimulation also can cause a transient hyperkalemia, as potassium follows glucose out of hepatic cells. This is followed by a longer hypokalemia, as β_2 stimulation then forces this extracellular potassium into red blood cells.[5] Because of the mechanism of action of the drug, care must be exercised in treating hypotension with epinephrine in patients who are concomitantly receiving α-antagonists. α-Blocking drugs, such as phentolamine, block the peripheral vasoconstricting effects of the α-agonism usually associated with epinephrine. This leaves the peripheral β_2 effects, which cause vasodilation, virtually unopposed.

Norepinephrine

Norepinephrine is known as a potent vasopressor. Although it is not as potent as epinephrine in stimulating α-receptors, it has little β_2 activity at low doses, and the end result is, for the most part, unopposed α stimulation. The chronotropic effect seen with β_1 stimulation is generally absent with norepinephrine because of the increase in systemic vascular resistance, which induces reflex vagal activity.

The aforementioned combination of adrenergic stimulation results in a decrease in vital organ flow; however, coronary artery perfusion may be increased because of the increase in diastolic pressure. Renal vascular resistance is increased, and urine output may fall. Simultaneous administration of dopamine has been recommended to correct the increase in renal vascular resistance seen with norepinephrine.[6] An increase in preload also may be seen because norepinephrine is a venoconstrictor.[7]

Norepinephrine is generally used in patients with adequate cardiac output but low systemic vascular resistance. In this group of patients, however, the underlying problem of peripheral tissue perfusion-oxygenation may be exacerbated by the intense norepinephrine-induced peripheral vasoconstriction, even if adequate blood pressure has been achieved.

Norepinephrine does have some generalized metabolic effects, such as a decrease in insulin production, but these metabolic effects are present to a lesser degree than those seen with epinephrine. Adverse effects are usually a result of the intense vasoconstriction that is associated with norepinephrine.

Dopamine

Dopamine is an endogenous central neurotransmitter that is derived from dopa in the chain of catecholamine synthesis. Pharmacologically, dopamine stimulates dopamine receptors, β-receptors, and α-receptors in a dose-dependent manner. Dopaminergic receptors are stimulated with low doses of less than 2 mcg/kg/min. At moderate doses of 2 to 5 mcg/kg/min, β effects are elicited, and α effects are seen with high infusion rates of greater than 10 mcg/kg/min. Dopamine also has an indirect sympathomimetic effect, eliciting the release of norepinephrine via β_1 stimulation.[8]

Dopamine is often the first inotropic agent chosen by the anesthetist presented with a patient in systemic shock. Some clinicians have found dopamine to have a poor response in cases of gram-negative sepsis, because of a down-regulation in which the sensitivity of β-receptors is diminished.[9,10]

During surgery and anesthesia dopamine is administered for its dopaminergic effect. The stimulation of dopamine receptors in the renal artery promotes an increase in renal blood flow and a resultant increase in glomerular filtration rate and urine output. Benefits, however, of so called "renal" dopamine are in doubt. Dopamine also inhibits aldosterone, resulting in an increase in sodium excretion and urine output.

Dopamine has been implicated in several cases of severe limb ischemia. If dopamine is administered through a peripheral line, increased vigilance in pediatric patients and in patients with any type of vascular disease such as diabetes, atherosclerosis, or Raynaud's phenomenon is advised. The presence of an arterial line in the affected limb also increases the incidence of limb ischemia with concurrent dopamine infusion. Other metabolic and central nervous system effects, similar to those seen with epinephrine but less extensive, have been attributed to dopamine administration.

The monoamine oxidase enzymes metabolize dopamine; therefore the effects of dopamine can be prolonged in patients who are receiving a monoamine oxidase inhibitor. Tricyclic antidepressants may also augment the activity of sympathomimetic drugs.

Isoproterenol

Isoproterenol is a synthetic catecholamine with the same underlying chemical structure as the endogenous catecholamines. It is a potent agonist of β_1- and β_2-receptors but has no agonistic activity at α-receptors and dopamine receptors. The uses of isoproterenol have been limited, and the drug is currently used in the treatment of bradycardia, which is characterized by hemodynamic instability that is unresponsive to atropine, and also in pediatrics for the management of status asthmaticus. Despite these two applications, other, more selective, drugs are frequently chosen for the treatment of these conditions.

The profound β_1 stimulation of isoproterenol results in both positive inotropic and chronotropic effects. In combination with the peripheral β_2-induced vasodilation and resultant drop in systemic vascular resistance, an increase in cardiac output is seen. However, the positive inotropic and chronotropic effects dramatically increase myocardial oxygen consumption, which may already be compromised by the β_2-induced peripheral vasodilation, causing a decrease in diastolic blood pressure and ultimately a decrease in coronary artery perfusion. Furthermore, the patient who is hypovolemic may become hypotensive as a result of the peripheral vasodilation.

Isoproterenol is also a potent bronchial dilator and pulmonary vasodilator. Initially this may cause a drop in arterial oxygen tension secondary to ventilation-perfusion mismatch if supplemental oxygen is not administered.

The detrimental effects of isoproterenol on the heart, such as excessive tachycardia, induction of myocardial ischemia, and arrhythmia production, are the major factors limiting its use to the treatment of significant heart block unresponsive to atropine. Other side effects are similar to those seen with epinephrine but occur to a lesser extent. One difference is that the profound β stimulation of the pancreatic islet cells increases insulin secretion and diminishes the degree of hyperglycemia.

Dobutamine

Dobutamine is a synthetic sympathomimetic amine. It is a modification of isoproterenol, but its use currently is much more widespread than that of isoproterenol. Dobutamine is a strong β_1-agonist with some β_2 effects and at high doses very weak if any α effects.[11] Consequently, dobutamine displays a strong inotropic response with minimal chronotropy. It also produces a slight drop in systemic vascular resistance, owing to peripheral vasodilation. However, the resultant increase in cardiac output compensates for the decrease in systemic vascular resistance, and the blood pressure is increased or at low doses relatively unchanged. Pulmonary artery pressure decreases, and an increase in left ventricular stroke work index is observed.[12]

The positive inotropic effects, coupled with the lack of chronotropy and maintenance of normal blood pressure, have made this agent a frequent choice in the treatment of acute congestive heart failure (CHF). Patients who do not have heart failure but do have coronary artery disease may develop myocardial ischemia if given dobutamine.[13] In hypovolemic patients, the decrease in systemic vascular response can become exacerbated, with a resultant drop in blood pressure. This decrease in blood pressure may also be seen in patients with sepsis.

Dobutamine enhances conduction through the atrioventricular node, necessitating that caution be exercised in patients with atrial fibrillation. Dobutamine-induced arrhythmias do occur, but the incidence is considerably less than that seen with the other sympathomimetic amines. Another potential side effect of dobutamine of interest to the anesthetist is platelet inhibition; however, the clinical significance of this inhibition is negligible.

DIRECT-ACTING α-Agonists

α_1-Agonists

Phenylephrine

Phenylephrine (Neo-Synephrine) and methoxamine (Vasoxyl) are the two most commonly employed pure α-agonists. Phenylephrine has strong α-stimulating effects, with virtually no β stimulation. A sharp rise in blood pressure is seen after administration; this rise is primarily the result of a significant increase in peripheral resistance secondary to the α_1 stimulation.

A reflex bradycardia can be elicited secondary to baroreceptor stimulation, and the anesthetist should allow for the return of an adequate baseline heart rate before using one of these agents. An antimuscarinic also can be used selectively in the treatment of bradycardia. Intravenous (IV) bolus administration of phenylephrine is frequently employed, but caution should be used because profound increases in blood pressure and decreases in heart rate can result. The onset of action of IV phenylephrine is immediate, with the duration of action ranging from 5 to 20 minutes. Phenylephrine is frequently used topically for the prevention of nosebleeds during nasal intubation because of its vasoconstricting effects.

Methoxamine

Methoxamine has a longer duration of action than phenylephrine because it is already O-methylated and therefore is not affected by catechol-O-methyltransferase or monoamine oxidase. Methoxamine does not have any β-stimulating effects and produces an intense arterial vasoconstriction but little venoconstriction.

α_2-Agonists

Clonidine

Clonidine (Catapres) is the α_2-agonist most frequently encountered by the anesthetist. Clonidine decreases blood pressure by acting as an agonist at peripheral presynaptic α_2-receptors and central postsynaptic α_2-receptors. Stimulation of the peripheral presynaptic α_2-receptors causes inhibition of catecholamine release, with subsequent vasodilation. Stimulation of the central postsynaptic α_2-receptors, which is considered the main antihypertensive mechanism of action, results in diminished sympathetic outflow and a resultant decrease in circulating catecholamines and renin activity. Rebound hypertension, which is seen after abrupt discontinuation of clonidine use, is a major concern. The resultant increase in catecholamine levels manifests as tachycardia and hypertension. Continuing the medication throughout the perioperative period is the desired approach. Tapering of the dose and discontinuation may occasionally be indicated. Patches may also be used during surgery to prevent withdrawal.

Clonidine is available in oral and transdermal forms. The transdermal form is frequently encountered and administered at a fixed rate for a period of 1 week. Use of clonidine as a premedicant has been advocated by some because of the sedative and analgesic qualities of the agent.[14] Clonidine also is used as a catecholamine suppression test in the diagnosis of pheochromocytoma. A newer α_2-agonist, dexmedetomidine (Precedex), has been introduced for sedation in critical care. It is an IV infusion drug for short-term use.

MIXED FUNCTION AGONISTS

Ephedrine is a synthetic noncatecholamine sympathomimetic commonly employed in anesthesia practice. It stimulates both α- and β-receptors via direct and indirect mechanisms of action. Ephedrine's effects are similar to those seen with epinephrine; however, they are lesser and not accompanied by a dramatic increase in serum glucose concentrations. The duration of action of ephedrine is also longer than that of epinephrine, owing to its lack of a basic catechol structure; this characteristic makes it resistant to metabolism by monoamine oxidase.

Ephedrine often is the first sympathomimetic chosen for alleviation of hypotension, because of the cardiac depressant effects of the anesthetic agents or vasodilation resulting from spinal anesthesia. Intravenously administered ephedrine, in doses ranging from 10 to 25 mg, has an immediate onset and a duration of action of 1 to 1.5 hours. This drug should be used cautiously in patients with questionable coronary perfusion because myocardial oxygen consumption may be more dramatically increased than is anticipated as a result of ephedrine's positive inotropic effect. In animal studies uterine perfusion has been found not to be diminished, and maternal blood pressure is predictably increased.[15] As with any indirect-acting agent, tachyphylaxis may develop with subsequent dosing because catecholamine stores become depleted. In addition, some authors believe that the tachyphylaxis seen with repeated dosing occurs because adrenergic receptors are still occupied; consequently, fewer receptors are available to bind with the drug.[16]

Ephedrine also may be administered by oral, intramuscular, or subcutaneous routes. Patients may receive long-term oral ephedrine for its bronchodilating effects secondary to β_2 stimulation.

Two other agents within this category are mephentermine (Wyamine) and metaraminol (Aramine). Mephentermine exhibits effects that are similar to those of ephedrine, and metaraminol elicits a greater α_1 response. The use of these agents has declined significantly in recent years.

SELECTIVE β_2-Agonists

The β_2-agonists include terbutaline (Breathine, Breathaire, Bricanyl), metaproterenol (Alupent, Metaprel), albuterol (Proventil, Ventolin), and salmeterol (Serevent). These "selective" β-agonists are effective in treating obstructive airway diseases such as asthma, chronic obstructive pulmonary disease, and acute bronchospasm.

The selectivity of these agents for β_2-receptors results in the desired response of bronchodilation and in the diminution of the undesired β_1 responses of tachycardia and arrhythmia. As a result these drugs are replacing epinephrine as the agent of choice for treatment of acute bronchospasm in anesthetic practice. All of these agents are available in aerosol form, and it is widely accepted that aerosol delivery is as effective as subcutaneous or other means of administration. Drugs of this class also have an increased duration of action because of their noncatecholamine structure; this renders them resistant to methylation by catechol-O-methyltransferase.

Two puffs of nebulized or metered-dose inhaler–administered terbutaline, albuterol, or salmeterol 10 to 15 minutes before exercise have been shown to have similar efficacy in preventing exercise-induced asthma. However, salmeterol provides protection against bronchospasm for up to 12 hours, whereas terbutaline and albuterol have 2- to 2.5-hour durations of action.[17]

Chronic use of these agents can result in tachyphylaxis secondary to down-regulation (i.e., diminished quantity) of β-receptors. Increased hyperresponsiveness of the airway also has been suspected with chronic use of these agents. Salmeterol, the newest agent in this class, has been indicated for long-term use. Some investigators[18] have found it to be an effective β_2-agonist for long-term use because its effect is not diminished over time[19]; others have found the opposite to be true.[20]

The β_2-agonists also are used for arresting premature labor. This is referred to as a *tocolytic effect*. Uterine relaxation is achieved through increases in the levels of cyclic adenosine monophosphate (cAMP); this decreases intracellular calcium levels and ultimately diminishes the level of actin-myosin coupling. Currently, terbutaline and ritodrine (Yutopar) are used. Ritodrine may first be administered intravenously, and maintenance doses are given orally. Terbutaline also is frequently employed.

The parturient who receives a β_2-agonist usually shows some degree of both β_1 and β_2 stimulation. Common findings include tachycardia and an increased cardiac output along with a widened pulse pressure because of a lower diastolic pressure. Increased renin levels diminish the degree of urinary excretion of sodium and water, potentially increasing the risk of pulmonary edema if fluids are not carefully titrated. Maternal hyperglycemia and hypokalemia also are seen. The total body potassium level is not altered, but an intracellular shift does occur. Ritodrine and terbutaline both freely cross the placenta. Contraindications to tocolytic therapy include fetal death or lethal abnormality, eclampsia, placental abruption, and proved chorioamnionitis. Relative contraindications are preeclampsia, severe chronic hypertension, renal disease, heart disease, fetal distress, and fetal growth retardation.[21]

Oral nicardipine has been found to be superior to magnesium sulfate as a tocolytic.[22] Patients already taking a calcium channel inhibitor should not receive nicardipine. Doses of selected vasoactive drugs are listed in Table 12-1.

α-Receptor Antagonists

The α-receptor antagonists are used for treatment of hypertension, benign prostatic hyperplasia, CHF, pheochromocytoma, Raynaud's phenomenon, toxicity, and ergot alkaloid toxicity.[23] Common side effects include orthostatic hypotension and baroreceptor-mediated reflex tachycardia, which may make their use in the treatment of hypertension somewhat difficult in the ambulatory patient. In addition, because of the significantly longer duration of action of the α-receptor antagonists, the direct vasodilators are considered more predictable in the treatment of emergent episodes of hypertension.

TABLE 12-1 Doses of Selected Vasoactive Drugs

Drug	Bolus Dose	Infusion Dose Rate	Comments
Calcium chloride ($CaCl_2$) or gluconate	500-1000 mg (chloride) 500-2000 mg (gluconate)		Onset: <1 min Peak effect: <1 min Duration: 10-20 min
Dobutamine (Dobutrex)		2-20 mcg • kg^{-1} • min^{-1}	Onset: 1-2 min Peak effect: 1-10 min Duration: 10 min
Dopamine (Intropin)		1-2 mcg • kg^{-1} • min^{-1} (renal doses) 2-10 mcg • kg^{-1} • min^{-1} (cardiac doses) 10-20 mcg • kg^{-1} • min^{-1} (vasopressor doses)	Onset: 2-4 min Peak effect: 2-10 min Duration: <10min
Ephedrine	5- to 10-mg incremental doses		Dilute to 5 or 10 mg • ml^{-1} Onset: <1 min Peak effect: 2-5 min Duration: 10-60 min
Epinephrine	10-100 mcg	0.01-0.03 mcg • kg^{-1} • min^{-1} (β doses) 0.03-0.15 mcg • kg^{-1} • min^{-1} (α and β doses) 0.15-0.3 mcg • kg^{-1} • min^{-1} (α doses)	Onset: <1 min Peak effect: 1-2 min Duration: 5-10 min
Fenoldopam		0.1-1.6 mg • kg • min	Onset: 4-5 min Peak effect: 7 min Duration: 15 min
Glucagon	1-5 mg over 2-5 min		
Isoproterenol (Isuprel)	1 ml over 1 min *after diluting* in 10 ml (= 0.02 mg • ml^{-1})	0.015-0.15 mcg • kg^{-1} • min^{-1}	Onset: <1 min Peak effect: 1 min Duration: 1-5 min
Methoxamine (Vasoxyl)	5-mg incremental doses		Onset: <1 min Peak effect: 1-2 min Duration: 15-60 min
Milrinone (Primacor)	50 mcg • kg^{-1}	0.375-0.75 mcg • kg^{-1} • min^{-1}	
Nesiritide ** (Natrecor)		0.01 mcg/kg/min	Onset: 15 min Peak effect: 1 hr Duration: 60 min
Norepinephrine (Levophed)		0.01-0.2 mcg • kg^{-1} • min^{-1}	Onset: <1 min Peak effect: 1-2 min Duration: 2-10 min
Phentolamine (Regitine)	5 mg (50-100 mcg • kg^{-1}) Repeat as required	1-10 mcg • kg^{-1} • min^{-1}	Onset: 1-2 min Peak effect: 2 min Duration: 10-15 min
Phenylephrine (Neo-Synephrine)	40-100 mcg	0.15-0.75 mcg • kg^{-1} • min^{-1}	Onset: <1 min Peak effect: 1 min Duration: 15-20 min
Sodium nitroprusside (Nipride, Nitropress)		0.1-10 mcg • kg^{-1} • min^{-1}	Onset: <1 min Peak effect: 1-2 min Duration: 1-10 min
Trimethaphan (Arfonad)		0.5-5 mcg • kg^{-1} • min^{-1}	Stored 2°-8° C Stable 14 days at 25° C Onset: <1 min Peak effect: 1-2 min Duration: 10-30 min

Phenoxybenzamine

Phenoxybenzamine (Dibenzyline) is a haloalkylamine with both α_1- and α_2-blocking activity. The α-receptors are irreversibly bound by phenoxybenzamine, and its action is terminated only by metabolism of the drug or by the generation of additional α-receptors. Clinically this drug is used preoperatively in patient with pheochromocytoma for diminishing the response to endogenous catecholamines. The preoperative course is started 1 to 3 weeks before surgery, with the maximum oral dosage being 40 to 120 mg in two to three divided doses given daily. Phenoxybenzamine also prevents the sympathomimetic response expected from phenylephrine. The response to norepinephrine is limited to its β_1-agonist activity, and epinephrine may show "epi-reversal," which is an enhanced β_2 response with a worsening of hypotension and tachycardia. Nasal stuffiness has been frequently associated with phenoxybenzamine use.

Phentolamine

Phentolamine (Regitine), an imidazole, is a competitive antagonist of α_1- and α_2-receptors. It has a rapid onset after IV administration and a much shorter duration of action when compared with phenoxybenzamine. It can be employed for the short-term control of hypertension in patients with pheochromocytoma. The recommended dose is 1 to 5 mg by slow IV push. Phentolamine has also been employed in the treatment of local infiltrations of vasoconstricting agents. Phentolamine (5 to 10 mg) can be mixed with 10 ml of normal saline and injected directly into the site of the infiltration. A related agent that may be encountered in neonatal patients with persistent pulmonary hypertension is tolazoline (Priscoline).

Prazosin and Others

Prazosin (Minipress), doxazosin (Cardura), and terazosin (Hytrin) are selective α_1-antagonists used in the chronic treatment of hypertension. Their lack of α_2-blocking activity indicates that they have no effect on norepinephrine levels. Therefore, selectivity for α_1-receptors leaves the inhibitory action of α_2-receptors on norepinephrine release intact, and less norepinephrine-induced tachycardia results than when a nonselective α-antagonist is used. Prazosin induces vasodilation in both arterioles and veins. Peripheral vascular resistance and cardiac preload are diminished. The diminished cardiac preload further minimizes the potential for increased heart rate and also results in a diminished cardiac output. The drugs are administered orally, and orthostatic hypotension can be a major side effect.

Droperidol

Droperidol (Inapsine), a butyrophenone, has been and continues to be used as an antiemetic and sedative agent in anesthesia practice. It also produces a minimal degree of α-adrenergic blockade and minimal reduction in blood pressure. Droperidol has proved to be useful clinically in the treatment of mild increases in blood pressure. Marked decreases in blood pressure in isolated patients may occur, especially in volume-depleted patients. The use of droperidol has decreased markedly as a result of the "black box warning" required by the U.S. Food and Drug Administration (FDA) as part of the package insert for this drug. Use of droperidol has been associated with prolongation of the corrected QT interval in certain patients, increasing the probability of the development of torsades de pointes, which has led to serious morbidity and death. There has been considerable debate regarding the relationship between the anesthetic administration of droperidol in very low doses as an antiemetic and the complications described.[24] Little doubt remains, however, that the potential for administrative and legal difficulties as well as the issues of patient safety have led to significant changes in the pattern of use of this drug.[25] A 12-lead electrocardiogram is required by the FDA prior to the use of droperidol. Off labeled use of low doses as an antiemetic may still be useful. Fortunately, the FDA has recently agreed to revisit the issue of the cardiac effects of droperidol and the ominous restrictions placed on its use. It is anticipated that these restrictions may be downgraded.

β-Adrenergic Blocking Agents

The β-blockers are drugs frequently encountered by the anesthesia provider. Common applications of agents of this pharmacologic class include the treatment of angina pectoris, essential hypertension, "fresh" myocardial infarctions, supraventricular tachycardias (including Wolff-Parkinson-White syndrome), and atrial fibrillation; the suppression of increased sympathetic activity (e.g., as occurs with intubation); the management of hypertrophic obstructive cardiomyopathies and CHF; and the preoperative preparation of hyperthyroid patients. Some authors also point out the effectiveness of β-blockers in the treatment of digitalis-induced arrhythmias (as an adjunct to phenytoin or lidocaine) and in the management of ventricular arrhythmias.[26] Evidence supports that the perioperative use of β-blocking may, in vascular and general surgery patients, reduce cardiac perioperative mortality by 8% and ischemic complications by 15%.[27]

The β-blockers are structurally related to isoproterenol. They bind β-receptors in a competitive manner and prevent the actions of catecholamines and other β-agonists. Because these agents are competitive antagonists, the law of mass action is applicable to their efficacy. If an agonist is present in sufficient concentration at the receptor, the blocking actions of the β-antagonists can be overcome.

The β-blockers are subdivided on the basis of their selectivity for cardiac β_1-receptors. Examples of cardioselective β_1-receptor antagonists include metoprolol (Lopressor), atenolol (Tenormin), acebutolol (Sectral), and esmolol (Brevibloc). Agents that block both β_1- and β_2-receptors include the prototype β-receptor antagonist propranolol (Inderal), as well as nadolol (Corgard), timolol (Blocadren), and pindolol (Visken). The degree of receptor selectivity is important because antagonism of β_1-receptors results in lowered heart rate, decreased myocardial contractility, and diminished atrioventricular conduction velocity; it also has beneficial effects with regard to decreasing myocardial oxygen consumption and the treatment of arrhythmias. However, antagonism of β_2-receptors can result in the nonbeneficial effects of bronchoconstriction and peripheral vasoconstriction. It is important to note that as the dose of the "selective" β-blockers is increased, the degree of selectivity is diminished.

Some of the β-blockers act as partial agonists and, as such, possess intrinsic sympathomimetic activity. A partial agonist does not stimulate β-receptors to the extent that a full agonist does, and in the presence of a full agonist the partial agonist acts as a competitive antagonist. It follows that β-blockers with intrinsic sympathomimetic activity competitively antagonize the effects of a full agonist (e.g., endogenous catecholamines released during times of maximal sympathetic tone) down to the activity level of its partial agonist component. Theoretically this would prevent patients who are teetering on the edge of cardiac failure from being "-blocked" into overt cardiac failure. Intrinsic sympathomimetic activity would also minimize the risk of bronchoconstriction in patients with reactive airway disease who require β-blockade. Pindolol, acebutolol, penbutolol, and carteolol are β-adrenergic blocking agents that possess intrinsic sympathomimetic activity.

Membrane-stabilizing activity is another property of some β-blockers. These agents diminish arrhythmogenicity by exerting a quinidine-like effect. However, membrane-stabilizing activity is seen only with high drug concentrations.[28] Propranolol and pindolol are two β-blockers with membrane-stabilizing activity. Bisoprolol has been shown to reduce the risk of myocardial infarction when administered before vascular surgery in high-risk patients.[29] Fifty-nine high-risk patients received 5 to 10 mg of bisoprolol versus placebo. A 3.4% mortality rate within 30 days occurred in the β-blocker–treated group versus 17% in the placebo group.

Some potential problems with β-adrenergic blocking agents have already been mentioned. β-Blockade can result in both bronchospasm and the development of overt cardiac failure in some patients with high doses or IV administration. Other potential problems arise with β_2-receptor blockade in patients with peripheral vascular disease and Raynaud's syndrome because of the possible potentiation of peripheral vasoconstriction. In diabetic patients, signs of hypoglycemia may be masked, and the patient's ability to increase serum glucose levels may be impaired. Serum potassium levels may also become elevated with β_2-blockade because uptake into skeletal muscle is inhibited. In patients whose heart-rate is controlled in order to maintain cardiac output, β-blockade may have a significant impact on blood pressure.

The β-receptors are considered to be "labile" receptors—that is, they are subject to up-regulation and down-regulation. Chronic therapy with β-blockers can lead to up-regulation of β-receptors or an increase in the absolute number of receptors. This phenomenon is suspected to be the underlying cause of the withdrawal syndrome seen with the abrupt discontinuation of β-adrenergic antagonist use. This syndrome is characterized by increased sympathetic activity for up to 2 days. Obviously, this means that the patient receiving β-blockers should continue to receive them without interruption throughout the perioperative period.

Propranolol and Esmolol

The two β-adrenergic blocking agents useful in the perioperative period are propranolol and esmolol. Propranolol may take up to 15 minutes to exert an effect. Its elimination half-life is approximately 4 hours, and its duration of action permits administration two to four times per day. The elimination of propranolol can be prolonged in patients with hepatic disease. IV administration of propranolol is 1 to 5 mg, but most clinical practitioners start with 0.25 to 0.5 mg intravenously and titrate upward, if needed. Esmolol has replaced propranolol in most instances of β-blocker application in anesthesia because of its short duration of action. Esmolol has an onset time of 2 minutes and an elimination half-life of approximately 9 minutes. Its rapid onset and short half-life, as well as its duration of action of 10 to 15 minutes, make it easily and reliably titratable in acute-care situations. The recommended IV loading dose of esmolol is 500 mcg/kg; this is followed by an infusion of 100 to 300 mcg/kg/min. Most anesthesia practitioners start with a bolus of 10 to 15 mg and continue administration according to patient response. Esmolol is metabolized by nonspecific plasma esterases found in the cytosol of red blood cells.

Labetalol

Labetalol (Normodyne, Trandate) is classified as a nonselective β-blocker but is unique in that it also possesses an α-blocking component. It provides β-blockade along with α-blockade in a ratio of 7:1. This action can be extremely beneficial in situations in which an acute rise in blood pressure could be devastating to the clinical outcome. The usual IV dose of labetalol is 0.25 mg/kg; this dose can be repeated every 10 minutes as indicated and followed by an infusion at a rate of 2 mg/min. In clinical practice, most practitioners use a bolus dose of labetalol (10 mg) and gauge follow-up administration on the basis of patient response. Labetalol can have a duration of action ranging from 2 to 18 hours depending on dose. Because labetalol provides both β- and α-blockade, an adequate heart rate must be present before labetalol can be employed in the acute management of hypertension. It should be noted that uterine blood flow is not affected in obstetric patients, even in the event of a dramatic decrease in systemic blood pressure.[30] Labetalol undergoes hepatic metabolism and renal elimination.[31] A new combined β- and α-blocker, Carvedilol, has been introduced. It is available as an oral formulation for the treatment of hypertension and CHF.

CHOLINERGICS

Cholinergic agents mimic the actions of the neurotransmitter acetylcholine but have been developed to differ in terms of comparative nicotinic and muscarinic activity and duration of action. Acetylcholine (Miochol) has no clinical application owing to its generalized enhancement of cholinergic effects throughout the body and its extremely short duration of action (approximately 1 ms), which is a result of its rapid metabolism by acetylcholinesterase.

Methacholine (Provocholine), carbachol (carbamylcholine chloride), and bethanechol (carbamylmethylcholine) are choline esters that have limited clinical applications. Methacholine can be used as an aerosol in the diagnosis of reactive airway disease, whereas carbachol, because of its significant muscarinic and nicotinic activity, is employed only as a topical ophthalmic solution in the treatment of narrow-angle glaucoma and for inducing miosis during diagnostic testing and surgery. Bethanechol is theoretically useful in instances of ileus and urinary retention, such as in postvagotomy and postpartum patients, respectively. Bethanechol's relative lack of nicotinic activity makes it the most attractive of these three agents, and it is the agent most frequently encountered in clinical practice. Pilocarpine, a natural alkaloid, also is a cholinergic agent that is employed as an ophthalmic solution in the treatment of glaucoma. Potential side effects of these agents include any cholinergic-induced response such as bradycardia, varying degrees of heart block, hypotension, bronchoconstriction, and an increase in gastric secretions.

ANTICHOLINERGICS

The anticholinergics are familiar agents in anesthesia practice and therefore are discussed only briefly. Atropine, scopolamine, and glycopyrrolate are the three anticholinergics employed in anesthesia practice. These agents are competitive antagonists of acetylcholine at muscarinic receptors. A comparison of the basic properties of the anticholinergic agents is given in Table 12-2.

Atropine

Atropine, a belladonna alkaloid, is the prototype anticholinergic. The anesthetist can use atropine for its antisialagogue effects, for the prevention or treatment of bradycardia, and concurrently with anticholinesterase agents in the reversal of muscle relaxants for preventing the resultant bradycardia from anticholinesterase-induced acetylcholine buildup. The usual adult IV dose for increasing heart rate during anesthesia is 0.4 to 0.6 mg, with the time to onset being 1 to 2 minutes. Atropine is a tertiary amine; this allows it to cross the blood-brain barrier freely, and may result in bradycardia when low doses are given. However, at usual clinical doses, significant central nervous system effects are rarely evident. Hepatic metabolism accounts for approximately half of a dose of atropine, with the remainder being eliminated unchanged in the urine. The elimination half-life of atropine is approximately 4 hours. Atropine should be avoided in patients with narrow-angle glaucoma, owing to its potential to increase intraocular pressure. Atropine poisoning or belladonna alkaloid toxicity manifests with extreme antimuscarinic effects, with potential progression to central nervous system depression and coma. The decades-old mnemonic, "red as a beet, blind as a bat, dry as a bone, mad as a hatter, and hot as a hare" was devised to be an easy way to remember the signs and symptoms of belladonna overdose. These include flushing ("red as a beet"); extreme mydriasis ("blind as a bat"); lack of secretions and dry mouth ("dry as a bone"); confusion ("mad as a hatter"); and hyperthermia ("hot as a hare").

Scopolamine

Scopolamine (hyoscine) also is a belladonna alkaloid with anticholinergic effects. Scopolamine is a tertiary amine. Compared with atropine, scopolamine has central nervous system effects that are much more pronounced at lower doses. Compared with atropine, it does not substantially increase heart rate. It can be used as a preoperative medication, with sedation and amnesia being a desirable effect. Scopolamine also is used to diminish the incidence of postoperative nausea and vomiting resulting from motion sickness. A scopolamine patch contains a total dose of 1.5 mg.

TABLE 12-2 Comparative Effects of Anticholinergic Drugs

Effect	Atropine	Scopolamine	Glycopyrrolate
Sedation	+	+++	0
Antisialagogue	+	+++	++
Increase heart rate	+++	+	++
Relax smooth muscle	++	+	++
Mydriasis, cycloplegia	+	+++	0
Prevent motion-induced nausea	+	+++	0
Decrease gastric hydrogen ion secretion	+	+	+

Glycopyrrolate

Glycopyrrolate (Robinul), a synthetic quaternary ammonium compound, has become the most frequently used anticholinergic in anesthesia practice. It has an excellent antisialagogue action,[32] with a longer duration of action than the belladonna alkaloids. It prevents bradycardia without inducing significant levels of tachycardia. The quaternary ammonium structure of glycopyrrolate prevents it from crossing the blood-brain barrier to any significant degree; therefore central nervous system effects are not seen. This property also makes it the agent of choice in obstetrics because it does not pass the placental barrier. Adult IV doses are generally 0.1 to 0.2 mg for antisialagogue activity and for the treatment of bradycardia. Onset of action is rapid, and the duration of action is up to 4 hours.

DIRECT VASODILATORS

Within this category, sodium nitroprusside, nitroglycerin, and hydralazine are the three drugs most commonly employed (Table 12-3). All three produce direct vasodilation. Sodium nitroprusside produces arterial and venous relaxation; nitroglycerin has a greater effect on venous than arterial relaxation; and hydralazine produces primarily arterial relaxation. The mechanism of action of all three agents is believed to be primarily an induced increase in the concentration of vascular nitric oxide, although that has not been confirmed with hydralazine.[33] It is important to note that none of the vasodilatory actions of these agents is the result of α-receptor antagonism.

Sodium Nitroprusside

Sodium nitroprusside is frequently used for the emergent control of hypertension, for inducing hypotension to decrease blood loss during surgical procedures, and for the treatment of acute pulmonary edema. Its rapid onset (within seconds) and its short duration of action (1 to 3 minutes) make it unique among agents for the rapid control of blood pressure. Sodium nitroprusside reduces both afterload and preload, and this results in a decrease in cardiac filling pressures and an increase in stroke volume and cardiac output. Left ventricular volumes are decreased, and diminished myocardial wall tension should contribute to a decrease in myocardial oxygen consumption.

Usually, sodium nitroprusside is started as an infusion at 0.5 mcg/kg/min and is titrated until a response occurs. An infusion rate of 3 mcg/kg/min is rarely exceeded, but young, normotensive patients may require up to 5 mcg/kg/min to achieve the desired response. A bolus dose of 1 to 2 mcg/kg has been found to be effective in blunting the hypertensive response to intubation.[34] Sodium nitroprusside is mixed with 5% dextrose in water, and the bottle and tubing are covered in a protective wrap because light causes the sodium nitroprusside to decompose. An infusion pump should always be used with sodium nitroprusside because of its potency and the associated risk of cyanide toxicity.

TABLE 12-3 Drugs Used in the Perioperative Management of Congestive Heart Failure

Drug	Mechanism	Preload Reduction	Afterload Reduction	Usual Dose
Renin Angiotensin System Antagonists				
Captopril	Inhibition of renal systemic and tissue generation of angiotensin II by ACE; decreased metabolism of bradykinin	++	++	6.25-50 mg PO q8h
Enalaprilat		++	++	2.5-10 mg PO q12h
Quinapril		++	++	0.5-2.0 mg IV q12h
Lisinopril		++	++	10-80 mg PO qd
Rampiril		++	++	2.5-50 mg PO q12-24h
Benazepril		++	++	10-40 mg in one or three doses
Fosinopril		++	++	10-40 mg in one or two doses
Moexepril		++	++	7.5-30 mg in one or two doses
Perindopril		++	++	4-8 mg in one or two doses
Trandolapril		++	++	1-4 mg in one dose
Losartan	Blockade of angiotensin II (AT_1) receptors	++	++	25-50 mg q12h
Candesartan		++	++	8-32 mg in one dose
Eprosartan		++	++	400-800 mg in one or two doses
Irbesartan		++	++	150-300 mg in one dose
Telmisartan		++	++	40-80 mg in one dose
Valsartan		++	++	80-320 mg in one dose
Introvasodilators				
Nitroglycerin	Nitric oxide donors	+++	+	0.2-10 mcg/kg/min IV, 5-6 mg transdermal
Isosorbide dinitrate		+++	+	10-60 mg qid
Nitroprusside		+++	+++	0.1-3 mcg/kg/min IV
Direct Vasodilator				
Hydrazaline	Unclear	+	+++	10-100 PO q6h
Calcium Channel Blocking Drug				
Amlodipine	Inhibition of L-type voltage-sensitive Ca^{2+} channels	+	+++	5-10 mg PO qd
Phosphodiesterase Inhibitors				
Amrinone	Inhibition of type II cAMP phosphodiesterase(s) and other mechanisms	++	++	0.5 mg/kg, then 2-20 mcg/kg/min IV
Milrinone		++	++	50 mcg/kg, then 0.25-1 mcg/kg/min IV
Sympathomimetics				
Dobutamine	Myocardial and vascular β-advenergic agonist	+	++	2-20 mcg/kg/min
Dopamine	Selective renal arterial vasodilation	–	– –	≤2 mcg/kg/min
Sympatholytics				
Prazosin (and other quinazoline derivatives)	α-Adrenergic receptor antagonist	++	++	1-5 mg PO q12h
Labetatol	Combined β- and α-adrenergic blockade	+	+	12.5-50 mg PO bid
Carvedilol		+	+	3.125-50 mg in two doses (titrate up every 2 wk)
Bucindolol	Additional mechanisms	+	++	6.25-100 mg PO bid

ACE, *Angiotensin converting enzyme;* bid, *twice a day;* IV, *intravenous;* PO, *oral;* qd, *every day;* qid, *four times a day.*

Cyanide Toxicity

Sodium nitroprusside contains five cyanide ions within its chemical structure, and its metabolism causes the release of these cyanide ions. One cyanide ion binds methemoglobin to form cyanomethemoglobin, whereas the other four cyanide ions undergo rhodinase-catalyzed conversion to thiocyanate in the liver, with the thiocyanate undergoing renal elimination. This conversion to thiocyanate requires the cofactor thiosulfate B_{12}. Cyanide toxicity results when this metabolism is overwhelmed. Various recommendations for preventing cyanide toxicity from sodium nitroprusside include maximum doses and lengths of administration. In general, infusions of 8 to 10 mcg/kg/min for periods of 3 hours or longer should be avoided, and chronic administration should not exceed 0.5 mcg/kg/min. Clinically the development of metabolic acidosis, increased mixed venous oxygen content, tachycardia, and tachyphylaxis during sodium nitroprusside use are signs of cyanide toxicity.

Treatment of cyanide toxicity consists of the discontinuation of the sodium nitroprusside infusion, the administration of oxygen, and the treatment of the metabolic acidosis. Sodium nitrite 3%, 4 to 6 mg/kg, can be administered over 3 to 5 minutes to promote the production of methemoglobin so that excess cyanide ions can be bound. Sodium thiosulfate, 150 to 200 mg/kg over 15 minutes, can be administered every 2 hours as needed; vitamin B_{12} also can be administered. If available, hydroxycobalamin can be used.

Nitroglycerin

Nitroglycerin is employed in the treatment of angina pectoris and ischemia with the patient under anesthesia and also can be used for lowering blood pressure. Nitroglycerin causes venodilation, with an increase in venous capacitance and a resultant decrease in preload.[35] This results in a lowering of cardiac filling pressures, a lessening of myocardial wall tension, and ultimately a decrease in myocardial oxygen requirements. Nitroglycerin's mechanism of action in the relief of angina is not an increase in coronary artery blood flow, which may actually be decreased during an infusion of nitroglycerin, but rather the aforementioned decrease in preload. Some of the larger coronary vessels may become dilated, with a resultant increase in blood flow to ischemic myocardium. At relatively high concentrations of nitroglycerin, arterial vasodilation also can occur.

Use of sublingual nitroglycerin (0.3-mg tablets), up to a total of three tablets, is the most efficient treatment for acute angina. Relief is generally achieved in 1 to 2 minutes and lasts up to 30 minutes. IV nitroglycerin also has an onset time of 1 to 2 minutes and a duration of action of up to 10 minutes. Nitroglycerin is extensively metabolized in the liver and has a half-life of only 3 minutes.[36] IV nitroglycerin is used for "unloading" of the heart in CHF and myocardial infarction. Nitroglycerin infusions are usually started at 5 to 10 mcg/min and titrated until effective. IV nitroglycerin can also be used for controlled hypotension but is not as potent in this regard as an infusion of sodium nitroprusside. Because nitroglycerin exerts its main effect on venous capacitance, any decrease in blood pressure is more volume dependent when compared with sodium nitroprusside–induced hypotension. Of note to the anesthesia provider is the ability of nitroglycerin to relax the smooth muscle of the biliary tract and provide relief from narcotic-induced biliary spasm. It also should be noted that nitroglycerin, as well as sodium nitroprusside, can cause cerebral steal in patients with cerebral injury.[37] Generally, 50 mg of nitroglycerin is mixed with 250 ml of dextrose 5% in water.[38] Nitroglycerin patches and ointments also are available for extended coverage (Tables 12-4 and 12-5).

TABLE 12-4 Pharmacologic Characteristics of Currently Available Nitrates

Agent	Dose	Dosing Interval	Onset of Action	Duration of Action
Nitroglycerin				
Sublingual	0.15-0.6 mg	Prn	1-5 min	10-30 min
Sublingual spray	0.4 mg/spray	Prn	2-5 min	10-30 min
Buccal	1-3 mg	Prn or q4-5 hr (while awake)	2-5 min	3-5 hr
Oral SR	2.6-13 mg	tid, qid	30-45 min	2-8 hr
Transdermal patches	2.5-15 mg/24 hr (1 patch)	qd (12 hr on/12 hr off)	30-60 min	8-14 hr
2% ointment	0.5-2 in	q6h (daytime)	20-60 min	3-8 hr
Isosorbide Dinitrate				
Sublingual	2.5-10 mg	Prn	3-15 min	1-2 hr
Chewable	5-10 mg	Prn	3-15 min	1-2 hr
Oral	5-40 mg	bid, tid	15-30 min	3-6 hr
Oral SR	40 mg	qd	30-60 min	6-10 hr
Isosorbide Mononitrate				
Oral	10-20 mg	bid	30 min	6-8 hr
Oral SR	60 mg	qd	30 min	6-10 hr

bid, *Twice a day;* Prn, *as needed;* qd, *every day;* qid, *four times a day;* tid, *three times a day.*

TABLE 12-5 Antihypertensive Drugs

Drug	Daily Adult Maintenance Dosage	Frequent or Severe Adverse Effects
Angiotension Converting Enzyme (ACE) Inhibitors		
Benazepril (Lotensin)	10-40 mg in one or two doses	Cough, hypotension, particularly with a diuretic or volume depletion; rash; acute renal failure with bilateral renal artery stenosis or stenosis of the artery to a solitary kidney; angioedema; hyperkalemia if also taking potassium supplements or potassium-sparing diuretics; loss of taste, usually not severe; blood dyscrasias and renal damage rare except in patients with renal dysfunction; increased fetal mortality with second- and third-trimester exposure; may decrease excretion of lithium
Captopril (Capoten)	12.5-150 mg in two or three doses	
Enalapril (Vasotec)	2.5-40 mg in one or two doses	
Fosinopril (Monopril)	10-40 mg in one or two doses	
Lisinopril (Prinivil or Zestril)	5-40 mg in one dose	
Moexipril (Univasc)	7.5-30 mg in one or two doses	
Perindopril (Aceon)	4-8 mg in one or two doses	
Quinapril (Accupril)	5-80 mg in one or two doses	
Ramipril (Altace)	1.25-20 mg in one or two doses	
Trandolapril (Mavik)	1-4 mg in one dose	
Angiotensin Receptor Antagonists		
Candesartan cilexetil (Atacand)	8-32 mg in one dose	Similar to ACE inhibitors but do not cause cough
Eprosartan (Teveten)	400-800 mg in one or two doses	
Irbesartan (Avapro)	150-300 mg in one dose	
Losartan (Cozaar)	25-100 mg in one or two doses	
Telmisartan (Micardis)	40-80 mg in one dose	
Valsartan (Diovan)	80-320 mg in one dose	
β-Adrenergic Blocking Drugs		
Atenolol (Tenormin)	25-100 mg in one or two doses	Fatigue; depression; bradycardia; decreased exercise tolerance; congestive heart failure; aggravate peripheral arterial insufficiency; aggravated allergic reactions; bronchospasm; mask symptoms of and delay in recovery from hypoglycemia; Raynaud's phenomenon; insomnia; vivid dreams or hallucinations; acute mental disorder; impotence; increased serum triglycerides
Betaxolol (Kerlone)	5-40 mg in one dose	
Bisoprolol (Zebeta)	5-20 mg in one dose	
Metoprolol (Lopressor)	50-200 mg in one or two doses	
(Toprol-XL)	50-400 mg in one dose	
Nadolol (Corgard)	20-240 mg in one dose	
Propranolol (Inderal)	40-240 mg in two doses	
Timolol (Blocadren)	10-40 mg in two doses	
β-Adrenergic Blocking Drugs with Intrinsic Sympathomimetic Activity		
Acebutolol (Sectral)	200-1200 mg in one or two doses	Similar to other β-adrenergic blocking drugs, but with less resting bradycardia and lipid changes; acebutolol has been associated with a positive antinuclear antibody test and occasional drug-induced lupus
Carteolol (Cartrol)	2.5-10 mg in one dose	
Penbutolol (Levatol)	20 mg in one dose	
Pindolol (Visken)	10-60 mg in two doses	
α- and β-Blockers		
Carvedilol (Coreg)	12.5-50 mg in two doses	Similar to other β-adrenergic blocking drugs, but more orthostatic hypotension; hepatotoxicity; do not affect serum lipids; labetolol has intrinsic sympathomimetic activity, carvedilol does not
Labetalol (Normodyne, Trandate)	200-1200 mg in two doses	
Thiazide-type Diuretics (Usually Once Daily)		
Chlorothiazide (Diuril)	125-500 mg	Hyperuricemia; hypokalemia, hypomagnesemia; hyperglycemia, hyponatremia; hyperglycemia; hypercholesterolemia; hyper-triglyceridemia; pancreatitis; rashes and other allergic reactions; sexual dysfunction; photosensitivity reactions; may decrease excretion of lithium
Hydrochlorothiazide (Esidrix, Microzide)	12.5-50 mg	
Chlorthalidone (Hygroton)	12.5-50 mg	
Indapamide (Lozol)	1.25-5 mg	
Metolazone (Zaroxolyn)	1.25-5 mg	
Loop Diuretics		
Bumetanide (Bumex)	0.5-5 mg in two or three doses	Dehydration; circulatory collapse; hypokalemia; hyponatremia; hypomagnesemia; hyperglycemia; metabolic alkalosis; hyperuricemia; blood dyscrasias; rashes; lipid changes as with thiazide-type diuretics
Ethacrynic acid (Edecrin)	25-100 mg in two or three doses	
Furosemide (Lasix)	20-320 mg in two or three doses	
Torsemide (Demadex)	5-20 mg in one or two doses	

TABLE **12-5** Antihypertensive Drugs—cont'd

Drug	Daily Adult Maintenance Dosage	Frequent or Severe Adverse Effects
Potassium-Sparing Diuretics		
Amiloride (Midamor)	5-10 mg in one or two doses	Hyperkalemia; GI disturbances; rash; headache
Spironolactone (Aldactone)	12.5-100 mg in one or two doses	Hyperkalemia; hyponatremia; mastodynia; gynecomastia; menstrual abnormalities; GI disturbances; rash
Triamtrene (Dyrenium)	50-150 mg in one or two doses	Hyperkalemia; GI disturbances; nephrolithiasis
Calcium Channel Blockers		
Diltiazem (Cardizem SR)	120-360 mg in two doses	Dizziness; headache; edema; constipation (especially verapamil); AV block; bradycardia; heart failure; lupus-like rash with diltiazem
(Cardizem CD)	120-360 mg in one dose	
(Dilacor)	120-480 mg in one dose	
(Diltia XT)	120-480 mg in one dose	
(Tiamate)	120-480 mg in one dose	
(Tiazac)	120-480 mg in one dose	
Verapamil (Calan)	120-480 mg in two or three doses	
(Calan SR)	120-480 mg in one or two doses	
(Isoptin SR)	120-480 mg in one or two doses	
(Verelan)	120-480 mg in one dose	
(Covera HS)	180-480 mg in one dose	
Dihydropyridines		
Amlodipine (Norvasc)	2.5-10 mg in one dose	Dizziness; headache; peripheral edema (more than with verapamil and diltiazem; more common in women); flushing; tachycardia; rash; gingival hyperplasia
Felodipine (Plendil)	2.5-10 mg in one dose	
Isradipine (DynaCirc)	5-10 mg in two doses	
(DynaCirc OR)	5-10 mg in one dose	
Nicardipine (Cardene)	60-120 mg in three doses	
(Cardene SR)	60-120 mg in two doses	
Nifedipine (Adalat CC)	30-90 mg in one dose	
(Procardia XL)	30-90 mg in one dose	
Nisoldipine (Sular)	10-60 mg in one dose	
α-Adrenergic Blockers		
Prazosin (Minipress)	First day: 1 mg at bedtime Maintenance: 1-2 mg in two or three doses	Syncope with first dose; dizziness and vertigo; headache; palpitations; fluid retention; drowsiness; weakness; anticholinergic effects; priapism
Terazosin (Hytrin)	First day: 1 mg at bedtime Maintenance: 1-20 mg in one dose	Both similar to prazosin, but with less hypotension after first dose
Doxazosin (Cardura)	First day: 1 mg at bedtime Maintenance: 1-6 mg in one dose	
Central α-Adrenergic Agonists		
Clonidine (Catapres)	0.1-0.6 mg in two or three doses	CNS reactions similar to methyldopa, but more sedation and dry mouth; bradycardia; heart block; rebound hypertension (less likely with patches); contact dermatitis from patches
(Catapres TTS)	One patch weekly (0.1-0.3 mg/day)	
Guanabenz (Wytensin)	4-64 mg in two doses	Similar to clonidine
Guanfacine (Tenex)	1-3 mg in one dose	Similar to clonidine, but milder
Methyldopa (Aldomet)	250 mg-2g in 2-4 doses	Drowsiness; sedation, fatigue; depression; dry mouth; heart block; autoimmune disorders, including colitis, hepatitis, hepatic necrosis; Coombs'-positive hemolytic anemia; lupus-like syndrome; thrombocytopenia; red cell aplasia; impotence
Direct Vasodilators		
Hydralazine (Apresoline)	40-200 mg in two to four doses	Tachycardia; aggravation of angina; headache; dizziness; fluid retention; nasal congestion; lupus-like syndrome; hepatitis
Minoxidil (Loniten)	2.5-40 mg in one or two doses	Tachycardia; aggravation of angina; marked fluid retention; pericardial effusion; hair growth on face and body
Peripheral Adrenergic Neuron Antagonists		
Guanadrel (Hylorel)	10-75 mg in two doses	Similar to guanethidine, but less diarrhea

AV, *atrioventricular;* CNS, *central nervous system;* GI, *gastrointestinal;* HDL, *high-density lipoprotein.*
From Drugs for Hypertension. Med Lett. *2001;43:17-20; and Drugs for hypertension. Treatment Guidelines.* Med Lett. *2003;1:33-40. With permission.*

Hydralazine

Hydralazine causes direct relaxation of arterial smooth muscle. It can be administered intravenously for the control of hypertension in doses ranging from 2.5 to 20 mg. Tachycardia frequently accompanies the decrease in blood pressure. It is important to remember that the onset of action can occur from 2 to 20 minutes after administration; therefore adequate time should be allowed before the initiation of repeat dosing so that profound decreases in blood pressure can be prevented. The elimination half-life in plasma is approximately 1 hour, but the duration of vasodilating action can be as long as 12 hours.[39-41] Hydralazine undergoes hepatic metabolism with renal excretion. Acetylation is partly responsible for the metabolism of hydralazine. Slow acetylators may be more prone to a drug-induced lupus syndrome that can result from high serum concentrations of hydralazine during chronic treatment.

CALCIUM ANTAGONISTS

The calcium antagonists have proved to be useful pharmacologic agents in the treatment of angina, hypertension, arrhythmias, peripheral vascular disease, esophageal spasm, and controlled hypotension and in the blocking of the stress response for intubation and skin incision.[42] The five calcium antagonists most likely to be encountered in clinical practice are of three chemical classes: nifedipine (Adalat, Procardia), nicardipine (Cardene), amlodipine (Norvasc), felodipine (Plendil), nisoldipine (Sular), and nimodipine (Nimotop) are 1,4-dihydropyridine derivatives; diltiazem (Cardizem) is a benzothiazepine derivative; and verapamil (Calan, Isoptin) is a phenylalkylamine derivative. In anesthesia practice, nifedipine and nicardipine, for the control of blood pressure, and verapamil, for the control of atrial tachyarrhythmias, are the most commonly employed calcium antagonists.

A discussion of the generalized mechanism of action of the calcium antagonists is necessary for a better understanding of their role. Depolarization of the sinoatrial and atrioventricular nodes is dependent on the inward flux of calcium during the phase 2 plateau of the cardiac action potential. Calcium antagonists "block" these channels, diminishing the inward flux of calcium and prolonging phase 2, and in this way exert a negative chronotropic effect on the heart. Ventricular pacemaker foci are dependent on the inward flux of sodium, which is minimally, if at all, affected by the calcium antagonists. It then follows that the calcium antagonists are effective in patients with atrial tachyarrhythmias but could be potentially detrimental if employed in patients with ventricular tachycardias. In clinical doses, verapamil exerts the greatest antiarrhythmic effect and has been found to be effective in treating atrial tachyarrhythmias, including Wolff-Parkinson-White syndrome, and in controlling the ventricular response to atrial fibrillation and flutter. Verapamil is not indicated for the treatment of atrial fibrillation associated with Wolff-Parkinson-White syndrome, nor is it indicated for the treatment of "simple" atrial tachycardia, for which β-blockers may be a better choice.

Calcium antagonists also exert a negative inotropic effect on the heart, which can be beneficial in patients with angina. Cardiac contractility is dependent on the influx of calcium into cardiac cells. The calcium binds with the regulatory protein troponin, neutralizing troponin's inhibitory influence on the interaction between the structural proteins actin and myosin. The greater the degree of interaction between actin and myosin, the greater the degree of cardiac contraction. It follows that the calcium antagonists, by diminishing the influx of calcium into cardiac cells, diminish the degree of cardiac contractility. This negative inotropic effect then leads to a decrease in myocardial oxygen consumption. However, it should be noted that a significant decrease in cardiac contractility could prove to be detrimental in patients with CHF.

The calcium antagonists also produce relaxation of vascular smooth muscle tone. Cytoplasmic calcium concentrations play an important role in the degree of vascular smooth muscle tension. Calcium antagonists, by diminishing the concentration of cytoplasmic calcium concentrations, induce vascular dilation or relaxation. This effect is more prominent on arteries than on veins. Peripheral arteries are affected with a resultant decrease in afterload and blood pressure, which contributes to an increase in cardiac output and a decrease in myocardial work and oxygen consumption. Coronary arteries also are affected, with an increase in coronary blood flow. The calcium antagonists have been found to be beneficial in the prevention of angina resulting from spasm of the coronary arteries, such as Prinzmetal's angina.

Most calcium antagonists induce vascular smooth muscle relaxation, except for verapamil, which has virtually no effect. Nimodipine has been found to be beneficial in the prevention of cerebral vasospasm associated with acute subarachnoid hemorrhage.[43]

Verapamil, 2.5 to 10 mg intravenously (dose can be repeated every 30 minutes), can be given for the treatment of atrial tachyarrhythmias. The onset time is up to 10 minutes, and the duration of action ranges from 2 to 4 hours. Verapamil is metabolized hepatically, has an elimination half-life of 4 to 7 hours, and is renally eliminated. Verapamil has been largely replaced by adenosine as the first-line drug of choice in the emergent treatment of atrial tachyarrhythmias. Orally administered nifedipine, 10 mg, is useful in the treatment of perioperative hypertension. Nifedipine has a time to onset of action of up to 20 minutes and a 2- to 3-hour duration of action. Nifedipine has an elimination half-life of 3 to 5 hours and undergoes hepatic metabolism and renal excretion. Nicardipine is also useful as an IV preparation for the treatment of hypertension or controlled hypotension under anesthesia.[44-46]

Varying degrees of atrioventricular block, myocardial depression, and hypotension are associated with the use of the calcium antagonists. An additive effect should be anticipated if the calcium antagonists are employed with other cardiodepressant agents. In addition, verapamil and nifedipine can increase serum digoxin levels by up to 30%.[47] Calcium antagonists may also potentiate muscle relaxants, but this effect is minimal at clinically relevant doses.[48] It is interesting to note that hemodynamic but not electrophysiologic effects of the calcium antagonists can be reversed with the administration of calcium (Table 12-6).[49]

ANGIOTENSIN CONVERTING ENZYME INHIBITORS

Angiotensin converting enzyme (ACE) inhibitors have proved useful in the treatment of hypertension and CHF and in the management of the post–myocardial infarction

TABLE 12-6 Drugs of Choice for Common Arrhythmias

Arrhythmia	Drug of Choice	Alternatives	Remarks
Atrial fibrillation or flutter	Verapamil, diltiazem, or a β-blocker to slow ventricular response	Digoxin to slow ventricular response Quinidine, procainamide, disopyramide, flecainide, propafenone, or sotalol for long-term suppression	Digoxin, verapamil, diltiazem, and possibly β-blockers may be dangerous for patients with Wolff-Parkinson-White syndrome. Amiodarone in low doses has also been effective for prevention. Radiofrequency catheter ablation has been used in selected patients.
Other supraventricular tachycardias	Adenosine or verapamil or diltiazem IV for termination	Esmolol, another β-blocker, or digoxin for termination	Direct current cardioversion or atrial pacing may be effective for some patients. Radiofrequency catheter ablation can cure many patients. Quinidine, procainamide, disopyramide, diltiazem, β-blockers, verapamil, flecainide, propafenone, or digoxin may be effective for long-term suppression.
Ventricular premature complexes or nonsustained ventricular tachycardia	No drug therapy indicated for asymptomatic patients Lidocaine for symptomatic patients	A β-blocker for symptomatic patients	There is no evidence that prolonged suppression with drugs prevents sudden cardiac death. For post-MI patients, treatment with a β-blocker has decreased mortality, and treatment with flecainide or moricizine has increased it.
Sustained ventricular tachycardia	Lidocaine for acute treatment	Procainamide, bretylium, amiodarone	Soltalol, other β-blockers, procainamide, quinidine, amiodarone, disopyramide, flecainide, propafenone, or mexiletine may be effective for long-term prevention.
Ventricular fibrillation	Lidocaine, amiodarone	Procainamide, bretylium	Specialized techniques such as programmed stimulation of the heart may be required to select long-term therapy, and some patients may be candidates for implanted cardioverter-defibrillators or radiofrequency catheter ablation.
Cardiac glycoside-induced ventricular tachyarrhythmias	Digoxin-immune Fab (digoxin antibody fragments—Digibind)	Lidocaine, phenytoin	Self-limited if short-acting digitalis stopped. Phenytoin can also be effective. Avoid cardioversion and bretylium, except for treatment of ventricular tachycardia. A β-blocker or procainamide can make heart block worse.
Torsades de pointes (acquired)	Magnesium sulfate	Cardiac pacing, isoproterenol	Causative agents (e.g., quinidine) should be discontinued. Magnesium sulfate in a dose of 1 g IV repeated once if necessary may be effective even in absence of hypomagnesemia. Potassium should be used to raise serum K to between 4 and 4.5 mEq/L.

IV, *intravenous*; MI, *myocardial infarction*.
Modified from Med Lett. *1996;38:75-82; Link MS, Homound M, Foote CB, et al.* J Cardiovasc Electrophysiol. *1996;7:653-670.*

patient.[50] These drugs exert their action by inhibiting the ACE peptidyl-dipeptidase. A brief description of the renin-angiotensin system is necessary for a full understanding of the actions of the ACE inhibitors (Figure 12-2).

Renin, a proteolytic protein, is released from the juxtaglomerular apparatus in response to diminished blood pressure. Renin is responsible for the conversion of angiotensinogen to the decapeptide angiotensin I. Angiotensin I is then converted to the octapeptide angiotensin II by peptidyl-dipeptidase, which is primarily located in the endothelial tissue of the lung. Angiotensin II is a potent vasopressor that also stimulates the release of endogenous norepinephrine and aldosterone. The end result is an increase in peripheral vasoconstriction with an increase in blood pressure and a resultant decrease in cardiac output. The increased aldosterone level results in increased sodium and water reabsorption, with concomitant secretion of potassium. Ultimately, angiotensin II is converted to angiotensin III via the activities of aminopeptidase. Angiotensin III retains most of the potency of angiotensin II[51] and is ultimately degraded to peptide fragments through the actions of angiotensinase. Peptidyl-dipeptidase also is responsible for the metabolism of bradykinin, which has potent vasodilatory effects. Of interest, the majority of people with hypertension do not have high serum levels of renin, but the ACE inhibitors have been shown to be effective in all patients with hypertension.[52]

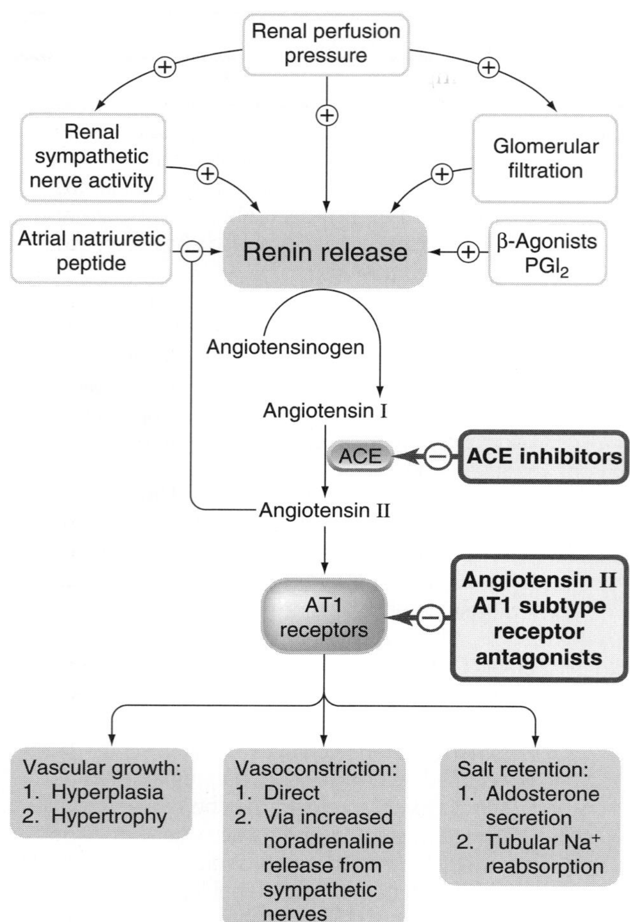

FIGURE **12-2**
Renin-angiotensin system. Angiotensin converting enzyme inhibitors block the conversion of angiotensin I to angiotensin II. Angiotensin receptor blockers act as antagonists at the (*AT1*) angiotensin receptors. (From Rang HP, Dale MM, Ritter JM, et al. *Pharmacology*. 5th ed. Edinburgh: Churchill-Livingstone; 2003:291.)

Common ACE inhibitors are listed in Table. 12-5. Enalapril and lisinopril usually require administration only once per day. Enalapril is a prodrug, and it undergoes hepatic metabolism to its active form of enalaprilat. Enalaprilat is currently the only ACE inhibitor available for IV administration, and it is used for perioperative hypertension. All of these agents are renally eliminated, and their elimination half-lives can be expected to be prolonged in renally compromised patients. Potential problems with the ACE inhibitors include cough, angioedema, hyperkalemia, neutropenia, and proteinuria. Drug-induced renal failure also can be seen, especially in patients with renal artery stenosis, which is usually reversible with discontinuation of ACE inhibitor therapy. Interaction between the anesthetic agents and the ACE inhibitors has been suspected to lead to bradycardia and hypotension during the perioperative period.[53] The patient receiving an ACE inhibitor also is frequently being treated with a β-blocker and a diuretic. The interaction of these three pharmacologic classes should be considered. ACE inhibitors have been associated with adverse outcomes in obstetric patients and are contraindicated.

ANGIOTENSIN II RECEPTOR ANTAGONISTS

Several new drugs have been introduced that block angiotensin II receptors (see Table 12-5 and Figure 12-2). These drugs interfere with binding of angiotensin II (AT_1) receptors and are effective for lowering blood pressure without the cough associated with the ACE inhibitors. ACE inhibitors, but not the angiotensin receptor blockers, prevent formation of angiotensin II, but angiotensin II is also formed by other enzymes. ACE inhibitors also prevent the breakdown of bradykinin and substance P, which accumulate and are thought to cause the troublesome cough response. This blockade, which the angiotensin II receptor antagonists do not produce, may also contribute to the cardiac and renal protective effects of the ACE inhibitors.[54]

CATECHOLAMINE-DEPLETING AGENTS

Catecholamine-depleting agents are rarely encountered in anesthesia practice, but the anesthetist should be familiar with their mechanism of action. The classic member of this group is reserpine. Reserpine blocks the uptake of catecholamines into storage vesicles within the presynaptic adrenergic neuron. This exposes the catecholamines to metabolism by monoamine oxidase in the axoplasm. This "catecholamine depletion" is responsible for reserpine's antihypertensive action.

TYROSINE HYDROXYLASE INHIBITORS

Metyrosine (Demser) is the only tyrosine hydroxylase inhibitor. Tyrosine hydroxylase is responsible for catalyzing the conversion of tyrosine to dopa and is considered the rate-limiting step in the synthesis of catecholamines. Inhibition of tyrosine hydroxylase results in a decrease in circulating catecholamine levels.

CATECHOL-*O*-Methyltransferase Inhibitors

Tolcapone (Tasmar) has recently been introduced for the treatment of Parkinson's disease as an adjunct to levodopa or carbidopa therapy. Tolcapone is a selective and reversible inhibitor of catechol-O-methyltransferase. It appears to enhance the action of levodopa and produces less fluctuation in drug response. There are concerns that this agent may interact with various cardiac drugs such as isoproterenol, dobutamine, and methyldopa. A reduction in the dose of these agents should be considered in patients receiving this drug.[55]

PHOSPHODIESTERASE III INHIBITORS

The phosphodiesterase III inhibitors, also known as *nonglycoside noncatecholamines*, include amrinone (Inocor)[56] and the newer, more potent, milrinone (Corotrope, Primacor).[57-59] They differ structurally and functionally from the catecholamines (see Table 12-3). They are generally used as alternatives or adjuncts to the standard inotropes.

The phosphodiesterase III inhibitors have several benefits over other inotropes currently in use. Their mechanism of action—the inhibition of phosphodiesterase III—allows for the buildup of intracellular cAMP and a subsequent increase in the uptake of intracellular calcium.[60] Because this result is directly achieved, adrenergic receptors are not used to achieve the inotropic effect. It follows that these drugs retain their inotropic effect even in the presence of β-blocking agents or the phenomenon of β-receptor down-regulation, situations frequently encountered in patients with heart failure. Phosphodiesterase III inhibitors also may be used, by virtue of their alternative pathway, to augment the effect of direct-acting β-agonists such as dobutamine or dopamine.[61]

These agents act as vasodilators because of the differential mechanism of cAMP in the smooth muscle versus its actions in the myocardium. In the smooth muscle cAMP causes an efflux of calcium, with a resultant relaxation of the muscle.[62] The clinical result is a decrease in both preload and afterload. Although this effect is desirable, caution must be exercised in treating the hypovolemic patient. This effect, along with the absence of an associated increase in heart rate, probably contributes to the absence of an increase in myocardial oxygen consumption seen in some patients with the use of these agents.[63]

IV amrinone has produced few notable side effects. Oral amrinone has been implicated in gastrointestinal disturbances; however, this effect is rarely seen with IV infusion. Amrinone-induced thrombocytopenia has achieved the greatest notoriety, but again the greater incidence occurs with administration of the oral form. Thrombocytopenia is usually dose related and reversible after discontinuation of the drug.[64]

Amrinone[65] and milrinone[66] both cause an increase in atrioventricular conduction when given within therapeutic dose ranges. The increase in cAMP also increases the automaticity of cardiac cells and can lead to calcium overload at high levels.[67] These effects can be arrhythmogenic. As previously noted, increases in heart rate are rare with the use of either amrinone or milrinone.

Amrinone and milrinone both have relatively long half-lives when compared with the catecholamines. They are metabolized by *N*-acetyltransferase. In the metabolism of amrinone, slow acetylators show a half-life of 4.4 hours, whereas fast acetylators demonstrate a half-life of 2.2 hours.[68] Elimination is via the kidney; therefore an extended half-life should be expected in patients with renal failure. The half-life of amrinone has also been shown to be prolonged in patients with CHF.[69] A loading dose of 0.75 mg/kg, followed by an infusion of 5 to 10 mcg/kg/min up to a daily maximum of 10 mg/kg, is recommended for amrinone.

Milrinone has demonstrated a 15-fold increase in inotropic potency compared with amrinone.[70,71] The current manufacturer's recommendation for the administration of milrinone is an IV loading dose of 50 mcg/kg, administered slowly over 10 minutes, followed by an infusion ranging from 0.375 to 0.75 mcg/kg/min, up to a total daily dose of 0.59 to 1.13 mg/kg.

CARDIAC GLYCOSIDES

Characterized by the digitalis preparations, the cardiac glycosides have been used to treat CHF for two centuries. The two most common preparations now employed are digoxin and digitoxin. The primary inotropic effect of digitalis is achieved by the binding to sodium-potassium adenosine triphosphatase in cardiac cells.[72,73] This allows the level of intracellular sodium to increase, which eventually results in an increase in the concentration of intracellular calcium. The increased intracellular calcium available to the sarcoplasmic reticulum is what causes the enhancement of myocardial contractility or inotropic effect. Electrophysiologically, enhancement of vagal tone, an indirect effect of digitalis, results in a slowing of the heart rate. This combination results in an increase in both diastolic filling and ejection fraction. Central venous pressure, ventricular end-diastolic volume, and pulmonary artery pressure are all reduced.[74] Because of its direct and indirect vagal effects, digitalis also is frequently used to control the ventricular response to atrial fibrillation and other atrial tachyarrhythmias. The digitalis-induced enhancement of vagal tone leads to a slowing of impulse conduction through the atrioventricular node and to a prolongation of the effective refractory period of the atrioventricular node.

Digitalis preparations have a narrow therapeutic index, great variability in action among patients, and several side effects. Hypokalemia greatly enhances the effects of digoxin, whereas hyperkalemia has the opposite effect.[75] A patient with hypokalemia whose digitalis level is within a therapeutic range may show toxic effects. All known arrhythmias have been attributed to digitalis preparations. Other signs and symptoms of digitalis toxicity include nausea, vomiting, diarrhea, headache, fatigue, and colored vision. Preoperatively the serum levels of potassium and digitalis must be closely monitored in patients receiving digitalis; additionally, electrocardiographic monitoring is required for the detection of arrhythmias.

CALCIUM

Calcium, through its interaction with actin and myosin, enhances myocardial contraction. Anesthetists usually use a bolus of calcium chloride (250 to 1000 mg) to improve cardiac output; calcium gluconate also is available. It is interesting to note that various studies have failed to show exogenous calcium to increase cardiac output significantly if the level of ionized calcium is normal or slightly depressed. However, exogenous calcium has been found to be beneficial if ionized calcium levels are significantly diminished (see Table 12-1 for doses).

GLUCAGON

Glucagon is an endogenous hormone produced by the α-cells of the pancreas and secreted in response to hypoglycemic states. It induces the release of catecholamines and has a direct inotropic effect. Exogenous glucagon can be administered as an inotrope in IV doses of 1 to 10 mg. Potential problems include tachycardia and hyperglycemia. In patients with inadequate glycogen stores, hypoglycemia may result from compensatory increases in serum insulin levels. Glucagon is not indicated for the maintenance of prolonged inotropy (see Table 12-1 for doses).

MANAGEMENT OF SPECIFIC DISEASES

In past decades the treatment of cardiovascular diseases under anesthesia was difficult and limited. The lack of specific cardiac drugs and the limited selection of anesthetic agents warranted symptomatic therapy designed to facilitate surgery until the patient was in the recovery room. Currently, with the vast

BOX 12-1

Clinical Predictors of Increased Perioperative Cardiovascular Risk (Myocardial Infarction, Heart Failure, Death)

Major Risk Factors

Unstable coronary syndromes
- Acute or recent myocardial infarction with evidence of important ischemic risk by clinical symptoms or noninvasive study*
- Unstable or severe angina (Canadian class III or IV)

Decompensated heart failure

Significant arrhythmias
- High-grade atrioventricular block
- Symptomatic ventricular arrhythmias in the presence of underlying heart disease
- Supraventricular arrhythmias with uncontrolled ventricular rate

Severe valvular disease

Intermediate Risk Factors

Mild angina pectoris (Canadian class I or II)

Previous myocardial infarction identified by history or pathologic Q waves

Compensated or previous heart failure

Diabetes mellitus (particularly insulin dependent)

Renal insufficiency

Minor Risk Factors

Advanced age

Abnormal ECG (left ventricular hypertrophy, left bundle-branch block, ST-T abnormalities)

Rhythm other than sinus (e.g., atrial fibrillation)

Low functional capacity (e.g., inability to climb one flight of stairs with a bag of groceries)

History of stroke

Uncontrolled systemic hypertension

ECG, *Electrocardiogram*

**The American College of Cardiology National Database Library defines recent myocardial infarction as having occurred more than 7 days previously, but less than or equal to 1 month (30 days); acute myocardial infarction is defined as having occurred within the last 7 days. May include "stable" angina inpatients who are unusually sedentary.*

From ACC/AHA Guideline Update for Perioperative Cardiovascular Evaluation for Noncardiac Surgery—Executive Summary: a Report of the American College of Cardiology/American Heart Association Task Force on Practice Guidelines (Committee to Update the 1996 Guidelines on Perioperative Cardiovascular Evaluation for Noncardiac Surgery). Circulation. *2002;105:10, 1257-1267.*

BOX 12-2

Cardiac Risk* Stratification for Noncardiac Surgical Procedures

High Risk (Reported Cardiac Risk Often Greater than 5%)
- Emergent major operations, particularly in the elderly
- Aortic and other major vascular surgery
- Peripheral vascular surgery
- Anticipated prolonged surgical procedures associated with large fluid shifts or blood loss

Intermediate Risk (Reported Cardiac Risk Generally Less than 5%)
- Carotid endarterectomy
- Head and neck surgery
- Intraperitoneal and intrathoracic surgery
- Orthopedic surgery
- Prostate surgery

Low Risk (Reported Cardiac Risk Generally Less than 1%)†
- Endoscopic procedures
- Superficial procedures
- Cataract surgery
- Breast surgery

**Combined incidence of cardiac death and nonfatal myocardial infarction.*

†These patients do not generally require further preoperative cardiac testing.

From ACC/AHA Guideline Update for Perioperative Cardiovascular Evaluation for Noncardiac Surgery—Executive Summary: a Report of the American College of Cardiology/American Heart Association Task Force on Practice Guidelines (Committee to Update the 1996 Guidelines on Perioperative Cardiovascular Evaluation for Noncardiac Surgery). Circulation. *2002;105:10, 1257-1267.*

array of cardiac drugs, the improved sophistication of anesthetic management, and monitoring that provides extensive hemodynamic information, the anesthetist is able to treat patients in a manner that is appropriate for management of their diseases. Therapies can be chosen that fit into a patient's plan of care. The anesthetic process can safely and effectively continue the care management of the individual patient. The American College of Cardiology and the American Heart Association have classified the cardiovascular and surgical risk to assist in predicting possible poor outcomes (Boxes 12-1 and 12-2).

The drugs listed for therapy of the cardiovascular disorders that follow are presented not so much for their specific intraoperative use but as a means of continuing the patient's current drug profile. Patient treatment mirrors general nonoperative indications and considerations. Anesthetic techniques take into account the combined effects of cardiac drugs and anesthetic agents when administered together.

Congestive Heart Failure

In the United States 4 to 5 million people have chronic CHF, with 400,000 to 700,000 new cases occurring each year. The incidences will undoubtedly increase as the population ages. Heart failure results in almost 1 million hospitalizations each year. It is the most common hospital discharge diagnosis in patients over age 65 years. More than 300,000 patients die as a direct or an indirect consequence of heart failure each year, a sixfold increase during the past 40 years. It is the only major cardiovascular disorder that is increasing in prevalence, with an estimated annual cost of 40 billion dollars. Once cardiac failure has been diagnosed, 5-year survival rates are typically 25% to 40%, similar to the survival rates for cancer.[76] The classification of heart failure is given in Box 12-3.

BOX 12-3

New York Heart Association Classification for Heart Failure

Class I
No limitation: ordinary physical exercise does not cause fatigue, dyspnea, or palpitations

Class II
Slight limitation of physical activity: comfortable at rest, but ordinary activity results in fatigue, palpitations, or dyspnea

Class III
Marked limitation of physical activity: comfortable at rest but less than ordinary activity results in symptoms

Class IV
Unable to carry out any physical activity without discomfort: symptoms of heart failure are present even at rest, with increased discomfort on any level of physical activity

CHF represents a significant risk factor for general anesthesia. Mortality estimates range from 3% to as high as 30% in patients undergoing abdominal surgery.[77] In patients with CHF and renal failure undergoing emergency surgery, mortality rates as high as 76% have been reported.

CHF is a complex syndrome resulting from a cardiac malfunction that impairs the ability of the heart's left ventricle to eject blood and meet the circulatory demands of the body. Until recently CHF was considered a disease of the hemodynamics of the cardiovascular system. This led to the view that goals for treatment should be to increase the pumping force of the heart with positive inotropes and unload the peripheral circulation with vasodilators and diuretics. It is now believed that the principal alteration in CHF is a change in the structure of the left ventricle called *left ventricular remodeling* and the resulting hormonal and physiologic consequences.[78] The chamber dilates, hypertrophies, and becomes more spherical. Substantial evidence suggests that activation of the body's endogenous neurohormonal systems, such as the renin-angiotensin system, plays an important role in cardiac remodeling and the progression of heart failure. Treatment is complex and tailored to the patient's age, current disease state, and associated concurrent disorders. It may involve a polypharmaceutical approach that includes digoxin,[79] diuretics, ACE inhibitors,[80-84] β-blockers,[85-87] and spironolactone.[88] Neutral endopeptidase (NEP) inhibitors block the metabolism of atrial natriuretic factor and are being tried as adjuncts to other agents for heart failure. Candoxatril and ecadotril are two new NEP inhibitors.[89] Recommendations for the management of CHF are given in Box 12-4.

In the perioperative period, anesthesia providers are faced with managing therapy for all degrees of severity of acute CHF. The goal can range from prevention of symptom

BOX 12-4

Recommendations for the Management of Congestive Heart Failure

Prevention of Heart Failure
- Control of coronary risk factors, including hypertension, hyperlipidemia, and smoking
- In patients with a recent myocardial infarction (MI), reperfusion and neurohormonal antagonism with an angiotensin converting enzyme (ACE) inhibitor and a β-blocker can reduce myocardial injury and the risk of subsequent events.
- In patients with asymptomatic left ventricular dysfunction, an ACE inhibitor and a β-blocker can produce complementary benefits

General Measures
- Maintenance of fluid balance by salt restriction and daily monitoring of body weight.
- Improved conditioning with encouragement of moderate exercise and avoidance of excessive bed rest.
- Control of atrial fibrillation and anticoagulation in high-risk patients and revascularization in selected patients.
- Avoidance of antiarrhythmic drugs, nonsteroidal antiinflammatory drugs, and most calcium channel blockers.

Diuretics
- Diuretics should be prescribed for all patients with symptoms of heart failure who have a predisposition to fluid retention. These drugs should not be used alone, even if they are effective in controlling symptoms.
- The goal of diuretic therapy is to eliminate symptoms as well as physical signs of fluid retention, such as jugular venous distention and edema.
- Measurement of body weight is the best way of monitoring when to initiate or titrate a diuretic regimen.
- Diuretics may alter the efficacy of ACE inhibitors and β-blockers.

ACE Inhibitors
- All patients—not some or most, but *all patients*—with heart failure resulting from left ventricular systolic dysfunction should receive an ACE inhibitor, unless they are intolerant of the drug or have a contraindication to its use. Treatment should not be delayed until symptoms are severe or resistant to other drugs.
- Alleviation of symptoms may be delayed, and disease progression may be modified, even if no symptomatic improvement occurs.
- Early side effects must not prevent long-term use.

β-Blockers
- All patients with stable New York Heart Association (NYHA) class II or III heart failure resulting from left ventricular systolic dysfunction should receive a β-blocker unless they are intolerant of the drug or have a contraindication to its use. Treatment should not be delayed until symptoms are severe or resistant to therapy.
- Alleviation of symptoms may be delayed and disease progression may be modified, even if no symptomatic improvement occurs.
- Early side effects must not prevent long-term use.

Continued

BOX 12-4

Recommendations for the Management of Congestive Heart Failure—cont'd

Digitalis
- Digitalis is recommended to improve symptoms of patients with heart failure resulting from left ventricular systolic dysfunction and should be used together with diuretics, ACE inhibitors, and β-blockers.
- Controversy exists about the proper dosing of digitalis, and it is unclear whether serum digoxin levels should be used to guide therapy.
- Digoxin is well tolerated, but there is some concern that the drug may be deleterious at levels within the therapeutic range.

Hydralazine-Nitrate Combinations
- Hydralazine-nitrate combinations should not be used in patients with no prior use of ACE inhibitors and should not be substituted for ACE inhibitors in patients who are tolerating ACE inhibitors without difficulty.
- Such combinations should be considered in patients who cannot tolerate ACE inhibitors because of hypotension or azotemia.
- Little evidence exists to support the use of nitrates alone or hydralazine alone in the treatment of heart failure.

Angiotensin and Aldosterone Antagonists
- Angiotensin receptor blockers should not be considered to be equivalent or superior to ACE inhibitors in the treatment of heart failure.
- Angiotensin receptor blockers should be used in patients with no prior use of ACE inhibitors and should not be substituted for ACE inhibitors in patients who are tolerating ACE inhibitors.
- These agents should be considered only in those patients who are unable to tolerate ACE inhibitors because of cough or angioedema.

Calcium Antagonists
- Calcium antagonists should not be used for the treatment of heart failure.
- Most calcium antagonists should be avoided in heart failure, even when used for the treatment of angina or hypertension. There is persuasive evidence, however, that amlodipine does not adversely affect survival.
- Until further data are available, amlodipine should not be used to prolong survival in patients with a nonischemic cardiomyopathy.

Antiarrhythmic Drugs
- Class I antiarrhythmic agents should not be used, except for immediately life-threatening ventricular arrhythmias.
- Some class III agents, such as amiodarone, do not appear to increase the risk of death and are preferred over class I agents.
- Amiodarone is not recommended with ACE inhibitors and β-blockers.
- Electrolyte deficiencies may cause arrhythmias and alter the efficacy and safety of antiarrhythmic drugs.

Inotropic Infusions
- Use of intermittent infusions of positive inotropic agents at home, in the physician's office, or in a short-stay unit cannot be recommended, even in patients with advanced heart failure.
- Continuous outpatient infusions may be considered, in order to improve the quality of life in the rare patient who cannot be weaned from inotropic therapy and in whom some relief of symptoms is worth the likelihood of an increased risk of death.

From Consensus recommendations for the management of chronic heart failure. On behalf of the membership of the advisory council to improve outcomes nationwide in heart failure. Am J Cardiol. *1999;83:1A-38A.*

progression to surviving the operation in life-threatening cases. Drugs, such as the inotropes, phosphodiesterase inhibitors, diuretics, and vasodilators, are commonly used. Some useful drugs for the treatment of heart failure during anesthesia are listed in Table 12-3.

Arrhythmias

The incidence of serious arrhythmias requiring intervention during general anesthesia is relatively low. A large multicenter study found that not counting simple tachycardia, bradycardia, or clinically minor rhythm disturbances, the frequency of serious arrhythmias was 1.6% in a series of more than 17,000 patients who underwent general anesthesia.[90] It is surprising that the incidence is not higher, because several contradictory factors are involved; most drugs given during anesthesia are cardiac depressants, therefore they tend to be antiarrhythmic. However, patients with multiple drug profiles in combination with the anesthetics may experience drug interactions that lead to rhythm disturbances. Add to these pharmacologic factors the stress of surgery and anesthesia, and a multitude of effects on cardiac rhythms may be expected.

In recent years new pharmacologic and nonpharmacologic management approaches for cardiac arrhythmias have emerged. New drugs, implantable cardiac devices, and ablation therapy are available for management of these disorders. The use of antiarrhythmic drugs in the United States is declining because of major trials indicating an increasing mortality rate with clinical use, proarrhythmic side effects, and the use of nondrug therapies. Some causes of intraoperative rhythm disturbances are listed in Box 12-5.

The goal of drug therapy for arrhythmias during anesthesia should be to treat immediate hemodynamic problems and to prevent progression of serious arrhythmias. Treatment is similar to that in the nonoperative setting, with the caveat that most therapies should be carefully titrated to avoid unexpected proarrhythmic or excessive hypotensive outcomes. Three cautionary statements should precede any discussion on the use of antiarrhythmic agents during anesthesia.[91]

BOX 12-5

Causes of Intraoperative Rhythm Disturbances

Structural Heart Disease
- Chronic coronary artery disease (infarction)
- Valvular and congenital heart disease
- Cardiomyopathies of diverse origins
- Sick sinus or long QT interval syndrome
- Wolff-Parkinson-White syndrome
- Hypertrophic, dilated, infiltrative, secondary to systemic disease (e.g., uremia, diabetes)

Transient Imbalance
- Stress: electrolyte or metabolic imbalance
- Laryngoscopy, hypoxia, hypercarbia
- Device malfunction, microshock
- Diagnostic or therapeutic intervention (pacemakers, cardioveter-defibrillators)
- Surgical stimulation
- Central vascular catheters

Adapted from Atlee JL. Perioperative dysrhythmias: diagnosis and management. Anesthesiology. *1997;86:1397-1424.*

TABLE 12-7 **Classification of Antiarrhythmic Drugs**

Class	Electrophysiologic Effect	Drug
I	Depression of phase 0 depolarization (block sodium channels)	
IA	Moderate depression and prolonged repolarization	Quinidine, procainamide, disopyramide
IB	Weak depression and shortened repolarization	Lidocaine, mexiletine, phenytoin, tocainide
IC	Strong depression with little effect on repolarization	Flecainide, propafenone, moricizine
II	β-Adrenergic blocking effects	Esmolol, propranolol, metoprolol, timolol, pindolol, atenolol, acebutolol, nadolol, carvedilol
III	Prolongs repolarization (blocks potassium channels)	Amiodarone, bretylium, sotalol, ibutilide, dofetilide
IV	Calcium channel blocking effects	Verapamil, diltiazem
Other		Adenosine, adenosine triphosphate, digoxin, atropine

- The cause of the arrhythmia should be explored before any treatment is instituted.
- Adequacy of ventilation, depth of anesthesia, acid-base balance, and fluid and electrolyte balance must be verified before appropriate therapy can be formulated.
- Multiple drug administration, which constitutes modern anesthesia practice, may result in unexpected drug interactions. Analysis of complex arrhythmias with the commonly used three- or five-lead electrocardiograph system during a surgical procedure is less than ideal for proper diagnosis and treatment. Nonetheless, rhythm disturbances that compromise hemodynamic stability or that may progress to more severe dysfunction must be addressed.

Classification of antiarrhythmic drugs is given in Table 12-7. The drugs of choice for the common arrhythmias are given in Table 12-6, and the dosage of the antiarrhythmic drugs are given in Table 12-8.

Hypertension

Hypertension is a major health problem in the United States; an estimated 50 million Americans have hypertension or should be monitored for elevated blood pressure.[92] The classification of hypertension has been recently revised and is given in Table 12-9. The optimal blood pressure is believed to be less than 120 systolic and less than 90 diastolic.[93,94] A new category, prehypertension, is included, and hypertension is classified as either stage 1 or 2. A number of drugs are available for the treatment of high blood pressure, including diuretics, β-blockers, calcium channel blockers, ACE inhibitors, and angiotensin receptor antagonists. Recommendations are that diuretics and β-blockers be first-line therapies in addition to combinations of other agents as warranted by patient characteristics and the concurrent presence of various target organ disease states. Drugs available for the treatment of hypertension are listed in Table 12-5. Antihypertensive drugs that are safe for use during pregnancy are listed in Table 12-10.

Manipulation of the patient's blood pressure is an ongoing task during anesthesia. Many drugs are available to increase and decrease blood pressure when indicated. Improved monitoring and sophistication of anesthetic techniques has made control of blood pressure almost routine.

The problem of hypertension has varying significance in preoperative, intraoperative, and postoperative situations. Some controversy has existed and still exists regarding the proper preoperative handling of patients with severe stage 2 hypertension. For a number of years some practitioners thought it was better to postpone an operation to stabilize the patient's blood pressure, whereas others believed acute treatment was sufficient. Several studies have been done with somewhat conflicting results.[95,96] At present what can be concluded is that blood pressure lability in the perioperative period is associated with postoperative morbidity.[97] Mild hypertension probably represents only a minor risk for anesthesia and surgery. Patients with more severe hypertensive episodes are at greater risk and will benefit from acute therapy combined with postoperative long-term follow-up. Hypertensive episodes during the perioperative period occur most often during emergence from anesthesia and may be associated with pain, airway stimulation, hypoxia-hypercarbia, hypothermia and shivering, bladder distention, withdrawal from preoperative medications, and intraoperative use of vasopressors. Drugs useful for the treatment of perioperative hypertension

TABLE 12-8 Doses and Therapeutic Concentrations for Antiarrhythmic Agents

Drug	USUAL DOSAGE RANGES				Time to Peak Plasma Concentration (Oral) (hr)	Effective Serum or Plasma Concentration (mcg/ml)	Elimination Half-Life (hr)	Bioavailability (%)	Major Route of Elimination
	Intravenous		Oral						
	Loading	Maintenance	Loading	Maintenance					
Quinidine	6-10 mg/kg at 0.3-0.5 mg/kg/min	—	800-1000 mg	300-600 mg q 6 hr	1.5-3.0	3-6	5-9	60-80	Liver
Procainamide	6-13 mg/kg at 0.2-0.5 mg/kg/min	2-6 mg/min	500-1000 mg	250-1000 mg q 4-6 hr	1	4-10	3-5	70-85	Kidneys
Disopyramide	1-2 mg/kg over 15-45 min*	1 mg/kg/hr		100-300 mg q 6-8 hr	1-2	2-5	8-9	80-90	Kidneys
Lidocaine	1-3 mg/kg at 20-50 mg/min	1-4 mg/min	N/A	N/A	N/A	1-5	1-2	N/A	Liver
Mexiletine	500 mg*	0.5-1.0 gm/24 hr	400-600 mg	150-300 mg q 8-12 hr	2-4	0.75-2.7	10-17	90	Liver
Phenytoin	100 mg q 5 min for ≤1000 mg		1000 mg	100-400 mg q 12-24 hr	8-12	10-20	18-36	50-70	Liver
Flecainide	2 mg/kg*	100-200 mg q 12 hr		50-200 mg q 12 hr	3-4	0.2-1.0	20	95	Liver
Propafenone	1-2 mg/kg		600-900 mg	150-300 mg q 8-12 hr	1-3	0.2-3.0	5-8	25-75	Liver
Moricizine	N/A	N/A	300 mg	100-400 mg q 8 hr	1-3	0.1	2	40	Liver
Propranolol	0.25-0.5 mg q 5 min to ≤0.20 mg/kg			10-200 mg q 6-8 hr	4	1-2.5	3-6	35-65	Liver
Amiodarone	15 mg/kg for 10 min, 1 mg/kg for 3 hr, 0.5 mg/kg thereafter	1 mg/min	800-1600 mg q.d. for 7-14 days	200-600 mg q.d.		0.5-1.5	56 days	25	Kidneys
Bretylium	5-10 mg/kg at 1-2 mg/kg/min	0.5-2 mg/min	N/A	4 mg/kg/day	2-4	0.04-0.90	8-14	20-50	Liver
Sotalol	10 mg over 1-2 min			80-320 mg q 12 hr	2.5-4	2.5	12	90-100	Kidneys
Ibutilide	1 mg over 10 min	N/A	N/A	N/A	N/A	N/A	6		Kidneys
Dofetilide	2-5 mcg/kg infusion	N/A	N/A	0.1-0.5 mg q 12 hr			7-13	90	Kidneys
Azimilide	N/A	N/A	N/A	100-200 mg q.d.		200-1000		90-100	Kidneys
Verapamil	5-10 mg over 1-2 min	0.005 mg/kg/min		80-120 mg q 6-8 hr	1-2	0.10-0.15	3-8	10-35	Liver
Adenosine	6-18 mg (rapidly)	N/A	N/A	N/A	N/A				
Digoxin	0.5-1.0 mg	0.125-0.25 mg q.d.	0.5-1.0 mg	0.125-0.25 mg q.d.	2-6	0.0008-0.002	36-48	60-80	Kidneys

**Intravenous use investigational.*

N/A = not applicable.

Results presented may vary according to doses, disease state, and intravenous or oral administration. From Braunwald E, Zipes DP, Libby P. Heart disease. *Vol 1. 6th ed. Philadelphia: Saunders; 2001; 712.*

TABLE 12-9 Classification and Management of Blood Pressure for Adults

Blood Pressure Classification	Systolic Blood Pressure (mm Hg)	Diastolic Blood Pressure (mm Hg)
Normal	<120	and <80
Prehypertension	120-139	or 80-89
Stage 1 hypertension	140-159	or 90-99
Stage 2 hypertension	≤160	or ≤100

From Joint National Committee on Prevention, Detection and Treatment of High Blood Pressure: Seventh Report of the National Committee on Detection, Evaluation and Treatment of High Blood Pressure (JNC-7), U.S. Department of Health and Human Services. National Institute of Health. National Heart, Lung and Blood Institute. National High Blood Pressure Education Program; May 2003. NIH publication number 03-5233.

are listed in Table 12-11. Figure 12-3 summarizes the mechanism of arterial blood pressure regulation and the sites of action of antihypertensive drugs.

Coronary Artery Disease

Coronary heart disease (CHD) is the most common cardiac disease encountered in the operating room. Approximately 12 million people in the United States have CHD. It is estimated that up to 208 deaths per 100,000 population result from significant coronary disease. The CHD death rate peaked in the mid 1960s and has declined in the general population over the past 35 years. This decline began in females in the 1950s and in males in the 1960s.[98]

High blood cholesterol is a major risk factor for CHD that can be modified. More than 50 million U.S. adults have blood cholesterol levels that require medical advice and treatment. More than 90 million adults have cholesterol levels that are higher than desirable. Experts recommend that all adults aged 20 years and older have their cholesterol levels checked at least once every 5 years to help them take action to prevent or lower their risk of CHD.[98]

The causes of coronary artery disease and management of patients with the disorder are discussed in detail in Chapters 21 and 22. The classification of angina pectoris is given in Table 12-12.

TABLE 12-10 Antihypertensive Drugs Used in Pregnancy*

Suggested Drug	Comments
Central α-agonists	Methyldopa is the drug of choice
β-Blockers	Atenolol, metoprolol, and labetalol
Diuretics	Diuretics are recommended for chronic hypertension, if prescribed before gestation or if patients appear to be salt sensitive; they are not recommended in patients with preeclampsia
Direct vasodilators	Hydralazine is the parenteral drug of choice based on its long history of safety and efficiency

**ACE inhibitors and angiotensin II receptor blockers should not be used. Fetal abnormalities and death have been reported.*
From Joint National Committee on Prevention, Detection and Treatment of High Blood Pressure: Seventh Report of the National Committee on Detection, Evaluation and Treatment of High Blood Pressure (JNC-7), U.S. Department of Health and Human Services. National Institute of Health. National Heart, Lung and Blood Institute. National High Blood Pressure Education Program. May 2003; NIH publication number 03-5233.

TABLE 12-11 Parenteral Drugs for Treatment of Severe Hypertension

Drug	Class	Route and Dose	Onset	Duration	Comments
Enalaprilat (Vasotec IV)	Angiotensin converting enzyme inhibitor	IV: 1.25-5 mg q6h	15 min	6-12 hr	Variable, sometimes excessive response
Fenoldopam (Corlopam)	Dopamine-1 receptor agonist	IV infusion pump: 0.1-1.6 mcg/kg/min	4-5 min	<10 min	May cause reflex tachycardia; may increase intraocular pressure
Labetalol (Trandate Normodyne)	α- and β-adrenergic blocker	IV: 20 mg initially, then 40-80 mg q10min (300 mg max)	5 min or less	3-6 hr	Not for patients with bronchospasm, congestive heart failure, first-degree heart block, cardiogenic shock, or severe bradycardia
Nicardipine (Cardene IV)	Calcium channel blocker	IV: 5 mg/hr, increased by 2.5 mg/hr q15min up to15 mg/hr	1-5 min	3-6 hr	May cause reflex tachycardia
Nitroglycerin (Nitro-Bid IV)	Venous arteriolar vasodilator	IV infusion pump: 5-100 mcg/min	2-5 min	5-10 min	Headache, tachycardia can occur; tolerance may develop with prolonged use
Sodium nitroprusside	Arteriolar and venous vasodilator	IV infusion pump: 0.3-10 mcg/kg/min	Seconds	3-5 min	Thiocyanate or cyanide toxicity with prolonged or too rapid infusion
Esmolol	β-blocker	IV: 500 mcg/kg/min for 1 min Titration to effect Usually 50 mcg/kg/min	1-2 min	5-10 min	Cardioselective; however, use with caution in patients with asthma

Medical Letter Treatment Guidelines. Cardiovascular drugs in the ICU. Med Lett. *2002;4:19-24.*

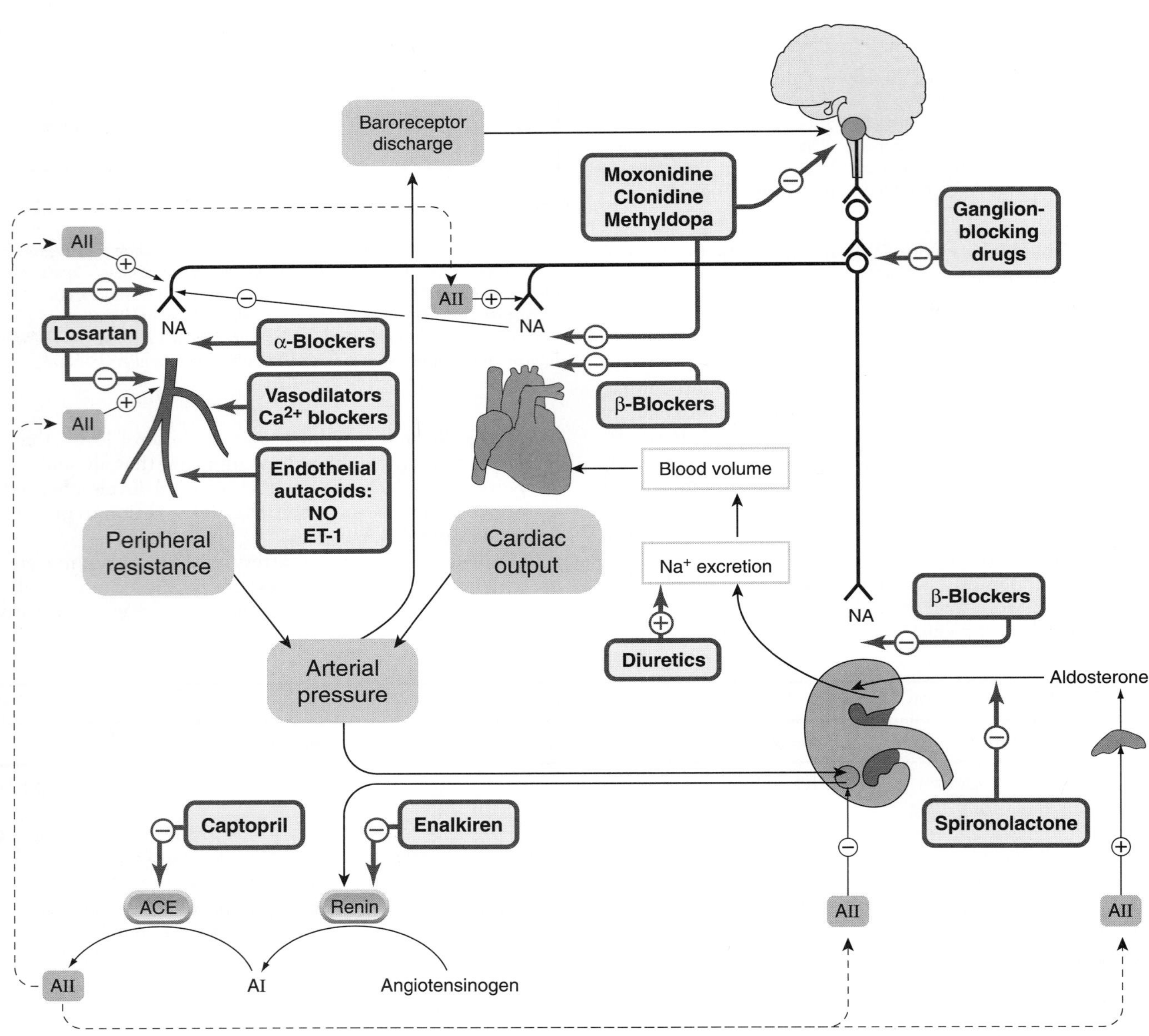

FIGURE **12-3**
Diagram showing the main mechanisms involved in arterial blood pressure regulation *(black lines)* and the sites of action of antihypertensive drugs *(boxes)*. (*ACE*, Angiotensin-converting enzyme; *AI*, angiotensin I; *AII*, angiotensin II; *NA*, noradrenaline; *NO*, nitric oxide; *ET-1*, endothelin-1). (From Rang HP, Dale MM, Ritter JM, et al. *Pharmacology*. 5th ed. Edinburgh: Churchill-Livingstone; 2003:299.)

TABLE 12-12 Classification of Angina Pectoris

Class	Canadian Cardiovascular Society Classification
I	Angina does not occur with ordinary physical activity (walking, climbing stairs) but may occur with strenuous, rapid, or prolonged exertion (work, recreation).
II	Slight limitation of ordinary activity. Angina may occur with walking or climbing stairs, after meals, in the cold, in the wind, or under emotional stress, walking uphill, walking more than two blocks on the level, and climbing one flight of stairs at a normal pace under normal conditions.
III	Marked limitation of ordinary physical activity. Angina may occur after walking one or two blocks on the level or climbing one flight of stairs in normal conditions at a normal pace.
IV	Inability to carry on any physical activity without discomfort. Angina may be present at rest.

From Campeau L. Grading of angina. Circulation. *1976;54:522-523.*

Pharmacotherapy includes nitrates, β-blockers, calcium channel blockers, aspirin, and "statin" drugs. Recent evidence suggests that ACE inhibitors may also provide a reduction in mortality and infarction rates. The β-blockers and calcium channel blockers are listed in Table 12-5. The nitrates and the HMG-CoA reductase inhibitors ("statins") are listed in Tables 12-4 and 12-13, respectively.

TABLE 12-13 HMG-CoA Reductase Inhibitors ("Statins")

Drug	Initial Dosage	Maximum Dosage	Comments
Atorvastatin (Lipitor)	10 mg once	80 mg once	Statins are generally tolerated better than other lipid-lowering drugs. Mild transient gastrointestinal disturbances, muscle pain, rash, and headache have occurred. Some patients have reported sleep disturbances. An increase in liver enzymes and creatine phosphokinase may occur with significant myalgia and muscle weakness.
Fluvastatin (Lescil)	20 mg once	40 mg bid	
Lovastatin (Mevacor)	20 mg once	80 mg once	
Pravastatin (Pravachol)	20 mg once	40 mg once	
Rosuvastatin (Crestor)	10 mg once	40 mg once	
Simvastatin (Zocor)			

Adapted from Med Lett. *1998;40:117-122; and Mosby's Drug Consult. St Louis: Mosby; 2004. With permission.*

PREOPERATIVE ADMINISTRATION OF CARDIAC DRUGS

Continuation of the patient's cardiac medications throughout the perioperative period is now considered routine practice. It is better to have the patient's disease state under proper control than to discontinue any medications before surgery and risk having the patient in unstable condition. Withdrawal after abrupt discontinuation of β-blockers and clonidine is especially severe. Some concern exists that the ACE inhibitors may precipitate significant hypotension during induction and that they should be withheld the morning of surgery.[99] Careful titration of induction agents and safe anesthesia has been performed in patients receiving these medications.

REFERENCES

1. Hoffman BB. Catecholamines, sympathomimetic drugs and adrenergic receptor antagonists. In: Hardman JG, Limbird LE, eds. *Goodman and Gilman's the pharmacological basis of therapeutics*. 10th ed. New York: McGraw-Hill; 2001:215-268.
2. Nitenberg A, Antony I. Coronary vascular reserve in humans: a critical review of methods of evaluation and of interpretation of the results. *Eur Heart J*. 1995;16:7-21.
3. Vergroesen I, Kal JE, van Wezel HB. Coronary vasodilating drug effects on normal coronary blood flow regulation? *J Cardiothorac Vasc Anesth*. 1998;450-456.
4. Mersmann HJ. Species variation in mechanisms for modulation of growth by beta-adrenergic receptors. *J Nutr*. 1995;125: 1777S-1782S.
5. Moss J, Renz CL. The autonomic nervous system. In: Miller RD, ed. *Anesthesia*. 5th ed. New York: Churchill Livingstone; 2000: 523-577.
6. Doggrell SA. The therapeutic potential of dopamine modulators on the cardiovascular and renal systems. *Exp Opin Investig Drugs*. 2002;11:631-644.
7. Mannelli M, Ianni L, Lazzeri C, et al. In vivo evidence that endogenous dopamine modulates sympathetic activity in man. *Hypertension*. 1999;34:398-402.
8. Zaritsky AL. Catecholamines, inotropic medications and vasopressor agents. In: Chernow B, Brater DC, Holaday, et al, eds. *The Pharmacological Approach to the Critically Ill Patient*. Baltimore: Williams & Wilkins; 1994.
9. Matsuda N, Hattori Y, Akaishi Y, et al. Impairment of cardiac beta-adrenoceptor cellular signaling by decreased expression of G (s alpha) is septic rabbits. *Anesthesiology*. 2000;93:1465-1473.
10. De Backer D, Creteur J, Silva E et al, Vincent JL. Effects of dopamine, norepinephrine, and epinephrine on the splanchnic circulation in septic shock: which is best? *Crit Care Med*. 2003;31:1659-1667.
11. Chatterjee K, De Marco T. Role of nonglycosidic inotropic agents: indications, ethics, and limitations. *Med Clin North Am*. 2003;87:391-418.
12. Rudis MI, Dasta JF. Vasopressors and inotropes in shock. In: Dipiro JT, et al, eds. *Pharmacotherapy: a pathophysiologic approach*. 5th ed. New York: McGraw-Hill; 2001:435-453.
13. Wang CH, Cherng WJ, Hung MJ. Dobutamine-induced hypotension is an independent predictor for mortality in patients with left ventricular dysfunction following myocardial infarction. *Int J Cardiol*. 1999;68:297-302.
14. Evers AS, Crowder CM. General anesthetics. In: Hardman JG, et al, eds. *Goodman and Gilman's the pharmacological basis of therapeutics*. 10th ed. New York: McGraw-Hill; 2001:337-366.
15. Ducros L, Bonnin P, Cholley BP, et al. Increasing maternal blood pressure with ephedrine increases uterine artery blood flow velocity during uterine contraction. *Anesthesiology*. 2002; 96:612-616.

16. Stoelting RK. Sympathomimetics. In: *Pharmacology and Physiology in Anesthetic Practice*. 3rd ed. New York: Lippincott; 1999:259-277.
17. Bartow RA, Brogden RN. Formoterol. An update of its pharmacological properties and therapeutic efficacy in the management of asthma. *Drugs*. 1998;55:303-322.
18. Kumar VH, Christian C, Kresch MJ. Effects of salmeterol on secretion of phosphatidylcholine by alveolar type II cells. *Life Sci.* 2000;66:1639-1646.
19. Kemp JP, et al. A 1-year study of salmeterol powder on pulmonary function and hyperresponsiveness to methacholine. *J Allergy Clin Immunol.* 1999;104:1189-1197.
20. Cheung D, et al. Long-term effects of a long-acting beta$_2$-adrenoreceptor agonist, salmeterol, on airway hyperresponsiveness in patients with mild asthma. *N Engl J Med.* 1992;327:1198-1203.
21. Gal P, Shaffer CL. Acute respiratory distress syndrome. In: Dipiro JT, et al, eds. *Pharmacotherapy: A Pathophysiologic Approach*. 5th ed. New York: McGraw-Hill; 2002:531-548.
22. Larmon JE, Ross BS, May WL, et al. Oral nicardipine superior to magnesium sulfate as a tocolytic. *Am J Obstet Gynecol.* 1999;181: 1432-1437.
23. *Mosby's Drug Consult* [CD-ROM]. St Louis: Mosby; 2004.
24. Kao LW, et al. Droperidol, QT prolongation, and sudden death: what is the evidence? *Ann Emerg Med.* 2003;41:546-558.
25. Arrhythmias from droperidol? *Med Lett.* 2002;44:53-54.
26. Sarkozy A, Dorian P. Advances in the acute pharmacologic management of cardiac arrhythmias. *Curr Cardiol Rep.* 2003;5:387-394.
27. Auerbach AD, Goldman L. Beta-blockers and reduction of cardiac events in noncardiac surgery: clinical applications. *JAMA.* 2002;287:1445-1447.
28. Miller JM, Zipes DG. Management of the patient with cardiac arrhythmias. In: Braunwald E, ed. *Heart Disease: A Textbook of Cardiovascular Medicine*. 6th ed. Philadelphia: Saunders; 2001: 700-766.
29. Poldermans D. Bisoprolol reduces risk of cardiac death in high-risk vascular surgery patients. *N Engl J Med.* 1999;341:1789-1794, 1838-1840.
30. Henderson NL, Mason RC. Juxtaglomerular cell tumor in pregnancy. *Obstet Gynecol.* 2001;98(pt 2):943-945.
31. Jouppilla P, Kirkinen P, Koivula A. Labetalol does not alter the placental and fetal blood flow or maternal prostanoids in preeclampsia. *Br J Obstet Gynaecol.* 1986;93:543-547.
32. Ali-Melkkila T, Kanto J, Iisalo E. Pharmacokinetics and related pharmacodynamics of anticholinergic drugs. *Acta Anaesthesiol Scand.* 1993;37:633-642.
33. Collard CL. Hypertension. Medication update. *South Med J.* 2001;94:1065-1070.
34. Patterson KW, Deb B, Kavanagh BP, et al. Inhaled nitric oxide potentiates actions of adenosine but not of sodium nitroprusside in experimental pulmonary hypertension. *Pharmacology*. 1999; 58:246-251.
35. Hatsuoka S, Sakamoto T, Stock UA, et al. Effect of L-arginine or nitroglycerine during deep hypothermic circulatory arrest in neonatal lambs. *Ann Thorac Surg.* 2003;75:197-203.
36. Kojda G, et al. Nitric oxide inhibits vascular bioactivation of glyceryl trinitrate: a novel mechanism to explain preferential venodilation of organic nitrates. *Mol Pharmacol.* 1998;53:547-554.
37. Hlatky R, Goodman JC, Valadka AB, et al. Role of nitric oxide in cerebral blood flow abnormalities after traumatic brain injury. *J Cereb Blood Flow Metab.* 2003;23:582-588.
38. Bauer JA, Nolan T, Fung HL. Vascular and hemodynamic differences between organic nitrates and nitrites. *J Pharmacol Exp Ther.* 1997;280:326-331.
39. Oates JA, Brown NJ. Antihypertensive agents and the drug therapy of hypertension. In: Hardman JG, et al, eds. *Goodman and Gilman's the pharmacological basis of therapeutics*. 10th ed. New York: McGraw-Hill; 2001:871-900.
40. Bang L, et al. Hydralazine-induced vasodilation involves opening of high conductance Ca^2-activated K^+ channels. *Eur J Pharmacol.* 1998;361:43-49.
41. Powers DR, Papadakos PJ, Wallin JD. Parenteral hydralazine revisited. *J Emerg Med.* 1998;16:191-196.
42. Pepine CJ, Handberg-Thurmond E, Marks RG, et al. Rationale and design of the International Verapamil SR/Trandolapril Study (INVEST): an Internet-based randomized trial in coronary artery disease patients with hypertension. *J Am Coll Cardiol.* 1998; 32:1228-1237.
43. Selman WR. Nimodipine in subarachnoid hemorrhage. *J Neurosurg.* 1999;91:520-521.
44. Epstein M. Role of a third generation calcium antagonist in the management of hypertension. *Drugs*. 1999;5:1-10.
45. Nishiyama T, Matsukawa T, Hanaoka K. Interactions between nicardipine and enflurane, isoflurane and sevoflurane. *Can J Anaesth.* 1997;44:1071-1076.
46. Cheung AT, et al. Nicardipine intravenous bolus dosing for acutely decreasing arterial blood pressure during general anesthesia for cardiac operations: pharmacokinetics, pharmacodynamics, and associated effects on left ventricular function. *Anesth Analg.* 1999;89:1116-1123.
47. Nolte CW, Jost S, Mügge A, et al. Protection from digoxin-induced coronary vasoconstriction in patients with coronary artery disease by calcium antagonists. *Am J Cardiol.* 1999;8: 440-442, A9.
48. Saitoh Y, Narumi Y, Fujii Y. Post-tetanic count and train-of-four response during neuromuscular block produced by vecuronium and infusion of nicardipine. *Br J Anaesth.* 1999;83:340-342.
49. Salhanick SD, Shannon MW. Management of calcium channel antagonist overdose. *Drug Saf.* 2003;26:65-79.
50. Nguyen T, El Salibi E, Rouleau JL. Postinfarction survival and inducibility of ventricular arrhythmias in the spontaneously hypertensive rat: effects of ramipril and hydralazine. *Circulation.* 1998;98:2074-2080.
51. Jackson EK. Renin and angiotensin. In: Hardman JG, et al, eds. *Goodman and Gilman's the pharmacological basis of therapeutics.* 10th ed. New York: McGraw-Hill; 2001:809-842.
52. Kaplan N. Treatment of hypertension: drug therapy. In: Kaplan N, ed. *Clinical Hypertension*. 5th ed. Baltimore: Williams & Wilkins; 1990:182.
53. Brown NJ, Vaughan DE. Angiotensin-converting enzyme inhibitors. *Circulation.* 1998;97:1411-1420.
54. Shusterman, N. Risk-benefit assessment of angiotensin II receptor antagonists. *Exp Opin Drug Saf.* 2002;1:137-152.
55. Tolcapone. In: *Mosby's Drug Consult.* St Louis: Mosby; 2004.
56. Rathmell JP, et al. A multicenter, randomized, blind comparison of amrinone with milrinone after elective cardiac surgery. *Anesth Analg.* 1998;86:683-690.
57. Kikura M, et al. The effect of milrinone on hemodynamics and left ventricular function after emergence from cardiopulmonary bypass. *Anesth Analg.* 1997;85:16-22.
58. Mehra MR, et al. Safety and clinical utility of long-term intravenous milrinone in advanced heart failure. *Am J Cardiol.* 1997;80:61-64.
59. Leier CV, Binkley PF. Parenteral inotropic support for advanced congestive heart failure. *Prog Cardiovasc Dis.* 1998;41:207-224.
60. Van der Zypp A, Rechtman M, Majewski H. The role of cyclic nucleotides and calcium in the relaxation produced by amrinone in rat aorta. *Gen Pharmacol.* 2000;34:245-253.
61. Okuno Y, Mashimo T, Takashina M, et al. Hemodynamic effects of amrinone combined with dopamine in patients undergoing living renal transplantation. *Masui.* 1997;46:87-94.
62. Matsuda F, Sugahara K, Sugita M, et al. Comparative effect of amrinone, aminophylline and diltiazem on rat airway smooth muscle. *Acta Anaesthesiol Scand.* 2000;44:763-766.
63. Ochiai Y, Morita S, Tanoue Y, et al. Effects of amrinone, a phosphodiesterase inhibitor, on right ventricular/arterial coupling immediately after cardiac operations. *J Thorac Cardiovasc Surg.* 1998;116:139-147.
64. Moazemi K, Chana JS, Willard Am, et al. Intravenous vasodilator therapy in congestive heart failure. *Drugs Aging.* 2003; 20:485-508.

65. Stump GL, Wallace AA, Gilberto DB, et al. Arrhythmogenic potential of positive inotropic agents. *Basic Res Cardiol.* 2000;95:186-198.
66. Varriale P, Ramaprasad S. Short-term intravenous milrinone for sever congestive heart failure: the good, bad, and not so good. *Pharmacotherapy.* 1997;17:371-374.
67. Whitehurst VE, Vick JA, Alleva FR, et al. Reversal of propranolol blockade of adrenergic receptors and related toxicity with drugs that increase cyclic AMP. *Proc Soc Exp Biol Med.* 1999; 221:382-385.
68. Kirsten R, Nelson K, Kirsten D, et al. Clinical pharmacokinetics of vasodilators. *Clin Pharmacokinet.* 1998;35:9-36.
69. Latifi S, Lidsky K, Blumer JL. Pharmacology of inotropic agents in infants and children. *Prog Pediatr Cardiol.* 2000;12:57-79.
70. Lindsay CA, Barton P, Lawless S, et al. Pharmacokinetics and pharmacodynamics of milrinone lactate in pediatric patients with septic shock. *J Pediatr.* 1998;132:329-334.
71. Southworth MR. Treatment options for acute decompensated heart failure. *Am J Health Syst Pharm.* 2003;60:S7-S15.
72. Digitalis Investigation Group. The effect of digoxin on mortality and morbidity in patients with heart failure. *N Engl J Med.* 1997;336:525-533.
73. Hauptman PJ, Kelly RA. Digitalis. *Circulation.* 1999;99:1265-1270.
74. Campbell TJ, MacDonald PS. Digoxin in heart failure and cardiac arrhythmias. *Med J Aust.* 2003;179:98-102.
75. Dominiak P. Pharmacotherapeutic strategy in heart failure. *Clin Nephrol.* 2002;58:S2-S6.
76. O'Connor CM, Hathaway WR, Bates ER, et al. Clinical characteristics and long-term outcome of patients in whom congestive heart failure develops after thrombolytic therapy for acute myocardial infarction: development of a predictive model. *Am Heart J.* 1997;133:663-673.
77. Aziz IN, Lee JT, Kopchok GE, et al. Cardiac risk stratification in patients undergoing endoluminal graft repair of abdominal aortic aneurysm: a single-institution experience with 365 patients. *J Vasc Surg.* 2003;38:56-60.
78. Francis GS, Tang WH. Pathophysiology of congestive heart failure. *Rev Cardiovasc Med.* 2003;4:S14-S20.
79. Fonarow GC. Pharmacologic therapies for acutely decompensated heart failure. *Rev Cardiovasc Med.* 2002;3:S18-S27.
80. Probstfield JL. How cost-effective are new preventive strategies for cardiovascular disease? *Am J Cardiol.* 2003;9:22G-27G.
81. Klein L, O'Connor CM, Gattis WA, et al. Pharmacologic therapy for patients with chronic heart failure and reduced systolic function: review of trials and practical considerations. *Am J Cardiol.* 2003;91:18F-40F.
82. Timmermans PB. Angiotensin II receptor antagonists: an emerging new class of cardiovascular therapeutics. *Hypertens Res.* 1999;22:147-153.
83. Sami M. Angiotensin-converting enzyme inhibitors and end-organ damage in heart failure. *Can J Cardiol.* 1999;15:19C-23C.
84. Manché A, Galea J, Busuttil W. Tolerance to ACE inhibitors after cardiac surgery. *Eur J Cardiothorac Surg.* 1999;15:55-60.
85. Krum H. Beta-blockers in heart failure. The 'new wave' of clinical trials. *Drugs.* 1999;58:203-210.
86. Eichhorn EJ. Medical therapy of chronic heart failure. Role of ACE inhibitors and beta-blockers. *Cardiol Clin.* 1998;16:711-725.
87. McGavin JK, Keating GM. Bisoprolol: a review of its use in chronic heart failure. *Drugs.* 2002;62:2677-2696.
88. Follath F. Do diuretics differ in terms of clinical outcome in congestive heart failure? *Eur Heart J.* 1998;19(suppl):P5-P8.
89. Northridge DB, et al. Comparison of the short-term effects of candoxatril, an orally active neutral endopeptidase inhibitor, and furosemide in the treatment of patients with chronic heart failure. *Am Heart J.* 1999;138:1149-1157.
90. Forrest J, et al. Multicenter study of general anesthesia. II. Results. *Anesthesiology.* 1990;72:262-268.
91. Niemann JT, Cairns CB. Hyperkalemia and ionized hypocalcemia during cardiac arrest and resuscitation: possible culprits for post-countershock arrhythmias? *Ann Emerg Med.* 1999;34:1-7.
92. Laird RD, Studenski SS. Management of hypertension for stroke prevention in older people. *Clin Geriatr Med.* 1999;15:663-684.
93. Joint National Committee on Prevention, Detection and Treatment of High Blood Pressure. Seventh Report of the National Committee on Detection, Evaluation and Treatment of High Blood Pressure (JNC-7), U.S. Department of Health and Human Services. National Institute of Health. National Heart, Lung and Blood Institute. National High Blood Pressure Education Program; May 2003. NIH publication number 03-5233.
94. Hansson L, Zanchetti A, Carruthers SG, HOT Study Group. Effects of intensive blood-pressure lowering and low-dose aspirin in patients with hypertension: principal results of the Hypertension Optimal Treatment (HOT) randomised trial. *Lancet.* 1998;351:1755-1762.
95. Prys-Roberts C, Meloche R, Fox P. Studies of anesthesia in relation to hypertension. I. Cardiovascular responses of treated and untreated patients. *Br J Anaesth.* 1971;43:122.
96. Ali MJ, Davison P, Pickett W, et al. ACC/AHA guidelines as predictors of postoperative cardiac outcomes. *Can J Anaesth.* 2000;47:10-19.
97. Mangano DT, et al. Association of perioperative stress myocardial ischemia with cardiac morbidity and mortality in men undergoing noncardiac surgery. *N Engl J Med.* 1990;323:1781.
98. Healthy People 2010. *Heart Disease and Stroke.* Hyattsville, Md: Centers for Disease Control and Prevention, National Center for Health Statistics; November 18, 2003.
99. Coriat, P et al. Influence of chronic angiotensin converting enzyme inhibition in anesthesia induction. *Anesthesiology.* 1994;81:299.

CHAPTER 13

Additional Drugs of Interest

John J. Nagelhout

Optimal anesthetic management requires a basic working knowledge of numerous nonanesthetic drugs that may have beneficial perioperative effects as well as adverse ones. Patients undergoing surgery and anesthesia have the full spectrum of available drugs in their preoperative drug profiles. Additional drugs with perioperative implications include antibiotics, antineoplastics, contrast dyes, and drugs used in the treatment of psychiatric disorders. The responsibility for antibiotic selection during surgery may not rest with the anesthesia provider, yet he or she may frequently be called on to administer these agents and must understand when prophylaxis is appropriate and what the inherent risks are.

PROPHYLACTIC ANTIBIOTICS

Postoperative surgical site infections remain a major source of illness and a cause of death (fortunately, less frequently) in surgical patients. Such infections number approximately 500,000 per year among an estimated 27 million surgical procedures and account for approximately one quarter of the estimated 2 million nosocomial infections in the United States. Infections result in longer hospitalization and higher costs.[1] The Centers for Disease Control and Prevention (CDCP) applies the following classifications to surgical site infections: incisional, organ, or other organs and spaces manipulated during an operation. Incisional infections are further divided into superficial infections (involving skin and subcutaneous tissue) and deep infections (involving deep soft tissue, muscle, and fascia). These definitions should be followed universally for surveillance, prevention, and control of surgical site infections.[2] Guidelines for the prevention of surgical site infections are summarized in Box 13-1. Appropriate surgical prophylaxis is a multifactorial enterprise that includes proper case selection, antibiotic selection, dosage and route of administration, duration of therapy, and, for lengthy procedures, intraoperative administration. Significant cost savings and improved infection rates have been shown to accrue with use of surgical antimicrobial prophylaxis. Laparoscopic procedures have a lower perioperative infection rate than open or combined open and laparoscopic surgery.[3,4]

A large percentage of antibiotics are administered to prevent infection rather than to treat established disease. Prophylactic antibiotics for various surgical procedures should ideally be administered before skin incision at induction of anesthesia or after cord clamping during delivery. If a tourniquet is used, antibiotics should be administered before inflation to ensure that drug has reached the tissues.[4-6] The antibiotic selected must be active against the most likely contaminating microorganisms.

Antibiotic prophylaxis should be used only in selected operative procedures for which there are data supporting its use. Unnecessary prophylaxis can lead to the development of more resistant flora as well as increasing the risk of toxicity and increasing expense. A number of studies indicate that it can be justified in cases of trauma and "dirty" or contaminated surgical procedures (Tables 13-1 and 13-2), such as surgery on the bowel, biliary tract, or vagina or head and neck surgery in which the esophageal lumen may be entered, resulting in a high incidence of wound infections. Exceptions are made when the procedure involves insertion of a prosthetic implant, such as an orthopedic device or a cardiac valve; although these are "clean" procedures, authorities agree that complications from infection can be devastating.[7]

Patients with valvular or congenital heart disease (except uncomplicated atrial septal defect), intracardiac prostheses, previous endocarditis, and mitral valve prolapse with holosystolic murmurs who are undergoing dental or surgical procedures that produce a high incidence of bacteremia should receive antibiotic prophylaxis to prevent bacterial endocarditis.[8-12] The most recent set of guidelines for bacterial endocarditis prophylaxis published by the American Heart Association stratifies cardiac conditions into high-, moderate-, and negligible-risk categories (Box 13-2, p.228), based on potential outcome if endocarditis develops.[9-11] Any procedure that involves a mucous membrane such as the oropharyngeal or gastrointestinal (GI) tract produces transient bacteremia with streptococci and enterococci, respectively. Staphylococci from the skin and genitourinary procedures also have a propensity to produce endocarditis, and chemoprophylaxis should be directed against these organisms. Specific guidelines recommended by the American Heart Association for prophylactic antibiotic use for prevention of subacute bacterial endocarditis during surgical procedures are listed in Box 13-3 on p.228 and Table 13-3 on p.229.[9,11] Major changes in the updated recommendations include the following: (1) procedures that may cause bacteremia are clearly specified; (2) the oral amoxicillin dose for oral and dental procedures is reduced to 2 g, and a follow-up dose is no longer recommended; and (3) erythromycin is no longer recommended for penicillin-allergic patients (instead, clindamycin and other alternatives are offered).

Penicillins

The basic structure of a penicillin is a thiazolidine ring connected to a β-lactam ring and a side chain that, when modified, results in the formation of a variety of penicillin compounds.[13-15] The bactericidal action of penicillins reflects the ability of these antibiotics to interfere with the synthesis of peptidoglycan, which is an essential component of cell walls of

BOX **13-1**

Hospital Infection Control Practices Advisory Committee Recommendations for the Prevention of Surgical Site Infection

Preparation of the Patient
- Treat remote infection before elective operation; postpone surgery until treated
- Do not remove hair from operative site unless necessary to facilitate surgery; if hair is removed, do so immediately before surgery, preferably with electric clippers or use of a depilatory
- Control serum blood glucose perioperatively
- Have patient stop tobacco use 30 days before surgery
- Do not withhold necessary blood products to prevent surgical site infection
- Patient should bathe with antimicrobial soap the night before an elective procedure
- Wash incision site before performing antiseptic skin preparation with approved agent
- Prepare skin in concentric circles from incision site
- Keep preoperative stay in hospital as short as possible

Before Surgery
- Perform surgical scrub for at least 5 minutes before first operation of day with an appropriate antiseptic
- Between consecutive operations perform surgical scrub for 2 to 5 minutes

Antimicrobial Prophylaxis
- Treat and control all bacterial infections before surgery and identify and treat all remote infections before elective surgery
- Select (if indicated) an antimicrobial agent with efficacy against expected pathogen
- Start administration of parenteral intravenous antimicrobial agents shortly before operation and discontinue shortly afterward; administer antimicrobial agents timed to ensure bactericidal serum and tissue levels when incision made
- Intravenous route is used to produce adequate serum levels during surgery and for at most a few hours after incision closed
- Before elective colorectal operations, in addition to parenteral agent, mechanically prepare the colon by use of enemas and cathartics; administer nonabsorbable oral antimicrobial agents in divided doses on the day before the operation
- Do not routinely use vancomycin for antimicrobial prophylaxis
- For cesarean sections in patients at high risk administer intravenous antimicrobial agent immediately after cord is clamped

From Mangram AJ, Horan TC, Pearson ML, Silver LC, Jarvis WR, the Hospital Infection Control Practices Advisory Committee. Guideline for prevention of surgical site infection 1999. Infect Control Hosp Epidemiol. *1999;20:247-280.*

susceptible bacteria.[14,15] Penicillins are classified according to their spectrums of antimicrobial activity (Table 13-4).

Penicillin G and its close congener penicillin V are highly active against sensitive strains of gram-positive cocci such as streptococci and pneumococci.[14,15] However, penicillin-resistant strains of *Streptococcus pneumoniae* and pneumococci are becoming more common. Such resistance is especially common in pediatric populations (e.g., children attending day care centers). Penicillin G and penicillin V are ineffective against most strains of *Staphylococcus aureus*.

The penicillinase-resistant penicillins (methicillin, nafcillin, oxacillin, cloxacillin, and dicloxacillin) are resistant to hydrolysis by staphylococcal penicillinase and are the agents of choice for treatment of most staphylococcal disease, despite the increasing incidence of methicillin-resistant microorganisms. Vancomycin is considered the agent of choice for such infections.[13,14]

Ampicillin, amoxicillin, and bacampicillin make up a group of penicillins whose antimicrobial activity is extended to include gram-negative microorganisms such as *Haemophilus influenzae*, *Escherichia coli*, and *Proteus mirabilis*. Unfortunately, hydrolysis by β-lactamases is rendering these microorganisms resistant with increasing frequency.

Carbenicillin, ticarcillin, azlocillin, mezlocillin, and piperacillin are classified as extended action penicillins. Their extended spectrum includes *Pseudomonas*, *Klebsiella*, *Enterobacter*, and *Proteus* species.[13,14]

Pharmacokinetics

Penicillins are widely distributed throughout the body; however, only low concentrations are found in prostatic secretions, cerebrospinal fluid (CSF) (1% of plasma levels when meninges are normal), and intraocular fluid. When inflammation is present, concentrations in CSF may increase to as much as 5%. Penicillins are eliminated rapidly by glomerular filtration and renal tubular secretion, so their half-lives are short. Serum half-life may be prolonged in patients with renal impairment, and dosage adjustment may be necessary.

Adverse Reactions

The most common adverse reaction is an allergic response, which is noted in 1% to 10% of patients treated with penicillins, making these antibiotics the most allergenic of all drugs.[13,15,16] The most common manifestations of allergy to penicillins are a maculopapular or urticarial rash and fever. In a few patients a life-threatening anaphylactic reaction (e.g., hypotension; bronchospasm; edema of the face, lips, tongue, and larynx) can occur. Less common manifestations of allergy include exfoliative dermatitis, positive result on Coombs' test, nephritis, drug-induced lupus nephritis, arthralgia, myalgia, and immune hemolytic anemias.[13-15,17]

Other rare adverse reactions to penicillins include convulsions, acute tubular necrosis, and potassium overdose that leads to asystole. Some penicillins, such as penicillin G, are potassium salts and contain 1.5 to 1.7 mEq of ionized potassium in every 1 million units.[15] Dosage should be adjusted in patients with renal impairment to avoid hyperkalemia and cardiac arrest.

Precautions and Contraindications

Before initiation of penicillin therapy, careful inquiry should be made concerning previous hypersensitivity

TABLE 13-1 Recommendations for Surgical Antimicrobial Prophylaxis in Adults

Type of Surgery	Recommended Regimen	Alternative Regimens[a]
Cardiothoracic	Cefazolin 1 g IV at induction of anesthesia and q8h for up to 72 hr[b,c]	Cefuroxime 1.5 g IV at induction of anesthesia and q12h for up to 72 hr, cefamandole 1 g IV at induction of anesthesia and q6h for up to 72 hr, vancomycin 1 g IV with or without gentamicin 2 mg/kg IV[d]
Gastrointestinal		
Gastroduodenal		
Procedures involving entry into the lumen of the gastrointestinal tract	Cefazolin 1 g IV at induction of anesthesia	
Highly selective vagotomy, Nissen's fundoplication, and Whipple's procedure	Cefazolin 1 g IV at induction of anesthesia	
Biliary tract		
Open procedure	Cefazolin 1 g IV at induction of anesthesia	
Laparoscopic procedure	None	
Appendectomy for uncomplicated appendicitis	Cefoxitin, cefotetan, or Cefmetazole 1-2 g IV at induction of anesthesia	Piperacillin 2 g IV at induction of anesthesia; if patient is allergic to penicillin, metronidazole 500 mg IV plus gentamicin 2 mg/kg IV at induction of anesthesia
Colorectal	Neomycin sulfate 1 g plus erythromycin base 1 g PO (after mechanical bowel preparation is completed at 19, 18, and 9 hr before surgery[e]); if oral route is contraindicated, cefoxitin, cefotetan, or cefmetazole 2 g IV at induction of anesthesia; for patients undergoing high-risk surgery (e.g., rectal resection), oral neomycin and erythromycin plus an IV cephalosporin	
Head and neck		
Clean	None	
With placement of prosthesis	Cefazolin 1 g IV at induction of anesthesia	
Clean-contaminated	Cefazolin 2 g IV at induction of anesthesia and q8h for 24 hr or clindamycin 600 mg IV at induction of anesthesia and q8h for 24 hr	Addition of gentamicin 1.7 mg/kg IV to clindamycin regimen or of metronidazole 500 mg IV q 8 hr to cefazolin regimen is controversial; single-dose regimens might be preferable, but this approach is controversial
Elective craniotomy or cerebrospinal fluid shunting	Cefazolin 1 g IV at induction of anesthesia	Oxacillin 1 g or nafcillin 1 g IV at induction of anesthesia; vancomycin 1 g IV[f]
Obstetric or gynecologic cesarean delivery[g]	Cefazolin 2 g IV immediately after clamping of umbilical cord	
Hysterectomy (vaginal, abdominal, or radical)	Cefazolin 1 g IV or cefotetan 1 g IV at induction of anesthesia	Cefoxitin 1 g IV at induction of anesthesia
Ophthalmic	Topical neomycin-polymyxin B-gramicidin 1-2 drops or tobramycin 0.3% or gentamicin 0.3% 2 drops instilled before procedure[h]	Addition of tobramycin 20 mg by subconjunctival injection is optional
Orthopedic		
Clean, not involving implantation of foreign materials[i]	None	
Hip fracture repair[j]	Cefazolin 1 g IV at induction of anesthesia and q8h for 24 hr	Vancomycin 1 g IV[f]
Implantation of internal fixation devices[k]	Cefazolin 1 g IV at induction of anesthesia and q8h for 24 hr	Vancomycin 1 g IV[f]
Total joint replacement	Cefazolin 1 g IV at induction of anesthesia and q8h for 24 hr	Vancomycin 1 g IV[f]

TABLE 13-1 Recommendations for Surgical Antimicrobial Prophylaxis in Adults—cont'd

Type of Surgery	Recommended Regimen	Alternative Regimens[a]
Urologic (high-risk patients only)[l]	Trimethoprim 160 mg with sulfamethoxazole 800 mg PO or lomefloxacin 400 mg PO 2 hr before surgery (if oral agents used) or cefazolin 1 g IV at induction of anesthesia (if injection preferred)	
Vascular[m]	Cefazolin 1 g IV at induction of anesthesia and q8h for 24 hr	Vancomycin 1 g IV with or without gentamicin 2 mg/kg IV[f]
Transplantation		
Heart	Cefazolin 1 g IV at induction of anesthesia and q8h for 48-72 hr[c]	Cefuroxime 1.5 g IV at induction of anesthesia and q12h for 48-72 hr, cefamandole 1 g IV at induction of anesthesia and q6h for 48-72 hr, or vancomycin 1 g IV with or without gentamicin 2 mg/kg IV[d]
Lung and heart-lung[n,o]	Cefazolin 1 g IV at induction of anesthesia and q8h for 48-72 hr	Cefuroxime 1.5 g IV at induction of anesthesia and q12h for 48-72 hr, cefamandole 1 g IV at induction of anesthesia and q6h for 48-72 hr, or vancomycin 1 g IV[f]
Liver	Cefotaxime 1 g IV plus Ampicillin 1 g IV at Induction of anesthesia and q 6 hr during procedure and for 48 hr beyond final surgical closure	Antimicrobials that provide adequate coverage against gram-negative aerobic bacilli, staphylococci, and enterococci may be appropriate
Pancreas and pancreas-kidney	Cefazolin 1 g IV at induction of anesthesia	
Kidney	Cefazolin 1 g IV at induction of anesthesia	

From American Society of Health-System Pharmacists. ASHP therapeutic guidelines on antimicrobial prophylaxis in surgery. Am J Health-Syst Pharm. *1999;56:1839-1888.*

IV, Intravenous; PO, *oral.*

[a]*If a short-acting agent is used, it should be readministered if surgery takes more than 3 hours. If surgery is expected to last more than 6 to 8 hours, it should be reasonable to administer an agent with a longer half-life and duration of action or to administer a short-acting agent at 3-hour intervals during the procedure. Readministration may also be warranted if prolonged or excessive bleeding occurs or there are factors that may shorten the half-life (e.g., extensive burns). Readministration may not be warranted in patients in whom the half-life is prolonged (e.g., patients with renal insufficiency or failure).*

[b]*Duration is based on expert panel consensus. Prophylaxis for 24 hours or less may be appropriate.*

[c]*There is currently no evidence to support continuing antimicrobial prophylaxis until chest and mediastinal drainage tubes are removed.*

[d]*According to Hospital Infection Control Practices Advisory Committee guidelines or American Heart Association recommendations for penicillin-allergic patients at high risk for endocarditis.*

[e]*Mechanical bowel preparation is required for nonobstructed patients undergoing elective operations.*

[f]*According to Hospital Infection Control Practices Advisory Committee guidelines.*

[g]*The American College of Obstetricians and Gynecologists (ACOG) considers the use of prophylaxis controversial in low-risk patients. ACOG does not routinely recommend prophylaxis in low-risk patients because of concerns about adverse effects, development of resistant organisms, and relaxation of standard infection-control measures and proper operative technique.*

[h]*According to ACOG guidelines, first-, second-, and third-generation cephalosporins can be used for vaginal, abdominal, and radical hysterectomies.*

[i]*The necessity of continuing topical antimicrobials postoperatively has not been established by data.*

[j]*Laminectomy and knee, hand, and foot surgeries. The evaluated studies did not include arthroscopy and did not identify specific procedures, like carpal tunnel release: however, arthroscopy and other procedures not involving implantation are similar enough to be included with clean orthopedic procedures not involving implantation.*

[k]*Procedures involving internal fixation devices (e.g., nails, screws, plates, wires).*

[l]*High risk is defined as prolonged postoperative catheterization, positive urine cultures, or hospital infection rate of greater than 20%.*

[m]*Prophylaxis is not indicated for brachiocephalic procedures. Although there are no data, patients undergoing brachiocephalic procedures involving vascular prostheses or patch implantation (e.g., carotid endartectomy) may benefit from prophylaxis.*

[n]*Patients undergoing lung transplantation with negative pretransplant cultures should receive antimicrobial prophylaxis as appropriate for other types of cardiothoracic surgeries.*

[o]*Patients undergoing lung transplantation for cystic fibrosis should receive 7-14 days of prophylaxis with antimicrobials selected according to pretransplant culture and susceptibility results. This may include additional antibacterial agents or antifungal agents.*

TABLE 13-2 Antimicrobial Regimens for Surgical Prophylaxis in Pediatric Patients[a]

Type of Surgery	Preferred Regimen[b]	Alternative Regimens[b]
Cardiothoracic	Cefazolin 20-30 mg/kg IV at induction of anesthesia and q8h for up to 72 hr[c,d]	Cefuroxime 50 mg/kg IV at induction of anesthesia and q8h for up to 72 hr, vancomycin 15 mg/kg IV with or without gentamicin 2 mg/kg IV[e]
Gastrointestinal		
Gastroduodenal procedures involving entry into the lumen of the gastrointestinal tract, highly selective vagotomy, Nissen's fundoplication, and Whipple's procedure)	Cefazolin 20-30 mg/kg IV at induction of anesthesia	
Biliary tract		
Open procedures	Cefazolin 20-30 mg/kg IV at induction of anesthesia	
Laparoscopic procedures	None	
Appendectomy for uncomplicated appendicitis	Cefoxitin 20-40 mg/kg IV, cefotaxime 25-50 mg/kg IV, or ceftizoxime 25-50 mg/kg IV at induction of anesthesia	Piperacillin 50 mg/kg IV at induction of anesthesia; if patient is allergic to penicillin, metronidazole 10 mg/kg IV plus gentamicin 2 mg/kg IV at induction of anesthesia
Colorectal	Neomycin sulfate 20 mg/kg plus erythromycin base 10 mg/kg PO (after mechanical bowel preparation is completed) at 19, 18, and 9 hr before surgery; if oral route is contraindicated, cefoxitin or cefotetan 30-40 mg/kg IV at induction of anesthesia; in patients undergoing high-risk surgery (e.g., rectal resection), oral neomycin and erythromycin plus an IV cephalosporin	
Head and neck		
Clean	None	
With placement of prosthesis	Cefazolin 20-30 mg/kg IV at induction of anesthesia and q8h for 24 hr or clindamycin 15 mg/kg IV at induction of anesthesia and q8h for 24 hr	Addition of gentamicin 2.5 mg/kg IV to clindamycin regimen or of metronidazole 10 mg/kg IV q8h to cefazolin regimen is controversial; single-dose regimens might be preferable, but this approach is controversial
Clean-contaminated		
Elective craniotomy or cerebrospinal fluid shunting	Cefazolin 20-30 mg/kg IV at induction of anesthesia	Vancomycin 15 mg/kg IV[f]
Obstetric or gynecologic cesarean delivery[g]	Cefazolin 2 g IV immediately after clamping of umbilical cord	Cefoxitin 1 g IV at induction of anesthesia
Hysterectomy (vaginal, abdominal, or radical)[h]	Cefazolin 2 g IV or cefotetan 1 g IV at induction of anesthesia	Cefoxitin 1 g IV at induction of anesthesia
Ophthalmic	Topical neomycin-polymyxin B-gramicidin 1-2 drops or tobramycin 0.3% or gentamicin 0.3% 2 drops instilled before procedure[i]	
Orthopedic		
Clean, not involving implantation of foreign materials	None	
Hip fracture repair,[j] implantation of internal fixation devices,[k] total joint replacement	Cefazolin 20-30 mg/kg IV at induction of anesthesia and q8h for 24 hr	Vancomycin 15 mg/kg IV[f]

TABLE 13-2 Antimicrobial Regimens for Surgical Prophylaxis in Pediatric Patients[a]—cont'd

Type of Surgery	Preferred Regimen[b]	Alternative Regimens[b]
Urologic procedures (high-risk patients only)[l]	Trimethoprim 6-10 mg/kg plus sulfamethoxazole 30-50 mg/kg PO 2 hr before surgery (if oral agents used) or cefazolin 20-30 mg/kg IV at induction of anesthesia (if injection preferred)	
Vascular procedures[m]	Cefazolin 20-30 mg/kg IV at induction of anesthesia and q8h for 24 hr	Vancomycin 15 mg/kg IV with or without gentamicin 2 mg/kg IV[f]
Transplantation		
Heart	Cefazolin 20-30 mg/kg IV at induction of anesthesia and q8h for 48-72 hr[d]	Cefuroxime 50 mg/kg IV at induction of anesthesia and q8h for 48-72 hr,[c,d] vancomycin 15 mg/kg with or without gentamicin 2 mg/kg IV[e]
Lung and heart-lung[n,o]	Cefazolin 20-30 mg/kg IV at induction of anesthesia and q8h for 48-72 hr[d]	Cefuroxime 50 mg/kg IV at induction of anesthesia and q8h for 48-72 hr,[d] vancomycin 15 mg/kg IV[f]
Liver	Cefotaxime 50 mg/kg IV plus ampicillin 50 mg/kg IV at induction of anesthesia and q6h for 48 hr after final surgical closure	Antimicrobials that provide adequate coverage against gram-negative aerobic bacilli, staphylococci, and enterococci may be appropriate
Pancreas and pancreas-kidney	Cefazolin 20 mg/kg IV at induction of anesthesia	
Kidney	Cefazolin 20 mg/kg IV at induction of anesthesia	

From American Society of Health-System Pharmacists. ASHP therapeutic guidelines on antimicrobial prophylaxis in surgery. Am J Health-Syst Pharm. *1999;56:1839-1888.*

IV, *Intravenous;* PO, *oral.*

[a]*The recommendations included in this table have been extrapolated from adult data. The pediatric dosages are approximately equivalent to the adult dosages listed in Table 13-1. With few exceptions (aminoglycosides), pediatric dosages should not exceed the maximum dosage recommended for adults. Adult dosages should be used for children who weigh more than 40-50 kg, because a dosage calculated on a milligram-per-kilogram basis will exceed the maximum recommended dosage for adults. Dosages for neonates (full-term and preterm) are not provided.*

[b]*If a short-acting agent is used, it should be readministered if surgery takes more than 3 hours. If surgery is expected to last more than 6 to 8 hours, it would be reasonable to administer an agent with a longer half-life and duration of action or to administer a short-acting agent at 3-hour intervals during the procedure. Readministration may also be warranted if prolonged or excessive bleeding occurs or there are factors that may shorten the half-life (e.g., extensive burns). Readministration may not be warranted in patients in whom the half-life is prolonged (e.g., patients with renal insufficiency or failure).*

[c]*Duration is based on expert panel consensus. Prophylaxis for 24 hours or less may be appropriate.*

[d]*There is currently no evidence to support continuing antimicrobial prophylaxis until chest and mediastinal drainage tubes are removed.*

[e]*According to Hospital Infection Control Practices Advisory Committee guidelines or American Heart Association recommendations for penicillin-allergic patients at high risk for endocarditis.*[32] *Pediatric cancer patients may require dosages greater than the standard dosage.*

[f]*According to Hospital Infection Control Practices Advisory Committee guidelines.*

[g]*The American College of Obstetricians and Gynecologists (ACOG) considers the use of prophylaxis controversial in low-risk patients. ACOG does not routinely recommend prophylaxis in low-risk patients because of concerns about adverse effects, development of resistant organisms, and relaxation of standard infection-control measures and proper operative technique.*

[h]*According to ACOG guidelines, first-, second-, and third-generation cephalosporins can be used for vaginal, abdominal, and radical hysterectomies.*

[i]*The necessity of continuing topical antimicrobials postoperatively has not been established by data.*

[j]*Laminectomy and knee, hand, and foot surgeries. The evaluated studies did not include arthroscopy procedures and did not identify specific procedures, like carpal tunnel release: however, arthroscopy and other procedures not involving implantation are similar enough to be included with clean orthopedic procedures not involving implantation.*

[k]*Procedures involving internal fixation devices (e.g., nails, screws, plates, wires).*

[l]*High risk is defined as prolonged postoperative catheterization, positive urine cultures, or hospital infection rate of greater than 20%.*

[m]*Prophylaxis is not indicated for brachiocephalic procedures. Although there are no data, patients undergoing brachiocephalic procedures involving vascular prosthesis or patch implantation (e.g., carotid endarterectomy) may benefit from prophylaxis.*

[n]*Patients undergoing lung transplantation with negative pretransplant cultures should receive antimicrobial prophylaxis as appropriate for other types of cardiothoracic surgeries.*

[o]*Patients undergoing lung transplantation for cystic fibrosis should receive 7-14 days of prophylaxis with antimicrobials selected according to pretransplant isolates and susceptibilities. This may include additional antibacterial or antifungal agents.*

BOX 13-2

American Heart Association Guidelines: Cardiac Conditions Associated with Endocarditis

Endocarditis Prophylaxis Recommended

High-Risk Category

Prosthetic cardiac valves, including bioprosthetic and homograft valves
Previous bacterial endocarditis
Complex cyanotic congenital heart disease (e.g., single-ventricle states, transposition of the great arteries, tetralogy of Fallot)
Surgically constructed systemic pulmonary shunts or conduits

Moderate-Risk Category

Most other congenital cardiac malformations (other than those listed previously and subsequently)
Acquired valvular dysfunction (e.g., rheumatic heart disease)
Hypertrophic cardiomyopathy
Mitral valve prolapse with valvular regurgitation, thickened leaflets, or both

Endocarditis Prophylaxis Not Recommended

Negligible-Risk Category (No Greater Risk Than the General Population)

Isolated secundum atrial septal defect
Surgical repair of atrial septal defect, ventricular septal defect, or patent ductus arteriosus (without residua beyond 6 months)
Previous coronary artery bypass graft surgery
Mitral valve prolapse without valvular regurgitation
Physiologic, functional, or innocent heart murmurs
Previous Kawasaki disease without valvular dysfunction
Previous rheumatic fever without valvular dysfunction
Cardiac pacemakers (intravascular and epicardial) and implanted defibrillators

Modified from Dajani A, Taubert KA, Wilson W, Bolger AF, Bayer A, et al. JAMA. *1997;277:1794-1801.*

BOX 13-3

Endocarditis Prophylaxis

Endocarditis Prophylaxis Recommended

Respiratory Tract

Tonsillectomy or adenoidectomy
Surgical operations that involve respiratory mucosa
Bronchoscopy with a rigid bronchoscope

*Gastrointestinal Tract**

Sclerotherapy for esophageal varices
Esophageal stricture dilation
Endoscopic retrograde cholangiography with biliary obstruction
Biliary tract surgery
Surgical operations that involve intestinal mucosa

Genitourinary Tract

Prostatic surgery
Cystoscopy
Urethral dilation

Dental Procedures

Extractions
Periodontal procedures, including surgery, scaling, and root planing and probing
Implant replacement and reimplantation of avulsed teeth
Endodontic (root canal) instrumentation or surgery only beyond the apex
Subgingival placement of antibiotic fibers or strips
Initial placement of orthodontic bands but not brackets
Intraligamentary local anesthetic injections
Prophylactic cleaning of teeth or implants if bleeding is anticipated

Endocarditis Prophylaxis Not Recommended

Respiratory Tract

Endotracheal intubation
Bronchoscopy with a flexible bronchoscope, with or without biopsy†
Tympanostomy tube insertion

Gastrointestinal Tract

Transesophageal echocardiography†
Endoscopy with or without gastrointestinal biopsy†

Genitourinary Tract

Vaginal hysterectomy†
Vaginal delivery†
Cesarean section

In Uninfected Tissue

Urethral catheterization
Uterine dilation and curettage
Therapeutic abortion
Sterilization procedures
Insertion or removal of intrauterine devices

Other Procedures

Cardiac catheterization, including balloon angioplasty
Implanted defibrillators, coronary stents
Incision or biopsy of surgically scrubbed skin
Circumcision

**Prophylaxis is recommended for high-risk patients, optional for medium-risk patients.*
†Prophylaxis is optional for high-risk patients.
Modified from Dajani A, Taubert KA, Wilson W, Bolger AF, Bayer A, et al. JAMA. *1997;277:1794-1801.*

reactions to penicillins and cephalosporins, because evidence exists of cross-allergenicity among β-lactams. Cephalosporins are often selected for treatment of patients who have a history of cutaneous reaction only; however, both penicillins and cephalosporins should be avoided if a history of anaphylactic-type reaction is obtained. Allergic reactions may occur in the absence of previous known exposure to any of the penicillins. This may reflect previous unrecognized exposure to penicillin, presumably in ingested foods.[17]

TABLE 13-3 American Heart Association Prophylactic Regimens for Dental, Oral, Respiratory Tract, Esophageal, Genitourinary, and Gastrointestinal Procedures

Situation	Agent	Regimen*
Prophylactic Regimens for Dental, Oral, Respiratory Tract, or Esophageal Procedures		
Standard general prophylaxis	Amoxicillin	Adults: 2 g Children: 50 mg/kg orally 1 hr before procedure
Unable to take oral medications	Ampicillin	Adults: 2 g IM or IV Children: 50 mg/kg IM or IV within 30 min before procedure
Allergic to penicillin	Clindamycin	Adults: 600 mg Children: 20 mg/kg orally 1 hr before procedure
	or Cephalexin† or cefadroxil†	Adults: 2 g Children: 50 mg/kg orally 1 hr before procedure
	or Azithromycin or clarithromycin	Adults: 500 mg Children: 15 mg/kg orally 1 hr before procedure
Allergic to penicillin and unable to take oral medications	Clindamycin	Adults: 600 mg Children: 20 mg/kg IV within 30 min before procedure
	or Cefazolin†	Adults: 1 g Children: 25 mg/kg IM or IV within 30 min before procedure
Prophylactic Regimens for Genitourinary and Gastrointestinal (Excluding Esophageal) Procedures		
High-risk patients	Ampicillin plus gentamicin	Adults: ampicillin 2 g IM or IV plus gentamicin 1.5 mg/kg (not to exceed 120 mg) within 30 min before procedure; 6 hr later, ampicillin 1 g IM or IV or amoxicillin 1 g orally Children: ampicillin 50 mg/kg IM or IV (not to exceed 2 g) plus gentamicin 1.5 mg/kg within 30 min before procedure; 6 hr later, ampicillin 25 mg/kg IV or IM or amoxicillin 25 mg/kg orally
High-risk patients allergic to ampicillin or amoxicillin	Vancomycin plus gentamicin	Adults: vancomycin 1 g IV over 1-2 hr plus gentamicin 1.5 mg/kg IV or IM (not to exceed 120 mg); complete injection or infusion within 30 min before procedure Children: vancomycin 20 mg/kg IV over 1-2 hr plus gentamicin 1.5 mg/kg IV or IM; complete injection or infusion within 30 min before procedure
Moderate-risk patients	Amoxicillin or ampicillin	Adults: amoxicillin 2 g orally 1 hr before procedure or ampicillin 2 g IM or IV within 30 min before procedure Children: amoxicillin 50 mg/kg orally 1 hr before procedure or ampicillin 50 mg/kg IM or IV within 30 min before procedure
Moderate-risk patients allergic to ampicillin or amoxicillin	Vancomycin	Adults: vancomycin 1 g IV over 1-2 hr; complete infusion within 30 min before procedure Children: vancomycin 20 mg/kg IV over 1-2 hr; complete infusion within 30 min before procedure

IM, *Intramuscular;* IV, *intravenous.*
**Total children's dose should not exceed adult dose. No second dose of vancomycin or gentamicin is recommended.*
†Cephalosporins should not be used in individuals with immediate-type hypersensitivity reaction (urticaria, angioedema, or anaphylaxis) to penicillins.
Modified from Dajani A, Taubert KA, Wilson W, Bolger AF, Bayer A, et al. JAMA. *1997;277:1794-1801.*

Management of Anaphylactic Reactions

If a severe hypersensitivity reaction occurs during penicillin therapy, the drug should be discontinued immediately, the patient should be oxygenated adequately, and appropriate interventions should be initiated, such as rapid administration of crystalloid or colloid, epinephrine 1:10,000 1 to 5 ml at 5- to 10-minute intervals, and corticosteroids. An epinephrine infusion should be started for treatment of cardiovascular collapse. Diphenhydramine and aminophylline may be appropriate ancillary agents for urticaria-angioedema and bronchospasm, respectively.[13,15,18]

Cephalosporins

The cephalosporins (Table 13-5) are semisynthetic β-lactam antibiotics structurally and pharmacologically related to the penicillins.[14] The bactericidal action of cephalosporins results from inhibition of cell-wall synthesis. All commercially available cephalosporins contain a β-lactam ring fused with a

TABLE 13-4 Parenteral Penicillins

Generic Name	Brand Name	Usual IV Adult Dose	Available Dosage Forms	Comments
Natural Penicillins				
Penicillin G benzathine	Bicillin L-A	Given IM (*never* IV) 1.2-2.4 million units (MU) as a single dose	300,000 units/ml	Provides low, long-lasting blood levels of penicillin G
Penicillin G benzathine and procaine combined	Bicillin C-R	Given IM (*never* IV) 2.4 MU as a single dose	300,00 units/ml (140,000 units each of penicillin G benzathine and penicillin G procaine)	Provides low, long-lasting blood levels of penicillin G
Penicillin G procaine	Wycillin	Given IM (*never* IV)	600,000 units/ml; 300,000-1,000,000 units/day as one or two doses per day	Indicated for infections that respond to low, long-lasting penicillin G blood levels
Penicillin G potassium	Pfizerpen	1-24 MU/day in divided doses q4h, depending on severity of infection and microbial sensitivity	Injection: 5 MU Frozen premixed bag: 1, 2, 3 MU Powder for injection: 1, 5, 10, 20 MU	Infuse over 1-2 hr; 250 mg = 400,000 units; sodium content of 1 MU = 2 mEq; potassium content of 1 MU = 1.7 mEq; often called *aqueous penicillin*
Broad-Spectrum Penicillins				
Ampicillin	Omnipen	1-12 g/day divided q4-6h	Powder for injection: 125, 250, 500 mg, 1, 2, 10 g	Infuse over at least 10-15 min
Ampicillin/sulbactam	Unasyn	1-12 g/day divided q4-6h	Powder for injection: 1.5 g (ampicillin 1 g + sulbactam 0.5 g), 3 g (ampicillin 2 g + sulbactam 1 g); 10 g	Infuse over 15-30 min
Ticarcillin	Ticar	4-24 g/day in divided doses q4-6h	Powder for injection: 1, 3, 5, 20, 30 g	Infuse over at least 30 min; sodium content of 1 g = 5.2-6.5 mEq; infuse over at least 30 min
Ticarcillin/clavulanate	Timentin	12-24 g/day in divided doses q4-6h	Powder for injection and frozen premixed bags; ticarcillin disodium 3 g + clavulanate potassium 0.1 g	Infuse over 30 min; sodium content of 1 g = 4.75 mEq; potassium content of 1 g = 0.15 mEq
Mezlocillin	Mezlin	6-24 g/day in divided dose q4-6h	Powder for injection: 1, 2, 3, 4, 20 g	Infuse over 30 min; sodium content = 1.85 mEq/g
Piperacillin	Pipracil	18-24 g/day divided q4-6h, depending on severity	Powder for injection: 2, 3, 4, 40 g	Infuse over at least 20 minutes; sodium content = 1.85 mEq/g
Piperacillin/tazobactam	Zosyn	3.375 g q6h or 4.5 g q8h	Powder for injection (piperacillin/tazobactam): 2/0.25, 3/0.375, 4 g/0.5 g, 36 g/4.5 g	Infuse over 30 min
Penicillinase-Resistant Penicillins				
Nafcillin	Unipen	500 mg: 2 g q4-6h	Powder for injection: 500 mg, 1, 2, 4, 10 g	Infuse over 30-60 min
Oxacillin	Bactocill, Prostaphlin	250 mg: 2 g q4-6h	Powder for injection: 250, 500 mg, 1, 2, 4, 10 g	By direct IV injection over 10 min

IM, *Intramuscular*; IV, *intravenous*
From Mosby's Drug Consult. *St Louis: Mosby; 2004. With permission.*

TABLE **13-5** Parenteral Cephalosporins

Generic Name (Generation)	Usual Adult Dose (g)	Adjust Dose for Renal Insufficiency	Comment
Cefazolin (1)	0.25-2 q6-12h	Yes	Commonly used for surgical prophylaxis
Cephapirin (1)	0.5-2 q4-6hr	Yes	
Cefamandole (2)	0.5-2 q4-8h	Yes	
Cefmetazole (2)	2 q6-12h	Yes	Intraabdominal infections
Cefonicid (2)	0.5-2 q24h	Yes	May be useful in outpatient therapy of endocarditis
Cefotetan (2)	1-2 q12-24h	Yes	Covers GI anaerobes
Cefoxitin (2)	1-2 q4-8h	Yes	Covers GI anaerobes
Cefuroxime (2)	0.75-1.5 q8h	Yes	Crosses blood-brain barrier
Cefepime (3)	0.5-2 q8-12h	Yes	
Cefoperazone (3)	1-2 q8-12h	No	
Cefotaxime (3)	1-2 q4-12h	Yes	Crosses blood-brain barrier
Ceftazidime (3)	0.5-2 q8-12h	Yes	
Ceftizoxime (3)	1-12 g/day divided q4-8h	Yes	Crosses blood-brain barrier
Ceftriaxone (3)	1-2 q12-24	No	Maybe useful in outpatient therapy of endocarditis; single-dose (250 mg IM) therapy for gonococcal genital and pharyngeal infections; crosses blood-brain barrier

GI, *Gastrointestinal;* IM, *intramuscular.*
From Mosby's Drug Consult. *St Louis: Mosby; 2004. With permission.*

six-membered dihydrothiazine ring instead of the five-membered ring of penicillins (Figure 13-1).[13] Addition of various groups at R1 and R2 of the cephalosporin nucleus results in derivatives with differences in antimicrobial activity, pharmacokinetic properties, or stability against hydrolysis by β-lactamases. Production of bacterial β-lactamase enzymes, which can cleave the β-lactam ring system and thereby cause complete loss of antibacterial activity, is a major mechanism of bacterial resistance to cephalosporins.

Currently available cephalosporins are generally divided into four groups based on their spectrums of activity: first, second, third, and fourth generations. The first-generation cephalosporins, typified by cefazolin, demonstrate good antimicrobial activity against gram-positive bacteria such as streptococci and methicillin-sensitive staphylococci. The second-generation cephalosporins are more active than the first-generation cephalosporins against certain gram-negative microorganisms, especially *Enterobacter*, *Proteus*, and *Klebsiella*.[13-15,17] The third-generation cephalosporins have the greatest activity against gram-negative microorganisms, with some having good activity against *Pseudomonas*, but less activity against the gram-positive microorganisms when compared with the first-generation agents.[13,17] Cefepime is the only available fourth-generation cephalosporin. The fourth-generation cephalosporins are more stable to hydrolysis by β-lactamases than other classes of cephalosporins and therefore are active against many *Enterobacteriaceae* that are resistant to other cephalosporins.

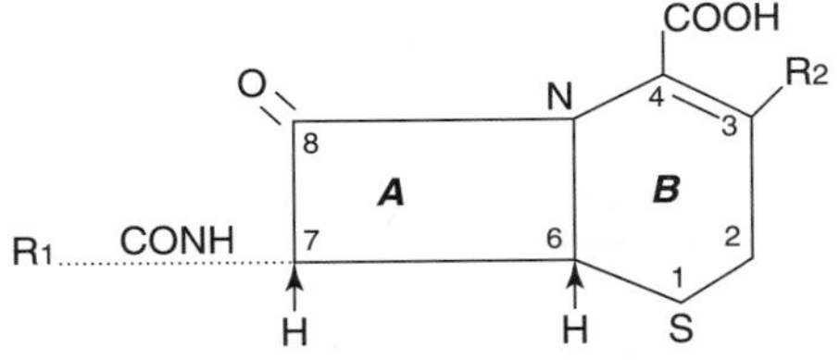

FIGURE **13-1**
Basic cephalosporin nucleus.

Pharmacokinetics

Most cephalosporins are widely distributed throughout the body, and several third-generation cephalosporins penetrate the CSF in therapeutic concentrations, especially if meninges are inflamed.[13-15] Cephalosporins cross the placenta. Individual cephalosporins differ significantly with respect to extent of absorption after oral administration and protein binding. Excretion of cephalosporins is principally by glomerular filtration and renal tubular section, which emphasizes the need to reduce dosage of the drugs in the presence of renal dysfunction.

Adverse Effects and Contraindications

The most common adverse reactions are hypersensitivity reactions ranging from maculopapular or urticarial rash to life-threatening anaphylaxis similar to that described with penicillin hypersensitivities.[13-15] Controversies exist as to whether cephalosporins should be administered to patients with a penicillin allergy because of the cross-tolerance that exists between the agents.[17] Allergic responses to cephalosporins occur in 5% to 10% of patients with known penicillin hypersensitivities. Some investigators recommend that cephalosporin use be avoided in patients with known anaphylactic reactions to penicillins.[16] However, cephalosporins are commonly used in patients with a penicillin allergy.

Aminoglycosides

The aminoglycosides (Box 13-4) contain one or two amino sugars glycosidically linked to an aminocyclitol nucleus.[13,15,19] Aminoglycosides are usually bactericidal in action and appear to inhibit protein synthesis in susceptible bacteria by irreversibly

BOX 13-4

Aminoglycosides

Amikacin (Amikin)
Gentamicin (Garamycin)
Kanamycin (Kantrex, Klebcil)
Neomycin (Mycifradin Sulfate, Myciguent)
Streptomycin
Tobramycin (Nebcin)

binding to 30S ribosomal subunits. Aminoglycosides are active against many aerobic gram-negative bacteria and some aerobic gram-positive bacteria. However, there are differences in spectrums of activity of the individual drugs. Aminoglycosides are inactive against fungi, viruses, and most anaerobic bacteria.

Aminoglycosides are active against *Acinetobacter, Citrobacter, Enterobacter, E. coli, Klebsiella, Proteus, Providencia, Pseudomonas, Salmonella, Serratia,* and *Shigella.* Most of these organisms are sensitive to amikacin, gentamicin, netilmicin, and tobramycin. Resistance is more common with kanamycin, streptomycin, and neomycin; therefore these agents are less commonly used.[13,15,19] Streptomycin and kanamycin are important second-line agents for the treatment of tuberculosis, particularly in cases of suspected multiple-drug resistance.

Aminoglycosides are used in the treatment of serious infections such as septicemia (including neonatal sepsis), bone and joint infections, skin and soft-tissue infections, respiratory tract infections, and intraabdominal infections. They are also effective for treatment of complicated recurrent urinary tract infections. Because of reported synergism, concomitant use of an extended-spectrum penicillin with antipseudomonal activity (carbenicillin, mezlocillin, piperacillin, and ticarcillin) is common in the treatment of *Pseudomonas* infections, especially in immunosuppressed patients.

Pharmacokinetics

Aminoglycosides are poorly absorbed from the GI tract and are usually given parenterally. They are well distributed into all body tissues, with the exception of the CSF.

A small portion of each dose accumulates and is tightly bound in the inner ear and kidney. These tissues become progressively saturated with aminoglycoside over the course of therapy, and it has been postulated that this accumulation may account for the ototoxicity and nephrotoxicity associated with aminoglycosides. The plasma elimination half-lives of aminoglycosides are usually 2 to 4 hours in adults with normal renal function. Plasma concentrations are higher and plasma elimination half-lives are more prolonged in patients with impaired renal function. In infants less than 1 month of age, plasma half-lives are also prolonged and are inversely proportional to birth weight and gestational age, probably reflecting renal immaturity. These drugs are not metabolized and are excreted almost entirely unchanged by the kidney.

Adverse Effects

Serious adverse systemic effects, including irreversible deafness, renal failure, and respiratory insufficiency from neuromuscular blockade, have been reported.[20-22] Ototoxicity and nephrotoxicity are most likely to occur in geriatric or dehydrated patients, patients with renal impairment, patients who are receiving high doses for long periods, and patients who are receiving other ototoxic or nephrotoxic drugs, such as ethacrynic acid, furosemide, torsemide, cisplatin, amphotericin B, vancomycin, methoxyflurane, or mannitol. Aminoglycosides produce varying degrees of neuromuscular blockade; neomycin and netilmicin are the most potent neuromuscular blocking agents of the currently available aminoglycosides. Neuromuscular effects are most likely to occur when aminoglycosides are administered to patients with neuromuscular disease (e.g., myasthenia gravis) or hypocalcemia, patients who are receiving general anesthetics or neuromuscular blocking agents, or patients receiving massive transfusions of citrated blood.[20,21,23] Drug-induced neuromuscular blockade is not easily reversed. Reversibility is thought to depend on the severity of the blockade, and mechanically assisted ventilation may be necessary. If an antibiotic muscle relaxant interaction is suspected to be causing residual paralysis postoperatively, the safest treatment is to leave the patient intubated, administer appropriate sedation to prevent a situation in which the patient is awake and paralyzed, let the drugs wear off. The efficacy of anticholinesterases in reversing aminoglycoside-induced neuromuscular blockade is highly variable. Hypersensitivity reactions occasionally have been reported, and cross-allergenicity has been demonstrated among the aminoglycosides.

Precautions and Contraindications

Renal function should be assessed before initiation of aminoglycoside therapy and should be monitored at regular intervals during therapy. Ototoxicity and nephrotoxicity may be related to high peak or high trough serum concentrations between doses. For gentamicin, netilmicin, and tobramycin, a commonly defined therapeutic range of serum concentrations is represented by peak serum levels of approximately 4 to 10 mcg/ml and trough concentrations of less than 2 mcg/ml; peak and trough serum concentrations of 15 to 40 mcg/ml and less than 5 to 10 mcg/ml, respectively, have been suggested for amikacin and kanamycin. Rapid intravenous infusion with corresponding high peak levels has also been associated with ototoxicity and nephrotoxicity; therefore intravenous administration should be slow (over approximately 30 minutes).

Dosage

Loading dose should be based on ideal body weight (Table 13-6). Maintenance dose should be selected (as a percentage of chosen loading dose) to continue peak serum concentrations indicated according to the desired dosing interval (Table 13-7) and the patient's creatinine clearance (CrCl).[13,15] Calculation of dose should be assisted by measured serum concentrations.

Equation 13-1

$$\text{CrCl (male)} = (140 - \text{Age/Serum creatinine})$$
$$\text{CrCl (female)} = 0.85 \times \text{CrCl (male)}$$

TABLE 13-6 Aminoglycoside Doses

Aminoglycoside	Usual Loading Doses	Expected Peak Serum Concentrations
Tobramycin	1-2 mg/kg	4-10 mcg/ml
Gentamicin	1-2 mg/kg	4-10 mcg/ml
Amikacin	5-7.5 mg/kg	15-30 mcg/ml
Kanamycin	5-7.5 mg/kg	15-30 mcg/ml

TABLE 13-7 Maintenance Dose According to Dosing Interval and Renal Status

Creatinine Clearance (ml/min)	Half-Life (hr)	8 hr (%)	12 hr (%)	24 hr (%)
90	3.1	84	—	—
80	3.4	80	91	—
70	3.9	76	88	—
60	4.5	71	84	—
50	5.3	65	79	—
40	6.5	57	72	92
30	8.4	48	63	86
25	9.9	43	57	81
20	11.9	37	50	75
17	13.6	33	46	70
15	15.1	31	42	67
12	17.9	27	37	61
10	20.4	24	34	56
7	25.9	19	28	47
5	31.5	16	23	41
2	46.8	11	16	30
0	69.3	8	11	21

Modified from McEvoy G, *ed.* American Hospital Formulary Service, Drug information 99. *Bethesda, Md: American Society of Hospital Pharmacists; 1999.*

Macrolide Antibiotics

The macrolide antibiotics (Table 13-8) inhibit protein synthesis in susceptible organisms by binding to 50S ribosomal units. These antibiotics are active against gram-positive bacteria (staphylococci and streptococci), *Mycoplasma*, and *Legionella*.[13,15,17,24,25] Although still relatively uncommon in most places, strains of streptococci that are resistant to erythromycin may be on the rise. Recently two new macrolides, azithromycin and clarithromycin, have become available. Similar to erythromycin in spectrum, these macrolides are better tolerated and also have more activity against *H. influenzae* and *Mycobacterium*.

TABLE 13-8 Macrolide Antibiotic Dosages

Macrolide Antibiotics	Usual Adult Dosage
Erythromycin	
Base (ERYC, PCE, E-mycin, Ery-Tab)	250 mg q6h or 333 mg q8h orally
Estolate (Ilosone)	250 mg q6h orally
Ethylsuccinate (EES, EryPed)	400 mg q6h orally
Gluceptate (Ilotycin)	15-20 mg/kg daily in divided doses q6h IV
Lactobionate (Erythrocin)	15-20 mg/kg daily in divided doses q6h IV
Azithromycin (Zithromax)	500 mg single dose on first day followed by 250 mg daily IV or orally
Clarithromycin (Biaxin)	250-500 mg q12h orally
Dirithromycin (Dynabac)	500 mg daily orally
Troleandomycin (TAO)	250-500 mg q6h orally

IV, Intravenous.

Pharmacokinetics

The bioavailability of the macrolides is variable, especially that of erythromycin, which depends on the particular erythromycin derivative, the formulation of the dosage form administered (e.g., erythromycin base must be enteric coated or it will be inactivated by gastric juices), and the presence of food in the GI tract. The macrolides are widely distributed throughout most bodily tissues except the brain and CSF. Erythromycin is concentrated in the liver and is excreted as the active form in the bile. Clarithromycin undergoes both renal and nonrenal elimination; it is metabolized in the liver to several metabolites, and 20% to 40% is excreted unchanged in the urine.

The exact biodisposition of azithromycin is still being elucidated. The drug probably undergoes some hepatic metabolism and biliary excretion.[13,15,24,25]

Adverse Effects

The most common adverse effects of erythromycin affect the GI tract and are dose related. Erythromycin stimulates smooth muscle and GI motility. Abdominal pain, cramping, nausea, vomiting, and diarrhea are common. Serious side effects are rare but can include eosinophilia, fever, urticaria, and cholestatic hepatitis (erythromycin estolate). Dosage alteration may be necessary in patients with liver impairment. Venous irritation and thrombophlebitis have occurred after intravenous administration of erythromycin gluceptate or lactobionate. Pain can be minimized if dilute solutions are administered over 20 to 60 minutes.

Precautions and Contraindications

Erythromycin, troleandomycin, and clarithromycin, via inhibition of the cytochrome P-450 microsomal enzyme systems, can reduce the hepatic metabolism of some drugs, including benzodiazepines and narcotics. Clearance of intravenous midazolam can be decreased by 54% after concomitant administration of oral erythromycin.[13] Patients should be observed carefully, and the dose should be adjusted in patients receiving these agents concomitantly. Concomitant administration of erythromycin, troleandomycin, and clarithromycin is contraindicated in patients receiving terfenadine, astemizole, cisapride, or pimozide, because macrolide antibiotics can impair metabolism of these drugs, resulting in QT prolongation and lethal dysrhythmias. Although azithromycin and dirithromycin appear to have no effect on the cytochrome P-450 system, it should be kept in mind that they have a pharmacology similar to that of other macrolides, and the possibility that similar drug interactions may occur cannot be ruled out pending further accumulation of data and experience.

Clindamycin

Clindamycin is a derivative of lincomycin and resembles erythromycin in antibacterial activity except that it is more active against many anaerobic bacteria.[13,15,17,24] Essentially all aerobic gram-negative bacilli are resistant. The mechanism of action is similar to that of erythromycin in that clindamycin binds to bacterial cell ribosomes at the 50S site and suppresses protein synthesis.

Pharmacokinetics

Although clindamycin is widely distributed in many fluids and tissues, including bone, significant concentrations are not achieved in the CSF. Clindamycin is partially metabolized to inactive and active metabolites, which are excreted into urine and bile. The serum half-life is 2 to 3 hours in adults and children with normal renal function.

Adverse Effects

Adverse GI effects such as nausea, vomiting, diarrhea, and abdominal pain frequently occur with clindamycin and may be severe enough to necessitate discontinuation of the drug. The high incidence of GI side effects limits its use to infections in which it is clearly superior to other antibiotics.[17] Clindamycin is occasionally associated with potentially fatal antibiotic-associated pseudomembranous colitis. If diarrhea occurs, clindamycin should be discontinued and vancomycin should be administered orally. Clindamycin may potentiate the neuromuscular blockade of nondepolarizing muscle relaxants.[20,21,26] Hypersensitivity reactions can also occur in patients treated with clindamycin.

Precautions and Contraindications

The drug is contraindicated in patients with a hypersensitivity to clindamycin or lincomycin.

Dosage

The usual parenteral dosage of clindamycin in adults is 0.9 to 2.7 g daily administered in two to four equally divided doses. The usual intravenous dosage of clindamycin for children older than 1 month of age is 15 to 40 mg/kg/day (not to exceed adult dose) administered in three or four equally divided doses.

Vancomycin

Vancomycin is a glycopeptide antibiotic that inhibits the biosynthesis of bacterial cell-wall formation and alters the cytoplasmic membrane. It is bactericidal for gram-positive cocci, including strains of *S. aureus* and *Staphylococcus epidermidis* that produce penicillinase or are resistant to methicillin.[13,15,17] *Streptococcus pyogenes*, *S. pneumoniae*, *Streptococcus viridans*, and most strains of *Enterococcus* are also highly susceptible.[24] Resistance to vancomycin has been reported in *Enterococcus faecalis* (formerly *Streptococcus faecalis*) and *Enterococcus faecium* (formerly *Streptococcus faecium*), and strains of vancomycin-resistant enterococci (VRE) have been reported with increasing frequency. According to CDCP surveillance data, approximately 0.3% of enterococci isolated from nosocomial infections in the United States in 1989 were resistant to vancomycin; in 1993 this percentage was 7.9%. Vancomycin is used parenterally to treat endocarditis, osteomyelitis, pneumonia, septicemia, and soft-tissue infections. The oral formulation is used to treat pseudomembranous colitis.

Pharmacokinetics

Oral absorption of vancomycin is poor. It is well distributed throughout the body, and therapeutic levels may be maintained up to 12 hours after administration. Vancomycin is principally excreted by the kidneys, with 90% of a dose being recovered unchanged in the urine.[17] Dosage adjustment in patients with renal impairment is necessary.

Adverse Effects

Rapid intravenous infusion (less than 30 minutes) has been associated with profound hypotension and even, rarely, cardiac arrest.[27-31] Hypotension is typically accompanied by signs of histamine release often characterized by intense facial and truncal erythema ("red man syndrome"). Intravenous administration should be slow (no faster than 1 g per hour) so that histamine release is minimized. Vancomycin may potentiate nondepolarizing neuromuscular blocking agents and may produce hypersensitivity reactions with associated hypotension, rash, and bronchospasm. The most significant untoward reactions to vancomycin have been ototoxicity and nephrotoxicity. Ototoxicity is associated with excessively high concentrations of the drug in plasma (more than 45 mcg/ml). Nephrotoxicity was formerly common but has become an unusual side effect when appropriate doses are used, as judged by renal function.

Precautions and Contraindications

Caution should be exercised when other ototoxic or nephrotoxic drugs such as aminoglycosides are administered concurrently. Renal function should be assessed before initiation of vancomycin therapy and should be monitored at regular intervals during therapy. Vancomycin should not be administered with other intravenous drugs, because it may cause precipitation or inactivation.

Dosage

The intravenous dose for adults with normal renal function is usually 1 g every 12 hours. For children older than 1 month of age with normal renal function, the manufacturers recommend an initial IV dose of 15 mg/kg followed by 40 mg/kg/day given in three or four divided doses daily. For meningitis, up to 60 mg/kg/day has been used. For specific information regarding other pediatric dosage regimens, such as for neonates younger than 1 month of age, specialized references should be consulted. Serum levels should be monitored to obtain troughs less than 5 to 10 mcg/ml for both adults and pediatric patients. For antibiotic-associated *Pseudomonas* colitis caused by *Clostridium difficile*, the usual adult dose is 500 mg every 6 hours, and the usual pediatric dose is 40 mg/kg/day given in three or four divided doses.

Quinolones

The quinolone antibiotics (Box 13-5), by virtue of their broad spectrum of antimicrobial activity against aerobic gram-negative bacilli, staphylococci, and gram-negative cocci, including penicillin-resistant *S. pneumoniae*, and their oral bioavailability are an important class of antibiotics.[32-35] Therapeutic uses

BOX **13-5**

Quinolones and Fluoroquinolones

- Cinoxacin (Cinobac)
- Ciprofloxacin (Cipro)
- Enoxacin (Penetrex)
- Gaitfloxacin (Tequin)
- Gemifloxacin (Factive)
- Levofloxacin (Levaquin)
- Lomefloxacin (Maxaquin)
- Moxifloxacin (Vigamox)
- Norfloxacin (Noroxin)
- Ofloxacin (Floxin)
- Sparfloxacin (Zagam)

include treatment of urinary tract infections, skin and soft-tissue infections, prostatitis, several sexually transmitted diseases, osteomyelitis, and bacterial diarrhea. Quinolones are not first-line agents for most respiratory tract infections because of poor activity against pneumococci.[13,15,36] Doses for selected quinolones are given in Table 13-9.

Pharmacokinetics

The quinolones are well absorbed after oral administration and are widely distributed in body tissues. Serum half-lives range from 3 to 5 hours for norfloxacin and ciprofloxacin and up to 10 to 11 hours for pefloxacin. Most quinolones are eliminated renally, and dose adjustments in patients with renal insufficiency are necessary. Pefloxacin is eliminated nonrenally and should not be used in patients with hepatic failure.

Adverse Effects

The quinolones and fluoroquinolones are generally well tolerated. The most common adverse effects are nausea, diarrhea, headache, and dizziness. Rashes, including photo-sensitivity reactions, also can occur. Sparfloxacin increases the risk of phototoxicity, so patients still get sunburned while using sunscreens or from sun exposure through glass. Patients should avoid sunlight while using sparfloxacin and for 5 days afterward.

Precautions and Contraindications

Quinolone antibiotics are not recommended for use in prepubertal children or during pregnancy because of their potential to produce arthropathy and degenerative articular changes in weight-bearing joints. Sparfloxacin, grepafloxacin, and trovafloxacin can prolong the QT interval and increase the risk of arrhythmias; trovafloxacin was removed from the U.S. market in late 1999 for this reason.[37] When sparfloxacin and grepafloxacin are indicated, they should not be combined with terfenadine, astemizole, certain antiarrhythmics, cisapride, erythromycin, pentamidine, tricyclic antidepressants, some antipsychotics, and other drugs that have similar effects on the QT interval, unless cardiac monitoring is available. Quinolones also inhibit cytochrome P-450 microsomal enzymes and reduce hepatic metabolism of other drugs metabolized via this route (e.g., theophylline) and result in toxicity.

Tetracyclines

The tetracyclines (Table 13-10) consist of four interconnected carbon rings with side chains on which various substitutions are made.[13,15,17] Tetracyclines inhibit protein synthesis by interfering with the bacterial cell ribosome (30S). They are broad-spectrum antibiotics with activity against aerobic and anaerobic gram-positive and gram-negative organisms, including rickettsiae (which cause Rocky Mountain spotted fever), mycoplasmas, and chlamydiae.[24] However, resistance to tetracyclines has reduced their clinical usefulness over the last decade.

Pharmacokinetics

The tetracyclines are widely distributed throughout the body, except the CSF. They are adequately but incompletely absorbed from the GI tract. Absorption is impaired by the presence of milk and antacids, presumably reflecting chelation. Tetracyclines are concentrated in the liver and excreted via bile; decreased hepatic function or obstruction of the common bile duct results in reduced biliary excretion. Tetracyclines, with the exception of doxycycline, also undergo glomerular filtration and renal tubular secretion and may accumulate significantly in the plasma of patients with renal failure.

TABLE 13-9 Parenteral Fluoroquinolones

Generic Name	Brand Name	Usual IV Adult Dose	Available Dosage Forms	Comments
Ciprofloxacin	Cipro	200-400 mg q12h	Injection: 200, 400 mg in glass vials and premixed bags	Infuse over 60 min
Gaitfloxacin	Tequin	200-400 mg q24h	Injection: 200, 400 mg; premixed bags; 400 mg/250 ml	Infuse over 60 min
Levofloxacin	Levaquin	500 mg q24h (for UTI, 250 mg q24h)	Injection: (24 mg/ml) 500, 750 mg; premixed bags; (5 mg/ml) 250, 500, 750 mg	*l*-Isomer of the racemate ofloxacin (another commercially available fluoroquinolone antibiotic); infuse over 60 min
Moxifloxacin	Avelox IV	400 mg q24h	Premixed bags	Infuse over 60 min
Ofloxacin	Floxin	200-400 mg q12h	Injection: 200, 400 mg	Not effective for syphilis; infuse over 60 min
Trovafloxacin	Trovan	200-300 mg qd	Injection: (as alatrofloxacin mesylate) (5 mg/ml) 250, 300 mg	IV formulation contains alatrofloxacin, a trovafloxacin prodrug; infuse over 60 min; case reports of fatal hepatic reactions; use only in cases of life- or limb-threatening infections, and begin therapy in inpatient setting

IV, *Intravenous;* UTI, *urinary tract infection.*
From Mosby's Drug Consult. *St Louis: Mosby; 2004. With permission.*

TABLE 13-10 Tetracycline Dosages

Tetracyclines	Adult Dosage	Pediatric Dosage (age 8-12 yr only)
Demeclocycline (Declomycin)	600 mg/day in divided doses orally	6-12 mg/kg/day in divided doses orally
Doxycycline (Vibramycin)	100 mg orally q12h × 2 doses, then 100 mg per day; or 100-200 mg/day IV in divided doses	Same as adult dose
Methacycline (Rondomycin)	600 mg/day in divided doses	Same as adult dose
Minocycline (Minocin)	200 mg orally or IV followed by 100 mg q12h	4 mg/kg/day orally in 2 divided doses or 4 mg/kg IV followed by 2 mg/kg q12h
Oxytetracycline (Terramycin)	1-2 g/day in four divided doses orally or 0.5-1 g IV per day in divided doses	25-50 mg/kg/day orally in divided doses
Tetracycline (Achromycin V, Panmycin, Robitet, Sumycin, Tetracyn)	1-2 g/day in divided doses orally or 250-500 mg IV q12h	25-50 mg/kg/day in divided doses orally or 10-20 mg/kg/day IV in two or three divided doses

IV, *intravenous*.

Adverse Effects

The most common adverse effects are gastrointestinal: diarrhea, nausea, vomiting, and flatulence. Phototoxicity, characterized by increased sensitivity of the skin to sunlight, can occur. Outdated tetracyclines have been associated with a form of Fanconi's syndrome (nausea, polyuria, polydipsia, or proteinuria), which emphasizes the importance of discarding unused supplies of the drug.[17] Intravenous administration of tetracycline frequently causes thrombophlebitis, especially when intravenous therapy is prolonged or a single vein is used for repeated infusions. Tetracyclines may potentiate neuromuscular blockade produced by neuromuscular blocking agents. An increase in muscular weakness has been reported in a few patients with myasthenia gravis, but a causal relationship has not been established.[13]

Precautions and Contraindications

Tetracyclines should not be administered to pregnant women or children less than 8 years of age. Tetracyclines are deposited in the enamel of teeth, including unerupted teeth, resulting in hypoplasia and brown discoloration of the tooth, presumably because of formation of a tetracycline orthophosphate–calcium complex.[15,17]

Antituberculosis Agents

Rifampin, isoniazid, and ethambutol are important first-line agents (Table 13-11) used in the treatment of tuberculosis. Successful treatment mandates the use of at least two drugs, such as isoniazid and rifampin, in combination for a period of 6 to 9 months, because resistance develops rapidly when a single agent is used. The treatment of tuberculosis has become even more of a challenge because of the emergence of multidrug-resistant organisms and because of the acquired immunodeficiency syndrome (AIDS) pandemic, which has been associated with a marked increase in tuberculosis. Patient noncompliance over the long course of therapy contributes to the development of microbial resistance. Single-agent therapy is used for prophylaxis in patients without apparent disease whose skin test has changed from negative to positive. Prophylaxis should be given for a period of 1 year. The mechanism of action of ethambutol is interference with cell metabolism. Isoniazid inhibits synthesis of the cell wall, and rifampin depresses the initiation of ribonucleic acid (RNA) chain synthesis.[13,15,38]

TABLE 13-11 Antituberculosis Agents

Agent	Adult Dosage
Ethambutol (Myambutol)	25 mg/kg/day orally
Isoniazid (INH)	300 mg/day orally
Rifampin (Rifadin, Rimactane)	600 mg/day orally

Pharmacokinetics

All of the antituberculosis drugs are absorbed adequately orally and are widely distributed into all body tissues and cells. Isoniazid is hepatically acetylated, and the metabolite is excreted in the urine. Rifampin undergoes deacetylation, and the resulting metabolite enters the bile. The elimination half-time is prolonged in patients with hepatic dysfunction. Ethambutol has a high renal clearance; up to 50% of a dose is excreted unchanged by the kidneys.[17]

Adverse Effects

Isoniazid increases the excretion of the B vitamin pyridoxine, resulting in peripheral neuritis and anemia. This effect can be minimized by prophylactic therapy with pyridoxine 10 mg daily. Isoniazid may precipitate seizures, and caution should be exercised with use of other medications such as enflurane or flumazenil, which can also precipitate seizures. Isoniazid significantly enhances defluorination of volatile anesthetics, presumably by inducing the necessary hepatic microsomal enzymes.[39] Isoniazid and ethambutol may cause optic neuritis, resulting in a decrease in visual acuity and loss of ability to perceive the color green. The incidence of this effect is dose related and occurs in less than 5% of patients who receive therapeutic doses.

The most common, and notable, side effect of rifampin is a red color to body secretions (tears, urine, saliva) of patients treated with this drug. Rifampin is a potent inducer of cytochrome P-450 microsomal enzymes, and its administration results in a decreased half-life for a number of compounds, including barbiturates, oral anticoagulants, oral contraceptives, benzodiazepines, propranolol, phenytoin, and digoxin.

Precautions and Contraindications

Patients receiving isoniazid, and to a lesser extent rifampin, should be carefully evaluated at intervals for symptoms of hepatitis (anorexia, malaise, fatigue, nausea, and jaundice) and warned to discontinue the drug if such symptoms occur. Some clinicians advocate determining serum aspartate aminotransferase levels at regular intervals.

DYES

Dyes (Table 13-12) are commonly administered perioperatively by anesthesia providers. Methylene blue is the intervention of choice for methemoglobinemia (decreased oxygen-carrying capacity and cyanosis).[40] Dyes are also given to color the urine so that disruptions in the urinary tract may be detected by the surgeon. Indocyanine is used in the measurement of cardiac output by the indicator-dilution method. Anesthesia providers can also administer dyes for diagnostic purposes, such as the confirmation of an aspiration by instillation of the agent down a tract of endotracheal tube or the filling of an endotracheal tube cuff with dye so that a perforation during laser surgery of the airway is readily apparent.[41] Dyes are also frequently added to succinylcholine intravenous infusions for identification purposes.

Isosulfan blue (Lymphazurin) is frequently administered during sentinel node biopsy in breast cancer patients to stain lymphatic channels for mapping as an aid to diagnosis and dissection. Preoperative lymphoscintigraphy is performed with technetium 99 m sulfur colloid followed by intraoperative isosulfan injection. Incidence of allergic reactions including anaphylaxis has been reported to be 0.7% to 1.6%.[42-44] Isosulfan dye may cause discoloration of the patient's serum, mimicking hypoxia on the pulse oximeter even though oxygenation is normal. Blue hives that transform to blue patches have also been noted.[45] Anaphylactic reactions quickly respond to standard treatment with antihistamines, corticosteroids, and epinephrine.[42,46] Isosulfan may also be used for liver and spleen scans and gastric emptying studies.

Radiocontrast media, which may be used during certain surgical procedures, cause allergic-like reactions in 5% to 10% of patients.[47] Urticaria (1%) and dyspnea (0.25%) may occur. Severe reactions (0.01%) are rare. The mechanism is unclear, and they are not IgE mediated. Skin testing is not helpful. A history of previous reaction, atopy, or asthma may signal a likeliness for reactions.

Pharmacokinetics

In patients with normal renal function, indigo carmine is cleared rapidly from the circulation after intravenous administration and has a plasma half-life of 4.5 minutes. It is excreted principally by the kidneys and usually appears in the urine within 10 minutes after intravenous injection.

TABLE 13-12 Dye Doses

Dye	Adult Dosage
Indigo carmine	5-40 mg IV
Indocyanine green	5 mg in 1 ml injected rapidly via cardiac catheter; 1-2 mg/kg IV for methemoglobinemia
Methylene blue	65-130 mg orally q8-12h as a urinary tract diagnostic aid

IV, *Intravenous*.

Indocyanine green is excreted rapidly unchanged in the bile, and it has a plasma half-life of 2 to 3 minutes. Methylene blue is excreted in the urine and via the bile.[13,15]

Adverse Effects

As mentioned previously, clinically used dyes have an important effect on pulse oximetry. Indigo carmine and indocyanine green can transiently decrease SaO_2. Methylene blue and isosulfan blue result in a more marked transient decrease in SaO_2. Occasional idiosyncratic reactions such as rash, pruritus, and bronchospasm may occur; these may be treated with diphenhydramine or epinephrine if needed. These reactions appear to be caused by a direct histamine-releasing effect rather than an allergic reaction. Indigo carmine has mild α pressor effects, and hypertension and reflex bradycardia lasting up to 30 minutes after injection can occur. Methylene blue may cause hypertension, nausea, and dizziness.

Precautions and Contraindications

Indocyanine green contains iodine, and caution should be used in patients with preexisting iodine allergy.

ANTINEOPLASTIC AGENTS

Chemotherapy is a therapeutic approach in which antineoplastic agents are used alone or, more commonly, in synergistic combinations with surgery or radiation for the eradication of malignant cells. The goal of cancer chemotherapy is to selectively kill malignant cells while sparing normal cells, because a single remaining cancer cell has the potential to proliferate, invade, or metastasize to distant sites. The chemotherapeutic agents are most effective for the treatment of rapidly proliferating cells; slow-growing malignant cells, such as carcinoma of the lung and colon, are often unresponsive to chemotherapeutic drugs. This rapid proliferation is characteristic of most malignancies, but some normal cells, such as hair follicles, bone marrow, lymphoid organs, and GI mucosa, also proliferate rapidly. The side effects commonly associated with the chemotherapeutic agents (bone marrow depression, leukopenia, thrombocytopenia, alopecia, nausea, vomiting, and stomatitis) are caused by susceptibility of these normal, rapidly dividing cells to the agents.[13,15,17,41,48]

The antineoplastic agents are commonly divided into several classifications, each having unique pharmacology, mechanisms of action, and side effects. Knowledge of drug-induced side effects and evaluation of appropriate laboratory tests are useful in the preoperative evaluation of patients being treated with chemotherapeutic drugs. Attention to asepsis is essential, because immunosuppression makes these patients susceptible to iatrogenic infection.

Alkylating Agents

Alkylating agents (Box 13-6) include the nitrogen mustards, alkyl sulfonates, and nitrosoureas. These chemotherapeutic drugs have the common property of undergoing electrophilic chemical reaction that results in alkylation with DNA. The result is miscoding of DNA information and damage to the DNA molecule. Cyclophosphamide is probably the most commonly used alkylating agent; its clinical spectrum of activity is broad, and it has been used in combination with other drugs in Hodgkin's disease, lymphosarcoma, acute lymphoblastic leukemia of childhood, carcinoma of the breast, and Burkitt's lymphoma.

BOX 13-6

Alkylating Agents

Nitrogen Mustards
Chlorambucil (Leukeran)
Cyclophosphamide (Cytoxan, Neosar)
Mechlorethamine (Mustargen)
Melphalan (L-Sarcolysin)
Uracil Mustard

Aziridinyl Derivative
Thiotepa

Alkyl Sulfonates
Busulfan (Myleran)

Nitrosoureas
Carmustine (BiCNU)
Lomustine (CeeNU)
Semustine (Methyl-CCNU)
Streptozocin

Triazines
Dacarbazine (DTIC-Dome)

Adverse Effects

In addition to the usual adverse effects of chemotherapeutic agents, pneumonitis and pulmonary fibrosis are potential adverse effects of alkylating drugs.[17] Inhibition of plasma cholinesterase activity may be responsible for prolonged skeletal muscle paralysis after administration of succinylcholine or mivacurium.[49] Hepatotoxicity is a possible side effect of cyclophosphamide, although it is much more common with streptozocin. Approximately 70% of patients who receive this drug develop hepatic or renal toxicity. Streptozocin can also induce hyperglycemia as a result of selective destruction of pancreatic β-cells.

Antimetabolites

Antimetabolites are chemotherapeutic agents (Box 13-7) that are structural analogs of normal metabolites required for normal cell function and replication. Methotrexate, for example, is a folic acid analog. Folic acid is an essential dietary factor that is essential for eventual synthesis of DNA and RNA. Normal cells can be protected from lethal damage by the folate antagonist methotrexate by concomitant administration of leucovorin rescue therapy.

BOX 13-7

Antimetabolites

Folic Acid Analogs
Methotrexate (Amethopterin)

Pyrimidine Analogs
Fluorouracil
Cytarabine

Purine Analogs
Mercaptopurine
Thioguanine

Adverse Effects

In addition to the usual adverse effects of myelosuppression, alopecia, nausea, and vomiting caused by chemotherapeutic agents, methotrexate can cause renal and hepatic toxicity. Occasionally, neurologic manifestations, including an acute cerebellar syndrome, have been reported with fluorouracil.

Vinca Alkaloids

The *Vinca* alkaloids (Box 13-8) are natural products derived from the periwinkle plant. These drugs block mitosis in rapidly dividing cells. The most important use of vinblastine is with other antineoplastics in the treatment of testicular tumors; lymphomas, including Hodgkin's disease, are also responsive.

Adverse Effects

Myelosuppression is more common with vinblastine. Alopecia and GI effects are more common with vincristine. Neuromuscular abnormalities occur in 5% to 20% of patients and include skeletal muscle weakness, ataxia, tremors, peripheral neuropathy, weakness of the extraocular muscles, and weakness of the larynx, which manifests as hoarseness.[17]

Antibiotic Antineoplastic Agents

The anthracycline antibiotics (Box 13-9) and their derivatives are among the most important antitumor agents. They are derived from fungus and differ only slightly in chemical structure. The antibiotic antineoplastic agents are effective against rhabdomyosarcoma; Wilms' tumor; Kaposi's sarcoma; leukemias; lymphomas; and breast, prostate, ovarian, endometrial, thyroid, cervical, and head and neck carcinomas. They are also beneficial in small cell carcinoma of the lung, Hodgkin's disease, and sarcomas. The clinical usefulness of these agents is limited by dose-dependent cardiomyopathy.

BOX 13-8

Vinca Alkaloids

Vinblastine
Vincristine (Oncovin)
Vindesine

BOX 13-9

Antibiotic Antineoplastic Agents

Dactinomycin (Actinomycin D)
Daunorubicin, daunomycin (Cerubidine)
Doxorubicin (Adriamycin)
Bleomycin (Blenoxane)
Plicamycin (Mithramycin)
Mitomycin

Adverse Effects

Cardiomyopathy is a unique characteristic of the anthracycline antibiotics, particularly daunorubicin and doxorubicin. Two types of cardiomyopathies may occur.[17,48,50] The first is an acute form that occurs in approximately 10% of patients and is characterized by abnormal electrocardiographic changes that include nonspecific ST-T changes, supraventricular tachydysrhythmias, and decreased QRS voltage and left-axis deviation. These abnormalities occur at all dose levels and, except for the decreased QRS voltage, resolve 1 to 2 months after discontinuation of therapy. A reversible reduction in ejection fraction occurs within 24 hours of a single dose. The second type of cardiomyopathy is a chronic, cumulative dose-related toxicity that occurs in 2% of patients; it manifests as a severe cardiomyopathy that can lead to irreversible congestive heart failure that may not respond to therapeutic interventions. A total dose as low as 250 mg/m^2 of body surface area can produce this myocardial toxicity. The risk increases markedly to more than 20% of patients at 550 mg/m^2 of body surface area, and this total dose should not be exceeded. Acute left ventricular failure 2 months after the cessation of treatment with doxorubicin has been described during general anesthesia.[51] Preoperative echocardiograms are useful in evaluating the extent of toxicity.

The most serious adverse effect of bleomycin is pulmonary toxicity in 5% to 10% of patients; 1% to 2% of all patients who receive bleomycin die from this complication.[17] The risk of toxicity is greatest in elderly patients and those who receive more than 400 U total dose.[13,15,17] Rales and rhonchi commonly precede radiographic changes, which usually reveal interstitial pneumonitis that may progress to pulmonary fibrosis generally appearing 4 to 6 weeks after the initiation of therapy. Patients treated with bleomycin may be at greater risk of developing postoperative adult respiratory distress syndrome.[52] One speculation is that increased concentration of oxygen facilitates production of superoxide and other free radicals in the presence of bleomycin, although this has never been proved. For this reason, it has been recommended that inhaled concentrations of oxygen during surgery be maintained below 30% in bleomycin-treated patients. Another recommendation is fluid replacement with colloids rather than crystalloids to prevent pulmonary interstitial edema. Hypersensitivity reactions ranging from chills and fever to anaphylactic reactions can also occur with bleomycin.

Fatal hemorrhagic diathesis may occur in 1% to 5% of patients treated with plicamycin.[13,15,17] This may reflect impaired synthesis of clotting factors in addition to thrombocytopenia. Partial thromboplastin time is frequently prolonged. Hepatic and renal toxicity may also occur.

Miscellaneous Drugs

Heavy Metal Complex

Cisplatin is a heavy metal inorganic complex that disrupts the DNA helix.[13,15,17] It is frequently used in combination with other drugs, especially in testicular and ovarian carcinomas.

Adverse Effects. Cisplatin is probably one of the most emetogenic of all cancer chemotherapeutic agents, and marked nausea and vomiting occur in almost all patients. Renal toxicity can occur, and hydration before and after the dose is indicated. Ototoxicity and myelosuppression have also been noted.

Hormones

Hormones and antagonists are also used in the treatment of neoplastic diseases. Most of these agents can cause fluid retention and hypercalcemia. Plasma calcium concentrations should be determined at intervals in patients receiving these hormones.

DRUGS USED IN THE TREATMENT OF PSYCHIATRIC DISORDERS

Psychiatric disorders and their associated drugs are classified in many ways. Frequently such drugs are referred to as *antipsychotics* when they have beneficial effects on mood and thought in acute psychosis or *neuroleptics* when used in patients who are not psychotic; *antidepressants*, or mood-elevating drugs; *mood-stabilizing* drugs; and *antianxiety* agents.

Antipsychotic Agents

The antipsychotic agents (Box 13-10) are used for treatment of psychosis. Schizophrenia is the disease most often associated with psychosis; however, psychotic symptoms may be evident in drug abuse, dementia of the Alzheimer's type, and certain types of depression. The clinical manifestations of psychosis are characterized by impairment of reality, hallucinations, delusions, impaired judgment, severe excitement, paranoia, and violent aggression. Some antipsychotic agents are also used in the treatment of intractable hiccups and antiemetic therapy.[13,15,41,53]

Phenothiazines and Thioxanthenes

Phenothiazines (e.g., chlorpromazine) and thioxanthenes were widely used in the past as antipsychotics. The quality of life was dramatically improved for schizophrenics in the 1950s when chlorpromazine was discovered. Phenothiazines and thioxanthenes provided symptomatic relief in 70% of schizophrenics.[53]

BOX 13-10

Antipsychotics

Phenothiazines
Acetophenazine maleate (Tindal)
Butaperazine maleate (Repoise)
Chlorpromazine hydrochloride (Thorazine)
Fluphenazine (Permitil, Prolixin)
Mesoridazine besylate (Serentil)
Perphenazine (Trilafon)
Prochlorperazine (Compazine)
Thioridazine hydrochloride (Mellaril)
Trifluoperazine hydrochloride (Stelazine)
Triflupromazine hydrochloride (Vesprin)
Thioxanthenes
Chlorprothixene (Taractan)
Thiothixene (Navane)
Butyrophenones
Haloperidol (Haldol)
Droperidol (Inapsine)
Atypical Antipsychotics
Clozapine (Clozaril)
Risperidone (Risperdal)
Olanzapine (Zyprexa)

However, a significant delay existed in their onset of action, with a therapeutic benefit often attained only after 4 to 8 weeks. These drugs are antagonists at acetylcholine, dopamine, serotonin, and norepinephrine receptors; however, their efficacy seems to depend on the ability of these drugs to disrupt dopaminergic neurotransmission in the basal ganglia and limbic system.[13,15,53]

Adverse Effects. Many side effects are an extension of the pharmacologic actions of these drugs and result from the blockade of several receptors. The antihistaminergic properties of these antipsychotics are probably responsible for producing the sedative effects, and they may have additive or synergistic effects with narcotics, barbiturates, and benzodiazepines. The antiadrenergic properties cause orthostatic hypotension, and reflex tachycardia and profound hypotension have occurred during spinal, epidural, and general anesthesia. The pressor effects of norepinephrine and other related drugs may also be blocked. The anticholinergic properties cause dry mouth, blurred vision, and urinary retention. These agents lower the seizure threshold; therefore, caution should be used with enflurane, ketamine, and flumazenil. Other side effects result from blockade of dopamine in specific brain regions. Extrapyramidal symptoms, including parkinsonian syndrome, characterized by bradykinesia and muscle rigidity; akathisia; and acute dystonic reactions are common. Tardive dyskinesia, characterized by involuntary and excessive oral-facial movements, can be disfiguring and can impair feeding.

An uncommon but potentially lethal side effect of antipsychotics is neurolept malignant syndrome (NMS), characterized by muscle rigidity, diaphoresis, and cardiovascular instability. Immediate intervention with administration of bromocriptine (a dopamine agonist), cessation of the agent causing the syndrome, and administration of dantrolene is necessary. An important distinction between NMS and malignant hyperthermia is that patients with NMS maintain normocapnia, in contrast to the increase in end-tidal CO_2 noted in patients with malignant hyperthermia.[54]

Butyrophenones

The butyrophenones haloperidol and droperidol, like phenothiazines, can reduce the anxiety of psychosis. Haloperidol has formerly been widely used as an antipsychotic agent; however, it shares the side effects and toxicities of the phenothiazines and thioxanthenes. Droperidol is commonly administered in the perioperative period for antiemetic therapy.

Atypical Antipsychotics

The clinical profile of the newer atypical antipsychotics differs from that of the typical antipsychotics in terms of side effects. The atypical ones are associated with a very low incidence of extrapyramidal symptoms and little or no tardive dyskinesia. The major adverse effect of clozapine therapy is agranulocytosis, characterized by leukopenia. Because agranulocytosis can be fatal, weekly blood cell counts must be performed in patients taking clozapine. The incidence of agranulocytosis associated with olanzapine and risperidone is no greater than with typical antipsychotics.[13,15,53,54]

Antidepressant Drugs

Tricyclic Antidepressants and Others

Tricyclic antidepressants (TCAs) (Box 13-11) have two benzene rings joined by a central seven-member ring. Imipramine is the prototype of the tricyclic antidepressants and was originally synthesized in 1948 as an antihistaminic sedative. It was noticed, however, that patients with signs and symptoms of depression showed a lessening of their depression. The most prominent action of TCAs is the blockade of reuptake of norepinephrine and serotonin from the synapse back into the nerve terminal without blocking the reuptake of dopamine. The nontricyclic antidepressant agents (Box 13-12) have the same mechanism of action as the tricyclic antidepressants and similar side effects that are somewhat less intense.

BOX 13-11

Tricyclic Antidepressants

Amitriptyline (Elavil, Endep, Enovil)
Amoxapine (Asendin)
Clomipramine (Anafranil)
Desipramine (Norpramin)
Doxepin (Adapin, Sinequan)
Imipramine (Tofranil)
Nortriptyline (Aventyl, Pamelor)
Protriptyline (Vivactil)
Trimipramine (Surmontil)

Adverse Effects. Numerous adverse effects are common with the TCAs. Anticholinergic effects such as sedation, nausea, vomiting, urinary retention, dry mouth, and blurred vision are troublesome for approximately 15% of patients. Other effects include hypotension and cardiac arrhythmias (often lethal in overdosage).

Monoamine Oxidase Inhibitors

The monoamine oxidase (MAO) inhibitors (Box 13-13) are used in the treatment of depression refractory to TCAs. They are as efficacious as TCAs (approximately 60% of patients respond to therapy), but MAO inhibitor therapy requires patient compliance with diet and concurrent medication use and it may cause hepatotoxicity. The MAO inhibitors inhibit the enzyme MAO, which is present at adrenergic nerve endings and is responsible for the degradation of epinephrine, norepinephrine, dopamine, and serotonin, and thereby cause an increase in the monoamine concentrations in the nerve terminal.

Adverse Effects. Adverse effects associated with MAO inhibitors include dry mouth, blurred vision, orthostatic hypoten-

BOX 13-12

Nontricyclic Antidepressants

Amoxapine (Asendin)
Bupropion (Wellbutrin)
Nefazodone (Serzone)
Trazodone (Desyrel)

Tetracyclics

Maprotiline (Ludiomil)
Mirtazapine (Remeron)
Venlafaxine (Effexor)

BOX 13-13

Monoamine Oxidase Inhibitors

Isocarboxazid (Marplan)
Phenelzine (Nardil)
Tranylcypromine (Parnate)

sion, and sedation. Toxic effects from overdosage can result in agitation, convulsions, hallucinations, hyperreflexia, and hyperpyrexia. A common recommendation is that MAO inhibitors be discontinued for a period of 14 to 21 days before elective surgery. It is now recognized that this approach may place patients at risk for psychiatric complications, including suicide. There is growing appreciation that anesthesia can be administered safely in the presence of chronic use of these drugs.[17]

Precautions and Contraindications. Meperidine is contraindicated with MAO inhibitor use and may result in an immediate severe reaction that manifests as excitation, hypertension, hyperthermia, sweating, and rigidity. Tyramine-containing foods (beer, cheese, wine, chicken liver), indirect-acting sympathomimetic agents (ephedrine, mephentermine), levodopa, methyldopa, guanethidine, and reserpine can cause hypertensive crisis in patients

Selective Serotonin Reuptake Inhibitors

Selective serotonin reuptake inhibitors (SSRIs) (Box 13-14) are newer antidepressants that are efficacious in the treatment of depression, obsessive-compulsive disorders, eating disorders, and personality disorders. SSRIs block the reuptake of serotonin at the synaptic cleft. The main advantage of the SSRIs compared with the MAO inhibitors and TCAs is their lower incidence of side effects, enhanced patient compliance resulting from once-daily dosing, and relative overdose safety.[8,13,15,17]

Adverse Effects. Nausea, headache, diarrhea, nervousness, insomnia, and sedation are relatively common problems with SSRIs. Impairment of sexual functioning can occur more frequently with some agents in this class than with others.

Precautions and Contraindications. SSRIs and selective norepinephrine reuptake inhibitors are highly protein bound, and caution should be exercised when other highly protein bound medications are given concomitantly. A case of serotonin syndrome was reported in a patient receiving sertraline (98% protein bound in serum), possibly because of displacement by lidocaine after an ankle block and sedation with fentanyl and midazolam, all highly protein-bound drugs.[54] Serotonin syndrome is a toxic hyperserotonergic state characterized by mental status changes, myoclonus, hyperreflexia, hyperpyrexia, hypertension, shivering, diaphoresis, restlessness, and tremor. Symptoms usually resolve with supportive treatment and cessation of the causative agent; however, at least five deaths have been reported. Rare cases of neuroleptic malignant syndrome have also been reported.[54]

BOX 13-14

Selective Serotonin Reuptake Inhibitors

Sertraline (Zoloft)
Fluoxetine (Prozac)
Venlafaxine (Effexor)
Paroxetine (Paxil)
Fluvoxamine (Luvox)
Citalopram (Celexa)
Escitalopram (Lexapro)
Reboxetine (Vestra)*

**Selective norepinephrine reuptake inhibitor.*

Lithium

Lithium is a mood-stabilizing drug, the treatment of choice for bipolar disorder (manic-depressive illness). Structurally, lithium is the lightest of the alkali metals, and the salts of this monovalent cation have characteristics similar to those of potassium and sodium. The mechanism of action of efficacy in bipolar disorder is unknown.[55]

The serum lithium level for treatment of acute mania is between 1 and 1.5 mEq/L, and for long-term control the desirable serum lithium level is 0.6 to 1.2 mEq/L.

Adverse Effects. The most common adverse effects from lithium are gastrointestinal and include nausea, vomiting, diarrhea, polyuria, polydipsia, and renal impairment. T-wave inversions may be seen on the electrocardiogram. Lithium toxicity is characterized by vomiting, diarrhea, coarse tremor, coma, ataxia, and convulsions. The neurologic manifestations of lithium toxicity may be irreversible, sometimes progressing to death. Dialysis should be considered for patients exhibiting symptoms of toxicity or in whom lithium concentrations are greater than 4 mEq/L.

Precautions and Contraindications. Potentiation of the effects of nondepolarizing and depolarizing muscle relaxants may occur.[13,15,17] Concentrations of lithium must be monitored to facilitate safe use of the drug because of a narrow therapeutic window. Toxicity may occur close to therapeutic levels (less than 2 to 3 mEq/L). Thiazide diuretics or sodium restriction may precipitate lithium toxicity.

REFERENCES

1. Nichols RL. Preventing surgical site infections: a surgeon's perspective. *Emerg Infect Dis*. 2001;7:220-224.
2. Center for Disease Control and Prevention. National Nosocomial Infections Surveillance (NNIS) report, data summary from October 1986-April 1996, issued May 1996. A report from the NNIS System. *Am J Infect Control*. 1996:24:380-388.
3. Burke JP. Maximizing appropriate surgical antibiotic prophylaxis: an update from LDS hospital. *Clin Infect Dis*. 2001;33(suppl 2): S78-S83.
4. Gaynes RP, Culver DH, Horan TC, et al. Surgical Site Infection (SSI) Rates in the United States, 1992-1998: The National Nosocomial Infection Surveillance System Basic SSI Risk Index. *Clin Infect Dis*. 2001;22(suppl 2):S69-S77.
5. Weed HG. Antimicrobial prophylaxis in the surgical patient. *Med Clin North Am*. 2003;87:59-75.
6. Martone WJ, Nichols RL. Recognition, prevention, surveillance, and management of surgical site infections: introduction to the problem and symposium overview. *Clin Infect Dis*. 2001;33(suppl 2) S67-S68.

7. Chambers H. Antimicrobial agents: general considerations. In: Hardman JG, Limbird LE, Goodman Gilman, A, eds. *Goodman and Gilman's the Pharmacological Basis of Therapeutics*. 10th ed. New York: McGraw-Hill; 2001:1143-1170.
8. Karchmen AW. Infective endocarditis. In: Braunwald E, et al, eds. *Harrison's Principles of Internal Medicine*. 15th ed. New York: McGraw-Hill; 2001:809-816.
9. Dajani A, et al. Prevention of bacterial endocarditis: recommendations by the American Heart Association. *JAMA*. 1997; 277:1794-1801.
10. Steckelberg JM, Wilson WR. Risk factors for infective endocarditis. *Infect Dis Clin North Am*. 1993;7:9-19.
11. Dajani AS, et al. Prevention of bacterial endocarditis. *JAMA*. 1990;264:2919-2922.
12. Ferrieri P, Gewitz MH, Gerber MA, et al. Unique features of infective endocarditis in childhood. *Circulation*. 2002;105: 2115-2127.
13. McEvoy G, ed. *American Hospital Formulary Service Drug Information*. Bethesda, Md: American Society of Health-System Pharmacist; 1999.
14. Petri W. Penicillins, cephalosporins, and other β-lactam antibiotics. In: Hardman JG, Limbird LE, Goodman Gilman, A, eds. *Goodman and Gilman's the Pharmacological Basis of Therapeutics*. 10th ed. New York: McGraw-Hill; 2001:1189-1218.
15. Antibiotics. In: *Mosby's Drug Consult*. St. Louis: Mosby; 2004.
16. Pallasch TJ. Principles of pharmacotherapy: III. Drug allergy. *Anesth Prog*. 1988;35:178-189.
17. Stoelting RK. *Pharmacology and Physiology in Anesthesia Practice*. Philadelphia: Lippincott; 1999:469-470.
18. Austen F. Allergies, anaphylaxis and systemic mastocytosis. In: Braunwald E, et al, eds. *Harrison's Principles of Internal Medicine*. 15th ed. New York: McGraw-Hill; 2001:1913-1921.
19. Chambers H. The aminoglycosides. In: Hardman J, et al, eds. *Goodman and Gilman's the Pharmacological Basis of Therapeutics*. 10th ed. New York: McGraw–Hill; 2001:1219-1238.
20. Pittinger C, Adamson R. Antibiotic blockade of neuromuscular function. *Annu Rev Pharmacol*. 1972;12:169-184.
21. Pittinger CP, Eryasa T, Adamson R. Antibiotic-induced paralysis. *Anesth Analg*. 1970;49:487-501.
22. Sladen RN. Renal physiology. In: Miller R, ed. *Anesthesia*. 5th ed. Philadelphia: Churchill Livingstone; 2000:686-687.
23. Snavely SR, Hodges GR. The neurotoxicity of antibacterial agents. *Ann Intern Med*. 1984;101:92.
24. Chambers H. Protein synthesis inhibitors and miscellaneous antibacterial agents. In: Hardman JG, Limbird LE, Goodman Gilman, A, eds. *Goodman and Gilman's the Pharmacological Basis of Therapeutics*. 10th ed. New York: McGraw-Hill; 2001:1239-1272.
25. Steigbigel NH. Macrolides and clindamycin. In: *Mandell, Douglas, and Bennett's Principles and Practice of Infectious Diseases*. 4th ed. London: Churchill Livingstone; 1995:334-346.
26. Morey TE, Guyton TS. Antibiotics. In: Atlee JL, ed. *Complications in Anesthesia*. Philadelphia: Saunders; 1999:194.
27. Lyon GD, Bruce DL. Diphenhydramine reversal of vancomycin-induced hypotension. *Anesth Analg*. 1988;67:1109-1110.
28. Mayhew JF, Deutsch S. Cardiac arrest following administration of vancomycin. *Can Anaesth Soc J*. 1985;32:65-66.
29. Miller R, Tausk HC. Anaphylactoid reaction to vancomycin during anesthesia. *Anesth Analg*. 1977;56:870-872.
30. Southorn PA, Plevak DJ, Wilson WR. Adverse effects of vancomycin administered in the perioperative period. *Mayo Clin Proc*. 1986;61:721-724.
31. Symons NLP, Hobbes AFT, Leaver HK. Anaphylactoid reactions to vancomycin. *Can Anaesth Soc J*. 1985;32:65-66.
32. Petri W. Sulfonamides, trimethoprim-sulfamethoxazole, quinolones, and agents for urinary tract infections. In: Hardman JG, Limbird LE, Goodman Gilman, A, eds. *Goodman and Gilman's the Pharmacological Basis of Therapeutics*. 10th ed. New York: McGraw-Hill; 2001:1171-1188.
33. Clement J, et al. In vitro and in vivo evaluations of A-80556, a new fluoroquinolone. *Antimicrob Agents Chemother*. 1994;38: 1071-1078.
34. Sanders CC. Ciprofloxacin: in vitro activity, mechanism of action, and resistance. *Rev Infect Dis*. 1988;10:516-527.
35. Hooper DC, Wolfson JS. Fluoroquinolone antimicrobial agents. *N Engl J Med*. 1991;324:384-394.
36. Levofloxacin. In: *Mosby's Drug Consult*. St Louis: Mosby; 2004.
37. Sparfloxacin. In: *Mosby's Drug Consult*. St Louis: Mosby; 2004.
38. Petri W. Drugs used in the chemotherapy of tuberculosis, *Mycobacterium avium* complex disease, and leprosy. In: Hardman JG, Limbird LE, Goodman Gilman, A, eds. *Goodman and Gilman's the Pharmacological Basis of Therapeutics*. 10th ed. New York: McGraw-Hill; 2001:1273-1294.
39. Mazze R, Woodruff RE, Heerdt ME. Isoniazid-induced enflurane defluorination in humans. *Anesthesiology*. 1982;57:5-8.
40. Stoelting R. *Handbook of Pharmacology and Physiology in Anesthetic Practice*. Philadelphia: Lippincott-Raven; 1995:131.
41. Sherbinski L, Nagelhout J. Additional drugs of interest. In: *Nurse Anesthesia*. Philadelphia: Saunders; 1997:491-510.
42. Sprung J, Tully MJ, Ziser A. Anaphylactic reactions to isosulfan blue dye during sentinel node lymphadenectomy for breast cancer. *Anesth Analg*. 2003;96:1051-1053.
43. Montgomery LL, Thorne AC, Van Zee JK, et al. Isosulfan blue dye reactions during sentinel lymph node mapping for breast cancer. *Anesth Analg*. 2002;95:385-388.
44. Lyew MA, Gamblin TC, Ayoub M. Systemic anaphylaxis associated with intramammary isosulfan blue injection used for sentinel node detection under general anesthesia. *Anesthesiology*. 2000;93:1145-1146.
45. Cimmino VM, Brown AC, Szocik JF, et al. Allergic reaction to isosulfan blue during sentinel node biopsy: a common event. *Surgery*. 2001;130:439-442.
46. Albo D, Wayne JD, Hunt KK. Anaphylactic reactions to isosulfan blue dye during sentinel lymph node biopsy for breast cancer. *Am J Surg*. 2001;182:393-398.
47. Dipiro JT, Ownby DR, Schlesselman LS. Allergic and pseudoallergic drug reactions. In: Dipiro JT, et al, eds. *Pharmacotherapy: A Pathophysiologic Approach*. New York: McGraw-Hill; 2002: 1585-1597.
48. Selvin BL. Cancer chemotherapy: implications for the anesthesiologist. *Anesth Analg*. 1981;60:425-434.
49. Zsigmond EK, Robins G. The effect of a series of anticancer drugs on plasma cholinesterase activity. *Can Anaesth Soc J*. 1972;19: 75-82.
50. Chabner B, et al. Antineoplastic agents. In: Hardman J, et al, eds. *Goodman and Gilman's the Pharmacological Basis of Therapeutics*. 10th ed. New York: McGraw-Hill; 2001:1389-1460.
51. Borgeat A, et al. Perioperative cardiovascular collapse in a patient previously treated with doxorubicin. *Anesth Analg*. 1988;67:1189-1191.
52. Goldiner PL, et al. Factors influencing postoperative morbidity and mortality in patients with bleomycin. *BMJ*. 1978;1:1664-1667.
53. Gudelsky G. Antipsychotic agents. In: Brody TM, Larner J, Minneman KP, eds. *Human Pharmacology: Molecular to Clinical*. 3rd ed. St Louis: Mosby; 1998:339-348.
54. Beauchamp C, Nagelhout J. Serotonin agonists and antagonists. *AANA J*. 1997;65:271-281.
55. Frazer A, Morilak DA. Drugs for the treatment of affective (mood) disorders. In: Brody TM, Larner J, Minneman KP, eds. *Human Pharmacology: Molecular to Clinical*. 3rd ed. St Louis: Mosby; 1998:349-363.

CHAPTER 14

CHEMISTRY AND PHYSICS

MICHAEL BOYTIM

Chemistry is the science that deals with structure and composition of matter. The study of physics investigates the behavior of atoms and molecules that make up elements of matter. For many years, these sciences made valuable contributions to the field of medicine.

The trend in the education of nurse anesthetists is not only to teach them to carry out tasks, but also to introduce them to the fundamental theory relating to these procedures. Knowledge of chemistry and physics serves as a basis for study of other sciences (e.g., anatomy and physiology, pathophysiology, pharmacology, and basic and advanced principles of anesthesia). As students progress through the anesthesia curriculum, the concepts of these courses are applied to the clinical decision-making process in the perioperative care of the anesthetized patient.

The following reasons have been cited for the study of chemistry and physics by anesthesia personnel:

1. It serves as a foundation for the study of other disciplines.
2. Its significant relationships with other courses help define the art of anesthesia.
3. It helps anesthesia personnel provide for the safety and comfort of patients and handle equipment appropriately.
4. It assists in development of an understanding of contributions made to the care of the sick, conquest of disease, and improvement of health.

PHYSICS

Relationship among Temperature, Pressure, and Volume

Temperature

Heat is a form of energy, and its intensity is by convention measured on one of three temperature scales: the Kelvin or absolute zero scale; the centigrade (Celsius) scale; and the Fahrenheit scale.[1] The Kelvin scale begins at absolute zero (−273.16° C) and moves only in an upward direction. The centigrade scale is based on the freezing and boiling points of water and allows 100° between the two to accommodate the decimal-based measurements of the metric system; the scale was set at base 0° (water's boiling point). In the Fahrenheit scale, water freezes at 32° and boils at 212°, a difference of 180°. The ratio (based on the freezing and boiling points of water) of the Fahrenheit scale to the centigrade scale is 180° to 100°, or 1.8:1. The temperature scales are illustrated in in Figure 14-1.

The ratio of freezing to boiling points of water from the Fahrenheit to the Celsius to the Kelvin scale is 1.8. Therefore the conversion factor among the scales is 1.8. Certain formulas are required for the conversion of temperatures from one scale to the next, as shown in the examples that follow.

Equation 14-1 Celsius to Fahrenheit

$$°F = (°C \times 1.8) + 32$$

For example,
$°F = (37° C \times 1.8) + 32$
$°F = 66.6 + 32$
$°F = 98.6$

Equation 14-2 Fahrenheit to Celsius

$$°C = (°F - 32)/1.8$$

For example,
$°C = (98.6° F - 32)/1.8$
$°C = 6.6/1.8$
$°C = 37$

Equation 14-3 Celsius to Kelvin

$$°K = °C + 273.16$$

For example,
$°K = 37° C + 273.16$
$°K = 310.16$

Equation 14-4 Kelvin to Celsius

$$°C = °K - 273.16$$

For example,
$°C = 310.16° K - 273.16$
$°C = 37$

Equation 14-5 Fahrenheit to Kelvin
First convert °F to °C
Then convert °C to °K

For example,
$°C = (98.6° F - 32)/1.8$
$°C = 37$
$°K = 37 + 273.16$
$°K = 310.16$

Equation 14-6 Kelvin to Fahrenheit
First convert °K to °C
Then convert °C to °F

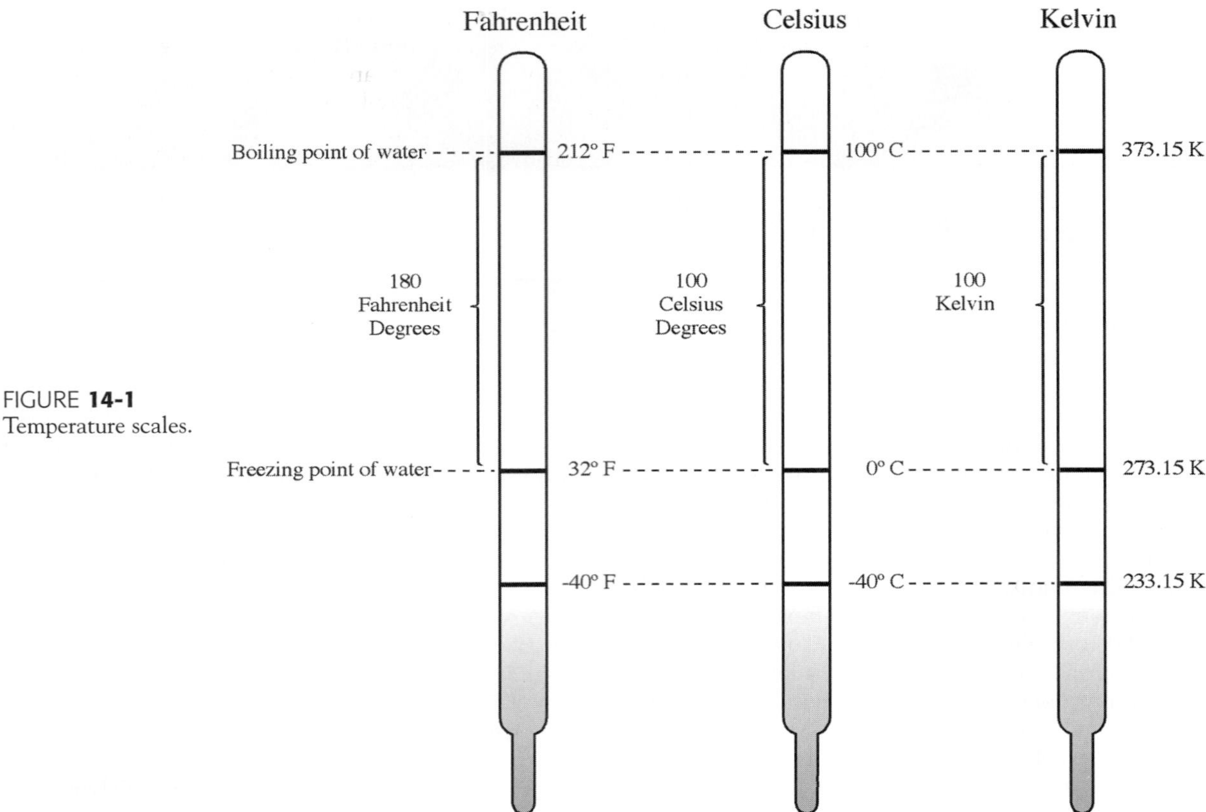

FIGURE **14-1**
Temperature scales.

For example,
°C = 310.16° K − 273.16
°C = 37
°F = (37 × 1.8) + 32
°F = 98.6

Transfer of Heat. The operating room environment presents a challenge to the nurse anesthetist with regard to temperature regulation of patients. Conditions in the operating room are conducive for hypothermia. Heat is transferred from areas of high to areas of low temperatures. The transfer of heat in the operating room occurs from patient to the physical environment because of the difference in their temperatures. Four mechanisms of heat transference can occur:

1. Conduction: transfer of heat from one molecule to another (10%)
2. Radiation: transfer of heat in electromagnetic waves (40%)
3. Convection: transfer of heat by air currents; operating room air currents turnover = 15/hour (30%)
4. Evaporation: transfer of heat through humidity (20%)

Conduction requires direct contact. Net energy movement is from warmer areas to cooler areas. Heat loss via conduction in the body is very slow. All objects emit electromagnetic radiation, and the amount is determined by the object's temperature and surface area. Warm and cool objects emit radiation at different rates. Radiation heat loss is from warmer areas to cooler areas. Evaporation heat loss occurs when water evaporates from the skin and respiratory tract at a rate of 30 cc/hour. In order for water to be converted to vapor, heat is required.[2]

In the operating room, heat is lost through cold intravenous (IV) fluids and air currents (convection); cold room temperature and surgical table (conduction); exposure of patients (radiation); and cold dry gases (evaporation). Vulnerable patient populations include children, whose large body surface area and lack of adequate body fat leads to potential temperature loss, and the elderly, who lack the ability to increase basal metabolic rate to increase heat production. Mechanisms to decrease heat loss include use of heating mattresses; heating of the room and IV fluids (conduction); use of warm blankets or forced air warmers (radiation and convection); and use of heat-moisture exchanges or humidifiers on anesthesia circuits (evaporation).

Pressure

Pressure is the force exerted by atoms and molecules. It is generated by kinetic energy. Movement of atoms and molecules is not uniform; the speed, direction, and movement vary. Gases can travel great distances and can expand indefinitely. Little intermolecular force is exerted between gas molecules. Gases can also be easily compressed. When molecules of gases collide, pressure is exerted. When gases are compressed, the sum of molecular forces occurs in a closed container and is called *cylinder pressure*. Cylinder pressure is measured in pounds-per-square-inch gauge (PSIG). When a cylinder of compressed gas is empty, the pressure inside the cylinder is equal to atmospheric pressure. A full tank (E cylinders) of oxygen measures 2200 PSIG; a full tank of nitrous oxide measures 745 PSIG.

A Bourdon gauge measures cylinder or pipeline pressures (PSIG) of anesthetic gases. This type of gauge is based on an aneroid type of measurement (without mercury). A hollow metal tube is bent into a curve, sealed, and linked into a clock-like mechanism.[3] One end is connected to the compressed gas source. As the pressure of the gas in the cylinder increases, the tube tends to straighten out, causing the gauge to read higher pressures. The American Society for Testing and Measuring

(ASTM) International for Bourdon type gauges standards include 38-mm diameter, lowest pressure between the 6 and 9 o'clock positions, and name and color of the gas marked on the gauge (Figure 14-2).

Pressure of a gas other than compressed gas may be measured in millimeters of mercury (mm Hg or torr) or centimeters of water (cm H_2O). The atmospheric pressure of gases at sea level is equal to 760 torr or 1034 cm H_2O.

Volume

Volume is the space occupied by an aggregate or collection of atoms and molecules. Volume is measured in centimeters or meters (solids) or milliliters or liters (liquids and gases). Liquids are measured by collecting the volume in a measured cylinder. Gases are measured by flowmeters (air, nitrous oxide, oxygen) or respirometers (exhaled tidal volume). A Wright respirometer measures exhaled tidal volumes by rotation of a vane, which causes gears to turn. It does not rotate when flow is reversed, such as during inspiration. It is therefore not used to measure continuous flow.

Newer electronic respirometers eliminate the need for mechanical gears and are more accurate. Beams of light are emitted across a vane to detectors. When an exhaled breath occurs, the vane spins, causing interruptions in the beam, which is converted to a digital readout of tidal volume.[4]

Gas Laws

There are two types of gas laws: ideal and general.

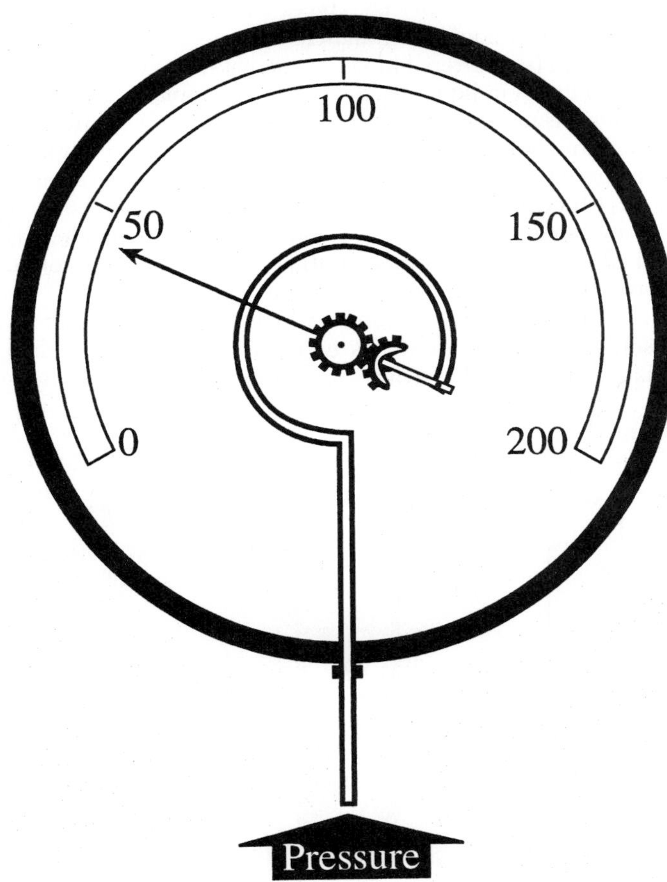

FIGURE 14-2
Bourdon pressure gauge.

Ideal Gas Laws

Ideal gas laws demonstrate the interrelationship among temperature, pressure, and volume. Ideal gas laws include Boyle's, Charles's, and Gay-Lussac's laws.

Boyle's law states that at a constant temperature, the volume of gas varies inversely with the pressure. It is written as P1V1 = P2V2. For example, at room temperature a volume of gas is 500 ml at sea level. What is the volume of gas at an atmospheric pressure of 380 torr?

Equation 14-7

$$(760)(500) = (380)(x)$$
$$(380000) = (380x)$$
$$(1000) = (x)$$

If the pressure is decreased by half, the volume is doubled.

Charles's law states that at a constant pressure a volume of gas is directly proportional to the temperature. It is written as V1/T1 = V2/T2. For example, at sea level a balloon of helium occupies a volume of 200 ml in a room with a temperature of 19° C. What is the volume of the helium balloon when it is taken outside at a temperature of 38° C?

Equation 14-8

$$200/19 = x/38$$
$$400 = x$$

If the temperature is doubled, the volume is doubled.

Gay-Lussac's law states that at a constant volume, the pressure of a gas is directly proportional to the temperature. It is written as P1/T1 = P2/V2. For example, a full cylinder of oxygen is placed on an anesthesia gas machine at a room temperature of 20° C. The room is accidentally heated to 40° C. What is the gauge pressure of oxygen in the tank?

Equation 14-9

$$2200/20 = x/40$$
$$4400 = x$$

If the temperature is doubled, the pressure is doubled.

General Gas Laws

Gases have a number of distinguishing properties. They expand easily and are readily compressed, have high velocity, weak intermolecular forces, and a high degree of random motion. These characteristics are addressed in several gas laws.

Fick's Law of Diffusion. Fick's law of diffusion states that the rate of diffusion of a gas is directly proportional to the surface area of the membrane through which the gas diffuses, the solubility of the gas, and the partial pressure gradient of the gas between two areas and is indirectly proportional to the square root of the molecular weight of the gas, the thickness of the membrane through which the gas travels, and temperature. It is written as follows:

Equation 14-10

$$\text{Vgas} = \frac{\text{Area} \times \text{Solubility} \times \text{Partial pressure difference}}{\text{Molecular weight} \times \text{Distance} \times \text{Temperature}}$$

The following factors affect the rate of diffusion of a gas according to Fick's law of diffusion.

1. A = Surface area:
   a. The greater the surface area, the greater the diffusion
   b. In patients with chronic obstructive pulmonary disease (COPD) and postoperative atelectasis, decrease A of alveolar capillary membrane
2. Distance (thickness):
   a. Increased distance, decreased diffusion
   b. In patients with pulmonary edema or fibrosis, increase distance of alveolar capillary membrane
3. Henry's law—the amount of gas dissolved in a liquid is:
   a. Directly proportional to the partial pressure of the gas over the liquid. Oxygen, which has a partial pressure of 100 torr in the alveoli at room air, diffuses from the alveoli to the pulmonary capillary, in which the partial pressure of oxygen is 40 torr. Carbon dioxide (CO_2), which has a partial pressure of 45 torr in the pulmonary capillary, diffuses from the capillary to the alveoli, in which the partial pressure of CO_2 is near zero. Henry's law is illustrated in Figure 14-3.
   b. Indirectly proportional to the temperature:
      - Increased temperature, decreased dissolved gas
      - Decreased temperature, increased dissolved gas
      - Hypothermic patients remain anesthetized longer
        - Febrile patients require more anesthesia
4. Graham's law—the rate of diffusion of a gas is:
   a. Indirectly proportional to the square root of the gram molecular weight (GMW) of the gas

Equation 14-11

$$CO_2 = 6.6 \text{ GMW}$$
$$O_2 = 5.5 \text{ GMW}$$

   b. Directly proportional to its solubility coefficient

Equation 14-12

$$CO_2 = 0.510$$
$$O_2 = 0.023$$

For example,

Equation 14-13

$$(CO_2)\ 0.510{:}6.6 = 0.023{:}5.5\ (O_2)$$
$$2.856 = 0.1518$$
$$20 = 1$$

CO_2 diffuses 20 × faster than O_2.
Both Henry's and Graham's laws are incorporated into Fick's law of diffusion.

5. **Dalton's law**—the total pressure exerted by a mixture of gases in a closed container at a given temperature is equal to the sum of the pressure that each gas exerts. The pressure of each individual gas is its partial pressure. For example, a cylinder of compressed air contains 21% oxygen and 79% nitrogen. Each gas therefore exerts it own partial pressure to equal 100%. Dalton's law is illustrated in Figure 14-4.

Solutions

A solution is a homogeneous mixture of 2 or more substances, which may or may not be present in equal proportions.

There are two parts to solutions: a solute, which is the dissolved substance, and the solvent, which is the substance into which the solute is placed. Types of anesthetic solutions include solid in liquid (e.g., muscle relaxant in sterile water), gas in liquid (e.g., arterial blood gases), gas in gas (e.g., N_2O in O_2), and liquid in liquid (neostigmine in atropine).

Solutions may be unsaturated, saturated, or supersaturated. An unsaturated solution permits the addition of more solute. A saturated solution does not allow the addition of more solute, which may result in precipitation of the solute. A supersaturated solution allows more solute to be added when heat is applied; cooling causes precipitation. The amount of solute dissolvable in a solvent is temperature dependent.

A suspension is a solution in which the solute cannot be dissolved. The solute remains intact as fine particles with a milky appearance (Diprivan). A colloid is a substance whose

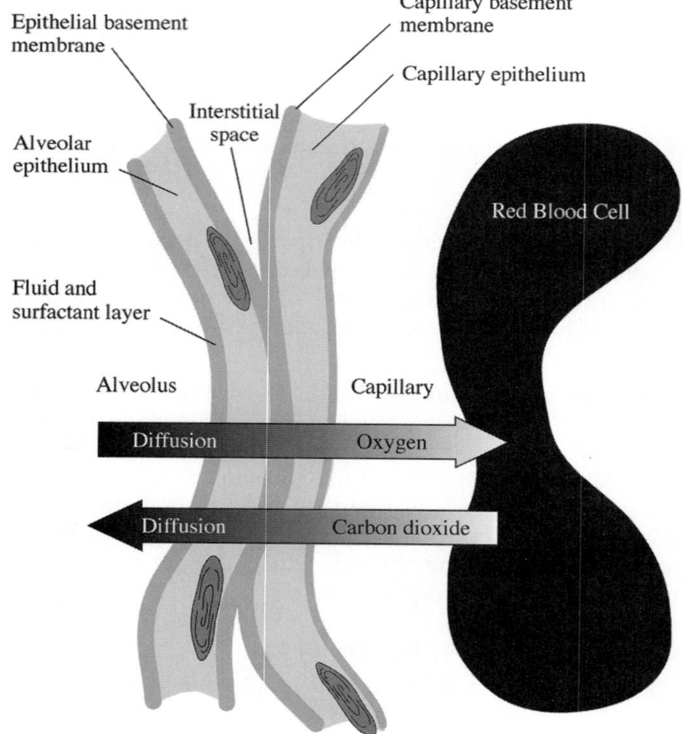

FIGURE **14-3**
Alveolar-capillary membrane.

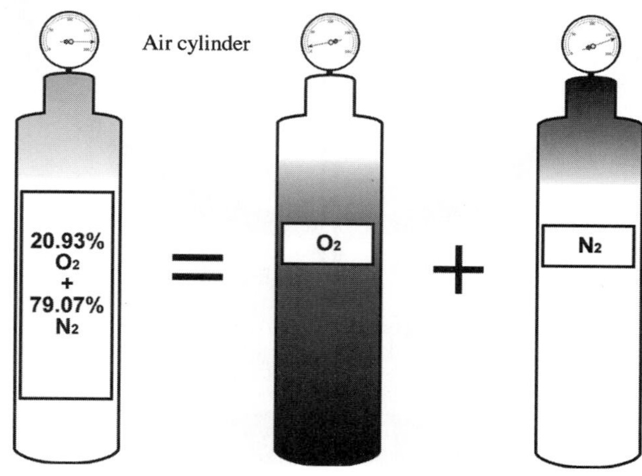

FIGURE **14-4**
Gas composition of air cylinder.

characteristics are between those of a solution and those of a suspension. It occurs when solutes are too small to be suspended and too large to dissolve in a solution.

Water is considered to be the universal solvent. It has a very low density of 1 g/ml. Water is altered by temperature. Heat increases density, whereas cooling decreases density. This is why ice floats.

One of the most valuable functions of water is its ability to dissolve many different substances. This ability is a result of the chemical nature of water. An individual water molecule is "bent" or **V**-shaped, with an H-O-H angle of 105 degrees.[5] The molecular configuration of water is shown in Figure 14-5.

The O-H bonds in the water molecule are covalent bonds formed by electron sharing between the oxygen and hydrogen atoms. The electrons are shared unequally between oxygen and hydrogen. Oxygen has a greater affinity for the electrons of hydrogen. Oxygen becomes slightly more negative, and hydrogen becomes slightly more positive. The "positive ends" of water become attracted to other negatively charged anions, and the "negative ends" become more attractive to positively charged cations. This process is called *hydration*. When ionic substances such as salt (NaCl) are added to water, they break up into individual cations (Na^+) and anions (Cl^-) and dissolve into a solution.

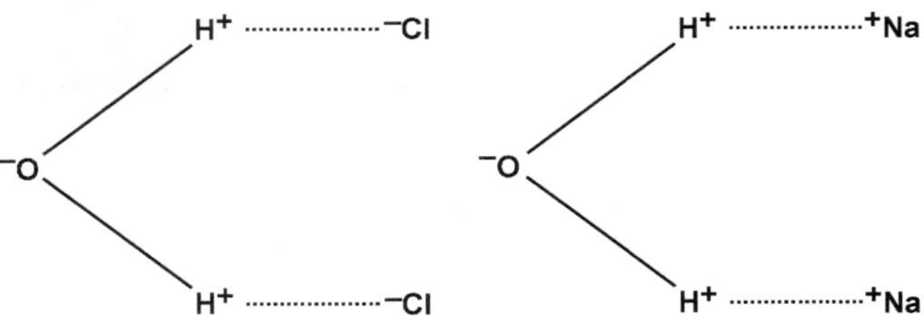

FIGURE **14-5**
Molecular configuration of water.

Movement of Solutions through Membranes

Solutions move through membranes by two methods: diffusion and osmosis. Diffusion is the movement of solute and solvent across a permeable membrane. Movement occurs from an area of high concentration to an area of lower concentration until concentrations are equal. The diffusion of sodium chloride and water is shown in Figure 14-6.

Osmosis is the movement of solvent only across a semipermeable membrane. The solvent, not solute, moves from an area of low concentration to an area of high concentration. Pressure that moves the solvent is called osmotic pressure (pulling pressure). Osmosis of water is shown in Figure 14-7.

Tonicity of Solutions

Any two fluids separated by a semipermeable membrane can be isotonic, hypertonic, or hypotonic relative to each other. Isotonic solutions exert equal osmotic pressures; no movement of solvent occurs. Examples are normal saline (0.9% NaCl) and red blood cells. Hypertonic solutions are solutions in which one solution has a higher osmotic pressure than the other. Examples are 3% normal saline and red blood cells. Hypertonicity causes solvent to be drawn out of the cell, resulting in crenation of the cell. Hypotonic solutions are solutions in which one solution has a lower osmotic pressure than the other. Examples are water and red blood cells. Water (low osmotic pressure) moves into the cell (higher osmotic pressure), causing the cell to rupture. This is often referred to as *hemolysis*. The tonicity of solutions between cells is illustrated in Figure 14-8.

Flow of Solutions through Tubes and Orifices

Anesthetic solutions (gases and liquids) are administered through a variety of circuits and tubing of different lengths and orifice sizes. A tube is defined as a pathway whose length is greater than its diameter, whereas an orifice is an opening whose diameter is greater than its length. Flow rates of solutions through tubes depend on the cross-sectional area of the tube, the pressure difference between the proximal and distal portions of the tube, the length of the tube, and the viscosity and density of the solution.

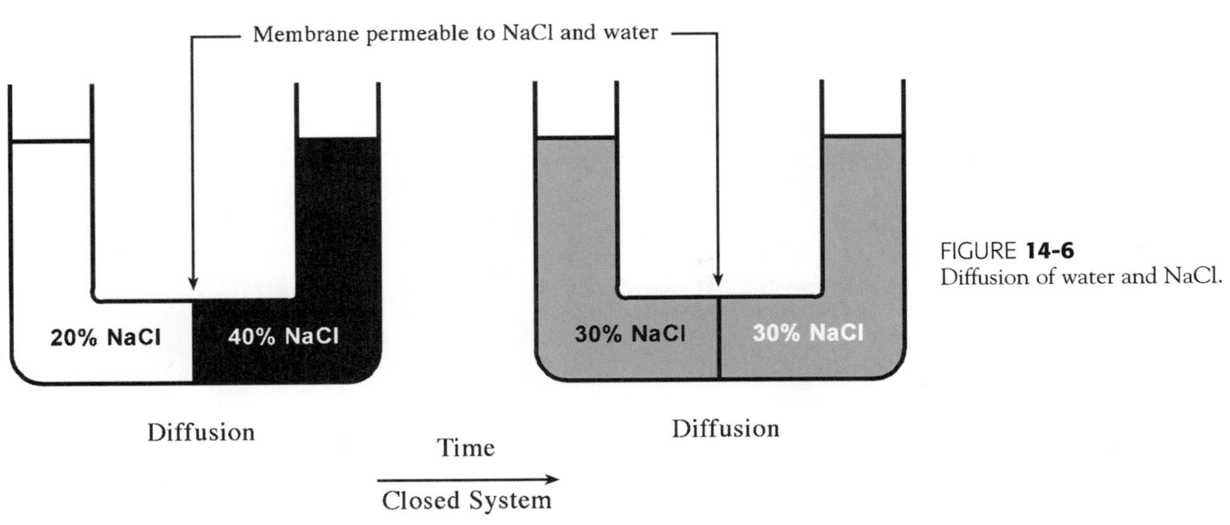

FIGURE **14-6**
Diffusion of water and NaCl.

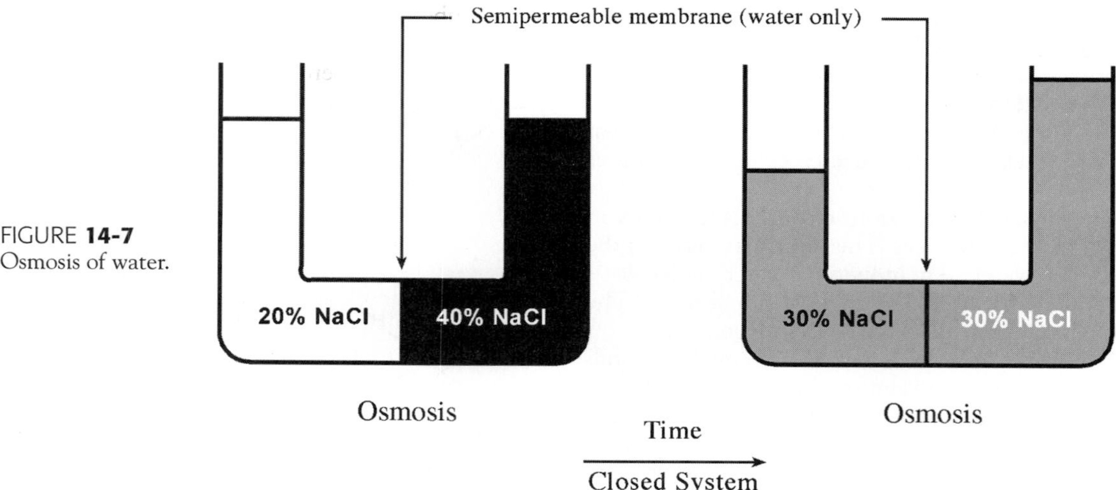

FIGURE **14-7**
Osmosis of water.

Three types of flow occur through tubes and orifices: laminar, turbulent, and transitional. Laminar flow is a type of flow in which all molecules of a gas or liquid travel in a parallel path within the tube. The molecules in the center of the tube encounter the least adhesive force with the walls of the tube and therefore move at a greater velocity than those closest to the walls.[6] True laminar flow only occurs in the smallest airways (terminal bronchioles). Laminar and turbulent airflow are illustrated in Figure 14-9.

Laminar flow is governed by Poiseuille's law:

Equation 14-14

$$\text{Flow} = \frac{\text{Pressure gradient} \times \text{radius to the fourth power of radius}}{\text{Viscosity} \times \text{Length}}$$

The greater the inflow is on one side of the tube (pressure gradient) than the outflow pressure is on the opposite side of the tube, the greater the flow.

Radius has the most dramatic effect on flow. A doubling of the radius results in a 16-fold increase in flow. A tripling of the radius increases flow 81-fold. A halving of the radius decreases flow by 1/16. Therefore flow through a 16-gauge angiocatheter is greater than 20 gauge. If the viscosity of solution is increased, flow decreases. Patients with polycythemia have decreased blood flow.

Increasing the length of a tube decreases flow because of decreased pressure difference. Decreasing the tube length by half results in a doubling of the flow. If the length of a tube is doubled, flow decreases by half. Clinical application of

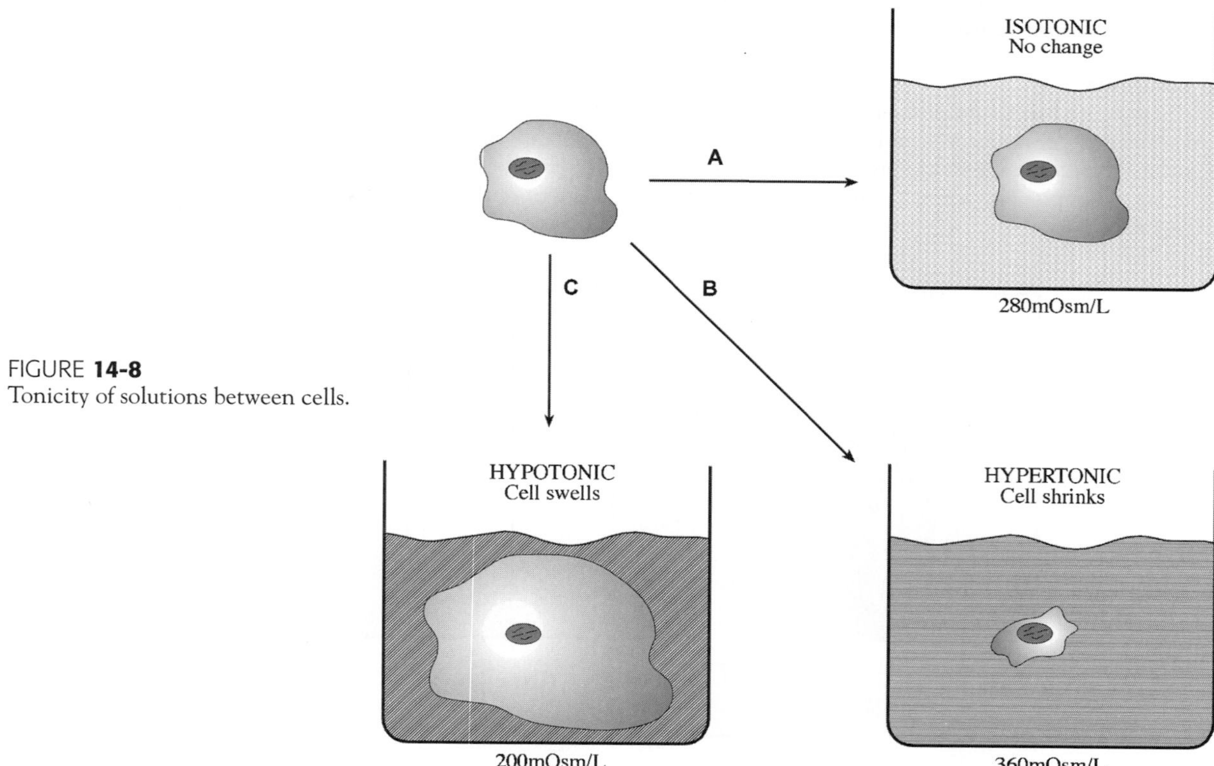

FIGURE **14-8**
Tonicity of solutions between cells.

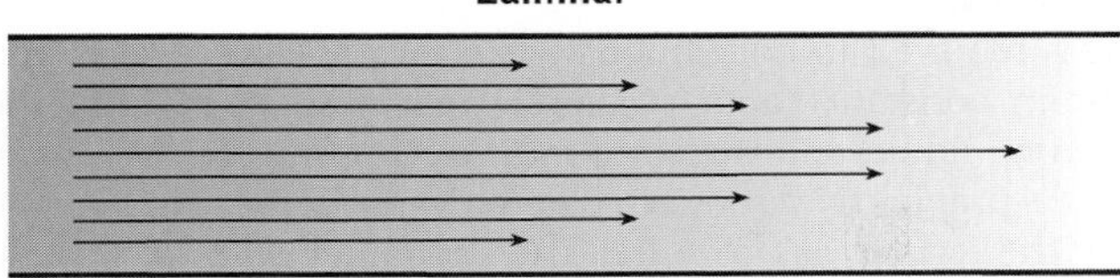

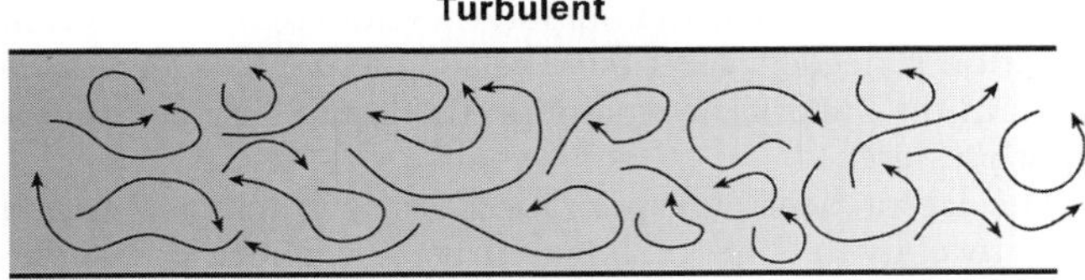

FIGURE **14-9**
Laminar and turbulent air flow in a tube.

Poiseuille's law in anesthesia is exemplified as follows. To run 1 unit of packed red blood cells quickly, a 16- to 18-gauge IV catheter (radius) is used, a pressure bag is placed on the packed red blood cells (pressure difference), and the packed red blood cells are diluted with normal saline (viscosity).

Turbulent flow results when molecules of a solution encounter the walls of the tube in a rough, tumbling pattern. Flow becomes turbulent when velocity of the flow is high, the tube wall is rough (corrugated), kinks or bends exist in the system (laminar flow becomes turbulent if the angle is >25 degrees), the density of a solution is increased, or the radius of the tube is large. Turbulent flow occurs in medium to large airways.

Turbulent flow is governed by Reynold's number; flow changes from laminar to turbulent when Reynold's number >2000. Reynold's number is directly proportional to the density of the solution, linear velocity of the flow, and tube diameter; flow is inversely proportional to fluid viscosity.

Transitional flow is a mixture of laminar and turbulent flow. It occurs at branch points (carina) or points distal to partial obstructions. Transitional flow is illustrated in Figure 14-10.

Another factor that governs flow of solutions is Bernoulli's law. This law states that when a solution flows through a constricted region of a tube, the velocity of flow increases and the lateral pressure exerted by the solution on the walls of the tube decreases. The Venturi mask and nebulizer are applications of this law. With the Venturi mask, room air is entrained through small holes as 100% oxygen flows through a constricted region of the tube. A specific fraction of inspired oxygen can therefore be delivered to the patient. In nebulization of a medication, as 100% oxygen flows past a constriction, medication is entrained into the system and hits a baffle (ball), where it is broken into fine droplets to be inhaled by the patient.

In anesthesia the flowmeter measures and indicates the rate of flow of a gas passing through it. Measurement of the flow of gases is based on the principle that flow past a resistance is proportional to pressure.[7] The flowmeter measures the drop in pressure when a gas passes through a resistance (the indicator or bobbin) and correlates this to the amount of gas delivered (e.g., 2 L, 5 L).

Flow meters in anesthetic gas machines are based on the Thorpe tube type, which has a variable orifice (tapered). The smallest diameter is at the bottom. Gas enters the base, which causes the indicator to rise. The anesthetic gas machine flow meter is shown in Figure 14-11.

The gas flows through an annular opening around the indicator. The annular opening increases in size as the height of the indicator rises up the tube. Therefore the height of the indicator is a measure of gas flow. The rate of flow through the flowmeter depends on the pressure drop across the constriction, the size of the annular opening, and the physical characteristics of the gas (gases that are denser need a wider tube). Therefore flowmeters can never be changed and used for another gas.

VAPORIZATION

Most of the inhalational anesthetic agents in use today are liquids and must be converted to vapor to be inhaled. Vapor is the gaseous phase of a substance that is otherwise liquid at room temperature and atmospheric pressure. Vaporization is the conversion of a liquid to a gas. A vaporizer is an instrument designed to facilitate the change of a liquid anesthetic into vapor. Vaporization depends on the vapor pressure of the agent, temperature of the environment, and amount of carrier gas used (nitrous oxide or oxygen).

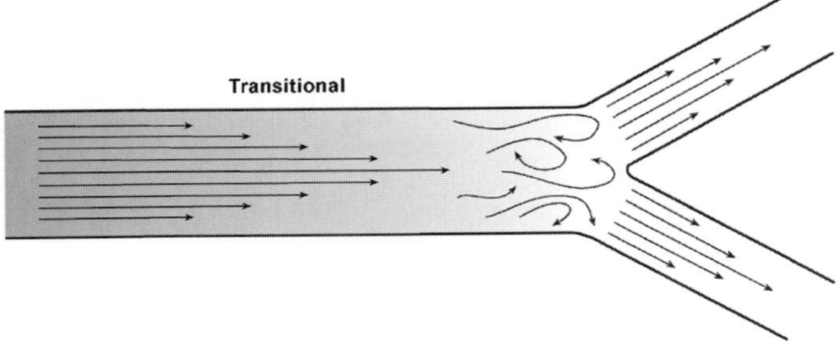

FIGURE **14-10**
Transitional air flow in a tube.

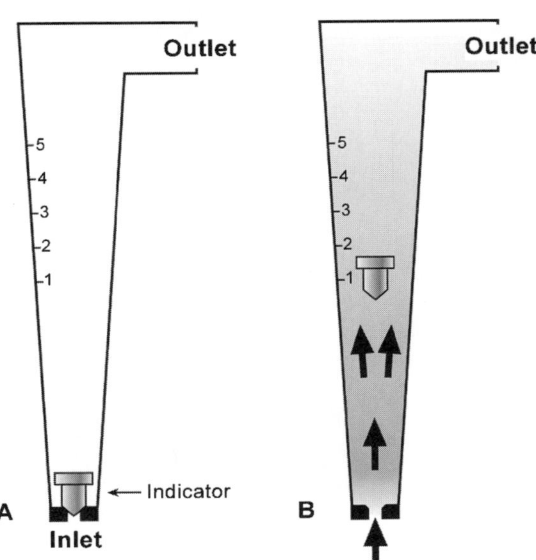

FIGURE **14-11**
Gas flow through anesthesia gas machine flow meter.

Vapor Pressure

When liquid is inside a closed container, molecules of liquid break away and enter the space above it to form a vapor. At a constant temperature the numbers of molecules entering and exiting the liquid phase become equal, and the number of molecules in the vapor phase remains constant. These molecules bombard the walls of the container, creating a pressure called the *saturated vapor pressure*. When the numbers of molecules entering and exiting the liquid phase become equal, the space above the liquid becomes saturated with vapor. An equilibrium is reached between the liquid and vapor phases at a constant temperature, creating vapor pressure of the liquid below.

A volatile anesthetic agent is a liquid that has an inherent tendency to change to a vapor at standard temperature and pressure; the higher the volatility of an agent, the stronger its tendency to enter the vapor phase and, therefore, the higher its vapor pressure.

Saturated vapor pressures (in torr) of common volatile anesthetic agents at standard temperature and pressure are as follows:

- Fluothane: 243
- Isoflurane: 238
- Desflurane: 660
- Sevoflurane: 160

Heat increases vapor pressure; more molecules enter the gas (vapor) phase than the liquid phase. Cooling decreases vapor pressure; more molecules enter the liquid phase than the gas phase. Passing a carrier gas (N_2O/O_2) over the liquid decreases vapor pressure. Phases of vapor pressure in any anesthetic vaporizer are shown in Figure 14-12.

Temperature

Heat is required to continuously vaporize volatile agents and maintain constant vapor pressure. Heat is supplied from the remaining liquid and the surroundings (housing of the vaporizer). As previously discussed, when a vaporizer is turned on to allow the carrier gas to enter the container to pick up and deliver anesthetic vapors to the patient, vapor pressure decreases. The liquid agent now generates more vapor to keep a constant vapor pressure. As vapor is generated, heat is lost. The temperature of the liquid and vaporizer structure decrease. This results in a decrease in vapor pressure of the volatile agent and a decrease in vaporizer output, therefore temperature compensation is needed. Heat must be supplied to the liquid anesthetic in the vaporizer to maintain the liquid temperature and vapor pressure.

The latent heat of vaporization is the amount of heat it takes to convert 1 ml of liquid to vapor. The following are latent heats of vaporization for the various volatile agents:

- Fluothane: 20° C, 68° F
- Isoflurane: 25° C, 77° F
- Desflurane: 39° C, 102° F
- Sevoflurane: not specified

The heat that is supplied to the volatile liquid anesthetic agent occurs through the thermal conductivity of the construction material of the vaporizer. Thermal conductivity is the ability to conduct heat from the environment, store it in the vaporizer body, and continuously supply it to the liquid anesthetic.[8] In order for the temperature of the liquid anesthetic to remain constant, modern vaporizers are constructed from materials of high thermal conductivity. The higher the

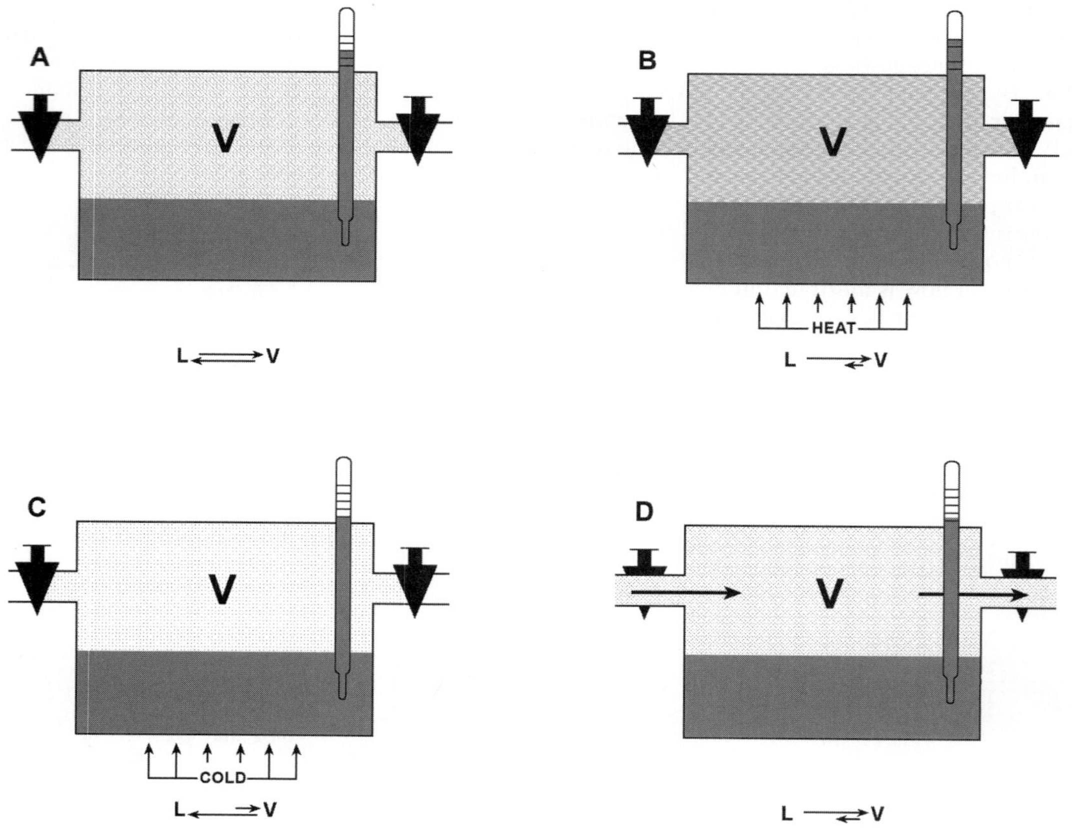

FIGURE **14-12**
Phases of vapor pressure in an anesthetic vaporizer.

thermal conductivity, the better the substance conducts heat. Some common construction materials for vaporizers include copper (Copper Kettle Vaporizer) in older vaporizers and bronze, stainless steel, and aluminum in newer vaporizers. In order to keep a constant vapor pressure of fluothane at 243 torr the vaporizer must continuously supply enough heat (temperature) to the liquid. The fluothane vaporizer must be maintained at 20° C. Because of this the vaporizer for fluothane is said to be temperature compensated.

Desflurane is the only volatile anesthetic agent whose vaporizer requires supplied heat. An electrical heater is used to supply heat to the vaporizer to maintain a constant temperature and vapor pressure. This is because desflurane is very volatile (vapor pressure of 660 torr) and changes quickly into a vapor phase. Because heat is needed to change desflurane from a liquid to a vapor, desflurane needs to be maintained at a higher temperature to prevent the liquid from cooling and to maintain a constant vapor pressure.

Boiling point is the temperature at which all of the liquid is in the vapor phase. Common boiling points of volatile agents are as follows:

- Fluothane: 50° C, 122° F
- Isoflurane: 48° C, 118° F
- Desflurane: 23° C, 73° F
- Sevoflurane: 58° C, 136° F

Because desflurane boils out at room temperature, it is supplied in a closed bottle that cannot be opened to air. It is filled directly into its vaporizer.

Specific heat is the amount of heat required to raise the temperature of a liquid 1° C. The higher the specific heat, the more heat required to raise the temperature of the liquid. The most volatile anesthetic agents possess low boiling points, high latent heats of vaporization, and high specific heats. Therefore desflurane is the most volatile anesthetic agent.

Amount of Carrier Gas

As previously discussed, when a vaporizer is turned on a carrier gas flows through its chamber to pick up and deliver anesthetic vapors to the patient. To produce clinically consistent output concentrations, a vaporizer must have one of two designs: concentrated calibrated (newer vaporizers) or measured flow (older vaporizers).

When a concentrated calibrated vaporizer is turned on, it directs a portion of the carrier gas entering the vaporizer into the vaporizing chamber in which the liquid anesthetic agent is contained. The remainder bypasses the chamber altogether. They are joined at the vaporizer outlet. The amount that enters the vaporizing chamber is determined by the dial on top of the vaporizer. For example, if the dial on a fluothane vaporizer is set to 2%, more carrier gas is directed into the vaporizing chamber than if the dial is set to 1%. Such vaporizers are referred to as *variable bypass* or *dial controlled* vaporizers and are described in Figure 14-13.

Measured flow vaporizers use a separate measured flow of a carrier gas (O_2) to pick up the anesthetic vapor. No dial is present to set the percentage of gas to be delivered into the vaporizing chamber. The vaporizer consists of the vaporizing body that holds the liquid anesthetic agent and a flowmeter assembly, which calculates how much oxygen (in liters per minute) is needed to bubble through the vaporizing body to pick up and deliver vapor to the patient. The percentage output of the agent delivered from the vaporizing body is calculated based on vapor pressure of the agent, total gas flow, and amount of carrier gas. Such vaporizers are often referred to as *Vernitrol* vaporizers. They are no longer available for sale.

Adding a volatile agent to the wrong vaporizer results in an output that is either higher or lower than dialed. A simple mnemonic to remember is *high-low-high* (HLH) or *low-high-low* (LHL).

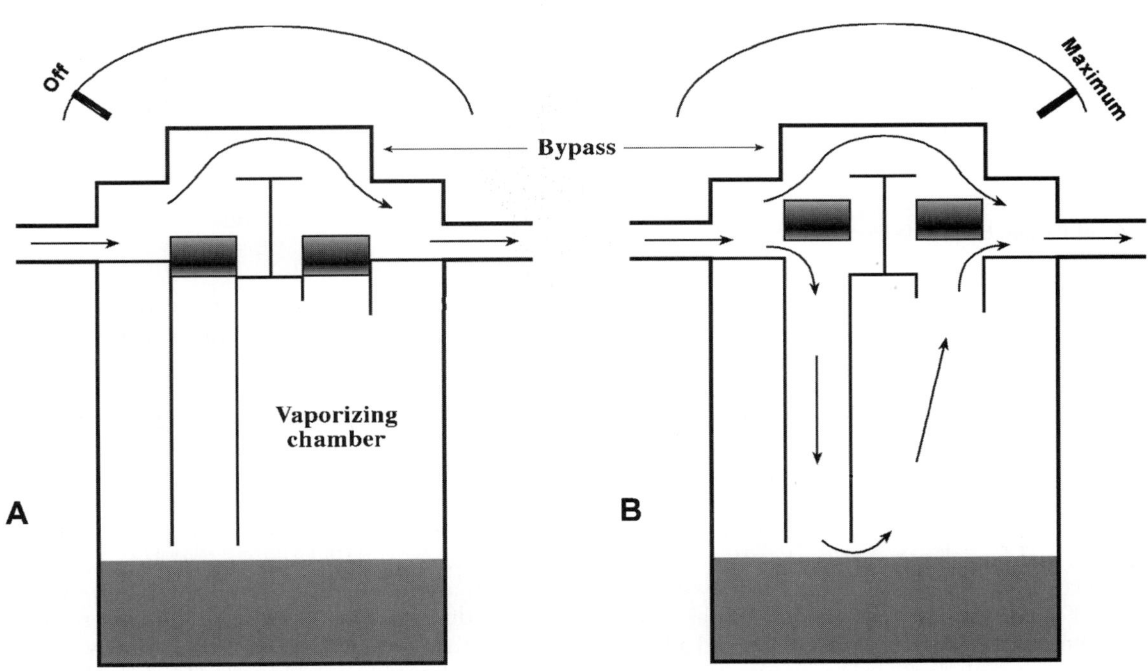

FIGURE **14-13**
Variable bypass vaporizer.

HLH If an agent with a higher vapor pressure is placed in a vaporizer of an agent with a lower vapor pressure, the concentration of agent delivered to the patient is higher than the dial setting.

LHL If an agent with a lower vapor pressure is placed in a vaporizer of an agent with a higher vapor pressure, the concentration of agent delivered to the patient is lower than the dial setting.

CARBON DIOXIDE ABSORPTION

A variety of anesthetic breathing systems are available. The most common is the circle absorption system. With this system, anesthetic gases flow in a circular pathway through separate inspiratory and expiratory channels. Components include a fresh gas source, unidirectional valves, Y-piece connector, corrugated inspiratory and expiratory breathing tubes, pop-off valve, reservoir bag, and CO_2 absorber.

Functions of the CO_2 absorber include complete removal of CO_2 from the circle system, and it employs the principle that a base (hydroxide) neutralizes an acid (CO_2); the end products are water, carbonates, and heat (exothermic).

CO_2-absorbent materials consist of a mixture of porous granules made up of bases (hydroxides).[9] Two types of absorbents are currently available: soda lime (Sodasorb) and barium hydroxide lime (Baralyme). Soda lime consists of: 4% NaOH, 1% KOH, 76% to 81% CaOH, and 14% to 19% H_2O. It consists of a mixture of large and small irregularly shaped granules of size 4 to 8 mesh (the higher the mesh number, the smaller the granule). Small granules offer a large surface area and increased resistance to flow, whereas large granules provide a small surface area and decreased resistance to flow. Moisture is added to prevent drying out, and silica is added for hardness. Barium hydroxide lime consists of 20% $Ba(OH)_2$ ($8H_2O$), and 80% CaOH. Small amounts of NaOH and KOH may be added. Granule size is 4 to 8 mesh. No hardening agent is needed. It is slightly less efficient than soda lime but less likely to dry out.

Equation 14-15 Chemical Reaction of Soda Lime

a. $CO_2 + H_2O \rightarrow H_2CO_3$

b. $2H_2CO_3 + 2NaOH \rightarrow NaCO_3 + 4H_2O + \text{Heat}$

$2KOH \rightarrow K_2CO_3$

c. $2Ca(OH)_2 + Na_2CO_3 \rightarrow 2CaCO_3 + 2NaOH + \text{Heat}$

$K_2CO_3 \rightarrow 2CaCO_3 + 2KOH$

where b = fast reaction, c = slow reaction; NaOH and KOH are regenerated.

Chemical Reaction of Barium Hydroxide Lime

a. $Ba(OH)_2\ (8H_2O) + CO_2 \rightarrow BaCO_3 + 9H_2O$

b. $9H_2O + 9CO_3 \rightarrow 9H_2CO_3$

c. $9H_2CO_3 + 9Ca(OH)_2 \rightarrow 9CaCO_3 + 18H_2O + \text{Heat}$

Indicators are added to absorbent to indicate exhaustion. They are organic dyes added to provide physical indication of absorbent function and do not affect absorption capacity. The most common is ethyl violet, which turns deep purple as pH falls below 10.3. The color may revert back to white if the absorbent remains idle (reactivation). This gives the user a false impression that the absorbent remains fully functional.

Each of the two canisters that hold the absorbent material contains approximately 1000 g of granules and has a volume of approximately 1500 cc. Each 100 g absorbs as much as 15 L of CO_2. The average production of CO_2 by anesthetized adults is 12 to 18 L/hr. Therefore each canister lasts approximately 8 to 10 hours. A certain amount of air space exists in each canister of absorbent material. Air space occupies 48% to 55% of canister volume. Two types of air space exist: void space (intergranular space, or the space between granules), which constitutes approximately 50% of the space for soda lime and barium hydroxide lime, and pore space (intragranular space, or the space within the pores of the granules), which constitutes approximately 8% to 10% of the space for both.

Each canister should be well filled with absorbent material and shaken to provide maximum function and absorption of CO_2. Soda lime degrades volatile anesthetic agents to some extent. Four times as much of sevofluorane breaks down in Baralyme as in soda lime. When degraded, sevoflurane also forms compound A, which has toxic renal and pulmonary effects. Therefore it is recommended that at least 2 L of fresh gas flow is used to prevent accumulation within the breathing system. Carbon monoxide has been known to accumulate in absorbers not used within 24 to 48 hours because of a slow reaction with the volatile agents and absorbent. Desflurane has the highest accumulation of carbon monoxide. For this reason it is recommended that the system be flushed with 100% oxygen for at least 15 minutes before use to purge the accumulated carbon monoxide.

ELECTRICAL SAFETY IN ANESTHESIA

Electrical devices in surgery have a potential to cause electrocution and burns in patients and personnel. Safety features are designed to reduce such risks. Three categories of surgical electrical devices exist: labor savers (e.g., operating room tables, drug administrations pumps); energy conversion devices (e.g., blood warmers, humidifiers); and information display systems (e.g., electrocardiograph, pulse oximeters).[10] The increased use of electrically powered devices resulting from advanced technology also increases the risk of electrocution and burns to the patient and surgical and anesthesia personnel.

Principles of Electricity

Ohm's law correlates the flow of electricity, the applied electrical pressure, and the resistance to this flow. It is written as follows:

Equation 14-16

$$\text{Electromotive forces (volts)} = \text{Current (amps)} \times \text{Resistance (ohms)}$$

or

Equation 14-17

$$E = I \times R$$

In order for electricity to occur, electrons need to move from an area of high concentration to an area of low concentration; a potential difference needs to exist between two points. This is expressed in volts.

In the United States 120 volts are emitted from the electrical power company. An ampere is the flow of electrons per second past a given point. When this happens, heat and light are produced. It is written as impedence = volts/resistance. Two types of current exist. Direct current (DC) is defined as the flow of electrons in the same direction (e.g., in a flashlight battery). In alternating current (AC) the flow of electrons occurs in one direction then reverses itself at a regular interval. A hertz is the number of times the AC reverses itself in one second. The United States has an AC of 60 Hz.

Resistance includes forces that oppose current flow, or impedance to flow. The higher the resistance, the less the

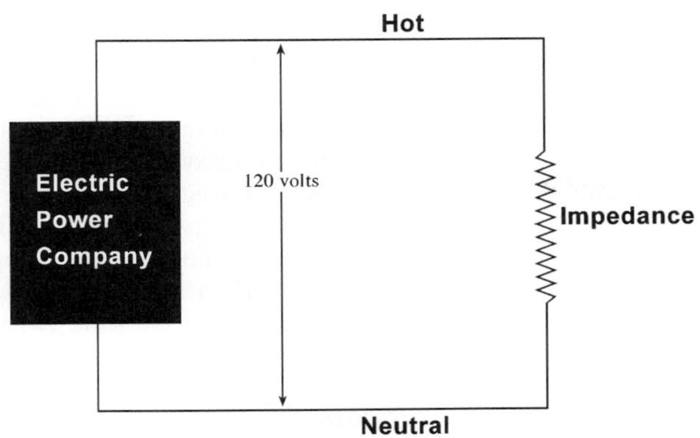

FIGURE **14-14**
Closed loop electrical current.

amount of current flow. A short circuit occurs with zero impedance.

A watt is a measure of electrical power (volts × current). It is the rate of energy expenditure or how much energy is needed. A 25-W light bulb uses less energy than a 75-W bulb and is therefore more energy efficient.

A complete circuit is a closed loop in which the voltage source drives the current through an impedance and the current is returned to the original source. Potential difference exists between a hot and a neutral wire, as shown in Figure 14-14.

An electrical shock occurs when the patient completes the circuit at two points, as identified in Figure 14-15. All components of the body are conductors of electricity. Muscle and blood are excellent conductors, whereas lungs are the poorest because they are air filled. Fat, bone, and dry skin are highly resistive. The severity of electrical shock depends on the patient's physical condition, duration of contact, and size of current. Injury is caused by two mechanisms: disruption of normal physiology (e.g., sustained muscle contraction, respiratory paralysis, ventricular fibrillation) and thermal injury.

There are two types of shock. *Macroshock* describes the effects of current applied to the body through intact skin. The flow of current takes the path of least resistance (great vessels, nerves, muscles). The units of measure associated with macroshock is the milliampere (mA). The following list

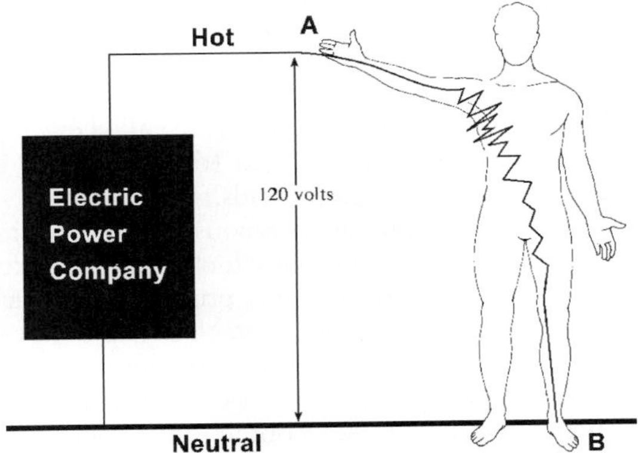

FIGURE **14-15**
Electrical shock.

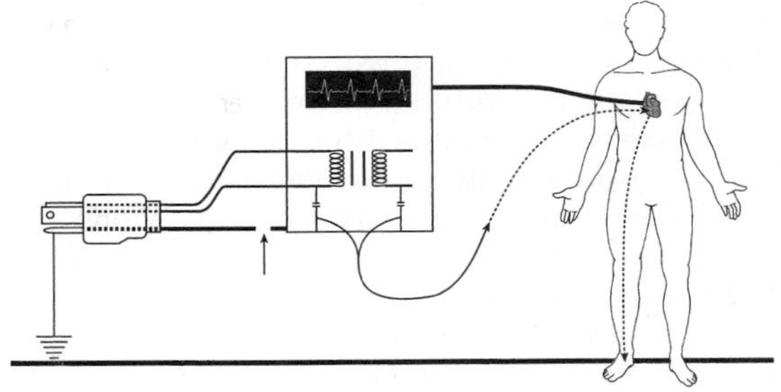

FIGURE **14-16**
Microshock.

describes the effects of certain levels of macroshock on the body.

Macroshock (mA)	Effect
1	Perception
5	Maximal harmless current
10 to 20	"Let-go" current
50	Loss of consciousness
100 to 300	ventricular fibrillation(v fib); respiratory center intact
6000	Complete physiologic damage

Macroshock is caused by exposure to current that arises as a result of equipment failure, unsafe design, or misuse.

Microshock results when an electrical current is accidentally supplied to an externalized conductor (e.g., saline-filled catheter or electrical pacing wire as shown in Figure 14-16). Microshock therefore concerns only the electrically susceptible patient. Measurement is in microamperes (μA). Very small amounts of current can cause damage (100 μA causes v fib).

Grounding is the intentional connecting of the power source or piece of equipment to earth ground. Electrical power in the United States is grounded. All utility companies ground the power. Power enters a home via two wires (hot and neutral) to the fuse box or circuit breakers. After leaving the circuit breaker, wires run through wall and supply outlets; in newer homes a ground wire (equipment) has been added and is attached to the neutral wire in fuse box. An equipment ground wire decreases the risk of electrical shock.

Electrical power in surgery is ungrounded, which provides an extra measure of safety from macroshock in surgery (in the United States). All surgical units use an isolation transformer to convert grounded electrical power from the utility company to ungrounded power in the operating room. The circuit in surgery has no direct connection to the ground. Energy from the utility company is coupled through a transformer, using electromagnetic induction, to two load supply conductors (lines 1 and 2) in the operating room. Neither line is hot or neutral with respect to ground. They are isolated from the grounded original source. Touching a line in the operating room does not result in shock, because the whole system is isolated from the grounded primary source. This protects surgical and anesthesia personnel from macroshock.

All hospital equipment is supplied with a ground wire. If an electrical fault occurs to the piece of equipment, surgical and anesthesia personnel are still prevented from incurring a macroshock, because the grounding wire carries the electrical current away. However, if this occurs, the operating room becomes grounded. Another faulty piece of equipment in the operating room would then greatly increase the potential for macroshock, because the entire system is grounded. The isolation system is equipped with an alarm that alerts surgical and anesthesia personnel that conversion to ground has occurred. The line isolation monitor is a device that monitors the integrity of the isolation power system and sounds an alarm when the isolated power is no longer isolated from the ground. The alarm occurs at 2 to 5 mA. This permits the offending device to be removed and changed to a new monitor.

Electrocautery is used in surgery to provide homeostasis by burning blood vessels via an electrical current (which produces heat) discharged from a machine to the patient. The energy is returned to the machine via a dispersive plate (often placed on patient's back or thigh) with a large surface area. If the device is faulty or improperly placed, the energy may bypass the dispersive plate and take the path of least resistance, through electrocardiographic electrodes, temperature probes, or stirrups. This may result in patient burn.

ORGANIC CHEMISTRY

Almost all drugs used during the administration of anesthesia are organic compounds (compounds formulated from a base of carbon atoms). The hydrocarbons are a group of compounds formed by the covalent bonding of carbon and hydrogen.[11] The simplest hydrocarbon is methane, which consists of one carbon atom surrounded by four hydrogen atoms. Ethane contains two carbon atoms that share one electron, with hydrogen filling the remaining binding sites. The list of hydrocarbons grows as the number of carbon atoms increases. Removing a hydrogen atom results in the formation of a hydrocarbon radical. Radicals are named by the conversion of the *-ane* of the parent hydrocarbon to an *-yl* ending.

Hydrocarbons are called *alkanes* or *saturated compounds* because only single bonds exist between carbon atoms. When double bonds (alkenes) or triple bonds (alkynes) exist between carbon atoms, the compound is said to be *unsaturated.* Compounds containing more than one double or triple bond are called *polyunsaturated.* Straight-chain alkanes are called *n-alkanes* (normal alkanes), and branching structures are their *isomers.* One way of naming branched hydrocarbons is assigning to the base the name of the longest straight portion of linked carbons and then separately naming the side chain based on its number of carbons. Carbon chains containing three or more carbons can be linked in a ring, forming a *cyclic compound.* Six-carbon cyclic compounds with alternating single and double bonds are called *aromatic*; these share the characteristics of benzene. Open-chain compounds and cyclic compounds that resemble the open-chain compounds are said to be *aliphatic* compounds.

Isomers

Compounds having the same molecular formula but different structural arrangements are called *isomers.* Enflurane and isoflurane are isomers with the same chemical formula and atomic weight. However, they have different structures and physical characteristics (vapor pressure, minimum alveolar concentration [MAC], blood-gas solubility). Compounds with identical structural formulas but different spatial arrangements are called *stereoisomers.* When the groups attached to the carbon atom differ from one another, polarized light passing through the substance is rotated; these molecules are called *optical isomers.* A *dextro*-isomer (*d*-isomer) rotates polarized light in one direction, whereas its *levo*-isomer (*l*-isomer) counterpart rotates polarized light in the opposite direction. These isomers paired in the same compound are mirror images of each other and are known as *enantiomers.* When equal amounts of *dextro-* and *levo*-isomers are mixed, the mixture is called *racemic.* Racemic epinephrine is a drug that is nebulized into the airway to reduce swelling of the airway mucosa. This synthetic stereoisomer mixture of the *d-* and *l*-forms of epinephrine is claimed to have adequate β_2 activity but less β_1 and (alpha) activity than that of natural epinephrine (which exists only in the *levo*-form).

Substituted Organic Compounds

Halogenation of hydrocarbons refers to the substitution of a halogen atom, such as fluorine, chlorine, or bromine, in the place of a hydrogen atom bound to the carbon. Although iodine is a halogen, the atom is too big for use in volatile anesthetics. Halogenation both decreases flammability and increases inhalational anesthetic potency. Halothane is ethane that is halogenated with fluorine, chlorine, and bromine.

Hydrocarbons in which a hydrogen is replaced by the -OH group (hydroxylation) are called *alcohols.* Substituting -OH for a hydrogen in methane produces methyl alcohol (methanol, which is the poisonous, so-called "wood alcohol"). Ethyl alcohol (ethanol, or "drinking alcohol") is derived from ethane. Ethanol given by IV administration has been used clinically for treating delirium tremens and halting premature labor, and it has been given by nebulization into the airway for reducing the foaming associated with pulmonary edema. Hydroxylation of benzene produces phenol, which was the first widely used antiseptic. Addition of the -OH group to the carbon atom at the end of a straight chain produces a substance classified as a primary alcohol. A secondary alcohol has the -OH group bound to a carbon atom, which is joined to two organic radicals. In a tertiary alcohol, a carbon atom is bound to an -OH group and three organic radicals.

Oxidation of a primary alcohol produces an aldehyde; oxidation of a secondary alcohol forms a ketone. These terms are sometimes abbreviated as RCHO (aldehyde) and RCOR (ketone), where R represents any radical (such as a methyl or ethyl group, although much larger and more complex radicals are possible).

Formaldehyde (a tissue preservative) and paraldehyde (a hypnotic drug) are examples of aldehydes encountered clinically. Acetone (a solvent commonly used for removing adhesive tape from the skin) is an example of a clinically useful ketone. Diabetic ketoacidosis results from increased ketone production when the body catabolizes fat as a result of inadequate insulin levels that prevent use of glucose.

Hydrocarbons in which one or more hydrogens have been replaced by a carboxyl (-COOH) group are called *organic acids.* Fatty acids, such as arachidonic acid (discussed later in this chapter), are examples of organic acids.

Amines are derived from hydrocarbons in which hydrogen is replaced by an $-NH_2$ group and for which the general formula is $R-NH_2$. Amines are divided into primary, secondary, and tertiary forms, just as alcohols are. Combining an amine with a structure that contains a benzene ring produces an aromatic amine. Catecholamines and many other sympathomimetics contain such a group. Amides contain the group $-CONH_2$. Many of the local anesthetics, including lidocaine and bupivacaine, are amides. Urea, the body's end product of protein catabolism, is also an amide. Urea condensed with malonic acid, a three-carbon dicarboxylic acid, is used in barbiturate synthesis. Amines differ from amides in that amines have hydrogen atoms or saturated carbon atoms attached to the nitrogen, whereas in amides the nitrogen is bound to a carbonyl radical. If the nitrogen is attached to four carbon radicals, the molecule is said to contain a quaternary ammonium and is ionized and therefore has difficulty passing through certain biologic barriers; the blood-brain barrier muscle relaxants, ganglionic blocking agents, and cholinergic drugs contain this important structure. Amino acids possess both an amine group (-NH_2) and an acid group (-COOH). Amino acids are covalently bound together during protein formation, as described later in this chapter.

Organic molecules that possess the general formula R-COO-R are classified as esters. Examples of clinically useful esters are succinylcholine and certain local anesthetics, such as procaine, chloroprocaine, and cocaine. All compounds broken down by esterases (e.g., mivacurium and esmolol) are also esters.

Ethers have the general formula R-O-R. The ethers originally associated with anesthetic practice were not halogenated and therefore were flammable and explosive. Isoflurane and desflurane are methyl ethyl ethers, whereas sevoflurane is a methyl ethyl ether.

When oxygen-containing molecules have their oxygen replaced by an atom of sulfur, they are called *thio compounds*. One group of thio compounds widely used in anesthesia induction is the *thiobarbiturates*, which include thiopental and thiamylal. Barbiturates, which have an oxygen atom in place of the sulfur bound to the barbituric acid ring, are designated as oxybarbiturates. In general, sulfuration increases lipid solubility and is associated with a greater hypnotic potency and a more rapid onset but a shorter duration of action. For instance, thiamylal has a more rapid onset and a shorter duration of action than its oxybarbiturate analogue, secobarbital. Addition of a methyl group to the nitrogen atom of the barbituric acid ring (e.g., with methohexital) also increases lipid solubility, thereby producing a compound with a short duration of action.

Biochemical Compounds

Water

Water is the most abundant compound in the human body, constituting 60% to 70% of the total body weight. Water is important to biochemical processes because it is a chemical source of hydrogen and oxygen. It is the medium in which materials are dispersed in the protoplasm of the cells. It is the solvent in which soluble materials are absorbed from the environment (e.g., in the absorption of inhaled anesthetic gases in the lungs). It plays an important role in the transport of foods, minerals, and other vital substances in living systems.

The predominantly aqueous body contains mineral salts as well as the four major types of compounds: carbohydrates, lipids, proteins, and nucleic acids. These molecules are an essential part of the structure of the human body and also function in its metabolism. Metabolism consists of the reactions that take place within the body. *Anabolism* refers to synthetic reactions, and *catabolism* describes degradation reactions (which are used during the production of energy or the elimination of waste materials).

Nucleic Acids

Nucleic acids constitute only a small portion of the organic material in the body. However, these molecules are essential for life because they are responsible for storage of genetic information and for its transmission from cell to cell. Nucleic acids also govern the intracellular formation of structural as well as enzymatic proteins. The nucleoside adenosine, contained in the molecule adenosine triphosphate (ATP), plays a vital role in bioenergetics.

The two types of nucleic acids are deoxyribonucleic acid (DNA) and ribonucleic acid (RNA). DNA molecules are responsible for storing genetic information, which is duplicated and then transmitted to the next generation of cells. RNA molecules are necessary for decoding this information into instructions that link a specific sequence of amino acids required in the synthesis of a specific protein. Messenger RNA copies some of the genetic information contained in the DNA and then is transported to the ribosomes, where it governs the sequencing of amino acids in protein formation. An important part of the ribosome is ribosomal RNA, where the information contained in the messenger RNA is translated into protein structure. Transfer RNA carries activated amino acids to the ribosomes, where they are joined together by peptide bonds (the linkage formed between amino acids during protein formation).

Nucleic acids are polymers composed of a linear sequence of subunits known as *nucleotides*. Each nucleotide consists of a phosphate group, a sugar, and a ring system known as a *base*. DNA contains the five-carbon sugar deoxyribose and four different bases, which are subgrouped into two categories: (1) the purines (adenine and guanine) and (2) the pyrimidines (thymine and cytosine). DNA consists of two chains of nucleotides coiled around each other in the form of a double helix and held together by hydrogen bonds. The bonds allow only adenine to bind with thymine and only guanine to bind with cytosine. This specificity of base pairing ensures the stability of the genetic information during duplication and transference. RNA consists of a single chain of nucleotides and contains the sugar ribose instead of deoxyribose. Additionally, the pyrimidine base thymine, which is present in DNA, is replaced by the pyrimidine uracil.

The high-energy compound ATP is used by the cells for the fueling of reactions such as muscle contraction, anabolism (the formation of a peptide bond between two amino acids requires the energy contained in three ATP molecules), and active transport across the cell membrane (as used by Na-K-ATPase). Other high-energy sources within the cell include creatine phosphate, which is formed by the enzyme creatine phosphokinase. The isoenzymes (enzymes with the same function but slightly different structures as a result of different tissues of origin) of creatine phosphokinase are fractionated to reveal sites of tissue injury, such as the brain, heart, or liver. The major source of ATP production is the breakdown of carbohydrates and lipids.

Carbohydrates

Carbohydrates exist as either monomers (monosaccharides) or polymers (oligosaccharides and polysaccharides). Monosaccharides consist of a single chain of carbon atoms that is between three and seven atoms long. The names of monosaccharides consist of a prefix that indicates the number of carbon atoms followed by the suffix *-ose* (e.g., hexoses contain six carbons). The most important monosaccharide is glucose, a hexose referred to as "blood sugar."

Carbohydrates that contain a number of monosaccharide subunits linked together with glycosidic bonds are called either *oligosaccharides* (having between two and 10 subunits) or *polysaccharides* (having more than 10 subunits). Disaccharides, such as sucrose and lactose, are the most common oligosaccharides, and starch and glycogen are the most important polysaccharides in the human body.

Excess glucose is stored mainly in the liver and skeletal muscle as the polymer glycogen, which is formed in a process called *glycogenesis*. Breakdown of glycogen (glycogenolysis) reforms glucose, which can be used as a quick source of energy.

Carbohydrate metabolism has several important implications for anesthetic practice. The three main pathways for glucose catabolism (glycolysis) are the Embden-Meyerhof pathway, the hexose monophosphate shunt, and the Krebs cycle. The Embden-Meyerhof pathway (the first step in glucose hydrolysis) consists of a series of reactions that are not oxygen dependent. Anaerobic glycolysis provides a limited source of energy when oxygen demand is greater than oxygen supply. The six-carbon glucose molecule is broken down and converted into a pair of three-carbon lactic acid molecules, hydrogen ions (which lower the pH), and only two ATP molecules (high-energy compound). Aerobic glycolysis of a glucose molecule feeds into the Krebs cycle, which breaks down the two-carbon molecules produced by glycolysis as well as by catabolism of fats, proteins, and nucleic acids. This process ultimately produces water and CO_2 molecules as the end products of metabolism as well as a total of 38 ATP molecules for each molecule of glucose used.

The increased ATP produced is mainly the result of the process known as *oxidative phosphorylation*, which uses the cytochrome electron transport chain. Oxidative phosphorylation is the oxygen-requiring, enzyme-mediated process in which relatively low-energy-containing adenosine diphosphate (ADP) is phosphorylated to form high-energy ATP. Aerobic metabolism is a much more efficient form of energy production. Although aerobic metabolism produces CO_2, which is converted to carbonic acid by use of the enzyme carbonic anhydrase, the carbonic acid is easily converted back into CO_2 and exhaled from the lungs.

Conversely, the lactic acid produced in anaerobic metabolism is nonvolatile. Both glycolytic pathways pass through 2,3-diphosphoglycerate (DPG) as a three-carbon intermediate product. Thus, when tissues are metabolically active and require large amounts of energy production, glycolysis is increased, and levels of end products as well as those of intermediates increase. The increase in 2,3-DPG level is associated with the shift of the oxyhemoglobin dissociation curve to the right. This shift decreases the affinity of the hemoglobin for the oxygen and allows more oxygen to be released to the metabolically active tissues. Anaerobic glycolysis causes a buildup of lactic acid, which is associated with muscle fatigue.

The hexose monophosphate shunt is an aerobic, enzyme-dependent sequence of reactions that are important for the synthesis of nucleic acids and fatty acids as well as for the balance of hydrogen ion production and use during the Embden-Meyerhof pathway and the Krebs cycle. One result of the hexose monophosphate shunt is the production of CO_2 without any oxygen use. The ratio of CO_2 production to oxygen use is called the *respiratory quotient*. Normal metabolism of the materials contained in a typical diet results in the production of approximately 200 ml of CO_2 per minute and the consumption of approximately 250 ml of oxygen per minute (for a 70-kg man at rest), resulting in a respiratory quotient of 0.8. When the diet contains excessive carbohydrate calories (as occasionally occurs during hyperalimentation), lipogenesis results, the hexose monophosphate shunt is used, and the respiratory quotient rises above 1. When metabolic studies of patients receiving hyperalimentation reveal a respiratory quotient of greater than 1, it is recommended that the hyperalimentation be reformulated to contain less carbohydrate and more lipid and protein calories to decrease lipogenesis. Lipogenesis is undesirable, especially in the critically ill patient, because it increases CO_2 production, minute ventilation, and work of breathing. Additionally, the newly formed lipid is initially stored in the liver, causing hepatomegaly, elevation of the diaphragm, and decreased pulmonary compliance at a time when increased minute ventilation is necessary.

Lipids

Lipids account for 40% of the organic matter of the body and are characterized as nonpolar, hydrophobic hydrocarbons. The main classes of lipids are triglycerides, phospholipids, and steroids. Most of the lipids in the human body are triglycerides, commonly referred to as fat. Phospholipids are similar in structure to triglycerides, except for the presence of a phosphate group, which renders that portion of the molecule hydrophilic (polar as a result of ionization); the remainder of the molecule is hydrophobic (nonpolar). Phospholipids are useful components of cell membranes, where they serve as barriers to the exchange of compounds with the surrounding extracellular fluid. Steroids constitute a large group of compounds that have in common a cyclic structure that contains four carbon rings. Examples of steroids include cholesterol, bile acids, adrenal corticosteroids, testosterone, estrogen, vitamin D, and even certain muscle relaxants, such as pancuronium.

Fats, like carbohydrates, consist almost exclusively of carbon, hydrogen, and oxygen. Fats, however, have a much lower proportion of oxygen than carbohydrates do. Free fatty acids are fairly long chains of carbon and hydrogen atoms (usually 14 to 18 carbon atoms long). If all of the carbon atoms in a fatty acid are joined by single bonds, the fatty acid is said to be *saturated*. When double bonds are present between the carbon atoms, the fatty acid is called *unsaturated*. If more than one double bond is present in the molecule, the fatty acid is said to be *polyunsaturated*. Three fatty acids combine with a three-carbon carbohydrate molecule (glycerol) to form triglycerides, which are neutral. Free (unbound) fatty acids are much more reactive and cause an increased permeability of the capillary endothelium.

Oleic acid (a type of free fatty acid) is sometimes administered as an infusion to experimental animals in order to produce a pulmonary injury that mimics adult respiratory distress syndrome. This phenomenon occurs because the oleic acid is carried to the pulmonary circulation, where it causes increased capillary leak, increased lung water, and decreased compliance of the lung. Massive trauma with long bone fractures can produce a clinical process called fat embolism, which impairs pulmonary function. The injury caused by fat embolism is similar to that caused by oleic acid infusion.

Fat ingested in the diet is absorbed through the wall of the intestine and is taken up by the circulation, where it is bound to carrier proteins, which decrease its toxicity. The portal system transports the fat to the liver, where it is further modified and detoxified before entering the systemic circulation. Fatty acids that are infused or suddenly liberated from traumatized tissue in large amounts cannot be detoxified by the liver's modifying effects and therefore produce their toxic effects in the pulmonary circulation.

Fat is important with regard to anesthesia because its presence in a cell membrane is the basis for one explanation of how inhaled anesthetics work. The Meyer-Overton theory of how an inhaled anesthetic works is based on the inhaled anesthetic's dissolving into the lipid membrane, causing membrane expansion and altering the pathways for ion flux (changing the ability of the cells to develop action potentials). The Meyer-Overton theory is based on the correlation between lipid solubility of inhaled anesthetics (oil-gas partition coefficient) and anesthetic potency (MAC). Anesthesia occurs when a sufficient number of anesthetic molecules dissolve (critical concentration) at the crucial hydrophobic sites, such as the lipid and cell membranes. This has been found to be true for short chain (up to four-carbon) molecules but not for larger molecules, even if they are highly lipophilic.

Metabolism of arachidonic acid (a polyunsaturated 20-carbon essential fatty acid) produces several products that have important anesthetic implications. Arachidonic acid is converted by the cyclooxygenase pathway into thromboxane, prostaglandins (endoperoxides), and prostacyclin.

Prostaglandins and their metabolites have several functions in the body, participating in platelet activities, hemostasis, vasomotor effects, uterine contractions, and pain mediation. Infusion of one certain prostaglandin (prostaglandin E_1) causes potent relaxation of the smooth muscle of the ductus arteriosus and preserves ductal patency in neonates with congenital heart disease, such as transposition of the great vessels or tetralogy of Fallot. Patency of the ductus arteriosus is necessary in these types of congenital heart diseases to allow blood to enter the pulmonary circulation until corrective surgery can be performed. A prostaglandin inhibitor (indomethacin) is given to otherwise normal neonates in order to close a patent ductus arteriosus.

The lipoxygenase pathway is used to convert arachidonic acid into leukotrienes. The actions of leukotrienes include bronchoconstriction, vasoconstriction, and increases in vascular permeability (leukotriene D was formerly called the "slow-reacting substance of anaphylaxis").

Nonsteroidal antiinflammatory drugs, such as aspirin, are used to reduce pain and fever. Aspirin also irreversibly blocks the production of thromboxane A in platelets; this causes intense local vasoconstriction and platelet activation, which leads to the formation of a platelet plug. Because the normal life span of platelets is approximately 10 days, elective surgery is usually delayed for 2 weeks after aspirin ingestion so that normal platelet levels are restored. Inhibition of the cyclooxygenase pathway by nonsteroidal anti-inflammatory drugs results in increased leukotriene production by the lipoxygenase pathway. This phenomenon may be an explanation for aspirin-induced asthma.

Proteins

Proteins account for approximately 50% of the organic material found in the human body and play a critical role in almost every physiologic process. They contain carbon, hydrogen, oxygen, nitrogen, and sometimes sulfur. Most proteins are very large molecules formed by the linking together of large numbers of amino acids (the basic subunit of protein). The 21 common amino acids are classified as either essential (synthesized in the body only slightly or not at all) or nonessential (easily formed by the body). During protein formation, amino acids are linked together by a polar covalent bond, the peptide bond.

The four levels of protein structure determine the shape, or configuration, of the molecule. The configuration is essential for proteins with special functions, such as enzymes or receptor sites. The sequence of amino acids composing a peptide chain constitutes the primary structure of the protein molecule. The secondary structure is the possible shape of the molecule, which results from hydrogen bonding within the molecule. These shapes include a coil-shaped helix, a random helix, and a so-called "pleated sheet" with hydrogen bonds between peptide chains. The tertiary structure results from various types of bonds between amino acid side chains, such as disulfide bridges, and causes the protein molecule to fold on itself. Quaternary structure is the joining of protein subunits to produce a complete protein, as is seen in hemoglobin, which has four peptide chains bound together, two alpha units and two beta units.

Structurally, proteins are classified as either fibrous or globular. Fibrous proteins, such as collagen and myosin, are composed of elongated filamentous chains. Globular proteins, such as antibodies and certain transport proteins, are somewhat spherical as a result of considerable folding of the long polypeptide chains. Proteins can be grouped according to function, as follows: (1) structural proteins; (2) contractile proteins; (3) antibodies; (4) blood and plasma proteins (hemoglobin and carrier proteins in the plasma); (5) the portion of an enzyme called the *apoenzyme* (an enzyme may also contain a nonprotein portion called the *coenzyme*); and (6) certain hormones. These hormones are further structurally categorized as long-chain polypeptides, such as insulin, or short-chain polypeptides, such as thyroxine or alcohol dehydrogenase. The third chemical category of hormones includes the nonprotein steroids, such as estrogen.

SUMMARY

Physical laws, chemical equations, and organic structures form the nucleus of our understanding of the physical and chemical world. Many phenomena associated with the practice of anesthesia are derived from roots in chemistry and physics, including the chemical structure of local anesthetics, the nomenclature of anesthetic solutions, the chemical reaction of soda lime and CO_2, the behavior of compressed gases, and the process of vaporization of gases. With the passing of the Vernitrol vaporizer into obsolescence, nurse anesthetists are rarely called on to perform physics-related calculations while administering anesthesia. However, a scientific understanding of the basic principles that govern our practice can provide nurse anesthetists information regarding the "tools of the trade" and the administration of safe, high-quality anesthesia.

REFERENCES

1. Zumdahl S. Atoms, molecules and ions. *Chemistry*. 2nd ed. Lexington, Ky: DC Heath and Company; 1986:112.
2. Kossick, MA. Clinical monitoring in anesthesia. In: Nagelhout J, Zaglaniczny K, eds. *Nurse Anesthesia*. Philadelphia: Saunders; 1997:287.
3. Ohmeda. *Explore! The Anesthesia System*. Madison, Wis: Ohmeda; 1996:6-32.
4. Dorsch J, Dorsch S. Vaporizers. *Understanding Anesthesia Equipment*. 4th ed. Baltimore: Williams & Wilkins; 1999:123.
5. Zumdahl S. Solution stoichiometry and chemical analysis. *Chemistry*. Lexington, Ky: DC Health and Company; 1986:115.

6. Levitsky M. Mechanics of breathing. *Pulmonary Physiology*. 5th ed. New York: McGraw-Hill; 1995:115.
7. Dorsch J, Dorsch S. Medical gas cylinders and containers. *Understanding Anesthesia Equipment*. 4th ed. Baltimore: Williams & Wilkins; 1999:6-32.
8. Kossick MA. Inhalation anesthetics. In: Nagelhout J, Zaglaniczny K, eds. *Nurse Anesthesia*. Philadelphia: Saunders; 1997:96.
9. Dorsch J, Dorsch S. Medical gas pipeline system. *Understanding Anesthesia Equipment*. 4th ed. Baltimore: Williams & Wilkins; 1999:32.
10. Lih L. Electrical safety in the OR. In: Miller R, ed. *Anesthesia*. 5th ed. Philadelphia: Churchill Livingstone; 2000:2693.
11. Brown, W. *Introduction to Organic and Biochemistry*. Monterey, Calif: Brooks/Cole; 1987:36.

CHAPTER 15

ANESTHESIA EQUIPMENT

MICHAEL P. DOSCH

Apparatus of reliable appearance engenders a strong sense of security which is often not supported by facts. A critical attitude often forestalls unpleasant surprises.

—*Lucien Morris*[1]

The incorporation of new technology into anesthesia care, particularly monitoring and ventilation technology, proceeds at a rapid pace. Gas machines manufactured in the last decade bear little resemblance to their ancestors. Much of the increase in patient safety in the specialty has been the result of education and of monitoring advances such as pulse oximetry and capnography. An equal but seldom appreciated increment in safety has resulted from advances in anesthesia gas machine design and manufacture. A practitioner accustomed to the current generation of anesthesia gas machines can barely imagine the inherent hazards and design flaws of older machines.[2,3] Collaboration among manufacturers, standards-writing bodies, and dedicated professionals has achieved a great deal.

Contemporary machines abound with features that contribute to safety and convenience. Yet these additional features carry problems of their own. In a simpler era, a schematic drawing of the pneumatic (gas-handling) systems of an anesthesia gas machine was straightforward. Now, such a diagram can be deciphered only with study. For experienced clinicians, confronting a new anesthesia gas machine, with its touch-sensitive screens and cable arms, can be daunting.[4-6] For a student, it may be even more intimidating. As a result, equipment usually is not the subject with which anesthetists feel the most confident. Many factors may contribute to this lack of confidence. For example, it is not always possible for the anesthetist to be available when department in-service education is conducted. Also, continuing education content may be too limited, or an opportunity to use new equipment soon after an educational session may not be available. Various pieces of new equipment are introduced frequently in the anesthesia work area. Although anesthesia equipment is designed to meet all legal and technical requirements, the designers of the equipment are not those who use it. Some designs may be recognized as flawed only when the devices are used clinically. Instructional materials accompanying equipment often are inadequate. For example, no matter how well written an instruction manual is, supplying one manual per *machine* is inferior to supplying one manual per *user*. The potential lack in equipment competency can be a safety problem.[7] Users may be legally obligated to know and follow manufacturer's instructions (operating manuals) and warnings, because these may contribute to the standard of care. Some courts have defined deviation from manufacturer's instructions as prima facie negligence.[8]

One way to ensure safe use of the anesthesia gas machine is conscientious performance of the U.S. Food and Drug Administration (FDA) apparatus checkout.[9,10] Each practitioner is obligated to check equipment in order to ensure that it is safe and ready for use for each patient.[11,12] Today, equipment is so reliable, and failures so seldom occur, that the clinician may be lulled into a false sense of security. A greater effort must be exerted by individuals to prevent patient injury resulting from the failure to check equipment or from unfamiliarity with equipment.[8]

This chapter discusses the anesthesia gas machine. A conceptual framework is presented to aid in proper use of the anesthesia gas machine. This framework is based on development of a clear understanding of how each component of the machine fits into the overall organization of the system. The framework encompasses systems that supply, process, deliver, and dispose of gases. The management of risks related to the anesthesia gas machine is discussed, including machine checkout, waste gases, and infection control. A major objective of this chapter is to help the practitioner gain skills in the use of the anesthesia gas machine. Therefore, throughout the chapter, explicit directions on how to use the machine safely are presented; these directions are solidly based on manufacturers' guidelines and are supplemented by reports of pitfalls from the anesthesia literature.

The last section of this chapter is devoted to selected clinical implications. Because of the variety of machines currently in use, no direction in this chapter can be considered universally applicable. The directions given here must be adapted to individual practice settings only after study of the manuals and appropriate local peer review.

Differences among gas machines are presented here if an understanding of these differences is important for safe use of the machine. The new ventilation modes are covered in detail, as are the new piston ventilators. Effects of electrical power failure on modern machines are discussed. New systems that support low-flow anesthesia are described (redesigned, low-volume breathing circuits; fresh gas decoupling). Finally, each section on basic components has been revised to reflect the computer-controlled pneumatic and monitoring systems now in place. Brief descriptions of newer gas machines (Datex-Ohmeda Aestiva and S/5 Anesthesia Delivery Unit [ADU]; Dräger Medical Fabius GS; and Narkomed 6000) are presented, and more detail is available in a companion web site (http://www.udmercy.edu/crna/agm/index.htm).

ORGANIZATION OF THE ANESTHESIA GAS MACHINE

Presenting the anesthesia gas machine as a litany of components does not promote retention, much less aid in the development of a solid conceptualization of the overall organization of the machine. An accurate presentation of the overall organization should help the reader understand the role of the individual components better, which should in turn promote correct use and therefore patient safety. This section presents the supply, processing, delivery, and disposal (SPDD) model.

Supply, Processing, Delivery, and Disposal Model

The SPDD model is depicted in Figure 15-1 and Box 15-1. This model is comprehensive in that the path of gases can be followed from their arrival in the operating room to their disposal from it. Most anesthesia gas machine components can be located easily within the overall scheme. Gas flows in the diagram proceed generally from left to right. The vertical bar separates components within the machine and proximal to the common gas outlet (left side) from external components downstream from the common gas outlet (right). The fact that nitrous oxide (N_2O) and air, unlike oxygen (O_2), have only one task in the machine is easy to appreciate. The five tasks of O_2 are easy to follow. Understanding the similarities and differences between the fail-safe and hypoxic guard systems is facilitated. The model makes clear that the scavenging system, rather than the patient, is the ultimate destination of gases. O_2 is central to the figure, because it is the most essential gas delivered. The reader should note that not every component of the SPDD model in Box 15-1 is depicted graphically in Figure 15-1. The reader should make frequent reference to the model while reading this chapter.

The model organizes the information on the basis of how components are used rather than on the pressures to which they are exposed. From that viewpoint, components are part of the high-, intermediate-, or low-pressure systems within (proximal to the common gas outlet) the gas machine (Box 15-2).

Introduction of new gas machines raises questions about the adequacy and safety of older equipment. One can begin the determination of whether current equipment is obsolete by considering how closely it matches current safety standards. Certain systems or components are required by the anesthesia workstation standard, which is a voluntary industry-group consensus standard (Box 15-3, p. 262).

SUPPLY

The concept of supply is concerned with the questions of how gases (and electrical power) come to the anesthesia gas machine and what are the likely faults and hazards.

Pipeline Supply

Configuration

O_2 is produced by the fractional distillation of liquid air. It is delivered to facilities and stored as a liquid, at a temperature of −150° to −175° C. Various components convert the liquid O_2 to a gas and supply it to hospital pipelines at a pressure of 50 psi (344 kPa). In the operating room suite, main and partial-area

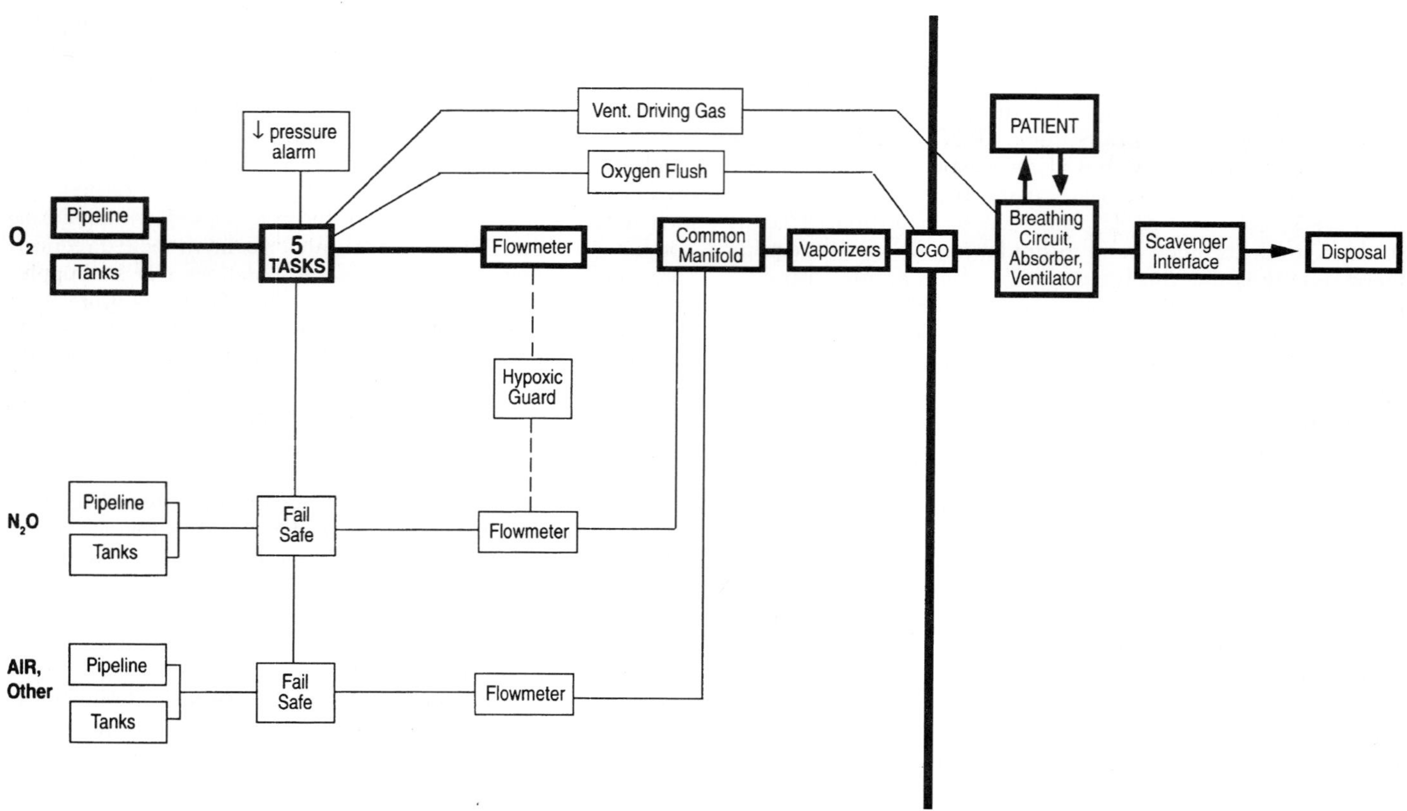

FIGURE **15-1**
Supply, processing, delivery, and disposal model. CGO, Common gas outlet. (Courtesy of Michael P. Dosch.)

BOX 15-1

Components in the Supply, Processing, Delivery, and Disposal Model

Supply

How Do Gases Come to the Anesthesia Gas Machine? (Site: Back of the Machine)

Pipeline
Wall outlets
Connecting valves and hoses
Filters and check valves
Pressure gauges
Cylinders
Hanger yokes (yoke block)
Filters and check valves
Pressure gauge
Pressure regulators

Processing

How Does the Anesthesia Gas Machine Prepare Gases before Their Delivery to the Patient? (Site: within the Machine, Proximal to Common Gas Outlet)

Fail-safe (oxygen pressure-failure devices)
Flowmeters (main, auxiliary, common gas outlet)
Oxygen flush
Low oxygen pressure alarms
Ventilator-driving gas
Proportioning systems (hypoxic guard)
Oxygen second-stage regulator (if present)
Vaporizers
Check valves distal to vaporizers (if present)
Common gas outlet

Delivery

How Is the Interaction of Gases with the Patient Controlled and Monitored? (Site: Breathing Circuit)

Gas delivery hose connecting common gas outlet and breathing circuit
Breathing circuits
- Nonrebreathing
- Circle

Carbon dioxide absorption
Ventilators
Integral monitors
- Oxygen analysis
- Disconnect
  - Spirometry (volumes and flows), capnography, airway pressure
- Ventilator alarms

Addition of positive end-expiratory pressure
Means of humidification

Disposal

How Are Gases Disposed of? (Site: Scavenger)

Scavenger systems
- Interface—closed (active and passive) or open
- Scavenger flowmeter

BOX 15-2

Components in the High-, Intermediate-, and Low-Pressure Pneumatic Systems

High-Pressure System (Exposed to Cylinder Pressure)

Hanger yoke
Yoke block with check valves
Cylinder pressure gauge
Cylinder pressure regulators

Intermediate-Pressure System (Exposed to Pipeline Pressure, about 50 psi)

Pipeline inlets, check valves, and pressure gauges
Ventilator power inlet
Oxygen pressure-failure devices
Flowmeter valve
Oxygen second-stage regulator (if present)
Flush valve

Low-Pressure System (Distal to Flowmeter Needle Valve)

Flowmeter tubes
Vaporizers
Check valves (if present)
Common gas outlet

shutoff valves are present to isolate sections with leaks, interrupt supply in case of fire, and allow repair work on subsections. Wall outlets or hoses dropped from the ceiling are finished with quick-connect couplers. These couplers are used so that the connection of gas machine supply hoses to wall outlets does not require tools. However, the springs and rubber gaskets (O-rings) that these couplers contain provide a connection that is less secure than a wrench-tightened connection; therefore they are a common source of leaks.[13-14]

Systems that process N_2O are similar in many respects. N_2O is delivered to the hospital in large (size H) cylinders that are connected to a manifold. Regulators reduce the pressure so that N_2O, like O_2, is supplied to the pipelines at 50 psi. Consequently, this is the normal working pressure of the anesthesia gas machine. Shutoff valves and wall outlets with quick-connect couplers are similar for N_2O and O_2. Delivery piping for both N_2O and O_2 uses the diameter index safety system (DISS) to prevent misconnections. In this system, gas piping connections are sized and threaded differently, so that cross-connection is difficult, although not impossible (Figure 15-2).[15]

Supply hoses connect the pipeline inlets on the back of the machine to the wall outlets. At the pipeline inlet, a filter, check valve, and pressure gauge are present. The check valve ensures unidirectional flow, so that a machine running on cylinder supplies, with the hoses disconnected at the wall outlet, does not leak (Figure 15-3). The filter is required by the current anesthesia workstation standard (ASTM-F1850), as it

BOX 15-3

Required Components of an Anesthesia Workstation

The current anesthesia gas machine (workstation) standard is ASTM F1850 (a standard promulgated by ASTM International [formerly the American Society for Testing and Materials]: *Standard Specification for Particular Requirements for Anesthesia Workstations and Their Components [F1850-00]*, Philadelphia: ASTM; 2000). The comparable European standard is EN740. F1850 specifies what is needed for an anesthesia workstation. The components are typically built into new gas machines, or they may be added to older machines. Requirements and required components include the following:

Battery backup for 30 minutes

Alarms
- Grouped into high, medium, and low priority
- High-priority alarms may not be silenced for more than 2 minutes
- Certain alarms and monitors must be automatically enabled, either by turning the machine on or by following the preuse checklist, and functioning before the machine is used: breathing circuit pressure, oxygen concentration, exhaled volume or carbon dioxide monitor (or both)
- A high-priority pressure alarm must sound if user-adjustable limits are exceeded, if continuing high pressure is sensed, or for negative pressure
- Disconnect alarms may be based on low pressure, exhaled volume, or carbon dioxide

Required monitors
- Exhaled volume
- Inspired oxygen, with a high priority alarm sounding within 30 seconds if oxygen falls below 18% (or a user-adjustable limit)
- Oxygen supply failure alarm
- A hypoxic guard system must protect against less than 21% inspired oxygen if nitrous oxide is in use
- Anesthetic vapor concentration must be monitored
- Pulse oximetry, blood pressure monitoring, and electrocardiogram are required

Pressure in the breathing circuit is limited to 12.5 kPa (125 cm H_2O)

The electrical supply cord must be nondetachable or resistant to detachment

Cylinder supplies
- The machine must have at least one oxygen cylinder attached
- The hanger yoke must be pin indexed, have a clamping device that resists leaks, and contain a filter; it must have a check valve to prevent transfilling and a cylinder pressure gauge
- Cylinder pressure regulators are required; the machine must use pipeline gas as long as pipeline pressure is greater than 345 kPa (50 psi)

Flowmeters
- Single control for each gas
- Each flow control next to a flow indicator
- Uniquely shaped oxygen flow control knob
- Valve stops (or some other mechanism) are required such that excessive rotation will not damage the flowmeter
- Oxygen flow indicator is to the right side of a flowmeter bank
- Oxygen enters the common manifold downstream of other gases
- An auxiliary oxygen flowmeter is strongly recommended

An oxygen flush is present, capable of 35-75 L/min flow, which does not proceed through any vaporizers

Vaporizers
- Concentration calibrated
- An interlock must be present
- Liquid level indicated, designed to prevent overfilling
- "Should" use keyed filler devices
- No discharge of liquid anesthetic occurs from the vaporizer even at maximum fresh gas flow

Only one common gas outlet, at 22-mm outer diameter, 15-mm inner diameter, which is designed to prevent accidental disconnection

Pipeline gas supply
- Pipeline pressure gauge
- Inlets for at least oxygen and nitrous oxide
- Diameter index safety system (DISS) protected
- In-line filter
- Check valve

Checklist must be provided (it may be electronic or may be performed manually by the user)

A digital data interface must be provided

may help prevent damage to the anesthesia gas machine from particulate matter present in the pipeline gas supply.[15]

Problems with Pipeline Supply

Some of the problems associated with pipeline use can be particularly dangerous because they are occult. Pressure loss, excess pressure, cross-connection of gas delivery pipelines, contamination, leaks, and theft of N_2O (for recreational use) have been reported.[2]

Loss of O_2 pipeline pressure is indicated by the pipeline pressure gauge. In addition, if pressure loss is profound, the O_2 low-pressure alarm sounds, and the fail-safe valves halt the delivery of all other gases. With the new electronic alarms, operator response may be delayed, because the electronic alarms lack the distinctive and familiar "whistle" of a pneumatic O_2 low-pressure alarm.[16]

With complete loss of O_2 pipeline pressure, the anesthetist should fully open the E cylinder of O_2, disconnect the pipeline, and consider the use of low fresh gas flows (FGFs) and manual ventilation (to conserve the emergency cylinder supply of O_2). If the E cylinder of O_2 is not opened fully, flow from it may end before the cylinder is empty. The pipeline is disconnected so that retrograde flow from within the machine to the pipeline is prevented. Retrograde flow occurs only if the pipeline inlet check valve fails simultaneously. Although this is unlikely, the author recommends disconnecting the hose at the quick-connect fitting for two reasons. First, it *must* be disconnected in the case of a cross-connection (which is more

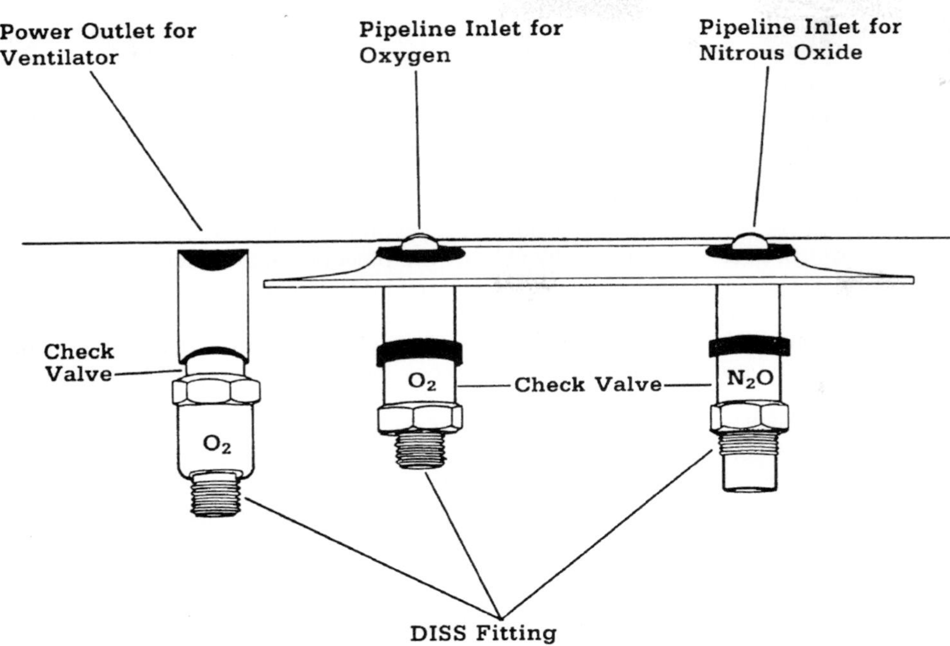

FIGURE **15-2**
Diameter index safety system for gas connections on the back of the anesthesia gas machine. (From Bowie E, Huffman LM. *The Anesthesia Machine: Essentials for Understanding*. Madison, Wis: Datex-Ohmeda; 1985:36.)

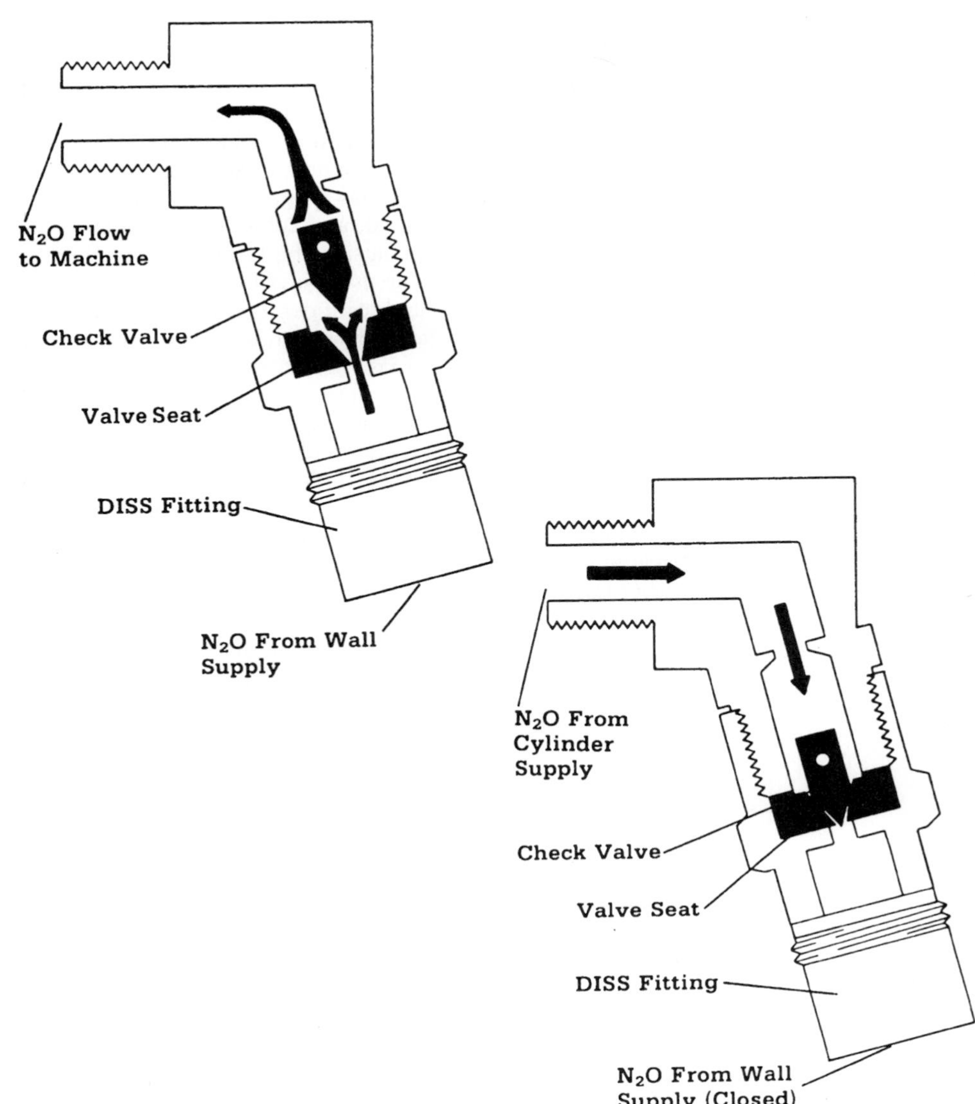

FIGURE **15-3**
Check valve in the nitrous oxide supply hose at the back of the anesthesia gas machine. (From Bowie E, Huffman LM. *The Anesthesia Machine: Essentials for Understanding*. Madison, Wis: Datex-Ohmeda; 1985:76)

fully described later in the chapter); otherwise the contents of the O_2 cylinder will not flow. Remembering one strategy that is effective for two reasonably similar problems is easier than remembering two different strategies. Second, if the loss of pipeline pressure is followed by the flow of contaminated contents from the O_2 pipeline, disconnecting when pipeline pressure is lost protects the patient from exposure to these contaminants.

Although excessive pipeline pressure does not trigger alarms in the machine, it should do so in the hospital's physical plant or engineering department. Excessive pressure can damage respiratory apparatus or machinery of various types connected to the pipeline, including the anesthesia gas machine.

Cross-connection of gases can occur anywhere from the liquid O_2 supply and piping to the wall outlets, hoses, and internal circuitry of the anesthesia gas machine. Incidents of cross-connection continue to be reported. Fatalities in which cross-connection was a factor have been reported as recently as 2002.[17-19] These fatalities have been associated with erroneous shipment to the hospital of liquid nitrogen instead of O_2 and liquid carbon dioxide instead of N_2O; the unintentional cross-connection of O_2 and N_2O pipelines during renovation of an operating room; and alteration of an O_2 flowmeter so that it would fit a N_2O outlet in a cardiac catheterization laboratory. A common factor associated with patient injury has been failure to use an O_2 analyzer.

Although not all incidents involve patients connected to anesthesia gas machines, cross-connections continue to be reported in anesthetized patients. In 1995 a case was described in which the nitrogen hose was discovered to be fitted with a quick-connect coupler for air (at the end that would be plugged into the wall outlet).[20] This did not result in patient injury, but would have allowed the delivery of 100% nitrogen had the machine been set to deliver air only. The consequences of this type of error in the O_2 wall outlet hose could be disastrous. In 1997 it was reported in the United States that two patients became hypoxemic as a result of delivery to the hospital of liquid nitrogen in a tank with O_2 fittings.[21] These incidents underscore the importance of O_2 analysis and proper response to O_2 analyzer alarms.

In the event of a suspected cross-over, the anesthetist must open the emergency cylinder O_2 supply, disconnect the pipeline, and consider the use of low FGFs and manual ventilation. If the pipeline is not disconnected, the pipeline gas will continue to flow, rather than the cylinder O_2 supply. This occurs because the pressure distal to the cylinder regulator is set at 45 psi (310 kPa), compared with the typical pipeline pressure of 50 psi (344 kPa). Lower pressure is intentionally set on the cylinder regulator, so that flow proceeds from the higher pressure pipeline source if a cylinder is inadvertently left open after the machine has been checked.[22] This is analogous to the situation with an intravenous main line and a piggyback line: the one that is held higher is the one that flows (greater hydrostatic pressure). In the case of cross-connection between O_2 and N_2O pipelines, the contents of the O_2 pipeline (now N_2O) continue to flow (because the pipeline pressure is 50 psi) whether or not the O_2 cylinder is open. Therefore, regardless of the problem with the pipeline supply (lack of pressure or cross-connection), the cylinder *must* be opened; I advocate disconnecting the pipeline in any instance of problems with the pipeline. If the pipeline is not disconnected and has pressure within it, the emergency supply of O_2 may not flow from the cylinder.

Pipeline supplies of gas have been reported to contain particulate, gaseous, and bacterial matter; other contaminants; and water.[2,23-25] In 1993 the National Fire Protection Association (NFPA) adopted more stringent testing standards.[23] Also in 1993 the Joint Commission on Accreditation of Healthcare Organizations (JCAHO) established standards that allow site visitors to randomly approach and question operating room and other hospital staff in order to ensure that they are aware of the location and function of shutoff valves and alarms related to gas supplies in their areas.[23]

Cylinder Supply

Cylinders are present on the anesthesia machine as reserves for emergency use. Therefore they should be open only when they are checked or when the pipeline supply is unavailable.[9] A fresh O_2 cylinder need not be obtained if at least one reserve cylinder on the machine has a pressure of 1000 psi.[9,26] Cylinders are labeled, marked, and color coded (Table 15-1). Anesthetists who practice outside the United States must be aware that the color scheme may differ from country to country.[27] Service pressure and cylinder contents are reported slightly differently in various sources; those given in Table 15-1 are from the Compressed Gas Association (CGA).[28] *Pin position* refers to the pin index safety system (PISS; Figures 15-4 and 15-5).[29] In this system each cylinder valve has a unique arrangement of pins that corresponds to its intended contents. The pin arrangement matches holes in the yoke, where the cylinder attaches to the machine. The PISS is thus another means of preventing misconnections. The system can be defeated if the pins are missing or removed or if more than one washer is used. Anesthetists should check both pins and washers whenever cylinders are replaced. Furthermore, they should be aware that not all E cylinders are of precisely the right size to fit properly on the machine. Installation of a longer aluminum cylinder has prevented an anesthesia gas machine from rolling.[30]

TABLE 15-1 E Cylinder Characteristics

Gas	Color, United States (International)	Service Pressure (psi [kPa])	Capacity (L)	Pin Position
Oxygen	Green (white)	1900 (13,100)	660	2-5
Nitrous oxide	Blue (blue)	745 (5100)	1590	3-5
Air	Yellow (black and white)	1900 (13,100)	625	1-5

Data from Standard Specification for Particular Requirements for Anesthesia Workstations and Their Components [F1850-00]. *Philadelphia: ASTM International; 2000; and* NFPA 99: Health Care Facilities. *Quincy, Mass: National Fire Protection Association; 1990:184. Note that slightly different values may be found in different sources.*

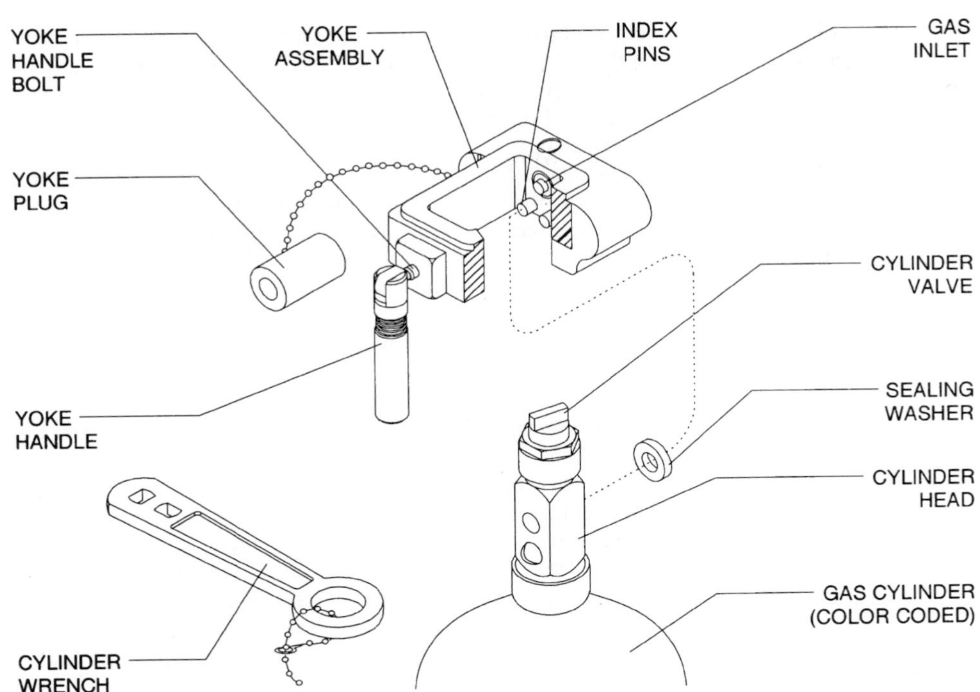

FIGURE **15-4**
Pin index safety system, cylinder valve, and yoke. (From Cicman J, Himmelwright C, Skibo V, Yoder J. *Operating Principles of Narkomed Anesthesia Systems*. Telford, Pa: North American Dräger; 1993.)

The cylinder valve is the most fragile part of the cylinder, so it must be protected during transport. The cylinder valve consists of a body, the port from which gas exits, a conical depression (opposite the port) for the securing screw, PISS pins, and safety relief devices. If a fire causes the temperature and pressure within the cylinder to increase, safety relief devices release cylinder contents in a controlled fashion rather than explosively. Manufacturers use one or more of the following on cylinder valves: a frangible disk that bursts under pressure, a valve that opens at extreme pressure, or a fusible plug made of Wood's metal (which melts at elevated temperatures).

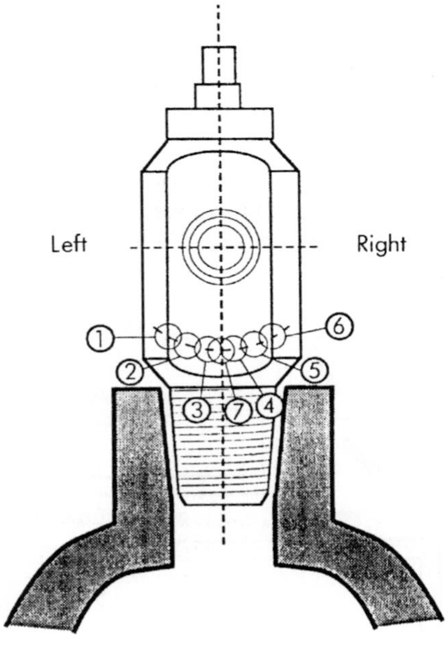

FIGURE **15-5**
Pin index safety system: pin positions. (Modified from Eichhorn JH, Ehrenwerth J. Medical gases: storage and supply. In: Ehrenwerth J, Eisenkraft JB, eds. *Anesthesia Equipment: Principles and Applications*. St Louis: Mosby; 1993:1-26.)

The hanger yoke serves three functions: it orients cylinders, provides a gastight seal, and ensures unidirectional flow. It also contains a filter that is required by standard.[15] The check valve within the hanger yoke minimizes the likelihood of transfilling or of leakage to the atmosphere (if a yoke is empty). It also allows cylinders to be replaced during use. If two cylinders are open, transfilling occurs when gas flows from the cylinder with higher pressure into the cylinder with lower pressure, rather than proceeding toward the flowmeters. This situation is a potential fire hazard because cylinder filling generates heat. The cylinder pressure gauge is a Bourdon-type gauge that indicates pressure within whichever of the two cylinders (if both are open) has the higher pressure (Figure 15-6).

Immediately distal to the hanger yoke for each gas is a regulator (Figure 15-7). Two diaphragms move together, connected by a rod. The smaller of the two diaphragms opens or closes the high-pressure inlet (from the cylinder). Gas entering the regulator exerts pressure on the larger diaphragm, whose movement tends to close the inlet. Therefore gas can enter the regulator only at a rate controlled by a feedback loop. The outlet pressure is adjustable with a screw and spring that bear on the inlet diaphragm. Therefore the regulator converts the high (but variable) cylinder pressure to a constant downstream pressure (45 psi), which is intentionally slightly less than pipeline pressure.[16,23,32,33] This prevents silent depletion of cylinder contents. Pipeline pressure varies, depending on the load that is placed on it throughout the facility. If a cylinder is left open, and pipeline pressure drops below 45 psi, gas flows from the cylinder. No alarm sounds to warn the user of this occurrence.[33] Furthermore, if the cylinder is left open after checking, and the pipeline fails, the operator is not alerted to the failure at the time it occurs, because gas simply begins to flow from the cylinder without alarms. If the

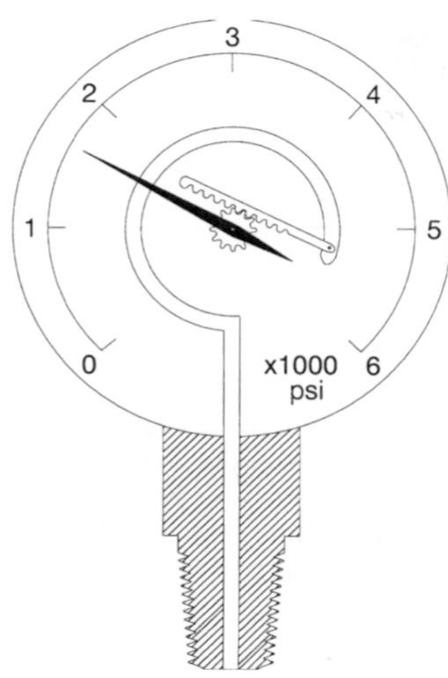

FIGURE **15-6**
Bourdon-type pressure gauges are aneroid gauges used for measuring cylinder (and pipeline) pressure. (From Cicman J, Himmelwright C, Skibo V, Yoder J. *Operating Principles of Narkomed Anesthesia Systems*. Telford, Pa: North American Dräger; 1993.)

mechanical ventilator is in use, a full E cylinder of O_2 may be depleted in as little as 1 hour, because the ventilator-driving gas often is O_2.[12] The low–O_2 supply failure alarm that rings subsequently announces the *end* of the emergency supply, instead of its beginning. This is the rationale for keeping cylinders closed after their presssure has been checked.[9]

The U.S. Department of Transportation issues regulations for the manufacture, handling, transport, storage, and disposal of cylinders. These regulations have binding legal force. Industry advisory groups such as the CGA and the NFPA also have a role in setting cylinder standards. Cylinders are constructed of steel approximately one-quarter inch in thickness. Nonferrous (aluminum) cylinders are available for the magnetic resonance imaging environment.

Anesthetists must be aware of the rules for the safe handling and use of cylinders.[2,34] Gas under pressure in cylinders has an enormous potential energy, which may be lethal if it is released in a rapid, uncontrolled fashion after the cylinder valve has been damaged. To avoid problems, the following suggestions are offered:

- Never stand a cylinder upright without support; instead, lay it on its side.
- Never leave empty cylinders on the machine.
- Never leave the plastic cover on the port while installing the cylinder.
- Never rely only on a cylinder's color for identification of its contents; read its labeling.
- Never oil valves.
- Never remove a cylinder from a yoke without filling the space with a yoke plug if available (see Figure 15-4), which is a backup strategy for guarding against check valve failure.

When installing a cylinder, check the labels, crack the valve, check that both PISS pins are present, check that only one washer is present, place the cylinder in the hanger yoke, observe for the absence of an audible leak, and check for proper gauge pressure. The valve is "cracked" in order to remove dirt from the port. This is done by opening the valve briefly and carefully before the cylinder is placed on the machine. While the valve is cracked, the cylinder is held securely; the port should not be pointed toward the operator or other personnel.

When relying on cylinder supplies in an emergency, one must be able to calculate how long an O_2 cylinder will last. The following relationship should be used:

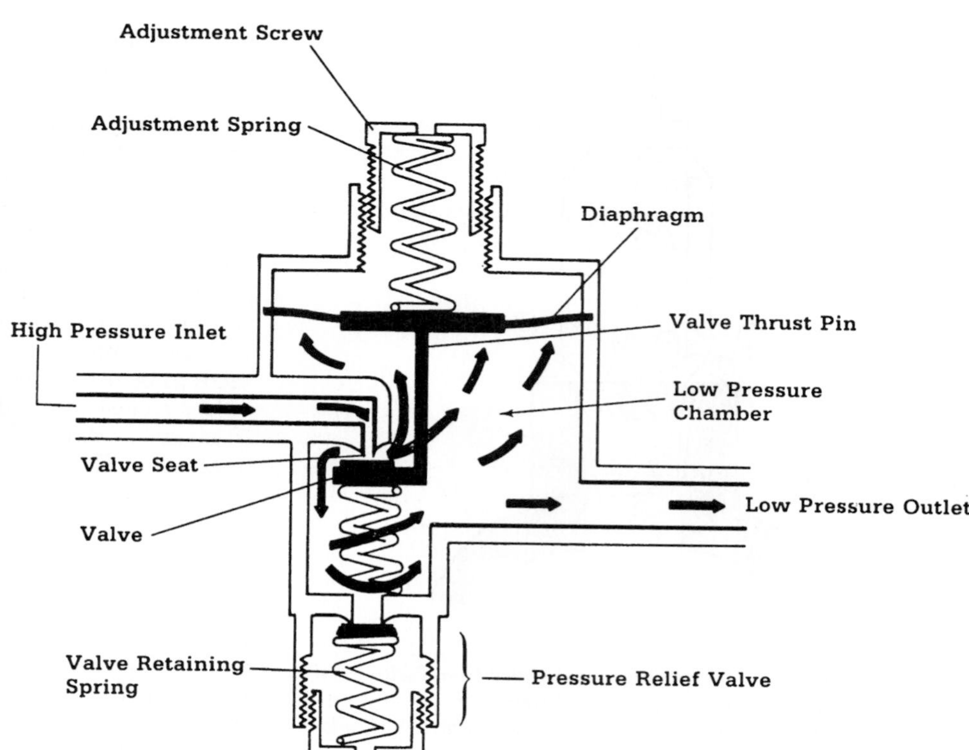

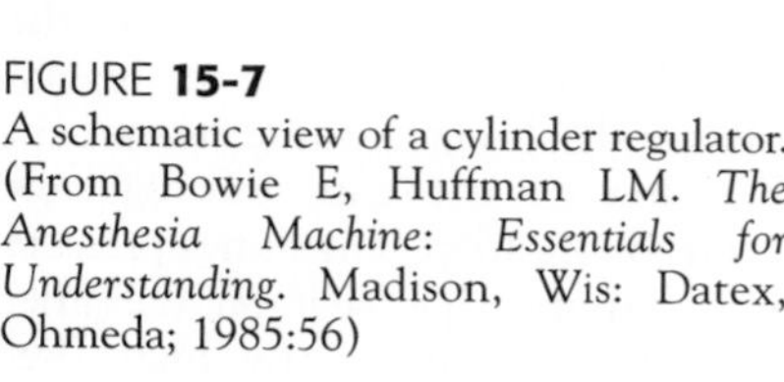
FIGURE **15-7**
A schematic view of a cylinder regulator. (From Bowie E, Huffman LM. *The Anesthesia Machine: Essentials for Understanding*. Madison, Wis: Datex, Ohmeda; 1985:56)

Equation 15-1

Capacity (L) ÷ Service pressure (psi) = Remaining contents (L) ÷ Gauge pressure (psi)

Remember to consider the O_2 flow rate set on the flowmeter when deciding how long the available liters will last. For example, if the O_2 flow is 2 L/min, and the cylinder's O_2 gauge pressure is 500 psi, how long will the cylinder last? From Table 15-1, we know that the service pressure is 1900 psi and that the capacity is 660 L. Substituting these values into the previous relationship, we obtain the following result:

Equation 15-2

$$660\ L \div 1900\ psi = X\ L \div 500\ psi$$
$$X = 174\ L$$

Because 2 L of O_2 flow each minute, the cylinder will last approximately 86 minutes (174 L ÷ 2 L/min). This type of calculation is not applicable to compressed gases stored as liquids (N_2O or carbon dioxide). It should be remembered that this calculation refers only to requirements at the flowmeters and assumes manual ventilation. Use of a mechanical ventilator consumes approximately a minute volume of driving gas each minute and therefore should be avoided in situations in which O_2 supply is limited to cylinders only.

The contents of cylinders must meet the purity requirements for medical gases established by the United States Pharmacopoeia. The contents are also regulated in the United States by the FDA. O_2 is used to power ventilators throughout the hospital because it is dry, readily available, and relatively inexpensive.

N_2O is stored as a liquid; therefore, the cylinder pressure of 745 psi represents the vapor pressure of liquid N_2O at room temperature. The N_2O cylinder pressure gauge remains at 745 psi until the liquid is gone; at that point, the cylinder is more than three-quarters empty. After that point the N_2O cylinder pressure swiftly declines with further use. Therefore N_2O cylinders should be changed if their pressure is less than 745 psi. Rapid removal (more than 4 L/min) from a cylinder may cause the formation of frost on its wall, or freezing of the valve, because of the loss of the latent heat of vaporization from the liquid N_2O. N_2O is nonflammable, but it does support combustion. Anesthesia personnel must be alert to the possibility of N_2O abuse.[35]

Compressed air is not entirely dry. Its composition varies from sample to sample, but its major constituents are nitrogen (78%), O_2 (21%), and argon (nearly 1%). Carbon dioxide (0.03%) and other gases are present in trace amounts.

Electrical Power Supply

Electrical power is supplied to the gas machine through a single power cord, which can become dislodged. Because of this possibility, as well as the possibility of loss of main electrical power, new gas machines must be equipped with battery backup sufficient for at least 30 minutes of limited operation.[15] Which functions remain powered during this period varies according to model, and users therefore must read the operator's manuals. For example, if the electrical power is disconnected from the S/5 ADU (Datex-Ohmeda, Madison, Wisconsin), it loses patient monitors (electrocardiogram, noninvasive blood pressure, gas analysis, pulse oximetry, and other monitors displayed on the right screen), but FGF, volatile agent delivery, and ventilation continue during the period that battery backup is used. Once battery power is lost, N_2O and agent delivery are cut off.

Convenience receptacles are usually found on the back of the machine so that monitors or other equipment can be plugged in. These convenience receptacles are protected by circuit breakers (usually) or fuses. It is a mistake to plug into these convenience receptacles devices that convert electrical power into heat (air or water warming blankets, intravenous fluid warmers) for two reasons.[36] First, these devices draw a lot of amperage (relative to other electrical devices), so they are more likely to cause a circuit breaker to open. Second, the circuit breakers are in nonstandard locations (so check for their location before the first case). In the Modulus SE they can be reset only by reaching from the front of the machine. If a circuit breaker opens, all devices that receive power there (such as monitors, and in some configurations the mechanical ventilator) may cease to function. If one is not familiar with the circuit breaker location, valuable time may be lost while a search is conducted.

Loss of Main Electrical Power

Devices (or techniques) that typically do not rely on wall outlet electrical power include spontaneous or manually assisted ventilation, mechanical flowmeters, scavenging, laryngoscope, flashlights, intravenous bolus or infusion, battery operated peripheral nerve stimulators or intravenous infusion pumps, monitoring using the anesthetist's five senses, and variable bypass vaporizers (Tec 4, Vapor 19).

Devices that typically require wall outlet electrical power include mechanical ventilators, physiologic monitors, room and surgical field illumination, digital flowmeter displays for electronic flowmeters, cardiopulmonary bypass pumps and oxygenators, air warming blankets, gas and vapor blenders (Suprane Tec 6), and vaporizers with electronic controls (Aladin cassettes in the S/5 ADU).

Generally, hospitals have emergency generators that supply operating room electrical outlets in the event that power is lost. But these backup generators are not completely reliable. A 90-minute interruption in power during cardiopulmonary bypass, complicated by almost immediate failure of the hospital generators, has been described.[37] One unanticipated hazard was injuries to personnel as they hurried to fetch lights and equipment.

With power failure in older gas machines, the principal problems were loss of room illumination and failure of mechanical ventilators and electronic patient monitoring. In general, new gas machines have battery backup sufficient for 30 minutes of operation—still, however, without patient monitors (electrocardiogram, pulse oximetry, gas analysis). Mechanical ventilation may or may not be powered by the backup battery (depending on the model). New flowmeters that are entirely electronic (Julian, Dräger Medical, Telford, Pennsylvania) require a backup pneumatic or mechanical flowmeter ("Safety O_2" flowmeter).[38] Mechanical flowmeters with digital display of flows may have a backup glass flow tube that indicates total FGF (S/5 ADU,[39] Datex-Ohmeda; Fabius GS,[40] Dräger Medical). New gas machines with mechanical needle valve flowmeters and variable bypass vaporizers (Fabius GS) have an advantage in that delivery of gases and agent can continue indefinitely.[40] However, in the event of generator failure, anesthesia would be limited to flashlight illumination and monitoring by the five senses. The Narkomed 6000 (Dräger Medical) and Julian provide gas and vapor delivery and integrated monitoring (O_2, breathing circuit volume and pressure, gas analysis) for 30 minutes if main electrical power is lost.[38,41]

Because of the growing differences among models, it remains important to understand and anticipate how each particular anesthesia gas machine type responds when main electrical power is lost. This information must be reviewed in the operator's manual.

PROCESSING

In this section, the various aspects of the anesthesia gas machine's preparation of gases before their delivery to the patient are discussed.

Manufacturers and Models

Two major manufacturers of anesthesia gas machines exist in the United States. Dräger Medical, Inc. (http://www.draeger.com/us/MT/mt.jsp) is the manufacturer of the Narkomed series (2A, 2B, 2C, 3, 4, 6000 and 6400, GS, MRI, and Mobile models), the Julian, and the Fabius GS. The Narkomed GS, MRI, Mobile, 6400, Julian, and Fabius GS are currently produced.

Datex-Ohmeda (http://www.datex-ohmeda.com/) is the manufacturer of the Modulus, Excel, Aestiva, Aestiva MRI, and S/5 ADU. The Aestiva, Aestiva MRI, and S/5 ADU are currently produced.

Gas machines that are not currently produced remain in widespread use. Currently produced models meet or exceed the specifications of the anesthesia workstation standard F1850.[16] The S/5 ADU, Julian, and Fabius GS were designed to the European anesthesia workstation standard (EN 740), so they are the most novel gas machines marketed in the United States. New gas machines have significant differences; therefore what one learns on one machine may not transfer very well to a different model. The differences are pointed out in this chapter when they are relevant to clinical practice or to demonstrate by comparison how systems function. This section continues with an overview of four new machines. The companion Web site for this chapter (http://www.udmercy.edu/crna/agm/) contains additional information and illustrations of the individual models (see "New Gas Machines" section).

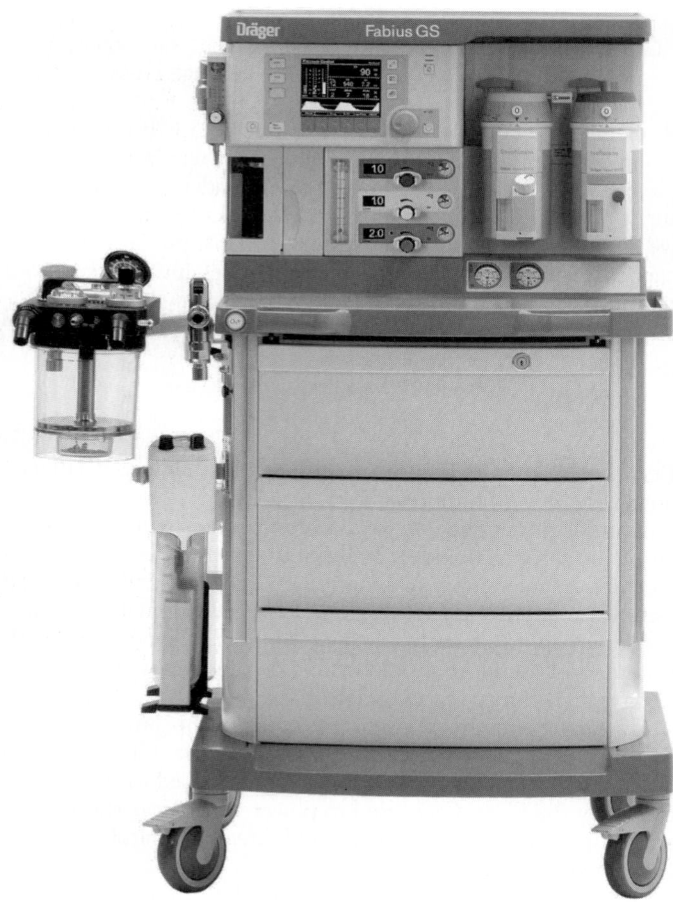

FIGURE **15-8**
Fabius GS, Dräger Medical. (Courtesy Draeger Medical, Inc., Telford, Pennsylvania.)

Dräger Fabius GS

The Fabius GS (Figure 15-8) includes volume, pressure, and inspired O_2 monitoring, but not physiologic monitors or gas analysis. The thermal anemometry ("hot wire") flow sensor in the breathing circuit is unique to this machine and the Julian. It may be sensitive to radio-frequency interference from electrosurgery units. The screen displays tidal and minute volume, respiratory rate, and a respiratory pressure waveform. The ventilator is piston driven, corrects tidal volume for compliance and leaks, and features pressure control mode (pressure-controlled ventilation [PCV]). The machine uses a manual FDA-style checklist with a few electronic self-tests (system, leaks, flow sensor, O_2 sensor). Therefore, with the Fabius GS, as with all the new models, users must review the operator's manual to check the machine correctly. The flowmeters are needle valves with electronic capture and display, with a common gas outlet flowmeter as backup. Variable-bypass vaporizers are used, and these may be removed without tools.

The Fabius GS breathing circuit is a lower-volume circuit (2.8 L, of which 1.5 L is absorbent volume). The absorber head is not warmed. Only loose carbon dioxide absorbent granules may be used. There is an open scavenger interface. Fresh gas decoupling causes the manual breathing bag to fluctuate during the mechanical ventilator cycle, which serves as a further disconnect alarm.

In case of electrical power failure, a 45-minute battery reserve is present, with fresh gas, vaporizers, integrated monitors, and ventilator operational. Patient monitors will not function, as they are not part of the gas machine. Several pneumatic functions remain after the battery is exhausted: vaporizers, hypoxic guard, adjustable pressure-limiting (APL or "popoff") valve, flowmeters, breathing pressure gauge, cylinder and pipeline pressure gauges, and common gas outlet flowmeter.

Dräger Narkomed 6000 and 6400

The Narkomed 6000 (Figure 15-9) includes volume, pressure, and inspired O_2 monitoring. It also includes gas monitoring (infrared agent and carbon dioxide) and an ultrasonic flow sensor in the breathing circuit (unique to this machine). An integrated patient monitoring module is available as an option, so that all parameters are displayed on the single touch screen.

The 6000 includes a piston ventilator (Divan) with tidal volume corrected for leaks, patient and breathing circuit compliance, and FGF (by fresh gas decoupling). The ventilator is capable of PCV and synchronized intermittent mandatory ventilation (SIMV) mode. Like the Fabius GS, there is no "bag-vent" switch, because changing of the ventilator mode is controlled electronically. It is accurate to very low tidal volume (range 10 to 1400 ml).

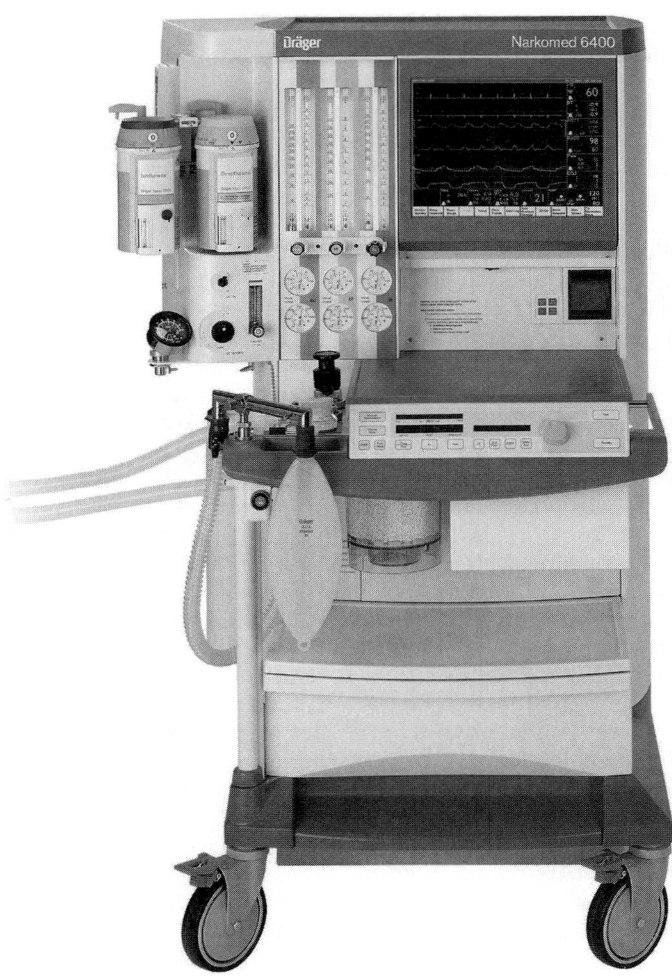

FIGURE **15-9**
Dräger Narkomed 6400. (Courtesy Draeger Medical, Inc., Telford, Pennsylvania.)

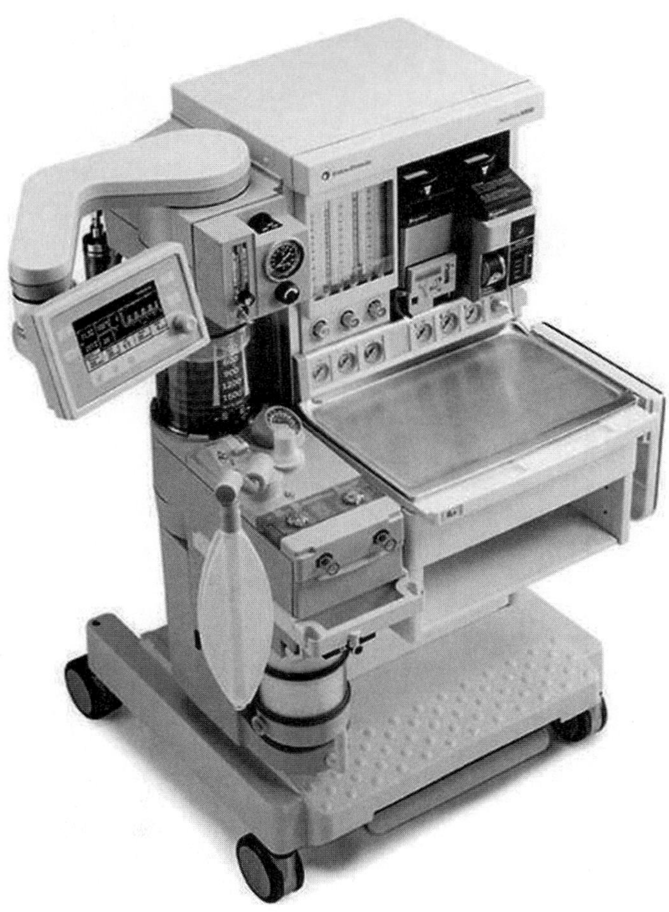

FIGURE **15-10**
Datex-Ohmeda Aestiva. (Courtesy of Datex-Ohmeda, Tewksbury, Massachusetts.)

From a cold startup, the machine performs a 1-minute power-on self-test, then a 5-minute ventilator self-test. One can bypass the ventilator test 10 days or 10 times only, after which the ventilator is unavailable until the self-test is performed. The machine checkout follows FDA guidelines, but some differences exist. For example, the manufacturer recommends breathing through each circuit limb to test unidirectional valves and disconnecting the O_2 wall hose to check the O_2 pipeline pressure-failure device.

Flowmeters are composed of needle valves and glass flowtubes, but electronic capture of FGFs has been added in the 6400. Variable-bypass vaporizers are used, and these may be removed without tools.

The breathing circuit is lower volume (1.5 L absorbent volume), and the absorber head is warmed. Only loose carbon dioxide absorbent granules may be used. An open scavenger interface or passive evacuation may be used. In case of power failure, the model has a 30-minute battery reserve, with fresh gas, vaporizers, monitors, and ventilator operational.

Datex-Ohmeda Aestiva

The Aestiva (Figure 15-10) is a gas machine of familiar size and design and includes volume, pressure, and inspired O_2 monitoring. Gas analysis and patient physiologic monitors must be added.

The ventilator uses a gas-driven standing bellows that is capable of PCV. The flow sensors compensate tidal volume for compliance losses and leaks in the absorber head and bellows, so the ventilator is accurate to very low tidal volumes. The variable orifice flow sensors have shown some sensitivity to moisture in the breathing circuit in the past. The "bag-vent" switch activates the mechanical ventilator in one step. The absorber head design allows for easier disassembly and cleaning than older models. The Aestiva uses a manual FDA-style checklist.

Flowmeters are traditional mechanical needle valves and glass flowtubes. No electronic capture of FGFs occurs. Variable-bypass vaporizers are used, and these may be removed without tools. The breathing circuit is of a relatively high volume (5.5 L, including dual canisters of 1.35 kg of absorbent each). Loose fill granules or prepackaged absorbent may be used. The machine is compatible with nonrebreathing circuits. The scavenger is available as a closed scavenger interface. The machine has a 30-minute battery reserve, with fresh gas, vaporizers, and ventilator operational. The Aestiva is also available in an MRI-compatible version.

Datex-Ohmeda S/5 Anesthesia Delivery Unit

The S/5 ADU (Figure 15-11) includes all monitoring: volume, pressure, inspired O_2, gas analysis (agent and carbon dioxide),

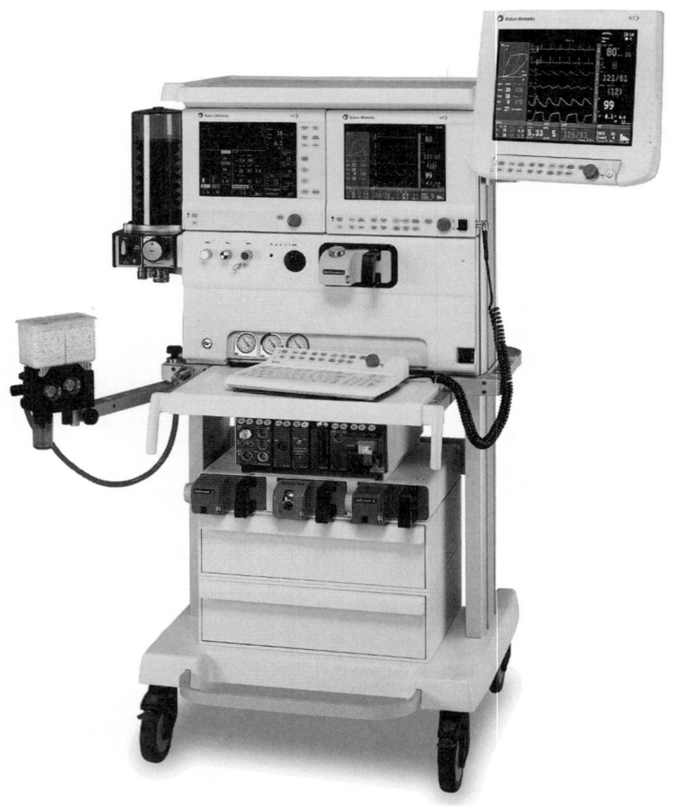

FIGURE **15-11**
Datex-Ohmeda S/5 Anesthesia Delivery Unit. Machine monitors are on the left screen (including video-screen display of fresh gas flow); patient monitors are on the left (including electrocardiograph and blood pressure). (Courtesy of Datex-Ohmeda, Tewksbury, Massachusetts.)

patient physiologic monitoring, and spirometry (flow-volume and pressure-volume respiratory loops).

The ventilator is a gas-driven standing bellows, with tidal volume corrected for leaks, compliance, and FGF (to the D-Lite sensor at the Y-piece). It is accurate to very low tidal volumes, and is capable of PCV and SIMV. The "bag-vent" switch activates the mechanical ventilator in one step.

The S/5 uses an almost completely automated checklist routine that conforms to FDA recommendations. Because the D-Lite sensor is removed from the breathing circuit during checkout, a high-pressure check of the breathing circuit must be performed after reassembly.

The flowmeters are mechanical needle valves. Flow is captured and displayed electronically, with a common gas outlet flowmeter as an optional backup. Variable-bypass vaporizers are used, and these may be removed without tools. The Aladin vaporizer cassettes may be tipped from the vertical during transport without any risk. The vaporizers are not interchangeable with any other model.

The breathing circuit has a very low volume (only 750 ml absorbent volume). Only the manufacturer's carbon dioxide absorbent canisters may be used, and these are single-use canisters or refillable with loose granules. Certain disposable accessories are available only from the manufacturer (spirometry tubing, D-Lite sensor, absorbent granule canisters). The machine is technically compatible with nonrebreathing circuits, but the need for them is questionable because the machine can ventilate patients who weigh as little as 3 kg. The scavenger interface is open. Scavenger suction adequacy is indicated on an optional glass flowmeter. The machine has a 30-minute battery reserve, with fresh gas, vaporizers, and ventilator operational. Patient monitoring (right screen) is lost unless main electrical power (or generator backup) is available, as is the case with most gas machines, new or old.

Path of Gases through the Machine

O_2, N_2O, and air follow similar paths through the anesthesia gas machine (see Figure 15-1). Each passes from its supply point to a flowmeter. All gases (except O_2) pass through a fail-safe valve before proceeding to their flowmeters. This valve is held open by pressure in the O_2 circuitry within the anesthesia gas machine. After passing through their respective flowmeters, the gases are joined for the first time in a common manifold. O_2 is always added to the common manifold downstream of other gases, so that the chance of hypoxic breathing mixtures is lessened (e.g., in the event that a flow tube has cracked).[42] The combined gases enter any vaporizer that is turned on and then pass through the common gas outlet. A delivery hose with a locking connection conducts gases from the common gas outlet to the breathing circuit.

The breathing circuit and ventilator (if used) transport gases to and from the patient. An amount equal to the FGF per minute (minus patient uptake, plus gases excreted) leaves the breathing circuit and is conducted to the scavenger interface. From there, it is disposed of in the hospital ventilation or suction systems.

Five Pathways of Oxygen

O_2 has five pathways in the anesthesia gas machine: (1) proceeds to the fresh gas flowmeter, (2) powers the O_2 flush, (3) activates fail-safe mechanisms, (4) activates O_2 low-pressure alarms, and (5) compresses the bellows of mechanical ventilators. The other gases supplied by the machine have only one pathway: they are transported via flowmeter and breathing circuit to anesthetize the patient (N_2O) or sustain life (the O_2 component in the air flowmeter).

Flowmeter

The first task of O_2 is to proceed through the flowmeter and on to the patient as a life-sustaining gas. Flowmeters have several components (Box 15-4). Control knobs are color and touch coded; therefore the O_2 flow control knob is distinguishable visually and tactilely from the control knobs for the other gases (Figure 15-12).[43] The needle valve, which controls gas flow through the flowmeter, can be damaged if it is closed with excessive force. Valve stops (Figure 15-13) are usually incorpo-

BOX **15-4**

Components of Flowmeters

- Knob
- Needle valve
- Valve stops
- Flowtube
- Indicator float
  - Rotating-ball (Dräger)
  - Plumb-bob (Datex-Ohmeda)

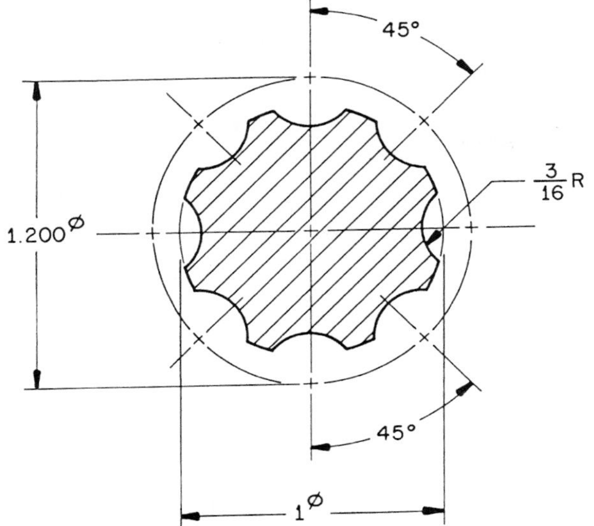

FIGURE **15-12**
Oxygen knobs are touch coded to make them more distinctive. (From Schreiber P. *Safety Guidelines for Anesthesia Systems*. Telford, Pa: North American Dräger; 1985.)

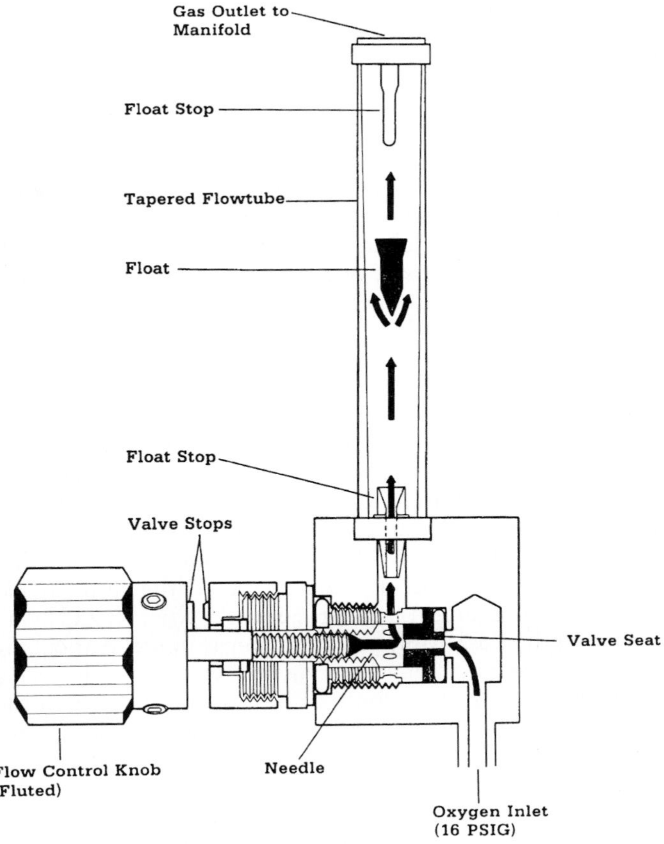

FIGURE **15-13**
Flowmeter components. (From Bowie E, Huffman LM. *The Anesthesia Machine: Essentials for Understanding*. Madison, Wis: Datex-Ohmeda; 1985.)

rated to prevent damage. Note that there are no valve stops in the ADU needle valves. Flow increases when the knob is turned counterclockwise. All current gas machines use mechanical needle valves except Kion (Siemens Medical, Malvern, Pennsylvania) and Julian (Dräger Medical), which use electronic controls for flow.

Display of Fresh Gas Flow. An indicator float in a glass flowtube is the classic way to capture and display FGF. Flowtubes (Thorpe tubes) are calibrated to 2% to 10% accuracy at room temperature and 760 mm Hg pressure.[22,31-33] They are specific for each gas and cannot be interchanged. The flowtube is tapered so that it is narrower at its bottom. Therefore it may be referred to as a "variable orifice flowmeter," because the annular opening around the float is larger at higher flows. If a gas has two tubes, they are connected in series with a single control valve (Figure 15-14). It is standard in the United States (but not in the United Kingdom) for the O_2 flowtube to be placed to the right of other flowtubes. Flowmeters on the Fabius GS are unique in that they are arranged vertically, rather than side by side (Figure 15-15). The flowtubes are the most fragile part of the machine. They are susceptible to breakage, leaks at their seals, and inaccuracy resulting from the presence of dirt or static electricity.

The Narkomed 6000, Mobile, MRI, and Aestiva use glass flowtube displays. Many newer gas machines capture flows electronically by means of a transducer and chamber of known volume. The chamber fills to a set pressure, and then the gas is allowed to proceed. The number of times this cycle occurs per minute can be converted to gas flow, which can be sent to automated record keepers. The ADU and Fabius GS dispense with glass flowtubes, displaying FGFs as colored bar graphs with numeric data on a computer screen. Both have as a backup at the common gas outlet a glass flowmeter that measures total FGF continuously and in the event of screen or electrical power failure. The Narkomed 6400 uses regular glass flowtubes for display of flows but can capture flows electronically.

Setting FGF on the Kion and Julian machines is quite different. The flowmeter controls and display are all electronic. The display is numeric, with an optional bar-graph display. The user sets the desired inspired O_2 concentration, the total FGF, and the carrier gas desired (N_2O, air).

Care of Flowmeters. Flowmeters should be turned off before pipelines are connected, cylinders are opened, or the machine is turned on. If a flowtube is left open, the float will shoot to the top of the flowtube and may damage it. Flowmeters should be included in visual monitoring sweeps. Never adjust a flowmeter without looking at it. Read ball-type indicator floats in their center (Dräger) and plumb bob–type floats at the top (Datex-Ohmeda). Remember to turn off flowmeters after each case and particularly at the end of the day. Failure to do so may contribute to premature drying of the carbon dioxide absorbent, which not only hastens its exhaustion, but also has been implicated in the increase of the degradation of volatile agent and in the generation of carbon monoxide in canisters.[44,45]

Other Flowmeters

Auxiliary Oxygen Flowmeters. Auxiliary O_2 flowmeters are an optional accessory currently offered on most models of gas machines. Useful for attaching a nasal cannula or other supplemental O_2 delivery devices, they are advantageous because the breathing circuit and gas delivery hose (between

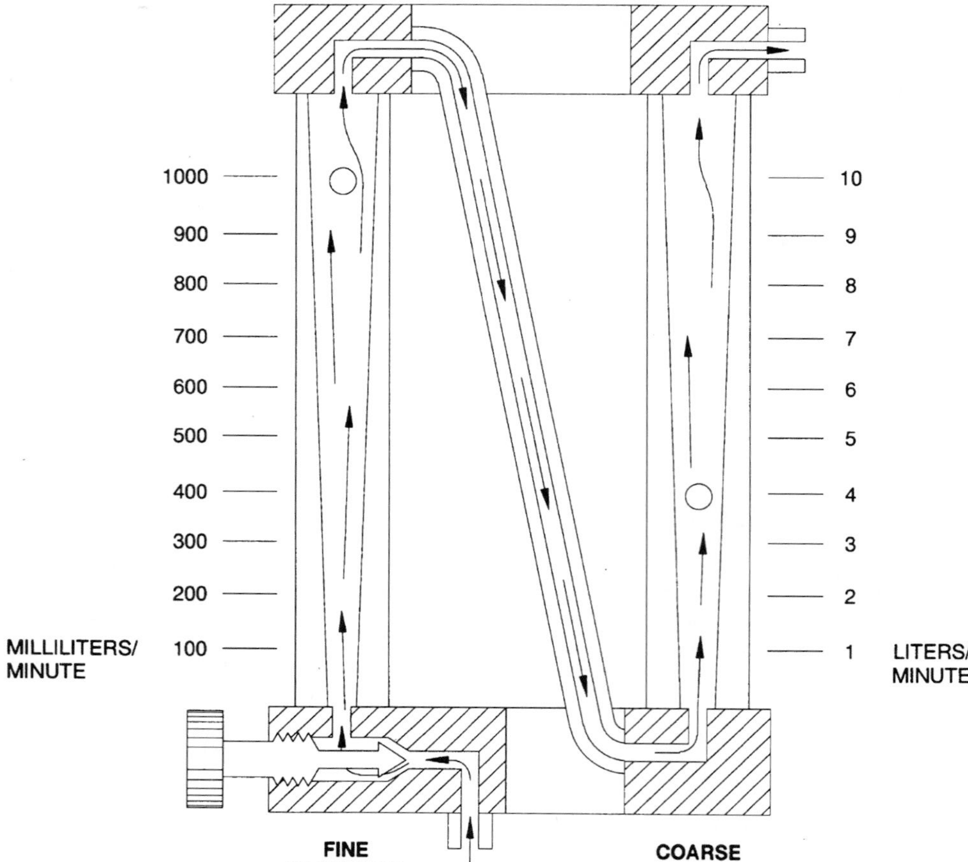

FIGURE **15-14**
When two flowmeters are present for one gas, they are arranged in series. (From Cicman J, Himmelwright C, Skibo V, Yoder J. *Operating Principles of Narkomed Anesthesia Systems*. Telford, Pa: North American Dräger; 1993.)

the common gas outlet and breathing circuit) remain intact while supplemental O_2 is delivered to a spontaneously breathing patient. Therefore if the anesthetist desires to switch from a nasal cannula to the circle breathing system during a case, this can be accomplished instantaneously and without the possibility of forgetting to reconfigure the breathing circuit properly. Another advantage is that an O_2 source is readily available for the Ambu bag if the patient needs to be ventilated manually for any reason during a case (for example, breathing circuit failure). One disadvantage is that the auxiliary flowmeter becomes unavailable if the pipeline supply has lost pressure or has been contaminated; this occurs because the auxiliary flowmeter is supplied by the same wall outlet and hose connection that supplies the main O_2 flowmeter. If users do not realize this, then time could be wasted while they attempt to make use of this potential O_2 source.[46]

Common Gas Outlet Flowmeters. Common gas outlet flowmeters (Figure 15-16) are used as backups on some gas machines that electronically capture and display flows on a computer screen (Fabius GS, ADU). If offered as an option, they are strongly recommended, as they are the only indication of O_2 flow if the computer display fails or in the case of power failure after battery backup is exhausted.

Scavenging Flowmeters. Most new machines use open scavenging interfaces. An indication that suction is adequate is mandatory with these systems in order to avoid exposure to waste anesthesia gases (see the discussion of disposal of scavenged and waste gases later in this chapter). Unfortunately, the suction indicator may not be visible from the operator's normal position. It is on the back of the machine, near the E cylinders, on the Fabius GS and Julian. It is behind and beneath the bellows block on the left side of the ADU (Figure 15-17). Even though scavenging flowmeters are desirable, they may be included not with the basic package, but only as an optional accessory (ADU).

Oxygen Flush

The second task of O_2 in the processing area of the machine is to supply the O_2 flush valve. The flush valve is required by standard to deliver from 35 to 75 L/min.[15,47] The nominal delivery is typically around 50 L/min or greater.[22,31,32,38-41,47,48] The flush valve is often protected by a rim that lessens the chance of accidental activation of the flush. Should this occur, barotrauma is a potential result. Users should avoid activating the flush while the ventilator is in use, particularly during the inspiratory phase, because the ventilator relief valve closes during this phase, preventing gas from exiting to the scavenger.[49] If flushing is necessary for filling of the ventilator bellows, it may be done with caution, in short bursts, during the expiratory phase.

The O_2 flush line proceeds directly from the gas supply source to the common gas outlet (see Figure 15-1). Therefore activation of the flush bypasses the vaporizers and adds 100% O_2 to the breathing circuit. If partial pressures of N_2O or volatile agent have already been established in the breathing circuit (during maintenance), excessive use of the O_2 flush

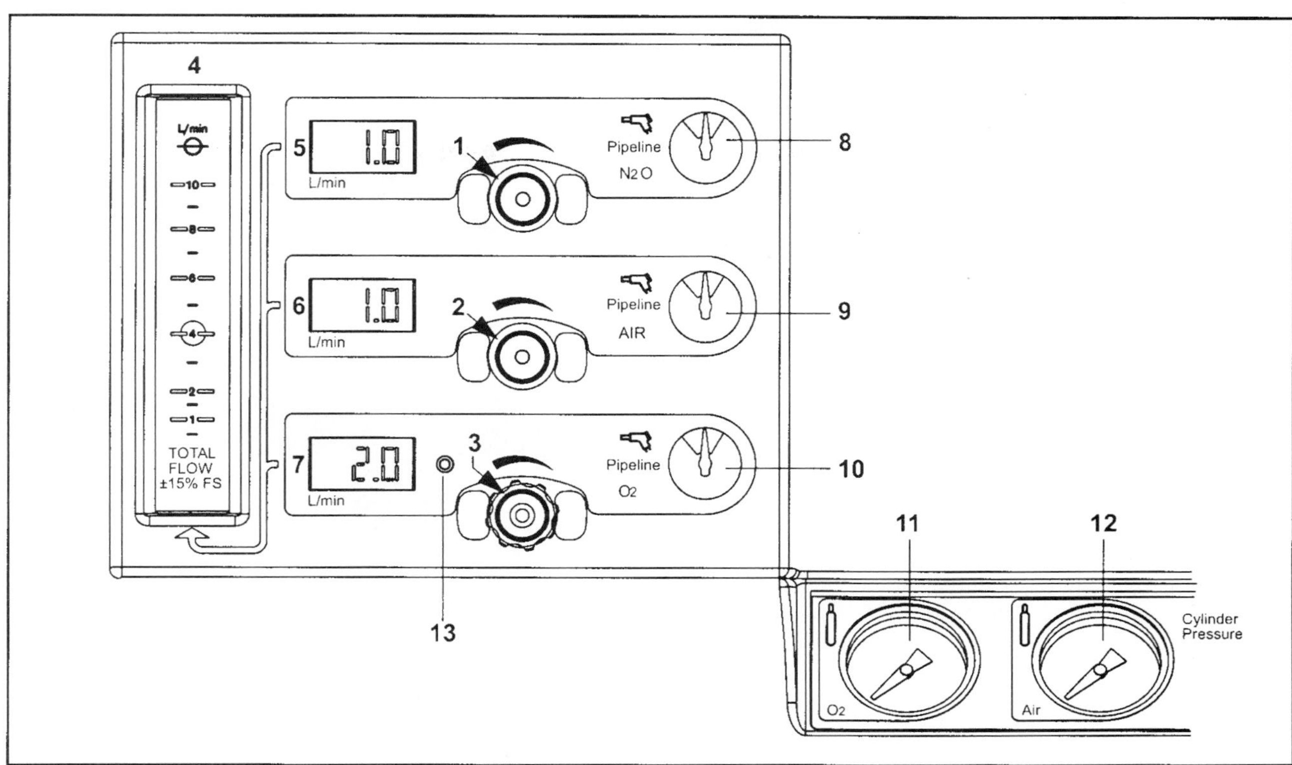

FIGURE **15-15**
Flowmeters on the Fabius GS are arranged vertically. The common gas outlet flowmeter is to the left *(5)*. Oxygen flowmeter is at the bottom of the bank, nitrous oxide at the top. To the left of each flow control knob is a digital display of flow; to the right is the pipeline pressure gauge for each gas. Cylinder gauges are to the right. (Courtesy Draeger Medical, Inc., Telford, Pennsylvania.)

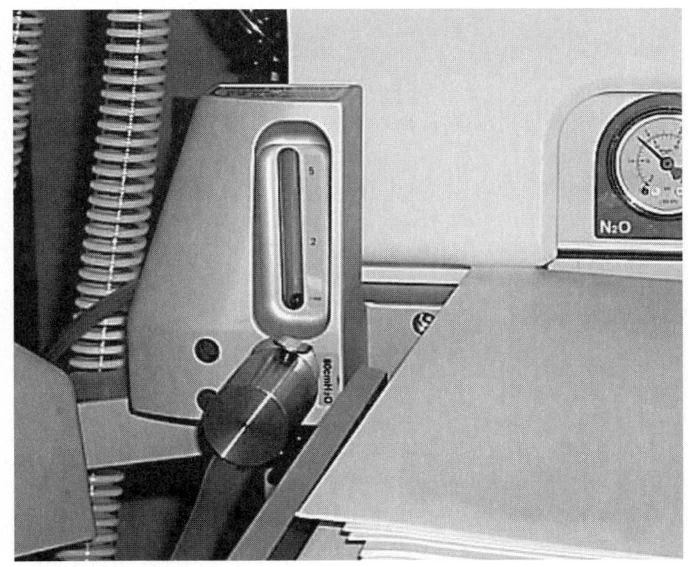

FIGURE **15-16**
The common gas outlet flowmeter on the ADU is located to the left of the writing surface. (From *Datex-Ohmeda. S/5 Anesthesia Delivery Unit User's Reference Manual.* Madison, Wis: Datex-Ohmeda; 2000. Catalog No. 8502304.)

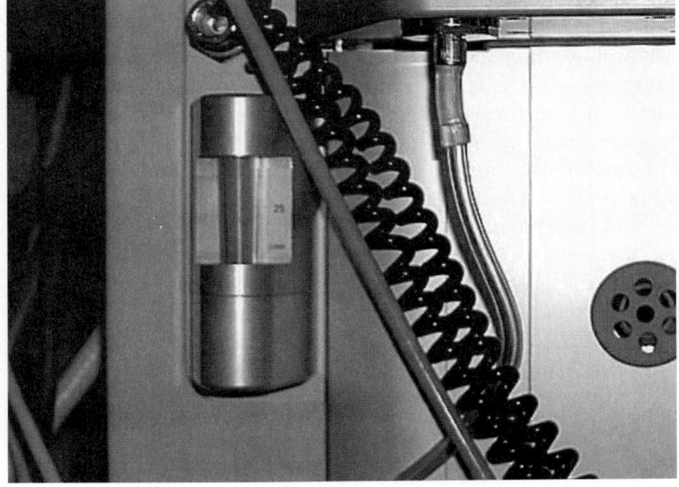

FIGURE **15-17**
Scavenger suction flowmeter on anesthesia delivery unit is located behind and beneath the bellows block, on the left side of the machine.

tends to dilute these inhaled agents and may lessen the depth of anesthesia.

Because of differences in design and the operating characteristics of their flush valves, not all anesthesia gas machines are suitable for effective transtracheal jet ventilation (via percutaneous cricothyrotomy with a small intravenous catheter). The Narkomed 2, 2A, 2B, and 3 machines and the Datex-Ohmeda Modulus II machines were tested in vitro and were found to perform adequately. The Datex-Ohmeda Modulus II Plus did not perform suitably on the same test.[50]

Fail-Safe Systems

If pipeline O_2 pressure were to fail while other gases such as N_2O continued to flow, the patient could receive a hypoxic gas mixture (less than 21% O_2). Therefore gas machines incorporate devices that halt the supply of all other gases in the event of O_2 supply pressure failure. These are called *fail-safe systems*. It is required by standard that the set concentration of O_2 at the common gas outlet does not decline if the pipeline pressure decreases.[15] This requirement is satisfied by the presence of gatelike fail-safe valves in the internal supply lines for all gases except O_2. The "gate" in each is held open by pressure in the O_2 line (Figure 15-18). Flow of all other gases in typical Datex-Ohmeda machines (Excel, Modulus) is shut off when pressure in the O_2 supply line decreases to 20 psi.[31,32,48] Datex-Ohmeda terms the shutoff device a *pressure sensor shutoff valve*.

On the Narkomed machines, the fail-safe gate valve is called the *oxygen failure protection device* (OFPD). This device reduces the supply of all other gases proportionally as O_2 supply pressure declines, finally halting the flow of N_2O and all other gases when O_2 supply pressure is approximately 12 psi.[51]

In summary, both types of fail-safe devices leave O_2 (however briefly) as the last gas flowing, because they interrupt the supply of all other gases before the flowmeters. For example, if a flow rate of 2 L/min is set on a machine for both N_2O and O_2, and the O_2 pipeline is disconnected, the N_2O float indicator would be seen to drop to zero first, and the O_2 float shortly thereafter.

Low-Pressure Alarms

The fourth task of O_2 is powering the low-pressure alarms, which signal the operator when pressure is lost in the O_2 circuitry. The older O_2 supply failure alarm (Datex-Ohmeda) is a container with a whistle at its outlet that is pressurized by O_2 when the anesthesia gas machine is turned on. When pipeline pressure decreases to 28 psi[32] or when the machine is shut off, a characteristic sound is heard as the container releases its contents. Newer models lack this distinctive alarm.[16]

Narkomed machines also sound an alarm when O_2 pipeline pressure reaches approximately 30 psi (older models)[22] to 37 psi (newer models).[33] A medium-priority alarm is displayed on the Narkomed central alarm display, and visible and audible alarms are activated on the main switch panel. The flowmeters on the Narkomed machines also indicate a reduction in all gas flows that is proportional to the decrease in pressure in the O_2 line. The proper response of the anesthetist to loss of pipeline pressure was discussed previously in the section covering supply.

Ventilator Driving Gas

The fifth task of O_2 in the anesthesia gas machine is compression of the ventilator bellows. All Datex-Ohmeda anesthesia ventilators use 100% O_2 as their driving gas.[39,52,53] The 7800 and 7900 may also use compressed air.[52,54] The ADU may use either, and switches from O_2 to air automatically if O_2 pressure is lost.[39]

The Dräger AV-E and AV-2 ventilators use the O_2 supply in a Venturi device, which augments the driving gas with entrained room air.[33] Room air enters through a shiny (chrome or stainless steel) cylindrical muffler, which may be seen at the back of some Narkomed models. If this muffler becomes dirty, insufficient gas may enter; the lack can potentially interfere with the ability of the ventilator to compress the bellows. If driving gas is prevented from exiting via the muffler, the bellows may remain compressed, and barotrauma results.

Piston ventilators use electric motors to compress the bellows and deliver tidal volume (Narkomed 6000 and 6400, Fabius GS).[40,41] Ventilator delivery of tidal volume is unaffected by variation in O_2 pipeline pressure. Piston ventilators may operate outside the operating room for prolonged periods with only cylinder supplies of gases, because they do not consume O_2 to drive the bellows.

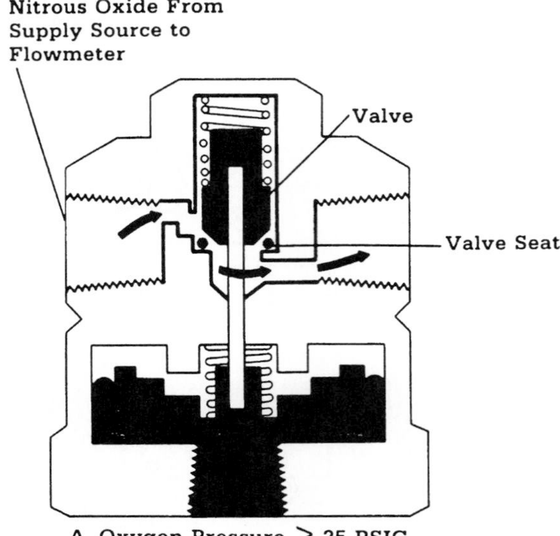

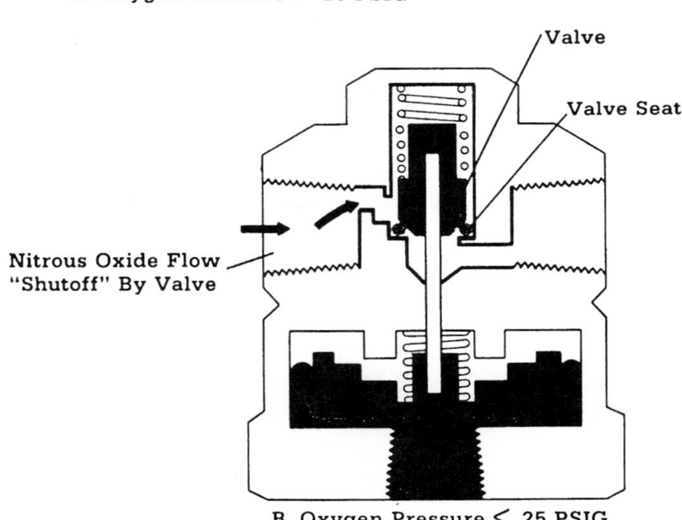

FIGURE **15-18**
Datex-Ohmeda pressure-sensor shutoff valve (fail-safe) in the nitrous oxide line. (From Bowie E, Huffman LM. *The Anesthesia Machine: Essentials for Understanding*. Madison, Wis: Datex-Ohmeda; 1985.)

Proportioning Systems

All current anesthesia gas machines incorporate hypoxic guard systems designed to prevent the delivery of hypoxic breathing mixtures. All link O_2 and N_2O so that final breathing mixtures are at least 25% ± 4% O_2.[32,33] The ratio of N_2O to O_2 is therefore not more than 3:1.

An example of a pneumatic-mechanical proportioning system is the Datex-Ohmeda Link-25 (Figure 15-19). In this system, the flowmeter control knobs are linked by a chain, so that O_2 flow is increased automatically when N_2O flow is increased. The Link-25 system also incorporates secondary regulators; therefore it has both pneumatic and mechanical components.

The Narkomed models incorporate the oxygen ratio monitor controller (ORMC) as their hypoxic guard system (later models use devices called *oxygen ratio controllers* [ORCs] or *sensitive oxygen ratio controllers* [S-ORCs]).[40,41] This system also maintains at least 25% O_2, but does so by limiting N_2O flow. Electronic alarms may be incorporated, so the system has pneumatic-mechanical and electronic components. As lower FGFs are used (associated with more rebreathing), the ORC increases the mandatory minimum O_2 concentration above 25%.[27]

It is important to recognize that hypoxic guard systems are not foolproof. Four situations in which a hypoxic breathing mixture can be delivered despite the use of hypoxic guard systems are listed in Box 15-5. Lack of O_2 in the O_2 pipeline may be detected with an O_2 analyzer. A system that is broken or defective should be detected in the preuse checklist, as should leaks downstream of the flowmeters. The most dangerous of these circumstances is the last, the administration of a third gas, especially that of an inert gas such as helium. It is not widely appreciated that the hypoxic guard systems link *only* N_2O and O_2. Perhaps because of the name, the assumption is made that *all* hypoxic breathing mixtures are prevented. These systems would not prevent the administration of a hypoxic mixture of a third inert gas (such as helium) and O_2. The proper use of an O_2 analyzer in each general anesthetic remains of vital importance.

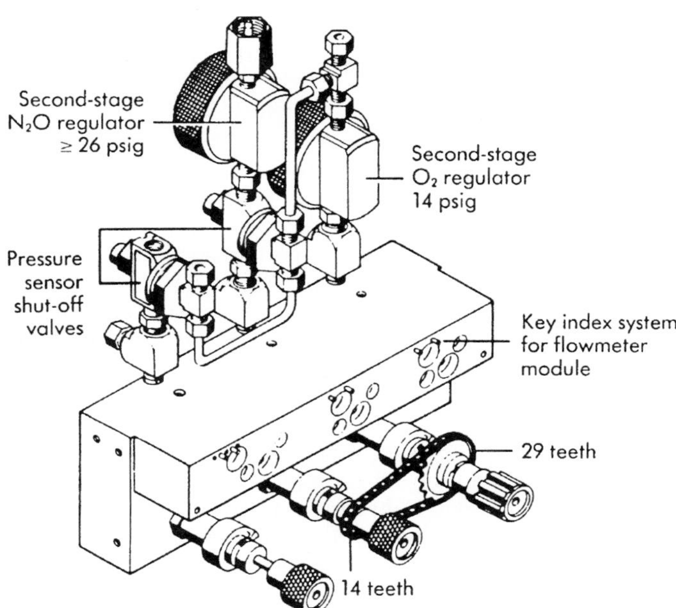

FIGURE **15-19**
Datex-Ohmeda Link-25 proportioning system. (Courtesy of Datex-Ohmeda, Madison, Wisconsin.)

BOX **15-5**

Circumstances under Which Hypoxic Guard Systems Can Permit Formation of a Hypoxic Mixture

- Wrong supply gas in oxygen pipeline or cylinder
- Defective pneumatics or mechanics
- Leaks downstream of flow control valves
- Inert gas administration (e.g., a third gas such as helium)

Many Narkomed machines in current use have a switch with two positions: "Nitrous Oxide–Oxygen" and "All Gases." In the "Nitrous Oxide–Oxygen" position, the ORMC and alarms (if present) are active, and only these two gases may flow. In the "All Gases" position, the ORMC and alarms are inactivated, and all gases (except N_2O) may flow without hypoxic guard system protection.

Vaporizers

Physics

A vapor is composed of molecules (in the gaseous phase) of a substance that is a liquid at room temperature and 1 atm of pressure. Vaporization proceeds at a rate that depends on the physical characteristics of the vaporizing liquid and the temperature. Different liquids evaporate at different rates. Elevated temperature increases the rate of evaporation of any liquid, whereas decreased temperature slows the rate. As evaporation proceeds, the remaining liquid and its container cool because heat energy is carried from the liquid with the energetic, mobile, evaporating molecules. Examples are the cooling effect of evaporating perspiration and the chilling effect of evaporating gasoline or ether on the hand. In both cases the molecules acquire the latent heat of vaporization from their surroundings. In the same way, one would expect an anesthetic vaporizer to cool as vaporization proceeds. This cooling limits the rate of further vaporization. To prevent this, materials such as copper are chosen for containing liquid anesthetics in current vaporizers. Copper has high thermal conductivity (transferring environmental heat easily to the liquid anesthetic) and high thermal capacity (acting as a thermal reservoir to help stabilize liquid anesthetic temperature).

The rate of vaporization depends only on the temperature, the vapor pressure of the liquid, and the partial pressure of the vapor above the evaporating liquid—not on the ambient pressure of the remaining gases present. For example, water at a constant temperature evaporates at the same rate into completely dry air whether it is at sea level, in a hyperbaric chamber, or at elevations far above sea level.

Classification and Design

Table 15-2 presents a comparison of older measured-flow (Vernitrol) vaporizers with the newer variable-bypass and heated-vapor types.[2,22,55-61] All vaporizers blend the combined flow of fresh gases from the flowmeters with sufficient vapor to form clinically useful concentrations. The problem is ensuring that the vapor concentration is appropriately limited. For example, a fully saturated isoflurane vapor consists of nearly 31% isoflurane (238 mm Hg, the saturated vapor pressure

TABLE 15-2 Classification of Vaporizers

Characteristic	Variable Bypass	Measured Flow	Injector
Example	Datex-Ohmeda Tec 4, 5, and 7, ADU Aladin; Dräger Vapor 19, 2000	Copper Kettle, Vernitrol	Datex-Ohmeda Tec 6 (Desflurane)
Splitting ratio (carrier gas flow)	Variable-bypass (vaporizer determines carrier gas split)	Measured-flow (operator determines carrier gas split)	Dual-circuit (carrier gas is not split)
Method of vaporization	Flow over	Bubble through	Gas or vapor blender (heat produces vapor, which is injected into fresh gas flow)
Temperature compensation	Automatic temperature compensation mechanism	Manual (i.e., by changes in carrier gas flow)	Electrically heated to a constant temperature (39° C; thermostatically controlled)
Calibration	Calibrated, agent specific	None; multiple agent	Calibrated, agent specific
Position	Out of circuit	Out of circuit	Out of circuit
Capacity	Tec 4: 125 ml Tec 5: 300 ml Vapor 19: 200 ml	200-600 ml (no longer manufactured)	390 ml

of isoflurane at 20° C, divided by the barometric pressure of 760 mm Hg). To limit vapor output to a clinically useful concentration, in measured-flow and variable-bypass vaporizers only a small amount of fresh gas is allowed to come into contact with the liquid and pick up anesthetic vapor.

The splitting ratio (gas entering the vaporizing chamber divided by total FGF) is automatically determined in a variable-bypass vaporizer by the internal resistance to flow; the operator merely has to set the control dial to the desired concentration (Figure 15-20). Setting the dial to a higher percentage increases the amount of flow sent through the vaporizing chamber. The small portion of the gas flow entering the vaporizing chamber ("carrier gas" or "chamber flow") flows over the liquid and picks up anesthetic vapor. Full saturation of the carrier gas is ensured by means of a series of wicks and baffles. This fully saturated, known concentration of carrier gas is then diluted with the balance of the fresh gas that bypassed the vaporizing chamber ("bypass flow"), to produce the desired final concentration.

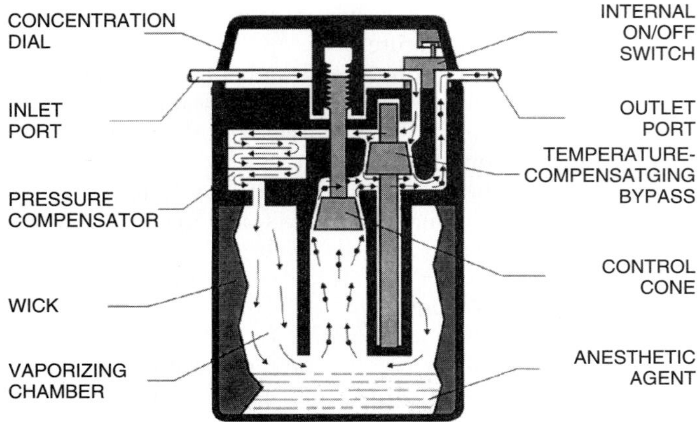

FIGURE 15-20
The Dräger Vapor 19 vaporizer. (From Cicman J, Himmelwright C, Skibo V, Yoder J. *Operating Principles of Narkomed Anesthesia Systems*. Telford, Pa: North American Dräger; 1993.)

A temperature compensation device is built into variable-bypass vaporizers, so that more gas is directed into the vaporizing chamber as the vaporizer cools. Variable-bypass vaporizers are calibrated for concentration and are agent specific. Like the measured-flow and heated Datex-Ohmeda Tec 6, variable-bypass vaporizers are "out of circuit," meaning that they are out of the breathing circuit. Their capacities for liquid agent are listed in Table 15-2. Variable bypass vaporizers in the ADU add microprocessor control of chamber flow based on inputs from pressure or temperature sensors at various sites (Figure 15-21).

In a measured-flow vaporizer, the operator determines how much gas should be bubbled through the anesthetic liquid by means of a formula; this amount is then set on a second O_2 flowmeter, marked "Oxygen for Vernitrol." If the vaporizer cools, the operator must recalculate and set a new chamber gas flow; this is called *manual temperature compensation*. These devices can be used with multiple agents and are out of circuit. It is possible to use them safely, but their design is not as inherently safe as that of more modern types.[62] Measured-flow vaporizers are no longer manufactured in the United States, and factory service for them is no longer available. The military still trains anesthetists in the use of these vaporizers,[43] and they may be seen overseas. They are not addressed in the current anesthesia gas machine standard.[15]

In the Datex-Ohmeda Tec 6 vaporizer, a completely different principle of operation is used (Figure 15-22): a heated, dual-circuit vaporizer.[57,60,64-67] FGF from the common manifold passes through the vaporizer in one circuit. This fresh gas never flows over or comes into contact with the liquid agent. Instead, an appropriate amount of vapor is prepared in the second circuit and added to the fresh gas flowing through the vaporizer. The second (vapor) circuit has two control points: one is the setting on the concentration control dial; the other is keyed to a transducer that is responsive to the amount of FGF. More vapor is delivered from the vapor circuit if either the desired volume percent setting is increased or the FGF is increased. To maintain a known vapor pressure in the second circuit, the Datex-Ohmeda Tec 6 is heated to 39° C; this produces a vapor pressure of approximately 1500 mm Hg. Desflurane is near boiling at room temperature; if it were placed in a variable-bypass vaporizer, it would constitute nearly

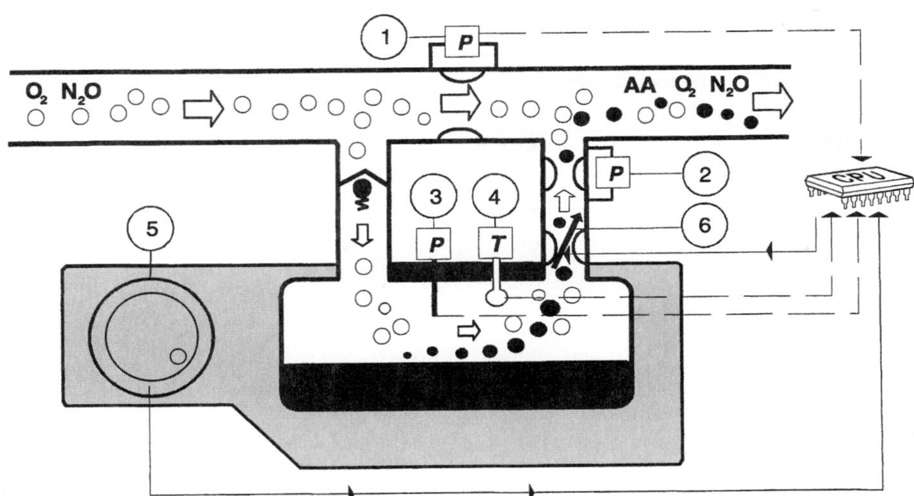

FIGURE **15-21**
The Anesthesia Delivery Unit (ADU) vaporizer. A microprocessor controls (6) and monitors (2) the vaporizer chamber flow based on inputs of bypass flow (*1*), vaporizing chamber pressure (*3*) and temperature (*4*), and the setting of the control dial (5). (From Datex-Ohmeda. *S/5 ADU User's Reference Manual.* Madison, Wis: Datex-Ohmeda; 2000. Catalog No. 8502304.)

100% of the output at first, and a hypoxic breathing mixture would result.[68]

The output of modern vaporizers may be influenced by extremes of FGF, extremes of temperature, or back pressure from the breathing circuit and ventilator. Current vaporizers function accurately over a wide range of settings at various ambient temperatures and FGFs[55,57,61] (Table 15-3). Furthermore, they are more resistant than previous models to the effects of intermittent back pressure, the so-called "pumping effect" that increases vaporizer output. This is because most incorporate unidirectional valves at the vaporizing chamber inlet or outlet or distal to the vaporizer.

Contemporary vaporizers are secured to the anesthesia machine in manifolds that hold two or three units. The operator is prevented from delivering more than one agent simultaneously by an interlock system. The interlock ensures that only one vaporizer is on, that gas enters only the one that is on, that all vaporizers are locked in so that leaks are decreased, and that trace vapor output is minimal when a vaporizer is off (Figure 15-23).[69]

Variable-bypass and Datex-Ohmeda Tec 6 vaporizers are all filled in a similar fashion. Funnel-type (Figure 15-24) and keyed-filler type (Figure 15-25) systems are permitted by standard.[15] Keyed-filler types are preferred because their use lessens the chance that filling with the wrong agent will occur.[70] The standard requires that overfilling be prevented in the normal operating position and that liquid level indicators be visible to the operator.[16] These indicators usually take the form of a sight glass with two etched lines corresponding to low and maximum liquid levels within the vaporizer. To fill either the funnel-type or keyed-filler vaporizers, the anesthetist should check the anesthetic liquid (to ensure that the agent and the vaporizer match) and then pour it in. The vaporizer is full when the liquid level reaches the maximum line on the sight glass. This is the method specified in the manuals for the Datex-Ohmeda Tec 4 and Tec 5 and for the Dräger Vapor 19.3 models.[55,56,61] It is a misconception that, while using the keyed-filler vaporizer, one should hold the bottle up until it stops bubbling. If the vaporizer is turned on or the keyed-filler device is not perfectly tight on the bottle, this method results

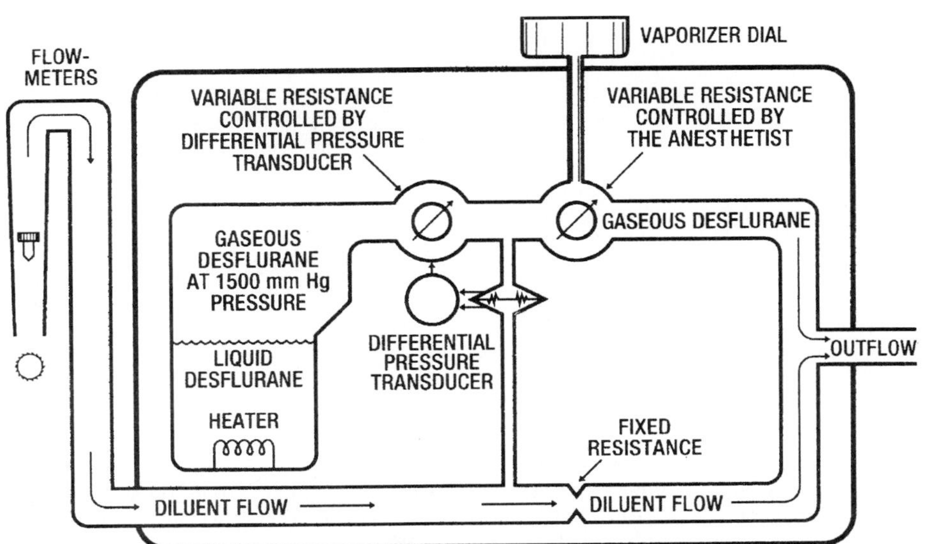

FIGURE **15-22**
Principle of operation of the Datex-Ohmeda Tec 6 vaporizer. (From *The Datex-Ohmeda Tec 6 Vaporizer: for the Administration of Suprane [Desflurane]* [brochure with prescribing information]. Liberty Corner, NJ: Anaquest; 1992.)

TABLE 15-3 Accuracy of Current Vaporizers*

Characteristic	Datex-Ohmeda Tec 4	Datex-Ohmeda Tec 5	Datex-Ohmeda Tec 6	Datex-Ohmeda Tec 7	Dräger Vapor 19.3	Datex-Ohmeda S/5 ADU
Fresh gas flow (L/min)	0.2-10	0.2-15	0.2-10	0.2-15	0.25-15	0.2-8
Temperature (°C)	20-35	17-35	18-30	18-35	15-35	18-25

ADU, Anesthesia delivery unit.
**The vaporizers listed function accurately within the ranges specified.*

in overfilling. Overfilling may result in discharge of liquid anesthetic from the vaporizer outlet, which has caused patient injuries.[2] The Tec 6 uses a similar system, but the desflurane bottle has a permanently attached, noninterchangeable spout. The sight glass on the Tec 6 is a liquid crystal display that indicates when the level of liquid is low enough to allow the addition of a full bottle, and it shows when the sump is full. The Tec 6 vaporizer is unique in that it can be filled while in operation.[57] All variable-bypass vaporizers must be shut off while they are being filled.[33,55,56,61] Before filling any vaporizer, the operator should carefully review procedures in the operator's manual.

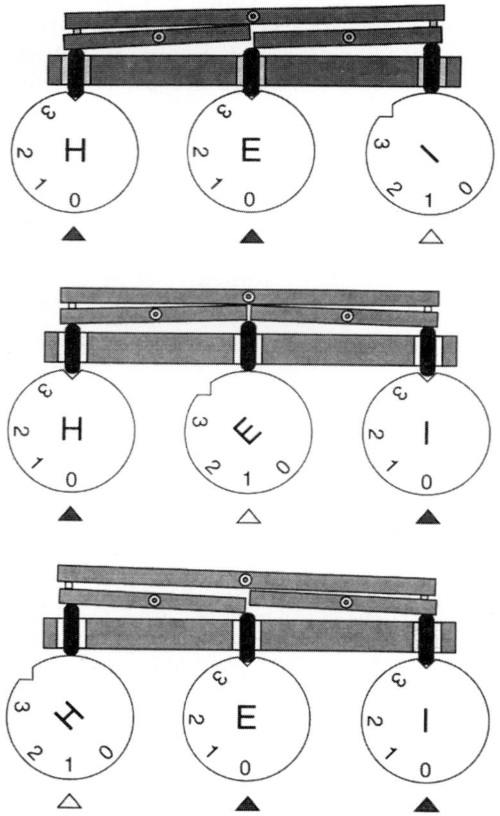

FIGURE **15-23**
Vaporizer interlock system. (From Cicman J, Himmelwright C, Skibo V, Yoder J. *Operating Principles of Narkomed Anesthesia Systems*. Telford, Pa: North American Dräger; 1993.)

Models

The Dräger Vapor 19 fits the Narkomed interlock system. If a vaporizer is removed from the machine, a short circuit block must be added to prevent leaks. The interlock continues to protect against simultaneous inhaled agent administration regardless of which vaporizer is removed. No check valve is present between the vaporizer outlets and the common gas outlet in Narkomed anesthesia gas machines. Like all contemporary vaporizers, the Dräger Vapor 19 has a button that must be depressed before the control dial can be turned on. All contemporary vaporizers are designed to increase agent concentration as the dial is turned counterclockwise (as viewed from above).

The Dräger Vapor 2000 (Figure 15-26) is similar to the Vapor 19 except that it is removable by hand. It has a "T" (transport) setting that allows the vaporizer to be tipped.

The Datex-Ohmeda Tec 4 (Figure 15-27) and Tec 5 are mated to an interlock system that holds two or three vaporizers. If three vaporizers are present, removal of the center vaporizer may disable the interlock system (machines delivered after 1995 have been redesigned to correct this problem). In this

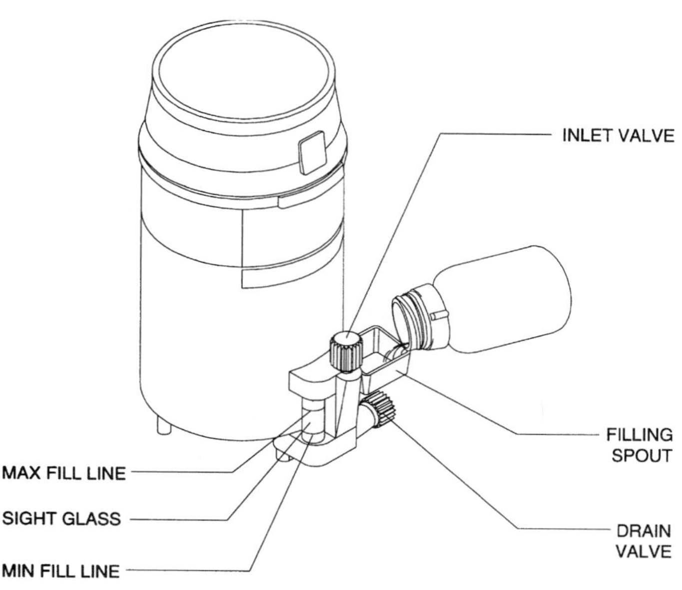

FIGURE **15-24**
Filling a vaporizer with a funnel-type filling system. (From *Narkomed 2C Anesthesia System—Setup and Installation Manual*. Telford, Pa: North American Dräger; 1994.)

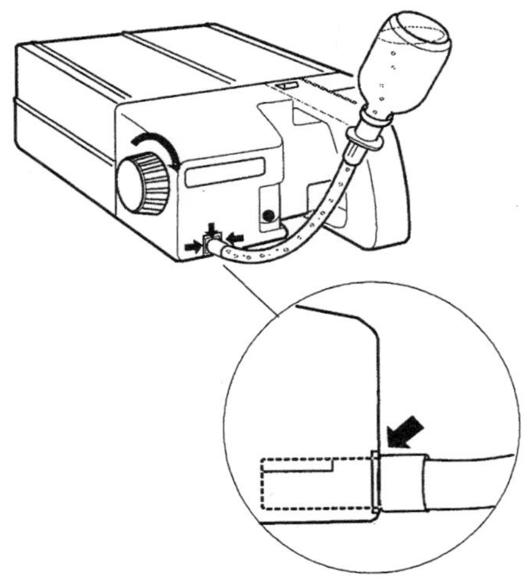

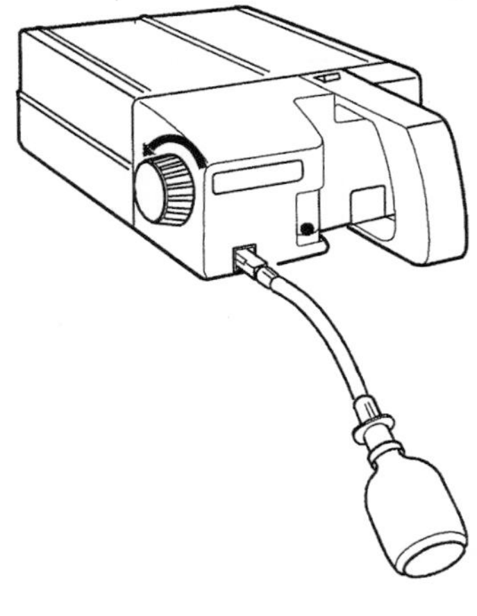

FIGURE **15-25**
Filling a vaporizer with a keyed-filler system. (From Datex-Ohmeda. *S/5 Anesthesia Delivery Unit User's Reference Manual.* Madison, Wis: Datex-Ohmeda; 2000. Catalog No. 8502304.)

case the two remaining vaporizers should be moved so that they are next to each other.

The Datex-Ohmeda Tec 7 is a variable-bypass vaporizer similar to the Tec 4 and 5. It is designed to need less frequent and less complicated service.

Use of the Datex-Ohmeda Tec 6 vaporizer is unique, as could be suspected from its unique principle of operation. However, it is not difficult to use. Filling the Tec 6 has been described in general terms. Further instructions are printed on the front of many vaporizers, as well as in the operator's manual. The operator must check the desflurane bottle to ensure that it is the right agent, push it into the vaporizer firmly, and rotate it upward until the display indicates that the vaporizer is full. The operator then rotates the bottle downward and holds it for an instant (to allow any drops to drain back into it). Finally, the operator supports the bottle while withdrawing it from the vaporizer (Figure 15-28).[57]

The operator turns the Tec 6 vaporizer on by turning the concentration control dial to the "On" position while depressing the dial release located opposite the zero indicator (which is on the front of the dial). The vaporizer requires electric power and a warm-up period of approximately 10 minutes before it can be used.[57]

The Tec 6 has several visual indicators that are grouped in a status display (Figure 15-29).[57] These include a light that indicates "Operational" status, a "No Output" indicator light (and audible alarm), a "Low Agent" light (and audible alarm), a "Warm-up" status light, and an "Alarm Battery Low" light. The "No Output" alarms are activated if the agent level is less than 20 ml, if the vaporizer is tilted more than 10 degrees from the vertical, if a power failure lasts longer than 10 seconds, or if an internal malfunction occurs. The cause of a "No Output" alarm may be sought if it occurs during a case; however, considering the rapid emergence that is characteristic with the use of desflurane, the operator should ensure the continuation of a surgical plane of anesthesia by switching to a different agent without delay.

FIGURE **15-26**
The Dräger Vapor 2000. Note the "T" (transport) setting to the right of "0." (Courtesy Draeger Medical, Inc., Telford, Pennsylvania.)

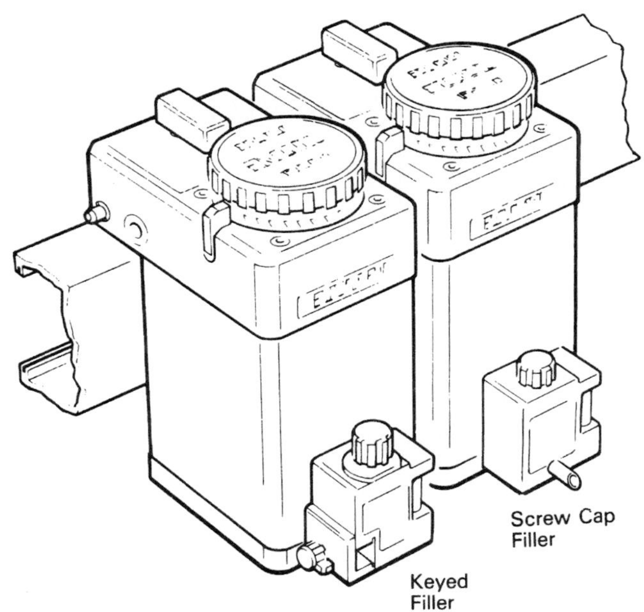

FIGURE **15-27**
Appearance of the Datex-Ohmeda Tec 4 vaporizer. The Tec 5 is similar in appearance. (Courtesy of Datex-Ohmeda, Madison, Wisconsin.)

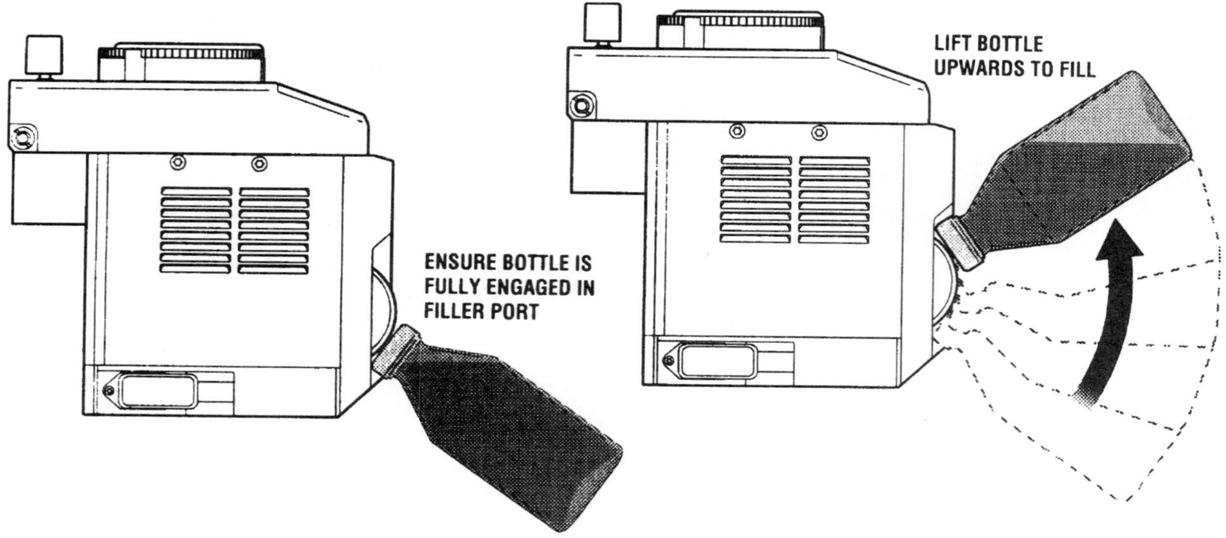

FIGURE **15-28**
Filling the Datex-Ohmeda Tec 6 vaporizer. (From Datex-Ohmeda. *Tec 6 Vaporizer: Operation and Maintenance Manual*. Madison, Wis: Datex-Ohmeda; 1993.)

Preoperative checkout for variable-bypass vaporizers is relatively straightforward. They are checked in order to determine whether they are turned off, whether they are full, and whether the interlock is functioning. The Datex-Ohmeda Tec 6 requires a more extensive checkout. After performing the appropriate leak test of the machine's low-pressure system, the operator checks the amber "Alarm Battery Low" indicator and replaces the battery if necessary. Next, the Tec 6 is turned on to at least 1%, and its electrical plug is disconnected. Within 15 seconds of disconnection, the "No Output" light and alarm should activate. If they do not, the battery must be replaced, and the vaporizer retested before use. If everything is functioning correctly, the operator reconnects the power and turns the dial to the "Off" position; the mute button is then pressed for 4 seconds to test all alarms and the display. When the mute button is pressed, all lights and the alarm should activate.[57]

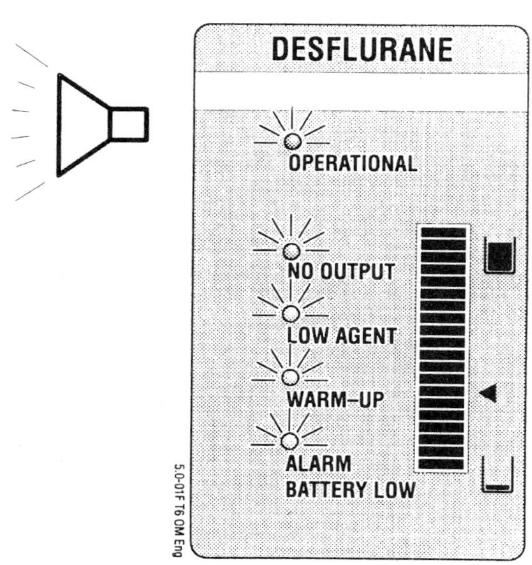

FIGURE **15-29**
Display panel of the Datex-Ohmeda Tec 6 vaporizer. (From Datex-Ohmeda. *Tec 6 Vaporizer: Operation and Maintenance Manual*. Madison, Wis: Datex-Ohmeda; 1993.)

The S/5 ADU vaporizer uses one central electronic control mechanism for all agents.[39] Cassettes containing the volatile liquid anesthetic are inserted into a port connected to these control mechanisms, which recognizes the contents of the cassette and dispenses agent into the stream of FGF (Figures 15-21 and 15-30). The cassettes and control mechanisms are checked as part of the electronic equipment checklist daily. The ADU does not deliver a volatile agent or N_2O without main power or battery backup and adequate O_2 pressure.

Hazards of Contemporary Vaporizers

Many of the hazards associated with the use of vaporizers have been corrected by advances in design. A few hazards remain (Box 15-6). Vaporizer contamination with incorrect agents

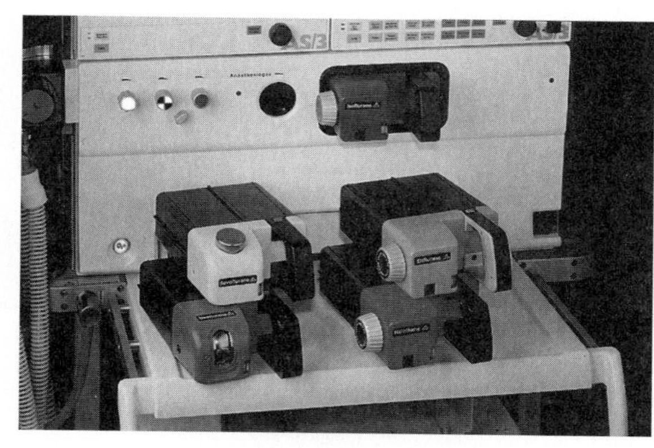

FIGURE **15-30**
Datex-Ohmeda S/5 Anesthesia Delivery Unit vaporizer cassettes. The isoflurane cassette is plugged into the vaporizer port and controls and may be adjusted with the control wheel to the left of the port. (Courtesy of Datex-Ohmeda, Tewksbury, Massachusetts.)

BOX 15-6

Hazards of Modern Vaporizers

Administration of incorrect agent
Tipping
Overfilling with agent
Simultaneous inhaled agent administration
Reliance on breath-by-breath gas analysis rather than preventive maintenance
Leaks
Electronic failures

continues to be noted.[70] Diligence during filling is not enough to prevent contamination. Departments should strongly consider replacing funnel-type with keyed-filler vaporizers in equipment purchases. If a vaporizer tips by more than 45 degrees from vertical, the operator's manual or a field service technician must be consulted. Tipping is hazardous because the entry of liquid agent into the control assembly at the top of the vaporizer can have unpredictable effects on its function. The vaporizer sump can be drained, and gas can be run through it for a specified time and at a specified concentration before the vaporizer is returned to use. For the recommended corrective action for a particular make and model, the operator's manual must be consulted.

Overfilling may be prevented by following the manufacturer's guidelines for filling (e.g., fill only to the top etched line on the liquid level indicator glass, fill only when the vaporizer is off).[70] Simultaneous agent administration should be preventable. The operator should remember to place Datex-Ohmeda vaporizers next to each other if the center vaporizer of three has been removed. Managers should not conclude, in this era of cost constraints, that breath-by-breath agent analysis can be substituted for regular preventive maintenance of vaporizers. Leaks are relatively common, often resulting from malposition of vaporizers on the back bar[71] or loss of gaskets, and these leaks may not be detected with the standard checklist unless the negative pressure check is performed. Tec 6 vaporizers can also leak liquid while being filled if the desflurane bottle is missing the white rubber O-ring near its tip. This situation can be mistaken for a defective vaporizer.[72] Finally, as vaporizers incorporate electronics, they are susceptible to electronic failure. Two case reports in 2000 detail ADU vaporizers failing because of "fresh gas unit failure," and from copious emesis soaking the machine.[73,74]

DELIVERY

How is the flow of gases to and from the patient controlled and monitored?

Breathing Circuits

Fundamental Considerations

Certain basic principles guide the design and use of all respiratory apparatus. The purpose of any anesthesia breathing circuit is the delivery of O_2 and anesthetic and the elimination of carbon dioxide. Carbon dioxide is eliminated from the breathing circuit by washout with adequate FGF or by absorption in soda lime.

Any type of breathing circuit creates some degree of resistance to gas flow. Resistance in a circuit may be minimized by reducing the circuit's length and increasing its diameter, by avoiding the use of sharp bends, by eliminating valves, and by maintaining laminar flow. It is important to decrease resistance to flow because added airway resistance is uncomfortable for the conscious patient. Furthermore, the unconscious or anesthetized patient challenged by an increased work of breathing may not be able to increase respiratory effort and therefore may hypoventilate. The resistance of the anesthesia breathing circuit is low—typically less than that of an endotracheal tube.

Rebreathing occurs with the use of anesthesia breathing circuits (as it does in space or submarine environments), but it is not found with other breathing circuits, such as those in the ventilators used in intensive care units. Rebreathing may be useful. Its advantages include cost reduction, an increase in tracheal warmth and humidity, and a decrease in the potential for exposure of operating room personnel to trace and waste gases (because of decreased rate of release of anesthetic gases into the environment). The degree of rebreathing in an anesthesia breathing circuit is increased as the FGF is decreased. Higher FGF is associated with less rebreathing in any type of circuit.

Patients under anesthesia may rebreathe any component of their exhalations—nitrogen, O_2, CO_2, N_2O, and volatile agent. The effects of rebreathing each of these components differ. The higher the FGF, the more quickly the composition of gas in the breathing circuit resembles that at the common gas outlet (the desired or dialed-in concentrations of agent, N_2O, and O_2). Rebreathing of exhaled nitrogen slows induction. Nitrogen that is not eliminated from the breathing circuit delays the establishment of the desired concentration of the agent; therefore high FGFs are appropriate during induction. Because higher flows reduce the discrepancy between desired concentrations and the concentrations actually inspired, they are appropriate during emergence as well. At the end of an anesthetic procedure, as the flow of volatile agent and N_2O is turned off, it is undesirable for exhaled agent and N_2O to be rebreathed, because this would delay emergence. In contrast, rebreathing of exhaled agent during maintenance is highly desirable because of cost and environmental considerations. Rebreathing of CO_2 has the undesirable effect of producing respiratory acidosis, so it is best avoided.

Dead space is increased to some degree with the use of any respiratory equipment. The effect of an increase in mechanical (apparatus) dead space is that rebreathing of exhaled CO_2 is more likely. This is one reason that ventilator tidal volumes are set much higher than the volume of a spontaneous breath. To avoid hypercarbia in the face of an acute increase in dead space, a patient must increase minute ventilation (V_E). Conversely, because alveolar ventilation is equal to the V_E minus dead space ventilation ($V_A = V_E - V_D$), if the patient's V_E is fixed, an increase in dead space decreases alveolar ventilation and increases arterial CO_2 tension.[75] Dead space ends where the inspiratory and expiratory gas streams diverge. In a circle system, dead space ends at the Y-piece. Use of a face mask is associated with greater dead space than is the use of an endotracheal tube.

The anesthesia gas machine uses dry gases so that the problems of internal corrosion and bacterial colonization are avoided. However, provision of completely dry gases to the patient's airway can cause various problems. It is common for anesthesia providers to use various means of humidifying and heating inspired gases, usually passively (with a heat and moisture exchanger and low FGF) or actively (with an electrically heated humidifier). Active humidification has become less common, because it is less effective at preventing hypothermia than heated air surface warming blankets, and because the added moisture can clog gas analysis lines and affect soda lime granules.

Finally, anesthesia breathing circuits are unique in the degree to which they allow manipulation of the inspired concentration of a variety of components for therapeutic benefit. Each component of the breathing mixture follows its own concentration gradient as it is made to wash in or out of the breathing system and to wash in or out of the breathing system into the patient's lungs. In the lungs gases flow down their concentration gradients, interchanging with pulmonary and blood gases. Understanding the pharmacokinetics of inhaled agent administration involves not only a knowledge of respiratory physiology, but also familiarity with the "physiology" of the patient-machine system. The concentration set on the dial differs from the concentrations in the breathing circuit, in the lungs, in the blood, and in the brain. Furthermore, the concentration differences are not constant but vary over time, depending on a number of patient- and machine-related factors. The concentration inspired most closely resembles that delivered from the common gas outlet when rebreathing is minimal or absent. This concentration is usually associated with high FGFs. Of course, it is desirable that the alveolar concentration differ from the inspired concentration at times. At the start of the emergence phase the inspired concentration of anesthetic is decreased so that anesthetic gas is washed out while ventilation is continued. Therefore emergence is very different from merely "waking up" and is as much an active process as induction.

Classification of Breathing Circuits

Table 15-4 gives a classification of breathing circuits that is based on whether a reservoir (breathing bag) is present and on the degree to which rebreathing occurs.[76] In open systems patients have access to the atmosphere; this is not true in semiopen, semiclosed, or closed systems. The reservoir is present in these three types to provide for the moments during the inspiratory phase when flow in the trachea is greater than FGF. Both nonrebreathing (Mapleson) systems and the circle system (at FGFs greater than VE) are semiopen.[12] If the FGF to the circle system is less than VE, some rebreathing must be occurring. In a closed system, rebreathing is total. The APL or "popoff" valve is closed, and the supply of O_2, N_2O, and agent just matches the patient's requirements.[77]

TABLE 15-4 Classification of Breathing Circuits

Type	Reservoir	Rebreathing	Example
Open	No	No	Open drop, insufflation, nasal cannula
Semiopen	Yes	No	Nonrebreathing circuit or a circle at high fresh gas flow
Semiclosed	Yes	Yes (partial)	Circle at fresh gas flow less than minute ventilation
Closed	Yes	Yes (complete)	Circle at extremely low fresh gas flow, with adjustable pressure-limiting valve closed

Nonrebreathing Circuits

Mapleson published a classification of nonrebreathing circuits in 1954; this classification is still used today.[78] A schematic drawing of his classification is presented in Figure 15-31. Currently, the Mapleson D circuit is in common use. Rebreathing is prevented in the Mapleson D system because during the expiratory pause fresh gas fills the corrugated limb, forcing the previous exhalation in a distal direction (toward the reservoir). If FGF is sufficient, no alveolar gas is rebreathed.

The Mapleson F circuit is also referred to as the "Jackson-Rees modification of Ayre's T-piece." The Bain system, shown at the bottom of the figure, often is referred to as a "modified" Mapleson D circuit because the arrangement of its components (entry point of fresh gas, reservoir bag, and APL valve) is similar to that of the Mapleson D. However, in the Bain system the fresh gas hose is directed coaxially within the corrugated limb, and this configuration gives the inhaled gases greater heat and humidity. Unfortunately, unrecognized kinking or disconnection of this relatively hidden fresh gas hose converts the entire corrugated limb into dead space. Users of Bain systems must test the circuit for these problems before the system is used. The Pethick test and a similar test are available and should be employed (see the discussion of clinical implications later in this chapter).[2]

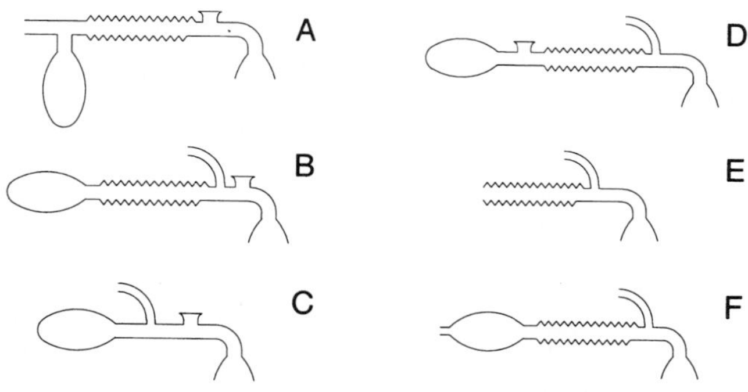

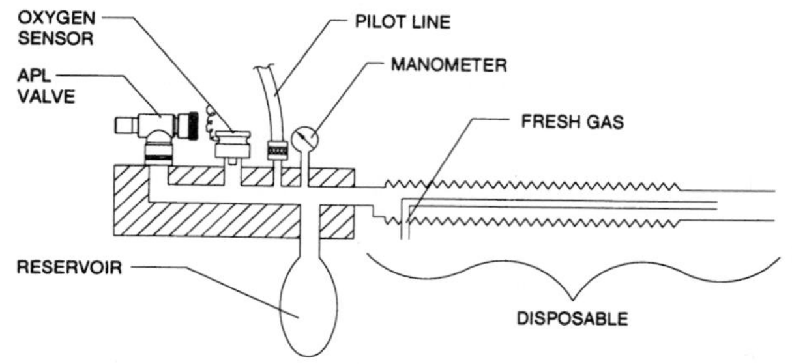

FIGURE 15-31
Mapleson's classification of breathing systems. (From Cicman J, Himmelwright C, Skibo V, Yoder J. *Operating Principles of Narkomed Anesthesia Systems*. Telford, Pa: North American Dräger; 1993.)

The common features of nonrebreathing systems are listed in Box 15-7. Often these circuits are used for children because they offer very low resistance to breathing. The popularity of these circuits is currently challenged by the availability of alternatives (low-compliance, disposable pediatric circle system hoses), because the high FGF required in nonrebreathing circuits cools children and is more costly.[79] Also, if a nonrebreathing circuit is used in the middle of a number of cases in which a circle system is used, some disassembly and reassembly is required, accompanied by the possibility of error. The small amount of resistance offered by the soda lime canisters and unidirectional valves of the circle system is deleterious only during spontaneous respiration, which is limited in duration in most general anesthesia for children. The minimum weight of a child in whom a pediatric circle would be suitable is approximately 10 to 20 kg. No single guideline applies to all situations, because the decision whether to use a pediatric circle system in a particular child depends on the type of circle system and hoses, the compliance of the corrugated breathing hoses, and the anticipated duration of unassisted respiration. The Mapleson circuits can be used for patients of almost any age, from premature infants to adults. The FGF required to prevent rebreathing is two to three times V_E.[2] In practice, this number can be calculated; however, many operators use at least 5 L/min of FGF.

The advantages and disadvantages of nonrebreathing circuits are presented in Box 15-8. Although they are convenient and in common use, nonrebreathing circuits are associated with loss of heat from the patient and with greater use of volatile agents, because they require relatively high FGF. The Fabius GS and Narkomed 6000 are not compatible with nonrebreathing circuits. With the increased accuracy at low tidal volumes in any new ventilator, the need for pediatric nonrebreathing circuits has lessened greatly.

Circle System

The circle system is the breathing circuit most commonly used in the United States because it prevents rebreathing of carbon dioxide while allowing rebreathing of all other gases. Gas flow during mechanical ventilator inspiration is shown in Figure 15-32, and with ventilator expiration in Figure 15-33.

A coaxial circle system is also available in which, as in the Bain system, the inspiratory limb is contained within the expiratory limb (Figure 15-34). It is checked and used like any circle system. Like the Bain, the coaxial circle is less bulky and is thought to provide greater heat and humidity to inhaled gases. Disadvantages include the potential for obstruction or lack of patency of either limb, which may cause respiratory acidosis or even mimic esophageal intubation.[80,81] This respiratory acidosis does not respond to increased V_E; if exhaled gases are not forced through the absorbent granules, no amount of ventilation will cleanse carbon dioxide from the exhaled gases. The tests for inner tube patency that can be used for a Bain circuit are not readily adaptable to the coaxial circle system.

Gas enters the circle system from the common gas outlet by way of the fresh gas delivery hose, and it exits the circle via the APL valve (or the ventilator relief valve if mechanical ventilation is employed) to the scavenger. The APL valve creates an adjustable leak during manual ventilation. If it is completely open and the bag is squeezed, all gas exits to the scavenger, because this is the path of least resistance. If the valve is completely closed, all gas ventilates the lungs. The setting of the APL is constantly adjusted during manual ventilation of the lungs so that a variable resistance sufficient to force gas to inflate the lungs is maintained.

Unidirectional valves enforce a pattern of gas flow by which exhalations are made to pass through the CO_2-absorbent granules (Figure 15-35). The valve leaflet (disk) is subject to damage, occlusion, foreign body contamination, and sticking as a result of collected moisture or absorbent dust, particularly on the expiratory valve disk.[82-84] Daily performance of the FDA Anesthesia Apparatus Checkout (Appendix 15-1) should enable the operator to detect most of these problems. Only two reasons for an increase in inspired CO_2 are common: absorbent granules have been exhausted, or unidirectional valves are faulty. Figure 15-36 on p. 286 shows that incompetence of an inspiratory or expiratory valve turns the entire corrugated limb into dead space.[85] This usually results in an increase in inspired and expired CO_2.

If inspired CO_2 of more than 1 to 3 mm Hg is detected on the capnograph (Figures 15-37 and 15-38, p. 286), the FGF should be increased to 5 to 8 L/min; this converts the system to a semiopen configuration in which rebreathing of exhaled gases is minimized. If this causes the inspired CO_2 to decrease substantially, the absorbent granules are exhausted and should be replaced at the end of the case (the ADU allows granules to be changed during the case, although it is not meant to function for more than brief periods without a canister attached). If elevated inspired CO_2 persists, the valves are likely to be incompetent. The operator should remove the expiratory valve,

BOX 15-7

Common Features of Nonrebreathing Systems

All lack unidirectional valves.
All lack soda lime carbon dioxide absorption.
Amount of rebreathing is highly dependent on fresh gas flow in all.
Amount of resistance is low in all (no unidirectional valves).

BOX 15-8

Nonrebreathing Systems: Advantages and Disadvantages

Advantages
Lightweight
Convenient
Easily sterilized and scavenged
Exhaled gases in corrugated limb may give heat and humidity to inhaled gas (Bain)

Disadvantages
Unrecognized disconnection or kinking of fresh gas hose in the Bain circuit (use Pethick test)
Pollution and increased costs of agents and gases resulting from need for higher flows
Loss of heat from patient
May require disconnection of circle fresh gas supply hose and scavenger connections for assembly; can be reassembled improperly

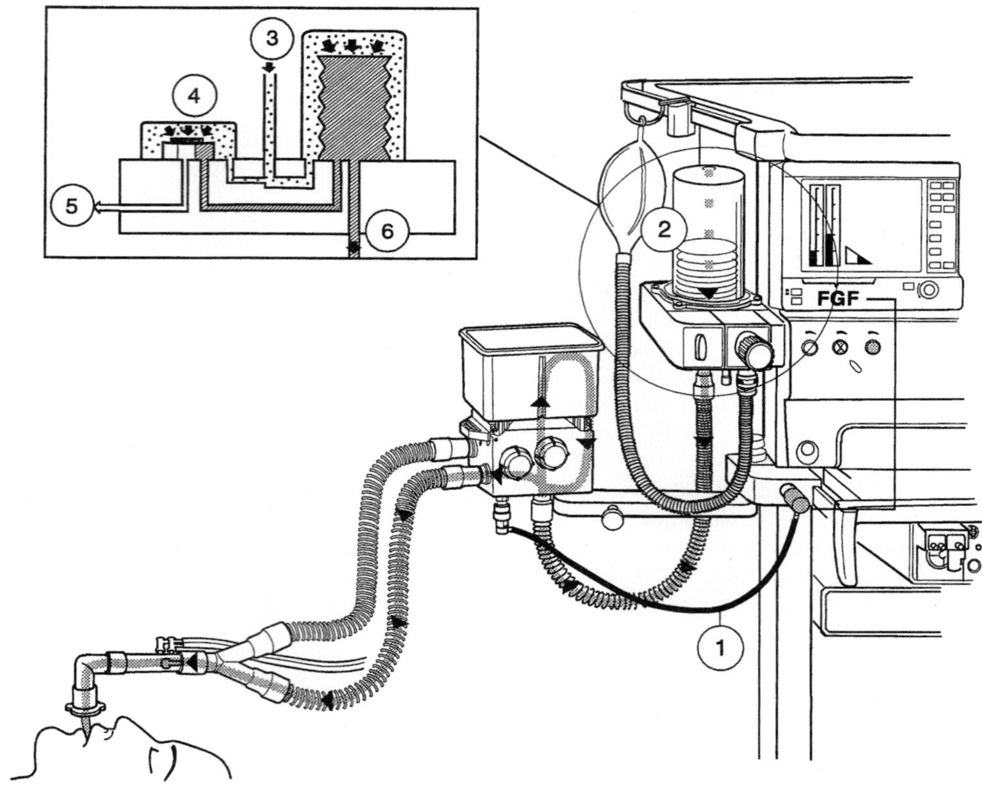

FIGURE **15-32**
Gas flow in a circle system during mechanical ventilator inspiration. *1,* Hose from common gas outlet to absorber head (which contains attachments for disposable breathing circuit hoses, inspiratory and expiratory unidirectional valves, and CO_2 absorbent granules). *2,* Bellows block with "Manual-Auto" switch, APL valve, and manual breathing bag. *3,* Ventilator driving gas. *4,* Ventilator relief valve (pathway to scavenging, which is closed during inspiration). *5,* Pathway for exhaled gas to scavenger interface. *6,* Pathway for gas to patient. (From Datex-Ohmeda. *S/5 Anesthesia Delivery Unit User's Reference Manual.* Madison, Wis: Datex-Ohmeda; 2000. Catalog No. 8502304.)

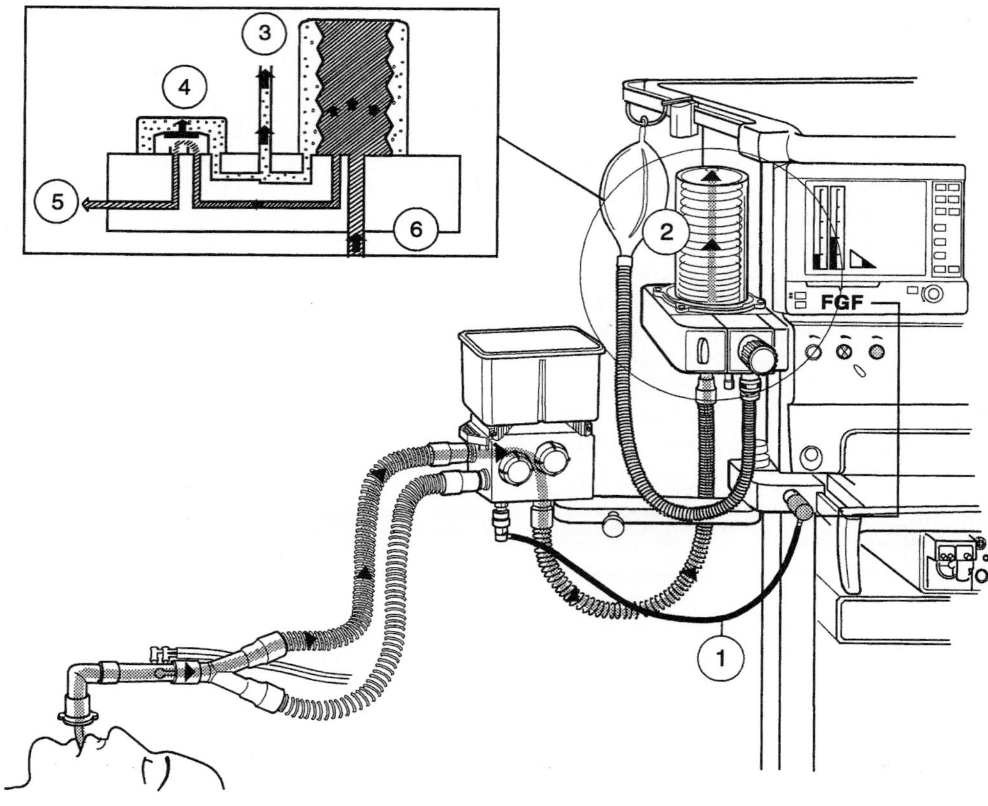

FIGURE **15-33**
Gas flow in a circle system during mechanical ventilator expiration. The ventilator relief valve was held shut during inspiration. When the driving gas flow ceases, the patient's exhalation fills the bellows. Once the pressure within the bellows reaches +2 to 3 cm H_2O, the ventilator relief valve opens, and any excess gas can exit to the scavenger. *1,* Hose from common gas outlet to absorber head. *2,* Bellows block (bellows refilling with patient's exhalation). *3,* Ventilator driving gas pressure is released and it leaves the upper section of the bellows. *4,* Ventilator relief valve (pathway to scavenging, open during expiration). *5,* Exhaled gas passing to scavenger interface. *6,* Gas from patient. (From Datex-Ohmeda. *S/5 Anesthesia Delivery Unit User's Reference Manual.* Madison, Wis: Datex-Ohmeda; 2000. Catalog No. 8502304.)

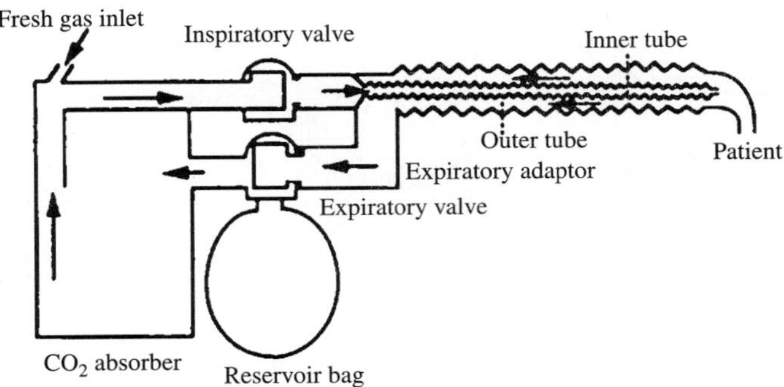

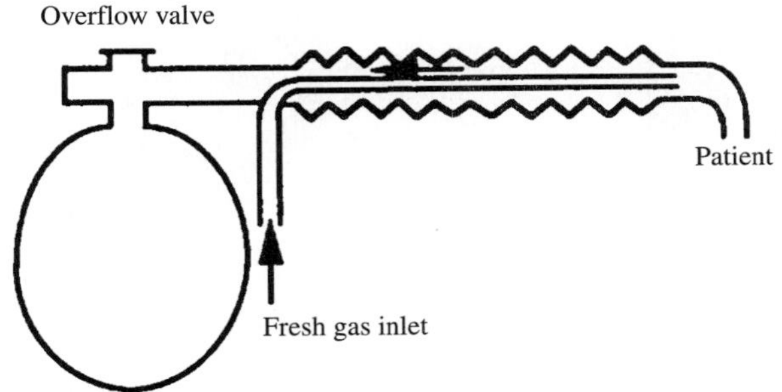

FIGURE **15-34**
In the coaxial circle system the inspiratory limb is contained within the expiratory limb.

inspect and dry it, and then reassemble it (while ventilating the patient with an Ambu bag).[2,83] Note that this may be more difficult with newer absorber heads (e.g., the ADU) than with older heads and is always more difficult when the user has never performed the task before. This emphasizes the importance of reading the operator's manual and practicing without a patient attached before the maneuver is attempted, because failure to reassemble the valve quickly results in a hypoventilated patient or one in whom anesthetic delivery has been interrupted. Perhaps the best recommendation is to bring a new gas machine into the room, because then any valve adjustment can take place without the pressure of the clinical situation and will not distract the anesthetist from patient care.

The daily check of the unidirectional valves[9] is done during the ventilator checkout (FDA Anesthesia Apparatus Checkout, step 12). A reservoir bag is placed on the elbow fitting at the patient's end of the Y-piece, and mechanical ventilation of this "artificial lung" is begun. The user carefully observes that the valves lift and fall during the appropriate phase of ventilation. Datex-Ohmeda recommends essentially the same test as that in the FDA Anesthesia Apparatus Checkout procedure.[39] North American Dräger suggests not only a similar test, but also breathing through each limb individually.[40,41,86] If the inspiratory limb is detached and occluded with one's palm, the operator should be able to exhale but *not* inhale through the expiratory limb. Similarly, if the inspiratory limb is replaced and the expiratory limb detached and occluded, the operator should be able to inspire but *not* expire through the inspiratory limb. This test is probably more sensitive than that recommended by the FDA. If the FDA Anesthesia Apparatus Checkout is performed daily, the capnograph is used properly, and the operator is aware of the steps that should be taken in the event of an increase in inspired CO_2, perhaps this more rigorous test must be performed only if unidirectional valve function is in doubt, particularly because it is problematic to perform the more rigorous test in a hygienic fashion. Nevertheless, it is required by the manufacturer.

Newer machines have electronic routines to check for leaks and compliance. This helps the ventilator accurately correct the delivered tidal volume. These checks must be repeated when the type of circuit is changed, for example, from adult to pediatric. Dräger does not recommend expandable breathing circuit hoses with the Narkomed 6000, because their volume and compliance may change after the leak and compliance testing is performed, which will degrade the accuracy of the delivered tidal volume.[41] With any newer gas machine, these hoses should be expanded before the leak and compliance test is initiated.

Maintenance of the circle system is detailed in the operator's manuals, which must be consulted before one disassembles and cleans the circle. Daily checkout of the circle is covered later in this chapter. The advantages and disadvantages of the circle system are listed in Box 15-9 on p. 287. One advantage of at least partial rebreathing is constancy of inspired concentrations. In a completely nonrebreathing circuit, each breath is fresh gas; therefore depth can vary much more quickly. The use of lower flows also reduces the rate of release of anesthetic agents into the environment. The circle conserves respiratory tract humidity. Misconnections, although a potential disadvantage, occur much less frequently now than in the past because the diameter of breathing hoses has been standardized to be different (22 mm) from the diameter of scavenger hoses (19 mm or 30 mm).[15] Nevertheless, misconnections continue to be reported.[87,88]

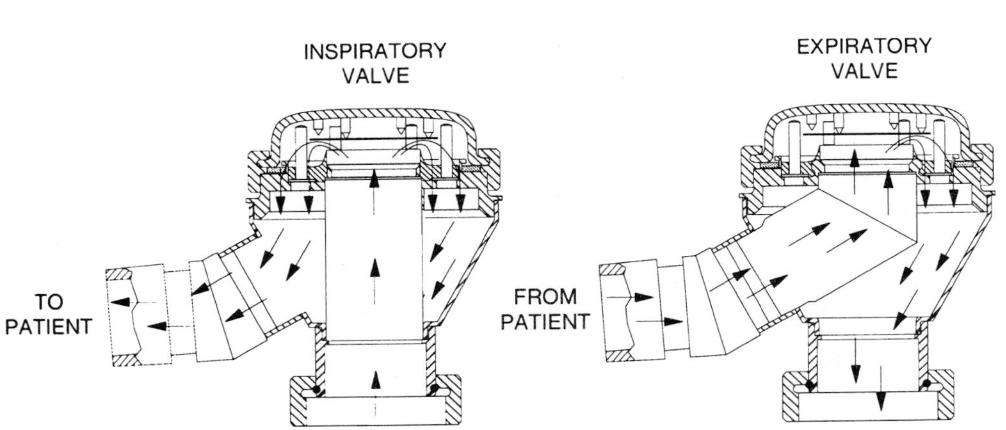

FIGURE **15-35**
Gas flows in inspiratory and expiratory unidirectional valves. (From Cicman J, Himmelwright C, Skibo V, Yoder J. *Operating Principles of Narkomed Anesthesia Systems*. Telford, Pa: North American Dräger; 1993.)

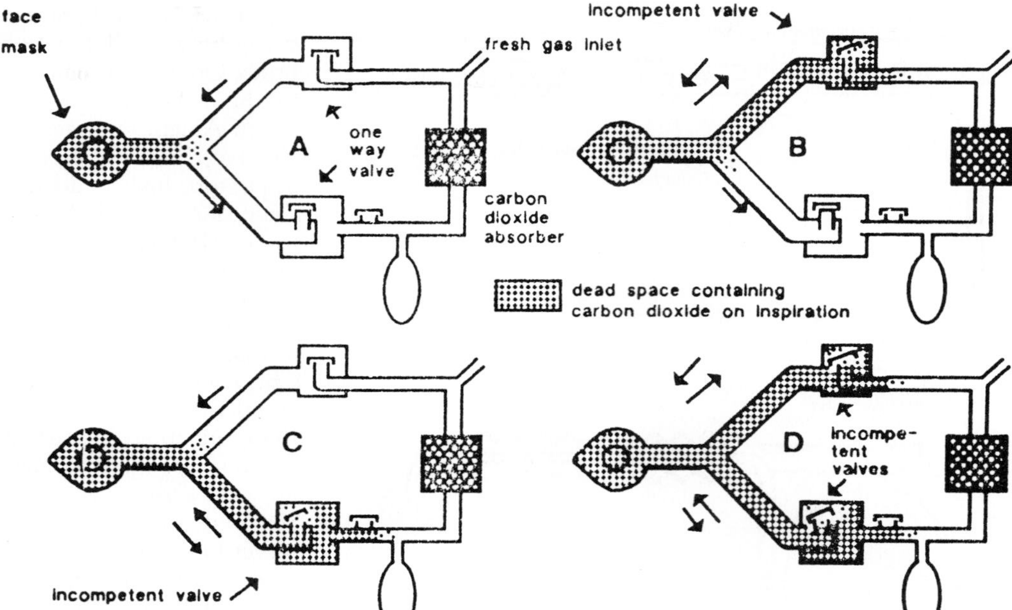

FIGURE **15-36**
Incompetence of a unidirectional valve. **A,** Normal function. Incompetence of an inspiratory valve **(B),** of an expiratory valve **(C),** or of both unidirectional valves **(D)** creates dead space (*stippled area*) that extends through the entire ipsilateral corrugated breathing hose. (Modified from Gravenstein JS, Paulus DA, Hayes TJ. *Capnography in Clinical Practice*. Boston: Butterworth; 1989.)

Several design changes in newer circle systems facilitate low flow anesthesia. Low FGF is desirable to reduce pollution and cost of using volatile agents and N_2O, preserve tracheal heat and moisture, prevent soda lime granules from drying, and preserve patient body temperature. Factors that enhance the safety and efficiency of low flows in modern circle breathing systems and ventilators are shown in Box 15-10. A traditional-sized absorber head like the Aestiva, which is similar to the Ohmeda GMS absorber head, has roughly twice the volume of any of the newer designs. Circles with smaller volumes have shorter time constants. The time constant equals capacity divided by flow and measures how quickly a breathing system reaches equilibrium with a change in the inflow. In a circle system with lower volume, changes in dialed concentration of agent are reflected more quickly in the inspired concentration at any flow rate, as compared with a circle system with a higher volume. In a nonrebreathing circuit, or a circle system at flows substantially higher than VE, each breath reflects the dialed concentration of agent precisely, because there is no rebreathing of exhaled gases in either. Therefore a circle system with higher flows is suitable when rapid changes are desired, such as at induction and emergence.

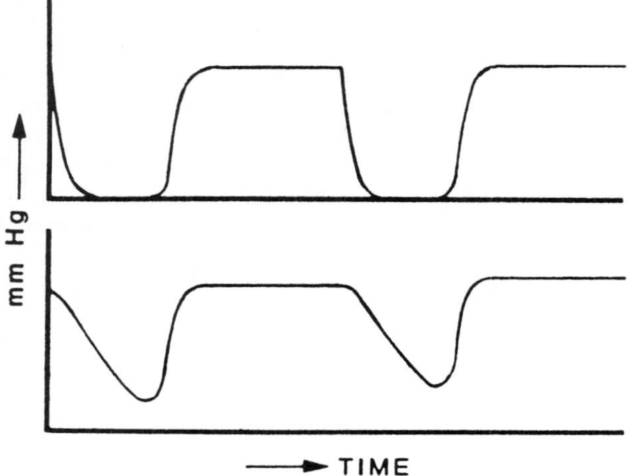

FIGURE **15-37**
Compared with a normal capnogram (*upper tracing*), a capnogram recorded when the inspiratory unidirectional valve is incompetent (*lower tracing*) shows increases in inhaled and exhaled carbon dioxide pressure and an abnormally prolonged downstroke. The prolonged downstroke during the inspiratory phase occurs because the patient inspires mixed alveolar and fresh gas from the inspiratory limb rather than fresh gas alone. (Modified from Gravenstein JS, Paulus DA, Hayes TJ. *Capnography in Clinical Practice*. Boston: Butterworth; 1989.)

Carbon Dioxide Absorption

Carbon dioxide absorption makes rebreathing of exhalations possible. Because of this it conserves agent and gases while preventing the respiratory acidosis that would result from the rebreathing of CO_2.

Gas flows set on the flowmeters determine the amount of rebreathing in the circle system. A circle system with FGFs of 0.3 to 0.5 L/min provides near-total rebreathing and full reliance on absorbent for prevention of rebreathing of CO_2. Use of a circle system with FGFs near or above VE (greater than 4 to 5 L/min for a traditional large dual-canister absorber head) has little, if any, reliance on absorbent granules.[12,86] This

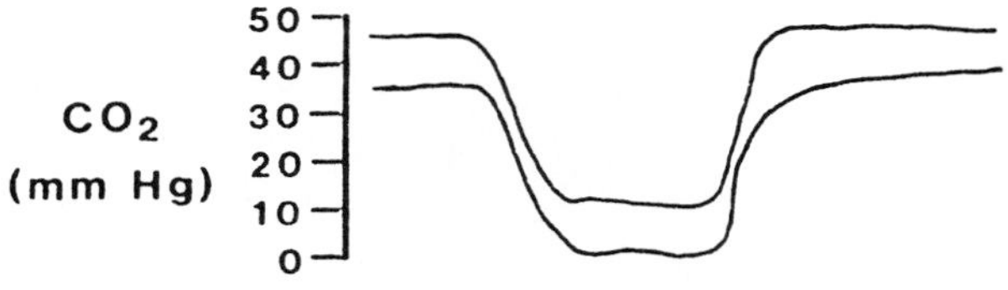

FIGURE **15-38**
Compared with a normal capnogram, a capnogram recorded with an incompetent expiratory unidirectional valve shows increases in inspired and expired carbon dioxide concentration but no changes in morphology. (Modified from Gravenstein JS, Paulus DA, Hayes TJ. *Capnography in Clinical Practice*. Boston: Butterworth; 1989.)

BOX 15-9

Circle System: Advantages and Disadvantages

Advantages
Constant inspired concentrations
Conservation of respiratory tract heat and humidity
Minimal operating room and environmental pollution
Useful for closed-system, low-flow, and semiopen configurations
Low resistance (less than the endotracheal tube; not as low as in nonrebreathing circuits)

Disadvantages
Relatively complex
Opportunities for misconnection or disconnection
Malfunctioning unidirectional valves cause serious problems
 Open: rebreathing
 Closed: occlusion
Less convenient and portable than nonrebreathing circuits
Increased dead space (true of all respiratory apparatus; extends to point where inspired and expired gas streams diverge, i.e., at Y-piece)

relationship can be confusing. When faced with exhausted granules, which cause an increase in expired (and inspired) CO_2, one may be tempted to increase VE. This approach is ineffective if the absorbent has been exhausted (even though it is the obvious response for controlling hypercarbia resulting from other causes), because the patient simply inspires more of a gas mixture containing CO_2. The correct response to hypercarbia associated with absorbent exhaustion is increasing FGF (the absorbent is changed at the end of the case).

Chemistry
The chemistry of soda lime and barium hydroxide lime (Baralyme) CO_2 absorption is shown in Box 15-11.[2,75] The

BOX 15-10

Breathing System and Ventilator Design Features that Support Low Flow Anesthesia

Compliance and leak testing, automatic leak detection
Fresh gas compensation or decoupling
Warmed absorber heads (Julian, Narkomed 6000)
Low volume absorber heads (allows faster equilibration of dialed and delivered agent concentration)
 Julian, Narkomed 6000, Fabius GS—1500-ml canister (Fabius GS volume is 2800 ml, including bag for entire breathing system)
 Aestiva—2700 ml in canisters alone
 S/5 ADU—750 ml canister
No mandatory minimum oxygen flows (the exception is Julian, with a minimum flow of 500 ml/min)
Electronic detection if bellows not filling (Julian)
Point in system at which fresh gas enters (distal to inspiratory unidirectional valve causes dialed changes to be reflected at airway more quickly at lower flows)

BOX 15-11

Chemistry of Carbon Dioxide Absorption*

Soda Lime
$CO_2 + H_2O \rightarrow H_2CO_3$
$H_2CO_3 + NaOH$ (or KOH) $\rightarrow Na_2CO_3$ (or K_2CO_3) $+ H_2O$ + Energy
Na_2CO_3 (or K_2CO_3) $+ Ca(OH)_2 \rightarrow CaCO_3\downarrow + NaOH$ (or KOH)

Barium Hydroxide Lime
$Ba(OH)_2 \cdot 8H_2O + CO_2 \rightarrow BaCO_3\downarrow + H_2O$ + Energy
$H_2O + CO_2 \rightarrow H_2CO_3$
Then by direct reactions and by NaOH and KOH, if present:
 $H_2CO_3 + Ca(OH)_2 \rightarrow CaCO_3\downarrow + H_2O$ + Energy

For soda lime, reaction 1 is also called the first neutralization reaction; *reaction 3 is also called the* second neutralization reaction *and the* regeneration of activator.
**It has been stated that not much carbonic acid forms at pH > 10. The reaction with sodium hydroxide is primarily with CO_2 in physical solution in water (Michael Clarke, PhD, personal oral communication, February 17, 2003).*

ionic reactions take place in the aqueous medium on the surface of the granules. An appropriate water content (10% to 20%) is important for the speed and efficiency of the reactions. Dry granules become exhausted much more quickly than moist granules. Activators (NaOH, KOH) are added to increase the speed of the reaction. They combine with carbonate ions or CO_2 in solution in a reversible reaction that produces water and energy. The absorption of 1 mol (gram molecular weight) of CO_2 produces 13,000 kcal of heat energy.[75] Absorbents contain ethyl violet as an additive. The ethyl violet serves as an indicator of absorbent pH. Fresh CO_2 absorbent has a caustic alkaline pH because of the sodium hydroxide. As the reactions proceed, the pH becomes less alkaline. At a critical pH of 10.3, the ethyl violet changes from colorless to bluish purple.

Neither soda lime nor barium hydroxide lime regenerate to any extent; in other words, they do not regain capacity to absorb CO_2 during periods when they are not in use. Whether they are used continuously or intermittently, their capacity is similar. However, they do exhibit some color reversion (a change in their appearance from bluish purple to white) during a rest period. The color of the absorbent at the beginning of the day may not reflect its remaining capacity because of this color reversion.[75] When a subsequent anesthetic case is begun, the color of absorbent that had not seemed exhausted initially may quickly change to bluish purple.[75] Therefore it is recommended that the user judge the degree of color change at the end of each case and, if necessary, change the canister before the next case.

Soda Lime
The characteristics of soda lime, barium hydroxide lime, and other absorbents are listed in Table 15-5. The main constituent of both is calcium hydroxide. Hardeners (silica and kieselguhr) may be added to soda lime. Soda lime is manufactured to have a water content between 14% and 19% by weight. The size of all absorbent granules is 4 to 8 mesh. This means that granules are approximately $\frac{1}{8}$ to $\frac{1}{4}$ inch in size. Compared with small granules, large granules have less resistance

TABLE 15-5 Characteristics of Absorbent

Component	Soda Lime	Baralyme	Medisorb	Drägersorb 800+	Amsorb
Ca(OH)2 %	94	80	70-80	80	83
NaOH %	2-4	—	1-2	2	—
KOH %	1-3	(May contain some)	0.003	2	—
$CaCl_2$ % (humectant)	—	—	—	—	1
$CaSO_4$ (hardener)	—	—	—	—	1
Polyvinylpyrrolidine % (hardener)	—	—	—	—	1
Water content %	14-19	As water of crystallization	16-20	Approximately 14	14.5
$Ba(OH)_2$-$8H_2O$%	—	20	—	—	—
Size (mesh)	4-8	4-8	4-8	4-8	4-8
Indicator	Yes	Yes	Yes	Yes	Yes

Data from Anesth Analg. *2001;93:221-225;* Anesthesiology. *2001;95:1205-1212; and* Anesth Analg. *2000;91:220-224.*
Numbers are approximations that may not total 100%.

to gas flow; however, they are also less efficient because their surface area is relatively small with respect to their mass. Fine granules or soda lime dust would have a great deal of resistance to gas flow, but the efficiency of such substances would be high because of their increased surface area. The selection of granule size involves a compromise between these two requirements.

Soda lime is absolutely incompatible with trichloroethylene, a flammable anesthetic. Soda lime degrades most current volatile agents to some extent,[39] with sevoflurane degraded most and desflurane least. Sevoflurane is unstable in soda lime, producing compound A. Compound A is lethal at 130 to 340 ppm and may cause renal injury at 25 to 50 ppm in rats. Compound A concentrations of 25 to 50 ppm are easily achievable in normal clinical practice. The incidence of toxic (hepatic or renal) and lethal effects in millions of humans are comparable to those seen with desflurane. The product insert does not recommend sevoflurane at total FGFs of less than 1 L/min for more than 2 MAC-hours.[89-93]

Carbon monoxide is produced by desflurane more than by isoflurane when these agents are in contact with absorbent granules. Halothane and sevoflurane produce little carbon monoxide, if any. Production of carbon monoxide is greatest in dry absorbent and is greater with Baralyme than with soda lime. It is recommended that O_2 be turned off at the end of each case, absorbents be changed regularly (particularly if FGF is left on over the weekend or overnight), and low flows be used (this tends to keep granules moist).[45,94-98] Current recommendations for avoiding problems with carbon monoxide are summarized in Box 15-12.

New Absorbents That Lack Strong Bases

The strong bases (activators NaOH, KOH) have been convincingly implicated in the carbon monoxide problem with the ethyl-methyl ethers and the generation of compound A by sevoflurane. Eliminating the activators produces an absorbent that has similar physical characteristics and carbon dioxide absorption efficiency (this is controversial) as compared with soda lime.[95,99] Amsorb (Armstrong Medical, Coleraine, Northern Ireland) was planned for introduction to the U.S. market in 2000 by Abbott, but it is not yet widely available. Lithium hydroxide is also an effective carbon dioxide absorbent.

Because of the controversial efficiency of absorbents like Amsorb that lack all strong bases, absorbents have been developed with reduced NaOH and KOH (see Table 15-5). The goal is to maintain efficiency while lessening the production of byproducts. Dräger Medical makes an absorbent with decreased amounts of NaOH and no KOH (Drägersorb 800 Plus). Datex-Ohmeda makes Medisorb, which has a similar composition. The canisters that fit on the S/5 ADU are filled with Medisorb.

Barium Hydroxide Lime

Barium hydroxide lime is similar to soda lime in many respects. The activator is barium hydroxide. No hardeners are added, because this absorbent is inherently less likely to produce dust during transport. It is slightly less efficient than soda lime, but it also is much less likely to dry out if it is stored under less than ideal conditions. This results from the water of crystallization, which is chemically bound to the barium hydroxide molecule. Barium hydroxide lime that has dried out completely may produce more carbon monoxide than dry soda lime[45]; however, this limitation is balanced by the lesser tendency of barium hydroxide lime to dry completely in clinical use.[100]

Using Carbon Dioxide Absorbents

Certain similarities are apparent with all absorbents. The resistance of filled canisters in a circle system is low (less than 1.5 cm H_2O at a flow rate of 100 L/min). Resistance of other

BOX 15-12

Recommendations for Maintaining Hydration in Canisters and Avoiding Carbon Monoxide Generation in Carbon Dioxide Absorbent Granules

Turn off oxygen flow at end of case.
Change canisters if oxygen flows have been left on overnight or over the weekend.
Consider changing canisters every Monday morning.
Use relatively low fresh gas flows for the majority of procedures.
Change flows from high to low as soon as practical in any given case (after the patient has attained maintenance levels of volatile anesthetic).

breathing circuit components, particularly the endotracheal tube, is greater.[75] Inhaled dust is caustic and is an irritant, and its presence may lead to laryngospasm, bronchospasm, and pneumonia.[75] A trap for water and dust that prevents the passage of dust toward the patient is often incorporated beneath the lower canister of circle systems. This trap must be emptied periodically. In addition, when the breathing circuit is pressurized for checkout, the pressure should be released through the APL valve rather than through the elbow at the patient's end. This technique (which is in accordance with the current FDA Anesthesia Apparatus Checkout) not only prevents the propulsion of dust toward the patient but also can be used to check APL valve function.[9]

Absorbent efficiency is decreased by channeling and the wall effect. The amount of CO_2 absorbed varies throughout the canister. The inside edge of the canister is a low-resistance pathway. Exhaled gas follows this pathway or other low-resistance pathways through the canister, forming channels whose capacity to absorb CO_2 is exhausted before the capacity of the bulk of the absorbent is used. Therefore the wall effect and channeling produce exhaustion of absorbent before its theoretic capacity has been reached. Methods for preventing these two effects include shaking of the canister before installation in the circle system to promote uniform packing throughout.[75]

Exhaustion and Replacement of Canisters

The clinical signs of absorbent exhaustion are shown in Box 15-13. Some of these signs—for example, hyperventilation—may be masked in the anesthetized patient. In practice, capnography and indicator color change are primary indications of exhaustion. It is unwise to rely on color change or canister temperature alone as a measure of exhaustion.[101] The process of canister replacement for old-style absorbers is illustrated in Figure 15-39, and the steps for replacement are shown in Box 15-14. Canister replacement for the ADU is shown in Figure 15-40. Do *not* change old-style canisters, or loose fill, in the middle of a case. If the new canister is placed in its clear plastic holder upside down or if for any other reason the circuit cannot be reassembled promptly, resumption of ventilation might be delayed. If granules do become exhausted, a safer alternative strategy is to change FGF to one to two times the VE; this approach should ensure that expired CO_2 is reduced to acceptable levels. The granules can then be replaced after the case.

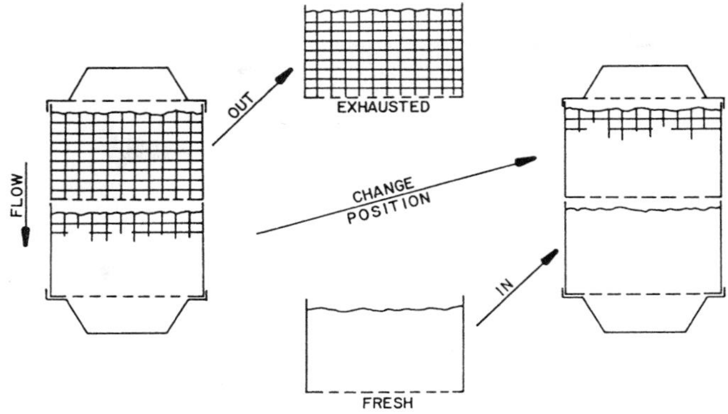

FIGURE **15-39**
Changing carbon dioxide absorber canisters. (From Schreiber P. *Safety Guidelines for Anesthesia Systems*. Telford, Pa: North American Dräger; 1985.)

Each canister (top or bottom) in an older-style absorber contains approximately 1 to 1.3 kg of granules that have a volume of 1400 to 1500 ml each. Each 100 g of granules can absorb as much as 15 L of CO_2 before the outlet concentration is 1% (7.6 mm Hg). This assumes that no channeling occurs. The average to maximum production of CO_2 by the anesthetized adult is 12 to 18 L/hr. Therefore when total rebreathing is occurring the top canister might be expected to last approximately 8 to 10 hours.[75] A much longer life is observed clinically, principally because higher flows are used (typically, 4 L/min of FGF). At these higher flows, both the dilution of exhaled CO_2 and the rate of washout of exhalations from the breathing circuit to the scavenger are greater. In one study in which FGFs of 4 L/min were employed, two canisters were used for 67 and 79 hours (anesthesia time) over 2.5 weeks without exhaustion, with a final minimum water content in some segments of 4% to 8.5%.[102] As lower flows become more common for economic and environmental reasons, anesthetists will need to become more aware of the signs of absorbent exhaustion and realize that absorbent must be changed more frequently.

The manufacturer of soda lime recommends that the absorbent be changed if it is left in the machine for longer than

BOX **15-13**

Clinical Signs of Carbon Dioxide Absorbent Exhaustion

- Increase in partial pressure of end-tidal carbon dioxide; may be accompanied by an increase in inspired carbon dioxide
- Increase (and later a decrease) in heart rate and blood pressure
- Hyperventilation
- Respiratory acidosis
- Arrhythmia
- Signs of sympathetic nervous system activation (flushed appearance, cardiac irregularities, sweating)
- Increased bleeding at surgical site
- Color of indicator at end of the case

BOX **15-14**

General Steps for Changing Carbon Dioxide Absorbent Canisters

- Protect eyes and skin with goggles and gloves.
- Note purple color, date, or both.
- Loosen clamp or screw.
- Remove and discard top canister.
- Remove plastic wrap and seals from new canister.
- Insert new canister on bottom and old bottom canister on top.
- Retighten screw.
- Check breathing circuit for leaks.

Do not change canister in the middle of a case; convert to semiopen with 5 L/min fresh gas flow.

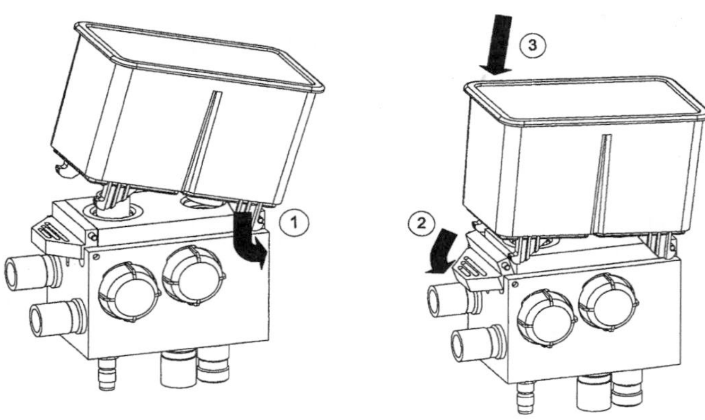

FIGURE **15-40**
Changing carbon dioxide cassette in the Anesthesia Delivery Unit. (From Datex-Ohmeda. *S/5 Anesthesia Delivery Unit User's Reference Manual*. Madison, Wis: Datex-Ohmeda; 2000. Catalog No. 8502304.)

48 hours.[75] This extremely cautious guideline is based on recognition of two problems that arise with extended use. First, the ethyl violet indicator present along the wall of the canister may be inactivated by gas flows or by intense light. Second, dehydration of the granules occurs over time, particularly if higher gas flows or an excessive amount of flushing with O_2 is employed. It is not uncommon for gases to be left flowing accidentally overnight or over the weekend. Dehydration of the granules reduces their efficiency. Dräger recommends that their loose-fill absorbent in the Fabius GS be changed if the machine has been idle for 48 hours, or at least each week on Monday.[40]

Abbott Laboratories has recently advised of a rare situation where fire or extreme heat in the respiratory circuit of anesthesia machines may occur when sevoflurane is used with desiccated CO_2 absorbent. The etiology is unknown; however, recommendations for prevention of this occurrence are listed in Box 15-15.

BOX **15-15**

Machine Fires when Sevoflurane is Used with Desiccated Carbon Dioxide Granules

Anesthesia providers should consider certain steps that might reduce the risk of these events occurring:

- If you suspect that the carbon dioxide (CO_2) absorbent may be desiccated because it has not been used for an extended period of time, it should be replaced.
- Although the exact conditions under which the CO_2 absorbent may become desiccated are not well defined, a low fresh gas flow rate over an extended period of non-use may contribute to unexpected desiccation of CO_2 absorbent materials on the anesthesia machine. Therefore, the anesthesia machine should be completely shut off at the end of clinical use or after any case when a subsequent extended period of non-use is anticipated.
- Turn off all vaporizers when not in use.
- Verify the integrity of the packaging of new CO_2 absorbents prior to use.
- Periodically monitor the temperature of the CO_2 absorbent canisters.
- Monitor the correlation between the Sevoflurane vaporizer setting and the inspired Sevoflurane concentration. An unusually delayed rise or unexpected decline of inspired Sevoflurane concentration compared to the vaporizer setting may be associated with excessive heating of the CO_2 absorbent canister.

In addition, please consider the following:

- The color indicator in the CO_2 absorbents does not necessarily change as a result of desiccation. Therefore, the lack of significant color change should not be taken as assurance of adequate hydration. Note the CO_2 absorbent canister, evaluate the clinical situation, and consider the following interventions to avoid or minimize possible patient injury:
  - Disconnect the patient for carbon monoxide exposure and possible chemical or thermal injury.
  - Shut off fresh gas flow to the breathing circuit or remove the CO_2 absorbent canister from the circuit.
  - Replace the CO_2 absorbent.
  - Monitor the patient for carbon monoxide exposure and possible chemical or thermal injury.
- The following findings have been reported in association with these events of fire and extreme heat:
  - Failed inhalation induction or inadequate anesthesia with Sevoflurane
  - Clinical signs or airway irritation, such as coughing
  - Oxygen desaturation, increased airway pressures, and difficult ventilation
  - Severe airway edema and erythema
  - Elevated carboxyhemoglobin levels
- Current information indicates that typically these cases of fire or extreme heat were the first case of the day for the specific anesthesia machine, and the domestically reported cases indicated Baralyme CO_2 absorbent was used. However, cases of extreme heat associated with desiccated soda lime have also been reported in Europe.
- When desiccated CO_2 absorbents are used with Sevoflurane under experimental conditions, flammable degradation products, including formaldehyde and methanol, may be present even in the absence of fire. The potential risk to patients receiving Sevoflurane anesthesia due to these breakdown products has not been evaluated.
- Clinicians should exercise caution in using potential ignition sources (e.g., electrocautery device) in an oxygen-rich environment near sites of potential gas leakage (e.g., open airway), including when using Sevoflurane.
- Halogenated anesthetics, including Sevoflurane, when exposed to desiccated CO_2 absorbents, can produce carbon monoxide.

McLeskey CH. *Dear health care professional letter.* Abbott Laboratories, Abbott Park, Ill. November 17, 2003.

Ventilators

Classification and Theory of Operation

Ventilators in current use may be classified with respect to a number of parameters (Box 15-15). Figures 15-32 and 15-33 show gas flow in the breathing circuit with mechanical ventilation. Similar to the anesthetist's hand squeezing a breathing bag to assist the patient's respiration, the mechanical ventilator uses the force of compressed gas (air or O_2) as the driving mechanism to compress the bellows. The bellows contains the gas inspired and expired by the patient, and it is surrounded by the driving gas.

The potential buildup of volume and pressure within the breathing circuit (and in the patient's lungs) from the continual addition of FGF is prevented by a ventilator relief valve (also known as the spill valve, or overflow valve) that remains open during the expiratory phase. During the inspiratory phase, driving gas closes this relief valve, thereby preventing gas within the bellows from exiting to the scavenger as the bellows is compressed. During early expiration a weight within the ventilator relief valve holds the pathway to the scavenger closed until the bellows has filled. This creates 2 to 3 cm H_2O of positive end-expiratory pressure (PEEP) within the breathing circuit when standing-bellows mechanical ventilation is employed.[33,52,53] Figures 15-32 and 15-33 shows a functional view of the ventilator relief valve. Note that the "Bag-Vent" switch, when set to "Vent" or "Auto," removes the reservoir bag and APL valve from the breathing circuit, so the APL valve can be open without causing a leak during mechanical ventilation.

Modern ventilators are multimode, double-circuit, electronically controlled, volume- or pressure-limited ventilators (see Box 15-16). Because they are electronically controlled, these ventilators do not operate without electrical power or a backup battery. They generally have ascending bellows (except for the Julian and the piston ventilators). To distinguish between ascending (standing) and descending (hanging) bellows, use the mnemonic, "Ascend and descend contain *e*'s, so look at the bellows during *e*xpiration to distinguish them." Ascending bellows are safer to use than descending bellows, because ascending bellows do not fill in the event of a disconnection.

The hanging design was chosen for the Julian for compactness and for ease of sterilization of the entire breathing circuit. The Julian hanging bellows housing, unlike previous designs, lacks an internal weight and senses when the bellows does not return to the full "down" position. These factors, plus the integration of disconnect alarms based on chemical (capnograph) and mechanical (pressure, volume, and flow sensors) detection, make hanging bellows designs safe. The placement of the hanging bellows below the writing surface makes visual detection of disconnects more difficult. It is also more difficult to determine if the patient is breathing spontaneously in addition to the rate set on the mechanical ventilator. The user must rely more on the pressure and capnography waveforms as opposed to the bellows. Water may gather in the bellows (lessening tidal volume and creating an infection risk), but this tendency should be opposed by the heated absorber head of the Julian.

Typical Ventilator Alarms

Most ventilators have safety alarms to protect the patient from a number of conditions (Box 15-17).

Choosing Ventilator Modes and Settings

Besides increased accuracy resulting from compliance and leak compensation (see subsequent discussion), the biggest improvement in current ventilators is their flexibility in modes of ventilation. PCV allows more efficient and safe ventilation for certain types of patients. The improvement in accuracy afforded by modern ventilators means that switching of circuits (e.g., to a nonrebreather for small children) is not as necessary. This helps avoid potential misconnects. Manufacturers will soon offer modes (pressure support) compatible with spontaneous ventilation, which has been seen in anesthesia with much greater frequency since the advent of the laryngeal mask airway.

BOX 15-16

Classification of Modern Ventilators

Power Source

Compressible bellows—compressed gas and electricity
Piston ventilator—electricity only

Drive Mechanism

Double-circuit (bellows compressed by driving gas) and pneumatically driven
 Driving gas is 100% oxygen or compressed air (Datex-Ohmeda) or Venturi mix of oxygen and room air (Dräger)
Piston ventilators (bellows compressed by electric motor)

Cycling Mechanism

Electronically time cycled

Modes

Controlled minute volume
Pressure-control ventilation
Synchronized intermittent mandatory ventilation
Other

Bellows Classification

All except the Julian have ascending (standing) bellows (mnemonic: "*Ascend* and *descend* have *e*'s, so look at the bellows during expiration")

Data from 7800 Ventilator: Operation and Maintenance Manual Software Revision 4. *Madison, Wis: Datex-Ohmeda; 1993;* 7000 Electronic Anesthesia Ventilator: Operation Maintenance. *Madison, Wis: Datex-Ohmeda; 1985; Andrews JJ. Understanding your anesthesia machine and ventilator. In:* 1989 Review Course Lectures. *Cleveland, Ohio: International Anesthesia Research Society; 1989; Cicman J, Himmelwright C, Skibo V, Yoder J.* Operating Principles of Narkomed Anesthesia Systems. *Telford, Pa: North American Dräger; 1993.*

Controlled Mandatory Volume. All ventilators offer controlled mandatory volume (CMV) ventilation. In this mode the volume is kept constant, and gas is delivered at a constant flow. The peak inspiratory pressure (PIP) is allowed to vary according to the patient's compliance and airway resistance. Rate and volume are adjusted for reasonable end-tidal carbon dioxide and PIP. Typical initial settings for CMV in an adult are tidal volume 10 ml/kg, rate 6 to 12 breaths per minute, and PEEP 0 cm H_2O to start.

Pressure Control Ventilation. Inspiratory pressure is controlled in PCV mode, rather than volume as with CMV. Inspired volume is allowed to vary with changes in compliance and airway resistance. The flow generated varies; high flow is

BOX 15-17

Typical Ventilator Alarms

Pressure
- High (isolated or continuing)
- Subatmospheric

Volume—low tidal or minute volume
Rate—high respiratory rate
Reverse flow (may indicate incompetence of expiratory unidirectional valve in the breathing circuit)
Apnea or disconnect alarms may be based on:
- Chemical monitoring (lack of end tidal carbon dioxide)
- Mechanical monitoring
  - Failure to reach normal inspiratory peak pressure
  - Failure to sense return of tidal volume on a spirometer
  - Failure of standing bellows to fill during mechanical ventilator exhalation
  - Failure of manual breathing bag to fill during mechanical ventilation (machines with fresh gas decoupling—the Julian, Fabius GS, Narkomed 6000)
  - Other—lack of breath sounds, etc
- Electronic monitoring
  - Failure of the hanging bellows to fill completely (infrared light sensor on the Julian)

needed at first, to produce the set pressure early in inspiration, and less flow is required to maintain this pressure through the inspiratory time. Target pressure and rate are adjusted to maintain a reasonable end-tidal carbon dioxide, and tidal volume is monitored. PCV, as compared with CMV, may result in increased tidal volume at a lower PIP, especially if PIP had been high when CMV was employed (for example, in laparoscopy).

PCV is indicated in patients for whom high inspiratory pressure is particularly dangerous (laryngeal mask airway,[103] emphysema, neonates and infants) and in patients with low compliance, where PCV can often produce higher tidal volumes than CMV (pregnancy, laparoscopic surgery, morbid obesity, or adult respiratory distress syndrome [ARDS]). Typical initial settings for PCV in an adult include pressure limit 20 cm H_2O, rate 6 to 12 breaths per minute, and PEEP 0 cm H_2O to start. PCV is available on the Datex-Ohmeda 7900.

Synchronized Intermittent Mandatory Ventilation and Other Modes for Spontaneous Ventilation. With the advent of the laryngeal mask airway, spontaneous unassisted breathing is much more common during general anesthesia. However, it is difficult to maintain a light enough plane of anesthesia to permit spontaneous ventilation while retaining sufficient depth for surgery to proceed. If the patient is maintained in a plane of anesthesia that is too deep, respiratory acidosis occurs; if anesthesia is too light, bucking and awareness are risks. Ventilation modes that could support a spontaneously breathing patient would be useful to provide normocapnia without bucking. Modes that might be useful include SIMV, pressure support ventilation (PSV), continuous positive airway pressure (CPAP), and airway pressure release ventilation (APRV).

Of these modes, only SIMV is currently available, and only on the S/5 ADU and the Narkomed 6000. SIMV is like CMV in that it is volume-controlled ventilation, but intermittent mandatory breaths are delivered that are triggered by the patient's spontaneous efforts. Typical initial settings include not only volume and rate, but also trigger window percent and sensitivity (Figure 15-41). Trigger window percent controls the amount of time during each expiratory cycle that the ventilator is sensitive to negative pressure generated by the patient's diaphragm, and sensitivity controls how much negative pressure the patient needs to produce before a breath is triggered.

New Features of Modern Ventilators

Piston Ventilators. Piston ventilators use an electric motor to compress the gas in the bellows during the inspiratory phase. They therefore use no driving gas and may be used without depleting the O_2 cylinder in case of O_2 pipeline failure.

In the Narkomed 6000 and 6400 the bellows is occult, being placed horizontally under the writing surface. Although it can be viewed by lifting the writing surface, the to-and-fro movement is not normally visible during mechanical ventilation. The anesthetist relies on pressure and capnography waveforms to guard against disconnects or other problems. The Fabius GS has a piston ventilator similar to the Divan, but the bellows travels vertically and the movement is continuously visible through a window to the left of the flowmeter bank.

The piston ventilator has positive and negative pressure relief valves built in. If the pressure within the piston reaches 75 ± 5 cm H_2O, the positive pressure relief valve opens. If the pressure within the piston declines to −8 cm H_2O, the negative pressure relief valve opens, and room air is drawn into the piston, protecting the patient from negative end-expiratory pressure (NEEP).

A piston ventilator has several advantages. It is quiet. There is no PEEP (2 to 3 cm H_2O are mandatory on standing bellows ventilators because of the design of the ventilator spill valve). Great precision exists in delivered tidal volume because of compliance and leak compensation, fresh gas decoupling, and the rigid piston design. Compliance losses are reduced with a piston, as compared with a flexible standing bellows compressed by driving gas. Measuring compliance and leaks with a transducer near the piston eliminates a bulky, costly sensor close to the patient's airway (such as the D-Lite sensor on the S/5 ADU). Electricity is the driving force for the piston, so if O_2 pipeline pressure fails and one must rely on O_2 from the

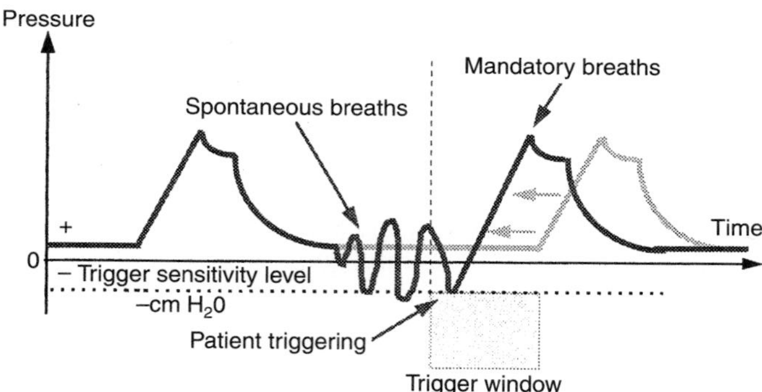

FIGURE 15-41
Trigger window and sensitivity must be set when choosing intermittent mandatory ventilation (IMV) mode. (From Datex-Ohmeda. *S/5 Anesthesia Delivery Unit User's Reference Manual.* Madison, Wis: Datex-Ohmeda; 2000. Catalog No. 8502304.)

emergency cylinder, mechanical ventilation may continue (without exhausting the cylinder O_2 simply to drive the bellows).

The piston design also has some disadvantages. The familiar visible behavior of a standing bellows is lost during disconnects or when the patient is breathing over and above the ventilator settings. Because the piston is quiet, it may be harder to hear its regular cycling. The piston ventilator design cannot easily accommodate nonrebreathing circuits, although this is also true of traditional absorber heads like the Ohmeda GMS or newer ascending bellows ventilators like the S/5 ADU. The piston has at least the potential for NEEP and dilution of the patient's inspired gas with room air.

Flexibility. PCV is a major advantage, allowing efficient ventilation of patients who are difficult to manage with control (CMV) mode, such as patients with ARDS or morbid obesity. PCV also increases safety for patients in whom excessive pressure must be strictly avoided, such as neonates, infants, and emphysematous patients. The future appearance of modes capable of supporting patients with spontaneous respirations will extend our capabilities further.

Accuracy at Lower Tidal Volumes. Factors contributing to a discrepancy between set and delivered tidal volumes are especially acute in pediatrics and include the large compression volume of the circle system relative to the infant's lung volume, leaks around uncuffed endotracheal tubes, the augmentation of delivered tidal volume produced by FGF, and the difficulty of setting a small tidal volume using an adult bellows assembly.

Modern ventilators have an unprecedented tidal volume range. This is because of the greatly increased accuracy in tidal volume delivery achieved through electronic compliance and leak testing, of which tidal volume is compensated for these factors. Modern ventilators are able to ventilate smaller patients much more accurately than any previous anesthesia ventilator could. This will undoubtedly lessen the need for nonrebreathing (Mapleson and Bain) circuits and make care safer, because anesthetists will no longer have to disassemble and reconfigure a nonrebreathing circuit for children between adult cases. However, it is mandatory to substitute a pediatric circuit for tidal volumes less than 200 ml with the Narkomed 6000 and the Fabius GS.[104] Smaller filters, a pediatric D-Lite sensor, and less-compliant circle breathing systems must be used on the S/5 ADU as well. The lower limit of accuracy for tidal volume is 10 ml for the Narkomed 6000; 20 ml for the Fabius GS, Aestiva, and S/5 ADU; and 50 ml for the Julian.

Compliance and Leak Testing. The accuracy comes with a price. An electronic leak and compliance test is part of the morning checklist, and it must be repeated be repeated every time the circuit is changed, particularly when changing to a circuit with a different configuration (adult circle to pediatric circle, or adult to long circuit).

The placement of the sensor used to compensate tidal volumes for compliance losses and leaks has some interesting consequences. The Aestiva flow sensors are placed between disposable corrugated breathing circuit limbs and the absorber head. Here they are able to compensate tidal volumes for FGF, compliance losses, and leaks internal to the machine and absorber head (but not in the breathing hoses).

The Datex-Ohmeda D-Lite sensor is placed just distal to the Y-piece. In this position it can compensate for all leaks and compliance losses out to the Y-piece (including the breathing circuit hoses). However, at this point it adds appreciable and perhaps objectionable bulk and weight close to the patient's face. This may make mask ventilation a bit more cumbersome. Furthermore, a sensor closer to the patient is exposed to more exhaled moisture, but the impact can be lessened with a heat and moisture exchanger between patient and sensor. Unfortunately, this adds further bulk and weight.

The Narkomed 6000 tests compliance and leaks of all components to the Y-piece via a pressure transducer within the internal circuitry near the bellows. Here the sensor is relatively protected from moisture.

Fresh Gas Decoupling versus Compensation. A final factor adding to the accuracy of modern ventilators is that they compensate delivered tidal volume for the FGF. In traditional ventilators the delivered tidal volume is the sum of the volume delivered from the ventilator and the fresh gas flowing during the inspiratory phase. Therefore delivered tidal volume may change as FGF is changed. For example, consider a patient with an FGF of 4 L/min, a respiratory rate of 10, an inspiratory to expiratory ratio of 1:2, and a tidal volume of 700 ml. During each minute the ventilator spends 20 seconds in inspiratory time and 40 seconds in expiratory time (1:2 ratio). During this 20 seconds, the FGF is 1320 ml (one third of 4000 ml/min FGF). So each of the 10 breaths of 700 ml is augmented by 132 ml of fresh gas flowing while the breath is being delivered, and the total delivered tidal volume is 832 ml per breath. This 19% increase is reasonably unimportant in an adult.

However, what happens if the FGF is decreased? Assume the same parameters, but with an FGF of 1000 ml/min. During each minute the ventilator spends 20 seconds in inspiratory time and 40 seconds in expiratory time (1:2 ratio). During this 20 seconds, the FGF is 330 ml (one third of 1000 ml/min FGF). Each of the 10 breaths of 700 ml, therefore, is augmented by 33 ml of fresh gas flowing while the breath is being delivered, making the total delivered tidal volume 733 ml/breath. This means that changing the FGF from 4000 ml/min to 1000 ml/min *without changing ventilator settings* has resulted in a 14% decrease in delivered tidal volume (832 to 733 ml). It would not be surprising if the end tidal carbon dioxide rose as a result.

The situation is more acute with a traditional anesthesia ventilator in children. Assume a 20-kg patient with an FGF of 4 L/min, a respiratory rate of 20, inspiratory to expiratory ratio of 1:2, and a tidal volume of 200 ml. During each minute the ventilator spends 20 seconds in inspiratory time and 40 seconds in expiratory time (1:2 ratio). During this 20 seconds, the FGF is 1320 ml (one third of 4000 ml/min FGF). Therefore each of the 20 breaths of 200 ml is augmented by 66 ml of fresh gas flowing while the breath is being delivered, making the total delivered tidal volume 266 ml/breath. This is a 33% increase over what is set on the ventilator.

Two approaches may be used for dealing with the problem. The Dräger Julian, Narkomed 6000, and Fabius GS use fresh gas decoupling (Figure 15-42). The fresh gas is not added to the delivered tidal volume. Therefore fresh gas decoupling helps ensure that the set and delivered tidal volumes are equal. This can be visualized most clearly by visiting the Virtual Fabius GS Simulation (http://www.simanest.org/). The action of the piston closes a one-way (check) valve, diverting FGF to the manual breathing bag during the inspiratory cycle. The visual appearance is unusual in that the manual breathing bag (normally quiescent during mechanical ventilation) moves with each breath. Furthermore, this manual breathing bag

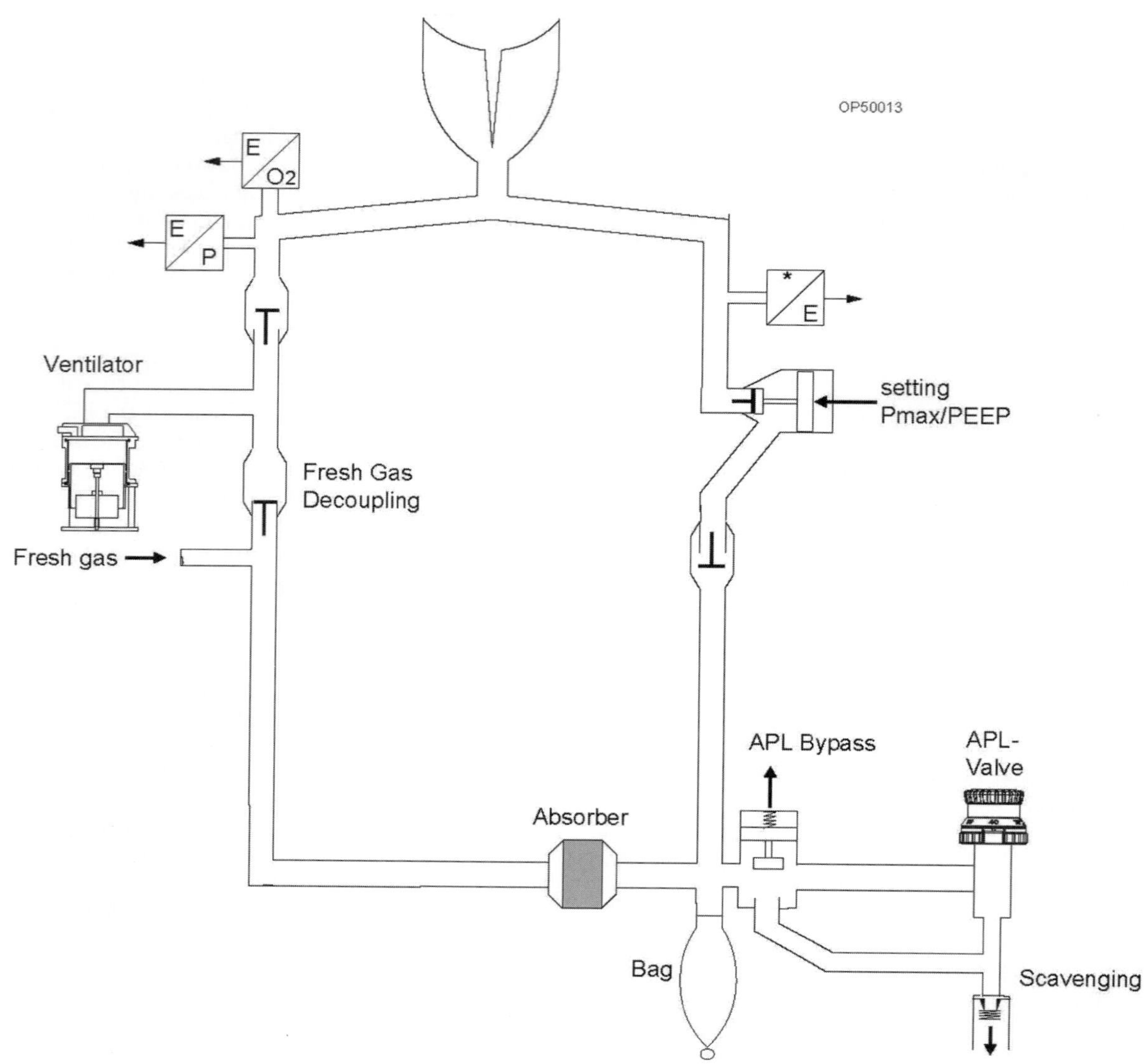

FIGURE **15-42**
Circle breathing system with fresh gas decoupling unidirectional valve. (Courtesy Draeger Medical, Inc., Telford, Pennsylvania.)

movement is opposite to the movement seen in a mechanical ventilator bellows, which empties during inspiration and fills during expiration. With fresh gas decoupling, the bag inflates during inspiration (because of FGF) and deflates during expiration as the contents empty into the absorbent and move on toward the patient. With fresh gas decoupling, if a disconnect occurs, the manual breathing bag rapidly deflates, because the piston retraction draws gas from it.

The second approach, fresh gas compensation, is used in the Aestiva and the S/5 ADU. The volume and flow sensors provide feedback that allows the ventilator to adjust the delivered tidal volume so that it matches the set tidal volume despite the total FGF or in case of changes in FGF.

Suitability for Low Flows. Low FGF is desirable to reduce pollution and the cost of volatile agents and N_2O, preserve tracheal heat and moisture, prevent soda lime granules from drying, and preserve patient body temperature. Factors that enhance the safety and efficiency of low flows in modern ventilators are shown in Box 15-10. A traditional-sized absorber head like the Aestiva, which is similar to the familiar Ohmeda GMS absorber head, has roughly twice the volume of any of the newer designs.

Newer ventilator designs

Datex-Ohmeda 7900 "SmartVent." The Datex-Ohmeda 7900 was designed to provide consistently delivered tidal volume (VT) despite changes in FGF, small leaks, and absorber or bellows compliance losses.[105] It uses flow sensors (in the inspiratory and expiratory limbs) and pressure sensors to accomplish this. Compliance losses in the breathing circuit corrugated hoses are not corrected for, but these are a relatively small portion of compliance losses.[105] Available modes include volume control and pressure control. PEEP is integrated and electronically controlled. It is found on a variety of machines including Aestiva, Modulus, and Excel.

Controls are similar to those of the older 7800 (Figure 15-43). Users should be vigilant for cracked tubing in the flow sensors,

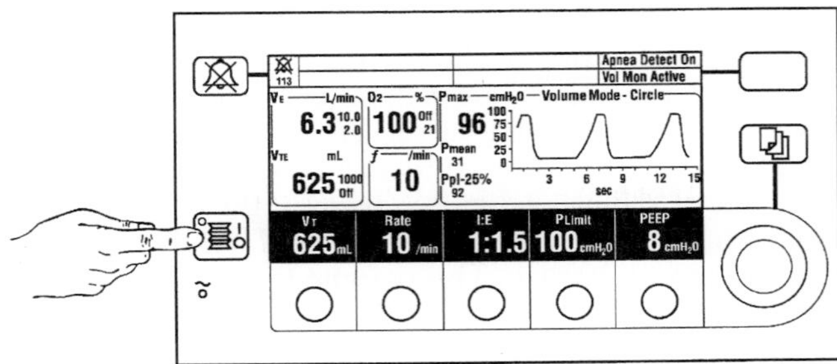

FIGURE **15-43**
Display and control panel of the Datex-Ohmeda 7900 ventilator. (From Ohmeda. *Ohmeda 7900 Ventilator Operation and Maintenance Manual.* Madison, Wis: Ohmeda; 1997.)

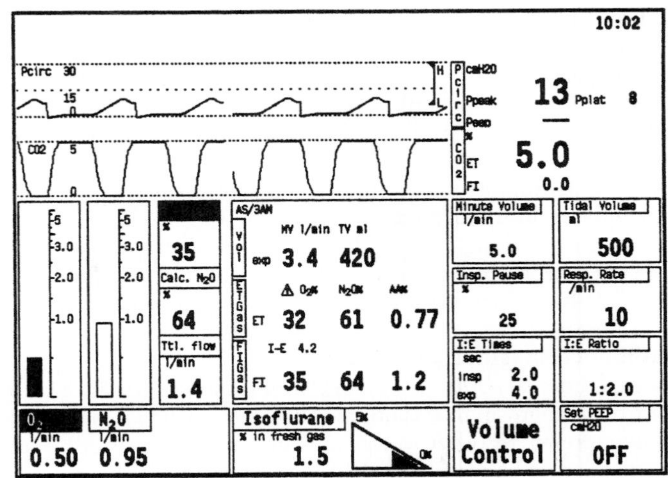

FIGURE **15-44**
Machine monitors and ventilator controls are on the left display screen of the Datex-Ohmeda S/5 ADU. (From Datex-Ohmeda. *Datex-Ohmeda AS/3 Anesthesia Delivery Unit User's Reference Manual.* Tewksbury, Mass: Datex-Ohmeda; 1998.)

which are located where the breathing circuit's corrugated hoses attach to the absorber head. Leaks here have been reported to cause inability to ventilate either mechanically or manually.[106,107] When these failures occur, the ventilator may indicate alarm messages such as "VT" or "Apnea," rather than "Check sensor." It has been reported that the sensors can be quite sensitive to humidity, causing ventilator inaccuracy or outright failure. The problem may be more likely to occur when active airway humidifiers are used.[108]

Datex-Ohmeda 7100. The 7100 model is similar to the 7900, except that the optional pressure control mode is not as robust. The 7100, like the 7900, features tidal volume compensation.

Datex-Ohmeda S/5 Anesthesia Delivery Unit Ventilator. The S/5 ADU ventilator was recently introduced to the North American market by its Finnish manufacturer. The design of the ventilator and gas machine system are superficially very different from the machines presently used in North America. The design has many innovative features.[39] The ventilator is activated by a single switch (setting the "Bag-Vent" switch to "Auto"). The ventilator can use either O_2 or air as a driving gas and switches automatically from one to the other if pipeline pressure is lost. Delivered VT is adjusted to compensate for changes in FGF and total (absorber head and corrugated limbs) breathing circuit compliance losses through the D-Lite sensor at the elbow. The patient's weight is entered, and appropriate ventilator settings are suggested. Volume control, PCV, manual-spontaneous, and SIMV modes are offered, along with integrated electronic PEEP. Flow-volume (resistance) or pressure-volume (compliance) loops may be displayed breath-by-breath. The controls are straightforward (Figure 15-44).

Users should exercise caution with regard to the displayed O_2 concentration. "Calc. O_2%," which is optionally displayed in the mid-lower left of the primary machine status screen, is based on the flowmeter settings only, unlike the O_2 analysis results displayed in the lower center area. The danger arises in a situation in which the pipeline O_2 supply is lost and is replaced with another gas (e.g., nitrogen). In this emergency, two sections of the same display offer conflicting information. Because it is based on flowmeter settings, "Calc. O_2%" indicates appropriate inspired O_2 concentration. The O_2 analyzer display simultaneously alarms, accurately showing a dangerous hypoxic mixture. Although the manual clearly warns of this problem, the design may confuse providers in this rare emergency situation, delaying the correct response, which might lead to patient injury.[39]

Dräger Divan Ventilator. The Divan ventilator is a modern piston ventilator found on the Narkomed 6000 and 6400. It offers PCV, volume control, manual-spontaneous, and SIMV modes. There is no mechanical "Bag-Vent" switch. Switching between modes is accomplished by electronic keypad. The ventilator corrects delivered tidal volume for compliance losses by measuring circuit compliance, and FGF by fresh gas decoupling. Electronic PEEP is integrated. The absorber head is warmed. The Divan is limited to a pressure of 70 cm H_2O, so like most ventilators it cannot ventilate patients in volume control mode beyond this pressure (but it is possible and perhaps preferable to ventilate the ARDS patient with PCV mode). It is accurate to very low tidal volumes (range 10 to 1400 ml). Use pediatric circle system (low compliance) hoses for tidal volumes less than 200 ml, and remember to repeat the ventilator self-test when changing circuits.

Unlike most other anesthesia ventilators, the Divan ventilator has no visible bellows. It is unique among current models in that it has a horizontal piston that is hidden within the writing surface of the gas machine. To provide a visible indication of lung inflation, fresh gas is diverted to the manual breathing bag, which inflates during mechanical ventilator inspiration and deflates during expiration.

The piston design avoids NEEP by entraining room air if pressure within the bellows is less than atmospheric pressure. The "Fresh gas low" error message warns of this condition.

Fabius GS Ventilator. The Fabius GS ventilator is another modern piston ventilator. It offers PCV, volume control, and manual-spontaneous modes. There is no mechanical "Bag-Vent" switch. Switching between modes is accomplished by electronic keypad. It corrects delivered tidal volume for compliance losses by measuring circuit compliance, and FGF by fresh gas decoupling. Electronic PEEP is integrated. One can view measured respiratory parameters or ventilator settings, but not both simultaneously, on the monitor screen. The ventilator is accurate to very low tidal volumes (range 20 to 1400 ml). Use pediatric circle system (low compliance) hoses for tidal volumes less than 200 ml, and remember to repeat the ventilator self-test when changing circuits.

The piston bellows movement is visible in a window to the left of the flowmeter bank. Like the Divan, the machine provides a visible indication of lung inflation and potential disconnects, in that fresh gas is diverted to the manual breathing bag, which inflates during mechanical ventilator inspiration and deflates during expiration.

The piston design avoids NEEP by entraining room air if pressure within the bellows is less than atmospheric pressure. The "Fresh gas low" error message warns of this condition.

Traditional Anesthesia Ventilators

Datex-Ohmeda 7000. The Datex-Ohmeda 7000 has a control mechanism that is unique (Figure 15-45)[53]: it is minute volume preset. In other words, the tidal volume cannot be set independently but rather is chosen on the basis of the control settings for minute volume and respiratory rate in accordance with the following relationship: minute volume = respiratory rate multiplied by tidal volume. Therefore if a constant minute volume of 10 L/min is chosen, a respiratory rate of 10 breaths per minute results in a tidal volume of 1000 ml. Keeping the minute volume at 10 L/min and increasing the frequency to 20 breaths per minute yields a tidal volume of 500 ml. Thus, alteration of the respiratory rate on the Datex-Ohmeda 7000 has little or no effect on alveolar ventilation and arterial CO_2 tension. Desired changes in arterial CO_2 can be produced only by changing the setting of the minute volume control knob.

The Datex-Ohmeda 7000 lacks several of the features now available on newer anesthesia ventilators. It has no display, no integral O_2 or exhaled volume monitoring, no pressure limit control, and no inspiratory flow control. Its internal battery has sufficient current only to sound a power failure alarm. It has a nonadjustable relief valve that halts the flow of driving gas if the pressure of the driving gas exceeds 65 cm H_2O.[53] This means that a patient who requires a higher PIP cannot be ventilated. Furthermore, a lower pressure limit (e.g., as would be needed in pediatric anesthesia) cannot be set. Disconnect monitoring is provided by the low airway pressure alarm, which creates audible and visible alarms if the pressure within the breathing circuit is not at least 6 cm H_2O during two or three consecutive breaths. This pressure is not adjustable. The driving gas is O_2 only (as opposed to air or air-O_2 mixtures). Although this ventilator is no longer sold, it is in common use and is effective, provided users understand its controls. Later models exceed it in capability, as well as in complexity.

Datex-Ohmeda 7800. The control panel of the Datex-Ohmeda 7800 is shown in Figure 15-46. It has a display panel that shows tidal volume, respiratory rate, minute volume, and inspired O_2 concentration. Alarm settings for these parameters are adjusted on the upper right of the panel. When the anesthesia gas machine is turned on, the alarms on the ventilator are enabled whether or not mechanical ventilation is on.[52] Apnea alarms keyed to exhaled volume cannot be disabled while the ventilator is active. If the operator wishes to disengage this alarm (e.g., between cases), the tidal volume control should be set to less than 300 ml.

Settings for mechanical ventilation with the Datex-Ohmeda 7800 are unlike those for the Datex-Ohmeda 7000. Tidal volume and respiratory rate may be adjusted independently. An increase in either leads to an increase in VE; a decrease in either decreases VE. An inspiratory flow control is provided. As inspiratory flow rate is increased, the bellows are compressed more quickly and forcefully; this shortens the duration of the inspiratory phase and decreases the inspiratory-expiratory ratio (i.e., from 1:2 to 1:3). An inspiratory pressure limit dial controls the maximum inspiratory pressure from 20 to 100 cm H_2O.[53] The sustained pressure alarm limit is responsive to this setting.[52]

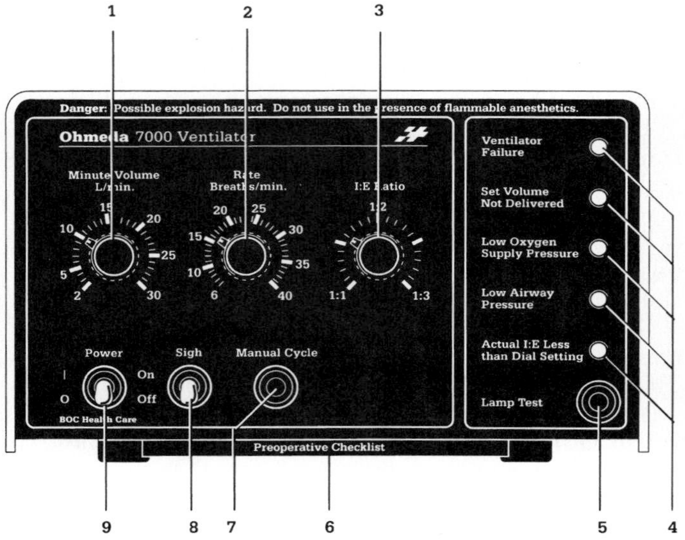

FIGURE **15-45**
Control panel of the Datex-Ohmeda 7000 ventilator. *1*, Minute volume. *2*, Rate. *3*, Inspiratory-expiratory ratio. *4*, Alarm light emitting diodes (LED)s. *5*, Lamp test button (test alarm LEDs). *6*, Preoperative checkout card. *7*, Manual cycle button. *8*, Sigh switch. *9*, Electrical power switch ("On-Off"). (From Datex-Ohmeda. *Datex-Ohmeda Excel Anesthesia System: Operation and Maintenance Manual.* Madison, Wis: Datex-Ohmeda; 1992.)

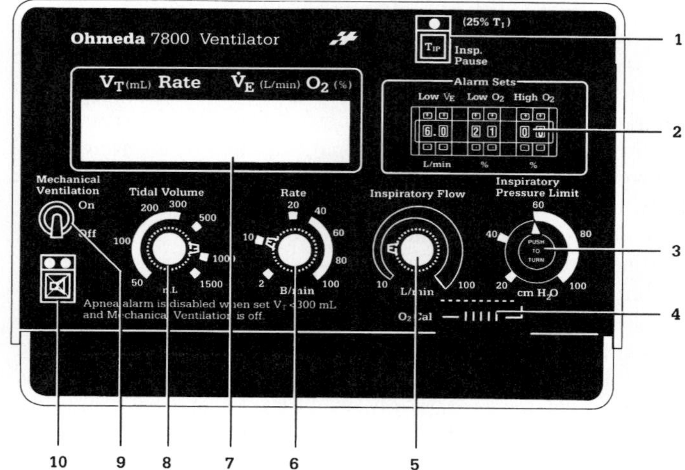

FIGURE **15-46**
Control panel of the Datex-Ohmeda 7800 ventilator. *1*, Inspiratory pause button. *2*, Alarm limits. *3*, Inspiratory pressure limit knob. *4*, Oxygen calibration limit adjustment. *5*, Inspiratory flow knob. *6*, Breath rate knob. *7*, Display. *8*, Tidal volume knob. *9*, Mechanical ventilation switch. *10*, Alarm silence button. (From Datex-Ohmeda. *Datex-Ohmeda Excel Anesthesia System: Operation and Maintenance Manual.* Madison, Wis: Datex-Ohmeda; 1992.)

The 7800 has a built-in suite of monitors. The O_2 monitor is a galvanic fuel cell–type monitor. The user calibrates the monitor by removing the sensor from the absorber and exposing it to room air for 3 minutes. At the end of this period, it should read 21%.[53] The exhaled volume monitor includes an apnea alarm that is activated automatically after breaths are sensed. Apnea alarms are always active during mechanical ventilation. The low-pressure (disconnect) alarm is activated if a pressure of 4 to 9 cm H_2O is not sensed with each ventilator breath. The driving gas for the 7800 is either O_2 or compressed air. A backup battery contained within the ventilator provides a minimum of 20 minutes of mechanical ventilation in the event of power failure.[53] In the case of power failure, the operator should manually ventilate the patient, if at all possible, to conserve battery power for monitoring functions.[38] The battery backup in the Datex-Ohmeda Modulus CD gas machine provides power for 1 hour if mechanical ventilation is employed and for 4 hours if it is not.[32]

Dräger AV-2 Ventilator. The AV-2 is much like the Datex-Ohmeda 7800. It is a volume-preset, time-cycled ventilator with electronic control. Its driving gas is a Venturi mix of O_2 and room air. All entrained room air enters the Venturi device through a muffler on the back of the machine. The Dräger gas machine backup battery has power sufficient for 30 minutes of ventilator use. Use of the ventilator creates a PEEP of 2 cm H_2O because of the ventilator relief valve.[33]

The controls of the Dräger AV-2 are shown in Figure 15-47. Tidal volume is set by the movement of a stop within the bellows housing. Respiratory rate and inspiratory-expiratory ratio have separate controls. Therefore, as with the 7800, increases in either the tidal volume or the respiratory rate increase the VE. The inspiratory flow control is set so that it provides flow sufficient to compress the bellows without deformation and so that no inspiratory pause occurs (unless desired).[33] The pressure limit control varies maximum inspiratory pressure between 15 and 120 cm H_2O.

When the main power switch of the gas machine is turned on, volume- and pressure-based apnea alarms enter standby mode. If breaths are sensed, these monitors and their alarms are activated. The apnea alarms also are enabled whenever the ventilator is turned on. When the ventilator is turned off, the volume- and pressure-related apnea alarms are placed on standby for 60 seconds and then reactivated.[33]

Addition of Positive End-Expiratory Pressure

Currently PEEP can be added to the breathing circuit in one of three ways: by using add-on adapters, by using devices built into the breathing circuit, or electronically. Risks are associated with each approach, although electronic approaches may be safer.

Add-on adapters come in different varieties, depending on how much PEEP is desired (e.g., 5 or 10 cm H_2O). They are intended to be placed between the expiratory limb of the breath-

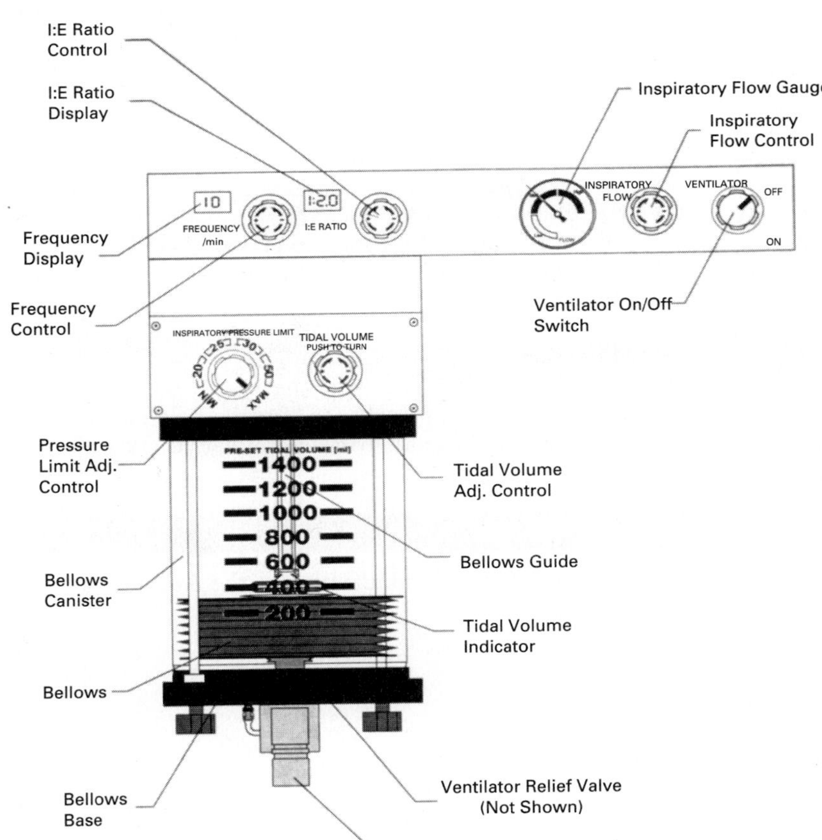

FIGURE **15-47**
Control panel of the Dräger AV-2 ventilator. *I:E*, Inspiratory-expiratory. (From North American Dräger. *Narkomed 2C Anesthesia System—Operator's Instruction Manual.* Telford, Pa: North American Dräger; 1994.)

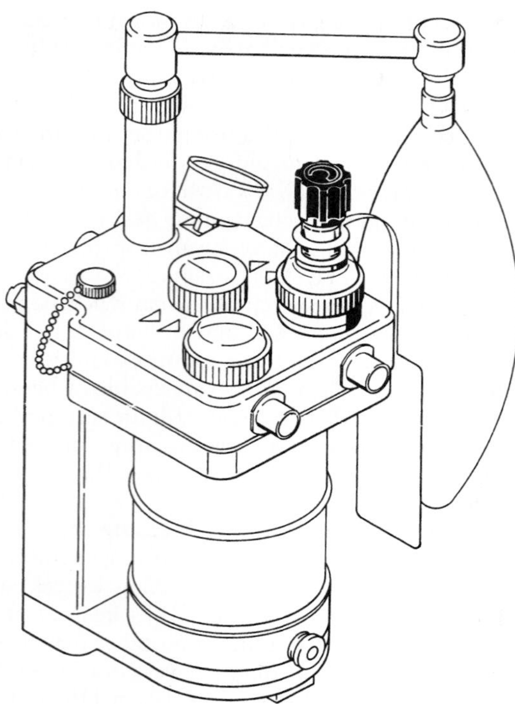

FIGURE **15-48**
The Datex-Ohmeda GMS PEEP valve in place on the absorber. (From Datex-Ohmeda. *GMS PEEP Valve: Operation and Maintenance Manual*. Madison, Wis: Datex-Ohmeda; 1991.)

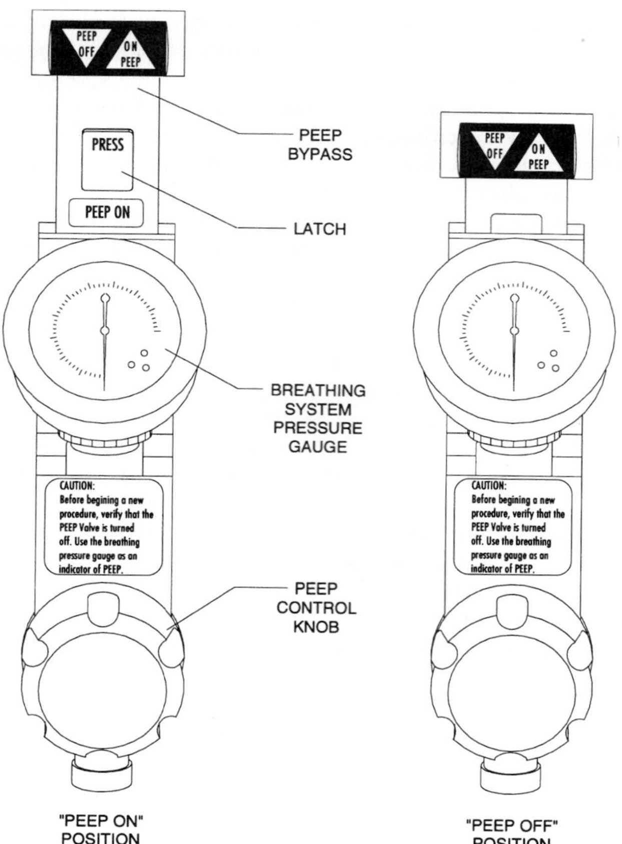

FIGURE **15-49**
Dräger PEEP valve. Note the latch (*above*), the adjustment dial (*below*), and the circle system analog pressure gauge. (From North American Dräger. *Narkomed 2C Anesthesia System—Operator's Instruction Manual*. Telford, Pa: North American Dräger; 1994.)

ing hoses and the expiratory unidirectional valve. They have been placed accidentally in the inspiratory limb, where they cause complete obstruction of flow in the breathing circuit.[110] Although it would not seem difficult to diagnose this fault immediately, in the "heat of the moment" with a patient who is already hypoxemic the clinician may become distracted and unable to focus effectively on the problem. This clinical "pearl" may prove helpful: when a change in a patient's condition is noticed, think back to the last alteration made to the equipment (or to the last drug *thought* to have been given) and determine whether it might have contributed to the change. Add-on PEEP adapters are inherently less safe than built-in valves.

The Datex-Ohmeda GMS PEEP valve is shown in Figure 15-48. This device replaces the disk and dome of the expiratory unidirectional valve.[110] It is not meant to be permanently installed on the absorber because of the risk of malfunction if the device is clogged with expired humidity or secretions. Problems associated with use of the device include mistaking the adjustment knob for the APL valve, inadvertent application of PEEP to a patient for whom it is not intended, potential clogging of the device with secretions, incorrect positioning or sticking of the valve disk, and decreased visibility of the motion of the expiratory unidirectional valve disk.[109,110]

The Narkomed absorber system also has an optional built-in PEEP adapter (Figure 15-49). The PEEP bypass enables or disables the PEEP valve. If the valve is enabled, the control knob can be adjusted to provide PEEP of 2 to 15 cm H_2O.[33] This valve is a better indicator that PEEP is enabled than the circuit pressure gauge alone. Although this valve cannot be disassembled or autoclaved, it can be cleaned (after the PEEP bypass has been latched in the "Off" position) and sterilized with ethylene oxide. It too can be mistaken for the adjustment knob of the APL valve, become clogged with secretions, or result in inadvertent application of PEEP to a patient for whom PEEP is not intended.

Finally, electronic PEEP control is present on all newer ventilators. It is easier to use and therefore probably safer than the older, mechanical approaches.

Humidification

Humidification is desirable with the use of any respiratory apparatus. Two basic approaches to humidification in anesthesia breathing circuits exist: passive and active (Box 15-18).

BOX **15-18**

Means of Adding Humidification to the Anesthesia Breathing Circuit

Passive
Low flows
Heat and moisture exchangers ("artificial nose")

Active—Heated Humidifiers
Flow-over, heated water bath
Heated-wire circuits (with or without wick)

Passive approaches have the advantages of greater economy and simplicity. The use of low flows during maintenance results in an increase in circuit humidity and a lower rate of use of volatile agents. Heat- and moisture-exchanging filters precipitate exhaled water vapor on their filter media. The next inhalation returns this water to the patient. These filters may slow the rate of heat loss from the patient because they decrease the rate of evaporation of water from the tracheal mucosa. They may also confer the benefit of bacterial and viral filtration.[111-113]

Heated (active) humidifiers are of two types; sometimes these types are combined. Flow-over heated water bath types usually require a minimum FGF; heated-wire circuit types do not. Both rely on a temperature sensor located near the Y-piece that controls the amount of heat generated. If water bath–type humidifiers are used (improperly) with low flows, any heat added at the water bath is radiated into the room before the gases reach the Y-piece. In this case, the device either continually sounds an alarm or malfunctions. Problems associated with heated humidifiers include overhydration, underhydration, hypothermia, hyperthermia, melting of disposable breathing circuits, aspiration, interference with gas analysis accuracy (clogged lines or sensors) and infection.[114] In addition, heated humidifiers are costly, and they may not produce as much humidification as is assumed.[116] No consensus exists regarding the efficacy of heated humidifiers for preventing or treating hypothermia.[115]

Causes and Prevention of Critical Incidents

Clinical experience with anesthesia ventilators and breathing circuits has identified several situations that lead (or could lead) to critical incidents. Vigilance directed toward situations that have the potential to cause patient injury may contribute to the prevention of future occurrences (Box 15-19). Failure to ventilate caused by disconnection has been called the most common preventable equipment-related cause of mishaps.[2] The most common site for disconnection is between the breathing circuit and the endotracheal tube (at the Y-piece). Disconnects can be partial or complete. The most important monitor for disconnection is continuous auscultation of breath sounds with a precordial or esophageal stethoscope (this is required by standard),[11] as well as direct visual observation of chest movement.[33] Electronic monitors for disconnection include capnography, as well as pressure-based and volume-based alarms (see Box 15-17).[32,33,52,116] Because electronic monitors may have alarms disabled either inadvertently or intentionally, because of artifacts, and because of monitor failure, there is no substitute for human vigilance.[117]

Failure to initiate or resume ventilation may be less likely in the future because of the incorporation of modern monitoring and gas machine standards in the newer models. All possess common features that add to patient safety.[39-41] They have a centralized data and alarm display, as well as alarms prioritized to warnings, cautions, and advisories. They provide electronic preuse checklists.[118] Furthermore, the apnea and disconnect alarms are typically placed on standby when the system's main power switch is activated, and the alarms are enabled after breaths are sensed. Therefore the anesthesia gas machine should alert the operator to a failure to turn on a mechanical ventilator after intubation or to a failure to resume ventilation after the ventilator is shut off either temporarily (e.g., in the middle of a case for radiography) or permanently (during emergence). The number of different alarm conditions programmed into a modern anesthesia gas machine with integrated monitoring is staggering. For machines of such complexity, it is absolutely necessary that the manuals be read.

Failure to close the APL when mechanical ventilation is initiated and misconnections of the breathing circuit are much less likely now than in the past because of improvements in design. However, occlusion, bellows leaks, failure of gas supply, failure of the ventilator relief valve, and application of suction are still possible causes of failure to ventilate or barotrauma.[119-126] Although equipment has improved dramatically, some of the underlying causes of failure to ventilate and of barotrauma will likely remain problems for the next decade (e.g., lack of knowledge or training and failure to use checklists).[127]

BOX 15-19

Some Causes of Critical Incidents

Underlying Causes of All Critical Incidents

- Improper or infrequent maintenance
- Inadequate in-service education
- Substandard equipment monitoring
- Failure to use checklists
- Lack of familiarity with equipment standards

Mechanisms of Critical Incidents

Failure to Ventilate

- Disconnection
  - Failure to initiate ventilation initially or after an interruption
  - Failure to close APL (applicable to older absorber systems that lack "Bag-Vent" switch)
- Misconnections of breathing circuit
- Occlusion or obstruction of breathing circuit
  - Kinking or plugging of endotracheal tube
  - Incorrect insertion of flow direction–sensitive components
    - Positive end-expiratory pressure valves
    - Cascade humidifiers
  - Kinking of fresh gas delivery hose
- Leaks
  - Failure or improper reassembly of bellows after cleaning
  - Damage to or disconnection of pressure monitoring hoses
- Failure of pipeline and tank oxygen supply
  - Driving a vent with cylinders (when pipeline is unavailable) causes rapid tank depletion
- Inadvertent application of suction to the breathing circuit
  - Failure of scavenger interface negative-pressure relief valve
  - Intubation of trachea with nasogastric tube, which is then connected to suction

Barotrauma

- Excess inflow to breathing circuit (flushing during ventilator inspiration)
- Ventilator relief valve may stick closed
- Control assembly problems

DISPOSAL

The final *D* of the SPDD model is concerned with a simple but vital question: How are gases disposed of?

BOX **15-20**

Components of the Scavenger System

Gas collection assembly—at APL valve and ventilator relief valve
Transfer tubing—19 mm or 30 mm, sometimes color coded yellow
Scavenging interface (most important part)
Gas disposal tubing
Gas disposal assembly—active disposal (common) or passive disposal

BOX **15-21**

Types of Scavenger Interface

Closed Interface (All Older Models)

Communicates to atmosphere only through valves
If used with passive disposal system, must have positive pressure relief
If used with active (suction) disposal system, must have positive *and* negative pressure relief

Open Interface (Most New Models)

No valves; open to atmosphere (both negative and positive pressure relief "built in")
Must be used *only* with active systems
Reservoir required
Safety
- Safer than closed interface for the patient; no barotrauma
- Less safe than closed interface for the care giver (if used improperly)

Disposal of Gases in Scavenging Systems

Scavenging is the collection of waste anesthetic gases from the breathing circuit and ventilator and their removal from the operating room. An amount equal to the FGF must be scavenged each minute.[128-130] Otherwise, the breathing circuit and the lungs either gain or lose volume, resulting in barotrauma or failure to ventilate. The components of the scavenger are listed in Box 15-20.

Standards for exposure to waste anesthetic gases are published by the U.S. Department of Labor's Occupational Safety and Health Administration (OSHA) as "technical instructions."[131] These instructions direct that no worker be exposed to more than 2 ppm of halogenated agents (0.5 ppm if used with N_2O) and no more than 25 ppm of N_2O, based on a time-weighted 8-hour average concentration. Levels in unscavenged anesthetizing locations may be as high as 7000 ppm (0.7%) N_2O and 85 ppm (0.009%) halothane.[13] The highest levels are found in the anesthetist's workstation and between the anesthesia gas machine and the wall.[14] Several variables determine the attainable reduction in waste anesthetic gases in the operating room, including the degree of room ventilation, the condition of anesthesia equipment, the effectiveness of the scavenger, and the anesthetic techniques of the user. However, with appropriate attention to these areas, trace gas levels within the operating room can meet OSHA requirements.[13]

The most important component of the scavenger system is the interface, because it protects the patient and breathing circuit from excessive buildup of positive pressure and from exposure to suction. Two types of interfaces exist: closed and open. The closed interface is found on older machines (Box 15-21).[132,133] A closed interface communicates with the atmosphere only through valves (Figure 15-50). Relief of positive pressure is mandatory for all closed interfaces. If the suction attached to the scavenger fails or if a hose distal to it becomes kinked, positive pressure relief valves operate before the pressure buildup within the scavenger is transmitted to the breathing circuit and the lungs. In this case the positive pressure relief valve opens and allows the release of accumulated gases into the operating room air. If the closed interface is attached to suction, a negative pressure relief valve opens to draw in room air when suction is excessive, preventing the emptying of gas from the patient circuit. Suction should be adjusted as FGFs change so that the scavenger reservoir bag is neither flat nor overdistended.[132,133]

Because the scavenger interface relief valves can fail,[134] an "open" scavenger interface is much more common on new machines. The open interface has large open holes or ports around the top (Figure 15-51). There are no valves to impede the flow of gases into or out of the reservoir,[33] such as are found in closed-interface systems. Each patient exhalation is led to the bottom of the open interface reservoir, where suction withdraws it before the next exhalation arrives. Use of the device with appropriate suction is critical to its proper function.[33] Yet, because the device is so different from the closed interface, errors in its use have already been reported. In one report, 10 of 10 newly purchased machines equipped

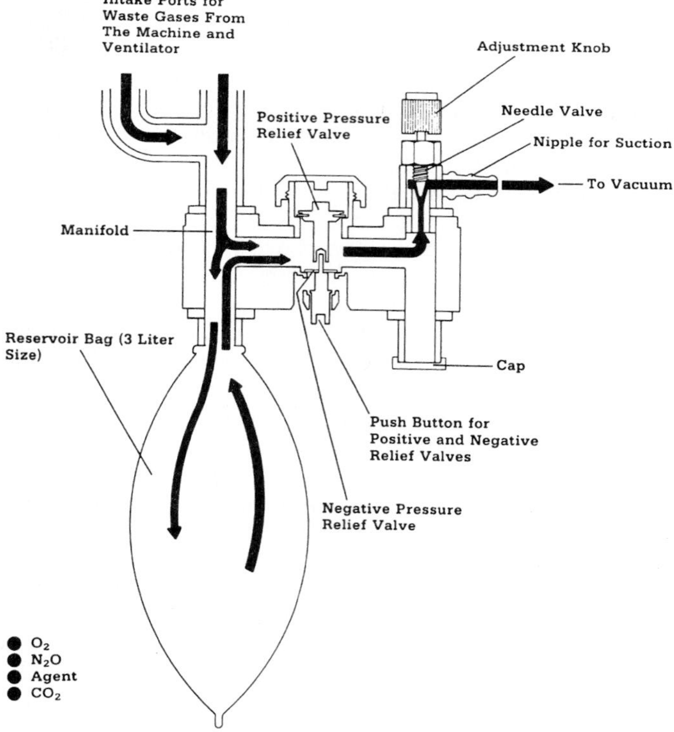

FIGURE **15-50**
Closed scavenger interface attached to suction. Note the reservoir, the positive and negative pressure relief valves, and the capped extra port. (From Bowie E, Huffman LM: *The Anesthesia Machine: Essentials for Understanding*. Madison, Wis: Datex-Ohmeda; 1985.)

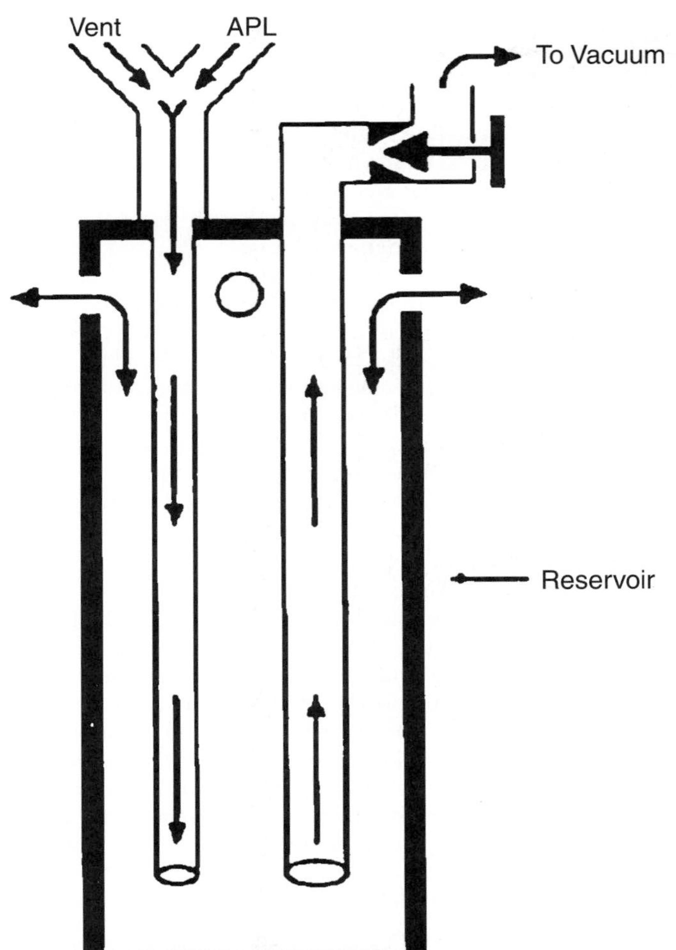

FIGURE **15-51**
Open interface scavenging system. (Courtesy Draeger Medical, Inc., Telford, Pennsylvania.)

with open interfaces had the suction to the scavenger turned off, resulting in the release of all patient exhalations into the operating room.[134] This error in use may be related to the sounds produced by the two different interfaces. When a closed interface is leaking gas into the room through the positive pressure relief valve, a soft, intermittent hiss is audible. The open interface, on the other hand, should hiss continuously when it has been properly adjusted. The open interface affords patient safety advantages. With the open interface, no chance exists of relief valve failure, which can cause barotrauma or the application of suction to the breathing circuit. The device is perhaps less safe for the operator who is unfamiliar with its use; however, the only danger is increased exposure to waste anesthetic gases. The smell of volatile agent during a case is abnormal, and its cause must be sought. The threshold for smelling volatile agents is variously stated as 5 to 300 ppm.[12,13,130,135] Therefore if any agent is smelled, the concentration is excessive (i.e., above that described in the OSHA standard).

Many factors in addition to the scavenger affect exposure to waste anesthetic gases. Guidelines for limiting exposure are listed in Box 15-22.[13,130,135-137] Some may be applied generally, whereas others (e.g., avoidance of N_2O) are not applicable to every practice setting.

BOX **15-22**

Means of Limiting Exposure to Waste Anesthetic Gases

- Check the scavenger according to Food and Drug Administration guidelines.
- Perform regular preventive maintenance of room ventilation systems.
- Perform regular preventive maintenance of all anesthesia equipment.
- Conduct personnel monitoring and ambient trace gas monitoring.
- Seek the source of the smell of anesthetics noted during a case.
- Keep a good mask fit.
- Avoid unscavengeable techniques (open drop, insufflation).
- Prevent flow from breathing system into room air.
- Turn on anesthetic gases only after mask is on the patient.
- Turn off anesthetic gases before suctioning.
- Wash out anesthetics at end of case.
- Do not spill liquid agent.
- Use cuffed endotracheal tubes.
- Use low fresh gas flows.
- Check the machine regularly for leaks.
- Disconnect nitrous oxide at wall outlet at end of day.
- Use total intravenous anesthesia.
- Avoid use of nitrous oxide.

RISK MANAGEMENT

Department-Level Aspects

Risk management is defined as a detection system designed to predict failures and ensure that precautions to prevent patient harm are taken.[12] Typical risk management components include preoperative and postoperative rounds, avoidance of indifferent treatment of patients, maintenance of vigilance and high standards of care, peer review, continuing education, and commitment to the delivery of high-quality and humane patient care. In terms of equipment, risk management includes cleanliness, daily performance of equipment checklists, familiarity with equipment manuals, and appropriate maintenance.[12,138]

The Safe Medical Device Act of 1990 requires hospitals to report instances in which medical devices cause or contribute to death, serious illness, or serious injury.[139,140] All medical personnel who become aware of a problem with a device must remove the equipment from contact with patients and report the problem to their supervisors. The hospital risk manager then conducts an investigation and reports the results to the FDA within 10 working days. The most common barrier to investigation of a critical incident and the degree to which anesthesia equipment may have contributed to it is alteration of the equipment (e.g., it has been cleaned, disassembled, or tested).[140] In the case of patient injury in which equipment may be at fault, it is most helpful if equipment (including wastebaskets and syringes in the anesthesia work area) is sequestered "as is" pending a forensic evaluation conducted by the representatives of the hospital, the manufacturer, and perhaps the patient.[140,141]

Equipment logs should be kept for each anesthesia machine and should include reports of maintenance, critical incidents, additions or alterations, pollution control, and vaporizer calibration. Preventive maintenance should be performed at intervals specified by the manufacturer (usually two to four times per year) by qualified, factory-trained technicians.[12]

Individual Risk Management

The department-level risk management plan requires the active involvement of all department members. In addition to participation in the department-level activities noted earlier, individuals play a vital role in three additional aspects: performance of the machine checklist before use, limitation of equipment-related disease transmission, and reduction of trace and waste gas exposure through alteration of work practices.

Anesthesia Gas Machine Checklist

Reports of equipment problems surfacing in the 1980s prompted governmental involvement in the development of a recommended anesthesia checklist.[141-143] Although equipment failures are rare, they often result from human error in the use of the equipment.[141] Failure to check anesthesia equipment adequately has been reported as a factor in up to 30% of critical incidents.[144,145] Checklists have been the focus of several studies of fault-detection ability[146-151] and much comment.[118,152-157] It is probable, but as yet unproved, that proper and consistent use of checklists not only prevents critical incidents but also helps teach and reinforce knowledge of the function and use of the anesthesia gas machine.

The new S/5 ADU prevents missed steps in the checklist by performing an electronic self-check routine. Although this checklist seems unfamiliar, it covers the functions tested by the FDA checklist and more; it can also detect leaks and breathing circuit compliance. If leaks are detected, check the tightness of all connections: respiratory and patient circuit tubing and bellows (bellows, bellows block, ventilator relief valve, and bellows chamber). Ensure the Y-piece is properly occluded, gas flows are closed, and the gas sampling lines in the D-Lite sensor are not still connected to the circuit. The Fabius GS, Julian, and Narkomed 6000 and 6400 have checklists that are partially electronic and partially manually performed by the user. All of these new machine checklists require that the circuit be occluded for compliance and leak testing, then reconfigured for use. Always perform a high-pressure check after the checklist is complete to ensure that all breathing circuit connections are gas-tight and that the circuit is not obstructed by mold flash or plastic wrapping.[158,159]

Appendix 15-1 shows the text of the current FDA anesthesia gas machine checklist (FDA Anesthesia Apparatus Checkout Recommendations).[9] The anesthetist should consider adding a few activities to the checklist. While performing steps 1 and 2 (checking the Ambu bag and cylinder O_2), he or she should walk around the machine, checking for suction and an extra circuit, the location of circuit breakers, and the presence of a cylinder wrench and head strap and whether gas analysis monitors are scavenged. The order of performance of steps 11 and 12 is arbitrary. Users should consider testing the ventilator and unidirectional valves (step 12) before checking for leaks of the breathing system (step 10). In this way, the relatively common fault of beginning a case with the "Bag-Vent" switch in the "Vent" mode can be avoided. The anesthetist also must check that vaporizers are off (step 14). Because the checklist calls for turning each of the vaporizers on during the low-pressure system leak test (step 5), it is possible that care of a patient could begin with the vaporizers inadvertently turned on.

Use of the negative pressure test (step 5) remains unfamiliar to users. This is unfortunate. The negative pressure test has been demonstrated to be the most effective test for leaks in the low-pressure system (that area within the machine distal to the flowmeters).[161] Leaks there may lead to hypoxic breathing mixtures or awareness under anesthesia.

No "minimum" test exists other than the FDA Anesthesia Apparatus Checkout. In administering an anesthetic for an emergency surgical procedure, one should always check the suction and pressure test the breathing circuit. In addition, the breathing bag should be evaluated for fluctuations during preoxygenation. This evaluation ensures that the patient is breathing, the mask fit is good, O_2 is flowing, and the "Bag-Vent" switch is in the "Bag" mode. A situation in which any of these conditions is absent requires immediate attention.

Disease Transmission

The Standards for Nurse Anesthesia Practice call on anesthetists to use safety precautions to minimize the risk of infection for the patient, the anesthetist, and other staff.[11] It is certain that anesthesia equipment (and providers) are contaminated with potential pathogens.[2,161-163] Furthermore, many of the surfaces of the anesthesia gas machine and monitors have been shown to be contaminated with blood.[164] It is therefore mandatory to ensure that departmental cleaning and sterilization programs are adequate, that "good housekeeping" during administration of anesthesia is practiced, and that universal precautions are observed. It is disappointing that recent evidence indicates that needle-stick injuries are still common, but full implementation of universal precautions is not.[165]

With regard to equipment, the American Association of Nurse Anesthetists advocates a classification system and specific equipment recommendations, which are published in their *Infection Control Guide*.[166] In addition, manufacturers include directions for cleaning and sterilizing equipment in their operation and maintenance manuals.

Trace and Waste Gases

Alterations of work practices can have a great impact on ambient levels of waste anesthetic gases. These have been discussed previously (see Box 15-21).

CLINICAL IMPLICATIONS

Description of the proper use of the anesthesia gas machine is explicit throughout the preceding sections of this chapter. This section presents selected clinical implications. The reader is encouraged to apply these ideas to clinical practice, bearing in mind that no prescription can be applied to each and every clinical situation or to every piece of equipment in current use. These suggestions are intended as a starting point for discussion with peers and department committees.

Decreased Inspired Oxygen

The algorithm for responding to an O_2 analyzer alarm that signals a hypoxic breathing mixture is as follows:

- Do *not* attempt to fix the monitor; it *must* be trusted until it can be proved wrong.
- Call for help.

- Open the cylinder *and* disconnect it from the pipeline at the wall outlet.
- If the fraction of inspired O_2 does not increase (with FGF adequate to wash in the O_2 quickly), ventilate the patient by Ambu bag with room air.
- If indicated, start cardiopulmonary resuscitation early, using a portable O_2 cylinder.

Pethick Test for the Bain Circuit

A unique hazard of the use of the Bain circuit is occult disconnection or kinking of the inner, fresh gas delivery hose. To perform the Pethick test, use the following steps:

- Occlude the patient's end of the circuit (at the elbow).
- Close the APL valve.
- Fill the circuit, using the O_2 flush valve.
- Release the occlusion at the elbow and flush. A Venturi effect flattens the reservoir bag if the inner tube is patent.

Sustained High Breathing Circuit Pressure

The algorithm for responding to sustained high pressure in the breathing circuit is as follows:

- Try manually ventilating the patient with the breathing circuit (in "Bag" mode).
- If the high pressure is relieved, it is likely that the ventilator relief valve is at fault; the ventilator is unusable until this valve is serviced.
- If circuit pressure is sustained during manual ventilation with the circuit, it is likely that the scavenger is obstructed or that its relief valves have failed.
- In either case, attempt to disconnect the scavenger gas collection tubing from the back of the APL, if possible.
- If the tubing cannot be disconnected, disconnect the patient from the breathing circuit and continue ventilation by Ambu bag.

Infection Control

Patients and caregivers can be protected when the anesthesia gas machine is used with an infected or immunocompromised patient. Cleaning the bellows is necessary after anesthesia has been provided to a patient with a disease transmitted by air or oral secretions. With a patient with acquired immunodeficiency syndrome (AIDS) or active respiratory disease, one or more of the following guidelines should be followed:

- Avoid using mechanical ventilators.
- Use bacterial and viral filters on each limb.
- Use a disposable soda lime assembly.
- Change soda lime after each case.

New Agents and Low Flows

Low FGFs should not be instituted too early when desflurane or sevoflurane is used. Induction at low flows would be extremely prolonged, creating the risk of awareness between propofol redistribution and the delayed onset of action of the volatile agent. Overpressure can be combined with low flows, but 18% of 2 L contains fewer desflurane molecules than 18% of 6 L, and it is the number of molecules presented to the brain per unit time that causes an increase in anesthetic tension within the brain.

Imagine a 1000-ml sink filled with water, with 100 ml/min inflow (of which 1 ml is methylene blue) and 100 ml/min outflow. The goal is to turn the initially colorless water in the sink as blue as the inflow solution. Now, imagine the effect of increasing the inflow to 500 ml/min (of which 5 ml is methylene blue) and increasing the outflow to 500 ml/min. Would the 1000 ml in the sink turn blue any faster in the second case? Of course it would, but not because the concentrations are different (both inflows are 1% methylene blue); rather, it would occur because the rate of inflow in the second example is a greater proportion of the capacity.

Wash-in is based on the concept of a time constant. One time constant (equal to capacity divided by flow) brings a system 63% of the way to equilibrium; two time constants, 86%; and three time constants, 95%. Therefore the first sink reaches 63% of equilibrium in 10 minutes (1000 ml ÷ 100-ml flow), whereas the second sink reaches this same degree of equilibrium in only 2 minutes (1000 ml ÷ 500-ml flow).

In the same way, the volume (capacity) of the functional residual capacity, hoses, and breathing circuit can be brought to equilibrium with the inflow more quickly as the rate of inflow increases. A rational approach for ensuring anesthesia that conserves volatile agents would include a nonrebreathing (semiopen) induction (FGF, 5 to 8 L/min), followed by a "low flow" maintenance (FGF, 1 to 2 L/min). This approach helps conserve tracheal heat and humidity, gases, and agent. Emergence, like induction, must occur at higher, nonrebreathing flows; otherwise, it will be unacceptably prolonged.

SUMMARY

Compared with its forebears, the anesthesia gas machine available today is a system of tremendous capability, power, safety, and complexity. The machine is a result both of improvements in design and of the integration of physiologic monitors and machine function monitors. Use of an anesthesia gas machine was more straightforward in the past, because all types of anesthesia machines contained simpler, similar elements. With the introduction of new designs, this is no longer the case. The days when a few "wizards" in an anesthesia department could specialize in equipment operation and maintenance and could instruct or troubleshoot for all of their co-workers have likewise passed. Equipment competency must be a part of everyone's toolkit of patient care skills. It is hoped that through study of this chapter, current equipment will be more widely understood and our future patients may "sleep" in safety, afforded the level of care that we all wish for ourselves and our loved ones.

REFERENCES

1. Morris LE. Vaporizer malfunction. In: Aldrete JA, Howe HJ, Virtue RW, eds. *Low Flow and Closed System Anesthesia*. New York: Grune & Stratton; 1979:251-256.
2. Dorsch JA, Dorsch SE. *Understanding Anesthesia Equipment*. 4th ed. Baltimore: Lippincott Williams & Wilkins; 1999.
3. Eisenkraft JB, Sommer RM. Hazards of the anesthesia delivery system. In: Ehrenwerth J, Eisenkraft JB, eds. *Anesthesia Equipment: Principles and Applications*. St Louis: Mosby; 1993:321-349.
4. Loeb RG, Jones BR, Leonard RA, Behrman K. Recognition accuracy of current operating room alarms. *Anesth Analg* 75: 499-505;1992.
5. Siker ES. A safety tutorial? *Anesth Patient Safety Found Newsletter*. 4:14;1989.
6. Pierce EC. Teaching safety while in touch with the patient. *Anesth Patient Safety Found Newsletter*. 1989;4:15.
7. Gravenstein JS. Is competency with our equipment a safety problem? *Anesth Patient Safety Found Newsletter*. 1992;7:20-21.

8. Peters JD. Products liability [and] anesthesia mishaps. In: *Anesthesiology and the Law*. Ann Arbor, Mich: Health Administration Press; 1983.
9. U.S. Food and Drug Administration. *Anesthesia Apparatus Checkout Recommendations, 1993*. Updated May 12, 1997. Available at: http://www.fda.gov/cdrh/humfac/anesckot.html. Accessed April 10, 2003.
10. FDA publishes final version of revised apparatus checkout. *Anesth Patient Safety Found Newsletter*. 1994;9:35.
11. Standard VIII. *Standards for Nurse Anesthesia Practice*. Park Ridge, Ill: American Association of Nurse Anesthetists; June 2002. Also available at: http://www.aana.com/crna/prof/scope.asp. Accessed April 10, 2003.
12. Petty C. *The Anesthesia Machine*. New York: Churchill Livingstone; 1987.
13. Kole TE: Environmental and occupational hazards of the anesthesia workplace. *AANA J*. 1990;58:327-331.
14. Bowie E, Huffman LM. *The Anesthesia Machine: Essentials for Understanding*. Madison, Wis: Datex-Ohmeda; 1985.
15. American Society for Testing and Materials. *Standard Specification for Particular Requirements for Anesthesia Workstations and Their Components* [F1850-00]. Philadelphia: ASTM; 2000.
16. Andrzejowski J, Freeman R. Oxygen failure alarms on modern anaesthetic machines. *Anaesthesia*. 2002;57:931-932.
17. Holland R. Another "wrong gas" incident in Hong Kong. *Anesth Patient Safety Found Newsletter*. 1991;6:9.
18. Sato T. Fatal pipeline accidents spur Japanese standards. *Anesth Patient Safety Found Newsletter*. 1991;6:14.
19. Morrell RC. Gas delivery mistakes continue to kill. *Anesth Patient Safety Found Newsletter*. 2002;17:4. Available at: http://www.gasnet.org//societies/apsf/newsletter/2002/spring/11gasdelivery.htm. Accessed July 7, 2003.
20. Bernstein DB, Rosenberg AD. Intraoperative hypoxia from nitrogen tanks with oxygen fittings. *Anesth Analg*. 1997;84:225-227.
21. Neubarth J. Another hazardous gas supply misconnection. *Anesth Analg*. 1995;80:206.
22. North American Dräger. *Narkomed 2A Anesthesia System—Specifications and Equipment*. Telford, Pa: North American Dräger; 1987.
23. Nagle TA. New standards focus on piped medical gas systems. *Anesth Patient Safety Found Newsletter*. 1993-1994;8:42-43.
24. Moss E. Medical gas contamination: an unrecognized patient danger. *Anesth Patient Safety Found Newsletter*. 1994;9:20-22.
25. Moss E. Danger seen possible from contaminated medical gases. *Anesth Patient Safety Found Newsletter*. 1993;8:6-7.
26. Good ML. Comments sought on new FDA preanesthesia checklist. *Anesth Patient Safety Found Newsletter*. 1992-1993;7:47-51.
27. North American Dräger. *Narkomed 2C Anesthesia System—Setup and Installation Manual*. Telford, Pa: North American Dräger; 1994.
28. National Fire Protection Association. *NFPA 99: Health Care Facilities*. Quincy, Mass: NFPA; 1990:184.
29. Eichhorn JH, Ehrenwerth J. Medical gases: storage and supply. In: Ehrenwerth J, Eisenkraft JB, eds. *Anesthesia Equipment: Principles and Applications*. St Louis: Mosby; 1993:1-26.
30. Andrews JJ, Johnston RV. Not all E cylinders were created equal. *Anesth Analg*. 1992;75:154.
31. Datex-Ohmeda. *Modulus II Anesthesia System: Operation and Maintenance Manual*. Madison, Wis: Datex-Ohmeda; 1985.
32. Datex-Ohmeda. *Modulus CD Anesthesia System: Operation and Maintenance Manual*. Madison, Wis: Datex-Ohmeda; 1991.
33. North American Dräger. *Narkomed 2C Anesthesia System—Operator's Instruction Manual*. Telford, Pa: North American Dräger; 1994.
34. Compressed Gas Association. *Handbook of Compressed Gases*. 3rd ed. New York: Van Nostrand Reinhold; 1990.
35. Yudenfreund-Sujka SM. Nitrous oxide abuse presenting as premature exhaustion of Sodasorb. *Anesthesiology*. 1990;73:580.
36. Chawla AV, Newton NI. Machine and monitoring failure from electrical overloading. *Anaesthesia*. 2002;57:1134-1135.
37. Troianos CA. Complete electrical failure during cardiopulmonary bypass. *Anesthesiology*. 1995;82:298-302.
38. *Julian anesthesia workstation operating instruction (software 3.n)*. Catalog No. 90 37 181. Telford, Pennsylvania: Dräger Medical Inc; 2000.
39. *S/5 anesthesia delivery unit user's reference manual*. Catalog No. 8502304. Madison, Wisconsin: Datex-Ohmeda; 2000.
40. Dräger Medical. *Fabius GS Operator's Instruction Manual*. Telford, Pa: Dräger Medical; 2002. Catalog No. 4117102-001.
41. Dräger Medical. *Narkomed 6000 Anesthesia Machine Operator's Instruction Manual*. Telford, Pa: Dräger Medical; 2000. Catalog No. 4114915-006.
42. Eger EI II, et al. Anesthetic flowmeter sequence: a cause for hypoxia. *Anesthesiology*. 1963;24:396.
43. Schreiber P. *Safety Guidelines for Anesthesia Systems*. Telford, Pa: North American Dräger; 1985.
44. Berry PD, Sessler DI, Larson MD. Severe carbon monoxide poisoning during desflurane anesthesia. *Anesthesiology*. 1999;90:613-616.
45. Fang ZX, Eger EI. Source of toxic CO explained: CF2 anesthetic dry absorbent. *Anesth Patient Safety Found Newsletter*. 1994;9:25, 28-30.
46. Haas RE. A simple technique to instantly convert from insufflation to positive-pressure ventilation. *AANA J*. 1992;60:526.
47. Petty C. Understanding your machine: O_2 flush valve key to safety. *Anesth Patient Safety Found Newsletter*. 1993;8:31.
48. Datex-Ohmeda. *Datex-Ohmeda Excel Anesthesia System: Operation and Maintenance Manual*. Madison, Wis: Datex-Ohmeda; 1992.
49. ECRI. Hazard: barotrauma from anesthesia ventilators. *Technol Anesth*. 1988;9:1-2.
50. Gaughan SD, Benumof JL, Ozaki GT. Can an anesthesia machine flush valve provide for effective jet ventilation? *Anesth Analg*. 1993;76:800-808.
51. North American Dräger. *Narkomed 3 Anesthesia System—Technical Service Manual*. Telford, Pa: North American Dräger; 1988.
52. Datex-Ohmeda. *7800 Ventilator: Operation and Maintenance Manual: Software Revision 4.XX*. Madison, Wis: Datex-Ohmeda; 1993.
53. Datex-Ohmeda. *7000 Electronic Anesthesia Ventilator: Operation Maintenance*. Madison, Wis: Datex-Ohmeda; 1985.
54. Datex-Ohmeda. *Ohmeda 7900 Ventilator Operation and Maintenance Manual*. Madison, Wis: Datex-Ohmeda; 1997. Catalog No. 1503-0211-000.
55. Datex-Ohmeda. *Operators Manual. Tec 4 Continuous Flow Vaporizers*. Madison, Wis: Datex-Ohmeda; 1986.
56. Datex-Ohmeda. *Tec 5 Continuous Flow Vaporizer: Operation and Maintenance Manual*. Madison, Wis: Datex-Ohmeda; 1990.
57. Datex-Ohmeda. *Tec 6 Vaporizer: Operation and Maintenance Manual*. Madison, Wis: Datex-Ohmeda; 1993.
58. Airco-Ohio Medical Products. *Compact Anesthesia Machine: Series 4000 Stand and Cart Models*. Madison, Wis: Airco-Ohio Medical Products; 1974. [Sales brochure.]
59. Airco-Ohio Medical Products. *Ohio Anesthesia Machine Accessories*. Madison, Wis: Airco-Ohio Medical Products; 1974. [Catalog.]
60. Anaquest. *The Datex-Ohmeda Tec 6 Vaporizer for the Administration of Suprane (Desflurane)*. Liberty Corner, NJ: Anaquest; 1992. [Brochure with prescribing information.]
61. Drägerwerk. *Dräger Vapor 19.n Anaesthetic Vaporizer: Instructions for Use*. Lübeck, Germany: Drägerwerk; 1991.
62. Schneider AJL. Older anesthesia machines targeted for component replacement. *Anesth Patient Safety Found Newsletter*. 1989;4:25-27.
63. Walter Reed Army Medical Center. *Ohmeda 885A Field Anesthesia Machine Use Tutor*. Available at: http://www.wramc.amedd.army.mil/fieldmed/885atutor/index.htm. Accessed July 12, 2003.
64. Miller D. The Tec 6 vaporizer: why desflurane needs to be heated. *AANA J*. 1994;62:527-531.
65. Andrews JJ, Johnston RV. The new Tec 6 desflurane vaporizer. *Anesth Analg*. 1993;76:1338-1341.

66. Eger EI. *Desflurane (Suprane): a Compendium and Reference*. Rutherford, NJ: Healthpress; 1993.
67. Johnston RV, et al. The effects of carrier gas composition on the performance of the Tec 6 desflurane vaporizer. *Anesth Analg*. 1994;79:548-552.
68. Andrews JJ, et al. Consequences of misfilling isoflurane vaporizers with desflurane. *Anesth Analg*. 1994;78:S7.
69. Petty C. Equipment safety: vaporizer exclusion or interlock systems. *Anesth Patient Safety Found Newsletter*. 1992;7:10.
70. Daniels D. Overfilling of vaporizers. *Anaesthesia*. 2002;57:288.
71. Macleod DM, McEvoy L. Report of vaporizer malfunction. *Anaesthesia*. 2002;57:299-300.
72. Rupani G. Refilling a Tec 6 desflurane vaporizer. *Anesth Analg*. 2003;96:1534-1535.
73. Aziz E, Sanders GM. Failure of Datex AS/3 anaesthesia delivery unit. *Anaesthesia*. 2000;55:1214-1215.
74. Macartney NJD, Cohen J. Another case of anaesthetic machine failure. *Anaesthesia*. 2000;55:1215.
75. *The Sodasorb Manual of Carbon Dioxide Absorption*. Lexington, Mass: WR Grace; Dewey and Almy Chemical Division; 1992.
76. Moyers J. A nomenclature for methods of inhalation anesthesia. *Anesthesiology*. 1953;14:609-611.
77. Forrester K. Cost savings associated with low flow anesthesia. *AANA J*. 1989;57:329-334.
78. Mapleson WW. The elimination of rebreathing in various semiclosed anaesthetic systems. *Br J Anaesth*. 1954;26:323-332.
79. Fritz MR. Safety danger in cost cutting discussed at ASA. *Anesth Patient Safety Found Newsletter*. 1995;9:46.
80. Jellish WS, Nolan T, Kleinman B. Hypercapnia related to a faulty adult co-axial breathing circuit. *Anesth Analg*. 2001;93:973-974.
81. Randhawa N, Semenov RA, Patel A. Coaxial breathing system outer tube occlusion: what goes in must come out. *Anaesthesia*. 2002;57:716-717.
82. Kitagawa H, et al. A new leak test for specifying malfunctions in the inhalation and exhalation check valve. *Anesth Analg*. 1994;78:611.
83. Aung SM, et al. An unusual cause of carbon dioxide rebreathing in a circle absorber system. *Anesth Analg*. 1994;78:1027-1028.
84. Dawood AMS, Digger T. An apparently normal looking valve as a cause of rebreathing. *Anaesthesia*. 2002;57:929-930.
85. Gravenstein JS, Paulus DA, Hayes TJ. *Capnography in Clinical Practice*. Boston: Butterworth; 1989.
86. North American Dräger. *Absorber System: Operator's Instruction Manual*. Telford, Pa: North American Dräger; 1988.
87. Croinin DFO, Keogh J. Connector mix-up on an anaesthetic machine. *Anaesthesia*. 2002;57:1137-1138.
88. Khorasani A, Saatee S, Khader RD, Nasr NF. Inadvertent misconnection of the scavenger hose: a cause for increased pressure in the breathing circuit. *Anesthesiology*. 2000;92:1501-1502.
89. Versichelen LFM, Bouche MPLA, Rolly G, et al. Only carbon dioxide absorbents free of both NaOH and KOH do not generate compound A during in vitro closed-system sevoflurane: evaluation of five absorbents. *Anesthesiology*. 2001;95:750-755.
90. Mchaourab A, Arain SR, Ebert TJ. Lack of degradation of sevoflurane by a new carbon dioxide absorbent in humans. *Anesthesiology*. 2001;94:1007-1009.
91. Kharasch ED, Powers KM, Artru AA. Comparison of Amsorb, sodalime, and Baralyme degradation of volatile anesthetics and formation of carbon monoxide and compound A in swine in vivo. *Anesthesiology*. 2002;96:173-182.
92. Yamakage M, Kimura A, Chen X, et al. Production of compound A under low-flow anesthesia is affected by type of anesthesia machine. *Can J Anaesth*. 2001;48:435-438.
93. Bouche MPLA, Versichelen LFM, Struys MMRF, et al. No compound A formation with Superia during minimal-flow sevoflurane anesthesia: a comparison with Sofnolime. *Anesth Analg*. 2002;95:1680-1685.
94. Wissing H, Kuhn I, Warnken U, et al. Carbon monoxide production from desflurane, enflurane, halothane, isoflurane, and sevoflurane with dry soda lime. *Anesthesiology*. 2001;95:1205-1212.
95. Lemmens HJM. Amsorb causes no less carbon monoxide formation than either "new" or "classic" sodalime. *Anesthesiology*. 2002;97:1038.
96. Knolle E, Heinze G, Gilly H. Small carbon monoxide formation in absorbents does not correlate with small carbon dioxide absorption. *Anesth Analg*. 2002;95:650-655.
97. Holak EJ, Mei DA, Dunning MB, et al. Carbon monoxide production from sevoflurane breakdown: modeling of exposures under clinical conditions. *Anesth Analg*. 2003;96:757-764.
98. Epstein RA. In my opinion: carbon monoxide: what should we do? *Anesth Patient Safety Found Newsletter*. 1995;9:39, 40-41.
99. Murray JM, Renfrew CW, Bedi A, et al. Amsorb A new carbon dioxide absorbent for use in anesthetic breathing systems. *Anesthesiology*. 1999;91:1342-1348.
100. Eger EI. CO researcher notes, compares CO production from different absorbents [letter to the editor]. *Anesth Patient Safety Found Newsletter*. 1995;9:41.
101. Pond D, Jaffe RA, Brock-Utne JG. Failure to detect CO_2-absorbent exhaustion: seeing and believing. *Anesthesiology*. 2000;92:1196-1198.
102. Strum DP, Eger EI. The degradation, absorption, and solubility of volatile anesthetics in soda lime depend on water content. *Anesth Analg*. 1994;78:340-348.
103. Brimacombe J, Keller C, Hörmann C. Pressure support ventilation versus continuous positive airway pressure with the laryngeal mask airway: a randomized crossover study of anesthetized adult patients. *Anesthesiology*. 2000;92:1621-1623.
104. Feldman JM, Smith J. Compliance compensation of the Narkomed 6000 explained. *Anesthesiology*. 2001;94:543-544.
105. Rothschiller JL, et al. Evaluation of a new operating room ventilator with volume-controlled ventilation: the Ohmeda 7900. *Anesth Analg*. 1999;88:39-42.
106. Shogase A, Mizutani K, Toyoda Y. Protecting Ohmeda 7900 ventilator flow sensor. *Anesth Analg*. 1999;88:234.
107. Krock JL, Padda GS, Moore JD. Ohmeda 7900 ventilator flow sensor failure. *Anesth Analg*. 1998;86:231-232.
108. Cantillo J, Domsky R, Gratz I, Goldberg ME. Ventilatory failures with the Datex-Ohmeda 7900 SmartVent. *Anesthesiology*. 2002;96:766-768.
109. Cooper JB. Unidirectional PEEP valves can cause safety hazards. *Anesth Patient Safety Found Newsletter*. 1990;5:28.
110. Datex-Ohmeda. *GMS PEEP Valve: Operation and Maintenance Manual*. Madison, Wis: Datex-Ohmeda; 1991.
111. Berry AJ, Nolte FS. An alternative strategy for infection control of anesthesia breathing circuits: a laboratory assessment of the Pall HME filter. *Anesth Analg*. 1991;72:651-655.
112. Gunn N. *Pall Technical Report: Nosocomial Infection from Anesthetic and Ventilation Equipment*. Portsmouth, England: Pall Biomedical Products; 1991.
113. Fargnoli JM, et al. Efficiency and importance of airway filters in reducing micro-organisms. *Anesth Analg*. 1992;74:S93.
114. ECRI. An overview of heated humidifiers. *Technol Anesth*. 1994;15:1-4.
115. Gilmour IJ, et al. The effect of heated wire circuits on humidification of inspired gases. *Anesth Analg*. 1994;79:160-164.
116. Epstein RA. The elusive disconnect alarm examined. *Anesth Patient Safety Found Newsletter*. 1988;3:39.
117. Bostek CC. Is it OK to read during OR cases [letter]? *Anesth Patient Safety Found Newsletter*. 1995;9:45.
118. Feldman JM, Blike G, Cheung KH. New electronic checklists aim at decreasing anesthetist errors. *Anesth Patient Safety Found Newsletter*. 1992;7:1-2.
119. Yassin K, Gibbons JJ. A hidden leak in the circle system. *Anesth Analg*. 1991;73:236.
120. Lee O, Sommer RM. Pressure monitoring hose causes leak in anesthesia breathing circuit. *Anesth Analg*. 1991;73:365.
121. Milliken RA, Bizzarri DV. An unusual cause of failure of anesthetic gas delivery to a patient circuit. *Anesth Analg*. 1984;63:1047-1048.

122. Johnstone R, Graf D. Bellows failure with Dräger anesthesia ventilator. *Anesth Analg.* 1993;76:685-686.
123. Chaney MA. Delivery of excessive airway pressure to a patient by the anesthesia machine. *Anesth Analg.* 1993;76: 1166-1167.
124. Sosis MB. Dräger ventilator failure on changing the respiratory rate setting. *Anesth Analg.* 1993;76:453-454.
125. Ananthanarayan C, Fisher JA. Dräger ventilator failure. *Anesth Analg.* 1993;77:638.
126. Bourke DL, Tolentino D. Inadvertent positive end-expiratory pressure caused by a malfunctioning ventilator relief valve. *Anesth Analg.* 2003;97:492-493.
127. Lees DE. Old anesthesia equipment target of study panel: ASA policy recommended. *Anesth Patient Safety Found Newsletter.* 1989;4:13-15.
128. Petty C. Scavenger is often a neglected safety device. *Anesth Patient Safety Found Newsletter.* 1992;7:28.
129. Huffman LM. Common problems in waste gas management. *AANA J.* 1991;59:109-112.
130. American Association of Nurse Anesthetists. *Management of Waste Anesthetic Gases.* Park Ridge, Ill: AANA; 1992.
131. *Waste Anesthetic Gases: Fact Sheet No. OSHA 91-38.* Washington, DC: Occupational Safety and Health Administration; 1991. US Department of Labor Publication No. 282-115/44392.
132. Datex-Ohmeda. *Waste Gas Scavenging Interface Valve Assembly: Operation and Maintenance Manual.* Madison, Wis: Datex-Ohmeda; 1991.
133. North American Dräger. *Scavenger Interface for Suction Systems: Operator's Instruction Manual.* Telford, Pa: North American Dräger; 1987.
134. Connell GR, Mangar D. Is your scavenger system functional? *Anesth Analg.* 1992;75:1075.
135. Kole TE. Reduce, reuse, and recycle in the anesthesia workplace. *AANA J.* 1992;60:109-112.
136. Troyer GT. Controlling the legal liabilities of anesthetic gases. *Health Care Strategic Manag.* 1985;3:11-15.
137. Ward BG. Monitoring toxic substances: protecting your employees and your institution. *Health Care Strategic Manag.* 1995;3: 16-17.
138. Karp D, Graham K. *Risk Management Guide for Certified Registered Nurse Anesthetists.* Park Ridge, Ill: American Association of Nurse Anesthetists; 1987.
139. Cooper JB. New law requires hospitals to report device-related injuries and deaths. *Anesth Patient Safety Found Newsletter.* 1991;6:13-17.
140. Huffman LM. Safe Medical Device Act: new law alters practice patterns. *Anesth Today.* 1992;3:7-11.
141. Spooner RB, Kirby RR. Equipment-related anesthetic incidents. *Int Anesthesiol Clin.* 1984;22:133-147.
142. Kumar V, Hintze MS, Jacob AM. A random survey of anesthesia machines and ancillary monitors in 45 hospitals. *Anesth Analg.* 1988;67:644-649.
143. Holley HS, Carroll JS. Anaesthesia equipment malfunction. *Anaesthesia.* 1985;40:62-65.
144. Craig J, Wilson MW. A survey of anaesthetic misadventures. *Anaesthesia.* 1981;36:933-936.
145. Cooper JB, Newbower RS, Kitz RJ. An analysis of major errors and equipment failures in anesthetic management: considerations for prevention and detection. *Anesthesiology.* 1984;60:34-42.
146. Henry DW. Examination of the efficacy of education concerning a standardized anesthesia machine checkout procedure upon the machine fault detection ability of anesthetists. *AANA J.* 1989;57:500-504.
147. Buffington CW, Ramanathan S, Turndorf H. Detection of anesthesia machine faults. *Anesth Analg.* 1984;63:79-82.
148. Biddle C. Report of controlled prospective study of students vs. practicing CRNAs on performance of routine gas machine maintenance and fault-detection ability [letter]. *AANA J.* 1985; 53:286-287.
149. March MG, Crowley JJ. An evaluation of anesthesiologists' present checkout methods and the validity of the FDA checklist. *Anesthesiology.* 1991;75:724-729.
150. Olympio MA, Goldstein MM, Mathes DD. Instructional review improves performance of anesthesia apparatus checkout procedures. *Anesth Analg.* 1996;83:618-622.
151. Manley R, Cuddeford JD. An assessment of the effectiveness of the revised FDA checklist. *AANA J.* 1996;64:277-282.
152. Lees DE. FDA preanesthesia checklist being evaluated, revised. *Anesth Patient Safety Found Newsletter.* 1991;6:25-27.
153. Chopra V, Bovill JG, Spierdijk J. Checklists: aviation shows the way to safer anesthesia. *Anesth Patient Safety Found Newsletter.* 1991;6:26-29.
154. Withiam-Wilson MJ. FDA pre-use equipment checklist spurred by accidents, studies. *Anesth Patient Safety Found Newsletter.* 1991;6:27.
155. Charlton JE. Checklists cited as contributing to safety. *Anesth Patient Safety Found Newsletter.* 1990;5:30-31.
156. Williams JR. What is the current status of the FDA checklist? *Nurse Anesth.* 1991;2:3-5.
157. Good ML. Comments sought on new FDA preanesthesia checklist. *Anesth Patient Safety Found Newsletter.* 1992-1993;7:47-51.
158. ECRI. Injuries—one fatal—highlight the need for pre-use testing of disposable breathing circuits. *Health Devices.* 2000;29:188-189.
159. Thorpe CM. Plastic in the anaesthesia circuit. *Anaesthesia.* 2002;57:85-86.
160. Myers JA, Good ML, Andrews JJ. Comparison of tests for detecting leaks in the low pressure system of anesthesia gas machines. *Anesth Analg.* 1997;84:179-184.
161. Tessler MJ, Grillas B, Gioseffini S. Bacterial counts on the hands of anesthetists and anesthesia technicians. *Anesth Analg.* 1994;78:1030-1031.
162. Crow S, Slaughter AL. Debunking the myths of anesthesia equipment processing. *Anesth Today.* 1991;2:7-10.
163. Huffman L. Cross-contamination during anesthesia: a serious threat to immunocompromised patients. *Anesth Today.* 1990; 1:14-16.
164. Hall JR. Blood contamination of anesthesia equipment and monitoring equipment. *Anesth Analg.* 1994;78:1136-1139.
165. Tait AR, Tuttle DB. Prevention of occupational transmission of human immunodeficiency virus and hepatitis B virus among anesthesiologists: a survey of anesthesiology practice. *Anesth Analg.* 1995;79:623-628.
166. American Association of Nurse Anesthetists. *Infection Control Guide.* Park Ridge, Ill: AANA; 1993.

APPENDIX 15-1: ANESTHESIA APPARATUS CHECKOUT RECOMMENDATIONS, 1993 (UPDATED MAY 12, 1997[9])

This checkout, or a reasonable equivalent, should be conducted before administration of anesthesia. These recommendations are valid only for an anesthesia system that conforms to current and relevant standards and includes an ascending bellows ventilator and at least the following monitors: capnograph, pulse oximeter, oxygen analyzer, respiratory volume monitor (spirometer), and breathing system pressure monitor with high- and low-pressure alarms. Users are encouraged to modify this guideline to accommodate differences in equipment design and variations in local clinical practice. Such local modifications should undergo appropriate peer review. Users should refer to the operator's manual for the manufacturer's specific procedures and precautions, especially the manufacturer's low-pressure leak test (step 5).

Emergency Ventilation Equipment

*1. **Verify backup ventilation equipment is available and functioning.**

High-Pressure System

*2. **Check oxygen cylinder supply.**
   a. Open O_2 cylinder and verify at least half full (approximately 1000 psi).
   b. Close cylinder.

*3. **Check central pipeline supplies.**
   a. Check that hoses are connected and pipeline gauges read approximately 50 psi.

Low-Pressure Systems

*4. **Check initial status of low-pressure system.**
   a. Close flow control valves and turn vaporizers off.
   b. Check fill level and tighten vaporizers' filler caps.

*5. **Perform leak check of machine low-pressure system.**
   a. Verify that the machine master switch and flow control valves are "off."
   b. Attach "Suction Bulb" to common fresh gas outlet.
   c. Squeeze bulb repeatedly until fully collapsed.
   d. Verify bulb stays fully collapsed for at least 10 seconds.
   e. Open one vaporizer at a time and repeat 'c' and 'd' above.
   f. Remove suction bulb, and reconnect fresh gas hose.

*6. **Turn on machine master switch and all other necessary electrical equipment.**

*7. **Test flowmeters.**
   a. Adjust flow of all gases through their full range, checking for smooth operation of floats and undamaged flowtubes.
   b. Attempt to create a hypoxic O_2-N_2O mixture and verify correct changes in flow and alarm.

Scavenging System

*8. **Adjust and check scavenging system.**
   a. Ensure proper connections between the scavenging system and both APL (pop-off) valve and ventilator relief valve.
   b. Adjust waste gas vacuum (if possible).
   c. Fully open APL valve and occlude Y-piece.
   d. With minimum O_2 flow, allow scavenger reservoir bag to collapse completely and verify that absorber pressure gauge reads approximately zero.
   e. With the O_2 flush activated allow the scavenger reservoir bag to distend fully, and then verify that absorber pressure gauge reads <10 cm H_2O.

Breathing System

*9. **Calibrate O_2 monitor.**
   a. Ensure monitor reads 21% in room air.
   b. Verify low O_2 alarm is enabled and functioning.
   c. Reinstall sensor in circuit and flush breathing system with O_2.
   d. Verify that monitor now reads greater than 90%.

10. **Check initial status of breathing system.**
   a. Set selector switch to "Bag" mode.
   b. Check that breathing circuit is complete, undamaged, and unobstructed.
   c. Verify that CO_2 absorbent is adequate.
   d. Install breathing circuit accessory equipment (e.g., humidifier, PEEP valve) to be used during the case.

11. **Perform leak check of the breathing system.**
   a. Set all gas flows to zero (or minimum).
   b. Close APL (pop-off) valve and occlude Y-piece.
   c. Pressurize breathing system to about 30 cm H_2O with O_2 flush.
   d. Ensure that pressure remains fixed for at least 10 seconds.
   e. Open APL (pop-off) valve and ensure that pressure decreases.

Manual and Automatic Ventilation Systems

12. **Test ventilation systems and unidirectional valves.**
   a. Place a second breathing bag on Y-piece.
   b. Set appropriate ventilator parameters for next patient.
   c. Switch to automatic ventilation ("Ventilator") mode.
   d. Fill bellows and breathing bag with O_2 flush and then turn ventilator "on."
   e. Set O_2 flow to minimum, other gas flows to zero.
   f. Verify that during inspiration bellows delivers appropriate tidal volume and that during expiration bellows fills completely.
   g. Set fresh gas flow to about 5 L/min.
   h. Verify that the ventilator bellows and simulated lungs fill and empty appropriately without sustained pressure at end expiration.
   i. Check for proper action of unidirectional valves.
   j. Exercise breathing circuit accessories to ensure proper function.
   k. Turn ventilator "off" and switch to manual ventilation ("Bag/APL") mode.
   l. Ventilate manually and assure inflation and deflation of artificial lungs and appropriate feel of system resistance and compliance.
   m. Remove second breathing bag from Y-piece.

Monitors

13. **Check, calibrate and set alarm limits of all monitors.**

Capnometer, pulse oximeter, oxygen analyzer, respiratory volume monitor (spirometer), pressure monitor with high and low airway alarms.

Final Position

14. **Check final status of machine.**
   a. Vaporizers off
   b. AFL valve open
   c. Selector switch to "Bag"
   d. All flowmeters to zero
   e. Patient suction level adequate
   f. Breathing system ready to use

---

*If an anesthesia provider uses the same machine in successive cases, these steps need not be repeated or may be abbreviated after the initial checkout.

CHAPTER 16

Clinical Monitoring in Anesthesia

Mark A. Kossick, E. Laura Wright

Monitoring of anatomic and physiologic variables during an anesthetic procedure enables anesthetists to enhance patient safety and meet established standards of care. Many different state-of-the-art monitors are commonly used to assist in the delivery of an anesthetic, and it is the responsibility of the anesthetist to assimilate the data provided by monitors and make appropriate clinical judgments. Consequently, sound physical assessment and critical thinking skills, appropriate selection and application of monitors, and vigilance are key requirements in the process of anesthesia monitoring.

Basic monitoring techniques include inspection, auscultation, and palpation. They provide essential subjective and objective data not available from technologic monitors and can alert the anesthetist to impending dangers in select patients. Inspection of the patient can provide information regarding adequacy of tissue oxygenation, fluid resuscitation, and patient positioning. Auscultation is used to verify correct placement of the endotracheal tube, assess arterial blood pressure, and continually monitor heart sounds and breath sounds. Palpation can aid the anesthetist in assessing the quality of the pulse and degree of skeletal muscle relaxation and in locating major vascular structures during the placement of central venous lines.

Critical thinking skills are cardinal prerequisites for successful monitoring of a patient's anesthetic. In addition, it is well known that errors in anesthesia care are minimized when anesthetists remain alert and vigilant. Not surprising, it is easy for anesthesia providers to experience occasional periods of inattentiveness because of the large number of anesthetic procedures that proceed without incident. This is partially the result of improvements that have been made in monitoring modalities and the development of drugs with more favorable pharmacokinetic and pharmacodynamic profiles. In addition, the large physiologic reserve most healthy patients possess helps to attenuate any errors made in monitoring secondary to an acute and transient physiologic insult. This chapter reviews the more commonly used noninvasive and invasive monitors in anesthesia practice.

PULMONARY ARTERY CATHETERIZATION

One of the most significant advances made in critical care medicine was the introduction of the pulmonary artery catheter (PAC) by Swan and Ganz in 1970.[1] Their development of the flow-directed right-sided heart catheter allowed for direct bedside assessment of pulmonary artery (PA) pressures, indirect assessment of left ventricular (LV) filling pressures and right-sided cardiac outputs, and calculation of pulmonary and SVRs, along with various cardiopulmonary indices. This section of the chapter reviews the interpretation of hemodynamic data obtained from a PAC, variables that can skew the data, and an extension of its use beyond the recording of vascular pressures and mixed venous oxygen saturation ($S\overline{V}O_2$) to calculation of oxygen delivery ($\dot{D}O_2$) and oxygen consumption ($\dot{V}O_2$).

An important question related to the use of the PAC is, "To what extent have morbidity and mortality been reduced when the PAC has been used to guide medical care?" It is evident that the literature in recent years has recommended that clinicians exercise greater discernment with regard to the decision to insert the PAC, because the benefits of its use remain controversial.[2-6] Factors that may contribute to the discrepancies in research findings include differences in patient populations and limitations in research methodology, such as retrospective analysis, lack of randomization, and double-blind techniques.[7,8] Another explanation for conflicting study results deals with competency levels in managing PAC data. This explanation was supported by a multicenter study conducted by Iberti and co-workers in 1990.[9] These investigators developed a questionnaire that covered four main topic areas (insertion techniques, cardiac physiology, interpretation of waveforms along with pressure-volume relationships, and application of PAC data in patient treatment) related to PAC use. Examinees from the departments of medicine, surgery, and anesthesiology scored an average of 67% (range 19% to 100%). It is surprising to note that the attending physicians from all departments scored a mean value of 69%. Statistically, examinees had the most difficulty in interpreting hemodynamic variables (e.g., 47% of 496 respondents were unable to correctly determine the PA occlusive pressure [PAOP] from a clear tracing) and applying PAC data for proper patient treatment. Anesthesia providers who specialize in cardiovascular anesthesia have also been shown to have difficulty in interpreting one of the cardinal waveforms derived from PAC; 39% of cardiovascular anesthesiologists could not correctly interpret a PAOP waveform.[10] Results from Iberti and Jacka studies suggest that the understanding of PAC data among patient care providers is extremely variable, and misinterpretation of PAC data may result in increased morbidity and mortality. Similarly, the 1988 prospective blinded study by Shoemaker and co-workers[11] supports the contention that PAC use per se does not improve patient outcome, but the way in which the physiologic information is interpreted and applied in patient care does. Such research findings have caused several groups to develop guidelines for the indications of a PAC, along with competency requirements for interpretation of data.[12,13]

Physiology and Morphology of Hemodynamic Waveforms

Essential to accurate interpretation of hemodynamic data derived from central venous lines is a solid foundation in what constitutes "normal" distances, pressures, and waveform morphology for central venous pressure (CVP), right ventricular (RV), PA, and PAOP recordings. Table 16-1 illustrates the approximate distances for reaching the junction of the venae cava and the right atrium (RA) from various distal anatomic sites. Table 16-2 lists the anticipated distances for reaching various cardiac and pulmonary structures from the right internal jugular vein. Advancement of a catheter 10 cm beyond these distances without the production of a characteristic waveform could indicate coiling of the central line. If this problem arises with a PAC, the balloon should be deflated and the catheter withdrawn. If any resistance is met during withdrawal, a chest radiograph should be taken to rule out knotting or entanglement with the chordae tendineae.

Right Atrial Pressure Waveform

In addition to familiarity with proper distances, knowledge of normal intracardiac pressures, pulmonary pressures (Table 16-3), and waveform morphology facilitates accurate interpretation of PAC data and placement of central lines. For example, under normal circumstances a CVP tracing generates mean RA pressures in the range of 1 to 10 mm Hg. The fidelity of the transducing system determines if discernible *a*, *c*, and *v* waves will be displayed once the distal tip of a central line lies just above the junction of the venae cavae and the RA (Figure 16-1). The *a* wave is produced by contraction of the RA, the *c* wave by closure of the tricuspid valve, and the *v* wave by passive filling of the RA (which encompasses a portion of RV systole). The reason the *a* wave is commonly larger than the *c* wave is based on the position of the catheter relative to the physiologic event responsible for the pressure change. In essence, RA systole and the subsequent increase in atrial pressure are directly sensed by a catheter positioned just above (or inappropriately within) the RA, whereas RV systole (a more distal physiologic event relative to the position of a CVP catheter) indirectly increases RA pressure by closure of the tricuspid valve.

Right Ventricular Pressure Waveform

Further advancement of a PAC (approximately 10 cm) produces dramatic changes in the morphology of the hemodynamic waveform. As shown in Figure 16-2, a brisk upstroke (isovolumetric contraction and rapid ejection or RV systole) and steep downslope (reduced ejection and isovolumetric relaxation or RV systole and diastole) are viewed on an oscilloscope when a PAC is advanced through the right intraventricular cavity. A PAC with the distal balloon inflated should remain in the RV for as short a time as possible to reduce the incidence of ventricular ectopy, or the development of a conduction defect such as bundle branch block. Because it is undesirable to leave the tip of a central line in the RV, pressures from this region of the heart should be indirectly assessed via the CVP (estimate of RV end-diastolic pressure [EDP] and preload) and PA systolic pressure (estimate of RV systolic pressure).

TABLE 16-1 Distance to the Junction of the Venae Cavae and Right Atrium from Various Distal Anatomic Sites

Location	Distance (cm)
Subclavian	10
Right internal jugular vein	15
Left internal jugular vein	20
Femoral vein	40
Right median basilic vein	40
Left median basilic	50

TABLE 16-2 Distance from the Right Internal Jugular Vein to Distal Cardiac and Pulmonary Structures

Location or Structure	Distance (cm)
Junction venae cava and right atrium	15
Right atrium	15-25
Right ventricle	25-35
Pulmonary artery	35-45
Pulmonary artery wedge position	40-50

TABLE 16-3 Normal Intracardiac and Pulmonary Pressures

Location	Absolute Value (mm Hg)	Range (mm Hg)
MRAP	5	1-10
RV	25/5*	15-30/0-8
PA S/D	25/10*	15-30/5-15
MPAP	15	10-20
PAOP	10	5-15
MLAP	8	4-12
LVEDP	8	4-12

**Values are systolic pressure/diastolic pressure.*
LVEDP, Left ventricular end-diastolic pressure; MLAP, mean left atrial pressure; MPAP, mean pulmonary artery pressure; MRAP, mean right atrial pressure; PA, pulmonary artery; PAOP, pulmonary artery occlusive pressure; RV, right ventricle; S/D, systolic/diastolic.

Pulmonary Artery Pressure Waveform

When a catheter enters the PA, the diastolic pressure is acutely increased with little change in systolic pressure. The upstroke of the PA tracing is produced by opening of the pulmonic

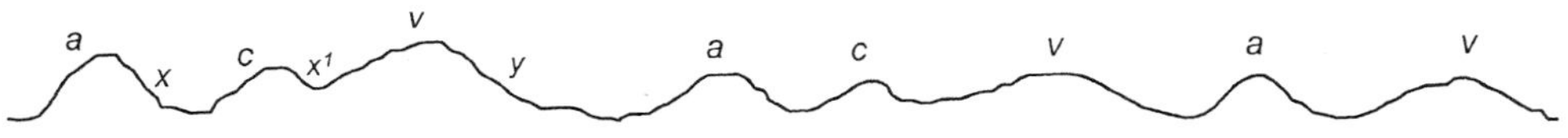

FIGURE 16-1
Positive and negative waveforms of a CVP tracing. The third cardiac cycle in this figure does not produce a c wave.

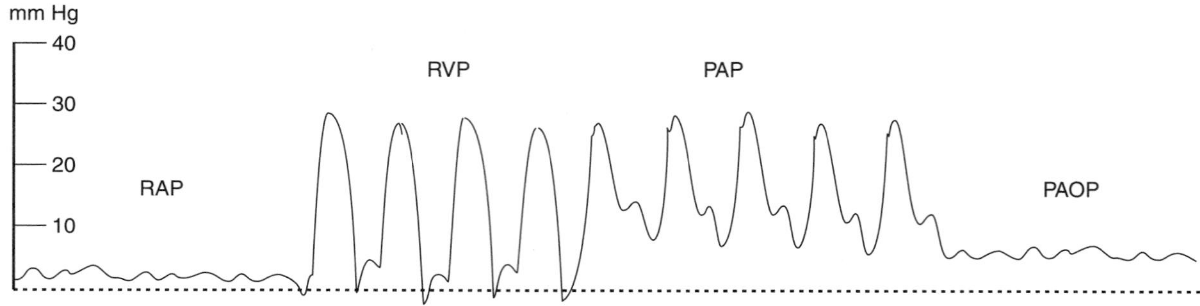

FIGURE **16-2**
Pressure waveforms during positioning of a PAC. *PAOP*, pulmonary artery occlusive pressure; *PAP*, pulmonary artery pressure; *RAP*, right atrial pressure; *RVP*, right ventricular pressure.

valve, followed by RV ejection. The downstroke contains the dicrotic notch, which is produced by sudden closure of the pulmonic valve leaflets (the beginning of diastole).

Pulmonary Artery Occlusive Pressure Waveform

Final advancement of a PAC by 5 to 10 cm should produce a PAOP tracing. This waveform is similar to a CVP (the *a* wave is produced by left atrial [LA] systole, the *c* wave by closure of the mitral valve, and the *v* wave by filling of the LA as well as upward displacement of the mitral valve during LV systole), except that the pressure values are higher. In addition, it is less common to detect a *c* wave on a PAOP tracing because retrograde transmission of LA pressure (produced by closure of the mitral valve) is significantly attenuated within the pulmonary circulation. The characteristic waveform morphologies of a PAOP tracing are illustrated in Figure 16-2.

Negative Waveforms

The descents that follow the *a*, *c*, and *v* waves of a CVP or PAOP tracing are labeled as *x*, x^1, and *y* (see Figure 16-1). The *x* descent corresponds to the start of atrial diastole (its terminal component [just before the upstroke of the *v* wave] with RVEDP and LVEDP), the x^1 descent is produced by downward pulling of the septum during ventricular systole, and the *y* descent corresponds to opening of the tricuspid valve.

Correlation of Pressure Waveforms and the Electrocardiogram

The interpretation of hemodynamic waveforms can be facilitated by correlating the pressure recordings with the electrocardiogram (ECG). The *a* waves of a CVP tracing, which is produced by atrial contraction, follow electrical activations of the atria (P waves on the ECG). The *c* and *v* waves occur after the beginning of ventricular depolarization (QRS complex), or the *v* wave may not appear until shortly after the T wave (Figures 16-3 and 16-4). Compared with the CVP tracing, the ECG shows a more pronounced temporal relationship with the PAOP recording, meaning there is a greater distance between ECG activity and the subsequent pressure waveform (e.g., the *a* wave of a PAOP tracing correlates with the QRS complex). Proper identification of abnormal waveforms is greatly facilitated by the use of the ECG; for example, without an ECG recording, large positive waveforms on a PAOP tracing can be diagnosed as either cannon *a* waves or large *v* waves.

Distortion of Pressure Waveforms

Dysrhythmias can produce significant alterations in hemodynamic waveforms. Atrial fibrillation, junctional rhythms, and premature ventricular contractions (PVCs) alter the shape of *a* waves. With atrial fibrillation no synchronized atrial contraction occurs. This results in some small fibrillatory *a* waves or, more commonly, the complete loss of *a* waves. Complete atrioventricular block and some forms of junctional dysrhythmias cause the atria to contract against a closed tricuspid valve, which produces large cannon *a* waves (Figure 16-5). Ventricular pacing can be associated with both the presence of cannon *a* waves and the loss of *a* waves. The former occurs if a patient does not have an atrioventricular sequential pacemaker; the latter occurs when ventricular pacing is used in the setting of atrial asystole. Valvular defects can also produce dramatic changes in the CVP and PAOP tracings, causing an increase in the amplitude of the *v* wave secondary to regurgitation (e.g., with mitral regurgitation a portion of the stroke volume is ejected retrograde into the pulmonary circuit because of an incompetent mitral valve). Recognition of such abnormalities is critical for accurate recording of pressure measurements and proper placement of central lines. Significant tricuspid regurgitation can cause a CVP recording to mimic an RV tracing, and mitral regurgitation can cause a PAOP recording to appear as a PA tracing. Specifically, large *v* waves become superimposed on *a* waves. For the indistinguishable PA and PAOP recording, an $S\overline{V}O_2$ sample can assist in making a differential diagnosis. The saturation will be

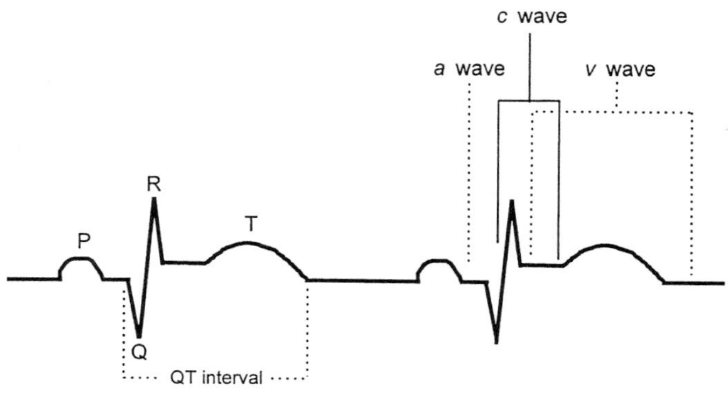

FIGURE **16-3**
Relationship between the electrocardiogram and hemodynamic waveforms.

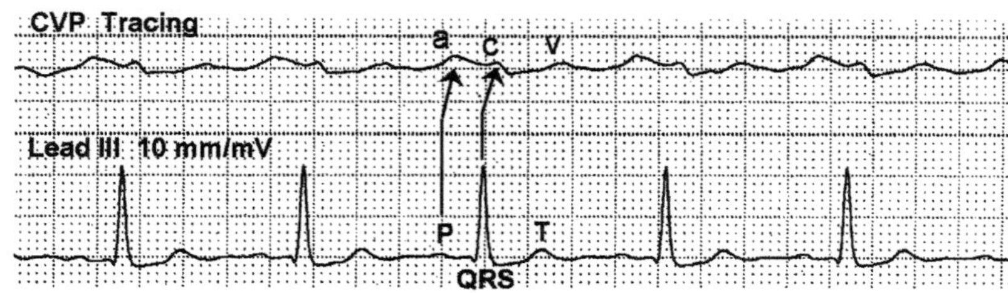

FIGURE **16-4**
Electrocardiographic recording with a concurrent central venous pressure tracing that shows the temporal relationship between atrial depolarization (P wave) and the production of an *a* wave, and the QRS complex and the *c* and *v* wave that follow.

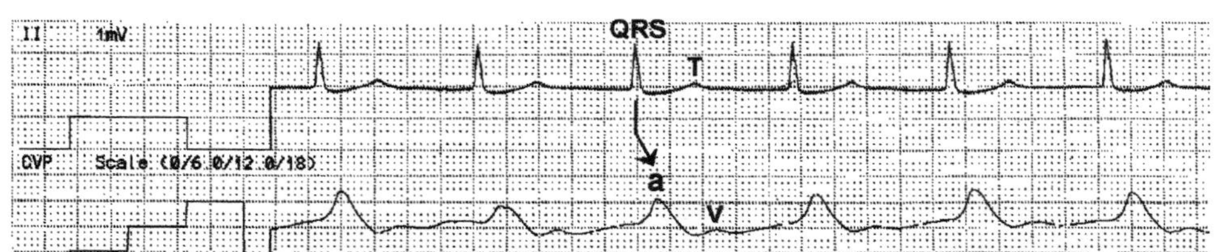

FIGURE **16-5**
Electrocardiographic recording of a junctional rhythm, specifically in which there is simultaneous retrograde atrial and antegrade ventricular depolarization (as evidenced by the lack of a P wave in each cardiac cycle). This results in the contracting of the right atrium against a closed tricuspid valve. As a consequence, the central venous pressure (CPV) tracing has cannon *a* waves.

elevated (greater than 77%) if the catheter is in a wedged position, assuming the distal tip is not in a region of the lung that is atelectatic or has pneumonia; both of these factors would produce a false-negative result (normal or low $S\bar{V}O_2$). As a precautionary measure, a catheter suspected of being in a wedged position should not be flushed with the fluid contained in the pressurized transducing system. Although the overall incidence of PA rupture is low (0.064%),[14] flushing of a wedged catheter (as well as balloon overinflation) can result in vascular damage ranging from minor endobronchial hemorrhage to massive hemoptysis.

Significant tricuspid regurgitation and mitral regurgitation may also be associated with normal CVP and PAOP tracings.

BOX **16-1**

Factors That Can Distort Central Venous Pressure and Pulmonary Artery Occlusive Pressure Tracings

Loss of a Waves or Only v Waves
- Atrial fibrillation
- Ventricular pacing (atrial asystole)

Giant a Waves—"Cannon" a Waves
- Junctional rhythms
- Complete AV block
- PVCs (simultaneous atrial and ventricular contraction)
- Ventricular pacing (asynchronous)
- Tricuspid or mitral stenosis
- Diastolic dysfunction
- Myocardial ischemia
- Ventricular hypertrophy

Large v Waves
- Tricuspid or mitral regurgitation
- Acute ↑ in intravascular volume

↑, *Increase; AV, atrioventricular; PVCs, premature ventricular contractions.*

These occur in patients with a low volume status and compliant atria. In addition, a poor correlation has been found between the size of the *v* wave and the degree of regurgitation. On the opposite end of this spectrum is the clinical situation in which a patient develops large *v* waves without significant regurgitation. This phenomenon can occur whenever an acute increase in preload occurs, which dynamically reduces atrial and pulmonary vascular compliance.[15]

Whenever large *v* waves are detected on a CVP or PAOP tracing, estimates of preload should be measured just before the upstroke of the *v* wave. This point on the pressure recording equates with the EDP, the moment just before ventricular systole that produces the large *v* waves; however, other sources claim that the apex of the *a* wave[16] or the point immediately after it[17] is the best representation of preload. Box 16-1 indicates how various rhythm disturbances, pacing, and valvular defects can distort the CVP tracing.

Implications of Abnormal Hemodynamic Values

The CVP serves as an estimate of RV preload (RVEDP). Box 16-2 lists the causes of an elevated CVP; a low CVP correlates with hypovolemia of any cause. As stated previously, RV pressures can be assessed indirectly from the CVP and PA pressure (PAP) recordings. RV values can be elevated secondary to pulmonary hypertension, ventricular septal defect, pulmonary stenosis, RV failure, constrictive pericarditis, or cardiac tamponade.

Like the RV waveform, the PA tracing occurs within the QT interval of the ECG. LVEDP can be estimated by measuring the pressure value that exists just before the upstroke of the PA waveform. See Box 16-2 for a list of causes of an increase in the PAP. A false high value can also be produced by a phenomenon called *catheter whip*, which is exaggerated oscillation of the PA tracing. This can occur with excessive catheter coiling if the tip of the PA catheter is near the pulmonic valve, or in patients with dilated pulmonary arteries. The latter may occur if pulmonary hypertension exists.

One of the most valuable hemodynamic parameters is the PAOP recording. Like the CVP, it indirectly assesses ventricular function and therefore has distinct limitations. To ensure that accurate pressure recordings are documented, the mean or diastolic pressure should always be determined at end-expiration (whether the patient is spontaneously breathing or receiving positive pressure ventilation). At this time pleural pressures usually become approximately equal to atmospheric pressures (except when positive end-expiratory pressure [PEEP] is being used). The rationale for this timing relates to the fact that vascular pressure recordings are calibrated relative to atmospheric pressure. As stated previously, the correct area on the pressure recording to determine preload (e.g., LVEDP) is just before the upstroke of the *v* wave (or *c* wave if present). Causes of an elevated PAOP are listed in Table 16-4.

Variables That Influence Hemodynamic Measurements

Essential for proper management of hemodynamic parameters is the recognition of how numerous variables can skew recorded pressure values. The foundation for understanding PAC data begins with the recognition that absolute numbers are generally not as important as trends. In addition, most of the data obtained from a PAC allow only an *indirect* assessment of cardiovascular function and pulmonary indices. For example, PA diastolic pressure (PADP) approximates PAOP, which approximates LA pressure, which approximates LVEDP, which estimates LV end-diastolic volume. Table 16-5 lists clinical factors that can skew these pressure and volume relationships. Obviously, reliance on indirect pressure measurements mandates that the anesthetist understand how to interpret these data, given such limitations. It should be assumed that for most patients who require a PAC or CVP, several, if not numerous, conditions (e.g., cardiovascular disease, pulmonary dysfunction) will skew the pressure-to-pressure and pressure-to-volume relationships.

Of the variables listed in Table 16-5, several require further discussion. Many of the factors listed can be viewed as disruptions or obstructions of the continuous column of blood that exists between the RA and LV. This is the case with valvular defects and pulmonary factors.

The goal for placement of a PAC is to have it reside in a West zone III[18] of the lung; this usually does occur, because the bulk of pulmonary blood flow lies within this region of the lung. In this position the PAP is greater than the pulmonary venous pressure, which is greater than the alveolar pressure. This zone corresponds to a complete circuit or conduit that allows for direct communication between the right-sided heart and pulmonary pressures and the left-sided intraventricular pressures. It is important to recall that each of the lung zones is physiologically, not anatomically, defined; therefore a zone III can change into a zone II (PAP > alveolar pressure > pulmonary venous pressure) or zone I (alveolar pressure > PAP > pulmonary venous pressure).

Factors that contribute to the dynamic state of zone III include the application of PEEP, significant diuresis, hemorrhage, and a change in patient position (e.g., supine to sitting). The influence of PEEP is contingent on the quantity applied, intravascular volume status, and pulmonary compliance. Normally, less than 50% of PEEP is transmitted to the microvasculature—even less if pulmonary compliance is poor (e.g., in patients with acute respiratory distress syndrome).[16] In contrast, patients with decreased volume status (e.g., LA pressure less than 5 mm Hg) who receive PEEP as low as 7.5 cm H_2O can have collapse of the pulmonary capillaries, which distorts the PAOP.[17] A PAC located in zone I or II produces marked variations in the PAOP waveform recording during the ventilatory cycle. In addition, *a* and *v* waves (cardiac influences) are lost, and the PAOP exceeds the PADP. This occurs in contrast to a PAOP recording produced by a catheter located in a true wedge position. The distinguishing criteria include the development of a characteristic waveform with balloon inflation and a PAOP reading less than or equal to the PADP. The latter criterion

TABLE 16-4 Potential Causes of Elevated Central Venous Pressure, Pulmonary Artery Pressure, and Pulmonary Artery Occlusive Pressure

CVP	PAP	PAOP
• RV failure • Tricuspid stenosis or regurgitation • Cardiac tamponade • Constrictive pericarditis • Volume overload • Pulmonary HTN • LV failure (chronic)	• LV failure • Mitral stenosis or regurgitation • L-to-R shunt • ASD or VSD • Volume overload • Pulmonary HTN • "Cathether whip"	• LV failure • Mitral stenosis or regurgitation • Cardiac tamponade • Constrictive pericarditis • Volume overload • Ischemia

ASD, atrial septal defect; CVP, central venous pressure; HTN, hypertension; L, left; LV, left ventricular; PAOP, pulmonary artery occlusive pressure; PAP, pulmonary artery pressure; R, right; RV, right ventricular; VSD, ventricular septal defect.

TABLE 16-5 Factors That Alter the Relationships among Central Cardiovascular Pressures and Volumes

CVP ≠ PADP	• Change in RV compliance (e.g., PS) • Tricuspid valve disease
PADP ≠ PAOP	• Pulmonary HTN • MR or AR • Lung zone I or II • Tachycardia • ARDS • RBBB
PAOP ≠ MLAP	• Juxtacardiac pressure (e.g., PEEP) • Lung zone I or II • Mediastinal fibrosis • RBBB
MLAP ≠ LVEDP	• Juxtacardiac pressure (e.g., PEEP) • Mitral valve disease • Change in LV compliance (e.g., AS)
LVEDP ≠ LVEDV	• Juxtacardiac pressure (PEEP) • Ventricular interdependence • Change in LV compliance (e.g., ischemia)

AR, Aortic regurgitation; ARDS, acute respiratory distress syndrome; AS, aortic stenosis; CVP, central venous pressure; HTN, hypertension; LVEDP, left ventricular end-diastolic pressure; LVEDV, left ventricular end-diastolic volume; MLAP, mean left atrial pressure; MR, mitral regurgitation; PADP, pulmonary artery diastolic pressure; PAOP, pulmonary artery occlusive pressure; PEEP, positive end-expiratory pressure; PS, pulmonic stenosis; PVR, pulmonary artery vascular resistance; RBBB, right bundle branch block; RV, right ventricle.

assumes that no valvular defect, which could also cause the mean PAOP to exceed the PADP, is present.

A rapid heart rate (HR) can also skew the relationship between PADP and the PAOP. Research has demonstrated that LA paced-induced tachycardia (increased HR from 74 to 124 beats per minute) can produce an 11– mm Hg gradient between the PADP and LVEDP. The increase in PADP and decrease in LVEDP result from the shortening of diastole, which reduces the amount of blood being transported from the pulmonary circulation to the LV.[19] Also, as HR increases, the LA begins to contract against a partially closed mitral valve.[20]

Another variable that significantly influences PAC data is a change in ventricular compliance. To illustrate this point, consider the fact that a high PAOP (or LVEDP) can exist in patients with an elevated preload with normal ventricular compliance and in patients with a low preload with poor ventricular compliance. A patient with reduced ventricular compliance (e.g., myocardial ischemia, LV hypertrophy, cardiac tamponade, ventricular interdependence) has a high PAOP or PADP that results in overestimation of LV end-diastolic volume (Figure 16-6) and underestimation of LVEDP. In the setting of poor compliance, PAOP is not a reliable index for LV end-diastolic volume.[21] In fact, it has been shown that during myocardial revascularization procedures, high PAOP values exist more than 50% of the time in conjunction with a low volume status (as determined by echocardiography), with patients responding favorably (despite a high PAOP) to an increase in intravascular volume.[22] As previously stated, one must be careful not to be misled by the wedge.[21]

To summarize, the PADP correlates poorly (by 5 mm Hg or more) with the PAOP under the following circumstances: when pulmonary vascular resistance (PVR) is elevated (e.g., in cases of chronic obstructive pulmonary disease, human papillomavirus infection, pulmonary embolus, acute respiratory distress syndrome, hypercarbia), when HR exceeds 130 beats per minute, when severe mitral or aortic regurgitation is present, or when a lung zone III has changed to a zone II or I (e.g., in cases of hypovolemia, PEEP). Increases in PVR and HR cause the PADP to exceed PAOP. Severe regurgitation and lung zone changes produce the opposite effect, with PADP being less than the PAOP; this may also hold true for right bundle branch block based on one researcher's findings of how this conduction defect caused the PADP (in the setting of normal PVR) to be up to 7 mm Hg less than the mean LA pressure.[23] A review of the gross interpretation of CVP and PAOP values is presented in Table 16-6.

Other Hemodynamic Indexes

Some authors encourage the use of calculated indexes to optimize the care of critical care patients. These indexes include the pulmonary vascular resistance index (PVRI), systemic vascular resistance (SVR) index (SVRI), and cardiac index (CI). The potential advantages and limitations of each index are reviewed here.

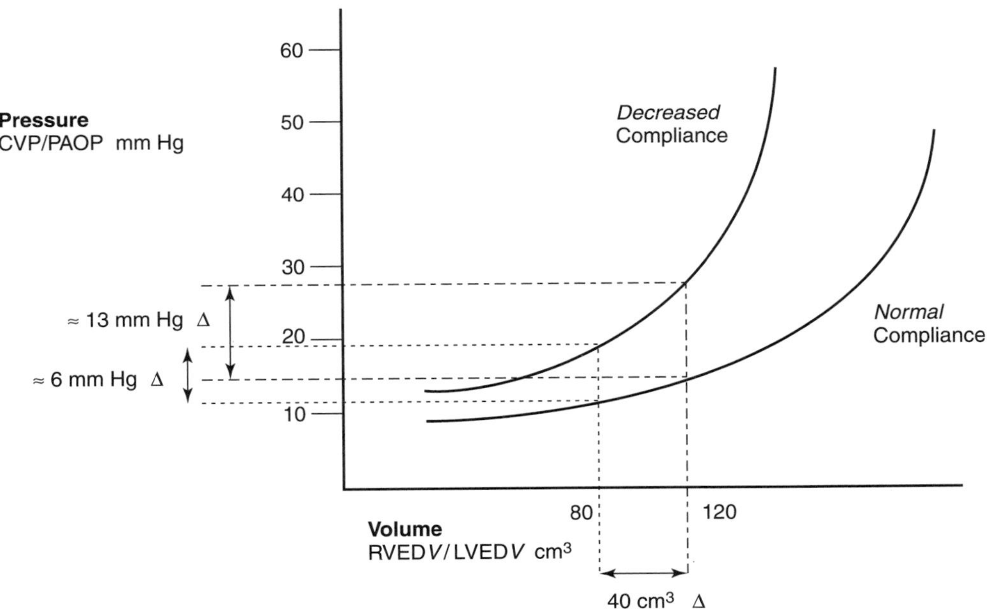

FIGURE **16-6**
Effect of changes in ventricular compliance on central venous pressure (which provides an estimate of right ventricular end-diastolic pressure) and pulmonary artery occlusive pressure (which provides an estimate of left ventricular end-diastolic pressure). The curve with decreased compliance distorts the relationship between pressure values and estimated ventricular volume. In this diagram, a preload of 80 cm^3 in a compliant versus noncompliant ventricle generates a pressure difference of approximately 6 mm Hg; note that this is the flat portion of each curve. On the steeper portion of both curves, the relationship between volume and pressure is skewed even more dramatically. A preload of 120 cm^3 generates a pressure difference of approximately 13 mm Hg, which can ultimately lead to a gross overestimation of ventricular preload. **Δ**, change; *RVEDP*, right ventricular end-diastolic pressure; *RVEDV*, right ventricular end-diastolic volume; *CVP*, central venous pressure; *LVEDP*, left ventricular end-diastolic pressure; *LVEDV*, left ventricular end-diastolic volume; *PAOP*, pulmonary artery occlusive pressure.

TABLE 16-6 Potential Clinical Diagnosis via the Use of Hemodynamic Values: Interpretation of Pulmonary Artery Catheter Data

CVP	PADP	PAOP	Interpretation
Low	Low	Low	Hypovolemia, transducer not at phlebostatic axis*
Normal or high	High	High	LV failure
High	Normal or low	Normal or low	RV failure, TR, or TS
High	High	Normal or low	Pulmonary embolism
High	High	Normal	Pulmonary HTN
High	High	High	Cardiac tamponade, ventricular interdependence, transducer not at phlebostatic axis*
Normal	Normal or high	High	LV myocardial ischemia or MR
Low	High	Normal	ARDS†

ARDS, Acute respiratory distress syndrome; CVP, central venous pressure; HTN, hypertension; LV, left ventricular; MR, mitral regurgitation; PAC, pulmonary artery catheter; PADP, pulmonary artery diastolic pressure; PAOP, pulmonary artery occlusive pressure; RV, right ventricular; TR, tricuspid regurgitation; TS, tricuspid stenosis.
**Phlebostatic axis is the fourth intercostal space midanteroposterior level (not midaxillary line); for the right lateral decubitus position, fourth intercostal space midsternum; for the left lateral decubitus position, fourth intercostal space at the left parasternal border.*
†ARDS patients commonly require initial fluid administration for hemodynamic stability.

The PVRI (PVR calculated with the CI instead of the cardiac output [CO]) is equal to the difference in pressure across the pulmonary circuit (mean PAP–PAOP) divided by flow (CI) times 80. This formula is taken from Ohm's law (with the variables mathematically manipulated) for electrical currents (R [Resistance] = V [Voltage] ÷ I [Current]). A normal value is considered to be 45 to 225 dynes • sec/cm^5 • m^2. Two limitations of extrapolating physiologic resistance from Ohm's law are that blood flow is pulsatile (not flowing continuously through a set of rigid pipes) and resistance is not uniform throughout the pulmonary circuit; the electrical counterpart describes resistance not in alternating currents, in but direct currents.[24]

When PVR is used clinically it is viewed as an *estimate* of RV afterload. Afterload is defined as systolic wall stress or the impedance the ventricle must overcome to eject its stroke volume. Vascular resistance is not synonymous with afterload but is used as an extension of the concept. Pulmonary vascular resistance, like SVR, can affect afterload, but neither formula accounts for changes in ventricular wall thickness or radius, which are components of afterload.

SVR is commonly used to provide guidance in the use of vasoconstrictors (e.g., phenylephrine infusion) or afterload reduction (e.g., intravenous nitroglycerine or sodium nitroprusside). The limitations described previously for PVR also hold true for SVR, although perhaps to a lesser extent because the systemic vasculature has lower compliance. Nevertheless, manipulation of SVRI to achieve normal or high values in shock syndromes (e.g., septic shock with low blood pressure, low blood flow, and low SVRI) has been shown not to correlate with survival, and the development of a low SVRI in shock syndromes does not correlate well with death.[25] In general, the use of vasoconstrictors to support afterload should be deferred until maximization of preload or the use of positive inotropes has proved ineffective. Indiscriminate use of α-adrenergic agonists can worsen microcirculatory blood flow by exaggerating existing nonuniform vasoconstriction; this can lead to a further deterioration in cellular oxygen debt.[26] The SVRI is calculated as the difference between systemic input pressure (mean arterial pressure [MAP]) minus the output pressure (RA pressure or CVP), divided by the CI times 80. The normal range is 1760 to 2600 dynes • sec/cm^5 • m^2.

Determination of CO assists critical care specialists in providing rational hemodynamic therapy; evaluating the response to therapy; and determining the adequacy of tissue perfusion, which is linked to maintenance of arterial blood pressure, the delivery of oxygen, and removal of wastes. It also permits the calculation of other hemodynamic indices (e.g., PVR and SVR). A normal CO value should be qualified by taking into account age differences, metabolic activity (declines with anesthesia and increases with hyperthermia), and patient size. This last factor may be adjusted for by converting a CO to a CI, which attempts to normalize CO for the large number of values found in the general population. However, CI adjusts only for the variables of height and weight; it does not address the lack of uniformity of predicted basal oxygen consumption and metabolic rates that results from differences in sex and age. In addition, the relationship between body surface area (BSA) and blood flow is indistinct.[27] CI is calculated by dividing CO by BSA. The plotting of height and weight on a body surface chart estimates the BSA in square meters (Figure 16-7). Commonly quoted "normal" values are 5 to 6 L/min for CO and 2.8 to 3.6 L/min • m^2 for CI.

The most commonly used technique for determining CO is thermodilution, whereby an analog computer calculates the CO by using the modified Stewart-Hamilton equation. This method was first used by Fegler in 1954.[28] It entails the injection of a known quantity of an indicator solution (most commonly 5% dextrose in water, although 0.9% normal saline has a similar density factor)[29] through the proximal port of a thermodilution PAC.[30] The injected solution is considered a thermal indicator because it is cold relative to body temperature. It rapidly mixes with the incoming blood and is carried through the RV until it is detected by the thermistor near the end of the catheter in the PA. The computer plots a time-temperature curve, with the area under the curve being inversely proportional to the CO; therefore larger curves are not desired. Variables that can influence recorded values include the computation constant (which varies with catheter

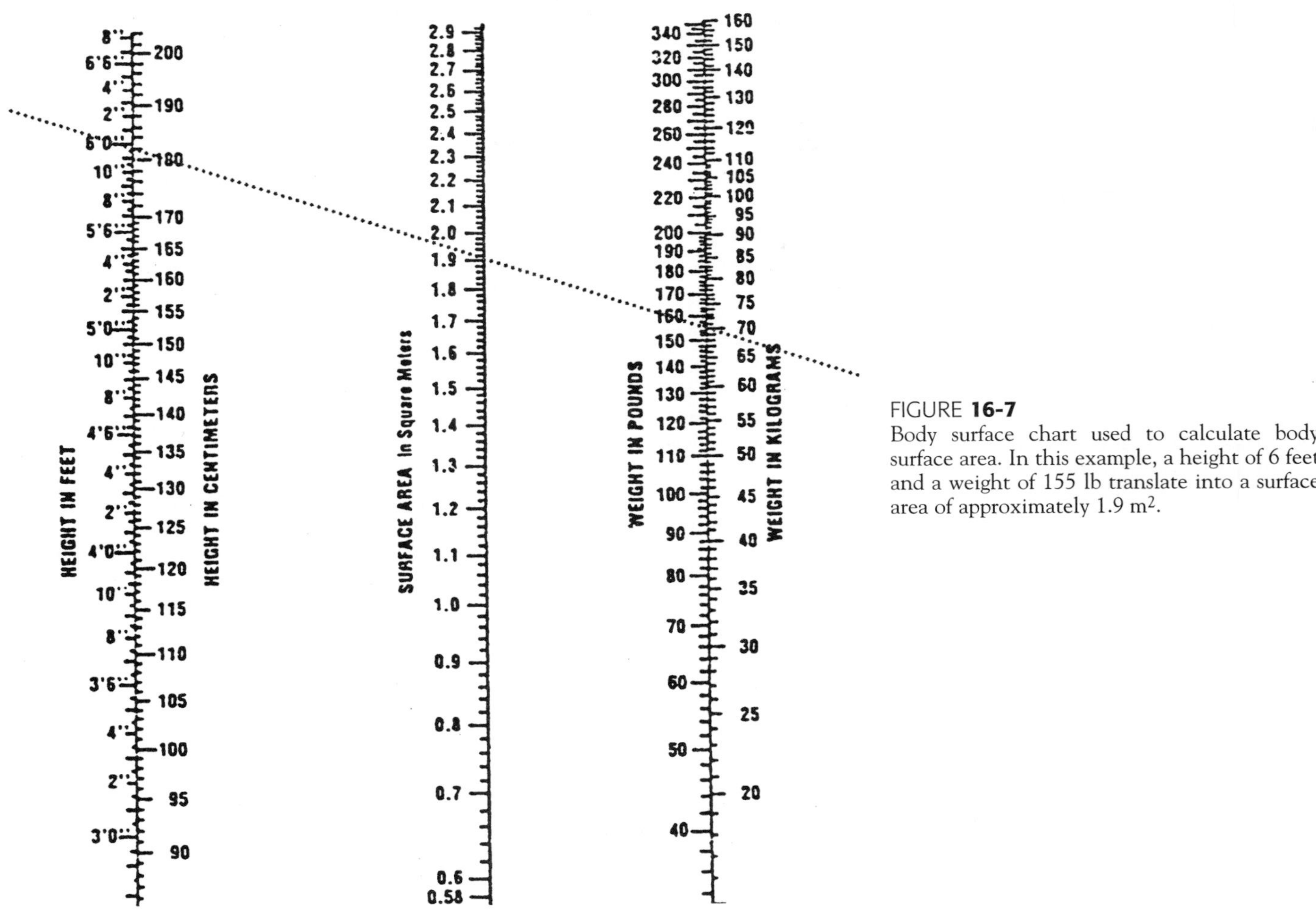

FIGURE **16-7**
Body surface chart used to calculate body surface area. In this example, a height of 6 feet and a weight of 155 lb translate into a surface area of approximately 1.9 m^2.

size, injectate volume, and temperature), temperature of the injectate (desired range of 0° C to 24° C), volume of injection,[29,31] speed of injection (should be completed in 4 seconds or less),[29,32] and the timing of injection (it should be consistent, i.e., at the same time during each respiratory cycle).[29,33,34] Iced injectants have not been shown to offer any significant advantage over room-temperature injectates.[29,31] In fact, cold indicator solutions injected rapidly into the RA have been shown to produce dysrhythmias, such as sinus bradycardia.[35,36] Research that has examined the impact of valvular or septal defects on thermodilution CO (TDCO) values has produced conflicting results.[37-39] A list of variables that can skew CO measurements is provided in Table 16-7.

The accuracy for TDCO (including TDCO in patients in the lateral position) is ±10%, and the reliability is ±5%.[40] These values are lower in the pediatric population,[41] in patients who have low CO,[42] and for measurements taken in the operating room.[43] Anesthetists should be careful not to overinterpret small changes (e.g., 5% to 10%) and should never express values beyond one decimal point. The common practice of averaging three CO values has also been shown to improve accuracy.[40]

A further advancement in the technology of the PAC has been achieved through the placement of a thermal filament in the RV portion of the PAC. A sophisticated computer algorithm permits for analysis of a thermal signal created by small quantities of heat being emitted from the PAC—a pulsed warm thermodilution technique. This heat signal is eventually transmitted by the blood to the distal thermistor, which permits for continuous cardiac output (CCO) assessment.[44] An adequate signal-to-noise

TABLE **16-7** Variables That Influence Thermodilution CO Values

Overestimates	Underestimates	Unpredictable
• Low injectate volume • Injectate that is too warm • Thrombus on the thermistor of the PAC • Partially wedged PAC	• Excessive injectate volume • Injectate solutions that are too cold	• Right-to-left ventricular septal defect • Left-to-right ventricular septal defect • Tricuspid regurgitation

CO, Cardiac output; PAC, pulmonary artery catheter.

ratio is necessary to produce accurate CCO measurements. Research has shown a low ratio (derived from a core body temperature >38.5° C) can result in inaccurate CCO values.[45] One advantage of a CCO catheter is the elimination of the time-consuming administration of a thermal injectate through the proximal port of the PAC. It also reduces the number of discrepancies in TDCO values that can occur because of inconsistent injectate administration relative to the respiratory cycle.

A significant drawback to the CCO device is the hysteresis in recording hemodynamic information. Although the monitor displays updated CO figures every 30 seconds, they nonetheless do not represent real-time data. Instead, the CCO values depict the average CO from the prior 3 to 6 minutes.[46] This can be a significant limitation in patients who develop acute hemodynamic changes in response to hemorrhage and resuscitation.[47] In this setting a standard bolus thermodilution technique is preferable. Manufacturers of CCO monitors have attempted to circumvent this limitation by developing "Fast-Filter" and "Urgent" modes to supplement the "Normal" mode of data processing. One investigation found a significant decline in the precision of CO measurements when the Fast-Filter and Urgent modes were employed.[48] The reliability and accuracy of the device with intensive care and surgical patients has been established with recordings taken in the supine position [45,49-52] and with the backrest elevated up to 45 degrees.[53] Nevertheless, some investigators have found the CCO technique to be less precise than iced bolus thermodilution.[54,55] In spite of reports in the literature of a positive clinical outcome based on the use of CCO,[56] future studies are required to establish whether CCO measurements reduce the length of hospitalization and improve morbidity and mortality rates.

Mixed Venous Oxygen Saturation

Since its introduction in 1981, use of $S\bar{V}O_2$ as an estimate of systemic oxygen delivery has generated controversy. The purported usefulness of monitoring $S\bar{V}O_2$ is based on the knowledge that it is determined by pulmonary function, cardiac function, oxygen delivery and tissue perfusion, oxygen consumption, and hemoglobin concentration. During the course of an anesthetic procedure (excluding cases of major trauma or hemorrhagic shock), it is not unusual for pulmonary function, hemoglobin content, and oxygen consumption to remain relatively stable. Therefore proponents of $S\bar{V}O_2$ monitoring state that it is reasonable to assume that a decrease in $S\bar{V}O_2$ reflects a change in oxygen delivery, presumably via a reduction in CO. However, numerous studies have shown that in the intensive care unit $S\bar{V}O_2$ values correlate poorly with CO,[57,58] causing some investigators to criticize its use. Nevertheless, other researchers that have found changes in $S\bar{V}O_2$ to parallel changes in CO,[59,60] as well as reduce hospital morbidity and mortality.[51,61-63] In addition, $S\bar{V}O_2$ monitoring may serve as a prognostic indicator in patients with acute myocardial infarction.[64]

Continuous mixed venous oximetry is measured with the use of fiberoptic reflectance spectrophotometry through two fiberoptics housed in the PAC. One fiberoptic transmits light-emitting diodes (narrow wavebands of light) to the distal catheter. The extent of light absorption and reflection is a function of the quantity of oxyhemoglobin and deoxyhemoglobin present in the PA.[65] The receiving fiberoptic transports the reflected light to a microprocessor, which interprets the signal and displays an $S\bar{V}O_2$ value. The normal range of $S\bar{V}O_2$ is 65% to 77%; sustained low values (e.g., 50%) merit investigation followed by appropriate intervention(s). Factors that increase $S\bar{V}O_2$ values include left-to-right shunts, hypothermia, sepsis, cyanide toxicity, a wedged PAC, and an increase in CO. $S\bar{V}O_2$ decreases with hyperthermia, shivering, seizures, reduced pulmonary transport of oxygen, hemorrhage, and decreased CO. It has also been demonstrated that some $S\bar{V}O_2$ monitoring systems adapt well to acute changes in hematocrit.[66] In addition, research with two-wavelength and three-wavelength $S\bar{V}O_2$ oximetry catheters has shown the systems to be comparable in accuracy.[67]

In conclusion, the cost-benefit ratio of using PACs that provide CCO or $S\bar{V}O_2$ measurements remains controversial.[46,68] The use of the PAC has the potential to promote health or cause harm; the major determinant is the clinician's ability to interpret and apply data from this sophisticated diagnostic tool.[69] The therapeutic strategies should be guided by a knowledge of the patient's underlying pathophysiology.

AUTOMATED ST-SEGMENT MONITORING

Recent years have seen the proliferation of ECG monitors for the operating room that include software to provide continuous real-time ST-segment analysis. The development of this ECG tool[70] correlates with the demographics of the general surgical population (approximately one third have risk factors for coronary artery disease [CAD]) and research that demonstrates that perioperative ischemia is associated with increased morbidity and mortality.[70-72] The overall incidence of perioperative ischemia in patients with CAD scheduled for cardiac or noncardiac surgery ranges from 20% to 80%.[73,74]

Because of its low cost, noninvasiveness, widespread availability, and designation as a standard of care for monitoring of all anesthetized patients, the ECG remains a common and required diagnostic tool in the operating room. Automated ST-segment monitors have also demonstrated good sensitivity (80% to 100%) in detecting myocardial ischemia[70,75,76] in one study, only transesophageal echocardiography had greater sensitivity.[77]

Although universal standards for an "ECG ischemic threshold" do not exist, acceptable ECG criteria suggestive of myocardial ischemia include the following: (1) ≥1 mm horizontal ST-segment depression; (2) ≥1 mm unsloping or downsloping ST-segment depression measured 60 ms (1.5 mm) or 80 ms (2 mm) from the J point; and (3) ≥1 mm ST-segment elevation (Figure 16-8).[78,79] The J point is used in analyzing depressed ST segments that are upsloped or downsloped. It is defined as the junction between the S wave and ST segment (Figure 16-9). The magnitude of ST-segment depression is determined by measuring a previously established horizontal distance (e.g., 60 ms) from the J point. For example, a vertical line is drawn at a distance of 60 ms from the J point, and the intersection of this line with the ST segment is noted. This point of intersection defines the degree of ST-segment deviation relative to the isoelectric line, which is referenced as the *iso point* (i.e., intersects the PR segment [see Figure 16-9]). A 60-ms distance measured from the J point is preferred with rapid HRs, because during tachyarrhythmias a shortened ST segment can result from encroachment of the T on the ST segment. The use of a J + 80 ms distance in this circumstance could actually lead to an ST point that intersects a T wave instead of the ST segment. Should this occur, the computer-derived ST-segment deviation value would reflect a false significant shift in the ST segment, suggesting myocardial

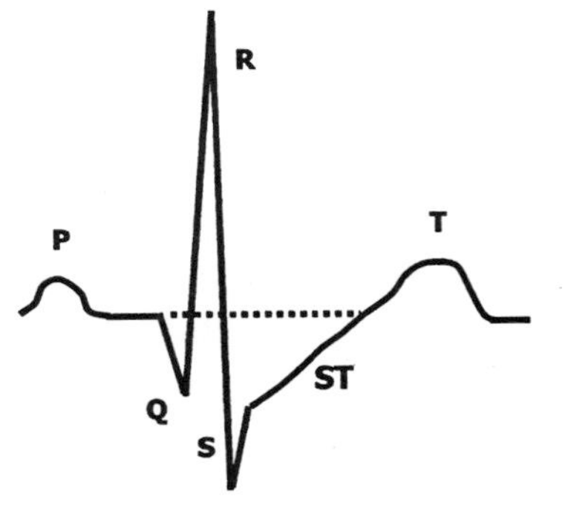

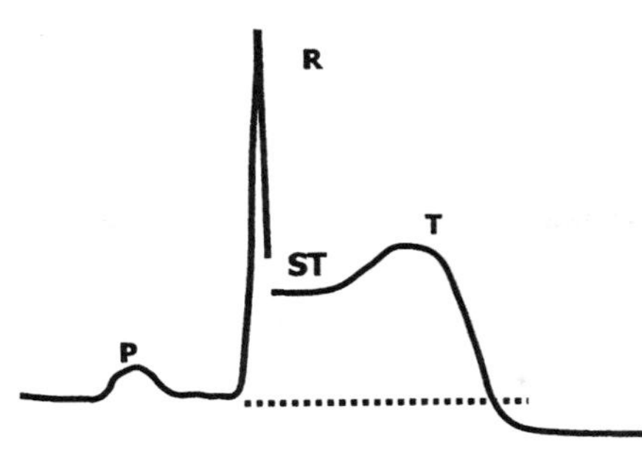

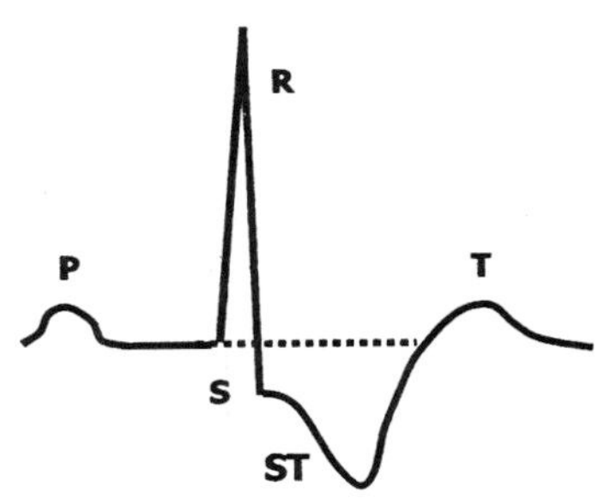

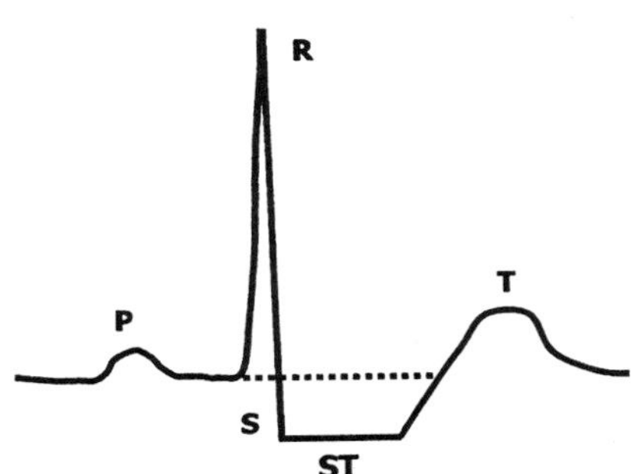

FIGURE **16-8**
Diagram illustrating the various forms of ST segment deviation that may occur as a result of myocardial injury. Depression of the ST segment correlates with subendocardial injury, and ST-segment elevation with transmural injury.

ischemia (Figure 16-10). Regarding the significance of the various forms of ST-segment depression, it is important to recall that a horizontal or downsloping depressed ST segment has greater specificity (fewer false positives) than an upsloping depressed ST segment. Adding upsloping ST-segment changes to ischemia diagnostic criteria does improve overall sensitivity but at a sacrifice to specificity and positive predictive value.[80,81]

Setting of the ST-Segment Parameters

Most manufacturers of automated ST-segment analysis monitors have sophisticated algorithms that allow fairly consistent and accurate placement of the ST measurement points. However, no system is perfect, which means anesthetists should periodically assess and change the ST measurement points as needed. Failure to do so could lead to iatrogenic injury by permitting false trends to be followed. In fact, manufacturers have incorporated software that permits the health-care provider to override the monitor's placement of the ST measurement points. A common technique for setting ST measurement points involves adjustment of three variables—iso point, J point, and ST point (Figure 16-11). Manipulation of a keypad on the ECG monitor permits the operator to scroll each of these "points" or vertical lines along a horizontal axis. Figures 16-12 and 16-13 illustrate the consequences when a monitor's programmed default settings places the ST-segment measurement points incorrectly (i.e., the display of inaccurate ST-segment deviation values). The application of an ST-segment deviation algorithm can reduce the occurrence of such mishaps and improve overall management of patients at risk for ischemic changes (Figure 16-14, p. 319).

Other significant variables to account for when monitoring patients at risk for ischemic events include ECG electrode placement, ECG lead selection, gain setting, and frequency bandwidth. Each of these is briefly reviewed here.

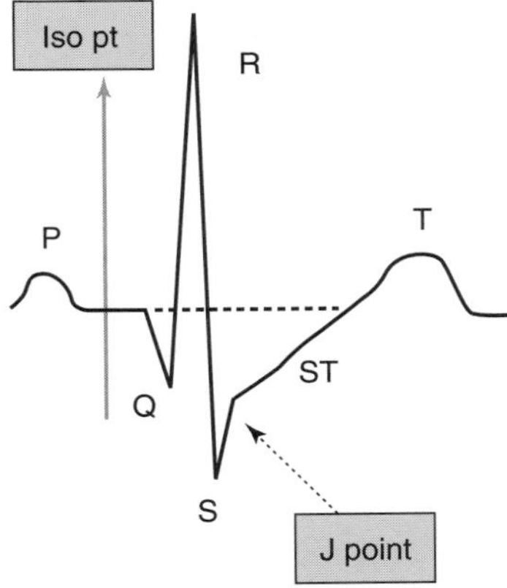

FIGURE **16-9**
A single cardiac cycle demonstrating a depressed ST segment that is upsloping. The junction between the S wave and ST segment defines the J point. The iso pt *(vertical line)* intersects the PR segment. The PR segment is measured from the end of the P wave to the beginning of the QRS complex. (Reprinted with permission from Kossick MA. Recognizing EKG evidence of ischemia, injury, and infarction. In: *EKG Interpretation: Simple, Thorough, Practical.* 2nd ed. Park Ridge, Ill: AANA Publishing; 1999:22.)

Electrocardiograph Electrode Placement

It is not uncommon to see ECG electrodes inaccurately placed on a patient in an attempt to "move an operating room schedule along." Many times in an American Society of

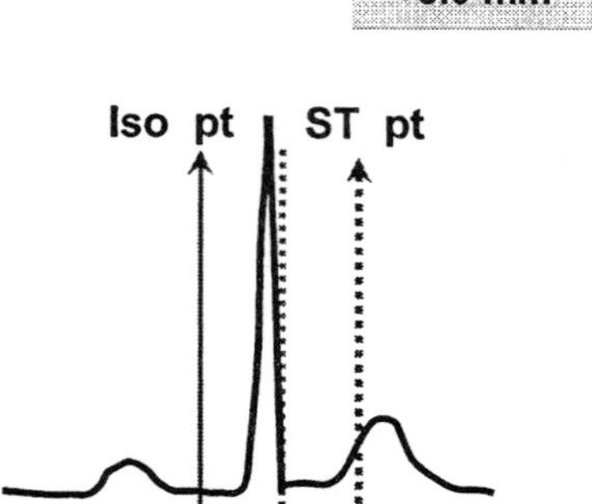

FIGURE **16-10**
A single cardiac cycle illustrating a shortened ST segment. Use of a J + 80 ms value to measure ST-segment deviation results in the intersection of the ST point with the T wave. The computer-derived ST-segment deviation value of 3 mm is predictably incorrect (falsely elevated).

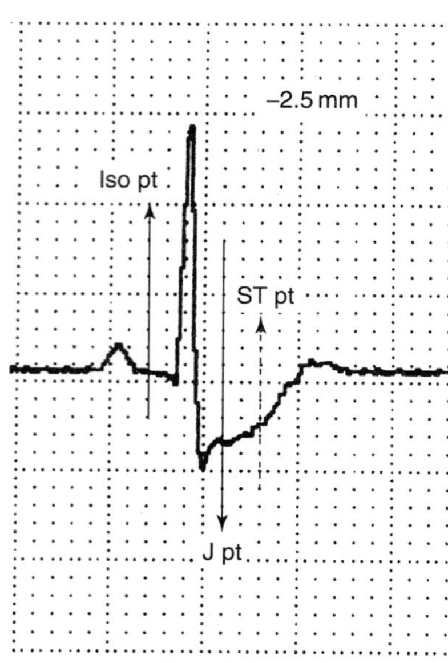

FIGURE **16-11**
Correct placement of the iso, J, and ST points. (Reprinted with permission from Kossick MA. Recognizing EKG evidence of ischemia, injury, and infarction. In: *EKG Interpretation: Simple, Thorough, Practical.* 2nd ed. Park Ridge, Ill: AANA Publishing; 1999:20.)

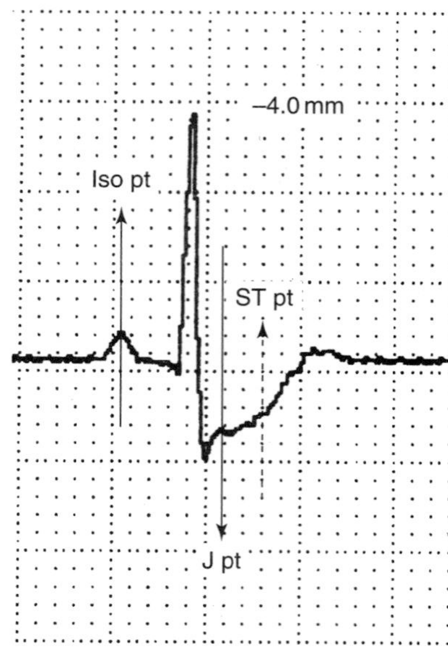

FIGURE **16-12**
Incorrect placement by an ECG monitor of the iso point on top of the P wave. This produces an exaggerated ST-segment deviation value. (Reprinted with permission from Kossick MA. Recognizing EKG evidence of ischemia, injury, and infarction. In: *EKG Interpretation: Simple, Thorough, Practical.* 2nd ed. Park Ridge, Ill: AANA Publishing; 1999:21.)

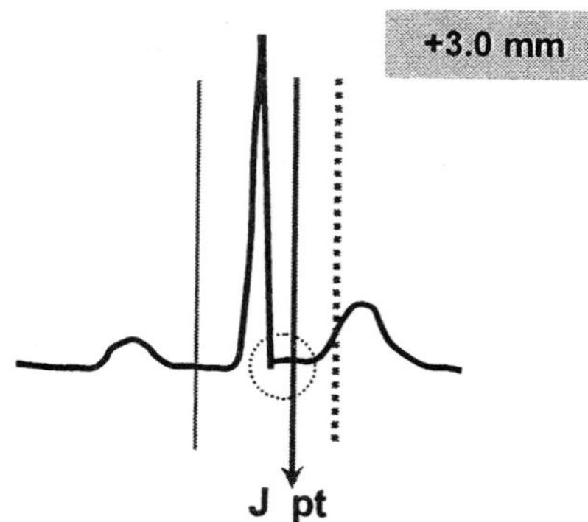

FIGURE **16-13**
Incorrect placement of the J point leads to an ST point that intersects on the T wave. (Reprinted with permission from Kossick MA. Recognizing EKG evidence of ischemia, injury, and infarction. In: *EKG Interpretation: Simple, Thorough, Practical.* 2nd ed. Park Ridge, Ill: AANA Publishing; 1999:21.)

Anesthesiologists Physical Status (ASA PS) I or II patient, correct ECG electrode placement is a moot point. However, in patients with risk factors for CAD, such inattentiveness can lead to iatrogenic injury by producing deviated ST segments or flipped T waves. Proper placement of the limb lead and chest lead electrodes is described in Table 16-8. For emphasis, the precordial leads should be placed via palpation of the costae, not by gross visual estimation of an intercostal space (Figure 16-15, p. 320). Understandably some surgical procedures do not permit the use of optimal ECG lead selection and placement; ECG electrode(s) can interfere with skin preparation and surgical incision. Under these circumstances a less than optimal ECG lead placement may be necessary.

Electrocardiographic Lead Selection

The selection of ECG lead(s) to be used during the course of an anesthetic procedure is extremely important. Improper selection can lead to unrecognized myocardial ischemia or injury. Research has validated that use of a single ECG lead for monitoring for ischemia in vulnerable patients is inadequate and that monitoring with multiple leads enhances patient safety.[82] In patients at risk for ischemic events, the maximum number of ECG leads (e.g., three) should be displayed for continuous and comprehensive assessment of ST-segment and T-wave changes (Figure 16-16, p. 320). Which lead(s) are best for detecting significant ST-segment changes remains somewhat controversial. First and foremost, if a baseline 12-lead ECG has been performed,

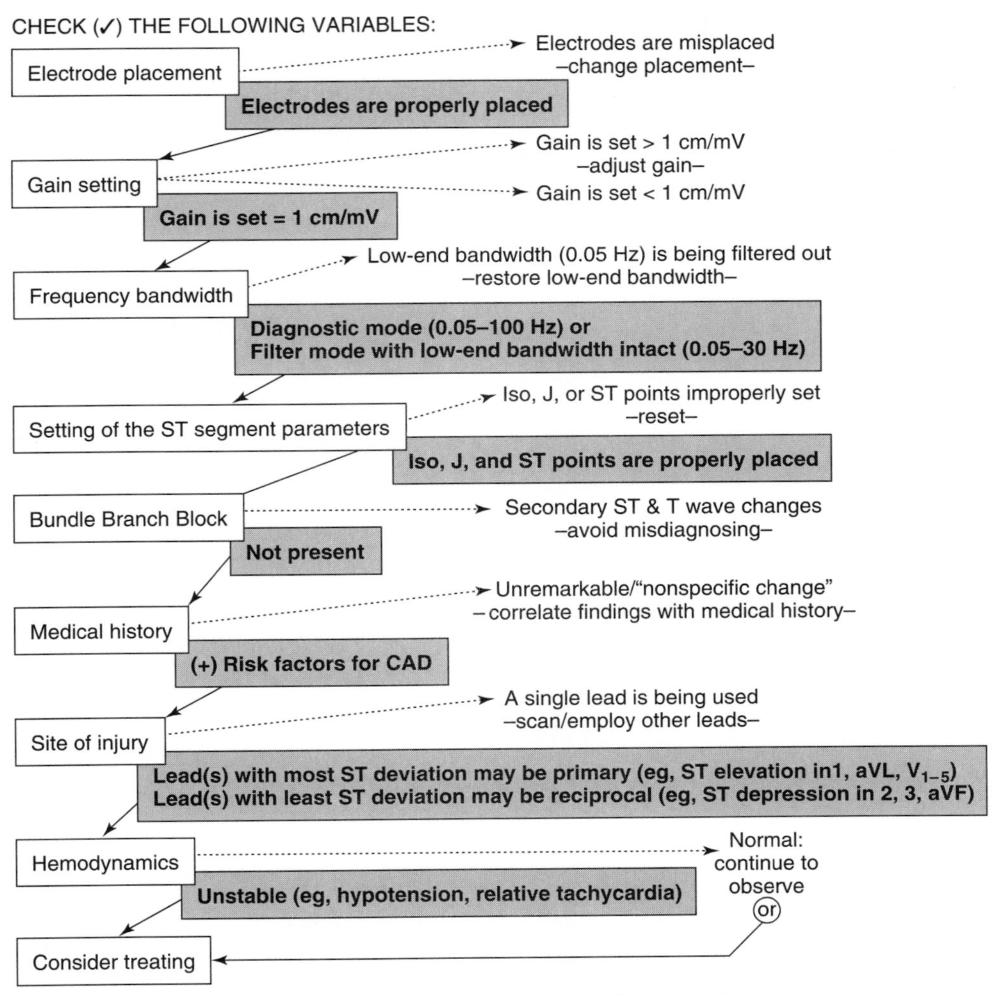

FIGURE **16-14**
An ST-segment deviation assessment and treatment algorithm (threshold of 1 mm elevation or depression). (Reprinted with permission from Kossick MA. Recognizing EKG evidence of ischemia, injury, and infarction. In: *EKG Interpretation: Simple, Thorough, Practical.* 2nd ed. Park Ridge, Ill: AANA Publishing; 1999:16.)

TABLE **16-8** Proper Placement of Electrocardiographic Electrodes for Monitoring Limb Leads and Chest Leads*

RA	Near the right shoulder directly the beneath clavicle
LA	Near the left shoulder directly beneath the clavicle
LL	Left lower abdomen
RL	At any convenient location
V1	Fourth intercostal space right of the sternal border
V2	Fourth intercostal space left of the sternal border
V3	Equal distance between V2 and V4
V4	Midclavicular line at the fifth intercostal space
V5	Horizontal to V4 on the anterior axillary line
V6	Horizontal to V5 on the midaxillary line

LA, Left arm electrocardiographic (ECG) electrode; LL, left leg ECG electrode; RA, right arm ECG electrode; RL, right leg ECG electrode.
**Placement of the LL electrode in a more superior location (e.g., near the left nipple) can affect the accuracy of ST-segment interpretation and dysrhythmia analysis.*

"fingerprinting" of this tracing should serve as the primary guide for lead selection intraoperatively. If a baseline 12-lead ECG shows significant primary ST-segment changes in leads 1, aVL, and V6, then this lead combination should be used for continuous ECG monitoring during the anesthetic.

For those patients who do not have a preoperative 12-lead ECG or who have a baseline 12-lead ECG that is essentially normal, the literature suggests the following leads be selected for continuous monitoring for ischemia. Chest lead V3, limb lead III, and lead II are recommended if the risk for ST-segment deviation favors elevation.[82,83] Leads V3 and III are sensitive for detecting supply ischemia and transmural myocardial injury (as seen during angioplasty procedures). Lead II is recommended for basic narrow QRS-complex rhythm assessment. If the anticipated change in ST segment is depression, which would correlate with subendocardial injury (demand or supply ischemia), then V5, limb lead II, and lead III may be most appropriate.[84] However, some researchers with strong internal validity in their study have found V5 and II to be insensitive leads for detecting ST-segment changes.[85]

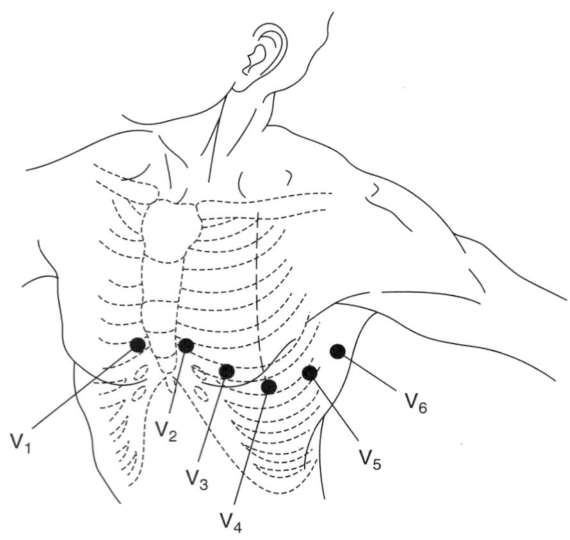

FIGURE **16-15**
Precordial electrodes positioned across the ventral-lateral aspect of the thorax. (Reprinted with permission from Kossick MA. Recognizing EKG evidence of ischemia, injury, and infarction. In: *EKG Interpretation: Simple, Thorough, Practical*. 2nd ed. Park Ridge, Ill: AANA Publishing; 1999:16.)

Given this information, it is prudent for anesthesia providers to monitor and assess multiple ECG leads in the operating room. This helps to optimize detection of regionalized myocardial ischemia. Many times this entails nothing more than changing the current lead selector switch or performing a multilead ECG. The latter produces an ECG recording of all six limb leads and a single chest lead, which permits the anesthetist to more comprehensively assess ECG data, including dysrhythmias, the mean QRS axis (limb leads 1 and aVF), T-wave morphology, ST-segment changes, and QT intervals.

With the introduction into clinical practice of the derived 12-lead system (EASI), nurses and physicians have a convenient method for global assessment of the overall well-being of the myocardium (Figure 16-17). This system provides a derived 12-lead ECG through a five-electrode configuration.[86] To monitor with this system, the five ECG electrodes are placed in the following locations: LA over the manubrium, chest (V) electrode over the lower body of the sternum, LL left midaxillary horizontal to the chest electrode, RA right midaxillary also horizontal to the chest electrode, and RL in any convenient location. Current and past research suggests that the derived 12-lead ECG is comparable to the standard 12-lead ECG for multiple cardiac diagnosis in adults and children (e.g., ST-segment changes, myocardial infarction, wide QRS-complex tachycardia).[83,86-91] For anesthetists who have ECG monitors configured with a derived 12-lead software option, its use could improve ischemic detection in patients with risk factors for CAD.

In summary, practitioners who limit ECG monitoring and assessment to a single or pair of leads *in patients at risk for ischemia* are potentially compromising patient safety by not using anesthesia monitors to their full capacity. For example, choosing not to display end-tidal CO_2 and arterial waveforms on a monitor that has this capability—and instead working only with numeric data—could lead to an error in anesthesia care (e.g., giving ephedrine to a patient with a systolic blood pressure recording of 70 mm Hg when the cause is a dampened waveform secondary to arm positioning). Unarguably, critical assessment of all available patient data will help anesthetists make more informed care decisions and potentially will improve anesthetic outcomes.

Gain Setting and Frequency Bandwidth

Two other potential problems with continuous ST-segment monitoring relate to the amplitude at which the ECG monitor has been set and whether filtering of the electrical signal is excessive. When ST-segment analysis is a priority during an

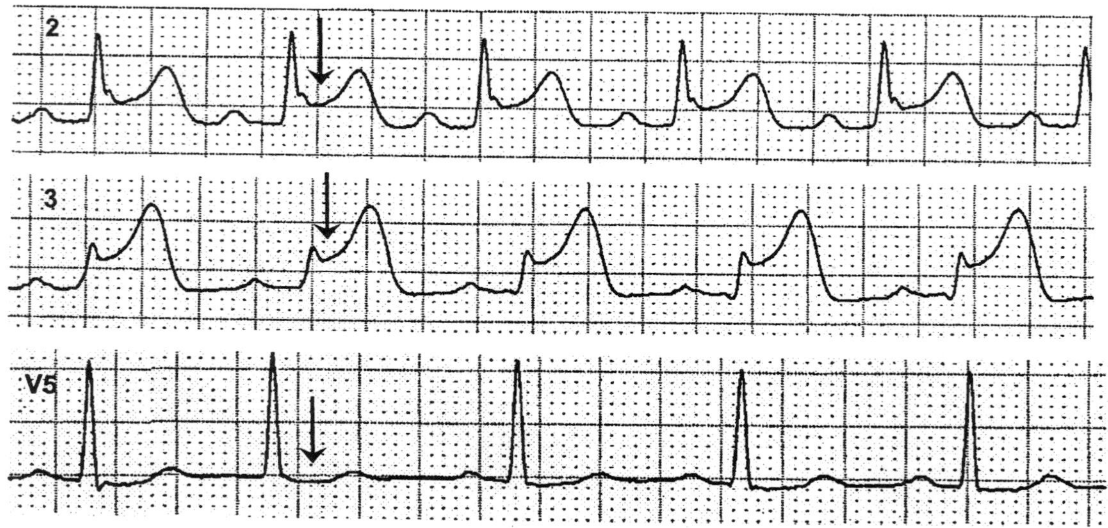

FIGURE **16-16**
Monitoring in 3 ECG leads during anesthetic administration captured significant ST-segment elevation. The greatest change in ST segments occurred in limb lead 3, followed by limb lead 2. Noteworthy was the failure of lead V5 to demonstrate any appreciable change in the ST segment. Postoperatively a cardiology consultation resulted in a diagnosis of Prinzmetals angina.

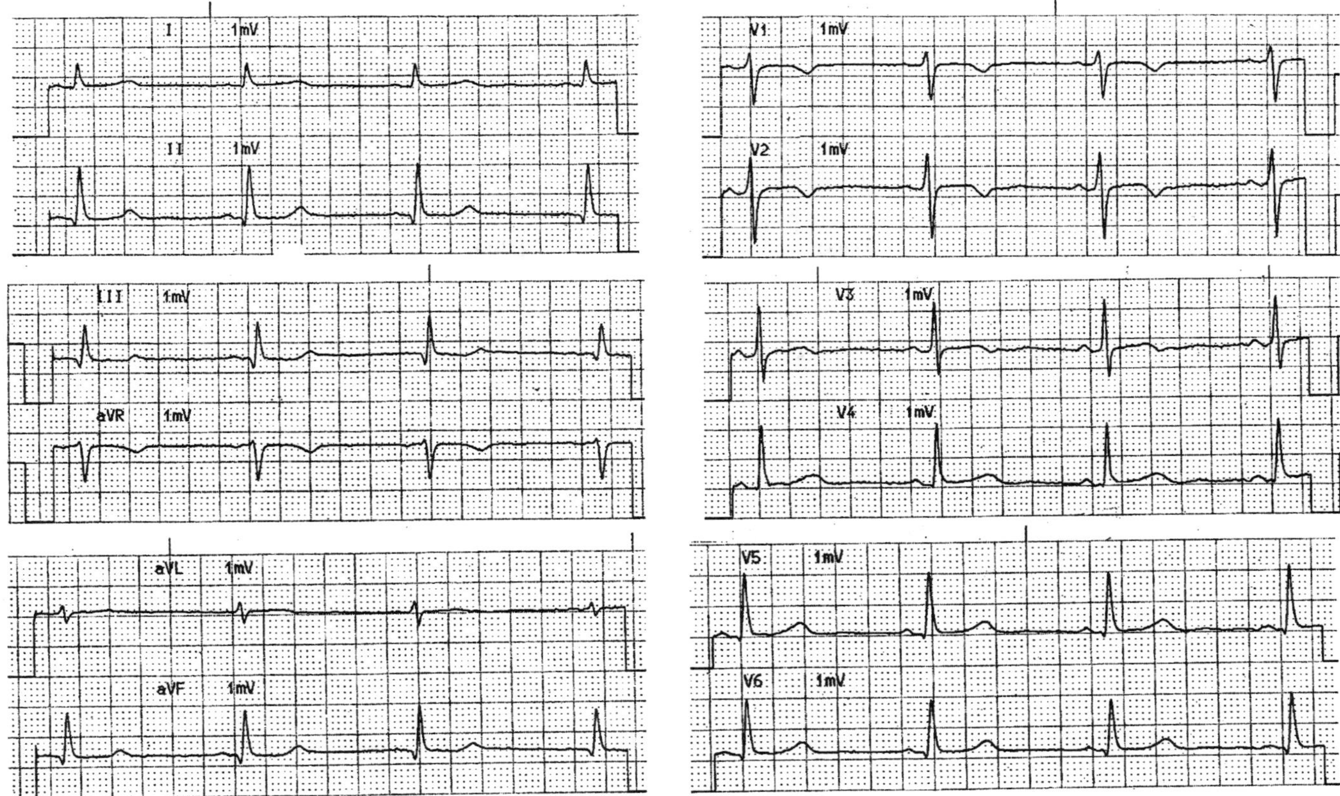

FIGURE **16-17**
A derived 12-lead electrocardiogram (ECG; EASI) recorded just before anesthetic induction in the operating room. On the existing ECG monitoring system, three ECG leads (e.g., V3, V5, III) can be continuously monitored during surgery for rhythm and ST-segment changes. A derived 12-lead can be calculated and displayed at any time during the case.

anesthetic, the gain of the ECG monitor should be set at standardization (i.e., a 1-mV signal delivered by the ECG monitor produces a 10-mm calibration pulse). This gain setting fixes the ratio of the ST-segment and QRS-complex size so that a 1-mm ST-segment change is accurately assessed (e.g., potential myocardial ischemia). Failure to recognize the use of other gain settings can lead to overdiagnosis or underdiagnosis of ischemic ST-segment changes. Figure 16-18 illustrates how changes in gain settings and improper lead placement can confound ST-segment assessment.

The filtering capacity of the ECG monitor is yet another potential source of artifact. Prior research has demonstrated that filtering out the low end of the frequency bandwidth (e.g., 0.05 to 0.5 to produce a new bandwidth range of 0.5 to 40 Hz) of the monitor's electrical signal can lead to distortion of the ST segment (elevation or depression).[77,92] For this reason in many (but not all) cases the diagnostic mode of an ECG monitor should be used when ST-segment analysis is a priority for an anesthetic case.

Clearly, the sensitivity and specificity of automated ST-segment analysis monitors is dependent on the ability of the anesthetist to critically analyze the large number of factors that influence ST-segment values. Attentiveness to such variables as the patient's physical status, ECG lead placement, type and total number continuously monitored, type of electronic filtering employed by the ECG monitor, and gain setting used can affect anesthetic outcome in patients at risk for ischemia.

ARTERIAL PRESSURE MONITORING

Arterial blood pressure monitoring gives information about LV volume, LV function, and SVR.[93] Because of its importance, arterial blood pressure should be measured at least every 5 minutes during anesthetic administration (and is so mandated as a "standard of care").[94]

Blood pressure monitoring falls into two categories: indirect (noninvasive) and direct (invasive). Noninvasive blood pressure monitoring is the most commonly used method during anesthesia administration and is generally accurate and safe. Sometimes, however, a direct method of blood pressure measurement is required and may be selected based on a patient's physical status, the surgeon's skills, and the type and length of surgical procedure. Accuracy and reliability of noninvasive and invasive methods are influenced by several factors, which are subsequently described.

Indirect Blood Pressure Monitoring

Indirect blood pressure monitoring was first described by Riva-Rocci in 1896.[95] He placed a pneumatic cuff around a person's arm and inflated the cuff while palpating the radial artery. The disappearance of the palpated arterial pulse correlated with systolic pressure. Korotkoff, in 1905, varied this technique by placing a stethoscope over the brachial artery and listening for changes in the sounds of pulsations as the cuff was deflated.[96] The first audible sound correlated with systolic pressure, and

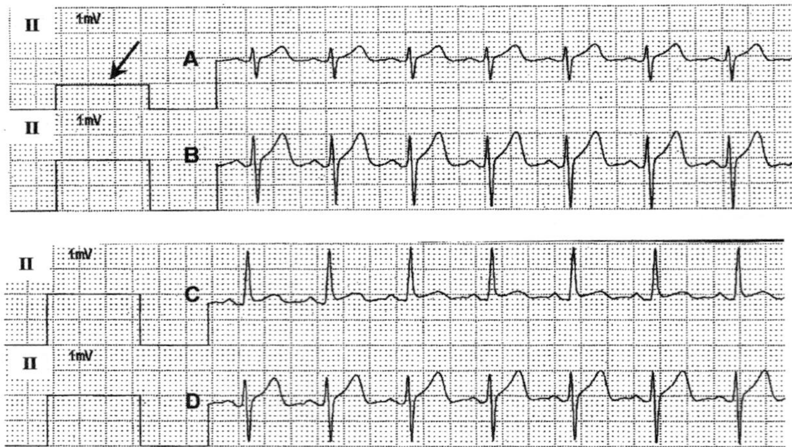

FIGURE **16-18**
This series of electrocardiographic (ECG) recordings illustrates how the gain setting and incorrect ECG electrode placement can lead to misinterpretation of ST-segment changes. In strip A, the gain setting *(arrow)* on the ECG monitor has been set at half standardization (1 mV = 5 mm); it grossly gives the appearance of a minor ST-segment change. When concurrent strip B is compared with strip A, it becomes apparent that use of smaller gain settings can mask ST-segment deviation. Therefore if a 0.5-mm ST-segment deviation in ECG strip A were to occur, it would equate with a 1-mm change. A similar error in assessment of ST-segment changes can occur secondary to misplaced ECG electrodes. ECG strip recording C has all limb lead electrodes properly placed and displays an ST-segment elevation of approximately 0.8 mm. In contrast, ECG strip D mistakenly has the left leg electrode placed in the second intercostal space, midclavicular line, and therefore is not a literal lead II. The end result is an ST segment that is falsely elevated (in excess of 2 mm), suggesting inferior myocardial ischemia. (Reprinted with permission from Kossick MA. Recognizing EKG evidence of ischemia, injury, and infarction. In: *EKG Interpretation: Simple, Thorough, Practical.* 2nd ed. Park Ridge, Ill: AANA Publishing; 1999:26-27.)

diastolic pressure correlated with the disappearance of the pulse sound. A commonly used measurement, MAP, correlated with a muffling of the pulse sound.

Today a manual (nonelectronic) blood pressure measurement may be obtained by two methods: the Korotkoff technique of measurement, which uses a mercury column sphygmomanometer, and the oscillometric (or aneroid) technique, which senses pressure changes underneath a pneumatic cuff as it is deflated. After the cuff is inflated, blood flow through the artery is occluded. Blood flow returns as the cuff is deflated, and oscillations occur. The first oscillation correlates with systolic pressure when an aneroid sphygmomanometer is used. As cuff pressure continues to be released, the oscillations become larger, peak, then decrease. The point at which oscillations peak correlates with MAP, and the point at which the oscillations cease correlates with diastolic pressure (Figure 16-19). The aneroid method, used by most automated (electronic) blood pressure systems, calculates diastolic pressure by a computer algorithm of analysis of cuff pressures and oscillations.[97] MAP is difficult to ascertain by the Korotkoff method but can be estimated with the following formula[98] :

Equation 16-1

$$\text{MAP} = \frac{1}{3}(\text{Systolic pressure} - \text{Diastolic pressure})$$

All three techniques are influenced by bladder cuff size. The recommended bladder cuff size is one that encircles 80% of the arm.[99] A bladder cuff that is too small for the extremity requires more pressure to occlude the artery beneath, yielding

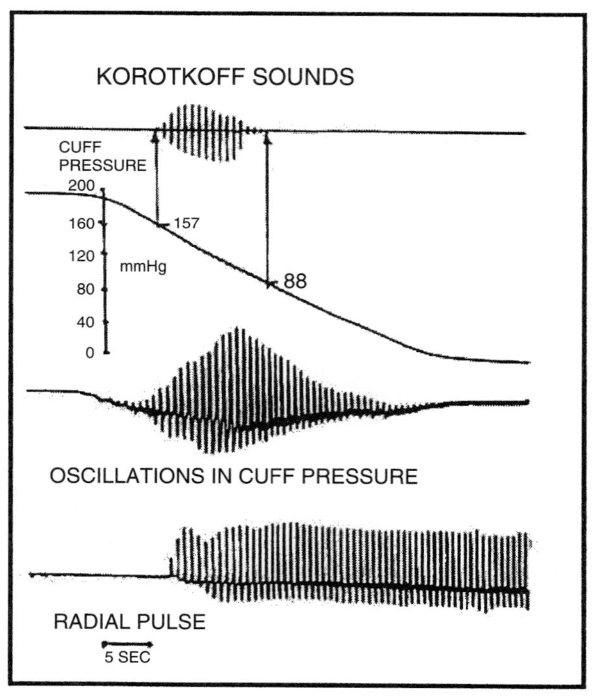

FIGURE **16-19**
Comparison of Korotkoff sounds, oscillations, and radial artery palpation. Note correlation between the onset of the first Korotkoff sound, the onset of oscillations in the cuff pressure, and the radial pulse wave. (Reprinted with permission from Reitan JA, Barash PG, eds. *Noninvasive Monitoring.* New York: Wiley; 1978.)

TABLE 16-9 Factors That Affect the Accuracy of Noninvasive Blood Pressure Monitoring

Falsely High Readings	Falsely Low Readings	Erroneous Readings (Falsely High or Low)
Small bladder cuff	Poor tissue perfusion	Improper cuff placement
Arterial stiffness	Large bladder cuff	Dysrhythmias
Hyperthermia	Failure to identify Korotkoff sounds	Rapid cuff deflation (optimal 2 mm Hg/sec)

a significantly false increase in recorded blood pressure. To a lesser degree, a bladder cuff that is too large may give a falsely decreased pressure measurement.[100]

One advantage of the noninvasive method is that it allows a cuff to be placed on any portion of a limb.[101] Common sites for measurements, other than the arm, include the forearm, thigh, and calf. MAP can even be measured with placement of a neonatal cuff on an adult finger.[102] Blood pressure measurements are also influenced by other factors such as deflation rate and hyperthermia[103,104] (Table 16-9).

Noninvasive blood pressure monitoring is safe and is associated with few complications. However, pain, ecchymosis, limb edema, venous stasis, thrombophlebitis, and nerve damage[105] can occur, especially if the cuff is misplaced. Nevertheless, even with the proper placement of the cuff, if the duration of measurements is prolonged and obtained frequently (e.g., every 5 minutes for a 10-hour procedure), the previously listed complications are more likely to occur. Similarly, a case of fascial compartment syndrome of the upper extremity has been cited when a cuff was wrapped too tightly at the beginning of the procedure.[106]

In summary, although the procedure is relatively safe, care must always be taken when a noninvasive blood pressure method is used. The anesthesia provider's responsibilities are to choose proper cuff size, to place the cuff appropriately, and to avoid excessive measurements, especially over prolonged anesthetic administration.

Direct Arterial Monitoring

Direct arterial pressure monitoring involves percutaneous insertion of a catheter into an artery, allowing one to obtain continuous real-time pressures and arterial blood samples when needed. Once inserted, the catheter is attached to a fluid-filled pressure system that consists of two elements: the transducer system, which captures the waveform and produces an electronic signal replicating the waveform, and the monitor electronics, which accept the electrical signal from the transducer and display it. Specifically, movement of the arterial pressure against the diaphragm in the transducer is converted to an electrical signal, and this signal is displayed as the arterial pressure waveform. The waveform is reproduced through Fourier analysis—a technique that re-creates the original complex pressure wave by summing a series of simpler sine waves of various amplitudes and frequencies.[107]

The goal is to have the displayed waveform accurately reproduce the arterial pressure. However, both parts of the monitoring system could distort the waveform as it is displayed. With modern monitor electronics, signal processing of the waveform for display can be accomplished by rapidly sampling the transducer's electrical output and mathematically processing it using a computer chip. With this type of instrumentation, the monitor electronics play only a minimal role in waveform distortion. Therefore, the physical properties of the catheter and the fluid-filled pressure transducer will control, to a greater extent, the accuracy of the waveform reproduction.

The catheter-transducer system is described as an underdamped second-order dynamic system that has three characteristic physical properties: elasticity, mass, and friction.[107,108] Specifically, movement through the catheter transducer system is influenced by the elasticity of its components (e.g., tubing and stopcocks) as well as the elasticity of the blood vessels.

The transducer system must have a natural frequency high enough to accommodate the harmonic content of the waveform (which minimally is equal to the HR). Decreasing the natural frequency of the system distorts the waveform, creating a resonating effect, also termed *overshoot* or *ringing*. The distortion produces extra displayed waveforms and results in an overestimation of blood pressure (Figure 16-20). An example of this is the addition of more compliant tubing, such as intravenous extension tubing, which lowers the natural frequency of the system. Similarly, tachycardias make it more

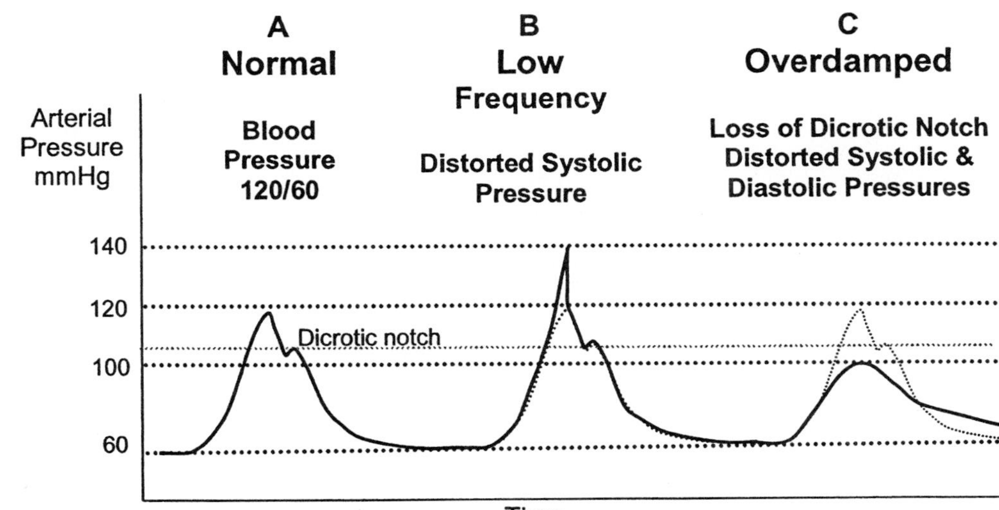

FIGURE 16-20 Distortion of direct arterial blood pressure readings. **A,** Normal waveform. **B,** False elevation of systolic pressure resulting from a lowered frequency of the system or decreased arterial compliance. **C,** False lowering of systolic pressure and elevation of diastolic pressure related to an increase in the damping of the system.

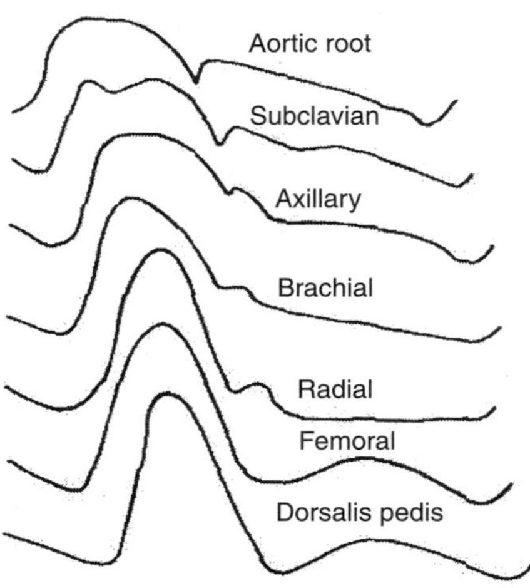

FIGURE **16-21**
Reflected blood pressures as they travel through the arterial tree from the aorta to the periphery. As the wave moves toward the periphery, the dicrotic notch occurs later and later in the waveform and eventually disappears. The reflected systolic pressures increase in size. (Reprinted with permission from Saidman LJ, Smith N. Noninvasive monitoring. In: Reitan JA Barash, PG, ed. *Monitoring in Anesthesia.* 2nd ed. London: Butterworth; 1984.)

difficult for the system to accurately reproduce the waveform because the natural frequency of the system is not always high enough to handle the greater harmonic content of fast HRs. Stiff arterial vessels can also distort the waveform by producing overshoot[108] (see Figure 16-20).

Damping refers to how rapidly a system comes to rest after being set into motion. If the system is overly damped, one will note loss of the dicrotic notch and other fine detail (see Figure 16-20). An underestimation of systolic blood pressure and an overestimation of diastolic pressure also occur with overdamping. Factors that increase damping include the presence of air bubbles in the tubing, thrombus formation in the catheter, and inadvertent kinking of the catheter. Although systolic and diastolic readings becomes distorted, MAP remains fairly accurate.[93]

When fluid travels through a system (e.g., blood flow through the arterial tree) the shape of reflected waveforms changes over time.[109] The systolic pressure wave increases, and the diastolic pressure wave decreases as the waves travel peripherally (Figure 16-21). Therefore the morphology of a reflected blood pressure of the brachial artery is different from that of a reflected blood pressure of the dorsalis pedis artery; again, MAP is not altered. The dicrotic notch in the waveform reflects closure of the aortic valve in diastole. Pressure recordings from arteries closer to the aorta display a prompt dicrotic notch, whereas those from more distal arteries have a delayed or an absent dicrotic notch. A patient with significant aortic regurgitation may have no dicrotic notch.

This direct arterial monitoring system measures pressure at the fluid-air interface in the transducer. Recorded pressure is influenced by gravity and the vertical location of the transducer. A zero reference point, equal to atmospheric pressure, is required for accurate measurements. Older monitoring systems required frequent calibration. However, most systems today have built-in calibrations, and therefore it is no longer necessary to calibrate during "setup."

Two steps are required for setting up the monitoring system. The first is establishment of a zero reference point. A stopcock is opened to air and a "zero" button on the monitor is pressed. This permits the recorded pressure waveform to reflect; which effectively eliminates the influence of atmospheric pressure.

The second step is "leveling" of the transducer because of gravitational effects on blood pressure. In a patient in the supine or sitting position the transducer is placed at the midaxillary line in the left fourth intercostal space (phlebostatic axis). The pressure then reflects the blood pressure in the heart and proximal aorta. In a patient in the left lateral decubitus position the transducer is placed at the midsternal line in the left 4th intercostal space, and in a patient in the right lateral decubitus position the transducer is placed at the left parasternal border in the left fourth intercostal space.[110]

In certain neurosurgical procedures it is important to monitor cerebral perfusion pressure. This is accomplished by placing the transducer at the tragus (of the ear); in a patient in the supine position the aortic and cerebral pressures are similar. However, in a patient in the sitting position the aortic pressure is higher than the cerebral pressure, reflecting the hydrostatic pressure difference between the heart and the brain (Figure 16-22).

Invasive blood pressure monitoring is relatively safe, although rarely it has been associated with serious complications including vascular compromise from occlusion of the catheter, development of an arterial aneurysm and the occurrence of significant blood loss from disconnection of tubing. Inadvertent intraarterial injection of medication, infection, and nerve damage have also been reported.[111]

Many arteries can be used for catheter placement, including the radial, femoral, dorsalis pedis, and axillary arteries. The radial artery is the most common for the following reasons: easy accessibility, minimal patient discomfort with insertion, and generally, excellent collateral circulation in the hand. Disadvantages of radial artery cannulation include its peripheral location from the aorta, which can slightly skew blood pressure recordings, and its small size, which can predispose it to catheter occlusion.[111]

The major collateral system of the radial artery in the hand is supplied by the ulnar artery, but occasionally the ulnar artery is inadequate for this purpose. The modified Allen's test helps detect adequacy of ulnar artery blood flow before radial artery cannulation. To perform the test the examiner compresses both the radial and ulnar arteries. The patient exsanguinates the blood from the hand by pumping a tight fist. The hand is then opened, and the examiner releases occlusion from the ulnar artery. If adequate circulation is present, hyperemia of the hand occurs within a few seconds. Poor collateral flow is indicated if the hand remains blanched for longer than 10 seconds.[112]

Blood pressure is an important hemodynamic parameter affected by all anesthetic techniques. When using any blood pressure monitoring method, careful consideration of advantages and limitations are important to ensure the safety of the patient and the accuracy of measurements.

NEUROLOGIC MONITORING

Electroencephalography

The electroencephalogram (EEG) is derived from electrical activity in the brain that is produced by nearly synchronous depolarization of cell bodies and dendrites as chemical activity is converted to electrical activity. Although anesthetics affect

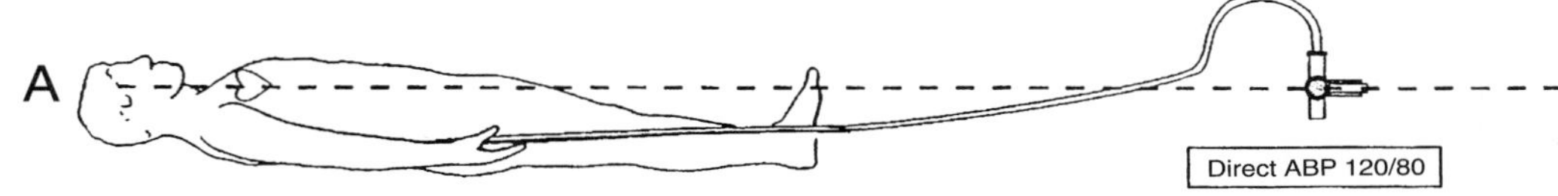

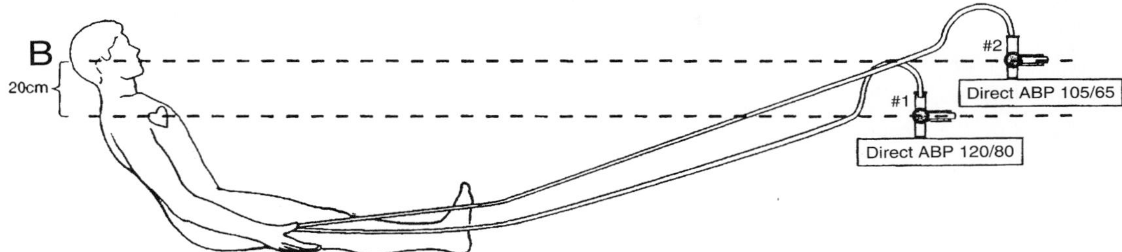

FIGURE **16-22**
The effect of pressure transducer level on measurement of blood pressure. **A,** With the patient supine, the level of the brain is considered to be at the same level as the heart, so directly measured blood pressure is considered to be the same at both sites. When the patient is placed in the sitting position, the brain is located above the heart. **B,** If the pressure transducer remains at the level of the heart, the recorded pressure remains unchanged, but if the transducer height is adjusted to the level of the brain, the recorded pressure is lower, reflecting the hydrostatic pressure difference between the head and heart, which equals approximately 20 cm H_2O. (From Mark JB. Direct arterial blood pressure monitoring. *Atlas of Cardiovascular Monitoring.* New York: Churchill Livingstone; 1998:121.)

the brain, EEG monitoring during anesthesia is rare, partly because EEGs are very sensitive to electrocautery artifact and are costly. Also, interpretation requires specialized training.[113,114] It is generally assumed that in the absence of pathologic conditions maintenance of adequate arterial pressure and cerebral oxygenation prevents injury to the brain. However, in some surgical procedures cerebral perfusion is altered and potentially decreased (e.g., cross-clamping of the carotid artery), and the EEG can rapidly detect potentially dangerous changes. Other uses for the EEG during anesthesia include monitoring of the degree of barbiturate coma or the occurrence of seizures.[115]

The raw EEG is obtained by placement of up to 21 electrodes on locations on the scalp.[116] The EEG wave is measured in millivolts and is recorded on a strip of paper moving at a speed measured in millimeters per second, producing a frequency range of 0.2 to 40 Hz. This frequency range is classically divided into bands that describe physiologic rhythms. The alpha rhythm is the most common wave produced on the EEG and is typically seen in the awake person who is resting with eyes closed. When the individual becomes excited or is concentrating and the eyes are open, the EEG waves become lower in amplitude and higher in frequency, resulting in a beta rhythm. Cortical depression, either from a pathologic condition or from anesthesia, leads to slower, higher-amplitude theta waves, with greater depression leading to the development of delta (sleep) waves (Table 16-10).

General anesthetics produce dose-dependent changes in the frequency of EEG waveforms.[115] Deepening anesthesia decreases the average EEG frequency and increases the average amplitude.[114] At a certain depth of anesthesia a pattern known as *burst suppression* develops. It is characterized by alternating periods of normal- to high-voltage activity changing to low voltage or even isoelectricity (rendering the EEG inactive in appearance). In the presence of pathologic states this pattern is indicative of a poor prognosis. However, during general anesthesia the isoelectrical state is associated with a decrease in cerebral metabolic oxygen demand, and this could provide cerebral (neuronal) protection against ischemia.[115]

TABLE **16-10** Frequency Bands of the Electroencephalogram

Band	Frequency Range
Beta	13-40 Hz
Alpha	8-12 Hz
Theta	4-7 Hz
Delta	1-3 Hz

Monitoring the Depth of Anesthesia

The Bispectral Index (BIS) monitor was developed to measure the depth of hypnosis and overcome disadvantages of EEG monitoring during anesthesia. Although it is not an EEG, the BIS monitor extrapolates its information from EEG parameters. This is accomplished through a high-order statistical analysis in which relationships between EEG data and states of consciousness have been noted. The BIS monitor averages information over a period of 15 seconds and derives a numerical value that correlates with the level of sedation.[114] The BIS number ranges from 0-100 (0 equating to an isoelectric EEG and 100 equating to an awake patient). See Figure 16-23 for a detailed description of the BIS range.

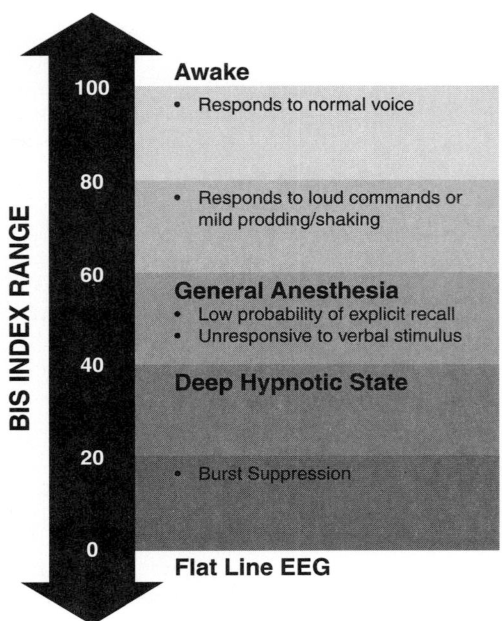

FIGURE **16-23**
Bispectral index (BIS) range guidelines. (Reproduced with permission from Apect MedicatSystems, Natick, Mass.)

Of concern to anesthesia providers is the occurrence of recall during general anesthesia. Incidences of recall range from 0.1% to 0.4% depending on patient population and type of surgery. The effects of intraoperative recall can be devastating. Patients can suffer from sleep disturbances, nightmares, and even posttraumatic stress disorder.[117-119] A benefit of monitoring depth of hypnosis is that it also correlates well with the incidence of recall. Recall is more likely to occur during periods of "light anesthesia," and until the development of the BIS monitor traditional methods of predicting probability of recall included skeletal muscle movement, increase in HR or blood pressure, pupillary changes, and perspiration.[119] Unfortunately, reliability of somatic signs is reduced by the use of neuromuscular blockers and autonomic nervous system changes caused by medications such as β-blockers and opioids.[117]

Deeper levels of anesthesia are associated with a lower incidence of recall.[119] BIS values within the general anesthesia range (40 to 70) correlate with low incidence of recall, whereas patients with higher BIS values (>70) are more likely to have recall.[120,121] However, a report has been made of patient recall with a BIS value of 47, which occurred without any autonomic or somatic evidence of light anesthesia.[122] This case report emphasizes the variability of patient response to anesthetics and encourages one not to rely on a single measurement to predict the possibility of recall. One must always assess the total clinical picture.

Hypnotic levels are also affected by anesthetic technique. Because BIS monitors only the hypnotic portion of an anesthetic procedure, use of a total opioid technique, which has little effect on hypnosis, produces a higher BIS number than a technique that uses potent volatile agents alone.[123,124] Similarly, nitrous oxide, when used as the sole anesthetic agent, has no effect on BIS.[125] In contrast, ketamine administration can transiently increase BIS values. The exact cause of this change is unknown.[126]

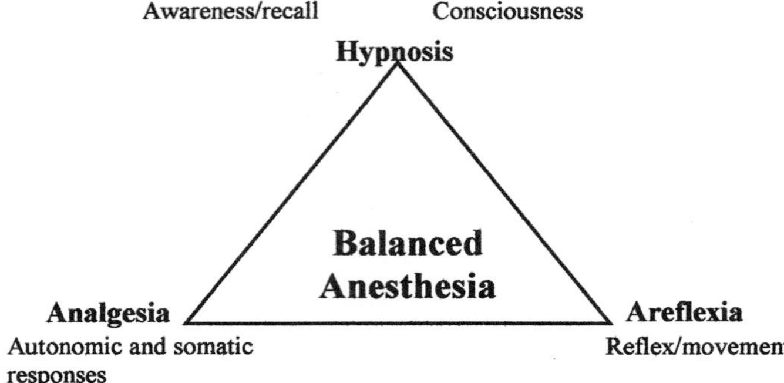

FIGURE **16-24**
The triad of balanced anesthesia: hypnosis, analgesia, and skeletal muscle relaxation. (Reproduced with permission from Apect MedicatSystems, Natick, Massachusetts.)

The BIS monitor allows more precise titration of anesthetic medications and therefore potentially more rapid patient emergence and recovery.[114,124,127] It also provides information to help guide anesthetic care. For example, an increase in HR or blood pressure during anesthesia is often interpreted as "light anesthesia" and treated by increasing the concentration of volatile agent or giving more opioids. However, if the BIS number is low in this setting (e.g., 50), deepening the anesthetic may not be the most suitable choice. A BIS value of 50 indicates that hypnosis is adequate. Therefore, it may be more appropriate to block the autonomic response through the use of a β-blocker.

Similar to EEG monitoring, the BIS monitor is susceptible to electrical interference. The use of unipolar electrocautery overloads BIS signal transmission and prevents the display of a BIS value. Similarly, electromyographic activity from a shivering patient,[128] the use of a forced air warmer placed over electrodes on the head, and pacemaker spikes can falsely elevate BIS readings.[129] As stated previously the BIS number is an average of information received over the prior 15 seconds. A sudden change in stimulation may cause an acute change in the level of hypnosis before the BIS value adjusts.

A new monitor call the *Patient Status Analyzer* (PSA) is currently undergoing clinical trials to judge its effectiveness as a monitor of depth of anesthesia. Operational principles are similar to those of the BIS monitor. However, the numerical values of the PSA uses a different scale, and interpretation is derived from four EEG channels as compared with one for the BIS monitor.[130]

Anesthesia balances amnesia, analgesia, skeletal muscle movement, and autonomic responses with surgical stimulation (Figure 16-24). Whatever method one chooses to monitor a patient's depth of anesthesia, it is necessary to take into consideration anesthetic technique, patient variability, and stimulation that arises from surgical manipulation.

TEMPERATURE MONITORING

In humans temperature is maintained between 36° and 37.5° C through a complex balance between heat loss and heat production.[131] Adverse physiologic effects are seen with temperatures above or below this range. Although both hyperthermia and hypothermia occur in the operative setting, hypothermia is much more common. Temperature monitoring can help detect hypothermia or hyperthermia, with the latter being a sign of malignant hyperpyrexia. Because of this, it is mandated by the American Association of Nurse Anesthetists that temperature be monitored during all general anesthetic cases lasting longer than 30 minutes and all pediatric anesthetic cases regardless of duration.[94]

The body can essentially be divided into two temperature zones: core temperature and peripheral temperature. Core temperature includes the trunk and major vessels, whereas the peripheral temperature includes the arms and legs. Temperature is maintained in the unanesthetized person through many physiologic and psychologic mechanisms that decrease heat loss and increase heat production. Physiologically, shivering is an example of heat production. Heat loss is decreased through peripheral vasoconstriction, which helps to keep vital organs normothermic.[132]

The perioperative setting contributes to the development of hypothermia. The cold environment of the operating room and the infusion of cold fluid promote heat loss. Both regional and general anesthetic techniques inhibit peripheral vasoconstriction. In addition, general anesthetics lower the hypothermic set point of the hypothalamus and inhibit behavioral mechanisms that normally prevent hypothermia.[133,134]

Effects of Hypothermia

Metabolic Rate

Hypothermia essentially affects all systems. It decreases metabolic rate. For this reason it is induced during certain neurosurgical and cardiac procedures for organ protection.[135-137] Most other effects are not beneficial and can be deleterious.

Cardiovascular Effects

As temperature decreases, initial sympathetic activation leads to an increase in HR, stroke volume, and peripheral vascular resistance, which increases myocardial oxygen demand.[138,139] As fluid shifts from the intravascular space, blood viscosity increases. If shivering occurs, oxygen demand can increase 400-fold.[140] Below 34° C the risk of ventricular dysrhythmias increases and bradycardia occurs, and at 32° C cardiac output begins to decline.[141,142]

Central Nervous System Effects

Hypothermia depresses membrane conduction and chemical processes. EEG waves begin to slow at a temperature of 35° C, with coma ensuing below a temperature of 32° C.[141,143] Cerebral blood flow and oxygen consumption decrease with hypothermia with a correlating decrease in anesthetic requirements.[144]

Coagulation Effects

Significant hypothermia produces a coagulopathy.[145] The coagulation cascade is an enzyme system, dependent on normothermia for proper function. Hypothermia decreases induction of the cascade, thereby inhibiting thrombin formation.[146] During hypothermia platelets are sequestered in the liver, and the function of circulating platelets is reduced.[145,147] The resulting relative thrombocytopenia contributes to the development of a coagulopathy.

Respiratory Effects

Initially, hypothermia stimulates the respiratory system, as evidenced by an increase in respiratory rate. Below 34° C respiratory rate decreases as the response to PCO_2 decreases. Respiratory drive, however, does not cease until 24° C. Hypoxic vasoconstriction is reduced, dead space can be increased through bronchodilation, and the oxyhemoglobin dissociation curve is shifted to the left.[148] All these factors lead to an increase in ventilation-perfusion mismatches.

Drug Metabolism and Elimination

Hepatic and renal blood flows are reduced during hypothermia. This causes a reduction in enzymatic activity in the liver and a decrease in glomerular filtration rate. The net result is a prolonged duration of action of many drugs.[149,150] Other effects of hypothermia include a decrease in wound healing[151] and an increase in the incidence of wound infections.

Core Temperature Monitoring

It is important to monitor core temperature during anesthesia, because peripheral and core temperatures may differ significantly. Sites for monitoring core temperature include the esophagus, nasopharynx, tympanic membrane, and PA. More peripheral sites include the skin, axilla, and rectum.

Maintaining Normothermia

The most effective means of preventing hypothermia during surgery is maintenance of an environmental temperature of at least 26° C.[152] This, however, is difficult to accomplish in the operating arena. Of all warming techniques available, the most commonly used are fluid warmers and forced air warmers. Of the two, the more efficacious is the forced air warmer.[153]

Maintaining patient normothermia during surgery can be a challenge for anesthesia providers. Monitoring patient temperature during an anesthetic procedure can help in detection and prevention of hypothermia and hyperthermia.

REFERENCES

1. Swan HJ, Ganz W, Forrester J, Marcus H, Diamond G, Chonette D. Catheterization of the heart in man with use of a flow-directed balloon-tipped catheter. *N Engl J Med.* 1970;283: 447-451.
2. Cruz K, Franklin C. The pulmonary artery catheter: uses and controversies. *Crit Care Clin.* 2001;17:271-291.
3. Jacka MJ, Cohen MM, To T, Devitt JH, Byrick R. The appropriateness of the pulmonary artery catheter in cardiovascular surgery [comment]. *Can J Anaesth.* 2002;49:276-282.
4. Sandham JD, Hull RD, Brant RF, et al. A randomized, controlled trial of the use of pulmonary-artery catheters in high-risk surgical patients [comment]. *N Engl J Med.* 2003;348:5-14.
5. de Jonge E, van Lieshout EJ, Vroom MB. The value of the pulmonary-artery catheter: not ruled out, but not proven either. *Ned Tijdschr Geneeskd.* 2003;147:792-795.
6. Handa F, Kyo SE, Miyao H. Reduction in the use of pulmonary artery catheter for cardiovascular surgery. *Masui.* 2003;52:420-423.
7. Rao TL, Jacobs KH, El-Etr AA. Reinfarction following anesthesia in patients with myocardial infarction. *Anesthesiology.* 1983;59:499-505.
8. Heyland DK, Cook DJ, King D, Kernerman P, Brun-Buisson C. Maximizing oxygen delivery in critically ill patients: a methodologic appraisal of the evidence. *Crit Care Med.* 1996;24:517-524.
9. Iberti TJ, Fischer EP, Leibowitz AB, Panacek EA, Silverstein JH, Albertson TE. A multicenter study of physicians' knowledge of

the pulmonary artery catheter. Pulmonary Artery Catheter Study Group. *JAMA*. 1990;264:2928-2932.
10. Jacka MJ, Cohen MM, To T, Devitt JH, Byrick R. Pulmonary artery occlusion pressure estimation: how confident are anesthesiologists [comment]? *Crit Care Med*. 2002;30:1197-1203.
11. Shoemaker WC, Appel PL, Kram HB, Waxman K, Lee TS. Prospective trial of supranormal values of survivors as therapeutic goals in high-risk surgical patients. *Chest*. 1988;94:1176-1186.
12. American College of Physicians/American College of Cardiology/American Heart Association Task Force on Clinical Privileges in Cardiology. Clinical competence in hemodynamic monitoring. *J Am Coll Cardiol*. 1990;15:1460-1464.
13. American Society of Anesthesiologists Task Force on Pulmonary Artery Catheterization. Practice guidelines for pulmonary artery catheterization. *Anesthesiology*. 1993;78:380-394.
14. Shah KB, Rao TL, Laughlin S, El-Etr AA. A review of pulmonary artery catheterization in 6,245 patients. *Anesthesiology*. 1984;61:271-275.
15. Pichard AD, Diaz R, Marchant E, Casanegra P. Large V waves in the pulmonary capillary wedge pressure tracing without mitral regurgitation: the influence of the pressure/volume relationship on the V wave size. *Clin Cardiol*. 1983;6:534-541.
16. Beique F, Ramsay JG. The pulmonary artery catheter: a new look. *Semin Anesth*. 1994;13:14-25.
17. Nadeau S, Noble WH. Misinterpretation of pressure measurements from the pulmonary artery catheter. *Can Anaesth Soc J*. 1986;33:352-363.
18. West JB, Dollery CT, Naimark A. Distribution of blood flow in isolated lung: relation to vascular and alveolar pressures. *J Appl Physiol*. 1964;19:713-724.
19. Enson Y, Wood JA, Mantaras NB, Harvey RM. The influence of heart rate on pulmonary arterial-left ventricular pressure relationships at end-diastole. *Circulation*. 1977;56:533-539.
20. Mitchell JH, Gilmore JP, Sarnoff SJ. The transport function of the atrium: factors influencing the relation between mean left atrial pressure and left ventricular end diastolic pressure. *Am J Cardiol*. 1962;9:237-247.
21. Raper R, Sibbald WJ. Misled by the wedge? The Swan-Ganz catheter and left ventricular preload. *Chest*. 1986;89:427-434.
22. Douglas PS, Edmunds LH, Sutton MS, Geer R, Harken AH, Reichek N. Unreliability of hemodynamic indexes of left ventricular size during cardiac surgery. *Ann Thorac Surg*. 1987;44:31-34.
23. Herbert WH. Pulmonary artery and left heart end-diastolic pressure relations. *Br Heart J*. 1970;32:774-778.
24. McGregor M, Sniderman A. On pulmonary vascular resistance: the need for more precise definition. *Am J Cardiol*. 1985;55:217-221.
25. Shoemaker WC, Appel P, Bland R. Use of physiologic monitoring to predict outcome and to assist in clinical decisions in critically ill postoperative patients. *Am J Surg*. 1983;146:43-50.
26. Shoemaker WC. Diagnosis and treatment of the shock and circulatory dysfunction. In: Shoemaker WC, Ayres SM, Grenvik A, Holbrook PR, eds. *Textbook of Critical Care*. 4th ed. Philadelphia: Saunders; 2000:92-114.
27. Reeves JT, Grover RF, Filley GF, Blount SG Jr. Cardiac output in normal resting man. *J Appl Physiol*. 1961;16:276-278.
28. Fegler G. Measurement of cardiac output in anesthetized animals by a thermodilution method. *Q J Exp Physiol*. 1954;39:153-164.
29. Hines R, Barash P. Pulmonary artery catheterization. In: Blitt C, Hines R, eds. *Monitoring in Anesthesia and Critical Care Medicine*. 3rd ed. New York: Churchill Livingstone; 1995:231-259.
30. Forrester JS, Ganz W, Diamond G, McHugh T, Chonette DW, Swan HJ. Thermodilution cardiac output determination with a single flow-directed catheter. *Am Heart J*. 1972;83:306-311.
31. Pearl RG, Rosenthal MH, Nielson L, Ashton JP, Brown BW Jr. Effect of injectate volume and temperature on thermodilution cardiac output determination. *Anesthesiology*. 1986;64:798-801.
32. Nelson LD, Houtchens BA. Automatic vs manual injections for thermodilution cardiac output determinations. *Crit Care Med*. 1982;10:190-192.
33. Synder JV, Powner DJ. Effects of mechanical ventilation on the measurement of cardiac output by thermodilution. *Crit Care Med*. 1982;10:677-682.
34. Stevens JH, Raffin TA, Mihm FG, Rosenthal MH, Stetz CW. Thermodilution cardiac output measurement. Effects of the respiratory cycle on its reproducibility. *JAMA*. 1985;253:2240-2242.
35. Weisel RD, Berger RL, Hechtman HB. Current concepts measurement of cardiac output by thermodilution. *N Engl J Med*. 1975;292:682-684.
36. Nishikawa T, Dohi S. Slowing of heart rate during cardiac output measurement by thermodilution. *Anesthesiology*. 1982;57:538-539.
37. Hamilton MA, Stevenson LW, Woo M, Child JS, Tillisch JH. Effect of tricuspid regurgitation on the reliability of the thermodilution cardiac output technique in congestive heart failure. *Am J Cardiol*. 1989;64:945-948.
38. Pearl RG, Siegel LC. Thermodilution cardiac output measurement with a large left-to-right shunt. *J Clin Monit*. 1991;7:146-153.
39. Heerdt PM, Pond CG, Blessios GA, Rosenbloom M. Inaccuracy of cardiac output by thermodilution during acute tricuspid regurgitation. *Ann Thorac Surg*. 1992;53:706-708.
40. Stetz CW, Miller RG, Kelly GE, Raffin TA. Reliability of the thermodilution method in the determination of cardiac output in clinical practice. *Am Rev Respir Dis*. 1982;126:1001-1004.
41. Maruschak GF, Potter AM, Schauble JF, Rogers MC. Overestimation of pediatric cardiac output by thermal indicator loss. *Circulation*. 1982;65:380-383.
42. Hillis LD, Firth BG, Winniford MD. Analysis of factors affecting the variability of Fick versus indicator dilution measurements of cardiac output. *Am J Cardiol*. 1985;56:764-768.
43. Fischer AP, Benis AM, Jurado RA, Seely E, Teirstein P, Litwak RS. Analysis of errors in measurement of cardiac output by simultaneous dye and thermal dilution in cardiothoracic surgical patients. *Cardiovasc Res*. 1978;12:190-199.
44. Yelderman M. Continuous measurement of cardiac output with the use of stochastic system identification techniques. *J Clin Monit*. 1990;6:322-332.
45. Luchette FA, Porembka D, Davis K Jr, et al. Effects of body temperature on accuracy of continuous cardiac output measurements. *J Invest Surg*. 2000;13:147-152.
46. Nelson LD. The new pulmonary artery catheters: continuous venous oximetry, right ventricular ejection fraction, and continuous cardiac output. *New Horiz*. 1997;5:251-258.
47. Poli de Figueiredo LF, Malbouisson LM, Varicoda EY, Carmona MJ, Auler JO Jr, Rocha e Silva M. Thermal filament continuous thermodilution cardiac output delayed response limits its value during acute hemodynamic instability. *J Trauma*. 1999;47:288-293.
48. Zollner C, Polasek J, Kilger E, et al. Evaluation of a new continuous thermodilution cardiac output monitor in cardiac surgical patients: a prospective criterion standard study. *Crit Care Med*. 1999;27:293-298.
49. Lazor MA, Pierce ET, Stanley GD, Cass JL, Halpern EF, Bode RH Jr. Evaluation of the accuracy and response time of STAT-mode continuous cardiac output. *J Cardiothorac Vasc Anesth*. 1997;11:432-436.
50. Medin DL, Brown DT, Wesley R, Cunnion RE, Ognibene FP. Validation of continuous thermodilution cardiac output in critically ill patients with analysis of systematic errors. *J Crit Care*. 1998;13:184-189.
51. Cariou A, Monchi M, Dhainaut JF. Continuous cardiac output and mixed venous oxygen saturation monitoring. *J Crit Care*. 1998;13:198-213.
52. Mihm FG, Gettinger A, Hanson CW 3rd, et al. A multicenter evaluation of a new continuous cardiac output pulmonary artery catheter system. *Crit Care Med*. 1998;26:1346-1350.

53. Giuliano KK, Scott SS, Brown V, Olson M. Backrest angle and cardiac output measurement in critically ill patients. *Nurs Res.* 2003;52:242-248.
54. Schmid ER, Schmidlin D, Tornic M, Seifert B. Continuous thermodilution cardiac output: clinical validation against a reference technique of known accuracy. *Intensive Care Med.* 1999;25:166-172.
55. Zollner C, Goetz AE, Weis M, et al. Continuous cardiac output measurements do not agree with conventional bolus thermodilution cardiac output determination. *Can J Anaesth.* 2001;48:1143-1147.
56. Forster MR, Ip-Yam PC. Pericardial injury following severe sepsis from faecal peritonitis—a case report on the use of continuous cardiac output monitoring. *Ann Acad Med Singapore.* 1998;27:857-859.
57. Norfleet EA, Watson CB. Continuous mixed venous oxygen saturation measurement: a significant advance in hemodynamic monitoring? *J Clin Monit.* 1985;1:245-258.
58. Magilligan DJ Jr, Teasdall R, Eisinminger R, Peterson E. Mixed venous oxygen saturation as a predictor of cardiac output in the postoperative cardiac surgical patient. *Ann Thorac Surg.* 1987;44:260-262.
59. Waller JL, Kaplan JA, Bauman DI, Craver JM. Clinical evaluation of a new fiberoptic catheter oximeter during cardiac surgery. *Anesth Analg.* 1982;61:676-679.
60. Krafft P, Steltzer H, Hiesmayr M, Klimscha W, Hammerle AF. Mixed venous oxygen saturation in critically ill septic shock patients. The role of defined events. *Chest.* 1993;103:900-906.
61. Ahrens T. Continuous mixed venous ($S\bar{v}O_2$) monitoring. Too expensive or indispensable? *Crit Care Nur Clin North Am.* 1999;11:33-48.
62. Tweddell JS, Hoffman GM, Fedderly RT, et al. Patients at risk for low systemic oxygen delivery after the Norwood procedure. *Ann Thorac Surg.* 2000;69:1893-1899.
63. Tweddell JS, Hoffman GM, Mussatto KA, et al. Improved survival of patients undergoing palliation of hypoplastic left heart syndrome: lessons learned from 115 consecutive patients. *Circulation.* 2002;106:182-189.
64. Sumimoto T, Takayama Y, Iwasaka T, et al. Mixed venous oxygen saturation as a guide to tissue oxygenation and prognosis in patients with acute myocardial infarction. *Am Heart J.* 1991;122:27-33.
65. Krouskop RW, Cabatu EE, Chelliah BP, McDonnell FE, Brown EG. Accuracy and clinical utility of an oxygen saturation catheter. *Crit Care Med.* 1983;11:744-749.
66. van Woerkens EC, Trouwborst A, Tenbrinck R. Accuracy of a mixed venous saturation catheter during acutely induced changes in hematocrit in humans. *Crit Care Med.* 1991;19:1025-1029.
67. Armaganidis A, Dhainaut JF, Billard JL, et al. Accuracy assessment for three fiberoptic pulmonary artery catheters for $S\bar{v}O_2$ monitoring. *Intensive Care Med.* 1994;20:484-488.
68. Pulmonary Artery Catheter Consensus Conference Participants. Pulmonary artery catheter consensus conference: consensus statement. *Crit Care Med.* 1997;25:910.
69. Squara P, Fourquet E, Jacquet L, et al. A computer program for interpreting pulmonary artery catheterization data: results of the European HEMODYN Resident Study. *Intensive Care Med.* 2003;29:735-741.
70. Kotrly KJ, Kotter GS, Mortara D, Kampine JP. Intraoperative detection of myocardial ischemia with an ST segment trend monitoring system. *Anesth Analg.* 1984;63:343-345.
71. Slogoff S, Keats AS. Does perioperative myocardial ischemia lead to postoperative myocardial infarction? *Anesthesiology.* 1985;62:107-114.
72. Mangano DT, Hollenberg M, Fegert G, et al. Perioperative myocardial ischemia in patients undergoing noncardiac surgery—I: incidence and severity during the 4 day perioperative period. The Study of Perioperative Ischemia (SPI) Research Group. *J Am Coll Cardiol.* 1991;17:843-850.
73. Coriat P, Harari A, Daloz M, Viars P. Clinical predictors of intraoperative myocardial ischemia in patients with coronary artery disease undergoing non-cardiac surgery. *Acta Anaesthesiol Scand.* 1982;26:287-290.
74. Sonntag H, Larsen R, Hilfiker O, Kettler D, Brockschnieder B. Myocardial blood flow and oxygen consumption during high-dose fentanyl anesthesia in patients with coronary artery disease. *Anesthesiology.* 1982;56:417-422.
75. Leung JM, Voskanian A, Bellows WH, Pastor D. Automated electrocardiograph ST segment trending monitors: accuracy in detecting myocardial ischemia. *Anesth Analg.* 1998;87:4-10.
76. Eagle KA, Berger PB, Calkins H, et al. ACC/AHA guideline update for perioperative cardiovascular evaluation for noncardiac surgery—executive summary: a report of the American College of Cardiology/American Heart Association Task Force on Practice Guidelines (Committee to Update the 1996 Guidelines on Perioperative Cardiovascular Evaluation for Noncardiac Surgery). *J Am Coll Cardiol.* 2002;39:542-553.
77. Slogoff S, Keats AS, David Y, Igo SR. Incidence of perioperative myocardial ischemia detected by different electrocardiographic systems. *Anesthesiology.* 1990;73:1074-1081.
78. Lehtinen R, Sievanen H, Turjanmaa V, Niemela K, Malmivuo J. Effect of ST segment measurement point on performance of exercise ECG analysis. *Int J Cardiology.* 1997;61:239-245.
79. Kossick MA. Recognizing EKG evidence of ischemia, injury, and infarction. In: *EKG Interpretation: Simple, Thorough, Practical.* 2nd ed. Park Ridge, Ill: AANA Publishing; 1999:18-29.
80. Ribisl PM, Liu J, Mousa I, et al. Comparison of computer ST criteria for diagnosis of severe coronary artery disease. *Am J Cardiology.* 1993;71:546-551.
81. Sansoy V, Watson DD, Beller GA. Significance of slow upsloping ST-segment depression on exercise stress testing. *Am J Cardiol.* 1997;79:709-712.
82. Mizutani M, Ben Freedman S, Barns E, Ogasawara S, Bailey BP, Bernstein L. ST monitoring for myocardial ischemia during and after coronary angioplasty. *Am J Cardiol.* 1990;66:389-393.
83. Horacek BM, Warren JW, Penney CJ, et al. Optimal electrocardiographic leads for detecting acute myocardial ischemia. *J Electrocardiol.* 2001;34:97-111.
84. Jain U. An electrocardiographic lead system for coronary artery bypass surgery. *J Clin Anesth.* 1996;8:19-24.
85. Smith JS, Cahalan MK, Benefiel DJ, et al. Intraoperative detection of myocardial ischemia in high-risk patients: electrocardiography versus two-dimensional transesophageal echocardiography. *Circulation.* 1985;72:1015-1021.
86. Drew BJ, Adams MG, Pelter MM, Wung SF. ST segment monitoring with a derived 12-lead electrocardiogram is superior to routine cardiac care unit monitoring. *Am J Crit Care.* 1996;5:198-206.
87. Drew BJ, Adams MG, Pelter MM, Wung SF, Caldwell MA. Comparison of standard and derived 12-lead electrocardiograms for diagnosis of coronary angioplasty-induced myocardial ischemia. *Am J Cardiol.* 1997;79:639-644.
88. Drew BJ, Pelter MM, Wung SF, et al. Accuracy of the EASI 12-lead electrocardiogram compared to the standard 12-lead electrocardiogram for diagnosing multiple cardiac abnormalities. *J Electrocardiol.* 1999;32(suppl):38-47.
89. Horacek BM, Warren JW, Stovicek P, Feldman CL. Diagnostic accuracy of derived versus standard 12-lead electrocardiograms. *J Electrocardiol.* 2000;33(suppl):155-160.
90. Rautaharju PM, Zhou SH, Hancock EW, et al. Comparability of 12-lead ECGs derived from EASI leads with standard 12-lead ECGs in the classification of acute myocardial ischemia and old myocardial infarction. *J Electrocardiol.* 2002;35 (suppl):35-39.
91. Pahlm O, Pettersson J, Thulin A, Feldman CL, Feild DQ, Wagner GS. Comparison of waveforms in conventional 12-lead ECGs and those derived from EASI leads in children. *J Electrocardiol.* 2003;36:25-31.

92. Berson AS, Pipberger HV. The low-frequency response of electrocardiographs, a frequent source of recording errors. *Am Heart J*. 1966;71:779-789.
93. Mark JB. Direct arterial blood pressure monitoring. In: *Atlas of Cardiovascular Monitoring*. New York: Churchill Livingstone; 1998:100-126.
94. Tunajek S, ed. *Standards of Care in Anesthesia Practice*. Park Ridge Ill: AANA Publishing; 2001.
95. Riva-Rocci S. Un sfigmomanometro nuovo. *Gazetta Medica di Torino*. 1896;47:981-986.
96. Shevchenko YL, Tsitlik JE. Ninetieth anniversary of the development by Nikolai S. Korotkoff of the auscultatory method of measuring blood pressure. *Circulation*. 1996;94:116-118.
97. Reitan JA, Barash BG, eds. *Noninvasive Monitoring*. New York: John Wiley & Sons; 1978.
98. Gilbert HC, Vender JS. Cardiovascular monitoring. In: Kirby RR, Gravenstein N, Lobato EB, Gravenstein JS, eds. *Clinical Anesthesia Practice*. 2nd ed. Philadelphia: Saunders; 2002:360-384.
99. Naqvi NH. Who was the first to monitor blood pressure during anaesthesia? *Eur J Anaesthesiol*. 1998;15:255-259.
100. Aylett M, Marples G, Jones K, Rhodes D. Evaluation of normal and large sphygmomanometer cuffs using the Omron 705CP. *J Hum Hypertens*. 2001;15:131-134.
101. Block FE, Schulte GT. Ankle blood pressure measurement, an acceptable alternative to arm measurements. *Int J Clin Monit Comput*. 1996;13:167-171.
102. Khan SQ, Wardlaw JM, Davenport R, Slattery J, Lewis S. Use of a neonatal blood pressure cuff to monitor blood pressure in the adult finger—comparison with a standard adult arm cuff. *J Clin Monit Comput*. 1998;14:233-238.
103. Yong P, Geddes L. The effect of cuff pressure deflation rate on accuracy in indirect measurement of blood pressure with the auscultatory method. *J Clin Monit Comput*. 1987;3:155.
104. Kerner T, Deja M, Ahlers O, et al. Monitoring arterial blood pressure during whole body hyperthermia. *Acta Anaesthesiol Scand*. 2002;46:561-566.
105. Lin CC, Jawan B, de Villa MV, Chen FC, Liu PP. Blood pressure cuff compression injury of the radial nerve. *J Clin Anesth*. 2001;13:306-308.
106. Sutin K, Longaker M, Wahlander S, Kasabian A, Capan L. Acute biceps compartment syndrome associated with the use of a noninvasive blood pressure monitor. *Anesth Analg*. 1996;83:1345-1346.
107. Davis P, Kenny G. *Basic Physics and Measurements in Anaesthesia*. 5th ed. Edinburgh: Butterworth Heinemann; 2002.
108. Gardner RM. Direct blood pressure measurement—dynamic response requirements. *Anesthesiology*. 1981;54:227-236.
109. Blitt CD, Hines RL. *Monitoring in Anesthesia and Critical Care Medicine*. 5th ed. New York: Churchill Livingstone; 1995.
110. Paolella L, Dorfman G, Cronan JJ, Hasan FM. Topographic location of the left atrium by computed tomography: reducing pulmonary artery catheter calibration error. *Crit Care Med*. 1988;16:1154-1156.
111. Shah N, Bedford RF. Invasive and noninvasive blood pressure monitoring. In: Lake CL, Hines RL, Blitt CD, eds. *Clinical Monitoring—Practical Applications for Anesthesia and Critical Care*. Philadelphia: Saunders ; 2001:181-203.
112. Allen E. Thromboangiitis obliterans: methods of diagnosis of chronic obstructive lesions distal to the wrist with illustrative cases. *Am J Med Sci*. 1929:178-237.
113. Bloom M. Electroencephalography and monitoring of anesthetic depth. In: Lake CL, Hines RL, Blitt CD, eds. *Clinical Monitoring—Practical Applications for Anesthesia and Critical Care*. Philadelphia: Saunders; 2001:92-101.
114. Rosow C, Manberg PJ. Bispectral index monitoring. *Anesthesiol Clin North Am*. 2001;19:xi, 947-966.
115. Rampil I. A primer for EEG signal processing in anesthesia. *Anesthesiology*. 1998;89:980-1002.
116. Jasper H. The ten-twenty electrode system of the International Federation. *Electroencephalogr Clin Neurophysiol*. 1958;10: 371-375.
117. Pete H, Spitellie PH, Holmes MA, Domino KB. Awareness during anesthesia. *Anesthesiol Clin North Am*. 2002;20:317-332.
118. Davidson AJ. Awareness and paediatric anaesthesia. *Paediatr Anaesth*. 2002;12:567-568.
119. Domino KB, Posner KL, Caplan RA, Cheney FW. Awareness during anesthesia: a closed claims analysis. *Anesthesiology*. 1999;90:1053-1061.
120. Glass PS, Bloom M, Kearse L, Rosow C, Sebel P, Manberg P. Bispectral analysis measures sedation and memory effects of propofol, midazolam, isoflurane, and alfentanil in healthy volunteers. *Anesthesiology*. 1997;86:836-847.
121. Kearse LA Jr, Rosow C, Zaslavsky A, Connors P, Dershwitz M, Denman W. Bispectral analysis of the electroencephalogram predicts conscious processing of information during propofol sedation and hypnosis. *Anesthesiology*. 1998;88:25-34.
122. Mychaskiw IG, Horowitz M, Sachdev V, Heath B. Explicit intraoperative recall at a bispectral index of 47. *Anesth Analg*. 2001;92:808-809.
123. Iselin-Chaves, Flaishon R, Sebel P. The effect of the interaction of propofol and alfentanil on recall, loss of consciousness, and the bispectral index. *Anesth Analg*. 1998;87:949-955.
124. Gan TJ, Glass PS, Windsor A, et al. Bispectral index monitoring allows faster emergence and improved recovery from propofol, alfentanil, and nitrous oxide anesthesia. BIS Utility Study Group. *Anesthesiology*. 1997;87(4):808-815.
125. Barr G, Jakobsso J, Owall A, Anderson R. Nitrous oxide does not alter bispectral index: Study with nitrous oxide as sole agent and as a adjunct to IV anaesthesia. *Br J Anaesth*. 1999;81: 827-830.
126. Sakai T, Singh H, Mi W, Kudo T, Matsuki A. The effect of ketamine on clinical endpoints of hypnosis and EEG variables during propofol infusion. *Acta Anaesthesiol Scand*. 1999;43:212-216.
127. Bard JW. The BIS monitor: a review and technology assessment. *AANA J*. 2001;69:477-483.
128. Bruhn J, Bouillon TW, Shafer SL. Electromyographic activity falsely elevates the bispectral index. *Anesthesiology*. 2000;92:1485-1487.
129. Hemmerling TM, Fortier JD. Falsely increased bispectral index values in a series of patients undergoing cardiac surgery using forced-air-warming therapy of the head. *Anesth Analg*. 2002;95:322-323.
130. Chen X, Tang J, White P, et al. Comparison of patient state index and bispectral index values during the perioperative period. *Anesth Analg*. 2002;95:1669-1674.
131. Wallace W. Normal temperature. *Br J Anaesth*. 1968;2:174.
132. Burton A. Human calorimetry: the average temperature of the tissues of the body. *J Nutr*. 1935;9:261-280.
133. Stoen R, Sessler DI. The thermoregulatory threshold is inversely proportional to isoflurane concentration. *Anesthesiology*. 1990;72:822-827.
134. Goto T, Matsukawa T, Sessler DI. Thermoregulatory thresholds for vasoconstriction in patients anesthetized with various 1-minimum alveolar concentration combinations of xenon, nitrous oxide and isoflurane. *Anesthesiology*. 1999;91:626-632.
135. Compagnoni G, Pogliani L, Lista G, Castoldi F, Fontana P, Mosca F. Hypothermia reduces neurological damage in asphyxiated newborn infants. *Biol Neonate*. 2002;82:222-227.
136. Wass CT, Lanier WL. Hypothermia-associated protection from ischemic brain injury: implications for patient management. *Int Anesth Clin*. 1996;34:95-111.
137. Ning XH, Chen SH, Xu CS, et al. Hypothermia preserves myocardial function and mitochondrial protein gene expression during hypoxia. *Am J Physiol Heart Circ Physiol*. 2003;285: 212-219.
138. Richards PG, Marath A, Edwards JM, Lincoln C. Management of difficult intracranial aneurysms by deep hypothermia and

elective cardiac arrest using cardiopulmonary bypass. *Br J Neurosurg*. 1987;1:261-269.
139. Frank S, Higgins M, Breslow M, et al. The Catecholamine, Cortisol, and Hemodynamic Responses to Mild Perioperative Hypothermia. 1995;82:83-93.
140. Bay J, Nunn J, Prys-Roberts C. Factors influencing arterial PO_2 during recovery from anaesthesia. *British Journal of Anaesthesia*. 1968;40:183-196.
141. Mattu A, Brady WJ, Perron AD. Electrocardiographic manifestations of hypothermia. *American Journal of Emergency Medicine*. 2002;20(4):314-326.
142. Groban L, Zapata-Sudo G, Lin M, Nelson TE. Effects of moderate and deep hypothermia on $Ca2+$ signaling in rat ventricular myocytes. *Cell Physiol Biochem*. 2002;12:101-110.
143. Harden A, Pampiglione G, Waterston DJ. Circulatory arrest during hypothermia in cardiac surgery: an EEG study in children. *Br Med J*. 1966;2:1105-1108.
144. Liu M, Hu X, Liu J. The effect of hypothermia on isoflurane MAC in children. *Anesthesiology*. 2001;94:429-432.
145. Schmeid J, Kurz A, Sessler DI, Kozek S, Reiter A. Mild intraoperative hypothermia increases blood loss and allogeneic transfusion requirements during total hop arthroplasty. *Lancet*. 1996;347:289-292.
146. Rohrer M, Natale A. Effect of hypothermia on the coagulation cascade. *Crit Care Med*. 1992;20:1402-1405.
147. Valeri R, Cassidy G, Khuri G, Feingold G, Ragno G, Altschule M. Hypothermia-induced reversible platelet dysfunction. *Ann Surg*. 1987;205:175-181.
148. Luginbuhl M, Schnider TW. Detection of awareness with the bispectral index: two case reports. *Anesthesiology*. 2002;96:241-243.
149. Heier T, Caldwell J, Sessler DI, Miller R. Mild intraoperative hypothermia increases duration of action and spontaneous recovery of vecuronium blockade during nitrous oxide-isoflurane anesthesia in humans. *Anesthesiology*. 1991;74:815-819.
150. Leslie K, Sessler DI, Bjorksten AR, Moayeri A. Mild hypothermia alters propofol pharmacokinetics and increases the duration of action of atracurium. *Anesth Analg*. 1995;80:1007-1014.
151. Kurz A, Sessler DI, Lenhardt R. A study of wound infection and temperature group: perioperative normothermia to reduce the incidence of surgical-wound infection and shorten hospitalization. *N Engl J Med*. 1996;334:1209-1215.
152. El-Gamal N, El-Kassabany N, Frank S, et al. Age-related thermoregulatory differences in a warm operating room environment (approximately 26° C). *Anesth Analg*. 2000;90:694-698.
153. Hynson J, Sessler DI, Christensen R, Turakhia M, Dechert M, Clough D. Intraoperative warming therapies: a comparison of three devices. *J Clin Anesth*. 1996;4:194-199.

CHAPTER 17

PREOPERATIVE EVALUATION AND PREPARATION OF THE PATIENT

REX A. MARLEY

A crucial element of the anesthesia provider's perioperative care of the patient includes a timely and thorough preoperative assessment. A fine-tuned approach to patient evaluation then enables appropriate interventions when required to properly prepare the patient for the upcoming anesthesia and surgery. For any patient scheduled to undergo anesthesia, preoperative evaluation is compulsory to help identify factors that increase the risk associated with anesthesia and the status of the patient relative to the proposed surgery. Essential goals of preoperative assessment and preparation of the patient include the following[1]:

1. Optimize patient care, satisfaction, comfort, and convenience.
2. Minimize perioperative morbidity and mortality by accurately assessing factors that influence the risk of anesthesia or that might alter the planned anesthetic technique.
3. Minimize surgical delays or preventable cancellations on the day of surgery.
4. Determine appropriate postoperative disposition of the patient (i.e., given the patient's status, whether the procedure is best performed on an ambulatory, inpatient, or intensive care basis).
5. Evaluate the patient's health status, thereby determining which, if any, preoperative investigations and specialty consultations are required.
6. Formulate a plan for the most appropriate perianesthetic care and postoperative supportive patient care.
7. Communicate patient management issues effectively among care providers.
8. Ensure time-efficient and cost-effective patient evaluation.

During the preoperative visit, patient assessment begins with a thorough review of the patient's medical records and patient interview, followed by the physical examination. A comprehensive medical history and physical examination are the cornerstones of a systematic approach to continued patient preparation. Information gathered from this evaluative process determines further individualized assessment (e.g., obtaining diagnostic tests, specialist consultation). The extent of this preoperative workup depends on the existing medical condition of the patient, the proposed surgical procedure, and the type of anesthesia. Significant findings from this initial evaluation enable the anesthesia provider to make adjustments in the patient's care (i.e., initiate specific treatment modalities to optimize the patient's condition for the proposed surgery and anesthesia).

An evolving challenge confronting anesthesia providers in the current managed care environment is the provision of high-quality patient care at a discounted cost. Changes designed to decrease costs include patient screening techniques (e.g., the preanesthesia assessment clinic) and intense scrutiny regarding the appropriate requisitioning of preoperative diagnostic testing. Important strategies for achieving high-quality, cost-effective patient evaluation include the following[2]:

1. Educating the practitioner (e.g., regarding the cost of diagnostic tests) and thereby modifying practice patterns
2. Developing and implementing practice guidelines
3. Using clinical pathways (interdepartmental teamwork required)
4. Disseminating information regarding protocols, thereby avoiding duplication of services
5. Performing economic analyses of services, including cost, effectiveness, and cost-benefit studies
6. Rendering efficient resource management
7. Providing for outcomes measurement

These concepts will become more familiar to practitioners as economic-based management.

PREANESTHESIA ASSESSMENT CLINIC

The preanesthesia assessment clinic has emerged as the most effective means of providing convenient "one-stop shopping" designed to (1) permit patient registration, (2) obtain a medical history and perform a physical examination, (3) promote patient teaching, (4) meet or schedule appointments with medical consultants, and (5) complete any required preoperative diagnostic testing. Successful preanesthesia assessment clinics have realized a reduction in patient anxiety,[3,4] last-minute surgical cancellations,[3] overall length of hospitalization after surgery,[4,5] and diagnostic testing,[6] as well as improvement in patient education[4] and a shift from inpatient to outpatient surgery status.[7] The preanesthesia assessment clinic allows patients scheduled for elective surgery to be evaluated and their condition optimized sufficiently in advance of the surgery.

Timing of Patient Assessment

Ideal preoperative assessment for surgery and anesthesia should take place well in advance of the proposed surgery to allow ample time for necessary risk assessment, preoperative testing, and specialty consultations. Patients with complex medical conditions should be evaluated at least 1 week before the scheduled procedure. Because of the present economic realities, patients undergoing more complex procedures and those who have complicated medical conditions (Box 17-1)[8] are frequently not admitted to the hospital before the day of surgery. Preoperative evaluation on the day of surgery can result in last-minute discoveries (e.g., of inappropriate fasting; suspected difficult airway; preexisting medical condition) that may result in surgical delay or cancellation. In one study no difference in the cancellation rate for ambulatory patients was observed between groups seen within 24 hours and groups seen within 1 to 30 days of the scheduled surgery.[9]

CHART REVIEW

To provide the basis for and direction of the patient interview and physical assessment, the patient's past and current medical records should be reviewed preoperatively. Ideally the anesthesia provider will have the opportunity to review the patient's medical records before the interview with the patient or caregiver.

Past Medical Records

For a patient who has undergone surgery at the same institution in the past, previous anesthesia records should be retrieved and reviewed, especially if complications are suspected. If past medical records are not available, the patient must provide details of significant anesthetic experiences. If this information suggests that the patient has an unusual condition (e.g., atypical plasma cholinesterase, susceptibility to malignant hyperthermia), surgery is delayed so that medical records can be obtained for review to provide further information that might affect patient care, or measures should be taken (e.g., avoidance of succinylcholine or mivacurium; provision of trigger-free anesthetic technique) to avoid consequences associated with the condition.

Patient Chart

A review of the current medical record includes verification of the surgical consent for accuracy and completeness. The names of the patient and surgeon, the date, and the proposed procedure should be matched with those on the operating room schedule. Demographic or baseline data, such as the age, height, and weight of the patient, can often be obtained from the admitting record. Vital sign trends and input-output totals are transcribed from graphic flow sheets, which may also contain pertinent data (e.g., daily blood glucose values for the diabetic patient).

Progress notes and consultation reports provide a valuable overview of the health history and physical status of the patient. Medical treatments, such as drug dosages and schedules, may be derived from these materials; diagnostic test results, conversely, should be obtained directly from their

BOX 17-1

Conditions that Require Early Preoperative Evaluation

General
- Medical conditions inhibiting ability to engage in normal daily activity
- Medical conditions necessitating continual assistance or monitoring at home within the past 6 months
- Admission within the past 2 months for acute episodes or exacerbation of chronic condition
- Use of medications (e.g., anticoagulants or monoamine oxidase inhibitors) for which modification of schedule or dosage might be required

Cardiocirculatory
- History of angina, coronary artery disease, myocardial infarction, symptomatic arrhythmias
- Poorly controlled hypertension (diastolic >110 mm Hg, systolic >160 mm Hg)
- History of congestive heart failure

Respiratory
- Asthma or chronic obstructive pulmonary disease that requires chronic medication, or acute exacerbation and progression of these diseases within the past 6 months
- History of major airway surgery, unusual airway anatomy, or upper or lower airway tumor or obstruction
- History of chronic respiratory distress requiring home ventilatory assistance or monitoring

Endocrinologic
- Non–diet-controlled diabetes (insulin or oral hypoglycemic agents)
- Adrenal disorders
- Active thyroid disease

Hepatic
- Active hepatobiliary disease or compromise

Musculoskeletal
- Kyphosis or scoliosis causing functional compromise
- Temporomandibular joint disorder with restricted mobility
- Cervical or thoracic spine injury

Oncologic
- Patients receiving chemotherapy
- Other oncologic process with significant physiologic residua or compromise

Gastrointestinal
- Massive obesity (>140% ideal body weight)
- Hiatal hernia
- Symptomatic gastroesophageal reflux

Modified from Pasternak LR. Preanesthesia evaluation of the surgical patient. In: Barash PG, ed.: ASA Refresher Courses in Anesthesiology. *Philadelphia: Lippincott; 1996:205-219.*

original sources. This retrieval of primary data prevents the possible misinterpretation of data that were transcribed incorrectly. Knowledge gleaned from a review of progress notes and consultative reports enables the anesthesia provider to formulate supplementary questioning, seek further specialist consultations, or obtain additional diagnostic testing as needed.

Baseline data concerning the patient, such as cultural diversity, coping mechanisms, or patient limitations (e.g., hearing impairment), can often be derived from nursing notes and can effectively guide the anesthesia provider in conducting a thorough preoperative interview. Increasingly the anesthetist must be able to appropriately interact with culturally diverse populations in order to properly evaluate and educate patients.[10]

A preanesthesia questionnaire is included on the patient's chart (Figure 17-1). This questionnaire should be part of the admission paperwork to be completed by the patient or the patient's caregiver and consists of a concise checklist regarding the patient's health history and medical care. When properly completed and readily available on the chart, the preanesthesia questionnaire allows the anesthesia provider's visit with the patient to be accomplished more efficiently. Interview questions and physical assessment are appropriately directed to abnormal findings and areas of concern.

PATIENT INTERVIEW

The preoperative interview may be conducted in person or by telephone. Although the personalized approach to the patient interview is preferred, for patients who are unable to visit the hospital setting (e.g., who live far from the hospital or have transportation constraints) an opportunity to participate in a telephone interview should be made available. Regardless of the location or approach used, the interview promotes a trusting relationship between the patient and anesthesia provider. When the interview is performed in a caring and unhurried manner, the degree of trust and confidence with anesthesia care is enhanced. Furthermore, compliance with perioperative instructions is increased when the patient is treated with respect; an example of such respect is addressing the patient using his or her surname unless instructed differently by the patient.

The title of the anesthesia provider and his or her specific role in the patient's perioperative care should also be defined. The patient is entitled to know whether the interviewer is a certified registered nurse anesthetist, student registered nurse anesthetist, anesthesiologist, or medical resident in anesthesiology. The professional appearance and attitude of the anesthesia provider also can create a positive impression during the preoperative visit.

The environment of the preoperative interview is staged to maximize the quality and effectiveness of the interaction. Adequate lighting enhances effective communication with the patient. Distractions, such as an operating television set, are eliminated. The anesthesia provider should ensure that the time and location of the interview, whether it occurs in person or by telephone, are convenient and private for the patient. A return visit or call may be necessary if the patient is eating or receiving medical therapy.

Because the preoperative interview is a private interaction between the patient and the anesthesia provider, visitors are requested to remain outside the interview area unless the patient wishes family members to be present. Otherwise, the patient may not volunteer confidential health information, such as a history of substance abuse or the sexual history. In certain situations, however, assistance from a family member or caregiver is required. The health history may be provided, for example, by the parent of a pediatric patient or by an interpreter for a patient with cognitive or language barriers.

The patient interview is designed to achieve specific objectives (Box 17-2, p. 338).[11] The interview process, along with patient education, yields beneficial consequences of reduced patient anxiety[12] and increased patient satisfaction.[13] A valuable step in preparing the patient or responsible caregivers (e.g., family members, legal guardian) for the scheduled surgery includes an educational process during which the staff counsels the patient concerning fundamental perioperative issues (Box 17-3, p. 338).[11] Reinforcing information to the patient verbally and in writing is essential to encourage patient compliance.[14] Coordinating the patient's visit to the preanesthesia assessment clinic to include educational time is ideal for the patient.

Patient History

The extent of a patient's health history depends partly on the amount of information available in the chart before surgery. If the surgeon has already documented a thorough medical history and physical examination, the interview can focus on confirming major findings and obtaining information that directly relates to the anesthetic management of the patient. The anesthesia provider must obtain and document a detailed health history, however, if one is unavailable in the chart during the preoperative visit.

The health history should be obtained in an organized and systematic way, as with the preanesthesia questionnaire, to minimize omission of important data. Open-ended and direct questions targeting each category of the checklist can be posed. With this approach, more detailed and graded responses are elicited from the patient. To avoid overwhelming or confusing a patient, questions are asked separately and formulated in comprehensible or layperson's terms.

Surgical History

The surgical history of a patient may be obtained from the chart or preoperative interview. Most patients vaguely recall surgical experiences, even from childhood operations. Information regarding complications related to previous operations, such as a peripheral nerve injury or uncontrolled blood loss, is elicited to determine the need for further investigation.

Anesthetic History

Past anesthetic experiences are often not as easily defined as the surgical history. It is important to determine the reaction of a patient to previously administered anesthetics. Adverse reactions to anesthetic agents and techniques, such as prolonged vomiting, difficult airway, malignant hyperthermia, postoperative delirium, anaphylaxis, and cardiopulmonary collapse, may simply be an annoyance to the patient or could be life threatening. Preoperative knowledge of these complications allows the anesthetic approach to be modified and the recurrence of the complication prevented. Causative factors are also thoroughly investigated in patients who note that a previous operation was aborted. Difficulties with airway management can alter the approach to endotracheal intubation, if indicated. Vague reports of fever and convulsions merit further investigation to rule out an episode of malignant hyperthermia.

QUESTION	YES	NO	COMMENTS
Height: ____ (cm) Weight: ____ (kg)			
Current Medications, Including Over-the-Counter & Herbal (dose & frequency):			
Allergies (include drugs, foods, & environmental items, i.e., latex):			
Previous Surgeries/Hospitalizations (list):			
Scheduled Surgery/Procedure:			
Anesthesia History			
Problems with anesthesia – self or blood relative?			
Respiratory			
Lung or breathing problems?			
Cough? If yes, do you bring up anything when you cough?			
Asthma? If yes, what is current treatment?			
Cold, flu, respiratory infection within the past 6 weeks?			
Diagnosed with sleep apnea? Do you snore?			
Ever required supplemental oxygen therapy?			
Abnormal chest x-ray?			
Smoke now or in past? If so, what type, how much, and for how many years?			
Exposed to passive smoke?			
Can you walk up two flights of stairs without getting short of breath?			
Do you have trouble walking one block?			
Cardiovascular			
Short of breath at night?			
Heart murmur?			
Heart attack, angina (with activity; @ rest), or chest pain related to your heart?			
Irregular heartbeat, or pacemaker?			
Congestive heart failure?			
Abnormal electrocardiogram?			
Problems with high blood pressure?			

FIGURE **17-1**
Preanesthesia questionnaire.

Continued

QUESTION	YES	NO	COMMENTS
Renal			
Kidney, bladder, or urine problems?			
Hepatic			
Jaundiced, now or in past?			
Liver problems, i.e., hepatitis?			
Use alcohol? If so, how much, how often, and when did you last use alcohol?			
Gastrointestinal			
Acid reflux, hiatal hernia, ulcer, or heartburn?			
Recent diarrhea?			
Neurologic			
Stroke, seizures, episodes of unconsciousness or fainting, or other neurological problems?			
Numbness or weakness in an arm or leg?			
Frequent headaches?			
Eye problem or problems with your vision?			
Hearing problems?			
Endocrine			
Diabetes or high blood sugar?			
Thyroid problems?			
Steroids (i.e., prednisone) during the past year?			
Musculoskeletal			
Back or neck problems?			
Arthritis?			
Physical disabilities?			
Hematologic			
Bleed easily?			
Anticoagulants (blood thinners) within the past month?			
Ever been anemic?			
Evaluated for sickle cell anemia?			
Object to blood products under any circumstances?			

FIGURE **17-1 cont'd**
Preanesthesia questionnaire.

QUESTION	YES	NO	COMMENTS
Cancer			
Diagnosed with cancer?			
Received treatment for cancer?			
Obstetrical			
Could you be pregnant? If yes, how many weeks?			
Airway			
Chipped or loose teeth, dentures, caps, bridgework?			
Problems with opening your mouth? Temporomandibular joint (TMJ) problems?			
Difficult airway management with previous anesthesia?			
Psychosocial			
Ever had mental health treatment?			
Taken prescribed psychiatric medications?			
Used "street" or "recreational" drugs? If so, when did you last use?			
Birth & Developmental (pediatrics)			
Child's delivery premature or at term?			
Neonatal complications?			
History of low heart rate or periods of low or absent respirations?			
Sudden infant death syndrome (SIDS) in your family?			
Do you have any medical problems that have not been discussed?			

FIGURE **17-1 cont'd**
Preanesthesia questionnaire.

Familial Anesthetic History

Numerous inheritable diseases involving metabolic derangements may affect a patient's reaction to stress and certain drugs, including the anesthetic agents. The patient is specifically asked whether any family member experienced an adverse reaction to anesthesia during surgery. Familial tendencies for diseases such as atypical plasma cholinesterase, malignant hyperthermia, porphyria, or glycogen storage diseases (e.g., glucose-6-phosphate deficiency) are then investigated. A diagnosis should be established before the surgery proceeds, because adjustments in the anesthetic management of the patient may be required.

Drug History

A preoperative drug history provides an excellent guide for the direction and depth of the patient interview and assessment. Drug dosages, schedules, and durations of treatment are reviewed. The patient is questioned about the purpose, as well as effectiveness, of his or her medications. An interview with a patient receiving β-adrenergic blockers, for example, can focus in greater detail on the cardiovascular system. Patients on medications for hypertension or angina pectoris require further investigation and possibly specialty consultation if they have not been recently evaluated.

Adverse Drug Effects and Interactions

Current drug therapy is carefully reviewed during the preoperative evaluation for side effects and potential interactions with anesthetic agents. Table 17-1 on pp. 339-340 lists selected drugs and their potential anesthetic interactions.[15] A drug management strategy is to discontinue particular drugs preoperatively in the hope of reducing the potential for adverse interactions. The therapeutic benefits of these drugs are weighed against the risks

BOX 17-2

Objectives of the Preoperative Interview

- Ensure that the goals of preoperative assessment are met.
- Provide preoperative education to the patient and family.
- Obtain informed consent.
- Acquaint the patient and family with the surgical process (to reduce stress and increase familiarity).
- Evaluate the patient's social situation with respect to surgery (e.g., support network).
- Motivate the patient to comply with preventive care strategies (e.g., smoking cessation, improvement of cardiovascular fitness).

Modified from Cassidy J, Marley RA. Preoperative assessment of the ambulatory patient. J Perianesth Nurs. *1996;11:334-343.*

BOX 17-3

Patient Education Objectives

- Promote interactive communication between patient and care provider.
- Encourage patient participation in making decisions about perioperative care.
- Maximize and enhance patient self-care skills and participation in continuing care during the postoperative phase.
- Increase the patient's ability to cope with his or her health status.
- Increase patient compliance with perioperative care.
- Provide individualized preoperative instructions regarding the following:

Where and when laboratory tests, consultations, and diagnostic procedures will be completed

Appropriate time at which the patient should cease ingestion of food and drink

Personal considerations (e.g., comfortable clothes to wear; no jewelry or makeup; what personal items to bring; leave valuables at home; bring favorite toy, comforter, or book)

Postoperative considerations and instructions (e.g., anticipated recovery course, discharge instructions, how to deal with complications)

Person to contact if the patient's physical conditions changes (e.g., upper respiratory tract infection, cancellation)

- Detail the process of arrival and registration on arrival to the surgical facility (i.e., time and location of arrival).
- Review advance directive information as required by law in some states.
- Explain the surgical facility policies to the patient and family.

Modified from Cassidy J, Marley RA. Preoperative assessment of the ambulatory patient. J Peri Anesth Nurs. *1996;11:334-343.*

of abrupt discontinuation. With occasional exceptions, the majority of medications are continued preoperatively. Should a decision be made to withhold a particular drug before surgery, sufficient time should be allowed for metabolic clearance (ideally three to five half-lives).[15]

Drug Allergies

A patient's drug history should include information regarding allergic reactions to certain foods and medications. Prior allergic responses are investigated so that they can be differentiated from adverse drug reactions. Use of certain antibiotics and opioids may be avoided because of gastrointestinal side effects. These do not represent a true allergic response, however. A distinction between allergic reactions and adverse effects is crucial, because an allergy to a drug is an absolute contraindication to its use. Medications within the same classification of a drug allergy should be avoided, and heightened awareness of a potential allergic reaction is required during the perioperative period.

Latex Sensitivity. Patient sensitivity to latex products has recently been identified as a frequent basis of allergic reaction. Up to 13% of intraoperative anaphylactic reactions have been attributed to latex sensitivity.[16] The preoperative questioning of patients should include inquiry regarding specific latex sensitivity or allergy. Patients at increased risk for latex sensitivity should be cared for in a no-latex setting and scheduled as the first case of the day to reduce the likelihood of aeroallergen latex exposure. The diagnosis of latex allergy is based on the findings of the history and physical examination, and if necessary, with in vivo (skin-prick test is the most sensitive) and in vitro testing. Patients at high risk for latex sensitivity include those with a history of the following[17,18]:

- Chronic exposure to latex-based products (e.g., workers in the natural rubber industry)
- Spina bifida, urologic reconstructive surgery
- Repeated surgical procedures (more than nine)
- Intolerance to latex-based products (e.g., balloons, rubber gloves, condoms, dental dams, rubber urethral catheters)
- Allergy to food and tropical fruits (e.g., banana, avocado, peach, passion fruit, kiwi, celery, chestnut)
- Intraoperative anaphylaxis of uncertain cause
- Working in health care, especially with a history of atopy or hand eczema

Social History

The addictive nature of tobacco and alcohol, as well as illegal drugs, exerts a detrimental influence on several aspects of life in the United States.

- More than 25% of Americans over age 15 years are physiologically dependent on at least one addictive substance.[19]
- Nearly one quarter of all deaths (75,000 annually)[20] in the United States are caused by addictive substances.[19]
- The economic burden of addiction (e.g., health-care expenditures, missed work, crime) is estimated at more than $400 billion annually.[19]

Certain drugs, despite their social or recreational application, may be associated with adverse and life-threatening consequences with long- or short-term use or overdose. The social history provides an excellent opportunity to explore the extent of self-medication. Open-ended questions, posed in a professional and nonjudgmental manner, are most likely to elicit detailed information from the patient. At this time the patient can also be educated about the adverse consequences of substance abuse, especially as such substances affect anesthetic care.

Tobacco Use

Many patients arrive for anesthesia and surgery with a history of tobacco smoking. In the United States some disturbing statistics are associated with this form of substance abuse:

TABLE 17-1 Potential Drug Interactions Affecting Perianesthesia Care

	PERIANESTHESIA CONCERN		
Drug Category	**Intraoperative Concerns**	**Management**	**Discontinuation Issues**
Drugs Affecting the Cardiovascular System			
Angiotensin converting enzyme (ACE) inhibitors	Hypotension with or without bradycardia; intolerance to hypovolemia	Maintain hydration; moderate doses of vasopressor	Brief interruption is well tolerated; continuation may improve regional blood flow and oxygen delivery and preserve renal function; consider withholding in patients taking amiodarone, on multiple (three or more) antihypertensives, or in whom even a brief period of hypotension is unacceptable
Diuretics	Hypokalemia; hypovolemia	Monitor potassium levels preoperatively; maintain hydration	Patients rarely become symptomatic if morning dose withheld; patients appreciate lack of urinary urgency while awaiting surgery; it might be desirable to continue in patients in whom diuretics are part of treatment for chronic renal failure
Antiarrhythmics	Cardiac depression; prolonged neuromuscular blockade; amiodarone—hypotension and atropine-resistant bradycardia requiring ventricular pacing	Monitor serum drug levels as needed; amiodarone—large doses of vasopressors or inotropes and pacemaker capability	Discontinuation rarely recommended because usually not prescribed for benign arrhythmias; amiodarone—impractical to discontinue because half-life is weeks to months; withhold concurrent medications (e.g., ACE inhibitors)
Drugs Affecting Hemostasis			
Nonsteroidal antiinflammatory drugs	Impaired platelet function; altered renal function; gastrointestinal bleeding		Unless the surgery puts the patient at particular risk for increased or catastrophic bleeding or impaired renal function, it is reasonable to continue up to morning of surgery
Anticoagulants (heparin, Coumadin)	Increased hemorrhage	May reverse heparin with IV protamine; may reverse Coumadin with vitamin K or fresh frozen plasma	Heparin—discontinue IV 4-5 hr before surgery and check PTT; Coumadin—discontinue 3-5 days before surgery and check PT
Fibrinolytic drugs (streptokinase, urokinase, tissue plasminogen activator)	Hemorrhage	Antifibrinolytic agent (aprotinin) may be indicated	Discontinuation usually not an option when administered for treatment of life-threatening conditions (e.g., acute myocardial infarction, massive pulmonary embolus)
Hypoglycemic Agents			
Insulin	Hyperglycemia; hypoglycemia	Monitor serum glucose; employ insulin supplementation protocol	Morning dose either withheld or reduced and adjustments in therapy based on periodic serum glucose determinations
Oral hypoglycemic agents	Hyperglycemia; hypoglycemia	Monitor serum glucose; avoid dehydration	Withhold oral hypoglycemic agents beginning on day of surgery

Continued

TABLE 17-1 Potential Drug Interactions Affecting Perianesthesia Care—cont'd

	PERIANESTHESIA CONCERN		
Drug Category	**Intraoperative Concerns**	**Management**	**Discontinuation Issues**
Drugs Affecting the Central Nervous System			
Monoamine oxidase inhibitors	Hypertension secondary to indirect-acting sympathomimetic drugs causing release of norepinephrine; excitatory state (from meperidine) or depressive phenomena secondary to opioid administration	Avoid known triggering agents such as meperidine and indirect-acting sympathomimetic agents (e.g., ephedrine)	Older, nonselective, irreversible monoamine oxidase inhibitors—discontinue for 2-3 wk with risk of serious psychiatric consequences; newer, reversible inhibitors of monoamine oxidase A—have short half-life, therefore discontinue drug on morning of surgery

IV, *Intravenous;* PT, *prothrombin time;* PTT, *partial thromboplastin time.*
Modified from Doak GJ. Discontinuing drugs before surgery. Can J Anaesth. *1997;44:R112-R117.*

- One in five deaths in the United States is related to smoking. Cigarette smoking is the leading cause of preventable premature death in the United States.[21]
- Of adults in the United States, 26% smoke. In 1994 in the United States 48 million adults were current smokers.[22]
- Teen smoking rates have increased by nearly one third from 1991 to 1997.[23]
- Smokers die almost 7 years earlier than nonsmokers.[24]
- Secondhand smoke is believed to cause 3000 deaths per year from lung cancer.[25]

The inhaled components of tobacco smoke lead to multiple pathophysiologic changes within the body (Box 17-4).[23,26-36] Nicotine and carbon monoxide are just two of the more than 2000 noxious components that have been identified in tobacco smoke.[37] Nicotine, a toxic alkaloid, produces ganglionic stimulant effects and is the tobacco component that affects the cardiovascular system.[38] Acute side effects of nicotine include increased heart rate, blood pressure, myocardial contraction, myocardial oxygen consumption, myocardial excitement, and peripheral vascular resistance. Net effects of nicotine's cardiovascular influence include impaired coronary blood flow and an adverse myocardial oxygen supply-demand ratio.[39] Carbon monoxide readily occupies the oxygen-binding sites of hemoglobin (approximately 250 to 300 times greater affinity for hemoglobin than oxygen).[40] Oxygen transport to the tissues and resultant oxygen use is thereby drastically reduced. In the heavy smoker, carboxyhemoglobin may be as high as 15%, which effectively reduces the patient's oxyhemoglobin percentage accordingly. The adverse effects of nicotine on the cardiovascular system and carbon monoxide on oxygen-carrying capacity are short lived (half-life of nicotine is 40 to 60 minutes[41,42]; half-life of carbon monoxide if room air is breathed is 130 to 190 minutes[43,44]). Patients should be instructed to stop smoking at least 12 hours before surgery. *Short-term (e.g., 12 hours) abstinence from tobacco smoke preoperatively reduces the deleterious effects of nicotine and carbon monoxide on cardiopulmonary function.*[45] Smoking cessation for even 1 night before surgery reduces heart rate, blood pressure, and circulating catecholamine levels[46] and allows carboxyhemoglobin values to return to normal levels.[47]

BOX 17-4

Risks Associated with Cigarette Smoking

Cardiovascular
Coronary artery disease (e.g., myocardial infarction), peripheral vascular occlusive disease, cerebrovascular disease, stroke

Respiratory
Chronic obstructive pulmonary disease, reduced lung function

Gastrointestinal
Peptic ulcer disease, esophageal reflux, gum disease, tooth loss

Cancer
Lung, oral cavity, larynx, esophagus, stomach, pancreas, kidney, urinary bladder, colon

Gestational
Perinatal—increases in miscarriage, stillbirth, low birth weight, and sudden infant death syndrome; impaired intellectual development
Maternal—increases in abruptio placentae and placenta previa

Ophthalmic
Macular degeneration, cataracts

Musculoskeletal
Osteoporosis, spinal disk disease

Reproductive
Infertility

Immune
Inhibited immune function

Dermatologic
Premature facial wrinkling

Patients who smoke have a higher incidence (a nearly sixfold increase[48]) of postoperative pulmonary complications (pneumonia and atelectasis).[49] Preoperative smoking cessation of at least 8 weeks is necessary before an appreciable improvement in pulmonary mechanics (e.g., enhanced ciliary function, decreased mucous secretion and small airway obstruction, and enhanced immune function) leads to a marked reduction in perioperative complications.[50-52] Patients who stopped smoking less than 2 months before surgery had nearly four times the pulmonary complications (e.g., purulent sputum, secretion retention, bronchospasm, pleural effusion, pneumothorax, segmental pulmonary collapse, pneumonia) of those who abstained from smoking for longer than 2 months.[52]

The influence of environmental tobacco smoke (also known as *secondhand* or *passive smoke*) on children has been found to produce disturbing respiratory consequences, including increased reactive airway disease,[53-55] abnormal results of pulmonary function tests,[56] and increased respiratory tract infections.[57] The perioperative complications in children exposed to smoke include laryngospasm,[58,59] coughing on induction or emergence,[59] breath holding,[59] and postoperative oxyhemoglobin desaturation.[60]

Alcohol Intake

An estimated 14 million Americans are dependent on alcohol, with 105,000 deaths annually attributed to alcohol abuse.[19] Information regarding the type and amount of alcohol regularly consumed and the frequency of consumption is important in the evaluation for anesthesia and surgery. Often an accurate assessment of a patient's alcohol intake may be difficult to obtain. A less confrontational and a reliable approach to evaluating a patient's potential for an alcohol problem uses the mnemonic CAGE, which refers to the following four questions[61]:

- Do you feel you should *c*ut down on your alcohol consumption?
- Have people *a*nnoyed you by criticizing your drinking habits?
- Have you felt *g*uilty about your drinking?
- Have you ever had a drink first thing in the morning to steady your nerves or get rid of a hangover (*e*ye-opener)?

A patient reporting more than two positive responses is at high risk for alcoholism and an increased likelihood of experiencing withdrawal symptoms.[62]

In the heavy drinker it is important to determine whether the patient has experienced seizures, abrupt withdrawal syndrome, or delirium tremens as a consequence of alcohol abuse. Clinical signs suggestive of alcohol withdrawal include increased hand tremors, autonomic hyperactivity (e.g., sweating, tachycardia, systolic hypertension), insomnia, anxiety, restlessness, nausea or vomiting, transient hallucinations (visual, tactile, or auditory), psychomotor agitation, and grand mal seizures.[62,63]

Chronic alcohol abuse results in the development of tolerance, physical dependence, and multisystem organ dysfunction. Tolerance to alcohol is evidenced by a resistance or cross-tolerance to other central nervous system (CNS) depressants. For example, the anesthetic requirement of hypnotics, opioids, and inhalation agents is increased in the chronic alcoholic[64,65]; however, exaggerated responses to anesthetic agents are likely during periods of acute intoxication or advanced alcoholism. This effect is attributed to the additive depressant effects of alcohol and anesthetic agents. Enzymatic function and plasma albumin concentrations may also be reduced in patients with alcoholic hepatic insufficiency. As a result, greater circulating concentrations of unbound intravenous agents (e.g., thiopental) may result in an exaggerated and prolonged drug effect.[66] This enhanced drug response has not been shown to occur with propofol in patients with moderate liver cirrhosis.[67,68]

An insidious progression of multisystem organ dysfunction is also characteristic of long-term alcohol abuse. Numerous illnesses are attributable to the toxic and malnutritional adverse effects of advanced alcoholism (Box 17-5).[69-86] Predictably, postoperative morbidity and mortality rates are increased in alcoholic patients as a result of poor wound healing, infection, bleeding, and further hepatic deterioration.[87]

Illicit Drug Use

Use of illicit drugs (e.g., cocaine, cannabis, "crack," lysergic acid diethylamide-25 [LSD], amphetamines) is a significant health-care issue in the United States. The most popular recreational drugs continue to be cocaine and marijuana. Approximately 13 million Americans used illicit drugs monthly in 1996.[88] The use of these substances increases the

BOX 17-5

Toxic Effects Associated with Chronic Alcohol Intake

Neurologic
Dementia
Diet related—Wernicke-Korsakoff syndrome, cerebellar degeneration, central pontine myelinosis

Cancer
Oropharynx, larynx, esophagus, liver, large intestine, breast

Cardiovascular
Cardiomyopathy, arrhythmias, hypertension, stroke, sudden death
Diet related—beriberi heart disease

Hematologic
Leukopenia, anemia, thrombocytopenia, coagulopathies
Diet related—macrocytic hyperchromic anemia

Metabolic
Increased high-density lipoprotein, hyperuricemia

Gastrointestinal
Acute and chronic gastritis, acute and chronic pancreatitis, esophageal varices
Diet related—malabsorption

Hepatobiliary
Fatty degeneration, acute hepatitis
Diet related—Laennec's cirrhosis

Gynecologic or Reproductive
Increased menstrual symptoms, increased infertility, increased spontaneous abortion, fetal damage

risk for adverse consequences and drug interactions during anesthesia. An accurate illicit drug history is often difficult to obtain because of the patient's fear of legal reprisal or refusal to believe a drug problem exists. During the physical examination the anesthesia provider should look for signs that indicate illicit drug use by the patient. A diagnosis of recent or continuing drug abuse should be suspected in patients exhibiting the following on physical examination[89,90]:

- Evidence of drug injection (e.g., track marks or scarring), thrombotic veins, phlebitis, tattoos (may be used to mask the sites), ablation of venous return leading to unilateral edema of the nondominant hand, subcutaneous skin abscesses
- Ophthalmologic changes, such as pupillary constriction from opioid use, pupillary dilation with amphetamine use, nystagmus from phencyclidine (PCP) use
- Lymphadenopathy secondary to nonspecific activation of the immune system as a result of repeated injections of impurities
- Malnourishment as a result of amphetamine abuse (opioid users tend to be well nourished)
- Poor dental care and bruxism (involuntary grinding and clenching of teeth) from amphetamine use
- Nasal perforation from cocaine abuse

Signs and symptoms of acute abuse of the more common substances are listed in Box 17-6.[89] *Elective surgery should be delayed or canceled in patients suspected of being under the influence of an illicit drug until further patient evaluation can be performed.* Suspicion of acute substance abuse should be followed up with a urine screen for drug identification.

BOX **17-6**

Signs and Symptoms of Acute Substance Abuse

Cannabis (Marijuana or Hashish)
Tachycardia, labile blood pressure
Euphoria, occasional anxiety and panic reactions, psychosis (rare)
Poor memory and decreased motivation with chronic use

Cocaine and Amphetamines
Tachycardia, labile blood pressure, hypertension
Excitement, delirium, hallucinations to psychosis
Hyperreflexia, tremors, convulsions, mydriasis, sweating, hyperpyrexia, exhaustion, coma with overdose

Hallucinogens: LSD, PCP
Sympathomimetic and weak analgesic effects
Altered perception and judgment; high doses may progress to toxic psychosis
PCP produces dissociative anesthesia with increasing doses

Opioids
Respiratory depression, hypotension, bradycardia, constipation
Euphoria (most marked with heroin)
Pinpoint pupils with overdose; decreased level of consciousness to coma

LSD, *Lysergic acid diethylamide-25*; PCP, *phencyclidine*.
Modified from Cheng DCH. The drug addicted patient. Can J Anaesth. *1997;44:R101-R106.*

Synthetic Androgens

Anabolic steroids are self-administered in an attempt to increase strength and muscle mass but can result in hepatic and endocrine system dysfunction. Risks associated with long-term androgen steroid supplementation include impaired liver function,[91] hepatic adenocarcinoma,[92] peliosis hepatis,[93] myocardial infarction (MI),[94] stroke,[95] hypertension,[96] dyslipidemia,[97] and psychiatric disturbances in susceptible patients.[98] The hepatotoxic effects have important implications for the anesthetic management of a chronic steroid abuser, particularly with agents metabolized by the liver, and such patients should undergo preoperative liver function testing.[99]

Herbal Dietary Supplements

Patients should be questioned regarding their use of nonprescription medications to determine the herb's name, the duration of herbal therapy, and the dose taken. Certain herbal products are known to influence blood clotting, affect blood glucose levels, produce CNS stimulation or depression, or interact with psychotropic drugs (Table 17-2).[100]

PATIENT EVALUATION: OVERVIEW OF SYSTEMS

Upper Airway

Assessment of the airway should be performed preoperatively in every patient, regardless of the plan of anesthetic management. It is important to evaluate the patient before anesthesia to identify those patients at risk for difficult airway management. The initial physical examination of the patient includes careful inspection of the teeth, inside of the mouth, mandibular space, and neck in a sequential fashion to determine predictors of airway management difficulties (Table 17-3).[101] Certain body structural features, metabolic disease states, and congenital or acquired structural anomalies are associated with difficult airway management (Box 17-7, p. 344).[102-215] The combination of subtle or minor physical anomalies may result in a difficult tracheal intubation, even when each factor, individually, is not expected to pose a problem.[131]

Tests for Prediction of Difficult Intubation

Several screening tests for predicting difficult endotracheal intubation are recommended as part of the preoperative patient evaluation. No single test should be relied on exclusively when the airway is evaluated; a combination of evaluative criteria should be employed to increase the predictive value for difficult intubation.[216]

Mallampati Classification. A popular technique for airway assessment is the modified Mallampati airway classification, which entails examination of tongue size relative to the oral cavity.[217] During the assessment for the Mallampati classification the patient is seated upright with the head in a neutral alignment, while the examiner sits opposite the patient at eye level. The patient is asked to open the mouth as wide as possible and maximally extrude the tongue. The patient is encouraged not to phonate during this maneuver because phonation may inappropriately elevate the soft palate. The airway is then classified based on the structures visible on direct examination of the oropharynx (Figure 17-2, p. 345).[217] Endotracheal intubation is generally easy in a patient with a Mallampati class I airway and can be expected to be difficult in a patient with a Mallampati class III or IV airway. The Mallampati airway classification has been criticized as not being a reliable or sensitive predictor of

TABLE 17-2 Anesthetic Considerations for Herbal Medicines

Clinical Effect	Herbal Drugs
Anticoagulant (discontinue 2 wk before elective surgery)	Alfalfa, chamomile, dong quai root, echinacea, feverfew, garlic, ginger, ginkgo, ginseng, goldenseal, guarana, horse chestnut, willow bark
Serum glucose alteration (monitor preoperative serum glucose level)	*Decrease*—akee fruit, alfalfa, aloe, argimony, artichokes, barley, bitter melon, burdock root, carrot oil, chromium, coriander, dandelion root, devil's club, eucalyptus, fenugreek seeds, fo-ti, garlic, ginseng, grape seed, guayusa, gymnena, juniper, neem seed oil, onions, periwinkle, yellow root *Increase*—ephedra
Central nervous system stimulation (consider potential vasoactive agent interactions)	Feverfew, goldenseal, gotu kola, guarana, ma huang, milk thistle, St. John's wort, yohimbine
Central nervous system depressant (may potentiate the central nervous system depressant effects of barbiturates, benzodiazepines, and opioids)	Hawthorn, kava, lavender, lemon balm, lemon verbena, mugwort, passion flower, rauwolfia, valerian
Antidepressant (use caution when coadministering with tricylic antidepressants, selective serotonin reuptake inhibitors, and monoamine oxidase inhibitors)	Ginseng, lemon balm, ma huang, mugwort, passion flower, St. John's wort, yohimbine

Modified from Zaglaniczny K. An introduction to herbal medicine and anesthetic considerations. Nurse Anesth Forum. *1999;2:4-5, 11.*

difficult intubating conditions.[218-221] Because of the unusually high incidence of false-positive and false-negative findings associated with the Mallampati classification system, it should not be used as the only means of screening for the difficult airway.

Thyromental Distance. Thyromental distance can also be quantified to enable prediction of difficulties with laryngoscopy. Thyromental distance represents the straight distance, with the neck fully extended and the mouth closed, between the prominence of the thyroid cartilage and the bony point of the lower mandibular border. In adults a thyromental distance of less than 7 cm is associated with difficult endotracheal intubation.[222] If the thyromental distance is less than 7 cm, which is approximately three adult fingerbreadths, the pharyngeal and laryngeal axes may not properly align, and difficult laryngoscopy can be anticipated.[131,222]

TABLE 17-3 Preoperative Airway Examinations, Acceptable Endpoints, and Significance of Endpoints

Preoperative Examination	Acceptable Endpoints	Significance of Endpoints
Length of upper incisors	Qualitative; short incisors	Long incisors—blade enters mouth in cephalad direction
Involuntary: maxillary teeth anterior to mandibular teeth	No overriding of maxillary teeth anterior to the mandibular teeth	Overriding maxillary teeth—blade enters mouth in a more cephalad direction
Voluntary: protrusion of mandibular teeth anterior to the maxillary teeth	Anterior protrusion of the mandibular teeth relative to the maxillary teeth	Test of temporomandibular joint function; indicates good mouth opening and jaw that will move anteriorly with laryngoscopy
Intercisor distance	>3 cm	2-cm phalange on blade can be easily inserted between teeth
Oropharyngeal class	Class II	Tongue is small in relation to size of oropharyngeal cavity
Narrowness of palate	Should not appear very narrow or highly arched	A narrow palate decreases the oropharyngeal volume and room for both blade and endotracheal tube
Mandibular space length (thyromental distance)	5 cm or three ordinary-size fingerbreadths	Larynx is relatively posterior to other upper airway structures
Mandibular space compliance	Qualitative palpation of normal resilience or softness	Laryngoscopy retracts tongue into the mandibular space; compliance of the mandibular space determines if tongue fits into mandibular space
Length of neck	Qualitative; a quantitative index is not yet available	A short neck decreases the ability to align the upper airway axes
Thickness of neck	Qualitative; a quantitative index is not yet available	A thick neck decreases the ability to align the upper airway axes
Range of motion of head and neck	Neck flexed on chest 35 degrees, plus head extended on neck 80 degrees = sniff position	The sniff position aligns the oral, pharyngeal, and laryngeal axes to create favorable line of sight

Modified from Benumof JL. The ASA difficult airway algorithm: new thoughts and considerations. Curr Rev Nurse Anesth. *1999;22:103-113.*

BOX 17-7

Conditions Associated with Difficult Airway Management

Head
Mass defects (e.g., encephalocele,[103] soft-tissue sarcoma[104])
Macrocephaly (e.g., severe hydrocephaly, Dandy Walker syndrome,[105,106] mucopolysaccharidoses[107,108] [Hurler syndrome])
Interference with airway access (e.g., thoracopagus conjoined twins,[109,110] stereotactic frame[111])

Facial Anomalies
Maxillary and mandibular deformities[112]
Maxillary hypoplasia (e.g., Apert syndrome,[112] Crouzon disease[113])
Mandibular hypoplasia, microgenia, micrognathia[114] (e.g., Pierre Robin syndrome,[106,115,116] Treacher Collins syndrome,[117] Goldenhar's syndrome,[118,119] cri du chat syndrome,[120] Nager syndrome[121])
Mandibular hyperplasia (e.g., cherubism[122])
Temporomandibular joint anomalies
Reduced mobility (e.g., arthrogryposis multiplex,[123] diabetes,[124,125] Dutch-Kentucky syndrome,[126] Hecht-Beals syndrome[127]), ankylosis[128-130] (inflammatory, congenital, traumatic, infectious)

Thoracoabdominal
Morbid obesity,[131] sleep apnea syndrome,[132-134] Prader-Willi syndrome[135]
Kyphoscoliosis
Prominent chest or large breasts
Full-term or near-term pregnancy

Mouth and Tongue Anomalies
Microstomia[136,137]
Congenital anomalies (e.g., Freeman-Sheldon [whistling face] syndrome[138,139])
Acquired anomalies (e.g., burn[140])
Stomatitis (e.g., noma[141,142])
Tongue disease
Macroglossia
Congenital (e.g., Beckwith-Wiedemann syndrome,[143] Down syndrome,[144,145] congenital hypothyroidism, Pompe disease)
Swelling (e.g., burns, trauma,[146] Ludwig's angina[147,148])
Tumors (e.g., hemangiomas,[149,150] lymphangioma[151])
Protruding upper incisors (e.g., Cockayne's syndrome[152])
Foreign body[153]

Nasal Pathology
Choanal atresia[154,155]
Tumors (e.g., encephaloceles,[156] gliomas,[157] foreign body[158])

Palate Pathology
Arch and cleft defects[159]
Soft-palate swelling and hematomas[160]

Pharynx
Adenoid and tonsillar disease
Hypertrophy[161]
Tumors and abscesses[162]
Lingual tonsils[163,164]
Pharyngeal wall pathology
Retropharyngeal and parapharyngeal abscesses[165]
Inflammatory disease[166] (e.g., epidermolysis bullosa, erythema multiforme bullosum)
Scarring (e.g., Behçet's syndrome)[167]

Laryngeal Pathology
Supraglottic
Laryngomalacia[168,169]
Supraglottis (epiglottitis)[170,171]
Glottic
Congenital lesions (vocal cord paralysis, laryngeal web, cyst, laryngocele)[172-174]
Papillomatosis[175,176]
Granuloma formation
Foreign body[177]
Subglottic
Congenital stenosis
Infectious (croup)[178]
Inflammatory (edema,[179,180] traumatic stenosis)

Tracheal and Bronchial Tree Pathology
Tracheomalacia[181] (e.g., Larsen syndrome[182,183])
Croup
Bacterial tracheitis[184]
Mediastinal masses[185,186]
Vascular malformation[187,188]
Foreign body aspiration[189,190]
Other (e.g., tracheal stenosis,[191,192] webbing, fistula,[193] diverticulum)

Neck
Mass lesions[194,195]
Lymphatic malformation,[196,197] hemangioma,[150,198] teratoma,[199] goiter,[200] abscess[201]
Skin contracture (postburn,[202,203] inflammatory [scleroderma, epidermolysis bullosa, erythema multiforme bullosum])
Webbed (e.g., Turner's syndrome[204])

Spine
Limited cervical spine mobility
Congenital (e.g., Klippel-Feil syndrome[205])
Acquired (e.g., surgical [fusion],[206,207] trauma [vertebral fracture], inflammatory [ankylosing spondylitis[208,209]])
Cervical spine instability
Congenital (e.g., Down syndrome,[210] Larsen syndrome,[183] Mobius' syndrome,[211] Morquio syndrome[212])
Acquired (e.g., trauma [subluxation, fracture],[213,214] inflammatory [rheumatoid arthritis[215]])

Modified from Gregory GA, Riazi J. Classification and assessment of the difficult pediatric airway. In: Riazi J, ed. Anesthesiology Clinics of North America: the Difficult Pediatric Airway. *Philadelphia: Saunders; 1998:729-741.*

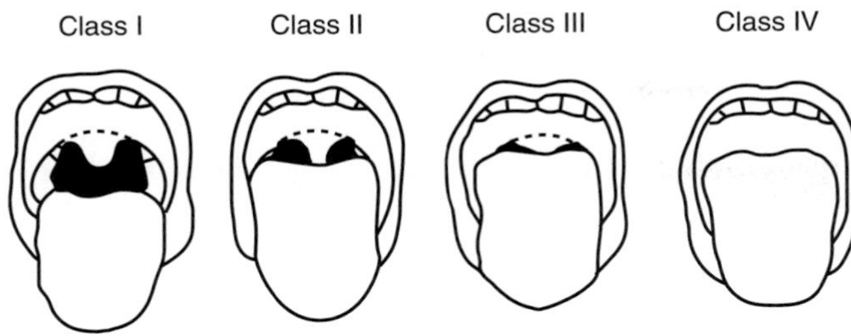

FIGURE **17-2**
Modified Mallampati classification of pharyngeal structures. *Class I*, Soft palate, tonsillar fauces, tonsillar pillars, and uvula visualized. *Class II*, Soft palate, tonsillar fauces, and uvula visualized. *Class III*, Soft palate and base of uvula visualized. *Class IV*, Soft palate not visualized. (From Samsoon GL, Young JR. Difficult tracheal intubation: a retrospective study. *Anaesthesia.* 1987;42:487-490.)

Sternomental Distance. The sternomental distance is measured as the straight distance, with the neck fully extended and the mouth closed, between the upper border of the manubrium sterni and the bony point of the lower mandibular border. The sternomental distance has been suggested as being more predictive of difficult intubation than the thyromental distance.[220] A sternomental distance of less than 13.5 cm is suggestive of intubation difficulty.[223]

Interincisor Distance. The degree of mouth opening, largely a function of the temporomandibular joint, is a vital component of the airway assessment. Limited temporomandibular joint movement is a well-recognized contributor to difficult endotracheal intubation. An adult should be able to open the mouth at least 4 cm, allowing two large fingers to be placed between the upper and lower incisors. An interincisor gap of less than two fingerbreadths is associated with difficulty in endotracheal intubation.[131,224] Some patients who are able to open their mouths sufficiently while awake experience limitations in temporomandibular joint mobility after anesthesia is induced. This limited movement renders the visualization of laryngeal structures difficult. Forward protrusion of the mandible can be attempted, in this situation, for opening the mouth adequately to allow direct laryngoscopy.[225]

Head and Neck Movement (Atlantooccipital Function). Moderate flexion of the neck on the chest and full extension of the atlantooccipital joint aligns the oral, pharyngeal, and laryngeal axes into the McGill, or "sniff," position. In this position, less tongue obscures the laryngeal view during laryngoscopy. Limitations to atlantooccipital joint extension, which are frequently attributed to cervical arthritis or a small C-1 gap, enhance the convexity of the neck and push the larynx anteriorly. This situation can impair laryngoscopy and render endotracheal intubation difficult.[131]

Dentition

The incidence of perianesthetic dental injury approximates 1:4500 and is associated with patients undergoing general anesthesia involving endotracheal intubation who have preexisting poor dentition and characteristics linked with difficult laryngoscopy and intubation (e.g., limited neck motion, previous head and neck surgery, craniofacial abnormalities, history of previous difficult tracheal intubation).[226] Because dental injuries account for one third of all anesthesia-related medicolegal claims in the United States,[227] a presurgical inspection of the teeth should be documented for each patient. Otherwise, fractured or missing teeth may be falsely attributed to damage occurring during airway instrumentation. The patient with protuberant or loose maxillary incisors should also be informed of the increased risk of tooth injury or loss with laryngoscopy. An informed consent to proceed with the anesthetic plan, despite this dental risk, must then be documented. If the patient is properly informed of the likelihood of dental damage, the anesthesia provider may not be held liable should dental injury occur.[228]

The location and condition of crowns, braces, and other significant dental work are also noted. Prosthetic devices, such as partial plates and dentures, are removed before surgery unless they significantly improve the mask fit. An extremely loose tooth may be extracted before laryngoscopy to prevent its aspiration during anesthesia.

Musculoskeletal System

Obesity

Evaluation of the musculoskeletal system usually begins with a general assessment of the size and stature of the patient. Baseline height and weight information can be obtained from the admission data or by direct questioning of the patient during the taking of the health history. Body weight is then compared with normal values for a given height in relation to the patient's age and gender. Ideal body weight, for example, can be determined for men and women (Box 17-8). The actual weight of the patient is compared with the calculated ideal body weight. Body weight that is 20% in excess of the ideal body weight at a particular height constitutes obesity. A body weight that is twice the ideal body weight is deemed to be morbid obesity.

A more scientific approach to describing weight in relation to height uses the measure of body mass index (BMI).[229] Box 17-8 presents the formula for calculating BMI and incorporates it into examples for an average and an overweight individual of the same height. The adult patient weight classification based on BMI is as follows: overweight—25 to 29.9 kg/m^2; obese—30 to 35 kg/m^2; and morbidly obese—greater than 35 kg/m^2.[230] More than half of the adult population in the United States is overweight or obese.[231] The prevalence of adult

BOX **17-8**

Calculation of Ideal Body Weight and Body Mass Index

Ideal Body Weight (IBW)
IBW (male) = 105 lb + 6 lb for each inch >5 ft
IBW (female) = 100 lb + 5 lb for each inch >5 ft

Body Mass Index (BMI)
BMI = Weight in kg/(Height in meters)^2
Example 1
70 kg/1.7 m^2 = 70 kg/2.89 m = 24 kg/m^2
Example 2
125 kg/1.7 m^2 = 125 kg/2.89 m = 43 kg/m^2

obesity (greater than 30 kg/m^2) in the United States increased from 12% in 1991 to 17.9% in 1998.[232] In 2003 the National Institute of Health estimates that 30.5% of adults are obese. This increase is partially due to change in the definition. Obese patients are at risk of illness from hypertension, dyslipidemia, type 2 diabetes, congestive heart failure, coronary heart disease, stroke, gallbladder disease, hiatal hernia, liver dysfunction, osteoarthritis, peripheral vascular disease, pseudotumor cerebri, sleep apnea and other respiratory disorders (e.g., asthma, chronic obstructive and restrictive pulmonary disease), and certain cancers (e.g., colorectal, biliary tract, prostate, breast, uterus, ovary).[233,234]

Particular attention is given to airway evaluation to determine the likelihood of difficult endotracheal intubation. If a problem is anticipated and an awake or fiberoptic tracheal intubation is planned, proper patient preparation, which includes a drying agent and proper upper airway anesthesia, should be planned.

The patient should be questioned about the use of antiobesity drugs, such as amphetamines, nonamphetamine schedule IV appetite suppressants, and antidepressants (e.g., fluoxitene, sertraline).[234] Additionally, use of dexfenfluramine and fenfluramine, alone or in combination, should be determined, because these agents have been associated with primary pulmonary hypertension and valvular heart disease.[235,236]

Ankylosing Spondylitis and Rheumatoid Arthritis

Disorders of the musculoskeletal system include degenerative disk disease (osteoarthritis), ankylosing spondylitis, and rheumatoid arthritis. The chronic pain and inflammation of spinal or extraspinal joints associated with these diseases limit the degree of patient mobility. Tolerance for positions required during surgery and regional anesthesia techniques should therefore be ascertained preoperatively. Aspirin, nonsteroidal antiinflammatory drugs, and corticosteroids may be included in pharmacologic regimens for such patients.[237] A careful family history and previous dental, obstetric, surgical, traumatic injury, transfusion, and drug histories should be elicited from patients taking these drugs to evaluate the propensity for bleeding. A history suggestive of a bleeding disorder (e.g., excessive bruising or prolonged bleeding) should lead to diagnostic testing that may include measurement of bleeding time, platelet count, prothrombin time, and activated partial thromboplastin time.[238] The preoperative bleeding time test is not a clinically reliable test for determining the risk of significant perioperative bleeding and should not be routinely used for this purpose in patients without a medical history or physical findings suggestive of a bleeding disorder.[238,239]

If the dosage and duration of corticosteroid therapy are considerable, perioperative supplementation may also be necessary in patients with a musculoskeletal disorder to avoid perioperative hemodynamic instability. Patients considered at risk for adrenal insufficiency include those who received hydrocortisone equivalent of more than 20 to 30 mg daily for longer than 2 weeks during the previous year and those who are receiving replacement corticosteroid treatment for adrenal insufficiency.[240] These patients should receive adequate perioperative steroid coverage (Table 17-4).[241]

Although less common than osteoarthritis, ankylosing spondylitis and rheumatoid arthritis have greater implications for anesthetic management. Systemic manifestations are extensive during the advanced stages of both disorders. Patients frequently have pain, inflammation, and limited mobility in affected joints, such as those in the back and the hands. Extreme ankylosis and joint deformity often make peripheral venous access and intraoperative positioning a challenge. On physical examination, limited range of motion of the temporomandibular joint and cervical spine can make tracheal intubation more difficult.[242] In rheumatoid arthritis this limitation is compounded by restrictions in vocal cord movement or tracheal stenosis caused by cricoarytenoid arthritis. These changes may be evidenced by preoperative hoarseness, stridor, painful speech, or dysphagia. During advanced stages of ankylosing spondylitis or rheumatoid arthritis, restrictive lung disease, polychondritis, pleural and pericardial effusions, and cardiac conduction abnormalities may be present.[240,243,244]

TABLE 17-4 Steroid Supplementation Regimen

Patients currently taking steroids	<10 mg prednisolone per day	Assume normal hormonal response	Additional steroid cover not required
	>10 mg prednisolone per day	Minor surgery	25 mg hydrocortisone at induction
		Moderate surgery	Usual preoperative steroids plus 25 mg hydrocortisone at induction plus 100 mg/day for 24 hr
		Major surgery	Usual preoperative steroids plus 25 mg hydrocortisone at induction plus 100 mg/day for 48-72 hr
	High-dose immunosuppression	Give usual immunosuppressive doses during perioperative period	
Patients who have stopped taking steroids	<3 mo	Treat as if on steroids	
	>3 mo	No perioperative steroids necessary	

Modified from Nicholson G, Burrin JM, Hall GM. Perioperative steroid supplementation. Anaesthesia. *1998;53:1091-1104.*

Neurologic System

The preoperative evaluation of the neurologic system includes the determination of CNS or peripheral nervous system dysfunction. An initial neurologic examination consisting of the following should be performed[245]:

- *Musculoskeletal (motor) system*: observe the patient's gait, ability to perform toe and heel walk, ability to maintain the arms held forward; evaluate the patient's grip strength
- *Sensory system*: physical distinction of vibration, pain, and light touch on the patient's hands, feet, and limbs
- *Muscle reflexes*: deep, superficial, and pathologic
- *Cranial nerve abnormalities*: obtained by patient medical history and by observation
- *Mental status and speech pattern*: appearance, mood, thought processes, cognitive function

Knowledge of clinical manifestations of neurologic disease is essential for the preoperative evaluation of patient with CNS or peripheral nervous system disorders. Signs and symptoms of increasing intracranial pressure and cerebral ischemia, for example, may include papilledema; unilateral mydriasis; headaches, made worse by coughing; nausea and vomiting; slurred speech, disorientation, and altered levels of consciousness; flaccid hemiplegia or hemiparesis; abducens or oculomotor palsy; neck rigidity; and respiratory disturbances. Hypertension, with corresponding decreases in heart rate, represents a physiologic attempt to enhance cerebral perfusion when intracranial pressure is high. The appearance of Q waves, deep and inverted T waves, prolonged QT intervals, and ST-segment elevations on the electrocardiogram (ECG) may reflect hypothalamic ischemia and sympathetic overactivity. These abnormalities are most often attributed to vasospasm after a subarachnoid hemorrhage, although myocardial ischemia should be ruled out before surgery.[246-248] Fever and leukocytosis can also follow a subarachnoid hemorrhage as a result of meningeal irritation by subarachnoid blood. The progression of neurologic dysfunction to coma, obtundation, and decerebrate rigidity worsens the overall prognosis of the patient with an intracranial mass or hemorrhage. This prognosis coincides that of a patient who has sustained an acute head injury. The patient with an initial Glasgow Coma Scale (Table 17-5)[249] score of less than 8 is considered comatose. Patients with a score of less than 7 usually require tracheal intubation and mechanical hyperventilation.[245]

Diagnostic reports should be reviewed so that the extent of neurologic and coexisting disease can be determined. These reports include the results of electromyography, conduction velocity study, electroencephalography, computed tomography (CT), magnetic resonance imaging (MRI), and cerebral arteriography studies. Consultation with a neurologist and a preoperative electromyography, for example, are recommended for patients with complaints of extremity weakness, pain, or paresthesia. This consultation is especially important in patients who are at greater risk for a peripheral neuropathy (e.g., patients with long-standing diabetes, patients with uremia, chronic alcoholics with nutritional deficits). Documentation of symptoms and reports of abnormal preoperative neurologic findings is important in these patients. Preoperative CT, whereby a 0.5-cm midline shift of the brain is significant, can also confirm suspicions of intracranial hypertension. The size and location of an intracerebral aneurysm are represented on cerebral arteriography. This information can facilitate the prediction of the surgical approach and can guide the evaluation of neurologic involvement. The degree of collateral circulation in the patient with cerebrovascular occlusive disease can also be determined from arteriographic films. In a patient with vertebral artery involvement, for example, extremes in head flexion, extension, and rotation are avoided. A thorough cardiac evaluation by a cardiologist, including 12-lead ECG and stress testing, is also advised for patients undergoing a carotid endarterectomy procedure, because of the associated risks of perioperative myocardial ischemia and infarction.[250]

TABLE 17-5 Glasgow Coma Scale

Response	Score
Eyes Open	
Spontaneously	4
To speech	3
To pain	2
Never	1
Best Motor Response	
Obeys commands	6
Localizes pain	5
Withdraws (flexion)	4
Abnormal flexion (decortication)	3
Extensor response (decerebration)	2
None	1
Best Verbal Response	
Oriented	5
Confused conversation	4
Inappropriate words	3
Incomprehensible sounds	2
None	1
Range of Scores	***3-15***

Modified from Teasdale G, Jennett B. Assessment of coma and impaired consciousness. A practical scale. Lancet. *1974;2:81-84.*

Information gained from the preoperative evaluation of neurologic function can facilitate the management of a patient with a CNS or peripheral nervous system disorder. For example, sedatives are avoided in patients with intracranial hypertension, especially when an altered level of consciousness accompanies it. Affected patients may be extremely sensitive to the CNS-depressant effects of such drugs as opioids.

Doses, schedules, and adverse effects of therapeutic regimens should also be considered before surgery. Serum concentrations of anticonvulsants, such as phenytoin and phenobarbital, are measured in order to determine whether levels are therapeutic. A complete blood cell count is also obtained for patients receiving prolonged phenytoin therapy because of the risk of agranulocytosis associated with this drug. As with anticonvulsant therapy, corticosteroid therapy is continued perioperatively in patients with a CNS tumor. Although the exact mechanism of the beneficial effects of corticosteroids is unknown, it is theorized to involve the reduction of cerebrospinal fluid production or cerebral edema as a result of capillary membrane stabilization. Blood glucose levels are also determined for the patient treated with either dexamethasone or methylprednisolone, because hyperglycemia frequently accompanies the use of these drugs. Heightened risks of pulmonary infection and gastrointestinal irritation are unlikely, however, with the patient undergoing only perioperative therapy.[251,252]

BOX 17-9

Clinical Predictors of Increased Cardiovascular Risk

Major Risk Factors
Unstable coronary syndromes
Recent myocardial infarction* with evidence of important ischemic risk by clinical symptoms or noninvasive study
Unstable or severe† angina (Canadian class III or IV)‡
Decompensated congestive heart failure
Significant arrhythmias
High-grade atrioventricular block
Symptomatic ventricular arrhythmias in the presence of underlying heart disease
Supraventricular arrhythmias with uncontrolled ventricular rate
Severe valvular disease

Intermediate Risk Factors
Mild angina pectoris (Canadian class I or II)
Prior myocardial infarction identified by history or pathologic Q waves
Compensated or prior congestive heart failure
Diabetes mellitus
Renal insufficiency

Minor Risk Factors
Advanced age
Abnormal electrocardiograph (left ventricular hypertrophy, left bundle branch block, ST-T abnormalities)
Rhythm other than sinus (e.g., atrial fibrillation)
Low functional capacity (e.g., inability to climb one flight of stairs with a bag of groceries)
History of stroke
Uncontrolled systemic hypertension

**The American College of Cardiology National Database Library defines recent myocardial infarction as having occurred more than 7 days but less than or equal to 30 days previously.*
†May include "stable" angina in patients who are unusually sedentary.
‡Campeau L. Grading of angina pectoris. Circulation. *1976;54:522-523.*
Modified from Eagle K, et al. ACC/AHA guideline update for perioperative cardiovascular evaluation for noncardiac surgery—executive summary. A report of the American College of Cardiology/American Heart Association task force on practice guidelines (committee to update the 1996 guidelines on perioperative cardiovascular evaluation for noncardiac surgery). Anesth Analg. *2002;94:1052-1064.*

TABLE 17-6 **New York Heart Association Functional Classification of Cardiovascular Disability**

Classification	Cardiovascular Status
Class I	*Patients with cardiac disease.* No functional limitations to physical activity, such as walking or climbing stairs. Ordinary physical activity is not associated with undue fatigue, palpitations, dyspnea, or anginal pain.
Class II	*Patients with cardiac disease who are comfortable at rest.* Slight functional limitations to physical activity, such as walking or climbing stairs rapidly, or during emotional stress. Patients are comfortable at rest. Ordinary physical activity results in fatigue, palpitation, dyspnea, or anginal pain.
Class III	*Patients with cardiac disease resulting in marked limitations to physical activity.* Patients are comfortable at rest. Less than ordinary physical activity causes fatigue, palpitations, dyspnea, or anginal pain.
Class IV	*Patients with cardiac disease resulting in inability to carry on any physical activity without discomfort.* Symptoms of cardiac insufficiency or of the anginal syndrome may be present even at rest. If any physical activity is undertaken, discomfort is increased.

Modified from Mangano DT. Preoperative assessment of cardiac risk. In: Kaplan JA, ed. Cardiac Anesthesia. *4th ed. Philadelphia: Saunders; 1999:3-39.*

Cardiovascular System

Evaluation of the cardiovascular system includes the determination of (1) preexisting cardiac disease (e.g., hypertension, ischemic heart disease, valvular dysfunction, cardiac arrhythmias, and cardiac conduction abnormalities, with or without evidence of ventricular failure); (2) disease severity, stability, and prior treatment; (3) comorbidity (e.g., diabetes mellitus, peripheral vascular disease, chronic pulmonary disease); and (4) the type of surgery to be performed (major abdominal, orthopedic, and vascular procedures are associated with high risk).[240] The prevalence and adverse consequences of cardiovascular disease make it a prime consideration in the overview of systems. Major cardiovascular risk factors that correlate with increased perioperative morbidity and mortality have been described by an American College of Cardiology and American Heart Association (ACC/AHA) task force (Box 17-9).[253]

A standard means of categorizing the degree of cardiovascular disability is the New York Heart Association classification (Table 17-6).[254] When the patient interview is conducted, specific inquiry should be made regarding the presence of dyspnea, chest pain, fatigability, syncope, palpitation, and the factors that predispose to angina. Whenever a patient has signs of cardiovascular disease, referral to a cardiologist is indicated if a recent workup has not been conducted.

Disorders of the Cardiovascular System

Hypertension. Hypertension, defined as a systolic blood pressure greater than 140 mm Hg or a diastolic pressure greater than 90 mm Hg,[255] is the most common circulatory derangement to affect humans (approximately 60 million in the United States) and is a major risk factor for coronary artery disease[256] and increased perioperative mortality.[257] All too often, patients undergoing surgery have uncontrolled stage 2 hypertension (systolic blood pressure greater than 160 mm Hg, diastolic pressure greater than 100 mm Hg, or both). This problem can be attributed to the lack or inadequacy of medical treatment or to patient noncompliance. In such a situation elective surgery is postponed until the preoperative blood pressure is normalized. Consultation with an internist can also be pursued for the medical evaluation and treatment of the patient with uncontrolled or newly diagnosed hypertension. These recommendations are aimed at reducing the occurrence of perioperative hemodynamic instability and consequently the incidence of myocardial ischemia. Both complications are more likely to occur when hypertension is not effectively treated before surgery.[257-259]

The practitioner taking the medical history should focus on identifying comorbid diseases, such as diabetes mellitus, and social risk factors (i.e., tobacco use, alcohol or caffeine consumption, illicit drug use [especially cocaine or amphetamines]).[260] The medications the patient takes to manage hypertension should be determined. In general the substances used affect the central and peripheral components of the sympathetic nervous system by altering the synthesis, release, biotransformation, or end-organ action of norepinephrine. Because the circulatory-depressant effects of general anesthesia may be additive, the combination of antihypertensive drugs and anesthetics is of concern. Complaints of syncope and dizziness are also investigated. These symptoms may be the clinical manifestations of cerebrovascular insufficiency, although a diagnosis of drug-induced orthostatic hypotension should be considered preoperatively. This diagnosis can be confirmed by a significant decrease in the blood pressure of the patient as he or she rises from the supine position. The lack of hemodynamic compensatory responses that normally accompany positional changes may then predict their absence during anesthesia and surgery.

The physical examination of the patient includes the following[260]:

- *Overall appearance*: truncal obesity with purpura and striae suggestive of Cushing's disease
- *Funduscopic examination*: hypertensive retinopathy
- *Neck*: carotid bruits, distended veins, or enlarged thyroid gland
- *Heart*: abnormal rhythm or size, murmurs, or heart sounds
- *Lungs*: rales or bronchospasm
- *Abdomen*: bruits, masses, enlarged kidneys, or abnormal aortic pulsation
- *Extremities*: delayed or absent femoral pulses secondary to aortic coarctation, or evidence of atherosclerosis
- *Neurologic evaluation*: see the discussion of the neurologic system earlier in this chapter

Ischemic Heart Disease. Myocardial ischemia occurs secondary to insufficient oxygen and nutrient supply (increased demand, reduced blood supply, or both) to meet the metabolic requirements of the myocardial cells. Nearly one third of the estimated 27 million patients undergoing surgery annually in the United States are at high risk for coronary artery disease or factors for cardiovascular disease.[261] Risk factors for ischemic heart disease include advanced age, smoking, diabetes mellitus, hypertension, pulmonary disease, previous MI, left ventricular wall motion dysfunction, and peripheral vascular disease.[262] The preoperative evaluation of a patient with known or suspected ischemic heart disease is aimed at determining the severity, progression, and functional limitations imposed by cardiovascular disease. Myocardial ischemia, cardiac arrhythmias, and left ventricular dysfunction are usually precipitating factors for patient symptomatology. Complaints of undue fatigue, angina pectoris, palpitations, syncope, or dyspnea should be thoroughly investigated. A 12-lead ECG is reviewed for evidence of myocardial ischemia or infarction, cardiac arrhythmias or conduction abnormalities, and ventricular hypertrophy. Signs and symptoms of myocardial ischemia may not be apparent at rest, however. Therefore the response of the patient to various activities, such as walking a certain distance or climbing several stairs, must be determined (see Table 17-6).

Anginal symptoms can also be classified according to the stability of precipitating factors, the frequency of the events, and the duration of pain. Stable angina (characterized as substernal discomfort brought on by exertion, relieved by rest or nitroglycerin or both in less than 15 minutes, and having a typical radiation to the shoulder, jaw, or the inner aspect of the arm[254]) poses no greater threat of MI perioperatively than the absence of anginal symptoms.[263] Unstable angina is defined as newly developed angina occurring within the past 2 months; angina that has progressively worsened, that occurs with increased frequency, intensity, or duration, that is less responsive to medicine, or that occurs when the patient is at rest; or angina that lasts longer than 30 minutes, exhibiting transient ST- or T-wave changes without development of Q waves or diagnostic elevation of enzymes.[254] Unstable angina is associated with the highest risk for perioperative MI.[264] In the patient with unstable angina, elective surgery is canceled until the cardiovascular status of the patient has been thoroughly evaluated and optimized. Advanced diagnostic techniques, such as coronary angiography and exercise ECG, may be used for determination of the extent and functional impairment of ischemic heart disease.

The overall risk of MI after general anesthesia is between 0.1% and 0.7% in the population at large. In patients known to have had an MI in the remote past (more than 6 months previously), the risk of perioperative reinfarction increases to approximately 6%. If MI occurred 3 to 6 months previously, the risk of reinfarction is 15%; within 3 months previously, 30%. If reinfarction occurs, the mortality rate is approximately 50%. The highest at-risk period appears to be within 30 days after an acute MI; therefore the ACC/AHA guidelines recommend waiting at least 4 to 6 weeks after an MI before a patient undergoes elective surgery.[253] Patients who have survived coronary revascularization and are asymptomatic are at lower risk of reinfarction when undergoing noncardiac surgery.[253]

Left Ventricular Dysfunction. Active left ventricular failure is the prominent cardiovascular risk factor for patients undergoing noncardiac surgery.[265] Patients with ischemic cardiomyopathy are at even greater risk for perioperative MI and ventricular dysfunction.[266] Prominent signs include moist rales in the lungs, often associated with tachypnea. These extraneous sounds may be confined to the bases, with mild degrees of left ventricular failure, or they may be generalized throughout the lungs, with acute pulmonary edema. As a result of sympathetic nervous system stimulation, resting tachycardia may also be present. A third heart sound (S_3) or ventricular gallop, jugular vein distention, and peripheral edema are significant. In the presence of congestive heart failure as confirmed by a chest radiograph, elective operations should be postponed until optimal ventricular performance can be achieved.

Valvular Heart Disease. Basic lesions of valvular heart disease may involve stenosis, incompetence, or both. In adults, aortic and mitral valve lesions are more common than those involving the tricuspid or pulmonic valve. Despite decreasing incidence, rheumatic heart disease is still the most common cause of adult valvular disease. Degenerative disorders (sclerosis, fibrosis) and congenital diseases are less common causes.

With stenosis, the chamber proximal to the obstruction must increase the work of maintaining a stroke volume; this eventually results in hypertrophy. Normal valves can episodically accommodate up to seven times the normal cardiac output—for example, in intense physical exercise in the normally active patient. Valvular stenosis usually is chronic and severe before cardiac output decreases. In valvular incompetence the chambers both proximal and distal to the lesions are involved, because regurgitant flow during one phase of the cardiac cycle is added to forward flow during subsequent systole. Because lesions are almost never entirely unitary, in stenosis some regurgitation is common, and vice versa. It is important to identify the type of valvular lesion before surgery. Evaluation of the clinical symptoms and cardiac catheterization data regarding valve area and gradients, combined with assessment of data from any prior surgical history (e.g., correction of congenital heart lesions), is an important component of the preoperative evaluation of patients with valvular heart disease.

Severe aortic stenosis poses the greatest patient risk for noncardiac surgery,[267,268] especially when the cross-sectional area of the aortic valve is less than 1 cm^2.[269,270] Severe aortic stenosis is associated with a 14-fold greater incidence of perioperative sudden death.[271] For patients in whom aortic stenosis is symptomatic, elective noncardiac surgery should be postponed until after cardiac surgical consultation.[253] Chapter 23 describes the perioperative care of patients with valvular heart disease.

Arrhythmias. Patients with cardiac arrhythmias must have an adequate preoperative evaluation for determination of the nature of the arrhythmia, associated underlying heart disease, and type of antiarrhythmic therapy. Whether symptoms of palpitations or dizziness have been relieved may be a sign of successful therapy or of continuing problems. Other cardiac symptoms such as dyspnea, angina, or syncope may suggest the worsening of associated cardiac disease. Treatment of the underlying disease preoperatively may aid in control of arrhythmia in the perioperative period. All patients with a history of symptomatic arrhythmias should undergo electrocardiography with rhythm strip before surgery. Other preoperative laboratory evaluations should include measurement of potassium and magnesium levels, determination of antiarrhythmic drug levels (if possible), and chest radiography (in the presence of structural cardiac disease).[272]

Ventricular arrhythmias are classified into three categories: benign ventricular arrhythmias (unifocal premature ventricular contractions); potentially malignant ventricular arrhythmias (patient has known organic heart disease and is on antiarrhythmic therapy); and malignant ventricular arrhythmias (patient has organic heart disease, hemodynamic compromise, and possibly a family history of sudden death).[272] Few data are available to help correlate the risk of arrhythmias and perioperative risk.[254] In the absence of cardiac disease, benign ventricular arrhythmias do not carry a significantly increased surgical risk.[273] In patients with severe coronary artery disease, recent MI, or peripheral vascular disease, arrhythmias may increase perioperative risk.[274,275]

Pacemaker. Anesthesia providers must be familiar with the different types of pacemakers, the indications for insertion, the evaluation of pacemaker function, and the perioperative management of patients with these devices. Too often, the presence of a permanent pacemaker is merely noted. Pacemakers can mask the toxicity of antiarrhythmic drugs, electrolyte disorders, and myocardial ischemia and irritability. In general the ECG should be examined for pacemaker malfunction, as evidenced by unexpected pauses. If the patient's heart rate is slower than the pacing rate, pacing spikes should appear on the ECG. To determine whether these pacing impulses are associated with myocardial contractions, the clinician should palpate a peripheral pulse. Evaluation of a pacemaker becomes more difficult when the patient's heart rate is faster than the pacing rate. A Valsalva maneuver slows the patient's rate so that pacing impulses appear on the ECG. Generally, because sensing is lost before pacing, the pacemaker is probably functioning normally if (1) it has been in place for fewer than 2 years, (2) chest radiography demonstrates that leads are intact, and (3) impulses do not appear on the ECG.[276] Chest radiography should provide information on electrode placement, the presence of electrode fracture, and even battery depletion.[277]

If each pacing impulse is not associated with a pulse, cardiologic consultation should be considered.[276] A cardiologic consultation should be sought when pacing impulses are not associated with a pulse and in a patient who has a return of the symptoms that led to pacemaker implantation. Anesthesia providers sometimes must decide whether a transvenous, temporary pacing wire should be inserted preoperatively. Persistent bradycardia not responsive to intravenous administration of atropine or exercise is one indication. Bifascicular block in a patient with a history of syncope suggests underlying, unrecognized complete heart block. Such patients can benefit from the availability of transvenous pacing.

It must also be determined whether exercising the muscles adjacent to the generator causes dizziness. The presence of this symptom, which indicates that myopotentials inhibit pacemakers, implies that muscle fasciculations caused by succinylcholine and shivering should be avoided.

Diagnostic Testing to Assess Cardiovascular Disease

Multiple tests are available to define the presence of cardiac disease. Preoperative cardiac testing should not be performed unless the results are likely to influence patient management.[278] The ACC/AHA guidelines include an algorithm for determining the appropriateness of preoperative testing (Figure 17-3).[253]

Exercise stress testing is designed to increase myocardial work and permit measurement of myocardial response to the increased workload. The exercise stress test not only is a standardized means of obtaining a functional history of angina but also provides excellent documentation of how ischemia manifests its effects on the cardiovascular system. By examining the stress test report, one can learn the extremes of blood pressure and heart rate that the patient can tolerate while awake (although exactly how these correlate with the anesthetized state is a matter of debate), the location of ischemic leads, and whether arrhythmias are associated with ischemia. Significant coronary disease is likely if ST-segment depression is greater than 0.2 mV, if ST depression occurs early in the test, if little increase in blood pressure or heart rate occurs at the time of ST depression, or if hypotension occurs. Hypotension is considered an ominous finding and usually prompts cardiac catheterization. Perioperative risk is considered low if exercise stress testing does not produce signs of myocardial ischemia at a reasonable workload (greater than 85% of predicted maximum heart rate).[279] Although it is useful in diagnosing coronary artery disease, its value as a preoperative test has been questioned.[266] Patients who are able to tolerate a good exercise

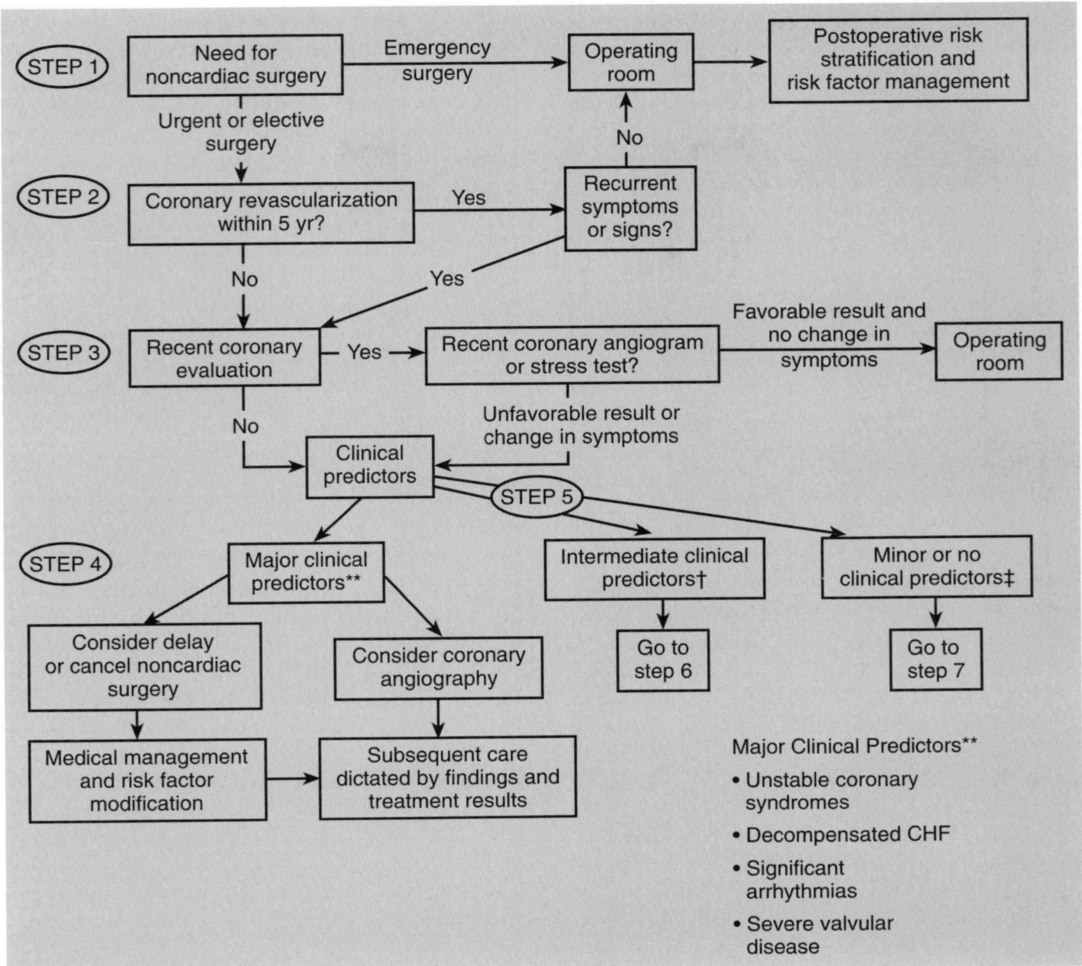

FIGURE **17-3**
Stepwise approach to preoperative cardiac assessment. *CHF*, Congestive heart failure. (From Eagle K, Berger PB, Calkins H, et al. ACC/AHA guideline update for perioperative cardiovascular evaluation for noncardiac surgery—executive summary. A report of the American College of Cardiology/American Heart Association task force on practice guidelines [committee to update the 1996 guidelines on perioperative cardiovascular evaluation for noncardiac surgery]. *Anesth Analg.* 2002;94:1052-1064.)

stress workload, even those with stable angina, are unlikely to have myocardial dysfunction.[280]

Pharmacologic stress testing can be performed in patients unable to exercise or in those who take digoxin. Two pharmacologic techniques, which incorporate either echocardiography or radionuclide scintigraphy, are used: (1) dipyramidole or adenosine, both of which cause a coronary steal phenomenon by redistributing coronary blood flow without direct negative inotropic effects, and (2) dobutamine for inotropic stress testing.[281]

Cardiac catheterization provides definitive information about the distribution and severity of coronary artery disease and may be indicated for patients with New York Heart Association class III or IV criteria who are undergoing high-risk surgical procedures.[279] Significant stenosis means narrowing of a major coronary artery by more than 70% or narrowing of the left main coronary artery by more than 50%. It is important to look beyond the coronary anatomy and concentrate on other findings that can guide perioperative decision-making. Three readily identifiable findings that indicate poor ventricular function are a cardiac index of less than 2.2 L/m^2, a left ventricular end-diastolic pressure of greater than 18 mm Hg, and an ejection fraction of less than 40%.[282] Taking note of ischemia-induced dysfunction of the papillary muscles can help in avoiding later confusion about the configuration of the pulmonary wedge pressure waveform and the significance of intraoperative changes in wedge pressure. Wall motion abnormalities should be noted. Areas of akinesis (no movement during systole) usually represent nonviable regions of myocardium and are relatively fixed deficits. In contrast, areas of hypokinesis (reduced contraction during systole) may represent ischemic but nonetheless viable regions of myocardium. This should alert anesthesia providers to a potentially dynamic situation in which alterations in the balance of myocardial oxygen supply and demand can either improve or worsen regional ischemia and associated contractility.

Respiratory System

A detailed evaluation of the respiratory system is crucial because of the relative frequency of and complications associated with respiratory disease. From an epidemiologic perspective, some form of lung disease is present in nearly 25% of the adult population. The most common problems are chronic obstructive pulmonary diseases (COPDs), such as chronic bronchitis, emphysema, and asthma, which are major predictors for postoperative pulmonary disorders.[283] In their acute or chronic forms the lung diseases are second only to coronary artery disease as a cause of death. Risk factors associated with increased postoperative respiratory morbidity and mortality rates include age (older than 60 years), history of smoking, comorbid diseases (e.g., cardiovascular disease, diabetes, American Society of Anesthesiologists [ASA] physical status class III or greater), chronic bronchitis, obesity (as little as 20% overweight), type of surgery (abdominal, thoracic), and prolonged duration of anesthesia (3 to 4 hours or longer).[48,284-290]

Emphysema and Chronic Bronchitis

The preparation of a patient with two forms of COPD—emphysema and chronic bronchitis—depends largely on the severity of the respiratory disease, as reflected by the preoperative history, physical examination, and diagnostic testing. Elective surgery is postponed, for example, when severe dyspnea, wheezing, pulmonary congestion, or hypercarbia ($PaCO_2$ greater than 50 mm Hg) is evident. The risk of postoperative respiratory failure in such circumstances is drastically increased. Consultation with a pulmonologist may be necessary for further evaluation and optimization of the respiratory status of the patient before anesthesia and surgery. Interventions to improve the pulmonary status of the patient with chronic bronchitis are the primary focus before surgery. Prophylactic measures that may reduce pulmonary risk are cited in Box 17-10.[290,291] Specific antibiotic therapy is initiated in patients with thick, purulent sputum and pulmonary infiltrates on the chest radiograph. Administration of prophylactic antibiotics to "sterilize" the sputum is not recommended. Secondary resistant infections may develop and complicate the perioperative management of the patient. To enhance the mobilization and clearance of pulmonary secretions, chest physiotherapy and adequate hydration can also be instituted. Instruction on incentive spirometric techniques, to lessen the incidence of postoperative atelectasis, is crucial in these patients.

The most reliable way to reduce the incidence of perioperative pulmonary complications is to have patients stop smoking cigarettes. Eight weeks after smoking cessation, the pulmonary complication rate correlates with that of nonsmokers.[50,52] This intervention may not be feasible when initial meetings with the patient occur within days or hours of the scheduled procedure.

Several diagnostic tests are used for clinically differentiating bronchitis and emphysema in patients in the advanced stages of COPD. Arterial blood gases, for example, may document the presence of preoperative hypoxemia or hypercarbia. An abnormally low partial pressure of arterial oxygen (PaO_2) value (less than 60 mm Hg), with or without partial pressure of arterial carbon dioxide ($PaCO_2$) retention, often reflects a state of chronic bronchitis. Over time the patient develops cor pulmonale because of the adverse effects of chronic hypoxemia on pulmonary vasculature. The diagnosis of COPD may be suggested by slight abnormalities on the chest radiograph, however, including emphysemic bullae and pulmonary hyperlucency, which reflect vascular deficiencies in the lung periphery. Diaphragmatic flattening and a vertical orientation of the cardiac silhouette are also characteristic. Chronic bronchitis, on the other hand, is rarely recognized through chest radiography unless secondary infections are apparent.

In addition to their role in categorizing patients with COPD, pulmonary function tests are occasionally used as diagnostic adjuncts for confirming the severity of air flow obstruction and its reversibility with bronchodilator therapy. In both chronic bronchitis and pulmonary emphysema, a decrease of the forced exhaled volume in 1 second (FEV_1) occurs in comparison to the forced vital capacity (FVC). FEV_1/FVC ratios of less than 80% indicate the presence of an obstructive process. Individual values of pulmonary function test results may be misleading. The FEV_1, for example, may already be low if the vital capacity is also decreased or the patient is uncooperative with the spirometric tests.

Numerous studies have found preoperative pulmonary function studies to be poor indicators of postoperative pulmonary complications.[292-294] The American College of Physicians offers guidelines for obtaining preoperative spirometric studies, although assessment of arterial oxygen desaturation is a more reliable predictor of perioperative morbidity (Table 17-7).[295] An emerging philosophy regarding preoperative spirometric studies limits their indication to patients scheduled to undergo lung resection or upper abdominal surgery and who have unexplained cough, dyspnea, or exercise intolerance.[296]

Asthma

Unlike other COPDs, asthma is characterized by a reversible airflow obstruction. Distal bronchoconstriction results from airway hyperreactivity to stimuli that have little or no effect on normal airways. Precipitating factors include allergens, exercise, upper respiratory tract infections (URTIs), emotional

BOX 17-10

Therapeutic Maneuvers to Decrease Risk of Pulmonary Complications

Preoperative

Instruction in respiratory maneuvers
Smoking cessation
Antibiotic treatment of pulmonary infection
Antibiotic treatment of chronic bronchitis
Psychologic preparation
Bronchodilator therapy for asthmatics
Maintenance of good nutrition
Chest physiotherapy

Postoperative

Minimization of postoperative opioid analgesia
Maximal inspiration maneuvers, incentive spirometry, chest physiotherapy
Early mobilization of elderly patients
Heparin prophylaxis in selected cases

Modified from Mohr DN, Lavender RC. Preoperative pulmonary evaluation. Identifying patients at increased risk for complications. Postgrad Med. *1996;100:241-256; and Marienau MES, Buck CF. Preoperative evaluation of the pulmonary patient undergoing nonpulmonary surgery.* J Peri Anesth Nurs. *1998;13:340-348.*

TABLE 17-7 American College of Physicians Recommendations for Preoperative Spirometry

Type of Surgery	Indication
Lung resection	All patients
Coronary artery bypass grafting	Smokers and patients with dyspnea
Upper abdominal surgery	Smokers and patients with dyspnea
Lower abdominal surgery	Uncharacterized pulmonary disease,* particularly if the surgical procedure will be prolonged or extensive
Head and neck, orthopedic	Uncharacterized pulmonary disease,* particularly in those who might require strenuous postoperative rehabilitation programs

**ACP defines uncharacterized pulmonary disease as pulmonary symptoms or history of pulmonary disease and no pulmonary function tests within 60 days.*
From American College of Physicians. Preoperative pulmonary function testing. Ann Intern Med. *1990;112:793-794.*

stressors, and unidentified triggers.[290] Pertinent data obtained from the medical history include the following[1]:

- The frequency of asthmatic attacks
- The severity of attacks (was endotracheal intubation required?)
- The time interval since the last attack
- How long since the patient was last hospitalized or treated in the emergency department for an asthmatic attack
- What triggers an asthmatic attack
- What works best for treating an acute asthmatic event

Information gleaned from these questions will help determine the nature and stability of the disease process. Patients with a history of coexistent cardiovascular disease, copious sputum production, previous perioperative complications from asthma, recurrent nocturnal awakenings from asthma, frequent or continuous systemic corticosteroid requirement, or a recent hospitalization or emergency department visit for asthma are considered to be at greater risk for perioperative aggravation of their asthma. Asthma should be under optimal medical management before a patient undergoes elective surgery and anesthesia. If the patient has a persistent cough, wheezing, or tachypnea on the day surgery is scheduled, it is best to reschedule surgery to allow for additional treatment of the asthma.

The need for diagnostic testing is based on the clinician's assessment of the severity of the disease and magnitude of the operative procedure. An ECG is indicated if right ventricular hypertrophy is suspected and generally implies long-standing insufficient therapy. A chest radiograph is considered only if the patient is suspected of having an acute infiltrative process (e.g., pneumonia) or if a recent change in the patient's physical status is suggestive of a worsening pulmonary condition. Arterial blood gases are usually indicated only when signs of chronic respiratory insufficiency (e.g., hypoxia, hypercarbia) are suspected or in patients with acute asthma who require emergency surgery. Spirometric evaluation, if age appropriate, consisting of a peak expiratory flow rate should be performed the morning of surgery if active disease is suspected, and the results compared with the patient's best value in recent weeks:

- Normal: 80% to 100% of baseline
- Moderate exacerbation: 50% to 80% of baseline
- Severe episode indicating the need for delay of surgery and more intensive therapy: less than 50% of baseline

Patient medications should be continued up to and on the day of surgery. Prophylactic β-adrenergic metered-dose inhalers should be used on the morning of surgery and should accompany the patient to the operating room. Oral medications (e.g., theophylline) may be taken with a sip (1 to 2 oz) of water up to 1 to 2 hours before surgery. Therapeutic serum theophylline levels, 10 to 20 mcg/ml, should be confirmed if theophylline is used. Supplemental stress doses of corticosteroids may be appropriate if the patient has recently taken corticosteroids. Antianxiety premedication should be considered, because psychologic triggers (e.g., anxiety) are common.

Ensure adequate hydration (e.g., minimize the fasting interval) to reduce airway desiccation and improve mobilization of secretions. If signs and symptoms of infection are present, surgery may be postponed while antibiotic therapy, based on sputum Gram stain and cultures, is initiated.

Upper Respiratory Tract Infection

Children with URTIs, particularly those younger than 1 year, have an increased risk (twofold to sevenfold increase) of respiratory-related adverse events intraoperatively and postoperatively (e.g., bronchospasm, laryngospasm, hypoxemia, atelectasis, croup, stridor). Signs and symptoms of URTI include sore throat; inflamed and reddened nasopharyngeal and oropharyngeal mucosa; sneezing; rhinorrhea (clear secretions) or mucopurulent nasal secretions; nasal congestion, including watery eyes; malaise; bulging, tender eardrums with associated inflammation; nonproductive cough; fever of 37.5° to 38.5° C (greater than 38° C associated with lower respiratory tract involvement); laryngitis or tonsillitis; viral ulcers in the oropharynx; and white blood cell count greater than 12,000 cells/mm^3 with a left shift. Positive chest findings such as pulmonary congestion and rales are usually associated with lower respiratory tract involvement.

Each case should be reviewed individually, and the decision to operate frequently depends on the urgency of the surgery, the duration and complexity of the surgery, and the need for instrumentation of the airway. It is important to obtain a specific history to distinguish a chronic state from an acute, superimposed infectious process, which has predictive value for morbidity. If the parents state that the child typically has a cold or chronic runny nose (clear rhinorrhea) and is in his or her optimal state (afebrile, without respiratory distress), short elective procedures may be considered. If the child has a productive cough from lower respiratory tract involvement or an infectious-appearing runny nose, elective surgery should be postponed. However, it may be necessary to schedule children who have chronic URTIs for procedures such as myringotomy with ventilation tube placement or tonsillectomies, because URTIs are commonly associated with these conditions. Exercise caution with children younger than 5 years old (consider postponing the procedure for children younger than 1 year old), because risks are increased. If the child is older than 1 year with resolving URTI, it is reasonable to proceed with minor procedures not requiring endotracheal intubation (intubation with URTI increases risk 11-fold).

Infectious nasopharyngitis (without lower respiratory tract involvement) requires postponing the surgery for approximately 2 weeks. If the child exhibits signs and symptoms of lower respiratory tract involvement, it is prudent to postpone an elective surgical procedure for 4 to 6 weeks, which is the time necessary to minimize airway hyperactivity.

Laboratory testing may consist of a complete blood count, including differential. The value of obtaining a preoperative white blood cell count has been questioned because it is of little value and rarely is a factor in determining whether to proceed with the surgery.[297] Nasal or throat cultures may be obtained if signs of an infectious process are observed. A chest radiograph is not warranted, especially if chest sounds are clear. Pulmonary function tests and arterial blood gas analysis rarely offer any useful information.

Gastrointestinal System

Evaluation of the gastrointestinal system includes preoperative determination of the presence of nausea and vomiting, diarrhea, occult or overt gastrointestinal bleeding, abdominal or referred pain, abdominal distention, palpable masses, dysphagia, or gastric hyperacidity, with or without reflux. The fluid and electrolyte status of the patient is reviewed, especially when gastrointestinal symptoms are associated with weight loss or malabsorption. Active bleeding requires the measurement of a preoperative hemoglobin concentration. The hematocrit value may be falsely elevated as a result of hemoconcentration in patients with acute or chronic bleeding. Radiographic and CT scans of the abdomen are reviewed for evidence of obstruction or masses. The presence of peptic ulcer disease or esophageal hiatus hernia is also ascertained. For affected patients, prophylactic measures to reduce the risk of aspiration and its adverse pulmonary sequelae (e.g., aspiration pneumonitis) are instituted before surgery.

Hepatobiliary System

The preoperative evaluation of the hepatobiliary system includes the determination of the presence of acute or chronic liver parenchymal disease, such as hepatitis or cirrhosis, or cholestatic liver disease. Because of the tremendous reserve of the liver, progression of hepatic disease is often insidious. Signs and symptoms may be inapparent or vague until physiologic functions of the hepatobiliary system (Box 17-11) are markedly affected. Liver function tests are also limited in their ability to reflect the acuity and extent of hepatobiliary disease.[298] Considerable damage to the liver may be evident before laboratory test results are altered.

During the early stages of hepatitis or cirrhosis, the clinical presentation ranges from one in which the patient is asymptomatic with normal liver function tests to one in which the patient has malaise, weight loss, abdominal discomfort, and mild jaundice with mild elevations in bilirubin levels. In cases of unexplained jaundice or elevated transaminase levels, suspicions of hepatobiliary dysfunction should be thoroughly investigated by a preoperative consultation with a gastroenterologist. Elective surgery is postponed until a definitive diagnosis and treatment are established, because further decompensation of hepatic function may follow anesthesia and surgery, notably after intraabdominal procedures.

Progression of hepatobiliary disease to overt hepatic failure may be evidenced by gross abnormalities of liver function test results, including coagulopathies; extreme jaundice with or without cyanosis; generalized tremors and increased deep tendon reflexes; ascites, spider nevi, and hepatosplenomegaly; hepatorenal failure; and signs of hepatic encephalopathy.[299] Elective surgery is avoided at this time, because surgery on a patient with hepatic failure is associated with an extremely high incidence of morbidity and mortality. Anesthesia may be required, however, for a patient who requires a palliative or emergent procedure. The placement of a portocaval shunt and the surgical control of hemorrhage from esophageal varices are common procedures, given the growing number of patients with advanced liver disease. Anesthetic management is supportive in such situations and aims to minimize the risk of further hepatobiliary deterioration. For example, administration of phytonadione (AquaMEPHYTON) and transfusion of fresh frozen plasma and cryoprecipitate may be required for the correction of preoperative coagulopathies. Sedative premedicants are avoided in the disoriented or somnolent patient in whom hepatic encephalopathy has been diagnosed. Because of the rapid development of hypoglycemia, the patient's blood glucose level is checked preoperatively. The acid-base balance,

BOX 17-11

Physiologic Functions of the Hepatobiliary System

Bilirubin Formation and Excretion

Conjugation of free bilirubin and secretion into bile

Carbohydrate Metabolism

Glycogenesis
Gluconeogenesis
Glycogenolysis

Fat Metabolism

Lipogenesis
Lipolysis

Protein Metabolism

Formation of proteins, such as albumin, prothrombin, transferrin, and glycoprotein
Synthesis of plasma cholinesterase
Deamination of proteins, such as hormones, into ammonia and urea

Hormone Metabolism Drug Detoxification

Conversion of lipophilic drugs into inactive hydrophilic substances
Hydrolysis of ester linkages by plasma cholinesterase

Vitamin Storage

Storage of fat-soluble vitamins A, D, E, and K
Storage of anti–pernicious anemia factor, vitamin B_{12}

Synthesis of Coagulation Factors

Synthesis of most clotting factors, including prothrombin; fibrinogen; and factors V, VII, IX, and X
Source of anticoagulant, heparin

Phagocytosis

Filtration and destruction of bacteria and debris in blood circulating through hepatic sinusoids by Kupffer's cells electrolyte status, and extent of hepatorenal reserve may also be determined by arterial blood gas analysis, serum multiphasic profiles, and liver function tests.[299]

The interpretation of liver function tests should be approached cautiously. Differential diagnosis of parenchymal versus cholestatic liver disease is limited by the insensitivity and nonspecificity of current measures, especially for determination of serum transaminase and alkaline phosphatase levels.[300] Aspartate transaminase (AST), or serum glutamic oxaloacetic transaminase (SGOT); alanine transaminase (ALT), or serum glutamic pyruvic transaminase (SGPT); and lactate dehydrogenase (LDH) are commonly measured hepatocellular enzymes that are also distributed throughout cells of the lungs, heart, kidneys, and skeletal muscles. Increases in their serum concentrations are therefore not always indicative of hepatobiliary disease. Greater specificity can be derived from isoenzyme-5 fractions of the enzymes, such as LDH.[301]

In cases of biliary obstruction or irritation, alkaline phosphatase enzymes may be released from the cells of bile ducts. Increases in the serum concentrations of these enzymes also facilitate the differentiation of hepatic dysfunction caused by parenchymal disease versus that caused by cholestasis. The interpretation of these results is again limited by the presence of extrahepatic stores of alkaline phosphatase. In this situation, cholestatic liver disease can be confirmed by high serum levels of conjugated (direct) bilirubin.[302] Causative factors are then determined from discussions with a gastroenterologist and from the results of ultrasound, CT, and endoscopic retrograde cholangiopancreatographic scans.

When acute parenchymal injury is evident, prolongation of prothrombin time offers the most rapid and reliable determination of liver dysfunction and is shown to have prognostic significance. It reflects the inability of the acutely damaged liver to synthesize clotting factors. Although the production of albumin is also affected, its plasma half-life exceeds that of prothrombin. Hypoalbuminemia may then be inapparent for days after an acute hepatocellular insult.[303]

Once a functional impairment of the liver has been established, the cause is investigated as part of the preoperative evaluation. Cirrhosis and hepatitis, for example, are frequently associated with long-standing alcohol abuse. The increasing consumption of alcohol in the United States parallels the rising incidence of liver disease. Exposure to hepatotoxic agents, such as carbon tetrachloride or vinyl chloride, in the workplace should also be ruled out. Hepatotoxic drugs may then be discontinued or avoided before surgery. These drugs commonly include acetaminophen and other nonsteroidal antiinflammatory drugs, aspirin, methyldopa, isoniazid, and rifampin.[304,305] Finally, a diagnosis of infectious hepatitis should be pursued in patients with hepatobiliary disease of unknown cause and in patients considered to be at high risk, which includes those with a history of hemodialysis, multiple blood transfusions, or intravenous drug abuse. Because of the virulent nature of the hepatitis viruses, care of an infected patient also poses an occupational hazard for anesthesia providers.[306] Maximum precautions must be consistently exercised, and, as recommended by the Centers for Disease Control and Prevention, vaccination with the hepatitis B virus should be performed.[307]

Renal System

Evaluation of the kidneys and urinary tract includes the preoperative determination of the patient's volume status and presence of polyuria; urinary incontinence or retention; microscopic or frank hematuria; recurrent infections in the form of glomerulonephritis, pyelonephritis, or cystitis; dysuria; and oliguria or anuria. Fluid balance is calculated from the patient's intake and output during the hospital stay. Preoperative dehydration may be evident, for example, in a patient receiving long-term diuretic therapy. Polyuria, when not attributed to diuretics, may reflect glycosuria or, rarely, inadequate secretion of antidiuretic hormone (diabetes insipidus). Urinary retention and other signs of neurogenic bladder may be caused by a spinal cord injury or long-standing diabetes mellitus. Frequent catheterizations are often necessary in such situations, which increases the patient's risk for development of chronic urinary tract infections. Preoperative urinalysis and culture are therefore required so that infection can be ruled out. Treatment and resolution should be accomplished before elective surgery is performed, especially for procedures involving the placement of a prosthetic graft for a mitral valve or total hip replacement. Problems with intraoperative bladder catheterization can be anticipated in patients with dysuria or voiding difficulties. In older men these problems are frequently attributed to chronic prostatism. Untreated prostatic hypertrophy, as well as renal calculi and congenital malformations of the ureters, results in obstructed urinary outflow. Over time these conditions may lead to a state of chronic renal insufficiency or failure.

Any suspicion of renal dysfunction should be investigated before surgery. Unfortunately, clinical evidence of renal insufficiency may not be apparent until at least 70% of nephrons are nonfunctional. Accurate diagnosis of renal insufficiency is further limited by the insensitivity of laboratory tests (Table 17-8).[308] Blood urea nitrogen (BUN) concentrations,

TABLE 17-8 Common Renal Function Tests

Test	Reference Range
Urea nitrogen	5-25 mg/dL
Creatinine	0.5-1.5 mg/dL
Sodium	133-147 mmol/L
Potassium	3.2-5.2 mmol/L
Chloride	94-110 mmol/L
CO_2	22-32 mmol/L
Uric acid	2.5-7.5 mg/dL
Calcium	8.5-10.5 mg/dL
Phosphorus	2.2-4.2 mg/dL
Urinalysis, routine	
Color	Straw-amber
Appearance	Clear-hazy
Protein	0 mg/dL
Blood	Negative
Glucose	0 mg/dL
Ketones	0 mg/dL
pH	4.5-8
Specific gravity	1.002-1.030
Bilirubin	Negative
Urinalysis, micro	
Red blood cells	0-3/high-power field
White blood cells	0-5/high-power field
Casts	0-2/low-power field

Modified from Miller ED Jr. Understanding renal function and its preoperative evaluation. In: Malhotra V, ed. Anesthesia for Renal and Genitourinary Surgery. *New York: McGraw-Hill; 1996:9.*

for example, do not accurately reflect glomerular filtration rate (GFR). Although urea is freely filtered at the glomerulus, it is reabsorbed to a large and variable extent through the tubules. BUN levels are also affected by the amount of protein ingested in the gastrointestinal tract and the amount of urea metabolized by the liver, as well as by the catabolic state of the patient. Because tubular reabsorption of creatinine does not occur, creatinine levels correlate more with the rate of glomerular filtration than do BUN concentrations. The serum levels of creatinine, a by-product of skeletal muscle metabolism, can reflect the muscle mass and catabolic state of each patient. This characteristic limits its precision in determining the magnitude of nephron loss. Normal serum creatinine levels may be higher, for example, in a muscular man than in a woman. Conversely, serum creatine levels can remain within the normal range in the elderly patient, despite a progressive decline in glomerular function,[309] because of the decrease in muscle mass associated with aging.

The most accurate reflection of renal reserve or GFR is creatinine clearance, which reflects the ability of glomeruli to excrete creatinine into the urine at a given blood concentration. The drawbacks of this assessment lie in the cost and time required for the collection of urine samples. As a general principle, urine is collected over a 24-hour period so that the creatinine clearance rate can be measured by the following equation:

Equation 17-1

$$\text{GFR (ml/min)} = UV/P$$

where U is the urinary concentration of creatinine (mg/dL), V is the volume of urine (ml/min), and P is the plasma concentration of creatinine (mg/dL).

Accurate measures of GFR can also be calculated from a 2-hour specimen.[310] Creatinine clearance or GFR values between 50 and 80 ml/min are indicative of mild renal dysfunction. Renal failure is otherwise evident when creatinine clearance levels decrease to less than 10 ml/min.

Practically all surgical patients with chronic renal failure are undergoing dialysis, usually hemodialysis performed at the hospital or renal facility. Others undergo continuous ambulatory peritoneal dialysis. The goal of dialysis therapy is to maintain a reasonable degree of homeostasis, although BUN and creatinine concentrations remain abnormal. The preoperative evaluation and preparation of the patient with chronic renal failure should therefore focus on fluid and electrolyte balance, as well as on the extent of concomitant diseases. Estimates of volume status are derived from the amount of weight gained between periods of dialysis. Fluid overload may also be evidenced by jugular vein distention, peripheral and periorbital edema, and bibasilar rales.

Preoperative measurement of serum potassium concentration is recommended, regardless of whether dialysis is performed, within 6 to 8 hours of surgery, because unexpected hyperkalemia, with its adverse cardiac effects, is known to occur rapidly. In cases in which the serum potassium level exceeds 5.5 mEq/L and congestive heart failure is apparent, elective surgery should be delayed until after dialysis. When postponement is not feasible, as with emergency surgery to relieve a pericardial effusion or procedures to revise a hemodialysis shunt, measures to reduce the serum potassium concentration are then instituted. These measures may include the infusion of a dextrose-insulin solution in the presence of tall, tented T waves on the ECG.

Although hemoglobin ranges from 5 to 8 mg/dL are not unusual in patients with chronic renal failure, a hemoglobin level should also be obtained as part of the preoperative evaluation. Chronic anemia is predominantly caused by decreases in renal erythropoietin production and enhanced fragility of red blood cells in the presence of uremia. It is further exacerbated by blood loss experienced with hemodialysis and chronic gastrointestinal bleeding. When extreme fatigue and pallor, limited exercise tolerance, and persistent tachycardia are evident before major surgery, the transfusion of packed red blood cells may be necessary. Because repeat transfusion and immunosuppression therapy are often required during the course of chronic renal failure, the patient is at greater risk for being infected with the hepatitis virus, human immunodeficiency virus (HIV), or both. Coagulopathies are also suspected. The most likely cause is a decrease in platelet adhesiveness secondary to the chronic state of metabolic acidemia. Hemodialysis can be effectively used for the correction of prolonged bleeding times before surgery in this situation.

Throughout the perioperative period, most therapeutic regimens for patients with chronic renal failure can be continued, including the administration of antihypertensives, digitalis preparations, corticosteroids, and insulin.[311] Requirements for preoperative sedation may be less than anticipated, and medications with prolonged durations, such as diazepam, are avoided.[312] Peripheral arteriovenous shunts should be assessed for patency and infection. Measurement of noninvasive blood pressures and application of intravenous lines are avoided in the limb of the graft. Administration of gastrointestinal preparations (e.g., antacids and gastrokinetic agents) and drainage of peritoneal dialysate, aimed at reducing the risks of regurgitation and pulmonary aspiration, are also instituted in order to prepare the patient with chronic renal failure for anesthesia and surgery.

Endocrine System

Endocrine diseases of concern in the preoperative evaluation include diabetes mellitus, thyroid gland disorders, and adrenocortical dysfunctions. End-organ effects of each of these diseases increase perioperative risk substantially. For example, morbidity and mortality rates are 5 to 10 times greater in diabetic patients with renal and autonomic nervous system involvement.[313]

Diabetes

Diabetes mellitus is the most common of endocrine disorders, affecting more than 2.4% of the population in the United States.[314] It represents a dysfunction in glucose metabolism that is caused by the impaired synthesis, secretion, or use of insulin.

Most patients with diabetes (80% to 90%) are not dependent on exogenous insulin for the regulation of blood glucose levels. As shown in Table 17-9,[315,316] the patient with non–insulin-dependent, or type 2, diabetes often benefits from diet modification, weight control, and exercise alone. An oral hypoglycemic agent (Table 17-10) may also be added to the patient's therapeutic regimen.[317] The remaining 10% to 20% of patients with diabetes are dependent on insulin preparations listed on Table 17-11 and are therefore classified as having insulin-dependent, or type 1, diabetes mellitus.[318] These patients are susceptible to periods of hyperglycemia and ketoacidosis. As a result of microvascular changes, they are also prone to the development of severe end-organ complications, including diabetic retinopathy and cataract formation, somatic and autonomic insufficiency (orthostatic hypotension,

TABLE 17-9 Distinguishing Features of Diabetes Mellitus

	Type 1	Type 2
Previous name	Insulin-dependent diabetes	Non–insulin-dependent diabetes
Age of onset	Childhood	Middle age or elderly
Timing of onset	Abrupt	Gradual
Predisposing factors	Genetic	Obesity, pregnancy, drugs
Prevalence	0.2%-0.3%	2%-4%
Insulin requirement	Always	Infrequent
Ketoacidosis	Common	Rare
Systemic complications	Frequent	Frequent

Modified from Sherwin RS. Diabetes mellitus. In: Goldman L, Bennett JC, eds. Cecil Textbook of Medicine. *21st ed. Philadelphia: Saunders; 2000:1263; and Larson CP Jr. Evaluation of the patient and preoperative preparation. In: Barash PG, Cullen BF, Stoelting RK, eds.* Clinical Anesthesia. *2nd ed. Philadelphia: Lippincott; 1992:553.*

TABLE 17-10 Oral Hypoglycemic Therapy

Drug Class	Drug Name	Onset	Duration of Action
First generation sulfonylureas	Tolbutamide	1 h	12 h
	Acetohexamide	3 h	24 h
	Tolazamide	4 h	16 h
	Chlorpropamide	2 h	24 h
Second generation sulfonylureas	Glyburide	30 min	24 h
	Glipizide	IR 30 min ER 2-4 h	IR 24 h ER 24 h
	Glimepiride	2-3 h	24 h
Biguanides	Metformin	1-3 h	17 h
Thiazolidinediones	Rosiglitazone	1-3 h	4 h
	Pioglitazone	2 h	N/A
Glinides	Repaglinide	30-90 min	4 h
Alpha-glucosidase inhibitor	Acarbose	2 h	4 h
	Miglitol	1 h	4 h

ER, *Extended release;* IR, *immediate release;* N/A, *not available.*
From Angelini G, Ketzler JT, Coursin DB. Perioperative care of the diabetic patient. In: Schwartz AJ, ed. ASA Refresher Courses in Anesthesiology. *Philadelphia: Lippincott; 2001:1-9.*

bradycardia, gastroparesis), and nephropathy. Hypertension, coronary artery disease (which may be silent), and peripheral vascular disease are more prevalent in patients with type 2 diabetes because of acquired abnormalities in the macrovasculature. MI or stroke is the cause of death in nearly 80% of patients with type 2 diabetes.[319] Careful upper airway evaluation should be performed, because the diabetic patient is at higher risk for difficulty in endotracheal intubation secondary to the stiff-joint syndrome.

The aim of an evaluation of a patient with diabetes, notably one with type 1 diabetes mellitus, is determining the degree of preoperative blood glucose control and the presence of major organ system dysfunction; renal and cardiovascular complications of diabetes substantially heighten perioperative morbidity and mortality. Early preoperative evaluation and workup of diabetic patients are important. This is especially true in patients who are noncompliant, patients whose blood glucose level is poorly controlled, and patients with newly diagnosed diabetes, because modifications in their care may be necessary before surgery. Early assessment of a patient allows for consultation with a medical internist in order to optimize the patient's preoperative condition before anesthesia and surgery. Elective surgery is also postponed in cases of extreme hyperglycemia and ketoacidosis. Aggressive fluid, electrolyte, and insulin therapy are initiated, and the cause of ketoacidosis must be investigated before surgery.

Consultation with a cardiologist may also help a practitioner evaluate and improve the preoperative cardiac status of a patient with diabetes, especially if the patient is undergoing a procedure associated with a greater risk of perioperative myocardial ischemia, such as a carotid endarterectomy or an abdominal aortic aneurysm resection. Exercise stress testing and a 12-lead ECG may be performed because of the high incidence of ischemic heart disease in this population. Orthostatic hypotension, resting tachycardia, and lack of respiratory

TABLE 17-11 Insulin Preparations

Insulin Type	Onset	Peak (hours)	Duration (hours)	Comments
Very Rapid Lispro	IV immediate SC 15-30 min	SC 1	SC 2-4	Newest agent Recombinant
Rapid acting Regular CZI	IV immediate	SC 2-4	SC 6-8	Most common in IV infusions
Intermediate NPH Lente	SC 2-3 hr	SC 6-12	SC 12-24	Often combined with regular insulin
Long acting	SC 4-8 hr	SC 12-24	SC 24-36	Perioperative use uncommon

IV, *Intravenous;* SC, *subcutaneous.*
From Graham GW, Unger BP, Coursin DB. Perioperative management of selected endocrine disorders. Int Anesth Clin. *2000;38:31-67.*

variability in cardiac rhythm may reflect autonomic neuropathy (20% to 40%). Abnormalities in autonomic function may also result in bladder atrophy and delayed gastric emptying times in 20% to 30% of diabetic patients.[320] A gastrokinetic agent, such as metoclopramide, should be administered before surgery to reduce the incidence of regurgitation and pulmonary aspiration during general anesthesia. Finally, the preoperative evaluation of patients with diabetes focuses on the assessment of the airway. Patients with type 2 diabetes are more often obese, and this condition in itself presents a challenge to endotracheal intubation. Joint stiffness, particularly in patients with type 1 diabetes, can limit cervical spine and temporomandibular joint mobility and makes laryngoscopy difficult.[124,125,321]

It is best to schedule surgery as early in the day as possible to minimize the fasting period. Just before surgery, diabetic patients who require insulin or oral hypoglycemic agents should have blood glucose checked. Depending on the type and length of surgery and the lability of diabetes, serum glucose levels are checked intraoperatively and in the postanesthesia care unit at 2- to 4-hour intervals. The goal of perioperative insulin therapy is to maintain the serum glucose level less than 180 mg/dL while avoiding hypoglycemia.[317] Several different regimens are available for the treatment of diabetic patients undergoing surgery and anesthesia. Consultation with the physician responsible for managing the diabetes is helpful in determining an acceptable range of serum glucose and when and what type of insulin therapy may be appropriate. Patients taking oral hypoglycemic agents should withhold the short half-life agents (e.g., repaglinide and acarbose) on the day of surgery and withhold the longer-lasting agents (e.g., chlorpropamide and glimepiride) for up to 48 hours. Fasting patients who are receiving insulin should have intravenous access established with a crystalloid solution containing 5% glucose. Insulin may then be administered to the patient intravenously (bolus or continuous infusion) or subcutaneously. The intravenous technique of administering regular insulin offers the advantage of providing a more predictable serum drug level and metabolic control. The intravenous route still has the risk of making the patient hyperglycemic or hypoglycemic if the glucose or insulin infusions become unbalanced.[322] The tighter the control of glucose levels, the more frequent the glucose monitoring. The subcutaneous route of insulin administration has been criticized as being too unpredictable in its absorption, especially perioperatively, with alterations in blood pressure and cutaneous blood flow.[323] In the patient with type I diabetes, a common approach, especially for brief procedures, is to subcutaneously administer a fraction (often one third to one half) of the patient's usual morning dose of intermediate- or long-acting insulin. For patients with either insulin-dependent or non–insulin-dependent diabetes, the most important goal of perioperative management is the prevention of hyperglycemia and especially hypoglycemia, as well as their adverse consequences, during surgical stress.

Thyroid Gland Disorders

Although disorders of the thyroid gland are relatively uncommon, the anesthesia provider may still encounter patients with hyperthyroidism or hypothyroidism who require surgery. Most have undergone adequate medical therapy before anesthesia and surgery are performed. Nevertheless, the anesthesia provider should be aware of the clinical manifestations of thyroid gland dysfunctions (Table 17-12).[324,325]

Hyperthyroidism. Hyperthyroidism is caused by an excess secretion of thyroid hormones, 3,5,3′-triiodothyronine (T_3) and tetraiodothyronine (thyroxine or T_4). It is evident in such conditions as Graves' disease, toxic goiter (multinodular, single), thyroid carcinoma, and pituitary tumors that oversecrete thyroid-stimulating hormone (TSH). Signs and symptoms reflect a hypermetabolic state with sympathetic overactivity resulting from the primary effects of thyroid hormones on the adenylate cyclase system.[324]

The preoperative preparation of the hyperthyroid patient is aimed at attaining a euthyroid state. This may be accomplished through administration of antithyroid drugs such as carbimazole or propylthiouracil for 4 to 6 weeks followed by iodine for 7 to 10 days.[324] Not only does it decrease the overall synthesis of thyroxine, propylthiouracil lessens its conversion into the more potent T_3. Reversible agranulocytosis is infrequently seen with long-term therapy.[326] A complete blood

TABLE 17-12 Clinical Features of Thyroid Gland Disorders

	Hyperthyroidism	Hypothyroidism
General	Heat intolerance, weight loss, tremor, sweating	Cold intolerance, arthralgia, alopecia, "strawberries and cream" complexion, gruff voice
Cardiovascular	Tachycardia, cardiac arrhythmias (atrial fibrillation), wide pulse pressure, heart failure	Bradycardia, cardiomegaly, cardiac failure, pericardial effusions
Respiratory	Dyspnea	Hypoventilation, sleep apnea
Gastrointestinal	Diarrhea, nausea, vomiting	Constipation
Neurologic	Anxiety, irritability, hyperactive reflexes, insomnia; depression and apathy in elderly	Fatigue, lethargy, slow mental function, hypoactive reflexes, myxedema coma
Musculoskeletal	Goiter, weight loss, proximal myopathy, bone resorption	Goiter, lethargy, large tongue, amyloidosis, peripheral neuropathy, muscle stiffness
Ophthalmic	Exophthalmos, lid lag, lid retraction, reduced blinking	
Renal		Impaired free water clearance

Modified from Edwards R. Thyroid and parathyroid disease. In: Desborough J, ed. International Anesthesiology Clinics: Endocrine Disorders and Anesthesia. *Philadelphia: Lippincott-Raven;1997:63-83; and Roizen MF. Anesthesia for the patient with endocrine disease (part I).* Curr Rev Clin Anesth. *1987;6:43.*

cell and platelet count should be determined preoperatively. β-Antagonist drugs, such as propranolol and esmolol, are also useful adjuncts in the management of hyperthyroidism. They ameliorate signs of sympathetic nervous system overstimulation such as tachycardia, diaphoresis, and tremors.[327,328]

All drugs used to manage hyperthyroidism, including propylthiouracil and propranolol, should be continued perioperatively, and elective surgery is postponed until the patient is rendered euthyroid. If emergency surgery cannot be delayed for a patient with symptomatic hyperthyroidism, a continuous infusion of esmolol (100 to 300 mcg/kg/min) may be initiated to control unwanted tachycardia.[329] Higher doses of preoperative anxiolytics and sedatives, such as benzodiazepines, may also be required. Anticholinergics are avoided because of their interference with normal heat-regulating mechanisms and their potentiation of tachyarrhythmias. Last, the preoperative evaluation should include a thorough assessment of the airway. Lateral radiographs or CT scans of the neck can be used to determine the extent of airway impingement by a large, immobile goiter.[330]

Hypothyroidism. Hypothyroidism represents several conditions, such as chronic thyroiditis or Hashimoto's disease, in which tissues are exposed to decreased circulating concentrations of T_3 and T_4. The cause of hypothyroidism may be primary, resulting from the destruction or hypofunction of the thyroid gland, or secondary, resulting from insufficient TSH production. The diagnosis of hypothyroidism is confirmed by decreased serum concentrations of T_3 and T_4, with or without secondary increases in TSH levels.[331]

The treatment of hypothyroidism consists of administration of T_4, levothyroxine sodium (Synthroid) replacement therapy, with the restoration of intravascular volume and electrolyte status. Elective surgery need not be delayed for patients with mild-to-moderate hypothyroidism. No difference in perioperative outcome has been noted between untreated hypothyroid patients and patients who are euthyroid.[332,333] However, the unusual susceptibility of hypothyroid patients to depressant drugs, such as opioids, should be taken into consideration.[334] Because of this, preoperative medications may be withheld until the patient is in a safely monitored area, such as the operating room. Last, a careful assessment of the airway is performed in hypothyroid patients because a large tongue and diffuse goiter may complicate laryngoscopy and endotracheal intubation.

Adrenocortical Disorders. Disorders of the adrenal cortex, ranging from hyperadrenocorticism to hypoadrenocorticism, are the result of primary disease of the adrenal cortex or pituitary gland, ectopic production of adrenocortical hormones by malignant tissue, or most commonly treatment with exogenous corticosteroids. Steroids are commonly used to treat bronchial asthma, autoimmune diseases, and connective tissue disorders, such as rheumatoid arthritis. Their high-dose administration for prolonged periods or their excess levels in circulating glucocorticoid hormones characteristically results in a syndrome referred to as *Cushing's syndrome*. This syndrome is clinically manifested as hypertension and hypovolemia, truncal obesity with an accumulation of interscapular fat ("buffalo hump"), abdominal and gluteal striae, plethoric facial appearance ("moon facies"), easy bruisability, osteoporosis, personality changes, and menstrual irregularities and hirsutism. Hyperaldosteronism—an excess of mineralocorticoid hormones—may also be manifested as hypertension in association with marked hypokalemia (plasma potassium [K] less than 3 mmol/L). Its major alterations involve sodium and water retention, potassium depletion, and metabolic alkalosis.

Adrenocortical insufficiency may be of a primary origin (Addison's disease) or may be caused by the secondary inhibition of adrenocortical function by prolonged exogenous steroid therapy. Clinical signs are less obvious than those of Cushing's disease and include skin hyperpigmentation, weight loss, muscle wasting, hypotension, intravascular volume depletion, hypoglycemia, hyponatremia, and hyperkalemia.[335]

The preoperative preparation of a patient with adrenocortical dysfunction includes the correction of fluid and electrolyte disturbances and the treatment of coexisting disorders, such as hypertension and diabetes mellitus. Glucocorticoid or mineralocorticoid replacement therapy is also continued perioperatively. Exogenous corticosteroids should be provided for patients who have been treated with steroids for more than 1 month within the previous year (see Table 17-4).[241] For patients currently receiving high-dose steroid therapy, such as those with chronic hypoadrenocorticism or Addison's disease, further supplementation of the daily maintenance doses is required. This recommendation is based on concerns that additional cortisol may not be released from the adrenal cortex as a result of its primary hypofunction or secondary suppression in response to surgical stress. Cardiovascular collapse may then ensue during major surgical procedures.

DIAGNOSTIC TESTING

Appropriate laboratory evaluations and diagnostic procedures should be obtained and the results considered to determine the patient's surgical and anesthetic risk, as well as the need for appropriate health-care modifications. The controversy lies in which tests are necessary and appropriate for specific settings. The rationale for performing "routine" tests has been under intense scrutiny, primarily because of recent and ongoing changes in health-care economics. A protocol that delineates the indications for testing should be established by each surgical facility and approved by the medical staff. When protocols are followed for the ordering of preoperative laboratory tests, the total number of tests performed has been reduced 50% to 60%, and the appropriateness of the tests has improved.[336] Based on 1990 dollars, this could result in a savings to the U.S. health-care system of 2.9 to 4.3 billion dollars annually.[337] A necessary step in the implementation process for preoperative testing guidelines is the education of the medical staff. Centralizing the test ordering process, such as in the preoperative assessment clinic, makes standardization and compliance more attainable.

Routine Diagnostic Testing

It has been traditional practice, even within the past decade, to order a "battery" of routine evaluative tests before a patient undergoes surgery and anesthesia. The routine ordering of preoperative diagnostic tests remains a common practice in many institutions. Until the early 1990s the rationale for obtaining preoperative diagnostic tests was rarely questioned. Tests were frequently ordered for a variety of reasons but were often unrelated to findings based specifically on the patient's history and physical examination. Reasons cited for ordering the standard battery of preoperative tests included the following[338-340]:

- To follow customary practice at an institution
- To adhere to institutional or legislative mandates that dictate the tests to be performed

- To further evaluate and determine the progress of a known disease or condition, because preexisting medical conditions have a greater risk for intraoperative and postoperative complications
- To detect asymptomatic yet modifiable conditions that could alter anesthetic and surgical care
- To detect asymptomatic but unmodifiable conditions that could alter anesthetic and surgical risk
- To screen for conditions unrelated to the planned surgery
- To acquire baseline results that might be useful in the perioperative period
- To protect against medicolegal involvement

When considering the value of preoperative tests, the following must be considered:

1. The diagnostic procedure should be cost effective—that is, the costs saved from knowing the results exceed the expense of performing the test.[341]
2. The diagnostic procedure should have a positive benefit-risk ratio—that is, the benefit derived from conducting the test outweighs the harm that might ensue from a false-positive result.[342]
3. Test results are available for interpretation and recuperative intervention before surgery.
4. Test results will yield information that could not be obtained from the history and physical examination.[342]
5. Abnormal test results in an asymptomatic patient would influence the patient care, the surgery, or the anesthesia management.[342]

Without any clinical sign, the likelihood of observing a significant anomaly is very small for diagnostic procedures such as ECG,[339] chest radiography,[339,343,344] or laboratory tests.[337,339,345] Asymptomatic disease is rarely of clinical concern in perioperative surgical care. In addition, unexpected abnormal findings from preoperative testing tend not to affect the upcoming surgery.[346] When a battery of routine preoperative tests are conducted, abnormal test results potentially alter patient care only 0.22% to 0.56% of the time.[339,345] A consistent conclusion of most studies is that routine preoperative laboratory screening is not cost-effective or predictive of postoperative complications.[338,347]

Limitations to Routine Preoperative Diagnostic Testing

It has been estimated that at least 10% of the more than 30 billion dollars spent on laboratory testing annually in the United States goes to preparing patients for surgery.[348] Although added health-care costs are the most apparent limitation to performing the routine battery of preoperative tests, additional factors can negatively affect the patient and care providers. The indiscriminant ordering of tests for diagnostic evaluation increases the likelihood that at least one test will be abnormal in a healthy patient.[340] False-positive, or even false-negative, test results can lead to additional medical evaluation and the potential for increased morbidity. Abnormal laboratory tests for continuous data are defined in probabilistic terms and assume a normal patient population distribution.[339,340] The endpoints of the bell-shaped distribution curve are arbitrarily set at 2.5%; therefore 5% of test results in normal patients are reported as abnormal. False-positive test results may lead to additional follow-up tests, which can place the patient at risk of increased morbidity.[341,349] Abnormal test results that were not further pursued and lack of documentation of the rationale for not investigating abnormal test results have increased the medicolegal risk for physicians.[350]

BOX 17-12

Indications for Diagnostic Procedures

Chest Radiograph

Previous abnormal results on chest radiography
History of malignancy in which pulmonary metastasis might alter the surgical therapy
History of tuberculosis or a positive skin test result for tuberculosis for which no treatment was given
History suggestive of pulmonary infection (e.g., new or chronic productive cough or blood-tinged or purulent-appearing sputum)
Suspected intrathoracic pathologic condition (e.g., tumors, vascular ring)
History of congenital heart disease
History of prematurity associated with residual bronchopulmonary dysplasia
Severe obstructive sleep apnea (patient may have cardiomegaly)
Down syndrome (patient may have asymptomatic subluxation of the atlantoaxial junction)
Symptomatic or debilitating asthma, chronic obstructive pulmonary disease, or cardiovascular disease

Electrocardiogram

Patients at risk for cardiovascular disease (e.g., because of cocaine abuse, hypertension, renal disease, circulatory disease, thyroid disease, diabetes mellitus [age ≥40 years], significant pulmonary disease)
History of previously unevaluated pathologic-sounding murmur or palpitation
Family history reveals possibility of inherited prolonged QT syndrome
Patients with history of moderate to severe sleep apnea or chronic anatomic airway obstruction (e.g., Pierre Robin syndrome) may be at risk for right-sided heart strain

Modified from Marley RA. Preoperative preparation. In: Zaglaniczny K, Aker J, eds. Clinical Guide to Pediatric Anesthesia. *Philadelphia: Saunders; 1999:29-45.*

Timing of Diagnostic Testing

In general, diagnostic testing results are deemed current within 60 days of the scheduled surgery, if the test results are normal and if the patient's current health status indicates no change has occurred since the test was performed.[351] However, specific tests require more current data analysis. A serum potassium level should be obtained within 7 days of surgery for patients receiving diuretics or digitalis, and blood glucose level determinations should be obtained on the day of surgery for patients with diabetes that is controlled by medication.[352]

Indications for Diagnostic Testing

A continuing point of controversy relates to agreement regarding which tests are appropriate for specific patients, surgeries, and conditions. Disagreement exists among and within medical specialties regarding which tests are appropriate.[353] Suggested guidelines for ordering various diagnostic tests based on results of the patient's history and physical examination have been offered for ordering diagnostic procedures (Box 17-12)[1] and laboratory tests (Box 17-13).[1]

BOX 17-13

Indications for Laboratory Testing

Complete Blood Count
Hematologic disorder
Vascular procedure
Chemotherapy
Unknown sickle cell syndrome status

Hemoglobin and Hematocrit
Age <6 mo (<1 yr if born prematurely)
Hematologic malignancy
Recent radiation or chemotherapy
Renal disease
Anticoagulant therapy
Procedure with moderate to high blood loss potential
Coexisting systemic disorders (e.g., cystic fibrosis, prematurity, severe malnutrition, renal failure, liver disease, congenital heart disease)

White Blood Cell Count
Leukemia and lymphomas
Recent radiation or chemotherapy
Suspected infection that would lead to cancellation of surgery
Aplastic anemia
Hypersplenism
Autoimmune collagen vascular disease

Blood Glucose Level
Diabetes mellitus
Current corticosteroid use
History of hypoglycemia
Adrenal disease
Cystic fibrosis

Serum Chemistry
Renal disease
Adrenal or thyroid disease
Chemotherapy
Pituitary or hypothalamic disease
Body fluid loss or shifts (e.g., dehydration, bowel prep)
Central nervous system disease

Potassium
Digoxin therapy
Diuretic therapy

Creatinine and Blood Urea
Nitrogen
Cardiovascular disease (e.g., hypertension)
Renal disease
Adrenal disease
Diabetes mellitus
Diuretic therapy
Digoxin therapy
Body fluid loss or shifts (e.g., dehydration, bowel prep)
Procedure requiring radiocontrast

Liver Function Tests
Hepatic disease
Exposure to hepatitis
Therapy with hepatotoxic agents

Coagulation Studies
Prothrombin Time and Partial Thromboplastin Time
Leukemia
Hepatic disease
Bleeding disorder
Anticoagulant therapy
Severe malnutrition or malabsorption
Platelet Count and Bleeding Time
Bleeding disorder
Abnormal hemorrhage, purpura, easy bruisability

Urinalysis
Not indicated as a routine screening test

Pregnancy Test
Possibility of pregnancy

Medication Levels
Monitor for medications (e.g., theophylline, phenytoin, digoxin, carbamazepine) if patient exhibits signs of ineffective therapy, potential drug side effects, or poor drug compliance or has recently changed medication therapy without documentation of the drug level

Modified from Marley RA. Preoperative preparation. In: Zaglaniczny K, Aker J, eds. Clinical Guide to Pediatric Anesthesia. *Philadelphia: Saunders; 1999:29-45.*

Pregnancy Testing

Routine preoperative pregnancy testing in women of childbearing age remains controversial. If a patient is uncertain of her status or if the physical examination or medical history suggests the possibility of pregnancy (e.g., because of information regarding sexually active status, time of last menstrual period, presence or absence of birth control methods), a preoperative pregnancy test should be performed.[2] Issues to address when deciding whether to test include the following:

- Policies of the hospital or health-care facility based on medical staff bylaws. The medical facility should have established guidelines that delineate when testing for pregnancy is appropriate.
- Patients should be advised of the fetal risk (e.g., spontaneous abortion) should anesthesia be performed during pregnancy. The incidence of congenital abnormalities is no greater in pregnant women who undergo surgery, however, than it is in those with a surgery-free pregnancy.[354] Despite this finding, patients are advised to postpone elective surgery until well after the first trimester, when fetal organogenesis is complete.
- Patients should be privately questioned about the possibility of pregnancy. Female staff should interview adolescent patients in the absence of family members.

Chest Radiography

A preoperative chest radiograph is of minimal predictive importance and is not cost effective as a screening test for postoperative respiratory problems, so it is not to be recommended without specific indications from the medical history and physical examination.[355,356] The risk of performing a routine preoperative chest radiograph in asymptomatic patients less than 75 years of age is greater than the benefit.[350]

Electrocardiography

Many medical facilities continue to use an age-specific criterion for acquiring a preoperative ECG regardless of indications, or lack of indications, based on the patient's medical history and physical examination. The recommended minimum age for routinely conducting a baseline ECG has gradually increased to 50 years or older,[2,8] older than 60 years,[357-359] and older than 75 physiologic years.[313] Inquiry has even been raised regarding the appropriateness of an age-only basis for preoperative ECG testing.[360]

The value of obtaining a routine preoperative 12-lead ECG in asymptomatic, low-risk patients has been questioned.[361,362] This rethinking of indications for when to order a preoperative ECG has been challenged for the following reasons:

- It has not been shown to be cost-effective.[346,363,364]
- It is a poor predictor of perioperative complications.[362,364,365]
- It is of limited value in detection of ischemia in asymptomatic individuals.[366,367]
- Abnormal preoperative ECGs rarely lead to alteration in patient care.[346,363,368]
- No evidence supports the value of a "baseline" ECG.[357,361,362]

FASTING CONSIDERATIONS

Part of the anesthesia provider's role in patient preparation involves the determination of an appropriate fasting interval. This requires knowledge of risk factors for pulmonary aspiration of gastric contents and the consequences of prolonged fasting in order to establish an appropriate fasting interval for the patient. The risk of perioperative pulmonary aspiration of gastric contents that results in morbidity or mortality is relatively low. The recommendations for the withholding of oral feeding before elective surgery have recently become much more liberal. When studies were conducted challenging the traditional fasting times (7 hours or greater) for clear liquids, the results appeared to show that a reduced fasting interval does not increase the risk of pulmonary aspiration in normal, healthy individuals.

The traditional policy of fasting after midnight fails to address three variables that influence gastric emptying for surgery: the time of the scheduled surgery, the time at which the patient retired for the night, and the variability in gastric emptying for solids and fluids among individuals. Prolonged fasting, especially in children, can be highly distressing in addition to causing physiologic alterations. Periods of long preoperative fasting have been shown to contribute to the following:

- Dehydration[369]
- Hypoglycemia (in smaller children)[370]
- Hypovolemia
- Increased irritability[370]
- Enhanced preoperative anxiety[371]
- Reduced compliance with preoperative fasting orders[369]
- Thirst[372] and related discomforts (e.g., hunger, headache, unhappiness)

Pulmonary Aspiration Risk

Recent ingestion of food and liquid before surgery contributes to an increased risk of pulmonary aspiration. Solid foods must be digested to a bolus diameter of less than 2 mm before the food can pass through the pylorus.[373] This process normally takes several hours for solids, whereas liquids pass through the pylorus in 1 to 2 hours. Historically, patients have been required to fast for extended periods in an attempt to ensure an empty stomach. However, sustained fasting does not guarantee that the stomach will be empty at the time of surgery.[374]

Part of the preoperative evaluation process identifies patients who are at risk for aspirating gastric contents into the lungs and developing aspiration pneumonitis. Factors associated with an increased risk of pulmonary aspiration of gastric contents are listed in Box 17-14.[375-384]

Fasting Interval

When the fasting interval is minimized, patients (especially children) are reported to be less irritable, less thirsty, and less hungry; to have fewer headaches; to be more comfortable; and generally to tolerate the preoperative phase better than patients who have fasted for longer periods of time. Modest amounts of clear liquids taken orally 2 hours[385-387] to 3 hours[388,389] preoperatively, when compared with a conventional fasting interval of "7 to 8 hours" or "after midnight," are acceptable and have been shown to lower residual gastric volume (stimulation of the gastric emptying reflex) and raise gastric pH in a majority of patients. Acceptable clear fluids (e.g., water, apple juice, black coffee, black tea, clear juice drinks, clear Jell-O, clear broth, ice Popsicles, Pedialyte) may be given to healthy, unpremedicated patients. In light of these recent findings, recommended fasting guidelines for otherwise healthy individuals have been liberalized (Box 17-15).[390,391]

BOX 17-14

Conditions that Increase the Risk of Regurgitation and Pulmonary Aspiration during Anesthesia

- Age extremes (<1 yr or >70 yr)
- Anxiety
- Ascites
- Collagen vascular disease (e.g., scleroderma)
- Depression
- Esophageal surgery
- Exogenous medications (e.g., opioids, premedication)
- Failed intubation or difficult airway history
- Gastroesophageal junction dysfunction (e.g., hiatal hernia)
- Mechanical obstruction (e.g., pyloric stenosis, duodenal ulcer)
- Metabolic disorders (e.g., hypothyroidism, chronic diabetes, hepatic failure, hyperglycemia, obesity, renal failure, uremia)
- Neurologic sequelae (e.g., those of developmental delays, head injury, hypotonia, seizures)
- Pain
- Pregnancy
- Prematurity with respiratory problems
- Type and composition of gastric contents (e.g., solid foods and milk products)

BOX 17-15

Fasting Guidelines for Healthy Patients (All Ages) Undergoing Elective Surgery

- No chewing gum or candy after midnight (foreign body aspiration concern)
- Clear liquids up to 2 hr before surgery*
- Breast milk until 4 hr before surgery
- No infant formula, nonhuman milk,† or light meal‡ for at least 6 hr before surgery
- Prescribed medications (e.g., premedication) administered with a sip of water or prescribed liquid mixture (up to 150 ml for adult; up to 75 ml for children) up to 1 hr before anesthesia

**Consider the possibility that the case may proceed earlier than scheduled.*
†Because nonhuman milk is similar to solids in gastric emptying time, the amount ingested must be considered when determining an appropriate fasting period.
‡A light meal typically consists of toast and clear liquids. Meals that include fried or fatty foods or meat may prolong gastric emptying time. Both the amount and type of foods ingested must be considered when determining an appropriate fasting period.

AMERICAN SOCIETY OF ANESTHESIOLOGISTS PHYSICAL STATUS CLASSIFICATION SYSTEM

With the conclusion of the preanesthesia assessment, assignment of an ASA physical status classification is made for each patient. The classification ideally represents a reflection of the patient's preoperative status and is not an estimate of anesthetic risk. For greater accuracy to be attained from its interpretation, the ASA status should also remain independent of the proposed surgical procedure.[392-395]

Advent and Purpose

In 1940 the American Society of Anesthetists developed a system "to classify the physical condition of a patient requiring anesthesia and surgery." This six-category classification was then revised by the ASA in 1961 to the current system of five categories (Table 17-13).[396] The purpose of the ASA classification, then and now, is to provide a consistent means of communication to anesthesia staff, within and among institutions, about the physical status of a patient.[396] Furthermore, it allows for a standardized interpretation of anesthesia outcome based on one criterion.

Despite rough correlations between patient physical status and postoperative outcome, *the ASA classification system does not represent an estimate of anesthesia risk*.[392-395] Although a patient in poor physical health is known to be at a greater risk for negative outcome, this does not account for other factors that influence perioperative morbidity and mortality. These factors include the duration and involvement of the surgical procedure, the degree of perioperative monitoring, and unfortunate circumstances, such as human error or equipment failure.

Definition

The current ASA classification system ranges from class I through V, with E denoting an emergent procedure. A classification of ASA status VI may also be assigned at some institutions to postmortem patients undergoing organ procurement procedures. By definition, a patient classified as ASA status I is a healthy individual except for the condition that has necessitated surgery. A healthy young woman about to undergo an emergency dilation and curettage for vaginal bleeding, for example, is classified as ASA status IE. At the other end of the spectrum, a 74-year-old man with hypertension, uncontrolled diabetes, and unstable angina who is scheduled for a coronary artery bypass graft procedure is classified as ASA status IV.[396]

Limitations of the Current System

Despite the numerous benefits of the ASA classification system, it has its shortcomings. Namely, the current system is not explicit enough in its categorization to account for every patient, and this can result in patient misclassification.[397] If the physical status classification system is used for statistical or reimbursement purposes within a department, overclassification is

TABLE 17-13 American Society of Anesthesiologists Physical Status Classification

Classification	Physical Status
ASA class I	No organic, physiologic, biochemical, or psychiatric disturbance *Example*: Healthy patient
ASA class II	Mild-to-moderate systemic disturbance *Examples*: Heart disease that slightly limits physical activity; essential hypertension; diabetes mellitus; chronic bronchitis; anemia; morbid obesity; age extremes
ASA class III	Severe systemic disturbance that limits activity *Examples*: Heart or chronic pulmonary disease that limits activity; poorly controlled essential hypertension; diabetes mellitus with vascular complications; angina pectoris; history of previous myocardial infarction
ASA class IV	Severe systemic disturbance that is life threatening *Examples*: Congestive heart failure; persistent angina pectoris; advanced pulmonary, renal, or hepatic dysfunction
ASA class V	Moribund patient undergoing surgery as a resuscitative effort despite a minimal chance for survival *Example*: Uncontrolled hemorrhage from a ruptured abdominal artery aneurysm
ASA class E	Emergency surgery is required *Example*: An otherwise healthy 30-year-old woman who requires a dilation and curettage for moderate but persistent hemorrhage is classified as ASA IE

ASA, *American Society of Anesthesiologists*.
Modified from American Society of Anesthesiologists. New classification of physical status. Anesthesiology. *1963;24:111*.

often the consequence. Overclassification of a patient also occurs when the proposed surgical procedure is incorporated into the assignment of ASA physical status. This improper classification, or overclassification, of patient status thereby limits the degree of accuracy attained from its original interpretation. As a result, correlations between preoperative status and postoperative outcome are skewed. Despite the shortcomings of the system, ASA physical status continues to be assigned to each patient as a summary of the preoperative evaluation.

PREVENTING OPERATIVE ERRORS

The Joint Commission on Accreditation of Healthcare Organizations (JCAHO) has endorsed a universal protocol for eliminating wrong site, wrong procedure, wrong patient surgeries. It has been endorsed by over 40 of the leading medical, nursing, and health care leadership organizations. The guidelines will be used in all hospitals, ambulatory care surgery centers, and office-based surgery sites, as shown in Box 17-16.

BOX **17-16**

Guidelines for Implementing the Universal Protocol for Preventing Wrong Site, Wrong Procedure, and Wrong Person Surgery

The following guidelines provide detailed implementation requirements, exemptions, and adaptations for special situations.

Preoperative verification process

Verification of the correct person, procedure, and site should occur (as applicable):

- At the time the surgery or procedure is scheduled
- At the time of admission or entry in the facility
- Any time the responsibility for care of the patient is transferred to another caregiver
- With the patient involved, awake and aware, if possible
- Before the patient leaves the preoperative area or enters the procedure/surgical room.

Before the start of the procedure begins, a preoperative verification checklist may be helpful to ensure availability and review of the following:

- Relevant documentation (e.g., history and physical, consent)
- Relevant images, properly labeled and displayed
- Any required implants and special equipment.

Marking the operative site

- Make the mark at or near the incision site. Do NOT mark any nonoperative site(s) unless necessary for some other aspect of care.
- The mark must be unambiguous (e.g., use initials or "YES" or a line representing the proposed incision; consider that "X" may be ambiguous).
- The mark must be positioned to be visible after the patient is prepped and draped.
- The mark must be made using a marker that is sufficiently permanent to remain visible after completion of the skin prep. Adhesive site markers should not be used as the sole means of marking the site.
- The method of marking and type of mark should be consistent throughout the organization.
- At a minimum, mark all cases involving laterality, multiple structures (fingers, toes, lesions), or multiple levels (spine). Note: In general spinal region, special intraoperative radiographic techniques are used for marking the exact vertebral level.
- The person performing the procedure should do the site marking.
- Marking must take place with the patient involved, awake and aware, if possible.
- Final verification of the site mark must occur during the "time out."
- A defined procedure must be in place for patients who refuse site markings.

Exemptions

- Single organ cases (e.g., Cesarean section, cardiac surgery).
- Intervention cases for which the catheter or instrument insertion site is not predetermined (e.g., cardiac catheterization).
- Teeth—But indicate operative tooth name(s) on documentation *or* mark the operative tooth (teeth) on the dental radiographs or dental diagram.
- Premature infants, for whom the mark may cause a permanent tattoo.

"Time out" immediately before starting the procedure

Must be conducted in the location where the procedure will be done, just before starting the procedure. It must involve the entire operative team, use active communication, be briefly documented (the type and amount of documentation) and must, at the least, include:

- Correct patient identity
- Correct side and site
- Agreement on the procedure to be done
- Correct patient position
- Availability of correct implants and any special equipment or special requirements.

The organization should have processes and systems in place for reconciling differences in staff responses during the "time out."

Procedures for non-operating room (OR) setting including bedside procedures

- Site marking must be done for any procedure that involves laterality, multiple structures, or levels (even if the procedure takes place outside of an OR).
- Verification, site marking, and "time out" procedures should be as consistent as possible throughout the organization, including the OR and other locations where invasive procedures are done.
- Exception: Cases in which the individual doing the procedure is in continuous attendance with the patient from the time of decision to do the procedure and consent from the patient to the execution of the procedure may be exempted from the site marking requirement. The requirement for a "time out" final verification still applies.

Guidelines for implementing the universal protocol to prevent wrong site surgery. JCAHO, *Chicago. Dec 2, 2003. Web site:* http://www.jcaho.org/accredited+organizations/patient+safety/universal+protocol/up+guidelines.pdf. *Accessed Jan. 12, 2004.*

SUMMARY

An important feature of patient care is a timely and thorough preoperative assessment to identify factors that increase the risk of anesthesia and surgery. The preoperative evaluation and preparation of the patient involve integration of information obtained from the patient interview, chart review, and physical examination and interpretation of the results from necessary diagnostic tests. The anesthesia provider can then assimilate the assessment data and devise and implement the most appropriate anesthetic plan for the patient.

REFERENCES

1. Marley RA. Preoperative preparation for the pediatric patient. In: Zaglaniczny K, Aker J, eds. *Clinical Guide to Pediatric Anesthesia*. Philadelphia: Saunders; 1999:29-45.
2. Fischer SP. Cost-effective preoperative evaluation and testing. *Chest*. 1999;115 (suppl):96S-100S.
3. Stokes-Roberts A. Pre-admission clinics. Smooth operators. *Health Serv J*. 1999;109:22-23.
4. Persaud DD, Dawe U. Effects of a surgical pre-operative assessment clinic on patient care. *Hospital Topics*. 1992;70:37-40.
5. Pollard JB, Garnerin P, Dalman RL. Use of outpatient preoperative evaluation to decrease length of stay for vascular surgery. *Anesth Analg*. 1997;85:1307-1311.
6. Power LM, Thackray NM. Reduction of preoperative investigations with the introduction of an anaesthetist-led preoperative assessment clinic. *Anaesth Intensive Care*. 1999;27:481-488.
7. Pollard JB, Garnerin P. Outpatient preoperative evaluation clinic can lead to a rapid shift from inpatient to outpatient surgery: a retrospective review of perioperative setting and outcome. *J Clin Anesth*. 1999;11:39-45.
8. Pasternak LR. Preanesthesia evaluation of the surgical patient. In: Barash PG, ed. *ASA Refresher Courses in Anesthesiology*. Philadelphia: Lippincott; 1996:205-219.
9. Pollard JB, Olson L. Early outpatient preoperative anesthesia assessment: does it help to reduce operating room cancellations? *Anesth Analg*. 1999;89:502-505.
10. Hanna K. Multicultural considerations for the advanced practice nurse anesthetist in the preoperative teaching area. *Nurs Admin Q*. 1997;21:55-60.
11. Cassidy J, Marley RA. Preoperative assessment of the ambulatory patient. *J Peri Anesth Nurs*. 1996;11:334-343.
12. Lichtor JL, Johanson CE, Mhoon D, et al. Preoperative anxiety: does anxiety level the afternoon before surgery predict anxiety level just before surgery? *Anesthesiology*. 1987;67:595-599.
13. Williams OA. Patient knowledge of operative care. *J R Soc Med*. 1993;86:328-331.
14. Malins AF. Do they do as they are instructed? A review of outpatient anaesthesia. *Anaesthesia*. 1978;33:832-835.
15. Doak GJ. Discontinuing drugs before surgery. *Can J Anaesth*. 1997;44:R112-R117.
16. Lexenaire MC. Drugs and other agents involved in anaphylactic shock occurring during anaesthesia. A French multicenter epidemiological inquiry. *Ann Fr Anesth Reanim*. 1993;12:91-96.
17. Holzman RS. Latex allergy: an emerging operating room problem. *Anesth Analg*. 1993;76:635-641.
18. Lebenbom-Mansour MH, et al. The incidence of latex sensitivity in ambulatory surgical patients: a correlation of historical factors with positive serum immunoglobin E levels. *Anesth Analg*. 1997;85:44-49.
19. McGinnis JM, Foege WH. Mortality and morbidity attributable to use of addictive substances in the United States. *Proc Assoc Am Physicians*. 1999;111:109-118, 1999.
20. Coleman P. Overview of substance abuse. *Prim Care*. 1993;20: 1-18.
21. Centers for Disease Control and Prevention. Smoking-attributable mortality and years of potential life lost—United States, 1990. *MMWR Morb Mortal Wkly Rep*. 1993;42:645-648.
22. Centers for Disease Control and Prevention. Cigarette smoking among adults—United States, 1994. *MMWR Morb Mortal Wkly Rep*. 1996;45:588-590.
23. Centers for Disease Control and Prevention. Selected cigarette smoking initiation and quitting behaviors among high school students—United States, 1997. *Morb Mortal Wkly Rep*. 1998;47:386-389.
24. Centers for Disease Control and Prevention. Annual smoking-attributable mortality, years of potential life lost, and economic costs—United States, 1995-1999. 2002;51(14). Web site: www.cdc.gov/tobacco/research_data/economics/mmwr5114.highlights.htm. Accessed Feb. 2, 2004.
25. US Environmental Protection Agency. *Respiratory Health Effects of Passive Smoking: Lung Cancer and Other Disorders*. Washington, DC: US Environmental Protection Agency, Office of Health and Environmental Assessment, Office of Research and Development; 1992. No. EPA/6-90/006F.
26. Benowitz NL. Tobacco. In: Goldman L, Ausiello D, eds. *Cecil Textbook of Medicine*. 22nd ed. Philadelphia: Saunders; 2004: 57-60.
27. Seddon JM, et al. A prospective study of cigarette smoking and age-related macular degeneration in women. *JAMA*. 1996;276:1141-1146.
28. Christen WG, et al. A prospective study of cigarette smoking and risk of age-related macular degeneration in men. *JAMA*. 1996;276:1147-1151.
29. DiFranza JR, Lew RA. Effect of maternal cigarette smoking on pregnancy complications and sudden infant death syndrome. *J Fam Pract*. 1995;40:385-394.
30. Gold DR, et al. Effects of cigarette smoking on lung function in adolescent boys and girls. *N Engl J Med*. 1996;335:931-937.
31. Law MR, Hackshaw AK. A meta-analysis of smoking, bone mineral density, and risk of hip fracture. *BMJ*. 1997;315:841-846.
32. Nieburg P, et al. The fetal tobacco syndrome. *JAMA*. 1985;253:2998-2999.
33. Wakschlag LS, et al. Maternal smoking during pregnancy and the risk of conduct disorders in boys. *Arch Gen Psychiatry*. 1997;54:670-676.
34. Kadunce DP, et al. Cigarette smoking: risk factor for premature facial wrinkling. *Ann Intern Med*. 1991;114:840-844.
35. Wewers MD, et al. Cigarette smoking in HIV infection induces a suppressive inflammatory environment in the lung. *Am J Respir Crit Care Med*. 1998;158:1543-1549.
36. McCrea KA, et al. Altered cytokine regulation in the lungs of cigarette smokers. *Am J Respir Crit Care Med*. 1994;150:696-703.
37. Nunn JE: Smoking. In: *Nunn's Applied Respiratory Physiology*. 4th ed. Boston: Butterworth-Heinemann; 1993:378-383.
38. Comroe JH Jr. The pharmacological actions of nicotine. *Ann N Y Acad Sci*. 1960;90:48-51.
39. Nicod PJ, et al. Acute systemic and coronary hemodynamic and serologic responses to cigarette smoking in long-term smokers with atherosclerotic coronary artery disease. *J Am Coll Cardiol*. 1984;4:964-971.
40. Nunn JE. Oxygen. In: *Nunn's Applied Respiratory Physiology*. 4th ed. Boston: Butterworth-Heinemann; 1993:247-305.
41. Kyerematen GA, et al. Pharmacokinetics of nicotine and 12 metabolites in the rat. Application of a new radiometric high performance liquid chromatography assay. *Drug Metab Dispos*. 1988;16:125-129.
42. Duan MJ, et al. Disposition kinetics and metabolism of nicotine-1′-N′ oxide in rabbits. *Drug Metab Dispos*. 1991;19:667-672.
43. Sasaki T. On half-clearance time of carbon monoxide hemoglobin in blood during hyperbaric oxygen therapy (OHP). *Bull Tokyo Med Dent Univ*. 1975;22:63-77.
44. Wagner JA, Horvath SM, Dahms TE. Carbon monoxide elimination. *Respir Physiol*. 1975;23:41-47, 1975.

45. Moller AM, Pedersen T. The effect of tobacco smoking on risks in connection with anesthesia and surgery. Development of complications and the preventive effect of smoking cessation. *Ugeskr Laeger*. 1999;161:4273-4276.
46. Pearch AC, Jones RM. Smoking and anesthesia: preoperative abstinence and perioperative morbidity. *Anesthesiology*. 1984;61:576-584.
47. Kambam JR, Chen SA, Hyman SA. Effect of short-term smoking halt on carboxyhemoglobin levels and P_{50} values. *Anesth Analg*. 1986;65:1186-1188.
48. Bluman LG, et al. Preoperative smoking habits and postoperative pulmonary complications. *Chest*. 1998;113:883-889.
49. Kaul HL, et al. Postoperative pulmonary complications in patients with preoperative lung disease. *Indian J Med Res*. 1993;98:55-60.
50. Warner MA, Divertie MB, Tinker JH. Preoperative cessation of smoking and pulmonary complications in coronary artery bypass patients. *Anesthesiology*. 1984;60:380-383.
51. Beckers S, Camu F. The anesthetic risk of tobacco smoking. *Acta Anaesthesiol Belg*. 1991;42:45-56.
52. Warner MA, et al. Role of preoperative cessation of smoking and other factors in postoperative pulmonary complications: a blinded prospective study of coronary artery bypass patients. *Mayo Clin Proc*. 1989;64:609-616.
53. Wright AL, et al. Relationship of parental smoking to wheezing and non-wheezing lower respiratory tract illnesses in infancy. *J Pediatr*. 1991;118:207-214.
54. Martinez FD, Cline M, Burrows B. Increased incidence of asthma in children of smoking mothers. *Pediatrics*. 1992;89:21-26.
55. Chilmonczyk BA, et al. Association between exposure to environmental tobacco smoke and exacerbation of asthma in children. *N Engl J Med*. 1993;328:1665-1669.
56. Sherrill DL, et al. Longitudinal effects of passive smoking on pulmonary function in New Zealand children. *Am Rev Respir Dis*. 1992;145:1136-1141.
57. Forastiere F, et al. Effects of environment and passive smoking on the respiratory health of children. *Int J Epidemiol*. 1992;21:66-73.
58. Lakshmipathy N, et al. Environmental tobacco smoke: a risk factor for pediatric laryngospasm. *Anesth Analg*. 1996;82:724-727.
59. Skolnick ET, et al. Exposure to environmental tobacco smoke and the risk of adverse respiratory events in children receiving general anesthesia. *Anesthesiology*. 1998;88:1144-1153.
60. Lyons B, et al. The effect of passive smoking on the incidence of airway complications in children undergoing general anaesthesia. *Anaesthesia*. 1996;51:324-326.
61. Kitchens JM. Does this patient have an alcohol problem? *JAMA*. 1994;272:1782-1787.
62. Lohr RH. Treatment of alcohol withdrawal in hospitalized patients. *Mayo Clin Proc*. 1995;70:777-782.
63. Erstad BL, Cotugno CL. Management of alcohol withdrawal. *Am J Health Syst Pharm*. 1995;52:697-709.
64. Han YH. Why do chronic alcoholics require more anesthesia? *Anesthesiology*. 1969;30:341-342.
65. Johnston RD, Kulp RA, Smith TC. The effects of acute and chronic ethanol administration on isoflurane requirement in mice. *Anesth Analg*. 1975;54:277-281.
66. Pandele G, et al. Thiopental pharmacokinetics in patients with cirrhosis. *Anesthesiology*. 1983;59:123-126.
67. Servin F, et al. Pharmacokinetics of propofol infusions in patients with cirrhosis. *Br J Anaesth*. 1990;65:177-183.
68. Costela JL, et al. Serum protein binding of propofol in patients with renal failure or hepatic cirrhosis. *Acta Anaesthesiol Scand*. 1996;40:741-745.
69. Ivan D, Jay CA. Alcoholism and alcohol abuse. In: Goldman L, Ausiello D, eds. *Cecil Textbook of Medicine*. 22nd ed. Philadelphia: Saunders; 2004:74-80.
70. Rehm J, Bondy S. Alcohol and all-cause mortality: an overview. *Novartis Found Symp*. 1998;216:223-232.
71. Peters TJ, Preedy VR. Metabolic consequences of alcohol ingestion. *Novartis Found Symp*. 1998;216:19-24.
72. Bradley KA, et al. Medical risks for women who drink alcohol. *J Gen Intern Med*. 1998;13:627-639.
73. Allebeck P, Olsen J. Alcohol and fetal damage. *Alcohol Clin Exp Res*. 1998;22(suppl 7):329S-332S.
74. Seitz HK, Poschl G, Simanowski UA. Alcohol and cancer. *Recent Dev Alcohol*. 1998;14:67-95.
75. Ringborg U. Alcohol and risk of cancer. *Alcohol Clin Exp Res*. 1998;22(suppl 7):323S-328S, 1998.
76. Yoshihara H, Noda K, Kamada T. Interrelationship between alcohol intake, hepatitis C, liver cirrhosis, and hepatocellular carcinoma. *Recent Dev Alcohol*. 1998;14:457-469.
77. Oslin D, et al. Alcohol related dementia: proposed clinical criteria. *Int J Geriatr Psychiatry*. 1998;13:203-212.
78. Hillbom M, Numminen H. Alcohol and stroke: pathophysiologic mechanisms. *Neuroepidemiology*. 1998;17:281-287.
79. Neiman J. Alcohol as a risk factor for brain damage: neurologic aspects. *Alcohol Clin Exp Res*. 1998;22(suppl 7):346S-351S.
80. Rosenqvist M. Alcohol and cardiac arrhythmias. *Alcohol Clin Exp Res*. 1998;22(suppl 7):318S-322S.
81. Richardson PJ, Patel VB, Preedy VR. Alcohol and the myocardium. *Novartis Found Symp*. 1998;216:35-45.
82. Kupari M, Koskinen P. Alcohol, cardiac arrhythmias and sudden death. *Novartis Found Symp*. 1998;216:68-79.
83. Friedman HS. Cardiovascular effects of alcohol. *Recent Dev Alcohol*. 1998;14:135-166.
84. Gaziano JM, Buring JE. Alcohol intake, lipids and risks of myocardial infarction. *Novartis Found Symp*. 1998;216:86-95.
85. Baraona E, Lieber CS. Alcohol and lipids. *Recent Dev Alcohol*. 1998;14:97-134.
86. Keil U, et al. Alcohol, blood pressure and hypertension. *Novartis Found Symp*. 1998;216:125-144.
87. Strunin I. Preoperative assessment of the patient with liver dysfunction. *Br J Anaesth*. 1978;50:25-34.
88. Iven VG. Recreational drugs. *Clin Sports Med*. 1998;17:245-259.
89. Cheng DCH. The drug addicted patient. *Can J Anaesth*. 1997;44:R101-R106.
90. Wang-Cheng R. Substance abuse. In: Cheng EY, Kay J, eds. *Manual of Anesthesia and the Medically Compromised Patient*. Philadelphia: Lippincott; 1990:620-630.
91. Ferner RE, Rawlins MD. Anabolic steroids: the power and the glory? *BMJ*. 1988;297:877-878.
92. Creagh TM, Rubin A, Evans DJ. Hepatic tumours induced by anabolic steroids in an athlete. *J Clin Pathol*. 1988;41:441-443.
93. McDonald EC, Speicher CE. Peliosis hepatis associated with administration of oxymetholone. *JAMA*. 1978;240:243-244.
94. McNutt RA, Ferenchick GS, Kirlin PC, Hamlin NJ. Acute myocardial infarction in a 22-year-old world class weightlifter using anabolic steroids. *Am J Cardiol*. 1988;62:164.
95. Frankle MA, Eichberg R, Zachariah SB. Anabolic androgenic steroids and a stroke in an athlete: case report. *Arch Phys Med Rehabil*. 1988;69:632-633.
96. Haupt HA, Rovere GD. Anabolic steroids: a review of the literature. *Am J Sports Med*. 1984;12:469-484.
97. Thompson PD, et al. Contrasting effects of testosterone and stanozolol on serum lipoprotein levels. *JAMA*. 1989;261:1165-1168.
98. Pope HG Jr, Katz DL. Affective and psychotic symptoms associated with anabolic steroid use. *Am J Psychiatry*. 1988;145:487-490.
99. Joyce JA. Anesthesia for athletes using performance-enhancing drugs. *AANA J*. 1991;59:139-144.
100. Zaglaniczny K. An introduction to herbal medicine and anesthetic considerations. *Nurse Anesth Forum*. 1999;2:4-5, 11.
101. Benumof JL. The ASA difficult airway algorithm: new thoughts and considerations. *Curr Rev Nurse Anesth*. 1999;22:103-113.
102. Gregory GA, Riazi J. Classification and assessment of the difficult pediatric airway. In: Riazi J, ed. *Anesthesiology Clinics of North America: the Difficult Pediatric Airway*. Philadelphia: Saunders; 1998:729-741.

103. Creighton RE, Relton JE, Meridy HW. Anaesthesia for occipital encephalocele. *Can Anaesth Soc J.* 1974;21:403-406.
104. Healy GB, et al. The role of surgery in rhabdomyosarcoma of the head and neck in children. *Arch Otolaryngol Head Neck Surg.* 1991;117:1185-1188.
105. Abouleish AE, Mayhew JF. Magnetic resonance imaging of the airway in an infant with micrognathia. *Anesth Analg.* 1998;86:964-966.
106. Selim M, et al. Intubation via LMA in pediatric patients with difficult airways. *Can J Anaesth.* 1999;46:891-893.
107. Sjogren P, Pedersen T, Steinmetz H. Mucopolysaccharidoses and anaesthetic risks. *Acta Anaesthesiol Scand.* 1987;31:214-218.
108. Walker RW, et al. Anaesthesia and mucopolysaccharidoses. A review of airway problems in children. *Anaesthesia.* 1994;49:1078-1084.
109. Diaz JH, Furman EB. Perioperative management of conjoined twins. *Anesthesiology.* 1987;67:965-973.
110. Hoshina H, et al. Thoracopagus conjoined twins: management of anesthetic induction and postoperative chest wall defect. *Anesthesiology.* 1987;66:424-426.
111. Bahk JH, Han SM, Kim SD. Management of difficult airways with a laryngeal mask airway under propofol anaesthesia. *Paediatr Anaesth.* 1999;9:163-166.
112. Perkins JA, et al. Airway management in children with craniofacial anomalies. *Cleft Palate Craniofac J.* 1997;34:135-140.
113. Sagehashi N. An infant with Crouzon's syndrome with a cartilaginous trachea and a human tail. *J Craniomaxillofac Surg.* 1992;20:21-23.
114. Skolimowski J, et al. Microgenia as a factor making endotracheal intubation impossible. *Anaesth Resusc Intensive Ther.* 1975;3:273-276.
115. Jones SE, Derrick GM. Difficult intubation in an infant with Pierre Robin syndrome and concomitant tongue tie. *Paediatr Anaesth.* 1998;8:510-511.
116. Osses H, Poblete M, Asenjo F. Laryngeal mask for difficult intubation in children. *Paediatr Anaesth.* 1999;9:399-401.
117. Bryden DC, Remington SA, Mason C. Treacher Collins syndrome and difficult intubation. *Br J Hosp Med.* 1995;53:419.
118. Madan R, et al. Goldenhar's syndrome: an analysis of anaesthetic management. A retrospective study of seventeen cases. *Anaesthesia.* 1990;45:49-52.
119. Johnson CM, Sims C. Awake fibreoptic intubation via a laryngeal mask in an infant with Goldenhar's syndrome. *Anaesth Intensive Care.* 1994;22:194-197.
120. Yamashita M, et al. Anesthetic considerations in cri du chat syndrome: a report of three cases. *Anesthesiology.* 1985;63:201-202.
121. Przybylo HJ, et al. Retrograde fibreoptic intubation in a child with Nager's syndrome. *Can J Anaesth.* 1996;43:697-699.
122. Maydew RP, Berry FA. Cherubism with difficult laryngoscopy and tracheal intubation. *Anesthesiology.* 1985;62:810-812.
123. Kimura F, et al. Difficult tracheal intubation and abnormal response to thiopental in a patient with arthrogryposis multiplex congenital. *Masui.* 1996;45:1022-1025.
124. Reissell E, et al. Predictability of difficult laryngoscopy in patients with long-term diabetes mellitus. *Anaesthesia.* 1990;45:1024-1027.
125. Salzarulo HH, Taylor LA. Diabetic "stiff joint syndrome" as a cause of difficult endotracheal intubation. *Anesthesiology.* 1986;64:366-368.
126. Vaghadia H, Blackstock D. Anaesthetic implications of the trismus pseudocamptodactyly (Dutch-Kentucky or Hecht Beals) syndrome. *Can J Anaesth.* 1988;35:80-85.
127. Nagata O, et al. Anaesthetic management of two paediatric patients with Hecht-Beals syndrome. *Paediatr Anaesth.* 1999;9:444-447.
128. Aiello G, Metcalf I. Anaesthetic implications of temporomandibular joint disease. *Can J Anaesth.* 1992;39:610-616.
129. Kawaguchi M, et al. Pseudoankylosis of the mandible after supratentorial craniotomy. *Anesth Analg.* 1996;83:731-734.
130. Arul A, Jacob R. A different under vision approach to a difficult intubation. *Paediatr Anaesth.* 1999;9:260-261.
131. Rose DK, Cohen MM. The airway: problems and predictions in 18,500 patients. *Can J Anaesth.* 1994;41:372-383.
132. Biro P, Kaplan V, Bloch KE. Anesthetic management of a patient with obstructive sleep apnea syndrome and difficult airway access. *J Clin Anesth.* 1995;7:417-421.
133. Hiremath AS, et al. Relationship between difficult tracheal intubation and obstructive sleep apnoea. *Br J Anaesth.* 1998;80:606-611.
134. Boushra NN. Anaesthetic management of patients with sleep apnoea syndrome. *Can J Anaesth.* 1996;43:599-616.
135. Dearlove OR, Dobson A, Super M. Anaesthesia and Prader-Willi syndrome. *Paediatr Anaesth.* 1998;8:267-271.
136. Temperley AD, Walker PJ. Blind nasal intubation by monitoring capnography in a neonate with congenital microstomia. *Anaesth Intensive Care.* 1995;23:490-492.
137. Diaz JH, Guarisco JL, LeJeune FE Jr. Perioperative management of paediatric microstomia. *Can J Anaesth.* 1991;38:217-221.
138. Munro HM, Butler PJ, Washington EJ. Freeman-Sheldon (whistling face) syndrome. Anaesthetic and airway management. *Paediatr Anaesth.* 1997;7:345-348.
139. Cruickshanks GF, Brown S, Chitayat D. Anesthesia for Freeman-Sheldon syndrome using a laryngeal mask airway. *Can J Anaesth.* 1999;46:783-787.
140. Kreulen M, et al. Surgical release for intubation purposes in postburn contractures of the neck. *Burns.* 1996;22:310-312.
141. Asai T, Matsumoto H, Shingu K. Awake tracheal intubation through the intubating laryngeal mask. *Can J Anaesth.* 1999;46:182-184.
142. Tassonyi E, et al. Fiberoptically guided intubation in children with gangrenous stomatitis (noma). *Anesthesiology.* 1990;73:348-349.
143. Suan C, et al. Anaesthesia and the Beckwith-Wiedemann syndrome. *Paediatr Anaesth.* 1996;6:231-233.
144. Kobel M, Creighton RE, Steward DJ. Anaesthetic considerations in Down's syndrome: experience with 100 patients and a review of the literature. *Can Anaesth Soc J.* 1982;29:593-599.
145. Bevilacqua S, et al. Difficult intubation in paediatric cardiac surgery. Significance of age. Association with Down's syndrome. *Minerva Anestesiol.* 1996;62:259-264.
146. Walls RM. Management of the difficult airway in the trauma patient. *Emerg Med Clin North Am.* 1998;16:45-61.
147. Shockley WW. Ludwig angina: a review of current airway management. *Arch Otolaryngol Head Neck Surg.* 1999;125:600.
148. Young P, Smith SP, Caesar H. Airway management in Ludwig's angina. *Br J Hosp Med.* 1995;54:239.
149. Bailey CM, Froehlich P, Hoeve HL. Management of subglottic haemangioma. *J Laryngol Otol.* 1998;112:765-768.
150. Batra RK, et al. Anaesthesia and the Sturge-Weber syndrome. *Can J Anaesth.* 1994;41:133-136.
151. Heindel DJ. Deep neck abscesses in adults: management of a difficult airway. *Anesth Analg.* 1987;66:774-776.
152. Cook S. Cockayne's syndrome. Another cause of difficult intubation. *Anaesthesia.* 1982;37:1104-1107.
153. Jacobus N, Kwok F, Lo C. The bamboo skewer: airway management in a patient with penetrating injury of the floor of mouth. *Can J Anaesth.* 1996;43:156-160.
154. Stack CG, Wyse RK. Incidence and management of airway problems in the CHARGE association. *Anaesthesia.* 1991;46:582-585.
155. Watanabe I, et al. Anesthetic management for bronchofiberscopy and esophageal mannometric study in a patient with CHARGE association. *Masui.* 1995;44:1010-1013.
156. Amata OA. Posterior encephalocoele: a case of difficult tracheal intubation. *West Afr J Med.* 1994;13:187-190.
157. Reilly JR, Koopman CF, Cotton R. Nasal mass in a pediatric patient. *Head Neck.* 1992;14:415-418.
158. Levitt MW, Collison JM. Difficult endotracheal intubation in a patient with pseudoxanthoma elasticum. *Anaesth Intensive Care.* 1982;10:62-64.

159. Gunawardana RH. Difficult laryngoscopy in cleft lip and palate surgery. *Br J Anaesth.* 1996;76:757-759.
160. Haselby KA, McNiece WL. Respiratory obstruction from uvular edema in a pediatric patient. *Anesth Analg.* 1983;62:1127-1128.
161. Shechtman FG, Lin PT, Pincus RL. Urgent adenotonsillectomy for upper airway obstruction. *Int J Pediatr Otorhinolaryngol.* 1992;24:83-89.
162. Parker GS, Tami TA. The management of peritonsillar abscess in the 90s: an update. *Am J Otolaryngol.* 1992;13:284-288.
163. Salvi L, et al. Hypertrophy of the lingual tonsil and difficulty in airway control. A clinical case. *Minerva Anestesiol.* 1999;65:549-553.
164. Cohle SD, Jones DH, Puri S. Lingual tonsillar hypertrophy causing failed intubation and cerebral anoxia. *Am J Forensic Med Pathol.* 1993;14:158-161.
165. Coulthard M, Isaacs D. Retropharyngeal abscess. *Arch Dis Child.* 1991;66:1227-1230.
166. Ames WA, Mayou BJ, Williams K. Anaesthetic management of epidermolysis bullosa. *Br J Anaesth.* 1999;82:746-751.
167. Turner ME. Anaesthetic difficulties associated with Behçet's syndrome. *Br J Anaesth.* 1972;44:100-102.
168. Antila H, et al. Difficult airway in a patient with Marshall-Smith syndrome. *Paediatr Anaesth.* 1998;8:429-432.
169. Baxter MR. Congenital laryngomalacia. *Can J Anaesth.* 1994;41:332-339.
170. Dark A, Armstrong T. Severe postoperative laryngeal oedema causing total airway obstruction immediately on extubation. *Br J Anaesth.* 1999;82:644-646.
171. Dixon J, Black JJ. Adult supraglottitis: an important cause of airway obstruction. *J Accid Emerg Med.* 1998;15:114-115.
172. Holinger PH, Brown WT. Congenital webs, cysts, laryngoceles and other anomalies of the larynx. *Ann Otol Rhinol Laryngol.* 1967;76:744-752.
173. Benjamin B. Chevalier Jackson lecture. Congenital laryngeal webs. *Ann Otol Rhinol Laryngol.* 1983;92:317-326.
174. Baruh S. Laryngeal web: a cause of difficult endotracheal intubation. *Anesthesiology.* 1982;57:123-125.
175. Hulme GJ, Blues CM. Acromegaly and papillomatosis: difficult intubation and use of the airway exchange catheter. *Anaesthesia.* 1999;54:787-789.
176. Theroux MC, et al. Juvenile laryngeal papillomatosis: scary anaesthetic! *Paediatr Anaesth.* 1998;8:357-361.
177. Lima JA. Laryngeal foreign bodies in children: a persistent, life-threatening problem. *Laryngoscope.* 1989;99:415-420.
178. Baugh R, Gilmore BB Jr. Infectious croup: a critical review. *Otolaryngol Head Neck Surg.* 1986;95:40-46.
179. Poppers PJ. Anaesthetic implications of hereditary angioneurotic oedema. *Can J Anaesth.* 1987;34:76-78.
180. Ishoo E, et al. Predicting airway risk in angioedema: staging system based on presentation. *Otolaryngol Head Neck Surg.* 1999;121:263-268.
181. Benjamin B. Tracheomalacia in infants and children. *Ann Otol Rhinol Laryngol.* 1984;93:438-442.
182. Tobias JD. Anesthetic implications of Larsen syndrome. *J Clin Anesth.* 1996;8:255-257.
183. Lauder GR, Sumner E. Larsen's syndrome: anaesthetic implications. Six case reports. *Paediatr Anaesth.* 1995;5:133-138.
184. Eckel HE, et al. Airway endoscopy in the diagnosis and treatment of bacterial tracheitis in children. *Int J Pediatr Otorhinolaryngol.* 1993;27:147-157.
185. Vas L, Naregal F, Naik V. Anaesthetic management of an infant with anterior mediastinal mass. *Paediatr Anaesth.* 1999;9:439-443.
186. Pullerits J, Holzman R. Anaesthesia for patients with mediastinal masses. *Can J Anaesth.* 1989;36:681-688.
187. McElhinney DB, et al. Compression of the central airways by a dilated aorta in infants and children with congenital heart disease. *Ann Thorac Surg.* 1999;67:1130-1136.
188. Chapotte C, et al. Airway compression in children due to congenital heart disease: value of flexible fiberoptic bronchoscopic assessment. *J Cardiothorac Vasc Anesth.* 1998;12:145-152.
189. Blazer S, Naveh Y, Friedman A. Foreign body in the airway. A review of 200 cases. *Am J Dis Child.* 1980;134:68-71.
190. Eyrich JE, Riopelle JM, Naraghi M. Elective transtracheal jet ventilation for bronchoscopic removal of tracheal foreign body. *South Med J.* 1992;85:1017-1019.
191. Mentzelopoulos SD, et al. Anesthesia for tracheal resection: a new technique of airway management in a patient with severe stenosis of the midtrachea. *Anesth Analg.* 1999;89:1156-1160.
192. Furimsky M, Aronson S, Ovassapian A. Case 6—1998. Perioperative anesthetic management of a patient presenting for resection of a tracheal mass. *J Cardiothorac Vasc Anesth.* 1998;12:701-704.
193. Au CL, White SA, Grant RP. A novel intubation technique for tracheoesophageal fistula in adults. *Can J Anaesth.* 1999;46:688-691.
194. Torsiglieri AJ Jr, et al. Pediatric neck masses: guidelines for evaluation. *Int J Pediatr Otorhinolaryngol.* 1988;16:199-210.
195. Liechty KW, et al. Intrapartum airway management for giant fetal neck masses: the EXIT (ex utero intrapartum treatment) procedure. *Am J Obstet Gynecol.* 1997;177:870-874.
196. Langer JC, et al. Cervical cystic hygroma in the fetus: clinical spectrum and outcome. *J Pediatr Surg.* 1990;25:58-61.
197. Tanaka M, et al. Anaesthetic management of a neonate with prenatally diagnosed cervical tumour and upper airway obstruction. *Can J Anaesth.* 1994;41:236-240.
198. Schwartz MZ, Silver H, Schulman S. Maintenance of the placental circulation to evaluate and treat an infant with massive head and neck hemangioma. *J Pediatr Surg.* 1993;28:520-522.
199. Miyoshi E, et al. Anesthetic management for newborn pharyngeal teratoma. *Masui.* 1999;48:884-887.
200. Wakeling HG, Ody A, Ball A. Large goiter causing difficult intubation and failure to intubate using the intubating laryngeal mask airway: lessons for next time. *Br J Anaesth.* 1998;81:979-981.
201. Pollard BA, El-Beheiry H. Pott's disease with unstable cervical spine, retropharyngeal cold abscess and progressive airway obstruction. *Can J Anaesth.* 1999;46:772-775.
202. Kreulen M, et al. Surgical release for intubation purposes in postburn contractures of the neck. *Burns.* 1996;22:310-312.
203. Karam R, et al. Severe neck burns and laryngeal mask airway for frequent general anesthetics. *Middle East J Anesthesiol.* 1996;13:527-535.
204. Divekar VM, Kothari MD, Kamdar BM. Anaesthesia in Turner's syndrome. *Can Anaesth Soc J.* 1983;30:417-418.
205. Daum RE, Jones DJ. Fibreoptic intubation in Klippel-Feil syndrome. *Anaesthesia.* 1988;43:18-21.
206. Lupien AE, Taylor C. Hybrid intubation technique for the management of a difficult airway: a case report. *AANA J.* 1995;63:50-52.
207. Penberthy A, Roberts N. Recurrent acute upper airway obstruction after anterior cervical fusion. *Anaesth Intensive Care.* 1998;26:305-307.
208. Defalque RJ, Hyder ML. Laryngeal mask airway in severe cervical ankylosis. *Can J Anaesth.* 1997;44:305-307.
209. Lin BC, Chen IH. Anesthesia for ankylosing spondylitis patients undergoing transpedicle vertebrectomy. *Acta Anaesthesiol Scand.* 1999;37:73-78.
210. Harley EH, Collins MD. Neurologic sequelae secondary to atlantoaxial instability in Down syndrome. *Arch Otolaryngol Head Neck Surg.* 1994;120:159-165.
211. Ferguson S. Moebius syndrome: a review of the anaesthetic implications. *Paediatr Anaesth.* 1996;6:51-56.
212. Tobias JD. Anesthetic care for the child with Morquio syndrome: general versus regional anesthesia. *J Clin Anesth.* 1999;11:242-246.

213. McGuire G, el-Beheiry H. Complete upper airway obstruction during awake fibreoptic intubation in patients with unstable cervical spine fractures. *Can J Anaesth*. 1999;46:176-178.
214. Wong JK, et al. Use of the intubating laryngeal mask airway to facilitate awake orotracheal intubation in patients with cervical spine disorders. *J Clin Anesth*. 1999;11:346-348.
215. Campbell RS, Wou P, Watt I. A continuing role for pre-operative cervical spine radiography in rheumatoid arthritis? *Clin Radiol*. 1995;50:157-159.
216. Randell T. Prediction of difficult intubation. *Acta Anaesthesiol Scand*. 1996;40:1016-1023.
217. Samsoon GL, Young JR. Difficult tracheal intubation: a retrospective study. *Anaesthesia*. 1987;42:487-490.
218. Karkouti KM, et al. Inter-observer reliability of ten tests used for predicting difficult tracheal intubation. *Can J Anaesth*. 1996; 43:554-559.
219. Tse JC, Rimm EB, Hussain A. Predicting difficult endotracheal intubation in surgical patients scheduled for general anesthesia: a prospective blind study. *Anesth Analg*. 1995;81:254-258.
220. Savva D. Prediction of difficult tracheal intubation. *Br J Anaesth*. 1994;73:149-153.
221. Oates JD, et al. Comparison of two methods for predicting difficult intubation. *Br J Anaesth*. 1991;66:305-309.
222. Frerk CM. Predicting difficult intubation. *Anaesthesia*. 1991;46:1005-1008.
223. Ramadhani SA, et al. Sternomental distance as the sole predictor of difficult laryngoscopy in obstetric anaesthesia. *Br J Anaesth*. 1996;77:312-316.
224. Block C, Brechnew VL. Unusual problems in airway management. II. The influence of the temporomandibular joint, the mandible, and associated structures on endotracheal intubation. *Anesth Analg*. 1971;50:114-123.
225. Wilson ME, et al. Predicting difficult intubation. *Br J Anaesth*. 1988;61:211-216.
226. Warner ME, et al. Perianesthetic dental injuries. Frequency, outcomes, and risk factors. *Anesthesiology*. 1999;90:1302-1305.
227. Chadwick RG, Lindsay SM. Dental injuries during general anaesthesia: can the dentist help the anaesthetist? *Dent Update*. 25:76-78, 1998.
228. Blumenreich GA. Res ipsa loquitur: dental damage during anesthesia. *AANA J*. 1997;65:33-36.
229. Gray DS, Fujioka K. Use of relative weight and body mass index for the determination of adiposity. *J Clin Epidemiol*. 1991; 44:545-550.
230. Allison DB, et al. Annual deaths attributable to obesity in the United States. *JAMA*. 1999;282:1530-1538.
231. Must A, et al. The disease burden associated with overweight and obesity. *JAMA*. 1999;282:1523-1529.
232. Mokdad AH, et al. The spread of the obesity epidemic in the United States, 1991-1998. *JAMA*. 1999;282:1519-1522.
233. NHLBI/NIDDK. Clinical guidelines on the identification, evaluation, and treatment of overweight and obesity in adults. National Institutes of Health, National Heart, Lung and Blood Institute Web site. Available at: http://www. nhlbi.nih.gov/guidelines/obesity/ob_home.htm. Accessed January 14, 2004.
234. Brodsky JB, Vierra MA. Anesthetic management of the obese patient. In: Lake CL, Rice LJ, Sperry RJ, eds. *Advances in Anesthesia*. Vol 17. St Louis: Mosby; 2000:149-171.
235. Jeffers LA. Anesthetic considerations for the new antiobesity medications. *AANA J*. 1996;64:541-544.
236. Rich JM, et al. Unusual hypotension and bradycardia in a patient receiving fenfluramine, phentermine, and fluoxetine. *Anesthesiology*. 1998;88:529-531.
237. Toussirot E, Wendling D. Current guidelines for the drug treatment of ankylosing spondylitis. *Drugs*. 1998;56:225-240.
238. Peterson P, et al. The preoperative bleeding time test lacks clinical benefit: College of American Pathologists' and American Society of Clinical Pathologists' position article. *Arch Surg*. 1998;133:134-139.
239. Gewirtz AS, Miller ML, Keys TF. The clinical usefulness of the preoperative bleeding time. *Arch Pathol Lab Med*. 1996;120:353-356.
240. MacKenzie CR, Sharrock NE. Perioperative medical considerations in patients with rheumatoid arthritis. *Rheum Dis Clin North Am*. 1998;24:1-17.
241. Nicholson G, Burrin JM, Hall GM. Perioperative steroid supplementation. *Anaesthesia*. 1998;53:1091-1104.
242. Sinclair JR, Mason RA. Ankylosing spondylitis: the case for awake intubation. *Anaesthesia*. 1984;39:3-11.
243. Tanoue LT. Pulmonary manifestations of rheumatoid arthritis. In: Matthay RA, ed. *Clinics in Chest Medicine. Thoracic Manifestations of the Systemic Autoimmune Diseases*. Philadelphia: Saunders; 1998:667-685.
244. Lee-Chiong TL Jr. Pulmonary manifestations of ankylosing spondylitis and relapsing polychondritis. In: Matthay RA, ed. *Clinics in Chest Medicine. Thoracic Manifestations of the Systemic Autoimmune Diseases*. Philadelphia: Saunders; 1998:747-757.
245. Fischer SP. Preoperative evaluation of the adult neurosurgical patient. In: Jaffe RA, Giffard RG, eds. *International Anesthesiology Clinics. Topics in Neuroanesthesia*. Boston: Little, Brown; 1996: 21-32.
246. Samra SK, Kroll DA. Subarachnoid hemorrhage and intraoperative electrocardiographic changes simulating myocardial ischemia—anesthesiologist's dilemma. *Anesth Analg*. 1985; 64:86-89.
247. White JC, Parker SD, Rogers MC. Preanesthetic evaluation of a patient with pathologic Q waves following subarachnoid hemorrhage. *Anesthesiology*. 1985;62:351-354.
248. Davies KR, et al. Cardiac function in aneurismal subarachnoid haemorrhage: a study of electrocardiographic and echocardiographic abnormalities. *Br J Anaesth*. 1991;67:58-63.
249. Teasdale G, Jennett B. Assessment of coma and impaired consciousness. A practical scale. *Lancet*. 1974;2:81-84.
250. Wilke HG II, Ellis JE, McKinsey JF. Carotid endarterectomy: perioperative and anesthetic considerations. *J Cardiothorac Vasc Anesth*. 1996;10:928-949.
251. Fishman RA. Steroids in the treatment of brain edema. *N Engl J Med*. 1982;306:359-360.
252. Miller JD, et al. Methylprednisolone treatment in patients with brain tumors. *Neurosurgery*. 1977;1:114-117.
253. Eagle K, et al. ACC/AHA guideline update for perioperative cardiovascular evaluation for noncardiac surgery—executive summary. A report of the American College of Cardiology/ American Heart Association task force on practice guidelines (committee to update the 1996 guidelines on perioperative cardiovascular evaluation for noncardiac surgery). *Anesth Analg*. 2002;94:1052-1064.
254. Mangano DT. Preoperative assessment of cardiac risk. In: Kaplan JA, ed. *Cardiac Anesthesia*. 4th ed. Philadelphia: Saunders; 1999:3-39.
255. The Joint National Committee on Prevention, Detection, Evaluation, and Treatment of High Blood Pressure. The seventh report of the Joint National Committee on Prevention, Detection, Evaluation, and Treatment of High Blood Pressure: the JNC 7 report. *JAMA*. 2003;289:2560-2572.
256. Pepine CJ. Systemic hypertension and coronary artery disease. *Am J Cardiol*. 1998;822:1H-24H.
257. Howell SJ, et al. Risk factors for cardiovascular death after elective surgery under general anaesthesia. *Br J Anaesth*. 1998; 80:14-19.
258. Kim HS, Kim CS, Yum MK. Abnormal cardiac autonomic activity and complexity in newly diagnosed and untreated hypertensive patients after general anesthesia. *Clin Exp Hypertens*. 21:1357-1372, 1999.
259. Howell SJ, et al. Predictors of postoperative myocardial ischaemia. The role of intercurrent arterial hypertension and other cardiovascular risk factors. *Anaesthesia*. 1997;52: 107-111.

260. Murray MJ. Perioperative hypertension: evaluation and management. In: *40th Annual Refresher Course: Lecture 221*. Park Ridge, Ill: American Society of Anesthesiologists; 1989.
261. Mangano D, Goldman L. Preoperative assessment of patients with known or suspected coronary disease. *N Engl J Med.* 1995;333:1750-1756.
262. Eagle KA, et al. Long-term survival in patients with coronary artery disease: importance of peripheral vascular disease. The Coronary Artery Surgery Study (CASS) Investigators. *J Am Coll Cardiol.* 1994;23:1091-1095.
263. Goldman L, et al. Multifactorial index of cardiac risk in noncardiac surgical procedures. *N Engl J Med.* 1977;297:845-850.
264. Shah KB, et al. Angina and other risk factors in patients with cardiac diseases undergoing noncardiac operations. *Anesth Analg.* 1990;70:240-247.
265. Detsky AS, et al. Cardiac assessment for patients undergoing noncardiac surgery. A multifactorial clinical risk index. *Arch Intern Med.* 1986;146:2131-2134.
266. Fleisher LA, Lehmann HP. Preoperative cardiac evaluation and perioperative monitoring for noncardiac vascular surgery. *JAMA.* 1995;274(24):1671-1672.
267. Skinner JF, Pearce ML. Surgical risk in the cardiac patient. *J Chronic Dis.* 1964;17:57.
268. Perlroth MG, Hultgren HN. The cardiac patient and general surgery. *JAMA.* 1975;232:1279-1280.
269. Carabello BA. Timing of surgery in mitral and aortic stenosis. *Cardiol Clin.* 1991;9:229-238.
270. Zile MR. Chronic aortic and mitral regurgitation. Choosing the optimal time for surgical correction. *Cardiol Clin.* 1991;9:239-253.
271. Goldman L. Multifactorial index of cardiac risk in noncardiac surgery: ten-year status report. *J Cardiothorac Anesth.* 1987;1: 237-244.
272. Royster R. Anesthesia and cardiac dysrhythmias. In: *40th Annual Refresher Course: Lecture 221*. Park Ridge, Ill: American Society of Anesthesiologists; 1989.
273. Belzberg H, Rivkind AI. Preoperative cardiac preparation. *Chest.* 115:82S-95S, 1999.
274. Schulze RA Jr, Strauss HW, Pitt B. Sudden death in the year following myocardial infarction. Relation to ventricular premature contractions in the last hospital phase and left ventricular ejection fraction. *Am J Med.* 1977;62:192-199.
275. Cooperman M, et al. Cardiovascular risk factors in patients with peripheral vascular disease. *Surgery.* 1978;84:505-509.
276. Vijayakumar E. Anesthetic considerations in patients with cardiac arrhythmias, pacemakers, and AICDs. *Int Anesthesiol Clin.* 2001;39:21-42.
277. Fleisher LA. Preoperative evaluation. In: Barash PG, Cullen BF, Stoelting RK, eds: *Clinical Anesthesia.* 4th ed. Philadelphia: Lippincott-Raven; 2000:473-490.
278. Hollenberg SM. Preoperative cardiac risk assessment. *Chest.* 1999;115:51S-57S.
279. Almany SL, Mileto L, Kahn JK. Preoperative cardiac evaluation. Assessing risk before noncardiac surgery. *Postgrad Med.* 1995;98:171-182.
280. Fleisher LA. Perioperative assessment of the patient with cardiovascular disease. *ASA Annu Refresher Course Lect.* 1999;1:125.
281. Hultman J. Pre-anaesthetic evaluation and management of patients with cardiovascular disease. *Acta Anaesthesiol Scand.* 1996;40:996-1003.
282. Caplan R. Preoperative evaluation of the patient with ischemic heart disease. In: *40th Annual Refresher Course: Lecture 221*. Park Ridge, Ill: American Society of Anesthesiologists; 1989.
283. Williams-Russo P, et al. Predicting postoperative pulmonary complications. Is it a real problem? *Arch Intern Med.* 1992;152: 1209-1213.
284. Robertson R, Cane RD. Perioperative management of the patient with respiratory disease. *Curr Rev Post Anesth Care Nurs.* 1993;13:103-110.
285. Lawrence VA, et al. Risk of pulmonary complications after elective abdominal surgery. *Chest.* 1996;110:744-750.
286. Hansen G, Drablos PA, Steinert R. Pulmonary complications, ventilation, and blood gases after upper abdominal surgery. *Acta Anaesthesiol Scand.* 1977;21:211-215.
287. Vodinh J, et al. Risk factors of postoperative pulmonary complications after vascular surgery. *Surgery.* 1988;105:360-365.
288. Marley RA. Postoperative oxygen therapy. *J Peri Anesth Nurs.* 1998;13:394-412.
289. Hayden SP, Mayer ME, Stoller JK. Postoperative pulmonary complications: risk assessment, prevention, and treatment. *Cleve Clin J Med.* 1995;62:401-407.
290. Marienau MES, Buck CF. Preoperative evaluation of the pulmonary patient undergoing nonpulmonary surgery. *J Peri Anesth Nurs.* 1998;13:340-348.
291. Mohr DN, Lavender RC. Preoperative pulmonary evaluation. Identifying patients at increased risk for complications. *Postgrad Med.* 1996;100:241-256.
292. De Nino LA, et al. Preoperative spirometry and laparotomy. Blowing away dollars. *Chest.* 1997;111:1536-1541.
293. Kocabas A, et al. Value of preoperative spirometry to predict postoperative pulmonary complications. *Respir Med.* 1996; 90:25-33.
294. Lawrence VA, et al. Risk of pulmonary complications after elective abdominal surgery. *Chest.* 1996;110:744-750.
295. American College of Physicians. Preoperative pulmonary function testing. *Ann Intern Med.* 1990;112:793-794.
296. Smetana GW. Preoperative pulmonary evaluation. *N Engl J Med.* 1999;340:937-944.
297. Tait AR, Malviya S. Anesthesia for the child with an upper respiratory tract infection. *Curr Rev Nurs Anesth.* 1999;21:170-175.
298. Schemel WH. Unexpected hepatic dysfunction found by multiple laboratory screening. *Anesth Analg.* 1976;55:810-812.
299. Ward ME, et al. Acute liver failure. Experience in a special unit. *Anaesthesia.* 1977;32:228-239.
300. Gitnick G. Assessment of liver function. *Surg Clin North Am.* 1981;61:197-207.
301. Viegas O, Stoelting RK. LDH_5 changes after cholecystectomy or hysterectomy in patients receiving halothane, enflurane, or fentanyl. *Anesthesiology.* 1979;51:556-558.
302. Stoelting RK, Dierdorf SF. Disease of the liver and biliary tract. In: Stoelting RK, Dierdorf SF, eds. *Anesthesia and Co-existing Disease.* 4th ed. New York: Churchill Livingstone; 2002:299-324.
303. O'Grady JG, et al. Early prognostic indicators in acute liver failure and application to selection for orthotopic liver transplantation. *Gastroenterology.* 1988;94:A578.
304. Tucker RA. Drugs and liver disease: a tabular compilation of drugs and the histopathological changes that can occur in the liver. *Drug Intell Clin Pharm.* 1982;16:569-580.
305. Kaplowitz N, et al. Drug-induced hepatotoxicity. *Ann Intern Med.* 1986;104:826-839.
306. Browne RA, Chernesky MA. Infectious diseases and the anaesthetist. *Can J Anaesth.* 1988;35:655-665.
307. Centers for Disease Control and Prevention. Protection against viral hepatitis. Recommendations of the Immunization Practices Advisory Committee (ACIP). *MMWR Morb Mortal Wkly Rep.* 1990;39:1-26.
308. Miller ED Jr. Understanding renal function and its preoperative evaluation. In: Malhotra V, ed. *Anesthesia for Renal and Genitourinary Surgery.* New York: McGraw-Hill; 1996:9.
309. Beck LH. Changes in renal function with aging. *Clin Geriatr Med.* 1998;14:199-209.
310. Sladen RN, Endo E, Harrison T. Two-hour versus 22-hour creatinine clearance in critically ill patients. *Anesthesiology.* 1987;67:1013-1016.
311. Weir PH, Chung FF. Anaesthesia for patients with chronic renal disease. *Can Anaesth Soc J.* 1984;31:468-481.
312. Stoelting RK, Dierdorf SF, McCammon RL. Renal disease. In: *Anesthesia and Co-existing Disease.* 4th ed. New York: Churchill Livingstone; 2002:341-372.

313. Roizen MF, Foss JF, Fischer SP. Preoperative evaluation. In: Miller RD, ed. *Anesthesia*. 5th ed. Philadelphia: Churchill Livingstone; 2000:824-883.
314. The Carter Center of Emory University. Closing the gap: the problem of diabetes mellitus in the United States. *Diabetes Care*. 1985;8:391-406.
315. Sherwin RS. Diabetes mellitus. In: Goldman L, Bennett JC, eds. *Cecil Textbook of Medicine*. 21st ed. Philadelphia: Saunders; 2000:1263.
316. Schwartz JJ, Rosenbaum SH, Graf GJ. Anesthesia and endocrine system. In: Barash PG, Cullen BF, Stoelting RK, eds. *Clinical Anesthesia*. 4th ed. Philadelphia: Lippincott-Raven; 2000:1119-1140.
317. Angelini G, Ketzler JT, Coursin DB. Perioperative care of the diabetic patient. In: Schwartz AJ, ed. *ASA Refresher Courses in Anesthesiology*. Philadelphia: Lippincott; 2001:1-9.
318. Graham GW, Unger BP, Coursin DB. Perioperative management of selected endocrine disorders. *Int Anesth Clin*. 2000;38:31-67.
319. Giugliano D, Ceriello A, Paolisso G. Oxidative stress and diabetic vascular complications. *Diabetes Care*. 1996;19:257-267.
320. Wright RA, Clemente R, Wathen R. Diabetic gastroparesis: an abnormality of gastric emptying of solids. *Am J Med Sci*. 1985;289:240-242.
321. Hogan K, Rusy D, Springman SR. Difficult laryngoscopy and diabetes mellitus. *Anesth Analg*. 1988;67:1162-1165.
322. McConaghy P, Kennedy N, Coleman D. Perioperative management of diabetes mellitus. *Br J Anaesth*. 1994;73:866-867.
323. Hjortrup A, et al. Effect of major surgery on absorption rate of NPH insulin injected SC. *Br J Anaesth*. 1990;64:741-742.
324. Edwards R. Thyroid and parathyroid disease. In: Desborough J, ed. *International Anesthesiology Clinics: Endocrine Disorders and Anesthesia*. Philadelphia: Lippincott-Raven; 1997:63-83.
325. Roizen MF. Anesthesia for the patient with endocrine disease (part I). *Curr Rev Clin Anesth*. 1987;6:43.
326. Cooper DS. Antithyroid drugs. *N Engl J Med*. 1984;311: 1353-1362.
327. Gittoes NJ, Franklyn JA. Hyperthyroidism. Current treatment guidelines. *Drugs*. 1998;55:543-553.
328. Pronovost PH, Parris KH. Perioperative management of thyroid disease. Prevention of complications related to hyperthyroidism and hypothyroidism. *Postgrad Med*. 1995;98:83-86, 96-98.
329. Thorne AC, Bedford RF. Esmolol for perioperative management of thyrotoxic goiter. *Anesthesiology*. 1989;71:291-294.
330. Melissant CF, et al. Lung function, CT-scan and x-ray in upper airway obstruction due to thyroid goiter. *Eur Respir J*. 1994;7:1782-1787.
331. Cooper DS. Subclinical hypothyroidism. *JAMA*. 1987;258: 246-247.
332. Weinberg AD, et al. Outcome of anesthesia and surgery in hypothyroid patients. *Arch Intern Med*. 1983;143:893-897.
333. Ladenson PW, et al. Complications of surgery in hypothyroid patients. *Am J Med*. 1984;77:261-266.
334. Murkin JM. Anesthesia and hypothyroidism: a review of thyroxine physiology, pharmacology, and anesthetic implications. *Anesth Analg*. 1982;61:371-383.
335. Sheeran P, O'Leary E. Adrenocortical disorders. In: Desborough J, ed. *International Anesthesiology Clinics: Endocrine Disorders and Anesthesia*. Philadelphia: Lippincott-Raven; 1997:85-98.
336. Nardella A, Pechet L, Snyder LM. Continuous improvement, quality control, and cost containment in clinical laboratory testing. *Arch Pathol Lab Med*. 1995;119:518-522.
337. Narr BJ, Hansen TR, Warner MA. Preoperative laboratory screening in healthy Mayo patients: cost-effective elimination of tests and unchanged outcomes. *Mayo Clin Proc*. 1991;66:155-159.
338. Velanovich V. Preoperative laboratory screening based on age, gender, and concomitant medical diseases. *Surgery*. 1994;115: 56-61.
339. Perez A, et al. Value of routine preoperative tests: a multicentre study in four general hospitals. *Br J Anaesth*. 1995;74:250-256.
340. Macpherson DS. Preoperative laboratory testing: should any tests be "routine" before surgery? *Med Clin North Am*. 1993;77:289-308.
341. Roizen MF. Cost-effective preoperative laboratory testing. *JAMA*. 1994;271:319-320.
342. Warner MA. Cost containment in anesthesia. *IARS Rev Course Lect* (suppl to *Anesth Analg*). 1995;82:48-53.
343. Archer C, Levy AR, McGregor M. Value of routine preoperative chest x-rays: a meta-analysis. *Can J Anaesth*. 1993;40: 1022-1027.
344. Charpak Y, et al. Prospective assessment of a protocol for selective ordering of preoperative chest x-rays. *Can J Anaesth*. 1988;35: 259-264.
345. Kaplan EB, et al. The usefulness of preoperative laboratory screening. *JAMA*. 1985;253:3576-3581.
346. Johnson H, et al. Are routine laboratory screening tests necessary to evaluate ambulatory surgical patients? *Surgery*. 1988;104:639-645.
347. Ransom SB, McNeeley SG, Hosseini RB. Cost-effectiveness of routine blood type and screen testing before elective laparoscopy. *Obstet Gynecol*. 1995;86:346-348.
348. Pasternak LR. Screening patients: strategies and studies. In: McGoldrick KE, ed. *Ambulatory Anesthesiology: A Problem-Oriented Approach*. Baltimore: Williams & Wilkins; 1995:2-19.
349. Sisson JC, Schoomaker EB, Ross JC. Clinical decision analysis. The hazard of using additional data. *JAMA*. 1976;236: 1259-1263.
350. Roizen MF, Cohn S. Preoperative evaluation for elective surgery: what tests are needed? *Adv Anesth*. 1993;10:25-47.
351. Roizen MF, Fischer SP. Preoperative evaluation: adults and children. In: White PF, ed. *Ambulatory Anesthesia and Surgery*. Philadelphia: Saunders; 1997:155-172.
352. Health Care Standards Committee. Ancillary studies screen for ambulatory surgery for Medicare patients. Glendale: Colorado Foundation for Medical Care;1990.
353. Bass EB, et al. Do ophthalmologists, anesthesiologists, and internists agree about preoperative testing in healthy patients undergoing cataract surgery? *Arch Ophthalmol*. 1995;113: 1248-1256.
354. Duncan PG, et al. Fetal risk of anesthesia and surgery during pregnancy. *Anesthesiology*. 1986;64:790-794.
355. Archer C, Levy AR, McGregor M. Value of routine preoperative chest x-rays: a meta-analysis. *Can J Anaesth*. 1993;40: 1022-1027.
356. Bouillot JL, et al. Are routine preoperative chest radiographs useful in general surgery? A prospective multicentre study in 3959 patients. *Eur J Surg*. 1996;162:597-604.
357. Callaghan LC, Edwards ND, Reilly CS. Utilisation of the preoperative ECG. *Anaesthesia*. 1995;50:488-490.
358. Wagner JD, Moore DL. Preoperative laboratory testing for the oral and maxillofacial surgery patient. *J Oral Maxillofac Surg*. 1991;49:177-182.
359. Haug RH, Reifeis RL. A prospective evaluation of the value of preoperative laboratory testing for office anesthesia and sedation. *J Oral Maxillofac Surg*. 1999;57:16-20.
360. Gloyna DF, et al. The incidence of an abnormal ECG in the surgical patient: is a positive history predictive? *Anesthesiology*. 1998;89:A1349.
361. Munro J, Booth A, Nicholl J. Routine preoperative testing: a systematic review of the evidence. *Health Technol Assess*. 1997;1:1-62.
362. Tait AR, Parr HG, Tremper KK. Evaluation of the efficacy of routine preoperative electrocardiograms. *J Cardiothorac Vasc Anesth*. 1997;11:752-755.
363. Turnbull JM, Buck C. The value of preoperative screening investigations in otherwise healthy individuals. *Arch Intern Med*. 1987;147:1101-1105.
364. Gold BS, et al. The utility of preoperative electrocardiograms in the ambulatory surgical patient. *Arch Intern Med*. 1992;152: 301-305.

365. Murdoch CJ, et al. The pre-operative ECG in day surgery: a habit? *Anaesthesia.* 1999;54:907-908.
366. Orkin FK, Gold B. Selection. In: Wetchler BV, ed. *Anesthesia for Ambulatory Surgery*. 2nd ed. Philadelphia: Lippincott; 1991: 81-129.
367. Margolis JR, et al. Clinical features of unrecognized myocardial infarction—silent and symptomatic. Eighteen year follow-up: the Framingham study. *Am J Cardiol.* 1973;32:1-7.
368. Golub R, et al. Efficacy of preadmission testing in ambulatory surgical patients. *Am J Surg.* 1992;163:565-570.
369. Hannallah R. Clear liquids before surgery offer ASCs more flexibility. *Same Day Surg.* 1991;15:105-108.
370. Dose VA, White PF. Effects of fluid therapy on serum glucose levels in fasted outpatients. *Anesthesiology*. 1987;66:223-226.
371. Sutherland AD, Stock JG, Davies JM. Effects of preoperative fasting on morbidity and gastric contents in patients undergoing day-stay surgery. *Br J Anaesth.* 1986;58:876-878.
372. Splinter WM, Stewart JA, Muir JG. The effect of preoperative apple juice on gastric contents, thirst, and hunger in children. *Can J Anaesth.* 1989;36:55-58.
373. Minami H, McCallum RW. The physiology and pathophysiology of gastric emptying in humans. *Gastroenterology*. 1984;86: 1592-1610.
374. Farrow-Gillespie A, Christensen S, Lerman J. Effect of the fasting interval on gastric fluid pH and volume in children. *Anesth Analg.* 1988;67:S59.
375. Cote CJ. Aspiration: an overrated risk in elective patients. In: Stoelting RK, ed. *Advances in Anesthesia.* St Louis: Mosby; 1992:1-26.
376. Yogendran S, Chung FF. How long should we fast our patients? *Soc Ambul Anesth Newslett.* 1992;7:10.
377. Simpson KH, Stakes AF. Effect of anxiety on gastric emptying in preoperative patients. *Br J Anaesth.* 1987;59:540-544.
378. Borland LM, Sereika SM, Woelfel SK, et al. Pulmonary aspiration in pediatric patients during general anesthesia: incidence and outcome. *J Clin Anesth.* 1998;10:95-102.
379. Nimmo WS. Drugs, diseases and altered gastric emptying. *Clin Pharmacokinet.* 1976;1:189-203.
380. Morgan M. Anaesthetic contribution to maternal mortality. *Br J Anaesth.* 1987;59:842-855.
381. Morrison JE Jr, Lockhart CH. Preoperative fasting and medication in children. *Anesthesiol Clin North Am.* 1991;9:731-743.
382. Cote CJ. Changing concepts in preoperative medication and "NPO" status of the pediatric patient. In: *ASA 1992 Annual Refresher Course Lecture*. Philadelphia: Lippincott; 1992:132.
383. Hinder RA, Kelly KA. Canine gastric emptying of solids and liquids. *Am J Physiol.* 1977;233:E335-E340.
384. Warner ME. Risks and outcomes of perioperative pulmonary aspiration. *J Peri Anesth Nurs.* 1997;12:352-357.
385. Read MS, Vaughan RS. Allowing preoperative patients to drink: effects on patients' safety and comfort of unlimited oral water until 2 hours before anaesthesia. *Acta Anaesthesiol Scand.* 1991;35:591-595.
386. Shevde K, Trivedi N. Effects of clear liquids on gastric volume and pH in healthy volunteers. *Anesth Analg.* 1991;72:528-531.
387. Splinter WM, Schaefer JD. Unlimited clear fluid ingestion two hours before surgery in children does not affect volume or pH of stomach contents. *Anaesth Intensive Care.* 1990;18:522-526.
388. Maltby JR, et al. Gastric fluid volume and pH in elective patients following unrestricted oral fluid until three hours before surgery. *Can J Anaesth.* 1991;38:425-429.
389. Splinter WM, Schaefer JD. Ingestion of clear fluids is safe for adolescents up to 3 h before anaesthesia. *Br J Anaesth.* 1991; 66:48-52.
390. Warner MA, et al. Practice guidelines for preoperative fasting and the use of pharmacologic agents to reduce the risk of pulmonary aspiration: application to healthy patients undergoing elective procedures. *Anesthesiology*. 1999;90:896-905.
391. Fasting S, Soreide E, Raeder JC. Changing preoperative fasting policies. *Acta Anaesthesiol Scand.* 1998;42:1188-1191.
392. Keats AS. The ASA classification of physical status—a recapitulation. *Anesthesiology*. 1978;49:233-236.
393. Keenan RL, Boyan CP. Cardiac arrest due to anesthesia. A study of incidence and causes. *JAMA.* 1985;253:2373-2377.
394. Marx GF, Mateo CV, Orkin LR. Computer analysis of postanesthesia deaths. *Anesthesiology*. 1973;39:54-58.
395. Vacanti CJ, VanHouten RJ, Hill RC. A statistical analysis of the relationship of physical status to postoperative mortality in 68,388 cases. *Anesth Analg.* 1970;49:564-566.
396. American Society of Anesthesiologists. New classification of physical status. *Anesthesiology*. 1963;24:111.
397. Owens WD, Felts JA, Spitznagel EL Jr. ASA physical status classifications: a study of consistency of ratings. *Anesthesiology*. 1978;49:239-243.

CHAPTER 18

FLUIDS, ELECTROLYTES, AND BLOOD COMPONENT THERAPY

EDWARD WATERS

Much effort in anesthesia is directed at maintaining the physiologic homeostasis of patients undergoing the stresses of surgery and anesthesia. Maintaining a physiologic balance of body fluids in both volume and composition is critical to maintaining overall homeostasis. The following discussion focuses on factors of fluid and electrolyte management and transfusion therapy that are of greatest consequence to the practicing anesthetist.

FLUID COMPARTMENTS

A prerequisite to understanding clinical fluid management is a fundamental appreciation of the role of fluids in the human body and the distribution of fluids and electrolytes among the fluid compartments of the body. The human body is in large part composed of fluid, ranging between 46% and 80% depending on the age and gender of the individual and the body's composition of fat relative to muscle. Compared with muscle, fat contains less fluid as a percentage of weight (Table 18-1).

TABLE 18-1 Approximate Values of Total Body Fluid as Percentage of Body Weight in Relation to Age and Sex

Age	Total Body Fluid (% of body weight)
Full-term newborn	70-80
1 year	64
Puberty to 39 years	Men: 60 Women: 52
40-60 years	Men: 55 Women: 47
>60 years	Men: 52 Women: 46

From Metheney *N.* Fluid and Electrolyte Balance: Nursing Considerations. *4th ed. Philadelphia: Lippincott; 2000;4.*

Total body water is partitioned into two principal compartments: the intracellular fluid (ICF) and the extracellular fluid (ECF). The extracellular compartment is further subdivided into intravascular fluid (IVF) and interstitial fluid (ISF) spaces. The fluid compartments are divided by water-permeable membranes[1]; the intracellular space is separated from the extracellular space by the cell membrane, and the extracellular space is divided into intravascular and interstitial spaces by the capillary membrane.

The ICF compartment contains approximately two thirds of the total body's fluid volume[2] and is characterized by high concentrations of potassium, phosphate, and magnesium. The adenosine triphosphatase (ATPase)–driven sodium-potassium pump (Na-K-ATPase pump) located in the cell membrane maintains the high concentration of potassium found in ICF.[3] (Figure 18-1 and Table 18-2). This mechanism exchanges three sodium ions for two potassium ions and offsets the tendency for sodium to diffuse into the intracellular space.

The ECF compartment contains approximately one third of the body's fluid volume[2] and contains high concentrations of sodium and chloride compared to the ICF compartment. The IVF (also known as *plasma*) space contains approximately one quarter of the ECF volume and has essentially the same composition and concentration of electrolytes as the ISF. The presence in the IVF of relatively high concentrations of osmotically active plasma proteins, of which albumin is most important, is a significant difference distinguishing the interstitial from intravascular space.[4] It should be noted that the capillary membrane is relatively impermeable to plasma proteins, which are therefore contained within the vascular space.

The properties of the membranes that separate the fluid compartments, as well as the relative concentration of osmotically active substances within each compartment, are in large part responsible for the movement of fluid (water and electrolytes) among compartments in the body. Because the intravascular space is the fluid compartment accessible to the clinician and the chief focus of fluid therapy, it is useful to understand the motion of fluid from the IVF space to the ISF space across the capillary membrane. Four forces known commonly as *Starling forces* determine the motion of fluids across the capillary membrane. The four forces that govern fluid dynamics in the microcirculation are: capillary pressure, ISF pressure, ISF colloid osmotic pressure, and plasma osmotic pressure.[2]

The plasma colloid osmotic pressure is significant to the anesthetist because this force is determined primarily by plasma protein concentration and serves to maintain the circulating fluid volume within the intravascular space. Plasma protein concentrations can be increased or decreased depending on the types and volumes of intravenous (IV) fluids the clinician administers.

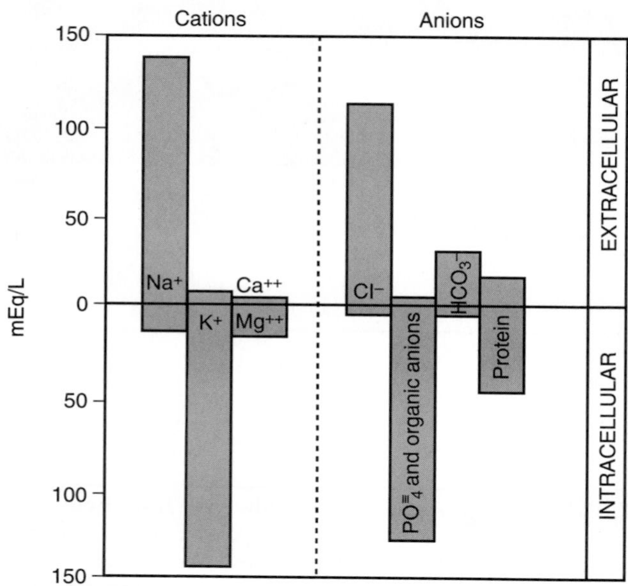

FIGURE **18-1**
Major cations and anions of the intracellular and extracellular fluids. (From Guyton AC, Hall JE. *Textbook of Medical Physiology*. 10th ed. Philadelphia: Saunders; 2000:266.)

INFLUENCES OF SURGERY AND ANESTHESIA ON FLUID BALANCE

Illness, surgery, and anesthetics can profoundly alter the fluid and electrolyte balance of patients during the perioperative period.

Preoperatively patients can become volume depleted and experience alterations of electrolyte balance because of several processes. Burns, vomiting, diarrhea, fever, and gastric suction can lead to hypovolemia before surgery.[5] If a large volume of fluid is lost from the gastrointestinal (GI) tract, careful evaluation of electrolytes and appropriate replacement is indicated.[4] Quite often preoperative hypovolemia is, at least in part, an iatrogenic phenomenon secondary to bowel preparation and preoperative fasting. Unless surgery is of the greatest urgency, preoperative fluid deficits and electrolyte abnormalities should be corrected before anesthetic induction to reduce the risk of hypotension and complications resulting from electrolyte imbalances.[6]

During the intraoperative period the effects of surgery and anesthesia combine to challenge fluid and electrolyte homeostasis. Surgery can lead to hemorrhage and a need to replace fluids or blood. Surgery can also lead to evaporative loss; this loss from exposed viscera is composed entirely of water (without electrolytes) and is most appropriately replaced with free water. Manipulation of tissues during surgery can lead to "third spacing" the redistribution of fluid from the intravascular space to the interstitial space, where it is nonfunctional. Replacement of fluid lost from the intravascular space in the phenomenon of third spacing is best carried out by balanced salt solutions, which have an electrolyte composition similar to ECF.[1,6] Absorption of electrolyte-free irrigation solutions during transurethral prostate surgery or endometrial ablation can result in a life-threatening hyposmolar state that must be addressed appropriately by the clinician.[7]

Anesthesia in and of itself can lead to derangements of fluid balance in surgical patients. The vasodilatory effects of both regional and general anesthesia can result in a relative hypovolemia, which may lead to hypotension on induction. General anesthesia increases the release of antidiuretic hormone, causing increased retention of water,[1,8] which can predispose the patient to hyponatremia.[9] Mechanical ventilation can increase

TABLE **18-2** Osmolar Substances in Extracellular and Intracellular Fluids

	Plasma (mOsm/L H_2O)	Interstitial Fluid (mOsm/L H_2O)	Intracellular Fluid (mOsm/L H_2O)
Na^+	142	139	14
K^+	4.2	4	140
Ca^{2+}	1.3	1.2	0
Mg^{2+}	0.8	0.7	20
Cl^-	108	108	4
HCO_3^-	24	28.3	10
HPO_4^-, $H_2PO_4^-$	2	2	11
SO_4^{2-}	0.5	0.5	1
Phosphocreatine	–	–	45
Carnosine	–	–	14
Amino acids	2	2	8
Creatine	0.2	0.2	9
Lactate	1.2	1.2	1.5
Adenosine triphosphate	–	–	5
Hexose monophosphate	–	–	3.7
Glucose	5.6	5.6	–
Protein	1.2	0.2	4
Urea	4	4	4
Others	4.8	3.9	10
Total mOsm/L	301.8	300.8	301.2
Corrected osmolar activity (mOsm/L)	282	281	281
Total osmotic pressure at 37° C (mm Hg)	5443	5423	5423

From Guyton AC, Hall JE. Textbook of Medical Physiology *10th ed. Philadelphia: WB Saunders; 2000;267.*

evaporative loss of water and decrease the release of atrial natruretic peptide, which results in conservation of sodium.[1]

The effects of surgery on fluid balance can persist into the postoperative period. Third-spaced fluids are typically mobilized (returned to the intravascular space) on the third postoperative day. The increased circulating volume may be poorly tolerated by patients with marginal renal or cardiovascular performance and can result in heart failure or pulmonary edema.[4,10]

FLUID VOLUME DISORDERS

Fluid volume disorders, particularly hypovolemia, are often encountered in patients undergoing surgery. Discussion of disorders of concentration and volume of body fluids is facilitated by careful consideration of the concepts of osmolarity, osmolality, and tonicity. Osmolarity is an expression of the number of osmoles of solute in a liter of solution, whereas osmolality expresses the number of osmoles of solute in a kilogram of solvent. Because of the dilute nature of body fluids, the difference between osmolarity and osmolality is minimal. Tonicity, related but not equivalent to osmolarity and osmolality, describes how a solution affects cell volume. Isotonic solutions have an effective osmolality close to that of body fluids (approximately 285 mOsm)[3]; therefore cells placed in an isotonic solution are not expected to swell or shrink.

Volume depletion, or *hypovolemia*, refers to the loss of ECF and is not to be confused with *dehydration*, which refers to a concentration disorder in which insufficient water is present relative to sodium levels.[3] Hypovolemia can result from an absolute loss of fluid from the body or a relative loss of bodily fluids in which water is redistributed within the body, leading to a reduced circulating volume. Causes of absolute fluid loss include loss of fluid from the GI tract, polyuria, and diaphoresis. Decreased intake of fluids is a common cause of absolute fluid deficit in surgical patients because of intolerance of oral intake and prolonged preoperative fasting. Relative fluid losses can be caused by conditions such as burns and third-space losses resulting from surgery. It should be noted that patient weight does not decrease in cases of relative fluid loss.

Because most cases of hypovolemia are caused by the loss of ECF, replacement with isotonic crystalloids (which have a composition similar to ECF) is appropriate.[3] Determination of the appropriate volume of fluids to administer for maintenance and replacement needs is discussed subsequently; however, in certain circumstances such as oliguria or hemodynamic instability a fluid bolus (also known as *fluid challenge*) may be warranted (Table 18-3). Estimated fluid and blood requirements based on the clinical presentation of a patient have been described by the American College of Surgeons (Table 18-4).

TABLE 18-3 Fluid Challenge Guideline Chart

BASELINE VALUES		
PAWP* (mm Hg)	**Challenge Volume**	**CVP* (mm Hg)**
<12	200 ml/10 min or 20 cc/min	<8
12-16	100 ml/10 min or 10 cc/min	8-13
>16-18	50 ml/10 min or 5 cc/min	>13

**References differ on CVP and PAWP range.*
- *Reprofile at the end of 10 minutes of fluid challenge.*
- *Discontinue challenge if PAWP increases >7 mm Hg or CVP increases >4 mm Hg.*
- *Repeat challenge if PAWP increases <3 mm Hg or CVP increases <2 mm Hg.*
- *Observe patient for 10 minutes and reprofile if PAWP increases >3 mm Hg but <7 mm Hg or CVP increases >2 mm Hg or <4 mm Hg.*

CVP, *Central venous pressure;* PAWP, *pulmonary artery wedge pressure; Adapted from Lichtenthal, PR.* Quick Guide to Cardiopulmonary Care. *Irvine, Calif: Edwards Lifesciences; 2002;60.*

Hypervolemia is an excess of fluid volume in an isotonic concentration. Hypervolemia is not usually encountered in surgical patients but can be seen if diseases such as congestive heart failure, renal failure, or cirrhosis of the liver are present. Iatrogenic causes of fluid overload include administration of steroids and excessive IV administration of isotonic fluids. Excessive consumption of sodium in the diet or in medications can lead to retention of water and hypervolemia. Treatment of hypervolemia may include sodium restriction, diuretics, and, in cases of renal failure, hemodialysis or ultrafiltration.

DISORDERS OF SODIUM BALANCE

Disorders of sodium balance are encountered frequently in anesthetic care and are of great clinical significance. Sodium is

TABLE 18-4 Advanced Trauma Life Support Estimates of Fluid and Blood Requirements in a 70-kg Man

	INITIAL PRESENTATIONS			
	Class I	**Class II**	**Class III**	**Class IV**
Blood loss (ml)	<750	750-1500	1500-2000	≥2000
Blood loss (% of blood volume)	<15	15-30	30-40	≥40
Pulse rate (bpm)	<100	>100	>120	≥140
Blood pressure	Normal	Normal	Decreased	Decreased
Pulse pressure (mm Hg)	Normal or increased	Decreased	Decreased	Decreased
Capillary blanch test	Normal	Positive	Positive	Positive
Respiratory rate	14-20	20-30	30-40	>35
Urine output (ml/hr)	30 or more	20-30	5-15	Negligible
CNS-mental status	Slightly anxious	Mildly anxious	Anxious and confused	Confused and lethargic
Fluid replacement	Crystalloid	Crystalloid	Crystalloid + blood	Crystalloid + blood

CNS, *Central nervous system.*
From Lichtenthal, PR. Quick Guide to Cardiopulmonary Care. *Irvine, Calif. Edwards Lifesciences, 2002;59.*

the most abundant electrolyte in the ECF and, along with its accompanying chloride anion, is responsible for most of the osmotic activity of the ECF. The physiologic significance of sodium can be appreciated when one considers that gain or loss of sodium is accompanied by a gain or loss of water.[3] Because sodium concentration in the ECF is much higher than the intracellular space (as a result of the action of the Na-K-ATPase pump in the cell membrane), alteration of sodium levels in the extracellular space greatly alters the osmotic relationship between intracellular and extracellular spaces, leading to movement of water across the cell membrane.

The clinical importance of sodium disorders is due largely to the influence of sodium on the water content in brain cells. The blood-brain barrier, unlike peripheral capillary beds, has only limited permeability to ionic solutes. The result of the limited permeability in the blood-brain barrier is prevention of equilibration of osmotically active ionic solutes between intravascular and interstitial spaces. This lack of permeability to sodium and consequent failure to equilibrate osmotically active solutes between the intravascular and interstitial spaces changes the osmotic gradients between fluid compartments, leading to the precedence of sodium over plasma proteins as the most important osmotically active substance influencing the water content of the brain tissues.[10,11]

Because sodium imbalances reflect impaired concentration between water and sodium, evaluation of sodium imbalance should take into consideration both the volume of the solvent (water) as well as the amount of solute (sodium) present in the solution. Likewise, treatment of sodium imbalances can involve restriction or expansion of water volume and enhanced elimination or supplementation of sodium.

Hyponatremia may have multiple causes (Box 18-1). Of particular interest to anesthetists is hyponatremia resulting from inappropriate secretion of antidiuretic hormone (SIADH), which is discussed in Chapter 31. Water intoxication resulting from the absorption of electrolyte-free irrigation solution during procedures such as transurethral resection of the prostate and endometrial ablation are discussed in Chapter 27. Water intoxication and SIADH lead to hyponatremia from an excess of water, not loss of sodium.[1,12]

Hyponatremia results in a state in which the intracellular environment is hyperosmolar relative to the ECF, leading to an influx of water into the intracellular space. Because the brain is contained within the fixed confines of the skull, cerebral edema is poorly tolerated.[13] Compensatory mechanisms can forestall the development of symptomatic cerebral edema for a period of time.[14] Over time the brain cells can maintain osmotic equilibrium without swelling by extruding intracellular solutes, thereby reducing intracellular osmolality to that of the plasma.[9,13] If the extrusion of solute by brain cells is inadequate to compensate for the hyposmolar influence of the ECF, an intracellular influx of water may lead to symptomatic cerebral edema, risking eventual tentorial herniation.[13]

Clinical studies have demonstrated that compared to men or postmenopausal women, menstruant women are at increased risk of brain damage resulting from hyponatremia.[3,13] It is believed that estrogen and progesterone inhibit the efficiency of the Na-K-ATPase pump, which is essential to the extrusion of intracellular solutes to maintain osmotic equilibrium in hyponatremia.[13] It is also believed that female sex hormones may facilitate movement of water into the brain through the mediation of ADH.[13]

BOX **18-1**

Hyponatremia (Serum Sodium <135)

Causative Factors and Classification

Isotonic Hyponatremia (Pseudohyponatremia)

Serum osmolality 280-285

- *Causes*: Hyperlipidemia, hyperproteinemia, infusion of isotonic nonelectrolytic substances (glucose, mannitol glycine)

Hypertonic Hypernatremia

Serum osmolality >285

- *Causes*: Hyperglycemia, infusion of hypertonic nonelectrolytic substances

Hypotonic Hyponatremia

Serum osmolality <280

Hypovolemic hypotonic hyponatremia

- *Causes*: Diuretics, salt losing nephropathy, ketonuria, third spacing, adrenal insufficiency, vomiting, diarrhea, third spacing of fluids

Isovolemic hypotonic hyponatremia

- *Causes*: SIADH, renal failure, hypothyroidism, drugs, water intoxication, drugs

Hypervolemic hypotonic hyponatremia

- *Causes*: Nephrotic syndrome, cirrhosis, congestive heart failure

Clinical Manifestations

Neurologic Manifestations

Seizure
Coma
Agitation
Confusion
Headache
Confusion
Cerebral edema

Gastrointestinal Manifestations

Anorexia
Nausea and vomiting

Muscular Manifestations

Cramps
Weakness

ADH, *Antidiuretic hormone;* SIADH, *inappropriate secretion of antidiuretic hormone;* U_{Na}, *urinary sodium.*

From Metheney N. Fluid and Electrolyte Balance: Nursing Considerations. *4th ed. Philadelphia: Lippincott; 2000;58-89; Ferri FF.* Practical Guide to the Care of the Medical Patient. *5th ed. St Louis: Mosby; 2001;594-601; Barash PG, Cullen BF, Stoelting RK.* Handbook of Clinical Anesthesia. *2nd ed. Philadelphia: Lippincott; 1993;95-96.*

Some controversy exists regarding how aggressively hyponatremia should be treated. (Figure 18-2). In chronically hyponatremic patients, rapid correction of serum sodium can lead to the neurologic disorder known as *myelinolysis*. Myelinolysis, originally known as *central pontine myelinolysis*, can lead to disorders of the upper neurons, spastic quadriparesis, pseudobulbar palsy, mental disorders, and in some cases death.[14] Patients at particular risk for myelinolysis are those who have been hyponatremic for more than 48 hours,[9,14] as well as individuals with who have had orthotopic liver transplantation or alcoholism.[14] Optimal treatment of hyponatremia must balance the risks of cerebral edema against the risks of myelinolysis.[12]

The risk of myelinolysis can be reduced by correcting serum sodium levels in a deliberate manner. It has been suggested that serum sodium concentrations should be increased by no more than 1 to 2 mEq/L/hr in symptomatic patients by infusing 3% saline at a rate of 1 to 2 ml/kg/hr. Once the patient is clinically stable, sodium administration should be slowed to raise serum sodium not more than 10 to 15 mmol/L in 24 hours.[9,12,14]

Hypernatremia can result from several causes (Figure 18-3 and Box 18-2) but is usually the result of impaired water intake.[12] Inadequate administration of free water to hospitalized patients can lead to an iatrogenic hypernatremia. Debilitated, mentally impaired, and intubated individuals are at particular risk for developing hypernatremia.[4,12] In cases of slow-onset hypernatremia the brain can adapt by conservation of intracellular solutes, which allows maintenance of normal intracellular volume. Rapidly occurring hypernatremia can be accompanied by rapid shrinking of the brain and concomitant traction on intracranial veins and venous sinuses, leading to intracranial hemorrhage.[7]

As with hyponatremia, overly aggressive treatment of chronic hypernatremia can lead to unwanted effects. In the case of hypernatremia, rapid correction of serum sodium may lead to cerebral edema.[7]

Correction of hypernatremia is carried out by replacement of the water deficit, which can be calculated by the formula shown in Box 18-3. If the hypernatremia is acute (i.e., less than 24 hours' duration), water deficits can be replaced rapidly with hypotonic solutions. If chronic hypernatremia accompanied by volume depletion is present, the volume disorder is corrected first with isotonic crystalloids. Once the circulating volume has been restored, hypotonic solutions are used to correct the water deficit. Correction of chronic hypernatremia, like treatment of chronic hyponatremia, calls for prudence. Plasma sodium should be decreased by 1 to 2 mEq/hr until the patient is clinically stable, followed by correction of serum sodium to normal levels over the subsequent 24 hours.[12]

DISORDERS OF POTASSIUM BALANCE

Potassium is the principal electrolyte of the ICF, where 98% of the body's supply of potassium is located. The ratio between

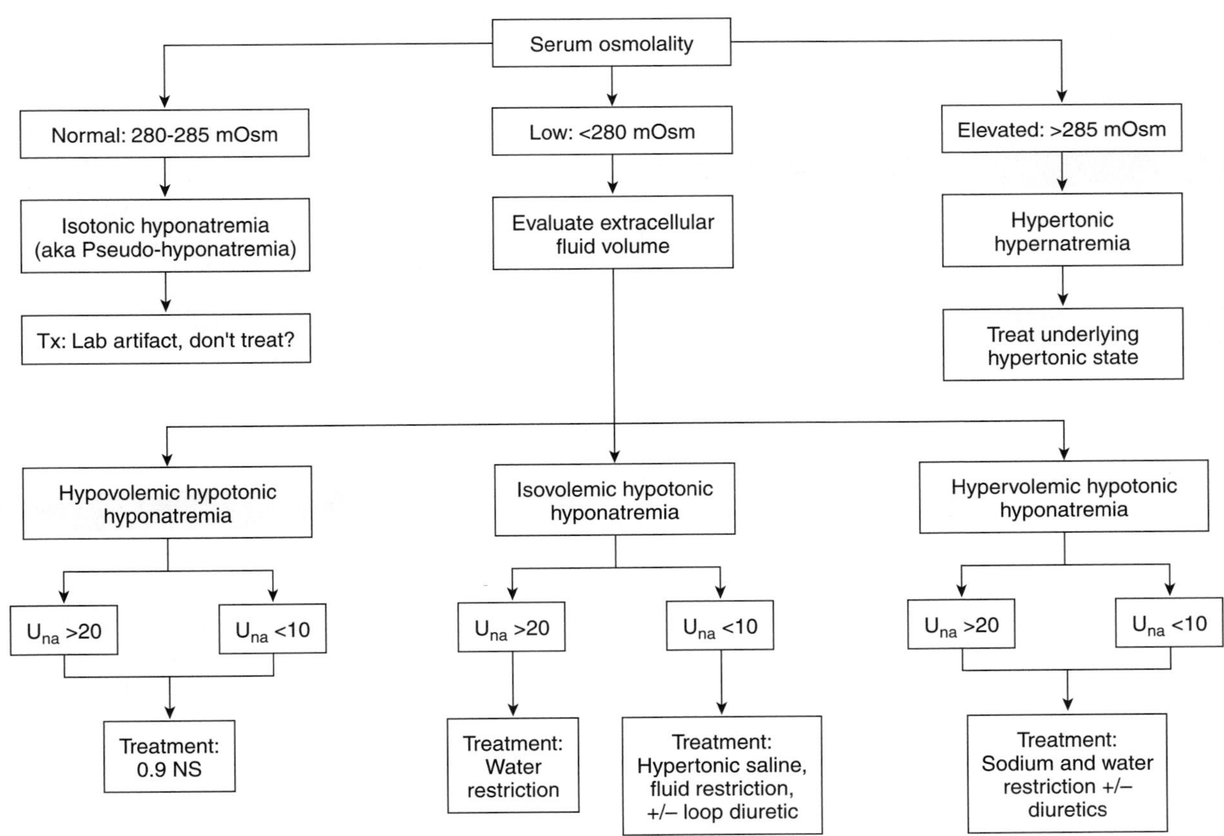

FIGURE **18-2**
Treatment of hyponatremia. (Adapted from Ferri, FF. *Practical Guide to the Care of the Medical Patient*. 5th ed. St. Louis: Mosby; 2001;595-598.) U_{na}, Urinary Sodium.

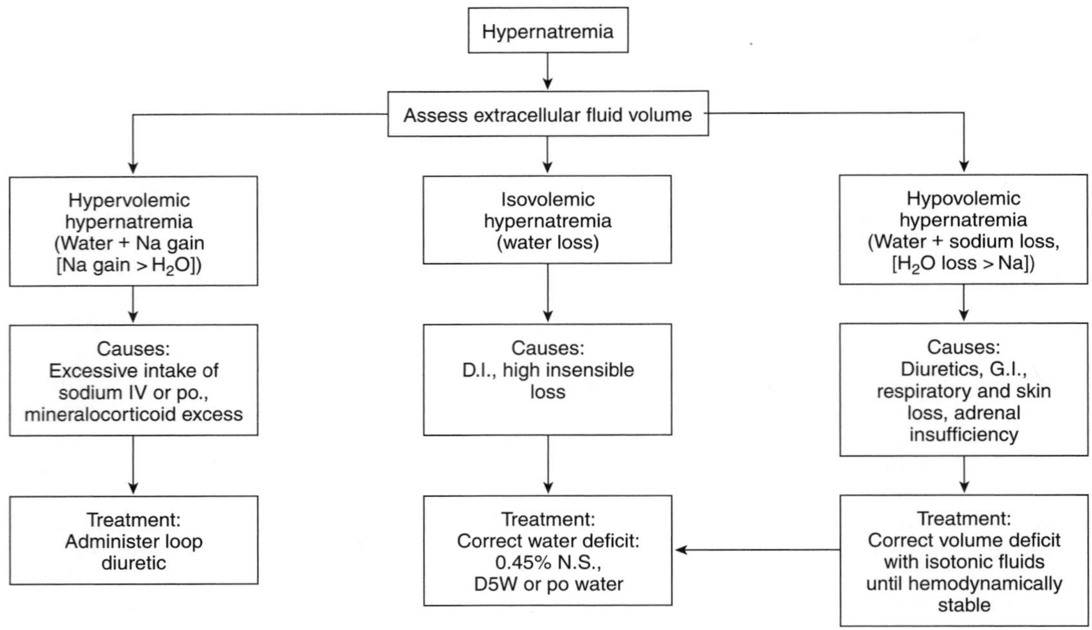

FIGURE **18-3**
Hypernatremia (serum sodium >145). (Ferri, FF. *Practical Guide to the Care of the Medical Patient.* 5th ed. St. Louis: Mosby; 2001;598-601; Morgan GE, Mikhail MS, Mung MJ. *Clinical Anesthesiology.* 3rd ed. New York: Lange Medical; 2002;606.) *D.I.* diabetes insipidus.

intracellular and extracellular potassium is, in large part, responsible for the resting membrane potential of the cell.[15] Potassium exists in a dynamic balance between the intracellular and extracellular compartments. Abnormal serum potassium levels may be the result of disturbances in the balance between intracellular and extracellular distribution of potassium or an abnormality in the total body store of potassium. β-Adrenergic stimulation, insulin, and alkalosis all promote movement of potassium into the intracellular space.[16] Evaluation and treatment of disorders of potassium homeostasis should address factors that can shift potassium into the cell, as well as total body levels of potassium. The symptoms associated with disorders of potassium homeostasis are largely a reflection of disorders of resting membrane potential. Clinically this is seen most clearly in the dysrhythmias associated with abnormal potassium levels (Box 18-4).

Hypokalemia, defined as plasma potassium of less then 3.5 mEq/L, can result from an absolute deficiency caused by GI loss or renal loss or from a poor intake of potassium (see Box 18-4). Redistribution of potassium from the extracellular to the intracellular compartment can also lead to hypokalemia.

BOX **18-2**

Clinical Manifestations of Hypernatremia (Serum Sodium >145)

Neurologic Manifestations
Thirst
Weakness
Seizure
Coma
Intracranial bleeding
Disorientation
Hallucinations
Irritability

Cardiovascular Manifestations
Hypovolemia

Renal Manifestations
Polyuria or oliguria
Renal insufficiency

Modified from Metheney N. Fluid and Electrolyte Balance: Nursing Considerations. *4th ed. Philadelphia: Lippincott; 2000;58-59; Ferri FF.* Practical Guide to the Care of the Medical Patient. *5th ed. St Louis: Mosby; 2001;594-601; Barash PG, Cullen BF, Stoelting RK.* Handbook of Clinical Anesthesia. *2nd ed. Philadelphia: Lippincott; 1993;97.*

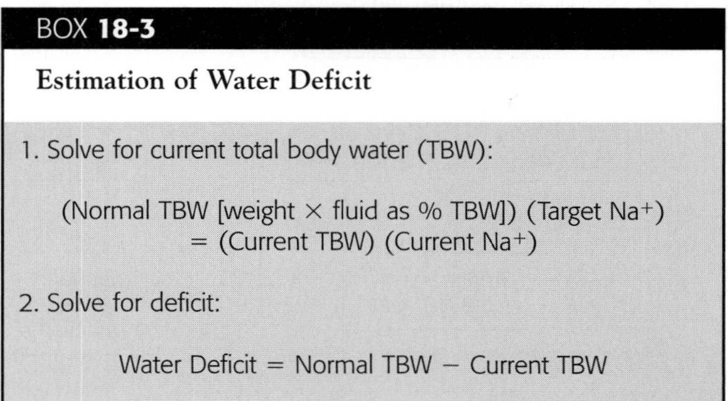
BOX **18-3**

Estimation of Water Deficit

1. Solve for current total body water (TBW):

$$(\text{Normal TBW [weight} \times \text{fluid as \% TBW]}) (\text{Target Na}^+) = (\text{Current TBW}) (\text{Current Na}^+)$$

2. Solve for deficit:

$$\text{Water Deficit} = \text{Normal TBW} - \text{Current TBW}$$

From Morgan GE, Mikhail MS, Mung MJ. Clinical Anesthesiology. *3rd ed. New York: Lange Medical; 2002.*

BOX **18-4**

Hypokalemia (Serum Potassium <3.5 mEq/L)

Causative Factors

Redistribution
Alkalosis
Insulin administration
β-Agonists
Increased Renal Excretion
Multiple drug use, especially potassium-losing diuretics, penicillin, aminoglycosides, corticosteroids
Hyperaldosteronism
Renal tubular acidosis
Magnesium deficiency
Gastrointestinal Loss
Diarrhea
Gastric suctioning
Villous adenoma
Fistulas
Inadequate Intake
Anorexia
Alcoholism
Debilitation

Clinical Manifestations

Cardiovascular Manifestations
ST-segment depression
Widened QRS complex
Flattened T waves
Ventricular ectopy
Neuromuscular Manifestations
Weakness
Decreased reflexes
Confusion
Renal Manifestations
Polyuria
Concentrating defect
Metabolic Manifestations
Glucose intolerance
Potentiation of hypercalcemia and hypomagnesemia

From Metheney N. Fluid and Electrolyte Balance: Nursing Considerations. *4th ed. Philadelphia: Lippincott; 2000;90-109; Ferri FF.* Practical Guide to the Care of the Medical Patient. *5th ed. St Louis: Mosby; 2001;601-606; Barash PG, Cullen BF, Stoelting RK.* Handbook of Clinical Anesthesia. *2nd ed. Philadelphia: Lippincott; 1993;97-99.*

Treatment of hypokalemia depends on the severity of the symptoms accompanying the potassium deficit. In the face of malignant dysrhythmias, aggressive IV administration of potassium is warranted.[15] IV replacement of potassium should be accomplished with the patient under continuous ECG monitoring. Rates of IV administration as fast as 40 mEq per hour have been reported,[16] although a maximum rate of 10 to 20 mEq/hr is usually recommended to avoid an iatrogenic hyperkalemia.[4,7]

Once symptoms such as respiratory muscle weakness or dysrhythmia have ceased, IV replacement can be discontinued in favor of oral supplementation.[16] It is recommended that IV potassium be replaced as a chloride, because the hypochloride state makes it difficult for the kidney to conserve potassium.[4] Furthermore, potassium chloride should be mixed in a dextrose-free solution to prevent stimulation of insulin leading to increased redistribution of potassium to the intracellular space.[7]

Some clinicians have questioned whether surgery should be canceled because of low serum potassium. In a study of 447 patients scheduled for cardiovascular surgery, Hirsch and co-workers used continuous electrocardiographic monitoring to evaluate the preoperative and intraoperative incidence of ectopy. They found no significant difference in frequent or complex ventricular ectopy between patients with normal serum potassium and those with mild to severe hypokalemia. The authors concluded that cancellation of surgery based on low serum potassium was not warranted.[17]

Hyperkalemia is less common than hypokalemia; if renal causes are excluded, the incidence is quite uncommon.[16] In addition to impaired renal excretion of potassium, causes of hyperkalemia include a high intake of potassium and a shift of potassium from the intracellular to the extracellular space. Movement of potassium from the intracellular to the extracellular compartment can result from lysis of cells as well as from acidemia and the administration of β-adrenergic blockers, which inhibit the Na-K-ATPase pump and disrupt movement of potassium into the cell (Box 18-5).

Treatment of hyperkalemia should be preceded by exclusion of pseudohyperkalemia, which is a laboratory artifact. Pseudohyperkalemia results from hemolysis of the blood sample, leukocytosis, thrombosis, or prolonged fist clenching during blood drawing. Treatment of hyperkalemia is based on the severity of the patient's presenting signs and symptoms (Figure 18-4).

DISORDERS OF CALCIUM BALANCE

Calcium is a divalent cation, 99% of which is found in the bone. Calcium has an important structural function, but perhaps most important to anesthetists is its role as a second messenger that couples cell membrane receptors to cellular responses. The action of calcium as a second messenger is critical to functions such as muscle contractions and release of hormones and neurotransmitters.[2,18] In addition to the second messenger function, calcium plays an important role in coagulation of blood and in muscle function.

Although most of the body's calcium is found in the bones, a small percentage is freely exchangeable with the ECF. Calcium in the ECF is found in three distinct fractions. Ionized calcium accounts for 50% of the calcium in the ECF and is the physiologically active portion of circulating calcium.[1] The

BOX **18-5**

Hyperkalemia (Serum Potassium >5.0)

Causative Factors	*Clinical Manifestations*
Redistribution	*Cardiovascular Manifestations*
Acidosis	Tall peaked T waves
Hypertonicity	Widened QRS complex
Hemolysis	Ventricular dysrhythmias
Tissue necrosis	Cardiac arrest
Rhabdomyolysis	*Neuromuscular Manifestations*
Decreased Renal Excretion	Muscle weakness
Renal insufficiency and failure	Confusion
Potassium-sparing diuretics	Paresthesias
Hypoaldosteronism	
Drugs (e.g., NSAIDS, β-blockers, ACE inhibitors)	
Excessive Potassium Intake	
IV or PO supplementation	
Excessive use of salt substitutes	
Rapid transfusion of banked blood	

ACE, *Angiotensin-converting enzyme;* IV, *intravenous;* NSAIDS, *nonsteroidal antiinflammatory drugs;* PO, *orally.*
From Metheney N. Fluid and Electrolyte Balance: Nursing Considerations. *4th ed. Philadelphia: Lippincott; 2000;90-109; Ferri FF.* Practical Guide to the Care of the Medical Patient. *5th ed. St Louis: Mosby; 2001;606-613; Barash PG, Cullen BF, Stoelting RK.* Handbook of Clinical Anesthesia. *2nd ed. Philadelphia: Lippincott; 1993;99-100.*

remainder of the circulating calcium is either bound to anions (10%) or bound to plasma proteins, primarily albumin (40%).[19] Changes in pH alter the extracellular distribution of calcium, with acidemia decreasing the protein-bound fraction and increasing the ionized fraction.[4]

Because the ionized fraction of calcium is clinically the most significant form and total serum calcium levels are largely dependent on albumin levels, direct measurement of ionized calcium is the preferred method in critically ill patients.[3] Mathematical formulas to "correct" total calcium measurement

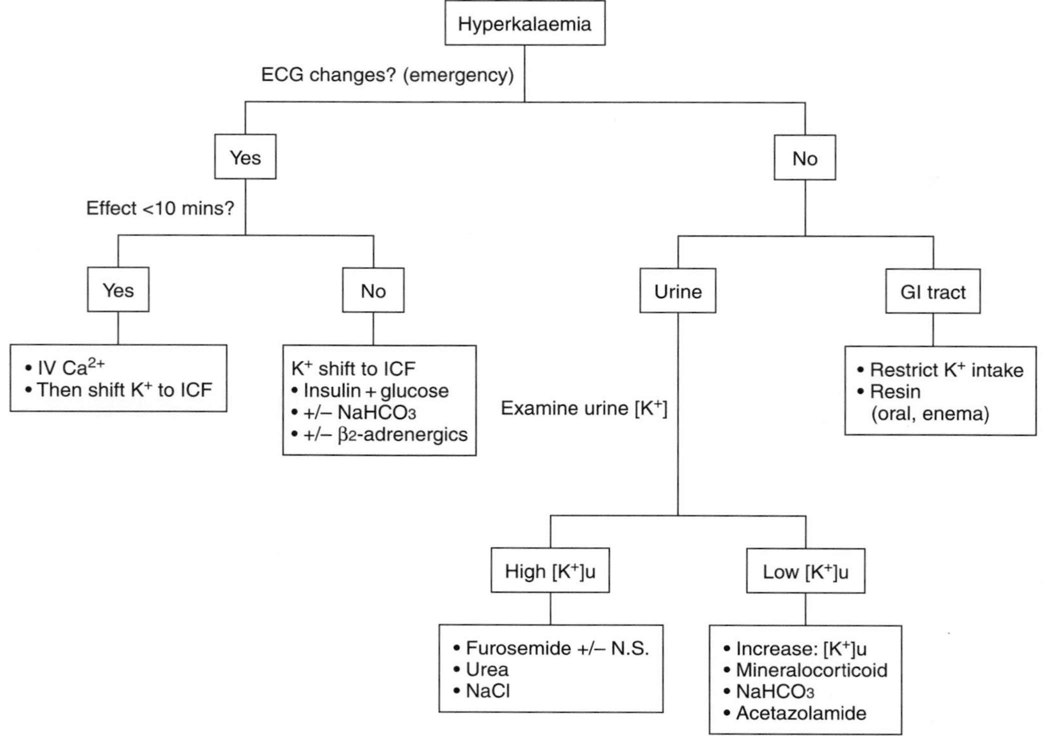

FIGURE **18-4**
Treatment of hyperkalemia. (From Halperin ML, Kamel KS. Potassium. *Lancet.* 1998;352;135-140.) *$[K^+]u$,* urine potassium.

BOX 18-6

Hypocalcemia (Serum Calcium <8.9 mg/dL, Ionized Calcium <4.6 mg/dL)

Causative Factors
Hypoparathyroidism (can be surgically induced)
Pseudohypoparathyroidism
Malabsorption
Acute pancreatitis
Malignancy
Alkalosis
Hyperphosphatemia
Rhabdomyolysis
Chronic renal insufficiency
Hypomagnesemia

Clinical Manifestations
Cardiovascular Manifestations
Dysrhythmia
Prolonged QT interval
T-wave inversion
Hypotension
Decreased myocardial contractility
Neuromuscular Manifestations
Cramps
Muscle weakness
Chvostek's sign
Trousseau's sign
Seizure
Numbness
Tingling
Pulmonary Manifestations
Laryngospasm
Bronchospasm
Hypoventilation

From Metheney N. Fluid and Electrolyte Balance: Nursing Considerations. 4th ed. Philadelphia: Lippincott; 2000;111-129; Barash PG, Cullen BF, Stoelting RK. Handbook of Clinical Anesthesia. 2nd ed. Philadelphia: Lippincott; 1993;100-102.

for albumin concentration are available but have been characterized as inaccurate.[4,19]

Hypocalcemia has numerous causes (Box 18-6), the most likely of which in the intraoperative period include hyperventilation and massive transfusion of citrated blood. Hyperventilation leads to an increased pH and an increased protein-bound fraction of calcium. Massive transfusion is discussed later in this chapter.

Treatment of acute hypocalcemia involves the infusion of calcium salts. Calcium chloride is the most bioavailable parenteral preparation of calcium and results in the most rapid correction of hypocalcemia; however, it is more irritating to the vein than calcium gluconate.[19] One technique for treatment of hypocalcemia calls for administration of 10 ml of 10% calcium gluconate (93 mg of elemental calcium) over 10 minutes, followed by an infusion of 0.3 to 2 mg/kg/hr of elemental calcium.[4]

Hypercalcemia typically results from a situation in which the influx of calcium from the bone to the ECF exceeds the ability of the kidney to excrete calcium (Box 18-7). Primary hyperparathyroidism accounts for more than half of all cases of hypercalcemia, with malignancy being the second most common cause.[19] Treatment of hypercalcemia involves volume expansion with normal saline (NS) (severely hypercalcemic patients are typically hypovolemic), which in and of itself increases renal excretion of calcium. Addition of a loop diuretic further enhances the renal excretion of calcium. Bisphosphonates, mithramycin, calcitonin, glucocorticoids, and phosphate salts have also been used in the treatment of hypercalcemia.[3]

BOX 18-7

Hypercalcemia (Serum Calcium >10.5 mg/dL, Ionized Calcium >5.6 mg/dL)

Causative Factors
Hyperparathyroidism
Malignancy
Thiazide diuretics
Thyrotoxicosis
Renal failure
Excessive intake of calcium supplements

Clinical Manifestations
Cardiovascular Manifestations
Hypertension
Heart block
Shortened QT interval
Dysrhythmia
Neuromuscular Manifestations
Muscle weakness
Decreased deep tendon reflexes
Sedation
Renal Manifestations
Hypercalcuria
Polyuria
Gastrointestinal Manifestations
Anorexia
Pancreatitis

Modified from Metheney N. Fluid and Electrolyte Balance: Nursing Considerations. 4th ed. Philadelphia: Lippincott; 2000;111-129; Barash PG, Cullen BF, Stoelting RK. Handbook of Clinical Anesthesia. 2nd ed. Philadelphia: Lippincott; 1993;102.

DISORDERS OF MAGNESIUM BALANCE

Magnesium is the second most abundant intracellular cation, second only to potassium. The physiologic importance of magnesium lies in its role as a cofactor in more than 300 enzymatic reactions, including those involving energy metabolism and the function of the Na-K-ATPase pump.[18]

Hypomagnesemia is common in hospitalized patients, especially critically ill patients.[1,7] Magnesium deficiency is usually the result of increased renal or GI loss or poor intake of the electrolyte[3] (Box 18-8). Thirty percent of alcoholics admitted to the hospital are hypomagnesemic because of poor dietary intake.[7] Severe hypomagnesemia can be treated with administration of 1 to 2 g of magnesium sulfate over 5 minutes while the ECG is monitored, followed by administration of 1 to 2 g/hr of magnesium sulfate.[3]

BOX 18-8

Hypomagnesemia (Serum Magnesium <1.7 mg/dL)

Causative Factors	***Clinical Manifestations***
Inadequate Intake	*Cardiovascular Manifestations*
Total parenteral nutrition without supplementation	Coronary vasospasm
Starvation	Dysrhythmia
Chronic alcoholism	Ventricular fibrillation
Increased Gastrointestinal Losses	Congestive heart failure
Diarrhea	QT and PR prolongation
Fistulas	QRS widening
Nasogastric suctioning	*Neuromuscular Manifestations*
Vomiting	Weakness
Increased Renal Losses	Chvostek's sign
Diuretics	Trousseau's sign
Aminoglycosides	*Miscellaneous Manifestations*
Changes in Distribution	Hypocalcemia
Pancreatitis	Hypokalemia
Insulin	Nausea
Glucose	Anorexia
Catecholamines	

Modified from Metheney N. Fluid and Electrolyte Balance: Nursing Considerations. *4th ed. Philadelphia: Lippincott; 2000;131-144; Ferri FF.* Practical Guide to the Care of the Medical Patient. *5th ed. St Louis: Mosby; 2001;608-609; Barash PG, Cullen BF, Stoelting RK.* Handbook of Clinical Anesthesia. *2nd ed. Philadelphia: Lippincott; 1993;103-104.*

Hypermagnesemia is most commonly the result of iatrogenesis (Box 18-9). Hypermagnesemia can result from the treatment of preeclampsia, preterm labor, ischemic heart disease, and cardiac dysrhythmias.[20] The symptoms of hypermagnesemia tend to reflect depression of the peripheral and central nervous systems and are dose related. Because magnesium potentiates the action of nondepolarizing neuromuscular relaxants, their use should be carefully monitored in patients with hypermagnesemia.[1] Treatment of hypermagnesemia involves discontinuation of the administration of magnesium and, in urgent situations such as bradycardia, heart block, and respiratory depression, the use of calcium as an antagonist.[7,21]

BOX 18-9

Hypermagnesemia (Serum Magnesium >2.5 mg/dL)

Causative Factors
Renal failure
Excessive magnesium administration
Adrenal insufficiency

Clinical Manifestations
Serum Magnesium Levels
3-5 Flushing, nausea and vomiting
4-7 Drowsiness, decreased deep tendon reflexes, weakness
5-10 Hypotension, bradycardia
7-10 Loss of patellar reflex
10 Respiratory depression
10-15 Respiratory paralysis, coma
15-20 Cardiac arrest

Modified from Metheney N. Fluid and Electrolyte Balance: Nursing Considerations. *4th ed. Philadelphia: Lippincott; 2000;131-144; Ferri FF.* Practical Guide to the Care of the Medical Patient. *5th ed. St Louis: Mosby; 2001;609; Barash PG, Cullen BF, Stoelting RK.* Handbook of Clinical Anesthesia. *2nd ed. Philadelphia: Lippincott; 1993;104.*

PARENTERAL FLUIDS

IV fluids are the primary means by which the anesthetist addresses a patient's need for fluid and electrolytes. Parenteral fluid therapy serves three principal purposes: provision of maintenance fluids, replacement of fluids lost as a result of surgery and anesthesia, and correction of electrolyte disturbances.[3] IV fluids fall into two main categories: crystalloids (Table 18-5) and colloids.

Crystalloid solutions, which consist of fluids and electrolytes, are the most commonly used fluids in the surgical setting. Balanced salt solutions are crystalloids formulated to consist of an electrolyte concentration similar to ECF.[1] Two balanced salt solutions commonly administered to patients undergoing surgery include NS (also known as *0.9% normal saline* or *0.9% NS*) and lactated Ringer's solution (LR).

Isotonic solutions such as NS and LR are commonly used in surgery to correct the hypovolemia resulting from surgery and anesthesia, because the bulk of fluid lost in surgery is isotonic. Excessive volumes of NS have been associated with hyperchloremic metabolic acidosis.[22] A study by Scheingraber and colleagues revealed that a significant acidosis was noted when NS but not LR was administered at a rate of 35 ml/kg/hr over a 2-hour period during the perioperative period.[23] Although large-volume administration of LR may not result in acidosis, metabolic alkalosis may result when lactate is metabolized into bicarbonate by the liver[6];

TABLE 18-5 Composition of Crystalloid Solutions

Solution	Tonicity (mOsm/L)	Na^+ (mEq/L)	Cl (mEq/L)	K^+ (mEq/L)	Ca^{2+} (mEq/L)	Mg^{2+} (mEq/L)	Glucose (g/L)	Lactate (mEq/L)
5% dextrose in water (D_5W)	Hypotonic (253)	–	–	–	–	–	50	–
Normal saline (NS)	Isotonic (308)	154	154	–	–	–	–	–
D5-$\frac{1}{4}$NS	Isotonic (355)	38.5	38.5	–	–	–	50	–
D5-$\frac{1}{2}$NS	Hypertonic (432)	77	77	–	–	–	50	–
D_5NS	Hypertonic (586)	154	154	–	–	–	50	–
Lactated Ringer's (LR) injection	Isotonic (273)	130	109	4	3	–	–	28
D_5LR	Hypertonic (525)	130	109	4	3	–	50	28
$\frac{1}{2}$NS	Hypotonic (154)	77	77	–	–	–	–	–
3% NaCL	Hypertonic (1026)	513	513	–	–	–	–	–

Modified from Morgan GE, Mikhail MS, Murray MJ. Clinical Anesthesiology. *3rd ed. New York: Lange Medical; 2002;629.*

furthermore, the potassium in LR can accumulate in patients with renal failure.

Hypertonic saline solutions (3% or 5% NaCl) have been used as low-volume solutions for fluid resuscitation. Because of its hyperosmolar characteristics, hypertonic saline draws water from the interstitium into the vascular space. However, hypertonic saline carries with it a risk of unwanted hyperchloremia, hypernatremia, and cellular dehydration and a limited intravascular duration. The principal role for hypertonic saline at the present is in the treatment of hyponatremia.[1]

Dextrose is often added to crystalloid parenteral solutions for a variety of reasons. Dextrose 5% in water (D_5W) is approximately isotonic and is often used to provide free water that is available to the body once the dextrose has been metabolized. Dextrose can also be used as a metabolic substrate but is not usually administered intraoperatively because of the risk of hyperglycemia, which, among other effects, can result in an osmotic diuresis. Intraoperative dextrose administration is warranted in patients such as neonates who have limited glycogen stores[24] and diabetic patients who have received insulin and are at risk of hypoglycemia and protein catabolism.[1]

Colloids are solutions containing osmotically active substances of high molecular weight that do not easily cross the capillary membrane and therefore draw fluid into the intravascular space and expand circulating volume.[3] Colloids can be manufactured from human blood or synthesized from nonanimal substances.

Normal human serum albumin is manufactured from pooled donor plasma and is available in 5% and 25% (salt-poor albumin) solutions. Albumin 5% replaces plasma loss in a 1:1 ratio, and, because of the presence of high–molecular-weight protein molecules, the fluid remains in the vascular space. Albumin 25% can expand intravascular volume up to five times the volume infused owing to its high osmotic pressure. Albumin 25% is well suited for use in patients with excessive ECF in need intravascular expansion.[1] Colloids formulated from human blood have at least a theoretic risk of disease transmission via pathogens such as prions,[25] and availability can be limited by donor supply.[26]

Synthetic colloids include dextran, gelatins, and hetastarch. Gelatins are generally not available for use in North America.[26] Dextrans are polysaccharides that are useful for volume expansion but are also associated with anticoagulation, which limits their application to settings such as vascular surgery, in which prevention of thrombosis is desired. Dextran is also associated with risk of anaphylaxis.[3]

Hetastarch is a synthetic colloid made from plant starch. Hetastarch has fluid expansion properties similar to those of albumin[3] and is far less expensive than albumin. Use of hetastarch 6% in saline has been limited by its impact on coagulation. Hetastarch can produce a dilutional dysfunction of coagulation like other colloids and crystalloids. Hetastarch also directly inhibits clot formation by movement into fibrin clots.[1] Because of the effect of hetastarch on coagulation it is generally not administered in volumes exceeding 20 ml/kg.

A recent formulation of hetastarch, Hextend, is a solution containing 6% hetastarch with balanced electrolytes, lactate buffer, and physiologic glucose. A study by Gan and colleagues evaluated hetastarch in saline versus the hetastarch in the buffered solution and found that patients with the newer formulation could receive the colloid in volumes exceeding 20 ml/kg without coagulopathy.[26]

Estimation of intraoperative fluid requirements is an imperfect science and is based on an understanding of patient fluid needs as well as the dynamics of fluid compartments. Fluid therapy in surgical patients should include administration of fluids to compensate for preoperative fluid deficit, maintenance fluids to compensate for evaporative losses and to provide solute for excretion of waste,[24] and fluids to replace surgical fluid losses (e.g., third-space loss and blood loss).

Hourly maintenance fluid requirements are estimated according to the 4-2-1-formula (Table 18-6). A shortcut for estimating hourly maintenance fluid requirements in patients who weigh more than 20 kg is to add weight in kilograms to 40 to arrive at an hourly infusion volume in milliliters. Fluid deficit is estimated by multiplying the hourly maintenance requirement by the number of hours the patient has been without oral or parenteral fluids. Calculation of the fluid deficit should also account for fluids lost through preoperative events such as nasogastric suctioning and bowel preparation.

Surgical fluid loss consists of blood loss, additional evaporative loss resulting from an open wound, and third-space losses resulting from fluid redistribution. Estimation of third-space loss is based on the degree of tissue trauma expected during the surgical procedure (Table 18-7) and can be substantial (e.g., as in major abdominal surgery). Estimation of blood loss is discussed in the section on transfusion therapy; blood volume loss

TABLE 18-6 Estimating Maintenance Fluid Requirements

Weight	Rate
For the first 10 kg	4 ml/kg/hr
For the next 10-20 kg	Add 2 ml/kg/hr
For each kg above 20 kg	Add 1 ml/kg/hr

Example
What are the maintenance fluid requirements of a 25-kg child?

Answer
40 + 20 + 5 = 65 ml/hr

From Morgan GE, Mikhail MS, Murray MJ. Clinical Anesthesiology. *3rd ed. New York: Lange Medical; 2002;631.*

TABLE 18-7 Redistribution and Evaporative Surgical Fluid Losses

Degree of Tissue Trauma	Additional Fluid Requirements
Minimal (e.g., in herniorrhaphy)	0-2 ml/kg
Moderate (e.g., in cholecystectomy)	2-4 ml/kg
Severe (e.g., in bowel resection)	4-8 ml/kg

From Morgan GE, Mikhail MS, Murray MJ. Clinical Anesthesiology. *3rd ed. New York: Lange Medical; 2002;633.*

can be replaced by crystalloids in a 3:1 or 4:1 ratio of crystalloid to blood. The 3:1 or 4:1 ratio has come into question recently because of the understanding that as crystalloids are infused, plasma osmotic pressure decreases, which leads to an increased loss of fluid from the intravascular to the interstitial space. This has led some authors to suggest replacement ratios of 7:1 or even 10:1.[27] Replacement of blood with crystalloid or colloid solutions replaces volume only and does not replace lost oxygen-carrying capacity or coagulation factors.

The rate at which fluids are administered intraoperatively is determined after summation of fluid requirements for surgical loss, deficit, and maintenance. Typically, maintenance and replacement fluids are administered to meet the hourly needs of the patient and the deficit is replaced within the first 3 hours after surgery. In clinical practice, induction of anesthesia frequently requires a fluid bolus to maintain blood pressure and often results in an initial infusion of IV fluids that exceeds what might be suggested by calculations.

Selection of IV fluid for therapy is based in large part on the purpose of the fluid and is the subject of much discussion. Maintenance needs are ideally met by fluids such as 5% dextrose and $\frac{1}{4}$% NS (D5-$\frac{1}{4}$NS), which provides free water to facilitate excretion of waste and replace evaporative loss.[24] IV therapy in the operating room is principally focused on replacement of fluids lost during surgery and utilizes balanced salt solutions such as NS or LR. Replacement needs can also be met by colloid solutions such as hetastarch.

The relative merits of LR versus NS as a replacement solution for trauma resuscitation was explored in an animal model by Healey and colleagues. They found that in cases of moderate hemorrhage NS and LR were both acceptable solutions.

TABLE 18-8 Advantages and Disadvantages of Crystalloid and Colloid Solutions for Fluid Resuscitation

Crystalloid	Colloid
Advantages	
Inexpensive	Causes sustained increase in plasma volume
Promotes urinary flow	Requires smaller volume for resuscitation
Restores third-space loss	Causes less peripheral edema
Used for extracellular fluid repletion	Tends to remain intravascular
Used for initial resuscitation	Causes more rapid resuscitation
	Useful in conditions of altered vascular permeability
Disadvantages	
Dilutes plasma proteins	Expensive
Causes reduction of capillary osmotic pressure	Can cause coagulopathy (dextran > hetastarch > Hextend)
Causes peripheral edema	Can cause anaphylactic reaction (dextran)
Has transient effect	Decreases Ca^{2+} (albumin)
Has potential for pulmonary edema	Can cause renal failure (dextran)
	Can cause osmotic diuresis
	Can cause impaired immune response (albumin)

However, in cases of massive hemorrhage LR was found to be superior to NS because of an absence of hyperchloremic metabolic acidosis.[28]

Whether crystalloids or colloids are superior as replacement fluids has been debated for decades. The relative merits and disadvantages of each fluid are well known (Table 18-8). The current literature has failed to demonstrate definitively that the choice of crystalloids over colloids or vice versa is significant with respect to mortality; however, several studies seem to suggest that use of colloids may be associated with increased mortality in critically ill and trauma patients.[27,29,30]

BLOOD COMPONENT THERAPY

Evaluation of blood volume, estimation of blood loss, and calculation of allowable blood loss are necessary elements of blood component therapy. Estimation of blood volume takes into account the patient's age, gender, and weight and is summarized in Table 18-9.

Once blood volume has been estimated, a clinician can then by a simple calculation determine the volume of blood loss that would decrease hematocrit to a target value. The formula for maximum allowable blood loss (MABL) is as follows:

Equation 18-1

$$\text{MABL} = \frac{\text{EBV} \times (\text{Starting hct} - \text{Target hct})}{\text{Starting hct}}$$

where EBV is estimated blood volume and hct is hematocrit.

TABLE **18-9** Average Blood Volumes

Age	Blood Volume
Neonates	
Premature	95 ml/kg
Full-term	85 ml/kg
Infants	80 ml/kg
Adults	
Men	75 ml/kg
Women	67 ml/kg

From Morgan GE, Mikhail MS, Murray MJ. Clinical Anesthesiology. *3rd ed. New York: Lange Medical; 2002;632.*

Unfortunately estimation of intraoperative blood loss is fraught with error because of a lack of practical objective measures. Intraoperative measurement of hematocrit can often be useful as a reflection of the ratio of formed elements to plasma but does not measure blood loss.[31] Intraoperative administration of replacement fluids can produce artificially lowered or elevated hemograms[32]; furthermore, rapid hemorrhage is not immediately reflected in changes in hemoglobin and hematocrit. Measure of net suction volume (amount of fluid suctioned minus amount of irrigant) and counting or weighing of sponges are common methods used in the determination of the volume of blood lost during surgery. A study by Orth and co-workers examined the accuracy of conventional, subjective techniques for estimation of blood loss by comparing the results with those derived from an objective technique (sodium fluorescein). They found a significant difference between subjective and objective techniques; in general, blood loss was underestimated by an average of approximately 300 ml. Some clinicians, however, overestimated blood loss, in one case by 100%.[33]

An alternative to estimation or measurement of blood loss and calculation of allowable blood loss is measurement of systemic oxygen delivery (DO_2). DO_2 integrates cardiac index, oxyhemoglobin saturation, and hemoglobin concentration to produce a global measure of DO_2, rather than one isolated parameter such as hemoglobin. Survival in high-risk patients is associated with a $DO_2 \geq 600$ ml O_2/min/m^2.[10,33]

A further prerequisite of blood component therapy is determination of blood compatibility. Because of the presence of antigens in red blood cell (RBC) membranes and circulating antibodies, a blood recipient can receive red cells only from a compatible donor (Table 18-10). Two blood groups deserve special attention. An individual with group AB blood possesses both A and B antigens on their RBCs and lacks anti-A and anti-B antibodies; therefore such individuals can receive blood from any ABO group and are known as *universal recipients*. Individuals with type O are known as *universal donors*, because their RBCs are devoid of any of the ABO antibodies.

The most important tests of blood compatibility are those used to determine ABO and Rh (also known as type D) blood groupings, because transfusion of ABO- or Rh-incompatible blood can result in serious hemolysis. Patients at risk of needing transfusion (as well as banked blood for transfusion) are "typed" to determine ABO and Rh status. To further reduce the risk of a transfusion reaction, patients and banked blood are screened for clinically significant antibodies. The ultimate test of blood compatibility is a type and cross-match, during which donor blood and recipient blood are mixed together in what is essentially a trial transfusion. In contemporary clinical practice patients are often prepared for surgery with only a type and screen, which predicts compatible transfusions 99.94% of the time; the addition of cross-matching increases the possibility of a compatible transfusion only one hundredth of 1%.[34]

TABLE **18-10** Relationship among Blood Groups, Antigens, Antibodies, and Blood Compatibility

Blood Group	Antigen on Red Blood Cell	Antibodies in Serum	Blood Group Compatibility
A	A	Anti-B	A, O
B	B	Anti-A	B, O
AB	A and B	–	AB, A, B, O
O	–	Anti-A and anti-B	O only
Rh positive	D	–	Rh positive and Rh negative
Rh negative	–	Anti-D if sensitized	Rh negative

In an emergency situation in which a patient's blood group is unknown, un–cross-matched type-O, Rh-negative blood can be given. If two or more units of O-negative whole blood have been given, the patient may not be able to receive transfusions of his or her own type (A, B, or AB) because of the risk of hemolysis.[34]

Currently in the United States, most donor blood is fractionated into its component parts (i.e., RBCs, plasma, and platelets). Because of fractionation, blood component therapy can be targeted to a specific patient need (e.g., diminished oxygen-carrying capacity). In addition, storage of blood as components rather than as whole blood has distinct advantages[35]; however, banked blood does undergo undesirable changes during storage (Box 18-10).

Deciding when to administer blood components is an important clinical judgment that should be based on sound evidence, not custom. In recent years critical attention has been directed to transfusion practices because of concerns regarding the expense, availability, and risks of transfusions. In 1996 the American Society of Anesthesiologists (ASA) convened a task force on blood component therapy to develop guidelines to help inform clinicians of the best practices in transfusion therapy.[32]

BOX **18-10**

Changes in Banked Blood

- Depletion of 2,3-diphosphoglycerate (DPG)
- Acidosis
- Altered red blood cell morphology
- Accumulation of microaggregates
- Hyperkalemia (as high as 17.2 mEq/L)
- Absence of viable platelets (after 2 days of refrigerated storage)
- Absence of factors V and VIII

From Corazza ML, Hranchook AM. Massive blood transfusion. AANA J. *2000;68:311-314.*

A single threshold for transfusion, a so-called *transfusion trigger*, has been the subject of much discussion and study. The literature, based largely on clinical experience with Jehovah's Witnesses, records the survival of patients with hemoglobin values as low as 1.8 g/dL, although significant mortality is associated with hemoglobin values of less than 5 g/dL.[25] Anemia can be partially compensated by increased cardiac output as well as improved blood flow because of the decreased viscosity of diluted blood.[36] The current consensus is that no single transfusion threshold exists and that decisions regarding RBC transfusions should be based on the specific clinical situation.

In practice, packed RBCs (PRBCs) are the component of choice for improvement of oxygen-carrying capacity. PRBC infusions are generally administered in a ratio of 1 ml for each 2 ml of blood loss (along with crystalloids or colloids for volume); a commonly used "rule of thumb" states that each unit of PRBCs increases hemoglobin 1 g/dL and hematocrit 2% to 3%.[31]

The ASA task force concluded that transfusion is "rarely" indicated in patients with hemoglobin ≥10 g/dL and "almost always" indicated when hemoglobin is >6 g/dL.[32] Transfusion of patients with a hemoglobin level of 6 to 10 g/dL is based on specific clinical factors. Factors that affect the selection of a transfusion threshold in individual patients include consideration of cardiopulmonary reserve, experienced and expected blood loss, O_2 consumption (reflected in indices such as arterial oxygen saturation and mixed venous oxygen saturation) and the presence or absence of atherosclerotic disease.[25,32]

Outcomes in patients whose transfusions were guided by restrictive transfusion triggers have been studied. A systematic review of 10 studies examining restrictive transfusion triggers by the Cochrane Injuries Group concluded that in patients without cardiovascular disease, renal failure, or hematologic disorders, withholding transfusions in patients with hemoglobin as low as 7 g/dL was a justifiable practice.[37] A compelling study by Hebert and colleagues randomized 838 critically ill patients to receive transfusions at a threshold of 7 or 10 g/dL. Hebert found that the more restrictive transfusion threshold was at least as effective and in some subsets superior to the more liberal transfusion threshold.[38]

Massive transfusion of RBCs, defined as replacement of estimated blood volume within 24 hours or 50% of blood volume within 3 hours or less or transfusion of more than 10 units of whole blood,[39] presents special concerns to anesthetists. Replacement of lost blood volume by PRBCs, often accompanied by crystalloids and colloids, does not provide coagulation factors and can lead to a dilutional coagulopathy or dilutional thrombocytopenia. Banked blood is typically anticoagulated by a solution containing citrate, which binds calcium, thereby preventing coagulation. Very rapid infusion of blood can reduce the level of ionized calcium.[34] This phenomenon, sometimes referred to as *citrate intoxication*, presents as acute hypocalcemia. Normothermic patients with normal kidney and liver function can metabolize the amount of citrate present in 20 units of banked blood per hour and are not likely to display citrate intoxication.[4]

Fresh frozen plasma (FFP) contains all coagulation factors[40] and is administered to provide coagulation factors that may be inadequate because of dilution or absolute loss (e.g., as occurs in hemorrhage). Indications for administration of FFP include reversal of the effects of warfarin, correction of known coagulopathy, correction of microvascular bleeding in the presence of elevated prothrombin time or partial thromboplastin time, and correction of microvascular bleeding in patients suspected of dilutional coagulopathy. FFP is usually administered in doses of 5 to 8 ml/kg for reversal of effects of warfarin reversal and 10 to 15 ml/kg for all other purpose.[32,40]

Platelets are essential to adequate hemostasis and may need to be transfused because of thrombocytopenia or abnormal function.[35] Platelets are available as platelet concentrates separated from one unit of whole blood or as apheresis platelets, which produce from a single donor the equivalent of approximately six platelet concentrates.[41] Transfusion of platelets is usually indicated when the count is <50,000/cc and not usually indicated when the platelet count is >100,000/cc. Platelet transfusions in patients with platelet counts of 50,000/cc to 100,000/cc are indicated when the patient displays microvascular bleeding or if the patient is at risk for more bleeding. The usual dose of platelets is one platelet concentrate per 10 kg of body weight and raises the platelet count for 6 to 7 days.[32,35]

A less frequently used blood component, cryoprecipitate, contains factor VIII, von Willebrand factor, and fibrinogen.[35] Cryoprecipitate is recommended for treatment of patients with von Willebrand's disease and in patients with documented or probable deficits in fibrinogen.[32]

Benefits of transfusion include increased oxygen-carrying capacity and improved coagulation. Unfortunately transfusion of blood and blood products is not without risk. Infectious and noninfectious complications are possible, and the risk of complications is increased by massive transfusion as well as the transfusion of blood that has been stored for a prolonged period.

Some of the most common serious complications of blood transfusion are due to incompatibility. In a survey of hematologists in the United Kingdom and Ireland (the serious hazards of transfusion [SHOT] initiative), reports of transfusion reactions over a 2-year period in the late 1990s were carefully examined. Clinicians participating in the SHOT initiative reported 366 cases of serious transfusion reactions, 191 of which were "wrong blood to patient" incidents.[42] The pathophysiologic result of transfusion to an incompatible recipient is an immune reaction, with the risk of intravascular hemolysis because of an interaction between the circulating antibodies of the recipient and the RBCs of the donor. Approximately half of all deaths from acute hemolytic reactions are caused by ABO-incompatible transfusions resulting from procedural or administrative error.[43] Volumes of donor blood as small as 10 ml may lead to hemolytic reactions, which may result in death for 20% to 60% of patients.[34] Complicating immune reactions is the fact that general anesthesia may obscure the symptoms associated with a hemolytic reaction.[32]

Incorrect transfusions in the SHOT study were typically the result of procedural errors that led to the misidentification of patients. In five cases the erroneous transfusion was the result of six errors; in one case seven errors preceded the transfusion. Almost 10% of the cases involved patients without identity wristbands.[42]

Other life-threatening immunologic interactions seen in the context of transfusion include transfusion-associated graft-versus-host disease and transfusion-related acute lung injury (TRALI). Transfusion-associated graft-verses-host disease results when donor lymphocytes incorporate themselves into the tissues of the recipient, leading the recipient's immune system to attack the embedded recipient tissues. Rash, leukopenia, and thrombocytopenia occur, with death and sepsis usually ensuing.[34]

TRALI, considered by some to be the second ranking cause of mortality from transfusion,[25] is believed to be the result of a complex reaction to particulate matter found in banked blood. TRALI manifests itself as an acute respiratory distress syndrome within a few hours of transfusion.[34,43]

Homologous transfusions have been implicated in immunosuppression of recipients, leading to unexpectedly early recurrences of cancer and higher than expected rates of postoperative infection. It is believed that the immunomodulatory effects of donor transfusions are related to exposure to leukocytes and can be reduced by the employment of techniques (e.g., filters, washing) to reduce the number of white blood cells in transfused blood.[32,35,43]

Nonhemolytic transfusion reactions are relatively common, occurring in 1% to 5% of all transfusions, and are associated with symptoms such as fever, chills, and urticaria. Like hemolytic reactions, these reactions are difficult to detect during general anesthesia.[32] Although not usually life threatening, febrile nonhemolytic and allergic reactions can cause concern and may lead to interruption of the transfusion.[34,44]

Despite enhanced safety of the blood supply, infectious complications remain a real, although perhaps overemphasized, possibility (Table 18-11).[42,45] The current rates of transmission of viral illness by transfusion are so low that mathematical models are now used to estimate risk.[43] Despite improved testing, transmission of viral disease can still occur and is believed to occur during a period commonly called a *window period*, during which the donor is infectious but screening tests used by the blood banks are insensitive. Polymerase chain reaction (PCR) assays have improved testing for antibodies and have shortened the window period to approximately 3 weeks in the case of hepatitis C.[46]

Bacterial contamination of blood remains a risk and increases with the length of time the blood is stored.[43] Platelets, contamination of which is of particular concern, are stored for a maximum of 5 days[47] at room temperature and carry a risk of bacterial contamination of 1 in 12,000.[43]

Concerns regarding cost and availability of and complications associated with blood and blood products have led to a great deal of interest in developing alternatives to conventional techniques of transfusion therapy.

Intraoperative blood salvage technology involves collection of blood shed into the surgical field, concentration of the RBCs, and washing of the shed blood to remove all debris, after which the RBCs are reinfused. Intraoperative blood salvage is contraindicated in contaminated wounds and in surgery in which malignant cells may be present in the shed blood. Cell washing devices can provide a volume equivalent to 10 units of blood per hour for transfusion in cases of massive blood loss.[48]

Donor directed blood transfusion is a homologous blood transfusion from a donor selected by the recipient. Donor directed blood transfusions are believed by some patients to decrease the risk of transmission of disease. Studies comparing the safety of donor directed blood with blood from anonymous donors do not support this belief.[31,41]

Autologous blood transfusion consists of the collection, storage, and reinfusion of an individual's own blood. Although this procedure may eliminate certain risks associated with transfusions, some risks remain, and other risks arise. Autologous donation and transfusion carries with it the risks of preoperative anemia and resultant myocardial ischemia, the risk of bacterial contamination, and the risk of administration of the wrong blood.[34] In addition to these patient risks, approximately half of autologously donated blood is discarded,[48] which contributes to waste.

Acute normovolemic hemodilution is a transfusion alternative involving the removal of whole blood from a patient immediately before or after the initiation of anesthesia and

TABLE 18-11 Risks of Blood Transfusions

Risk Factor	ESTIMATED FREQUENCY Per Million Units	Per Actual Unit	No. of Deaths per Million Units
Infection Viral*			
Hepatitis A	1	1/1,000,000	0
Hepatitis B	7-32	1/30,000-1/250,000	0-0.14
Hepatitis C	4-36	1/30,000-1/150,000	0.5-17
HIV	0.4-5	1/2,000,000-1/2,000,000	0.5-5
HTLV types I and II	0.5-4	1/240,000-1/2,000,000	0
Parvovirus B19	100	1/10,000	0
Bacterial contamination			
Red cells	2	1/500,000	0.1-0.25
Platelets	83	1/12,000	21
Acute hemolytic reactions	1-4	1/250,000-1/1,000,000	0.67
Delayed hemolytic reactions	1000	1/1000	0.4
Transfusion-related acute lung injury	200	1/5000	0.2

*HIV, *Human immunodeficiency virus*; HTLV, *human T-cell lymphotropic virus*.
Goodnough LT, Brecher ME, Kanter MH, AuBuchon JP. Transfusion medicine. First of two parts—blood transfusion. N Engl J Med. *1999;340: 438-447.*

surgery and replacement of volume with crystalloid or colloid solutions. Reinfusion of the whole blood is initiated when intraoperative loss of blood has stopped or earlier if the patient's condition warrants it. Advocates of acute normovolemic hemodilution state that hemodilution, compared with autologous donation, eliminates the expense of testing, risks of bacterial contamination, and opportunity for wrong unit transfusion, because the whole blood remains in the operating room.[48]

The search for a "blood substitute" has evolved over time into efforts to develop "oxygen therapeutics," which involves use of technology to increase the oxygen-carrying capacity of the circulating volume.[49] Main areas of concentration in this field include development of cell-free hemoglobin solutions to carry oxygen, development of perfluorochemicals to carry dissolved oxygen in a manner similar to that of plasma, and development of drugs to enhance the amount of oxygen released to the tissues by hemoglobin.[48,49]

SUMMARY

Surgery and anesthesia challenge the body's ability to maintain the dynamic balance of fluids and electrolytes necessary for proper function. Skillful management of fluids and electrolytes in the perioperative period is one of the most challenging and important tasks of the anesthetist and requires knowledge of both basic sciences and clinical research.

A subject intimately related to fluid and electrolyte management is transfusion therapy. An expanding body of evidence addressing transfusion therapy is better informing the clinician, who must evaluate risks versus benefits in the process of clinical decision-making.

REFERENCES

1. Kaye AD, Grogono AW. Fluid and electrolyte physiology. In: Miller RD, ed. *Anesthesia*. 5th ed. Philadelphia: Churchill Livingstone; 2000:1586-1612.
2. Guyton AC, Hall JE. The microcirculation and the lymphatic system: capillary fluid exchange, interstitial fluid and lymph flow. *Textbook of Medical Physiology*. 10th ed. Philadelphia: Saunders; 2002.
3. Metheney N. *Fluid and Electrolyte Balance: Nursing Considerations*. 4th ed. Philadelphia: Lippincott; 2000.
4. Prough DS, Mathra M. Acid-base, fluids, and electrolytes. In: Barash PG, Cullen BF, Stoelting RK, eds. *Clinical Anesthesia*. 4th ed. Philadelphia: Williams & Wilkins; 2001.
5. Kreimeier U. Pathophysiology of fluid imbalance. *Crit Care*. 2000;4(suppl 2):S3-S7.
6. Rosenthal MH. Intraoperative fluid management—what and how much? *Chest*. 1999;115(suppl 5):106S-112S.
7. Kapoor M, Chan G. Fluid and electrolyte abnormalities. *Crit Care Clin*. 2001;7:503-529.
8. Gold MS. Perioperative fluid management. *Crit Care Clin*. 1992;8:409-421.
9. Kumar S, Berl T. Sodium. *Lancet*. 1998;352:220-228.
10. Prough DS, Svens C. Current concepts in perioperative fluid management. *Anesth Analg*. 2001;92(suppl):70-77.
11. Zornow MH, Todd MM, Moore SS. The acute cerebral effects of changes in plasma osmolality and oncotic pressure. *Anesthesiology*. 1987;67:936-941.
12. Fried F, Palevsky PM. Hyponatremia and Hypernatremia. *Med Clin North Am*. 1997;81:585-609.
13. Fraser CL, Arieff AI. Epidemiology, pathophysiology, and management of hyponatremic encephalopathy. *Am J Med*. 1997;102:67-77.
14. Laureno R, Karp BI. Myelinolysis after correction of hyponatremia. *Ann Intern Med*. 1997;126:57-62.
15. Halperin ML, Kamel KS. Potassium. *Lancet*. 1998;352:135-140.
16. Mandal AK. Hypokalemia and hyperkalemia. *Med Clin North Am*. 1997;81:611-639.
17. Hirsch IA, Tomlinson DL, Slogoff S, Keats AS. The overstated risk of preoperative hypokalemia. *Anesth Analg*. 1988;67:131-136.
18. Malloch A, Bodenham AR. Regulation of blood volume and electrolytes. In: Hemmings HC, Hopkins PM, eds. *Foundations of Anesthesia: Basic and Clinical Sciences*. London: Mosby; 2000:571-581.
19. Bushinsky DA, Monk RD. Electrolyte quintet: Calcium. *Lancet*. 1998;352:306-311.
20. Weisinger JR, Bellonin-Font E. Magnesium and phosphorus. *Lancet*. 1998;325:391-396.
21. Tolksdorf W. Electrolyte disorders relevant to anesthesia. *Acta Anaesthesiol Scand Suppl*. 1997;111:328-329.
22. Prough DS, Bidani A. Hyperchloremic metabolic acidosis is a predictable consequence of intraoperative infusion of 0.9% saline. *Anesthesiology*. 1999;90;1247-1249.
23. Scheingraber S, Rehm M, Sehmisch C. Fisterer U. Rapid saline infusion produces hyperchloremic acidosis in patients undergoing gynecological surgery. *Anesthesiology*. 1999:90;1265-1270.
24. Culpepper TL. AANA Journal course; update for nurse anesthetists—intraoperative fluid management for the pediatric surgical patient. *AANA J*. 2000;68:531-538.
25. Goldhill D, Boralessa H, Boralessa H. Anaemic and red cell transfusion in the critically ill. *Anaesthesia*. 2002;57:527-529.
26. Gan TJ, Bennett-Guerrero E, Phillips-Bute B, et al. Hextend, a physiologically balanced plasma expander for large volume use in major surgery: a randomized phase III clinical trial. Hextend Study Group. *Anesth Analg*. 1999;88:992-998.
27. Rizoli SB. Crystalloids and colloids in trauma resuscitation: a brief overview of the current debate. *J Trauma*. 2003;54(suppl 5):S82-S88.
28. Healey MA, Davis RE, Liu FC, Loomis WH, Hoyt DB. Lactated ringer's is superior to normal saline in a model of massive hemorrhage and resuscitation. *J Trauma*. 1998;45:894-899.
29. Choi PT, Yip G, Quinonez LG, Cook Dj. Crystalloids vs. colloids in fluid resuscitation: a systematic review. *Crit Care Med*. 1999;27:200-210.
30. Cochrane Injuries Group Albumin Reviewers. Human albumin administration in critically ill patients: systematic review of randomized controlled trials. *BMJ*. 1998;317:235-240.
31. Morgan GE, Mikhail MS, and Murray MJ. *Clinical Anesthesiology*. 3rd ed. New York: Lange Medical; 2002.
32. American Society of Anesthesiologists Task Force on Blood Component Therapy. Practice guidelines for blood component therapy. *Anesthesiology*. 1996;84:732-747.
33. Orth VH, Rehm M, Thiel M, et al. First clinical implications of perioperative red cell volume measurement with a nonradioactive marker (sodium fluorescein). *Anesth Analg*. 1998;87:1234-1238.
34. Miller RD. Transfusion therapy. In: *Anesthesia*. 5th ed. Philadelphia, Churchill Livingstone; 2000:1613-1644.
35. Carrico CJ, Miteski WJ and Kaplan HS. Transfusion, auto transfusion and blood substitutes. In: Mattox KL, Feliciano DV, Moore EE, eds. *Trauma*. 4th ed. New York: McGraw-Hill; 2000.
36. Leone BJ, Spahn DR. Anemia, hemodilution, and oxygen delivery. *Anesth Analg*. 1992;75:651-653.
37. Hill SR, Carless PA, Henry DA, et al. Transfusion thresholds and other strategies for guiding allogenic red blood cell transfusion. *Cochrane Database of Systemic Reviews*. 2003;3.
38. Hebert PC, Wells G, Blachman MA, et al. A multicenter, randomized, controlled clinical trial of transfusion requirements

in critical care. Transfusion requirements in Critical Care Investigators, Canadian Critical Care Trials Group. *N Engl J Med*. 1999;340:409-417.
39. Corazza ML, Hranchook AM. Massive blood transfusion. *AANA J*. 2000;68:311-314.
40. Manino PL. *The ICU Book*. 2nd ed. Philadelphia: Lippincott Williams & Wilkins; 1998.
41. Menitore JE. Blood transfusion. In: Stein JH, ed. *Internal Medicine*. 5th ed. St Louis: Mosby; 1998;572-576.
42. Williamson LM, Lowe S, Love EM, et al. Serious hazards of transfusion (SHOT) initiative; analysis of the first two annual reports. *BMJ*. 1999;319:16-19.
43. Goodnough LT, Brecher ME, Kanter MH, AuBuchon JP. Transfusion medicine. First of two parts—blood transfusion. *N Engl J Med*. 1999:340:438-447.
44. Perrotta PL, Synder EL. Non-infectious complications of transfusion therapy. *Blood Rev*. 2001;15:69-83.
45. Boraless H, Rao MP, Morgan C, et al. A survey of physicians attitudes to transfusion practice in critically ill patients in the UK. *Anesthesia*. 2002;57:584-588.
46. Lauer GM, Walker BD. Hepatitis C virus infection. *N Engl J Med*. 2001;345:41-52.
47. Snyder EL, Rinder HM. Platelet storage—time to come in from the cold? *N Engl J Med*. 2003;2032-2033.
48. Goodnough LT, Brecher ME, Kaner MH, AuBuchon JP. Transfusion medicine—blood conservation—second of two parts. *N Engl J Med*. 1999;340:525-533.
49. Wahr JA. Clinical potential of blood substitutes or oxygen therapeutics during cardiac surgery. *Anesthesiol Clin North Am*. 2003;21:553-568.

CHAPTER 19

Positioning for Anesthesia and Surgery

Elizabeth J. Monti-Seibert, Lyle Dorman, Don Hill

Surgical positions are a compromise among the needs of the patient, the surgeon, and the anesthetist. Positioning has three goals. First, the position must allow maximum exposure to the surgical area while preventing patient injury and maintaining adequate function of all physiologic systems. Second, the position must allow the anesthetist access to the patient for assessment, maintenance of ventilation, infusion of drugs, and institution of appropriate monitoring. Finally, positioning must allow the patient to achieve a satisfactory surgical result that permits a rapid return to preoperative levels of health and activity without injury.

Awake patients are unable to tolerate the uncomfortable positions required for many surgical procedures. Conscious individuals move if a position becomes uncomfortable. Unconsciousness induced by anesthesia prevents patients from complaining about distortions of body alignment and posture produced by positions used for many surgical procedures.

During a procedure the anesthetist usually has the greatest opportunity to assess the effects of surgical positioning on ventilation, circulation, and peripheral nerves. Although all members of the surgical team are responsible for proper patient positioning, the anesthetist and surgeon bear overall responsibility for protecting the patient and preventing injury resulting from improper or poorly conceived surgical positions. Anticipation of potential problems and prevention through proper planning are necessary to prevent harm to patients.

Injuries that occur as a result of improper positioning are often assumed to be preventable, although the causes of some postoperative complications are increasingly recognized as multifactorial.[1-3] Optimum patient outcomes require careful planning of all aspects of the procedure by all team members. Anesthetists must be familiar with the surgical procedure being performed and recognize the potential for injury associated with various positions. Communication among the surgeon, anesthetist, and operating room team is vital to the anticipation and prevention of position-related complications.

Injuries associated with positioning run the gamut from minor skin abrasions and backache to events with serious morbidity (Table 19-1). Position-related injuries include damage to eyes, ears, skin, genitalia, muscles, nerves, and blood vessels. Complications of these injuries can lead to tissue necrosis, infection, renal failure, neurologic dysfunction, loss of limbs, and even loss of life.[4-9] Patients injured because of poor positioning face a potentially prolonged hospital stay and recovery, psychologic trauma, and perhaps permanent disability. Hospitals, medical personnel, and patients and their families incur increased costs as a result of these adverse outcomes. Liability for perioperative injuries may be assigned to the anesthetist even if appropriate standards of care have been followed.[1,10] Prevention and adherence to standards of care are the keys to reducing position-related injuries.

Specific complications are associated with certain positions. Examples are air embolism related to the sitting position and hypotension resulting from vena cava compression associated with the lateral position. Anesthesia providers incorporate preventive measures into the anesthesia plan when known complications can occur. However, complications can result from unexpected events despite the employment of standard preventive measures.[1,10] Closed claim studies and case reports attest to the fact that patient injury occurs from surgical positions despite the best intentions of providers. Anesthetists must be aware of factors that place patients at risk for the development of position-related injuries and plan accordingly.

Quantifying the precise incidence of position-related complications positions is difficult, because the frequency of such events is low. Data from closed claims studies and case reports are not representative samples and probably underestimate the incidence of injuries. Literature searches easily identify case reports of position-related complications, but these reported events are probably the "tip of the iceberg." Anesthetists may also be unaware of complications that are reported only in specialty surgical publications. Although surgeons and anesthetists have a professional obligation to report new and known complications of surgical and anesthetic procedures, fear of litigation or damage to one's professional reputation may prevent timely reporting in the scientific literature.[11] For example, the possibility of venous air embolism (VAE) when the patient is in the prone position is confirmed by many anesthesiologists in personal communications but is poorly reported in the literature.[12,13] Others note that few reports of quadriplegia or unintentional vascular compromise resulting from positioning exist in the literature.[6,14]

CAUSES OF POSITION-RELATED INJURIES

Injuries to soft tissue, nerves, and vascular structures occur when pressure is applied over a body surface for a period of time. Externally generated pressure (compression) limits fluid movement into and out of the capillaries. Normally, fluid moves at the microcapillary level because of small differences between hydrostatic and colloid osmotic pressures in the capillary and interstitial tissues.[15] At the arterial end of the capillary the net effect is the movement of fluid from the capillary to the interstitium, whereas the reverse is true on the venous side of the capillary.

TABLE **19-1** Potential Position-Related Injuries

System	Potential Injury
Head, eyes, ears, nose, and throat	Blindness Corneal abrasion Facial edema Vocal cord edema
Cardiovascular	Vascular occlusion Deep vein thrombosis Ischemic injuries
Respiratory	Atelectasis Endobronchial intubation
Neurologic	Peripheral neuropathy Quadriplegia Decreased cerebral blood flow Increased intracranial pressure
Genitourinary	Myoglobinuria Acute renal failure
Musculoskeletal	Amputation Backache Compartment syndrome Rhabdomyolysis
Integumentary	Abrasion Alopecia Decubiti

Arterial inflow pressures are slightly higher than those on the venous side. Compression increases tissue resistance to venous capillary outflow, causing a rise in venous capillary pressure and a decrease in the pressure gradient between capillary and tissue. If mean hydrostatic pressures are low and tissue pressures are high, an ischemic condition can result that ultimately results in tissue edema and cellular breakdown. The arterial-venous pressure gradient is also reduced, decreasing flow to tissues along the capillary. If venous and tissue pressures continue to rise, arterial inflow is eventually occluded, and ischemia results.

The underlying cause of all tissue damage—whether to muscles, nerves, or organs—is lack of perfusion. Ischemia results from many causes including occlusion of major vascular structures, emboli, tissue edema, or inhibition of perfusion at the capillary level. Despite the absence of blood flow, metabolism continues, and its acidic byproducts accumulate in the tissues. Eventually membrane ion pumps fail, normal metabolic processes are interrupted, and sodium accumulates intracellularly, creating an osmotic pressure gradient. Water follows sodium into the cells, intracellular volume is increased, and tissue edema occurs.[16] A vicious cycle of ischemia ensues as tissue pressures increase, preventing the movement of fluid and nutrients from the capillaries into the cells.

COMPARTMENT SYNDROME

Compartment syndrome is a potentially life-threatening complication that causes damage to neural and vascular structures from swelling of tissues within a muscular compartment. Prolonged operative procedures, surgical positions, elevation of extremities, intraoperative hypotension, increasing age, and extremes of body habitus are reported to contribute to the development of compartment syndrome in surgical patients.[17-22] Compartment syndrome can be precipitated by intraoperative hypotension in conjunction with leg elevation that causes low flow states as blood pressure decreases by 0.75 mm Hg per centimeter change in height.[23] Pneumatic compression boots and fluid extravasation into tissues have also been linked to the syndrome.[20,24,25]

Unless the syndrome is promptly diagnosed and treated, permanent neuromuscular damage ensues.[22] Fasciotomy is generally considered the definitive treatment, as less aggressive therapies will not release the constricted compartments. If untreated the syndrome progresses to tissue necrosis with myoglobinuria and acute renal failure.[5,17] Amputation and even death can occur.[17,22]

Compartment syndrome is the result of increased tissue pressures and decreased perfusion within a muscle with tight fascial borders (Figure 19-1). Although compartment syndrome occurs most often in the extremities, it can occur in any area of the body in which fascia and bone form a relatively closed compartment around a muscle.[26] Compartment syndrome has been dubbed a *reperfusion injury*, as tissue swelling typically occurs when blood flow returns after a period of ischemia. Cellular membranes are disrupted because of ischemia, and reperfusion of the area results in tissue edema that compresses neural and vascular structures.[26,27]

Both internal and external compression can cause compartment syndrome[27] (Box 19-1). Trauma, embolic phenomena,

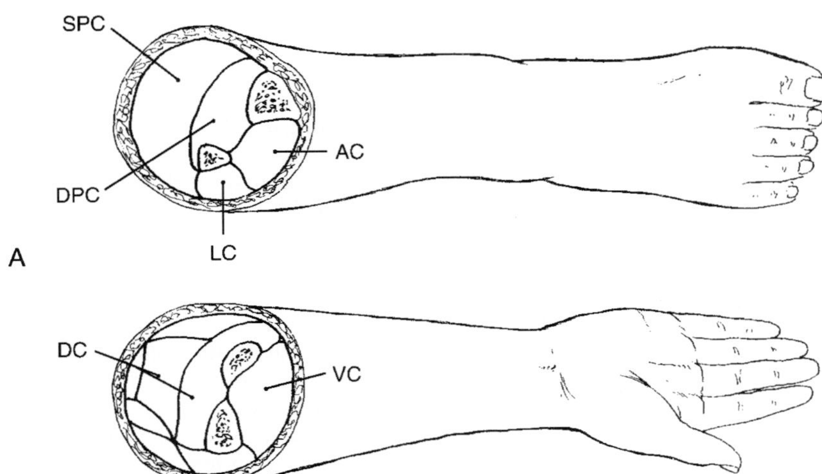

FIGURE **19-1**
Compartments of the upper and lower extremities. **A,** Four compartments of the lower extremity: the anterior compartment *(AC)*, the lateral compartment *(LC)*, the superficial posterior compartment *(SPC)*, and the deep posterior compartment *(DPC)*. **B,** Two compartments of the forearm: the volar compartment *(VC)* and the dorsal compartment (DC). (Modified from Matsen FA III. *Compartmental Syndromes.* New York: Grune & Stratton; 1980:82.)

BOX 19-1

Causes of Compartmental Ischemia

I. Remote perfusion failure
  A. Vascular obstruction
  B. Systemic hypotension
II. Increased compartmental resistance
  A. Decrease in compartment size
    1. Constriction by tight dressings or casts
    2. Tight repair of surgical wounds
    3. Local pressure
  B. Increase in compartment volume
    1. Bleeding and coagulopathies
    2. Increased capillary permeability
      a. Reperfusion edema (postischemic swelling)
      b. Exercise (seizures and eclampsia)
      c. Trauma and burns
      d. Intraarterial drugs
    3. Increased capillary pressure
      a. Exercise
      b. Venous obstruction
    4. Decreased oncotic pressure
    5. Infiltrated infusions
    6. Muscle hypertrophy

From Martin JT. Compartment syndromes: concepts and perspectives for the anesthesiologist. Anesth Analg. *1992;75:276.*

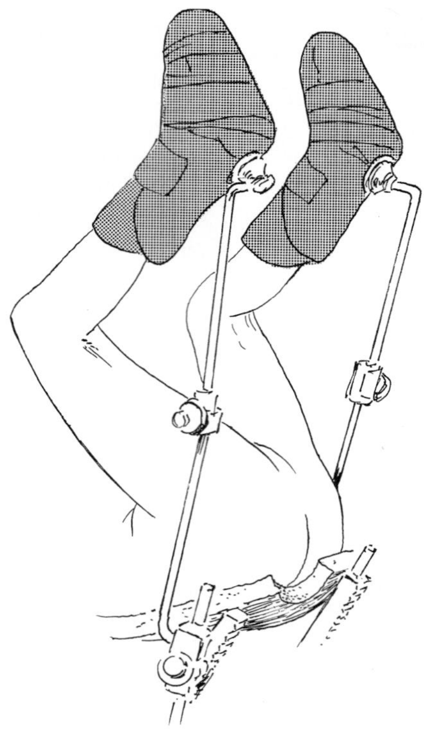

FIGURE **19-2**
The exaggerated lithotomy position. The hips and lower back are elevated, and the legs are suspended in boot-type stirrups. (Modified from Angermeier KW, Jordan GH. Complications of the exaggerated lithotomy position: a review of 177 cases. *J Urol.* 1994;151:867.)

tumors, and vascular insufficiency are additional common causes of compartment syndrome. Other predisposing perioperative factors include tight wound closures, expanding hematomas, prolonged surgical procedures, and external pressure generated by positioning devices, compression stockings,[20,25] and body weight. A higher incidence has been reported in patients undergoing surgery in the lithotomy and lateral decubitus positions.[17,22,28] Although anesthetic technique has not been implicated as causing compartment syndrome, general and regional anesthesia can contribute to intraoperative hypotension and impaired blood flow. Controversy exists regarding whether regional anesthesia contributes to delayed diagnosis of the syndrome.[17,19,22,29]

NERVE INJURY

General Mechanisms

Peripheral nerve injury occurs frequently after anesthesia and surgery.[1,3,30] Nerves that are most susceptible to damage are those that are superficial, have a long course, and are poorly covered by overlying tissues. Each peripheral nerve has anatomic sites at which its vulnerability is the greatest.[31] The most commonly injured nerves are the ulnar and brachial plexus in the upper extremity and the common peroneal nerve in the lower extremity.[1,30]

Perioperative peripheral nerve damage during surgery results from transection or mechanical factors such as compression, traction or stretch, and angulation or kinking.[30] Direct nerve injury can be caused by transection by surgical instruments intraoperatively or by needles during the performance of regional blocks. Compression occurs from pressure on a nerve either against a bony prominence or a hard surface such as the operating room table. An example of a short-term compression effect is numbness in the foot resulting from pressure on the peroneal nerve caused by the crossing of the legs at the knees.[32] Traction or stretch injuries occur when nerves such as the sciatic nerve or brachial plexus have a long course across many structures. Stretch injuries cause internal disruption of neural tissue and its vascular supply. Sciatic nerve stretch injury has been reported after the exaggerated lithotomy position, in which the legs are flexed and elevated above the torso (Figure 19-2). Ischemia is a common component of all these injuries, as interruption of the vascular supply from compression or edema, disruption of the nerve tissue, or cessation of blood flow because of stretch limits perfusion.[3]

For many years postoperative peripheral nerve injuries have been attributed to incorrect surgical positioning, but more recent evidence indicates that multiple factors are involved.[1,30,33,34] Position-related factors that contribute to the development of nerve injuries include ancillary positioning devices, the length of the procedure, and anesthetic techniques. Patient-related factors include gender, age, body habitus, and preexisting medical conditions (Box 19-2). It should be emphasized that the precise mechanism of nerve injury in many reported cases is unclear and that more research is needed to identify causative factors.[1,33,35]

Contributing Factors

Positioning Devices

The list of injuries attributable to positioning devices is almost endless. Ancillary positioning devices, such as straps used to restrain the patient or an extremity, can cause pressure and temporary injury if excessively tightened. The lateral femoral cutaneous nerve in the thigh is susceptible to injury from tight table straps or the leg-holding device used for knee arthroscopy.[36]

BOX **19-2**

Causes of Positioning Injuries

Positioning Devices
Table straps
Leg holders and stirrups
Axillary roll
Bolsters
Fracture table post
Shoulder braces
Positioning frames
Headrests
Ether screen

Length of Procedure
Longer than 4-5 hr

Body Habitus
Obesity
Malnutrition
Bulky musculature

Preexisting Pathophysiology
Diabetes mellitus
Peripheral vascular disease
Liver disease
Peripheral neuropathies
Alcoholism
Limited joint mobility
Smoking

Anesthetic technique
General anesthesia
Hypotensive techniques
Neuromuscular blockade

Common peroneal nerve injury is frequently attributed to the use of crutch-type stirrups. Brachial plexus injury has been caused by a damaged arm board falling off the operating room table.[37] The use of shoulder braces with a steep Trendelenburg position is associated with postoperative brachial plexus injury.[1] Compression injury of the radial nerve has been reported after the intraoperative use of tourniquets and blood pressure cuffs and after compression between the humerus and a firm surface, such as a positioning device.[32,38] Improper placement of an axillary roll can cause compartment syndrome and compression of neural and vascular structures. It should be noted that most reports of injuries related to positioning devices are isolated case reports. Few large studies have examined complications after the use of specific devices, and the findings are often contradictory.

Length of Procedure

Prolonged surgical procedures contribute to postoperative positioning complications. The weight of the body on the operating table results in external compression of dependent muscles and nerves and states of low perfusion.[5] The longer this situation persists, the higher the potential for injury. Surgery longer than 4 to 5 hours has been implicated in multiple reports of nerve injuries and compartment syndrome associated with a variety of procedures and positions.[4,39,40] Rhabdomyolysis and acute renal failure have also been reported after lengthy procedures.[5,6] However, nerve injury can occur even during short procedures if compression, traction, or stretch occurs.

Anesthetic Techniques

Anesthetic techniques are factors in the development of position-related injuries. Patients who receive general anesthesia cannot move in response to painful stimuli generated by uncomfortable body positions. The constraints of the procedure or surgeon may limit movement even when patients are receiving sedation. Muscle relaxation resulting from neuromuscular blocking drugs or volatile anesthetics can contribute to nerve injuries by allowing increased mobility of joints.[3] Subsequently nerves can be more susceptible to stretch or traction. Hypotensive techniques accentuate decreases in perfusion pressures in the extremities associated with prolonged procedures and the lithotomy and Trendelenburg positions and in hypertensive individuals. Recognition of postoperative neuropathies has been delayed by the attribution of patient symptoms to the residual effects of local anesthetics.

Surgical Procedures

Ulnar and brachial plexus injuries are frequent complications of cardiac procedures performed with median sternotomy. In this instance ulnar neuropathies result from injury to the brachial plexus. Cephalad placement of the sternal retractor with subsequent depression or fracture of the first rib, compressing the plexus, is thought to be one cause[41] (Figure 19-3). Excessive spread of the retractor or asymmetric elevation of the thorax for internal mammary dissection can also play a role.[3] Patients with a preexisting asymptomatic ulnar neuropathy may be more susceptible to injury.[41,42]

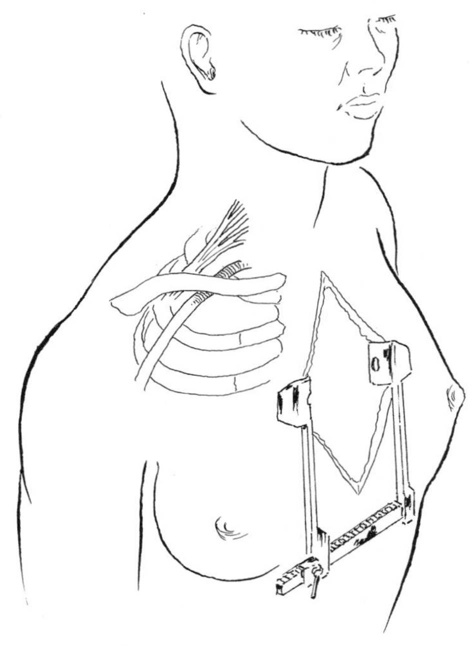

FIGURE **19-3**
Opening the sternal retractor pinches the medial cord of the brachial plexus between the middle third of the clavicle and the fixed first rib. (Modified from Casscells CD, Lindsey RW, Ebersole J, Li B. Ulnar neuropathy after median sternotomy. *Clin Orthop*. 1993;291:263.)

Patient-Related Factors

Deviations from normal nutritional status and body habitus are correlated with an increased incidence of positioning complications.[5,6,40] Individuals who are underweight can develop decubiti or nerve damage because of lack of adequate adipose tissue over bony prominences.[40] For example, thin patients may be at higher risk for sciatic nerve damage when the opposite buttock is elevated.[30] Obesity increases morbidity from positioning because large tissue masses place increased pressure on dependent body parts; in addition, adipose tissue is poorly perfused. For example, in the lateral position a heavy superior extremity can interfere with perfusion by exerting substantial pressure on the inferior extremity. Extreme flexion of heavy thighs onto the abdomen can also compromise ventilation. Muscular individuals are reportedly at increased risk of compartment syndrome and median nerve injury. Neuromuscular blockade can overcome limited elbow extension from tight biceps muscles and allow the arms to be extended flat with subsequent stretch of the median nerve.[3]

Preexisting pathophysiologic conditions increase the potential for postoperative position-related injuries. Hypertension, diabetes mellitus, peripheral vascular disease, peripheral neuropathies, and alcoholism can exacerbate the physiologic effects of various positions. Nerve injury and preexisting neuropathies are more common in patients with diabetes.[30] Diabetes is the most common metabolic cause of spontaneous isolated femoral neuropathy.[43] A history of smoking within 1 month of the surgical procedure has been identified as a risk factor for nerve injury.[40] Individuals with subclinical ulnar nerve entrapment, which may not be apparent to the patient or anesthetist, are also at risk for nerve injuries.[2,42]

Ulnar neuropathies are reported to occur more often in men—particularly those over age 50—than in women.[33] Gender-related anatomic variations may explain this difference. The cubital tunnel may be narrower in men, and the ulnar nerve may be unusually mobile.[30] The coracoid process is larger in men than in women, and men have less subcutaneous tissue over the ulnar nerve in this region.[3]

THE SUPINE POSITION (DORSAL RECUMBENT)

General Considerations

The supine position is most frequently used for surgical procedures on the abdomen, head, neck, extremities, and chest because of the favorable exposure it allows. When the patient is positioned supine, the patient's head should be maintained in a neutral position on a small pad, pillow, or dougnnut. If the patient has severe arthritis or decreased mobility of the head and neck, the head is best placed in the position favored by the patient before induction. Because alopecia of the occiput can occur after prolonged procedures, the head should be massaged and repositioned at intervals. Gel-type dougnnuts can more evenly distribute pressure on the scalp. However, the head should not be turned laterally when the arms are abducted on arm boards, because brachial plexus stretch can occur.[44]

A small support such as a folded sheet or bag of intravenous fluid can be placed under the spine to prevent postoperative back pain resulting from abolition of the normal lumbosacral curve. Conscious individuals cross their legs to alleviate lumbosacral strain in the supine position. The legs must be uncrossed once the patient is anesthetized, because pressure of the superior extremity can damage the superficial peroneal nerve in the dependent leg and the sural nerve in the superior leg. Placing the table in a slight "lounge chair" position with the hips and knees flexed and the trunk slightly elevated increases patient comfort. If the procedure is prolonged, the heels should be elevated off the mattress to prevent pressure sores; however, using too large a support to elevate the heels can cause hyperextension of the knees and postoperative pain. Gel pads or mattresses more evenly distribute the patient's body weight and prevent reddened areas after prolonged procedures.

The arms can be placed in several positions. One or both arms can be either tucked at the sides or abducted on padded arm boards that are level with the top of the table. If the arms are tucked, the elbow must not be allowed to hang over the edge of the operating table, or ulnar nerve damage can occur (Figure 19-4). When the arms are tucked, the hands should be parallel to the legs and trunk. Placement of the hands under the buttocks can result in compression of the fingers and hands. If the arms are secured on arm boards, the forearm should be supinated, as pronation is postulated to cause ulnar nerve compression at the cubital tunnel at the elbow[2] (Figure 19-5). The arms should be abducted less than 90 degrees, and the head should be maintained in a neutral position to avoid brachial plexus injuries. Turning the head to the side when the arms are abducted can cause stretching and compression of the contralateral brachial plexus beneath the clavicle.[44] The humeral head can also compress the plexus when the arms are tucked.

Cardiovascular Considerations

Changing from the erect to the supine position has several effects on the cardiovascular system in conscious individuals. Venous return is increased when blood that pools in the extremities because of gravity is returned to the right side of the heart. A subsequent increase in preload stimulates atrial

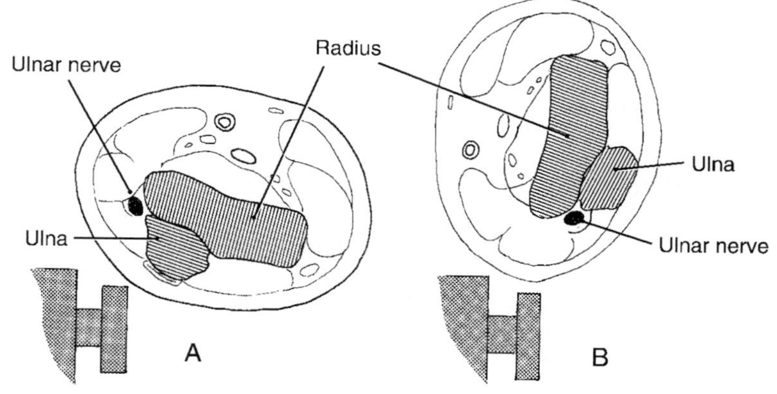

FIGURE **19-4**
Cross-sections of the right upper extremity, viewed distally at the level of the ulnar groove with the patient lying supine on the operating table. **A,** With the patient's hand supinated, the ulnar groove is at the posteromedial aspect of the elbow, and the ulnar nerve is vulnerable to pressure from the equipment rail of the table if the elbow slips out of the restraint. **B,** Pronating the patient's hand rotates the ulnar groove outward, protecting the ulnar nerve. (From Dornette WH. Compression neuropathies: medical aspects and legal implications. *Int Anesth Clin.* 1986;24:215.)

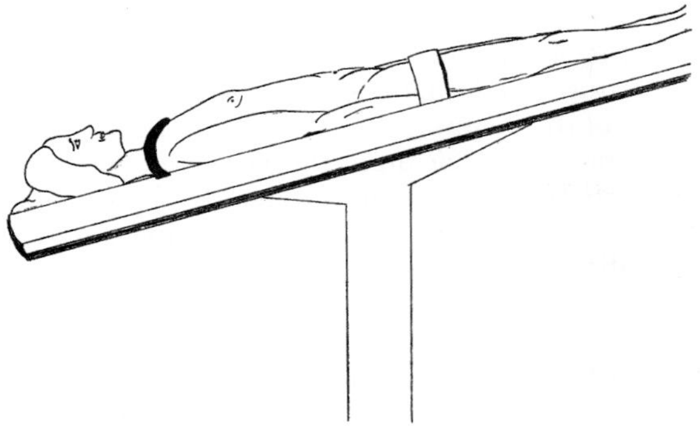

FIGURE **19-5**
In a supine patient, pronating the forearm places the ulnar nerve in contact with supporting surfaces. Placing the forearm with the palm up (supination) rotates the ulnar nerve away from compressive surfaces.

stretch receptors and the sinoatrial node and heart rate increases. Myocardial contractility increases to disperse the increased venous return. As a result, cardiac output and blood pressure are transiently increased. Baroreceptors in the great vessels respond to increased blood pressure by decreasing the sympathetic output of the vasomotor center in the medulla. The heart rate slows in response, and vasodilatation occurs, returning the blood pressure to normal.[16] Unfortunately, these normal compensatory mechanisms are depressed or attenuated by the administration of general anesthesia.

Respiratory Considerations

Ventilatory changes associated with the supine position have been well documented. Functional residual capacity (FRC) and total lung capacity are significantly reduced in patients in the supine position compared with sitting patients.[45] A cephalad shift of the dependent diaphragm caused by pressure of the abdominal viscera has been proposed to cause this decrease[46] (Figure 19-6). Changes in the elastance and resistance of the diaphragm and abdomen occur when a patient shifts from the sitting to the supine position. These changes have little effect on movement of the chest wall in healthy individuals but can have an effect in persons with conditions that predispose to abnormalities of lung function.[47] Expansion of the rib cage is not limited by the supine position; however, the elastic recoil of the chest wall and its anterior-posterior diameter are decreased in the anesthetized state. Regardless of the cause the decline in FRC is augmented by general anesthetics and neuromuscular blocking drugs.[46]

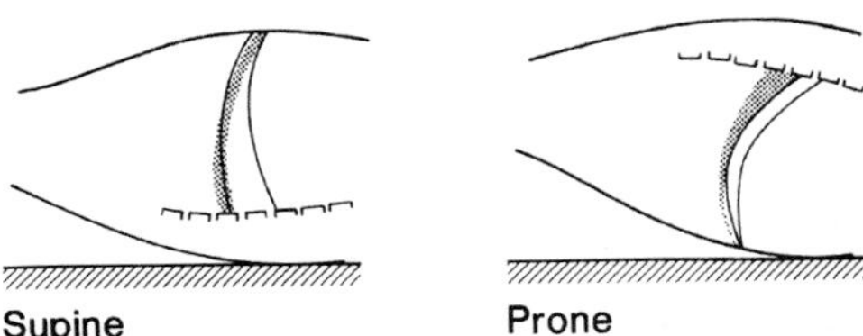

FIGURE **19-6**
Position of the diaphragm in supine and prone subjects. Solid lines represent end-expiratory and end-inspiratory diaphragm positions during spontaneous breathing while the patient is awake. Stippled areas represent diaphragm excursions during mechanical ventilation for anesthesia paralysis. (Modified from Krayer S, Rehder K, Vettermann J, Didier EP, Ritman EL. Position and motion of the human diaphragm during anesthesia-paralysis. *Anesthesiology*. 1989;70:895.)

Patients are vulnerable to several airway problems in the supine position. Flexion of the head on the neck can result in downward displacement of an endotracheal tube into the right mainstem bronchus, causing inadvertent one-lung ventilation.[48] Extreme degrees of flexion can cause kinking of the endotracheal tube with difficulty in ventilation. Use of a wire-reinforced tube is recommended when extreme flexion is anticipated. Extreme flexion can also contribute to postoperative airway obstruction from supraglottic edema or macroglossia.[49,50]

THE PRONE POSITION

General Considerations

The prone position provides optimal exposure for various spinal procedures and has also been advocated for posterior fossa procedures because of the decreased risk of VAE compared with the sitting position. Many modifications of the prone position exist (Figure 19-7).[51] The anesthetist must become familiar with the various methods of securing the

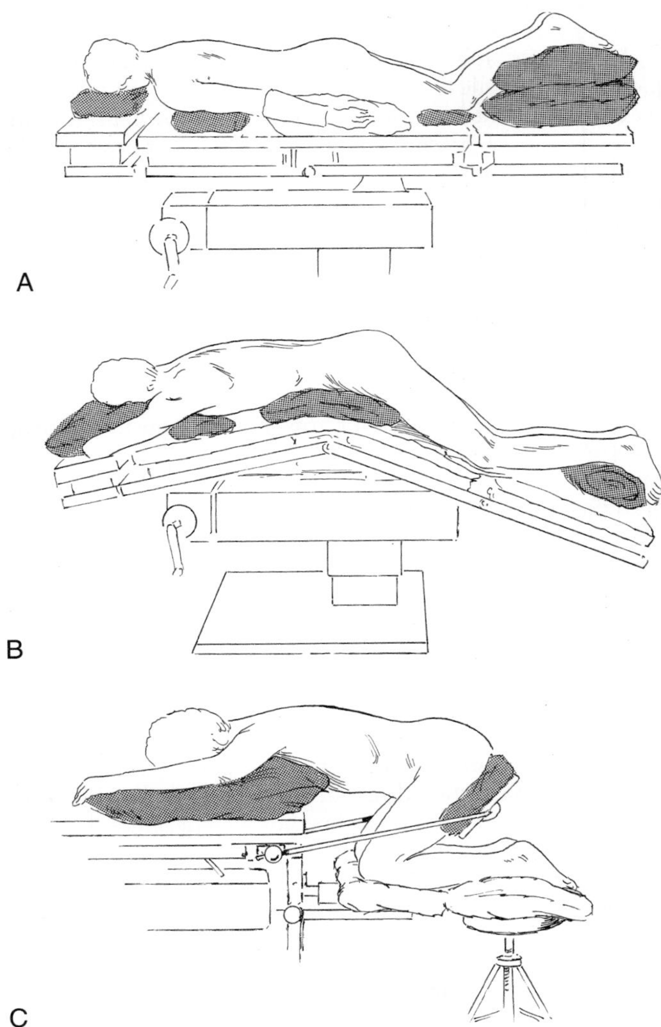

FIGURE **19-7**
Variations of the prone position. **A,** The classic prone position with the torso supported on chest rolls. **B,** The jackknife position. **C,** The sitting prone position. (Modified from Martin JT. The prone position: anesthesiologic considerations. In: Martin JT, ed. *Positioning in Anesthesia and Surgery*. 2nd ed. Philadelphia: Saunders; 1987:192-196.)

patient in the prone position and recognize the potential hazards of each variation or device.

In the prone position the body is typically supported at the chest with a frame or with rolls placed parallel to the chest. Alternatively, supports can be placed crosswise at the pelvis and shoulders. The lower legs are supported with pillows, and the upper extremities are secured parallel to the body or on arm boards. Care must be taken to pad pressure points at elbows, knees, ankles, and genitalia. Breasts must be positioned to limit pressure on the nipples.

When the patient is turned to or from the prone position, particular care must be taken to maintain alignment of the head and neck. The head should be supported in a neutral position with pillows or a head-holding device. Hyperextension or lateral rotation of the neck should be avoided, as either can compromise spinal cord blood flow, especially in elderly individuals who have narrowing of the spinal canal because of osteoarthritis.[52] To avoid hyperextension, the clinician should place the patient's shoulders higher than the head.[52] If the patient is unable to turn the head laterally, devices specifically intended to maintain the face-down position may be indicated to avoid cervical strain and prevent ocular trauma.

Meticulous attention must be paid to protection of the patient's eyes while he or she is being turned, as injuries can easily occur. Blindness can follow occlusion of the central retinal artery because of pressure on the globe from poor positioning or head-holding devices.[53] Several devices are available that allow the head to be placed in a neutral position while the eyes are kept free of pressure. Three-point skull fixation, a horseshoe headrest, foam cushions, pillows, dougnnuts, towels, and other devices can be used to support the head. The three-prong Mayfield headrest is preferable to the padded horseshoe headrest, which can allow the head to slip or rotate.[53] Even if adequately padded, the horseshoe head-rest can apply sufficient pressure over the face to cause skin damage.

Head, neck, shoulder, and arm mobility must be assessed preoperatively, as arm placement can be limited by ankylosis of shoulder or elbow joints.[51] Depending on the variation of the prone position used, the arms can be tucked parallel to the trunk with a draw sheet or supported on armboards. If tucked, the arms should be pronated and the elbows padded to avoid injury if one of the arms slips over the edge of the table. Plastic or metal arm "sleds," with sufficient padding, can be used to protect the arms and vascular access sites from compression by the bodies of the surgical team. If the arms are not tucked at the sides, they should be carefully rotated into position. The preferred arm placement is slightly abducted and lower than the shoulders, with the forearms and hands adequately supported. The arms should rest at a comfortable height on the arm boards and should not support the weight of the shoulders. Padding the elbow against pressure from the arm support can prevent ulnar nerve damage. Care must be taken to avoid pressure against the inner aspect of the upper arm by positioning devices or the operating room table.

Cardiovascular Considerations

Cardiac output is decreased in the prone position, although other hemodynamic variables do not change significantly.[54] Devices that increase abdominal pressure or impede venous return via the vena cava and femoral veins can contribute to decreased cardiac output. Extreme flexion of the hips in some variations of the prone position can occlude the femoral vessels and contribute to decreased venous return and compartment syndrome.

A primary goal of use of the prone position is to avoid pressure over the abdomen that impedes venous return, increases venous pressures, and interferes with ventilation by inhibiting movement of the diaphragm.[9,55] Valves are not present in the intervertebral veins that drain the vertebral and spinal cord venous plexuses into the lumbar veins.[56,57] External abdominal pressure is transmitted to the vena cava and communicated to the lumbar epidural veins (Figure 19-8). Fragile, engorged epidural veins are easily traumatized, and the ensuing blood loss decreases surgical exposure and contributes to hypotension.[56] Positioning devices that allow the abdomen to hang freely are associated with greater decreases in inferior vena cava (IVC) pressures than those that compress the abdomen[55] and therefore prevent engorgement of spinal venous plexuses.

Respiratory Considerations

Ventilation of the anesthetized patient in the prone position is affected by compliance of the rib cage and abdominal wall, diaphragmatic excursion, and ventilation-perfusion ratios. The rib cage contributes less to ventilation in the prone position than in the sitting position because of limitations in anterior chest expansion.[45] However, lung and chest wall compliance in sitting and supine patients are not different because increases in thoracic compliance are paralleled by reductions in the collateral abdominal compartment.[58] Diaphragmatic excursion can be limited by the abdominal viscera if the abdomen is compressed by the weight of the body or positioning devices (see Figure 19-6). If the abdomen hangs free, gravity allows the abdominal contents to shift anteriorly, reducing interference with diaphragmatic movement.[59]

The degree to which pulmonary mechanics are altered is suggested to be frame dependent and not dependent on body habitus.[59] Use of the Jackson table resulted in the smallest change in pulmonary compliance and peak airway pressures when compared with use of the Wilson frame and chest rolls. It is hypothesized that these differences result from the abdomen's hanging freely, which allows better diaphragmatic excursion and lower intraabdominal and intrathoracic pressures.[59]

Conflicting evidence exists regarding the effect of the prone position on FRC. FRC has been found to be decreased when compared to the sitting position, although less so than as compared to the supine position.[45] Others have found an increase in FRC.[58] Oxygenation is significantly improved despite changes in FRC.[58]

Improvement in ventilation-perfusion ratios has been postulated as the cause of improved oxygenation.[60] More lung volume is present posteriorly than anteriorly, where anterior mediastinal structures occupy significant space; as a consequence, posterior lung segments are better ventilated. Ventilation is more uniform, and ventilation-perfusion matching is better, in the prone position than in the supine position.[61] Improvements in FRC, lung compliance, and oxygenation are also reported in obese patients in the prone position.[62]

Complications of the Prone Position

Complications associated with the prone position include eye injury, VAE, macroglossia, and neurologic injuries. Although corneal abrasion is the most common eye injury,[63,64] visual loss is a feared complication of the prone position.[65,66] Both peripheral nerve injuries and spinal cord damage have been reported after procedures in the prone position.

The cause of visual loss after undergoing surgery in the prone position is unknown, although several theories have been

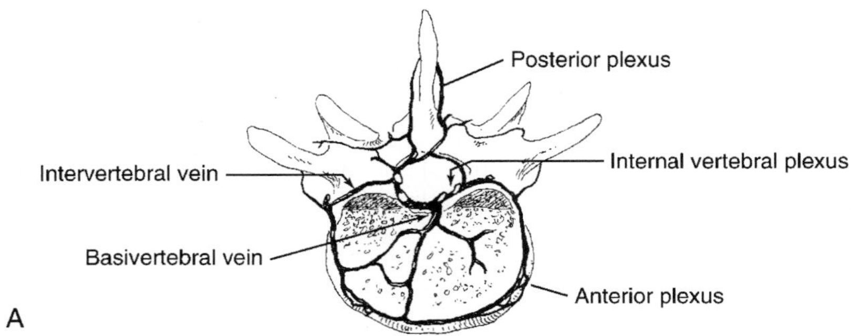

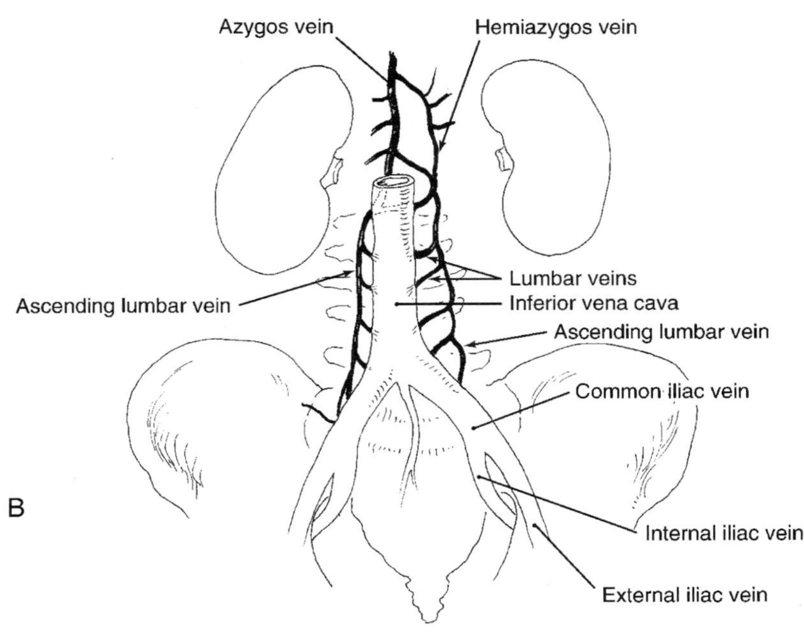

FIGURE **19-8**
Venous drainage of the lumbar epidural space. **A,** Internal and external venous plexuses communicate with the intervertebral veins, posterior branches of the lumbar veins. **B,** The lumbar veins anastomose with the iliac veins, vena cava, or azygos veins. (Modified from Williams PL, Bannister LH, Berry MM, eds. *Gray's Anatomy*. 37th ed. London: Churchill Livingstone; 1989:809-811.)

proposed.[67] The basic mechanism of injury is thought to be ischemia of the optic nerve after alterations in perfusion pressure have occurred. Ocular perfusion pressure is defined as mean arterial pressure minus intraocular pressure (MAP − IOP). General anesthesia in itself causes a decrease in both MAP and IOP, whereas the prone position increases IOP compared with the supine position.[67] Perfusion pressure is also decreased by hypotension, hypovolemia, emboli, and increased IOP from pressure on the globe. Increased IOP has also been associated with massive fluid replacement, dependent positioning of the head in relationship to the body, prolonged surgical procedures, and facial edema.[68] Therefore factors that can contribute to vision loss include intraoperative hypotension with resultant optic nerve ischemia, increases in IOP, and occlusion of the central retinal artery because of pressure on the eye from poor positioning or head-holding devices.[53,67,69]

Although not reported as frequently as in the sitting position, VAE is also a complication of the prone position.[12,13,70] Although the lumbar epidural veins are not held open by bone, as the diploic veins of the skull are, negative pressures can still develop if the surgical site is higher than the heart. Pooling of blood in the extremities or abdominal viscera in the prone position is postulated to contribute to the development of VAE. The relative hypovolemia that ensues results in a gradient between the right side of the heart and the surgical site. Maintaining filling pressures with aggressive fluid replacement can result in hypervolemia and the need for diuresis when the patient is returned to the supine position. Sequential compression devices have been advocated to increase venous return; however, these techniques can also contribute to compartment syndrome. Wound irrigation with hydrogen peroxide has been identified as a factor that contributes to VAE.[71]

Entrained air enters the right atrium through the IVC in the prone position; therefore, central venous pressure (CVP) catheters placed at the junction of the superior vena cava and right atrium may not aspirate air emboli when the patient is prone. Central venous catheter placement or Doppler devices have not traditionally been advocated for management of procedures performed in prone patients; if a CVP catheter is placed in a patient in the prone position, the catheter should be positioned at the junction of the IVC and right atrium.[70] Doppler probes require adequate padding for prevention of excessive pressure on the chest and can be difficult to position correctly with the patient in the prone position.

The brachial plexus is vulnerable to injuries from arm malposition in the prone position (Figure 19-9), although few reports of brachial plexus neuropathy exist in the literature.[72] Inadequate support of the shoulders allows them to sag anteriorly, causing traction on the plexus. Extending the arms over the head compresses the plexus against the clavicle and first rib. Abduction of the arms laterally at right angles to the body places strain on the shoulder capsule as well as the brachial plexus.

Neurologic deficits after cervical laminectomy and fusion with patients positioned on chest rolls have been reported.[9]

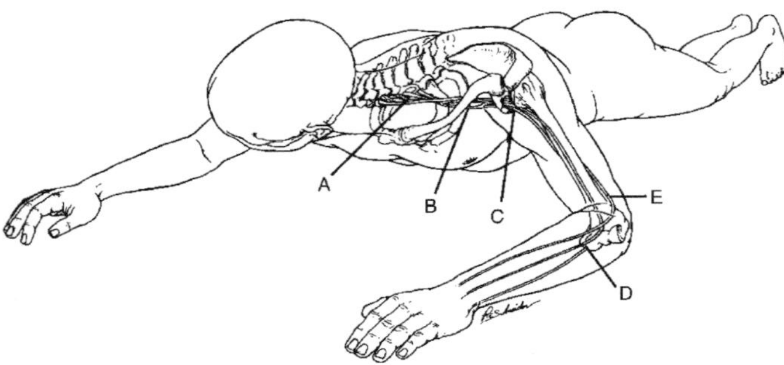

FIGURE **19-9**
Sources of potential injury to the brachial plexus and its peripheral components in a pronated patient. **A,** Head position stretching the plexus. **B,** Clavicle trapping the neurovascular bundle against the first rib with the patient's arms at sides and cephalad end of chest roll compression of the clavicle. **C,** Head of humerus thrust into the neurovascular bundle with nonrelaxation of arm and axilla. **D,** Compression of ulnar nerve at the elbow. **E,** Area of vulnerability of the radial nerve to lateral compression above the elbow. (From Martin JT. The prone position: anesthesiologic considerations. In: Martin JT, ed. *Positioning in Anesthesia and Surgery*. 2nd ed. Philadelphia: Saunders; 1987:215.)

The events were theorized to result from spinal cord ischemia caused by moderate hypotension and increased venous pressures from the chest rolls.

Mild facial edema is not uncommon after prone positioning. However, severe swelling of the face, tongue, and oropharyngeal structures that can occlude the airway after extubation can also occur.[49,73] Extreme flexion of the head and neck combined with a dependent position of the head contributes to decreased venous return with subsequent edema. Oral airways are also associated with this complication. At least two fingerbreadths should be allowed between the lower jaw and sternal notch and the patient checked frequently throughout the procedure for evidence of edema. Use of a bite block is recommended instead of an oral airway.[49]

THE LITHOTOMY POSITION

General Considerations

The lithotomy position is used for surgical procedures that require access to any perineal structure. In the typical lithotomy position, the legs are held in flexion and abduction above the level of the torso by a leg-holding device (Figure 19-10). The position is termed *low, standard, high,* or *exaggerated* lithotomy depending on the distance the legs are elevated above the torso (Figure 19-2). In the low position the legs are almost level with the torso, whereas in the exaggerated lithotomy position the legs are suspended with boots or stirrups so that the feet are well above the body. A hemilithotomy position, with one leg elevated, is used for some orthopedic procedures (Figure 19-10).

The arms are usually positioned as for the supine position, either tucked at the sides or abducted on arm boards. In the hemilithotomy position, one arm can be secured across the chest. The cautions applied when positioning the upper extremity in the supine position also apply in the lithotomy position. Additionally, care must be taken to avoid injury to the fingers if the arms are tucked and extend over the edge of the table, where they can be trapped when the foot section is raised.

Cardiovascular Considerations

The central blood volume is increased in the lithotomy position because of autotransfusion from elevation of the legs above the trunk. The blood volume of the legs has been estimated to be 100 to 250 ml per leg.[74] Passive leg raising in healthy, conscious, normovolemic adults produces transient small increases in blood pressure with no change in cardiac output or stroke volume. CVP, pulmonary artery pressure (PAP), and pulmonary capillary wedge pressure (PCWP) are increased and cardiac output decreased when the Trendelenburg position is added to the lithotomy position.[75] Therefore the combination of the lithotomy position and a head-down tilt can have a detrimental effect on myocardial function in patients with coronary artery disease.

The lithotomy position can pose a risk for individuals with peripheral vascular disease. Elevating the legs above the level of the heart decreases blood pressure by 0.75 mm Hg per centimeter. This reduction in pressure can cause hypoperfusion and ischemia, particularly if tissue compartment pressures are high because of compression.[76,77] Perfusion can be reduced further by preexisting hypovolemia, intraoperative hypotension, and use of intermittent sequential pressure devices. Leg holders that support the foot combined with a low lithotomy position are preferable in individuals with vascular disease.

Hypovolemia may not be recognized with the lithotomy position, particularly when the position is augmented by the Trendelenburg position. Lowering of the legs and a resumption of the supine position are accompanied by a redistribution of blood volume. Severe hypotension can occur if volume

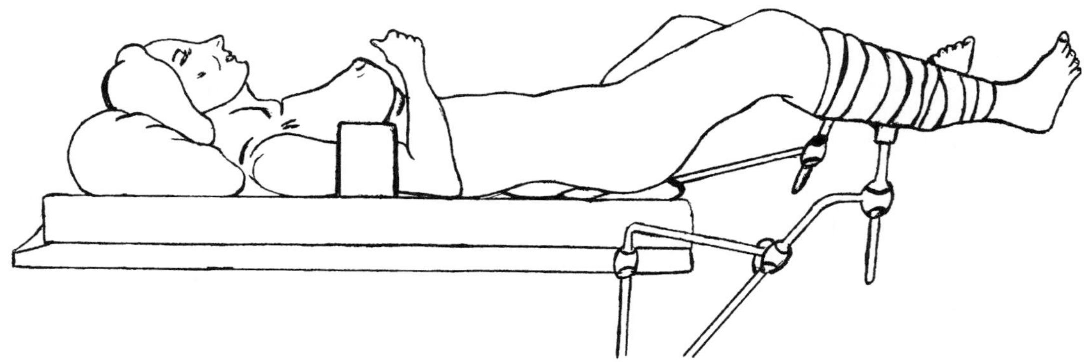

FIGURE **19-10**
The legs are supported by leg cradles in the Lloyd-Davies variation of the lithotomy position.

replacement has been inadequate or compensatory mechanisms have been abolished by general or regional anesthesia.

Respiratory Considerations

The ventilatory changes associated with the lithotomy position are similar to those associated with the supine position. FRC is not reduced further in the lithotomy position, nor does the diaphragm shift further cephalad.[74] However, the concomitant use of the Trendelenburg position can cause an additional decrease in FRC. In spontaneously breathing individuals the lithotomy position can restrict diaphragmatic movement and tidal volume. Ventilation and perfusion ratios are unchanged in normal individuals receiving epidural anesthesia in the lithotomy position, but obese individuals and patients under general anesthesia demonstrate reductions in ventilation-perfusion ($\dot{V}/\dot{Q}$) ratios and lung aeration.[74] Lithotomy position has little effect on the compliance of the respiratory system in healthy, conscious volunteers.[47]

Complications of the Lithotomy Position

Many neurologic and vascular complications occur in the lithotomy position because of the position of the leg and hip. Both legs should be elevated and flexed at the hip simultaneously when they are placed in a leg-holding device, as raising the legs separately can cause hip dislocation or postoperative back and hip pain. Acute abduction and external rotation of the hips can also cause femoral nerve or lumbosacral plexus stretch injuries. Flexion of the hips more than 90 degrees in the lithotomy position can cause kinking or compression of femoral neurovascular structures under the tight inguinal ligament with subsequent arterial or venous occlusion and nerve palsy.[78] Extreme flexion of the knee can obstruct the popliteal vein and impede venous outflow from the extremity. Leg holders that support the leg under the knee can also compromise vascular structures in the popliteal space.

Peroneal nerve injury is frequently associated with the lithotomy position regardless of the type of leg-holding device used.[39] Its superficial course and fixation against the fibular head posteriorly and inferiorly render the peroneal nerve susceptible to injury at the knee (Figure 19-11). Depending on the type of leg holder used, the nerve can be injured by compression against the upright bar or against the supporting cradle of the leg holder. Care must be taken to adequately pad any points of potential compression.

The type of leg holder used also has a direct bearing on the development of compartment syndrome, which is frequently described after various procedures performed using the lithotomy position.[17,19,25,28,35,79] The syndrome has also occurred in the well leg when the hemilithotomy position is used.[80] The fascia of the muscles of the lower extremity provide a potentially closed compartment (see Figure 19-1). Stirrups that support the calf of the lower extremity can generate sufficient external pressure to significantly decrease differences between mean arterial and tissue pressures.[77] Suspension-type leg holders that support the foot are preferable to those that cradle the lower extremity. The use of compression devices or tight straps or other devices to secure the legs can augment the external pressures applied by the leg-holding device.

Compartment syndrome is best prevented by keeping the legs at the level of the heart, limiting the time spent in the lithotomy and Trendelenburg positions, avoiding the use of sequential compression devices and leg-holding devices that support the calf, and maintaining normotension.[4,76,81]

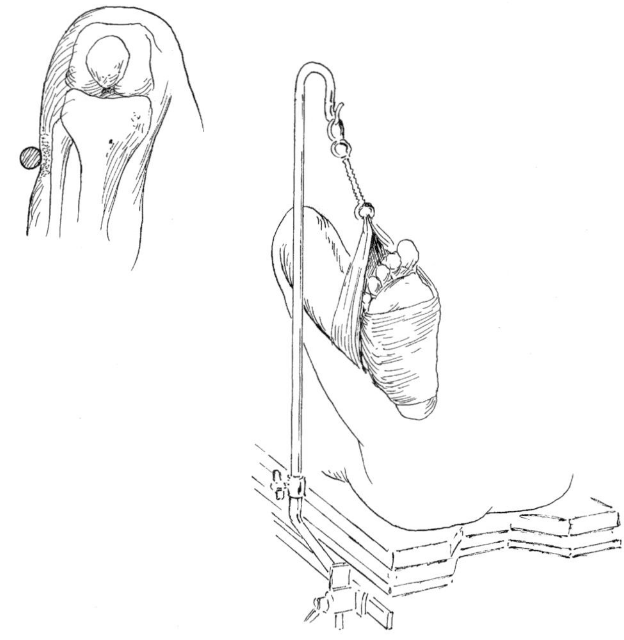

FIGURE **19-11**
Compression of the common peroneal nerve by the upright post of the leg holder. (From Smith BE. Unusual patients: obstetrics. In: Martin JT, ed. *Positioning in Anesthesia and Surgery*. 2nd ed. Philadelphia: Saunders; 1987:275.)

Repositioning the patient between segments of an extensive procedure that uses a combined abdominal-lithotomy approach is preferable for minimization of the time spent in the lithotomy position. The anesthetist and surgeon should discuss the possibility of repositioning the patient between the two stages, particularly if a prolonged procedure is anticipated and the patient has preexisting conditions that predispose to development of compartment syndrome.

At present the only method of monitoring the lower extremities for the development of compartment syndrome is the measurement of compartment pressures.[81] The procedure is reported to be of low risk but is invasive and represents an additional cost to the patient. Placing a pulse oximeter on a toe has also been suggested as another method of monitoring the lower extremity.[82] Observation of the amplitude of the oximeter waveform might give some indication of the adequacy of lower extremity perfusion, but pulses can be present despite significant ischemia of compartmental tissues. Theoretically desaturation would also indicate a decrease in lower extremity perfusion; however, desaturation would seem to be a late sign that occurs when the syndrome is already well advanced.

THE LATERAL DECUBITUS POSITION

General Considerations

The lateral decubitus position is often used for surgeries involving the thorax and kidneys when the supine position cannot provide sufficient lateral or posterior-lateral exposure. The lateral position is also useful for procedures involving the posterior or lateral spine and craniotomies that require access to the lateral or posterior cranium. Orthopedic procedures involving the hips, shoulders, or upper or lower extremities can require this position for better access to be gained to the surgical site. When a nephrectomy is performed using a lateral approach, exposure of the kidney can be facilitated by elevating the kidney rest beneath the dependent iliac crest and flexing the operating table to so that the operative flank is higher than the upper torso or legs (Figure 19-12*B*).[83,84]

Initially the patient is placed supine for induction of anesthesia and intubation. If a beanbag is used to support the torso, it is placed flat on the operating table before the patient arrives. Before the patient is positioned, the endotracheal tube, breathing circuit, intravenous and monitoring lines, and any other devices should be secured so that none are beneath the body after the turn. The anesthetist should control the airway, head, and neck as well as coordinate the turn.

Particular attention should be paid to body alignment in the lateral position. The shoulders, hips, head, and legs are maintained in the same plane and turned simultaneously to avoid stress and twisting of the torso and spine. The head and neck remain in a neutral position aligned with the spine. The head should be supported on pillows, dougnnuts, or unwrinkled, folded blankets and not allowed to hang, tilt laterally, hyperflex, or hyperextend (Figure 19-12*A*). Extreme neck angulation places the patient at risk for occlusion of the vertebral or carotid arteries, compromise of perfusion to the head, impairment of jugular venous drainage, and increase in intracranial pressure. Angulation of the head and neck also places tension on the brachial plexus, which can cause postoperative neuropathies.[84,85] The anesthetist should make sure the dependent eye and ear are free of pressure. A doughnut head holder is useful for keeping the dependent ear suspended and pressure free.

Padding and pillows are required at bony prominences and between extremities to prevent nerve compression, to pad cutaneous pressure points, and to promote venous drainage.[85] Once the patient is in the lateral position, flexing the knee and hip of the dependent leg stabilizes the patient. The nondependent leg remains straight and is supported by a pillow placed between the lower extremities. Positioning the legs in this manner prevents bony prominences of the legs from resting on each other and reduces compression of the inferior leg by the superior extremity (Figure 19-12*A*). The peroneal nerve of the lower leg is padded to protect it from external pressure against the table.

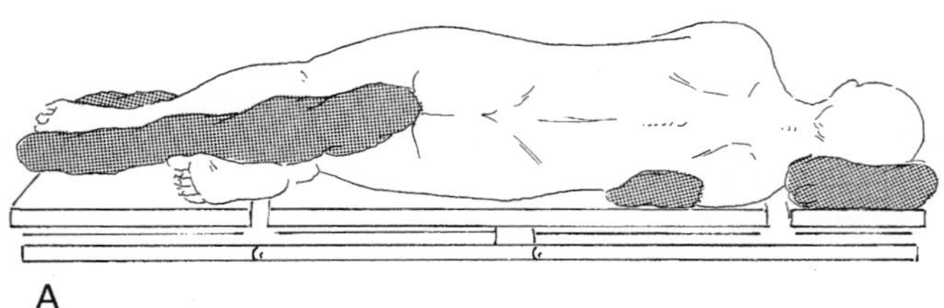

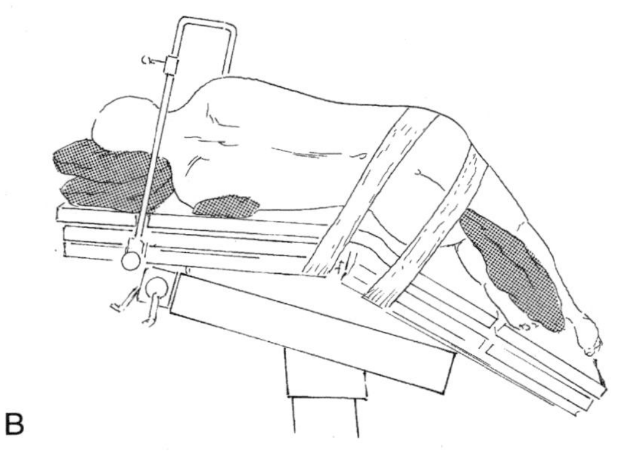

FIGURE **19-12**
A, The standard right lateral decubitus position. **B,** The flexed lateral position with the kidney rest properly elevated under the iliac crest. (Modified from Lawson NW. The lateral decubitus position: anesthesiologic considerations. In: Martin JT, ed: *Positioning in Anesthesia and Surgery*. 2nd ed. Philadelphia: Saunders;1987:155-156.)

The dependent arm is positioned on a padded arm board perpendicular to the torso or flexed no more than 90 degrees at the elbow.[30] The nondependent arm is placed to avoid interference with surgical exposure—usually parallel to the dependent arm and level with the shoulder. It can be supported with a well-cushioned arm-holding device or with pillows or blankets between the arms. Caution must be taken with the use of folded blankets or pillows because they can obstruct the anesthetist's view of the inferior arm. Padding both elbows may prevent ulnar nerve compression in the cubital tunnel. Perfusion to the upper extremities, especially the dependent arm, should be periodically assessed by palpating the radial artery and checking capillary refill.

The dependent shoulder and upper extremity are susceptible to compression in the lateral position. An axillary support is placed under the dependent side of the thorax, slightly caudad to but not directly in the axilla, to decompress the shoulder, axillary vessels, and brachial plexus of the dependent arm.[86,87] Posterior displacement of the shoulder should not occur because of the risk of brachial plexus stretch and injury.[86]

Ancillary positioning devices such as "bean bags," pillows, sandbags, braces, and adhesive tape aid in securing the patient and preventing rotation of the trunk. If tape or straps are used to stabilize the torso, they should be placed just caudal to the axilla to reduce the risk of brachial plexus injury.[85] Placement across the ribs can impair ventilation. Care must be taken to prevent overtightening to avoid soft-tissue injury.

Cardiovascular Considerations

Cardiovascular changes—in particular blood pressure changes—are usually minimal in the lateral position. Transesophageal echocardiography (TEE) has revealed that ejection fraction, blood pressure, and heart rate were unchanged in the lateral position in patients undergoing nephrectomies.[88] Hypotension is likely to be pronounced with positions that use extreme flexion—such as the right lateral decubitus—or elevation of the kidney rest, as compression of the great vessels in the abdomen by flexion reduces venous return and the legs are lower than the heart.[54,85] Therefore a slow, subtle assumption of the flexed position is most beneficial. Improper placement of the kidney rest at the flank instead of at the iliac crest can cause further vena caval compression. Facial swelling and increased intracranial pressure because of venous pooling in the head also can occur with the flexed position.

Several techniques are useful for prevention of hypotension with the flexed lateral position. Intravascular volume loading before positioning can reduce or eliminate hypotension. Volume replacement must be done cautiously because excessive fluid can lead to volume overload when the patient is returned to supine position.[85] Hemodynamic changes are reduced or absent with a lighter level of anesthesia (less than 0.5 minimum alveolar concentration [MAC]) for positioning or if a deeper level of anesthesia is achieved slowly.[85] Compensatory mechanisms to increase heart rate when hypotension occurs are diminished or absent in the patient anesthetized with greater than 0.5 MAC isoflurane.[54]

Respiratory Considerations

The effect of the patient's position or posture on ventilation is caused by mechanical interference with the chest wall, diaphragm, and belly wall.[47] The mediastinum shifts toward the dependent lung in the lateral position, decreasing FRC in that lung and increasing it in the nondependent lung.[89] Vital capacity and tidal volume are reduced in awake and anesthetized individuals in the lateral position. Vital capacity in an awake, spontaneously breathing patient is reduced by 10%; elevation of the kidney rest produces an additional 5% reduction.[85] Similar reductions in tidal volume occur in anesthetized, mechanically ventilated patients.

In the lateral decubitus position ventilation and perfusion are greater in the dependent lung than in the nondependent lung in an awake, spontaneously breathing patient. With the induction of anesthesia the abdominal contents force the hemidiaphragm of the dependent lung cephalad, thereby decreasing ventilation in the dependent lung and reducing its compliance. In the nondependent lung, ventilation is greater and compliance increased in the anesthetized patient because of the caudal shift of the upper hemidiaphragm that allows unrestricted lung excursion.

A gravitational effect on gas and blood flow is theorized to result in differences in ventilation and perfusion in different lung segments. Nongravitational factors such as the distance that blood must flow to reach a site are also thought to play a factor.[89] In both awake and anesthetized patients, gravitational forces create a gradient that favors perfusion in dependent portions of the lungs. This causes pulmonary perfusion to be the greatest in the dependent lung.[85] Positive pressure ventilation abolishes the gravitational effects of ventilation in anesthetized patients.[89]

Ventilation-perfusion mismatching while the patient is in the lateral decubitus position affects patient oxygenation, especially with procedures requiring one-lung ventilation. Hypoxic pulmonary vasoconstriction in the unventilated lung further redistributes blood flow to the dependent lung to improve ventilation.[89] Patients are susceptible to atelectasis in the lateral position as closing volumes occur above FRC, with closing occurring earlier in the dependent than in the nondependent lung. Tidal volumes of 10 to 12 ml/kg and an FIO_2 of 0.5 or higher have been suggested to compensate for V/Q mismatch in the lateral position; however, excessive tidal volumes can cause barotrauma, decrease hypoxic vasoconstriction, and reduce oxygenation in patients in the lateral position.[89] Tidal volumes of 5 to 7 ml/kg and higher respiratory rates cause smaller declines in oxygenation. Although positive end expiratory pressure (PEEP) applied to both lungs can increase ventilation to the dependent lung,[74] controversy exists regarding whether PEEP selectively applied to the dependent lung increases or decreases ventilation to that lung.[89] Application of 2 to 5 cm H_2O of continuous positive airway pressure (CPAP) to the dependent lung can significantly improve oxygenation during one-lung ventilation.[89,90]

Complications of the Lateral Position

Meticulous care must be taken to prevent nerve injury when positioning the patient in the lateral decubitus position. Compression and stretching of nerves are the usual cause of injury. The most common sites of injury are the brachial plexus and the ulnar and peroneal nerves.[30]

Brachial plexus injury with the lateral decubitus position is most commonly the result of excessive stretching, usually because of arm abduction greater than 90 degrees, external rotation, extension and lateral flexion of the head, and posterior shoulder displacement.[30] Injuries to the brachial plexus and the musculocutaneous and ulnar nerves have occurred with shoulder arthroscopies in which the lateral decubitus position was used and traction was applied to the arm to improve joint visualization; manual traction is preferable to mechanical.[36] The humeral head of the dependent arm can also compress the plexus against the thorax, therefore warranting the use of a support placed just below the axilla.[85] If the nondependent arm is to be suspended on an arm holder, abduction of less than 90 degrees should be maintained.

Because of its superficial path along the medial epicondyle of the humerus, injury occurs more commonly to the ulnar nerve than to the brachial plexus.[30] This makes the nerve vulnerable to compression within the cubital tunnel against the operating table or positioning devices. Padding of both elbows is recommended, but injuries have occurred despite appropriate padding.[1]

The common peroneal nerve is the most commonly injured nerve in the lower extremity. Injury occurs as a result of compression of the nerve between the operating table and the head of the fibula. Padding should be placed along the lateral aspect of the dependent leg extending from the knee to the heel to protect against injury.[30]

Damage to the dependent eye can occur in lateral decubitus position if the eye is not adequately protected. Permanent blindness can result from retinal artery thrombosis resulting from pressure on the eye when the head is improperly placed on a headrest or pillow.[85] Intraoperative hypotension can further reduce retinal artery perfusion pressure and potentiate ischemia from compression. It is important that care be taken when positioning the head so that the eyes remain pressure free.

Rhabdomyolysis has been reported after use of the lateral decubitus position. The condition was attributed to positioning devices inappropriately placed against muscle rather than bony prominences during a total hip arthroplasty.[8] Prolonged operating time and pressure of the operating table against gluteal and flank muscles have also been described as contributory factors. The anesthetist, as well as the entire operating team, should ensure that the operating table is well padded and that positioning devices are properly placed. Furthermore, prolonged or excessive hypotension should be avoided to ensure adequate tissue perfusion.

THE SITTING POSITION

General Considerations

The term *sitting position* commonly refers to any position in which the torso is elevated from the supine position and is higher than the legs. Depending on the surgical procedure the amount of elevation of the head above the heart can vary greatly. A true sitting position, in which the torso is elevated at 90 degrees to the legs, is rarely used. The modified sitting position in which the torso is elevated 45 degrees, the head is flexed, and the legs are at the level of the heart is probably most familiar to anesthetists. This position is variously described as the *lounging, lawn chair,* or *beach chair* position.

The sitting position offers advantages to the surgeon and anesthetist.[23] Although its use is reported to be decreasing in popularity, some neurosurgeons favor the sitting position for procedures in the posterior fossa and cervical spine because it allows excellent visualization of intracranial structures and facilitates drainage of blood and cerebral spinal fluid from the wound. Plastic surgeons favor the sitting position for mammoplasty and breast reconstruction because it allows visualization of the breasts in the natural, upright position. During shoulder arthroplasty and arthroscopy the sitting position reduces brachial plexus stretch and aids surgical exposure and manipulation of the arm and shoulder.[1,91] Access to the airway and monitoring devices is easier for the anesthetist with the sitting position.

Placement of the patient in the sitting position involves flexion of the operating room table, elevation of the backrest, and head-down rotation. The degree of torso elevation desired determines the amount of operating table manipulation required. For neurosurgical procedures a pin head-holding device is generally used to secure the head. The device provides better head stabilization compared with horseshoe-type headholders and avoids eye compression, but jugular venous obstruction can occur if the head is held too flexed on the neck. At least two fingerbreadths of space should be allowed between the neck and mandible. Endobronchial intubation can also occur when the head is flexed, as the endotracheal tube moves downward with flexion. Care must be taken when fixing the head in the three-point head holder, as sharp skull pins can lacerate or perforate ears and eyelids. Additionally, incorrect placement of the head holder and direct contact of its metal bars with the nose or skin can cause pressure necrosis.

A horseshoe headrest is often used to support the head for shoulder procedures performed in the sitting position. Straps or adhesive tape secures the head to the headrest. The anesthetist should be aware that vigorous surgical manipulation of the arm and shoulder can move the patient's body toward the operative side of the table. If the head is firmly secured to the headrest, excessive traction or stretch can be placed on the neck. If the restraining straps are loose, the head can become partially or completely dislodged from the headrest, introducing the potential for cervical spine injury. Accidental extubation can occur if the endotracheal tube is secured by a supporting device and the head is displaced. Profound hypotension and bradycardia from activation of the Bezold-Jarisch reflex occurs frequently when shoulder surgery is performed under an interscalene block.[91]

Cardiovascular Considerations

Profound hemodynamic effects and the risk of VAE are often cited as reasons for avoiding the sitting position. Hypotension is a frequent occurrence but can be minimized by elevating the knees, wrapping the legs, and applying flexion at the hips.[23] Anesthetic techniques can affect the degree of hypotension; decreases in MAP are less with nitrous-narcotic techniques than with inhalation techniques.[92] Cardiac index (CI), CVP, and pulmonary artery wedge pressure decrease significantly and systemic vascular resistance (SVR) increases when the patient is in the seated position as compared to supine.[92,93] The amount of decrease in hemodynamic parameters depends on the degree of elevation of the torso. Cardiovascular changes are minimal if the patient is placed 45 degrees in a head-up position, but cardiac output decreases 20% if the patient is raised to 90 degrees because of pooling of venous blood in the extremities. In healthy patients MAP is maintained by compensatory increases in heart rate and SVR, but elderly patients and those with preexisting diseases can be less adaptive.

Intracranial perfusion can be threatened by the sitting position. Because MAP decreases 0.75 mm Hg per centimeter of elevation, cerebral perfusion can be reduced considerably, particularly if intracranial pressure is increased.[23] Anesthetic reductions in blood pressure combined with hypocarbia and limited fluid intake to decrease intracranial pressure can excessively decrease cerebral perfusion.[23] Balanced anesthetic techniques allow use of lower concentrations of volatile agents to reduce hemodynamic changes and greater provide greater cardiovascular stability. In procedures in which cerebral perfusion is a concern, invasive arterial blood pressure monitoring should be instituted, with the transducer placed at the level of the circle of Willis.[23]

Respiratory Considerations

The effect of the sitting position on the respiratory system varies depending on the relationship among the chest, abdomen, and lower extremities. The sitting position is more favorable for ventilation and has less effect on lung volumes than other positions. The more the torso is elevated, the smaller the effect on lung mechanics. FRC and forced vital capacity are within normal parameters in the seated position.[45] The abdominal contents shift caudally and anteriorly, causing less interference with diaphragmatic movement and allowing greater expansion of dependent lung regions.[47] Compared with the supine position, in which the abdominal muscles are used for breathing, the rib cage contributes more to ventilation in the sitting position.[45]

Respiratory benefits of the sitting position are attenuated when the sitting position is modified to minimize cardiovascular effects. Flexion of the lower extremities at the hip and elevation of the legs causes abdominal contents to shift cephalad against the diaphragm. The sitting position then more closely resembles the supine position, limiting diaphragmatic excursion and decreasing FRC and closing volumes.[23] External compression devices (G-suit) to prevent VAE can compound this effect.

Complications of the Sitting Position

Serious complications associated with the sitting position are among the reasons that the position is falling out of favor. Among the potential sequelae are VAE, pneumocephalus, quadriplegia, and peripheral nerve injuries.

VAE is a well-known consequence of the sitting position; air can enter the venous system because of the negative pressure gradient that exists between the right atrium and veins at the operative site.[94] The precise incidence of VAE is unknown but is variously estimated at between 1% and 76%.[94-99] Differences in estimates result from variations in the sensitivity of monitoring devices used and the type of surgical procedure.[23,95,97,98] Complications of VAE are proportional to both the volume of air entrained and its rapidity. Sequelae range from no effect for minimal amounts of air to hypotension, arrhythmias, and cardiac arrest with larger volumes.[94,95,97-99] Air that enters the right side of the heart can limit gas exchange in the lungs as it displaces blood in the pulmonary vasculature.

Paradoxic air embolism (PAE) can occur in the patient with a patent foramen ovale (PFO) or when right atrial pressures are higher than left atrial pressures. Studies in vivo and in cadavers indicate that the incidence of PFO can be as high as 35% in the general population.[95,96,100] In the patient with PFO, air can enter the systemic circulation when right atrial pressure is greater than left atrial pressure, a reversal of the normal pressure gradient. Very small amounts of air in the arterial system can result in severe cardiovascular and neurologic complications. PEEP and other conditions that elevate right atrial pressure can also predispose to PAE.[23]

In addition to the use of standard anesthetic monitoring tactics, monitors are chosen for patients in the sitting position to detect and treat VAE. At a minimum, monitoring techniques should include noninvasive blood pressure monitoring, an electrocardiogram, an esophageal stethoscope is used to monitor both breath sounds and temperature, capnography, a Foley catheter, and a peripheral nerve stimulator.[23] An arterial catheter is generally accepted as offering a good risk-benefit ratio. A multiorifice central venous catheter placed in the right atrium at the junction of the superior vena cava is recommended for most patients undergoing surgery for monitoring of blood volume and aspiration of entrained air.[23] The risks of central venous catheter placement, the potential for VAE, and the cardiopulmonary risks of the sitting position must be weighed against the benefits of fluid volume management and air recovery.

Because VAE and PAE are results of surgical intervention and carry the potential for serious consequences, much attention has been placed on identifying individuals at risk for these complications. Preoperative TEE with contrast is the gold standard for detection of PFO in patients scheduled for surgery in the sitting position.[96,97] If PAE is detected, surgery can be performed using the prone or park-bench position.[96,97] The cost of TEE is thought to be justified because it is a low-risk, semiinvasive procedure and the sequelae of PAE are severe; however, the low incidence of VAE and PAE in some types of procedures may not justify the expense.[101] In addition, PFO can be present and PAE can occur despite negative preoperative TEE.[95] Because echocardiography is uncomfortable for patients and has rare but serious complications, transcranial Doppler studies are recommended as an alternative approach for detection of PFO.[96]

TEE, Doppler ultrasonography, capnography, and pulmonary artery catheterization vary in their ability to detect VAE. Having the ability to identify emboli as small as 0.05 ml/kg, TEE is the most sensitive monitor for VAE detection, but it is not specific for gas emboli.[23,94,97] The precordial Doppler is placed over the third to sixth intercostal spaces to the right of the sternum. It is equally as sensitive as TEE, and less expensive and cumbersome, but does not have the advantage of localizing entrained air within the cardiac chambers. Although TEE is the gold standard for VAE detection and can be used to position right atrial catheters, disadvantages are that it requires specialized training, considerable time, and experience to use and may not provide a continuous monitor of cardiovascular events. The precordial Doppler is sensitive to electrical interference from other operating room equipment, and its effectiveness can be reduced by auditory fatigue in the anesthetist. False positives can be generated by rapid infusion of fluid or flushing transducers.

Both TEE and Doppler detect changes resulting from VAE at smaller air volumes than either capnography or measurement of PAP.[23] Because VAE increases dead space and contains nitrogen, capnography reveals a drop in end-tidal CO_2 and the presence of end-tidal nitrogen. The esophageal stethoscope, EKG, and pulse oximeter can also be used to detect changes caused by VAE. A "mill-wheel murmur" is a characteristic of VAE that can be heard through the esophageal stethoscope.[23] Unfortunately, many anesthesia providers are unfamiliar with the rumbling sound of a mill wheel. Air in the coronary arteries can cause ischemic electrocardiographic changes, and air in the pulmonary vessels can result in an increase in PAP and hypoxia. These signs occur later than changes detected by TEE, Doppler, or capnography and are indicative of PAE or large emboli.

Controversy exists regarding the inclusion of nitrous oxide in the anesthetic management of patients susceptible to VAE. Nitrous oxide is theorized to increase the size of air bubbles and reduce the lethal dose of air. The use of nitrous oxide has been advocated as it decreases the amount and subsequently the hemodynamic effects of other anesthetic agents and allows a more rapid return to consciousness. However, no differences in awakening were observed in neurosurgical patients anesthetized with and without nitrous oxide.[102] Several investigators described no difference in the incidence of VAE or postoperative pneumocephalus whether or not nitrous oxide was included in the anesthetic technique.[7,102] However, TEE was not used in these studies to evaluate differences in the size of intraoperative emboli between groups. The investigators postulated that because standard anesthetic practice is to discontinue nitrous oxide and administer 100% oxygen when VAE is detected or the dura is being closed, the air-filled cavity or bubble would rapidly decrease in size as nitrous oxide rapidly diffuses out.

Intravascular volume expansion, PEEP, leg wraps, and the antigravity-suit (G-suit) have been advocated to reduce the negative incision-to-heart pressure gradient and the incidence of VAE. The G-suit was ineffective in preventing VAE and hypervolemia, and PEEP are no longer recommended as a means of reducing the chance of VAE.[23] PEEP was postulated to decrease VAE by increasing right atrial pressure and decreasing venous return from cerebral and intrathoracic veins.[99] However, studies of canine cerebral venous pressures in the sitting position found no change in cerebral venous pressure when PEEP of up to 20 cm H_2O was applied.[103] A similar incidence of VAE was found in patients who received controlled ventilation without PEEP and those who received PEEP of 10 cm H_2O.[93] Valves located at the thoracic inlet of the jugular veins prevent retrograde blood flow when intrathoracic pressures are increased.[103] Significant levels of PEEP may actually increase the incision-heart pressure gradient by decreasing atrial pressures.[95] PEEP can also worsen right-to-left shunts in patients with PFO and cause systemic VAE. The release of PEEP has been demonstrated to cause a recurrence of VAE in patients who had intraoperative episodes of intracardiac air.[99]

Quadriplegia is a dreaded complication of procedures performed using the sitting position. The postulated mechanism of injury is stretch of the spinal cord when the head is flexed, coupled with ischemia resulting from loss of spinal cord autoregulation under general anesthesia in the sitting position.[14] The spinal cord stretches when the head is flexed on the neck, causing a decrease in the caliber of spinal cord vessels. Somatosensory evoked potentials are useful in identifying position-related changes in spinal cord function.[104]

Pneumocephalus is a frequent occurrence after neurosurgical procedures performed using the sitting or supine positions and is typically a benign condition.[7,105,106] Gravity is the most important factor in the development of pneumocephalus. Opening of the dura, drainage of cerebrospinal fluid, and surgical decompression allow relaxation of the brain and entrance of air, which rises to the top of the cranial vault. Contributing factors are those that decrease brain volume such as the use of diuretics, hypocarbia, the presence of intraventricular shunts, and gross hydrocephalus.[106,107] Tension pneumocephalus, on the other hand, rarely occurs, but its advent requires immediate intervention to prevent rapid deterioration of the patient. The onset of tension pneumocephalus manifests as restlessness, deterioration of consciousness, convulsions, or other changes in neurologic status.[106,107] Definitive diagnosis is made by the presence of air on computed tomographic scan. Prompt evacuation of the air collection through twist drill holes is indicated.[7,106]

TRENDELENBURG POSITION

General Considerations

Use of the Trendelenburg or reverse Trendelenburg position often augments surgical exposure. The Trendelenburg position was first described in the 1860s but was used before then.[108] The position used today bears little resemblance to the original, which entailed suspension of the patient's legs over the shoulders of an assistant to improve exposure of the pelvic organs. (Figure 19-13). Today the term *Trendelenburg* refers to any position in which the head is lower than the rest of the body; *reverse Trendelenburg* indicates a head-up tilt. Physiologic alterations vary greatly depending on the degree of tilt.

Cardiovascular Considerations

The Trendelenburg position is often used in the treatment of hypotension because it is assumed to increase venous return and MAP. However, studies have demonstrated variable effects of the Trendelenburg position on cardiovascular parameters. Changes in intrathoracic blood volume of 2% to 3% in unanesthetized normovolemic individuals are reported with the Trendelenburg position.[109,110] CVP can be increased in the head-down position, but this increase may not reflect changes in stroke volume or MAP.[110,111] MAP was unchanged or decreased despite increases in CVP, mean PAP (MPAP), and CI. Hypotensive patients demonstrated no increase in MAP, an increase in SVR, and a decrease in CI. Similar results have been obtained by others.[112] Normotensive individuals compensate for increases in CVP and PAP with vasodilatation and a decrease in heart rate from stimulation of baroreceptor reflexes; hypotensive individuals may not respond in the same manner.

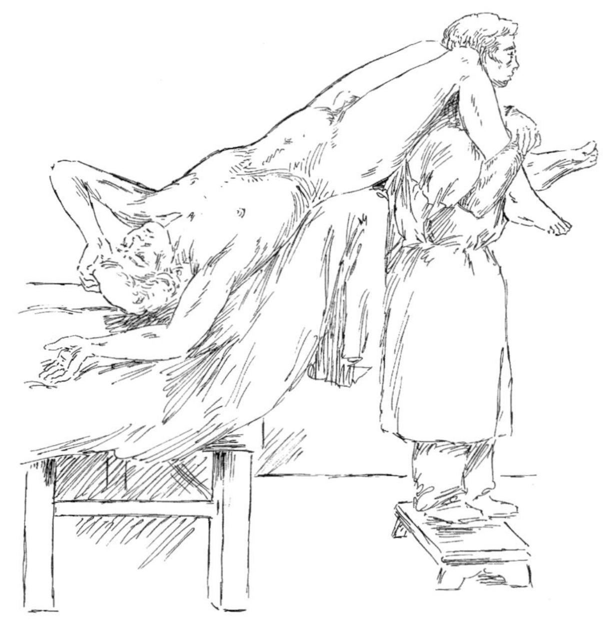

FIGURE **19-13**
Pelvic elevation for urologic surgery: the Trendelenburg position according to Meyer. (From Meyer W. Über die Nachbehandlung des hohen Steinschnittes sowie. Über Verwendbarkeit desselben zur Operation von Blasenscheidenfisteln. *Arch Klin Chir.* 1885;31:49.)

Increased filling pressures with the Trendelenburg position can be detrimental to patients with coronary artery disease. The position may increase myocardial work by increasing central blood volume, cardiac output, and stroke volume. Individuals with very poor cardiac function can have decreased cardiac output if the increased central blood volume moves them to a worse position on the Frank-Starling curve.

Hypovolemia can be unrecognized in the Trendelenburg position, as MAP can remain normal despite volume deficit. Volume replacement can be assessed as adequate until acute hypotension occurs when the patient is returned to the horizontal position. An additive effect can occur if the Trendelenburg position is used to supplement the lithotomy position. In addition, a relative state of hypoperfusion can exist in the lower extremities because of their elevation above the heart and increases in SVR to maintain central blood pressure. Individuals with peripheral vascular disease can be at risk of ischemia in this situation.

Although the Trendelenburg position may not augment venous return, venous pressure can be increased in the upper body with resultant swelling of the face and pharyngeal and orbital structures. Intracranial pressure can be elevated as venous pressures are transmitted to the head and intracranial structures through the valveless jugular system. Cerebral blood flow can be decreased as inflow is limited by venous congestion in intracranial structures. Although these changes are usually not harmful in normal individuals, they can exacerbate intracranial pathology.

Respiratory Considerations

The Trendelenburg position exacerbates the deleterious ventilatory effects of the various positions. The diaphragm is displaced cephalad, and its excursion is limited by shifting of the abdominal contents, decreasing the FRC progressively as the degree of Trendelenburg increases. Movement of the mediastinum toward the head moves the carina closer to the endotracheal tube and can result in preferential ventilation of one lung if the tube moves into the right mainstem bronchus.[48,113,114] This complication also occurs in the reverse Trendelenburg position during laparoscopic procedures, in which the diaphragm is displaced in a cephalad direction by pressurized gas.

The risk of aspiration is generally assumed to increase with the Trendelenburg position as gastric pressure is increased and secretions accumulate in the oropharynx and nasopharynx. However, increases in gastric pressure are offset by increases in lower esophageal sphincter pressure, minimizing the potential for passive regurgitation.[115]

Complications of the Trendelenburg Position

Various complications, many transient, have been observed as a result of the Trendelenburg position. Many are the result of devices designed to prevent the patient from moving in a steep Trendelenburg or reverse Trendelenburg position. Wristlets used to restrain the patient can cause traction on the arm and stretch of the brachial plexus. Improperly positioned shoulder braces can also injure the brachial plexus. Placement of the shoulder brace in a position that is either too lateral or too medial can result in depression of underlying bony structures and compression or stretching of the plexus.[1] Shoulder braces should be avoided if at all possible. The arms are vulnerable to injury in the Trendelenburg position, particularly if they are positioned on arm boards and inadequately restrained, as the arms can slip off, hyperextend, and abduct above the level of the shoulder, stretching the plexus. Suspension of the patient by ankle restraints can cause sore knees or hips. When too tight, table straps used to prevent the patient from sliding in the reverse Trendelenburg position have resulted in lower extremity neuropathies.[116] Use of a foot board is preferable to the overzealous tightening of the table strap if the use of a steep reverse Trendelenburg position is anticipated.

SUMMARY

Surgical positioning disturbs normal cardiovascular and respiratory physiology. These positional changes can be augmented by anesthetic techniques, patient pathophysiology, and body habitus. The implications of physiologic changes associated with each position should be considered when the procedure is planned, when positioning is initiated, and when the patient is returned to the supine posture. Anesthetists must recognize and anticipate both the publicized complications and the potential for damage inherent in each surgical position. Prevention is the best method for decreasing both the incidence of position-related injuries and the associated physical, psychologic, and economic costs to the patient.

REFERENCES

1. Cheney FW, Domino K, Caplan RA, Posner K. Nerve injury associated with anesthesia: a clinical closed claims analysis. *Anesthesiology*. 1999;90:1062-1069.
2. Stoelting RK. Postoperative ulnar nerve palsy—is it a preventable complication? *Anesth Analg*. 1993;76:7-9.
3. Warner MA. Perioperative neuropathies. *Mayo Clin Proc*. 1998;73:567-574.
4. Fowl RJ, Akers DL, Kempczinski RF. Neurovascular lower extremity complications of the lithotomy position. *Ann Vasc Surg*. 1992;6:357-361.
5. Ali H, Nieto JG, Rhamy RK, Chandarlapaty SKC, Vaamonde CA. Acute renal failure due to rhabdomyolysis associated with the extreme lithotomy position. *Am J Kidney Dis*. 1993;22:865-869.
6. Guzzi LM, Mills LM, Greenman P. Rhabdomyolysis, acute renal failure, and the exaggerated lithotomy position. *Anesth Analg*. 1993;77:635-637.
7. Hernandez-Palazon J, Martinez-Lage JF, de la Rosa-Carrillo VN, Tortosa JA, Lopez F, Poza M. Anesthetic technique and development of pneumocephalus after posterior fossa surgery in the sitting position. *Neurocirugia (Astur)*. 2003;14:216-221.
8. Mathes D, Assimos D, Donofrio P. Rhabdomyolysis and myonecrosis in a patient in the lateral decubitus position. *Anesthesiology*. 1996;84:727-729.
9. Bhardwaj A, Long DM, Ducker TB, Toung TJK. Neurologic deficits after cervical laminectomy in the prone position. *J Neurosurg Anesthesiol*. 2001;13:314-319.
10. Liang BA. Ulnar nerve injury after abdominal surgery. *J Clin Anesth*. 1997;9:671-674.
11. Schwartz RO. Complications of laparoscopic hysterectomy. *Obstet Gynecol*. 1993;81:1022-1024.
12. Albin MS, Ritter RR, Pruett CE, Kalff K. Venous air embolism during lumbar laminectomy in the prone position: report of three cases. *Anesth Analg*. 1991;73:346-349.
13. Albin MS, Ritter RT, Bunegin L. Venous air embolism during spinal instrumentation and fusion in the prone position. *Anesth Analg*. 1992;75:141-156.
14. Wilder BL. Hypothesis: the etiology of midcervical quadriplegia after operation with the patient in the sitting position. *Neurosurgery*. 1982;11:530-531.
15. Stoelting RK. *Pharmacology and Physiology in Anesthetic Practice*. 3rd ed. Philadelphia: Lippincott-Raven; 1999.
16. Guyton AC, Hall JE. *Textbook of Medical Physiology*. Philadelphia: Saunders; 2000.
17. Goldsmith AL, McCallum MI. Compartment syndrome as a complication of the prolonged use of the Lloyd-Davies position. *Anaesthesia*. 1996;51:1048-1052.
18. Martin JT. Compartment syndromes: concepts and perspectives for the anesthesiologist. *Anesth Analg*. 1992;75:275-283.
19. Tuckey J. Bilateral compartment syndrome complicating prolonged lithotomy position. *Br J Anaesth*. 1996;77:546-549.
20. Verdolin MH, Toth AS, Schroeder R. Bilateral lower extremity compartment syndromes following prolonged surgery in the low lithotomy position with compression stockings. *Anesthesiology*. 2000;92:1189-1191.
21. Aschoff A, Steiner H-H. Lower limb compartment syndrome following lumbar discectomy in the knee chest position. *Neurosurg Rev*. 1990;13:155-159.
22. Warner ME, LaMaster LM, Thoeming AK, Marienau ME, Warner MA. Compartment syndrome in surgical patients. *Anesthesiology*. 2001;94:705-708.
23. Porter JM, Pidgeon C, Cunningham AJ. The sitting position in neurosurgery: a critical appraisal. *Br J Anaesth*. 1999;82:117-128.
24. Kaper BP, Carra CF, Shirreffs TG. Compartment syndrome after arthroscopic surgery of the knee: a report of two cases managed nonoperatively. *Am J Sports Med*. 1997;25:123-125.
25. Mulhall JP, Drezner AD. Postoperative compartment syndrome and the lithotomy position: a report of three cases and analysis of potential risk factors. *Connecticut Medicine*. 1993;57:129-133.
26. Azar FM. Traumatic disorders. In: Canale ST, ed. *Campbell's Operative Orthopedics*. 10th ed. St Louis: Mosby; 2003.
27. Tuncer R, Zorludemir U. Lower limb compartment syndrome following urethroplasty. *Br J Urol*. 1997;79:646.
28. Schwartz LB, Stahl RS, DeCherney AH. Unilateral compartment syndrome after prolonged gynecologic surgery in the dorsal lithotomy position: a case report. *J Reprod Med*. 1993;56:469-471.
29. Venkatesh R, Ralston SJ, Parr NJ. Compartment syndrome. *Br J Urol*. 1996;78:964-965.
30. Sawyer RJ, Richmond MN, Hickey JD, Jarrratt JA. Peripheral nerve injuries associated with anaesthesia. *Anaesthesia*. 2000;55:980-991.
31. Fuller G. Focal peripheral neuropathies. *Neurology in Practice*. 2003;74(suppl):ii20-ii24.
32. Lundborg G, Dahlin LB. The pathophysiology of nerve compression. *Hand Clin*. 1992;8:225-227.
33. Warner MA, Warner DO, Matsumoto JY, Harper CM, Schroeder DR, Maxson PM. Ulnar neuropathy in surgical patients. *Anesthesiology*. 1999;90:54-59.
34. Schinsky MF, Macaulay W, Parks ML, Kiernan H, Nercessian OA. Nerve injury after primary total knee arthroplasty. *J Arthroplasty*. 2001;16:1048-1054.
35. Angermeier KW, Jordan GH. Complications of the exaggerated lithotomy position: a review of 177 cases. *J Urol*. 1994;151:866-868.
36. Rodeo SA, Forster RA, Weiland AJ. Neurological complications due to arthroscopy. *J Bone Joint Surg. Am*. 1993;75:917-926.
37. Wong DH, Ward MG. A preventable cause of brachial plexus injury. *Anesthesiology*. 2003;98:798.
38. Lowe J, Sen S, Mackinnon S. Current approach to radial nerve paralysis. *Plast Reconstr Surg*. 2000;110:1099-1112.
39. Jacobs D, Azagra JS, Delauwer M, Bain H, Vanderheyden JE. Unusual complication after pelvic surgery: unilateral lower limb crush syndrome and bilateral common peroneal nerve paralysis. *Acta Anaesthesiol Belg*. 1994;43:139-143.

40. Warner MA, Martin JT, Schroeder DR, Offord KP. Lower-extremity motor neuropathy associated with surgery performed on patients in a lithotomy position. *Anesthesiology*. 1994;81:6-12.
41. Casscells CD, Lindsey RW, Ebersole J, Li B. Ulnar neuropathy after median sternotomy. *Clin Orthop*. 1993;291:259-265.
42. Alvine FG, Schurrer ME. Postoperative ulnar nerve palsy. *J Bone Joint Surg Am*. 1987;69-A:255-259.
43. Sharma K, Cross J, Santiago F, Avyar D, Burke G. Incidence of acute femoral neuropathy following renal transplantation. *Arch Neurol*. 2002;59:541-545.
44. Coppieters MW, Van de Velde M, Stappaerts KH. Positioning in anesthesiology: Toward a better understanding of stretch-induced perioperative neuropathies. *Anesthesiology*. 2002;97:75-81.
45. Lumb AB, Nunn JF. Respiratory function and ribcage contribution to ventilation in body positions commonly used during anesthesia. *Anesth Analg*. 1991;73:422-426.
46. Krayer S, Rehnder K, Vetterman J, Didier EP, Ritman EL. Position and motion of the human diaphragm during anesthesia-paralysis. *Anesthesiology*. 1989;70:891-898.
47. Barnas GM, Green MD, Mackenzie CF, et al. Effect of posture on lung and regional chest wall mechanics. *Anesthesiology*. 1993;78:251-259.
48. Yap SJ, Morris RW, Pybus DA. Alterations in endotracheal tube position during general anaesthesia. *Anaesth Intensive Care*. 1994;22:586-588.
49. Sinha A, Agarwal A, Gaur A, Pandey CK. Oropharyngeal swelling and macroglossia after cervical spine surgery in the prone patient. *J Neurosurg Anesthesiol*. 2001;13:237-239.
50. Kuhnert SM, Faust RJ, Berge K, Piepgras DG. Postoperative macroglossia: report of a case with rapid resolution after extubation of the trachea. *Anesth Analg*. 1999;88:220-223.
51. Martin JT. The prone position: anesthesiologic considerations. In: Martin JT, ed. *Positioning in Anesthesia and Surgery*. 2nd ed. Philadelphia: Saunders; 1987:191-222.
52. Anderton JM. The prone position for the surgical patient: a historical review of the principles and hazards. *Br J Anaesth*. 1991;67:452-463.
53. Hoski JJ, Eismont FJ, Green BA. Blindness as a complication of intraoperative positioning. *J Bone Joint Surg Am*. 1993;75:1231-1232.
54. Yokoyama M, Ueda W, Hirakawa. Haemodynamic effects of the lateral decubitus position and the kidney rest lateral decubitus position during anaesthesia. *Br J Anaesth*. 2000;84:753-757.
55. Lee T-C, Yang L-C, Chen H-J. Effect of patient position and hypotensive anesthesia on inferior vena caval pressure. *Spine*. 1998;23:941-947.
56. Park CK. The effect of patient positioning on intraabdominal pressure and blood loss in spinal surgery. *Anesth Analg*. 2000;91:552-557.
57. Chaynes P, Verdic JC, Moscovici J, Zadeh J, Vaysse P, Becue J. Microsurgical anatomy of the internal vertebral venous plexuses. *Surg Radiol Anat*. 1998;20:47-51.
58. Pelosi P, Croci M, Calappi E, et al. The prone positioning during general anesthesia minimally affects respiratory mechanics while improving functional residual capacity and increasing oxygen tension. *Anesth Analg*. 1995;80:955-960.
59. Palmon SC, Kirsch JR, Depper JA, Toung TJK. The effect of the prone position on pulmonary mechanics is frame-dependent. *Anesth Analg*. 1998;87:1175-1180.
60. Mure M, Lindahl SGE. Prone position improves gas exchange—but how? *Acta Anaesthesiol Scand*. 2001;45:150-159.
61. Mure M, Domino K, Lindahl SGE, Hlastala MP, Altemeier WA, Glenny RW. Regional ventilation-perfusion is more uniform in the prone position. *J Appl Physiol*. 2000;88:1076-1083.
62. Pelosi P, Croci M, Calappi E, et al. Prone positioning improves pulmonary function in obese patients during general anesthesia. *Anesth Analg*. 1996;83:578-583.
63. Cucchiara RF, Black S. Corneal abrasion during anesthesia and surgery. *Anesthesiology*. 1988;69:978-979.
64. Roth S, Thisted RA, Erickson JP, Black S, D. Schreider BD. Eye injuries after nonocular surgery. *Anesthesiology*. 1996;85:1020-1027.
65. Stoelting RK. APSF survey results identify safety issues priorities. *Anesth Patient Saf Found Newsletter*. 1999;14:6-7.
66. Lee LA, Lam AM. Unilateral blindness after prone lumbar spine surgery. *Anesthesiology*. 2001;95:793-795.
67. Cheng MA, Todorov A, Tempelhoff R, McHugh T, Crowder CM, Lauryssen C. The effect of prone positioning on intraocular pressure in anesthetized patients. *Anesthesiology*. 2001;95:1551-1555.
68. Lee LA. Postoperative visual loss data gathered and analyzed. *ASA Newsletter*. 2000;64.
69. Wolfe SW, Lospinuso MF, Burke SW. Unilateral blindness as a complication of patient positioning for spinal surgery. *Spine*. 1992;17:600-605.
70. Horlocker TT, Wedel DJ, Cucchiara RF. Venous air embolism during spinal instrumentation and fusion in the prone position. *Anesth Analg*. 1992;75:141-156.
71. Dubey PK, Singh AK. Venous oxygen embolism due to hydrogen peroxide irrigation during posterior fossa surgery. *J Neurosurg Anesthesiol*. 2000;12:54-56.
72. Goettler CE, Pryor JP, Reilly PM. Brachial plexopathy after prone positioning. *Crit Care*. 2002;6:540-542.
73. Drummond JC. Macroglossia, deja vu. *Anesth Analg*. 1999;89:534-535.
74. Reber A, Bein T, Hogman M, Khan ZP, Nilsson S, Hedenstierna G. Lung aeration and pulmonary gas exchange during lumbar epidural anaesthesia and in the lithotomy posision in elderly patients. *Anaesthesia*. 1998;53:854-861.
75. Hirvonen EA, Nuutinen LS, Kauko M. Hemodynamic changes due to Trendelenburg positioning and pneumoperitoneum during laparoscopic hysterectomy. *Acta Anaesthesiol Scand*. 1995;39:949-955.
76. Halliwill JR, Hewitt SA, Joyner MJ, Warner MA. Effect of various lithotomy positions on lower-extremity blood pressure. *Anesthesiology*. 1998;89:1373-1376.
77. Meyer RS, White KK, Smith JM, Groppo ER, Mubarak SJ, Hargens AR. Intramuscular and blood pressures in legs positioned in the hemilithotomy position: clarification of risk factors for well-leg acute compartment syndrome. *J Bone Joint Surg Am*. 2002;84:1829-1835.
78. Al Hakim M, Katirji MB. Femoral mononeuropathy induced by the lithotomy position: a report of 5 cases with a review of the literature. *Muscle Nerve*. 1993;16:891-895.
79. Adler LM, Loughlin JS, Morin C J, Haning RV Jr. Bilateral compartment syndrome after a long gynecologic operation in the lithotomy position. *Am J Obstet Gynecol*. 1990;162:1271-1272.
80. Mathews PV, Perry JJ, Murray PC. Compartment syndrome of the well leg as a result of the hemilithotomy position: a report of two cases and review of the literature. *J Orthop Trauma*. 2001;15:580-583.
81. Scott JR, Daneker G, Lumsden A. Prevention of compartment syndrome associated with the dorsal lithotomy position. *Am Surg*. 1997;63:801-806.
82. Horgan AF, Geddes S, Finlay IG. Lloyd-Davies position with Trendelenburg—a disaster waiting to happen? *Dis Colon Rectum*. 1999;42:916-919.
83. Matin S, Novick A. Renal dysfunction associated with staged bilateral partial nephrectomy: the importance of operative positioning. *J Urol*. 2001;165:880-881.
84. Battillo JA, Hendler MA. Effects of patient positioning during anesthesia. *Int Anesthesiol Clin*. 1993;31:67-86.
85. Lawson NW, Meyer DJ. Lateral positions. In: Warner MA, ed. *Positioning in Anesthesia and Surgery*. Philadelphia: Saunders; 1997:127-152.
86. Della Valle A, Salonia-Ruzo P, Peterson MGE, Salvati EA, Sharrock NE. Inflatable pillows as axillary support devices

during surgery performed in the lateral decubitus position during epidural anesthesia. *Anesth Analg.* 2001;93:1338-1343.
87. Alexander CM, Vandam LR. Positioning of patients for operation. In: Longnecker DE, Tinker JH, Morgan GE, eds. *Principles and Practice of Anesthesiology*. St Louis: Mosby; 1998:680-699.
88. Fahy BG, Hasnain JU, Flowers JL, Plotkin JS, Odonkor P, Ferguson MK. Transesophageal echocardiographic detection of gas embolism and cardiac valvular dysfunction during laparoscopic nephrectomy. *Anesth Analg.* 1999;88:500-504.
89. Dunn PF. Physiology of the lateral decubitus position and one-lung ventilation. *Int Anesth Clin.* 2000;38:25-53.
90. Hogue CW. Effectiveness of low levels of nonventilated lung continuous positive airway pressure in improving arterial oxygenation during one-lung ventilation. *Anesth Analg.* 1994;79:364-367.
91. D'Alessio JG, Weller RS, Rosenblum M. Activation of the Bezold-Jarisch reflex in the sitting position for shoulder arthroscopy using interscalene block. *Anesth Analg.* 1995;80:1158-1162.
92. Buhre W, Weyland A, Buhre K, et al. Effects of the sitting position on the distribution of blood volume in patients undergoing neurosurgical procedures. *Br J Anaesth.* 2000;84:354-357.
93. Giebler R, Kollenberg B, Pohlen G, Peters J. Effect of positive end-expiratory pressure on the incidence of air embolism and on the cardiovascular response to the sitting position during neurosurgery. *Br J Anaesth.* 1998;80:30-35.
94. Duke DA, Lynch JJ, Harner SG, Faust RJ, Ebersold MJ. Venous air embolism in sitting and supine patients undergoing vestibular schwannoma resection. *Neurosurgery*. 1998;42:1282-1287.
95. Papadopoulos G, Kuhly P, Brock M, Rudolph KH, Eyrich K. Venous and paradoxical air embolism in the sitting position. A prospective study with transesophageal echocardiography. *Acta Neurochir (Wien)*. 1994;126:140-143.
96. Stendel R, Gramm H-J, Schroder K, Lober C, Brock M. Transcranial doppler ultrasonography as a screening technique for detection of a patent foramen ovale before surgery in the sitting position. *Anesthesiology*. 2000;93:971-975.
97. Girard F, Ruel M, McKenty S, et al. Incidences of venous air embolism and patent foramen ovale among patients undergoing selective peripheral denervation in the sitting position. *Neurosurgery*. 2003;53:316-320.
98. Lobato EB, Paige GB, Brown MM, Bennett B, Davis JD. Pneumoperitoneum as a risk factor for endobronchial intubation during laparoscopic gynecologic surgery. *Anesthesia & Analgesia*. 1998;86:301-303.
99. Schmitt HJ, Hemmerling TM. Venous air emboli occur during release of positive end-expiratory pressure and repositioning after sitting position surgery. *Anesth Analg.* 2002;94:400-403.
100. Lieutaud T, Bodonian C, Lak F, Salord F, Artru F. Transesophageal echocardiography and air embolism during posterior fossa neurosurgery: interest and limits of preoperative detection of foramen ovale. *Ann Fr Anesth Reanim.* 2001;20:631-634.
101. Cucchiara RF, Bechtle PS. Incidences of venous air embolism and patent foramen ovale among patients undergoing selective peripheral denervation in the sitting position [comment]. *Neurosurgery Online*. 2003;53:320.
102. Losasso TJ, Muzzi DA, Dietz NM, Cucchiara RF. Fifty percent nitrous oxide does not increase the risk of venous air embolism in neurosurgical patients operated upon in the sitting position. *Anesthesiology*. 1992;77:21-30.
103. Toung TJK, Aizawa H, Traystman RJ. Effects of positive end-expiratory pressure ventilation on cerebral venous pressure with head elevation in dogs. *J Appl Physiol.* 2000;88:655-661.
104. Deinsberger W, Christophis P, Jodicke A, Heesen M, Boker DK. Somatosensory evoked potential monitoring during positioning of the patient for posterior fossa surgery in the semisitting position. *Neurosurgery*. 1998;43:36-40.
105. Prabhakar H, Bithal PK, Garg A. Tension pneumocephalus after craniotomy in supine position. *J Neurosurg Anesthesiol.* 2003;1:278-281.
106. Satapathy GC, Dash HH. Tension pneumocephalus after neurosurgery in the supine position. *Br J Anaesthesia.* 2000;84:115-117.
107. Suri A, Mahapatra AK, Singh VP. Posterior fossa tension pneumocephalus. *Child's Nerv Syst.* 2000;16:196-199.
108. Wilcox S, Vandam LD. Alas, poor Trendelenburg and his position: a critique of its uses and effectiveness. *Anesth Analg.* 1988;67:574-578.
109. Bivins HG, Knopp R, dos Santos PA. Blood volume distribution in the Trendelenburg position. *Ann Emerg Med.* 1985;14:641-643.
110. Hofer CK, Zalunardo MP, Klaghofer R, Spahr T, Pasch T, Zollinger A. Changes in intrathoracic blood volume associated with pneumoperitoneum and positioning. *Acta Anaesthesiol Scand.* 2002;46:303-308.
111. Sibbald WJ, Paterson NA, Holliday RL, Baskerville J. The Trendelenburg position: hemodynamic effects in hypotensive and normotensive patients. *Ann Emerg Med.* 1979;7:218-224.
112. Sing RF, O'Hara D, Sawyer MA, Marino PL. Trendelenburg position and oxygen transport in hypovolemic adults. *Ann Emerg Med.* 1994;23:564-567.
113. Brimacombe J. Endobronchial intubation during upper abdominal laparoscopic surgery in the reverse Trendelenburg position. *Anesth Analg.* 1994;78:601.
114. Inada T, Uesugi F, Kawachi S, Takubo K. Changes in tracheal tube position during laparoscopic cholecystectomy. *Anaesthesia.* 1996;51:823-826.
115. Heijke SA, Smith G, Key A. The effect of the Trendelenburg position on lower oesophageal sphincter tone. *Anaesthesia.* 1991;46:185-187.
116. Johnston RV, Lawson NW, Nealon WH. Lower extremity neuropathy after laparoscopic cholecystectomy. *Anesthesiology*. 1992;77:835.

CHAPTER 20

Airway Management

Anthony Chipas, Wayne Ellis, Karen L. Zaglaniczny

As airway experts, anesthetists are responsible for managing the airway in a wide variety of settings. It is imperative that anesthesia providers acquire the requisite knowledge and skills associated with different airway management techniques. Outcomes related to airway management have focused on injury to the airway and management of the difficult airway. In a review of 266 closed claims related to airway injury, 87 involved the larynx, with the most common lesions being vocal cord paralysis, granulomas, arytenoid dislocation, and hematomas.[1] Of laryngeal injuries, 80% were associated with a routine (nondifficult) tracheal intubation and only 17 were associated with a difficult intubation.[1] Airway injuries placed fourth (6%) behind three other major types of outcomes: death (32%), spinal cord or peripheral nerve damage (16%), and brain damage (12%). Outcomes related to difficult airway claims included death (46%), brain damage (11%), airway injury (34%), and aspiration (7%).[1] The Difficult Airway Algorithm, introduced in 1992, established a structure for the management of expected and unexpected difficult airways.[2] These practice guidelines have improved the assessment and management of potentially difficult airways. Recent advances in equipment, technology, and monitoring have significantly improved airway management options and outcomes. This chapter describes the anatomy and physiology, patient assessment, anesthetic considerations, and techniques related to airway management.

ANATOMY AND PHYSIOLOGY OF THE AIRWAY

Numerous anatomy texts contain full descriptions of the tissues and structures of the respiratory system.[3,4] The airway is divided into two sections: upper and lower. Various anatomists divide the upper from the lower airway at the cricoid cartilage. The upper airway includes the nose, mouth, pharynx, hypopharynx, and larynx. The lower airway consists of the trachea, bronchi, bronchioles, terminal bronchioles, respiratory bronchioles, and alveoli. This section reviews primary structures, innervation, blood supply, and normal and abnormal function of the upper airway structures.

Nose

The nose and mouth are the external openings to the respiratory tree. The large surface area of the nasal mucosa warms and humidifies inspired air. The nose is the primary passage by which air enters the lungs. Because of the surface area over the turbinates and the sinuses, the nasal passages are well suited for the task of humidification of the air and primary filtration. As the air passes through the nose it meets the turbinates, which cause directional changes in the airflow. Branches of three arteries—the maxillary (sphenopalatine), ophthalmic, and facial (septal)—provide a rich supply of blood to the nasal mucosa. The innervation of the nose is from the nasopalatine and ethmoidal branches of the facial nerve. These nerves also supply the nasopharynx, nasal septum, and palate. Sensory nerve supply to the nasal mucosa is from the ophthalmic and maxillary divisions of the trigeminal nerve. Parasympathetic innervation arises from the seventh cranial nerve and pterygopalatine ganglion. Sympathetic innervation is derived from the superior cervical ganglion. Sympathetic stimulation results in vasoconstriction and shrinkage of the nasal tissue. Depression of the sympathetic nervous system, as occurs with general anesthesia, may cause engorgement of the nasal tissues, increasing the likelihood of bleeding with manipulation from nasal airways or endotracheal tubes.

Mouth

The oral cavity is separated from the nasal passages by the hard and soft palates. The hard palate is stationary and remains positionally unchanged. The soft palate covers the posterior third to half of the oral cavity. The palate rises during eating to prevent food and liquids from passing from the mouth into the nose and thereby decreases the chance of aspiration. With age, obesity, and other conditions, this structure may stretch and become more movable. When an individual is asleep or paralyzed, as with general anesthesia, this structure can fall back against the nasal passages, blocking air movement and causing symptoms of sleep apnea. The tongue is a large muscular organ that fills most of the oral cavity and is involved in the tasting and ingestion of food. It relaxes when the individual is either asleep or paralyzed, which increases the potential for airway obstruction. The passage from the oral cavity into the oropharynx is "guarded" by the uvula. This pendulous piece of tissue extends from the posterior edge of the middle of the soft palate into the oral cavity. If swollen, enlarged, or injured, it can be a cause of airway obstruction. The tonsils are walnut-shaped structures that sit on both sides of the posterior opening of the oral cavity. They are partially buried in the soft tissue at the base of the tongue and are protected by the anterior and posterior tonsillar pillars.

Pharynx

The pharynx is divided into three compartments—the nasopharynx, oropharynx, and hypopharynx (laryngopharynx)—and extends from the base of the skull to the level of the cricoid cartilage. The nasopharynx lies anterior to C1 and is bound superiorly by the base of the skull and inferiorly by the soft palate. The openings to the auditory (eustachian) tubes and the adenoids are found in the nasopharynx. Sensory innervation of the mucosa is derived from the maxillary nerve. The oropharynx lies at the C2 to C3 level and is bound superiorly by the soft palate and inferiorly by the epiglottis. It opens into the mouth anteriorly, through the anterior and posterior tonsillar pillars. The hypopharynx lies posterior to the larynx and is bound by the superior border of the epiglottis and the inferior border of the cricoid cartilage at the C5 to C6 level. The upper esophageal sphincter lies at the lower edge of the hypopharynx and arises from the cricopharyngeous muscle. This muscle acts as a barrier to regurgitation in the conscious patient.

Numerous nerves supply motor and sensory fibers to the airway. The glossopharyngeal, vagus, and spinal accessory nerves share nuclei in the medulla and innervate all of the muscles of the pharynx, larynx, and soft palate. Afferent (sensory) stimuli elicited when the posterior wall of the pharynx is touched are carried by the glossopharyngeal nerve to the medulla, where they synapse with nuclei of the vagus nerve and the cranial portion of the spinal accessory nerve. The efferent response returns primarily through the vagus nerve, resulting in the gag reflex as the muscles of the pharynx elevate and constrict.

Two branches of the vagus nerve innervate the hypopharynx: the superior laryngeal nerve and the recurrent laryngeal nerve (RLN; Figure 20-1). The superior laryngeal nerve divides into the internal and external branches. The internal branch of the superior laryngeal nerve provides sensory input to the hypopharynx above the vocal folds (cords). The external branch provides motor function to the cricothyroid muscle of the larynx.

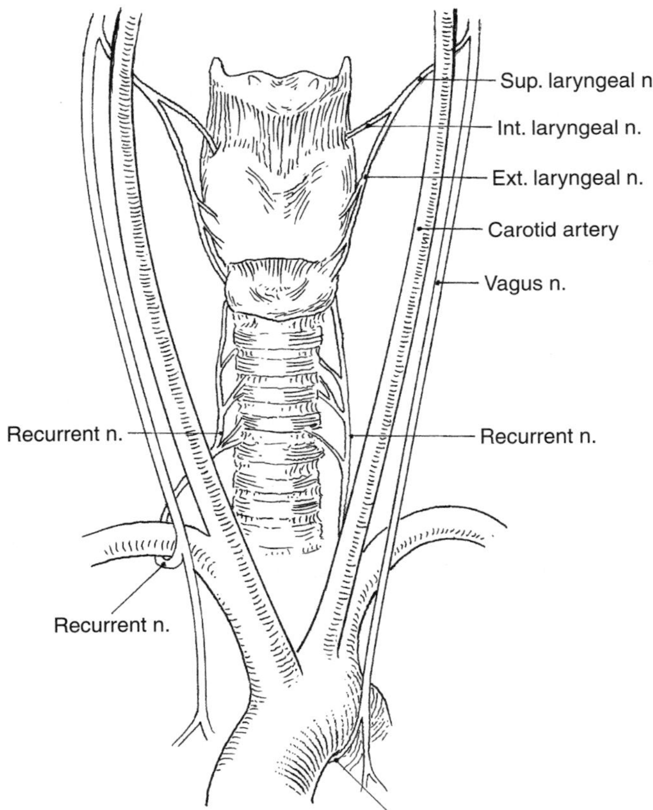

FIGURE **20-1**
Anatomy of the superior laryngeal and recurrent laryngeal nerves.

The RLN provides sensory innervation to the subglottic area and to the trachea. The motor component of the RLN provides motor function to all the muscles of the larynx except the cricothyroid muscle.

The superior laryngeal nerve and the RLN may be damaged by surgery, neoplasms, and neck trauma. Dissecting aortic arch aneurysms and mitral stenosis place traction on the RLN, causing hoarseness. Unilateral injury to the RLN usually results in hoarseness but does not compromise respiratory status. The vocal cords compensate by shifting the midline toward the uninjured side. In the acute phase of bilateral injury to the RLN, unopposed tension and adduction of the vocal cords result in stridor, which may deteriorate into severe respiratory distress and possibly death. Patients with chronic injury develop compensatory mechanisms that allow for normal respiration and gruff or husky speech. Injury to the superior laryngeal nerve does not usually cause respiratory distress.

Larynx

The larynx begins with the epiglottis and extends to the cricoid cartilage. It is composed of three single cartilages, three paired cartilages, and intrinsic and extrinsic muscles connected by ligaments and membranes. These structures function intricately together to protect the airway from aspiration, provide airflow between the hypopharynx and trachea, provide cough and gag reflexes, and produce phonation (Figure 20-2). The larynx begins between the third and fourth cervical vertebrae and ends in the adult at the cricothyroid muscle, at the level of the sixth cervical vertebrae. The anterior and lateral larynx is formed by the thyroid cartilage. This cartilage fuses anteriorly and is identified by the thyroid notch. Posteriorly, the thyroid cartilage rises toward the hyoid bone at the base of the tongue as the posterior horns or cornu. The thyroid cartilage is connected to the hyoid bone by the thyrohyoid fascia and muscle. The posterior border of the larynx is formed by the posterior portion of the cricoid cartilage. Internal to the larynx are the articulating cartilages, the arytenoids, and the epiglottis. The epiglottis is a single cartilage that is leaflike in shape. It sits above the glottic opening and closes during swallowing. The space between the epiglottis and the base of the tongue is known as the *superior vallecula.* Applying upward force on this area results in "lifting" or pulling of the epiglottis away from the glottic opening. This tissue is very delicate in the infant

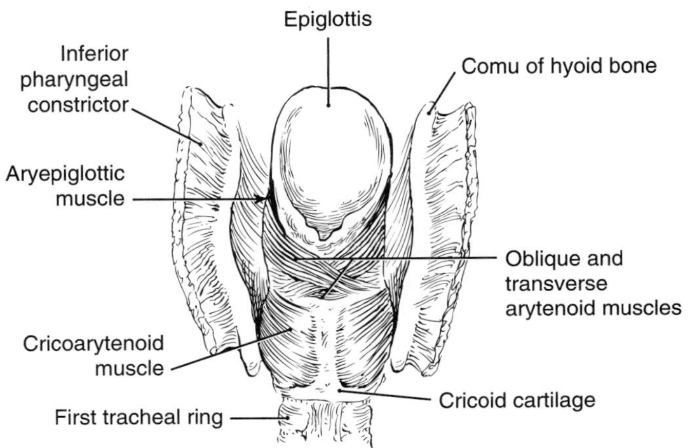

FIGURE **20-2**
Larynx.

TABLE 20-1 Intrinsic Muscles of the Larynx

Muscle	Action
Posterior cricoarytenoid	Separates the vocal cords (abducts) and opens the glottis
Lateral cricoarytenoid	Closes the glottis (adducts)
Arytenoids	Closes the glottis, especially posterior
Cricothyroid	Produces tension and elongates the vocal cords
Thyroarytenoid	Shortens and relaxes the vocal cords

TABLE 20-2 Extrinsic Muscles of the Larynx

Muscle	Action
Sternohyoid	Draws hyoid bone inferiorly
Sternothyroid	Draws thyroid cartilage caudad
Thyrohyoid	Pulls hyoid bone inferiorly
Omohyoid	Pulls hyoid bone caudad

and child, and pressures exerted to lift the epiglottis can result in damage to the tissues of the vallecula, bleeding, edema, and airway obstruction. The inferior vallecula is between the inferior edge of the epiglottis and the true vocal cords.

The intrinsic muscles of the larynx control the tension of the vocal cords and the opening and closing of the glottis (Table 20-1). The extrinsic muscles connect the larynx with the hyoid bone and other neighboring structures (Table 20-2). Their primary function is to adjust the position of the trachea and other structures during phonation, breathing, and swallowing.

Branching from the external carotid, the superior thyroid artery gives rise to the superior laryngeal artery. This artery supplies the supraglottic region of the larynx. The infraglottic region is supplied by the inferior laryngeal artery, a terminal branch of the inferior thyroid artery.

Trachea

The trachea originates at the inferior border of the cricoid cartilage and extends to the carina (Figure 20-3). It is approximately 10 to 20 cm long in adults. The cricoid cartilage is the only cartilage of the trachea that is a complete ring. The remainder of the trachea is composed of 16 to 20 C-shaped cartilaginous rings. The posterior side of the trachea lacks cartilage, thereby accommodating the esophagus during the act of swallowing. The cartilaginous rings and plates continue until the bronchi reach 0.6 to 0.8 mm in size. At this point the cartilage disappears and the bronchi are termed *bronchioles*. The function of the bronchi is to provide humidification and warming of the air as it passes to the alveoli.

The angle of bifurcation of the right mainstem bronchus is approximately 25 to 30 degrees. The bifurcation to the right upper lobe is approximately 2.5 cm from the carina. The angle of the left mainstem bronchus is 45 degrees. The left mainstem bronchus is approximately 5 cm long before it bifurcates into the left superior and inferior lobe bronchi.

The tracheobronchial trees receive sympathetic innervation from the first through fifth thoracic ganglia. Parasympathetic innervation is derived from branches of the vagus nerve. The carina is richly innervated, making it sensitive to sensory stimulation.

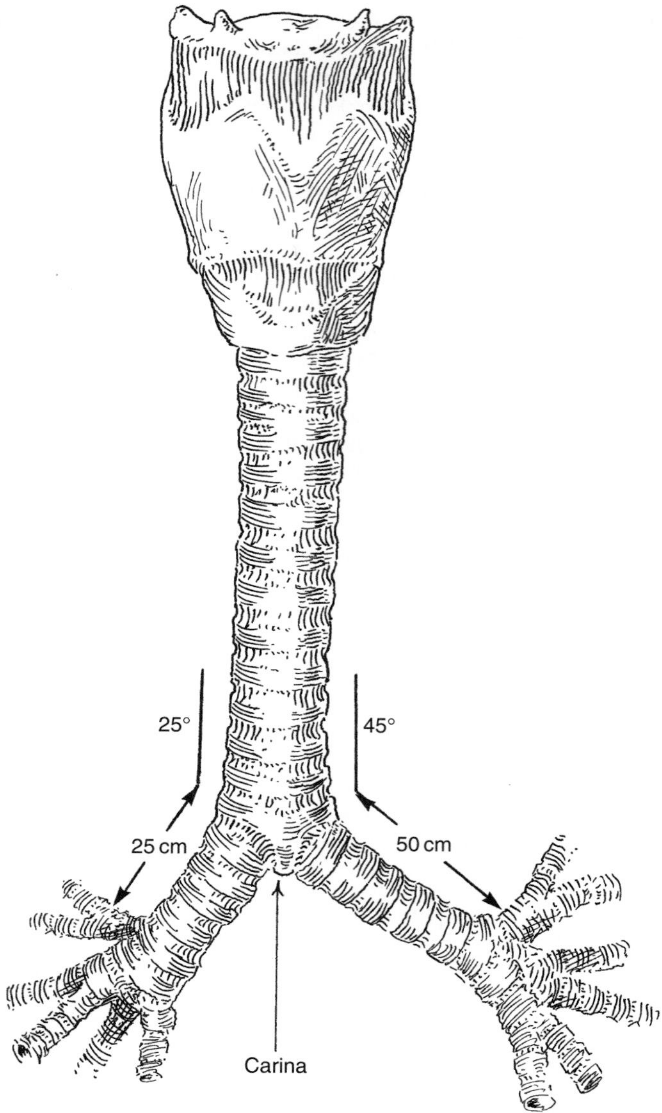

FIGURE **20-3**
Trachea.

AIRWAY ASSESSMENT

A complete airway assessment and physical examination should be done in the preoperative period. This assessment includes evaluation of multiple patient physical characteristics to identify potential airway problems indicative of the unanticipated difficult airway. Criteria that can be assessed to identify potentially difficult airways include interincisor distance, thyromental distance, head and neck extension, Mallampati classification, body weight, and a past history of difficult airway. Evaluation of the length of the upper incisors, visibility of the uvula, shape of the palate, compliance of the mandibular space, and length and thickness of the neck provides further assessment.[2] The most prominent factors that are predictive of a difficult airway are obesity, decreased head and neck

TABLE 20-3 Acute and Chronic Diseases and Syndromes Associated with Difficult Airways

Category	Diseases and Syndromes
Congenital	Pierre Robin, Treacher Collins, Down, choanal atresia
Physical	Large, protruding teeth; thick neck; spinal malformations ("humpback," scoliosis); large tongue; micrognathia; maxillary overbite
Traumatic	Oral or airway burns, facial trauma, head and neck injuries, mandibular fracture, dislocation of the temporal mandibular joint
Chronic diseases	Rheumatoid or degenerative arthritis, diabetes mellitus, obesity, supraglottic tumors, acromegaly
Acute disorders	Peritonsillar or retropharyngeal abscess, epiglottitis, postoperative airway bleeding, Ludwig's angina

TABLE 20-4 Airway Classification

Classification	Description	Ease of Intubation
1	Soft palate, fauces, uvula, and anterior and posterior tonsillar pillars seen	Easy
2	Same as 1, except tonsillary pillars hidden by tongue	Possibly difficult
3	Only base of uvula seen	Probably difficult
4	Even uvula not visualized	Very difficult

From Mallampati SR. Clinical signs to predict difficult tracheal intubation. Can Anaesth Soc J. *1983;30:429-434.*

movement, decreased jaw movement, receding mandible, and buck teeth.[5] In determination of the probability of a difficult airway, no ideal method exists that is highly sensitive and specific, with minimal false-positive or false-negative reports.[6-9] In an attempt to standardize the physical examination, it is recommended that all tests be completed with the patient in the sitting position with head in full extension, mouth opened wide, and tongue extruded and with phonation. The history should focus on prior airway management problems, acute or chronic diseases, and syndromes associated with difficult airways (Table 20-3).

During the airway physical examination, findings that may indicate a difficult airway are integrated into the proposed airway management. Normally the interincisor distance should be at least 4 cm; less than 3 cm indicates a potential problem. If the mouth is narrow it may be difficult to get the 2-cm flange of the laryngoscope blade and the endotracheal tube into the mouth while maintaining good visualization of the cords. The thyromental distance is measured from the thyroid notch to the inner border of the mandible when the patient's head is extended. A thyromental distance less than 6 cm or three ordinary fingerbreadths is associated with a higher incidence of difficult intubation. The full range of flexion-extension of the neck varies from 90 to 165 degrees, decreasing approximately 20% between ages 16 and 75 years. The atlantooccipital joint is capable of extending up to 35 degrees and provides the highest degree of mobility in the neck. When extension is reduced to 23 degrees, visualization may become difficult.[10] Patients should be able to touch the tip of the chin to the chest.

The Mallampati classification is an indirect method of relating the size of the base of the tongue to the oral cavity (Table 20-4, Figure 17-2). It is based on the theory that the tongue is singularly the largest obstacle to direct visualization of the glottis.[11] The incidence of grades III and IV laryngoscopic views varies throughout the literature. Variability in observation, years of experience, and definitions of airway categories results in differences in reporting statistics. Approximately 15% to 18% of patients have a grade III view requiring multiple intubation attempts. Approximately 1% to 4% have a grade IV view, and approximately 0.0001% to 0.02% fit into the "cannot intubate, cannot ventilate" category.[12] Difficult direct laryngoscopy occurs in 1.5% to 8.5% of general anesthetic procedures, and difficult intubation occurs with a similar incidence. Failed intubation occurs in 0.13% to 0.3% of general anesthetic procedures.[13]

TRACHEAL INTUBATION

Intubation of the trachea can be performed by means of a variety of techniques and equipment for the administration of anesthesia and for emergency airway conditions. Competency with various intubation techniques and equipment is primarily related to the skill and expertise of the provider. The challenge of a "can't intubate, can't ventilate" situation can arise, requiring the prompt initiation of various airway management strategies. Tracheal intubation is recommended in the following situations: compromise or inaccessibility of the patient's airway; long surgical procedures; surgical procedures involving the head, neck, abdomen, or chest; need for controlled positive pressure ventilation; inability to maintain airway with a mask or airway device; disease process involving the airway; risk of aspiration from a full stomach; and pregnancy.

Proper positioning of the head is essential to facilitate success with mask ventilation and tracheal intubation. The use of the "sniffing position" requires the head to be flexed forward 35 degrees and extended 80 degrees. This position allows for better alignment of the oral, pharyngeal, and tracheal axis and promotes optimal conditions (Figures 20-4 and 20-5). Techniques for routine laryngoscopy and intubation are detailed in basic anesthesia texts.

With the patient under general anesthesia, if the first attempt is unsuccessful, the patient should be evaluated for adequate muscle relaxation and repositioned. The type and length of the laryngoscope blade may need to be changed. Use of optimal external laryngeal pressure during laryngoscopy may improve the view of the vocal cords. This is accomplished by applying pressure in a posterior-cephalad direction sequentially over the thyroid, hyoid, and cricoid cartilages with the right hand during laryngoscopy. Subsequent intubation attempts

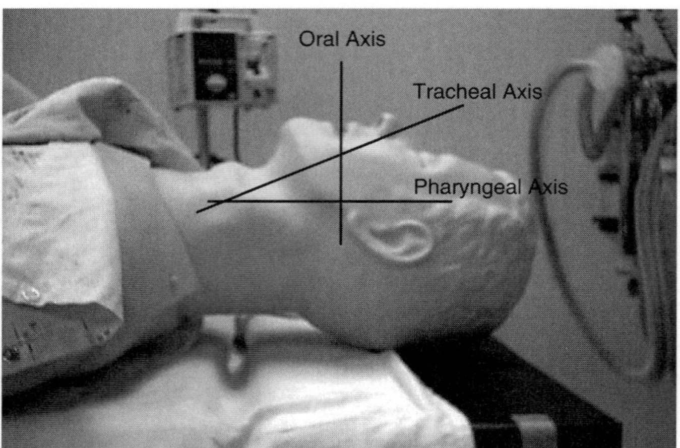

FIGURE **20-4**
Axis with head flat.

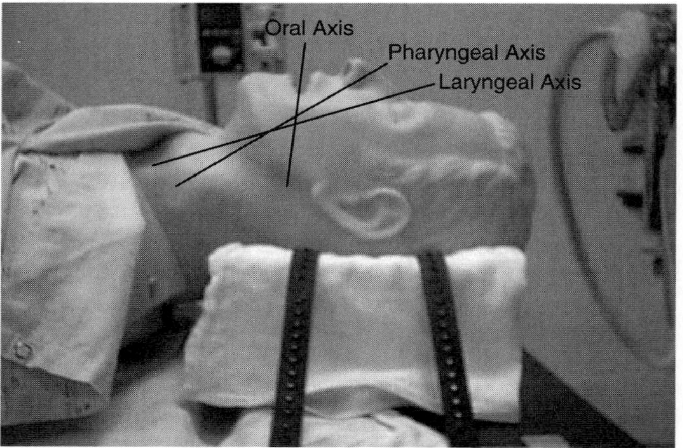

FIGURE **20-5**
Axis with sniffing position.

should adhere to practice guidelines, with prompt consideration of waking up the patient.

Management of the Difficult Airway

The Difficult Airway Algorithm established the standardized approach to the management of the anticipated or unanticipated difficult airway (Figure 20-6). The practice guidelines were updated in 2003 to reflect current management strategies.[2] The airway algorithm provides guidelines to manage difficult face mask ventilation, difficult laryngoscopy, difficult tracheal intubation, and failed intubation. An organized plan should be initiated when a difficult airway is encountered. All departments have a dedicated difficult airway cart or box (Box 20-1) that must be readily available and well stocked. This cart should be checked on a routine basis to ensure that all materials are available and all devices are working. Team members should know their responsibilities and be ready to react calmly.

Devices and techniques used for difficult intubation and ventilation may include different laryngoscopes blades, fiberoptic scope, light wand, Bullard scope, laryngeal mask airway (LMA), intubating stylet, retrograde intubation kit, Eschmann stylet, transtracheal jet ventilation (TTJV), and Combitube. A commercial kit is available for retrograde intubation, or the practitioner can choose to insert either a "J-wire" or #2 Mersiline suture via a cricothyrotomy and pass the device into the oropharynx. Adjunct airway equipment should be routinely used in nonemergent or practice situations to increase familiarity with the equipment and facilitate ease of use in emergent situations.

Failure to acknowledge that the patient cannot be intubated or ventilated and reluctance to accept the fact that the endotracheal tube is in the esophagus contribute to adverse outcomes. These include brain injury, death, cardiopulmonary arrest, unnecessary tracheotomy, airway trauma, and damage to teeth.[2] Continued attempts at intubation and exertion of unnecessary force can cause bleeding and edema of the mucous membranes. Ventilation can become progressively more difficult, leading to morbidity from hypoxemia and hypercarbia.

The patient with a potentially difficult airway should be optimally positioned. Pillows and blankets should be built up under the head and shoulders to afford the optimal "sniffing" position. This also provides more space for introduction of the laryngoscope blade into the mouth. Locating and marking the cricoid cartilage or cricothyroid ligament enables the assistant applying cricoid pressure to easily find the correct position and identify landmarks should a surgical airway be needed.

Preoxygenation is an essential component with the difficult airway to delay arterial desaturation during subsequent apnea. It increases the oxygen content and eliminates much of the nitrogen (79% of room air) from the functional residual capacity (FRC). Adequate preoxygenation should include having the patient breathe at normal tidal volumes for 3 to 5 minutes with a fresh gas flow of no less than 5 L and a tight mask fit.[11] This is easily accomplished by applying the face mask as soon as the patient arrives in the operating room, before the application of other monitors. If time is limited, "fast-track" preoxygenation, in which the patient takes four vital capacity breaths in 30 seconds, can be used before induction of anesthesia. This does not completely denitrogenate the blood but is useful in the emergent situation.[14]

Alternative anesthetic management options exist if a difficult airway is anticipated, including use of monitored anesthesia care (MAC) and regional anesthesia. The selection of MAC or regional anesthesia does not obviate the need to plan for management of the difficult airway. Failure of the regional block or complications resulting from placement may require emergent intubation under less than desirable conditions. It is not recommended that regional anesthesia be used for conditions in which the patient is unwilling to cooperate, the surgery cannot be quickly terminated, or access to the airway is lost.

Awake Intubation

In many situations an oral or nasal intubation while the patient is awake is the preferred method of intubating the trachea. Examples of such situations include patients with anticipated difficult airway, unstable neck fractures, halo devices, or small or limited oral openings and intubation of awake patients in the critical care setting. With proper patient preparation and a sufficiently anesthetized airway, an awake intubation can be accomplished quickly and with minimal discomfort to the patient.

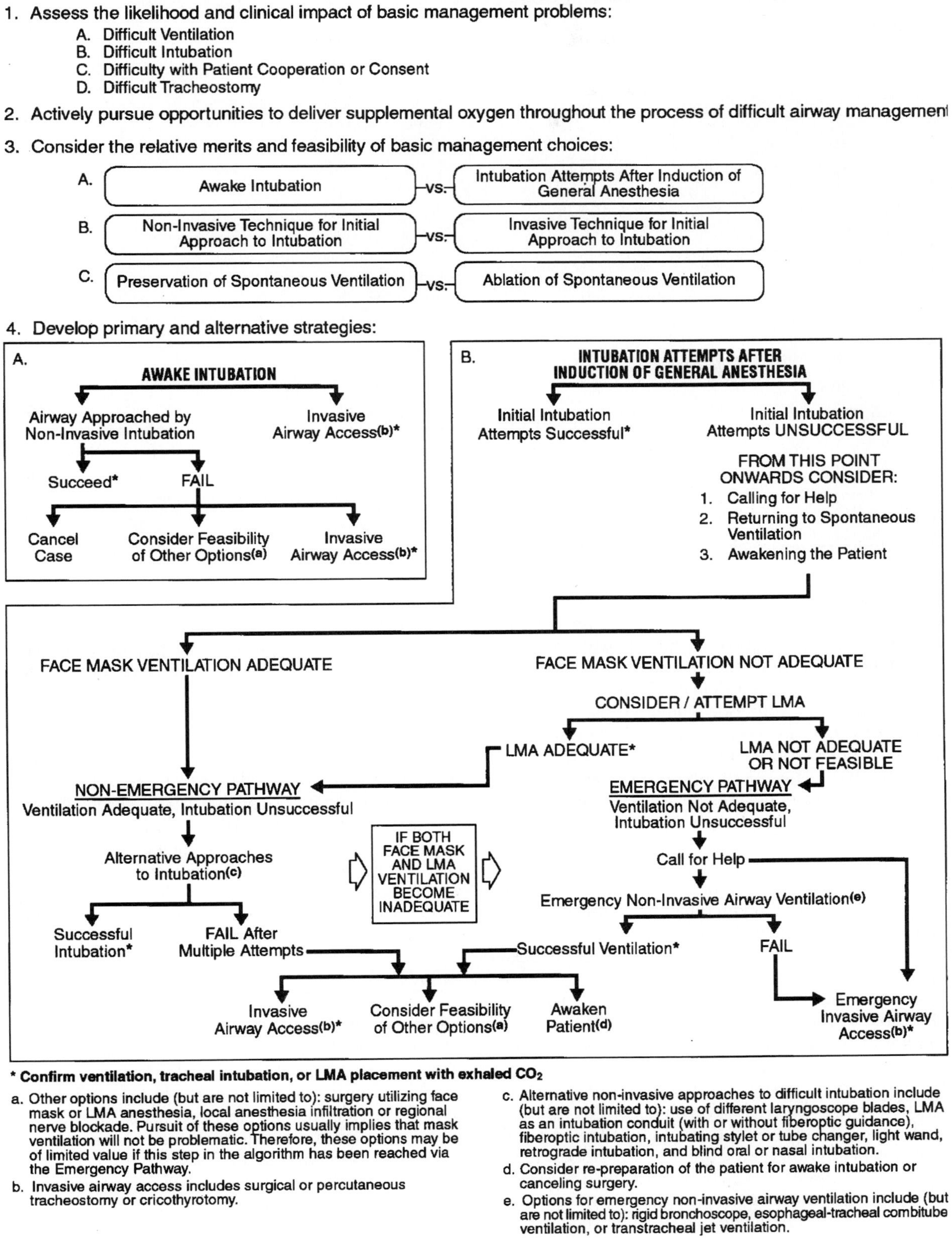

1. Assess the likelihood and clinical impact of basic management problems:
A. Difficult Ventilation
B. Difficult Intubation
C. Difficulty with Patient Cooperation or Consent
D. Difficult Tracheostomy
2. Actively pursue opportunities to deliver supplemental oxygen throughout the process of difficult airway management
3. Consider the relative merits and feasibility of basic management choices:
A. Awake Intubation vs. Intubation Attempts After Induction of General Anesthesia
B. Non-Invasive Technique for Initial Approach to Intubation vs. Invasive Technique for Initial Approach to Intubation
C. Preservation of Spontaneous Ventilation vs. Ablation of Spontaneous Ventilation
4. Develop primary and alternative strategies:
A.
AWAKE INTUBATION
Airway Approached by Non-Invasive Intubation
Invasive Airway Access(b)*
Succeed*
FAIL
Cancel Case
Consider Feasibility of Other Options(a)
Invasive Airway Access(b)*
B.
INTUBATION ATTEMPTS AFTER INDUCTION OF GENERAL ANESTHESIA
Initial Intubation Attempts Successful*
Initial Intubation Attempts UNSUCCESSFUL
FROM THIS POINT ONWARDS CONSIDER:
1. Calling for Help
2. Returning to Spontaneous Ventilation
3. Awakening the Patient
FACE MASK VENTILATION ADEQUATE
FACE MASK VENTILATION NOT ADEQUATE
CONSIDER / ATTEMPT LMA
LMA ADEQUATE*
LMA NOT ADEQUATE OR NOT FEASIBLE
NON-EMERGENCY PATHWAY
Ventilation Adequate, Intubation Unsuccessful
EMERGENCY PATHWAY
Ventilation Not Adequate, Intubation Unsuccessful
Alternative Approaches to Intubation(c)
IF BOTH FACE MASK AND LMA VENTILATION BECOME INADEQUATE
Call for Help
Emergency Non-Invasive Airway Ventilation(e)
Successful Intubation*
FAIL After Multiple Attempts
Successful Ventilation*
FAIL
Invasive Airway Access(b)*
Consider Feasibility of Other Options(a)
Awaken Patient(d)
Emergency Invasive Airway Access(b)*
* Confirm ventilation, tracheal intubation, or LMA placement with exhaled CO2
a. Other options include (but are not limited to): surgery utilizing face mask or LMA anesthesia, local anesthesia infiltration or regional nerve blockade. Pursuit of these options usually implies that mask ventilation will not be problematic. Therefore, these options may be of limited value if this step in the algorithm has been reached via the Emergency Pathway.
b. Invasive airway access includes surgical or percutaneous tracheostomy or cricothyrotomy.
c. Alternative non-invasive approaches to difficult intubation include (but are not limited to): use of different laryngoscope blades, LMA as an intubation conduit (with or without fiberoptic guidance), fiberoptic intubation, intubating stylet or tube changer, light wand, retrograde intubation, and blind oral or nasal intubation.
d. Consider re-preparation of the patient for awake intubation or canceling surgery.
e. Options for emergency non-invasive airway ventilation include (but are not limited to): rigid bronchoscope, esophageal-tracheal combitube ventilation, or transtracheal jet ventilation.

FIGURE **20-6**
The American Society of Anesthesiologists (ASA) Difficult Airway Algorithm. (From ASA Task Force on Management of the Difficult Airway. Practice guidelines for management of the difficult airway: an updated report. *Anesthesiology*. 2003;98:1269-1277.)

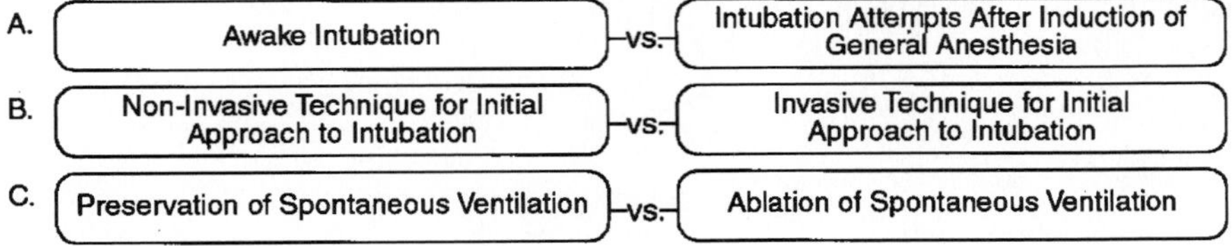

BOX **20-1**

Components of a Difficult Airway Cart

Airways—oral and nasal—various sizes
- Tongue blades
- Flexible stylets
- Endotracheal tubes—cuffed and uncuffed—2.5, 3.0, 3.5, 4.0, 4.5, 5.0, 5.5, 6.0, 7.0, 8.0 (two of each size)
- Miller laryngoscope blades—sizes 0, 1, 2, 3, 4
- Macintosh laryngoscope blades—sizes 2, 3, 4
- Laryngoscope handles—regular and stubby
- Extra laryngoscope batteries and bulbs
- Magill forceps
- Syringes—3, 5, 10, and 20 ml (three or four of each size)
- Angiocatheters—14, 16, 18, 20 gauge (three each)
- Xylocaine jelly 2%
- Surgilube
- Salem sump—16 and 18 French
- Suction catheters—10, 12, 14 French
- Nebulizer
- Atomizer
- Oxygen mask
- Nasal cannula
- Oxygen with 15 L/min regulator

Alternate airway devices
- Laryngeal mask airways—sizes 3, 4, 5
- Intubating laryngeal mask airway
- Combitube
- Lighted stylet (Trachlite) (two)
- Eschmann stylet
- Tube exchanger—small, medium, large
- Ventilating stylet
- Needle cricothyrotomy set
- Retrograde intubation set
- Melker percutaneous dilational cricothyrotomy set

Transtracheal jet ventilator

Ambu bag

Bullard or Upsher Scope

Intubating bronchoscope
- Tongue clamp
- Light source
- Endoscopy mask
- Ovassapian intubating airway

Lidocaine—4% topical, 2% for injection

Patient Preparation

For maximum cooperation to be elicited from the patient, the procedure must be clearly explained and consent obtained. It is difficult if not impossible to proceed if the patient is uncooperative or unwilling to participate. Depending on the situation and the patient's condition, judicious use of anxiolytics and narcotics may be considered. Administration of antisialogogues to dry secretions can also maximize the view of the laryngeal structures. The risk of aspiration must always be considered when the airway reflexes have been anesthetized. Initiation of aspiration prophylaxis protocols may be warranted.

The most widely used local anesthetic for anesthetizing the airway is lidocaine in various forms and concentrations. Cocaine 4%, benzocaine 20%, and tetracaine are also effective anesthetics. Peak serum lidocaine levels are highest 30 minutes after instillation. Use of lidocaine within the recommended dosage keeps serum lidocaine levels well within the acceptable range.[15,16] Vasoconstrictors are commonly used to decrease bleeding associated with nasal intubation. Cocaine 4% or solutions containing oxymetazoline 0.05% should be used before insertion of local anesthetic gels into the nares.

The nares and nasopharynx are easily anesthetized by insertion of 5 ml of lidocaine viscous down each naris. The solution "melts" and drips down the back of throat. The nares and oral pharynx may also be anesthetized by adding 2% lidocaine to either a hand-held nebulizer or a nebulizer attached to a face mask. As the patient breathes through the nose and mouth, small droplets of local anesthetic are deposited on the mucous membranes. This method also is effective for anesthetization of subglottic tissue.

Anesthetization of the mouth and oral pharynx helps decrease the gag reflex and coughing associated with awake intubations. Benzocaine spray is a topical anesthetic with a quick onset and short duration. Flavored sprays may increase salivation. A lidocaine lollipop can be made by coating the tip of a tongue blade with lidocaine ointment and then placing it on the back of the tongue to provide anesthesia to the oropharynx. Another method is to have the patient swish and gargle for 2 minutes with 2% lidocaine viscous.

Anesthetizing the vocal cords may be accomplished by instilling local anesthetic directly onto the cords or through transtracheal blocks. After the nares have been anesthetized, a nasal airway or endotracheal tube is passed and positioned in close approximation to the vocal cords. The patient is instructed to take a deep breath. On inspiration, 5 ml of 2% lidocaine are inserted down the lumen of the nasal airway. This causes the patient to cough, indicating that local anesthetic was deposited on the vocal cords. If a fiberoptic scope is to be used, local anesthetic may be administered through the injection port onto the vocal cords under direct visualization.

AIRWAY BLOCKS

Superior Laryngeal Nerve Block

The superior laryngeal nerve block is easily performed and provides a dense block of the supraglottic region. To perform the block, the practitioner locates the hyoid bone and displaces it toward the side that is being injected (Figure 20-7). This stabilizes the bone and eases identification of structures and injection of the local anesthetic. The inferior border of the cornu is palpated, and the needle is inserted perpendicular to the skin, approximately 0.25 inch caudad and 0.25 inch medially. This approximates the site at which the superior laryngeal nerve pierces the thyrohyoid membrane. Just below the subcutaneous tissue the tip of the needle may be felt to "bounce" on the thyrohyoid membrane. One to 2 ml of local anesthetic are deposited above this membrane, then the membrane is "popped through," and 2 ml of local anesthetic are deposited just below the membrane. Aspiration is performed before

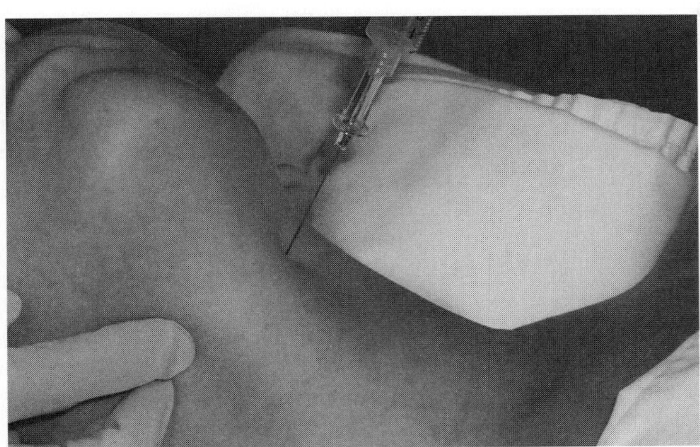

FIGURE **20-7**
Superior laryngeal nerve block.

injection of the local anesthetic. If air is obtained, the needle has been placed too deep and is in the pharynx. The tip of the needle is withdrawn and repositioned. The block is repeated on the other side.

Transtracheal Block

The transtracheal block is accomplished by injecting local anesthetic through the cricothyroid membrane (Figure 20-8). To administer the block, the practitioner attaches a 23-gauge needle or a 24-gauge angiocatheter to a syringe containing 5 ml of 2% lidocaine. While aspiration is constantly performed, the needle is advanced in a caudad direction through the cricothyroid membrane. When air bubbles up through the solution, the tip of the needle is in the tracheal lumen.

The patient usually coughs when this occurs. The patient is then instructed to take a deep breath. On inspiration the local anesthetic is injected into the tracheal lumen. This causes the patient to cough, spraying the local anesthetic onto the vocal cords. Care must be taken to stabilize the needle so as not to tear the tracheal mucosa when the patient coughs. Use of the softer angiocatheter may decrease trauma.

Glossopharyngeal Block

The lingual branch of the glossopharyngeal nerve block supplies sensory innervation to the back of the tongue (Figure 20-9). To block the lingual branch, the practitioner has the patient open his or her mouth and displaces the tongue to the opposite side with a tongue blade; this forms a gutter. Where the gutter meets the base of the palatoglossal arch, a 26-gauge spinal needle is inserted approximately 1 quarter inch. If air is obtained on aspiration, the needle has been placed too deep. If blood is obtained, the needle must be withdrawn and repositioned more medially. One to 2 ml of 2% lidocaine are injected, and the block is repeated on the other side.

CRICOID PRESSURE

The practice of using cricoid pressure in patients with full stomachs is considered the standard of care in the anesthesia community. Debate and controversy exist regarding the effectiveness of routine use of cricoid pressure in actual practice. Sellick described cricoid pressure as the posterior displacement of the cricoid cartilage against the cervical vertebrae.[17] The most recent recommendation is that cricoid pressure as a requirement for rapid sequence induction may be beneficial as long as the procedure is performed properly and does not impede effective airway management.[18]

This procedure occludes the esophagus, thereby preventing aspiration of gastric contents and insufflation of the stomach during positive pressure ventilation. However, errors are commonly made when cricoid pressure is

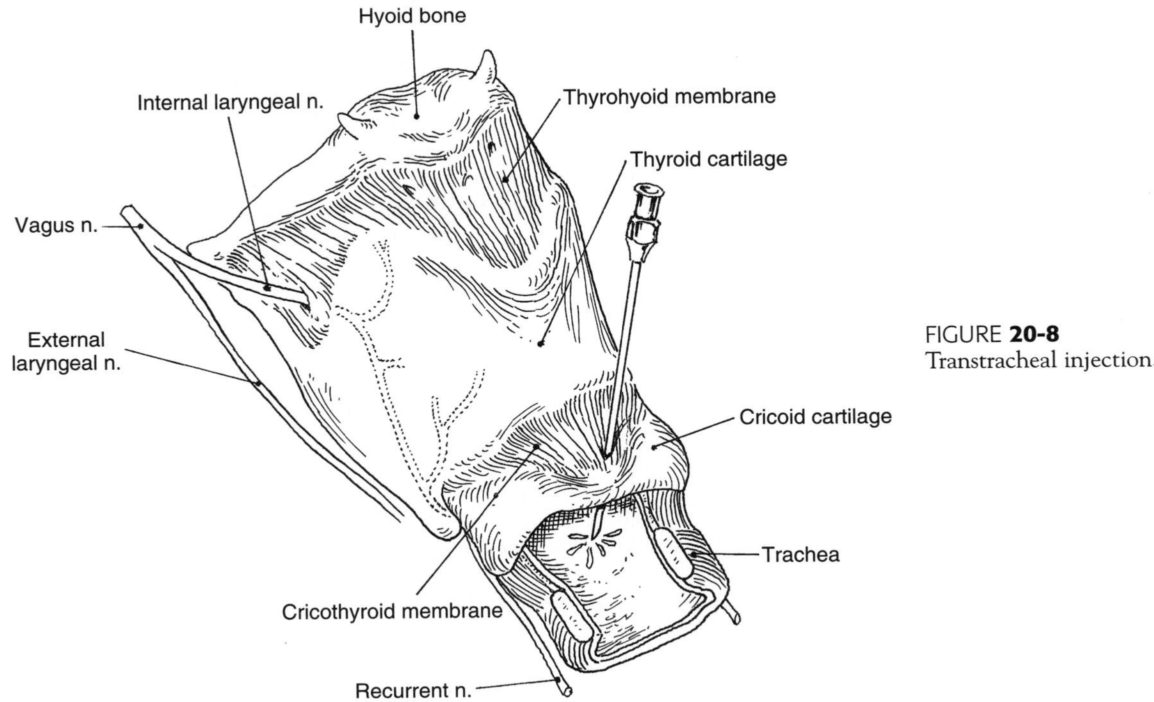

FIGURE **20-8**
Transtracheal injection.

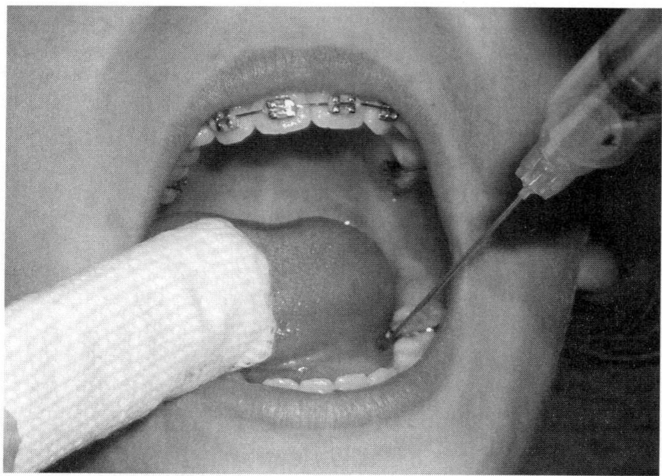

FIGURE **20-9**
Glossopharyngeal nerve block.

applied.[19,20] Inadequate force applied at the wrong anatomic position and improper timing contribute to the decreased effectiveness of cricoid pressure and put the patient at increased risk for aspiration. Application of cricoid pressure may also cause flexion of the neck and distort or deviate the trachea from midline. If pressure is applied too forcefully, difficulty in ventilation and passing of the endotracheal tube may be encountered.

The upper and lower esophageal sphincters serve as barriers to aspiration when the patient is awake. On loss of consciousness, the upper esophageal sphincter relaxes and allows for passive flow of gastric contents into the hypopharynx. Use of neuromuscular blockers further exacerbates relaxation of the upper esophageal sphincter. If aspiration is to be prevented, cricoid pressure must be applied before loss of consciousness. The recommended pressure to be exerted before loss of consciousness is 20 N, or approximately 2 kg of pressure. On loss of consciousness the pressure exerted must be increased to 44 N, or approximately 4 kg of pressure.[20] Required pressures are independent of age and sex. Also, the force applied declines steadily after 30 seconds. In the management of a difficult airway, recovery from induction drugs and neuromuscular blockers may take a significant amount of time, during which the maintenance of adequate cricoid pressure is necessary.

To add to the risk of aspiration, the lower esophageal pressure is also affected by the force of cricoid pressure. Mechanoreceptors in the esophagus are stimulated by the pressure of a bolus of food. Cricoid pressure mimics this pressure, decreasing lower esophageal pressure by 9 to 12 mm Hg.[21] Insufflation of air into the stomach during forceful mask ventilation and use of succinylcholine increase intragastric pressures, increasing the risk that the gastric contents will be expelled into the esophagus.

Assistants who apply cricoid pressure should be instructed regarding the required force of application and location of correct anatomic landmarks in noncritical situations. Inappropriately applied pressure can result in difficulty in ventilating the patient or inserting the endotracheal tube and displacement of the esophagus lateral to the larynx with no compression of the esophagus. The assistant holding cricoid pressure must be instructed to not release pressure until placement of the endotracheal tube is verified and the tube is secured in place.

When a difficult airway is anticipated, the cricoid cartilage can be marked before induction of anesthesia. Marking the cricothyroid ligament may be of additional value if a surgical airway must be established.

ADJUNCT AIRWAY EQUIPMENT AND TECHNIQUES

Over the past decades alternative airway devices and techniques have been developed and implemented for use in airway management. The devices include the LMA, endotracheal tube guides, lighted stylets, rigid laryngoscopes, indirect rigid fiberoptic laryngoscopes, and supraglottic ventilatory devices. Special airway techniques include flexible fiberoptic intubation.

Laryngeal Mask Airway

Since its introduction in the United States in 1991 the LMA has been used extensively in the administration of anesthesia. Its development has been hailed as one of the most significant advances in airway management since the endotracheal tube.[22] The LMA is a valuable airway tool in the management of the difficult airway. The literature contains anecdotal reports of the successful use of the LMA for the establishment of an airway and the provision of a conduit for intubation of the trachea.[22-24]

The LMA was used extensively in Europe, primarily in England, before its introduction in the United States. Several variations of the LMA exist, including the classic and Pro-Seal devices. In daily clinical use this airway can be used in place of mask ventilation. It is inserted blindly into the posterior pharynx until resistance is felt. At that point the LMA is positioned in the hypopharynx below the base of the tongue and above the epiglottis. If the appropriately sized LMA is selected, the resistance denotes placement of the LMA's tip in the hypopharynx, and the black line on the tubing will be even with the upper lip. The cuff is then inflated, sealing the airway over the larynx. The esophageal opening at the base of the hypopharynx has no seal. If the cuff is overinflated, it can actually open the upper esophageal sphincter. The Pro-Seal LMA is designed with a second posterior cuff that inflates, closing the hypopharynx. The LMA is designed with a second tube so that a gastric tube can be inserted into the esophagus without passing through the hypopharynx.

Familiarity with the LMA, its ease and speed of insertion, and its high likelihood of success in difficult airway situations makes it an extremely valuable rescue device. One of the concerns with the LMA is the possibility of aspiration during insertion or when the LMA is in place. The LMA devices do not prevent inflation of the stomach, regurgitation, or aspiration if the inflation pressure is too high. If ventilation is accomplished using positive pressure greater than 25 torr within the airway, the stomach becomes inflated. The device can also be malpositioned or the cuff overinflated, resulting in failure to ventilate the patient. Both malpositioning of the airway and overinflation of the cuff result in additional pressure to the sidewalls of the pharynx and pressure on the posterior wall of the larynx. When this pressure is generated, the epiglottis can be folded back against the glottic opening, sealing the airway. Pathology at or below laryngeal level may make the LMA ineffective as a supraglottic device. In obstetric anesthesia the LMA is used when tracheal intubation has failed and ventilation with face mask is difficult or impossible. Attempted use of the LMA should precede a cricothyroidotomy.

Fastrach

The Fastrach (Figure 20-10) is a new model of the LMA specifically designed to improve blind endotracheal intubation through a laryngeal mask.[24-26] It has been used successfully in the "can't intubate, can't ventilate" scenario, as well as in situations in which difficult intubation is anticipated. The design of the Fastrach allows for reasonable control of the airway throughout the intubation process, first with the laryngeal mask, then with endotracheal intubation. Most practitioners are familiar with the insertion of the LMA and adapt readily to insertion of the Fastrach. As with all adjunct airway equipment, the Fastrach should be used in routine cases to ensure familiarity with the technique before its use is attempted in an emergent situation or with a difficult airway.

Combitube

The Combitube (Figure 20-11) is a double-lumen airway device that is inserted blindly into the hypopharynx. Irrespective of where the tip is placed, the lungs may be ventilated.[27] The usual placement of the tip is into the esophagus. This blind insertion is easily accomplished, and the patient's head can be kept in the neutral position. With the cuffs of both lumens inflated, the Combitube may offer some protection from aspiration. The Combitube is a supraglottic device, and pathology at or below the laryngeal level may make the Combitube ineffective. The esophageal lumen offers a way to further decompress the stomach. To successfully insert the Combitube, cricoid pressure must be released. Reported complications include esophageal rupture. In 2002 King Systems introduced the King LT, a minimally invasive airway device similar to the Combitube. This device is inserted in a manner similar to insertion of the Combitube but has only one ventilation port.

Trachlite

The Trachlite (Figure 20-12) is a recent adaptation of the light wand or lighted stylet that uses transillumination of the neck to accomplish endotracheal intubation.[28] Because the placement of the glottic opening is anterior to the esophagus, as the light source enters the trachea a well-defined, circumscribed glow is noticed below the thyroid prominence and can be readily seen on the anterior neck. Placement of the light wand in the esophagus results in much more diffuse transillumination of the neck without this circumscribed glow. The Trachlite has a bright light source that does not require low ambient light to use. In addition, it has a retractable stylet that increases the success rate for intubation.

The success rate of the Trachlite is similar to that of conventional direct laryngoscopy. It is less affected by anterior placement of the larynx, is less stimulating than conventional laryngoscopy, and is associated with a lower incidence of sore throat. It can be used in both the anticipated and the unanticipated difficult airway in which conventional laryngoscopy has failed. Intubation of the trachea can be accomplished with a small oral opening and minimal neck manipulation.

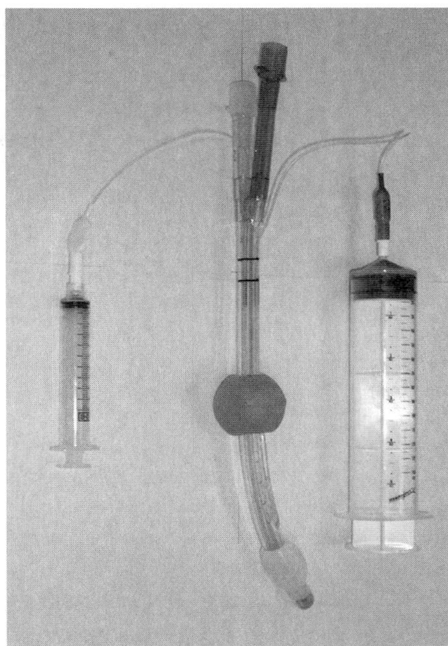

FIGURE **20-11**
Combitube.

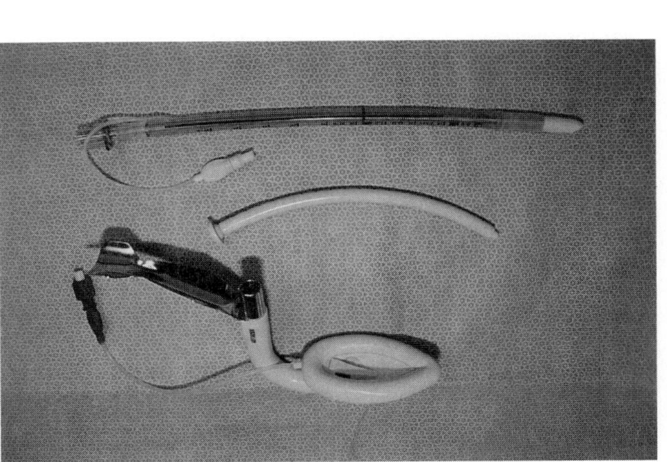

FIGURE **20-10**
Fastrach.

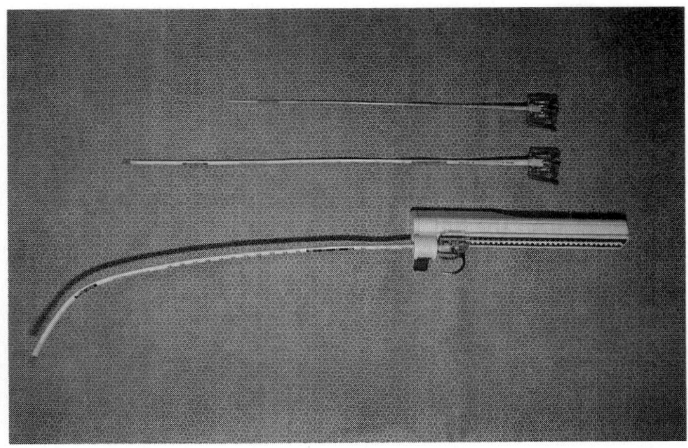

FIGURE **20-12**
Trachlite.

Because the Trachlite is inserted blindly using transillumination, risk of injury or failure is increased when the device is used in patients with any upper airway anomaly, such as foreign body, tumor, polyps, or soft-tissue injuries. If these anomalies exist, other airway adjuncts should be used. In addition, it may be more difficult to accurately place the Trachlite in patients with short, thick necks or redundant soft tissue.

Eschmann Stylet (Gum Elastic Bougie)

The Eschmann stylet (Figure 20-13) is a flexible stylet with a bent tip that can be useful when the glottic opening is difficult to visualize. The stylet is placed into the glottic opening. An endotracheal tube is inserted over the stylet and slid into place into the trachea.

Transtracheal Jet Ventilation

In the "can't intubate, can't ventilate" scenario a means to deliver oxygen must be made available if hypoxemia and other adverse outcomes are to be avoided. This can be accomplished quickly and easily with TTJV[29-32] (Figure 20-14). TTJV is a technique used to provide oxygenation using high-pressure delivery systems. TTJV systems have been used widely in anesthesia practice for surgical procedures on the airway. A large-bore intravenous (IV) catheter is inserted through the cricothyroid membrane in a caudad direction (Figure 20-15). The lungs are ventilated using a high-pressure oxygen source and a regulating valve to control oxygen flow through noncompliant tubing attached to the IV catheter. As high-flow oxygen is introduced through the catheter, air is also entrained (Venturi effect) through the upper airway. At a delivered pressure of 50 psi, a 20-gauge catheter delivers approximately 400 ml of oxygen per second, a 16-gauge catheter delivers 500 ml of oxygen per second, and a 14-gauge catheter delivers 1600 ml of oxygen per second.[33] High-pressure oxygen is delivered reliably through central wall outlets and high-flow (50 to 100 psi) tank regulators. The flush valve on anesthesia machines with a one-way outlet check valve between the vaporizer and the flush valve also delivers an adequate minute volume.[34,35] Noncompliant tubing must be placed between the catheter and the common gas outlet. Use of corrugated tubing or other compliant tubing decreases the minute volume delivered. Multiple devices are available for use in the operating room, including the Cook Emergency Cricothyrotomy kit.

Complications associated with the use of TTJV include barotrauma, tissue emphysema, and exhalation difficulties. Exhalation occurs passively through the upper airway. Obstructions to passive exhalation or excessively large tidal volumes result in hyperinflation. Placement of bilateral nasal airways or an oral airway facilitates exhalation. Use of an in-line pressure gauge and inspiration to expiration ratios of 1:2 or 1:3 decreases the incidence of barotrauma. Bilateral breath sounds should be confirmed frequently to rule out pneumothorax and subcarinal placement or dislodgment of the catheter.

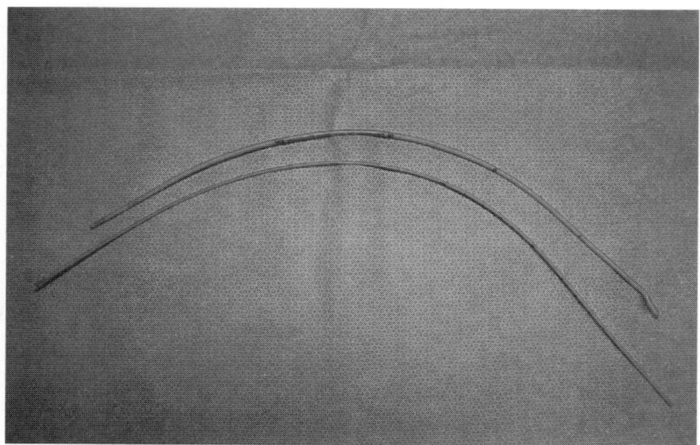

FIGURE **20-13**
Eschmann stylet.

Fiberoptic Laryngoscope

The fiberoptic bronchoscope can be used to evaluate the airway, ease intubation of the patient with a difficult airway, check placement of endotracheal tubes, change endotracheal tubes, and perform pulmonary toilet and postextubation evaluations.[36] The flexible fiberoptic laryngoscope consists of multiple strands of tiny glass fibers that carry light. These fibers are bound together inside a rubberized coating that allows for flexibility. Within the scope are working channels that can act as suctions ports or be used to instill local anesthetic or carry oxygen. The

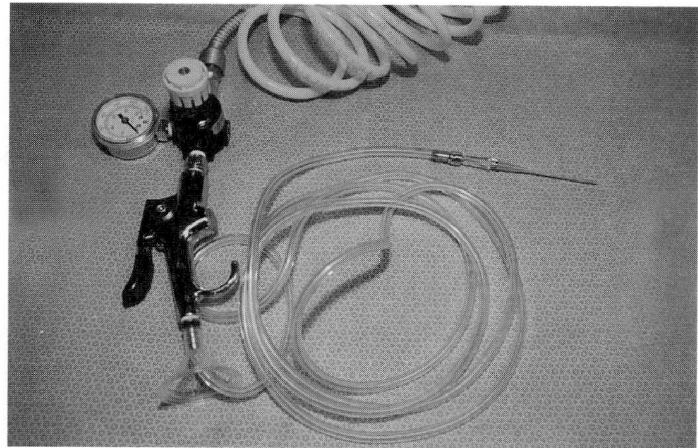

FIGURE **20-14**
Transtracheal jet ventilation.

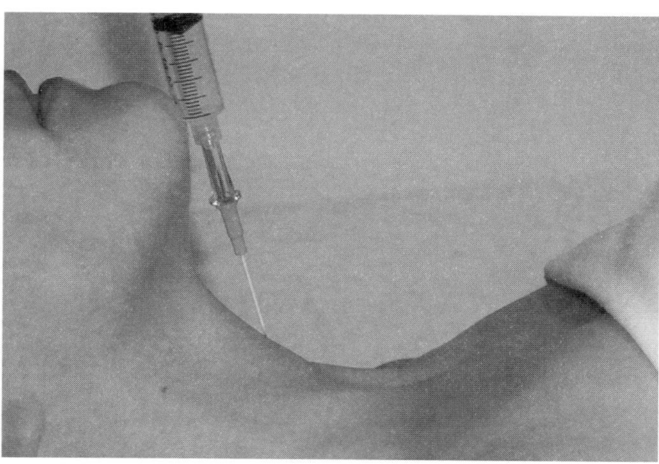

FIGURE **20-15**
Insertion of needle for transtracheal jet ventilation.

handle contains an eyepiece for viewing and a lever for controlling the distal end of the scope through one plane. The second plane is navigated by turning the scope. Light is supplied by an external light source or most recently by battery.

Limitations of the fiberoptic laryngoscope include the following:

1. The scope can become fogged, especially if it is cold. Soaking the scope in warm saline before use may help prevent this.
2. Limitation of view can result when multiple fiberoptic strands are broken or damaged. The scope should never be banged or dropped and should always be stored flat in a protective case or cart.
3. Vision can be obstructed by secretions or blood. This can be prevented with the instillation of 10 to 15 L of oxygen per minute through one of the side channels.

The fiberoptic bronchoscope can be used for oral or nasal intubation with the patient either awake or asleep. For awake intubation, instillation of local anesthesia or nerve blocks should be accomplished as previously described. With oral intubations, a bite block should be used to prevent damage to the fibers caused by the patient's biting of the scope.

When the fiberoptic bronchoscope is prepared for use, a cart should be dedicated to the equipment. The light source and extension cord should be securely mounted to the cart, along with any outlet adapters required, suction devices, and oxygen delivery systems. Oral airways, irrigation catheters, and suction catheters or devices, as well as other equipment used in the management of the airway, should be placed on the cart and labeled. Practitioners should use the equipment frequently to ensure that they are comfortable with it and to verify that the devices are functionally ready for use.

A Yankauer suction device must be available and set up whenever the fiberoptic bronchoscope is used. Medications used in airway management should be readily available. These include local anesthetics, resuscitation drugs, induction agents, and muscle relaxants. If the equipment is to be used outside of the operating room, the appropriate monitors should be on the cart as well. This cart can become the central location for all emergency airway devices including the TTJV and LMAs.

Debate and controversy exist regarding the administration of drying agents and sedation. Atropine or glycopyrrolate may be administered 5 to 20 minutes before the beginning of the procedure. Administration of light sedation (midazolam 0.04 mg/kg) to the patient may help reduce the patient's stress and provide for a more relaxed environment for the practitioner. Some practitioners routinely administer narcotics as an adjunct to midazolam, although this practice must be a cautious choice whenever control of the airway is in doubt. The most widely used sedation-analgesia technique seems to be administration of fentanyl and midazolam, carefully titrated in small bolus doses. A short-acting and easily titratable opioid such as remifentanil is an alternative choice for the intensely stimulating, but usually brief, airway manipulation during fiberoptic nasotracheal intubation.[37]

The fiberoptic scope is first inserted through the endotracheal tube and is then inserted through either the mouth or the nose and advanced to the posterior pharynx. Care must be taken to keep the tube and scope in the midline while the tip is advanced toward the epiglottis. Instillation of oxygen through the suction port not only aids in the oxygenation of the patient but also helps keep the optics clear. The anesthetist can manipulate the scope in two planes by rotating the lever on the right side of the handle back and forth and by rotating the scope laterally. The tip of the scope is slipped through the epiglottis and advanced until the tracheal rings come into view. The endotracheal tube is slipped downward, with the scope used as a stylet, and then through the cords. Care must be taken to ensure that the tube does not damage the rubber coating of the scope.

One way to gain experience with the device is to use it routinely to secure the airway in controlled intubation procedures in class I and II airway patients. After the induction of anesthesia and the securing of the airway, the evaluation of the airway and tube placement can be accomplished using the fiberoptic bronchoscope. Use of the fiberoptic bronchoscope to observe airway landmarks in the pharynx and the epiglottis can help the practitioner become acquainted with the anatomy. Additionally, intubation mannequins made by Laerdal and Ambu can be used to practice intubation techniques with this equipment.

Suctioning is almost impossible through the suction port. A more advantageous use of this channel is to provide the patient with supplemental oxygen. A 2- to 4-L flow through this port provides the patient with up to 26% oxygen insufflation and keeps debris from collecting on or near the port and lens. Another use of this port can be the administration of local anesthesia through an epidural catheter that is threaded down the port.

The fiberoptic bronchoscope is contraindicated in patients with epiglottis, laryngotracheitis, or bacterial tracheitis. The manipulation of the fiberoptic bronchoscope through the glottis may cause enough stimulation to convert a partial obstruction into a total obstruction of the airway. Caution should be strictly exercised in patients with airway burns because of the restricted size and the hyperirritability of the airway. Special care should be used in patients who have been irradiated. Radiation can cause fibrosis and loss of mucous-producing glands, so drying of the airway can be extensive with the use of either glycopyrrolate or atropine. The use of the fiberoptic bronchoscope is very limited in airway trauma. The presence of blood and mucus in the airway obscures the lens and makes visualization impossible. If significant soft-tissue trauma is present, the edema of the tissues can prevent adequate visualization of the larynx and trachea.

Additionally, all personnel who will be using the device should be trained in its care and cleaning. The fibers in the bronchoscope are very fragile. Bending, curling, or any other type of kinking of the scope will break the fibers. Cleaning is very important. All of the channels, suction and injection, must be cleaned thoroughly after each use. This requires flushing with warm saline immediately after use. The manufacturers will indicate which detergent and sterilizing solution they recommend. Instructions regarding solution, dilution, soak times, and rinsing must be closely followed to ensure the integrity of the equipment. After external washing is performed, a small bottle brush is used to clean the channels. This brush is usually supplied with the device, but it does not hurt to buy several extras. Flushing with warm water after cleaning is mandatory.

Retrograde Intubation

This procedure is performed by inserting a 14- to 18-gauge IV catheter or a Cook needle through the cricothyroid membrane and directing it cephalad. A wire or suture is inserted through the needle and passed cephalad until it can be seen and passed through the mouth or nose. The distal end of the wire is secured with a clamp to prevent the wire from being pulled into the trachea prematurely. An endotracheal tube can be directed over the wire and passed into the trachea. As the tube enters the larynx, tension is increased on the wire or suture. When this occurs, the distal wire is cut at the level of the skin and permitted to pass into the trachea. The tube is passed into the trachea and secured in place. This is not an emergent process and often can be completed by a skilled practitioner in 5 to 7 minutes.

Percutaneous Cricothyrotomy

Percutaneous cricothyrotomy allows emergency oxygenation through insertion of a 14-gauge IV catheter through the cricothyroid membrane. Oxygen can be instilled by inserting the barrel of a 3-ml syringe into the proximal end of the IV needle and connecting this to an oxygen supply via the connector from a 7-mm endotracheal tube. The oxygen flow must be provided through TTJV or a rigid bronchoscope. A needle cricothyrotomy can provide a patient with oxygenation for 30 minutes while a tracheotomy is performed.

An incision can also be made at the level of the cricothyroid membrane, and a small endotracheal tube inserted to ventilate the patient. The midline of the cricothyroid membrane is relatively avascular for approximately 0.5 cm on either side of the midline. This distance is also the approximate size of a #20 knife blade.

Tracheotomy

An additional technique for securing the airway in the patient with airway problems is the tracheotomy. This surgical intervention is not a procedure that is performed by an anesthetist. In certain cases, such as patients with facial and neck trauma when a difficult airway is anticipated, a surgical consultation should be requested as part of the patient assessment and anesthesia plan. The standard tracheotomy is performed at the level of the fourth to sixth tracheal ring, below the isthmus of the thyroid gland. This procedure can take up to 30 minutes. If a need to perform a tracheotomy exists, then the airway should be secured first, or the procedure performed with the patient under a local anesthetic.

Extubation

Extubating the trachea at the completion of surgery depends on a number of factors, which including the type of airway anatomy encountered during induction, the type of surgery, and the potential for bleeding or severe airway edema. Criteria for extubation provide guidelines for safe removal of the endotracheal tube. The same care taken to secure the airway should be exercised when control of the airway is returned to the patient. Extubation may occur when the patient is in a deep plane of anesthesia, awakening, or fully awake. Extubation criteria commonly used in patients undergoing general anesthesia with neuromuscular blockers include an adequate tidal volume and rate; ability to open eyes widely on command with no diplopia; demonstration of sustained protrusion and purposeful movement of the tongue; ability to swallow effectively; completion of sustained head or leg lift for at least 5 seconds (in small children a strong knee to chest movement is equivalent); demonstration of a strong, constant hand grip; presence of effective cough; adequate vital capacity of at least 15 ml/kg; and inspiratory force of at least 25 to 30 cm H_2O negative pressure. The neuromuscular monitor must also identify a sustained tetanic response to 50 Hz for 5 seconds, train-of-four ratio >0.90 with no fade, and no fade to double burst stimulation.

The patient who was difficult to ventilate or intubate should be fully awake, able to follow commands, and have all protective reflexes present before extubation. Guidelines for extubating patients with a difficult airway are noted in the American Society of Anesthesiologists (ASA) Difficult Airway Algorithm.[2] One of the suggestions is the use of a device over which the endotracheal tube is removed, such as a fiberoptic bronchoscope, a jet stylet, or a gum-elastic bougie. Because these devices may not be suitable in very small infants, the use of a guide wire from the Cook airway exchange catheter (CAEC; Cook, Inc., Bloomington, Indiana) has been described. This guide wire is 0.018 inch and permits the use of the 8 Fr CAEC, over which a 3.0 endotracheal tube can be passed. This technique of leaving a device in the trachea in the patient with a difficult airway has proved useful in a number of reports.

COMPLICATIONS OF TRACHEAL INTUBATION

Airway Mishaps

Complications from intubation can occur at any point during management of the airway (Table 20-5). Intubation attempts during light anesthesia, numerous attempts at intubation, or prolonged intubations are only a few of the reasons complications occur.[38] Gentle manipulation of the airway, adequate preparation, and vigilance are all required to decrease the incidence and severity of complications. Laryngeal swelling can be caused by placement of an endotracheal tube (ETT) that significantly contributes to the increment of laryngeal resistance. Laryngeal resistance increases because of anatomic narrowing of the laryngeal aperture (anatomic mechanisms) or imbalance between the abductor and adductor of the vocal cords (neural mechanisms). The increased laryngeal resistance may not manifest clinical symptoms in subjects with normal preoperative laryngeal function. However, the results should be taken seriously, prompting routine airway management procedures with ETTs, particularly in patients with preoperative laryngeal

TABLE 20-5 Causes of Injury and Complications of Intubation

Cause of Injury	Complications of Intubation
Physical	
Tube induced	Nasal mucosal damage; turbinate fractures; dissection of the posterior pharyngeal wall; sore throat; hoarseness; granulomas; tracheal mucosa damage leading to scarring and strictures; endobronchial intubation; pressure injuries to the recurrent laryngeal, laryngeal, or hypoglossal nerves
Laryngoscopy	Hypertension, tachycardia, bradycardia, dental trauma, spinal cord trauma, aspiration, corneal abrasion
Mechanical	
Obstruction resulting from kinking, dried secretions	Negative pressure pulmonary edema, hypoxia, hypercarbia
Disconnect	Hypoxia, hypercarbia
Airway fire	Airway burns, pulmonary edema

narrowing and small children who may have no clinical symptoms preoperatively.

Esophageal Intubation

Unrecognized esophageal intubation can lead to catastrophic complications from hypoxia. Signs of an esophageal intubation include absence of breath sounds over the lung fields, a gurgling over the epigastrum with progressive distention of the abdomen, and lack of sustained end-tidal CO_2 on the capnogram. Signs of hypoxemia may not readily appear because of preoxygenation of the patient. Once an esophageal intubation has been recognized and corrected, the stomach should be decompressed to decrease the risk of aspiration.

Endobronchial Intubation

When the endotracheal tube is placed too deeply, it may migrate into a mainstem bronchus. In adults endobronchial intubation most commonly occurs in the right mainstem bronchus. The distance to the right upper lobe is short, and a right mainstem intubation may also occlude the right upper lobe.

Signs of an endobronchial intubation include increased peak inspiratory pressures, uneven chest excursion, decreased breath sounds on the unventilated side, a drop in the end-tidal CO_2 concentration, tachycardia, and hypoxemia. If endobronchial intubation is suspected, the balloon on the endotracheal tube should be deflated and withdrawn until bilateral breath sounds are heard. The fiberoptic scope may be used to confirm placement of the tube.

Risks of Intubation

Trauma to the structures of the upper and lower airway and the neck can occur during placement of the endotracheal tube.[38] Careful positioning, proper depth of anesthesia, and gentle manipulation of the airway limit the incidence of injury.

The endotracheal tube is often a cause of injury. The larger the diameter of the tube and the longer it is left in place, the greater the incidence of injury. Most susceptible to injury are the arytenoids, the posterior half of the vocal cords, and the posterior tracheal wall (Figure 20-16). The natural curve of the endotracheal tube rests on these structures and can cause desquamation, inflammation, and ulceration of the tissue. Formation of scar tissue over areas of ulceration may lead to tracheal stenosis. Granuloma formation on scar tissue most often occurs on the posterior wall of the trachea (Figure 20-17). The most common injuries are as follows:

1. Injuries to lips, gums, and soft tissues of the oral cavity caused by insertion of the laryngoscope.
2. Dental trauma from the laryngoscope, causing teeth to be chipped, broken, or loosened. All possible attempts should be made to find the missing fragments so that they are not aspirated. If not all fragments are found, radiographs of the chest and abdomen must be taken to check for aspiration.
3. Nasal intubation can result in nosebleed. This can be prevented by progressive dilation of the nasal passage with progressively larger, well-lubricated nasal airways. Use of a vasodilator such as NeoSynephrine or Afrin is recommended.
4. Puncture or tearing of the trachea can result when a stylet is used. The tip should never protrude beyond the end of the endotracheal tube or through the Murphy's eye.

Nasal intubation carries the additional risks of turbinate fractures, hemorrhage, laceration of the nasal mucosa, and dissection of the adenoids. Prolonged intubation may contribute to infection of the paranasal sinuses.

Endotracheal Tube Obstruction

The endotracheal tube can become obstructed by foreign materials or mechanically obstructed by the patient. The obstruction can be partial or complete. Obstruction may be more troublesome with spontaneous ventilation because positive-pressure ventilation overcomes some of the increased resistance. This obstruction, especially in young, healthy patients, can lead to negative pressure pulmonary edema (NPPE). NPPE is caused by the movement of fluid from the interstitial space of the lung into the plural cavity. Treatment includes administration of diuretics and positive pressure ventilation.

Some of the possible causes of obstruction include the following:

1. *Biting.* A partially anesthetized patient may react to the presence of an endotracheal tube by biting down. This action may partially or totally occlude the endotracheal tube. This can be prevented by insertion of an oral airway or bite block.
2. *Kinking.* Kinks are one of the most common causes of endotracheal tube obstruction and may occur anywhere along the length of the tube. The tube may be kinked because of the patient's position or because increased weight distal to the patient causes the tube to kink at the patient's mouth. If the anesthetist does not have immediate access to the airway

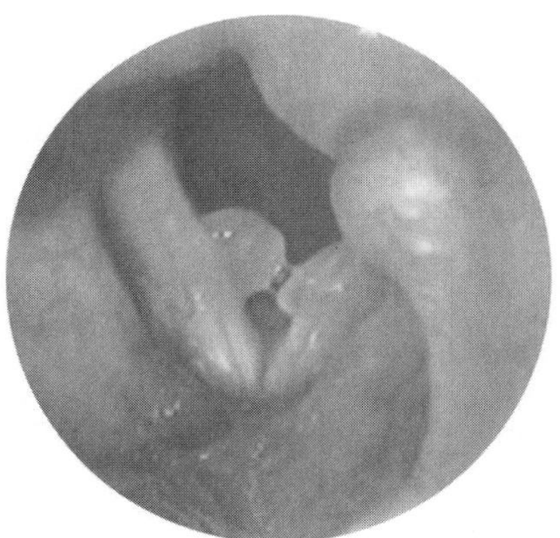

FIGURE **20-16**
Fiberoptic view of vocal cord polyps.

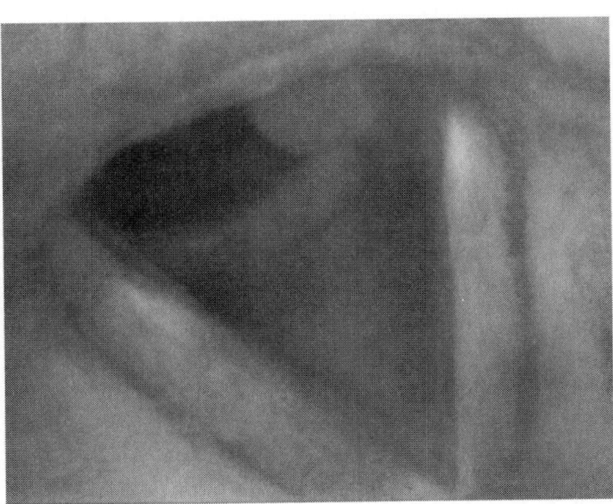

FIGURE **20-17**
Fiberoptic view of granuloma.

because of surgical positioning, use of an armored or reinforced endotracheal tube should be considered.

3. *Foreign materials.* As the endotracheal tube passes through the pharynx, any number of substances can be picked up and cause obstruction. These substances include mucus, blood, pus, and tissue.

Endotracheal Tube Ignition

With the use of lasers becoming common in laryngeal surgery, the possibility of tracheal tube fires has increased. Direct penetration of the tube (combustible material) with the laser (ignition source) in the presence of an oxygen-rich environment (O_2 greater than 21%) (Oxidizer) involves all of the three components required for fire. Special endotracheal tubes, avoidance of nitrous oxide, and use of lower oxygen concentrations are recommended anytime.

Sore Throat

Sore throat is the most common postoperative anesthesia complaint. It usually is transient and not severe. Factors contributing to a sore throat include endotracheal tube size, difficulty with the intubation, use of a nasogastric tube, female gender, and a history of smoking. The use of local anesthetic lubricants has not been shown to be effective in prevention and may in fact increase the incidence of a sore throat. The best prevention is a careful, gentle technique when inserting the endotracheal tube and the placement of as few tubes as possible through the pharynx.

Laryngospasm

Forceful, involuntary spasm of the laryngeal musculature occurs through sensory stimulation of the superior laryngeal nerve and afferent responses from the RLN. Laryngospasm can be caused by either secretions or stimulation of the larynx while the patient is in a light plan of anesthesia. In the awakening patient, it can be lessened by extubation when the patient is either in a deeper plane of anesthesia or fully awake. Extubation should occur during a full tidal volume breath as the patient exhales, so that any secretions are projected out of the airway.

Laryngospasm consists of two phases—a "shutter" mechanism that results in partial airway obstruction, followed by a "ball-valve" mechanism in which complete obstruction occurs.[39] The shutter mechanism reflects adduction of the vocal cords, whereas the ball-valve mechanism entails constriction of the false vocal cords and supraglottic soft tissue. Treatment of a partial or shutter laryngospasm includes the administration of gentle positive-pressure ventilation with 100% oxygen (10 to 20 cm H_2O pressure). Care must be taken not to force air into the esophagus or stomach, causing gastric distention. If the condition persists, administration of lidocaine or succinylcholine 0.1 mg/kg IV may be necessary. The treatment of a full or ball-valve laryngospasm requires an intubating dose of succinylcholine (1 to 2 mg/kg IV or 4 mg/kg administered intramuscularly).

Croup

Croup can be caused by postintubation edema around the glottic and subglottic regions. Croup is more common in children than in adults because children have smaller airways. This condition is often associated with multiple intubation attempts, a large endotracheal tube without an air leak, or exaggerated movement of the patient's head. Croup usually occurs within 3 hours of extubation. Symptoms include respiratory stridor and a barking cough. Treatment is aimed at reducing swelling by inhalation of cool, moist oxygen, dexamethasone 0.1 to 0.5 mg/kg, and inhalation of racemic epinephrine (0.5 ml of a 2.25% solution in 2.5 ml of normal saline).

DIFFICULT AIRWAY IN OBSTETRIC ANESTHESIA

Case Presentation

A healthy primigravida has developed sustained fetal bradycardia. The decision is made to proceed with an emergency cesarean section. Anesthesia is induced with sodium thiopental and succinylcholine. The laryngoscopic view is grade III, and a blind attempt at intubation is made. It is immediately apparent that the endotracheal tube is in the esophagus. The tube is removed, the head is repositioned, and a second attempt is made, resulting in another esophageal intubation. Mask ventilation has become increasingly difficult, and the SaO_2 is 80 and falling. What is the next step?

Defining the Problem

This case demonstrates the challenges of providing obstetric anesthesia care. Maternal mortality in the United States has remained approximately 7.5 maternal deaths per 100,000 live births over the last 15 years.[40] Anesthesia-related problems are the sixth leading cause of maternal mortality. General anesthesia carries a higher risk than regional anesthesia in obstetric patients, primarily because airway management is more difficult in obstetric patients. Airway problems are by far the most common cause of anesthesia-related death. The incidence of failed intubation in obstetric patients is 1:280, whereas the incidence of failed intubation in the general operating room is 1:2230.[41] The primary causes of maternal death are related to aspiration, complications from failed or difficult intubations, local anesthetic toxicity, and high regional blocks.

The Obstetric Airway

Because of the dynamic nature of obstetrics, a thorough airway examination should be performed on every parturient who requests anesthesia services. A stable patient may quickly deteriorate and require emergent interventions. Obstetric patients have classic changes of the airway. By virtue of their age they are likely to have full dentition. Edema of the airway structures and soft tissues may limit visualization and access to the laryngeal opening. In addition to weight gain, breast tissue is enlarged and engorged and may interfere with the introduction of the laryngoscope into the patient's mouth or with the practitioner's vision during laryngoscopy. The gravid uterus pushes up against the diaphragm, making full diaphragmatic excursion difficult and decreasing the FRC of the lungs. Oxygen consumption is increased by approximately 20% during pregnancy. During active labor it is increased an additional 23%. These factors contribute to rapid desaturation once oxygen delivery is interrupted, as it is during laryngoscopy.

Aspiration Syndrome

Hormonal changes during pregnancy delay emptying of the stomach and increase gastric volume and acid content. It is estimated that 45% of pregnant patients at term have reflux corresponding to moderate to severe heartburn. A gravid uterus can increase intragastric pressures up to 17 cm H_2O. Multiple gestations, polyhydramnios, and obesity can increase intragastric pressures up to 40 cm H_2O. Medications commonly used in anesthesia, such as narcotics, benzodiazepines, and anticholinergics, decrease the lower esophageal sphincter tone, further increasing aspiration risk.

After a failed intubation attempt, intermittent mask ventilation is necessary to provide oxygenation. Positive pressure ventilation may result in gastric insufflation, further increasing intragastric pressure. Peak airway pressures less than 15 cm H_2O rarely cause gastric insufflation. As higher pressures are required for ventilation (greater than 25 cm H_2O), gastric insufflation occurs. Cricoid pressure (Sellick maneuver) is used universally to decrease the incidence of passive regurgitation and to prevent gastric insufflation. Application of appropriate cricoid pressure allows the use of peak airway pressures up to approximately 45 cm H_2O.

Aspiration Prophylaxis

Aspiration remains a significant cause of morbidity and mortality in obstetrics. Interventions should be taken to prevent the occurrence of this potentially catastrophic complication. Whenever possible, regional anesthesia should be considered for cesarean delivery. Methods to reduce the acidity and volume of gastric contents may reduce maternal morbidity should aspiration occur. The administration of nonparticulate antacids such as sodium citrate in a 30-ml dose 10 to 20 minutes before induction of anesthesia effectively raises gastric pH. A histamine blocking agent (e.g., ranitidine) administered preoperatively either orally or IV is effective in raising gastric pH. Metoclopramide (10 mg) accelerates gastric emptying. Although the onset of action after IV administration occurs within minutes, sufficient time must be given for gastric emptying to be complete. In a synthesis of the data from several large-scale clinical studies and revised practice recommendations, revisions in the standard practices with regard to aspiration prophylaxis were noted.[42] These included the following:

1. The use of gastric fluid volume of >0.4 ml/kg (25 ml/70 kg) and pH <2.5 should be abandoned as surrogate end points for aspiration risk.
2. Cricoid pressure as a requirement for rapid sequence induction may be beneficial as long as it is performed properly and does not impede effective airway management.
3. Patients should be ventilated during a rapid sequence induction. There is no evidence that smooth, controlled light ventilation increases the incidence of aspiration. Prolonged periods of apnea should be abandoned.

SUMMARY

Airway management is a critical component of anesthesia practice. Knowledge of anatomy, equipment, and techniques is paramount if safe airway management is to be provided. Adherence to established standards and protocols including the Difficult Airway Algorithm could minimize complications. Competence and skill with a variety of airway management techniques will facilitate the appropriate management when a difficult airway situation occurs.

REFERENCES

1. Miller CG. Management of the difficult intubation in closed malpractice claims. ASA Newsletter. 2000;64:1-6. Available at: http://www.asahq.org/Newsletters/2000/06_management0600.html. Accessed Feb. 17, 2004.
2. Practice guidelines for management of the difficult airway: an updated report by the American Society of Anesthesiologists Task Force on Management of the Difficult Airway. *Anesthesiology*. 2003;98:1269-1277.
3. Gray H. *Anatomy of the Human Body*. 30th ed. Philadelphia: Lea & Febiger; 1984.
4. Moore K. *Clinically Oriented Anatomy*. 3rd ed. Philadelphia: Williams & Wilkins; 1992.
5. Wilson ME, Spiegelhalter D, Robertson JA, Lesser P. Predicting difficult intubation. *Br J Anaesth*. 1988;61:211-216.
6. Yamamoto K, Tsubokawa T, Shibata K, et al. Predicting difficult intubation with indirect laryngoscopy. *Anesthesiology*. 1997;86:316-321.
7. Khan ZH, Kashfi A, Ebranhimkhani B. A comparison of the upper lip bite test with the Mallampati classification in predicting difficult airway in endotracheal intubation: a prospective double blind study. *Anesth Analg*. 2003;96:595-599.
8. Karkouti K, Rose DK, Wigglesworth D, et al. Predicting difficult intubation: a multivariate analysis. *Can J Anaesth*. 2000;47:730-739.
9. Karkouti K, Rose DK, Ferris LE, Wigglesworth DF, Meisami-Fard T, Lee H. Inter-observer reliability of ten tests used for predicting difficult tracheal intubation. *Can J Anaesth*. 1996;43:554-559.
10. Frerk CM, Till CB, Bradley AJ. Difficult intubation: thyromental distance and the atlanto-occipital gap. *Anaesthesia*. 1996;51:738-740.
11. Mallampati SR, et al. A clinical sign to predict difficult tracheal intubation: a prospective study. *Can J Anaesth*. 1985;32:429-434.
12. Domino KB, Posner KL, Caplan RA, Cheney FW. Airway injury during anesthesia: a closed claims analysis. *Anesthesiology*. 1999;91:1703-1711.
13. Crosby ET, Cooper RM, Douglas MJ, et al. The unanticipated difficult airway with recommendations for management. *Can J Anaesth*. 1998;45:757-776.
14. Nimmagadda U, Chiravuri SD, Salem MR, et al. Preoxygenation with tidal volume and deep breathing techniques: the impact of duration breathing and fresh gas flow. *Anesth Analg*. 2001;92:1337-1341.
15. Parkes SB, Butler CS, Muller R. Plasma lignocaine concentration following nebulization for awake intubation. *Anaesth Intensive Care*. 1997;25:369-371.
16. Milman N, Laub M, Munch EP, Angelo HR. Serum concentrations of lignocaine and its metabolite monoethylglucinexylidide during fiber-optic bronchoscopy in local anaesthesia. *Respir Med*. 1998;92:40-43.
17. Sellick BA. Cricoid pressure to control regurgitation of stomach contents during induction of anesthesia. *Lancet*. 1961;2:404-406.
18. Herman NL, Carter B, Van Decar TK. Cricoid pressure: teaching the recommended pressure. *Anesth Analg*. 1996;83:859-863.
19. Tournadre JP, et al. Cricoid cartilage pressure decreases lower esophageal sphincter tone. *Anesthesiology*. 1997;86:7-9.
20. Lichtwarck-Aschoff M, Helmer A, Kawati R, et al. Good short-term agreement between measured and calculated tracheal pressure. *Br J Anaesth*. 2003;91:239-248.
21. Asai T, Morris S. Cricoid pressure impedes placement of the laryngeal mask airway. *Br J Anaesth*. 1995;74:521-525.
22. Tanaka A, et al. Laryngeal resistance before and after minor surgery: endotracheal tube versus laryngeal mask airway. *Anesthesiology*. 2003;99:252.
23. Cook TM, McCormick B, Asai T. Randomized comparison of laryngeal tube with classic laryngeal mask airway for anaesthesia with controlled ventilation. *Br J Anaesth*. 2003;91:373-378.
24. Joo H, Rose K. Fastrach—a new intubating laryngeal mask airway: successful use in patients with difficult airways. *Can J Anaesth*. 1998;45:253-256.
25. Ferson DZ, Rosenblatt WH, Johansen MJ, et al. Use of the intubating LMA-Fastrach in 254 patients with difficult-to-manage airways. *Anesthesiology*. 2001;95:1175-1181.
26. Fukutome T, et al. Tracheal intubation through the intubating laryngeal mask airway (LMA Fastrach) in patients with difficult airways. *Anaesth Intensive Care*. 1998;26:387-391.

27. Blostein PA, Koestner AJ, Hoak S. Failed rapid sequence intubation in trauma patients: esophageal tracheal Combitube is a useful adjunct. *J Trauma*. 1998;44:534-537.
28. Sdrales L, Benumof JL. Prevention of kinking of a percutaneous transtracheal intravenous catheter. *Anesthesiology*. 1995;82:288-291.
29. Petty WC. Establish the airway; use percutaneous high-pressure transtracheal jet ventilation in an emergency [letter]. *AANA J*. 1993;61:349.
30. Somerson SJ, Sicilia MR. AANA journal course: update for nurse anesthetists—beyond the laryngoscope; advanced techniques for difficult airway management. *AANA J*. 1993;61:64-71.
31. Biro P, Moe KS. Emergency transtracheal jet ventilation in high-grade airway obstruction [letter]. *J Clin Anesth*. 1997;9:604-607.
32. Smith RB, Albin MS, Williams RL. Percutaneous transtracheal jet ventilation [letter]. *J Clin Anesth*. 1996;8:689-690.
33. Gaughan SD, Ozaki GT, Benumof JL. A comparison in a lung model of low and high flow regulators for transtracheal jet ventilation. *Anesthesiology*. 1992;77:189-199.
34. Ho AM. A simple anesthesia machine driven transtracheal jet ventilation system. *Anesth Analg*. 1994;78:405-406.
35. Gaughan SD, Benumof JL, Ozaki GT. Can an anesthesia machine flush valve provide for effective jet ventilation? *Anesth Analg*. 1993;76:800-808.
36. Liem EB, Bjoraaker DG, Gravenstein D. New options for airway management: intubating fiberoptic stylets. *Br J Anaesth*. 2003;91:408-418.
37. Machata AM, Gonano C, Holzer A, et al. Awake nasotracheal fiberoptic intubation: patient comfort, intubating conditions, and hemodynamic stability during conscious sedation with remifentanil. *Anesth Analg*. 2003;97:904-908.
38. Weber S. Traumatic complications of airway management. *Anesthesiol Clin North Am*. 2002;20:265-274.
39. Landsman IS. Mechanism and treatment of laryngospasm. *Anesthesiol Clin North Am*. 2002;20:67-73.
40. Hawkins JL. Maternal mortality: anesthetic implications. *Int Anesthesiol Clin*. 2002;40:1-11.
41. Ross BK. ASA closed claims in obstetrics: lessons learned. *Anesthesiol Clin North Am*. 2003;21:183-197.
42. Nagelhout JJ. AANA Journal Course Update for Nurse Anesthetists Aspiration prophylaxis: is it time for some changes in our practice? *AANA J*. 2003;71:299-303.

CHAPTER 21

Cardiovascular Anatomy, Physiology, and Pathophysiology

Sass Elisha

CARDIOVASCULAR SYSTEM

Knowledge of anatomy and physiology of the cardiovascular system is essential to anesthesia practice. Every anesthetic agent has either a direct or an indirect effect on the cardiovascular system. Therefore, whether the nurse anesthetist is concerned about a sympathectomy and a decrease in blood pressure during neuroaxial blockade or myocardial depression during inhalation anesthesia, a thorough understanding of these effects and their implications with regard to human physiology is vital if competent anesthesia care is to be provided.

The cardiovascular system is composed of the heart and the vasculature that carries blood to provide nutrients to all cells in the body. In addition, the cardiovascular system transports substances such as hormones and electrolytes from one part of the body to another.

At the center of this network is the heart. The heart pumps unoxygenated blood to the lungs and then supplies oxygenated blood to all parts of the body. This chapter describes the anatomic and physiologic characteristics of the cardiovascular system.

Heart

Gross Anatomy

The heart is bound anteriorly by the sternum and the costal cartilages of the third, fourth, and fifth ribs and inferiorly by the diaphragm. It is positioned with the apex projecting anteriorly and inferiorly toward the left fifth intercostal space. At this location the apex may be palpated. This is known as the *point of maximal impulse*, and the first heart sound (S_1) is best auscultated in this area. A third (S_3) or fourth (S_4) heart sound, if present, can also be heard in this location.

Cardiac Silhouette

The superior aspect of the cardiac silhouette is formed by the transverse and ascending aorta. The right lateral border is composed of the right atrium (RA), and the mass of the right ventricle (RV) constitutes most of the inferior border. The left ventricle (LV) makes up most of the apex and the lower left lateral border. The left atrial appendage lies superior to the LV and to one side of the pulmonary artery. This left atrial appendage may be seen radiographically between the LV and the pulmonary outflow tract. The heart is rotated on its base such that the anterior surface is almost entirely made up of the RV. The base of the heart is the most superior portion of the cardiac silhouette.

Pericardium

The heart is situated within the mediastinum and is surrounded by a fibrous, double-walled sac called the *pericardium*,[1] which envelops the heart and the roots of the great vessels. It consists of a visceral portion, which is in intimate contact with the outer surface of the heart (epicardium), and an outer parietal portion, which is adherent to the fibrous pericardium (Figure 21-1).

The fibrous pericardium is pierced superiorly by the aorta, the pulmonary trunk, and the superior vena cava. The base of the fibrous pericardium is fused with the central tendon of the diaphragm. The visceral pericardium and parietal pericardium are separated by a thin potential space known as the *pericardial cavity*. This space normally contains approximately 10 to 25 ml of serous fluid, which provides lubrication for the free movement of the heart within the mediastinum. In disease states the pericardial space can fill with blood, compress the heart, and decrease cardiac output (CO). In acute cardiac tamponade the volume rapidly increases, producing myocardial dysfunction. In contrast, in chronic cardiac tamponade the degree of pressure exerted on the heart occurs slowly because of stretching of the pericardial sac. However, the pressure may eventually increase as much as tenfold before symptoms of cardiac tamponade occur.[2]

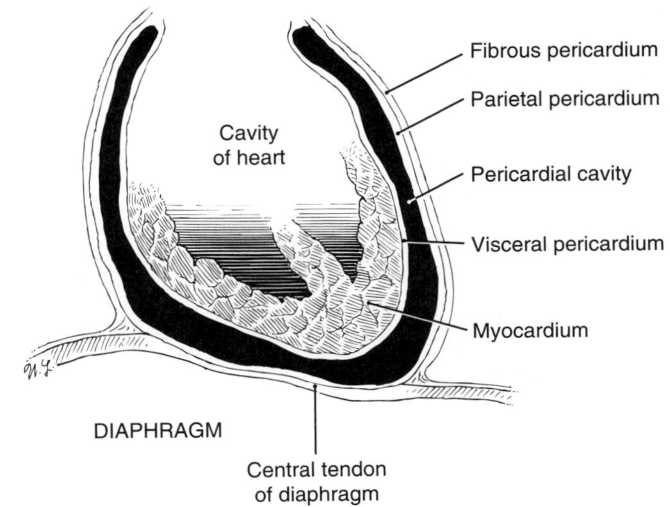

FIGURE **21-1**
The pericardium.

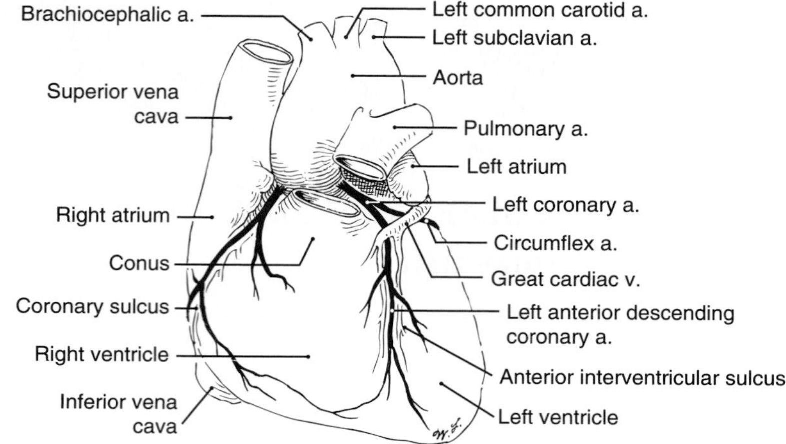

FIGURE **21-2**
Surface anatomy of the heart (anterior view).

The pericardium receives its arterial blood supply from the branches of the internal thoracic arteries and through the bronchial, esophageal, and superior phrenic arteries. Venous drainage from the pericardium occurs through the azygos system as well as the pericardiophrenic veins, which anastomose with the internal thoracic veins. Nervous innervation to the pericardium is derived from the vagus nerve, the phrenic nerves, and the sympathetic trunks.

Surface Anatomy

The atria are separated from the ventricles by the coronary sulcus (atrioventricular [AV] sulcus; Figure 21-2). The right coronary artery travels within sulcus. The circumflex artery arises from the left coronary artery and travels in the coronary sulcus until it ramifies posteriorly. The RV and LV are separated by the interventricular sulci, which descend from the coronary sulcus to the apex. The interventricular sulci are composed of an anterior interventricular sulcus and a posterior interventricular sulcus. The anterior interventricular sulcus contains the left anterior descending (LAD) artery, which courses over the interventricular septum and continues in the posterior interventricular sulcus.

The crux of the heart is the place at which the coronary and the posterior interventricular sulci meet. Internally, it is where the atrial and ventricular septa meet (Figure 21-3). This anatomic crux is important in order to determine coronary artery dominance.

Cardiac Skeleton

Essential to a discussion of the chambers of the heart is a description of the fibrous skeleton, the annulus fibrosus (Figure 21-4). Tough fibrous rings surround the AV valves and act as points of attachment for the valves. Two additional fibrous annuli develop in relation to the bases of the aorta and the pulmonary trunk. The aortic fibrous annulus is connected to the pulmonary annulus by a fibrous band, called the *tendon of the conus*. The aortic annulus is connected to the AV annuli by the small left fibrous trigone and the larger right fibrous trigone, also called the *central fibrous body*. The four annuli and their interconnections constitute the fibrous cardiac skeleton.

The annulus fibrosus is the fixation point for the cardiac musculature and plays an important role in the structure, function, and efficiency of the heart. The annulus acts as an insulator to prevent aberrant electrical conduction from the atria to the ventricles so that AV conduction moves through one pathway only: the AV node to the bundle of His. This element increases the electromechanical efficiency of the heart and helps prevent dysrhythmias.

Chambers of the Heart

Right Atrium. The atria act as the priming chambers for the ventricles. As such, the RA acts as a reservoir for the RV and has unique anatomic characteristics. It has a muscle wall thickness of approximately 2 μm.

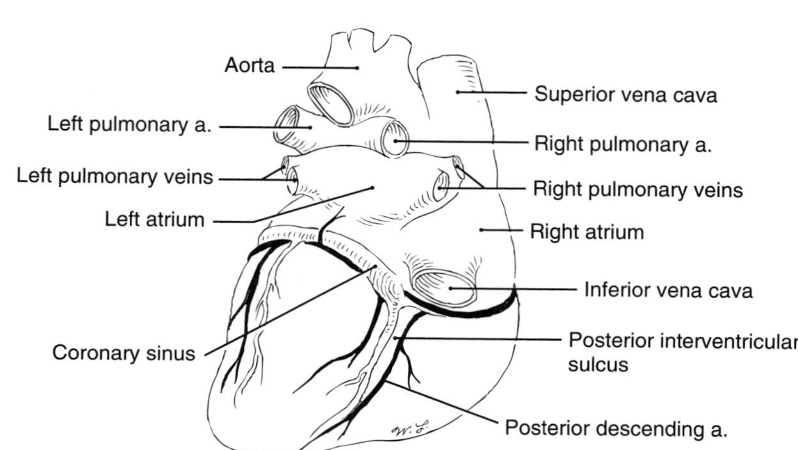

FIGURE **21-3**
Surface anatomy of the heart (posterior view).

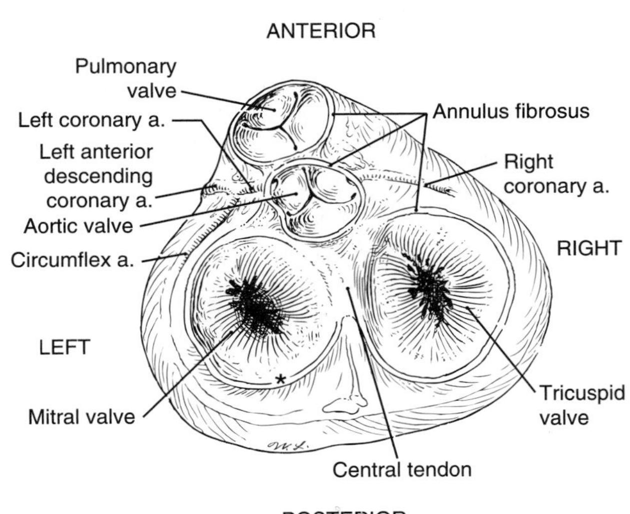

FIGURE **21-4**
The annulus fibrosus.

The RA receives blood from several sources: the superior vena cava, the inferior vena cava, and the coronary sinus (Figure 21-5). The RA consists of two parts: an anterior, thin-walled trabeculated portion and a posterior, smooth-walled portion called the *sinus venarum*. The sinus venarum receives blood from the venae cavae and the coronary sinus. The auricle projects to the left from the root of the superior vena cava and overlaps the root of the ascending aorta.

The superior vena cava returns blood to the RA from the upper part of the body. The inferior vena cava returns blood to the RA from the lower part of the body. The entrance of the inferior vena cava into the RA is protected by a rudimentary valve called the *eustachian valve*.[3]

The entrance from the coronary sinus into the RA is located between the AV orifice and the valve of the inferior vena cava. This opening is protected in part by a rudimentary valve of the coronary sinus, called the *thebesian valve*.[4] Other distinguishing structures in the RA include the interatrial septum and, within the septum, the fossa ovalis cordis, which is the remnant of the fetal foramen ovale.

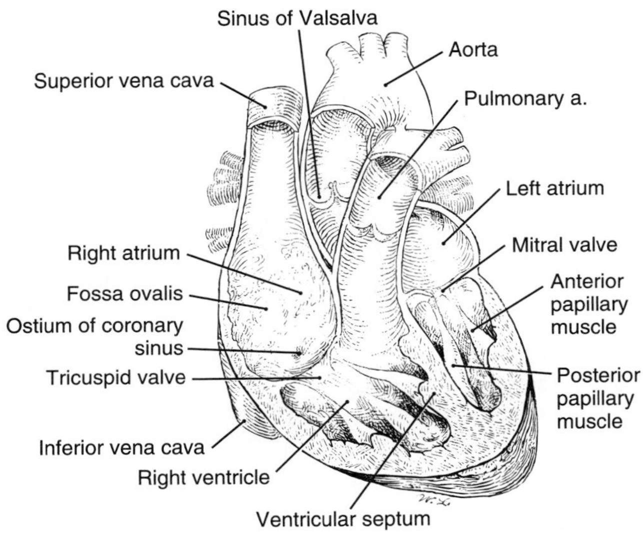

FIGURE **21-5**
Internal anatomy of the heart chambers.

Right Ventricle. The RV ejects blood into the pulmonary arteries for oxygenation and removal of carbon dioxide by the lungs. The RV communicates with the RA through the AV orifice, which is guarded by the tricuspid valve. The RV also communicates with the pulmonary outflow tract through the pulmonary orifice, which is guarded by the pulmonic valve (see Figure 21-5).

The walls of the RV are much thicker (4 to 5 mm) than those of the RA because of the increased pressures that are required to generate forward blood flow into the pulmonary circulation. The superior portion of the RV as it approaches the pulmonary orifice has a conical appearance and is called the conus arteriosus or infundibulum.[5]

The inner wall of the conus is smooth, but the remainder of the right ventricular wall has a rough appearance because of the presence of several irregular muscular bundles, called the *papillary muscles* and the *trabeculae carneae*. One of the trabeculae carneae (the moderator band) crosses the cavity of the ventricles and carries the right branch of the AV bundle. The papillary muscles have attachments to the ventricular walls and to the chordae tendineae. The chordae tendineae are attached to the cusps of the tricuspid valve and, in conjunction with the papillary muscles, they help to prevent the eversion of the tricuspid valve into the RA during ventricular systole.[6]

Left Atrium. The left atrium (LA) acts as a reservoir for oxygenated blood from the pulmonary veins and also as a pump during ventricular diastole. It provides a 20% to 30% increase in left ventricular end-diastolic volume (LVEDV), which is known as the *atrial kick*. A person who has normal myocardial performance does not rely on this increase in ventricular filling in order to achieve adequate CO. However, in certain cardiovascular or respiratory pathologic conditions, compromised patients rely on this atrial kick to maintain an adequate CO. The LA is located superiorly and posteriorly to the other cardiac chambers. The walls of the LA are slightly thicker (3 μm) than those of the RA. The LA connects to the LV through the left AV orifice, which contains the mitral valve. The atrial septum is smooth but may contain a central depression that corresponds to the location of the fossa ovalis cordis.

Left Ventricle. The apex of the LV is positioned within the mediastinum in an anterior and inferior orientation. The LV receives blood from the LA and ejects it into the aorta. Left ventricular wall thickness is approximately 8 to 15 mm, or two to three times the thickness of the RV. This additional muscle mass is required to overcome the systemic vascular resistance (SVR) or afterload in order to maintain CO.

The ventricular septum separates the right and left ventricular cavities.[7] The upper third of the septum is smooth endocardium. The remaining two thirds of the septum and the rest of the ventricular wall are covered with trabeculae carneae.

Two large papillary muscles are present within the LV. The anterior papillary muscle attaches to the anterior part of the left ventricular wall, and the posterior papillary muscle arises from the posterior aspect of the inferior wall. The chordae tendineae of each muscle are attached to the cusps of the mitral valve and prevent eversion of the valve during ventricular systole.

Myocardium

Cardiac musculature consists of three distinct layers: an outer epicardium, a middle muscular myocardium, and an inner endocardium. The epicardium is composed of mesothelium, connective tissue, and fat. The middle muscular myocardium consists of two muscle layers—a superficial and a deep layer. These layers are arranged in a spiral fashion and appear on cross-section to run at right angles to each other. It has been postulated that the superficial and deep layers of the myocardium are not two separate layers but one tortuous and continuous layer. The arrangement of the muscle layers provides strength during contraction of the myocardium and efficient propulsion of blood toward the semilunar valves. The endocardium consists of endothelium and a layer of connective tissue.

Valves

The cardiac valves increase the efficiency of the heart by ensuring a one-way flow of blood through the circuit. They open and close in response to pressure gradients that exist above or below the valves. These valves may be categorized as AV or semilunar in configuration.

One of the most accurate ways to determine the presence of valvular pathology is by calculation of valve area. The standard method for determining valve area is by cardiac catheterization. A cardiologist is able to determine valve gradients by calculation with Gorlin's formula or its correction, which can provide information regarding the degree of pathology that exists.[8] Echocardiography has also found a place in the determination of valve area and is used in the diagnosis of valvular disease.

Atrioventricular Valves

Tricuspid Valve. The tricuspid valve is situated within the right AV orifice, which lies between the RA and the RV. The tricuspid leaflets are thinner and more translucent than the mitral valve and are more easily separated into well-defined leaflets. Three leaflets of unequal size exist and include the anterior, septal, and posterior leaflets. The leaflets are attached to the chordae tendineae, which are attached to the papillary muscles.[9] The normal tricuspid valve area is approximately 7 cm^2. Symptoms of tricuspid insufficiency occur when the valve area is less than 1.5 cm^2.

Mitral Valve. The mitral valve is situated in the left AV orifice between the LA and the LV. Two major leaflets, the anteromedial leaflet and the posterolateral leaflet, are connected by commissural tissue. The normal mitral valve area is 4 to 6 cm^2. When the surface area of the valve is decreased by half, clinical symptoms may appear. Like the tricuspid valve the mitral valve has papillary muscles and chordae tendineae attached to the leaflets to prevent eversion of the valve during ventricular systole.[10]

Semilunar Valves

The configuration of the aortic and pulmonary valves is similar. The cusps of the aortic valve are slightly thicker because it is subjected to greater pressures, which are created by left ventricular ejection. The semilunar valves are situated within the outflow tracts of their corresponding ventricles. Each valve is composed of three cusps. Above the aortic valve is a dilation known as the *sinus of Valsalva*, which allows the valve to open efficiently without occluding the ostia or openings that communicate with the coronary arteries. Eddy currents form behind the valve leaflets and prevent contact between the valve leaflets and the walls of the aorta. The normal valve area of the aortic valve is 1 to 3 cm^2. Reduction of the valve area by one third to one half is associated with an increase in the symptoms of valvular disease.

Coronary Circulation

The heart is an aerobic organ that depends on a constant supply of oxygen to meet its high metabolic demand. It requires an elaborate arterial and venous network to ensure that myocytes are adequately supplied with oxygen. The arterial system consists of epicardial and subendocardial vessels. The epicardial vessels are located superficially and most commonly become obstructed at areas of bifurcation where the blood flow is turbulent rather than laminar. Significant obstruction (50% reduction in luminal diameter) can result in myocardial ischemia or infarction as a result of increased resistance to flow across the stenotic areas.

Coronary Arteries. The ostia of the two coronary arteries are located behind the aortic cusps near the superior part of the sinus of Valsalva. The ostium of the left coronary artery is superior and posterior to the right coronary ostium. The coronary arteries act as end arteries, and each supplies blood to its respective capillary bed[11] (Figure 21-6).

Left Main Coronary Artery. The left main coronary artery travels anteriorly, inferiorly, and leftward from the left coronary sinus to emerge from behind the pulmonary trunk. Within 2 to 10 μm of its emergence the left main coronary artery divides into two or more branches of near-equal diameter. The branches include the LAD artery, the left circumflex coronary artery, and possibly the diagonal branch.

Left Anterior Descending Coronary Artery. The LAD is a continuation of the left main coronary artery. The branches of this vessel include the first diagonal branch, the first septal perforator, the right ventricular branches (not always observed), other septal perforators, and other diagonal branches. The LAD provides blood flow to the anterior two thirds of the interventricular septum, the right and left bundle

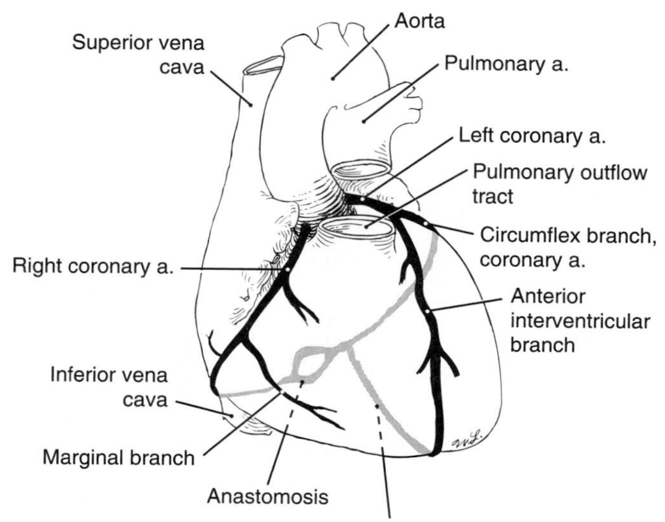

FIGURE **21-6**
The coronary arterial circulation.

branches, the anterior and posterior papillary muscles of the mitral valve, and the anterior lateral and apical walls of the LV. The LAD also provides collateral circulation to the anterior wall of the RV.

Left Circumflex Coronary Artery. The left circumflex artery arises from the left main coronary artery at an obtuse angle and is directed posteriorly as it travels around the left side of the heart within the left AV sulcus. Branches are variable and may include the sinus node artery (40% to 50% of the population), the left atrial circumflex artery, the anterolateral marginal artery, the distal circumflex artery, one or more posterolateral marginal arteries, and the posterior descending artery (10% to 15% of the population). The circumflex artery supplies blood to the left atrial wall, the posterior and lateral LV, the anterolateral papillary muscle, the AV node in 10% of the population, and the sinoatrial (SA) node in 40% to 45% of the population.

Right Coronary Artery. The right coronary artery supplies blood to the SA and AV nodes, the RA and RV, the posterior third of the interventricular septum, the posterior fascicle of the left bundle branch, and the interatrial septum. In approximately 90% of the population the right coronary artery leaves the right coronary sinus and descends in the right AV groove. At the crux the right coronary artery courses inferiorly in the posterior AV groove and terminates as a left ventricular branch.

The branches of the right coronary artery include the conus artery, the sinus node artery (50% to 60% of the population), several anterior right ventricular branches, the right atrial branches, the acute marginal branch, the AV node artery (90% of the population), the proximal bundle branches, the posterior descending artery, and the terminal branches to the LA and LV.

Coronary Artery Dominance. Dominance of one coronary artery is determined by the coronary artery that crosses the crux and provides blood flow to the posterior descending artery. The dominant coronary artery in 50% of the general population is the right coronary. In addition, 10% to 15% of the general population are left coronary dominant, and 35% to 40% of the general population have mixed right and left dominance.

Venous Drainage. An extensive venous system exists in the heart. The three major systems include the coronary sinus, the anterior cardiac veins, and the thebesian veins (Figure 21-7).

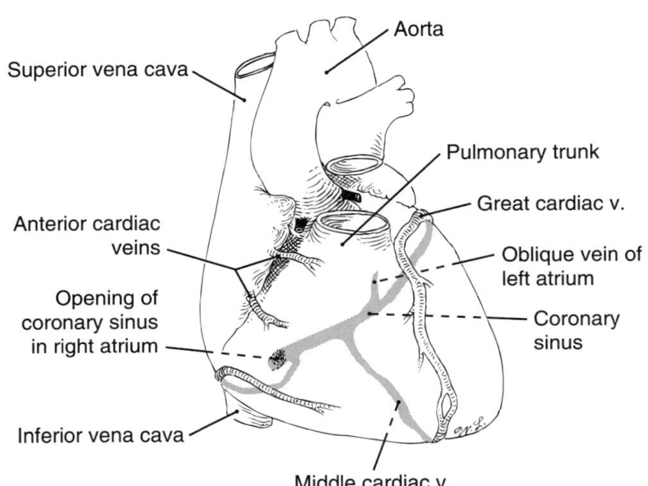

FIGURE **21-7**
The coronary venous system.

The coronary sinus is located in the posterior AV groove near the crux. It collects approximately 85% of the blood from the LV, and for this reason it is catheterized when metabolic studies of the LV are performed. It may also be cannulated during cardiopulmonary bypass in order to deliver cardioplegia. The coronary sinus receives blood from the great, middle, and small cardiac veins; the posterior left ventricular veins; and the left atrial vein of Marshall.

Two to four anterior cardiac veins drain the anterior right ventricular wall. These veins may enter the RA directly, or they may empty into the coronary sinus.

The thebesian veins traverse the myocardium and drain into the various chambers, especially the RA, the RV, and, to a lesser extent, the LV. The thebesian veins may carry up to 40% of the blood that is returned to the RA.

Cardiac Innervation

The innervation of the heart originates from the autonomic nervous system as well as from sensory fibers. The myocardium also has a specialized conduction system that is discussed in this chapter.

The sympathetic nervous system increases the rate and the strength of myocardial contraction. Sympathetic nervous system activation results in the mobilization of myocardial glycogen for energy use by the myocardial cells. The preganglionic sympathetic nervous system fibers originate from the cells in the intermediolateral columns of the higher thoracic segments of the spinal cord and synapse in the upper four to five thoracic paravertebral ganglia. The postganglionic fibers then travel as the superior, middle, and inferior cardiac nerves, as well as the thoracic visceral nerves. These fibers form an epicardial plexus and are distributed over the entire ventricular myocardium.

Some of these postganglionic sympathetic fibers also join with the postganglionic parasympathetic fibers from the cardiac plexus and innervate the SA and AV nodes and the atrial myocardium. Suppression or blockade of this thoracic portion of the spinal cord by regional anesthesia causes bradycardia and hypotension as a result of the blockade of these sympathetic ganglia.

The preganglionic parasympathetic fibers originate in the dorsal motor nucleus of the medulla. Short postganglionic fibers innervate the SA and AV nodes and the atrial muscle fibers. The function of the parasympathetic nervous system is primarily to slow the heart rate (HR) and secondarily to decrease contractility. In fact, maximal vagal (parasympathetic) stimulation reduces contractility by only 30%, whereas maximal sympathetic stimulation increases contractility by 100%.

Sensory innervation of the heart originates in the nerve endings in the walls of the heart, the coronary artery adventitia, and the pericardium. These nerve endings synapse with ascending fibers in the posterior gray columns of the spinal cord, where the fibers synapse with second-order neurons. From these neurons the fibers ascend in the ventral spinothalamic tract and terminate in the posteroventral nucleus of the thalamus.

Cardiac Conduction System

Within the myocardium lies the specialized conduction system whose purpose is to automatically initiate and coordinate the cardiac rhythm. The cells of this system differ from the other myocardial cells because they are more variable in shape, contain fewer myofibrils, and have a characteristic pale staining of the cytoplasm. The conductive system consists of the following components: the SA node, the internodal tracts, the AV node, the AV bundle, and the Purkinje system (Figure 21-8).

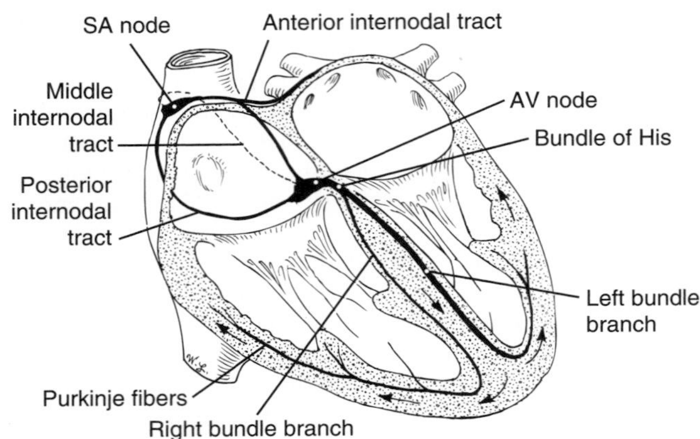

FIGURE **21-8**
The cardiac conduction system. *AV*, Atrioventricular; *SA*, sinoatrial.

Sinoatrial Node. The SA node (the Keith-Flack node) is a small mass of specialized cells and collagenous tissue located along the epicardial surface at the junction of the superior vena cava and the RA. The SA node has a prominent central artery that is a branch of the right coronary artery.

The SA node is derived from the junction of the right horn of the sinus venosus and the primitive atrium. The SA node consists of two cell types—P cells (pacemaker cells), which are pale and ovoid with large round nuclei, and intermediate or transitional cells, which are elongated. These transitional cells are intermediate between ovoid and ordinary cells. They conduct impulses within and away from the SA node.

Internodal Tracts. The internodal tracts are found within the atria and are the preferential conduction pathways between the SA and the AV nodes. They contain a mixture of closely packed parallel myocardial fibers and large pale-staining cells with a perinuclear clear zone. They have large nuclei and sparse myofibrils that resemble the Purkinje cells. Like the SA node, the internodal tracts contain P cells and transitional cells.

Three major internodal tracts exist—the anterior, middle, and posterior internodal tracts. The anterior internodal tract, or Bachmann's bundle, sends fibers to the LA and then travels down through the atrial septum to the AV node. The middle internodal tract, or Wenckebach's tract, curves behind the superior vena cava before descending to the AV node. Finally, the posterior internodal tract, or Thorel's tract, continues along the terminal crest to enter the atrial septum and then passes to the AV node.

Atrioventricular Node. The AV node is located beneath the endocardium on the right side of the atrial septum, anterior to the opening of the coronary sinus. The AV node is supplied by an abundance of nerve endings as well as vagal (ganglionic) cells. The AV node causes a delay in the transmission of the action potential. This delay may be attributed to several factors, such as the size of the AV nodal cells (smaller than the surrounding atrial cells), the resting membrane potential (which is less negative than the normal resting membrane potentials of the surrounding cells), and the paucity of gap junctions. Greater resistance to the transmission of an action potential exists within the AV node.

Atrioventricular Bundle. The AV bundle (bundle of His) extends from the lower end of the AV node and enters the posterior part of the ventricle and the Purkinje system. This AV bundle is the preferential channel for the conduction of the action potential from the atria to the ventricles.

Purkinje System. The Purkinje system consists of the bundle branch system and its terminal branches. The left bundle branch spreads out under the endocardium and forms several fascicles, which branch out to various parts of the LV. The anterior fascicle innervates the anterolateral wall of the LV and the anterior papillary muscle. The posterior fascicle innervates the lateral and posterior ventricular wall and the posterior papillary muscle. The anterior and posterior fascicles join to form the septal fascicle, which innervates the lower ventricular septum and the apical wall of the LV.

The right bundle branch travels under the endocardium along the right side of the ventricular septum to the base of the anterior papillary muscle.

Structural and Regulatory Proteins. The myocardium has characteristics of both skeletal and smooth muscle. Like smooth muscle, it acts as a syncytium for the coordinated contraction and the "all or none" response of the muscle mass.

The myocardial cell is similar to skeletal muscle in that it is made of sarcomeres (Figure 21-9). These sarcomeres contain all the microfilaments and structures that have become familiar in descriptions of skeletal muscle sarcomere. The sarcomere stretches from Z line to Z line. The A bands consist of the actin filaments, which contain a bilayer filament of F-actin and tropomyosin. Along the actin filament, many active sites exist that can attach to the head of the myosin molecule. A troponin complex that is necessary for the mobilization of the active sites is present on the tropomyosin filament.

The other microfilament in the cardiac muscle is the *myosin* molecule. This molecule is made up of two major parts—a light meromyosin chain and a heavy meromyosin chain. The heavy meromyosin chain consists of two hinged ends and a head that plays a role in the "ratchet theory" of muscle contraction.[12]

Some evidence indicates that the troponin-tropomyosin complex inhibits the binding of the heads of the myosin filaments with the active sites on the actin molecule. During the initiation of contraction, calcium is released from the

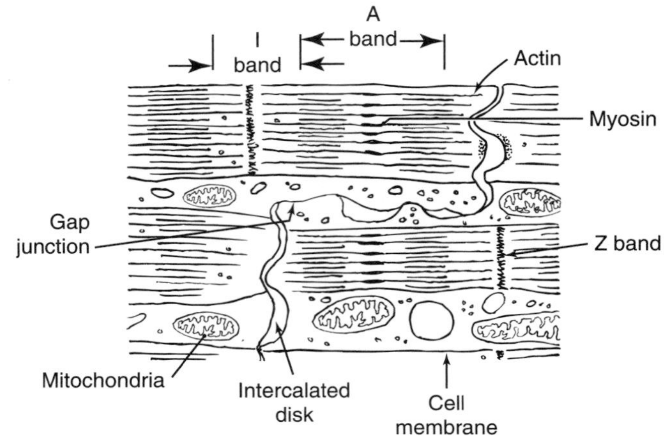

FIGURE **21-9**
The myocardial sarcomere.

sarcoplasmic reticulum. This calcium binds to the troponin-tropomyosin complex and causes a conformational change so that the active binding sites become uncovered. When the active sites are uncovered, the heads of the myosin filaments move along the actin filament by alternately attaching and detaching from the active sites, thereby causing shortening of the Z lines. Cellular energy or adenosine triphosphate (ATP) is required for excitation-contraction coupling to occur.

Similar length-force relationships exist within the myocardium and in skeletal muscle. The resting sarcomere length at which the muscle cell is most efficient is 2 to 2.4 μm. At greater lengths the interdigitation of the actin and the myosin is compromised, and at shorter lengths the sarcomere is unable to generate an efficient contraction.

Clinically, this concept is demonstrated by the ideal filling pressure of the LV that is necessary for achieving efficient CO. Filling pressures are used to reflect the filling volumes of the ventricles and, indirectly, the amount of stretch on the ventricular muscle at rest. Filling pressures are measured by the use of the pulmonary capillary wedge pressure (PCWP) or the pulmonary artery diastolic pressure. It has been demonstrated that at excessively high filling pressures (as in congestive heart failure) and at excessively low filling pressures (as in hypovolemia) the CO can be compromised as a result of either excessive or inadequate stretch of the left ventricular myocardium. This concept is the basis for the Frank-Starling law of the heart, which is discussed later in this chapter.

Differences between Skeletal and Cardiac Muscle Cells. Several differences exist between the myocardial muscle cells and the skeletal muscle cells (see Figure 21-9). At the junctions between the fibers in the myocardial muscle mass, many branching interconnected fibers are intercalated disks and gap junctions, or nexi. Areas of low resistance exist that facilitate the conduction of the action potential from one myocardial cell to another.

The myocardial sarcomeres also contain higher concentrations of mitochondria (sarcosomes) than do other types of muscle cells. The cardiac cells are aerobic and cannot tolerate oxygen deficiency. Skeletal muscles can function both aerobically and anaerobically.

The myocardial sarcomere system has a rich capillary supply (one capillary per fiber) that allows for efficient diffusion and perfusion. The T-tubular system and the sarcoplasmic reticulum are extensive within the cardiac sarcomere. This situation allows for the rapid release and reabsorption of calcium from the cells. It also serves to highlight the important role that extracellular calcium plays in the contractile process of the myocardial cell.

Generation of Membrane Potentials

Resting Membrane Potentials. The myocardial sarcomere is not merely a contractile entity. It also possesses properties that are common to neural tissue, such as the generation of a resting membrane potential, the ability to generate an action potential, and the conduction of the action potential from one sarcomere to the next.

The resting cell membrane is relatively permeable to potassium and relatively impermeable to both sodium and calcium. The resting membrane potential is caused by a chemical force, an electrostatic counterforce, and the sodium-potassium active transport pump.

TABLE 21-1 Equilibrium Potential of Various Ions

Ion	Intracellular Concentration (mmol)	Extracellular Plasma Concentration (mmol)	Equilibrium Potential E_m (mV)
Na^+	10	145	60
K^+	135	4	−94
Cl^-	4	114	−97
Ca^{2+}	10^{-4}	2	132

The chemical force relies on the potential difference in ion concentration between one side of the cell membrane as compared with the other. The ions primarily responsible for this force are sodium, potassium, and calcium.[13]

The electrostatic counterforce results from the negative potential of the interior of the cell that is generated by the ion difference. This force can pull ions into the cell, especially potassium.

The sodium-potassium pump requires an energy source (active transport) and involves the enzyme magnesium-dependent adenosine triphosphatase located in the cell membrane. Three molecules of sodium are pumped out of the cell into the extracellular fluid for every two molecules of potassium pumped into the intracellular fluid.

Calculation of the equilibrium potential (E_m, measured in millivolts) has been accomplished by examination of the concentration of an ion inside the cell versus outside the cell (see the following equation [the Nernst equation]). Table 21-1 lists the equilibrium potentials of the most interesting ions. The ion most responsible for the resting membrane potential is potassium.

Equation 21-1

$$E_m = (-RT/FZ) \times \log[K]_i/[K]_o$$

where R is a gas constant, T is temperature in K, F is Faraday's constant, $[K]_i$ is the intracellular concentration of potassium, and $[K]_o$ is the extracellular concentration of potassium.

If a temperature of 310° K is assumed for a living human, the Nernst equation reduces to the following in a human heart:

Equation 21-2

$$E_m = (-61.5/Z) \times \log[K]_i/[K]_o$$

The Nernst potential is useful only in discussions of a single ion. The membrane potentials are generated because the cell membrane is permeable to several different ions. Three factors affect the calculation of the effect of these different ions on the resting membrane potential: the electrical charge of each ion, the permeability of the membrane to each ion, and the concentration gradient across the membrane. The following equation, the Goldman-Hodgkin-Katz equation, is a modification of the Nernst equation that accounts for these factors.

Equation 21-3

$$EMF = 61.5 \times \log([Na]_iP_{Na} + [K]_iP_K + [Cl]_oP_{Cl})/([Na]_oP_{Na}\ [K]_oP_K\ [Cl]_iP_{Cl})$$

where $[K]_i$ is the intracellular ion concentration of potassium, $[K]_o$ is the extracellular ion concentration of potassium, and P_K is the membrane permeability of potassium.

Ventricular Muscle Fiber Action Potential

Gate Theory. Several electrostatic gates have been elucidated for the various ions. These gates open (activate) and close (inactivate), depending on the electrical potential of the cell membrane. An electrostatic gate exists for each of the major cardiac ions (sodium, potassium, calcium, and chloride).

Phases of the Action Potential. The action potentials of the various parts of the conduction system vary according to their locations and functions.[14] The action potential of the ventricular muscle fiber is separated into five phases (Figure 21-10). Phase 0, or depolarization, involves the fast sodium channels. The fast sodium channel activation gates (M gates) open between −70 and −65 mV (threshold potential). At 0 mV both the activation and the inactivation gates (H gates) are open. The rapid upstroke velocity of phase 0 gives a relative indication of the conductivity of the myocardial cell.

At phase 1, or initial repolarization (+2 to +30 mV), the inactivation gates close, thereby stopping the influx of sodium into the cell. During phase 1 the rapid influx of sodium is halted and the slower influx of calcium begins.

One of the characteristics of the action potential of the ventricular muscle mass is phase 2, or plateau. The plateau phase exists because the slow calcium channels open at −30 to −40 mV and allow an influx of calcium. This inward calcium flux delays repolarization and prolongs the absolute refractory period. Toward the end of phase 2, a decreased permeability to potassium occurs that accounts for a small outward leakage of potassium, balanced by the calcium and sodium influx that maintains a membrane potential near 0 mV. The terminal repolarization phase, phase 3, is initiated as the slow calcium channels become inactivated, and this phenomenon is sustained by an accelerated potassium efflux. These events return the transmembrane potential to its resting membrane value. The sodium-potassium pump then reestablishes the proper intracellular-to-extracellular ionic concentrations during phase 4 (diastolic phase). Phase 4 lasts from the completion of repolarization to the next action potential.

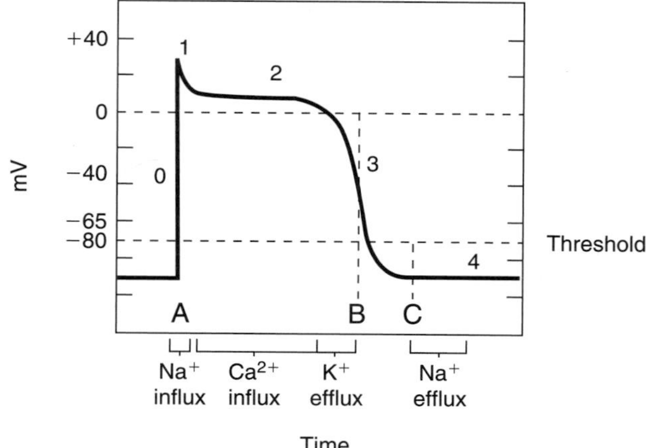

FIGURE **21-10**
The ventricular muscle action potential. *A* to *B*, Absolute refractory period; *B* to *C*, relative refractory period; *0*, depolarization; *1*, overshoot; *2*, plateau; *3*, repolarization (rapid); *4*, repolarization (complete).

Refractory Periods. The extended duration of the action potential of the myocardial cell protects it against premature excitation. This period of quiescence is known as the *refractory period* and can be divided into absolute and relative periods. The refractory periods are a result of the properties of the sodium channels during the action potential.

The absolute refractory period is the time during the action potential when no membrane response occurs to a second stimulus. This period lasts from phase 0 to the middle of phase 3, when the membrane potential drops below −60 mV. The relative refractory period is the time during the action potential when a second stimulus can result only in an action potential with decreased amplitude, upstroke velocity, and conduction velocity. The relative refractory period extends from this middle part of the phase 3 range to the beginning of phase 4, when the membrane potential is from −60 to −90 mV. The term *effective or absolute refractory period* is used to describe the time during which a conducted action potential may not be evoked, even if an active response is elicited by a stimulus at the cellular level.

Sinoatrial Node Action Potential. The myocardium has among its characteristics contractility, automaticity, and conductivity. Each of the various myocardial masses has its own intrinsic automaticity and rate of action potential initiation. The SA node is the primary pacemaker of the heart and has several unique characteristics (Figure 21-11). The membranes of SA node cells, as a result of their higher resting membrane potentials, are more permeable to sodium than other atrial myocardial cells. This "leakiness" gradually raises the membrane potential closer to threshold (−55 to −60 mV), at which point an action potential may be initiated. Therefore the action potential originating within the SA node differs from the action potential that is generated within the ventricular muscle mass.

The SA node and the other automatic cells exhibit only phase 4, phase 0, and phase 3 of the action potential. Because rapid depolarization does not occur, the phase 1 or phase 2 (plateau phase) does not occur.

If the SA node fails, the area of the heart with the next highest intrinsic rate, the AV node, replaces the SA node as the pacemaker of the heart. If both the SA and the AV nodes fail, the ventricular cells take over and become automatic, firing at a rate of 15 to 30 beats per minute.

Physiology of the Heart

Cardiac Cycle. In order to understand the cardiac cycle, one must have a firm understanding of the basics of the

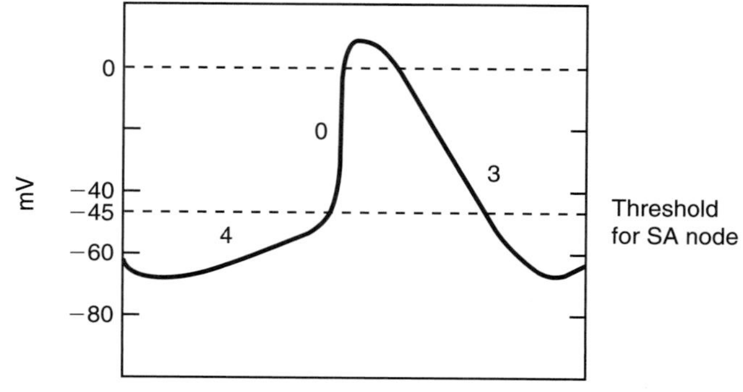

FIGURE **21-11**
The sinoatrial nodal action potential.

anatomy of the heart and the pressures and volumes that are generated within the various chambers during the cardiac cycle. An appreciation for the valves and their positions during the phases of the cycle is essential (Figure 21-12).

The cardiac cycle is the period from one ventricular contraction to the next. It may be divided into two main phases—systole and diastole. Usually the cardiac cycle is described in relation to the left side of the heart. However, similar conclusions about the function of the right side of the heart may be drawn in the absence of active disease or cardiopulmonary pathology.

Diastole. During ventricular systole the atria fill with blood returning from the venous system to the right side of the heart and from the pulmonary circulation to the left side of the heart. The first phase of diastole is the period of isovolumetric relaxation. The ventricular muscle mass relaxes, and the aortic and the mitral valves are closed as long as the ventricular pressure remains higher than the atrial pressure. The true filling phase is divided into three periods: rapid inflow, or diastasis or reduced inflow, and atrial systole. Once the ventricular pressure drops below atrial pressure, the mitral valve opens and the period of rapid inflow to fill the ventricle begins. The second period of diastole is diastasis, in which minimal changes occur in volume and in pressure.

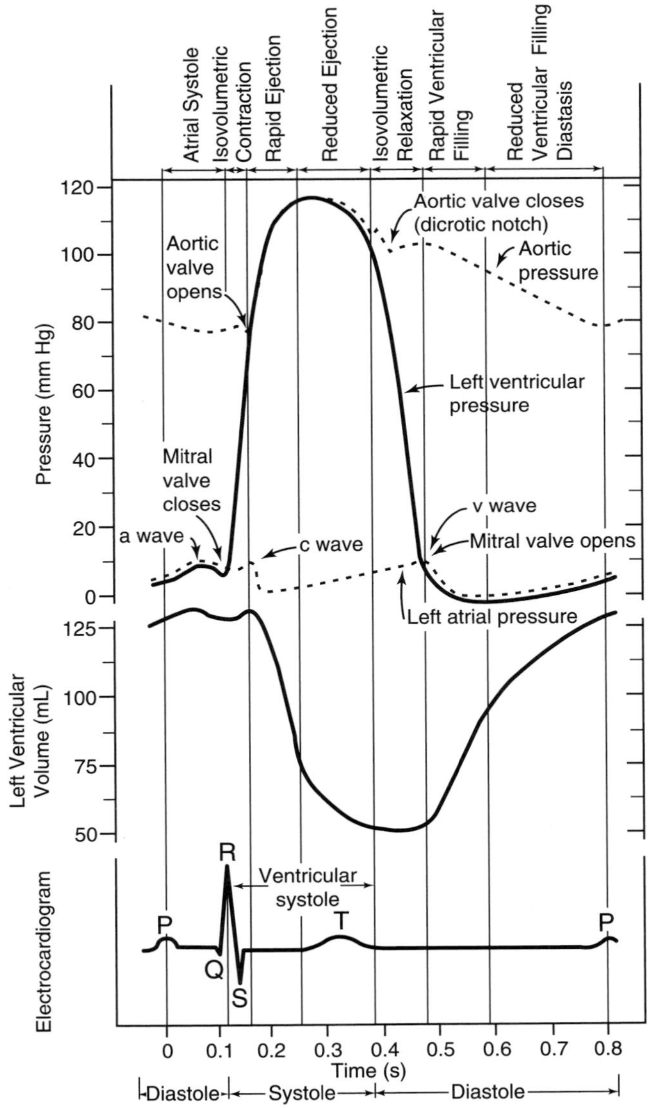

FIGURE **21-12**
The cardiac cycle.

Atrial systole provides another period of rapid filling that is commonly referred to as the *atrial kick*. This phenomenon has been noted to increase ventricular filling by 20% to 30%.

In patients who have severe mitral stenosis, the atrial kick may be responsible for up to 40% of the ventricular filling. A healthy person at rest does not rely on the atrial kick to maintain CO. However, during periods of strenuous exercise or in patients with many pathologic conditions such as shock or congestive heart failure the additional ventricular filling is critical in order to maintain CO.

Systole. After atrial systole the isovolumetric phase, or isovolumetric contraction, which is the phase at the beginning of ventricular contraction, occurs. The myocardial fibers shorten, and pressure is generated within the ventricle but only enough to close the mitral valve. Therefore during this period an increase in left ventricular pressure occurs without a change in ventricular diastolic volume. Isovolumetric contraction begins with closure of the mitral valve and lasts until opening of the mitral valve.

True systole begins with the opening of the aortic valve and occurs when the ventricular pressure exceeds the aortic pressure. Systolic ejection is divided into two periods, with the period of rapid ejection taking the first third of systole and the period of reduced ejection taking the last two thirds of systole. During rapid ejection, ventricular systolic pressures reach their maximum and the largest amount of volume is ejected. Therefore systole is composed of isovolumetric contraction, rapid ejection, and reduced ejection. The dicrotic notch or incisura on the arterial pressure tracing occurs within the period of isovolumetric relaxation. This segment represents retrograde blood flow back into the LV before aortic valve closure. Three waveform segments are present on the left atrial pressure tracing: the *a* wave, *c* wave, and *v* wave. The specific waveforms correspond to their position within the cardiac cycle. The *a* wave represents atrial systole as it ends just before the mitral valve closure. The *c* wave represents ventricular contraction and is produced by bulging of the mitral valve caused by increasing left ventricular pressure. The *v* wave represents increased pressure in the LA caused by blood return from the pulmonary artery before mitral valve opening (see Figure 21-12.)

Physiology of Coronary Circulation. The anatomy of the coronary circulation has already been discussed. A description of the physiologic determinants of coronary blood flow follows.

Coronary Blood Flow. As in all hemodynamics, flow equals change in the pressure divided by resistance of the system. Alterations of the radius of a vessel change the flow to the fourth power of the radius. This phenomenon is an extension of Poiseuille's law, which determines the flow of a fluid through a tube.

At rest, approximately 4% to 5% of the CO, or 225 ml/min of blood, passes through the coronary vasculature. Phasic changes have been documented in the coronary blood flow. A greater amount of coronary flow in the LV occurs during diastole. During systole, left coronary artery blood flow ceases to the subendocardium as a result of compression of the subendocardial vessels by the myocardium. The flow through the epicardial vessels is not affected during systole to this extent.

The flow to the left coronary artery is greatest during diastole as a result of the decreased resistance to flow that occurs as the intracavitary pressure decreases.

Control of Coronary Circulation and Oxygen Supply and Demand. Coronary blood flow is regulated by intrinsic and extrinsic factors that affect coronary artery tone. Intrinsic factors include the anatomic arrangement and the perfusion pressure of the coronary vessels. Extrinsic factors include compressive factors within the myocardium as well as metabolic, neural, and humoral factors. The blood flow through the coronary circulation is primarily controlled by the factors that determine oxygen demand and oxygen supply. Myocardial oxygen supply is determined by arterial blood content; diastolic blood pressure; diastolic time as determined by HR; oxygen extraction; and coronary blood flow. Myocardial oxygen demand is determined by preload, afterload, contractility, and HR (Figure 21-13).

Because at rest the myocardium extracts 65% to 70% of the available oxygen, the only way to increase the oxygen delivery to the myocardium is by increasing blood flow. Several vasodilator substances have been identified and are released from the myocardium in response to decreased oxygen delivery or concentration. Among these substances are adenosine, adenosine phosphate compounds, potassium ions, hydrogen ions, carbon dioxide, bradykinin, and prostaglandin. Many authors believe that adenosine is the primary substance responsible for coronary vasodilator. See Box 21-1.

The determinants of myocardial oxygen consumption include myocardial contractility, myocardial wall tension (preload), HR, and mean arterial pressure (MAP; afterload). Oxygen extraction is determined by measurement of the difference between the oxygen tension in the pulmonary artery blood and that in the coronary sinus.

Oxygen supply relies on the blood oxygen content (see following equation), which is affected by both the oxygen carried on the hemoglobin (Hb) molecule (1.34 ml of oxygen per gram of hemoglobin) and, to a lesser extent, the oxygen that is dissolved in the plasma (0.003 ml of oxygen per milliliter of plasma).

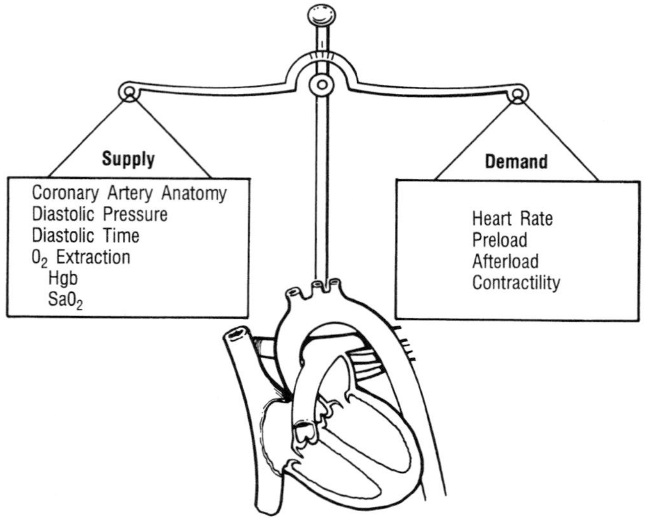

FIGURE **21-13**
The heart's supply of and demand for oxygen must be balanced by the practitioner, who should increase the former and reduce the latter. *Hgb,* Hemoglobin; *SaO_2,* saturation with oxygen, arterial blood.

BOX **21-1**

Normal Physiologic Parameters

Heart size	230-280 g (female) 280-340 g (male)
Coronary blood flow	225-250 ml/min or 4%-7% total cardiac output
Myocardial O_2 consumption	65%-70% extraction 8-10 ml O_2/100 g per min
Normal autoregulation	50-120 mm Hg (MAP)
Coronary filling	80%-90% during diastole

MAP, *Mean arterial pressure.*

Equation 21-4

$$O_2 \text{ content (ml } O_2\text{/ml plasma)} = (Pao_2 \times 0.003) + (\text{Hb content} \times \text{Hb-}O_2 \text{ saturation \%})$$

Other factors that have an influence on coronary circulation include the direct and indirect effects of the sympathetic nervous system and the effect of certain substrates of cardiac metabolism.

Autoregulation. Under normal physiologic conditions the coronary circulation, like other tissue beds in the body, exhibits *autoregulation,* which is the ability to maintain coronary blood flow through a range of MAPs. The coronary blood flow is maintained at a constant rate through a MAP range of 50 to 120 mm Hg. When arterial blood pressure is less than or exceeds these pressure limits, coronary blood flow becomes pressure dependent. Therefore during hypotension, when the coronary arteries are maximally dilated, the coronary blood flow is determined by the MAP minus the right atrial pressure. Coronary perfusion pressure (CPP) is calculated by subtracting left ventricular end diastolic pressure (LVEDP) from diastolic pressure (DBP), that is, CPP = DBP − LVEDP.

Coronary vascular reserve is the difference between the maximal flow and the autoregulated flow. The closer these two values, the lower the coronary reserve of the patient.

The concept of "coronary steal" has emerged, especially in reference to the use of agents such as nitroglycerin and isoflurane. If vasodilator treatment is used in a patient who has both an ischemic area of the heart that is supplying a stenotic vessel with collateral flow and another area that has an intact autoregulated vessel, only the autoregulated vessel dilates further and has the ability to increase its flow. Therefore only the areas of the heart with intact autoregulation respond to vasodilators and receive preferential flow over the stenotic area. The existence of this phenomenon is questionable. Agnew and colleagues have determined that as long as adequate CPP is maintained, coronary steal and myocardial ischemia caused by isoflurane do not occur.[15,16] A second factor that could result in this phenomena is coronary steal–prone anatomy. This has been defined as complete occlusion of one coronary artery and at least 50% occlusion of a second coronary artery that supplies collateral blood flow to the area in which the complete occlusion exists.[15] In addition, recent evidence suggests that isoflurane produces myocardial protection during periods of ischemia in humans by decreasing the formation of free radicals, preserving myocardial ATP stores, and inhibiting increased intracellular calcium.[16,17]

Cardiac Output. CO is the amount of blood that is ejected from the LV during 1 minute. The comparison of COs among several patients requires a method for calculating output in relation to the size of the patient. The CO is measured in liters per minute. CO is indexed because a CO of 3.5 L/min may be adequate for a patient who is 5 ft tall and weighs 95 lb, but it is less than optimal for a patient who is 6 ft 7 in tall and weighs 300 lb. The average CO is 5 L/min, and the average cardiac index (CI) is 2.5 L/min or more per square meter of body surface area (BSA). The formula for this relationship is CI = CO/BSA.

The primary determinants of CO are stroke volume (SV) and HR. CO is derived by using the equation CO = HR × SV. The SV is the amount of blood that is ejected from the LV with each beat. The average SV is approximately 70 ml. If the average HR is 70 to 80 beats per minute, a CO of 5 L/min results.

Several key factors affect the SV, including preload, afterload, and myocardial contractility. Preload is the effective tension of the blood on the ventricle or the wall tension at the end of diastole. Preload can either be passive (the flow of blood from the atria to the ventricles during diastole) or active (the volume that is contributed by the atrial kick). Preload may be described by the Frank-Starling law of the heart, which states that the greater the wall tension, the greater myocardial contractility becomes until overdistension of the heart occurs. Clinically the preload can be estimated by pressure. The pressures that are often monitored are the PCWP and the pulmonary artery diastolic pressure. In patients with normal mitral valve function and ventricular muscle function, either of these measures provides an estimate of the preload or left ventricular end-diastolic pressure and volume.

The CO can be determined indirectly by applying the Fick principle (see Equation 21-5). Assuming normal respiratory function, CO is equal to the amount of oxygen absorbed by the lungs divided by the arteriovenous oxygen difference.

Equation 21-5

$$\text{CO (L/min)} = \frac{\text{Oxygen absorbed per minute by the lungs (ml/min)}}{\text{Arteriovenous oxygen difference (ml/L of Blood)}}$$

The right-sided heart pressures (central venous pressure) that are obtained clinically can be estimates of left ventricular volumes in patients with good left ventricular function.[18]

Afterload is the wall tension that the myocardium needs to overcome in order to eject the CO. It is the pressure within the LV during peak systole. Factors affecting the afterload of the LV include the ventricular chamber and the vasculature. The shape, size, and wall thickness of the ventricle play an important role in afterload. The vascular component of the afterload includes the SVR and the MAP as it relates to the vascular compliance of the aorta.

Afterload is most often estimated clinically by determination of the SVR. The SVR may be calculated once the CO and the difference between the MAP and the central venous pressure (CVP) are known (see equation). The normal SVR is 800 to 1500 dynes/s/cm^{-5}.

Equation 21-6

$$\text{SVR} = (\text{MAP} \times \text{CVP})/\text{CO} \times 80$$

The problem with equating afterload with SVR is that ventricular wall tension, which is an integral part of the afterload, is not considered.

Contractility of the myocardium is the state of inotropy that is independent of either preload or afterload. It may be altered by many cardiovascular disease states. Factors such as rate of pressure changes over time (dP/dt), force-velocity or Starling ventricular function curves, pressure-volume loops, ejection fraction (EF), and velocity of circumferential fiber shortening have all been used to estimate contractility.

Left ventricular dP/dt measurements require a high-fidelity recording system, and for this reason these measures are not readily available in the clinical setting. Such a wide range of normal values exists (800 to 1700 mm Hg/sec) that making intrapatient comparisons is difficult. Assessment of the acute change in contractility of a single patient over time is still the common method of using this measurement.

Ventricular function curves[19] (Figure 21-14) define the relationship between the left ventricular filling pressure (left ventricular diastolic pressure, left atrial pressure, PCWP) and the left ventricular stroke work index (LVSWI), which is calculated by use of the following equation:

Equation 21-7

$$\text{LVSWI (in gm/m}^2\text{ per beat)} = 0.0136 \times \text{SVI} \times (\text{MAP} - \text{PCWP})$$

where SVI = CI/HR.

Each left ventricular function curve has a steep upstroke that has a plateau at higher filling pressures. Symptoms may be elicited by either high or low filling pressures. At high filling pressures, dyspnea may be seen, whereas at low pressures, signs of shock may be elicited. The clinical determination of LVSWI is worthwhile because it contains many of the factors that

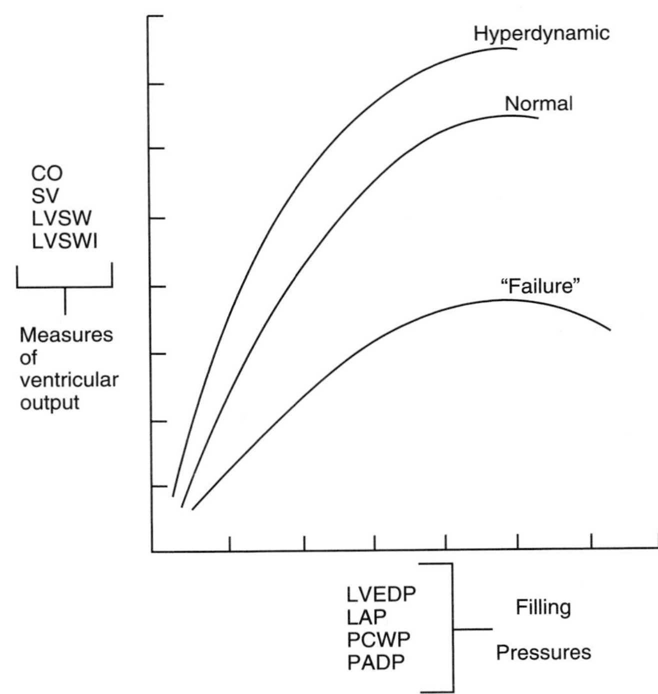

FIGURE **21-14**
The ventricular function curve. CO, Cardiac output; *LAP*, left atrial pressure; *LVEDP*, left ventricular end-diastolic pressure; LVSW, left ventricular stroke work; *LVSWI*, left ventricular stroke work index; *PADP*, pulmonary artery diastolic pressure; *PCWP*, pulmonary capillary wedge pressure; *SV*, stroke volume.

contribute to CO and it gives measures of both systolic and diastolic performance.

Pressure-volume loops have been mentioned before as indexes of the cardiac cycle. They may also be used as tools to determine myocardial performance. Pressure-volume loops simultaneously measure chamber pressures and the resultant volumes (Figure 21-15). The loop is a cycle divided into four phases. Phase I corresponds to diastolic filling; phase II is isovolumetric contraction; phase III is systolic ejection; phase IV is isovolumetric relaxation. The interior of the curve is representative of SV. SV may be determined by use of these curves or the EF; see equation.

Equation 21-8

$$EF = (EDV \times ESV)/\ EDV \times 100$$

or

Equation 21-9

$$EF = (SV/EDV) \times 100$$

(NOTE: EDV = end diastolic volume and ESV = end systolic volume.)

The EF is the percentage of the end-diastolic volume that is ejected during systole. The normal EF is 60% to 70%. An EF of less than 40% is associated with significant left ventricular impairment.

Another value used to estimate contractility is the velocity of circumferential fiber shortening. Measuring both the mean and the maximum requires sophisticated equipment; for this reason this measurement is almost exclusively used as a research tool.

A clinically useful tool is two-dimensional transesophageal echocardiography (TEE). When this technology is appropriately used, real-time movement of all four chambers of the heart, as well as that of the valves, may be visualized.

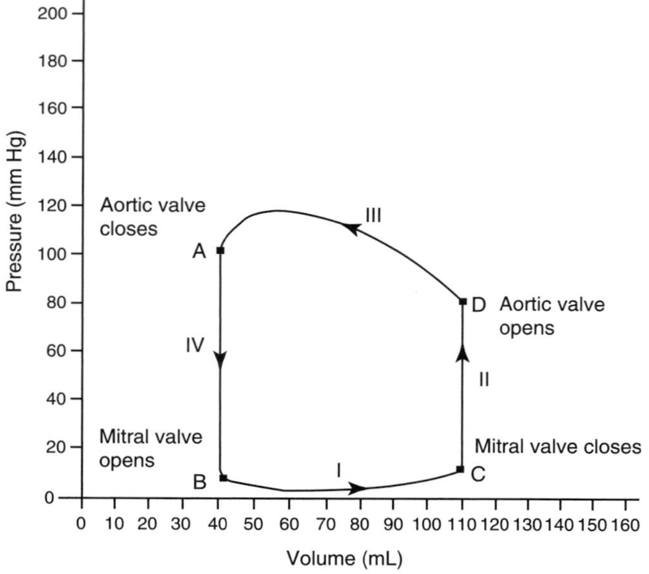

FIGURE **21-15**
The pressure-volume loop denotes interventricular pressure and volume changes during cardiac cycle. Period I = ventricular filling (diastole); period II = isovolumetric contraction (systole); period III = ventricular action (systole); period IV = isovolumetric relaxation (diastole).

TEE can be used to detect valvular function and blood flows in both regurgitant and stenotic lesions. It is also useful in determining areas of hypokinesis, dyskinesis, or akinesis caused by myocardial infarction, ischemia, or injury. It can be useful in determining myocardial contractility, and it is a more direct measure of intraventricular volume status than pulmonary artery catheter pressure measures. TEE has also proved useful in direction of fluid and pharmacologic therapy in patients who have undergone coronary bypass and other surgical procedures. Ventricular dysfunction or reperfusion injury as well as the presence of intraventricular air can be determined with TEE. This diagnostic tool is fast becoming the "gold standard" in the treatment of cardiac patients. The practical problems associated with the clinical use of TEE consist of acquiring the skills necessary for accurate interpretation of the visual data, the possibility of esophageal rupture, and the cost associated with its use.

Cardiac Output Regulation. A direct interplay exists between CO and venous return. Maintenance of a constant return of blood flow to the heart ensures an adequate CO as long as neither the contractility nor the HR is compromised. The body's regulation of CO depends on its ability to regulate HR and contractility of the myocardium as well as constriction and distention of the vascular tree.

Many of the factors that affect CO also affect the MAP and are addressed in the section on regulation of MAP. Some of the more common reflexes that can alter the CO are described in this section or in the section on regulation of MAP.

Valsalva's Maneuver. The Valsalva maneuver is forced expiration against a closed glottis. The reflex is mediated through the baroreceptors located at the bifurcation of the internal and external carotid arteries (carotid sinus) and the aortic arch. The afferent pathway is through Hering's nerve and either the glossopharyngeal nerve (carotid sinus) or the vagus nerve (aortic arch). Stimulation of either of these areas inhibits the vasomotor center in the medulla. The response inhibits the sympathetic nervous system and stimulates the parasympathetic nervous system, producing a decrease in HR, a decrease in myocardial contractility and vasodilatation, produces vasodilation that results in a decrease in blood pressure. The Valsalva maneuver also increases intrathoracic pressure, which decreases venous return as a result of pressure on the vena cava, and thereby decreases CO.

Oculocardiac Reflex. Traction on the extraocular muscles, conjunctiva, or orbital structures causes hypotension and a reflex slowing of the HR, as well as arrhythmias. The oculocardiac reflex may also be elicited during retrobulbar block, ocular trauma, or pressure on the tissue that remains after enucleation. The afferent path of the reflex is mediated by the long and short ciliary nerves to the ciliary ganglion of the oculomotor nerve and then the ophthalmic division of the trigeminal nerve (cranial nerve V) to the gasserian ganglion. The efferent branch of the reflex is mediated by the vagus nerve (cranial nerve X). This reflex may be blunted by the administration of an anticholinergic agent (atropine or glycopyrrolate), the use of retrobulbar block, or the release of the offending stimulus.

Celiac Reflex. The celiac reflex is elicited by traction on the mesentery or the gallbladder or stimulation of the vagus nerve in other areas of the body, such as the thorax and abdominal cavity. Stimulation of this reflex causes bradycardia, apnea, and hypotension.

TABLE 21-2 Cardiac reflexes

Reflex	Stimulus	Response
Baroreceptor reflex	Hypertension resulting in baroreceptor stimulation. Carotid baroreceptors send afferent response via Hering's and glossopharyngeal nerves (CN IX). Aortic baroreceptors send afferent response via the vagus nerve (CN X).	Decreased heart rate, decreased contractility, peripheral vasodilation from efferent response via the vagus nerve (CN X)
Valsalva maneuver	Forced expiration against a closed glottis mediated via baroreceptors. See Baroreceptor reflex for afferent pathways.	Decreased heart rate, decreased blood pressure as a result of decreased vascular tone
Cushing's reflex	Increased intracranial pressure resulting in cerebral ischemia.	Cushing's triad—hypertension, bradycardia respiratory variability
Chemoreceptor reflex	Decreased oxygen saturation, increased carbon dioxide, increased hydrogen ion concentration. Chemoreceptors located in the carotid body and aortic arch. See Baroreceptor reflex for afferent pathways.	Increased respiratory drive, increased blood pressure
Atrial stretch reflex (Bainbridge reflex)	Hypervolemia, increased venous return causes stimulation of atrial stretch receptors.	Decreased heart rate, decreased blood pressure, decreased systemic vascular resistance
Oculocardiac reflex	Traction on the extraocular muscles (especially medial rectus) or pressure on the globe causes an afferent response via the trigeminal nerve (CN V) and results in an efferent vagal response via the vagus nerve (CN X).	Bradycardia, hypotension, and arrhythmias
Celiac reflex	Traction or pressure on structures within the peritoneal and thoracic cavity causes vagal nerve stimulation.	Bradycardia, hypotension, and apnea

CN, *Cranial nerve*.

Bainbridge Reflex. The Bainbridge reflex is elicited by stretch on the atria, specifically stretch on the SA node. This stretch increases the HR by 10% to 15%. The afferent limb from the vagus nerve travels to the medulla, and the efferent limb is mediated by the vagus and the sympathetic nerves. This maneuver helps to prevent sequestering of the blood in the veins, atria, and pulmonary circulation and thereby increases CO.

Other cardiovascular reflexes are described later in this chapter. Table 21-2 provides a summary of the cardiovascular reflexes.

VASCULAR SYSTEM

Anatomy

Vascular Anatomy

The vascular circulation is divided into the pulmonary circulation and the peripheral systemic circulation (Figure 21-16). Several functional parts of this vascular system exist.

Arteries

Arteries transport blood to the tissues under high pressure. Arteries have an average diameter of 4 mm and a wall thickness of 1 mm. They have a thick layer of elastic tissue, smooth muscle, and fibrous tissue. Arteries are able to maintain the flow of blood because of their large internal diameter.

Arterioles

Arterioles are the last small branches of the arterial system, and they act as control valves for the release of blood into the capillary beds. Arterioles have an average diameter of 30 μm and a wall thickness of 20 μm. Like arteries, arterioles have a thick layer of elastic tissue, smooth muscle, and fibrous tissue. Constriction of the arterioles, compared with that of other structures within the vascular system, causes the greatest increase in SVR. Because of this contribution, arterioles exhibit the greatest pressure drop in the vascular system across the length of their vessels.

Capillaries

The exchange of fluids, nutrients, electrolytes, hormones, and other substances occurs between the blood and the interstitial

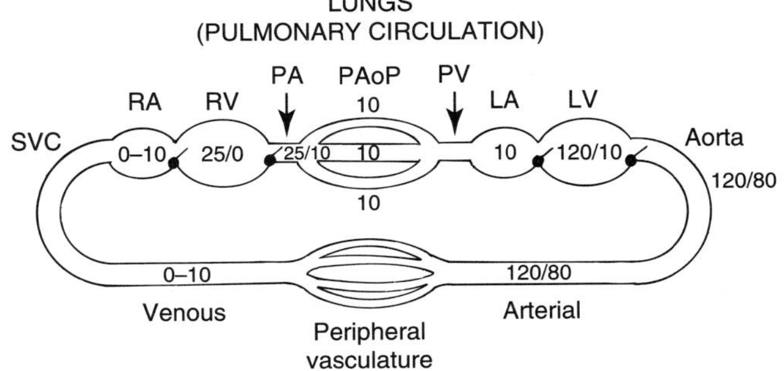

FIGURE 21-16
The vascular circuit. *PA*, Pulmonary artery; *PAOP*, pulmonary artery occlusion pressure; *RA*, right atrium; *RV*, right ventricle; *SVC*, superior vena cava.

fluids in the capillaries. Capillaries have an average diameter of 8 μm and a wall thickness of 1 μm. The walls of capillaries are only one cell thick and have no elastic tissue, smooth muscle, or fibrous tissue. The capillary cell membrane is semipermeable to water and other small molecules.

Venules

Venules collect blood from capillaries and gradually coalesce into progressively larger veins. Venules have an average diameter of 20 μm and a wall thickness of approximately 0.5 mm. They do not have an elastic or smooth muscle layer but have a thin fibrous layer.

Veins

Veins act as conduits for the transport of blood back to the heart. They also act as a large reservoir because they are very distensible. They have an average diameter of 30 mm and a wall thickness of 1.5 mm. The venous system contains approximately 60% of the blood volume, as opposed to the 20% contained within the arteries (Figure 21-17). The elastic tissue

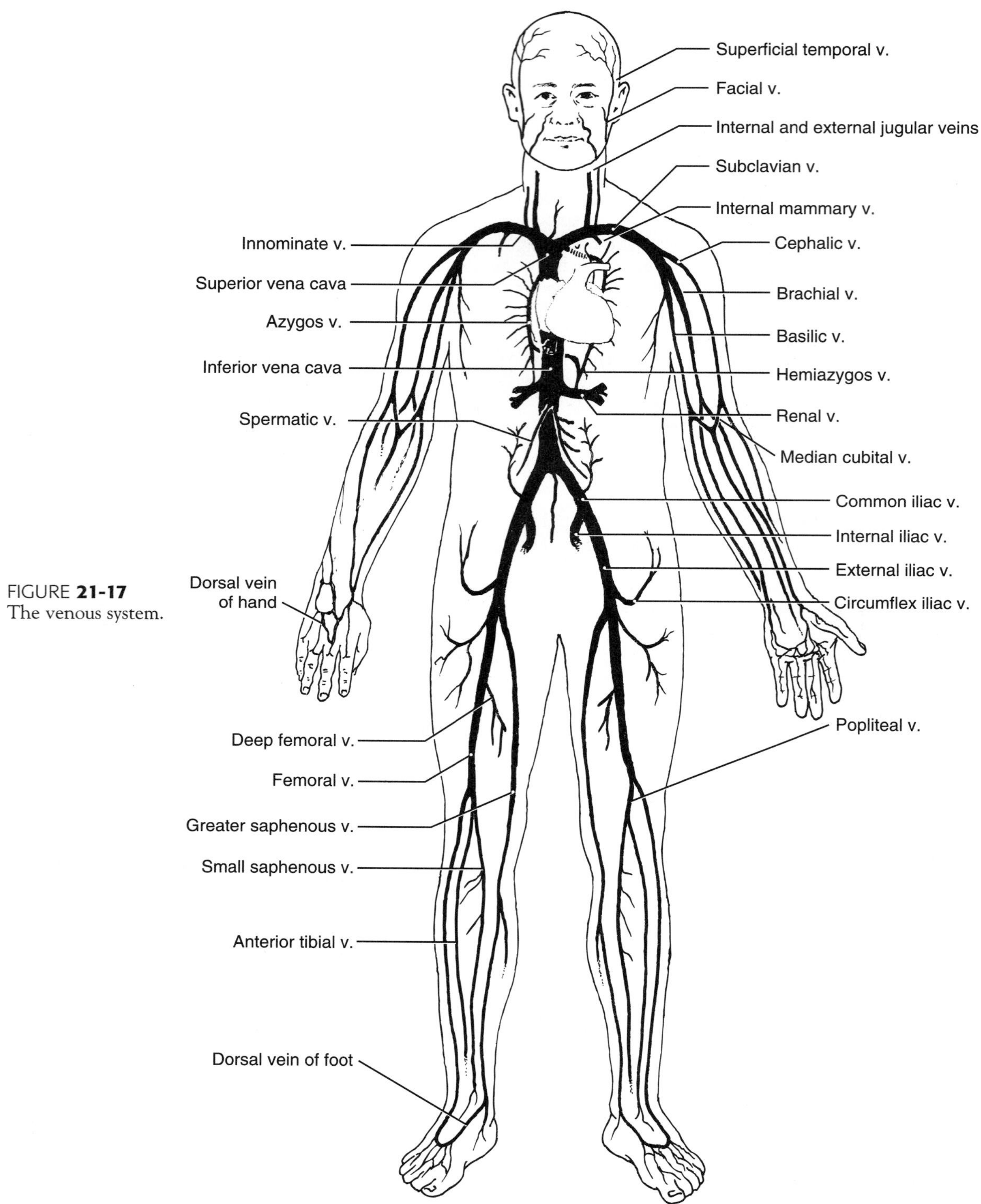

FIGURE **21-17** The venous system.

and the fibrous tissue layers are similar in size to those of the arterioles, but the smooth muscle layer in the veins is smaller than that in the other large vessels.

Arterial Circulation

Knowledge of the anatomy of the arterial circulation is an important part of anesthesia practice. Such information is essential for obtaining intraarterial access, assessing HR and pulse quality, understanding the anatomic relationships for the purpose of regional blocks, and understanding the physiologic implications of blood flow in shock states.

Microscopic Anatomy of the Arterial Circulation. Arteries are classically divided into two types: conducting or elastic arteries and distributing or muscular arteries. Conducting arteries include the major arteries, such as the aorta, and their major branches, such as the brachial, radial, and ulnar arteries. The walls of the arteries are thicker than the walls of veins and consist of three major layers—the tunica intima, the tunica media, and the tunica adventitia.

Thoracic Aorta. The thoracic aorta is divided into three sections: the ascending aorta is the portion that leaves the LV; the transverse aorta, or arch, is the portion that levels off; and the descending aorta is the portion that descends into the thorax. After the thoracic aorta penetrates the diaphragm, the vessel is called the abdominal aorta (Figure 21-18).

The first branches of the ascending aorta are the right and left coronary arteries. From this point, three major branches of the thoracic aorta exist: the brachiocephalic (innominate) artery, the left common carotid artery, and the left subclavian artery.

The brachiocephalic artery branches and becomes the right common carotid artery and the right subclavian artery. The left and right common carotid arteries branch into internal and external carotid arteries. The external carotid arteries supply blood to the face and neck, and the major branches are the superior thyroid artery, the lingual artery, the facial artery, the posterior auricular artery, the maxillary artery, the transverse facial artery, the middle temporal artery, and the superficial temporal artery (Figure 21-19).

The internal carotid arteries supply blood to the brain via the circle of Willis and to the eyes via the ophthalmic arteries (Figure 21-20). The circle of Willis also receives a major part of its blood supply from the vertebral branches of the subclavian artery.

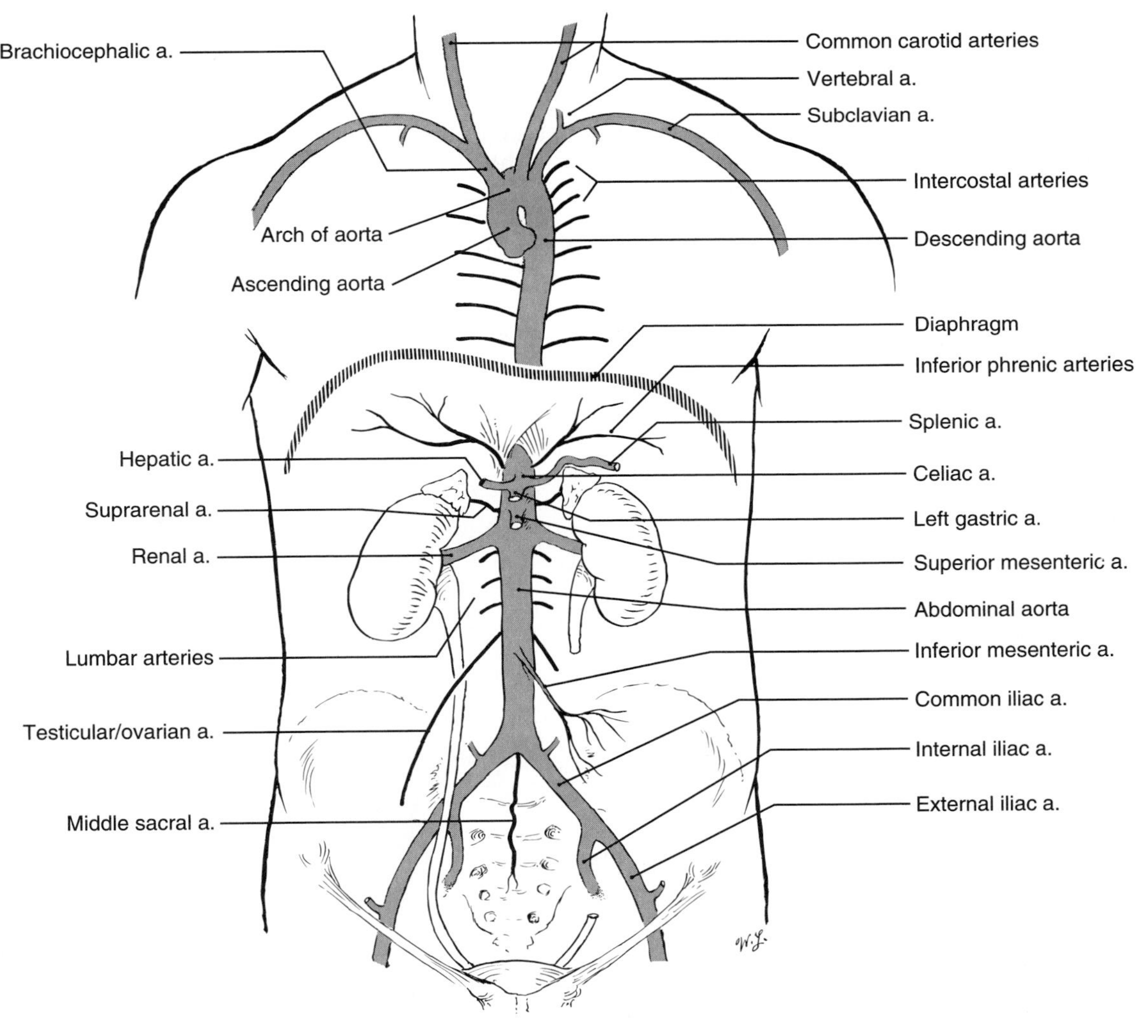

FIGURE **21-18**
Thoracic aorta and abdominal aorta and their branches.

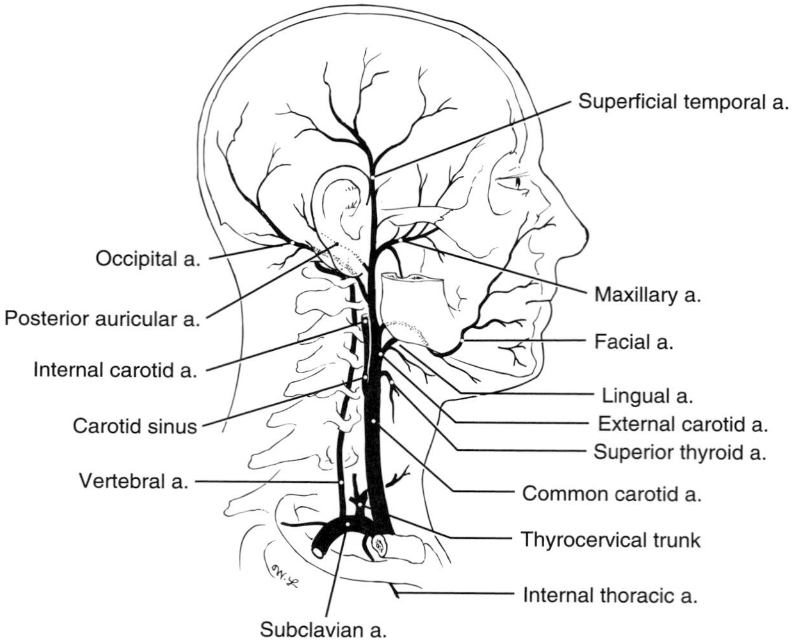

Superficial temporal a.
Occipital a.
Maxillary a.
Posterior auricular a.
Facial a.
Internal carotid a.
Lingual a.
Carotid sinus
External carotid a.
Superior thyroid a.
Vertebral a.
Common carotid a.
Thyrocervical trunk
Internal thoracic a.
Subclavian a.

FIGURE **21-19**
Arterial supply to the face.

Upper Extremity Arteries. The subclavian arteries branch before entering the upper arm. These branches include the vertebral arteries, as noted earlier; the thyrocervical trunk, which supplies blood to the thyroid gland as well as other structures in the neck; the internal thoracic artery, which supplies blood to the anterior chest; and the costocervical trunk, which supplies blood to the first two intercostal spaces and the muscles of the neck.

The subclavian artery continues at the border of the first rib as the axillary artery (Figure 21-21). Branches from the axillary artery supply blood to the axillary region and include the highest thoracic artery, the thoracoacromial artery, the lateral thoracic artery, the subscapular artery, and the anterior and posterior circumflex humoral arteries.

The brachial artery begins at the terminal end of the axillary artery at the inferior border of the teres major muscle. The artery continues until the neck of the radius, where it ends by dividing into the radial and ulnar arteries. The radial artery forms the deep palmar arch, and the ulnar artery supplies blood to the superficial palmar arch.

Descending Thoracic Aorta. The descending thoracic aorta passes caudad through the posterior mediastinum on the left side and, at the level of the twelfth thoracic vertebra, passes through the aortic opening in the diaphragm and becomes the abdominal aorta. Branches of the descending thoracic aorta include the lower nine posterior intercostal arteries, the subcostal arteries, the pericardial arteries, the esophageal arteries, and the bronchial arteries.

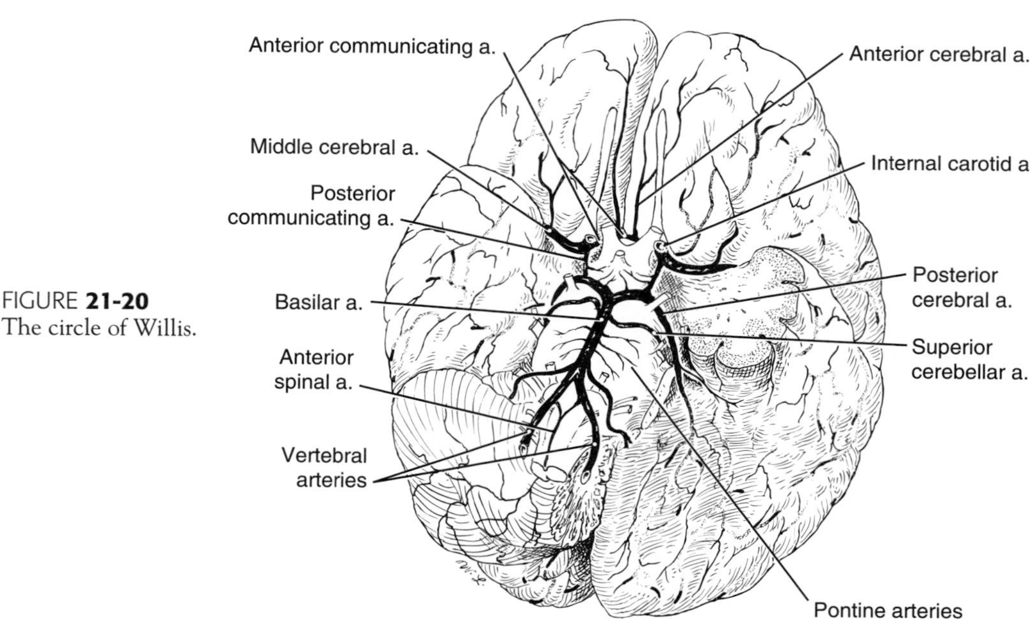

FIGURE **21-20**
The circle of Willis.

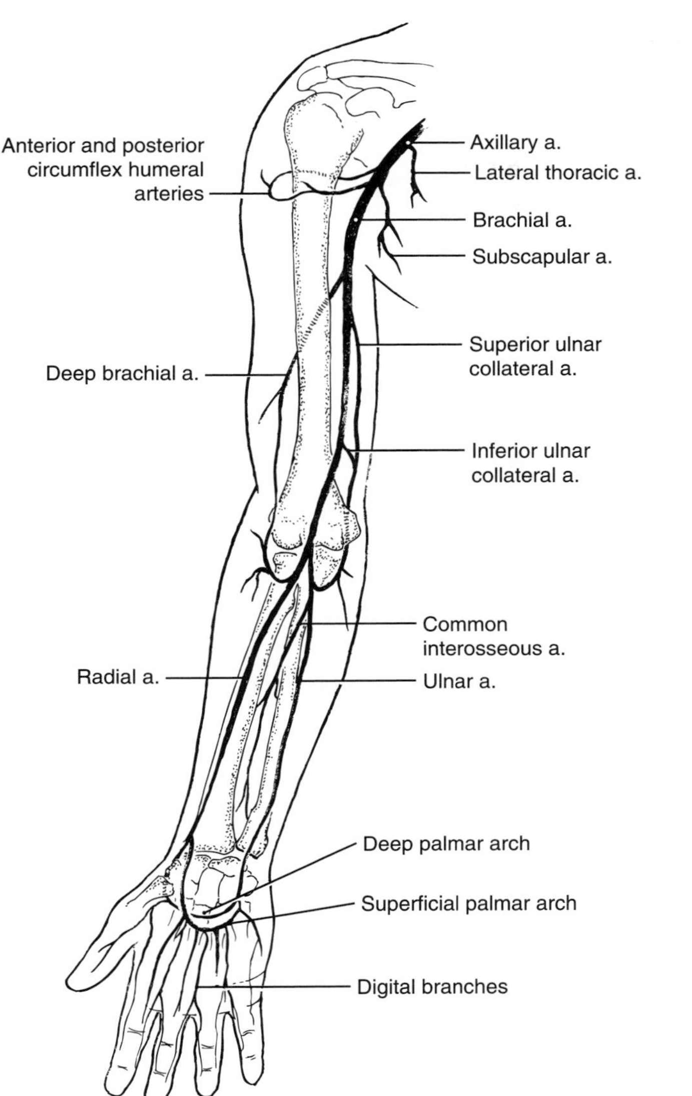

FIGURE **21-21**
Arterial supply to the upper extremity.

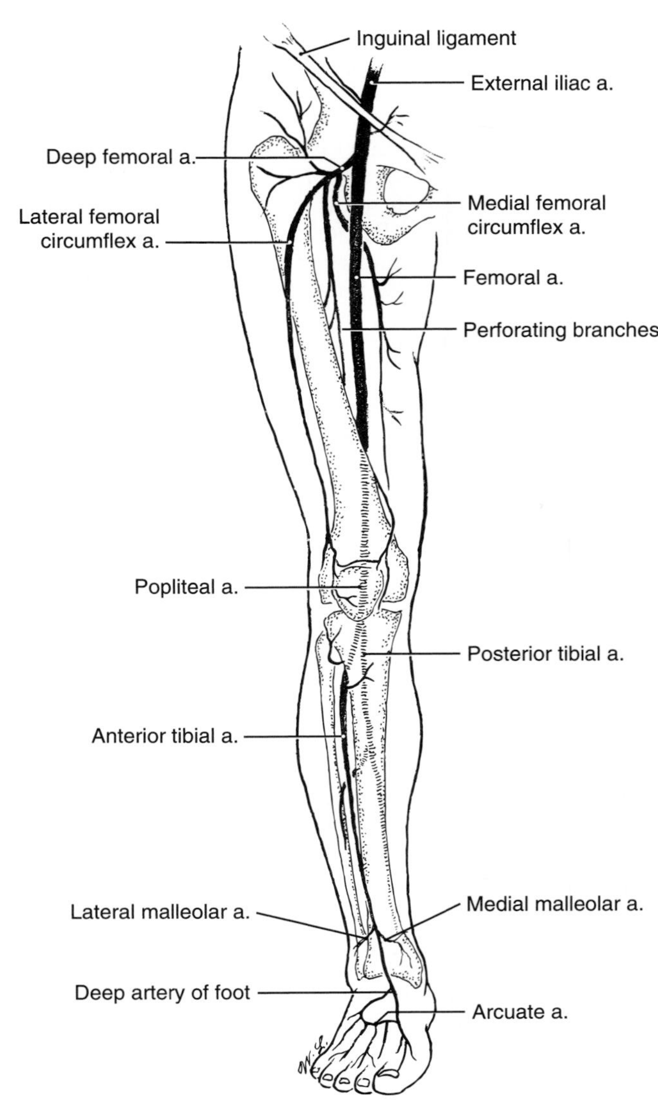

FIGURE **21-22**
Arterial supply to the lower extremity.

Abdominal Aorta. As the thoracic aorta passes through the aortic hiatus of the diaphragm, it becomes the abdominal aorta. The first branches of the abdominal aorta are the inferior phrenic arteries, which supply blood to branches to the underside of the diaphragm and to the adrenal glands (see Figure 21-18).

The next major branch of the abdominal aorta is the celiac trunk, which supplies blood to many of the organs in the upper abdomen. Its branches include the splenic artery, the left gastric artery, the gastroduodenal artery, and the hepatic artery. The cystic artery, which supplies blood to the gallbladder, is a branch of the hepatic artery.

Below the celiac trunk of the aorta lies the superior mesenteric artery. The superior mesenteric artery arises at the level of L1. This artery supplies blood to the jejunum, the ileum, and the transverse colon by means of an anastomosis with the middle colic artery. The jejunal and ileal branches unite to form the arterial arcades of the colon.

Below the superior mesenteric artery are the right and left renal arteries. The right renal artery branches to the right adrenal gland called the middle *suprarenal artery*. Below the renal arteries are the testicular or ovarian arteries.

Below the level of the renal arteries lies the inferior mesenteric artery. This artery has branches to the transverse colon, the descending colon, and the sigmoid colon and rectum.

Iliac Arteries. The abdominal aorta terminates at the common iliac arteries in the pelvis. These arteries divide into internal and external iliac arteries. The internal iliac arteries supply blood to structures within the pelvis, whereas the external iliac arteries supply blood to the legs.

Lower Extremities. The external iliac continues as the femoral artery and the deep femoral artery (Figure 21-22). The femoral artery becomes the popliteal artery behind the knee and then divides into the anterior and posterior tibial arteries. The anterior tibial artery continues as the dorsal artery of the foot. The posterior tibial artery continues and supplies blood to the plantar arches. Clinically, the dorsal artery of the foot is not only an important landmark for the assessment of lower extremity circulation but can also be used for arterial cannulation if the radial artery is not available.

Venous Circulation

An understanding of the anatomy of the venous system is essential in the practice of anesthesia, not only for vascular access but also for identification of significant landmarks for the location of nerve bundles for nerve blocks. Evaluation of venous distention is an important assessment tool for fluid overload and cardiovascular dynamics.

Head and Neck. In the head and neck venous drainage returns to the heart via the internal and external jugular veins. The drainage from the brain comes from the sagittal, transverse, and sigmoid sinuses. These sinuses drain into the internal jugular vein, whereas the more superficial structures of the face and head drain into the external jugular vein.

Upper Extremities. Superficial veins of the upper extremities include those that drain into the axillary vein, the cephalic vein laterally, and the basilica vein medially. The axillary vein drains into the subclavian vein on the right and then into the right brachiocephalic vein. The left subclavian vein drains into the left brachiocephalic vein. The right and left brachiocephalic veins empty into the superior vena cava and account for the venous drainage that occurs from the upper extremities.

Thorax. Venous drainage of the chest comes from the branches of the superior and inferior vena cava and the azygous and hemiazygous systems. These systems are an important alternative blood return route if a major obstruction of the inferior vena cava occurs. These vessels include the intercostal vessels, the bronchial veins, and the pericardial veins.

Abdomen, Pelvis, and Lower Extremities. The deep femoral and femoral veins receive superficial and deep venous drainage from the legs and join to form the external iliac veins. The internal iliac veins drain blood from the pelvis. The common iliac vessels receive blood from the internal and external iliac veins and drain into the inferior vena cava. In this region, the common iliac vessels are joined by branches from the abdomen and the hepatic portal system.

Microcirculation

The function of the microcirculation is to control the delivery of nutrients to the capillary tissue beds, remove waste products, maintain ionic concentrations, and transport hormones to the tissues.

Anatomy. In general, a main nutrient artery enters an organ, where it branches six to eight times until the vessels are small enough to be called *arterioles* (<20 μm in diameter). Arterioles then branch two to five times and reach diameters of 5 to 9 μm, small enough to supply blood to the capillary bed.

In the capillary bed, the blood enters through an arteriole that has a muscular coat. Arterioles are connected to metarterioles, which have many interconnections to the true capillaries and whose branches are protected by precapillary sphincters. These sphincters can control blood flow through the capillary bed.

The capillary wall is a unicellular layer of endothelium that is surrounded by a basement membrane. The total wall thickness is 0.5 μm, and the diameter of the capillaries is 4 to 9 μm. In the capillary membrane, intercellular clefts allow the diffusion of water-soluble ions and small solutes. Plasmalemma vesicles exist and form channels in the cell membrane.

The diffusion of substances through the cell membrane is determined by several factors: lipid solubility, water solubility, size of the molecule, and concentration difference from one side of the membrane to the other.[12]

Movement of fluid volume from the plasma and the interstitial fluid is determined by four factors: capillary pressure, interstitial fluid pressure, plasma colloid osmotic pressure, and interstitial fluid colloid osmotic pressure. Excess fluid from the interstitial space is transported through the lymphatic system, which plays an important role in the prevention of pulmonary edema formation when pulmonary artery pressures are elevated.

Local Control of Capillary Blood Flow. The blood flow to the various capillary beds is regulated in response to tissue requirements for nutrition. Therefore capillary blood flow may be controlled by the delivery of oxygen and other nutrients, the removal of end products of metabolism, or the maintenance of ionic balance of pH in the tissues.

Two major theories of capillary blood flow include the vasodilator theory and the oxygen demand theory. According to these theories the vessels dilate to increase the blood flow as a result of either hypoxemia or release of a vasodilator substance in response to hypoxemia. Some of the vasodilator substances that have been suggested are adenosine, carbon dioxide, lactic acid, adenosine phosphate compounds, histamine, potassium ions, and hydrogen ions. These theories indicate that an active microcirculatory process exists that responds to tissue metabolic needs.

Certain tissue capillary beds do not function as explained by the vasodilator and the oxygen demand theories of microcirculatory blood flow. Blood flow to the skin is dependent on external temperature and dissipation of body heat, whereas blood flow to the kidneys is dependent on the amount of fluid and sodium that needs to be excreted.

Autoregulation is another process that is demonstrated by certain organ tissues to keep the blood flow through the capillary bed constant, despite the normal changes in MAP. Autoregulation has been demonstrated in such tissues as the brain, the kidney, and the coronary circulation. Autoregulation keeps the blood flow to an organ constant by vasodilation or vasoconstriction as occurs in response to fluctuations in MAP.

A substance that causes the secondary vasodilation of the large arteries in response to increased flow has been isolated and is called the *endothelium-derived relaxing factor*,[20] or more commonly referred to as *nitric oxide*. This factor is synthesized by the endothelial lining of the arterioles and the small arteries. Shear stress on the walls of the vessels accelerates the release of this substance and allows larger vessels to dilate when blood flow to the tissues increases.

Growth of Collateral Circulation

Microcirculation is a good example of vascular growth that can occur to provide collateral circulation. The growth of new vessels results in part from angiogenesis and the release of angiogenic factors. These substances are released from ischemic tissues, rapidly growing tissues, and tissues with high metabolic rates.

Several angiogenic factors have been identified, including endothelial cell growth factor,[21] fibroblast growth factor,[22] and angiogen.[23] These factors act by the dissolution of the basement membrane of the endothelial cells, followed by the rapid dissolution of new endothelial cells that stream out of the vessels into cords. The cells in these cords divide and then gradually fold over into a tube. The tubes then connect with other tubes to form a vascular network.

Vascular flow is dependent on neurologic as well as hormonal regulation. Some vasoconstrictor hormones include epinephrine and norepinephrine from the central nervous system (CNS) and the adrenal medulla; angiotensin from the adrenal cortex; and vasopressin from the posterior pituitary. Some vasodilator substances include bradykinin, serotonin, histamine, and the prostaglandins. Various other ionic and chemical factors can produce vasoconstriction and vasodilation as well and have an effect on the flow of blood that is delivered to tissues.

Blood Pressure

Pressure, Flow, and Resistance Interrelationships

Ohm's Law. Ohm's law correlates the flow of electricity (current), the applied electrical pressure (voltage), and the resistance to this flow (resistance). A modification of this law is used in medicine to describe the flow of a fluid (blood) through a tube (blood vessel), even though the vessels are dynamic rather than static. Ohm's law and fluid flow are described by the following equation:

Equation 21-10

$$Q = (P_1 \times P_2)/R$$

where the flow through a cylinder (Q) is equal to the change in pressure from one end of the tube to the other ($P_1 \times P_2$) divided by the resistance (R) of the tube. Therefore either a decrease in resistance or an increase in pressure change across the tube increases the flow of fluid through the tube.

Blood Flow. Blood flow is the quantity of blood that passes a given point in a given amount of time. Clinically, CO may be inserted into the equation as blood flow. Two types of flow exist: laminar and turbulent (Figure 21-23).

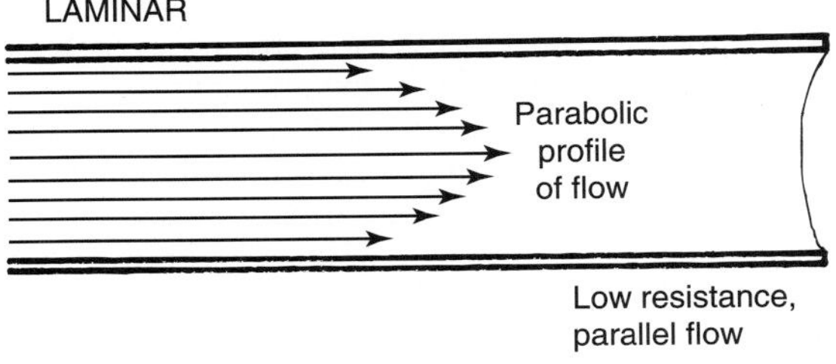

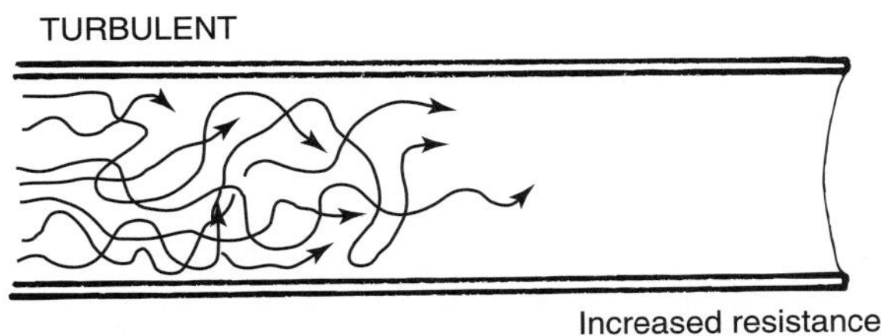

FIGURE **21-23**
Laminar and turbulent flow.

Laminar flow has a parabolic profile that illustrates the parallel movement of molecules. Conversely, turbulent flow is described as a whirlpool and does not move as easily, thereby increasing resistance to flow. Reynold's number (Re) is a means of determining the type of flow in a tube and uses the diameter of the blood vessel (d) and the velocity (v), density (ρ), and viscosity (n) of the fluid to determine whether or not turbulence occurs.

The formula for calculating Reynold's number includes the velocity of blood flow in centimeters per second multiplied by the diameter of the tube in centimeters, multiplied by the density of the fluid in grams per cubic centimeter, divided by the viscosity (see equation). A Reynold's number below 200 indicates laminar flow. A Reynold's number of 200 to 400 indicates that turbulence occurs at bends in the tube, and a Reynold's number above 2000 indicates turbulent flow, even in straight smooth vessels.

Equation 21-11

$$Re = (v \times d \times \rho)/n$$

Reynold's number demonstrates that in large vessels with high velocities, such as the aorta and large arteries, turbulent flow occurs even in the straight portions of these vessels.

Poiseuille's Law. Poiseuille's law (see equation) describes the amount of fluid flowing through a tube (Q) in relation to the pressure drop across the tube ($P_1 - P_2$), the radius of the tube (r), the length of the tube (l), and the viscosity of the fluid (n):

Equation 21-12

$$Q = ([P_1 - P_2]\, r^4)/(8 \times n \times 1)$$

One of the most important factors in determining fluid flow is the radius of the vessel.

Clinical applications of Poiseuille's law include selection of intravenous catheter size and endotracheal tube size and determination of vascular distention and constriction in response to pharmacologic agents.

Resistance. Resistance is the impediment to blood flow in a blood vessel. Clinically it cannot be measured directly but is calculated from measures of blood flow (CO) and pressure differences in the vessels.

The units of measure that are most commonly used in the clinical area are the centimeter-gram-second units. The normal SVR is 800 to 1500 dyne/sec per centimeter^{-5}, and the normal pulmonary vascular resistance is approximately one tenth of that number, or between 50 and 150 dyne/sec per centimeter^{5}.

Resistance of Systems. Resistance is calculated for two major systems (Figure 21-24). In a series system, such as the systemic vasculature, the total resistance (R_T) is equal to the sum of the resistances for the individual tissue beds within the system (see equation):

Equation 21-13

$$R_T = R_1 + R_2 + R_3 + \ldots R_n$$

In a parallel system, such as a capillary bed, the total resistance is less than any of the individual resistances (see equation).

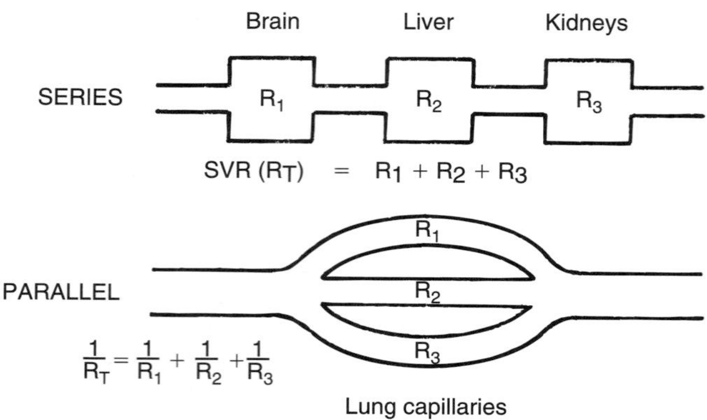

FIGURE **21-24**
Resistance in series and parallel systems. *R*, Resistance; *SVR*, systemic vascular resistance.

Therefore the blood flow through a capillary bed such as the pulmonary capillaries is less than the resistance through any of the individual capillaries of the pulmonary system.

Equation 21-14

$$1/R_T = 1/R_1 + 1/R_2 + 1/R_3 + \ldots 1/R_n$$

Regulation of Mean Arterial Blood Pressure

Regulation of arterial blood pressure is an important function in the maintenance of the homeostasis of the patient receiving anesthesia. MAP is an important indicator of the perfusion of the tissue beds.

Blood pressure regulation can be categorized as either short term or long term. The choice of category depends on the onset of action, the duration of action, and the intensity of action to return the MAP to normal values.

Short-Term Regulation. The short-term blood pressure regulators are those that respond to rapid changes in MAP and attempt to rapidly (within 30 minutes) return the MAP back to normal range. These reflexes rely on an intact nervous system, and this interaction is responsible for the rapid onset of action of these blood pressure regulators.

The short-term blood pressure regulators include the baroreceptors, the CNS ischemic mechanisms, and the chemoreceptors. All are initiated within 10 minutes of the change in MAP.

It is important to understand the role of the cardiovascular (vasomotor) center that is located in the medulla and pons. This center regulates four basic actions: vasoconstriction, vasodilation, cardiac excitation, and cardiac inhibition. These areas activate the sympathetic and parasympathetic nervous systems in response to certain stimuli. Under normal conditions the vasoconstrictor area sends out impulses to maintain a certain degree of peripheral vascular tone.

The baroreceptors are located in most of the major vessels within the head and neck. However, they are densely distributed within the aortic and carotid sinuses. They are spray-type nerve endings that increase impulse production when they are stretched. Impulses from the baroreceptors affect the inhibitory centers of the vasomotor center. At MAP of less than 60 mm Hg, the baroreceptors do not transmit impulses. However, as the MAP increases to between 60 and 180 mm Hg, the impulses sent to the inhibitory area of the vasomotor center increase. The baroreceptors are most efficient in responding to rapid changes in blood pressure. They are not as efficient in long-term blood pressure regulation because they adapt to the higher pressures, in effect by being reset. Therefore the baroreceptors act as a buffer system to prevent wide short-term swings in blood pressure. Two clinically significant examples of stimulation of the baroreceptor reflex during surgery include carotid sinus manipulation during carotid endarterectomy and aortic baroreceptor stimulation from pressure exerted on the aortic arch during mediastinoscopy.

Chemoreceptors are chemosensitive cells that are located within the carotid and aortic bodies. Each area is supplied by a small nutrient artery and thereby maintains constant contact with the internal environment. Chemoreceptors send impulses to excite the vasomotor center in response to decreases in PaO_2. Chemoreceptors play a greater role in respiratory system regulation than in blood pressure regulation.

Low-pressure receptors, or stretch receptors, are located in many areas of the vasculature, especially within the atria and pulmonary arterial tree. They act in conjunction with the baroreceptors to buffer changes in the blood pressure that are caused by changes in volume status.

Included with these low-pressure receptors are several other atrial reflexes. Stretching of the atria caused by an increase in volume results in a slight dilation of the peripheral arterioles, which decreases SVR, MAP, and CO.

Another atrial reflex that is stimulated in response to hypervolemia involves the release of the atrial natriuretic factor by the atria as a result of increased stretch.[24] This factor causes a reflex dilation of afferent arterioles in the kidney, a phenomenon that increases the glomerular filtration rate and decreases the secretion of antidiuretic hormone via signals to the hypothalamus. The combination of these events causes an increase in urine formation and an attempt to change the MAP by decreasing vascular volume.

The CNS ischemic mechanisms are another rapidly acting blood pressure control system. These mechanisms are initiated in an attempt to restore the MAP to adequate levels for CNS perfusion and especially for perfusion to the vasomotor center. When the vasomotor area becomes ischemic as a result of hypotension (MAP <50 mm Hg), maximal stimulation of the vasomotor center occurs. The stimulation persists for approximately 10 minutes, by which time either the ischemia has been relieved or the vasomotor center has infarcted, and the stimulation ceases.

Another special type of CNS ischemic mechanism is Cushing's reflex, which is triggered by an elevation of the intracranial pressure to a value greater than the MAP, thereby decreasing cerebral perfusion and causing ischemia. An intense response from the vasomotor center is initiated. Cushing's reflex results in the most powerful sympathetic vasoconstrictor response within the human body. These compensatory physiologic changes attempt to restore adequate cerebral perfusion. However, if cerebral ischemia is not relieved, cerebral infarction results. See Table 21-2 for a summary of cardiac reflexes.

Several hormones are instrumental in the short-term regulation of MAP. The onset of action is not as rapid as that of neural control mechanisms, but activation occurs within a short time of stimulation. Norepinephrine and epinephrine are released from the adrenal medulla during times of sympathetic stimulation and cause vasoconstriction.

Angiotensin I is converted to angiotensin II in the lung by angiotensin-converting enzyme. This substance is one of the most potent vasoconstrictive substances secreted by the body. It takes approximately 20 minutes to become fully activated. Angiotensin II also plays a role in the secretion of aldosterone from the adrenal cortex. Aldosterone has a role in the long-term regulation of MAP.

The antidiuretic hormone vasopressin has both short-term and long-term effects on blood pressure control. The short-term effect of antidiuretic hormone causes potent and direct vasoconstriction. The long-term control effects of antidiuretic hormone decrease urine output from the kidneys.

Two short-term systems for maintenance of blood pressure that could be classified as intermediate mechanisms are the capillary fluid shift and the stress-relaxation mechanism. Both of these mechanisms depend on an intact vascular system.

The capillary fluid shift is a simple mechanism. As the hydrostatic pressure (MAP) increases within the capillaries, a larger movement of fluid occurs across the capillary membrane as increased pressure. This phenomenon lowers the fluid volume within the vasculature and results in a decrease in MAP.

The stress-relaxation mechanism is an example of the ability of the vasculature to compensate for hypervolemia and hypovolemia as a result of alterations of smooth muscle tone within the vasculature. When the fluid volume increases, tension on the blood vessels results in dilation of the vasculature to compensate for increased volume. Conversely, as the blood volume decreases, the vessels constrict to compensate for the decreased volume in order to maintain MAP.

Long-Term Regulation. Long-term regulation of MAP includes mechanisms that eventually regulate blood volume to within normal range. The renal body fluid system is one of the major long-term regulators of MAP. Renal homeostasis of blood pressure occurs as the kidneys preferentially excrete sodium and water in order to maintain a normal fluid balance.

It is important to understand the concept of fluid balance and its effect on arterial blood pressure. A chronic increase in blood volume leads to increases in mean filling pressure, venous return, CO, and SVR. The combination of an increased CO and an increased SVR can increase the arterial blood pressure by more than 30%. This causes an increase in myocardial oxygen demand.

Several factors govern the effectiveness of the renal body fluid system, including the renin-angiotensin system, aldosterone secretion, and the nervous system. As fluid intake and blood pressure increase, the secretion of renin by the kidneys decreases. This decreased renin secretion causes a reduced secretion of aldosterone as a result of the decreased secretion of angiotensin II. A decrease in sympathetic nervous system response to the kidney also occurs. The net effect is an increased renal output of sodium and water.

Physiology of the Venous System

In the past the venous system has been described as simply the return conduit for the arterial system. The venous system was not thought to play a very active role in the maintenance of circulation and CO. The modern view gives the venous system an integral role in the support of the circulation.[25]

The venous system's ability to accommodate large volume changes helps to buffer the intravascular volume during periods of hypervolemia or hypovolemia and thereby helps to maintain CO. In addition, the venous system is well innervated by the autonomic nervous system and therefore has the ability to respond to the wide variations in intravascular volume that occur over the course of long surgical procedures and during times of intensive fluid resuscitation.

Knowledge of the anatomy and physiology of the cardiovascular system is essential for the safe practice of anesthesia. This section has discussed issues of concern to the anesthesia provider and has provided reference material for the integration of that knowledge into clinical practice.

HYPERTENSION

Extent, Definition, and Etiology

The pathophysiologic cardiovascular condition that is most commonly encountered in patients who require surgery is hypertension. Hypertension affects approximately 60 million people in the United States, and the frequency at which it occurs increases with age. Almost two thirds of people over the age of 65 years have hypertension. It is vital for the anesthesia provider to understand the pathophysiology of the condition and its relation to the cardiovascular system and other body systems. Only then can a comprehensive anesthesia plan be constructed.

Patients frequently do not exhibit signs or symptoms associated with hypertension. Chronic uncontrolled hypertension affects specific target organs, including the heart, brain, and kidney. Hypertension accelerates and exacerbates the onset of atherosclerotic changes in the arterial vessels of the target organs. It is a primary risk factor for the development of coronary artery disease. Hypertension is a significant cause of congestive heart failure and cardiomyopathy because of increased afterload from chronic vasoconstriction. Because hypertension increases the likelihood of the development of atherosclerosis, it has been implicated as a causative factor that is responsible for the development of stroke and renal failure.[26]

Hypertension is classified on the basis of its causes. Essential (primary) hypertension, which has no identifiable cause, accounts for 95% of all cases of the disease, and its diagnosis is determined on the basis of exclusion. Remedial (secondary) hypertension has an identifiable and potentially curable cause. Sources of secondary hypertension include pheochromocytoma, coarctation of the aorta, renal artery stenosis, primary renal diseases (e.g., pyelonephritis, glomerulonephritis), primary aldosteronism (Conn's disease), and hyperadrenocorticism (Cushing's disease).

Recently updated guidelines regarding blood pressure values that constitute hypertension have been published by the National Institutes of Health (NIH). The classification of hypertension is listed in Table 21-3. In order to determine accurate blood pressure measurements, two readings taken 5 minutes apart with the patient in the sitting position are necessary. Because of new information that states that the risk of cardiovascular disease doubles with each increment of 20/10 mm Hg above 115/75 mm Hg, the NIH has coined the term *prehypertension* to refer to those patients who would benefit from lifestyle modifications in order to decrease the likelihood of developing the pathophysiologic changes associated with hypertension.[27] It is estimated that the implementation of antihypertensive therapy is associated with a 25% decrease in cardiovascular complications and a 38% decrease in stroke.[28] If lifestyle modifications are not successful in decreasing blood pressure to acceptable levels, then antihypertensive

TABLE 21-3 Classification of Blood Pressure for Adults Age 18 Years and Older

Category	Systolic (mm Hg)		Diastolic (mm Hg)
Normal	<120	and	<80
Prehypertension	120-139	or	80-89
Hypertension, stage 1	140-159	or	90-99
Hypertension, stage 2	≥160	or	≥100

From Seventh Report of the Joint National Committee on Prevention, Detection, Evaluation and Treatment of High Blood Pressure. National Institutes of Health, National Heart, Lung and Blood Institute; National High Blood Pressure Education Program, Bethesda, MD. 2003. NIH publication no. 03-5233;3.

therapy should be prescribed.[29] In many instances, patients may have developed advanced atherosclerotic vascular disease or target-organ dysfunction before the start of treatment for hypertension.[30,31]

Pathophysiology

Systemic blood pressure is regulated by interactive feedback mechanisms involving the sympathoadrenal axis and baroreceptors in the heart and great vessels. It is accepted that some degree of sympathetic dysfunction is responsible for essential hypertension. Dysfunction of the sympathetic nervous system leads to a state of chronic vasoconstriction. In an attempt to maintain normal intravascular volume, the renal juxtaglomerular apparatus secretes renin. All the vascular and hormonal effects of renin are caused by its conversion of angiotensin I to angiotensin II. Angiotensin II is the major stimulus for the secretion of aldosterone by the adrenal cortex.

Anesthesia Management for the Patient with Hypertension

Preoperative Evaluation

The most important issues to be addressed in the preoperative evaluation of the hypertensive patient are the identification and the adequacy of treatment. A number of otherwise healthy patients scheduled for elective procedures are determined to have hypertension, even though they had no prior need for medical treatment. The goal of antihypertensive therapy is to maintain normotension on a consistent basis. Effective antihypertensive therapy that renders the patient normotensive on a routine basis may not necessarily prevent episodes of perioperative hypertension. However, patients whose condition is optimized before surgery have a more stable perioperative course and a lower incidence of cardiovascular system–related morbidity. As long as perioperative diastolic blood pressure is maintained below 110 mm Hg, the risk of perioperative cardiac morbidity does not increase significantly.[26,32]

It is imperative for anesthesia providers to have an adequate understanding of the pharmacology and side effects of the drugs used for treating hypertension. For a complete discussion of antihypertensive drugs see Chapter 12. Some of the drugs used to treat hypertension block or depress homeostatic sympathetic reflexes. The depression of these reflexes may prevent homeostatic compensatory mechanisms from functioning at normal levels during the course of anesthesia. Subsequently, compensatory mechanisms (tachycardia and vasoconstriction) associated with blood loss may be diminished or may not occur. Patients treated with antihypertensive medication do not lose their responsiveness to vasoactive drugs but instead may respond to these substances in an exaggerated manner. Even with depression of the sympathetic reflexes, no predominance of the parasympathetic system occurs. A review of all the medications used for treatment of hypertension is beyond the scope of this chapter.

The clinician should carefully obtain a thorough history of the cardiovascular system to elicit any symptoms of ischemic cardiovascular disease. Hypertension is a major risk factor for coronary artery disease. Any symptoms related to coronary artery disease should be further investigated. In addition to being a risk factor for coronary artery disease, hypertension directly affects myocardial function. The chronic increase in myocardial wall tension caused by long-standing hypertension results in left ventricular hypertrophy (LVH; Figure 21-25). Ventricular diastolic dysfunction occurs before the development of hypertrophy. This diastolic dysfunction is not clinically apparent, and the patient may appear to have normal cardiac function except under stressful physiologic conditions. A delayed rate of passive ventricular filling is evidence of ventricular diastolic dysfunction. The rate of ventricular filling from atrial contraction becomes predominant in the hypertensive patient. This represents the inverse of the normal ventricular filling patterns.

LVH is a consequence of chronic hypertension and increased afterload. LVH results in an enlargement of myocardial mass, which leads to an increase in myocardial oxygen demand. Hypertrophy that occurs in response to chronic increases in pressure is termed *concentric hypertrophy*. Ventricular hypertrophy also may produce subendocardial ischemia at perfusion pressures that would normally be adequate in a healthy ventricle. Concomitant development of

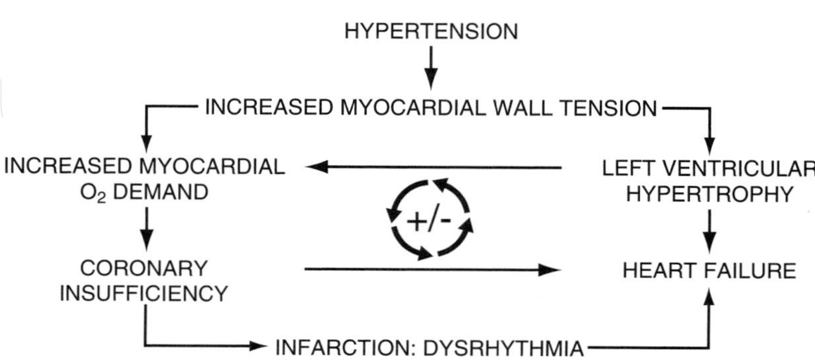

FIGURE **21-25**
Schematic representation of the relationship between hypertension and heart failure. (Modified from Stoelting RK, Dierdorf SF. *Anesthesia and Co-Existing Disease*. 3rd ed. New York: Churchill Livingstone; 1993:21-102.)

coronary artery disease coupled with increased myocardial oxygen demand hastens and exacerbates the development of ischemic symptoms. As a rule, all patients with chronic hypertension should be suspected of having some degree of coronary artery disease.

Hypertensive cardiomyopathy and systolic ventricular dysfunction are the direct result of the pathophysiologic changes associated with chronic hypertension. This hypertensive cardiomyopathy manifests as a decrease in both EF and SV. Increasing diastolic dysfunction results in ventricular dilation in conjunction with systolic dysfunction. The subsequent replacement of myocardial cells with fibrous tissue results in a cardiomyopathy.[3]

Long-standing hypertension that has remained either untreated or inadequately controlled has adverse consequences on brain and kidney function, and patients with such long-standing disease have a higher incidence of strokes than do patients whose blood pressure has been controlled.[3] Inadequate control of hypertension can lead to alterations in cerebrovascular and coronary artery autoregulation. For example, normal physiologic coronary artery autoregulation occurs at a MAP between 50 and 120 mm Hg. However, a patient with chronic hypertension and coronary artery disease may develop ischemic changes at a MAP of 50 mm Hg. The cerebral and coronary autoregulation curves are shifted to the right in patients with chronic hypertension, necessitating higher perfusion pressures to ensure adequate organ blood flow. Therefore cerebral and myocardial ischemia may occur with significant decreases in MAP in patients with hypertension and coronary artery disease. This phenomenon makes insufficiently treated patients more susceptible to cerebrovascular ischemia at MAPs that would be of no consequence in the normotensive patient.[31] Chronic untreated hypertension can cause nephrosclerosis, which can impair renal function. The nephrosclerosis can produce proteinuria and a gradual decrease in renal function. Early treatment of hypertension results in little change in renal function and spares the kidneys. Signs of target organ involvement must be investigated in the hypertensive patient who is to undergo anesthesia.

Anesthesia Management

In order to maintain a stable intraoperative course, administration of antihypertensive medications should be continued on schedule until the time of surgery. All oral medications can be given with one or two sips of water without increased risk of aspiration.[30] It should be noted that acute hypertensive rebound can occur with abrupt cessation of clonidine therapy. Angina, hypertension, and tachycardia can result from interruption of therapy with β-blockers and calcium channel–blocking agents. These drugs should be discontinued with caution and only after utmost discretionary review of the patient's physiologic status.

The determination of whether to proceed with elective surgery in a patient in whom hypertension is untreated or poorly controlled remains controversial. However, evidence suggests that patients with diastolic blood pressures of 110 mm Hg or greater have a significantly increased risk of perioperative cardiac morbidity.[31] This caveat may be modified in patients with hypertension in whom diastolic blood pressures of 110 mm Hg or greater occur frequently despite aggressive antihypertensive drug therapy (e.g., patients with end-stage renal disease).

Mild preoperative sedation may be indicated for such patients with hypertension when there exists the possibility that any degree of anxiety in the patient could initiate sympathetic response. Establishing control of the blood pressure before induction should result in a more stable hemodynamic course during the induction, maintenance, and emergence from anesthesia.

Induction of Anesthesia

Patients with hypertension react in an exaggerated manner to induction agents and the stimulation associated with laryngoscopy and tracheal intubation. Such patients are hypovolemic, either as a result of renal-compensatory mechanisms or because of medical therapy. Increased vasoconstriction as a consequence of hypertension results in volume contraction and a greater susceptibility to hypotension from the vasodilating effects of anesthetic agents. Etomidate, propofol, or sodium pentothal induction agents can be used in patients with hypertension. It is not uncommon to see exaggerated and precipitous decreases in blood pressure when standard doses of these agents are administered. This hypotension results from relative hypovolemia coupled with the vasodilation and potential myocardial depression produced by most intravenous induction agents.

The stimuli of laryngoscopy and tracheal intubation can result in an exaggerated hypertensive response despite postinduction hypotension. An existing hypertensive state is further compounded by intense stimulation caused by airway manipulation. In order to suppress the exaggerated hypertensive response to intubation, a greater depth of anesthesia must be achieved. However, the depth of anesthesia at induction necessary to suppress this response may produce a more profound hypotensive state. Administration of adjunct medications before induction such as blocker or arterial dilators can reduce the hyperdynamic sympathetic response to tracheal intubation. Hypotensive episodes can be treated with fluid administration, decrease in anesthetic depth, and administration of vasoconstrictors. Numerous strategies have been suggested for the management of this hyperdynamic response. Stoelting and Dierdorf demonstrated that the pressor response to laryngoscopy and intubation could be significantly reduced by laryngotracheal or intravenous administration of lidocaine. They also proposed that reducing the duration of airway manipulation to 15 seconds or less may be helpful. Use of a β-blocker before induction has been shown to reduce the hyperdynamic sympathetic responses, as may the administration of sodium nitroprusside before laryngoscopy.[30] Administration of fentanyl (2 to 3 mcg/kg) just before induction also helps reduce pressor response.

Certainly, with regard to suppression of marked hemodynamic responses, no substitute exists for a smooth induction followed by a rapid and atraumatic intubation. The maintenance of an adequate depth of anesthesia at induction that produces extreme hypotension may be more detrimental to both coronary and cerebral perfusion than the hypertensive response it was intended to prevent. Because the hypertensive patient is frequently hypovolemic as compared with the normotensive patient, adequate hydration before induction may help to prevent postinduction hypotension.[26,30]

Most standard intravenous induction agents are appropriate for the hypertensive patient. The propensity for these agents to cause vasodilation in a comparatively hypovolemic patient is a concern. In light of this a combination of low doses of more than one agent in addition to titration of medications may prove a better choice than a full dose of a single agent. In emergency cases in which securing the airway is of paramount importance, the choice of agents may be limited, and hyperdynamic pressor responses become a secondary issue.

Maintenance of Anesthesia

The goal of anesthetic management of the hypertensive patient undergoing general anesthesia is to maintain blood pressure stability within 20% of the normal mean pressure. Intraoperative events that cause wide fluctuations in blood pressure should be anticipated and treated immediately. The most common event precipitating intraoperative hypertension is the painful stimulus of surgery. This induces increased sympathetic tone via a neurohormonal reflex and represents the stress-induced response of surgical stimulation. Volatile and opioid agents given alone and in combination have the ability to attenuate this response.[26,30,31] Altering the depth of anesthesia to suppress maximal surgical stimulation may not be adequate for achieving rapid and complete control of hypertensive responses. The adjunct use of drugs such as β-antagonists, nitroprusside, angiotensin-converting enzyme inhibitors (e.g., enalapril), α_2-agonists (e.g., clonidine), calcium-channel blockers (e.g., nifedipine), and α_1-blockers (e.g., droperidol) may be necessary for achieving control. These drugs offer the advantage of continued control of hypertensive response in the immediate postanesthesia recovery period.

The onset of profound hypotension during anesthesia maintenance should be immediately recognized, diagnosed, and treated. Prolonged severe hypotension has predictive significance in perioperative cardiac morbidity.[32] Treatment of hypotension may require reduction of the amount of volatile agent used and infusion of adequate volume. Should these measures prove inadequate or untimely, a rapid-acting vasopressor such as phenylephrine or ephedrine may be administered as a temporizing measure until the cause of the hypotension can be diagnosed. It is important to realize that hypertensive patients may have exaggerated responses to vasopressor agents. The goal of intraoperative anesthesia management is maintenance of hemodynamic stability, which includes anticipation of intraoperative events that may affect cardiovascular stability and thereby prevent extreme fluctuations in blood pressure.

Postoperative Considerations in the Hypertensive Patient

Termination of anesthesia results in hyperdynamic, hypertensive responses, even in patients with well-controlled hypertension. Intraoperative control of blood pressure should continue into the immediate postoperative period. Initiation of adjunct administration of antihypertensive medications should be anticipated early in the postoperative period. Adequate control of pain represents a primary antihypertensive consideration. The hypertensive patient is more susceptible to perioperative cardiac morbidity than the normotensive patient during the postoperative period. Adequate control of blood pressure in the postoperative period reduces the incidence of cardiovascular complications.[26,33] Mangano and associates studied the effects of atenolol administered to patients who had confirmed or were at risk for the development of coronary artery disease. Atenolol was administered preoperatively, postoperatively, and throughout the hospital stay. The results in the atenolol study group showed a 65% reduction in mortality caused by adverse cardiac events. In addition, patients in the atenolol study group had a 67% decrease in mortality within 1 year of surgery and a 48% decrease in mortality in the 2 years after surgery.[34]

Pericardial Disease

In reviewing the anesthetic management of patients with pericardial disease, this section focuses on the pathophysiology, clinical presentation, and anesthetic implications of three primary disease processes: acute pericarditis, constrictive pericarditis, and cardiac tamponade.

The pericardium stabilizes the heart to its anatomic position, concomitantly reducing contact between it and surrounding structures. It consists of an inner visceral layer, which envelops the surface of the heart, and an outer parietal layer. The pericardial space between these layers usually contains 20 to 25 ml of clear fluid, which under normal circumstances can accommodate gradual volume fluctuations. Rapid accumulation of pericardial fluid in the pericardial space can result in cardiac tamponade and cardiovascular collapse.[35]

Acute Pericarditis

Acute inflammation of the pericardium is caused by a number of disorders.[35] The most common cause of acute pericarditis is viral infection. Postmyocardial infarction syndrome (Dressler's syndrome), postcardiotomy, metastatic disease, irradiation, tuberculosis, and rheumatoid arthritis represent the remaining primary predisposing conditions that cause the development of this process.[36]

Pathophysiology. It is common for a serofibrinous inflammatory reaction associated with a small intrapericardial exudative effusion to evolve. This may result in adherence of the two layers of the pericardium. The sequelae are largely dependent on the severity of the reaction as well as on the specific cause. Most often when the condition is left untreated or undiagnosed, complete resolution is the end result. Infrequently, however, extended organization of fibrinous exudate within the pericardial sac may lead to encasement of the heart by dense fibrous connective tissue (chronic constrictive pericarditis) or to the accumulation of a large amount of pericardial fluid and consequent cardiac tamponade, usually when fluid levels exceed 1 L. Constrictive pericarditis and cardiac tamponade result in impaired diastolic filling and subsequent diminution of CO.[35,36]

Clinical Presentation. The principal symptom associated with acute pericarditis is chest pain with sudden onset. Although similar in nature to that experienced during myocardial infarction, this pain is differentiated from it by the inclusion of a pleural component, which includes increased discomfort associated with postural changes and relief on sitting or leaning forward. Other signs that are characteristic of acute pericarditis include fever with a pericardial friction rub, absence of elevation of cardiac enzymes levels, and diffuse ST-segment elevation in two or three limb leads and in most of the precordial leads (Figure 21-26). Echocardiography is another reliable method for diagnosing pericarditis and pericardial effusion.

Anesthetic Management. Acute pericarditis in the absence of an associated pericardial effusion or scarring does not alter cardiac function. Specific considerations for anesthetic management are directed toward the underlying illness.

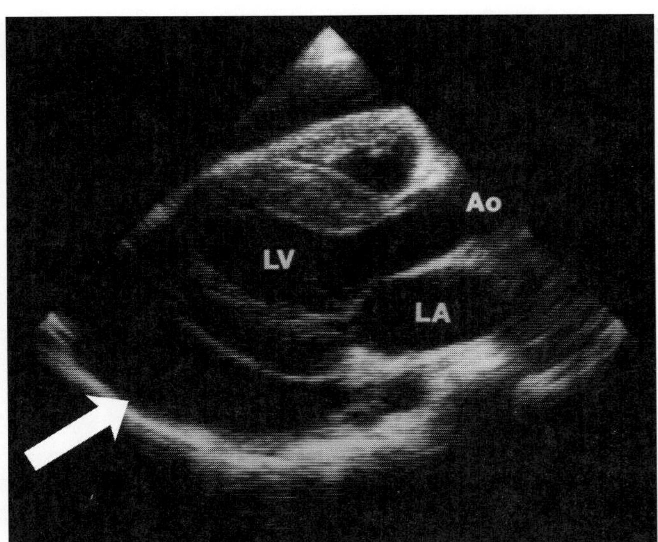

FIGURE **21-26**
Echocardiogram demonstrating a large pericardial effusion (*arrow*). *Ao*, Aorta; *LA*, left atrium; *LV*, left ventricle.

Chronic Constrictive Pericarditis

Chronic constrictive pericarditis results from pericardial thickening and fibrosis. In the past, tuberculosis was the most common cause of pericardial constriction. Currently the most common causes are idiopathic in nature and include complications following cardiac surgery, neoplasia, uremia, radiation therapy, and rheumatoid arthritis.[36,37]

Pathophysiology. Stiff, fibrous tissue encircles the heart and limits its ability to expand during diastole. The fundamental hemodynamic abnormality in chronic constrictive pericarditis is abnormal diastolic filling. The reduced myocardial compliance impairs filling of both ventricles. Consequently, filling pressures increase, and as a result, pulmonary and peripheral congestion occurs. SV and CO can also be decreased. Equilibration of pulmonary artery diastolic pressure, PCWP, and right atrial pressure commonly occurs. Initially, ventricular systolic function is normal. However, over time the underlying myocardial tissue may atrophy, and systolic function may decrease.

Clinical Presentation. Clinical features representative of constrictive pericarditis include gradually increasing fatigue and dyspnea. Typical signs of increasing venous pressure and congestion are engorgement of neck veins, hepatomegaly, ascites, and peripheral edema. In approximately 50% of patients the fibrous enclosure becomes calcified and is visible on a chest radiograph.[30] The electrocardiogram may reveal diffuse low-voltage QRS complexes, T-wave inversion, and notched P waves. As many as 25% of patients have atrial dysrhythmias because of the involvement of atrial conduction pathways. Diagnosis is confirmed by demonstration of pericardial thickening with echocardiography or computed tomography.

The treatment used for patients with hemodynamically significant constrictive pericarditis is pericardiectomy. Unfortunately, the surgical removal of adherent pericardium may precipitate malignant cardiac dysrhythmias and massive bleeding. Consequently, pericardiectomy is associated with relatively high perioperative morbidity and mortality rates, ranging from 6% to 19%.[38,39]

Anesthetic Management. Large-bore intravenous lines must be established preoperatively because of the potential for sudden, rapid hemorrhage. A cardiopulmonary bypass circuit should be readily available. Invasive hemodynamic monitoring is essential. Arterial catheterization allows beat-to-beat blood pressure monitoring and assists in the evaluation of significant cardiac dysrhythmia. A pulmonary artery catheter is useful because it permits measurement of filling pressures on both the right and left sides of the heart as well as determination of CO.

The anesthetic agents chosen for management of patients with constrictive pericarditis should preserve myocardial contractility, HR, preload, and afterload. Among these parameters, HR is of greatest concern. CO is dependent on HR in patients with constrictive pericarditis. As a consequence of limited ventricular diastolic filling, bradycardia is poorly tolerated and reflects a decrease in SV that can lead to hypotension. Therapy with drugs that maintain HR, such as pancuronium or ketamine, has a practical application in these patients. Potent inhalation agents that cause myocardial depression should be avoided. The use of opioids and etomidate, benzodiazepines, and nitrous oxide for the induction and maintenance of anesthesia is suitable in this setting. The clinician should be aware that vigorous positive-pressure ventilation may cause a decrease in venous return to the heart and result in a further decrease in CO.[40]

Immediate hemodynamic improvement may not occur after removal of the constricting tissue. Consistently low CO after pericardiectomy may be secondary to diffuse atrophy of myocardial muscle fibers or myocardial damage from the underlying disease. Intensive postoperative care with inotropic support and awareness of the potential for dysrhythmia or bleeding are integral components of the anesthetic management plan.

Cardiac Tamponade

Cardiac tamponade is a syndrome caused by the impairment of diastolic filling of the heart because of continuous increases in intrapericardial pressure.[41] Slow accumulation of fluid in the pericardial space can cause minute increases in intrapericardial pressure. This is a result of the pericardium's ability to stretch to accommodate this increase in volume. If the pericardial fluid accumulates rapidly, the presence of a few hundred milliliters may cause a significant increase in intrapericardial pressure that will result in cardiac tamponade.

A simple classification of the causes of cardiac tamponade includes (1) trauma, including sharp or blunt trauma to the chest and dissecting aortic aneurysms; (2) causes associated with cardiac surgery; and (3) expansion of pericardial effusions after any form of pericarditis.[42]

Pathophysiology. Normal intrapericardial pressure is subatmospheric. Accumulation of pericardial fluid leads to an increase in intrapericardial pressure. As a result, diastolic expansion of the ventricles decreases. As in constrictive pericarditis, poor ventricular filling develops and leads to peripheral congestion and a decrease in SV and CO. The decrease in SV stimulates compensatory mechanisms for maintaining CO (tachycardia, vasoconstriction, and an increase in venous pressure). If these mechanisms fail, cardiac collapse can occur.[43]

Clinical Presentation. In addition to obvious indications of cardiac distress, specific signs of cardiac tamponade include Beck's triad: hypotension, jugular venous distention, and distant muffled heart sounds.[44] Another common finding is pulsus paradoxus, an exaggeration (i.e., >10 mm Hg) of a decrease in systolic blood pressure that normally occurs with inspiration. Other conditions that may result in pulsus paradoxus are chronic obstructive pulmonary disease, obesity, and congestive heart failure. Jugular venous distention that occurs because of decreased forward blood flow through the heart may also be present.

In cardiac tamponade, chest radiography may show enlargement of the cardiac silhouette. The electrocardiogram usually demonstrates a decrease in voltage across all leads or electrical alterations of either the P wave or the QRS complex.[45] Echocardiography is the most sensitive, noninvasive method for detection of pericardial effusion and exclusion of tamponade. Use of a pulmonary artery catheter may reveal equilibration of right and left atrial pressures and right ventricular end-diastolic filling pressures at approximately 20 mm Hg.[46]

The definitive treatment for cardiac tamponade is pericardiocentesis, performed either percutaneously or through a subxiphoid pericardial window. In contrast to patients with constrictive pericarditis, in patients with cardiac tamponade immediate hemodynamic improvement occurs once the pericardium is opened. However, despite this fact, pulmonary edema, acute right and left ventricular dysfunction, and circulatory collapse can occur.[39]

Anesthetic Management. Preoperatively the patient's clinical status should be optimized. This includes expansion of intravascular fluid volume, use of positive inotropic agents, and correction of acidosis. The degree to which these measures are instituted depends on the hemodynamic state of the patient. Severely compromised patients require immediate medical therapy, and therefore emergency pericardiocentesis is indicated. Invasive hemodynamic monitoring should be established before the procedure. Intraarterial and central venous pressure catheters are required for frequent drawing of blood, continuous blood pressure monitoring, and assessment of intravascular fluid status.

Local infiltration anesthesia is the technique of choice for operative correction of cardiac tamponade.[47] Many reports exist of severe hypotension and cardiac arrest after induction of general anesthesia in patients with tamponade.[48,49] The potential for decompensation that is associated with the use of general anesthetics is attributed to direct myocardial depression and vasodilation in patients with established impairment of cardiac filling. The use of positive-pressure ventilation in such patients may result in a decrease of venous return to the heart and can further decrease CO.[50] After percutaneous pericardiocentesis and the improvement of hemodynamic status, induction of general anesthesia and initiation of positive-pressure ventilation are sufficient for further surgical exploration.

When it is not possible to relieve intrapericardial pressure that causes cardiac tamponade before the induction of anesthesia, the same anesthetic principles that are applied to the anesthetic management of patients with constrictive pericarditis should be used, including the use of anesthetic agents that preserve myocardial contractility, HR, preload, and afterload. Because of the sympathomimetic effects of ketamine, this drug has been advocated for the induction and maintenance of anesthesia.[45,47] However, many combinations of anesthetic agents that preserve the previously mentioned determinants of CO have been used safely.[40,47,49]

BOX 21-2

Hemodynamic Goals for Cardiac Tamponade

Preload	Maintain or increase
Afterload	Maintain
Contractility	Maintain or increase
Heart rate	Maintain
Heart rhythm	Normal sinus rhythm
Treatment	Pericardiocentesis, pericardial window

Postoperative continuous monitoring of blood pressure, central venous pressure, and chest tube drainage is necessary. Possible complications after pericardiocentesis include the reaccumulation of pericardial fluid, coronary laceration, cardiac puncture, and pneumothorax. Box 21-2 lists hemodynamic goals in patients with cardiac tamponade.

Acquired Valvular Heart Disease

The cardiac valves are membranous leaflets that separate the chambers of the heart. When open, they allow blood flow between the chambers and great vessels. When the valves are closed, they prevent regurgitant blood flow between the chambers or backflow from the great vessels. A valve orifice of normal size presents a small degree of flow obstruction and thereby creates a hemodynamically insignificant gradient. Primary dysfunction of the mitral and aortic valves represents the most common and most severe hemodynamic derangement. Acquired primary dysfunction of the tricuspid or pulmonic valves is extremely rare and therefore is not addressed in this chapter.

Valvular disease is classified according to the type of lesion that exists—stenosis, insufficiency, or mixed lesions. Valvular stenosis is a stenotic narrowing of the valvular orifice, which restricts flow through the orifice when the valve is open. This situation creates an increase in flow resistance and increases turbulent blood flow. Valvular insufficiency results in regurgitation secondary to incomplete or partial valve closure, which allows blood to flow back through the valve into the previous chamber. In patients with mixed lesions (stenosis with insufficiency, or insufficiency with stenosis) one type of dysfunction is considered dominant over the other on the basis of the severity of clinical symptoms.

Valvular dysfunction is classified as either primary or secondary. In primary valvular dysfunction the valve leaflets or the anchoring and supporting structures are damaged or do not function properly. In secondary valvular dysfunction the valve is not directly damaged. However, normal valve function is altered secondary to another pathophysiologic entity. Causes of this type of manifestation include ventricular dilation, which produces mitral insufficiency; retrograde aortic dissection, which creates aortic insufficiency (AI); and papillary muscle infarction, which causes mitral insufficiency.[51,52]

Cardiac Output. The primary components of CO are preload, afterload, contractility, compliance, and HR.[52-54] Blood flow may increase due to an increase in HR or an increase in SV. Because blood viscosity decreases with decreasing hematocrit and increasing flow rate, normovolemic anemia reduces cardiac afterload, thereby facilitating the augmentation of

CO. This sequence of events occurs as long as intravascular volume is maintained and cardiac reserve is ample. The amount of afterload that is present determines the degree of tension that cardiac fibers must develop before systolic ejection can occur.[55]

Evaluation of the Patient with Acquired Valvular Heart Disease. Evaluation of the patient with valvular heart disease should focus on the pathophysiologic derangements and their effects on cardiac function. The systematic evaluation of primary valvular dysfunction should include the following:

1. Category of valvular dysfunction
   - Stenosis (progressive narrowing of the valve orifice)
   - Insufficiency (incomplete valve closure that causes backflow through the valve)
   - Mixed (regurgitant and stenotic dysfunction)
2. Status of left ventricular loading
   - Left ventricle (LV) overload from mitral or aortic regurgitation (AR)
   - Pressure overloading from aortic stenosis
   - Volume underloading from mitral stenosis
3. Acute versus chronic evolution of the dysfunction
   - Acute lesions have severe and precipitous hemodynamic consequences
4. Cardiac rhythm and its effects on ventricular diastolic filling time
5. Left ventricular function
   - Poor left ventricular function places the patient at a higher risk for perioperative cardiac morbidity
6. Secondary effects on the pulmonary vasculature and right ventricular function
   - Secondary pulmonary hypertension from valvular lesions can significantly affect right ventricular function
7. HR
   - Changes in HR (either bradycardia or tachycardia) can significantly alter the hemodynamic manifestations of a specific valvular lesion
   - Bradycardia occurring with regurgitant lesions can result in a significant increase in the regurgitant fraction
   - Tachycardia is detrimental in patients with stenotic lesions because it shortens the time of ejection and increases myocardial oxygen demand.[24-26,30,31]

Clinical Symptomatology of Valvular Heart Disease. The most frequent clinical symptoms and signs of valvular dysfunction are congestive heart failure, dysrhythmias, syncope, and angina pectoris. Symptoms commonly associated with congestive heart failure include dyspnea, orthopnea, and fatigue. The severity of left ventricular dysfunction can be related to the patient's activity level before the onset of cardiac symptoms.[32]

Patient Evaluation: Compensatory Mechanisms. In order to maintain cardiac function despite progressive valvular dysfunction, sympathetic activity increases as a compensatory mechanism. A decrease in sympathetic tone that occurs during anesthesia can cause severe myocardial dysfunction. Evaluation of the patient should include recognition of sympathetic compensatory mechanisms and management strategies to maintain hemodynamic stability. Despite maximum medical therapy, patients with severe valvular dysfunction may remain in congestive heart failure.

The evaluation should also focus on associated organ dysfunction. CO that is decreased by chronic myocardial failure can cause significant major organ dysfunction, including renal and hepatic insufficiency as well as poor cerebral perfusion, which can produce an altered level of consciousness, restlessness, agitation, and lethargy.

Diagnostic Modalities for the Evaluation of Valvular Heart Disease. The most valuable diagnostic modalities used to evaluate valvular heart disease include electrocardiography, chest radiography, color flow Doppler imaging, echocardiography, and cardiac catheterization of both the right and left chambers of the heart. Electrocardiography can be used for evaluation of ventricular hypertrophy, atrial enlargement, and axis deviation and, most important, for determining cardiac rhythm. Chest radiography demonstrates the size of the cardiac silhouette and signs of pulmonary vascular congestion. Color flow Doppler imaging can be used to determine the valvular area, transvalvular gradients, degree of regurgitation, and flow velocity and direction and can measure cardiac function. Cardiac catheterization can be used directly to measure transvalvular gradients, estimate the degree of regurgitation, visualize the coronary arteries, and determine intracardiac pressures.[56-60]

Mitral Stenosis

In mitral stenosis the mitral valve orifice becomes progressively narrowed. This narrowing reduces flow from the LA into the LV during diastole. The narrowing of the mitral valve orifice has two significant hemodynamic consequences. First, a gradient develops across the valve orifice. This change represents a compensatory response directed at maintaining adequate flow. Second, as the cross-sectional area of the orifice decreases and the gradient increases, flow is restricted and left ventricular volume is decreased. The clinical symptomatology of severe mitral stenosis results in pulmonary congestion and decreased CO. Pulmonary congestion occurs as a result of increases in left atrial pressure. Decreased SV is caused by decreased left ventricular volume. LV filling is dependent on the length of diastole, the gradient between the LA and LV, and the surface area of the mitral valve. As the valve area narrows to less than 1 cm^2, the prolonged diastolic filling time and elevated mean left atrial pressure are incapable of maintaining normal LVEDV, and decreases in left ventricular volume occur.[52] Atrial systole accounts for 20% to 30% of LVEDV. Because mitral stenosis presents a fixed resistance to ventricular inflow, most of the pressure generated during atrial systole is used to overcome the resistance caused by the stenotic valve rather than for producing forward flow. As the HR increases to greater than 90 beats per minute and diastolic time intervals are shortened, LVEDV is decreased. This is demonstrated by Gorlin's equation, which relates flow rate (CO divided by diastolic filling time) divided by valve area to the square root of the pressure gradient. Any subsequent increase in flow rate or decrease in diastolic filling time reflects an increase in the pressure gradient between the LA and the LV. As the diastolic time interval shortens, the pressure gradient increases by the square of the increase in flow rate. Therefore any marked increase in HR can result in an increase in left atrial pressure, which can precipitate a rise in pulmonary artery pressures and ultimately leads to pulmonary edema.[61]

Left atrial hypertrophy and distention result as a consequence of elevated left atrial pressures. This distention of the LA can lead to atrial dysrhythmias (most commonly, atrial fibrillation). The atrial systolic "kick" is lost during atrial fibrillation; this implies that diastolic filling can be maintained only by a further increase in left atrial pressure. Mean left atrial pressure is limited by the development of pulmonary congestion at pressures greater than 25 mm Hg. Elevation of left atrial pressures to greater than 25 mm Hg leads to pulmonary congestion and, eventually, pulmonary edema. Pulmonary hypertension develops in patients with chronic mitral stenosis because of continuous elevations in left atrial pressure.

Pulmonary Vascular Changes in Right Ventricular Function. The pulmonary vasculature and eventually the RV are adversely affected by the chronic elevation of the left atrial pressure that occurs with mitral stenosis. As mitral stenosis progresses, chronic elevation of left atrial pressure causes increased blood volume in the pulmonary vascular circuit. This can cause perivascular edema, and changes in pulmonary vascular resistance may ensue. These changes in pulmonary vascular resistance result in an increase in RV afterload. As a compensatory response, right ventricular hypertrophy occurs; however, because the RV is not capable of generating high pressures, it eventually begins to fail.[52-54] As the disease progresses, overt signs of biventricular failure such as low CO with poor systemic perfusion become evident. Peripheral edema, hepatic congestion, and marked venous distention are signs of right ventricular failure. The deterioration of right ventricular function decreases adequate left ventricular filling and therefore causes further deterioration in CO.

Anesthetic Considerations in Mitral Stenosis. Any anesthetic technique should be based on the thorough understanding of the pathophysiology of mitral stenosis as well as of the cardiovascular effects of the anesthetic agents employed. The following goals should be achieved in the anesthetic management of the patient with mitral stenosis:

1. Maintenance of sinus rhythm
2. HR between 70 and 90 beats per minute
3. LVEDV high enough to maintain adequate CO without increasing pulmonary congestion
4. Avoidance of extreme decreases in contractility
5. Reduction in both right ventricular and left ventricular afterload may improve hemodynamics; this must be done in a controlled manner and with careful monitoring; the extent of the surgical procedure and the degree and severity of mitral stenosis determine the level of monitoring that is necessary

The LVEDV is normal in approximately 85% of patients with mitral stenosis. An increased LVEDV in patients with mitral stenosis should alert the anesthesia provider to the presence of mitral or aortic insufficiency or primary coronary artery disease. Most patients with moderate mitral stenosis also have low-to-normal SV and therefore may have a normal EF. Approximately 33% of patients with mitral stenosis have an EF below normal (normal, 0.67 ± 0.08).[53] When the mitral valve is narrowed to less than 1 cm^2 (severe mitral stenosis), a mean left atrial pressure of 25 mm Hg is necessary in order to maintain even an adequate resting CO.

MITRAL REGURGITATION AND INSUFFICIENCY

Pathophysiology

During ventricular systole the mitral valve is closed, preventing blood flow from the LV back into the LA. However, if for any reason the two leaflets of the mitral valve are not in opposition to each other, then a portion of systolic ventricular flow regurgitates back through this incompetent (insufficient) valve. Therefore the LV has a double outlet for systolic ejection. Ejection into the aorta is a high-impedance outlet, and regurgitation back through the mitral valve into the LA is a low-impedance outlet. This condition is termed *mitral regurgitation* (MR) or *mitral insufficiency*. The degree of regurgitation (quantitatively), called the *regurgitant fraction*, is determined by four factors, which include:

1. Size of the regurgitant valve orifice (surface area measured in square centimeters)
2. The pressure gradient between the LA and the LV
   - Inotropic state of the LV (peak systolic pressure)
   - Compliance of the LA and pulmonary veins
3. Time available for regurgitation (systole); the systolic interval determines the length of time during which regurgitation can occur; the length of the systolic time interval is inversely proportional to the HR
4. Aortic outflow impedance SVR; the regurgitant fraction can be significantly influenced by changes in impedance to aortic blood flow

The major pathophysiologic derangement associated with MR is volume overload of the LV. This occurs because the regurgitant fraction (blood ejected into the LA) delivers an increased diastolic volume to the LV. This increase in LVEDV results in ventricular dilation.[41,52,61] Acute MR and chronic MR have substantially different pathophysiologic manifestations. The primary determinant of these pathophysiologic adaptations is left atrial compliance. If acute MR is caused by papillary muscle rupture the mortality rate approaches 75% within 24 hours and 95% within 48 hours.[62] Chronic MR produces a dilated compliant LA, whereas the long-standing and gradual elevation of left atrial pressure results in left atrial dilation. This consequently facilitates containment of relatively large end-diastolic volumes while reflecting relatively low increases in LA pressures. With chronic MR, hypertrophic changes occur in response to a continual increased left ventricular volume by increasing the left ventricular chamber size. This type of hypertrophic change is called *eccentric hypertrophy*.

In contrast, in acute MR the LA is small and noncompliant, but over time eccentric hypertrophic changes occur. In this situation a small regurgitant volume bolus can generate deflections or *v* waves that appear in the PCWP tracing. This *v* wave appears as a result of a systolic jet (ejection) back through the incompetent mitral valve. The pressure wave produced by this jet is transmitted upstream into the pulmonary artery. This pressure wave is designated as a *pathologic* v *wave*. The time delay for this pressure wave to be transmitted results in its appearance at the time interval in which the normal *v* wave (passive atrial filling) occurs.[52] The height of the *v* wave in MR does not represent a measurement of regurgitant volume but rather of left atrial compliance in relationship to the regurgitated volume. The hypertrophic LA accommodates a larger regurgitant volume, which results in small increases in pressure. The dilated and compliant LA allows the pulmonary vascular circuit to be buffered from the excessive left atrial volume. However, chronic MR causes pulmonary venous congestion, which creates pulmonary vascular reactive changes that eventually result in pulmonary artery hypertension. Distention of the LA may lead to atrial fibrillation, a common arrhythmia that is associated with MR.

Pulmonary Vasculature and Right Ventricular Function Associated with Mitral Regurgitation

In acute MR the pulmonary circuit is exposed to immediate and marked elevation of left atrial pressure because of a small and noncompliant LA. Pulmonary vascular congestion is precipitous and results in almost immediate development of pulmonary edema. An acute rise in left atrial pressure and congestion of the pulmonary circuit creates an increased right ventricular workload. This immediate increase in right ventricular afterload results in ventricular dilation and consequently may lead to right ventricular failure. In chronic MR, elevation of baseline pulmonary pressures is much more gradual, occurring over a prolonged period. This allows secondary pulmonary artery hypertension via intimal fibroelastosis generated by chronic perivascular edema. If the patient has coexisting mitral stenosis, pulmonary vascular resistance and right ventricular pressures may be excessively elevated.[41,52,61]

Effects of Afterload Reductions Associated with Mitral Regurgitation

The path of least resistance for blood flow during left ventricular systole is retrograde into the LA. Reduction of SVR via arterial vasodilatation reduces impedance to systolic outflow into the aorta and increases forward flow. Conversely, increases in SVR have marked effects on the reduction in forward flow and the increase in the regurgitant fraction. A 20% increase in MAP raises LA pressure by 50% and reflects a 120% increase in regurgitant flow concurrent with a 16% decrease in forward flow.[52]

Anesthetic Management of Patients with Mitral Regurgitation

An otherwise healthy patient with stable and controlled MR undergoing an ambulatory or uncomplicated surgical procedure has a minimal increase in risk of adverse hemodynamic fluctuations. Patients with cardiovascular disease who undergo major vascular, intrathoracic, intraabdominal, neurosurgical, orthopedic, or emergency procedures may have a 25% to 50% higher mortality risk than patients without the disease process. Controversy exists regarding whether the duration of surgery correlates with perioperative cardiac morbidity.[32,51,52]

Kinetics

Preoperative assessment is essential in order to determine the degree of cardiac compensation (Table 21-4). Anesthetic management of the patient with MR should focus on the following hemodynamic goals: decreasing regurgitant blood flow to enhance CO by decreasing afterload; maintaining or increasing preload; and maintaining cardiac contractility. Bradycardia or dysrhythmias that cause a loss of atrial kick can result in pulmonary congestion, left atrial and left ventricular overload, and a significant decrease in CO.[51-53]

Another anesthetic consideration of MR includes decreasing SVR or afterload. Cautiously lowering SVR via an arterial vasodilator such as sodium nitroprusside improves forward flow. However, extreme reductions in blood pressure, and especially diastolic pressure, can lead to decreased coronary artery blood flow and decreased CO.

Selection of the anesthetic technique should take into consideration the adverse effects associated with changes in HR and SVR. General anesthesia is the technique of choice in patients with MR. Regional anesthesia (spinal or epidural) is not contraindicated; however, the potential for profound and precipitous decreases in blood pressure via sympathetic blockade can result in severe decreases in blood pressure. Induction of general anesthesia can be safely achieved with any of the presently available agents. Hemodynamic goals include avoiding bradycardia and significant increases in SVR. The use of muscle relaxants does not present a significant risk as long as the resulting changes in HR do not cause severe bradycardia. Because of the vagolytic properties of pancuronium, this drug may help to maintain HR. Maintenance of anesthesia can be accomplished with nitrous oxide and a volatile agent. Any changes in vascular resistance induced by nitrous oxide are frequently offset by the pulmonary vasodilatation produced by the volatile agent. No volatile agent has been proved to be superior in patients with MR. Isoflurane may be an ideal choice because of its significant vasodilatory effects, causing an increased HR. Because all volatile agents induce some degree of myocardial depression, they may be detrimental in patients with severe ventricular dysfunction caused by MR. In this instance, the use of a high-dose opioid technique may provide for a more effective hemodynamic profile. Anesthetic management should attempt to avoid bradycardia or increases in SVR.[52] See Table 21-4 for anesthetic goals for management of mitral lesions.

TABLE 21-4 Anesthetic Goals for Management of Mitral lesions

Parameter	Mitral Regurgitation	Mitral Stenosis
Heart rate	Increase	Decrease
Rhythm	Maintain normal sinus rhythm	Maintain normal sinus rhythm
Systemic vascular resistance	Decrease	Maintain normal
Pulmonary vascular resistance	Avoid increases	Avoid increases
Left ventricular preload	Normal to increased	Normal to increased

AORTIC STENOSIS

Etiology and Pathophysiology

The most common causes of aortic stenosis include a congenital defect resulting in a bicuspid aortic valve (especially in males) and the sequelae of rheumatic valvular heart disease. Isolated aortic valvular dysfunction in patients with rheumatic heart disease is rare. Commonly, rheumatic valvular disease is associated with mitral valve involvement. Whatever the cause, the pathophysiology remains the same and results in the need for increased left ventricular systolic pressure to overcome the left ventricular outflow tract obstruction caused by a narrowed aortic valve orifice.

An understanding of the flow rates through a normal aortic valve orifice is needed for gaining an appreciation of ventricular pressure overload. A normal aortic valve area of 2.5 to 3.5 cm^2 and a SV of approximately 80 ml result in a flow rate of 250 ml/min during the interval of ventricular systole (80 ml/sec × 0.32 sec − systolic time interval). The flow rate through a normal orifice results in a minimal gradient (2 to 4 mm Hg). The normal left ventricular systolic pressure of 100 to 130 mm Hg is sufficient to generate flow rates of 250 to 300 ml/sec. To ensure normal flow rates and therefore CO through the narrowed orifice, the velocity of systolic ejection must increase. For systolic ejection to be increased, ventricular systolic pressure increases dramatically depending on the degree of valvular pathology. The LV must compensate for gradually increasing mechanical impedance to ejection. This results in LVH, which allows the heart to generate high ventricular systolic pressure and overcome impedance to ejection. The elevation of systolic ejection pressure produces a gradient between the left ventricular cavity and the aorta. The valve area must be constricted by at least 50% before the gradient becomes significant to the point that symptoms occur at rest. An aortic valve area of less than 1 cm^2 produces a clinical triad of symptoms, including angina (even in the absence of significant coronary artery disease), syncope, and congestive heart failure.[61] An aortic valve area of less than 1 cm^2 represents severe aortic stenosis and should be a cause of concern in planning anesthetic management, because of the associated increase in perioperative cardiac morbidity.[32] An aortic valve area less than 0.7 cm^2 is associated with sudden death.[63] For adequate assessment of the degree of valvular stenosis, both the flow rate across the valve and the pressure gradient should be evaluated, either by cardiac catheterization or echocardiography.[59,60]

Left Ventricular Function

Left ventricular concentric hypertrophy is the hallmark of aortic stenosis. It results in several hemodynamic adaptations that are unique to aortic stenosis and present a challenge and a dilemma with regard to anesthesia management. The consequence of LVH in aortic stenosis is a decrease in ventricular compliance, hypertrophic remodeling, and an eventual decrease in the intrinsic contractility of the myocardium.[64] The reduction in ventricular compliance affects normal hemodynamics as follows:

I. Higher filling pressures are needed to produce the same amount of ventricular work.
II. To achieve adequate left ventricular filling, normal sinus rhythm must be maintained in order to ensure adequate LVEDV from the atrial kick.
III. Concentric ventricular hypertrophy causes alterations in myocardial oxygen balance.
   A. Myocardial oxygen consumption is increased.
      1) Myocardial mass is increased.
      2) Pressure generation (isovolumetric contraction) uses more energy than left ventricular ejection, because a high intracavitary pressure must be generated to maintain CO.
      3) The ejection phase is prolonged.
   B. Myocardial oxygen supply is decreased.
      1) CPP is decreased as a result of an increase in LVEDP.
      2) Systolic coronary flow is absent because left ventricular systolic pressure exceeds aortic systolic pressure.
      3) Prolonged systolic ejection reduces the coronary perfusion interval.
      4) Subendocardial capillaries are compressed by hypertrophic myocardium.[41,51,52]

Pulmonary Circuit and Right Ventricular Responses

To maintain CO in the presence of a noncompliant and hypertrophic ventricle, left atrial pressures increase to accommodate left ventricular filling. Left atrial pressures of greater than 18 mm Hg can cause an increase in pulmonary artery pressure, resulting in passive pulmonary venous congestion. Eventually pulmonary fibroelastosis occurs, causing pulmonary artery hypertension. If the ventricular EF is decreased to less than 40% in association with aortic stenosis, CO can be maintained only with increases in left atrial pressures. These pressures increase to 25 to 30 mm Hg, which results in increased mean pulmonary artery pressure. Elevated mean pulmonary artery pressure increases pulmonary vascular resistance, which can cause right ventricular failure. Decreasing left ventricular preload in association with significant aortic stenosis can result in decreases in CO.

Goals of Anesthetic Management

The goals of anesthesia management include maintaining hemodynamic stability without causing significant alterations in compensatory mechanisms. Anesthetic management of patients with aortic stenosis should focus on the following hemodynamic factors:

1. Maintenance of sinus rhythm at a normal rate (70 to 90 beats per minute)
2. Assurance of sufficient preload (LVEDV) to maintain CO
3. Assurance of adequate coronary perfusion, through maintenance of diastolic blood pressure levels
4. Avoidance of myocardial depression

Anesthesia Technique

General anesthesia is the preferred technique for major surgical procedures involving patients with aortic stenosis because of the ability to manipulate hemodynamic parameters, especially diastolic blood pressure. Central neural blockade (spinal or epidural) is not contraindicated. However, these techniques must be used with extreme caution, as precipitous reductions in blood pressure associated with a sympathectomy decrease SVR. The heart may not be able to compensate for increase CO for generalized systemic vasodilatation. Successful cardiopulmonary resuscitation is virtually impossible because of the mechanical left ventricular outflow obstruction associated with this type of valvular pathology. The pressure necessary to overcome outflow obstruction and produce adequate coronary artery perfusion and CO cannot be generated with closed chest compressions. Furthermore, short periods of hypotension may lead to a decrease in coronary perfusion. Because of the increased oxygen demands of the LV, irreversible myocardial ischemia and cardiovascular collapse can occur if hypotension is not promptly and aggressively treated.

Intraoperative control of HR and rhythm is a major goal of the anesthetic management of patients with aortic stenosis. Tachycardia can be detrimental because it decreases diastolic filling time, resulting in a reduction of left ventricular preload. The reduced time interval for coronary artery perfusion reduces oxygen supply to the myocardium. In patients with HRs of greater than 110 beats per minute, systolic ejection time and CO are decreased.[52,53] Bradycardia (60 or fewer beats per minute) is detrimental in aortic stenosis. Prolonged diastolic filling time, which occurs as a result of bradycardia, causes ventricular distention, which can further decrease CPP, especially to the subendocardium.[41,51,52]

Monitoring and Premedication

It is prudent to titrate preoperative sedatives while vital signs can be continuously monitored. In addition to standard intraoperative monitoring, complete invasive monitoring may be required for patients with aortic stenosis, even for routine procedures. Any significant change in basic hemodynamic variables (i.e., HR and heart rhythm, LVEDV, CPP) can rapidly cause irreversible myocardial deterioration. It is imperative that these variables be monitored closely and appropriate interventions be performed to prevent adverse hemodynamic consequences. The complexity of hemodynamic monitoring modalities is dependent on the physical status of the patient, the severity of aortic stenosis, the extent of the surgical procedure, and the ability of anesthesia provider to use and interpret hemodynamic values.

The use of intraarterial monitoring for direct beat-to-beat blood pressure assessment allows the anesthesia provider to rapidly treat undesirable hemodynamic changes. Pulmonary artery catheterization provides the ability to monitor all the hemodynamic parameters necessary in order to diagnose and treat adverse hemodynamic events. Absolute criteria for intraoperative invasive monitoring for patients with aortic stenosis are controversial. However, clinical judgment, experience, and the ability to appropriately use the pulmonary artery catheter must be considered before implementation.[63,65]

Maintenance of Anesthesia

Any of the standard induction agents may be used as long as caution is exercised. Tracheal intubation can be performed with any of the available muscle relaxants. However, caution must be exercised to avoid histamine release, as this situation can dramatically increase HR. Anesthetic maintenance can be accomplished with the use of a volatile agent in conjunction with nitrous oxide, opiates, or both. The adverse cardiovascular effects of the volatile agents must be considered before these drugs are used. Higher concentrations of inhaled agent result in greater degrees of myocardial depression and vasodilatation. Volatile agents must be used with extreme caution, as the myocardial depressant effect can be deleterious in patients with impaired ventricular function. The use of high-dose opioid-based agents (fentanyl, 50 to 100 mcg/kg, or sufentanil, 5 to 30 mcg/kg) is an alternative anesthetic approach that may help achieve cardiovascular stability by not causing a significant amount of myocardial depression. Finally, a combination of inhaled agents and narcotics has been used safely to provide anesthesia for patients with aortic stenosis. Despite the anesthetic technique that is chosen, immediate and aggressive treatment of adverse changes that occur in HR and rhythm, SVR, blood pressure, and LVEDV is paramount if successful anesthetic outcomes are to be achieved in patients with aortic stenosis.[63,65]

AORTIC INSUFFICIENCY

AI, also known as *aortic regurgitation*, can be classified as acute or chronic and as primary or secondary, depending on the cause. Primary chronic AI is caused by rheumatic valvular disease and almost always involves the mitral valve to some degree. Primary acute AI usually is caused by infective endocarditis, which is caused by direct damage to the valve cusps. Acute secondary (functional) AI results from aortic root dissection caused either by trauma or aneurysm and results in a mechanical and functional impairment of functional aortic valve closure.

Pathophysiology

The major hemodynamic aberration related to AI occurs during diastole. A portion of the blood volume that is ejected from the LV into the aorta regurgitates back into the ventricle because of incomplete closure of the aortic valve. AI causes volume overload of the LV. Chronic ventricular overload causes eccentric ventricular hypertrophy and chamber dilation. The degree of regurgitation depends on three factors: the diastolic time available for regurgitation to occur, the diastolic pressure gradient between the aorta and the LV, and the degree of incompetence of the aortic valve.[61,63]

Diastolic time and diastolic pressure can be manipulated during the course of anesthesia so that the amount of regurgitant flow is decreased and the amount of forward flow is increased. A HR of 90 to 110 beats per minute and decreases in diastolic time interval occur and thereby reduce the time available for regurgitation. Reducing SVR reduces aortic diastolic pressure and thereby decreases the gradient between the aorta and the LV. Unique pathophysiologic adaptations differentiate chronic AI from the acute form. In chronic AI the LV has had time to compensate for the increased volume. In time the LV hypertrophies and is able to tolerate significant increases in volume without dramatic decreases in EF.[41,52] In situations in which the onset of AI is acute, the LV has inadequate time to adapt to volume overload, which renders compensatory mechanisms ineffective. Frequently left ventricular failure, pulmonary edema, and cardiovascular collapse occur. LVEDP rises precipitously in acute AI because of the inability of the LV to alter its compliance.

Patients with chronic AI can remain asymptomatic for long periods. Except during times of stress the clinical symptoms associated with chronic AI are usually not incapacitating. End-stage AI is characterized by myocardial failure with decreased CO and precipitous elevation of LVEDV with evidence of pulmonary congestion. As long as ventricular hypertrophy and dilation do not affect the mitral valve, the pulmonary circulation is not affected by the pathophysiologic changes associated with AI. Increased myocardial oxygen consumption occurs because of the development of eccentric hypertrophy. The decrease in aortic diastolic pressure that results from AI reduces coronary flow and can cause subendocardial ischemia. In acute AI, a precipitous increase in LVEDP with a decrease in aortic diastolic pressure can severely compromise coronary blood flow and result in acute myocardial ischemia. The RV and pulmonary vascular circuit usually are spared in chronic AI until secondary (functional) MR occurs. This results in dilation of the mitral valve annulus. A gradual increase in LA pressure and pulmonary artery pressure caused by functional MR eventually causes pulmonary hypertension right ventricular failure can occur if pulmonary hypertension becomes severe. In acute AI functional MR is poorly tolerated because of noncompliance of the LA. This situation leads to immediate pulmonary vascular congestion and pulmonary edema. Patients with asymptomatic AI have a 0.2% annual mortality rate as compared with symptomatic patients, who have a greater than 10% mortality rate per year.[66] Therefore when evidence suggests that increases in left ventricular volume result in left ventricular dysfunction, aortic valve replacement is recommended.

Anesthesia Management

The goals for anesthesia management are to increase forward flow and decrease the degree of regurgitation.

HR should be maintained slightly higher than normal (80 to 110 beats per minute). SVR (especially diastolic pressure) should be decreased, and significant myocardial depressants should be avoided.[51] Central neural blockade is an appropriate anesthetic choice, depending on the invasiveness of the surgical procedure. Reduction in SVR resulting from sympathetic blockade may reduce the degree of regurgitation. The potential for immediate and uncontrolled hypotension during spinal anesthesia is a concern. However spinal and epidural anesthesia has been used successfully for patients with AI. Induction of general anesthesia can be accomplished with any of the available intravenous agents. Tracheal intubation can be achieved with the use of available nondepolarizing muscle relaxants. Pancuronium is a preferred agent because its vagolytic properties may increase HR. Succinylcholine may be used, but its potential to cause bradycardia (although rarely) must be considered. Maintenance of anesthesia can be achieved with nitrous oxide and a volatile agent. Isoflurane, with its ability to increase HR and decrease SVR, produces little myocardial depression, and therefore its use is preferred over use of other volatile agents. If significant ventricular dysfunction exists, a high-dose opioid technique may be preferable.[26,52,53]

Monitoring and Premedication with Aortic Insufficiency

Unless end-stage AR or significant preoperative ventricular dysfunction exists, aggressive invasive monitoring is not warranted. However, if the surgical procedure is extensive or if vasodilators or inotropes are being used, then an arterial line and a pulmonary artery catheter should be used for assessment of the results and efficacy of these therapeutic agents. Premedication should be tailored to the patient's clinical condition. In elderly or debilitated patients a conservative amount of premedication should be titrated until effective in a monitored environment.

Appropriate anesthetic management of the patient with valvular heart disease requires a basic knowledge of cardiac physiology and the pathophysiologic changes that occur with valvular dysfunction. The cardiovascular effects of all the agents, techniques, and adjunct pharmacologic agents used during anesthesia must be integrated into the anesthetic plan. A thorough understanding of the use of invasive monitoring along with other sophisticated diagnostic modalities enables the clinician to continuously monitor hemodynamic parameters. Contemporary anesthesia practice has allowed patients with severe valvular dysfunction to undergo surgical procedures that would not have been performed a decade ago.[63] See Table 21-5 for anesthetic goals for management of aortic lesions.

TABLE 21-5 Anesthetic Goals for Management of Aortic Lesions

Parameter	Aortic Insufficiency (Regurgitation)	Aortic Stenosis
Heart rate	Moderate increase	Normal to slow
Heart rhythm	Maintain normal sinus rhythm	Maintain normal sinus rhythm
Systemic vascular resistance	Decrease	Moderate to increased
Pulmonary vascular resistance	Maintain	Maintain
Left ventricular preload	Normal or slight increase	Increased

HYPERTROPHIC CARDIOMYOPATHY

Cardiomyopathy is a compensatory enlargement of the heart. Hypertrophic cardiomyopathy, a genetically transmitted disease, is a form of myocardial dysfunction that can cause coronary artery disease, valvular dysfunction, and hypertension. Obstructive hypertrophic cardiomyopathy has previously been referred to as *idiopathic hypertrophic subaortic stenosis*. Currently the preferred term is *hypertrophic cardiomyopathy with or without left ventricular outflow obstruction*.[67]

The myocardial defect that is associated with hypertrophic cardiomyopathy is related to the contractile mechanism. An increase in the density of calcium channels appears to lead to myocardial hypertrophy. Asymmetric hypertrophy of the interventricular septum of the LV occurs. The asymmetric hypertrophy of the intraventricular septum causes a left outflow tract obstruction, and therefore the hemodynamic consequences are similar to those that are characteristic of aortic stenosis. Hypertrophic cardiomyopathy is the most common cause of sudden death in the pediatric and young adult populations.[68]

Pathophysiology of Cardiomyopathy

Myocardial hypertrophy is the pathophysiologic abnormality that precipitates the hemodynamic derangements associated with dilated cardiomyopathy and is caused by left ventricular outflow obstruction. Left ventricular myocytes are hypertrophic and chaotically arranged. Coronary arterial walls are narrowed because of the presence of collagen. If the entire myocardium is involved, then a disproportionate hypertrophy of the intraventricular septum exists. The contraction of the hypertrophied septum bulging into the subaortic area of the left ventricular outflow tract creates a dynamic gradient. The left ventricular outflow tract is bounded anteriorly by the intraventricular septum and posteriorly by the anterior leaflet of the mitral valve. The rapid acceleration of blood traveling through the narrowed outflow tract creates a Venturi effect, which pulls the anterior mitral valve leaflet into the outflow tract. The systolic anterior motion of the anterior mitral valve leaflet further obstructs left ventricular outflow. The valve leaflet may even contact the septum and further compromise left ventricular outflow.[67]

The pathophysiologic abnormalities related to hypertrophic cardiomyopathy include the presence of systolic and diastolic dysfunction. A loss of diastolic compliance results in an abnormally elevated LVEDP in the presence of low-normal end-diastolic volume. Loss of left ventricular diastolic compliance requires a greater contribution of volume from atrial contraction. As a result congestive heart failure may ensue as left atrial pressures continue to increase.[68] Maintenance of normal sinus rhythm is vital, because as much as 75% of left ventricular preload comes from the LA. The increase in LVEDP, which results from a noncompliant LV, decreases CPP to the hypertrophic LV. Altered coronary perfusion and the presence of left ventricular hypertrophy decreases myocardial blood supply and increases myocardial oxygen demand, respectively.

Hypertrophic cardiomyopathy with obstruction is characterized by its dynamic nature. Three basic hemodynamic parameters can affect the degree of outflow obstruction. Manipulation of these parameters can exacerbate or ameliorate the hemodynamic consequences of outflow obstruction. These three parameters include preload, afterload, and

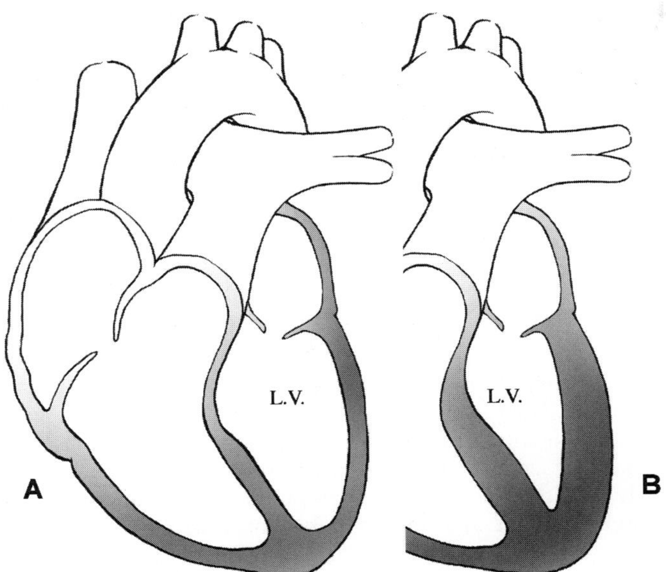

FIGURE **21-27**
A, Normal left ventricular outflow tract. **B,** Hypertrophic cardiomyopathy with an enlarged interventricular septum. A further decrease of left ventricular outflow is caused by migration of the anterior mitral leaflet toward the septum.

contractility.[30] Increasing myocardial contractility in patients with dilated cardiomyopathy exacerbates the obstruction by increasing septal wall contraction and decreasing CO. Increased blood flow velocity causes a greater degree of systolic anterior motion of the mitral valve's anterior leaflet, creating further obstruction. Decreased preload changes left ventricular geometry and thereby brings the anterior leaflet of the mitral valve into closer proximity of the hypertrophied septum. Increases in left ventricular contractility cause the LV to empty more completely and increase the degree of septal contractility, which results in a greater degree of obstruction.[67]

In hypertrophic cardiomyopathy with obstruction, conditions that impair ventricular function under normal physiologic conditions improve cardiac function. This implies that factors that normally impair contractility, such as myocardial depression, increased end-diastolic volume, and increased SVR, improve forward flow and diminish the degree of obstruction. See Figure 21-27 for pathology related to hypertrophic cardiomyopathy.

Anesthetic Management of Patients with Hypertrophic Cardiomyopathy

Anesthetic management should focus on strategies that alleviate and do not increase left ventricular outflow obstruction. It is imperative that adequate or slightly elevated left ventricular volume be maintained. Measures that decrease venous return and interfere with adequate ventricular preload should be avoided. Factors that increase myocardial contractility should be avoided. Inadequate depth of anesthesia that causes sympathetic nervous system stimulation may be detrimental. In the event that hypotension occurs, adequate perfusion pressure should be maintained by increasing preload with fluid administration and increasing SVR with phenylephrine.

BOX 21-3

Desired Hemodynamic Goals for Dilated Cardiomyopathy

Preload	Maintain
Afterload	Maintain to increase
Contractility	Decrease
Heart rate	Maintain
Heart rhythm	Normal sinus rhythm

Pharmacologic therapy used to treat hypertrophic cardiomyopathy (including β-blockers and calcium channel blockers) should be continued until the time of surgery. β-Blockers may be administered intraoperatively in order to reduce HR and contractility. Dysrhythmias must be avoided and immediately treated if they occur, as the atrial contribution to left ventricular volume is necessary to achieve CO.[65,67] Box 21-3 lists hemodynamic goals for patients with dilated cardiomyopathy.

Anesthesia Techniques

Anesthetic management must focus on maintaining left ventricular preload, decreasing myocardial contractility, and maintaining SVR. Regional anesthesia is not contraindicated in patients with dilated cardiomyopathy. Decreases in blood pressure must be treated immediately. Hypovolemia must be avoided and expeditiously treated if it occurs. Deep general anesthesia with a volatile agent is preferred in patients with hypertrophic cardiomyopathy and obstruction. Because halothane is the most potent myocardial depressant inhaled agent in use today, it the ideal choice of anesthetic agent.[69]

The potential for hemodynamic deterioration because of increasing subaortic obstruction along with secondary MR necessitates aggressive hemodynamic monitoring. Invasive monitoring via a pulmonary artery catheter allows for maintenance of adequate LVEDV. Because of reduced diastolic compliance associated with hypertrophic cardiomyopathy, PCWP does not correlate directly with LVEDV. The PCWP should be maintained at approximately 18 to 25 mm Hg. If hemodynamic status deteriorates and exacerbation of outflow obstruction is suspected, β-blocking drugs (propanolol or esmolol) should be administered. In addition, vasoconstrictors such as phenylephrine should be used in order to increase SVR.[30]

MITRAL VALVE PROLAPSE

Description and Etiology

The incidence of mitral valve prolapse, which was thought to be present in 5% to 15% of the VS population, is presently estimated at 1.6% to 2.4% of adults.[70] A familial predisposition exists, and women are three times more likely than men to develop mitral valve prolapse. Other conditions frequently associated with mitral valve prolapse include pectus excavatum and kyphoscoliosis. Symptoms are general and include weakness, dizziness, syncope, atypical chest pain, and palpitations. Atrial and ventricular dysrhythmias are common

BOX 21-4

Desired Hemodynamic Goals for Mitral Valve Prolapse

Preload	Maintain or increase
Afterload	Maintain
Contractility	Maintain
Heart rate	Maintain or increase
Heart rhythm	Normal sinus rhythm

findings in asymptomatic patients. A diagnosis of mitral valve prolapse is confirmed through echocardiography. Most patients with this condition remain undiagnosed. Despite its benign nature, mitral valve prolapse can produce potentially life-threatening complications. Ventricular premature contractions are the most common dysrhythmia associated with mitral valve prolapse. Prolonged periods of ventricular tachycardia occur in approximately 21% of patients with mitral valve prolapse. Mitral valve prolapse is also the most common cause of isolated MR. Supraventricular tachyarrhythmias and bradycardia associated with AV block may occur. Medical therapy for mitral valve prolapse consists primarily of the use of β-blocking drugs, which are thought to inhibit an autonomic imbalance that exists in women with mitral valve prolapse. Additionally, β-blocking drugs may increase end-diastolic volume and thereby decrease the degree of prolapse. The majority of patients with mitral valve prolapse do not require medical or pharmacologic management, which reflects the asymptomatic nature of this relatively common valvular abnormality (see Box 21-4).[30,65]

Pathophysiology and Unique Problems

The pathophysiologic changes that occur in mitral valve prolapse primarily affect the cusps and the chordae tendineae. Involved is a myxomatous degeneration of the valve cusps that replaces normal fibrous tissue. Also, this myxomatous degeneration affects the chordae tendineae and causes them to become pliable and elongated. The valve leaflets become supple and redundant, as the valve everts into the LA during systole.[69]

Mitral valve prolapse is undiagnosed in the majority of patients. Manifestation commonly occurs as an unexpected dysrhythmia (premature ventricular contractions) in a healthy patient who is receiving anesthesia. Many dysrhythmias resolve spontaneously. Lidocaine does not always terminate the premature ventricular contractions in mitral valve prolapse. β-Blockers are the best choice for control of arrhythmias in patients with mitral valve prolapse. Hemodynamic events and certain positions tend to exacerbate the degree of mitral valve prolapse and dysrhythmias. Hemodynamic changes that cause a decrease in ventricular preload and increase the incidence of eversion of the mitral valve are caused by increased myocardial contractility, decreased SVR, head-up or sitting positions, use of drugs that decrease ventricular preload (e.g., nitroglycerin and sodium nitroprusside), and hypovolemia.

Pharmacology

Preoperative anxiety stimulates the sympathetic nervous system and can increase the degree of mitral valve prolapses, especially dysrhythmias. Decreasing anxiety can reduce the sympathetically mediated responses and improve the hemodynamic profile that is characteristic of mitral valve prolapse. Anticholinergics can cause tachycardia and should therefore be omitted from the preoperative regimen.

Anesthetic Technique

No contraindication to providing regional anesthesia exists, although SVR should be maintained slightly above normal even in the presence of sympathetic blockade. General anesthesia is an appropriate choice and may be preferred in many instances. Whichever technique is chosen, it is important that preload be maintained. Induction of anesthesia can be accomplished with any of the available intravenous agents. Ketamine, with its ability to stimulate the sympathetic nervous system, should not be used in patients with mitral valve prolapse. Use of a volatile agent alone or in combination with opioids is appropriate for maintenance of anesthesia. Muscle relaxants that have a stable cardiovascular profile can be used. Because of the vagolytic effects of pancuronium, tachycardia and stimulation of the sympathetic nervous system can occur. These cardiovascular effects can be minimized if the drug is administered slowly.[69] Antibiotic prophylaxis is recommended for patients with mitral valve prolapse because of the potential for endocarditis. Currently the American Heart Association has guidelines for antibiotic prophylaxis in surgical patients with valvular disease. All patients who have valvular dysfunction or prosthetic valves are candidates for antibiotic prophylaxis.[24,57] These guidelines are provided in Chapter 13.

REFERENCES

1. Freeman GL. The effects of the pericardium on function of normal and enlarged hearts. *Cardiol Clin.* 1990;8:579-586.
2. Shabetai R. Acute pericarditis. *Cardiol Clin.* 1990;8:639-644.
3. Powell EDU, Mullaney JM. The Chiari network and the valve of the inferior vena cava. *Br Heart J.* 1960;22:579-584.
4. Hellerstein HK, Orbison TL. Anatomic variations of the orifice of the human coronary sinus. *Circulation.* 1951;3:514-523.
5. Dell'Italia LJ. The right ventricle: anatomy, physiology and clinical importance. *Curr Probl Cardiol.* 1991;26:658-720.
6. Farb A, Burke AP, Virmani R. Anatomy and pathology of the right ventricle (including acquired tricuspid and pulmonic valve disease). *Cardiol Clin.* 1992;10:1-21.
7. Rosenquist GC, Sweeny LJ. The membranous ventricular septum in the normal heart. *Johns Hopkins Med J.* 1974;135:9-16.
8. Cannon SR, Richards KL, Crawford M. Hydraulic estimation of stenotic orifice area: a correction of the Gorlin formula. *Circulation.* 1985;71:1170.
9. O'Rourke RA, Rackley CE, Edwards JE, Karp RB, Katy NM. Tricuspid valve, pulmonic valve and multivalvular disease. In: Hurst JW. *The Heart.* 9th ed. New York: McGraw-Hill; 1998:1833-1850.
10. Rahimtoola SH, et al. Mitral valve disease. In: Hurst JW. *The Heart.* 9th ed. New York: McGraw-Hill; 1998:1789-1820.
11. Goldbert AH, Warltier DC. The coronary circulation: implications for anesthesiologists. *Semin Anesth.* 1990;9: 232-244.
12. Guyton AC. *Textbook of Medical Physiology.* 10th ed. Philadelphia: Saunders; 2000:195-209, 221.
13. Wostczak JA. Basic cellular electrophysiology of the heart. In: Thys DM, Kaplan JA, eds. *The ECG in Anesthesia and Critical Care.* New York: Churchill Livingstone; 1987:109.

14. Little RC, Little WC. *Physiology of the Heart and Circulation*. 4th ed. Chicago: Yearbook; 1989:53.
15. Agnew NM, Pennefather SH, Russell GN. Isoflurane and coronary heart disease. *Anaesthesia*. 2002;57:338-347.
16. Teo A, Koh KF. Isoflurane and coronary steal. *Anaesthesia*. 2003;58:95-96.
17. Roscoe AK, Christensen J, Lynch C. Isoflurane but not halothane, induces protection of human myocardium via adenosine A1 receptors and adenosine triphosphate sensitive potassium channels. *Anesthesiology*. 2000;92:1692-1701.
18. Tuman KJ, Gilbert CC, Ivankovich AD. Pitfalls in interpretation of pulmonary artery catheter data. *J Cardiothorac Anesthesiol*. 1989;3:625-641.
19. Sarnoff SJ. Myocardial contractility as described by ventricular function curves: observations on Starling's law of the heart. *Physiol Rev*. 1955;35:107.
20. Johns RA. Endothelium-derived relaxing factor: basic review and clinical implications. *J Cardiothorac Vasc Anesth*. 1991; 5:69.
21. Hoover GA. Endothelial cell growth factors in atherogenesis. CMAJ. 1990;143:1035.
22. Schelling ME. FGF medication of coronary angiogenesis. *Ann N Y Acad Sci*. 1991;638:467-469.
23. Klagsbrun M. Angiogenic factors: regulators of blood supply-side biology. FGF, endothelial cell growth factors and angiogenesis: a keystone symposium. *New Biol*. 1991;3:745-749.
24. deBold AJ. Atrial natriuretic factor: a hormone produced by the heart. *Science*. 1985;230:767.
25. Rothe CF. Physiology of venous return. *Arch Intern Med*. 1986;146:977.
26. Zweiten PA, Wetzel HB. Antihypertensive drug treatment in the perioperative period. *J Cardiothorac Vasc Anesth*. 1993;7: 213-226.
27. Seventh Report of the Joint National Committee on Prevention, Detection, Evaluation and Treatment of High Blood Pressure. National Institutes of Health, National Heart, Lung and Blood Institute; National High Blood Pressure Education Program. 2003. US Government Printing Office, Washington, DC. NIH publication no. 03-5233.
28. Wallis EJ, Ramsay LE, Jackson PR. Cardiovascular and coronary risk estimation in hypertensive management. *Heart*. 2002;88:306-312.
29. Hopkins TJ. US guidelines say blood pressure of 120/80 mm Hg is not "normal." *Br Med J*. 2003;326:1104.
30. Stoelting RK, Dierdorf SF. *Anesthesia and Co-existing disease*. 3rd ed. New York: Churchill Livingstone; 1993:21.
31. Ross AF, Gomez MN, Tinker JH. Anesthesia for adult cardiac procedures. In: Tinker JH, Morgan GE, Longnecker DE, eds. *Principles and Practice of Anesthesiology*. 2nd ed. St Louis: Mosby; 1998:1659-1698.
32. Mangano DT. Perioperative cardiac morbidity. *Anesthesiology*. 1990;72:151-165.
33. Frohlich ED, Chobanran AV, Devereaux RB. The heart of hypertension. *N Engl J Med*. 1992;327:998-1008.
34. Mangano DT, Layug EL, Wallace A, Tateo I. Effect of atenolol on mortality and cardiac morbidity after noncardiac surgery. *N Engl J Med*. 1996;23:1713-1720.
35. Agner RC, Gallis HA. Pericarditis: differential diagnostic considerations. *Arch Intern Med*. 1979;139:401-412.
36. Robertson R. Constrictive pericarditis with particular reference to etiology. *Circulation*. 1982;65:525.
37. Spodick DH. Pericarditis, pericardial effusion, cardiac tamponade, and constriction. *Crit Care Clin*. 1989;5:455-476.
38. Seifert FC, et al. Surgical treatment of constrictive pericarditis: analysis of outcome diagnostic error. *Circulation*. 1985;72: 264-273.
39. Hoit BD. Management of effusion and constrictive pericardial disease. *Circulation*. 2002;105:2939-2942.
40. Konchigeri HN, Levitsky S. Anesthetic considerations for pericardectomy in uremic pericardial effusion. *Anesth Analg*. 1976;55:378-382.
41. Guyton AC. Cardiac tamponade. In: *Textbook of Medical Physiology*. 10th ed. Philadelphia: Saunders; 2000:214.
42. Williams C, Soutter L. Pericardial tamponade. *Arch Intern Med*. 1954;94:571.
43. Shabetai R, Fowler NO, Guntheroth WG. The hemodynamics of cardiac tamponade and constrictive pericarditis. *Am J Cardiol*. 1970;26:480-489.
44. Beck CA. Two cardiac compression triads. *JAMA*. 1935;104:715.
45. Lake CL. Anesthesia and pericardial disease. *Anesth Analg*. 1983;62:431-443.
46. Weeks KR, Chatterjee K, Block S. Bedside hemodynamic monitoring: its value in the diagnosis of tamponade complicating cardiac surgery. *J Thorac Cardiovasc Surg*. 1976;71:250-252.
47. Stanley TH, Weidauer HE. Anesthesia for the patient with cardiac tamponade. *Anesth Analg*. 1973;52:110-114.
48. Cyna AM, Rogers RC, McFarlane H. Hypotension due to unexpected pericardial tamponade. *Anaesthesia*. 1990;45: 140-142.
49. Murray BR, Robertson DS. Anaesthesia for mitral valvotomy complicated by hypotension due to pericardial effusion. *Br J Anaesth*. 1964;36:256-258.
50. Guntheroth WG, Morgan BC. Effect of respiration on venous return and stroke volume in cardiac tamponade. *Circ Res*. 1967;20:381-390.
51. Mastropietro C. Anesthesia for cardiac and peripheral vascular surgery. In: Waugaman WR, Foster SD, Rigor BM, eds. *Principles and Practice of Nurse Anesthesia*. Norwalk, Conn: Appleton & Lange; 1992:705.
52. Swartz AJ, Maddi R. Anesthesia for cardiac surgery. In: Liu PL, ed. *Principles and Procedures in Anesthesiology*. Philadelphia: Lippincott; 1992:339.
53. Wray-Roth DL, Rothstein P, Thomas SJ. Anesthesia for cardiac surgery. In: Barash PG, Cullen BF, Stolting RK, eds. *Clinical Anesthesia*. 3rd ed. Philadelphia:1997 Lippincott; 835.
54. Lake CL. Cardiovascular anatomy and physiology. In: Barash PG, Cullen BF, Stoelting RK, eds. *Clinical anesthesia*. 3rd ed. Philadelphia. 1997. Lippincott. p 805.
55. Mohrman DE, Heller LJ. *Cardiovascular Physiology*. 3rd ed. New York: McGraw-Hill; 1991:175.
56. Thrush DN, et al. Blood pressure after cardiopulmonary bypass: which technique is accurate? *J Cardiothorac Vasc Anesth*. 1994;8:269-272.
57. Church JA, et al. Incidence of cerebral air embolism during left atrial catheter insertion in cardiopulmonary bypass patients. *Anesthesiology*. 1993;79:52.
58. Edwards Critical Care Division. *Invasive Hemodynamic Monitoring: Physiologic Principles and Clinical Applications*. Santa Ana, Calif: Baxter Healthcare; 1989:1.
59. Kato M, et al. Does transesophageal echocardiography improve postoperative outcome in patients undergoing coronary artery bypass surgery? *J Cardiothorac Vasc Anesth*. 1993;7: 285-289.
60. Sutton DC, Calahan MK. Transesophageal echocardiography is routine in anesthesia for cardiac surgery. *J Cardiothorac Vasc Anesth*. 1993;7:357-360.
61. Jackson MJ, Thomas SJ. Valvular heart disease. In: Kaplan JA, ed. Cardiac Anesthesia. 3rd ed. Philadelphia: Saunders; 1993:629.
62. Iung B. Management of ischemic mitral regurgitation. *Heart*. 2003;89:459-464.
63. Shanewise JS, Hug CC. Anesthesia for adult cardiac surgery. In: Miller RD, ed. *Anesthesia*. 5th ed. New York: Churchill Livingstone; 2000:1753.
64. Zile MR, Gaasch WH. Heart failure in aortic stenosis—improving diagnosis and treatment. *N Engl J Med*. 2003;348: 1735-1736.

65. Mark JB, Slaughter TF, Reves JG. Cardiovascular monitoring. In: Miller RD, ed. *Anesthesia*. 5th ed. New York: Churchill Livingstone; 2000:1117.
66. Hicks GL, Massey TH. Update on indications for surgery in aortic insufficiency. *Curr Opin Cardiol*. 2002;17:172-178.
67. Ammar T, Reich DL, Kaplan JA. Uncommon cardiac diseases. In: Benumof JL, ed. *Anesthesia and Uncommon Diseases*. 4th ed. Philadelphia: Saunders; 1998:70.
68. Maron B. Hypertrophic cardiomyopathy: a systematic review. *JAMA*. 2002;287:1308-1320.
69. Oliver WC, De Castro, MA, Strickland RA. Uncommon diseases and cardiac anesthesia. In: Kaplan JA, ed. *Cardiac Anesthesia*. 3rd ed. Philadelphia: Saunders; 1993:819.
70. Pellerin D, Brecker S, Veyrat C. Degenerative mitral valve disease with emphasis on mitral valve prolapse. *Heart*. 2002;88:20-28.

CHAPTER 22

CARDIAC ANESTHESIA

CHARLENE V. BROUILLETTE

Care of the patient with cardiac compromise is a complex undertaking and requires knowledge of basic cardiac physiology, mechanics of circulation, requirements of myocardial oxygen supply and demand, and the basics of pharmacologic and hemodynamic management. Perioperative evaluation and preparation of the patient are important facets of the anesthetic plan of care. Intraoperatively, anesthetic maintenance is often achieved in corroboration with the perfusionist during bypass procedures and in conjunction with the minute-to-minute needs of the surgeon during off-pump procedures. Postoperative management begins at cessation of the pump run on bypass procedures and with completion of anastomoses during off-pump cases. The postoperative care includes temperature management and prevention and control of coagulopathies as well as regulation of hemodynamic stability and pain management.

The first recorded open cardiac procedure was performed on April 15, 1952. Dr. R. E. Gross of Children's Hospital in Boston was able to close an atrial septal defect under direct vision. In October of that year in Detroit Dr. Dodril used right-sided heart bypass to perform an open pulmonary valvotomy. In May of 1953 in Philadelphia Dr. Gibbon used a heart-lung machine to close an atrial septal defect. Also in 1953 the Mayo Clinic was the site of the first series of open-heart surgeries using a heart-lung machine.[1] This was a prototype for the coronary artery bypass grafting procedures familiar to practitioners today.

Coronary artery disease is the predominant cause of death in patients in the fourth and fifth decades and the most common cause of *premature* death in men aged 35 to 45 years. Annually approximately 1.5 million individuals endure some level of myocardial insult. There are more than 519,000 adult coronary artery surgeries yearly—80% of all adult heart operations performed in the United States.[2]

CORONARY ARTERY DISEASE

The coronary arteries arise from the aorta. Coronary artery perfusion pressure is mainly determined by aortic diastolic pressure and left ventricular[3] end diastolic pressure. Coronary artery disease alters coronary blood flow, decreases coronary reserve, and increases the incidence of coronary artery vasospasm. Risk factors associated with the progression of coronary artery disease include age, gender, genetic predisposition, obesity, hyperlipidemia, hypertension, stress, diabetes mellitus, and smoking. Exacerbating the effects of coronary artery disease are combinations of peripheral vascular disease, carotid disease, and a compromised pulmonary system.

Atherosclerosis is a disease process in which fatty lesions are deposited on the intimal layer of the arteries. These fatty deposits are called *atheromatous plaques* and begin as crystals of cholesterol that adhere to the intima and smooth muscle layer of the arteries. This disease rarely involves small arteries and should not be confused with arteriosclerosis, which is considered relatively benign. The cholesterol crystals develop and form a larger matrix that stimulates fibrous tissue and smooth muscle growth to create additional layers on which larger plaques grow. Eventually the plaques mature and develop into obstructive lesions or contribute to the formation of fibroblasts, which eventually deposit dense connective tissue, resulting in sclerosis (fibrosis). Atheromatous plaque and the resulting sclerotic lesions lead to loss of arterial distensibility and tissue degeneration and ulceration of the arterial wall. Inherent in this process are thrombi, which form and embolize, causing blood flow obstruction and distal tissue ischemia.[4]

Patients with atherosclerotic coronary disease become symptomatic when 75% of the coronary vessel is occluded, resulting in a decrease in coronary blood flow. Ischemia depresses myocardial function and causes severe chest pain referred to as *angina pectoris*. In addition to pain, cells are subject to increased irritability and become increasingly vulnerable to fibrillation, alterations in the conduction pathways, and thrombus formation.

SYSTEMS AFFECTED BY CARDIOPULMONARY BYPASS

Pulmonary System

Cardiopulmonary bypass (CBP) can precipitate morphologic changes known as *pump lung*. This acute lung injury can result in diffuse congestion, edema in the alveolar and interstitial regions, and hemorrhagic atelectasis. One theory regarding this phenomenon is that microemboli of protein aggregates, disintegrated platelets, damaged fibrin, and fat particles contribute to the development of pump lung. Acute lung injury can also be caused by complement activation, inflammatory response, hemodilution, lung hypoxia, and elevated pulmonary artery (PA) pressure. Hypothermia and topical cooling contribute to instances of phrenic nerve dysfunction that can play a role in alterations in pulmonary function.[5] CPB has a negative influence on ventilation-perfusion parameters. Gas distribution occurs preferentially to nondependent areas of the lung, thereby producing hypoventilation of dependent lung sections, which can result in postoperative atelectasis.

Various approaches for prevention of atelectasis have been proposed and studied (e.g., delivery of positive-pressure ventilation, intermittent sighs, or static inflation (continuous positive airway pressure [CPAP]) during CPB), but none has demonstrated a definitive or reliable effect. It is recommended that a reduction of microemboli proliferation (using blood filtration), prevention of pulmonary vascular distention, and hemodilution along with steroids and vasodilator prostaglandins may preclude the onset of this problem.

Central Nervous System

The predominant postoperative neurologic complication after open-heart surgical procedures on CPB is stroke. The word *stroke* refers to a sudden onset of focal deficit of the central nervous system (CNS) that lasts more than 24 hours. Up to 50% of patients demonstrate postoperative neurophysiologic dysfunction in the postoperative period after CPB.[6] Cerebrovascular sequelae indicators include visual impairment, hemiparesis, aphasia, and sensory impairment. Other neurologic deficits include abnormal reflexes, loss of the sensation of vibration, impaired locomotion, and impaired visual acuity associated with retinal lesions or infarction. The incidence of cerebrovascular insult is related to age, valvular repair or replacement, the extent of aortic calcification, and preexisting cerebrovascular disease. The presence of preoperative cerebrovascular disease indicates the need to maintain higher perfusion pressures during CPB. A recent history of stroke should be considered a contraindication for anticoagulation therapy necessary in CPB-dependent procedures.

The CNS is sensitive to hypoxemia and is at risk when cerebral hypoperfusion occurs. At a mean arterial pressure (MAP) between 50 and 150 mm Hg (autoregulatory plateau) cerebral blood flow (CBF) is maintained at approximately 50 ml/100 g/min because of changes in cerebrovascular tone. Maintenance of adequate CBF may decrease the incidence of arterial hypoperfusion, which could result in stroke.[7] Cerebral autoregulation is dependent on CBF and MAP and is established at a lower plateau with hypothermia. Global ischemia is possible with rapid hypoperfusion of collaterals, lost autoregulation in profound hypothermia, or circulatory arrest of longer than 1 minute.[8]

Changes in arterial blood pressure and blood flow may be precipitated as a result of hypothermic responses, hypocarbia, venous congestion arising from superior vena caval obstruction, or emboli. Sources of emboli include aortic atheroma from the aortic clamp, intraventricular thrombi, valve calcification, air during open chamber procedures, aortic cannulation, bubble oxygenators, nitrous oxide administered before bypass, or factors associated with a long pump run (CPB). Pump runs longer than 90 minutes are considered an independent risk factor, in which the risk of cognitive dysfunction is greatly increased.[9] Avoidance of nitrous oxide decreases the possibility of remobilization. The use of nitrous oxide can increase the size of gaseous emboli.

Hyperglycemia may intensify global and focal insults to the CNS. Strict glucose control is essential, because evidence suggests that hyperglycemic states increase the magnitude and extent of neurologic injury that ensues during ischemia.[10] Solutions containing glucose are to be avoided, and patients who are diabetic must be monitored closely to maintain tight control of glucose status. Although it may be necessary to institute insulin therapy to manage hyperglycemia in some patients, insulin resistance develops during CPB in part because of increased endogenous catecholamines, which increase the incidence of refractory hyperglycemia.

Cerebral protection techniques include metabolic suppression with hypothermia, administration of medications such as thiopental or propofol, and the use of calcium channel blockers to reduce the incidence of vasospasm.[7] In addition, deep hypothermic circulatory arrest can be employed for arch reconstruction and for treatment of giant aneurysms. This technique necessitates core and external cooling to temperatures of 15° to 20° C, selective cerebral perfusion, pH management, and intermittent or low-flow perfusion (as in pediatric hearts for aortic arch procedures). Cerebral protection techniques during cardiopulmonary bypass are listed in Box 22-1.

BOX 22-1

Cerebral Protection Techniques Used during Cardiopulmonary Bypass

- Maintain mean arterial pressure >50 mm Hg after start of rewarming
- Maintain euglycemia
- Maintain mild hypothermia (nasopharyngeal temperature <37° C at rewarming)
- Perform pharmacologic metabolic suppression:
  - Thiopental
  - Propofol
  - Calcium channel blockers
  - Aprotinin (associated with decreased incidence of stroke)

Gastrointestinal Tract

GI tract morbidity in the postoperative CPB patient is a significant complication of bypass procedures. According to current studies, risk factors that increase the incidence of gastrointestinal (GI) complications include advanced age, prolonged CPB, open chamber procedures, and immunosuppressive therapies,[11,12] the same risk factors as those proposed for emboli formation.

Renal Function

Impairment of renal function is not uncommon in patients undergoing surgical procedures requiring CPB. Studies have demonstrated that renal dysfunction of varying degrees is related to length of time on bypass (longer than 3 hours), cardiac output (CO), infection, type of procedure (valve surgery has higher incidence of renal dysfunction), excessive blood loss, increased use of vasopressors, perioperative myocardial infarction (MI), use of intraaortic balloon pump (IABP), and massive transfusion.[13] Independent risk factors for postoperative renal failure include use of IABP, deep hypothermic circulatory arrest, low CO syndrome, advanced age, and low urinary output during the pump run. CPB by itself is a less-problematic risk factor.[14]

Serum creatinine levels are accepted predictors of morbidity. Normal creatinine is 1.8 mg/100 ml or less; values ranging from 1.9 to 5 mg/11 ml are considered abnormal. Creatinine levels in excess of 5 mg/100 ml indicates renal failure, and the patient requires dialysis. Preoperative serum creatinine levels are directly proportional to predicted mortality rate and postoperative renal failure and inversely related to the preoperative cardiac index (CI).

Hypothermia during CPB depresses renal tubular function; however, hemodilution, administration of mannitol (CPB prime), and maintenance of glomerular filtration rate result in adequate urinary output. The standard for measurement of perfusion is a urinary output of at least 1 ml/kg/hr.[13] Perfusion pressure is a primary determinant of urinary output during CPB. Hypothermia does not seem to have a great influence on urinary output during bypass. Studies have shown no difference in urinary output (renal function) among cases in which hypothermic versus normothermic CPB is used.[15]

Nondiabetic hyperglycemia during CPB is largely the result of increased glucose reabsorption by the kidneys. Even small amounts of glucose introduced during CPB have been shown to precipitate hyperglycemia. This is problematic because hyperglycemia is detrimental to the brain as well as the renal tubules.

Catecholamines rise progressively during CPB. The release and circulation of vasopressin (antidiuretic hormone; ADH) are thought to occur in response to low atrial pressures, hypotension, and nonpulsatile flow. Reduction in urinary output may be the result of renal vasoconstriction stimulated by high levels of vasopressin. Hemodilution has a significant impact in counteracting the effects of vasopressin by increasing perfusion to the outer cortex of the kidney, thereby stimulating renal plasma flow and the clearance of free water and potassium. Perioperative administration of low-dose dopamine (2 to 5 mcg/kg/min) may protect renal perfusion while increasing urinary output.[14]

Urinary output is the single most important intraoperative monitor of the renal system during coronary artery bypass grafting (CABG) procedures using CPB. Anuria is not uncommon during CPB, and approximately one third of patients may experience acute renal failure. It is thought that the nonpulsatile flow of the extracorporeal circuit interferes with autoregulation of renal blood flow. Maintenance of good urinary flow (0.5 to 1 ml/kg/hr) during the pump run ensures that free water can be eliminated. Evaluation of electrolyte status is recommended before and after termination of CPB. Levels of cations such as potassium and calcium may have to be adjusted postoperatively.

METABOLIC FACTORS RELATED TO HYPOTHERMIA

Hypothermia is an integral aspect of CPB and has a profound impact on enzyme systems and the coagulation cascade. Activated clotting time (ACT), prothrombin time (PT), and partial thromboplastin time (PTT) are prolonged, and platelets become nonfunctional as the body temperature is lowered to approximately 28° C. Cellular potassium uptake is increased and may result in hypokalemia.

The beneficial aspects of hypothermia include a reduced basal metabolic rate, improved myocardial protection, tissue and organ preservation, and reduced oxygen consumption. The metabolic requirement for O_2 is reduced by 50% for each 7° C drop in core body temperature. However, it may not be possible to convert heartbeat to normal sinus rhythm until the rewarming core temperature is 34° C.

ANESTHESIA CONSIDERATIONS

The goals of anesthetic management for coronary revascularization are directed toward producing analgesia, amnesia and muscle relaxation; abolishing autonomic reflexes; maintaining physiologic homeostasis; and providing myocardial and cerebral protection. The avenues available to accomplish these goals include an effective preoperative evaluation, administration of modest doses of sedation and pain medication before any attempt at line placement is made; and use of O_2 in the preoperative setting. Administration of a balanced anesthetic with opioid, inhalation agents, sedative-hypnotics, and muscle relaxant provides a stable hemodynamic state for the difficult cardiovascular patient.

Preoperative Assessment

A thorough preoperative assessment of the patient who will undergo cardiac surgery should include comprehensive review of systems, airway status, and laboratory data; physical examination; review of surgical history; and review of current medications. Actual reports of diagnostic procedures such as cardiac catheterization, echocardiogram, and Doppler studies should be reviewed by the anesthesia care provider. Figure 22-1 illustrates the cascade of preoperative assessment used for preoperative planning.

Airway assessment in cardiac patients is necessary, because such patients are unable to compensate for a reduced oxygen supply. Often patients who undergo cardiac revascularization procedures are oxygen compromised because of body habitus, pulmonary disease, age, and general physical condition. These patients cannot tolerate decreases in oxygen supply. Careful evaluation and preparation for airway management is very important.

Myocardial Ischemia

Prevention of myocardial ischemia in patients undergoing myocardial revascularization procedures is paramount if the procedures are to be successful. Ischemia can be precipitated by hemodynamic alterations, which can occur at any time during the perioperative period. Alterations such as tachycardia, hypertension, hypotension, and ventricular distention can cause myocardial ischemia. Treatment of ischemia is directed at stabilization of hemodynamic parameters. A patient who is subjected to perioperative ischemia is three times more likely to suffer an MI.[16]

Perioperative hypertension may be responsible for myocardial ischemia, ventricular failure, intracerebral hemorrhage, pulmonary edema, or aortic dissection. Continuation of antihypertensive therapy is recommended during the preoperative preparation of cardiac patients. Patients should be instructed to take any antihypertensive or cardiac medications until the day of surgery. Providing sedation during the invasive placement and induction lessens the possibility of hypertension from sympathetic stimulation.

Intraoperative events that are known to precipitate ischemia are illustrated in Box 22-2. The goal of anesthetic management is to reduce or obtund responses to these stimuli to reduce exposure to ischemia. Treatment of ischemia is based on four modes of support: oxygen administration, stabilization of hemodynamic parameters, inotropic support, and mechanical support when indicated.[17]

Coexisting Disease States

Preoperative risk factors include age, cigarette smoking (which contributes to development of atherosclerosis), peripheral vascular and cerebral vascular disease, hypertension, angina, congestive heart failure (CHF), previous MI, and diabetes mellitus.

Angina pectoris is classified by degree of severity based on factors promoting the onset, duration, and response to symptomatic treatment with vasodilator therapy (nitroglycerin). Angina is defined as stable if there has been no change in frequency, precipitating event, or duration for the previous 2 months. Unstable angina (crescendo angina) is defined as angina of new onset that lasts longer than 30 minutes and is associated with ST- or T-segment changes. Unstable angina often does not respond to rest or medication.[18,19]

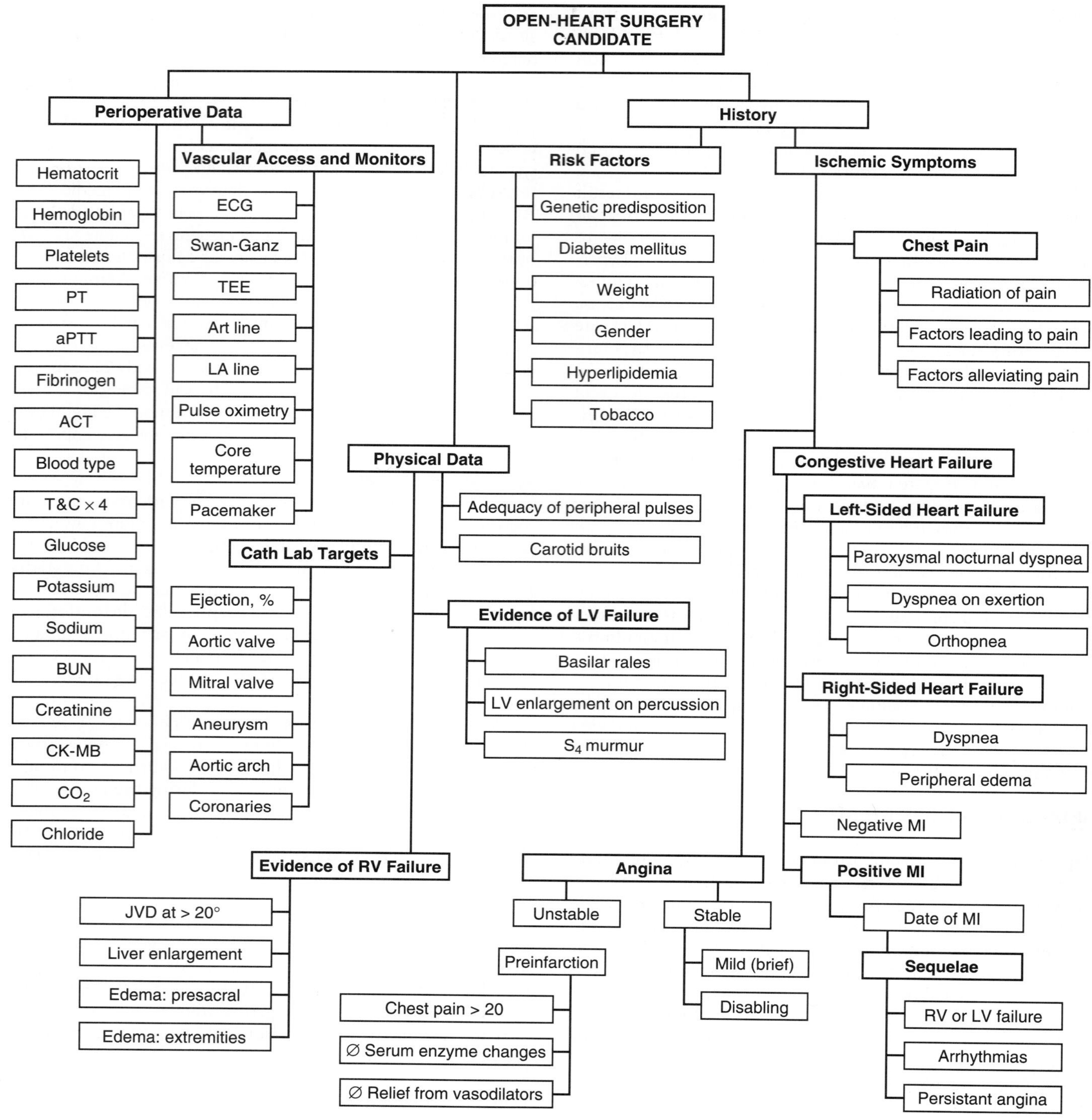

FIGURE **22-1**
Preoperative assessment of patients with myocardial ischemia. *ACT*, Activated coagulation time; *aPTT*, activated partial thromboplastin time; *BUN*, blood urea nitrogen; *CK-MB*, creatinine phosphokinase myocardial band; *ECG*, electrocardiography; *JVD*, jugular venous distention; *LA*, left atrial; *LV*, left ventricular; *MI*, myocardial infarction; *PT*, prothrombin time; *RV*, right ventricular; *T&C*, type and cross-match; *TEE*, transesophageal echocardiography.

Previous cardiac surgery results in an increase in blood loss because of reoperation through adhesions from a previous sternotomy. Anticipation of excessive blood loss may indicate the use of antihyperfibrinolytic agents and implementation of a cell saver device. The sternotomy is a cause for significant concern because scar tissue formation may have led to anatomic distortion or superficial attachment of the pericardium to the anterior chest wall, which presents a potential hazard for laceration of the myocardium or great vessels. It may become necessary for the anesthesia care provider to heparinize the patient

BOX **22-2**

Perioperative Events That May Elicit Ischemia

- Coronary spasm
- Endotracheal intubation
- Sympathetic stimulation
- Sternal split
- Light anesthesia
- Cannulation
- Initiation of bypass
- Incomplete revascularization
- Tachycardia
- Atherosclerotic plaque
- Hypertension
- Air or particulate thrombus formation
- Manipulation of heart
- Fibrillation

earlier than anticipated to allow for percutaneous femoral artery cannulation for bypass. Blood products and heparin bolus must be immediately available should this extremely emergent situation occur.

Because of the frequent need for PA catheterization or central venous pressure monitoring, prior surgery that has distorted the vascular and anatomic features of the neck and upper thorax must be noted. Of particular importance is a history of radical neck dissection, subclavian bypass procedures, ligation of the internal jugular (IJ) vein, or carotid artery surgery, which should be evaluated for impact on intubation and line placement.

For cardiac surgery involving recent or concomitant endarterectomy of carotid artery lesions, reinstitution of normal perfusion pressure may result in edema and hemorrhage. The inability of capillary beds to vasoconstrict and regulate flow, leads some areas of the brain to exhibit a mismatch of CBF to metabolic ratio.[20] Cerebral perfusion is dependent on autoregulation to maintain constant blood flow regardless of changes in perfusion pressure or CO. Chronic hypoperfusion related to carotid stenosis may lead to maximal dilation of the cerebral vessels, compromising compensatory mechanisms normally available for tolerance of low-pressure or low-flow states.[19] In cases in which this condition remains uncorrected before cardiac surgery, systemic arterial pressure must be maintained at a level that ensures adequate cerebral perfusion.

Hemodynamic Status

Evaluation of cardiovascular status includes a discussion with the patient regarding his or her functional status. One method of qualifying the functional status is to determine by interview which activities of daily living the patient is able to perform. If a patient is unable to climb one flight of stairs without difficulty, then the anesthesia care provider can plan for a patient with reduced ability to handle the hemodynamic changes inherent to induction and maintenance of anesthesia.

Cardiac catheterization may be used for diagnostic assessment, electrophysiologic evaluation, or direct intervention in patients in cardiogenic shock. The catheterization report provides significant information regarding patient cardiac performance. The catheterization evaluation provides information about pressures and oxygen saturations of the four chambers of the heart, PA pressure, systemic pressure, body surface area, CI (liters per minute per square meter), stroke index (milliliters per beat per square meter), left ventricular ejection fraction (EF), degree of stenosis in coronary vessels, and coronary dominance (Table 22-1).

TABLE **22-1** Normal Intracardiac Pressures

	Notation	Range (mm Hg)
Central venous pressure	CVP	0-8
Right atrial pressure	RAP	0-8
Right ventricular end-systolic pressure	RVESP	15-25
Right ventricular end-diastolic pressure	RVEDP	0-8
Pulmonary artery pressure (systolic)	PAP systolic	15-25
Pulmonary artery pressure (diastolic)	PAP diastolic	8-15
Pulmonary artery pressure (mean)	PAP	10-20
Pulmonary capillary wedge pressure (PCWP); pulmonary artery occlusion pressure	PAOP (PCWP)	6-12

EF is the end-diastolic volume (EDV) minus the end-systolic volume (ESV), divided by the EDV:

Equation 22-1

$$EF = (EDV - ESV)/EDV$$

Tables 22-2 and Table 22-3 summarize cardiac formulas that are useful in clinical practice. An EF of 50% or greater in a patient with normal valve function is acceptable. If the patient has mitral regurgitation, an EF of 50% to 55% is considered to indicate left ventricular dysfunction. An EF of less than 50% reflects a moderate reduction of ventricular function. Poor cardiac function relates to an EF below 30% and may stem from ventricular hypokinesis, akinesis, or dyskinesis. Echocardiography is used to evaluate ventricular function by measuring wall motion during systole. It can permit a qualitative and quantitative assessment and reflects the four types of abnormal wall function described previously.[21] Single photon emission computed tomography (SPECT) scan is another diagnostic tool used in the preparation of patients for cardiac surgery. It is a noninvasive procedure that makes use of a radionuclide tracer to provide a three-dimensional picture of heart structures and function. It is capable of producing a measurement of rate and volume of blood flow, size and location of blockages or narrowing of vessels, and more accurate diagnosis of heart disease in women.[22]

Right Ventricular Function

Patients with right coronary artery disease may be susceptible to right ventricular ischemia and infarction when right ventricular distention or increased afterload results in diminished cardiac performance and reduced right coronary perfusion pressure. The interrelationships among aortic end-diastolic pressure, afterload volume, coronary perfusion pressure, and pulmonary vascular resistance play a significant role in the management of right-sided cardiac performance. Assessment of these variables before treatment is essential if compromise of function is to be avoided.

TABLE 22-2 Cardiac Formulas

Parameter	Notation	Formula	Normal Range
Stroke volume	SV	SV = CO ÷ HR	60-90 ml/beat
Stroke index	SI	SI = SV ÷ BSA	40-60 ml/beat/m^2
Cardiac output	CO	CO = SV × HR	5-6 L/min
Cardiac index	CI	CI = CO ÷ BSA	2.5-4 L/min/m^2
Mean arterial pressure	MAP	MAP = diastolic pressure + one third pulse pressure	80-120 mm Hg
Systemic vascular resistance	SVR	SVR = (MAP − CVP) ÷ (CO × 80)	700-1400 dyne/sec/cm^5
Pulmonary vascular resistance	PVR	PVR = (PAP − PCWP) ÷ (CO × 80)	50-300 dyne/s/cm^5
Left ventricular stroke work index	LVSWI	LVSWI = 0.0136 × (MAP − PCWP) × SI	40-60 g • m/beat/m^2
Coronary perfusion pressure	CPP	CPP = DIA BP − LVEDP	mm/hg
Ejection fraction	EF	EF = (EDV − ESV) ÷ EDV	55%-70%
Rate-pressure product	RPP	RPP = SYS BP × rate	>15,000
Triple index	TI	TI = SYS BP × rate × PCWP	>180,000

BSA, *Body surface area;* DIA BP, *diastolic blood pressure;* EDV, *end-diastolic volume;* ESV, *end-systolic volume;* HR, *heart rate;* LVEDP, *left ventricular end-diastolic pressure;* PCWP, *pulmonary capillary wedge pressure;* SI, *stroke index;* SYS BP, *systolic blood pressure.*

TABLE 22-3 Hemodilution

Circulating Blood Volume

Patient	Estimated Red Blood Count
Male	80 ml/kg
Female	65 ml/kg
Pediatric	85-105 ml/kg

Hemodilutional Hematocrit

	Notation	Formula
Estimated red blood cell count	ERBC	Determined by age and gender
Circulating blood volume	CBV	ERBC × weight (kg)
Red blood cell volume	RBCV	CBV × HCT
Total circulating volume	TCV	CBV + prime volume
Dilutional hematocrit	Dilutional HCT	RBCV ÷ TCV

Common treatment for systemic hypotension before initiation of CPB incorporates the use of phenylephrine, an α_1-adrenergic agonist. The primary indication for use is hypotension induced by a reduction in systemic vascular resistance (SVR) as opposed to compromised CO. The perceived advantage of the use of phenylephrine is its effect of increasing coronary perfusion pressure with minimal chronotropic side effects.[23]

Pulmonary Function

Risk factors of note for the pulmonary system include a history of cigarette smoking, dyspnea, and wheezing. Patients with chronic obstructive pulmonary disease and dyspnea or wheezing have two to six times more pulmonary complications in the postoperative phase of cardiac surgery. A recent respiratory infection predisposes to postoperative atelectasis and pneumonia.[24]

Diabetes Mellitus

Patients with diabetes mellitus are at increased risk intraoperatively and postoperatively because of the increased risk of silent ischemia and MI. These patients have peripheral as well as autonomic neuropathies. With autonomic neuropathy they are at an increased risk of aspiration and sudden death. Patients on NPH insulin have the added risk of allergic reaction to protamine, necessitating the possibility that heparin may have to be metabolized instead of being reversed. Investigational substances may be available in the future to safely reverse heparin in these allergic patients. Heparinase I has been introduced as an alternative to protamine. It is a carbohydrate-modifying enzyme that cleaves heparin at specific sites that are important for anticoagulation. This agent fractionates heparin into small inactive fragments with no apparent adverse hemodynamic changes.[25]

Laboratory Data

Laboratory examinations for patients with ischemic heart disease involving two or more associated risk factors (diabetes, obesity, family history, and smoking) should include complete blood count; electrolytes, cardiac enzymes (including enzyme fraction for creatinine phosphokinase), serum creatinine, cholesterol; and coagulation screening profile.[26]

Coagulation function studies include platelet count, PT, and activated PTT (aPTT). PTT and ACT are used to monitor patients receiving heparin therapy, and PT and international normalized ratio (INR) are used to monitor patients receiving warfarin products.[27] Platelet inhibitors are often part of the drug regimens of patients who need cardiac surgery. These agents are associated with the risk of excess bleeding. However, no evidence suggests that surgery is contraindicated in this situation. It is recommended that 24 to 48 hours should elapse before surgery is performed after these drugs are discontinued. The platelet inhibitors (glucoprotein IIb/IIIa receptor inhibitors) in use at this time include abciximab (ReoPro), eptifibatide (Integrilin), and tirofiban (Aggrastat).[28] It should be emphasized that long-term heparin therapy results in prolonged bleeding times and may affect calculations of loading doses of heparin required for CPB.[29] Other issues related to the cause and treatment of adverse bleeding are discussed later in this chapter.

Long-Term Use of Medications

Prevention of rebound hypertension and reduction of perioperative hemodynamic stress are primary considerations for continuation of antihypertensive therapy until the morning of surgery. Potential drug interactions with anesthetic agents should be anticipated and evaluated, and treatment should proceed accordingly.

Calcium-channel blockers are used widely to control hypertension, angina, and arrhythmias in patients with cardiovascular disease. Their continued use up to the day of surgery is a common practice and provides the advantage of controlling dysrhythmias and preventing coronary spasm. Potential hazards associated with continued therapy include a reduction in patient responses to inotropes and vasopressors and atrioventricular conduction problems.

β-Adrenergic receptor–blocking agents such as propranolol must be continued up to and during the preinduction period. β-Blockers allow for reduction in myocardial oxygen consumption by providing an overall decrease in sympathetic stimulation and catecholamine release. Because the heart rate is slowed, diastolic filling is improved. These drugs are helpful in controlling anginal symptoms, hypertension, tachycardia, and myocardial ischemia. Bronchospasm and decreased inotropic response to β stimulants in conjunction with greater vasoconstriction in response to sympathomimetics are potential disadvantages to continuation of β-blockade up to the time of surgery.

Digitalis therapy may be continued until the morning of surgery if it is used to treat rapid ventricular response to atrial fibrillation or flutter; otherwise, it may be discontinued, because other inotropes with greater efficacy may be given preoperatively if needed. If potassium is used, its effects must be carefully monitored.

It is recommended that antidysrhythmics be continued until the day of surgery except for disopyramide, encainide, and flecainide, which should be discontinued except in the presence of the most life-threatening dysrhythmias. These agents have been associated with increased mortality, and postbypass MI has been noted with their continuance. Disopyramide has been noted to cause difficulty in termination of CPB.

Antidepressants provide no advantage if continued up to the day of surgery and may interact negatively with sympathomimetics. However, as noted previously, it is important to give sedation and anxiolysis to these patients during the preoperative phase.

ANESTHESIA MONITORING

Electrocardiography and Noninvasive Blood Pressure

Leads II and V_5 can help in the diagnosis of dysrhythmias, ischemia, conduction defects, and electrolyte disturbances. None of the standard leads can detect posterior wall ischemia. The noninvasive blood pressure cuff must be placed on the same side as the arterial line to allow for correlation of blood pressure. This is a backup monitor.

Radial Arterial Line

Sternal retraction may play a role in distorting the radial artery waveform. The right radial artery is usually selected in cases in which the left internal mammary artery is dissected for anastomosis and because radial arterial line monitoring may show a false low number because of compression of the subclavian artery at the retractor. The brachial artery is contraindicated because it is an end artery of the arm. Some authors evaluate results of an Allen's test because it screens for patients with inadequate palmar collateral flow from the ulnar artery. Reduced collateral flow is a relative contraindication to the use of a radial artery catheter.

Other Arterial Line Sites

Use of the brachial artery for monitoring is most commonly dismissed because it provides the bulk of circulation for the lower arm and is considered an end artery. The femoral artery is superficial and offers access to the central arterial tree. It also provides appropriate access should an IABP placement be necessary. However, if the femoral artery is used, it should be noted that an alternative site may become necessary if use of IABP is instituted. The dorsalis pedis arteries may have a more distorted wave form and are not recommended for patients with aortoiliac or peripheral vascular disease. The axillary artery is not commonly cannulated because of an increased risk of cerebral air embolus and because it has a tendency to bleed more easily. The ulnar artery can be cannulated for monitoring, but an Allen's test of the ulnar artery is necessary before placement, and the risk of problems with placement on the same extremity as a radial attempt must be taken into consideration. The complications inherent to arterial line placement include ischemia, thrombosis, infection, and bleeding.

Central Venous Pressure

Use of the of the right internal jugular (IJ) vein is recommended, as cannulation of the left internal jugular (IJ) vein increases the risk of laceration of the left brachiocephalic vein. Relative contraindications to right IJ cannulation include carotid disease, recent cannulation (increases the risk of thrombosis), contralateral diaphragmatic dysfunction, thyromegaly, and prior major neck surgery. Central venous pressure (CVP) lines may be used for monitoring, to provide a central line for fluid and drugs, and in situations in which a PA catheter is not used.[30,31]

Pulmonary Artery Catheter

The PA catheter was historically used for all CABG procedures, but it is associated with complications and now has a more narrow range of uses (Box 22-3). It is indicated for use in high-risk patients with an EF of less than 40%.[31] It is a flexible catheter constructed with a balloon at the tip that, when inflated, facilitates flotation to the PA (Table 22-4).

Inflation of the positioned balloon occludes the PA pressure and reflects left chamber pressures of the heart. This catheter also allows simultaneous monitoring of central venous pressure and pulmonary arterial blood temperature. The thermistor on the PA catheter allows calculation of derived parameters such

BOX 22-3

Complications of Pulmonary Artery Catheters

- Tachyarrhythmias
- Right bundle branch block
- Complete heart block
- Cardiac perforation
- Pulmonary infarction and prolonged wedge times
- Pulmonary artery rupture
- Endocarditis
- Knotting of catheter
- Pulmonic valve insufficiency

TABLE 22-4 Pulmonary Artery Catheter Insertion Sites

Location	Distance to Vena Cava-Right Atrium Junction (cm)
Internal jugular vein	15-20
Superior vena cava	10-15
Femoral vein	30
Right antecubital fossa	40
Left antecubital fossa	50

Modified from Headley JM. Invasive Hemodynamic Monitoring: Physiological Principles and Clinical Applications. *Irvine, Calif: Baxter Healthcare; 1989.*

as CO via the thermodilution method, SVR, CI, and stroke volume (SV). This hemodynamic tool is used to monitor demand factors such as preload, afterload, heart rate, and contractility.

During systole with the balloon deflated the catheter transduces right ventricular systolic pressure. During diastole with the balloon deflated the catheter transduces PA diastolic pressure, which also represents left atrial pressure. During ventricular diastole with the balloon inflated the pulmonary catheter is said to be *wedged* and reflects left ventricular filling pressure. During ventricular systole with the balloon wedged the catheter reflects left atrial filling pressure.[32] Types of PA catheters include the venous infusion port (with a third port for administration of intravenous [IV] solutions), pacing PA catheter, mixed venous saturation catheters, EF catheters, and PA catheters capable of measuring continuous CO, which is valuable during off-pump cardiac procedures.

Transesophageal Echocardiography

Transesophageal echocardiography (TEE) allows continuous monitoring of the chambers of the heart, ascending and descending aorta, valvular function, chamber filling, and wall contractility and motion. Detection of gaseous or particulate emboli, identification of intracardiac shunting, diagnosis of aortic dissection, evaluation of saphenous vein graft flow, and confirmation of left ventricular dimension (filling) during weaning are other potential applications for this monitoring method. TEE may predict or suggest myocardial ischemia as defined by regional wall motion abnormalities, valve replacement procedures, cardiac aneurysms, intracardiac tumors, aortic dissection, and repair of complex congenital lesions.[33]

Relative contraindications to the use of TEE include dysphagia, mediastinal radiation, upper GI surgery or bleeding, esophageal stricture, tumor, varices, and recent chest trauma. In conjunction with the increased use of TEE, certain complications have been reported to occur during open-heart surgery. Cardiac arrhythmias, bronchospasm, and esophageal laceration are rare. Guidelines for the indications and use of TEE have been established. The Society of Cardiovascular Anesthesiologists has published guidelines for the perioperative use of TEE.[34]

Monitoring of Core Temperature

Accurate monitoring of core temperature is essential in order to control target hypothermia as well as to reestablish normothermia. The most accurate indicator of core temperature is at the thermistor of the PA catheter. Brain temperature is reflected in nasopharyngeal measurement, but a lag time occurs on rewarming. The probe should be inserted before heparinization to a depth of 7 to 10 cm through the nares. Tympanic temperature may also lag behind brain rewarmed temperature and is no better for monitoring of this parameter. Bladder or rectal temperature measurement is today considered inaccurate when renal and splanchnic blood flow is decreased.[26] Brain temperature should not drop below 20° C, as profound hypothermia (15° to 20° C) appears to cause a loss of cerebral autoregulation.[8]

Cerebral Monitoring

In addition to the monitoring of brain temperature, electrophysiologic monitoring is often employed. EEG is not an effective method for monitoring subtle changes, but any asymmetric EEG activity is considered a problem. Bispectral analysis (BIS) monitoring *may* correlate with the depth of anesthesia; it is actually a derived parameter to assess the degree of wakefulness. BIS does not measure brain function or the adequacy of oxygenation of the brain.[35,36]

Evoked potentials are another electrophysiologic monitor, but some anesthetics interfere with somatosensory evoked potentials and motor evoked potentials. Transcranial Doppler blood flow monitoring is not accurate because of artifact noise. Cerebral perfusion pressure can be determined by CVP because this parameter reflects intracranial pressure.

Monitoring of glucose is important in cerebral preservation because hyperglycemia increases the extent and degree of any ischemia that may occur. Glucose is considered an independent risk factor for aggravation of ischemia. Hyperglycemia prevents the increase of adenosine, which is responsible for cerebrovasodilatation, thereby preventing the brain from protecting itself from ischemic damage.[37]

PERFUSION PRINCIPLES

The goal of CPB is to provide a motionless heart in a bloodless field while the vital organs continue to be adequately oxygenated. The CPB pump provides respiration (oxygenation and elimination of CO_2), circulation (maintenance of perfusion pressure), and regulation of temperature (hypothermia to preserve myocardium). Initiation of CPB subjects the circulating blood of the patient to significant physiologic and physical changes. Anesthetic and perfusion management must address the impact of low flow indices, reduced metabolic requirements, changing viscosity of the patient's circulating volume, and postoperative inflammatory response. Multiple factors interact to create a substantially new environment for physiologic homeostasis. Hemodynamic abnormalities that occur during CPB include endothelial dysfunction ("total body systemic inflammatory response"), which causes symptoms similar to those in patients with sepsis or trauma.[38,39] Other abnormalities include persistent heparin effect, platelet dysfunction or loss, coagulopathy, fibrinolysis, and hypothermia.

Rapid recirculation of the total blood volume during CPB subjects blood and tissue components to a foreign environment that invites cellular trauma. The patient experiences tremendous alterations in core temperature, hematocrit (in the form of hemodilution), the coagulation cascade, and perfusion pressures (nonpulsatile perfusion). Clinical and experimental evidence indicates that CPB significantly alters the plasma and cellular constituents of blood, affecting both platelet count and function. As a result of excessive hemodilution, the platelet count decreases rapidly to 50% of the preoperative level but usually remains above 100,000 per microliter. Bleeding time is greatly prolonged, and platelet aggregation and function are impaired. Reductions occur in the plasma concentrations of coagulation factors II, V, VII, IX, X, and XII and are attributed to hemodilution.[40]

Extracorporeal Circuit

The CPB (pump) circuit consists of separate disposable components bioengineered to interface with perfusion pumps, fluid-based thermoregulating systems, air-oxygen blenders, anesthetic vaporizers, pressure transducers, temperature monitors, and in-line oxygen and blood-gas analyzers. The pump components include venous cannulas from the right atrium or vena cava, which are usually fenestrated at the tip and reinforced. Venous tubing includes the venous return for the blood drained to the machine from the left ventricle. The venous drainage to the venous reservoir depends on gravity, patient intravascular volume, and the position of and resistance from the venous cannula. The table height can affect venous drainage to the pump. Drainage collects in the venous reservoir, where air bubbles are removed and drainage from other reservoirs is mixed together. If a low volume is allowed here, air can be entrained into the arterial circulation.[41] Blood suctioned from the heart, pericardium, and pleural spaces drains to the cardiotomy reservoir.

The pump's oxygenator can be of the bubble type or the membrane type. Bubble-type oxygenators are implicated in gas embolisms because of incomplete removal of bubbles. Membrane oxygenators made of artificial polypropylene remove CO_2 independently of oxygenation. Membrane oxygenators have a higher resistance to flow and are placed after the pump. A heat exchanger cools or rewarms blood and is located in the venous reservoir or oxygenator.[40] An arterial cannula returns oxygenated blood from the pump to the patient. Blood pressure is usually reduced at the time of arterial cannulation so that blood does not spray from this high-pressure site.

The CPB circuit pushes blood forward and returns blood under pressure to the patient by means of either rollers (most common) or a centrifugal (vortex) pump. The roller-type pump can deliver blood to the body at a constant rate or in a pulsatile fashion. The centrifugal pump is affected by pressure downstream and will stop if air is present in the pump (Figure 22-2).

Various safety mechanisms are included to alert the operator of low venous operating reserve, high arterial line pressures, disconnection from air supply, and introduction of air embolus into the arterial line. As an extension of the extracorporeal circuit, the cardioplegia delivery system provides and maintains hypothermic and pharmacologic arrest of the heart during revascularization. Ultrafiltration and red blood cell–sequestering devices may be incorporated into the circuit to counteract hemodilution by removing excess volume through dialysis or centrifugal separation of fluid and plasma components from the circulating blood volume.

Prime

A significant factor is the amount of crystalloid solution required to prime the tubing, reservoir, filters, and oxygenator. Establishment of an air-free circuit is essential for unimpaired fluid volume transport and prevention of air embolism. Most circuits require at least 2000 ml of a solution such as Normosol, Plasmalyte A, or Isolyte S, with pH and electrolytes closely matching the composition of whole blood. Added to this base solution are heparin, sodium bicarbonate, mannitol, hetastarch, albumin, and possibly corticosteroids or antihyperfibrinolytic agents. This addition can result in priming volumes in excess of 2000 ml, which, when transfused to the patient at the onset of CPB, can cause a hemodilutional bolus of 30% to 50% of the patient's circulating blood volume (see Table 22-3).

Vascular Transport

The heart and lungs are isolated and bypassed from systemic blood flow. This function is accomplished by right atrial or vena caval cannulation with subsequent diversion of venous blood that is returning to the heart. The venoatrial cannulas are connected to polyvinyl chloride tubing that extends from the surgical field to the venous reservoir situated at a level well below the patient's heart to facilitate gravity exsanguination. Blood from the reservoir is propelled by roller or centrifugal pump to the oxygenator, where it becomes arterialized by interfacing with a membrane oxygenator. A heat exchanger mounted on the oxygenator provides for control of blood temperature. Oxygenated blood passes through an arterial filter and an in-line arterial gas monitoring device.

Aortic cannula placement is distal to the sinus of Valsalva and proximal to the brachiocephalic (innominate) artery. The arterial line pressure of the extracorporeal circulation (ECC) depends on flow and resistance but usually is maintained below 300 mm Hg.[41]

Myocardial Protection Techniques

Injury to the myocardium is a complex occurrence and may result from numerous physiologic events. Tachycardia, hypertension or hypotension, and ventricular distention can all play a role in the events that produce an oxygen supply-demand imbalance. Contractile function deteriorates rapidly after the initial insult of ischemia. Rapid cardioplegia-induced cardiac arrest, decompression of the ventricles, and hypothermia are the underlying techniques used to ensure myocardial protection during CPB. The duration of aortic cross-clamping time, collateral coronary blood supply, frequency of cardioplegia delivery, and composition of cardioplegia are factors that influence the extent of reperfusion injury.[42] Intermittent doses of cold crystalloid cardioplegia help to maintain cardiac arrest, hypothermia, and pH, counteract edema, wash out metabolite, and provide oxygen and substrate for aerobic metabolism.

Cardioplegia

Cardioplegia is a potassium solution administered into the coronary circulation to provide diastolic arrest. It is composed of potassium (15 to 30 mEq/L), calcium to prevent ischemic contracture (stone heart), albumin or mannitol for osmolarity correction, and glucose or simple amino acids as a metabolic substrate. The cardioplegia delivers oxygen and nutrients, removes waste products, and cools or rewarms the heart. It is administered in an antegrade manner into the aortic root, from which it distributes to the coronaries and into the myocardium. It may also be administered in a retrograde fashion into the coronary sinus, from which it distributes through veins, venules, and capillaries of the myocardium.

The cardioplegia composition is blood or crystalloid based. Blood-based cardioplegia is oxygenated blood that is diluted with fluid at a 4:1 ratio. It has a hematocrit of 16% to 18% and is given at 4° to 14° C. Crystalloid-based solutions do not contain hemoglobin; therefore they deliver dissolved O_2 only. Because of this, crystalloid solutions can be used only with myocardial hypothermic techniques. Intracellular cardioplegia

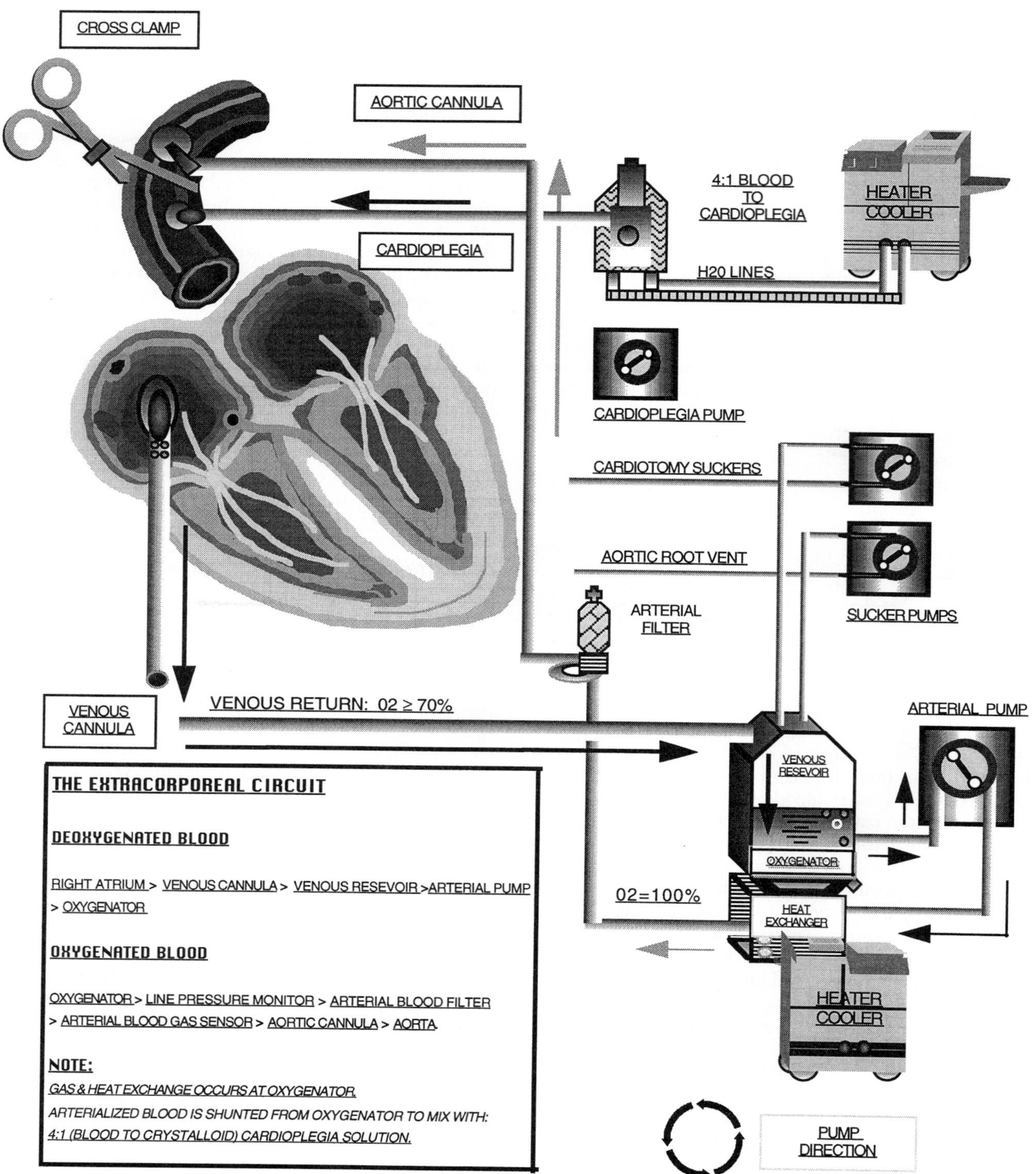

FIGURE **22-2**
The extracorporeal circuit and anatomic cannulation sites. The average amount of crystalloid required to prime this circuit is 2000 ml. Heparin, mannitol, $NaHCO_3^-$, albumin, corticosteroids, and antifibrinolytics such as aminocaproic acid are also added, depending on institutional preferences. Most circuits incorporate in-line arterial and venous blood-gas monitoring, line pressure manometers, anesthetic vaporizers, temperature monitoring systems, and numerous safety devices with computerized override mechanisms to be used in the event of mechanical failure or operator error.

has a low sodium content to produce loss of membrane potential by eliminating the sodium gradient across the membrane. Extracellular solutions produce diastolic arrest by depolarization of the membrane with high potassium concentrations.[43]

COAGULATION

Coagulation Cascade

Intrinsic Pathway

The coagulation cascade is initiated when blood becomes traumatized by exposure to a foreign surface (Figure 22-3). In the initiation of CPB, contact with the polyvinylchloride tubing used in the extracorporeal circuit, the squeezing mechanism of the roller head pump, and various filtering devices can cause lysis of the blood cells. This leads to activation of factor XII (Hageman factor), also known as the *contact factor*.[44]

Activated factor XII is a proteolytic enzyme that stimulates the production of factor XI. This reaction is mediated by high–molecular-weight kininogen and is accelerated by prekallikrein. Platelets are damaged because of adherence to collagen or secondarily to damage associated with the extracorporeal circulation. Platelet disruption mediates the release of platelet phospholipids containing platelet factor III, which is a lipoprotein that plays a role in subsequent clotting reactions.

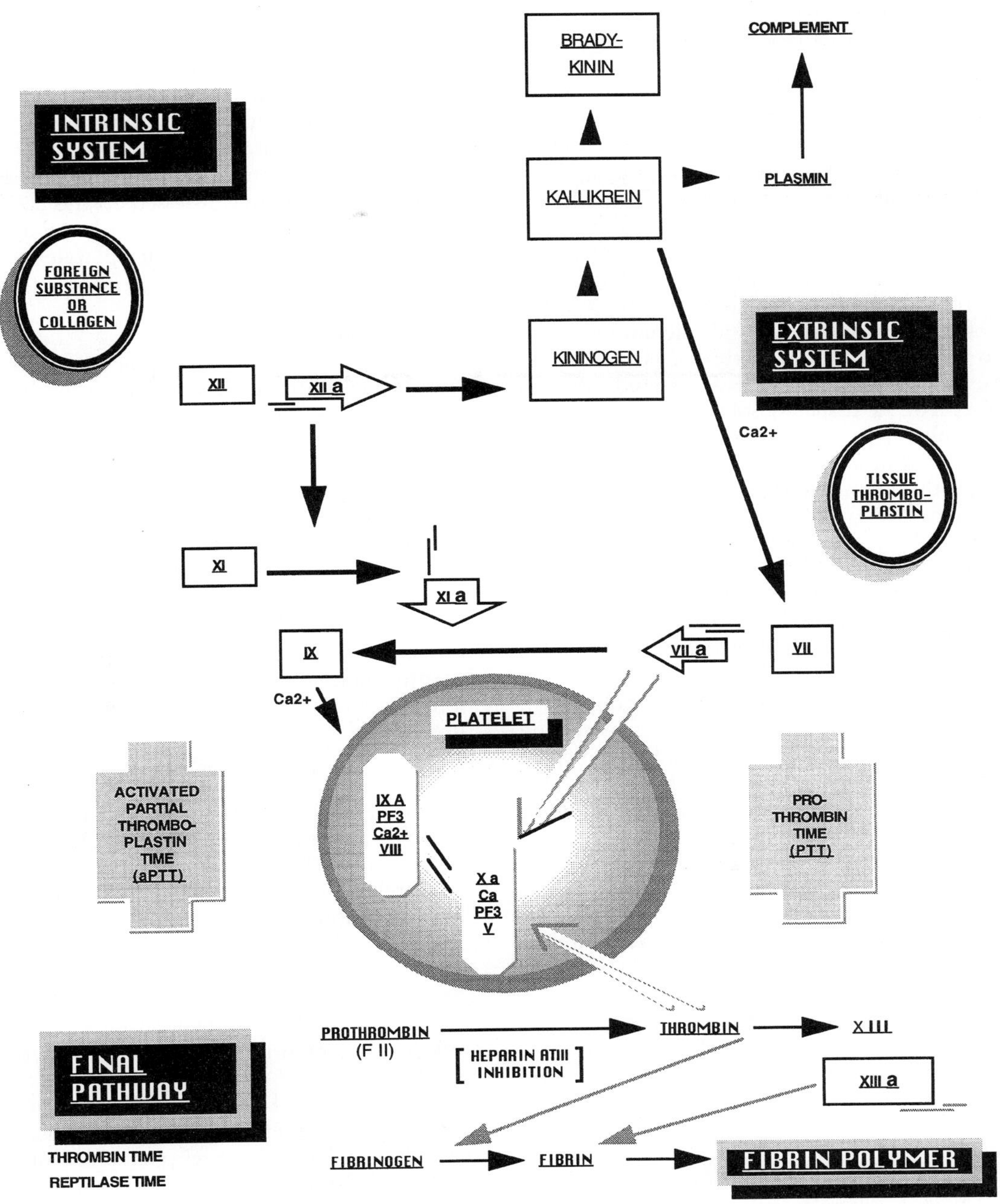

FIGURE **22-3**
Coagulation cascade. The coagulation cascade illustrated here provides an explanation of the interplay of each component. Absence or dysfunction of any of these factors precipitates a bleeding problem.

Activated factor XI, factor VIII, and platelet factor III interact to activate factor X, which initiates the common pathway for both intrinsic and extrinsic coagulation mechanisms. An acute deficiency in either factor VII (hemophilia) or platelets (thrombocytopenia) results in a clotting deficiency.

Activated factor X combines with factor V and platelet or tissue phospholipids to form a complex called *prothrombin activator*, which cleaves prothrombin to form thrombin. This process and subsequent processes are mediated by the presence of calcium ions. Thrombin facilitates the conversion of fibrinogen to a fibrin monomer that polymerizes into long fibrin threads to form the reticulum of the clot. Clot is composed of a meshwork of fibrin threads extending in all directions, entrapping blood cells, platelets, and plasma. The fibrin threads adhere to damaged surfaces of blood vessels (or a foreign surface) and prevent further blood loss.[44]

Extrinsic Pathway

The extrinsic mechanism for coagulation is activated when blood comes into contact with traumatized vascular wall or extravascular tissues. Traumatized tissue releases a complex of factors called *tissue thromboplastin* (see Figure 22-3). Of particular interest are the phospholipids (derived from tissue membranes) and a lipoprotein complex containing a glycoprotein that functions as a proteolytic enzyme. This lipoprotein complex of tissue thromboplastin interacts with factor VII and, in the presence of tissue phospholipids and calcium ions, converts factor X to its activated form. Activated factor X complexes with either the tissue phospholipids released from the tissue thromboplastin or the tissue phospholipids released from platelets and, in combination with factor V, forms a new complex called *prothrombin activator*. Within seconds, prothrombin activator splits prothrombin to form thrombin, and the clotting process begins.[44]

Common Pathway

The endpoint of activity for both the extrinsic and intrinsic coagulation pathways is the activation of factor X. Reactions beyond this point are common to both pathways and involve the combining of activated factor X with procoagulants (factor II, factor V, calcium ions, and platelet phospholipids) to form a prothrombinase complex. This complex catalyzes the conversion of circulating prothrombin to thrombin, which in turn converts circulating fibrinogen to insoluble fibrin. The coagulation process is terminated by the stabilization of fibrin via the activation of factor XIII.[45]

Blood Components

Fibrinogen

Fibrinogen is a high–molecular-weight protein present in the plasma in quantities of 100 to 700 mg/dL. In the presence of calcium ions it becomes the precursor for fibrin threads, the foundation of the blood clot. For replacement therapy a target value of 150 mg/dL may be achieved with the administration of blood products such as cryoprecipitate or fresh-frozen plasma (FFP).[46,47]

Fresh-Frozen Plasma

FFP contains the same concentrations of plasma proteins present in the donor's plasma. Therefore fibrinogen and all other factors are not concentrated. When some deficiency of a factor is present, a considerable amount of FFP is required to raise levels back to normal. Fibrinogen is accepted as the protein most critical in the coagulation cascade. Considering the fact that each unit of FFP is approximately 250 ml and that the patient's circulating blood volume averages 5000 ml or greater, the FFP usually is diluted in the patient's own plasma and has little effect in raising overall plasma fibrinogen concentrations.[48,49]

Platelets

The normal platelet concentration in blood is 150,000 to 300,000 platelets per microliter. Changes in platelet count and function can be associated with CPB. The circulating platelet count declines to approximately 50% of prebypass levels, partially as a result of hemodilution, adhesion to the surface of the oxygenator and bypass circuit, sequestration to the spleen, and platelet aggregation.[44] Platelet count rarely drops below 100,000 per microliter, but this decrease in count does explain the bleeding abnormalities found after CPB. Platelet dysfunction may occur because of hypothermia, trauma-induced activation, fibrinolysis, or drug-related causes. Heparin, nitrates, phosphodiesterase inhibitors, and protamine can all affect platelet function. Platelet function cannot be appropriately assessed on the basis of count alone. The properties required for adhesion and aggregation may be diminished or nonexistent in platelets that have been subjected to ECC.

Anticoagulation

Initiation of CPB requires systemic heparinization to establish a safe level of anticoagulation. The currently accepted regimen is 300 units of heparin per kilogram of patient weight. The heparin dose is usually calculated to maintain an ACT of 400 seconds (the normal range is 130 seconds or less). Heparin is a catalyst and binds with circulating antithrombin (AT III) and potentiates its natural anticoagulant properties (see Figure 22-3). Heparin is administered intravenously through the central venous port. Its peak effect occurs within 2 minutes, and verification is based on the ACT, which should be established 5 to 10 minutes after administration. Special circumstances such as long-term heparinization, antithrombin III deficiency, heparin-induced thrombocytopenia, and excessive hemodilution may cause "heparin resistance," which alters the algorithm for calculating the loading dose. The surgeon, anesthesia provider, and perfusion teams should consider these circumstances.

Management of a patient with heparin-associated thrombocytopenia and thrombosis (HATT or HIT) presents a particular challenge. HIT is evident after exposure to heparin because the platelet count suddenly falls. The onset can be as soon as 2 days or as long as 5 days after institution of heparin therapy. Surgery should be postponed if at all possible, and heparin must be eliminated from the patient's medication regimen until the platelets are normal and do not aggregate in response to heparin. A polysulfated glycosaminoglycan (danaparoid) as well as a thrombin inhibitor (hirudin) have been used safely for CPB.[44]

Heparin should be a part of the resuscitation protocol for cardiac surgery patients. If the patient undergoes cardiac arrest during the induction or prebypass phase of the case, heparin can be given and the patient placed on bypass as a resuscitative measure.

Anticoagulation is imperative for CPB used during cardiac surgery. It is imperative in all patients that the ACT is at least 350 before CPB is performed.

Coagulation Tests

Treatment for coagulopathy depends on the cause. A review of tests for assessing functions of coagulation are included as a guide to management.

Activated Clotting Time

ACT is a standardized measurement of the patient's procoagulation or anticoagulation level. The unit of measurement is the time (in seconds) required for an ACT counter to detect the formation of blood clot in a 2- to 3-ml sample of whole blood. Normal ACT levels range from 100 to 130 seconds. Because this test is a crude measure of clotting, CPB requires anticoagulation levels of 400 seconds or more. Patients may show significant variability in the reaction as a result of different rates of metabolism of heparin. Hypothermia and hemodilution are factors associated with CPB that directly affect the ACT. Hypothermia has the most profound effect in terms of prolonging intraoperative values.[43]

Whole Blood Heparin Concentration

The whole blood heparin concentration method of assessing anticoagulation is usually followed by use of an automated protamine titration (Medtronic HemoTec). However, the amount of heparin necessary for this technique is increased, and any benefit may be at the expense of greater platelet activation, which could confound platelet dysfunction after CPB.[44]

Other Anticoagulation Monitors

Because ACT and heparin concentration testing is less than perfect, other tests are being investigated. aPTT and thrombin time are too sensitive to be useful in CPB monitoring.

Thromboelastogram

The thromboelastogram assesses clot function from the time of initial activation, to clot formation, through the acceleration phase, clot strengthening phase, and retraction phase, until eventual lysis. It examines the entire life cycle of a clot in a rather gross manner and does not isolate the subsegments of procoagulant precursors and their individual contributions to clot dynamics. It is capable of indicating abnormalities in formation and lysis of clots. Its primary function is to examine clot strength. This coagulation test is finding utility in the diagnosis of fibrinolysis for liver transplants.[44]

PROPHYLAXIS AND TREATMENT OF COAGULOPATHY

Antifibrinolytics

Patients for CABG procedures on CPB receive an antifibrinolytic. First-time patients are treated with aminocaproic acid. Patients undergoing subsequent surgeries, those with renal failure, those at high risk of bleeding, and Jehovah's Witnesses are treated with aprotinin.

ε-Aminocaproic Acid and Tranexamic Acid

Aminocaproic acid (Amicar) was initially proposed for the treatment of fibrinolysis associated with prostate and cardiac surgery. Tranexamic acid is considered to be more potent than aminocaproic acid. Antifibrinolytics are hemostatic agents given as an IV loading dose and then by continuous infusion before CPB. The loading dose of aminocaproic acid is 100 to 150 mg/kg, followed by an infusion dose of 10 to 15 mg/kg/hr. The dose of tranexamic acid is 10 to 15 mg/kg loading with an infusion of 1 to 1.5 mg/kg/hr. The drug has renal excretion and a plasma half-life of approximately 80 minutes. These drugs have proven effective in reducing bleeding after bypass.[44]

Aprotinin

Aprotinin (Trasylol) is a serine inhibitor extracted from the bovine lung and has demonstrated efficacy in reducing blood loss in cardiac surgery.[50] A loading dose of aprotinin must be preceded by a test dose of 1 ml (1.4 mg), followed by 20 ml over 20 minutes starting before the skin incision. The remainder of the dose is administered at 0.5 million units/hr, which should run the duration of the CPB. Aprotinin inhibits the intrinsic pathway of coagulation and causes an increased minimal acceptable celite ACT to be 750 seconds. A kaolin ACT demonstrates resistance to interference, and normal parameters are used. Anaphylactoid reactions are a risk associated with reexposure within 6 months. Administration of aprotinin is delayed until the surgical team is ready for immediate conversion to CPB.

Desmopressin

Desmopressin acetate (DDAVP) is a synthetic analog of vasopressin, which releases a variety of hemostatically active substances from the vascular endothelium. It is administered in doses of 0.3 mcg/kg intravenously, intranasally, or subcutaneously. It has a half-life of 55 minutes (with clinical effects lasting from 5 to 6 hours) and results in an approximately fourfold increase in circulating levels of factor VIII, prostacycline, tissue plasminogen activator, and von Willebrand factor. The overall effect of desmopressin is hemostatic. DDAVP has also been used to treat uremia, cirrhosis, platelet disorders, and mild or moderate cases of hemophilia A (von Willebrand's disease). Current evidence does not support the broad administration of DDAVP to cardiac surgical patients as prophylaxis for bleeding.[44]

PHARMACOLOGIC APPROACHES TO BLOOD PRESSURE CONTROL

Blood pressure control during the perioperative phase may be accomplished with the use of pharmacologic agents independently or in combination. Vasodilators such as hydralazine, nitroglycerine, and nitroprusside are useful for control of blood pressure and improving peripheral blood flow.

α-Adrenergic agonists (like clonidine) reduce stress-mediated neurohumoral responses to induction and CPB. They decrease heart rate and blood pressure and have sedative and antinociceptive characteristics, which may reduce opioid requirements without respiratory depression. They can be used independently or in conjunction with IV induction agents and opioids; they help to reduce the amount of agent required.

Careful use of β-blockers can decrease heart rate, contractility, and blood pressure, which works to reduce oxygen use. These drugs increase the duration of diastole to allow for a more complete oxygenation of the left ventricle. They act synergistically with nitroglycerin and blunt tachycardia and decrease ischemia of the myocardium. They have the ability to reduce catecholamine-induced ventricular arrhythmias. The disadvantage associated with β-blockers is that they may precipitate bradyarrhythmias, heart block, or bronchospasm. β-blockers available in IV form for use during cardiac surgery include esmolol, labetalol, metoprolol, and propranolol. Reversal of the effects of β-blockers can be achieved through use of β-agonists (isoproterenol) and cardiac pacing (unless emergent CPB initiation is possible).

Vasodilator therapy includes direct vasodilators (hydralazine, nitroglycerin, or nitroprusside), α-adrenergic blockers (labetalol, phentolamine), angiotensin-converting enzyme (ACE) inhibitors (enalaprilat IV), central α-agonists clonodine, or calcium channel blockers (nicardipine IV, verapamil, or diltiazem). Disadvantages include slow onset of action or long duration of action, reflex tachycardias, and toxicity reactions. The drug therapy is to be selected individually for each patient and situation and administered judiciously for the desired effect.

Vasopressor therapy includes agents with selective direct effects (methoxamine, phenylephrine), α_1-agonist mixed agents (dopamine, ephedrine, epinephrine, noradrenaline), or vasopressin (direct peripheral vasoconstriction with no β-adrenergic effects).[51,52] Other drugs that work indirectly to increase blood pressure include the positive inotropic drugs (e.g., dobutamine, dopamine, amrinone, and milrinone).[52] Calcium reverses hypotension associated with the use of halogenated agents, calcium-channel blockers, hypocalcemia, β-blockers, and CPB. When administered intravenously by central line, it can increase blood pressure as well as reverse the cardiac effects of toxicity resulting from hyperkalemia.[53]

PREOPERATIVE PERIOD

Considerations during the preoperative period include sedation and monitoring of the patient while placement of appropriate invasive monitoring lines ensues. All equipment should be available and invasive lines inserted before the patient is brought to the operating room. Invasive monitors are useful during induction and should be placed before induction except in emergency situations like ruptured aneurysms, cardiac tamponade, or ventricle rupture.

Premedication should provide anxiolysis and amnesia as well as some degree of pain relief for the insertion of invasive lines. Midazolam (0.05 to 0.1 mg/kg) IV titrated or lorazepam (15 to 20 mcg/kg) titrated with morphine, fentanyl (10- to 20-mcg increments IV) or sufentanil (5- to 10-mcg increments) titrated until effective work well in compensated patients. For patients who are poorly compensated a titrated low dose of lorazepam or midazolam is sufficient.[54] Oxygen should be administered to these medicated patients during line placement and until preoxygenation for induction ensues.

Extensive preparation and setup is required for heart surgery. Each institution has specific setup guidelines with regard to medication and equipment needs. It is advisable that patients be intubated with an endotracheal tube that is as large as possible, because they may remain intubated and mechanically ventilated for several hours after surgery in some situations.

Induction

Hemodynamic alterations occur at induction of anesthesia. The induction plan should take into consideration left ventricular function.[54] No single technique has been demonstrated as superior with regard to the prevention of postoperative MI by intraoperative ischemia. It is important to control heart rate because this parameter is most likely to produce myocardial ischemia.[54] Prevention of myocardial ischemia is a primary concern. Two factors associated with myocardial ischemia include inadequate oxygen supply to the myocardium from localized coronary lesions and excessive oxygen demand because of the increased hemodynamic workload associated with increased heart rate and blood pressure or adrenergic stimulation. On induction, myocardial ischemia can be detected through the electrocardiogram (ECG), TEE, or PA wedge pressure readings.

TABLE 22-5 Common Opioid Doses for Maintenance during Cardiopulmonary Bypass

	Loading Dose	Infusion Rate	Additional Bolus
Sufentanil	0.5-2 mcg/kg	0.5-1.5 mcg/kg/hr	2.5-10 mcg
Fentanyl	4-20 mcg/kg	2-10 mcg/kg/hr	25-100 mcg
Remifentanil	1-2 mcg/kg	0.1-1 mcg/kg/min	0.1-1 mcg/kg

Methods for diminishing the incidence of ischemia include therapeutic interventions such as preoxygenation before induction, reduction of wall tension with nitroglycerin, control of heart rate with β-adrenergic blocking agents, reduction of the work of the myocardium through control of myocardial depression with increased anesthetic levels, and maintenance of coronary perfusion pressure through the use of a nonchronotropic agent such as phenylephrine. Many cardiac patients have low circulating blood volume because of hypertensive vasoconstriction. A reduced plasma volume may necessitate fluid loading or prophylactic treatment with pressors such as phenylephrine before induction. Hypovolemia should be anticipated and can be monitored by observation of blood pressure alterations and CVP.

High or low CO has a significant effect on the pharmacokinetics of anesthetic agents. The anesthetic ideally should not interfere with heart rate or metabolic demand for oxygen. Patients with disease of the left main coronary artery are more susceptible to insult during induction. Hemodynamic changes in these patients precipitate extension of already present ischemic effects. A slow, methodic, balanced technique with combinations of midazolam, fentanyl or sufentanil, etomidate, thiopental, or propofol and a nondepolarizing muscle relaxant reduces hemodynamic changes and meets the goals of diminishing workload on the myocardium. Typical opioid maintenance doses are shown in Table 22-5.

INTRAOPERATIVE PERIOD

Incision to Bypass

After induction the skin incision and sternal split constitute two very stimulating steps in the process of preparation for CPB. A patient in whom anesthesia is adequate will show minimal response to these steps, thereby reducing the need for additional adjuncts. A continuous opioid infusion with "background" volatile agent or continuous infusion of propofol may help to maintain blood pressure and ensure amnesia as well as provide a smooth transition toward CPB. The list of adjuncts that are available for immediate use are listed in Table 22-6.

During sternotomy, for approximately 15 to 20 seconds, the lungs must be deflated to prevent laceration or puncture. In most cases the left internal mammary artery is dissected and mobilized for anastomosis to the left anterior descending artery. This requires placement of an internal mammary artery retractor on the left side of the operating table. When there is a left radial arterial line, careful attention to positioning of the wrist ensures that the arterial waveform is not damped. When only saphenous vein grafts are to be harvested, the pace of the

TABLE 22-6 Sample Adjunct Drugs for Cardiac Procedures

Type of Drug	Drug Name	Method of Administration
Prepared		
Vasopressor	Phenylephrine	Titrate 50-100 mcg
Vasodilator	Nitroglycerin or Nitroprusside	Titrate as infusion or bolus; Titrate as infusion
Available		
β-blocker	Esmolol	Titrate as bolus or infusion
Inotrope	Milrinone, amrinone, epinephrine, dopamine, dobutamine	Titrate as infusion; usually facility or surgeon specific
Calcium chloride		Infusion or bolus
Vagolytic (anticholinergic)	Atropine	Bolus
Antiarrhythmic	Lidocaine, adenosine, diltiazem or verapamil, procainamide, amiodarone, magnesium	Titrate

operation may increase significantly, and cannulation of the aorta and right atrium may occur earlier.

Once the internal mammary and saphenous grafts are mobilized or harvested, the patient requires heparinization before cannulation of the aorta and right atrium. Bolus administration of heparin is administered in a central line and *may* decrease arterial pressure 10% to 20%. Anticoagulation is measured with ACT approximately 3 to 5 minutes after heparin administration. The ACT should be approximately 400 seconds before it is safe to institute CPB.

Aortic cannulation is associated with a hypertensive response, probably because of direct stimulation of sympathetic nerves in the aortic arch. Reduction of MAP assists aortic cannulation and prevents laceration of the aorta. As a result of manipulation of the heart during cannula placement, venous cannulation (right atrium) may lead to fluctuations in arterial pressure. Right atrial cannulation drains the superior and inferior venae cavae; ventricular tachyarrhythmias may occur, and CO and blood pressure may decrease. If additional cannulation of the coronary sinus for retrograde cardioplegia delivery is required, severe hypotension may ensue and necessitate administration of volume by the perfusionist via the aortic cannula. Once the patient has been placed on extracorporeal support and adequate perfusion flow and pressure have been achieved, most surgeons prefer to stop ventilation in order to deflate the lungs and optimize surgical conditions. Some surgeons prefer to continue ventilation until the myocardium is motionless. CPB should not commence unless all of the parameters for institution of bypass have been addressed by the anesthesia care provider (Box 22-4).

BOX 22-4

Checklist for "Going on Pump"

- Heparin administered
- ACT checked and at least 350-400
- Muscle relaxant adequate (or infusion turned on to maintain)
- Inotropic infusions turned off
- Pupil symmetry assessed for later comparison (unilateral dilation may indicate unilateral carotid perfusion on cardiopulmonary bypass)
- Pulmonary artery catheter (if used) pulled back 5 cm
- Urinary output emptied before bypass (start anew with initiation of bypass)
- Proper functioning of all monitors ensured

Initiation of Bypass

Multiple events occur simultaneously and can cause a significant drop in blood pressure at the initiation of CPB. Hemodilution decreases blood viscosity and dilutes catecholamines in the plasma, contributing to the drop in pressure. Rapid cooling of the patient occurs to a target temperature of 28° C. When the target temperature is reached or spontaneous hypothermic fibrillation of the heart occurs, the aorta is cross-clamped. At times the myocardial arrest may require retrograde administration of cardioplegia via the coronary sinus.

Cerebral and renal protection are important during CPB. Techniques of cerebral protection include metabolic suppression, which can be accomplished with hypothermia, burst suppression, use of calcium channel blockers to reduce the incidence of vasospasm, and decrease in intraoperative bleeding attained through use of aprotinin (or other antifibrinolytic). The perfusionist also plays a central role in providing cerebral protection. As core temperature is lowered, the pH rises, placing the patient in an alkalotic state. The alpha-stat system represents alkalotic management of cerebral perfusion, but pH-stat relies on hypercarbia to manage CBF. The essential difference is that alpha-stat management represents CBF that is not dependent on MAP and does not mandate the addition of exogenous CO_2 to maintain pH in the normal range.

Renal protection is best maintained by the preservation of renal blood flow and monitoring of urine production. Risk factors for renal dysfunction after CPB include prolonged bypass time (greater than 3 hours) and low CO. Osmotic diuretics, low-dose dopamine, and fenoldopam are used during CPB in patients at risk for development of acute renal failure. Prevention of renal insufficiency postoperatively includes control of hypertension, control of hyperglycemia, reduction of "pump" time, maintenance of fluids, and the use of medications that promote urinary output.[55] Urinary output is considered satisfactory if it measures 1 ml/kg/hr during CPB.

Bypass

During bypass, anesthesia is maintained with an opioid drip as described in Table 22-5 as well as the addition of volatile agent on the perfusion circuit. Controversy exists regarding an acceptable mean blood pressure (BP) range during CPB. Keep in mind that CBF is autoregulated, as is flow to other organs. Because of hypothermia the lower limit of autoregulation is further decreased. This fact, coupled with the presence of high perfusion pressures, can result in an increase in the possibility of emboli and bleeding on the surgical field; the use of 50 to 70 mm Hg is promoted as a practical norm in most facilities.[55-57]

ACT is checked every 20 to 30 minutes by the perfusionist and is maintained at greater than 400 seconds with the addition of heparin to the pump as necessary. Because of hemodilution the hematocrit frequently falls to approximately 20 g/dl, which is an acceptable level in most patients. Hypokalemia can be problematic, and the perfusionist checks electrolytes frequently during the pump run. Fluids are kept to a minimum during the bypass phase, and the perfusionist often makes adjustments. It is important to have open communications with the perfusionist, surgeon and anesthesia care provider during CPB so that coagulation, pressure maintenance, and adjustment of electrolyte imbalances are carefully regulated.

Weaning from Bypass

When a patient is weaned from CPB, considerations should include the ventricular function of the heart before bypass and the length of time the aorta was cross-clamped. If the ventricle was in good condition before bypass and the cross-clamp time was less than 60 minutes, the initiation of inotropes is probably not necessary. Otherwise, an inotrope should be chosen in consultation with the surgeon. Additional parameters that should be verified include patient temperature, heart rhythm, monitor status, and adequacy of perfusion. During weaning the perfusionist partially occludes the venous line to increase right atrial pressure, blood flows into the right ventricle and out through the PA, and pressures become pulsatile (Box 22-5).

The rate of rewarming must be limited to 1° C per 3 to 5 minutes to prevent formation of gaseous emboli in the circulatory system or the ECC. Rewarming begins slightly before removal of the aortic cross-clamp, when the last distal anastomosis begins in multiple graft procedures, or when the valve sutures have been placed during valve replacement procedures. The temperature gradient between arterial and venous blood should be maintained below 10° C, and the time frame for rewarming is usually 30 minutes.[58]

Many tasks are required at this time. Laboratory values including arterial blood gases, electrolytes, and hematocrit should be obtained. Patient ventilation is reinstituted. An infusion of calcium chloride (1 g/100 ml 5% dextrose in water [D_5W]) is administered via a central line. After most of the calcium chloride has been given, a small test dose of protamine, usually 10 mg, is administered to test for an unexpected reaction before infusion. If the patient remains stable, protamine administration is initiated slowly over approximately 20 minutes to avoid hypotension. Protamine is given in a calculated dose that is approximately a 1:1 ratio of the initial heparin dose (Box 22-6). When one third of the dose of protamine has been given, notify the perfusionist to stop collecting blood via suction from the operative field, as this would clot the pump. Small increments of phenylephrine may be administered to maintain blood pressure within desired ranges. The surgeon can restart bypass throughout the weaning process as necessary.

BOX 22-5

Checklist for Weaning from the Pump

- Patient is warm (at least 35° C).
- Heart rhythm has returned.
- All monitors are functioning; electrocardiogram, pulmonary artery tracing, arterial line tracing, central venous pressure reflect heart filling.
- Heart rate is 70-100 (<60 means reduced cardiac output; >120 is detrimental to left ventricular filling).
- Infusions are prepared as necessary.
- Inflate lungs (but keep them out of the surgeon's field).
- Pressures become pulsatile as ventricles fill.
- Draw blood for measurement of electrolytes, hematocrit, arterial blood gases, and activated clotting time.
- Surgeon clamps venous drain and removes cannula.
- Patient is off pump.

BOX 22-6

Protamine Reversal of Heparin

- 10 mg protamine reverses 1000 units heparin
- 10 mg protamine = 1 ml of protamine
- 1 ml of protamine reverses 30 ml heparin (an average initial dose)
- *Protamine reversal is 1:1 ratio with heparin dose.*

Communication is vital during the weaning process. The possibility always exists that the patient will have to be returned to bypass. Notify the surgeon when the protamine has been completely administered, and recheck the ACT. Recheck CO and pressures to establish postoperative baselines.

When bypass is completely discontinued, check ACT values and institute treatment if they are elevated. Bypass may have to be reinstituted if severe hypotension, excessive bleeding, or a persistently low CO is present. If the protamine is completely administered and a return to bypass is required, heparin (300 U/kg) may be readministered. At times an IABP may be required.

In anticipation of the increased metabolic uptake associated with this phase of the operation, administration of amnestic agents and muscle relaxants to maintain appropriate anesthetic levels should be instituted. When the aortic cross-clamp is removed, reperfusion to the myocardium allows the heart to rewarm and flushes residual cardioplegic solution and accumulated metabolic byproducts out of the coronary vessels. Hypotension should be anticipated. Plasma levels of atrial natriuretic factor have been shown to decrease with the onset of aortic cross-clamping and either decrease or increase significantly when the cross-clamp is removed. Studies have demonstrated that this factor increases glomerular filtration, inhibits renin release, reduces aldosterone concentrations, and antagonizes endogenous vasoconstrictors, resulting in a reduction in blood pressure.[59]

Sweating during the rewarming phase of CPB represents a normal thermoregulatory response that can be associated with cutaneous dilation that is caused by elevated skin temperatures. Anesthetic agents depress vasoconstriction and shivering while increasing the propensity for sweating. Postoperative shivering should be avoided to prevent increased oxygen demand and carbon dioxide production.

Protamine Administration

Protamine sulfate is the drug of choice for heparin reversal. It inactivates heparin by binding with it to form an inert salt. At the conclusion of CPB the residual amount of heparin is assessed and appropriately neutralized. Protamine is initiated after a test dose of 1 mg in 100 ml over 10 minutes before heparinization. It binds and inhibits the anticoagulation effects to circulating heparin. Adverse cardiopulmonary responses to protamine have been observed. Suggested risk factors include valvular heart disease (mitral), preexisting pulmonary hypertension, infusion rates greater than 5 mg/min, diabetes with prior exposure to NPH insulin, and vasectomy. Adverse reactions to protamine include histamine-releasing reactions, true anaphylaxis mediated by a specific antiprotamine antibody, or reactions in which release of thromboxane leads to pulmonary vasoconstriction or bronchoconstriction. In the presence of increased risk factors, heparinase I may be given.[60] In a small study by Heres and colleagues, heparinase I was found to result in no adverse hemodynamic changes when given to patients after heparinization for CPB in coronary artery surgery.[25]

Separation from Cardiopulmonary Bypass

Preexisting ventricular dysfunction or myocardial insult associated with CPB complicates the process of weaning the patient from extracorporeal support. Separation from bypass presents a tremendous challenge in providing appropriate pharmacologic and mechanical support sufficient for the recovery of ventricular function. The major pharmacologic interventions include the use of both inotropic and vasodilator treatment of systolic or diastolic dysfunction.

Regardless of the therapeutic technique employed, the focus on basic hemodynamic and physiologic goals should be maintained when one selects an anesthetic regimen for termination of bypass. Tachycardia and arrhythmias must be prevented, arterial blood pressure maintained, and myocardial contractility promoted, while constraints on oxygen demand are maintained. The ideal regimen for pharmacologic therapy includes drugs that have rapid onset and termination, have a neutralizing effect on ischemia, and are nontoxic to the myocardium.

A primary therapeutic consideration for patients not previously in atrial fibrillation is to establish an atrioventricular sequence. Altered ventricular compliance necessitates optimal loading conditions for nondynamic ventricles. Patients who are dependent on atrial kick for ventricular filling experience a serious compromise in CO in the presence of atrial fibrillation or supraventricular tachycardia. Impaired diastolic function may be managed by treating hypertension and decreasing ventricular load with vasodilator therapy. Nitric oxide–based drugs (nitroglycerin, sodium nitroprusside) are commonly used agents that promote vasodilation, counteract the vasoconstrictive effects of circulating catecholamines, and reduce ventricular distention by relieving myocardial wall tension. The aim of administration of vasodilators is treatment of specific hemodynamic conditions such as increased arterial blood pressure, left atrial pressure, pulmonary capillary wedge pressure, and rising central venous pressure. The intent is to optimize ventricular loading conditions and, in combination with inotropic support, provide adequate CO while minimizing demand on the revascularized myocardium.

Catecholamines have variable effects on heart rate, rhythm, and metabolism. Amrinone, milrinone, epinephrine, norepinephrine, dobutamine, dopamine, and isoproterenol are selected based on targeted functions. Dopamine increases pulmonary vascular resistance, PA pressure, and left ventricular filling pressures; however, chronic heart failure can lead to a depletion of neurotransmitters, making indirect-acting catecholamines such as dopamine less effective. The impact of high-dose dopamine on renal perfusion cannot be ignored, and low (renal dose) levels may be required if concern for α-adrenergic-mediated constriction of renal or tissue beds exists.

Calcium may be beneficial on termination of CPB and should be administered just before weaning, when ionized calcium levels are deficient and inotropic assistance is required. Phosphodiesterase inhibitors such as amrinone may be helpful in providing prophylactic inotropic support in anticipation of ventricular failure. In conjunction with decreased left ventricular wall tension, amrinone promotes cardiac function without increasing myocardial oxygen demand. This drug may be administered with a loading dose of 0.75 mg/kg per minute in 2 to 3 minutes given when the aortic cross-clamp is released, followed by an infusion of 10 mcg/kg per minute. Amrinone and milrinone are similar to dobutamine in their effects on myocardial contractility, myocardial oxygen consumption rate, SVR, and pulmonary vascular resistance; however, they are less susceptible to biochemical changes in neurohumoral regulation that may reduce the efficacy of β-agonists.[53]

Blood from the pump is sequestered into the cell saver device and concentrated to be returned to the patient via IV infusion after separation from CPB. This will assist in bolstering the blood pressure without the administration of large amounts of crystalloid or pressors. In addition, colloid may be included to decrease the incidence of hypotension. Monitoring devices should be recalibrated before separation from the CPB, and the lungs should be expanded and mechanical ventilation instituted before weaning. This is done to assess the possibility of atelectasis, pneumothorax, and hydrothorax.

Pacing

Usually on rewarming, fibrillation of the myocardium occurs with a gradual progression to normal sinus rhythm. If defibrillation does not occur spontaneously, antiarrhythmic therapy, electrical cardioversion, or both are used. Control of heart rate and rhythm may be effected through the use of atrial, ventricular, atrioventricular (AV) sequential, or overdrive pacing in addition to necessary antiarrhythmic drugs. Epicardial electrode placement on the wall of the atrium is routine for cardiac surgery. Pacemakers allow for rapid adjustment of decreased CO when the conduction pathway is damaged or highly irritable.

Atrial contraction determines CO by controlling the volume of blood ejected into the ventricle. Atrial volume, ventricular volume and compliance, and the pattern of atrial contraction influence ventricular filling. If ventricular pacing is used alone, CO may decrease because of loss of the atrial "kick," but atrioventricular pacing alters the AV interval in relation to the PR interval, thereby improving CO.[61,62] (See Table 22-7 for an explanation of types of pacemakers.)

Left Ventricular Dysfunction

Left ventricular dysfunction may be indicated by a rise in PA pressure in conjunction with depressed systemic arterial blood pressure. The causes of left ventricular failure can be varied and may include preoperative markers such as a diminished left ventricular EF and left ventricular hypokinesis or akinesis. TEE is an invaluable tool for confirming and isolating hypodynamic ventricular wall motion. If depressed contractility results from lack of appropriate inotropic and pharmacologic support, this should be remedied immediately.

TABLE 22-7 Pacemaker Codes and Function

I Chamber Paced	II Chamber Sensed	III Response Mode	IV Program Function	V Special Function
A = Atrial V = Ventricular D = Dual Chamber	Atrium Ventricle Both	I = Inhibited T = Triggered D = Dual 0 = None R = Reverse	P = Program M = Multiprogram C = Communicating	B = Bursts N = Norm Rate S = Scanning E = External
Assigned Function				
DDD	Atrial and ventricular sensing and pacing			
VDD	Programmable AV interval: senses both chambers, paces ventricle			
DVI	Programmable AV interval: senses R wave, paces atrium			
VVT	Programmable escape interval: senses ventricle, paces ventricle			
VVI	Inhibited output from sensed ventricle: demand ventricular pacing			
VOO	Asynchronous ventricular pacing			
AAT	Programmable escape interval: senses atrium, paces atrium			
AAI	Inhibited output from sensed atrium: demand atrial pacing			
AOO	Asynchronous atrial pacing			

AV, *Atrioventricular.*

In some cases the myocardium may be "stunned" and may require additional support through the reengagement of CPB, resting of the heart, and examination of the anastomosis for leaks and the grafts for air emboli or kinking. In the event that cardiac depression remains unresolved or worsens, a mechanical assist device such as an IABP may be percutaneously introduced to provide diastolic augmentation and decreased afterload.

Right Ventricular Dysfunction

An inflammatory mediated response from the ECC or acute anaphylactic reaction caused by protamine sulfate or blood product transfusion may lead to increased pulmonary vascular resistance, resulting in depressed right ventricular function. Pharmacologic intervention to reduce pulmonary vasoconstriction includes nitric oxide–based vasodilators and β_2-adrenergic agonists and may include, in cases in which conventional treatment fails, the use of prostaglandin E_1. Left atrial injection of norepinephrine has been demonstrated to increase systemic pressures while avoiding the first-pass effects on the pulmonary vascular system. When right ventricular failure is unrelated to pulmonary vascular resistance, cyclic adenosine monophosphate–specific phosphodiesterase inhibitors may be beneficial for resolving the condition while avoiding the vasodilatory effects of prostaglandins and β-adrenergic blockers.[53]

Failure to Wean

The quality of the surgical correction and the quality of myocardial preservation are important determinants of the success in weaning from CPB. Failure to wean can be attributed to multiple factors including heart block or ventricular dysfunction resulting from hyperkalemia, interruption of coronary flow (because of air, fat, or particulate emboli), extended CPB and aortic cross-clamp times, and arrhythmias associated with reperfusion injury.

Failure to wean on the primary attempt may lead to significant damage or distention of the heart. Systemic hypotension may promote metabolic acidosis and organ damage or failure. Additional inotropic support may be required for returning to bypass under these conditions and may result in the additional administration of blood products, as a result of excessive hemodilution.[63] If return to CPB becomes necessary, an additional heparin bolus may be required. These situations are always emergent and require extreme caution in ensuring that the patient is being ventilated and adequately anticoagulated and that anatomic reconnection to ECC is achieved before bypass is reengaged. Preparations should include an avenue for mechanical support (e.g., IABP, ventricular assist device) should the need arise.

Intraaortic Balloon Pump

In the event of left ventricular failure or myocardial hypokinesia resulting from CPB or ischemic insult, insertion of an intraaortic balloon may be necessary to provide diastolic counterpulsation for the patient. The intraaortic balloon is a distensible polyurethane catheter that is percutaneously inserted through the femoral artery using the Seldinger technique for large-diameter catheter placement. The tip of the catheter allows aortic pressure monitoring and is threaded to the descending thoracic aorta with the tip at the distal aortic arch. The balloon (size 34, 40, or 50 ml) is inflated with helium or carbon dioxide gas. Balloon deflation can be triggered by the R wave of the electrocardiograph or by the arterial pressure waveform, atrial pacing mode, AV sequential pacing mode, or internal asynchronous timing (not recommended).[64]

Inflation of the intraaortic balloon is timed to occur during diastole, forcing blood into the coronary arteries and periphery. It deflates during systole to promote ventricular ejection. Diastolic augmentation is achieved during inflation and results in increased coronary perfusion pressure as well as increased flow to the great vessels arising from the aorta. In most instances this diastolic augmentation results in pressures greater than the patient's systolic pressure. Afterload reduction results when the balloon is rapidly deflated before ventricular ejection, reducing ventricular wall tension and therefore myocardial oxygen demand.

Ventricular Assist Devices

The placement of a ventricular assist device is an option when termination of bypass cannot be tolerated by the patient and no other options to ensure survival exist. This effort in most cases represents a bridge to cardiac transplantation or allows for additional resting time to promote recovery of severely compromised cardiac contractile function. Most institutions have established protocols and criteria for considering a patient as a candidate for this device. Age, pulmonary function, and organ system viability are factors in this selection process.

CPB is reinstituted to prepare the circuit and cannulation sites for transfer from the ECC to a centrifugal assist device. Cannulation depends on which ventricle requires support and represents a mechanically assisted atrial-aortic shunt of blood flow to circumvent the impaired ventricle.[41] This is a simple circuit with no oxygenator or heating element component; therefore, during the transfer from the ECC to the mechanical assist device, the patient must be ventilated. Appropriate pharmacologic support is essential.

EXTUBATION

The current trend is toward early extubation of the postoperative cardiac surgical patient. Controversy surrounds the efficacy of extubation within 2 to 4 hours of closure. However, "fast-tracking," a term used to describe early extubation and discharge from the intensive care unit, has become popular as a cost-effective technique associated with this major surgical procedure. The patient population for fast-track cardiac anesthesia must be a "less sick" group to prevent precipitation of hypertensive episodes and increased postoperative myocardial ischemia. Ideally the fast-track candidate is under 70 years of age, has normal ventricular and valvular function and an uncomplicated surgery, and is free of renal, neurologic, and coagulation disorders in the immediate postoperative period.

The selection of agents for fast-tracking starts in the preinduction phase with agents that have a short duration of action. Lower doses of opioids are supplemented with low-dose inhalation agents and propofol infusions. α-agonists are used as adjuncts because of their ability to blunt neurohumoral stress responses. Postoperative analgesia can be accomplished with the use of low-dose morphine, nonsteroidal antiinflammatory drugs, patient-controlled analgesia, and thoracic epidurals with short acting opioids.[65]

Extubation criteria include a warm patient, low-dose or no inotropic drugs or vasoactive drips, no balloon pump, and bleeding less than 100 ml/hr.[66-68] The patient must be awake, pain free, and hemodynamically stable and must meet all conventional metabolic criteria for extubation. Regardless of the anesthetic technique employed, the key to optimizing patient recovery is postoperative pain management, which facilitates early mobility and nutritional intake.[69,70]

UNIQUE SITUATIONS IN CARDIAC ANESTHESIA

Automatic Internal Cardioverter Defibrillator

Automatic implantable cardioverter defibrillators are surgically implanted to prevent sudden cardiac death from malignant ventricular tachyarrhythmias. These are self-contained diagnostic devices that continuously monitor the patient's heart rate and electrocardiographic activity. They sense potentially lethal ventricular arrhythmias and treat them with electrical discharges. Whereas pacemakers use low-energy impulses measured in microjoules, these defibrillators release an electrical discharge of approximately 30 J after sensing periods of fibrillation lasting approximately 20 seconds. Most devices can now be programmed to reconfirm ventricular tachycardia or ventricular fibrillation after charging to prevent inappropriate shock therapy.[71]

Patients considered for implantation are those who have had minimal success with standard antiarrhythmic drug therapy. The majority of patients have severe coronary artery disease with reduced left ventricular function, ischemic cardiomyopathy, or idiopathic cardiomyopathy.

Anesthetic management is best handled by general anesthesia because of testing that is necessary to properly place and program this device. Prolonged periods of asystole are at times encountered and can cause cerebral and myocardial ischemia. Vasoactive drugs are helpful for blood pressure stabilization. If ventricular tachycardia occurs before clinical induction, lidocaine treatment should be avoided because it may result in the inability to induce ventricular tachycardia on demand during testing.

Minimal monitoring includes ECG leads II and V_5 along with an arterial line. Although some institutions suggest IV sedation for these patients, the stress associated with testing and the amount of sedation necessary for the procedure suggest that general anesthesia with a controlled airway would be a better choice. Patients undergoing extracorporeal shock wave lithotripsy are a special problem in that the automatic implantable cardioverter defibrillator (AICD) may discharge. The shock waves themselves are capable of damaging the pacemaker components. In order to reduce the risk of life-threatening arrhythmias, the shock waves are synchronized to the R wave of the ECG. In situations in which the AICD is involved, the manufacturer should be contacted to determine if it is better to reprogram the device or use a magnet.[72]

Deep Hypothermic Circulatory Arrest

Hypothermic circulatory arrest is indicated for aortic arch lesions and in infants and children with small hearts. Exposure is improved when no multiple cannulas exist and no blood is present in the operative field. The margin of safe time for circulatory arrest under these conditions is unknown. The primary purpose of this process is cerebral and major organ preservation. A gradient of no more than 10° C is allowed between the patient and the perfusate at initial institution of bypass for cooling. Core cooling is gradual, with a target temperature of 18° to 20° C.

Anesthetic considerations include prevention of prebypass respiratory alkalosis. During the circulatory arrest time frame, the perfusate is maintained at 28° C while CPB is off. At the time of rewarming, phentolamine is administered in the pump and phenylephrine is administered to the patient to maintain perfusion pressure at 30 to 50 mm Hg. The maximum acceptable temperature for deep hypothermia circulatory arrest is below 40° C.[73-75]

Cardiac Tamponade

Cardiac tamponade is a rare but potentially lethal consequence of open-heart surgery. For the cardiac surgical patient it is usually related to a leaking anastomosis that requires surgical reexploration. It can also occur as a result of infection, uremia, trauma, CHF, rheumatoid arthritis, and anticoagulant therapy. Clinical diagnosis of this condition is made on the basis of decreasing systolic blood pressure accompanied by pulsus paradoxus, jugular venous distention, tachycardia, and an enlarged cardiac silhouette.

Pericardial effusion can lead to cardiac tamponade after open-heart bypass. This condition can be relieved using either percutaneous pericardiocentesis or subxiphoid pericardiotomy. Percutaneous pericardiocentesis in conjunction with two-dimensional echocardiography has been demonstrated to be successful in preventing cardiac puncture. Patients require only local anesthetic and are placed in the supine position with the head slightly raised.[76]

MINIMALLY INVASIVE CORONARY ARTERY BYPASS TECHNIQUES

Port-Access Coronary Artery Bypass Grafting

To minimize postoperative pain and to speed recovery, some cardiovascular surgeons have used a port access method of coronary artery bypass (PACAB). In these procedures multiple ports are placed in the chest wall for video surgery in addition to performance of a minithorocotomy in some patients. PACABs take advantage of the nonbeating heart on CPB. The Heartport system necessitates the femoral artery approach and uses an endoaortic balloon occlusion for instillation of cardioplegia. One-lung ventilation is necessary during the IMA dissection, and monitoring is extensive. The heart is not viewed directly; rather, it is viewed through echocardiography, video (endoscopy), and fluoroscopy. This makes the procedure somewhat cumbersome and tedious for the surgeon.

Anesthetic techniques include all monitors and considerations for CPB as well as the need for one-lung ventilation. Patients benefit from this port-access technique because they experience less postoperative pain, a reduced ICU stay, an accelerated recovery time, improved postoperative pulmonary function, and a reduced need for inpatient cardiac rehabilitation.[77] Aortic atherosclerotic disease is a contraindication. Heartport has a long bypass run for single vessel CABG, which maximizes the risk of stroke even though the sternotomy is eliminated.

Procedures that benefit from port access include multivessel CABG, mitral valve procedures, aortic valve replacements, and some congenital heart defect procedures. Some concern remains about aortic dissection as well as stroke and embolism, because the surgeon does not have direct access to the surgical field and cannot directly suction air from the heart. Patient selection is an important factor in safety of the procedure.

Minimally Invasive Direct Coronary Artery Bypass

Minimally invasive direct coronary artery bypass (MIDCAB) follows the basics of conventional CABG procedures but does not require CPB, cardioplegia, or a large incision. Through a small incision (10 to 12 cm) and under direct vision the graft is anastomosed while the heart is still beating. This procedure is beneficial to the patient because of the smaller incision, that absence of CPB and its inherent complications, and the reduced need for blood transfusions. The disadvantages include the fact that it is limited to use for only one or two arteries and that one-lung ventilation often is requested by the surgeon. Because the heart continues to beat, the anastomoses are difficult to suture and significant ischemia may occur, precipitating hemodynamic compromise of the patient. At times urgent conversion to coronary bypass is necessary, and the perfusionist and equipment for this must be immediately available.[78] Anesthetic management is closely related to that for off-pump coronary artery bypass procedures with normal sternotomies.

Off-Pump Coronary Artery Bypass

CABG procedures without CPB were attempted in Canada in the 1950s. These were single-vessel procedures only.[1] Surgical techniques in this area, along with advances in equipment, allow multivessel procedures with median sternotomy to be performed. Because CPB is not used, hearts of patients undergoing off-pump coronary artery bypass (OPCAB) are normothermic, and maintenance of coronary perfusion and hemodynamic stability are absolutely necessary. Communication between the surgeon and the anesthesia care provider is of paramount importance. The anesthesia provider is a crucial member of the team who should be as observant of the surgical field as the surgeon. Unlike CPB cases, during OPCAB procedures the grafting phase requires involvement and vigilance on the part of the anesthesia provider.

The hearts of patients undergoing OPCAB are anesthetized with the intent of "early" extubation. A modified fast-track approach that avoids ischemia while facilitating early extubation is desirable. The choice of an anesthetic must take into consideration that a slow heart rate facilitates the surgical procedures and reduces myocardial oxygen demand. A narcotic oxygen muscle relaxant technique facilitates minute-to-minute control of hemodynamics. Maintenance of the systolic pressure promotes hemodynamic stability when the heart position is changed during exposure of the different vessels. It is recommended that the systolic pressure be maintained above 100 mm Hg.[79] Prudent volume loading and positioning of the patient in the Trendelenburg position with a right rotation promote recovery of blood pressure when retraction is used in exposure of the posterior pericardium.

Extensive invasive monitoring is indicated, along with a large-bore peripheral IV and a right IJ triple-lumen catheter capable of handling continuous thermodilution CO and transvenous pacing. Multiple central ports must be available for continuous infusion of various vasoactive medications. Temperature monitoring is vital. It is necessary to maintain fluids and any other drips or instillations at warm temperatures, to use a forced air-warming device on the head and neck, and to maintain a warm room temperature.[80] If the grafts are completely arterial, as is often the case in OPCAB procedures, the possibility of placing a forced air warmer on the patient's lower extremities should be investigated.

The muscle relaxant chosen should be one without histamine-releasing effects. Some anesthesia care providers insist that a neuromuscular blocker like pancuronium, which independently causes tachycardia, should be avoided.[81] However, when potent narcotics such as sufentanil are used, the synergistic effects of these two drugs is to be considered and used. A target heart rate of not greater than 70 beats per minute can be achieved with the addition of an esmolol drip. Because surgical manipulation itself precipitates arrhythmias, antiarrhythmic medications (lidocaine, magnesium, or amiodarone)[82] for treatment of these problems must be readily available. In addition to drugs, it is appropriate to let the surgeon know what impact surgical manipulations have on the myocardium and to ask the surgeon to stop temporarily, if possible, when the situation warrants it. If bradycardia becomes a problem, treatment with medications or epicardial or transvenous pacing may be necessary.

The use of antifibrinolytics is controversial, because some surgeons are concerned about graft thrombosis associated with the use of these agents.[81] Anticoagulant therapy is facility specific but usually directed at a target ACT of 300 seconds and incomplete reversal. When protamine is given it is usually at a reduced dose to achieve an anticoagulation level 25% to 50% above the control ACT. When instilling protamine check the ACT one third and two thirds of the way through the dose to avoid overshooting the target ACT. In off-pump procedures the coagulation system is normal because it has not been exposed to the ECC and its effects; therefore the possibility of pulmonary embolus, graft clotting, and so on exists just as in other major vascular procedures.

For OPCAB patients to be extubated, they must be warm, awake, and pain free and receiving no or low-dose inotropes and vasoactive drugs; no balloon pump must be in use; bleeding must be less than 100 ml/hr; patients must be hemodynamically stable and meet conventional metabolic and mechanical criteria for extubation.

PEDIATRIC APPROACHES

A limited discussion of pediatric cardiac anesthesia is presented here because of the extent of information required to apply appropriate anesthetic techniques for the many types of anomalies present in pediatric patients. An entire career can be and usually is devoted to pediatric cardiac anesthesia. Only basic information is presented here.

Pediatric physiology requires revised anesthetic approaches that take into consideration the fetal circulatory system, neonatal response to stress, and developmental alterations in anatomy and hemodynamics. Although requiring the clinician to have excellent judgment, pediatric cardiac anesthesia is an anesthetic challenge. Pathophysiology such as coronary artery disease and associated life-threatening arrhythmias are not common problems in pediatric patients.[83]

Maturation of the fetal circulatory system may be incomplete in some newborns. They may have a patent ductus arteriosus or incomplete closure of the foramen ovale, resulting in arteriovenous shunting. In most circumstances the ductus arteriosus closes within 15 hours to 4 days after birth, and the foramen ovale structurally closes within 1 month.

Neonates are less susceptible to anesthetic techniques traditionally applied to adults for increasing SV and myocardial contractility. CO in neonates is more dependent on heart rate than it is on SV. The parasympathetic tone is greater than the sympathetic tone in neonates, making them more prone to bradycardia after stimulation of the parasympathetic nervous system.[83] Infants with congenital heart disease are more susceptible to cerebral insult or injury than adults. Depending on the type of malformation, the defect may represent a 10% morbidity from cerebral injury.

Principles of Intracardiac Shunts

In the presence of a congenital defect of the cardiac septum or great vessels in which a communication is present between the left and right cardiac structures, blood flow is diverted from the area of greater resistance to the chamber or vessel of lower resistance. As a result, part of the blood that characteristically flows from the right side of the cardiac structure through the pulmonary system may be shunted back to the venous side of the heart because of greater left heart pressures. This condition is referred to as a *left-to-right* shunt and is most commonly associated with a congenital lesion such as an atrial septal defect or a ventricular septal defect. If left unresolved, the left-to-right shunt results in right atrial enlargement as a compensatory mechanism for the increased volume and workload associated with the shunt. Pathologic changes occur in the pulmonary system because of this increase in blood flow and are eventually reflected as an extension of the muscle layer into peripheral vessels, resulting in medial hypertrophy of the lung. The subsequent development of pulmonary hypertension ultimately results in right ventricular hypertrophy, which in time elevates right cardiac pressures to a point at which the shunt is reversed (right-to-left). When outflow tract resistance exceeds SVR, the result is reduced pulmonary blood flow, a condition that is commonly referred to as *Eisenmenger's syndrome*.[84]

Anesthetic Considerations

Because more than 40 cardiac malformations are known, manifesting as isolated or combined lesions, the anesthesia care provider should tailor the therapeutic approach to the physiologic consequences associated with the specific condition. Cardiac defects are be classified according to their effect in precipitating CHF, cyanosis, or a combination of the two. The key points for anesthetic assessment center on the net effect of the intracardiac or extracardiac shunts, the status of ventricular function, pulmonary vascular compliance and flow, and whether or not an obstructive lesion is involved.[83]

Cyanosis in newborns represents inadequate pulmonary blood flow as a result of right ventricular outflow tract obstruction, intracardiac right-to-left shunting, a common ventricle, or transposition of the pulmonary and aortic arteries. In severe cases pulmonary blood flow may be diminished to less than 50% of the CO. This condition is immediately treated with a continuous infusion of prostaglandin to prevent closure of the ductus arteriosus. Cyanotic lesions result in polycythemia, a condition that may lead to dehydration, thrombosis, and elevations in pulmonary vascular resistance and SVR resulting from increased blood viscosity.[84] Survival of these patients is contingent on the existence of a systemic-to-pulmonary shunt and usually requires palliative surgery to create a temporary shunt. This allows the newborn time to develop sufficiently for future corrective cardiac surgery.

CHF in the newborn may result from a combination of lesions that contribute to increased pulmonary flow, with concomitant outflow tract obstruction. These patients have left-to-right shunts through an existing atrial or ventricular septal defect or patent ductus arteriosus. Aortic coarctation, endocardial defects, transposition of the great vessels, anomalous pulmonary venous return, truncus arteriosus, and formation of a single ventricle are congenital defects that may lead to the development of CHF. Initial surgery is most often directed toward the correction of the pathology that caused the development of CHF; this allows the eventual repair of other, coexisting malformations.

Premedication depends on the type of lesion and symptoms. Infants who are cyanotic, dyspneic, or less than 6 months old should not be premedicated before surgery. For pediatric patients undergoing corrective surgery for congenital lesions, induction should not be focused simply on prevention of hemodynamic or circulatory deterioration. Rather, it should be directed at improvement of circulatory performance and oxygen transport. If CO is not depressed, the decreased oxygen consumption associated with general anesthesia should result in overall improvement in mixed venous oxygen saturation. This improvement should be reflected in increased arterial saturations as a result of intracardiac shunting.

In neonates or infants with complex lesions, high-dose opiate anesthetic agents may be useful because of the ability of these agents to maintain cardiovascular stability. Continued use of opioids during the operation offers additional benefit by reducing the stress response associated with CPB, decreasing ventricular arrhythmias after bypass, and allowing hemodynamic stabilization during and after CPB. Volatile anesthetic agents may be less suitable because of the myocardial depression associated with their use. The myocardium of infants less than 2 years of age is immature and potentially more sensitive to these negative inotropic effects. Increases in pulmonary vascular resistance (PVR) may exacerbate cyanosis and must be avoided. Conditions that may increase pulmonary vascular resistance include light anesthesia, positive end-expiratory pressure, hypoxia, hypercarbia, acidosis, and hypothermia.[83]

When an intracardiac shunt is present, the anesthetic technique employed should minimize drops in SVR to prevent an increase in right-to-left shunting. Pretreatment with a vasoconstrictor such as phenylephrine or methoxamine may offset the reduction of SVR associated with induction. The administration of ketamine at a dose of 1 to 2 mcg/kg has been shown to have no significant impact on systemic or pulmonary vascular resistance in children and therefore causes no major fluctuations with regard to their shunts.[83] This ability to maintain systemic blood pressure makes ketamine a suitable choice for induction of anesthesia in pediatric patients with right-to-left shunts.[85]

REFERENCES

1. Hessel EA II. History of cardiac surgery and anesthesia. In: Estefanous FG. *Cardiac Anesthesia Principles and Clinical Practice.* Philadelphia: Lippincott Williams & Wilkins; 2001:4.
2. American Heart Association. *Heart Disease and Stroke Statistics—2003 Update.* Dallas: American Heart Association; 2002:38.
3. Norton JM. Toward consistent definitions for preload and afterload. *Adv Physiol Educ.* 2001;25:53-61.
4. Le Winter MM, Osol G. Normal physiology of the cardiovascular system. In: Fuster V, Alexander RW, O'Rourke RA, eds. *Hurst's the Heart.* 10th ed. New York: McGraw-Hill; 2001:1:63-94.
5. Maccherini M, Davoli G, Sani G, et al. Warm heart surgery eliminates diaphragmatic paralysis. *J Cardiac Surg.* 1995;10:257.
6. Roach GW, Newman MF, Murkin JM, et al. Ineffectiveness of burst suppression therapy in mitigating perioperative cerebrovascular dysfunction. Multicenter Study of Perioperative Ischemia (McSPI) Research Group. *Anesthesiology.* 1999;90:1255-1264.
7. Arrowsmith JE, Grocott HP, Reves JG, et al. Central nervous system complications of cardiac surgery. *Br J Anaesth.* 2000;84: 3:378-393.
8. Murkin JM, Baird DL, Martzke JS, et al. Cognitive dysfunction after ventricular fibrillation during implantable cardioverter/defibrillator procedures is related to duration of the reperfusion interval. *Anesth Analg.* 1997;84:1186-1192.
9. Arrowsmith JE, Sroscott H, Reves JG, et al. Central nervous system complications of cardiac surgery. *Br J Anaesth.* 2000;84:378-383.
10. Murkin JM. Intraoperative tight glucose control improves outcome in cardiovascular surgery: pro. *J Cardiothorac Vasc Anesth.* 2000;14:475-478.
11. Yilmaz AT, Arslan M, Demirkilc U, et al. Gastrointestinal complications aftercardiac surgery. *Eur J Cardiothorac Surg.* 1996;10:763-767.
12. Huddy SP, Joyce WP, Pepper JR. Gastrointestinal complications in 4473 patients who underwent cardiopulmonary bypass surgery. *Br J Surg.* 1991;78:293-296.
13. Mangano CM, Diamondstone LS, Ramsay JG, et al. Renal dysfunction after myocardial revascularization: risk factors, adverse outcomes, and hospital resource utilization. The Multicenter Study of Perioperative Ischemia Research Group. *Ann Intern Med.* 1998;128:194-203.
14. Picca S, Principato F, Mazzera E, et al. Risks of acute renal failure after cardiopulmonary bypass surgery in children: a retrospective 10 year case control study. *Nephrol Dial Transplant.* 1995;10:630.
15. Regragui IA, Izzat MB, Birdi I, et al. Cardiopulmonary bypass perfusion temperature does not influence perioperative renal function. *Ann Thorac Surg.* 1995;60:160.
16. Solina A, Ginsberg SH, Horrow JC, Hensley FA Jr. Anesthetic management for myocardial revascularization. In: Hensley FA, Martin DE, Gravlee GP, eds. *A Practical Approach to Cardiac Anesthesia.* 3rd ed. Philadelphia: Lippincott Williams & Wilkins; 2003:273-301.
17. Reich DL, Bodian CA, Krol M, et al. Intraoperative hemodynamic predictors of mortality, stroke, and myocardial infarction after coronary artery bypass surgery. *Anesth Analg.* 1999;89:814-822.
18. Noronha B, Duncan E, Byrne JA. Optimal medical management of angina. *Curr Cardiol Rep.* 2003;5:259-265.
19. Suematsu Y, Nakano K, Sasako Y, et al. Strategies for CABG patients with carotid artery disease and perioperative neurological complications. *Heart Vessels.* 2000;15:129-134.
20. Joshi S, Ornstein E, Young WL. Cerebral and spinal cord blood flow. In: Cottrell JE, Smith DS. *Anesthesia and Neurosurgery.* 4th ed. St Louis: Mosby; 2001:36.
21. Mantha S, Roizen MF, Barnard J, et al. Relative effectiveness of four preoperative tests for predicting adverse cardiac outcomes after vascular surgery: a metaanalysis. *Anesth Analg.* 1994;79:422-433.
22. Soman P, Parsons A, Lahiri N, Lahiri A. The prognostic value of a normal Tc-99m sestamibi SPECT study in suspected coronary artery disease. *J Nucl Cardiol.* 1999;6:252-256.
23. Riedel BJ. Ischemic injury and its prevention. on right ventricular function in patients undergoing myocardial revascularization. *J Cardiothorac Vasc Anesth.* 1995;9:2-8.
24. Martin DE, Chambers CE, Luck JC, Hensley FA. The cardiac patient. In: Hensley FA, Martin DE, Gravlee GP, eds. *A Practical Approach to Cardiac Anesthesia.* 3rd ed. Philadelphia: Lippincott Williams & Wilkins; 2003:23-26.
25. Heres EK, Horrow JC, Gravlee GP, et al. A dose determining trial of heparinase I (Neutralase) for heparin neutralization in coronary artery surgery. *Anesth Analg.* 2001;93:1446-1452.
26. Merin RG. Preoperative preparation of the patient with myocardial ischemia. *Anesthesiol Clin North Am.* 1999;9:555-563.
27. Whit GC. Approach to the bleeding patient. In: Colman RW, et al, eds. *Hemostasis and Thrombosis.* Philadelphia: Lippincott; 1994.
28. Crouch MA, Nappi JM, Cheang KI. Glycoprotein IIb/IIIa receptor inhibitors in percutaneous coronary intervention and acute coronary syndrome. *Ann Pharmacother.* 2003;37:860-875.
29. Hirsh J, Fuster V. Guide to anticoagulant therapy. Part 1. Heparin, American Heart Association. *Circulation.* 1994;89:1449-1468.
30. Grock H, Gabriel C, Bibl D, et al. Monitoring intravascular volumes for postoperative volume therapy. *Eur J Anaesthesiol.* 2003;19:288-294.
31. Godje O, Peyerl M, Seebauer T, et al. Central venous pressure, pulmonary capillary wedge pressure and intrathoracic blood volumes as preload indicators in cardiac surgery patients. *Eur J Cardiothorac Surg.* 1998;13:533-539; 539-540 [discussion].
32. Baxter Healthcare Corporation, Edwards Critical Care Division. *Invasive hemodynamic monitoring: physiologic principals and clinical applications.* Santa Anna, Calif: Baxter Healthcare; 1989:1.
33. Shanewise JS, Savage R, Aronson S, Thys DM. Transesophageal echocardiography. In: Hensley FA, Martin DE, Gravlee GP, eds. *A Practical Approach to Cardiac Anesthesia.* 3rd ed. Philadelphia: Lippincott, Williams & Wilkins; 2003.
34. American Society of Anesthesiologists and the Society of Cardiovascular Anesthesiologists Task Force on Transesophageal Echocardiography. Practice guidelines for perioperative transesophageal echocardiography. *Anesthesiology.* 1996;84:986-1006.

35. Lehmann A, Karzau J, Boldt J, et al. Bispectral index-guided anesthesia in patients undergoing aortocoronary bypass grafting. *Anesth Analg*. 2003;96:336-343.
36. Heck M, Kumle B, Boldt J, et al. Electroencephalogram bispectral index predicts hemodynamic and arousal reactions during induction of anesthesia in patients undergoing cardiac surgery. *J Cardiothorac Vasc Anesth*. 2000;14:693-697.
37. Newfield P, Cottrell JE. *Handbook of Neuroanesthesia*. 3rd ed. Philadelphia: Lippincott Williams & Wilkins; 1999:60.
38. Hall RI, Smith MS, Rocker G. The systemic inflammatory response to cardiopulmonary bypass: pathophysiologic, therapeutic and pharmacologic considerations. *Anesth Analg*. 1997;85:766-782.
39. Asimakopoulas G. Systemic inflammation and cardiac surgery: an update. *Perfusion*. 2001;16:353-360.
40. Michelsen LG. Cardiopulmonary bypass. In: Kirby RR, Gravenstein N, Logato EB, Gravenstein JS, eds. *Clinical Anesthesia Practice*. 2nd ed. Philadelphia: Saunders; 2002:329-350.
41. Brodie JE, Johnson BB. *The Manual of Clinical Perfusion*. Augusta, Ga: Glendale Medical Corporation; 1994.
42. Buckberg, GD. Recent progress in myocardial protection during cardiac operations. In: McGoon DC, ed. *Cardiac Surgery*. 2nd ed. Philadelphia: FA Davis; 1987:291.
43. Rinder CS, Bohnert J, Rinder HM, et al. Platelet activation and aggregation during cardiopulmonary bypass. *Anesthesiology*. 1991;75:388-393.
44. Shone-Lessersen L, Gravlee GP, Horrow JC. Coagulation management during and after cardiopulmonary bypass. In: Hensley FA, Martin DE, Gravlee GP, eds. *A Practical Approach to Cardiac Anesthesia*. 3rd ed. Philadelphia: Lippincott Williams & Wilkins; 2003:491-493.
45. Guyton AC. Hemostasis and blood coagulation. In: *Textbook of Medical Physiology*. 9th ed. Philadelphia: Saunders; 1990:463.
46. Hunt BJ, Parratt RN, Segal HC, et al. Activation of coagulation and fibrinolysis during cardiothoracic operations. *Ann Thorac Surg*. 1998;65:712-718.
47. Tanaka K, Takao M, Yada I, et al. Alterations in coagulation and fibrinolysis associated with cardiopulmonary bypass during open heart surgery. *J Cardiothorac Anesth*. 1989;3:181-188.
48. Wilhelmi M, Franke U, Cohnert T, et al. Coronary artery bypass grafting surgery without the routine application of blood products: is it feasible? *Eur J Cardiothorac Surg*. 2001;19: 657-661.
49. Kasper SM, Giesecke, T, Limpers P, et al. Failure of autologous fresh frozen plasma to reduce blood loss and transfusion requirements in coronary artery bypass surgery. *Anesthesiology*. 2001;95:81-86; 6A [discussion].
50. Alvarez JM, Quincy NF, McMillan D, et al. The use of ultra–low-dose aprotinin to reduce blood loss in surgery. *J Cardiothorac Vasc Anesth*. 1995;9:29-33.
51. Chugh SS, Larie Kg, Lindner KH. Pressor with promise. Using Vasopressin in cardiac arrest. *Circulation*. 1997;96:2453-2454.
52. The American Heart Association in collaboration with the International Liaison Committee on Resuscitation (ILCOR) Guidelines 2000 for cardiopulmonary resuscitation and emergency cardiovascular care. Part 6: advanced cardiovascular life support, section 6: Pharmacology II: agents to optimize cardiac output and blood pressure. *Circulation*. 2000;102:I-129–I-135.
53. Balser JR, Butterworth J. Cardiovascular Drugs. In: Hensley FA, Martin DE, Gravlee GP, eds. *A Practical Approach to Cardiac Anesthesia*. 3rd ed. Philadelphia: Lippincott Williams & Wilkins; 2003:34-97.
54. Kaplan JA, Wynands JE. Anesthesia for myocardial revascularization. In: Kaplan JA. *Cardiac Anesthesia*. 4th ed. Philadelphia: Saunders; 1999:702.
55. Michelsen LG. Cardiopulmonary bypass. In: Kirby RR, Gravenstein N, Logato EB, Gravenstein JS, eds. *Clinical Anesthesia Practice*. 2nd ed. Philadelphia: Saunders; 2002:342.
56. Gold J, Charlson M, Williams-Russo P, et al. Improvement of outcomes after coronary artery bypass: a randomized trial comparing intraoperative high versus low mean arterial pressure. *J Thorac Cardiovasc Surg*. 1995;110:1302.
57. Cartwright CR, Mangano CM. Con: during cardiopulmonary bypass for elective coronary artery bypass grafting, perfusion pressure should not routinely be greater than 70 mm Hg. *J Cardiothorac Vasc Anesth*. 1998;12:36.
58. Thomas SJ, Davis RF. Termination of cardiopulmonary bypass. In: Gravlee GP, Davis RF, Kurusz M, Utley JR, eds. *Cardiopulmonary Bypass*. Principles and Practice. 2nd ed. Baltimore: Lippincott Williams & Wilkins; 2000:613-632.
59. Morgan GE, Mikhail MS, Murray MJ. Cardiovascular physiology and anesthesia. In: *Clinical Anesthesiology*. 3rd ed. New York: McGraw-Hill; 2002:671.
60. Strong M, Bennett JA, Gravlee GP, et al. Efficacy and pharmacokinetics of neutralase in CABG. *Int Anesth Res Soc*. 1998;86;28SCA.
61. Atlee JL, Bernstein AD. Cardiac rhythm management devices. Part I, indications, device selection and function. *Anesthesiology*. 2001;95:1265-1280.
62. Atlee JL, Bernstein AD. Cardiac rhythm management devices. Part II. Perioperative management. *Anesthesiology*. 2001:95: 1492-1506.
63. Kikura M, Levy JH, Michelsen LG, et al. The effect of milrinone on hemodynamics and left ventricular function after emergence from cardiopulmonary bypass. *Anesth Analg*. 1997;85:16.
64. Harter RL, Michler RE. Circulatory assist devices. In: Hensley FA, Martin DE, Gravlee GP, eds. *A Practical Approach to Cardiac Anesthesia*. 3rd ed. Philadelphia: Lippincott Williams & Wilkins; 2003.
65. Scott NB, Tunfrey DJ, Ray D, et al. A prospective randomized study of the potential benefits of thoracic epidural anesthesia and analgesia in patients undergoing coronary artery bypass grafting. *Anesth Analg*. 2001;93:528-535.
66. Leslie K, Sessler D. The implications of hypothermia for early extubation following cardiac surgery. *J Cardiothorac Vasc Anesth*. 1998:12(suppl 2):30-34.
67. Montes F, Sanchez S, Giraldo J, et al. The lack of benefit of tracheal extubation in the operating room after coronary artery bypass surgery. *Anesth Analg*. 2000;91:776-780.
68. Cheng D, Darshi J, Peniston C, et al. Early tracheal extubation after coronary artery bypass graft surgery reduces costs and improves resources use. *Anesthesiology*. 1996;85:1300-1310.
69. Hardy JF. Cardiac anesthesia: perspective 1990s. *Can J Anaesth*. 1993;9:1115-1119.
70. Cheng D. Fast-track cardiac surgery: economic implications in postoperative care. *J Cardiothorac Vasc Anesth*. 1998;12:72-79.
71. Trankina MF. Automatic implantable cardioverter-defibrillator. In: Fause RJ, Cucchiara RF, Rose SH, et al. *Anesthesiology Review*. 3rd ed. New York: Churchill-Livingstone; 2002.
72. Vijayakumar E. Anesthetic considerations in patients with cardiac arrhythmias, pacemakers, and AICDs. *Int Anesthesiol Clin*. 2001;39:21-42.
73. Hennein HA. Cardiopulmonary bypass/deep hypothermia circulatory arrest. PediHeart Organization's Practitioner Website 1998. Available at: http://anes01.wustl.edu/all-net/english/cardpage/operate/bypass/cpb-19.htm. Accessed May 5, 2003.
74. Caldarone CA, Abonassaly C. Hypothermic circulatory arrest and cardiopulmonary bypass. E-medicine 2002. Available at: http://www.emedicine.com/ped/topic2813.htm. Accessed April 2, 2003.
75. Kuimral E, Yuksel M, Buket S, et al. Neurologic complications with deep hypothermic circulatory arrest. *Tex Heart Inst J*. 2001;28:83-88.
76. Valley VT. Cardiovascular pericarditis and cardiac tamponade. MedWebPlus Website. *E-med J*. 2001;2. Available at: http://www.emedicine.com/EMERG/topic412.htm. Accessed April 2, 2003.
77. Ribakove GH, Grossi EA, Steinberg BM, Ursomanno P, Colvin SB, Galloway AC. Port-access minimally invasive CABG: techniques and results. 2000;15:296-302.

78. Ganapathy S. Anaesthesia for minimally invasive cardiac surgery. *Best Pract Res Clin Anaesthesiol.* 2002;16:63-80.
79. Chassot PG, Van Der Linden P, Zaugg M, Mueller XM, Spahn DR. Off-pump coronary artery bypass surgery: physiology and anaesthetic management. 2004;92:400-413.
80. Shanewise JS, Ramsay JG. Off-pump coronary surgery: how do the anesthetic considerations differ? *Anesthesiol Clin North America.* 21:613-623, 2003.
81. Barnes RD. Off pump coronary artery bypass and minimally invasive direct coronary artery bypass. In: Faust RJ, Cucchiara RT, Ross SH, et al. *Anesthesiology Review.* 3rd ed. New York: Churchill-Livingstone; 2002.
82. Huss MG, Wasnick JD. Magnesium and off pump coronary artery bypass. *J Cardiac Thorac Vasc Anesth.* 1999;13: 374-375.
83. Stratford MA. Cardiovascular physiology. In: Motayama EK, Davis PJ, eds. *Smiths' Anesthesia for Infants and Children.* 6th ed. St Louis: Mosby; 1996:69.
84. Bell C, Kain ZN. *The Pediatric Anesthesia Handbook.* 2nd ed. St Louis: Mosby; 1997:540.
85. Reid RW, Burrows FA, Hickey PR. In: Cote CJ, Todres ID, Goudsouzian NG, Ryan JF. *A Practice of Anesthesia for Infants and Children.* 3rd ed. Philadelphia: Saunders; 2001:397.

CHAPTER 23

Vascular Surgery

Sass Elisha

PERIPHERAL VASCULAR DISEASE

Atherosclerosis is the most common cause of occlusive disease in the arteries of the lower extremities. This degeneration involves the formation of atheromatous plaques that may obstruct the vessel lumen and thereby cause a reduction in distal blood flow. The pathophysiologic processes that affect the arteries include plaque formation, which obstructs the lumen (stenosis); thrombosis, which results in acute ischemia; and weakening of the arterial wall with aneurysm formation.[1] The most common risk factors associated with atherosclerosis appear in Box 23-1. Cigarette smoking and diabetes mellitus are major risk factors in the pathogenesis of atherosclerosis in the peripheral vascular system.[1] Typical symptoms of peripheral occlusive disease include claudication, skin ulcerations, gangrene, and impotence.[1] The extent of disability is primarily influenced by the development of collateral blood flow. Initially, collateral blood flow sufficiently meets tissue oxygen demands. As the disease process progresses, supply is unable to meet demand, and limb ischemia becomes symptomatic, requiring therapeutic intervention. The mortality rates associated with peripheral vascular disease are 30% at 5 years and 70% at 10 years.[2]

Treatment for peripheral occlusive disease may range from pharmacologic therapy to surgery. Surgical therapy includes transluminal angioplasty, endarterectomy, thrombectomies, and multiple bypass procedures. Examples of common surgical maneuvers used for bypassing occlusive lesions are aortofemoral, axillofemoral, femorofemoral, and femoropopliteal bypass techniques. Bypass techniques may be classified as *inflow* or *outflow* procedures, depending on the level of the obstruction, with the dividing axis being at the level of the groin. Temporary occlusion of the operative artery is mandatory when bypass procedures are used. The response to aortic cross-clamping in patients with aortoiliac occlusive disease is of less magnitude than in patients with aneurysmal disease. The presence of collateral circulation provides the cardiovascular stability observed in patients with occlusive disease.[3,4]

BOX **23-1**

Risk Factors Related to the Development of Atherosclerotic Lesions

- Hypercholesterolemia
- Cigarette smoking
- Physical inactivity
- Type A behavior
- Hypertension
- Diabetes mellitus
- Obesity
- Heredity

From Zarins CK, Graham HM. Aorta and arterial disease of the lower extremity. In: Miller TA, ed. Physiologic Basis of Modern Surgical Care. *St Louis: Mosby; 1988:837.*

Preoperative Evaluation

The atherosclerotic process in occlusive disease is not limited to the peripheral arterial beds and should be expected to be present in the coronary, cerebral, and renal arteries. More than half of the mortality associated with peripheral vascular disease results from adverse cardiac events.[5] Szilagyi and co-workers[6] reported that 60% of late deaths that follow reconstructive operations for aortoiliac occlusive disease in 1647 patients were the result of atherosclerotic heart disease. The identification and management of CAD in the preoperative period should follow the same progression as that described for patients undergoing abdominal aortic reconstruction. Similarly, the presence of concurrent pulmonary, renal, neurologic, and endocrine dysfunction should be identified, and actions should be taken to improve organ function.

Monitoring

The extent of perioperative monitoring should be based on the presence of coexisting disease processes. Clearly the detection of myocardial ischemia should be a primary objective in patients with vascular disease. Methods for assessing cardiac function include the monitoring of pulmonary artery pressure and transesophageal echocardiography. Direct intraarterial blood pressure monitoring allows for near–real-time determination of blood pressure values and is warranted because dramatic fluctuations frequently occur during anesthesia.

Anesthetic Selection

The anesthetic technique chosen for vascular surgery depends on the type of surgical procedure to be performed and the presence of coexisting disease. In certain instances infiltration

BOX 23-2

Benefits of the Epidural Technique in Vascular Surgery

Endocrine
Inhibits surgical stress response
Inhibits adrenaline and cortisol release
Inhibits hyperglycemia
Inhibits lymphopenia and granulocytosis
Causes nitrogen sparing
Blocks sympathetic tone

Cardiovascular
Decreases myocardial oxygen demand and afterload
Decreases myocardial infarct size (experimental model)
Increases endocardial perfusion at ischemic zone
Causes fewer sympathetic blood pressure swings
Causes less blood loss
Requires less general anesthesia depressant medication
Redistributes blood to the lower extremities

Pulmonary
Decreases FVC, FEV_1, and PEFR
Requires less shunting oxygen consumption
Improves atrioventricular oxygen differentiation
Causes fewer pulmonary infections
Causes fewer thromboembolisms

Renal
Increases blood flow in the renal cortex
Causes less renovascular constriction

Geriatric
Causes less cardiorespiratory trespass
Improves postoperative mental status

Miscellaneous
Allows earlier extubation, ambulation, and discharge
Achieves greater postoperative pain control

FEV_1, *forced expiratory volume in 1 second;* FVC, *forced vital capacity;* PEFR, *peak expiratory flow rate.*
Modified from Raggi R, Dardik H, Mauro AL. Continuous epidural anesthesia and postoperative epidural narcotics in vascular surgery. Am J Surg. *1987;154:192-197.*

of local anesthetic and intravenous sedation may be sufficient, whereas other situations may require the use of general anesthesia. Regional anesthesia for surgery on the lower extremities may decrease the overall morbidity and mortality associated with this patient population. In a review of 912 patients who underwent peripheral vascular reconstruction, Baron and associates[7] documented the safety of a continuous epidural anesthetic technique for patients who had received heparin; these investigators identified specific advantages of this technique. Similarly, Raggi and co-workers[8] documented favorable consequences of the use of epidural anesthesia during vascular surgery in 85 patients (Box 23-2). Specific anesthetic techniques and their contribution to postoperative complications remain controversial. For example, Underwood and associates[9] report a higher frequency of cardiac complications in patients who underwent peripheral vascular surgery while receiving epidural anesthesia; however, all patients studied were over 69 years of age.

Postoperative Considerations

Postoperative pain management is an important issue related to peripheral vascular surgery. Most clinicians agree that postoperative administration of narcotics not only provides patient comfort but also contributes to cardiac stability. The use of epidural opioid and local anesthetics in patients recovering from vascular surgery is an important component of postoperative care, as pain can greatly enhance sympathetic nervous system stimulation. Raggi and co-workers[8] describe the benefits of this technique, which were previously discussed. Despite a decrease in discomfort during the postoperative course, these patients must be monitored in an appropriate surgical unit that is capable of detecting possible adverse events, such as myocardial infarction or respiratory depression, which could be attributed to the administration of epidural opioids and local anesthetics.

ABDOMINAL AORTIC ANEURYSMS

Incidence

The incidence of abdominal aortic aneurysms has increased since the 1970s[10] and has risen over the last 5 decades from 12.2 to 36.2 per 100,000 surgical procedures.[11] This increase may partially be the result of the detection of asymptomatic aneurysms by noninvasive diagnostic modalities, such as computed tomography (CT), magnetic resonance imaging (MRI), and ultrasonography. The occurrence of abdominal aortic aneurysms has increased because of the increased age of the general population and the vascular changes that occur as a result of aging.[10] Aortic aneurysms can be identified in approximately 1% to 4% of the population older than 50 years and in approximately 5% of the population older than 60 years.[12-14] Aneurysms are more common in men than in women and in whites than in blacks.[10,13,15,16]

Risk Factors

Atherosclerosis is thought to be the primary cause of abdominal aortic aneurysms in more than 90% of patients.[16] However, this traditional theory has been challenged by some who speculate that aneurysmal development may result from proteolysis of elastin and collagen within the vessel wall and that atherosclerosis may be an incidental finding in the pathogenesis of aneurysm development.[10,17] Hypertension is present in 60% of patients with aneurysmal lesions.[16] In cigarette smokers the incidence of abdominal aortic aneurysms increases eightfold.[10,16,18] Although investigators have demonstrated a correlation between aneurysms and these factors, aneurysms can also be observed in normotensive nonsmokers.[10] Perhaps it may be safer to suggest that hypertension and cigarette smoking increase the potential for the development of aneurysms.[10] Genetics may also contribute to the predisposition for aneurysmal development.[17,19] Obesity, although not an independent risk factor, may mask the signs and symptoms of an abdominal aortic aneurysm until complications arise.[15,16]

Mortality

Mortality rates for elective abdominal aortic aneurysmectomies have decreased since the 1970s. The present mortality rate ranges from 1% to 11%, although most commonly estimated at 5%, as compared with the mortality rates in the 1950s of 18% to 30%.[15,16,19-23] Advanced detection capabilities, earlier surgical intervention, extensive preoperative preparation, refined surgical techniques, better hemodynamic monitoring, improved anesthetic techniques, and aggressive postoperative management have all contributed to this improvement in surgical outcomes. Unfortunately, the mortality rates for ruptured aortic aneurysms have not followed this trend. Estimates of mortality resulting from ruptured aneurysms vary from 35% to 94%.[12,15,24-26] The 5-year mortality rate for individuals with untreated aortic aneurysms is 81%, and the 10-year mortality rate is 100%.[21] Because rupture leads to an increased incidence of mortality, early detection and elective surgical intervention are advisable.

Diagnosis

Frequently, asymptomatic aneurysms are detected incidentally during routine examination or abdominal radiography. Smaller aneurysms are often undetected on routine physical examination. Diagnostic techniques, such as ultrasonography, CT scan, and MRI, may identify vascular abnormalities in these patients. Such noninvasive techniques not only reveal the presence of aneurysms but also provide information about aneurysm size, vessel wall integrity, and adjacent anatomic definition.[27] Invasive techniques, including contrast-enhanced CT scan, contrast angiography, and digital subtraction angiography, can provide additional information and more detailed representations of arterial anatomy. Digital subtraction angiography is the best method of evaluating suprarenal aneurysms because this method provides superior definition of the aneurysmal relationship to the renal arteries.[28]

ABDOMINAL AORTIC RECONSTRUCTION

Patient Selection

As a result of recent advances in surgical and anesthetic techniques, the mortality associated with elective repair of abdominal aortic aneurysms is fairly low as compared with nonsurgical management. Most patients with abdominal aneurysms, including octogenarians, are considered surgical candidates. Although advancing age contributes to an increased incidence of morbidity and mortality, age alone is not a contraindication to elective aneurysmectomies.[29] Mortality in patients who undergo elective aortic reconstruction has been reported to be 5.6% for patients younger than 75 years and 11.3% for those older than 75 years.[30] However, physiologic age is more indicative than chronologic age of increased surgical risk. Contraindications to elective repair include intractable angina pectoris, recent myocardial infarction, severe pulmonary dysfunction, and chronic renal insufficiency.[3] Table 23-1 lists characteristics that define high-risk patients; however, in most cases the presence of an abdominal aortic aneurysm warrants surgical intervention.[21]

The dimensions of an aneurysm can change over time. Abdominal aortic aneurysms grow approximately 4 mm/yr.[17]

TABLE 23-1 Criteria for High Risk in Abdominal Aortic Aneurysm Repair

Parameter	Criterion
Age	85 yr
Pulmonary	Home oxygen, Pa_{O_2} <50 mm Hg, FEV_1 <1 L/s
Renal	Serum creatinine level (3 mg/dL)
Cardiac	Class III-IV angina
	Resting LVEF <30%
	Recent congestive heart failure
	Complex ventricular ectopy
	Large left ventricular aneurysm
	Severe valvular disease
	Recurrent congestive failure or angina after CABG
	Severe, noncorrectable CAD

CABG, *Coronary artery bypass grafting;* CAD, *coronary artery disease;* FEV_1, *forced expiratory volume in 1 second;* LVEF, *left ventricular ejection fraction;* Pa_{O_2}, *partial pressure of arterial oxygen.*
Modified from Pairolero PC. Repair of abdominal aortic aneurysms in high-risk patients. Surg Clin North Am. *1989;69:765-774.*

Aneurysmal vessel dimensions correspond to the law of Laplace:

Equation 23-1

$$T = P \times r$$

where T = wall tension, P = transmural pressure, and r = vessel radius.

As the radius of a vessel increases, the wall tension increases. Therefore the larger the aneurysm, the more likely the risk of spontaneous rupture. Generally, aneurysms measuring greater than 4 to 5 cm in diameter require surgical intervention.[15] Aneurysms measuring less than 4 to 5 cm in diameter should not be considered benign, because an aneurysm has the potential to rupture regardless of its size. On postmortem examination, Darling and associates[31] reported that 18% of ruptured aneurysms were less than 5 cm in diameter.

Patient Preparation

Preoperative volume loading and restoration of intravascular volume are perhaps the most important techniques used in the enhancement of cardiac function during abdominal aortic aneurysmectomies. Reliable venous access must be secured if volume replacement is to be accomplished. Large-bore intravenous lines and central lines can be used to infuse fluids or blood. Massive hemorrhage is an ever-present threat; therefore the availability of blood and blood products should be ensured. Provisions for rapid transfusion and intraoperative blood salvage should be confirmed.

Routine Monitoring

Standard monitoring methods include electrocardiography with display of lead II, for detection of dysrhythmias and the precordial V_5 lead for analysis of ischemic ST-segment changes, pulse oximetry, and capnography. An esophageal stethoscope allows for continuous auscultation of heart and breath sounds as well as temperature determination. Placement of an indwelling urinary catheter is necessary for the continuous measurement of urinary output and renal function. Neuromuscular function is also routinely monitored.

Invasive Monitoring

The maintenance of cardiac function is crucial for a successful surgical outcome, and cardiac function should be closely monitored during abdominal aortic reconstruction. Invasive blood pressure monitoring permits beat-to-beat analysis of the blood pressure, immediate identification of hemodynamic alterations related to aortic clamping, and access for blood sampling.

Pulmonary artery catheters can be used in abdominal aortic reconstruction for monitoring left-sided filling pressures as a guide for fluid replacement. Correlations between central venous pressure and PAOP have been demonstrated in both coronary revascularization[56] and aortic surgery.[57] This correlation is predictable only in patients with adequate ventricular function (ejection fraction 0.5).[56] Pulmonary artery catheterization not only provides clinical indices that reflect intravascular volume, but also facilitates calculations of stroke volume, cardiac index, and left ventricular stroke work index. Myocardial ischemia can be detected by analysis of pulmonary artery catheter tracings. Finally, some pulmonary artery catheters allow for measurement of mixed venous oxygen saturation.

By detecting changes in ventricular wall motion, two-dimensional transesophageal echocardiography provides a sensitive method for assessing regional myocardial perfusion. Thys and associates[58] reported a positive correlation between hemodynamic indices obtained by invasive monitoring and those derived by two-dimensional echocardiography. Wall motion abnormalities also occur much sooner than electrocardiographic changes during periods of reduced coronary blood flow.[59] Because myocardial ischemia poses the greatest risk of mortality after abdominal aortic reconstruction, such a form of intraoperative monitoring may enable earlier detection and intervention during ischemic cardiac events.

Aortic Cross-Clamp Application

Abdominal aortic reconstruction may be one of the most challenging situations for the anesthetist. Patients with abdominal aortic aneurysms tend to be elderly and have varying degrees of coexisting disease. In addition to the risks associated with any major surgical procedure, these patients also experience physiologic changes that are specific to abdominal aortic aneurysmectomies. Perhaps the most dramatic physiologic change occurs with the application of an aortic cross-clamp. Temporary aortic occlusion produces various hemodynamic and metabolic alterations.

Hemodynamic Alterations

The hemodynamic effects of aortic cross-clamping depend on the application site along the aorta, the patient's preoperative cardiac reserve, and the patient's intravascular volume. The most common site for cross-clamping is infrarenal because most aneurysms appear below the level of the renal arteries. Less common sites of aneurysm development are the juxtarenal and suprarenal areas.

When aortic cross-clamping is used, hypertension occurs above the cross-clamp and hypotension occurs below the cross-clamp. Organs proximal to the aortic occlusion may experience a redistribution of blood volume.[32] There is an absence of blood flow distal to the clamp in the pelvis and lower extremities.[3] Increases in afterload cause myocardial wall tension to increase. Mean arterial pressure (MAP) and systemic vascular resistance (SVR) also increase. Cardiac output may decrease or remain unchanged. Pulmonary artery occlusion pressure (PAOP) may increase or display no change. Table 23-2 summarizes the cardiac function observed during aortic cross-clamping and release as measured by radionuclide angiography.

TABLE 23-2 Responses of 23 Patients Undergoing Abdominal Aortic Aneurysm Resection with Aortic Occlusion

	RESPONSE	
Parameter	**Application of Clamp**	**Release of Clamp**
LVEF	↓ (0.56-0.48)	↑ (0.51-0.58)
EDV	↑ (171-225 ml)	↓ (205-187 ml)
ESV	↑ (85-127 ml)	↓ (105-94 ml)
MAP	↑ (82-91 mm Hg)	↓ (84-69 mm Hg)
ESWS	↑ (53-67 10^3 dyne/cm^2)	↓ (67-46 10^3 dyne/cm^2)

↑, *Increased;* ↓, *decreased;* EDV, *end-diastolic volume;* ESV, *end-systolic volume;* ESWS, *end-systolic wall stress.* LVEF, *left ventricular ejection fraction;* MAP, *mean arterial pressure.*
Modified from Harpole DH, Clements FM, Quill T, Wolfe WG, Jones RH, McCann RL. Right and left ventricular performance during and after abdominal aortic aneurysm repair. Ann Surg. *1989;209:356-362.*

Table 23-3 lists the percentages of change in cardiovascular indexes at different levels of aortic occlusion.

Patients with adequate cardiac reserve commonly adjust to sudden increases in afterload without the occurrence of adverse cardiac events. However, patients with ischemic heart disease or ventricular dysfunction are unable to fully compensate as a result of the hemodynamic alterations. The increased wall stress attributed to aortic cross-clamp application may contribute to decreased global ventricular function and myocardial ischemia. Clinically, these patients experience increases in PAOP in response to aortic cross-clamping. Aggressive pharmacologic intervention is required for restoration of cardiac function during this time.

TABLE 23-3 Change in Cardiovascular Variables at Different Levels of Aortic Occlusion as Assessed by Two-Dimensional Transesophageal Echocardiography

	CHANGE AFTER OCCLUSION AT DIFFERENT LEVELS (PERCENT INCREASE OR DECREASE)		
Variable	**Infrarenal**	**Suprarenal Infraceliac**	**Supraceliac**
Mean arterial pressure	↑ 2	↑ 5	↑ 54
Pulmonary artery occlusion pressure	0	↑ 10	↑ 38
End-diastolic area	↑ 9	↑ 2	↑ 28
End-systolic area	↑ 11	↑ 10	↑ 69
Ejection fraction	↓ 3	↓ 10	↓ 38
Number of Patients Affected			
Patients with wall motion abnormality	0	33	92
New myocardial infarction	0	0	8

Modified from Roizen MF, Beaupre PN, Alpert RA, et al. Monitoring with two-dimensional transesophageal echocardiography: comparison of myocardial function in patients undergoing supraceliac, suprarenal-infraceliac, or infrarenal aortic occlusion. J Vasc Surg. *1984;1:300-305.*

Metabolic Alterations

After the application of an aortic cross-clamp, the lack of blood flow to distal structures makes these tissues prone to developing hypoxia. In response to hypoxia, metabolites, such as lactate, accumulate. Gelman and co-workers[33] demonstrated that the reduction in cardiac output during aortic cross-clamping might be partly the result of metabolic alterations, such as decreased oxygen consumption. Gold and co-workers[34] found that plasma catecholamine levels increase significantly during application of the aortic cross-clamp. Both epinephrine and norepinephrine stimulate myocardial β_1-receptors that can increase heart rate and increase myocardial oxygen demand.

The release of arachidonic acid derivatives may also contribute to the cardiac instability that is observed during aortic cross-clamping. Thromboxane A_2 synthesis, which is accelerated by the application of an aortic cross-clamp, may be responsible for the decrease in myocardial contractility and cardiac output that occurs. Numerous studies have attempted to determine if cyclooxygenase inhibition caused by the administration of aspirin or ibuprofen before elective aneurysmectomies can preserve myocardial function. Pretreatment with ibuprofen has been shown to have positive results; however, its effectiveness in stabilizing cardiac function remains unclear.[35,36]

Traction on the mesentery is a surgical maneuver used for exposing the aorta. Gottlieb and associates[37] and Seltzer and colleagues[38] described the mesenteric traction syndrome associated with this procedure. Decreases in blood pressure and SVR, tachycardia, increased cardiac output, and facial flushing are common responses to mesenteric traction. Although the cause of this syndrome is unknown, it has been associated with high concentrations of 6-ketoprostaglandin F_1, the stable metabolite of prostacyclin at the time of mesenteric traction.[37] The 6-ketoprostaglandin F_1 levels and hemodynamic stability returned to preclamp values as reperfusion occurs. Pretreatment with cyclooxygenase inhibitors may reduce the incidence of mesenteric traction syndrome, although the effectiveness of these agents remains unclear.

The neuroendocrine response to major surgical stress is believed to be mediated by cytokines such as interleukin (IL)-1B, IL-6, and tumor necrosis factor, as well as plasma catecholamines and cortisol.[39] These mediators are thought to be responsible for triggering the inflammatory response that results in increased body temperature, leukocytosis, tachycardia, tachypnea, and fluid sequestration. Norman and colleagues[40] demonstrated that patients who had an exaggerated plasma stress mediator release had longer operative and cross-clamp times and required a greater number of blood transfusions (see Table 23-3).

Effects on Regional Circulation

Structures distal to the aortic clamp are underperfused during aortic cross-clamping. Renal insufficiency and renal failure have been reported to occur after abdominal aortic reconstruction. Suprarenal and juxtarenal cross-clamping may be associated with a higher incidence of altered renal dynamics; however, reductions in renal blood flow can occur with any level of clamp application. Infrarenal aortic cross-clamping is associated with a 38% decrease in renal blood flow and a 75% increase in renal vascular resistance.[3] These effects may lead to acute renal failure, which is fatal in 50% to 90% of patients who have undergone aneurysmectomies.[41] Preoperative evaluation of renal function is one of the most significant predictors of postoperative renal dysfunction. Therefore a complete evaluation of renal function is required in the preoperative period.

Spinal cord damage is associated with aortic occlusion. Interruption of blood flow to the greater radicular artery (artery of Adamkiewicz) in the absence of collateral blood flow has been identified as a causative factor in paraplegia. The incidence of neurologic complications increases as the aortic cross-clamp is positioned in a higher or more proximal area. Somatosensory evoked potential (SSEP) monitoring has been advocated as a method of identifying spinal cord ischemia. However, SSEP monitoring reflects dorsal (sensory) spinal cord function and does not provide information regarding the integrity of the anterior (motor) spinal cord.[3] Motor evoked potential (MEP) monitoring is capable of determining anterior cord function but relies on intact neuromuscular function for analysis, which limits its use in abdominal aortic aneurysmectomies. Alternative methods for reliable evaluation of spinal cord ischemia are still under investigation.[42]

Ischemic colon injury is a well-documented complication that is associated with abdominal aortic resections. Ischemia of the colon is most frequently attributed to manipulation of the inferior mesenteric artery, which supplies the primary blood supply to the left colon. This vessel is often sacrificed during surgery, and blood flow to the descending and sigmoid colon depends on the presence and the adequacy of the collateral vessels. Mucosal ischemia occurs in 10% of patients who undergo abdominal aortic aneurysm repair. In less than 1% of these patients, infarction of the left colon necessitates surgical intervention.[41]

Aortic Cross-Clamp Release

While the aorta is occluded, metabolites that are liberated as a result of anaerobic metabolism, such as serum lactate, accumulate below the aortic cross-clamp and induce vasodilation and vasomotor paralysis. As the cross-clamp is released, SVR decreases, and blood is sequestered into previously dilated veins, which decreases venous return. Reactive hyperemia causes transient vasodilation secondary to the presence of tissue hypoxia, the release of adenine nucleotides,[41] and the liberation of an unnamed vasodepressor substance that acts as a myocardial depressant and a peripheral vasodilator.[43] This combination of events results in decreased preload and afterload. The hemodynamic instability that may ensue after the release of an aortic cross-clamp is called *declamping shock syndrome*.[43] Evidence demonstrates that venous endothelin (ET)-1 may be partially responsible for the hemodynamic alterations that accompany declamping shock syndrome. Venous ET-1 has a positive inotropic effect on the heart as well as a vasoconstricting and vasodilating action on blood vessels. Fukuda and colleagues[44] found that venous ET-1 is released in response to tissue ischemia, which is associated with the release of the aortic cross-clamp. Table 23-4 summarizes the most frequently observed hemodynamic responses to aortic declamping.

TABLE 23-4 Hemodynamic Consequences of Aortic Declamping

Clinical Indexes	Responses to Clamp Release
Mean arterial pressure	Decrease
Systemic vascular resistance	Decrease
Cardiac output	No change or increase
Pulmonary artery occlusion pressure	Decrease

The magnitude of the response to unclamping the aorta may be manipulated. Although SVR and MAP decrease, intravascular volume may influence the direction and the magnitude of change in cardiac output. Restoration of circulating blood volume is paramount in the provision of circulatory stability before release of the aortic clamp.[4,41,43-45] The site and the duration of cross-clamp application, as well as the gradual release of the clamp, influence the magnitude of circulatory instability.

Surgical Approach

The standard approach for elective abdominal aortic reconstruction is the transperitoneal incision. The advantages of this route include exposure of infrarenal and iliac vessels, ability to inspect intraabdominal organs, and rapid closure.[46] Unfavorable consequences associated with this approach include increased fluid losses, prolonged ileus, postoperative incisional pain, and pulmonary complications.

The retroperitoneal approach has gained popularity as an alternative to the standard route. Its advantages include excellent exposure (especially for juxtarenal and suprarenal aneurysms), decreased fluid losses, less incisional pain, and fewer postoperative pulmonary and intestinal complications.[46] In addition, the retroperitoneal approach does not elicit mesenteric traction syndrome.[46] The reported limitations of this approach are unfamiliarity of surgeons with this technique, poor right distal renal artery exposure, and inability to inspect abdominal contents. Table 23-5 compares these two surgical approaches.

Management of Fluid and Blood Loss

Extreme loss of extracellular fluid and blood should be expected with abdominal aortic aneurysmectomies. Evaporative losses and third spacing occur, with the magnitude of loss depending on the surgical approach, the duration of the surgery, and the experience of the surgeon. Most blood loss occurs because of back bleeding from the lumbar and inferior mesenteric arteries after the vessels have been clamped and the aneurysm is opened.[41,47] The use of heparin also contributes to blood loss. Excessive bleeding, however, can occur at any point during surgery, and blood replacement is commonly administered during abdominal aortic resections.

Because of the heightened awareness of transfusion-related morbidity, the use of autologous blood has generated increasing interest. Presently, three options are available for the use of autologous transfusions: preoperative deposit, intraoperative phlebotomy and hemodilution, and intraoperative blood salvage. Preoperative deposit is becoming more feasible because asymptomatic aneurysms are being detected with greater frequency. Ideally, patients donate their own blood in order to minimize the intraoperative use of homologous blood products and the subsequent risk of transfusion-related viruses. Autotransfusion systems may be used for replacement of intraoperative blood loss. In a study at the Mayo Clinic in which intraoperative autologous red-cell salvage was used, 75% less banked blood was transfused.[47] In a prospective study of 100 patents who underwent elective abdominal aortic resections, 80% of the patients received only their own blood.[47]

Presence of Concurrent Disease

Preoperative Management

The presence of underlying coronary artery disease (CAD) in patients with vascular disease has been well documented. CAD is reported to occur in more than 50% of patients who require abdominal aortic reconstruction and is the single most significant risk factor influencing long-term survivability.[4,5,11,48,49] Myocardial infarctions are responsible for 40% to 70% of all fatalities that occur after aneurysm reconstruction.[4,5,20,49] In the presence of such threatening mortality rates the extent of CAD and the subsequent functional limitations must be clearly defined and cardiac function optimized preoperatively before elective aortic vascular reconstruction is performed.

Preoperative cardiac evaluation begins with the identification of risk factors that may contribute to adverse cardiac events and subsequent death. When preoperative CAD exists, an increased incidence of postoperative adverse cardiac complications has been demonstrated.[50] Goldman and co-workers[51] described the cardiac risk index, which is used to predict the likelihood of adverse cardiac complications and death in patients undergoing noncardiac surgery. Advanced age, cardiac history, aberrations on physical examination, electrocardiographic abnormalities, and previous surgical procedures are identifiable factors in the cardiac risk index that contribute to

TABLE 23-5 Comparison of Transperitoneal and Retroperitoneal Approaches

Transperitoneal	Retroperitoneal
Advantages	
Familiarity	Exposure for juxtarenal and suprarenal aneurysms
Access to infrarenal aorta and iliac vessels	Decreased fluid loss
Visualization of intraabdominal viscera	Improved postoperative respiratory function
Rapid opening and closure	Better-tolerated incisional pain avoids formation of intraabdominal adhesions
Versatility	Mesenteric traction syndrome, non-elicited
Disadvantages	
Increased fluid losses	Inaccessibility to distal right renal artery complications
Less postoperative ileus	
More frequent postoperative respiratory complications	
Increased postoperative incisional pain	

Modified from Sicard GA, Allen BT, Munn JS, et al. Retroperitoneal versus transperitoneal approach of repair of abdominal aortic aneurysms. Surg Clin North Am. *1989;69:795-806.*

cardiac complications. Cooperman and associates[52] used similar risk factors, which include angina, congestive heart failure, dysrhythmias, myocardial infarction, cerebrovascular accidents, and abnormal electrocardiograph findings to derive an equation for computing the possibility of cardiac complications in patients undergoing vascular surgery. Although the reliability of multivariate risk factor analysis in the prediction of adverse cardiac events has been disputed, these systems are applicable to all patients and can serve as the initial evaluation of cardiac risk for patients undergoing elective aneurysmectomies.

Initially, controversy existed regarding which diagnostic modality should be used in the evaluation of patients undergoing elective vascular surgery. Patients with unremarkable medical histories and normal physical examinations, exercise testing, electrocardiography, and laboratory studies have a decreased surgical risk. Some centers advocated the use of routine coronary angiography in all candidates for elective aortic revascularization.[53] This was the experience at the Cleveland Clinic until more recent studies suggested that this method had little influence on surgical outcomes. Currently, investigators advocate the use of coronary angiography in selected patients who have positive findings on the initial cardiac evaluation.[5,11,48]

Patients with symptomatic CAD require more extensive cardiac evaluation. Dipyridamole thallium testing is perhaps one of the most reliable methods for evaluating the extent of myocardial dysfunction associated with CAD and for predicting coronary events after vascular surgery.[3,13,20,54] In addition to its sensitivity in detection of myocardial dysfunction, dipyridamole thallium testing does not rely on exercise for detection of areas of myocardial hypoperfusion. Techniques capable of evaluating left ventricular performance, such as echocardiography, are of some value in the prediction of adverse cardiac events. Ambulatory electrocardiographic monitoring has also been very successful in the identification of postoperative cardiac complications.[55] Finally, coronary angiography provides the most reliable definition of coronary anatomy and the extent of CAD.

The endpoint of any method of preoperative cardiac evaluation for aneurysmectomy is identification of functional cardiac limitations. Depending on the degree of cardiac dysfunction, preoperative optimization of cardiac function may range from simple pharmacologic manipulation to surgical intervention. Some centers advocate the use of cardiac revascularization for reversible CAD before abdominal aortic aneurysm repair is performed and demonstrate reduced mortality rates for elective aneurysmectomies.[5,21,53] On the other hand, the risk associated with cardiac revascularization and the potential for aneurysmal rupture add credibility to approaches that proceed to aneurysmectomies in patients with reversible CAD.[11] Percutaneous transluminal coronary angioplasty may provide an alternative method of restoring oxygen supply to the myocardium; however, the advantages of this technique have not been established. Figure 23-1 is an algorithm for the evaluation and treatment of CAD for patients with abdominal aortic aneurysms.

Hypertension, chronic obstructive pulmonary disease, diabetes mellitus, renal impairment, and carotid artery disease are frequently observed in patients with abdominal aortic aneurysms. Table 23-6 lists the frequency rates of coexisting disease in patients who require abdominal aortic aneurysm repair. Each of these disease entities deserves attention in the preoperative period. Measures must be taken to optimize organ function, because each of these disease states contributes to postoperative complications. Preoperative renal dysfunction deserves special consideration because aortic cross-clamping produces alterations in renal dynamics. The degree of preoperative renal insufficiency contributes to the extent of any postoperative renal damage.[41]

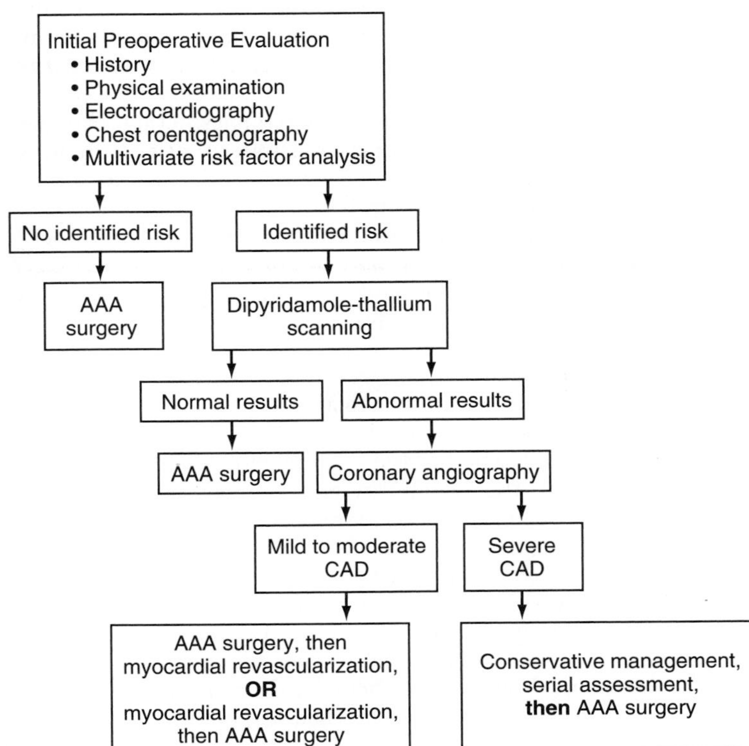

FIGURE **23-1**
Algorithm for patient management and surgical selection for abdominal aortic aneurysm (AAA) resection. *CAD*, Coronary artery disease.

TABLE 23-6 Occurrence of Coexisting Disease in Abdominal Aortic Resections

Disease	Percent of Patients
Hypertension	50-60
Heart disease	40-50
Chronic obstructive pulmonary disease	25-50
Diabetes mellitus	9-12
Renal impairment	5-17
Carotid artery disease	6-16

Data from Graor RA. Preoperative evaluation and management of coronary and carotid artery occlusive disease in patients with abdominal aortic aneurysms. Surg Clin North Am. *1989;69:737-743; and Cunningham AJ. Anesthesia for abdominal aortic surgery. I: a review.* Can J Anaesth. *1989;36:426-444.*

Intraoperative Management

Anesthetic Selection

Many anesthetic techniques are available for abdominal aortic resections. Although each technique has its advantages and disadvantages, a superior technique has not been identified. The anesthetic selection should be based on the following objectives: provision of analgesia and amnesia, facilitation of relaxation, maintenance of hemodynamic stability, and minimization of morbidity and mortality.

Inhalation Agents

Circulatory stability is desirable for patients undergoing abdominal aortic aneurysm reconstruction, especially for those with CAD. All inhalation anesthetics may depress the myocardium and cause hemodynamic instability. Potential organ toxicity and lack of postoperative analgesia may be additional limitations to the use of these agents. Beneficial effects attributed to the use of inhalation agents include the ability to alter autonomic responses, reversibility, rapid emergence, and potentially earlier extubation.

Narcotic Technique

A balanced technique using a combination of high-dose narcotics with nitrous oxide can be used as the anesthetic for major vascular surgery. The cardiovascular stability provided by opioids has been well documented, and this feature is especially attractive for patients with ischemic heart disease and ventricular dysfunction. Provision of intense analgesia for the initial postoperative period after major abdominal vascular surgery, via the administration of neuraxial opioid, does not alter the combined incidence of major cardiovascular, respiratory, and renal complications.[60]

Regional Anesthesia

The use of epidural anesthesia for abdominal aneurysmectomies has gained renewed interest. Hessel[45] and Yeager and co-workers[61] identified several benefits of epidural use, including decreased preload and afterload, preserved myocardial oxygenation, reduced stress response, excellent muscle relaxation, decreased incidence of postoperative thromboembolism, and increased graft flow to the lower extremities. However, Underwood and associates[9] reported more postoperative complications in the epidural group than in the general anesthetic group in 66 elderly patients who underwent vascular surgery.

Hypotension may also be a significant unfavorable result of an epidural technique. In fact, this technique requires the administration of approximately 1600 to 2000 ml more intravenous fluid than is usual with general anesthetic.[45] The controversy regarding hematoma formation after heparinization during epidural techniques is still noteworthy. Rao and El-Etr[62] investigated the neurologic consequences of 3164 epidural anesthetics and 847 subarachnoid blocks; only 20 patients experienced neurologic complications, all of which were self-limiting and resolved with time, demonstrating that the simultaneous use of epidural anesthesia and low-dose heparinization rarely produces complications.

Postoperative pain control is vital in order to maintain hemodynamic stability and to alleviate patient suffering. Epidural narcotics have been shown to decrease pain after major surgery.[63] Because of the high incidence of CAD in patients presenting for abdominal aortic reconstruction, severe postoperative pain can result in increased heart rate and blood pressure, which may contribute to cardiac-related morbidity and mortality. Pain relief may decrease respiratory splinting and decrease the likelihood of hypoxemia.[64]

Combination Techniques

Combining anesthetic techniques for major vascular surgery is more popular than using them alone because the advantages of each technique contribute to a smoother anesthetic. A balanced technique supplemented by low-dose inhalation agents maintains cardiovascular hemodynamics and controls momentary autonomic responses to surgical stimulation. Similarly, epidural anesthesia combined with light general anesthesia provides the benefits of epidural anesthesia plus the ability to provide amnesia and controlled ventilation.

A combined spinal and epidural anesthetic has been used successfully for infrarenal abdominal aortic aneurysmectomy using an endovascular approach. Aadahl and associates[65] found that a lumbar epidural catheter at L2-L3 followed by a spinal block at L3-L4 using isobaric bupivacaine provided excellent muscle relaxation and hemodynamic stability during surgery. These patients were able to ambulate after the first postoperative day.

In summary, all the aforementioned anesthetic techniques can be used safely and can demonstrate positive outcomes. More important than the anesthetic selection is the clinical management of each patient. Observation, accurate interpretation, and immediate intervention during the anesthetic process reduce morbidity and mortality to a much larger extent than does selection of the superior anesthetic technique.

Fluid Management

The maintenance of intravascular volume may be an extreme challenge during abdominal aortic resections. Controversy exists regarding whether the administration of crystalloids or colloids affects the overall incidence of morbidity and mortality. Crystalloids may be used for replacing basal and third-space losses at an approximate rate of 10 ml/kg/hr.[45] Blood losses initially can be replaced with crystalloids at a ratio of 3:1. The combination of crystalloid and colloid administration is also acceptable. Regardless of the choice of fluid, volume replacement must be dictated by physiologic parameters. Fluid replacement should be sufficient for the maintenance of normal cardiac filling pressures, cardiac output, and urine output of 1 ml/kg/hr.[4]

Hemodynamic Alterations

Hemodynamic changes are likely to occur throughout the anesthesia process. Adequate preoperative sedation should be given before placement of invasive monitoring equipment. Momentary fluctuations in heart rate and blood pressure should be anticipated during induction and intubation. Preoperative replacement of fluid deficits prevents exaggerated responses to vasodilating induction agents. For patients with adequate left ventricular function, hemodynamic stability can be preserved with a "slow" induction using opioids and β-adrenergic blocking agents. The response to mesenteric traction (discussed previously in this chapter) is also associated with momentary hemodynamic changes.

Application of the aortic cross-clamp produces various hemodynamic responses. Patients without underlying ischemic heart disease usually demonstrate slight changes in PAOP when the aorta is occluded, requiring minimal intervention. However, patients with a history of CAD may experience an increase in PAOP and a decrease in cardiac output, indicating left ventricular decompensation. Although several different pharmacologic agents may be used, nitroglycerin appears to be the drug of choice because of its primary pharmacologic effect of decreasing preload and thereby decreasing myocardial oxygen demand .[4,45] Inotropic agents, such as dopamine and dobutamine, may improve cardiac output, whereas pharmacologic agents that decrease afterload, such as sodium nitroprusside and isoflurane, may decrease SVR. The more proximal the application of the aortic cross-clamp, the greater the magnitude and the severity of these responses.

When the aortic cross-clamp is released, declamping shock syndrome may occur. Severe hypotension and reduction in cardiac output may ensue. These conditions can be prevented by volume loading and raising of the central venous pressure 3 to 5 mm Hg[4] or raising the PAOP 3 to 4 mm Hg[4,36,45] just before the clamp is released. If severe acidosis is present, sodium bicarbonate may be administered.[45] Temporarily increasing minute ventilation may also be useful for the control of acidosis.

Renal Preservation

Alterations in renal dynamics during intrarenal cross-clamping may continue up to 1 hour after the clamp is released. Such alterations can be profound and can extend into the postoperative period. Mechanisms for the preservation of renal function during aortic cross-clamping include maintenance of cardiac output and intravascular volume. Prevention of hypovolemia is the best prophylaxis against renal failure.[4] Administration of mannitol 20 to 30 minutes before aortic clamping may help preserve renal function.[3,45] Further intervention includes intravenous administration of low-dose dopamine at 3 to 5 mcg/kg/min and use of loop diuretics.[45]

Postoperative Considerations

Cardiac, respiratory, and renal failure are the most common complications observed postoperatively in patients recovering from abdominal aortic reconstruction. Cardiovascular function must be closely monitored in the intensive care unit (ICU) for at least 24 hours after surgery. Maintenance of adequate blood pressure, intravascular fluid volume, and myocardial oxygenation is paramount during this period. Because myocardial infarction so often contributes to postoperative morbidity and mortality, serial cardiac enzyme analysis may be justified. Pharmacologic agents used in the treatment of hypertension must also be available.

Most patients require ventilatory assistance during the postoperative period. Vigilant monitoring of respiratory function is mandatory, especially when epidural catheters are used for postoperative analgesia. Yeager and colleagues[61] demonstrated fewer postoperative complications and improved pain control when epidural analgesia was provided postoperatively.

Finally, renal function must be continuously evaluated in the postoperative phase. Urine output should be maintained at 1 ml/kg/hr. Administration of fluid, maintenance of physiologic hemodynamics, and concurrent administration of pharmacologic agents should be considered for the improvement of urinary output.

Juxtarenal and Suprarenal Aortic Aneurysms

Although most abdominal aortic aneurysms occur below the level of the renal arteries, 2% extend proximally and involve the renal or visceral arteries.[13,14] Juxtarenal aneurysms are located at the level of the renal arteries, but they spare the renal artery orifice. More proximal suprarenal aneurysms include at least one of the renal arteries and may involve visceral vessels. The effects of aortic cross-clamping for juxtarenal or suprarenal aneurysms are similar to those for infrarenal aortic occlusions; however, the magnitude of hemodynamic alterations increases as the aorta is clamped more proximally.

Preoperative preparation includes a thorough evaluation of coexisting disease, with an emphasis on cardiac function. As the aorta is clamped more proximally, left ventricular afterload increases, and, consequently, myocardial ischemia is more likely to occur.[15] Diligent cardiac monitoring is necessary, and direct intraarterial blood pressure assessment, cardiac filling pressure monitoring, and transesophageal echocardiography are advocated in order to detect cardiac dysfunction and allow for immediate pharmacologic intervention.

Renal failure, although possible during infrarenal aortic cross-clamping, occurs more frequently as a result of suprarenal aortic occlusion. Maintaining adequate intravascular volume and administering osmotic and loop diuretics may minimize renal ischemia and dysfunction. If the ischemic episode persists for longer than 45 minutes, renal cooling is suggested. Renal cooling consists of flushing the kidney with an iced electrolyte perfusate that contains heparin and glucose.[14,41]

Paraplegia is possible when the blood supply to the spinal cord is interrupted by aortic cross-clamping at or above the level of the diaphragm. Increasing the MAP or decreasing the cerebrospinal fluid (CSF) pressure may be used as a means to increase spinal cord perfusion pressure.[4,13,14] Box 23-3 summarizes the complications that may result from juxtarenal or suprarenal aortic occlusion.

Ruptured Abdominal Aortic Aneurysm

A high mortality rate of up to 94% is associated with a ruptured abdominal aortic aneurysm.[15,16,25] A wide range of morbidity rates has been reported. One explanation for the discrepancies may be the parameters used for the definition of "rupture." Centers that have reported lower mortality rates may not be truly assessing rupture as intraperitoneal hemorrhage. Rutherford and McCroskey[26] attempted to identify mortality rates related to hemodynamic status. Their results are summarized in Table 23-7. This information further demonstrates the need for earlier detection of aneurysms and aggressive surgical intervention.

BOX 23-3

Potential Complications of Juxtarenal or Suprarenal Aortic Occlusion

- Renal failure
- Hemorrhage
- Distal arterial occlusion
- Infarction
- Pulmonary or cardiac dysfunction
- Impotence
- Paraplegia
- Thrombosis
- Pseudoaneurysm formation
- Aortoenteric fistula

From Hollier LH, Moore WM. Surgical management of juxtarenal and suprarenal aortic aneurysms. Acta Chir Scand. *1990;555(suppl):117-122.*

TABLE 23-7 Mortality Rates for Ruptured Aortic Aneurysms Related to Hemodynamic Status at Time of Presentation

Hemodynamic Status	Mortality Rate (%)
Normal blood pressure	20
Hypotensive, but responding to resuscitation	40
Hypotensive, incompletely responding to resuscitation	60
Hypotension recurs with induction (unstable), incompletely responding to resuscitation	60
Hypotension recurs with induction (unstable), no urinary output	80

Data from Rutherford RB, McCroskey BL. Ruptured abdominal aortic aneurysms. Surg Clin North Am. *1989;69:859-868.*

The most common symptoms of ruptured abdominal aortic aneurysms are abdominal discomfort with a pulsatile mass, back pain, and hypotension.[24,26,66] Hypotension and a history of cardiac disease are two factors associated with the poorest prognosis.[12,25] Patients with these symptoms should be immediately transferred to the operating room for surgical exploration. When hypotension is absent, more time is available for a comprehensive CT scan to search for other causes of abdominal discomfort. Figure 23-2 provides a plan for the evaluation and treatment of the patient with a symptomatic but unruptured aneurysm.

Once the patient arrives in the operative suite, a brief preoperative evaluation, the establishment of venous access, and provisions for fluid and blood product administration can be completed. Induction of anesthesia should follow the principles of trauma anesthesia. Hemodynamic stability must be the primary objective, and anesthetic induction and maintenance agents must be selected on a case-by-case basis.

Cardiovascular resuscitation is the anesthetist's primary focus until blood loss from the proximal aorta is controlled by surgical intervention. Fluid resuscitation can begin with crystalloids, and blood products can be administered as they become available. Intraoperative blood salvage provisions should be secured. If large amounts of blood products are given, coagulation studies and ionized calcium values should be calculated. The use of fresh frozen plasma has been shown to decrease the total transfusion requirements and the incidence of coagulopathies.[12] The ability to administer platelets may also be necessary.

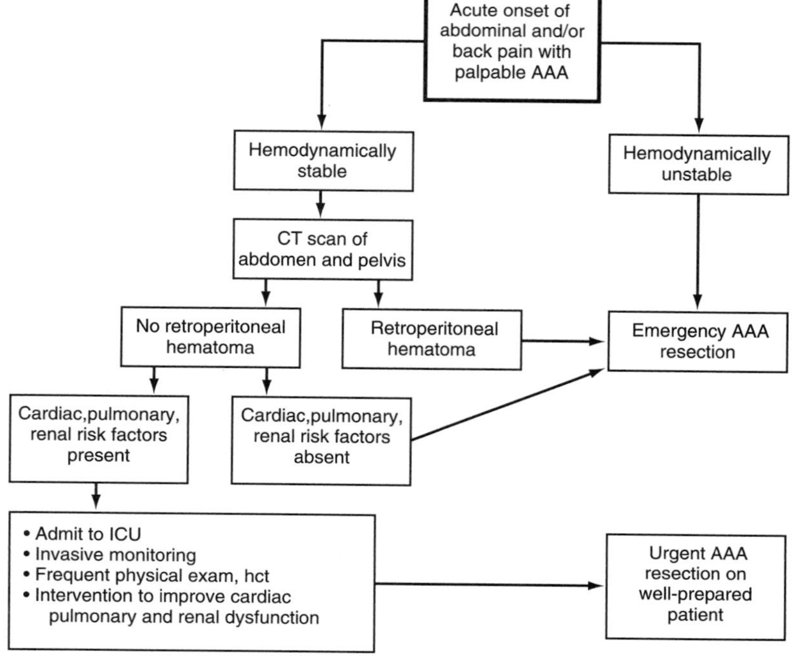

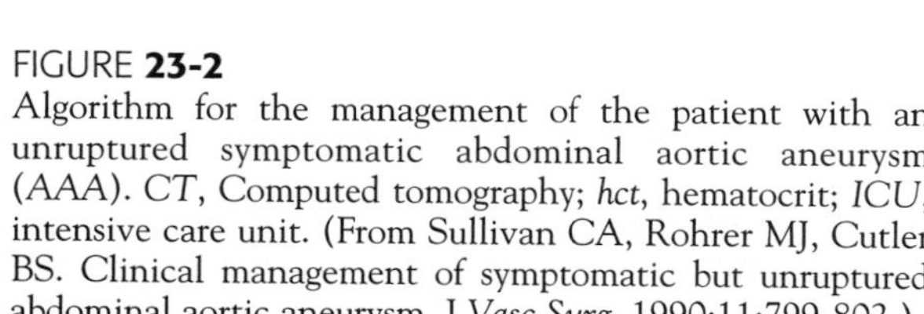
FIGURE **23-2**
Algorithm for the management of the patient with an unruptured symptomatic abdominal aortic aneurysm (AAA). *CT*, Computed tomography; *hct*, hematocrit; *ICU*, intensive care unit. (From Sullivan CA, Rohrer MJ, Cutler BS. Clinical management of symptomatic but unruptured abdominal aortic aneurysm. *J Vasc Surg.* 1990;11:799-802.)

After initial resuscitation has been performed and hemodynamic stability has been ensured, direct arterial blood pressure monitoring must be instituted. A central venous or pulmonary artery catheter may be inserted. The hemodynamic effects of aortic cross-clamping and release are similar to those for elective surgery; however, responses may be extreme, especially if hypotension exists when the clamp is released. Measures for ensuring the adequacy of renal circulation, such as administering mannitol, should be incorporated. Because most patients require large amounts of fluid and blood replacement, postoperative mechanical ventilation is recommended.

THORACIC AORTIC ANEURYSMS

The mortality associated with thoracic aneurysms is well established. Patients with aortic dissections have only a 3-month survival if they do not undergo surgical repair, because the incidence of rupture is high.[67] Aneurysms have been described in the literature for hundreds of years, but not until 1951 did the development of the arterial prosthesis lead to successful bypass options.[68] The refinement of synthetic grafts, surgical and perfusion techniques, and intraoperative management has contributed to improved surgical outcomes. Today the early mortality rate is thought to be less than 10%, demonstrating that elective surgical intervention is an acceptable means of treating thoracic aortic aneurysms.[69,70]

Classification

Aneurysms of the thoracic aorta may be classified with respect to type, shape, and location. Typically, aneurysms involving all three layers of the arterial wall, tunica adventitia, tunica media, and tunica intima, are considered to be *true aneurysms*. In comparison, aneurysms that solely involve the adventitia are termed *false aneurysms*. The shape of the lesion can also serve as a means of characterizing aneurysms. Fusiform aneurysms have a spindle shape and result in dilation of the aorta. Saccular aneurysms are spherical dilations and are generally limited to only one segment of the vessel wall. Aortic dissection is the result of a spontaneous tear within the intima that permits the flow of blood through a false passage along the longitudinal axis of the aorta. Aneurysms can also be classified according to their location within the aortic arch, as illustrated in Figure 23-3. In addition, thoracoabdominal aneurysms can be classified into four types on the basis of their location, as shown in Figure 23-4.

Etiology

Atherosclerosis is the most common cause of aneurysmal pathology. Atherosclerotic lesions occur most often in the descending and distal thoracic aorta and are most often classified as fusiform. Less common causes include the histologic contributions of cystic medial necrosis observed in patients with Marfan's syndrome, infective and inflammatory processes within the vessel wall, and Takayasu's arteritis.[71,72] Finally, aneurysms that were once related to syphilitic aortitis are now rarely observed, as a result of the advent of early diagnosis and treatment of syphilis. The various causes of arterial aneurysms are classified in Box 23-4.

Diagnosis

The symptomatology of thoracic aneurysms is often related to the site of the lesion and its compression on adjacent structures. Pain, stridor, and cough may result from compression of thoracic structures. Symptoms related to aortic insufficiency may be observed in aneurysms of the ascending aorta. An upper mediastinal mass may be an incidental finding on conventional chest radiography in an asymptomatic patient. Further investigation with noninvasive methods, such as CT scan and MRI, can describe the configuration and location of the aneurysm. Invasive aortography, although associated with a higher risk of complications, provides the most information,

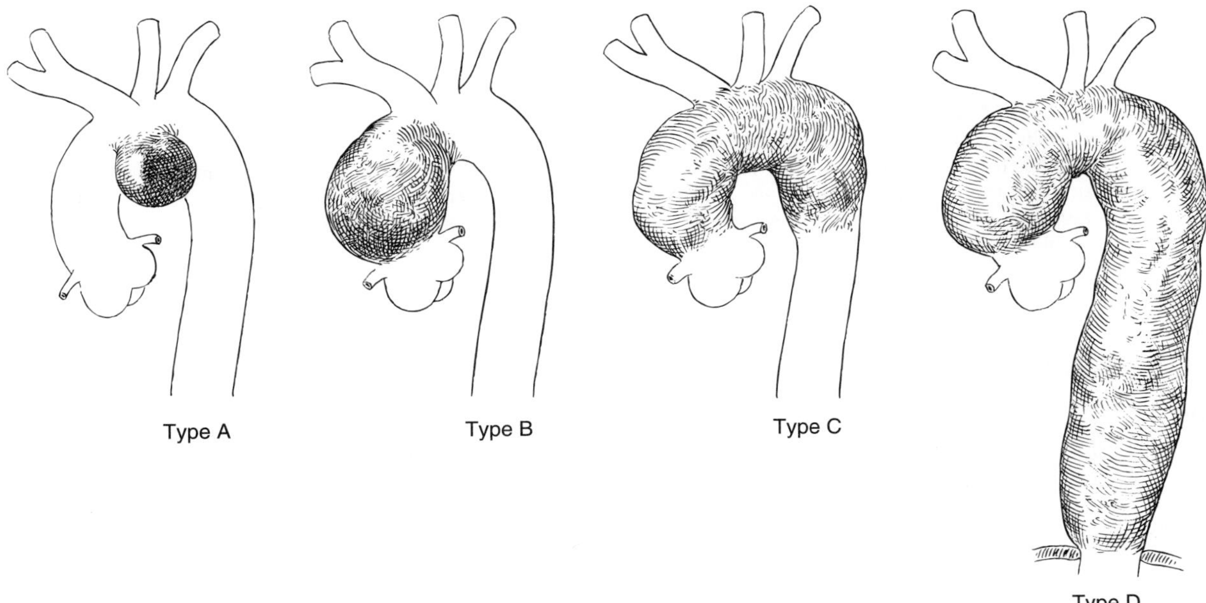

FIGURE **23-3**
Cooley classification of aortic arch aneurysms. *Type A*, Saccular transverse arch. *Type B*, Fusiform ascending aorta and proximal arch. *Type C*, Fusiform aneurysm extending into the proximal aorta. *Type D*, Fusiform aneurysm involving the entire aorta.

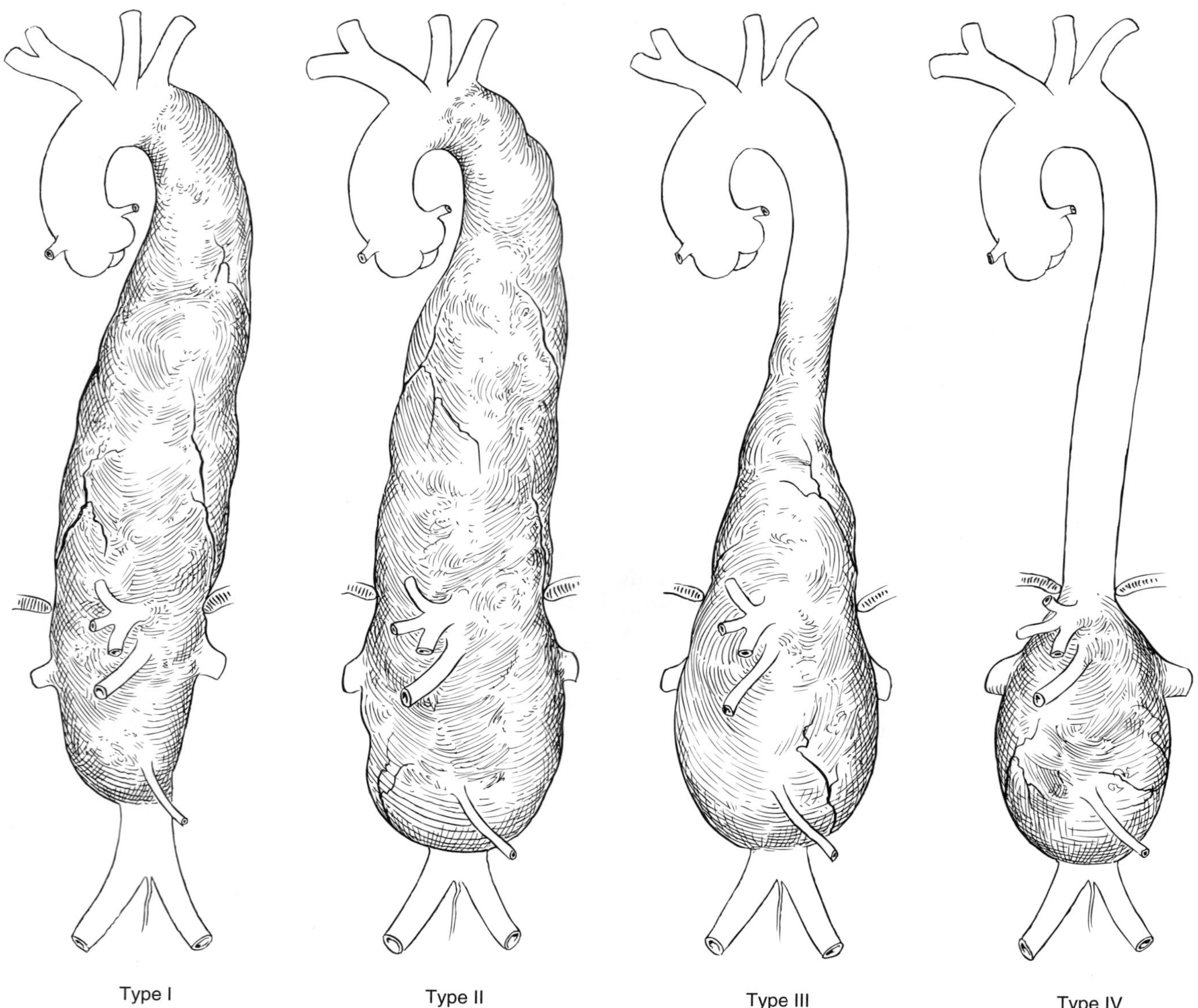

FIGURE **23-4**
Classification of thoracoabdominal aneurysms. *Type I*, Begins distal to the subclavian artery and extends to involve visceral artery orifices. *Type II*, Involves most of the descending aorta and most or all of the abdominal aorta. *Type III*, Involves the distal descending thoracic aorta and varying segments of the abdominal aorta. *Type IV*, Involves most or all of the abdominal aorta, including segments of visceral vessel origins.

because it allows evaluation of the coronary vessels and branches of the aortic arch.

Treatment

As previously described, a high mortality rate is associated with a rupture of thoracic aneurysms. Crawford and DeNatale[73] investigated the survival of 94 patients who did not undergo surgery for thoracoabdominal aneurysms. The investigators reported that only 24% of the patients survived 2 years after detection of the lesion and that 50% of the deaths were the result of aortic rupture. Therefore early detection and surgical intervention have made a significant contribution to long-term survival.

Surgical approach and mode of resection vary according to the location of the lesion within the thoracic aorta. Resection of the ascending aorta and graft replacement necessitate the use of cardiopulmonary bypass. The aortic valve may also require replacement. Surgical resection of lesions in the transverse arch compromises cerebral perfusion, although various bypass techniques combined with profound hypothermia and circulatory arrest have been used.[74] Aneurysms of the descending aorta may be resected by application of an aortic cross-clamp. However, perfusion to distal organs can be compromised during this procedure.

ENDOVASCULAR AORTIC ANEURYSM REPAIR

Over the last decade a new and less invasive approach to aortic aneurysm repair has been established. Endovascular aortic aneurysm repair involves deployment of an endovascular

BOX 23-4

Classification of Arterial Aneurysms by Cause

Congenital (Developmental)
Ehlers-Danlos syndrome
Marfan's syndrome

Mechanical (Hemodynamic)
Poststenotic
Arteriovenous fistula-associated

Traumatic
Blunt or penetrating trauma

Inflammatory (Noninfectious)
Takayasu's disease
Behçet's disease
Kawasaki's disease
Microvascular disorder (e.g., polyarteritis)
Periarterial inflammatory disease (e.g., pancreatitis)

Infectious
Bacterial
Fungal
Spirochetal

Degenerative
Nonspecific (commonly considered arteriosclerotic), dysplastic

Anastomosis
Postarteriotomy

Adapted from Johnston KW, Rutherford RB, Tilson MD, Shah DM, Hollier L, Stanley JC. Suggested standards for reporting on arterial aneurysms: Subcommittee on Reporting Standards for Arterial Aneurysms, Ad Hoc Committee on Reporting Standards, Society for Vascular Surgery and North American Chapter, International Society for Cardiovascular Surgery. J Vasc Surg. *1992;13:452-458.*

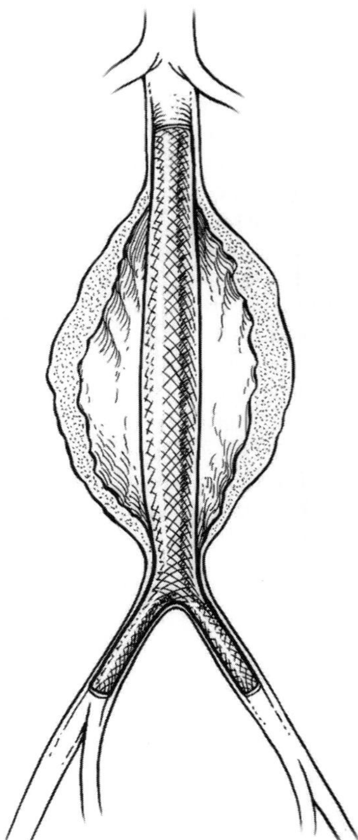

FIGURE **23-5**
Aortic endovascular graft.

stent graft within the aortic lumen. The graft restricts blood flow to the portion or the aorta in which the aneurysm exists. This procedure can be performed for patients who have descending thoracic aortic aneurysms or abdominal aortic aneurysms. Cannulation of both femoral arteries is performed. A guide wire is threaded through the iliac artery to the level of the aneurysm. Next a sheath is inserted over the guide wire and positioned at the aneurysm location through use of fluoroscopy. The proximal end of the sheath must extend beyond the aneurysm. The graft is composed of a Dacron skin that surrounds a stainless steel skeleton. Once the sheath is deployed, hooks on the sheath become embedded into the aortic wall in order to prevent migration. See Figure 23-5.

Endovascular abdominal aortic aneurysm repair was initially intended for patients with severe coexisting disease, however, its popularity has increased as the success of the procedure has improved. Neuroaxial blockade or local anesthesia and sedation are techniques that are commonly employed.[75] In addition, the procedure frequently takes place in an interventional radiology suite. Thoracic aortic aneurysm repair requires general anesthesia, and the procedure is performed in the operating room. Advantages of the endovascular approach as compared with the conventional surgical method include improved hemodynamic stability, decreased incidence of embolic events, reduced stress response, decreased incidence of renal dysfunction, and decreased postoperative discomfort.[76,77] Plasma catecholamine concentrations and mediators of the systemic immune response were decreased in patients who underwent the endovascular approach as compared with those in patients who underwent the conventional repair.[78,79] A serious complication that can occur as a result of this procedure is termed *endoleak*, defined as blood flow between the endovascular graft and the aortic aneurysm. This complication has been reported to occur in 15% to 52% of patients as diagnosed by postoperative CT scan.[80] Other complications that can arise as a result of endovascular aortic aneurysm repair include endograft thrombosis, migration or rupture, graft infection, iliac artery rupture, and lower extremity ischemia.[81] Long-term results of endovascular aortic aneurysm repair have demonstrated that this procedure yields good results, but the overall durability of conventional surgical techniques is superior.[82]

In the future minimally invasive aortic aneurysm surgery will continue to be used. Improvements in surgical techniques, imaging, and graft devices will allow a greater number of patients to experience the technical and physiologic advantages of endovascular aortic aneurysm repair.

AORTIC DISSECTION

As mentioned previously, aortic dissection is characterized by a spontaneous tear of the vessel wall intima, which permits the passage of blood along a false lumen. Although the cause of the dissection is unclear, lesions that were thought to be related to cystic necrotic processes may actually be caused by variations in wall integrity. Hypertension is the most common factor that contributes to the progression of the lesion. Manipulation of the ascending aorta during cardiac surgery may be associated with aortic dissection.[83] The symptoms of aortic dissection are the result of the interruption of blood supply to vital organs. The most serious complication is aneurysm rupture. Diagnosis can be accomplished by the previously mentioned noninvasive techniques; however, aortography appears to be most reliable. Simon and associates[84] evaluated the efficacy of transesophageal echocardiography as a diagnostic tool for the detection and analysis of aortic dissections in 32 patients. The authors concluded that this bedside modality allows for the reliable, expedient diagnosis and classification of thoracic lesions, thereby allowing urgent surgical intervention.

Treatment of dissecting aortic lesions depends on their location within the thoracic aorta. Figure 23-6 illustrates the location of dissecting aortic lesions. Type A lesions have the highest incidence of rupture and require immediate surgical intervention. Type B lesions may initially be managed medically, with the administration of arterial dilating and β-adrenergic blocking agents. However, some authors suggest that surgical intervention contributes to an improved long-term survival rate.[60] Studies have shown a survival rate of 94% to 95% for repair of dissecting aortic aneurysm by investigators using the newer techniques.[60,85]

In summary, surgical resection of thoracic aortic lesions enhances long-term survival. As a result of the refinement of surgical techniques and the improvement in perfusion technology, mortality rates of less than 10% have been demonstrated. The surgical method used is dependent on the location of the aortic lesion. Anesthesia for aneurysms of the ascending and transverse aorta requires cardiopulmonary bypass.

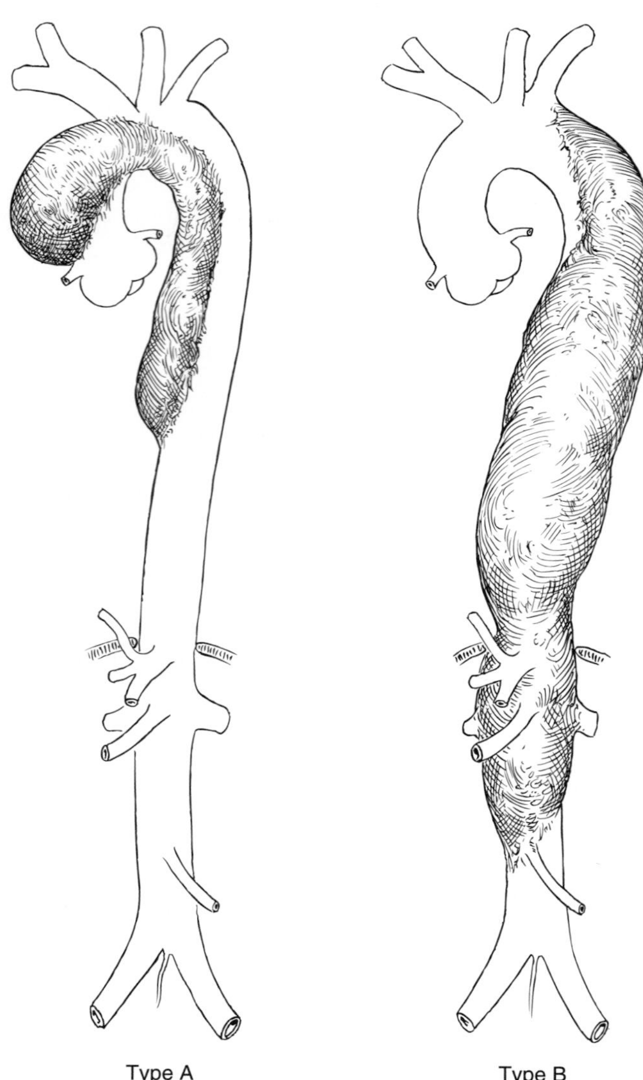

FIGURE **23-6**
Types of aortic dissection. Type A involves the ascending aorta and may extend into the aortic arch. Type B starts at the proximal descending aorta and extends distally.

DESCENDING THORACIC AND THORACOABDOMINAL ANEURYSMS

Preoperative Management

Assessment

Patients who undergo major vascular surgery are frequently elderly and have varying degrees of concurrent disease. Crawford and colleagues[70] described the frequency with which atherosclerotic occlusive disease, heart disease, chronic obstructive pulmonary disease, hypertension, and renal insufficiency occurred in 605 patients who had thoracic aortic aneurysms. In this study advancing age, chronic obstructive pulmonary disease, renal artery occlusive disease, atherosclerotic heart disease, and renal insufficiency were associated with diseases that most often contributed to early death. Hollier and Moore[86] identified risk factors associated with thoracoabdominal aneurysms in a smaller group consisting of 101 patients. Risk factors identified for patients undergoing thoracoabdominal aneurysmectomies are listed in Table 23-8.

The importance of a thorough preoperative evaluation cannot be overemphasized in this patient population. Special

TABLE **23-8** Risk Factors Identified in 101 Patients Undergoing Thoracoabdominal Aneurysm Repair

Risk Factors	Incidence (%)
Smoking history	90
Coronary artery disease	67
Chronic lung disease	42
Renal insufficiency	38
Strokes or transient ischemic attacks	12
Diabetes mellitus	6

Adapted from Hollier LH, Moore WM. Avoidance of renal and neurologic complications following thoracoabdominal aortic aneurysm repair. Acta Chir Scand. *1990;55(suppl):129-135.*

TABLE 23-9 Early Causes of Death in 54 Patients after Thoracoabdominal Aneurysm Repair

Cause	Incidence (%)
Cardiac	44
Renal	37
Pulmonary	18
Sepsis	19
Stroke	9
Hemorrhage	9
Pulmonary embolus	7
Gastrointestinal bleeding	7

Modified from Hollier LH, Symmonds JB, Pairolero PC, Cherry KJ, Hallett JW, Gloviczki P. Thoracoabdominal aortic aneurysm repair: analysis of postoperative morbidity. Arch Surg. *1988;123:871-875.*

attention should be directed toward cardiac, renal, and neurologic function. Although most fatalities related to thoracic aortic surgery are cardiac in origin, renal and neurologic dysfunction contribute to poor surgical outcomes.[70] Table 23-9 lists the causes of early death after thoracoabdominal aneurysm repair. Preoperative renal dysfunction is directly related to postoperative renal failure and is thought to be one of the strongest contributors to renal deterioration after surgery.[70,86] Neurologic function should be carefully assessed in the preoperative phase. Because paraplegia is one of the most devastating consequences of thoracic aortic surgery, any alteration in lower-extremity function should be noted. Hoarseness related to compression of the recurrent laryngeal nerve should be assessed and documented. Bilateral recurrent laryngeal nerve compression or damage can result in respiratory compromise.

Monitoring

Intraoperative monitoring devices used for thoracoabdominal aneurysm resection are the same as those used for abdominal aneurysmectomies. Direct intraarterial (right radial) blood pressure and pulmonary artery pressure monitoring is mandatory. Use of two-dimensional transesophageal echocardiography is suggested for cardiac monitoring in patients with myocardial dysfunction. An indwelling urinary catheter is used for assessing renal function. To facilitate exposing the descending thoracic aorta, a double-lumen endotracheal tube is inserted to allow for one-lung ventilation. As a result careful monitoring of oxygenation is mandatory. Pulmonary artery catheters equipped with fiberoptics are useful for the measurement of mixed venous oxygen. Routine use of pulse oximetry may be limited if the left subclavian artery is manipulated; therefore the right hand, the ear, or the nasal passages should be used for monitoring oxygen saturation. Finally, a lumbar intrathecal catheter is inserted in order to access CSF. SSEPs or MEPs may be used to detect neurologic dysfunction; however, their clinical usefulness remains uncertain.[86-89]

Aortic Cross-Clamping

Simple aortic cross-clamping and graft replacement is an acceptable method for surgical repair of descending thoracic or thoracoabdominal aortic aneurysms.[70] Application of a simple cross-clamp has eliminated the need for shunts and extracorporeal circulation. However, the consequences of this maneuver include myocardial compromise and occlusion of blood flow to distal structures. The hemodynamic alterations produced by the application of an aortic clamp have previously been discussed. Similar responses are observed during proximal aortic occlusion; however, the magnitude of these responses is extreme. When the aorta is occluded, afterload and therefore myocardial workload increase. As a result, increases occur in left ventricular end-diastolic pressure, left ventricular stroke work index, and myocardial oxygen consumption.[69,90-92] When oxygen demands are not accompanied by an increase in oxygen supply, ischemia results, and myocardial failure can occur. Although methods have been instituted to decrease myocardial afterload (e.g., partial bypass and shunts), the use of sodium nitroprusside appears to be the most effective means of decreasing afterload during cross-clamp application.[69,90] Administration of nitroglycerin may be required in order to decrease preload during aortic occlusion.[90]

Hemodynamic Alterations

The hemodynamic consequences of releasing the aortic cross-clamp are similar to those of abdominal aortic occlusion, but they are of greater magnitude. Metabolites that have accumulated during aortic cross-clamping are released into circulation. The combination of reactive hyperemia and sequestration of blood volume within hypoperfused areas can lead to severe hypotension. Restoration of blood volume, guided by left-sided filling pressures, before the gradual release of the clamp can minimize hemodynamic alterations. Increasing ventilation and the administration of sodium bicarbonate may control carbon dioxide increases at the time of declamping.

Spinal Cord Ischemia

Neurologic dysfunction is a serious complication of thoracic aortic reconstruction. The incidence of paraplegia is reported to be approximately 20% after elective surgery and as high as 40% after surgery for dissecting and ruptured aneurysms.[86,91,92] Neurologic deficits are the result of hypoperfusion to the spinal cord during thoracic aortic reconstruction. The artery of Adamkiewicz, or the greater radicular artery, arises from an intercostal branch between T8 and L2 and provides the majority of the blood flow to the anterior spinal artery. The anterior spinal artery perfuses the ventral aspect of the spinal cord, which is responsible for motor control.[86] Although attempts have been made to reimplant the intercostal branches that contribute blood flow to the spinal cord, these efforts do not always decrease the incidence of paraplegia.[86,93] The duration of aortic occlusion also contributes to spinal cord ischemia. Jex and co-workers[94] suggest that damage to the spinal cord can occur in as little as 34 minutes of unprotected aortic occlusion, as is illustrated in Figure 23-7.

Several techniques have been described in an attempt to decrease the incidence of neurologic dysfunction after thoracic aortic surgery. However, few techniques have been proved to decrease spinal cord ischemia. Systemic hypothermia and selective cooling of the spinal cord may lengthen ischemic time intervals; however, the clinical benefits of these methods are unclear.[90,95] The use of various bypass mechanisms and distal shunts may minimize the length of aortic occlusion time; however, the risks associated with the implementation of these techniques could be greater than the potential benefits.

One method that has been successful is CSF drainage. McCullough and associates[92] reported a decrease in the incidence of paraplegia when CSF was drained before the thoracic aorta was cross-clamped in animal models. CSF drainage involves manipulation of spinal cord perfusion pressure during

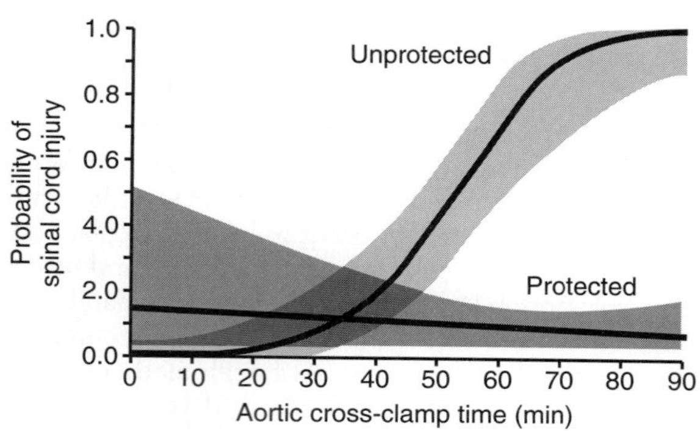

FIGURE **23-7**
Relationship between probability of spinal cord injury and length of aortic occlusion. Note that the risk of spinal cord injury increases substantially after 45 minutes of aortic occlusion for patients without protection of distal circulation. No such relationship between probability of spinal cord injury and length of aortic occlusion was noted for patients with protection of distal circulation. Shaded areas indicate the 70% confidence limits. (From Jex RK, et al. Early and late results after repair of dissections of the descending thoracic aorta. *J Vasc Surg*. 1986;3:226-237.)

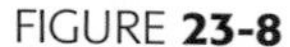

aortic clamping. Spinal cord perfusion pressure can be defined as the arterial pressure minus the CSF pressure. During aortic clamping, CSF pressure increases while arterial pressure decreases distal to the clamp. The spinal cord perfusion pressure can therefore be manipulated by alteration of arterial blood pressure and draining of CSF through the intrathecal catheter.[94,95] Hollier and Moore[86] reported no cases of paraplegia in more than 50 patients who underwent thoracic or thoracoabdominal aneurysm repairs in which CSF drainage was used.

Recently several studies have attempted to identify metabolic markers that are predictors of spinal cord ischemia. Drenger and colleagues[96] found that during and after thoracic aortic occlusion a dramatic increase occurs in CSF lactate levels. Patients who became paraplegic had higher CSF lactate levels compared with those who were neurologically intact postoperatively. Van Dongen and colleagues[97] observed that S-100 protein, which is only found in glial and Schwann cells, is released during acute damage to the central nervous system. Increases in S-100 protein concentration occurred after aortic cross-clamping despite normal SSEP and MEP monitoring values.

Methods for detecting spinal cord ischemia were previously discussed. The intraoperative use of SSEPs and MEPs can provide early identification of neurologic dysfunction; however, these monitoring modalities do not ensure spinal cord integrity. Factors that contribute to the development of neurologic deficit include level of aortic clamp application, ischemic time, embolization or thrombosis of a critical intercostal artery, failure to revascularize intercostal arteries, and urgency of surgical intervention.[69,70] Neurologic dysfunction has also been reported to occur in the postoperative phase. Delayed paraplegia may be the result of reperfusion injury, although this mechanism of injury has not been proved.[69,92,98] Figure 23-8 summarizes the events that contribute to permanent spinal cord injury and various interventions to halt the progression of the injury.

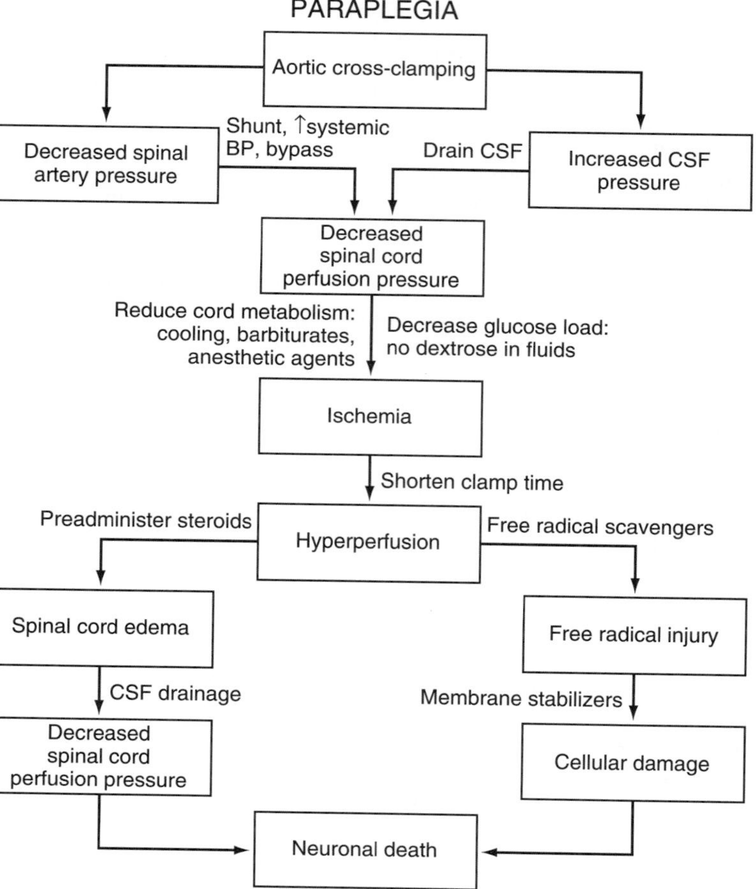

FIGURE **23-8**
Diagrammatic representation of the pathophysiologic events that contribute to permanent spinal cord injury and the methods of intervention for interruption of the neurologic injury cascade. BP, Blood pressure; CSF, cerebrospinal fluid. (Modified from Hollier LH, Moore WM. Avoidance of renal and neurologic complications following thoracoabdominal aortic aneurysm repair. *Acta Chir Scand Suppl*. 1990;555: 129-135.)

Renal Dysfunction

The incidence of renal dysfunction after thoracoabdominal aortic resection is estimated to be between 30% and 50%; the possibility of permanent renal failure requiring hemodialysis is estimated to be between 2% and 12%.[86] The cause of renal insufficiency is ischemia, which is related to aortic occlusion. Crawford and colleagues[70] identified preoperative renal dysfunction as one of the most significant factors that contributes to postoperative renal failure. These investigators also showed that renal artery perfusion with cold lactate solution demonstrated no apparent benefit with regard to renal function. Intraoperative hypotension has been identified as an independent predictor of postoperative renal dysfunction.[69] Maintenance of intravascular volume and stable circulatory status appears to be the most reliable method of minimizing renal dysfunction. Preoperatively, volume status should be corrected with non–glucose-containing crystalloid solutions. Intraoperative volume replacement should be guided by invasive monitoring. Pharmacologic adjuncts to produce diuresis, such as mannitol and furosemide, should be given approximately 20 to 30 minutes before clamp application.[90] Low-dose dopamine is also advocated as a means of increasing renal perfusion.

In summary, neurologic and renal dysfunction are devastating consequences of thoracic and thoracoabdominal aortic resections. A complete preoperative evaluation, identification of risk, optimization of organ function, and use of the suggested methods to minimize the consequences of ischemia all contribute to optimal surgical outcomes. Additional complications of thoracoabdominal aortic reconstruction are listed in Box 23-5.

BOX **23-5**

Complications after Thoracoabdominal Aortic Aneurysm Repair

Early Complications

Hemorrhage
Cardiac dysfunction
Spinal cord ischemia
Embolization
Pulmonary insufficiency
Distal artery occlusion
Thrombosis
Visceral ischemia
Sexual dysfunction
Infection
Renal failure
Cerebrovascular accident

Late Complications

Graft thrombosis
Aortoenteric fistula
False aneurysm
Aortocaval fistula
Graft infection

From Hollier LH, Moore WM. Avoidance of renal and neurologic complications following thoracoabdominal aortic aneurysm repair. Acta Chir Scand. *1990;555(suppl):129-135.*

Anesthetic Management

The principles of perioperative management of thoracic or thoracoabdominal aneurysms are similar to those previously discussed for abdominal aortic aneurysmectomies. Anesthetic selection should be based on the presence of concomitant disease processes, with the objective of maintenance of cardiovascular stability and the minimization of morbidity and mortality. Intraoperative monitoring should focus on detection of myocardial, neurologic, and renal ischemia. The hemodynamic consequences of aortic cross-clamping should be attenuated by the use of pharmacologic adjuncts. Restoration of circulating blood volume, as guided by left-sided filling pressure, minimizes the hemodynamic alterations caused by the release of the aortic clamp. Unique to thoracic aortic surgery is the use of one-lung ventilation. The highest degree of vigilance must be employed in order to detect potential inadequacies in ventilation and oxygenation. Extreme blood loss should be anticipated. Venous access and blood product availability should be confirmed during the preoperative phase. Methods of minimizing the use of homologous blood products, such as perioperative blood salvage, can be used. Coagulopathy is a constant threat that results from the administration of blood products. The close monitoring of coagulation parameters and the administration of fresh-frozen plasma, platelets, or specific coagulation factors can minimize the incidence and severity of coagulopathies.

Postoperative Considerations

After surgery is completed, if a double-lumen endotracheal tube was used, it must be replaced with a standard endotracheal tube to provide a secure airway, as postoperative ventilatory assistance is usually required. Anatomic landmarks may have become edematous during surgery, causing difficulty with reintubation. Under these circumstances, the double-lumen endotracheal tube may be left in place. Replacement, guided by fiberoptic evaluation, can proceed in the postoperative period after the airway edema has dissipated.

Close observation of circulatory and pulmonary status is warranted in the postoperative phase. Hemodynamic control is vital to maintain perfusion to vital organs without creating excessive demands on the heart or the aortic graft. Administration of dopamine may be continued during this time. Careful monitoring of respiratory status aided by arterial blood gas analysis is important. Epidural analgesia using local anesthetics, narcotics, or both can be administered for pain relief.

CEREBRAL INSUFFICIENCY AND CAROTID ENDARTERECTOMY

Cerebrovascular accidents, or strokes, are the third leading cause of death in the United States and account for a yearly cost of 14 billion dollars in medical expenses and lost productivity.[99,100] Most strokes occur as a result of carotid atherosclerotic disease; subintimal fatty streaks that give rise to fibrous plaques increase in size and compromise the vascular lumen. Ultimately the plaques rupture and release, a phenomenon that leads to abrupt occlusion of the lumen or rupture of the plaque, which can result in embolus formation. In each scenario an abrupt decrease in cerebral blood flow (CBF) leads to transient ischemic attacks (TIAs) or strokes.

More than half of all strokes are heralded by a TIA. The Framingham study reported that the risk of a stroke was 30% 2 years after a TIA and approximately 55% 12 years after a TIA had occurred.[101] It is this increased risk of stroke associated with TIA that provides the rationale for use of carotid endarterectomy, the surgical procedure in which the carotid artery is incised and the carotid arterial lumen reopened as a result of removal of plaque.

Indications

The first carotid endarterectomy was performed in 1954 on a 66-year-old woman with intermittent, right-sided hemiplegia associated with left carotid stenosis. Since that time the specific indications for and expected outcomes of carotid endarterectomy have been the subject of heated debate. The initial indication for carotid endarterectomy was symptomatic stenosis but not complete occlusive carotid disease.[99] This presentation occurs in most patients who undergo carotid surgery. Some centers have extended the indications to include evolved (nondense), nonhemorrhagic strokes and asymptomatic severe stenosis or lesser stenosis associated with contralateral occlusive disease.[99] The North American Symptomatic Carotid Endarterectomy Trial concluded that carotid endarterectomy for patients with recent hemispheric TIAs and high-grade stenosis (70% to 99%) had a risk reduction of 65% for the development of an ipsilateral stroke 2 years after surgery as compared with patients whose condition was medically managed.[102] The Executive Committee for Asymptomatic Carotid Atherosclerosis Study demonstrated that asymptomatic patients with carotid artery stenosis of at least 60% who underwent carotid endarterectomy had a 53% lower 5-year risk of ipsilateral stroke than patients who were treated medically.[103]

Morbidity and Mortality

The surgical outcomes reported for carotid endarterectomy remain inconclusive because of differences in patient populations and varying degrees of surgical expertise. Other variables that cannot be stratified in studies but that may affect outcome include the state of collateral flow through the circle of Willis, the presence of concurrent atherosclerotic disease in the cerebral vasculature, the size and morphology of the offending plaque, the specific presenting symptoms, and the presence of concurrent cardiovascular disease.[104] If this information is obtained, the recommended acceptable perioperative stroke rates should be limited to less than 3% in asymptomatic patients, less than 5% in symptomatic patients, and 10% or less in patients with recurrent disease or existing strokes.[105] Morbidity rates related to carotid endarterectomies have been reported to be at or below these recommended limits.[105,106] The perioperative myocardial infarction rate of 2% to 5% illustrates the global nature of atherosclerotic disease and may represent the greatest contribution to overall morbidity. The perioperative mortality rates for carotid endarterectomies are approximately 0.5% to 2.5%,[107,108] and the long-term postoperative stroke incidence ranges from 1% to 3% per year.[99,109]

Patient Selection

Criteria for the best candidates for carotid artery surgery remain unclear. The risks associated with having surgery and the possibility of a stroke must be measured against the risks associated with not having surgery and undergoing medical management. As mentioned previously, the Framingham study identified the incidence of stroke after TIAs and demonstrated the increased risk of stroke in untreated disease. In a study of 561 patients who underwent carotid endarterectomy during a 10-year period, Sieber and associates[110] attempted to identify the preoperative and intraoperative risk factors associated with stroke. Preoperative neurologic dysfunction was found to be the most significant factor for predicting postoperative stroke incidence (4%). Several conditions that can increase the risk of perioperative complications include severe preoperative hypertension, carotid endarterectomy (CEA) performed in preparation for coronary artery bypass, angina, internal carotid artery stenosis near the carotid siphon, age older than 75 years, and diabetes mellitis.[111] Box 23-6 identifies various factors that contribute to morbidity during carotid endarterectomy. Because carotid endarterectomies are performed prophylactically, it would seem prudent that patient selection be based on the risks associated with the neurologic and myocardial ischemia of surgery, as opposed to risks associated with the neurologic sequelae of nonsurgical management.

Diagnosis

The neurologic symptoms of cerebral vascular dysfunction, such as TIAs and strokes, are most frequently related to decreased CBF. Asymptomatic carotid bruits may be a sign of the possibility of carotid artery disease. Amaurosis fugax or monocular blindness occurs in 25% of patients with high-grade carotid artery stenosis. This syndrome is believed to be caused by microthrombi that travel into the internal carotid artery and that decrease the blood supply of the optic nerve via the ophthalmic artery. Duplex ultrasonography, a noninvasive diagnostic modality that combines ultrasound and Doppler analysis, is currently one of the most sensitive noninvasive techniques capable of evaluating extracranial occlusive disease.[99] Arteriography may be performed if surgery is being contemplated and can provide anatomic details of arterial vessels. CT scan or MRI may be useful in patients with a neurologic deficit, in whom an alternative diagnosis may be discovered.

BOX **23-6**

Factors Contributing to Morbidity during Carotid Endarterectomy

- History of stroke or infarction on computed tomographic scan
- Early operation after stroke
- Significant medical problems
- Age
- Contralateral carotid artery disease
- Progressing stroke
- Hypercapnia
- Bilateral surgery
- Ulcerative lesion
- Low stump pressures
- Hemodynamic failure or hypoperfusion
- Surgery without intraoperative monitoring
- Surgery with shunt
- Surgery without shunt
- Vein patch closure
- Primary closure

Modified from Schroder T. How to predict which patient with carotid atherosclerosis is "high risk." Acta Chir Scand. *1990;555(suppl):209-222.*

Preoperative Assessment

The presence of concurrent CAD and carotid stenosis is well documented. Although stroke is a devastating consequence of carotid endarterectomy, myocardial infarction contributes more frequently to poor surgical outcomes than stroke. Callow and Mackey[105] reported on myocardial infarction as a cause of late mortality in 49% of patients who underwent carotid endarterectomy. The stroke-related fatality was 15%. The prevalence of cardiac disease and related risk factors is summarized in Table 23-10.

Hertzer and co-workers[53] performed coronary angiography in 1000 patients who underwent elective peripheral reconstruction as a means of identifying the presence of CAD. In this report the authors identified severe correctable CAD in 26% of the 195 patients with cerebrovascular disease. Although coronary angiography may not be justified in all patients undergoing carotid endarterectomy, a systematic approach to the identification of CAD and its subsequent risks should be performed before elective surgery. Figure 23-9 illustrates a stepwise approach to the evaluation and management of CAD.

Patients with no significant medical history, normal physical examination and normal electrocardiography should proceed directly to surgery, because these patients have low surgical risks. When abnormal cardiac information is obtained, further evaluation should be performed. Radionuclide imaging is highly sensitive in diagnosing CAD. Redistribution demonstrated on dipyridamole-thallium imaging is very suggestive of increased risk of adverse cardiac events. In these patients coronary angiography is suggested as a means of quantifying CAD and selecting an appropriate therapeutic intervention.

The progression of surgical intervention when CAD accompanies carotid artery disease is controversial. Most agree that in cases of mild CAD, patients may undergo carotid endarterectomy with a low degree of risk. However, in cases of moderate-to-severe CAD, the direction of surgical intervention is unclear. One option is the simultaneous performance of carotid endarterectomy and coronary revascularization. The safety of combined procedures has been addressed in the literature. Although some authors dispute the benefit of concomitant coronary and cerebral revascularization, most seem to advocate this combination in a select group of individuals within the population that have severe CAD and significant carotid artery occlusion.[112,113] A combined carotid endarterectomy and coronary artery bypass surgery (CABG) may decrease the operative mortality rate and does not appear to put the patient at increased surgical risk.[114,115] However, Brown and associates[116] state that there is a high overall mortality rate of 17.7% when CABG and carotid endarterectomy are performed as a combined procedure. It is doubtful that strict conclusions will soon be drawn regarding the appropriate surgical management of concomitant CAD and carotid artery disease. Until more specific information is available, decisions should be guided by the individual's symptoms, the associated risk factors, and the center's experience.

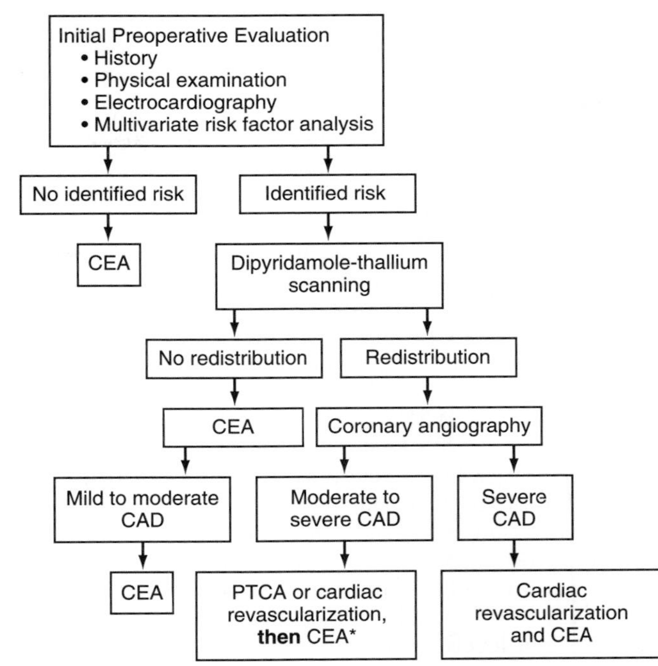

FIGURE **23-9**
Algorithm for the management and the surgical selection of patients with concurrent carotid artery disease (*CAD*). Asterisk indicates that some may suggest reversing the order of these events. *CEA*, Carotid endarterectomy; *PTCA*, percutaneous transluminal coronary angioplasty.

TABLE 23-10 Prevalence of Cardiac Disease and Associated Risk Factors in 614 Patients Undergoing Carotid Endarterectomy

Risk Factor	Incidence (%)
Cigarette smoking	62
Hypertension	62
Abnormal electrocardiographic results	34
Prior myocardial infarction	24
Angina	21
Diabetes mellitus	20
Hyperlipidemia	12

Modified from MacKey MC, O'Donnell TF, Callow AD. Cardiac risk in patients undergoing carotid endarterectomy: impact on perioperative and long-term mortality. J Vasc Surg. *1990;11:226-234.*

Anesthetic Management

The anesthetic objectives for vascular surgery are similar to those for any type of elective procedure: to provide analgesia and amnesia, to facilitate surgical intervention, and to minimize operative morbidity and mortality. Goals that are specific to carotid endarterectomy include provision of cerebral and myocardial protection. However, it may be difficult to maintain the integrity of one system without adversely affecting the other. For example, raising the arterial blood pressure to augment cerebral perfusion can increase myocardial oxygen demand, which may lead to ischemia. In addition, significantly decreasing blood pressure can lead to cerebral hypoperfusion. Therefore the anesthetic goal is to optimize perfusion to the brain, minimize myocardial workload, ensure cardiovascular stability and allow for rapid emergence. An understanding of the physiology of the cerebrovascular system is important if the principles of management for carotid endarterectomy are to be understood. This knowledge enables the selection of appropriate monitoring and anesthetic techniques that will protect and improve cerebral and myocardial perfusion.

Cerebral Physiology

CBF can remain relatively constant at different cerebral perfusion pressures as a result of cerebrovascular autoregulation. Cerebral perfusion pressure can be expressed as the difference between MAP and intracranial pressure. During carotid endarterectomy, intracranial pressure is usually not elevated; therefore MAP plays the predominant role in determining cerebral perfusion pressure. When MAP is maintained between 60 and 160 mm Hg, CBF remains constant. However, the adverse effects of chronic systemic hypertension shifts the patient's cerebral autoregulatory curve to the right, and therefore a higher than normal MAP may be required to ensure adequate cerebral perfusion. CBF is also influenced by arterial carbon dioxide and oxygen levels as well as by inhalation agents.

Normal CBF is approximately 50 ml/100 g per minute. Neuronal function is generally maintained at levels greater than 25 ml/100 g per minute. Levels less than this critical value jeopardize cellular function. Decreased perfusion and ischemia can be reflected in changes in consciousness. Cellular death occurs at levels less than 6 ml/100 g per minute, as evidenced by flattening seen on an electroencephalogram.

Carotid occlusive disease jeopardizes the cerebral perfusion pressure in the ipsilateral artery. Ischemia leads to the disruption of autoregulation and compensatory vasodilation, and thus blood flow becomes pressure dependent. During carotid endarterectomy the anesthetic goals must focus on improvement and protection of CBF and diligent monitoring of brain function.

Monitoring

In addition to standard monitoring, direct intraarterial pressure is continuously assessed in order to evaluate near–real-time values. During the administration of anesthetic agents, blood pressure fluctuation commonly occurs in patients who have a history of hypertension. Because of the high incidence of CAD and neurovascular disease in this patient population, prompt treatment of blood pressure values below 20% of preoperative values is imperative. Pulmonary artery catheterization is not warranted in most individuals unless the presence of concurrent cardiac disease justifies its use. Carbon dioxide has a potent effect on cerebrovascular tone. Both hypocapnia and hypercapnia directly affect CBF; therefore maintenance of normocapnia is paramount.

During repair the carotid artery cross-clamp is applied. Various monitoring techniques have been proposed for the assessment of the adequacy of CBF during this maneuver. Carotid stump pressure has been used as a means of assessing collateral flow.[117] After the carotid cross-clamp is placed, the distal pressure in the internal carotid artery is measured. A carotid stump pressure of less than 40 to 50 mm Hg reflects neurologic hypoperfusion and is a criterion for shunt placement. However, there is no correlation between stump pressures and electroencephalographic changes.[106] In a study by Harada and associates,[118] a carotid stump pressure of less than 50 mm Hg had a positive predictive value of only 36% of patients who exhibited ischemic EEG changes during carotid artery cross-clamping.

Regional CBF can be measured by the inhalation or by direct administration of radioactive xenon 133 (^{133} Xe). In the operating room intraarterial carotid injections of xenon 108 (^{108}Xe) are more feasible as compared with inhalation anesthetic, and the reliability of the injection technique has been well demonstrated. Intravenous methods have been recently proposed as a new means of measuring regional CBF for patients undergoing general anesthesia. Young and colleagues[119] demonstrated a positive correlation between intracarotid and intravenous ^{133}Xe methods in determining regional CBF.

The use of SSEP monitoring can be used to identify inadequate CBF during cross-clamping. Lam and co-workers[120] compared the efficacy of SSEP monitoring and electroencephalography (EEG) and concluded that these two monitoring techniques were similar. SSEP monitoring is a feasible alternative to conventional EEG for predicting neurologic deficits; however, false-positive results can occur. In addition, SSEPs are a measure of the integrity of the dorsal or sensory portion of the spinal cord. Therefore a motor deficit can occur despite a normal SSEP waveform.

Electroencephalographic monitoring constitutes the gold standard in the identification of neurologic deficits related to carotid artery cross-clamping.[120] EEG has demonstrated reliability in the monitoring of cortical electrical function.[121] Loss of β-wave activity, loss of amplitude, and emergence of slow-wave activity all are indicative of neurologic dysfunction.

Transcranial Doppler velocity monitoring has been used as a method of detecting adverse cerebral events during carotid endarterectomy. McDowell and associates[122] used intraoperative transcranial Doppler monitoring during 238 carotid endarterectomies. They concluded that this method was more reliable than EEG for assessment of interior integrity of the cerebral hemispheres.

Anesthetic Selection

In an attempt to decrease the incidence of perioperative stroke during carotid endarterectomy, individual anesthetic techniques have been investigated. Many authors have reported the advantages and disadvantages of both general and regional anesthesia; however, no consensus indicates that a particular technique is more effective in decreasing overall perioperative morbidity and mortality. Therefore anesthetic selection must be based on the anesthetist's familiarity and competence with a specific technique as well as the patient's condition and the surgeon's preference.

Regional Anesthesia

A regional anesthetic technique during carotid endarterectomy can be accomplished by local infiltration or by superficial and deep cervical plexus block. Perhaps the greatest advantage of regional anesthesia is the anesthetist's ability to directly assess neurologic function in an awake individual. Assessing level of consciousness is perhaps the most effective method of detecting cerebral ischemia. In fact, assessment of consciousness in the awake patient may be more sensitive than conventional EEG in detection of cerebral ischemia. Corson and colleagues[123] reviewed data from 399 patients who underwent carotid endarterectomy in which general and regional techniques were used. The authors concluded that perioperative strokes occurred less frequently when a regional anesthetic was provided, especially in high-risk patients. McCarthy and colleagues[124] compared middle cerebral artery blood flow velocity using transcranial Doppler monitoring in patients undergoing carotid endarterectomy with either local or general anesthesia. It was determined that preservation of cerebral circulation was better maintained in patients who received local anesthesia. In addition, 67% of the general anesthesia group and 15% of the local anesthesia group received shunts. However, despite these

TABLE 23-11 **Comparison of Hospital Costs in Patients Undergoing Carotid Endarterectomy with General or Regional Anesthetic Techniques**

	REGULAR HOSPITAL		
	ICU Stay (d)	Bed Stay (d)	Total Cost
General	1.2	6.1	$4547
Regional	0.1	4.1	$2067

Modified from Godin MS, Bell WH III, Schwedler M, Kerstein MD. Cost effectiveness of regional anesthesia in carotid endarterectomy. Am Surg. *1989;55:656-659.*

seemingly physiologic advantages, no differences occurred in outcomes between the local and general anesthesia groups. The use of regional anesthesia has been associated with shorter operative times, less frequent cardiopulmonary complications, and shorter postoperative hospitalization. In addition, a significant decrease occurs in routine carotid artery shunting.[125] Other studies have had similar results.[126-128]

When complications are prevented and favorable surgical outcomes are demonstrated, health-care economics may be improved. Use of a regional technique during carotid endarterectomy has been associated with economic savings. In a prospective study, Godin and colleagues[129] examined hospital costs in a comparison of general versus regional techniques (Table 23-11). These investigators computed that the use of regional anesthesia saved $2480 per patient and $124,000 total in their series without an increase in morbidity or mortality. Considering that carotid endarterectomy is the second most common vascular operation performed in the United States (the first being coronary revascularization), the cost-effectiveness associated with regional anesthesia is tremendous.

The limiting factor for use of a regional technique is patient acceptance. Because these individuals are awake, their cooperation during surgery is mandatory. Anxiety and fear related to being awake during surgery compound the problem. Fear and apprehension can initiate sympathetic stimulation, and as a result extreme hemodynamic response can occur. Pharmacologic adjuncts required in the apprehensive patient may confound the neurologic assessment and therefore negate the advantages of a regional technique. Furthermore, converting to a general anesthetic technique once surgery has begun can be problematic.

General Anesthesia

Although the use of regional anesthesia has a number of advantages, general anesthesia is commonly used during carotid endarterectomies. Perhaps the greatest benefit of this technique is that it counters the most cited disadvantage of regional anesthesia: lack of patient cooperation. General anesthesia promotes a calmer environment for surgery. In addition, inhalation agents may provide hemodynamic stability and may have beneficial effects on cerebral circulation.[130]

Comparison of inhaled agents with narcotic-based techniques yields no scientific evidence to suggest that patient outcome is improved. In studies of inhalation agents the critical regional CBF (the blood level below which electroencephalographic signs of ischemia occur) during isoflurane anesthesia was less than when other volatile anesthetic were used.[130,131] Isoflurane also contributed to fewer adverse cardiac events when compared with enflurane and halothane in 2223 patients who underwent carotid endarterectomy at the Mayo Clinic.[132] The effects of sufentanil on cerebral hemodynamics were similar to those of isoflurane.[133] The inhalation agents may alter the monitoring methods used for detecting cerebral ischemia, such as EEG and SSEP monitoring. In these cases general anesthetic techniques may require modification, and direct communication is required between the anesthetist and the surgical team. The use of nitrous oxide during carotid endarterectomy can potentially increase the incidence of a clinically significant pneumocephalus. During shunt placement and carotid artery cross-clamp release, microbubbles can be entrained into carotid artery blood flow. If nitrous oxide is used, some believe that it should be discontinued before the carotid artery cross-clamp.[134]

In summary, no scientific consensus supports the idea that one anesthetic technique is superior in terms of decreasing perioperative morbidity and mortality. Palmer[135] investigated the type of anesthetic technique employed and the associated morbidity and mortality in more than 200 patients. He concluded that no significant differences existed among all possible techniques. Furthermore, he recommended that the choice of anesthetic technique be governed by the preferences of the surgeon and the operative team. However, anesthetic agents should be selected that allow for a rapid assessment of neurologic function at the completion of surgery.

Cerebral Protection

The major objective during carotid artery revascularization is to maintain CBF and decrease cerebral ischemia. Prevention of cerebral ischemia can be accomplished in one of two ways: by increasing the collateral flow (placement of intraluminal shunt) or by decreasing the cerebral metabolic requirements (pharmacologic adjunct).

Temporary Shunt Placement. When the carotid artery is clamped, CBF is compromised. Therefore maintenance of CPP is dependent on collateral blood flow for adequate cerebral perfusion. The EEG changes that are associated with cerebral ischemia can be reversed when an intraluminal shunt is inserted. The shunt acts as a temporary conduit that allows for arterial blood flow during the time the surgeon is dissecting plaque from the intima of the carotid artery. Although some surgeons routinely insert shunts during carotid artery cross-clamping, others do not use shunts or use shunts only in a select group of patients. Studies have demonstrated successful surgical outcomes when carotid endarterectomy was performed without the use of intraoperative shunting.[110,121] Schroder[109] reported a 5% incidence of stroke in patients who underwent carotid endarterectomy. In this group of 561 patients, neither the use of a shunt or cross-clamp nor administration of glucose was identified as a primary determinant of stroke severity.[110] The application of a shunt imposes the risk of embolic complications and intimal dissections.[109] Cerebral ischemic events are most often the result of embolic complications rather than hemodynamic instability.[108,136] It has been suggested that 65% to 95% of neurologic deficits that occur as a result of CEA are related to thromboembolic events that are unrelated to the carotid artery cross-clamping.[137] Therefore surgeons more frequently reserve the use of shunts for patients with impaired contralateral cerebral circulation or an unstable neurologic history. However, Hankey and colleagues[138] state that inconclusive evidence exists, as reported by randomized controlled trials comparing routine or selective shunting and the overall mortality rate. The need for shunt placement can be based on information obtained using intraoperative monitoring techniques, which determine CBF. Stump pressures and EEG measurements are the intraoperative monitoring modalities most frequently used to determine the need for shunt placement.

A new, less invasive surgical approach for treatment of carotid artery stenosis is carotid artery angioplasty and stenting. The procedure is performed with the patient under local anesthesia and makes use of angiographic techniques to precisely determine the degree and characteristics of the stenotic lesion. Balloon angioplasty and deployment of a stent keep the lumen of the carotid artery patent. Controversy exists regarding the degree of success that this procedure affords as an alternative to carotid endarterectomy. Stanovic and associates[139] in a study of 100 patients undergoing carotid artery stenting conclude that this procedure is a safe, effective, and reliable method of treating carotid artery disease. However, other researchers have stated that this procedure is associated with an increased stroke rate, poor durability of carotid angioplasty and stenting as evidenced by restenosis, and increased procedural costs.[140,141]

Cerebral Metabolism. Barbiturates have the capability of decreasing cerebral metabolism to 40% of normal values.[95] During transient focal ischemia, barbiturates decrease the cerebral metabolic rate of oxygen consumption, which results in cerebral protection. The disadvantages of administering barbiturates during carotid endarterectomy surgery include myocardial depression and delayed emergence. The surgeon may request that thiopental be given before the carotid artery is cross-clamped.

Hypothermia is also associated with decreases in cerebral metabolic rates and oxygen consumption. When core temperature has been reduced to 12° to 20° C, the safe duration of ischemia is 30 to 60 minutes.[95] Hypothermic techniques were initially advocated; however, the risks associated with these techniques outweigh the clinical usefulness.

Blood Pressure Control

The presence of hypertension in patients with cerebrovascular disease is well known. Therefore one of the most challenging aspects of care associated with anesthesia for carotid endarterectomy is blood pressure control. Patients with cerebral insufficiency are vulnerable to perioperative blood pressure instability. Hypotension occurs in 10% to 50% of patients who undergo carotid endarterectomy and is believed to be the result of carotid sinus baroreceptor stimulation.[142] Conversely, 10% to 66% of patients experience hypertension, which is attributed to surgical manipulation of the carotid sinus.[142] Preoperative blood pressure control, volume status, and depth of anesthesia can also contribute to intraoperative hemodynamic instability.

Blood pressure control must begin in the preoperative phase. Mangano and associates[143] studied the effects of atenolol administered to patients who had confirmed or were at risk for CAD. Atenolol was administered preoperatively, postoperatively, and throughout the patients' hospital stays. Overall the atenolol study group had a 65% reduction in mortality secondary to adverse cardiac events. In addition, patients in the atenolol study group had a 67% decrease in mortality within 1 year of surgery and a 48% decrease in mortality 2 years after surgery. All patients should continue taking their antihypertensive medications until the time of surgery. Additional pharmacologic adjuncts may be required in the preoperative period, especially during the insertion of intravenous and intraarterial catheters, in order to reduce increases in heart rate and blood pressure. The induction of anesthesia, the initial incision, the dissection, the manipulation of the carotid sinus, and the emergence from anesthesia are all events that precipitate blood pressure fluctuations. The use of pharmacologic adjuncts, such as short-acting β-adrenergic blockers, may stabilize blood pressure during induction and emergence. Continuous intravenous use of nitroglycerin or sodium nitroprusside should be available for hypertension. Patients with chronic hypertension are predisposed to dramatic decreases in blood pressure after the induction of general anesthesia. This condition must be treated promptly and can be successfully managed through provision of intravenous fluids or administration of a vasoconstrictor, such as phenylephrine hydrochloride. Hypotension and bradycardia, which result from carotid sinus baroreceptor manipulation, can be inhibited by infiltration with local anesthetic. Although this maneuver is a fairly common practice during carotid endarterectomy, one series demonstrated no benefit from the prophylactic administration of local anesthetic to the carotid sinus nerve. These investigators suggested that this technique might be detrimental because it can cause hypertension.[142]

Postoperative Considerations

Perhaps the most common problem experienced in the postoperative period is hypertension. Although its cause remains unclear, postoperative hypertension may be related to events or conditions that alter cerebral autoregulation, such as use of halogenated hydrocarbons, diabetes mellitus, and cerebral hypoperfusion.[144] Hypertension in the postoperative period occurs in 29% to 69% of patients undergoing carotid endarterectomy.[144] A systolic blood pressure greater than 180 mm Hg is associated with an increased incidence of TIA, stroke, or myocardial infarction.[111] Those patients with systolic blood pressures of 145 mm Hg or less had fewer postoperative complications.[102]

Although an uncommon complication, carotid artery hemorrhage can occur in the postoperative phase. Hemorrhage is a devastating event that requires immediate surgical intervention. Initial manifestations of hemorrhage may be those of upper airway obstruction, which may make reintubation difficult or impossible because of tracheal deviation. Emergency management of a patient with airway compromise as a result of carotid artery hemorrhage includes immediate evacuation of the hematoma. In addition, recurrent laryngeal nerve damage can occur and routinely manifests as inspiratory stridor. However, respiratory insufficiency can occur in patients who have preexisting respiratory conditions. Lastly, cerebral hyperperfusion syndrome (CHS) can occur and results from an increased blood flow to the brain as a result of a loss of cerebral vascular autoregulation. The mechanism of action causing this phenomena is unknown; however, it is hypothesized that CHS may occur as a result of chronic cerebral ischemia. Signs and symptoms of CHS include severe headache, visual disturbances, altered level of consciousness, and seizures. CHS may occur more often in patients who have had a contralateral carotid endarterectomy within the last 3 months and undergo a second carotid endarterectomy for occlusion on the ipsilateral side.[145]

The incidence of postoperative stroke after carotid endarterectomy was discussed previously. Unfortunately, even after successful revascularization of the carotid artery, occlusion can recur at a rate of 3% per year.[108] Although symptoms occur in only a small percentage of patients (3% to 5%), the incidence of recurrent carotid stenosis may be much larger

TABLE 23-12 Cranial Nerve Assessment for the Carotid Endarterectomy Patient

Cranial Nerve	Function	Assessment
VII (Facial)	Muscles of facial expression, saliva secretion	Smile, frown
IX (glossopharyngeal)	Swallowing, pharyngeal muscle	Pharyngeal reflexes, swallowing
X (vagus)	Pharyngeal and laryngeal muscles	Speech
XII (hypoglossopharyngeal)*	Muscles of tongue	Stick tongue out, move tongue side to side

**This nerve traverses the internal carotid artery.*
From Drain CB. Perianesthesia Nursing. *4th ed. Philadelphia: Saunders; 2003:500.*

than that reported because asymptomatic cases may be overlooked.[146] Clinical assessment of cranial nerve function is performed as noted in Table 23-12.

Perioperative Cost Containment

During the past few decades, a dramatic change has occurred in the way surgical care is delivered. For patients undergoing carotid endarterectomy, efforts to curtail hospital costs have led to changes in preoperative evaluations and anesthetic techniques and reductions in the length of stay.

Contrast arteriography, which has been the standard technique for determination of the degree of carotid artery stenosis, usually does not provide any additional information, as compared with carotid duplex scanning, in a patient without atypical neurologic symptoms.[147] The cost of contrast arteriography is in excess of $4000, whereas the cost of carotid duplex scanning is $160. As discussed previously, a significant cost savings is associated with the use of regional anesthesia. The dramatic cost difference is the result of decreased ICU use, decreased length of stay, and reduced costs for pharmacologic agents.[148] A carotid endarterectomy protocol in which patients are discharged 1 day postoperatively has been evaluated. In a prospective study by Friedman and colleagues,[149] 72 patients were evaluated preoperatively on an outpatient basis, and hospital admission took place on the day of surgery. General anesthesia was administered to all patients in the study group. A total of 66 (88%) patients were discharged on the first postoperative day. The average length of stay was 1.13 days, and no complications were attributed to early discharge.

REFERENCES

1. Zarins CK, Graham HM. Aorta and arterial disease of the lower extremity. In: Miller TA, ed. *Physiologic Basis of Modern Surgical Care*. St Louis: Mosby; 1988:837.
2. Panetta TF, Veith FJ. Aortoiliac occlusive disease. In: Cameron JL, ed. *Current Surgical Therapy*. 4th ed. St Louis: Mosby; 1992.
3. Cunningham AJ. Anesthesia for abdominal aortic surgery. I. A review. *Can J Anaesth*. 1989;36:426-444.
4. Stenseth R. Advances in anesthesiological management of aortic surgery. *Acta Chir Scand*. 1990;155:123-128.
5. DeBakey ME, Lawrie GM. Combined coronary artery and peripheral vascular disease: recognition and treatment. *J Vasc Surg*. 1984;1:605-607.
6. Szilagyi DE, Elliott JP Jr, Smith RF, et al. A thirty-year survey of the reconstructive surgical treatment of aortoiliac occlusive disease. *J Vasc Surg*. 1986;3:421-435.
7. Baron HC, La Raja RD, Rossi G, Atkinson D. Continuous epidural analgesia in the heparinized vascular surgical patient: a retrospective review of 912 patients. *J Vasc Surg*. 1987;6:144-146.
8. Raggi R, Dardik H, Mauro AL. Continuous epidural anesthesia and postoperative epidural narcotics in vascular surgery. *Am J Surg*. 1987;154:192-197.
9. Underwood PS, Kepes E, Hollinger I. A comparison of epidural versus general anesthesia for elderly patients undergoing peripheral vascularization. *Anesthesiology*. 1988;6:A105.
10. Reilly JN, Tilson MD. Incidence and etiology of abdominal aortic aneurysms. *Surg Clin North Am*. 1989;69:705-711.
11. Hall, SW. Endovascular repair of abdominal aortic aneurysms. *AORN J*. 2003;77(3):630-648.
12. Lambert ME, Baguley P, Charlesworth D. Ruptured abdominal aortic aneurysms. *J Cardiovasc Surg*. 1986;27:256-261.
13. Hollier LH, Moore WM. Surgical management of juxtarenal and suprarenal aortic aneurysms. *Acta Chir Scand*. 1990;555:117-122.
14. Budden J, Hollier LH. Management of aneurysms that involve the juxtarenal or suprarenal aorta. *Surg Clin North Am*. 1989; 69:837-844.
15. Quill DS, Colgan MP, Sumner DS. Ultrasonic screening for the detection of abdominal aortic aneurysms. *Surg Clin North Am*. 1989;69:713-720.
16. Thurmond AS, Semler HJ. Abdominal aortic aneurysm: incidence in a population at risk. *J Cardiovasc Surg*. 1986;27:457-459.
17. Dobrin PB. Pathophysiology and pathogenesis of aortic aneurysms. *Surg Clin North Am*. 1989;69:687-703.
18. Brady AR, Thompson SG, Greenhalgh RM. *Br J Surg*. 2003; 90:492-493.
19. Webster MW, St Jean PL, Steed DL, Ferrell RE, Majumder PP. Abdominal aortic aneurysm: results of a family study. *J Vasc Surg*. 1991;13:366-372.
20. Graor RA. Preoperative evaluation and management of coronary and carotid artery occlusive disease in patients with abdominal aortic aneurysms. *Surg Clin North Am*. 1989;69:737-743.
21. Pairolero PC. Repair of abdominal aortic aneurysms in high-risk patients. *Surg Clin North Am*. 1989;69:755-763.
22. Johansen K. Treatment options for aneurysms in high-risk patients. *Surg Clin North Am*. 1989;69:765-774.
23. Hertzer NR, et al. The risk of vascular surgery in a metropolitan community. *J Vasc Surg*. 1984;9:13-19.
24. Sullivan CA, Rohrer MJ, Cutler BS. Clinical management of symptomatic but unruptured abdominal aortic aneurysm. *J Vasc Surg*. 1990;11:799-802.
25. Wakefield TW, et al. Abdominal aortic aneurysm rupture: statistical analysis of factors affecting outcome of surgical treatment. *Surgery*. 1982;91:586-595.
26. Rutherford RB, McCroskey BL. Ruptured abdominal aortic aneurysms. *Surg Clin North Am*. 1989;69:859-868.
27. Bandyk DF. Preoperative imaging of aortic aneurysms: conventional and digital subtraction angiography, computed tomography scanning, and magnetic resonance. *Surg Clin North Am*. 1989;69:721-735.
28. Vowden P, Wilkinson D, Ausobsky JR, Kester RC. A comparison of three imaging techniques in the assessment of an abdominal aortic aneurysm. *J Cardiovasc Surg*. 1989;30:891-896.
29. Glock Y, Smile E, Dalous P, et al. Abdominal aortic aneurysmectomy in octogenarian patients. *J Cardiovasc Surg*. 1990;31:71-76.

30. Plecha FR, Bertin VJ, Plecha EJ, et al. The early results of vascular surgery in patients 75 years of age and older: an analysis of 3259 cases. *J Vasc Surg*. 1985;2:769-774.
31. Darling RC, Messina CR, Brewster DC, Ottinger LW. Autopsy study of unoperated abdominal aortic aneurysms: the case for early resection. *Circulation*. 1977;56:161-164.
32. Gelman S, Khazaeli MB, Orr R, Henderson T. Blood volume redistribution during cross-clamping of the descending aorta. *Anesth Analg*. 1994;78:219-224.
33. Gelman S, McDowell H, Varner PD, et al. The reason for cardiac output reduction after aortic cross-clamping. *Am J Surg*. 1988;155:578-586.
34. Gold MS, DeCrosta D, Rizzuto C, Ben-Harari RR, Ramanathan S. The effect of lumbar epidural and general anesthesia on plasma catecholamines and hemodynamics during abdominal aortic aneurysm repair. *Anesth Analg*. 1994;78:225-230.
35. Huval WV, Lelcuk S, Allen PD, Mannick JA, Shepro D, Hechtman HB. Determinants of cardiovascular stability during abdominal aortic aneurysmectomy (AAA). *Ann Surg*. 1984; 199:216-222.
36. Galt SW, Bech FR, McDaniel MD, et al. The effect of ibuprofen on cardiac performance during abdominal aortic cross-clamping. *J Vasc Surg*. 1991;13:876-883.
37. Gottlieb A, Skrinska VA, O'Hara P, Boutros AR, Melia M, Beck GJ. The role of prostacyclin in the mesenteric traction syndrome during anesthesia for abdominal aortic reconstructive surgery. *Ann Surg*. 1989;209:363-367.
38. Seltzer JL, Ritter DE, Starsmic MA, Marr AT. The hemodynamic response to traction on the abdominal mesentery. *Anesthesiology*. 1985;63:96-99.
39. Naito Y, Tamai S, Shingu K, et al. Responses of adrenocorticotropic hormone, cortisol, and cytokines during and after upper abdominal surgery. *Anesthesiology*. 1992;77:426-431.
40. Norman JG, Fink GW. The effects of epidural anesthesia on the neuroendocrine response to major surgical stress: a randomized prospective trial. *Am Surg*. 1997;63:75-80.
41. Hermreck AS. Prevention and management of surgical complications during repair of abdominal aortic aneurysms. *Surg Clin North Am*. 1989;69:869-894.
42. Mongan PD, Peterson RE, Williams D. Spinal evoked potentials are predictive in a porcine model of aortic occlusion. *Anesth Analg*. 1994;78:257-266.
43. Damask MC, Weissman C, Rodrigues J, Askanazi J, Rosenbaum SH. Abdominal aortic cross-clamping: metabolic and hemodynamic consequences. *Arch Surg*. 1984;119:1332-1337.
44. Fukuda S, Taga K, Tanaka T, et al. Relationship between tissue ischemia and venous endothelin-1 during abdominal aortic aneurysm surgery. *J Cardiothorac Vasc Anesth*. 1995;9:510-514.
45. Hessel EA. Intraoperative management of abdominal aortic aneurysms: the anesthesiologist's viewpoint. *Surg Clin North Am*. 1989;69:775-793.
46. Sicard GA, Allen BT, Munn JS, Anderson CB. Retroperitoneal versus transperitoneal approach of repair of abdominal aortic aneurysms. *Surg Clin North Am*. 1989;69:795-806.
47. Hallett JW. Minimizing the use of homologous blood products during repair of abdominal aortic aneurysms. *Surg Clin North Am*. 1989;69:817-826.
48. Roger VL, Ballard DJ, Hallett JW Jr, Osmundson PJ, Puetz PA, Gersh BJ. Influence of coronary artery disease on morbidity and mortality after abdominal aortic aneurysmectomy: a population-based study, 1971-1987. *J Am Coll Cardiol*. 1989;14:1245-1252.
49. Pasternack PF, Imparato AM, Bear G, et al. The value of radionuclide angiography as a predictor of perioperative myocardial infarction in patients undergoing abdominal aortic aneurysm resection. *J Vasc Surg*. 1984;1:320-325.
50. Mangano DT, Brower WS, Hollenburg M. Association of perioperative myocardial ischemia with cardiac morbidity and mortality in men undergoing noncardiac surgery. *N Engl J Med*. 1990;323:1781-1787.
51. Goldman L. Multifactorial index of cardiac risk in noncardiac surgery: ten-year status report. *J Cardiothorac Anesth*. 1987;1: 237-244.
52. Cooperman M, Pflug B, Martin EW Jr, Evans WE. Cardiovascular risk factors in patients with peripheral vascular disease. *Surgery*. 1978;84:505-509.
53. Hertzer NR, Beven EG, Young JR, et al. Coronary artery disease in peripheral vascular patients: a classification of 1000 coronary angiograms and results of surgical management. *Ann Surg*. 1984;199:223-233.
54. Pohost GM. Dipyridamole thallium test: is it useful for predicting coronary events after vascular surgery? *Circulation*. 1991;84: 931-932.
55. Raby KE, Goldman L, Creager MA, et al. Correlation between preoperative ischemia and major cardiac events after peripheral vascular surgery. *N Engl J Med*. 1989;321:1296-1300.
56. Mangano DT. Monitoring pulmonary arterial pressure in coronary artery disease. *Anesthesiology*. 1980;53:364-370.
57. Rice CL, Hobelman CF, John DA, et al. Central venous pressure or pulmonary capillary wedge pressure as the determinant of fluid replacement in aortic surgery. *Surgery*. 1978;84:437-440.
58. Thys DM, Hillel Z, Goldman ME, Mindich BP, Kaplan JA. A comparison of hemodynamic indices derived by invasive monitoring and two-dimensional echocardiography. *Anesthesiology*. 1987;67:630-634.
59. Clements FM, deBruijn NP. Perioperative evaluation of regional wall motion by transesophageal two-dimensional echocardiography. *Anesth Analg*. 1987;66:249-261.
60. Fleron MH, Weiskopf RB, Bertrand M, et al. A comparison of intrathecal opioid and intravenous analgesia for the incidence of cardiovascular, respiratory, and renal complications after abdominal aortic surgery. *Anesth Analg*. 2003;97:2-12.
61. Yeager MP, Glass DD, Neff RK, Brinck-Johnson T. Epidural anesthesia and analgesia in high-risk surgical patients. *Anesthesiology*. 1987;66:729-736.
62. Rao TL, El-Etr AA. Anticoagulation following placement of epidural and subarachnoid catheters: an evaluation of neurological sequelae. *Anesthesiology*. 1981;55:618-620.
63. Gold MS, Rockman CB, Riles TS. Comparison of lumbar and thoracic epidural narcotics for postoperative analgesia in patients undergoing abdominal aortic aneurysm repair. *J Cardiothorac Vasc Anesth*. 1997;11:137-140.
64. Major CP Jr, Greer MS, Russell WL, Roe SM. Postoperative pulmonary complications and morbidity after abdominal aneurysmectomy: a comparison of postoperative epidural versus parenteral epidural analgesia. *Am Surg*. 1996;62:45-51.
65. Aadahl P, Lundbom J, Hatlinghus S, Myhre HO. Regional anesthesia for endovascular treatment of abdominal aortic aneurysms. *J Endovasc Surg*. 1997;4:56-61.
66. Bower TC, Cherry KJ, Pairolero PC. Unusual manifestations of abdominal aortic aneurysms. *Surg Clin North Am*. 1989;69: 745-754.
67. Crawford ES, Svensson LG, Coselli JS, Safi HJ, Hess KR. Aortic dissection and dissecting aortic aneurysms. *Ann Surg*. 1988;208:254-273.
68. Piotrowski JJ, McCroskey BL, Rutherford RB. Selection of grafts currently available for repair of abdominal aortic aneurysms. *Surg Clin North Am*. 1989;69:827-836.
69. Hollier LH, Symmonds JB, Pairolero PC, Cherry KJ, Hallett JW, Gloviczki P. Thoracoabdominal aortic aneurysm repair: analysis of postoperative morbidity. *Arch Surg*. 1988;123:871-875.
70. Coselli JS, Conklin LD, LeMaire SA. Thoracoabdominal aortic aneurysm repair: review and update of current strategies. *Ann Thorac Surg*. 2002;74:S1881-S1884.
71. Johnston KW, Rutherford RB, Tilson MD, Shah DM, Hollier L, Stanley JC. Suggested standards for reporting on arterial aneurysms: Subcommittee on Reporting Standards for Arterial Aneurysms, Ad Hoc Committee on Reporting Standards, Society for Vascular Surgery and North American Chapter,

International Society for Cardiovascular Surgery. *J Vasc Surg.* 1991;13:452-458.
72. Bickerstaff LK, Pairolero PC, Hollier, et al. Thoracic aortic aneurysms: a population-based study. *Surgery.* 1982;92:1103-1108.
73. Crawford ES, DeNatale RW. Thoracoabdominal aortic aneurysms: observations regarding the natural course of the disease. *J Vasc Surg.* 3:578-582.
74. Crawford ES, Svensson LG, Coselli JS, Safi HJ, Hess KR. Surgical treatment of aneurysm and/or dissection of the ascending aorta, transverse aortic arch, and ascending aorta and transverse aortic arch: factors influencing survival in 717 patients. *J Thorac Cardiovasc Surg.* 1989;98:659-673.
75. Buth J, Harris P, Hop W, Riambau V, Laheiji R. Outcome of endovascular abdominal aortic aneurysm repair in patients with conditions considered unfit for an open procedure. *J Vasc Surg.* 2002;35:211-221.
76. Carpenter JP, Baum RA, Barker CF, Golden MA, Velazquez OC, Mitchell ME. Durability of benefits of endovascular versus conventional abdominal aortic aneurysm repair. *J Vasc Surg.* 2002;35:222-228.
77. Boyle JR, Goodall S, Thompson MM. *Br J Surg.* 1999;86:23.
78. Thompson JP, Boyle JR, Thompson NM, Strupish J, Bell PR, Smith G. Cardiovascular and catecholamine responses during endovascular and conventional abdominal aortic aneurysm repair. *J Vasc Surg.* 1999;17:326-333.
79. Sweeny KJ, Evoy D, Sultan C, et al. Endovascular approach to abdominal aortic aneurysms limits the postoperative systemic immune response. *Eur J Vasc Surg.* 2002;23:303-308.
80. Brewster DC. Presidential address: What would you do if it was your father? Reflections of endovascular abdominal aortic aneurysm. *J Vasc Surg.* 2001;33:1139-1147.
81. Fairman RM, Velazquez O, Baum R, et al. Endovascular repair of aortic aneurysms: critical events and adjunctive procedures. *J Vasc Surg.* 2001;33:1226-1232.
82. Dattilo JB, Brewster DC, Fan C, et al. Clinical failures of endovascular abdominal aortic aneurysm repair: incidence, causes and management. *J Vasc Surg.* 2002;35:1137-1144.
83. Murphy DA, Craver JM, Jones EL, Bone DK, Guyton RA, Hatcher CR Jr. Recognition and management of ascending aortic dissection complicating cardiac surgical operations. *J Thorac Cardiovasc Surg.* 1983;85:247-256.
84. Simon P, Owen AN, Havel M, et al. Transesophageal echocardiography in the emergency surgical management of patients with aortic dissection. *J Thorac Cardiovasc Surg.* 1992;103: 1113-1117.
85. Svensson LG, Crawford ES, Hess KR, Coselli JS, Safi HJ. Dissection of the aorta and dissecting aortic aneurysms: improved early and long-term surgical results. *Circulation.* 1990;82:24-38.
86. Hollier LH, Moore WM. Avoidance of renal and neurologic complications following thoracoabdominal aortic aneurysm repair. *Acta Chir Scand.* 1990;555(suppl):129-135.
87. Svensson LG, Patel V, Robinson MF, Ueda T, Roehm JO Jr, Crawford ES. Influence of preservation or perfusion of intraoperatively identified spinal cord blood supply on spinal motor evoked potentials and paraplegia after aortic surgery. *J Vasc Surg.* 1991;13:355-365.
88. Laschinger JC, Owen J, Rosenbloom M, Cox JL, Kouchoukos NT. Direct noninvasive onitoring of spinal cord motor function during thoracic aortic occlusion: use of motor evoked potentials. *J Vasc Surg.* 1988;7:161-171.
89. Grubbs PE Jr, Marini C, Toporoff B, et al. Somatosensory evoked potentials and spinal cord perfusion pressure are significant predictors of postoperative neurologic dysfunction. *Surgery.* 1988;104:216-223.
90. Stenseth R, Myhre HO. Anesthesia in surgery for aneurysm of the descending thoracic or thoracoabdominal aorta. *Acta Chir Scand.* 1988;154:147-150.
91. Coles JG, Wilson GJ, Sima AF, et al. Intraoperative management of thoracic aortic aneurysm: experimental evaluation of perfusion cooling of the spinal cord. *J Thorac Cardiovasc Surg.* 1983;85:292-299.
92. McCullough JL, Hollier LH, Nugent M. Paraplegia after thoracic aortic occlusion: influence of cerebrospinal fluid drainage. *J Vasc Surg.* 1988;7:153-160.
93. Naslund TC, Hollier LH. Thoracoabdominal aneurysm. In: Cameron JL, ed. *Current Surgical Therapy.* 4th ed. St Louis: Mosby; 1992:676.
94. Jex RK, Schaff HV, Piehler JM, et al. Early and late results following repair of dissections of the descending thoracic aorta. *J Vasc Surg.* 1986;3:226-237.
95. Hollier LH. Protecting the brain and spinal cord. *J Vasc Surg.* 1987;5:524-528.
96. Drenger D, Parker SD, Frank SM, Beattie C. Changes in cerebrospinal fluid pressure and lactate concentrations during thoracoabdominal aortic aneurysm surgery. *Anesthesiology.* 1997;86:41-47.
97. van Dongen EP, Ter Beek HT, Boezeman EH, Schepens MA, Langemeijer HJ, Aarts LP. Normal serum concentrations of S-100 protein and changes in cerebrospinal fluid concentrations of S-100 protein during and after thoracoabdominal aortic aneurysm surgery: is S-100 protein a biochemical marker of clinical value in detecting spinal cord ischemia? *J Vasc Surg.* 1998;27:344-346.
98. Naslund TC, Hollier LH, Money SR, Facundus EC, Skenderis BS II. Protecting the ischemic spinal cord during aortic clamping: the influence of anesthetics and hypothermia. *Ann Surg.* 1992;215:409-415.
99. Mackey WC. Extracranial cerebral vascular disease. In: Cameron JL, ed. *Current Surgical Therapy.* 4th ed. St Louis: Mosby; 1992:684.
100. Warlow C. Surgical versus medical treatment for symptomatic carotid atherosclerosis. *Acta Chir Scand.* 1990;555(suppl): 223-224.
101. Wolf PA, Kannel WB, Dawber TR. Transient ischemic attacks and the risk of stroke: the Framingham study. *Circulation.* 1979;60:98.
102. Massachusetts Medical Society. Beneficial effect of carotid endarterectomy in symptomatic patients with high-grade carotid stenosis. *N Engl J Med.* 1991;325:445-453.
103. Executive Committee for the Asymptomatic Carotid Atherosclerosis (ACAS) Study. Endarterectomy for asymptomatic carotid artery stenosis. *JAMA.* 1995;273:1421-1428.
104. Wheeler HB. Presidential address: common sense and carotid endarterectomy. *J Vasc Surg.* 1990;11:735-744.
105. Callow AD, Mackey WC. Optimum results of the surgical treatment of carotid territory ischemia. *Circulation.* 1991;83(suppl 1): 190-195.
106. Callow AD, Mackey WC. Long-term follow-up of surgically managed carotid bifurcation atherosclerosis. *Ann Surg.* 1989;210:308-315.
107. Hsia DC, Krushat WM, Moscoe LM. Epidemiology of carotid endarterectomies among Medicare beneficiaries. *J Vasc Surg.* 1992;16:201-208.
108. Ackroyd N, Lane R, Appleberg M. Carotid endarterectomy long-term follow-up with specific reference to recurrent stenosis: contralateral progression, mortality and recurrent neurological episodes. *J Cardiovasc Surg.* 1986;27:418-425.
109. Schroder T. How to predict which patient with carotid atherosclerosis is "high risk." *Acta Chir Scand.* 1990;555(suppl). 209-222.
110. Sieber FE, Toung TJ, Diringer MN, Wang H, Long DM. Preoperative risks predict neurological outcome of carotid endarterectomy related strokes. *Neurosurgery.* 1992;30:847-854.
111. Young B, Moore WS, Robertson JT, et al. An analysis of perioperative surgical mortality and morbidity in the asymptomatic carotid atherosclerosis study: ACAS investigators: Asymptomatic Carotid Atherosclerosis Study. *Stroke.* 1996;27:2216-2224.
112. Cambria RP, Ivarsson BL, Akins CW, Moncure AC, Brewster DC, Abbott WM. Simultaneous carotid and coronary disease: safety of the combined approach. *J Vasc Surg.* 1989;9:56-64.

113. Perler BA, Burdick JF, Minken SL, Williams GM. Should we perform carotid endarterectomy synchronously with cardiac surgical procedures? *J Vasc Surg*. 1988;8:402-409.
114. Chang BB, Darling RC III, Shah DM, Paty PS, Leather RP. Carotid endarterectomy can be safely performed with acceptable mortality and morbidity in patients requiring coronary artery bypass grafts. *Am J Surg*. 1994;168:94-96.
115. Ricotta JJ, Char DJ, Cuadra SA, et al. Modeling stroke risk after coronary artery bypass and combined coronary artery bypass graft and carotid endarterectomy. *Stroke*. 2003;34:1212-1217.
116. Brown KR, Kresowik TF, Chin MH, Kresowik RA, Grund SL, Hendel ME. Multistate population-based outcomes of combined carotid endarterectomy and coronary artery bypass graft. *J Vasc Surg*. 2003;37:32-39.
117. Dared M. Carotid endarterectomy: anesthesia and monitoring. *Acta Anaesthesiol Belg*. 1988;39(suppl 2):271-273.
118. Harada RN, Comerota AJ, Good GM, Hashemi HA, Hulihan JF. Stump pressure, electroencephalographic changes, and the contralateral carotid artery: another look at selective shunting. *Am J Surg*. 1995;170:148-153.
119. Young WL, Prohovnik I, Schroeder T, Correll JW, Ostapkovich N. Intraoperative ^{133}Xe cerebral blood flow measurements by intravenous versus intracarotid methods. *Anesthesiology*. 1990;73:637-643.
120. Lam AM, Manninen PH, Ferguson GG, Nantau W. Monitoring electrophysiologic function during carotid endarterectomy: a comparison of somatosensory evoked potentials and conventional electroencephalogram. *Anesthesiology*. 1991;75:15-21.
121. Redekop G, Ferguson G. Correlation of contralateral stenosis and intraoperative electroencephalogram change with risk of stroke during carotid endarterectomy. *Neurosurgery*. 1992;30:191-194.
122. McDowell HA Jr, Gross GM, Halsey JH. Carotid endarterectomy monitored with transcranial Doppler. *Ann Surg*. 1992;215:514-519.
123. Corson JD, Chang BB, Shah DM, Leather RP, DeLeo BM, Karmody AM. The influence of anesthetic choice on carotid endarterectomy outcome. *Arch Surg*. 1987;122:807-812.
124. McCarthy RJ, Nasr MK, McAteer P, Harrocks M. Physiological advantages of cerebral blood flow during carotid endarterectomy under local anesthesia: a randomized trial. *Eur J Vasc Surg*. 2002;24:215-221.
125. Allen BT, Anderson CB, Rubin BG, et al. The influence of anesthetic technique on perioperative complications after carotid endarterectomy. *J Vasc Surg*. 1994;19:834-842.
126. Mashiah M, Soroker D, Pasik S, Mashiah T. Carotid surgery under local anesthesia in the elderly. *J Am Geriatr Soc*. 1988;36:545-547.
127. Zuccarello M, Yeh H, Tew JM. Morbidity and mortality of carotid endarterectomy under local anesthesia: a retrospective study. *Neurosurgery*. 1988;23:445-450.
128. Slutzki S, Behar M, Negri M, Hod G, Zaidenstein L, Bogokowsky H. Carotid endarterectomy under local anesthesia supplemented with neuroleptic analgesia. *Surg Gynecol Obstet*. 1990;170:141-144.
129. Godin MS, Bell WH III, Schwedler M, Kerstein MD. Cost effectiveness of regional anesthesia in carotid endarterectomy. *Am Surg*. 1989;55:656-659.
130. Messick JM Jr, Casement B, Sharbrough FW, Milde LN, Michenfelder JD, Sundt TM Jr. Correlation of regional cerebral blood flow (rCBF) with EEG changes during isoflurane anesthesia for carotid endarterectomy: critical rCBF. *Anesthesiology*. 1987;66:344-349.
131. Michenfelder JD, Sundt TM, Fode N, Sharbrough FW. Isoflurane when compared to enflurane and halothane decreases the frequency of cerebral ischemia during carotid endarterectomy. *Anesthesiology*. 1987;67:336-340.
132. Cucchiara RF, Sundt TM, Michenfelder JD. Myocardial infarction in carotid endarterectomy patients anesthetized with halothane, enflurane of isoflurane. *Anesthesiology*. 1988;69:783-784.
133. Young WL, Prohovnik I, Correll JW, et al. A comparison of the cerebral hemodynamic effects of sufentanil and isoflurane in humans undergoing carotid endarterectomy. *Anesthesiology*. 1989;71:863-869.
134. Herrick IA, Gelb AW. Occlusive cerebrovascular disease: anesthetic considerations. In: *Anesthesia and Neurosurgery*. Cottrell JE, Smith DS, eds. St Louis: Mosby; 2001.
135. Palmer M. Comparison of regional and general anesthesia for carotid endarterectomy. *Am J Surg*. 1989;157:329-333.
136. Welton RJ, Eikelboom BC. Technical details in carotid endarterectomy. *Acta Chir Scand*. 1990;555:205-208.
137. Wilke HJ, Ellis JE, McKinsey JF. Carotid endarterectomy: perioperative and anesthetic considerations. *J Cardiothorac Vasc Anesth*. 1996;10:928-949.
138. Hankey GJ, Bond R, Rerkasem K, Rothwell PM. Routine or selective carotid artery shunting for carotid endarterectomy. *Stroke*. 2003;34:824-825.
139. Stankovic G, Liistro F, Moshiri S, Briguori C, Corvaja N, Gimelli G. Carotid artery stenting in the first 100 consecutive patients: results and follow up. *Heart*. 2002;88:381-386.
140. Leger AR, Neale M, Harris JP. Poor durability of carotid angioplasty and stenting for treatment of recurrent artery stenosis after carotid endarterectomy: an institutional experience. *J Vasc Surg*. 2001;33:1008-1014.
141. Kilaru S, Korn P, Kasirajan K, et al. Is carotid angioplasty and stenting more cost effective than carotid endarterectomy? *J Vasc Surg*. 2003;37:331-339.
142. Elliott BM, Collins GJ Jr, Youkey JR, Donohue HJ Jr, Salander JM, Rich NM. Intraoperative local anesthetic injection of the carotid sinus nerve: a prospective, randomized study. *Am J Surg*. 1986;152:695-699.
143. Mangano DT, Layug EL, Wallace A, Tateo I. Effect of atenolol on mortality and cardiac morbidity after noncardiac surgery. *N Engl J Med*. 1996;23:1713-1720.
144. Skydell JL, Machleder HI, Baker JD, Busuttil RW, Moore WS. Incidence and mechanism of post-carotid endarterectomy hypertension. *Arch Surg*. 1987;122:1153-1155.
145. Ascher E, Markevich N, Schutzer RW, Kallakuri S, Theresa P, Hingorani A. Cerebral hyperperfusion syndrome after carotid endarterectomy: predictive factors and hemodynamic changes. *J Vasc Surg*. 2003;37:769-777.
146. Edwards WH Jr, Edwards WH Sr, Mulherin JL Jr, Martin RS III. Recurrent carotid artery stenosis: resection with autogenous vein replacement. *Ann Surg*. 1989;209:662-668.
147. Kraiss LW, Kilberg L, Critch S, Johansen KJ. Short-stay carotid endarterectomy is safe and cost-effective. *Am J Surg*. 1995;169:512-515.
148. Ricotta JJ, Hargadon T. Cost management strategies for carotid endarterectomy. *Am J Surg*. 1998;176:188-192.
149. Friedman SG, Tortolani AJ. Reduced length of stay following carotid endarterectomy under general anesthesia. *Am J Surg*. 1995;170:235-236.

CHAPTER 24

Respiratory Anatomy, Physiology, and Pathophysiology

John J. Nagelhout

Knowledge of the respiratory system is essential to the practice of anesthesia. A large percentage of the major malpractice awards are related to respiratory system difficulties such as inability to intubate, hypoventilation, and esophageal intubation. Improved monitors for evaluating the function of the respiratory system, such as capnographs and pulse oximeters, greatly increase the safety of anesthesia while reducing the incidence of injury. In humans, air enters and leaves the lungs by the same route; therefore a significant part of anesthesia care involves the securing and maintenance of this airway.

The functions of the respiratory system include gas exchange, acid-base balance, phonation, pulmonary defense, and metabolism (synthesis and breakdown of bioactive materials). The respiratory system takes oxygen (O_2) from the atmosphere and supplies it to the cells while removing carbon dioxide (CO_2) from the body. The ventilatory muscles respond to impulses generated by the respiratory centers in the brain stem. These muscles generate forces that increase the volume of the chest cavity, causing atmospheric air to be inspired through the conducting airways into the lungs. Peripheral chemoreceptors sense the O_2, CO_2, and hydrogen ion (H^+) levels in the arterial blood, whereas the central chemoreceptors monitor CO_2 and H^+ levels in the cerebrospinal fluid and brain. Both sets of chemoreceptors affect the control of breathing by the brain-stem respiratory centers.

Movement of air over the vocal cords produces sounds by means of a process known as *phonation*. Injury of the vocal cords and other laryngeal structures necessary for speech can occur during endotracheal intubation, resulting in hoarseness or "loss of voice." The larynx and other structures in the airway also have an important role in the defense of the lungs. Laryngeal reflexes help prevent aspiration of food or liquid as it is being swallowed. Airway structures also help to filter and remove particles from the inspired air (Figure 24-1). The cells of the lung have an active metabolic role, producing materials such as surfactant, which is necessary for normal pulmonary function. The cells of the pulmonary circulation can metabolize many substances in the blood, such as angiotensin I, which the lung's angiotensin-converting enzyme modifies into the more physiologically active angiotensin II.

ANATOMY OF THE RESPIRATORY SYSTEM

A knowledge of airway anatomy is not only necessary for understanding respiratory physiology but also essential for anesthesiology practice. The airway consists of the nose, pharynx, larynx, trachea, and lower airways.

The components of the respiratory system are the conducting airways, the lungs, the portions of the central nervous system responsible for control of the muscles of ventilation, and the chest wall. The chest wall contains the muscles of ventilation (diaphragm and intercostal muscles) as well as the ribs, sternum, and vertebrae; accessory muscles of ventilation include muscles of the neck and abdomen. Also see Chapters 20 and 36 for discussions of airway anatomy, physiology, and function.

Nose

Inhaled air enters the body through the nose or mouth. Air passing through the nose is filtered, heated to body

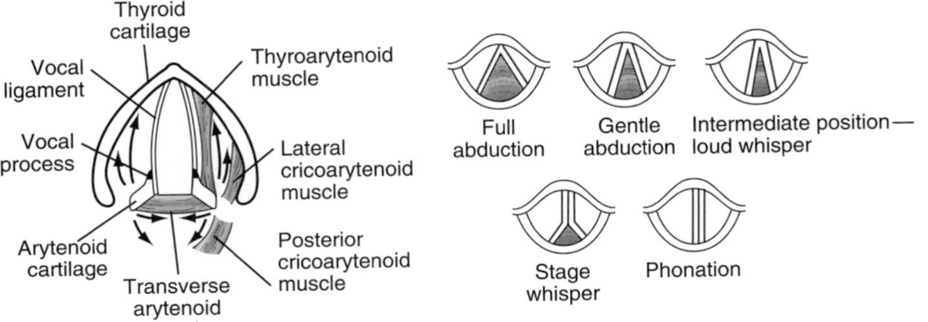

FIGURE **24-1** **A,** Anatomy of the throat. **B,** Laryngeal function in phonation showing the positions of the vocal folds during different types of phonation. (From Guyton AC, Hall JE. *Textbook of Medical Physiology*. 10th ed. Philadelphia: Saunders; 2001:442.)

temperature, and humidified. The two nostrils are the beginning of the nasal passages. The external nose is only a small part of the nasal air passageway, the major portion of which underlies the face.

Each nostril (anterior naris) opens directly into the vestibule, which is the slightly forwardly expanded portion of the nasal cavity. The vestibule is lined with cutaneous epithelium and in its lower half has hairs and sebaceous glands. The floor of the nose is at a level higher than the opening of the nostril; therefore during nasal intubation the apex of the nose should be pushed superiorly with steady gentle pressure while the tube is inserted parallel to the roof of the mouth. The tube should not be directed upward into the turbinates (conchae). Prolonged nasotracheal intubation is associated with obstruction of the nasal sinuses, sinus infection, and fever. Intranasal infections can produce intracranial infection via vascular connections, as discussed later in this section.

The anterior portion of the external nose, the vestibule, expands above and behind into triangular spaces, or fossae. The fossae are separated from each other by the nasal septum, which also separates the two nostrils. These nasal fossae usually communicate freely with the paranasal air sinuses. They open into the pharynx by the posterior nares (also known as *choanae*) and are bordered medially by the nasal septum and laterally by three turbinate scrolls (nasal conchae) arranged one above the other. Choanal atresia is a birth defect that results in the obstruction of the airway of the obligate nose-breathing newborn.

The conchae are more or less horizontally situated ledges projecting from the lateral walls that have their free margins directed downward and inward. The spaces that these conchae overlie and partly shut off from the nasal cavity are the superior, middle, and inferior meatus (which contain the openings to the paranasal sinuses).[1]

The superior concha is by far the smallest of the three, and the middle concha extends forward much farther than the superior. The inferior concha, which lies along the lower part of the lateral wall of the nasal cavity, is in the pathway of airflow in the nose. It is the one most commonly injured during nasal intubation. It extends to within approximately 2 cm of the middle of the anterior naris, and its posterior tip lies approximately 1 cm in front of the pharyngeal orifice of the eustachian tube. Eustachian drainage can become obstructed when the inferior concha or adenoid tonsils become inflamed. Such obstruction can lead to middle ear disease.

The nasal cavities are lined with mucous membranes that are continuous with those of the pharynx. The mucosa can be divided into respiratory and olfactory areas because it not only lines the tracts followed by respired air but also covers the cells that act as the receptors for smell. The respiratory mucosal tract lines the lower two thirds of the nose and consists of ciliated epithelial cells and mucous glands. The direction of motion of the cilia is toward the exterior of the nasal cavity, and the amount of mucus produced can often be copious. The olfactory epithelium occupies the apical third of the nasal cavity and consists of specialized sensory cells. The principal arterial supply of the nasal fossae comes from the ophthalmic arteries through the anterior and posterior ethmoid branches and from the internal maxillary artery through the sphenopalatine arteries. Because of the location of the interior maxillary artery, it is sometimes ligated for the treatment of persistent nosebleed. The veins accompany the arteries; the ethmoid veins open into the superior sagittal sinus, and the nasal veins drain into the ophthalmic veins and then into the cavernous sinuses. Infections in the nose can result in meningitis because of this venous communication between the intracranial and intranasal circulation. The lymphatic drainage from the cavities of the nose is via the deep cervical lymph nodes adjacent to the internal jugular vein.

The afferent fibers from the olfactory nerves (cranial nerve I) pierce the openings of the cribriform plate of the ethmoid bone then reach the rhinencephalon of the brain. The sensory nerves from the upper respiratory tract come from the ophthalmic nerve (a branch of cranial nerve V) and the maxillary nerve (another branch of cranial V).

Functions of the nose include the heating, humidification, and filtration of inspired air as well as olfaction. The inspired air is warmed very efficiently because of the rich vascular supply of the nasal mucosa. As long as the incoming air is not extremely cold, the nose itself can warm the inspired air to nearly body temperature. Inspired air is moistened to nearly 100% relative humidity.

The heating and humidifying functions of the nose are affected by general anesthesia. The inspiration of cold, dry gas often dries the nasal and pharyngeal passageways, causing sore throat even if no manipulation of the airway takes place. The hairs at the entrance to the nostrils are of minor importance to filtration because they remove only large particles. Much more important is the removal of particles by turbulent precipitation. Air passing through the nasal passageways hits many obstructions—the septum, the turbinates, and the pharyngeal wall. When the inspired air is forced to change direction, the inhaled particles cannot change course as rapidly, and they become embedded in the sticky mucus-covered surfaces of these processes. The particles trapped in the mucus are moved by the cilia either to the nostril or posteriorly to the pharynx to be either expectorated or swallowed. This nasal mechanism for removing particles from the air is so effective that almost no particle greater than approximately 6 mm in size is allowed to enter the trachea.[2]

Pharynx

The pharynx is a wide muscular tube that is a part of both the respiratory tract and the alimentary tract. Its upper border is the base of the skull, and it extends to the level of the C6 vertebra, where it becomes continuous with the esophagus. At this level ingested foreign bodies, such as coins, are frequently lodged. The pharynx is lined by a musculomembranous coat and is divided into three parts: the nasopharynx, which extends from the posterior nares (choanae) to the end of the soft palate; the oropharynx, which is bounded superiorly by the soft palate and anteriorly by the tonsillar pillars and oral cavity and which extends inferiorly to the tip of the epiglottis; and the laryngopharynx, which extends from the tip of the epiglottis to the level of C6.

The pharyngeal region includes the tonsils, which are composed of three aggregations of lymphoid tissue: the palatine tonsils (major tonsils), which lie in the tonsillar fossae at the boundary of the oral cavity and oropharynx; the lingual tonsils, which extend across the tongue from the base of each palatine tonsil; and the pharyngeal tonsils (adenoids), which lie on the lateral walls of the nasopharynx. The lymphoid tissue of the tonsils forms Waldeyer's tonsillar ring, which acts as a first line of defense against bacterial invasion of the nasal and buccal passages.

TABLE 24-1 The Nine Cartilages of the Larynx

UNPAIRED CARTILAGES		PAIRED CARTILAGES	
Number	**Name**	**Number**	**Name**
1	Epiglottic	4 and 5	Arytenoids
2	Thyroid	6 and 7	Corniculates
3	Cricoid	8 and 9	Cuneiforms

Blood supply to the entire mouth and pharyngeal region is from branches of the external carotid artery. Venous drainage is via the facial vein and the external jugular vein. The nerve supply to the inner mouth is from cranial nerves VII, IX, X, and XII. The lymphatic circulation is abundant, draining into the cervical lymph nodes located under and anterior to the sternocleidomastoid muscle (this configuration accounts for lumps in the neck that accompany a sore throat).

Larynx

The adult larynx extends from vertebrae C3 to C6 and is a protective structure that prevents aspiration during swallowing; vocalization evolved secondarily. The larynx consists of one bone, nine pieces of cartilage (Table 24-1), ligaments, muscles, and membranes. (Also see Chapter 36, Table 36-1).

The hyoid bone is the chief support for the larynx. Its anterior aspect can be easily palpated. The thyroid cartilage and the cricoid cartilage make up the principal part of the framework of the larynx, whereas the epiglottis guards its entrance.

The complete circle of the cricoid cartilage can form a seal against the endotracheal tube; therefore a cuffed tube is usually unnecessary in children. In adults the space between the vocal cords (glottis) is smaller than the inside of the cricoid cartilage; therefore a cuffed tube is necessary for a seal to form for positive-pressure ventilation.

Laryngeal Cartilages

The epiglottic cartilage lies closest to the root of the tongue and is vertical to the opening of the larynx. It is attached to the body of the thyroid cartilage by the thyroepiglottic ligament just above the vocal cords and to the base of the tongue by the glossoepiglottic folds. The thyroid cartilage is the largest cartilage of the larynx, formed by two quadrangular plates or laminae (wings) fused near the midline anteriorly. It has great strength and affords a great deal of protection to the larynx. The thyroid cartilage forms the Adam's apple.

The cricoid cartilage is palpable just below the thyroid gland, and its level corresponds to the beginning of the trachea and the esophagus. It is the only true ring of cartilage encircling the airway. Anteriorly, the cricoid cartilage lies below the thyroid cartilage. The arytenoid cartilages articulate on the superior posterior aspect of the cricoid cartilage, which is slanted forward. The paired arytenoid cartilages are attached to the posterior ends of the vocal cords. The paired corniculate (median) and cuneiform (more lateral) cartilages are embedded in the aryepiglottic folds and give support to these structures. These cartilages cause the two bumps seen in the aryepiglottic folds, which are mistakenly called the "arytenoids" when visualized during difficult intubation.

In adults the narrowest portion of the laryngeal cavity is the area between the vocal cords; in children younger than 10 years of age, the narrowest part is just below the cords at the cricoid cartilage. This anatomic difference is of clinical significance: when small children are intubated, a tube may pass through the cords but will be unable to pass through the cricoid ring.[3]

Membranes of the Larynx

The thyrohyoid membrane suspends the larynx from the hyoid bone. The conus elasticus or cricothyroid membrane lies between the cricoid and the thyroid cartilages. The easiest and most rapid laryngotomy can be performed through this membrane. Cricothyrotomy is recommended for the emergency establishment of an airway when both endotracheal intubation and mask ventilation are unsuccessful. The so-called "transtracheal block" also can be performed through the cricothyroid membrane.

Interior of Larynx

The cavity of the larynx is divided into three compartments by the false vocal cords and the true vocal cords. The supraglottic area extends from above the false cords to the tip of the epiglottis. On each side of this area is located a pharyngeal sinus (the pyriform sinus). This recess or sinus is important because it is likely to be a place at which foreign bodies that enter the pharynx become lodged. The second component of the larynx is the area between the false cords and the true cords known as the *laryngeal ventricles*. The third area is the infraglottic region below the true cords and above the beginning of the trachea. The rima glottidis (glottic slit) is the space between the true cords.

Movements of the Vocal Cords

The true vocal cords are fibromembranous folds attached anteriorly to the thyroid cartilage and posteriorly to the arytenoids. The focal points of movement are the arytenoid cartilages, which rotate and slide up and down on the sloping cricoid cartilage. The muscles controlling laryngeal movement (Box 24-1) are most conveniently thought of as pairs having opposing actions. (Also see Chapter 36, Table 36-1.) The laryngeal inlet is closed by the aryepiglottic muscle and opened by the thyroepiglottic muscle. The glottic slit is dilated by the posterior cricoarytenoid muscles and is closed by the interarytenoid muscles, assisted by the lateral cricoarytenoid muscles. The cricothyroid muscles lengthen the true vocal cords, and the *thyroarytenoid muscles* shorten them. Both sets of muscles can alter the tension on the vocal cords and are important for determining the pitch of the voice.[4]

BOX 24-1

Intrinsic Muscles of the Larynx

Laryngeal Inlet

Closed by the aryepiglottic muscle
Opened by the thyroepiglottic muscle

Glottic Slit

Dilated by the posterior cricoarytenoid muscles
Closed by the interarytenoid muscle and the lateral cricoarytenoid muscles

True Vocal Cords

Lengthened by the cricothyroid muscles
Shortened by thyroarytenoid muscles

Nerve Supply to the Larynx

Both the superior and inferior laryngeal nerves are branches of the vagus nerve. The superior laryngeal nerve arises from the ganglion nodosum of the vagus and divides into two branches, the internal and external. The external segment gives a branch to the inferior constrictor muscle of the pharynx and also to the cricothyroid muscles. These muscles change the position of the cricoid and thyroid cartilages and, in doing so, lengthen or increase the tension of the vocal cords. If these muscles are paralyzed, the voice becomes weak, rough, and easily fatigued. The internal branch enters the larynx and then the thyrohyoid membrane and is distributed to the mucous membranes of the larynx and epiglottis. It provides sensation from the laryngeal side of the epiglottis down to the true cords (the tongue side of the epiglottis is innervated by the glossopharyngeal nerve). The internal branch also innervates the interarytenoid muscles, which are important in phonation.

The inferior (or recurrent) laryngeal nerves arise from the two vagus nerves at different levels. The left nerve descends with the vagus and then loops around the arch of the aorta to come back up to the neck. The right nerve travels with the vagus nerve as far as the subclavian artery; it loops around this artery and then comes back up the neck. The recurrent laryngeal nerve supplies sensation to the larynx below the level of the vocal cords and innervates all the muscles of the larynx except the cricothyroid and part of the interarytenoid muscles. (See Chapter 36, Table 36-1.)

The blood supply to the larynx is provided by the superior thyroid artery (a branch of the external carotid artery) and by the inferior thyroid artery (a branch of the thyrocervical trunk, which arises from the subclavian artery).[5]

Trachea

The trachea is lined by ciliated columnar epithelium, and it extends from the inferior larynx to the carina, where it bifurcates into the two mainstem bronchi. In adults of normal size the distances are fairly constant: the distance from the incisors to the larynx is approximately 13 cm, as is that from the larynx to the carina. Therefore the distance from the incisors to the carina is approximately 26 cm (note the distance marks on endotracheal tubes). The trachea is formed of rings of cartilage that open posteriorly, extending down to the level of T4 to T5, where the carina is located. This posterior T4-T5 level corresponds anteriorly to the angle of Louis on the sternum, which is the articulation of the second rib. The trachea is not a "fixed" structure—that is, it moves with head or neck movement. If a patient flexes the neck, the trachea moves upward; as a result the endotracheal tube moves downward and endobronchial intubation is possible. Similarly, the trachea moves upward if the patient turns the head to the left or the right. During extension of the head and neck the trachea moves downward, the endotracheal tube moves upward, and extubation can occur.

The blood supply to the trachea is through the inferior thyroid artery, which comes from the thyrocervical branch of the subclavian artery. The trachea is innervated by the vagus nerve.

The diameter of the trachea approximates that of the index finger. The bronchi do not branch off at the same angle, the right bronchus being more nearly in line with the trachea. Also, the right mainstem bronchus is wider and shorter than the left one. Because the right bronchus is more nearly vertical than the left, the tendency for endotracheal tubes, suction catheters, or aspirated foreign materials to enter it is much greater. Additionally, if an endotracheal tube is inserted too far, its beveled tip makes right-sided intubation more likely. The hole (Murphy's eye) on the nonbeveled edge of the tube allows the delivery of gas to the left mainstem bronchus if the tip of the tube is on the carina.

The right mainstem bronchus ends only 1.5 cm from the carina before giving rise to the right upper lobe bronchus. The other divisions of the right mainstem bronchus are the right middle lobe bronchus and the right lower lobe bronchus. The left mainstem bronchus is narrower than the right and nearly 5 cm in length. It terminates by bifurcating into the left upper lobe bronchus and the left lower lobe bronchus. The left upper lobe bronchus divides into halves, an upper half and a lower half (the lingular branch).

Each mainstem bronchus divides into segmental bronchi that deliver ventilation to the various bronchopulmonary segments of the lung. Each subsegmental bronchus divides several times, giving rise to many bronchioles that still possess cartilaginous support. These bronchioles divide two or more times before losing their cartilaginous support; those without such support are called *terminal bronchioles*. The terminal bronchioles are the last structures perfused by the bronchial circulation and are the end of the conducting airways (anatomic dead space, as discussed later). The terminal bronchioles divide into the respiratory bronchioles, which are perfused by the pulmonary circulation and are the first place in the airway at which alveoli appear and where exchange of gas with the blood occurs. The respiratory bronchioles divide into several alveolar ducts, which lead to circular spaces called *atria*. Each atrium opens into two to five alveolar sacs, which are spaces lined by alveoli or air sacs.

The lungs have a dual blood supply: (1) the bronchial arteries (usually one on the right and two on the left), which arise from the descending aorta and which in general provide nutrients to the lungs and the bronchi; and (2) the pulmonary arteries, which bring unoxygenated blood to the lungs. The flow through the pulmonary artery is the entire output of the right ventricle; in contrast, the flow through the bronchial artery is only approximately 2% to 3% of the output of the left ventricle. The pulmonary vessels meet and anastomose with the bronchial vessels at the junction of the terminal and respiratory bronchioles. The venous bronchopulmonary anastomoses are an important part of the normal anatomic shunt (the addition of unoxygenated blood to the left chambers of the heart).

When a patient is on complete bypass during cardiac surgery, blood enters the left atrium even though all blood is shunted from the right ventricle by the venous cannula. This is because blood flow continues through the bronchial vessels, which anastomose with the pulmonary veins, which in turn ultimately drain into the left atrium—one reason why a ventricular drain may be inserted during the surgery to prevent overdistention of the heart.

The lungs are divided into lobes and segments (Box 24-2). As stated earlier, the right lung is subdivided into the right upper lobe, the right middle lobe, and the right lower lobe. The left lung has only upper and lower lobes. The right lung has 10 bronchopulmonary segments, whereas the left has eight. Segments whose names contain the word *basal* are located adjacent to the diaphragm.

The nerve supply to the bronchi and lungs arises chiefly from the sympathetic nerves and the vagus nerve, which supplies sensory and parasympathetic innervation. All conduits to

BOX 24-2

Lung Lobes and Segments

- I. Right lung
  - A. Right upper lobe (3 segments)
    1. Apical
    2. Anterior
    3. Posterior
  - B. Right middle lobe (2 segments)
    1. Medial
    2. Lateral
  - C. Right lower lobe (5 segments)
    1. Superior
    2. Anterior basal
    3. Posterior basal
    4. Lateral basal
    5. Medial basal
- II. Left lung
  - A. Left upper lobe (4 segments)
    1. Apical posterior
    2. Anterior
    3. Superior lingular
    4. Inferior lingular
  - B. Left lower lobe (4 segments)
    1. Superior
    2. Anteromedial basal
    3. Posterior basal
    4. Lateral basal

the lung pass through the hilum, which is the connection of the mediastinum to the pedicle of each lung. The structures in each hilum include the mainstem bronchus, pulmonary artery and vein, bronchial arteries and veins (which drain into the azygous system), lymphatics, lymph nodes, pulmonary nerve plexuses, and pulmonary ligament. All of this is surrounded by connective tissue. The double-walled serous membrane covering the lung is called the pleura. Its two layers are the visceral pleura, which is tightly adherent to the lung surface, and the parietal pleura, which lines the interior of the chest wall and the diaphragm. These two layers meet at the hilum. Between these two layers is a potential space called the *pleural cavity*. The touching surfaces of the two layers of pleura are kept slippery by a small amount of serous fluid. Certain conditions can result in the occupation of the pleural space by liquids or gas (Table 24-2) and may affect ventilation and lung expansion. Infected intrapleural blood can clot and organize to form a

TABLE 24-2 Conditions That Affect the Pleural Space

Material in Pleural Space	Medical Name
Air	Pneumothorax
Air under pressure	Tension pneumothorax
Blood	Hemothorax
Serous fluid	Pleural effusion
Lymph	Empyema or pyothorax
Organized blood clot	Fibrothorax

fibrothorax, which must be peeled from the surface of the lung (in a procedure called *lung decortication*) so that the lung can reexpand.[4]

Mediastinum

The mediastinum is the region between the two pleural sacs. It lies roughly in the center of the thoracic cavity but is slightly displaced to the left by the presence of the heart. Therefore the left lung represents 45% of the total lung capacity (TLC), whereas the right lung provides 55%. Perforation of the larynx, trachea, pharynx, or esophagus, which sometimes occurs during esophagoscopy, bronchoscopy, or traumatic intubation, can produce mediastinitis, a life-threatening infection of an area containing the trachea, esophagus, and major blood vessels and nerves.

MECHANICS OF BREATHING

Contraction of the muscles of inspiration lowers intrathoracic pressure and causes the volume of the thoracic cavity to increase as air enters from the atmosphere. The diaphragm and internal intercostals are the muscles that contract during normal breathing (eupnea). Normally, eupneic expiration results from passive recoil of the chest wall and does not require muscular contraction. Accessory breathing muscles in the neck are required for forced inhalation. During forceful inspiration the sternocleidomastoid and scalene muscles contract in conjunction with the diaphragm and intercostals. During forced exhalation (e.g., with coughing and the clearing of secretions), the abdominal muscles—that is, the rectus abdominis, the transversus abdominis, and the external and internal oblique muscles of the abdomen—are active. The diaphragm is the principal muscle of eupneic inspiration and is innervated by the phrenic nerve, which arises from the third, fourth, and fifth cervical spinal nerve roots.

The muscles of ventilation are attached to the cartilaginous and bony components (ribs, sternum, and vertebrae) of the chest wall. The two diaphragms are dome-shaped muscles with central tendons located at the bottom of each hemithorax. They separate the thoracic and abdominal cavities and function separately, such that injury to a phrenic nerve results in paralysis in the diaphragm on that side. When the diaphragm contracts during spontaneous inspiration, it flattens and moves the abdominal contents downward, raising intraabdominal pressure while lowering intrathoracic pressure. Pressure within the alveoli becomes slightly negative with respect to atmospheric pressure, and gas flows inward through the conducting airways to expand the lungs. When the diaphragm is paralyzed, it cannot contract; therefore it moves upward from its normal position owing to the effects of the intraabdominal pressure and negative intrapleural pressure. When the normal diaphragm contracts (moving downward), the paralyzed diaphragm moves upward, and when the normal diaphragm relaxes (moving upward), the paralyzed diaphragm moves downward, resulting in paradoxic movements.

The diaphragms have a surface area of approximately 250 cm^2. They descend approximately 1 to 2 cm during eupneic breathing and as much as 10 cm during forceful breathing. For air to move into the alveoli, alveolar pressure must be less than atmospheric pressure. This can be achieved either through an increase in atmospheric pressure (as in positive-pressure ventilation) or a reduction in alveolar pressure, as during spontaneous ventilation (negative-pressure breathing). During anesthesia, respiratory therapy, and cardiopulmonary resuscitation, the air or gas mixtures are delivered to the alveoli by means of an increase of the pressures at the nose and mouth or endotracheal tube to greater than alveolar pressure (positive-pressure ventilation).[6]

Lung Compliance

Compliance is defined as the change in volume divided by the change in pressure (V/P). For a certain change in pressure, a more compliant lung has a greater change in volume than a less compliant one. Figure 24-2 shows pressure-volume relationships for a lung. Note that the inspiratory pressure-volume curve is different from the expiratory pressure-volume curve. This difference between the inflation curve and deflation curve is called *hysteresis* and indicates energy loss. Each individual alveolus does have its own compliance characteristics; however, each alveolus is considered as being somewhere on the pressure-volume curve for the whole lung.

Static compliance is the pressure-volume relationship for a lung when the air is not moving. Static compliance is decreased by conditions that make the lung difficult to inflate, such as fibrosis, obesity, vascular engorgement, edema, and external compression (e.g., that caused by tight dressings or a surgeon's leaning on the chest). Static compliance is increased by emphysema, which destroys the elastic tissue of the lung. This makes the emphysematous lung easier to inflate. The problem with emphysema is not inflation but rather deflation, because the loss of elastic tissue results in airway collapse as the lung deflates; this causes gas trapping. It is important to note that compliance changes as lung volume changes. In other words, compliance is volume dependent. Figure 24-2 shows that the lung is less compliant both at very high lung volumes and at very low lung volumes. Alveoli require greater pressure changes to be inflated and deflated when they are almost empty or almost full, respectively. When an alveolus is collapsed, a great increase in pressure is necessary for inflation to begin.

Dynamic compliance is the compliance of the lung while the air is moving. Here the forces involved in static compliance are added to the effects of airway resistance. Airway obstruction (e.g., that caused by bronchospasm or the presence of foreign bodies in the airway) can greatly decrease dynamic compliance.[7]

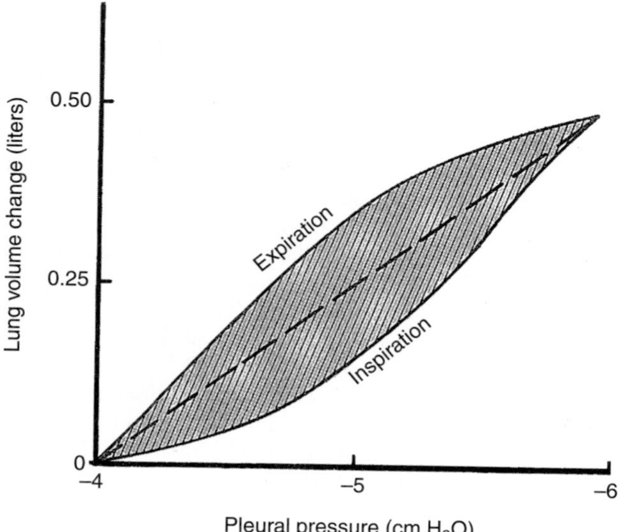

FIGURE **24-2**
Pressure-volume curve. (From Guyton AC, Hall JE. *Textbook of Medical Physiology*. 10th ed. Philadelphia: Saunders; 2001:434.)

Lung Elastic Recoil

The forces that cause elastic recoil of the lung are responsible for emptying the lung during exhalation and have a large role in determination of lung compliance. In addition to actual elastic fibers, the surface tension of the liquid film that lines the alveoli causes elastic recoil of the lung. Surface tension occurs at a gas-liquid interface and is generated by the cohesive forces among the molecules of the liquid. Surface tension is what causes water to bead and form droplets. The liquid lining the alveolar surface that faces the alveolar air has special characteristics that increase lung compliance.

If the alveolar interface were lined with water, surface tension would be high, making the lung harder to inflate. Laplace's law ($P = T/r$) states that if surface tension (T) is constant, pressure (P) would increase as radius (r) decreases. This does not occur in the lungs because as alveolar radius decreases, surface tension also decreases, so that pressure remains the same. This occurs because of a substance secreted by alveolar type II cells and known as *pulmonary surfactant*, which consists mainly of the phospholipid, dipalmitoyl lecithin. Pulmonary surfactant lowers the surface tension of the alveolar lining and decreases the work of breathing.

Additionally, the alveoli do not obey Laplace's law because surfactant preferentially lowers the surface tension in the small alveoli, thereby stabilizing the alveolar unit. Without surfactant, alveoli would all have the same surface tension and would obey Laplace's law. Smaller alveoli would empty into larger alveoli because pressure would be greater in the smaller alveoli. This would result in the eventual collapse of the smaller alveoli and in the impairment of gas exchange.

Surfactant is not produced by the fetal lung until approximately 28 weeks to 32 weeks of gestation and does not reach mature levels until approximately 35 weeks' gestation. Formation of surfactant can be hastened by the administration of glucocorticoids to the parturient. This is done when premature delivery is threatened or imminent. Low surfactant levels are a major factor in infant respiratory distress syndrome. The administration of synthetic surfactant to the airways of premature newborns has greatly reduced the incidence of this syndrome. Amniocentesis is sometimes performed in order to determine whether mature surfactant levels are present in the fetus when elective cesarean section is scheduled to be performed. The ratio of lecithin to sphingomyelin (the L/S ratio) indicates the amount of mature surfactant (dipalmitoyl lecithin) in proportion to the amount of surfactant precursor (sphingomyelin).

The chest wall is pulled in by the elastic forces of the lung. At the end of eupneic exhalation, the outward recoil of the chest wall is balanced by the inward elastic recoil of the lung. This is called the *resting end-expiratory point*. These opposing forces produce the negative intrapleural pressure of the space surrounding the lung. If air enters the pleural space via a rupture in the lung or a hole in the chest wall (pneumothorax), the lung on that side collapses because of its elastic recoil.[7]

Resistance to Breathing

In addition to the static elastic recoil of the lung and chest wall, frictional resistance of lung tissues and chest wall (inertia), as well as resistance to air flow, opposes inflation of the lung.

Certain characteristics of air flow affect its ability to pass through conducting airways. Laminar flow is an orderly movement, with the gas in the center of the tube moving faster than that closer to the wall. During turbulent flow, resistance greatly increases. True laminar flow occurs in smaller airways, where linear velocity is very low. (Linear velocity is inversely proportional to cross-sectional area for any flow rate.) In the airways both laminar and turbulent flow occur, depending on an index called Reynold's number for the particular segment of airway under consideration. Laminar flow changes to turbulent flow when Reynold's number exceeds 2000. Turbulence caused by sudden narrowing or branching of the airways produces the breath sounds heard on auscultation. Laminar flow follows Poiseuille's law ($R = 8\eta l/r^4$, where η equals viscosity). Resistance (R) to laminar air flow is directly proportional to the length (l) of the tube and inversely proportional to the fourth power of the radius (r). Therefore doubling the radius of the tube decreases resistance $16(2^4)$ times. Normally, approximately 40% of the total airway resistance resides in the upper airways (nasal cavity, pharynx, and larynx). Although resistance to air flow is greatest in individual small airways, the net total resistance to air flow of the small airways is very low because they represent a huge number of parallel pathways. Under normal circumstances the greatest resistance to air flow resides in medium-sized bronchi, whose smooth muscle tone greatly affects airway resistance.

The autonomic nervous system affects the tone of the bronchial smooth muscle. The sympathetic nervous system as well as sympathomimetic drugs (e.g., norepinephrine, epinephrine, and isoproterenol) produce bronchodilation. The parasympathetic nerves as well as parasympathomimetic drugs (e.g., acetylcholine) cause bronchoconstriction. Parasympatholytic drugs (e.g., atropine and ipratropium) therefore cause bronchodilation. Irritation of the airway by foreign bodies or inhaled irritants causes reflex bronchoconstriction. During lung inflation, increasing lung volumes exert retractive forces on the airways, resulting in a reduction in airway resistance. During forced expiration, dynamic compression of the airways increases airway resistance and may even cause airway collapse (most likely in small airways with no cartilaginous support).

The amount of O_2 consumed by the ventilatory muscles during eupneic breathing is usually less than 5% of the total body O_2 uptake. This percentage can greatly increase during exercise or with lung disease. For this reason controlled ventilation is sometimes used in very ill patients in order to increase the availability of O_2 for other body functions.

The two major categories of lung disease are obstructive and restrictive. Pulmonary function tests reveal increased airway resistance in patients with obstructive lung disease (e.g., asthma, emphysema, and bronchitis). Airway obstruction can cause gas trapping (e.g., emphysematous blebs), which in turn can result in a barrel chest and increased lung volume. The time necessary for exhalation is increased in obstructive lung disease. Normally, approximately 80% of the vital capacity can be exhaled in 1 second. In severe obstructive lung disease, expiratory flow rates are greatly decreased. Although obstructive lung disease restricts air flow through the airways, it is different from restrictive lung disease (as in pulmonary fibrosis, scoliosis, and obesity), which decreases lung compliance and lung volumes. Unfortunately, a patient can have both obstructive and restrictive disease simultaneously.[8]

Lung Volumes

The following discussion of lung volumes gives the parameters of a normal 70-kg male (Table 24-3). The amount of air that enters and leaves the body with each eupneic breath contains approximately 500 ml of air and is called the *tidal volume* (V_T). The minute volume (7500 ml) equals the rate of breathing (15 breaths per minute) multiplied by V_T. The amount of alveolar ventilation in a minute equals V_T minus the volume of the conducting airways (anatomic dead space, which is approximately 1 ml per pound of body weight) multiplied by the ventilatory rate. The residual volume (RV) is the volume of gas left in the lung after a maximal exhalation (1.5 L). The RV cannot be removed from the lungs voluntarily and is important because it provides air to the alveoli for

TABLE **24-3** Glossary for Static Lung Volumes and Capacities

Measurement	Symbol	Definition	Capacity (mm)
Volumes			
Residual volume	RV	The volume of air remaining in the lungs after maximum expiration	1200
Expiratory reserve volume	ERV	The maximum volume of air expired from the resting end-expiratory level	1100
Tidal volume	V_T	The volume of air inspired or expired with each breath during quiet breathing	500
Inspiratory reserve volume	IRV	The maximum volume of air inspired from the resting end-inspiratory level	3000
Capacities			
Inspiratory capacity	$IC = IRV + V_T$	The maximum volume of air inspired from the end-expiratory level (the sum of IRV and TV)	3500
Vital capacity	$VC = IRV + V_T + ERV$	The maximum volume of air expired from the maximum inspiratory level	4500
Functional residual capacity	$FRC = RV + ERV$	The volume of air remaining in the lungs at the end expiratory level (the sum of RV and ERV)	2300
Total lung capacity	$TLC = IRV + V_T + ERV + RV$	The volume of air in the lungs after maximum inspiration (the sum of all volume compartments)	5800

aeration of the blood, even between breaths. The expiratory reserve volume is the volume of gas that is expelled from the lungs during a maximal forced exhalation, starting at the end of a normal tidal exhalation. The inspiratory reserve volume is the volume of gas inhaled into the lungs during a maximal forced inhalation, starting at the end of a normal tidal inspiration (2.5 L).

The sum of the four basic lung volumes is the TLC. Several types of lung capacity measures exist, each of which is the sum of two or more lung volumes. TLC is the volume of air in the lungs after a maximal inspiratory effort (approximately 6 L in a 70-kg adult). The vital capacity is the amount of air that can be forcibly exhaled from the lungs after a maximal inspiratory effort (approximately 4.5 L). The functional residual capacity (FRC) is the volume of gas contained in the lungs after normal quiet expiration. It is the sum of the RV and expiratory reserve volume (approximately 3 L). The inspiratory capacity is the volume of air inhaled into the lungs during a maximal inspiratory effort that begins at FRC (approximately 3 L).

Closing volume is that phase of expiration that occurs as nitrogen-rich alveoli at the lung apexes continue to empty after closure of the small airways in the base of the lungs (which are exposed to greater intrapleural pressures and have less alveolar elastic recoil traction). The closing volume increases from approximately 30% of the TLC at age 20 years to approximately 55% at age 70 years. The closing volume may exceed the FRC in elderly people, which suggests that they may have airway closure and poorly ventilated or unventilated alveoli at resting lung volumes, which would contribute to intrapulmonary shunt.[8]

Respiratory Pressure

During normal inspiration intraalveolar pressure becomes slightly negative with respect to atmospheric pressure (normally by less than 1 mm Hg); this causes air to flow inward. During expiration intraalveolar pressure increases to 1 mm Hg above atmospheric pressure, and air flows outward. Therefore very little pressure is applied during eupneic ventilation. During maximal expiration with a closed glottis (such as during coughing), intraalveolar pressure may be greater than 100 mm Hg, whereas during maximal inspiration it may be reduced to as low as −90 mm Hg. Even a newborn can attain an intraalveolar pressure from −40 to −60 mm Hg during the first few breaths of life.

Dead Space

The volume of the conducting airways is called the *anatomic dead space* and normally equals approximately 1 ml per pound of body weight. The conducting airways are considered to be dead space because their relatively thick walls do not allow the gas that they contain to be exchanged with the gas contained in the blood. Alveoli that are ventilated but not perfused are known as *alveolar dead space* and contribute nothing to gas exchange with the blood. The sum of the anatomic dead space plus the alveolar dead space is the physiologic dead space (VDS). This is calculated with the Bohr equation:

Equation 24-1

$$\%VDS = (PaCO_2 - PECO_2)/PaCO_2$$

where $PaCO_2$ is the arterial partial pressure of CO_2 as determined from arterial blood gas (ABG) measurement, and $PECO_2$ is the PCO_2 of mixed expired gas as determined with a CO_2 meter. Certain pathologic conditions, such as pulmonary embolus, increase the alveolar dead space and can abruptly decrease the end-tidal CO_2 levels monitored with capnography.

Distal to the anatomic dead space the lung has 14 million alveolar ducts from which arise approximately 300 million alveoli perfused by 280 billion pulmonary capillaries. The average alveolar diameter is approximately 250 μm; therefore the total surface area available for gas exchange is 60 to 80 m^2.[9]

Regional Distribution of Alveolar Ventilation

In the normal upright lung the alveoli at the bottom of the lung increase their volume more with each inspiration and decrease their volume more with each expiration during eupnea (from FRC) than do those alveoli at the top. This is because at FRC the dependent alveoli are more compliant. If lung volumes were decreased, upper alveoli would be more compliant and receive more ventilation, and the dependent alveoli would be emptier or even collapsed. Review of the compliance curve (see Figure 24-2) reveals that alveoli become less compliant at higher volumes (e.g., in upper alveoli at high lung volume) and also at lower volumes (e.g., in independent alveoli at low lung volumes).

Alveolar Oxygen and Carbon Dioxide Levels

The levels of O_2 and CO_2 in the alveolar gas are determined by several factors. These include the amount of alveolar ventilation, the inspired concentrations of O_2 and CO_2, the flow of mixed venous blood to the lungs, and the body's consumption of O_2 and production of CO_2. Each breath brings approximately 350 ml of fresh air (21% of which is O_2) into the alveoli, which already contain approximately 3 L of gas (the FRC). Each exhalation removes approximately 350 ml of gas consisting of 5% to 6% CO_2. Every minute approximately 250 ml of O_2 diffuses from the alveoli into the pulmonary capillary blood, whereas approximately 200 ml of CO_2 diffuses from the pulmonary capillary blood into the alveoli. The ratio of the amount of CO_2 produced to the quantity of O_2 consumed is called the *respiratory quotient* (RQ = 200 ml CO_2 produced/250 ml O_2 consumed = 0.8).

Approximately 21% of dry atmospheric air is O_2; therefore at the standard barometric pressure of 760 mm Hg, PO_2atm equals 0.21 × 760 mm Hg, or 160 mm Hg. Only 0.04% of atmospheric air is CO_2, so PCO_2atm = 0.3 mm Hg. As the inspired air passes through the upper airways, it is heated to body temperature and humidified to a relative humidity of nearly 100%. The partial pressure of water vapor at body temperature is a fairly constant 47 mm Hg. The PO_2 of inspired air (PIO_2) saturated with water vapor at standard atmospheric pressure equals 0.21 × (760 mm Hg – 47 mm Hg), or 149 mm Hg.

The inspired gas mixes with the gas already in the alveoli (FRC) and rapidly equilibrates with the pulmonary capillary blood. The alveolar PO_2 (PAO_2) can be calculated with the alveolar air equation:

Equation 24-2

$$PAO_2 = PIO_2 - (PACO_2/RQ)$$

Thus during the breathing of atmospheric air, when $PACO_2$ is 40 mm Hg and the RQ is 0.8, then PAO_2 = (0.21 × [760 mm Hg − 47 mm Hg]) − 40 mm Hg/0.8 = 99 mm Hg. Therefore, using the alveolar air equation, one can calculate the PAO_2 if the atmospheric pressure, inspired O_2 concentration, and $PACO_2$ (which is approximately equal both to the end-tidal PCO_2 and the arterial PCO_2 [$PaCO_2$]) are known because water vapor pressure and RQ are fairly constant. If the inspired O_2 concentration differs from that of room air, then that fraction replaces the 0.21.

The alveolar air equation works because the RQ represents the ratio of the amount of O_2 removed to the quantity of CO_2 delivered to the alveoli by the pulmonary capillary blood flow. PAO_2 is less than PIO_2 because the CO_2 is delivered to the alveoli by the pulmonary blood flow at the same time that O_2 is taken up from the alveoli. Therefore $PACO_2$ divided by the RQ approximates the amount of O_2 that was removed from the alveoli by the pulmonary capillary blood flow.

Effects of Alveolar Ventilation on Carbon Dioxide and Oxygen

Within certain limits $PACO_2$ is inversely proportional to alveolar ventilation. If alveolar ventilation is doubled, then $PACO_2$ and $PaCO_2$ are reduced by half (if CO_2 production remains unchanged).

As alveolar ventilation increases, PAO_2 also increases slightly. However, doubling alveolar ventilation does not double PAO_2; according to the alveolar air equation, reduction of the $PACO_2$ raises the PAO_2, bringing PAO_2 closer to the PIO_2.

PULMONARY BLOOD FLOW

The lung receives blood from two sources. The bronchial circulation branches off from the aorta and supplies the conducting airways as far distal as the terminal bronchioles. It receives approximately 2% of the output of the left ventricle. The pulmonary circulation provides blood flow to the structures distal to the terminal bronchioles. These distal airways are the site of gas exchange between alveolar air and the pulmonary capillary blood. The mean pulmonary transit time is approximately 4 to 5 seconds, with the blood spending approximately 0.75 second in the pulmonary capillaries. It usually takes only 0.25 second for equilibration to occur between the alveolar air and the pulmonary capillary blood.

Anatomy of Pulmonary Circulation

The wall of the main pulmonary artery is much thinner than that of the aorta. The pulmonary arteries rapidly subdivide into terminal branches, which have thinner walls, much less smooth muscle, and greater internal diameters than corresponding branches of the systemic arterial tree. Pulmonary vessels are also much shorter than systemic vessels (and, according to Poiseuille's law, a decrease in length decreases resistance). Subsequently, pulmonary vascular resistance is very low, being approximately one eighth of systemic vascular resistance. Pulmonary vascular resistance is fairly evenly distributed among the arteries, capillaries, and veins, whereas most of the resistance in the systemic circulation is in the muscular arteries. Although pulmonary vascular resistance is very low, it can decrease further when blood flow increases. This is because of passive changes in resistance caused by recruitment and distensibility of the pulmonary vessels. Recruitment is the opening to perfusion of pulmonary vessels that were previously not perfused. Distensibility is an increase in diameter of a pulmonary vessel that is already being perfused, and it results from the vessel's compliance. The sympathetic nervous system has some influence on pulmonary vascular resistance, as do certain substances circulating in the pulmonary blood. Pulmonary vascular resistance is increased by norepinephrine, serotonin, histamine, hypoxia, and hypercapnia, and it is decreased by acetylcholine and isoproterenol.

Hypoxic Pulmonary Vasoconstriction

Blood flow to hypoxic, hypercarbic, or atelectatic alveoli is actively diverted at a precapillary site by a process known as *hypoxic pulmonary vasoconstriction*. This decreases blood flow to focal diseased areas of the lung and improves matching of ventilation and perfusion.

Distribution of Pulmonary Blood Flow

In the normal upright lung a greater portion of the blood flow goes to the bottom (dependent) portion because of the effects of hydrostatic pressure and greater distention of dependent lung vessels. The variation in blood flow to the different regions of the lung allows the lung to be divided into zones (Figure 24-3). In the upper parts of the lung, alveolar pressure can be greater than pulmonary artery pressure (PAP), so that no blood flow occurs in this region. This is called *zone 1* and is alveolar dead space because the region is ventilated but not perfused. Normally, no zone 1 is present during spontaneous ventilation, but the use of high airway pressures during mechanical ventilation can produce it.

The bottom portion of the lung, where both pulmonary artery and venous pressures exceed alveolar pressure, is known as *zone 3*. The middle portion of the lung, where PAP exceeds alveolar pressure, is *zone 2*. However, because alveolar pressure is greater than pulmonary venous pressure, the gradient for blood flow is decreased.[10]

Pulmonary Edema

The normal distance for diffusion from the alveolar air space into the pulmonary capillary blood cells is less than 0.5 mm. The gas must traverse the surfactant layer, the flat alveolar type I cells, the interstitial space, the endothelial cells that make up the wall of the pulmonary capillary, the plasma, and then,

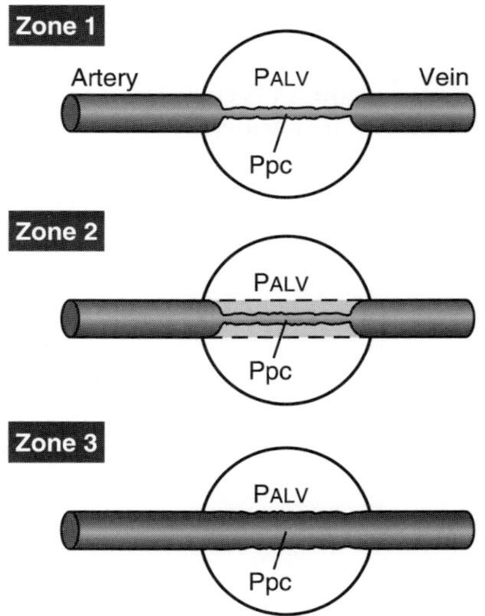

FIGURE **24-3**
Mechanics of blood flow in the three blood flow zones of the lung. *Zone 1, no flow,* Alveolar air pressure (*PALV*) is greater than arterial pressure. *Zone 2, intermittent flow,* Systolic arterial pressure rises higher than alveolar air pressure, but diastolic arterial pressure falls below alveolar air pressure. *Zone 3, continuous flow,* Arterial pressure and pulmonary capillary pressure (*Ppc*) remain greater than alveolar air pressure at all times. (From Guyton AC, Hall JE. *Textbook of Medical Physiology*. 10th ed. Philadelphia: Saunders; 2001:446.)

finally, the membrane of the red blood cell. Pulmonary vascular congestion causes increased capillary leakage into the interstitium, which can increase the distance for gas diffusion. If the capillary leak is sufficiently great, then the fluid may even fill the entire alveolar air space. Pulmonary edema affects oxygenation more than CO_2 excretion because CO_2 is 20-fold more diffusible than O_2. Many conditions can result in pulmonary edema. The high capillary pressures associated with heart failure or the excessive administration of intravenous fluids can increase lung water content. The size of the pulmonary capillary pores can be increased by sepsis, smoke inhalation, and other toxic conditions. Brain trauma can produce an intense sympathetic discharge, resulting in neurogenic pulmonary edema. A condition that occasionally occurs during emergence from anesthesia is negative-pressure pulmonary edema. After extubation the patient experiences laryngospasm and then attempts forceful inhalation against the closed glottis. The drastic decrease in intrathoracic pressure pulls fluid from the pulmonary capillaries. Treatment for this condition may require an increase in inspired O_2, continuous positive airway pressure (CPAP), and diuretics; however, the problem usually resolves within 24 hours.

Ventilation-Perfusion Relationships in the Lung

Normally, ventilation ($\dot{V}$) is approximately 4 L/min whereas pulmonary blood flow ($\dot{Q}$) is approximately 5 L/min. Therefore the ventilation-perfusion ratio ($\dot{V}/\dot{Q}$) for the whole lung is 0.8. However, $\dot{V}$ and $\dot{Q}$ must be matched at the alveolocapillary level for gas exchange with the blood to occur in the lung.

Dependent portions of the lung receive relatively more blood flow than nondependent portions because of the effects of gravity. Additionally, ventilation goes to the more compliant portions of the lung. Normally at FRC the dependent regions of the lung are more compliant, and the alveoli of the nondependent portions are more inflated and less compliant. Therefore relatively more ventilation and perfusion go to the dependent portions; this results in optimal gas exchange.

Although distribution of ventilation normally decreases going from dependent to nondependent regions of the lung, the accompanying decrease in perfusion is even greater; therefore $\dot{V}/\dot{Q}$ increases, going up the lung (Figure 24-4). $\dot{V}/\dot{Q}$ varies: in alveoli that are ventilated but not perfused, $\dot{Q}$ equals 0, so $\dot{V}/\dot{Q}$ equals infinity (i.e., dead space); in alveoli that are perfused but not ventilated, $\dot{V}$ equals 0, so $\dot{V}/\dot{Q}$ equals 0 (i.e., a shunt). Similarly, alveoli that are ventilated but poorly perfused are described as "dead space–like," whereas alveoli that are perfused but poorly ventilated are termed "shuntlike"; the latter contribute to the $\dot{V}/\dot{Q}$ mismatch of the lung. Shuntlike alveoli (low $\dot{V}/\dot{Q}$) have relatively low PO_2 and high PCO_2 when compared with dead space–like alveoli (high $\dot{V}/\dot{Q}$), which have relatively high PO_2 and low PCO_2.

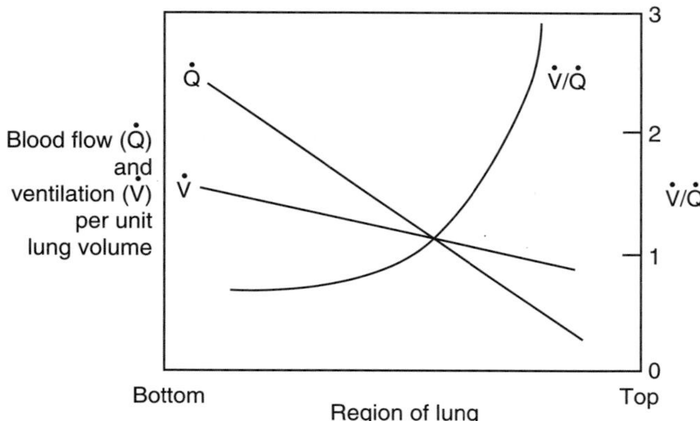

FIGURE **24-4**
Ventilation-perfusion relationships.

$\dot{V}/\dot{Q}$ mismatch can result from a number of causes. A pulmonary embolus of clots, air, or other material that passes through the pulmonary artery to obstruct blood flow through the pulmonary capillaries creates alveolar dead space. Likewise, very high airway pressure can produce alveoli that are ventilated but not perfused. Furthermore, very low cardiac output (CO) results in low pulmonary blood flow and therefore in dead space. This is reflected by a low end-tidal CO_2 pressure on capnography and a wide gradient between the end-tidal and the arterial $PaCO_2$.

Total pulmonary venous admixture (unoxygenated blood delivered to the left chambers of the heart) is the sum of the shunt and shuntlike states. It can be calculated with the shunt equation, which is discussed below. Bronchopulmonary anastomoses are a cause of normal anatomic shunt along with thebesian veins, which drain into the left side of the heart and usually account for less than 2% of the CO. Airway obstruction, alveolar collapse (atelectasis), and alveolar filling processes, such as pneumonia, also produce shunt.

A lung scan after a single breath of xenon 133 (^{133}Xe) gas can be used to determine the location of poorly ventilated areas in the lung. A lung scan after intravenous injection of dissolved ^{133}Xe reveals areas of the lung that are poorly perfused. Angiography (radiography with injection of a dye that is opaque) of the pulmonary vasculature shows if any pulmonary blood vessels are obstructed.[4]

Effects of General Anesthesia on Respiratory Physiology

General anesthesia affects the matching of ventilation and perfusion in several ways. Changing position from upright to supine and induction of general anesthesia produce a significant decrease in the FRC. See Chapter 25, Respiratory Anesthesia: Thoracic Surgery. The distribution of ventilation becomes more uniform, so that both the dependent and nondependent alveoli receive about the same amount of ventilation. At the same time the gradient for perfusion becomes greater, so that nondependent alveoli might receive no blood flow at all. General anesthesia usually causes a significant decrease in the CO; this decrease is exacerbated by positive-pressure ventilation, especially if it is accompanied by positive end-expiratory pressure (PEEP). As a result the dependent alveoli may receive excess perfusion for the amount of ventilation, and a shuntlike state can occur. In contrast, the nondependent alveoli receive little perfusion in proportion to the amount of ventilation producing dead space. Therefore $\dot{V}/\dot{Q}$ mismatch is increased.

Although hypoxic pulmonary vasoconstriction is partially effective in diverting blood flow away from poorly ventilated, unventilated, or atelectatic lung regions, most inhaled anesthetics (as well as potent vasodilators, such as nitroprusside and nitroglycerin) further decrease the effectiveness of hypoxic pulmonary vasoconstriction, but most intravenous anesthetics do not. The inhibition of hypoxic pulmonary vasoconstriction contributes to the decrease in PaO_2 and the increase in the alveolar-arterial PO_2 difference usually seen with inhaled general anesthetic agents.

Although general anesthesia, particularly when administered in combination with muscle relaxants, tends to increase chest wall compliance, the decrease in FRC actually produces a large decrease in the compliance of the respiratory system. Laryngoscopy and endotracheal intubation can increase airway resistance by stimulating airway irritant receptors, thereby decreasing dynamic compliance. However, most inhaled anesthetics (except for nitrous oxide [N_2O]) act as bronchodilators. Also, general anesthesia depresses the ventilatory response to CO_2, metabolic acidosis, and hypoxia (as discussed later in this chapter).[11,12]

Oxygen and Carbon Dioxide Exchange

When an individual is at rest, it takes approximately 0.75 second for a blood cell to traverse a pulmonary capillary. Normally the gas in the pulmonary capillary blood reaches equilibrium with the alveolar gas in approximately 0.25 second. During exercise CO may be so greatly increased that the time a blood cell spends in a pulmonary capillary can be reduced to 0.25 second. This decreased time available for diffusion has a much greater effect on exchange of O_2 than on that of CO_2 because CO_2 diffuses approximately 20-fold more rapidly than O_2 does. Diffusivity is defined as the solubility divided by the square root of the molecular weight. CO_2 is a slightly heavier molecule than O_2, but it is 24-fold as soluble in body fluids as O_2.[4]

Oxygen Transport

The blood carries O_2 in two ways: (1) O_2 can be physically dissolved in the blood, and (2) O_2 can be chemically bound to the hemoglobin (Hb) in the red blood cells. Normally most of the O_2 carried is bound to the Hb. Without Hb the cardiovascular system could not transport sufficient O_2 to meet the metabolic demands of the tissues. The ratio of the volume of the blood cells to the total volume of blood (expressed as a percentage) is called the *hematocrit*.

There is 0.003 ml of O_2 per 1 mm Hg of PO_2 physically dissolved in 100 ml of whole blood. Therefore with a PaO_2 of 100 mm Hg, only 0.3 ml of O_2 is transported physically dissolved in 100 ml of blood. Hb rapidly and reversibly combines with O_2, allowing the O_2 to be released to the tissues. Each gram of Hb can combine with approximately 1.34 ml of O_2; therefore if the level of Hb is 10 g/100 ml, then at 100% saturation 13.4 ml of O_2 is bound to Hb per 100 ml of blood. Note that an Hb level of 10 g/100 ml of blood corresponds to a hematocrit of 30%, because the hematocrit is approximately equal to Hb level multiplied by three.

The normal hematocrit for a man is approximately 45% (an Hb of 15 g/dL) and for a woman is approximately 39% (an Hb of 13 g/dL). Centrifugation of the blood in a capillary tube separates the cells from the plasma. A thin layer called the *buffy coat* separates the plasma and the red blood cells (erythrocytes). This thin layer (approximately 1% of the volume of the blood) consists of white blood cells and platelets.[4]

Oxyhemoglobin Dissociation Curve

The relationship between the PO_2 of the plasma and the percent Hb saturation is represented by the oxyhemoglobin (HbO_2) dissociation curve (Figure 24-5). This relationship between PO_2 and HbO_2 is not linear; rather, it is described by an **S**-shaped curve that is steep at lower PO_2 values and nearly flat when the PO_2 is greater than 70 mm Hg. As the PO_2 of the plasma increases, the amount of O_2 bound to the Hb also increases, but not in a linear manner. This is because each of the four Hb subunits combines with O_2, and each combination facilitates the next. Similarly, when the O_2 is being unloaded at the peripheral tissues, each dissociation facilitates the next. Therefore, this **S**-shaped curve is extremely important physiologically. Interaction between O_2 and Hb is also influenced by the pH, PCO_2, temperature, and 2,3-diphosphoglycerate (a metabolite of glucose hydrolysis) levels.

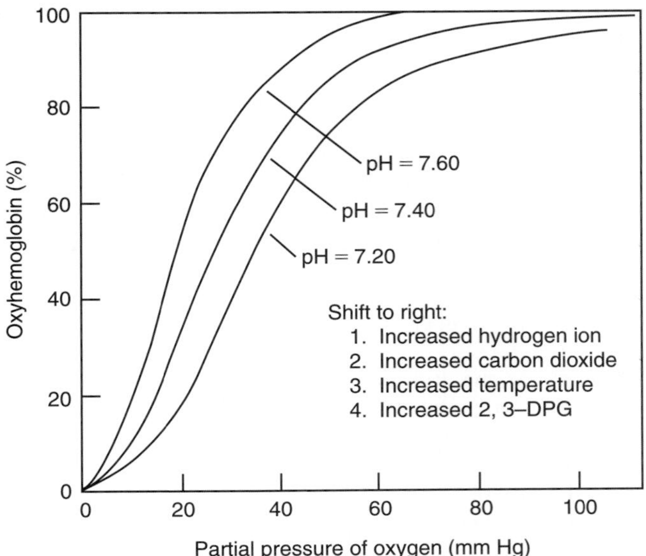

FIGURE **24-5**
Oxyhemoglobin dissociation curve.

The changing affinity of Hb for O_2 facilitates loading at the pulmonary capillaries and unloading of the O_2 at the peripheral tissues. The **S**-shaped HbO_2 dissociation curve is displaced to the left of the normal curve by hypocapnia, a decrease in temperature, alkalosis, and a decrease in 2,3-diphosphoglycerate levels, resulting in an increased affinity of the Hb for O_2 (a higher saturation for a given PO_2). When exposed to increased temperature, hypercapnia, acidosis, and elevated 2,3-diphosphoglycerate levels, the affinity of Hb for O_2 decreases. Therefore the O_2 is given up to the tissues; this results in a shift of the HbO_2 dissociation curve to the right. Note that the conditions that favor the release of O_2 from the Hb to the tissues are likely to be associated with increased tissue metabolism, which would increase the tissue's O_2 demand. The influence of pH and PCO_2 on the HbO_2 dissociation curve is referred as the *Bohr effect*. The P_{50} is the PO_2 at which 50% of the Hb is saturated. Under normal conditions adult human blood has a P_{50} of 26 to 27 mm Hg. If the HbO_2 dissociation curve shifts to the right, then the P_{50} increases; if it shifts to the left, then the P_{50} decreases.

Other factors that affect O_2 transport include carbon monoxide poisoning and methemoglobinemia. Carbon monoxide binds to Hb (forming carboxyhemoglobin) with 240 times the affinity of O_2. The carbon monoxide binds with Hb at the site that O_2 would occupy, making the carboxyhemoglobin unable to transport O_2.

Methemoglobin is Hb with its iron in the ferric state (Fe^{3+}) instead of the normal ferrous state (Fe^{2+}). In the ferric state, the Hb iron atoms do not combine with O_2. Methemoglobinemia can be caused by nitrate poisoning (nitroglycerin overdose) or toxic reactions to oxidant drugs, such as the local anesthetic prilocaine. Methemoglobinemia is treated with O_2 therapy and methylene blue at a dose of 1 to 2 mg/kg intravenously over 5 minutes.[4]

Oxygen Content Calculations

Values for the amount of O_2 in arterial blood are yielded by the O_2 content equation:

Equation 24-3

$$CaO_2 = (0.003 \times PaO_2) + (1.34 \times Hb \times \%\ \text{arterial Hb saturation})$$

where CaO_2 is the arterial O_2 content, and PaO_2 and percent of Hb saturation are obtained from ABG analysis. CaO_2 is normally approximately 20 ml of O_2 per 100 ml of arterial blood (when Hb is 15 g/dL and PaO_2 is 90 mm Hg).

The amount of O_2 in mixed venous blood is calculated with the following equation:

Equation 24-4

$$C\bar{v}O_2 = (0.003 \times P\bar{v}O_2) + (1.34 \times Hb \times \%\ \text{mixed venous Hb saturation})$$

where $C\bar{v}O_2$ is the mixed venous O_2 content, and $P\bar{v}O_2$ and percent of Hb saturation are obtained from mixed venous blood gas analysis of blood drawn from the distal lumen of a Swan-Ganz catheter placed in the pulmonary artery (the only site in the body with truly mixed venous blood). $C\bar{v}O_2$ is normally approximately 15 ml of O_2 per 100 ml of mixed venous blood when Hb is 15 g/dL and $P\bar{v}O_2$ is 40 mm Hg.

Subtraction of $C\bar{v}O_2$ from CaO_2 yields the arterial-venous O_2 content difference. This difference is useful in determination of the relationship between O_2 delivery to the body's tissues and the tissues' O_2 demand. Normally the difference is approximately 5 ml/dL of blood. A difference greater than 5 ml/dL of blood can be associated with low CO because the blood takes longer to traverse the capillaries in the tissues; therefore more O_2 is extracted. A difference of less than 5 ml/dL of blood can be associated with systemic arteriovenous shunts, which allow blood to bypass the tissue capillaries; such shunts occur during hyperdynamic sepsis.

The amount of O_2 in pulmonary capillary blood is calculated with the following equation:

Equation 24-5

$$CpcO_2 = (0.003 \times PpcO_2) + (1.34 \times Hb \times \%\ \text{pulmonary capillary Hb saturation})$$

where $CpcO_2$ is the pulmonary capillary O_2 content, and $PpcO_2$ is given by the alveolar air equation described earlier in this chapter. $CpcO_2$ is normally approximately 21 ml of O_2 per 100 ml of pulmonary capillary blood (when Hb is 15 g/dL and $PpcO_2$ is 99 mm Hg). The percent of pulmonary capillary Hb saturation is obtained from the HbO_2 dissociation curve. The CaO_2, $C\bar{v}O_2$, and $CpcO_2$ are used in the shunt equation:

Equation 24-6

$$\dot{Q}S/\dot{Q}T = (CpcO_2 - CaO_2)/(CpcO_2 - C\bar{v}O_2)$$

In this equation, $\dot{Q}S$ is the shunt blood flow, $\dot{Q}T$ is the total blood flow (CO), $CpcO_2$ is the pulmonary capillary O_2 content, CaO_2 is the arterial O_2 content, and $C\bar{v}O_2$ is the mixed venous O_2 content.[12]

Transport of Carbon Dioxide

The blood carries CO_2 in three forms: (1) in physical solution, (2) chemically combined with the amino acids of blood proteins, and (3) as bicarbonate ions. Approximately 5% to 10% of the total CO_2 transported in the blood is carried in physical solution. Chemical combination of CO_2 with the terminal amine groups of blood proteins forms carbamino compounds. The reaction occurs rapidly and does not require enzymes. Carbamino compounds constitute another 5% to 10% of the blood's total CO_2 content. The remaining 80% to 90% of the CO_2 in the blood is carried as bicarbonate. In the presence of carbonic anhydrase, CO_2 combines with water to form carbonic acid. The carbonic acid can dissociate into a bicarbonate ion and H according to the following chemical reaction:

Equation 24-7

$$CO_2 + H_2O \xrightarrow{\text{carbonic anhydrase}} H_2CO_3 \rightarrow H^+ + HCO_3^-$$

When HCO_3^- leaves the blood cells, chloride ions enter to maintain electrical neutrality (the so-called "chloride shift").[13]

Carbon Dioxide Dissociation Curve

As expected, decreases in the PCO_2 of the blood correspond to a decrease in the total CO_2 content of the blood. This is because of corresponding decreases in the levels of bicarbonate and carbamino compounds. When the PCO_2 falls, the amount of the total CO_2 decrease is affected by the presence of O_2 in the blood. When blood contains mainly HbO_2, the CO_2 dissociation curve shifts to the right; when the blood contains mostly deoxyhemoglobin, the curve shifts to the left. This is known as the *Haldane effect*, and it allows the blood to load more CO_2 at the tissues, where more deoxyhemoglobin is present. CO_2 is unloaded at the lung, where more HbO_2 is present.

The fact that deoxyhemoglobin is a weaker acid than HbO_2 accounts for the Bohr and Haldane effects. Deoxyhemoglobin more readily accepts the H^+ produced by the dissociation of carbonic acid. This permits more CO_2 to be carried in the form of bicarbonate ions (Haldane effect). Conversely, the association of H^+ with the amino acids of Hb lowers the affinity of Hb for O_2, shifting the HbO_2 dissociation curve to the right at low pH or high PCO_2 (Bohr effect).[14]

ACID-BASE BALANCE

The respiratory system has an important role in maintaining a normal pH balance in the body. It works along with the kidneys and the buffer systems to balance the acids and the bases of the blood and other body tissues, allowing them to function normally. Hydrogen ions interact with negatively charged regions of other molecules, such as proteins, altering their structural conformation and, in doing so, altering their behavior. As previously mentioned, pH affects the HbO_2 dissociation curve and the activity of enzymes, thereby changing metabolic functions in all body tissues. The severe metabolic acidosis that results from prolonged cardiopulmonary arrest must be treated with sodium bicarbonate, because protein receptor sensitivity and other enzymatic functions must be restored before epinephrine can be effective in resuscitation.

Metabolism of the substances that are ingested as food produces mainly acidic metabolic waste products. Under normal conditions a tremendous amount of the acid produced daily can be removed from the body by the respiratory system as exhaled CO_2. The acidic products are known as *volatile acids* because they can be converted into carbonic acid gas that is exhaled at a rate of approximately 24,000 mEq/day. A much smaller amount of nonvolatile or fixed acids also is produced during normal metabolic breakdown of food at a rate of approximately 50 mEq/day; these acids are primarily removed by the kidneys.

In addition to the efforts of the respiratory system and kidneys to regulate pH levels, buffers in the human body maintain pH in the physiologic range. The buffers consist mainly of bicarbonate, phosphate, and proteins. A buffer is a mixture of substances that usually consists of a weak acid and its conjugate base. When a strong acid or base is added to a buffer system, the changes in H^+ concentration are much smaller than those that would occur if the same amount of acid or base were added to pure water or another nonbuffered solution.[15]

Interpretation of Arterial Blood Gases

Analysis of ABGs can provide useful information concerning the relationship of acid production and acid removal by the lungs and kidneys. Acid-base disturbances can be categorized into four major groups: respiratory acidosis, metabolic acidosis, respiratory alkalosis, and metabolic alkalosis.

Although it may seem that a great number of acid-base states are possible, actually only 11 conditions exist (Table 24-4). Blood gases in a normal individual have a pH in the range of 7.35 to 7.45, $PaCO_2$ ranges from 35 to 45 mm Hg, and bicarbonate concentration is approximately 25 mEq/L.

Acidosis

Any process that leads to an elevation in $PaCO_2$ tends to lower the arterial pH, resulting in respiratory acidosis. An acute change in $PaCO_2$ of 10 mm Hg is associated with a change in pH of 0.08 units. An increase in $PaCO_2$ with a normal bicarbonate level is termed *uncompensated respiratory acidosis*.

Metabolic acidosis should more properly be referred to as "nonrespiratory acidosis" because it does not always involve alterations in metabolism. Causes of this condition include ingestion (poisoning), infusion, production of a fixed acid (lactic acidosis), and decreased excretion of acid by the kidneys. A base change of 10 mEq/L is associated with a pH change of 0.15 unit (in the absence of a change in $PaCO_2$). Therefore if the bicarbonate level increases by 10 mEq/L, then the pH also increases by 0.15 unit. A decrease in bicarbonate level when the PCO_2 remains at approximately 40 mm Hg is termed *uncompensated metabolic acidosis*. The combination of respiratory acidosis and metabolic acidosis is termed *mixed acidosis* and can produce a drastically decreased arterial pH.[16]

Alkalosis

When alveolar ventilation exceeds that necessary to keep up with CO_2 production in the body, both $PACO_2$ and $PaCO_2$ decrease to below 35 mm Hg. This hyperventilation results in respiratory alkalosis. A decrease in $PaCO_2$ in the presence of a normal bicarbonate level is termed *uncompensated respiratory alkalosis*. The relationship between alveolar ventilation and CO_2 production that results in hyperventilation can occur because of an increase in alveolar ventilation or a decrease in CO_2 production, as occurs with hypothyroidism or hypothermia if alveolar ventilation is maintained at normal levels.

Metabolic alkalosis occurs when fixed acid loss is increased or when the intake of bases is abnormally high. Above-normal increases in the bicarbonate level when the PCO_2 is maintained at approximately 40 mm Hg is termed *uncompensated metabolic alkalosis*. The combination of respiratory alkalosis and metabolic alkalosis produces mixed alkalosis, in which the arterial pH is markedly elevated.

TABLE 24-4 Acid-Base States

Physiologic State	pH	$PaCO_2$ (mm Hg)	HCO_3^- (mEq/L)	Examples
Normal	7.40 ± 0.05	40 ± 5	25 ± 1	
Uncompensated respiratory acidosis	↓↓	↑↑	↑	Acute hyperventilation (such as during neurosurgery)
Uncompensated respiratory alkalosis	↑↑	↓↓	↓	Acute hypoventilation (such as during an asthma attack)
Uncompensated metabolic acidosis	↓↓	↔	↓↓	Metabolic acidosis with controlled mechanical ventilation (respiratory compensations not possible)
Uncompensated metabolic alkalosis	↑↑	↔	↑↑	Metabolic alkalosis with controlled mechanical ventilation
Compensated respiratory acidosis	↓	↑↑	↑↑	Chronic hypoventilation (as in chronic obstructive pulmonary disease)
Compensated respiratory alkalosis	↑	↓↓	↓↓	Chronic hyperventilation (as in chronic increased intracranial pressure)
Compensated metabolic acidosis	↓	↓↓	↓↓	Renal failure or diabetic ketoacidosis
Compensated metabolic alkalosis	↑	↑↑	↑↑	Long-term hypokalemia or bicarbonate ingestion
Mixed respiratory and metabolic acidosis	↓↓↓	↑↑	↓↓	Respiratory and circulatory arrest
Mixed respiratory and metabolic alkalosis	↑↑↑	↓↓	↑↑	"Overresuscitation" (hyperventilation and excess bicarbonate administration)

Compensatory Mechanisms

The respiratory system can rapidly compensate for metabolic acidosis or alkalosis by altering alveolar ventilation. It normally occurs because changes in blood H^+ concentrations affect the chemoreceptors, which in turn increases or decreases alveolar ventilation, altering $PaCO_2$ within minutes. The kidneys can compensate for respiratory acidosis and metabolic acidosis of nonrenal origin by excreting fixed acid and retaining bicarbonate. Conversely, the kidneys compensate for respiratory alkalosis or metabolic alkalosis of nonrenal origin by decreasing H^+ excretion and decreasing retention of bicarbonate. Renal compensatory mechanisms act more slowly than do respiratory mechanisms and may take several days.

TREATMENT OF BLOOD GAS ABNORMALITIES

For the patient being mechanically ventilated, respiratory acidosis and respiratory alkalosis can be treated with a simple increase or decrease in the amount of alveolar ventilation. Mild-to-moderate metabolic acidosis can be treated with hyperventilation and correction of shock in order to restore a stable spontaneous circulation. Certain types of severe metabolic acidosis (pH <7.20) may be treated with sodium bicarbonate. The total body bicarbonate deficit equals the base deficit (in mEq/L) that is obtained from the blood gas values: the patient's bicarbonate level is subtracted from the normal bicarbonate level; the difference is multiplied by the patient's weight (in kilograms) and then by 0.3 (which is equal to the extracellular fluid compartment and the volume of distribution for bicarbonate). Complete correction of the base deficit is not indicated; only half of the calculated dose of bicarbonate is used. Severe lactic acidosis is treated with bicarbonate, but the acidosis associated with renal failure is better treated with dialysis. The hyperosmolarity and high sodium content of bicarbonate are usually contraindicated for renal failure patients. Manipulation of the blood's volume and electrolyte composition is used in the treatment of certain types of metabolic acidosis or alkalosis.

Hypoxemia is treated with an increase in the inspired O_2 concentration (FIO_2), PEEP, and correction of atelectasis (e.g., with bronchoscopy for the removal of foreign bodies in the airway). As previously mentioned, increasing alveolar ventilation usually has only a modest effect on PaO_2.

Control of Breathing

The respiratory centers in the brain stem control breathing by automatically generating a cycle of inspiration and expiration. This spontaneously generated cycle of inspiration and expiration can be modified by reflexes or by higher centers in the brain. The respiratory centers affect the nerves of the spinal cord, which innervate the muscles of respiration (the cervical branches of the spinal nerves C3, C4, and C5 form the phrenic nerves, which innervate the diaphragm). The spontaneous respiratory rhythm is generated by the medullary respiratory center, which is found in the reticular formation of the medulla under the floor of the fourth ventricle. The pons, which is the portion of the brain stem immediately above the medulla, contains the apneustic center (in the lower pons) and the pneumotaxic center (in the upper pons), both of which modify the output of the medullary respiratory center. See Figure 24-6.

The activity of the brain stems breathing centers is modulated by information received from afferent spinal nerves and higher brain centers, as occurs in voluntary control of breathing. Additionally, a great number of sensors in the lungs, cardiovascular system, muscles, tendons, skin, and viscera can affect the control of breathing by eliciting reflex changes. Stimulation of stretch receptors in the lungs can elicit three respiratory reflexes: the Hering-Breuer inflation reflex, the Hering-Breuer deflation reflex, and the paradoxic reflex of Head. The Hering-Breuer inflation reflex may help prevent overdistention of the alveoli at high lung volumes by inhibiting large V_Ts and may decrease the frequency of the inspiratory efforts by causing a transient apnea. The Hering-Breuer deflation reflex may be responsible for the increased ventilation elicited when the lungs are deflated abnormally, such as in pneumothorax, or it may have a role in the periodic spontaneous deep breaths (sighs) that help to prevent atelectasis. The paradoxic reflex of Head results during partial block of the phrenic nerves, such that lung inflation results in further deep inspiration instead of the apnea expected when the vagus nerve is fully functional. This reflex may be involved in generating the first breath of the newborn baby. Chemical or mechanical irritation of the airways may elicit a reflex cough or sneeze, hyperpnea, bronchoconstriction, and increased blood pressure. The vagus nerves provide afferent pathways for all of the airway's irritant receptors, except for the nasal mucosa receptors, which send information centrally by means of the trigeminal and olfactory tracts. Pulmonary embolism (PE) typically causes rapid, shallow breathing, whereas pulmonary vascular congestion causes hyperpnea. The vascular receptors that initiate these responses are named *J receptors* (for "juxtapulmonary capillary"). Stimulation of receptors in the muscles, tendons, and joints can also increase ventilation during exercise. Elevated blood pressure stimulates the arterial (carotid and aortic) baroreceptors, resulting in apnea and bronchodilation. Somatic pain tends to cause hyperpnea, whereas visceral pain usually causes apnea or decreased ventilation. Stimulation of the arterial chemoreceptors by decreased PO_2, increased PCO_2, or low pH tends to increase lung inflation and cause hyperpnea, bronchoconstriction, and an increase in blood pressure.[17] Table 24-5 summarizes the respiratory control reflexes.

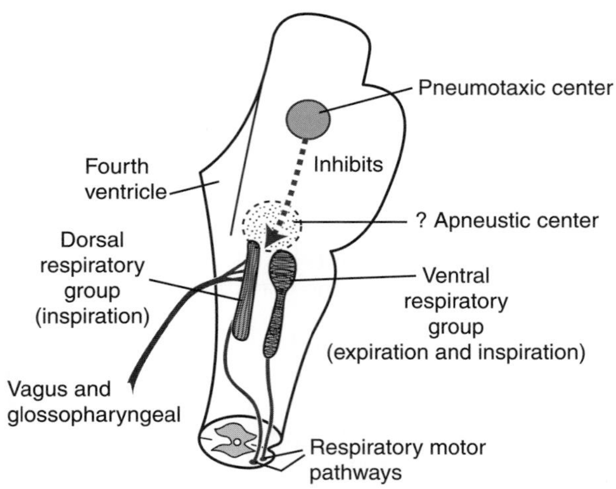

FIGURE **24-6**
Organization of the respiratory center. (From Guyton AC, Hall JE. *Textbook of Medical Physiology*. 10th ed. Philadelphia: Saunders; 2001:475.)

TABLE **24-5** Reflex Mechanism of Respiratory Control

Stimulus	Reflex	Receptor	Afferent Pathway	Effects
Lung inflation	Hering-Breuer inflation reflex	Stretch receptors within smooth muscles of large and small airways	Vagus	Respiratory—cessation of inspiratory effort, apnea, or decreased breathing frequency; bronchodilation Cardiovascular—increased heart rate; slight vasoconstriction
Lung deflation	Hering-Breuer deflation reflex	Possibly J receptors, irritant receptors in lungs, or stretch receptors in airway	Vagus	Respiratory—hyperpnea
Lung inflation	Paradoxic reflex of head	Stretch receptors in lungs	Vagus	Respiratory—inspiration
Negative pressure in upper airway	Pharyngeal dilator reflex	Receptors in nose, mouth, upper airways		Respiratory—contraction of pharyngeal dilator muscles
Mechanical or chemical irritation of airways	Cough	Receptors in upper airways, tracheobronchial tree	Vagus	Respiratory—cough; bronchoconstriction
	Sneeze	Receptors in nasal mucosa	Trigeminal, olfactory	Respiratory—sneeze; bronchoconstriction Cardiovascular—increased blood pressure
Face immersion	Diving reflex	Receptors in nasal mucosa and face	Trigeminal	Respiratory—apnea Cardiovascular—decreased heart rate; vasoconstriction
Pulmonary embolism		J receptors in pulmonary vessels	Vagus	Respiratory—apnea or tachypnea
Pulmonary vascular congestion		J receptors in pulmonary vessels	Vagus	Respiratory—tachypnea, possible sensation of dyspnea
Specific chemicals in the pulmonary circulation	Pulmonary chemoreflex	J receptors in pulmonary vessels	Vagus	Respiratory—apnea or tachypnea; bronchoconstriction

Modified from Levitzky MG. Pulmonary Physiology. *6th ed. New York: McGraw-Hill; 2003:196-197.*

CHEMICAL CONTROL OF BREATHING

The arterial and cerebrospinal fluid partial pressures of CO_2 are probably the most important inputs to the brain stem centers for establishing the ventilatory rate and VT. Hypoxemia potentiates the ventilatory response to CO_2. Its effect is that, for any particular $PaCO_2$, ventilatory response becomes greater as the PaO_2 decreases. Narcotics and anesthetic drugs (Figure 24-7) may profoundly depress the ventilatory response to CO_2. Chronic obstructive lung disease (COLD) also depresses the ventilatory response to hypercapnia, so that the hypoxic drive may be solely responsible for maintaining spontaneous breathing in these patients. Administration of high FIO_2 may halt the spontaneous ventilatory efforts of these patients. Metabolic acidosis shifts the CO_2 curve to the left, so that for any particular PCO_2 ventilation is increased during metabolic acidosis.

A depressed or abnormal response to CO_2 during sleep may be involved in central sleep apnea (characterized by pauses of

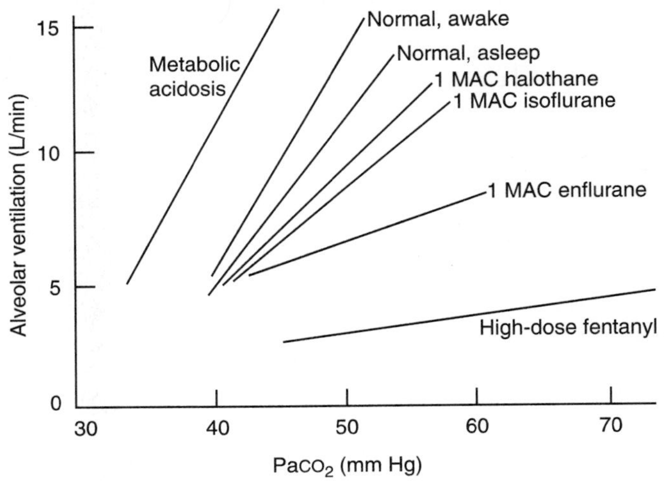

FIGURE **24-7**
Carbon dioxide response curve.

2 minutes' duration between breaths). Central sleep apnea, which possibly is caused by a defect in the chemoreceptors or brain stem respiratory controller, may be an important contributor to sudden infant death syndrome.

Increased $PaCO_2$ and decreased PaO_2 and arterial pH stimulate the arterial (peripheral) chemoreceptors, with the carotid bodies apparently exerting a much greater influence on the medullary respiratory centers than the aortic bodies. The afferent nerve from the carotid body is Hering's nerve, a branch of the glossopharyngeal nerve; the afferent pathway from the aortic body is the vagus nerve. The central chemoreceptors are in contact with cerebrospinal fluid but are not directly exposed to the arterial blood (because of the blood-brain barrier). CO_2 is rapidly diffusible through the blood-brain barrier; therefore changes in $PaCO_2$ are rapidly transmitted to the cerebrospinal fluid, taking less than 2 minutes. Hydrogen ions and bicarbonate ions are slowly diffusible through the blood-brain barrier, so that changes in arterial pH that do not result from changes in PCO_2 take considerably longer to affect the cerebrospinal fluid. The central chemoreceptors are located just beneath the surface of the medulla. They are not stimulated by hypoxia; their activity may even be suppressed by it. Although the central chemoreceptors are almost solely responsible for determining the resting ventilatory level and long-term response to and maintenance of blood CO_2 levels, the peripheral chemoreceptors may be more important in short-term responses to CO_2.[18]

CHRONIC OBSTRUCTIVE PULMONARY DISEASE

The American Thoracic Society defines chronic obstructive pulmonary disease (COPD) as a "disorder characterized by abnormal tests of expiratory flow that does not change markedly over periods of several months of observation." Although the intent of this qualification is the differentiation of COPD from asthma, other definitions do not separate asthma from COPD.[18,19] The terminology can be confusing, because asthma, chronic bronchitis, and emphysema are all common obstructive diseases characterized by decreased air flow through the tracheobronchial tree and small airways.

The terms *chronic obstructive pulmonary disease* and *chronic obstructive lung disease* are widely used as synonyms for the combination of chronic bronchitis and emphysema. Because of the prevalence of cigarette smoking, the combination of these two entities is encountered much more commonly than either of the two in its "pure" form. As a rule the combination of chronic bronchitis and emphysema is seen in those who smoke heavily, and the disease process takes 30 years or longer to manifest.

Definition

The term *chronic bronchitis* refers to "the condition of subjects with chronic or recurrent excess [mucous] secretion into the bronchial tree." In this definition, *chronic* means "occurring on most days for at least 3 months of the year for at least 2 successive years."[19] A critical element is the presence of airway obstruction of expiratory air flow. A glossary of static lung volumes and capacities is presented in Table 24-3.

Emphysema is defined as "a condition of the lung characterized by abnormal permanent enlargement of the air spaces distal to the terminal bronchiole, accompanied by destruction of their walls and without obvious fibrosis."[18] Destroyed alveolar tissue is largely incapable of regeneration, and therefore the changes that occur in emphysema are irreversible.[20] Classification of COPD and suggested therapies for each stage are given in Table 24-6. Differential diagnosis of COPD compared with other common lung disorders is noted in Table 24-7.

Incidence and Outcome

COPD affects an estimated 15 to 20 million Americans and is the fifth leading cause of death in the United States, accounting for approximately 60,000 deaths each year. Chronic bronchitis and emphysema are the most common causes of COPD.[21]

The social and economic impacts of COPD are enormous. Patients in advanced stages of obstructive lung diseases are unable to work and frequently cannot participate in activities of daily living. Even in milder cases, activities often are restricted. The prognosis for patients with chronic bronchitis is poor, with death often occurring within 5 years after the first episode of acute respiratory failure.[22] Acute respiratory failure is defined as a functional disturbance of physiologic mechanisms characterized by a significant reduction in a patient's partial pressure of arterial O_2 (PaO_2) from his or her usual baseline or by an increase in the partial pressure of arterial CO_2 ($PaCO_2$) with concomitant acidosis.[23] In the subset of patients with severe COPD and acute respiratory failure who require tracheal intubation the presence of pulmonary infiltrates on chest radiography has been associated with diminished likelihood for survival.[24,25]

Etiology

The principal factor that predisposes a patient to the development of COPD is cigarette smoking.[24,26] Environmental pollution appears to have some role, but its effects are minor compared with those of cigarette smoking. Additionally, emphysema may develop in some patients because of a genetic predisposition to an imbalance between protease and antiprotease activities in the lungs.[27]

Pathophysiology

The dominant feature of the natural history of COPD is progressive air flow obstruction, as reflected by a decrease in forced expiratory volume in 1 second (FEV_1). Three causes of decreases in FEV_1 are as follows:

1. A decrease in the intrinsic size of bronchial lumina
2. An increase in the collapsibility of bronchial walls (this cause is the most difficult to quantify)
3. A decrease in elastic recoil of the lungs[22]

Emphysema may develop in some patients because of an imbalance between protease and antiprotease activities in the lungs. α_1-Antitrypsin deficiency results in the unopposed degradation of pulmonary interstitial elastin fibers by the enzyme elastase and in the early development of emphysema.[27]

Bullae, a form of emphysema, are air-containing spaces greater than 1 cm in diameter that result from the destruction and dilation of air spaces distal to terminal bronchioles. Their walls consist of attenuated and compressed parenchyma, are confined by connective tissue septa of the lung, and are deep to the internal elastic layer of the visceral pleura.[28]

Blebs are collections of air within the pleura. Because blebs do not involve the acinus, they are not a form of emphysema. If the definition of blebs included the presence of collections of air in the interstitium as well as in the pleura, interstitial emphysema could be referred to more appropriately as "multiple blebs." Pulmonary interstitial emphysema occasionally is seen in adults as a complication of assisted ventilation or if air from other sites has dissected backward into the lung[28] (Figures 24-8 and 24-9).

TABLE 24-6 Therapy at Each Stage of Chronic Obstructive Pulmonary Disease

Stage	Characteristics	Recommended Treatment	
All		Avoidance of risk factors; influenza vaccination	
0: At risk	Chronic symptoms (cough, sputum); exposure to risk factors; normal spirometry		
I: Mild COPD	$FEV_1/FVC < 70\%$; $FEV_1 \geq 80\%$ predicted; with or without symptoms	Short-acting bronchodilator when needed	
II: Moderate COPD	IIA: $FEV_1/FVC \geq 70\%$; $50\% \leq FEV_1 < 80\%$ predicted; with or without symptoms	Regular treatment with one or more bronchodilators; rehabilitation	Inhaled glucocorticosteroids if significant symptoms and lung function response
	IIB: $FEV_1/FVC < 70\%$; $30\% \leq FEV_1 > 50\%$ predicted; with or without symptoms	Regular treatment with one or more bronchodilators; rehabilitation	Inhaled glucocorticosteroids if significant symptoms and lung function response or if repeated exacerbations
III: Severe COPD	$FEV_1/FVC < 70\%$; $FEV_1 < 30\%$ of predicted or presence of respiratory failure or right heart failure	Regular treatment with one or more bronchodilators; inhaled glucocorticosteroids if significant symptoms and lung function response or if repeated exacerbations; treatment of complications; rehabilitation; long-term oxygen therapy if respiratory failure; consider surgical treatments	

COPD, *Chronic obstructive pulmonary disease;* FEV_1, *forced expiratory volume in 1 second;* FVC, *forced vital capacity.*
Modified from Pauwels RA, Buist S, Calverley PM, et al. Global strategy for the diagnosis, management, and prevention of chronic obstructive pulmonary disease. Am J Respir Crit Care Med. *2001;163:1256-1276.*

TABLE 24-7 Differential Diagnosis of Chronic Obstructive Pulmonary Disease

Diagnosis	Suggestive Features*
COPD	Onset in midlife; symptoms slowly progressive; long-term smoking history; dyspnea during exercise; largely irreversible airflow limitation
Asthma	Onset early in life (often childhood); symptoms vary from day to day; symptoms occur at night or in early morning; allergy, rhinitis, or eczema also present; family history of asthma; largely reversible airflow limitation
Congested heart failure	Fine basilar crackles on auscultation; chest radiograph shows dilated heart, pulmonary edema; pulmonary function tests indicate volume restriction, not airflow limitation
Bronchiectasis	Large volumes of purulent sputum; commonly associated with bacterial infection; coarse crackles or clubbing on auscultation; chest radiograph or CT scan shows bronchial dilation, bronchial wall thickening
Tuberculosis	Onset at all ages; chest radiograph shows lung infiltrate or nodular lesions; microbiologic confirmation; high local prevalence of tuberculosis
Obliterative bronchiolitis	Onset at younger age, in nonsmokers; may have history of rheumatoid arthritis or fume exposure; CT scan taken on expiration shows hypodense areas
Diffuse panbronchiolitis	Most patients are male and nonsmokers; almost all have chronic sinusitis; chest radiograph and HRCT scan show diffuse small centrilobular nodular opacities and hyperinflation

COPD, *Chronic obstructive pulmonary disease;* CT, *computed tomography;* HRCT, *high-resolution computed tomography.*
**These features tend to be characteristic of the respective diseases but do not occur in every case. For example, a person who has never smoked can develop COPD (especially in developing countries, where other risk factors may be more important than cigarette smoking); asthma can develop in adult and even elderly patients.*
Modified from Pauwels RA, Buist AS, Calverley PMA, et al. Global strategy for the diagnosis, management, and prevention of chronic obstructive pulmonary disease: NHLBI/WHO global initiative for chronic obstructive lung disease (GOLD) workshop summary. Am J Respir Crit Care Med. *2001;163:1256-1276.*

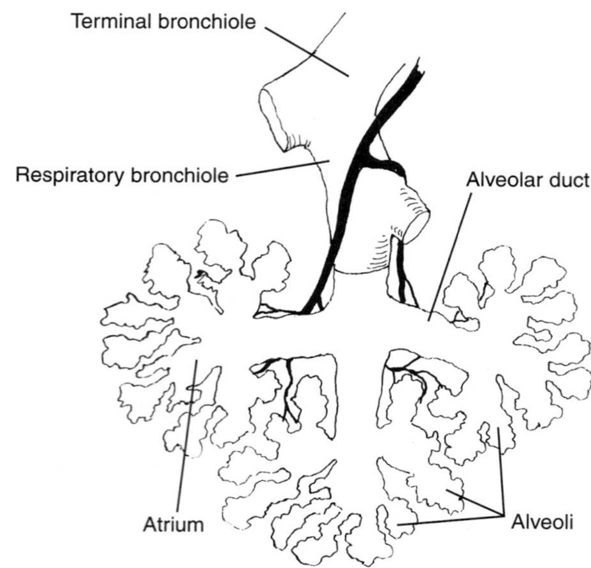

FIGURE **24-8**
The respiratory lobule. (Redrawn from Miller WS. *The Lung.* Springfield, Ill: Charles C Thomas; 1950.)

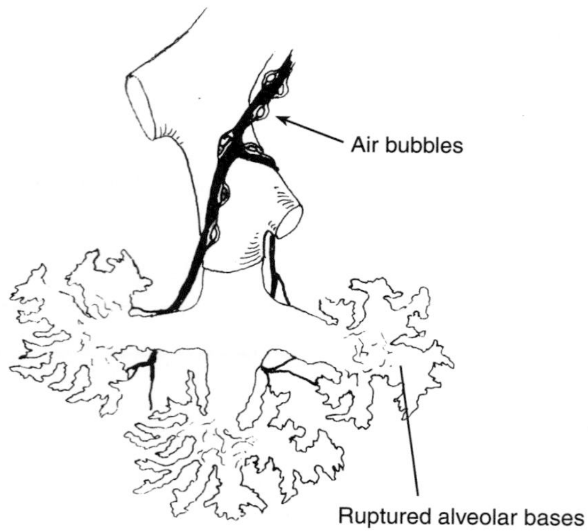

FIGURE **24-9**
Artist's conception of the development of interstitial emphysema. (Redrawn from Samuelson WM, Fulkerson WJ. Barotrauma in mechanical ventilation. In: Fulkerson WJ, MacIntyre NR, eds. *Problems in Respiratory Care: Complications of Mechanical Ventilation.* Philadelphia: Lippincott; 1991:58.)

Distinct morphologic changes can be found in the airways of patients exposed to an ongoing inflammatory challenge. In chronic bronchitis there occurs a proliferation of the compound tracheobronchial mucous glands in the subepithelial layers of the airway wall. The presence of excessive airway mucus and thickened airway walls cause a narrowing of the functional air flow channel. Approximately 25% of patients with COPD also have enhanced airway reactivity. In these patients, an increased amount of airway muscle is noted; this increase also may contribute to airway narrowing.[29]

The defense system of a patient with COPD is disrupted by the excessive production of mucus and by paralysis of the mucociliary transport system, which leads to microbial colonization. However, the presence of microbial organisms in the airway secretions of patients with chronic bronchitis is common and does not necessarily imply the presence of active infection.[29]

1. Destruction of lung connective tissue, which normally provides elastic pull on the outsides of bronchi and bronchioles, reduces the tethering of airways of the pulmonary interstitium, leads to premature collapse of the airways from external pressure, and increases the unevenness of distribution of inspired air to different regions of the lungs. Consequently, the exchange of CO_2 and O_2 between the blood and alveolar air is impeded. Compensation for lower diffusion of gases is partly achieved via collateral ventilation by diffusion across alveolar walls.[30]
2. Injury and inflammation of the bronchial tubes and alveoli increase the resistance to air flow during both inspiration and expiration. More forceful breaths or quicker breaths are needed for maintaining even normal levels of ventilation.[31]
3. Lung compliance increases with the tissue damage, and the airways' narrowing and greater collapsibility impede the ability of the ventilatory muscles to empty the lung completely. Hyperinflation results, raising the resting end-expiratory position of the lungs. Because the lung is more expanded, the inspiratory muscles operate from a shorter initial length and produce less force when foreshortened.
4. The more horizontally placed diaphragm is less able to lift the rib cage. The diaphragm may contract ineffectively such that the abdomen moves inward rather than outward with each inspiration.[32]
5. Because of the increased demands for work output placed on the respiratory muscles, the energy requirement of these muscles escalates. A greater proportion of the CO goes to these muscles. If hypoxemia is present and increased ventilation is required (e.g., as in exercise), the energy supply of the muscles may become inadequate, and respiratory muscle fatigue ultimately is produced.[33]
6. The expansion of the lung and thorax also misaligns the intercostal muscles and accessory respiratory muscles. To compensate, patients may assume special postures, such as leaning forward.[34]
7. Inflammation allows noxious agents in the air to reach the more deeply located tissues in the lung and to gain access to blood vessels, macrophages, mast cells, and nerves in the lung. Airway irritation increases; as a result, asthmatic episodes occur, as the introduction of noxious agents causes the release of spasmogenic agents from tissue cells and nerve endings.[34]

General Characteristics

The ability of compensatory mechanisms to preserve ventilation and ABG tensions varies. Ventilation usually is very well protected, even more than is gas exchange. CO_2 is 20 times more soluble than O_2 and therefore is more diffusible.[35] Also, if hypercapnia should occur, pulmonary ventilation is stimulated. Minute ventilation (Ve) in COPD generally is normal to above normal. Usually, $PaCO_2$ does not increase beyond normal levels in COPD until FEV_1 is less than 1 L. In comparison, PaO_2 is not appreciably restored by an increase in either e or depth of breathing, and even slight variations in $\dot{V}/\dot{Q}$ ratios in the lung adversely affect oxygenation.[19,36] O_2 delivery (DO_2) to the tissues is preserved as much as possible by an increase in CO, a greater extraction of O_2 from the blood, polycythemia, or some combination of these three factors. Consequently, respiratory muscle work is greater than normal and O_2 use by the muscles is increased.[37]

Associated Conditions

Cigarette Smoking

Cigarette smoking has been firmly established as the primary environmental risk factor associated with emphysema and bronchitis.[26] Its pathogenic mechanism is not known. The unchecked protease hypothesis holds that emphysema is caused by damage to elastic fibers because of an imbalance between elastase and antielastases in the lung.[38] Also, evidence that oxidants have a role in lung damage is increasing. The lungs of cigarette smokers are subject to an enhanced oxidant burden. Oxidants are highly reactive electron acceptors capable of removing electrons from a variety of molecules. The process of oxidation may reversibly or irreversibly damage compounds of all chemical classes, including nucleic acids; proteins and free amino acids; lipids and lipoproteins; and carbohydrates. In this regard oxidants can damage cells and extracellular matrix components critical for normal lung function. Cigarette smoke and activated lung phagocytes generate an increase in the level of oxidants.[39] Additionally, excess sputum production and hyperplasia of the mucous glands of the trachea and large bronchi are linked to cigarette smoking.[19,39]

Chronic hyperinflation results in diaphragmatic shortening and a decrease in the length of each sarcomere. Over time the decrease in the number of sarcomeres impairs diaphragmatic contraction and contractile force.[40,41]

Peripheral Circulation in Chronic Obstructive Pulmonary Disease

COPD can change the determinants of systemic venous return through alteration of the mechanical characteristics of either the heart or lungs. When a patient adapts a forced expiratory breathing pattern (e.g., during exercise), very positive pressure swings occur during expiration. The positive swings cyclically decrease systemic venous return, leading to an exaggeration of respiratory variation in arterial blood pressure or to pulsus paradoxus.[42] Pulsus paradoxus is present in two thirds of patients with severe COPD, and its severity correlates with the degree of air flow obstruction.[43] Increases in lung volume may directly impede systemic venous return through compression of the vena cava or heart. Normally, inspiration augments systemic venous return because of a decrease in right atrial pressure.[44]

Patients with COPD often have an increase in CO mediated by an increase in catecholamine levels and by a redistribution of blood flow and volume from the high-capacitance splanchnic regions to the lower-capacitance cardiac, cerebral, and muscle regions.[44]

A characteristic enhanced heart rate response also has been identified. Four parameters of airway obstruction (forced vital capacity [FVC], the ratio of FEV_1 to FVC [%FEV_1], the ratio of RV to TLC [RV/TLC], and %RV) have been correlated with the heart rate response to hypoxia. This increased response appears to be the result of an unknown mechanism of diseased lung tissue.[45]

Fluid Retention in Chronic Obstructive Pulmonary Disease

It appears that patients with hypoxic and hypercapnic respiratory failure from emphysema or chronic bronchitis, or from both, have impaired renal function, with reduced renal plasma flow and decreases in glomerular filtration.[46]

Note that cardiac responses to chronic and acute pressure increases are not the same. Chronic pressure overload causes right ventricular hypertrophy , whereas acute pressure changes cause right ventricular dilation.

Clinical Features and Diagnosis

The clinical presentation of COPD varies markedly, and crippling changes for one person may be a minor incapacity for another. Chronic productive cough and progressive exercise limitation are the hallmarks of COPD. Spirometric evaluation in accordance with the standards of the American Thoracic Society establishes the diagnosis of COPD. See Table 24-6.

Diagnostic Testing

Pulmonary Function Tests. It is desirable to perform spirometry in all patients with unexplained dyspnea and in those in whom COPD is suspected. A decrease in FEV_1/FVC on spirometry is characteristic of expiratory air flow obstruction. FEV_1 is typically less than 80% of FVC in the presence of COPD (Figure 24-10). Measurement of the FEV_1 alone may be misleading, as this value may be low if the vital capacity (VC) also is low or if the patient is uncooperative. Measurement of lung volumes demonstrates an increased RV and often an increased FRC (Figure 24-11). Slowing of expiratory flow and gas trapping behind prematurely closed airways is responsible for the increase in RV.[47] The advantage of increased RV and

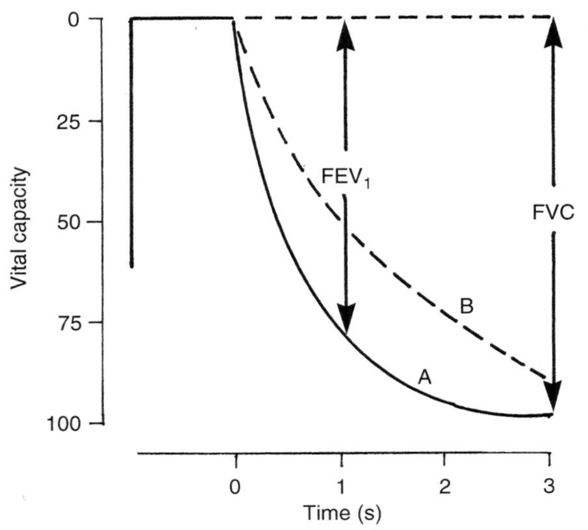

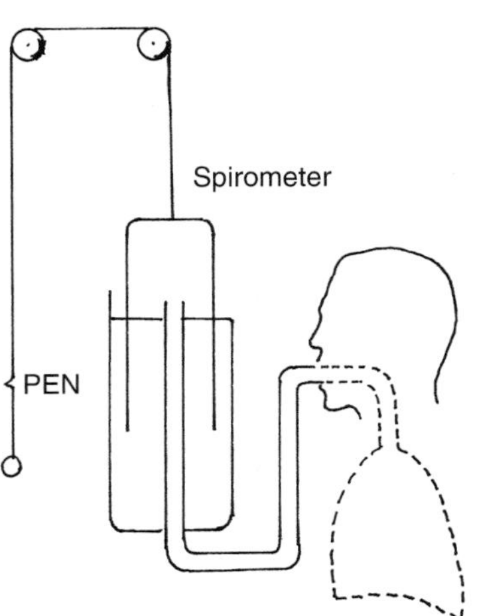

FIGURE **24-10**
Schematic diagram of the forced expiratory volume in 1 second (FEV_1) and forced vital capacity (FVC). The total volume of air exhaled in the first second should be equivalent to at least 80% of the FVC *(A)*. In the presence of obstructive airway disease the FEV_1 is less than 80% of the FVC *(B)*. (Modified from Stoelting RK, Miller RD. Chronic pulmonary disease. In: Stoelting RK, Miller RD, eds. *Basics of Anesthesia*. 2nd ed. New York: Churchill Livingstone;1989:288.)

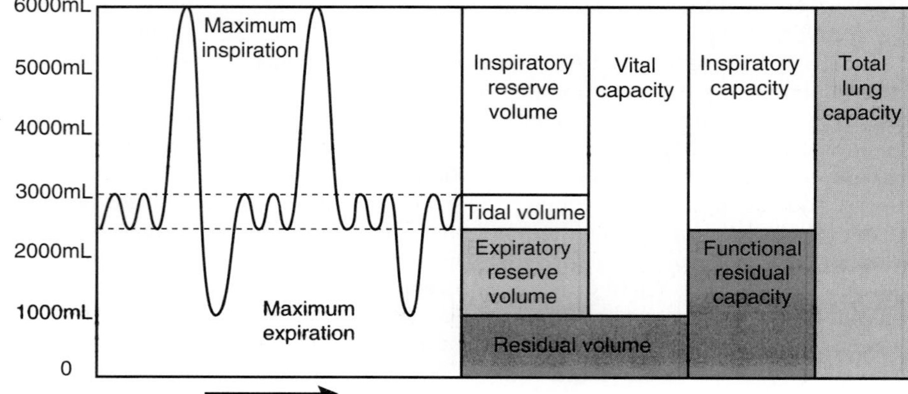

FIGURE **24-11**
Respiratory volumes and capacities. (From Applegate EJ. *The Anatomy and Physiology Learning System*. Philadelphia: Saunders; 1995:313.)

FRC in the patient with significant COPD is enlargement of airway diameter with greater radial support and elastic recoil for exhalation (compared with a patient with a smaller airway diameter, not with one who has a healthy airway and preservation of lung connective tissue). The cost to the patient is the need for greater work of breathing owing to the higher lung volumes.

Sputum examination may be helpful for guiding antimicrobial therapy during exacerbations.

Arterial Blood Gas Analysis. ABG analysis, which is often performed in patients with advanced COPD, helps in the categorization of patients as either "pink puffers" (PaO_2 greater than 60 mm Hg, $PaCO_2$ normal) or "blue bloaters" (PaO_2 less than 60 mm Hg, $PaCO_2$ greater than 45 mm Hg, and presence of cor pulmonale). Pink puffers usually have severe emphysema, whereas blue bloaters are more likely to have chronic bronchitis.[18] Cyanosis reflects the concentration of deoxygenated Hb (not the percentage of deoxygenated Hb) but not the amount of oxygenated Hb, because the dark blue color of deoxygenated blood masks the red color of oxygenated blood. Cyanosis is present if the arterial blood contains more than 5 g of deoxygenated Hb per deciliter of blood.[48]

Pulmonary artery hypertension that leads to cor pulmonale is a likely development in bronchitic patients with arterial hypoxemia and hypercarbia. Conversely, loss of pulmonary capillaries from the destruction of alveoli in emphysema is manifested by a decrease in the diffusing capacity of carbon monoxide (DLCO). In addition, pulmonary vasoconstriction also is a late consequence, because arterial hypoxemia is not prominent in emphysema until the disease's very late stages (Tables 24-8 and 24-9).[22]

Chest Radiography and Computed Tomography. Radiographic abnormalities may be minimal, even in the presence of advanced COPD.[47] Hyperlucency of the lungs (caused by arterial vascular deficiency in the lung periphery) and hyperinflation (flattening of the diaphragm with loss of the silhouette)

TABLE **24-8** Clinical Hallmarks: Predominant Bronchitis versus Predominant Emphysema

	Blue Bloater, Predominant Bronchitis	Pink Puffer, Predominant Emphysema
General appearance	Overweight; dusky; warm extremities	Thin, often emaciated; pursed-lip breathing; anxious; prominent use of accessory muscles; normal-to-cool extremities
Age (y)	40-55	50-75
Onset	Cough	Dyspnea
Cyanosis	Marked	Slight to none
Cough	More evident than dyspnea	Less evident than dyspnea
Sputum	Copious	Scanty
Upper respiratory infections	Common	Occasional
Breath sounds	Moderately diminished	Markedly diminished
Cor pulmonale and right-sided heart failure	Common	Only during bouts of respiratory infection, and terminally
Radiographic features	Normal diaphragm position; cardiomegaly; lungs normal or with increased bronchovascular markings	Small pendulous heart; low, flat diaphragm; areas of increased radiolucency
Course	Ambulatory but constantly on verge of right-sided heart failure and coma	Incapacitation of breathlessness punctuated by life-threatening bouts of upper respiratory infections; prolonged course culminating in right-sided heart failure and coma

Modified from Fishman AP. The spectrum of chronic obstructive disease of the airways. In: Fishman AP, ed. Update: Pulmonary Diseases and Disorders. *2nd ed. New York: McGraw-Hill; 1988:1165.*

TABLE 24-9 **Functional Hallmarks: Predominant Bronchitis versus Predominant Emphysema**

	Blue Bloater, Predominant Bronchitis	**Pink Puffer, Predominant Emphysema**
FEV_1/FC	Reduced	Reduced
FRC	Mildly increased	Markedly increased
TLC	Normal-to-slight increase	Considerably increased
RV	Moderately increased	Markedly increased
Lung compliance	Normal or high	Normal or low
Recoil pressure	Normal or high	Low
MVV	Moderately decreased	Markedly decreased
Airway resistance	Increased	Normal to slightly increased
DLCO	Normal or low	Low
PaO_2	Moderate-to-severe decrease	Mildly to moderately reduced
Arterial hypercapnia	Often present	Present during an acute respiratory infection
Hematocrit	Generally high; may reach 70%	Normal or slightly high; uncommon exceeds 55%
Pulmonary arterial pressure	Generally increased	Normal or slightly increased

DLCO, *Diffusing capacity of carbon monoxide;* FEV_1, *forced expiratory volume in 1 second;* FRC, *functional residual capacity;* MVV, *maximum voluntary ventilation;* PaO_2, *partial pressure of arterial oxygen;* RV, *residual volume;* TLC, *total lung capacity;* VC, *vital capacity.*
Modified from Fishman AP. The spectrum of chronic obstructive disease of the airways. In: Fishman AP, ed. Update: Pulmonary Diseases and Disorders. *2nd ed. New York: McGraw-Hill; 1988:1166.*

suggest the diagnosis of emphysema.[49] If bullae also are present, the diagnosis of emphysema is virtually certain; however, only a small percentage of patients who have emphysema have bullae. Chronic bronchitis can be detected only on chest radiography. Computed tomography (CT) can delineate the pulmonary parenchyma much better than standard chest radiography. CT may also be used to quantitate the amount of air trapping.

Operative Treatment

Preoperative Evaluation

The surgical site and the preoperative status of the patient are critical factors in determining the incidence of postoperative complications. Multiple factors are predictive of postoperative respiratory difficulties, but no preoperative pulmonary function test establishes absolute contraindications to surgery. The preoperative evaluation of patients with COPD should determine the severity of the disease and identify treatments for reducing inflammation, improving secretion clearance, treating underlying infection, and increasing airway caliber that can ensure the best surgical outcome. Supplemental administration of O_2 usually is recommended if the PaO_2 is less than 60 mm Hg, if the hematocrit is greater than 55%, or if evidence of cor pulmonale is present.[18]

The causes of acute exacerbations of COPD are multiple and may be explained only partially by airway infection or inflammation. Multiple contributing factors, including bronchitis, underlying airway hyperresponsiveness, inhalation of noxious agents, mucous plugging, pneumonitis, cardiovascular disease, congestive heart failure (CHF), and generalized systemic inflammation, must be considered.[25] Signs of COPD may be subtle.[50] The clinician must assess for increased respiratory effort, altered breathing patterns, abnormal breath sounds, and a productive cough.[51] A consensus statement by the American Thoracic Society defines dyspnea as "a term used to characterize a subjective experience of breathing discomfort that is comprised of qualitatively distinct sensations that vary in intensity. The experience derives from interactions among multiple physiological, psychological, social and environmental factors, and may induce secondary physiological and behavioral responses."[52,53]

In evaluation of the patient for dyspnea, a visual analogue scale is commonly used (Figure 24-12).

A history or the presence of atopy (predisposition to allergies), childhood respiratory impairment, high serum immunoglobulin E (IgE) levels, and eosinophilia are suggestive of asthmatic bronchitis, which is generally more responsive to treatment than is smoking-induced COPD. The clinician should perform ABG analysis or pulse oximetry (or both) for those patients with FEV_1 less than 1.5 L and should document the changes that occur with O_2 treatment. Pulmonary function tests should be repeated after bronchodilator or steroid treatment (or both) so that airway disease reversibility can be evaluated. Although β-agonists are the mainstay of treatment, increasing emphasis on the inflammatory component of reactive airway disease has resulted in an increase in the use of steroids.[50]

VISUAL ANALOGUE SCALE FOR DYSPNEA

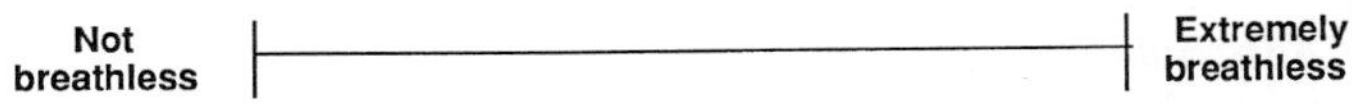

FIGURE **24-12**
Visual analogue scale, such as the horizontal one shown here, can be used for measuring dyspnea during an activity (e.g., exercise testing) or in response to questions. Such scales may be depicted vertically as well. On request the subject marks a point on the line in response to a question (e.g., "How short of breath are you right now?"). The score is determined by the length of the line from "not breathless" to the point marked by the patient. The scales are usually 10 cm long to facilitate scoring, and electronic scales may be used to allow online scoring (e.g., during exercise testing). Instructions about what is meant by the terms used to describe a sensation (e.g., "extremely breathless") must be clear and must be presented in a uniform fashion to provide meaningful results. (From Murray JF, Nadel JA. *Textbook of Respiratory Medicine*. 3rd ed. Philadelphia: Saunders; 2000:545.)

Conditions that predispose a patient to infectious complications include dehydration, decreased ability to cough, immobility, decreased level of consciousness, microatelectasis and macroatelectasis, decreased mucociliary clearance of inhaled particles and microbial organisms, pain, analgesia, and supplemental O_2 therapy. Optimal control of airway inflammation may require a course of broad-spectrum antimicrobial therapy preoperatively. A patient with an acute exacerbation of chronic bronchitis may have fatigue, chest tightness, increased cough, and dyspnea.[29]

The patient may observe a change in sputum volume, color, or consistency. Viruses are frequently causative organisms in acute exacerbations of chronic bronchitis and may be responsible for 25% to 50% of acute infections. In contrast to bacteria, viruses do not colonize the airways, and, when identified, they signify an active infective process.[29] Acute infection is associated with epithelial desquamation and correlates with airway hyperreactivity that may persist for 3 to 6 weeks after the resolution of symptoms.[53] The clinician should consider performing pulmonary function tests because they are useful for confirming the presence, severity, and reversibility of air flow obstruction, as well as for monitoring the progression of the disease. Surgery is not likely to be withheld on the basis of a decrease in ventilatory capacity, because patients with FEV_1 in the low range of 0.3 to 1 L often undergo surgery and anesthesia successfully.[54] It should be recognized that decreased pulmonary function as reflected by FEV_1 correlates with coronary artery disease and increased total mortality; the reason for this relationship has yet to be determined. Measures to improve respiratory skeletal muscle strength include good nutrition and balanced fluid and electrolyte intake. Bronchodilators should be used if the patient exhibits some degree of airway obstruction (coughing may temporarily increase in frequency as greater quantities of sputum are removed). Some commonly used bronchodilators are listed in Table 24-10.

An increased plasma concentration of bicarbonate in the presence of a low or normal $PaCO_2$ suggests that acute hyperventilation is masking chronic CO_2 retention. If the $PaCO_2$ has been chronically elevated, it is important that the hypercarbia not be corrected too quickly. Sudden decreases in $PaCO_2$ can result in alkalemia because the kidneys cannot instantly excrete the excess bicarbonate.

Patients arriving for surgery who are already undergoing mechanical ventilation may require a ventilator that is more powerful than that on the anesthesia machine. High airway pressures (i.e., those greater than 60 cm H_2O) create impedance to the high compressible volume of the anesthesia circuit, preventing adequate ventilation.[50] Finally, the patient with COPD who arrives for an emergency operation presents a further challenge because of an increased risk for mortality.[55] The anesthetist must attempt to provide optimal care despite less than optimal conditions.

Anesthesia Management

The presence of COPD does not dictate the use of specific drugs or techniques for the management of anesthesia. It is crucial to realize that COPD patients are susceptible to the development of acute respiratory failure during the postoperative period. Therefore, continued intubation of the trachea and mechanical ventilation of the lungs may be necessary, particularly after thoracic and upper abdominal surgery. Postoperative ventilation is more likely to be needed in those patients with low PaO_2 and dyspnea at rest.

Regional Anesthesia

Regional anesthesia is useful if sedation is not needed, and it may be safer than general anesthesia. Anesthetists must avoid complacency if they use regional rather than general anesthesia, monitoring for potential adverse side effects (pneumothorax, impaired muscle function). Regional anesthetic techniques that produce sensory anesthesia above T6 are not

TABLE 24-10 Commonly Used Bronchodilator Drugs

Drug*	Metered-Dose Inhaler (mcg)†	Nebulizer (mg)	Oral (mg)	Duration of Action (h)
β_2-Agonists				
Fenoterol	100-200	0.5-2	—	4-6
Salbutamol (albuterol)‡	100-200	2.5-5	4	4-6
Terbutaline	250-500	5-10	5	4-6
Formoterol	12-24	—	—	12+
Salmeterol	50-100	—	—	12+
Anticholinergics				
Ipratropium	40-80	0.25-0.5	—	6-8
Tiotropium (Spiriva)	18 (dry powder)	—	—	24-72
Methylxanthines§				
Aminophylline(SR)	—	—	225-450	Variable, up to 24
Theophylline (SR)	—	—	100-400	Variable, up to 24

**Not all products are available in all countries.*

†Doses: β_2-agonists refer to average dose given up to 4 times daily for short-acting and 2 times daily for long-acting preparations; anticholinergics are usually given 3 to 4 times daily.

‡Name in parentheses refers to North American generic term.

§Methylxanthines require dose titration depending on side effects and plasma theophylline levels.

Modified from Pauwels RA, Buist S, Calverley PM, et al. Global strategy for the diagnosis, management, and prevention of chronic obstructive pulmonary disease. Am J Respir Crit Care Med. *2001;163:5, 1256-1276.*

recommended because of the potential for decreasing expiratory reserve volume, impairing cough effort, and creating anxiety-provoking weakness.[56]

General Anesthesia

General anesthesia often is provided with a volatile anesthetic (for facilitating bronchodilation) and humidification (for preventing the drying of secretions). Maintenance of adequate anesthesia in patients with significant lung disease presents a challenge. General anesthesia often is associated with an increase in the alveolar-arterial difference in PO_2 ($PAO_2 - PaO_2$). Causes include a fairly consistent 20% decrease in FRC when neuromuscular relaxants are used, as well as airway closure, for which signs will lessen. Atelectasis in dependent lung regions has been found to worsen with muscle paralysis and prolonged surgical duration.[57] It is interesting to note that patients with chronic hyperinflation appear to be less likely to develop atelectasis than subjects with healthy lungs, possibly because of airway closure before alveolar collapse or because of resistance to early alveolar collapse from long-standing lung hyperinflation, which prevents prompt formation of atelectasis.[58]

If N_2O is used, bullae may enlarge and rupture; therefore their presence is a contraindication to the use of N_2O.[59] The anesthetist should provide adequate hydration to prevent excessive drying of secretions. The major limitation to gas movement in tissues is diffusion through tissue water. The impairment of gas exchange worsens during anesthesia.[60,61] Patients with COPD have slower diffusion and therefore may have longer induction and emergence times. The anesthetist should have the patient produce sighs during anesthesia; this has been found to improve the $PAO_2 - PaO_2$ significantly, ultimately improving oxygenation.[61] The capnograph should be monitored for expiratory air flow obstruction (Figure 24-13). Patients generally require an increased V_T; gas exchange is very dependent on V_T in some patients who require an increase in V_T for the improvement of gas exchange at the periphery of the lobule. This response varies among patients.[62]

Positive End-Expiratory Pressure

Severe air flow obstruction prevents full lung decompression at end-expiration; as a result inspiration begins at volumes at which the respiratory system exhibits positive recoil pressure, or auto or intrinsic PEEP (PEEPi).[63,64] Patients must generate pressure sufficient to overcome PEEPi before inspiratory flow can start.[64] In the past, external PEEP (PEEPe) was generally not used in patients with COPD because hypoxemia often is improved with increases in the fraction of inspired O_2 (FIO_2) and because the risk of barotrauma resulting from further hyperinflation was deemed too great. However, more recent studies suggest that a PEEPe that is less than the PEEPi in the presence of expiratory flow limitation may assist patients in overcoming the inspiratory mechanical load of PEEPi, ultimately decreasing the work of breathing and eliminating or decreasing atelectatic areas.[57,64] Patients whose peak cycling pressures remain essentially unaffected by PEEPe experience the greatest improvement and the least hazard.[65] In the operating room the clinician can best diagnose PEEPi by assessing whether exhalation is still taking place when the next inhalation starts.[50]

Clinical judgment must dictate the judicious use of PEEPe because the results of PEEPe are largely unpredictable.[63] PEEPe that is less than 85% of PEEPi has been found helpful, whereas PEEPe greater than 85% of PEEPi can cause further hyperinflation and may compromise hemodynamics and gas exchange. When PEEPe is added, it should be titrated in 2.5- to 5-cm H_2O increments while peak cycling pressures are closely monitored. The inspiratory-expiratory ratio is adjusted so that expiration is prolonged and the decrease in PEEPi is facilitated.[64]

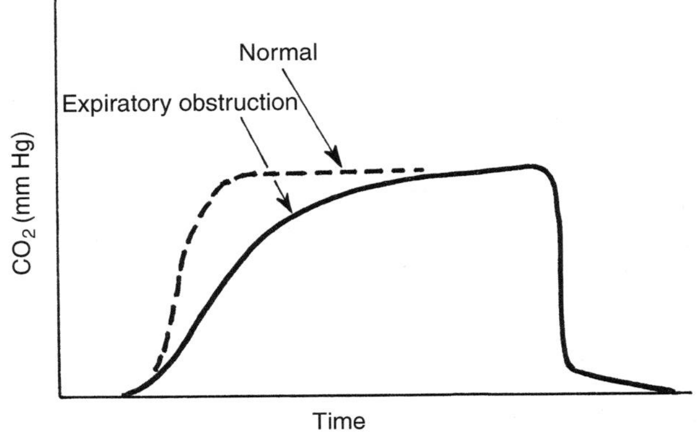

FIGURE **24-13**
Capnograph of a patient with expiratory airway obstruction. (Modified from Morgan GE, Mikhail MS. Anesthesia for patients with respiratory disease. In: Morgan GE, Mikhail MS, eds. *Clinical Anesthesiology*. 3rd ed. Norwalk, Conn: Appleton & Lange; 1996:444.)

Postoperative Care

Postoperative care of patients with COPD is directed at minimizing the incidence and severity of pulmonary complications, as such patients are at increased risk for the development of acute respiratory failure.[51] Postoperative pulmonary complications most often are characterized by atelectasis, followed by pneumonia and decreases in PaO_2.[50] These patients require close monitoring; worsening $\dot{V}/\dot{Q}$ mismatch after extubation may not be detected by ABG analysis, possibly because of changes in breathing pattern and cardiovascular function. In fact, e may not change, but often respiratory rate increases and V_T decreases after the termination of mechanical ventilation.[65] The choice of drugs or techniques for producing anesthesia does not seem to alter predictably the incidence of postoperative pulmonary infections. Whether a relationship exists between the duration of anesthesia and the incidence of postoperative pulmonary complications is not clear.

Ambulation should be encouraged in order to increase FRC and improve oxygenation via $\dot{V}/\dot{Q}$ matching. Incentive spirometry with maintenance of peak inflation for 3 to 5 seconds reexpands collapsed alveoli.[53] Expiratory maneuvers (e.g., floating of balls on an expiratory spirometer) generate pleural pressures that exceed airway pressures and thereby can cause alveolar collapse.[51,66]

ASTHMA

Definition

Asthma is a chronic inflammatory disorder of the airways characterized by increased responsiveness of the tracheobronchial tree to a variety of stimuli. Many cells and cellular elements play a role—in particular, mast cells, eosinophils, T lymphocytes, neutrophils, and epithelial cells. In susceptible individuals this inflammation causes recurrent episodes of wheezing, breathlessness, chest tightness, and cough, particularly at night and in the early morning. These episodes are usually associated with widespread but variable airflow obstruction that is often reversible either spontaneously or with treatment.[67]

Various subtypes of asthma exist. The most important consideration is the identification of exacerbating factors whenever possible. A well-known system classifies asthmas as either extrinsic or intrinsic. Although this system is conceptually helpful, its two groups are not mutually exclusive. Extrinsic asthma (or allergic asthma) most commonly affects children and young adults and involves infectious, environmental, psychologic, or physical factors, whereas intrinsic asthma (or idiosyncratic asthma) usually develops in middle age without specifically identifiable attack-provoking stimuli. The term *atopy*, which refers to a hereditary, IgE-mediated, clinical hypersensitive state, is often used when extrinsic asthma is described.

Incidence and Outcome

Up tc 15 million persons in the United States have asthma. It is the most common chronic disease of childhood, affecting an estimated 4.8 million children. People with asthma collectively have more than 100 million days of restricted activity and 470,000 hospitalizations annually. More than 5000 people die of asthma each year.[67]

Pathogenesis and Pathophysiology

Our contemporary understanding of asthma is that it is not a single entity, but rather a heterogeneous clinical syndrome characterized by episodes in which airways are hyperresponsive, interspersed with symptom-free periods.[68] Bronchoconstriction is a factor long associated with the asthmatic symptom complex, but asthma is much more than bronchoconstriction. Airway inflammation and a nonspecific hyperirritability of the tracheobronchial tree are now recognized as being central to the pathogenesis of even mild cases of asthma. Permanent changes in airway anatomy, referred to as *airway remodeling*, magnify the inflammatory response.[68,69]

Allergic asthma (atopic or immunologic disease) is triggered by antigens that provoke a T-lymphocyte–generated, IgE-mediated immune response.[70] It is often associated with a personal or familial history of allergic disease.

In susceptible patients exposure to even minute amounts of an offending agent can cause activation of lymphocytes and cytokine release, setting into motion an immune-mediated inflammatory response. Endobronchial biopsy specimens, even from asymptomatic patients, frequently show an active inflammatory process. Eosinophils, mast cells, neutrophils, and macrophages are prominent features in asthmatic airways, and their activation and degranulation fuel the proinflammatory cascade.

Potent biochemical mediators released from proinflammatory and airway epithelial cells promote vasoconstriction, increased smooth muscle tone, enhanced mucous secretion, submucosal edema, increased vascular permeability, and inflammatory cell chemotaxis. Leukotrienes have been identified as especially potent spasmogenic and proinflammatory substances. Released molecules that are toxic to the airway epithelium cause patchy desquamation, exposing cholinergic nerve endings and compounding the bronchoconstrictive and hyperresponsive response.

The asthmatic diathesis creates airways that are inflamed, edematous, and hypersensitive to irritant stimuli, and the degree of airway hyperresponsiveness and bronchoconstriction appears to parallel the extent of inflammation.[71-73] When airway reactivity is high, asthmatic symptoms are generally more severe and unrelenting, and the amount of therapy required to control the episode is greater.[68] Table 24-11 lists some of the chemical mediators involved in asthmatic episodes and their physiologic effects.

The mechanisms underlying idiosyncratic asthma (nonimmunologic disease) are less clearly defined. Nonimmunologic asthma occurs in patients with no history of allergy and normal serum IgE. These patients typically develop asthmatic symptoms in response to some provocative or noxious stimulus such as cold air, airway instrumentation or irritation, climate changes, or an upper respiratory illness. Recent upper respiratory infection may precipitate bronchospasm in any patient, but the risk is higher in patients with a history of asthma. The increased bronchomotor tone associated with viral respiratory infections may persist for as long as 5 weeks.[74] Nonasthmatic children with an upper respiratory infection are two to seven times more likely to experience an adverse event perioperatively and are more prone to postoperative desaturation.[75] Asthmatic children can be considered to be at a similar if not greater risk. Enhanced parasympathetic nervous system tone can contribute to the airflow obstruction.

TABLE 24-11 Inflammatory Mediators and Asthma

Inflammatory Mediator	Source	Effects
Histamine	Mast cells	Bronchoconstriction
Leukotrienes (LTB_1, LTC_4, LTD_4, LTE_4)	Mast cells, basophils, eosinophils, neutrophils, macrophages, monocytes	Chemotaxis, bronchoconstriction, mucous hypersecretion, edema
Platelet-activating factor	Mast cells, basophils, eosinophils, neutrophils, macrophages, monocytes, platelets, endothelial cells	Eosinophil recruitment, bronchoconstriction, airway hyperresponsiveness
Proteases	Enzymes	Bronchial hyperresponsiveness
Prostaglandins ($PGF_{2\alpha}$, PGD_2, PGF_2, PGI_2)	Mast cells, endothelial cells	Bronchoconstriction, mucous secretion
Major basic protein	Eosinophils	Epithelial damage
Thromboxanes (TXA_2)	Macrophages, monocytes, platelets	Bronchoconstriction, mucous secretion

Modified from Bigby TD, Wasserman SI. Asthma. In: Stein JH, ed. Internal Medicine. *5th ed. St Louis: Mosby; 1998:1185-1193; and Blake K. Asthma. In: Jerfindal ET, Gourley DR, eds.* Textbook of Therapeutics. *7th ed. Philadelphia: William & Wilkins; 2000:727-764.*

Immune mechanisms appear to be causally related or contributory to the development of asthma in over 50% of cases, but many patients with asthma have disease mechanisms from both categories. Asthma that has its onset in childhood tends to have a strong allergic component, whereas asthma that arises in adults tends to be nonallergic or to have a mixed cause.[68,76] As a general rule, nonallergic mechanisms are more prevalent in the perioperative period.[77] It is of significance that the clinical features of idiosyncratic asthma are essentially indistinguishable from the immune-mediated response.

IgE-mediated asthma occurs after initial antigen exposure has resulted in IgE antibody formation. On reexposure, in the presence of IgE, mast cells release multiple mediators as noted in Table 24-11. These mediators directly constrict small and large airways, increase capillary permeability, stimulate vasoconstriction, and increase mucous gland secretion, which contributes to mucous plugging.

The mechanism of exercise-induced asthma is unknown. One popular theory suggests that a high minute ventilation (Ve) and the low temperature or low H_2O content of inspired gas (which requires greater heat and water transfer from the mucosal surface to the inspired gas) generates a bronchoconstrictive response. Another theory proposes that the evaporation of water from respiratory mucosa and the resultant increase in the osmolarity of the surface-lining fluid induces the degranulation of mast cells. A third theory suggests that reactive hyperemia of the bronchial mucosa occurs with rewarming, resulting in airway narrowing.[78] Regardless of the mechanism, most symptoms last less than 1 hour and are usually quickly reversed with administration of β_2-adrenergic receptor agonists.[79]

Occupational asthma develops when irritants directly stimulate vagal nerve endings in the airway epithelium. Infection-induced asthma with acute inflammation of the bronchi may be caused by viral, bacterial, or mycoplasmal infections. Aspirin-induced asthma occurs when, in some predisposed persons, cyclooxygenase promotes an increase in leukotriene levels via the arachidonic acid pathway, thereby triggering the asthma attack. This peculiar response can occur with the use of other nonsteroidal antiinflammatory agents. The aspirin-induced asthma variant is not IgE mediated or allergic in nature; furthermore, it is clinically associated with nasal polyps.

Clinical Features

Key hallmarks of asthma in the awake patient include the following[71]:

- Wheezing
- Dyspnea (may parallel the severity of expiratory airflow obstruction)
- Cough (productive or nonproductive; frequently at night or early morning)
- Labored respirations with accessory muscle use
- Tachypnea (a respiratory rate >30 breaths per minute and a heart rate of 120 suggests severe bronchospasm)
- Chest tightness
- Prolonged expiratory phase of respiration
- Fatigue

Clinical classification of asthma is noted in Table 24-12. Typically attacks are short-lived, lasting minutes to hours. Between attacks the asthmatic patient may be entirely symptom free; however, underlying airway remodeling is still evident.[69,70] Severe obstruction persisting for days or weeks is known as *status asthmaticus*. Use of accessory muscles of respiration and the increased work of breathing associated with a protracted asthmatic episode can result in respiratory muscle fatigue and respiratory failure.

During exacerbations, pulmonary function tests may reflect acute expiratory airflow obstruction (↓ forced expiratory flow $[FEF]_{25\%-75\%}$; ↓ FEV_1/FVC). Viscid mucous secretion may compound the airway narrowing and produce airway collapse.[80]

The asthmatic episode produces not only airflow obstruction, but also gas exchange abnormalities. The resulting low $\dot{V}/\dot{Q}$ state produces arterial O_2 desaturation.[81] Hypoxemia is common, but in most patients with acute bronchospasm, CO_2 elimination is relatively well preserved until $\dot{V}/\dot{Q}$ abnormalities are severe. An increased arterial CO_2 tension may indicate impending respiratory failure in the acutely ill asthmatic patient. Chronic asthma may eventually lead to irreversible lung destruction, loss of lung elasticity, pulmonary hypertension (PH), and lung hyperinflation.

Anesthetized Patients

In anesthetized patients prominent manifestations of the asthmatic episode are wheezing, mucous hypersecretion, high inspiratory pressures, a blunted expiratory CO_2 waveform, and hypoxemia.

Mechanical ventilation and positive airway pressure are associated with a higher incidence of air-trapping and lung hyperinflation, and the associated barotrauma can result in a pneumothorax.[81] Additionally, alveolar overdistention may lead to decreased venous return and diminution of CO. The combination of impaired ventilation and hypoxia can precipitate increased pulmonary vascular resistance, enhanced right ventricular afterload, and finally hemodynamic collapse.

The onset of an asthmatic episode may occur abruptly in surgical patients. Airway manipulation, acute exposure to allergens, or the stress of surgery can provoke wheezing in a patient who was previously asymptomatic. The lability of the disease makes assiduous observation crucial.

Wheezing often suggests potentially reversible bronchoconstriction, but the extent or degree of wheezing is a notoriously poor indicator of the degree of airway obstruction.[82] In addition, care must be taken to differentiate wheezing of asthmatic origin from other causes of wheezing such as pneumothorax, endotracheal tube obstruction, endobronchial intubation, anaphylaxis, pulmonary edema, and pulmonary aspiration.[83,84]

Diagnostic Testing

Pulmonary Function Tests

Lung function testing should routinely be performed in asthmatic patients. Pulmonary function tests allow the clinician to assess the degree of impairment and the reversibility of airway limitation (see Table 24-12). Spirometry is based on a VC or FVC maneuver, with volume recorded as a function of time. The FVC maneuver requires total patient effort; a lack of effort may produce faulty results.[85]

The FVC is divided into several time intervals, of which the FEV_1 is the most reproducible. Patients with increased airway resistance exhibit decreased FEV_1 and FEV_1/FVC ratios. FEV_1 is extremely useful and reliable, and the technique for its determination is noninvasive and easy to perform.[85]

Respiratory activity represented by the midportion of the FVC curve is the most effort independent and the most sensitive indicator of small airway disease. This parameter is the $FEF_{25\%-75\%}$. The normal $FEF_{25\%-75\%}$ of 4 to 5 L/s may decrease markedly in pulmonary disease, with early changes evident sooner in patients with obstructive disease than in those with

TABLE 24-12 Clinical Asthma Classification and Associated Pharmacotherapy

	Clinical Characteristics before Therapy	Pharmacologic Treatment*
Step 1—Mild intermittent asthma	Signs and symptoms occur twice per week or less frequently Patients generally asymptomatic with normal peak flows between exacerbations Exacerbations brief, although intensity may vary Nighttime symptoms occur twice per month or less frequently FEV_1 or PEFR ≥80% of predicted value	Short-acting bronchodilator, as needed: inhaled β_2-agonists are the first-line selection
Step 2—Mild persistent asthma	Signs and symptoms occur more than twice per week but less than once per day Exacerbations may affect activity Nighttime symptoms occur more than twice per month FEV_1 or PEFR ≥80% of predicted value	Long-term antiinflammatory medication: inhaled corticosteroid (low dose) Cromolyn or nedocromil, particularly in children Sustained-release theophylline is an alternative Zafirlukast or zileuton may be considered for patients ≥12 years old
Step 3—Moderate persistent asthma	Daily symptoms Daily use of short-acting β_2-agonist Exacerbations that affect activity occur at least twice a week and may last for days Nighttime symptoms occur more than once per week FEV_1 or PEFR 60% of 80% of predicted value	Long-term control medications: medium-dose inhaled corticosteroids or low- to medium-dose inhaled corticosteroids plus long-acting bronchodilator (inhaled or oral β_2-agonist, sustained-release theophylline), especially for treatment of nocturnal symptoms
Step 4—Severe persistent asthma	Continuous signs and symptoms, frequently exacerbated Frequent nighttime symptoms Limited physical activity FEV_1 or PEFR ≤60% of predicted value	High-dose inhaled corticosteroids Long-acting bronchodilators, as indicated in step 3 Systemic corticosteroids (e.g., prednisone)

FEV_1, *Forced expiratory volume in 1 second;* PEFR, *peak expiratory flow rate.*
**For all severity steps, β_2-agonists are used for quick relief of acute symptoms.*
Modified from National Heart, Lung, and Blood Institute National Asthma Education and Prevention Program. Expert Panel Report 2. Guidelines for the diagnosis and management of asthma. Bethesda, Md: US Department of Health and Human Services; 1997. NIH publication no. 97-4051; Galant SP. Pharmacotherapeutic options for the management of asthma. Formulary. *1998;33:343-356; and Kaiser Permanente Care Management Program.* Asthma Successful Practice Guidelines. *Pasadena, Calif: Kaiser Permanente; 2003:1-14.*

restrictive disease. The value of $FEF_{25\%-75\%}$ is computed electronically.[86]

RV, FRC, and TLC all increase because of an increase in volume of the gas trapped beyond closed airways, and lung deflation is less because of airway obstruction. Comparison of current and prior pulmonary function test results is useful. Tolerance of activities is used for classifying the degree of dyspnea.[87] The patient in remission may have negative results on all parameters of pulmonary function and may be tested with a cholinergic agonist for bronchial provocation. A typical abnormality is an increase in the FEV_1 of more than 15% in response to a bronchodilator. Episodes of severe airway obstruction may not respond to bronchodilator treatment, and cessation of wheezing may occur with the worsening of obstruction (i.e., the "ominously silent chest"). Although the diagnosis of asthma does not require the measurement of lung volumes, knowledge of these volumes is helpful in assessing the severity of the disease.

Arterial Blood Gas Analysis

Increased diffusibility of CO_2 (compared with that of O_2) in combination with an often increased respiratory rate generally produces ABG analysis results that reflect the presence of respiratory alkalosis. Even slight hypercapnia may indicate severe air trapping and potential impending respiratory failure.

Chest Radiography

Because nearly 75% of asthma patients have a normal chest radiograph, chest radiography is not helpful in diagnosing or determining the severity of asthma. Hyperinflation with flattening of the diaphragm may be evident. Chest radiography is more helpful in detection of complications.

Electrocardiography

Changes evident on electrocardiography (ECG), such as ST-segment changes, right ventricular strain, and right axis deviation, usually manifest only in severe attacks and generally are of little significance with regard to the asthmatic condition.

Sputum Analysis

Eosinophilia, which is common in asthmatic patients, may be manifested as the production of grossly purulent sputum. Microscopic evaluation may reveal Curschmann's spirals and Charcot-Leyden crystals rather than polymorphic neutrophils associated with infection.

Serum Values

Eosinophilia (defined as more than 275 eosinophils per cubic millimeter of blood) is common in asthmatic patients with active IgE-mediated bronchial asthma, but its presence does not serve to differentiate extrinsic from intrinsic asthma. Asymptomatic patients with asthma generally have a total blood eosinophil count that is less than 50/mm^3, with an increasing count often signaling the acceleration of bronchial asthma even before such patients experience symptoms. Determination of an increased eosinophil value in the absence of signs and symptoms of asthma requires that a differential analysis be undertaken. Tests for detection of IgE antibodies are performed only if an identifiable and avoidable substance is suspected. In this instance, consultation with a physician skilled in testing for allergic disease may be indicated.

Anesthesia Management

Several important anesthetic considerations and risk reduction strategies have been reported.

Preoperatively

A careful preoperative history and physical examination are essential to the discernment of the current disease status and medication profile. Frequent nocturnal awakenings because of respiratory difficulty, recent increases in medication use, and signs of viral infection may signal an increased likelihood of intraoperative difficulties.[88-90] Elective procedures in patients who are exhibiting significant respiratory symptoms should be postponed, and the condition of such patients should be normalized as much as possible.[90]

The predictive value of routine pulmonary function testing remains controversial.[89-93] FEV and peak expiratory flow rate, which can be measured with inexpensive hand-held devices, may be helpful in assessment of current respiratory status. Values that fall 30% to 50% below expected baseline values indicate a moderate episode of bronchoconstriction. Values below 50% of normal indicate a severe episode.[88]

Pretreatment with systemic corticosteroids has been advocated in asthma patients undergoing surgical procedures. Kabalin and co-workers[94] studied the administration of corticosteroids in asthmatic surgical patients. Of the 89 subjects in the study, 86 had no postoperative wheezing when given either prednisone or hydrocortisone preoperatively. Complications of steroid therapy such as delayed wound healing, infection, or adrenocortical insufficiency were not noted. Ensuring that a patient who is currently receiving inhaled or systemic steroids receives them immediately before surgery is a prudent course.

Routine preoperative medications should be given to allay anxiety. The anticholinergics atropine and glycopyrrolate exhibit mild bronchodilating effects, and, as noted earlier, asthmatics experience an increased parasympathetic tone. These agents are most effective as prophylactic drugs given 20 to 30 minutes preoperatively rather than for acute therapy.[95] Caution must be exercised when administering narcotics to patients whose respiratory difficulties are evident or when using narcotics associated with histamine release, such as morphine. Fentanyl and the other phenylpiperidine analogues commonly used in anesthesia have been widely used and are safe.[89,95,96] The use of histamine-2 (H_2)–receptor blocking agents such as cimetidine and ranitidine to reduce gastric volume and acidity should be avoided.[75,95] Bronchospasm after their use has been reported, possibly resulting from loss of inhibitory feedback control via presynaptic H_2 autoreceptor blockade, resulting in increased histamine release. Usual drug therapy for asthma is listed in Table 24-13. Some suggested risk reduction strategies for use in the perioperative period are listed in Table 24-14.

Intraoperative Management

Despite a lack of definitive controlled clinical studies, regional anesthetic techniques are generally felt to be safer than general anesthesia.[97,98] Spinal or epidural levels to the midthoracic area or higher however, decrease FRC, expiratory reserve volume, and the ability to cough and should be avoided.

All of the common induction drugs—thiopental, propofol, etomidate, and ketamine—have been used successfully in asthmatic patients; however, some differences exist. Ketamine is the only induction drug with bronchodilating properties, which makes it the agent of choice in patients with active asthmatic symptoms who require emergency surgery. Thiopental and the other barbiturates may cause histamine release in a small percentage of patients; however, when higher doses are used the rapidly produced deep levels of anesthesia are a primary factor in blunting this problem. Pizov and colleagues[99] compared thiopental, thiamylal, methohexital, and propofol in a double-blind randomized study in patients with and without asthma. None of the asthmatic patients who received propofol exhibited wheezing 2 and 5 minutes after intubation. Wheezing after intubation occurred in 26% to 45% of the patients who received one of the three barbiturates. These authors suggested that propofol is advantageous for routine induction in asthmatic patients.

The potent inhalation agents produce bronchial relaxation and have all been successfully used in asthmatic patients after administration of an intravenous induction drug. Isoflurane and desflurane, however, are both mild respiratory irritants, which may be a consideration during emergence. It is common practice to blunt this effect with the administration of opiates. Sevoflurane has been shown to be effective for inhalation induction in children.[100,101] Other anesthesia-related medications that should be avoided in asthmatic patients include atracurium and mivacurium, because of histamine release, and esmolol and labetalol, which as β-receptor blockers produce bronchoconstriction. Many practitioners avoid long-acting muscle relaxants and the associated possibility of residual muscle weakness in patients with asthma. Ketorolac and other nonsteroidal antiinflammatory agents should be avoided in patients with aspirin-intolerant asthma.[102]

If an episode of bronchospasm occurs during anesthesia the following steps are recommended: (1) deepen the level of anesthesia with a volatile agent, ketamine, propofol, lidocaine, or a combination that rapidly increases anesthetic depth; (2) administer 100% O_2; (3) administer a β_2-agonist; (4) in severe cases administer epinephrine intravenously or subcutaneously; (5) administer intravenous corticosteroids; (6) consider intravenous aminophylline if long-term postoperative mechanical ventilation is planned. Theophylline has little efficacy for the treatment of acute bronchoconstrictive episodes.[103]

A strategy for mechanical ventilation that avoids lung hyperinflation and barotrauma while allowing for longer expiratory times should be chosen. A reduction in Ve, by limitation of inspiratory times and prolongation of expiratory times, and moderate permissive hypercapnia have been suggested.[104-106]

Emergence

The primary issue during emergence is when to extubate. Some authors suggest deep extubation to avoid the mechanical stimulation from the endotracheal tube on awakening. Others fear that the loss of a secure airway before patient awakening may present a greater difficulty than the presence of the endotracheal tube. Either way, a judgment must be made as to

TABLE 24-13 Drug Therapy for Asthma

Drug Group	Specific Agent	Dose
Antiinflammatory drugs, corticosteroids, mast cell–inhibiting agents	Hydrocortisone, intravenous	4-mg/kg bolus followed by infusion of 0.5 mg/kg/h
	Methylprednisolone, intravenous	0.8 mg/kg bolus followed by infusion of 0.1 mg/kg/h
	Beclomethasone dipropionate (Beclovent, Vanceril) (MDI)	42 mcg/puff; 2 puffs 4 times per day or 4 puffs twice per day
	Budesonide (Pulmicort Turbuhaler)	1-2 inhalations twice per day
	Flunisolide (AeroBid) (MDI)	250 mcg/puff; 2-4 puffs twice per day
	Fluticasone propionate (Flovent)	44 mcg/puff ; 2-4 puffs twice per day
	Triamcinolone (Azmacort) (MDI)	100 mcg/puff; 2 puffs 3-4 times per day or 4 puffs twice per day
	Cromolyn sodium (Intal) (MDI)	100 mcg/puff; 2-4 puffs twice per day; 2-4 puffs 4 times per day
	Nedocromil (Tilade)	1.75 mg/puff; 2 puffs every 6 h
Bronchodilators, $beta_2$-selective adrenergic drugs	Albuterol (Proventil, Ventolin) (MDI)	90 mcg/puff; 2 puffs every 4-6 h (nebulized solution, 2.5 mg every 1-4 h)
	Bitolterol mesylate (Tornalate) (MDI)	370 mcg/puff; 2-3 puffs every 4-6 h (nebulized solution, 1.5-3.5 mg every 4-6 h)
	Salmeterol xinafoate (Serevent) (MDI)	21 mcg/puff; 2 puffs every 12 h
	Pirbuterol (Maxair)	200 mcg/puff; 2 puffs every 4-6 h
	Terbutaline (Brethine, Bricanyl) subcutaneous	0.25 mg (may repeat once after 15-30 min; maximum dose, 0.5 mg in 4 h)
	Levalbuterol (Sepracor)	0.63 mg every 6-8 h nebulized as needed
Antimuscarinic	Ipratropium bromide (Atrovent)	18 mcg/puff; 2 puffs 4 times per day maximum, 12 puffs in 24 h
Methylxanthine	Theophylline (Theo-Dur, and others)	Extended-release capsules or tablets, 300-600 mg/d Intravenous: 5-6 mg/kg loading; 0.9-1 maintenance via slow infusion
Leukotriene modifiers	Montelukast (Singulair)	10-mg tablet once per day
	Zafirlukast (Accolate)	20-mg tablet twice per day
	Zileuton (Zyflo)	600-mg tablet twice per day
Anti-IgE antibody	Omalizumab (Xolair)	150-300 mg every 4 weeks to 225-375 mg every 2 weeks subcutaneous injection

Modified from Nagelhout JJ, Zaglaniczny KL. Nurse Anesthesia. *2nd ed. Philadelphia: Saunders; 2000:529; Drugs for Asthma.* Med Lett. *2000;42: 19-24; and Omalizumab (Xolair): an anti-IgE antibody for asthma.* Med Lett. *2003;45:67-69.*

when to extubate the patient, with the understanding that the earliest possible time is advantageous for prevention of mechanical bronchial stimulation. Administration of lidocaine and small non–respiratory-depressing doses of opiates may help diminish airway sensitivity.

The use of anticholinesterase reversal agents has also been an area of concern. If their administration can be avoided by the use of short-acting nondepolarizing muscle relaxants, this should be considered. When they are necessary, a small increase in the coadministered dose of atropine or glycopyrrolate to ensure total blockade of parasympathomimetic side effects is suggested.

Asthma and the Pregnant Surgical Patient

Treatment for pregnant asthmatic patients undergoing surgery is generally the same as for nonpregnant patients. Inhaled β-agonists, corticosteroids, and theophylline have been safely used in pregnant patients; however, parenteral β-agonists should be avoided. Maintaining proper maternal oxygenation is essential to the health of the fetus. Some anesthetic considerations for the pregnant asthmatic patient are given in Table 24-15.[107-109]

PULMONARY HYPERTENSION

Definition

PH usually represents an advanced stage of a large number of cardiovascular diseases.[110] The mortality rate associated with PH is high. Pulmonary arterial hypertension exists if the mean level of PAP increases by 5 to 10 mm Hg or if pulmonary artery systolic pressure exceeds 30 mm Hg and mean PAP exceeds 20 mm Hg.[111,112]

Incidence and Outcome

PH may be (1) primary or idiopathic (unexplained) or (2) secondary to an associated condition. In young adults the female-to-male incidence of primary PH (PPH) is 4:1; this incidence is similar to that in older groups of men and women. PPH is a rare disorder, and its true incidence is unknown; however, it is found on autopsy in 1% of patients in whom cor pulmonale had been diagnosed.[112]

Etiology

PH may be caused by many associated conditions, including pulmonary venous hypertension caused by left atrial outflow

TABLE 24-14 Risk Reduction Strategies for Anesthetization of Patients with Asthma

Preoperative
Encourage cessation of cigarette smoking for at least 8 weeks.
Aggressively treat airflow obstruction.
Administer antibiotics and delay surgery if respiratory infection is present.
Begin patient education regarding lung-expansion maneuvers.
Intraoperative
Limit duration of surgery to less than 3 hours.
Use regional anesthesia when possible.
Avoid the use of long-acting neuromuscular blocking agents.
Use laparoscopic procedures when possible.
Substitute less ambitious procedure for upper abdominal or thoracic surgery when possible.
Postoperative
Encourage deep-breathing exercises or incentive spirometry.
Use continuous positive airway pressure.
Use intercostal nerve blocks and local anesthesia infiltration of incisional area for pain when appropriate.

Modified from Smetana GW. Current concepts: preoperative pulmonary evaluation. N Engl J Med. *1999;340:937-944; and Hurford WE. The bronchospastic patient.* Int Anesthesiol Clin. *2000;38:77-89.*

TABLE 24-15 Anesthetic Considerations in the Pregnant Asthmatic Patient

Avoid nonemergency surgery until after delivery.
Postpone semiemergent surgery until after the first trimester.
Administer higher than normal oxygen concentrations.
Use antacids but not histamine$_2$-receptor blockers for gastric preparation.
Use uterine displacement, generous fluid replacement, compression stockings, or leg elevation to minimize hypotension.
If a vasopressor is necessary, use ephedrine.
Avoid nitrous oxide.
Shield the fetus from radiographic exposure when possible.
Use inhaled but not parenteral β_2-receptor agonists.
Use fetal monitoring and ultrasound when feasible.

Modified from Karlet M, Nagelhout J. Asthma: an anesthetic update. AANA J. *2001;69:317-324.*

obstruction or pulmonary venous occlusive disease; and pulmonary arterial hypertension caused by hyperdynamic circulation (e.g., secondary to burns or sepsis), vasoconstriction, viscosity, obstruction, and reactive vascular disease.[112]

PPH is characterized by a rapidly progressive course with a 79% mortality rate within 5 years of clinical diagnosis.[113] The degree of increase in pressure in the pulmonary circulation has an important influence on the patient's life expectancy.[114] Resistant PH has long been identified as a major cause of early death.[115] Prognosis is largely determined by right ventricular integrity.[116]

Pathophysiology

The normal pulmonary circulation is mostly passive, of low resistance, and highly distensible.[111] PH is characterized by an increase in vascular tone and the growth and proliferation of pulmonary vascular smooth muscle. Initial reversible vasoconstriction may progress to muscle hypertrophy and irreversible degeneration.[112]

Pulmonary vasoconstriction appears to occur in some (but not all) patients with PH. Some speculate that the disease progresses from vasoconstriction to fixed obstruction of the pulmonary vascular bed. Pathologic changes associated with a fixed resistance are the presence of intimal sclerosis, plexiform (resembling a plexus or network) lesions, and the obliteration of as many as 90% or more of the small vessels within the lung.[117] Other reported abnormalities include impairment of endothelium-dependent vasodilation.[118]

Clinical Features and Diagnosis

PH may be either acute or chronic. In almost all patients with PH, dyspnea and exercise intolerance usually are the first complaints.[116,119] Patients also may have angina. PH associated with chest pain was reported as early as 1891; however, whether PH actually causes anginal chest pain is uncertain. Many cases of this combination have been reported, suggesting that PH may be associated with chest pain and electrocardiographic changes typical of myocardial infarction even in the absence of coronary artery disease. Some clinicians propose that the source of the chest pain is (1) an increase in right ventricular myocardial O_2 demand secondary to an increase in wall stress, or (2) a decrease in coronary blood flow because of a decrease in flow in the arteries supplying the right ventricle during systole.[120]

Right atrial hypertrophy or right ventricular hypertrophy (or both) may be evident on ECG. Chest radiography may demonstrate an enlarged pulmonary artery.[121] Cardiac catheterization combined with pulmonary angiography is most informative in assessment of PH, cardiac reserve, and the effects of pulmonary vasodilator therapy.[112] Vasodilator therapy is attempted when a vasoconstrictor component is identified. Vasodilator challenge may be performed with cardiac catheterization using a rapid and effective pulmonary vasodilator such as nitroglycerin, isoproterenol, nifedipine, prostaglandin E_1, prostacyclin, prostaglandin E_2, hydralazine, nitroprusside, or adenosine for evaluation of the reversibility of PH.[115] Frequently, open-lung biopsy is performed for assessment of the histopathologic composition of small pulmonary arteries.[122] Noninvasive evaluation includes Doppler echocardiography for measurement of the velocity of tricuspid regurgitation (which correlates well with invasive PAP measurements) and pulmonic peak flow velocity.[123,124]

Anesthesia Management

Attempts to alleviate pulmonary hypertensive disease states have had varied success.[125] Vasodilator agents are used most commonly and may be helpful in patients with reversible vasoconstriction. A list of vasodilators used in PH is given in Table 24-16. Possible beneficial effects of pulmonary arterial dilation are preservation of lung function, prevention of right ventricle deterioration, and, it is hoped, improved survival.

The principal objectives during anesthesia in patients with PH are prevention of increases in PH and avoidance of major hemodynamic changes.[114] Considerations that apply to the care of patients with cor pulmonale also apply to those with PH. Information regarding PH and intravenous induction agents is

TABLE 24-16 Drug Treatment Options for Patients with Pulmonary Hypertension

Drug or Drug Class	Rationale	Potentially Responsive Types of Pulmonary Hypertension	Limitations
Anticoagulants	Reduce risk of pulmonary thromboembolism	Primary and that secondary to acute pulmonary thromboembolism, chronic pulmonary thromboembolism, and anorectic drugs	For primary hypertension, concomitant vasodilator treatment also required
Vasodilators			
Calcium antagonists	Inhibit influx of calcium into smooth muscle cells with elevated vasomotor tone; preferentially act on pulmonary vasculature	Primary and that secondary to connective tissue vascular disease and COPD	Initial treatment in specialized centers recommended to avoid severe adverse outcomes such as negative inotropic effects
Epoprostenol (Flolan)—prostacyclin	May replace deficiencies in endogenous prostacyclin; also inhibits smooth muscle proliferation and platelet aggregation	Primary, persistent pulmonary hypertension of the neonate and that secondary to ARDS, crises after heart surgery in infants, and connective tissue disease in adults	Peripheral adverse effects occur when administered by continuous IV infusion
Nitric oxide	Interferes with endogenous vasoconstrictor mechanisms	Primary, persistent pulmonary hypertension of the neonate and that secondary to corrective cardiac surgery in children, lung or lung-heart ransplant surgery in adults, and COPD	Potential adverse effects include increased bleeding times, negative inotropic effects, and formation of potentially toxic products (e.g., nitrogen dioxide, methemoglobin)
Alprostadil (prostaglandin E_1)	Interferes with endogenous vasoconstrictor mechanisms	Secondary to ARDS	Impaired pulmonary metabolism may result in systemic hypotension
Bosentan (Tracleer)	Oral endothelin receptor antagonist	Severe pulmonary hypertension	Hepatotoxicity
Treprostinil (Remodulin)	Prostacyclin analogue	Primary pulmonary hypertension; class II–IV	Given by continuous infusion via wearable infusion pump
Inhibitors of Vasoconstriction			
α-Adrenoceptor antagonists	Inhibit the formation of the vasoconstrictor angiotensin II	Persistent pulmonary hypertension of the neonate (especially preterm infants) and that secondary to COPD	Can cause severe systemic adverse effects
ACE inhibitors	Inhibit the formation of the vasoconstrictor angiotensin II	Secondary to connective tissue disease, effects of high altitude, and congestive heart failure	Prolonged treatment required to obtain an effect

ACE, *Angiotensin-converting enzyme;* ARDS, *acute respiratory distress syndrome;* COPD, *chronic obstructive pulmonary disease;* IV, *intravenous. Modified from Different types of pulmonary hypertension require different treatment strategies.* Drug Ther Perspect. *1999;14:5-8; and Treprostinil (Remodulin) for pulmonary arterial hypertension.* Med Lett. *2002;44:80-82.*

lacking; however, most agents either have little effect on pulmonary vascular resistance (PVR) or decrease it.[112] Ketamine, which causes an increase in PVR, may be the exception.[126]

COR PULMONALE

Definition

The term *cor pulmonale* or *pulmonary heart disease* refers to patients exhibiting PH resulting in progressive right ventricular hypertrophy, dilation, and eventual cardiac decompensation. This arises from disorders that affect ventilatory drive or musculoskeletal respiratory mechanics; pulmonary airway, infiltrative, fibrotic, or vascular diseases; and diseases that are primarily cardiac but affect the pulmonary circulation and the lungs (Table 24-17).

Incidence and Outcome

In individuals older than 50 years of age, cor pulmonale is the third most common cardiac disorder (after ischemic heart disease and hypertensive cardiac disease). The male-to-female ratio of incidence of the disease is 5:1; 10% to 30% of patients admitted to the hospital with coronary heart failure exhibit cor pulmonale.[127]

Prognosis is determined by the pulmonary disease responsible for the increased PVR. In patients with COPD in whom PaO_2 can be maintained at near-normal levels, the prognosis is favorable. However, cor pulmonale associated with hypoxic lung disease is associated with a 70% rate of mortality within 5 years after onset of associated peripheral edema.[128] Prognosis is poor for those patients in whom cor pulmonale is the result of gradual obstruction of pulmonary vessels by intrinsic pulmonary

TABLE 24-17 Classification of Pulmonary Hypertension

Passive
Left ventricular systolic pump failure
Decreased left ventricular diastolic compliance, elevated left atrial pressure
Mitral stenosis
Idiopathic
Hyperkinetic
Dietary or ingestive pulmonary hypertension
Obstructive
Obliterative
Vasoconstrictive
Reflex secondary to chronic pulmonary venous or capillary hypertension
Hypoxic

Modified from Murray JF, Nadel JA. Textbook of Respiratory Medicine. *3rd ed. Philadelphia: Saunders; 2000:1641.*

vascular disease or pulmonary fibrosis. These anatomic changes cause irreversible alterations in the pulmonary vasculature, resulting in fixed elevations of PVR.

Etiology

COPD is associated with the functional loss of pulmonary capillaries and the subsequent arterial hypoxemia; these events initiate pulmonary vasoconstriction, which is the leading cause of chronic cor pulmonale. The World Health Organization has proposed a classification of conditions associated with cor pulmonale. Diseases associated with hypoxic pulmonary vasoconstriction include the following:

- COPD
- Bronchiectasis
- Chronic mountain sickness
- Cystic fibrosis
- Idiopathic alveolar hypoventilation
- Obesity-related hypoventilation syndrome
- Neuromuscular disease
- Kyphoscoliosis
- Pleuropulmonary fibrosis
- Upper airway obstruction

Diseases that produce obstruction or obliteration of the pulmonary vasculature include the following:

- PE
- Pulmonary fibrosis
- Pulmonary lymphangitic carcinomatosis
- Idiopathic PH
- Progressive systemic sclerosis
- Sarcoidosis
- Intravenous drug abuse
- Pulmonary vasculitis
- Pulmonary venoocclusive disease[129]

Pathophysiology

Sustained pulmonary vasoconstriction produces hypertrophy of the smooth muscle in the tunica media and an irreversible increase in the PVR.[130] In the presence of chronically elevated pulmonary capillary pressure the lungs are increasingly resistant to pulmonary edema, because lymph vessels expand and their ability to carry fluid away from the interstitial spaces increases. The lymphatic pumping action creates a suction effect, which results in a negative pleural pressure.[131] The rate at which right ventricular dysfunction develops depends on the magnitude of pressure increase in the pulmonary circulation and on the rapidity with which this increase occurs. For example, PE may result in right ventricular failure in the presence of a mean PAP as low as 30 mm Hg. By contrast, when PH occurs gradually, as it does in COPD, right ventricular compensation occurs; CHF rarely occurs before mean PAP exceeds 50 mm Hg.

The normal pulmonary circulation can accommodate a maximal right ventricular output with minimal increase in pulmonary pressure via distention of existing vessels or recruitment of unused vessels. However, patients with COPD have larger-than-normal increases in PAP when executing maneuvers that increase pulmonary blood flow (e.g., exercise, even if resting hemodynamic status is normal).[132] In COPD, derangements in intrapulmonary gas exchange are the major factors involved in the hemodynamic changes. Namely, alveolar hypoxia appears to mediate locally the vasoconstriction of precapillary pulmonary vessels. Acidosis and hypercarbia potentiate this effect.[133]

The compensatory mechanism for pressure overload on the right ventricle involves enhancement of contractility and an increase in preload, which result in an increase in right ventricular end-diastolic volume.[134] In response to chronic pressure overload imposed by the PH, right ventricular hypertrophy occurs (chronic leads to hypertrophy). Preterminally a bout of intolerable hypoxia often exaggerates the PH and imposes an acutely rising afterload on the right ventricle, which accommodates by dilating (acute leads to dilation). Although acute hypercapnia does not directly affect pulmonary circulation, it does cause and potentiate PH if it causes acidosis.[133] Acute hypercapnia stimulates ventilation, dilates cerebral vessels, and elicits central nervous system disturbances.[135]

Right ventricular hypertrophy is characterized by increased firmness of the myocardium and increased thickness of its wall, most prominently in the pulmonary outflow tract. The papillary muscles and the trabeculae carneae may be twice as thick as normal. The thickness of individual muscle fibers also is greater than normal and may approximate that of left ventricular myofibers.

Clinical Features and Diagnosis

Clinical manifestations of cor pulmonale often are nonspecific and obscured by coexisting COPD. Right-sided heart catheterization usually is required for diagnosis. Cardiac catheterization combined with pulmonary angiography provides the most definitive information on the degree of PH, cardiac reserve, and the effects of pulmonary vasodilator treatment.[130]

Symptoms of cor pulmonale are retrosternal pain, cough, dyspnea on exertion, weakness, fatigue, early exhaustion, and hemoptysis.[130] Occasionally hoarseness secondary to left recurrent laryngeal nerve compression by the enlarged pulmonary artery is present. Syncope on effort may occur, reflecting the inability of the right ventricular stroke volume to increase in the presence of a fixed elevation of PVR.

Physical signs of cor pulmonale include the following:

- Elevation of jugular venous pressure
- Cardiac heave or thrust along the left sternal border and S_3 gallop
- Presence of an S_4 secondary to significant right ventricular hypertrophy
- A widely split S_2

- Possible murmur of pulmonic and tricuspid insufficiency
- Hepatomegaly, ascites, and lower-extremity edema (late signs)

Testing

Electrocardiography

Right atrial displacement, right ventricular hypertrophy, right atrial hypertrophy, and right atrial enlargement may be observed. Patients may develop concomitant supraventricular tachycardiac arrhythmias (i.e., tachycardiac atrial fibrillation, sinus tachycardia, and paroxysmal atrial tachycardia).

Chest Radiography

On chest radiography, enlargement of the pulmonary arteries is observed, followed by right ventricular hypertrophy.

Doppler Echocardiography

Enlargement, dilation, or thickening of the right ventricle, with or without tricuspid valve regurgitation, and a pulmonary artery systolic pressure estimated to be increased all suggest that at least acute or possibly chronic PH is present.

Treatment

The goals of treatment are decreasing the workload of the right ventricle, reducing PVR, preventing increases in PAP, and avoiding major hemodynamic changes. Improvement of gas exchange is the primary focus of treatment in COPD patients with cor pulmonale.[130,136] Treatment includes supplemental administration of O_2 in order to maintain a PaO_2 of greater than 60 mm Hg or an arterial O_2 saturation of greater than 90%. O_2 is the only vasodilator with a selective effect on pulmonary vessels that is not associated with a risk of worsening hypoxemia.[137] See Table 24-16.

Heart-Lung Transplantation

A heart-lung transplantation may ultimately be needed when cor pulmonale progresses despite the provision of maximal medical therapy.

In general, preoperative preparation of the patient with cor pulmonale includes the following:

- Elimination and control of acute or chronic pulmonary infections
- Reversal of bronchospasm
- Improvement in clearance of secretions
- Expansion of collapsed or poorly ventilated alveoli
- Hydration
- Correction of any electrolyte imbalance

Anesthesia Management

Regional anesthesia technique may be appropriate as long as a high sensory level of anesthesia is not required, because any decrease in systemic vascular resistance in the presence of a fixed PVR may produce undesirable degrees of systemic hypotension.[127]

General Anesthesia

Volatile agents decrease PVR. Studies have demonstrated that PAP is not affected by halothane or enflurane, whereas both PAP and PVR are decreased by isoflurane. N_2O has been shown to increase PVR in patients with PPH. Intravenous agents, with the exception of ketamine, appear to have little effect on PVR.[138] During all stages of anesthesia, manipulations that increase PAP must be avoided. Five key principles should be followed:

- Keep the patient well oxygenated
- Avoid acidosis
- Avoid the use of exogenous and endogenous vasoconstrictors
- Avoid presenting stimuli that increase sympathetic tone
- Avoid hypothermia[130]

PULMONARY EMBOLISM

Definition

PE is the impaction of a dislodged thrombus into the pulmonary vascular bed.

Incidence and Outcome

PE is a major source of morbidity and mortality, claiming the lives of over 50,000 patients in the United States annually. It is the third most common cause of cardiovascular death after myocardial infarction and stroke. PEs originate from deep vein thrombosis (DVT) of the iliofemoral vessels in approximately 90% of patients, and the clinical course depends on the size of the clot. Evidence suggests that at least five million episodes of DVT occur annually in the United States, with approximately 10% leading to PE. Of those resulting in PE, approximately 10% are fatal.[139]

Etiology

PE is considered by some to be a clinical manifestation of DVT rather than a separate entity. As noted previously, most emboli (90%) arise in the proximal deep veins of the lower extremities, with the remainder originating from pelvic veins. DVT at proximal sites is more likely to cause symptoms. Three major factors promote the formation of venous thrombi: stasis of blood flow, venous injury, and hypercoagulation states. Other, less common causes of PE include air, tumor, bone, fat, catheter fragments, and amniotic fluid. Fillers used in illicit drug preparations by intravenous drug abusers also may cause PE. Of particular concern to anesthesia providers are air emboli caused by the opening of venous structures during surgery or by disconnected intravenous lines.

Most pulmonary emboli resolve within 8 to 21 days of the initial presentation; 10% to 20% are estimated to develop into unresolved emboli, and 0.5% to 4% lead to the development of chronic PH. Chronically unresolved emboli that lodge in major pulmonary arteries may become incorporated into the vascular walls and obstruct blood flow. Patients with such emboli are surgical candidates, representing approximately 1000 cases in the United States each year.[139]

Pathophysiology

Once a thrombus has formed, it rarely remains static. It can be dissolved through fibrinolysis, become "organized" into a vessel wall, or be released into the circulation. Because thrombi are most friable early in their development, it is then that the greatest risk for embolism exists.

Once the fragment has been released from its site of formation, it can be rapidly swept into one of the pulmonary arteries. It may pass through the vasculature completely, break up, and block several smaller pulmonary vessels, or, if the thrombus is sufficiently large, it may impact against one or both pulmonary arteries and cause pulmonary collapse, massive infarction, and ultimately cardiac arrest.[140] Emboli are most often seen in the lower lung lobes, which receive the greatest amount of blood flow. Fortunately, these lower lung lobes also tend to receive the least ventilation, so much of the $\dot{V}/\dot{Q}$ ratio is preserved in patients with small- to moderate-sized emboli.

Within the pulmonary capillaries, hemorrhage is frequently seen distal to the site of the embolism. The alveolar structures

TABLE 24-18 Virchow's Triad: Clinical States Predisposing to Venous Thrombosis

Stasis	Immobility Bed rest Anesthesia Congestive heart failure or cor pulmonale Prior venous thrombosis
Hypercoagulability	Malignancy Anticardiolipin antibody Nephrotic syndrome Essential thrombocytosis Estrogen therapy Heparin-induced thrombocytopenia Inflammatory bowel disease Paroxysmal nocturnal hemoglobinuria Disseminated intravascular coagulation Protein C and S deficiencies Antithrombin III deficiency
Vessel wall injury	Trauma Surgery

Modified from Fishman AP, et al. Pulmonary thromboembolic diseases. In: Fishman AP, Elias JA, Fishman JA, Grippi MA, Kaiser LR, Senior RM. Manual of Pulmonary Disease and Disorders. *New York:McGraw-Hill; 2002:462.*

in this area can remain viable for a period of time.[140] However, if the clot does not dissolve or if it is not quickly squeezed through the vasculature, the alveolar structure will be permanently damaged. Bronchial circulation limits this consequence of pulmonary infarction, and substantial damage is unusual unless an embolus completely blocks a large artery or preexisting lung disease is present.[141] In fact, less than 10% of emboli actually cause any type of infarction.[142] The three components of Virchow's triad—stasis, hypercoagulability, and vessel wall injury—lead to venous thrombosis (Table 24-18).

Pulmonary Function

Pulmonary Circulation. Normally the pulmonary circulation has a very large reserve capacity. However, when PAPs increase, previously unfilled capillaries are recruited, and distention occurs. This allows for obstruction of at least half of the pulmonary circulation before a substantial increase in PAP becomes manifest.[140]

Occlusion of approximately 70% of the pulmonary vascular bed results in PH with subsequent right ventricular failure, increased end-diastolic pressures, and development of arrhythmias and possibly of tricuspid valve incompetence.[141] Pulmonary edema may follow.[140,143] Acute pulmonary edema may develop when hyperperfusion from intact circulation to the perfused lung results in extravasation of fluid into the alveoli. If the clot breaks up and passes quickly or if the affected area is minimal, the PAPs gradually decrease with embolus resolution by fibrinolysis or transformation onto the vessel wall as a scar.[141]

Mechanism. When a pulmonary artery is occluded, ventilation distal to the obstruction is decreased. This is a result of the direct effect of alveolar PCO_2 ($PACO_2$) on the smooth muscle of the local small airways, which is bronchoconstriction. The reduction of air flow to the unperfused lung reduces the amount of wasted ventilation. This mechanism is very short lived, with distribution of ventilation returning to normal within several hours.[140,142] The elastic properties of the embolized region may change some hours after the event; localized atelectasis is believed to result from a loss of pulmonary surfactant, the rapid turnover of which requires adequate blood flow.[142]

Gas Exchange. An embolus can have a significant impact on gas exchange. Moderate hypoxemia without CO_2 retention is often seen after PE as both physiologic shunt and dead space increase. In spontaneously breathing patients $PACO_2$ is maintained at the normal level after PE by increasing the respiratory rate. The resultant increase in ventilation may be substantial because of the large physiologic dead space. The anesthetized patient obviously cannot increase his or her ventilation; as a result, the $PACO_2$ builds up and O_2 saturation decreases more quickly.[142,144]

The difference between $PACO_2$ and end-tidal PCO_2 ($PETCO_2$) is a very useful indicator in PE.[140] The mixed $PACO_2$ tends to be low because of the high $\dot{V}/\dot{Q}$ ratio in the embolized region; because little uneven ventilation occurs with this disease, the $PETCO_2$ is an accurate and immediate indicator of the status of alveolar blood gas exchange. In anesthetized patients the $PACO_2$ continues to increase more quickly because of this increase in shunt without ventilatory compensation.[141] If the embolus does not completely occlude the vessel, the discrepancy between $PETCO_2$ and $PACO_2$ may not be as great.[140]

Clinical Features and Diagnosis

The patient's clinical presentation depends largely on the size of the embolus. Signs and symptoms of PE vary, and the differential diagnosis according to size of emboli may be difficult (Table 24-19). Dyspnea of sudden onset appears to be the

TABLE 24-19 Differential Diagnosis of Acute Pulmonary Embolism

Myocardial infarction (unstable angina)
Pericarditis
Congestive heart failure ("left sided")
Pneumonia, bronchitis, chronic, obstructive pulmonary disease exacerbation
Asthma
Chronic obstructive pulmonary disease
Pneumothorax
Pleurodynia
Pleuritis from collagen vascular disease
Thoracic herpes zoster (shingles)
Rib fracture pneumothorax
Primary or metastatic intrathoracic cancer
Infradiaphragmatic processes (e.g., acute cholecystitis, splenic infarction)
Hyperventilation syndrome
Cardiomyopathy (global)
Primary pulmonary hypertension
Intrathoracic cancer
Costochondritis, musculoskeletal pain
Anxiety

From Tapson VF. Pulmonary embolism. In: Goldman L, Ausiello D, eds. Cecil's Textbook of Medicine. *22nd ed. Philadelphia: Saunders; 2004:561; and Goldhaber SZ. Pulmonary embolism. In: Braunwald E, Zipes DP, Libby P, eds.* Heart Disease. *6th ed. Philadelphia: Saunders; 2001:1890.*

TABLE 24-20 Most Common Symptoms and Signs among the 2454 Patients in the International Cooperative Pulmonary Embolism Registry

Symptom or Sign	Percent
Dyspnea	82
Respiratory rate >20 breaths per minute	60
Heart rate >100 beats per minute	40
Chest pain	49
Cough	20
Syncope	14
Hemoptysis	7

Modified from Braunwald E, Fanci AS, Kasper DL, et al. In: Harrison's Principles of Internal Medicine. *15th ed. New York: McGraw-Hill; 2001:1889.*

only common historical complaint. Hypoxia is a constant feature of PE, possibly owing to intrapulmonary shunting. Several clinical features can be associated with emboli of varying sizes.

Small emboli frequently go unrecognized; uncommonly, however, multiple small emboli can produce extensive obstruction of the pulmonary capillary bed, possibly causing PH and cardiac failure. Generally, however, small thromboemboli are incorporated into the arterial wall and have little effect on either parenchyma or the circulation. Patients may complain of dyspnea on exertion that may lead to syncope; sometimes, a right ventricular "heave" or a split-second heart sound can be detected on examination. For patients with chronic embolization, medical therapy with anticoagulant, thrombolytic, or vasodilating drugs does not alter the prognosis.

Patients with medium-sized emboli may present with pleuritic pain accompanied by dyspnea, a slight fever, and a productive cough that yields blood-streaked sputum. These patients usually are tachycardic. A small pleural effusion can develop and mimic the appearance of pneumonia.

Massive emboli can produce sudden cardiac collapse. Preceding symptoms range from pallor, shock, and central chest pain to sudden loss of consciousness. In patients with cardiac collapse the pulse becomes rapid and weak, blood pressure decreases, neck veins become engorged, and cardiogenic shock may be present or impending. Also, a decrease in $\mathrm{PETCO_2}$ and an increase in $\mathrm{PACO_2}$ occur, with the difference between the values for these two indexes increasing as conditions worsen. If a pulmonary artery catheter is in place, PAPs are observed to increase rapidly; also, the ECG may begin to show right ventricular strain. The prognosis for these patients is very poor. The most common clinical signs are noted in Table 24-20.[140]

Diagnostic Testing

Few of the common preoperative tests indicate the presence of PE. A number of imaging and laboratory tests are now available for diagnosis, and the advantages and disadvantages are given in Table 24-21. Echocardiographic and electrocardiographic signs are noted in Box 24-3. In the patient with PE, ABG analysis generally reveals hypoxemia and increased differences between $\mathrm{PACO_2}$ and $\mathrm{PaCO_2}$, which result from ventilation of unperfused alveoli.[144] Massive PE is associated with severe hypoxemia and hypocapnia. An initial difference between $\mathrm{PACO_2}$ and $\mathrm{PETCO_2}$ is common early during the embolic event.[142]

Treatment

Aggressive efforts at prevention have been successful in reducing the incidence of DVT in surgical patients. Some suggested preventative measures are noted in Table 24-22. Treatment mainly is aimed at prevention of further embolism and at provision of ventilatory support.[145] Use of graded compression stockings, intermittent pneumatic compression, administration of various anticoagulants and thrombolytics, and ambulation are typical measures for preventing embolus formation. It must be remembered that PE is a mechanical disease caused by acute pulmonary obstruction in a previously healthy patient.

Treatment requires rapid intervention before vital signs are affected by hypoxia and mechanical failure of the heart. Treatment for PE is summarized in Table 24-23 on p. 547.

TABLE 24-21 Advantages and Disadvantages of Diagnostic Tests for Suspected Pulmonary Embolism

Diagnostic Test	Advantages	Disadvantages
Plasma D-dimer ELISA	A normal result makes PE exceedingly unlikely	Level is elevated in many systemic illnesses that mimic PE; unless a rapid assay is available, the turnaround time will be long
ECG	Universally available; may indicate acute cor pulmonale	Acute cor pulmonale on ECG is not specific for PE; not a sensitive test
Impedance plethysmography	Portable, inexpensive, easy to use	Inaccurate, with failure to detect major nonobstructive proximal DVT
Chest radiograph	Usually has minor abnormalities but occasionally pathognomonic; may suggest alternative diagnoses; may guide workup toward chest CT rather than lung scan	Not specific
Venous ultrasonography	Excellent for detection of symptomatic proximal DVT; surrogate for PE	Cannot image iliac vein thrombosis; imaging of calf is operator dependent; DVT may have embolized completely, resulting in a normal result

TABLE 24-21 Advantages and Disadvantages of Diagnostic Tests for Suspected Pulmonary Embolism—cont'd

Diagnostic Test	Advantages	Disadvantages
Nuclear venography	Used to image pelvic and calf veins and differentiate acute versus chronic DVT	Limited experience with this test
Contrast venography	Used to be gold standard; excellent for calf veins	Can cause chemical phlebitis; uncomfortable; costly; may fail to result in diagnosis of massive DVT because veins are filled with thrombus and cannot be opacified
Lung scanning	Standard initial imaging test for PE; high-probability scans are reliable for detecting PE; normal or near-normal scans are reliable for precluding PE	Most scans are neither high probability nor normal or near normal; ventilation scans are falling out of favor; most test results are equivocal
Chest CT	Excellent for PE in the proximal pulmonary arterial tree	Insensitive for important but distal PE
MRI	Excellent for anatomy and cardiac function	In preliminary use; not widely available; experience very limited
Echocardiography	Excellent for identifying right ventricular dilatation and dysfunction that is not obvious clinically, thereby providing an early warning of potentially adverse outcome	Not specific; many patients with PE have normal echocardiograms; the test cannot reliably differentiate causes of right ventricular dysfunction
Pulmonary angiography	Considered the gold standard for diagnosis	Invasive, costly, uncomfortable

CT, *Computed tomography;* DVT, *deep-vein thrombosis;* ECG, *electrocardiogram;* ELISA, *enzyme-linked immunosorbent assay;* MRI, *magnetic resonance imaging;* PE, *pulmonary embolism.*
Modified from Goldhaber SZ. Pulmonary embolism. In: Braunwald E, Zipes DP, Libby P. Heart Disease. *6th ed. Philadelphia: Saunders; 2001:1896.*

Surgery

Surgical intervention often is indicated for patients who are unresponsive to other measures. Procedures that used to be the mainstay of this intervention, such as ligation of the inferior vena cava, are now rarely performed. Currently the most common surgical procedure for patients with PE is placement of an umbrella filter, which traps thromboemboli. It is estimated that 30,000 to 40,000 patients receive such filters annually in the United States. Indications for vena cava filters are listed in Box 24-4. The filter is placed in the inferior vena cava under fluoroscopic guidance, usually below the renal veins at the level of the L2 to L3. Suprarenal placement is required when a thrombus directly involves the renal veins or has propagated above the level of the renal veins.

The presence of an infrarenal filter in a pregnant woman may place her and her fetus at risk because of the possibility that the filter will come into contact with the gravid uterus. Suprarenal placement prevents this risk.

Thromboendarterectomy is the treatment of choice for chronic large vessel thromboembolic PH.[146] Desired results include decreased PVR, improved CO, restoration of exercise tolerance, and resolution of hypoxemia. Improvements in RV function and hemodynamics may be prompt, whereas improvements in gas exchange occur over weeks to months.

Although the role of pulmonary embolectomy remains controversial, in the few patients who do not benefit from optimal medical therapy, it remains an acceptable procedure.[147]

BOX 24-3

Electrocardiographic and Echocardiographic Signs of Pulmonary Embolism

- Incomplete or complete right bundle branch block
- S in lead I and aV_L >1.5 mm
- Transition zone shift to V_5
- Qs in leads III and aV_F but not in lead II
- QRS axis >90 degrees or indeterminate axis
- Low limb-lead voltage
- T-wave inversion in leads III and aV_F or in leads V_1-V_4
- Direct visualization of thrombus (rare)
- Right ventricular dilatation
- Right ventricular hypokinesis (with sparing of the apex)
- Abnormal interventricular septal motion
- Tricuspid valve regurgitation
- Pulmonary artery dilatation
- Lack of decreased inspiratory collapse of inferior vena cava

Modified from Sreeram N, Cheriex EC, Smeets JLRM, et al. Value of the 12-lead electrocardiogram at hospital admission in the diagnosis of pulmonary embolism. Am J Cardiol. *1994;73:298.*

Anesthesia Management

Anesthesia for patients at risk for PE is aimed at supporting vital organ function and minimizing anesthetic-induced myocardial depression. The use of a high FIO_2 aids in prevention of pulmonary vasoconstriction, and the monitoring of PAP helps the anesthesia provider optimize right-sided heart function and assess the effects of anesthetic management on PVR.[143] Many anesthesia providers choose not to place pulmonary artery catheters because of concerns about the possibility that these catheters dislodge clots in the right side of the heart.

Intravenous fluid infusion must be adjusted so that right ventricular stroke volume is optimized in the presence of

TABLE 24-22 Prevention of Venous Thromboembolism

Condition	Strategy
Total hip or knee replacement; hip or pelvis fracture	Warfarin (Coumadin) (target INR 2-2.5) × 4-6 weeks
	Low–molecular-weight heparin (e.g., enoxaparin [Lovenox], 30 mg SC twice daily)
	IPC ± warfarin
Gynecologic cancer surgery	Warfarin (Coumadin) (target INR 2-2.5) IPC
	Unfractionated heparin, 5000 U q8h ± IPC
	Dalteparin (Fragmin) 2500 U once daily ± IPC
	Enoxaparin 40 mg SC once daily
Urologic surgery	Warfarin (Coumadin) (target INR 2-2.5) ± IPC
Thoracic surgery	IPC *plus* unfractionated heparin, 5000 U q8h
High-risk general surgery (e.g., prior VTE, current cancer, or obesity)	IPC *or* GCS *plus* unfractionated heparin, 5000 U q8h
General, gynecologic, or urologic surgery (without prior VTE) for noncancerous conditions	GCS *plus* unfractionated heparin 5000 U q12h
	Dalteparin 2500 U SC once daily
	Enoxaparin 40 mg SC once daily
	IPC alone
Neurosurgery, eye surgery, or other surgery when prophylactic anticoagulation is contraindicated	GCS ± IPC
Medical conditions	Graded-compression stockings ± heparin, 5000 U q12h
	IPC alone
	Enoxaparin (Lovenox) 40 mg SC once daily
Orthopedic surgery	Enoxaparin 30 mg twice daily
	Enoxaparin 40 mg once daily*
	Dalteparin 5000 U once daily*
	Danaparoid 750 U twice daily*
	Warfarin (target INR = 2-3)
	GCS plus IPC
General surgery	Enoxaparin 40 mg daily
	Dalteparin 2500 or 5000 U once daily
	GCS plus IPC
Pregnancy	Enoxaparin 40 mg daily
	Dalteparin 5000 U daily
Medical patients	Enoxaparin 40 mg daily
	GCS plus IPC

GCS, *Graduated compression stockings;* INR, *international normalized ratio;* IPC, *intermittent pneumatic compression;* SC, *subcutaneous;* VTE, *venous thromboembolism.*

**Approved only for total hip replacement prophylaxis.*

Modified from Goldhaber SZ. Pulmonary thromboembolism. In: Braunwald E, Fauci AS, Kasper DL, et al. Harrison's Principles of Internal Medicine. *15th ed. New York: McGraw-Hill; 2001:1508-1513; and Goldhaber SZ. Pulmonary embolism. In: Braunwald E, Zipes DP, Libby P, eds.* Heart Disease: Textbook of Cardiovascular Medicine. *6th ed. Philadelphia: Saunders; 2001:1903.*

marked increase in afterload. A continuous catecholamine infusion may be needed to enhance cardiac contractility.

Induction is often performed with etomidate or ketamine (for maintenance of hemodynamic stability), but ketamine must be titrated judiciously as it may increase PVR.[142]

The use of N_2O is generally believed to be acceptable. However, this may not be possible with the use of a high FIO_2.[142] Use of N_2O should be discontinued if PVR increases. Obviously the use of N_2O is contraindicated in patients with venous air embolism.[141] Patients with moderate to severe PE often are experiencing acute right-sided heart failure. Cardiac function can be optimized by the use of minimally depressing cardiac agents such as narcotics.[143]

Persistent severe hypotension, such as that accompanying a massive PE, may necessitate the use of a cardiotonic agent. The goal is preservation of perfusion to the brain and heart until cardiopulmonary bypass is started and surgical removal of the clot attempted.[143] As always, heparin should be readily available, and when needed it should be administered into a central line while blood aspiration is verified before and after injection. Reports of operative mortality during pulmonary embolectomy range from 11% to 55%, with much higher rates among patients experiencing cardiac arrest.[148]

Detection of Pulmonary Embolism during Anesthesia. In the intubated patient under general anesthesia, combinations of the symptoms may occur. A decreasing $PETCO_2$ and tachycardia usually are the first symptoms seen in PE.[142,144] These can be followed by a decrease in SaO_2 and the generation of ABG values that indicate unexplained arterial hypoxemia. Increased PAP and central venous pressure (CVP) can be seen in combination with a decrease in systolic and diastolic blood

TABLE **24-23** Guidelines for the Treatment of Pulmonary Embolism

1. Treat DVT or PTE with therapeutic levels of unfractionated intravenous heparin, adjusted subcutaneous heparin, or low–molecular-weight heparin for at least 5 days and overlap with oral anticoagulation for at least 4 to 5 days. Consider a longer course of heparin for massive PTE or severe iliofemoral DVT.
2. In most patients heparin and oral anticoagulation can be started together and heparin discontinued on day 5 or 6 if the INR has been therapeutic for 2 consecutive days.
3. Continue oral anticoagulant therapy for a least 3 months with a target INR of 2.5 (range 2 to 3).
4. Patients with reversible or time-limited risk factors can be treated for 3 to 6 months. Patients with a first episode of idiopathic DVT should be treated for at least 6 months. Patients with a first episode of idiopathic DVT should be treated for at least 6 months. Patients with recurrent venous thrombosis or a continuing risk factor such as cancer, inhibitor deficiency states, or antiphospholipid antibody syndrome should be treated indefinitely.
5. Isolated calf vein DVT should be treated with anticoagulation for at least 3 months.
6. The use of thrombolytic agents continues to be highly individualized, and clinicians should have some latitude in using these agents. Patients with hemodynamically unstable PTE or massive iliofemoral thrombosis are the best candidates.
7. Inferior vena caval filter placement is recommended in the presence of a contraindication to or failure of anticoagulation, for chronic recurrent embolism with pulmonary hypertension, and with concurrent performance of surgical pulmonary embolectomy or pulmonary endarterectomy.

DVT, *Deep vein thrombosis;* INR, *international normalized ratio;* PTE, *pulmonary thromboembolism.*
Modified from Goldhaber SZ. Pulmonary thromboembolism. In: Braunwald E, Fauci AS, Kasper DL, eds. In: Harrison's Principles of Internal Medicine. *15th ed. New York: McGraw-Hill; 2001:1511.*

BOX **24-4**

Indications for Inferior Vena Caval Filters

Anticoagulation Contraindicated and PE Documented
Active bleeding that might cause exsanguination (e.g., gastrointestinal)
Feared bleeding that might be catastrophic (e.g., postoperative craniotomy)
Ongoing complications of anticoagulation (e.g., heparin-associated thrombocytopenia)
Planned intensive cancer chemotherapy (with anticipated pancytopenia or thrombocytopenia)

Anticoagulation Failure despite Documentation of Adequate Therapy (e.g., Recurrent PE)
Extensive or progressive venous thrombosis
In conjunction with catheter-based or surgical pulmonary embolectomy
Severe pulmonary hypertension or cor pulmonale

PE, *Pulmonary embolism.*
Modified from Braunwald E, Fauci AS, Kasper DL, et al. Harrison's Principles of Internal Medicine. *15th ed. New York: McGraw-Hill; 2001:1899.*

pressures.[144] Bronchospasm may occur.[141] Finally, ECG changes that indicate right axis deviation, incomplete or complete right bundle branch block, or peaked T waves may be observed in the presence or absence of an accompanying systolic ejection murmur.[140,144]

Intraoperative Management

Several measures can be taken to support the anesthetized patient with suspected PE. First and most important, an airway must be established by intubation if the patient is not already intubated. Second, delivery of the anesthetic agent must be discontinued, and administration of a 100% FIO_2 initiated.[142] Next, the circulatory system should be supported with the infusion of intravenous fluids or blood (or both) as needed, and the use of sympathomimetics (e.g., dobutamine or dopamine) initiated if necessary. Dysrhythmias should be treated with intravenous administration of lidocaine, and the patient should receive PEEP for optimization of O_2 transport across the alveolar membrane.[141]

Pulmonary embolectomy may be necessary. Severe hemodynamic difficulty should be anticipated and resuscitative efforts continued. Patients with PE are extremely sensitive to any anesthetic agent and are likely to require femoral bypass under local anesthesia with partial cardiopulmonary bypass before induction. Again, it is critical to have heparin ready to infuse into a central line (if available). Although separation from bypass is beyond the scope of this chapter, the anesthetist must realize that difficulties may be encountered. Depending on the insult to the right ventricle, pulmonary vasodilation and catecholamine infusions may be indicated. Simultaneous left atrial and right atrial pressure monitoring is helpful.

Patients with PE present particular management challenges in their postoperative course, including reperfusion edema, persistent hypoxemia, pericardial effusion, psychiatric disorders, and pulmonary blood flow steal. The areas of the lung to which pulmonary artery flow has been restored are subject to development of reperfusion pulmonary edema, presumably as a manifestation of oxidant- and protease-mediated acute lung injury. Other possible causes are extracorporeal circulation, anticoagulation, and an increase in perfusion pressure in a previously obstructed pulmonary artery. Complications include immediate pulmonary hemorrhage and respiratory disturbance, and death may occur.[148] This syndrome may develop 3 to 5 days after surgery.[149] Olman and associates have observed that, after pulmonary thromboendarterectomy for relief of chronic thromboembolic PH, perfusion lung scans frequently reveal new perfusion defects in segments served by undissected pulmonary arteries. This phenomenon has been labeled *pulmonary blood flow steal* and is believed to be caused by postoperative redistribution of regional PVR and not by rethrombosis or embolism.[150]

RESTRICTIVE PULMONARY DISEASES

Definition

Restrictive pulmonary disease is defined as any condition that interferes with normal lung expansion during inspiration. Typically, it includes disorders that increase the inward elastic recoil of the lungs or chest wall (Table 24-24). Consequently, the alteration in pulmonary dynamics results in decreases in lung volumes and capacities and in lung or chest wall compliance. Some restrictive diseases produce ventilation abnormalities and $\dot{V}/\dot{Q}$ mismatching, whereas others lead to impairment of diffusion. FEV_1 and FVC are both decreased owing to a reduction in TLC or a decrease in chest wall compliance or muscle strength However, the FEV_1/FVC ratio is normal or elevated.

Impairment-producing restrictive pulmonary diseases can be classified as (1) acute intrinsic, (2) chronic intrinsic, or (3) chronic extrinsic. Acute intrinsic disorders are primarily caused by the abnormal movement of intravascular fluid into the interstitium of the lung and alveoli secondary to the increase in pulmonary vascular pressures occurring with left ventricular failure, fluid overload, or an increase in pulmonary capillary permeability. Examples of acute intrinsic disorders include pulmonary edema, aspiration pneumonia, and acute respiratory distress syndrome (ARDS). Chronic intrinsic diseases are characterized by pulmonary fibrosis. Conditions that produce fibrosis of the lung include idiopathic pulmonary fibrosis (IPF), radiation injury, cytotoxic and noncytotoxic drugs exposure, O_2 toxicity, autoimmune diseases, and sarcoidosis. Chronic extrinsic diseases can be defined as disorders that inhibit the normal lung excursion. They include flail chest, pneumothorax, atelectasis, and pleural effusions. They also include conditions that interfere with chest wall expansion, such as ascites, obesity, pregnancy, and skeletal and neuromuscular disorders.

The pulmonary system and its functions are directly manipulated by the administration of anesthesia. The impact of intraoperative pulmonary insult or preexisting pulmonary disease on respiratory function during anesthesia and the postoperative period is predictable: greater degrees of pulmonary impairment lead to marked alterations in intraoperative respiratory status and higher rates of occurrence of postoperative pulmonary complications. This section illustrates the pathophysiologic changes involved in these clinical disorders and discusses their clinical presentation, diagnosis, treatment, and anesthetic implications.

Pulmonary Edema

Pulmonary edema is not itself an independent disease entity, but rather the result of a variety of disease processes. Simply stated, pulmonary edema is the accumulation of excess fluid in the interstitial and air-filled spaces of the lung. The mechanisms responsible for its development include an increase in hydrostatic pressure within the pulmonary capillary system, an increase in the permeability of the alveolocapillary membrane, and a decrease in intravascular colloid oncotic pressure.[151]

Before one can understand the etiology and pathophysiology of pulmonary edema, the Starling forces and Starling's law of transcapillary fluid exchange must be clearly understood. The pulmonary capillary endothelium is thought to be semipermeable. Pulmonary interstitial fluid pressures, both hydrostatic (P_{if}) and osmotic (π_{if}), along with the hydrostatic pressure in the pulmonary capillaries (P_c) and the osmotic pressure of the plasma (π_p), are the primary determinants that balance fluid exchange across this semipermeable barrier.[152] These factors, which ultimately determine the amount of fluid that actually leaves the pulmonary vascular space, are incorporated into what is known as the *Starling equation*. A simplified version of this equation is as follows:

Equation 24-8

$$\dot{Q} = k[(P_c - P_{if}) - (\pi_p - \pi_{if})]$$

where $\dot{Q}$ is the total amount of fluid that transverses the endothelial membrane and k is the fluid filtration coefficient, which describes quantitatively the permeability of the membrane.[151,152]

The P_c, the force favoring fluid movement out of the vessel wall, is in direct opposition to the P_{if}. The P_{if}, when positive, tends to force fluid inward through the capillary membrane; when it is negative, it tends to force fluid outward.[36] The π_p and P_{if} also oppose each other, with the π_{if} keeping fluid within the capillary and the π_{if} pulling it outward into the interstitium. Overall the balance of forces shown in the Starling equation favors fluid filtration into the interstitial space. Fluid that is filtered out into the alveolar interstitial space does not enter the alveoli, because under normal conditions the alveolar epithelium is composed of very tight junctions that prevent fluid and protein from entering the alveolar air spaces. The fluid moves to the extravascular interstitial space, where the lymphatics remove all of the filtered fluid and return it to the systemic circulation.[153]

Pulmonary edema can occur if any variable in the Starling equation is altered in the direction favoring increased fluid

TABLE 24-24 Causes of a Restrictive Pattern

Disease Process	Anatomic Location of Lesion	Etiology of Pulmonary Function Test Abnormality
Primary parenchymal disease	Pulmonary parenchyma	Loss of lung tissue → reduced volumes and flows
Surgical removal of lung disease	Pulmonary parenchyma	Loss of lung tissue → reduced volumes and flows
Diseases of pleura and chest wall	Pleura, chest wall	Limited expansion of thoracic cavity → reduced volumes and flows
Reduced generation of expiratory force	Central nervous system, peripheral nerves, neuromuscular junction, muscles of respiration	Reduced muscle tension → reduced expiratory flow rates, atelectasis

Modified from Fishman AP. The spectrum of chronic obstructive disease of the airways. In: Fishman AP, ed. Update: Pulmonary Diseases and Disorders. *2nd ed. New York: McGraw-Hill; 1988:2510.*

filtration. High pressure (P_c) and increased permeability (k) are the two most important components of the Starling equation that are altered in states of pulmonary edema. Because of this, pulmonary edema is classified as being either cardiogenic (high pressure, hydrostatic) or noncardiogenic (permeability is increased).

Cardiogenic pulmonary edema occurs whenever the P_c is increased. Increased P_c is the most common form of pulmonary edema. Cardiogenic pulmonary edema is initiated by some type of left-sided heart incompetence or failure. The term *left ventricular failure* implies that a decrease has occurred in left ventricular contractility, which ultimately leads to a reduction in both stroke volume and CO. Incomplete left ventricular emptying elevates left ventricular end-diastolic volume, which in turn elevates left ventricular end-diastolic pressure. Increased left ventricular end-diastolic pressure is "reflected back," causing elevation of the left atrial, pulmonary venous, and pulmonary capillary pressures. When pulmonary capillary pressure reaches levels of 20 to 25 mm Hg (normal range, 10 to 16 mm Hg), the rate of fluid transudation often exceeds lymphatic drainage capacity, and alveolar flooding occurs.

Coronary artery disease, hypertension, cardiomyopathies, mitral regurgitation, and mitral stenosis are a few of the cardiac conditions that may increase pulmonary intravascular hydrostatic pressure (P_c) and predispose a patient to the development of pulmonary edema. Although an elevated left ventricular end-diastolic pressure is the major cause of an increase in P_c, and therefore pulmonary edema, it is important to realize that several noncardiac problems also may increase P_c. These include pulmonary venoocclusive disease, fibrosing mediastinitis, head trauma, cerebrovascular accident, exposure to high altitudes, and overhydration.

Noncardiogenic pulmonary edema is associated with an increase in endothelial permeability caused by an insult that disrupts the barrier function of the blood-tissue interface. Unlike cardiogenic pulmonary edema, in which the capillary endothelium remains intact and no leakage of protein is noted, noncardiogenic pulmonary edema is associated with the leakage of both fluid and protein from the vascular space.[152] Because this respiratory membrane disruption cannot be easily or directly measured, noncardiogenic pulmonary edema is said to exist when suspicious chest radiographic evidence coexists with insufficient hemodynamic basis. The presence of a pulmonary wedge pressure less than 12 mm Hg and the absence of a significant history of cardiac disease generally suffice for exclusion of a hemodynamic mechanism.[151]

Although a multitude of disorders are associated with noncardiogenic pulmonary edema, the most commonly encountered cause is systemic sepsis that leads to ARDS (Box 24-5). Other clinical conditions associated with noncardiogenic pulmonary edema include the aspiration syndromes, inhalation of toxic fumes and gases, and the embolization phenomena.

Pulmonary edema is nearly always associated with some type of preexisting disease state or insult. If a patient with pulmonary edema has a history of CHF, hypertension, or ischemic heart disease, the presence of cardiogenic pulmonary edema can be assumed. In addition to systemic sepsis, anaphylaxis, pancreatitis, disseminated intravascular coagulation, trauma, multiple transfusions, and near-drowning can all result in noncardiogenic pulmonary edema.

Neurogenic Pulmonary Edema

Neurogenic pulmonary edema begins with a massive outpouring of sympathetic nervous system stimulation triggered by central nervous system insult. This centrally mediated central nervous system overactivity typically occurs in the hypothalamic area.[154] Excessive sympathetic activation induces remarkable hemodynamic alterations—primarily systemic and pulmonary vasoconstriction. The left ventricle fails because of the inordinate pressure work imposed by the systemic hypertension, and pulmonary blood volume increases because of the functional imbalance between the failing left ventricle and the normal right ventricle.[152] Although this sequence seems to parallel that of hemodynamic pulmonary edema, a permeability component exists as evidenced by the high protein concentration found in the pulmonary secretions of affected patients.

Uremic Pulmonary Edema

Uremic pulmonary edema is seen in those patients with renal insufficiency or failure. Overhydration and expansion of the circulating blood volume lead to increases in pulmonary capillary pressures. Again, a "leaky" component exists because of the metabolic abnormalities associated with uremia. Reducing the circulating blood volume of these patients via hemodialysis promotes the resolution of this type of pulmonary edema.[152]

High Altitude–Related Pulmonary Edema

High altitude–related pulmonary edema can occur in the absence of left ventricular failure whenever an individual overexerts before acclimating to a high altitude. The pathogenesis of this form of pulmonary edema is unclear, but it may be the result of intense hypoxic pulmonary arterial vasoconstriction or massive sympathetic discharge triggered by cerebral hypoxia.[154]

Pulmonary Edema Caused by Upper Airway Obstruction

Pulmonary edema resulting from upper airway obstruction is caused by the prolonged, forced inspiratory effort against an obstructed upper airway. The most common cause of this type of pulmonary edema in adults is laryngospasm after extubation

BOX **24-5**

Common Causes of Restrictive Lung Disease

Cause	Example
Interstitium	
Interstitial fibrosis, infiltration	Asbestosis
Pulmonary edema	Left ventricular failure
Pleura	
Pleural disease	Fibrothorax
Thoracic Cage and Abdomen	
Neuromuscular disease	Poliomyelitis
Skeletal abnormalities	Severe kyphoscoliosis
Marked obesity	Gross obesity
Pulmonary Vascular Disease	
Pulmonary hypertensive disorders	Primary pulmonary hypertension

Modified from Fishman AP. Approach to the Patient: Fishman's Manual of Pulmonary Disease and Disorders. *New York: McGraw-Hill; 2002:10.*

and general anesthesia. In children, pulmonary edema after obstruction caused by croup, epiglottitis, and laryngospasm also is well documented. Vigorous inspiration against obstruction creates high negative intrathoracic, transpleural, and alveolar pressures, enlarging the pulmonary vascular volume and subsequently the interstitial fluid volume. The capacity of the lymphatics becomes overwhelmed, and interstitial fluid transudes into the pulmonary alveoli. Hypoxia causes a massive sympathetic discharge that results in systemic vasoconstriction and a translocation of fluid from the systemic circulation to the already expanding pulmonary vascular and interstitial spaces. Hypoxia also increases pulmonary capillary pressures. Because hypoxia alters myocardial activity, left atrial function and left ventricular function are reduced.

During obstruction, vigorous inspiratory efforts are unsuccessful because of the airway obstruction. Unsuccessful expiration produces an increase in intrathoracic and alveolar pressures. Intrinsic PEEP also is produced during this stage. Relief of the obstruction results in cessation of intrinsic PEEP.

The consequence of these events is the sudden massive transudation of fluid from the pulmonary interstitium into the alveoli, which results in pulmonary edema. The malignity of pulmonary edema is determined by the extent of prior alveolar and capillary damage and the immensity of hemodynamic and cardiovascular alterations.

Not all of those who experience an acute airway obstruction develop pulmonary edema, and no specific risk factors for its occurrence have been identified. Factors that may predispose to its formation after obstruction include youth, male gender, long periods of obstruction, overzealous perioperative fluid administration, and the presence of preexisting cardiac and pulmonary disease.

Treatment includes prompt recognition of the condition, the securing of a patent airway, supportive therapy with oxygenation, and the administration of diuretics. Although the onset of pulmonary edema after laryngospasm usually is immediate, cases have been reported of the occurrence of pulmonary edema several hours after laryngospasm. Therefore it is recommended that patients who develop laryngospasm be observed postoperatively longer than the typical 60 to 90 minutes. The diagnosis of pulmonary edema and its differentiation into cardiogenic and noncardiac categories requires the taking of a detailed medical history, physical examination, chest radiography, and ABG analysis.

Physical examination reveals an increased work of breathing. As water accumulates, the lungs become heavy and noncompliant, and a decrease in FRC occurs. This increase in the volume of extravascular lung fluid provides a potent stimulus for surrounding interstitial stretch receptors (J-receptors), the activation of which results in tachypnea. Tachypnea is not relieved by the administration of O_2 and the return of PaO_2 to normal. Intercostal retractions and use of accessory muscles are apparent on physical examination. Signs of sympathetic stress stimulation such as hypertension, diaphoresis, and tachycardia often are noted. The expectoration of pink, frothy sputum signals that alveoli have been flooded.[153]

The detection of basilar crackles on auscultation is the traditional hallmark of early pulmonary edema. In reality, by the time these crackles become audible, excess water has already flooded the alveoli and overflowed into the terminal bronchioles.[150] It is in the bronchioles, not in the alveoli, that the crackles of pulmonary edema are generated. The earliest and most often disregarded clinical sign is rapid, shallow breathing.

In cardiogenic pulmonary edema, heart size may be increased. High CVPs, an S_3 or S_4 gallop, and jugular venous distention often are observed.[151] Chest radiography is still the most reliable and expedient tool for early detection of pulmonary edema.[152] In cardiogenic pulmonary edema the cardiac silhouette may appear abnormal or enlarged; in noncardiogenic pulmonary edema it can be enlarged or remain normal. Interstitial edema can be observed before the alveoli flood and the onset of clinical signs occurs. Pleural effusions are common, and a "whited-out" or "butterfly" appearance may be noted.[152]

ABG analysis reveals hypoxemia secondary to $\dot{V}/\dot{Q}$ abnormalities. When right-to-left shunting is great, the PaO_2 can be affected by any change in the central venous O_2 content. Increases in O_2 consumption or decreases in CO further reduce the PaO_2. The $PaCO_2$ may be low, normal, or elevated. The initial hypocarbia is related to tachypnea and high minute volumes; at later stages hypercarbia is frequently secondary to muscle fatigue and exhaustion. Changes in pH usually reflect changes in $PaCO_2$, but metabolic or lactic acidosis or both may occur from tissue O_2 deficiency, low CO, or sepsis.

Anesthetic Management

Pulmonary edema is considered a medical emergency, and immediate intervention is required for treatment of the underlying disease, support of other failing organ systems, and optimization of O_2 delivery.[151] O_2 should be administered either by nasal cannula, face mask, or endotracheal tube. If oxygenation does not improve with the administration of high FIO_2, positive-pressure ventilation with either PEEP or CPAP must be initiated. Institution of positive-pressure mechanical ventilation in patients with acute pulmonary edema usually results in a prompt increase in oxygenation and, in some cases, in CO. Improvement occurs because of superior inflation and $\dot{V}/\dot{Q}$ matching. Amelioration of left ventricular function (CO) may occur secondary to four possible mechanisms: (1) improvement in arterial oxygenation and therefore improvement of myocardial O_2 supply; (2) reduction in the extreme pleural pressure swings present with spontaneous ventilation and, hence, reduction in afterload on the left ventricle; (3) decrease in the workload of the failing heart because of a reduction in work of breathing (and, therefore, a reduction in O_2 requirement) effected by a mechanical ventilator; and (4) decrease in preload (and a subsequent reduction in venous return) occurring secondary to the use of positive-pressure ventilation.

Pharmacologic therapy includes the use of vasodilators, inotropes, steroids, and diuretics. For more than 50 years morphine sulfate has been used in the treatment of cardiogenic pulmonary edema because of its venodilatory and preload-reducing properties.[153] Nitroprusside is a very effective preload and afterload reducer. By reducing systemic blood pressure, nitroprusside decreases the afterload on the left ventricle; this may result in better cardiac function, with a subsequent lowering of left atrial pressures. Inotropic agents such as dopamine or dobutamine improve myocardial contractility and lower cardiac filling pressures. In patients with chronic CHF and pulmonary congestion, digitalis augments contractility and promotes decreases in left atrial and ventricular filling pressures. (The use of steroids is discussed later in this chapter in the section on ARDS.)

Fluid balance is managed with both fluid restriction and diuresis. This therapy helps achieve a "negative" fluid balance in hydrostatic pulmonary edema, in which P_c is high. Even in permeability pulmonary edema, in which P_c is thought to be low, any decrease in the hydrostatic pressure further reduces the net movement of pulmonary microvascular fluid outward.[151] Potent diuretics such as furosemide not only lower left atrial filling pressure by decreasing systemic venous tone but also induce diuresis of the expanded extravascular volume.

The type of fluid, whether crystalloid or colloid, that should be used in the presence of pulmonary edema remains controversial. Regardless of type used, it is generally agreed that administration should proceed slowly.

ASPIRATION PNEUMONIA

Definition

Aspiration is a rare yet serious complication of general anesthesia. Much effort is expended to prevent this untoward occurrence and to minimize sequelae if it does occur. It can occur at any time during the course of anesthesia administration, and if it is severe a multitude of serious complications may follow. Mendelson's laboratory investigations led him to the conclusion that two entirely separate clinical aspiration disorders existed. One followed the aspiration of solid food and produced a picture of laryngeal or bronchial obstruction, whereas the other resulted from direct acid injury to the lung and produced the "asthmalike" syndrome that now carries his name.[155] By definition, pulmonary aspiration has two components. First, gastric contents escape from the stomach into the pharynx, and, second, they enter the lungs. This results from preexisting disease, airway manipulation, and the inevitable compromise in protective reflexes that accompanies the anesthetic process. Aspirates are commonly categorized as contaminated, acidic, particulate, and nonparticulate. Less than half of all aspirations lead to pneumonia. Pneumonia occurs most often in patients with pulmonary ingestion of virulent material or who are immunocompromised. Ingestion of highly acidic or particulate aspirate may cause severe respiratory damage without an infectious component. Patients who initially show no signs of infection, however, may develop pneumonia over the long term because of the severity of the lung injury and prolonged respiratory support.[156]

Incidence and Outcome

Several major reviews have been published regarding the incidence of aspiration during anesthesia. Olsson and co-workers[157] retrospectively studied 185, 358 anesthetic procedures in Sweden and found 83 cases of aspiration, constituting an incidence of 4.7 per 10,000 cases. Fifty-three percent of the patients required no treatment; the diagnosis in 47% was confirmed by x-ray examination. Of this 47%, 17% required mechanical ventilation, and four patients died. Factors associated with significant morbidity were emergency procedures, pregnancy, obesity, gastrointestinal disease, elevated intracranial pressure, extremes of age, and airway difficulties. The investigators concluded that clinically significant aspiration occurs in 1 of 35,000 anesthetic procedures.

In a multicenter, prospective study in France involving infants and children the aspiration incidence rate was 5 cases in 40, 240 anesthetic procedures. High status according to the American Society of Anesthesiologists (ASA) guidelines and emergency procedures were noted as risk factors.[158] The Anesthetic Incidence Monitoring Study database in New Zealand noted 133 cases of aspiration out of 5000 reported anesthesia incidents.[159] Five deaths occurred. Aspiration was confirmed by clinical signs or radiography. Predisposing factors included abdominal pathology, obesity, diabetes, neurologic deficit, lithotomy position, difficult intubation, reflux disease, hiatal hernia, and inadequate anesthesia leading to straining and bucking.

In an interesting study researchers looked at general anesthesia by mask in obstetric patients who required surgery immediately after vaginal delivery.[160] Procedures included placental extraction; repair of vaginal, cervical, and perineal tears; and uterine manipulation. This database in Israel involved 1705 anesthetic procedures with one case of mild aspiration diagnosed by observation and follow-up chest x-ray examination.

Warner and colleagues[161] from the Mayo Clinic reviewed 215,488 general anesthetics. Pulmonary aspiration defined by particulates visualized in the tracheobronchial tree or radiographic confirmation occurred in 67 patients. Forty-two (63%) did not develop symptoms and were discharged the same day. Of the 24 (36%) who did develop symptoms 13 required mechanical ventilatory support for more than 6 hours. Three of these patients died. The overall mortality was 1 of 71,829 anesthetic procedures. Several of their findings were interesting. Complications developed in equal percentages among those who received and those who did not receive pharmacologic acid aspiration prophylaxis. Patients who aspirated did not develop problems and could be discharged within 2 hours of the incident if they did not develop symptoms that included a new cough or a wheeze; if no decrease in oxygen saturation as measured by pulse oximetry (SpO_2) of $\geq$10% of preoperative levels occurred while the patient breathed room air; and if no radiographic evidence of pulmonary aspiration was present. Not surprisingly, the largest number of aspirations occur during induction and intubation or on emergence within 5 minutes of extubation. They found no serious morbidity from pulmonary aspiration in nearly 120,000 elective procedures in ASA class I or II.

In a later study the same group reported on the incidence of aspiration in infants and children.[162] Unlike other researchers they found no increased incidence in young patients. They noted 24 aspirations in a series of 63,180 general anesthetic procedures. Fifteen of the 24 children did not develop symptoms within 2 hours, and no treatment was required. Five children required respiratory support, three for more than 48 hours. No deaths occurred. Common risk factors for aspiration are given in Box 24-6.

Etiology

Although vomiting and gastroesophageal reflux are common clinical events, aspiration usually occurs only when normal protective reflexes (swallowing, coughing, gagging) fail.[161] Three broad categories of failure include the following: (1) depression of reflex protection, (2) alteration in anatomic structures, and (3) iatrogenic disorder. Reflex responses to aspiration are automatically blunted with depression of consciousness. The most common setting for depression of reflex protection occurs during anesthesia induction and emergence.[161]

Three aspiration syndromes have been identified: (1) chemical pneumonitis (Mendelson's syndrome); (2) mechanical obstruction; and (3) bacterial infection. Because acute chemical pneumonitis poses the greatest difficulty to anesthesia providers, the pathophysiology, presentation, and anesthetic implications of Mendelson's syndrome are discussed.

BOX 24-6

Risk Factors for Aspiration

- Emergency surgery
- Full stomach
- Obstetrics
- Gastrointestinal obstruction
- Ascites
- Diabetic gastroparesis
- Gastroesophageal reflux
- Hiatal hernia
- Peptic ulcer disease
- Difficult airway management
- High gastric pressure or lower esophageal sphincter tone
- Impaired reflexes
- Head injury
- Depression of consciousness
- Seizures
- Obesity
- Scleroderma
- Trauma or stress
- Nausea and vomiting
- Opioids
- Cricoid pressure
- Cardiac arrest, severe hypotension

The triphasic sequence of (1) immediate respiratory distress combined with bronchospasm, cyanosis, tachycardia, and dyspnea followed by (2) partial recovery and (3) a final phase of gradual return of function is characteristic of Mendelson's syndrome.[163] This acute chemical pneumonitis is caused by the irritative action of hydrochloric acid, which is quite damaging to the lungs.

Pathophysiology

The pathophysiology of aspiration pneumonia often is characterized according to the pH, volume, and type of gastric material aspirated. It has long been felt that gastric fluid volume (GFV) >0.4 ml/kg (25 ml/70 kg) and a pH <2.5 are significant indicators of risk for aspiration sequelae. In 1974 Roberts and Shirley[164] published a classic article advocating these arbitrarily defined surrogate end-points in patients undergoing cesarean section. These markers became widely accepted in clinical practice, and efforts to reach these levels preoperatively in many patient groups included insertion of nasal gastric tubes as well as multidrug pharmacologic intervention. Questions are being raised as to the validity of the data behind these recommendations, with the suggestion that a reappraisal is in order.[163] Because GFVs >0.4 ml/kg are common, even with fasting, and aspiration rarely accompanies these higher levels, the use of this marker seems less than realistic. In a recent report comparing gastric content differences in healthy obese versus lean patients, GFV >25 ml and pH <2.5 were noted in 26.6% of obese and 42% of lean patients.[165] These data suggest that healthy obese patients do not exhibit delayed gastric emptying and that many patients routinely fall into the surrogate range of GFV >25 ml and pH <2.5 without aspiration. Acidity plays a role in aspiration-induced lung damage; however, preoperative pharmacologic manipulation of gastric pH has not been proved to be clinically effective.[161,162,166] It has been suggested that the focus be shifted away from GFV and pH and toward patient characteristics, patient condition, and anesthetic practices that place the patient at risk of pulmonary aspiration.

When aspiration is severe, damage to the entire alveolocapillary barrier, including the basement membranes and capillary endothelial cells, may occur. Damage to these structures causes an increase in the permeability of the pulmonary blood vessels followed by a profound capillary leak syndrome. This capillary leak produces flooding of the interstitium and alveolar spaces with a protein-rich fluid (permeability pulmonary edema). If a sufficient amount of intravascular fluid is lost, hypotension and a decrease in CO may develop. In addition to the inactivation of surfactant by the gastric aspirate itself, the loss of protein through the impaired capillary wall can cause changes in surfactant production and in turn can contribute to a loss of lung compliance. Mucus rapidly buffers the acidic fluid entering the lungs. Despite this, initial contact with highly acidic material has still been shown to increase the vascular permeability in a very predictable fashion.

Hypoxia occurs secondary to a shunting effect. Initially $PaCO_2$ tends to be low because of hyperventilation from hypoxic drive and because of the mechanical and irritative stimuli to the large airways and parenchyma. Hypercarbia associated with hypoventilation occurs from either acute or chronic lung obstruction and is a negative prognostic sign.

Clinical Features and Diagnosis

Arterial hypoxemia, the hallmark sign of aspiration pneumonia, may not be suspected until after surgery, when unanticipated instability occurs in otherwise healthy patients. Signs to alert the anesthetist include tachypnea, dyspnea, tachycardia, hypertension, and late cyanosis.

Diagnosis may be difficult to establish unless the aspiration is witnessed or gastric contents are visualized directly in the airway or suctioned from an endotracheal tube. ABG analysis and chest radiography are needed for evaluation. Infiltrates in perihilar and basilar regions along with pulmonary edema are the most common findings on radiography; however, aspiration pneumonitis may not be revealed for up to 6 to 12 hours after insult.[155] Determination of tracheal aspirate pH, once advocated, has proved to be an inaccurate means of detection owing to the neutralization of secretions by mucus.

Anesthetic Management

Preoperative Management

When dealing with aspiration, "an ounce of prevention is worth a pound of cure." Avoiding the use of general anesthesia is the most effective means of preventing aspiration. However, regional and local sedation anesthesia is unrealistic for many procedures and in certain patient populations. When the use of general anesthesia is unavoidable, taking the following steps may help minimize the risk of aspiration, or at least limit its consequences.

Pharmacologic prophylaxis for aspiration has been common practice for many years. Much of the concern arose from the finding that large volumes of acidic gastric contents, if aspirated, caused lung damage and increased the risk of serious morbidity and mortality. Agents such as gastrokinetics, histamine blockers, anticholinergics, antacids, proton pump inhibitors, and antiemetics are all used alone or in various combinations to raise gastric pH and lower volume. Recent evidence questioning the benefit of this practice of routine administration of these agents

TABLE 24-25 Fasting Guidelines

Ingested Material	Minimum Fasting Period (hr)
Clear liquid	2
Breast milk	4
Infant formula	6
Nonhuman milk	6
Light meal	6

Modified from Practice guidelines for preoperative fasting and the use of pharmacologic agents to reduce the risk of pulmonary aspiration: application to healthy patients undergoing elective surgery. Anesthesiology. 1999;90:896-905.

in healthy patients without an increased aspiration risk has led to new practice guidelines. A task force appointed by the ASA has reviewed data with an evidence-based approach to the current fasting guidelines and drug prophylaxis.[167] Their fasting guidelines are given in Table 24-25, and drug prophylaxis guidelines are in Table 24-26. Evidence does not support the practice of routine preoperative administration of these gastric-related agents. Use in patients believed to exhibit risk factors should be continued.

The administration of clear nonparticulate antacids such as sodium citrate has been shown to be clinically effective in increasing the pH of gastric contents. Desired onset of action occurs within 15 minutes, and duration of action is 1 to 3 hours. Intravenous administration of the H_2-receptor blockers cimetidine, ranitidine, and famotidine 45 to 60 minutes before surgery can raise gastric pH. Metoclopramide stimulates gastric emptying, increases lower esophageal pressure, and acts as an antiemetic. When this agent is used in combination with the H_2-receptor blockers or antacids, the resultant reduction in gastric volume and acidity may be helpful in reducing aspiration risk.

TABLE 24-26 Drug Prophylaxis for Anesthesia

Medication Type	Common Examples	Recommendation
Gastrointestinal stimulants	Metoclopramide	No routine use*
Gastric acid secretion blockers	Cimetidine Famotidine Omeprazole Lansoprazole	No routine use*
Antacids	Sodium citrate Sodium bicarbonate Magnesium trisilicate	No routine use*
Antiemetics	Droperidol Ondansetron	No routine use*
Anticholinergics	Atropine Scopolamine Glycopyrrolate	No use†
Combinations of the medications above		No routine use*

**The routine preoperative use of these medications to decrease aspiration risk in patients with no apparent increased risk is not recommended.*

†The use of anticholinergics to decrease aspiration risk is not recommended.

Modified from American Society of Anesthesiologists. Practice guidelines for preoperative fasting and the use of pharmacologic agents to reduce the risk of pulmonary aspiration: application to healthy patients undergoing elective surgery. Anesthesiology. 1999;90:896-905.

Intraoperative Management

If intubation is not expected to be difficult, a rapid-sequence induction (rather than awake endotracheal intubation) is indicated. If awake or rapid-sequence intubation is indicated for decreasing the risk of aspiration, awake extubation is needed. Premature extubation before the patient is fully awake, manifests reflexes, and can follow commands may place him or her at risk for aspiration and laryngospasm.

If vomiting or aspiration occurs during induction, immediate treatment includes tilting of the patient's head downward or to the side, rapid suctioning of the mouth and pharynx, and intubation. Warner and colleagues[161] noted that patients could be discharged if they did not develop symptoms within 2 hours of the incident. Their criteria were as follows: (1) patients did not develop symptoms that included a new cough or a wheeze; (2) no decrease in SpO_2 of greater than or equal to 10% of preoperative levels occurred while the patient was breathing room air; (3) patients did not exhibit an A-a gradient of greater than or equal to 300 mm Hg; and (4) no radiographic evidence of pulmonary aspiration was present. For patients who experience more severe aspirations, endotracheal intubation should be performed quickly and the cuff inflated so that further aspiration is prevented. Before 100% O_2 is administered and positive pressure ventilation initiated, the endotracheal tube should be suctioned. This measure has been advocated in order to avoid the pushing of aspirated material further down the tracheobronchial tree. A nasogastric tube should be placed for emptying of the stomach. If aspiration is severe, surgery may be postponed. ABG analysis should be performed for determination of the extent of hypoxia. Early application of PEEP is recommended for improving pulmonary function.[163] Bronchoscopy should be reserved for those patients who are suspected of having aspirated solid material. Pulmonary lavage is not recommended unless conducting airways are obstructed. Again, the use of steroids is controversial, and the routine use of antibiotics is not recommended.[167]

ACUTE RESPIRATORY DISTRESS SYNDROME

Definition

The term *acute respiratory failure* is often used synonymously with *acute* (formerly *adult*) *respiratory distress syndrome* (ARDS). Although ARDS may be caused by or associated with a variety of clinical conditions, most patients with this disease demonstrate similar clinical and pathologic features regardless of the cause of lung injury. Common features include the following: (1) a history of a preceding noxious event that served as a trigger for the subsequent development of ARDS; (2) an interval from hours to days of relatively normal lung function after the insult; and (3) the rapid onset and progression over several hours of dyspnea, severe hypoxia, diffuse bilateral pulmonary infiltration, and stiffening and noncompliance of the lungs.[168] The consensus definition is given in Table 24-27.

Incidence and Outcome

Risk factors for the development of ARDS appear to be additive. Taylor reported the incidence of occurrence to be 25%

TABLE 24-27 American-European Consensus Conference on ARDS: Recommended Criteria For Acute Lung Injury and Acute Respiratory Distress Syndrome

Criteria	Timing	Oxygenation	Chest Radiography	P wedge
Acute lung injury	Acute onset	Pa_{O_2}/F_{IO_2} <300 mm Hg (regardless of PEEP level)	Bilateral infiltrates	<18 mm Hg or no clinical evidence left atrial hypertension
Acute respiratory distress syndrome	Acute onset	Pa_{O_2}/F_{IO_2} <200 mm Hg (regardless of PEEP level)	Bilateral infiltrates	<18 mm Hg or no clinical evidence of left atrial hypertension

F_{IO_2}, *Fraction of inspired oxygen;* Pa_{O_2}, *partial pressure of oxygen in arterial blood;* PEEP, *positive end-expiratory pressure;* P wedge, *pulmonary capillary wedge pressure.*

From Bernard GR, Artigas A, Brigham KL, et al. The American-European Consensus Conference on ARDS: definitions, mechanisms, relevant outcomes, and clinical trial coordination. Am J Respir Crit Care Med. *1994;149:818-824.*

with the presence of one risk factor, 42% with the presence of two, and 85% with the presence of three.[169] The mortality rate for ARDS remains high, ranging from 50% to 70%.[170] However, the mortality rate often exceeds 90% when gram-negative septic shock precedes ARDS development.[171]

Etiology

Events and risk factors associated with the development of ARDS include the following: (1) shock (septic, cardiogenic, or hypovolemic); (2) trauma; (3) pulmonary infection (e.g., with *Pneumocystis carinii* or *Escherichia coli*); (4) disease states that result in the release of inflammatory mediators (e.g., extrapulmonary infections, disseminated intravascular coagulation, anaphylaxis, coronary bypass grafting, and transfusion reactions); (5) exposure to various agents (e.g., narcotics, barbiturates, and O_2); (6) diseases of the central nervous system; (7) aspiration (e.g., of gastric contents or as in drowning); and (8) metabolic events (e.g., pancreatitis and uremia) (Box 24-7).[168]

BOX 24-7

Clinical Disorders Associated with Acute Respiratory Distress Syndrome

Sepsis Trauma
Fat emboli
Lung contusion
Nonthoracic trauma

Liquid Aspiration
Gastric contents
Fresh and salt water (drowning)
Hydrocarbon fluids

Drug Associated
Heroin
Methadone
Propoxyphene
Barbiturates
Colchicine
Ethchlorvynol
Aspirin
Hydrochlorothiazide

Inhaled Toxins
Smoke
Oxygen (high concentration)
Corrosive chemicals (NO_2, Cl_2, NH_3, phosgene)

Shock from Any Cause
Hematologic disorders
Massive blood transfusion
Disseminated intravascular coagulation

Metabolic
Acute pancreatitis
Uremia

Miscellaneous
Lymphangiography
Reexpansion pulmonary edema
Increased intracranial pressure
After cardiopulmonary bypass
Eclampsia
Air emboli
Amniotic fluid embolism
Ascent to high altitude

Primary Pneumonias
Viral
Bacterial
Mycobacteria
Tuberculosis
Fungal
Pneumocystis carinii

From Matthay MA, Matthay RA. Pulmonary edema: cardiogenic and noncardiogenic. In: George RB, Light RW, Matthay MA, Matthay RA, eds. Chest Medicine: Essentials of Pulmonary and Critical Care Medicine. *2nd ed. Baltimore: Williams & Wilkins; 1990:446.*

Pathophysiology

As with pulmonary edema and aspiration pneumonitis, the pathophysiology of ARDS is centered around severe damage and inflammation to the alveolocapillary membrane. Irrespective of the cause of acute respiratory failure, the lung's structural response to injury and subsequent repair occurs in a similar fashion.[169] Although the exact mechanisms of this response and repair remain unclear, research has focused on the release of cytokines and membrane-bound phospholipids from the capillary endothelium and the activation of leukocytes and macrophages (via the complement system) within the lungs.[170]

Phospholipids are converted into prostaglandins and leukotrienes by the enzymes cyclooxygenase and lipoxygenase, respectively. It is believed that prostaglandin metabolites mediate pulmonary vasoconstriction, alter vascular reactivity (i.e., decrease hypoxic pulmonary vasoconstriction), and cause airway constriction.[172]

In addition, microembolus formation is a common manifestation of ARDS. Complement system activation and the release of thromboplastin from soft-tissue injury can trigger the coagulation cascade. Microemboli contribute to the severity of lung injury and are often found during autopsy.[173]

Clinical Features and Diagnosis

The clinical presentation of ARDS resembles that of pulmonary edema and aspiration pneumonitis. Patients are dyspneic, hypoxic, and hypovolemic and often require intubation and mechanical ventilation. Findings on histologic examination are similar to those of aspiration pneumonitis, with the exception that fibrosis of lung is more pronounced. Recovery of lung function is unpredictable. Milder cases resolve quickly, whereas others progress to fibrosis and death.

Treatment

Because lung infections (e.g., *P. carinii* pneumonia) mimic ARDS, antibiotic therapy often is initiated before the cause of respiratory failure is known. Maintenance of tissue oxygenation and replacement of lost intravascular fluids are the main goals of therapy. Preservation of end-organ perfusion is of utmost importance. Treatment is supportive and includes correction of hypoxia, preload and afterload reduction, and inotropic support as indicated.

Anesthetic Management

Anesthetic preparation includes evaluation of the patient's respiratory, cardiac, and renal status. Ventilator settings should be noted and special attention devoted to peak inspiratory pressures and PEEP levels. If the anesthesia ventilator cannot accommodate these settings, then arrangements must be made to bring the patient's ventilator into the operating room. The nature of lung sounds and amount of secretions should be noted. The presence of excess secretions should alert the anesthetist to the potential risk of airway obstruction. The degree of barotrauma from prolonged mechanical ventilation with high levels of PEEP can be assessed by the presence of chest tubes and subcutaneous emphysema secondary to pneumothorax. The effectiveness of therapy with bronchodilators should be assessed, because the use of these drugs may be initiated preoperatively and continued intraoperatively if effective. An arterial line should be placed preoperatively and ABG analysis performed. If possible, lactic acid values should be determined.

Volume status should be evaluated closely because patients with ARDS often are hypovolemic. Invasive monitoring via central venous lines and pulmonary artery catheters often is available, and cardiac filling pressures along with CO values should be assessed. Patients requiring inotropic support may arrive for surgery with infusions of dopamine or dobutamine. For all procedures renal function should be monitored with a bladder catheter. Antibiotic therapy should be continued intraoperatively and continuation of steroid preparations should be considered if patients were receiving these medications preoperatively.

Because patients with ARDS often are hemodynamically unstable, careful titration of anesthetic agents and adjunct agents is necessary. Owing to the multisystemic involvement characteristic of ARDS, drug metabolism and elimination should be carefully considered.

Transport should be carefully planned so that complications are minimized and safe arrival in the intensive care unit is ensured. Patients should undergo pulse oximetry, ECG, and blood pressure transport monitoring (by arterial line or noninvasively) before departure from the operating room. Breath sounds should be continually assessed with a precordial stethoscope. A full tank of O_2 and PEEP adapter valves should be available for transport. The potential need for emergency medications and a defibrillator should be considered. If the patient's ventilator needs to be returned to the intensive care unit, plans should be made so that it arrives there before the patient does. Finally, if possible, another member of the anesthesia team should accompany the patient during transport. Pulmonary dysfunction is the most common cause of postoperative complications after the administration of general anesthesia. To minimize pulmonary derangement the anesthesia provider must identify those patients who are at risk for the development of pulmonary impairment and must have a thorough understanding of the preexisting lung dysfunction. Some common modes of positive pressure ventilation are shown in Table 24-28.

NONCYTOTOXIC AND CYTOTOXIC DRUG-INDUCED PULMONARY DISEASE

Currently, more than 100 pharmacologic agents are known to produce adverse effects on the lung parenchyma, the pleura, and the airway. Drug-induced pulmonary injury occurs in several hundred thousand people each year in the United States. Knowledge of doses and the potential adverse effects of the prescribed medications may prevent or minimize drug-induced damage.

Mechanism

The mechanism of drug-induced pulmonary injury is not well defined. It has been shown that cytotoxic drugs used in the treatment of cancer cause pulmonary insult by a combination of the direct toxic effects of a drug or its metabolite and of their indirect effects—that is, the enhancement of inflammation or immune processes. The clinical features produced by different cytotoxic agents are similar, but chronic pneumonitis and fibrosis are the most commonly associated clinical syndromes. Table 24-29 lists various chemotherapeutic agents that may produce pulmonary toxicity. The pathogenesis of pulmonary toxicity is uncertain but has been found to include disruption of the endothelial cells and changes in calcium homeostasis that lead to toxic injury. The mechanisms of drug-induced pulmonary injury associated with noncytotoxic drugs are less well defined but may involve changes in pulmonary homeostasis.

TABLE 24-28 Modes of Positive Pressure Ventilation

Mode	Description	Advantages and Disadvantages
Controlled mechanical ventilation (CMV)	Ventilator f, inspiratory time, V_T (and therefore V_E) preset	May be used with sedation or paralysis; ventilator cannot respond to ventilatory needs
Assisted mechanical ventilation (AMV) or assisted-control mechanical ventilation	Ventilator V_T and inspiratory time preset, but patient can increase f (and therefore V_E)	Ventilator may respond to ventilatory needs; ventilator may undertrigger or overtrigger, depending on sensitivity
Intermittent mandatory ventilation (IMV)	Ventilator delivers preset V_T, f, and inspiratory time, but patient also may breathe spontaneously	May decrease asynchronous breathing and sedation requirements; ventilator cannot respond to ventilatory needs
Synchronized intermittent mandatory ventilation (SIMV)	Same as IMV, but ventilator breaths delivered only after patient finishes inspiration	Same as IMV, and patient not overinflated by receiving spontaneous and ventilator breaths at same time
High-frequency ventilation (HFV)	Ventilator f is increased and, V_T may be smaller than V_D	May reduce peak airway pressure; may cause auto-PEEP
Pressure-support ventilation (PSV)	Patient breathes at own f; V_T determined by inspiratory pressure and CRS	Increased comfort and decreased work of breathing; ventilator cannot respond to ventilatory needs
Pressure-control ventilation (PCV)	Ventilator peak pressure, f, and respiratory time preset	Peak inspiratory pressures may be decreased; hypoventilation may occur
Inverse ratio ventilation (IRV)	Inspiratory time exceeds expiratory time to facilitate inspiration	May improve gas exchange by increasing time spent in inspiration; may cause auto-PEEP
Airway pressure release ventilation (APRV)	Patient receives CPAP at high and low levels to stimulate V_T	May improve oxygenation at lower airway pressure; hypoventilation may occur
Proportional assist ventilation (PAV)	Patient determines own f, V_T, pressures, and flows	May amplify spontaneous breathing; depends entirely on patient's respiratory drive

CPAP, *Continuous positive airway pressure;* CRS, *respiratory system compliance;* f, *respiratory rate;* PEEP, *positive end-expiratory pressure;* V_D, *dead space;* V_E, *minute ventilation;* V_T, *tidal volume.*
Modified from Luce JM. Ventilator management in the intensive care unit. In: Goldman L, Ausiello D, eds. Cecil Textbook of Medicine. *22nd ed. Philadelphia: Saunders; 2004:604.*

Noncytotoxic agents can induce the development of numerous clinical syndromes. Several commonly implicated agents are discussed in the following sections.

Noncytotoxic Drug-Induced Pulmonary Disease

Amiodarone

Amiodarone (Cordarone) is a potent and effective agent used primarily in the long-term management of refractory, life-threatening arrhythmias—predominantly ventricular tachycardia and fibrillation. Despite its therapeutic benefits it is considered to be the drug of last resort because of the numerous adverse effects with which it is associated—in particular, severe pulmonary toxicity.[174] Acute administration is common during life support protocols for arrhythmias. Toxicity is rare when given acutely.

Pulmonary complications associated with amiodarone therapy are reported to occur in no patients to 61% of patients and are associated with an estimated mortality rate of 1% to 33%; however, patients with pulmonary complications usually have concomitant cardiac disease. Amiodarone has been found to accumulate in the lung. Kachel and associates have shown that α-tocopherol, a naturally existing antioxidant, offers protection against the effects of amiodarone.[175] According to Dusman and associates, clinical diagnosis of amiodarone-induced pulmonary toxicity is based on the presence of two or more of the following signs and symptoms:

1. New onset of pulmonary symptoms, such as dyspnea, cough, or pleuritic chest pain
2. Detection of new chest radiographic abnormalities, such as an interstitial or alveolar infiltrate
3. A decrease in DLCO of 20% from the pretreatment value; if no pretreatment values are available, then a value equal to less than 80% of the predicted value
4. Abnormal gallium-67 uptake by the lungs
5. Characteristic histologic changes of lung tissue obtained by bronchoscopic or open-lung biopsy[176]

Two syndromes of amiodarone-induced pulmonary toxicity are recognized. The more common syndrome is characterized by an insidious onset with nonproductive cough, dyspnea, weight loss, and occasional fever. Hypoxemia is common. Chest radiographs demonstrate parenchymal infiltrates with a predominant diffuse interstitial pattern that may progress to fibrosis. Pleural thickening and effusions also have been reported. Onset usually occurs after 2 months and with a dose of 400 mg/d or greater.[174] Case reports have shown favorable responses with and without the use of corticosteroids.[177]

The second syndrome has a more acute or explosive onset and accounts for 25% to 33% of cases. Presenting signs include rapidly progressive dyspnea, high fever, and hypoxemia. Chest radiographs show a predominant alveolar pattern with a patchy distribution that often involves the peripheral areas of the lung. The acute form is associated with a higher mortality rate than the insidious form, and prompt recognition and treatment are essential for a favorable recovery.

Pulmonary function tests performed at the onset of pulmonary toxicity reveal abnormalities typical of restrictive lung disease. Findings include a decrease in FVC and TLC, an elevation in FEV_1/FVC, and diffusion abnormalities.[176]

TABLE 24-29 Classification of Drug-Induced and Related Pulmonary Diseases by Type of Medication

Chemotherapeutic	***Cardiovascular***
Cytotoxic	Amiodarone*
Azathioprine inhibitors	Angiotensin-converting enzyme
Bleomycin*	Anticoagulants
Busulfan	β-Blockers*
Chlorambucil	Dipyridamole
Cyclophosphamide	Flecainide
Etoposide	Protamine*
Interleukin-2	Tocainide
Melphalan	
Mitomycin C*	***Inhalant***
Nitrosamines	Aspirated oil
Procarbazine	Oxygen
Tumor necrosis factor	
Vinblastine	***Intravenous***
Zinostatin	Blood*
Noncytotoxic	Ethanolamide maolate (sodium morrhuate)*
Bleomycin*	Ethiodized oil (lymphangiogram)
Cytosine arabinoside*	Talc
Methotrexate*	
Procarbazine*	***Miscellaneous***
	Bromocriptine
Antibiotic	Dantrolene
Amphotericin B*	Hydrochlorothiazide*
Nitrofurantoin	Methysergide
Acute*	Tocolytic agents*
Chronic	Tricyclics*
Sulfasalazine	L-Tryptophan
	Radiation
Antiinflammatory	Systemic lupus erythematosus (drug induced)
Acetylsalicylic acid*	Complement-mediated leukostasis*
Gold	
Methotrexate	
Nonsteroidal antiinflammatory agents	
Penicillamine	
Analgesic	
Heroin*	
Methadone*	
Naloxone*	
Placidyl*	
Propoxyphene*	
Salicylates*	

**Typically manifests as acute or subacute respiratory insufficiency.*
Modified from Murray JF, Nadel JA. Textbook of Respiratory Medicine. *3rd ed. Philadelphia: Saunders; 2000:1973.*

Therapeutic options are limited. Drug withdrawal is mandatory. Resolution is gradual because the drug's half-life is approximately 40 to 70 days; therefore serum and tissue levels of amiodarone are measurable long after discontinuation of therapy. Radiographic clearing occurs within 2 months. However, as signs and symptoms of pulmonary toxicity abate, so does the therapeutic benefit. The underlying arrhythmia commonly returns during the same period. At times, reduction of the dose may be successful in decreasing toxicity while control of the dysrhythmia is maintained. This strategy may be the only option. The impression that corticosteroids are efficacious in this syndrome is unsubstantiated.

Gold

The administration of gold salts is common in the treatment of rheumatoid arthritis. Unfortunately, their use has been implicated in the development of hypersensitivity lung disease, interstitial pneumonitis, and pulmonary fibrosis.[178] The incidence of pulmonary insult occurs in fewer than 1% of patients who receive gold therapy. Several possible mechanisms of injury have been proposed, but none has been proved. Symptoms may occur as early as 6 hours to 1 month after administration of the last dose of gold salts, and they usually are seen within 4 months after the initiation of therapy. Rarely the presentation may be acute and characterized by fever, wheezing, and cough. More commonly it is insidious and manifested by progressive dyspnea and nonproductive cough. Fever and eosinophilia are present in 40% and 33% of patients, respectively.[177] Although chest radiography demonstrates the presence of an interstitial process, this process may predominate in the upper lung zones. Pulmonary function abnormalities show a restrictive ventilatory defect and impairment of diffusion. Discontinuation of therapy with gold salts after their causal role has been suspected is the most important treatment measure. Corticosteroids have been used with equivocal results.

Cytotoxic Drug-Induced Pulmonary Disease

Three clinical syndromes are associated with cytotoxic drug-induced pulmonary injury: (1) chronic pneumonitis and fibrosis, (2) acute hypersensitivity lung disease, and (3) noncardiogenic pulmonary edema.[174] These syndromes may coexist.

Chronic Pneumonitis and Fibrosis

Interstitial pneumonitis and fibrosis is the most frequently encountered pattern in drug-induced pulmonary injury. The mechanism of injury is a direct cytotoxic effect of a drug or its metabolites on the endothelial, interstitial, or alveolar epithelial cells. On lung parenchyma the cytotoxic effect elicits an inflammatory response characterized by the proliferation of macrophages, lymphocytes, and other inflammatory cells. This inflammatory response leads to the deposition of fibrin within the alveoli, which produces interstitial inflammation and fibrosis.

Interstitial pneumonitis can be classified as acute, subacute, or chronic; the chronic form is the most frequently encountered. Common manifestations of these subgroups include dyspnea, dry cough, low-grade fever, fatigue, and malaise that develop over several weeks to months. Chest radiography demonstrates diffuse interstitial infiltrates. Bleomycin is the causative agent most frequently implicated in interstitial pneumonitis. Treatment includes discontinuation of the offending agent with or without institution of corticosteroid therapy; prognosis is variable.

Hypersensitivity Syndrome

Hypersensitivity lung disease has been associated with the cytotoxic agents bleomycin, methotrexate, L-asparaginase, and procarbazine. Common pulmonary manifestations include a nonproductive cough, dyspnea, and chest pain. The systemic allergic response is manifested as fever, urticaria, arthralgias, hypotension, and eosinophilia. Chest radiography may reveal pneumonitis, pleuritis, and pleural effusion. Suspicion of a hypersensitivity drug reaction should be followed by prompt withdrawal of the agent. Corticosteroid use may or may not be indicated, and prognosis is generally favorable.

Noncardiogenic Pulmonary Edema

The development of noncardiogenic pulmonary edema is an acute but rare phenomenon that occurs after the administration of some antineoplastic agents. Cytotoxic drugs that contribute to its development include methotrexate, cytosine arabinoside (cytarabine), and cyclophosphamide. One major difference between the noncardiogenic pulmonary edema caused by cytotoxic agents and that produced by noncytotoxic ones is prognosis. The latter form usually is fully reversible on discontinuation of the offending agent. Patients with cytotoxic pulmonary insult have a variable prognosis, and survivors may show residual pulmonary dysfunction.

Numerous pharmacologic agents used in the treatment of cancer have been implicated in the development of toxic pulmonary side effects. The agents most commonly implicated in pulmonary insult include bleomycin, busulfan, carmustine, and methotrexate. Pulmonary toxicity in the use of antineoplastic agents is defined as the development of clinical signs and symptoms of pulmonary distress that were not present during the pretreatment studies. The prevalence of diffuse pulmonary infiltration occurring as a result of drug toxicity is reported to be as high as 20%.

Bleomycin. Bleomycin, an antitumor antibiotic, is the most common chemotherapeutically induced potentiator of pulmonary injury. It is used primarily in the treatment of lymphomas, testicular tumors, and squamous cell carcinomas of the head and neck. Despite the benefits of bleomycin therapy, the development of pulmonary toxicity is the limiting factor of its use.[179]

The most common adverse effect of bleomycin is the development of interstitial fibrosis. The incidence of pulmonary fibrosis is approximately 20%, with a 1% mortality rate. Anesthesia-related problems occur postoperatively and are associated with exposure to high O_2 concentrations. Those factors associated with an increased risk for bleomycin-related pulmonary toxicity include the following:

1. Therapy with a cumulative dose greater than 450 to 500 mg; however, cases of pulmonary toxicity occurring with doses of 100 mg have been well documented
2. Prior or concomitant irradiation to the thorax, which increases the incidence of toxicity to 35% to 55% and the mortality rate to over 50%
3. Age greater than 70 years
4. Smoking, which increases the release of hydrogen peroxide and other reactive oxidative metabolites into the surrounding lung tissue, potentiating impairment of respiratory function
5. Treatment with multiple antineoplastic agents, especially cyclophosphamide
6. Hyperoxia and retention of carbon monoxide

Because bleomycin is predominantly excreted via the kidneys, impairment of renal function impedes the rate of elimination and may contribute to injury.

Concentration of bleomycin is preferentially in the skin, causing ulcerations. In the lungs it produces interstitial fibrosis. The cause of the adverse pulmonary effects induced by bleomycin is thought to be the generation of reactive oxidative metabolites. Pulmonary damage appears in two clinical syndromes: acute and chronic. The acute pattern is rare and occurs with lower doses of bleomycin.[180] The chronic form is more common; its severity is related to dose, and it develops within weeks to months of the initiation of therapy. Approximately 15% of patients who receive a cumulative dose greater than 450 mg develop clinical pulmonary dysfunction.[174]

Symptoms of toxicity initially include a dry hacking cough and dyspnea on exertion. Progression of lung disease is associated with dyspnea at rest, tachypnea, fever, and cyanosis. Changes on chest radiography usually occur later and manifest as bibasilar reticular infiltrates that may progress to frank consolidation.

Several investigators have suggested that patients undergoing general anesthesia who have a concurrent history of bleomycin therapy should receive the lowest possible O_2 concentrations that allow maintenance of adequate PO_2.[181,182] They also have suggested that excessive administration of crystalloid solutions be avoided; however, data that demonstrate the superiority of colloid solution administration in these patients are unavailable. Treatment is supportive therapy and discontinuation of bleomycin treatment. The use of steroids has been effective in some patients. Prognosis for these patients is poor.[180]

Anesthetic Management of Bleomycin-Treated Patients. Although universally accepted guidelines for the management of bleomycin-treated patient undergoing general anesthesia are lacking, the following suggestions have been made:

1. O_2 saturation should be monitored continuously and ABG analysis performed intermittently.
2. Immediately before anesthesia 100% O_2 should be administered for 1 to 4 minutes.
3. After induction a target PaO_2 should be chosen and the FIO_2 maintained at the lowest level that allows adequate oxygenation.
4. The use of PEEP should be considered.
5. Crystalloid solutions should be administered carefully and the use of colloid solutions considered if large fluid volumes are required.
6. The patient should be informed of the possible need for postoperative ventilation.
7. Postoperatively the FIO_2 should be kept at the lowest possible setting that maintains the target PaO_2.

The choice of anesthetic technique varies, but as with all surgical procedures, careful evaluation and management are essential. There are no reports suggesting the superiority of regional anesthesia in patients treated with bleomycin.

Methotrexate. Methotrexate is an analogue of folic acid that inhibits cellular reproduction by causing an acute intracellular deficiency of folate coenzymes. Methotrexate is used in the treatment of malignant and benign conditions, including leukemia, osteogenic sarcoma, choriocarcinoma, polymyositis, psoriasis, and connective tissue disorders (particularly rheumatoid arthritis). Regardless of the route of administration, pulmonary toxicity has been reported to occur with all forms of delivery, with an incidence of 7.6%. Clinically, the onset of pulmonary dysfunction may be chronic, but more commonly it is acute. Several cases of acute noncardiogenic pulmonary edema have been reported after intrathecal administration. The majority of reported methotrexate-induced pulmonary reactions occur in children with acute lymphocytic leukemia. The syndrome often develops over 7 to 14 days and is characterized by fever, dry cough, dyspnea, hypoxemia, and bilateral pulmonary infiltrates. Improvement may begin 10 to 14 days after onset.

No precipitating factors—including age, total dose, duration of therapy, and underlying disease—have been conclusively implicated. In addition, no injury has been reported in individuals receiving less than 20 mg of methotrexate per week.[181]

The mechanism of pulmonary injury in humans is consistent with a hypersensitivity response and includes the presence of fever, eosinophilia, and occasionally granuloma and multinucleated giant cells in histopathologic specimens. Cytologic examination of bronchoalveolar lavage specimens reveals a lymphocytic alveolitis with a disproportionately high ratio of helper T lymphocytes to suppressor T lymphocytes, which suggests the presence of an immunologic disorder.[183]

As with injury by most agents that have toxic effects, the earlier the response is identified, the more likely it is that the damage will resolve fully. Treatment consists of the withdrawal of methotrexate. Corticosteroid use may be advantageous in severe cases.[181,183] Despite a mortality rate of 1%, the majority of patients return to their pretreatment status.

PULMONARY OXYGEN TOXICITY

Etiology

The administration of O_2 for the treatment of hypoxemia is a common practice. As with all prescribed drugs, the risks of the adverse effects of O_2 administration must be considered, despite its beneficial effects. The prolonged use of high concentrations of O_2 (greater than 50% for longer than 24 hours) is potentially toxic and may result in irreversible lung damage.[180] Injury to the lung affects the upper airways mildly; the predominant damage occurs in the lower respiratory tract, particularly in the alveolar structures.[181,182] The rate of development of O_2 toxicity is directly related to the partial pressure of inspired O_2.[183]

Normobaric hyperoxia can result in four clinical syndromes, as follow: (1) acute tracheobronchitis, (2) absorption atelectasis, (3) acute alveolar lung injury (ARDS), and (4) bronchopulmonary dysplasia.[183] When nitrogen is replaced with O_2, absorption atelectasis occurs in the alveoli that are poorly ventilated. The loss of the so-called "nitrogen splint" promotes alveolar collapse.

Pathophysiology

The pathogenesis of pulmonary O_2 toxicity is linked to the excessive production of free O_2 radicals. Free radicals are molecules that contain one or more unpaired electrons.[183] Free radicals are highly reactive metabolites of O_2 (e.g., superoxide anion, hydrogen peroxide, and hydroxyl radical) that overwhelm antioxidant systems, including cellular enzymatic defenses (superoxide dismutase, catalase, glutathione peroxidase) and nonenzymatic scavengers (α-tocopherol acetate). Free radicals exert their toxic effect on cell and organelle membranes; they interfere with vital cellular functions, causing inactivation of enzymes and transport proteins, membrane lipid peroxidation, and inhibition of cell growth and division.[184]

Five common risk factors have been described in the development of O_2 toxicity. First is an increased propensity for toxicity with use of increasing concentrations. This cumulative dose effect also has been noted with the use of the antineoplastic agents bleomycin, busulfan, and carmustine. The second risk factor is age. As an individual ages, a decrease in the antioxidant defense system may occur. Bleomycin and methotrexate administration in the elderly augments the risk of pulmonary toxicity. The third risk factor is previous or concurrent radiotherapy to the thorax. The production of superoxides secondary to gamma irradiation is believed to cause a synergistic reaction with bleomycin, busulfan, and mitomycin. The fourth factor is O_2 therapy concurrent with the use of various chemotherapeutic agents. Cytotoxic chemicals such as bleomycin, cyclophosphamide, and mitomycin either alter antioxidant defense mechanisms or generate oxidants, causing further pulmonary insult. The fifth factor is use of a combination chemotherapy regimen. Agents associated with an increased likelihood of lung damage include carmustine, mitomycin, cyclophosphamide, bleomycin, and methotrexate.

Pulmonary injury induced by hyperoxia has two phases: exudative and proliferative.[184] The exudative or acute phase is characterized by injury to alveolar type I cells and capillary endothelial cells; this injury increases the permeability of

TABLE 24-30 Approximate Sequence of Pulmonary Changes during 100% Oxygen Breathing

Duration of Exposure (h)	Manifestation
>12	Decreased tracheobronchial clearance; cough; chest pain; decreased vital capacity
>24	Depressed protein synthesis; altered endothelial function
>36	Decreased CL and DL; increased $P_{AO_2} - Pa_{O_2}$
>48	Increased alveolar epithelial permeability; alveolar edema; surfactant inactivation
>60	Acute respiratory distress syndrome

CL, *Lung compliance;* DL, *maximum diffusing capacity of lung;* PAO_2, *alveolar partial pressure of oxygen;* PaO_2, *arterial partial pressure of oxygen. From Fisher AB. Pulmonary oxygen toxicity In: Fishman AP, ed.* Pulmonary Diseases and Disorders. *2nd ed. New York: McGraw-Hill; 1988:2334.*

membranes to water, electrolytes, and proteins. Progression of damage causes interstitial and alveolar edema and alveolar hemorrhage, which are consistent with noncardiogenic pulmonary edema. These events of pulmonary insult usually occur within 24 to 72 hours, depending on the concentration and duration of hyperoxia. The proliferative or chronic phase is characterized by hyperplasia of alveolar type II cells, deposition of collagen and elastin in the interstitium, and the formation of hyaline membrane. Eventually, interstitial fibrosis develops.

Clinical Features and Diagnosis

The earliest manifestations are related to the effects on the tracheobronchial mucosa (Table 24-30). Symptoms may occur after 6 hours of O_2 exposure and include substernal chest pain that is prominent with inspiration, tachypnea, and a nonproductive cough. By 24 hours, paresthesia, anorexia, nausea, and headache occur. Physiologic changes include a decrease in tracheal mucous velocity, VC, pulmonary compliance, and diffusing capacity and increased $PAO_2 - PaO_2$. Some individuals develop signs of mild airway obstruction. Chest radiography demonstrates an alveolar and interstitial pattern. Respiratory failure and death ensue if O_2 poisoning persists.

Management

Both hyperoxia and hypoxemia have undesirable effects. Therefore deciding whether to administer O_2 requires mature clinical judgment. The goal is to deliver the lowest level of FIO_2 needed for maintenance of adequate arterial O_2 saturation (generally, a PaO_2 of greater than 90 mm Hg, as determined by ABG analysis). Measures such as PEEP should be used for decreasing the need for high FIO_2. Corticosteroid therapy reduces antioxidant enzyme activity and may be useful during the exudative phase.

AUTOIMMUNE DISORDERS

Autoimmune diseases, connective tissue diseases, collagenosis, and *rheumatologic diseases* are terms used interchangeably in clinical medicine. These entities are frequently characterized by multiple-organ involvement and inflammation. On the whole these disorders have unknown causes; however, the inflammatory process is immunologically mediated, as evidenced by the presence of autoantibodies, rheumatoid factor, and immune complexes, as well as by elevation of the sedimentation rate and the observation of certain clinical characteristics. Pulmonary manifestations are common and often assume a major role in the disease process. Characteristic restrictive lung changes may result if pulmonary impairment is sufficiently severe. Table 24-31 lists pulmonary manifestations of various collagen vascular diseases.

Sarcoidosis

Sarcoidosis is a multisystemic disorder characterized by the presence of noncaseating epithelioid-cell granulomata. It is described as an intense interaction of activated lymphocytes and macrophages that results in tissue injury. The disease most frequently involves the lungs, reticuloendothelial system, skin, eyes, and myocardium. The prevalence of disease in the United States is 10 to 40 persons per 100,000, with blacks being more commonly affected than whites (12:1 ratio). In whites the distribution among men and women is equal; in blacks, however, the female-to-male ratio is 2:1. The disease predominantly occurs in those aged 20 to 40 years.[185] The cause of sarcoidosis is unclear, as no organic or inorganic causative agent has been consistently found. The route of transmission also is uncertain.

Most sarcoid granulomata resolve spontaneously, leaving no scar; others persist for a longer duration, with little or no fibrosis; still others become hyalinized and fibrotic areas that cause tissue damage. Pulmonary involvement is primarily in regions rich in lymphatic vessels, such as the subpleural, perivascular, and peribronchial areas. Frequently, adjacent nonspecific inflammatory changes as well as alveolitis with cellular infiltrates are noted.[186]

Parenchymal infiltration and fibrosis result in a decrease in lung compliance, impairment of diffusing capacity, and a reduction in lung volumes. Many patients exhibit a reduced FEV_1/FVC and increased airway resistance. $\dot{V}/\dot{Q}$ imbalance and an increase in PaO_2 occurs in response to a nonuniform decrease in lung compliance. An obstructive pattern resulting from endobronchial disease or peribronchial fibrosis may occur simultaneously. Cor pulmonale may develop in the presence of severe pulmonary fibrosis. Clinical presentation is varied and may be categorized as asymptomatic (occurring in 20% of individuals investigated and based on the detection of abnormality of chest radiography) or symptomatic (characterized by nonspecific features ranging from fever, fatigue, anorexia, weight loss, chills, and night sweats to dyspnea and blindness).

The lung is the most commonly affected organ, with pulmonary involvement occurring in more than 90% of individuals with sarcoidosis. Respiratory symptoms are those typical of interstitial involvement and include dyspnea, dry cough, and retrosternal chest pain (35% to 50% of patients). Less common symptoms include wheezing, hemoptysis, pleural effusion, and clubbing of the fingers. Sarcoidosis is one of the few chest diseases that concurrently involve lymph nodes in the lung (hilar) and the mediastinum.[187] On radiography, intrathoracic involvement has been classified into three categories: stage I is characterized by bilateral, symmetric, hilar adenopathy; stage II by hilar adenopathy and diffuse pulmonary changes; and stage III by diffuse pulmonary infiltrates without adenopathy. Stage I is associated with the most favorable prognosis, and stage III with the worst.

TABLE 24-31 Pulmonary Manifestations of Some Collagen Vascular Diseases

Rheumatoid Arthritis	***Polymyositis–Dermatomyositis***
Pleural disease (effusions)	Interstitial pneumonitis
Diffuse interstitial pneumonitis	Aspiration pneumonia
Necrobiotic nodules	Respiratory myositis
Caplan's syndrome	Pulmonary hypertension
Pulmonary hypertension (arteritis)	Bronchiolitis obliterans organizing pneumonia
Apical fibrobullous disease	
Bronchiolitis obliterans with and without organizing pneumonia	***Mixed Connective Tissue Disease***
Cricoarytenoid arthritis	Diffuse interstitial lung disease
	Pulmonary hypertension (vasculitis)
Systemic Lupus Erythematosus	Pleural disease
Pleural disease (pleuritis, effusions)	Diaphragmatic muscle dysfunction
Atelectasis	
Acute lupus pneumonitis	***Sjögren's Syndrome***
Diffuse interstitial lung disease	Respiratory mucosal dryness
Pulmonary hemorrhage	Pleurisy
Respiratory muscle dysfunction	Chronic airway disease
	Lymphocytic interstitial pneumonia
Progressive Systemic Sclerosis	Pseudolymphoma
Diffuse interstitial fibrosis	Lymphoma
Pulmonary vascular disease	Amyloid
Aspiration pneumonia	Pulmonary hypertension (vasculitis)
Chest wall restrictions secondary to thoracic skin sclerosis	
Pleural disease	

The distribution of extrathoracic involvement is as follows: peripheral lymphatic, 50% to 75%; skin, 25% to 70%; liver, 60% to 80%; eye, 25%; spleen, 20% to 30%; bone, 1% to 35%; salivary glands, 5%; heart, 5%; nervous system, 5%. Laryngeal involvement occurs in 1% to 5% of patients and may make insertion of an adult-sized tracheal tube difficult.[188] In patients with diffuse pulmonary involvement, a transbronchial approach that includes fiberoptic bronchoscopy is the procedure of choice.[187]

The diagnosis of sarcoidosis is typically based on the presence of a combination of clinical, radiographic, and histologic criteria, as follows: (1) a compatible clinical or radiologic picture; (2) the presence of noncaseating granulomas, and (3) negative results on bacterial and fungal studies of biopsied tissue and sputum. The overall prognosis in sarcoidosis is good. The acute onset usually is followed by a self-limiting course of approximately 2 years' duration with spontaneous resolution; sarcoidosis of insidious onset may be followed by progressive disease characterized by pulmonary fibrosis.[189] Approximately 15% to 20% of cases remain active or recur. Treatment with corticosteroids is frequently employed and produces relief of symptoms, clinical remissions, and suppression of inflammation and granuloma formation. Conversely, because spontaneous and permanent remissions occur in 50% of patients, the use of corticosteroids in these individuals is controversial. Pulmonary disease is the most frequent indication for corticosteroid therapy in systemic disease.[190] Other treatment options include the use of antiinflammatory agents, antimalarials, radiation therapy, and immune system–modulating drugs.[191]

The mortality rate for patients with sarcoidosis after 5 years is approximately 4% to 10% and is attributed to respiratory failure, azotemia from renal injury caused by chronic hypercalciuria, cardiac arrest resulting from myocardial involvement, and massive hemoptysis because of colonization of bullae by *Aspergillus fumigatus*.

FLAIL CHEST

Flail chest, a condition that results from chest trauma and multiple rib fractures, is reported to occur in 5% of patients who sustain thoracic injury (Figure 24-14).[192] The hallmark of flail chest is paradoxic movement of the chest wall at the site of the fracture. During inspiration the chest wall is drawn inward owing to the negative intrathoracic pressure; its outward movement during expiration occurs when the intrathoracic pressure increases above atmospheric pressure (Figure 24-15). Inefficient lung inflation caused by rib fracture and paradoxic breathing limits alveolar ventilation and may progress to hypoventilation, hypercapnia, and progressive alveolar collapse.[193] Treatment includes pain control with measures such as intercostal nerve block with a local anesthetic or insertion of an epidural catheter with a local anesthetic or a narcotic; incentive spirometry to reduce the risk of atelectasis; and, in severe cases, tracheal intubation with mechanical ventilation and PEEP (Box 24-8). Ventilator settings are adjusted so that wide swings in pleural pressure are decreased or avoided. Surgical fixation of the rib cage may be indicated in some patients. The mortality rate is directly related to the underlying and associated injuries and is reported to be between 8% and 35%.[192]

PNEUMOTHORAX

Pneumothorax can be subdivided into three categories, depending on whether air has direct access to the pleural cavity.

Simple Pneumothorax

In simple pneumothorax no communication exists with the atmosphere (Figure 24-16). Additionally, no shift of the mediastinum or hemidiaphragm results from the accumulation of air

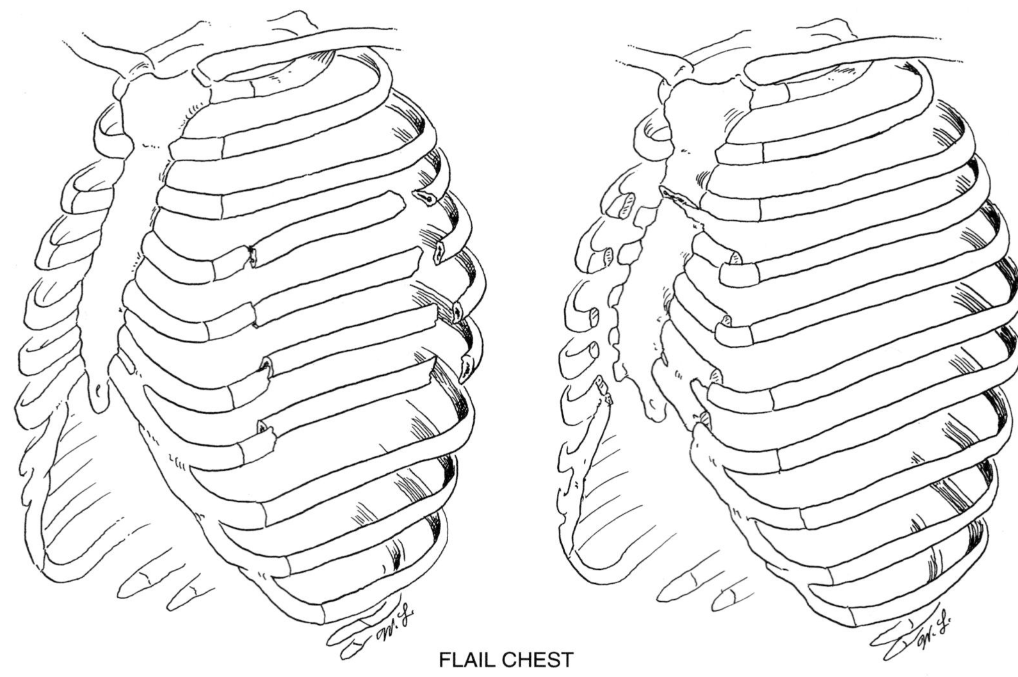

FIGURE **24-14**
Fracture of several adjacent ribs in two places with lateral flail or central flail segments. (Redrawn from Eckstein M, Henderson S, Markovchick V. Thorax. In: Marx JA, Hockberger RS, Walls RM, eds. *Rosen's Emergency Medicine: Concepts and Clinical Practice*. 5th ed. St Louis: Mosby; 2002:385.)

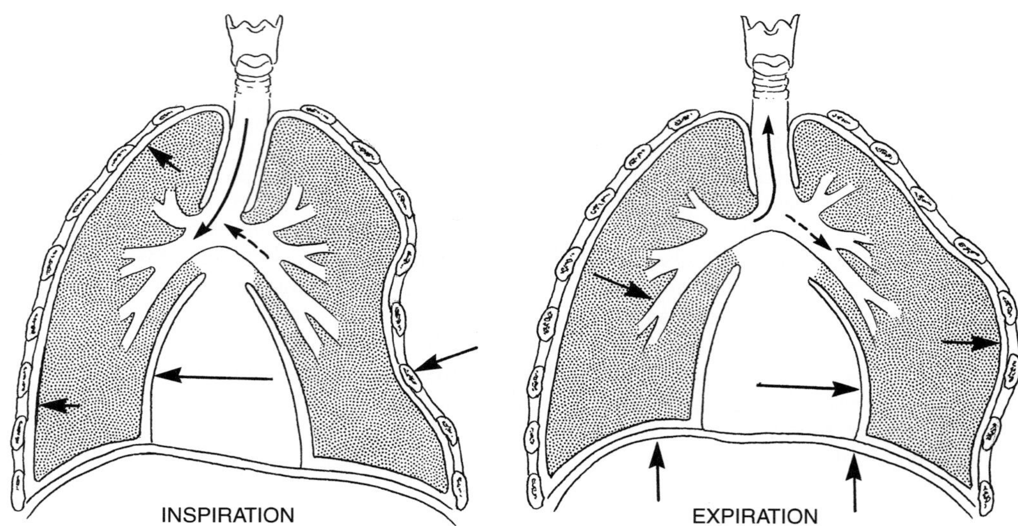

FIGURE **24-15**
On inspiration, flail section sinks in as chest expands, impairing ability to produce negative intrapleural pressure to draw in air. Mediastinum shifts to uninjured side. On expiration, flail segment bulges outward, impairing ability to exhale. Mediastinum shifts to injured side. Air may shift uselessly from side to side in severe flail chest *(broken arrows)*. (Redrawn from Eckstein M, Henderson S, Markovchick V. Thorax. In: Marx JA, Hockberger RS, Walls RM, eds. *Rosen's Emergency Medicine: Concepts and Clinical Practice*. 5th ed. St Louis: Mosby; 2002:389.)

BOX **24-8**

Indications for Treatment of Flail Chest with Mechanical Ventilation

Respiratory Failure Manifested by One or More of the Following Criteria:

Clinical signs of respiratory fatigue
Respiratory rate >35/min or <8 min
$Pa{O_2}$ <60 min Hg at $F{I}{O_2}$ ≥0.5
$Pa{CO_2}$ <55 min Hg at $F{I}{O_2}$ ≥0.5
Alveolar-arterial oxygen gradient >450
Clinical evidence of severe shock
Associated severe head injury with lack of airway control or need to ventilate
Severe associated injury necessitating surgery

in the intrapleural space. The severity of pneumothorax is graded on the basis of the degree of collapse: collapse of 15% or less is small; collapse of 15% to 60% is moderate; and collapse of greater than 60% is large. Treatment of a simple pneumothorax is determined by the size and cause of injury and may include catheter aspiration or tube thoracostomy; close observation of the patient with simple pneumothorax is essential.

Communicating Pneumothorax

In communicating pneumothorax, air in the pleural cavity exchanges with atmospheric air through a defect in the chest wall (Figure 24-17). Because the exchange of air may often be heard through the site of injury, this entity is commonly known as a "sucking chest wound." Communicating pneumothorax represents a severe ventilatory disturbance because the affected lung collapses on inspiration and expands slightly on expiration. The exchange of air in and out of the wound

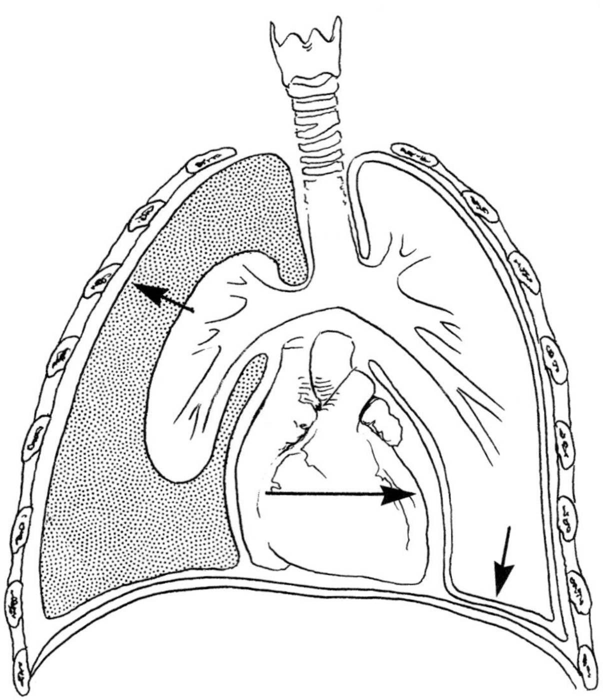

FIGURE **24-16**
Closed pneumothorax. Simple pneumothorax is present in the right lung, with air in the pleural cavity and collapse of right lung. (Redrawn from Eckstein M, Henderson S, Markovchick V. Thorax. In: Marx JA, Hockberger RS, Walls RM, eds. *Rosen's Emergency Medicine: Concepts and Clinical Practice*. 5th ed. St Louis: Mosby; 2002:388.)

results in a large functional dead space and a decrease in the efficacy of ventilation.

The wound should be covered with an occlusive dressing immediately. Development of tension pneumothorax is possible (see next section). The injury should never be packed during inspiration, because the negative pressure could suck the dressing into the chest cavity. Treatment measures include administration of supplemental O_2, tube thoracostomy, and intubation; mechanical ventilation may be indicated.

Tension Pneumothorax

Tension pneumothorax develops when air progressively accumulates under pressure within the pleural cavity (Figure 24-18). If the pressure becomes too great, the mediastinum shifts to the opposite hemithorax, and this causes compression of the contralateral lung and great vessels. Subsequently venous return is decreased, and air enters the pleural space but cannot exit. Respiratory and cardiac disturbances ensue, exhibited by a decrease in CO, a decrease in blood pressure, an increase in CVP, and a shunting of blood to nonventilated areas. The hallmark signs of tension pneumothorax are hypotension, hypoxemia, tachycardia, increased CVP, and increased airway pressure. Other findings include absence of breath sounds on the affected side, asymmetric chest wall movement, tracheal shift, displacement of the cardiac impulse, and hyperresonance to percussion in the affected hemithorax. Also, the patient may exhibit extreme anxiety.

Tension pneumothorax is potentially lethal; therefore immediate treatment is essential. Decompression of the chest can be performed with the insertion of a 16- or 18-gauge angiocatheter into the second or third interspace anteriorly or the fourth or fifth interspace laterally. A rush of air is heard when decompression occurs. The angiocatheter must be covered if the sucking of more air into the pleura is to be prevented.

Hemothorax

A hemothorax is the accumulation of blood in the pleural cavity. It usually is a result of trauma (Figure 24-19), but other causes include the rupture of small blood vessels in the presence of inflammation, pneumonia, tuberculosis, or erosion by tumors.

The treatment of hemothorax consists of airway management as necessary, restoration of circulating blood volume, and evacuation of the accumulated blood. Thoracostomy may be indicated if the initial bleeding rate is greater than 20 ml/kg/hr. If bleeding subsides but its rate remains greater than 7 ml/kg/hr, if chest radiograph worsens, or if hypotension persists after initial blood replacement and decompression, thoracostomy is indicated.

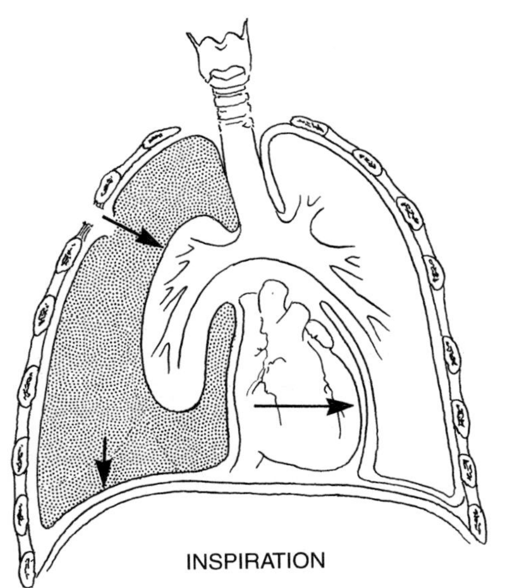

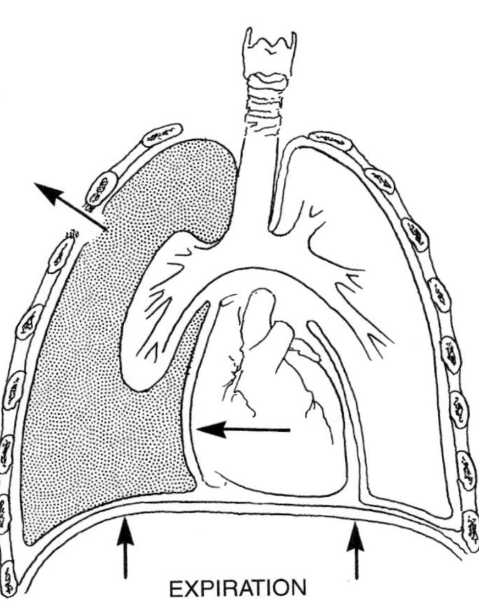

FIGURE **24-17**
Communicating pneumothorax. The right lung has collapsed, and air is present in the pleural cavity, with communication to the outside through the defect in the chest wall. In sucking chest wounds, lung volume is greater with expiration. (Redrawn from Eckstein M, Henerson S, Markovchick V. Thorax. In: Marx JA, Hockberger RS, Walls RM, eds. *Rosen's Emergency Medicine: Concepts and Clinical Practice*. 5th ed. St Louis: Mosby; 2002:389.)

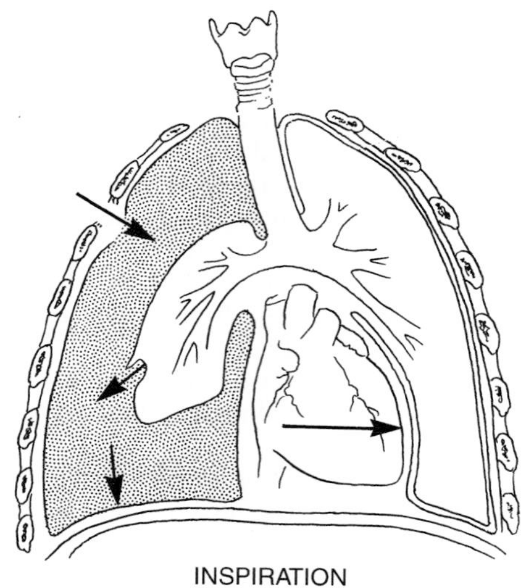

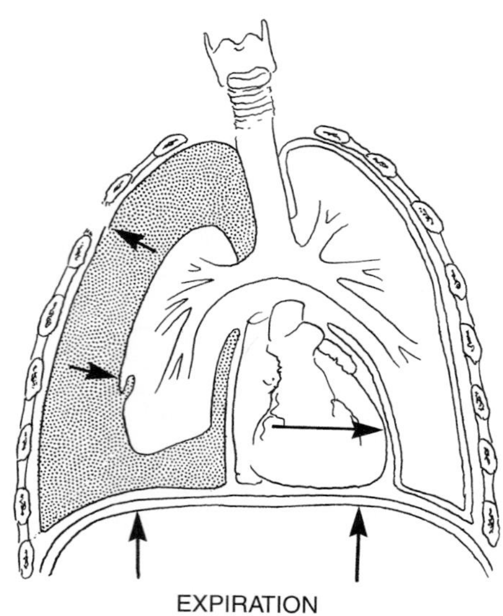

FIGURE **24-18**
Tension pneumothorax. Shown are right pneumothorax under tension, total collapse of right lung, and shift of mediastinal structures to left. (Redrawn from Eckstein M, Henderson S, Markovchick V. Thoracic trauma. In: Marx JA, Hockberger RS, Walls RM, eds. *Rosen's Emergency Medicine: Concepts and Clinical Practice*. 5th ed. St Louis: Mosby; 2002:389.)

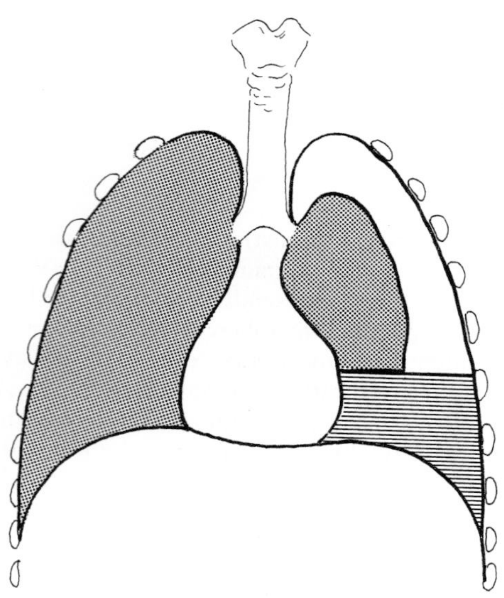

FIGURE **24-19**
Hemopneumothorax. Note that the fluid level produces a straight line as opposed to a meniscus when pneumothorax is present with the pleural fluid. (From Roberts RR, Hedges JR, eds. *Clinical Procedures in Emergency Medicine*. 2nd ed. Philadelphia: Saunders; 1991:129.)

Pathogenesis

Different presentations may be distinguished, according to the mechanism of injury.

Spontaneous. Hemothorax usually is caused by rupture of alveoli near the pleural surface of the lung after a forceful sneeze or cough. This mechanism is most common in individuals with a long narrow chest and in those with emphysema.

Traumatic. Hemothorax, pneumothorax, and flail chest may occur after blunt chest trauma; however, they most frequently occur after rib fracture. Hemopneumothorax also may occur with penetrating injury.

Iatrogenic. Hemothorax, pneumothorax, and flail chest may occur after any of the following:

1. Subclavian central line insertion (incidence, 2% to 16%)
2. Supraclavicular block to the brachial plexus (incidence, 1%; hemothorax, pneumothorax, and flail chest can be complications of interscalene block but are rare with intercostal block)
3. Barotrauma (resulting from overdistention of the alveoli by PEEP; an abrupt deterioration of P_{AO_2} and cardiovascular function during PEEP administration should arouse suspicion of pulmonary barotrauma, especially pneumothorax)
4. Exposure to high airway pressures (e.g., during mechanical ventilation)
5. Other surgical procedures (e.g., mediastinoscopy, radical neck dissection, mastectomy, or nephrectomy)

Nitrous Oxide and Pneumothorax

The blood-gas partition coefficient of N_2O (0.47) is 34 times greater than that of nitrogen (0.014). This differential solubility means than N_2O can leave the blood to enter an air-filled cavity 34 times more rapidly than nitrogen can leave the cavity and enter the blood. As a result, the volume or pressure of the air-filled cavity surrounded by a compliant wall increases. In an animal model the inhalation of 75% N_2O doubles the volume of a pneumothorax in 10 minutes.[194] N_2O is acceptable for use if the chest tube is patent and functioning. A closed pneumothorax is a contraindication to the administration of N_2O. Decreased pulmonary compliance (increased pulmonary inspiratory pressure) during administration of anesthesia to patients with a history of chest trauma may reflect the expansion of an unrecognized pneumothorax.

ATELECTASIS

Definition

Atelectasis is an abnormal condition characterized by a collapse of pulmonary tissue that prevents the respiratory exchange of CO_2 and O_2. Atelectasis can involve a small localized area or an entire lung. The two most common causes of atelectasis are obstruction of the airway and lack of surfactant.[195]

BOX 24-9

Risk Factors for Postoperative Pulmonary Complications

Factors Related to the Patient
Chronic obstructive pulmonary disease
Advanced age
Extensive (and recent) smoking history
Obesity
High physical status category according to American Society of Anesthesiologists guidelines

Factors Related to the Surgery
Thoracic and upper abdominal procedures
Emergency surgery
Prolonged anesthesia time (>3 hr)
Large intraoperative blood transfusion requirements

Etiology and Pathophysiology

Atelectasis results from a blockage or obstruction of many small bronchi or of a major bronchus. Absorption atelectasis may occur if lung tissue is pliable and allows alveolar collapse. However, if lung tissue is unable to collapse, absorption of air from the alveoli creates a tremendous negative pressure within the alveoli; this negative pressure pulls fluid from the pulmonary interstitium into the alveoli, causing alveolar edema. This condition, called *massive collapse* of the lung, occurs when the entire lung becomes atelectatic because the stability of the chest wall and mediastinum allows reduction in lung volume to one-half normal, rather than causing complete collapse. The remaining volume is filled with fluid.

Massive collapse of the lung causes physiologic changes in pulmonary function. An increase in PVR occurs from compression of the pulmonary vessels as lung volumes diminish. Hypoxia in the collapsed alveoli causes further vasoconstriction. Despite the vasoconstriction, blood is shunted to the aerated lung; this usually produces moderate compromise and mild O_2 desaturation.

Incidence and Outcome

Atelectasis occurs most frequently after thoracic and upper abdominal procedures, with rates of incidence reaching 80% (Box 24-9). It is the most common postoperative cause of respiratory dysfunction. Postoperative atelectasis most often is subclinical and resolves spontaneously within 24 to 48 hours. No recent data support that atelectasis predisposes one to the development of pneumonia.

Treatment

Standard postoperative measures for improving pulmonary function include incentive spirometry, deep breathing, intermittent positive-pressure breathing, and administration of CPAP, with the last of these offering the greatest superiority by increasing FRC. Intraoperatively an increase in V_T, a decrease in respiratory rate, and periodic sighs occur.

PLEURAL EFFUSION

Pleural effusion is the abnormal accumulation of fluid in the pleural space. It usually is an indication of disorders or disease complications in the surrounding structures. Possible causes of effusion are the following: (1) blockage of lymphatic drainage from the pleural cavity; (2) cardiac failure, which causes an increase in pulmonary capillary pressures and eventual movement of fluid into the pleural cavity; (3) reductions in plasma colloid osmotic pressure; and (4) infection or any other inflammatory process of the pleural membranes that alters capillary membrane permeability.

Treatment modalities include tube thoracostomy, thoracentesis, and pleurodesis. Pleurodesis is a procedure used to prevent the reaccumulation of pleural fluid. Inflammation is produced with injection of a sclerosing agent, usually tetracycline, into the chest tube; adhesion formation and fusion of the pleural membranes result.

SKELETAL DISORDERS

The primary pathophysiology of skeletal disorders is an alteration in the structure of the thorax that diminishes chest wall excursion. Disorders commonly producing this restriction of breathing include sternal deformities, kyphoscoliosis, and ankylosing spondylitis (AS).

Pectus Deformities

Pectus Excavatum

Pectus excavatum, also referred to as *funnel chest*, is the most common chest wall deformity, occurring in 1 in 400 children.[196] It is a congenital abnormality characterized by depression of the sternum (usually above the xiphisternal junction) and symmetric or asymmetric prominence of the ribs on either side. Pectus excavatum is the most common chest wall deformity, but its origin is unknown; however, it is thought that excessive diaphragmatic traction on the lower sternum or displacement of the heart into the left hemithorax is largely responsible.[197] Family history of some type of anterior thoracic deformity is present in 37% of patients. If uncorrected, the disease usually worsens at adolescence. Self-limiting deformities are either gone or vastly improved by the age of 3 years.[198]

Clinically the majority of patients are asymptomatic unless pectus excavatum is extreme. Patients with pectus excavatum have reduced chest cavities and TLC compared with normal subjects; however, pulmonary function often is normal except in severe cases, in which VC, TLC, and maximum breathing capacity may be diminished. The indications for repair of pectus excavatum are the subject of controversy. Conflicting data have been presented regarding whether the repair of pectus excavatum is performed only for cosmetic purposes or whether it actually improves cardiorespiratory function and exercise tolerance.[199] Some clinicians suggest that pectus excavatum should be corrected in childhood—ideally when patients are between the ages of 4 and 6 years—to relieve the structural compromise of the chest, to allow normal growth of the thorax, to prevent pulmonary and cardiac dysfunction in teens and adults, and to improve cosmetic appearance.[200] Others have found that surgery does not significantly improve pulmonary function and that exercise tolerance and cardiorespiratory function during exercise do not benefit significantly from surgical correction.[201] Patients with Marfan's syndrome have a high incidence of chest wall deformities; they usually are seen in their most severe form and often are accompanied by scoliosis. Other musculoskeletal diseases that may be present in patients with pectus excavatum are listed in Table 24-32. Congenital heart disease, mitral valve prolapse,

TABLE 24-32 Musculoskeletal Abnormalities Identified in 133 of 704 Cases of Pectus Excavatum

Abnormality	Number of Cases
Scoliosis	107
Kyphosis	4
Myopathy	3
Poland's syndrome	3
Marfan's syndrome	2
Pierre Robin syndrome	2
Prune belly syndrome	2
Neurofibromatosis	3
Cerebral palsy	4
Tuberous sclerosis	1
Congenital diaphragmatic hernia	2

From Shields TW. General Thoracic Surgery. *Philadelphia: Lea & Febiger; 1994.*

and asthma also occur more frequently in patients with pectum excavatum. Electrocardiographic abnormalities are common and attributable to the abnormal chest wall configuration and to the displacement and rotation of the heart into the left thoracic cavity. A systolic ejection murmur of grades II to III or IV frequently is identified.

Pectus Carinatum

Pectus carinatum is characterized by a longitudinal protrusion of the sternum. It is the second most common chest deformity, occurring in 1 or 2 persons per 1000. A familial tendency exists, and the disorder is more frequent in males than in females (4:1). The pathogenesis is unclear, and the disorder may be congenital or acquired. The development of pectus carinatum is thought to result from the overgrowth of the costal cartilages, which results in displacement of the sternum. The development of pectus carinatum has also been associated with severe childhood asthma and rickets.[202] The physiologic effects are probably related to the restriction of thoracic excursion. Patients with pectus carinatum have an increased incidence of congenital heart disease, including ventricular septal defect, patent ductus arteriosis, atrial-septal defects, and mitral valve abnormalities.[203]

Three classifications of pectus carinatum exist. Type I—pigeon breast or keel chest—consists of symmetric protrusion of the sternum and costal cartilages. Type II—pouter pigeon breast or Currarino-Silverman syndrome—is characterized by protrusion of the manubrium of the first two sternal cartilages, backward arching of the sternal body, and anterior displacement of the xiphoid process. Type III—lateral pectus carinatum—is manifested by unilateral protrusion of the anterior chest wall.[204]

Surgery is the only effective treatment for pectus carinatum and is performed to alleviate possible cardiopulmonary dysfunction and to prevent progressive postural deformities, as well as for cosmetic reasons.

KYPHOSCOLIOSIS

Definition

Kyphosis is a deformity marked by an accentuated posterior curvature. Scoliosis is a lateral curvature of the spine. Kyphoscoliosis results when both kyphosis and scoliosis occur concomitantly, causing a lateral bending and rotation of the vertebral column. Scoliosis alone, despite its severity, does not cause sensory or motor impairment. In contrast, kyphosis and kyphoscoliosis may induce cord damage because of the sharp angulation of the spine. Respiratory dysfunction is associated with scoliosis, significant kyphosis, and severe kyphoscoliosis.

Incidence and Outcome

Scoliosis is the most common spinal deformity, with an incidence of 4 persons per 1000.[205] The etiologic classification of scoliosis is composed of five categories: idiopathic, congenital, neuropathic (e.g., poliomyelitis, cerebral palsy, syringomyelia, and Friedreich's ataxia), myopathic (e.g., muscular dystrophy and amyotonia), and traumatic. Idiopathic scoliosis is the most common deformity, accounting for 80% of all cases. On the basis of the time of onset, idiopathic scoliosis is divided into the following two categories: (1) the rare infantile form (male-to-female ratio, 6:4); and (2) the common adolescent form (male-to-female ratio, 1:9). The children in the adolescent group are born with a straight spine; however, at some point during the growth period, the spine begins to bend and deform, with deformation progressively worsening until growth ends. However, conflicting studies by Collis and Ponseti have demonstrated that curvatures tend to progress throughout life rather than to stop progressing at the end of growth.[206] In general, curves associated with adolescent idiopathic scoliosis are convex and deviated to the right, whereas those related to other disease may be deviated to the left. The presence of cervical scoliosis should alert anesthesia personnel to potential difficulties in airway management. Any significant curvature involving the thoracic spine may alter lung function. Unless deformity is severe, patients with kyphosis are able to maintain normal pulmonary function; in contrast, even mild forms of scoliosis can result in impaired ventilatory function.

A long-term study of pulmonary function tests performed 20 years apart in patients with unfused scoliosis (nonoperated) demonstrated that respiratory failure occurred in patients with a VC less than 45% of that predicted during initial testing who had an angle of curvature greater than 110 degrees. Results also showed that the initial VC was the strongest predictor of the development of respiratory failure (magnitude of the scoliotic angle was the second strongest indicator).[207]

Severe thoracic deformity may result in respiratory alterations during sleep. Several types of breathing abnormalities have been documented, including obstructive apnea and hypopnea. The lowest HbO_2 saturations occurred during rapid–eye-movement sleep.[208]

Respiratory mechanics in anesthetized young patients with kyphoscoliosis are characterized by an increase in mean total respiratory elastance, chest wall elastance, and respiratory flow resistance during corrective spinal surgery for kyphoscoliosis that may have resulted from rib cage trauma and changes in airway caliber, with microatelectasis and uneven distribution of mechanical properties within the lung. Spinal correction results in immediate and short-term deterioration of respiratory mechanics in anesthetized patients.[209]

Clinical Features and Diagnosis

Diminution of pulmonary function occurs with curvatures of greater than 60 degrees, and pulmonary symptoms develop with curvatures greater than 70 degrees (as measured by the Cobb technique; Figure 24-20). Curvatures greater than 100 degrees

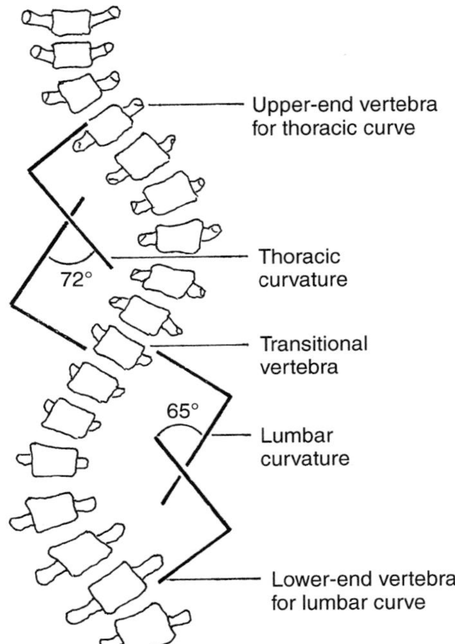

FIGURE **24-20**
Cobb method of measuring scoliosis curves. First, the "end vertebrae" of the curve are identified. These are the vertebrae that have the maximum tilting toward the curve to be measured. Then, horizontal lines are drawn at the superior border of the superior end vertebra and at the inferior border of the inferior end vertebra. Then, perpendicular lines are erected from each of the horizontal lines. The angle between the intersecting perpendicular lines is the angle of curvature. (From Prakash UB. Pulmonary manifestations in systemic diseases. In: Baum GL, Wolinsky E, eds. *Textbook of Pulmonary Diseases*. Vol 2. 5th ed. Boston: Little, Brown; 1993:1692.)

may be associated with significant gas exchange impairment.[210] In general, the greater the curvature, the greater the loss of pulmonary function. Because of this, mechanical ventilation becomes inefficient; this inefficiency is the major factor causing respiratory embarrassment.[211] At the time of diagnosis, it often is possible to document a reduction in lung capacity. The characteristic deformity seen in scoliosis causes one hemithorax to become relatively smaller than the other.

Skeletal chest wall deformity in kyphoscoliosis leads to a reduction in lung volumes and the pulmonary vascular bed.[212] Ventilatory failure associated with severe kyphoscoliosis produces a lung size that is 30% to 65% of normal. As the patient ages, the chest wall becomes less compliant; this increases the work of breathing and leads to hypoventilation and respiratory muscle weakness.

The main features of lung mechanics in the patient with early-stage scoliosis are reduced lung volumes (VC, TLC, FRC, and RV) and reduced chest wall compliance; in the late stages of disease, $\dot{V}/\dot{Q}$ mismatching with hypoxemia (attributed to alveolar hypoventilation because of a decrease in V_T), increased PAP, hypercapnia, abnormal response to CO_2 stimulation, increased work of breathing, and cor pulmonale occur and eventually lead to cardiorespiratory failure.[212] Reduction in VC to 60% to 80% of the predicted value is a typical finding.[210] FEV_1/FVC is normal unless other pulmonary diseases are present. Although normocarbia prevails for most of the clinical course, an elevated $PACO_2$ signifies the onset of respiratory failure. The severity of hypercapnia most closely correlates with the patient's age and inspiratory muscle strength.

Associated Conditions

Scoliosis may be associated with several cardiovascular abnormalities, of which mitral valve prolapse is the most common. If mitral regurgitation is present, antibiotic prophylaxis is indicated before surgical manipulation. Other common changes include an increase in PVR and ensuing PH, which leads to the development of right ventricular hypertrophy. Several contributing factors are thought to be responsible for the development of increased PVR. First, arterial hypoxemia results in pulmonary vasoconstriction. Second, changes in the pulmonary arterioles consequent to the increased pulmonic pressure may cause narrowing and result in irreversible PH. Third, a compressed chest wall may increase vascular resistance in affected areas. Fourth, development of scoliosis at an early age inhibits growth of the pulmonary vascular bed. Alveolar multiplication is nearly complete by 2 years of age but continues until the age of 8 years. During the first few years lung growth occurs primarily by enlargement of existing alveoli. Olgiati and coworkers have supported this argument by showing that a decrease in diffusion capacity results from partial failure of alveolar enlargement because of the thoracic deformity rather than any atrophy of the alveoli or pulmonary vasculature.[212]

Treatment

The management of scoliosis may include the following: (1) observation of the problem without active medical treatment; (2) treatment by nonoperative methods that include the use of braces or electronic stimulators; and (3) operative methods such as anterior or posterior spinal fusion and instrumentation, such as Harrington rod insertion.[213] The largest studies by Nachemson and Nilsonne have shown that the mortality rate among persons with untreated scoliosis is twice that of the normal population and the rate for those with thoracic curvatures alone was fourfold that of the normal population.[214,215] Patients with congenital thoracic scoliosis are particularly at risk for cor pulmonale.[215]

Anesthetic Management

Preoperative Evaluation

Preoperatively a thorough review of systems is essential. The severity of scoliosis and of any underlying conditions must be noted. Any reversible pulmonary involvement such as pneumonia should be corrected before elective surgery. Laboratory data should include complete blood count; prothrombin time; partial thromboplastin time; values for electrolytes, blood urea nitrogen, and creatinine; ECG; chest radiography; and routine pulmonary function test values. ABG analysis may be indicated if the results of the pulmonary function tests reflect significant impairment or if the surgical procedure dictates its need. Because these procedures can potentially involve large blood losses, young healthy asymptomatic patients may donate autologous blood. Blood typing and cross-match also are required.

When sedatives are used in the preoperative area, care must be taken to ensure that respiratory status is not depressed. The need for intraoperative monitoring is dictated by the type of surgery and the physical status of the patient. No specific anesthetic techniques have been shown to be superior in patients with scoliosis; however, N_2O may increase PVR by direct vasoconstrictive effects on the pulmonary vasculature. It has been suggested that scoliosis is associated with an increased incidence of malignant hyperthemia.[216] Ventilation should be adjusted so that adequate arterial oxygenation and normocarbia are maintained.

Patients undergoing surgery for correction of the spinal curvature should be informed preoperatively of the possible need for the "wake-up" test; once the patient is able to move both feet on request and surgical correction has been achieved, anesthesia can be quickly reinstituted. The use of somatosensory evoked potentials may require an alteration in anesthetic technique. All anesthetic agents depress somatosensory evoked potentials to a varying degree. Administration of volatile anesthetics should not exceed a minimum alveolar concentration of 1. An N_2O–continuous infusion opioid technique often is preferred. Communication between the technician and anesthetist is essential.

Intraoperative Management

Considerable fluid and blood loss may occur during surgery. The surgeon may request the institution of deliberate hypotension. Deliberate hypotension can be produced with the use of one or more of the following: potent inhalation anesthetics; vasodilators (e.g., sodium nitroprusside, nitroglycerin) or β-adrenergic blocking agents (e.g., propranolol and esmolol). The risks and potential benefits should be weighed against the effects of deliberate hypotension. The mean arterial blood pressure should be maintained at no lower than 60 to 65 mm Hg. Cell Saver blood is often used. Interventions for prevention of hypothermia, such as use of a hot air warming blanket or heated humidifiers, should be employed. Careful positioning is essential.

Postoperative Care

The decision whether to use mechanical ventilation postoperatively is based on the severity of scoliosis and intraoperative events. Most patients with mild to moderate pulmonary dysfunction are able to undergo safe extubation in the operating room. Those with severe deformity should be weaned slowly.

ANKYLOSING SPONDYLITIS

Definition

AS, also known as *rheumatoid spondylitis* and *Marie-Strumpell disease*, is a chronic inflammatory disorder that primarily affects the spine and sacroiliac joints and produces fusion of the spinal vertebrae and the costovertebral joints.

Etiology and Incidence

The cause of AS remains unclear. However, it is strongly associated with the histocompatibility antigen HLA-B27, the presence of which is detected in more than 90% of whites with the disease.[217,218] It is a disease of adults younger than 40 years, and it demonstrates a predilection for males (male-to-female ratio, 9:1). The disease is rare in nonwhites.

Clinical Features and Diagnosis

AS is diagnosed on the basis of clinical criteria that include (1) chronic low back pain with limitation of spinal motion (less than 4 cm as measured by the Schober test); (2) radiographic evidence of bilateral sacroiliitis; and (3) limitation of chest wall expansion (less than a 2.5-cm increase in chest circumference measured at the fourth intercostal space). Extraskeletal manifestations of this disease include iritis, cardiovascular involvement (cardiac conduction defects, aortitis, and aortic insufficiency in 20% of individuals), peripheral arthritis, fever, anemia, fatigue, weight loss, and fibrocavitary (fibrobullous) disease of the apexes of the lungs. The most limiting factors associated with the disease are pain, stiffness, and fatigue.

Complications

Pulmonary complications are reported to occur in 2% to 70% of patients with AS, although 1 large review of 2080 AS patients found the frequency to be less than 2%.[219] Apical fibrosis is the most commonly occurring abnormality, followed by aspergilloma and pleural effusion with nonspecific pleuritis. In apical fibrosis the pulmonary lesion begins with apical pleural thickening and patchy consolidation of one or both apexes and often progresses to dense bilateral fibrosis and air space enlargement. Patients with apical fibrosis usually have advanced AS. Stewart and colleagues suggest that impaired thoracic cage excursion caused by AS results in a greater impairment of apical ventilation and that this may be one factor in the pathogenesis of apical fibrosis.[220]

The most common thoracic complication is fixation of the thoracic cage as a result of costovertebral ankylosis, which can lead to pulmonary dysfunction.[218] In patients with this complication, motion of the thoracic cage is restricted because of fusion of the costovertebral joints; this restriction leads to a decrease in thoracic excursion. Respiratory function typically demonstrates a restrictive pattern with mild diminution of TLC, VC, and DLCO and normal or slightly increased RV and FRC. Pulmonary compliance, diffusion capacity, and ABG values usually are normal.[217] Despite having abnormal pulmonary function, the majority of patients with AS are able to perform normal physical activities without pulmonary symptoms. It has been suggested that patients who exercise regularly and thus improve cardiovascular fitness could maintain a satisfactory work capacity.[221]

Bone ankylosis may occur in the numerous joints around the thorax (the thoracic vertebrae and the costovertebral, costotransverse, sternoclavicular, and sternomanubrial joints), resulting in limitation of chest wall movement. Patients with AS rarely complain of respiratory symptoms or functional impairment unless they have coexisting cardiovascular or respiratory disease. Progressive kyphosis is equivalent to progressive rigidity of the thorax. Increased diaphragmatic function compensates for decreased thoracic motion, allowing lung function to be well preserved. Patients with advanced disease may have an entirely diaphragmatic respiration.[221] Regional lung ventilation in patients with AS is normal unless they have preexisting apical fibrosis.

Cervical spondylosis affects levels C5 to C6 and C6 to C7 most often, and less frequently C4 to C5, C7 to T1, and C3 to C4. The degenerative changes may result in nerve root entrapment by foraminal encroachment. The phrenic nerve, which innervates the diaphragm, is supplied primarily by the C4 nerve root, and to a lesser extent, by the C3 and C5 nerve roots. A case of hemidiaphragmatic paralysis secondary to C4 nerve root compression has been reported.[222]

Cricoarytenoid involvement may exist and can lead to respiratory dysfunction and upper airway obstruction. Cricoarytenoid dysfunction can manifest as a hoarse, weak voice. Respiratory failure from cricoarytenoid ankylosis has necessitated therapeutic tracheostomy. In all reported cases, laryngeal symptoms were present before cricoarytenoid arthritis caused airway compromise. A case of acute respiratory failure and cor pulmonale resulting from cricoarytenoid arthritis has also been reported in a patient with AS.[223]

Treatment

Medical therapy for adult patients with AS is supportive and preventive. Most patients with AS are asymptomatic. Depending on the severity of disease involvement, management may consist of the use of corticosteroids and nonsteroidal antiinflammatory agents. Patients should refrain from smoking tobacco.

Anesthetic Management

Patients with AS have specific anesthetic requirements.[224] Management of the upper airway is the priority because of the potential for obstruction. Cervical spine involvement may result in limitation of movement. The ankylosed neck is more susceptible to hyperextension injury, and cervical fracture may occur. Intubation awake with or without the use of a fiberoptic bronchoscope is indicated. In rare situations tracheostomy must be performed with the patient under local anesthesia before anesthesia can be induced. A regional anesthetic technique may not be feasible because of skeletal involvement that precludes access or because of neurologic complications such as spinal cord compression, cauda equina syndrome, focal epilepsy, vertebral basilar insufficiency, and peripheral nerve lesions. Patients with cardiovascular system involvement may require antibiotic coverage, treatment of heart failure, or insertion of a temporary pacemaker before surgery. Restriction of chest expansion and, rarely, pulmonary fibrosis necessitate performance of a thorough preoperative assessment and immediate postoperative mechanical ventilation. Careful attention to positioning is essential.

REFERENCES

1. Norton ML, Brown A. *Atlas of the Difficult Airway*. St Louis: Mosby; 1991:11.
2. Ellis H, Feldman S. *Anatomy for Anaesthetists*. London: Blackwell; 1988:7.
3. Whitten C. *Anyone Can Intubate*. San Diego: KW Publications; 1997:12.
4. Guyton AC, Hall JE. *Textbook of Medical Physiology*. 10th ed. Philadelphia: Saunders; 2001:432-443.
5. Miller RD. *Anesthesia*. 5th ed. New York: Churchill Livingstone; 2000:414.
6. Ackerman U. *Essentials of Human Physiology*. St Louis: Mosby; 1999:53.
7. Levitzky MG. *Pulmonary Physiology*. 4th ed. New York: McGraw-Hill; 1996:12.
8. Nunn JF. *Nunn's Applied Respiratory Physiology*. 4th ed. Oxford: Butterworth-Heinemann; 1993:36.
9. Weible ER. Design and structure of the human lung. In: Fishman AP, ed. *Pulmonary Disease and Disorders*. Vol 1. New York: McGraw-Hill; 1980.
10. Reynolds HY. Respiratory structure and function. In: Goldman L, Ausiello D, eds. *Cecil's Textbook of Medicine*. 22nd ed. Philadelphia: Saunders; 2004:495.
11. Murray JF. *The Normal Lung*. 2nd ed. Philadelphia: Saunders; 1986.
12. West JB. *Pulmonary Pathophysiology*. 4th ed. Baltimore: Williams & Wilkins; 1992:3.
13. Kaplan JA. *Thoracic Anesthesia*. 2nd ed. New York: Churchill Livingstone; 1991:143.
14. West JB. *Ventilation: Blood Flow and Gas Exchange*. 5th ed. Oxford, United Kingdom: Blackwell Scientific; 1990.
15. West JB. *Respiratory Physiology—the Essentials*. 4th ed. Baltimore: Williams & Wilkins; 1990.
16. Rose BD. *Clinical Physiology of Acid-Base and Electrolyte Disorders*. 4th ed. New York: McGraw-Hill; 1994:261.
17. Levitzyk MG, Cario JM, Hall SM. *Introductions to Respiratory Care*. Philadelphia: Saunders; 1990.
18. Crystal RG, West JB. *The Lung Scientific Foundations*. New York: Raven; 1991:1307.
19. American Thoracic Society. Standards for the diagnosis and care of patients with chronic obstructive pulmonary disease (COPD) and asthma. *Am Rev Respir Dis*. 1987;136:225-243.
20. Ciba Guest Symposium Report. Terminology, definitions, and classification of chronic pulmonary emphysema and related conditions. *Thorax*. 1959;14:286-299.
21. Campbell EJ, Senior RM. Emphysema. In: Fishman AP, ed. *Update: Pulmonary Diseases and Disorders*. New York: McGraw-Hill; 1991:37.
22. Pauwels RA, Buist S, Calverley MA, et al. Global strategy for the diagnosis, management, and prevention of chronic obstructive pulmonary disease. *Am J Respir Crit Care Med*. 2001;163:1256-1276.
23. Fishman AP. The spectrum of chronic obstructive disease of the airways. In: Fishman AP, ed. *Pulmonary Diseases and Disorders*. 2nd ed. New York: McGraw-Hill; 1988:1164.
24. Sherman CB, Osmanski JP, Hudson LD. Acute exacerbations in COPD patients. In: Cherniak NS, ed. *Chronic Obstructive Pulmonary Disease*. Philadelphia: Saunders; 1991:449.
25. American Thoracic Society. Standards for the diagnosis and care of patients with chronic obstructive pulmonary disease, *Am J Respir Crit Care Med*. 152:S77-120, 1995.
26. Rieves RD, Bass D, Carter RR, Griffith JE, Norman JR. Severe COPD and acute respiratory failure: correlates for survival at the time of tracheal intubation. *Chest*. 1993;104:854-860.
27. US Public Health Service. The health consequences of smoking. A report of the Surgeon General. Washington, DC: US Government Printing Office; 1972. US Department of Health, Education, and Welfare publication HSM 72-7516.
28. Carrell RW, Jeppsson JO, Laurell CB, et al. Structure and variation of human α-1-antitrypsin. *Nature*. 1982;298:329-334.
29. Murphy DM, Fishman AP. Bullous disease of the lung. In: Fishman AP, ed. *Pulmonary Diseases and Disorders*. 2nd ed. New York: McGraw-Hill; 1988:1219.
30. Drain CB. Anesthesia care of the patient with reactive airways disease, *CRNA*. 7:207-212, 1996.
31. Luijendijk SCM, deVries WR, Zwart A. Collateral ventilation by diffusion across the alveolar walls and the exchange of inert gases in the lung. *Eur Respir J*. 1991;4:1228-1236.
32. Cherniack NS, Milic-Emili J. Mechanical aspects of loaded breathing. In: Roussos C, Macklem PT, eds. *Thorax*. New York: Marcel Dekker; 1985:751.
33. Bellemare F, Grassino A. Force reserve of the diaphragm in patients with chronic obstructive pulmonary disease. *J Appl Physiol*. 1983;55:8-15.
34. Jardim J, Farkas G, Prefaut C, Thomas D, Macklem PT, Roussos C. The failing inspiratory muscles under normoxic and hypoxic conditions. *Am Rev Respir Dis*. 1981;124:274-279.
35. Kim CS, Eldridge MA, Wanner A. Airway responsiveness to inhaled and intravenous carbachol in sheep: effect of airway mucus. *J Appl Physiol*. 1988;65:2744-2751.
36. Guyton AC. Physical principles of gaseous exchange: diffusion of oxygen and carbon dioxide through the respiratory membrane. In: Guyton AC, Hall JE, eds. *Textbook of Medical Physiology*. 10th ed. Philadelphia: Saunders; 2000:452-461.
37. Burrows B, Kettel LJ, Niden AH, Rabinowitz M, Diener CF. Patterns of cardiovascular dysfunction in chronic obstructive lung disease. *N Engl J Med*. 1972;286:912-917.

38. Rochester DF. Effects of COPD on the respiratory muscles. In: Cherniak NS, ed. *Chronic Obstructive Pulmonary Disease*. Philadelphia: Saunders; 1991:1135.
39. Janoff A. Elastases and emphysema: current assessment of the protease-antiprotease hypothesis. *Am Rev Respir Dis*. 1985;132: 417-433.
40. Hoidal JR, McCusker KT, Marshall BC, Rao NV. Oxidative damage and COPD. In: Cherniak NS, ed. *Chronic Obstructive Pulmonary Disease*. Philadelphia: Saunders; 1991:45.
41. Thurlbeck WM. Chronic airflow obstruction: correlation of structure and function. In: Petty T, ed. *Chronic Obstructive Pulmonary Disease*. 2nd ed. New York: Marcel Dekker; 1985:1985.
42. Cherniak NS. Control of breathing in COPD. In: Cherniak NS, ed. *Chronic Obstructive Pulmonary Disease*. Philadelphia: Saunders; 1991:118.
43. Natarajan TK, Wise RA, Karam M, Permutt S, Wagner HN Jr. Immediate effect of expiratory loading on left ventricular stroke volume. *Circulation*. 1987;75:139-145.
44. Bilgi C, Jones RL, Sproule BJ. Relation between pulsus paradoxus and pulmonary function in patients with chronic airways obstruction. *CMAJ*. 1977;117:1389-1392.
45. Wise RA. COPD and the peripheral circulation. In: Cherniak NS, ed. *Chronic Obstructive Pulmonary Disease*. Philadelphia: Saunders; 1991:168.
46. Miyamoto K, Nishimura M, Akiyama Y, Yamamoto H, Kishi F, Kawakami Y. Augmented heart rate response to hypoxia in patients with chronic obstructive pulmonary disease. *Am Rev Respir Dis*. 1992;145:1384-1388.
47. Kilburn KH. Fluid retention associated with pulmonary insufficiency and respiratory failure. In: Cherniak NS, ed. *Chronic Obstructive Pulmonary Disease*. Philadelphia: Saunders; 1991:187.
48. Fraser RG, Pare JA. Pulmonary emphysema. *Diagn Dis Chest*. 1979;3:11.
49. Guyton AC. Respiratory insufficiency-pathophysiology, diagnosis, oxygen therapy. In: Guyton AC, Hall JE, eds. *Textbook of Medical Physiology*. 10th ed. Philadelphia: Saunders; 2001: 484-492.
50. Flenley DC. The diagnosis of emphysema. In: Cherniak NS, ed. *Chronic Obstructive Pulmonary Disease*. Philadelphia: Saunders; 1991:352.
51. Bishop MJ. The patient with respiratory disease: evaluation, preparation and timing of surgery. *ASA Annu Refresher Course Lect*. 1992;246:1-7.
52. Gass GD, Olsen GN. Preoperative pulmonary function testing to predict postoperative morbidity and mortality. *Chest*. 1986;89:127-135.
53. American Thoracic Society. Dyspnea. Mechanisms, assessment, and management: a consensus statement. *Am J Respir Crit Care Med*. 1999;159:321-340.
54. Hirshman CA, Bergman NA. Factors influencing intrapulmonary calibre during anesthesia. *Br J Anaesth*. 1990;65:30-42.
55. Nunn JF, Milledge JS, Chen D, Dore C. Respiratory criteria for fitness for surgery and anesthesia. *Anesthesia*. 1988;43:543-551.
56. Fowkes FGR, Lunn JN, Farrow SC, Robertson IB, Samuel P. Epidemiology in anesthesia III: mortality risk in patients with coexisting physical disease. *Br J Anaesth*. 1982;54:819-825.
57. Coursin DB, Croy S, Goelzer SL. Pulmonary disorders. In: Cheng EY, Kay J, eds. *Manual of Anesthesia and the Medically Compromised Patient*. Philadelphia: Lippincott; 1990.
58. Hedenstierna G. Gas exchange during anesthesia. *Br J Anaesth*. 1990;64:507-514.
59. Gunnarsson L, Tokics L, Lundquist H, et al. Chronic obstructive pulmonary disease and anesthesia: formation of atelectasis and gas exchange impairment. *Eur Respir J*. 1991;4:1106-1116.
60. Slinger P. Anesthesia for lung resection. *J Anaesth*. 1990;37:Sxv-Sxxiv.
61. Rehder K, Knopp TJ, Sessler AD, Didier EP. Ventilation-perfusion relationship in young healthy awake and anesthetized-paralyzed man. *J Appl Physiol*. 1979;47:745-753.
62. Wagner PD, Dantzker DR, Dueck R, Clausen JL, West JB. Ventilation-perfusion inequality in chronic obstructive pulmonary disease. *J Clin Invest*. 1977;59:203-216.
63. Bates DV. The lung in transition between health and disease. In: Macklem PT, Permutt S, eds. *Lung Biology in Health and Disease*. Vol 12. New York: Marcel Dekker; 1979.
64. Pepe PE, Marini JJ. Occult positive end-expiratory pressure in mechanically ventilated patients with airflow obstruction: the auto-PEEP effect. *Am Rev Respir Dis*. 1982;126:166-170.
65. Rossi A, Gottfried SB, Zocchi L, et al. Measurement of static compliance of the total respiratory system in patients with acute respiratory failure during mechanical ventilation: the effect of intrinsic positive end-expiratory pressure. *Am Rev Respir Dis*. 1985;131:672-677.
66. Torres A, Reyes A, Roca J, Wagner PD, Rodriguez-Roisin R. Ventilation-perfusion mismatching in chronic obstructive pulmonary disease during ventilator weaning. *Am Rev Respir Dis*. 1989;140:1246-1250.
67. National Heart, Lung, and Blood Institute. National Asthma Education and Prevention Program, Expert Panel Report 2. Guidelines for the diagnosis and management of asthma. Bethesda, Md: US Department of Health and Human Services; 1997. NIH publication no. 97-4051.
68. McFadden ER Jr. Asthma. In: *Diseases of the Respiratory System*. Chapter 252. Available at: http://www.harrisonsonline.com. Accessed February 25, 2003.
69. Laitnen LA, Laitnen A, Haahtela T. Airway mucosal inflammation even in patients with newly diagnosed asthma. *Am Rev Respir Dis*. 1993;147:697-704.
70. Beach JR. Immunologic versus toxicologic mechanisms in airway responses. *Occup Med*. 2000;15:455-470.
71. Bigby TD, Wasserman SI. Asthma. In: Stein JH, ed. *Internal Medicine*. 5th ed. St Louis: Mosby; 1998:1185-1193.
72. Gibson PG, Saltos N, Borgas T. Airway mast cells and eosinophils correlate with clinical severity and airway hyperresponsiveness in corticosteroid-treated asthma. *J Allergy Clin Immunol*. 2000;105:752-759.
73. Kaliner M, Lemanske R. Rhinitis and asthma. *JAMA*. 1992;268:2807-2828.
74. Hall WJ, Douglas RG, Hyde RW, et al. Pulmonary mechanics after uncomplicated influenza A infection. *Am Rev Respir Dis*. 1976;113:141.
75. Moudgil GC. The patient with reactive airways disease. *Can J Anaesth*. 1997;44:R77-R83.
76. Boulet L-P, Laviolette M, Turcotte H, et al. Bronchial subepithelial fibrosis correlates with airway responsiveness to methacholine. *Chest*. 1997;112:45-52.
77. Geer RT. Pulmonary complications of anesthesia. In: Longnecker DE, Tinker JH, Morgan GE, eds. *Principles and Practice of Anesthesiology*. St Louis: Mosby; 1998:232-241.
78. Argyros GJ, Phillips YY, Rayburn DB, Rosenthal RR, Jaeger JJ. Water loss without heat flux in exercise-induced bronchospasm. *Am Rev Respir Dis*. 1993;147:1419-1424.
79. Anderson SD, Daviskas E. The airway microvasculature and exercise-induced asthma. *Thorax*. 1992;47:748-752.
80. McFadden ER. Asthma. In: Braunwald E, et al. *Harrison's Principles of Internal Medicine*. 15th ed. New York: McGraw-Hill; 2001:1456-1462.
81. Dietzel DP, Ciullo JV. Spontaneous pneumothorax after shoulder arthroscopy: a report of four cases. *Arthroscopy*. 1996;12: 99-102.
82. Roizen MF. Anesthetic implications of concurrent diseases. In: Cucchiara RF, Miller ED, Reves JG, Roizen MF, Savarese JJ, eds. *Anesthesia*. New York: Churchill Livingstone; 2000:903-1015.
83. Stoelting RK, Dierdorf SF. Bronchial asthma. In: Stoelting RK, Dierdorf SF, eds. *Anesthesia and Co-Existing Disease*. New York: Churchill Livingstone. 4th ed, 2002;193-204.
84. Hepner DL. Sudden Bronchospasm on intubation: Latex anaphylaxis? *J Clin Anesth*. 2000;12:162-166.

85. Cherniack RM. Pulmonary function testing. In: Mitchell RS, Pety TL, Schwarz MI, eds. *Synopsis of Clinical Pulmonary Disease*. 4th ed. St Louis: Mosby; 1988.
86. Macklem PT. Tests of lung mechanics. *N Engl J Med*. 1975;293:339.
87. Roizen MF. Preoperative evaluation of patients with diseases that require special preoperative evaluation and intraoperative management. In: Miller RD, ed. *Anesthesia*. 5th ed. New York: Churchill Livingstone; 2000:824.
88. Stoelting RK, Miller RD. Chronic pulmonary disease. In: Stoelting RK, Miller RD, eds. *Basics of Anesthesia*. 4th ed. New York: Churchill Livingstone; 2002:177-192.
89. Hurford WE. The bronchospastic patient. *Int Anesthesiol Clin*. 2000;38:77-89.
90. Wong DH, Weber EC, Schell MJ, Wong AB, Anderson CT, Barker SJ. Factors associated with postoperative pulmonary complications in patients with severe chronic obstructive pulmonary disease. *Anesth Analg*. 1995;80:276-284.
91. Smetana GW. Current concepts: preoperative pulmonary evaluation. *N Engl J Med*. 1999;340:937-944.
92. Gass GD, Olsen GN. Preoperative pulmonary function testing to predict postoperative morbidity and mortality. *Chest*. 1986;89:127-135.
93. Kocabas A, Kara K, Ozgur G, Sonmez H, Burut R. Value of preoperative spirometry to predict postoperative pulmonary complications. *Respir Med*. 1996;90:25-33.
94. Kabalin CS, Yarnold PR, Grammer LC. Low complication rate of corticosteroid-treated asthmatics undergoing surgical procedures. *Arch Intern Med*. 1995;155:1379-1384.
95. Gal TJ. Bronchial hyperresponsiveness and anesthesia: physiologic and therapeutic perspectives. *Anesth Analg*. 1994;78: 559-573.
96. Karlet M, Nagelhout J. Asthma: an anesthetic update. Part 3, *AANA J*. 69:317-324, 2001.
97. Christopherson R, Beattie C, Frank SM, et al. Perioperative morbidity in patients randomized to epidural or general anesthesia for lower extremity vascular surgery. *Anesthesiology*. 1993;79:422-434.
98. Yeager MP, Glass DD, Neff RK, Brink-Johnsen T. Epidural anesthesia and analgesia in high-risk surgical patients. *Anesthesiology*. 1987;66:729-736.
99. Pizov R, Brown RH, Weiss YS, et al. Wheezing during induction of general anesthesia in patients with and without asthma. A randomized, blinded trial. *Anesthesiology*. 1995;82:1111-1116.
100. Habre W, Scalfaro P, Sims C, Tiller K, Sly PD. Respiratory mechanics during sevoflurane anesthesia in children with and without asthma. *Anesth Analg*. 1999;89:1177-1181.
101. Rooke GA, Choi JH, Bishop MJ. The effect of isoflurane, halothane, sevoflurane and thiopental/nitrous oxide on respiratory system resistance after tracheal intubation. *Anesthesiology*. 1997;86:1294-1299.
102. Blake K. Asthma. In: Herfindal ET, Gourley DR, eds. *Textbook of Therapeutics*. Philadelphia: William & Wilkins; 2000:727-764.
103. Treatment Guidelines from The Medical Letter. Drugs for Asthma, *The Medical Letter*. 2002;1:7-12.
104. Levy BD, Kitch B, Fant CH. Medical and ventilatory management of status asthmaticus. *Intensive Care Med*. 1998;24:105-117.
105. Jain S, Hanania NA, Guntupalli KK. Ventilation of patients with asthma and obstructive lung disease. *Crit Care Clin*. 1998;14:685-705.
106. Corbridge TC, Hall JB. The assessment and management of adults with status asthmaticus. *Am J Respir Crit Care Med*. 1995;5:1296-1316.
107. Rosen MA. Management of anesthesia for the pregnant surgical patient. *Anesthesiology*. 1999;91:1159-1161.
108. Koren G, Pastusak A, Ito S. Drug therapy: drugs in pregnancy. *N Engl J Med*. 1998;338:1128-1137.
109. Manthous CA. Management of severe exacerbations of asthma. *Am J Med*. 1995;99:298-308.
110. Salvaterra CG, Brundage BH, Rubin LJ. Is the early diagnosis of pulmonary hypertension possible, useful, and cost-effective? In: Weir EK, Archer SL, Reeves JT, eds. *The Diagnosis and Treatment of Pulmonary Hypertension*. Mt Kisco, NY: Futura; 1992.
111. Fishman AP. Pulmonary hypertension and cor pulmonale. In: Fishman AP, ed. *Pulmonary Diseases and Disorders*. 2nd ed. New York: McGraw-Hill; 1988:159.
112. Armstrong P. Thoracic epidural anesthesia and primary pulmonary hypertension. *Anesthesia*. 1992;47:496-499.
113. Rostagno C, Prisco D, Abbate R, Poggesi L. Pulmonary hypertension associated with long-standing thrombocytosis. *Chest*. 1991;99:1303-1305.
114. Gassner A, Sommer G, Fridrich L, Magometschnigg D, Priol A. Differential therapy with calcium channel antagonists in pulmonary hypertension secondary to COPD: hemodynamic effects of nifedipine, diltiazem, and verapamil. *Chest*. 1990;98: 829-834.
115. Costard-Jackle A, Fowler MB. Influence of preoperative pulmonary artery pressure on mortality after heart transplantation: testing of potential reversibility of pulmonary hypertension with nitroprusside is useful in defining a high-risk group. *J Am Coll Cardiol*. 1992;19:48-54.
116. Rozkovec A, Montanes P, Oakley CM. Factors that influence the outcome of primary pulmonary hypertension. *Br Heart J*. 1986;55:449-458.
117. Reeves JT, Groves BM, Turkevich D. The case for treatment of selected patients with primary pulmonary hypertension. *Am Rev Respir Dis*. 1986;134:342-346.
118. Uren NG, et al. Response of the pulmonary circulation to acetylcholine, calcitonin gene-related peptide, substance P and oral nicardipine in patients with primary pulmonary hypertension. *J Am Coll Cardiol*. 1992;19:834-841.
119. Laskey WK, Ferrari VA, Palevsky HI, Kussmaul WG. Pulmonary artery hemodynamics in primary pulmonary hypertension. *J Am Coll Cardiol*. 1993;21:406-412.
120. Morrison DA, Klein C, Welsh CH. Relief of right ventricular angina and increased exercise capacity with long-term oxygen therapy. *Chest*. 1991;100:534-539.
121. Speich R, Jenni R, Opravil M, Pfab M, Russi EW. Primary pulmonary hypertension in HIV infection. *Chest*. 1991;100: 1268-1271.
122. Moser KM, Bloor CM. Pulmonary vascular lesions occurring in patients with chronic major vessel thromboembolic pulmonary hypertension. *Chest*. 1993;103:685-692.
123. Abramson SV, Burke JF, Kelly JJ Jr, et al. Pulmonary hypertension predicts mortality and morbidity in patients with dilated cardiomyopathy. *Ann Intern Med*. 1992;116:888-895.
124. Eysmann SB, Palevsky HI, Reichek N, Hackney K, Douglas PS. Echo/Doppler and hemodynamic correlates of vasodilator responsiveness in primary pulmonary hypertension. *Chest*. 1991;99:1066-1071.
125. Rich S, Kaufmann E. High-dose titration of calcium channel blocking agents for primary pulmonary hypertension: guidelines for short-term drug testing. *J Am Coll Cardiol*. 1991;18: 1323-1327.
126. Hickey PR, Hansen DD, Cramolini GM, Vincent RN, Lang P. Pulmonary and systemic hemodynamic responses to ketamine in infants with normal and elevated pulmonary vascular resistance. *Anesthesiology*. 1985;62:287-293.
127. Stoelting RK, Dierdorf SF. Cor pulmonale In: Stoelting RK, Dierdorf SF, eds. *Anesthesia and Coexisting Disease*. 4th ed. New York: Churchill Livingstone; 2002:127-134.
128. Morgan JM, Griffiths M, du Bois RM, Evans TW. Hypoxic pulmonary vasoconstriction in systemic sclerosis and primary pulmonary hypertension. *Chest*. 1991;99:551-556.
129. Weir EK, Reeves JT. *Pulmonary Hypertension*. Mt Kisco, NY: Futura; 1984:292.
130. Armstrong P. Thoracic epidural anaesthesia and primary pulmonary hypertension. *Anesthesia*. 1992;47:496-499.

131. Guyton AC, Hall JE. Pulmonary circulation; pulmonary edema; pleural fluid. In: Guyton AC, Hall JE, eds. *Textbook of Medical Physiology*. 10th ed. Philadelphia: Saunders; 2000:444-450.
132. Burrows B, et al. Patterns of cardiovascular dysfunction in chronic obstructive lung disease. *N Engl J Med*. 1972;286:912-918.
133. Enson Y, et al. The influence of hydrogen ion concentration and hypoxia on the pulmonary circulation. *J Clin Invest*. 1964;43:1146.
134. Salvaterra CG, Brundage BH, Rubin LJ. Is the early diagnosis of pulmonary hypertension possible, useful, and cost-effective? In: Weir EK, Archer SL, Reeves JT, eds. *The diagnosis and Treatment of Pulmonary Hypertension*. Mt Kisco, NY: Futura; 1992.
135. Weitzenblum E. Acute respiratory failure in the patient with obstructive airways disease. In: Fishman AP. *Pulmonary Diseases and Disorders*. 2nd ed. New York: McGraw-Hill; 1988:2292.
136. Ingram R. Chronic bronchitis, emphysema, and chronic airways obstruction. In: Braunwald E, ed. *Harrison's Principles of Internal Medicine*. 15th ed. New York: McGraw-Hill; 2001:1491-1498.
137. Cooper CB, Howard P. An analysis of sequential physiologic changes in hypoxic cor pulmonale during long-term oxygen therapy. *Chest*. 1991;100:76-80.
138. Bovill JG, Sebel PS, Stanley TH. Opioid analgesics in anesthesia: with special reference to their use in cardiovascular anesthesia. *Anesthesiology*. 1984;61:731-755.
139. Berqvist D, Lindblad B. A 30-year survey of pulmonary embolism verified at autopsy: an analysis of 1274 surgical patients. *Br J Surg*. 1985;72:105-108.
140. West JB. Vascular diseases. In: West JB, ed. *Pulmonary Pathophysiology: the Essentials*. 5th ed. Baltimore: Williams & Wilkins; 1997:95.
141. Roizen MF. Anesthetic implications of concurrent diseases. In: Miller RD, ed. *Anesthesia*. 5th ed. New York: Churchill Livingstone; 2000:903.
142. Donegan J. *Manual of Anesthesia for Emergency Surgery*. New York: Churchill Livingstone; 1987.
143. McCarren JP. Respiratory diseases. In: Benumof J, ed. *Anesthesia and Uncommon Diseases: Pathophysiologic and Clinical Correlates*. 4th ed. Philadelphia: Saunders; 1998:51.
144. Brown M. ICU: critical care. In: Barash PG, Cullen BF, Stoelting RK, eds. *Clinical Anesthesia*. 4th ed. Philadelphia: Lippincott; 2001:1463-1484.
145. Moser KM. Thromboembolic disease therapy. In: Bordow RA, Moser KM, eds. *Manual of Clinical Problems in Pulmonary Medicine*. 4th ed. Boston: Little, Brown; 1996:296.
146. Magnant JG, Walsh DB, Juravsky LI, Cronenwett JL. Current use of inferior vena cava filters. *J Vasc Surg*. 1992;16:701-706.
147. Arcelus JI, Caprini JA, Monreal M, Suarez C, Gonzalez-Fajardo J. The management and outcome of acute venous thromboembolism: a prospective registry including 4011 patients. *J Vasc Surg*. 38:916-922, 2003.
148. Buchalter SE, Groves RH, Zorn GL. Surgical management of chronic pulmonary thromboembolic disease. *Clin Chest Med*. 1992;13:17-22.
149. Daily PO, Dembitsky WP, Iversen S. Risk factors for pulmonary thromboendarterectomy. *J Thorac Cardiovasc Surg*. 1990;99: 670-678.
150. Olman MA, Auger WR, Fedullo PF, Moser KM. Pulmonary vascular steal in chronic thromboembolic pulmonary hypertension. *Chest*. 1990;98:1430-1434.
151. Perel A. Pulmonary edema. In: Civetta JM, Taylor RW, Kirby RR. *Critical Care*. Philadelphia: Lippincott; 1988:1043.
152. Fishman AP. Pulmonary edema. In: Fishman AP, ed. *Pulmonary Diseases and Disorders*. 2nd ed. New York: McGraw-Hill; 1988:919.
153. Matthay MA, Matthay RA. Pulmonary edema: cardiogenic and noncardiogenic. In: George RB, Light RW, Matthay MA, Matthay R, eds. *Chest Medicine: Essentials of Pulmonary and Critical Care Medicine*. 2nd ed. Baltimore: Williams & Wilkins; 1990:439.
154. Stoelting RK, Dierdorf SF, McCammon RL. Restrictive Lung Disease. *Anesthesia and Coexisting Disease*. 4th ed. New York: Churchill Livingstone; 2002:205-216.
155. Goodwin SR. Aspiration syndromes. In: Civetta JM, Taylor RW, Kirby RR, eds. *Critical Care*. Philadelphia: Lippincott; 1988:1081.
156. Cassiere HA. Aspiration pneumonia: current concepts and approach to management. *Medscape*. 1998;2:1-11.
157. Olsson GL, Hallen B, Hambraeus-Jonzon K. Aspiration during anaesthesia: a computer-aided study of 185 385 anaesthetics. *Acta Anaesthesiol Scand*. 1986;30:84-92.
158. Tiret L, Nivoche Y, Hatton F, et al. Complications related to anaesthesia in infants and children. A prospective survey of 40240 anaesthetics. *Br J Anaesth*. 1986;61:263-269.
159. Kluger MT, Short TG. Aspiration during anaesthesia: a review of 133 cases from the Australian Anaesthetic Incident Monitoring Study (AIMS). *Anaethesia*. 1999;54:19-26.
160. Ezri T, Szmuck P, Stein A, et al. Peripartum general anaesthesia without tracheal intubation: incidence of aspiration pneumonia. *Anaesthesia*. 2000;55:5:421-426.
161. Warner MA. Warner ME, Weber JG. Clinical significance of pulmonary aspiration during the perioperative period. *Anesthesiology*. 1993;78:56-62.
162. Warner MA. Warner ME, Warner DO, et al. Perioperative pulmonary aspiration in infants and children. *Anesthesiology*. 1999;90:66-71.
163. Schreiner MS. Gastric fluid volume: is it really a risk factor for pulmonary aspiration? *Anesth Analg*. 1998;87:874-876.
164. Roberts RB, Shirley MA. Reducing the risk of acid aspiration during cesarean section. *Anesth Analg*. 1974;53:6:859-868.
165. Harter RL, Kelly WB, Kramer MG, et al. A comparison of the volume and pH of gastric contents of obese and lean surgical patients. *Anesth Analg*. 1998;86:147-152.
166. Stoelting RK, "NPO" and aspiration: new perspectives. *ASA Refresher Course Lect*. 2002;274:1-6.
167. American Society of Anesthesiologists. Practice guidelines for preoperative fasting and the use of pharmacologic agents to reduce the risk of pulmonary aspiration: application to healthy patients undergoing elective surgery. *Anesthesiology*. 1999;90: 896-905.
168. Smith RM, Spragg RG. Adult respiratory distress syndrome. In: Bordow RA, Moser KM, eds. *Manual of Clinical Problems in Pulmonary Medicine*. 3rd ed. Boston: Little, Brown; 1991:263.
169. Taylor RW. The adult respiratory distress syndrome. In: Kirby RR, Taylor RW, eds. *Respiratory Failure*. Chicago: Year Book; 1986:208.
170. Epstein PE. Acute respiratory failure in the surgical patient. In: Fishman AP, ed. *Manual of Pulmonary Diseases and Disorders*. 3rd ed. New York: McGraw-Hill; 2002:1034-1043.
171. Ranieri VM, Giunta F, Suter PM, Slutsky AS. Mechanical ventilation as a mediator of multisystem organ failure in acute respiratory distress syndrome. *JAMA*. 2000;284:43-44.
172. Morgan GE, Mikhail MS. Anesthesia for patients with respiratory disease. In: *Clinical Anesthesiology*. 3rd ed. East Norwalk, Conn: Appleton & Lange; 2002:511-521.
173. Brown M. ICU: critical care. In: Barash PG, Cullen BF, Stoelting RK, eds. *Clinical Anesthesia*. 4th ed. Philadelphia: Lippincott; 2001:1463-1484.
174. Muzaffar A, Demeter SL. Drug-induced pulmonary disease. In: Baum GL, Wolinsky E, eds. *Textbook of Pulmonary Diseases*. Vol 1. 5th ed. Boston: Little, Brown; 1993:775.
175. Kachel DL, Moyer TP, Martin WJ. Amiodarone-induced injury of human pulmonary artery endothelial cells: protection by α-tocopherol. *J Pharmacol Exp Ther*. 1990;254:1107-1112.
176. Dusman RE, Stanton MS, Miles WM, et al. Clinical features of amiodarone-induced pulmonary toxicity. *Circulation*. 1990; 82:51-59.
177. Suarez LD, Poseroso JJ, Elsner B, Bunster AM, Esteva H, Bellotti M. Subacute pneumopathy during amiodarone therapy. *Chest*. 1983;83:566-568.
178. Cooper JA, White DA, Matthay RA. Drug-induced pulmonary disease: part 2. noncytotoxic drugs. *Am Rev Respir Dis*. 1986;133:488-505.

179. Kawai K, Akaza H. Bleomycin-induced Pulmonary Toxicity in Chemotherapy for Testicular Cancer. *Expert Opin Drug Saf.* 2003 Nov;2(6):587-96.
180. Bowden DH. Unraveling pulmonary fibrosis: the bleomycin model [editorial]. *Lab Invest.* 1984;50:487-488.
181. Weiss RB, Muggia FM. Cytotoxic drug-induced pulmonary disease: update 1980. *Am J Med.* 1980;68:259-266.
182. Clark JM, Lambertsen CJ. Pulmonary oxygen toxicity: a review. *Pharmacol Rev.* 1971;23:37-133.
183. Fisher AB. Pulmonary oxygen toxicity. In: Fishman AP, ed. *Pulmonary Diseases and Disorders.* Vol 3. 2nd ed. New York: McGraw-Hill; 1988:2331.
184. Muzaffar A, Demeter SL. Drug-induced pulmonary disease. In: Baum GL, Wolinsky E, eds. *Textbook of Pulmonary Diseases.* Vol 1. 5th ed. Boston: Little, Brown; 1993:775.
185. Donat SM, Levy DA. Bleomycin associated pulmonary toxicity: is perioperative oxygen restriction necessary? *J Urol.* 1998;160: 1347-1352.
186. Auger WR. Pulmonary oxygen toxicity. In: Bordow RA, Moser KM, eds. *Manual of Clinical Problems in Pulmonary Medicine with Annotated Key References.* 3rd ed. Boston: Little, Brown; 1991:282.
187. Cooper JA, White DA, Matthay RA. Drug-induced pulmonary disease: Part 1. Cytotoxic drugs. *Am Rev Respir Dis.* 1986; 133:321-340.
188. Sharma OP. Sarcoidosis. In: Kelley WN, ed. *Textbook of Internal Medicine.* 2nd ed. Philadelphia: Lippincott; 1993:1742.
189. Johns CJ. Sarcoidosis. In: Fishman AP, ed. *Pulmonary Diseases and Disorders.* 2nd ed. New York: McGraw-Hill; 1988:619.
190. Reynolds HY, Matthay RA. Diffuse interstitial and alveolar inflammatory diseases. In: George RB, et al, eds. *Chest Medicine: Essentials of Pulmonary and Critical Care Medicine.* 2nd ed. Baltimore: Williams & Wilkins; 1990:231.
191. Wills MH, Harris MM. An unusual airway complication with sarcoidosis. *Anesthesiology.* 1987;66:554-555.
192. James DG. Clinical picture of sarcoidosis. In: Schwarz MI, King TE, eds. *Interstitial Lung Diseases.* 2nd ed. St Louis: Mosby; 1993:159.
193. Sharma OP. Pulmonary sarcoidosis and corticosteroids. *Am Rev Respir Dis.* 1993;147:1598-1600.
194. Tozman EC. Sarcoidosis: clinical manifestations, epidemiology, therapy, and pathophysiology. *Curr Opin Rheumatol.* 1991;3:155-159.
195. Eckstein M, Henerson S, Markovchick V. Thorax. In: Marx JA, Hockberger RS, Walls RM, eds. *Rosen's Emergency Medicine: Concepts and Clinical Practice.* 5th ed. St Louis: Mosby; 2002:381-414.
196. Cheitlin MD, Trunkey DD. Chest trauma. In: Saunders CE, Ho MT, eds. *Emergency Diagnosis and Treatment.* 4th ed. East Norwalk, Conn: Appleton & Lange; 1992:266.
197. Stoelting RK, Miller RD. *Basics of Anesthesia.* 3rd ed. New York: Churchill Livingstone; 1994:457.
198. Guyton AC, Hall JE. Respiratory insufficiency: pathophysiology, diagnosis, oxygen therapy. In: Guyton AC, Hall JE, eds. *Textbook of Medical Physiology.* 10th ed. Philadelphia: Saunders; 2001:484-492.
199. Lukanich JM, Sugarbaker DJ. Chest wall and pleura. In: *Sabiston Textbook of Surgery: the Biological Basis of Modern Surgical Practice.* 17th ed. Philadelphia: Saunders; 2004:1711-1734.
200. Prakash UB. Skeletal diseases. In: Baum GL, Wolinsky E, eds. *Textbook of Pulmonary Diseases.* Vol 2. 5th ed. Boston: Little, Brown; 1993:1691.
201. Welch KJ, Shamberger RC. Chest wall deformities. In: Shields TW, ed. *General Thoracic Surgery.* 3rd ed. Philadelphia: Lea & Febiger; 1989:515.
202. Castile RG, Staats BA, Westbrook PR. Symptomatic pectus deformities of the chest. *Am Rev Respir Dis.* 1982;126:564-568.
203. Haller JA Jr, Scherer LR, Turner CS, Colombani PM. Evolving management of pectus excavatum based on a single institutional experience of 664 patients. *Ann Surg.* 1989;209: 578-582.
204. Wynn SR, Driscoll DJ, Ostrom NK, et al. Exercise cardiorespiratory function in adolescents with pectus excavatum: observations before and after operation. *J Thorac Cardiovasc Surg.* 1990;99:41-47.
205. Dudley FR, Findley LJ. Neuromuscular and skeletal disease. In: Murray J, ed. *Pulmonary Complications of Systemic Disease.* New York: Marcel Dekker; 1992:333.
206. Chidambaram B, Mehta AV. Currarino-Silverman syndrome (pectus carinatum type 2 deformity) and mitral valve disease. *Chest.* 1992;102:780-782.
207. Robicsek F, Cook JW, Daugherty HK, Selle JG. Pectus carinatum. *J Thorac Cardiovasc Surg.* 1979;78:52-61.
208. Prakash UB. Pulmonary manifestations in systemic diseases. In: Baum GL, Wolinsky E, eds. *Textbook of Pulmonary Diseases.* Vol 2. 5th ed. Boston: Little, Brown; 1993:1691.
209. Collis DK, Ponseti IV. Long-term follow-up of patients with idiopathic scoliosis not treated surgically. *J Bone Joint Surg.* 1969;51A:425-445.
210. Pehrsson K, Bake B, Larsson S, Nachemson A. Lung function in adult idiopathic scoliosis: a 20-year follow up, *Thorax.* 1991; 46:474-478.
211. Guilleminault C, Kurland G, Winkle R, Miles LE. Severe kyphoscoliosis, breathing, and sleep: the "Quasimodo" syndrome during sleep. *Chest.* 1981;79:626-630.
212. Baydur A, Swank SM, Stiles CM, Sassoon CS. Respiratory mechanics in anesthetized young patients with kyphoscoliosis: immediate and delayed effects of corrective spinal surgery. *Chest.* 1990;97:1157-1164.
213. Zayas V. Scoliosis. In: Yao FS, Artusio JF, eds. *Anesthesiology: Problem-Oriented Patient Management.* 3rd ed. Philadelphia: Lippincott; 1993:708.
214. Jones RS, et al. Mechanical inefficiency of the thoracic cage in scoliosis. *Thorax.* 1981;36:456-461.
215. Boffa P, Stovin P, Shneerson J. Lung developmental abnormalities in severe scoliosis. *Thorax.* 1984;39:681-682.
216. Winter R, Lonstein J, Chou S. Scoliosis, kyphosis, and lordosis. In: Youmans JR, ed. *Neurosurgical Surgery.* Vol 4. 3rd ed. Philadelphia: Saunders; 1990.
217. Nachemson A. A long-term follow-up study of nontreated scoliosis. *Acta Orthop Scand.* 1968;39:466-576.
218. Nilsonne U, Lundgren KD. Long-term prognosis in idiopathic scoliosis. *Acta Orthop Scand.* 1968;39:456-465.
219. Kafer ER. Respiratory and cardiovascular functions in scoliosis and the principles of anesthetic management. *Anesthesiology.* 1980;52:399-351.
220. Dickey BF, Myers AR. Pulmonary manifestations of collagen-vascular diseases. In: Fishman AP, ed. *Pulmonary Diseases and Disorders.* Vol 1. 2nd ed. New York: McGraw-Hill; 1988:645.
221. King TE. Connective tissue disease. In: Schwarz MI, King TE, eds. *Interstitial Lung Diseases.* 2nd ed. St Louis: Mosby; 1993:271.
222. Rosenow FC III, Strimlan CV, Muhm JR, Ferguson RH. Pleuropulmonary manifestations of ankylosing spondylitis. *Mayo Clin Proc.* 1977;52:641-649.
223. Stewart RM, Ridyard JB, Pearson JD. Regional lung function in ankylosing spondylitis. *Thorax.* 1986;31:433-437.
224. Fisher LR, Cawley MID, Holgate ST. Relation between chest expansion, pulmonary function, and exercise tolerance in patients with ankylosing spondylitis. *Ann Rheum Dis.* 1990;49:921-925.
225. Buszek MC, et al. Hemidiaphragmatic paralysis: an unusual complication of cervical spondylosis. *Arch Phys Med Rehabil.* 1983;64:601-603.
226. Libby DM, Schley WS, Smith JP. Cricoarytenoid arthritis in ankylosing spondylitis. *Chest.* 1981;5:641-643.
227. Sinclair JR, Mason RA. Ankylosing spondylitis. *Anesthesia.* 1984;39:3-11.

CHAPTER 25

RESPIRATORY ANATOMY: THORACIC SURGERY

JOHN J. NAGELHOUT

Thoracic anesthesia has evolved as a specialty since the development of bronchial blockers and double-lumen endobronchial tubes. The anesthetist can safely and selectively ventilate one lung to create a quiet field for the surgeon. Patients undergoing thoracic surgery have varying degrees of respiratory disease and may experience profound changes in ventilation and blood flow through the lungs. A thorough understanding of this complex physiology is required.

PREOPERATIVE PREPARATION

Resection of affected lung tissue in bronchogenic carcinoma offers a better prognosis than radiation and chemotherapy. Because most patients have many risk factors for respiratory disease, evaluation of respiratory function and prediction of postresection function are necessary for as many patients as possible to benefit from surgery.[1]

Preoperative assessment of patients in need of pulmonary resection surgery should address two questions. First, is the likelihood of a postoperative complication so high that the surgery should not be performed? Second, will postoperative pulmonary function be sufficient to allow reasonable quality of life? Because most pulmonary resection surgery is performed with the hope of curing lung cancer, the risks of postoperative complications would have to be extraordinarily high before they would preclude the operation.

Fear of creating pulmonary insufficiency by lung resection is an important concern, and numerous studies have been designed to find the lowest limit of pulmonary function that will allow surgery to be safely performed. The data are unclear as to the value of preoperative evaluations in making this decision.

Studies performed to predict postoperative pulmonary complications after lung resection show that patients develop both pulmonary and cardiac complications such as arrhythmias, myocardial infarction, pulmonary embolism, pneumonia, and empyema. These complications influence the duration of mechanical ventilation and outcome; however, none of these complications can be accurately predicted by preoperative studies of pulmonary function. No consensus exists with regard to what should be included in a preoperative evaluation for lung resection. See Box 25-1 for commonly used preoperative criteria for lung resection.[2,3]

Lung resection surgeries are now being performed on patients who have "end-stage" chronic obstructive pulmonary disease (COPD), and postoperative respiratory failure has not been a problem in these patients. Newer data are necessary to determine which preoperative tests are useful in predicting outcome and which tests are cost effective.

BOX **25-1**

Patient Characteristics Identifying Postoperative Disability

Factors That Identify "Low-Risk" Patients

FEV_1 >2 L
MVV >50% predicted
Predicted postoperative FEV_1 >0.8 L and 40% predicted
Absence of cardiac disease

Proposed Factors That Identify "High-Risk" Patients

PCO_2 >45
PO_2 <50
Predicted postoperative FEV_1 <0.7 L and/or 40% of predicted value
Age >70
Poor exercise performance

FEV_1, *Forced expiratory volume in 1 second;* MVV, *maximum voluntary ventilation;* PCO_2, *partial pressure of carbon dioxide;* PO_2, *partial pressure of oxygen.*
Reilly JJ. Evidence-based preoperative evaluation of candidates for thoracotomy. Chest. *1999;116:474S-476S.*

Changes in surgical techniques, especially the use of video-assisted laparoscopy, have markedly decreased the incidence of postoperative pulmonary complications and will necessitate a reevaluation of the testing required for preoperative assessment.[4] For smaller lung resections minimal preoperative evaluations of cardiac disease, gas exchange, and oxygenation may suffice. Given the large physiologic changes that occur after pneumonectomy, complete pulmonary function testing as well as cardiac testing may still be reasonable in these patients.

Preoperative Evaluation

History and Physical Examination

Cancer patients who undergo lung resection typically have a history of multiple risk factors and signs of respiratory disease. Risk factors include cigarette smoking, air pollution, and industrial chemical exposure. Patients must be evaluated for exertional dyspnea, productive cough, hemoptysis, cyanosis, poor exercise tolerance, and chest pain. Difficulty breathing in the supine position can result from COPD or from compression of the airway by a mediastinal mass. Lung cancer patients should be assessed for mass and metabolic effects, metastasis, and medications, as noted in Table 25-1.

TABLE 25-1 Anesthetic Considerations in Lung Cancer Patients (the "4 Ms")

Mass effects	Obstructive pneumonia, lung abscess, SVC syndrome, tracheobronchial distortion, Pancoast's syndrome, recurrent laryngeal nerve or phrenic nerve paresis, chest wall or mediastinal extension
Metabolic effects	Lambert-Eaton syndrome, hypercalcemia, hyponatremia, Cushing's syndrome
Metastases	Particularly to brain, bone, liver, and adrenals
Medications	Chemotherapy-induced lung changes

SVC, *Superior vena cava syndrome.*
Modified from Slinger PP, Johnston MR. Preoperative assessment and management. In: Kaplan JA, Slinger PD, eds. Thoracic Anesthesia. *3rd ed. Philadelphia: Churchill Livingstone; 2003:16.*

TABLE 25-2 Initial Preanesthetic Assessment for Thoracic Surgery

Patient Type	Assessments
All patients	Assess exercise tolerance, estimate ppoFEV_1%*, discuss postoperative analgesia, recommend discontinuation of smoking
Patients with PPO FEV_1 <40%	DLCO, $\dot{V}/\dot{Q}$ scan, $\dot{V}O_2$max
Patients with cancer	Consider the "4 Ms": mass effects, metabolic effects, metastases, medications (Table 25-1)
Patients with COPD	Arterial blood gas analysis, physiotherapy, bronchodilators
Patients with increased renal risk	Measure creatinine and blood urea nitrogen

COPD, *Chronic obstructive pulmonary disease;* DLCO, *diffusing capacity for carbon monoxide;* FEV_1, *forced expiratory volume in 1 second;* PPO, *predicted postoperative;* $\dot{V}O_2$max, *maximum oxygen consumption;* $\dot{V}/\dot{Q}$, *ventilation-perfusion ratio.*
**PPO FEV_1% = Preoperative FEV_1 % × (1 − % functioning lung tissue removed/100). For values >40%, postoperative complications are rare; for values between 30% and 40%, postoperative problems are possible; for values <30%, postoperative ventilation is likely to be required.*
Modified from Slinger PP, Johnston MR. Preoperative assessment and management. In: Kaplan JA, Slinger PD, eds. Thoracic Anesthesia. *3rd ed. Philadelphia: Churchill Livingstone; 2003:17.*

A history of COPD is common. The chest radiograph of the patient with COPD shows hyperinflation, increased anteroposterior diameter, and increased vascular markings. Increased pulmonary vascular resistance (PVR) resulting from compression of the vascular bed increases the likelihood of right ventricular failure.

The patient should be evaluated for ischemic and valvular heart disease. A high index of suspicion should be maintained for hormonal abnormalities because some tumors secrete endocrine-like substances such as adrenocorticotropic hormone, antidiuretic hormone, serotonin, parathyroid hormones, and insulin, causing a variety of metabolic abnormalities (Table 25-2 and Box 25-2).

BOX 25-2

Evidence-Based Preoperative Evaluation of Candidates for Thoracotomy

1. All patients considered for thoracotomy should have preoperative spirometry.
2. Patients who meet the following criteria should also have quantitative radionuclide perfusion scanning: significant obstructive lung disease (FEV_1 <60% predicted); known or suspected endobronchial obstruction; significant hilar disease (mass or adenopathy); significant pleural disease; prior resection.
3. Patients believed to be at high risk on the basis of predicted postoperative FEV_1 should be considered for exercise assessment.
4. If exercise assessment is performed, an $M\dot{V}O_2$ of <10-15 ml/kg/min or a predicted postoperative $M\dot{V}O_2$ <10 ml/kg/min identifies a patient at very high risk for complications and mortality.
5. Limited available data support the use of preoperative risk indexes to identify patients at high risk.
6. Lung volume reduction surgery may provide new approaches in selected patients with significant obstructive lung disease and concomitant lung cancer.

$M\dot{V}O_2$, *Maximal oxygen uptake.*
Modified from Reilly JJ. Evidence-based preoperative evaluation of candidates for thoracotomy. Chest. *1999;116:474S-476S.*

Diagnostic Data

Chest Radiograph. Anteroposterior and lateral projections show hyperinflation and increased vascular markings in patients with COPD. Bullae of emphysema may be present. Infection or pleural effusions may be noted preoperatively and treated to improve the postoperative course.

The locations of masses can be identified. In some patients it can be ascertained whether lesions compress mediastinal structures, cause tracheal shift, or invade the airway. Chest radiography is done to predict whether intubation will be difficult, whether induction of anesthesia could cause collapse of the airway, or whether surgical dissection may be difficult or bloody.[5]

Electrocardiogram. Pulmonary disease can cause right ventricular hypertrophy and strain. In such a case the electrocardiogram (ECG) shows low-voltage QRS waves and poor R-wave progression over the precordial leads. Right ventricular hypertrophy causes an R/S ratio greater than 1 in lead V_1, along with a shift toward right-axis deviation.[6] Right atrial hypertrophy causes the initial component of a biphasic P wave in lead V_1 to be larger than the second component.[7] Increased PVR and right ventricular strain could preclude pneumonectomy because of the added resistance produced by clamping the vasculature of one lung.

Arterial Blood Gases. Measurement of preoperative room air arterial blood gases is useful in guiding the weaning of O_2 and ventilation postoperatively. Carbon dioxide (CO_2) retention with an arterial partial pressure ($PaCO_2$) greater than 45 mm Hg is a predictor of increased risk of perioperative pulmonary complications.[3]

Exercise Testing. Evaluation of the exercise tolerance of patients before thoracic surgery can be useful in predicting which patients are at increased risk for pulmonary complications postoperatively. Markos and colleagues[8] found that a fall of more than 2% in arterial oxygen saturation (SaO_2) with exercise is predictive of complications in patients undergoing lobectomy. Berchard and Wetstein studied 50 thoracotomy patients using cycle ergometry and exercised them to the point of exhaustion or dyspnea. They found that a maximum oxygen (O_2) consumption of less than 10 ml/kg per minute correlated with an increased incidence of pulmonary complications. In this group the investigators found a 29% incidence of mortality and a 43% incidence of morbidity.[9]

Pulmonary Function Tests. Multiple studies have been done to identify which preoperative pulmonary function tests are good indicators of postoperative complications. Patients at high risk of complications include those with a forced vital capacity (FVC) less than 50% of the predicted value, a forced expiratory volume in 1 second (FEV_1) less than 2 L, FEV_1/FVC less than 50%, a lung carbon monoxide diffusing capacity (DLCO) less than 50% of the predicted value, and $PaCO_2$ greater than 45 mm Hg.[1] Specific parameters of lung volumes and flows correlate poorly with postoperative morbidity and mortality.[10,11,12]

When the preoperative lung function tests indicate that the patient is at increased risk for perioperative complications, split lung function tests of ventilation and perfusion are valuable in the prediction of postresection lung function. Removal of a diseased portion of lung may not decrease overall lung function. Ventilation can be measured by having the patient inhale one vital capacity breath of a radioisotope and measuring isotope counts with multiple scanners placed over the chest wall. Radioisotope injected intravenously and imaged shows the distribution of perfusion to all areas of the lung. Calculations can then be made to estimate postresection function.

Markos and colleagues[8] compared predicted postoperative (PPO) function tests with actual results measured at 3 and 12 months postoperatively. They found a very good correlation between PPO values and actual postoperative measures of FEV_1, FVC, total lung capacity (TLC), and DLCO. In an extensive study of thoracic surgery patients they found that the PPO FEV_1 and DLCO are valuable in prediction of postoperative morbidity and mortality. They suggest that a PPO FEV_1 at least 40% of predicted is a good criterion for safe lung resection, and in their study no deaths occurred in this group. A PPO FEV_1 less than 40% was associated with a mortality rate of 50%. DLCO values reflect the adequacy of gas exchange. A PPO DLCO less than 40% was associated with high morbidity and mortality.

In study by Nakahara and associates, all of 10 thoracic surgery patients with a PPO FEV_1 less than 30% needed mechanical ventilation postoperatively. Six of these patients died. A high incidence of pulmonary complications was associated with a PPO FEV_1 less than 60%.[13]

Lung Scanning Techniques and Pulmonary Artery Occlusion. Differential lung function can be measured by xenon radiospirometry. This technique involves the intravenous injection of radioactive xenon 133 (^{133}Xe) that has been dissolved in sodium chloride. Radionuclide perfusion lung scanning is considered an acceptable and simple method with which to predict postoperative function.[2,14,15]

Although differential lung function tests may provide an indication of who will do poorly after lung resection, they cannot predict this outcome with complete accuracy. Pulmonary arterial pressure measurements, with occlusion of the pulmonary artery supplying the lung to be resected, appear to give a better indication of which patients will not tolerate lung resection. A resting mean pulmonary arterial pressure of 22 mm Hg implies a grave prognosis, and a mean pulmonary arterial pressure of more than 30 mm Hg during exercise also has been associated with high postoperative mortality.[16]

Patient Optimization

Aggressive treatment of acute or reversible components of respiratory disease greatly decreases the risk of postoperative complications. Treatable preoperative conditions include infections, excess bronchial secretions, bronchospasm, dehydration, electrolyte imbalance, cigarette smoking, alcohol abuse, and malnutrition (Figure 25-1).

Monitoring

The purpose of monitoring during thoracic surgery is the quick recognition of sudden and severe changes in ventilation and hemodynamics that can accompany positioning, one-lung

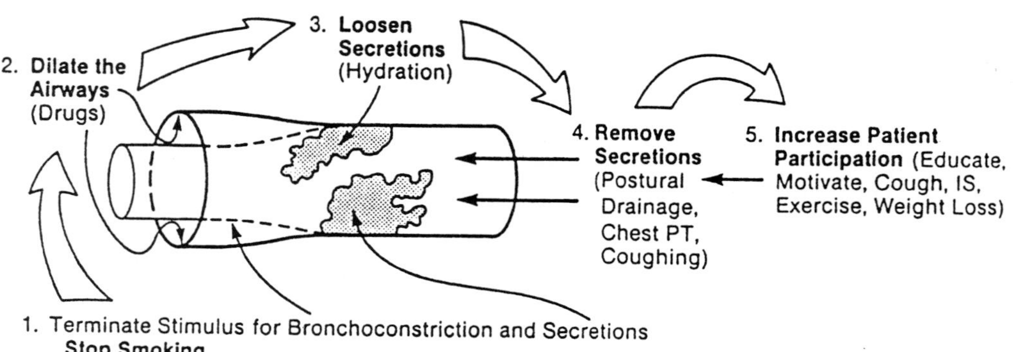

FIGURE **25-1**
A full, aggressive preoperative respiratory preparation regimen consists of a five-pronged attack. *1*, Require the patient to stop smoking. *2*, Dilate the airways. *3*, Loosen secretions. *4*, Remove secretions. *5*, Increase patient participation. *IS*, Incentive spirometry; *PT*, chest physiotherapy. (From Benumof JL, Alfery DD. Anesthesia for thoracic surgery. In: Miller RD, ed. *Anesthesia*. 5th ed. Philadelphia: Churchill Livingstone; 2000:1673.)

ventilation (OLV), and surgical manipulation of the airway and thoracic structures. All patients require continuous monitoring of the ECG. Leads II and V_5 detect more than 85% of ischemia.[1] Esophageal stethoscopes, temperature monitoring, and pulse oximetry are routine. An airway pressure monitor helps detect changes in airway compliance and assists in the identification of the proper placement of double-lumen tubes (DLTs). Capnography is useful for determining whether ventilation is adequate when one lung is deflated.

Arterial Pressure Monitoring

Arterial blood pressure monitoring instantly identifies acute hypotension with surgical manipulation. It also allows for frequent sampling of arterial blood for gas analysis. For thoracotomies the arterial cannula is generally placed in the dependent arm, where it is more easily stabilized. For mediastinoscopy an arterial line placed on the right detects compression of the innominate artery and helps detect a decrease in cerebral blood flow. A pulse oximeter probe placed on a digit of the right hand also detects compression of the innominate artery during mediastinoscopy.

Central Venous Pressure Monitoring

Central venous pressure monitoring is not required for routine thoracotomies but may be indicated if the patient's volume status is unclear or if large fluid shifts are anticipated. In addition, it provides large-bore access for rapid infusion and an access site should transvenous pacing or pulmonary artery pressure monitoring become necessary.

The central venous pressure line can be inserted via the external or internal jugular veins or the subclavian veins. An external jugular line is more easily kinked in the lateral position. One should remain alert to the possibility of pneumothorax with the insertion of central lines. A pneumothorax on the ventilated side can lead to severe hypoxemia during OLV. If a subclavian puncture is planned, the insertion site should be on the same side as the thoracotomy.

Pulmonary Artery Pressure Monitoring

Monitoring of the pulmonary artery pressure is indicated in the presence of a history of severe cardiovascular disease, valvular heart disease, or significant pulmonary hypertension. In these circumstances the normal correlation of right and left ventricular pressures may be disturbed. Pulmonary artery pressure monitoring allows estimation of left ventricular pressures and provides information of use in the improvement of cardiac performance with fluids and cardiovascular drugs.

The use of pulmonary artery catheters has limitations during OLV. More than 90% of pulmonary artery catheters float into the right lung.[17] During right thoracotomy, then, the catheter will likely be in the nondependent, collapsed lung and will give a false-low reading for cardiac output; consequently the values for pulmonary artery pressure may not reflect left ventricular performance.[18]

LATERAL DECUBITUS POSITION

The most frequent position chosen for surgical exposure during thoracotomy is the lateral decubitus position. A roll is placed beneath the torso just caudal to the axilla to prevent compression of the neurovascular bundle. Hyperabduction of the arms is prevented to keep the brachial plexus from stretching against the humeral head. Arms can be separately padded and placed on arm rests or tables in front of the patient's face. Pulse oximetry or frequent palpation of the radial pulse ensures the integrity of circulation to the hand.[19]

The head is supported on pillows to maintain alignment of the head and neck with the spine. Lateral flexion of the neck can cause compression of the jugular veins or vertebral arteries, compromising cerebral circulation. The dependent ear can be compressed by the weight of the head. Careful padding or use of a foam doughnut relieves this pressure. The eyes should be checked for pressure to prevent corneal abrasion and retinal ischemia.

Physiology of the Lateral Decubitus Position

Positional changes and changes in chest wall integrity produce significant alterations in ventilation and perfusion of the lungs during thoracic surgery.

Upright Position

The distribution of perfusion in the lungs depends on gravity in relation to the level of the heart and on pressures transmitted through alveoli. In a spontaneously breathing, upright patient, blood perfusion increases linearly from the apex to the base of the lung (Figure 25-2). Flow reaches very low rates in the apex and is greatest at the base of the lung.

Pleural pressure is most negative at the apex of the lung, and this keeps alveoli distended (Figure 25-3). Dependent alveoli are distended less and are more compliant. Therefore most of a tidal breath is distributed to the dependent alveoli (Figure 25-4). The higher ventilation matches the higher perfusion in the dependent lung, making gas exchange efficient.[20]

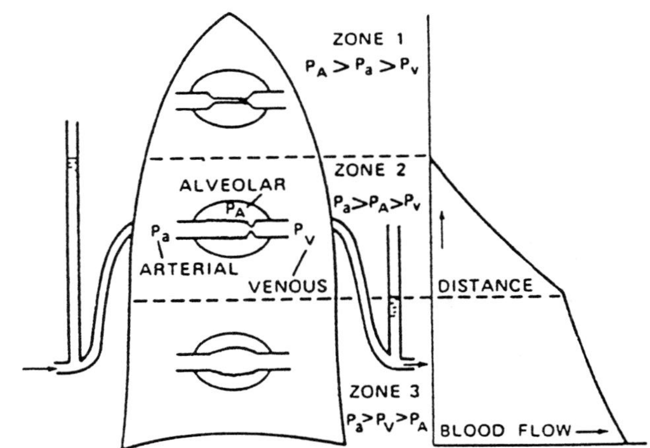

FIGURE **25-2**
The lung is divided into three zones according to the relative magnitudes of the pulmonary arterial, venous, and alveolar pressures (*Pa, Pv,* and *PA*, respectively). In zone 1, alveolar exceeds arterial pressure, so the collapsible vessels are held closed and there is no flow. In zone 2, arterial exceeds alveolar pressure, but alveolar exceeds venous pressure. Under these conditions a constriction occurs at the downstream end of each collapsible vessel, and the pressure inside the vessel at this point is equal to alveolar pressure, so that the pressure gradient causing flow is arterial-alveolar. This gradient increases linearly with distance down the lung, and therefore so does blood flow. In zone 3, venous exceeds alveolar pressure, and the collapsible vessels are held open. Now the pressure gradient causing flow is arterial-venous, and this is constant down the zone. (From West JB. Distribution of blood flow in isolated lung; relation to arterial, venous and alveolar pressures. *Respiratory Physiology: the Essentials.* 4th ed. Baltimore: Williams & Wilkins; 1990:41.)

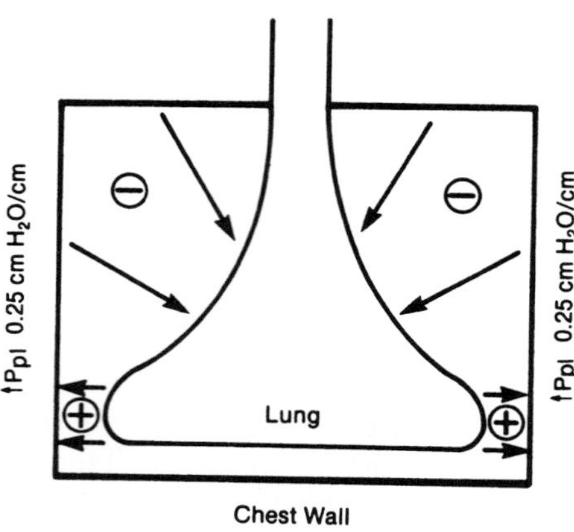

FIGURE **25-3**
Schematic diagram of the lung within the chest wall, showing the tendency of the lung to assume a globular shape because of its viscoelastic nature. The tendency of the top of the lung to collapse inward creates a relatively negative pressure at the apex, and the tendency of the bottom of the lung to spread outward creates a relatively positive pressure at the base. Therefore pleural pressure *(Ppl)* increases by 0.25 cm H_2O per centimeter of lung dependency. (From Triantafillou AN, Benumof JL, Lecamwasam HS. Physiology of the lateral decubitus position, the open chest, and one-lung ventilation. In: Kaplan JA, Slinger PD, eds. *Thoracic Anesthesia.* 3rd ed. Philadelphia: Churchill Livingstone; 2003:73.)

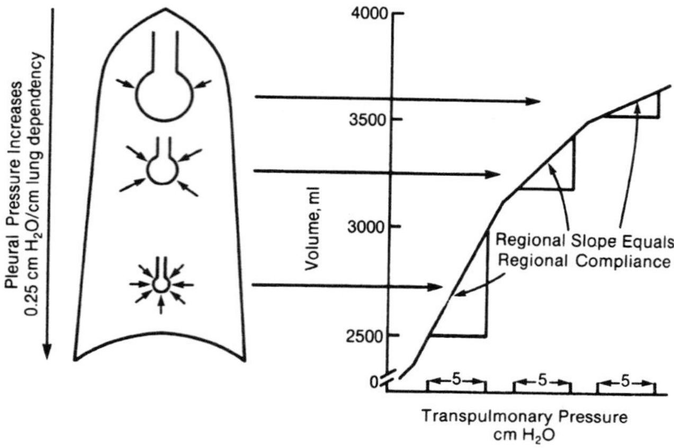

FIGURE **25-4**
Pleural pressure increases by 0.25 cm H_2O with each centimeter down the lung. The increase in pleural pressure causes a fourfold decrease in alveolar volume. The caliber of the air passages also decreases as lung volume decreases. When regional alveolar volume is translated over to a regional transpulmonary pressure-alveolar volume curve, small alveoli are on a steep *(large slope)* portion of the curve, and large alveoli are on a flat *(small slope)* portion of the curve. Because the regional slope equals regional compliance, the dependent small alveoli normally receive the largest share of the tidal volume. Over the normal tidal volume range (lung volume increases by 500 ml from 2500 [normal FRC] to 3000 ml), the pressure-volume relationship is linear. Lung volume values in this diagram relate to the upright position. (From Triantafillou AN, Benumof JL, Lecamwasam HS. Physiology of the lateral decubitus position, the open chest, and one-lung ventilation. In: Kaplan JA, Slinger PD, eds. *Thoracic Anesthesia.* 3rd ed. Philadelphia: Churchill Livingstone; 2003:74.)

Awake Lateral Position

Less vertical distance is present to cause differences in the intrapleural pressure and blood pressure gradients in the lateral position (Figure 25-5). Abdominal contents displace the diaphragm in a cephalad direction on the dependent side. During inspiration, contraction of the diaphragm causes more of the tidal volume (VT) to fill the dependent lung. Because perfusion is dependent on gravity, perfusion in the lateral position is greatest in the dependent lung (Figure 25-6). Overall the relationship of greater ventilation and perfusion in the dependent lung is unchanged, and gas exchange remains efficient.

Anesthetized Lateral Position, Chest Closed, with Spontaneous Ventilation

A change in the distribution of ventilation is seen with the induction of anesthesia. Functional residual capacity (FRC) decreases in both lungs with anesthesia. The weight of the mediastinum and the cephalad displacement of the diaphragm by abdominal contents further decrease FRC in the dependent lung. Lower volumes in each lung shift their place on the compliance curve. The lungs are less compliant when they are either at a very high volume (distended alveoli) or a very low volume (atelectasis). As the upper lung loses FRC, its lower volume results in improved compliance. The upper lung moves from a flat, noncompliant portion of the compliance curve to a more compliant position. As the lower lung loses FRC, its volume becomes so low as to decrease its compliance. It shifts to a less compliant, flatter portion of the curve (Figure 25-7). Ventilation is preferentially distributed to the upper lung while gravity-dependent blood flow preferentially goes to the dependent lung, resulting in a mismatch of ventilation and perfusion.

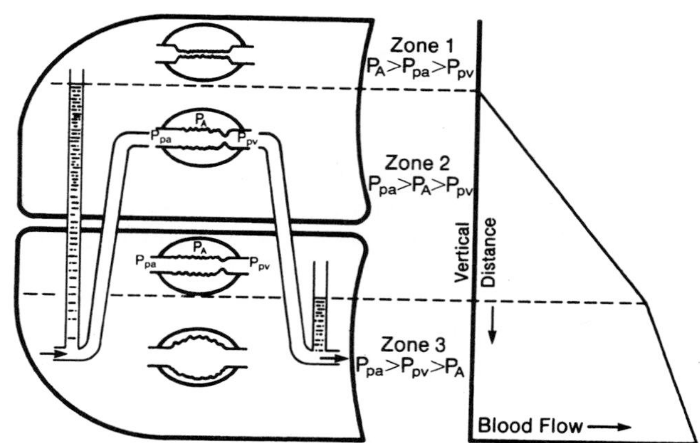

FIGURE **25-5**
Schematic representation of the effects of gravity on the distribution of pulmonary blood flow in the lateral decubitus position. The vertical gradient in the lateral decubitus position is less than in the upright position. Consequently blood flow in zones 2 and 3 is less in the lateral decubitus position than in the upright position. Nevertheless, pulmonary blood flow increases with lung dependency and is greater in the dependent lung than in the nondependent lung. *P*A, Alveolar pressure; *Pa*, pulmonary artery pressure; *P*V, pulmonary venous pressure. (From Triantafillou AN, Benumof JL, Lecamwasam HS. Physiology of the lateral decubitus position, the open chest, and one-lung ventilation. In: Kaplan JA, Slinger PD, eds. *Thoracic Anesthesia.* 3rd ed. Philadelphia: Churchill Livingstone; 2003:76.)

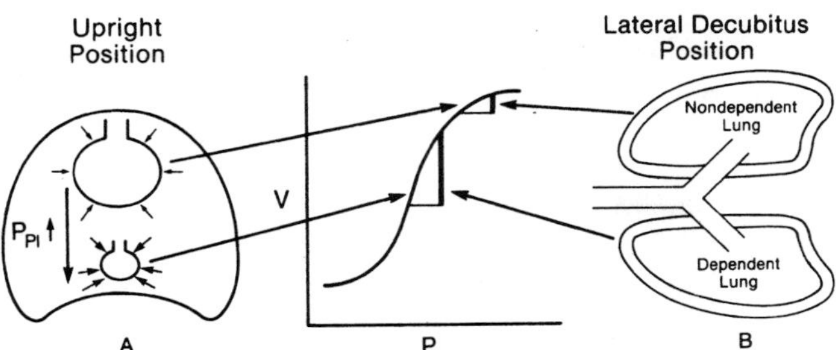

FIGURE **25-6**
Pleural pressure *(Ppl)* in the awake upright patient **(A)** is most positive in the dependent portion of the lung, and alveoli in this region are therefore most compressed and have the lowest volume. Pleural pressure is least positive (most negative) at the apex of the lung, and alveoli in this region are therefore least compressed and have the highest volume. When these regional differences in alveolar volume are translated in to a regional transpulmonary pressure-alveolar volume curve, the small dependent alveoli are on a steep (large-slope) portion of the curve, and the large nondependent alveoli are on a flat (small-slope) portion of the curve. In this diagram regional slope equals regional compliance. Therefore for a given and equal change in transpulmonary pressure, the dependent part of the lung receives a much larger share of the tidal volume than does the nondependent lung. In the lateral decubitus position **(B)**, gravity also causes pleural pressure gradients and therefore affects the distribution of ventilation similarly. The dependent lung lies on a relatively steep portion and the nondependent lung lies on a relatively flat portion of the pressure-volume curve. Therefore in the lateral decubitus position the dependent lung receives the majority of the tidal ventilation. *V*, Alveolar volume; *P*, transpulmonary pressure. (From Triantafillou AN, Benumof JL, Lecamwasam HS. Physiology of the lateral decubitus position, the open chest and one-lung ventilation. In: Kaplan JA, Slinger PD, eds. *Thoracic Anesthesia*. 3rd ed. Philadelphia: Churchill Livingstone; 2003:76.)

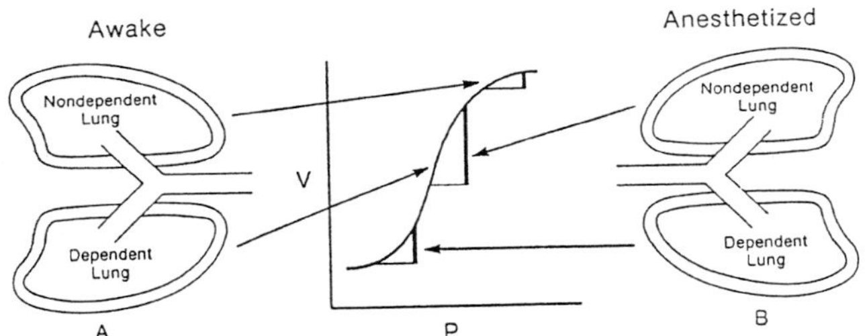

FIGURE **25-7**
Schematic diagram showing **(A)** the distribution of ventilation in the awake patient in the lateral decubitus position and **(B)** the distribution of ventilation in the anesthetized patient in the lateral decubitus position. The induction of anesthesia has caused a loss of lung volume in both lungs, with the nondependent lung moving from a flat, noncompliant portion to a steep, compliant part of the pressure-volume curve. Therefore the anesthetized patient in the lateral decubitus position has the majority of the tidal ventilation in the nondependent lung (where there is the least perfusion) and the minority of the tidal ventilation in the dependent lung (where there is the greatest perfusion). *V*, Alveolar volume; *P*, transpulmonary pressure. (From Triantafillou AN, Benumof JL, Lecamwasam HS. Physiology of the lateral decubitus position, the open chest, and one-lung ventilation. In: Kaplan JA, Slinger PD, eds: *Thoracic Anesthesia*. 3rd ed. Philadelphia: Churchill Livingstone; 2003:77.)

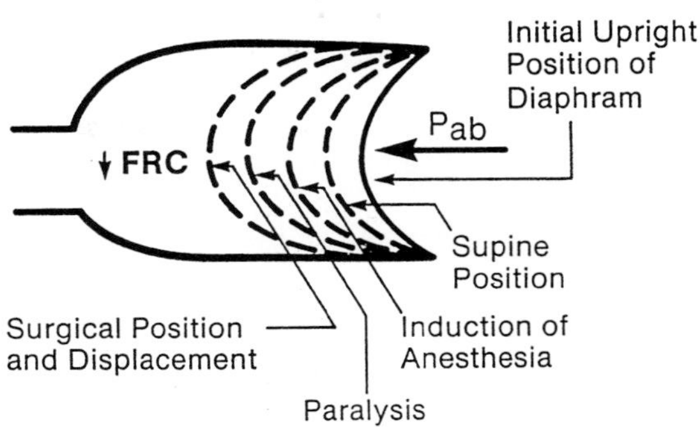

FIGURE **25-8**
Anesthesia and surgery may cause a progressive cephalad displacement of the diaphragm. The sequence of events involves assumption of the supine position, induction of anesthesia, causation of paralysis, assumption of several surgical positions, and displacement by retractors and packs. The cephalad displacement of the diaphragm results in a decreased function residual capacity *(FRC)*. P_{ab}, Pressure of the abdominal contents. (From Benumof JL. *Anesthesia for Thoracic Surgery*. 2nd ed. Philadelphia: Saunders; 1995:100.)

Anesthetized, Paralyzed, Mechanically Ventilated Patient

The ventilation-perfusion relationship further deteriorates as more and more ventilation goes to the upper part of the lung. The diaphragm no longer contributes to ventilation of the lower lung, and FRC further declines (Figure 25-8). The addition of positive end-expiratory pressure (PEEP) to mechanical ventilation may help restore FRC and improve the ventilation-perfusion ratio.

Anesthetized Open-Chest Patient

The open chest causes further loss of ventilation to the dependent lung. The mediastinum shifts downward because of loss of negative intrapleural pressure in the nondependent lung. Ventilation to the dependent lung is decreased in proportion to the displacement of the lung by the mediastinal structures. Compression of the great vessels may cause a decrease in cardiac output and circulatory compromise. In addition, paradoxic movement of air occurs on inspiration from the open-chest lung into the dependent lung, which has the greater negative intrapleural pressure. On expiration gas exits the dependent lung and enters both the trachea and the open-chest lung, causing the lung to expand (Figure 25-9). Paradoxic respiration compromises fresh gas exchange in the dependent lung as part of the VT moves to and fro between the lungs.[21] Positive pressure ventilation diminishes the effects of mediastinal shift and paradoxic respiration. During mechanical ventilation the open chest provides no resistance, and the increased compliance of that lung allows a higher proportion of ventilation to go to the more poorly perfused upper part of the lung. The less-ventilated, better-perfused dependent lung contributes to physiologic shunt.

ONE-LUNG VENTILATION

Indications for Lung Separation

With the use of endobronchial blockers or DLTs it is possible to separate ventilation of the lungs to improve surgical exposure or to protect one lung from material in the

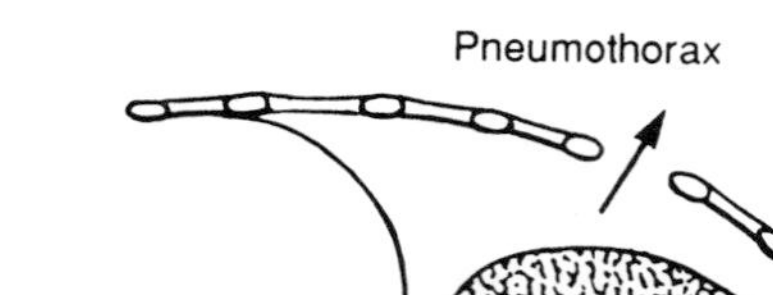
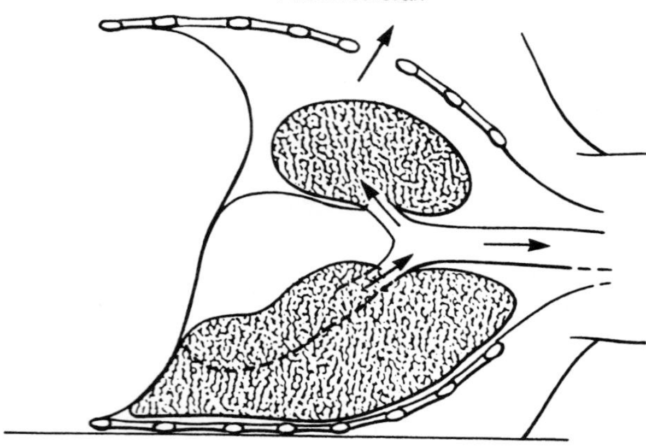

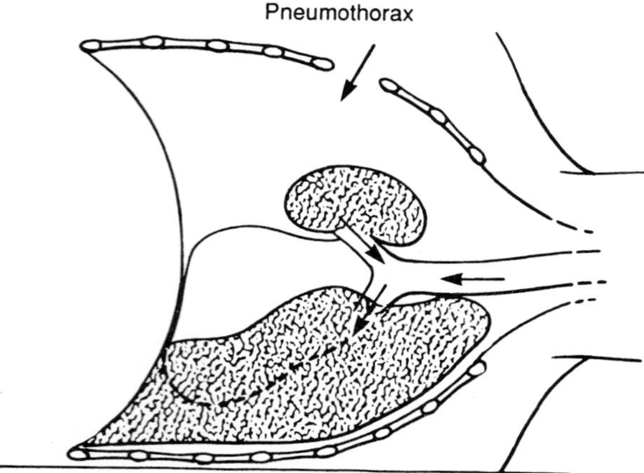

FIGURE **25-9**
Paradoxic respiration in the spontaneously breathing patient lying on the side. (From Tarhan S, Moffitt EA. Principles of thoracic anesthesia. *Surg Clin North Am*. 1973;53:813.)

other lung. Indications for the use of a DLT are noted in Box 25-3.

Methods of Lung Separation

Several devices have been developed to enable isolation of one lung and ventilation of the other. The single-lumen endobronchial tube was developed in 1931 to isolate an infected lung. A 7.5-mm, 32-cm endotracheal tube can be advanced over a fiberoptic scope to intubate one bronchus. A disadvantage to use of a single-lumen tube for OLV is that the ability to ventilate or suction the other lung is lost. Another disadvantage is that use of a single-lumen tube in the right lung would probably occlude the right upper lobe orifice. However, in an emergent situation, use of a single-lumen tube advanced blindly down the right bronchus or placed into the left bronchus aided by a bronchoscope can be life saving. A single-lumen tube placed in the trachea can be used in pediatric thoracic cases via an apneic technique in which the surgeon works on the lung during a period of apnea and then waits while the patient is hyperventilated.

BOX **25-3**

Indications for One-Lung Ventilation

Surgical Procedures
- Lung resection (lobectomy, segmental resection, pneumonectomy)
- Drainage of lung abscess or cyst
- Video-assisted thoracoscopic surgery under general anesthesia
- Bronchopleural fistula
- Bronchial tumors
- Lung transplant
- Esophageal surgery
- Anterior approach to the thoracic spine
- Bronchopulmonary lavage (unilateral)
- Pericardial procedures
- Select open-heart procedures
- Repair of thoracic aortic aneurysm
- Pulmonary artery rupture or embolism
- Pleural procedures (pleurectomy, decortication)

Improved Patient Outcome
- Restrict infection or bleeding to one lung
- Desire to differentially ventilate each lung such as with bronchopleural fistula, tracheobronchial mass, or trauma or postoperatively

Bronchial blockers were developed in the mid 1930s. These generally consist of catheters with an inflatable balloon that blocks the bronchus. A separate endotracheal tube is then placed into the trachea. Bronchial blockers are very useful in patients in whom the securing of the airway is anticipated to be difficult. These devices are appropriate for patients already intubated in whom changing to another tube would be too dangerous. They can also be advanced down a nasally intubated patient or used for pediatric video-assisted thoracoscopy procedures.[22] The use of bronchial blockers has declined because of the risk of slippage and obstruction of the trachea. Placement is difficult and requires use of a bronchoscope.

The Univent tube was developed in Japan in the 1980s. It consists of an endotracheal tube with a second lumen for a movable endobronchial blocker. After intubation of the trachea has been performed, the blocker is advanced into the bronchus with the aid of the fiberoptic bronchoscope. This tube is as easy to pass into the trachea as a single-lumen tube, making it a good choice in patients with difficult airways. Postlaryngectomy patients can also benefit from this tube, because it is easily advanced through the stoma.

DLTs consist of two bonded catheters, each with its own lumen; one lumen is used for ventilating the trachea and the other for ventilating the bronchus. Several types of DLTs have been used in thoracic surgery. The Carlens tube is a left-sided DLT with a carinal hook to aid in stabilization of the tube. Insertion is difficult, and the hook can cause vocal cord damage. A White tube is a right-sided DLT with a carinal hook. See Table 25-3.

The Robertshaw DLT was developed in 1962. This tube is available as a right- or left-sided DLT without a carinal hook (Figure 25-10). The original tubes are reusable red rubber tubes

TABLE 25-3 Types of Double-Lumen Tubes

Name	Bronchus Intubated	Carinal Hook
Carlens	Left	Yes
White	Right	Yes
Robert-Shaw	Right or left	No

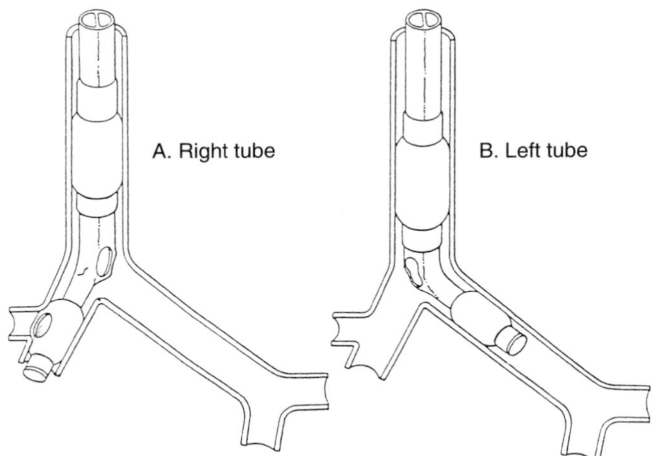

FIGURE **25-10**
The correct positions of a right- and a left-sided double-lumen tube. (From Morgan GE, Mikhail MS. Anesthesia for thoracic surgery. In: *Clinical Anesthesiology*. East Norwalk, Conn: Appleton & Lange; 3rd ed, 2002:531.)

in sizes of small, medium, and large. Disposable polyvinyl chloride tubes are available in French sizes 41, 39, 37, 35, and 28. These correspond, respectively, to internal lumen diameters of 6.5, 6, 5.5, 5, and 4.5 mm. DLTs are not used for small children; the external diameter of the 28 Fr DLT is 9 mm.[23]

When a right-sided DLT is placed, slight movements in the tube's position can dislodge the bronchial lumen into the trachea or cause obstruction of the right upper lobe by the bronchial cuff. This happens because the distance from the carinal bifurcation to the beginning of the right upper lobe is 2 cm, as compared with a 5-cm left mainstem bronchus (Figure 25-11).

Modifications have been made in right-sided tubes to allow ventilation through a slot in the endobronchial cuff. It is thought that a greater margin of safety is associated with the use of a left-sided DLT for all right and left thoracotomies unless a left-sided tube is contraindicated. Contraindications to the use of DLTs include internal lesions of the trachea or main bronchi, compression of the trachea or main bronchi by an external mass, or the presence of a descending thoracic aortic aneurysm, which can compress or erode the left main bronchus. In these circumstances, it may be possible to use a DLT with the bronchial lumen on the unaffected side. An increased risk of aspiration may exist with the use of a DLT, because it takes longer to place, and to verify its placement, compared with a single-lumen tube. Another contraindication is a difficult airway in which direct laryngoscopy is impossible. The use of a DLT may be precluded in a critically ill patient who arrives with a single-lumen tube if it is judged that the patient cannot tolerate a short period of extubation.[1] Recommendations for placement of the various lung separation devices are given in Table 25-4.

Placement of Double-Lumen Tubes

The DLT has two curves along its length to aid in its placement. A stylet aids placement through the larynx. Some practitioners prefer the Macintosh blade for intubation because it offers greater clearance for the tube and may decrease the chance of balloon rupture from the teeth.[23] For laryngoscopy the lubricated DLT is advanced with the distal curve concave anteriorly until the vocal cords are passed. The stylet is removed. The tube is then rotated 90 degrees toward the bronchus to be intubated and advanced until resistance is met. The tracheal cuff

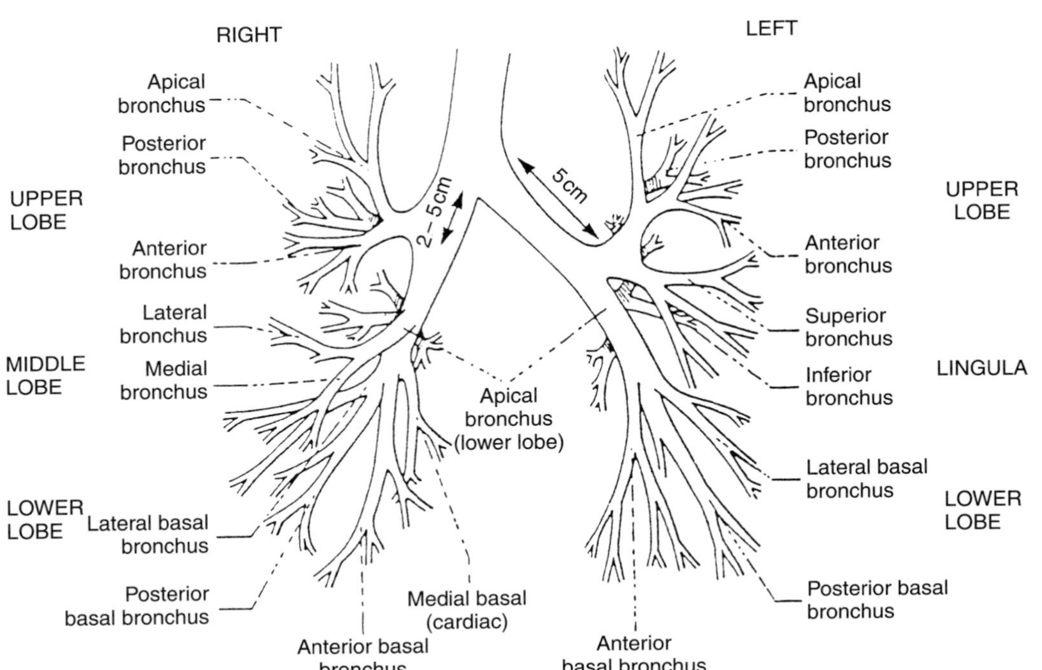

FIGURE **25-11**
Anatomy of the tracheobronchial tree, illustrating the difference between the lengths of the right and left mainstem bronchi. (From Gothard JWW, Branthwaite MA. *Anaesthesia for Thoracic Surgery*. Cambridge, England: Blackwell Scientific; 1982.)

TABLE 25-4 Summary of Lung Separation Devices and Recommendations for Placement

Device	Indication	Tube Size	Placement and Confirmation
Left-sided DLT	Majority of elective left or right thoracic surgical procedures	Determined by measurements of the tracheal width from chest radiograph	Fiberoptic bronchoscopy
Right-sided DLT	Left bronchus—distorted anatomy; left pneumonectomy		Fiberoptic bronchoscopy with guided technique
Fogarty occlusion catheter	Critically ill patient; small bronchus; difficult airway; nasotracheal intubation	Standard endotracheal tube at least 6 mm in diameter	Fiberoptic bronchoscopy
Univent blockers	Selective lobar blockade; difficult airway requiring lung separation		Fiberoptic bronchoscopy
WEB blockers	Critically ill patients; selective lobar blockade; difficult airway; nasotracheal intubation requiring lung separation	Standard endotracheal tube at least 8 mm in diameter	Fiberoptic bronchoscopy with guided technique

DLT, *Double-lumen endotracheal tube*; WEB, *wire-guided endobronchial blocker*.
From Campos JH. Lung separation techniques. In: Kaplan JA, Slinger PD, eds. Thoracic Anesthesia. *3rd ed. Philadelphia: Churchill Livingstone; 2003:172.*

requires 5 to 10 ml (up to 20 ml) of air, and the bronchial cuff requires 1 to 2 ml of air. Overinflation of the bronchial cuff can cause its lumen to be narrowed or occluded and increases the risk of tearing the bronchus. Adapters are attached to the two lumens for interface with the anesthesia circuit. Breath sounds should be auscultated with use of a systematic method to verify the proper position of each lumen (Box 25-4). Note the difference in airway pressure when one lung is ventilated.

BOX 25-4

Auscultation of Breath Sounds after Placement of a Double-Lumen Tube

- Inflate the tracheal cuff.
- Verify bilaterally equal breath sounds. If breath sounds are present on only one side, both lumens are in the same bronchus. Deflate the cuff and withdraw the tube 1 to 2 cm at a time until breath sounds are equal bilaterally.
- Inflate the endobronchial cuff.
- Clamp the endobronchial lumen and open its lumen cap proximal to the clamp.
- Verify breath sounds in the correct lung and the absence of breath sounds in the opposite lung.
- Verify that breath sounds are equal at the apex of the lung and at the lateral lung. If the apex is diminished, withdraw the tube until upper lung sounds return.
- Verify the absence of air leakage through the opposite lumen cap.
- Unclamp the endobronchial lumen and verify bilateral breath sounds.
- Clamp the tracheal lumen and open its cap.
- Verify breath sounds on the side opposite the lung with the endobronchial lumen and the absence of breath sounds on the other.
- When absolute lung separation is needed, as in bronchopulmonary lavage, connecting a clamped lumen to an underwater drainage system will show air bubbles if a leak is present.

Flexible fiberoptic bronchoscopy is essential to verify placement of the DLT (Figure 25-12). Fiberoptic bronchoscopy has revealed a 38% to 83% incidence of malpositioning of DLTs that were judged by auscultation to be properly placed.[24,25] If the bronchial lumen is found to be in the wrong bronchus, the flexible bronchoscope can be used as a stylet to guide the tube into the proper bronchus. Placement of the tube should again be verified by bronchoscopy after the patient is repositioned laterally. A fiberoptic bronchoscope of 4.9 mm external diameter can be lubricated and passed through an endobronchial tube of size 37 Fr or larger. A fiberoptic bronchoscope of 3.6 mm can pass through a 35 Fr tube.[5]

Complications of Double-Lumen Tubes

Placement of DLTs carries the same risks as laryngoscopy and intubation with endotracheal tubes. In addition, there exists a risk of hypoxemia with malpositioning of the tube (Figure 25-13). Rupture of a thoracic aneurysm is possible with a left DLT if the aneurysm compresses the left mainstem

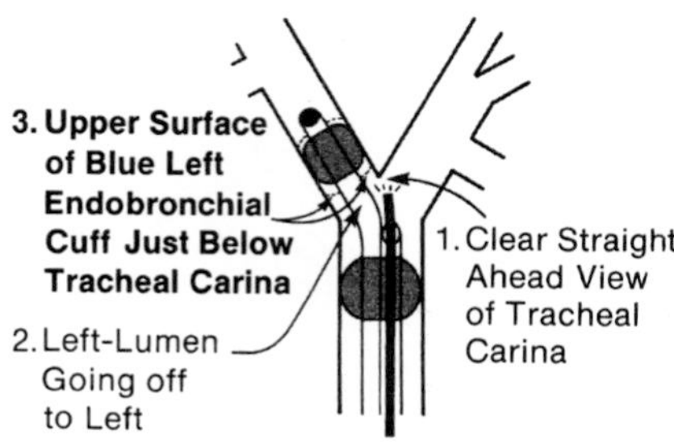

FIGURE 25-12
The fiberoptic bronchoscope is placed down the right lumen to determine precise left-sided double-lumen tube position. The endoscopist should see a clear straight-ahead view of the tracheal carina *(1)*, the left lumen going off into the left mainstem bronchus *(2)*, and, most important, the upper surface of the blue left endobronchial cuff just below the tracheal carina *(3)*. (From Benumof JL. *Anesthesia for Thoracic Surgery*. 2nd ed. Philadelphia: Saunders; 1995:352.)

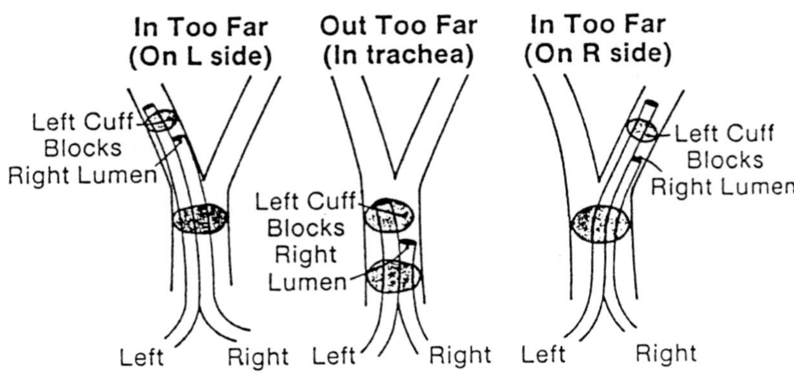

Procedure	Breath Sounds Heard		
	In Too Far (on Left Side)	Out Too Far (in Trachea)	In Too Far (on Right Side)
Clamp Right Lumen Both Cuffs Inflated	Left	Left and Right	Right
Clamp Left Lumen Both Cuffs Inflated	None or Very ↓↓	None or Very ↓↓	None or Very ↓↓
Clamp Left Lumen Deflate Left Cuff	Left	Left and Right	Right

FIGURE **25-13**
In each of these three malpositions of the endobronchial tube, the left cuff when fully inflated can completely block the right lumen. (From Benumof JL. *Anesthesia for Thoracic Surgery*. 2nd ed. Philadelphia: Saunders; 1995.)

bronchus. Damage to the vocal cords or arytenoid cartilages is possible from a carinal hook. A carinal hook can also break off, requiring retrieval with a bronchoscope. Bronchial rupture, which was thought to be caused by overinflation of the bronchial cuff, has been reported[26,27] An incident was reported in which pulmonary artery exsanguination occurred on extubation after a Carlen DLT had been inadvertently sutured to the artery through the wall of the trachea.[28]

Physiology of One-Lung Ventilation

During two-lung ventilation, blood flow to the dependent lung averages approximately 60% (Figure 25-14). When one lung is allowed to deflate and OLV is started, any blood flow to the deflated lung becomes shunt flow, causing the PaO_2 to decrease. Without autoregulation of pulmonary blood flow a 40% shunt would be anticipated. The lungs have a compensatory mechanism of increasing vascular resistance in hypoxic areas of the lungs, and this diverts some blood flow to areas of better ventilation and oxygenation. This mechanism is termed *hypoxic pulmonary vasoconstriction* (HPV). HPV is an intrapulmonary reflex-feedback mechanism in inhomogeneous lungs to improve gas exchange and arterial oxygenation.

Recent work suggests an important role for pulmonary arteriolar smooth muscle cell O_2-sensitive voltage-dependent potassium channels in HPV. Inhibition of these channels by decreased PO_2 inhibits outward potassium current, causing membrane depolarization, and calcium entry through voltage-dependent calcium channels. Endothelium-derived vasoconstricting and vasodilating mediators modulate this intrinsic smooth muscle cell reactivity to hypoxia.[4,29,30]

HPV during OLV is effective in decreasing the cardiac output to the nonventilated lung to 20% to 25% (Figure 25-15).[31] Shunt flow changes from 10% during two-lung ventilation to 27% during OLV. This increase in shunt decreases the mean PaO_2 from greater than 400 mm Hg during two-lung ventilation to slightly less than 200 mm Hg during OLV when the fraction of inspired O_2 (FIO_2) is 1.[23]

HPV occurs whether the lung is rendered hypoxic by atelectasis or by ventilation with a hypoxic mixture. HPV improves arterial oxygenation when the amount of hypoxic lung is between 30% and 70%, which is the condition during OLV. When less than 30% of the lung is hypoxic, the total amount of shunt is not significant; when more than 70% of the lung is hypoxic, HPV increases PVR, but the amount of well-perfused lung is not sufficient to accept shunt flow to maintain arterial oxygenation. This increase in PVR increases the work of the right side of the heart and can cause right ventricular strain and failure.[23]

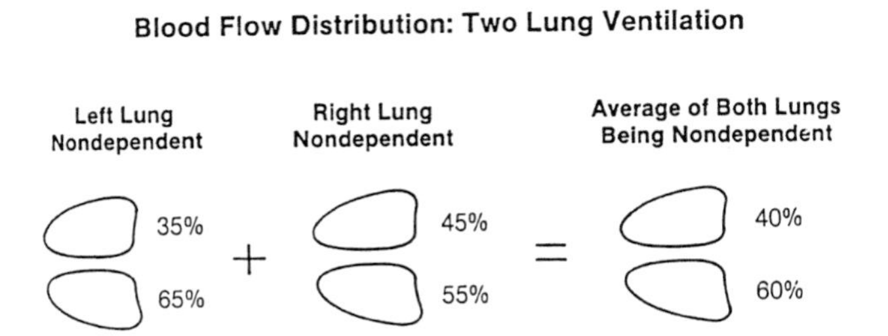

Blood Flow Distribution: Two Lung Ventilation

Left Lung Nondependent: 35% / 65% + Right Lung Nondependent: 45% / 55% = Average of Both Lungs Being Nondependent: 40% / 60%

FIGURE **25-14**
When the left lung is the nondependent lung, the distribution of the blood flow between the nondependent and dependent lungs is 35%/65%. When the right lung is the nondependent lung, the blood flow distribution between the nondependent and dependent lungs is 45%/55%. The average one-lung ventilation blood flow distribution consists of a nondependent-dependent ratio of 40%/60%. (From Benumof JL. *Anesthesia for Thoracic Surgery*. 2nd ed. Philadelphia: Saunders; 1995:314.)

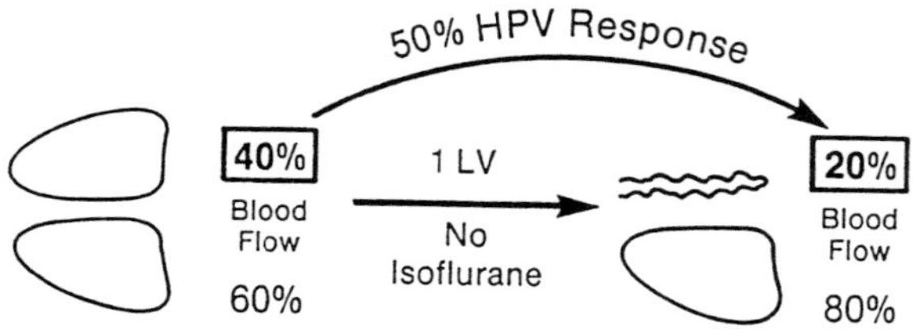

FIGURE **25-15**
The two-lung ventilation nondependent-dependent lung blood flow ratio is 40%/60%. When two-lung ventilation is converted to one-lung ventilation *(1 LV)*, the hypoxic pulmonary vasoconstriction *(HPV)* response decreases the blood flow to the nondependent lung by 50% so that the nondependent-dependent lung blood flow ratio becomes 20%/80%. (From Benumof JL. *Anesthesia for Thoracic Surgery*. 2nd ed. Philadelphia: Saunders; 1995:316.)

Because HPV is effective in decreasing shunt flow, avoidance of drugs or events that inhibit the mechanism is important. Inhalation agents have been studied extensively to determine their effect on HPV. Inhaled anesthetics have been reported to inhibit HPV in a variety of in vitro experimental preparations. In studies in which animal lungs were isolated from the body, inhalation agents have been found to decrease the vasoconstrictor response to hypoxic lung segments. However, when the same agents are used in intact specimens, human and animal, no change or very little change is seen in PaO_2, shunt flow, or regional blood flow. In patients, higher concentrations than minimal alveolar concentration are needed to inhibit HPV.[30] The intact body has autoregulatory mechanisms (e.g., baroreceptor reflexes, humeral influences, and changes in cardiac output) that probably account for the difference in inhibition of HPV between in vitro and intact in vivo specimens.[32]

The influence of various intravenous agents on HPV has also been investigated. In vitro and in vivo studies have revealed no change in HPV with fentanyl, pentazocine, ketamine, droperidol, diazepam, thiopental, or pentobarbital.[33] When propofol was administered after the institution of OLV, no change in venous admixture or PaO_2 was found.[34]

Several vasodilating drugs inhibit HPV, including nitroglycerin, nitroprusside, dobutamine, some calcium antagonists, and some β_2-agonists. Vasoconstrictive drugs, including dopamine, epinephrine, and phenylephrine, may preferentially constrict normally oxygenated pulmonary vessels and increase shunt flow.[31]

Elevations in pulmonary vascular pressure or cardiac output can cause recruitment of constricted vessels and inhibit HPV. Hypocapnia, alkalosis, and acidosis decrease HPV. Hypothermia causes pulmonary vasoconstriction and can shunt blood away from the ventilated lung.[1]

Management of One-Lung Ventilation

Choice of Anesthetic

On the basis of the preceding discussion, clinical doses of potent inhalation agents do not significantly alter the mechanism of HPV. Inhalation agents offer several benefits in thoracic surgery. They allow the use of a high FIO_2 to help prevent hypoxemia during OLV. They produce bronchodilatory effects and decrease airway irritability in patients to be subjected to direct manipulation of lung tissue. In contrast, the dose of narcotics required to obtund airway reflexes could depress ventilation and necessitate postoperative ventilation. Inhalation agents are rapidly eliminated at the end of surgery and allow for early extubation. For these reasons inhalation agents are usually chosen as the primary anesthetics during thoracic surgery.

Nitrous oxide is generally avoided in favor of 100% O_2 to prevent hypoxia and any significant increase in PVR. Nitrous oxide increases PVR in cardiac patients whose baseline PVR is within normal limits, from a mean of 112 to 130 dynes • sec^{-1} • cm^{-5}. Nitrous oxide raises PVR much more markedly in patients whose PVR is already elevated from mitral valve stenosis, from a mean of 357 to 530 dynes • sec^{-1} • cm^{-5}.[34] This is cause for even greater clinical concern with concurrent right ventricular dysfunction. Nitrous oxide should also be avoided in patients with bullous or emphysematous lungs because it may increase the volume of trapped airspace.

Ventilation during One-Lung Ventilation

The primary goal during OLV is maintenance of adequate arterial oxygenation. Two-lung ventilation should be maintained as long as possible, and the time of OLV minimized. In the past, large VTs of 10 ml/kg (range 8 to 15 ml/kg) were recommended to prevent atelectasis in the dependent lung and maintain an adequate FRC. Recent data suggest that most patients during OLV develop auto-PEEP and have an increased FRC.[35,36] The use of a large VT in a lung that is starting at an increased volume can lead to end-inspiratory lung volumes that approach the theoretic limits associated with ventilator-induced lung injury. Because of this concern, clinicians have backed down from the traditional large VTs for one-lung anesthesia and are using more physiologic volumes (e.g., 5 ml/kg), adding PEEP to those patients without auto-PEEP and limiting plateau inspiratory pressures to <25 cm H_2O.[36,37]

An appropriate air-O_2 mixture, at times as high as an FIO_2 of 1, is necessary to maximize the PaO_2. The respiratory rate is adjusted to maintain a normal $PaCO_2$. The relationship between $PaCO_2$ and end-tidal CO_2 is not altered by OLV.

Should hypoxemia occur during OLV, one or more of the following interventions will help improve PaO_2. PEEP applied to the dependent, ventilated lung acts to increase PaO_2 by recruiting collapsed airways, increasing compliance of the lung, and increasing FRC. If atelectasis is the mechanism of hypoxia during OLV, PEEP will improve FRC and PaO_2. Under different conditions, PEEP can exert pressure on small pulmonary vessels, causing more shunt to the unventilated lung and decreasing PaO_2.[38]

Continuous positive airway pressure (CPAP) to the nondependent, nonventilated lung is almost 100% efficacious in increasing PaO_2. In a 1992 study by Lewis and colleagues, a PaO_2 of less than 80 mm Hg developed in 28.5% of patients during OLV with an FIO_2 of 1. In 37% of these instances hypoxia was transient and responded to suctioning, brief lung reinflation, DLT repositioning, VT adjustment, or final unclamping of the DLT. In the remaining 63% of these patients some combination of PEEP and CPAP was required. When PEEP alone was added, PaO_2 rose above 80 mm Hg in only 40% of cases. CPAP was used alone in six patients and raised the PaO_2 above 80 mm Hg in all patients. PEEP plus CPAP raised the PaO_2 to higher than 80 mm Hg in all but one patient.[23]

The application of 5 to 10 cm H_2O of CPAP during the deflation phase of a VT breath maintains patency and distention of small airways and allows some O_2 exchange in the operative lung. These low levels of CPAP distend the lung to a volume of 50 to 100 ml, which is generally not a hindrance to the surgeon.[21] When the chest is open, CPAP does not significantly alter hemodynamics or shunt flow.[39]

Other methods of improving oxygenation during OLV include (1) combining PEEP and CPAP and (2) early ligation of the pulmonary artery in pneumonectomy patients. Communication with the surgical team is vital throughout the procedure, especially during the evaluation and correction of hypoxia.

ANALGESIA FOR THORACIC SURGERY

Pain after thoracic surgery causes splinting, decreased respiratory effort, hypoxemia, and respiratory acidosis. Aggressive management of pain is aimed at seeking a balance between comfort and respiratory depression in patients with decreased lung function. Residual pain exists in half of thoracotomy patients after 1 year and in one third of patients after 4 years.[40]

Several options can be considered in management of postoperative pain. Patients can titrate intravenous patient-controlled analgesia to obtain a more constant level of analgesia than that provided by intermittent intramuscular injections.[1] Intercostal nerve blocks can be placed at the level of the incision plus one or two intercostal interspaces above and below the site. Rapid intravascular absorption of the local anesthetic is possible in this highly vascular area.

Cryoanalgesia is performed by applying a cryoprobe cooled to −60° C to nerves in intercostal spaces two to three spaces above and below the incision, disrupting nerve activity for 1 to 3 months. Local anesthesia may be instilled in a catheter placed in the intrapleural space by the surgeon. Thoracic epidural catheters may be placed preoperatively (T6 to T8) and infused with epidural opioids or dilute solutions of local anesthetics to provide analgesia postoperatively.

COMPLICATIONS AFTER THORACOTOMY

Significant factors associated with acute lung injury (ALI) after pulmonary resection include right pneumonectomy, intraoperative overhydration with high vascular volume, high intraoperative airway pressure during one-lung ventilation and preoperative alcohol abuse. Other factors that have been suggested are mediastinal lymphatic damage, administration of fresh frozen plasma, serum cytokines, O_2 toxicity, and an increased postoperative urine output. Fortunately, the incidence of postoperative pneumonia and atelectasis is declining. Minimizing pulmonary intravascular pressures by intraoperative fluid restriction is advocated to decrease postoperative complications. Surgical requirements for proper hydration and tissue perfusion must be balanced with the desire to prevent high postoperative intravascular pressures and possible pulmonary edema. Avoidance of fluid overload in pneumonectomy patients is especially important.[36]

Several preoperative patient comorbidities such as chronic alcoholism and respiratory diseases are associated with increased susceptibility to ALI because they reduce lung defense mechanisms, restrict capillary volume, and enhance the inflammatory response against injurious agents. During and after surgery the effects of lung hyperinflation, surgical trauma, ischemia, and reperfusion induce the release of inflammatory mediators and a combination of insults at the alveolar-endothelial barrier. The result is lung edema and eventual organ dysfunction. In addition, stretching of capillaries by overzealous fluid administration (or impaired pulmonary venous return) may cause stress failure within microvessels, which further aggravates permeability disturbances.[37,41-43]

Implementation of risk-reduction strategies for the occurrence of ALI, particularly in patients undergoing pneumonectomy and in those with underlying lung diseases, is important. Such strategies may include withdrawal of alcohol for a safe period of abstinence and correction of nutritional deficits before elective surgery; intraoperative application of pressure-controlled ventilation with small VTs and with air-O_2 mixtures to prevent barotrauma or volume-trauma and oxidative damages; limitation of fluid intake for the first 24 to 48 hours after surgery while maintaining tight control of hemodynamics; and implementation of monitoring tools to assess cardiac preload, intrathoracic blood volume, and pulmonary artery pressure (e.g., stroke volume or pressure variation, transpulmonary thermo-dye dilution technique, and echocardiography) that allow early detection of pulmonary hypertension and interstitial lung edema. These conditions can be treated with diuretics, inhaled nitric oxide, and noninvasive positive pressure ventilatory techniques.[37]

Low cardiac output in the early postoperative period can be caused by several factors, including blood loss, herniation of the heart through a pericardial defect, right-sided heart failure, and dysrhythmias. Generally, blood entering the pleural space drains into chest tubes at a rate of less than 500 ml per day. Chest tube drainage greater than 200 ml per hour necessitates surgical reexploration. An obstructed chest tube can conceal bleeding in a hemothorax. Hypotension, unexplained tachycardia, and decreasing hematocrit are other signs of bleeding.

If the pericardium has been opened to gain exposure to hilar blood vessels, the heart may herniate through the pericardial defect. Acute cardiovascular collapse can occur if the great vessels are kinked and obstructed. Immediate surgery is required to repair the pericardial defect. Temporary measures to regain stability include positioning the patient with the operative side up to allow the heart to reenter the sac, discontinuing chest tube suction, discontinuing PEEP, and maintaining spontaneous ventilation if possible.[44,45]

Loss of pulmonary vasculature with lung resection can result in increased PVR and right-sided heart failure. Pneumonectomy patients have greater changes in the ejection fraction than lobectomy patients. The ejection fraction in lobectomy patients changed from 40% to 36%, compared with a change from 41% to 29% in pneumonectomy patients.[46] Conditions that increase the likelihood of right-sided heart failure include postoperative pneumonia, hypercarbia, and acidosis. Vasodilating agents such as nitroglycerin, sodium nitroprusside, calcium channel blockers, and hydralazine have been used to dilate the pulmonary vasculature to decrease PVR. Amrinone or dobutamine can be administered if an inotrope is also needed.[1]

Dysrhythmias are relatively common after thoracotomy because of hypoxemia, vagal irritation, atrial inflammation, preexisting cardiac disease, pulmonary hypertension, or right atrial or ventricular dilation. In a review of 236 pneumonectomy patients, 22% experienced cardiac dysrhythmias, most commonly atrial fibrillation, supraventricular tachycardia, and atrial flutter.[47] Morbidity and mortality rates in patients with supraventricular tachydysrhythmias are high, with 20% of the total associated with hypotension and 25% associated with death within 30 days postoperatively, despite institution of aggressive treatment. No correlation between the incidence of dysrhythmias and preoperative pulmonary function or age was found. The incidence of dysrhythmias in association with intrapericardial dissection and pulmonary edema was higher than expected. Administration of more than 2000 ml of fluids intraoperatively may increase the risk of pulmonary infiltration and the incidence of dysrhythmias.

Administration of a β-blocking agent can help prevent atrial dysrhythmias. Jakobsen and co-workers[48] administered 100 mg of oral metoprolol preoperatively and daily postoperatively. The incidence of atrial tachycardia lasting longer than 30 seconds was 6.7% compared with 40% in the placebo group.

Digitalis, adenosine, calcium channel blockers, and β-blockers are used to treat supraventricular tachydysrhythmias. Cardioversion may become necessary if a patient is hemodynamically unstable.

The increased PVR and right-sided heart pressures after lung resection can cause a right-to-left shunt through a patent foramen ovale. Treatment is aimed at correction of hypoxemia, acidosis, and hypercarbia; use of pulmonary vasodilators; and treatment of infection to lower right-sided pressures and functionally close the defect.

Respiratory complications in the early postoperative period include atelectasis, pneumonia, respiratory failure, bronchopleural or bronchocutaneous fistula, pneumothorax, torsion of remaining lobes necessitating surgical correction, and pulmonary edema resulting from high fluid administration. Aggressive respiratory care is needed to prevent deterioration and allow weaning from ventilation. Blood, blood clots, or thick secretions can cause airway obstruction. Tracheal suction or bronchoscopy may be needed to clear the lungs.

Disruption of the bronchial stump repair creates a communication between the bronchus and the pleural space. The escape of gas causes massive bubbling in the chest tube drainage system if it is patent or a potential tension pneumothorax with mediastinal shift if the chest tube is occluded. A large portion of the V_T can be lost to this low-resistance pathway, compromising gas exchange. Any fluid present in the pleural space can enter the defect and contaminate the healthy lung.[21] A small leak may heal with conservative medical management, including placement of a chest tube and ventilatory support if needed. High-frequency ventilation has been used with varying results to allow the defect to heal. Surgical interventions to close the defect include endoscopic application of sealing agents, closure with vascular tissue or muscle flaps, and further lung resection.[49]

If the leak from the bronchopleural fistula is so large that it interferes with adequate ventilation, the placement of a DLT facilitates ventilation of the healthy lung and prevents further contamination. Until the DLT is placed, the patient should be positioned so that the lung with the fistula is dependent, and the patient should maintain spontaneous respiration. The endobronchial lumen should be in the healthy lung before positive pressure ventilation is begun.[21]

Thoracic duct injury is possible during a left thoracotomy or the placement of left-sided central lines. A chylothorax may occur in either thorax after removal of lymph nodes during thoracotomies. Creamy chyle may be noted in the chest tube drainage or may be suspected weeks later with weight loss and recurrent sepsis. Thoracic duct injury necessitates ligation of the duct or pleuroperitoneal shunting.[50]

Nerve injuries that may follow thoracic surgery include damage to the phrenic nerve as it passes through the mediastinum and damage to the left recurrent laryngeal nerve, which is vulnerable during dissection of aortopulmonary lymph nodes and mediastinal procedures.[51] Spinal cord injury is a possibility if an intercostal artery supplying a major radicular artery is injured or if an epidural hematoma is created by surgical dissection between the pleura and the epidural space.

MEDIASTINAL MASSES

Masses in the mediastinum can compress vital structures and cause changes in cardiac output, obstruction to air flow, atelectasis, or central nervous system changes. Masses can include benign or cancerous tumors, thymomas, substernal thyroid masses, vascular aneurysms, lymphomas, and neuromas.

Tumors within the anterior mediastinum can cause compression of the trachea or bronchi, increasing resistance to air flow. Changes in airway dynamics with supine positioning, induction of anesthesia, and positive pressure ventilation can cause collapse of the airway with total obstruction to flow. Manipulation of tissue intraoperatively, edema, and bleeding into masses can increase their size and effects on airways or vasculature. Total airway obstruction can occur at any phase of anesthesia, positioning, induction, intubation, emergence, or recovery. Positive pressure ventilation may be impossible even with a properly placed endotracheal tube. Maintenance of spontaneous ventilation retains normal airway-distending pressure gradients and can maintain airway patency when positive pressure will not.[52,53]

Signs and symptoms of respiratory tract compression should be sought preoperatively. Wheezing may represent air flow past a mechanical obstruction rather than bronchospasm. Shortness of breath at rest or with exertion and coughing are other symptoms. Symptoms may be positional, worsening in the supine or other position. A chest radiograph may show airway compression or deviation. Computed tomography and magnetic resonance imaging further delineate the size and effects of masses. Subclinical airway obstruction may be revealed by flow-volume loops, which demonstrate changes in flow rates at different lung volumes. Decreased maximal inspiratory or expiratory flow rate alerts the anesthetist to increased risk of obstruction perioperatively. Comparison of flow rates obtained with the patient in the upright and supine positions can reveal whether the supine position will exacerbate obstruction intraoperatively (Figure 25-16).[54]

If any sign of respiratory obstruction is present, surgery for the biopsy of masses should be performed with the patient under local anesthesia whenever possible. Radiation to decrease mass bulk in radiosensitive tumors is recommended before surgery to reduce the risk of airway obstruction.[55]

The use of a helium-O_2 mixture can improve air flow during partial obstruction. The use of this low-density gas decreases turbulence past a stenotic area, improving flow and decreasing the work of breathing.[56]

Awake fiberoptic bronchoscopy and intubation enables the anesthetist to evaluate the large airways for obstruction and to place the endotracheal tube beyond the obstruction while maintaining spontaneous ventilation. The effect of positional changes can be checked with the bronchoscope.[57] If general anesthesia is required in a patient with a significant airway obstruction, the means for cardiopulmonary bypass should be immediately available in the sterile field.[58]

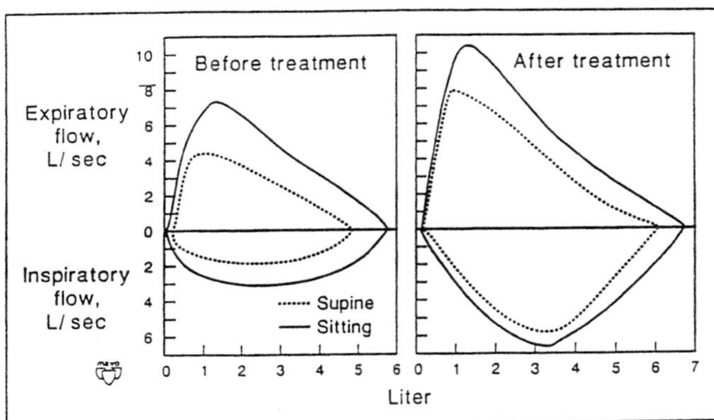

FIGURE **25-16**
Flow-volume curves obtained in supine and upright positions before *(left)* and 4 weeks after *(right)* two courses of chemotherapy in a patient with mediastinal Hodgkin's lymphoma. (From Prakash UB, Abel MD, Hubmayer RD. Mediastinal mass and tracheal obstruction during general anesthesia. *Mayo Clin Proc.* 1988;63:1004-1011. By permission of the Mayo Foundation.)

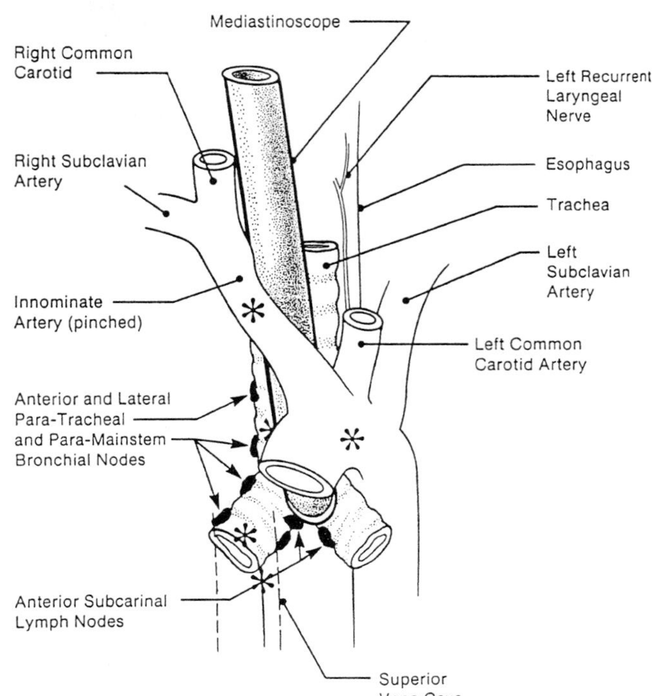

FIGURE **25-17**
Placement of a mediastinoscope into the superior mediastinum. The mediastinoscope passes in front of the trachea but behind the thoracic aorta. Anatomic structures that can be compressed by the mediastinoscope *(asterisks)* leading to major complications are the thoracic aorta (rupture, reflex bradycardia), innominate artery (decreased right carotid and right subclavian flow), trachea (inability to ventilate), and vena cava (risk of hemorrhage with superior vena cava syndrome). (From Benumof JL. *Anesthesia for Thoracic Surgery.* 2nd ed. Philadelphia: Saunders; 1995:505.)

Masses can also cause compression of great vessels or cardiac chambers. Compression of the pulmonary artery is rare because it is a higher-pressure vessel than the pulmonary vein and is somewhat protected by the arch of the aorta. Compression of this vessel, however, can lead to sudden hypoxemia, hypotension, or cardiac arrest.[59] Patients with any cardiac or great vessel involvement should receive only local anesthesia whenever possible, remain in the sitting position, and maintain spontaneous respirations.[60] If general anesthesia is required, the means for cardiopulmonary bypass should be immediately available.[61]

Superior vena cava syndrome is venous engorgement of the upper body caused by compression of the superior vena cava by a mass. It leads to the following signs and symptoms: dilation of collateral veins of the upper part of the thorax and neck; edema and rubor of the face, neck, and upper torso and airway; edema of the conjunctiva with or without proptosis; shortness of breath; and headache, visual distortion, or altered mentation.[54] Placement of intravenous lines in the lower extremities is preferred because insertion in sites above the superior vena cava could delay the drug effect as a result of slow distribution. Fluids should be administered with caution, because large volumes can worsen symptoms.

Mediastinoscopy

Mediastinoscopy involves passing a scope into the mediastinum via an incision above the suprasternal notch. The scope is passed anterior to the trachea in close proximity to the left common carotid artery, the left subclavian artery, the innominate artery, the innominate veins, the vagus nerve, the left recurrent laryngeal nerve, the thoracic duct, the superior vena cava, and the aortic arch. Complications of mediastinoscopy include pneumothorax, hemorrhage resulting from tearing of major vessels, arrhythmias, bronchospasm resulting from manipulation of the airway, laceration of the esophagus, and chylothorax secondary to laceration of the thoracic duct.[60,62] Large-bore intravenous lines should be in place, and blood should be immediately available in the event of a tear in a major blood vessel. Air embolism is also a risk if a venous tear is present. Arrhythmias such as bradycardia are possible with manipulation of the aorta or trachea during blunt dissection.

The mediastinoscope can place pressure on the innominate artery as it passes through the upper thorax, causing a decrease in blood flow to the right common carotid artery and the right vertebral artery and a decrease in subclavian flow to the right arm (Figure 25-17).[63] The decrease in cerebral flow could be detrimental, especially if the patient has a history of cerebrovascular disease. Monitoring perfusion to the right arm with a pulse oximeter or radial artery catheter can detect decreased flow to the right arm and signal concurrent loss of flow to the brain via the innominate artery. Repositioning of the mediastinoscope is required to reestablish flow to the brain. A noninvasive blood pressure cuff placed on the left arm enables continued monitoring of systemic blood pressure during periods of innominate artery compression.

THORACOSCOPY

Advances in videoscopic technology have led to the increased use of thoracoscopy. The uses of the thoracoscope and anesthetic techniques are still being expanded and refined. The procedure used most commonly involves placing the patient in the lateral decubitus position. A trocar is usually introduced at the fourth to fifth or fifth to sixth intercostal space to allow passage of the thoracoscope. Additional trocars and cannulas can be passed to insert suction, cautery, or other instruments.[64]

Drainage and examination of the pleural space, débridement of an empyema, removal of foreign bodies, instillation of talc or chemotherapeutic agents into the pleural space, stapling of blebs, diagnostic biopsies and staging, and evaluation of bronchopleural fistulas are some of the procedures possible with thoracoscopy.[65-67]

General anesthesia with a double-lumen endobronchial tube offers several advantages for thoracoscopy. The airway is secured before lateral positioning. This avoids the need to change to general anesthesia under less-than-optimal conditions should local anesthesia or sedation techniques fail.[64] It allows for deflation of the lung before the introduction of the trocar. CPAP and PEEP can be applied as needed to improve oxygenation. Controlled ventilation helps prevent paradoxic respiration and mediastinal shift, and the lung can be actively reinflated at the end of the procedure.[68] The anesthetist should be prepared for a switch to an open thoracotomy should the surgeon be unable to complete the procedure by thoracoscopy.

An arterial line is generally placed for thoracoscopy except in selected healthy patients. Patients for thoracic procedures are generally at risk for cardiopulmonary morbidity. OLV alters respiratory physiology, necessitating the ability to rapidly obtain arterial blood gas analysis.

Thoracoscopic sympathectomy for hyperhydrosis is an outpatient procedure. A DLT is preferred over a bronchial blocker because the procedure is bilateral. Positioning the DLT once at the beginning of the case so that each lung can be deflated one at time is much easier than repositioning a bronchial blocker into the opposite bronchus once one side has been completed. The patient is in the supine position, and no chest tubes are inserted. Air and O_2 are preferred carrier gases.

Pain after a thoracoscopy is generally more easily managed than after an open thoracotomy. The incision length is smaller, and spreading of the ribs is avoided. Adequate pain relief is commonly obtained with the use of oral analgesics or nonsteroidal antiinflammatory drugs. More extensive procedures such as decortication or pleurodesis often require parenteral narcotics. Intercostal block may also be used to treat pain from manipulation of the thoracoscope in the camera port.[68]

BULLAE

Bullae are air-filled spaces of lung tissue resulting from the destruction of alveolar tissues. They offer low resistance to inspiration and tend to increase in size with positive pressure ventilation. A valvelike mechanism may be present that causes air trapping on expiration. Enlarging bullae compress normal lung tissue and vasculature to the point of causing hypoxemia, polycythemia, and cor pulmonale. Overdistended bullae can rupture and cause pneumothorax or tension pneumothorax with cardiopulmonary collapse, requiring insertion of a chest tube. A chest tube may show a large, continuous air leak, and ventilation may be difficult.[69]

A DLT is indicated when a thoracotomy is planned to resect bullous tissue. This allows for separate ventilation of each lung and the ability to use adequate VTs on the healthy lung. In the event of a pneumothorax the unaffected lung can be ventilated while a chest tube is placed or the incision is made. When the surgery is nearing completion, each lung can be separately checked for air leaks.

During general anesthesia for bullous disease, spontaneous ventilation is desirable until the chest is opened. Patients with severe cardiopulmonary disease may not be able to ventilate adequately under general anesthesia, however, and positive pressure ventilation may be required. Small VTs, high respiratory rates, and high FIO_2 can be delivered by gentle manual ventilation to keep airway pressures below 10 to 20 cm H_2O.[69] An alternative to positive pressure ventilation is high-frequency jet ventilation, used to decrease the chance of barotrauma. Normandale[70] describes jet ventilation with settings of a respiratory rate of 250 per minute, a volume of driving gas of 18 L/min, and inspiratory time of 3% of the total respiratory cycle with an FIO_2 of 0.8.

Nitrous oxide should be avoided in bullous disease because it rapidly enlarges the air-filled space. The choice of other anesthetic agents depends on the patient's cardiopulmonary status and the anesthetist's desire to maintain spontaneous ventilation. Hasenbon and Gielen described a combination general-epidural technique using epidural bupivacaine with epinephrine and a light general anesthetic. Bupivacaine 0.25% with epinephrine 1:200,000, 8 ml, resulted in an anesthetic block of T2 to T10. After induction with intravenous anesthetics the vocal cords were anesthetized with 10% lidocaine topically, and a DLT was placed. Spontaneous ventilation was maintained, occasionally with manual assistance. The catheter was then used for postoperative epidural analgesia.[71]

After excision of the bulla, normal lung tissue rapidly expands, and compliance and gas exchange rapidly improve. Care must still be taken with positive pressure ventilation if some unresectable bullae remain.

SUMMARY

Anesthetizing a patient for thoracic surgery requires intricate coordination of multiple factors. The patient may have cardiac or respiratory diseases, masses, bullae, and other problems. Working knowledge of respiratory physiology, respiratory pathophysiology, and the physiology of OLV is required. Special equipment such as DLTs and fiberoptic bronchoscopes must be understood. A thorough understanding of the properties of anesthetic drugs is necessary so that the most beneficial combination of agents can be selected to manage the patient's anesthesia.

ACKNOWLEDGMENT

I would like to thank Jim Baer, CRNA, MS, for his expert review and suggestions during the preparation of this chapter.

REFERENCES

1. Weiss SJ, Aukburg SJ. Thoracic anesthesia. In: Longnecker DE, Tinker JH, Morgan GE, eds. *Principles and Practice of Anesthesiology*. 2nd ed. St Louis: Mosby; 1998:1736-1840.
2. Pate P, Tenholder MF, Griffin JP, et al. Preoperative assessment of the high-risk patient for lung resection. *Ann Thorac Surg*. 1996;61:1494-1500.
3. Slinger PP, Johnston MR. Preoperative assessment and management. In: Kaplan JA, Slinger PD. *Thoracic Anesthesia*. 3rd ed. Philadelphia: Churchill Livingstone; 2003:1-23.

4. Tassi G, Marchetti G. Minithoracoscopy: a less invasive approach to thoracoscopy. *Chest*. 2003;124:1975-1977.
5. Eisenkraft JB, Cohen E, Neustein SM. Anesthesia for thoracic surgery. In: Barash PG, Cullen BF, Stoelting RK, eds. *Clinical Anesthesia*. 4th ed. Philadelphia: Lippincott; 2001:813-852.
6. Marriot HJL. Chamber enlargement. In: *Practical Electrocardiography*. Baltimore: William & Wilkins; 1988:50-62.
7. Dubin D. Hypertrophy. In: *Rapid interpretation of EKGs*. 6th ed. Tampa, Fl: Cover; 2000:243-258.
8. Markos J, Mullan BP, Hillman DR, et al. Preoperative assessment as a predictor of mortality and morbidity after lung resection. *Am Rev Respir Dis*. 1989;139:902-910.
9. Berchard D, Wetstein L. Assessment of exercise oxygen consumption as preoperative criterion for lung resection. *Ann Thorac Surg*. 1987;44:344-349.
10. Wyser C, Stulz P, Soler M, et al. Prospective evaluation of an algorithm for the functional assessment of lung resection candidates. *Am J Respir Crit Care Med*. 1999;159:1450-1456.
11. Pate P, Tenholder MF, Griffin JP, et al. Preoperative assessment of the high-risk patient for lung resection. *Ann Thorac Surg*. 1996;61:1494-1500.
12. Reilly JJ. Evidence-based preoperative evaluation of candidates for thoracotomy. *Chest*. 1999;116:474S-476S.
13. Nakahara K, Ohno K, Hashimoto J, et al. Prediction of postoperative respiratory failure in patients undergoing lung resection for lung cancer. *Ann Thorac Surg*. 1988;46:549-552.
14. Ali MK, Mountain C, Miller JM, et al. Regional pulmonary function before and after pneumonectomy using 133 Xenon. *Chest*. 1975;68:288-296.
15. Ali MK, Mountain CF, Ewer MS, et al. Predicting loss of pulmonary function after pulmonary resection for bronchogenic carcinoma. *Chest*. 1980;77:337-342.
16. Wiener-Kronish JP, Albert RK. Preoperative evaluation. In: Murray JF, Nadel JA. *Textbook of Respiratory Medicine*. 3rd ed. Philadelphia: Saunders; 2000:883-894.
17. Bowdle TA. Complications of invasive monitoring. *Anesthesiol Clin North Am*. 2002;20:571-588.
18. Ehrenwerth J, Urban MK. Monitoring during thoracic surgery. *Probl Anesth*. 1990;4:306-325.
19. Lawson NW, Meyer J. Lateral decubitus positions. In: Martin JT, Warner MA, eds. *Positioning in Anesthesia and Surgery*. 3rd ed. Philadelphia: Saunders; 1997:124-145.
20. West J. *Respiratory Physiology: the Essentials*. Baltimore: Williams & Wilkins; 1990:31-50.
21. Benumof JL. Special respiratory physiology of the lateral decubitus position, the open chest and one lung anesthesia. In: *Anesthesia for Thoracic Surgery*. 2nd ed. Philadelphia: Saunders; 1995:123-151.
22. Takahashi M, Yamada M, Honda I, et al. Selective lobar-bronchial blocking for pediatric video-assisted thoracic surgery. *Anesthesiology*. 2001;94:170-172.
23. Lewis JW, et al. The utility of a double-lumen tube for one-lung ventilation in a variety of noncardiac thoracic surgical procedures. *J Cardiothorac Vasc Anesth*. 1992;6:705-710.
24. Campos JH. Lung isolation techniques. *Anesthesiol Clin North Am*. 2001;19:455-474.
25. Klein U, et al. Role of fiberoptic bronchoscopy in conjunction with the use of double-lumen tubes for thoracic anesthesia. *Anesthesiology*. 1998;88:346-350.
26. Gilbert TB, Goodsell CW, Krasna MJ. Bronchial rupture by a double-lumen endobronchial tube during staging thoracoscopy. *Anesth Analg*. 1999;88:1252-1253.
27. Yuceyar L, Kaynak K, Canturk E, et al. Bronchial rupture with a left-sided polyvinylchloride double-lumen tube. *Acta Anaesthesiol Scand*. 2003;47:622-625.
28. Dryden GE. Circulatory collapse after pneumonectomy (an unusual complication from the use of a Carlen's catheter): case report. *Anesth Analg*. 1977;56:451-452.
29. Weir EK, Archer SL. The mechanism of acute hypoxic pulmonary vasoconstriction: the tale of two channels. *FASEB J*. 1995;9:183-189.
30. Hillier SC, Graham JA, Hanger CC, Godbey P, Glenny RW, Wagner WW. Hypoxic vasoconstriction in pulmonary arterioles and venules. *J Appl Physiol*. 1997;82:1084-1090.
31. Benumof JL. One-lung ventilation and hypoxic pulmonary vasoconstriction: implications for anesthetic management. *Anesth Analg*. 1985;64:821-833.
32. Eisenkraft J. Effects of anesthetics on the pulmonary circulation. *Br J Anaesth*. 1990;65:63-78.
33. Schulte-Sasse U, Hess W, Tarnow J. Pulmonary vascular responses to nitrous oxide in patients with normal and high pulmonary vascular resistance. *Anesthesiology*. 1982;57:9-13.
34. Van Keer L, Van Aken H, Vandermeersch E, Vermaut G, Lerut T. Propofol does not inhibit hypoxic pulmonary vasoconstriction in humans. *J Clin Anesth*. 1989;1:284-288.
35. Slinger P, Kruger M, McRae K, Winton T. Relation of the static compliance curve and positive end-expiratory pressure to oxygenation during one-lung ventilation. *Anesthesiology*. 2001;95:1096-1102.
36. Slinger PD. Acute lung injury after pulmonary resection: more pieces of the puzzle. *Anesth Analg*. 2003;97:1555-1557.
37. Licker M, De Perrot M, Spiliopoulos A, et al. Risk factors for acute lung injury after thoracic surgery for lung cancer. *Anesth Analg*. 2003;97:1558-1565.
38. Cohen E, Eisenkraft JB, Positive end-expiratory pressure during one-lung ventilation improves oxygenation in patients with low arterial oxygen tensions. *J Cardiothorac Vasc Anesth*. 1996;10:578-582.
39. Cohen E, Eisenkraft JB, Thys DM, Kirschner PA, Kaplan JA. Oxygenation and hemodynamic changes during one-lung ventilation: effects of $CPAP_{10}$, $PEEP_{10}$, and $CPAP_{10}/PEEP_{10}$. *J Cardiothorac Anesth*. 1988;2:34-40.
40. Tippana E, Nilsson E, Kalso E. Post-thoracotomy pain after thoracic epidural analgesia: a prospective follow-up study. *Acta Anaethesiol Scand*. 2003;47:433-438.
41. Acute Respiratory Distress Syndrome Network. Ventilation with lower tidal volumes as compared with traditional tidal volumes for acute lung injury and the acute respiratory distress syndrome. *N Engl J Med*. 2000;342:1301-1308.
42. Brodsky JB, Fitzmaurice B. Modern anesthetic techniques for thoracic operations. *World J Surg*. 2001;25:162-166.
43. Matthay MA. Conference summary: acute lung injury. *Chest*. 1999;116:119S-126S.
44. Higgins T. Postthoracotomy complications. In: Kaplan JA, Slinger PD, eds. *Thoracic Anesthesia*. 3rd ed. Philadelphia: Churchill Livingstone; 2003:383-396.
45. Mascotto G, Bizzarri M, Messina M, et al. Prospective randomized, controlled evaluation of the preventive effects of positive end-expiratory pressure on patient oxygenation during one-lung ventilation. *Eur J Anaesthesiol*. 2003;20:704-710.
46. Boldt J, Muller M, Uphus D, Padberg W, Hempelmann G. Cardiorespiratory changes in patients undergoing pulmonary resection using different anesthetic management techniques. *J Cardiothorac Vasc Anesth*. 1996;10:854-859.
47. Krowka MJ, Pairolero PC, Trastek VF, Payne WS, Bernatz PE. Cardiac dysrhythmia following pneumonectomy: clinical correlates and prognostic significance. *Chest*. 1987;91:490-495.
48. Jakobsen CJ, Bille S, Ahlburg P, Rybro L, Hjortholm K, Andresen EB. Perioperative metoprolol reduces the frequency of atrial fibrillation after thoracotomy for lung resection. *J Cardiothorac Vasc Anesth*. 1997;11:746-751.
49. Baumann MH, Sahn SA. Medical management and therapy of bronchopleural fistulas in the mechanically ventilated patient. *Chest*. 1990;97:721-728.
50. Milsom JW, Kron IL, Rheuban LS. Chylothorax: an assessment of surgical management. *J Thorac Cardiovasc Surg*. 1985;89:221-227.
51. Gallagher C, Sladen RN, Lubarsky D. Thoracotomy: postoperative complications. *Probl Anesth*. 1990;4:393-415.
52. Mackie AM, Watson CB. Anaesthesia and mediastinal masses: a case report and review of the literature. *Anaesthesia*. 1984;39:899-903.

53. Rendina EA, Venuta F, Giacoma T. Biopsy of anterior mediastinal masses under local anesthesia. *Ann Thorac Surg*. 2002;74: 1720-1722; 1722-1723 [discussion].
54. Pullerits J, Holzman R. Anaesthesia for patients with mediastinal masses. *Can J Anaesth*. 1989;36:681-688.
55. Piro AJ, Weiss DR, Hellman S. Mediastinal Hodgkin's disease: a possible danger for intubation anaesthesia. *Int J Radiat Oncol Biol Phys*. 1976;1:415-419.
56. Mizrahi S, Yaari Y, Lugassy G, Cotev S. Major airway obstruction relieved by helium/oxygen breathing. *Crit Care Med*. 1986;14: 986-987.
57. Prakash UBS, Abel MD, Hubmayer RD. Mediastinal mass and tracheal obstruction during general anesthesia. *Mayo Clin Proc*. 1988;63:1004-1011.
58. Neuman GG, Weingarten AE, Abramowitz RM, Kushins LG, Abramson AL, Ladner W. The anesthetic management of the patient with an anterior mediastinal mass. *Anesthesiology*. 1984;60:144-147.
59. Levin H, Bursztein S, Heifetz M. Cardiac arrest in a child with a mediastinal mass. *Anesth Analg*. 1985;64:1129-1130.
60. Keon TP. Death on induction of anesthesia for cervical node biopsy. *Anesthesiology*. 1981;55:471-472.
61. Goh MH, Liu XY, Goh YS. Anterior mediastinal masses: an anaesthetic challenge. *Anaesthesia*. 1999;54:670-674.
62. Roberts JT, Gissen AT. Management of complications encountered during anesthesia for mediastinoscopy. *Anesthesiol Rev*. 1979;6:31-35.
63. Plummer S, Hartley M, Vaughan RS. Anaesthesia for telescopic procedures in the thorax. *Br J Anaesth*. 1998;80:223-234.
64. Fair J. Anesthesia for thoracoscopy: an overview. *AANA J*. 1994;62:133-138.
65. Conacher ID. Anaesthesia for thoracoscopic surgery. *Best Pract Res Clin Anaesthesiol*. 2002;16:53-62.
66. Allen MS, Deschamps C, Jones DM, Trastek VF, Pairolero PC. Video-assisted thoracic surgical procedures: the Mayo experience. *Mayo Clin Proc*. 1996;71:351-359.
67. Berrisford RG, Page RD. Video assisted thoracic surgery for spontaneous pneumothorax. *Thorax*. 1996;51:523-528.
68. Horswell JL. Anesthetic techniques for thoracoscopy. *Ann Thorac Surg*. 1993;56:624-629.
69. Cohen E, Kirschner PA, Benumof JL. Case 1—1990. A 59 year old, oxygen dependent man with severe giant bullous emphysema is admitted for pulmonary angiography and pulmonary bulla resection. *J Cardiothorac Vasc Anesth*. 1990;4:119-129.
70. Normandale JP. Bullous cystic lung disease. *Anaesthesia*. 1985;40: 1182-1185.
71. Hasenbon MA, Gielen MJ. Anesthesia for bullectomy: a technique with spontaneous ventilation and extradural blockade. *Anaesthesia*. 1985;40:977-980.

CHAPTER 26

Neuroanatomy, Neurophysiology, and Neuroanesthesia

John Aker

This chapter reviews the organization of the central nervous system (CNS), electrophysiology, cerebral blood supply, role of neurotransmitters, and effects of selected anesthetic agents on cerebral physiology. This chapter also provides recommendations for the management of specific neurologic procedures.

ORGANIZATION OF THE CENTRAL NERVOUS SYSTEM

Cells of the Central and Peripheral Nervous Systems

Nerve tissue is organized into the CNS, which includes the brain and spinal cord, and the peripheral nervous system, which consists of the cranial and spinal nerves and their receptors and effector endings. The peripheral nervous system is divided into the somatic and autonomic nervous systems. The somatic nervous system contains sensory neurons for the control of skin, muscles, and joints. The autonomic nervous system, which consists of the sympathetic, parasympathetic, and enteric subdivisions, is responsible for involuntary innervation of various organ systems.

The CNS is derived from two primary cell types: neurons and neuroglial (or glial) cells. The neuron is the basic functional cell of the CNS and consists of a cell body (perikaryon) and specialized cytoplasmic processes, dendrites, and a single axon (Figure 26-1). A single axon emerges from the cell body at the axon hillock. The axon may branch to form collateral nerves at a point distal to the neuron cell body. Axon diameters range from 0.2 to 20 μm. Most of the axons in the brain are only a few millimeters long, although the axons that run from the spinal cord may be as long as 1 m. Stimulation of the dendrites produces antegrade impulse conduction (toward the neuron cell body) with subsequent conduction away from the neuron cell body by way of the axon.

Neuron cell bodies vary in size and shape and are classified as unipolar, bipolar, pseudounipolar, or multipolar. Unipolar neurons are found only in lower invertebrates. Bipolar neurons are found in the retina, the ear, and the olfactory mucosa. Pseudounipolar neurons have one cytoplasmic process that exits the cell and divides into two branches, one serving as the dendrite, the other as the axon. Pseudounipolar neurons are present in the dorsal root ganglia and cranial ganglion cells. Pseudounipolar neurons enable sensory impulses to travel from the dendrite directly to the axon without passing through the cell body. Multipolar neurons have multiple dendritic processes but only one axon and constitute the majority of the CNS neurons.

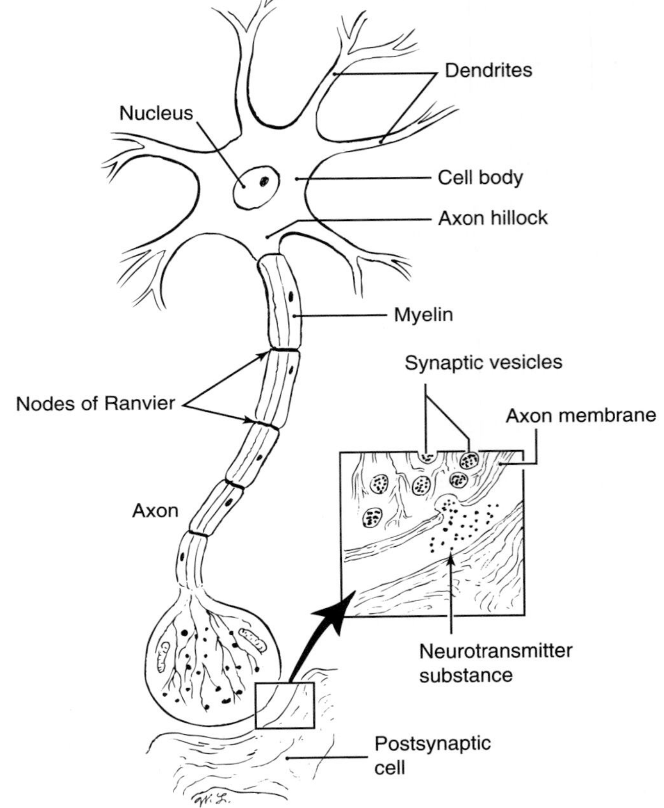

FIGURE **26-1**
Neuron and chemical synapse.

The gray matter of the CNS is composed of neuron cell bodies in the CNS, and the white matter is composed of myelinated axons. Regions of concentrated cell bodies within the peripheral nervous system form the cranial, spinal, and autonomic ganglia.

Neurons may be classified according to their specific function and are motor neurons, sensory neurons, or interneurons. Motor neurons are multipolar and innervate and control effector tissues such as muscles and glands. Sensory neurons are pseudounipolar and receive exteroceptive, interoceptive, or proprioceptive input. Interneurons are pseudounipolar and connect adjacent neurons.

The neuron is bounded by a bilaminar lipoprotein membrane derived from phospholipid molecules arranged with their fatty acid chains facing one another, producing an inner hydrophobic membrane. The membrane surface in contact with the extracellular fluid contains polar hydrophilic groups of phospholipid molecules. The neuronal membrane contains integral membrane proteins, which form ionic pumps, ion channels, enzymes (adenylate cyclase as an example), receptor proteins, and structural proteins.

The neuron contains a number of common cellular organelles including a well-developed nucleus, mitochondria (distributed throughout the cell body), and cytoplasmic processes. Ribosomes, endoplasmic reticulum, lysosomes, and Golgi complexes are also found. Neurotubules and neurofilaments extend through the cytoplasm from the dendrites to the axon terminal and provide structural support as well as a pathway for intracellular transport of neurotransmitters.

The second major cell type found within the CNS is the neuroglial, or glial, cell (Table 26-1). Four types of glial cells are found within the CNS: astrocytes, oligodendrocytes, microglial cells, and ependymal cells. Most neoplasms of the CNS arise from glial cells (astrocytes). Glial cells are smaller, outnumber neuronal cells, and lack dendritic and axonal processes. Although they do not participate in neuronal signaling, glial cells are essential for neuronal function. The role of neuroglia includes the maintenance of a proper ionic environment, the modulation of nerve cell electrical conduction, control of reuptake of neurotransmitters, and repair after neuronal injury.

The astrocyte is the predominant glial cell. Astrocytes provide structural neuronal support, group and pair neurons and nerve terminals, regulate the metabolic environment, and are active in repair after neuronal injury.

Two distinct types of astrocytes exist: fibrous astrocytes, found in the white matter, and protoplasmic astrocytes, concentrated in the gray matter. Astrocytes have multiple processes that radiate from the cell, producing a star-shaped appearance. Some of these processes (astrocytic feet) terminate on the surfaces of blood vessels within the CNS (perivascular feet). The contact of the cerebral endothelium by astrocytes has been proposed to be essential in the development of the blood-brain barrier.[1]

Oligodendrocytes have fewer branches than astrocytes (*oligo*—few; *dendro*—branches). Oligodendrocytes form the myelin sheath of axons in the brain and spinal cord and are capable of myelinating more than one axon. However, oligodendrocytes are incapable of division and fail to regenerate after injury.

TABLE 26-1 Glial Cells

Type	Major Functions
Astrocytes	Support (for neurons) Metabolic and nutritive functions
Ependymal cells	Probable role in cerebrospinal fluid production
Microglia	Phagocytosis
Oligodendrocytes	Insulation—form myelin sheath in the brain and spinal cord
Schwann cells	Insulation—form myelin sheath in the peripheral nerves

The velocity of nerve impulse conduction in an unmyelinated axon increases with the square root of the diameter of the axon. Accordingly, a doubling of impulse conduction requires that the axon be doubled in size. One could only imagine the size of the peripheral nervous system without the presence of myelin. Myelin is essential to increase the velocity of impulse conduction and minimize the size of the axon.

Myelin is formed in the vertebral peripheral nervous system by modified glial cells termed *Schwann cells*.[2] Unlike the oligodendrocyte, the Schwann cell myelinates only one axon, surrounding the axon and forming successive layers of plasma membrane. The resultant thickness is variable in different axons. The junction between adjacent Schwann cells is devoid of myelin at 1-mm intervals along the length of the axon. This nonmyelinated portion of the axon, the node of Ranvier, is the site of electrical impulse propagation. Impulses in myelinated axons travel from one node of Ranvier to another (saltatory conduction), bypassing the area between the nodes and increasing the velocity of conduction (see Figure 26-1). Wallerian degeneration results in the distal degeneration of the axon after peripheral nerve injury. Proximal axon degeneration may also occur. Within 1 week of the initial injury, Schwann cells proliferate to form a tube into the area of degeneration, forming a scaffold to direct axon regeneration. Myelin regeneration precedes axon regeneration, with the myelin eventually reaching its previous thickness.

Microglial cells are the smallest neuroglial cells and are scattered throughout the CNS. Microglial cells are transported throughout the CNS to sites of neuronal injury or degeneration, where they proliferate and develop into large macrophages that phagocytize neuronal debris.

Ependymal cells line the roof of the third and fourth ventricles of the brain and the central spinal canal. Ependymal cells form the cuboidal epithelium (choroid plexus), which secretes cerebrospinal fluid (CSF).

Blood-Brain Barrier

The injection of an intravenous dye causes most of the body tissues and internal organs to be stained, yet the brain and spinal cord remain unblemished. This finding led to the discovery of the blood-brain barrier, which effectively isolates the brain and spinal cord extracellular compartment from the intravascular compartment.

The endothelial cells of the CNS form tight junctions between adjacent cells, preventing the transport of polar substances from the intravascular to the cerebral extracellular fluid compartment. CNS endothelial cells lack transport mechanisms, so little intracellular transport takes place. A number of midline brain structures receive neurosecretory products from the blood and therefore lack a blood-brain barrier. These structures, the circumventricular organs, include the area postrema, pituitary gland, pineal gland, choroid plexus, and portions of the hypothalamus.

The blood-brain barrier is incompletely developed in the newborn. The high vascular content of bile pigments in jaundiced newborns may enter the basal ganglia, producing kernicterus. Blood-brain barrier disruption can be caused by traumatic head injury, subarachnoid or intracerebral hemorrhage, or cerebral ischemia. The development of mass lesions may also produce blood-brain barrier disruption. Osmotically active substances may penetrate the brain or spinal cord after blood-brain barrier disruption. Intentional intracarotid injection of a hyperosmolar solution shrinks the endothelial cells, opens tight junctions, and disrupts the blood-brain barrier. This technique allows the delivery of chemotherapeutic drugs through the blood-brain barrier for the treatment of neural malignancy.[3]

ANATOMY OF THE CENTRAL NERVOUS SYSTEM

Cerebral Structures

The cerebral hemispheres are the most intricately developed and largest regions of the brain (Figures 26-2 and 26-3, Table 26-2). The cerebral hemispheres contain the cerebral cortex, hippocampal formation, amygdala, and basal ganglia. The cerebral cortex consists of the outer 3-mm layer of the cerebral hemispheres. The surface of the cerebral cortex is convoluted, increasing the surface area of the cerebral hemispheres. Elevated convolutions called *gyri* are separated by shallow grooves called *sulci* and by deeper grooves called *fissures*.

The medial longitudinal fissure divides the cerebral hemispheres into right and left halves. The lateral fissure of Sylvius and the central sulcus of Rolando divide each hemisphere into four lobes, which are named for the cranial bones that overlie each area. The frontal lobe, essential for motor control, and the parietal lobe, essential for the senses of pain and touch, are separated by the central sulcus. Voluntary muscle activity is controlled by the motor cortex located in the precentral gyrus, or Brodmann's area (see Figure 26-3). The sensations of touch, pain, and limb position, as well as the sensory perception of grasped objects, are controlled by the somatic sensory cortex located in the postcentral gyrus of the parietal lobe. The temporal lobe, which contains the auditory cortex, is separated from the frontal and parietal lobes by the sylvian fissure. The occipital lobe lies posterior to the parietooccipital sulcus. Here the visual cortex lies within the walls of the calcarine fissure on the medial brain surface.

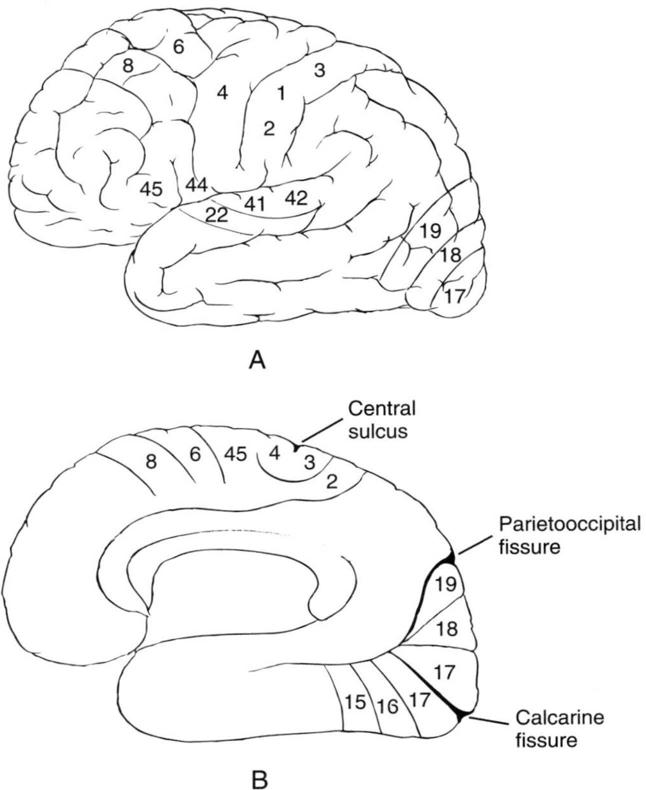

FIGURE **26-2**
Cerebral cortex. **A,** Gyri, sulci, and fissures of the surface of the brain. **B,** Some functional areas of the cerebral cortex. *Inf.*, Inferior; *Mid.*, middle; *Sup.*, superior. (Modified from Guyton AC. *Basic Neuroscience: Anatomy and Physiology*. Philadelphia: Saunders; 1991:12.)

The corpus callosum lies deep in the longitudinal fissure and contains commissural fibers, which interconnect the cerebral hemispheres. These fibers arise from neurons in one hemisphere and synapse with neurons in the corresponding area of the adjacent hemisphere. The remaining major structures of the cerebral hemispheres include the basal ganglia, the amygdala, and the hippocampal formation. The basal ganglia are involved in the control of movement. The amygdala functions in the regulation of emotional behavior and appetite and is essential in formation of the organism's response to stressors. The hippocampal formation is essential for memory formation and learning.

The diencephalon is located in the midline between the two cerebral hemispheres and contains two important structures—the thalamus and the hypothalamus. The oval-shaped thalamus integrates and transmits sensory information to various cortical areas of the cerebral hemispheres via separate thalamic nuclei. The hypothalamus is composed of several nuclei, including the mamillary bodies. The hypothalamus is the master neurohumoral organ.

The midbrain, pons, and medulla form the brain stem. The brain stem contains the reticular activating system, which functions to maintain consciousness and alertness. The pons is anterior to the cerebellum, separated by the fourth ventricle, connecting the medulla oblongata and the midbrain (Figure 26-4). The pons contains ascending and descending fiber tracts and the nuclei of the trigeminal nerve (cranial nerve V) and the facial nerve (cranial nerve VII).[4] The medulla extends from the pons to the foramen magnum, where it becomes continuous with the spinal cord (see Figure 26-4). In addition to ascending and descending fiber tracts, the medulla contains respiratory and cardiovascular control centers and the vestibulocochlear nerve (cranial nerve VIII), the glossopharyngeal nerve (cranial nerve IX), the vagus nerve (cranial nerve X), the spinal accessory nerve (cranial nerve XI), and the hypoglossal nerve (cranial nerve XII) nuclei.[4] The cerebellum is convoluted in appearance and lies below the occipital lobe of the cerebral cortex and posterior to the pons and medulla. Structurally it resembles the cerebral cortex, containing an outer layer of gray matter and an inner core of white matter with several nuclei embedded within. The cerebellum can be divided into three functional areas. The flocculonodular lobe (archeocerebellum) is active in the maintenance of equilibrium, and the paleocerebellum (anterior lobe and part of vermis) regulates muscle tone. The neocerebellum (posterior lobe plus most of the vermis) is the largest subdivision of the cerebellum and is essential in the coordination of voluntary muscle activity. The cerebellum integrates information received from other areas of the CNS and the peripheral nervous system. Information from the cerebellum is transmitted to the cerebral cortex and to lower motor neurons involved in the maintenance of muscle tone, equilibrium, and voluntary muscle activity.[4]

Meninges

The brain and spinal cord are enveloped by three meningeal layers: the dura mater, the arachnoid mater, and the pia mater (Figure 26-5). The dura mater, the thickest of the meningeal

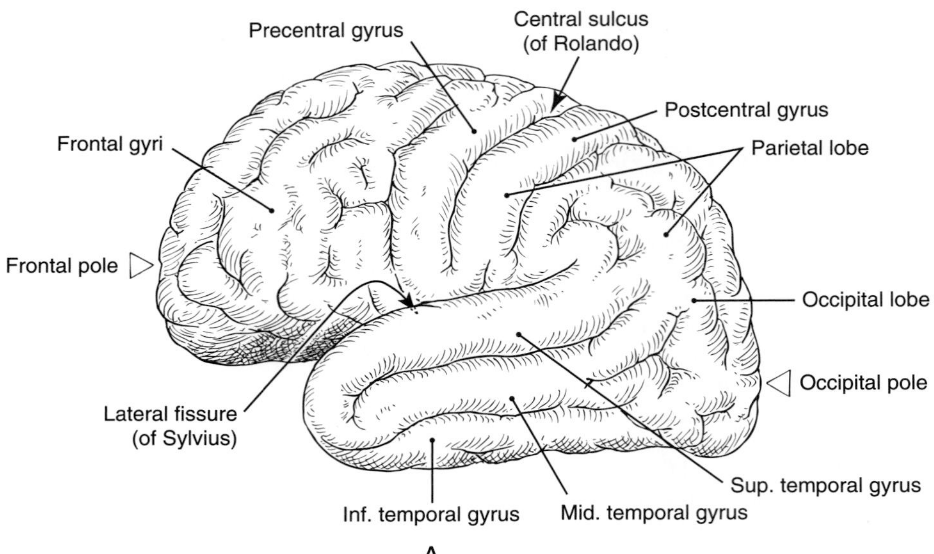

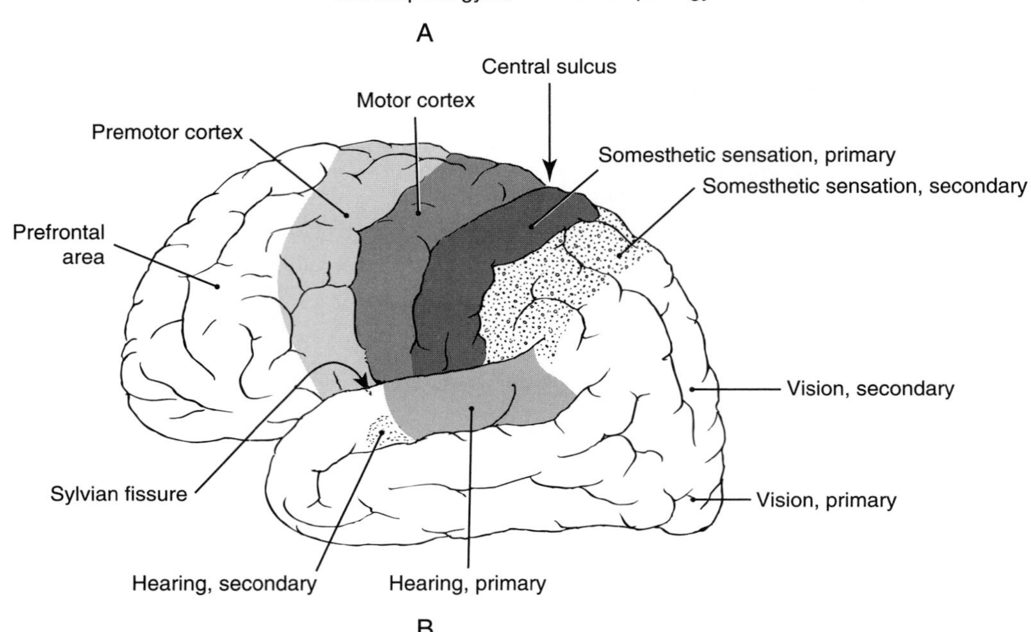

FIGURE **26-3**
Brodmann's areas of the cerebral cortex. (Modified from Carpenter MD. *Core Text of Neuroanatomy*. Baltimore: Williams & Wilkins; 1991:286.)

TABLE **26-2** **Divisions of the Brain**

Division	Major Structures	Division	Major Structures
Telencephalon	Cerebral hemispheres Basal ganglia (globus pallidus, putamen, caudate)	Mesencephalon	Tectum Corpora quadrigemina Tegmentum
Diencephalon	Most of the third ventricle Thalamus		Red nucleus Nuclei of CN III and CN IV
	Subthalamus Medial geniculate body	Pons	Ascending and descending fiber tracts Nuclei of CN V and CN VII
	Lateral geniculate body Epithalamus Habenula	Medulla oblongata	Ascending and descending tracts Respiratory and cardiovascular control centers Nuclei of CN VIII through CN XII
	Pineal body Optic nerves and chiasm	Cerebellum	

CN, *Cranial nerve*.

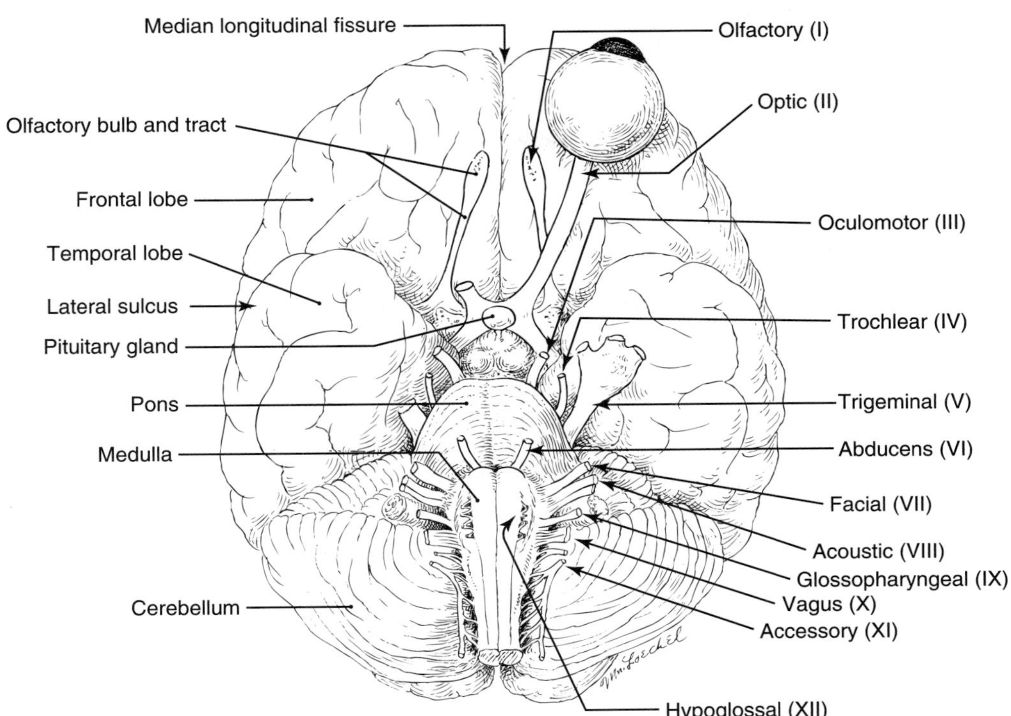

FIGURE **26-4**
The pons and medulla and the origin of the cranial nerves.

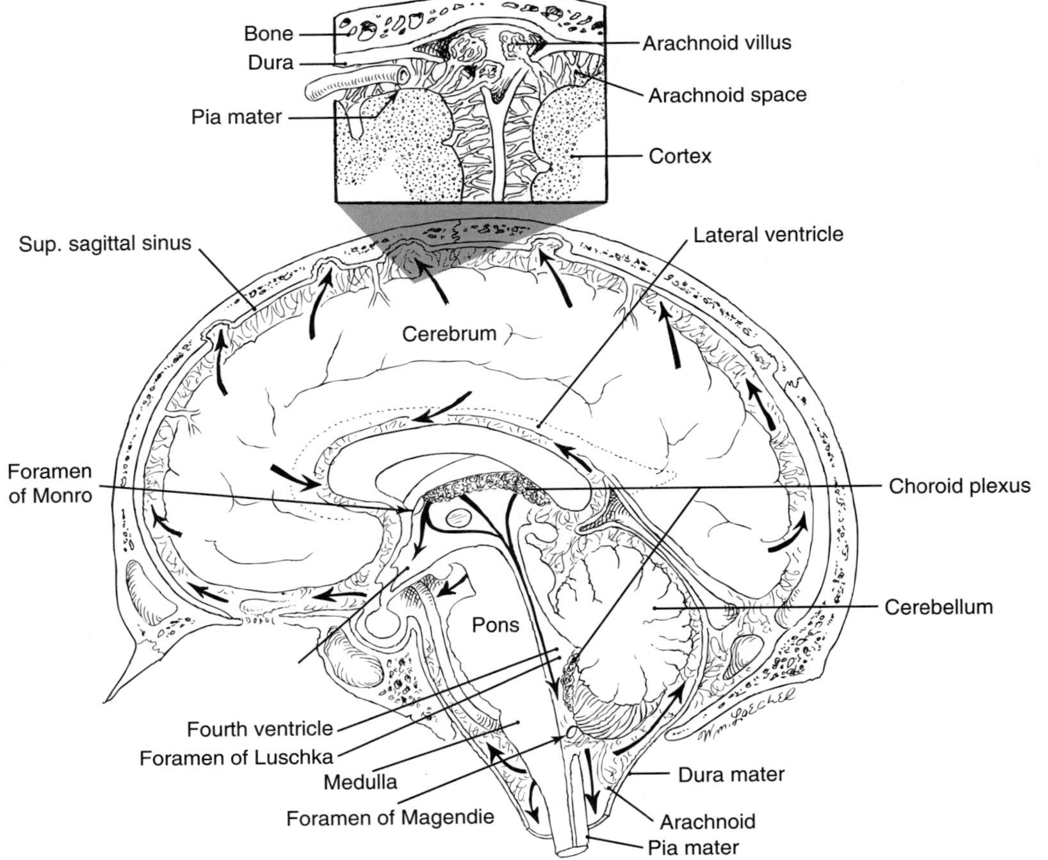

FIGURE **26-5**
Meninges and the flow of cerebrospinal fluid through the ventricular system.

layers, overlies the cerebral hemispheres and brain stem and is functionally separated into an outer periosteal layer (adherent to the inner cranium) and an inner meningeal layer. The dura mater forms a fold, the falx cerebri, which functionally separates the cerebral hemispheres. A similar fold, the tentorium cerebelli, separates the occipital lobe and the cerebellum. The dura mater of the spinal cord is continuous with the meningeal layer of the cranial dura mater and the perineurium of the peripheral nerves. Innervation of the dura mater is provided by the first three cervical roots and the trigeminal nerve. During awake craniotomy the patient may complain of pain "behind the eye" when traction is applied to the dura.

The arachnoid mater is a thin, avascular membrane joining the dura mater. The subdural space, a potential space between the dura mater and the arachnoid mater, is of clinical importance. The unintentional injection of local anesthetic during spinal anesthesia into the subdural space produces patchy, asymmetric block. In addition, injury to a blood vessel in the subdural space can create bleeding (subdural hematoma), requiring surgical intervention.

The pia mater is a thin avascular membrane adherent to the brain and spinal cord. The subarachnoid space lies between the arachnoid mater and the pia mater. In the spinal cord the subarachnoid space extends to the S2 to S3 level and is filled with CSF. In addition, the vasculature that overlies the CNS is located within the subarachnoid space. Injury to the vascular structures may produce subarachnoid hemorrhage and hematoma.

The spinal epidural space is located outside the dura but inside the spinal canal. The epidural space contains a venous plexus and epidural fat that provides protection of the neural structures. The distance from the skin to the epidural space may be as little as 3 cm or as large as 8 cm.

Cerebrospinal Fluid

CSF is contained within the ventricles of the brain, the cisterns surrounding the brain, and the subarachnoid space of the brain and spinal cord (see Figure 26-5). The total volume of cranial and spinal CSF in the adult is approximately 150 ml. The specific gravity is 1.002 to 1.009, and the pH is 7.32. CSF bathes the brain and spinal cord, cushioning these delicate structures, and controls and maintains the extracellular milieu for neurons and glial cells.

CSF is secreted by the ependymal cells of the choroid plexus within the ventricular system at a rate of approximately 30 ml/hr. Although CSF is isotonic with plasma, it is not a plasma filtrate. CSF concentrations of potassium, calcium, bicarbonate, and glucose are lower and concentrations of sodium, chloride, and magnesium are higher than their respective plasma concentrations. The entire CSF volume is replaced every 3 to 4 hours. Normal CSF pressure is between 5 and 15 mm Hg. CSF flows from the lateral ventricles of the cerebral hemispheres through the foramen of Monro into the third ventricle, through the aqueduct of Sylvius in the midbrain, into the fourth ventricle. CSF enters the subarachnoid space through the medial foramen of Magendie and the paired lateral foramina of Luschka, openings in the roof of the fourth ventricle.

The cisterna magna, located between the medulla and the cerebellum, is formed from the separation of the arachnoid mater from the pia mater and is filled with CSF. Two additional cisterns exist, the cisterna pontis and the cisterna basalis. CSF drains into the venous blood via the superior sagittal sinus and is absorbed by arachnoid granulations.

Spinal Cord

The spinal cord extends from the medulla at the foramen magnum to the filum terminale, a threadlike connective tissue structure that attaches to the first segment of the coccyx. Thirty-one pairs of spinal nerves carry motor and sensory information: 8 cervical, 12 thoracic, 5 lumbar, 5 sacral, and 1 coccygeal. The first pair of cervical nerves exits the spinal cord between the base of the skull and the first cervical vertebrae (atlas), and the remaining 30 pairs exit between adjacent vertebrae. All of the exiting spinal nerves are covered with pia mater. Because the spinal cord is approximately 25 cm shorter than the vertebral canal in which it is enclosed, the lumbar and sacral nerves have relatively long roots (the cauda equina).

The spinal cord is divided into dorsal, lateral, and ventral regions by the entering dorsal sensory root fibers and the outgoing ventral motor root fibers. Neuron cell bodies and unmyelinated fibers lie in the **H**-shaped central gray region of the cord surrounded by fiber tracts that form the white matter. Although it does not have a uniform appearance, this general arrangement continues throughout the entire spinal cord.

The spinal gray matter is divided into the ventral and dorsal gray commissures. The ventral projections of gray matter are called the *gray horns* or *columns*; the posterior projections are called the *posterior gray horns* or *columns*. Intermediolateral gray horns or columns are found between T1 and L2. The gray matter has been subdivided into 10 (I through X) laminae of Rexed. Laminae I through VI are located in the dorsal (posterior) horn and contain cell bodies that receive sensory information from the periphery. Projections from the laminae form afferent tracts. A large number of interneurons are found in laminae V, VI, and X. Laminae VII, VIII, and IX make up the ventral (anterior) horn and contain motor neurons and interneurons involved in motor functions. The gray matter is enlarged in two areas of the spinal cord, C5 to C7 and L3 to S2. The cervical enlargement contains neuron cell bodies that innervate the upper extremities; the lumbosacral enlargement contains neuron cell bodies that innervate the lower extremities.

The tracts or fascicles that make up the white matter are highly organized, similar to the organization of the cerebral cortex and other areas of the brain. The dorsal white matter is composed almost exclusively of ascending sensory fiber tracts. The lateral and ventral white matter contains descending motor tracts. Commonly, fiber tracts at some level in the spinal cord or brain decussate, or cross over to the other side. As in the brain, spinal cord fiber tracts can be projection tracts connecting the spinal cord and brain, or they can be association (intersegmental, fasciculi proprii) tracts that originate and terminate entirely within the spinal cord. The association tracts play an important role in spinal reflexes.[4-7]

Shortly after leaving the spinal cord, the meningeal coverings of the peripheral nerves merge with the connective tissue layers that cover the peripheral nerve. The outermost covering of the peripheral nerve is called the *epineurium*. The bundles or fascicles of axons in each nerve are covered by the perineurium, and each axon in a fascicle is surrounded by the endoneurium.

Peripheral nerves may be classified according to their diameter. Recall that the larger the diameter, the faster the conduction velocity; therefore A alpha fibers, the fibers with the largest diameters, have the fastest conduction velocity, and C fibers, which have the smallest diameter, have the slowest conduction velocity. Between the two extremes lie A beta, A gamma, A delta, and B fibers, in

TABLE 26-3 Peripheral Nerves

Fiber Type	Location	Information Conveyed
General somatic afferent	CN V, CN VII, CN IX, CN X, all spinal nerves	Pain, touch, temperature, pressure, and proprioception from muscles, tendons, and joint capsules
General visceral afferent	CN V, CN VII, CN IX, CN X, all spinal nerves	Conscious pain sensations
Special somatic afferent	CN II, CN VIII	Sight; hearing
Special visceral afferent	CN I, CN IX, CN X, CN VII (intermediate branch)	Olfaction; taste
Special visceral efferent	CN V, CN VII, CN IX, CN X, CN XI	Mastication; facial expressions
General somatic efferent	CN III, CN IV, CN VI, CN VII, all spinal nerves	Voluntary muscles (trunk and extremities); extrinsic muscles of eye; muscles of the tongue
General visceral efferent	CN III, CN VII, CN IX, CN X, spinal nerves T1 through L2 or L3, S2, S3, S4	Smooth muscle; cardiac muscle; some glands

CN, *Cranial nerve*.

decreasing order of size and conduction velocity. Table 26-3 lists cranial and peripheral nerve fiber types, locations, and functions.

PERIPHERAL NERVOUS SYSTEM

The peripheral nervous system is divided into the somatic and autonomic nervous systems (Figure 26-6). The somatic system contains sensory neurons for the control of skin, muscles, and joints. Somatic motor fibers arise from motor neurons in the ventral horn, their axons exiting the spinal cord via the ventral root. A few centimeters after leaving the spinal cord, the somatic motor fibers join with incoming sensory fibers carrying information from afferent receptors (muscles, skin, tendons, and joints) to form a mixed nerve. As a mixed nerve approaches its site of innervation, the motor and sensory fibers separate.

Cranial nerves emerge from the cranium. Cranial nerves provide sensory and motor innervation for the head and neck. The sensory cranial nerves include the olfactory nerve (cranial nerve I), optic nerve (cranial nerve II), and vestibulocochlear nerve (cranial nerve VIII); the motor cranial nerves include the oculomotor, trochlear, abducens, spinal accessory, and hypoglossal nerves; and four mixed cranial nerves that have both sensory and motor function are the trigeminal nerve (cranial nerve V), facial nerve (cranial nerve VII), glossopharyngeal nerve (cranial nerve IX), and vagus nerve (cranial nerve X).

The autonomic nervous system controls involuntary visceral functions and is composed of three subdivisions: the sympathetic, parasympathetic, and enteric nervous systems. The sympathetic nervous system (SNS) and the parasympathetic nervous system (PNS) are functionally antagonistic.[5,8] The SNS and PNS originate within the CNS and require two efferent neurons—a preganglionic neuron originating within the CNS and a postganglionic neuron terminating within the effector organ (smooth muscle, cardiac muscle, or sweat gland). Autonomic fibers originating in the brain arise from cell bodies located in the brain stem. PNS fibers supplying the lower gastrointestinal tract and genitourinary systems arise from the sacral portion of the spinal cord.

Sympathetic Nervous System

Preganglionic neurons of the SNS originate in the intermediolateral gray horn of the spinal cord between the first thoracic (T1) and second or third lumbar vertebra (L2 or L3). The myelinated preganglionic axons (preganglionic fibers of the preganglionic neurons) exit the spinal cord via the anterior (ventral) nerve root. These processes leave the spinal cord by way of a small trunk, the white rami communicans. A series of paired paravertebral ganglia is located bilaterally along the spinal cord (Figure 26-7). All of the paired segmental paravertebral ganglia are connected, forming the sympathetic trunks. These ganglia may contain the cell body of the second efferent neuron (postganglionic neuron). The preganglionic fibers of the preganglionic neuron enter the white rami communicans and may synapse with the second efferent neuron located within the ganglion. The postganglionic fiber of the postganglionic neuron may either exit the gray ramus to enter a spinal nerve or may extend through a connection between the paravertebral ganglion and one of the three (celiac, superior, or inferior) mesenteric ganglia. The postganglionic fibers then synapse with the smooth muscle of the digestive tract and other abdominal organs. SNS preganglionic axons secrete acetylcholine at their ganglionic synapses, and postganglionic fibers secrete norepinephrine.

Usually one paravertebral ganglion is present for each spinal nerve, except in the cervical area, where they fuse to form two or three ganglia. On entering the sympathetic chain the preganglionic fiber may synapse at the entry level or travel up or down the ganglionic chain before forming a synapse. Some preganglionic axons pass through the sympathetic chain without synapsing and after leaving the chain form a distinct nerve (e.g., splanchnic nerve) before synapsing in prevertebral ganglia, such as the superior or inferior mesenteric ganglia. Some preganglionic axons in the sympathetic trunk synapse with several postganglionic neurons located in several chain ganglia. This arrangement explains the manner in which a central SNS discharge spreads over several segments. After synapsing in the sympathetic chain, the postganglionic axons, which are unmyelinated, enter the spinal nerve through the gray ramus communicans and travel to the periphery.

The cervical ganglia are divided into superior, medial, and inferior cervical ganglia. The inferior cervical ganglion fuses with the first thoracic ganglion to form the stellate ganglion. Stimulation of SNS fibers from the superior cervical ganglion produces contraction of the radial muscle of the iris (mydriasis), relaxation of the ciliary muscle of the eye, and constriction of the blood vessels of the head (see Figure 26-6). Destruction of the superior cervical ganglion, central SNS

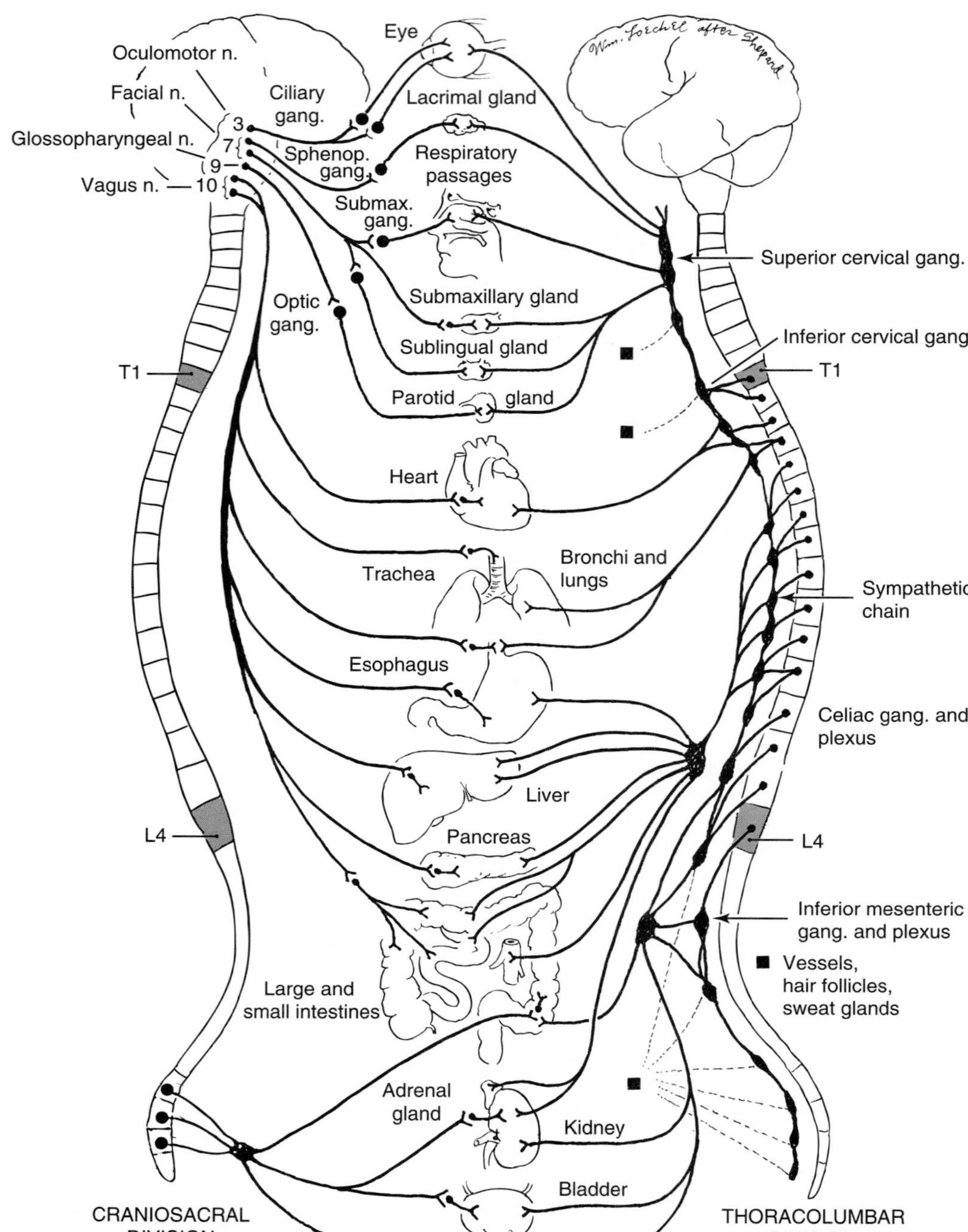

FIGURE **26-6**
Both divisions of the autonomic nervous system. *gang.*, Ganglion, *n.*, nerve.

damage, or injury to other cervical paravertebral ganglia produces Horner's syndrome, clinically distinguished by miosis, anhydrosis (absence of sweating), and ptosis on the affected side. Ptosis is incomplete because the primary innervation to the levator palpebrae superioris muscle of the eyelid is through the oculomotor nerve, and only a few SNS fibers innervate this muscle.

Postganglionic fibers from the upper thoracic chain ganglia (stellate to T4 to T5) innervate the heart and lungs. β-receptor stimulation produces an increased heart rate (positive chronotropic effect), an increase in conduction (positive dromotropic effect), and an increase in myocardial contractility (positive inotropic effect). Myocardial α-receptor stimulation produces coronary vasoconstriction. The resultant pulmonary effects also depend on the receptor type that is stimulated; bronchial dilation follows β_2-receptor stimulation, and bronchoconstriction follows α-receptor stimulation.

The SNS fibers supplying abdominal and pelvic viscera (T5 through L3) pass through the chain ganglia forming the greater and lesser splanchnic nerves, which subsequently terminate in preterminal ganglia. Postganglionic fibers from the prevertebral ganglia, such as the superior and inferior mesenteric ganglia, travel to the abdominal and pelvic viscera. Stimulation of these SNS fibers activates liver glycogenolysis and gluconeogenesis, decreases secretions from pancreatic acinar cells and β-cells, initiates lipolysis, decreases the tone and motility of

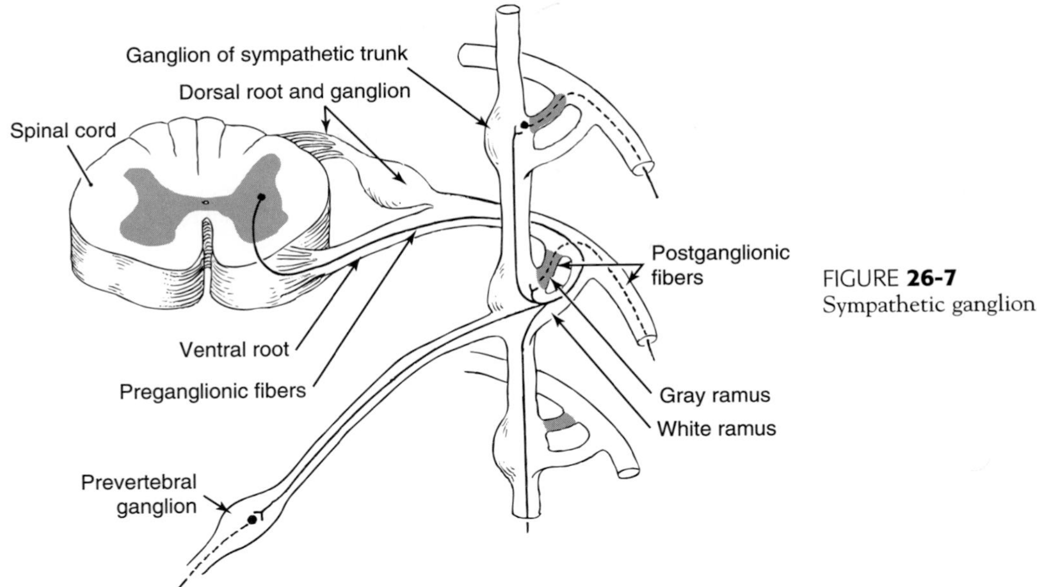

FIGURE **26-7**
Sympathetic ganglion.

the gastrointestinal tract, contracts gastrointestinal sphincters, relaxes urinary smooth muscle, and increases renin secretion from the kidney.

Parasympathetic Nervous System

The efferent neurons of the parasympathetic subdivision are located in the gray matter of the midbrain and medulla. The preganglionic fibers exit the brain via cranial nerves II, VII, IX, and X. The remainder of the cell bodies of the first efferent neurons arise from the lateral horn of the sacral portion of the spinal cord (S2 through S5). Acetylcholine is secreted by both parasympathetic preganglionic and postganglionic fibers (see Figure 26-6).

The second efferent neuron (postganglionic neuron) of the parasympathetic subdivision may be located in a small ganglion adjacent to the innervated organ, or within the organ itself. Preganglionic axons travel with the vagus to ganglia located near the organ they innervate. The postganglionic axons innervate the bronchioles, the heart, the coronary arteries, the stomach, and the large intestine up to the left colic flexure. PNS postganglionic fibers to the descending colon and the genitourinary systems are supplied by parasympathetic fibers from sacral segments of the spinal cord. Most of the parasympathetic preganglionic fibers originate at the S3 and S4 segments. Shortly after exiting the spinal cord with the spinal nerves, the preganglionic fibers form the pelvic nerves (nervi erigentes), which synapse in ganglia in close proximity to the innervated organ.

VASCULATURE OF THE CENTRAL NERVOUS SYSTEM

The brain and spinal cord are dependent on an uninterrupted blood supply to deliver the essential fuels, oxygen and glucose (Figure 26-8). The brain receives 15% of the cardiac output, or approximately 50 ml/100 g/min. The brain's blood supply originates from two arterial circulations that receive blood from two distinct systemic arteries: the anterior circulation receives

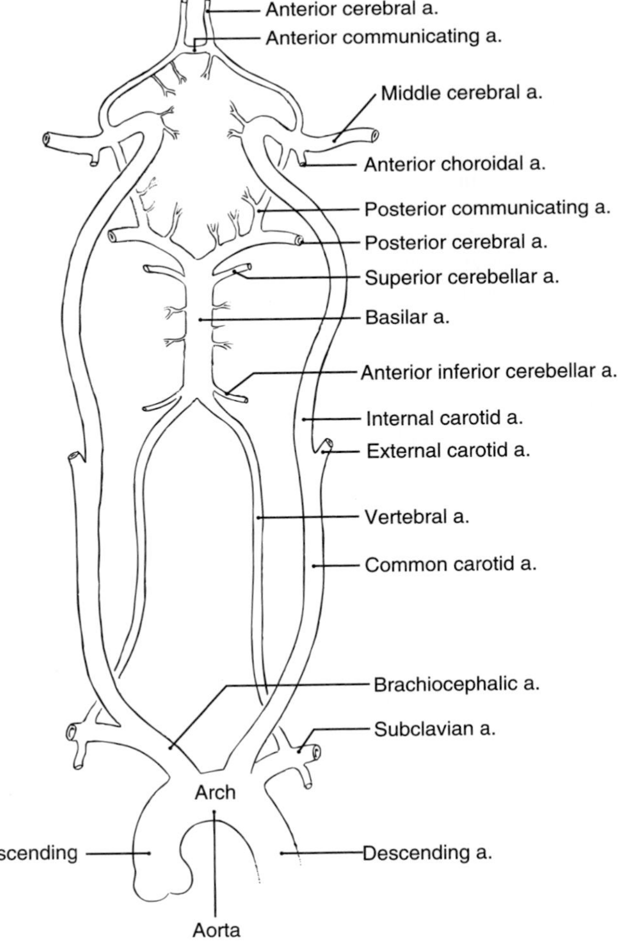

FIGURE **26-8**
Cerebral vasculature.

blood from the carotid arteries, and the posterior circulation receives blood from the vertebral arteries. These arterial systems communicate through arterial anastomoses that form the circle of Willis. The paired anterior, middle, and posterior cerebral arteries originate from the circle of Willis. Although these arterial communications exist, under normal conditions little mixing of blood flow occurs. Intraarterial contrast studies demonstrate that the carotid artery supplies the ipsilateral cerebral hemisphere and the vertebrobasilar system supplies the structures of the posterior fossa.

The internal carotid arteries enter the skull through the foramen lacerum and bifurcate near the lateral border of the optic chiasm, forming the anterior and middle cerebral arteries. The anterior cerebral arteries supply the medial surface of the cerebral hemispheres, and the middle cerebral arteries supply the lateral surface of the hemispheres. The striate arteries, which are branches of the middle cerebral arteries, supply the internal capsule and its motor tracts. Cerebrovascular accidents commonly involve the striate arteries. Communicating arteries provide connections between the two anterior cerebral arteries of each hemisphere (anterior communicating arteries) and between the middle and posterior cerebral arteries (posterior communicating arteries).

The vertebral arteries, branches of the subclavian artery, enter the cranium through the foramen magnum and, in the vicinity of the pons, join to form the basilar artery. Branches of the vertebral and basilar arteries supply a wide area, including the cervical region of the spinal cord, the brain stem, the cerebellum, the vestibular apparatus and cochlea of the inner ear, parts of the diencephalon, and the occipital and temporal lobes of the cerebral hemispheres.

Venous blood exits the brain via two separate systems. The blood from the cerebral and cerebellar cortex flows through veins on the surface and empties into overlying dural venous sinuses. Venous blood from the basal portions of the brain empties into the great vein of Galen and the straight sinus. These sinuses empty into the internal jugular veins. The superficial veins of the scalp are linked to the dural sinuses by the emissary veins.[4,5]

Like the brain, the spinal cord receives blood from two arterial sources: the anterior and posterior spinal arteries, which are branches of the vertebral artery, and the radicular arteries, which are branches of segmental vessels (cervical, intercostal, and lumbar). The spinal cord blood supply is not continuous along its length, and although each spinal cord segment is perfused, blood is delivered preferentially by one of the supply sources. The cervical cord is supplied by the vertebral and radicular arteries, and the thoracic and lumbar cord is supplied by the radicular arteries arising from this respective region (intercostal and lumbar). Of particular importance is the radicular artery, the artery of Adamkiewicz, which enters the cord at approximately T7 and supplies the lumbosacral segment. Spinal cord segments that receive blood from one source are particularly prone to ischemic injury if this blood supply is interrupted. Interruption of the blood flow from the artery of Adamkiewicz results in paraplegia.

ELECTROPHYSIOLOGY

The physiologic basis for the propagation of a nerve impulse lies in the structural nature of the axolemma and the differential concentration of electrolytes within the axolemma and the extracellular space, and the semipermeability of the axolemma to these specific ions. The resting nerve cell has a potential difference, or voltage, created by the asymmetric distribution of sodium and potassium ions. Sodium ions are tenfold richer in the extracellular medium, and potassium ions are tenfold richer in the intracellular medium. The resting membrane potential is created through the excess positive charges on the extracellular surface and excess negative charges on the interior of the cell membrane. The nerve cell is said to be *polarized* in the resting state.

In the resting state the cell membrane permeability to sodium ions is low, so little movement of extracellular sodium ions to the cell interior occurs. Although larger than sodium ions, potassium ions are freely permeable through the axolemma, and their movement creates a net deficit of positive ions within the interior of the axolemma. This ionic asymmetry is maintained by the sodium-potassium adenosine triphosphate (ATP) pump. The distribution of ions outside the cell produces a negative resting membrane potential of approximately –60 to –90 mV.

Nerve impulses are transmitted through action potentials that are generated with membrane alterations in permeability of the axolemma to sodium and potassium ions. Depolarization occurs when a stimulus of sufficient intensity (threshold potential) increases membrane permeability to sodium ions, facilitating the passage of a greater number of sodium ions into the cell interior than potassium ions to the cell exterior. The lowering of the voltage difference of the axolemma occurs as a result of "gating," or the opening or closing of integral membrane proteins. Gating occurs in response to voltage differences across the axolemma (voltage-gated channel) or after the binding of a specific molecule to a receptor or channel protein (chemically gated channel, e.g., the binding of acetylcholine to the neuromuscular junction). Sodium channels open when the threshold potential is reached, facilitating a rapid influx of sodium into the axolemma interior and producing depolarization (Figure 26-9). The initial flow of sodium ions results in the opening of additional sodium channels. The action potential develops as the cell interior undergoes a transition from negative to positive. At the peak of depolarization the electrical potential is 30 to 40 mV higher than the cell exterior, and sodium channels close. The action potential develops as a result of the change from the resting potential of –60 to –90 mV to a peak of 30 to 50 mV at the completion of depolarization. The action potential cannot occur without the delivery of a stimulus, or critical threshold potential. For myelinated mammalian nerves the threshold potential is 20 to 30 mV less than the resting potential. This threshold potential can be modified by a variety of factors, including pH, partial pressure of oxygen (PO_2), and partial pressure of carbon dioxide (PCO_2). Alkalosis increases neuronal excitability, and hypoxemia and acidosis depress neuronal excitability.

After depolarization, cell repolarization is initiated with the closing of sodium channels and the opening of potassium channels, allowing the flow of potassium ions to the exterior of the axolemma to return the axon to the resting potential of –60 to –90 mV. The sodium pump is active in the reestablishment of this ionic asymmetry. During repolarization the axon is refractory, or unable to respond to an additional stimulus, no matter how strong (it will not respond to an action potential). In the later phases of repolarization, the axolemma is in a state of ready refractoriness, that is, depolarization can be initiated only by a stimulus with an intensity greater than that which produced the original depolarization.

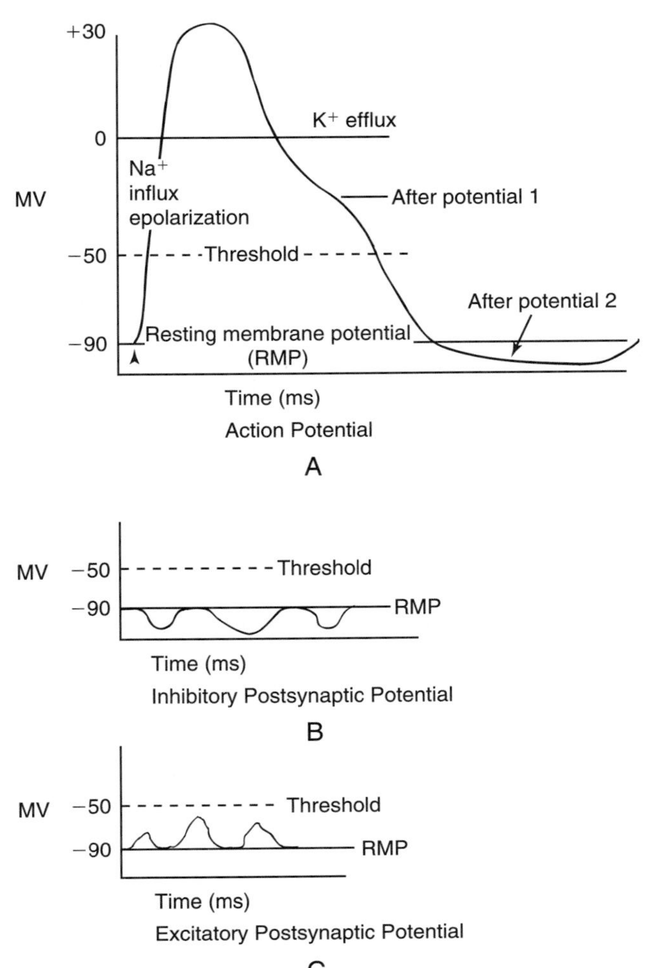

FIGURE **26-9**
A, Phases of the action potential (AP) and major ionic movements during the AP. **B** and **C,** Subthreshold changes in the resting membrane potential.

Chemical, mechanical, and electrical stimulation may elicit an action potential. Mechanical stimulation via pinching or crushing increases the membrane's permeability to sodium ions. The resulting change in ion permeability determines whether the postsynaptic neuron is either excited or inhibited.

Tissues whose sodium channels are not completely closed at rest (cardiac and smooth muscle) have a constant leak of sodium inside the cell, and excitation occurs by electrical stimulation to produce an action potential. Because these tissues repetitively discharge, they are described as having *rhythmicity*. The resting membrane potential of cells displaying rhythmicity is usually −60 to −70 mV. After stimulation a wave of depolarization is transmitted to the axon terminal. At electrical synapses the wave of depolarization crosses the 2-nm synaptic space and spreads to the postsynaptic cell (neuron or muscle cell).

Synaptic Transmission

After depolarization the flow of information is transmitted to adjacent neurons at specialized membrane sites called *synapses* (see Figure 26-1). Synapses are present on dendrites and axons. Synapses may be present on axon terminals of specific neurons in contact with endocrine glands (e.g., salivary glands) or skeletal muscle. The neuron sending the information is the presynaptic neuron, and the receiving neuron is the postsynaptic neuron. Separating the presynaptic and postsynaptic neurons is a small intracellular space (the synaptic cleft). The majority of synaptic transmission occurs in the direction from the presynaptic to the postsynaptic neuron, but retrograde nerve impulse conduction is known to occur and modulates the strength of synaptic connections.

Synaptic transmission may be electrically or chemically mediated. Electrically mediated synapses are large compared with chemically mediated synapses. Electrical synapses have direct cytoplasmic continuity and no synaptic delay. Electrical synapses are excitatory in nature and are located in the CNS, peripherally in smooth muscle, and in cardiac muscle. Synaptic delays (delayed synaptic transmission) occur in chemically mediated transmission because of the transit time of the chemical mediator (specific neurotransmitter) from the presynaptic terminal to the postsynaptic membrane.

The majority of CNS neurons have chemically mediated synapses. The presynaptic neuron releases a neurotransmitter, a low–molecular-weight compound that diffuses across the synaptic cleft and binds to specific receptors on the postsynaptic membrane. Depolarization stimulates the uptake of calcium by the nerve terminal, fusing intracellular vesicles that contain the neurotransmitter to the presynaptic membrane. The neurotransmitters are subsequently released into the synaptic cleft. The neurotransmitter diffuses across the synaptic cleft, interacting with a specific postsynaptic receptor. Neurotransmitters that increase the permeability of the axolemma to sodium ions are excitatory (e.g., acetylcholine, glutamate); neuroinhibitory neurotransmitters (e.g., γ-aminobutyric acid [GABA], glycine) hyperpolarize the membrane by increasing the permeability to chloride ions. The neurotransmitter serotonin excites some neurons and inhibits others. The attachment of the neurotransmitter to the postsynaptic receptor can produce either an immediate (fraction of millisecond) or a delayed (from a few milliseconds up to seconds) effect on the postsynaptic membrane. The delayed transmission involves second messengers, such as cyclic adenosine monophosphate and cyclic guanosine monophosphate, which are activated when the neurotransmitter attaches to the postsynaptic membrane.

NEUROTRANSMITTERS

Neurotransmitters are molecules contained within the presynaptic neuron that are discharged in a calcium-dependent manner after presynaptic depolarization and interact with specific receptors on the postsynaptic membrane. More than 100 molecules meet these criteria. Acetylcholine is an excitatory neurotransmitter that interacts with both nicotinic and muscarinic receptors. Additional neurotransmitters include biogenic amines (epinephrine, norepinephrine, dopamine, serotonin, histamine), amino acids (aspartate, glycine, GABA, glutamate), neuropeptides (substance P, the opioids, several hormones), and the second messenger nitric oxide (Table 26-4).

The synthesis of neurotransmitters occurs within the presynaptic neuron terminal. The neuron regulates the synthesis, packaging, release, and degradation of the synthesized neurotransmitter. The enzymes essential for neuron transmitter synthesis are obtained by axonal transport and taken into the nerve terminal by transport proteins. The synthesized neurotransmitter is then packaged into synaptic vesicles by membrane transport proteins.

TABLE 26-4 Common Neurotransmitters

Class	Neurotransmitter
Monoamines	Epinephrine
	Norepinephrine
	Dopamine
	5-Hydroxytryptamine (serotonin)
Amino acids	γ-Aminobutyric acid
	Glycine
	Glutamate
Peptides	Hypothalamic-releasing hormones (thyrotropin-releasing hormone, somatostatin)
	Posterior pituitary hormones (vasopressin, oxytocin)
	Substance P
	Opioids (β-endorphin, enkephalins, dynorphin)
	Insulin
	Glucagon
	Neurokinin A
Other	Acetylcholine
	Nitric oxide

Acetylcholine

Acetylcholine is an excitatory neurotransmitter with a widespread distribution. Acetylcholine is the predominant neurotransmitter within the CNS, at the neuromuscular junction, within all autonomic nervous system preganglionic fibers and postganglionic parasympathetic fibers, and within postganglionic sympathetic fibers innervating sweat glands. Acetylcholine is synthesized in the presynaptic nerve terminal from acetic acid, coenzyme A, and choline in the presence of the enzymes acetyl kinase and choline acetylase. Acetylcholine is packaged in vesicles and stored in the presynaptic terminal. Calcium uptake into the presynaptic terminal is required for acetylcholine release, and magnesium (Mg^{2+}) and manganese (Mn^{2+}) block the uptake of Ca^{2+} and the subsequent release of acetylcholine. Acetylcholine interacts with the postsynaptic receptor for a few milliseconds before being hydrolyzed by acetylcholinesterase to acetic acid and choline. Both the acetic acid and the choline are taken up by the presynaptic nerve terminal and are recycled.

Cholinergic receptors are classified as either nicotinic or muscarinic. Nicotinic receptors are found in autonomic ganglia and at the neuromuscular junction. Muscarinic receptors are found on smooth muscle, cardiac muscle, and sweat glands. Acetylcholine is the neurotransmitter at cranial nerve nuclei and motor neurons of the ventral horn of the spinal cord that include various collateral nerves to Renshaw cells (interneurons). Acetylcholine may be interactive in neuronal circuits involved with pain reception. Acetylcholine may also act as a sensory transmitter in thermal receptors and taste bud endings.

Biogenic Amines

The biogenic amines include epinephrine, norepinephrine, dopamine, serotonin, and histamine. The catecholamines epinephrine, norepinephrine, and dopamine are synthesized in a series of hydroxylation, decarboxylation, and methylation reactions from the amino acids phenylalanine and tyrosine. The adrenal medulla secretes both epinephrine (75%) and norepinephrine (25%). Postganglionic adrenergic neurons secrete norepinephrine; norepinephrine and dopamine are probably neurotransmitters within the CNS. Amacrine cells of the retina and some neurons of the intrinsic nervous system of the intestine secrete dopamine. As with acetylcholine, the release of norepinephrine, epinephrine, and dopamine is calcium dependent. One notable difference from acetylcholine is that norepinephrine and dopamine act by means of second messengers (slow synaptic transmission), whereas most of the actions of acetylcholine are directly on ion channels (fast synaptic transmission). The duration of effect of catecholamines is regulated by presynaptic reuptake. Enzymatic breakdown of catecholamines by monoamine oxidase and catechol-O-methyltransferase within the liver is primarily responsible for the termination their effects.

Dopamine is an inhibitory neurotransmitter and is the predominant biogenic amine within the CNS. Dopamine is concentrated within the basal ganglia. Dopamine's inhibitory effects occur through action on adenylate cyclase, which is dopamine sensitive.

Norepinephrine is concentrated in the reticular activating system and the hypothalamus. Norepinephrine acts as an inhibitory neurotransmitter, inhibiting impulses to the cerebral cortex.

Serotonin is an inhibitory neurotransmitter that influences behavior and mood. Histamine is also an inhibitory neurotransmitter concentrated within the hypothalamus and the reticular activating system. Histamine requires the second messenger cyclic adenosine monophosphate to mediate its inhibitory effects.

Amino Acids

Glutamate is the primary excitatory transmitter found within the cerebral cortex, the hippocampus, and the substantia gelatinosa of the spinal cord.[9] Glutamate plays a formidable role in learning and memory (perhaps interactive in memory formation during awareness during anesthesia) and the appreciation of pain. Glutamate has also been implicated in excitotoxic neuronal injury after ischemic or traumatic brain injury.

Glutamate is formed from the deamination of glutamine supplied by the Krebs cycle. Glutamate may activate either an inotropic or a metabotropic amino acid receptor. *N*-methyl-D-aspartate (NMDA) receptors are ligand-gated inotropic receptors that produce a conformational change in the receptor, opening a sodium channel, which results in the depolarization of the postsynaptic membrane. The metabotropic receptor is an integral transmembrane receptor that regulates intracellular second messenger systems.

GABA is the major inhibitory neurotransmitter found in the CNS. It is concentrated in the basal ganglia, cerebral cortex, cerebellum, and spinal cord. Activation of the GABA receptor opens neuronal membrane chloride channels, producing hyperpolarization (the hyperpolarized neuron is resistant to excitation). GABA is important in antagonizing the excitatory effects of amino acid neurotransmitters.

Glycine is the primary inhibitory neurotransmitter in the spinal cord. In the past glycine irrigation was employed during transurethral resection of the prostate. Postoperative visual impairment after the intravascular absorption of glycine suggests that glycine may act as an inhibitory neurotransmitter within the retina.

Neuropeptides

Neuropeptides are either excitatory or inhibitory. Common neuropeptides include the opioids, substance P, and many pituitary and pancreatic islet hormones.

Substance P is an excitatory neurotransmitter found in the striatum and substantia nigra of the basal ganglia, the hypothalamus, the brain stem (raphe nuclei), and the dorsal root ganglia of the spinal cord. Substance P is released by pain fiber terminals that synapse with the substantia gelatinosa of the spinal cord.

The opioid neuropeptides include β-endorphin, enkephalins, and dynorphin. They act at opiate receptors distributed throughout the brain and spinal cord. Three classes of opiate receptors have been identified—delta, kappa, and mu. Dynorphin is a potent agonist at kappa receptors, and the enkephalins are agonists at delta and mu receptors. Opiate alkaloids, like morphine, interact with mu receptors. Morphine-like agents block slow pain pathways, raise the pain threshold, and modify the response to pain. Other effects, such as miosis and respiratory depression, result from the actions of these agents on opiate receptors located in the parts of the brain that control these functions.[2,7,10]

SENSORY PATHWAYS

Sensory or afferent pathways transmit pain, temperature, pressure, touch, vibratory sense, and proprioceptive information to the CNS. Sensory pathways also include the special senses of vision, taste, hearing, smell, and equilibrium.

Receptors for pain and temperature are located in the epidermis and the dermis; those for pressure, touch, vibratory sense, and proprioception are located in the dermis. Receptors can be classified as (1) exteroceptors, which are located near the surface of skin and oral mucosa, and (2) proprioceptors, which are located in deeper skin layers, joint capsules, ligaments, tendons, muscles, and periosteum. Several types of receptors exist. Pacinian corpuscles are receptors for vibration and pressure. Free nerve endings, Ruffini's corpuscles, muscle spindles, and Golgi tendon organs are involved in movement sense. The receptors for light (or crude) touch sensations include Merkel's disks, Meissner's corpuscles, and the nerve plexuses surrounding some hair roots. Fibers travel from these receptors to a ganglion, where they synapse with first-order neurons, the fibers of which continue to the CNS. Fibers from receptors in the trunk and extremities travel to the dorsal root ganglion, where they synapse with first-order neurons. Most of the sensory fibers from the head, excluding those from the special sense organs (hearing, equilibrium, vision, taste, and smell), synapse in first-order neurons located in the semilunar or trigeminal ganglion.[7,8]

Pain and Temperature Pathways

Pain and temperature fibers from the head synapse in the trigeminal ganglion and enter the pons, forming the trigeminal nerve (cranial nerve V) (Figure 26-10). These fibers subsequently synapse with second-order neurons in the nucleus of the descending tract of cranial nerve V. The second-order axons cross to the ventrolateral side and ascend as the ventral

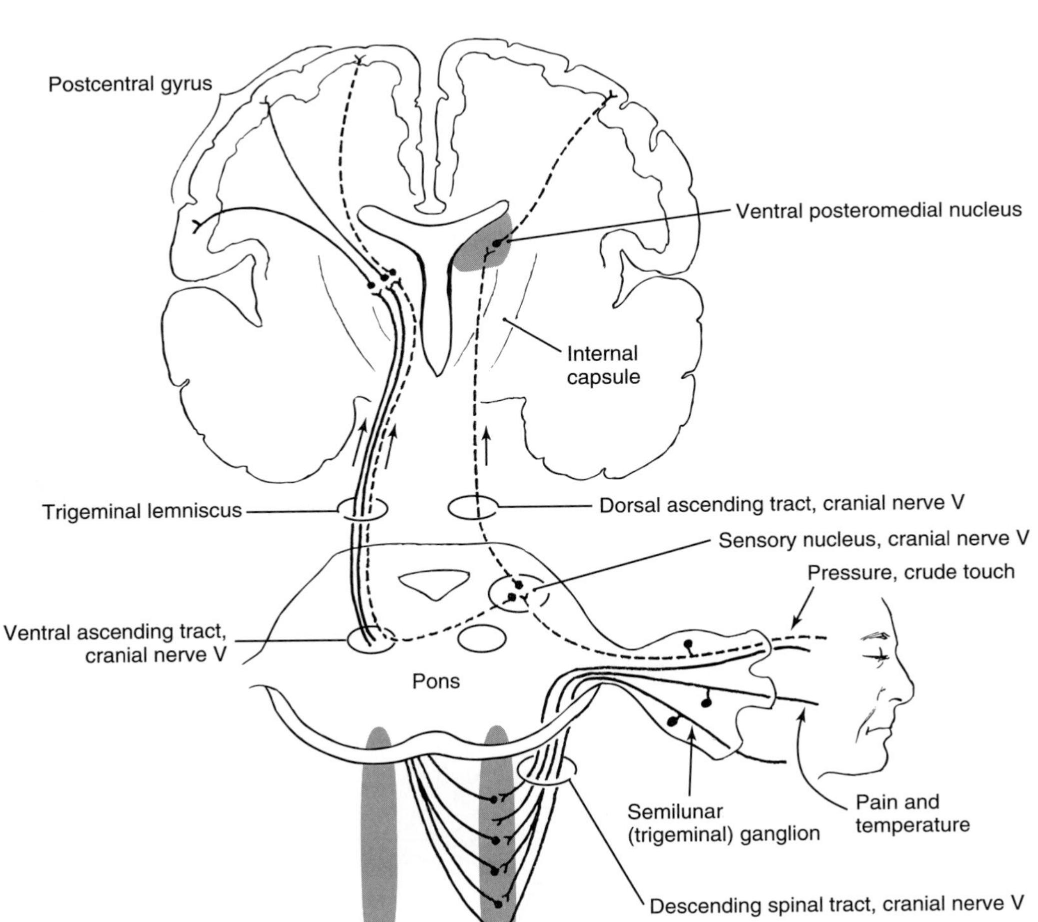

FIGURE **26-10**
Sensory pathways from the head and neck. (Modified from Liebman M. *Neuroanatomy Made Easy and Understandable*. Gaithersburg, Md: Aspen; 1991:19. Copyright © 1991, Michael Liebman.)

trigeminal tract to the ventral posteromedial nucleus of the thalamus, where they synapse with third-order neurons. From the ventral posteromedial thalamic nucleus, third-order axons ascend in the internal capsule and end in the postcentral gyrus of the cerebral cortex, which is the primary somatic sensory area of the brain. Pain and temperature receptors in the skin of the trunk and extremities send fibers to the dorsal root ganglion, where they synapse with first-order neurons (Figure 26-11). The first-order axons enter the dorsal horn gray matter of the spinal cord and synapse with second-order neurons. Axons from the second-order neurons decussate (cross) in the ventral white commissure and enter the lateral white columns before ascending as the lateral spinothalamic tract to the ventral posterolateral thalamic nucleus, where they synapse with third-order neurons. Axons from the third-order neurons travel in the posterior limb of the internal capsule and ultimately synapse in the postcentral gyrus, where sensations of pain, temperature, touch, and pressure are interpreted and responses to the sensations are initiated.

Some pain and temperature fibers in the dorsal horn give off branches that synapse with internuncial (messenger) neurons. The internuncial neurons have axons that synapse with motor neurons in the ventral horn, which are not necessarily at the same level of the spinal cord. The axons can cross over and travel up or down the spinal cord before synapsing. These circuits are part of the reflex response to pain, which results in a rapid, automatic response to nociceptive stimuli.

The afferent fibers from each dorsal root ganglion come from a relatively limited area of the skin termed a *dermatome*. Some overlap exists, so if a spinal nerve that supplies a certain dermatome is severed, pain and temperature sensations from that dermatome are supplied by adjacent dermatome fibers. For example, if T6 is severed, T5 and T7 sensory neurons carry pain and temperature sensations from the skin area supplied by T6. Axons entering the dorsal horn from the dorsal root ganglion send branches to one spinal segment above and one segment below in the dorsolateral column of Lissauer.[2,6,8,11]

Pressure and Crude Touch

Pressure and crude (light) touch fibers from the head synapse with first-order neurons in the trigeminal ganglion. From the trigeminal ganglion, first-order axons travel to the pons, where they synapse with second-order neurons in the sensory nucleus of cranial nerve V (see Figure 26-11). From the sensory nucleus of cranial nerve V, second-order axons form the dorsal trigeminal tract, which has both crossed and uncrossed fibers. The second-order fibers terminate in the ventral posteromedial nucleus of the thalamus. Third-order axons from the ventral posteromedial nucleus subsequently terminate in the postcentral gyrus of the cerebral cortex.

After leaving the dorsal root ganglion, crude touch and pressure fibers from the extremities and trunk enter the dorsal white column on the ipsilateral side and bifurcate (Figure 26-12). One branch immediately enters the dorsal gray horn and synapses with second-order neurons. The other branch ascends for up to 10 spinal segments before synapsing with the second-order neurons in the dorsal horn. Second-order axons from both branches cross over and enter the ventral white column, forming the ventral spinothalamic tract, which ascends to the thalamus and synapses with third-order neurons in the ventral posterolateral nucleus. Tertiary axons travel through the internal capsule to the postcentral gyrus.

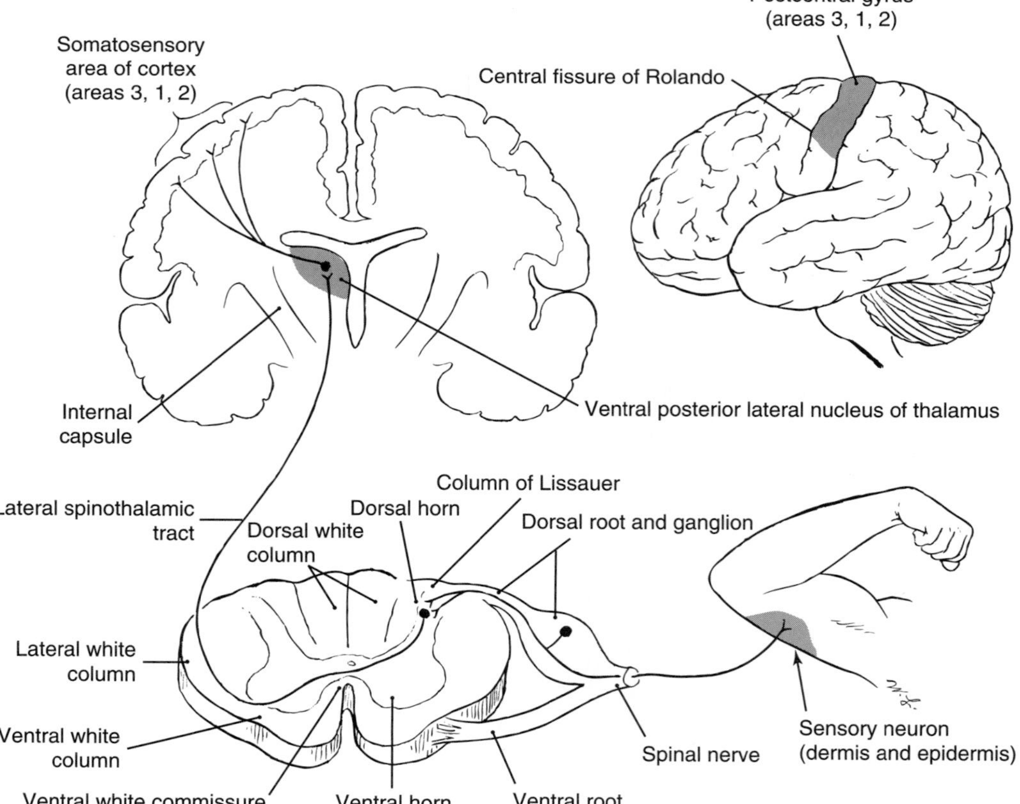

FIGURE **26-11**
Pain and temperature pathways from the trunk and extremities. (Modified from Liebman M. *Neuroanatomy Made Easy and Understandable*. Gaithersburg, Md: Aspen; 1991:11. Copyright © 1991, Michael Liebman.)

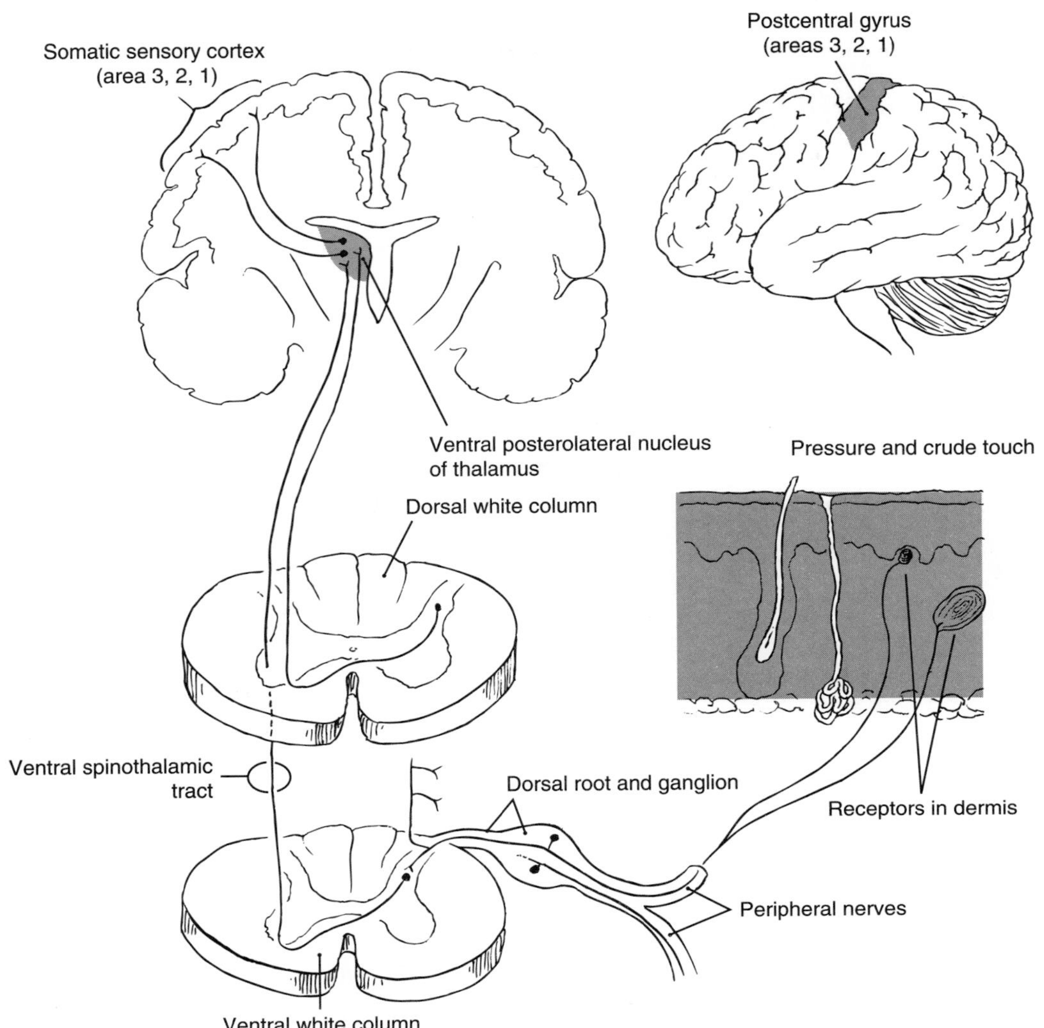

FIGURE **26-12**
Crude touch and pressure sensations from the extremities and trunk. (Modified from Liebman M. *Neuroanatomy Made Easy and Understandable*. Gaithersburg, Md: Aspen; 1991:14. Copyright © 1991, Michael Liebman.)

Owing to the branching arrangement of the first-order fibers from the trunk and extremities, injuries to the spinal cord rarely result in the total loss of these two sensations. Each cerebral cortex receives both crossed and uncrossed pressure and light touch fibers from the face, and, as a result, damage to the postcentral gyrus on one side does not result in loss of pressure and crude touch sensations to the face, even though these sensations are lost on the trunk and extremities of the contralateral side.[2,7,8,11]

Vibratory Sense, Proprioception, and Discriminatory Touch

Proprioceptive fibers from muscles of the face involved in facial expression and mastication synapse in cell bodies located in the mesencephalic nucleus of the midbrain. Little is known about the rest of the pathway.

Fibers from the trunk and extremities carrying proprioceptive, vibratory, and discriminatory (fine) touch sensations synapse with neuron cell bodies in the dorsal root ganglion. From the dorsal root ganglion, first-order axons enter the dorsal white column and ascend to the medulla (Figure 26-13). The fibers are somatotopically organized in the white columns. Axons from the lumbar and sacral parts of the spinal cord travel medially in the fasciculus gracilis, and fibers from the cervical and thoracic areas of the cord are located laterally in the fasciculus cuneatus of the dorsal white column of the spinal cord. Each fasciculus terminates in its respective medullary nucleus; for example, the fasciculus gracilis terminates in the nucleus gracilis. Second-order axons decussate after leaving their medullary nucleus and form a bundle termed the *medial lemniscus*, which terminates in the ventral posterolateral thalamic nucleus. Third-order fibers from the ventral posterolateral nucleus terminate in the postcentral gyrus.[2,7,8,11]

Pupillary light and accommodation reflexes are mediated through the Edinger-Westphal nucleus and cranial nerve III. Pupillary dilation is produced by postganglionic sympathetic fibers from the superior cervical ganglion that travel with branches of the internal carotid artery to the radial muscle of the iris.[2,7,8,11]

MOTOR PATHWAYS

Motor, or efferent, pathways transmit information from the brain to the voluntary muscles of the body, to smooth and cardiac muscles, and to some glands. The corticospinal tracts supply the voluntary muscles of the trunk and extremities; nine cranial nerves supply the voluntary muscles of the head and neck. Autonomic preganglionic fibers arise in the brain

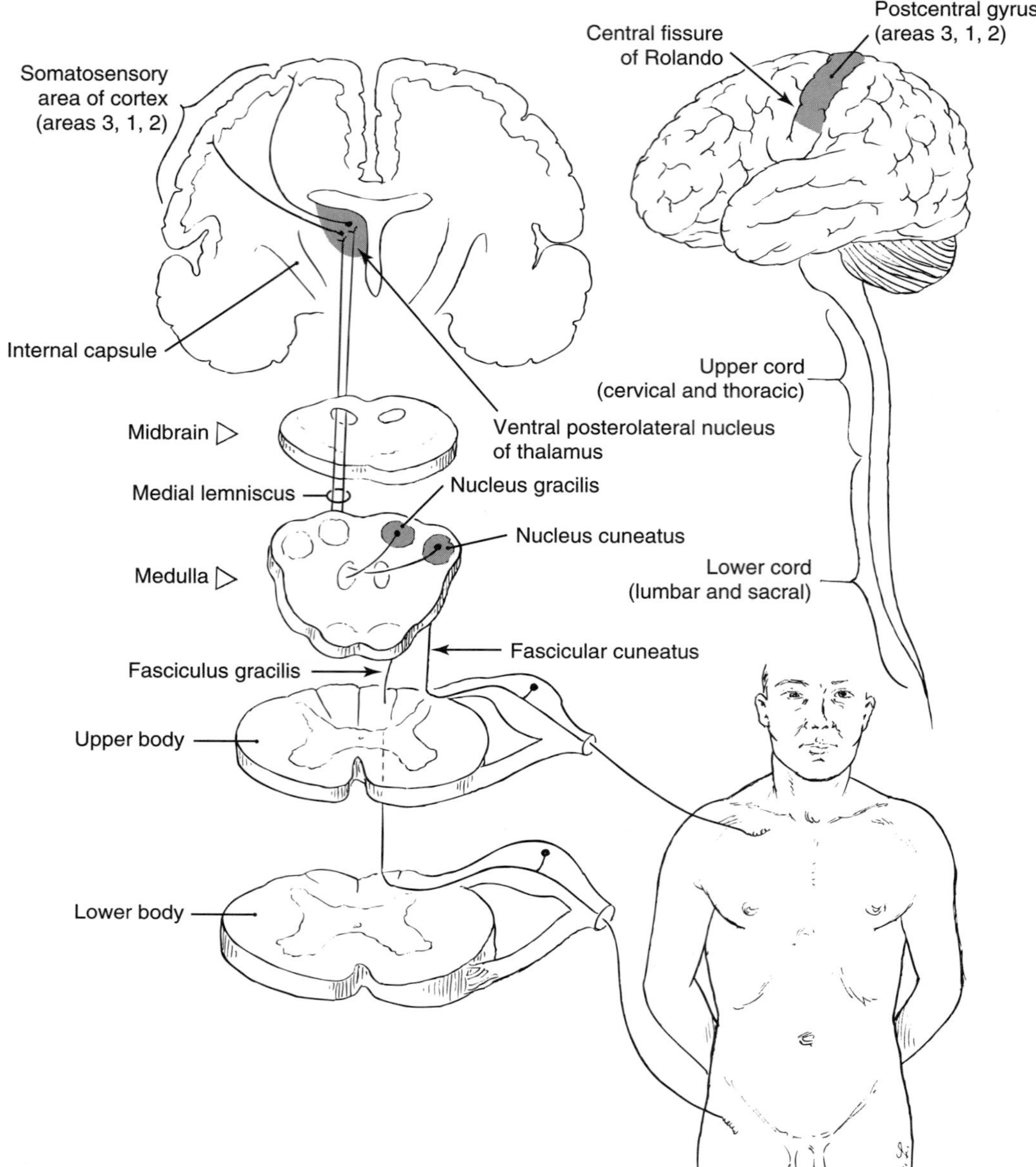

FIGURE **26-13**
Proprioceptive, fine touch, and vibratory sensations from the extremities and trunk. (Modified from Liebman M. *Neuroanatomy Made Easy and Understandable*. Gaithersburg, Md: Aspen; 1991:16. Copyright © 1991, Michael Liebman.)

and spinal cord and transmit efferent signals to smooth muscle, cardiac muscle, and some glands (lacrimal, bronchial).

Corticospinal Tract

The corticospinal tract originates in large, upper motor neurons located in the precentral gyrus of the frontal lobe (Figure 26-14). These neurons are arranged in a specific manner. Neurons supplying voluntary muscles of the head are found in the precentral gyrus near the lateral fissure of Sylvius, and those innervating the legs and feet are found in an area of the gyrus near the median longitudinal fissure. All parts of the body are represented in the gyrus. However, areas that perform complex movements (such as the hands when writing, typing, or playing the piano) have a larger area in the gyrus than other parts of the body not involved in intricate movements. Many of the upper motor neurons are pyramid shaped.

Axons travel from the pyramidal cells through the internal capsule, the major pathway for ascending and descending fibers between the cortex and other sites in the CNS. The internal capsule has three parts: the anterior limb, the posterior limb, and the genu, which lies between the anterior and posterior limbs. Fibers in the internal capsule are highly organized. Motor fibers to all parts of the body except the face are located in the anterior limb and part of the posterior limb. Fibers supplying the face are located in the genu. From the internal capsule the axons travel through the midbrain (basis pedunculi) to the medulla, where approximately 90% of the fibers decussate, forming the pyramids of the medulla. The corticospinal tract is frequently called the *pyramidal tract*, either because of the shape of the upper motor neurons or because of the site at which the fibers decussate in the medulla. The fibers that cross over form the lateral corticospinal tract. Axons from the lateral corticospinal tract continue their descent to the spinal cord. At each level of the cord, some fibers leave the lateral corticospinal tract and enter the ventral horn gray matter, where they synapse with lower motor neurons. The fibers that do not decussate (approximately 10%) in the medulla continue to the spinal cord as the ventral corticospinal tract. The ventral corticospinal tracts cross

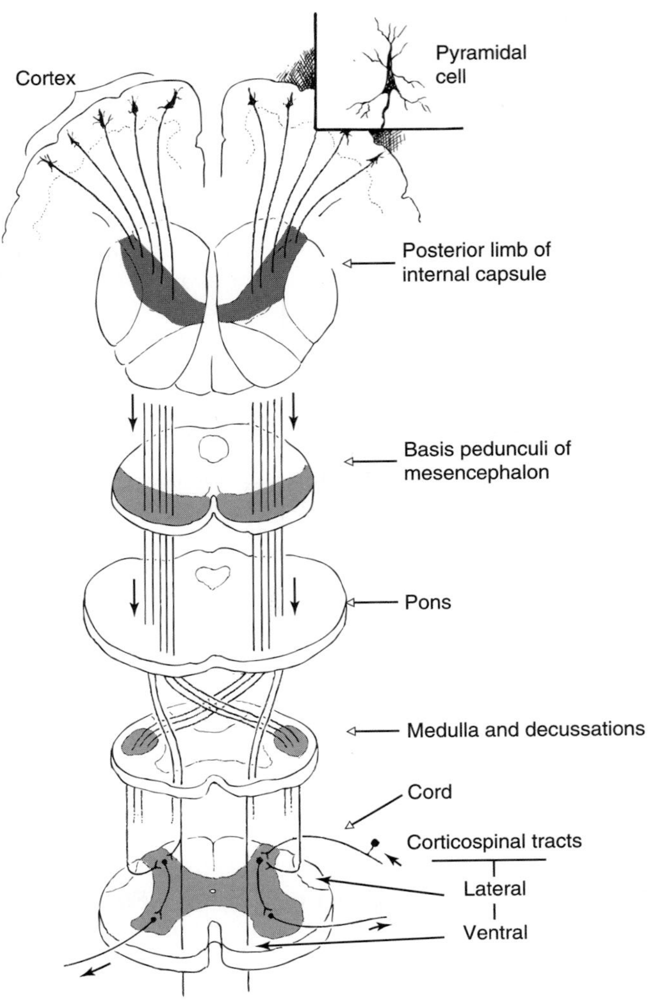

FIGURE **26-14**
Corticospinal tracts. (Modified from Guyton AC. *Basic Neuroscience: Anatomy and Physiology*. Philadelphia: Saunders; 1991:212.)

over before synapsing with lower motor neurons in the gray matter. Axons from the lower motor neurons travel in the spinal nerves to innervate voluntary muscle.

A few corticospinal tract neurons are located anterior to the precentral gyrus. Axons from these neurons have an inhibitory effect on the lower motor neurons because they prevent them from discharging excessively. Damage to these suppressor fibers can stimulate the lower motor neurons either to overfire, resulting in hyperreflexia, or to discharge simultaneously, causing spasticity. Damage to the corticospinal tract anywhere along its route to the spinal cord can cause upper motor neuron paralysis. If the injury occurs above the decussation in the medulla, the paralysis is on the opposite side of the body; the paralysis occurs on the same side of the body if the damage occurs below the medulla. With upper motor neuron paralysis, reflexes are intact, but the suppressor fiber activity is impeded, and, as a result, hyperreflexia is present and the upper motor neuron paralysis is spastic. Damage to lower motor neuron cell bodies in the ventral horn or ventral root fibers produces lower motor neuron paralysis, a flaccid type of paralysis. Cerebral palsy and amyotrophic lateral sclerosis are diseases that affect the corticospinal tracts.

Motor Innervation to the Head

Upper motor neurons whose axons supply the voluntary muscles of the head are found in the precentral gyrus next to the lateral fissure of Sylvius. The cell bodies, whose axons supply the extrinsic muscles of the eye, are located in the middle frontal gyrus. Axons from both areas form the corticobulbar tracts, which travel through the genu of the internal capsule to the brain stem, where they synapse with neurons located in nuclei spread throughout the brain stem. Axons from these neurons form many of the cranial nerves.

Axons originating from neurons located in the midbrain form the oculomotor and trochlear nerves (Figure 26-15). The oculomotor nerve innervates most of the external muscle of the eye (inferior oblique and the inferior, medial, and superior rectus muscles), along with the levator palpebrae superioris muscle, which raises the upper eyelid. The trochlear nerve innervates the external oblique muscle of the eye. Three other groups of

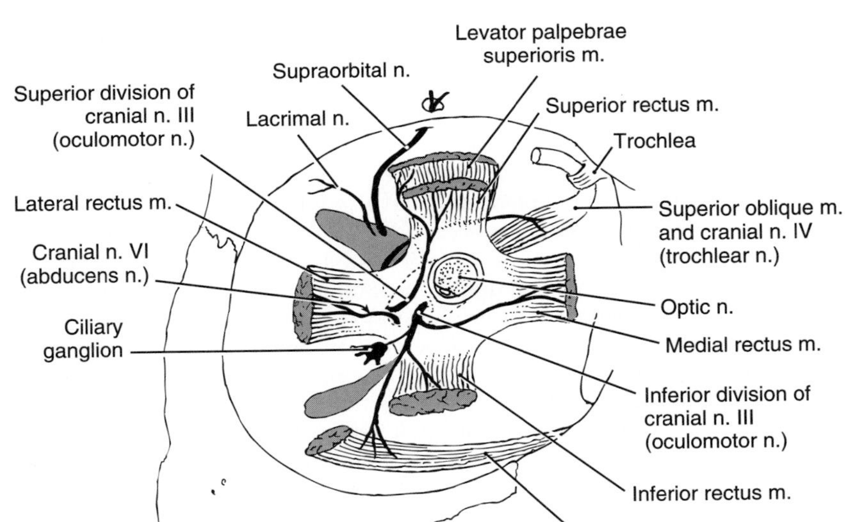

FIGURE **26-15**
Frontal view of the posterior orbit with its motor nerves and the extraocular muscles.

nuclei have neurons whose axons form the trigeminal, abducens, and facial nerves. The trigeminal nerve innervates part of the soft palate and all of the muscles of mastication. The abducens innervates the lateral rectus muscle of the eye, and the facial nerves supply all of the muscles involved in facial expression.

Axons from neurons located in medullary nuclei form the glossopharyngeal, vagal, accessory, and hypoglossal nerves. Both the glossopharyngeal and vagal nerves arise from the ambiguous nucleus. The glossopharyngeal nerve supplies the stylopharyngeal muscle of the pharynx, and the vagal nerve innervates the muscles of the throat that are involved in swallowing and phonation. All of the tongue muscles are supplied by the hypoglossal nerve. The accessory nerve innervates the trapezius and sternocleidomastoid muscles of the neck. With the exception of the facial and hypoglossal nerves, the remaining nerves receive information from both the right and the left corticobulbar tracts. The nuclei of facial nerve fibers to the upper part of the face receive axons from the left and right corticobulbar tracts; the facial nerve nuclei whose fibers supply the lower part of the face receive fibers only from the contralateral corticobulbar tract. The nuclei from the origin of the hypoglossal nerves receive innervation from only the contralateral corticobulbar tract.[2,7,8,11]

Subcortical Motor Areas

Several motor areas in the brain are outside the cerebral cortex. For the most part these are relatively primitive motor areas that have a modulating influence on motor function. Included in the subcortical motor areas are the basal ganglia, the nucleus of Luys, the red nucleus (nucleus ruber), the substantia nigra, and the reticular formation.

The basal ganglia lie deep within the cerebral hemispheres at the level of the internal capsule. They are composed of three nuclei: the globus pallidus, the putamen, and the caudate, which are collectively termed the *corpus striata.* The globus pallidus and the putamen are sometimes termed the *lentiform nucleus.* The globus pallidus makes up the paleostriatum, and the other two nuclei are part of the neostriatum.

The globus pallidus receives input from the motor cortex and from the other basal ganglia; it sends fibers to the subcortical motor areas. The globus pallidus is connected to the thalamus by two tracts, the ansa lenticularis and the lenticular fasciculus, which merge as they enter the thalamus to form the thalamic fasciculus. The thalamus forms a feedback process by sending fibers to the caudate nucleus and motor cortex. In this way the motor activity of the basal ganglia can be influenced by the motor cortex without the presence of direct connections between the two structures. Dopamine, an important neurotransmitter in the basal ganglia, is produced in the substantia nigra of the midbrain and then travels by axonal transport to the caudate nucleus and the putamen.

The subthalamic nucleus of Luys is located in the diencephalon and is connected to other subcortical motor areas. Lesions in this nucleus result in a suppression of motor activity.

Three motor areas are located in the midbrain: the red nucleus, the substantia nigra, and the reticular formation. The red nucleus is located at the level of the corpora quadrigemina and gives rise to the crossed rubrospinal tract. When stimulated this tract excites alpha and gamma flexor motor neurons and inhibits extensor motor neurons. The reticular formation consists of a diffuse collection of neurons found throughout the brain stem and into the diencephalon. Two major tracts arise from the reticular formation. One tract is the uncrossed medial reticulospinal tract, which excites alpha and gamma extensor motor neurons and inhibits flexor motor neurons when stimulated. The second tract is the lateral reticulospinal tract, which contains crossed and uncrossed fibers and activates alpha and gamma flexor motor neurons and inhibits extensor motor neurons when stimulated.

Lesions in the subcortical motor areas produce diseases characterized by disturbed muscle tone and dyskinesia (abnormal involuntary movements). In Parkinson's disease the globus pallidus and substantia nigra are affected. Huntington's chorea involves atrophy of the caudate nucleus and putamen, as well as degeneration of cortical neurons. Other diseases that involve subcortical motor nuclei include athetosis, dystonia, ballismus, and Sydenham's chorea.

NEUROANESTHESIA

Neuroanesthesia is the application of anesthetic pharmacologic principles to the intraoperative care of patients with CNS pathology. A comprehensive discussion of the clinical aspects of neuroanesthesia (e.g., cerebral ischemia and protection, evoked-potential and electroencephalographic monitoring, surgical intervention in epileptic patients) is beyond the scope of this chapter. The intention of this section is not to present a dogmatic view of the approach to the neurosurgical patient, but to provide a broad overview of the effects of anesthetic agents on cerebral blood flow (CBF), cerebral metabolic rate for oxygen ($CMRO_2$), and intracranial pressure (ICP). The remainder of this chapter provides a general discussion of the preoperative, intraoperative, and immediate postoperative care for common intracranial surgical procedures.

Effects of Anesthetic Agents on Cerebral Physiology

Although inhalation and intravenous anesthetic agents are often selected to minimize cardiovascular insult, appropriate drug selection must include consideration of underlying pathology. Physiologic parameters such as CBF, cerebral blood volume (CBV), ICP, $CMRO_2$, and cerebral compliance all must be considered in concert with pharmacologic principles in the design of a neurosurgical anesthetic regimen (Table 26-5). This section highlights the effects of the inhalation and intravenous anesthetics, neuromuscular relaxants, and antihypertensives on cerebral physiology.

Inhalation Agents

All anesthetic agents influence ICP by decreasing cerebrovascular resistance through cerebrovascular dilation and by dose-dependent impairment of autoregulation, producing increases in ICP, CBV, and CBF and a decrease in $CMRO_2$. The changes in ICP are generally greater in patients who have an underlying increase in ICP.[12,13] The potent inhalation agents decrease mean arterial pressure (MAP) and increase ICP, reducing cerebral perfusion pressure (CPP).[14-16] Halothane produces the greatest increases in CBF and ICP, followed by isoflurane, sevoflurane, and desflurane. Additional increases in ICP after halothane administration in patients with increased ICP may be attenuated with hyperventilation for at least 10 minutes before halothane administration; however, this may not be successful if ICP is markedly increased.[12,17-19]

CBF in humans is unaltered with isoflurane inspired concentrations of 0.6 to 1.1 minimum alveolar concentration (MAC); however, 1.6 MAC isoflurane doubles CBF. Animal studies have shown that isoflurane may enhance the carbon dioxide (CO_2) reactivity of the cerebral vessels. Cerebral

TABLE 26-5 Effects of Anesthetics on Cerebral Dynamics

Drug	Cerebral Blood Flow	$CMRO_2$	Intracranial Pressure	Cerebral Perfusion Pressure
Inhalation				
Nitrous oxide	↑	↑↓	0	↓
Halothane	↑↑	↓	↑	↓
Sevoflurane	↑	↓	↑	↓
Isoflurane	↑	↓	↑	↓
Desflurane	↑	↓	↑	↓
Intravenous				
Barbiturates	↓↓	↓↓	↓↓	0/↓
Etomidate	↓↓	↓↓	↓	0
Propofol	↓	↓	↓	↓
Ketamine	↑↑	↑	↑↑	↓
Benzodiazepines	↓	↓	↓	0/↓
Morphine	0/↓	0/↓	↓	↑↓
Fentanyl	0/↓	0/↓	↓	0/↓
Alfentanil	0/↓	0/↓	↓	↓
Sufentanil	0/↓	0/↓	↓	↓
Remifentanil	0/↓	0/↓	↓	↓

$CMRO_2$, *Cerebral metabolic rate of oxygen.*
From Aker J. Neuroanesthesia. In: Zaglaniczny K, Aker J, eds. Clinical Guide to Pediatric Anesthesia. *Philadelphia: Saunders; 1999:176.*

autoregulation is impaired with concentrations exceeding 1 MAC.[20,21] $CMRO_2$ is depressed to a greater extent with isoflurane than with halothane, and progressive metabolic depression occurs with concentrations of isoflurane greater than 1 MAC until the electroencephalograph (EEG) becomes isoelectric at approximately 2.5 MAC.[22,23] These properties suggest that clinically relevant doses *may* provide a neuroprotective effect against ischemic insults, as demonstrated in human studies of critical regional CBF during carotid clamping.[24] Although isoflurane has been referred to as "cerebral protective", no contemporary evidence suggests that isoflurane is uniquely protective in the setting of cerebral ischemia versus other volatile anesthetic agents. The high concentrations of isoflurane necessary for abolishing cortical activity have no toxic effect on cerebral metabolic pathways; in contrast, high concentrations of halothane induce cerebral acidosis.[23,25] The majority of human studies show that inspired concentrations of isoflurane of less than 1% have little effect on ICP and that any increase in ICP is attenuated by hyperventilation. An exception to this generalization is that some patients with malignant brain tumors may show increases in ICP despite prior hyperventilation, particularly if computed tomography shows a midline shift.[26-28]

Desflurane is unique among the potent inhalation agents in that its low blood-gas solubility facilitates a rapid emergence, which may be useful for immediate postoperative neurologic evaluation. Desflurane has effects on EEG, CBF, and $CMRO_2$ that are similar to those of isoflurane. Young[29] and Ornstein and co-workers[30] compared the effects of desflurane and isoflurane on CBF at two concentrations (1 MAC and 1.5 MAC) in an air-oxygen mixture during hypocapnia and reported no difference between isoflurane and desflurane at the two different MAC levels. However, the results of ICP studies are not as definitive. Muzzi and colleagues[31] reported that desflurane 1 MAC in an air-oxygen mixture with an arterial CO_2 tension ($PaCO_2$) of 26 mm Hg resulted in sustained increases in ICP until the dura was incised. A similar study reported no appreciable change in ICP before or after 0.5 MAC of either isoflurane or desflurane in 50% nitrous oxide (N_2O).[32]

The physiologic effects of sevoflurane are similar to those of other inhalation anesthetics. Like other anesthetics it produces cerebral vasodilation, but its effect appears to be less than that of isoflurane.[33,34]

In summary, all of the potent inhalation agents are known to increase CBF, CBV, and ICP, and with respect to cerebral physiology no one agent is known to be better than another. Hyperventilation attenuates these dose-dependent increases in ICP. These agents are thought to be acceptable in all patients except those with marked intracranial hypertension with midline shift.

N_2O continues to be administered in neuroanesthesia despite a growing call for its abandonment. Its ease of administration and short elimination half-life are advantageous in neurosurgical patients. N_2O is more soluble than nitrogen and expands closed gas spaces. This may have particular relevance in patients with pneumocephalus.[35] Some practitioners abandon N_2O administration before closure of the dura to attenuate the development of iatrogenic pneumocephalus. Although this reduces ICP at the conclusion of the surgical procedure, continuous N_2O administration throughout the intraoperative period provides for equilibration with air before closure of the dura.

Most anesthetists generally regard N_2O as an innocuous anesthetic. However, N_2O is a potent cerebral vasodilator and can produce increases in both CBF and ICP (after cerebral vasodilatation) equal to or greater than those produced by the volatile anesthetic agents themselves. N_2O also may increase $CMRO_2$. Concomitant hyperventilation or the administration of one of several intravenous anesthetics (barbiturates, propofol, benzodiazepines, opioids) can reduce the increases in CBF and $CMRO_2$ during N_2O administration. However, the combination of N_2O and the volatile anesthetics behave much differently. The administration of a volatile anesthetic in low doses (below 1 MAC) may decrease CBF and $CMRO_2$. The addition of 50% N_2O with less than 1 MAC of the volatile anesthetic produces increases in both CBF and $CMRO_2$. The cerebral vasodilatation produced by N_2O is greater when increasing doses (greater than 1 MAC) of the volatile anesthetic are administered. N_2O may increase CBF by 100% or more at approximately 0.5 MAC. Even when it is added to a background of 1 MAC halothane, a threefold increase in CBF is noted. It is interesting to note that N_2O appears to produce nonuniform changes in CBF, increasing flow in anterior regions and decreasing flow in posterior brain regions. N_2O is not thought to affect CBV or CSF dynamics.[36]

Is N_2O neurotoxic? The data are conflicting. Some data suggest that N_2O may reduce the tolerance of neurons to survive ischemic insults. In contrast, studies using animal models of ischemic injury have failed to find increases in neuronal injury with N_2O administration. Even more recent studies suggest that N_2O may antagonize the NMDA receptor. Some neuroanesthesiologists have advocated that N_2O should no longer be administered in neurosurgical patients. The vast clinical experience of N_2O in thousands of neurosurgical patients, with little documentation of adverse neurologic events, argues against N_2O as having major neurotoxic effects. The reader should appreciate that N_2O has been administered to thousands of neurosurgical patients and that no controlled studies outlining adverse neurologic events exist.

When should the anesthetist consider the avoidance of N_2O? The practitioner should consider the elimination of N_2O in the following clinical circumstances:

- In the presence of intracranial air (recent craniotomy, cranial-facial trauma)
- When signal quality during intraoperative evoked-potential monitoring is inadequate
- When the patient has clinical evidence of moderate to severe increases in ICP
- When a "tight-brain" is clinically appreciated during the intraoperative period

Intravenous Agents

Barbiturates. Barbiturates are beneficial neuroanesthetic agents because of their ability to decrease $CMRO_2$. This occurs as a result of a reduction in CNS neuronal activity that, in turn, leads to a coupled reduction in CBF and ICP. However, barbiturates decrease CBF only in normal regions. Because of vasomotor paralysis, vessels within injured or ischemic zones fail to react and remain maximally dilated. The result is the shunting of blood from normal to ischemic areas (termed *inverse steal*). CSF production and absorption are not affected. However, a dose-dependent depression of the CNS does occur; this depression is reflected as progressively slowing EEG activity.[36] A reduction in the metabolic requirement for EEG permits this energy to be used for neuronal basal metabolic needs. When the EEG is isoelectric, neuronal energy consumption is decreased approximately 50%.

Additional benefits of barbiturate administration include the reduction of free radical formation, which may prevent further injury in ischemic zones, reduction of ATP depletion, effective anticonvulsant activity; and decreasing cytotoxic cerebral edema, often seen after incomplete ischemia. Barbiturates may be clinically useful for the control of ICP in patients with head injury when standard therapy is ineffective.[15,36,37]

Propofol. Propofol is a popular induction and maintenance agent for neurosurgical patients. The cerebral effects are similar to those found after barbiturate administration, with a dose-dependent reduction in CBF and $CMRO_2$ producing an isoelectric EEG. CPP may decrease because of reductions in blood pressure after bolus induction doses; however, the reduction in CBF appears to be independent of systemic hemodynamic changes.[38] The dose of propofol required to maintain isoelectricity is 500 mcg/kg/min. However, reductions in systemic blood pressure produce corresponding reductions in CPP. Very high doses (beyond that required to produce an isoelectric EEG) may produce an increase in CBF (direct cerebral vasodilatation).

Etomidate. Etomidate, like the barbiturates, has similar cerebrovascular and metabolic effects, reducing $CMRO_2$, CBF, and ICP in normal brains and in situations of reduced intracranial compliance. Etomidate has a rapid elimination compared with barbiturates, allowing a more prompt postoperative neurologic evaluation. In addition to the indirect effect of reduced cerebral metabolism on blood flow, etomidate has a direct vasoconstricting effect. Unlike barbiturates, etomidate does not produce clinically significant cardiovascular depression, resulting in an unchanged or mildly increased CPP.[39-41] Major disadvantages include a high incidence of nonpurposeful movements, thrombophlebitis, and suppression of the adrenocortical response to stress.[41,42] Small doses of etomidate may elicit seizure activity in patients with an underlying seizure disorder. Renal toxicity may develop from the accumulation of propylene glycol after continuous intravenous infusions.

Opioids. Opioid-based anesthetic techniques are popular for neurosurgical procedures because they provide a steady hemodynamic course and predictable emergence. The synthetic opioids fentanyl, sufentanil, alfentanil, and remifentanil have all been successfully used for neuroanesthesia. These opioids produce dose-related reductions in CBF (decrease to 25 ml/100 g/min) and $CMRO_2$ (40% to 50%).[43-46] Later investigations in patients after acute head injury or those undergoing supratentorial craniotomy noted increases in ICP and decreases in CPP after administration of induction doses of fentanyl, sufentanil, and alfentanil.[47] These opioid-induced changes in ICP have been suggested to occur secondarily to an autoregulatory response to decreases in MAP.[48]

Fentanyl decreases the resistance to CSF absorption and results in a 10% reduction in CBV.[35,42,43] Sufentanil is 5 to 10 times more potent than fentanyl and has the highest therapeutic index of the clinically used opiates. Of the synthetic opiates, alfentanil produces the greatest decreases in MAP and CPP.[35,42,44] High-dose opioid administration has been reported to produce seizures in humans.[49] Meperidine should probably be avoided in the neurosurgical patient because its metabolite, normeperidine, is a well-known convulsant.

Judiciously titrated doses of naloxone reverse opioid-induced respiratory depression and normalize both CBF and $CMRO_2$. The abrupt reversal of opioid-induced respiratory depression should be avoided in neurosurgical patients. Naloxone administered in this fashion is associated with hypertension, cardiac dysrhythmias, pulmonary edema, and intracranial hemorrhage.[50,51]

Benzodiazepines. The benzodiazepines midazolam, diazepam, and lorazepam are useful anesthetic adjuncts employed for their anxiolytic, anticonvulsant, and amnesic effects. Benzodiazepines produce dose-dependent decreases in $CMRO_2$ and reductions in CBF; however, their effects on ICP are minimal.

Flumazenil, the benzodiazepine-specific antagonist, has no effect on cerebral dynamics when administered alone. High-dose midazolam anesthetic in the canine was associated with rebound increases in CBF and ICP to values greater than baseline when abrupt reversal was accomplished with flumazenil.[52] Flumazenil may produce seizures when large doses are administered.

Ketamine. Ketamine has limited usefulness in neuroanesthesia. The dissociative mechanism of action and resultant stormy emergence from anesthesia are both undesirable after neurosurgical procedures. The primary advantage of ketamine is the stable hemodynamic course in the face of hypovolemia that may occur in the head-injured patient with multisystem trauma. However, ketamine is known to produce untoward alterations in cerebral physiology, increasing CBF by 60% to 80% and elevating ICP. Ketamine also increases the resistance to CSF reabsorption, which over time may increase ICP beyond that produced by increases in CBF alone. Cerebral metabolic rate is unchanged, but regional differences may exist.[35] A renewed interest in ketamine has been prompted because of its noncompetitive antagonism of the glutamine NMDA receptor. Similar compounds have been demonstrated to afford some degree of neuroprotection. Current studies are inconclusive regarding the neuroprotective effects. Because of the aforementioned emergence problems, ketamine continues to be an unpopular drug for neuroanesthesia.

Neuromuscular Relaxants. The selection of a neuromuscular relaxant must take into account the resultant cardiovascular and intracranial effects of individual agents. Nondepolarizing neuromuscular relaxants do not appear to have clinically significant direct effects on CBF or $CMRO_2$, provided that MAP is not altered after administration.[53] However, the depolarizing agent succinylcholine in select circumstances may produce elevations in ICP, CBF, and $CMRO_2$.

Upper motor neuron disease may alter the peripheral-nerve–stimulating response of nondepolarizing neuromuscular relaxants. Generally the twitch response shows relative resistance to muscle relaxants on the hemiparetic or hemiplegic side compared with the unaffected side or respiratory muscles.[54,55] This effect can also be bilateral but is usually less pronounced on the hemiplegic side. Decreased sensitivity to nondepolarizing muscle relaxants is most exaggerated in the first 3 weeks of upper motor neuron disease. Therefore monitoring of neuromuscular blockade is preferentially performed on the unaffected side. Patients on chronic anticonvulsant therapy may be more resistant to long-acting nondepolarizing muscle relaxants.[56] Patients receiving chronic phenytoin therapy have an increased dosage requirement and reduced duration of action for the nondepolarizing neuromuscular relaxants, with the exception of atracurium and *cis*-atracurium.

Succinylcholine increases ICP through an increase in muscle spindle activity and increased cerebral stimulation with coupled increases in CBF.[42] Despite the use of thiopental and accompanying hyperventilation during induction, greater increases in ICP have been noted with succinylcholine than with pancuronium. Succinylcholine is contraindicated in patients with neurologic or denervated muscle because of the potential for life-threatening hyperkalemia.[35,41] Succinylcholine should be avoided in patients with cerebrovascular accident, upper and lower motor neuron lesions, coma, encephalitis, and closed head injury and after severe burns and prolonged bed rest.

Succinylcholine has had great utility in facilitating rapid-sequence induction for emergency neurosurgical procedures in patients with little or no preoperative preparation. The availability of suitable nondepolarizing alternatives such as rocuronium (1 mg/kg intubating dose) facilitates endotracheal intubation within 60 to 90 seconds and avoids the known complications attendant on the administration of succinylcholine.

Antihypertensives. β-Adrenergic antagonists have great utility for the control of the inotropic and chronic effects of sympathetic stimulation that attend laryngoscopy, endotracheal intubation, and endotracheal extubation. Esmolol is a rapid-onset, short-acting selective β_1-adrenergic receptor antagonist. Administration of 0.5 to 1 mg/kg 2 minutes before laryngoscopy and endotracheal intubation attenuates the predictable increases in heart rate and blood pressure. Its effects on ICP are thought to be negligible. Labetalol is a selective α_1-adrenergic antagonist and nonselective β_1- and β_2-adrenergic antagonist (ratio of β-blockade to α-blockade is 7:1 for intravenous preparation). Labetalol spares presynaptic α_2-receptors, and consequently, released norepinephrine produces further inhibition of catecholamine release via a negative feedback from the stimulation of α_2-receptors. Labetalol administration in a canine model with and without intracranial hypertension failed to alter ICP despite reductions in MAP of up to 38%.[57] However, esmolol may be preferred for the control of emergence hypertension after intracranial procedures. In this study patients treated with labetalol experienced a higher incidence of bradycardia in the immediate postoperative period.[58]

The smooth muscle relaxants, sodium nitroprusside and nitroglycerin, produce increases in CBV and ICP. Sodium nitroprusside is a direct-acting cerebrovasodilator, increasing CBV after dilation of cerebral capacitance vessels.[53,59] Deliberate hyperventilation and the administration of a barbiturate may attenuate the cerebrovasodilation. Patients with decreased intracranial compliance may better benefit from β-blockade, barbiturate administration, and opioid administration before laryngoscopy and endotracheal intubation. Nitroglycerin causes an increase in CBF and ICP that may be greater than the increase produced by sodium nitroprusside.[60-62] With respect to these two agents, sodium nitroprusside may be more efficacious in the control of hypertension during craniotomy.

The calcium channel–blocking agents not only have been used for the control of blood pressure during the perioperative period, but also have been studied for their potential cerebral protectant effects. Nimodipine is commonly used to prevent vasospasm after neurologic trauma or hemorrhage. The available calcium channel–blocking agents have been shown to increase ICP.[63,64]

INTRACRANIAL PRESSURE

In its simplest definition, *intracranial pressure* refers to the supratentorial CSF pressure. The supratentorial pressure may be measured within the lateral ventricle or within the subarachnoid space over the convexity of the cerebral cortex. CSF pressure may vary markedly in different areas within the cranium, and, similarly, CSF pressure in the cranial subarachnoid space may differ from that in the spinal subarachnoid space. In an individual free of neurologic pathology in the recumbent position, the CSF pressure measured at the lumbar cistern accurately reflects ICP. However, many factors, including the assumption of the upright position, can alter the relationship between cranial and spinal CSF pressures. In addition, in the presence of intracranial mass lesions infratentorial CSF pressure (as measured in the cisterna magna or lumbar cistern) often decreases, whereas supratentorial pressure increases. Therefore the measurement of supratentorial CSF pressure is a useful clinical concept.[15,65]

Determinants of Intracranial Pressure

The brain is enclosed within a rigid container (the cranium), and because the brain is not compressible, any increase in total intracranial volume produces an accompanying increase in ICP. Increased ICP may have a detrimental effect on the well-being of the brain. The intracranial contents consist of the brain (12%), intracellular water (78%), CSF (approximately 75 ml), and blood (approximately 50 ml), for a combined volume of approximately 1200 to 1500 ml.[66] Recall that the brain is surrounded by the dura mater rigidly encased in the bone of the calvaria and skull base. In the strictest sense the intracranial space, volume, and pressure are defined by the limits of the encasing bone; however, should the skull become disrupted, the remaining intracranial contents may be subject to the potential for abnormal pressure accumulation because of the restrictions imposed by an intact dura mater. The same dural restrictions also may contribute to regional ICP gradients in patients with intracranial mass lesions and an intact cranial vault.[67] Intracranial hypertension may lead to global reductions in CPP (CPP = MAP − ICP) from compression-induced ischemia or may produce shifting of intracranial contents, resulting in compression of the brain against the falx, the tentorium, or the foramen magnum.

The ICP is approximately 5 to 15 mm Hg in adults; lower values are recorded in children and infants. This pressure is determined by the relationship between the volume allowed by the structures that limit intracranial volume and the actual volume of the intracranial space. Individuals without intracranial pathology maintain normal ICP, despite transient increases that develop with coughing or during a Valsalva maneuver, because of the normal elastance of the intracranial contents. Small increases in intracranial volume do not produce abrupt increases in ICP. This normal elastance exists because the limits of the intracranial contents have not been reached. However, once the growing mass, be it blood or tumor, has increased intracranial volume to its limit, dramatic increases in ICP may occur.[68] This relationship is depicted in Figure 26-16. Although this ICP-volume curve is commonly used to explain these relationships, Todd and colleagues[69] suggest that the x-axis be relabeled as the volume "of the growing mass," because this axis does not really represent total intracranial volume. The initial portion of the curve in Figure 26-16 is relatively flat because the total intracranial volume does not change with early periods of bleeding or tumor growth. This portion of the curve reflects the phenomenon of spatial compensation. As the mass (blood or tumor) increases, the volume of the intracranial compartments must decrease to maintain normal ICP. In most cases the CSF compartment decreases; that is, CSF is absorbed by the arachnoid granulations or shunted to the spinal subarachnoid space to compensate for the increasing intracranial volume. Compensation is exhausted when the CSF compartment cannot decrease further in size, and total intracranial volume increases, accounting for the increase in ICP. In summary, an increase in total intracranial volume increases ICP.

Measurement of Intracranial Pressure

ICP monitoring is facilitated by ventriculostomy, subdural bolt, epidural transducer, or subdural fiberoptic catheter placed in a supratentorial location (Figure 26-17). Access to the subarachnoid space facilitates the removal of CSF for assistance in the control of increased ICP.[70,71]

Intracranial Hypertension

Intracranial hypertension occurs with a sustained increase in ICP above 15 to 20 mm Hg. Intracranial hypertension develops with expanding tissue or fluid mass, interference with normal CSF absorption, excessive CBF, or systemic disturbances promoting brain edema. Often, multiple factors are responsible for the development of intracranial hypertension. For example, tumors in the posterior fossa usually produce some degree of brain edema and readily obstruct CSF flow by compressing the fourth ventricle.[72]

Although many patients with intracranial hypertension are initially asymptomatic, all eventually develop characteristic signs and symptoms, including headache, nausea, vomiting, papilledema, focal neurologic deficits, altered ventilatory function, decreasing consciousness, seizures, and coma. When ICP exceeds 30 mm Hg, CBF progressively decreases, and a vicious cycle is established: ischemia produces brain edema, which in turn increases ICP, precipitating further ischemia. If this cycle remains unchecked, progressive neurologic damage or catastrophic herniation may result.[15,72,73]

Intracranial Pressure Reduction

Box 26-1 lists the major methods for the treatment of elevated ICP. Selective application of these methods often results in ICP reduction accompanied by clinical improvement. A patent airway, adequate oxygenation, and hyperventilation provide the foundation for neuroresuscitative care in acute intracranial

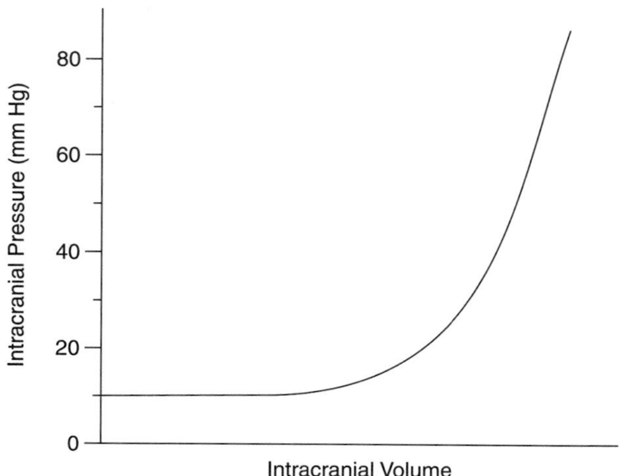

FIGURE **26-16**
Intracranial pressure-volume curve. (From Newfield P, Cottrell JE, eds. *Neuroanesthesia: Handbook of Clinical and Physiologic Essentials.* 2nd ed. Boston: Little, Brown; 1991:14.)

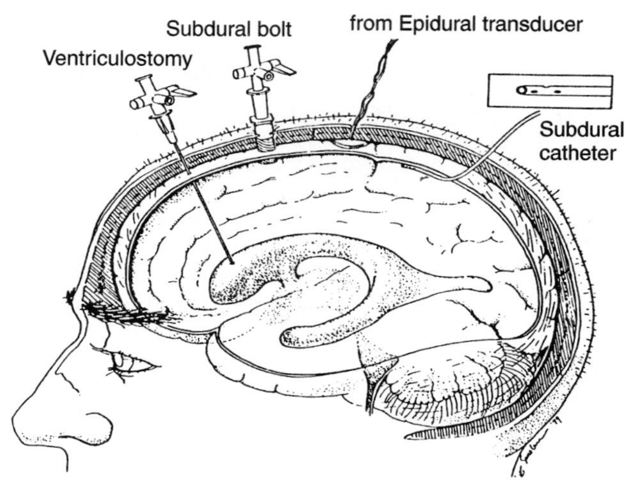

FIGURE **26-17**
Representation of sites for placement of intracranial pressure monitors. (From Shapiro HM. Neurosurgical anesthesia and intracranial hypertension. In: Miller RD, ed. *Anesthesia.* 3rd ed. New York: Churchill Livingstone; 1991:1749.)

BOX 26-1

Methods for the Treatment of Elevated Intracranial Pressure

- Apply hyperventilation on demand ($Paco_2$ 30 to 35 mm Hg)
- Administer diuretics (osmotic mannitol 0.25-1 g/kg^{-1} IV) (may repeat if serum osmolarity <320 mOsm • 1^{-1} and patient is euvolemic) or furosemide
- Perform cerebrospinal fluid drainage (if available)
- Avoid overhydration; target normovolemia
- Elevate patient's head; position to improve cerebral venous return; avoid neck vein compression
- Insert intracranial pressure monitor; Sjo_2, $AVDo_2$, and CBF monitoring recommended
- Optimize hemodynamics: mean arterial pressure, central venous pressure, pulmonary capillary wedge pressure, heart rate, and cerebral perfusion pressure; consider antihypertensive therapy as needed
- Administer corticosteroids (dexamethasone)
- Surgical decompression; consider decompressive craniectomy if hematoma is present
- Cerebral vasoconstriction (thiopental, propofol)
- Consider mild hypothermia

$AVDo_2$, *Arteriovenous difference in oxygen content;* CBF, *cerebral blood flow;* IV, *intravenous;* Sjo_2, *jugular bulboxyhemoglobin saturation.*

hypertensive states. Frequently overlap occurs among causes of increased ICP, and this may necessitate simultaneous application of a number of different therapeutic modalities.[47]

Hyperventilation

Lowering $PaCO_2$ increases cerebrovascular resistance, reducing CBV and ICP. The exact mechanism by which CO_2 exerts its effect on cerebral vessels is not completely understood. The prevailing theory is that changes in CO_2 produce alterations in the pH of the CSF surrounding the arterioles, although this is still controversial. This alteration occurs because CO_2 crosses the blood-brain barrier freely, whereas bicarbonate fails to cross. Therefore decreases in $PaCO_2$ increase pH in the CSF and arteriolar walls. Because bicarbonate ions cross the blood-brain barrier, changes in CSF pH and CBF that result from alterations in $PaCO_2$ last only a few hours. After this time, CBF returns to prehyperventilation values, despite continuing hypocapnia or hypercapnia.[65]

In cooperative patients, voluntary hyperventilation is encouraged just before induction of anesthesia. When this is not possible, airway control is obtained as early as possible after anesthetic induction, and hyperventilation is rapidly initiated. In emergency neuroresuscitative care, hyperventilation is the first step when acute decompensation occurs.[47] In previously normocapnic patients, acute hyperventilation to a $PaCO_2$ range of approximately 30 mm Hg probably provides maximum intracranial decompression with minimal risk of cerebral ischemia.

Pharmacologic Manipulation of Intracranial Pressure

Diuretics

Loop Diuretics. Loop diuretics (furosemide, bumetanide, ethacrynic acid) produce a general diuresis, decrease the rate of CSF production, and decrease cerebral edema. Osmotic diuretics are effective in decreasing the water content of the brain. Mannitol is the most widely used osmotic diuretic for acute control of intracranial hypertension. Rapid administration may produce vasodilation, an increase in CBF, a transient rise in ICP, and a transient increase in circulating blood volume. Increases in circulating blood volume may prove to be detrimental to patients with underlying cardiac dysfunction. Prior administration of intravenous furosemide may minimize these potential complications. Decreases in ICP begin shortly after mannitol administration and may continue for up to 6 hours. The typically prescribed dose of mannitol is 0.25 to 1 g/kg. Continued use of mannitol may produce hyperosmolality and electrolyte imbalance, which may be attenuated with concurrent administration of a loop diuretic.[74-77]

Corticosteroids

Glucocorticoids penetrate the blood-brain barrier and decrease edema associated with mass lesions. In the absence of mass lesions, glucocorticoid administration may produce pseudotumor cerebri (increased ICP when no mass lesion exists) and papilledema. Additional complications ascribed to the continuous use of steroids in neurosurgical patients include hyperglycemia, glucosuria, gastrointestinal bleeding, electrolyte abnormalities, and an increase in the incidence of infection. Evidence remains contradictory regarding the efficacy of high-dose steroids for head injury.[78,79] Steroids, even when clinically efficacious, require many hours for their ICP decompression effects to become apparent.[47]

Barbiturates

A bolus injection of 1.5 to 5 mg of thiopental per kilogram has been shown to be effective in reducing ICP. Although the CPP in most patients increases because the magnitude of the decrease in ICP exceeds the magnitude of the decrease in MAP, close monitoring of both pressures is indicated. In situations in which either hypotension or hypovolemia is present, lidocaine, 1.5 mg/kg, may be useful in reducing ICP while maintaining MAP. Failure of intracranial hypertension to respond to barbiturates usually indicates a poor prognosis.[77]

Surgical Decompression

Surgical decompression may be used for uncontrollable increases in ICP. Internal decompression involves the excision of brain tissue, reduction in ICP, and reduction of the potential for brain-stem displacement or herniation. External decompression involves excision of the skull overlying the site of either an epidural or a subdural hematoma. Decompressive surgery is generally considered to be a last resort in patients with persistent, intractable increases in ICP.[41]

Cerebrospinal Fluid Drainage

Intracranial hypertension may be reduced by a surgical CSF diversion. The long-term effectiveness of this therapeutic alternative depends on the cause of the increased ICP. When brain edema produces elevation of ICP, CSF drainage may provide only transient abatement of intracranial hypertension. If external drainage is continued in this circumstance, ventricular collapse can occur and can prevent further venting of CSF. Successful chronic control of high ICP caused by hydrocephalus can be achieved with implanted CSF shunts.[47]

ANESTHETIC CONSIDERATIONS FOR SPECIFIC PROCEDURES

Supratentorial Surgery

The majority of intracranial neurosurgical procedures are performed for supratentorial mass lesions. Intracranial masses may be congenital, neoplastic (benign, malignant, or metastatic), infectious (abscess or cyst), or vascular (hematoma or malformation). Although the underlying pathology may be different for different lesions, the anesthetic considerations are the same. Procedures performed by means of minimally invasive techniques are listed in Box 26-2.

Preoperative Evaluation

The clinical signs of a supratentorial mass include seizures, hemiplegia, and aphasia. The clinical signs of infratentorial masses include cerebellar dysfunction (ataxia, nystagmus, dysarthria) and brain stem compression (cranial nerve palsies, altered consciousness, abnormal respiration). When ICP increases, frank signs of intracranial hypertension can also develop.[72]

Preanesthetic evaluation should attempt to establish the presence or absence of intracranial hypertension. Computed tomography or magnetic resonance imaging data should be reviewed for evidence of brain edema, midline shift greater than 0.5 cm, and ventricular size. A neurologic assessment should evaluate the current mental status and any existing neurologic deficits. Medications prescribed for the control of ICP (corticosteroids, diuretics) and anticonvulsant therapy should be reviewed to determine whether they have been properly administered. Laboratory evaluation should rule out corticosteroid-induced hyperglycemia and electrolyte disturbances that may develop secondary to diuretic therapy.

The decision regarding what and when premedication is administered should be made only after a thorough patient evaluation. Benzodiazepines produce respiratory depression and hypercapnia. Premedication should be omitted in patients with a large mass lesion, a midline shift, and abnormal ventricular size. Opioids are universally avoided. If premedication is desired in those patients deemed appropriate, careful titration of intravenous midazolam may begin once the patient has been delivered to the preoperative holding area. In an attempt to help control ICP in patients with mass lesions, the head of the bed should be elevated 15 to 30 degrees during transport to the preoperative holding area and the operating room.

BOX 26-2

Minimally Invasive Neurosurgery

Radiosurgery	Arteriovenous malformation (AVM) ablation, Parkinson's disease
Stereotactic	MRI and CT guidance
	Frameless stereotaxy
Endoscopic techniques	Hydrocephalus, choroid plexus cauterization, third ventriculostomy tumor biopsy, myeloscopy, fenestration of colloid, arachnoid cysts and the septum pellucidum
	Transphenoidal approach to suprasellar masses
	Acoustic neuroma
	Thoracoscopic diskectomy
	Lumbar laminectomy
	Hematoma or abscess removal

CT, *Computed tomography*; MRI, *magnetic resonance imaging*.
From Johnson J. Anesthesia for minimally invasive surgery. Anesthesiol Clin North Am. *2002;20:2-3.*

Intraoperative Monitoring

Routine monitors for supratentorial procedures include continuous electrocardiography (ECG), cuff measurement of blood pressure, precordial stethoscope, monitoring of the fraction of inspired oxygen, pulse oximetry, temperature, peripheral nerve stimulation, end-tidal CO_2 monitoring, and indwelling urinary catheterization. For patients with ischemic heart disease, use of a modified V_5 ECG lead is recommended. An arterial line placed either before or immediately after anesthetic induction provides for uninterrupted blood pressure monitoring and easy access for blood sampling for laboratory analysis (Box 26-3). Somatosensory evoked potentials (SSEPs) may be assessed. The effect of various anesthetics on SSEPs is given in Box 26-4. Methods for cerebral oxygenation monitoring are listed in Box 26-5.

Fluid Management

Preoperative fluid deficits and intraoperative blood and fluid losses must be adequately replaced during neurosurgical procedures. Judicious fluid administration minimizes the occurrence

BOX 26-3

Intraoperative Monitoring

- Electrocardiography
- Direct intraarterial blood pressure monitoring
- End-tidal CO_2, pulse oximetry, arterial blood gas analysis
- Peripheral nerve stimulation
- Central venous pressure measurement
- Body temperature measurement
- Urinary output
- Electroencephalography or somatosensory evoked potentials
- Cerebral oxygen monitoring

BOX 26-4

Effects of Anesthetics on Somatosensory Evoked Potentials

Drug	Latency	Amplitude
Isoflurane	↑	↓
Sevoflurane	↑	↓
Halothane	↑	↓
Nitrous oxide	↑	↓
Desflurane	↑	↓
Thiopental	↑	↓
Fentanyl	Slight ↑	Slight ↓
Propofol	↑	No change
Ketamine	↑	↑
Etomidate	↑	↑

BOX **26-5**

Cerebral Oxygenation Monitoring

Monitor	Abbreviations	Comments
Jugular venous bulb oxygen saturation	$SjvO_2$	A lack of a "gold standard" for comparison; invasive; monitors global not regional ischemia and hypoxia
Transcranial cerebral oximetry	rSO_2	Lack of definition of brain tissue being monitored; trend monitor; patients act as their own control, technology rapidly changing
Cerebral oxygen tension monitors	$Pbto_2$	Highly invasive; reserved for severe head injuries; cerebral perfusion pressure must be at least 60 mm Hg

Modified from Smyth PR, Samra S. Monitors of cerebral oxygenation. Anesthesiol Clin. *2002;20:3-7.*

of cerebral edema and ICP, reduced CPP, and worsened cerebral ischemia. In most neurosurgical patients, fluids that contain sodium in a concentration similar to that of serum (e.g., lactated Ringer's solution or 0.9% saline) are administered in a volume that is sufficient for the maintenance of peripheral perfusion but that avoids hypervolemia (0.5 to 1 ml/kg/hr). Traditionally, less fluid is given than would be administered for nonneurologic surgery, although new recommendations indicate that patients should be kept isovolemic, isotonic, and isooncotic[80-83] (Box 26-6).

The brain is entirely dependent on a continuous supply of glucose to maintain energy requirements. Glucose is administered in an attempt to prevent hypoglycemia, provide energy substrates, replace water that is lost during the nothing-by-mouth period, conserve protein, and prevent ketosis by preventing gluconeogenesis. However, glucose is a "double-edged sword," because too much may produce hyperglycemia, delayed gastric emptying, osmotic diuresis, increased CO_2 production, and hyperglycemia-associated intracellular lactic acidosis. Emerging evidence questions the rationale of routine administration of glucose, particularly in situations in which cerebral ischemia may occur, because if the hypoxic brain is exposed to glucose, a poor neurologic outcome may result.

The association between preischemic glucose administration and poor neurologic outcome has been validated in a number of animal models. The specific mechanism of neurologic injury resulting from increased plasma glucose concentrations has not been elucidated. The current hypothesis of neurologic injury is as follows. Cerebral hypoxia or ischemia results in the failure of cerebral oxidative metabolism. Glycolysis ensues, with the development of lactate. In combination with intracellular acidosis, intracellular lactate concentrations increase and intracellular pH decreases. This produces a disruption in cell function and may lead to cell death. It is important to note that the greatest neurologic damage in animal models has been shown to occur when hyperglycemia occurs immediately before the ischemic event.

The relationship between plasma glucose concentrations and poor neurologic outcome has not been completely elucidated in humans, although retrospective data indicate that increased plasma glucose concentrations may be detrimental.[84] The role of glucose in the case of focal cerebral ischemia (ischemia that follows the disruption of CBF in a major intracranial vessel) is not known. Animal research has presented mixed information regarding an adverse neurologic effect after glucose administration. Notwithstanding the obvious adverse effects of glucose administration, indications for glucose administration are clear in particular clinical circumstances in which hypoglycemia may develop. Such situations include diabetic patients who receive insulin preoperatively, individuals who are receiving glucose-containing parenteral infusions, and infants and young children, who have a greater tendency to become hypoglycemic with fasting.

BOX **26-6**

Fluid Management Considerations for Neurosurgical Patients

- Avoid dextrose-containing solutions.
- Limit volume of lactated Ringer's solution, and use colloid and normal saline for volume resuscitation.
- Limit hetastarch to 1 to 1.5 L to avoid coagulopathy.
- Maintain hematocrit at 30% to 35%.
- Mild volume expansion for aneurysm clipping may help reduce vasospasm.
- Keep patients isovolemic, isotonic, and isooncotic.

From Mears SL, Sperry RJ. Fluid management. In: Sperry RJ, Stirt JA, Stone DJ, eds. Manual of Neuroanesthesia. *Philadelphia: Decker; 1989:106.*

Fluid therapy is most challenging during prolonged surgical procedures or in the surgical management of multiple trauma. If tissue trauma is severe or if hemorrhage has been prolonged, patients develop a marked reduction in functional extracellular volume as a result of the internal redistribution of fluids (third-space losses). Although the extent of tissue manipulation in most routine neurosurgical procedures is small, third-space fluid losses during prolonged surgery and in patients with severe associated systemic trauma can be sufficient to decrease intravascular volume, reduce peripheral perfusion, and impair renal function. The sequestered extracellular fluid can be cautiously replaced with lactated Ringer's solution or with 0.9% saline. In the absence of diuretic therapy a urinary output of 0.5 to 1 ml/kg/hr suggests adequate replacement, as do hemodynamic stability and cardiac filling pressures within the normal range. Although some clinicians prefer to use colloid-containing solutions in neurosurgical patients, such solutions appear to exert negligible effects on brain water and ICP.[80,82]

Anesthetic Induction and Maintenance

Although induction of anesthesia for patients undergoing craniotomy can be performed with various agents, a smooth and gentle induction of general anesthesia is more important than the drug combination used. No evidence indicates that one technique or set of drugs is better than another. A reasonable induction sequence would combine preoxygenation, thiopental (2 to 4 mg/kg) or propofol (1 to 2 mg/kg), and a nondepolarizing muscle relaxant. No evidence suggests that any of the induction agents (midazolam, etomidate, propofol, methohexital) is superior to thiopental. The hemodynamic response to intubation may be blunted with the administration of fentanyl (10 to 15 mcg/kg total dose) or lidocaine (1.5 mg/kg) administered 3 minutes before laryngoscopy. The dose of these induction agents may need to be adjusted according to the patient's age and physical status. Whatever agents are selected, the induction should be accomplished without the development of sudden hypertension or hypotension.

Frontal, temporal, and parietooccipital craniotomies are performed with the patient in the supine position. The head typically is elevated from 15 to 30 degrees to facilitate venous and CSF drainage. The head may also be turned to the side to facilitate exposure. Excessive neck flexion may impede jugular venous drainage and increase ICP. The endotracheal tube should be stabilized with the anesthetist's hand during positioning. After positioning is complete, the chest should be auscultated to ascertain proper endotracheal tube position. The endotracheal tube follows the position of the chin: with extension of the neck the chin and endotracheal tube move cephalad; the chin and endotracheal tube move caudad with neck flexion. The anesthesia circuit connections must be firmly secured by simultaneously pushing and twisting to seat the plastic connectors. The risk of unrecognized disconnections may be increased because the operating table is usually turned 90 to 180 degrees away from the anesthetist, and both the patient and the breathing circuit are almost completely covered by surgical drapes.[72]

Maintenance of anesthesia may be accomplished with an oxygen-N_2O-opioid technique, with a selected potent inhalation agent, or with oxygen-N_2O and a continuous infusion of propofol. After endotracheal intubation, mechanical hyperventilation is begun, decreasing end-tidal CO_2 to 25 to 30 mm Hg, confirmed through arterial blood gas analysis. The patient should be covered with blankets or a forced air warming blanket to maintain core body temperature.

An opioid-based anesthetic technique with N_2O in oxygen with low-dose (less than 1%) isoflurane is a popular choice. Incremental administration of fentanyl, sufentanil, or alfentanil or an infusion of remifentanil is acceptable. Alternatively, sufentanil, 0.5 to 1 mcg/kg load, followed by either incremental boluses (not to exceed 0.5 mcg/kg/hr) or an intravenous infusion of 0.25 to 0.5 mcg/kg/hr in combination with less than 1% isoflurane in oxygen may be used. Sufentanil administration should be discontinued approximately 45 minutes before the end of surgery to ensure that the patient awakens promptly. The primary advantage of remifentanil is rapid awakening. If the patient experiences hypertension or tachycardia near the end of surgery, the practitioner should consider giving either labetalol or esmolol, not additional opioids.[85]

A volatile agent (preferably isoflurane or sevoflurane) with little or no opioid supplementation can also be used for maintenance of anesthesia. If isoflurane is used, the concentration should remain less than 1%. Hyperventilation in combination with less than 1% isoflurane generally results in stable intracranial dynamics.[85]

N_2O may be used in an anesthetic regimen if it is deemed desirable. However, if the patient is suspected to have a pneumocephalus or if the potential for air embolism exists, N_2O use is contraindicated. N_2O expands both the pneumocephalus and the air embolus. A tension pneumocephalus acts like an expanding mass lesion. A large air embolus can cause cardiovascular collapse.[85]

Hyperventilation is an important adjunct to any neuroanesthetic technique. Hypocapnia decreases ICP before opening of the dura and attenuates the vasodilation produced by the volatile anesthetic agents. Optimal hyperventilation during surgery would yield a $PaCO_2$ of 25 to 30 mm Hg.

Skeletal muscle relaxation prevents patient movement at inappropriate times. It may decrease ICP by relaxing the chest wall, decreasing intrathoracic pressure, and facilitating venous drainage. In choosing an agent for muscle relaxation, the length of the procedure and the impact of the drug on ICP should be considered.[85]

Emergence

Most patients who undergo craniotomy can be extubated at the end of the procedure as long as intracranial hypertension is no longer present. Patients left intubated should remain sedated, paralyzed, and hyperventilated. Like induction, emergence must be slow and controlled. Straining or bucking on the endotracheal tube may precipitate intracranial hemorrhage or worsen cerebral edema. A brief period of coughing or gagging is probably not detrimental provided the blood pressure is optimally controlled. Uncontrolled hypertension during emergence is associated with increased incidence of postoperative intracranial hemorrhage.[86] Judicious titration of short-acting antihypertensives (esmolol, labetalol) has great clinical utility in controlling the blood pressure during emergence. After the head dressing is applied and full access to the patient is regained, the use of anesthetic gases is discontinued and the muscle relaxant is reversed. Intravenous lidocaine (1.5 mg/kg) can be given just before suctioning for cough suppression before extubation. Rapid awakening facilitates immediate neurologic assessment and can generally be expected after a pure opioid-N_2O technique. Delayed awakening may result from residual opioid or remaining end-tidal concentrations of potent inhalation agent. Residual opioid may be carefully antagonized when necessary with naloxone in 40-mcg increments to attain a respiratory rate of 12 to 16 breaths per minute. After extubation the patient is transported to the intensive care unit postoperatively for continued monitoring of neurologic function.[72]

Posterior Fossa Surgery

Neuropathology within the posterior fossa may impair control of the airway, respiratory function, cardiovascular function, autonomic function, and consciousness. The major motor and sensory pathways, the primary cardiovascular and respiratory centers, the reticular activating system, and the nuclei of the lower cranial nerves are all concentrated in the brain stem. All these vital structures are contained in a tight space with little room for edema, tumor, or blood.

Venous Air Embolus

In addition to the previously mentioned monitoring modalities, monitoring during posterior fossa surgery requires consideration of patient position (generally the seated position) and the potential for venous air embolus (VAE). Although a number of physiologic consequences are related to the seated position, additional clinical considerations involve the choice of anesthetic technique and monitoring devices for the detection of VAE. The potential for VAE has been traditionally associated with neurosurgical anesthesia. Clinical situations that contribute to the occurrence of VAE are listed in Box 26-7. Air may also be entrained from the cranial pin sites of the Mayfield

BOX 26-7

Clinical Situations Contributing to the Occurrence of Venous Air Embolism

- Patient positioning (seated, prone, steep Trendelenburg)
- Transfusion therapy
- Intravenous therapy
- Central venous catheterization
- Hepatic surgical procedures
- Urologic surgical procedures
- Posterior spinal procedures
- Epidural or caudal catheter insertion
- Bone marrow harvesting
- Laparoscopy
- Radical pelvic surgery

head holder and from improperly connected vascular lines (arterial, central, and intravenous).

The occurrence of VAE depends on the development of a negative pressure gradient between the operative site and the right side of the heart. As the gradient between the cerebral veins and the right atrium increases, the potential for air entry increases. The estimated incidence of VAE during neurosurgical procedures ranges from 5% to 50%, with an increased incidence in the seated position.[86,87]

The physiologic consequences of VAE depend on both the volume and the rate of air entrainment. In the canine model large cumulative doses of air produce sudden cardiac arrest and death; smaller cumulative doses produce less profound physiologic consequences, including increased pulmonary artery and central venous pressure, decreased cardiac output with accompanying hypotension, progressive hypotension, and dysrhythmias.[88] Despite the potentially devastating effects of VAE, a retrospective review of neurosurgery patients who had appropriate monitoring for the detection of VAE found that VAE contributed to patient morbidity or mortality in only six instances (0.4%).[89-91]

Paradoxic Air Embolism

Paradoxic air embolism develops with the entry of air into the systemic circulation. Individuals with an existing anatomic connection between the right and left sides of the heart (atrial or ventricular septal defect, probe patent foramen ovale) are particularly at risk. A patent foramen ovale may exist in 30% to 35% of the population.[92] If right-sided heart pressures exceed left-sided pressures (a situation that may occur in fluid-restricted neurosurgical patients), systemic air may embolize and enter the arterial circulation through a probe patent foramen ovale.

Patients who require a seated position for a neurosurgical procedure should be carefully evaluated with echocardiograms if the history suggests the presence of an intracardiac defect (presence of heart murmur) or probe patent foramen ovale. The presence of a probe patent foramen ovale may be elicited with the injection of contrast material before, during, and after the patient produces a Valsalva maneuver. If a probe patent foramen ovale is identified, the surgical procedure should be accomplished in an alternative position.

Detection of Venous Air Embolus

The entrainment of air into the vascular system is usually of little consequence because the lungs serve as effective blood filters.[93] Small bubbles of air are absorbed into the blood or enter the alveoli, where they are eliminated during exhalation. However, the efficient filtering capacity of the lung may be breached by a large bolus of air or after the administration of a pulmonary vasodilator (e.g., aminophylline), which acts to widen the venous-arterial barrier. Air enters the venous circulation as small bubbles that pass through the right side of the heart, entering the pulmonary arterioles. A reflexive sympathetic pulmonary vasoconstriction is produced after the release of endothelial mediators, which are ultimately responsible for the clinical manifestations (pulmonary hypertension, hypoxemia, CO_2 retention, increased dead-space ventilation, and decreased end-tidal CO_2). The continued entry of air produces an airlock within the right ventricle, producing right ventricular failure and decreased cardiac output. Altered ventilation-perfusion relationships parallel the hemodynamic changes. Obstructed pulmonary blood flow increases dead-space ventilation, resulting in decreased end-tidal CO_2. The entry of a large volume of air in the alveoli may be detected by the sudden appearance of end-tidal nitrogen.

The selection of appropriate monitoring for the detection of VAE is based on the various sensitivities of the available monitoring modalities. Figure 26-18 lists the sensitivity of VAE detection devices. Precordial Doppler monitoring can detect air entrainment at rates as small as 0.0021 ml/kg/min.[94] The Doppler probe is affixed over the right side of the heart along the right sternal border between the third and sixth intercostal spaces. Proper positioning over the right atrium is confirmed if a change in Doppler signal is elicited when a 10-ml bolus of saline is injected rapidly into a previously placed right central venous catheter.[94-96] The placement of a right atrial or pulmonary artery catheter affords the means for diagnosis and recovery of intravenous air and also reflects cardiac preload. When a right atrial catheter is placed, it is recommended that either radiographic confirmation or ECG confirmation of proper placement of the catheter tip be obtained.[94] Advantages and disadvantages of select monitors for detection of venous air embolism (VAE) are noted in Table 26-6.

Capnography complements the capabilities of the Doppler device, because small, hemodynamically insignificant air emboli detected with the Doppler device can be differentiated from emboli that may produce arterial hypotension. Capnography is virtually as sensitive as pulmonary artery pressure monitoring but has the added advantage of being noninvasive.[97]

Transesophageal echocardiography is the most sensitive method of air embolism detection, but it is also the most expensive. With transesophageal echocardiography, it is possible to observe both cardiac contractility and air bubbles as they pass through the heart.[98] The detection of a "mill-wheel" murmur via precordial or esophageal stethoscope is a late sign of air entrainment.

Treatment of Venous Air Embolus

Detection of VAE should prompt the following steps. The surgeon should be notified and N_2O should be immediately discontinued, 100% oxygen delivered, and the right atrial catheter aspirated.[99] The surgeon should flood the surgical field with irrigation or pack the area with saline-soaked sponges. A Valsalva maneuver or bilateral compression of the jugular veins for 5 to 10 seconds increases the cerebral venous

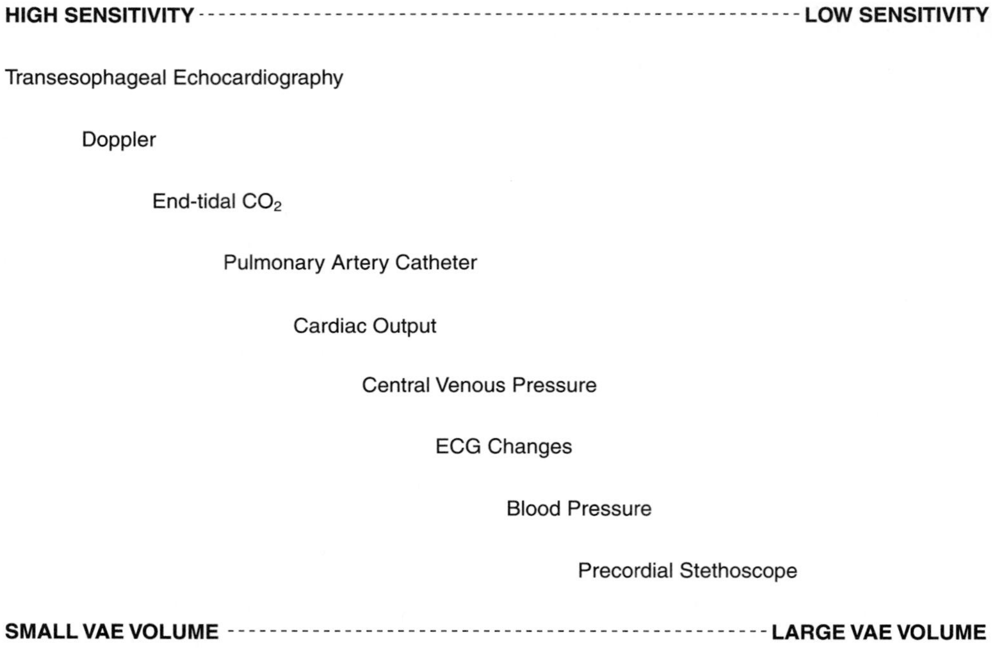

HIGH SENSITIVITY ---------- LOW SENSITIVITY

Transesophageal Echocardiography

Doppler

End-tidal CO_2

Pulmonary Artery Catheter

Cardiac Output

Central Venous Pressure

ECG Changes

Blood Pressure

Precordial Stethoscope

SMALL VAE VOLUME ---------- LARGE VAE VOLUME

FIGURE **26-18**
Sensitivity of venous air embolus *(VAE)* detection devices. (From Aker JG. Clinical dilemmas in neuroanesthesia. *CRNA Clin Forum Nurse Anesthetist.* 1995;6:13.)

TABLE **26-6** **Monitors for Detection of Venous Air Embolism**

Monitor	Advantages	Disadvantages
Precordial Doppler	Noninvasive Most sensitive noninvasive monitor Earliest detector (before air enters pulmonary circulation)	Nonquantitative May be difficult to place in obese patients, patients with chest wall deformity, or patients in the prone or lateral position False negative result if air does not pass beneath ultrasonic beam (approximately 10% of cases) Useless during electrocautery IV mannitol may mimic intravascular air
Pulmonary artery (PA) catheter	Quantitative slightly more sensitive than $ETCO_2$ Widely available Placed with minimum difficulty in experienced hands Can detect right-atrial pressure more easily than pulmonary capillary wedge pressure	Small lumen, less air aspiration than with right-atrial catheter Placement for optimal air aspiration may not allow pulmonary capillary wedge pressure measurement Nonspecific for air
Capnography ($ETCO_2$)	Noninvasive Sensitive Quantitative Widely available	Nonspecific for air Less sensitive than Doppler, PA catheter Accuracy affected by tachypnea, low cardiac output, chronic obstructive pulmonary disease
End-tidal nitrogen (ETN_2)	Specific for air Detects air earlier than ($ETCO_2$)	May not detect subclinical air embolism May indicate air clearance from pulmonary circulation prematurely Accuracy affected by hypotension
Transesophageal echocardiography (TEE)	Most sensitive detector of air Can detect air in left side of heart and aorta	Invasive, cumbersome Expensive Monitor must be observed continuously Not quantitative May interfere with Doppler

$ETCO_2$, *End-tidal carbon dioxide;* IV, *intravenous.*
Modified from Smith DS, Osborne I. Posterior fossa: anesthetic considerations. In: Cottrell JE, Smith DS. Anesthesia and Neurosurgery. *4th ed. St Louis: Mosby; 2001:343.*

pressure and induces bleeding. The addition of positive end-expiratory pressure also slows air entry. However, 10 to 15 cm H_2O may be required to effectively elevate venous pressure when the head is elevated. The head should be lowered to decrease air entrainment. This may be accomplished by placing the operating table in the Trendelenburg position. If air entrainment continues, the anesthetist should ask for an assistant. A second pair of hands allows simultaneous jugular vein compression and central catheter aspiration.[100,101]

Supportive therapy is required for hemodynamic compromise. Administration of ephedrine, 10 to 20 mg intravenously, and an intravenous fluid bolus improves the blood pressure. If these measures do not restore blood pressure, additional vasopressors (epinephrine) may be required (Box 26-8).

Anesthetic agent and technique may influence the rate of air entrainment and the resulting physiologic consequences. The anesthetist should recall the role N_2O may play in the patient at risk for VAE, because N_2O is known to increase the volume of embolized air. Munson and Merrick[99] demonstrated that the expansion of an intravascular air bubble is proportional to the delivered concentration of N_2O. A 50% concentration doubles the initial air bubble volume, and a 70% concentration quadruples the air bubble volume.

General endotracheal anesthesia with controlled ventilation is thought to be protective in patients experiencing VAE. Durant and colleagues demonstrated the appearance of a respiratory "gasp" with the onset of VAE in dogs who were spontaneously ventilating. This reflexive gasp may worsen VAE, because additional air is entrained into the venous system with the gasping respiration.[102]

Surgical Positioning

Although most posterior fossa explorations may be performed with the patient in either the lateral or the prone position, the sitting position is occasionally preferred because the enhanced CSF and venous drainage facilitates surgical exposure. The use of this position, however, has declined dramatically because of the potential for serious complications.[103] The patient is semirecumbent in the standard seated position (Figure 26-19), with the back elevated to 60 degrees and the legs elevated (with the knees flexed) to the level of the heart. The latter is important for prevention of venous pooling and for reduction of the risk of venous thromboembolism. The head is fixed in a three-point head holder with the neck in flexion, and the arms remain at the sides with the hands resting on the lap.[72]

BOX 26-8

Therapy for Venous Air Embolism

- Notify surgeon on detection (flood surgical field with saline, and wax bone edges).
- Discontinue nitrous oxide administration. Administer 100% oxygen.
- Perform a Valsalva maneuver or compression of jugular veins.
- Aspirate air from atrial catheter.
- Support blood pressure with volume and vasopressors.
- Reposition patient in left lateral decubitus position with a 15 degree head-down tilt if blood pressure continues to decrease.
- Modify the anesthetic as needed to optimize hemodynamics.

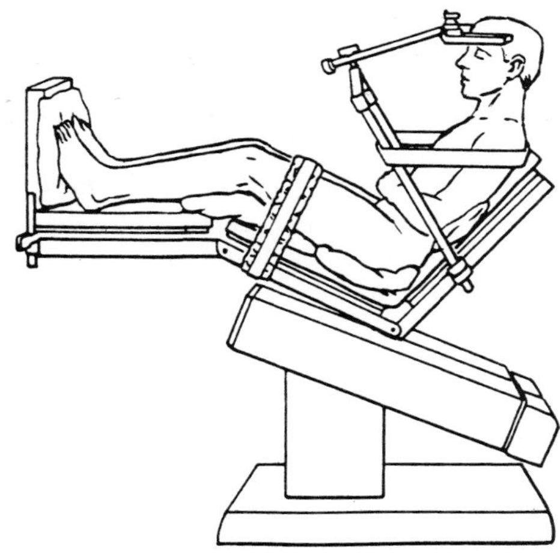

FIGURE **26-19**
Representation of a patient properly positioned for seated posterior fossa operation with the knees at heart level and the neck not hyperflexed. (From Morgan GE, Mikhail MS, eds. *Clinical Anesthesiology*. Norwalk, Conn: Appleton & Lange; 1992:434.)

Careful positioning is essential to prevent iatrogenic injury. Pressure points such as the elbows, ischial spines, and forehead must be protected with foam padding. Excessive neck flexion has been associated with swelling of the upper airway (venous obstruction) and, rarely, quadriplegia resulting from compression of the cervical spinal cord and decreased cervical cord perfusion with elevation of the neck above the heart. Preexisting cervical spinal stenosis probably predisposes to the latter injury.[72]

Anesthetic Induction, Maintenance, and Emergence

Increased ICP, although common in patients with supratentorial lesions, is less common in patients with posterior fossa lesions. However, obstructive hydrocephalus is more typical because CSF outflow is occluded at the level of the aqueduct of Sylvius or fourth ventricle. This can be readily identified preoperatively by magnetic resonance imaging or computed tomography. This may be corrected before definitive surgical intervention with the placement of a ventricular catheter. Premedication is contraindicated in patients with obstructive hydrocephalus.

Anesthetic management for posterior fossa procedures is essentially the same as that for supratentorial surgery. Induction should be slow and deliberate to avoid changes in cerebral perfusion and the aggravation of increased ICP. Because the head is generally flexed and fixed in this position, a wire-reinforced endotracheal tube may prevent intraoperative kinking. However, these tubes may become permanently kinked if the patient is lightly anesthetized and bites the tube. Intravenous fluid administration during posterior fossa surgery should be limited to the infusion of deficit and maintenance quantities of a balanced salt solution. Major volume resuscitation can be accomplished with the infusion of blood, colloid, or crystalloid solutions.

Emergence from anesthesia should be as smooth and gentle as possible. The intraoperative use of opioids facilitates a smooth emergence without significant coughing or bucking. The administration of lidocaine 1.5 mg/kg intravenously decreases the airway irritation of the endotracheal tube.[100]

The decision to remove the endotracheal tube should be made after the anesthetic course and the surgical procedure are reviewed. Intraoperative air embolism may be followed by the development of pulmonary edema. Although this condition is often self-limiting, continued mechanical ventilation is the treatment of choice. Consideration must also be given to the possibility of cranial nerve damage during the operative procedure. Provided the patient is safely extubated, continued vigilant observation is essential because airway compromise may develop after injury to cranial nerves IX, X, and XI. If during the surgical dissection the patient experienced episodes of sudden bradycardia, tachycardia, or hypertension, endotracheal extubation should be delayed, and the patient should be delivered to the intensive care unit and mechanical ventilation continued (Box 26-9).

Pituitary Surgery

Approximately 10% of intracranial neoplasms are found in the pituitary gland and come to clinical attention because of their mass effects or the hypersecretion of pituitary hormones. These tumors are rarely metastatic and produce local symptoms via bone invasion, hydrocephalus, and compression of a cranial nerve (most often the optic nerve). Frontal-temporal headache and bitemporal hemianopsia are the most common nonendocrine symptoms of enlarging pituitary lesions. Nonsecretory pituitary tumors account for approximately 20% to 50% of lesions in this area and are classified as chromophobe adenomas.[103]

Tumors that secrete excess growth hormone produce acromegaly. Increased growth hormone increases the size of the skeleton, particularly the bones and soft tissues of the hands, feet, and face. The enlarged facial structures may increase the likelihood of difficult intubation. Excess growth hormone may also contribute to the development of coronary artery disease, hypertension, and cardiomyopathy. Hyperglycemia is also a common finding, reflecting a growth hormone–induced glucose intolerance.[104]

Surgical Approach

Medical and surgical therapies exist for both functional and nonfunctional pituitary tumors. Cushing introduced the oronasal midline rhinoseptal transsphenoidal approach to the pituitary in 1910. In 1962 Hardy helped reintroduce the procedure with the introduction of the surgical microscope and microsurgical dissection techniques. These advances simplified tumor removal by making it easier to distinguish tumor from normal gland.[105]

BOX **26-9**

Postoperative Considerations with Posterior Fossa Surgery

- Central apnea
- Impaired swallowing
- Hypertension
- Cardiac dysrhythmias
- Delayed awakening (brain stem compression)

From Barash PG, Cullen BF, Stoelting RK, eds. Handbook of Clinical Anesthesia. *3rd ed. Philadelphia: Lippincott; 1997:392.*

Transsphenoidal surgery offers several advantages over the intracranial approach. Statistically, morbidity and mortality rates are reduced because of a decrease in blood loss and less manipulation of brain tissue. In addition, the risk of inducing panhypopituitarism is reduced, and the incidence of permanent diabetes insipidus is lower. For patients with large tumors (greater than 10 mm), tumors of uncertain type, and tumors that have substantial extrasellar extension, the transsphenoidal approach is inadequate and a bifrontal intracranial approach is required for successful removal[105] (Figure 26-20).

Preoperative Evaluation

Patients undergo transsphenoidal operations for the treatment of hypersecreting pituitary tumors. Clinical symptoms of pituitary tumors include amenorrhea, galactorrhea, Cushing's disease, and acromegaly.

Each preoperative condition has its own constellation of systemic disorders and accompanying effects on intracranial dynamics that must be considered when an anesthetic technique is selected. Pituitary tumors can damage decussating nasal optic fibers, producing blindness in the temporal half of the visual field of both eyes (bitemporal heteronymous hemianopia). Occasionally, an aneurysm of one of the internal carotid arteries may produce nasal hemianopia on the affected side. Patients who have Cushing's disease may also be affected by hypertension, diabetes, osteoporosis, obesity, and friability of skin and connective tissue. Patients who have acromegaly may have hypertension, cardiomyopathy, diabetes, and osteoporosis, as well as prognathism, cartilaginous and soft tissue hypertrophy of the larynx, and enlargement of the tongue, which may complicate intubation of the trachea. Patients who have panhypopituitarism may exhibit hypothyroidism, requiring preoperative thyroid supplementation.

The transsphenoidal approach usually necessitates that the head and back be elevated 10 to 20 degrees. The patient's head is supported by a three-point pin head holder and centered within a C-arm fluoroscopy unit for radiographic control during surgery. The patient's arms are placed at the sides and padded so that injury to the ulnar nerves is avoided. The patient's airway is shared with the surgeon; therefore, great attention must be directed to the proper securing of the endotracheal tube and anesthesia circuit to prevent unintended extubation and

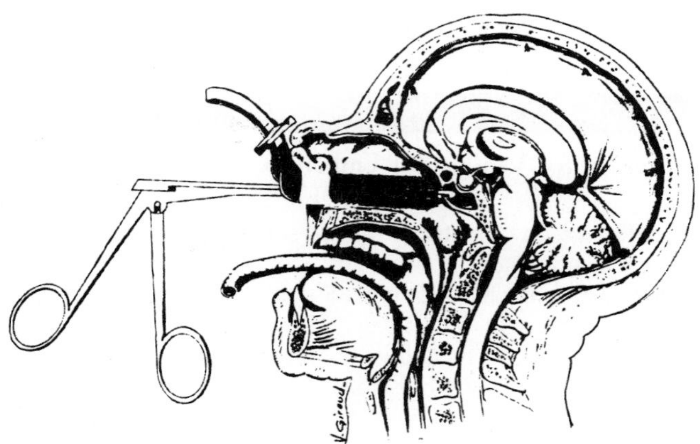

FIGURE **26-20**
Transsphenoidal approach to the pituitary gland. (From Wilkins RH, Rengachary SS, eds. *Neurosurgery*. New York: McGraw-Hill; 1985:892. Used with permission of the publisher.)

anesthesia circuit disconnect. Hyperventilation is avoided after anesthetic induction because reductions in ICP result in retraction of the pituitary into the sella, making surgical access difficult. The anesthetist should also consider the potential for massive hemorrhage because the carotid arteries lie adjacent to the suprasellar area and may be inadvertently injured. Massive bleeding from the carotid artery would probably be fatal.

Postoperative endocrine dysfunction may occur, namely diabetes insipidus when the resection involves the suprasellar area. Diabetes insipidus that occurs after most transsphenoidal procedures is usually self-limited and resolves within 1 week to 10 days.[105] Although the onset is usually on the first or second postoperative day, diabetes insipidus may develop during the perioperative period or in the immediate recovery period. Intraoperative diagnosis is made with the sudden onset of diuresis. The diagnosis may be confirmed with concurrent urine and serum osmolalities. If diabetes insipidus persists or if it becomes difficult to match urinary losses, the patient may receive aqueous vasopressin (Pitressin) or desmopressin (DDAVP). Intravenous DDAVP is longer acting and is not associated with the coronary vasoconstriction that follows administration of aqueous vasopressin.

Anesthetic Induction, Maintenance, and Emergence

After anesthetic induction and intubation the endotracheal tube is typically moved to the left corner of the patient's mouth and secured to the chin with adhesive and tape. A right-angled endotracheal tube may be effective, because such tubes are prebent and curve along the mandible when exiting the mouth. The esophageal stethoscope and temperature probe are inserted and secured on the lower left as well, leaving the upper lip totally free. An orogastric tube is placed, aspirated, and then put to gravity drainage during the procedure. The oropharynx is then packed with moist cotton gauze. The eyes are first taped closed and then covered with cotton-padded adhesive patches to prevent corneal abrasion and seepage of cleansing solution and blood into the eyes.

Thiopental, propofol, an opioid (either fentanyl, sufentanil, alfentanil, or remifentanil), and a neuromuscular relaxant (either succinylcholine or a nondepolarizing neuromuscular relaxant for intubation, followed by a selected nondepolarizing agent) with a combination of N_2O and oxygen is a commonly used anesthetic combination for this procedure. Isoflurane may be added in low concentrations for blood pressure control; alternatively it may be used as the primary anesthetic drug (after the establishment of hyperventilation). Halothane is contraindicated because of its potential for inducing ventricular dysrhythmias after infiltration of the oral and nasal mucosa with epinephrine-containing local anesthetics and the application of cocaine-soaked pledgets.[106]

The topical use of cocaine and the oral and nasal submucosal injection of local anesthetic solutions containing epinephrine help constrict gingival and mucosal vessels and dissect the nasal mucosa away from the cartilaginous septum. Epinephrine use may produce hypertension or dysrhythmias or both; cocaine interferes with the intraneuronal uptake of catecholamines and can augment both the hypertensive and dysrhythmogenic properties of epinephrine. However, the use of epinephrine is relatively safe if (1) halothane is avoided, (2) ventilation is adequate, (3) epinephrine is given in combination with lidocaine instead of saline, (4) epinephrine concentrations of 1:100,000 to 1:200,000 are used, and (5) total dose does not exceed 10 ml of 1:100,000 solution in 10 minutes for a 70-kg adult. A total dose of 200 mg of cocaine should not be exceeded. Persistent dysrhythmias may require treatment with lidocaine or possibly a β-blocker. Hypertension may be controlled with an increased concentration of the selected inhalation agent or with small intravenous doses of hydralazine, labetalol, or esmolol.[106,107]

In some cases it may be necessary to insert a catheter into the lumbar subarachnoid space to facilitate the injection of preservative-free saline to delineate the suprasellar margins. If air is injected, N_2O must be discontinued from the anesthetic mixture because of rapid diffusion into the air now present in the closed cranial vault.[107]

Emergence from anesthesia should be conducted as described for the previously discussed procedures. Intravenous lidocaine, 1.5 mg/kg given approximately 3 minutes before suctioning and extubation, decreases coughing, straining, and hypertension. Postoperatively, patients should be responsive to commands in the recovery room. Steroid therapy is continued throughout this period and is tapered over time if appropriate.

Cerebrovascular Surgery

Cerebral Aneurysms

Cerebral aneurysms are abnormal, localized dilations of the intracranial arteries. They are classified as berry or saccular, mycotic, traumatic, fusiform, neoplastic, or atherosclerotic. Rupture of a saccular aneurysm is a leading cause of subarachnoid hemorrhage.[108-110]

Approximately 5 million people in North America have cerebral aneurysms, with approximately 30,000 new cases of subarachnoid hemorrhage occurring annually. The peak age for rupture of a cerebral aneurysm is 55 to 60 years. A slight female predilection also exists, with aneurysmal rupture occurring in three women for every two men.[111]

More than one third of patients with subarachnoid hemorrhage die or develop significant and lasting neurologic disabilities before they receive any treatment. A small bleed occurs in approximately 50% of patients and is often tragically ignored or misdiagnosed. Even in patients who receive prompt care, only half remain functional survivors; the remainder die or develop serious neurologic deficits.[109]

Aneurysms may arise at any point in the circle of Willis. The most common locations for the occurrence of aneurysms are shown in Table 26-7. Most aneurysms are broad based and located in the middle cerebral system. Traumatic aneurysms develop as a result of direct trauma to an artery with injury to the wall.

TABLE 26-7 Location and Occurrence of Cerebral Aneurysms

Location	Occurrence (%)
Internal carotid	38
Anterior cerebral system	36
Anterior communicating junction	30
Internal carotid at posterior communicating junction	25
Middle cerebral system	21
Vertebrobasilar system	5

From Frost AEM. Management of neurosurgical anesthesia: aneurysms. Curr Rev Clin Anesth. *1991;11:125-132. Used with permission of* Current Reviews.

TABLE 26-8 Hunt's Classification of Patients with Intracranial Aneurysms According to Surgical Risk

Grade	Perioperative Criterion	Mortality Rate (%)
I	Asymptomatic or minimal headache and slight nuchal rigidity	0-5
II	Moderate to severe headache, nuchal rigidity, no neurologic deficit, possible cranial nerve palsy	2-10
III	Drowsiness, confusion, or mild focal deficit	10-15
IV	Stupor, moderate to severe hemiparesis, possibly early decerebrate rigidity and vegetative disturbances	60-70
V	Deep coma, decerebrate rigidity, moribund appearance	70-100

From Hunt WE, Hess RM. Surgical risk as related to time of intervention in the repair of intracranial aneurysms. J Neurosurg. *1968;28:14.*

Mirror aneurysms of the internal carotid system are common, and other combinations of locations occur. The site of the bleeding aneurysm is best located by computed tomographic studies, evidence of vasospasm in the immediate vicinity, and lobulation of the aneurysm wall on angiographic studies.[110]

Diagnosis of Subarachnoid Hemorrhage

Subarachnoid hemorrhage produces an abrupt intense headache in 85% of patients, and transient loss of consciousness may be seen in up to 45% of patients. Nausea and vomiting, photophobia, fever, meningismus, and focal neurologic deficits are not uncommon. The severity of a subarachnoid hemorrhage can be graded clinically with the use of classifications developed by either Botterell or Hunt (Table 26-8). Although surgical mortality rates vary somewhat among institutions, patients with a neurologic grade I subarachnoid hemorrhage generally undergo surgical clipping with a low mortality rate (less than 5%), whereas grade V patients generally do not survive.[109]

General Considerations

Hypertension often accompanies acute subarachnoid hemorrhage and is postulated to develop secondary to autonomic hyperactivity, which may increase transmural pressure in the aneurysmal sac. Transmural pressure is defined as the differential pressure between MAP and ICP and represents the stress applied to the aneurysm's wall[109] (Figures 26-21 and 26-22).

Increases in blood pressure directly increase the transmural pressure and the likelihood of bleeding; conversely, reductions in blood pressure reduce transmural pressure. Caution should be exercised when purposefully reducing transmural pressure because cerebral autoregulation may be impaired after subarachnoid hemorrhage, and a reduction in blood pressure may induce or aggravate cerebral ischemia, particularly if vasospasm is present. To balance these opposing concerns, many neurosurgeons attempt to maintain systolic blood pressure between 120 and 150 mm Hg before clipping of the aneurysm.[109]

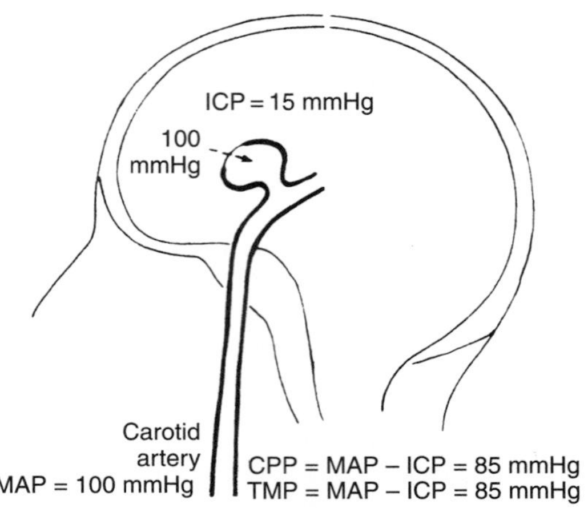

FIGURE **26-21**
Transmural pressure (*TMP*) of the aneurysm. TMP is the same as the cerebral perfusion pressure (*CPP*) and is equal to the difference between mean arterial pressure (*MAP*) and intracranial pressure (*ICP*). (From Newfield P, Cottrell JE, eds. *Neuroanesthesia: Handbook of Clinical and Physiologic Essentials*. 2nd ed. Boston: Little, Brown; 1991:195.)

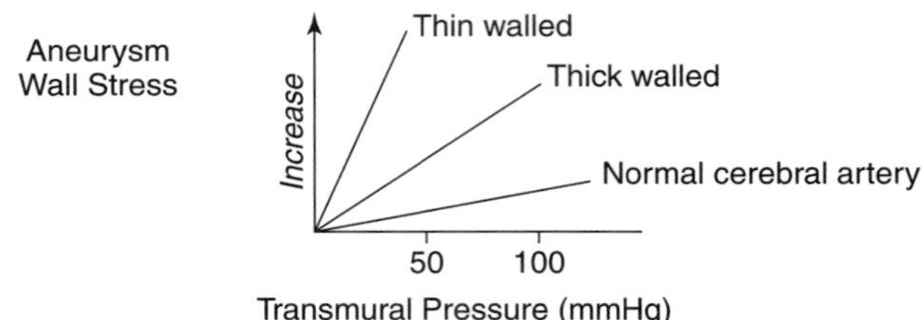

FIGURE **26-22**
Aneurysm wall stress. Wall tension divided by wall thickness equals aneurysm wall stress. The relationship between transmural pressure and wall stress is linear: the thinner the wall, the greater the wall stress at any given pressure. (From Newfield P, Cottrell JE, eds. *Neuroanesthesia: Handbook of Clinical and Physiologic Essentials*. 2nd ed. Boston: Little, Brown; 1991:195.)

Electrocardiographic changes are common after subarachnoid hemorrhage and have been reported to occur in 50% to 80% of patients. The most common changes involve the T wave or the ST segment, but other changes such as the presence of a U wave, QTc-interval prolongation, and dysrhythmias may be present. Whether such changes in the ECG represent myocardial injury has long been debated. In the majority of patients these changes do not appear to be associated with adverse neurologic or cardiac outcomes.[109,111]

Rebleeding from a previously ruptured aneurysm is a life-threatening complication. The incidence of rebleeding is approximately 50% in the first days after subarachnoid hemorrhage, and rebleeding is associated with an 80% mortality rate. The chance of rebleeding from an unsecured aneurysm declines over time, and by 6 months the risk stabilizes at approximately 3% per year. Approaches used to decrease the risk of rebleeding include early surgical clipping, the use of antifibrinolytic agents, and blood pressure control.[108,109,112]

Vasospasm

Vasospasm is reactive narrowing of cerebral arteries after subarachnoid hemorrhage. Although arterial narrowing may be detected with angiography in 60% of patients, only half of these patients develop clinical symptoms. The accompanying neurologic deterioration, arising from impaired cerebral perfusion, ischemia, and secondary infarction of the brain, peaks between the fourth and ninth day after subarachnoid hemorrhage and resolves over the next 2 to 3 weeks.[108]

Vasospasm and the ensuing delayed ischemic deficit are thought to result from several factors. First, direct trauma to vessels or mechanical distortion or displacement from the hemorrhage itself produces localized, short-lived spasm. Second, spasmogenic substances, such as oxyhemoglobin, may be present in the subarachnoid blood; the effects of these substances may be mediated by free radicals. Because of their high serotonin content, platelets are also spasmogenic.[113] Third, prostaglandins synthesized by platelets and brain tissue as a response to injury are known to produce prolonged arterial constriction when given intrathecally to laboratory animals. Fourth, mediators of the inflammatory response (eicosanoids, circulating immune complexes, complement activators) may have a role in vasospasm.[114]

Successful treatment of vasospasm depends on the maintenance of adequate CPP (CPP = MAP − ICP). This is accomplished with expansion of the intravascular volume, which augments blood pressure and cardiac output; avoidance of hyponatremia; and preservation of relative hemodilution (hematocrit approximately 32%).[114] Because of the risk of rebleeding, both hypertension and hypervolemia are used with caution in the period preceding surgical correction. Deliberate intraoperative hypotensive techniques are common. Postoperative hypertension is not treated aggressively and at times is encouraged.

Pharmacologic vasodilation of spastic vessels has been ineffective, because vasospasm involves a structural alteration in the vessel wall rather than just a spastic contracture or failure of relaxation of the smooth muscle cells in the media of the vessels. Nimodipine and nicardipine, calcium channel blockers, are currently in wide use for prevention of delayed neurologic deficit after subarachnoid hemorrhage. They diminish the level of myoplasmic calcium in smooth muscle cells and impede the entry of extracellular calcium necessary for the contraction of the smooth muscle[115-117] (Box 26-10).

Timing of Surgery

The presence or absence of vasospasm on angiographic studies has frequently determined the timing of aneurysmal surgery. However, current neurosurgical practice suggests that a good outcome is achieved with early operation (within 24 to 48 hours) in patients who are neurologically intact (grades I or II), regardless of whether vasospasm has been demonstrated. Such emergency intervention decreases the likelihood of rebleeding. However, only 53% of grade III patients achieve a good outcome after early surgery; this indicates that the gross neurologic condition preoperatively is the best prognostic indicator of intact survival.[110,118]

In the first few days after hemorrhage the brain is swollen, soft, hyperemic, and prone to contusion and laceration. Impaired autoregulation may decrease cerebral tolerance to brain retraction. Although removal of a subarachnoid clot probably decreases the incidence and severity of delayed arterial narrowing, clearly, operative management clearly may be hazardous. In more severely injured patients (grades III through V) surgery is often delayed in anticipation of resolution of vasospasm and improvement in neurologic status.[110,119]

BOX 26-10

Treatment of Vasospasm

- Maintenance of cerebral perfusion
- Augmentation of blood pressure and cardiac output
- Administration of inotropes (dopamine, dobutamine)
- Administration of nimodipine or nicardipine
- Intravascular volume expansion
- Relative hemodilution (hematocrit 32%)
- Correction of hyponatremia
- Transluminal angioplasty

From Newfield P. Perioperative management of intracranial pressure. ASA Annu Refresher Course Lect. *1993;21:13.*

Preoperative Evaluation

The baseline neurologic status must be ascertained. The level of consciousness may vary from perfect alertness to deep coma and is an important prognostic factor for the postoperative state. Evidence of increased ICP should be elicited preoperatively so that it can be managed appropriately. Focal motor and sensory signs may indicate intracerebral extension of subarachnoid hemorrhage, vasospasm, or cerebral edema.[109]

Pulmonary complications, such as pneumonia, neurogenic pulmonary edema, and atelectasis, are not uncommon and are potentially treatable. Patients often have an increased risk of aspiration because of their depressed level of consciousness, and measures should be taken to reduce gastric acidity and volume preoperatively. The use of prophylactic hypervolemia also increases the likelihood of pulmonary edema.[109]

The hemodynamic status of the patient should be assessed, with particular attention paid to the relationship between neurologic deterioration and blood pressure changes. Continuous arterial blood pressure monitoring is essential. Serious dysrhythmias or evidence of ventricular dysfunction should be diagnosed preoperatively so that appropriate monitoring and management can be instituted.[120]

The syndrome of inappropriate antidiuretic hormone and diabetes insipidus can occur in patients with subarachnoid hemorrhage.

The presence of blood in the subarachnoid space may produce a 1° to 2° C elevation of body temperature. Temperature elevation increases cerebral oxygen requirements and therefore should be treated in order to prevent an increase of cerebral ischemia.[108,109]

Preoperative sedation is rarely necessary in these patients. Depression of ventilation associated with opioids, barbiturates, and benzodiazepines may result in hypercapnia with resultant increases in CBF and ICP. Additionally, the reduced level of consciousness preoperatively and postoperatively may make clinical assessment difficult. Preoperative anxiety is not a problem in patients with a depressed level of consciousness (grades III through V), and sedation is not required in these patients. In awake patients a reassuring preoperative visit usually allays anxiety. If preoperative sedation is considered necessary, a small dose of a benzodiazepine (midazolam) with continued observation after its administration is probably the best choice.

Anesthetic Induction, Maintenance, and Emergence

The maintenance of adequate intravascular volume requires two large-bore intravenous cannulas. Intraoperative monitoring includes continuous ECG (V_5), arterial pressure monitoring, peripheral nerve stimulator, central venous pressure monitoring, end-tidal CO_2 monitoring, pulse oximetry, and monitoring of temperature and fluid balance.[121]

The anesthetic induction should be slow and deliberate. The anesthetic depth should be sufficient to avoid the hypertensive responses that accompany laryngoscopy and endotracheal intubation. Anesthesia is induced with titrated doses of either thiopental or propofol. The addition of an opioid (5 to 10 mcg/kg of fentanyl or 1 to 2 mcg/kg of sufentanil) and intravenous lidocaine (1.5 mg/kg) further blunts the patient's response to sympathetic stimulation of laryngoscopy and intubation. An additional dose of opioid or thiopental is required for the placement of the three-point pin head holder. Prior injection of local anesthetic minimizes the associated sympathetic stimulation. Epinephrine should not be included with the local anesthetic, because delayed absorption (up to 30 minutes after injection) may produce significant increases in blood pressure. Isoflurane may be introduced after hyperventilation before laryngoscopy to increase the depth of anesthesia. Ventilation is controlled with administration of 100% oxygen to achieve a $PaCO_2$ of 35 to 40 mm Hg with normal intracranial compliance. Mild hyperventilation (end-tidal carbon dioxide [$ETCO_2$] 25 to 30 mm Hg) is instituted when intracranial compliance is impaired.[109]

Succinylcholine produces moderate increases in ICP.[122-124] Elevation of serum potassium sufficient to produce lethal dysrhythmias has been reported in comatose, nonparetic, head-injured patients and in patients after subarachnoid hemorrhage who received succinylcholine. Alternatively, intubation can be accomplished with 1 mg of rocuronium per kilogram.

The patient is placed in one of several positions, depending on the site of the aneurysm. Aneurysms that arise from the anterior part of the circle of Willis require that the patient be supine for a frontotemporal approach. The lateral position for a temporal approach is required for aneurysms that arise from the posterior aspect of the basilic artery. Aneurysms that arise from the vertebral artery or from the lower basilic artery require a sitting or prone position for a suboccipital approach. Aneurysms that arise from the anterior communicating artery are usually approached from the right, and those from the middle cerebral and posterior communicating arteries are approached from the side on which the aneurysm is located.[125]

Anesthesia is maintained with air and oxygen or N_2O in oxygen, with incremental titrated dosages of an opioid (fentanyl, alfentanil, or sufentanil) or an infusion of remifentanil and a muscle relaxant. Isoflurane may also be added in inspired concentrations not to exceed 1%. Patients who have intracranial aneurysms require precise intraoperative control of blood pressure for prevention of rebleeding and counteraction of vasospasm.[126] In addition, controlled hypotension is commonly used intraoperatively to make aneurysms softer and more pliable at the time of clipping, as well as to minimize blood loss should aneurysmal rupture occur at this time.[111] Sodium nitroprusside and an inhalation anesthetic agent are the drugs most widely used for induction of hypotension.[126]

The safe limit of controlled hypotension has not been definitively established. Because autoregulation is maintained to a MAP of 50 to 60 mm Hg, some argue that this limit should not be exceeded. In addition, because patients with poor-grade aneurysms may not have intact autoregulation, some argue that a lower limit of 60 mm Hg should be adopted. Limits of autoregulation are shifted to higher pressures in patients with preexisting hypertension, so decreases in MAP should probably be limited to no more than 40% of preoperative values.[109] Many neurosurgeons now routinely use temporary proximal occlusion of the parent vessel rather than induced hypotension to facilitate clip-ligation of the neck of the aneurysm.[127]

At the conclusion of the anesthetic procedure, patients with good-grade aneurysms may be extubated in the operating room, although care must be exercised so that coughing, straining, hypercarbia, and hypertension are avoided. Propofol, lidocaine, or small doses of alfentanil may be used for short-term anesthesia as the procedure is being finished and for reducing the hemodynamic responses to extubation. Although the residual depressant effects of opioids may be reversed with judicious titrated dosages of naloxone, larger doses of naloxone can be hazardous because they may cause sudden, violent awakening of the patient and marked increases in systemic blood pressure. Endotracheal tubes should be retained in patients with poor-grade aneurysms and in those who have had intraoperative complications; these patients will probably require postoperative ventilation.[108]

Postoperative Care

Postoperative care is directed at the prevention of vasospasm via the maintenance of intravascular volume expansion and moderate hypertension (MAP of 80 to 120 mm Hg). Changes in the level of consciousness and the development of focal neurologic deficits are usually early signs of vasospasm. These clinical signs should be aggressively managed with hypertensive hypervolemic hemodilution and the use of dopamine for blood pressure support. Computed tomography should be used for ruling out other causes of neurologic deterioration, including rebleeding, infarction, and hydrocephalus.[108]

Aneurysmal Rupture

Intraoperative aneurysmal rupture can be catastrophic. An abrupt increase in blood pressure during or after induction of anesthesia may indicate that an aneurysm has bled. The use of 100 to 200 mg of thiopental or 0.5 to 1 mcg of sodium nitroprusside per kilogram decreases the transmural pressure of the aneurysm, although hypotension can be detrimental at this juncture. Intraoperative aneurysmal rupture necessitates maintenance of the MAP between 40 and 50 mm Hg or lower to facilitate surgical control of the neck of the aneurysm or the parent vessel. Alternatively, one or both carotid arteries may be compressed for up to 3 minutes to produce a bloodless field. Blood that is lost should be continuously replaced with whole blood, blood products, or colloid solution so that intravascular volume is maintained.[108]

Although barbiturates have been used for protection against focal cerebral ischemia, their efficacy has not been demonstrated in this clinical situation. However, some practitioners advocate the administration of thiopental (3 to 5 mg/kg) before temporary clipping.[13]

Arteriovenous Malformation

Arteriovenous malformations are congenital, intracerebral networks in which arteries flow directly into veins. Patients with these malformations generally are younger than those with aneurysms. Patients may have bleeding or seizures or, less commonly, ischemia resulting from "steal" from normal areas or occurring with high-output congestive heart failure.[128]

The anesthetic problems parallel those associated with patients undergoing aneurysm surgery. Notably, arteriovenous malformations do not autoregulate their blood flow. The operation is likely to be longer and bloodier than that of aneurysm clipping. Surgery may be preceded by an attempt at embolization by the neuroradiologist in order to diminish the risk of surgery. The neurologic examination should be repeated after embolization to document new deficits that otherwise might be attributed to anesthesia and surgery.[128]

Head Trauma

Head injuries are a contributory factor in up to 50% of deaths resulting from trauma. Most patients with head trauma are young, and many (10% to 40%) have associated intraabdominal injuries, long bone fractures, or both. The significance of a head injury is dependent not only on the extent of the irreversible neuronal damage at the time of injury but also on the occurrence of any secondary insults. These additional insults include systemic factors such as hypoxemia, hypercapnia, and hypotension; the formation and expansion of an epidural, subdural, or intracerebral hematoma; and sustained intracranial hypertension (Box 26-11). Studies suggest that sustained increases in ICP of approximately 60 mm Hg result in irreversible brain edema. Surgical and anesthetic management of these patients is directed at preventing these secondary insults[72] (Figure 26-23).

BOX **26-11**

Peripheral Sequelae of Head Trauma

Cardiopulmonary
Abnormal breathing patterns
Airway obstruction
Hypoxia
Shock
Adult respiratory distress syndrome
Neurogenic pulmonary edema
Electrocardiographic changes

Hematologic
Disseminated intravascular coagulation

Endocrinologic
Diabetes insipidus
Syndrome of inappropriate antidiuretic hormone

Skeletal
Cervical spine injury
Maxillofacial injuries

Modified from Newfield P, Cottrell JE, eds. Neuroanesthesia: Handbook of Clinical and Physiologic Essentials. *2nd ed. Boston: Little, Brown; 1991:301.*

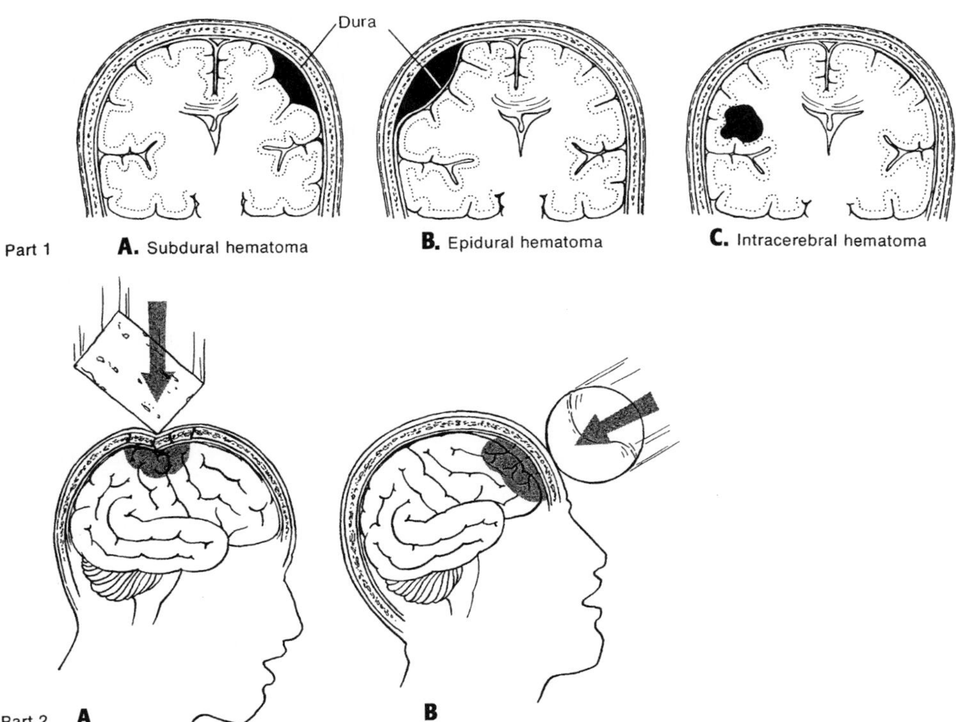

FIGURE **26-23**
Care of the neurosurgical patient. Types of hematomas. Part 1: **A,** Subdural hematoma. **B,** Epidural hematoma. **C,** Intracerebral hematoma. Part 2: Mechanisms of head injury. **A,** Direct injury resulting in depressed skull fracture and compression injury. **B,** Blow to skull resulting in tearing of blood vessels. Shaded areas represent cerebral contusion. (Part 1 from Clochesy J, Breu C, Cardin S, et al. *Critical Care Nursing.* 2nd ed. Philadelphia: Saunders; 1996. Part 2 from Luckman J, Sorensen KC. *Medical-Surgical Nursing: A Psychophysiologic Approach.* 3rd ed. Philadelphia: Saunders; 1987.)

TABLE 26-9 Glasgow Coma Scale Scoring System

Parameter	Score
Eye Opening	
Spontaneously	4
To command	3
To pain	2
No response	1
Motor Response	
Obeys verbal command	6
Localizes pain	5
Flexion withdrawal	4
Decorticate rigidity	3
Decerebrate rigidity	2
No response	1
Verbal Response	
Oriented and converses	5
Disoriented and converses	4
Inappropriate words	3
Incomprehensible words	2
No response	1

TABLE 26-10 Modified Coma Scale for Infants

Response	Score
Eye Opening	
Spontaneous	4
To speech	3
To pain	2
None	1
Verbal Response	
Coos, babbles	5
Irritable cries	4
Cries to pain	3
Moans to pain	2
None	1
Motor Response	
Normal spontaneous movement	6
Withdraws to touch	5
Withdraws to pain	4
Abnormal flexion	3
Abnormal extension	2
None	1

Preoperative Management

Emergency therapy for head injury should begin before hospital admission, because a large proportion of deaths occur in the prehospital phase. Therapy is based on prevention of secondary brain injury resulting from hypoxia, hypercapnia, hypotension, and expanding intracranial masses.

Airway Management

Measures to ensure airway patency, adequacy of ventilation and oxygenation, and the correction of systemic hypotension should be instituted simultaneously with neurologic evaluation. Airway obstruction and hypoventilation are common. Up to 70% of head-injured patients have concurrent hypoxemia, which may be complicated by pulmonary contusion, fat emboli, or neurogenic pulmonary edema. All patients must be assumed to have a cervical spine injury (10% incidence) until disproved by radiography. Axial traction to maintain the head in a neutral position should be used during airway instrumentation. Fiberoptic intubation may be preferred for airway management in some cases. Patients with obvious hypoventilation, the absence of the gag reflex, or a persistent total score below 7 on the Glasgow Coma Scale (Table 26-9) require tracheal intubation and hyperventilation. A modified coma scale for infants is given in Table 26-10. Box 26-12 outlines

BOX 26-12

Respiratory Patterns

Pattern	Description	Location of Injury and Other Causes
Cheyne-Stokes respiration	Regular increase in the rate and depth of breathing that peaks and is followed by a decreasing rate and depth of breathing, which progresses to apnea; then the cycle repeats itself	Bilateral dysfunction of cerebral hemispheres Midbrain and upper pons
Central neurogenic hyperventilation	Deep, rapid, and regular pattern of breathing	Low midbrain and upper pons Increased intracranial pressure with head trauma
Apneusis breathing	A pause at full inspiration occurs; may see prolonged inspiratory pause alternating with prolonged expiratory pause	Mid and low pons Hypoglycemia, anoxia, and meningitis
Cluster breathing	Periodic breathing with frequent apneic episodes	Low pons and high medulla
Ataxic breathing	Irregular breathing with shallow, deep respirations and irregular apneic episodes; usually slow	Medulla

From Hawkins VC, Hawkins JK. Care of the neurosurgical patient. In Drain CB, ed. Perianesthesia Nursing. *4th ed. St Louis: Saunders; 2003:534.*

respiratory patterns seen with various neurologic injuries. All other patients should be carefully observed for deterioration. The Glasgow Coma Scale score generally correlates well with the severity of injury and outcome.[72]

When intubation is indicated, the oral route provides the most efficient means of safely securing the airway. When possible a modified, rapid-sequence endotracheal intubation should be performed; that is, it should be preceded by a period of 100% oxygen administration and hyperventilation supplemented by continuous cricoid pressure.[129,130] Nasal intubation should be avoided in the presence of suspected basilar skull fracture, bleeding diathesis, suspected upper airway foreign body, or severe facial fractures.[130] If a difficult intubation is anticipated, awake intubation, fiberoptic techniques, or tracheostomy may be necessary.

Cardiovascular Assessment

Multisystem trauma frequently accompanies head injury. Hypotension results from intravascular loss from associated injuries. These injuries must be identified and treated early in the resuscitative period. Fluid resuscitation is facilitated by the administration of isotonic fluid, either normal saline or lactated Ringer's solution, or colloids if blood is not readily available. Glucose in water should not be used, because it decreases serum osmolality and can aggravate the cerebral swelling. The ideal replacement fluid, of course, is blood. Because the cerebral vessels are already dilated from hypotension, rapid restoration of the normal arterial pressure precipitates brain swelling. It is extremely valuable to insert an ICP monitor during resuscitation for the monitoring of both systemic arterial pressure and ICP. Dysrhythmias and ECG abnormalities in the T wave, U wave, ST segment, and QT interval are common after head injuries but are not necessarily associated with cardiac injury.[72]

Coagulopathies

Severe brain injury initiates the outpouring of tissue thromboplastin and activation of the complement system, causing disseminated intravascular coagulopathy and fibrinolysis and precipitating the development of the adult respiratory distress syndrome. Recognition of abnormal prothrombin and partial thromboplastin times and prompt therapy with fresh frozen plasma, cryoprecipitate, whole blood, and, if necessary, platelets may abort the development of full-blown disseminated intravascular coagulopathy.[131,132]

Increased Intracranial Pressure

The clinical appreciation of elevated ICP is difficult in unconscious patients. Therefore initial therapy is directed toward lowering ICP or at least toward preventing further increases in ICP. Simple maneuvers such as use of a head-up tilt of 15 to 20 degrees that keeps the head in the midline position and not rotated to either side (for maintenance of jugular vein patency), avoidance of overhydration, maintenance of normovolemia, and maintenance of normal (rather than increased) arterial pressure all help control ICP.[133]

In patients in whom intracranial hypertension is suspected, either from an epidural or subdural hematoma or from diffuse brain swelling, emergency treatment directed at reducing ICP is the rational course. Ideally a definitive study for identifying the cause of clinical deterioration is performed before therapy. The first and most rapidly effective therapy is hyperventilation. In a patient who has multiple trauma and reduced blood volume, care must be taken during controlled ventilation to avoid increasing the intrathoracic pressure, decreasing venous return, and producing secondary hypotension. Corticosteroids (dexamethasone or methylprednisolone) are of little benefit in trauma, and these drugs must not be relied on to lower the ICP rapidly.[133]

Although mannitol effectively lowers the ICP minutes after administration, its use remains controversial. The drug is indicated, however, when either elevated ICP or a mass and herniation are responsible for the patient's deteriorating state. The risk of increasing the size of a hematoma is negligible compared with the disastrous effects of untreated progressive uncal herniation. If decompression of transtentorial herniation is delayed, secondary hemorrhage into the brain stem can occur and cause irreversible neurologic deficit. Once mannitol is given and the ICP is reduced, the specific intracranial disorder must be identified as soon as possible if a recurrence of the patient's deterioration is to be prevented.[133]

Neurodiagnostic Evaluation

The choice between operative and medical management of head trauma is based on radiographic and clinical findings. Patients should be stabilized before any computed tomographic or angiographic studies are performed. Critically ill patients should be closely monitored during such studies. Restless or uncooperative patients may require general anesthesia if these diagnostic examinations are to be accomplished. Sedation without control of the airway should be avoided because of the risk of further increases in ICP from hypercapnia or hypoxemia. In the event of neurologic deterioration before completion of these studies, intravenous administration of mannitol should be considered.[72] Reductions of $PaCO_2$ levels may, by decreasing CBF, allow better angiographic studies. The introduction of computed tomography and magnetic resonance imaging has greatly facilitated neuroradiologic diagnosis. Serial computed tomography is an aid in prediction of the outcome of patients with severe head injury. New findings after the initial study are associated with poorer outcomes.[134]

Intraoperative Management

Operative treatment is reserved for depressed skull fracture; depressed fractures associated with underlying brain injury; and evacuation of epidural, subdural, and some intracerebral hematomas.

Monitoring during anesthesia is generally similar to that for other mass lesions associated with intracranial hypertension. Intraarterial and central venous (or pulmonary artery) pressure monitoring should be established if it is not already present, but it should not delay surgical decompression in a rapidly deteriorating patient.[72,133] Monitors for cerebral oxygenation are noted in Box 26-5.

Anesthetic Induction, Maintenance, and Emergence

Intubation must be accomplished as expeditiously as possible with the use of small, incremental doses of thiopental, rocuronium, (assuming the airway can be instrumented), lidocaine, and labetalol (for the treatment of systemic hypertension) with concurrent cricoid pressure. Hyperkalemia may be induced with succinylcholine in a patient with closed head injury without paresis; therefore use of this drug should be avoided.[135] Blood loss and diuretic therapy cause hypovolemia, but this state may not initially cause hypotension because the victim generally has a healthy vasculature that compensates. Intracranial damage is usually associated with hypertension. The true state of hydration may be realized for the first time after induction, when catastrophic hypotension may occur if fluid replacement is inadequate or barbiturate dosage is excessive.

Ventilation should be controlled. A $PaCO_2$ of 25 to 30 mm Hg promotes brain relaxation for surgical exposure without producing ischemia from hypocapnic vasoconstriction. A higher $PaCO_2$ (30 to 35 mm Hg) is recommended for patients who require burr holes for evacuation of chronic subdural hematomas, particularly after decompression, because a slack brain may encourage recurrence.[77]

The choice of anesthetic drugs for a patient with head injury is determined by the patient's condition. If the patient is unconscious in the absence of a drug overdose, the ICP is probably elevated. In this case a barbiturate and an opioid in combination with oxygen or air in oxygen and a muscle relaxant are appropriate. A similar technique is indicated in the patient whose computed tomographic scan demonstrates obliteration of basal cisterns, dilation of the fourth or lateral ventricles, or a midline shift of 10 mm.[77]

Although hyperventilation attenuates the increase in ICP when inhalation anesthetics are used, in patients with head injury cerebral vasoconstriction in response to hypocapnia is not a dependable indicator. The introduction of inhalation agents in such patients may increase ICP and exacerbate the formation of edema. The administration of inhalation anesthetics in low inspired concentrations may have a role in the treatment of intraoperative hypertension.[77]

Patients who have chronic subdural hematoma and are alert and responsive may have burr holes placed for evacuation of accumulated blood under local anesthesia with sedation. Depressed skull fractures may also be elevated while the patient is awake and under local anesthesia with sedation. This technique must be used cautiously when the patient placed in the three-point pin head holder has a full stomach.[77]

Fluid replacement should be with glucose-free solutions. Hypovolemia results in systemic hypotension, an unstable anesthetic course, and, by decreasing cerebral oxygen delivery, increased cerebral vasodilation. Rheologic conditions are optimal at hematocrit levels of 30% to 32%.[133]

The decision of whether to extubate the trachea at the conclusion of the surgical procedure depends on the severity of the injury, the presence of concomitant abdominal or thoracic injuries, preexisting illnesses, and the preoperative level of consciousness. The incidence of postoperative complications is high with neurosurgical procedures. A recent study noted that up to 54.5% of patients had an adverse event after surgery.[136] Occurrence of nausea, vomiting, and respiratory and cardiac problems was significantly more likely than in patients undergoing routine surgical procedures. Young patients who are conscious preoperatively may be extubated after the removal of a localized lesion, whereas patients with diffuse brain injury should remain intubated. Moreover, persistent intracranial hypertension requires continued paralysis, sedation, hyperventilation, and possibly a pentobarbital infusion postoperatively.[72]

REFERENCES

1. Davson H, Oldendorf WH. Transport in the central nervous system. *Proc R Soc Med.* 1967;60:326-329.
2. Snell RS. Nerve fibers and peripheral nerves. In: *Clinical Neuroanatomy for Medical Students*. Philadelphia: Lippincott-Raven; 1997:90-92.
3. Rapoport SI, Hori M, Klatzo I. Testing of a hypothesis for osmotic opening of the blood-brain barrier. *Am J Physiol.* 1972;223:323-331.
4. deGroot J. The brain stem and cerebellum. In: *Correlative Neuroanatomy*. 21st ed. Norwalk, Conn: Appleton & Lange; 1991:55-72.
5. Romero-Sierra C. Spinal cord and its coverings. In: *Neuroanatomy: a Conceptual Approach*. New York: Churchill Livingstone; 1986:69-88.
6. de Groot J. The spinal cord. *Correlative Neuroanatomy*. 21st ed. Norwalk, Conn: Appleton & Lange; 1991:27-42.
7. Guyton AC, Hall JE. Motor functions of the spinal cord: the cord reflexes. *Textbook of Medical Physiology*. 10th ed. Philadelphia: Saunders; 2000:622-632.
8. Marieb E. The autonomic nervous system. In: *Human Anatomy and Physiology*. 4th ed. Menlo Park, Calif: Benjamin Cummings; 1998:494-512.
9. Hudspith MJ. Glutamate: a role in normal brain function, anesthesia, analgesia and CNS injury. *Br J Anaesth.* 1997;78:731-747.
10. Gustein HB, Akil H. Opioid analgesics. In: Hardman JG, Limbird LE, eds. *Goodman & Gilman's the Pharmacological Basis of Therapeutics*. 10th ed. New York: McGraw-Hill; 2001:569-620.
11. Wilson DR, Florete OG, Rowe, DS. Chronic and interventional pain management. In: Cucchiara RF, Black S, Michenfelder JD, eds. *Clinical Neuroanesthesia*. New York: Churchill Livingstone; 1998:623-642.
12. Jennett WB, Barker J, Fitch W, McDowall DG. Effect of anaesthesia on intracranial pressure in patients with space-occupying lesions. *Lancet.* 1969;1:61-64.
13. Sloan TB. Anesthetics and the brain. *Anesthesiol Clin North Am.* 2002;20:265-292.
14. Albin MS. Anesthesia for neurosurgical procedures. In: Grossman RG, Hamilton WJ, eds. *Principles of Neurosurgery*. New York: Raven; 1991:1-17.
15. Baker AJ. Management of the severely head injured patient. *Can J Anaesth.* 1999;46:R35-R45.
16. Steen PA. Inhalational versus intravenous anesthesia: cerebral effects. *Acta Anaesthesiol Scand.* 1982;75:32-35.
17. Fitch W, McDowal DG. Effect of halothane on intracranial pressure gradients in the presence of intracranial space-occupying lesions. *Br J Anaesth.* 1971;43:904-911.
18. Adams RW, Gronert GA, Sundt TM Jr, Michenfelder JD. Halothane, hypocapnia, and cerebrospinal fluid pressure in neurosurgery. *Anesthesiology.* 1972;37:510-517.
19. McGrath BJ, Matjasko MJ. Anesthesia and head trauma. *New Horiz.* 1995;3:523-533.
20. Drummond JC, Todd MM. The response of the feline cerebral circulation to $PaCO_2$ during anesthesia with isoflurane and halothane and during sedation with nitrous oxide. *Anesthesiology.* 1985;62:268-273.
21. Van Aken H, Fitch W, Graham DI, Brussel T, Themann H. Cardiovascular and cerebrovascular effects of isoflurane-induced hypotension in the baboon. *Anesth Analg.* 1986;65:565-574.
22. Todd MM, Drummond JC. A comparison of the cerebrovascular and metabolic effects of halothane and isoflurane in the cat. *Anesthesiology.* 1984;60:274-282.
23. Oshima T, Karasawa F, Okazaki Y, et al. Effects of sevoflurane on cerebral blood flow and cerebral metabolic rate of oxygen in human beings: a comparison with isoflurane. *Eur J Anaesthesiol.* 2003;20:543-547.
24. Michenfelder JD, et al. Isoflurane when compared to enflurane and halothane decreases frequency of cerebral ischemia during carotid endarterectomy. *Anesthesiology.* 1987;67:336-340.
25. Michenfelder JD, Theye RA. In vivo toxic effects of halothane on canine cerebral metabolic pathways. *Am J Physiol.* 1975;229:1050-1055.
26. Adams RW, Cucchiara RF, Gronert GA, Messick JM, Michenfelder JD. Isoflurane and cerebrospinal fluid pressure in neurosurgical patients. *Anesthesiology.* 1981;54:97-99.
27. Campkin TV. Isoflurane and cranial extradural pressure. *Br J Anaesth.* 1984;56:1083-1087.

28. Sponheim S, Skraastad O, Helseth E, et al. Effects of 5.0 and 1.0 MAC isoflurane, sevoflurane and desflurane on intracranial and cerebral perfusion pressures in children. *Acta Anaesthesiol Scand.* 2003;47;932-938.
29. Young WL. Effects of desflurane on the central nervous system. *Anesth Analg.* 1992;75:s32-s37.
30. Ornstein E, Young WL, Fleischer LH, Ostapkovich N. Desflurane and isoflurane have similar effects on cerebral blood flow in patients with intracranial mass lesions. *Anesthesiology.* 1993;79:498-502.
31. Muzzi DA, Losasso TJ, Dietz NM, Faust RJ, Cucchiara RF, Milde LN. The effect of desflurane and isoflurane on cerebrospinal fluid pressure in humans with supratentorial mass lesions. *Anesthesiology.* 1992;76:720-724.
32. Fraga M, Rama-Maceiras P, Rodino S, Aymerich H, Pose P, Belda J. The effects of isoflurane and desflurane on intracranial pressure, cerebral perfusion pressure, and cerebral arteriovenous oxygen content difference in normocapnic patients with supratentorial brain tumors. *Anesthesiology.* 2003;98:1085-1090.
33. Matta BF, Heath KJ, Tipping K, Summors AC. Direct cerebral vasodilatory effects of sevoflurane and isoflurane. *Anesthesiology.* 1999;91:677-680.
34. Summors AC, Gupta AK, Matta BF. Dynamic cerebral autoregulation during sevoflurane anesthesia: a comparison with isoflurane. *Anesth Analg.* 1999;88:341-345.
35. Boos DL, Stirt JA. Pharmacology. In Sperry RJ, Stirt JA, Stone DJ, eds. *Manual of Neuroanesthesia.* Philadelphia: Decker; 1989:37-66.
36. Smith AL, Marque JJ. Anesthetics and cerebral edema. *Anesthesiology.* 1976;45:64-72.
37. Baughman VL. Brain protection during neurosurgery. *Anesthesiol Clin North Am.* 2002;20:vi,315-327 .
38. Ramani R, Todd MM, Warner DS. A dose-response study of the influence of propofol on cerebral blood flow, metabolism, and the electroencephalogram of the rabbit. *Neurosurg Anesthesiol.* 1992;4:110-119.
39. Moss E, Powell D, Gibson RM, McDowell DG. Effect of etomidate on intracranial pressure and cerebral perfusion pressure. *Br J Anaesth.* 1979;51:347-352.
40. Milde LN, Milde JH, Michenfelder JD. Cerebral functional, metabolic, and hemodynamic effects of etomidate in dogs. *Anesthesiology.* 1985;65:371-377.
41. Alves S, Yermal S. Assessment of the neurological systems of the adult. In: Waugaman WR, Foster SD, Rigor BM, eds. *Principles and Practice of Nurse Anesthesia.* 3rd ed. Norwalk, Conn: Appleton & Lange; 1999:224-226.
42. Bendo AA, Kass IS, Hartung I, et al. Anesthesia for neurosurgery. In: Barash PG, Cullen BF, Stoelting RK, eds. *Clinical Anesthesia.* 4th ed. Philadelphia: Lippincott; 2001:743-790.
43. Keykhah MM, Smith DS, Carlsson C, Safo Y, Englebach I, Harp JR. Influence of sufentanil on cerebral metabolism and circulation in the rat. *Anesthesiology.* 1985;63:274-277.
44. McPherson RW, Krempasanka E, Eimerl D, Traystman RJ. Effects of alfentanil on cerebral vascular reactivity in dogs. *Br J Anaesth.* 1985;57:1232-1238.
45. Ostapkovich ND, Baker KZ, Fogarty-Mack P, Sisti MB, Young WL. Cerebral blood flow and CO_2 reactivity is similar during remifentanil/N_2O and fentanyl/N_2O anesthesia. *Anesthesiology.* 1998;89:358-363.
46. Paris A, Scholz J, von Knobelsdorff G, Tonner PH, Schulte am Esch J. The effect of remifentanil on cerebral blood flow velocity. *Anesth Analg.* 1998;87:569-573.
47. Drummond JC, Patel PM. Neurosurgical anesthesia. In: Miller RD, ed. *Anesthesia.* 5th ed. New York: Churchill Livingstone; 2000:1895-1933.
48. Vesely R, Hoffman WE, Gil KS, Albrecht RF, Miletich DJ. The cerebrovascular effects of curare and histamine in the rat. *Anesthesiology.* 1987;66:519-523.
49. Rao TLK, Mummaneni N, Elt AA. Convulsions: an unusual response to intravenous fentanyl administration. *Anesth Analg.* 1982;61:1020-1021.
50. Prough DS, Roy R, Bumgarner J. Acute pulmonary edema in healthy teenagers following conservative doses of intravenous naloxone. *Anesthesiology.* 1984;60:485-486.
51. Estilo AE, Cottrell JE. Naloxone, hypertension and ruptured cerebral aneurysm. *Anesthesiology.* 1981;54:352.
52. Fleisher JE, Milde JH, Moyer TP. Cerebral effects of high-dose midazolam and subsequent reversal with Ro 15-1788 in dogs. *Anesthesiology.* 1988;68:234-242.
53. Stirt JA, Maggio W, Haworth C, Minton MD, Bedford RF. Vecuronium: effect on intracranial pressure and hemodynamics in neurosurgical patients. *Anesthesiology.* 1987;67:570-573.
54. Shayevitz JR, Matteo RS. Decreased sensitivity to metocurine in patients with upper motor neuron disease. *Anesth Analg.* 1985;64:767-772.
55. Iwasaki H, Namiki A, Omote K, Omote T, Takahashi T. Response differences of paretic and healthy extremities to pancuronium and neostigmine in hemiplegic patients. *Anesth Analg.* 1985;64:864-866.
56. Hans P, Bonhomme V. Muscle relaxants in neurosurgical anaesthesia: a critical appraisal. *Eur J Anaesthesiol.* 2003;20: 600-605.
57. Van Akne H, Puchstein C, Schweppe ML, Heinecke A. Effect of labetalol on intracranial pressure in dogs with and without intracranial hypertension. *Acta Anaesthesiol Scand.* 1982;26: 615-619.
58. Muzzi DA, Black S, Losasso TJ, Cucchiara RF. Labetalol and esmolol in the control of hypertension after intracranial surgery. *Anesth Analg.* 1990;70:68-71.
59. Griswold WR, Reznik V, Mendoza SA. Nitroprusside-induced intracranial hypertension. *JAMA.* 1981;246:2679-2680.
60. Marsh ML, Shapiro HM, Smith RW, Marshall LF. Changes in neurologic status and intracranial pressure associated with sodium nitroprusside administration. *Anesthesiology.* 1979;51:336-338.
61. Dohi S, Matsumoto M, Takahashi T. The effects of nitroglycerin on cerebrospinal fluid pressure in awake and anesthetized humans. *Anesthesiology.* 1981;54:511-514.
62. Cottrell JE, Gupta B, Rappaport H, Turndorf H, Ransohoff J, Flamm ES. Intracranial pressure during nitroglycerin-induced hypotension. *J Neurosurg.* 1980;53:309-311.
63. Bedford RF, Dacey R, Winn HR, Lynch C III. Adverse impact of calcium entry-blocker (verapamil) on intracranial pressure in patients with brain tumors. *J Neurosurg.* 1983;59:800-802.
64. Gaab MR, Czech T, Korn A. Intracranial effects of nicardipine. *Br J Pharmacol.* 1985;20(suppl 1):67S-74S.
65. Ass IS. Physiology and metabolism of the brain and spinal cord. In: Newfield P, Cottrell JE, eds. *Handbook of Neuroanesthesia.* 3rd ed. Philadelphia: Lippincott Williams & Wilkins; 1999: 3-19.
66. Lanier WL, Weglinski MR. Intracranial pressure. In: Cucchiara RF, Michenfelder JD, eds. *Clinical Neuroanesthesia.* New York: Churchill Livingstone; 1990:77-115.
67. Weaver DD, Winn HR, Jane JA. Differential intracranial pressure in patients with unilateral mass lesions. *J Neurosurg.* 1982;56:660-665.
68. Miller JD, Garibi J, Pickard JD. Induced changes of cerebrospinal fluid volume. *Arch Neurol.* 1973;28:265-269.
69. Todd MM, Maktabi M, Warner DS. Neuroanesthesia: a critical review. In: Longnecker D, Tinker J, Morgan GE, eds. *Principles and Practice of Anesthesiology.* Baltimore: Mosby; 1998:1615.
70. Jenkinson JL. Neuroanesthesia. In: Nimmo WS, Smith G, eds. *Anaesthesia.* Oxford: Blackwell Scientific; 1989:576-593.
71. Pavlin EG. Emergency anaesthesia and trauma. In: Nimmo WS, Smith G, eds. *Anaesthesia.* Oxford: Blackwell Scientific; 1989:687-692.
72. Morgan GE, Mikhail MS. Anesthesia for neurosurgery. In: *Clinical Anesthesiology.* 3rd ed. New York: Lange Medical; 2003:567-570.
73. Miller JD, Sullivan HG. Severe intracranial hypertension. *Int Anesthesiol Clin.* 1989;17:19-75.

74. Cottrell JE, Robustelli A, Post K, Turndorf H. Furosemide- and mannitol-induced changes in intracranial pressure and serum osmolality and electrolytes. *Anesthesiology*. 1977;47:28-30.
75. Albright AL, Latchaw RE, Robinson AG. Osmotic and oncotic therapy in experimental cerebral edema. *J Neurosurg*. 1984;60:481-489.
76. Cote CJ, Greenhow DE, Marshall BE. The hypotensive response to rapid intravenous administration of hypertonic solutions in man and in the rabbit. *Anesthesiology*. 1979;50:30-35.
77. Sakabe T. Anesthetic management of head trauma. In: Newfield P, Cottrell JE, eds. *Handbook of Neuroanesthesia*. 3rd ed. New York: Lippincott Williams & Wilkins; 1999:129-145.
78. Kobrine AL, Kempe LG. Studies in head injury: part II. Effect of dexamethasone on traumatic brain swelling. *Surg Neurol*. 1973;1:38.
79. Braakman R, Schouten HJ, Blaauw-van Dishoeck M, Minderhoud JM. Megadose steroids in severe head injury: results of a prospective double-blind clinical trial. *J Neurosurg*. 1983;58:326-330.
80. Mears SL, Sperry RJ. Fluid management. In: Sperry RJ, Stirt JA, Stone DJ, eds. *Manual of Neuroanesthesia*. Philadelphia: Decker; 1989:107-118.
81. Tommasino C. Fluid management. In: Newfield P, Cottrell JE, eds. *Handbook of Neuroanesthesia*. 3rd ed. New York: Lippincott Williams & Wilkins; 1999:368-384.
82. Prough DS, Johnson JC, Stump DA, Stullken EH, Poole GV Jr, Howard G. Effects of hypertonic saline versus lactated Ringer's solution on cerebral oxygen transport during resuscitation from hemorrhagic shock. *J Neurosurg*. 1986;64:627-632.
83. Tommasino C. Fluids and the neurosurgical patient. *Anesthesiol Clin North Am*. 2002;20:329-346.
84. Pulsinelli WA, et al. Moderate hyperglycemia augments ischemic brain damage: a neurological study in the rat. *Neurology*. 1982;32:1239-1246.
85. Ravussin PA, Wilder-Smith, O. General anaesthesia for supratentorial neurosurgery. *CNS Drugs*. 2001;15:527-535.
86. Michenfelder JD, Miller RH, Gronert GA. Evaluation of an ultrasonic device (precordial Doppler) for the diagnosis of venous air embolus. *Anesthesiology*. 1972;36:164-167.
87. Voorhies RM, Frasier RAR, Van Poznak A. Prevention of air embolism with positive-end expiratory pressure. *Neurosurgery*. 1983;12:503-506.
88. Adornato DC, Gildenberg PL, Ferrario CM, Smart J, Frost EA. Pathophysiology of intravenous air embolism in dogs. *Anesthesiology*. 1978;49:120-127.
89. Standiferd M, Bay JW, Truso R. The sitting position in neurosurgery: a retrospective analysis of 488 cases. *Neurosurgery*. 1984;14:649-659.
90. Matjasko J, Petrozza P, Cohen M, Steinberg P. Anesthesia and surgery in the seated position: analysis of 554 cases. *Neurosurgery*. 1985;17:695-702.
91. Young ML, Smith DS, Murtagh F, Vasquez A, Levitt J. Comparison of surgical and anesthetic complications in neurosurgical patients experiencing venous air embolism in the sitting position. *Neurosurgery*. 1986;18:157-161.
92. Perkins-Pearson NAK, Marshall WK, Bedford RF. Atrial pressures in the seated position: implications for paradoxical air embolism. *Anesthesiology*. 1982;57:493-498.
93. Butler BD, Hills BA. The lungs as a filter for microbubbles. *J Appl Physiol*. 1979;47:537-543.
94. Todd MM. Monitoring in neuroanesthesia. In: Saidman L, Smith T, eds. *Monitoring in Anesthesia*. 3rd ed. Boston: Butterworth-Heinemann; 1993:180.
95. Culley DJ, Crosby G. Anesthesia for posterior fossa surgery. In: Newfield P, Cottrell JE, eds. *Handbook of Neuroanesthesia*. 3rd ed. New York: Lippincott Williams & Wilkins; 1999:165-174.
96. Tinker JH. Detection of air embolism: a test for positioning of right atrial catheter and Doppler probe. *Anesthesiology*. 1975;43:104-106.
97. Bedford RF, Marshall WK, Butler A, Welsh JE. Cardiac catheters for diagnosis and treatment of venous air embolism: a prospective study in man. *J Neurosurg*. 1981;55:610-614.
98. Cucchiara RF, Nugent M, Seward JB, Messick JM. Air embolism in upright neurosurgical patients: detection and localization by two-dimensional transesophageal echocardiography. *Anesthesiology*. 1984;60:353-355.
99. Munson ES, Merrick HC. Effect of nitrous oxide on venous air embolism. *Anesthesiology*. 1966;27:783-787.
100. Cottrell JE, Smith DS. Posterior fossa: anesthetic considerations. In: *Anesthesia and Neurosurgery*. 4th ed. St Louis: Mosby; 2002:335-352.
101. Colohan AR, Perkins NA, Bedford RF, Jane JA. Intravenous fluid loading as prophylaxis for paradoxical air embolism. *J Neurosurg*. 1985;62:839-842.
102. Durant TM, Long J, Oppenheimer MJ. Pulmonary (venous) air embolism. *Am Heart J*. 1947;33:269.
103. Liutkus D, Gouraud JP, Blanloeil Y. The sitting position in neurosurgical anaesthesia: a survey of French practice. *Ann Fr Anesth Reanim*. 2003;22:296-300.
104. Porter JM, Pidgeon C, Cunningham AJ. The sitting position in neurosurgery: a critical appraisal. *Br J Anaesth*. 1999;82:117-128.
105. Matijasko MJ. Neuroendocrine procedures. In: *Handbook of Neuroanesthesia*. 3rd ed. New York: Lippincott Williams & Wilkins; 1999:207-213.
106. Cucchiara RF, Benefiel DJ, Matteo RS, DeWood M, Albin MS. Evaluation of esmolol in controlling increases in heart rate and blood pressure during endotracheal intubation in patients undergoing carotid endarterectomy. *Anesthesiology*. 1986;65:528-531.
107. Matjasko MJ. Anesthetic Consideration in Patients with Neuroendocrine disease. In: Cottrell JE, Smith DS. *Anesthesia and Neurosurgery*. 4th ed. St Louis: Mosby; 2002:591-610.
108. Newfield P. Perioperative management of intracranial aneurysms. *ASA Annu Refresher Course Lect*. 1993;22:13-26.
109. Guy J, Gelb AW. Perioperative management of intracranial aneurysms. *Curr Rev Clin Anesth*. 1993;14:1-8.
110. Frost E. Management of neurosurgical anesthesia: aneurysms. *Curr Rev Clin Anesth*. 1991;11:125-132.
111. Herrick LA, Gelb AW. Anesthesia for intracranial aneurysm surgery. *J Clin Anesth*. 1992;4:73-85.
112. Kalfas IH, Little JR. Postoperative hemorrhage: a survey of 4992 intracranial procedures. *Neurosurgery*. 1988;23:343-347.
113. Macdonald RL, Weir BK, Runzer TD, et al. Etiology of cerebral vasospasm in primates. *J Neurosurg*. 1991;75:415-424.
114. Chyatte D. Anti-inflammatory agents and cerebral vasospasm. *Neurosurg Clin North Am*. 1990;1:433-450.
115. Petruk KC, West M, Mohr G, et al. Nimodipine treatment in poor-grade aneurysm patients: results in a multicenter double-blind placebo-controlled trial. *J Neurosurg*. 1988;68:505-517.
116. Pickard JD, Murray GD, Illingworth R, et al. Effect of oral nimodipine on cerebral infarction and outcome after subarachnoid haemorrhage: British aneurysm nimodipine trial. *BMJ*. 1989;298:636-642.
117. Meyer FB. Calcium antagonists and vasospasm: cerebral vasospasm. *Neurosurg Clin North Am*. 1990;1:367-376.
118. Taneda M. Effect of early operation for ruptured aneurysms on prevention of delayed ischemic symptoms. *J Neurosurg*. 1982;57:622-628.
119. Solomon RA, Fink ME, Lennihan L. Early aneurysm surgery and prophylactic hypervolemic hypertensive therapy for the treatment of aneurysmal subarachnoid hemorrhage. *Neurosurgery*. 1988;23:699-704.
120. Davies KR, Gelb AW, Manninen PH, Boughner DR, Bisnaire D. Cardiac function in aneurysmal subarachnoid hemorrhage: a study of electrocardiographic and echocardiographic abnormalities. *Br J Anaesth*. 1991;67:58-63.
121. Keane JF, Lam AM, Manninen PH. Monitoring of brain stem auditory evoked potentials during induced hypotension for

cerebral aneurysm surgery. *Can Anaesth Soc J.* 1984;31: 584-585.
122. Brown MM, Parr MJ, Manara AR. The effect of suxamethonium on intracranial pressure and cerebral perfusion pressure in patients with severe head injuries following blunt trauma. *Eur J Anaesthesiol.* 1996;13:474-477.
123. Minton MD, Stirt JA, Bedford RF. Intracranial pressure after atracurium in neurosurgical patients. *Anesth Analg.* 1985;64:113-116.
124. Clancy M, Halford S, Walls R, Murphy M. In patients with head injuries who undergo rapid sequence intubation using succinylcholine, does pretreatment with a competitive neuromuscular blocking agent improve outcome? A literature review. *Emerg Med J.* 2001;18:373-375.
125. Yasargil MF, Fox JL. The microsurgical approach to intracranial aneurysms. *Surg Neurol.* 1975;3:7-14.
126. Lagerkranser M. Controlled hypotension in neurosurgery. *J Neurosurg Anesthesiol.* 1991;3:150-152.
127. Charbel FT, Ausman JI, Diaz FG, Malik GM, Dujovny M, Sanders J. Temporary clipping in aneurysm surgery: technique and results. *Surg Neurol.* 1991;36:83-90.
128. Dodson BA. Interventional neuroradiology and the anesthetic management of patients with arteriovenous malformations. In Cottrell JE, Smith DS, eds. *Anesthesia and Neurosurgery.* 4th ed. St Louis: Mosby; 2001:399-424.
129. Gopinath SP, Robertson C. Management of severe head injury. In: Barash PG, Cullen BF, Stoelting RK, eds. *Clinical Anesthesia.* 4th ed. Philadelphia: Lippincott; 2001:663-692.
130. Grande CM, Barton CR, Stene JK. Appropriate techniques for airway management of emergency patients with suspected spinal cord injuries [letter]. *Anesth Analg.* 1988;67:714-715.
131. Becker P, Zieger S, Rother U, Lutz H, Osswald PM. Complement activation following head and brain trauma. *Anaesthetist.* 1987;36:301-305.
132. Konig SA, Schick U, Dohnert J, Goldammer A, Vitzthum HE. Coagulopathy and outcome in patients with chronic subdural haematoma. *Acta Neurol Scand.* 2003;107:110-116.
133. Bendo AA. Head trauma: management. In: Barash PG, Cullen BF, Stoelting RK, eds. *Clinical Anesthesia.* 4th ed. Philadelphia: Lippincott; 2001:398-408.
134. Kobayashi S, Nakazawa S, Otsua T. Clinical value of serial computed tomography with severe head injury. *Surg Neurol.* 1983;20:25-29.
135. Frankville DD, Drummond JC. Hyperkalemia after succinylcholine administration in a patient with closed head injury without paresis. *Anesthesiology.* 1987;67:264-266.
136. Manninen PH, Raman SK, Boyle K, elBeheiry H. Early postoperative complications following neurosurgical procedures. *Can J Anesth.* 1999;46:7-14.

CHAPTER 27

Renal Anatomy, Physiology, and Pathophysiology

Sandra Maree Ouellette, Sherry Owens

The kidneys are paired organs that lie retroperitoneally on both sides of the vertebral column. They function to excrete the end products of bodily metabolism and thereby control the concentration of constituents of body fluids. A rich blood supply to these vital organs, coupled with the physiologic processes of filtration, reabsorption, secretion, and excretion, maintains homeostasis of the fluid that bathes each cell. For management of anesthetized patients to be optimal, the anesthetist must be familiar with physiologic mechanisms that allow the kidneys to control the body's intracellular and extracellular environments.

This chapter addresses the impact of anesthesia and surgery on the normal and the diseased kidney. After a discussion of the anatomic structure and physiologic mechanisms of the kidney, the effects of anesthesia on normal renal function are addressed. Pathophysiologic mechanisms associated with acute and chronic renal failure are discussed. Preoperative renal assessment and anesthetic considerations for patients with impaired renal function are emphasized, and pertinent anesthetic considerations for common urologic procedures are identified.

STRUCTURE OF THE KIDNEY

The kidneys are bean-shaped, reddish-brown organs that are located in the posterior part of the abdomen on both sides of the vertebral column (Figure 27-1). These organs extend from the twelfth thoracic vertebra to the third lumbar vertebra; each organ weighs approximately 125 to 170 g in men and 115 to 155 g in women. Each kidney is approximately 11.25 cm long, 5 to 7.5 cm wide, and 2.5 cm thick. The right kidney is slightly lower than the left one because of hepatic displacement. The kidneys and their vessels are embedded in fatty tissue (perirenal fat) and are enclosed in renal fascia. Renal fascia and large vessels hold the kidneys in position.

The anterior and posterior surfaces, upper and lower poles, and lateral margin of the kidney have convex contours. The medial margin is concave because of the presence of the hilus. Structures that enter or leave the kidney through the hilus include the renal artery and vein, nerves, lymphatics, and ureters.

A longitudinal section of the kidney reveals two distinct regions—the outer cortex and the inner medulla (Figure 27-2). The medulla is divided into 8 to 18 triangular wedges called *pyramids*. The base of each pyramid is directed toward the renal cortex, and the apexes converge toward the renal pelvis. Pyramids have a striated appearance because they contain the loop of Henle and collecting ducts of the nephron. The apex of each pyramid, called the *papilla*, is composed of many collecting ducts. Papillary ducts empty into a cup-shaped structure known as the *minor calyx*. Several minor calyces join to form major calyces, which come together as the renal pelvis. The renal pelvis is the major reservoir for urine. Ureters connect the renal pelvis to the bladder.

Nephron

The functional unit of the kidney is the nephron. Approximately 1,250,000 of these units are present in each kidney. The shape of the nephron is unique, unmistakable, and admirably suited for its function. Each area of the nephron is selective with regard to its performance. Nephrons hold the filtrate that has been filtered from the blood. End products of metabolism are excreted, and metabolically important substances, such as water, are reabsorbed as needed.

The nephron (Figure 27-3) begins in the cortex at the glomerulus and ends where the tubule joins the collecting tubule at the papilla. The glomerulus is a tuft of capillaries derived from the afferent arteriole. Blood is brought to the glomerulus by the afferent arteriole; blood that is not filtered returns to the circulation by way of the efferent arteriole. The filtrate from the glomeruli enters Bowman's capsule, flows through a tortuous tube, or proximal convoluted tubule, and then goes to the loop of Henle, distal convoluted tubule, and collecting duct.

The nephron, which changes in shape and direction as it follows its course, is contained partly in the renal cortex and partly in the medulla (Figure 27-4, p. 635). The cortex contains Bowman's capsule, the glomerulus, and the proximal and distal tubules. The thin, descending loop of Henle comes from the proximal tubule and dips toward the pyramid. At some point it bends on itself and forms an enlarged, ascending loop of Henle. The ascending limb joins the distal convoluted tubule.[1]

The kidneys have two kinds of nephrons: cortical nephrons, which extend only partially into the medulla, and juxtamedullary nephrons, which lie deep in the cortex and extend deep into the medulla. One fifth to one third of the nephrons are juxtamedullary and play an important role in concentration of urine.

Renal Blood Supply

To understand how the kidneys function, it is essential to know how blood is brought to them. The kidneys are highly vascular. Although they represent only 0.5% of body weight, they receive 1100 to 1200 ml of blood per minute, or 20% to 25% of the cardiac output. Blood reaches these organs through the

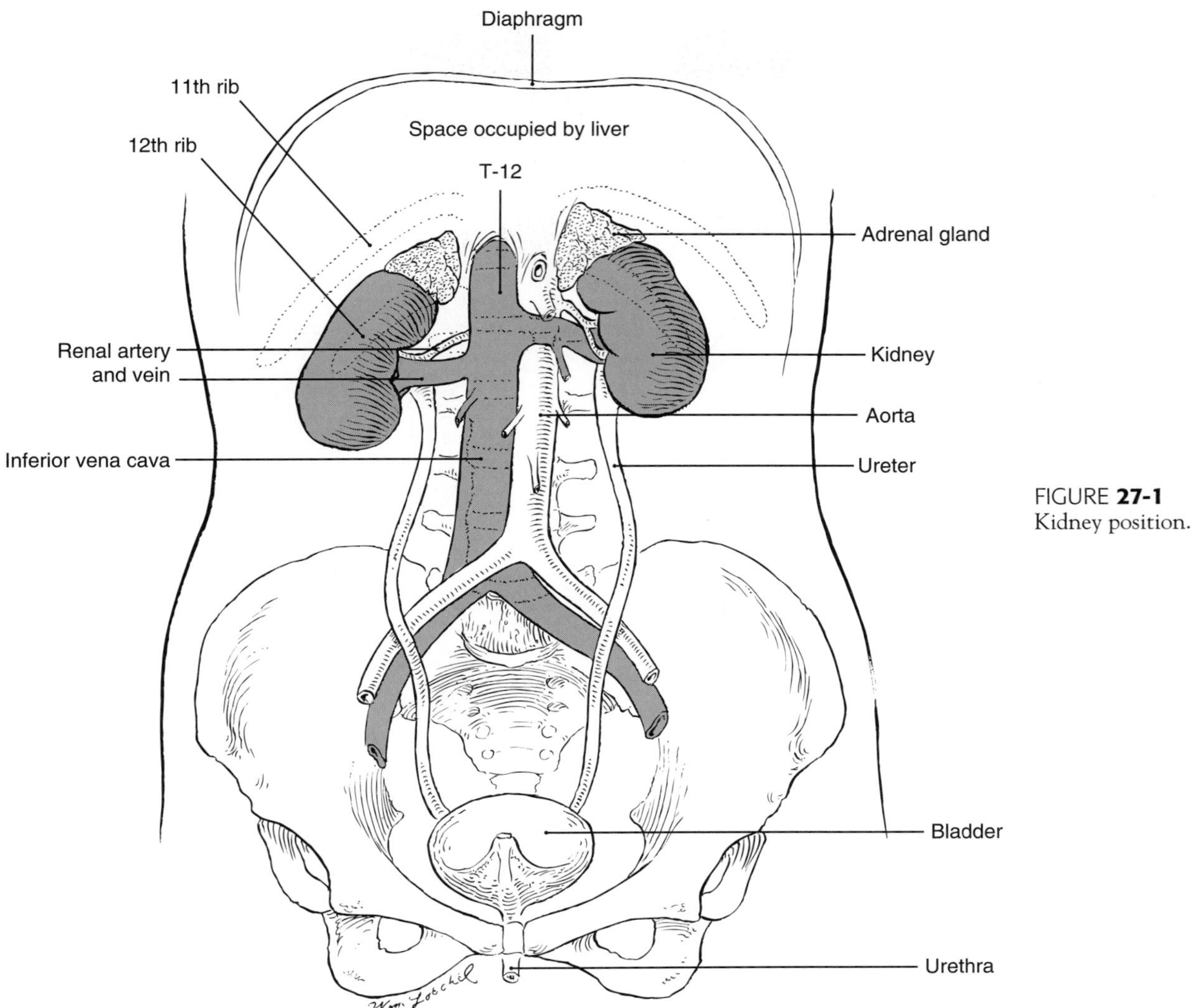

FIGURE **27-1**
Kidney position.

renal arteries. At the hilus of the kidney the renal artery divides into several lobar arteries and then subdivides again into interlobar arteries, which run between the pyramids. When these vessels reach the corticomedullary zone, they make well-defined arches over the bases of the pyramids. These vessels, known as *arcuate arteries*, give off a series of vessels known as *interlobular arteries*. An interlobular artery may terminate as an afferent arteriole or as a nutrient artery to the tubule.

The afferent arterioles form the high-pressure capillary bed within Bowman's capsule called the *glomerulus*. Because little or no oxygen is removed in the glomerulus, the blood that is not filtered begins its passage to the venous system via the efferent arteriole. The efferent arteriole is smaller than the afferent arteriole, thereby affording some resistance to blood flow. The efferent vessel soon becomes a plexus of capillaries again, and this low-pressure bed is known as the *peritubular capillary*. The peritubular capillary bed winds and twists around the proximal and distal tubule. At one point a few hairpin loops called *vasa recta* dip down among the loops of Henle. Anatomic arrangements of these capillary beds and the renal tubules set the stage for filtration, reabsorption, and concentration of urine.

After leaving the peritubular capillary, blood returns to the central circulation via the veins. Renal veins are named in reverse order of the arteries, and therefore are the interlobular, arcuate, interlobar, lobar, and renal veins. The renal vein leaves the kidney at the hilus and empties into the inferior vena cava.

The portion of the cardiac output that passes through the kidney is called the *renal fraction*. Because cardiac output in a 70-kg man is approximately 5600 ml/min and blood flow through both kidneys is 1200 ml/min, the normal renal fraction is 21%. This flow may vary from 12% to 30%. Distribution of renal blood flow is to the renal cortex and the medulla, with the cortex receiving the larger amount. Values obtained from dogs indicate that 3 to 5 ml/g/min are distributed to the cortex, 1 to 2 ml/g/min to the outer medulla, and 0.3 to 0.6 ml/g/min to the inner medulla. Only a small portion of blood (1% to 2%) flows through the vasa recta in the medulla.

Regulation of Renal Blood Flow

Blood flow to any organ is determined by the arteriovenous pressure difference across the vascular bed and is given by the following relationship:

Equation 27-1

$$\text{Renal blood flow} = (\text{MAP} - \text{VP}) \times \text{VR}$$

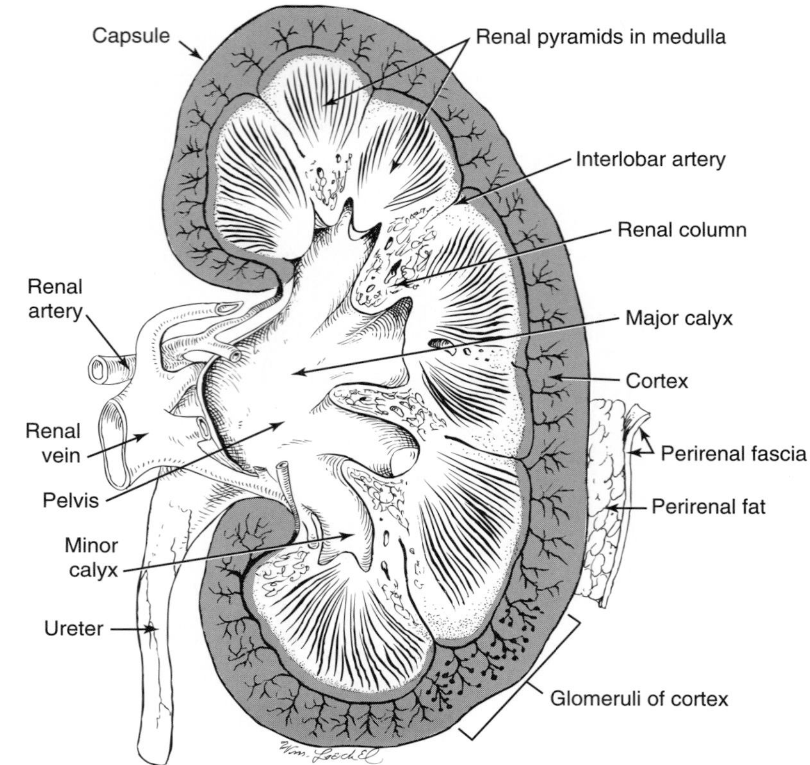

FIGURE **27-2**
Longitudinal section of the kidney.

where MAP is the mean arterial pressure, VP is the venous pressure, and VR is the vascular resistance. Renal blood flow is regulated by intrinsic autoregulation and neural regulation.

Autoregulation of renal blood flow implies that blood flow remains normal despite a considerable change in pressure. With a MAP between 75 and 160 mm Hg, renal blood flow to both kidneys remains 1200 ml/min. If mean systemic blood pressure falls below 60 mm Hg, filtration ceases. Afferent arteriole vasodilation and myogenic mechanisms are responsible for autoregulation.

When renal blood flow decreases, glomerular filtration is reduced. A reduction in glomerular filtration leads to dilation of the afferent arteriole. An increase in blood flow to the glomerulus returns glomerular filtration to normal.

Myogenic mechanisms also play a role in renal autoregulation. When arterial pressure rises, the arterial wall is stretched, the vessel constricts, and blood flow remains normal. When arterial pressure decreases, the opposite effect occurs. Therefore renal blood flow remains constant over a wide range of pressure changes.

Neural regulation also has a role in renal blood flow. The sympathetic nervous system innervates both the afferent and efferent arterioles. Although autoregulation overrides the adrenergic system with mild stimulation, acute sympathetic stimulation with its associated vasoconstriction can decrease renal blood flow substantially. The parasympathetic nervous system is not physiologically significant.

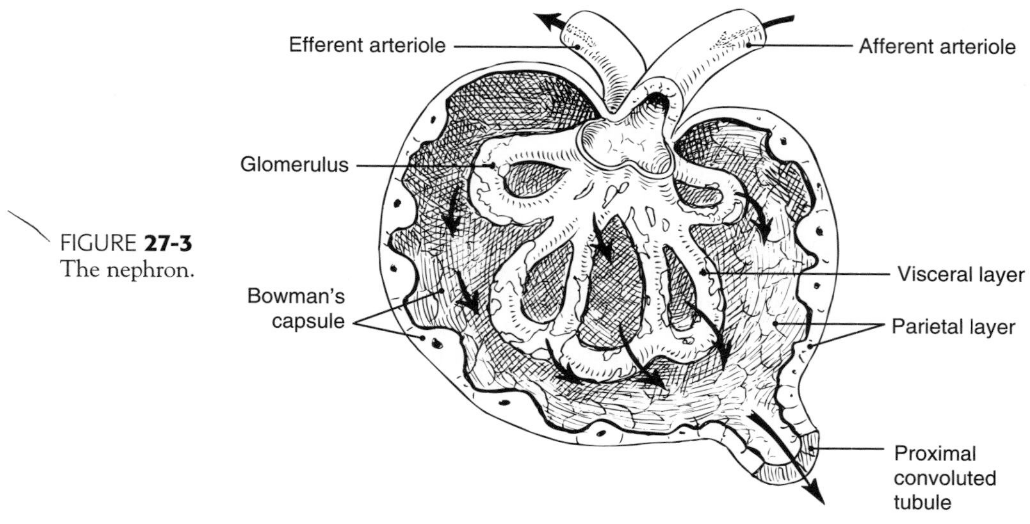

FIGURE **27-3**
The nephron.

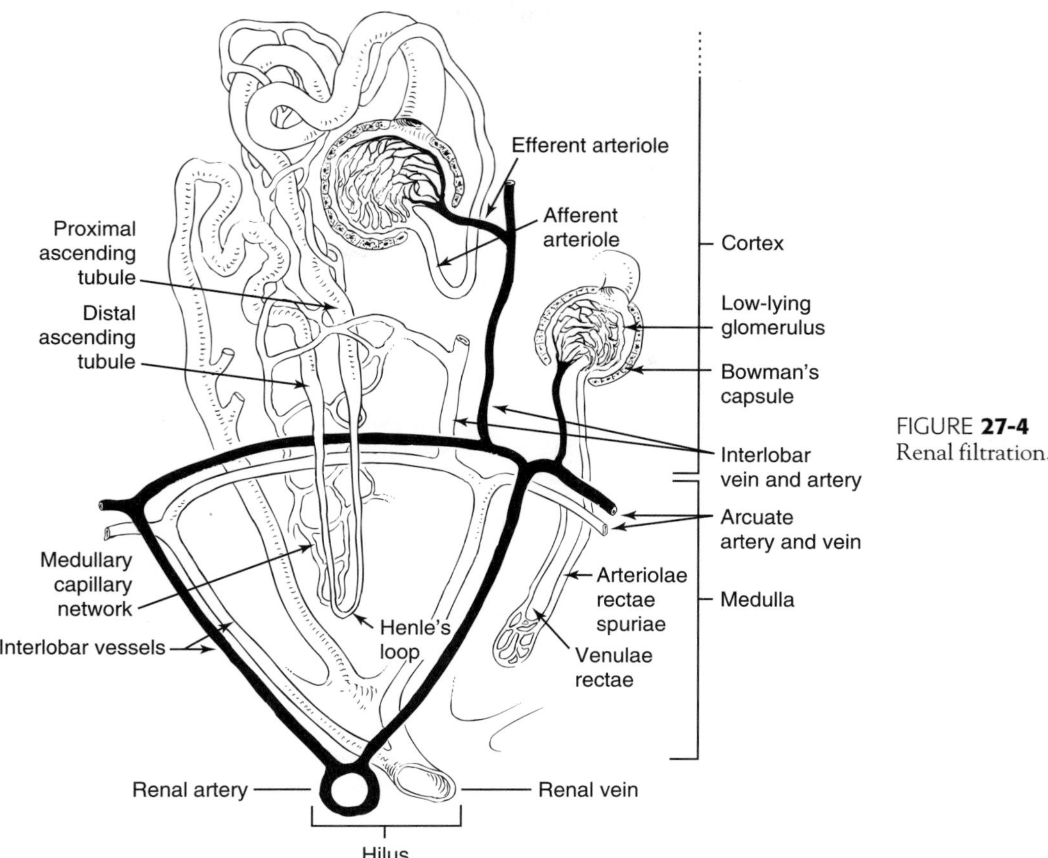

FIGURE **27-4**
Renal filtration.

RENAL PHYSIOLOGY

The kidneys maintain a steady state that is essential to life. This is accomplished by three major mechanisms: filtration, reabsorption, and tubular secretion. What is filtered or secreted but not reabsorbed is excreted as urine.

Filtration

Filtration, which results from pressures that force fluids and solutes through the glomerulus, is the first step in the formation of urine. The quantity of glomerular filtrate formed each minute in all nephrons is called the *glomerular filtration rate* (GFR). The filtration fraction is the quantity of renal plasma flow that becomes filtrate and is defined as GFR divided by the flow to one kidney. Because the GFR is approximately 125 ml/min and the flow to one kidney is 650 ml/min, the filtration fraction is 125/650, or 19% (approximately one fifth) of plasma flow. Of the 125 ml/min, or 180 L/day, of this protein-free filtrate that is made, 99% is reabsorbed from the renal tubules, and the remaining small portion is excreted as urine.

Regulation of Glomerular Filtration Rate

Glomerular filtration is also dependent on several physiologic factors:

- The pressure inside the glomerular capillaries
- The pressure in Bowman's capsule
- The colloid osmotic pressure of the plasma proteins

The pressure inside the high-pressure glomerulus (60 mm Hg) is an outward force, whereas the colloid osmotic pressure created by proteins in the glomerulus (28 mm Hg) is an inward force that tends to hold fluid within the glomerulus. Pressure in Bowman's capsule (18 mm Hg) opposes filtration. As illustrated in Figure 27-4, filtration pressure is the pressure that forces fluid through the glomerular membrane. It is equal to the glomerular pressure minus the sum of the glomerular colloid osmotic pressure and the capsular pressure. With the values given, the normal filtration pressure is 10 mm Hg. Several factors can alter GFR. Increased renal blood flow, dilation of the afferent arteriole, and increased resistance in the efferent arteriole increase GFR. Afferent arteriole constriction and efferent arteriole dilation tend to decrease GFR.

A special structure called the *juxtaglomerular complex* regulates GFR. At the juxtaglomerular complex the distal convoluted tubule lies between the afferent and efferent arterioles. Cells of the distal tubule coming in contact with the arterioles are dense and therefore are referred to as the *macula densa.* Smooth muscle cells of both the afferent and efferent arterioles consist of juxtaglomerular cells, which contain renin. Anatomically this structure is arranged to allow fluid in the distal tubule to alter afferent or efferent arteriolar tone and thus regulate GFR.

Decreased glomerular filtration causes overabsorption of sodium ions (Na^+) and chloride ions (Cl^-) in the ascending limb of the loop of Henle and therefore a reduction in the delivery of these ions to the macula densa. Decreases in the concentrations of sodium and chloride cause afferent arterioles to dilate and thus increase renal blood flow and GFR. Sympathetic stimulation and decreased delivery of sodium and chloride to the macula densa also cause the juxtaglomerular cells to release renin. Renin clears angiotensinogen from the liver to form angiotensin I. In the lung angiotensin I is changed into angiotensin II under the influence of a converting enzyme. In addition to having a generalized vasoconstricting effect, angiotensin II causes constriction of the efferent arteriole. This causes the pressure in the glomerulus to increase and the GFR to return to normal.

Filtrate Composition

Although permeability at the glomerulus is 100- to 500-fold greater than that of most capillaries, filtration at the glomerulus is a selective process. The process by which some substances are filtered and others are not is not completely understood. It is thought that the glomerular capillary contains pores that are negatively charged. These pores, which are 70 to 100 nm in size, are freely permeable to water, some ions, and small molecules. Molecules with diameters up to 80 nm that do not have a negative charge are easily filtered. The glomerulus is almost impermeable to all plasma proteins but highly permeable to most other dissolved substances. Glomerular filtrate is therefore similar to plasma, except that it lacks significant amounts of proteins.

Tubular Reabsorption and Secretion

Conversion of glomerular filtrate to urine is the result of filtration at the glomerulus, tubular reabsorption or transport from the tubular lumen to the renal cell, and secretion or transport from the renal cell to the filtrate. Of all that is filtered or secreted, 99% is reabsorbed as the filtrate moves along the nephron.

Tubular reabsorption permits conservation of essential substances such as water, glucose, amino acids, and electrolytes. Some substances, such as water and sodium, are reabsorbed throughout the nephron, whereas others, such as glucose, are completely reabsorbed when plasma concentrations are low. Certain substances have a reabsorption maximum value. After it is reached, excess filtered material is excreted regardless of plasma concentration. This maximum value is termed *maximum transport*. Maximum transport occurs because of saturation of a carrier for a particular substance.

By the time the blood has reached the peritubular capillary, one fifth of the plasma has been filtered into Bowman's capsule. The hydrostatic pressure in this low-pressure capillary bed has dropped to 13 mm Hg, whereas the osmotic pressure has increased to 30 to 32 mm Hg. The peritubular capillaries are extremely porous in comparison with those in other body tissues, and their proximity to the proximal and distal tubule sets the stage for movement of water and solutes from the tubule to the peritubular capillary bed. Anatomic location and the colloid osmotic pressure of the plasma proteins account for the rapid absorption required in this area.

Transport Mechanisms

Basic mechanisms of transport through the tubular membrane can be divided into active transport and passive transport. Active transport is the net movement of particles across a membrane against an electrochemical gradient, generally at the cost of metabolic energy. Passive transport involves the movement of substances across membranes that relies on concentration or chemical gradients. Active transport can be further divided into primary active transport, which requires energy, and secondary active transport, which does not require energy. Most primary active transport is for sodium. Secondary active transport is a result of the movement of sodium from the tubular lumen to the interior of the cell. For example, the active transport of sodium pulls glucose and amino acids with it. Because a carrier protein in the membrane combines with sodium and glucose, the process is termed *cotransport*. In addition to glucose and amino acids, chloride, phosphate, calcium, magnesium, and hydrogen ions are cotransported.

Some substances are secondarily actively secreted into the renal tubule. Hydrogen, potassium, and urate ions are secreted in this manner. Hydrogen or potassium is generally secreted in exchange for sodium in a process termed *countertransport*.

When substances are actively transported from the tubule to the peritubular capillary bed, a concentration gradient that causes passive absorption of water by osmosis is established. When positive ions are actively transported, negative ions follow to maintain electrical neutrality. Chloride ions and urea are examples of substances that are passively absorbed.

Proximal Tubule

Each portion of the renal nephron is selective with regard to what is reabsorbed or secreted. Active transport of sodium is the primary function of the proximal tubule. Water, most electrolytes, and organic substances are cotransported with sodium. The osmotic force generated by active sodium transport promotes passive diffusion of water out of the tubules into the peritubular capillaries. Passive transport of water is further enhanced by the elevated osmotic pressure of the blood in the peritubular capillaries. Reabsorption of water leaves an increased concentration of urea within the tubular lumen, thereby creating a gradient for its passive diffusion into the peritubular plasma. As positively charged sodium ions leave the tubular lumen, negatively charged chloride ions passively follow to maintain electroneutrality. Hydrogen ions are actively secreted in exchange for sodium. Secretory transport of sodium also occurs in the proximal tubule.

As the filtrate passes along the proximal tubule, 60% to 70% of filtered sodium and water, 50% of urea, and potassium, calcium, phosphate, uric acid, and the bicarbonate (HCO_3) form of carbon dioxide (CO_2) have been reabsorbed. Glucose, proteins, amino acids, acetoacetate ions, and vitamins are completely or almost completely reabsorbed by active processes. Because protein molecules are too large to be reabsorbed by normal mechanisms, a special mechanism called *pinocytosis* is used to save proteins. In this process the tubular membrane engulfs the protein and internalizes it. Once inside the cell the protein is digested into amino acids that can then be absorbed into the interstitial fluid.

Loop of Henle

The primary function of the loop of Henle is the establishment of a hyperosmotic state within the medullary area of the kidney, a mechanism vital to conservation of salt and water. Water conservation and the production of a concentrated urine involve a countercurrent exchange system in which a concentration gradient causes fluid to be exchanged across parallel pathways. The fluid moves up and down the parallel sides of the hairpin loop of Henle in the medulla. The longer the loop, the greater the concentration gradient, because the gradient increases from the cortex to medulla. Sluggish blood flow in the vasa recta helps maintain the gradient.

Countercurrent exchange begins in the thick ascending limb of the loop of Henle with the active transport of sodium and chloride out of the tubular lumen and into the medullary interstitium. Because the lumen in this area is impermeable to water, water cannot follow. The tubular fluid becomes hypo-osmotic, and the medullary interstitium hyperosmotic. The descending limb of the loop is highly permeable to water but does not actively transport sodium and chloride. Sodium and chloride diffuse into the interstitium, the hypertonic interstitium causes water to move out, and the remaining fluid in the descending loop becomes concentrated at the tip of the medulla. As the tubular fluid rounds the loop and enters the ascending limb, water is retained and sodium and chloride are removed. The filtrate, therefore, is very dilute as it reaches the distal tubule. The thick segment of the loop of Henle has a powerful role in renal mechanisms for diluting or concentrating the urine.

Late Distal Tubule

In the late distal tubule, sodium, under the influence of aldosterone, is reabsorbed. In this area, potassium is secreted into the lumen in exchange for sodium. It is mainly by this means that the potassium concentration is controlled in the extracellular fluids of the body.

The late distal tubule also secretes hydrogen against a concentration gradient. This function has a role in acid-base balance and the final degree of urine acidification. The late distal tubule reabsorbs 10% of filtered water. This area is permeable to water only in the presence of antidiuretic hormone (ADH).

Collecting Duct

The permeability of the collecting duct to water also is controlled by ADH. When this neurohypophyseal hormone is present, water is reabsorbed into the medullary interstitium, and the urine volume is reduced and concentrated. The collecting duct can also secrete hydrogen and therefore has a role in acid-base balance. Figure 27-5 illustrates renal blood flow, filtration, reabsorption, and secretion.

Renal Secretion

In addition to renin, hydrogen, and potassium, the kidneys release erythropoietin. Erythropoietin, a glycoprotein, stimulates red blood cell production in the bone marrow. Any condition that causes the quantity of oxygen transported to the tissues to decrease stimulates the release of erythropoietin, production of red blood cells, and correction of hypoxia. When both kidneys are destroyed by renal disease, the person invariably becomes very anemic.

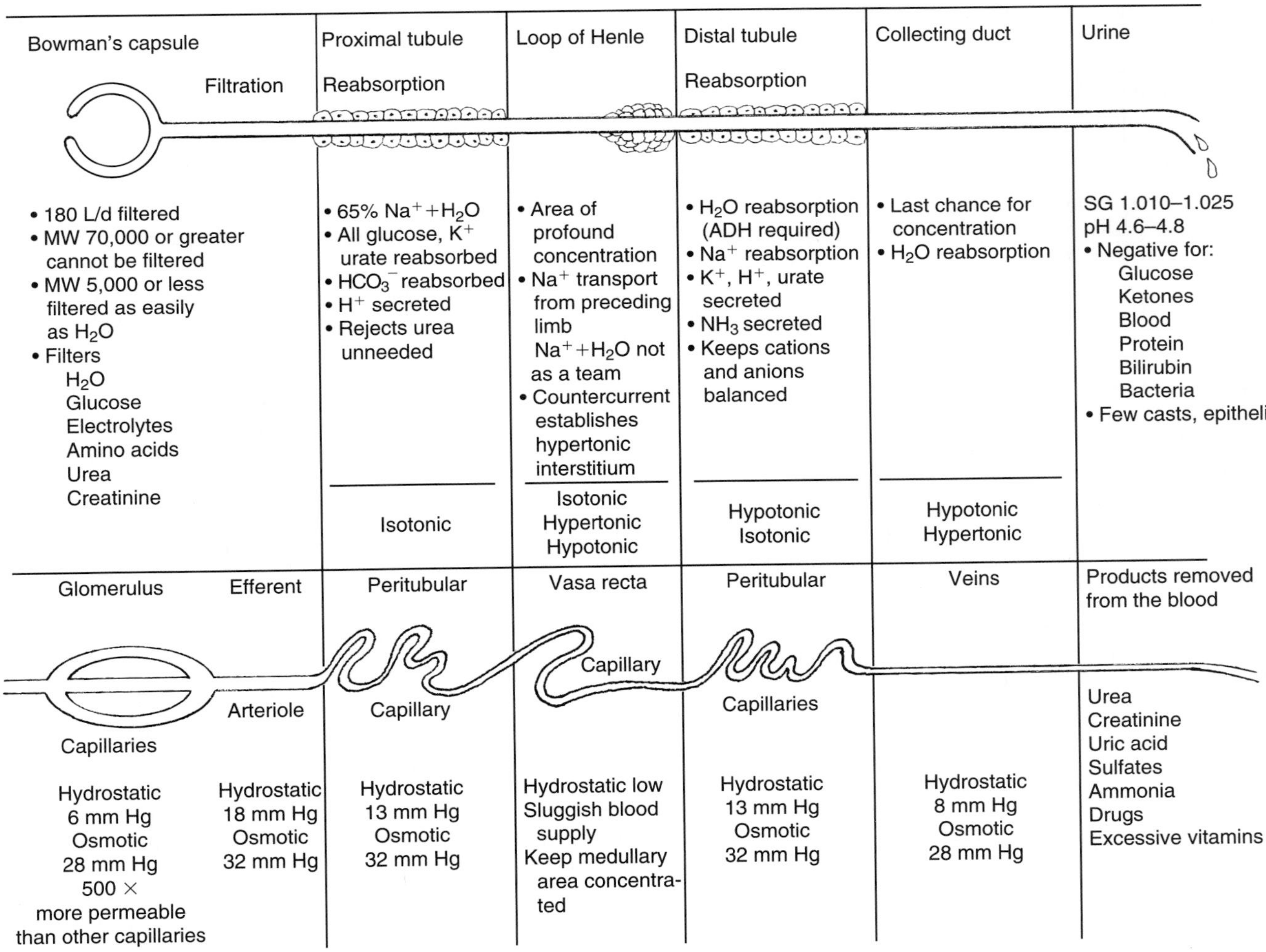

Bowman's capsule — Filtration	Proximal tubule — Reabsorption	Loop of Henle	Distal tubule — Reabsorption	Collecting duct	Urine
• 180 L/d filtered • MW 70,000 or greater cannot be filtered • MW 5,000 or less filtered as easily as H_2O • Filters H_2O Glucose Electrolytes Amino acids Urea Creatinine	• 65% $Na^+ + H_2O$ • All glucose, K^+ urate reabsorbed • HCO_3^- reabsorbed • H^+ secreted • Rejects urea unneeded	• Area of profound concentration • Na^+ transport from preceding limb $Na^+ + H_2O$ not as a team • Countercurrent establishes hypertonic interstitium	• H_2O reabsorption (ADH required) • Na^+ reabsorption • K^+, H^+, urate secreted • NH_3 secreted • Keeps cations and anions balanced	• Last chance for concentration • H_2O reabsorption	SG 1.010–1.025 pH 4.6–4.8 • Negative for: Glucose Ketones Blood Protein Bilirubin Bacteria • Few casts, epithelial cells
	Isotonic	Isotonic Hypertonic Hypotonic	Hypotonic Isotonic	Hypotonic Hypertonic	

Glomerulus — Capillaries	Efferent Arteriole	Peritubular Capillary	Vasa recta Capillary	Peritubular Capillaries	Veins	Products removed from the blood
Hydrostatic 6 mm Hg Osmotic 28 mm Hg 500 × more permeable than other capillaries	Hydrostatic 18 mm Hg Osmotic 32 mm Hg	Hydrostatic 13 mm Hg Osmotic 32 mm Hg	Hydrostatic low Sluggish blood supply Keep medullary area concentrated	Hydrostatic 13 mm Hg Osmotic 32 mm Hg	Hydrostatic 8 mm Hg Osmotic 28 mm Hg	Urea Creatinine Uric acid Sulfates Ammonia Drugs Excessive vitamins

FIGURE **27-5**
Renal blood flow, filtration, reabsorption, and secretion. *ADH*, Antidiuretic hormone; *SG*, specific gravity.

Renal Hormones

Aldosterone

A number of hormones affect renal function. Aldosterone, the chief mineralocorticoid produced by the adrenal cortex, affects the distal segment of the nephron, causing the reabsorption of sodium and water. Several physiologic control systems regulate aldosterone release: potassium concentration in extracellular fluid; the renin-angiotensin system; and the extracellular fluid sodium concentration. Of these, potassium is the stronger release, followed by renin and then sodium.

Antidiuretic Hormone

ADH, a hormone synthesized in the hypothalamus but released from the neurohypophysis, also has the distal nephron as its target tissue. Because the distal tubule and collecting ducts are almost totally impermeable to water in the absence of ADH, water is not reabsorbed and is lost in the urine. In the presence of ADH, tubular permeability is increased and water is reabsorbed. The release of ADH is controlled by the osmotic concentration of the extracellular fluids. Osmoreceptors located near the hypothalamus sense extracellular fluid concentration and release ADH accordingly. ADH is inhibited by stretch of atrial baroreceptors.

Angiotensin

Angiotensin is a hormone that has a direct renal effect as well as a general systemic effect. As previously discussed, renin is a small protein enzyme released by the kidneys. Stimuli for the release of renin include β-adrenergic stimulation, decreased perfusion to the afferent arterioles, and reduction in sodium delivery to the distal convoluted tubule. Once released, renin acts on hepatic angiotensinogen to form angiotensin I. Angiotensin I is converted by an enzyme in the lung to form angiotensin II. In addition to causing powerful vasoconstriction, angiotensin II stimulates the release of aldosterone from the adrenal cortex. Aldosterone increases salt and water retention by the kidneys. Both of these actions increase arterial pressure.[2]

Atrial Natriuretic Factor

Atrial natriuretic factor (ANF) is a peptide hormone synthesized, stored, and secreted by the cardiac atria.[3] It acts on the kidney to increase urine flow and sodium excretion, and it may enhance renal blood flow and GFR. In addition, ANF antagonizes both the release and end-organ effects of renin, aldosterone, and ADH. The stimulus for ANF release is atrial distention, stretch, or pressure.[4] It is one of the most potent diuretics known. Inhibition of plasma renin, angiotensin, and aldosterone can produce a dose-dependent decrease in blood pressure.

Vitamin D

Vitamin D, along with parathyroid hormone and calcitonin, has a vital role in calcium metabolism. Vitamin D or cholecalciferol is obtained in the diet or synthesized by the action of ultraviolet radiation on cholesterol in the skin. To become active, cholecalciferol is hydroxylated in the kidney, first to 25-hydroxycholecalciferol, and then to 1,25-dihydroxycholecalciferol. Patients with advanced renal disease often have abnormal serum calcium levels.

Prostaglandins

Prostaglandins (PGs) such as PGE_2 and thromboxane A_2 modulate the renal effects of other hormones. PGE_2 is a vasodilator, and thromboxane A_2 produces contraction of vascular smooth muscle. Renal PGs influence renal excretion.

Renal Regulation of Acid-Base Balance

The kidneys, along with the body's fluid buffers and respiratory system, play a major role in the regulation of acid-base balance. Epithelial cells of the proximal tubules, thick portion of the loop of Henle, distal tubules, and collecting ducts secrete hydrogen into the tubular fluid. This secretory process actually begins with CO_2 in the epithelial cells. CO_2, under the influence of carbonic anhydrase, combines with water to form carbonic acid (H_2CO_3). H_2CO_3 dissociates into HCO_3 and hydrogen ions, and hydrogen ions are actively secreted into tubular fluid in exchange for sodium ions. This exchange maintains appropriate electrical balance between anions and cations in the tubular fluid.

An increase in HCO_3 in alkalosis means that the amount of HCO_3 filtered exceeds the amount of hydrogen secreted. Because excess HCO_3 must react with hydrogen ($HCO_3^- + H^+ \rightarrow H_2CO_3 \rightarrow CO_2^- + H_2O$) and be absorbed as CO_2, excess HCO_3 ions are lost in the urine along with sodium. In this way, sodium and excess HCO_3 are removed from the extracellular fluid.

In acidosis the concentration of hydrogen ions increases to a level that is far greater than that of HCO_3 in the tubules. Excess hydrogen ions are lost in the urine through the phosphate or ammonia (NH_3) buffer system.

The phosphate buffer is composed of hydrogen phosphate (HPO_2^-) and dihydrogen phosphate (H_2PO_4). Both of these ions become concentrated in the tubular fluid because of poor reabsorption. The quantity of HPO_2^- is normally fourfold greater than that of H_2PO_4. Excess hydrogen ions entering the tubules combine with monohydrogen phosphate to form H_2PO_4, which is lost in the urine. A sodium ion is absorbed into the extracellular fluid in exchange for hydrogen. It combines with HCO_3, which was formed in the process of secretion of the hydrogen, and sodium bicarbonate is added to the extracellular fluid.

NH_3, which is synthesized by all epithelial cells except those in the thin segment of the loop of Henle, is also secreted into the tubules. NH_3 reacts with hydrogen to form the ammonium ion (NH_4). Ammonium ions are lost in the urine with chloride and other tubular anions.

The kidneys control extracellular fluid hydrogen concentration by excreting an acidic or basic urine. Excretion of acidic urine removes excess acid from the extracellular fluid, whereas loss of basic urine removes base from the extracellular fluid.

Concentration and Dilution of Urine

The kidneys have the ability to respond to the changing tonicity of body fluids by excreting a dilute or concentrated urine. This function involves a countercurrent exchange system in which a concentration gradient causes fluid to be exchanged across parallel pathways (Figure 27-6). In a countercurrent exchanger, reversal of flow in one stream results in the formation of a gradient that allows water and solutes to be exchanged along the length of the tube. The countercurrent exchanger in the kidney is the descending and ascending loop of Henle. The concentration gradient increases from the cortex to the tip of the medulla. The anatomic arrangement of this part of the nephron and sluggish blood flow in the vasa recta help maintain the gradient.

Plasma water filtered at the glomerulus is isotonic with plasma. The daily urinary output is approximately 1.5 L/day,

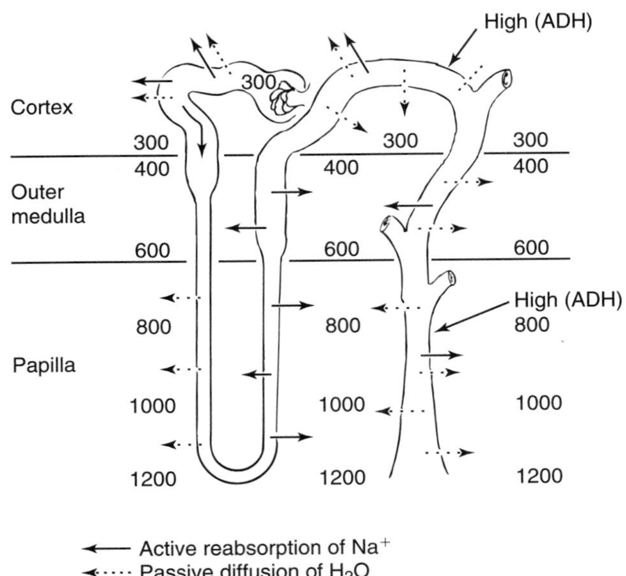

FIGURE **27-6**
The countercurrent mechanism.

and its osmolarity may vary from 40 to 1400 mOsm/L, depending on water intake or loss. This is possible because of the countercurrent mechanism.

Approximately two thirds of the tubular fluid is reabsorbed between the glomerulus and the end of the proximal tubule. The tonicity of the filtrate in this area is the same as that of the surrounding tissue, or 300 mOsm. As the filtrate leaves the proximal tubule, it passes through an increasingly more concentrated medulla. Changes in the thick ascending limb of the loop of Henle are responsible for the hypertonicity.

The thick ascending limb of the loop of Henle is responsible for the active transport of sodium and chloride into the medullary interstitium. In contrast to the descending limb of the loop of Henle, the tonicity of which is in equilibrium with that of the interstitium, the ascending loop has a low permeability to water. The active transport of sodium and chloride produces a gradient between the ascending loop of Henle on one side and the descending loop and interstitium of the renal medulla on the other. The descending limb is highly permeable to water but does not actively transport sodium and chloride. The hyperosmotic interstitium causes water to move out of the descending limb, and the filtrate in the descending tubule is concentrated to 1200 mOsm at the tip of the medulla. As the tubular fluid rounds the loop and enters the ascending limb, active transport of sodium and chloride and retention of water create a hypoosmotic fluid of 100 mOsm at the distal tubule.

The hypoosmotic fluid of the distal tubule is delivered to the collecting duct, where the final adjustments of urine volume and concentration take place. In the absence of ADH water permeability is low, and water is not reabsorbed. Because Na^+ and Cl^- can be reabsorbed, the osmolality decreases to below that of the distal tubule, and the urine is dilute. When the need for water conservation develops, ADH is secreted, permeability of the collecting duct increases, and water diffuses out of the duct into the hyperosmolar environment of the medullary extracellular fluid. In this way urine is concentrated and its volume is reduced.

A sluggish blood supply of the vasa recta in the medulla allows blood to flow through the medullary tissue without disturbing the osmotic gradient. If blood flow were rapid, the medullary concentration gradient and the ability to concentrate the urine would be lost.

EFFECTS OF ANESTHESIA ON NORMAL RENAL FUNCTION

Before considering anesthetic implications for patients with renal disease, it is important to review the effects of anesthesia and surgery on normal renal function. Numerous studies have attempted to identify the effects of anesthesia on renal function. Although some have contributed to a better understanding of this area, differences among the studies in premedication, depth of anesthesia, fluid regimens, and other aspects of the experimental protocol allow only the broadest comparisons.

Anesthetic Effects

General anesthesia is associated with a temporary depression of renal blood flow, GFR, urinary flow, and electrolyte excretion. Although similar changes occur after spinal and epidural anesthesia, the magnitude of change tends to parallel the degree of sympathetic block and blood pressure depression. This consistent and generalized depression of renal function has been attributed to a number of factors, including type and duration of surgical procedure, physical status of the patient, volume and electrolyte status, depth of anesthesia, and choice of agent.[5]

Anesthesia may alter renal function by direct or indirect effects. Indirect effects are mediated through changes in the circulatory, endocrine, or sympathetic nervous system. Anesthetic drugs alter the circulatory system by decreasing renal perfusion, increasing renal VR, or a combination of both. Drugs associated with catecholamine release lead to vasoconstriction, an increase in renal VR, a decrease in renal blood flow, and a decrease in renal function. Volatile agents such as halothane and isoflurane cause a mild to moderate increase in renal VR as a compensatory response to decreased perfusion pressure secondary to alterations in cardiac output or systemic VR.[6-10] Desflurane has been shown to produce hemodynamic effects comparable to those produced by isoflurane.[11] It increases heart rate and decreases both MAP and systemic VR while maintaining cardiac output. In some studies, but not all, desflurane maintains arterial pressure and systemic VR to a greater degree than equianesthetic concentrations of isoflurane. Otherwise, desflurane and isoflurane have similar effects on most vascular beds, including the renal circulation. Although earlier studies suggested that renal blood flow was reduced with sevoflurane, no renal functional or morphologic defects were noted after administration of this agent. Issues regarding the renal effects of the release of free fluoride ion associated with sevoflurane metabolism have been debated. Historically, high fluoride ion concentrations in the range of 60 to 90 mmol/L after methoxyflurane metabolism have led to nephrotoxicity characterized by polyuria. Sevoflurane has not acted in the same way as methoxyflurane. Intrarenal production of inorganic fluoride may be a more important factor than hepatic metabolism for the nephrotoxicity that causes increased serum fluoride concentration. Sevoflurane is not associated with nephrotoxicity.[12,13]

Changes in renal function during barbiturate, opiate, and nitrous oxide anesthesia are similar to those observed during the administration of low-dose volatile anesthesia.[14] Preoperative hydration, lower concentrations of volatile anesthetics, and maintenance of normal blood pressure attenuate reductions in renal blood flow and GFR.[15]

High levels of spinal or epidural anesthesia can impair venous return, diminish cardiac output, and reduce renal perfusion.[16] Epidural blocks at thoracic levels with epinephrine-containing local anesthetics cause moderate reductions in renal blood flow and GFR that parallel the decrease in mean blood pressure.[17] Epidural blocks performed with epinephrine-free solutions generate little change in systemic hemodynamics and only a small decrease in renal blood flow and GFR in animal models.[18]

In summary, virtually all anesthetics have the potential to alter the cardiovascular system and affect renal blood flow, GFR, and urinary output. Although arterial blood pressure may not fall below 80 to 90 mm Hg, renal blood flow may be decreased by 30% to 40% after the administration of various anesthetics. This suggests impairment of autoregulation. In most cases changes in renal function are transient and reversible. If they persist into the postoperative period, the cause is often a combination of factors such as preexisting renal or cardiovascular disease, severe fluid imbalance, or mismatched blood, and the importance of the anesthetic is decreased.

Physiologic Responses

The renal vasculature is richly innervated by the sympathetic nervous system. Drugs or perioperative events that stimulate this system cause an increase in renal VR and a decrease in renal blood flow and glomerular filtration. Surgical stress may also alter autonomic and neuroendocrine responses. Norepinephrine from sympathetic postganglionic fibers and epinephrine and norepinephrine from the adrenal medulla shift blood away from the cortical nephrons; this results in decreases in renal blood flow, GFR, electrolyte excretion, and urinary output. Catecholamines also stimulate the release of renin, which ultimately leads to the production of angiotensin II, a potent vasoconstrictor.

Endocrine changes associated with anesthesia and surgical stress involve ADH, aldosterone, and the renin-angiotensin-aldosterone system. Although the perioperative period is associated with high circulating levels of ADH and aldosterone, it is not clear whether anesthetics stimulate the release or whether the release is secondary to a stress response. General anesthetics and narcotics are thought to be minor stimuli of the release of ADH, but the results of studies in this area are inconsistent.[19] Clinical studies have shown that induction of anesthesia with thiopental, nitrous oxide, and halothane does not elicit a significant release of ADH, but that blood loss and traction on abdominal viscera result in large elevations in blood levels.[20] Other investigations have shown that ADH levels do not change after the induction of anesthesia but do change in lightly anesthetized patients.[21]

It is clear that ADH release is modulated by blood volume changes that are sensed by stretch receptors in the atrial wall. Hemorrhage, positive pressure ventilation, and the upright position increase ADH release.[22] A decrease in arterial pressure stimulates ADH release. Distention of a balloon in the atrium, negative pressure ventilation, and immersion in water up to the neck decrease ADH release.

Renin-angiotensin levels may be elevated during the perioperative period, but the role of anesthetics and stress is not clear. Some studies have reported large increases in plasma renin levels associated with the use of anesthetics, whereas others reported only small increases.[23-26] The influence of renin-angiotensin on the renal effects of anesthetic agents needs further clarification. Renin levels have been shown to increase during halothane or enflurane anesthesia when sodium depletion is present. Preoperative hydration is thought to be important in the intraoperative release of renin.

Aldosterone is a hormone released from the adrenal gland, which is responsible for the precise control of sodium excretion. It is not known whether anesthetic agents act directly on the adrenal gland to cause aldosterone release. They probably act indirectly through the neuroendocrine system and the renin-angiotensin-aldosterone system. Stimulation of the sympathetic nervous system causes renal vasoconstriction, which is a trigger for the renin-angiotensin-aldosterone system. Aldosterone leads to sodium and water reabsorption and can be associated with decreased urinary output.

Nephrotoxicity of Anesthetic Agents

The kidneys are extremely vulnerable to toxicity because of their rich blood supply and the increase in the concentration of excreted compounds that occurs in the renal tubules during the process of reabsorption. Medullary hyperosmolality encourages concentration of all substances, including toxins. The amount of renal damage associated with nephrotoxic agents depends on the concentration of the toxins, the degree of toxin binding to plasma proteins and nonrenal versus renal tissue, and the length of exposure of the kidneys to the toxin. The nephrotoxicity of anesthetic agents became fully appreciated in 1966, when vasopressin-resistant polyuria renal insufficiency was reported in patients receiving prolonged methoxyflurane anesthesia for abdominal surgery.[27] Evidence gathered indicated that the release of the inorganic fluoride ions (F^-) in the metabolism of this fluorinated anesthetic was the causative agent in nephrotoxicity.

Fluoride Ion Toxicity

Fluoride alters renal concentration mechanisms by interfering with active transport of sodium and chloride in the medullary portions of the loop of Henle. It also acts as a potent vasodilator, resulting in increased blood flow in the vasa recta and washout of medullary solute. Fluoride is a potent inhibitor of many enzyme systems, including those involving ADH, and it is necessary for distal nephron reabsorption of water. Proximal tubular swelling and necrosis associated with fluoride ions also contribute to nephrotoxicity. Signs and symptoms of fluoride nephrotoxicity include polyuria, hypernatremia, serum hyperosmolality, elevations in blood urea nitrogen (BUN) and serum creatinine levels, and decreased creatine clearance. The extent of nephrotoxicity in general surgical patients has been correlated with dosage or maximum allowable concentration hours (MAC-hours), duration, and peak fluoride concentrations.[28]

Methoxyflurane

Methoxyflurane was the first anesthetic associated with serious nephrotoxicity. The serum fluoride concentration after methoxyflurane anesthesia showed positive correlation with the degree of renal dysfunction.[29] Vasopressin-resistant polyuria similar to that seen after methoxyflurane anesthesia was later produced in Fischer 344 rats injected with sodium fluoride.[30] After 2.5 to 3 MAC-hours of methoxyflurane anesthesia, fluoride concentration was 50 to 80 mmol, and subclinical toxicity evidenced by a delayed return to maximum preoperative urine osmolarity and decreased urate clearance were noted. At 5 MAC-hours, fluoride concentration was 90 to 120 mmol, and mild nephrotoxicity with serum hyperosmolality, hypernatremia, polyuria, and urinary hypoosmolality was noted. At 7 to 9 MAC-hours, fluoride concentration was 175 mmol, and marked nephrotoxicity was noted. Patients vary in nephrotoxic susceptibility, with genetic heterogeneity, preexisting renal disease, and drug interactions all contributing to toxicity. For example, the combination of methoxyflurane and aminoglycoside antibiotics encourages toxicity.[31]

Enflurane

Enflurane defluorination may occasionally result in serum fluoride concentrations great enough to produce mild renal impairment. This has been well documented in animal studies; the only controlled human study that showed mild renal dysfunction with enflurane included 29 healthy volunteers.[32] After 9.6 MAC-hours of enflurane, maximum urinary osmolality after ADH was reduced from 1050 to 800 mOsm/kg, and mean serum fluoride level was 33 mmol. These changes were associated with mild impairment of renal concentrating ability but not with hypernatremia, serum hyperosmolality, or increases in serum creatinine or urea levels.[33]

Although surgical patients almost never show renal dysfunction after enflurane anesthesia, serum fluoride ion concentrations are occasionally elevated. In one study peak serum fluoride concentration averaged 22.2 mmol in nine patients after 2.7 MAC-hours of enflurane anesthesia. Although some concern exists that patients with preexisting renal disease may develop additional dysfunction after enflurane anesthesia, this concern is generally without merit. Patients with mild-to-moderate renal insufficiency have shown no clinically significant difference in renal function after enflurane or halothane anesthesia.[34] It appears that storage of fluoride in bone offsets the effect of decreased GFR on clearance and prevents sustained exposure of the renal tubules to fluoride.

Although rare, postoperative renal dysfunction has been reported after enflurane anesthesia in patients with renal disease.[35] After 6 hours of uneventful enflurane anesthesia in one patient, the serum inorganic fluoride concentration reached 93 mmol, a level indicative of renal failure. Because that patient had received enflurane 6 weeks previously, the possibility of enzyme induction and accelerated metabolism was suggested.[36] Because volatile anesthetics are defluorinated by the cytochrome P-450 system in the liver, drugs that induce this system may lead to greater fluoride production and nephrotoxicity. Animal studies suggest that chronic treatment with isoniazid before enflurane anesthesia may result in higher than expected fluoride concentrations and transient concentrating defects.[37] Surgical patients chronically treated with isoniazid before enflurane anesthesia had higher fluoride concentrations than predicted. However, the levels were not high enough or sustained long enough to produce clinically significant renal impairment.[38] Obese patients have higher serum fluoride levels after methoxyflurane and enflurane anesthesia than do nonobese patients. Renal dysfunction is not increased after administration of these drugs to obese patients.[39,40]

Isoflurane

Isoflurane is metabolized only slightly and defluorinated much less than enflurane. In one report of nine surgical patients, mean peak serum fluoride concentration measured 6 hours after anesthesia was only 4.4 mmol.[41] Clinical experience has indicated that renal toxicity is unlikely after the administration of isoflurane.[42]

Desflurane

The metabolism of desflurane has been assessed in both animals and humans with the measurement of the appearance of fluoride metabolites (fluoride ion, nonvolatile organic fluoride, trifluoroacetic acid) in blood and urine. Administration of desflurane to rats that were either pretreated or not pretreated with phenobarbital or ethanol for 3.2 MAC-hours, as well as to swine for 5.5 MAC-hours, produced fluoride levels in blood that were almost indistinguishable from values measured in control animals.[43] In human studies, desflurane administered to patients for 3.1 MAC-hours and volunteers for 7.3 MAC-hours resulted in postanesthesia serum fluoride concentrations that did not differ from background fluoride concentrations. Similarly, postanesthesia urinary excretion rates of fluoride and organic fluoride in volunteers was comparable with preanesthetic excretion rates.[44-46] Small but statistically significant increases in the levels of trifluoroacetic acid were found in both the serum and urine of volunteers after exposure to desflurane. Although these increases in trifluoroacetic acid were statistically significant, they were approximately one tenth the levels seen after exposure to isoflurane. Desflurane strongly resists biodegradation, and only a small amount is metabolized in animals and humans.[47]

Sevoflurane

Sevoflurane undergoes approximately 5% metabolism, and the primary metabolites are fluoride and hexofluro-2-propranolol (HFIP). The oxidative defluorination of sevoflurane in the liver with the liberation of free fluoride ions raised concerns that sevoflurane, like methoxyflurane, might impair the ability of the kidneys to concentrate urine. Earlier research indicated that with methoxyflurane, renal dysfunction was likely to occur when plasma fluoride levels exceeded 50 uM. The same does not appear to be true with sevoflurane.

Preliminary investigations with sevoflurane found that some adult patients receiving the drug had plasma fluoride levels that exceeded 50 uM. However, renal function, assessed by BUN, creatinine, and decrease in urine osmolality, was not different from that in patients receiving similar amounts of other fluorinated anesthetics. In one study, serum fluoride levels averaged 29 uM after 1 to 7 MAC-hours of anesthesia. The fluoride levels peaked 2 hours after the end of anesthesia and decreased by 50% within 8 hours.[48] The fast decline in plasma fluoride levels was attributed to insolubility and rapid pulmonary elimination of sevoflurane.

Numerous published reports indicate the absence of renal toxicity after sevoflurane anesthesia.[49-52] An explanation for the absence of fluoride-induced nephrotoxicity may be that intrarenal production of fluoride ion is important in the pathogenesis of this complication. The intrarenal metabolism of methoxyflurane is four times greater than that of sevoflurane.[13]

Studies of surgical patients receiving intermediate-duration sevoflurane with high and low fresh gas flow and long-duration sevoflurane with high fresh gas flow included sensitive measures of renal function or injury. These studies also indicate the absence of renal toxicity after sevoflurane anesthesia.[53-58]

In addition to release of inorganic fluoride ion resulting from biotransformatoin, CO_2 absorbents degrade sevoflurane, resulting in production of a vinyl ether called *compound* A. Factors associated with the generation of higher levels of compound A during administration of sevoflurane to patients include (1) a high concentration of agent, (2) fresh Baralyme,

(3) increased temperature in the CO_2 absorbent, (4) low fresh gas flow rates, and (5) increased states of CO_2 production. The potential for compound A nephrotoxicity exists, particularly in the animal mode.

Because the potential for renal injury exists with sevoflurane, studies in volunteers have raised the question of whether it is important to apply more sensitive measures of renal function in evaluation of this drug. Such tests have included urine concentrations or excretion of enzymes, albumin, protein, and glucose and creatinine clearance.[59] Two studies of volunteers receiving prolonged sevoflurane anesthesia with fresh gas flow no greater than 2 L/min concluded that the potential for adverse renal effects of sevoflurane may exist.[60,61] However, other studies of volunteers did not.[62-65]

A number of reports describe instances in which sevoflurane has been given to patients with renal dysfunction and other conditions that might enhance renal injury. Such conditions include patients who are hypotensive, hypertensive, elderly, or obese or who have renal insufficiency.[66-73] The only proved direct toxic effect of any anesthetic agent is the fluoride-related toxicity of methoxyflurane.[74]

Because the amount of compound A produced increases with lower gas flows, the package insert at one time recommended flows of 2 L/min or more. Several studies indicate no effect of low-flow sevoflurane on renal function, even those with moderate renal insufficiency.[75,76] Today the U.S. Food and Drug Administration recommends the use of sevoflurane with fresh gas flow rates of at least 1 L/min for exposures up to 1 hour and at least 2 L/min for exposures greater than 1 hour.[77] Other countries have not recommended such limitations on the use of sevoflurane, and problems have not been noted.

ACUTE RENAL FAILURE

Acute renal failure (acute tubular necrosis, vasomotor neuropathy, lower nephron necrosis) is defined as the sudden inability of the kidneys to vary urine volume and content appropriately in response to homeostatic needs. Perioperative acute renal failure accounts for half of all patients who require dialysis and is associated with a 50% mortality rate.[78,79]

Classification

Acute renal failure is classified according to its predominant cause or on the basis of urine flow rates. As illustrated in Table 27-1, the cause of acute renal failure has prerenal, renal, or postrenal origins. Prerenal failure results from hemodynamic or endocrine factors that impair renal perfusion; renal failure results from tissue damage; and postrenal failure results from urinary tract obstruction. Prerenal or postrenal failure is reversed with attention to hemodynamics or relief of obstruction. Acute renal failure caused by parenchymal disease or damage is more serious and often requires hemodialysis.

Failure classified according to urine flow rates is known as *oliguric*, *nonoliguric*, or *polyuric* failure. Oliguria is defined as a urinary flow rate less than 0.5 ml/kg/hr in a patient subjected to acute stress. This rate is higher than that seen in unstressed patients because acutely stressed patients cannot maximally concentrate urine. Polyuric failure is associated with elevations of blood urea, nitrogen, and serum creatinine levels and is characterized by urine flow rates that exceed 2.5 L/day.

Conditions that lead to prerenal oliguria include acute reductions in GFR, excessive reabsorption of salt or water, or both. Increases in circulating levels of catecholamines, ADH, or aldosterone are physiologic factors that can decrease urinary output. Hypotension may or may not be present in the initiation of acute renal failure. If not reversed, prerenal oliguria may progress to parenchymal damage and tubular necrosis.

TABLE 27-1 Systemic Effects of Renal Disease

System	Effects
Cardiovascular	Hypertension Congestive heart failure Peripheral and pulmonary edema Pericarditis Coronary artery disease
Hematologic	Normochromic, normocystic anemia Platelet dysfunction Leukocyte, immunologic dysfunction
Neurologic	Encephalopathy Peripheral and autonomic neuropathy
Endocrine	Hyperparathyroidism Adrenal insufficiency
Respiratory	Pneumonitis Pulmonary edema
Gastrointestinal	Bleeding Nausea, vomiting Delayed gastric emptying
Metabolic	Acidosis Electrolyte imbalance

Acute tubular necrosis may be produced by a variety of factors that interfere with glomerular filtration or tubular reabsorption. The pathogenesis of acute tubular necrosis may be divided into an initiation period, a maintenance period, and a recovery period. Renal hypoperfusion or a nephrotoxic insult may initiate renal failure. Surgical patients with external and internal fluid losses or sepsis may have renal hypoperfusion. The renal medulla, with its sluggish blood supply and active transport mechanisms, is especially susceptible to even moderate renal ischemia.

The initiating insult culminates in the development of one or more maintenance factors, such as decreased tubular function, tubular obstruction, and sustained reductions in renal blood flow and glomerular filtration. Urine flow and solute excretion are reduced. Once the maintenance period has begun, pharmacologic interventions to improve renal blood flow do not reverse the failure.

Prerenal oliguria is associated with physiologic mechanisms that conserve salt and water. In this case urine has low sodium levels and high osmolality. Patients with parenchymal disease have trouble concentrating the urine. Urine sodium levels are high, and osmolality is low. Renal damage is also associated with a progressive rise in serum urea, creatinine, uric acid, and polypeptide levels. Serum potassium levels may increase by 0.3 to 3 mEq/L/day, and a decrease occurs in the serum levels of sodium, calcium, and proteins such as albumin. Assessment of renal dysfunction perioperatively is difficult. Arterial blood gas analysis, which allows the anesthetist to detect pulmonary dysfunction quickly, has no renal equivalent. Exogenous factors may alter BUN level, and subtle changes in serum creatinine concentration are easily ignored. The creatinine clearance remains the single most helpful test in defining renal status and predicting the prognosis in cases of severe renal dysfunction.

Risk Factors

A number of conditions may place patients at high risk for acute renal failure (Box 27-1). Renal reserve decreases progressively with age. For each year after 50 years of age, creatinine clearance decreases by 1.5 ml and renal plasma flow by 8 ml. Older patients are less able to cope with fluid and electrolyte imbalance and are more prone to renal damage. Overall mortality rates associated with acute renal failure increase from 50% for those younger than age 40 years to 80% for those older than age 60 years.

Patients with preexisting renal dysfunction are also at high risk. Cardiac and hepatic failure are associated with abnormal renal hemodynamics. Cortical redistribution of blood flow, salt and water retention, and reduced GFR are all increased by anesthetics, stress, and hypovolemia, and therefore the incidence of postoperative renal failure increases. Bilirubin is nephrotoxic, and levels greater than 8.5 mg/dL are associated with elevated levels of endotoxin that may cause renal dysfunction.

Certain surgical procedures are associated with a higher risk of acute renal failure. Although cardiac surgery has only a 2% to 4% incidence of this complication, the risk increases in patients with preoperative ventricular dysfunction or bacterial endocarditis, in those undergoing emergency procedures, and in those who have procedures in which cardiopulmonary bypass lasts longer than 2 hours. Postoperative bleeding with reexploration and low cardiac output requiring use of the intraaortic balloon pump also carry a higher incidence of failure.

A ruptured abdominal aortic aneurysm implies hypovolemia, shock, and the need for a high aortic cross-clamping. Of these patients, 40% have renal damage, and 11% develop acute renal failure with an associated mortality rate of 80%. Renal dysfunction after elective surgery is less profound if attention is given to adequate hydration and if a brisk diuresis is established before and is maintained during aortic cross-clamping. The proximity of the aortic clamp to the renal arteries is critical. Aortic arteriography performed just before surgery also increases risk. Predisposing factors are preexisting renal disease with serum creatinine levels greater than 3 mg/dL, proteinuria, diabetes, and hypovolemia. Risk is reduced by minimizing the amount of dye given, maintaining hydration, and using diuretics such as mannitol to promote diuresis. Acute postoperative renal failure is a common complication of thoracic aorta, thoracoabdominal aorta, and aortic arch surgeries. It is observed in 6% to 18% of such surgical procedures. Predisposing factors for this complication include age older than 50, preoperative renal dysfunction, duration of renal ischemia, and amount of blood transfused.[80]

Mechanical obstruction by calculi or prostatic disease is the most common cause of obstructive uropathy. Risk is increased by the frequent presence of hypovolemia and electrolyte imbalance and by preoperative diagnostic studies that involve the use of dye.

Hypovolemia, hemolysis, disseminated intravascular coagulopathy, and acidosis are key factors in the development of acute renal failure in septic patients. The use of vasoconstrictive adrenergic agonists and antibiotics with nephrotoxic potential compounds the problem. Complications of pregnancy such as hemorrhage, amniotic fluid embolus, and toxemia carry a high risk of renal failure. Because patients are usually young and healthy, mortality in this group is reduced.

BOX 27-1

Preoperative Assessment and Preparation of the Patient with End-Stage Renal Disease

I. Clinical history
   A. Document central nervous system deficits.
   B. Review cardiovascular history; look for significant hypertension, accelerated atherosclerosis, pericarditis, tamponade; assess extent, stability, and management of coronary artery disease.
   C. Look for history of excessive bleeding; if present consider use of desmopressin.
   D. Assess intravascular volume; correlate body weight changes with changes in blood pressure and heart rate before and after dialysis.
   E. Review pulmonary history.
   F. Dialyze 24 hr or less before surgery; ideal weight preoperatively is 1-2 kg above "dry" weight.
II. Physical examination
   A. Locate and check patency of arteriovenous fistula or shunt.
   B. Evaluate vessels for venous or arterial access.
   C. Look for signs of congestive heart failure, pericarditis, or cardiac tamponade.
   D. Look for evidence of noncardiogenic pulmonary edema or aspiration.
III. Laboratory tests
   A. Electrocardiography, chest radiography
   B. Blood urea nitrogen, creatinine
   C. Complete blood count with platelet count
   D. Bleeding time; prothrombin time; partial thromboplastin time
   E. Hematocrit; red blood cell index
   F. Electrolytes (especially potassium)
   G. Acid-base status
   H. Hepatitis antigen status

Prevention and Management

The old saying that an ounce of prevention is worth a pound of cure is especially true with regard to acute renal failure, because prevention is far more successful than management. Prevention can be based on the following generalizations:

1. The most common cause of failure is prolonged renal hypoperfusion.
2. Prophylaxis reduces mortality more effectively than dialytic therapy.
3. The duration and magnitude of the initiating renal insult are critical in determining the severity of failure.

A key strategy in reducing the incidence of renal failure is limiting the magnitude and duration of renal ischemia. Prevention begins in the preoperative period.

Preoperative Strategies

In the preoperative preparation of surgical patients, high-risk patients and procedures should be identified. Reversible renal dysfunction should be sought, and fluid losses and hypovolemia should be corrected by intravenous fluids. Perioperative ADH and renin-angiotensin-aldosterone secretion can be minimized with adequate hydration before anesthetic induction. Administration of saline rather than solutions low in sodium is helpful in prevention of aldosterone secretion, hyponatremia, and oliguria.

Oliguria often signals inadequate systemic perfusion, and prevention of acute renal failure requires its rapid recognition through adequate monitoring. In addition to standard monitors and a urinary catheter, monitors for patients with questionable cardiac and pulmonary function should include a direct arterial line for blood pressure monitoring and a central VP or Swan-Ganz catheter, when appropriate, for assessment of cardiac function and volume status. The hemodynamic endpoint should be adequate cardiac output and renal perfusion, not pulmonary dysfunction (e.g., pulmonary edema). Pulmonary edema can be supported with mechanical ventilation and is associated with a lower mortality rate than is acute renal failure.

Perioperative Strategies

Use of a urinary catheter is the only means of monitoring renal function in the operating room. A fluid challenge is necessary if hourly urinary output decreases to below acceptable levels.

The use of diuretics in the face of inadequate urinary output must be carefully evaluated. Although the administration of furosemide (Lasix) and mannitol decreases experimental renal failure in animals subjected to fixed insults, it worsens hypoperfusion and renal ischemia in hypovolemic patients.[81-83] Although diuretics may not be effective during the initiation of failure, large doses of furosemide can convert oliguric renal failure into nonoliguric failure, which is easier to manage.[84] In the maintenance phase, doses of furosemide in excess of 1 g may be required to convert oliguric failure to nonoliguric failure.[85] Little evidence suggests that doses smaller than 100 mg alter the course of renal failure. Diuretic therapy must be associated with aggressive monitoring and intravascular volume expansion. Prophylactic administration of mannitol and/or furosemide might prevent renal damage in hydrated patients.

Although the mechanism is unknown, prophylactic administration of mannitol in well-hydrated patients protects renal function. Loop diuretics may also prevent acute renal failure. Mechanisms for protection include the inhibition of sodium reabsorption and the prevention of tubular obstruction through the maintenance of high flow and pressure within the tubules and the reversal of intrinsic renal vasoconstriction. Prophylactic use of diuretics may be of benefit in the case of jaundice in surgical patients, excessive exposure to contrast media, hyperuricemia, or the presence of pigment in the urine. Fenoldopam, a dopamine receptor agonist also may be helpful.

Management of Acute Renal Failure

If acute renal failure develops, it progresses through four distinct phases: onset, the oliguric phase, the diuretic phase, and the recovery phase. Onset, or the initiation phase, precedes actual necrotic injury and correlates with a major alteration in renal hemodynamics. The oliguric phase reflects four pathophysiologic processes:

1. Obstruction of tubules by cellular debris, tubular casts, or tissue swelling
2. Total reabsorption or backleak of urine filtrate through damaged tubular epithelium and into the circulation
3. Tubular cell damage with leakage of adenosine triphosphate (ATP) and potassium and edema
4. Continuation of renal vasoconstriction

The diuretic phase signifies that tubular function is returning. It is marked by large daily urinary output (more than 3 L) secondary to the osmotic diuretic effect produced by an elevated BUN and impaired ability of tubules to conserve sodium and water. The recovery phase is characterized by gradual improvement of renal function over 3 months to 1 year.

After renal failure is established, the primary consideration in management is the maintenance of fluid and electrolyte balance. The early use of hemodialysis for the prevention of severe fluid and electrolyte imbalance is necessary during the oliguric and diuretic phases. The most common complication that results in death is infection.[86] Once identified, infection must be aggressively treated with antibiotics.

CHRONIC RENAL FAILURE

Chronic renal failure is a slow, progressive, irreversible condition characterized by diminished functioning of nephrons and a decrease in renal blood flow, GFR, tubular function, and reabsorptive capacity. Although many conditions may lead to renal failure, primary causes include glomerulonephritis, pyelonephritis, diabetes mellitus, vascular or hypertensive insults, and congenital defects.

The general course of progressive renal failure may be divided into three stages: decreased renal reserve, renal insufficiency, and end-stage renal failure or uremia. As the number of functioning nephrons declines, the signs, symptoms, and biochemical abnormalities become more severe.

Clinical signs or laboratory evidence of renal disease are absent until less than 40% of normal-functioning nephrons remain. Loss of nephron function without symptoms is known as the *decrease in renal reserve*. Renal insufficiency occurs when only 10% to 40% of nephrons are functioning adequately. Nocturia occurs secondary to a decrease in concentrating ability. Although affected patients seem well compensated when excretory capacity is unstressed, little renal reserve is present. Elimination of a large protein load or excretion of certain drugs is impaired, and preservation of remaining nephron function is a major goal. Toxic substances such as aminoglycosides potentiate existing damage, and aminoglycoside toxicity is enhanced in the presence of either volume depletion or arterial hypotension.[87] Radiocontrast exposure in patients with chronic renal insufficiency often causes further reversible decreases in renal function in those with either myocardial failure or diabetes mellitus.[88]

As renal function deteriorates further, end-stage renal disease develops. In this stage concentrating and diluting properties of the kidney are severely compromised, and electrolyte, hematologic, and acid-base disturbances are common. The loss of 95% of functioning nephrons culminates in uremia, which is associated with volume overload and congestive heart failure. Uremia, which can be viewed as urine in the blood, adversely affects almost every organ system. Death occurs unless dialysis is performed.

Dialytic Therapy

Approximately 72,000 people in the United States today require chronic dialysis.[89] Thirty patients per 1 million population receive dialysis for acute renal failure per year, and half of these patients require treatment early in the postoperative period.[78]

Dialysis Techniques

Dialysis is a general term used to describe therapy in which solute moves from blood through a semipermeable membrane into a chemically prescribed solution. The movement of solute, which is called *diffusive transport*, depends on differences in molecular concentration between the blood compartment and the dialysate. *Ultrafiltration* is a technique in which a hydraulic pressure difference across a semipermeable membrane causes the bulk removal of fluid and solute by convective transport.

Major types of dialysis include hemodialysis and peritoneal dialysis. In hemodialysis, blood moves through a device that exposes it to an individually prescribed dialysate solution across a semipermeable membrane. The hollow fiber type of dialyzer provides a membrane area of 0.8 to 2 m^2. Blood flow occurs through multiple channels and runs in a direction opposite to the flow of the dialysate. Both convective and diffusive movement of solute occurs. Hemodialysis requires systemic or regional anticoagulation.

In peritoneal dialysis the blood compartment is the peritoneal microvasculature, and the semipermeable membrane is the peritoneal lining. The dialysate is infused into and withdrawn from the abdominal cavity. Movement of water occurs down an osmotic gradient from blood to dialysate and may be increased with an increase in the glucose concentration of the dialysate. Diffusive transport is influenced by the solute concentration within the dialysate.

Physiologic Effects

Dialysis and ultrafiltration are associated with a number of physiologic effects and complications. Major systems involved include the nervous system, cardiovascular system, and respiratory system. The disequilibrium syndrome is the most severe central nervous system (CNS) effect of dialysis. This syndrome is associated with a rapid increase in brain intracellular volume as serum sodium and BUN levels are reduced. Predisposing factors include a BUN concentration greater than 150 mg/dL, hypernatremia, severe acidemia, and preexisting brain disease. The syndrome may be mild or may progress to seizures, stupor, and coma. The incidence is reduced by the avoidance of high rates of hemodialysis therapy in high-risk patients.

Hemodialysis is associated with a 30% incidence of hypotension. Contributing factors include reduced plasma volume and blunted sympathetic nervous system response associated with uremia. Acetate from the dialysate moves into the blood and contributes to the hypotension by causing vasodilation and cardiac depression.

The incidence of hypotension with dialysis is less in patients who have fasted than in those who have not. Fasting prevents the contribution to hypovolemia of increased gastrointestinal blood flow and the secretion of isotonic intestinal juices. Anemia should be corrected if the hematocrit is less than 20%. Leg elevation, a decrease in dialyzer transmembrane pressure, or the use of volume expanders or vasoconstrictors usually corrects hypotension. Substitution of HCO_3 for acetate in the dialysate decreases the incidence.

Hypoxemia is a common side effect of hemodialysis and may be seen during peritoneal dialysis.[90,91] During hemodialysis arterial oxygen tension often decreases by 5 to 20 mm Hg. Pulmonary leukostasis and extracorporeal loss of CO_2 with a reduction in minute ventilation have been implicated. Hypoxemia is managed by increasing the inspired oxygen concentration during dialysis. The use of HCO_3 in place of acetate limits extracorporeal losses of CO_2 and reduces the incidence of hypoxemia.

Muscle cramping is the most common neuromuscular complication of dialysis. It is seen almost exclusively with hemodialysis and results from the rapid reduction of intravascular volume and serum sodium level. Intravenous administration of hypertonic saline relieves muscle cramping.

The nutritional depletion that is common in dialysis-dependent patients may be caused by the primary disease, dietary restrictions, or the loss of protein associated with peritoneal dialysis. Protein depletion may produce hypoalbuminemia and immunocompromise. The large quantities of hypertonic glucose solutions absorbed with peritoneal dialysis contribute to obesity, hyperglycemia, and hyperlipidemia. Insulin controls hyperglycemia, and exercise limits hyperlipidemia.

PREOPERATIVE RENAL ASSESSMENT

Preoperative assessment of the patient with suspected or known renal dysfunction must include the taking of a thorough history and a physical examination, as well as appropriate laboratory evaluation. The medical history is the single most important source of information in establishing the presence or absence of renal disease. Poorly controlled hypertension, trauma to the urinary system, prior renal surgery, or systemic disease (e.g., diabetes) may be associated with renal impairment. A history that arouses suspicion should lead to a more thorough evaluation of renal function.

Although abnormalities are commonly found on urinalysis, the quality of urinalysis results obtained by dipstick technique varies.[92-94] Because abnormal results on urinalysis usually fail to lead to a change in management, the test is generally omitted. If the test is available, attention should be directed to the following:

1. *Specific gravity*. Specific gravity, a measurement of solutes in the urine, indicates the ability of the kidney to excrete concentrated or dilute urine. It is a reflection of tubular function and normally varies from 1.003 to 1.030, depending on fluid intake and the presence or absence of high–molecular-weight substances such as glucose or mannitol. In the absence of such substances a specific gravity of 1.018 or greater after overnight dehydration indicates reasonable function. A low specific gravity is meaningless if the condition under which the sample was collected is not known.
2. *Urine osmolality*. Osmolality, or the number of moles of solute (measured in osmoles) per kilogram of solvent, is more specific than specific gravity. Excretion of concentrated urine (specific gravity, 1.030; 1400 mOsm/kg) indicates excellent tubular function, whereas urinary osmolality fixed to that of plasma (serum gravity, 1.010; 290 mOsm/kg) suggests tubular concentrating defects. Urinary diluting mechanisms are present after concentrating ability is lost.
3. *Proteinuria*. Proteinuria exists when more than 150 mg of protein is excreted per day. Massive proteinuria or the renal loss of more than 750 mg/day is always abnormal and usually is indicative of severe glomerular damage. In addition to its association with glomerular damage, proteinuria may also be present with abnormal plasma proteins or increased concentrations of normal proteins or when the renal tubules fail to reabsorb the small amount of protein that may be filtered. Patients can have proteinuria without renal disease under conditions of stress, fever, dehydration, exercise, or congestive heart failure. Patients who have significant proteinuria are more likely to develop acute renal failure postoperatively than those who do not. The incidence of hypoalbuminemia and its consequences is increased in patients with severe proteinuria. In a concentrated urine sample, trace or 1+ proteinuria is a nonspecific finding, whereas 3+ or 4+ proteinuria suggests glomerular disease.

The kidneys share regulation of acid-base balance with the lungs. Because they provide the sole pathway for the excretion of the 60 mEq of hydrogen ions produced per day, urinary pH is a reflection of the ability of the kidneys to acidify urine. The inability to excrete an acid urine in the presence of systemic acidosis is indicative of renal insufficiency.

Laboratory Tests for Renal Function

Patients with suspected or known renal disease should be tested preoperatively to evaluate GFR and renal tubular function. Although urine specific gravity (1.003 to 1.030), urine osmolarity (65 to 1400 mOsm/L), and urine sodium concentration (130 to 260 mEq/day) reflect renal tubular function, BUN concentration (10 to 20 mg/dL), plasma creatinine level (0.7 to 1.5 mg/dL), and creatinine clearance (110 to 150 ml/min) are necessary for the evaluation of GFR.

Blood Urea Nitrogen

Urea, the chief end product of protein metabolism, is formed in the liver. It is excreted by glomerular filtration, but significant amounts of urea are reabsorbed along the renal tubule. Although the normal range for BUN level is 10 to 20 mg/dL, it is altered by a variety of factors, including ingestion of protein, anabolic and catabolic states, GFR, state of hydration, and reabsorption of urea by the nephrons. Because of the numerous extrarenal factors that can influence BUN, it is a better indicator of uremic symptoms than of GFR. Levels below 8 mg/dL suggest overhydration or underproduction of urea, whereas those between 20 and 40 mg/dL suggest dehydration, high nitrogen levels, or decreased GFR. Levels higher than 50 mg/dL almost always indicate decreased glomerular filtration. Elevations of BUN level in the presence of normal serum creatinine concentration suggest a nonrenal cause of the elevation. In general, BUN level is a late indicator of renal disease because it does not increase in most patients until the GFR is reduced by more than 50%.

Serum Creatinine

Creatinine is a metabolite of creatine, a major muscle constituent. The daily rate of production of creatinine is constant and determined by skeletal muscle mass. Because body creatinine is eliminated almost entirely by glomerular filtration, its steady-state concentration in the serum has been used as a marker of glomerular function. Normal values range from 0.7 to 1.5 mg/dL, but the serum concentration can be lower in the elderly or in women who have reduced muscle mass. Patients with muscle wasting have lower levels, whereas those who are heavily muscled or those in acute catabolic states have higher values because of more rapid muscle breakdown. Because the production and release of creatinine are relatively stable throughout the day and from day to day, serum levels are inversely related to GFR if a steady state exists. In other words, for every 50% reduction in GFR, creatinine level doubles. Excretion of drugs dependent on glomerular filtration may be significantly decreased despite only a slight elevation in serum creatinine level.

An elevation of both BUN and serum creatinine levels provides more information than an elevation of either level alone. The usual ratio of urea nitrogen to creatinine in the serum is 10:1. Increased ratios are seen with increased urea input, decreased circulatory blood volume, and obstructive uropathy. Decreased ratios are seen with decreased urea input, increased creatinine production, and volume expansion.

Creatinine Clearance

Creatinine clearance is a specific test of GFR and is the most reliable assessment tool for renal function. This test measures the ability of the glomeruli to excrete creatinine into the urine for a given plasma creatinine concentration. Although it does not depend on corrections for age or the presence of a steady state, a disadvantage of this test is the need for accurate 24-hour urine specimens.

Creatinine clearance is calculated according to the following formula:

Equation 27-2

$$\text{GFR} = (\text{Urine creatinine} \times \text{Urine volume}) \times \text{Serum creatinine}$$

A 2-hour urine sample collected through a urinary catheter permits acceptable accuracy. In the absence of urine volume, creatinine clearance can be approximated with use of the following formula:

Equation 27-3

$$\text{GFR} = \frac{([140 - \text{Age}] \times \text{Lean body weight})}{(72 \times \text{Serum creatinine})}$$

where weight is expressed in kilograms. To compensate for smaller muscle mass, when values for women are calculated the weight should be multiplied by 0.8.[95]

The normal range for creatinine clearance is 95 to 150 ml/min. Mild renal dysfunction is present when creatinine clearance is 50 to 80 ml/min, and moderate dysfunction is present at values below 25 ml/min. In patients with dysfunction the administration of drugs that depend on renal excretion should be reduced, and fluid and electrolyte balance should be carefully monitored. Patients with creatinine clearance less than 10 ml/min are anephric and require dialysis for fluid and water hemostasis.

Other Tests

Advanced renal disease affects most organ systems. Additional tests that may be useful in patients with advanced renal disease include chest radiography, electrocardiography, complete blood count, serum electrolytes, and acid-base studies.

Systemic Abnormalities and Advanced Renal Disease

Renal failure is characterized by a wide variety of biochemical disturbances. Although most organ systems are involved (see Table 27-1), only those most relevant to anesthetic management are discussed in this section.

Cardiovascular Alterations

Cardiovascular disease accounts for approximately 50% of all deaths in patients on hemodialysis.[96] Hypertension and congestive heart failure often accompany end-stage renal disease. Ninety percent of the hypertension is volume dependent and related to sodium and water retention. The remainder can be attributed to high circulatory levels of renin. The combination of hypertension, anemia, hypoalbuminemia, and circulatory overload secondary to salt and water retention contributes to peripheral and pulmonary edema and to an increased risk of congestive heart failure.

In nonsurgical settings ischemic heart disease is the most common cause of death in patients with chronic renal failure. Multiple risk factors such as hypertension, hyperlipidemia, and abnormal carbohydrate metabolism contribute to this high incidence of ischemic heart disease.[97] The anesthetist should assume that clinically significant coronary artery disease exists and should evaluate the extent and stability of the disease. Several uncontrolled studies suggest that correction of coronary lesions with coronary artery bypass grafting is associated with better outcomes than coronary angioplasty in patients on hemodialysis.[98] Improvement of symptoms is common after coronary artery bypass grafting. A rate of restenosis of 80% within 6 months is seen with coronary angioplasty.[99]

A fibrous pericarditis is clinically evident in approximately 50% of patients with severe uremia. Signs and symptoms may include pain on deep inspiration or when lying down and a friction rub over the pericardium. An enlarged cardiac silhouette on chest radiography indicates pericardial effusion. Patients with uremic pericarditis occasionally develop a massive hemorrhagic effusion and cardiac tamponade, especially when anticoagulants are used for hemodialysis.

Uremic patients exhibit a wide range of hemodynamic abnormalities when studied during hemodialysis.[100,101] The striking feature of these studies is that the peripheral vasculature responds abnormally to hypovolemia induced by dialysis. Hypovolemia decreases arterial pressure without increasing heart rate. Peripheral VR is unchanged or decreased, and cardiac output is increased.

Because the potential for significant cardiovascular complications exists, patients with advanced renal disease should undergo chest radiography and electrocardiography preoperatively. Administration of antihypertensive drugs should be continued, blood pressure should be monitored, and signs and symptoms of cerebrovascular disease should be recorded. The blood pressure should be normal or slightly elevated before induction. Because adequate intravascular volume is necessary for hemodynamic stability, the patient's weight should ideally be 1 to 2 kg more than dry weight at the end of the last dialysis before anesthetic induction.

Hematologic Changes

Normochromic, normocytic anemia is an inevitable finding in advanced renal disease. Hematocrit levels often decrease to the 20% to 30% range and generally parallel the degree of azotemia. The primary reason for anemia is a decrease in erythrocyte formation secondary to a decrease in production by the failing kidney.[102] Also, some evidence suggests that uremic toxins may inactivate erythropoietin or suppress the response of the bone marrow to its action. A second factor that contributes to the anemia in uremic patients is reduction of the life span of the erythrocyte because of an increase in hemolysis secondary to the presence of an abnormal chemical environment. Additionally, blood loss from frequent sampling for laboratory tests, loss in hemodialysis tubing, and a tendency for gastrointestinal bleeding further aggravate anemia.

Hematocrit and red blood cell indexes should be measured preoperatively, and their values should be checked against dialysis records to ensure that no acute changes have occurred. Preoperative hematocrit levels that are similar to those of a patient maintained on dialysis suggest that the patient can withstand the chronic anemia, and routine transfusion of blood preoperatively is not recommended for these patients. If transfusion is necessary because of acutely decreased or poorly tolerated hematocrit values, no need exists to withhold red blood cell transfusions for fear of sensitization to histocompatibility antigens.[103]

Exogenous administration of human recombinant erythropoietin corrects the anemia associated with chronic renal failure.[104-106] Adequate iron stores and good dialysis are essential if the response to recombinant erythropoietin or epoetin is to be maximized.[107] Endogenous erythropoietin levels and hematocrit values increase to normal after successful renal transplantation.[108]

Patients with chronic uremia have a tendency to bleed excessively. Although platelet counts are only mildly reduced, a defect in platelet function appears to be responsible for a prolonged bleeding time and a tendency for excessive bleeding.[109] Dialysis partially corrects platelet dysfunction, and dialysis 24 hours or less before surgical intervention is recommended.[110,111]

Desmopressin is known to shorten bleeding time and increase circulating levels of factor VIII, the von Willebrand antigen, in uremic patients. Desmopressin is the agent of choice because of its rapid onset and minimal side effects.[112,113] Repeated doses over time may increase bleeding time between treatments. Cryoprecipitate and conjugated estrogens also shorten bleeding time and may reduce blood loss.[114,115]

Gastrointestinal Effects

Patients on dialysis have a high incidence of gastrointestinal mucosal inflammatory changes and are at high risk of gastrointestinal bleeding perioperatively. The use of histamine-2 (H_2) blocking drugs or antacids is recommended throughout the perioperative period for decreasing the incidence of stress ulcers.[116,117]

Infections

Infectious complications are common in patients with renal failure and represent a leading cause of death in dialysis-dependent patients. Protein malnutrition and abnormalities in neutrophil, monocyte, and macrophage function contribute to this problem.[118-120] Mechanisms that lead to leukocyte dysfunction and increased susceptibility to infection are not known but may be related to uremia, immunosuppressive therapy, and increased exposure to invasive therapy. Frequent exposure to blood and blood products increases the risk of infection with hepatitis B and C and the human immunodeficiency viruses. Universal precautions are mandatory for the protection of both patients and health-care providers.[121]

Neurologic Effects

Neurologic symptoms associated with end-stage renal disease roughly parallel the degree of azotemia. Early symptoms include apathy, decreased mental acuity, and lethargy. Fatigue and weakness are early complaints, and untreated patients eventually become confused and comatose. Seizures may be associated with hypertensive encephalopathy. Peripheral and autonomic nervous system neuropathy is common. Autonomic neuropathy is associated with delayed gastric emptying and places the patient at risk for aspiration pneumonitis.

Endocrine Abnormalities

Endocrine abnormalities in patients with end-stage renal disease include hyperparathyroidism and adrenal insufficiency. Hypocalcemia is common in patients with advanced renal disease, and hyperparathyroidism represents an appropriate compensatory increase in parahormone in response to a reduction in serum calcium levels. Adrenal insufficiency often is secondary to exogenous steroid administration.

Respiratory Effects

Respiratory complications associated with renal failure include pneumonitis and the "uremic lung." Chest radiographs of the uremic lung reveal bilateral, butterfly-shaped infiltrates indicative of pulmonary edema. Pulmonary congestion and edema usually are related to volume overload.

Electrolyte Abnormalities

Abnormalities of water, electrolyte, and acid-base balance become more common as the degree of renal failure increases. With a normal diet the kidneys typically excrete 40 to 60 mEq of hydrogen ions per day to prevent acidosis. Impaired ability of the kidney to excrete hydrogen ions with renal failure results in metabolic acidosis characterized by decreases in plasma pH and HCO_3 concentration. Acidosis is usually moderate, but symptoms of anorexia, nausea and vomiting, and lethargy, which are common in uremic patients, may be partly related to acidosis.

Sodium ion excretion by the kidney normally varies according to intake. Patients with chronic renal failure lose this flexibility and have sodium wasting or retention. In early renal insufficiency with polyuria an increased solute load for each intact nephron results in sodium wasting. In renal failure the patient is more likely to retain sodium. Salt and water retention leads to circulatory overload, hypertension, edema, and congestive heart failure.

Although the ability to excrete magnesium is reduced in uremic patients, hypermagnesemia is generally not a serious problem. Magnesium intake is usually reduced because of anorexia, reduced protein intake, and decreased absorption from the gastrointestinal tract.

Calcium balance is controlled by parathyroid hormone, calcitonin, and vitamin D. Vitamin D, or cholecalciferol, is inactive until it has been hydroxylated in the liver and kidney. Inability of the diseased kidney to hydroxylate 25-hydroxycholecalciferol to 1,25-dihydroxycholecalciferol (active vitamin D) results in hypocalcemia. Patients with chronic renal failure have skeletal disorders or osteodystrophy, and defective mineralization of bone predisposes patients to fractures. Special precautions should be taken when these patients are moved and positioned.

Potassium imbalance is one of the most serious disturbances that occurs in patients with renal failure. Although hypokalemia may be associated with the polyuria of renal insufficiency, end-stage renal disease invariably leads to hyperkalemia. Although the major mechanism for hyperkalemia is the inability of distal nephrons to secrete potassium in exchange for calcium, systemic acidosis also contributes to potassium imbalance. Acidosis causes potassium ions to shift from intracellular to extracellular fluid.

Fatal dysrhythmias or cardiac standstill can occur when serum potassium levels reach 7 to 8 mEq/L. Dialysis is the most effective means of managing perioperative hyperkalemia, and hemodialysis is indicated when serum potassium exceeds 6 mEq/L. Other techniques for treating hyperkalemia include insulin in glucose infusions (25 to 50 g of glucose with 10 to 20 units of regular insulin) and HCO_3 administration. These measures promote rapid translocation of extracellular potassium to the intracellular space during hyperkalemic emergencies. Hyperventilation of the lungs with respiratory alkalosis lowers serum potassium concentration by approximately 0.5 mEq/L for every 10–mm Hg change in arterial CO_2 tension. Life-threatening cardiac dysrhythmias are treated with intravenous administration of calcium chloride. A typical dose may be 1 g in adults. Although calcium does not change the serum concentration of potassium, it antagonizes the cardiotoxic effects of hyperkalemia.

Unexpected hyperkalemia can develop rapidly, and it is important to measure potassium even when dialysis has been performed within 6 to 8 hours of surgery. Hyperkalemia occurs early postoperatively and is the primary reason patients with renal failure require dialysis within the first 24 hours after surgery.[122]

Surgical procedures are becoming increasingly more common in anephric patients. The perioperative course of these patients may be complicated by a high incidence of untoward events that increase morbidity and mortality. These complications are related to the abnormal physiology of the anephric state. They are predictable and can be minimized by preoperative evaluation and preparation. Pertinent points in the preoperative assessment and preparation of patients with end-stage renal disease are listed in Box 27-1.

ANESTHETIC MANAGEMENT OF PATIENTS WITH ADVANCED RENAL DISEASE

Preoperative preparation of patients with advanced renal disease should include an evaluation of recent laboratory measurements, coexisting diseases, and current medications. Patients with end-stage renal disease should undergo determination of BUN and serum creatinine levels, complete blood count, bleeding time measurement, and electrolyte studies preoperatively. Special attention should be given to serum potassium, the type of and schedule for dialysis, and volume status.

Discussions regarding premedication should take into consideration unexpected sensitivity to CNS depressants and delayed gastric emptying. Benzodiazepines are useful as premedicants because of their oral route of administration and hepatic metabolism. Diazepam has active and long-lasting metabolites, and its action is prolonged in renal failure. Midazolam has virtually no active metabolites, and its half-life is only slightly prolonged in renal failure. Although this drug is useful when it is carefully titrated, patients with renal disease may be more susceptible to the sedative-hypnotic effects of this benzodiazepine than those without renal dysfunction.[123]

Reduced protein binding may be responsible for increased sensitivity to these drugs in these patients. Protein binding of morphine (Table 27-2) decreases by 10% in the presence of chronic renal failure.[124] This alters the free fraction only slightly, because morphine generally is protein bound to such a small extent. Because morphine is almost completely metabolized in the liver to the inactive glucuronide, premedicant doses in patients with renal failure should not cause prolonged depression. However, one report has described severe respiratory and cardiovascular depression in a patient with renal failure who received 8 mg of morphine.[125] Excessive depression in these patients is thought to result from high brain levels of metabolites. These metabolites are pH dependent, and their concentration does not increase with respiratory alkalosis. Morphine is not removed by dialysis.

Meperidine is more lipophilic than morphine. It is 60% protein bound and is metabolized to renally eliminated compounds that are less potent respiratory depressants than morphine. Meperidine can cause convulsions when used in high concentrations, and it cannot be removed by dialysis.[126] Meperidine should be avoided in patients with renal failure.

Approximately 20% to 50% of a dose of atropine or glycopyrrolate is recovered unchanged in the urine, so the dose should be reduced.[127] Although only one tenth as much scopolamine is recovered from the urine, CNS effects prohibit its use when large or repeated doses of an anticholinergic are required.

TABLE 27-2 Protein Plasma Binding of Some Important Anesthetic Drugs

Drug	Percent Bound
Alfentanil	92
Atropine	39
Bupivacaine	95
Etidocaine	95
Etomidate	71-75
Fentanyl	84
Ketamine	26
Lidocaine	60-80
Remifentanil	66-93
Meperidine	42-60
Methohexital	73
Midazolam	94
Morphine	35
Pancuronium	11-29
Propofol	98
Ropivacaine	95
Sufentanil	93
Thiopental	80-84
Vecuronium	30

From Bovill JG, Howie MB. Clinical pharmacology for anaesthetists. *London: Saunders; 1999.*

Gastric hyperacidity and gastrointestinal bleeding are common in patients with renal failure. H_2 blockers and magnesium-free antacids should be considered. Cimetidine has been used, but renal elimination accounts for 80% of total elimination, and elimination is impaired with reduced renal function. Although newer H_2 antagonist are now available, all H_2-receptor blockers are very dependent on renal excretion. Metoclopramide is partly excreted unchanged in the urine and will accumulate in patients with renal failure.

Intraoperative Monitoring

The selection of monitors for a patient with diminished or absent renal function is based on the physiologic status of the patient and the proposed surgical procedure. Frequent measurements of blood pressure and continuous recording of temperature and heart rate and rhythm are essential. Electrocardiography may allow early detection of hyperkalemia.

Because these patients are often chronically anemic, a further reduction in oxygen delivery secondary to hypoxia can be extremely hazardous. Pulse oximetry is helpful for the early detection of arterial desaturations. Pulse oximetry and capnography are useful and required in all patients. Minor surgical procedures in stable patients can be monitored noninvasively.

The decision to use invasive monitors depends on the patient's functional cardiac reserve and the severity and control of hypertension. Continuous monitoring of intraarterial blood pressure is helpful when major surgical procedures are performed. A femoral or dorsalis pedis artery is sometimes used for cannulation because vessels in the upper extremities may be needed later for vascular shunts. Vascular volume and fluid replacement can be guided by central VP or pulmonary artery catheter monitoring. A pulmonary artery catheter is useful if interpretation of the central VP is questionable or cardiac disease is present.

Vascular shunts and fistulas must be protected. Patency is easily monitored with Doppler imaging. Because of the immunocompromised state of these patients, strict aseptic technique is required during the placement of vascular catheters.

Regional Anesthesia

Regional anesthesia is tolerated by patients with advanced renal disease, provided no significant coagulation disorder is present and MAP is maintained. Regional techniques avoid most of the pharmacokinetic and pharmacodynamic problems associated with general anesthetics and sedative drugs. Major concerns regarding this type of anesthesia include psychologic intolerance, coagulation abnormalities, the presence of peripheral neuropathies, difficulty in making intravascular volume adjustments, and risk of infection.

Arteriovenous shunts or fistulas may be surgically created with the use of local infiltration or brachial plexus block. In addition to providing analgesia, brachial blocks improve surgical conditions by providing maximum vascular vasodilation and abolishing vasospasm. Studies have shown that brachial plexus block is associated with greater brachial artery blood flow than local anesthesia, but this effect is not significant enough for the technique to be recommended over another.[128] Both brachial plexus block and local infiltration are good alternatives to general anesthesia for creation of arteriovenous fistula. Age, American Society of Anesthesiologists (ASA) class, and cardiac status were the determining factors for choice of anesthetic technique.[129]

The duration of brachial plexus block has been reported to be shortened by 40% in patients with chronic renal failure.[130] The reason for this reduction was thought to be an elevation in tissue blood flow secondary to an increase in cardiac output and a more rapid clearance of local anesthetics from active sites. A shortened duration of action would support the use of a longer-acting local anesthetic, such as bupivacaine, especially if prolonged surgery is anticipated. However, data suggest a similar duration of anesthesia with brachial plexus blocks in patients with renal failure and normal renal function.[131] High-dose mepivacaine has been used for brachial plexus block in patients with end-stage chronic renal failure. Brachial plexus anesthesia with 650 mg of plain mepivacaine did not result in serious systematic toxicity in these patients despite high mepivacaine plasma concentrations.[132] Levobupivacaine 0.5%, 50 to 60 ml, has also been used for axillary brachial plexus block in patients with renal disease and was well tolerated.[133]

With regard to spinal or epidural anesthesia, patients with long-standing renal disease often have undergone multiple procedures and prefer general anesthetic techniques. In addition to the history, the bleeding time, platelet count, prothrombin time, partial thromboplastin time, and fibrinogen level should be evaluated before subarachnoid or epidural catheters are placed in uremic patients. Paraplegia secondary to hematoma formation with spinal anesthesia has been reported in patients with chronic renal failure and clotting abnormalities.[134] A case of epidural hematoma in a surgical patient with chronic renal failure and epidural postoperative analgesia has been reported. The only risk factor for development of epidural hematoma was a history of chronic renal failure. High-risk patients should be monitored closely for early signs of cord compression such as severe back pain and motor or sensory deficits. An opioid or opioid and local epidural solution rather than local solution alone allows continuous monitoring of neurologic function. If spinal hematoma is suspected, the patient should undergo immediate magnetic resonance imaging or computed tomographic scan, and decompressive laminectomy should be performed without delay.[135]

Peripheral neuropathies should be discussed with the patient and documented before regional anesthesia is undertaken. The incidence of hypotension with subarachnoid or epidural blockade may be increased because of effects of chronic hypertension or hypovolemia related to recent dialysis. Correction of hypovolemia postoperatively is hazardous. Recession of the sympathetic block in patients who cannot undergo diuresis may lead to pulmonary edema. One must weigh the advantages of fluid infusion against the effects of pressor drugs with these factors in mind.

Patients with end-stage renal disease are often acidotic, and local anesthetic toxicity may be increased with acidosis. The onset and duration of blocks have also been shown to vary in these patients. Subarachnoid blockade induced with 3 ml of 0.75% bupivacaine developed more rapidly, attained a greater level, and was of shorter duration in patients with renal failure than in control patients.[136] The slower onset of epidural anesthesia is of advantage in these patients.

General Anesthesia

Intravenous Drugs

Intravenous anesthetics can be used in patients with advanced renal disease, but the response of these patients may be more variable than normal. Variability arises from a complex interplay among changes in volume of distribution (which is often increased), protein binding (which may be low), low pH, and dependence on renal excretion for the parent drug or metabolites.

The action of many drugs is potentiated by metabolic abnormalities associated with renal failure. Highly protein-bound drugs (see Table 27-2) have more target organ effect in the presence of hypoalbuminemia. The acidemic state associated with renal failure increases the proportion of the agent that is unionized and unbound and therefore more available to target tissue. Anemia associated with renal failure increases cardiac output and enhances delivery to the brain. Uremia alters the blood-brain barrier; this also increases the sensitivity to intravenous drugs.

From 75% to 85% of sodium thiopental is normally bound to albumin. It may have an exaggerated effect in renal failure because of decreased protein binding and an altered blood-brain barrier.[137] Ketamine and benzodiazepines are less heavily protein bound. The sympathomimetic effects of ketamine are frequently associated with an increase in blood pressure and cardiac output, which may be deleterious in hypertensive patients who are at risk for coronary artery disease or decreased left ventricular function. In addition, metabolites of ketamine depend on renal excretion and can accumulate in patients with renal failure.

The pharmacokinetic profile of narcotics can be altered in the presence of renal disease. Fentanyl is metabolized in the liver, and 85% of it appears in the urine and feces as inactive metabolites. Its slow elimination half-life is the result of a large volume of distribution. The effect is exaggerated in renal failure. Chronic renal failure is associated with a decrease in alfentanil plasma protein binding, but it does not change plasma clearance of the drug. The volume of distribution at steady state is greater in patients with renal failure. Altered protein binding of alfentanil must be considered in patients with renal failure.[138] Although the pharmacokinetics of sufentanil do not appear to be altered in patients with advanced renal disease, clearance and half-life are more variable in this group. Sufentanil should be carefully administered to these patients.[139] Remifentanil, which is metabolized by nonspecific plasma esterases and is not dependent on renal function for elimination, is a logical choice for renally compromised patients.

Propofol has gained wide acceptance for both induction and maintenance of anesthesia and appears to be safe. Induction doses of 2.5 mg/kg in patients with normal renal function or renal failure resulted in no significant difference between the groups in quality of induction or hemodynamics.[140] Studies suggest, however, that patients with end-stage renal disease require a higher dose to achieve hypnosis. A hyperdynamic circulation in these anemic patients may be responsible.[141] The half-life did not differ significantly between the groups, although the values were longer with propofol in patients with renal failure. Propofol has been used for induction and maintenance for 3- to 8-hour kidney transplant procedures. No accumulation of the drug occurred, and no unusual hemodynamic effects were observed. Emergence was rapid, and resumption of diuresis was satisfactory. The pharmacokinetics of propofol do not appear to be significantly altered in patients undergoing kidney transplantation.[142]

Uremic patients are generally anemic and may require high inspired oxygen concentrations. Because intravenous anesthesia is often supplemented with nitrous oxide, the inspired concentration of oxygen is reduced. Volatile agents are more reliable in controlling hypertension, and their action is more easily reversed. For these reasons inhalation agents may be preferable for general anesthesia.

Volatile Anesthetic Agents

Inhalation agents offer some advantage in patients with renal failure. Although biotransformation of some agents may produce renally excreted metabolites, elimination of volatile agents does not rely on renal function. Volatile agents potentiate neuromuscular blocking drugs, allowing administration of reduced doses. Although the potency of these agents allows them to be administered without nitrous oxide, excessive depth of anesthesia may lead to a depression of cardiac output. Reductions in cardiac output and tissue blood flow must be avoided in these anemic patients if tissue oxygen delivery is to be maintained.

A disadvantage of inhalation agents relates to their biotransformation and nephrotoxic potential. The nephrotoxic threshold for fluoride of 50 mmol is rarely reached with current agents. Excessive plasma fluoride elevations do not occur in anephric patients receiving enflurane because storage of fluoride in bone offsets renal excretion.[143] Fluoride levels after isoflurane anesthesia increased by only 1 to 2 mmol, and desflurane is metabolized approximately one tenth as much as isoflurane. It is the least metabolized of the currently available volatile agents. In studies of patients and volunteers administered desflurane for prolonged periods, no evidence of renal, hepatic, or hematologic toxicity was observed.[144]

Some practitioners may avoid use of sevoflurane in patients with renal dysfunction because of the potential for nephrotoxicity. Studies do not support this concern. One study compared renal function after long-duration low-flow (<1 L/min) sevoflurane and isoflurane anesthesia in surgical patients with normal renal function. Postoperative renal function was no different as assessed by serum creatinine and BUN levels and urinary excretion of protein and glucose, suggesting that low-flow sevoflurane is as safe as low-flow isoflurane.[145] Another study concluded that prolonged low-flow sevoflurane anesthesia had the same effect on renal and hepatic function as high-flow sevoflurane and low-flow isoflurane anesthesia. During low-flow sevoflurane, intake of compound A reached 277 ppm/hr, but the effect on the kidney and liver was the same in high-flow sevoflurane and low-flow isoflurane anesthesia.[146]

In summary, both regional and general anesthesia have been used successfully in patients with advanced renal disease. Advantages and disadvantages of both techniques are listed in Table 27-3.

Neuromuscular Blocking Drugs

The appropriate use of neuromuscular blocking drugs in patients with advanced renal disease has received much attention over the years. At one time, caution was advised in all cases of the use of a muscle relaxant in patients with renal disease. Because these drugs are ionized, water-soluble compounds freely filtered at the glomerulus, it was believed that their action would be prolonged. It was further theorized that as the anticholinesterase or relaxant antagonist level decreased, the patient would be at risk of "recurarization," or reappearance of neuromuscular blockade. It is now known that renal excretion is of major importance for cholinesterase inhibitors as well. Approximately 50% of neostigmine and 70% of edrophonium and pyridostigmine are excreted in the urine.[147-149] Excretion of all cholinesterase inhibitors is delayed to the same extent as, or to a greater extent than, muscle relaxants in patients with renal impairment.

Succinylcholine. Several problems have been associated with the use of succinylcholine in patients with renal failure.

TABLE 27-3 Regional versus General Anesthesia

Technique	Advantages	Disadvantages
Regional	Patient responsiveness Minimal changes in renal hemodynamics	Presence of peripheral neuropathy Tendency for bleeding Patient anxiety Prolonged procedures Hypotension with sympathetic block; may cause reluctance to expand volume
Volatile anesthetics	Good airway control Blood pressure control Duration not dependent on urinary excretion Less neuromuscular blocking with drugs required FiO_2 can be increased because N_2O not necessary	Alterations in renal hemodynamics Decreased cardiac output Hypotension Biodegradation and potential nephrotoxicity; halothane 15%-20%; sevoflurane 5%; isoflurane 0.2%; desflurane 0.02%
Intravenous anesthetics	Hemodynamic stability	Unpredictable response Hypertension Greater need for N_2O and neuromuscular blockers

FiO_2, *Fraction of inspired oxygen;* N_2O, *nitrous oxide.*

Succinylcholine is metabolized by hepatic-derived pseudocholinesterase to succinic acid and choline. A metabolic precursor of these two compounds is succinylmonocholine, which has nondepolarizing blocking activity and is eliminated by the kidneys. Large doses administered over prolonged periods of time, as may be seen with succinylcholine infusions, may lead to accumulation of the metabolite. Introduction of newer drugs eliminates the risk of prolonged blockade from succinylcholine infusions.

When succinylcholine is given after anticholinesterase administration, the action of succinylcholine is prolonged. An explanation for this prolongation is the alteration in pharmacokinetics of both drugs in patients with renal failure and their prolonged duration of action. Patients with renal failure who require muscle relaxants are at greater risk for prolonged succinylcholine blockade than normal individuals if they have recently undergone anticholinesterase-induced reversal of neuromuscular blockade.[150] Prolongation of succinylcholine has also been associated with depressed levels of pseudocholinesterase in uremic patients who require hemodialysis. Newer methods of hemodialysis have no effect on cholinesterase levels.[151,152]

Serum potassium increases by approximately 0.5 mEq/L in both normal patients and those with renal failure. This elevation in extracellular potassium is not prevented by pretreatment with a nondepolarizing muscle relaxant. The rise in serum potassium level is particularly dangerous in uremic patients who are hyperkalemic. The use of succinylcholine is inadvisable unless a patient has undergone dialysis within 24 hours before surgery and the potassium concentration is less than 5.5 mEq/L. Succinylcholine is safe in normokalemic patients who have recently undergone dialysis.[153-155]

Pancuronium. Approximately 40% to 50% of pancuronium is excreted in the urine. Biliary excretion accounts for much of the nonrenal elimination.[156,157]

With pancuronium a significant portion that is excreted renally occurs after biotransformation to a less active metabolite.[158,159] Pancuronium has a prolonged terminal elimination half-life in patients with reduced renal function and should be administered cautiously.

Atracurium and *cis*-Atracurium. Atracurium and vecuronium were introduced into clinical practice in the late 1980s. Initial reports indicated that the action of neither atracurium nor vecuronium was prolonged in patients with decreased renal function; however, it now appears that this is true only for atracurium.[160-162] Atracurium and *cis*-atracurium are broken down by enzymatic ester hydrolysis and by nonenzymatic alkaline hydrolysis or Hoffman elimination to inactive products. This process is not dependent on renal excretion for termination of action. Onset, duration, and recovery are the same in patients with and without renal disease, and it is the drug of choice in patients with renal failure. Metabolism of atracurium and to a lesser extent *cis*-atracurium produces the CNS excitant laudanosine, which is renally excreted and accumulates in patients with renal failure.[163] The clinical significance of this finding is yet to be determined.

Vecuronium. Vecuronium is excreted renally, and the duration of neuromuscular blockade is longer in patients with renal failure than in those without renal failure.[164] This accumulation is presumed to be the result of the gradual saturation of peripheral storage sites.[165] Prolonged neuromuscular block may result from the use of an infusion or from large doses of vecuronium in patients with severely impaired renal function.[166] An 81-year-old patient with renal failure and subclinical, chronic hepatic cirrhosis remained paralyzed for 13 days after vecuronium infusion.[167] Prolonged blockade with vecuronium has also been reported in an 11-day-old infant with renal failure. In this case an initial dose of 97 mg/kg was followed by complete neuromuscular blockade for 210 minutes.[168] If vecuronium is used, a low dose is recommended, and repeated administration should be avoided. Neuromuscular blockade is rapidly reversible with dialytic treatment.[169,170]

Doxacurium. Doxacurium, pipecuronium, and mivacurium were introduced in the 1990s. Doxacurium has a long duration of action and is devoid of cardiovascular effective doses. Renal excretion of unchanged drug is an important elimination route for doxacurium; therefore doxacurium has a longer duration of action in patients with liver or kidney failure. The duration of action in patients with renal dysfunction can be expected to be prolonged and be more variable.[171,172]

Pipecuronium. Pipecuronium bromide is another long-acting, nondepolarizing neuromuscular blocking drug that is free of cardiovascular effects. Pharmacokinetic studies suggest that plasma clearance of the drug is reduced and its elimination half-life increased in patients with renal dysfunction. The volume of distribution for pipecuronium is greater, its clearance lower, and its duration of action more variable in patients with renal failure than in those with normal renal function.[173] It is less suitable for use in patients with renal failure than is atracurium or vecuronium.

Mivacurium. Mivacurium is a nondepolarizing muscle relaxant with a shorter duration of action than either atracurium or vecuronium. It has minimal cardiovascular side effects and is metabolized by plasma cholinesterase to substances devoid of neuromuscular action. It does not rely on renal excretion for its inactivation, but studies have shown that the action is prolonged in anephric patients, although not to a great extent. The longer duration of action was thought to result from a decrease in plasma cholinesterase level rather than from changes in elimination.[174,175]

Rocuronium. Rocuronium bromide is a nondepolarizing neuromuscular blocking drug released for clinical use. It has a rapid onset of action, and in humans it produces good to excellent conditions for tracheal intubation in 60 to 90 seconds.[176] It has one fifth to one sixth the potency of vecuronium, few to no cardiovascular effects, and an intermediate duration of action.[177,178] Studies indicate that the pharmacokinetics and the onset of action of twice the effective dose to produce 95% response (ED_{95}) dose of rocuronium are not altered in patients with renal failure who are undergoing renal transplantation. Whether these results can be applied to patients with renal failure who undergo surgery other than renal transplantation is unknown. It is suitable for patients with renal failure who undergo renal transplantation and may be particularly desirable in those patients in whom rapid onset of neuromuscular blockade is desired.[179] A rapid onset is particularly attractive in these patients because they are subject to autonomic neuropathy and delayed gastric emptying.

INTRAVENOUS FLUID MANAGEMENT

Perioperative management of fluids and electrolytes in patients with renal disease is critical. The state of hydration affects renin, aldosterone, and antidiuretic levels. Dehydration and hypovolemia lead to elevations in these hormones and to a decline in urinary output.

Perioperative Renal Function

Surgical patients at high risk for acute renal failure or those with advanced disease who do not require hemodialysis present unique challenges. Preservation of renal function intraoperatively is a major goal. Preservation of renal function is dependent on the maintenance of intravascular volume and cardiovascular stability and on the avoidance of events that cause renal vasoconstriction. Preoperative hydration with 10 to 20 ml of balanced salt solution per kilogram may be helpful. Intraoperatively, urinary output is the only time monitor for renal function. A urinary output of 0.5 to 1 ml/kg/hr intraoperatively and postoperatively is recommended in these patients.

Although urinary output seems to be a reasonable reflector of renal function intraoperatively, its value as a sole indicator of adequate volume resuscitation in patients undergoing aortic surgery has been questioned. In one study intraoperative urinary output was not predictive of postoperative changes in renal function.[180] In this study pulmonary artery occlusion pressure and blood pressure were maintained in the normal range with the infusion of fluids and blood. If urinary flow decreased to below 0.125 mg/kg/hr, the patient was treated with crystalloid solution, mannitol, furosemide, or nothing. Postoperative BUN and serum creatinine levels were similar among treatment groups and did not correlate with intraoperative urinary flow rates. Serum creatinine rose by 0.5 mg/dL in 21 patients, 17 of whom had preoperative renal dysfunction. This study highlighted the increased risk of renal dysfunction in patients with preexisting disease and emphasized that maintenance of intravascular volume guided by adequate hemodynamic monitoring is as important as maintaining an arbitrary urinary flow rate.

Renal Pathology

Decreased Renal Reserve

Patients with renal disease progress through several stages: decreased renal reserve, renal insufficiency, renal failure, and uremia. The goal of fluid management in patients with decreased renal reserve is the maximization of renal perfusion. Basal fluids should be replaced; 5% dextrose in water (D_5W) with 50 to 70 mEq of Na^+ per liter is appropriate. Potassium should be administered as needed to sustaining a normal plasma level. Deficit and intraoperative losses should be replaced as for a normal patient. Third-space losses can be replaced with balanced salt solution. Although it is better to err on the side of excess with respect to volume replacement in these patients, if the ratio of replacement crystalloid solution to lost blood exceeds 3:1, consideration should be given to the use of a colloid solution. The administration of huge volumes of crystalloid solution may be associated with pulmonary edema as fluids are mobilized. This generally occurs on the second to the fourth postoperative day.

Renal Insufficiency

In patients with renal insufficiency, volume deficits should be replaced preoperatively, as in normal patients. Basal fluids must be carefully regulated, because these patients cannot tolerate much deviation. Overall basal fluid requirements must be related to metabolic rate and be designed to provide an overall fluid balance that allows an isotonic urine to carry excreted electrolytes and waste products. Intraoperative losses greater than 10% to 15% of the blood volume should be replaced with colloid solution on a 1:1 basis after red blood cell losses are corrected. Smaller losses can be replaced with the usual 3:1 ratio of crystalloid infusion to blood loss. Third-space losses are ideally replaced initially with crystalloid solution without potassium or excess chloride. Initial third-space losses should be replaced with crystalloid solution at a rate of 2 to 3 ml/kg/hr. The critical goal in patients with renal insufficiency is sustaining blood volume. Monitoring of colloid osmotic pressure and hemoglobin can guide the choice between crystalloid and colloid infusions. If hemoglobin and colloid osmotic pressure are increasing, crystalloid solution is clearly indicated. If they are decreasing, crystalloid solution should be withheld in favor of colloid solution. Close monitoring of blood pressure, heart rate, central VP, pulmonary artery occlusion pressure, and cardiac output also guides fluid titration. This is especially true in patients with cardiac or respiratory compromise.

End-Stage Renal Disease

With regard to perioperative fluid management, patients with end-stage renal disease who are hemodialysis dependent require special attention. Although these patients are similar to normal patients in terms of fluid deficit, basal, and third-space requirements, they have a narrow margin of safety. The patient's ability to compensate for either fluid excess or fluid deficiency progressively declines as renal function is lost.

Fluid deficits must be replaced preoperatively in patients with end-stage renal disease. If deficits exceed 10% to 15% of the blood volume, invasive monitoring is justified. Dialysis is recommended on the day before anesthesia to allow time for equilibration of fluid and electrolyte shifts that are common with dialysis. Electrolyte levels must be checked before anesthesia.

Basal fluids in patients with end-stage renal disease should be replaced in a manner similar to that for patients with renal insufficiency. Volume restriction is recommended for intraoperative losses. Third-space losses should be replaced with a balanced salt solution that contains no potassium and small amounts of chloride. Close monitoring of hemoglobin and cardiac filling pressures is indicated for all major procedures. Patients with end-stage renal disease generally require dialysis within 24 to 36 hours after major surgery.

Uremia

Deficit replacement in patients with uremia must be guided by hemodynamic monitoring. Basal fluids should be replaced with red blood cells, fresh frozen plasma, or colloid solutions. Third-space losses are best replaced with crystalloid solutions in association with frequent monitoring of hemoglobin and cardiac filling pressures. A moderate degree of volume overload is not a grave problem. Many uremic patients require dialysis within 24 to 36 hours for the removal of mobilized fluid and the control of hypertension.

Although volume overload is most often emphasized in patients with end-stage renal disease, complications of hypovolemia are also serious. Hypotension associated with hypovolemia increases the risk of thrombosis of the arteriovenous fistula and predisposes to cardiac and cerebral ischemia. Hemodynamic goals include the avoidance of hypotension and gross fluid overload. This can be accomplished only through careful titration with the patient well monitored.

ANESTHESIA FOR RENAL TRANSPLANTATION

Transplantation Procedure

Renal transplantation has been performed for nearly a century and is an accepted means of replacing kidney function in patients with end-stage renal disease who are on maintenance dialysis. In this procedure the donor kidney is placed extraperitoneally in the recipient's iliac fossa. The renal artery is anastomosed to the internal iliac artery, the renal vein to either the external or the common iliac vein, and the ureter to the bladder. The anesthesia provider plays a vital role in management of the viability of the transplanted kidney. Three interrelated variables affect surgical outcomes: management of the donor, preservation of the harvested organ, and perioperative care of the transplant recipient.[181] Additionally, improved surgical and immunosuppressive techniques have contributed to better outcomes in terms of graft survival.[182]

Harvested Organ Preservation

Ischemic time, beginning with the clamping of the donor's renal vessels and ending with the vascular anastomosis in the recipient, is a crucial factor in graft preservation. When renal ischemic time is less than 30 minutes, diuresis begins quickly, but if it is 2 hours or longer, a variable period of oliguria or anuria may occur according to the following ischemic times:

Warm	Cold
Begins: Clamping of donor vessels; initial placement in recipient	Perfusion of harvested organ with cold preservation solution; storage at 4° C
Ends: Vascular anastomosis in recipient; interrupted with perfusion of cold preservation solution	Perfusion by recipient

Donor Preparation

Choice of anesthesia for the living, related donor is not critical. Adequate amounts of balanced salt solution should be administered to ensure a brisk diuresis from the donor kidney and to offset reduced venous return resulting from use of the flank position.[181] The greatest risk to the donor is hemorrhage. Adequate intravenous access and blood must be available in the event that transfusion becomes necessary.

If the donor kidney is obtained from a brain-dead patient, preservation of graft function is the highest priority. The loss of sympathetic tone after brain death may produce mild hypotension despite adequate volume replacement. Many patients with irreversible cerebral dysfunction are hypovolemic and require vigorous fluid resuscitation. If pharmacologic support of the cardiovascular system is necessary, a dopamine infusion at a rate of 1 to 3 mcg/kg/min is recommended. Renal vasoconstrictive properties of high-dose vasopressors reduce immediate allograft function and increase the risk of kidney damage. Maintenance of urinary output is paramount and may warrant the use of diuretics and a low-dose dopamine infusion.[181,183]

Recipient Preparation

Because cadaveric kidneys can be preserved for 36 to 48 hours with cold perfusion, time is sufficient for optimal preparation of the transplant recipient (Box 27-2). The recipient should be

BOX 27-2

Anesthesia for Renal Transplantation

I. Preoperative assessment and preparation
  A. Clinical evaluation
    1. Evaluate status of coexisting diseases.
      a. Diabetes mellitus
      b. Hypertension
      c. Cardiac disease
      d. Hyperparathyroidism
      e. Pericardial tamponade
    2. Perform dialysis within 24 hr of transplantation; check weight.
    3. Evaluate tolerance to chronic anemia.
  B. Laboratory evaluation
    1. Complete blood count with platelet count
    2. Prothrombin time, partial thromboplastin time, bleeding time
    3. Blood urea nitrogen, creatinine, calcium, fluid balance
    4. Electrocardiography; chest radiography
  C. Type and cross-match 2 U of washed packed red blood cells
  D. Determine current drug regimen
  E. Premedication
    1. Benzodiazepines, narcotics
    2. Antacids, histamine-2 antagonist, metoclopramide
II. Monitors
  A. Electrocardiography
  B. Indirect or direct blood pressure measurement
  C. Precordial, esophageal stethoscopy
  D. Neuromuscular blockade evaluation
  E. Foley catheter
  F. Central venous, pulmonary capillary wedge pressure measurement, if required
III. Anesthetic management
  A. Regional techniques
    1. Continuous spinal or epidural
    2. Advantages
      a. No need for muscle relaxants
      b. Potential respiratory tract infection from intubation is avoided
      c. Amount of local anesthetic required is small
      d. Patients are awake and comfortable postoperatively
    3. Disadvantages
      a. Patient anxiety
      b. Uncomfortable surgical positions, especially for donor
      c. Coagulation abnormalities present
      d. Fluid management with sympathetic blockade a challenge
      e. Unprotected airway in patients with delayed gastric emptying
  B. General anesthesia
    1. Induction with thiopentapropofol or etomidate
    2. Maintenance with volatile anesthetic (halothane, isoflurane, or desflurane) or narcotic-based technique
    3. Neuromuscular blockers
      a. Succinylcholine
      b. Atracurium and *cis*-atracurium
      c. Vecuronium
IV. Miscellaneous drugs
  A. Mannitol or furosemide
  B. Prednisone or methylprednisolone
  C. Azathioprine
  D. OKT3
  E. Cyclosporine

free of acute illness and infections because of the likelihood of their spread during immunosuppressive therapy. Acute alterations in fluid and electrolyte balance should be corrected with dialysis carried out 24 hours before transplantation. Postdialysis laboratory values should be checked, and serum potassium (K^+) level should be below 5.5 mEq/L. Coagulation studies and acid-base status should be normal. Serum creatinine concentration should be below 10 mg/dL, and BUN level below 60 mg/dL after dialysis.

Chronic anemia is common, and transfusion is not required if oxygen delivery is adequate. Because of the danger of volume overload, anemia should be corrected during dialysis with transfusion of packed red blood cells. It was formerly thought that multiple blood transfusions increased the risk of kidney rejection secondary to sensitization of the human leukocyte antigen system, but this belief has been disproved. Studies have shown a lower survival rate for transplanted kidneys in nontransfused patients and in those receiving leukocyte-poor blood.[184]

Abnormal platelet function, as well as ineffective production of factor VIII and von Willebrand factor, accounts for the syndrome of uremic coagulopathy seen in patients with renal failure. Correction of coagulation abnormalities has been accomplished through dialysis and administration of conjugated estrogen and desmopressin (see following chart).[185]

Treatment	Effect
Dialysis	Improves platelet formation
Conjugated estrogen	
Desmopressin	Increases factor VIII and von Willebrand factor

Acceptance of kidney transplantation in patients with type I diabetes mellitus is widespread. This is not the case, however, in patients with type II diabetes, as this condition brings increased risk for poor postoperative outcomes, largely because of the propensity for associated coexisting disease in such patients. One researcher found that patients with type II diabetes who had a history of stroke or myocardial infarction had a poorer prognosis than those patients without coexisting vascular disease.[186]

Patients should fast for 6 to 8 hours if possible. Premedication may include narcotics or benzodiazepines in usual to reduced doses, depending on the status of the patient. The use of antacids, H_2 antagonists, and metoclopramide should be considered if gastric emptying is delayed; however, reduced doses should be considered, as these drugs depend on the kidney for excretion, and metoclopramide is partially excreted unchanged in the urine.[181]

In addition to routine monitors a Foley catheter is inserted for the assessment of graft function. Although central VP lines are not routinely inserted, their use may indirectly improve graft function by improving the assessment of hydration status. A pulmonary artery catheter is useful if cardiac compromise is suspected or if the kidney is expected to have delayed graft function. Protection of vascular access and fistula patency is of prime importance with the use of blood pressure cuffs or if arterial cannulation is necessary. Sterile precautions during insertion of invasive lines are extremely important because transplant patients are immunocompromised. Strict adherence to aseptic technique is mandatory in the management of these lines, catheters, and endotracheal tubes. Commitment to aseptic technique on the part of the entire team may make the difference between safe transplantation and death for the patient.

Fluid management may be generous or conservative. Fluid replacement should be with normal saline or with dextrose in saline, generally at a maintenance infusion rate. Immediate function of the transplanted kidney cannot be guaranteed, and excessive intraoperative fluid replacement can lead to pulmonary edema and swelling of the grafted kidney.

Anesthesia

Regional Anesthesia

Both regional and general anesthesia have been used successfully for renal transplantation. Spinal and epidural anesthesia are both satisfactory, and because the procedure is extraperitoneal and in the lower half of the abdomen, the block can be kept low.[187,188] Advantages of regional anesthesia include a more aseptic technique, avoidance of the use of muscle relaxants and other drugs excreted by the kidney, and the fact that endotracheal intubation is not required. Intubation may increase the risk of nosocomial pneumonia. Pulmonary infection occurs in 10% to 15% of transplant recipients and is associated with a high mortality rate.[189] An additional advantage of regional anesthesia is postoperative analgesia.

Disadvantages of regional anesthesia techniques in these patients include hypotension associated with sympathetic blockade, the length of the procedure, and heparinization of the kidney. Sympathetic blockade can make control of blood pressure difficult in patients who may be hypovolemic. Because transplantation procedures may last several hours, large amounts of sedation may be needed to supplement regional techniques. Because local heparinization of the kidney is often employed, the use of continuous regional techniques may be contraindicated. For these reasons, general anesthesia is now the preferred approach in patients who undergo transplantation.

General Anesthesia

Volatile Agents. When general anesthesia is used, nitrous oxide combined with volatile agents, particularly isoflurane, or short-acting opiates is well tolerated. The skeletal muscle relaxant properties and minimal metabolism make isoflurane an attractive choice. Reductions in cardiac output secondary to the negative inotropic effects of volatile drugs must be minimized if suboptimal tissue oxygenation is to be avoided in these anemic patients.

Although no studies describe use of sevoflurane during kidney transplantation, researchers have reported on its effects on the kidney with impaired function. Evidence of increased plasma fluoride concentrations has been the predominant finding.[190,191] Also, compared with isoflurane, no significant difference in other renal function markers was found.[191] Although limited by a small sample size of chronic renal failure patients, Nishiyama and colleagues[192] found that these patients had significantly lower levels of urine fluoride than control subjects. The data suggest that fluoride kinetics in patients with chronic renal failure might be different from fluoride kinetics in patients with normal renal function.[192] These findings may facilitate further research in this area.

Muscle Relaxants. The choice of muscle relaxant must take into consideration the unpredictable nature of renal function after transplantation. Relaxants that are independent of renal function for plasma clearance, such as atracurium and *cis*-atracurium, are excellent for this patient population.[159,160] *cis*-Atracurium, one of 10 isomers of atracurium, represents approximately 15% of the total atracurium mixture.[193] It is three times more potent than atracurium. The process of Hoffman elimination and ester hydrolysis is the elimination pathway for both drugs. No significant differences have been found in the duration of action of *cis*-atracurium between patients with and those without renal failure. However, variability in recovery times has been seen in patients with renal failure.[193-195] The pharmacokinetics of anticholinesterase drugs used for antagonizing nondepolarizing muscle relaxants is unchanged within 1 hour after renal transplantation.[148] Succinylcholine can be used to facilitate intubation if serum K^+ level is normal.

Other Drugs. Mannitol is included in many transplant protocols. It does not depend on renal tubular concentrating mechanisms to promote urinary formation, and it facilitates urinary output and a reduction in tissue and intravascular volume. The effect of low-dose dopamine administration on cadaver graft function has also been evaluated. An infusion rate of 1 to 3 mcg/kg/min preoperatively does not affect early or late graft function. These findings are true in normovolemic, hemodynamically stable patients without severe vascular disease. Patients who do not receive kidneys subjected to prolonged hypertension, preservation, or anastomotic times can also benefit from low-dose dopamine infusion. In normovolemic and hemodynamically stable patients without severe vascular disease or in patients who do not receive kidneys subjected to prolonged hypertension, preservation, or anastomotic times, infusion of dopamine at a rate of 1 to 3 mcg/kg/min perioperatively does not affect early or late graft function. In these circumstances, early graft function is dependent on ischemic changes, and late graft function is dependent on the management of rejection.[196]

Cardiac arrest has been reported after completion of the renal artery anastomosis to the transplanted kidney.[197] Arrest occurred at the time the occlusion clamp was released and was attributed to hyperkalemia from washout of the K^+-containing solutions used to preserve the kidney. If clamping of the external iliac artery is necessary during the procedure, K^+ can be released from the ischemic limb.[198] Unclamping may also result in hypotension from the release of vasodilating substances from ischemic limbs and the subsequent increase in vascular capacity.

Immunosuppressants

Azathioprine. Immunosuppression is critical for graft survival, and most patients receive several immunosuppressive drugs. Azathioprine (Imuran) is a bone marrow–toxic derivative of 6-mercaptopurine. Although its mechanism of action is unknown, a single dose of 5 mg/kg is administered intravenously at the time of transplantation. The drug is added to an intravenous drip chamber and administered over 10 to 30 minutes. Maintenance doses of 2 mg/kg/day are used thereafter if the leukocyte count is greater than 4000. Imuran is associated with dose-dependent neutropenia and occasionally with thrombocytopenia.

OKT3. OKT3 is a mouse monoclonal antibody to the T3 antigen or human lymphocyte. It is administered daily by slow intravenous injection. A standard dose in patients who weigh more than 25 kg is 5 mg given by slow intravenous push. This drug is given only intravenously and is administered for 14 days. Patients receiving OKT3 are given antibiotics to minimize the risk of opportunistic infection. Risks associated with the use of this drug include anaphylaxis, pulmonary capillary leak, and fluid overload.

Cyclosporine. Cyclosporine is a fungal metabolite that suppresses interleukin II production and amplification of cell-mediated immunity. Side effects include nephrotoxicity, hypertension, hirsutism, tremor, and anaphylaxis. Use of the drug early after transplantation delays recovery of allograft function. It is not administered until renal allograft function has reduced serum creatinine level to half of the admission value. The induction dose is 12 mg/kg in two divided doses, and plasma levels are maintained by periodic intravenous or oral doses. The anesthetic action of drugs may be altered in individuals who receive even a single dose of cyclosporine. Several animal studies have shown that a single dose of this immunosuppressant increases the hypnotic effects of phenobarbital and the analgesic effect of fentanyl.[199] The drug also enhances the neuromuscular blockade produced by vecuronium and atracurium.[200]

Steroids. Steroid administration is common in patients who undergo renal transplantation. Both prednisone and methylprednisolone sodium succinate (Solu-Medrol) have potent antiinflammatory and immunosuppressive effects. They are also associated with impaired fibroblast proliferation and function and with impaired wound healing. Prednisone administration is initiated with a dose of 2 mg/kg given daily and slowly tapered to maintenance doses. Adjustments in the dosage of prednisone must be made according to the clinical situation. Methylprednisolone is used prophylactically in a dose of 2 mg/kg intravenously. It is also used for treatment of acute allograft rejection at a dose of 0.5 to 1 g/day for 3 days. The maximum dose is 6 g.

EXTRACORPOREAL SHOCK-WAVE LITHOTRIPSY

Extracorporeal shock-wave lithotripsy (ESWL), developed in Munich between 1974 and 1980, was first used in the United States in 1984. It is a technique that uses high-energy shock waves to fragment renal calculi into small particles. A biplanar fluoroscopy unit is used to focus the shock wave on the target stone. The shock wave is repeated several thousand times and causes the stone to disintegrate.

Water Immersion Effects

The original ESWL procedure required patients to be strapped in a chair in a semireclining position, followed by submersion in water up to the clavicle. The focused, reflected shock wave passed through the water and entered the body through the flank. Immersion in water has significant physiologic effects on cardiovascular and respiratory function and on temperature regulation (Box 27-3). Studies of healthy volunteers after immersion in water up to the neck demonstrated an increase in central blood volume of up to 700 ml and an increase in preload, stroke volume, and cardiac output. Although significant increases in central VP and pulmonary artery pressures occur, no changes in heart rate or arterial pressure occur.[201-203] Increased cardiac filling pressures may precipitate cardiac failure in patients with cardiac compromise.

Hydrostatic pressure on the chest estimated at 20 cm H_2O decreases functional residual capacity by 30% to 35%. Similar changes are noted in expiratory reserve volume and expiratory lung volumes. These changes encourage ventilation-perfusion mismatch. If spontaneously ventilating, awake patients are sedated while immersed, the likelihood of a reduction in oxygen saturation is increased. Supplemental oxygen is recommended.

Because the lungs are filled with air, they present a different acoustic impedance to the shock wave. If not protected the lungs may be injured. A thick sheet of Styrofoam should be placed between the shock wave and lung tissue. Observation of fluoroscopy during ventilation ensures that the lungs are not in the path of the shock wave.

Diuresis, natriuresis, and kaliuresis have been observed after patients have been immersed in the water bath. These changes are thought to be related to ADH suppression or an increase in renal PG levels. If the patient is well hydrated before immersion, the diuresis that follows vasopressin suppression is reduced.

Immersion lithotripsy units require that the entire body except the head and neck be submerged. Changes in the temperature of the water bath affect the patient's temperature. Both general and epidural anesthesia are associated with vasodilation and loss of shivering. This loss encourages heat transfer between the patient and the water. Both hypothermia and hyperthermia have been reported.[204,205] The temperature of the water bath should be maintained at 35° to 37° C and should be continuously monitored. Newer second- and third-generation lithotriptors do not require the patient to be submerged in water. Although they do use water for the production of shock waves, a membrane over the shock-wave generator encapsulates the fluid. Transmission of shock waves to the patient is ensured by the use of coupling gel between the patient and the generator membrane.[206]

BOX 27-3

Side Effects Associated with Extracorporeal Shock Wave Lithotripsy

- Hypothermia, hyperthermia
- Cardiac dysrhythmias
- Hemorrhagic blisters of skin
- Renal edema
- Renal hematoma
- Lung injury
- Flank pain
- Hypertension, hypotension
- Autonomic hyperreflexia
- Nausea, vomiting

Patient Monitoring

Electrocardiography, automated cuff measurement of blood pressure, and pulse oximetry are indispensable during lithotripsy. The electrocardiograph must be of good quality because the R wave is used to trigger the shocks. Synchronization of the shock wave to the electrocardiograph has reduced the incidence of cardiac dysrhythmias but has not totally eliminated them. These dysrhythmias are attributed to mechanical stimulation of the heart. Supraventricular premature complexes and premature ventricular complexes are the most common dysrhythmias noted. Atropine or glycopyrrolate may be given to increase the heart rate and thus the shock-wave rate.[207]

Patient Movement

For lithotripsy to be most effective, the stone must remain at the focal point. Because patient movement and patterns of respiration can change kidney and stone position, movement must be minimized and ventilation carefully controlled. The number and intensity of shock waves can be reduced when stone movement is minimized.[208]

Although high-frequency jet ventilation (HFJV) has been used to decrease stone movement during this procedure, its effectiveness is controversial.[209] Benefits of HFJV include less stone movement, less tissue trauma, and less stone disintegration, but its use is not without risk. Complications associated with HFJV include air trapping, bronchoconstriction, failure to adequately ventilate patients, and inaccurate delivery of anesthetic gases.[210,211] Heart-synchronized ventilation, by which the electrocardiograph signal from the patient has been used to trigger both the inspiratory cycle of the ventilator and the firing of shock waves, has improved the HFJV technique.[212] Conventional mechanical ventilation with respiratory rates of 20 to 80 breaths per minute and smaller tidal volumes has also been used for reducing stone movement.

Anesthetic Techniques

Various anesthetic techniques have been employed for ESWL. General anesthesia is advantageous because of its rapid onset and control of patient movement. It also allows the use of HFJV. Other techniques include spinal or epidural anesthesia, patient-controlled analgesia (PCA), monitored anesthesia care, and topical anesthesia with eutectic local anesthetics. Continuous infusions of propofol, methohexital, ketamine, and alfentanil have been used alone or with midazolam for ESWL anesthesia.[213-215]

Spinal anesthesia has the advantage of a rapid onset, but its disadvantages could be troublesome. Hypotension, spinal headache, and the inability to reinforce the block are drawbacks to use of this technique. Use of intrathecal opioids has also been evaluated. Lau and co-workers[215] compared 5% lidocaine with sufentanil 20 mcg and found no differences in pain perception between groups of patients who received the two agents. However, they also noted earlier discharge times in the sufentanil group.[216] Data from a study by Eaton and colleagues[217] yielded similar results. Patients in the sufentanil group were discharged 52 minutes earlier than those who received lidocaine. The magnitude of hypotension was less in the sufentanil group, yet pruritus, at times intractable, was a common side effect.[216-218]

Although epidural anesthesia is associated with a slower onset, hypotension is less, and the block can be reinforced as needed. A dermatomal level of T6 or T4 must be achieved to ensure patient comfort. Air bubbles in Micropore foam tape used to secure epidural catheters, as well as within the catheter itself, have been associated with attenuation of shock-wave energy at the stone and with a reduction in success rate.[219] Changes in compliance in the epidural vicinity of air bubbles or epidural catheters have been blamed for failure of epidural anesthesia on subsequent ESWL treatments.[219,220] Studies comparing general and regional anesthesia indicate that no differences exist with regard to morbidity with ESWL.[221] Both methods have been found to be effective techniques, with general anesthesia producing more rapid recovery.[221] Zeitlin and Roth[222] found no differences in the long-term effectiveness of ESWL, comparing epidural and general anesthesia with conventional low-volume ventilation or HFJV. Epidural opiates have also been used successfully as an alternative to general anesthesia or in combination with traditional epidural anesthesia.[222,223]

ESWL has evolved with several modifications to the original Dornier HM3 machine. The intensity of the shock wave is lower, immersion is not necessary, and the procedure can be performed with less anesthesia on awake patients.[224] Subsequently, machine modification has been associated with changes in anesthetic technique.[225] Kovac[226] evaluated general risk and outcome in the recovery room among four different anesthetic techniques (general, spinal, epidural, and monitored anesthesia care) associated with the Dornier HM3 and the modified HM3. Both machines and all anesthetic techniques were associated with good outcomes. A gender-related difference was associated with the procedure: with general anesthesia and monitored anesthesia care, female patients experienced a rate of flank pain and nausea and vomiting that was approximately twice the frequency in males.[226,227]

Eutectic mixture of local anesthetics (EMLA) is a local anesthesia cream that contains a mixture of lidocaine and prilocaine. Monk and colleagues[228] investigated the efficacy of EMLA in minimizing the pain associated with shock waves and found that EMLA significantly decreased the pain produced by test shocks greater than 15,000 V. Hemodynamic responses were comparable in EMLA cream and placebo groups. EMLA cream was significantly more effective in men than in women, possibly because of differences in pain perception, skin thickness, or dermal penetration.[228] Other investigators have concluded that, although cutaneous anesthesia with lidocaine-prilocaine cream has significant effects on pain during ESWL, it does not eliminate the need for analgesic sedation. It can be used, however, for reducing the dose of analgesic and sedative drugs during ESWL performed with regional or general anesthesia and an unmodified Dornier HM3 lithotriptor.[229]

The effectiveness of PCA with and without the use of EMLA cream has been studied. Alfentanil has been used alone or in combination with midazolam or propofol. Although patient satisfaction scores were high, increased incidences of desaturation, bradypnea, and increased end-tidal CO_2 levels were found.[230] Ganapathy and co-workers[231] reported no difference in pain perception between groups treated with alfentanil PCA combined with EMLA cream and those treated with placebo. They also reported that the inclusion of EMLA cream did not facilitate early discharge from the postanesthesia care unit.[231] Schelling and colleagues[232] found a gender-based relationship in patients treated with alfentanil PCA alone: men were found to have a higher pain tolerance than women.

PERCUTANEOUS NEPHROLITHOTOMY

Removal of kidney stones 25 mm or smaller can also be accomplished through percutaneous nephrolithotomy. This procedure requires general anesthesia and postoperative hospitalization. Stones are removed via a rigid operating scope inserted in the lower calyx of the kidney under fluoroscopy. Once located, calculi are pulverized by using laser, electrohydraulic, or ultrasound probes placed directly on the stones. The procedure is performed with the patient in the prone position; therefore associated anesthetic considerations apply (see following chart of complications of percutaneous nephrolithotomy).

Minor	Major
Pain	Septicemia
Fever	Bleeding
Urinary tract infection	Pelvic or ureteral tears
Renal colic	Pneumothorax
	Hemothorax
	Anaphylaxis secondary to contrast dye

TRANSURETHRAL RESECTION OF PROSTATE

Surgical Technique

Transurethral resection of the prostate (TURP) is one of the most commonly performed surgical procedures in men older than 60 years of age. These patients are often at greater anesthetic risk because they are more likely to have cardiovascular or pulmonary problems. The procedure consists of opening the outlet channel from the bladder with the use of a resectoscope in the urethra for electrically cutting away the obstructing median and lateral lobes of prostate tissue. Bleeding is controlled with a coagulation current. For visualization of the area the bladder is distended, and continuous irrigation is used to wash away blood and dissected prostatic tissue.

Various types of irrigating fluid have been used. Although distilled water is associated with the least optical impairment, hemolysis of red blood cells is an unacceptable side effect. Normal saline or lactated Ringer's solution is highly ionized and promotes dispersion of high current from the resectoscope. For these reasons, irrigating solutions typically consist of sorbitol (2.70 g) and mannitol (0.54 g) in 100 ml of water (Cytal) or glycine 1.5%.[233,234] Glycine is slightly hypoosmolar to the blood but is used widely because of its low cost.

Complications

Fluid Absorption

A number of complications are associated with resection of the prostate (Box 27-4). Large amounts of irrigating solution can be absorbed through venous sinuses. The amount absorbed and the rate of absorption depend on the size of the gland to be resected, the congestion of the gland, the duration of resection, the pressure of the irrigating solution, the number of sinuses open at any one time, and the experience of the resectionist.[235] An average of 10 to 30 ml of fluid can be absorbed per minute of resection time, and 6 to 8 L can be absorbed in cases that last up to 2 hours.[236,237] In general, limiting resection time to 1 hour is desirable.

Complications specifically related to absorption of irrigating fluid include volume overload with pulmonary edema and dilutional hyponatremia. As fluid enters the vascular compartment, intravascular pressure and myocardial work increase. The fluid dilutes plasma proteins and electrolytes, and the change in intravascular pressure favors movement of fluid from the vascular to the interstitial compartment. This is poorly tolerated by patients with a high incidence of cardiovascular disease.

BOX 27-4

Complications of Transurethral Resection of the Prostate

- Hypervolemia
- Hyponatremia
- Bladder perforation
- Hemorrhage
- Glycine toxicity
- Ammonia toxicity
- Electrical hazards
- Hypothermia
- Bacteremia

Absorption of irrigating fluid also leads to dilutional hyponatremia. Sodium is a major cation of extracellular fluid, and it is responsible for the depolarization of excitable cells and the production of action potentials. CNS symptoms associated with hyponatremia range from restlessness, headache, irritability, and confusion to blindness, coma, and seizures. Cardiac dysrhythmias may also develop.

Serum sodium (Na^+) concentrations of 120 mEq/L appear to be borderline for the development of severe reactions. Electrocardiographic changes characterized by widening of the QRS complex and ST-segment elevation are seen when the serum level decreases to 115 mEq/L. At levels less than 100 mEq/L, ventricular tachycardia and fibrillation can occur.[238] CNS symptoms associated with hypovolemia include restlessness, confusion, nausea, vomiting, coma, and convulsions. These symptoms can be detected more easily in patients receiving regional anesthesia. CNS symptoms are hidden under general anesthesia. Progressive increases in blood pressure, central VP, or pulmonary artery wedge pressure (when monitored) suggest hypervolemia.

Hyponatremia in such cases results from water excess rather than from Na^+ loss. Hypertonic saline (3% to 5% sodium chloride) and diuretics (furosemide, 0.15 to 0.5 mg/kg) are useful.

Bladder Perforation

Perforation of the bladder is another complication of prostatic surgery.[239] Symptoms vary, depending on whether the rupture is intraperitoneal or extraperitoneal (Box 27-5). These symptoms are better recognized when the patient has regional anesthesia if the regional technique does not produce a high block. With general anesthesia, only the surgeon can appreciate the inability to recover bladder fluid as a sign of perforation. Intraperitoneal fluid will be excreted by the kidney. However, if hemodynamic embarrassment occurs, suprapubic drainage is effective for removal of excess intraperitoneal fluid.

Glycine Absorption

Absorption of glycine has been associated with toxicity. Glycine, an amino acid normally found in the body, is a major inhibitory transmitter. Toxic effects have been produced in animals and humans. Signs and symptoms include nausea, vomiting, fixation and dilation of the pupils, weakness, and

BOX 27-5

Bladder Perforation

Extraperitoneal
Periumbilical, inguinal, or suprapubic pain
Lower abdominal distention
Pain

Intraperitoneal
Abdominal rigidity, distention, pain
Referred shoulder pain
Hiccup, shortness of breath
Tachycardia
Hypotension or hypertension
Diaphoresis
Vomiting

muscle incoordination. Transient blindness after TURP has been attributed to edema of the cortex, atropine, and hyponatremia.[240-242] Ovassapian and co-workers[243] reported five cases of transient blindness that they thought were attributable to glycine toxicity. Glycine may also result in CNS toxicity as a consequence of its biotransformation to NH_3.[244,245] NH_3 toxicity results in encephalopathy and delayed awakening in the postoperative period. NH_3 yields glutamine, which is metabolized to the inhibitory neurotransmitter serotonin. Hyperammonemia also decreases the production of dopamine and norepinephrine, which are central excitatory neurotransmitters.[246] Animal studies suggest that both glycine and NH_3 reduce the amplitude of the visual evoked potential and therefore have CNS effects.[247]

Skin Burns

The use of high voltage for cutting and coagulation during TURP may result in skin burns. Electrocardiography pads may be placed at other sites so that potential burns are avoided. Many patients who undergo TURP have pacemakers. These devices must be converted to a fixed rate unless they are designed to operate in the presence of applied currents.[248]

Blood Loss

Blood loss during TURP generally is related to the weight of the resected tissue, operating time, and skill of the surgeon.[249-251] Assessment of blood loss is difficult because of the dilution of blood in irrigating fluid. Hematocrit may be increased, decreased, or unchanged, depending on the amount of fluid in the intravascular space at the time. Blood transfusion should be based on preoperative hematocrit, the duration and difficulty of resection, and a general assessment of the patient.

Anesthesia

Spinal anesthesia and general anesthesia have both been used for TURP procedures. Some clinicians believe that spinal anesthesia is ideal because with it the signs and symptoms of hypervolemia and bladder perforation are more easily detected. As a result, a T10 sensory level is necessary for adequate anesthesia. Pain impulses from the bladder neck and prostate are propagated by afferent parasympathetic fibers originating primarily from the second and third sacral roots in concert with the pelvic splanchnic nerves. The sympathetic nerves via the hypogastric plexus, which is derived from T11 to L2 nerve roots, transmit sensation from the bladder.[252] Although general anesthesia may mask early complications, it may be desirable in patients who require pulmonary support or who cannot tolerate a fluid load for compensation of a loss of sympathetic tone. All inhalation agents have been used successfully.

REFERENCES

1. Guyton AC. *Textbook of Medical Physiology*. 10th ed. Philadelphia: Saunders; 2000:279-284.
2. Mirenda JV, Grisson TE. Anesthetic implications of the renin-angiotensin system and angiotensin converting enzyme inhibitors. *Anesth Analg*. 1991;72:667-683.
3. Ballermann BJ, Brenner BM. Role of arterial peptides in body fluid homeostasis. *Circ Res*. 1986;58:619-630.
4. Mcloughlin TM, Watkins DW. Atrial natriuretic peptide: the state of the art. *Semin Anesth*. 1988;7:243-250.
5. Sladen RN. Renal physiology. In: Miller R, ed. *Anesthesia*. 5th ed. New York: Churchill Livingstone; 2000:663-694.
6. Price HL, Linde HW, Jones RE. Sympathoadrenal responses to general anesthesia in man and their relation to hemodynamics. *Anesthesiology*. 1959;20:563-575.
7. Cousins MJ, Greenstein LR, Hitt BA, Mazze RI. Metabolism and renal effects of enflurane in man. *Anesthesiology*. 1976;44:44-53.
8. Mazze RI, Schwartz FD, Slocum HC, Barry KG. Renal function during anesthesia and surgery. I. The effects of halothane anesthesia. *Anesthesiology*. 1963;24:279-284.
9. Deutsch S, Goldberg M, Stephen GW, Wu WH. Effects of halothane anesthesia on renal function in normal man. *Anesthesiology*. 1966;27:793-804.
10. Mazze RI, Cousins MJ, Barr GA. Renal effects and metabolism of isoflurane in man. *Anesthesiology*. 1974;40:536-542.
11. Warltier DC, Pagel PS. Cardiovascular and respiratory actions of desflurane: is desflurane different from isoflurane? *Anesth Analg*. 1992;75:S17-S31.
12. Stoelting RK, Dierdorf SF. *Renal Disease and Coexisting Diseases*. 4th ed. New York: Churchill Livingstone; 2002:362.
13. Kharasch ED, Hankins DC, Thummel KE. Human kidney methoxyflurane and sevoflurane metabolism: intrarenal fluoride production as a possible mechanism of methoxyflurane nephrotoxicity. *Anesthesiology*. 1995;90:505-508.
14. Deutsch S, Bastron RD, Pierce EC Jr, Vandam LD. The effects of anaesthesia with thiopentone, nitrous oxide, narcotics, and neuromuscular blocking drugs on renal function in normal man. *Br J Anaesth*. 1969;41:807-815.
15. Barry KG, Mazze RI, Schwartz FD. Prevention of surgical oliguria and renal hemodynamic suppression by sustained hydration. *N Engl J Med*. 1964;270:1371-1377.
16. Monk TG, Weldon BC. The renal system and anesthesia for urologic surgery. In: *Clinical Anesthesia*. 3rd ed. Philadelphia: Lippincott; 1996:943-972.
17. Kennedy WF Jr, Sawyer TK, Gerbershagen HY, Cutler RE, Allen GD, Bonica JJ. Systemic cardiovascular and renal hemodynamic alterations during peridural anesthesia in normal man. *Anesthesiology*. 1969;31:414-421.
18. Sivarajan M, Amony DW, Lindblood LE. Systemic and regional blood flow during epidural anesthesia without epinephrine in the rhesus monkey. *Anesthesiology*. 1976;45:300-310.
19. Bachman L. The antidiuretic effect of anesthetic agents. *Anesthesiology*. 1955;16:939-949.
20. Moran WH Jr, Miltenberger FW, Shuayb WA, Zimmermann B. The relationship of antidiuretic hormone secretion to surgical stress. *Surgery*. 1964;56:99-108.

21. Philbin D, Coggins CH. Plasma antidiuretic hormone levels in cardiac surgical patients during morphine and halothane anesthesia. *Anesthesiology*. 1978;49:95-98.
22. Kharasch ED, Yeo KT, Kenny MA, Buffington CW. Atrial natriuretic factor may mediate the renal effects of PEEP ventilation. *Anesthesiology*. 1988;69:862-869.
23. Pettinger WA. Anesthetics and the renin-angiotensin-aldosterone axis. *Anesthesiology*. 1978;48:393-396.
24. Miller ED Jr, Bailey DR, Kaplan JA, Rogers PW. The effect of ketamine on the renin-angiotensin system. *Anesthesiology*. 1975;42: 503-505.
25. Miller ED, Longnecker DE, Peach MJ. The regulatory function of the renin-angiotensin system during general anesthesia. *Anesthesiology*. 1978;48:399-403.
26. Udelsman R, Norton JA, Jelenich SE, et al. Responses of the hypothalamic-pituitary-adrenal and renin-angiotensin axes and the sympathetic system during controlled surgical and anesthetic stress. *J Clin Endocrinol Metab*. 1987;64:986-994.
27. Crandell WB, Pappas SG, MacDonald A. Nephrotoxicity associated with methoxyflurane anesthesia. *Anesthesiology*. 1966;27: 591-607.
28. Cousins MJ, Mazze RI. Methoxyflurane nephrotoxicity: a study of dose response to man. *JAMA*. 1973;225:1611-1616.
29. Mazze RI, Shue GL, Jackson SH. Renal dysfunction associated with methoxyflurane anesthesia: a randomized prospective clinical evaluation. *JAMA*. 1971;216:278-283.
30. Mazze RI, Cousins MJ, Kosek JC. Dose-related methoxyflurane nephrotoxicity in rats: a biochemical and pathologic correlation. *Anesthesiology*. 1972;36:571-587.
31. Mazze RI, Cousins MJ. Combined nephrotoxicity of gentamicin and methoxyflurane anesthesia in man: a case report. *Br J Anaesth*. 1973;45:394-397.
32. Barr GA, Cousins MJ, Mazze RI, Hitt BA, Kosek JC. A comparison of the renal effects and metabolism of enflurane and methoxyflurane in Fischer 344 rats. *J Pharmacol Exp Ther*. 1974; 188:257-264.
33. Mazze RI, Calverley RK, Smith NT. Inorganic fluoride nephrotoxicity: prolonged enflurane and halothane anesthesia in volunteers. *Anesthesiology*. 1977;46:265-271.
34. Mazze RI, Sievenpiper TS, Steveson J. Renal effects of enflurane and halothane in patients with abnormal renal function. *Anesthesiology*. 1984;60:161-163.
35. Loehning RW, Mazze RI. Possible nephrotoxicity from enflurane in a patient with severe renal disease. *Anesthesiology*. 1974;40: 203-205.
36. Eichhorn JH, Hedley-Whyte J, Steinman TI. Renal failure following enflurane anesthesia. *Anesthesiology*. 1976;45:557-560.
37. Rice SA, Sbordone L, Mazze RI. Metabolism by rat hepatic microsomes of fluorinated ether anesthetics following isoniazid administration. *Anesthesiology*. 1980;53:489-495.
38. Mazze RI, Woodruff RE, Hurdt ME. Isoniazid-induced enzyme defluorination in humans. *Anesthesiology*. 1982;57:5-8.
39. Young SR, Stoelting RK, Peterson C, Madura JA. Anesthetic biotransformation and renal function in obese patients during and after methoxyflurane or halothane anesthesia. *Anesthesiology*. 1975;42:451-457.
40. Bentley JB, Vaughan RW, Miller MS, Calkins JM, Gandolfi AJ. Serum inorganic fluoride levels in obese patients during and after enflurane anesthesia. *Anesth Analg*. 1979;58:409-412.
41. Hitt BA, Mazze RI, Cousins MJ, Edmunds HN, Barr GA, Trudell JR. Metabolism of isoflurane in Fischer 344 rats and man. *Anesthesiology*. 1974;40:62-67.
42. Davidkova T, Kikuchi H, Fujii K, et al. Biotransformation of isoflurane: urinary and serum fluoride ion and organic fluorine. *Anesthesiology*. 1988;69:218-222.
43. Koblin DD, Eger EI II, Johnson BH, Konopka K, Waskell L. I-653 resists degradation in rats. *Anesth Analg*. 1988;67:534-538.
44. Jones RM, Koblin DD, Cashman JN. Biotransformation and hepatorenal function in volunteers after exposure to desflurane (I-653). *Br J Anaesth*. 1990;64:482-487.
45. Sutton TS, Koblin DD, Gruenke LD, et al. Fluoride metabolites after prolonged exposure of volunteers and patients to desflurane. *Anesth Analg*. 1991;73:180-185.
46. Smiley RM, Ornstein E, Pantuck EJ, Pantuck CB, Matteo RS. Metabolism of desflurane and isoflurane to fluoride ion in surgical patients. *Can J Anaesth*. 1991;38:965-968.
47. Koblin DD. Characteristics and implications of desflurane metabolism and toxicity. *Anesth Analg*. 1992;75:510-516.
48. Frink EJ Jr, Ghantous H, Malan TP, et al. Plasma inorganic fluoride with sevoflurane anesthesia: correlation with indices of hepatic and renal function. *Anesth Analg*. 1992;74:231-235.
49. Blanco E, Vidal MI, Blanco J, Fagundo S, Campana O, Alvarez J. Comparison of maintenance and recovery characteristics of sevoflurane–nitrous oxide and enflurane–nitrous oxide anaesthesia. *Eur J Anaesthesiol*. 1995;12:517-523.
50. Goldberg ME, Cantillo J, Larijani GE, Torjman M, Vekeman D, Schieren H. Sevoflurane versus isoflurane for maintenance of anesthesia: are serum inorganic fluoride ion concentrations of concern? *Anesth Analg*. 1996;82:1268-1272.
51. Newman PJ, Quinn AC, Hall GM, Grounds RM. Circulating fluoride changes and hepatorenal function following sevoflurane anaesthesia. *Anaesthesia*. 1994;49:936-939.
52. Wiesner G, Wild K, Schwurzer S, Merz M, Hobbhahn J. Serum fluoride concentrations and exocrine kidney function with sevoflurane and enflurane. An open, randomized, comparative phase III study of patients with healthy kidneys. *Anaesthetist*. 1996;45:31-36.
53. Matsumura C, Kemmotsu O, Kawano Y, Takita K, Sugimoto H, Mayumi T. Serum and urine inorganic fluoride levels following prolonged low-dose sevoflurane anesthesia combined with epidural block. *J Clin Anesth*. 1994;6:419-424.
54. Highiyama T, Hirasakai A. Effects of sevoflurane anaesthesia on renal function—duration of administration and area under the curve and rate of decrease of serum inorganic fluoride. *Eur J Anaesthesiol*. 1995;12:477-482.
55. Bito H, Ikeuchi Y, Ikeda K. Effects of low-flow sevoflurane anesthesia on renal function: comparison with high-flow sevoflurane anesthesia and low-flow isoflurane anesthesia. *Anesthesiology*. 1997;86:1231-1237.
56. Kobayashi Y, Ochiai R, Takeda J, Sekiguchi H, Fukushima K. Serum and urinary inorganic fluoride concentrations after prolonged inhalation of sevoflurane in humans. *Anesth Analg*. 1992;74:753-757.
57. Higuchi H, Arimura S, Sumikura H, Satoh T, Kanno M. Urine concentrating ability after prolonged sevoflurane anaesthesia. *Br J Anaesth*. 1994;73:239-240.
58. Higuchi H, Sumikura H, Sumita S, et al. Renal function in patients with high serum fluoride concentrations after prolonged sevoflurane anesthesia. *Anesthesiology*. 1995;83:449-458.
59. Frink EJ Jr, Isner RJ, Malan TP Jr, Morgan SE, Brown EA, Brown BR Jr. Sevoflurane degradation product concentrations with soda lime during prolonged anesthesia. *J Clin Anesth*. 1994;6:239-242.
60. Eger EI II, Gong D, Koblin DD, et al. Dose-related biochemical markers of renal injury after sevoflurane versus desflurane anesthesia in volunteers. *Anesth Analg*. 1997;85:1154-1163.
61. Eger EI II, Koblin DD, Bowland T, et al. Nephrotoxicity of sevoflurane versus desflurane anesthesia in volunteers. *Anesth Analg*. 1997;84:160-168.
62. Frink EJ Jr, Malan TP Jr, Isner RJ, Brown EA, Morgan SE, Brown BR Jr. Renal concentrating function with prolonged sevoflurane or enflurane anesthesia in volunteers. *Anesthesiology*. 1994;80: 1019-1025.
63. Munday IT, Stoddart PA, Jones RM, Lytle J, Cross MR. Serum fluoride concentration and urine osmolality after enflurane and sevoflurane anesthesia in male volunteers. *Anesth Analg*. 1995;81: 353-359.
64. Ebert TJ, Frink EJ Jr, Kharasch ED. Absence of renal and hepatic toxicity after four hours of 1.25 minimum alveolar anesthetic concentration sevoflurane anesthesia in volunteers. *Anesth Analg*. 1998;86:662-667.

65. Ebert TJ, Frink EJ, Kharasch ED. Absence of biochemical evidence for renal and hepatic dysfunction after 8 hours of 1.25 minimum alveolar concentration sevoflurane anesthesia in volunteers. *Anesthesiology*. 1998;88:601-610.
66. Frink EJ Jr, Malan TP Jr, Brown EA, Morgan S, Brown BR Jr. Plasma inorganic fluoride levels with sevoflurane anesthesia in morbidly obese and nonobese patients. *Anesth Analg*. 1993;76: 1333-1337.
67. Bedford RF, Ives HE. The renal safety of sevoflurane. *Anesth Analg*. 2000;90:505-508.
68. Rooke GA, Ebert T, Muzi M, Kharasch ED. The hemodynamic and renal effects of sevoflurane and isoflurane in patients with coronary artery disease and chronic hypertension. Sevoflurane ischemic study group. *Anesth Analg*. 1996;82:1159-1165.
69. Conzen PF, Nuscheler M, Melotte A, et al. Renal function and serum fluoride concentrations in patients with stable renal insufficiency after anesthesia with sevoflurane or enflurane. *Anesth Analg*. 1995;81:569-575.
70. Nishiyama T, Aibiki M, Hanaoka K. Inorganic fluoride kinetics and renal tubular function after sevoflurane hemodialysis. *Anesth Analg*. 1996;83:574-577.
71. Tsukamoto N, Hirabayashi Y, Shimizu R, Mitsuhata H. The effects of sevoflurane and isoflurane anesthesia on renal tubular function in patients with moderately impaired renal function. *Anesth Analg*. 1996;82:909-913.
72. Artu AA. Renal effects of sevoflurane during conditions of possible increased risk. *J Clin Anesth*. 1998;10:531-538.
73. Hara T, Fukusaki M, Nakamura T, Sumikawa K. Renal function in patients during and after hypotensive anesthesia with sevoflurane. *J Clin Anesth*. 1998;10:539-545.
74. Burchardi H, Kaczmarczyk G. The effects of anaesthesia on renal function. *Eur J Anaesthesiol*. 1994;11:163-168.
75. Higuchi H, Adachi Y, Wada H, Kanno M, Satoh T. The effects of low-flow sevoflurane and isoflurane anesthesia on renal function in patients with stable moderate renal insufficiency. *Anesth Analg*. 2001;92:650-655.
76. Conzen PF, Kharasch ED, Czerner SF, et al. Low-flow sevoflurane compared with low-flow isoflurane anesthesia in patients with stable renal insufficiency. *Anesthesiology*. 2002;97: 578-584.
77. Gentz BA, Malan TP. Renal toxicity with sevoflurane in storm in a teacup? *Drugs*. 2001;61:2155-2162.
78. Kasiske BL, Kjellstrand CM. Perioperative management of patients with chronic renal failure and postoperative acute renal failure. *Urol Clin North Am*. 1983;10:35-50.
79. Hou SH, Bushinsky DA, Wish JB, Cohen JJ, Harrington JT. Hospital-acquired renal insufficiency: a prospective study. *Am J Med*. 1983;74:243-248.
80. Godet G, Fleron MH, Vicaut E, et al. Risk factors for acute postoperative renal failure in thoracic or thoracoabdominal aortic surgery: a prospective study. *Anesth Analg*. 1997;85: 1227-1232.
81. Hanley MJ, Davidson K. Prior mannitol and furosemide infusion in a model of ischemic acute renal failure. *Am J Physiol*. 1981;241:556-574.
82. De Torrente A, Miller PD, Cronin RE, Paulsin PE, Erickson AL, Schrier RW. Effects of furosemide and acetylcholine in norepinephrine-induced acute renal failure. *Am J Physiol*. 1978;235: F131-F136.
83. Burke TJ, Cronin RE, Duchin KL, Peterson LN, Schrier RW. Ischemia and tubule obstruction during acute renal failure in dogs: mannitol in protection. *Am J Physiol*. 1980;238:F305-F314.
84. Kleinknecht D, Ganeval D, Gonzalez-Duque LA, Fermanian J. Furosemide in acute oliguric renal failure: a controlled trial. *Nephron*. 1976;17:51-58.
85. Brown CV, Ogg SC, Cameron JS. High dose furosemide in acute renal failure: a controlled trial. *Clin Nephrol*. 1981;15:90-96.
86. Wilson LM. Acute renal failure. In: *Pathophysiology: Clinical Concepts of Disease Processes*. 4th ed. St Louis: Mosby; 1992: 704-710.
87. Moore RD, Smith CR, Lipsky JJ, Mellits ED, Lietman PS. Risk factors for nephrotoxicity in patients treated with aminoglycosides. *Ann Intern Med*. 1984;100:352-357.
88. Shafi T, Chou SY, Porush JL. Infusion intravenous pyelography and renal function: effect in patients with chronic renal insufficiency. *Arch Intern Med*. 1978;138:1218-1221.
89. Prough D, Foreman A. Anesthesia and the renal system. *Clinical Anesthesia*. 3rd ed. Philadelphia: Lippincott; 1992:1134.
90. Sherlock J, Ledwith J, Letteri J. Determinants of oxygenation during hemodialysis and related procedures: a report of data acquired under varying conditions and a review of the literature. *Am J Nephrol*. 1984;4:158-168.
91. Ganella S, Chang BS. Hemodialysis associated hypoxemia. *Am J Nephrol*. 1984;4:273-279.
92. Turnbull JM, Buck C. The value of preoperative screening investigations in otherwise healthy individuals. *Arch Intern Med*. 1987;147:101-105.
93. Lawrence VA, Kroenke K. The unproven utility of preoperative urinalysis: clinical use. *Arch Intern Med*. 1988;148: 1370-1373.
94. Gold BD, Wolfersberger WH. Findings from routine urinalysis and hematocrit on ambulatory oral and maxillofacial surgery patients. *J Oral Surg*. 1980;38:677-678.
95. Morgan GE Jr, Mikhail MS, Murray MJ, Larson CP Jr. Anesthesia for patients with renal disease. In: *Clinical Anesthesiology*. New York: Lange Medical; 2002:680.
96. Ifudu O. Care of patients undergoing hemodialysis. *N Engl J Med*. 1998;339:1054-1062.
97. Rostand SG, Gretes JC, Kirk KA, Rutsky EA, Andreoli TE. Ischemic heart disease in patients with uremia undergoing maintenance hemodialysis. *Kidney Int*. 1979;16:600-611.
98. Owen CH, Cummings RG, Sell TL, Schwab SJ, Jones RH, Glower DD. Coronary artery bypass grafting in patients with dialysis-dependent renal failure. *Ann Thorac Surg*. 1994;58: 1729-1733.
99. Kahn JK, Rutherford BD, McConahay DR, Johnson WL, Giorgi LV, Hartzler GO. Short- and long-term outcome of percutaneous transluminal coronary angioplasty in chronic dialysis patients. *Am Heart J*. 1990;119:484-489.
100. Endou K. Hemodynamic changes during hemodialysis. *Cardiology*. 1978;63:175-187.
101. Kinet J. Hemodynamic study of hypotension during hemodialysis. *Kidney Int*. 1982;21:868-876.
102. Eschbach JW. Correction of the anemia of the end-stage renal disease with recombinant erythropoietin: results of a combined phase I and II clinical trial. *N Engl J Med*. 1987;316:73-78.
103. Opelz G. Blood transfusion: current relevance of the transfusion effect in renal transplantation. *Transplant Proc*. 1985;27: 1015-1022.
104. Erslev A. Erythropoietin coming of age. *N Engl J Med*. 1987; 316:101.
105. Eschbach JW. Treatment of the anemia of progressive renal failure with recombinant human erythropoietin. *N Engl J Med*. 321:158, 1989.
106. Eschbach JW. Recombinant human erythropoietin in anemic patients with end-stage renal disease: results of a phase III multicenter clinical trial. *Ann Intern Med*. 1989;111:992-999.
107. Ifudu O, Feldman J, Friedman EA. The intensity of hemodialysis and the response to erythropoietin in patients with end-stage renal disease. *N Engl J Med*. 1996;334:420-425.
108. Sun CH. Serum erythropoietin levels after renal transplantation. *N Engl J Med*. 1989;321:151-157.
109. Gafter U. Platelet count and thrombopoietic activity in patients with chronic renal failure. *Nephron*. 1987;45:207-209.
110. DiMinno G. Platelet dysfunction in uremia: multifaceted defect partially corrected by dialysis. *Am J Med*. 1985;79: 552-559.
111. Remuzzi G. Bleeding in renal failure: altered platelet function in chronic uremia only partially corrected by haemodialysis. *Nephron*. 1978;22:347-353.

112. Kentro TB, Lottenberg R, Kitchens CS. Clinical efficacy of desmopressin acetate for hemostatic control in patients with primary platelet disorders undergoing surgery. *Am J Hematol.* 1987;24:214-218.
113. Mannucci PM. 1-Desamino-8-D-arginine vasopressin shortens the bleeding time in uremia. *N Engl J Med.* 1983;308:8-11.
114. Janson PA. Treatment of the bleeding tendency in uremia with cryoprecipitate. *N Engl J Med.* 1980;303:1318-1321.
115. Livio M. Conjugated estrogens for the management of bleeding associated with renal failure. *N Engl J Med.* 1986;315:731-735.
116. Margolis DM. Upper gastrointestinal disease in chronic renal failure: a prospective evaluation. *Arch Intern Med.* 1978;138: 1214-1217.
117. Shuman RB, Schuster DP, Zuckerman GR. Prophylactic therapy for stress ulcer bleeding: a reappraisal. *Ann Intern Med.* 1987;106:562-566.
118. Young GA. Anthropometry and plasma valine, amino acids, and proteins in the nutritional assessment of hemodialysis patients. *Kidney Int.* 1992;21:492-497.
119. Lewis SL, Van Epps DE. Neutrophil and monocyte alterations in chronic dialysis patients. *Am J Kidney Dis.* 1987;9:381-395.
120. Ruiz P, Gomez F, Schreiber AD. Impaired function of macrophage Fc receptors in end-stage renal disease. *N Engl J Med.* 1990;322:717-720.
121. Zeldis JB. The prevalence of hepatitis C virus antibodies among hemodialysis patients. *Ann Intern Med.* 1990;112:958-960.
122. Pinson CW, Schuman ES, Gross GF, Schuman TA, Hayes JF. Surgery in long-term dialysis patients: experience with more than 300 cases. *Am J Surg.* 1986;151:567-571.
123. Vinik RH, Reves JG, Greenblatt DJ. The pharmacokinetics of midazolam in chronic renal failure patients. *Anesthesiology.* 1983;59:390-392.
124. Olsen GD, Bennett WM, Porter GA. Morphine and phenytoin binding to plasma proteins in renal and hepatic failure. *Clin Pharmacol Ther.* 1975;17:677-681.
125. Don HF, Dieppa RA, Taylor P. Narcotic analgesics in anuric patients. *Anesthesiology.* 1975;42:745-747.
126. Kay J. Renal disorders. In: *Manual of Anesthesia and the Medically Compromised Patient.* Philadelphia: Lippincott; 1990:244-264.
127. Gosselin RE, Gabourel JD, Willis JH. The fate of atropine in man. *Clin Pharmacol Ther.* 1960;1:597-603.
128. Mouquet C, Bitker MO, Bailliart O, et al. Anesthesia for creation of a forearm fistula in patients with endstage renal failure. *Anesthesiology.* 1989;70:909-914.
129. Alsalti RA, el-Dawlatly AA, al-Salman M, et al. Arteriovenous fistula in chronic renal failure patients: comparison between three different anesthetic techniques. *Middle East J Anesthesiol.* 1999;15:305-314.
130. Bromage PR, Gertel M. Brachial plexus anesthesia in chronic renal failure. *Anesthesiology.* 1972;36:488-493.
131. Martin R, Beauregard L, Tetrault JP. Brachial plexus blockade and chronic renal failure. *Anesthesiology.* 1988;69:405-406.
132. Rodriquez J, Quintela O, Lopez-Rivadulla M, Barcena M, Diz C, Alvarez J. High doses of mepivacaine for brachial plexus block in patients with end-stage chronic renal failure: a pilot study. *Eur J Anaesthesiol.* 2001;18:171-176.
133. Crews JC, Weller RS, Moss J, James RL. Levobupivacaine for axillary brachial plexus block: a pharmacokinetic and clinical comparison in patients with normal renal function or renal disease. *Anesth Analg.* 2002;95:219-223.
134. Grejda S, Ellis K, Arino P. Paraplegia following spinal anesthesia in a patient with chronic renal failure. *Reg Anesth.* 1989;14: 155-157.
135. Basta M, Sloan P. Epidural hematoma following epidural catheter placement in a patient with chronic renal failure. *Can J Anaesth.* 1999;46:271-274.
136. Orko R, Pitkanen M, Rosenberg PH. Subarachnoid anesthesia with 0.75% bupivacaine in patients with chronic renal failure. *Br J Anaesth.* 1986;58:605-609.
137. Ghoreim MM, Pandya H. Plasma protein binding of thiopental in patients with impaired renal or hepatic function. *Anesthesiology.* 1975;42:545-548.
138. Chauvin M, Lebrau M, Leuron JC. Pharmacokinetics of alfentanil in chronic renal failure. *Anesth Analg.* 1987;66:53-56.
139. Davis PJ, Stiller RL, Cook DR, Brandom BW, Davin-Robinson KA. Pharmacokinetics of sufentanil in adolescent patients with chronic renal failure. *Anesth Analg.* 1988;67:268-271.
140. Morcos WE, Payne JP. The induction of anaesthesia with propofol compared in normal and renal failure patients. *Postgrad Med J Suppl.* 1985;61:62-63.
141. Goyal P, Puri GD, Pandey CK, Srivastva S. Evaluation of induction dose of propofol: comparison between endstage renal disease and normal renal function patients. *Anaesth Intensive Care.* 2002;30:584-587.
142. Reiter V, Fay R, Pire JC, Lamiable D, Rendoing J. Continuous flow propofol during kidney transplantation in the adult. *Can J Anesthesiol.* 1989;37:23-31.
143. Carter R, Heerdt M, Acchiardo S. Fluoride kinetics after enflurane anesthesia in healthy and anephric patients and in patients with poor renal function. *Clin Pharmacol Ther.* 1977;20:565-570.
144. Litz RJ, Hubler M, Lorenz W, Meier VK, Albrecht DM. Renal responses to desflurane and isoflurane in patients with renal insufficiency. *Anesthesiology.* 2002;97:1133-1136.
145. Kharasch ED, Frink EJ Jr, Artru A, Michalowski P, Rooke GA, Nogami W. Long-duration low-flow sevoflurane and isoflurane effects on postoperative renal and hepatic function. *Anesth Analg.* 2001;93:1511-1520.
146. Obata R, Bito H, Ohmura M, et al. The effects of prolonged low-flow sevoflurane anesthesia on renal and hepatic function. *Anesth Analg.* 2000;91:1262-1268.
147. Cronnelly R, Stanski DR, Miller RD, Sheiner LB, Sohn YJ. Renal function and the pharmacokinetics of neostigmine in anesthetized man. *Anesthesiology.* 1979;51:222-226.
148. Cronnelly R, Stanski DR, Miller RD, Sheiner LB. Pyridostigmine kinetics with and without renal function. *Clin Pharmacol Ther.* 1980;28:78-81.
149. Morris RB, Cronnelly R, Miller RB. Pharmacokinetics of edrophonium in anephric and renal transplant patients. *Br J Anaesth.* 1983;53:131-134.
150. Bishop MJ, Hornbein TF. Prolonged effect of succinylcholine after neostigmine and pyridostigmine administration in patients with renal failure. *Anesthesiology.* 1983;58:384-386.
151. Thomas JL, Holmes JH. Effects of hemodialysis on plasma cholinesterase. *Anesth Analg.* 1970;49:323-325.
152. Ryan DW. Preoperative serum cholinesterase concentration in chronic renal failure. *Br J Anaesth.* 1977;49:945-949.
153. Desmond JW, Gordon RA. The effect of haemodialysis on blood volume and plasma cholinesterase levels. *Can Anaesth Soc J.* 1969;16:292-301.
154. Miller RD, Way WL, Hamilton WK, Layzer RB. Succinylcholine-induced hyperkalemia in patients with renal failure? *Anesthesiology.* 1972;36:138-141.
155. Koide M, Waud BE. Serum potassium concentrations after succinylcholine in patients with renal failure. *Anesthesiology.* 1972;36: 142-145.
156. Meijer DKF, Weitering JG, Vermeer GA, Scaf HA. Comparative pharmacokinetics of *d*-tubocurarine and metocurine in man. *Anesthesiology.* 1979;51:402-407.
157. Matteo RS, Brotherton WP, Nishitateno K, Khambatta HJ, Dias J. Pharmacodynamics and pharmacokinetics of metocurine in humans: comparison to *d*-tubocurarine. *Anesthesiology.* 1982;57: 183-190.
158. Miller RD, Agoston S, Booij LH, Kersten UW, Crul JF, Ham J. The comparative potency and pharmacokinetics of pancuronium and its metabolites in anesthetized man. *J Pharmacol Exp Ther.* 1978;207:539-543.
159. Agoston S, Vermeer GA, Kertsten UW, Meijer DK. The fate of pancuronium bromide in man. *Acta Anaesthesiol Scand.* 1973;17: 267-275.

160. Hughes R, Chapple DJ. The pharmacology of atracurium: a new competitive neuromuscular blocking agent. *Br J Anaesth.* 1981;53:31-44.
161. Fahey MR, Rupp SM, Fisher DM, et al. The pharmacokinetics and pharmacodynamics of atracurium in patients with and without renal failure. *Anesthesiology.* 1984;61:699-702.
162. Fahey MR, Morris RB, Miller RD. Pharmacokinetics of ORG NC 45 (Norcuron) in patients with and without renal failure. *Br J Anaesth.* 1981;53:1049-1053.
163. Fahey MR, Rupp SM, Fisher DM. Effects of renal failure on laudanosine excretion in man. *Br J Anaesth.* 1985;57:1049-1051.
164. Lynam DP, Cronnelly R, Castagnoli KP, et al. The pharmacodynamics and pharmacokinetics of vecuronium in patients anesthetized with isoflurane with normal renal function or with renal failure. *Anesthesiology.* 1988;69:231-277.
165. Bevan DR, Donati F, Gyasi H. Vecuronium in renal failure. *Can Anaesth Soc J.* 1984;31:491-496.
166. Slater RM, Pollar BJ, Doran BRH. Prolonged neuromuscular blockade with vecuronium in renal failure. *Anaesthesia.* 1988;43: 250-251.
167. Lagasse RS, Katz RI, Petersen M, Jacobson MJ, Poppers PJ. Prolonged neuromuscular blockade following vecuronium infusion. *J Clin Anesth.* 1990;2:269-271.
168. Haynes SR, Morton NS. Prolonged neuromuscular blockade with vecuronium in a neonate with renal failure. *Anaesthesia.* 1990;45:743-745.
169. Rollino C, Visetti E, Borsa S, et al. Is vecuronium toxicity abolished by hemodialysis? A case report. *Artif Organs.* 2000;24: 386-387.
170. Sakamoto H, Takita K, Kemmotsu O, Morimoto Y, Mayumi T. Increased sensitivity to vecuronium and prolonged duration of its action in patients with end-stage renal failure. *J Clin Anesth.* 2001;13:193-197.
171. Cashman JN, Luke JJ, Jones RM. Neuromuscular block with doxacurium in patients with normal absent renal function. *Br J Anaesth.* 1990;64:186-192.
172. Cook DR, Freeman JA, Lai AA, et al. Pharmacokinetics and pharmacodynamics of doxacurium in normal patients and in those with hepatic or renal failure. *Anesth Analg.* 1991;72: 145-150.
173. Caldwell JE, Canfell PC, Castagnoli KP, et al. The influence of renal failure on the pharmacokinetics and duration of action of pipecuronium bromide in patients anesthetized with halothane and nitrous oxide. *Anesthesiology.* 1989;70:7-12.
174. Phillip BJ, Hunter JM. Use of mivacurium chloride by constant infusion in the anephric patient. *Br J Anaesth.* 1992;68: 492-498.
175. Cook DR, Freeman JA, Lai AA, et al. Pharmacokinetics of mivacurium in normal patients and in those with hepatic or renal failure. *Br J Anaesth.* 1992;69:580-585.
176. Bartkowski RR, Witkowski TA, Azad S, Lessin J, Marr A. Rocuronium onset of action: a comparison with atracurium and vecuronium. *Anesth Analg.* 1993;77:574-578.
177. Foldes FF, Nagashima H, Nguyen HD, Schiller WS, Mason MM, Ohta Y. The neuromuscular effects of ORG 9426 in patients receiving balanced anesthesia. *Anesthesiology.* 1991;75:191-196.
178. Agoston S, Vandenbrom RH, Wierda JM. Clinical pharmacokinetics of neuromuscular blocking drugs. *Clin Pharmacokinet.* 1992;22:94-115.
179. Szenohradszky J, Fisher DM, Segredo V, et al. Pharmacokinetics of rocuronium bromide (ORG 9426) in patients with normal renal function or patients undergoing cadaver renal transplantation. *Anesthesiology.* 1992;77:899-904.
180. Alpert RA, Roizen MF, Hamilton WK, et al. Intraoperative urinary output does not predict postoperative renal function in patients undergoing abdominal aortic revascularization. *Surgery.* 1984;95:707-711.
181. Sprung J, Kapural L, Bourke DK, O'Hara JF Jr. Anesthesia for kidney transplant surgery. *Anesthesiol Clin North Am.* 2000;18:919-951.
182. Tilney NL, Milford EL, Araujo JL, Strom TB, Carpenter CB, Kirkman RL. Experience with cyclosporine and steroids in clinical renal transplantation. *Ann Surg.* 1984;200:605-613.
183. Opelz G, Terasaki PI. Poor kidney survival in recipients with frozen blood transfusions or no transfusions. *Lancet.* 1974;2: 696-698.
184. Borland LM, Cook DR. Anesthesia for organ transplantation. In: *Advances in Anesthesia.* Chicago: Year Book; 1986:1-36.
185. Linke CL, Merin RG. A regional anesthetic approach for renal transplantation. *Anesth Analg.* 1976;55:69-73.
186. Hirsche MM. Renal transplantation in patients with type II diabetes mellitus. *Nephrol Dial Transplant.* 1995;10:58-60.
187. Strunin L. Some aspects of anaesthesia for renal homotransplantation. *Br J Anaesth.* 1966;38:812-822.
188. Katz J, Kountz SL, Cohn R. Anesthetic considerations for renal transplant. *Anesth Analg.* 1967;55:69-73.
189. Munda R, Alexander JW, First MR, Gartside PS, Fidler JP. Pulmonary infections in renal transplant recipients. *Ann Surg.* 1978;187:126-133.
190. Conzen PF, Nuscheler M, Melotte A, et al. Renal function and serum fluoride concentrations in patients with stable renal insufficiency after anesthesia with sevoflurane or enflurane. *Anesth Analg.* 1995;81:569-575.
191. Tsukamoto N, Hirabayashi Y, Shimizu R, Mitsuhata H. The effects of sevoflurane anesthesia on renal tubular function in patients with moderately impaired renal function. *Anesth Analg.* 1996;82:909-913.
192. Nishiyama T, Aibiki M, Hanaoka K. Inorganic fluoride kinetics and renal tubular function after sevoflurane anesthesia in chronic renal failure patients receiving hemodialysis. *Anesth Analg.* 1996;83:574-577.
193. Bluestein LS, Stinson LW Jr, Lennon RL, Quessy SN, Wilson RM. Evaluation of cisatracurium, a new neuromuscular blocking agent, for tracheal intubation. *Can J Anaesth.* 1996;43:925-931.
194. Pollard BJ. Rocuronium and cisatracurium. *Br J Hosp Med.* 1997;57:346-348.
195. Schmith VD, Fiedler-Kelly J, Phillips L, Grasela TH Jr. Dose proportionality of cisatracurium. *J Clin Pharmacol.* 1997;37:625-629.
196. Kadieva VS, Friedman L, Margolivs LP. The effect of dopamine on graft function in patients undergoing renal transplantation. *Anesth Analg.* 1993;76:362-365.
197. Hirschman CA, Edelstein G. Intraoperative hyperkalemia and cardiac arrests during renal transplantation in an insulin dependent diabetic patient. *Anesthesiology.* 1979;51:161-162.
198. Hirschman CA, Leon D, Edelstein G, et al. Risk of hyperkalemia in recipients of kidneys preserved with an intracellular electrolyte solution. *Anesth Analg.* 1980;59:283-286.
199. Cirella VN, Pantuck CB, Lee YJ, Pantuck EJ. Effects of cyclosporine on anesthetic action. *Anesth Analg.* 1987;66: 703-706.
200. Gramstad L, Gjerlow JA, Hysing ES, Rugstad HE. Interaction of cyclosporin and its solvent, Cremophor, with atracurium and vecuronium: studies in the cat. *Br J Anaesth.* 1986;58:1149-1155.
201. Behnia R, Moss J, Graham JB, Linde HW, Roizen MF. Hemodynamic and catecholamine responses associated with extracorporeal shock wave lithotripsy. *J Clin Anesth.* 1990;2:158-162.
202. Gissen D. Anesthesia for extracorporeal shock wave lithotripsy. *Semin Anesth.* 1987;6:57-60.
203. Behnia R, Shanks CA, Ovassapian A, Wilson LA. Hemodynamic responses associated with lithotripsy. *Anesth Analg.* 1987;66: 354-356.
204. Malhortra V. Hyperthermia and hypothermia as complications of extracorporeal shock wave lithotripsy. *Anesthesiology.* 1987; 67:448.
205. Higgins TL, Miller EV, Roberts J. Accidental hyperthermia as a complication of ESWL under general anesthesia. *Anesthesiology.* 1987;66:389-391.
206. Vandeursen H, Tjandramaga B, Verbesselt R, Smet G, Baert L. Anesthesia-free extracorporeal shock wave lithotripsy in patients with renal calculi. *Br J Urol.* 1991;68:18-24.

207. Warner MA, Warner ME, Buck CF, Segura JW. Clinical efficacy of high frequency jet ventilation during extracorporeal shock wave lithotripsy of renal and ureteral calculi: a comparison with conventional mechanical ventilation. *J Urol.* 1988;139: 486-487.
208. Schulte AM, Esch J, Kochs E, Meyer WH. Use of high frequency jet ventilation in extracorporeal shockwave lithotripsy. *Anaesthesist.* 1985;34:294-298.
209. Perel A, Hoffman B, Poeleh D. High frequency positive pressure ventilation during general anesthesia for extracorporeal shock wave lithotripsy. *Anesth Analg.* 1968;65:1231-1234.
210. Berger JJ, Boysen PG, Gravenstein JS, Banner MJ, Carlson CA. Failure of high frequency jet ventilation to ventilate patients adequately during extracorporeal shock-wave lithotripsy. *Anesth Analg.* 1987;66:262-263.
211. Jansson L, Bengtson M, Carlsson C. Heart synchronized ventilation during general anesthesia for extracorporeal shock wave lithotripsy. *Anesth Analg.* 1988;67:706-709.
212. Harries A, Bagley G, Lim M. Anesthesia for extracorporeal shock wave lithotripsy: a comparison of propofol and methohexitone infusions during high frequency jet ventilation. *Anaesthesia.* 1988;43:100-105.
213. Burmeister MA, Brauer P, Wintruff M, Graefen M, Blanc I, Standl TG. A comparison of anaesthetic techniques for shock wave lithotripsy: the use of a remifentanil infusion alone compared to intermittent fentanyl boluses combined with a low dose propofol infusion. *Anaesthesia.* 2002;57:877-881.
214. Monk TG, Rater JM, White PF. Comparison of alfentanil and ketamine infusion in combination with midazolam for outpatient lithotripsy. *Anesthesiology.* 1991;74:1023-1028.
215. Lau WC, Green CR, Faerber GJ, Tait AR, Golembiewski JA. Intrathecal sufentanil for extracorporeal shock wave lithotripsy provides earlier discharge of the outpatient than intrathecal lidocaine. *Anesth Analg.* 1997;84:1227-1231.
216. Eaton MP, Chhibber AK, Green DR. Subarachnoid sufentanil versus lidocaine spinal anesthesia for extracorporeal shock wave lithotripsy. *Reg Anesth.* 1997;22:515-520.
217. Eaton MP, Kristensen EA. Subarachnoid sufentanil for extracorporeal shock lithotripsy. *Reg Anesth.* 1997;22:86-88.
218. Pandit SK, Powell RB, Crider B, McLaren ID, Rutter T. Epidural fentanyl is not effective for analgesia for extracorporeal lithotripsy (ESWL). *Anesthesiology.* 1988;68:176-177.
219. Korbon GA, Lynch C III, Arnold WP, Ross WT, Hudson SB. Repeated epidural anesthesia for extracorporeal shock-wave lithotripsy is unreliable. *Anesth Analg.* 1987;66:669-672.
220. Kelly RE, Binion M, Malhotra V, Artusio JF Jr. Pulmonary function after extracorporeal shock wave lithotripsy: a comparison of general and regional anesthesia. *Can J Anaesth.* 1989;36:137-140.
221. Richardson MG, Dooley JW. The effects of general versus epidural anesthesia for outpatient extracorporeal shock wave lithotripsy. *Anesth Analg.* 1998;86:1214-1218.
222. Zeitlin GL, Roth RA. Effect of three anesthetic techniques on the success of extracorporeal shock wave lithotripsy in nephrolithiasis. *Anesthesiology.* 1988;68:272-276.
223. Kwa AM, Murray WB, Foster PA. Low dose epidural lidocaine/sufentanil is effective for outpatient lithotripsy. *Middle East J Anesthesiol.* 1995;13:71-78.
224. Graff J, Schmidt A, Pastor J, Herberhold D, Rassweiler J, Hankemeier U. New generator for low pressure lithotripsy with the Dornier HM3: preliminary experience of 2 centers. *J Urol.* 1988;139:904-907.
225. Duvall JO, Griffith DP. Epidural anesthesia for extracorporeal shock wave lithotripsy. *Anesth Analg.* 1985;64:544-546.
226. Kovac AL. Recovery room risk and outcome associated with renal extracorporeal shock wave lithotripsy. *J Clin Anesth.* 1993;5:364-368.
227. Gravenstein D. Extracorporeal shock wave lithotripsy and percutaneous nephrolithotomy. *Anesthesiol Clin North Am.* 2000;18: 953-972.
228. Monk TG, Ding Y, White PF. Analgesic efficacy of EMLA during outpatient shock wave lithotripsy. *Anesth Analg.* 1992;74:S213.
229. Tiselius HG. Cutaneous anesthesia with lidocaine-prilocaine cream: a useful adjunct during shock wave lithotripsy with analgesic sedation. *J Urol.* 1993;149:8-11.
230. Uyar M, Uyar M, Ugar G, Bilge S, Ozyar B, Ozyurt C. Patient-controlled sedation and analgesia during SWL. *J Endourol.* 1996;10:407-410.
231. Ganapathy S, Razvi H, Moote C, et al. Eutectic mixture of local anaesthetics is not effective for extracorporeal shock wave lithotripsy. *Can J Anaesth.* 1996;43:1030-1034.
232. Schelling G, Weber W, Mendl G, Braun H, Cullmann H. Patient controlled analgesia for shock wave lithotripsy: the effect of self-administered alfentanil on pain intensity and drug requirement. *J Urol.* 1996;155:43-47.
233. Desmond J. Serum osmolality and plasma electrolytes in patients who develop dilutional hyponatremia during transurethral resection. *Can J Surg.* 1970;13:116-121.
234. Hesbit TE. The use of glycine in transurethral prostatic surgery. *J Urol.* 1948;59:1212-1216.
235. Desmond J. Complications of transurethral prostatic surgery. *Can Anaesth Soc J.* 1970;17:25-36.
236. Hagstrom RS. Studies on fluid absorption during transurethral prostatic resection. *J Urol.* 1955;73:852-859.
237. Henderson DJ, Middleton RG. Coma from hyponatremia following transurethral resection of the prostate. *Urology.* 1980;15:267-271.
238. Aasheim GM. Hyponatremia during transurethral surgery. *Can Anaesth Soc J.* 1973;20:274-280.
239. Kenyon HR. Perforation of the transurethral operations: technique for immediate diagnosis and management of extravasation. *JAMA.* 1950;142:798-801.
240. Harrison RH, Boren JS, Robison JR. Dilutional hyponatremic shock: another concept of the transurethral prostatic resection reaction. *J Urol.* 1956;75:95-110.
241. Defalque KJ, Miller DW. Visual disturbances during transurethral resection of the prostate. *Can Anaesth Soc J.* 1975;22:620-621.
242. Gooding JM, Holcomb MC. Transient blindness following intravenous administration of atropine. *Anesth Analg.* 1977;56: 872-873.
243. Ovassapian A, Joshi CW, Brunner EA. Visual disturbance: an unusual symptom of transurethral prostatic resection reaction. *Anesthesiology.* 1982;57:332-334.
244. Hoekstra PT, Kahnoski R, McCamish MA, Bergen W, Heetderks DR. Transurethral prostatic resection syndrome: a new perspective: encephalopathy with associated hyperammonemia. *J Urol.* 1983;130:704-707.
245. Roesch RP, Stoelting RK, Lingeman JE, Kahnoski RJ, Backes DJ, Gephardt SA. Ammonia toxicity resulting from glycine absorption during a transurethral resection of the prostate. *Anesthesiology.* 1983;58:577-579.
246. James JH, Ziparo V, Jeppsson B, Fischer JE. Hyperammonaemia, plasma aminoacid imbalance, and blood-brain aminoacid transport: a unified theory of portal-systemic encephalopathy. *Lancet.* 1979;2:772-775.
247. Wang JM, Wong KC, Creel DJ, Clark WM, Shahangian S. Effects of glycine on hemodynamic responses and visual evoked potentials in the dog. *Anesth Analg.* 1985;64:1071-1077.
248. Kellow NH. Pacemaker failure during transurethral resection of the prostate. *Anaesthesia.* 1993;48:136-138.
249. Madsen RE, Madsen PO. Influence of anesthesia form on blood loss in transurethral prostatectomy. *Anesth Analg.* 1967;46:330-332.
250. Perkins JB, Miller HC. Blood loss during transurethral prostatectomy. *J Urol.* 1969;101:93-97.
251. Levin K, Nyren O, Pompeius R. Blood loss, tissue weight, and operating time in transurethral prostatectomy. *Scand J Urol Nephrol.* 1981;15:197-200.
252. Malhotra V. Transurethral resection of the prostate. *Anesthesiol Clin North Am.* 2000;18:883-898.

CHAPTER 28

Hepatobiliary and Gastrointestinal Disturbances

Timothy J. Palmer

Several symptomatic manifestations are characteristic of gastrointestinal disease. A common finding is pain, which may be localized or referred and variable in intensity. Common symptoms include nausea and vomiting, abdominal distention, bloating, constipation, diarrhea, fever, and malaise. Clinical signs of gastrointestinal disease may range from occult, painless rectal bleeding to frank hemorrhage via the rectum or esophagus. Other signs of gastrointestinal disease include increased abdominal girth, petechiae, dehydration, jaundice, and evidence of malnutrition. Secondary organ system dysfunction caused by gastrointestinal disease is evidenced by decreases in urinary output, alterations in cardiac rhythm, peripheral edema, pulmonary edema, perturbations in electrolyte balance, alterations in hemostatic function, and sepsis.

The planning for and delivery of anesthesia in patients with gastrointestinal disease must take into consideration whether the illness is acute or chronic. This assessment is for appraisal of the patient's compensatory status, particularly if secondary organ system involvement is apparent. The presence of preexisting acquired or age-related disease processes must also be determined in the patient's preanesthetic assessment. An anesthetic technique that preserves the patient's preexisting compensatory capabilities can therefore be chosen.

Certain procedures have benefited from advances in technology and technique, to the ultimate benefit of patients. Laparoscopic surgical methods have allowed formerly extensive open procedures to be performed on an outpatient basis or with an abbreviated postoperative hospital stay. The negative effects of open surgical techniques have consequently been significantly reduced. Anesthesia delivery methods for these procedures have concomitantly been modified to accommodate the goal of shorter patient hospital stays. Anesthetists must be familiar not only with the scope and ramifications of gastrointestinal disease in acutely and in profoundly ill patients but also with the new directions in diagnostic and surgical management of chronic or subacute disease.

The purpose of this chapter is to give an overview of the pathophysiologic processes in the hepatobiliary and gastrointestinal system that are commonly encountered by the anesthetist. Fundamental anesthetic considerations are elucidated, and the reader is encouraged to consult chapters in this book that specifically address certain management issues in greater detail (e.g., endocrine disease, morbid obesity, trauma, oncology, and electrolyte imbalance). Other resources that further elaborate on the topics discussed in this chapter may be found in the reference section.

PANCREATIC DISEASE

Physiologic Overview

The pancreas functions in both an endocrine and an exocrine hormonal capacity. Exocrine function consists primarily of the daily, continuous secretion of 1500 to 3000 ml of pancreatic juice, which is normally clear and colorless and has a pH of 8.3. The ionic composition consists largely of sodium, potassium, bicarbonate, and chloride, with smaller concentrations of phosphate, sulfate, zinc, and calcium. The principal function of pancreatic juice is to adjust the pH of the duodenal contents in order to promote optimal activity of pancreatic enzymes.

Arrival of acidic chyme into the duodenum and jejunum stimulates the release of the hormones cholecystokinin-pancreozymin (CCK-PZ) and secretin. Both hormones are produced in the duodenum, jejunum, and ileum. Secretin is responsible for stimulating the pancreas to release bicarbonate and water, and CCK-PZ, which is released in response to the presence of fats and partially digested proteins in the duodenum, stimulates elaboration of the pancreatic enzymes necessary for further intestinal digestive processes. Trypsinogen, which is produced by pancreatic cells, is converted to the active enzyme trypsin in response to the release of enterokinase by the gastric mucosa. Trypsin is responsible for the conversion of large ingested proteins into smaller peptides and amino acids in preparation for intestinal absorption. The major pancreatic enzyme groups are listed in Table 28-1.

Although control of pancreatic secretion is primarily hormonal, evidence suggests that a parasympathetic influence also exists. Administration of vagolytic agents, such as atropine and glycopyrrolate, or ganglionic blocking agents, along with physical interruption of the vagus nerve, may induce a decreased response to the hormone secretin. Vagotomy has also been shown to result in a decrease in the release of pancreatic bicarbonate in response to duodenal acidity.

Other factors influence pancreatic secretion. Fasting results in a decreased secretion of pancreatic lipase and amylase. In protein malnutrition, as occurs in starvation and hypoalbuminemic states, a decrease in the secretion of pancreatic peptidases is typically seen. Severe protein-calorie malnutrition causes structural and functional changes within the pancreas. In general, acinar cell atrophy occurs, zymogen granules decrease, and the overall

TABLE 28-1 Major Pancreatic Enzyme Groups*

Enzyme group	Enzyme, proenzyme, or precursor
Proteolytic	Trypsinogen (trypsin), chymotrypsinogen (chymotrypsin), procarboxypeptidase A (carboxypeptidase A), procarboxypeptidase B (carboxypeptidase B), proaminopeptidase (aminopeptidase), proelastase (elastase)
Amylolytic	α-Amylase
Lipolytic	Lipase, prophospholipase A_2 (phospholipase A_2), carboxylesterase lipase, procolipase (colipase)
Nucleolytic	Deoxyribonuclease, ribonuclease
Other:	Trypsin inhibitor

**Precursor molecules are listed, with products in parentheses.*

enzymatic activities of pancreatic juice decrease.[1] Therefore digestion of fat and protein is impaired.

The endocrine function of the pancreas consists primarily of regulation of the plasma glucose level. To do this the pancreas releases hormones from the islets of Langerhans. Three types of these cells exist:

1. Beta cells are responsible for the secretion of insulin, facilitate use of carbohydrates, and suppress fat metabolism. Insulin enhances anabolism, inhibits catabolic processes (e.g., glycogenolysis, ketogenesis, and gluconeogenesis), and promotes glycogenesis and triglyceride storage.
2. Alpha cells are responsible for the secretion of glucagon, which basically acts in opposition to the effects of insulin.
3. Delta cells secrete the inhibitory hormone somatostatin (growth hormone–releasing inhibitory factor), which is responsible for controlling the plasma levels of both insulin and glucagon.

α-Adrenergic stimulation has been shown to be inhibitory to insulin secretion. β-Adrenergic and cholinergic blockade are inhibitory to insulin secretion as well. Arterial hypoxemia, hypothermia, traumatic stress, and surgical stress all suppress insulin secretion through α-adrenergic stimulation. Insulin secretion is enhanced by vagal stimulation, β_2-adrenergic activation, and cholinergic drug administration.

Anesthetic considerations in patients with derangements in pancreatic endocrine function, such as diabetes mellitus, are not within the scope of this chapter. The present discussion is directed toward anesthetic considerations that are germane to patients with inflammatory or neoplastic disease of the pancreas.

Acute Pancreatitis

The cause of pancreatitis is multifactorial. Common causes include alcohol abuse, direct or indirect trauma to the pancreas, ulcerative penetration from adjacent structures (e.g., the duodenum), infectious processes, biliary tract disease, metabolic disorders (e.g., hyperlipidemia and hypercalcemia), and certain drugs (e.g., corticosteroids, furosemide, estrogens, and thiazide diuretics). Patients who have undergone extensive surgery involving mobilization of the abdominal viscera are at risk for development of postoperative pancreatitis, as are patients who have undergone procedures involving cardiopulmonary bypass. Patients who have received large doses of calcium intraoperatively, particularly after cardiopulmonary bypass, have also been shown to be at risk for development of postoperative pancreatitis.[1] A reasonable hypothetical pathophysiologic mechanism involves the imposition of a syndrome of induced autodigestion. Indeed, acute pancreatitis is characterized as a severe chemical burn of the peritoneal cavity.[2] Aberrant activation or release of pancreatic enzymes or injury to the acinar cells caused by one or more of the aforementioned etiologic factors produces a syndrome that results in hemorrhage, edema, and necrosis of the pancreas.

Enzymes implicated as major culprits in the syndrome of pancreatitis are those activated by trypsin, enterokinase, and bile acids. These enzymes are necessary for proteolysis, elastolysis, and lipolysis. The inappropriate elaboration of these enzymes results in pancreatic inflammation, which is caused by vascular breakdown, coagulation necrosis, fat necrosis, and parenchymal necrosis. Cardiovascular complications of acute pancreatitis can lead to pericardial effusions, alterations in cardiac rhythmicity, signs and symptoms mimicking acute myocardial infarction, thrombophlebitis, and cardiac depression. Acute pancreatitis also predisposes patients to the development of acute respiratory distress syndrome and disseminated intravascular coagulopathy.[3]

Pain is the foremost symptom of acute pancreatitis and may be variable in quality. Pain may be localized or radiating, dull and tolerable, or severe and unremitting. Pancreatic pain may radiate from the midepigastric to the periumbilical region and may be more intense when the patient is in the supine position. Causes of pancreatitis include (1) obstruction and distention of the pancreatic ducts; (2) edema, with stretching of the pancreatic capsule; (3) edematous duodenal obstruction; (4) biliary tract obstruction; (5) inflammatory exudates, blood, and enzymes in the retroperitoneum; and (6) chemical peritonitis. Abdominal distention is often seen and is largely attributable to the accumulation of intraperitoneal fluid and paralytic ileus. Nausea and vomiting and fever are common symptoms. Hypotension is seen in 40% to 50% of patients and is attributable to hypovolemia secondary to the loss of plasma proteins into the retroperitoneal space. Acute renal failure secondary to dehydration and hypotension may occur.

Hypocalcemia frequently develops in patients with acute pancreatitis, and this condition obviates monitoring the electrocardiogram (ECG) for cardiac rhythm disorders (e.g., lengthened QT interval with possible reentry dysrhythmias). The clinician must also be observant for signs of tetany. Clinical shock may develop that is largely secondary to the effects of vasoactive kinin peptides (e.g., bradykinin) released during the inflammatory process; these peptides enhance vasodilation, vascular permeability, and leukocyte migration. Furthermore, the inappropriate release of pancreatic kinin peptides stimulates smooth muscle contraction and causes impairment in myocardial contractility.[4]

Elevated serum amylase levels are often present but do not necessarily indicate primary pancreatic disease; other intraabdominal disease processes result in such elevations, including biliary tract disease, tuboovarian disease, peptic ulcer disease, and acute bowel disease, including obstruction, inflammation, and ischemia.[5] Elevated serum lipase levels may also be observed. Disruption in the parenchymal integrity of the pancreas allows passage of enzymes into the venous blood and lymphatic stream. Passage of enzymes into the peritoneal cavity may occur, resulting in subsequent absorption into the general circulation. Compressive obstruction of the common bile duct by an edematous head of the pancreas contributes to elevations in serum bilirubin and alkaline phosphatase levels.

Radiographic and ultrasonographic findings aid in the differential diagnosis of pancreatic disease. Evidence of free intraperitoneal air by radiography suggests the presence of a perforated viscus. Pancreatic calcification also may be observed. Ultrasonography is useful in determination of the presence of concurrent (and perhaps causative) cholelithiasis, cholecystitis, and biliary obstruction caused by stone or tumor. Computed tomography (CT) is highly effective in the diagnosis of an enlarged, edematous pancreatic head, which is typically seen in patients with pancreatitis.[5]

Supportive therapy is initially undertaken in acute pancreatitis. This regimen usually includes intensive care unit admission and may involve implementation of invasive monitoring, fluid and hemodynamic resuscitation, and interventions necessary for the preservation of perfusion and function of the abdominal viscera.[4] Severely ill, malnourished patients are often given parenteral nutritional support. Pain is controlled with the use of synthetic opioids, such as fentanyl, which are preferable to morphine. Morphine-induced spasms of Odds' sphincter may exacerbate bile obstruction and stasis. The metabolite of meperidine, normeperidine, which causes analeptic activity, makes meperidine unattractive in pain management in these patients. Epidural analgesia may be selectively appropriate.

If the cause of pancreatitis is obstructive biliary disease caused by the presence of a stone in the common bile duct or by inflammation of the gallbladder, cholecystectomy and possibly common bile duct exploration are indicated. The choice of anesthetic technique and the extent to which monitoring modalities are used are based on an assessment of the patient's history, the acuity of disease, and the degree of preexisting physical compensation. Special attention is directed toward the correction of significant intravascular volume deficits. The presence of labile hemodynamics and alterations in hepatic function must also be discerned, and appropriate accommodating modifications must be made to the anesthetic plan, for example, ensuring stable arterial pressure, using anesthetic agents and adjuvants that require minimal hepatic biotransformation, ensuring adequate oxygenation, and replacing electrolytes and blood volume.

Chronic Pancreatitis

Chronic alcoholism is a common etiologic factor in chronic pancreatitis. This condition is strongly suggested by the classic diagnostic triad of steatorrhea, pancreatic calcification (evidenced radiographically), and diabetes mellitus. Individuals with chronic pancreatitis are often malnourished and emaciated. They are more often male than female. Other conditions besides chronic alcohol abuse that are associated with the development of chronic pancreatitis include significant and usually chronic biliary tract disease and the effects of pancreatic injury sustained at an earlier age.[3]

Formation of a pseudocyst occurs in up to 8% of alcoholic patients after resolution of a bout of acute pancreatitis. Pancreatic abscess occurs in 3% to 5% of patients with acute pancreatitis but is present in 90% of patients dying as a result of acute pancreatitis.[5] Pancreatic pseudocyst is best evidenced through CT and may be continuous with the pancreatic ductal system. This collection of pancreatic fluid is not totally surrounded by an epithelial lining and therefore is not a true cyst. The mass consists of a collection of proteolytic enzymes that pose a potentially lethal danger to the patient should erosion or rupture occur with consequent spillage into the abdominal cavity or other proximal intraperitoneal structures.

The clinical picture may also include hepatic disease, as evidenced by jaundice, ascites, esophageal varices, derangements in coagulation factors, serum albumin, and transferase enzymes. Perturbation in pancreatic exocrine function with consequent enzymatic insufficiency results in malabsorption of fats and proteins in the intestine. Patients with chronic pancreatitis also have a predisposition for the development of pericardial and pleural effusions.[4]

Pancreatic abscesses develop from infected peripancreatic collections of fluid. Abscesses are usually secondary manifestations of chronic pancreatitis and warrant surgical drainage in order to prevent spread of the infectious contents to the subphrenic and pericolic spaces. Fistula formation is possible, particularly into the transverse colon. Severe intraabdominal hemorrhage is also possible as a result of erosion into major proximal arteries.

Surgical Therapy for Pancreatitis

Surgical drainage of a pancreatic pseudocyst is usually undertaken after a period of maturation of the cyst (usually 6 weeks). The procedure consists of formation of either a cystogastrostomy, cystojejunostomy, cystoduodenostomy, or possibly distal pancreatectomy. The location of the pseudocyst dictates the extent and type of procedure used for the provision of drainage of cystic contents into the gastrointestinal tract. Percutaneous external drainage, guided by CT, is reserved for cases in which the pseudocyst is particularly friable.[6] Spontaneous resolution of pseudocysts may be expected in 20% or more of patients who have undergone surgical drainage.[6]

Pancreatic Tumors

Adenocarcinoma of the pancreas arises most often from the ductal system (90%) and less frequently from the acini.[6] Patients with pancreatic carcinoma are typically 50 to 80 years of age, and the incidence is equal in men and women. Causation is multifactorial, but adenocarcinoma of the pancreas is associated with familial or genetic predisposition. Other etiologic factors include chronic diabetes, alcoholism, chronic pancreatitis, and heavy tobacco and caffeine use.

Because the head of the pancreas is most often the locus of the tumor, biliary obstruction is likely, resulting in progressive jaundice. The patient may have symptoms that are vague and nonspecific and include dull, aching midepigastric or back pain. Anorexia and fatigue are often present and are associated with weight loss. Laboratory studies usually show elevated bilirubin and alkaline phosphatase levels. Radiographic evidence is generally nonspecific; needle biopsy during CT is most helpful in achieving diagnosis. Percutaneous transhepatic cholangiography and endoscopic retrograde cholangiopancreatography are useful diagnostic modalities. Endoscopic retrograde cholangiopancreatography is the most useful modality for defining lesions of the body and tail of the pancreas or of the duodenum and ampulla.[6]

Neoplastic involvement of beta cells is referred to as *insulinoma*. Hypersecretion of insulin is a major manifestation of this disease and results in profound hypoglycemia, which may lead to mental depression, seizures, and coma. Treatment of this disease is surgical excision, except in patients with advanced metastatic disease, and involves distal pancreatectomy, subtotal pancreatectomy, or removal of all but a small portion of pancreatic tissue around the rim of the duodenum (Child's procedure).[6]

If neoplastic disease is determined to be resectable, that is, without involvement of mesenteric vessels or infiltration into the mesenteric arterial root or hepatobiliary structures, a pancreaticoduodenectomy (or a modification of this procedure) may be performed. This procedure involves excision of the antrum of the stomach with the duodenum, distal bile duct, and pancreatic head, along with reconstruction via choledochostomy and pancreaticogastrojejunostomy (Whipple's procedure).[7]

Gastrinoma (Zollinger-Ellison syndrome) is associated with hypersecretion of gastrin, resulting in excessive stimulation of gastric acid secretion. Severe peptic ulcer disease is therefore a possibility, with marked potential for perforation and erosion into adjacent structures, a condition that results in severe hemorrhage. Diarrhea or steatorrhea is typical in this disease process. The culpable lesion is typically a non–beta-cell pancreatic tumor. These lesions are usually occult, slow growing, late metastasizing, and resistant to medical and surgical therapy. Surgical excision of the lesion is the treatment of choice in patients without metastatic disease. Total gastrectomy is infrequently performed because of the proven efficacy of histamine-2 (H_2) antagonists in the medical management of peptic ulcer disease.[5]

Anesthetic Considerations in Pancreatic Disease

The patient undergoing surgical treatment of pancreatic disease exhibits a variable clinical picture: the patient may be jaundiced and stable with a painless pancreatic mass or may be severely ill with multiorgan system involvement.

Patients may have severe, acute abdominal pain with possible intestinal obstruction or ileus. Aspiration precautions should be in effect during induction of anesthesia and emergence from anesthesia. Perioperative assessment of serum glucose level and institution of appropriate control measures are warranted because these patients are likely to be diabetic (secondary to beta-cell dysfunction) or hypoglycemic (as in the case of insulinoma). Derangements in fluid and electrolyte balance must also be anticipated. Rigorous blood product and crystalloid resuscitation may be necessary throughout the perioperative period and likely will necessitate the placement of invasive hemodynamic lines in order to guide therapy and to monitor central pressures.

Potential electrolyte disorders include hypocalcemia, hypomagnesemia, hypokalemia, and possibly hypochloremic metabolic alkalosis. The serum hematocrit value may be falsely increased secondary to hemoconcentration, or it may be decreased secondary to the presence of a bleeding diathesis. Coagulation parameters, including platelet count, prothrombin time (PT), activated partial thromboplastin time (PTT), and fibrinogen level, should be assessed at regular intervals perioperatively. Preservation of renal function mandates the preoperative assessment of blood urea nitrogen, serum creatinine, and 24-hour creatinine clearance (if possible); urinalysis should also be performed. Intraoperatively a urine output of at least 0.5 to 1 ml/kg/hr hour should be maintained.

A significant incidence of postoperative respiratory morbidity associated with upper abdominal surgery, as well as the possible preexisting debilitated state of the patient, mandates a thorough assessment of preexisting pulmonary status. This assessment includes arterial blood gas analysis, chest radiography, and, when appropriate, pulmonary function tests. The pulmonary assessment assumes added importance because of the high incidence of pleural effusion secondary to pancreatic disease and secondary to the potential history of heavy tobacco use.

Cardiovascular assessment should assimilate related findings from the assessment of other organ systems so that the degree to which functional hemodynamic impairment may need to be corrected is fully appreciated. Correction of preexisting hemodynamic disturbances entails restitution of plasma volume and the oxygen-carrying capacity of the blood. Ischemic changes noted on the ECG must be treated promptly. ECG changes mimicking myocardial ischemia are often seen in pancreatitis.

General endotracheal anesthesia is the technique of choice. Preoperative placement of an epidural catheter allows greater flexibility in the intraoperative management of pain and in the provision of postoperative pain control. Patients undergoing extensive pancreatic surgery often require postoperative ventilatory support and intensive care unit monitoring because of the magnitude and the length of the procedure, as well as the patient's preexisting cardiopulmonary status. Pancreatic transplants are discussed later in this chapter.

LIVER DISEASE

Physiologic and Pathophysiologic Considerations

The basic functional unit of the liver is the hepatic lobule. This structure is composed of cylindrically arranged hepatocytes that envelop a central vein, which empties into hepatic veins and ultimately into the vena cava. Hepatic lobules number between 50,000 and 100,000 in the normal liver. Primary blood supply to the liver is furnished by the hepatic artery and the portal vein. The combined blood from both sources joins in the hepatic sinusoidal channels lying between the layer of cells in the lobule. These channels serve as capillaries. Endothelial cells and Kupffer's cells line the sinusoids. Bile canaliculi are located between hepatocytes; these canaliculi empty into terminal bile ducts. A coalescence of central veins from hepatic lobules forms the hepatic veins, which empty into the inferior vena cava. An extensive arcade of lymphatic vessels is also present within the layer of cells.[7]

The liver is responsible for an enormous number of complex and interrelated functions. Because the liver possesses a large functional reserve, significant disease must be present before clinically apparent manifestations are seen. Hepatic dysfunction after anesthesia and surgery is therefore uncommon and, when discovered, is often related to preexisting hepatic disease processes.

The liver receives approximately 1500 ml of blood per minute, 25% to 30% from the hepatic artery and 70% to 75% from the portal vein. This represents 25% to 30% of the cardiac output.[3] The fact that most of the hepatic blood supply is derived from the gut permits speculation on the adequacy of hepatic oxygenation. Adequacy in hepatic oxygen delivery is not seen to be a prominent issue in the normal liver, given the large percentage of cardiac output that perfuses the liver, the great permeability of the hepatic sinuses, and the close proximity of the hepatic sinuses to hepatic cells; therefore the processes of oxygenation, nutrient supply, and carbon dioxide and metabolic waste removal are greatly facilitated.

The filtering function of the liver has a prominent physiologic role. Blood from the gut contains large quantities of colonic bacilli; it is cleansed of more than 99% of the bacterial load by Kupffer's cells (macrophages) that line the hepatic sinuses.[7] Endothelial cells that line the hepatic sinuses permit diffusion of large plasma proteins and other substances into the extravascular spaces in the liver. This phenomenon results in a large quantity of lymph, which is nearly equal in protein concentration to plasma.

The low resistance of the hepatic sinusoids (7 to 10 mm Hg) to portal blood flow allows the liver to function as a circulatory reservoir. Up to 350 ml of blood may be delivered into the circulation in time of need, such as during hemorrhage. Splanchnic blood flow vessels, which provide the blood supply to the liver, gallbladder, omentum, spleen, and pancreas, are innervated by the splanchnic nerves derived from spinal nerves T3 through T11. Both α- and β-receptors are present in the hepatic arterial circulation, but only α-receptors are noted in the portal circulation. Hepatic arterial flow is autoregulated in accordance with metabolic demand, that is, oxygen consumption. Portal blood flow is dependent on the combined venous outflow from the spleen and gastrointestinal tract. A decrease in either portal or arterial blood flow is seen to affect a compensatory increase in blood flow delivered by the other system.[3]

Increased sympathetic nervous system outflow caused by factors such as hypotension, hypovolemia, hypoxia, hypercarbia, and light anesthesia produces hepatic arterial vasoconstriction. Abdominal surgery is recognized as the most profound etiologic factor that results in decreased hepatic blood flow, particularly if the liver is directly involved.

All volatile anesthetics are implicated in reduction of hepatic blood flow. Hepatic blood flow may be reduced as much as 25% with the use of halothane.[8] Although this impairment in hepatic blood flow is largely attributable to decreased systemic blood pressure, halothane is known to directly impair hepatic blood flow even further through abolition of the vasoconstrictor response to hypercarbia.[9] These changes reflect drug- or technique-induced alterations in splanchnic circulatory tone, perfusion pressure, or both. Indeed, hepatic blood flow may be reduced up to 30% in the absence of surgical stimulation when sympathectomy that results from regional lower extremity anesthesia (i.e., subarachnoid or epidural) is present.

Essential physiologic functions of the liver include bile production, protein synthesis, glycogen storage, protein metabolism, insulin clearance, lactate conversion into glucose, and drug metabolism and transformation. Glycogen, a storage form of glucose, is formed by the process of gluconeogenesis from lactate. Other substrates from which the liver manufactures glycogen include amino acids (particularly alanine) and glycerol. Glucose levels are maintained to relatively normal levels by the liver through glycogenolysis during periods of fasting. Hypoglycemia may therefore be encountered in patients with severe liver disease caused by derangements in insulin clearance, a decrease in glycogen capacities, and impairment in gluconeogenesis.

Bile is the primary secretion of the liver and is normally formed at a rate of approximately 1 L/day. Hepatocytes in each lobule continuously secrete fluid, which contains phospholipids, cholesterol, conjugated bilirubin (the end product of hemoglobin metabolism), bile salts, and other substances. Bile is stored and concentrated in the gallbladder. In response to the intestinal hormone CCK, bile is released by the gallbladder. The presence of fat and protein in the duodenum. Contraction of the gallbladder causes bile to flow via the common bile duct through the relaxed Oddi's sphincter and into the duodenum to assist in the absorption of fat and fat-soluble vitamins (vitamins A, D, E, K). The metabolic end products of many drugs are also removed via the bile. Liver disease therefore may result in impaired bile production or flow, leading to steatorrhea, vitamin K deficiency, and delayed removal of active drug metabolites.

A deficiency in vitamin K results in coagulopathy as a result of impaired production of clotting factors II (prothrombin), VII, IX, and X. Indeed, all clotting factors are produced by the liver except for factor VIII, which is produced in endothelial cells. Although only 50% of normal factor activity is necessary for normal clotting, liver disease often results in derangements in coagulation. Hepatocellular disease therefore results in decreased clotting factor levels and abnormal bile production. A perturbation in bile production ultimately manifests as impaired production of vitamin K–dependent clotting factors.

Intrahepatic obstruction of blood flow ultimately results in the development of portal hypertension. A consequence of the resultant transmission of backward pressure is congestive splenomegaly. Thrombocytopenia results from this condition as a consequence of platelet sequestration. Therefore severe liver disease with portal hypertension induces coagulopathy not only as a result of impairment in hepatic coagulation factor production but also as a result of diminution in circulating functional platelets. In the presence of biliary deficiency, parenteral vitamin K administration helps correct coagulopathy. However, significant hepatocellular disease may dictate the need for fresh frozen plasma (FFP) for immediate correction of coagulation factor deficits.

The use of subarachnoid and epidural blockade should be avoided in the presence of frank coagulopathy. Derangements in parameters such as PT, activated PTT, and platelet count are a relative contraindication to these techniques as well. Instrumentation of the nasopharynx, as well as invasive procedures, must be performed cautiously and carefully in the presence of increases in PT and activated PTT, a low platelet count, or other laboratory signs that arouse suspicion of coagulopathy.

With the exception of the immunoglobulins the liver is responsible for the production of proteins. Therefore decreased plasma oncotic pressure and impairment in drug binding are a consequence of severe liver disease. In addition, overexpansion of the interstitial space and third spacing secondary to derangements in plasma oncotic pressure results in a large increase in the volume of distribution of clinically used medications. Clinical concerns should therefore focus on the potential for an exaggerated effect with a given dose of drug, particularly a drug that is highly protein bound. Exaggeration of effect is particularly true with barbiturates. The amount of nondepolarizing muscle relaxant may also need to be increased in order to achieve a given level of blockade. This is secondary to an increased volume of distribution of the drug. Plasma cholinesterase, which is produced in the liver, may also be deficient, a condition that may prolong the effects of succinylcholine and mivacurium as well as enhance the potential toxicity of ester local anesthetics.

Other roles in protein metabolism performed by the liver include synthesis of lipoproteins (important for lipid transport in the blood), deamination of amino acids into carbohydrates and fats for production of adenosine triphosphate (ATP) through citric acid cycle oxidation, and production of urea for the removal of ammonia, which is formed by hepatic deamination processes and by bacteria in the gut.

The liver plays a prominent role in the biotransformation of many exogenous substances, in particular, most drugs. The end products of these processes are the result of deactivation and transformation of these substances into benign by-products that are capable of being excreted in the bile or urine. Two types of biotransformative processes are predominant:

- Phase I reactions, which use oxidation, reduction, deamination, dealkylation, methylation, sulfoxidation, and hydrolysis to alter reactive chemical constituents. This phase is particularly important in the metabolism of most anesthesia-related drugs.

- Phase II reactions, which involve conjugation of the substance with glycine, sulfate, taurine, or glucuronide. Once conjugated the substance is ready for elimination in bile or urine.

Increased tolerance to certain drugs results from overproduction of enzymes within hepatic enzyme systems, including the cytochrome P-450 system. Drugs that are capable of inducing this process include ethanol, benzodiazepines, ketamine, barbiturates, and phenytoin. The result is an increased requirement for certain clinically used drugs, such as sedatives, opioids, and muscle relaxants such as vecuronium and rocuronium.

Hyperactivity of hepatic enzyme systems results in a state of increased pharmacokinetic tolerance or cross-tolerance to other drugs that are metabolized by the same enzyme system. Certain drugs, such as cimetidine and chloramphenicol, are noted to decrease the activity of these enzymes, thereby increasing the effects of other drugs.[10] This effect assumes greater importance with the use of certain drugs known to yield metabolites that exert greater activity than the parent substrate drug or are potentially cytotoxic after phase I hepatic metabolism. Such properties are associated with the drugs isoniazid, acetaminophen, and halothane.[10]

Certain drugs, such as lidocaine, morphine, meperidine, and propranolol, are highly dependent on hepatic extraction from the circulation for sufficient metabolism. Decreased blood flow to the splanchnic circulation, which occurs during hypotensive states and even during uneventful laparotomy, may decrease metabolic clearance of these drugs.

In addition to degradation of insulin, the liver is also responsible for the metabolism of other hormones, as well as vitamins and minerals. Triiodothyronine, the more active of the thyroid hormones, is produced from thyroxine in the liver. Degradation of thyroid hormone, steroid hormones (including aldosterone, cortisol, and estrogen), antidiuretic hormone, and glucagon is also primarily a function of the liver. The hepatocytes also function in the storage of vitamins A, B_{12}, E, and D. Metabolism of iron is affected through the hepatic synthesis of transferrin and haptoglobin. Ceruloplasmin produced in the liver is a necessary component in the process of copper metabolism.

TABLE 28-2 Liver Function Tests (Normal Ranges)

Test	Normal Range
Protein	
Total	60-85 g/L
Albumin	35-50 g/L
Globulin	22-35 g/L
Enzymes	
Aspartate aminotransferase (AST)	0-4 U/L
Alanine aminotransferase (ALT)	2-22 U/L
Alkaline phosphatase (ALP)	30-115 U/L
Lactic dehydrogenase (LDH)	60-200 U/L
γ-Glutamyl transferase (GGT)	8-78 U/L
5′-Nucleotidase	1-11 U/L
Bilirubin	
Total	3-20 μmol/L
Conjugated	<8 μmol/L
Prothrombin time (always compared to a control; abnormal >3 seconds over control)	12-13 sec
Porphyrins (urine)	
Coproporphyrin	24-190 nmol/24 hr
Uroporphyrin	<36 nmol/24 hr
Ammonia (serum)	11-35 μmol/L
Ceruloplasmin	1.8-2.5 μmol/L
Immunoglobulins	
IgG	7.23-15.85 g/L
IgA	0.69-3.82 g/L
IgM	0.63-2.77 g/L
IgE (adult)	10,000-150,000 U/L

From Strunin L, Eagel CJ. Hepatic diseases. In: Anesthesia and Uncommon Diseases. *4th ed. Philadelphia: Saunders; 1998:149.*

Laboratory Evaluation of Liver Function

No single laboratory test reliably assesses liver function. As indicated previously, the huge capacity and functional reserve of the liver allow for the presence of significant disease processes before evidence of liver failure is reflected through abnormal laboratory findings. Abnormalities reflected in laboratory findings, however, aid in differentiation of parenchymal from obstructive disorders. Parenchymal disorders reflect dysfunction at the hepatocellular level, whereas obstructive disorders reflect disease processes caused by dysfunctional bile excretion. Table 28-2 lists laboratory tests commonly used in the diagnosis of liver disease. Table 28-3 lists diagnostic uses of liver function tests.

Effects of Anesthesia on Liver Function

Both general and regional anesthetic techniques have been identified as inducing a reduction in hepatic blood flow. Both the direct effects of the anesthetics and the indirect sequelae of related adjunctive anesthetic activities, such as ventilatory techniques, have been implicated as contributing factors in a reduction of hepatic blood flow. Some locations of surgery, particularly the upper abdomen, have also been implicated as a cause of decreased hepatic blood flow.[8]

All of the volatile anesthetics have also been shown to reduce hepatic blood flow. Halothane has been shown to cause the greatest reduction, and isoflurane the smallest. The use of desflurane has been shown to have hepatic effects similar to those of isoflurane.[8] Sevoflurane appears to undergo hepatic biotransformation, rendering organic and inorganic fluoride ion. In human subjects levels of serum inorganic fluoride ion secondary to sevoflurane metabolism are generally below nephrotoxic levels but may approach previously documented problematic levels with prolonged use of higher concentrations. Studies continue with sevoflurane in order to determine the influence of biotransformation on renal and hepatic function; however, no significant clinical toxicity has been reported.[11]

The reduction in mean arterial pressure and cardiac output frequently seen with the use of volatile anesthetics proportionately reduces hepatic blood flow. Another factor that impairs hepatic blood flow is the vasoconstrictive response of the splanchnic circulation; this response occurs as a sympathetic reflex to reduced mean arterial pressure. Isoflurane increases hepatic blood flow through direct vasodilatory properties. This effect is likely offset, however, by a reduction in portal blood flow. Hypotension secondary to regional anesthetic–induced sympathectomy (e.g., epidural or subarachnoid blockade) principally accounts for the reduced splanchnic blood flow associated with the use of these techniques.

Increased airway pressures associated with controlled mechanical ventilation may adversely affect venous delivery to the right atrium. Increased airway pressures also result in reduced cardiac output, with a consequent reduction in hepatic blood flow. Positive end-expiratory pressure further exacerbates this condition. Impairment in hepatic blood flow

TABLE **28-3** Diagnostic Uses of Liver Function Tests

Enzyme	Clinical Considerations
Transaminases (AST; ALT)	Grossly raised in drug-induced, viral, and ischemic hepatitis; nonspecific and not prognostic alone; may fall when liver failure occurs
Alkaline phosphatase (ALP)	Raised in cholestasis; measure 5′-nucleotidase and γ-GT to distinguish hepatic ALP from nonhepatic origin (e.g., bone)
Glutathione-*S*-transferase	May be sensitive marker for effects of volatile anesthetics
γ-Glutamyl transferase (γ-GT)	Used to assess alcohol-, barbiturate-, and phenytoin-induced liver damage
Lactate dehydrogenase (LDH)	LDH-5 is said to be liver specific, but like isocitrate dehydrogenase (ICD), LDH is of limited use; both are elevated in hepatitis and hepatoma
α-Fetoprotein	Present in 70%-90% of patients with hepatoma; a glycoprotein responsible for copper transport; is low

ALT, *Alanine aminotransferase;* AST, *aspartate aminotransferase.*
From Strunin L, Eagel CJ. Hepatic diseases. In: Anesthesia and Uncommon Diseases. *4th ed. Philadelphia: Saunders; 1998:149.*

under these conditions may result from increased hepatic venous pressure from increased intrathoracic pressure and from increased reflex sympathetic tone caused by reduced cardiac output. Hypercapnia and acidosis have vasodilatory effects on the hepatic circulation that result in increased blood flow, whereas hypocapnia and alkalosis exert vasoconstricting effects that result in decreased flow. The interplay of various intraoperative variables (e.g., surgical site, ventilatory mode, direct and indirect effects of anesthetics used, physiologic responses to intraoperative events) influences the degree to which hepatic blood flow is compromised.

Other effects of anesthetics on hepatic function include a limited attenuation of the stress response that is usually associated with surgical trauma. With both general and regional techniques the effects of increased levels of circulatory catecholamines, glucagon, and cortisol are partially blunted (all of which may compromise hepatic blood flow and metabolic activity).

New opioids have been implicated in causing spasm of Oddi's sphincter, with a resultant increase in biliary pressure. Judicious titration of opioids minimizes this occurrence. Opioids can be ranked in terms of their spasm-causing ability as follows, from greatest to least effect: fentanyl, alfentanil, sufentanil, remifentanil (morphine > meperidine > butorphanol > nalbuphine).[12] Spasm of Oddi's sphincter may cause biliary colic, or it may cause a false-positive result on intraoperative cholangiography.

Although the use of opioids is not discouraged, morphine is the opioid that is most associated with spasm and is best avoided with the preferential use of synthetic opioids. Spasm is low (3%) even when a fentanyl-based anesthetic is used. The cause of the spasm is unclear, and the spasm may have causes other than the anesthetic, such as surgical manipulation, cold irrigating solutions, and the irritant effect of contrast dye. The treatment of suspected spasm of Oddi's sphincter involves increases in the concentration of the volatile agent in use and administration of atropine or glycopyrrolate, glucagon, nitroglycerin, and naloxone or nalbuphine (if the spasm is related to prior opioid administration). Although direct inhibition in the metabolism of certain drugs (e.g., warfarin, ketamine, and phenytoin) occurs with the use of halothane, it is most likely the reduction of hepatic blood flow that indirectly causes altered drug metabolism through reduced drug delivery to appropriate hepatic enzyme systems.

Mild hepatic dysfunction in the postoperative period, as evidenced by increased plasma lactic dehydrogenase and transaminase levels, is common. This development is most likely the result of such factors as sympathetic stimulation, decreased splanchnic blood flow, the surgical site, and the procedure performed.

Significant and persistent postoperative hepatic dysfunction may be caused by preexisting liver disease, sepsis, drug reaction, surgical complications, and viral hepatitis (resulting from blood product transfusion). Postoperative jaundice results from red-cell hemolysis that may be related to transfusion reaction and hematoma reabsorption. Postoperative jaundice also results from biliary obstruction. Causality must be determined through review of intraoperative events to include adverse sequelae from the administration of blood products.

The cause and incidence of halothane hepatitis continue to generate investigation. Liver damage after intraoperative exposure to halothane traditionally occurs most frequently in middle-aged, obese women of childbearing age. It is most common with repeat exposure within the 28 days.[3,8] The incidence of hepatitis after halothane exposure is relatively low in octogenarians and children. Laboratory differentiation between halothane hepatitis and other forms of hepatitis has been inconclusive. An estimated 1 in 10,000 patients develops postoperative jaundice after halothane exposure. In this population a viral source of infection is more likely to be the cause, for instance, as occurs as a complication of intraoperative blood transfusion. According to epidemiologic studies a mild form of halothane hepatitis may occur secondary to 20% of all halothane administrations. The incidence of fatal, hepatic necrosis is only 1:35,000.[8]

Reduced hepatic perfusion related to halothane exposure results in hepatocyte hypoxia. This condition results in the conversion of the normal oxidative hepatic pathway for halothane metabolism to reductive pathways. As a result, potentially hepatotoxic metabolites are produced.

The presence of a hypersensitive immune response secondary to halothane exposure has also been implicated as an etiologic factor in the development of halothane-related hepatitis. An overabundance of antibodies that attack the hepatocytes is produced. Genetic susceptibility has also been theorized to be responsible for the development of halothane hepatitis.

Prevention of halothane hepatitis may be facilitated by the following:

- Limiting the use of halothane to prepubescent children
- Avoiding the use of halothane in patients with evidence or a history of liver dysfunction
- Avoiding the use of halothane in patients who have received it within the past month

The spectrum of the severity of halothane hepatitis may extend from a mild increase in hepatic transaminase enzyme levels to fulminant hepatic failure. In the differential diagnosis of halothane hepatitis, pathogenic sources, such as viral hepatitis (types A, B, and C), Epstein-Barr virus, herpetic viruses, and cytomegalovirus, must first be excluded. The introduction of sevoflurane has essentially made the modern use of halothane obsolete in the United States and most parts of the world. In recent years it was generally avoided in adults and used for inhalation inductions in children; however, sevoflurane is a safe and effective alternative.

Hepatitis

Acute Hepatitis

Acute hepatitis presents a variable clinical picture. Manifestations may extend from mild inflammatory increases in serum transaminase levels to fulminant hepatic failure. The cause of this syndrome is usually exposure to an infectious virus. Other causes include exposure to hepatotoxic substances and adverse drug reactions.

Viral hepatitis may be attributable to exposure to one of a number of viruses, including hepatitis viruses (A, B, C [formerly referred to as *non-A, non-B*], D [delta virus], E [enteric non-A, non-B]), Epstein-Barr virus, herpes simplex virus, cytomegalovirus, and coxsackievirus. The most common culprits are hepatitis A, hepatitis B, and hepatitis C. Hepatitis A and E are transmitted by the oral-fecal route, and hepatitis B and C are transmitted by contact with body fluids and physical contact with disrupted cutaneous barriers.

The common clinical course of viral hepatitis begins with a 1- to 2-week prodromal period, the signs and symptoms of which include fever, malaise, and nausea and vomiting. Progression to jaundice typically occurs, with resolution within 2 to 12 weeks. However, serum transaminase levels often remain increased for up to 4 months. If hepatitis B or C is the cause, the clinical course is often more prolonged and complicated. Cholestasis may manifest in certain cases. Fulminant hepatic necrosis in certain individuals is also possible. Table 28-4 lists the major characteristics of hepatitis types A, B, C, D, and E.

Acute viral hepatitis may evolve into a chronic active syndrome, which develops in 3% to 10% of cases involving hepatitis B and in 10% to 50% of cases involving hepatitis C.[13] Many patients become asymptomatic infectious carriers of hepatitis B and C. These patients include many who are immunosuppressed or require chronic hemodialysis.

The B surface antigen (HBsAg) has been seen to persist in the blood of 0.3% to 30% of all patients previously infected with hepatitis B and C. Approximately 1% of patients infected with hepatitis C remain asymptomatic infectious carriers.[10] Avoiding exposure to blood and body fluids from high-risk patients (e.g., intravenous drug abusers, homosexual men, hemodialysis patients, patients residing in group homes, immunosuppressed patients) is an unreliable means of preventing exposure to hepatitis viruses in view of the large number of asymptomatic and unrecognized carriers. It therefore behooves all health-care personnel to adhere to universal precautions in the performance of patient care. Hepatitis vaccination is strongly recommended. Successful vaccination against hepatitis B (transmitted by parenteral and percutaneous routes) confers a limited measure of protection from hepatitis D, which requires hepatitis B for its expression.

Drug-Induced Hepatitis

Drug-induced hepatitis results from an idiosyncratic drug reaction, from direct hepatic toxicity, or from a combination of the two. Clinically its manifestations resemble those of viral hepatitis, thereby complicating diagnosis. Alcoholic hepatitis is probably the most common form of drug-induced hepatitis and results in fatty infiltration of the liver (causing hepatomegaly), with impairment in hepatic oxidation of fatty acids, lipoprotein synthesis and secretion, and fatty acid esterification.[3] Box 28-1 lists drugs and substances that are associated with the development of hepatitis.

Chronic Hepatitis

Chronic hepatitis does not occur in hepatitis A infections but does occur in 1% to 10% of acute hepatitis B infections and in 10% to 40% of hepatitis C infections.[3] Patients are classified as having one of three distinct syndromes, based on liver biopsy:

- Chronic persistent hepatitis
- Chronic lobular hepatitis
- Chronic active hepatitis

Chronic persistent hepatitis is relatively benign and is confined to portal areas. Hepatic cellular integrity is preserved,

TABLE 28-4 Five Causes of Acute Viral Hepatitis

Hepatitis Virus	Size (nm)	Genome	Route of Transmission	Incubation Period (Days)	Fatality Rate	Chronic Rate	Antibody
A	27	RNA	Fecal-oral	15-45 (mean = 25)	1%	None	Anti-HAV
B	45	DNA	Parenteral Sexual	30-180 (mean = 75)	1%	2%-7%	AntiHBs Anti-HBc Anti-HBe
C	60	RNA	Parenteral	15-150 (mean = 50)	<0.1%	70%-85%	Anti-HCV
D (delta)	40	RNA	Parenteral Sexual	30-150	2%-10%	2%-7% 50%	Anti-HDV
E	32	RNA	Fecal-oral	30-60	1%	None	Anti-HEV

HAV, *hepatitis A virus;* HCV, *hepatitis C virus;* HBs, *hepatitis B surface;* HBe, *hepatitis B e antigen;* HBc, *hepatitis B core;* Anti-HDV, *hepatitis D virus antibody;* Anti-HEV, *hepatitis E virus antibody.*

From Hoofnagle JH, Lindsay KL. Acute viral hepatitis. In: Goldman L, Ausiello D, eds. Cecil's Textbook of Medicine. *22nd ed. Philadelphia: Saunders; 2004:912.*

BOX **28-1**

Drugs and Substances Associated with Hepatitis

Toxic
Alcohol
Acetaminophen
Salicylates
Tetracycline
Trichloroethylene
Vinyl chloride
Carbon tetrachloride
Yellow phosphorus
Poisonous mushrooms
Amanita
Galerina

Idiosyncratic
Volatile anesthetics
Halothane
Phenytoin
Sulfonamides
Rifampin
Indomethacin

Toxic and Idiosyncratic
Methyldopa
Isoniazid
Sodium valproate
Amiodarone

Primarily Cholestatic
Chlorpromazine
Chlorpropamide
Oral contraceptives
Anabolic steroids
Erythromycin estolate
Methimazole

From Morgan GE, Mikhail MS. Anesthesia for patients with liver disease. In: Morgan GE, Mikhail MS. Clinical Anesthesiology. *3rd ed. Norwalk, Conn: Appleton & Lange; 2002:725.*

and progression to cirrhosis is rare. Chronic lobular hepatitis involves recurrent exacerbations of acute inflammation, but, as in persistent hepatitis, progression to cirrhosis is rare.

The most serious form of chronic hepatitis is chronic active hepatitis, which is progressive and results in hepatocyte destruction, cirrhosis, and ultimately hepatic failure. Death often results from related manifestations of hepatic failure, such as hemorrhage from esophageal varices, multiorgan system failure (e.g., hepatorenal syndrome), and encephalopathy. The typical etiologic agent is hepatitis B or hepatitis C virus. Autoimmune disorders (e.g., systemic lupus erythematosus) and exposure to certain drugs (e.g., methyldopa, isoniazid, and nitrofurantoin) have been implicated as etiologic factors, as well.

Marked fatigue and jaundice are common in chronic hepatitis. Arthritis, neuropathy, myocarditis, thrombocytopenia, and glomerulonephritis may also be present. Plasma albumin levels are usually decreased, and PT is often prolonged.

Anesthetic Considerations in Hepatitis

Increased perioperative mortality (10%) and morbidity (12%) rates have been reported with surgery, particularly laparotomy, in patients with acute viral hepatitis. Operative procedures performed in patients with alcohol intoxication are also likely to be associated with increased perioperative complications. Surgery performed in those undergoing alcohol withdrawal is associated with a mortality rate as high as 50%.[10] With the acutely intoxicated alcoholic patient, certain anesthetic issues must be kept in mind: (1) less anesthetic is needed, (2) aspiration precautions must be implemented, (3) surgical bleeding may be increased as a result of interference with platelet aggregation, (4) the brain is less tolerant of hypoxia, and (5) the level of circulating catecholamines is increased, as evidenced by lability in vital signs and exaggerated responses to drugs and stimuli (probably indicating decreased neurotransmitter uptake).[3]

It is therefore prudent to postpone elective surgical procedures until liver function has been normalized. Surgery and anesthesia greatly increase the risk for further hepatic decompensation in patients with hepatitis; this risk may be compounded by the development of renal failure (hepatorenal syndrome), encephalopathy, and the decompensation of other organ systems.

If urgent or emergency surgery is necessary, as thorough a preoperative history as possible must be obtained. If serious time constraints are imposed, the preoperative evaluation should focus on signs and symptoms (e.g., encephalopathy, bleeding diatheses, jaundice, ascites, and hemodynamic findings) and on the results of laboratory studies (e.g., levels of electrolytes, blood urea nitrogen, creatinine, serum glucose, hemoglobin, hematocrit, liver enzymes, and bilirubin, as well as arterial blood gas determinations and coagulation studies). Other pertinent studies include chest radiography and ECG. If not previously ordered, blood typing and cross-matching are warranted, depending on the magnitude of the planned procedure. Any history of hospitalizations and anesthetic use should also be obtained. In general, as much pertinent information as possible should be procured and recorded.

Dehydration and electrolyte derangements should be anticipated and corrected before surgery. Metabolic alkalosis and hypokalemia are often present as a result of vomiting. The presence of hypomagnesemia predisposes to the development of perioperative dysrhythmias. Elevated enzyme (e.g., alkaline phosphatase, alanine aminotransferase [ALT], aspartate aminotransferase [AST]) and serum bilirubin levels are nonspecific with regard to the degree of hepatic necrosis. Alcoholic hepatitis and obstructive hepatitis are commonly associated with an elevation in AST. Viral hepatitis and drug-induced hepatitis often reflect elevated ALT levels. The highest measured levels of AST are seen in viral hepatitis or in fulminant hepatic failure.

PT is the best indicator of the liver's ability to synthesize coagulation factors. Severe hepatic dysfunction results in a persistent prolongation of PT, even after the administration of vitamin K. Evaluation of serum albumin level is warranted, although deficiencies in serum albumin, as well as in all proteins synthesized by the liver (i.e., coagulation factors), are manifestations of severe hepatic dysfunction and malnutrition.

Preoperative medication (e.g., sedation) may best be avoided, so that exacerbation of preexisting encephalopathy or respiratory embarrassment is prevented. Administration of FFP, vitamin K, and packed red blood cells may be necessary for the correction of coagulopathy and red-cell deficiency

TABLE 28-5 Child-Turcote-Pugh Score of Severity of Liver Disease

Points	1	2	3
Encephalopathy	None	1-2	3-4
Ascites	Absent	Slight	Moderate
Bilirubin (mg/dl)	<2	2-3	>3
For PBC/PSC	<4	4-10	>10
Albumin (g/dl)	<3.5	2.8-3.5	>2.8
PT (INR)	<1.7	1.7-2.3	>2.3

INR, *International normalized ratio;* PBC, *Primary biliary cirrhosis;* PSC, *Primary sclenosing cholangitis.*

before surgery. Premedication with benzodiazepines and thiamin may be necessary for alcoholic patients in impending withdrawal. Child's classification system (Table 28-5) is useful in conjunction with other available assessment parameters for determining the degree to which liver disease influences surgical and anesthetic risk.

Cirrhosis

Cirrhosis is a progressive and ultimately fatal syndrome of hepatic failure. Chronic alcoholism is the most common cause of cirrhosis (Laënnec's cirrhosis) in the United States. Cirrhosis is also caused by biliary obstruction, chronic hepatitis, right-sided heart failure, α_1-antitrypsin deficiency, Wilson's disease, and hemochromatosis. Anatomic alterations secondary to hepatocyte necrosis are the primary cause of the deterioration that occurs in liver function. Over time the liver parenchyma is replaced by fibrous and nodular tissue, which distorts, compresses, and obstructs normal portal venous blood flow. Portal hypertension develops and impairs the ability of the liver to perform various metabolic and synthetic processes.

Obstructive engorgement of vessels within the portal system ultimately results in transmission of increasing back pressure within the splanchnic circulation. Therefore splenomegaly, esophageal varices, and right-sided heart failure ensue in addition to deterioration in liver function.

The development of esophageal varices places the patient at risk for spontaneous, severe upper gastrointestinal hemorrhage. Fluid sequestration resulting from ascites causes consequent alteration in intravascular fluid dynamics and alteration in the renin-angiotensin system. Subsequent reduction in renal perfusion results in eventual renal failure in conjunction with hepatic failure (hepatorenal syndrome). Failure of the liver to clear nitrogenous compounds (ammonia) from the blood contributes to the development of progressive mental status changes (caused by encephalopathy), ultimately leading to coma.

It is interesting to note that the clinical manifestations of cirrhosis may not be strongly correlated with the severity of the disease process. Patients may have severe liver disease without overt jaundice and ascites. However, the eventual development of jaundice and ascites is observed in most patients. Other signs of severe liver disease include gynecomastia, spider angiomata, palmar erythema, and asterixis.[10]

Hepatic fibrosis results from the presence of other diseases; portal hypertension ensues, along with its sequelae. These diseases include Budd-Chiari syndrome (vena cava or hepatovenous obstruction), idiopathic portal fibrosis (Banti's syndrome), schistosomiasis, and certain rare congenital fibrotic disorders. Venous occlusive disease secondary to metastases, primary hepatic neoplasia, or thromboembolism is also associated with portal hypertension.[10]

Perioperative Considerations in Liver Disease

Preoperative Assessment

The preoperative assessment of a patient with hepatic disease or insufficiency begins with a thorough history and proceeds in a systematic manner to include physical examination and laboratory studies. Incidences of jaundice, ascites, hepatitis, blood transfusion, or substance abuse are important factors, as is an alternative lifestyle (if the patient offers such information). Patients living in group or communal settings (e.g., special homes or halfway houses) are also at greater risk for hepatitis. History and outcome of prior anesthetic use are also important.

Physical signs, such as petechiae, jaundice, ascites, dependent edema, altered mental status, and asterixis, suggest the presence of significant liver disease. Laboratory assessment includes the following:

- Albumin (normal, 3.5 to 5 g/dL)
- Complete blood count
- Coagulation studies
- Serum electrolyte and glucose levels
- Serum liver enzyme levels: ALT and AST (pathologic above 40 international units per liter), alkaline phosphatase (pathologic above 115 international units per liter), lactic dehydrogenase (pathologic above 300 international units per liter), γ-glutamyl transpeptidase (pathologic above 85 international units per liter; often seen in chronic ethanol abuse)
- Blood type and screen

Serum ammonia level is a useful indicator of hepatic dysfunction and, along with other parameters, aids in the determination of the presence of encephalopathy. A preoperative ECG is warranted, as are arterial blood gas determinations and pulmonary function tests in patients with suspected respiratory impairment. A toxicology screen is also useful in the presence of suspected substance abuse to aid in detection of intoxication and to assess the potential for acute withdrawal.

In patients without overt signs of hepatic disease but with a history of chronic intravenous or ingested drug abuse or alcohol abuse, the issue of enzyme induction must be considered relative to clinical dosages of drugs necessary to achieve and maintain anesthesia. This is particularly true for sedatives, barbiturates, and opioids. These patients often require increased amounts of sedatives and anesthetic agents, which are judiciously titrated to attain a therapeutic effect.

Patient history and preexisting physical status dictate the degree to which preoperative assessment should proceed, as well as the intensity with which perioperative monitoring modalities are instituted. Generally the preoperative degree of liver dysfunction is a major determinant of the patient's postoperative outcome. The greater the severity of liver disease, the greater the risk of exceeding the limited preexisting functional reserve. A greater potential for postoperative hepatic failure, therefore, exists in patients with compromised hepatic function who undergo major surgery.

Liver Disease and Other Organ Systems

Perioperative Considerations

Cardiovascular System. Increased levels of endogenous vasodilators such as vasoactive intestinal peptide, ferritin glucagon, and others result in a hyperdynamic circulatory state, especially in the presence of cirrhotic liver disease. A high cardiac output and a decreased systemic vascular resistance are present. Decreased blood viscosity and anemia contribute to the hyperdynamic circulatory state. The development of arteriovenous shunting occurs as a result of the development of extensive systemic collateral vessels. These vessels develop secondary to increased back pressure reflected backward as a result of impaired hepatic circulation (portal hypertension). These collateral and frequently engorged vessels are well represented in the splanchnic circulation. Proliferation of collateral vessels also occurs in the lungs, skin, and musculature. Esophageal varices are a good example of this phenomenon. Chronic alcohol abuse predisposes a patient not only to hepatic cirrhosis but also to cardiomyopathy. Both conditions place the patient at risk for developing perioperative congestive heart failure.[10]

Hematologic Considerations. Anemia is a common finding and usually results from hemorrhage, hemolysis, nutritional deficiencies, and bone marrow suppression. Congestive splenomegaly contributes to the development of thrombocytopenia and leukopenia. Failure of hepatic synthetic processes results in clotting factor deficiencies, decreased blood viscosity, and enhanced fibrinolysis caused by the decreased clearance of fibrinolytic factors.

The decision to transfuse blood products must be weighed against certain clinical considerations. Excessive blood transfusion may exacerbate encephalopathy as a result of the breakdown of red blood cells and the subsequent increase of protein-rich by-products in the plasma; these by-products are ordinarily metabolized by hepatocytes. When indicated, FFP, platelet, and cryoprecipitate transfusion should be undertaken to correct coagulation deficiencies before surgery. An acceptable preoperative hematocrit value in patients with liver disease is 30%. A platelet count of less than 100,000/mm^3 should be corrected before surgery, particularly when major blood loss is anticipated.[14]

Respiratory Considerations. Derangements in ventilatory mechanics and pulmonary gas exchange are commonly encountered in patients with liver disease. Right-to-left shunting secondary to arteriovenous shunting attributable to increased circulating vasoactive substances normally metabolized by the liver effects a hypoxemia that may involve up to 40% of the cardiac output. Impaired diaphragmatic descent resulting from ascites results in the eventual development of a restrictive ventilatory defect; this defect causes decreased functional residual capacity and atelectasis with subsequent alveolar hypoventilation.

Arterial blood gas determinations and chest radiographs are valuable additions to the preoperative assessment when the potential for perioperative respiratory embarrassment exists. Patients with a history of chronic alcoholism may also have a history of heavy tobacco use, suggesting the possible presence of obstructive pulmonary disease.

Fluid Balance and Renal Considerations. Ascites and edema offer distinct evidence of the presence of derangements in fluid balance in patients with liver disease. Hypoalbuminemia, sodium retention, and distortion in splanchnic intravascular hydrostatic pressure secondary to portal hypertension all contribute to alterations in renal perfusion, usually secondary to a state of hypoperfusion. The result is a progressive decline in renal function, as evidenced by decreased free water clearance, with resultant dilutional hyponatremia and hypokalemia.

Perioperative concerns focus on judicious correction of preexisting intravascular volume and electrolyte imbalances. Diuresis should be performed in a methodic and judicious manner, and ample time should be taken to prevent hypotension and further electrolyte derangements. Perioperative preservation of adequate renal perfusion is of the utmost importance. Water restriction, controlled isotonic intravenous fluid administration, and potassium replacement may be necessary components of the preoperative plan of fluid therapy.

Intraabdominal ascites exerts a profound influence on many organ systems, including the renal system. Cirrhotic liver disease results in the development of excessive hydrostatic pressure within the hepatic venous and lymphatic systems. This phenomenon, coupled with impaired albumin synthesis, results in decreased plasma oncotic pressure within the liver parenchyma. An exudative process occurs across interstitial barriers and serosal liver surfaces, resulting in systemic edema, accumulation of protein-rich fluid within the peritoneum, and eventual electrolyte derangements. Ongoing exudation establishes an osmotic gradient for ongoing intraperitoneal filling, a relative intravascular hypovolemia, and sodium retention. Intraoperatively a sudden release of the tamponade effect of the ascitic abdomen during laparotomy can induce profound hypotension.

Sodium retention is explained by two theories. The underfilling theory describes sodium retention in terms of a discrepancy between total extracellular and plasma volumes and "effective" plasma volume. In this condition an increased splanchnic vascular volume with resultant ascites causes a relative hypovolemia and consequent hyperaldosteronism. The cause is an imbalance in Starling's forces brought about by a leakage of protein-rich fluid into the peritoneal cavity. The overflow theory establishes the cause of sodium retention as a primary event in the kidney in the presence of abnormal Starling's forces, with ascites resulting from expansion of fluid volume. Leakage into the peritoneum then occurs via previously described exudative processes.[5]

Hepatorenal syndrome may occur as a consequence of gastrointestinal hemorrhage, sepsis, or surgery or as a result of aggressive diuretic therapy, all of which place patients at risk for derangements in renal perfusion. Characteristic signs include progressive ascites, azotemia, oliguria, and eventually multisystem organ failure. Institution of supportive therapy is undertaken until hepatic transplantation can be performed. Hepatic transplantation remains the only definitive treatment for this ultimately fatal syndrome.

Correction of volume status should be undertaken with attention to central filling pressures, electrolyte and coagulation status, and maintenance of adequate urinary output. Diuresis, after adequate cardiac preload is established, is usually performed with the administration of mannitol (1 to 2 g/kg), furosemide (0.3 to 4 mg/kg), or low-dose dopamine infusion (1 to 4 mcg/kg/min). Alternative diuretic agents include the loop diuretics ethacrynic acid and bumetanide and the potassium-sparing diuretics spironolactone, triamterene, and amiloride. Potentially nephrotoxic drugs should be avoided. These include nonsteroidal antiinflammatory drugs (NSAIDs), which inhibit renal prostaglandin synthesis. Interference with the production of prostaglandins results in renal artery and glomerular constriction, as well as interference with tubular sodium-potassium exchange.

Central Nervous System Considerations. Encephalopathy is the most dramatic manifestation of central nervous system involvement during hepatic failure. Alterations in the function of the central nervous system are progressive and consist of neuromotor abnormalities, such as asterixis and hyperreflexia, and mental status changes. Ultimately the development of coma portends irreversible central nervous system failure and death. The degree of neurologic severity, however, correlates with the amount of portal blood entering the systemic circulation that is deprived of the cleansing processes of the liver.

Toxins delivered from the gastrointestinal tract that are implicated in the development of encephalopathy are substances normally metabolized by the hepatocytes. These nitrogenous substances include ammonia, aromatic amino acids, phenols, and short-chain amino acids (mercaptans). Buildup of these substances within the cerebral circulation contributes to the erosion of the blood-brain barrier. A markedly increased level of γ-aminobutyric acid is also noted, as are decreased levels of branched-chain amino acids.

The preoperative attenuation of encephalopathy is often undertaken through the administration of enteral lactulose or neomycin. These agents reduce the absorption of ammonia from the gastrointestinal tract. By altering the pH of the colon, lactulose enhances fecal elimination of ammonium, which is a poorly absorbable conversion product of ammonia. Neomycin interferes with the buildup of ammonia (converted from urea by bacterial ureases) by decreasing the amount of colonic bacteria. Potential precipitating factors associated with the development of encephalopathy should be corrected. These factors include gastrointestinal bleeding, metabolic alkalosis (e.g., from nausea and vomiting), infectious processes, progressive hepatic dysfunction, and a high level of dietary protein. Cerebral uptake of benzodiazepines is greatly enhanced as a result of a theoretically increased number of receptors or breakdown of the blood-brain barrier. Preoperative medication may be omitted altogether in the presence of encephalopathy.[5,8]

Intraoperative Anesthetic Considerations

Preoperative sedatives should be administered with caution or possibly omitted altogether. Full-stomach aspiration precautions should be used in patients with liver disease, even in patients who have had nothing by mouth for an extended time. Patients with liver disease and concomitant ascites frequently have decreased gastric motility. Hiatal hernia also is common in these patients. Intravenous metoclopramide, ranitidine, and oral sodium citrate may be used for chemical prophylaxis before surgery. In the induction of general endotracheal anesthesia, aspiration precautions should be taken through the use of a rapid-sequence technique.

Standard monitoring procedures may be supplemented with more invasive modalities based on the perceived intraoperative risk of further decompensation, which the patient's preoperative assessment has disclosed. Pulmonary artery catheterization and central venous pressure monitoring add a greater sensitivity to volume and cardiopulmonary support. Arterial cannulation allows not only beat-to-beat arterial pressure assessment but also access through which laboratory studies can be readily performed and sent.

Hypoxic injury to the liver occurs during surgery and anesthesia as a result of disturbances in oxygen supply-and-demand relationships. These disturbances are caused by inadequate ventilation, excessive bleeding, hypovolemia, hypotension, inadequate cardiac output, and iatrogenic disturbances in hepatic metabolic processes. Furthermore, a reduction in splanchnic perfusion normally occurs during the anesthetized state. Therefore efforts to attenuate these phenomena are directed toward optimization of cardiovascular and pulmonary function, including central and systemic perfusion pressures.

Arterial hypotension induces increased oxygen extraction by the tissues. This condition can have particularly deleterious consequences on the diseased liver, which is functioning with a limited reserve and is particularly vulnerable to further decompensation under hypoxic conditions. Reductions in cardiac output and arterial hypotension therefore warrant prompt correction.

Anesthetic Technique and Medication Choices

Regional anesthesia is used effectively for peripheral procedures if coagulation status is normal. Local anesthetic infiltration with judicious sedation may be used for selected procedures. Certain medications, such as benzodiazepines and barbiturates and some opioids, are highly protein bound, so that reduced concentrations of blood proteins call for a reduction in the usual dose. Patients with severe disease are theorized to have increased numbers of central benzodiazepine receptors, a phenomenon that also magnifies the effect of an administered dose. Therefore all sedatives, induction agents, and drugs known to depress organ and system function should be titrated judiciously to achieve a therapeutic effect.

The use of succinylcholine during induction is acceptable; however, a prolonged effect is possible secondary to decreased levels of plasma cholinesterase, which is synthesized in the liver. Prolongation of effect must be expected in muscle relaxants that require hepatic clearance (e.g., vecuronium and rocuronium), making *cis*-atracurium, which is relatively devoid of hepatic metabolic clearance mechanisms, an attractive choice.[3] The rapid-onset, nondepolarizing muscle relaxants such as rocuronium and the short-duration, nondepolarizing muscle relaxant mivacurium are also capable of exhibiting prolongation of effect in patients with hepatic dysfunction.[3,15] Halothane is best avoided because of its association with postoperative hepatic dysfunction, halothane-associated hepatitis, and the fact that it causes the greatest impairment in hepatic perfusion of all the commonly used volatile anesthetics. Although reports have been published of hepatic dysfunction with the use of isoflurane, this agent may be used effectively. The alleged possibility of hepatic dysfunction secondary to the use of the anesthetics is recognized as being a lesser risk than the spontaneous attack of viral hepatitis. The nearly nonexistent metabolism of desflurane makes this agent an unlikely cause of postoperative hepatic dysfunction. The use of sevoflurane has not been accompanied by reports of overt hepatic dysfunction. However, the metabolic by-products of sevoflurane, including free fluoride ion, may make this agent less attractive.

The use of nitrous oxide is not associated with an increased risk of postoperative hepatic dysfunction. The sympathomimetic effect of nitrous oxide, however, may induce a variable degree of hepatic vasoconstriction and may limit its use in patients with hepatic impairment.

Opioids are used effectively for providing anesthesia in patients with liver disease. Fentanyl has relatively few deleterious effects on hepatic blood flow, oxygen supply, and oxygen consumption. Isoflurane and fentanyl exhibit equal effects on hepatic oxygen supply and demand. For this reason, isoflurane used with small doses of fentanyl provides an appropriate and effective anesthetic technique. Sufentanil, alfentanil, and remifentanil are other alternatives. Morphine may be less appropriate because it is the opioid most closely associated with spasm of Oddi's sphincter and it has the potential for causing histamine release. Opioids generally undergo hepatic metabolism. Therefore prolongation of effect, including potential side effects such as respiratory depression and hypotension, is possible even with small-to-moderate doses in this patient population. However, remifentanil, an ultra–short-acting opioid, possesses the advantage of nonspecific plasma esterase metabolism. It is therefore an attractive agent for use by infusion in patients with hepatic disease.

Anesthetic management of patients undergoing hepatic surgery is often complicated by coagulopathy. This condition is caused by splenomegaly-induced thrombocytopenia and by decreased synthesis of clotting factors secondary to hepatic parenchymal destruction. This situation can occur in patients with liver disease undergoing nonhepatic surgery as well. Yet another issue in the coagulopathic process in these patients involves the interaction of instilled blood in the peritoneal cavity with the collagen procoagulants found in peritoneal fluid. The result is a consumptive process involving platelets and fibrinogen. The clots formed are lysed by tissue plasminogen activator. A similar process results from exposure of ascitic fluid to blood in the general circulation. A clinical picture resembling disseminated intravascular coagulopathy results, with increased PT and PTT, decreased platelet count, decreased fibrinogen level, and increased levels of fibrin degradation products.[16]

Treatment of perioperative coagulopathy is accomplished by blood product replacement that includes FFP, platelets, cryoprecipitate, and packed red blood cells, as indicated. Other therapeutic options include the use of antifibrinolytic agents, such as aminocaproic acid and aprotinin. Activities performed by the anesthetist in anticipation of major blood loss include establishment of large-bore intravenous lines suitable for rapid transfusion and blood typing and cross-matching for an appropriate number of homologous units of packed red blood cells. Blood salvage techniques effectively minimize homologous blood product use.

Maintenance of normocarbia is important for ensuring optimal hepatic function, organ perfusion, and oxygen extraction. Hypothermia is particularly deleterious to coagulation processes. Warming the intravenous fluids and breathing circuit through the use of warming blankets and increasing the ambient room temperature help maintain intraoperative normothermia.

Therapeutic Modalities for Portal Hypertension

Pharmacologic management of the patient with portal hypertension and acute variceal bleeding is considered secondary to endoscopic treatment and traditionally consists of intravenous infusion of vasopressin or somatostatin. Vasopressin is a splanchnic vasoconstrictor but may also induce undesirable systemic vasoconstriction. Infusion of vasopressin is initiated at 0.1 to 0.4 U/min. Concurrent infusion of nitroglycerin, titrated at around 40 mcg/min, may be used to control systolic blood pressure at 100 to 110 mm Hg.[17] In the presence of profound variceal exsanguination and hemodynamic instability, vasopressin may be used in conjunction with mechanical compression of bleeding esophageal varices provided by insertion of a triple-lumen Sengstaken-Blakemore tube. Use of this device also requires endotracheal intubation for airway support and for prevention of pulmonary aspiration.

Octreotide, a somatostatin analog, has been shown to be equally as effective as vasopressin in pharmacologic control of variceal bleeding. Infused at 50 mcg/hr, octreotide acts as a potent and reversible inhibitor of gastrointestinal peptide hormone activity, thereby decreasing gut motility and venous return to the portal circulation. Octreotide has also been shown to be equally as efficacious as sclerotherapy in acute treatment of variceal hemorrhage.[18]

Endoscopic sclerotherapy, usually performed with the patient under intravenous titrated sedation, has been recognized as the treatment of choice in definitive correction of variceal bleeding. Sclerotherapy is accomplished endoscopically by injection of a thrombosing agent either directly into the variceal bleeder or through creation of a fibrotic overlayer over the varix, accomplished by injection of the sclerosing agent proximal to the paravariceal mucosa. A course of treatments is usually necessary to reduce the incidence of rebleeding. Rebleeding, however, continues to be problematic in this subset of patients, with an incidence of up to 60%.[19]

SURGICAL DECOMPRESSION PROCEDURES

Transjugular intrahepatic portosystemic shunt (TIPS) is an interventional radiologic procedure that accomplishes portal decompression without surgery. It is generally considered when endoscopy and drug therapies are unsuccessful as alternatives to surgery.

Portosystemic shunt procedures are considered either selective or nonselective, based on the degree to which portal venous blood is diverted from the diseased liver.

A nonselective shunt diverts all portal blood from the liver. Examples of this kind of shunt are the portacaval shunt (end-to-side and side-to-side), mesocaval shunt (anastomosis of the mesenteric vein to the vena cava), and the splenorenal shunt (anastomosis of the proximal splenic vein to the renal vein). An example of a selective portosystemic shunt is the Warren shunt, or distal splenorenal shunt. The significant feature of this shunt is that portal venous blood supply is preserved. It is therefore the preferred surgical shunt procedure.[20]

Anesthetic considerations in portosystemic shunt procedures include all perioperative accommodations made for patients with liver disease. Particular concern focuses on the likelihood of considerable blood loss compounded by a variable degree of preexisting coagulopathy. These procedures are usually lengthy, necessitating close monitoring of the patient's hematologic parameters (hemoglobin, hematocrit, platelet count), coagulation status (PT, activated PTT), plasma osmolality, fibrinogen level, electrolyte levels, serum glucose level, and acid-base status. Urine output also must be meticulously monitored. Hemodynamic assessment is best performed by means of information derived from an intraarterial line, as well as measures to determine central filling pressures and systemic perfusion (central venous pressure line and possibly pulmonary artery catheter). The partial pressure of arterial carbon dioxide ($PaCO_2$) should be kept at 40 mm Hg or slightly above to optimize portal blood flow. Nitrous oxide is avoided in order to prevent bowel distention and maximize partial pressure of oxygen (PaO_2). This also serves to attenuate the effect of intrapulmonary shunting and ventilation-perfusion mismatch commonly found in patients with severe liver disease.

Controversy exists regarding the choice of crystalloid intravenous solutions. Patients with hepatic failure may have preexisting metabolic alkalosis that may theoretically be exacerbated by the use of lactated Ringer's solution, which is metabolized into bicarbonate in the liver. Sodium retention is common in patients with hepatic disease and ascites. Therefore intravenous saline solutions should be used judiciously, with periodic measurement of serum and urinary sodium levels. Other isotonic, isoosmolar intravenous solutions such as Plasma-Lyte warrant consideration. Urinary output less than 50 ml/hr warrants the use of mannitol to induce osmotic diuresis. The potential for precipitation or exacerbation of acid-base and electrolyte derangements, as well as hepatorenal syndrome, justifies avoidance of furosemide and loop diuretics.

The TIPS procedure is an effective alternative method of hepatic decompression that significantly decreases morbidity and mortality associated with the previously described surgical decompressive procedures. The procedure has been accepted as an effective method for management of variceal bleeding. The technique consists of establishment of an artificial channel between a branch of the portal vein and the systemic circulation within the liver parenchyma. This technique has been recognized as being hemodynamically equivalent to a side-to-side portacaval anastomosis.[21]

In the TIPS procedure, percutaneous placement of a catheter through the internal jugular vein into the vena cava and into a branch of the hepatic vein is performed under fluoroscopy. The procedure is preferably performed with the patient under local anesthesia with sedation. Numerous clinical studies attest to the efficacy and safety of the TIPS procedure in indicated patients.

Encephalopathy is the principal complication of the TIPS procedure and does not occur as frequently as with surgical portosystemic shunts. Stenosis or occlusion of the shunt within the first 6 months is also problematic. Major intraprocedural complications include liver capsular laceration, perforation of the gallbladder, oliguric renal failure secondary to contrast dye injection, and embolization of the stent to the pulmonary vascularature.[22] Use of the TIPS procedure is therefore becoming increasingly recognized as a temporizing measure in the advent of definitive hepatic transplantation.[23]

DISEASES OF THE BILIARY TRACT

Biliary tract disease is usually a symptomatic expression of the presence of gallstones. Gallstone formation is most likely caused by physicochemical derangements in the formation of bile. Approximately 90% of gallstones appear as radiolucent structures composed of hydrophobic cholesterol crystals. Calcium bilirubinate generally accounts for the composition of the remaining percentage. Stones composed of calcium bilirubinate are usually seen in patients with cirrhosis and hemolytic anemia. An estimated 15 to 20 million adults in the United States have biliary tract disease, as evidenced by the presence of gallstones.[24]

Anatomic and Physiologic Overview

The biliary tract is the excretory conduit for the liver. It is composed of (1) the intrahepatic ducts, which collect bile from the liver segments; (2) the coalescence of the intrahepatic ducts and the right and left hepatic ducts; (3) the common hepatic duct, which is formed by the junction of the right and left hepatic ducts in the liver hilum; (4) the gallbladder, which serves as a reservoir of bile; (5) the cystic duct, which joins the gallbladder to the common bile duct; and (6) the common bile duct, which begins at the junction of the cystic duct and the common hepatic duct and terminates in the lumen of the duodenum.[24]

The gallbladder is attached to the liver in a shallow fossa that lies at the junction of the right and left hepatic lobes. On gross examination the gallbladder is a pear-shaped organ that is capable of holding 30 to 50 ml of fluid. The cystic duct is usually 2 to 3 cm long and arises from the narrow end (or infundibulum) of the gallbladder. The common bile duct is usually approximately 6 mm in diameter, and it passes behind the duodenum to the right of the gastroduodenal artery, traversing the head of the pancreas before entering the second part of the duodenum. The common bile duct shares a channel with the main pancreatic duct. At the termination, these ducts are enveloped in smooth muscle (Oddi's sphincter). Oddi's sphincter provides a barrier to intestinal bacteria for the sterile environment of the biliary tract. At this point biliary tract obstruction can occur from a pancreatic tumor. Both the biliary and the pancreatic tracts empty into the duodenum via the ampulla of Vater (Figure 28-1).

Arterial blood supply is furnished by the cystic artery, which is a branch of the right hepatic artery. The biliary ducts receive their blood supply from collateral branches of the hepatic artery and from small retroperitoneal vessels. Venous drainage flows into the portal vein. Lymphatic drainage flows into a cystic duct node that is located between the cystic duct and the common hepatic duct.

The gallbladder and Oddi's sphincter are innervated by neurons of the enteric nervous system. This system is a hybrid of the sympathetic and parasympathetic nervous systems and is composed of neurons with cell bodies that lie in gut ganglia. The neurons in this system are activated by neuropeptides, which are released under the influence of preganglionic fibers of both the sympathetic and the parasympathetic nervous systems. Reflex control of the gallbladder and sphincter is mediated by afferent fibers of the enteric nervous system.

Another structure, the porta hepatis, consists of an area bounded by the common bile duct, the cystic duct, and the undersurface of the liver. This area is known as the *cystohepatic triangle* (*Calot's triangle*) and is a critical region that contains the cystic artery, the right hepatic artery, the cystic node, and sometimes an aberrant right segmental bile duct. This area must be carefully dissected during cholecystectomy so that damage to these important structures is avoided.

The gallbladder mucosa secretes mucus, an action that prevents damage by bile salts. After food is ingested, the gallbladder contracts, emptying its contents (bile) into the duodenum in order to assist in the digestive processes. Regulation of gallbladder contraction is primarily hormonal, through the action of cholecystokinin. The release of cholecystokinin from duodenal cells is mediated by the presence of intraluminal amino acids and fat. Vagal stimulation also serves a role (secondary to the role of cholecystokinin). Indeed, vagotomy is associated with impaired gallbladder contraction and increased prevalence of gallstones.

Bile, the combined secretory product of the hepatocyte and biliary tract epithelial cell, has three main functions: (1) to emulsify and enhance absorption of ingested fats and fat-soluble vitamins; (2) to provide an excretory pathway for bilirubin, drugs and toxins, and immunoglobulin A (IgA); and (3) to maintain duodenal alkalization. The combined output of the ductal cells and hepatocytes is 500 to 1500 ml/day. The hepatocytes secrete bilirubin (the metabolic waste product of heme metabolism), cholesterol, bile salts, lecithin, water, and electrolytes. The epithelial cells contribute water and electrolytes. Vagal stimulation, secretin, cholecystokinin, and gastrin stimulate

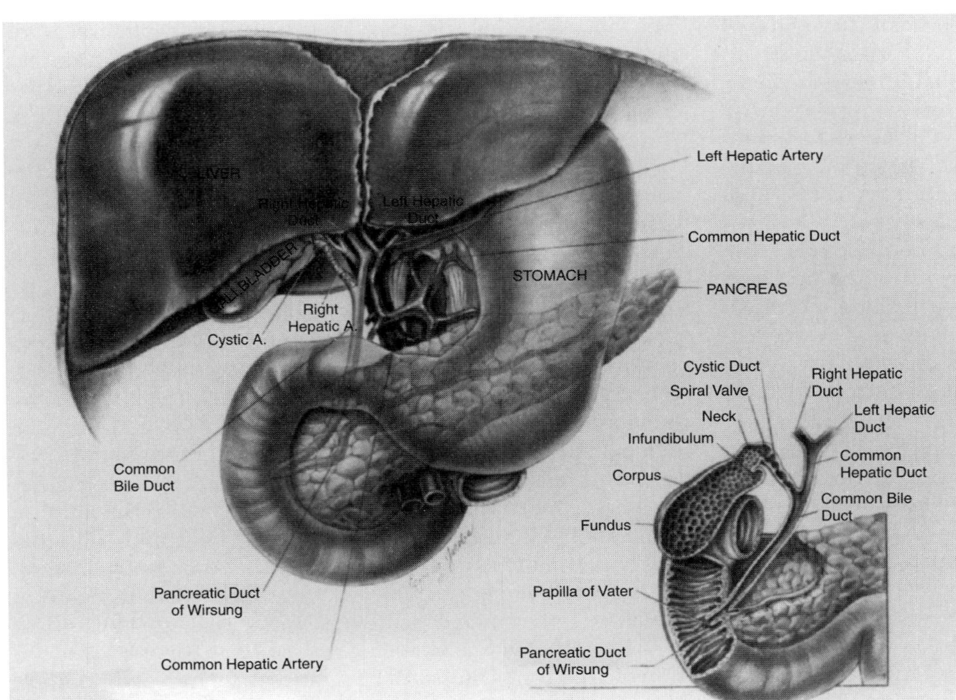

FIGURE **28-1**
Anatomy of the biliary tract. A, artery. (From Orloff MJ. The biliary system. In: Sabiston DC, ed. *Davis-Christopher Textbook of Surgery*. Philadelphia: Saunders; 1981:1230.)

ductular cell secretion and increase bile flow. In addition, bile acids furnish a positive-feedback mechanism in the elaboration of hepatocyte and ductular secretion. Gallbladder filling during fasting occurs with relaxation and contraction of Oddi's sphincter. Vasoactive intestinal peptide produces relaxation, whereas somatostatin, an inhibitory peptide, produces contraction. In states of prolonged fasting the risk of gallstone formation increases as a result of the lack of cholecystokinin stimulation and consequent biliary stasis.[24]

Cholecystitis

Obstruction of the cystic duct by gallstones results in acute, severe midepigastric pain, typically radiating to the right abdomen. Inspiratory effort usually accentuates the pain (Murphy's sign). Increases in plasma bilirubin, alkaline phosphatase, and amylase levels frequently occur. Ileus and localized tenderness may indicate perforation with peritonitis. Leukocytosis and fever are often present. The presence of jaundice indicates complete obstruction of the cystic duct. Symptoms are frequently confused with those of myocardial infarction. Differential diagnosis is accomplished through serial ECG evaluations and laboratory analysis of serum enzymes that are specific to cardiac muscle. Cholescintigraphy (a contrast study that evaluates gallbladder excretion of a radiographically labeled substance) and ultrasonography are often used for clinical confirmation of the diagnosis.

Patients with symptoms indicative of acute cholecystitis are often volume depleted as a result of intolerance of oral intake, vomiting, and possible preoperative nasogastric evacuation of gastric contents. Dehydration warrants preoperative intravenous fluid replacement. Gastric suction may be warranted in the presence of ileus. The presence of free abdominal air, as determined by abdominal radiography or symptoms of an acute abdomen (fever, ileus, rigid and painful abdomen, vomiting, dehydration), suggests the presence of a ruptured viscus, possibly including perforation of the gallbladder. Under these circumstances emergency exploratory laparotomy is undertaken.

Cholelithiasis and Choledocholithiasis

Acute obstruction of the common bile duct often produces symptoms similar to those seen in patients with cholecystitis. Recurrent bouts of acute cholecystitis induce the development of fibrotic changes in gallbladder structure, thereby impeding the ability of the gallbladder to adequately expel bile. The presence of Charcot's triad (fever and chills, jaundice, upper quadrant pain) aids in establishing the differential diagnosis in acute ductal obstruction. Weight loss, anorexia, and fatigue complete the symptomatology. Diagnostic modalities include radiography, transhepatic cholangiography, ultrasonography, cholescintigraphy, and CT scan. A dilated common bile duct and biliary tree are typically observed in these studies.

Anesthetic Considerations in Gallbladder and Biliary Tract Disease

Removal of gallstones is undertaken not only for relief of symptoms but also for prevention of further sequelae, including cholecystitis, cholangitis, jaundice, pancreatitis, and peritonitis, all of which may result from stasis or impediment to bile flow. Diversity among patients who undergo biliary surgery is common; patients may range from otherwise healthy individuals with a history of recurrent bouts of cholecystitis to those who are desperately ill.

Cholecystectomy is now commonly performed as an elective procedure through laparoscopy. Open cholecystectomy is usually reserved for patients who are emergently ill or in whom laparoscopy poses a particularly formidable technical challenge, for example, in cases of morbid obesity. Another relative contraindication may be a suspicion of the presence of intraperitoneal adhesions. The use of abdominal carbon dioxide insufflation to effect adequate exposure of anatomic structures mandates general endotracheal intubation anesthesia to effectively seal the airway and prevent passive aspiration of gastric contents. Abdominal insufflation displaces the abdominal viscera and diaphragm in a cephalad direction, placing extra pressure on the lower esophageal sphincter (LES) and thereby increasing the risk of gastric reflux.

Insufflation of the abdomen with carbon dioxide also impedes diaphragmatic excursion, thereby causing a decrease in functional residual capacity, closing capacity, and increased peak inspiratory pressure. A relative hypercarbia, as evidenced by increased end-tidal and arterial carbon dioxide levels, reflects uptake of insufflated carbon dioxide. Controlled ventilation is therefore necessary in order to minimize the development of atelectasis and to prevent progressive hypercarbia. The use of a reverse Trendelenburg position during laparoscopic cholecystectomy may induce a variable degree of hemodynamic compromise by impeding venous return. Occult hemorrhage is also possible and may go undetected.

Patients who undergo open cholecystectomy often experience more complications as a result of preexisting pathologic medical conditions and the greater likelihood of severe postoperative pain and respiratory splinting (caused by the use of a right subcostal or upper abdominal midline incision). Full-stomach precautions should be used during the induction of and emergence from anesthesia and in the presence of abdominal distention and ileus. Patients with jaundice require a more thorough preparation because the likelihood of hepatic dysfunction makes them more susceptible to hemorrhage, exaggerated drug effects, and fluctuation in hemodynamics. Institution of invasive hemodynamic monitoring and preparation for blood product transfusion are influenced by the patient's clinical status.

No strong evidence has contraindicated the use of nitrous oxide during laparoscopic surgery. However, reports of increased postoperative nausea and intraoperative expansion of bowel gas associated with its use are considerations. In the presence of hepatic dysfunction, isoflurane, desflurane, and sevoflurane are safe. The choice of muscle relaxant depends on the patient's ability to tolerate possible side effects of the drug (e.g., pancuronium-induced tachycardia), the drug's dependence on hepatic clearance, and the length of the procedure to be performed.[25,26]

Common bile duct exploration may be carried out in conjunction with cholecystectomy, if necessary. Patients who require this intervention are often more ill and older; therefore a 1.5-times greater incidence of morbidity and mortality exists in patients who require this procedure in addition to cholecystectomy.[24] Severe postoperative pain may be reduced by patient-controlled analgesia, intercostal nerve blocks, or neuraxial opioid administration.

DISEASES OF THE ESOPHAGUS

Anatomic and Physiologic Overview

The esophagus originates at the pharynx at approximately the level of the sixth cervical vertebra and extends to the stomach. It can be divided into three functional zones: the upper esophageal sphincter (UES), the esophageal body, and the LES. The esophageal wall consists of an inner circular muscular layer, which consists of smooth and striated muscle, and an outer longitudinal layer, which is devoid of serosal covering. The mucosal lining consists of squamous epithelium except for the distal 1 to 2 cm, which is composed of columnar epithelium. The esophagus traverses a hiatus that is created by the right crus of the diaphragm in order to reach the abdomen. Intraabdominal length is variable.

The inferior thyroid arteries provide the blood supply to the cervical region of the esophagus, and the aorta and esophageal branches from the bronchial arteries supply the thoracic region. The esophagus is well endowed with lymphatics, which run longitudinally along the esophageal wall before perforating the muscular layers to reach the regional lymphatics.

The esophagus has both intrinsic and extrinsic innervation. The intrinsic enteric innervating system consists of two interconnected plexuses, the myenteric (Auerbach's plexus) and the submucosal (Meissner's plexus). This system is a continuum that extends from the esophagus to the anus. Extrinsic innervation of the esophagus is derived from the sympathetic, parasympathetic, and somatic nervous systems. Parasympathetic stimulation by means of cranial nerves IX, X, and XI causes esophageal muscular contraction, but it also causes relaxation of the LES. Sympathetic fibers act on the myenteric plexus to modulate rather than control motor activity.

At rest the UES is closed, as is the LES. Excitatory stimulation of UES tone consists of inspiration, esophageal distention, gagging, Valsalva maneuver, and acidity of gastroesophageal contents. Distention, belching, and vomiting reduce UES tone. Swallowing initiates peristaltic activity, which consists of a maximum pressure of 150 mm Hg with an average velocity of 3 to 4 cm/sec. The exact mechanisms responsible for peristaltic activity, which include production, propagation, and regulation, remain controversial. It is clear, however, that peristaltic activity is highly integrated and involves central and local mechanisms that are mediated largely through excitatory cholinergic neuronal activity.

The UES and upper portions of the esophageal body are composed of striated muscle, whereas the bulk of the LES and the esophageal body consist of smooth muscle. The tone of the LES is maintained at 20 mm Hg through a combination of intrinsic myogenic and excitatory neural mechanisms. Vagal mediation of the neuronal component is predominant. β-Blockade is seen to increase LES tone, an effect that suggests adrenergic inhibitory tone. Ingestion of a meal or increased intraabdominal pressure increases LES tone via vagal afferent pathways. Swallowing decreases LES tone within 1.5 to 2.5 seconds and is maintained for the duration of the peristaltic wave (approximately 6 to 8 seconds).[20]

Esophageal Disorders

A common symptom found in esophageal disease is dysphagia. The presentation of this disorder initiates pursuit of the underlying cause, often through barium contrast studies (e.g., barium swallow) and through endoscopic examination of the esophagus and stomach with procurement of cytology and biopsy specimens, when indicated.[27]

Chronic alcoholism is associated with impaired esophageal peristalsis and LES hypotonia. Degeneration of Auerbach's plexus is closely associated with this condition. Achalasia often develops secondary to systemic disease states, including diabetes, stroke, amyotrophic lateral sclerosis, and certain connective tissue diseases, such as amyloidosis and scleroderma. A progressive inability to swallow is the salient symptom of this syndrome. Regurgitation of food and liquid is common and places these patients at high risk for aspiration.

The formation of Barrett's esophagus occurs when normal squamous epithelium changes to metaplastic columnar epithelium. Chronic exposure to acidic gastric contents because of reflux is a major etiologic mechanism. Other etiologies include chronic alcohol abuse and tobacco use. Esophagitis and hiatal hernia are also precipitating factors. Development of Barrett's esophagus is closely correlated with the eventual development of carcinoma of the esophagus. A Mallory-Weiss tear most commonly occurs at the gastroesophageal junction because of persistent retching, most often secondary to chronic alcohol abuse. Pain and bloody vomitus may be noted with its presence.[28] Surgical repair is usually not indicated.[28]

Esophageal dilation is moderately successful in the correction of achalasia. Sublingual nifedipine has been used successfully to alleviate symptoms in some patients. Operative correction, consisting of esophagomyotomy with fundoplasty, is associated with a reasonable success rate and is the definitive treatment for this syndrome.[29]

Anesthetic Considerations in Esophageal Disease

Symptomatic patients who have peptic esophagitis associated with hiatal hernia or LES incompetence often take oral antacids or H_2 antagonists, such as cimetidine, ranitidine, nizatidine, and famotidine. A history of symptoms that indicate the presence of gastric reflux warrants aspiration prophylaxis during induction of and emergence from general anesthesia. The safe maintenance of general anesthesia mandates the use of an endotracheal tube in order to effect a sealed airway so that the risk from passive regurgitation and aspiration is minimized. When general anesthesia is used, a rapid-sequence induction technique should be used with the application of cricoid pressure. The patient must be fully awake and have demonstrated control of airway reflexes, that is, swallowing and sustained head lift for 5 seconds, before extubation. Awake intubation also is an option before the induction of general anesthesia. In selected procedures, regional anesthesia may be used effectively. A sealed, secured airway in which a cuffed endotracheal tube is placed provides the safest method for providing ventilatory support during general anesthesia.

For elective procedures administration of an H_2 antagonist on the evening before surgery and in the morning at least a half hour before surgery helps increase gastric pH. In urgent and emergency situations preoperative oral administration of a clear, nonparticulate antacid, such as sodium citrate increases gastric pH. Gastric volume may be slightly increased, but the gastric pH is raised as well. Administration of a gastrokinetic agent, such as metoclopramide, in conjunction with an H_2 antagonist, stimulates gastrointestinal motility, which aids in the emptying of gastric contents, an effect that H_2 antagonists alone do not promote.

Use of anticholinergic drugs must be judicious. Theoretically these drugs could decrease LES tone, thereby enhancing the possibility of silent regurgitation. Succinylcholine increases LES pressure. Barrier pressure (LES pressure minus gastric pressure), however, is unchanged, because muscle fasciculations increase gastric pressure.[3] Sedatives and opioids must be administered cautiously for preoperative anxiolysis in these patients so that obtundation of airway reflexes is prevented.

Hiatal Hernia

A hiatal hernia consists of a defect in the diaphragm that allows a portion of the stomach to migrate upward into the thoracic cavity. Two types of esophageal hiatal hernias are the sliding type (type I), which is formed by the movement of the upper stomach through an enlarged hiatus, and the paraesophageal type (type II), in which the esophagogastric junction remains in normal position but all or part of the stomach moves into the thorax and assumes a paraesophageal position. A third type of hiatal hernia (type III) has been identified that combines the features of a sliding and a paraesophageal hernia (Figure 28-2). A fourth type of hiatal hernia (type IV) occurs when other organs, such as the colon or small bowel, are contained in the hernia sac that is formed by a large paraesophageal hernia.[29] Hiatal hernia and peptic esophagitis often exist concurrently, although one does not cause the other. The major symptom is retrosternal pain of a burning quality that commonly occurs after meals. It is assumed that patients with a hiatal hernia are predisposed to developing peptic esophagitis, thereby providing a rationale for surgical correction of this condition. Most patients with hiatal hernia do not have symptoms of reflux esophagitis, however, and do not require H_2-agonist and oral antacid therapy. Nevertheless, implementation of aspiration precautions on induction of general anesthesia and emergence is still strongly recommended.

The primary goal in the surgical correction of hiatal hernia consists of reestablishment of gastroesophageal competence. This usually entails repair of the sliding hernia, reduction by 2 cm or more of the tubular distal esophagus below the diaphragm, and valvuloplasty. An abdominal, a thoracic, or a thoracoabdominal surgical approach may be selected. Common procedures for correction of hiatal hernia include the Nissen, Belsey, and Hill operations. Laparoscopic fundoplication techniques are also more commonly being used. A gastroplasty may be performed (the Collis procedure) in association with repair of the hiatal hernia when indicated, usually in patients with a shortened esophagus. If a thoracic approach is selected, the patient must be assessed for ability to tolerate one-lung anesthesia, because this method may be used to enable surgical exposure.[29]

Esophageal Diverticula

Esophageal diverticula place the patient at risk for pulmonary aspiration of regurgitated food; another risk is posed from food and fluids ingested but sequestered within the diverticular pouch. Surgical correction may be performed in two stages, with the first stage involving mobilization of the pouch and the second stage consisting of excision of the diverticulum with esophageal repair. Esophageal diverticula are classified according to location. These classifications are epiphrenic (located near the LES), traction (in the midesophagus), and Zenker's (upper esophagus). Zenker's diverticulum places the patient at greater risk of pulmonary aspiration.[30]

Esophageal Carcinoma

Patients undergoing surgical procedures for esophageal malignancy are often of advanced age, cachectic, malnourished, and suffering from disease processes that are both age related and relevant to other organ systems. Therefore consideration is given to adequate preoperative multisystem assessment and preparation to ensure safe and effective anesthesia in patients who undergo a curative or palliative procedure for this malady.

Patients with esophageal carcinoma often have a significant associated history of alcohol and tobacco use. Therefore the presence of a variable degree of obstructive pulmonary disease and alcohol-related hepatic disease should be considered in the anesthetic plan for these patients. Furthermore, by the time the differential diagnosis of esophageal carcinoma is determined, metastases to adjacent lymph nodes and structures may have

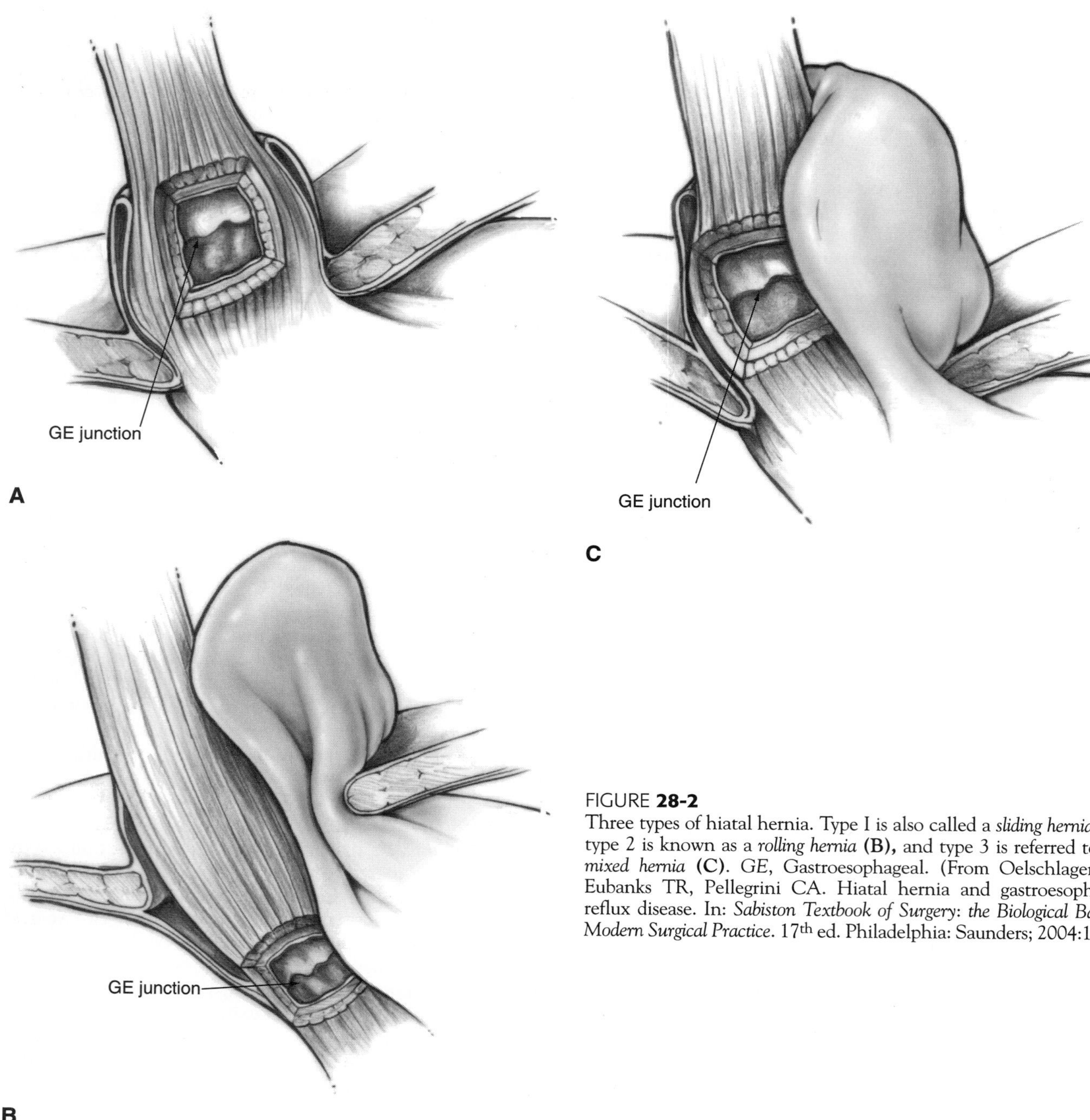

FIGURE **28-2**
Three types of hiatal hernia. Type I is also called a *sliding hernia* **(A)**, type 2 is known as a *rolling hernia* **(B)**, and type 3 is referred to as a *mixed hernia* **(C)**. GE, Gastroesophageal. (From Oelschlager BK, Eubanks TR, Pellegrini CA. Hiatal hernia and gastroesophageal reflux disease. In: *Sabiston Textbook of Surgery: the Biological Basis of Modern Surgical Practice*. 17th ed. Philadelphia: Saunders; 2004:1154.)

occurred. The absence of a serosal esophageal layer and the presence of abundant lymphatic networks facilitates rapid metastatic spread to the lungs and liver from a primary esophageal site. Preoperative radiation and chemotherapy also introduce a variable into the anesthetic planning: the side effects of those treatments. These effects often include bone marrow depression, fibrosis, and increased friability of the tissues. These situations predispose the patient to intraoperative bleeding problems. Other side effects, particularly those related to chemotherapy, include induced cardiomyopathy (which is associated with daunorubicin and doxorubicin [Adriamycin] therapy) and pulmonary fibrosis (which is associated with bleomycin therapy). Chemotherapy-induced lung pathology results in a restrictive lung defect and an increased potential for oxygen toxicity.

A curative procedure may be attempted in a patient whose preresection physical condition and tumor characteristics indicate the potential for long-term survival. This procedure involves en bloc resection of the esophagus for tumors in the lower third of the thoracic esophagus, along with reestablishment of gastrointestinal continuity through left colon interposition. This procedure involves a combined laparotomy and anterior thoracotomy.[28]

DISEASES OF THE STOMACH

Anatomic and Physiologic Overview

The stomach is essentially composed of two sections. The thin-walled and distensible fundus is located in the upper abdomen and has primarily a storage function. The thick-walled, distal

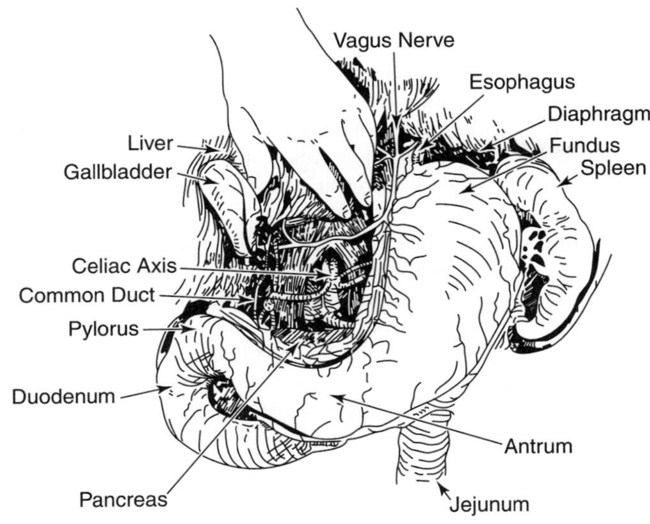

FIGURE **28-3**
Position of the stomach relative to the other principal organs of the upper abdomen. (From Moody GF, Miller TA. Stomach. In: Schwartz SI, Shires GT, Spencer FC, eds. *Principles of Surgery*. 6th ed. New York: McGraw-Hill; 1994:1124.)

portion of the stomach is responsible for the mixing of food and its slow release through the pyloric sphincter into the duodenum. The liver is positioned right and ventral and the spleen left and lateral to the stomach. The biliary tract courses posterior to the stomach (Figure 28-3).

The blood supply of the stomach consists primarily of four major arteries: the right and left gastric arteries and the right and left gastroepiploic arteries (Figure 28-4). An extensive submucosal arterial arcade is also present. Major autonomic innervation is

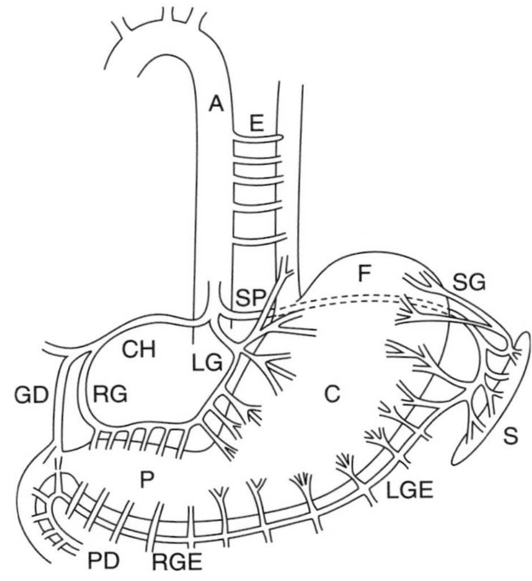

FIGURE **28-4**
Blood supply to the stomach. A, Aorta; C, cardia; *CH*, common hepatic artery; *E*, esophageal arteries; *F*, fundus; *GD*, gastroduodenal artery; *LG*, left gastric artery; *LGE*, left gastroepiploic artery; *P*, pylorus; *PD*, pancreaticoduodenal artery; *RG*, right gastric artery; *RGE*, right gastroepiploic artery; *S*, spleen; *SG*, short gastric arteries; *SP*, splenic artery. (Courtesy of KR Larsen, PhD; from Moody GF, Miller TA. Stomach. In: Schwartz SI, Shires GT, Spencer FC, eds. *Principles of Surgery*. 6th ed. New York: McGraw-Hill; 1994:1124.)

furnished by two branches of the vagus nerve: the right posterior (celiac) branch and the left anterior (hepatic) branch.

The gastric wall consists of an external serosal layer, which covers an inner oblique, a middle circular, and an outer longitudinal layer of smooth muscle. The submucosa and mucosa provide a continuous inner integument that is separated by a thin sheet of muscularis mucosae (smooth muscle).

Within the gastric mucosa reside the glands responsible for the significant physiologic role played by the stomach during the digestive processes. Within the fundic mucosa lie mucus-secreting glands that provide a protective barrier to the acid outflow of the parietal cells, which are located in the same region of the stomach. The endocrine function of the stomach is apparent through the secretions (pepsinogen) of the chief cells and the secretions (serotonin) of other cells. Within the antrum are cells that secrete mucus (surface epithelial cells and mucous cells) and gastrin (G cells). The two important sphincters are the LES at the gastroesophageal junction and the pyloric sphincter at the gastroduodenal junction.

The stomach normally stores food for up to 4 hours. The sight and smell of food stimulates acid and pepsinogen production. Gastrin is released by the G cells in response to gastric distention, which stimulates parietal cell acid (hydrochloric acid) secretion. Both the duodenum and the upper jejunum also secrete a small amount of gastrin. Luminal acid suppresses gastrin feedback (negative feedback).

Pepsinogen and gastrin release are vagally mediated. Acid in duodenal contents induces the release of secretin, an effect that inhibits gastrin release even more and inhibits further acid production. Pancreatic bicarbonate release is also stimulated by duodenal acidity.

The acidic secretion of the parietal cells occurs through a hydrogen/potassium (H^+/K^+) exchange pump, which requires ATP. Release is mediated by vagal stimulation (from acetylcholine), gastrin, and histamine. Administration of H_2 antagonists such as cimetidine and ranitidine, H^+/K^+–ATP inhibitors such as omeprazole, and prostaglandins inhibits acid secretion. Vagotomy greatly diminishes parietal cell response to gastrin and histamine. Anticholinergic agents, however, have only a minor influence on parietal cell secretion.

Other gastric functions include the provision of a barrier against ingested pathogens. This goal is accomplished through the maintenance of a highly acidic environment and through a functional role in immunosurveillance. The stomach heats or cools ingested substances as needed for the maintenance of normothermia. Furthermore, parietal cells also secrete intrinsic factor (in addition to hydrochloric acid), which facilitates ileal vitamin B_{12} absorption.

Peptic Ulcer Disease

Vagal stimulation causes elaboration of gastrin from antral cells. Gastrin, after entering the circulation, induces parietal cell hydrochloric acid secretion. Secretion of hydrochloric acid is also caused by H_2-receptor activation. A chronic overabundance of hydrochloric acid and pepsin (from various causes) results in erosion of the protective mucous layer of the stomach and duodenum. Subsequent ulceration occurs in time, with lesions extending beyond the mucosal barrier into the submucosa and muscularis epithelial layers and sometimes into the serosal layer. In the case of LES incompetence, ulcerative involvement of the esophagus may occur.

A chronic ulcerative lesion in the duodenum constitutes duodenal ulcer disease. Because of similarity of symptoms and responses to therapy, this classification is also placed on lesions that occur before the pylorus in the lower antrum of the stomach. Men 45 to 65 years of age and women older than 55 years of age have the highest incidence of duodenal ulcer disease. Chronic use of NSAIDs is the second most common cause of ulcer disease after *Helicobacter pylori* infection. Alcohol and corticosteroids are relatively minor etiologic factors.[3] Affected patients possess twice the number of acid-secreting parietal cells.[3]

H. pylori has been identified as a major etiologic factor of gastritis-associated disease, as well as gastric and duodenal ulcers and gastric carcinoma. Epidemiologic findings indicate a higher prevalence of this organism in older adults, individuals of lower socioeconomic status, and those born outside the United States. Infected patients undergoing stress are at greatest risk for exacerbation of the infection, with potential development of gastric and duodenal ulceration. At present, despite the numerous exposures of anesthesia providers to possible oral and ambient routes of transmission, *H. pylori* has not been recognized as a serious occupational hazard.[31]

Gastric mucosal acidosis has been commonly reported in critically ill patients; patients undergoing prolonged, complex surgical procedures; and patients undergoing cardiopulmonary bypass. Gastritis associated with gastric mucosal acidosis is associated with increased perioperative morbidity and mortality. The splanchnic viscera is particularly vulnerable to decreased circulatory blood flow, with the potential for breakdown of intestinal barrier function. This occurrence results in translocation of bacteria and endotoxin into the bloodstream, with consequent systemic sepsis. Ischemia and acidosis of the gut is the primary causative factor for erosion of gut barrier function. Studies using gastric tonometry have correlated measurement of gastric mucosal pH (pHi) with indexes of systemic acid-base balance.[32]

The attractiveness in pHi measurement of the gut is threefold. First, the splanchnic circulation is reduced during stress in an effort to preserve more vital myocardial and cerebral circulation. Second, the gut villus is particularly susceptible to reduced blood flow. Third, the gut is readily accessible for regional monitoring via transesophageal or rectal probe. Measurement of gut pHi has been recognized as an earlier indicator of perturbations in acid-base balance than conventional blood gas analysis. Numerous studies have also demonstrated improvement in outcome in acutely ill patients who received pHi-directed therapy.[33] However, controversy persists regarding how therapy should be guided and what pHi values are acceptable. Therefore until the various clinical controversies are resolved and suitable technology developed that is adaptable to the needs of perioperative monitoring, efforts should be directed toward optimizing systemic perfusion. This is accomplished through optimization of hemodynamics and assurance of adequate oxygen-carrying capacity.

Patients in intensive care units who experience acute major illness or sustain major traumatic injury are at high risk for the development of acute, typically painless, erosive gastritis (Curling's ulcer). This lesion is associated with a significant mortality rate as a result of the consequent severe hemorrhagic diathesis that often accompanies it. Other disease entities previously implicated as etiologic factors in gastritis and peptic ulcerative disease include hepatic cirrhosis, hyperparathyroidism, obstructive airway disease, and rheumatoid arthritis. Lifestyle-related factors such as emotional stress and alcohol consumption have been shown to be weak correlates with the development of peptic ulcer disease.[24] Therefore the role of gastric hyperacidity in and of itself in predisposing a patient to duodenal ulcer disease is controversial.

A condition of reduced duodenal buffering, as is seen in biliary diversion away from the duodenum, has a greater likelihood of predisposing a patient to duodenal ulceration. Another example of reduced duodenal buffering with the potential for inducing ulcer formation in the duodenum occurs in a reduction in the flow of alkaline pancreatic juice, as would occur in a patient with chronic pancreatitis or pancreatic resection.[34]

Therapeutic Options in Peptic Ulcer Disease

Oral antacids, H_2-receptor antagonists, proton pump inhibitors, sucralfate, and antibiotics are the major medical therapies used for the control of peptic ulcer disease. The proton pump inhibitor omeprazole is now being used in duodenal ulcer management. Surgical treatment is reserved for patients who continue to experience intractable symptoms despite aggressive medical therapy and for treatment of complications such as gastrointestinal hemorrhage, perforation into adjacent structures such as the pancreas, and obstruction.

The use of antacids in the medical treatment of peptic ulcer disease has potential complications that are of interest to the anesthetist. Antacids may produce an acid rebound in which gastric acid secretion may increase after acid is neutralized by calcium-containing antacids. Another condition that may result from antacid therapy is the milk-alkali syndrome. In this condition, hypercalcemia, alkalosis, and an elevated blood urea nitrogen level may develop from the daily ingestion of large quantities of calcium-containing antacids and milk. Manifestations of this syndrome include skeletal muscle weakness and polyuria. Ingestion of large quantities of aluminum-containing antacids may result in acute hypophosphatemia caused by increased binding of intestinal phosphorus. Skeletal muscle weakness and fatigue result with chronic overuse, resulting in pathologic fractures and osteoporosis.

The secretion of hydrochloric acid is blocked by H_2 antagonists, thereby promoting the healing of duodenal ulcers. A noteworthy side effect is seen in the alteration of cytochrome P-450 enzyme activity in the liver; this alteration may result in prolongation of the effects of concurrently administered drugs that rely on hepatic metabolism and elimination by means of this mechanism. Famotidine is the H_2 antagonist that is least likely to cause this effect.[34] Other side effects include decreased hepatic blood flow, leukopenia and thrombocytopenia, mental confusion, interstitial nephritis, hepatitis, bradycardia, and hypotension.[3]

The proton pump inhibitors are the most effective antisecretory agents and are listed in Table 28-6. Sucralfate, the aluminum salt of sulfated sucrose, not only binds to ulcers but also increases the gastric mucous layer, thereby promoting healing processes. It has been shown to be equally efficacious when used with H_2 antagonists and antacids and is relatively devoid of side effects.

Misoprostol is a synthetic prostaglandin and may be used as a secondary therapy to prevent ulcers in patients taking NSAIDs. *H. pylori* is a species of gram-negative spiral bacteria that are sensitive to combination therapy with a variety of antibiotics. Laparoscopic repair is indicated when medical therapy is unsuccessful.

Gastric Ulcer Disease

Gastric ulcers develop as a result of degeneration of the stomach's mucosal barrier to gastric acid. In patients with this condition, normal acid secretion and hypochlorhydria are present, phenomena that differentiate this condition from duodenal ulcer disease. Pain and anorexia predispose the patient to metabolic derangements and weight loss. Surgery, consisting of

TABLE 28-6 Proton Pump Inhibitors

Generic Name	Trade Name	Adult Dosage Range	Available Dosage Forms*	Dose Adjustment in Renal Dysfunction	Drug Interactions and Comments
Esomeprazole	Nexium	20 mg qd	Capsule: 20, 40 mg	No	Cefuroxime, cefpodoxime, digoxin, dihydropyridine calcium channel blockers, iron salts, itraconazole, ketoconazole, sucralfate
Lansoprazole	Prevacid	15-30 mg qd or bid	Capsule: 15, 30 mg	No	Same as esomeprazole plus theophylline
Omeprazole	Prilosec	20-40 mg qd or bid	Capsule: 10, 20, 40 mg	No	Same as esomeprazole plus benzodiazepines, cilostazol, citalopram, clarithromycin, cyclosporine, disulfiram, methotrexate, phenytoin, sulfonylureas, theophylline, warfarin
Pantoprazole	Protonix, Protonix IV	40-80 mg qd	Tablet: 40 mg; Injection: 40 mg/vial	No	Same as esomeprazole
Rabeprazole	Aciphex	20 mg qd	Tablet: 20 mg	No	Same as esomeprazole plus cyclosporine

**All oral forms are delayed release.*
Data from Mosby's Drug Consult. *St Louis: Mosby; 2004.*

antrectomy with pyloroplasty and vagotomy, is undertaken if the patient's condition does not respond to medical therapy.

Parietal cell vagotomy is another surgical option. In this procedure selective sectioning of vagal fibers of the gastric fundus and parietal cells is performed while the fibers innervating the antrum are preserved. However, mixed results regarding the efficacy of the procedure have been reported.

Gastric Neoplastic Disease

Most gastric neoplasms are malignant. The incidence of these neoplasms according to type is adenocarcinoma, 95%; lymphoma, 4%; and leiomyosarcoma, 1%. Signs and symptoms, such as anorexia and weight loss, may occur late; these serve as poor prognostic indicators of curative surgical treatment because of probable metastases to adjacent peritoneal organs and structures.[35]

Gastric carcinoma is treated primarily through either total or subtotal gastrectomy. In addition, omentectomy, lymph node dissection, and splenectomy are considered to depend on the extent of spread, the patient's condition, and the preference of the surgeon.

Gastrinoma, a neoplasm arising from the pancreas or duodenum, releases overabundant quantities of gastrin, resulting in the secretion of massive quantities of hydrochloric acid from the parietal cells (Zollinger-Ellison syndrome). This condition is associated with severe, intractable ulcer pain. If other neoplasias are present, that is, thyroid and parathyroid adenoma, pituitary adenoma, and insulinoma, the condition is referred to as *multiple endocrine neoplasia type I*.

Definitive therapy for gastrinoma is surgical excision. During anesthetic induction for excision of gastrinoma, a rapid-sequence technique is recommended because of the likelihood of a large volume of stagnant, acidic intragastric fluid. Electrolyte and intravascular volume derangements (e.g., from severe diarrhea) should be anticipated and corrected before surgery. Attention should also be given to intraoperative monitoring of electrolyte and fluid balance. Hypokalemia and metabolic alkalosis are likely to be present if the patient has been vomiting and is dehydrated. Furthermore, preparations for the treatment of patients with known or suspected derangements in endocrine function must be included in the anesthetic plan, for example, blood glucose monitoring; vigilance for and timely correction of swings in vital signs and physiologic parameters; maintenance of normothermia and normocarbia; maintenance of an appropriately anesthetized state; and maintenance of renal function.

Anesthetic Considerations in Gastric Disease

Patients undergoing surgery for gastric disease are generally either acutely ill and require emergency surgery, as in the case of a bleeding gastric ulcer, or stable and require elective surgical treatment of gastric carcinoma or intractable ulcer disease. Many procedures are performed laparoscopically. Acutely ill patients are more likely to be hemodynamically unstable and dehydrated. Elective surgical patients may have a variable degree of debilitation and anemia. Aspiration precautions in both groups are warranted during anesthesia.

Hypovolemia should be corrected with the administration of appropriate colloid, crystalloid, or blood products before the induction of anesthesia. Clinical anemia and coagulopathy should be corrected with packed red blood cells and appropriate blood products (FFP, cryoprecipitate, platelets). The degree to which invasive monitoring (i.e., that using a pulmonary artery catheter, central venous pressure line, or arterial line) is used is determined by the presence of preexisting, age-related, or acquired compromise in the function of other organ systems. Preparations for the perioperative transfusion of blood products must be undertaken before anesthesia and surgery. Potential postoperative complications include hemorrhage, hypovolemia, hypothermia, atelectasis, and ileus. A postoperative stay in the intensive care unit may be necessary.

The anesthetic technique used in gastrectomy may include preoperative epidural catheter placement for intraoperative use, for instance, as an adjunct to general endotracheal anesthesia. Postoperative analgesia is also administered through an epidural catheter.

Procedures other than total and partial gastrectomy performed for gastric disease include the following:

- Billroth I: resection of the distal stomach with reconstruction via end-to-end gastroduodenostomy
- Billroth II: resection of the distal stomach with reconstruction via end-to-side gastrojejunostomy
- Laparotomy with oversewing of the ulcer and application of an omental patch

Vagotomy is usually performed during gastric ulcer surgery in order to decrease gastric acid secretion.

Postgastrectomy Syndromes

Surgical procedures are undertaken for the treatment of peptic ulcer disease to reduce the acid-secreting capabilities while preserving antral function and the gastric reservoir of the stomach. Untoward side effects of these procedures may result from loss of pyloric sphincter function, from loss of the stomach's reservoir function, and as a secondary result of parasympathetic denervation. These sequelae may occur in combination or alone and are termed *postgastrectomy syndromes*.

Recurrent ulcer disease after operation for duodenal ulcer is occasionally seen in patients in whom vagotomy has been performed without partial gastrectomy (e.g., antrectomy). Symptoms include onset of typical ulcer pain, and diagnostic confirmation is made through endoscopic examination. Other causes of recurrent ulcer disease may be an unrecognized gastrinoma, the presence of an excessively long afferent limb after gastroenterostomy, or the retention of acid-secreting antral tissue at the duodenal stump (causing hypergastrinemia).[36] Initial treatment is with H_2-receptor blocking agents, followed by repeat vagotomy with antrectomy if medical interventions fail.

In the most commonly occurring postgastrectomy syndrome, early postprandial dumping occurs. The syndrome consists of gastrointestinal signs and symptoms that include nausea, cramping abdominal pain, weakness, and explosive diarrhea occurring within the first half-hour after ingestion of a meal. Diaphoresis, dizziness, flushing, and palpitations indicate vasomotor instability. The syndrome results from rapid gastric emptying of hyperosmolar chyme from the residual stomach into the small intestine. Osmotic movement of fluid from the extracellular spaces into the intestine in order to achieve isotonicity is theorized to be responsible for the vasomotor aberrations that occur in patients with the syndrome. Increased proximal small-intestine hormone release brought about by distention probably accounts for the other clinical signs; this hormone release induces the facial flushing, increased small-intestine motility, and explosive diarrhea.[36] Many patients with this syndrome may be treated effectively without surgery. In other patients, surgery may be necessary, including revision of the gastroenterostomy, typically to a Roux-en-Y reconstruction. A Roux-en-Y gastroenterostomy provides a peristaltic conduit for drainage of pancreatic and biliary secretions into the jejunum and significantly attenuates the incidence of reflux.

Late postprandial dumping syndrome occurs less commonly than the early postprandial syndrome. Diaphoresis, tremulousness, and dizziness usually occur 1 to 3 hours after ingestion of a high-carbohydrate meal. The symptoms occur secondary to rapid gastric emptying and absorption of a high-carbohydrate load in the intestine, with resultant hyperglycemia. Overshoot of insulin release occurs in response to the development of hypoglycemia. Symptoms similar to insulin shock may become clinically manifest. Treatment is primarily medical.

Intermittent or complete obstruction of the afferent limb of a gastroenteric anastomosis (as seen in gastrectomy with a Billroth II reconstruction) may result in distention of the loop and a subsequent increase in hepatobiliary and pancreatic secretion. This condition, termed *afferent loop syndrome*, occurs after ingestion of a meal and is relieved by projectile, bilious vomiting. The vomitus typically lacks ingested food content because the food passes into the intestine and is absorbed. Definitive treatment of this condition is surgical reconstruction of the afferent limb, that is, creation of a long-limb Roux-en-Y.[34]

Excessive reflux may occur from the intestinal tract into the stomach after gastrectomy and gastroenterostomy. A high incidence of excessive reflux is seen after gastrojejunostomy. Signs and symptoms include epigastric pain, bilious vomiting, anemia, and weight loss. Under these circumstances, conversion of the previous reconstruction to a Roux-en-Y has a high success rate.

Anesthetic considerations for postgastrectomy syndrome must include a thorough appreciation of the patient's nutritional and metabolic status. Involvement of the stomach remnant in the disease process may result in anemia as a result of insufficient secretion of intrinsic factor. Measures for the prevention of aspiration (i.e., full-stomach precautions) should be in effect perioperatively. Aggressive preoperative and intraoperative fluid and electrolyte replacement may be necessary and should be anticipated.

Gastrostomy

Gastrostomy consists of the surgical placement of a tube through the abdominal wall for the purpose of gastric decompression and feeding. Patients who require placement of a gastrostomy tube (permanent or temporary) are often neurologically incapacitated and are likely to have compromised command of their airway reflexes. This situation places them at greater risk for aspiration.

Gastrostomy placement is performed percutaneously with endoscopic guidance or through a small laparotomy incision. A gastrostomy tube may also be placed during a laparotomy performed for another purpose. Sedation and local anesthesia may be used, although general endotracheal anesthesia is indicated in patients who require laparotomy in conjunction with endoscopic placement and in those in whom endoscopic placement is not possible.

PERITONEUM

The peritoneum consists of two double-layered sheets of cells with separately derived neural innervation. The visceral peritoneum is adherent to the intraabdominal organs, with the parietal peritoneum covering the inner surface of the abdominal wall. Innervation of the visceral peritoneum consists of autonomic sympathetic and parasympathetic fibers. Pain perceived is nonspecific, dull, and cramping and is mediated by C fibers. Parietal visceral innervation consists of somatic spinal fibers originating at levels T7 through L2. Pain transmitted is sharp and exquisite, mediated by A delta fibers.

Most intraabdominal organs are insensitive to many forms of stimulation (e.g., cutting, electrical) except for distention, stretch, torsion, and compression. Ischemic and inflammatory pain may be diffuse and nondistinct. Only when the visceral stimulation becomes transmural or affects the parietal peritoneum does pain become localized. Pain from visceral structures may be referred to another intraperitoneal region because a common nerve plexus is shared. An example is seen in pain originating from the kidneys, ureters, or bladder. These structures not only have visceral autonomic innervation, but also fibers from the celiac plexus, the thoracic and lumbar splanchnic nerves, and the intermesenteric and superior hypogastric plexus.[37]

Peritonitis

The peritoneal circulation not only cleans contaminants from the peritoneal cavity, but may also facilitate transmission of pathologic substances to other regions of the abdomen. The peritoneum is secretory, hence the role the peritoneum serves in the development of ascites and its utility in peritoneal dialysis. Only the surface of the diaphragm is absorptive. Ventilatory mechanics power fluid absorption via lacunae (channels of small openings) into subphrenic lymphatic channels. In this manner pathologic processes, including dissemination of infectious and metastatic substances, may occur.

Peritonitis (inflammation of the peritoneal cavity) may be either primary or secondary. Primary peritonitis is the rarer of the two types, with immunocompromised individuals and those with cirrhotic liver disease at highest risk. Primary peritonitis results from direct bacterial contamination of the peritoneum. Secondary peritonitis is usually a result of perforation of the gut, with translocation of bacterial flora and toxins into the normally sterile peritoneal cavity. Events responsible for secondary peritonitis include inflammation, neoplasia, ischemia, and trauma.[38]

DISEASES OF THE INTESTINAL TRACT

Anatomic and Physiologic Overview of the Small Intestine

The small intestine has three functional anatomic and physiologic subdivisions. In adults the first division, the duodenum, has a length of approximately 20 cm. The duodenum is followed by the second division, the jejunum, which has a length of approximately 100 to 110 cm. The third and longest division of the small intestine is the ileum, which has a length of approximately 150 to 160 cm. The jejunoileum extends from the ligament of Treitz (at the duodenojejunal junction) to the ileocecal valve. The jejunum is larger and thicker than the ileum and possesses a less extensive blood supply (one or two vascular networks versus four or five in the ileum).

The mesentery, which is rich in lymphatics and blood vessels, tethers the small intestine. The superior mesenteric artery provides the primary arterial supply to the jejunum and ileum and to the proximal transverse colon. The mesentery supplies a vast network of collateral arterial supply as well. Venous drainage is primarily furnished by the superior mesenteric vein. This vessel joins the splenic vein posterior to the pancreas, which is joined into the portal vein. Lymphatic drainage from the bowel wall originates from the central bowel wall lacteal and continues through the superior mesenteric nodes into the cisterna chyli and, ultimately, the thoracic duct.

Histologic composition of the small bowel consists of a serosal outermost layer that is composed of visceral peritoneum. This layer is formed in the jejunum, ileum, and anterior duodenum. The muscular layer consists of an outer longitudinal layer and a thin circular layer, both composed of smooth muscle. Auerbach's (myenteric) plexus, which primarily controls gastrointestinal motility, lies between the two muscular layers. The strongest component of the bowel wall is the submucosa, which consists of fibroelastic connective tissue. Within it lies Meissner's plexus, which controls local blood flow and gastrointestinal secretions. The innermost layer, the mucosa, is composed of transverse folds with millions of villi. These intraluminal projections greatly increase the absorptive surface of the small intestine.

The mucosa is further subdivided into three distinct layers:

1. Muscularis mucosae: the deepest layer, composed of a thin muscular sheet.
2. Lamina propria: a continuous connective tissue layer between the muscularis mucosae and the epithelium. This layer serves as a support epithelium and immunogenic barrier. Constituents of this layer include plasma cells, macrophages, fibroblasts, lymphocytes, eosinophils, and smooth muscle.
3. Epithelial layer: covers the villi and lines Lieberkühn's crypts (which contain mucus-producing goblet cells, enterochromaffin [endocrine] cells, zymogen granules [Paneth's cells], and basal undifferentiated cells). Cell turnover takes 3 to 7 days. The villi contain goblet, absorptive, and endocrine cells. Absorptive cells contain digestive enzymes and specific absorption receptors.[38]

Innervation of the small intestine is essentially parasympathetic through the vagus nerve and celiac ganglia. Parasympathetic stimulation is responsible for motility and secretion. Splanchnic nerves from the celiac plexus provide sympathetic innervation, which controls secretion, vascular integrity, and bowel motility. Sympathetic nerve tracts are also responsible for carrying pain afferents.[39] Physiologic functions of the small intestine are summarized in Box 28-2.

The intestinal mucosa provides a barrier to the entry of pathogens. The lamina propria provides a rich reservoir of IgA (the secretory immunoglobulin) and plasma cells (responsible for synthesis of IgA). IgA antigen binding initiates mucous secretion, which prevents intestinal bacterial and viral uptake. Furthermore, IgA binds with, incapacitates, and facilitates enzymatic destruction of bacteria. Binding with and preventing entry of toxins is another role of IgA. Lymphocytes, which are instrumental in the elaboration of a specific antibody to a given antigen, are found in Peyer's patches, which are located in the intestinal wall.[38]

The mucosa of the small intestine provides a rich supply of hormones that regulate gastrointestinal function. An overview of the major gastrointestinal hormones is noted in Table 28-7.

A basic electrical rhythm in the longitudinal smooth muscle layer initiates action potentials in the circular muscular layers of the small intestine after feeding. This activity sets forth the muscular contractions that constitute small-bowel motility. Both segmental contractions, which mix chyme with digestive enzymes and expose it to absorptive surfaces, and peristaltic (propulsive) contractions are noted.

Autonomic functions have a major influence on intestinal motility. Sympathetic influence generally inhibits motility, whereas parasympathetic activity increases it. The intestinal inhibitory reflex responds to abnormal distention by decreasing motility proximal to the locus of distention. This reflex may have significant indirect clinical implications (e.g., aspiration risk).[39]

Malabsorption Syndromes

Numerous disorders of the small intestine manifest as derangements in absorption. Primary clinical signs include unexplained weight loss, steatorrhea, and diarrhea. These disorders

BOX 28-2

Synopsis of Physiologic Functions (Digestion and Absorption) of the Small Intestine

Protein
Initiated in the stomach
Completed in the duodenum and jejunum; further hydrolysis (via intracellular peptidases) of peptides to free amino acids occurs before entry into the portal vein (approximately 90% of intact peptides)

Carbohydrates
Initiated by salivary amylase
Digested by pancreatic amylase in the duodenum; absorption completed by brush border of the intestinal microvilli (through conversion of monosaccharides into absorbable hexoses)

Fats
Digestion and absorption of lipid (primarily triglycerides) occurs almost entirely in the small intestine by two processes:
- Lipolysis
- Formation of micelles

Facilitated by pancreatic bicarbonate and bile salts

Water and Electrolytes
10 L of water enters the small bowel daily; most of this volume is absorbed
Net absorption of water is facilitated primarily via osmosis; another mechanism involves passive diffusion through luminal pores under the influence of hydrostatic pressure
Sodium absorption occurs essentially in conjunction with bulk flow of water (primarily in the jejunum); this process occurs with concomitant hydrogen ion extrusion
Bicarbonate secretion and chloride ion absorption occur in conjunction with sodium absorption
Electrical neutrality is maintained
Calcium ion absorption (facilitated by an acidic environment) occurs primarily in the duodenum and jejunum via active transport; enhanced by vitamin D and parathyroid hormone
Passive potassium absorption occurs primarily in the jejunum
Absorption of iron occurs primarily in the duodenum

Other Vitamins and Minerals
Ascorbic acid—absorbed in the ileum and coupled to sodium
Cobalamin (vitamin B_{12})—absorbed in the distal ileum and linked to glycoprotein carrier molecules (especially intrinsic factor)
Folate—absorbed in the proximal jejunum in conjunction with sodium
Biotin—absorbed in the proximal small bowel as a result of sodium-linked active transport
Thiamine (vitamin B_1)—absorbed predominantly in the duodenum
Vitamin B_6—absorbed in the proximal small bowel
Niacin, pantothenate, and riboflavin—absorbed passively (mechanism incompletely understood)

Modified from Evers MB, Townsend CM, Thompson JC. Small intestine. In: Schwartz SI, et al, eds. Principles of Surgery. *7th ed. New York: McGraw-Hill; 1999:1217-1229.*

affect the absorption of the major constituents of ingested nutrients, including amino acids, carbohydrates, and fats. Gluten-sensitive enteropathy is a disorder of malabsorption formerly referred to as *celiac sprue* and *tropical sprue*. It is characterized by the eventual development of megaloblastic anemia, fatigue, and weight loss and is managed through regulation of the diet (i.e., removal of dietary gluten) and administration of steroids (i.e., prednisone). Complications of gluten-sensitive enteropathy include small-bowel ulceration and a predisposition to malignancy as well as megaloblastic anemia, fatigue, and weight loss. Treatment of this disorder is with administration of folic acid and antibiotics.[3]

Fat malabsorption results in deficiency of fat-soluble vitamins (vitamins A, D, E, and K). Deficiency in vitamin K manifests through hypoprothrombinemia. This condition is often evidenced through bleeding dyscrasia. Vitamin B_{12} deficiency results in anemia (which may also be encountered in patients with impaired iron absorption), neuropathy, and glossitis. Protein malabsorption may result in the development of peripheral edema and ascites. Tetany, osteomalacia, and pathologic fractures result from calcium deficiency caused by vitamin D malabsorption.[39]

The cause of malabsorption syndromes is multifactorial. The basic underlying defect is either disruption of intestinal mucosal integrity, such as from disease processes, or loss of absorptive surface area caused by surgical resection of the small intestine. With regard to alterations in small-intestine absorption secondary to surgical resection, the particular part of the small bowel resected and the amount removed have a significant bearing on the degree to which deficiencies in minerals, vitamins, and electrolytes are clinically manifested.

Maldigestion Syndromes

Maldigestion syndromes are generally caused by derangements or deficiencies in pancreatic secretion. Diseases more likely to result in malabsorption syndromes may be differentiated from those responsible for maldigestion. The hallmark of maldigestion is steatorrhea. Significant pancreatic disease is usually present when a maldigestion syndrome is present, because the pancreas has a large functional reserve in normal as well as in disease states. Chronic pancreatitis is the major and most common cause of pancreatic insufficiency. Cystic fibrosis, fistulas, gallstones, and neoplastic disease processes, however, are also etiologic factors.[39]

Anatomic and Physiologic Considerations of the Large Colon

The large colon is approximately 3 to 5 feet long and may be recognized not only by its size and position but also by the presence of three strips of longitudinal muscle and the numerous outpouchings (haustrations) throughout its length. The arterial supply essentially consists of the superior mesenteric artery (which perfuses the right to the midtransverse colon), the inferior mesenteric artery (which perfuses the midtransverse colon

TABLE 28-7 Gastrointestinal Hormones

Hormone	Location	Major Stimulants of Peptide Secretion	Primary Effects	Diagnostic and Therapeutic Uses
Gastrin	Antrum, duodenum (G cells)	Peptides, amino acids, antral distention, vagal and adrenergic stimulation, gastrin-releasing peptide (bombesin)	Stimulates gastric acid and pepsinogen secretion; stimulates gastric mucosal growth	Gastrin analogue (pentagastrin) used to measure maximal gastric acid secretion
CCK	Duodenum, jejunum (I cells)	Fats, peptides, amino acids	Stimulates pancreatic enzyme secretion; stimulates gallbladder contraction; relaxes sphincter of Oddi; inhibits gastric emptying	Biliary imaging of gallbladder concentration
Secretin	Duodenum, jejunum (S cells)	Fatty acids, luminal acidity, bile salts	Stimulates release of water and bicarbonate from pancreatic ductal cells; stimulates flow and alkalinity of bile; inhibits gastric acid secretion and motility and inhibits gastrin release	Provocative test for gastrinoma; measurement of maximal pancreatic secretion
Somatostatin	Pancreatic islet (D cells), antrum, duodenum	Gut: Fat, protein, acid, other hormones, (e.g., gastrin, CCK) Pancreas: Glucose, amino acids, CCK	Universal "off" switch; stimulates release of all GI secretion and motility; stimulates gastric acid secretion and release of antral gastrin; stimulates growth of intestinal mucosa and pancreas	Treatment of carcinoid; diarrhea and flushing; decreases secretion from intestinal fistulas (particularly pancreatic fistulas); ameliorates symptoms associated with hormone-overproducing endocrine tumors; treatment of esophageal variceal bleeding
Gastrin-releasing peptide (mammalian equivalent of bombesin)	Small bowel	Vagal stimulation	Universal "on" switch; stimulates release of all GI hormones (except secretin); stimulates GI secretin; stimulates growth of intestinal mucosa and pancreas	
Gastric inhibitory polypeptide	Duodenum, jejunum (K cells)	Glucose, fat, protein adrenergic stimulation	Inhibits gastric acid and pepsin secretion; stimulates pancreatic insulin release in response to hyperglycemia	
Motilin	Duodenum, jejunum	Gastric distention, fat	Stimulates upper GI tract motility; may initiate the migrating motor complex	
Vasoactive intestinal peptide	Neurons throughout GI tract	Vagal stimulation	Primarily functions as a neuropeptide; potent vasodilator	
Neurotensin	Small bowel (N cells)	Fat	Stimulates pancreatic and intestinal secretion; inhibits gastric acid secretion; stimulates growth of small and large bowel mucosa	
Enteroglucagon	Small bowel (L cells)	Glucose, fat	Glucagon-like peptide-1: Stimulates insulin release; inhibits pancreatic glucagon release; Glucagon-like peptide-2: Potent enterotrophic factor	
Peptide YY	Distal small bowel, colon	Fatty acids, CCK	Inhibits gastric and pancreatic secretions; inhibits gallbladder contraction	

CCK, *cholecystokinin;* GI, *gastrointestinal.*
From Evers MB. Small intestine. In: Sabiston Textbook of Surgery. *17th ed. Philadelphia: Saunders; 2004:1333.*

to the superior rectum), and the internal iliac artery (which perfuses the middle and lower rectum). Venous drainage basically parallels arterial drainage, with the middle and superior veins contributing to the portal venous system. Sympathetic innervation is derived from T10 to T12 (right colon), L1 to L3 (left colon), and the presacral nerves arising within the preaortic plexuses (rectum). Parasympathetic innervation is primarily from the vagus nerve (right and transverse colon) and from nerve fibers arising from S2 to S4 (descending colon, sigmoid colon, and rectum). A rich endowment of lymphatics is present throughout the length of the colon and the rectum.

The function of the large colon is primarily to store and expel waste products. Another function that is performed largely in the right colon is the absorption of sodium and water. Most of the 1 to 2 L of ileal effluent presented to the large colon per day is absorbed, with the exception of 100 to 200 ml.

Sodium absorption occurs through active transport against a gradient and is enhanced by minerals, corticoids, glucocorticoids, and fatty acids that are produced by indigenous bacteria. Potassium is passively absorbed and secreted, whereas chloride is absorbed in exchange for bicarbonate. Potassium is lost through passive diffusion in the colonic mucoid secretions. Significant potassium loss is likely to occur, therefore, in the presence of colitis and villous adenoma, two disease processes that are notable for mucoid stools. The colon is also involved in the enterohepatic circulation of bile acids (the greater degree of which occurs in the ileum). The colonic role in this process assumes a greater importance in the presence of ileal disease or decreased ileal absorptive area. Conversion of primary bile acids to secondary bile acids also occurs in the colon.[40]

Conservation of sodium is so efficient in the large colon that a normal individual may require only 5 mEq/day in order to remain in sodium balance. Therefore the presence of an ileostomy necessitates a greater intake of sodium (80 to 100 mEq/day) in order to approximate the high sodium content present as ileal effluent. The loss of the normal colonic reabsorption of sodium chloride and water (e.g., after colectomy) may eventually exceed the small intestine's capacity to increase absorption and result in clinical derangements in electrolyte balance.[41]

Inflammatory Bowel Disease

In the United States between 200,000 and 300,000 individuals have inflammatory bowel disease, and approximately 30,000 new cases are diagnosed each year.[39] The two major types of inflammatory bowel disease are Crohn's disease and ulcerative colitis, which have different clinical features and manifestations (Table 28-8).

Crohn's disease involves primarily the distal ileum and large colon in approximately 50% of patients. The remainder of patients experience disease that is localized to either the colon or portions of the small intestine (regional enteritis). The deeper layers of the intestinal mucosa are typically involved, a situation that leads to derangements in colonic absorption. Owing to the loss of functional absorptive surfaces in the large colon, patients with Crohn's disease are often deficient in magnesium, phosphorus, zinc, and potassium. They also have deficiencies secondary to the loss of absorptive capability in portions of the small intestine. Protein-losing enteropathy is often encountered, as is anemia resulting from occult blood loss and deficiencies in vitamin B_{12} and folic acid. Iron deficiency secondary to insufficient intestinal absorption also contributes to development of an anemic state. Involvement of the distal ileum in the disease

TABLE 28-8 Diagnosis of Crohn's Colitis versus Ulcerative Colitis

Observation	Crohn's Colitis	Ulcerative Colitis
Symptoms and Signs		
Diarrhea	Common	Common
Rectal bleeding	Less common	Almost always
Abdominal pain (cramps)	Moderate to severe	Mild to moderate
Palpable mass	At times	No (unless large cancer)
Anal complaints	Frequent (<50%)	Infrequent (<20%)
Radiologic Findings		
Ileal disease	Common	Rare (backwash ileitis)
Nodularity, fuzziness	No	Yes
Distribution	Skip areas	Rectum extending upward and continuously
Ulcers	Linear, cobblestone, fissures	Collar-button
Toxic dilation	Rare	Uncommon
Proctoscopic Findings		
Anal fissure, fistula, abscess	Common	Rare
Rectal sparing	Common (50%)	Rare (5%)
Granular mucosa	No	Yes
Ulceration	Linear, deep, scattered	Superficial, universal

From Evers MB. Small intestine. In: Sabiston Textbook of Surgery: the Biological Basis of Modern Surgical Practice. *17th ed. Philadelphia: Saunders; 2004:1347.*

process results in deficiencies in vitamin B_{12} and in nutrients that are dependent on bile acids for absorption. Disturbance in the enterohepatic circulation of bile in the terminal ileum is reflected in complex nutrient deficiencies, including proteins, zinc, magnesium, phosphorus, fat-soluble vitamins, and vitamin B_{12}. This state is typical of patients with chronic Crohn's disease. Folate deficiency may also be present in patients with Crohn's disease who receive sulfasalazine preparations.

Fistulas often develop between inflamed portions of the intestine and adjacent abdominal structures. Abdominal and pelvic abscesses, rectocutaneous fistulas, and perirectal abscesses have a high incidence in these patients. Increased calcium oxalate absorption in the terminal ileum frequently occurs, resulting in a high rate of renal calculi and cholelithiasis.

Medical therapy for Crohn's disease includes sulfasalazine (Azulfidine), an aminosalicylate, as first line therapy. Other sulfasalazine-like drugs such as mesalamine (Pentasa; Asacol) and olsalazine (Dipentum) are also commonly used.

Systemic corticosteroids such as prednisone are used for anti-inflammatory purposes. Other common medications include antimicrobial agents, such as metronidazole and immunosuppressive agents, such as azathioprine and 6-mercaptopurine. Cyclosporine, methotrexate and tacrolimus have been shown to be efficacious in the treatment of active disease and in maintenance of remission in preliminary trials. Monoclonal antibodies with cytokinin and anticytokinin activity have recently shown promising results. Severe weight loss, cachexia, and malnutrition indicate the need for parenteral nutritional support.

Surgery is warranted when medical treatment fails or when complications supervene. Although effective in the relief of complications, surgical resection of the diseased colon and ileum does not alter the progression of the disease. The primary principle of surgical management is to limit the operation to the correction of the presenting complication, which could include bowel obstruction, fistulas, abscesses, and symptoms that indicate widespread symptomatic disease (for which total colectomy and ileal resection may be warranted).

Most patients with Crohn's disease undergo surgery, and a large number require repeat or continued procedures. The recurrence rate at 10 years after surgery is 50%. A high likelihood of repeat surgery involves areas of the remaining bowel proximal to the area of a previous anastomosis. Patients with a history of Crohn's disease are also shown to have a higher prevalence of bowel carcinoma.[42,43]

Ulcerative colitis is an inflammatory disease, primarily of the mucosa of the rectum and distal colon. It is a chronic disease that is fraught with remissions and exacerbations. It affects female patients more frequently than male patients and has a bimodal age distribution that shows a first peak incidence between ages 15 and 20 years and a second, smaller, peak between ages 55 and 60 years. The disorder is speculated to have a strong familial genetic predisposition, but psychologic factors have also been implicated in its cause.[40]

Symptoms usually include abdominal pain, fever, and bloody diarrhea. Ulcerative colitis is typically chronic, with relatively low-grade symptoms, such as bloody stools, malaise, diarrhea, and pain. In approximately 15% of patients, however, ulcerative colitis that has acute, fulminating characteristics may occur. Under this circumstance, severe abdominal pain, profuse rectal hemorrhage, and high fever are seen. Associated symptoms include nausea and vomiting, anorexia, and profound weakness. Physical signs usually include pallor and weight loss.

Associated with an acute onset of fulminating ulcerative colitis is toxic megacolon, which is characterized by severe colonic distention that causes shock. In patients with this condition the distended bowel lumen provides an environment that is conducive to bacterial overgrowth. This condition, coupled with erosive intestinal inflammation and perforation, allows for the systemic release of bacteria-produced toxins. Clinical signs and symptoms of toxic megacolon include fever, tachycardia, abdominal distention, pain, ileus, and dehydration. Electrolyte derangements, anemia, and hypoalbuminemia are also commonly present.[44]

Patients with ulcerative colitis are at increased risk for the development of carcinoma of the colon. An increased incidence of large-joint arthritis is seen in patients when the disease is clinically active. Concomitant liver disease, as evidenced by fatty infiltrates and pericholangitis, may also complicate the clinical picture. Other extracolonic manifestations of ulcerative colitis include iritis, erythema nodosum, and ankylosing spondylitis.[44]

Therapy for ulcerative colitis is initially medical. As with Crohn's disease, sulfasalazine preparations, antidiarrheal agents, and corticosteroids are the cornerstones of medical therapy. Both Crohn's disease and ulcerative colitis result in systemic disorders, such as anemia and nutritional deficiencies, which are handled in the same supportive manner. In both diseases, surgical resection is reserved for patients with intractable complications. Whereas surgery for Crohn's disease is nondefinitive and complication oriented, proctocolectomy with ileostomy is generally curative for ulcerative colitis.[44]

Anesthetic Considerations in Inflammatory Bowel Disease

Anesthetic management of patients with inflammatory bowel disease begins with a thorough, systematic patient history, and particular attention is paid to the patient's fluid and electrolyte status. Possible extracolonic complications (e.g., sepsis, liver disease, anemia, arthritis, hypoalbuminemia, and other metabolic derangements) must also be considered during planning and perioperative management. Efforts to optimize the medical condition of such patients before elective surgery are strongly recommended.

Prophylactic steroid coverage is likely to be indicated, particularly in patients receiving long-term steroid therapy. Nitrous oxide should be avoided so that the possibility of intraoperative bowel distention is minimized. Awareness of complications from parenteral nutritional therapy (e.g., hyperglycemia or hypoglycemia, increased carbon dioxide production, renal or hepatic dysfunction, nonketotic hyperosmolar hyperglycemic coma, and hyperchloremic metabolic acidosis) is also necessary for patients receiving total or partial parenteral nutritional support. The severity of extracolonic influence on the function of other organ systems dictates appropriate technique and drug selection, as well as the extent to which invasive monitoring is used. Correction of fluid, electrolyte, and hematologic derangements may be necessary before surgery. Increased intraluminal pressure caused by the administration of anticholinesterases (for reversal of neuromuscular blockade) has been shown to have no effect on colonic suture lines. No particular anesthetic technique is mandated; however, the use of a combined technique (epidural and general anesthesia) is attractive for both intraoperative use and postoperative analgesia needs.[45,46]

Diverticulitis and Diverticulosis

Diverticulosis of the colon is characterized by the presence of numerous mucosal outpouchings in the large colon, with the highest prevalence noted in the sigmoid colon (65%). Structural weakness of the colonic wall and increased intracolonic pressures are two mechanisms theorized to be responsible for the development of diverticulosis. Diverticulitis is inflammation of diverticula; this syndrome manifests as abdominal pain with ileus and other symptoms that indicate an acute abdomen, such as nausea, vomiting, rigid abdominal distention, and dehydration. Inflamed diverticula may be localized or more widespread and may involve the mesentery and other abdominal organs. Abscess formation and visceral perforation indicate the need for urgent surgical intervention.

Surgical treatment of diverticulosis is reserved for symptoms that are refractory to aggressive medical therapy. Intravenous corticosteroids, antibiotics, and fluid replacement are attempted initially. Exploratory laparotomy with colectomy may be necessary under emergent conditions of acute bleeding, recurrent bleeding that fails to cease spontaneously, or sepsis. The goals of surgical exploration include fecal diversion and abscess drainage, as well as resection of the diseased colon.

Complications of diverticulitis, which occur in up to 25% of patients, frequently necessitate surgical intervention. Such complications include bowel obstruction, fistulas, and abscesses. Abscess formation after colonic obstruction and perforation may involve such structures as the abdominal wall and the subdiaphragmatic spaces. Abscess formation may be extensive; it may include the deep pelvic organs and the hip and thigh.[47]

Diverticulitis occurs in only 1% of patients with diverticulosis. Clinical symptoms of diverticulitis include abdominal pain, diarrhea, and fever. Progression of symptoms may lead to hypovolemia, hypokalemia, and shock. The presence of free intraperitoneal air, as evidenced on radiographic abdominal films, suggests perforation. Air in the retroperitoneum may be indicative of paracolic abscess. Both conditions require urgent surgical exploration.[5,47]

Bleeding is uncommon in patients with diverticular disease. When present, however, it often defies localization through endoscopy and even laparotomy. A bleeding diathesis in diverticular disease may be either occult or massive and is caused by erosion of the vessels adjacent to the diverticulum. Elective colon resection is usually considered in patients with recurrent episodes of acute diverticulitis. After a second attack of acute diverticulitis the prevalence of complications associated with the disease approaches 50%, and the associated mortality rate is twice that of an initial attack.[3,47] Diverticulitis, when present in the right colon or cecum, often mimics acute appendicitis. Surgery for appendectomy, therefore, may uncover the presence of an inflamed diverticulum or diverticulitis, necessitating extension of the procedure so that colonic resection can be performed.

The clinical symptoms of diverticulitis may also be confused with those of Crohn's colitis in middle-aged and elderly patients. Some indications for surgery (e.g., obstruction and abscess) are similar in both diseases. Examination of the resected specimen differentiates the diagnoses. The patient may therefore be spared ineffective medical therapy for inflammatory bowel disease when a segmental colonic resection is potentially curative.[48]

Abdominal Compartment Syndrome

Increased abdominal pressure imposes profound effects on the circulation and systemic perfusion. Normal intraabdominal pressure is less than 10 mm Hg. At 10 mm Hg, hepatic arterial blood flow significantly decreases. Cardiovascular perturbations occur at 15 mm Hg. Oliguria occurs at 15 to 20 mm Hg, and anuria at 40 mm Hg. The etiology of abdominal compartment syndrome (ACS) is multifactorial, and the condition may be acute or insidious. Cases of acute ACS include intestinal obstruction, mesenteric arterial thrombosis, and ruptured abdominal aortic aneurysm. Increased abdominal pressure may also result from postoperative or posttraumatic complications. Causes of chronic ACS include ascites, pregnancy, and intraabdominal tumors.

Cardiac output is decreased secondary to decreased cardiac preload (venous return), elevated systemic vascular resistance, and elevated intrathoracic pressure. Reflex tachycardia is a baroreptor-mediated response to decreased preload with resultant diminished diastolic filling and coronary perfusion. Decreased thoracic compliance and decreased lung volumes result from impaired diaphragmatic descent. The result is increased pulmonary shunt fraction and atelectasis. Impairment in renal function results from compression of the kidney and diminished glomerular perfusion.[49]

Treatment of ACS is undertaken urgently with decompressive laparotomy. Affected patients often have myriad medical problems that may influence outcome significantly. Provision of anesthesia care can be extremely challenging. Intraoperative monitoring is directed toward maintenance of hemodynamic stability. This includes knowledge of the patient's preoperative hemodynamic profile. Inclusion of monitors such as an invasive arterial line and pulmonary artery catheter may be appropriate for perioperative management. Opioids and inhalation agents are used with discretion in accordance with patient tolerance. Provision for adequate muscle relaxation and amnesia with a benzodiazepine or scopolamine assumes prominence in pharmacologic anesthetic management of the physiologically labile patient. Other vasoactive agents are included as necessary for hemodynamic support. These patients may not tolerate abdominal closure after surgery. This is usually a result of intraabdominal edema. It is common for these patients to return to the operating room for dressing changes and for definitive correction of lesions bypassed because of resuscitative priorities in the initial procedure. This implies the likelihood of aggressive perioperative supportive care along with further modifications of anesthesia delivery in order to attenuate further erosion of the patient's compensatory powers.

Opening of the abdomen releases intraabdominal pressure and may have profound consequences on systemic perfusion. This results from release of the tamponade on a vast visceral bed and a resultant reperfusion syndrome. Reperfusion washout of by-products of anaerobic metabolism releases an array of cardiac depressant and vasodilatory mediators into the general circulation. Proper preparation is mandated. Preparation for this event includes optimization of intravascular volume, acid-base status, and arterial oxygenation.[50]

Mortality rate in ACS approaches 42%, with most patients succumbing to secondary systemic inflammatory response syndrome, sepsis, and multiple organ dysfunction syndrome. Other causes of death include the consequences of added stress imposed on cardiac function in susceptible patients.[51]

Colonic Polyps

Four categories of gastrointestinal polyps are recognized: neoplastic, inflammatory, hamartomatous, and unclassified. Neoplastic polyps are tubulovillous or villous adenomas or tubular adenomas. The potential for malignancy increases as the polyp size exceeds 1 cm. If pedunculated and limited to the mucosa, polyps may be removed while the patient is sedated in the outpatient setting via colonoscopy. If the lesion is sessile, colon resection is indicated, because the potential for malignancy is greater.[29]

Inflammatory polyps are typically small and have low potential for malignancy. The lesions are usually caused by chronic colitis. Hamartomatous polyps are usually small juvenile polyps that have minor-to-nonexistent neoplastic potential (Peutz-Jeghers syndrome). Unclassified polypoid disorders include familial adenomatous polyposis coli. This disease is a genetic autosomal dominant disorder that is characterized by the presence of multiple adenomatous polyps. This disease has a very high neoplastic potential. Total colectomy with ileostomy is the treatment of choice in patients with this condition. Other familial polypoid disorders include Turcot syndrome (colonic polyps with central nervous system tumors) and Gardner's syndrome (colonic polyposis with cutaneous tumors and osteosarcoma).[3,15]

A common presenting sign in the diagnosis of polypoid colonic disease is painless frank or occult rectal bleeding. Such bleeding has the potential for causing anemia. Cramping abdominal pain may be present, particularly in children.

Anesthetic Considerations in Elective Surgery of the Colon

To prevent wound infection and facilitate healing of colorectal anastomoses, preoperative elimination of fecal mass and reduction of bacterial flora are undertaken, usually while the patient is in the hospital the evening before surgery or at home (by the patient) the night before admission. Lavage with isotonic and isosmotic solutions may be performed by the patient orally or instilled via nasogastric tube. Cleansing enemas may also be ordered. These techniques often are used for elective procedures in conjunction with dietary changes that emphasize the intake of fluids and low-residue foodstuffs and that culminate in the intake of only clear liquids for 24 to 48 hours before surgery. Intravenous and oral antibiotics used for bowel cleansing commonly include drugs of the aminoglycoside family (e.g., neomycin, erythromycin) and/or a combination of the cephalosporins and metronidazole.

The anesthetist must be aware of this preoperative preparation in patients who undergo elective surgery. Aggressive preoperative bowel preparation predisposes a patient to water and electrolyte imbalance that may have a deleterious influence on perioperative cardiovascular function, hemodynamics, and systemic organ perfusion, particularly if the patient is elderly or debilitated. Depending on the chronicity of the disease process, anemia resulting from frank or occult bleeding may be present. Malnutrition with hypoalbuminemia may also be present before surgery.

The presence of an adynamic colon or obstruction commonly necessitates evacuation of stagnant stomach and upper intestinal contents via nasogastric drainage. This preoperative intervention may be superimposed on a dehydrated patient or one who is electrolyte depleted. Fluid and electrolyte derangements therefore may be of sufficient magnitude to require postponement of the procedure until volume and electrolyte resuscitation has been accomplished.

Carcinoma of the Colon

Cancer of the colon is a highly treatable and often curable disease when localized to the bowel. It is the second most frequently diagnosed malignancy in the United States as well as the second most common cause of cancer death. Surgery is the primary treatment and results in cure in approximately 50% of patients. Recurrence after surgery is a major problem and often is the ultimate cause of death. The prognosis of patients with colon cancer is clearly related to the degree of penetration of the tumor through the bowel wall and the presence or absence of nodal involvement.[52] Carcinoma of the colon accounts for approximately 60,000 deaths annually, and more than 140,000 new cases are diagnosed annually. The etiology is multifactorial and includes a strong correlation with diet, such as a high red meat intake and a low dietary fiber intake, as well as a genetic predisposition. Inflammatory bowel disease is usually associated with a greater predisposition to colonic carcinoma. Occult stool testing for blood is a standard screening method. Rectal examination and colonoscopic examination with biopsy are important diagnostic modalities.

Right-sided colonic lesions often cause symptoms that may indicate the presence of an obstructive lesion because of their concentric characteristics. Right-sided lesions are also associated with a higher incidence of anemia and fatigue. Bleeding is usually less profuse than in patients with diverticular disease.[3]

Volvulus of the Colon

Obstruction of blood supply with subsequent necrosis may affect a given length of redundant bowel, which rotates and twists around the mesentery. This condition usually affects a freely mobile colonic segment and a fixed point or set of points about which the colon twists. Approximately 75% of colonic volvulus affects the sigmoid colon.[40]

Symptoms usually suggest the presence of acute bowel obstruction (e.g., acute, severe, colicky abdominal pain and distention). Acute strangulation of the bowel is suggested by generalized severe abdominal pain, hypovolemia, and fever. Initial therapy is attempted through endoscopic reduction via proctoscopy with rectal tube placement. This treatment has a high success rate (70% to 80%) and permits elective resection of the involved dysfunctional segment of the sigmoid colon with primary anastomosis at a later date. Failure of nonoperative detorsion necessitates surgical intervention. If gangrene is discovered on laparotomy, resection is carried out with the formation of an end colostomy and a mucous fistula (Hartmann's procedure).[40]

Many patients with this condition are elderly or debilitated individuals and are referred from long-term care facilities. Associated disease processes include Alzheimer's disease, Parkinson's disease, multiple sclerosis, paralysis, pseudobulbar palsy, chronic schizophrenia, and dementia. Medications taken on a long-term basis by these patients may include neuropsychotropic drugs, which are known to alter bowel motility.[39]

Pseudomembranous Colitis

Pseudomembranous colitis is associated with inflammatory bowel disease, uremia, intestinal ischemia, Hirschsprung's disease, and shigellosis. It is characterized by mucosal exudate and plaque formation within the colon. It is also associated with antibiotic therapy, particularly with clindamycin and lincomycin.

Antibiotic-associated pseudomembranous colitis is usually caused by infection of the colonic mucosa caused by *Clostridium difficile* enterotoxin. Clinical manifestations include fever, diarrhea, abdominal pain, distention, and shock caused by dehydration and systemic bacterial dissemination.

Therapy begins with termination of the offending antibiotic. Supportive therapy and institution of antibiotic therapy, such as oral vancomycin or oral or parenteral metronidazole, directed against C. *difficile* often results in prompt clinical resolution. A 10% to 30% mortality rate is seen, however, in seriously ill patients.[39]

Ischemic Bowel Disease

Ischemic injury to the bowel occurs under numerous circumstances, including advanced atherosclerosis, shock, vasculitis, hypercoagulopathy, and amyloidosis. Surgical iatrogenic causes, such as interruption of the inferior mesenteric artery as a result of aortic cross-clamping during abdominal aortic surgery, are also culpable. The extent, severity, and prognosis of the syndrome of ischemic bowel disease are variable. Localized or segmental ischemia is often present. Differentiation of ischemic colitis from infectious processes, diverticulitis, or inflammatory bowel disease may be difficult. Definitive diagnosis depends on endoscopic examination with biopsy. Exclusion of bowel perforation in the differential diagnosis is made through radiographic examination of the abdomen for the presence of free air.

Patients with ischemic bowel disease are usually of advanced age. Symptoms typically consist of fever, vomiting, rectal bleeding, and abdominal cramping pain and may be present for weeks or months. The development of sudden rectal bleeding associated with left-sided abdominal pain and peritoneal signs strongly suggests the presence of this disease process. Concomitant ischemic heart disease and peripheral vascular disease are often present in these patients.[3,29]

Supportive measures are initially undertaken if bowel necrosis is not suspected. This includes antibiotic therapy and fluid resuscitation. In patients in whom perforation or necrosis is suspected, emergency laparotomy is indicated, with possible bowel resection and temporary or permanent colostomy. Stable patients may be candidates for vascular reconstructive procedures.[3]

Diseases of the Rectum and Anus

Diseases of the anorectal region may include neoplastic lesions. If biopsy findings are consistent with localized adenocarcinoma, abdominal-perineal resection of the rectum and sigmoid colon with permanent colostomy may be curative. Squamous cell carcinomas of the rectum are effectively treated with chemotherapy and radiation, as well as local excision. Surgical proctectomy is another treatment option.

Other rectal diseases include rectal prolapse (repaired with rectosigmoidectomy or proctopexy), which is seen most often in the elderly. Perirectal disease may be manifested by abscess formation that requires drainage, which may be performed on either an inpatient or an outpatient basis.

Perirectal fistulas typically develop secondary to infectious disease processes that cause abscess formation. Four types are generally recognized: extrasphincteric, suprasphincteric, transsphincteric, and intersphincteric. Initial therapy is incision and drainage with delayed fistulectomy in order to facilitate healing of the abscess.

Hemorrhoidal disease is characterized by dilation of the perianal submucosal venous plexus. Internal hemorrhoids are often bleeding prolapsed veins and are usually painless. Treatment is usually by rubber band ligation or surgical excision. External hemorrhoids are associated with a greater tendency to thrombose and are typically painful. Surgical excision is the treatment of choice.[53]

Anesthesia for most perirectal and perianal procedures may be effectively provided by regional techniques, such as spinal subarachnoid block or epidural blockade, as well as by local anesthesia infiltration with sedation. In some cases general endotracheal anesthesia may be necessary. Anesthetic considerations must include the influence of patient position (e.g., prone or lithotomy position) on intraoperative cardiovascular and respiratory dynamics.

Radiation Enteritis

The colon is highly susceptible to radiation injury because of the normal rapid renewal of the intestinal epithelial lining. Radiation injury results from radiation therapy, usually for malignant disease of the bladder, uterus, ovaries, and cervix. Mucosal inflammation and atrophy cause symptoms similar to those seen in patients with idiopathic ulcerative colitis, and corticosteroid therapy may have only limited success. Strictures, obstruction, and secondary ulceration may develop in the colon; these conditions may require diverting colostomy or bowel resection for relief of symptoms, sometimes under emergent conditions. The presence of adhesions and the induced increased friability of the intestinal tissues predispose affected patients to increased intraoperative bleeding and tissue third spacing.

Appendicitis

The appendix arises from the cecum and is normally 5 to 10 cm long. It possesses a separate mesoappendix and derives its blood supply from an appendicular artery and vein, which are branches of the ileocolic vessels. The appendix may assume any of a number of positions that influence the quality of symptoms and the site of pain when inflammation occurs.

Appendicitis occurs most often in individuals in their late teens and early twenties. A slight prevalence for male patients over female patients exists. Obstruction of the appendiceal lumen is the usual cause. Obstruction is often the result of hyperplasia of lymphoid follicles, of which the lumen of the appendix is richly endowed. A fecalith is often the cause of obstruction as well, occurring in 35% of cases. The presence of foreign bodies, inflammatory strictures, and other rare factors (e.g., appendiceal carcinoma and Meckel's diverticulum) can mimic the symptoms of appendicitis.[53]

Obstruction of the appendiceal lumen results in stasis of mucus secreted within the lumen. Bacterial overgrowth occurs secondarily and results in proliferation of secreted exotoxins and endotoxins that damage the epithelium. This condition leads to inflammation, ulceration, and eventual perforation. Depending on the time interval during which these events take place, either a walled-off abscess is formed or infective exudate is released into the peritoneum, resulting in generalized peritonitis. The latter condition, in which numerous intraperitoneal abscesses are formed, predisposes the patient to the development of systemic sepsis. The development of adhesions with bowel obstruction is also associated with peritonitis after rupture of an inflamed appendix.[54]

Symptoms of appendicitis include localized rebound lower right quadrant pain, fever, nausea, and vomiting. Leukocytosis is a common but nonspecific finding.

Other common clinical conditions with symptomatologies similar to that of appendicitis include such gynecologic conditions as salpingitis, ovarian torsion, ruptured ovarian cyst, and ectopic pregnancy. In males, epididymitis and testicular torsion may mimic appendicitis. Other confounding clinical conditions include ureteral stones, cystitis, ruptured peptic ulcer, and mesenteric adenitis.[55,56]

Given the potentially life-threatening nature of the sequelae of untreated acute appendicitis, the diagnosis is made liberally. It is recognized, therefore, that 10% to 15% of patients exhibiting accepted clinical symptomatology that is indicative of appendicitis are revealed to have a normal appendix at operation. If negative findings exist, other causes for the clinical symptoms are sought. This may necessitate further exploration and possibly extension of the laparotomy.

Definitive treatment of appendicitis is appendectomy, which may be performed with general or regional anesthesia. Laparoscopic techniques performed with the patient under general anesthesia also are now commonly employed.[38] Patients are frequently dehydrated and may be febrile, thereby requiring preoperative volume replacement. Antibiotic therapy is usually initiated before surgery. If general anesthesia is selected, aspiration precautions that include a rapid-sequence induction should be considered.

SPLENIC DISEASE

Anatomic and Physiologic Overview

The spleen is located in the left upper quadrant of the abdomen and is surrounded by the fundus of the stomach (medially), the splenic flexure of the colon (inferiorly), the left kidney and adrenal gland (posteriorly), and the diaphragm (superiorly). Attachment to these organs via suspensory ligaments, which are vascular except for the gastrosplenic ligament, provides protection and support of this organ.

The splenic artery arises from the celiac plexus. The splenic vein joins the superior mesenteric vein to contribute to portal venous blood flow. The parenchyma of the spleen is divided into three zones, which are surrounded by a 1- to 2-mm capsule.

These zones consist of (1) the red pulp, which consists of large, thin-walled, branching vessels, also known as the *splenic sinusoids*; (2) the white pulp, which consists of end-arterial branches of the central arteries and contains lymphocytes, plasma cells, and macrophages; and (3) the marginal zone, which is an ill-defined vascular space that connects the white pulp with the red pulp.

Total splenic blood flow is approximately 300 ml/min. The splenic artery divides into several branches within the splenorenal ligament before entering the splenic hilum, where they branch again into these trabeculae as they enter the splenic pulp. Small arteriolar branches leave the trabeculae, and their adventitial coat becomes replaced by a sheath of lymphatic tissue that accompanies the vessels and their branches until they divide into capillaries. It is these lymphatic sheaths that make up the white pulp of the spleen and that are interspersed along the arteriolar vessels as lymphatic follicles. The central arteries branch into vessels that enter the marginal zone and red pulp, ultimately collecting in the splenic sinusoid. From this juncture, blood flows via pulp veins, traverses the trabecular veins, and enters into the main splenic vein.

The spleen functions in several physiologic capacities, including hematopoiesis in the fetus, blood filtering, and immune processing of blood-borne foreign antigens. In filtering the blood the splenic sinusoids remove nuclear remnants and excess cell membrane found in immature erythrocytes. Abnormal blood cells, such as those found in sickle cell disease and spherocytosis, are filtered and removed by macrophages and other cells of the reticuloendothelial system. Aged red blood cells (older than 120 days) are removed by the same processes.

The spleen has an important role in specific and nonspecific immune responses. Macrophages and specialized histiocytes engulf and remove foreign cells, particularly those with a layer of affixed antibody. The production of specific antibody (immunoglobulin M [IgM]) is facilitated in the white pulp through the processing of foreign antigens.

The spleen has a minor role as a reservoir of platelets. This function, however, is important in only a few pathologic conditions. No significant reservoir function of red blood cells is performed by the spleen.[41]

Correction or amelioration of certain hematologic and immunologic disorders may be attempted through splenectomy. Despite its important and myriad functions, the spleen is not essential for life. Commonly accepted medical disease processes for which splenectomy is considered include idiopathic thrombocytopenic purpura, thrombotic thrombocytic purpura, Hodgkin's disease, lymphoma, certain leukemias, hereditary spherocytosis, hereditary hemolytic anemia, idiopathic autoimmune hemolytic anemia, and hypersplenism. Splenectomy may also be performed in treatment of thalassemia and sickle cell disease when these diseases are refractory to medical management and when hypersplenism supervenes. The development of primary (having no identifiable underlying cause) or secondary (having a known cause) hypersplenism may warrant splenectomy. Symptoms of hypersplenism include fatigue, malaise, recurrent infection, and easy or prolonged bleeding. These symptoms occur from a hyperfunctional spleen that removes and destroys normal blood cells. In portal hypertension, transmitted back pressure results in hypersplenism, which leads to congestive failure of splenic function. Treatment of the primary disease process usually provides relief of symptoms. Splenectomy, however, is often a necessary part of therapy; particularly with long-standing disorders.[57,58]

Splenic Trauma

Blunt or penetrating abdominal trauma may involve the richly vascular spleen, thereby necessitating splenectomy as part of resuscitative measures, such as control of hemorrhage. Any patient who has sustained blunt abdominal trauma and who has left upper quadrant pain should be suspected of having sustained splenic injury. Conservative, nonoperative treatment (with avoidance of splenectomy) may be elected in minor splenic injury. Splenectomy is generally avoided in children because of the greater importance of splenic function (i.e., immunologic function) in growth and development in patients of this age-group.[59]

In the presence of impending shock, emergency exploratory laparotomy is carried out to diagnose and treat all injuries to the abdominal viscera, including the spleen. Anesthetic management in these cases is directed by considerations given all unstable patients undergoing emergency laparotomy. A paramount consideration is the maintenance of physiologic hemoglobin and hematocrit levels as well as arterial blood pressure. Hemoglobin and hematocrit are decreased in the emergent setting not only by hemorrhagic diathesis, but also from dilution secondary to aggressive volume resuscitation with crystalloid solutions. These considerations assume an integral part in the decision to implement perioperative blood product transfusion.

Anesthetic Considerations in Elective Splenectomy

Elective splenectomy necessitates a thorough hematologic assessment in the patient's preoperative history. For example, precautions to prevent sickling crisis are an important part of the anesthetic plan in patients with sickle cell disease. Likewise, patients receiving bone marrow–suppressant drugs as in cases of malignancy may also exhibit derangements in physiologic levels of blood constituents.

Often these patients are in generally good health apart from the primary disease. The ability to transfuse blood products when indicated should be accommodated with the insertion of at least one large-bore intravenous line for this purpose. The extent of monitoring modalities is dictated by the patient's preexisting condition and anticipated perioperative course.

Patients who have been receiving chemotherapy for diseases such as Hodgkin's and non-Hodgkin's lymphoma, leukemia, or myeloid metaplasia may exhibit peripheral neuropathies (e.g., those associated with vincristine and cisplatin), hepatotoxicity (associated with methotrexate), and nephrotoxicity (associated with methotrexate and cisplatin). All derangements noted preoperatively must be noted and documented. Appropriate measures must also be implemented intraoperatively to prevent any further deterioration in preexisting function. These measures include careful patient positioning, administration of appropriate intravenous fluids, maintenance of adequate urine output, monitoring of hemoglobin and hematocrit levels, and avoidance of anesthetics and adjuvants that place an extra metabolic burden on the renal or hepatic system.

CARCINOID TUMORS AND CARCINOID SYNDROME

Carcinoid tumors consist of slow-growing malignancies composed of enterochromaffin cells usually found in the gastrointestinal tract. Approximately 75% are gastrointestinal and 22% are in the lung. They have also occurred in the pancreas, thymus, and liver. A high incidence of carcinoid tumor is found in the appendiceal region. Symptoms can therefore be confused with acute appendicitis. Carcinoid tumors have also been noted

TABLE 28-9 Secretory Products of Carcinoid Tumors

Amines	Tachykinins	Peptides	Other
5-HT	Kallikrein	Pancreatic polypetide (40%)	Prostaglandins
5-HIAA (88%)	Substance P (32%)	Chromogranins (100%)	
5-HTP	Neuropeptide K (67%)	Neurotensin (19%)	
Histamine		HCG_a	
Dopamine		Motilin (14%)	

HCG_a, *human chorionic gonadotropin.*

From Evers MB. Small intestine. In: Sabiston Textbook of Surgery: the Biological Basis of Modern Surgical Practice. *17th ed. Philadelphia: Saunders; 2004:1359.*

to occur in the bronchi and rarely from an ovarian site. Carcinoid tumors release vasoactive substances such as serotonin, bradykinin, histamine, tachykinins, kallikrein, adrenocorticotrophic hormone, prostaglandins, vasoactive peptide, and others (Table 28-9). These substances are capable of producing profound deleterious effects on cardiovascular homeostasis, although under normal circumstances the effects of the release of these substances are usually insignificant because of their hepatic metabolism. In the event that hepatic metastatic disease or processes cause impairment in liver function, the ability of the liver to clear these substances may be compromised and overwhelmed. This results in manifestations of the carcinoid syndrome (Box 28-3). Approximately 5% to 10% of patients with carcinoid tumors develop carcinoid syndrome.[60]

Vasoactive peptides released from carcinoid tumors located in the bronchi and ovaries exert a faster effect because of their direct drainage into the portal vein. Carcinoid tumors are also functionally autonomous. Two factors that enhance release of carcinoid hormones are direct physical manipulation of the tumor and β-adrenergic stimulation.[61] Secretory products of carcinoid tumors are listed in Table 28-9.

BOX 28-3

Signs and Symptoms of Carcinoid Syndrome

- Episodic cutaneous flushing (kinins, histamine)
- Diarrhea (serotonin, prostaglandins E and F)
- Heart Disease
  - Tricuspid regurgitation, pulmonic stenosis
  - Supraventricular tachydysrhythmias (serotonin)
- Bronchoconstriction (serotonin, bradykinin, substance P)
- Hypotension (kinins, histamine)
- Hypertension (serotonin)
- Abdominal pain (small bowel obstruction)
- Hepatomegaly (metastases)
- Hyperglycemia
- Hypoalbuminemia (pellagra-like skin lesions resulting from niacin deficiency)

Modified from Stoelting RK, Dierdorf SF. Diseases of the gastrointestinal system. In: Anesthesia and Co-Existing Disease. *4th ed. New York: Churchill Livingstone; 2002:333.*

Bronchospasm occurs in response to carcinoid hormonal activity on histamine receptors. Patients with carcinoid tumors are also known to be at greater risk for the development of supraventricular tachydysrhythmias and atrial ectopy. Distortion of the cusps of the tricuspid valve or pulmonic valve results in failure in valvular function, with development of deleterious sequelae, such as valvular regurgitation. Flushing, diarrhea, and edema may be in evidence, as well as hypotension and decreased cardiac output. These signs and symptoms are caused by the exaggerated level of bradykinin activity. Abdominal pain and diarrhea are indicative of increased serotonin levels. Serotonin mimics epinephrine in its role in stimulating glycogenolysis and gluconeogenesis, thereby resulting in hyperglycemia. Clinical hypoalbuminemia may be present as a result of the diversion of tryptophan from protein synthesis to serotonin production.[3]

Patients with carcinoid syndrome may undergo primary resection of the carcinoid tumor. Examples of other procedures that these patients often undergo include cardiac valve replacement and hepatic resection (e.g., lobectomy) for excision of metastases.

Particular discretion should be exercised in the use of drugs requiring significant hepatic biotransformation and elimination, particularly for patients with hepatic neoplasia or metastases who exhibit signs of carcinoid syndrome. Consideration is also given to patients with tumors in areas that drain into the portal circulation (e.g., the mesentery and spleen).

Many anesthetic techniques have been used successfully in the treatment of patients with carcinoid syndrome. Preoperative preparation of the patient requires correction of deficiencies in circulating volume and electrolyte levels. Use of histamine-releasing agents, such as morphine, thiopental, atracurium, and mivacurium, should be avoided. Fasciculations may induce release of carcinoid hormones and are therefore prevented by avoidance of succinylcholine, although it has been used successfully many times, especially for rapid sequence induction.

Etomidate may be used for induction, but thiopental should be avoided because of associated histamine release. Propofol in both bolus and infusion doses has also been frequently used. Because it may produce hypotension, judicious use is advised. Vecuronium and *cis*-atracurium may be safely used for neuromuscular blockade. Rocuronium is an attractive alternative when rapid onset is desired.

Vecuronium, *cis*-atracurium, and rocuronium are virtually devoid of activity that invokes histamine release or hemodynamic changes. The piperidine-derivative opioids fentanyl, sufentanil, alfentanil, and remifentanil are suitable for use because of their lack of histamine-releasing properties and their innocuous effect on hemodynamics. Isoflurane, desflurane, and sevoflurane may all be safely used. No one anticholinesterase neuromuscular relaxant reversal agent is thought to have advantage over any other. However, glycopyrrolate, used as an adjunct to attenuate vagolysis, may be more desirable than atropine if a significantly increased heart rate is to be avoided. Ketamine activates the sympathetic nervous system, and catecholamine release may activate the kallikreins and other vasoactive substances and therefore should be avoided. The desire to avoid the use of sympathomimetics such as ephedrine to treat hypotension makes the use of regional anesthesia controversial. Epidural anesthesia, cautiously administered, may be a reasonable technique for lower extremity and abdominal procedures. Severe and possibly refractory hypotension resulting from sympathectomy makes spinal anesthesia relatively contraindicated for use in carcinoid patients.

Octreotide, a somatostatin analogue, is used to blunt the vasoactive and bronchoconstrictive effects of carcinoid tumor products. Octreotide mimics the inhibitory action of somatostatin on the release of several gastrointestinal hormones, as well as those derived from carcinoid tumors. Treatment for 2 weeks preoperatively with a dose of 100 mcg subcutaneously three times a day is standard. If prior therapy was not used a dose of 50 to 150 mcg subcutaneously is given preoperatively. Intraoperative infusion may be continued at 100 mcg/hr. Bolus doses of 100 to 200 mcg given intravenously may be used for intraoperative carcinoid crises.

Aprotinin, an inhibitor of kallikrein, has been reported to be effective in reversal of carcinoid-induced bronchospasm and hypotension. Used in conjunction with octreotide and methylprednisolone, aprotinin (2,000,000 kallikrein inactivation units [kIU] bolus; 50,000 kIU/hr infusion) has been reported to be effective prophylaxis for hypotension in a carcinoid patient undergoing cardiac surgery.[62]

Hypotension should be treated with an α-adrenergic agonist (e.g., phenylephrine infusion) in order to avoid hormone release by β-adrenergic stimulation. Bronchospasm resulting from histamine or bradykinin release has been shown to be resistant to ketamine and inhalation anesthetics. Low-dose β_2-agonists are effective in bronchodilation and have relatively little influence on carcinoid hormone release. In the presence of high levels of serotonin in carcinoid syndrome, adjustments in anesthetic selection and dosage must be considered if further compromise of cardiovascular function is to be prevented.[63,64] Anesthetic management is reviewed in Box 28-4.

BOX **28-4**

Anesthetic Considerations in Carcinoid Syndrome

- The most common clinical signs are flushing, wheezing, blood pressure and heart rate changes, and diarrhea.
- Preoperative assessment should include complete blood count, measurement of electrolytes, liver function tests, measurement of blood glucose, electrocardiogram (echocardiogram if indicated), and determination of urine 5-HIAA levels.
- Optimize fluid and electrolyte status and pretreat with octreotide as noted. Continue octreotide throughout the postoperative period. Interferon-α has shown success in controlling some symptoms.
- Both histamine-1 and histamine-2 receptor blockers must be used to fully counteract histamine effects.
- Avoid histamine-releasing agents such as morphine, thiopental, atracurium, and mivacurium. Avoid sympathomimetic agents such as ketamine and ephedrine.
- Treat hypotension with an α-receptor agonist such as phenylephrine.
- General anesthesia is preferred over regional anesthesia. Patients with high serotonin levels may exhibit prolonged recovery; therefore desflurane and sevoflurane, which have rapid recovery profiles, may be beneficial.
- Aggressively maintain normothermia to avoid catecholamine-induced vasoactive mediator release.
- Monitor intraoperative plasma glucose, as these patients are prone to hyperglycemia. Treat with insulin as is customary.

HIAA, *5-hydroxy-indoleacetic acid.*
Modified from Vaughan DJ, Brunner MD. Anesthesia for patients with carcinoid syndrome. Int Anesthesiol Clin. *1997;35:129-142.*

TRANSPLANTATION

Liver Transplantation

Orthotropic liver transplantation (OLT) has emerged as a definitive treatment option for patients with end-stage hepatic disease. This is largely attributable to advances in surgical technique, immunosuppressive therapy, and donor organ procurement. Other contributing factors that have greatly attenuated the previously formidable morbidity and mortality associated with this procedure include advances made in technologic and perioperative management.

Patients with end-stage hepatic disease who experience progressive life-threatening complications that become increasingly refractory to medical intervention are the usual candidates for OLT.[65] Transplantation may also be considered a therapeutic option in patients with certain viral infections who respond poorly to medical management and who are nevertheless deemed physiologically salvageable. In the adult population postnecrotic (nonalcoholic) cirrhosis constitutes the most common indication for OLT, followed by (in decreasing occurrence) primary biliary cirrhosis, sclerosing cholangitis, and primary hepatic neoplasia. In the pediatric population the most common indicator for OLT is biliary atresia, followed by various inborn errors of metabolism (Wilson's disease, Crigler-Najjar syndrome, 1-antitrypsin deficiency) and postnecrotic cirrhosis. Transplantation in patients with a history of alcoholic cirrhosis is performed but is a matter of considerable ethical debate. Current recommendation is to have the patient refrain from alcohol consumption for at least 6 months before surgery. Recidivism to active alcoholism after transplantation is the major stimulating factor in the ongoing controversy; although studies have shown that only 7% of those who refrain from alcohol for 6 months return to active alcoholism.[66]

The refinement of immunosuppressant therapy has been instrumental in the increasingly impressive survival rates in patients undergoing OLT. Key to this has been the use of cyclosporine, which interferes with helper T-cell activity and inhibits interleukin (IL)-2 and other proinflammatory cytokines. Cyclosporine is often used concurrently with azathioprine and corticosteroids. Anti-OKT3, a monoclonal antibody directed toward lymphocytes, has also shown efficacy in prevention of acute rejection, particularly if it is steroid refractory. Tacrolimus (FK-506) has demonstrated efficacy as an alternative to cyclosporine.[67,68] Technical refinements in the procedure resulting from experience and research, as well as development of more precise support modalities (e.g., venovenous bypass and rapid infusion technology), have also contributed to an overall improved outcome in patients undergoing OLT.

Anesthesia-related concerns for patients undergoing OLT are consistent with those related to patients undergoing major surgery with severe cirrhosis. The multisystem effects of cirrhosis are underscored. Profound hemodynamic derangements may be preexistent and are likely to be exacerbated secondary to the numerous stressors imposed during particular phases of the procedure. These include hemodynamic consequences resulting from clamping and unclamping of the portal vein and vena cava as well as alterations in metabolism. Hyperkalemia and venous air embolism may be encountered with perfusion of the emplaced graft.

Frequently, optimal preoperative preparation of the patient is not possible. Priorities are therefore established and adhered to. Patients with severe cirrhosis are typically coagulopathic to a variable extent (deficient in coagulation factors and thrombocytopenic). Massive blood loss should be anticipated. Red blood cells, FFP, platelets, and cryoprecipitate should be readily available. Blood-salvaging technology should also be employed. Infusion of antifibrinolytics such as aprotinin and ϵ-aminocaproic acid may also be useful perioperatively in efforts to control hemorrhagic diatheses.

Invasive monitoring modalities are mandatory for OLT. These include intraarterial pressure monitoring and central venous or pulmonary artery catheterization. Owing to the profound fluid shifts and blood loss encountered in these procedures, direct measurement of central filling pressures assumes paramount importance for guiding volume and blood product replacement. Large bore (14- to 16-gauge) intravenous catheters and possibly an antecubital 8.5 F catheter may also be employed for administration of volume, which may be performed via a rapid infusion device. All administered fluids should be warmed to prevent hypothermia and its attendant affects on coagulation and metabolic processes. Other measures to maintain normothermia include forced-air surface warming and possibly increased ambient room temperature. All airway gases should be humidified. Urinary output, as measured via indwelling urinary catheter, should be maintained at a minimum of 0.5 ml/kg/hr.

Serial laboratory measurements are performed throughout surgery. These include measurements of arterial blood gases, electrolytes, and hemoglobin and hematocrit levels and metabolic studies assessing ionized calcium and serum glucose. Coagulation parameters are also closely assessed via activated PTT, PT, fibrinogen, and platelet count. Another useful monitoring modality for assessment of overall clotting capability, fibrinolysis, and platelet quality is thromboelastography (TEG).[69] Changes in commonly monitored parameters are shown in Table 28-10.

TABLE 28-10 Relative Changes in Various Parameters during Liver Transplantation

Variable	Preanhepatic	Anhepatic	Neohepatic
Glucose	+	−/+	+ +
Hemoglobin	−/− −	−	−/− −
Platelets	−	−	−
Urine output	+ +	− −	+/+ +
Cardiac index	+ +	+	+ + +
Systemic vascular resistance	− −	+ +	− − −
Peripheral vascular resistance	+	− −	+
Mean arterial blood pressure	−	− −	− − −/− followed by +
Lactate	+	+	+/+ +
K	+	+	+ + + followed by +
Ca	−	− −	−
Mg	−	− −	−
Na	+	+	+
Temperature	−	− − −	+

From Amand MS, Al-Sofayan M, Ghent C, et al. Liver transplant. In: Sharpe MD, Gelb AW. Anesthesia and Transplantation. *Boston: Butterworth-Heinemann; 1999:190.*

No single anesthetic technique is indicated for OLT. Patients undergoing OLT are considered at marked risk for aspiration of stomach contents because of the likelihood of abdominal distention or history of upper gastrointestinal bleeding. General anesthesia is therefore induced via rapid sequence technique with cricoid pressure. Premedication may be administered but may be curtailed in the presence of marked encephalopathy. Sodium thiopental, ketamine, propofol, and etomidate are all suitable hypnotic agents, but the requisite doses may be modified based on the patient's preexisting mental and hemodynamic status. Succinylcholine is used for rapid onset of neuromuscular blockade; however, rocuronium may also be employed if no difficulty with intubation is anticipated. Maintenance of anesthesia is accomplished through the use of a volatile agent (e.g., isoflurane) and an intravenous opioid (usually sufentanil or fentanyl) by bolus administration or infusion. Patients with severe encephalopathy may have increased intracranial pressure, therefore requiring hyperventilation. The minimum alveolar concentration of volatile agent should also be reduced in these patients. The use of nitrous oxide is limited or avoided because of concerns pertaining to its capability to expand air bubbles that may reside in the nonperfused donor liver. Bowel distention is also a consideration with prolonged usage. Choice of neuromuscular relaxant is a relatively minor issue and is subject to individual preference. Patients undergoing OLT typically remain intubated and mechanically ventilated in the intensive care unit postoperatively. Typical drugs used during liver transplant procedures are listed in Table 28-11.

Intraoperative anesthetic management is strongly influenced by the various hemodynamic manifestations presented during the three major phases of the procedure. During the preanhepatic (dissection) phase, a wide subcostal incision is used to provide optimal surgical exposure. Prior abdominal surgeries may have resulted in adhesion formation, thereby potentially increasing blood loss. The liver is still attached to the portal vein, inferior vena cava, biliary tract, and hepatic artery. During the anhepatic phase the vena cava is clamped above and below the liver. The portal vein, common bile duct, and hepatic artery are also ligated. Total excision is then undertaken. Venovenous bypass is generally reserved for patients with pulmonary hypertension or significant cardiovascular disease. Removal of the liver may result in hypocalcemia because of loss of the liver's role in the metabolic removal of citrate from blood products that may have been administered. Hypocalcemia may also result in cardiac depression. Ionized calcium levels should be regularly assessed and should guide exogenous replacement (200 to 500 mg). Loss of hepatic clearance of acid metabolites from the gastrointestinal tract results in progressive acidosis. Sodium bicarbonate is administered judiciously to prevent hypernatremia, hyperosmolality, and metabolic alkalosis. Should large amounts of sodium bicarbonate be needed, tromethamine should be considered as an alternative. Hyperglycemia may be encountered more commonly than hypoglycemia because of the large glucose load presented from large amounts of transfused blood products. In general, dextrose-containing intravenous fluids are avoided. Air emboli may result from air entrapped in venous sinusoids and released when the donor liver is reperfused. The incidence of air embolism is reduced by infusing cold crystalloid solution (e.g., Normosol, Plasma-Lyte) through the venous structures as the raft is being anastomosed. After the portal and suprahepatic caval anastomoses but before infrahepatic caval anastomosis is completed, the liver

TABLE 28-11 Drugs Typically Used during a Liver Transplantation

Drug	Induction	Preanhepatic	Anhepatic	Posthepatic
Aprotinin	2 million KIU	150,000 KIU/hr	150,000 KIU/hr	140,000 KIU/hr
Vasopressin	—	0.5 mcg/kg/hr	0	0
Fentanyl	4-6 mcg/kg	4-6 mcg/kg	—	4-6 mcg/kg
Midazolam	10-40 mcg/kg	0-1 mg	0-1 mg	0-1 mg
Thiopental	4-6 mg/kg	—	—	—
Furosemide	—	10-20 mg	—	—
Mannitol 20%	—	1-1.5 g/kg	—	—
Methylprednisolone	—	—	500 mg	—
Magnesium	—	2-4 g	—	—
Calcium chloride	—	2-4 g	1 g	—
Sodium bicarbonate	—	—	0-100 mEq	—
Protamine	—	—	—	0.50 mg
Phenylephrine boluses	—	—	80 mcg/bolus	80 mcg/bolus
Dopamine (renal)	—	0-2.5 mcg/kg/min	0-2.5 mcg/kg/min	0-2.5 mcg/kg/min
Dopamine vasopressor	—	2.5-10 mcg/kg/min	2.5-10 mcg/kg/min	2.5-10 mcg/kg/min

KIU, *kallikrein inactivation units.*
From Amand MS, Al-Sofayan M, Ghent C, et al. Liver transplant. In: Sharpe MD, Gelb AW. Anesthesia and Transplantation. *Boston: Butterworth-Heinemann; 1999:188.*

is flushed by portal blood through the incomplete infrahepatic anastomosis.

Caval clamping is associated with profound hemodynamic changes, particularly decreased cardiac output and hypotension. Renal perfusion may be adversely affected as well. Increased venous back pressure may also increase bleeding as well as impair splanchnic perfusion. The technique of venovenous bypass consists of cannulation of the inferior vena cava and portal vein and an axillary vein with the intention of diverting blood away from the liver and delivering it directly to the heart. Venovenous bypass is employed to minimize hypotension, maintain renal and splanchnic perfusion, and prevent gut edema and ischemia. Heparinization is not necessary because of circuit design technology. Venovenous bypass is associated with an element of risk, however. Venovenous bypass may lengthen operative time as well as subject the patient to increased risk of air embolic and thromboembolic events. Brachial plexus injury and hypothermia are also recognized side effects. Cannulation of the internal jugular vein rather than the axillary vein as a return circuit has also been employed and has been shown to attenuate a number of the side effects of venovenous bypass. Percutaneous methods for establishment of venous bypass have also been described. Prophylactic measures for preservation of renal perfusion include the use of mannitol and low-dose dopamine infusion (2 to 3 mcg/kg/min). Other agents that show promise in the promotion of renal protection include the dopaminergic receptor agonist (DA1 and DA2 with β_2-receptor agonist) dopexamine.[70] Another agent, commercially available, is the DA1 receptor agonist fenoldopam.[71] The lack of DA1, α-adrenergic, and β-adrenergic activity seen with the use of this agent makes it particularly attractive. Ultimately, renal perfusion as well as overall systemic organ perfusion is best accomplished through optimization of cardiac output and systemic blood pressure. For this, any of a number of vasoactive and inotropic agents should be available and used as needed.

The consequent hypocalcemia and myocardial depression associated with removal of the liver is managed with the periodic administration of calcium chloride (200 to 500 mg), which is guided by assessment of serum ionized calcium concentration. Hyperkalemia may be a consequence of the progressive acidosis frequently encountered during the anhepatic stage. Symptomatic hyperkalemia may lead to cardiac dysrhythmias and refractory asystole. Treatment consists of the administration of calcium chloride, sodium bicarbonate, and glucose and insulin and the application of hyperventilation. Attenuation of the magnitude of hyperkalemia is assisted through maintenance of an adequate diuresis throughout surgery.

Fluid management presents a formidable perioperative challenge because of its unpredictability and variability. This is influenced in large part by the extent and magnitude of portal hypertension, the challenges in dissection, and the coagulation status. Ongoing goals are to maintain normovolemia, sustain organ system perfusion, and optimize oxygen-carrying capacity. Selection of crystalloid is based on these goals as well as that of preservation of electrolyte and acid-base balance. Lactated Ringer's solution may increase serum lactate levels and contribute to hyperkalemia. Normal saline may impose a hyperchloremic metabolic acidosis. Isotonic solutions with greater compatibility to normal osmolality are therefore preferred. Rapid-transfusion devices that allow the infusion of large volumes of warmed fluids and blood products should be used. Correction of acidosis may be accomplished through optimization of systemic perfusion, hyperventilation, and sodium bicarbonate. Excessive sodium bicarbonate may result in hyperosmolality, hypernatremia, central pontine myelinolysis, and metabolic acidosis. Before reperfusion of the grafted donor liver, correction of electrolyte and acid-base abnormalities should be undertaken. Central filling pressures should also be allowed to increase, and hyperventilation should be instituted. Preparation for rapid infusion of warmed blood products (e.g., salvaged blood and packed red blood cells) as well as for administration of indicated inotropic and vasoactive agents allows prompt retrieval of hemodynamic parameters secondary to reperfusion hypotension. During the postanhepatic (revascularization-biliary reconstruction) phase the venous anastomoses are completed, and circulation to the new liver is accomplished via the anastomosed hepatic artery. A Roux-en-Y choledochojejunostomy connects the bile duct to the recipient gastrointestinal tract. The reperfusion phenomenon can result in acidosis, hypotension, and electrolyte abnormalities; particularly hyperkalemia.[69]

Electrocardiographic aberrations may be noted; typically bradycardia. Management is largely supportive and consists of volume restoration by colloid or crystalloid (as directed by laboratory findings, central filling pressures and urinary output), calcium chloride, and sodium bicarbonate. Inotropic and vasoactive support may be indicated. This may entail a polypharmacologic approach because of the recipient's possible attenuated response to vasoactive agents. For optimization of the activity of these agents, existing acidosis must be corrected. A postperfusion coagulopathy is commonly encountered after reperfusion. This may be attributable to the release of sequestered heparin in the donor liver, which is administered during retrieval or by activity of an endogenous heparinoid. Hyperfibrinolysis is frequently encountered and is attributable to increased release of tissue plasminogen activator inhibitor during the anhepatic phase. The use of TEG furnishes a method for accurate detection of fibrinolysis and abnormalities in platelet activity and is valuable, in addition to laboratory findings, in direction of blood and blood component resuscitation. Platelets should be available as well as FFP. Cryoprecipitate may also be used for restoration of an adequate fibrinogen level in the presence of fibrinolysis. Desmopressin (DDAVP) may be administered to help improve platelet function. Overtransfusion with blood components and crystalloid should be avoided in order to prevent pulmonary edema, decreased oxygenation, peripheral edema, and prolonged intubation and ventilation and their attendant risks (e.g., pneumonia). Some common intraoperative complications and their management are noted in Table 28-12.

TABLE 28-12 Intraoperative Complications and Management

Complication	Management
Hypothermia	Use heat exchanger, fluid warmer, warming blanket, forced-air units, postoperative ventilation, warm blood flush
Hyperkalemia	Administer binding resins; perform diuresis, dialysis, hyperventilation; administer sodium bicarbonate, calcium chloride, insulin, or glucose
Hypocalcemia	Administer calcium chloride or gluconate by central line
Oliguria	Maintain adequate volume; increase renal perfusion pressure; administer mannitol, furosemide, and ethacrynic acid; avoid vasopressor use
Hypotension	Maintain adequate volume; check calcium and magnesium; rule out cardiac dysfunction; administer vasopressors; transfuse blood products if anemia or coagulopathy is present
Hypertension	Maintain adequate anesthetic depth; reduce filling pressures; avoid long-acting agents that are used to treat hypertension
Postreperfusion syndrome	Anticipate; ensure that volume loading is not excessive; administer calcium, vasopressors

From Amand MS, Al-Sofayan M, Ghent C, et al. Liver transplant. In: Sharpe MD, Gelb AW. Anesthesia and Transplantation. *Boston: Butterworth-Heinemann; 1999:191.*

Postoperative problems may include persistent hemorrhage, volume overload, metabolic and electrolyte abnormalities (e.g., hyperglycemia, hyperkalemia, metabolic alkalosis), and infection. Neurologic complications include encephalopathy, seizures, cyclosporine neurotoxicity, and cerebrovascular hemorrhage. Surgical complications that may require return to the operating room for correction include anastomotic leak or strictureof the biliary reconstruction or dehiscence or thrombosis of the hepatic or portal vessels. Prophylactic antibacterial and antifungal agents are administered in addition to the immunosuppressive agents. The incidence of infection is high. The locus of infection may be an intraabdominal source, an indwelling catheter, the surgical wound, the urinary tract, or an intrapulmonary source. Numerous infective entities may be causative. Commonly encountered are fungi (e.g., *Candida* and *Aspergillus* species), gram-negative bacteria, viruses (e.g., cytomegalovirus), and parasites (e.g., *Pneumocystis*). Postoperative hepatitis may be caused by herpesvirus, Epstein-Barr virus, cytomegalovirus, andenovirus, or hepatitis B or C virus. Reactivation of a preexisting viral infection is also a causative possibility. The possibility of rejection is closely monitored and is differentially determined by live biopsy. The most common period in which rejection occurs is during weeks 1 to 6 after transplant. Laboratory findings usually reflect a prodromal period before this occurs.

Considerations in addition to those for patients with hepatic failure apply to patients who undergo retransplantation. These patients are immunosuppressed and are sensitized to antibodies, which makes type-matching and cross-matching more complex. These patients may have acquired a variable degree of renal insufficiency and hypertension secondary to cyclosporine toxicity. Patients who undero retransplantation are also considered steroid dependent and require steroid supplementation before surgery (e.g., methylprednisolone, 500 mg). Aseptic technique is mandatory and must be strictly adhered to.

Pancreatic Transplantation

Pancreatic transplantation is increasingly becoming an efficacious option in patients with insulin-dependent diabetes mellitus refractory to medical management. One-year graft and patient survival rates are currently 70% and 91%, respectively. The most common procedures include simultaneous pancreas and kidney transplant for uremic patients, pancreas after kidney transplant for immunocompromised patients (e.g., secondary to antirejection therapy), and pancreas transplantation alone for nonuremic patients.[72]

Preoperative screening is meticulous and thorough. One of the numerous laboratory-screening procedures is measurement of basal and stimulated C peptide. C peptide is the portion of the precursor insulin molecule used in production of circulating insulin. Functional pancreatic beta cells secrete C peptide in conjunction with insulin. The absence of C peptide serves as a strong marker for loss of endogenous insulin production and confirms absolute insulin deficiency (i.e., type 1 diabetes). Other assessment measures include evaluation of the magnitude of other secondary diabetic complications and, most prominently, determination of the presence of ischemic cardiac disease and renal insufficiency. Ischemic cardiac disease is common in diabetic patients who are considered candidates for pancreatic transplantation. The presence of silent coronary disease should be considered, particularly in candidates with preexisting peripheral neuropathy and uremia. Cardiac disease, the chief cause of morbidity and mortality in patients with end-stage renal disease, may often not be detected by means of ECG or the standard preoperative history and physical examination. Other complications of type 1 diabetes detected during the preoperative assessment that require strong consideration of modification of the anesthetic plan include peripheral vascular disease, ketoacidosis, chronic hypertension, chronic hyperglycemia, gastroparesis, and retinopathy. The reader is referred to Chapter 31 for greater detail with regard to specific anesthetic and perioperative considerations for patients with secondary complications from type 1 diabetes mellitus.

Airway evaluation should be given special priority. Diabetic patients may pose a particular challenge with regard to intubation. The exact cause of increased difficulty in intubation of diabetic patients is not known. Contributing factors, however, may be contractures and general joint stiffness known to occur in diabetic patients. Joint stiffness involves the joints of the patient's head and neck, particularly those joints of the atlantooccipital axis. Neuropathy, both autonomic and systemic, is common in pancreatic transplant recipients and places affected patients at risk for wide swings in hemodynamic lability perioperatively. Denervation hypersensitivity of cardiac acetylcholine receptors may develop in diabetic patients and may place them at risk for severe refractory bradycardia—a strong consideration when anticholinesterase reversal agents are used. Autonomic neuropathy may also affect patients' response to hypoxia, thereby placing them at risk for pulmonary embarrassment. This could be of particular concern in the postoperative setting. Vagal neuropathy promotes gastroparesis, which places the patient at risk for aspiration of gastric contents. Motor and sensory neuropathy resulting from diabetes or uremia increases the risk of hyperkalemia subsequent to succinylcholine administration. Risk of postoperative neuropraxias must also be considered when preexisting deficits have been documented preoperatively. In order for the magnitude of autonomic dysfunction to be determined, the preoperative history should include history of nausea, diarrhea and bloating (indicative of intestinal involvement), hypotension on initiation of dialysis, esophageal dysfunction, and dizziness with position change. Orthostatic blood pressures and heart rate change also must be noted.[73]

Metabolic status by laboratory assay is also necessary preoperatively. Laboratory studies include baseline blood glucose, electrolytes, blood urea nitrogen, and creatinine and may include a liver function panel (i.e., bilirubin and transaminases). Hematologic and coagulation studies as well as a type and screen should also be included. If severe hyperglycemia (blood glucose >500 mg/dl) is present, the blood and urine should be analyzed for the presence of ketones, and an arterial blood gas evaluation should be performed in order to determine whether ketoacidosis is present. Surgery may be delayed in order for the patient's metabolic status to be stabilized. With the high incidence of renal insufficiency in pancreatic transplant patients, many of these patients will be receiving hemodialysis. It is important to determine when dialysis was last performed. The presence of hyperkalemia (serum potassium >5.5 mmol/L) should be assessed and appropriate corrective measures undertaken, such as administration of insulin (in the presence of hyperglycemia), with ion exchange resins (e.g., kayexalate) or with dialysis.

Pancreatic transplantation, particularly when associated with renal transplantation, is a lengthy procedure. General anesthesia is administered in a standard manner with modifications in agent selection and administration consistent with planned preservation of the patient's hemodynamic status. Agents with a minimal direct depressant effect on cardiac function (e.g., etomidate, opioids) and with minimal organ dependence on renal metabolism and elimination (e.g., *cis*-atracurium, vecuronium) should be selected. Maintenance of general anesthesia is accomplished with volatile agents (e.g., isoflurane, sevoflurane, desflurane), low-dose opioids, and muscle relaxants. Aspiration precautions during induction and intubation should be in effect. Adjunctive airway devices should be readily available in the event of an anticipated or unanticipated difficult airway. Standard monitoring intraoperatively may be supplemented by the use of an arterial catheter for rapid detection of blood pressure changes and for laboratory sampling. A central venous catheter is also useful for administering immunosuppressive drugs, for inotropic support, and for assessment of central filling pressures.

Metabolic monitoring intraoperatively consists of regular measurement of serum glucose. Hyperglycemia is often encountered intraoperatively secondary to the metabolic stress response as well as from the hyperglycemic effect of administered corticosteroids or cyclosporine. Glucose determinations should be performed every half-hour after allograft anastomosis is completed and reperfusion established. This is mandatory not only for optimization of the glucose level but also for determination of the level of function of the islet cells. Along with periodic monitoring of serum electrolytes and hemoglobin, periodic blood gas analysis is also recommended because of the common occurrence of metabolic acidosis in pancreatic transplant patients. This not only occurs as a result of systemic hypoperfusion but also may also be attributed to ketosis or renal insufficiency. Many patients with renal failure live with a compensated metabolic acidosis such that a mild acidosis may be tolerable and treatable with increased ventilation. Significant acidosis may require intravenous administration of sodium bicarbonate.[74]

It is imperative that hemodynamic status be optimized both before anastomosis of the allograft and after reperfusion has been established. A significant incidence of graft thrombosis and subsequent failure is attributed to hypotension. Vascular expansion must be directed judiciously, particularly in patients known to have cardiac insufficiency. In these patients the use of a pulmonary artery catheter may be necessary to guide volume administration. Overzealous vascular expansion, particularly with crystalloid, may result in allograft edema, which may also result in vascular insufficiency, thrombosis, and failure. Prevention of graft edema and thrombosis may be accomplished by emphasizing colloid (including packed red blood cells for a hemoglobin less than 10 g/dl) rather than crystalloid transfusion and by administering sodium mannitol (25 g) before reperfusion. All patients receive antibiotics, usually broad spectrum. Low-dose heparin is usually administered at the discretion of the surgeon before the clamping of major vessels. Cyclosporine is most commonly started after surgery. Immunosuppression is often initiated intraoperatively with the use of agents such as tacrolimus (FK506), OKT3, azathioprine, prostaglandin E1 (PGE_1) and methylprednisolone. Hypotension and pulmonary edema are potential complications with the use of the immunosuppressant OKT3.[75]

Postoperative extubation is accomplished only after reversal of neuromuscular blockade when the patient is hemodynamically stable and demonstrates control of airway reflexes. Monitoring of laboratory parameters (serum glucose, electrolytes, arterial blood gases, and hemoglobin) continues throughout the postanesthesia period. Infusions initiated intraoperatively, (such as insulin for serum glucose management, supplemental dextrose, and vasoactive medications) should be adjusted as needed in accordance with metabolic and hemodynamic findings. Supplemental bicarbonate may be necessary for correction of acidosis secondary to losses of bicarbonate from pancreatic secretions into the urine and bladder. Pancreatic rejection is assessed via determinations of serum glucose and urinary amylase levels. Abdominal pain and distention serve as indicators of possible acute rejection syndrome, as well as other indicators such as hemodynamic compromise and signs and symptoms consistent with sepsis (e.g., fever and refractory hyperglycemia and ketosis). Under these circumstances graft pancreatectomy is indicated, as is graft nephrectomy if necessary.[76]

Small Bowel Transplantation

Currently, small bowel transplantation (SBT) is performed at a limited number of centers. This procedure is still considered experimental. SBT may be considered an alternative therapy for select individuals with no prognosis for independence from total parenteral nutrition (TPN). The high morbidity and mortality associated with long-term TPN (e.g., because of infections, vascular occlusions, hepatobiliary dysfunction) may serve to make SBT an attractive option.[77]

Conditions that warrant chronic TPN are frequently those associated with short-gut syndrome (SGS). The causes of SGS differ to an extent between adults and children. In children SGS may result from necrotizing enterolysis, intestinal atresia, midgut volvulus, gastroschisis, and Hirschsprung's disease. Crohn's disease eventually also may cause SGS in older children. Other syndromes associated with promotion of SGS in children include Gardner's syndrome with associated desmoid retroperitoneal tumors (causing abdominal vascular compression) and amilial microvillous inclusion disease.

In adults Crohn's disease and conditions that result in vascular occlusive disease in the gut, particularly of the superior mesenteric artery, are common causative factors in the development of SGS. In children and adults a primary cause of SGS is surgical resection of the small bowel. Depending on the magnitude of affiliation of the disease process on the small bowel, resection varies in terms of extent of resection and the episodes in which it is necessarily undertaken. Complications of SGS are basically the result of malabsorption and maldigestive syndrome resulting from loss of absorptive surface area. These syndromes may eventually result not only in malnutrition but also in metabolic bone disease, electrolyte derangements, bile salt deficiency, anemia, biliary lithiasis, and nephrolithiasis.

Preoperative assessment must take numerous issues into consideration. These include the degree of debilitation of the patient, which factors prominently in determination of the function and compensation of other organ systems (e.g., cardiopulmonary, renal, hematologic). Hepatobiliary function also requires careful assessment, particularly if the patient has been receiving long-term TPN. A combined liver transplant and SBT may be undertaken in patients with significant hepatic dysfunction. Adequate vascular access must be established. This may require central venous access because of obliteration of peripheral veins secondary to previous access attempts. Routine monitors are employed, with consideration given to more aggressive hemodynamic monitoring (e.g., arterial, central venous, pulmonary arterial) if deemed appropriate. General anesthesia is used, with agent selection (e.g., muscle relaxants) taking into consideration the deficiencies assessed in the function of organ systems necessary for a particular drug's metabolism and elimination. A rapid sequence induction is indicated.

Intraoperatively, central filling pressures are carefully monitored to facilitate maintenance of renal perfusion and hemodynamic stability. A balanced anesthetic technique is used, involving a volatile agent of low solubility and an opioid. Nitrous oxide may be avoided because of the long duration of the procedure and associated potential for bowel distention. Episodes of hemodynamic liability may be seen intraoperatively because of caval clamping during anastomosis and at the time of reperfusion of the graft after anastomosis. These periods may closely mimic those seen during resection of an abdominal aortic aneurysm and should be anticipated. Good communication among members of the anesthesia and surgical teams is requisite. Careful monitoring of electrolyte, hematologic, and metabolic (i.e., glucose) status should be performed. Blood loss may not be as great as that seen during liver transplantation but could be significant if there have been previous laparotomies with resultant significant peritoneal adhesion formation. Consideration should also be given to the patient's serum albumin status, which can have consequences that affect not only intravascular volume status but also the amount of available unbound circulating administered drugs. Optimization of intravascular volume status and central filling pressures is accomplished with the use of crystalloid (e.g., lactated Ringer's solution), albumin (especially in the presence of low serum albumin), and pentastarch (e.g., Hespan, Hextend).[78]

Immunosuppression is usually initiated intraoperatively with OKT3 IV. A continuous infusion of PGE_1 is usually started at the time of reperfusion. PGE_1 is a potent vasodilator and is employed to enhance graft perfusion. Renal protection from the toxic effects of immunosuppressants is also alleged to occur with the use of PGE_1. Measures to prevent hypothermia are also of paramount importance. The major consequences of graft reperfusion on cardiac function are dysrhythmias and asystole, which result from acute hyperkalemia and hypothermia. Ionized serum calcium should be monitored and corrected if necessary. Metabolic acidosis is corrected by maintaining adequate perfusion pressures, optimizing ventilatory status, and judiciously using sodium bicarbonate. Hemodynamic stability assures adequate graft perfusion.[79,80]

Postoperatively patients are closely monitored in the intensive care unit. Derangements in metabolic, electrolyte, and volume status are corrected. A variable time of assisted positive-pressure ventilation is usually necessary because of the length of the procedure and secondary to edema from a large graft placed in a restrictive cavity (i.e., the abdomen). Analgesia is achieved via intravenous narcotics and eventually patient-controlled methods. Epidural catheter analgesia may be avoided because of possible coagulopathy in patients with hepatic insufficiency. Extubation of the trachea is performed only when the patient has attained adequate respiratory parameters and demonstrates control of airway reflexes.

REFERENCES

1. Lobo DN, Memon MA, Allison SP, Rowlands BJ. Evolution of nutritional support in acute pancreatitis. *Br J Surg*. 2000;87: 695-707.
2. Michel M, Murr NJ. Acute pancreatitis. In: Greenfield LJ, Mulholland MW, et al, eds. *Surgery: Scientific Principles and Practice*. 3rd ed. Philadelphia: Lippincott Williams & Wilkins; 2001:863-872.
3. Stoelting RK, Dierdorf SF. Diseases of the gastrointestinal system. In: Stoelting RK, Diredorf SF, eds. *Anesthesia and Co-existing Diseases*. 4th ed. New York: Churchill Livingstone; 2002:210-284.
4. Yeo CJ, Cameron JL. Exocrine pancreas. In: Townsend CM, Beauchamp RD, et al, eds. *Sabiston Textbook of Surgery: the Biological Basis of Modern Surgical Practice*. 16th ed. Philadelphia: Saunders; 2001:1116-1124.
5. Sharp KW, Pofahl WE. Pancreas. In: Lawrence PF, et al, eds, *Essential of General Surgery*. 3rd ed. Philadelphia: Lippincott Williams & Wilkins; 2000:333-334.
6. Pitchumoni CS, Agarwal N. Pancreatic pseudocysts. When and how should drainage be performed? *Gastroenterol Clin North Am*. 1999:28;615-639.
7. Babineau TJ, Bothe A, Steele G. The liver. In: Sabiston DC, Lyerly HK, eds. *Sabiston Essential of Surgery*. 2nd ed. Philadelphia: Saunders; 1994:362-363.
8. Mushlin PS, Gelman S. Liver dysfunction after anesthesia. In: Benumof JL, Saiman LJ, eds. *Anesthesia and Perioperative Complications*. 2nd ed. St Louis: Mosby; 1999:441-470.
9. Gelman S, Fowler K, Smith LR. Liver circulation and function during isoflurane and halothane anesthesia. *Anesthesiology*. 1984;61:726-730.
10. Morgan GE, Mikhail MS, Murray M. *Clinical Anesthesiology*. 3rd ed. Norwalk, Conn: Appleton & Lange; 2002:708-717.
11. Nishiyama T, et al. Inorganic fluoride kinetics and renal and hepatic function after repeated sevoflurane anesthesia. *Anesth Analg*. 1998;87:468-473.
12. Stoelting RK. Opioid agonists and antagonists. In: Stoelting RK, ed. *Pharmacology and Physiology in Anesthetic Practice*. 3rd ed. Philadelphia: Lippincott; 1999:77-112.
13. Shaw BW, Rakesh SK, Heffron TG. Diagnostic considerations in liver disease. In: Baker RJ, Fischer JE, eds. *Mastery of Surgery*. 4th ed. Philadelphia: Lippincott Williams & Wilkins; 2001: 1060-1071.
14. Potts JR, Chapman WC. Liver. In: Lawrence PF, et al, eds. *Essentials of General Surgery*. 3rd ed. Philadelphia: Lippincott Williams & Wilkins; 2000:343-347.
15. Organon. *Rocuronium Bromide: Product Information*. West Orange, NJ: Organon; 1995.
16. Kelly DA, Tuddenham EGD. Haemostatic problems in liver disease. *Gut*. 1986;27:339-349.
17. Jenkins SA, Baxter JN, Corbett W, Devitt P, Ware J, Shields R. A prospective randomized controlled trial comparing somatostatin and vasopressin in controlling acute variceal hemorrhage. *BMJ*. 1985;290:270-278.
18. Burroughs A, McCormick P, Hughes M, Sprengers D, D'Heygere F, McIntyre N. Randomized, double blind, placebo-control and prevention of early variceal rebleeding. *Gastroenterology*. 1990;99:1388.
19. Saari A, KL Vilaakso E, Ingberg M, et al. Comparison of somatostatin and vasopressin in bleeding esophageal varies. *Am J Gastroenterol*. 1990;85:804.
20. Westaby D, Williams R. Status of sclerotherapy for variceal bleeding in 1990. *Am J Surg*. 1990;160:32-37.
21. Pivalizza EG, Gottschalk LI, Cohen A, Middelbrook M, Soltes G. Anesthesia for transjugular intrahepatic portosystemic shunt placement. *Anesthesiology*. 1996;85:946-947.
22. Chong WK, Malisch TA, Mazer MJ, Lind CD, Worrell JA, Richards WO. Transjugular intrahepatic portosystemic shunt: US assessment with maximum flow velocity. *Radiology*. 1993:189; 789-793.
23. Sahagun G, Benner KG, Saxon R, Barton RE, Rabkin J, Keller FS, Rosch J. Outcome of 100 patients after transjugular intrahepatic portosystemic shunt for variceal hemorrhage. *Am J Gastroenterol*. 1997:92;1444-1452.
24. Ahrendt SA, Pitt HA. Biliary tract. In: *Sabiston Textbook of Surgery*. Philadelphia: Saunders; 2001:1076-1111.
25. Jones RM, et al. Incidence of choledochoduodenal sphincter spasm during fentanyl-supplemented anesthesia. *Anesth Analg*. 1981; 60:638-640.
26. Leonard IE, Cunningham AJ. Anaesthetic considerations for laparoscopic cholecystectomy. *Best Pract Res Clin Anaesthesiol*. 2002;16:1-20.
27. Castell DO. Approach to the patient with dyspagia. In: Yamada T, et al, eds. *Textbook of Gastroenterology*. Philadelphia: Lippincott; 1991:562-572.
28. Zwischenberger JB, Savage C, Bhutani M. Esophagus. In: *Sabiston Textbook of Surgery: the Biological Basis of Modern Surgical Practice*. 17th ed. Philadelphia: Saunders; 2004:1041-1050.
29. Peters JH, DeMeester TR. Esophagus and diaphragmatic hernia. In: Schwartz SI, et al, eds. *Principles of Surgery*. 7th ed. New York: McGraw-Hill; 1998:1081-1180.
30. Duranceau A. The esophagus. In: Sabiston DC, Lyerly HK, eds. *Sabiston's Essentials of Surgery*. 2nd ed. Philadelphia: Saunders; 1994:258-260.
31. Shelley KH, Haddadhin AS. Is *Helicobacter pylori* infection an occupational hazard for anesthesiologists? *Anesth Analg*. 1998;87:973.
32. Fiddian-Green RG. Gastric intramucosal pH, tissue oxygenation and acid-base balance. *Br J Anesth*. 1995;74:591-606.
33. Creteur J, DeBacker D, Vincent J. Monitoring gastric mucosal carbon dioxide using gas tonometry: in vitro and in vivo validation studies. *Anesthesiology*. 1997;87:504-510.
34. Ashley SW, Evoy D, Daly J. Stomach. In: Schwartz SI, et al, eds. *Principles of Surgery*. 7th ed. New York: McGraw-Hill; 1998:1181.
35. Bianchi-Porro G, Dicenta C, Cook T, Humphries TJ. Review of an extensive worldwide study of a new H_2 receptor antagonist, famotidine, as compared to ranitidine in the treatment of acute duodenal ulcer. *J Clin Gastroenterol*. 1987;2:14-19.
36. Mercer DW, Robinson EK. Stomach. In: *Sabiston Textbook of Surgery: the Biological Basis of Modern Surgical Practice*. 17th ed. Philadelphia: Saunders; 2004:1265-1322.
37. Sittig KM, Rohr M, McDonald J. Abdominal wall, umbilicus, peritoneum, mesenteries, omentum and retroperitoneum. In: *Sabiston Textbook of Surgery: the Biological Basis of Modern Surgical Practice*. 16th ed. Philadelphia: Saunders; 2001:769-782.
38. Hallak A. Spontaneous bacterial peritonitis. *Am J Gastroenterol*. 1989;84:345.
39. Evers BM. Small intestine. In: *Sabiston Textbook of Surgery: the Biological Basis of Modern Surgical Practice*. 17th ed. Philadelphia: Saunders; 2004:1323-1380.
40. Mahmoud N, Rombeau J, Ross HM. The colon and rectum. In: *Sabiston Textbook of Surgery: the Biological Basis of Modern Surgical Practice*. 17th ed. Philadelphia: Saunders; 2004:1401-1482.
41. Guyton SC. *Textbook of Medical Physiology*. 10th ed. Philadelphia: Saunders; 2001:718-726.
42. Trnka YM, Glotzer DJ, Kasdon EJ, Goldman H, Steer ML, Goldman LD. The long-term outcome of restorative operation in Crohn's disease. *Ann Surg*. 1982;196:345-354.
43. Olaison G, Smedh K, Sjodahl R. Natural course of Crohn's disease after ileocolic resection: endoscopically visualized ideal ulcers preceding symptoms. *Gut*. 1992;33:331-335.
44. Stark ME, Tremaine WJ. Medical care of the inflammatory bowel disease patient. In: Quigley EM, Sorrell MF, eds. *The Gastrointestinal Surgical Patient*. Baltimore: Williams & Wilkins; 1994:421-423.
45. Yellin AE, Newman J, Conovan AJ. Neostigmine-induced hyperperistalsis: effects on security of colonic anastomoses. *Arch Surg*. 1973;106:779-781.
46. Steinbrook RA. Epidural anesthesia and gastrointestinal motility. *Anesth Analg*. 1998;86:837-844.

47. Canver CC, Freier, DT. Management of cecal diverticulitis. *Am J Gastroenterol.* 1986;81:1104-1106.
48. Elfrink RJ, Miedema BW. Colonic diverticula: when complications require surgery and when they don't. *Postgrad Med.* 1992;92:92-98, 101-102.
49. Jones RS, Claridge JA. Acute abdomen. In: *Sabiston Textbook of Surgery: the Biological Basis of Modern Surgical Practice.* 17th ed. Philadelphia: Saunders; 2004:1219-1241.
50. Wilmore DW, Smith RJ, O'Dwyer ST, Jacobs DO, Ziegler TR, Wang XD. The gut: a central organ after surgical stress. *Surgery.* 1988;104:917-922.
51. Aranow JS, Fink MPL. Determinants of intestinal barrier failure in critical illness. *Br J Anesthesiol.* 1997;77:71-81.
52. McLeod HL, Murray GI. Tumour markers of prognosis in colorectal cancer. *Br J Cancer.* 1999;79:191-203.
53. Mazier WP. Hemorrhoids, fissures, and pruritus ani. *Surg Clin North Am.* 1994;74:1277-1292.
54. Shelton T, McKinlay R, Schwartz RW. Acute appendicitis: current diagnosis and treatment. *Curr Surg.* 2003;60:502-505.
55. Arnbjornsson E. Management of appendiceal abscess. *Curr Surg.* 1984;41:4.
56. Lally KP, Cox Jr CS, Andrassy RJ. Appendix. In: *Sabiston Textbook of Surgery: the Biological Basis of Modern Surgical Practice.* 17th ed. Philadelphia: Saunders; 2004:1381-1401.
57. Akwari OE, Itani KM, Coleman RE, Rosse WF. Splenectomy for primary and recurrent immune thrombocytopenia purpura (ITP). *Ann Surg.* 1987;206:529-541.
58. Vevon PA, Ellison EC, Carey LC. Splenectomy for hematologic disease. *Adv Surg.* 1989;22:105-140.
59. Lucas CE. Splenic trauma. *Ann Surg.* 1991;213:98-112.
60. Vaughan DJ, Brunner MD. Anesthesia for patients with carcinoid syndrome. *Int Anesthesiol Clin.* 1997;35:129-142.
61. Kinney MA, Warner ME, Nagorney DM, et al. Perianaesthetic risks and outcomes of abdominal surgery for metastatic carcinoid tumors. *Br J Anaesth.* 2001;87:447-452.
62. Neustein S, Cohen E. Anesthesia for aortic and mitral valve disease in a patient with carcinoid heart disease. *Anesthesiology.* 1995;82:1067-1070.
63. Marsh MH, Martin JK Jr, Kvols LK, et al. Carcinoid crisis during anesthesia: successful treatment with somatostatin analogue. *Anesthesiology.* 1987;66:89-91.
64. Jenset RT, Norton JA. Carcinoid tumors and the carcinoid syndrome. In: DeVita VT, Hellman S, Rosenberg SA, eds. *Cancer Principles and Practice of Oncology.* 5th ed. Philadelphia: Lippincott-Raven; 1997.
65. Rosen HR, Shackleton CR, Martin P. Indications for and timing of liver transplantation. *Med Clin North Am.* 1996;80:1069-1102.
66. Diehl AM. Alcoholic liver disease: natural history. *Liver Transpl Surg.* 1997;3:206-211.
67. Otte JB. History of pediatric liver transplantation. Where are we coming from? Where do we stand? *Pediatr Transplant.* 2002;6:378-387.
68. Herbert MF, Wacher VJ, Roberts JP, Benet LZ. Pharmacokinetics of cyclosporine pre- and post-liver transplantation. *J Clin Pharmacol.* 2003;43:38-42.
69. Murakawa M. Coagulation monitoring and management during liver transplantation. *J Anesth.* 2003;17:77-78.
70. Kaisers U, Pappert D, Langrehr JM, Undi H, Neuhaus P, Rossaint R. Dopamine, dopexamine and dobutamine in liver transplant recipients: a comparison of their effects on hemodynamics, oxygen transport and hepatic venous oxygen saturation. *Transpl Int.* 1996:9:214-220.
71. Mathur VS. The role of DA1 receptor agonist fenoldopam in the management of critically ill, transplant, and hypertensive patients. *Rev Cardiovasc Med.* 2003;4(suppl 1):S35-S40.
72. Cicalese L, Giacomoni A, Rastellini C, et al. Pancreatic transplantation: a Review. *Int Surg.* 1999;84:305-312.
73. Stratta RJ, Larsen JL, Cushing K. *Pancreas transplantation for diabetes mellitus. Annu Rev Med.* 1995:46:281-298.
74. Sutherland DE, Gruessner AC, Gruessner RW. Pancreas transplantation: a review. *Transplant Proc.* 1998;30:1940-1943.
75. Dubernard JM, Tajra LC, Lefrancois N, et al. Pancreas transplantation: results and indications. *Diabetes Metab.* 1998;24:195-199.
76. Stratta RJ, Taylor RJ, Larsen JL, Cushing K. Pancreas transplantation. *Ren Fail.* 1995;17:323-337.
77. Grant D. Intestinal transplantation: 1997 report of the International Registry. Intestinal Transplant Registry. *Transplantation.* 1999:67:1061-1064.
78. Abu-Elmagd K, Reyes J, Bond G, et al. Clinical intestinal transplantation: a decade of experience at a single center. *Ann Surg.* 2001;234:404-417.
79. Thompson JS. Intestinal transplantation. Experience in the United States. *Eur J Pediatr Surg.* 1999;9:271-273.
80. Asfar S, Zhong R, Grant D. Small bowel transplantation. *Surg Clin North Am.* 1994;74:1197-1210.

CHAPTER 29

Anesthesia for Laparoscopic Surgery

Edward Waters

The word *laparoscopy* is derived from two Greek words: *laparo*, meaning "flank," and *skopein*, meaning "to examine."[1] Indeed, laparoscopy can be defined as the process of examining the contents of the abdominal cavity using a specially designed endoscope.[2] An important trend in surgery in recent decades has been the expanded use of laparoscopy by surgeons of many subspecialties as a tool in the diagnosis and treatment of many conditions.

Laparoscopic surgical techniques are central to the current emphasis on minimally invasive surgery. Surgeons in gynecologic, urologic, and general surgical disciplines currently employ laparoscopic approaches to surgery. Common surgical applications of laparoscopy are noted in Box 29-1.

The advantages of laparoscopic surgery as compared with open techniques are numerous and include better aesthetic results (because the incisions are small), earlier postoperative mobility, and shorter hospital stays.[3-6] Many of the benefits of laparoscopic surgery are attributed to the reduced tissue trauma seen in laparoscopic surgery as compared with open surgery.[7] Studies of patients undergoing laparoscopic cholecystectomy have demonstrated significant improvement in postoperative pain as compared with patients undergoing open cholecystectomy, as well as superior postoperative pulmonary function.[5,8]

BOX 29-1

Applications of Laparoscopy

General Surgery
Diagnosis
Evaluation of abdominal trauma
Lysis of adhesions
Cholecystectomy
Appendectomy
Inguinal hernia repair
Bowel resection
Esophageal reflux surgery
Splenectomy
Adrenalectomy

Gynecologic Surgery
Diagnosis
Lysis of adhesions
Fallopian tube surgery (sterilization, ectopic pregnancy surgery)
Fulguration of endometriosis
Ovarian cyst surgery
Laparoscopic-assisted hysterectomy

Urologic Surgery
Nephrectomy

Modified from Soper, Brut Kerbl, 1994; Smith, 2001; Ruurda, Van Vroonhoven, Broders, 2002; and Zupi, Marconi, Sbracia, et al, 2000.

The history of laparoscopy began in 1901 in Germany when Kelling insufflated the abdominal cavity of a dog with air and used a cystoscope to view the viscera. Kelling later expanded his technique to human subjects.[9] Early laparoscopists focused on gynecologic diagnostic procedures. The first operative laparoscopy, a lysis of adhesions, was performed in 1933.[10] Kalk advanced laparoscopic technology by introducing a two-trocar technique. The two-trocar technique allowed access to the abdomen for a laparoscope as well as surgical instruments and facilitated more sophisticated procedures such as biopsies.[9] In the 1950s glass fiber illumination became available, which permitted the use of a light source external to the patient, resulting in a reduced rate of visceral burns and better illumination for the operator.[9]

The 1980s marked the beginning of a revolution in laparoscopic surgery. Before the 1980s, surgeons relied on a monocular laparoscope, which provided a direct view of the abdomen.[11] The union of a small video camera with a laparoscope during the 1980s allowed many improvements in laparoscopic surgery. Use of a video camera allowed much better ergonomics for the operator and, perhaps more significantly, allowed the entire surgical team to view and assist in the surgery. More complicated surgeries involving multiple assistant surgeons became possible and were facilitated by an ever-expanding variety of surgical instruments.[2,11]

An early result of the improved technology for laparoscopic surgery was the increased use of laparoscopy by general surgeons. The first four-trocar laparoscopic surgery, a laparoscopic cholecystectomy, was performed in France in 1987.[9,12] As general surgeons developed skills in laparoscopic cholecystectomies and other abdominal surgeries a significant change in the patient population for laparoscopic surgery occurred.[1] No longer were laparoscopic cases of brief duration and reserved for women of childbearing age. Laparoscopic procedures were now of greater duration and complexity and were performed on elderly, debilitated patients, sometimes in unusual positions such as the reverse Trendelenburg position.[13,14]

CREATION OF THE PNEUMOPERITONEUM

One constant in laparoscopic surgery has remained over the years: the need to establish and maintain a pneumoperitoneum. The pneumoperitoneum is essential to the surgeon performing laparoscopic surgery. It provides the exposure necessary for the operator to view the operative site and allows room for the surgeon to move instruments.[14] The pneumoperitoneum is the distinguishing feature of laparoscopic surgery as far as the anesthetist is concerned. The establishment of a pneumoperitoneum brings with it the risk of severe acute injury to the patient. The presence of a pneumoperitoneum is accompanied by physical stress to the patient, and the residual effects of a pneumoperitoneum can persist into the immediate postoperative period, leading to patient morbidity.

Clinical experience shows that the patient who undergoes laparoscopic surgery is at the highest risk for serious complications during the initial establishment of the pneumoperitoneum.[15] At present, initial access to and insufflation of the abdominal cavity are accomplished in one of two manners: an "open" or a "closed" technique.

The older of the two techniques, the closed technique, involves the use of a spring-loaded needle, introduced by the Hungarian surgeon Veress in 1939, to pierce the abdominal wall at its thinnest point—the infraumbilical region.[9] The position of the Veress needle is confirmed by the injection of 10 ml of saline through the needle. The needle is assumed to be correctly placed if the surgeon is unable to aspirate the saline. An appropriate gas, usually carbon dioxide (CO_2), is then passed through the needle to create a space between the abdominal wall and organs. After insufflation of the abdomen a trocar is blindly inserted to allow the surgeon to pass instruments into the abdominal cavity.[16]

Hasson first described the so-called "open technique" in 1971. Hasson's technique involves a small (1.5 to 3 cm) incision made immediately inferior to the umbilicus, through the skin and fascia. The surgeon then directly incises the peritoneum, and a trocar, the Hasson cannula, is placed. Once the Hasson cannula is placed the abdomen is insufflated and the catheter sutured in place.[15]

The relative merits of the open technique versus the closed technique for establishment of the pneumoperitoneum have been a source of debate among surgeons for some time. Proponents of the open technique argue that Hasson's technique, while not totally eliminating risk, minimizes the risk of major vascular injury on induction of pneumoperitoneum, a grave complication.[17]

Investigators comparing open and closed techniques suggest that the open technique does have distinct practical advantages, such as faster insufflation, which leads to a shorter operative time, as well as a lower rate of complications.[15,18] A review of the literature examining the incidence of complications on establishment of pneumoperitoneum concluded that visceral injuries were less frequent when an open technique was used, but not at a level of statistical significance.The same review found a statistically significantly reduction of major vascular injuries when Hasson's technique was employed to establish pneumoperitoneum rather than a Veress needle.[19]

The potential for injury to the patient early in the course of a laparoscopic surgery is apparent when one considers the anatomic structures in close proximity to the infraumbilical puncture and incision site. The inferior vena cava, aorta, and iliac arteries and veins, as well as the bladder, bowel, and uterus, are near the infraumbilical site. A subset of patients are at increased risk of injury during the establishment of the pneumoperitoneum because of anatomic variations such as obesity, a very thin body habitus, adhesions, or distortion of the viscera as a result of masses such as neoplasms.[16] Iatrogenic injury of the patient during the establishment of the pneumoperitoneum can result from trauma to vascular structures, gas embolism, injury to abdominal and pelvic organs, and the migration of gas to extraperitoneal spaces.[20]

Vascular injury early in the intraoperative period resulting from trauma to the epigastric vessels is often minor[6]; however, major vascular injuries occur in 0.02 to 0.9% of cases.[15] *Major vascular injury* refers to injury to the aorta, inferior vena cava, right renal artery, iliac arteries and veins, or mesenteric vessels. Estimates of mortality related to injury to these major vessels are as high as 15%.[15] Remarkably, trauma to major vessels may be occult, because these vessels lie in the retroperitoneal space, which can contain significant hemorrhage. A case report[21] documented an incident in which a patient showed signs of cardiovascular decompensation; observation of the abdominal cavity via the laparoscope failed to detect signs of bleeding, and it was only on laparotomy that a large retroperitoneal hematoma resulting from laceration of the common iliac artery and vein was observed. In addition to concealed bleeding in the retroperitoneum, some authors state that venous bleeding may not be observed intraoperatively because of a tamponading effect resulting from the pneumoperitoneum-induced increase in intraabdominal pressure.[22]

A potentially catastrophic complication of laparoscopic surgery is gas embolism. Gas embolism is quite rare, having a reported incidence of 1 occurrence in 77,604 cases[3] or 15 occurrences in more than 100,000 laparoscopies.[14] Gas embolism is most likely to occur during the initial insufflation of the abdomen.[22,23] The gas embolism can result from the erroneous placement of a Veress needle or trocar into the lumen of an intraabdominal vessel or vascular organ (e.g., uterus or liver) and insufflation through that needle or trocar.[22] In the case of laparoscopic cholecystectomy the patient is also at risk for gas embolism as the gall bladder is dissected away from the liver bed.[23]

Small gas bubbles can enter the pulmonary circulation, leading to pulmonary hypertension, right ventricular failure, and pulmonary edema. If the gas bubble is large enough, it can result in a "gas-lock" phenomenon, which obstructs right ventricular outflow.[22] Fortunately, catastrophic gas embolism that leads to cardiac arrest is exceedingly rare.[21]

Signs of a significant gas embolism include hypotension, dysrhythmia, and a distinctive "mill wheel" murmur, as well as cyanosis and pulmonary edema.[21] Management of gas embolism includes halting the insufflation of gas, elimination of nitrous oxide (N_2O) from the anesthetic gases, release of the pneumoperitoneum, placement of the patient in the left lateral decubitus position (Durant's maneuver), and aspiration of the gas through a central venous catheter.[22] It should be noted that low central venous pressure (CVP) increases the risk of venous gas embolism[23]; adequate hydration should therefore be provided for the patient undergoing laparoscopy. Box 29-2 lists the signs, symptoms, and treatment of gas embolism.

Visceral injuries can lead to significant morbidity and mortality in patients who undergo laparoscopy. The incidence of visceral injuries in patients in whom a pneumoperitoneum is created via the closed technique is in the range of 0.1% to 0.4%.[6,15] Trocar insertion has been associated with gastrointestinal tract

BOX 29-2

Gas Embolism

Signs and Symptoms
Hypotension
Dysrhythmia
Cyanosis
Hypoxia
Pulmonary edema
"Mill wheel" murmur

Treatment
Discontinue gas insufflation
Discontinue nitrous oxide
Administer 100% oxygen
Release pneumoperitoneum
Position patient in left lateral decubitus position
Attempt to aspirate gas via central venous catheter

Modified from Noga, Fredman, Olsfanger, Jedekin, 1997; Beck, McQuillan, 1994; and Brimacomb, Orland, 1994.

perforation as well as hepatic and splenic tears.[13] Urinary bladder catheterization and nasogastric suction are often employed in patients who undergo laparoscopy to reduce the risk of trauma to the bladder and stomach, respectively.[10,13,24]

Visceral lesions sustained during laparoscopic surgery are of particular concern because they are not always recognized at the time of surgery and tend to become symptomatic only after a period of time has elapsed postoperatively. Intraabdominal injuries can result in sepsis, fistulas, peritonitis, and abscesses.[3,15] Supporters of the open technique for creation of the pneumoperitoneum contend that the use of this technique reduces the incidence of visceral trauma and has the advantage of causing lesions that are more easily recognized at the time of surgery.[15]

Another serious complication of the pneumoperitoneum is pneumothorax. A retrospective review of 968 cases revealed an incidence of pneumothorax or pneumomediastinum in 1.9% of patients.[25] A subset of patients at increased risk for pneumothorax includes patients undergoing laparoscopic surgery for esophageal reflux disease.[23] Gas can enter the thoracic cavity by two mechanisms. In some cases gas from a properly induced pneumoperitoneum can pass from the peritoneal cavity to the thoracic cavity via weak points in the esophageal or aortic hiatus.[26] Alternatively a pneumothorax can result from barotrauma secondary to the increased airway pressures and decreased pulmonary compliance typical of pneumoperitoneum.[27] Pneumothorax caused by CO_2 insufflation (perhaps more properly called *capnothorax)* may rapidly resolve both clinically and radiographically without intervention.[26,28] Pneumothorax resulting from barotrauma, such as a ruptured bleb, typically requires thoracentesis.[26]

A relatively minor complication of laparoscopic surgery is subcutaneous emphysema that occurs independently from a pneumothorax. Subcutaneous emphysema can be the result of trocar or Veress needle misplacement in subcutaneous tissue[23,29] and is characteristically manifested as crepitus.

The ideal gas for the creation and maintenance of pneumoperitoneum would demonstrate several properties; among these properties are colorlessness, lack of flammability in the presence of electrocautery, physiologic inertness, and excretion via a pulmonary route.[13] Several gases have been investigated in the search for the ideal gas for use in surgical peritoneum. The earliest laparoscopists used air[9] to create a pneumoperitoneum; unfortunately air supports combustion and is poorly absorbed from the circulation, which leads to an unacceptably high risk of embolism.[24] N_2O is three times more soluble than nitrogen; however, it supports combustion.[13] Helium was evaluated as a gas for abdominal insufflation. The potential suitability of helium lay in its inert physiochemical properties, but helium is not absorbable and could prove very dangerous if present in a gas embolism.[30]

The gas most commonly used in laparoscopic surgery today is CO_2. Although not an ideal gas for pneumoperitoneum, CO_2 is readily available and inexpensive, does not support combustion, and is rapidly absorbed from the vascular space[7] as well as easily excreted by the respiratory system. CO_2 does have disadvantages when used in a pneumoperitoneum. These disadvantages include an increased risk of hypercarbia (and subsequent respiratory acidosis) and the fact that CO_2 causes peritoneal and diaphragmatic irritation, which has been implicated in postoperative shoulder pain.[3,7,24]

PHYSIOLOGIC EFFECTS OF PNEUMOPERITONEUM

As laparoscopic surgery has progressed from simple gynecologic surgeries in a young, healthy population to more complicated surgical procedures in a population with increased incidence of systemic disease[2,31] the need for an improved understanding of the physiologic impact of laparoscopic surgery has grown.

Patient response to laparoscopic surgery varies depending on the interplay of numerous factors. The impact of pneumoperitoneum on the patient differs depending on several factors, including the degree of intraabdominal pressure generated by the gas, the presence or absence of preexisting cardiopulmonary disease, intravascular volume status, and the duration of the surgery.[13] It is believed that pneumoperitoneum affects the body by means of three mechanisms: a direct mechanical effect, the presence of neurohumoral responses to the pneumoperitoneum, and the effects of absorbed CO_2.[5,23] In addition to experiencing pneumoperitoneum-induced physiologic changes the patient undergoing laparoscopic surgery is affected by the anesthetic and ventilatory techniques used by the anesthetist, intraoperative positioning, and the surgical conditions (e.g., the presence of retractors and packing).[13,32]

A consistent finding in studies of the hemodynamic effects of pneumoperitoneum is increased systemic vascular resistance (SVR).[32] In animal models (dogs) pneumoperitoneum-induced intraabdominal pressure as low as 8 torr leads to increased SVR.[33] Increases in SVR in healthy human subjects have been documented at intraabdominal pressures of 14 torr.[24] Increases in SVR of as high as 65% have been documented in healthy human laparoscopy patients.[34]

Mechanical factors such as the compression of the abdominal arteries as well as humoral factors are implicated in the increased afterload observed in patients undergoing laparoscopic surgery.[5,24] The persistence of increased SVR observed in patients immediately after the release of pneumoperitoneum has been attributed to the action of humoral mediators. In healthy patients the persistent influence of humoral mediators resolves within 30 minutes of the release of the pneumoperitoneum.[24]

The opinions of investigators regarding the influence of pneumoperitoneum on cardiac filling pressures are mixed. A study of swine in which a pneumoperitoneum of 15-torr pressure was created resulted in reports of increased pulmonary artery pressures.[12] Healthy human subjects undergoing laparoscopic surgery have demonstrated increased venous return when intraabdominal pressure was in the 14- to 20-torr range.[24,26] Although venous return improved in healthy gynecologic surgery patients with modestly elevated intraabdominal pressures, increasing the intraabdominal pressure to greater than 20 torr was found to decrease CVP. Motew reported a similar effect: an increased CVP in patients with an intraabdominal pressure of 20 torr and a decrease in CVP when intraabdominal pressure was 30 torr.[37]

Confounding factors such as the vasodilating actions of anesthesia[5] and the effects of intraoperative positioning can alter cardiac preload. The reverse Trendelenburg position, so often used in laparoscopic cholecystectomy, tends to decrease venous return,[5] whereas the Trendelenburg position customarily used in gynecologic laparoscopy increases venous return.[24]

Two mechanisms have been proposed as reasons for the elevated filling pressures sometimes observed during laparoscopy. One theory proposes that increased intraabdominal pressure leads to compression of the abdominal venous beds, leading to a redistribution of blood to the central circulation. Another explanation suggests that the increased cardiac filling pressures are the result of increased intrathoracic pressure caused by elevated intraabdominal pressure. The increase in intrathoracic and cardiac filling pressures occurs in the absence of increased circulating volume.[5,35] The decreased filling pressures observed with grossly elevated intraabdominal pressures (e.g., >30 torr) have been explained as the result of compression of the vena cava.[14]

Reports of the effects of pneumoperitoneum on stroke volume uniformly record a reduction in stroke volumes.[14,24,35,36] In both human and animal studies stroke volume was observed to decrease when intraabdominal pressure was in the range of 14 to 15 torr.[12,24] Decreases in stroke volume have been attenuated by interventions that increase the patient's circulating volume. Interventions to minimize the decrease in stroke volume include institution of the Trendelenburg position,[24] hydration with parenteral fluids, and compression of lower extremity veins.[36] Despite preoperative expansion of intravascular volume and the wrapping of legs with elastic bandages,[35] the stroke volume in laparoscopic cholecystectomy patients (under general anesthetic and in reverse Trendelenburg) has been observed to decrease approximately 30%. Observations of laparoscopic cholecystectomy patients immediately after the release of pneumoperitoneum and return to the supine position (from reverse Trendelenburg) typically find an increase in the stroke volume. This postpneumoperitoneum increase in stroke volume has been attributed to a return of blood to the systemic circulation from the lower extremities.[35]

The relationship of pneumoperitoneum to cardiac output (CO) and cardiac index (CI) is complex because of the multiplicity of variables that influence CO. With a few exceptions investigators report reduction of CO in the presence of pneumoperitoneum.[32,34] In a canine model decreased CO was noted at intraabdominal pressures of 8 to 12 torr, although significant reduction in CO was not observed until intraabdominal pressure reached 16 torr.[33] In pigs a combination of intraabdominal pressure of 16 torr and an elevation of the head of the bed resulted in a 70% to 80% reduction in CO.

Patients undergoing laparoscopic gynecologic surgery have demonstrated decreases in CO associated with intraabdominal pressures in excess of 20 torr.[37,38] In patients undergoing laparoscopic cholecystectomy, decreases in CO of 50% have been observed.[36] A technique involving optimization of intravascular volume and wrapping of the legs in elastic bandages has been shown to reduce the degree of decrease in CO in patients undergoing laparoscopic cholecystectomy. Healthy laparoscopic cholecystectomy patients with corrected hypovolemia and wrapped legs experienced a 20% drop in CO, as compared with a 50% decrease in control patients.[24,35,36]

In clinical studies of human subjects an initial decrease in CO is typically observed early in the course of surgery. This initial decrease is attributed to the mechanical effects of the pneumoperitoneum as well as any superimposed positional changes, such as the reverse Trendelenburg position, that may reduce venous return.[32] Five to ten minutes after this initial decrease the CO tends to increase, partially reversing the initial reduction in CO.[5,32] This biphasic response is believed by some to be mediated by a neurohumoral response.[5] Aside from neurohumoral factors an increased heart rate, usually observed in laparoscopy patients, helps reduce the decrease in CO that results from the diminished stroke volume seen in patients with pneumoperitoneum.[24]

Arterial blood pressure has been observed to rise in patients with intraabdominal pressures as low as 14 torr.[24] Some investigators have reported a 35% increase in mean arterial pressure associated with peritoneal insufflation.[34] The rise in arterial pressure observed in laparoscopy patients has been attributed to the increased afterload observed in patients with pneumoperitoneum.[5,34] Box 29-3 lists expected hemodynamic changes associated with pneumoperitoneum.

Humoral factors have been implicated in the increased afterload observed in patients with CO_2 pneumoperitoneum. Elevated levels of dopamine, vasopressin, epinephrine, norepinephrine, renin, and cortisol have been noted in laparoscopic cholecystectomy patients.[5,36] Vasopressin has been identified as a particularly significant mediator of hemodynamics in patients undergoing laparoscopy.[23] Catecholamine levels in laparoscopy patients have been noted to be mildly elevated and may be related to a generalized stress response.[23] In animal models catecholamine levels (epinephrine and norepinephrine) are unchanged at intraabdominal pressures of 10 torr but

BOX **29-3**

Hemodynamic Changes Associated with Pneumoperitoneum

- Central venous pressure ↑ or ↓
- Mean arterial pressure ↑
- Stroke volume ↓
- Cardiac output ↑, ↓, or without change
- Systemic vascular resistance ↑
- Heart rate ↑

↑, *Increased;* ↓, *decreased.*
Modified from Wahba, Beique, Kleiman, 1995; Coskum, Salman 2001; Nuzzo, et al, 1997; Koivusalo, Lindgren, 2000; Sharma, Brandstetter, Brensilver, Jung, 1996; O'Leary, Hubbard, Tormey, Cunningham, 1997; Hirvonen, Nuutinen, Kauho, 2000; and Motew, Ivankovich, Bieniarz, Albrecht, Zahed, Scommegna, 1973.

increase significantly at a pressure of 20 torr.[39] The increases in catecholamines observed in swine undergoing intraperitoneal insufflation appear to be directly related to increased intraabdominal pressure because of the fact that equivalent results are noted whether N_2O, air, or CO_2 is used.[39]

An important cardiovascular effect of pneumoperitoneum is related to distension of the vagus nerve during insufflation. As the vagus is distended, bradycardia is sometimes observed in patients undergoing laparoscopic cholecystectomy.[23]

At an intraabdominal pressure of 14 torr a reduction of lower extremity blood flow velocity has been observed similar to that seen in parturients and patients with ascites.[8] The effect of decreased venous blood flow on the risk for thromboembolic events is not clear. One opinion holds that the laparoscopic technique in cholecystectomy has the net effect of reducing emboli by facilitating early ambulation.[8] Another commentator on this topic reports a lower incidence of deep vein thrombosis in gynecologic surgery and a higher incidence in laparoscopic surgery and attributes this difference to the lithotomy and Trendelenburg positions used in gynecologic surgery, as contrasted with the reverse Trendelenburg position used in laparoscopic cholecystectomy surgery.[40]

When compared with healthy patients, patients with significant comorbidity may exhibit exaggerated hemodynamic responses to pneumoperitoneum.[5] Specifically the cumulative effects of CO_2 pneumoperitoneum and the reverse Trendelenburg position seen in laparoscopic cholecystectomy can result in moderate decreases in CO as well as significant increases in filling pressures and afterload in sick patients.[41] A study by Safran[14] found that in American Society of Anesthesiologists (ASA) class III and IV patients an IAP of 15 torr resulted in significantly decreased CO and significantly increased MAP and SVR. The increased sensitivity of sick patients to the hemodynamic effects of pneumoperitoneum warrants careful intraoperative monitoring as well as preoperative attention to the patient's intravascular volume status.[5]

The relationship among intraabdominal, intrathoracic, and filling pressures in the presence of pneumoperitoneum was discussed previously. Serious reservations have been expressed regarding the use of direct measures of filling pressures to estimate intravascular volume. Several authors warn that measurements of CVP and pulmonary artery occlusion pressure are distorted in the presence of increased intraabdominal pressure.[35,36] One solution to this pressure-induced distortion is to calculate a transmural right atrial pressure (right atrial pressure [RAP] − extracardiac pressure) rather than relying on a directly measured−RAP as an indication of preload.[35] Another approach involves echocardiographic observation of ventricular wall motion for signs of cardiac decompensation.[36] A pulmonary artery catheter may be of increased utility and its use more valid if serial measurements of CO and mixed venous oxygen saturation are carefully evaluated for signs of decreased cardiac performance.[5,24]

Compared with open surgery, laparoscopic surgery, and in particular laparoscopic cholecystectomy, has the advantage of a decreased incidence of postoperative pulmonary complications. However, relative to patients who undergo open surgery, those who undergo laparoscopic surgery are subjected to increased levels of intraoperative pulmonary dysfunction because of the mechanical effects of pneumoperitoneum and the introduction of exogenous CO_2 into the peritoneal space.[24]

CO_2 pneumoperitoneum is characteristically associated with increases in the partial pressure of arterial CO_2 ($PaCO_2$) and end tidal CO_2 ($EtCO_2$) with or without acidosis.[14] The increase in $PaCO_2$ seen in CO_2 pneumoperitoneum is attributed primarily to absorption of the gas from the peritoneal surface.[14,31,42] Attribution of increased $PaCO_2$ levels to the presence of intraabdominal CO_2, not increased metabolism, is supported by studies that failed to find increased levels of oxygen consumption in animals undergoing abdominal insufflation.[14] Increased intraabdominal pressure in and of itself as a cause of hypercarbia was excluded by the findings of a study in which a helium pneumoperitoneum failed to increase $PaCO_2$.[5]

Maximum absorption of CO_2 is noted with an intraabdominal pressure of 10 torr.[23] $PaCO_2$ levels are noted to reach a plateau approximately 40 minutes after the induction of the peritoneum.[23]

Compared with intraperitoneal insufflation of CO_2, extraperitoneal insufflation has been associated with an unusually rapid increase in $PaCO_2$ as well as exceptionally high levels of CO_2.[43,44] CO_2 can be inadvertently insufflated extraperitoneally because of a misplaced trocar, or the insufflation can be deliberate as in herniorrhaphy and selected urologic procedures.[24,45] Researchers comparing laparoscopic hernia surgery and laparoscopic cholecystectomy have proposed that the increased $PaCO_2$ observed in patients undergoing extraperitoneal insufflation can be explained by fact that the lack of containment of CO_2 by the peritoneum leads to an increased area for gas exchange.[46]

Mild hypercarbia (45 to 50 torr) is not believed to be clinically significant.[14] Hypercarbia in the range of 50 to 70 torr is associated with physiologic effects such as increased cerebral blood flow, peripheral vasodilation, pulmonary vasoconstriction, and increased risk of cardiac dysrhythmia.[5,10,24]

The mechanical effects of peritoneal insufflation inhibit ventilation. Insufflation of the peritoneum displaces the diaphragm in a cephalad direction.[5] The resulting compression of the basilar lobes of the lungs results in atelectasis,[23] decreased functional residual capacity (FRC), decreased vital capacity, and increased dead space ventilation.[14] Increased intraabdominal pressure also affects pulmonary compliance; in supine patients pulmonary compliance has been observed to be reduced by 43%.[5] Pulmonary changes associated with pneumoperitoneum are listed in Box 29-4.

An additive effect is observed when general anesthesia, which in and of itself reduces FRC and pulmonary compliance, is combined with pneumoperitoneum.[5] Intraoperative positioning can either aggravate or attenuate pneumoperitoneum-induced

BOX **29-4**

Pulmonary Function Changes Associated with Pneumoperitoneum

- Positive inspiratory pressure (PIP) ↑
- Pulmonary compliance dV/dP ↓
- Vital capacity ↓
- Functional residual capacity ↓
- Intrathoracic pressure ↑

dV/dP, Change in volume/change in pressure; ↑, increased; ↓, decreased. Modified from Safran, Orlando, 1994.

pulmonary changes. The Trendelenburg position increases the effects of pneumoperitoneum on pulmonary mechanics. In laparoscopic hysterectomy, pulmonary compliance decreased 20% when the head of the bed was depressed and an additional 30% with peritoneal insufflation.[42] In contrast, the reverse Trendelenburg position partially counteracts the effects of the pneumoperitoneum on the diaphragm and improves diaphragmatic function.[13]

One of the most common complications of pneumoperitoneum, endobronchial intubation, has been attributed to the cephalad displacement of the diaphragm caused by pneumoperitoneum. A study of 50 patients with an intraabdominal pressure of 15 torr and in the reverse Trendelenburg position found a 6% rate of right mainstem bronchial intubation.[47] Verification of bilateral breath sounds after insufflation is considered prudent practice by some authors.[40]

Controlled mechanical ventilation provides anesthetists a method for maintaining CO_2 homeostasis in patients undergoing laparoscopic surgery with CO_2 peritoneum. Studies of patients with pneumoperitoneum in the Trendelenburg position reveal that a 20% to 30% increase in minute volume is necessary if $PaCO_2$ is to be maintained at preperitoneum levels.[42,48] Preinsufflation $PaCO_2$ levels in patients who underwent surgery in the reverse Trendelenburg position were maintained by increasing minute volume by a factor of 12% to 16%.[48] Clinical studies of patients undergoing laparoscopic surgeries indicate that increasing the minute volume by preferentially increasing tidal volume rather than respiratory rate is the most effective way to speed CO_2 elimination.[42,48] The preference for increasing tidal volume rather than respiratory rate is based on a belief that increased lung volumes recruit lung tissues that previously constituted nonfunctional anatomic dead space.[42]

Laparoscopic surgical patients who have marginal cardiopulmonary function are at risk of decompensation when faced with the stress introduced by increased intraabdominal pressure and exogenous CO_2. Patients particularly vulnerable to the effects of CO_2 peritoneum are those with increased metabolic rates (as in sepsis), large ventilatory dead space, and decreased CO.[14] Patients with pulmonary emphysema warrant special consideration. Studies in animals as well as clinical studies in humans indicate that whereas healthy patients experience minor changes in $PaCO_2$ and $EtCO_2$ when confronted with CO_2 peritoneum, patients with obstructive lung disease have significantly increased levels of CO_2 retention that may lead to decreases in arterial pH.[13,30]

The high incidence of CO_2 retention observed in patients with chronic obstructive pulmonary disease warrants careful intraoperative monitoring of CO_2 levels in individuals at risk during laparoscopic surgery. Healthy, mechanically ventilated patients demonstrate a proportional relationship between $EtCO_2$ and $PaCO_2$; consequently, continuous $EtCO_2$ monitoring is widely accepted as a method for clinical monitoring.[5,13] Patients with preexisting lung disease present challenges to clinicians responsible for intraoperative monitoring. In individuals with elevated $EtCO_2$ the relationship between $EtCO_2$ and $PaCO_2$ becomes inaccurate, with $EtCO_2$ underestimating $PaCO_2$.[24,48] A similar effect, in which $EtCO_2$ underestimates $PaCO_2$, is seen in patients with obstructive lung disease.[30,31] Direct measurement of $PaCO_2$ by serial arterial blood gas measurements may be warranted in patients with cardiopulmonary disease.[13]

Pulmonary dysfunction has been observed to persist into the immediate postoperative period in patients recovering from laparoscopic surgery. A slight restrictive breathing pattern in the postoperative period has been observed. Explanations for this aberrant breathing pattern include the residual effects of anesthesia, pain, and diaphragmatic dysfunction induced by stretching or reflex inhibition.[8] Furthermore, the postoperative patient may be subjected to an elevated CO_2 load. In the circumstance of prolonged CO_2 insufflation, CO_2 not excreted is stored in skeletal muscle and bone. It may take hours for this excess CO_2 to be excreted from the patient.[12,24]

The impact of abdominal insufflation on the kidneys often manifests as oliguria, probably because of three mechanisms: compression of the kidneys (including the renal vasculature); compression of the inferior vena cava (with concomitant reduction in CO); and increased levels of antidiuretic hormone.[23] Significant reduction of renal blood flow was noted in pigs when intraabdominal pressure reached 24 torr.[49] In addition to the direct mechanical effects on the kidneys observed during pneumoperitoneum, humoral factors have an important effect on renal function. In laparoscopic cholecystectomy patients, plasma vasopressin levels were noted to be three times higher than preoperative levels at 30 minutes after insufflation and 20 times higher at 1 hour after insufflation.[50] Renin and aldosterone levels are also typically elevated in laparoscopic surgeries, with a fourfold increase noted in laparoscopic cholecystectomy patients.[32]

The effects of increased intraabdominal pressure on hepatic and splanchnic blood flow have been the subject of both human and animal studies. In swine an intraabdominal pressure of 16 torr and elevated head-of-bed position was associated with a 68% decrease in hepatic blood flow.[7] Use of low insufflation pressure has been demonstrated to attenuate the impact of CO_2 pneumoperitoneum on hepatic circulation. In a study of five healthy human subjects splanchnic blood flow was not disrupted when intraabdominal pressure was maintained at 11 to 13 torr for 30 to 60 minutes.[50]

ANESTHETIC MANAGEMENT

Laparoscopic surgeries have been performed using local, regional, and general anesthetic techniques. The choice of technique is in large part dependent on the specifics of the surgery.

Local anesthesia with sedation has been used in patients undergoing minor gynecologic laparoscopic surgical procedures such as diagnostic laparoscopy or sterilization.[2,13] The use of local anesthesia is facilitated by surgical techniques such as the use of only one port (as in diagnostic laparoscopy) and small diameter laparoscopes.[24,51] A randomized, controlled trial studied 164 women undergoing diagnostic laparoscopy for evaluation of infertility. Compared with patients who received general anesthetics, patients who received local anesthesia had shorter hospital stays and a reduction in anesthetic costs. The investigators did report limitations on the use of local anesthesia with sedation for laparoscopic surgery. In patients initially treated with local anesthesia, 5.5% required conversion to general anesthesia for completion of the surgery; furthermore, surgical exposure in patients who received local anesthesia with sedation was inferior to the surgical exposure in patients who received general anesthesia.[51]

Like the use of local anesthesia, the use of regional anesthesia for laparoscopic surgery tends to be limited to minor gynecologic surgical procedures. Shoulder and chest discomfort resulting from the pneumoperitoneum is not well managed by means of regional techniques.[27]

General anesthesia is the most practical technique for many, if not most, laparoscopic procedures.[2] General anesthesia facilitates the management of the patient discomfort associated with pneumoperitoneum[13] and intraoperative positions such as a steep Trendelenburg position. General anesthesia also has the advantage of facilitating controlled ventilation[13] and the use of muscle relaxants,[5] which may help minimize, respectively, hypercapnia and abdominal insufflation pressure.

Use of the laryngeal mask airway (LMA) in patients receiving general anesthesia for laparoscopic surgery has been the subject of some controversy. Several authors have expressed concerns that the increased intraabdominal and intrathoracic pressures characteristic of pneumoperitoneum place the patient at increased risk of gastroesophageal reflux and pulmonary aspiration.[13,14]

Resistance to gastroesophageal reflux is quantified by the barrier pressure, which is the difference between the lower esophageal sphincter pressure and the gastric pressure.[52,53] A study examining the effect of laparoscopy on barrier pressure has shown that in endotracheally intubated patients undergoing gynecologic laparoscopy an increase in intraabdominal pressure was accompanied by an adaptational increase in lower esophageal pressure, resulting in a net increase in barrier pressure.[53] However, concerns have been raised that use of LMAs impairs lower esophageal sphincter pressure, thereby reducing barrier pressure. Rabey and others, in a study of general and orthopedic surgery patients, did in fact observe reductions in lower esophageal sphincter pressures when an LMA was used as an airway in general anesthesia.[52]

Researchers have conducted studies to evaluate the safety and efficacy of LMAs in gynecologic laparoscopy. Authors of a retrospective study of 1469 gynecologic laparoscopies concluded that use of the LMA "appears safe."[54] A prospective study using direct fiberoptic examination of the laryngopharynx in 91 patients undergoing gynecologic laparoscopy with an LMA in place failed to identify a single incidence of regurgitation.[38] The efficacy of the LMA was evaluated in a randomized controlled trial that compared the performance of the LMA to endotracheal intubation (ETT) in 209 women undergoing gynecologic laparoscopy. The LMA compared favorably with ETT, with no statistical difference found in SpO_2, $EtCO_2$, or stomach size changes.[55]

Authoritative sources suggest that under certain circumstances LMA use may be appropriate during laparoscopy Guidelines for use of the LMA in laparoscopy are given in Box 29-5. Brimacomb and Brain recommend that clinicians who use the LMA during laparoscopy should, among other considerations, be experienced and adhere to the "15" rule, which requires that the surgery not exceed 15 minutes duration, the tilt of the bed be less than 15 degrees, and the intraabdominal pressure be less than 15 cm H_2O.[56] Although evidence can be presented to support the use of the LMA in pelvic surgery, research to support employment of the LMA in upper abdominal surgery is lacking. A consensus of clinicians fail to recommend the use of the LMA in upper abdominal surgeries such as laparoscopic cholecystectomy.[2,54,56]

Use of N_2O in laparoscopic surgery has been a source of controversy because of beliefs that N_2O contributes to bowel distension and increases the incidence of nausea and vomiting. The effect of N_2O on bowel distension has been examined in two studies. A randomized controlled trial involving 50 patients undergoing laparoscopic surgery was conducted; surgeons were asked to determine, based on their observation of the bowel, whether or not the anesthetist was using N_2O. The surgeons, blinded to anesthetic technique, were unable to reliably detect the use of N_2O based on observation of the gut.[57] A similar study was conducted in 150 patients undergoing open colon surgery; again, surgeons blinded to anesthetic technique were unable to identify patients receiving N_2O based on clinical observation.[58]

BOX 29-5

Some Guidelines for Use of the Laryngeal Mask Airway during Laparoscopy

- Ensure that clinician is an experienced LMA user.
- Select patients carefully (e.g., fasted, not obese).
- Use correct size of LMA.
- Make surgeon aware of use of LMA.
- Use total IV anesthetic technique or volatile agent.
- Adhere to "15" rule: <15 degree tilt; <15 cm H_2O intraabdominal pressure; <15 min duration.
- Avoid inadequate anesthesia during surgery.
- Avoid disturbance of the patient during emergence.

IV, *Intravenous;* LMA, *laryngeal mask airway.*
Modified from Maltby, Beriault, Watson, Liepert, Fick, 2003.

Nausea and vomiting are common postoperative complaints from patients who have undergone laparoscopic surgery; some investigators report incidences of nausea and vomiting in postoperative laparoscopy patients to be as high as 50% to 62%.[23,59] The question of N_2O's role in postoperative nausea and vomiting remains controversial and is beyond the scope of this discussion. However, a brief review of studies examining the use of N_2O and postoperative nausea and vomiting in laparoscopy patients is in order. Three separate randomized controlled trials involving gynecologic laparoscopies enrolling a total of 640 patients failed to demonstrate a statistically significant increase in the rate of nausea and vomiting in patients receiving N_2O as compared with patients not receiving N_2O.[60,61]

Postoperative pain after laparoscopic surgery is typically of a visceral quality on the day of surgery, with shoulder pain predominating on the first postoperative day.[62] Postoperative pain in laparoscopy patients is believed to be primarily the result of the pneumoperitoneum rather the incisions used to introduce trocars into the peritoneal space.[63] The pneumoperitoneum is believed to induce pain through both mechanical and chemical means. Insufflation of the abdomen is associated with distension of the peritoneum and abdominal wall, leading to traction of the nerves and trauma to blood vessels.[62] CO_2, commonly used as an insufflation gas, contributes to postoperative pain by decreasing intraperitoneal pH to as low as 6 in the immediate postoperative period.[63] The CO_2-induced intraperitoneal acidosis is believed to contribute to irritation of the phrenic nerve, which is manifested as shoulder pain typically seen in postoperative laparoscopy patients.[47,62,63]

Management of postoperative pain in laparoscopy patients typically involves a multimodal approach including opioids, nonsteroidal antiinflammatory drugs (NSAIDs), and local anesthetics.[2] In a randomized controlled trial of laparoscopic cholecystectomy patients the use of a multimodal technique was demonstrated to decrease levels of postoperative pain and nausea as well as speed discharge.[59]

The use of NSAIDs in the management of postoperative laparoscopic pain has been demonstrated to be of value. The efficacy of NSAIDs in the management of postoperative laparoscopic pain has been repeatedly studied; in all cases NSAIDs were demonstrated to be superior to placebo, although not always at a level of statistical significance.[62] Although NSAIDs are insufficiently potent to control laparoscopic pain as a single agent, they are often used in combination with opioids, with the resulting synergism leading to decreased opioid consumption.[62,63]

The efficacy of peripherally administered local anesthetics in the management of postoperative laparoscopy pain is a complicated question. A systematic review by Moiniche and colleagues evaluated 41 randomized controlled trials that studied pain control using local anesthesia in intraperitoneal and port site infiltration as well as mesosalpinx and fallopian tube block. Moiniche concluded, after reviewing 11 studies of port site infiltration, that the technique was without major effect. Evaluation of 12 trials of mesosalpinx and fallopian tube blockade concluded that the treatment was of significant yet short-lasting value.[64] Evaluation of studies of intraperitoneal local anesthesia injection characterized the intervention as statistically significant but questioned the clinical significance of the treatment effect.[64]

THE FUTURE OF LAPAROSCOPIC SURGERY

The dramatic growth in laparoscopy seen in the 1980s and early 1990s has reached a plateau, and the procedure has entered a period of incremental development.[9] Recent innovations in technology that have advanced laparoscopy include systems such as EndoAssist and AESOP, which are computer-controlled laparoscopic camera holders.[11,65] Efforts to eliminate the need for pneumoperitoneum have led to the development of "gasless" laparoscopy. The gasless laparoscopy technique creates a working space for the surgeon by inserting a fan-shaped device into the abdomen to lift the abdominal wall away from the viscera. Gasless laparoscopic techniques have significant limitations, including the need to make multiple skin incisions to insert the lifting device, an increased risk of injury to the abdominal wall, and a quality of surgical exposure that is inferior to that associated with pneumoperitoneum.[20,63]

Current technology limits laparoscopists in several ways. For example, two-dimensional television limits depth perception, and movement of contemporary laparoscopic instruments is counterintuitive (i.e., to move an instrument within a patient to the left, the operator moves his or her hand to the right).[4] New technologies have the potential to allow surgeons to operate far more intuitively and with greater dexterity than traditional laparoscopic techniques.

Robotic surgery, perhaps more properly termed *telemanipulation* or *computer-assisted surgery*, may permit surgeons to overcome some of the limitations imposed by present laparoscopic technology. A surgeon using telerobotic technology controls surgical instruments from a control console that may be immediately adjacent to the patient or at a site hundreds of miles away from the operating room. An important feature of telerobotic technology is three-dimensional imaging, which permits superior depth perception.[65] The robot arms manipulated by the surgeon facilitate delicate surgery by simulating the motion of the human wrist and by permitting scaling of the surgeon's movement (i.e., translation of the movement of a surgeon's hand into a finer movement of the instrument). The surgeon's dexterity is further improved by the robotic system's ability to factor out tremor.[4] Robotic surgery offers the surgeon improved ergonomics, superior dexterity, and the ability to use traditional open surgical skills for laparoscopic operations. Surgeries using telerobotic technology have been performed in cardiac, general, gynecologic, and urologic surgical disciplines.[4]

As technology advances, one can anticipate even broader application of laparoscopy and other minimally invasive surgical techniques in the future. Provision of safe and effective anesthetic care demands that the anesthetist understand the unique concerns of laparoscopic surgery, in particular the impact of abdominal insufflation on the physiology of the patient undergoing surgery.

REFERENCES

1. Soper NJ, Brut LM, Kerbl K. Medical progress: laparoscopic general surgery. *N Engl J Med.* 1994;330:409-419.
2. Smith I. Anesthesia for laparoscopy with emphasis on outpatient laparoscopy. *Anesthesiol Clin North Am.* 2001;19:21-42.
3. Deziel DJ, Millikan KW, Econonmou SG, Doolas A, Ko ST, Arian MC. Complications of laparoscopic cholecystectomy: a national survey of 4,292 hospitals and an analysis of 77,604 cases. *Am J Surg.* 1993;165:9-14.
4. Ruurda JP, Van Vroonhoven TJ, Broeders IA. Robot-assisted surgical systems: a new era in laparoscopic surgery. *Ann R Coll Surg Engl.* 2002;84:223-226.
5. Wahba RWM, Beique F, Kleiman SJ. Cardiopulmonary function and laparoscopic cholecystectomy. *Can J Anaesth.* 1995;42:51-63.
6. Lee VS, Chari RS, Cucchiaro G, Meyers WC. Complications of laparoscopic cholecystectomy. *Am J Surg.* 1993;165:527-532.
7. Chiu PT, Gin T, Oh TE. Anesthesia for laparoscopic general surgery. *Anaesth Intensive Care.* 1993;21:163-174.
8. Goodale RL, Beebe DS, McNevin MP, et al. Hemodynamic, respiratory and metabolic effects of laparoscopic cholecystectomy. *Am J Surg.* 1993;166:533-537.
9. Vecchio R, MacFayden V, Palazzolo F. History of laparoscopic surgery. *Panminerva Med.* 2000;42:87-90.
10. Coskun F, Salman M. Anesthesia for operative endoscopy. *Curr Opin Obstet Gynecol.* 2001;13:371-376.
11. Sackier JM, Wang Y. Robotically assisted laparoscopic surgery. *Surg Endosc.* 1994;8:63-66.
12. Ho H, Gunter R, Wolfe M. Intraperitoneal carbon dioxide insufflation and cardiopulmonary function. *Arch Surg.* 1992;127:928-933.
13. Cunningham AJ, Brull SJ. Laparoscopic cholecystectomy: anesthetic implications. *Anesth Analg.* 1993;76:1120-1133.
14. Safran DB, Orlando R. Physiologic effects of pneumoperitoneum. *Am J Surg.* 1994;167:281-286.
15. Nuzzo G, et al. Routine use of open technique in laparoscopic operations. *J Am Coll Surg.* 1997;184:58-62.
16. Rosen DM, Lam AM, Chapman M, Carlton M, Cairo GM. Methods of creating pneumoperitoneum: a review of techniques and complications. *Obstet Gynecol Surv.* 1998;53:167-174.
17. Hanney RM, Carmalt HL, Merrett N, Tait N. Use of the Hasson cannula producing major vascular injury at laparoscopy. *Surg Endosc.* 1999;13:1238-1240.
18. Sigman HH, Fried GM, Garzon J, et al. Risks of blind verses open approach to celiotomy for laparoscopic surgery. *Surg Laparosc Endosc.* 1993;3:296-299.
19. Bonjer HJ, Hazebroek EJ, Kazemier G, Giuffrida MC, Meijer WS, Lange JF. Open versus closed establishment of pneumoperitoneum in laparoscopic surgery. *Br J Surg.* 1997;84:599-602.
20. Canestrelli M, Canni M, Mori R, Blanc B, Trompeo P. New techniques of gynaecologic laparoscopy, gasless, open Hasson, optic trocar. *Panminerva Med.* 1999;41:371-377.

21. Noga J, Fredman B, Olsfanger D, Jedekin R. Role of the anesthesiologist in the early diagnosis of life threatening complications during laparoscopic surgery. *Surg Laparosc Endosc.* 1997;7:63-65.
22. Beck DH, McQuillan PJ. Fatal carbon dioxide embolism and severe haemorrhage during laparoscopic salpingectomy. *Br J Anaesth.* 1994;72:243-245.
23. Koivusalo A, Lindgren L. Effects of carbon dioxide pneumoperitoneum for laparoscopic cholecystectomy. *Acta Anaesthesiol Scand.* 2000;44:834-841.
24. Sharma KC, Brandstetter RD, Brensilver JM, Jung LD. Cardiopulmonary physiology and pathophysiology as a consequence of laparoscopic surgery. *Chest.* 1996;110:810-815.
25. Murdock CM, Wolff AJ, VanGreen T. Risk factors for hypercarbia, subcutaneous emphysema, pneumothorax and pneumomediastinum during laparoscopic surgery. *Obstet Gynecol.* 2000;95: 704-709.
26. Batra MS, Driscoll JJ, Coburn WA, Marks WM. Evanescent nitrous oxide pneumothorax after laparoscopy. *Anesth Analg.* 1983;62:1121-1123.
27. Collins L, Vaghadia H. Regional anesthesia for laparoscopy. *Anesthesiol Clin North Am.* 2001;19:43-55.
28. Hasel R, Arona SK, Hickey DR. Intraoperative complications of laparoscopic cholecystectomy. *Can J Anaesth.* 1993;40:459-464.
29. Lew JKL, Gin T, Oh TE. Anaesthetic problems during laparoscopic cholecystectomy. *Anaesth Intensive Care.* 1992;20:91-92.
30. Fitzgerald SD, Andrus CH, Baudendistel LJ, Dahms TE, Kaminski DL. Hypercarbia during carbon dioxide pneumoperitoneum. *Am J Surg.* 1992;163:186-190.
31. Kendall AP, Bhatt S, Oh TE. Pulmonary consequences of carbon dioxide insufflation for laparoscopic cholecystectomy. *Anaesthesia.* 1995;50:286-289.
32. O'Leary E, Hubbard K, Tormey W, Cunningham AJ. Laparoscopic cholecystectomy; haemodynamic and neuroendocrine responses after pneumoperitoneum and changes in position. *Br J Anaesth.* 1997;76:640-644.
33. Ishizaki Y, et al. Safe intraabdominal pressure of carbon dioxide pneumoperitoneum during laparoscopic surgery. *Surgery.* 1993; 114:549-554.
34. Joris JL, Noirot DP, Legrand MJ, Jacquet JN, Lamy ML. Hemodynamic changes during laparoscopic cholecystectomy. *Anesth Analg.* 1993;76:1067-1071.
35. Hirvonen EA, Nuutinen LS, Kauho M. Hemodynamic changes due to Trendelenburg positioning and pneumoperitoneum during laparoscopy. *Surg Endosc.* 2000;14:272-277.
36. McLaughlin JG, Scheeres DE, Dean RJ, Bonnell BW. The adverse hemodynamic effects of laparoscopic cholecystectomy. *Surg Endosc.* 1995;9:121-124.
37. Motew M, Ivankovich AD, Bieniarz J, Albrecht RF, Zahed B, Scommegna A. Cardiovascular effects and acid-base and blood gas changes during laparoscopy. *Am J Obstet Gynecol.* 1973;115: 1002-1012.
38. Bapat PP, Verghese C. Laryngeal mask airway and the incidence of regurgitation during gynecological laparoscopies. *Anesth Analg.* 1997;85:139-143.
39. Mikami O, Fujise K, Matsumoto S, Shingu K, Ashida M, Matsuda T. High intra-abdominal pressure increases plasma catecholamine levels during pneumoperitoneum for laparoscopic procedures. *Arch Surg.* 1998;133:39-43.
40. Rosen DM. Femoral venous flow during laparoscopic gynecologic surgery. *Surg Laparosc Endosc Percutan Tech.* 2000;10:158-162.
41. Fox LG, Hein HAT, Gawey BJ, Hellman CL, Ramsay MAE. Physiological changes during laparoscopic cholecystectomy in ASA III and IV patients. *Anesthesiology.* 1993;79:A55.
42. Hirvonen EA, Nuutinen LS, Kanko M. Ventilatory effects, blood gas changes and oxygen consumption during laparoscopic hysterectomy. *Anesth Analg.* 1995;80:961-966.
43. Wolf JS, Clayman RV, Monk TG, McClennan BL, McDougall EM: Carbon dioxide absorption during laparoscopic pelvic operation. *J Am Coll Surg.* 1995;180:555-560.
44. Burton A, Steinbrook RA. Precipitous decrease in oxygen saturation during laparoscopic surgery. *Anesth Analg.* 1993;76: 1177-1178.
45. Mellinger JD, Ponsky JL. Recent publications in laparoscopic surgery: an overview. *Endoscopy.* 1996;28:441-451.
46. Liem MS, Kallewaard JW, deSmet AM, van Vroonhoven TJ. Does hypercarbia develop faster during laparoscopic herniorrhaphy then during conventional laparoscopic cholecystectomy? *Anesth Analg.* 1995;81:1243-1249.
47. Brimacomb JR, Orland H. Endobronchial intubation during upper abdominal laparoscopic surgery in the reverse Trendelenburg position. *Anesth Analg.* 1994;78:607.
48. Wahba RWM, Mamazza J. Ventilatory requirements during laparoscopic cholecystectomy. *Can J Anaesth.* 1993;40:206-210.
49. Hashikura Y, Kawasaki S, Munakata Y, Hashimoto S, Hayashi K, Makuuchi M. Effects of peritoneal insufflation on hepatic and renal blood flow. *Surg Endosc.* 1994:8;759-761.
50. Odeberg S, Ljunqvist O, Sollevi A. Pneumoperitoneum for laparoscopic cholecystectomy is not associated with compromised splanchnic circulation. *Eur J Surg.* 1998:164;843-848.
51. Zupi E, Marconi D, Sbracia M, et al. Is local anesthesia an affordable alternative to general anesthesia for mini laparoscopy? *J Am Assoc Gynecol Laparosc.* 2000;7:111-114.
52. Rabey PG, et al. Effects of the laryngeal mask airway on lower oesophageal sphincter pressure in patients during general anesthesia. *Br J Anaesth.* 1992;69:346-348.
53. Jones MJ, Mitchess RW, Hindocha N. Effects of increased intra-abdominal pressure during laparoscopy on the lower esophageal sphincter. *Anesth Analg.* 1989;68:63-65.
54. Verghese C, Brimacombe JR. Survey of laryngeal mask airway usage in 11,910 patients: safety and efficacy for conventional and non-conventional usage. *Anesth Analg.* 1996;82:129-133.
55. Maltby JR, Beriault MT, Watson NC, Liepert DJ, Fick GH. LMA-Classic and LMA-ProSeal are effective alternatives to endotracheal intubation for gynecological laparoscopy. *Can J Anaesth.* 2003;50:71-77.
56. Brimacomb JR, Brain AIJ. *The Laryngeal Mask Airway. A Review and Practical Guide.* London: Saunders; 1996.
57. Taylor E, Feinstein R, White PF, Soper N. Anesthesia for laparoscopic cholecystectomy: is nitrous oxide contraindicated? *Anesthesiology.* 1992;76:541-543.
58. Krogh B, Jom Jensen P, Henneberg SW, Hole P, Kronborg O. Nitrous oxide does not influence operating conditions or postoperative course in colonic surgery. *Br J Anaesth.* 1996;72:55-57.
59. Michaloliakou C, Chung F, Sharma S. Preoperative multimodal analgesia facilitates recovery after ambulatory laparoscopic cholecystectomy. *Anesth Analg.* 1996;82:44-51.
60. Arellano RJ, Pole ML, Rafuse SE, et al. Omission of nitrous oxide from a propofol based anesthetic does not affect the recovery of women undergoing outpatient gynecologic surgery. *Anesthesiology.* 2000;93:332-339.
61. Sukhani R, Lurie J, Jabamoni R. Propofol for ambulatory gynecological laparoscopy: does omission of nitrous oxide alter postoperative sequelae and recovery? *Anesth Analg.* 1994;78:831-835.
62. Alexander JI. Pain after laparoscopy. *Br J Anesth.* 1997;79:369-378.
63. Mouton W, Bessell JR, Otten KT, Madden GJ. Pain after laparoscopy. *Surg Endosc.* 1999;13:445-448.
64. Moiniche S, Jorgensen H, Wetterslev J, Dahl JB. Local anesthetic infiltration for postoperative pain relief after laparoscopy. *Anesth Analg.* 2000;90:899-912.
65. Ballantyne GH. Robotic surgery, telerobotic surgery, telepresence and telementoring. Review of early clinical results. *Surg Endosc.* 2000;16:1389-1402.

CHAPTER 30

Musculoskeletal System: Anatomy, Physiology, and Pathophysiology

Mary C. Karlet

MUSCULOSKELETAL ANATOMY AND PHYSIOLOGY

Motor Unit

Somatic musculature is broadly classified into two compartments, skeletal or smooth, based on the muscles' anatomic and functional roles. Skeletal muscle is under voluntary control and is striated in appearance. Smooth muscle is found in most internal organs (except the heart), is under nonvoluntary autonomic control, and is nonstriated. The focus of this chapter is skeletal muscle, its function, and its neurologic control.

Skeletal muscle tissue includes muscles of the tongue and the soft palate, the extrinsic eye muscles, the muscles that move the scalp, all muscles attached to the skeleton, and the muscles in the pharynx and the upper one third of the esophagus. Some skeletal muscles, such as those of the lips and the anus, serve as sphincters. Skeletal muscle is innervated by myelinated efferent motor nerve fibers (α motor neurons). These fast-conducting somatic fibers arise from cell bodies located in the ventral horn of the spinal cord gray matter (Fig. 30-1).

The motor nerve axon exits through the spinal cord ventral root and travels uninterrupted to the muscle through a mixed peripheral nerve. Inputs to the motor nerve cell body are both excitatory and inhibitory. The inputs include neurons from the brain, neurons from other spinal cord segments, and afferent neurons from various sensory receptors (Fig. 30-2). A motor neuron fires an action potential when the sum of the excitatory and inhibitory inputs depolarizes the nerve cell body to its critical threshold potential. Threshold depolarization of the cell body produces local electrical currents that spread to adjoining regions of the nerve membrane, leading to depolarization and action potential propagation down the axon.

At the muscle, each motor nerve divides into branches that enter the muscle and end on individual muscle cells, called *muscle fibers*. A single motor neuron and all the muscle fibers it innervates are collectively called a *motor unit* (Fig. 30-3). When a motor nerve fires, all the fibers within a single motor unit contract simultaneously.

Motor units exhibit considerable variability and each unit usually contains between 100 and 200 muscle fibers. However, the motor unit may contain as few as two muscle fibers for fine, delicate movements or as many as a thousand for coarse movements.[1,2]

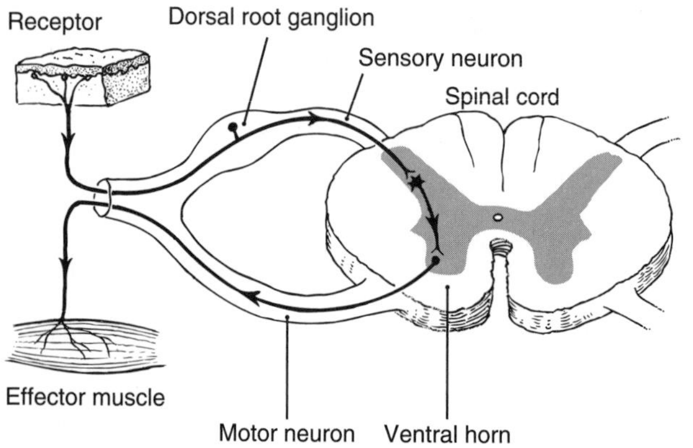

FIGURE **30-1**
Spinal reflex arc. Sensory information from the skin is relayed to the motor neuron in the ventral horn of the spinal cord gray matter.

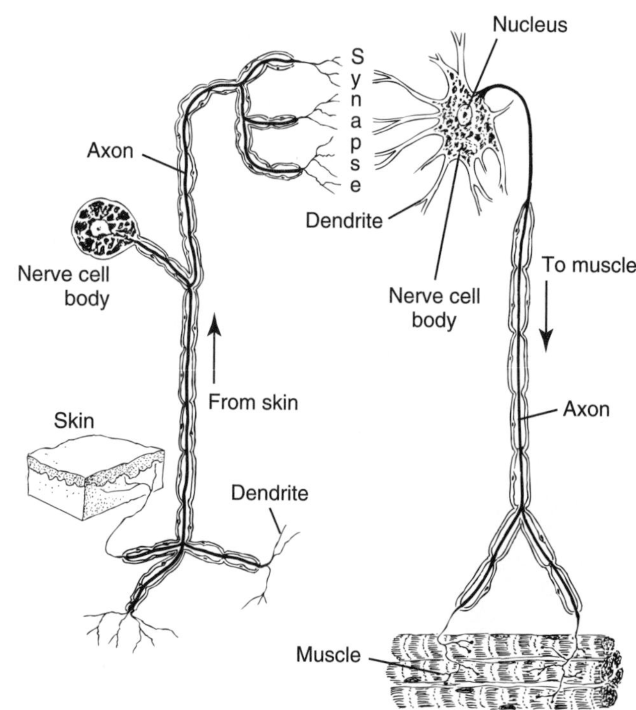

FIGURE **30-2**
A sensory neuron synapsing with a motor neuron.

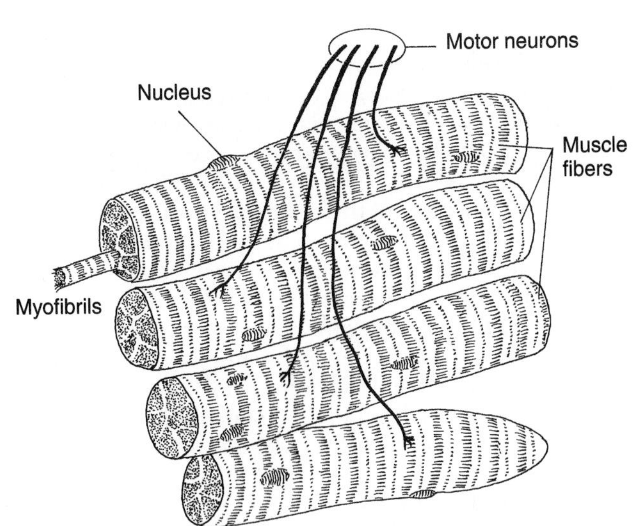

FIGURE **30-3**
A motor unit. One motor neuron can synapse with several muscle fibers, which contract as a unit.

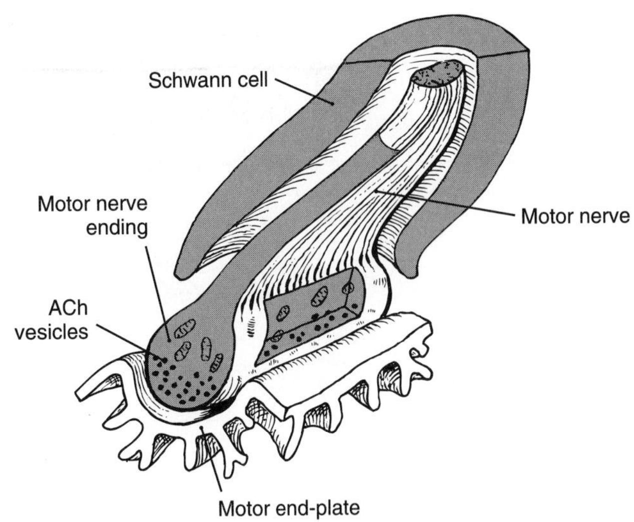

FIGURE **30-4**
A cross-section of the neuromuscular junction. A Schwann cell covers the motor nerve ending, which is nonmyelinated. Acetylcholine (ACh) vesicles aggregate close to the nerve membrane.

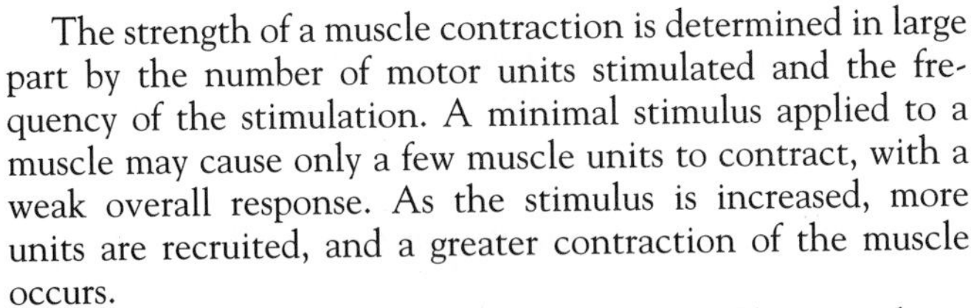

The strength of a muscle contraction is determined in large part by the number of motor units stimulated and the frequency of the stimulation. A minimal stimulus applied to a muscle may cause only a few muscle units to contract, with a weak overall response. As the stimulus is increased, more units are recruited, and a greater contraction of the muscle occurs.

Activation of nerve cell bodies in the ventral horn produces depolarization of the smallest motor units first. As the excitatory input into the motor neuron pool increases, larger motor units fire. The smaller motor units that are recruited first are resistant to fatigue. The larger motor units are less excitable, but they allow for more forceful contractions.[1,2]

Overview of Neuromuscular Transmission

Skeletal muscles are normally relaxed and do not contract without nervous stimulation. At rest, the electrical potential difference across the muscle membrane is approximately −90 mV (inside negative). There is a high potassium ion (K^+) concentration inside the muscle cell and a high sodium ion (Na^+) concentration outside the cell.

The process of muscle contraction begins when the electrical activity of a *presynaptic* motor neuron communicates across a *junctional cleft*, or *synaptic gap*, to *postsynaptic* skeletal muscle fibers. The specialized conduction area, or *synapse*, where the axon of a motor neuron ends on a skeletal muscle fiber is called the *neuromuscular junction*, or *myoneural junction* (Fig. 30-4). Each skeletal muscle fiber usually has only one neuromuscular junction, a notable exception being extraocular muscles that have multiple innervations per cell. The mediator substance that chemically transduces the axon's electrical message across the synaptic gap to the muscle is the neurotransmitter *acetylcholine* (ACh).[2,3]

Muscle contraction develops when the propagated action potential of the presynaptic motor neuron induces expulsion of the chemical mediator ACh into the junctional cleft. ACh binds to specialized receptors on the postsynaptic muscle membrane. If released from the axon nerve ending in sufficient quantity, ACh-receptor (AChR) occupation induces a transient change in the electrical property of the skeletal muscle membrane, and an action potential and muscle contraction follow.[2]

In the overall process of neuromuscular transmission, an action potential in the motor neuron induces the release of ACh into the junctional cleft, which evokes an action potential in the muscle, followed by muscle contraction.[4]

Neuromuscular Junction

Motor nerve endings develop in intimate and precise proximity to skeletal muscle. The motor axon terminal is separated from the muscle cell it innervates by a synaptic gap of only 20 to 50 nm. A carbohydrate-rich, filamentous material in the synapse holds the nerve ending and its associated muscle cell in close alignment. This anatomic alliance increases the likelihood for prompt receptor activation after transmitter release.[2,4]

The synaptic gap is contiguous with the extracellular fluid, which provides a route for drugs or toxins to gain access to the neuromuscular junction. Botulinum toxin, for example, gains access to the junction through the extracellular fluid and produces its depressive neuromuscular effects by inhibiting ACh release from the nerve ending.

Both sides of the neuromuscular junction, the presynaptic motor axon and the postsynaptic muscle cell, serve specialized functions (Fig. 30-5). As it nears the neuromuscular junction, the motor nerve axon loses its myelin sheath and divides into many smaller nerve fibers, which terminate as *end-feet*.

The motor nerve end-foot is distinct from the rest of the nerve. It is rich in mitochondria and the materials and support structures necessary for the synthesis, storage, mobilization, and release of the neurotransmitter ACh. Small clear vesicles or granules are particularly numerous in the part of the nerve ending closest to the junctional gap. Each of these vesicles contains a small packet, or *quantum*, of ACh molecules. The ACh vesicles concentrate along the junctional surface of the nerve end-feet in areas called "active zones."[4]

At the neuromuscular junction each motor nerve ending closely approximates with a thickened and highly convoluted portion of the postsynaptic membrane called the *motor end*

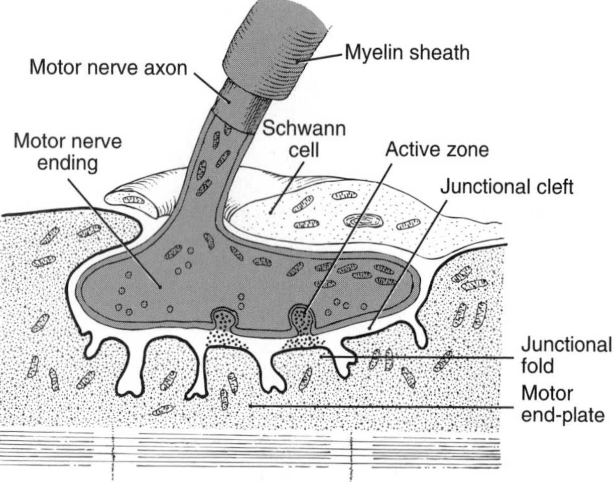

FIGURE **30-5**
A longitudinal view of the neuromuscular junction. Nerve ending "active zones" are located opposite the junctional folds of the motor end plate. The motor end plate is distinct from the muscle contractile machinery. At the active zones, the ACh vesicles are shown discharging their ACh into the junctional cleft.

plate. The motor end plate is physically and functionally demarcated from the surrounding muscle membrane. The many membrane convolutions at the end plate are known as *junctional folds*. ACh receptors are concentrated near the shoulders of the junctional folds. The receptors lie near the ACh release sites, which ensures little transmitter waste and direct coupling of nerve signal and muscle response.[5]

Acetylcholine Release

Physiologic transmission of the nerve message to the muscle begins with a calcium ion (Ca^{2+})–dependent mechanism for ACh release from the nerve terminal. When a nerve impulse arrives at a motor nerve ending, the action potential causes a transient increase in Ca^{2+} conductance by activating voltage-dependent Ca^{2+} channels in the nerve membrane. Both "fast" and "slow" Ca^{2+} channels appear to open, but it is primarily the fast ("N-type" and "P/Q-type") Ca^{2+} channels that are involved in depolarization-induced transmitter release.[6,7,8] Calcium enters the nerve terminal, flowing down its electrochemical gradient. The influx of Ca^{2+} causes ACh vesicles to fuse with the nerve plasma membrane, rupture, and then expel their content into the synaptic cleft.[9] The amount of ACh released is influenced by the amount of Ca^{2+} that enters the nerve terminal during nerve stimulation.

The number of ACh vesicles or quanta released with each nerve impulse is about 200 to 400. Each quantum in turn contains 2000 to 10,000 molecules of the neurotransmitter. This amount of ACh and the number of postjunctional receptors at each neuromuscular junction readily ensures muscle activation. A considerable safety margin exists in the synaptic transmission. With each nerve impulse, excess ACh is released and excess ACh receptors are available for occupation.[5,10,11]

Small concentrations of other divalent cations can limit Ca^{2+} influx into the nerve ending, decreasing ACh release and impairing neuromuscular transmission. When administered intravenously, magnesium sulfate, for example, can produce muscle weakness by inhibiting ACh release.[12]

Certain antibiotics, particularly the aminoglycosides, inhibit ACh release from the nerve terminal and can enhance neuromuscular blockade when administered concomitant with clinical dosages of neuromuscular blocking agents.

Calcium channel blockers block Ca^{2+} conductance through so-called "slow" ("L-type") channels. Their primary action is on the slow Ca^{2+} channels of the heart and blood vessels, but they can potentially inhibit prejunctional Ca^{2+} influx. The large safety margin inherent in normal neuromuscular transmission obscures any clinically detectable effect these drugs may have on neuromuscular transmission. However, with disorders associated with impaired neuromuscular transmission, such as myasthenia gravis, the Ca^{2+} channel blocker's prejunctional attenuation of ACh release may be unmasked, and neuromuscular transmission may be further weakened.[13]

Acetylcholine Synthesis

Neurons that release the neurotransmitter ACh are called *cholinergic neurons*. Active cholinergic motor neurons replenish their ACh stores by resynthesizing the neurotransmitter. Many enzymes and other proteins needed by the nerve ending to synthesize, store, and release ACh are made in the motor nerve cell body and are transported distally to the nerve ending by axonal transport.

In the axoplasm of the motor nerve ending, the enzyme *choline acetyltransferase* (CAT) catalyzes the reaction of two substrates, *acetyl coenzyme* A (acetyl CoA) and *choline*, to form ACh, as seen in Equation 30-1.

Equation 30-1

$$\text{Choline} + \text{Acetyl CoA} \xrightarrow{\text{CAT}} \text{Acetylcholine} + \text{CoA}$$

Choline is obtained locally by a Na^{+}-linked uptake into the cholinergic nerve ending. Acetyl CoA is synthesized from pyruvate in neuronal mitochondria. Mitochondria and other metabolic machinery used to synthesize ACh are abundant in the nerve ending (Fig. 30-6).

About 80% of the newly synthesized ACh is stored within synaptic vesicles at the nerve terminal, positioned for release. Each nerve ending contains more than 300,000 of these vesicles; the remainder of the ACh is stored in a nonvesicular axoplasmic reserve.[2]

The ACh vesicles are released through exocytosis in response to action potential stimulation, but only a small fraction of the available vesicles are used to send each signal.[2]

Postjunctional End Plate

The binding of ACh molecules to postsynaptic receptor proteins causes a transient increase in conductance in chemically gated cation channels at the postjunctional motor end plate. The cation flow at the end plate produces a net inward Na^{+} and Ca^{2+} current and a net outward K^{+} current. The previously polarized end plate membrane (resting membrane potential of approximately -90 mV) becomes transiently "depolarized." The resulting postjunctional membrane voltage change is called the *end plate potential* (EPP).[4]

The EPP does not begin until 0.5 milliseconds after the arrival of the action potential at the presynaptic nerve ending. This *synaptic delay* arises from the relatively slow liberation and diffusion of ACh across the junctional cleft.[2,4]

There is a distinction between the postjunctional cation channels of the muscle end plate and the cation channels of

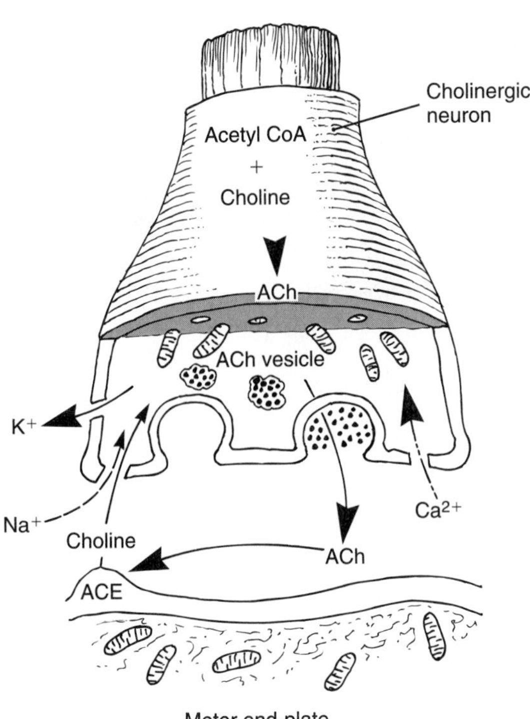

FIGURE **30-6**
ACh synthesis from choline and acetylcoenzyme A (acetyl CoA) in the motor nerve ending. Calcium ion entry into the nerve ending causes the ACh vesicles to release their contents. Acetylcholinesterase (ACE) on the postjunctional membrane destroys ACh. Choline is recycled into the nerve ending by a sodium ion–linked transport mechanism.

the nerve membrane. Motor end plate cation channels are gated (opened or closed) by the action of a chemical (i.e., the channels are ligand gated), whereas cation channels of nerves are gated by electrical changes in the membrane (i.e., the channels are voltage gated).[4]

EPPs vary in strength according to the quantity of ACh released. The more ACh released, the greater the postsynaptic end plate voltage change. In other words, EPPs do not adhere to the "all-or-none" principle. EPPs can be summed, and their magnitude depends on the strength of the summed stimuli (i.e., ACh).

With a typical motor neuron's action potential, the end plate potential produced at the muscle end plate is usually sufficient to create an action potential at the muscle membrane, and muscle contraction is regularly produced.

Perijunctional Area

The postjunctional end plate membrane does not fire action potentials. After it is depolarized by ACh-receptor occupation, the current sink created by the local EPP depolarizes the *adjacent* muscle membrane. If the depolarizing input is great enough (i.e., reaches threshold potential), action potentials are fired from either side of the end plate in both directions along the muscle fiber (Fig. 30-7).

The transition zone where the potential developed at the end plate is converted to an action potential is called the *perijunctional area.* A demarcation exists between the chemically sensitive AChR channels of the end plate and the chemically insensitive but electrically sensitive Na^+ channels in the perijunctional area of the muscle membrane. The membrane in the perijunctional area is rich in Na^+ channels, and this fea-

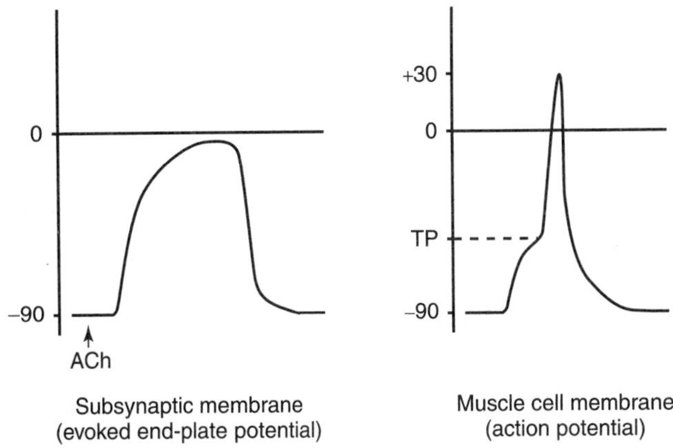

FIGURE **30-7**
Depiction of the depolarization characteristics (the end plate potential) at the postsynaptic membrane in response to ACh and the depolarization and action potential response at the adjacent, electrically excitable muscle membrane. *TP*, threshold potential.

ture enhances its capacity to respond to an end plate potential and transform it to an action potential.

Acetylcholine Receptor

Postjunctional neuromuscular ACh receptors have been extensively purified and studied in detail.[14] An estimated 50 million tightly packed nicotinic AChR sites are at each neuromuscular junction.

In fetal muscle, the ACh nicotinic receptor is a protein composed of five polypeptide subunits: two identical alpha (α) subunits, a beta (β) subunit, a gamma (γ) subunit, and a delta (δ) subunit.[15] Figure 30-8 shows the receptor subunits organized in a pentagonal array around a central ion channel. Without ACh occupation, the central channel is closed; when open, small cations are allowed to pass through the channel down their electrochemical gradients.

In adults, the AChR protein structure is unaltered, except that the fetal γ subunit is replaced by an epsilon (ϵ) subunit. The subunit's change produces an adult cholinergic receptor that has an increased cation conductance and a shortened open time.

As noted earlier, the ACh receptors are located at the crests of the motor end plate junctional folds, which approximate with nerve terminal release sites. In active adults, only the end

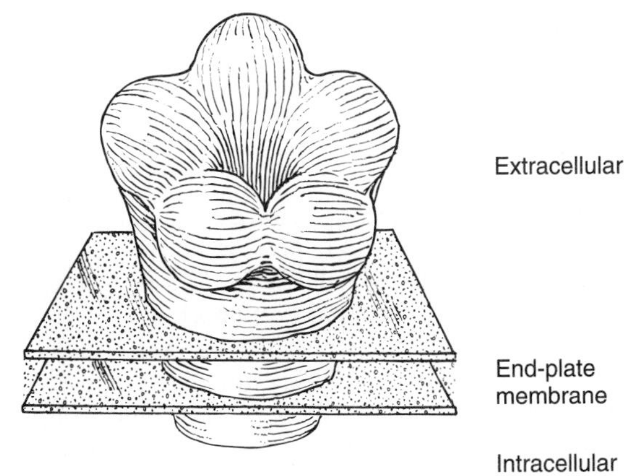

FIGURE **30-8**
The ACh receptor. Five polypeptide subunits surround a central ion channel.

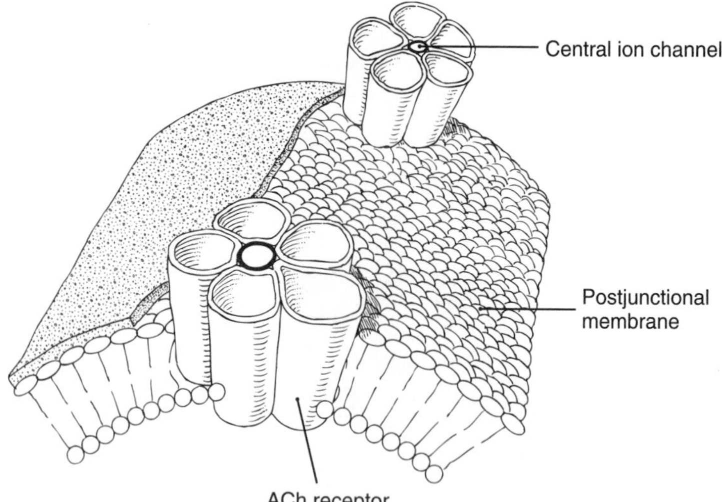

FIGURE **30-9**
Two ACh receptors embedded in the postjunctional membrane.

plate region of the muscle contains ACh receptors. As little as 200 μm away from the end plate, the muscle membrane becomes practically devoid of receptors.

The ACh receptors are synthesized in the muscle cells and then incorporated into the end plate membrane as integral membrane proteins. They are deeply embedded into the hydrophobic matrix of the muscle membrane. The extracellular or junctional face of the receptor protrudes from the surface of the end plate membrane; the cytoplasmic surface of the receptor is more flush to the plasma membrane surface (Fig. 30-9).

Activation of the postjunctional AChR and opening of the cation channel require simultaneous ACh occupation at each of the two α receptor subunits. If only one α subunit site is occupied by the agonist, the channel remains closed. The binding of two ACh molecules causes a conformational change in the α polypeptides, and the protein conformational change causes the central ion channel to open.[2] As described earlier, the open channel increases the conductance to cations, particularly Na^+, an effect that produces the net depolarizing potential, the EPP. When even one ACh molecule leaves the α subunit, the channel snaps shut and the current stops.

The α subunits are the sites of competition between the cholinergic agonist ACh and receptor antagonists, such as nondepolarizing neuromuscular blocking agents. The outcome of the competition, neuromuscular transmission or neuromuscular blockade, depends on the concentration of ACh and the relative concentration and binding properties of the antagonist involved.[3,12] Nondepolarizing muscle relaxants produce neuromuscular blockade, in part because they bind to one or both α subunit sites and, in so doing, prevent ACh from binding to both sites and opening the channel.

Prejunctional Receptors

Cholinergic receptors are also present at the prejunctional motor nerve ending. It is postulated that ACh, in addition to mediating nerve transmission at postjunctional receptor sites, also acts on prejunctional receptors to modulate its mobilization and release. Prejunctional cholinergic receptor occupation may transform the ACh pool from a reserve store to a readily releasable store so that transmitter output can keep pace with transmitter demand.[16]

All the nondepolarizing muscle relaxants used in anesthesia practice compete with ACh for postjunctional cholinergic receptor sites to produce neuromuscular blockade. Receptor antagonist effects at prejunctional receptors may augment nondepolarizing blockade by diminishing ACh output as well. Herein also lies an explanation for the *fade* that is observed with nondepolarizing muscle relaxation. Fade of tetanic and train-of-four stimulation may reflect the blockade of prejuctional ACh receptors by the muscle relaxant and failure of ACh release to keep pace with rapid stimulation.[17,18] This property of the nondepolarizer muscle relaxants is not entirely elucidated.

Acetylcholinesterase

As noted earlier, the combination of ACh with its muscle end plate receptor causes a transitory depolarization of the end plate. The end plate potential is short lived because the depolarizing action of ACh is quickly abated by the neurotransmitter's hydrolysis to choline and acetate.[4] The removal of ACh from the junctional cleft is critical for the continued muscle contractile response. The ACh must be off the muscle end plate receptor in order for the perijunctional muscle membrane to repolarize, or "reset," in anticipation of further activation.

The hydrolysis of ACh to choline and acetate is rapid and efficient (Equation 30-2). Most ACh is destroyed less than 1 millisecond after it is released into the junctional cleft. The enzyme *acetylcholinesterase*, also known as *true* or *tissue cholinesterase*, catalyzes the hydrolysis.

Equation 30-2

$$\text{Acetylcholine} \xrightarrow{\text{Acetylcholinesterase}} \text{Choline} + \text{Acetate}$$

Much of the choline released by hydrolysis is efficiently drawn back within the prejunctional nerve terminal for use in the synthesis of new ACh. Acetylcholinesterase is present in high concentrations on the external surface of the postjunctional membranes. The acetylcholinesterase protein is a localized, balloonlike structure and is loosely associated with the muscle end plate basement membrane by thin stalks of collagen.

Without acetylcholinesterase, the concentration of ACh would become extremely high in the junctional cleft. Under these circumstances, acetylcholine would maintain the muscle end plate in a state of persistent depolarization as ligand-gated cation channels remained open; yet paradoxically, the muscle itself would be paralyzed.[3] The reason for this seemingly illogical behavior (ACh-receptor occupation, end plate depolarization, yet no muscle contraction) is that in the face of persistent end plate depolarization, the Na^+ channels of the perijunctional muscle membrane do not reactivate or reset; these membrane ion channels remain closed, prohibiting muscle membrane depolarization. Thus, even with persistent end plate depolarization, muscle contraction is prohibited, and clinical weakness follows. A cyclic muscle membrane depolarization/repolarization sequence is necessary for normal muscle contraction to occur.

The mechanism of depolarizing muscle relaxants can, at least in part, be explained by a similar mechanism. Depolarizing muscle relaxants, such as succinylcholine, activate the muscle end plate in a manner similar to that of ACh, but they have a more protracted end plate depolarizing response because they are less rapidly metabolized. AChR occupation by a depolarizing muscle relaxant causes a prolonged depolarization of the end plate, prohibits activation of perijunctional channels, and produces a depolarizing block.[3,12]

Reversal of a nondepolarizing neuromuscular block may be accomplished by the use of cholinesterase inhibitors. Anticholinesterase agents inhibit the breakdown of ACh and, in so doing, increase the amount of ACh at the neuromuscular junction. The abundance of ACh in the synaptic gap changes the agonist-antagonist ratio and enables the agonist (ACh) to bind to the ACh receptor with a greater frequency than the antagonist (nondepolarizing muscle relaxant). Hence, a higher ACh concentration can overcome the receptor occupation by the muscle relaxant, and neuromuscular transmission can be restored (see Chapter 11, Neuromuscular Blocking Agents, Reversal Agents, and Their Monitoring).

Various other esterases, in addition to acetylcholinesterase, are present throughout the body. One that is found in the plasma is *pseudocholinesterase*, or *nonspecific cholinesterase*. Like acetylcholinesterase, pseudocholinesterase is capable of hydrolyzing ACh, but it also has properties distinct from those of acetylcholinesterase. One distinction from acetylcholinesterase that is particularly relevant to anesthesia practice is the ability of pseudocholinesterases to metabolize the depolarizing muscle relaxant succinylcholine and the nondepolarizing relaxant mivacurium chloride.

Extrajunctional Receptors

In utero, before muscle innervation occurs, the muscle cells of a fetus synthesize *extrajunctional receptors*. These fetal receptors are inserted over the entire length of the muscle cell. As the fetal neuromuscular junction develops, increasing motor nerve activity appears to have a trophic effect in restricting the ACh receptors specifically to the neuromuscular junction.[11,12] By the age of 2 years, the nerve-muscle contact is fully mature and active, and the extrajunctional receptors disappear from the peripheral part of the muscle. If neural activity is reduced or abolished and the neural trophic influence is lost, the muscle resorts to fetal-like synthesis of extrajunctional cholinergic receptors.[15]

Several situations, including stroke, spinal cord transection, thermal trauma, direct muscle damage, and prolonged immobility, have been associated with the accelerated spread of cholinergic receptors from the end plate region to large areas of the skeletal muscle membrane. These so-called *denervation injuries* result in an abnormal excitability of the muscle and an increase in muscle sensitivity to ACh, a condition that is called *denervation hypersensitivity*.[2] The extrajunctional receptors may develop within 48 hours after diminution of nerve activity. Eventually, the number of aberrant receptors per muscle fiber may increase 5- to 32-fold.[15,19] These receptors disappear and the muscle sensitivity returns to normal if neural input is reestablished. Extrajunctional and end plate cholinergic receptors are similar in many ways, but an important distinction that is pertinent to anesthesia practice is their differing response to receptor agonists and antagonists.[15]

Clinically, extrajunctional receptors demonstrate a resistance to nondepolarizing muscle relaxants. Hence, larger doses of nondepolarizing relaxants may be necessary to induce neuromuscular blockade—for example, in an immobilized limb or in parts of the body affected by a stroke.[15,20,21] Monitoring a nondepolarizing neuromuscular block with a peripheral nerve stimulator in a paretic limb may result in an underestimation of the magnitude of neuromuscular blockade in nonparetic muscles.[20]

Conversely, extrajunctional receptors are more easily activated by agonists, such as ACh or succinylcholine, than are junctional receptors. Moreover, each extrajunctional channel stays open about four times longer than junctional receptors, allowing more ions to flow (primarily Na^+ into the muscle cell and K^+ out) in response to agonist-induced depolarization.[22]

The clinical significance of denervation injuries and the proliferation of extrajunctional receptors becomes evident with the administration of succinylcholine, which can produce alarmingly high levels of plasma K^+ in these patients.[23] Succinylcholine-induced hyperkalemia reflects the extensive proliferation of extrajunctional receptors along the entire muscle membrane and their prolonged and exaggerated depolarization response to agonists. Succinylcholine stimulates the aberrant cholinergic receptors; triggers a protracted opening of the cation channels; and admits excess Na^+ movement into the cell and excess K^+ movement out, down their respective gradients.

Dangerous levels of succinylcholine-induced hyperkalemia have been observed within 4 days of denervation injury with doses of succinylcholine as low as 20 mg. The pronounced release of K^+ in response to succinylcholine cannot be circumvented by the prior administration of nonparalyzing doses of nondepolarizing muscle relaxants.

Muscle Physiology

Skeletal muscle constitutes the greatest mass of somatic musculature. Skeletal muscle is composed of bundles of multinucleated, long, cylindrical cells; because their length is much greater than their width, these cells are called *muscle fibers*. Each muscle fiber is a single cell surrounded by an electrically polarized cell membrane, the *sarcolemma*, which separates the extracellular space from the *myoplasm* or intracellular space of the muscle fiber.

Individual skeletal muscle cells are parallel to the muscle body and have no anatomic or functional bridges between them. The parallel arrangement helps maximize shortening capacity and velocity. The cells function independently so that the force of contraction of the total muscle is equal to the sum of individual fibers. This contrasts with smooth and cardiac muscle, in which the muscle cells are interdependent and are mechanically coupled to adjacent cells.[1,2,24]

Bundles of cylindrical filaments, called *myofibrils*, run along the axis of the muscle fiber. Each muscle fiber contains several hundred myofibrils, which are composed of contractile proteins that impart a striking, repetitive, light and dark banding pattern along the entire fiber length. The repeating unit, called a *sarcomere*, is the basic contractile unit of the skeletal muscle. The alternating light and dark banding pattern is responsible for the classification called *striated muscle*. Cardiac muscle is also classified as striated muscle because it also has the repetitive pattern of light and dark bands.[24] The arrangement of the muscle fibers, myofibrils, and sarcomeres is diagrammed in Figure 30-10.

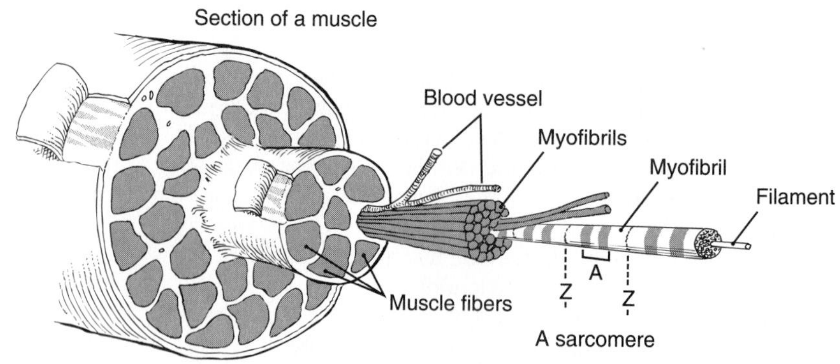

FIGURE **30-10**
The structural arrangement and organization at each level of the muscle assembly. The skeletal muscle is composed of muscle fibers that contain long, cylindrical myofibrils. Each myofibril is made up of precisely arranged thick and thin filaments that form repeating dark and light bands called *sarcomeres*.

Most skeletal muscles bridge two skeletal attachment points and are recruited to generate force and movement in actions ranging from chewing to walking. A muscle contraction that involves shortening of the muscle length to perform work is an *isotonic contraction*; a muscle contraction that produces an increased tension but no appreciable decrease in length is an *isometric contraction*.

Structure of the Contractile Apparatus

The repeating, striated arrangement of the myofibril arises from the contractile filaments that compose the sarcomere: the *thick filaments* and the *thin filaments*.

The thick filaments, which are composed of the protein *myosin*, are in the central region of the sarcomere in a dark-colored area termed the *A band*. A densely staining *M line* in the middle of the A band contains proteins that link the thick filaments. The thin filaments are about half the diameter of the thick filaments and are composed of the proteins actin, troponin, and tropomyosin. Thin filaments, connected to *Z lines* or *Z disks*, normally interdigitate with the thick filaments in the relaxed muscle and to an even greater degree in the contracted muscle. The less dense areas of the sarcomere, which contain only thin filaments, are referred to as *I bands*. Two adjacent Z lines delimit each repeating sarcomere unit. The diagram of the sarcomere units in Figure 30-11 may warrant careful study.

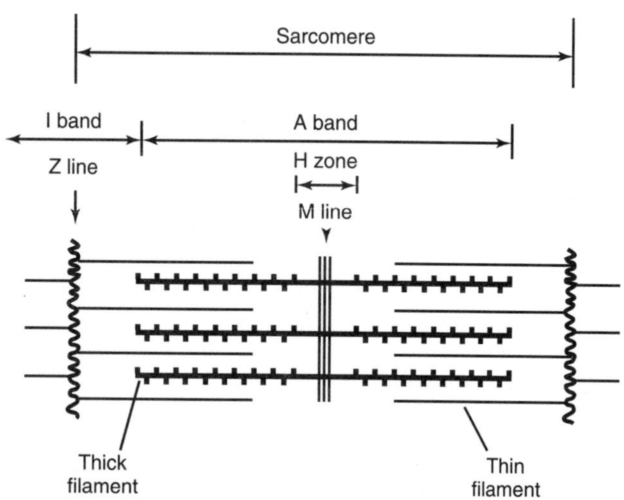

FIGURE **30-11**
Longitudinal diagram of a sarcomere showing the arrangement of the thick filaments (myosin) and the thin filaments (primarily actin). (Redrawn from Squire JM: *The Structural Basis of Muscular Contraction*, New York, 1981, Plenum Press.)

Cross-sections of the myofibril reveal that each thick filament is surrounded by a hexagonal arrangement of six thin filaments. The myosin and actin filaments are arranged to slide over one another, overlap, and create shortening of the sarcomere and the muscle.[2,24] (Fig. 30-12).

Thin Filament. The three major proteins that compose the thin filament, (1) actin, (2) tropomyosin, and (3) troponin, each play a different role in the contractile process. Each thin filament includes two beadlike chains of polymerized *actin* twisted into a double helix. About 40 to 60 *tropomyosin* molecules are located along the groove between the two actin chains. Each rod-shaped tropomyosin molecule covers about six or seven individual actin proteins. The most important protein in the regulation of the contractile process is *troponin*.[24] As depicted in Figure 30-13, one molecule of troponin is bound to each tropomyosin molecule.

Thick Filament. Myosin, the primary protein component of the thick filament, is a very large protein containing three pairs of polypeptides: one pair of heavy chains and two pairs of light chains. The six different polypeptides assemble to form the myosin protein, and each protein contains a long tail with two globular heads.

The tail regions of several hundred myosin molecules aggregate to form one thick filament. The globular heads laterally project out from the thick filament at regular intervals toward the six thin filaments surrounding it. In the relaxed muscle, the myosin heads are oriented toward but are not attached to the thin filaments. The thick filament's globular projections are termed *cross-bridges* because they can link the thick and the thin filaments. The cross-bridges in each half of the sarcomere

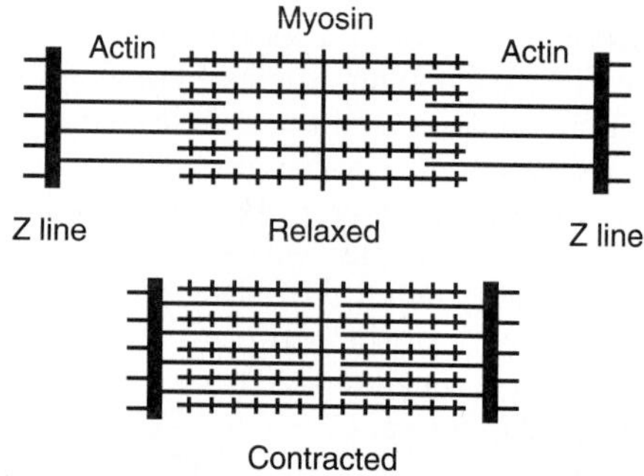

FIGURE **30-12**
Sliding of the actin filament over the myosin filament during muscle contraction. (Redrawn from Ganong WF: Excitable tissue: muscle. In Ganong WF, editor: *Review of Medical Physiology*, ed 17, Stamford, Connecticut, 1991, Appleton & Lange.)

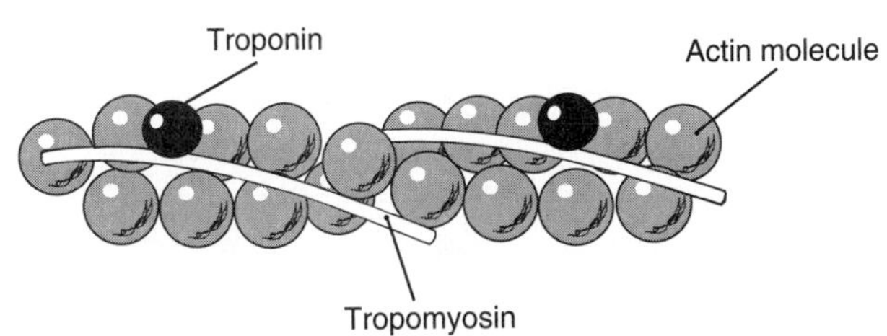

FIGURE **30-13**
A thin filament. Globular actin molecules polymerize into a two-stranded, twisted filament. Rod-shaped tropomyosin molecules occupy the grooves between the two actin chains. The regulatory protein troponin binds to the tropomyosin component.

are oriented in opposite directions away from the midpoint of the filament, which is important for their functional role in sarcomere shortening and muscle contraction.[24] The cross-bridge components are arranged as shown in Figure 30-14.

The myosin head and tail have a jointlike attachment, permitting a certain degree of movement. When muscle contraction is activated and myosin and actin link, the ability of the myosin head to swivel enables the attached actin filaments to slide over the thick myosin filaments (Fig. 30-15).

Cross-Bridge Interaction and Cycling

Sliding Filament Mechanism. Physiologic contraction of striated muscle occurs when muscle fibers are depolarized to a mechanical threshold for action potential formation. The excited muscle then transforms the chemical energy stored in adenosine triphosphate (ATP) directly into mechanical energy. The depolarizing wave initiated by AChR occupation at the motor end plate is carried along the muscle membrane surface from one Na^+ channel to the next. Action potential depolarization of the sarcolemma spreads rapidly to the muscle cell's interior through a reticular network of intracellular tubules that are contiguous with the cell membrane.

This network, composed of *transverse tubules* or *T tubules*, forms a grid around the intracellular myofibrils and closely associates with the intracellular sarcoplasmic reticular membranes. The T tubules rapidly transmit the action potential from the sarcolemma to the myoplasm.

The *sarcoplasmic reticulum* is an irregular, closed membrane structure that weaves throughout the myoplasm of the muscle cell and contains large amounts of Ca^{2+}. The sarcoplasmic reticular membrane is active in sequestering Ca^{2+} by way of numerous high-affinity Ca^{2+} active transport carriers in its membrane. These pumps maintain a high sarcoplasmic reticular store of Ca^{2+} and a very low resting myoplasmic Ca^{2+} concentration.[2,24]

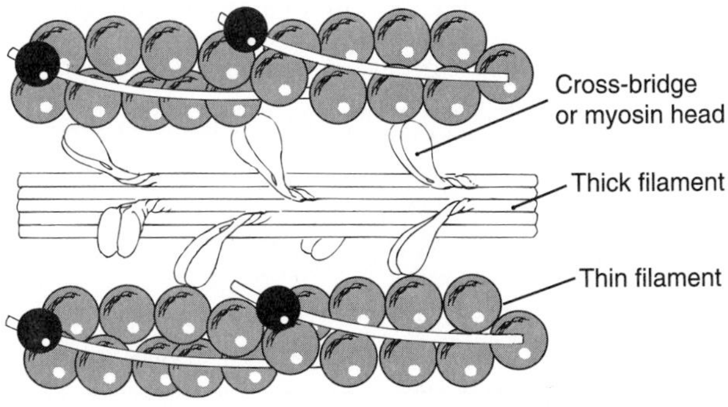

FIGURE **30-14**
The tail regions of many myosin molecules intertwine to form a thick filament. The myosin heads, or cross-bridges, project out laterally toward the actin in the surrounding thin filaments.

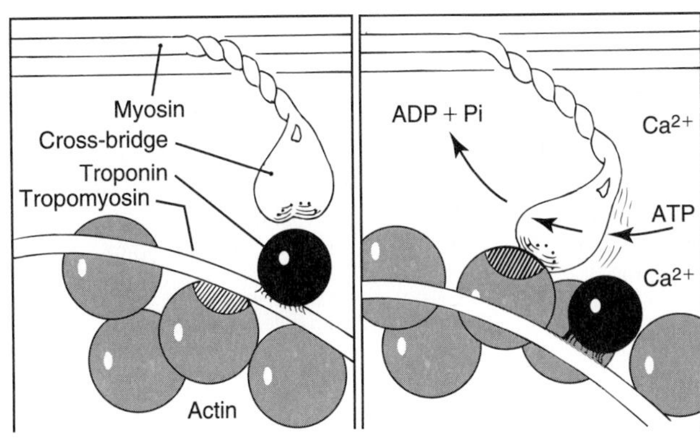

FIGURE **30-15**
Formation of the actomyosin complex. Hydrolysis of adenosine triphosphate (ATP) leads to tipping of the myosin heads. *ADP*, adenosine diphosphate; *P*, phosphate.

The transit of an action potential along the sarcolemma and into the T-tubule system is detected by voltage sensors, which trigger Ca^{2+} efflux from the sarcoplasmic reticular stores into the myoplasm. The myoplasmic Ca^{2+} concentration rises several fold from a resting value of less than 0.1 mmol. The overall effect is the discharge of Ca^{2+} into the myoplasm by the transit of an action potential.

The Ca^{2+} released into the myoplasm binds to troponin, which acts as a switch that changes the conformation of the tropomyosin to which it is bound. The conformational change in the rod-shaped tropomyosin exposes myosin binding sites on the underlying actin. The myosin heads react by binding to the exposed thin filament sites, forming a reversible complex with actin—the *actomyosin complex*. The process of myosin-actin binding in response to elevated myoplasmic Ca^{2+} is *cross-bridge formation*.[24]

The myosin filaments' heads contain not only an actin binding site but also a catalytic adenosine triphosphatase (ATPase) site that hydrolyzes ATP to adenosine diphosphate (ADP) and phosphate. Binding of a myosin head with an actin molecule is associated with ATP hydrolysis and energy release. ATP is essential for the sliding of the filaments and for muscle contraction. The energy yielded by the ATP breakdown is harnessed to tilt the myosin heads, which draws the thin actin filaments with them. The pull of the actin filaments accentuates the overlap of the thick and thin filaments, causes the shortening of the sarcomere, and culminates in muscle contraction (Fig. 30-16).

The actomyosin complex is stable and can be broken only by a renewed binding of ATP to each myosin head. With the binding of ATP, the actomyosin cross-bridge dissociates, and the myosin heads are repositioned for another round of cross-bridge formation. If the intracellular Ca^{2+} concentration is still sufficiently high, which mainly depends on the frequency of incoming action potentials, the cycle begins again: myosin links to actin, swivels, detaches, and reconnects at the next actin site.

A single sliding cycle or myosin "rowing stroke" shortens the sarcomere's length by 1%, causing the entire muscle fiber, which consists of a serial arrangement of sarcomeres, to also shorten by 1%. The sliding cycle has to be repeated about 50 times for full shortening of the muscle. The cycle continues until it is interrupted by the active removal of Ca^{2+} from the

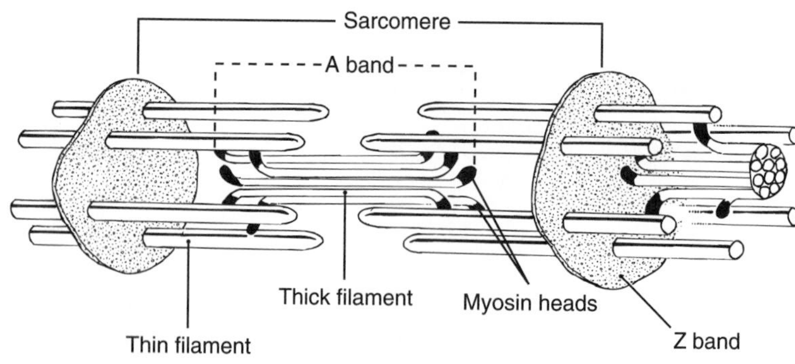

FIGURE **30-16**
The basic contractile unit. The myosin heads at each end of the thick filament are oriented in opposite directions. With cross-bridge formation, tilting of the myosin heads pulls the thin filaments along with them and causes sarcomere shortening.

myoplasm or until the ATP is exhausted. Active Ca^{2+} removal from the cytoplasm back into the sarcoplasmic reticulum causes troponin, tropomyosin, and actin to return to a configuration that prohibits myosin binding, and the muscle relaxes.

The overall process by which depolarization of the muscle fiber causes Ca^{2+} release from the sarcoplasmic reticulum into the myoplasm to cause cross-bridge cycling is called *excitation-contraction coupling*.

Box 30-1 summarizes the excitation-contraction coupling events. Box 30-2 summarizes the events leading to skeletal muscle relaxation.

Grading Contractile Force. Two major mechanisms grade skeletal muscle contractile force. One determining factor of muscle force is the number of motor units activated or recruited. With increasing voluntary effort, more and more motor units are recruited, and an increasing muscle force develops.[24]

The other mechanism by which skeletal muscle tension is graded is by varying the frequency of the action potential discharge to the muscle. A single action potential invariably liberates sufficient Ca^{2+} ions to activate skeletal muscle contraction. However, the Ca^{2+} ions are rapidly transported back into the sarcoplasmic reticulum before the muscle has time to develop maximal tension. The brief contraction that results from a single action potential is called a *twitch*.[2]

Unlike cardiac muscle, skeletal muscle does not have a refractory period. Because of this property, rapidly repeated electrical impulses can cause summation of contractions and greatly increase the muscle tension. Repetitive action potentials maintain a high Ca^{2+} concentration in the myoplasm. The greater the myoplasmic Ca^{2+} concentration, the more cross-bridge sites exposed and the stronger the force of the contraction. Maximal and sustained muscle tension, without relaxation, produced by the fusion and summation of successive twitch responses is a *tetanus*.[2]

Figure 30-17 shows the time course and the relationship between a single action potential, the myoplasmic Ca^{2+} rise, and the resulting twitch response. The action potential lasts about 2 to 4 milliseconds. The twitch begins about 2 milliseconds after the start of the muscle membrane depolarization; the duration of the twitch varies with the type of muscle stimulated.

BOX **30-1**

Outline of Neurohumoral Transmission and Excitation-Contraction Coupling

An action potential reaches the motor nerve ending.
Ca^{2+} enters the nerve ending; ACh is released into the synaptic cleft.
ACh binds to a postsynaptic cholinergic receptor at the motor end plate.
The motor end plate membrane depolarizes (the EPP); depolarization spreads to the surrounding muscle membrane.
An action potential is generated at the perijunctional muscle membrane; the action potential spreads along the muscle membrane and inward to the transverse tubules.
Depolarization of the T tubules causes Ca^{2+} release from the sarcoplasmic reticulum.
Ca^{2+} triggers actomyosin complex cross-bridge formation; the sarcomere shortens; the muscle contracts.

Ach, *acetylcholine;* EPP, *end plate potential;* T, *transverse*.

BOX **30-2**

Outline of Skeletal Muscle Relaxation

ACh is hydrolyzed by acetylcholinesterase in the synaptic cleft.
The end plate and muscle membrane repolarize to their resting potentials.
Ca^{2+} is actively pumped back into the sarcoplasmic reticulum.
The muscle relaxes.

Slow Versus Fast Muscle

Skeletal muscle fibers are classified as type I ("slow fibers") or type II ("fast fibers"). Different myosin isoenzymes distinguish the two types. The two fiber types differ in their metabolic demands, their myosin ATPase activity, and their cross-bridge cycling rates. Muscles usually contain a mixture of both types of fibers, but one type often predominates.[25]

Slow (type I) muscle fibers are adapted for powerful, gross, sustained movements, such as maintaining posture. They have

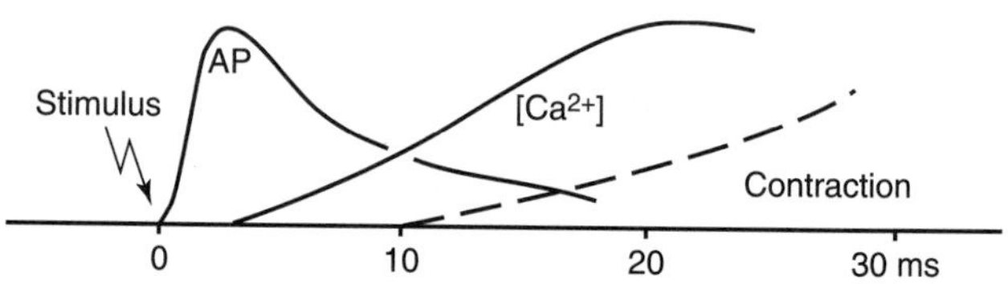

FIGURE **30-17**
The electrical, ionic, and mechanical responses of a skeletal muscle to a single maximal stimulus. *AP*, action potential.

twitch durations of up to 100 milliseconds and have relatively modest metabolic demands.[2] Type I muscle is called "red" muscle because its high myoglobin content imparts a dark, rubrous color.

Fast (type II) muscle fibers usually predominate in "white" muscle and are primarily concerned with rapid and precise movement. They have twitch durations as short as 7.5 milliseconds and are easily fatigued. Muscles specialized for fine, skilled movement, such as extraocular muscles and some muscles of the hand, are in this category.

Infants have a tendency toward respiratory failure in part because only 25% of their diaphragm is composed of type I fatigue-resistant fibers, compared to 50% in the adult. Before 37 weeks' gestational age, type I fibers make up less than 10% of the total diaphragm muscle content.[25]

Energy Sources for Skeletal Muscle

Muscle contraction requires a continual supply of energy at a rate proportionate to its energy consumption.[24] The energy consumed by skeletal muscle is used for cross-bridge cycling during muscle contraction, sarcoplasmic reticular resequestration of Ca^{2+} during muscle relaxation, rephosphorylation of creatine to replenish creatine phosphate energy stores, and resynthesis of muscle glycogen.

Muscle cells derive energy from three basic metabolic systems: (1) creatine phosphate hydrolysis, (2) anaerobic glycolysis, and (3) aerobic glycolysis and oxidative phosphorylation.

Creatine Phosphate. The energy-rich phosphate bonds in muscle creatine phosphate supply a limited amount of energy. The anaerobic hydrolysis of creatine phosphate to creatine and phosphate is an extremely rapid reaction. The high-energy phosphate product is directly transferred to ADP, which generates a rapid source of ATP energy. Creatine phosphate provides a stored source of energy that is used at the very beginning of muscle contraction while other, more sustainable, energy-regenerating systems are being turned on.[24]

Anaerobic Glycolysis. With intense muscle exertion, muscle oxygen consumption may outpace oxygen supply. When the oxygen supply is inadequate, muscles meet their energy demands from a process called *anaerobic glycolysis*, the metabolism of glucose or glycogen to lactate. Anaerobic glycolysis is a rapid process, but it has a relatively small ATP yield and is limited by the cellular stores of glycogen, which can be quickly depleted. Additionally, the accumulation of lactate in the muscle produces an enzyme-inhibiting acidosis and causes the anaerobic pathway to be self-limiting.[2]

Aerobic Glycolysis and Oxidative Phosphorylation. When adequate glucose and oxygen are available to skeletal muscle, the breakdown of glucose to pyruvate generates energy. This process is called *aerobic glycolysis*. In the presence of oxygen, pyruvate enters the mitochondrial citric acid cycle, liberating CO_2, water, and energy-rich ATP.

When glucose is scarce but oxygen is still plentiful, the skeletal muscle takes up free fatty acids, or other substrates such as amino acids or ketone bodies, and efficiently oxidizes them to CO_2, water, and ATP in the muscle fiber mitochondria; this is an energy-yielding process called *oxidative phosphorylation*. The oxidation of free fatty acids is a slow process, but it is usually sufficient to meet the more modest energy demands of the most frequently used skeletal muscle. Free fatty acids are the primary energy substrate for most skeletal muscle.[2,24]

MUSCULOSKELETAL PATHOPHYSIOLOGY AND ANESTHESIA

Musculoskeletal diseases have a wide variety of causes, ranging from autoimmune destruction of tissue to genetically determined defects in muscle membrane protein to pharmacologically induced alterations in calcium (Ca^{2+}) metabolism. Musculoskeletal defects may reside in the neuromuscular junction, the muscle infrastructure, or the skeletal support structures.

Understanding the pathophysiologic characteristics of the disease, the clinical presentation, and the supporting laboratory studies is essential for the safe management of the anesthesia for patients with musculoskeletal abnormalities. A thorough preoperative assessment of the patient helps determine the extent of muscle, respiratory, and cardiac reserve and aids in the anesthetic selection and the planning for postoperative care.

Management of cases of musculoskeletal pathology must take into account preoperative drug therapy for the disease and the potential impact that the drug therapy may have on anesthetic agents and muscle relaxants. The anesthetic agents' margin of safety is often reduced in these patients; therefore, fixed dosage regimens should be avoided.

MYASTHENIA GRAVIS

Myasthenia gravis, a chronic disease of the neuromuscular junction, is manifested by increasing skeletal muscle weakness, fatigability on effort, and at least partial restoration of function after rest.

Incidence

In the United States at least 1 in 7500 people have myasthenia gravis. In individuals younger than 50 years, the ratio of women to men with the disease is 3:2; however, in those older than 50 years, the disease is equally distributed between the sexes. Myasthenia gravis can begin spontaneously at any age, but it occurs most frequently at about the age of 30 years. The onset may be abrupt or insidious, and the course is fluctuating, marked by periods of exacerbation and remission.[26] Spontaneous remissions that do occur sometimes persist for years.

Pathophysiology

Electron microscopic examination of the neuromuscular junction of the patient with myasthenia gravis shows a decrease in the number of functional postsynaptic ACh receptors. The AChR lesion appears to be caused by immune-mediated destruction, blockage, or inactivation. The prejunctional ACh pool is normal.[26]

Myasthenia gravis is a prototype autoimmune disease. Circulating antibodies react with myoneural AChR proteins, leading to varying degrees of dysfunction. Anti-AChR antibodies are found in the sera of 85% to 90% of patients with myasthenia gravis, but the antibody level does not necessarily correlate with severity of disease.[27,28,29] Most patients in clinical remission continue to show elevated serum levels of AChR antibodies.

The initiating stimulus for the production of antiAChR IgG antibodies is still unclear. A genetic cause or induction by microbial antigens has been postulated. The thymus gland seems to play a central role in the pathogenesis.[27,28,29]

Pregnancy exacerbates the symptoms of myasthenia gravis in 40% of pregnant women with the disease; however, other patients with this disease experience remission or no change in symptoms during pregnancy.[30] Anti-AChR antibodies that pass across the placenta may produce transitory symptoms of weakness in approximately 15% of infants born to mothers with myasthenia gravis. Signs of weakness (e.g., difficulty with breathing, ptosis, facial weakness) in the affected infant are usually present within the first few hours after birth. The condition lasts as long as 21 days, mirroring the half-life of the IgG antibodies.[27,29]

Clinical Manifestations

The clinical hallmarks of myasthenia gravis include a generalized muscle weakness, which improves with rest, and an inability to sustain or repeat muscular contractions. Enhanced effort produces enhanced weakness. The severity of myasthenia gravis can range from mild (slight ptosis only) to severe (respiratory failure). Environmental, physical, and emotional factors seem to affect the disease process, although unpredictably.[30]

Mouth, eyes, pharynx, proximal limb, and shoulder girdle musculature are most often affected. Visual symptoms (ptosis and diplopia) from extraocular muscle weakness occur in more than 50% of patients with myasthenia gravis.[28] The disease is restricted to the extraocular muscles in 20% of patients. Sensation and cognition are not affected by the disease process.[29]

Thymus gland abnormalities are detectable in about 75% of patients with myasthenia gravis.[29] Autoimmune disorders, such as thyroid disease, collagen vascular diseases, polymyositis, and rheumatoid arthritis, occur more frequently in patients with myasthenia gravis.[27,29]

Myocarditis may complicate myasthenia gravis, especially in patients with thymomas. Microscopic lesions of myasthenic cardiac muscles are similar to skeletal muscle lesions, indicating a common pathogenesis. The myocardial inflammation produces dysrhythmias, particularly atrial fibrillation and atrioventricular block.[31]

Treatment

Therapy for patients with myasthenia gravis is directed toward improving neuromuscular transmission and includes cholinesterase inhibitors, corticosteroids and other immunosuppressants, plasmapheresis, intravenous immunoglobulin, and thymectomy.[27,30]

Treatment with cholinesterase inhibitors can dramatically reduce the symptoms of myasthenia gravis by inhibiting the hydrolysis of ACh and therefore increasing the neurotransmitter's concentration at the neuromuscular junction. Increasing the synaptic concentration of ACh enhances the possibility of postsynaptic AChR occupation, which is critical for the production of a threshold-reaching end plate potential for muscle contraction. Anticholinesterase treatment is particularly successful in patients with milder disease.[26] The most commonly used anticholinesterase agent in the United States is oral pyridostigmine. A 60-mg oral dose of pyridostigmine lasts 3 to 4 hours and is equivalent to an intramuscular or intravenous dose of 2 mg of pyridostigmine or 1 mg of neostigmine.[32]

Titration of the anticholinesterase dose is challenging. Underdosing does not sufficiently retard the muscle weakness and can result in *myasthenic crisis*, a severe exacerbation of myasthenic symptoms. Overmedicating with a cholinesterase inhibitor can produce a surplus of ACh at the myoneural junction, causing a depolarizing block and augmenting skeletal muscle weakness. This situation is called *cholinergic crisis*. Muscarinic side effects (e.g., abdominal cramping, diarrhea, salivation, bradycardia, and miosis) predominate in a cholinergic crisis.

Corticosteroid therapy produces an 80% remission rate in patients with myasthenia gravis, in part by reducing AChR antibody levels. The use of steroid therapy is limited by the severe side effects (e.g., osteoporosis, gastrointestinal bleeding, suppression of endogenous cortisol release, cataracts, increased susceptibility to acute infections, hypertension, and glucose intolerance) observed with long-term administration.

In patients with more debilitating, widespread disease, the antimetabolite azathioprine (Imuran) may induce remission by interfering with the production of AChR antibodies.[26] Side effects of azathioprine include severe hemopoietic depression; infection; and, in rare cases, malignancy.

Excision of the thymus gland is recommended for adults with generalized disease and for patients with thymomas, thymus gland hyperplasia, or drug-resistant myasthenia gravis.[28,29] Thymectomy effectively arrests or reverses the myasthenic process by removing a major source of antibody production. Clinical improvement of myasthenic symptoms is seen in 75% to 96% of patients within weeks to months after surgery.[32]

Plasmapheresis (plasma exchange) arrests severe refractive myasthenia gravis by reducing the concentration of circulating antibodies. It is used primarily as a short-term treatment because the improvement that it produces in symptoms is generally short lived. Intravenous immunoglobulin may also be used for short-term control of symptoms prior to surgery.[26,27]

Anesthetic Implications

Several days before the operation and again immediately prior to surgery, the surgical candidate with myasthenia gravis should be evaluated for disease control and, if applicable, for stabilization of anticholinesterase dose.

The use of anticholinesterase medication in the immediate preoperative period is controversial.[33,34,35,36] Some experts feel that an awareness of drug mechanisms can enable anticholinesterase therapy to be safely continued into the preoperative period, especially in patients who depend on this therapy for their well-being. Others recommend discontinuing or tapering anticholinesterase medication before surgery in order to avoid complicating the anesthetic management. Patients with mild myasthenia gravis can usually tolerate the temporary disruption in treatment.[34]

The presence of cholinesterase inhibitors may potentiate vagal responses and becloud both the intraoperative administration of muscle relaxants and the differential diagnosis and treatment of postoperative muscle weakness.

Emotional stress and surgery may precipitate or worsen skeletal muscle weakness. Pharyngeal and laryngeal muscle weakness, difficulty in eliminating oral secretions, and risk of pulmonary aspiration should be considered in the anesthesia plan of care. Swallowing and respiratory muscle dysfunction account for much of the morbidity and potential mortality in patients with myasthenia gravis.[30]

Regional or local anesthesia with careful monitoring are the preferred anesthetic techniques when appropriate. If general anesthesia is indicated, the respiratory depressant effects of barbiturates, sedatives, narcotics, and volatile anesthetic agents, compounded by the presence of an already weakened respiratory system, must be carefully considered.[36,37] Additionally, administration of calcium channel antagonist drugs or aminoglycoside antibiotics in large doses is capable of exacerbating myasthenic neuromuscular weakness.[13,26]

In many patients the relaxant effects of a volatile anesthetic in combination with the patient's preexisting skeletal muscle weakness are sufficient to facilitate intubation of the trachea.[34,36] Enhanced muscle relaxation may be seen with the administration of all the potent volatile anesthetics.[37]

Succinylcholine may be used to facilitate tracheal intubation, but the response may be unpredictable.[30] Untreated patients with myasthenia gravis appear to be two to three times more resistant to succinylcholine. Normal dosages of succinylcholine may not effectively depolarize the end plate because of the deficiency of viable AChRs. On the other hand, patients treated with cholinesterase inhibitors exhibit a normal or prolonged response to succinylcholine. Cholinesterase inhibitors block the effects of plasma cholinesterase, as well as those of true cholinesterase; hence, succinylcholine and other medications metabolized by plasma cholinesterase (e.g., ester local anesthetics) may have a delayed hydrolysis and a prolonged duration of action.[34,38] Mivacurium also is hydrolyzed by plasma cholinesterase, but it has been used successfully, with careful titration, in myasthenic patients.[39] The ester hydrolysis of atracurium is independent of plasma cholinesterase activity.

The deficient number of functioning AChRs in patients with myasthenia gravis produces an extraordinary sensitivity to nondepolarizing muscle relaxants. Small doses of nondepolarizing agents can produce a profound block with a prolonged effect, even in patients being treated with cholinergic drugs.[36] In one study of 11 myasthenic patients, the average ED_{95} value for vecuronium was 72% less in the myasthenic patient group than in the control group (12 mcg/kg versus 49 mcg/kg).[40] Some patients require no medication for surgical muscle relaxation at all.[41]

Generally, muscle relaxant requirements are widely variable in patients with myasthenia gravis, a characteristic that makes neuromuscular blockade monitoring an essential and integral part of the anesthetic management. The orbicularis oculi muscle may overestimate the degree of muscle relaxation in patients with myasthenia gravis.[42] This site may be the most ideal site to monitor neuromuscular blockade to avoid the possibility of undetected residual muscle weakness. When needed, the use of smaller doses (one half to two thirds the normal dose) of shorter-acting nondepolarizing relaxants is the prudent choice.[27,43]

Reversal of neuromuscular blockade with an acetylcholinesterase inhibitor should be performed cautiously in patients with myasthenia gravis. Overtreatment with an anticholinesterase agent can precipitate a cholinergic crisis and aggravate rather than reverse the muscle weakness. In many circumstances the neuromuscular block can be titrated to allow complete spontaneous recovery, avoiding the use of reversal.

Complete, sustained return of muscle strength must be demonstrated before extubation and resumption of spontaneous ventilation. The patient should be informed that postoperative tracheal intubation and ventilatory support may be required. Skeletal muscle strength may appear to be adequate shortly after surgery but may deteriorate a few hours later. For patients undergoing transsternal thymectomy, duration of the disease longer than 6 years, a daily pyridostigmine dose greater than 750 mg, the presence of chronic obstructive pulmonary disease, and a preoperative vital capacity less than 2.9 L predict a higher likelihood for postoperative ventilation.[43]

DUCHENNE'S MUSCULAR DYSTROPHY

Muscular dystrophy is a heterogeneous set of diseases that includes fascioscapulohumeral dystrophy, limb-girdle dystrophy, Becker's muscular dystrophy, Duchenne's muscular dystrophy, and others. *Duchenne's muscular dystrophy*, also known as *pseudohypertrophic muscular dystrophy*, is the most common and most severe form.

Incidence

Duchenne's muscular dystrophy (DMD) is an inherited, sex-linked recessive disease. The disease presents in early childhood between 2 and 6 years of age. It is clinically evident in males and has an incidence of 1 in 3500 live male births.[44] Females are generally unaffected but are carriers of the disorder. Mental retardation, of varying degrees, occurs in about 30% of patients with Duchenne's muscular dystrophy.[45] Death often occurs in late adolescence or early adulthood and is usually caused by respiratory failure.

Pathophysiology

Patients with Duchenne's muscular dystrophy experience an infiltration of fibrous and fatty tissue into the muscle, followed by a progressive and painless degeneration and necrosis of muscle fibers. Muscle weakness ends with muscle destruction.

In 1987 the abnormal gene responsible for DMD was identified. This gene is located on the X chromosome and is errant in coding for a vital protein called *dystrophin*. Dystrophin, unique to muscle cells, is normally bound to a complex of glycoproteins as a structural component of the muscle fiber sarcolemma.[46] Patients with Duchenne's muscular dystrophy have an absence or a severe deficiency of the dystrophin protein, which alters sarcolemma integrity or stability.[45,47] The protein is present in low amounts or is structurally altered in Becker's muscular dystrophy, a similar disorder that follows a milder, less progressive course than the Duchenne type.[46,47]

In the early stages of DMD, increased permeability of the sarcolemma and skeletal muscle necrosis are mirrored by elevated serum levels of the enzyme creatine kinase (CK) (formerly referred to as *creatine phosphokinase*). Serum CK levels are often 30 to 300 times normal levels (normal level, 0 to 200 IU), but as muscle is lost to the destructive process, CK levels decrease.

Clinical Manifestations

Duchenne's muscular dystrophy is characterized by an unremitting weakness and a steady deterioration of the proximal muscle groups of the pelvis and shoulders. The child exhibits a clumsy, waddling gait and falls frequently. Weakness of the pelvic girdle leads to the classic finding of Gowers' sign, in which patients use their hands to climb up their legs in order to arise from the floor. A steady deterioration of muscle strength forces most of these boys to be wheelchair bound by the ages of 8 to 12 years.[48]

Skeletal muscle atrophy is usually preceded by fat and fibrous tissue infiltration, resulting in pseudohypertrophy. The infiltrative process is most apparent in the calf muscles, which become particularly enlarged.

Degeneration of respiratory muscles occurs and leads to a restrictive type of ventilatory impairment. Unopposed action by healthy, nondystrophic axial muscles predisposes these patients to kyphoscoliosis, which further decreases the pulmonary reserve. Decreasing muscle strength also results in ineffective cough, impaired swallowing, and inability to mobilize secretions.[48]

More progressive forms of the disease affect not only skeletal muscle but also smooth muscle of the alimentary tract and cardiac muscle. Alimentary tract involvement can lead to intestinal hypomotility, delayed gastric emptying, and gastric dilation.[49,50]

Myocardial involvement occurs in almost all patients with progressive disease.[51] Studies by Nigro and coworkers[52] established the presence of preclinical cardiac disease in 25% of patients with Duchenne's muscular dystrophy who were younger than 6 years of age and in 59% of those between the ages of 6 and 10 years. Myocardial pathology includes fibrotic changes localized primarily to the left ventricle (LV). Echocardiography can effectively evaluate LV function in patients with DMD.[53] Clinical symptoms of heart failure do not usually appear unless the patient is severely stressed or until advanced stages of the disease.

Electrocardiographic (ECG) changes characteristic of preclinical cardiomyopathy include a large or polyphasic R wave in lead V_1, deep Q waves in the lateral precordial leads (V_4 through V_6), premature beats (atrial and ventricular), and labile sinus or atrial tachycardia.[54]

Although often severe, the compromised cardiac and respiratory conditions may be masked by the limited activity imposed by the patient's skeletal myopathy. Added stress, such as that produced by surgery and anesthesia, may suddenly increase cardiorespiratory demand and uncover the weakened cardiac and respiratory states.

Anesthetic Implications

Patients with Duchenne's muscular dystrophy are susceptible to untoward anesthesia-related complications. When possible, local or regional anesthesia should be considered.[55]

Generalized muscle weakness, especially in the advanced stages of muscular dystrophy, makes these patients exquisitely sensitive to the respiratory depressant properties of opioids, sedatives, and general anesthetic agents. Preoperative sedation should be minimal, and the smallest possible amounts of anesthetic agents should be used.[56]

Preoperative and postoperative respiratory therapy can help maximize the patient's pulmonary condition. In patients with more advanced disease, arterial blood gas determinations and preoperative pulmonary function studies may elucidate the extent of respiratory involvement and the amount of respiratory reserve. A forced vital capacity of less than 35% of that predicted indicates a risk for postoperative pulmonary complications.[56]

The effects of nondepolarizing muscle relaxants must be scrupulously monitored. There is increased muscle relaxant sensitivity and recovery may be prolonged to three to six times the normal duration in patients with DMD.[57] Short-acting nondepolarizing muscle relaxants that are carefully titrated with the use of a nerve stimulator are recommended.

Assiduous attention to respiratory function must be continued into the postoperative period. Delayed pulmonary insufficiency, as late as 36 hours after surgery, has been reported. At least 24 hours of observation should be instituted after the patient undergoes anesthesia.

Their decreased cardiac reserve makes these patients sensitive to the myocardial depressant effects of general anesthetic agents, sedatives, and narcotics. Cardiac arrests associated with inhalation anesthetics have been reported. A carefully titrated intravenous "balanced" technique may help provide a smoother cardiovascular course. Ketamine has been used successfully for anesthesia during diagnostic muscle biopsy in patients with DMD.[58] Judicious administration of intravenous fluids is warranted. The sudden occurrence of tachycardia during anesthesia may herald heart failure.

The potential for delayed gastric emptying, plus the presence of weak laryngeal reflexes, dictates that the anesthesia plan of care include measures for guarding against aspiration of stomach contents.[56] Gastrokinetic agents and the prophylactic use of a nasogastric tube are recommended to avoid gastric dilation.[50]

Succinylcholine and the potent inhalational agents should not be used in patients with muscular dystrophy, as the altered sarcolemma can lead to rhabdomyolysis with their administration.[59] The resultant massive breakdown of muscle fibers produces a profound hyperkalemia that requires extensive and tenacious treatment with hyperventilation, calcium chloride, sodium bicarbonate, and glucose and insulin. Several cases of ventricular fibrillation or cardiac arrest occurring during anesthetic induction have been associated with succinylcholine or potent inhalational agent administration.[60,61] Additionally, DMD is included among the myopathies that may be associated with malignant hyperthermia (MH).[62] The anesthetist should avoid MH-triggering agents and vigilantly observe for signs and symptoms of MH when these children undergo surgery. Dantrolene and other treatment modalities for MH should be readily available.[63]

MALIGNANT HYPERTHERMIA

Epidemiology/Incidence

Malignant hyperthermia is an uncommon, life-threatening, hypermetabolic disorder of skeletal muscle triggered in susceptible individuals by potent inhalation agents, including sevoflurane, desflurane, isoflurane, and halothane, and the depolarizing muscle relaxant succinylcholine.[64,65,66] A review of published cases of MH by Strazis and Fox reported that about 52% of cases occur in patients under age 15, with a mean age of 18.3 years.[67] The exact incidence of MH is unknown but the rate of occurrence has been estimated to be 1 in 50,000 in adults and 1 in 15,000 in children.[64,65] High incidence areas in the United States include Wisconsin, West Virginia, and Michigan.[66]

MH susceptibility is inherited in some families as an autosomal dominant pattern with variable penetrance.[64,66] A single defective gene is the basis for the underlying problem for many families, but in other families the genetic pattern has not been established.

The first formal case report of MH was of an Australian family, described by Denborough and Lovell over 40 years ago in the journal *Lancet*.[68] Since that time a great deal has been learned about the biochemical and physiologic components of the disease. Nonetheless, many questions remain regarding the pathophysiology, the diagnosis, and the significance of some clinical manifestations.

Pathophysiology

Although the cause of MH is not yet known with certainty, it is generally agreed that MH is an inherited disorder of skeletal muscle in which a defect in calcium regulation is expressed by exposure to triggering anesthetic agents; intracellular hypercalcemia results. The ryanodine receptor modulates calcium release from channels in the sarcoplasmic reticulum, and much attention has been focused on this receptor as a site of the MH defect.[69] There is no evidence for a primary defect in cardiac or smooth muscle cells.

Malignant hyperthermia is initiated when specific triggering agents induce increased concentrations of calcium in the muscle cells of malignant hyperthermia–susceptible (MHS) patients. Actomyosin cross-bridging, sustained muscle contraction, and rigidity result.[70] Energy-dependent reuptake mechanisms attempt to remove excess calcium from the muscle cells, increasing muscle metabolism twofold to threefold. The accelerated cellular processes increase oxygen consumption, augment carbon dioxide and heat production, deplete ATP stores, and generate lactic acid. Acidosis, hyperthermia, and ATP depletion cause sarcolemma destruction, producing a marked egress of potassium, myoglobin, and creatine kinase to the extracellular fluid.[66,70] Skeletal muscle constitutes 40% to 50% of our body mass, so relatively small changes in muscle metabolism may produce the dramatic systemic biochemical changes observed with MH.

Clinical Presentation

Not all cases of MH are fulminant, but rather there is a spectrum or continuum of severity, ranging from an insidious onset with mild complications to an explosive response with pronounced rigidity, temperature rise, arrhythmias, and death.[64,71]

Although MH may present in several ways, a typical MH episode begins while the patient is under general anesthesia (GA) with a volatile anesthetic. Succinylcholine may or may not precede the MH episode.[64,70] The onset of MH symptoms may occur immediately after induction of anesthesia or several hours into the surgery.[71] Succinylcholine appears to accelerate the onset and increase the severity of the MH episode.[64,70] The presentation of MH may follow a dose-dependent response, with lower concentrations of volatile anesthetics resulting in a more protracted onset of hypermetabolic symptoms.[71,72] Rarely, MH occurs in the recovery room, usually within 1 hour after general anesthesia.[70]

The clinical features of MH reflect increased intracellular muscle Ca^{2+} concentration and the greatly increased body metabolism (Box 30-3). Common signs of MH include tachycardia, tachypnea, skin mottling, cyanosis, and total body or jaw muscle rigidity. Muscle rigidity is clinically apparent in 75% of cases.[70] The most sensitive indicator of MH is an unanticipated increase in end-tidal carbon dioxide ($ETCO_2$) levels out of proportion to minute ventilation. The increased $ETCO_2$ may be abrupt or it may rise gradually over the course of the anesthetic. Hyperthermia, which may climb at a rate of 1° to 2° C every 5 minutes and exceed 43.3° C (110° F), is often a late but confirming sign of MH.[64]

The combination of acidosis, hyperkalemia, and hyperthermia lead to cardiac irritability, a labile blood pressure, and arrhythmias that can rapidly progress to cardiac arrest. Laboratory findings mirror the muscle breakdown and include myoglobinuria and increased serum potassium and CK. CK levels peak 12 to 24 hours after the onset of MH.[70] Myoglobin appears in the plasma within minutes of the muscle injury response. Arterial and venous blood gas analysis reveals decreased oxygen tension and mixed metabolic and respiratory acidosis. Late complications may include cerebral edema, myoglobinuric renal failure, consumptive coagulopathy, hepatic dysfunction, and pulmonary edema.[64]

The variable time course and the nonspecific clinical features and laboratory findings can make the diagnosis of MH difficult. Insufficient anesthetic depth, hypoxia, neuroleptic malignant syndrome, thyrotoxicosis, pheochromocytoma, and sepsis can share several characteristics with MH, making the clinical picture ambiguous and the differential diagnosis challenging to even the most experienced practitioner[73] (Box 30-4). Surgical procedures performed of necessity in a

BOX **30-3**

Clinical Events and Laboratory Findings During Malignant Hyperthermia

Clinical Events During MH

Unexplained, sudden rise in end-tidal CO_2
Unexplained tachycardia, tachypnea, labile blood pressure, or arrhythmias
Masseter muscle or generalized muscle rigidity
Unanticipated respiratory or metabolic acidosis
Rising patient temperature
Cola-colored urine (myoglobinuria)
Mottled, cyanotic skin, decreased SaO_2

Laboratory Findings Consistent with MH

Arterial blood gases: $PCO_2 > 60$ mm Hg, base excess more negative than −8 mEq/L, pH <7.25
Potassium ion > 6 mEq/L CK > 10,000 IU/L after anesthetic without succinylcholine
Serum myoglobin > 170 mcg/L
Urine myoglobin > 60 mcg/L

BOX **30-4**

Manifestations That Mimic MH—Signs and Symptoms

Tachycardia

Hypoxia
Hypercarbia
Hypovolemia
Insufficient anesthetic depth
Anticholinergics, sympathomimetics, cocaine
Pheochromocytoma

Hyperpyrexia

Heatstroke
Blood transfusion reaction
Infection
Drug reaction
Neuroleptic malignant syndrome, serotonin syndrome
Hypermetabolic states (sepsis, thyroid storm, pheochromocytoma)

Tachypnea, Hypercapnia

Congestive heart failure, pulmonary edema
Hypermetabolic states
Intraperitoneal carbon dioxide insufflation
Airway obstruction, pneumothorax
Excess dead space, low minute volume

Masseter Muscle Rigidity

Insufficient neuromuscular blockade
Temporomandibular joint syndrome
Neuroleptic malignant syndrome
Myotonia

darkened operating room can further compromise the practitioner's diagnostic acumen.

In addition to being a trigger of MH, succinylcholine may also induce a hyperkalemic-mediated cardiac arrest in children with occult myopathies.[61,74,75] As such, most anesthetists use nondepolarizing muscle relaxants or deep inhalational anesthesia for elective intubation in children and reserve the use of succinylcholine for treatment of laryngospasm or emergency airway management. In 1994 the package insert for succinylcholine was modified to warn against the routine use of succinylcholine in children.

Preoperative Assessment and Prevention

Patients who are MH susceptible may be otherwise healthy and completely unaware of their risk until exposed to a triggering anesthetic.[67,76] Furthermore, not everyone who has the MH gene develops an MH episode upon each exposure to triggering anesthetics. It is estimated that about 21% of MHS patients have at least one uneventful anesthetic prior to having an MH episode.[67,70] Although MH susceptibility cannot be ruled out by history alone, every surgical patient should be questioned about:

- Family or personal history of muscle disorders
- Family history of unexpected intraoperative complications or deaths
- Family or personal history of muscle rigidity/stiffness or high fever under anesthesia
- Personal history of dark or cola-colored urine following surgery

Because MH is considered an inherited disorder, all members of a family in which MH has occurred must be considered MHS unless proven otherwise. Moreover, the absence of a positive family history does not preclude MH susceptibility.

There are certain disorders that should alert the anesthetist to an increased possibility of MH susceptibility. A clear genetic association between MH and the inherited myopathy central core disease has been demonstrated. Case reports have also linked MH to Duchenne's and Becker's muscular dystrophy and forms of periodic paralysis and myotonia.[70] MH triggering agents should not be administered to patients with these disorders.[77] This caveat is especially consequential in patients undergoing outpatient procedures who will have limited postoperative observation and same-day discharge.

Weglinski and others report that 50% of patients with unexplained CK elevation test positive for MH on biopsy.[67,78] However, as a diagnostic test for MH, CK levels are imprecise and nonspecific. Stress, fever, prior exercise, and cocaine and alcohol ingestion have been implicated as causal factors, but it is debated whether these factors cause, exacerbate, or have no effect on MH triggering in humans.[70,79,80]

Treatment

Enhanced patient monitoring, earlier diagnosis and treatment, and the introduction of dantrolene are responsible for the dramatic decrease in mortality from nearly 80% 20 years ago to less than 10% today.[64,70] Clearly, the nurse anesthetist plays a critical role in the early recognition and treatment of MH.

In 1975 dantrolene sodium (Dantrium) was introduced as a treatment for MH. Since that time, dantrolene has contributed greatly to the dramatic decline in death and disability associated with MH. Dantrolene is a unique muscle relaxant that works by reducing the release of calcium from skeletal muscle sarcoplasmic reticulum, counteracting the abnormal intracellular calcium levels accompanying MH.[81] It does not work at the neuromuscular junction as do standard neuromuscular blocking drugs. At clinical concentrations, dantrolene does not render the muscle totally flaccid and without tone, but it may cause significant muscle weakness and respiratory insufficiency, especially in patients with preexisting muscle disease.

Dantrolene pretreatment for the MHS surgical patient is no longer routine, but it may be used prophylactically in specific surgical patients who cannot tolerate hypermetabolic states (e.g., the MHS patient with severe cardiac or cerebrovascular disease) or myoglobinuria (e.g., the MHS patient with renal disease). A single intravenous dose (2.5 mg/kg) immediately before induction is recommended.[75] Dantrolene should not be used with calcium channel blockers, since the combination may induce life-threatening hyperkalemia and myocardial depression.[77]

The Malignant Hyperthermia Association of the United States (MHAUS) provides an "Emergency Therapy for MH" poster that should be posted in every surgical site. The following treatment sequence is recommended for an acute MH episode:

- Call for help and alert the surgeon to conclude the procedure promptly.
- Discontinue the volatile anesthetic and succinylcholine.
- Hyperventilate with 100% oxygen at high flows (at least 10 L/min) to improve tissue oxygenation and eliminate CO_2.
- Administer 2.5 mg/kg dantrolene IV bolus and repeat as necessary until symptoms abate. Occasionally, a total dose greater than 10 mg/kg may be needed.
- Dysrhythmias will usually respond to treatment of acidosis or hyperkalemia. Treat persistent or life-threatening arrhythmias with standard antiarrhythmic agents (avoid calcium channel blockers).
- If fever is present, initiate cooling by lavage (orogastric, bladder, open cavities), administration of chilled intravenous normal saline and surface cooling (hypothermia blanket; ice packs to the groins, axillae, and neck).
- Determine arterial blood gases, serum electrolytes, and blood sugar every 15 minutes until the syndrome stabilizes. Correct metabolic acidosis with sodium bicarbonate. Baseline values for coagulation studies, CK, myoglobin, and liver enzymes should be established.
- Treat hyperkalemia with hyperventilation, bicarbonate, and intravenous insulin and glucose (10 units regular insulin in 50 mL 50% glucose) titrated to potassium level. Life-threatening hyperkalemia may be cautiously treated with calcium administration.
- Maintain urine output greater than 2 mL/kg/hr by hydration and mannitol (300 mg/kg) and/or furosemide (0.5 to 1.0 mg/kg). Large losses of intravascular volume should be anticipated. Consider central venous or pulmonary artery hemodynamic monitoring.

Bissonnette and Ryan report that the $ETCO_2$ should start to abate about 6 minutes after dantrolene administration. They recommend continuing intensive therapy if there are any signs or symptoms of MH after 45 minutes.[75] Dantrolene must be reconstituted with sterile water, and its poor water solubility makes it very time consuming to mix and administer the requisite doses. During an MH emergency, the full-time efforts of additional medical personnel should be enlisted. Documentation of an MH episode should include patient responses, personnel involved, medications, interventions, and patient outcomes.

Anesthesia for the MH-Susceptible Patient

Standard intraoperative monitoring for the MHS surgical patient includes blood pressure, ECG, pulse oximetry, capnography, and continuous measurement of core body temperature (nasopharyngeal, distal esophageal, tympanic, or pulmonary artery). A cooling water mattress should be placed under the MHS patient at the start of the procedure. Inconsistent reports of emotional stress or anxiety predisposing a patient to MH have led to recommendations that anxiolytic agents be included in the premedication.[71]

If the surgical site permits, a regional or local anesthetic technique is preferable for the MHS patient. Local anesthetics (both amide and ester) are nontriggering drugs. Nontriggering general anesthetics can also be administered safely in concert with close monitoring of appropriate vital functions. The list of "nontriggering" anesthetic agents is comprehensive enough to meet most anesthetic requirements (Box 30-5). The volatile inhalation anesthetics and succinylcholine are MH triggers and should not be administered to the MHS patient. Potassium salts can depolarize the muscle membrane and are considered unsafe for the MHS patient.[64]

Not all drugs have been thoroughly screened as potential MH triggers, but it is clear that the vast majority of prescription and nonprescription drugs are safe, including antibiotics, antihypertensive agents, and drugs used in the treatment of gastrointestinal disorders. Keys to successful perioperative outcome include the following:

- Avoidance of MH-triggering medications
- Preparation of an anesthesia machine by changing the soda lime and breathing circuits, removing or inactivating vaporizers, and flushing with oxygen or air at 10 L/min for at least 20 minutes or 10 minutes if the fresh gas hose is also replaced
- Assiduous perioperative observation for the signs of MH, including continuous intraoperative monitoring of the patient's end-tidal carbon dioxide concentration, arterial oxygen saturation, and central temperature
- A full appreciation of a preestablished treatment protocol by all perioperative medical personnel

A machine to manufacture ice or the ready availability of ice and the ability to crush it, and a refrigerator containing at least 3000 mL of cold intravenous solution, should be available. Because early arterial blood gas analysis is an integral part of MH diagnosis and treatment, some MH experts recommend that every facility where MH-triggering agents are administered have ready access to blood gas analysis.

Ambulatory surgery can be safely performed in most MHS patients, provided that appropriate monitoring is employed and an adequate supply of dantrolene is available.[82] Yentis and others reviewed the medical records of 303 children labeled as MHS who underwent surgery with nontriggering anesthetics between 1981 and 1990. None of the children developed MH, and on the basis of their retrospective analysis the authors concluded that admission to the hospital solely on the basis of the MHS label is not warranted.[83] Outpatient surgical cases for the MHS patient are best scheduled early in the day to allow for adequate recovery and at least 4 hours of observation time after surgery.[82,83] As with any ambulatory procedure, patient selection for outpatient surgery should be individualized. Patients known or suspected of having MH should be assessed well before their date of outpatient surgery, so that anesthesia records and MH testing center reports (if available) can be collected to corroborate the history. Some experts recommend conservative management with overnight hospital admission for patients who have survived a previous fulminant or severe MH episode or when dantrolene prophylaxis is utilized.[70]

All locations where general anesthesia is administered should contain a fully stocked MH cart with drugs and supplies, including 36 vials of dantrolene. Because minutes count in an MH emergency, a dantrolene supply should never be shared with a nearby facility, but rather it should be kept in or very close to the operating room so that it is available immediately if MH occurs.

BOX 30-5

Triggering and Nontriggering Agents

Triggering Agents

All volatile inhalation anesthetics (halothane, desflurane, isoflurane, sevoflurane)
Succinylcholine
Potassium salts

Nontriggering Agents

Local anesthetics
Opioids
Nitrous oxide
Barbiturates, propofol, ketamine, etomidate
Benzodiazepines
Nondepolarizing skeletal muscle relaxants (vecuronium, atracurium, cisatracurium, pancuronium, mivacurium, rocuronium, doxacurium, pipecuronium)
Digoxin, tricyclic antidepressants, magnesium
Anticholinesterase agents
Anticholinergic agents

Diagnostic Testing

The most accurate and commonly accepted test available for determining MH susceptibility is the caffeine halothane contracture test (CHCT). This test involves taking a biopsy of skeletal muscle from the patient's thigh and measuring its contractile response to caffeine, halothane, or both. Normal muscle contracts in response to caffeine or halothane, but this is augmented in the patient with MH. The test is available at eight medical centers in North America; because it must be completed within hours after muscle biopsy, the patient must travel to the testing site. The test has a sensitivity of 92% and a specificity of 78%.[75] Patients who have survived an unequivocal episode of MH are considered MHS. The CHCT is indicated for family members of an MHS patient or for patients who have had a previous suspicious but undiagnosed reaction to anesthesia.

Intensive investigations have focused on identifying the gene or genes responsible for MH. Less than 50% of MHS patients appear to have an abnormality in the gene(s) that encode the ryanodine receptor protein. For other MHS patients, the molecular genetic basis for the disease may be more heterogeneous, involving mutations at various sites on different chromosomes.[69,75,84] Once the gene(s) for MH are identified, a simpler noninvasive DNA-based diagnostic test can be a realistic expectation.

Postoperative Care

The patient who has experienced an acute MH episode should be observed in an ICU for at least 24 hours. Recrudescence of an intraoperative episode may occur in 25% of cases.[85] Dantrolene treatment is continued for a minimum of 24 hours after control of the episode.

For the MHS patient who has undergone an uneventful surgical course, close observation and assiduous monitoring should continue into the postanesthesia care unit (PACU). Malignant hyperthermia can first manifest in the recovery room after uneventful surgery and anesthesia. Most MHS patients undergoing outpatient surgery may be discharged on the day of surgery, but each case should be individualized.

Masseter Muscle Rigidity

Masseter muscle rigidity (MMR) or trismus is a sustained and forceful contracture of the masseter muscle following the use of succinylcholine. The contracture may be severe enough to make opening the jaw impossible ("jaws of steel"). A mild increase in masseter muscle tone or incomplete jaw relaxation following succinylcholine is fairly common and may be a normal response.[75] However, severe jaw tightness that interferes with intubation may portend an episode of MH. If trismus is further accompanied by generalized body rigidity, MH is highly likely.[64,77]

Masseter muscle rigidity occurs most often in children, with an incidence reported as high as 1% in children undergoing a halothane-succinylcholine anesthetic.[70]

Management of trismus in the surgical patient is a contentious issue, and experts are divided on how to proceed after MMR.[75,86,87] Some experts recommend cautiously continuing the anesthetic with nontriggering agents after an episode of MMR, while monitoring for rhabdomyolysis and signs and symptoms of MH.[87] Others maintain that the safer course is to assume that trismus is a harbinger of MH, discontinue the anesthetic, and cancel elective surgery until results of a muscle biopsy are available.[75,77]

Because of the likelihood of rhabdomyolysis, as well as the possibility of undiagnosed myopathy, the surgical patient should be admitted to the hospital and observed for at least 24 hours following MMR.[75] Myoglobinuria may be apparent in the recovery room, and inducing a brisk urine output may lessen the risk of myoglobinuric renal damage.[88] Studies indicate that following MMR, if the CK is greater than 20,000 IU and a concomitant myopathy is not present, the diagnosis of MH is likely.[64] Patients who have experienced MMR should be counseled concerning the possibility that they are MHS and should be referred to a well-informed primary or specialty care physician or genetic counselor for further investigation.

Information Resources

The Malignant Hyperthermia Association of the United States (MHAUS) is a nonprofit organization that provides educational and technical information to patients and health care providers. Information is available via fax-on-demand 1 (800) 440-9990 or on the World Wide Web at http://www.mhaus.org. An MH hotline may be consulted for MH emergencies 24 hours a day at 1 (800) MH-HYPER [1 (800) 644-9737]. Health care providers are encouraged to report MH episodes to the North American MH Registry at 1 (888) 274-7899.

MYOTONIC DYSTROPHY

The myotonias are a group of hereditary degenerative muscle diseases that include myotonic dystrophy, myotonia congenita (Thomsen's disease), and paramyotonia congenita. A symptom common to all myotonias is the inability of skeletal muscles to relax after chemical or physical stimulation.[88]

Myotonic dystrophy, also known as *Steinert's disease*, *myotonia atrophica*, or *myotonia dystrophica*, is the most common and the most severe form of the myotonias. It is characterized by skeletal muscles that are hypoplastic, dystrophic, and weak yet prone to persistent contraction. Although muscles are primarily affected, myotonic dystrophy is distinguished from nondystrophic myotonias by being a multisystem disease.[88,89]

Incidence

Myotonic dystrophy is inherited as an autosomal dominant trait. In most cases an affected person has one affected parent. The onset of symptoms can occur at any age, but usually occurs in the second to third decade of life. A slow, progressive deterioration of skeletal, cardiac, and smooth muscle occurs, resulting in death by the sixth decade.[88] An estimated 1 in 20,000 people worldwide have the disorder, with an equal occurrence in males and females. The severity of clinical symptoms usually increases with transmission to subsequent generations.[90,91] Myotonic dystrophy is the most common and severe inherited muscular dystrophy of adulthood.

Pathophysiology and Treatment

Myotonic dystrophy is a disorder of muscle membrane excitability that results in self-sustaining runs of depolarization. Electrophysiologic studies show a lowered resting membrane potential in muscle cells from patients with myotonic dystrophy. Therapeutic agents used to treat the myotonic contractures include quinine, procainamide, and phenytoin. These agents delay the return of membrane excitation by blocking rapid Na^+ influx into muscle cells. Regional anesthesia and muscle relaxants do not prevent or relieve the recalcitrant contraction.[92] Dantrolene has also been ineffective in reversing myotonia.[93] Warming the ambient temperature or injecting local anesthetics into the involved muscles may induce relaxation.[94] Steroids and inhalation anesthetic agents may also attenuate the contraction in some patients. No treatment is available for the muscle weakness that develops with myotonic dystrophy.

Clinical Manifestations

A wide variety of symptoms are characteristic of myotonic dystrophy. Facial weakness ("expressionless facies"), ptosis, and sternocleidomastoid muscle and distal limb weakness are prominent features of the disease.[88,91] Frontal balding, cataracts, and testicular atrophy in males form a frequently recognized triad of characteristics. Endocrine abnormalities, such as diabetes mellitus and thyroid disease, occur with a greater frequency in this patient group than in the general population.

Myotonia, the inability to relax a muscle, occurs in most symptomatic patients and may be worsened by pressure, touch, cold or shivering.[91] Insidious muscle atrophy, particularly of the face, neck, pharynx, and distal limbs, causes severe muscle debility in the later stages of the disease. Myotonic symptoms usually precede the atrophy and weakness.[88]

Cardiac disturbances occur in most patients with myotonic dystrophy, often manifesting as conduction defects and arrhythmias.[91] Conduction defects were present in about 50% of the patients in one series.[95] First-degree atrioventricular block is the most common finding, but greater degrees of heart block are also seen.[92] Arrhythmias include sinus bradycardia, atrial flutter or fibrillation, and ventricular extrasystoles.[95,96] Respiratory muscle weakness may be disproportionately greater than weakness elsewhere.[88,92] Weakening of the thoracic muscles, including the diaphragm, reduces the respiratory reserve and the vital capacity. A restrictive type of ventilatory impairment develops with progression of the disease. Central sleep apnea and hypersomnolence cause hypoventilation and decreased ventilatory response to carbon dioxide.

Anesthetic Implications

Any drug that has the potential to depolarize skeletal muscle may produce an exaggerated contraction in patients with myotonia dystrophica. Administration of succinylcholine to patients with myotonic dystrophy should be avoided, since it can produce an intense generalized myotonic contracture that makes ventilation and intubation difficult or impossible. Agents associated with myoclonus (methohexital, etomidate) have the potential to produce similar effects.[92]

Nondepolarizing muscle relaxants may be used in these patients, as long as the degree of muscle wasting and weakness is appreciated. The dose of the nondepolarizer should be reduced according to the degree of muscle impairment, and the neuromuscular block should be monitored closely with a peripheral nerve stimulator.

An abnormal swallowing mechanism resulting from palatal, pharyngeal, and esophageal muscle involvement and gastrointestinal hypomotility renders these patients vulnerable to pulmonary aspiration of gastric contents.[88,92]

Reversal of neuromuscular blockade with anticholinesterase agents may theoretically precipitate skeletal muscle contraction by producing an ACh-induced depolarizing block.[97] Shorter-acting nondepolarizing muscle relaxants have the obvious advantage of being less likely to require reversal.

Hypothermia and shivering should be avoided by raising the room temperature, warming inhaled gases and intravenous fluids, and provision of a forced air thermal blanket.

Underestimating the severity of respiratory compromise is not uncommon in these patients. Preoperative arterial blood gas determinations and pulmonary function results may serve as useful baselines. The respiratory depressant effects of barbiturates, opioids, and volatile anesthetics may compromise already weakened respiratory musculature and may lead to unexpected decompensation.[98] Even small doses of short-acting anesthetic agents may be associated with an exaggerated and prolonged anesthetic effect. Speedy[99] reported on a typical case in which a 31-year-old man with myotonic dystrophy remained unconscious and unable to maintain a patent airway for 4 hours after receiving an anesthetic that consisted of 50 mg of propofol, 0.5% isoflurane, and 50% nitrous oxide in oxygen. Completely uneventful responses to anesthesia in myotonic patients have also been reported.

Assiduous monitoring of cardiovascular parameters should be maintained intraoperatively and postoperatively. Cardiac function that was clinically normal preoperatively may become unacceptably depressed as a result of the administration of general anesthetic agents. The ECG should be examined closely for indications of atrioventricular conduction blocks and other arrhythmias. The patient should be questioned preoperatively about syncope or presyncope to help ascertain the need for cardiac pacing. It may be wise to assume that even asymptomatic patients have some degree of cardiac involvement.

Pregnancy may exacerbate the symptoms of myotonia. Uterine atony, postpartum hemorrhage, and retained placenta have accompanied delivery in patients with myotonic dystrophy. Increased progesterone levels are linked to the deleterious effects.[100]

MH triggering agents should be avoided in these patients, since associations between some forms of myotonia and MH have been described.[77,101]

LAMBERT-EATON MYASTHENIC SYNDROME

Incidence

Lambert-Eaton myasthenic syndrome (LEMS), is a rare autoimmune disease that classically occurs in patients with malignant disease, particularly small cell carcinoma of the bronchi. One third to one half of patients, however, have no evidence of carcinoma.[102,103] Most patients with myasthenic syndrome are men between the ages of 50 and 70 years.

Pathophysiology

The basic defect associated with LEMS appears to be an autoantibody-mediated derangement in presynaptic Ca^{2+} channels leading to a reduction in Ca^{2+}-mediated exocytosis of ACh at neuromuscular and autonomic nerve terminals.[104] The decreased release of ACh quanta from the cholinergic nerve endings produces a reduced postjunctional response. Unlike in myasthenia gravis, the number and the quality of postjunctional AChRs remain unaltered, and the end plate sensitivity is normal. The neuromuscular junction abnormality of LEMS resembles that of Mg^{2+} intoxication or botulism poisoning, in which the release of presynaptic ACh is attenuated.

Clinical Manifestations and Treatment

Muscle weakness, fatigue, hyporeflexia, and proximal limb muscle aches are the dominant features of LEMS. The diaphragm and other respiratory muscles are also involved. Autonomic nervous system dysfunction is often present and is manifested as impaired gastric motility, orthostatic hypotension, and urinary retention.

Patients with LEMS experience a brief increase in muscle strength with voluntary contraction, distinguishing it from myasthenia gravis. Tetanic stimulation results in a progressive augmentation in muscle strength as the frequency of the stimulation is increased. Posttetanic potentiation is also enhanced.

There is no cure for LEMS. Treatment is aimed at improving muscle strength and reversing autonomic deficits.[105,106] 3,4-Diaminopyridine is used in some patients to improve muscle strength. It acts presynaptically to promote Ca^{2+} influx and increase the number of ACh quanta that are liberated by a single nerve action potential. Anticholinesterase agents, plasmapheresis, corticosteroids, intravenous immunoglobulin,[107] and immunosuppressive drugs provide improvement for some patients with LEMS. Patients being treated with aminopyridine derivatives should have their medication continued into the preoperative period.[30]

Anesthetic Implications

An index of suspicion for LEMS should be maintained in patients undergoing surgery with suspected or diagnosed carcinoma of the lung. Patients with LEMS are extremely sensitive to the relaxant effects of both depolarizing and nondepolarizing muscle relaxants. Inhalational anesthetics alone may provide adequate relaxation, but if muscle relaxants are required, their dosages should be reduced and the neuromuscular blockade closely monitored.[108] Neuromuscular reversal with an anticholinesterase agent may be used. Prolonged ventilatory assistance may be required postoperatively.

RHEUMATOID ARTHRITIS

Rheumatoid arthritis (RA) is a chronic inflammatory polyarthropathy with myriad degrees of systemic involvement. The disease is multifactorial, and the clinical picture varies widely in severity, extent of involvement, and symptoms. The capricious course of the disease may be persistent and debilitating or relapsing and remitting.[109] With each successive exacerbation, new joints may become involved.

Incidence

Rheumatoid arthritis is the most common form of inflammatory arthritis, affecting approximately 1% of the United States population.[110,111] The onset of RA can occur at any age, but most cases are diagnosed in patients between the ages of 35 and 50 years.[110] RA is two to three times more likely to develop in women than in men.[111] Patients with RA have a reduced life expectancy ranging from 3 to 7 years.[110]

Etiology

The exact cause of RA remains elusive; heredity plays some role in increasing a person's susceptibility to RA.[110,111] Impaired immunity, stress, and other environmental factors may precipitate or aggravate the disease.[110,112]

A viral or a bacterial infection that alters the immune system in a genetically susceptible host may play a role in the etiology.[110,112] The invading microbe may mimic or produce a protein similar to those in the body's own tissue, particularly joint tissue. To destroy the antigen, the immune system may mistakenly mount an autoimmune response and direct its attack against its own tissue. Circulating autoantibodies called *rheumatoid factors* are detectable in 70% to 80% of patients with RA.

Clinical Manifestations

Joint Involvement. Inflammation and destruction of synovial tissues are responsible for most of the symptoms and chronic disability associated with RA. Joint involvement progresses in three main stages: (1) inflammation of the joint synovial membrane and infiltration by polymorphonuclear leukocytes; (2) rapid division and growth of cells in the joint (synovial proliferation and pannus formation); and (3) liberation of osteolytic enzymes, proteases, and collagenases, which damage small blood vessels, cartilage, ligaments, tendons, and bones. Collapse of normal cortical and medullary architecture leads to erosion and dislocation of bone that is contiguous with the inflammatory cell mass.

The onset of symptoms is most often insidious, evolving over a period of weeks to months. The most common sites of onset are the hands, wrists, and feet. There is often symmetric joint involvement. Swelling, warmth, and pain in the affected joints are caused by the inflammatory process. Morning stiffness, weight loss, and fatigue are noted early in the disease course.

Dissolution of bone and disuse atrophy of bone (osteoporosis) are found in all seriously affected areas. Pain, inflammation, and erosion of bone and tissue may permanently limit the joint's full range of motion. Later stages of the disease are characterized by severe pain, joint instability, and crippling deformities.[110]

Nerve entrapment may occur at any site where peripheral nerves pass near the inflamed joint. Carpal tunnel syndrome is a common peripheral neuropathy.

Synovitis in the temporomandibular joint may limit jaw motion. An estimated 30% to 70% of patients with RA have involvement of the temporomandibular joint. As the disease progresses, flexion contractures and soft tissue swelling may lead to a marked limitation in the patient's ability to open the jaw.

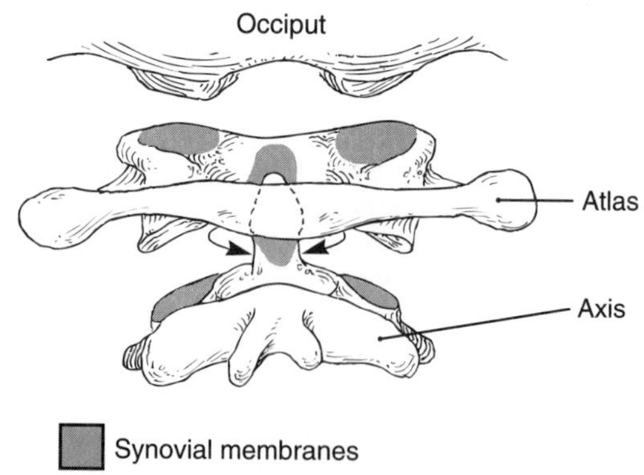

FIGURE **30-18**
The relationship between the occiput, the atlas (C1), and the axis (C2). The atlas supports the head and rotates about the odontoid process of the axis. The occipitoatlantoaxial articulations are lined by synovial membranes and are firmly supported by surrounding ligaments (not shown).

Although the thoracic and lumbar spine are usually spared, involvement of the cervical spine may be extensive and can lead to limited movement or deformity of the neck and to severe laryngeal deviation.[113,114] The most common site of cervical spine synovitis is C1-C2 (Fig. 30-18).[113] Atlantoaxial (C1-C2) instability results from erosion and collapse of bone and from destruction of supporting cervical ligaments. Symptoms occur when excessive motion between C1 and C2 exerts pressure on the spinal cord (Fig. 30-19). Additionally, separation of the atlanto-odontoid articulation may allow the odontoid process of the axis to impinge on the spinal cord, leading to neurologic damage.[114] The atlantoaxial subluxation may also exert pressure and impair blood flow through the vertebral arteries (Fig. 30-20).

Arthritis extends to the cricoarytenoid joint of the larynx in 40% of patients with severe RA.[115] The joint may become swollen, inflamed, and fixed in a position that obstructs air flow.[116] Vocal cord nodules and polyps may also be present. Symptoms of cricoarytenoid arthritis include tenderness over the larynx, hoarseness, pain on swallowing with radiation to the ear, and dyspnea or stridor. Patients with no overt clinical symptoms may also have significant disease.

Systemic Involvement. Although the effects of RA are most clearly seen in joints, the disease is systemic. The immune-mediated destructive process affects a wide variety of

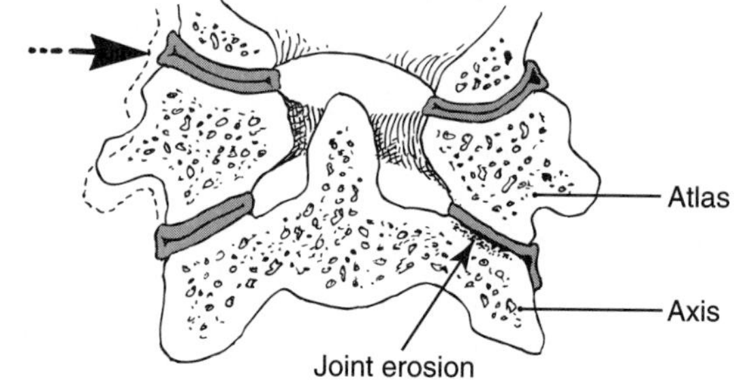

FIGURE **30-19**
Erosion and collapse of C1 and C2 articular surfaces can lead to a shifting of the atlas over the axis. If the subluxation is pronounced, spinal cord compression may occur.

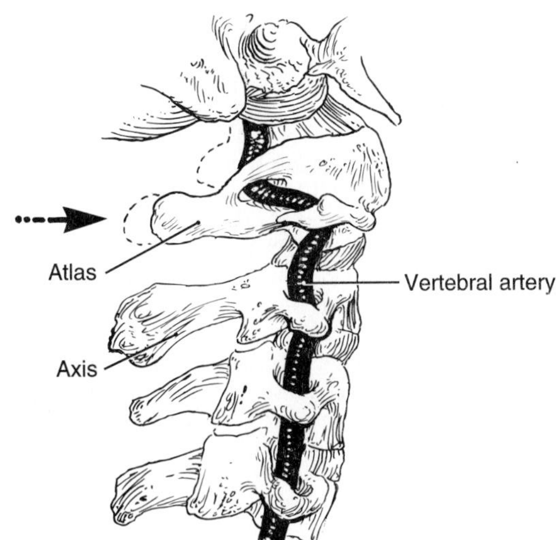

FIGURE **30-20**
Vertebral artery compression may result from atlantoaxial subluxation.

organs, including the heart, the lungs, muscle, the vasculature, and the eyes. The occurrence of extraarticular manifestations is usually associated with more active, erosive articular disease.

Firm, painless subcutaneous nodules occur in approximately 20% to 40% of patients with RA. The nodules usually occur over pressure points, such as the occiput, the sacrum, the ulna, or the Achilles tendon, and may be associated with pressure ulcerations. Rheumatoid nodules can also occur in most visceral organs, including the lungs and the heart. Dural nodules can cause spinal cord compression and neurologic complications.

Pericarditis and pericardial effusion may accompany severe progressive RA and impair cardiac performance. Rheumatoid nodules have been isolated from the cardiac conduction system and may be associated with conduction defects, including complete heart block.[117]

Pulmonary involvement manifests as pleural effusion, pneumonitis, or interstitial fibrosis.[110,118] Decreased lung volume and decreased vital capacity may result from the lung alterations.

Rheumatoid myositis, which is characterized by muscle weakness and eventual muscle necrosis and atrophy, may accompany RA. Inflamed, painful, and underused joints contribute to the skeletal muscle atrophy.

Lacrimal duct and salivary gland destruction may result in dryness of the eyes and the mouth (Sjögren's syndrome) in about 10% of patients with rheumatoid arthritis.[110]

Treatment

Medical therapy is directed toward relief of pain, nonspecific suppression of the inflammatory process, immunosuppression, prevention and correction of deformity, and control of systemic involvement.

Most patients, including those with mild-to-moderate disease, obtain some relief of symptoms with rest, joint immobilization, and use of nonsteroidal antiinflammatory drugs (NSAIDs). NSAIDs relieve joint pain, stiffness, heat, and swelling, in part by blocking cyclooxygenase and inhibiting prostaglandin, thromboxane, and prostacyclin synthesis. Despite their potent antiinflammatory properties, they do not alter the underlying disease process.[110,119]

Corticosteroids are potent antiinflammatory drugs that suppress many symptoms of RA. Long-term side effects (osteoporosis, predisposition to infection, suppression of endogenous cortisol release, cataracts, gastrointestinal bleeding, hypertension, and hyperglycemia), however, limit their use to isolated flares of the disease or to adjunctive, rather than primary, treatments.

Disease-modifying antirheumatic drugs (DMARDs) can arrest the underlying disease process.[120,121] Newer agents, such as the immunosuppressants etanercept (Enbrel), adalimumab (Humira), and infliximab (Remicade), work by interfering with the proinflammatory cytokine tumor necrosis factor.[122,123,124] Biologic agents such as interleukin-1 receptor antagonists offer the potential for more effective treatment of RA.[125] Leflunomide (Arava) is a DMARD that reduces inflammation and slows disease progression of rheumatoid arthritis. Leflunomide may be associated with liver enzyme elevation and liver disease.

The antimetabolite methotrexate (Rheumatrex) is widely used as an effective DMARD for patients with aggressive RA. Bone marrow suppression, oral ulcerations, pneumonitis, and hepatic damage are potential side effects of methotrexate.[126] Gold salts, sulfasalazine, antimalarial drugs, and penicillamine are effective DMARDs used when more conservative measures fail to retard symptoms.[110,120] Immunosuppressive drugs such as cyclophosphamide (Cytoxan) and cyclosporin (Sandimmune) and antimetabolites such as azathioprine (Imuran) are effective agents, generally reserved for more refractory cases.

Surgical interventions for relief of pain or for correction or prevention of deformities include total joint replacement, synovectomy, and tenolysis.

Anesthetic Management

Overall, no individual anesthetic agent or mode of anesthesia is substantially safer than another for the patient with RA. Preoperative examination of individual patients' disease course and medication history are likely to reveal specific features that affect the anesthesia or surgical course.

Long-term NSAID ingestion may result in platelet dysfunction and prolongation of bleeding time. Mild anemia, a common finding in patients with RA, may be secondary to the disease process or to drug therapy. NSAID therapy may exert harmful effects on the liver or kidney and exacerbate allergic rhinitis or asthma; these effects may influence the choice of anesthesia. NSAIDs with preferential inhibition of cyclooxygenase 2 offer a better safety profile over nonspecific cyclooxygenase inhibiting agents.[119]

Patients receiving long-term corticosteroid therapy may develop hypophyseal-pituitary axis suppression, which may require perioperative steroid supplementation. Long-term administration of corticosteroids may increase the patient's susceptibility to infection by inhibiting normal host defense mechanisms. The newer tumor necrosis factor inhibitors are also associated with serious infections. Assiduous attention to sterile techniques should be maintained.

A thorough preoperative assessment of the airway is essential. Particular attention should be directed to the temporomandibular joints, the cervical spine, and the cricoarytenoid joints.

Range of motion of the temporomandibular joint must be assessed before anesthesia is induced. Patients with severe temporomandibular joint involvement may be able to open their mouths only 1 to 2 cm. In such cases, the use of the flexible fiberoptic bronchoscope for tracheal intubation is of proven value.[113]

A thorough neurologic assessment and a radiographic evaluation of the cervical spine should be performed, especially for patients with advanced disease.[127] Some patients with significant radiographic evidence of atlantoaxial or subaxial instability may be entirely asymptomatic.[113,127]

Neck pain is an early symptom of cervical spine instability. Paresthesias into the shoulders and arms, muscle weakness, paresis, and bowel or bladder dysfunction are some of the clinical manifestations of spinal cord compression secondary to atlantoaxial or subaxial subluxation. Compression on the vertebral arteries, with embarrassment of vertebral artery blood flow, may lead to symptoms such as nausea, vomiting, dysarthria, dysphagia, blurred vision, or transient loss of consciousness.

Altered cervical spine anatomy or laryngeal deviation can make intubation of the trachea an extreme challenge. Deviation of the larynx can frequently be detected preoperatively by palpating the location of the larynx in relation to the sternal notch. Flexion, extension, and rotation of the neck must be avoided in the presence of cervical instability. Such circumstances dictate fiberoptic-guided intubation of the trachea in the awake patient.

Hoarseness in a patient with RA should alert the anesthetist to possible cricoarytenoid joint involvement. A smaller endotracheal tube may be necessary because of narrowing of the glottic opening. Laryngoscopy can assess normal cord motion and glottic patency. The patient should be observed closely for signs of airway obstruction after extubation.

Generalized demineralization of bone may increase the risk of fractures in patients with RA. Proper patient positioning and padding of pressure points prevent nerve palsies, skin ulcerations, and further structural damage to the joints.

REFERENCES

1. Murphy RA: Skeletal muscle physiology. In Berne RM, Levy MN, editors: *Physiology*, St. Louis, 1998, Mosby, p 282.
2. Guyton A, Hall J: Contraction of skeletal muscle. In *Textbook of Medical Physiology*, Philadelphia, 2000, Saunders, p 67.
3. Bevan DR, Donati F: Muscle relaxants. In Barash PG, editor: *Clinical Anesthesia*, Philadelphia, 2001, Lippincott-Raven, p 419.
4. Kutchai HC: Synaptic transmission. In Berne RM, Levy MN, editors: *Physiology*, St. Louis, 1998, Mosby, p 43.
5. Guyton A, Hall J: Excitation of skeletal muscle. In *Textbook of Medical Physiology*, Philadelphia, 2000, Saunders, p 80.
6. Katz E Protti DA, Ferro PA, Rosata Siri MD, Uchitel OD: Effects of Ca^{2+} channel blocker neurotoxins on transmitter release and presynaptic currents at the mouse neuromuscular junction, *Br J Pharmacol* 121:1531-1540, 1997.
7. Losavio A, Muchnik S: Spontaneous acetylcholine release in mammalian neuromuscular junctions, *Am J Physiol* 273:C1835-C1841, 1997.
8. Lin MJ, Lin-Shiau SY: Multiple types of Ca^{2+} channels in mouse motor nerve terminal, *Eur J Neurosci* 9:817-823, 1997.
9. Sheng ZH, Westenbrock RE, Catteral WA: Physical link and functional coupling of presynaptic calcium channels and the synaptic vesicle docking/fusion machinery, *J Bioenerg Biomembr* 30:335-345, 1998.
10. Paton WM, Waud DR: The margin of safety of neuromuscular transmission, *J Physiol* 191:59-90, 1967.
11. Ruff RL: Electrophysiology of postsynaptic activation, *Ann N Y Acad Sci* 841:57-70, 1998.
12. Haspel KL, Ali HH: Physiology of neuromuscular transmission and mechanism of action of neuromuscular blocking agents. In Longnecker DE, Tinker JH, Morgan GE: *Principles and Practice of Anesthesiology*, St Louis, 1998, Mosby, p 755.
13. Pina Latorre MA, Cobeta JC, Rodilla F, Navarro N, Zabala S: Influence of calcium antagonist drugs in myasthenia gravis in the elderly, *J Clin Pharm Ther* 23:399-401, 1998.
14. Lindstrom J: Nicotinic acetylcholine receptors in health and disease, *Mol Neurobiol* 15:193-222, 1997.
15. Goudsouzian NG, Standaert FG: The infant and the myoneural junction, *Anesth Analg* 65:1208-1217, 1986
16. Singh S, Prior C: Prejunctional effects of the nicotinic ACh receptor agonist dimethylphenylpiperazinium at the rat neuromuscular junction, *J Physiol (Lond)* 511:451-460, 1998.
17. Prior C, Tian L, Dempster J, Marshall G: Prejunctional actions of muscle relaxants: synaptic vesicles and transmitter mobilization as sites of action, *Gen Pharmacol* 26:659-666, 1995.
18. Storella RJ, Ackerman TS, Katul ZJ: Tetanic fade and acetylcholine release, *Anesthesiology* 79:A923, 1993.
19. Almon RR, Appel SH: Cholinergic sites in skeletal muscles: denervation effects, *Biochemistry* 15:3662-3667, 1976.
20. Moorthy SS, Hilgenberg JC: Resistance to non-depolarizing muscle relaxants in paretic upper extremities of patients with residual hemiplegia, *Anesth Analg* 59:624-627, 1980.
21. Gronert GA: Disuse atrophy with resistance to pancuronium, *Anesthesiology* 55:547-549, 1981.
22. Sastry BVR: Nicotinic receptor, *Anaesth Pharmacol Rev* 1:6-13, 1993.
23. Gronert GA: Use of suxamethonium in cord patients—whether and when, *Anaesthesia* 53:1035-1036, 1998.
24. Murphy RA: Contractile mechanisms of muscle cells. In Berne RM, Levy MN, editors: *Physiology*, St Louis, 1998, Mosby, p 269.
25. Keens TG, Bryan AC, Levison H, Ianuzzo CD: Developmental pattern of muscle fiber types in human ventilatory muscles, *J Appl Physiol Resp* 44:909-913, 1978.
26. Drachman DB: Myasthenia gravis and other diseases of the neuromuscular junction. In Braunwald E et al, editors: *Harrison's Principles of Internal Medicine*, New York, 2001, McGraw-Hill, pp. 2515-2519.
27. Baraka A: Anaesthesia and myasthenia gravis, *Can J Anaesth* 39:476-486, 1992.
28. Zweiman B, Levinson AI: Immunologic aspects of neurological and neuromuscular diseases, *JAMA* 268:2918-2922, 1992.
29. Dalakas MC: Diseases of muscle and the neuromuscular junction, *Scientific American*, November 1-14, 1997.
30. Dierdorf SF: Anesthesia for patients with rare and co-existing diseases. In Barash PG, Cullen BF, Stoelting RF, editors: *Clinical Anesthesia*, Philadelphia, 2001, Lippincott, p 491.
31. Hofstad H, Ohm OJ, Mork SJ, Aarli JA: Heart disease in myasthenia gravis, *Acta Neurol Scand* 70:176-184, 1984
32. Lindberg C, Andersen O, Larsson S, Oden A: Remission rate after thymectomy in myasthenia gravis when the bias of immunosuppressive therapy is eliminated, *Acta Neurol Scand* 86:323-328, 1992.
33. Ceremuga TE, Xiang-Lan Y, McCabe JT: Etiology, mechanisms, and anesthesia implications of autoimmune myasthenia gravis. *AANA J* 70:301-310, 2002.
34. Miller JD, Rosenbaum H: Muscle disorders. In Benumof JL, editor: *Anesthesia and Uncommon Diseases*, Philadelphia, 1998, Saunders, p 316.
35. Froelich J: Anaesthetic management of a patient with myasthenia gravis and tracheal stenosis, *Can J Anaesth* 43:84-89, 1996.
36. Rusa R, Ulatowski JA: The patient with neurologic disorder. In *Problems in Anesthesia*, Philadelphia, 1997, Lippincott-Raven, p 221.
37. Nilsson E, Muller K: Neuromuscular effects of isoflurane in patients with myasthenia gravis, *Acta Anaesthesiol Scand* 34: 126-131, 1990.
38. Baraka A: Suxamethonium block in the myasthenic patient: Correlation with plasma cholinesterase, *Anaesthesia* 47:217-219, 1992.

39. Paterson IG, Hood JR, Russell SH, Weston MD, Hirsch NP: Mivacurium in myasthenic patient, *Br J Anaesth* 73:494-498, 1994.
40. Nilsson E, Meretoya OA: Vecuronium dose-response and maintenance requirements in patients with myasthenia gravis, *Anesthesiology* 73:28-32, 1990.
41. Tortosa JA, Hernandeq-Palazon J: Anaesthesia for laparoscopic cholecystectomy in myasthenia gravis: a non-muscle relaxant technique. *Anaesthesia* 52:807-808, 1997.
42. Itoh H, Shibata K, Yoshida M, Yamamoto K: Neuromuscular monitoring at the orbicularis oculi may overestimate the blockade in myasthenic patients, *Anesthesiology* 93:1194-1197, 2000.
43. Leventhal SR, Orkin FK, Hirsh RA. Prediction of the need for postoperative mechanical ventilation in myasthenia gravis, *Anesthesiology* 53:26-30, 1980.
44. Brown RH, Mendell JR: Muscular dystrophies and other muscle diseases. In Braunwald E et al, editors: *Harrison's Principles of Internal Medicine*, New York, 2001, McGraw-Hill, pp 2529-2540.
45. Evans BK, Gayne C: Duchenne's muscular dystrophy: review and recent scientific finding, *Am J Med Sci* 303:118-123, 1991.
46. Carlson CG: The dystrophinopathies: an alternative to the structural hypothesis, *Neurobiol Dis* 5:3-15, 1998.
47. Michalak M, Opas M: Functions of dystrophin and dystrophin associated proteins, *Curr Opin Neurol* 10:436-442, 1997.
48. Curran MJ: Muscular dystrophies and myotonic syndromes: anesthesia and musculoskeletal disorders. In Lui ACP, Crosby ET, editors: *Problems in Anesthesia*, Philadelphia, 1991, Lippincott, p 124.
49. Staiano A, Del Giudice E, Romano A, et al: Upper gastrointestinal tract motility in children with progressive muscular dystrophy, *J Pediatr* 121:720-724, 1992.
50. Chung BC, Park HJ, Yoon SB, et al: Acute gastroparesis in Duchenne's muscular dystrophy, *Yonsei Med J* 39:175-179, 1998.
51. Sasaki K, Sakata K, Kachi E, Hirata S, Ishihara T, Ishikawa K: Sequential changes in cardiac structure and function in patients with Duchenne type muscular dystrophy: a two-dimensional echocardiographic study, *Am Heart J* 135:937-944, 1998.
52. Nigro G, Comi LI, Politano L, Bain RJ: The incidence and evolution of cardiomyopathy in Duchenne's muscular dystrophy, *Int J Cardiol* 26:271-277, 1990.
53. Corrado G, Lissoni A, Beretta S, et al: Prognostic value of electrocardiograms, ventricular late potentials, ventricular arrhythmias, and left ventricular systolic dysfunction in patients with Duchenne muscular dystrophy, *Am J Card* 89:838-841, 2002.
54. Perloff JK, Roberts WC, de Leon AC Jr, O'Doherty D: The distinctive electrocardiogram of Duchenne's progressive muscular dystrophy, *Am J Med* 42:179-188, 1967.
55. Maccani RM, Wedel DJ, Melton A, Gronert GA: Femoral and lateral femoral cutaneous nerve block for muscle biopsies in children, *Paediatr Anaesth* 5:223-227, 1995.
56. Miller JD, Rosenbaum H: Muscle disorders. In Benumof JL, editor: *Anesthesia and Uncommon Diseases*. Philadelphia, 1998, Saunders, p 316.
57. Ririe DG, Shapiro F, Sethna NF: The response of patients with Duchenne's muscular dystrophy to neuromuscular blockade with vecuronium, *Anesthesiology* 88:351-354, 1998.
58. Ramchandra DS, Anisya V, Gourie-Devi M: Ketamine monoanaesthesia for diagnostic muscle biopsy in neuromuscular disorders in infancy and childhood: floppy infant syndrome, *Can J Anaesth* 37:474-476, 1990.
59. Obata R, Yasumi Y, Suzuki A, Nakajima Y, Sato S: Rhabdomyolysis in association with Duchenne's muscular dystrophy. *Can J Anaesth* 46:564-565, 1999.
60. Larsen UT, Juhl B, Hein-Sorensen O, de Fine Olivarius B: Complications during anesthesia in patients with Duchenne's muscular dystrophy, *Can J Anaesth* 36:418-422, 1989.
61. Larach MG, Rosenberg H, Gronert GA, Allen GC: Hyperkalemic cardiac arrest during anesthesia in infants and children with occult myopathies, *Clin Pediatr (Phila)* 36:9-16, 1997.
62. Rosenberg H: Death during anesthesia in children: malignant hyperthermia or muscular dystrophy? *Myasthenia Gravis (M G) Assoc Bull* 11:1-4, 1993.
63. Karan SM, Colonna-Romano P, Rosenberg H: Evaluation of the patient with neuromuscular disease. In Longnecker DE, Tinker JH, Morgan GE, editors: *Principles and Practice of Anesthesiology*, St Louis, 1998, Mosby, p 272.
64. Rosenberg H, Fletcher JE, Seitman J: Malignant hyperthermia and other pharmacogenetic disorders. In Barash PG, Cullen BF, Stoelting RK, editors: *Clinical Anesthesia*, Philadelphia, 2001, Lippincott-Raven, p 521.
65. Patel R, Leith P, Hannallah R: Evaluation of the difficult pediatric patient: ambulatory anesthesia, *Anesth Clin North Am* 14:753-767, 1996.
66. Malignant Hyperthermia Association of the United States. *Managing MH: Clinical Update Online Brochure*. Available at http://www.info@mhaus.org. Accessed on July 17, 2003.
67. Strazis KP, Fox AW: Malignant hyperthermia: a review of published cases, *Anesth Analg* 77:297-304, 1993.
68. Denborough MA, Forster JF, Lovell RR, Maplestone PA, Villiers JD: Anaesthetic deaths in a family, *Br J Anaesth* 34:395, 1962.
69. Manning BM, Quane KA, Ording H, et al: Identification of novel mutations in the ryanodine receptor gene (RYR1) in malignant hyperthermia: genotype-phenotype correlation, *Am J Hum Genet* 62:599-609, 1998.
70. Allen GC: Malignant hyperthermia susceptibility, *Anesth Clin North Am* 12:513-535, 1994.
71. Smith CA, Carvill KA, Eckert T: Suspected malignant hyperthermia in a 13-month-old: today's "typical" episode—a case report, *AANA J* 65:247-249, 1997.
72. Michalek-Sauberer A, Fricker R, Gradwohl I, Gilly H: A case of suspected malignant hyperthermia during desflurane administration, *Anesth Analg* 85:461-462, 1997.
73. Stuebing VL: Differential diagnosis of malignant hyperthermia: a case report, *J AANA* 63:455-460, 1995.
74. Sullivan M, Thompson WK, Hill GD: Succinylcholine-induced cardiac arrest in children with undiagnosed myopathy, *Can J Anaesth* 41:497-501, 1994.
75. Bissonnette B, Ryan JF: Temperature regulation: normal and abnormal (malignant hyperthermia). In Cote CJ, Ryan JF, Todres ID, Goudsouzian NG, editors: *A Practice of Anesthesia for Infants and Children*, Philadelphia, 2001, Saunders, p 610.
76. Bendixen D, Skorgaard LT, Ording H: Analysis of anesthesia in patients suspected to be susceptible to malignant hyperthermia before diagnostic in vitro contracture test, *Acta Anesthesiol Scand* 41:480-484, 1997.
77. Malignant Hyperthermia Association of the United States: *Managing MH: Clinical Update Online Brochure*. Available at www.info@mhaus.org. Accessed July 17, 2003.
78. Weglinilski MR, Wedel DJ, Engel AG: Malignant hyperthermia testing in patients with persistently increased serum creatine kinase levels, *Anesth Analg* 84:1038-1041, 1997.
79. Haggendal J, Jonsson L, Carlsten J: The role of sympathetic activity in initiating MH, *Acta Anaesthesiol Scand* 34:677-682, 1990.
80. Britt BA: Combined anesthetic- and stress-induced malignant hyperthermia in two offspring of malignant hyperthermic-susceptible parents, *Anesth Analg* 67:393-399, 1988.
81. Nelson TE, Lin M, Zapata-Sudo G, Sudo RT: Dantrolene sodium can increase or attenuate activity of skeletal muscle ryanodine receptor calcium release channel, *Anesthesiology* 84:1368-1379, 1996.
82. McGoldrick K: Is malignant hyperthermia a contraindication for outpatient surgery? *Soc Ambul Anesth News* 7:11, 1992.
83. Yentis SM, Levine MF, Hartley EJ: Should all children with suspected or confirmed malignant hyperthermia susceptibility be admitted after surgery? A ten-year review, *Anesth Analg* 75:345-350, 1992.

84. Reuter DA, Anetseder M, Muller R, Roewer N, Hartung EJ: The ryanodine contracture test may help diagnose susceptibility to malignant hyperthermia, *Can J Anaesth* 50:643-648, 2003.
85. Greenberg C: Diagnosis and treatment of hyperthermia in the post anesthesia care unit, *Anesth Clin North Am* 8:377-397, 1990.
86. Orr RJ, Ramamoorthy C: Controversies in pediatric ambulatory anesthesia, *Anesth Clin North Am* 14:767-779, 1996.
87. O'Flynn RP, Shutack JG, Rosenberg H, Fletcher JE: Masseter muscle rigidity and malignant hyperthermia susceptibility in pediatric patients: An update on management and diagnosis. *Anesthesiology* 80:1228-1233, 1994.
88. Curran MJ: Muscular dystrophies and myotonic syndromes: anesthesia and musculoskeletal disorders. In Lui ACP, Crosby ET, editors: *Problems in Anesthesia*, Philadelphia, 1991, Lippincott, p 124.
89. Ptacek LJ, Johnson KJ, Griggs RC: Genetics and physiology of the myotonic muscle disorders, *N Engl J Med* 328:482-489, 1993.
90. Bruner HG, Jansen G, Nillesen W: Brief report: reverse mutation in myotonic dystrophy, *N Engl J Med* 328:476-480, 1993.
91. Barahn RJ: Muscle diseases. In Goldman L, Ausiello D, editors: *Cecil Textbook of Medicine*, Philadelphia, 2004, Saunders, pp 2379-2386.
92. Miller J, Rosenbaum H: Muscle diseases. In Benumof JL, editor: *Anesthesia and Uncommon Diseases*, Philadelphia, 1998, Saunders, p 316.
93. Phillips DC, Ellis RF, Exley KA, Ness MA: Dantrolene sodium and dystrophia myotonica, *Anaesthesia* 39:568-573, 1984.
94. Cope DK, Miller JN: Local and spinal anesthesia for cesarean section in a patient with myotonic dystrophy, *Anesth Analg* 65:687-690, 1986.
95. Tokgozoglu LS, Ashizawa T, Pacifico A, Armstrong RM, Epstein HF, Zoghbi WA: Cardiac involvement in a large kindred with myotonic dystrophy. Quantitative assessment and relation to size of CTG repeat expansion, *JAMA* 13:813-819, 1995.
96. Hawley RJ, Milner MR, Gottdiener JS, Cohen A: Myotonic heart disease: a clinical follow-up, *Neurology* 41:259-262, 1991.
97. Stoelting RK, Dierdorf SF: Skin and musculoskeletal diseases. In Stoelting RK, Dierdorf SF, editors: *Anesthesia and Co-existing Disease*, New York, 2002, Churchill Livingstone, p 505.
98. White RJ, Bass S: Anaesthetic management of a patient with myotonic dystrophy. *Paediatric Anaesth* 11:494-497, 2001.
99. Speedy HL: Exaggerated physiological responses to propofol in myotonic dystrophy, *Br J Anaesth* 64:110-112, 1990.
100. Blumgart CH, Hughes DG, Redfern N: Obstetric anaesthesia in dystrophia myotonica, *Anaesthesia* 45:26-29, 1990.
101. Lehmann-Horn F, Iaizzo PA: Are myotonias and periodic paralyses associated with susceptibility to malignant hyperthermia? *Br J Anaesth* 65:692-697, 1990.
102. Leonovicz B, Gordon EA, Wass CT: Paraneoplastic syndromes associated with lung cancer: A unique case of concomitant subacute cerebellar degeneration and Lambert-Eaton myasthenic syndrome, *Anesth Analg* 93:1557-1559, 2001.
103. Gutman L, Phillips HG II: Trends in the association of Lambert-Eaton myasthenic syndrome with carcinoma, *Neurology* 42: 848-850, 1992.
104. Leys K, Lang B, Johnston I, Newsom-Davis J: Calcium channel autoantibodies in the Lambert-Eaton myasthenic syndrome, *Ann Neurol* 29:307-314, 1991.
105. Telford RJ, Hollway TE: The myasthenic syndrome: anaesthesia in a patient treated with 3,4 diaminopyridine, *Br J Anaesth* 64:363-366, 1990.
106. Oh SJ, Kim DS, Head TC, Claussen GC: Low-dose guanidine and pyridostigmine: relatively safe and effective long-term symptomatic therapy in Lambert-Eaton myasthenic syndrome, *Muscle Nerve* 20:1146-1152, 1997.
107. Muchnik S, Losavio AS, Vidal A, Cura L, Mazia C: Long-term follow-up of Lambert-Eaton syndrome with intravenous immunoglobulin, *Muscle Nerve* 20:674-678, 1997.
108. Itoh H, Shibata K, Nitta S: Neuromuscular monitoring in myasthenic syndrome. *Anaesthesia* 56:562-567, 2001.
109. Eberhardt K, Fex E: Clinical course and remission rate in patients with early rheumatoid arthritis: relationship to outcome after 5 years, *Br J Rheumatol* 37:1324-1329, 1998.
110. Lipsky PE: Rheumatoid arthritis. In Braunwald E et al, editors: *Harrison's Principles of Internal Medicine*, New York, 2001, McGraw-Hill, pp 1928-1936.
111. Shiozawa S, Hayashi S, Tsukamoto Y, et al: Identification of the gene loci that predispose to rheumatoid arthritis, *Int Immunol* 10:1891-1895, 1998.
112. Jeffries WM: The etiology of rheumatoid arthritis, *Med Hypotheses* 51:111-114, 1998.
113. Keenan MA, Stiles CM, Kaufman RL: Acquired laryngeal deviation associated with cervical spine disease in erosive polyarticular arthritis, *Anesthesiology* 58:441-449, 1983.
114. Bourke DL, Yates Jr AJ, Yates HM: Evaluation of the patient with musculoskeletal disease. In Longnecker DE, Tinker JH, Morgan GE, editors: *Principles and Practice of Anesthesiology*, St Louis, 1998, Mosby, p 287.
115. Khanan T: Anaesthetic risks in rheumatoid arthritis, *Br J Hosp Med* 52:320-325, 1994.
116. Vetter TR: Acute airway obstruction due to arytenoiditis in a child with juvenile rheumatoid arthritis, *Anesth Analg* 79:1198-1200, 1994.
117. Ahern M, Lever JV, Cosh J: Complete heart block in rheumatoid arthritis, *Ann Rheum Dis* 42:389-397, 1983.
118. Tanoue LT: Pulmonary manifestations of rheumatoid arthritis, *Clin Chest Med* 19:667-685, 1998.
119. Simon LS, Weaver AL, Graham DY, et al: Anti-inflammatory and upper gastrointestinal effects of celecoxib in rheumatoid arthritis: a randomized controlled trial, *JAMA* 282:1921-1928, 1999.
120. Mest CG: Osteoarthritis and rheumatoid arthritis. In Arcangelo V, Peterson AM, editors: *Pharmacotherapeutics for Advanced Practice*, Philadelphia, 2001, Lippincott, p 515.
121. Rich E, Moreland LW, Alarcon GS: Paucity of radiographic progression in rheumatoid arthritis treated with methotrexate as the first disease-modifying antirheumatic drug, *J Rheumatol* 26:259-261, 1999.
122. Lipsky PE, Desiree MFM, van der Heijde MD: Infliximab and methotrexate in the treatment of rheumatoid arthritis. *N Engl J Med* 343:1594-1602, 2000.
123. Bathon JM, Martin RW, Fleischmann RM: A comparison of etanercept and methotrexate in patients with early rheumatoid arthritis. *N Engl J Med* 343:1586-1593, 2000.
124. Adalimumab (Humira) for rheumatoid arthritis. In Abramowick M, editor: *The Medical Letter on Drugs and Therapeutics* 45:25-28, 2003.
125. Bresnihan B, Alvaro-Gracia JM, Cobby M, et al: Treatment of rheumatoid arthritis with recombinant human interleukin-1 receptor antagonist, *Arthritis Rheumatol* 41:2196-2204, 1998.
126. Hakim NS, Kobienia B, Benedetti E, Bloomer J, Payne WD: Methotrexate-induced hepatic necrosis requiring liver transplantation in a patient with rheumatoid arthritis, *Int Surg* 83:224-225, 1998.
127. Kwek TK, Lew TW, Thoo FL: The role of preoperative cervical spine X-rays in rheumatoid arthritis. *Anaesth Intensive Care* 26:636-641, 1998.

CHAPTER 31

THE ENDOCRINE SYSTEM

MARY C. KARLET

GENERAL PRINCIPLES OF ENDOCRINE PHYSIOLOGY

Body homeostasis is controlled by two major regulating systems: (1) the nervous system and (2) the endocrine or hormonal system. Both of these systems communicate, integrate, and organize the body's response to a changing internal or external environment.[1]

Organs that secrete hormones are called *endocrine glands*; collectively, these glands make up the *endocrine system*. The purpose of the endocrine system is regulation of behavior, growth, metabolism, fluid status, development, and reproduction. To accomplish these complex processes, multiple hormones interact to produce precise biochemical and physiologic responses.[2]

Endocrine glands secrete their hormone products directly into the surrounding extracellular fluid. This distinguishes them from *exocrine glands*, such as salivary or sweat glands, whose products are discharged through ducts. Important endocrine glands include the pituitary gland, the thyroid gland, the parathyroid glands, the adrenal glands, the pancreas, the ovaries and testes, and the placenta.

Hormones

Endocrine function is mediated by hormones. Hormones are the signaling molecules or chemical messengers that transport information from one set of cells (endocrine cells) to another (target cells). *Hormaein*, the original Greek term for the word *hormone* means "to set in motion" or "to excite." Hormones are released from endocrine glands into body fluids in minute quantities but exert powerful control over most metabolic functions.[3]

Transmission of a hormonal signal through the bloodstream to a distant target cell (e.g., pituitary gland to the adrenal gland) is called an *endocrine function*. If a hormone signal acts on a neighboring cell of a different type (e.g., pancreas α-cells to pancreas β-cells), the interaction is termed a *paracrine function*. If the secreted hormone acts on the producer cell itself or on neighboring identical cells, the interaction is called an *autocrine function*.[1,2]

Types of Hormones. Hormones can be classified into three major categories: (1) proteins or peptides, (2) amines or amino acid derivatives, and (3) steroids.[1]

Peptide or Protein Hormones. Most hormones have a peptide or protein structure. This group of hormones includes insulin, growth hormone, vasopressin (antidiuretic hormone), angiotensin, prolactin, erythropoietin, calcitonin, somatostatin, adrenocorticotropic hormone (ACTH), oxytocin, glucagon, and parathyroid hormone. Peptide hormones are synthesized in endocrine cells as prehormones and prohormones. They are processed by the cell and stored in secretory granules within the endocrine gland.[1,2] The proper stimulus to secretion causes exocytosis of the peptide or protein hormone into the extracellular fluid.

Hormones, such as insulin, erythropoietin, and growth hormone, can now be synthesized for therapeutic purposes by recombinant deoxyribonucleic acid (DNA) techniques.

Amine- or Amino Acid–Derivative Hormones. Several hormones are amino acid or amine compound derivatives. Serotonin, important for its central nervous system effects, is synthesized from the naturally occurring amino acid tryptophan.[2] Thyroid hormones and catecholamine hormones (dopamine, epinephrine, and norepinephrine) are derived from the amino acid tyrosine. Thyroid hormones and catecholamine hormones are stored in the thyroid gland and adrenal medulla, respectively, and are released by the appropriate stimulation.[1]

Steroid Hormones. All steroid hormones are derived from cholesterol or have a chemical structure similar to that of cholesterol. Common steroid hormones include hormones of the adrenal cortex (e.g., cortisol, aldosterone) and reproductive hormones (e.g., estrogen, progesterone, testosterone). Active metabolites of vitamin D are also steroid hormones. In contrast to most other hormones, steroid hormones are not stored in discrete secretory granules, but are compartmentalized within the endocrine cell and released into the extracellular fluid by simple diffusion through the cell membrane.[1,2]

Circulating steroid and thyroid hormones are bound to *transport proteins*, whereas circulating catecholamine hormones and most protein hormones are not bound to carriers. Plasma protein binding protects hormones from metabolism and renal clearance.[2] The circulating half-life of steroid and thyroid hormones is therefore typically longer than that of peptide and catecholamine hormones. For example, T_4, which is 99.95% protein bound, has a plasma half-life of 6 days, whereas insulin, which has essentially no plasma protein binding, has a half-life of about 7 minutes.[1]

The major sites of hormone degradation and elimination are the liver and the kidneys. Some hormone degradation also occurs at target cell sites.[1,2,3]

Hormone Receptors

Binding to a specific target cell receptor is the primary event that initiates a hormone response.[2] The hormone receptor displays high specificity and affinity for the proper hormone ligand, and the location of the receptor directs the hormone to the proper target organ or target cell site.[4] Some hormones, such as insulin and growth hormone, act on widespread target sites; others, such as thyroid-stimulating hormone (TSH), act on one target tissue.[5] After binding, the hormone-receptor complex induces a cascade of intracellular events that produce specific physiologic responses in the target cell.[2]

Hormone Receptor Activation. Hormone receptors are located either on the surface of cells or inside cells.[3] Receptors for protein, peptide, and catecholamine hormones are located in or on the surface of the target cell membrane. Hormone binding to a cell membrane receptor triggers a response by activating enzyme systems in or near the plasma membrane bilayer. The activated enzymes generate intracellular signals, called *second messengers*, which carry the hormone's message within the intracellular space.

Several different second-messenger systems operate in response to cell membrane receptor-hormone binding. Probably the most widely described second-messenger system is the *cyclic adenosine monophosphate (cAMP) system*. This hormone transduction mechanism is initiated when receptor occupation activates the plasma membrane enzyme *adenyl cyclase*. The membrane-bound adenyl cyclase then catalyzes the intracellular conversion of adenosine triphosphate (ATP) to cAMP. cAMP, in turn, becomes the hormone's intracellular messenger, activating intracellular enzymes, modifying cell membrane permeability or transport, and altering cellular gene expression.[1] The enzyme phosphodiesterase catalyzes the hydrolysis of cAMP and terminates its intracellular actions. Hormones that utilize cAMP as their second messenger include TSH, vasopressin, parathyroid hormone, glucagon, some catecholamines, corticotropin, follicle-stimulating hormone (FSH), and luteinizing hormone (LH).

Other intracellular second messengers include calcium, diacylglycerol, inositol triphosphate, and cyclic guanosine monophosphate. The primary intracellular messenger has not been determined for many hormones.

In contrast to peptide and catecholamine hormones, thyroid and steroid hormones produce the desired target cell response chiefly by interacting with specific intracellular hormone receptors.[1] Thyroid and steroid hormones are small lipophilic molecules that enter target cells by simple diffusion or by special transport mechanisms. Once within the cell, these hormones occupy specific intracellular receptors.[2] In combination with their receptors, these hormones interact with DNA in the cell nucleus to enhance or suppress gene transcription or translation.[1,2]

Thyroid and steroid hormones enable the cell to alter gene expression, protein formation, and cell activity in response to environmental and developmental stimuli.[2]

Every hormone has a specific onset and duration of action.[3] Hormones that act by binding to cell membrane receptors (peptide, protein, and catecholamine hormones) usually generate a hormonal effect in seconds to minutes.[1,3] Hormones that bind to intracellular receptors and activate the transcription processes of specific genes (thyroid and steroid hormones) may require several hours or even days to generate a hormonal response.[1,3]

Hormone Receptor Regulation. Receptors are dynamic molecules that are constantly being destroyed and replaced.[2] The receptor for insulin, for example, has a normal half-life of only about 7 hours.[2] Hormone receptor destruction may be part of a normal endocrine response or may be part of an acquired or genetic disease state.

In many instances the hormone receptor number is inversely related to the concentration of the circulating hormone. A sustained elevation of the plasma level of a given hormone may cause the target site to decrease the number of receptors per cell. This *downregulation* of receptor number serves to decrease the responsiveness of a target cell to hormone excess.[1] The insulin resistance observed in obesity and type 2 diabetes mellitus may be partly explained by downregulation of the insulin receptors in response to chronically high levels of circulating insulin.[2]

Conversely, a low circulating hormone concentration may cause the target gland to increase the number of hormone receptors per cell.[2] This *upregulation* of hormone receptor number amplifies the cell's sensitivity to hormone stimulation.[1,2]

The number of receptors in a target cell usually changes from day to day.[3] Regulation of receptor turnover, and thus hormone receptor number, is a mechanism by which hormone activity can be modulated.[1]

Regulation of Hormone Secretion. The synthesis and secretion of hormones by endocrine glands is regulated by three general control mechanisms: neural controls, biorhythms, and feedback mechanisms.

Neural control can evoke or suppress hormone secretion. Pain, emotion, smell, touch, injury, stress, sight, and taste can alter hormone release through neural mechanisms.[1] Glucagon, cortisol, antidiuretic hormone, and catecholamines, for example, are all stimulated by the stress response to anesthesia, surgery, and trauma.

The secretion of many hormones is governed by genetically encoded or acquired *biorhythms*. These intrinsic hormonal oscillations may be circadian (e.g., the daily variability in glucocorticoid secretion), weekly (e.g., the menstrual cycle), or seasonal (e.g., thyroxine production).[1,4] The biorhythms may also vary at different stages of life (e.g., growth hormone secretion).[6]

Feedback control is another sophisticated mechanism through which a hormonal response is controlled. Many endocrine disorders arise from the breakdown of feedback loops.[2] *Negative feedback* acts to limit or terminate the production and secretion of a given hormone, once the appropriate response has occurred. Negative feedback of a target cell product to the hormone producer (the endocrine gland) limits or prevents hormone excess. When concentrations of the product are low, feedback inhibition to the endocrine gland is lessened and hormone secretion enhanced.

Virtually all hormones are controlled by some type of negative feedback mechanism.[3,4] For example, parathyroid hormone is controlled by calcium, insulin and glucagon are controlled by glucose, and vasopressin is controlled by serum osmolarity.[5] The negative feedback mechanism is a very important factor in the regulation of hormones of the hypothalamus and pituitary gland. Hypothalamic hormones stimulate the release of pituitary hormones from the pituitary gland. The pituitary hormones, in turn, may stimulate an output of product from peripheral target cells. Product from peripheral target tissues may initiate feedback to the pituitary gland or the hypothalamus to inhibit pituitary or hypothalamic hormone synthesis and discharge.[1]

Positive feedback is a less common hormone regulating mechanism, in which a given hormone response initiates signals amplifying hormone release. The surge in LH that precedes ovulation is stimulated by LH; this is an example of positive feedback.[2]

PITUITARY GLAND

Relationship Between Pituitary Gland and Hypothalamus

The *pituitary gland*, or *hypophysis*, is known as the "master endocrine gland." It secretes hormones that have far-reaching effects on various homeostatic, developmental, metabolic, and reproductive functions of the body. The pituitary is a small endocrine gland (only 500 mg in weight and about the size of a pea) centrally located at the base of the brain. It is enclosed within a bony cavity of the sphenoid bone called the *sella turcica*.[5,6] The pituitary gland is connected to the overlying hypothalamus by the *hypophyseal stalk (pituitary stalk)*. The hypothalamus is located below the thalamus, behind the optic chiasm, and between the optic tracts. The pituitary, hypothalamus, and some of the surrounding structures are shown in Figure 31-1.

The brain, via the hypothalamus, is an important regulator of pituitary gland secretion.[6] The hypothalamus collects and integrates information (pain, emotions, energy needs, water balance, olfactory sensations, electrolyte concentrations) from almost all parts of the body and uses this information to control the secretion of vital pituitary hormones.[5,6] Pituitary hormone secretion also is regulated by feedback control from peripheral target organ hormones or other target organ products.[5]

Functionally and histologically, the pituitary gland is divided into two distinct portions: the *anterior lobe (adenohypophysis)* and the *posterior lobe (neurohypophysis)*.[6] The anterior pituitary lobe is embryologically derived from an upward invagination of pharyngeal epithelial cells. The posterior pituitary lobe develops from a downward outpouching of ectoderm from the brain.[5] Blood supply to the anterior pituitary lobe is principally from the superior hypophyseal artery, which is a branch of the internal carotid artery. Blood supply to the posterior pituitary lobe is via the inferior hypophyseal artery.[5]

Anterior Pituitary Lobe

The anterior pituitary lobe, which constitutes about 80% of the pituitary gland by weight, secretes six primary hormones.[6] Target sites for the anterior pituitary hormones are shown in Figure 31-2.

1. *Growth hormone* promotes skeletal development and body growth and regulates protein and carbohydrate metabolism.
2. *Adrenocorticotrophic hormone (ACTH)* regulates the growth of the adrenal cortex and the release of cortisol and androgenic hormones from the adrenal gland. ACTH possesses mild melanocyte-stimulating properties, resulting in skin pigmentation at high levels.
3. *TSH* controls the growth and metabolism of the thyroid gland and the secretion of thyroid hormones, which regulate the rates of most chemical reactions in the body.[5,6]
4. *FSH* stimulates ovarian follicle development in females and spermatogenesis in males.
5. *LH* induces ovulation and corpus luteum development in females and stimulates the testes to produce testosterone in males.
6. *Prolactin* promotes mammary gland development and milk production (lactogenesis) by the breasts. Prolactin also exerts an effect on reproductive function by inhibiting the synthesis and secretion of LH and FSH. Prolactin synthesis is markedly increased during pregnancy.[5]

Several other less important or less well-defined hormones also are secreted from the anterior pituitary lobe.[6]

Anterior pituitary hormones are synthesized and secreted by at least five distinct cell types within the gland: *somatotrophs (acidophils)* synthesize growth hormone; *gonadotrophs* synthesize the two gonadotropic hormones, LH and FSH; *thyrotrophs* synthesize TSH; *corticotrophs* synthesize ACTH; and *lactotrophs (mammotrophs)* synthesize prolactin. About 40% to 50% of the anterior pituitary cells are somatotrophs and about 20% are corticotrophs.[5]

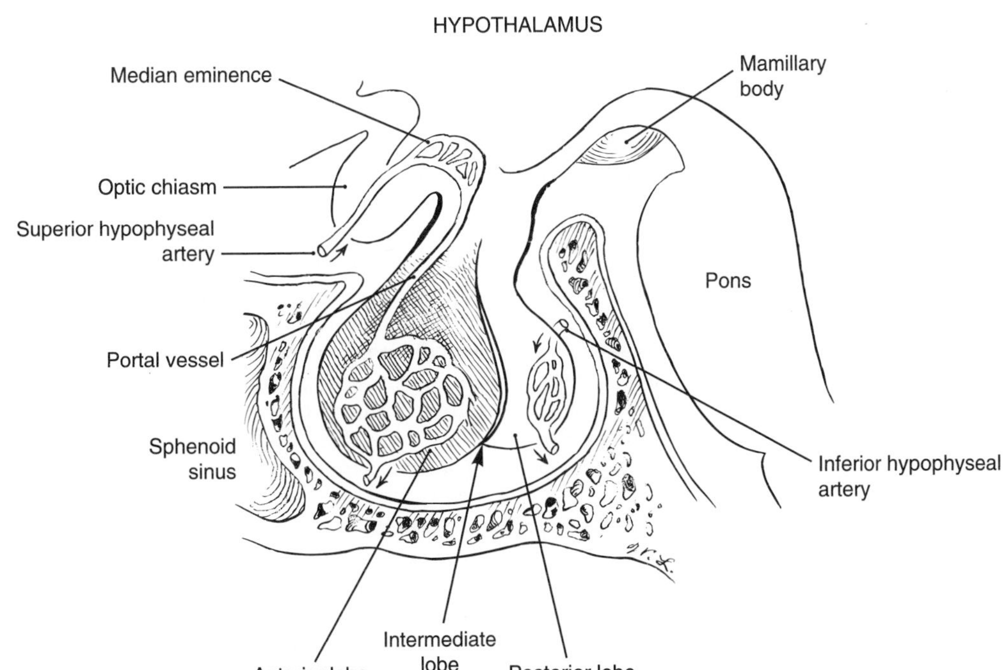

FIGURE **31-1** The pituitary gland is located at the base of the brain, enclosed within a cavity of the sphenoid bone called the *sella turcica*. It is connected to the overlying hypothalamus by the pituitary stalk.

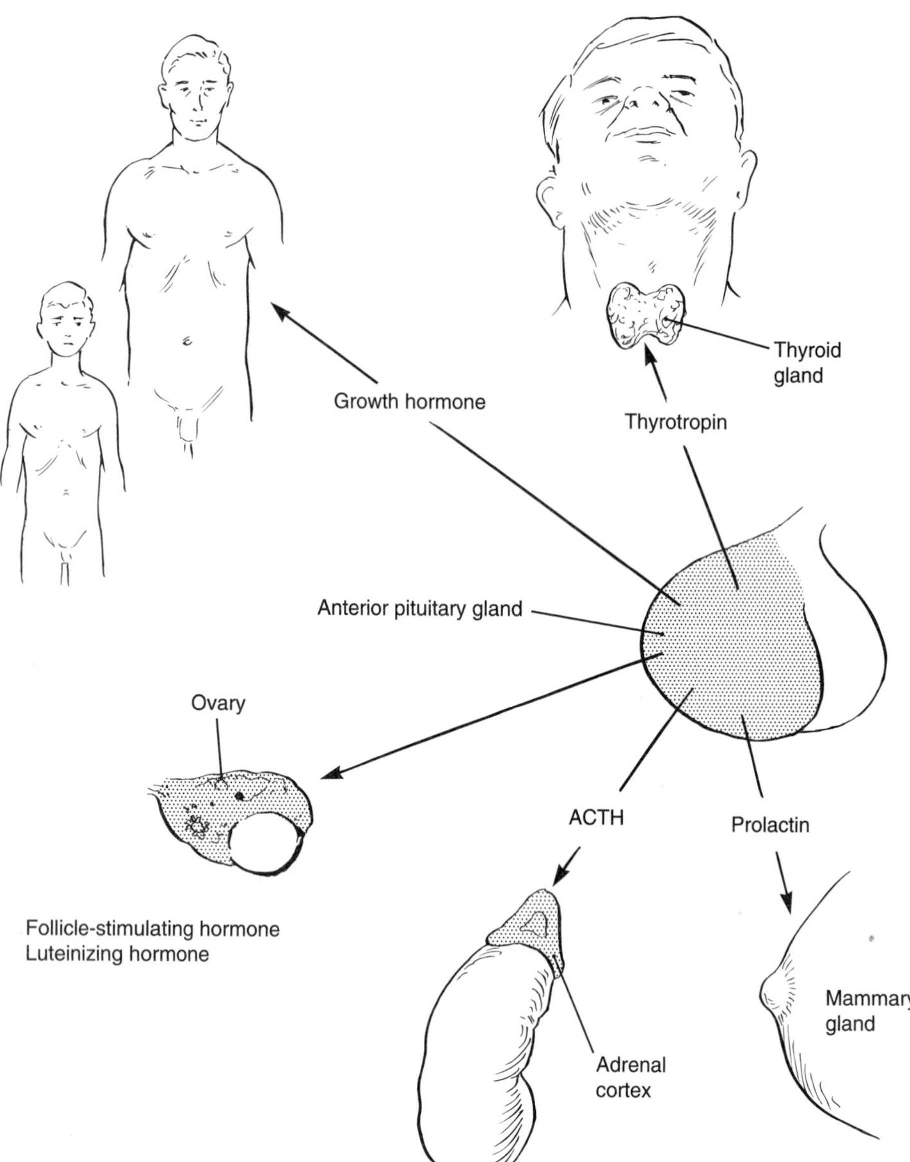

FIGURE **31-2**
Major target sites for anterior pituitary hormones. *ACTH*, adrenocorticotropic hormone.

Control of Anterior Pituitary Lobe's Hormone Secretion. Synthesis of anterior pituitary hormones is controlled by signals from the hypothalamus. Neurosecretory cells in various hypothalamic nuclei respond to input from the body by synthesizing specific neurohormones. Each hypothalamic neurohormone has a corresponding anterior pituitary target cell type(s).[6]

Hypothalamic neurohormones are released into a capillary bed of the hypothalamus in an area called the *median eminence*. The hypothalamic hormones travel from the capillary plexus of the median eminence, down the pituitary stalk, in a specialized vascular system called the *hypothalamic-hypophyseal portal vessels*. At the anterior pituitary lobe, the hypothalamic hormones are released in high concentrations into capillary sinuses located among the glandular cells.[6] The hypothalamic hormones then locate and bind to their specific target cell type.

Specific hypothalamic hormones have either an inhibitory or a stimulatory effect on their corresponding anterior pituitary target cells. Synthesis and release of most anterior pituitary hormones depend on a positive stimulatory signal from a given hypothalamic hormone. Some anterior pituitary cells are subject to both inhibitory and stimulatory control by more than one hypothalamic neurohormone.[5]

Synthesis of prolactin from anterior pituitary lactotroph cells is unique in that it is tonically restrained by an inhibitory hormonal signal (dopamine) from the hypothalamus. In essence, dopamine serves as a "physiologic brake" for lactotroph growth and prolactin synthesis. The inhibitory effect of dopamine agonists, such as bromocriptine, is exploited therapeutically for suppressing undesired nursing or for inhibiting pathologic production of prolactin from pituitary tumors.[5] Table 31-1 outlines the major hypothalamic releasing or inhibiting hormones and their corresponding anterior pituitary target sites.

Anterior Pituitary Disorders

Hyposecretion. Anterior pituitary hyposecretion may occur when large pituitary tumors (usually chromophobe adenomas) compress and destroy normal anterior pituitary cells. Postpartum shock (Sheehan's syndrome), irradiation, trauma, and hypophysectomy are other causes of anterior pituitary

TABLE 31-1 Hypothalamic Hormones and Corresponding Anterior Pituitary Hormones

Hypothalamic Releasing/ Inhibiting Hormones	Anterior Pituitary Target Cell Type	Anterior Pituitary Hormone Produced	Hormone Target Site
Thyrotropin-releasing hormone	Thyrotroph	Thyroid-stimulating hormone (TSH, thyrotropin)	Thyroid gland
Corticotropin-releasing hormone	Corticotroph	Adrenocorticotropic hormone (ACTH, corticotropin)	Adrenal gland
Gonadotropin-releasing hormone	Gonadotroph	Follicle-stimulating hormone Luteinizing hormone	Gonads (testes, ovaries)
Prolactin-releasing factor Prolactin-inhibitory factor (dopamine, PIF)	Lactotroph (mammotroph)	Prolactin	Breasts
Growth hormone–releasing hormone Growth hormone–inhibitory factor (somatostatin)	Somatotroph	Growth hormone	All tissues

hormone deficiency states.[7,8] Generalized pituitary hypofunction (*panhypopituitarism*) is more common than reduced output of a single anterior pituitary hormone.[9]

Important effects of panhypopituitarism include a decrease in thyroid function because of a reduction in levels of TSH, depression of glucocorticoid production by the adrenal cortex because of the lowering of ACTH levels, and suppression of sexual development and reproductive function because of deficient gonadotropic hormone secretion.[6,10] In addition, large pituitary tumors (macroadenomas) may extend into or compress the surrounding brain tissue, producing diplopia, visual loss, facial numbness, facial pain, or (rarely) seizures.

Surgical intervention may be implemented to control bleeding or for decompression or removal of the pituitary tumor. Surgical patients with hypopituitary disorders may require thyroid hormone replacement and corticosteroid coverage in the perioperative period.[11] Because of the possibility of diabetes insipidus after removal of the tumor, vasopressin should also be available.

Most pituitary adenomas are operated on via a transsphenoidal approach, and this route is generally well tolerated by most patients.[12,13] A transfrontal approach may be used for tumors with suprasellar extension.[14] Serious complications from transsphenoidal pituitary surgery occur in less than 1.5% of cases.

For transsphenoidal pituitary surgery, the surgeon may request that the patient be placed in a half-sitting position. Occasionally the approach and exposure of the tumor are associated with significant blood loss. The surgeon may use submucosal injection of epinephrine-containing solutions or topical cocaine to assist in hemostasis. Preparing the patient preoperatively for awakening with nasal packing is important. An anesthetic technique that allows for smooth extubation and rapid neurologic assessment is desirable.

Hypersecretion. The hypersecretion of anterior pituitary hormones usually is caused by a hyperfunctioning pituitary adenoma. The three most common hypersecreting pituitary tumors are those that produce prolactin, ACTH, and growth hormone. Tumors that secrete gonadotropin and thyrotropin hormones are rare.

Prolactin-secreting tumors commonly produce symptoms of galactorrhea, amenorrhea, and infertility in women, and decreased libido and impotence in men. The dopamine agonist bromocriptine is usually effective in controlling prolactin levels, decreasing the tumor size, and restoring normal gonadal function. Patients who have a suboptimal response to medical therapy benefit from microsurgical removal of the pituitary tumor.[12,13]

Preparation of the patient awaiting pituitary surgery is guided in part by the results of preoperative endocrine tests. Hypersecreting pituitary tumors may become so large that they compress and destroy normal anterior pituitary cells, producing a deficiency in some anterior pituitary hormones. Specific anesthetic management implications for patients with excess ACTH (Cushing's disease) and excess growth hormone (acromegaly) are described later in this chapter.

Growth Hormone. *Growth hormone (somatotropin)* is synthesized and secreted by somatotroph cells of the anterior pituitary lobe and is under dual control by the hypothalamus.[6] Growth hormone–releasing hormone stimulates growth hormone release, and growth hormone–inhibiting hormone (somatostatin) is a powerful inhibitor of growth hormone release.[5] Pulsatile fluctuations of the hypothalamic releasing and inhibiting hormones regulate somatotroph activity throughout the day.[5]

The growth hormone secretion rate is generally increased in childhood, followed by a further increase in adolescence, a plateau in adulthood, and declining values in old age. In addition, growth hormone secretion is stimulated by stress (including anesthesia and surgery), hypoglycemia, exercise, and deep sleep. Growth hormone release is inhibited by hyperglycemia and increased plasma free fatty acids. The normal fasting growth hormone concentration in adults is 1 to 5 ng/mL.

Unlike the other anterior pituitary hormones, growth hormone does not exert its principal effects through a specific target gland but functions through all or almost all tissues of the body. Growth hormone promotes the growth and development of most tissues that are capable of growing.[6] Skeletal muscle, the heart, skin, and visceral organs undergo hypertrophy and hyperplasia in response to growth hormone.

Growth hormone's most obvious effect is on the skeletal frame. It produces linear bone growth by stimulating the epiphyseal cartilage or growth plate at the ends of long bones.[5,6] Throughout childhood, under the influence of growth hormone, bones elongate at the epiphyseal plate, and the skeletal frame enlarges. After puberty, the growth plates unite with the shaft of the bone, and bone lengthening stops. Growth hormone then has no further capacity to increase the bone length.[6]

Growth hormone supports growth by increasing amino acid transport into cells and enhancing protein synthesis in the cell. It also decreases the catabolism of existing proteins by stimulating lipolysis and mobilizing free fatty acids for energy use, a protein-sparing effect.[6]

In addition to its growth-promoting activities, growth hormone is said to be a "diabetogenic hormone." It increases blood glucose levels by decreasing the sensitivity of the cell to insulin and by inhibiting glucose uptake into the cell.[6]

As is true of other anterior pituitary hormones, growth hormone secretion is subject to negative feedback control. Somatomedins (growth factors) and growth hormone itself exert negative feedback control on the hypothalamus and the pituitary to inhibit growth hormone secretion.

Hyposecretion. Deficient growth hormone production in childhood can result in insufficient bone maturation and short stature, a condition known as *dwarfism*. Mild obesity, decreased lean body mass, and hypoglycemia are common in growth hormone–deficient dwarfs. Puberty usually is delayed. Symptoms of growth hormone deficiency may be the result of hypothalamic dysfunction, pituitary disease, failure to generate normal somatomedins, or growth receptor defects.[6]

The biosynthesis of human growth hormone by recombinant DNA techniques has enhanced the outlook for patients with growth hormone deficiency. Treatment of these patients with growth hormone leads to a positive nitrogen balance, accretion of lean body mass, and an improvement in metabolic homeostasis.[15]

Hypersecretion. Growth hormone hypersecretion, usually caused by a growth hormone–secreting pituitary adenoma (99% of cases), can produce a highly distinctive syndrome in adults called *acromegaly*. Acromegaly is produced by sustained hypersecretion of growth hormone after adolescence. The condition occurs with equal frequency in both sexes.[16,17] If hypersecretion of growth hormone occurs before puberty—that is, before closure of the growth plates—the individual grows very tall (8 to 9 feet), a rare condition known as *gigantism*.

The excessive production of growth hormone associated with acromegaly does not induce bone lengthening but rather enhances the growth of periosteal bone. Periosteal growth causes new bone to be deposited on the surface of existing bone.[6] The unrestrained bone growth in patients with acromegaly produces bones that are massive in size and thickness. Bones of the hands and feet (*acral*) become particularly large. Overgrowth of vertebrae may cause kyphoscoliosis and arthritis.

Soft tissue changes are also prominent with growth hormone hypersecretion. The patient develops coarsened facial features (*acromegalic facies*) including a large, bulbous nose; supraorbital ridge overgrowth; dental malocclusion; and a prominent prognathic mandible.[16] The changes in appearance are insidious, and many patients do not seek treatment until the diagnosis is obvious and the disease course advanced.[16,18]

Overgrowth of internal organs is less apparent clinically but no less serious. The liver, heart, spleen, and kidneys become enlarged. Lung volumes increase, which may lead to ventilation-perfusion mismatch. Exercise tolerance may be limited because of increased body mass and skeletal muscle weakness.[16]

Cardiomyopathy, hypertension (28% of cases), and accelerated atherosclerosis in patients with acromegaly can lead to symptomatic cardiac disease (congestive heart failure, arrhythmias).[16,18] Echocardiography often shows left ventricular hypertrophy.[8] Resting electrocardiograms are abnormal in 50% of acromegalic patients. ST-segment and T-wave depression, conduction defects, and evidence of prior myocardial infarction may be present.[16]

The insulin antagonistic effect of growth hormone produces glucose intolerance in up to 50% of patients with acromegaly, and frank diabetes mellitus in 10% to 25% of patients.[16]

Clinical manifestations resulting from the local effects of the expanding tumor may include headaches (55%), which reflect extrasellar extension of the tumor; papilledema; and visual field defects (19%), which are caused by compression of the optic nerves and chiasm. Significant increases in intracranial pressure are uncommon. Compression or destruction of normal pituitary tissue by the tumor may lead to panhypopituitarism.[16,17] Common features of acromegaly are summarized in Box 31-1.

Treatment for acromegaly is aimed at restoring normal growth hormone levels. The preferred initial therapy for active acromegaly is microsurgical removal of the pituitary tumor with preservation of the gland.[12,18] The surgical approach to the pituitary tumor most often is via a transsphenoidal route.[18] Surgical ablation is usually successful in rapidly reducing tumor size, inhibiting growth hormone secretion, and alleviating some symptoms.[16,17,18] Administration of octreotide (a long-acting somatostatin analogue) or bromocriptine and gland irradiation are treatment options for patients who are not surgical candidates; these are useful adjunctive forms of therapy.[12]

Anesthetic Implications of Acromegaly. Preanesthetic assessment of patients with acromegaly should include a careful examination of the airway. Facial deformities and the large nose may hamper adequate fitting of an anesthesia mask.[9,19] Endotracheal intubation may be a challenge because of these patient's large and thick tongue (macroglossia), enlargement of the thyroid, obstructive teeth, hypertrophy of the epiglottis, and general soft tissue overgrowth in the upper airway.[11,19] Subglottic narrowing and vocal cord enlargement may dictate the use of a smaller-diameter endotracheal tube.[20] Nasotracheal intubation should be approached cautiously because of possible turbinate enlargement.[9] Muchler and colleagues reported intubation difficulties in 31% of the acromegalic patients studied.[21] Preoperative dyspnea, stridor, or hoarseness should alert the anesthetist to airway involvement.[9] Indirect laryngoscopy and neck radiography may be performed for thorough assessment. If

BOX **31-1**

Common Features of Acromegaly

- Skeletal overgrowth (enlarged hands and feet, prominent prognathic mandible)
- Soft tissue overgrowth (enlarged lips, tongue, and epiglottis; distortion of facial features)
- Visceromegaly
- Osteoarthritis
- Glucose intolerance
- Peripheral neuropathy
- Skeletal muscle weakness
- Extrasellar tumor extension (headache, visual field defects)

difficulties in maintaining an adequate airway are anticipated, a fiberoptic-guided intubation in an awake patient is of proven value.[20,22] The endotracheal tube should remain in place until the patient is fully awake and has total return of reflexes. The predisposition to airway obstruction in these patients makes assiduous postoperative monitoring of the patient's respiratory status a wise precaution.

The frequent occurrence of cardiac arrhythmias, coronary artery disease, and hypertension in acromegalic patients warrants a thorough preanesthetic cardiac evaluation. The increased risk of diabetes mellitus in these patients mandates careful perioperative monitoring of blood glucose and electrolyte levels.

If preoperative assessment reveals impairment of the adrenal or thyroid axis, stress-level glucocorticoid therapy and thyroid replacement should be implemented in the perioperative period.

Entrapment neuropathies, such as carpal tunnel syndrome, are common in patients with acromegaly. An Allen test should be performed before placement of a radial artery catheter as hypertrophy of the carpal ligament may cause inadequate ulnar artery flow.[9]

Posterior Pituitary Lobe

The posterior pituitary lobe secretes two important peptide hormones: *antidiuretic hormone* (*vasopressin* or *ADH*) and *oxytocin*. Oxytocin and ADH are structurally very similar, but they have quite different actions. ADH controls water excretion and reabsorption in the kidney and is a major regulator of serum osmolarity. Oxytocin stimulates contraction of myoepithelial cells of the breast for milk ejection during lactation. It also powerfully stimulates uterine smooth muscle contraction, and it may play a role in parturition.[6] Oxytocin and its derivatives are used clinically for inducing labor and decreasing postpartum bleeding.

In contrast to the anterior pituitary lobe, which communicates with the hypothalamus via a vascular system, the posterior pituitary lobe communicates with the hypothalamus through a neural pathway. Unlike anterior pituitary hormones, posterior pituitary hormones are not synthesized within the pituitary gland itself but rather within two large nuclei of the hypothalamus, called the *supraoptic nucleus* and the *paraventricular nucleus*. ADH is largely synthesized in the supraoptic nucleus, and oxytocin is chiefly synthesized in the paraventricular nucleus.[6] As shown in Figure 31-3, nerve fibers arising from these hypothalamic nuclei transport ADH and oxytocin down the pituitary stalk by axoplasmic flow to the posterior pituitary lobe. There, the hormones are stored in secretory granules at the nerve terminals. With proper excitation, nerve impulses, originating in the cell bodies of the supraoptic or paraventricular nucleus, are transmitted down the pituitary stalk and stimulate the release of ADH or oxytocin from the posterior pituitary lobe. The hormones are picked up by nearby blood vessels and are transported to their distant target sites.

Antidiuretic Hormone. ADH is the body's principal preserver of water balance. It acts on renal collecting ducts to increase the absorption of solute-free water from kidney tubules, thereby conserving water in the body and supporting normal body fluid osmolarity. Without ADH, the collecting ducts are impermeable to water reabsorption; in this setting, water loss in the urine is excessive and serious dehydration is provoked.[6]

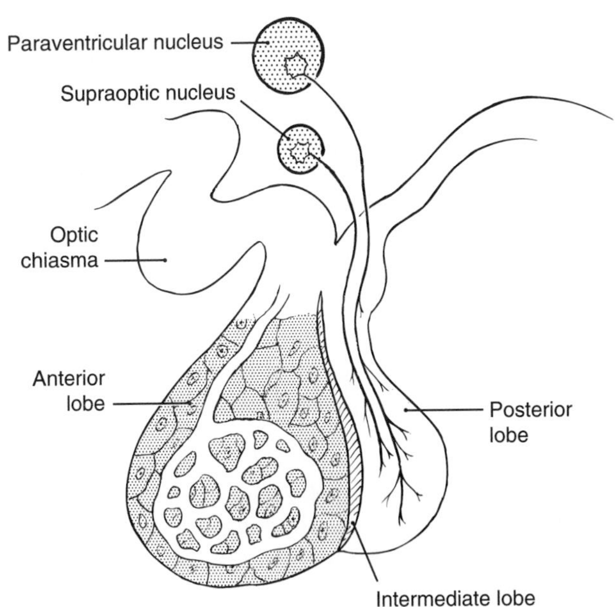

FIGURE **31-3**
Nerve fibers, arising from the supraoptic nucleus and the paraventricular nucleus, transport antidiuretic hormone and oxytocin to the posterior pituitary.

ADH acts primarily to increase urine osmolarity, decrease serum osmolarity, and increase blood volume.[6] Additionally, high levels of ADH cause potent systemic vasoconstriction, especially in coronary, splanchnic, and renal vascular beds. ADH-induced vasoconstriction of splanchnic beds has been exploited therapeutically for the control of hemorrhage caused by esophageal varices. ADH also promotes hemostasis by increasing circulating levels of von Willebrand factor and factor VIII. Desmopressin (DDAVP), an arginine analogue of ADH, is used to reverse coagulopathy associated with platelet adhesion defects.

Consonant with its role of maintaining normal fluid homeostasis, ADH is secreted in response to an increase in plasma osmolarity or plasma sodium ion concentration, a decrease in blood volume, or a decrease in blood pressure.

The osmolarity of body fluids is the main variable controlling ADH secretion. Serum osmolarity changes, as small as 1% to 2%, are sensed by hypothalamic *osmoreceptors*, which in turn alter ADH synthesis and secretion. The plasma *osmotic threshold* for ADH release is about 285 mOsm/L. When the plasma tonicity reaches this level, healthy individuals release ADH into the blood.

The interplay between ADH and water is controlled by a delicate negative feedback loop. Water deprivation (increased plasma osmolarity) initiates signals in the hypothalamic osmoreceptors that cause ADH release from the pituitary gland to increase three- to fivefold. ADH, in turn, enhances renal tubular water reabsorption, dilutes the extracellular fluid, and restores normal osmotic composition.[6] Conversely, water ingestion (decreased plasma osmolarity) suppresses the osmoreceptor signal for ADH release.

A 5% to 15% decrease in blood volume or blood pressure also provokes ADH release.[23] Changes in blood volume are sensed in peripheral baroreceptors (especially in the great veins and pulmonary vessels) and atrial stretch receptors. When these baroreceptors sense underfilling (volume depletion), they transmit afferent signals through vagal and glossopharyngeal nerves to the hypothalamus.[23] The hypothalamus responds by increasing ADH synthesis and stimulating ADH release.

The perioperative period is characterized by enhanced ADH secretion.[7] Pain, emotional stress, nausea, hemorrhage, and various drugs can be potent stimuli to ADH release. Positive-pressure ventilation enhances ADH release by reducing central blood volume.[7] The mild hyponatremia sometimes observed postoperatively may be at least partly explained on the basis of ADH action. Box 31-2 lists common stimulators of ADH release.

Thirst provides a second line of defense of water balance. It is stimulated when plasma osmolarity reaches the *thirst threshold* (about 290 mOsm/L).[23]

Deficient Antidiuretic Hormone and Anesthetic Implications. Inadequate ADH secretion from the posterior pituitary lobe or the inability of renal collecting duct receptors to respond to ADH (impaired receptor sensitivity) results in a disorder called *diabetes insipidus (DI)*. The former disorder is termed *neurogenic DI*, and the latter is called *nephrogenic DI*.

Common causes of neurogenic DI include severe head trauma, neurosurgical procedures (trauma to the median eminence, pituitary stalk, or posterior pituitary lobe), infiltrating pituitary lesions, and brain tumors.[7,23] Diabetes insipidus that develops after pituitary surgery is usually transient, and often resolves in 5 to 7 days.[14]

Nephrogenic DI may be an X-linked inherited trait, or it may occur in association with hypercalcemia, hypokalemia, and medication-induced nephrotoxicity.[23] Ethanol, phenytoin, chlorpromazine, and lithium all inhibit the action of ADH or its release.

The hallmark of DI is polyuria. The inability to produce a concentrated urine results in dehydration and hypernatremia. Most patients have incomplete DI and retain some capacity to concentrate their urine and conserve water. The polyuria is characterized by a urine osmolarity less than 300 mOsm/L, urine specific gravity less than 1.010, and urine volumes greater than 30 mL/kg each day. The tremendous urinary water loss produces serum osmolarities greater than 290 mOsm/L and serum sodium concentrations greater than 145 mEq/L. Neurologic symptoms of hypernatremia may be present and include hyperreflexia, weakness, lethargy, seizures, and coma.[11,23]

BOX 31-2

Stimulators of Antidiuretic Hormone Release

Increased plasma sodium ion concentration
Increased serum osmolarity
Decreased blood volume
Decreased blood pressure
Pain
Stress
Nausea
Various medications (morphine, nicotine, cyclophosphamide)
Angiotensin II
Positive-pressure ventilation

The thirst mechanism assumes a primary role in maintaining water balance in patients with DI. Ingestion of large volumes of water prevents serious hyperosmolarity and life-threatening dehydration.[14]

Treatment protocols for DI depend on the degree of ADH deficiency. Significant deficiency may be treated with various ADH preparations. Aqueous vasopressin is commonly used for short-term therapy and desmopressin is useful for long-term control.[11,14] Caution is advised when administering these drugs to patients with coronary artery disease and hypertension because of the arterial constrictive action of ADH.[7,23] The surgical patient with DI receiving ADH replacement therapy should be monitored for ECG changes indicative of myocardial ischemia. Desmopressin (5 to 10 mcg/d intranasally, or 0.5 to 1 mcg twice daily, subcutaneously) is often a preferred agent because it has less pressor activity, a prolonged duration of action (6 to 24 hours), and enhanced antidiuretic properties.[11]

Mild cases (incomplete DI) are treated with medications that either augment the release of ADH or increase the receptor response to ADH. These drugs may include chlorpropamide (sulfonylurea hypoglycemic agent), carbamazepine (anticonvulsant), and clofibrate (hypolipidemic agent).[14] Perioperative administration of vasopressin is usually not necessary in the patient with partial DI, unless plasma osmolarity levels increase above 290 mOsm/L.[14]

The surgical patient with a total lack of ADH (complete DI) may be managed with a continuous intravenous infusion of vasopressin intraoperatively (0.1 to 0.2 U/h).[7,14] Plasma osmolarity, urine output, and serum sodium concentration should be measured hourly during surgery and in the immediate postoperative period. Isotonic fluids can generally be administered safely during the intraoperative period. If, however, the plasma osmolarity rises above 290 mOsm/L, hypotonic fluids should be considered and the vasopressin infusion increased above 0.2 U/h.[14]

Preoperative assessment of the patient with DI includes careful appraisal of plasma electrolytes (especially serum sodium), renal function, and plasma osmolarity.[11] Dehydration will make these patients especially sensitive to the hypotensive effects of anesthesia agents. Intravascular volume should slowly be restored preoperatively, over a period of at least 24 to 48 hours.

Hypersecretion of Antidiuretic Hormone and Anesthetic Implications. The *syndrome of inappropriate antidiuretic hormone (SIADH)* secretion is a disorder characterized by a high circulating vasopressin level relative to plasma osmolarity and serum sodium concentration. With SIADH, the kidneys, under ADH stimulation, continue to reabsorb water from the renal tubules despite the presence of hyponatremia (<130 mEq/L) and plasma hypotonicity (<270 mOsm/L).[14] Hormone-induced water reabsorption causes expansion of intracellular and extracellular fluid volumes, hemodilution, and weight gain. The urine is hypertonic relative to the plasma, and urine output is typically low.[7] An assay of high ADH levels in the blood confirms the diagnosis of SIADH.

Clinical features of SIADH reflect water intoxication, dilutional hyponatremia, and resulting brain edema. The swelling of brain cells may cause lethargy, headache, nausea, and mental confusion, especially if the plasma osmolarity declines below 250 mOsm/L or if the serum sodium concentration falls below 125 mEq/L.[24] Symptoms may progress to seizures and coma, particularly if the hyponatremia is severe and of rapid onset.

Hypertension and peripheral edema are not common. Surgical patients may exhibit delayed awakening from anesthesia.[14]

Inappropriate hypersecretion of ADH can result from various pathologic processes, including hypothyroidism, pulmonary neoplasia, head trauma or infection, intracranial tumors, and pulmonary infection.[7,9] Secretion of ADH by neoplasms, especially small cell carcinomas of the lung, is a common cause of SIADH.[14] The ectopic ADH produced by these tumors is identical to the ADH of hypothalamic origin.[14] Certain drugs are associated with enhanced ADH secretion or response; these include morphine, chlorpropamide, cyclophosphamide, nicotine, clofibrate, thiazide diuretics, and phenothiazines.[3,20,32]

The patient with mild SIADH not associated with symptoms of hyponatremia are often managed effectively with fluid restriction.[9] Patients with profound hyponatremia (plasma $Na^+ <115$ to 120 mEq/L) and acute neurologic symptoms may require more aggressive treatment with a slow intravenous infusion of hypertonic (3%) saline and intravenous furosemide.[7,11,24] In order to prevent acute loss of brain water and possible permanent neurologic damage, *central pontine demyelination syndrome*. General recommendations are that the plasma sodium concentration be corrected slowly; not greater than 0.5 to 0.7 mEq/L per hour, or 6 to 8 mEq/L per day.[9,25,26]

Demeclocycline, a tetracycline antibiotic, has been used successfully in SIADH patients to antagonize the effects of vasopressin on the renal tubules.[14,24] Definitive treatment for SIADH is directed at the underlying disorder.

Stress and surgery may initiate or potentiate an inappropriate release of ADH. Clinical assessment of the patient's volume status is an essential part of the preoperative evaluation. Perioperative fluid management of the surgical patient with SIADH can usually be accomplished with fluid restriction that involves the use of isotonic solutions.[14] Estimation of the central volume status on the basis of central venous pressure or pulmonary artery catheter measurements can help guide fluid replacement. Frequent determinations of urine output, urine osmolarity, plasma osmolarity, and serum sodium concentrations can also help direct fluid management. Nausea should be prevented, as it is a potent stimulus of ADH release.

PARATHYROID GLAND

Calcium Regulation

The adult human body contains about 1000 g of the divalent cation calcium.[27] Approximately 99% of the calcium exists in the bony skeleton and about 1% is in the extracellular space and soft tissues.[7,27]

The concentration of the total serum calcium is tightly regulated within a range of 8.8 to 10.4 mg/dL. Serum calcium exists in three different forms (Fig. 31-4):

1. Approximately 10% of the serum calcium exists in a nonionized, chelated form. This calcium is bound to diffusible anions such as citrate, bicarbonate, and phosphate.
2. Approximately 40% of the serum calcium is combined with plasma proteins (primarily albumin) in a nonionized, nondiffusible complex.
3. Approximately 50% of the blood calcium exists in an ionized and diffusible form (normal level 4.7 to 5.2 mg/dL).

Only the free, ionized form of calcium exerts physiologic effects, and measurement of serum ionized calcium levels provides the most clinically relevant determination.[7,27,28] Ionized calcium performs a wide range of vital physiologic functions, including hemostasis (platelet aggregation, blood coagulation), muscle contraction, neurotransmission, bone formation, cell division, and many other aspects of cell function.[27]

Total blood calcium levels may not always reflect the ionized calcium status. Changes in serum protein levels can alter total blood calcium levels without altering ionized calcium values. The changes in total calcium levels usually parallel the serum albumin.[28] A decrease in serum albumin of 1 gm/dL, for instance, causes an associated decrease in total serum calcium of about 0.8 mg/dL.[7]

Alterations in the pH of blood affect ionized calcium levels. Plasma proteins are more ionized in an alkaline pH, and as such, provide an increase in the number of anion binding sites for the positively charged calcium. Alkalosis, such as that occurring with hyperventilation, decreases the ionized portion of serum calcium by increasing protein-calcium binding. Acidosis, on the other hand, increases the ionized portion of serum calcium.[28,29]

Three principal hormones operate in concert to regulate the plasma concentration of calcium: vitamin D, parathyroid hormone (PTH), and calcitonin. Vitamin D and PTH serve to raise serum calcium, whereas calcitonin lowers it.[30] Of these, PTH has by far the strongest effect on calcium regulation.

Vitamin D. Vitamin D compounds, which are ingested from food or formed by the action of ultraviolet light on the skin, are inactive prohormones.[28] Inactive vitamin D, called cholecalciferol, is converted by a series of reactions in the liver and kidneys to an active metabolite. The in vivo conversion of inactive vitamin D to an active product, *1,25-dihydroxycholecalciferol*, is shown in Figure 31-5. The final step in the conversion of vitamin D to an active form is controlled in the kidneys by PTH.

Active vitamin D increases plasma calcium and phosphate ion concentrations by promoting their absorption across the intestinal epithelium to the extracellular fluid.[27,30]

Inadequate vitamin D intake or absorption, or insufficient exposure to sunlight, can lead to poor intestinal absorption of calcium. In children, the resulting calcium deficiency leads

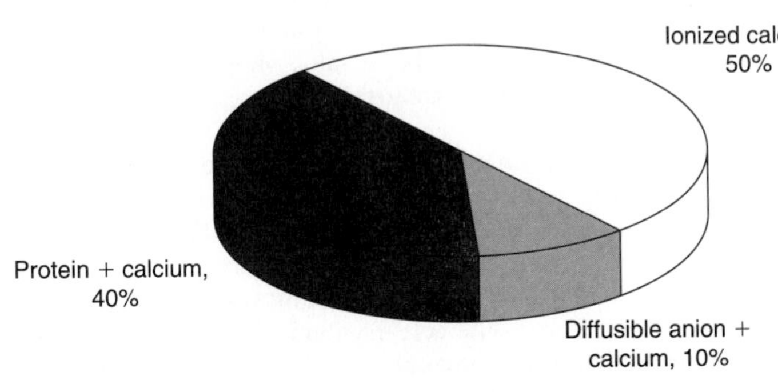

FIGURE **31-4**
Serum calcium exists in three different forms: ionized, bound to serum proteins, and bound to diffusible anions. Only the ionized form of calcium exerts physiologic effects.

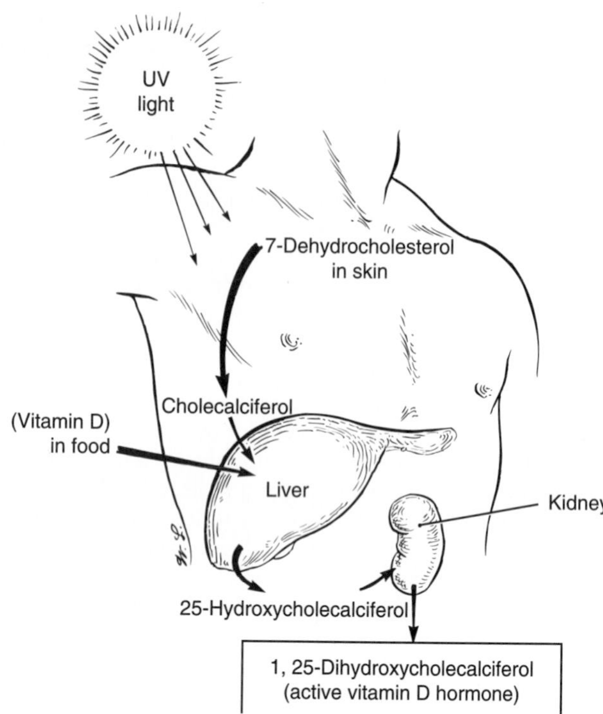

FIGURE **31-5**
Conversion of cholecalciferol or vitamin D to an active form, 1,25-dihydroxycholecalciferol, involves hydroxylation in the liver and the kidneys. Active vitamin D is important in transporting calcium across the gastrointestinal tract. *UV*, ultraviolet.

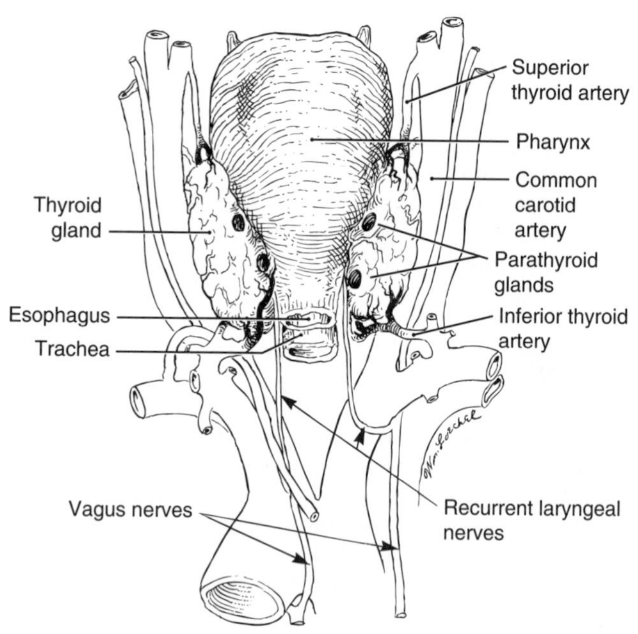

FIGURE **31-6**
The four parathyroid glands are located on the posterior poles of the thyroid gland.

to a defective mineralization of bone, a condition known as *rickets*.[27,28]

Parathyroid Hormone. The parathyroid glands are small (approximately 3 × 6 × 2 mm) oval bodies located on the posterior surface of the thyroid gland (Fig. 31-6). Most individuals have four parathyroid glands, one on each pole of the thyroid, but approximately 6% of individuals have five glands and 13% have only three.[31] Blood supply is via the inferior thyroid arteries.

PTH is secreted from *chief cells* of the parathyroid gland in response to a low serum ionized calcium concentration. Hyperphosphatemia (indirect effect) and acute hypomagnesemia also stimulate PTH secretion.[7,29]

PTH is the body's major hormonal regulator of calcium and phosphate metabolism. In PTH, the body possesses an extremely potent negative feedback agent for controlling serum calcium levels. In general, PTH increases the extracellular calcium concentration and decreases the extracellular phosphate concentration. A small decline in the level of circulating ionized calcium produces a rapid increase in PTH secretion from the parathyroid glands. A sustained deficit in serum calcium levels (lactation, pregnancy) produces hypertrophy of the parathyroid glands, sometimes fivefold or greater, in order to maintain adequate PTH output.[27]

An elevation in serum calcium ion concentration produces an abrupt decline in PTH synthesis and output. Conditions associated with chronic elevations of serum calcium (immobility, malignancy, Paget's disease) provoke a blunted PTH secretion response and a diminution in gland size. Parathyroid gland function and PTH secretion are inhibited by severe and chronic hypomagnesemia.[29]

The increase in serum calcium level and the decline in serum phosphate level in response to PTH secretion are the result of the hormone's effect on bone, the kidney, and the intestinal tract.

Effect on Bone. Bone is a living tissue that is constantly being remodeled.[28] In the healthy adult, bone-forming cells, called *osteoblasts*, are balanced by bone-destroying cells, called *osteoclasts*.[27] Exchangeable calcium in bone serves as a large, rapid buffer that plays a vital role in extracellular fluid calcium homeostasis.

When ionized serum calcium levels decline, PTH is released and acts directly on bone to mobilize skeletal calcium stores.[28] PTH promotes the activation and proliferation of osteoclasts, stimulating rapid absorption of calcium (and phosphate) from bone tissue to the extracellular fluid. Over time, abnormally high levels of circulating PTH can produce extensive absorption of calcium from the bone matrix.[27]

The reservoir of calcium in bone is about 1000 times greater than the amount of calcium in the extracellular fluid. Only after sustained PTH activation, therefore, does bone erosion and destruction become apparent. With protracted PTH stimulation, however, the bones eventually become severely depleted of calcium.[27]

An increase in extracellular fluid calcium causes PTH levels to decline. Decreased PTH levels stimulate rapid deposition of calcium and phosphate bone salts, an effect that lowers serum calcium levels back to normal.

Effect on the Intestinal Tract. Parathyroid hormone indirectly enhances both calcium and phosphate absorption from the intestines by promoting the formation of 1,25-dihydroxycholecalciferol, or active vitamin D. When the plasma calcium level is low, PTH acts to stimulate the formation of 1,25-dihydroxycholecalciferol. The active vitamin D, in turn, increases the intestinal absorption of calcium. [28]

PTH stimulates the final step in vitamin D conversion to an active form in the kidney. In the absence of PTH, or in the presence of severe kidney disease, 1,25-dihydroxycholecalciferol is not formed, and vitamin D's effect on calcium and phosphate regulation is lost.

Patients with chronic renal failure often suffer from hypocalcemia, in part because the diseased kidneys lose their ability to form active vitamin D. Consequently, these patients are unable to absorb a sufficient amount of calcium from the gastrointestinal tract.[30]

Effect on the Kidney. PTH has two major effects on the kidney: (1) it increases calcium reabsorption, and (2) it increases phosphate excretion. PTH elevates serum calcium level by augmenting the reabsorption of calcium from nephron tubules to the extracellular fluid. The major site of PTH-mediated calcium reabsorption is the distal convoluted tubule.[27,32]

Accompanying calcium reabsorption is enhanced phosphate excretion. PTH promotes phosphaturia by reducing phosphate ion reabsorption from the proximal convoluted tubule. The PTH-mediated phosphate loss from the kidney is generally strong enough to overcome the PTH-induced phosphate absorption from bone and intestines.[27]

Calcitonin. Calcitonin is a hormone secreted from the thyroid *parafollicular cells*, or *C cells*, in response to an elevation of serum ionized calcium.[28] Calcitonin has an effect opposite that of the PTH system, lowering the serum ionized calcium concentration. Calcium levels are reduced by a calcitonin-mediated inhibition of bone osteoclasts, which shifts the balance toward osteoblasts and bone deposition.[28]

The serum calcium–lowering effect of calcitonin is weak in adults.[27] More of the hormone is secreted in children, possibly to aid in skeletal development.

Calcitonin acts chiefly as a short-term regulator of calcium ion concentration. Its effect in lowering serum calcium is rapidly outweighed by the more powerful activity of PTH. Therefore, over an extended period, the level of calcium ions in the extracellular fluid is determined almost completely by the parathyroid system. The rather weak effect of calcitonin is demonstrated by the observation that removal of the thyroid gland causes no significant alterations in bone density or long-term serum calcium levels.[27,28]

Parathyroid Gland Dysfunction

Hypoparathyroidism. Hypoparathyroidism is a disorder characterized by inadequate secretion of PTH or a peripheral resistance to its effect.[9] Patients with hypoparathyroidism typically have low serum calcium levels. The blood phosphate concentration may be elevated because of the decreased renal excretion of phosphate.

Inadvertent removal of parathyroid tissue, parathyroid gland injury from irradiation or autoimmune destruction, and chronic severe magnesium deficiency (alcohol abuse, poor nutrition, malabsorption) are possible causes of hypoparathyroidism.[29,33] Clinical signs of hypoparathyroidism reflect the degree of hypocalcemia and the rapidity of calcium decline. A sudden drop in ionized calcium usually produces more severe symptoms than does a slow decline.[29] Treatment of chronic hypoparathyroidism includes vitamin D and calcium supplementation.

The decreased serum calcium ion concentration accompanying hypoparathyroidism produces hyperexcitability of nerve and muscle cells by lowering the threshold potential of excitable membranes. Cardinal features of the neuromuscular excitability are muscle spasms and hypocalcemic tetany. Symptoms vary in severity and may take the form of muscle cramps, perioral paresthesias, numbness in the feet and toes, or hyperactive deep tendon reflexes.[29,33,34] The patient may feel restless or hyperirritable. Life-threatening laryngeal muscle spasm may occur, producing stridor, labored respirations, and asphyxia.

Two classic manifestations of latent hypocalcemic tetany are *Chvostek's sign* and *Trousseau's sign*. Chvostek's sign is a contracture or twitching of ipsilateral facial muscles produced when the facial nerve is tapped at the angle of the jaw. Trousseau's sign is elicited by the inflation of a blood pressure cuff slightly above the systolic level for a few minutes. The resultant ischemia aggravates the muscle irritability in hypocalcemic states and causes flexion of the wrist and thumb with extension of the fingers (*carpopedal spasm*).[29] Figure 31-7 illustrates some of the clinical manifestations of hypoparathyroidism and hypocalcemia.

Anesthesia Implications for Hypoparathyroidism. Temporary hypocalcemia often is observed after successful parathyroid surgery for hyperparathyroidism.[29] This may occur within a few hours after surgery or 1 to 2 days postoperatively.[28] The transient postoperative hypocalcemia is the result of parathyroid gland suppression (by preoperative hypercalcemia) and rapid bone uptake of calcium ("hungry bone syndrome").[29] Inadvertent removal of all parathyroid gland tissue induces a decline in the serum calcium concentration from a normal level to 6 to 7 mg/dL. Even a small amount of remaining parathyroid tissue usually is capable of sufficient hypertrophy to preserve normal calcium-phosphate balance.[27]

Assiduous observation for signs of musculoskeletal irritability and frequent measurement of serum ionized calcium levels should be performed following parathyroid surgery. The threshold for the development of signs of hypocalcemia is variable; however, manifestations of neuromuscular compromise often are observed at serum calcium levels of 6 to 7 mg/dL.[27]

Laryngeal muscles are especially sensitive to tetanic spasm, and laryngospasm may cause life-threatening airway compromise in the hypocalcemic patient.[27] Respiratory distress following parathyroid surgery may be secondary to laryngeal muscle spasm, edema or bleeding in the neck, or bilateral recurrent laryngeal nerve injury. Unilateral recurrent laryngeal nerve injury produces hoarseness and usually requires only close observation. Bilateral recurrent laryngeal nerve injury causes aphonia and requires immediate airway support and intubation.

Hypocalcemia may be apparent on electrocardiographic tracings as a prolonged QT interval, reflecting delayed ventricular repolarization and a predisposition to ventricular dysrhythmias.[9] The cardiac rhythm usually remains normal. Decreased cardiac contractility and hypotension may occur.[29,34] Congestive heart failure, although rare, is a danger.

Circulating levels of ionized calcium can decline abruptly in the perioperative period. Precipitous increases in the circulating levels of anions such as bicarbonate, phosphate, and citrate lower ionized calcium levels.[29] Hyperventilation, the rapid transfusion of citrated blood, or the rapid administration of bicarbonate may induce overt tetany in a previously asymptomatic hypocalcemic patient. Vigorous diuresis can augment calcium loss. Patients with hypocalcemia may have an altered response to muscle relaxants.[11]

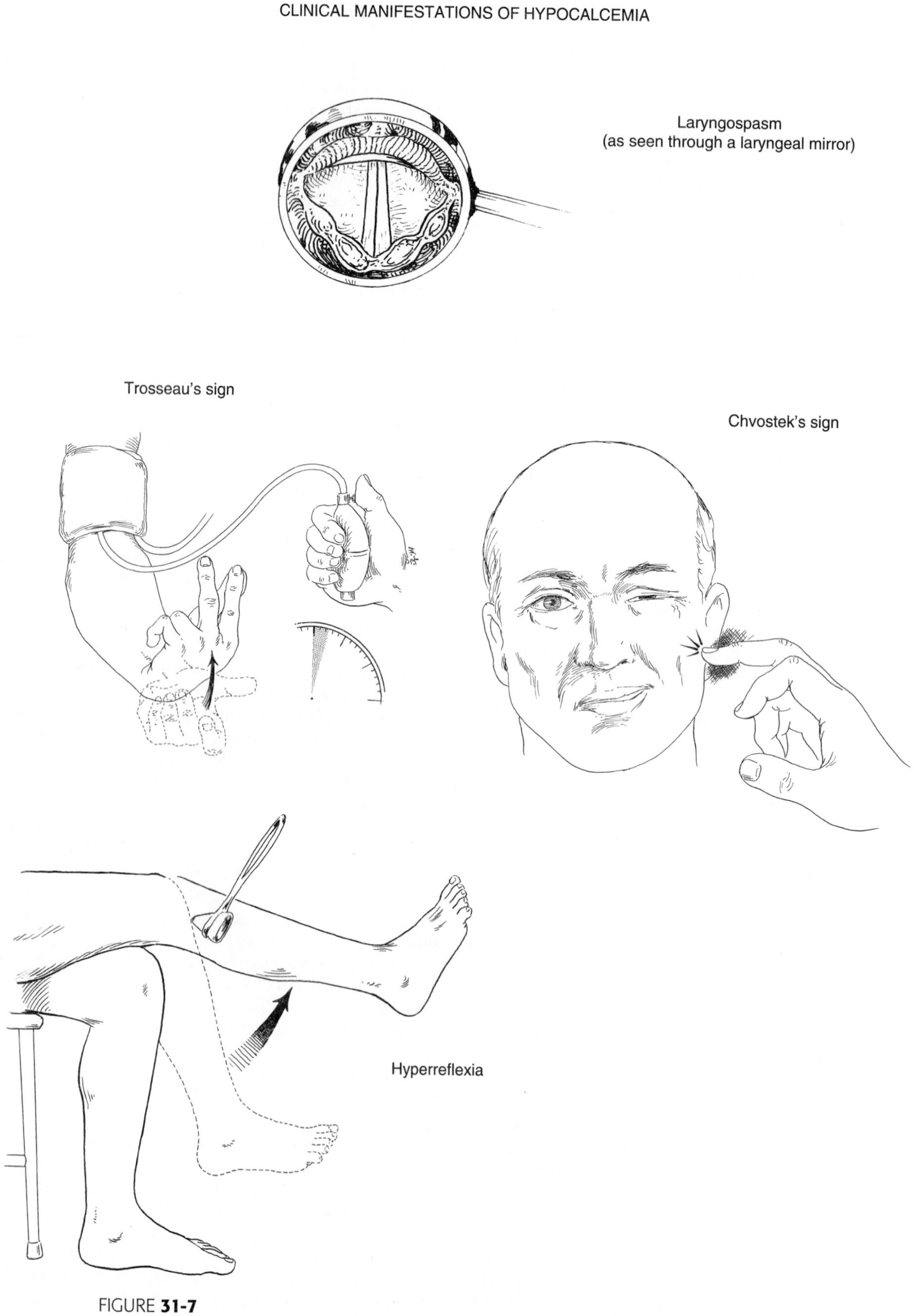

CLINICAL MANIFESTATIONS OF HYPOCALCEMIA

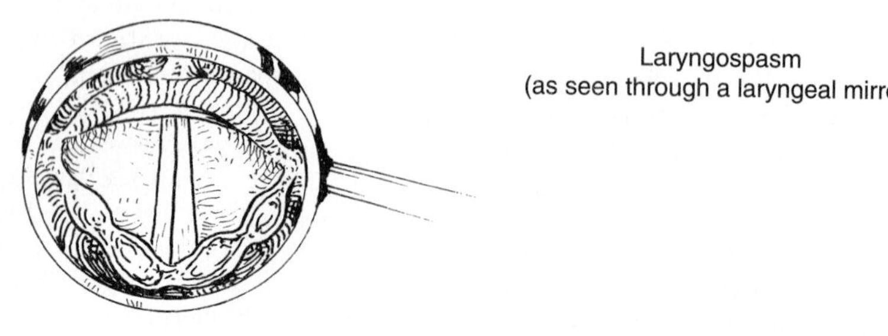

Trosseau's sign

Chvostek's sign

Hyperreflexia

FIGURE **31-7**
Hypocalcemia produces hyperexcitability of nerve and muscle cells. Chvostek's sign and Trousseau's sign are two classic manifestations of hypocalcemic tetany. Deep tendon reflexes may be hyperactive; laryngeal muscles are also sensitive to tetanic spasm.

Patients with confirmed, symptomatic hypocalcemia require prompt therapy.[29,33] Acute hypocalcemia can be treated with an initial intravenous bolus of 100 to 200 mg of elemental calcium administered over 10 minutes (10 mL of 10% calcium gluconate = 93 mg elemental calcium; 10 mL of 10% calcium chloride = 272 mg elemental calcium). Relief of symptoms is usually prompt but may be transient.[29] For maintenance of normal levels, the initial bolus may be followed by an infusion of 1 to 2 mg/kg per hour of elemental calcium, diluted in 50 to 100 mL of saline. Calcium, magnesium, phosphate, potassium, and creatinine levels should be monitored diligently during calcium replacement.[7]

HYPERPARATHYROIDISM

Primary hyperparathyroidism is characterized and diagnosed by the presence of elevated serum PTH levels despite high serum calcium levels. Primary hyperparathyroidism may result from a parathyroid adenoma, gland hyperplasia, or parathyroid cancer.[35] In 85% to 90% of the cases, hyperparathyroidism is caused by hypersecretion of a single parathyroid adenoma.[32,34,36] Hyperplasia of one or more parathyroid glands accounts for about 10% of the cases. Carcinoma of the parathyroid gland is found in less than 1% of patients and is associated with particularly high serum calcium levels.[9,35,36] Hyperparathyroidism may also exist as part of a multiple endocrine neoplastic (MEN) syndrome.

The incidence of primary hyperparathyroidism in the United States is approximately 5 cases per 10,000 people per year, with a higher occurrence in females and the elderly.[36] Stimulation of the parathyroid gland during pregnancy or lactation, prior neck irradiation, or a family history of parathyroid disease are predisposing factors.[35]

Sustained overactivity of the parathyroid glands is characterized by high serum calcium levels. Most patients re- main asymptomatic until the total serum calcium level rises above 11 to 12 mg/dL.[7] A concentration greater than 14 mg/dL may be life threatening and demands immediate treatment.[7,11,34]

High levels of PTH lead to exaggerated osteoclast activity in bone, resulting in diffuse osteopenia, subperiosteal erosions, and elevated extracellular calcium levels. As osteoblasts attempt to reconstruct the ravaged bone, they secrete large amounts of the enzyme *alkaline phosphatase*. A heightened serum alkaline phosphatase level, therefore, is a significant diagnostic feature of hyperparathyroidism.[36]

The effect of hyperparathyroidism on bone becomes clinically apparent when osteoclastic absorption of bone overwhelms osteoblastic deposition. With severe and protracted disease, the weakened bones become filled with decalcified cavities, making them painful and susceptible to fracture. The destructive bone disease associated with sustained hyperparathyroidism is called *osteitis fibrosa cystica*.

Many of the nonskeletal manifestations of primary hyperparathyroidism are related to the accompanying hypercalcemia.[36] Sustained hypercalcemia may produce deleterious effects in the pancreas (pancreatitis), in the kidney (nephrolithiasis, nephrocalcinosis, polyuria), in blood vessels (hypertension), in the heart (shortened ventricular refractory period, bradyarrhythmias, bundle branch block, heart block), and in the acid-producing areas of the stomach (peptic ulcer).[34,36,37] The mnemonic "stones, bones, and groans" summarizes features of advanced, untreated hyperparathyroidism. Profound muscle weakness, anorexia, confusion, nausea, vomiting, and lethargy are additional features of the disorder. Figure 31-8 illustrates some of the clinical features of hyperparathyroidism.

Despite an increased mobilization of phosphorus from bone, serum phosphate concentration usually is normal or low in hyperparathyroidism as a result of increased urinary excretion.

Patients with chronically low levels of serum calcium, such as those with chronic renal failure and gastrointestinal malabsorption, may develop compensatory parathyroid gland hyperplasia or *secondary hyperparathyroidism* in response to the hypocalcemia. Their clinical course is marked by the same PTH-mediated skeletal assault seen in the primary form of the disorder, but because it is an adaptive response, secondary hyperparathyroidism is seldom associated with hypercalcemia.[28,34] Table 31-2 compares common clinical manifestations of hyperparathyroidism and hypoparathyroidism.

Anesthesia Implications for Hyperparathyroidism. The usual treatment for symptomatic primary hyperparathyroidism is surgical removal of abnormal parathyroid tissue. Surgical treatment for asymptomatic hyperparathyroidism is more controversial.[7] Parathyroidectomy is commonly performed with the patient under general anesthesia, although a cervical plexus block technique has been utilized, especially for elderly and medically compromised patients.[37,38]

Parathyroid tissue resembles brown fat, and this can occasionally make it difficult for the surgeon to locate parathyroid tissue. Further, parathyroid tissue is sometimes footloose and can be found in such ectopic places as the deep recesses of the mediastinum, the carotid sheath or the thymus gland.[28,39] Blood loss from parathyroid surgery is usually minimal, and advanced monitoring is not required based on the surgical procedure. Serum calcium, magnesium, and phosphorous levels should be monitored in the postoperative period until stable. In most cases, serum calcium levels return to normal within 3 to 4 days after surgery.[7,9]

With current methods of detection, most patients with hyperparathyroidism are asymptomatic; however, erosive effects of elevated PTH on bone and the systemic effects of chronic hypercalcemia should be considered in the anesthetic plan for these patients.

Severely hypercalcemic (>14 mg/dL) or symptomatic patients should be controlled preoperatively. Isotonic saline hydration and loop diuretics (furosemide, 40 to 80 mg every 2 to 4 hours) can rapidly decrease serum calcium levels by 2 to 3 mg/dL.[9,34] Less frequently, drugs that inhibit osteoclastic bone resorption (mithramycin, bisphosphonates, calcitonin) are used.[34,40] Loop diuretics promote calciuresis by decreasing tubular reabsorption of calcium.[40] Thiazide diuretics increase renal tubular calcium reabsorption and will not effectively correct hypercalcemia.[31,35]

The hypercalcemic patient may be dehydrated because of anorexia, vomiting, and the impaired ability of the kidneys to concentrate urine.[40] Hydration with non–calcium-containing solutions should be maintained throughout the perioperative period to dilute serum calcium, maintain adequate glomerular filtration and calcium clearance, and ensure adequate intravascular volume. Vigorous hydration dictates the use of bladder catheterization, central venous pressure monitoring, and frequent determinations of serum electrolytes.[7]

Elevated calcium levels may depress the central and peripheral nervous systems.[27,32] The use of preoperative sedatives in the hypercalcemic patient who appears lethargic or confused

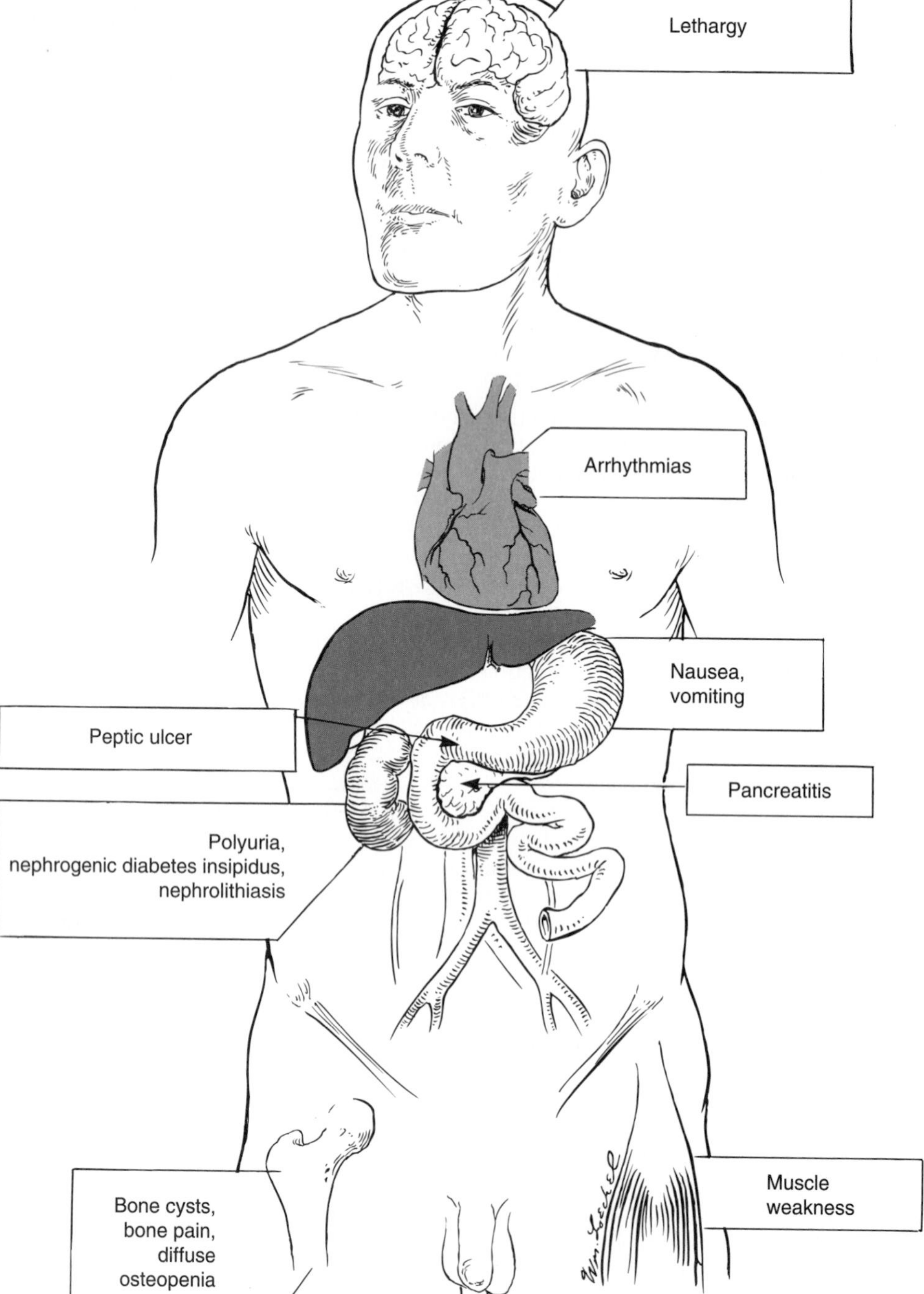

FIGURE **31-8**
The patient with hyperparathyroidism may exhibit manifestations of hypercalcemia, in addition to skeletal destruction.

TABLE **31-2** Clinical Features of Hyperparathyroidism and Hypoparathyroidism

System	Hyperparathyroidism	Hypoparathyroidism
Cardiovascular	Hypertension, cardiac conduction disturbances, shortened QT interval	Prolonged QT interval, hypotension, decreased cardiac contractility
Musculoskeletal	Bone pain, pathologic fractures, muscle weakness, muscle atrophy	Neuromuscular excitability
Neurologic	Somnolence, cognitive impairment, depression, hypotonia	Tetany, paresthesias, numbness in fingers and toes, seizures
Gastrointestinal	Anorexia, nausea, vomiting, constipation, abdominal pain, pancreatitis, peptic ulcer	None significant
Renal	Tubular absorption defects, diminished renal function, kidney stones, polyuria	None significant

should be avoided. General anesthetic requirements may be decreased as well.[9]

Careful review of the patient's renal status is especially crucial in patients with secondary hyperparathyroidism. Associated complications of renal impairment (volume overload, anemia, electrolyte derangements) may affect anesthetic medication dosages and selection.[32,41]

Cardiac conduction disturbances such as a shortened QT interval and a prolonged PR interval are observed with hypercalcemia.[9] Dysrhythmias and hypertension may respond to calcium channel antagonists (e.g., verapamil, 5 to 10 mg intravenously).

Awareness of the effects of pH on the ionized portion of plasma calcium is important. Alkalosis protects against hypercalcemia by shifting the ionized calcium to the protein-bound form.[33] Periodic determinations of serum ionized calcium levels help guide management.

The response to neuromuscular blockade may be unpredictable.[9,32] Muscle weakness, hypotonia, and muscle atrophy may increase the patient's sensitivity to nondepolarizing skeletal muscle relaxants. Careful titration of muscle relaxants with use of a peripheral nerve stimulator is prudent.[9] The surgeon may sometimes request no muscle relaxation to facilitate identification of the recurrent laryngeal nerve during parathyroid surgery.

Enhanced osteoclastic bone resorption produces clinically significant bone disease in 10% to 15% of patients with hyperparathyroidism. These patients are susceptible to fractures, and care must be exercised in positioning and padding.[7]

Hyperparathyroid patients are prone to postoperative nausea and vomiting.[42] Prophylactic antiemetic medications are advisable.

Pancreas

The *pancreas* is a flattened, elongated, retroperitoneal organ that has both exocrine and endocrine functions. *Acinar cells*, which make up the exocrine portion of the pancreas, account for 98% to 99% of the gland's weight. Acinar cells synthesize and secrete digestive enzymes and bicarbonate into the pancreatic ducts to aid the digestive process.

Islets of Langerhans. The *islets of Langerhans*, which make up 1% to 2% of the pancreas's weight, constitute the endocrine pancreas. The islets are microscopic collections of cells scattered throughout the gland. They produce hormones that do not enter ducts but are secreted directly into capillary blood vessels. Each islet cell has an abundant blood supply. Venous blood from the islets drains into the hepatic portal vein and then into the general circulation.[43]

At least three distinct cell types are found in the islets of Langerhans, identified as α, β, and δ cells. Each cell type secretes a different peptide hormone. The *β-cells* account for 60% to 70% of the islet mass and secrete the hormone *insulin*. The *α-cells* constitute about 25% of the islet cells and secrete the hormone *glucagon*. The *δ-cells* represent about 10% of total cells and secrete the hormone *somatostatin*.[44]

Insulin and glucagon are crucial in regulating carbohydrate, fat, and protein metabolism. Their secretion is part of a hormonal regulatory system that accommodates repeated periods of feast and fasting throughout the day. Somatostatin may play a role in regulating gastrointestinal function by restraining the rate at which nutrients are digested and absorbed.[44] Somatostatin also is distributed throughout the central nervous system and is a hypothalamic inhibitor of anterior pituitary growth hormone release.

Energy Balance. Glucose is the body's most abundant circulating fuel. The breakdown of glucose into simpler compounds releases energy, which the body uses for cellular metabolism. The energy-yielding breakdown of glucose to pyruvate or lactate is called *glycolysis* or the *Embden-Meyerhof pathway*.

Despite daily fluctuations between feeding and fasting states, plasma glucose concentration is maintained within a narrow range. This is accomplished by the counterbalancing effect of multiple hormones that control the storage of glucose and other nutrient fuels after meals and that regulate fuel mobilization during fasting.

In a healthy person an overnight fast usually lowers the blood glucose to 80 to 90 mg/dL. This concentration increases briefly to 120 to 140 mg/dL after a meal, before returning to control levels. In a person with diabetes mellitus, the fasting blood sugar is almost always above 110 mg/dL.[44]

Certain metabolic processes ensure the efficient storage of nutrients so that they can be available for later use. *Glycogenesis*, or the storage of glucose as glycogen, occurs primarily in the liver and muscle. *Lipogenesis*, which represents the formation and storage of fat as triglycerides, occurs primarily in adipose tissue.

Other metabolic processes work in the opposite direction, providing adequate energy sources during times of fasting. *Gluconeogenesis* is the formation of glucose from lactate, pyruvate, amino acids, and glycerol; it is an important glucose production mechanism during fasting and starvation and occurs in the liver. *Glycogenolysis*, the breakdown of glycogen into glucose, occurs primarily in the liver. *Lipolysis*, the breakdown of stored triglycerides to free fatty acids and glycerol, is stimulated by the enzyme *hormone-sensitive lipase*.

The rates of glycogenesis, lipogenesis, gluconeogenesis, glycogenolysis, and lipolysis are determined largely by the actions of insulin and the opposing actions of so-called "counterregulatory hormones" (growth hormone, cortisol, epinephrine, and glucagon). Insulin plays an important role as an *anabolic hormone*. It promotes growth and the constructive phase of metabolism. The potent anabolic effects of insulin are balanced by the opposing *catabolic actions* of the counterregulatory hormones. These hormones mobilize fuel substrates from protein, carbohydrate, and fat stores to meet the energy demands of various tissues.[43]

The "push and pull" effect of these two hormone systems helps maintain normal glucose concentrations in the healthy individual. In diabetes, when insulin concentrations are low or absent, the unopposed counterregulatory hormones begin to exert more prominent metabolic effects.

Obligate Versus Facultative Tissue. Different tissues have different glucose requirements and some tissues are able to adapt to alternative sources of fuel when glucose is scarce. Muscle and most other tissues in the body are said to be *facultative glucose organs*. They use glucose for energy when it is available, but they can also shift to alternative sources of fuel (amino acids or fat) in the absence of glucose.

The brain is unique in that it is one of the few organs that uses only glucose for energy. It is said to be an *obligate glucose organ*.[44] Erythrocytes and the adrenal medulla also depend on glucose as their sole source of energy. Unlike most other tissues, such as muscle, obligate glucose organs cannot immediately switch to alternative fuels when glucose levels fall. The brain's absolute, uninterrupted requirement for glucose dictates that the blood glucose concentration be maintained above a critical level. The central nervous system accounts for about 70% of total body glucose utilization, and normal cerebral function requires the delivery of about 125 to 150 g of glucose per day. During prolonged starvation ketone bodies can substitute for glucose as cerebral fuel.

Insulin. Of the hormones secreted from the islet cells, insulin is of the greatest physiologic importance. In 1922 Banting and Best first isolated this critical hormone from the pancreas in its pure form. The clinical importance of this event is demonstrated by insulin's history of lifesaving effects in diabetes, a previously uniformly fatal disease.

Insulin was the first mammalian peptide hormone produced in bacteria with the use of recombinant DNA techniques. Genetically engineered insulin does not differ in biologic or chemical characteristics from pancreatic human insulin.

Storage and Release. Insulin is synthesized within the β-cells of the pancreas, and it is packaged and stored in membrane-lined vesicles within the β-cell cytoplasm. About 200 units of insulin are stored in the pancreas in this form. On β-cell stimulation, insulin is released via exocytosis from the β-cell to the surrounding capillaries, where it enters the portal circulation. In the first pass through the hepatic circulation, the liver removes 50% of the insulin that is delivered to it. Total daily insulin secretion is estimated to be about 60 units, but the total daily peripheral delivery is about 30 units.[43]

Insulin circulates unbound to any carrier protein. The circulating half-life of insulin is only 5 to 8 minutes, and the biological half-life is about 20 minutes.[43] Almost all tissues in the body can metabolize insulin, but the major sites of hormone degradation are the liver and the kidney.[44] Very little insulin is excreted unchanged in the urine.

Metabolic Effects. Insulin is a hormone of energy or fuel storage. It is important to many cellular mechanisms related to growth, and it is intimately involved in the regulation of carbohydrate, fat, and protein metabolism.

Following ingestion of a meal, insulin levels increase sharply in response to stimulation by abundant circulating nutrient substrates. Insulin promotes the storage of carbohydrate, fat, and protein for future use when substrate supply is low.[44] Figure 31-9 outlines the effects of insulin on nutrient substrates.

The peripheral effects of insulin are initiated by a reversible binding to specific cell membrane insulin receptors. Most cells in the body have insulin receptors, but the major targets of insulin action are the liver, muscle, and adipose tissue.[43]

Effects on Carbohydrate Metabolism. Insulin is the body's key hormone in controlling glucose removal from the plasma. It facilitates the disposition of glucose by stimulating its uptake into liver, muscle, and adipose tissue. The brain is one of the few tissues in the body that does not require insulin for glucose transport into its cells.[44]

In the liver, and to a lesser extent in muscle cells, insulin promotes the efficient storage of excess glucose in the form of glycogen (glycogenesis).[43] Under normal circumstances, about 60% of the glucose ingested with a meal is stored in the liver as glycogen. In addition to promoting hepatic glucose storage, insulin limits hepatic glucose output by inhibiting enzymes responsible for gluconeogenesis.[43,44]

Between meals, when the blood glucose and blood insulin levels decrease, the stored glucose can be released back into the blood (through gluconeogenesis and glycogenolysis) and

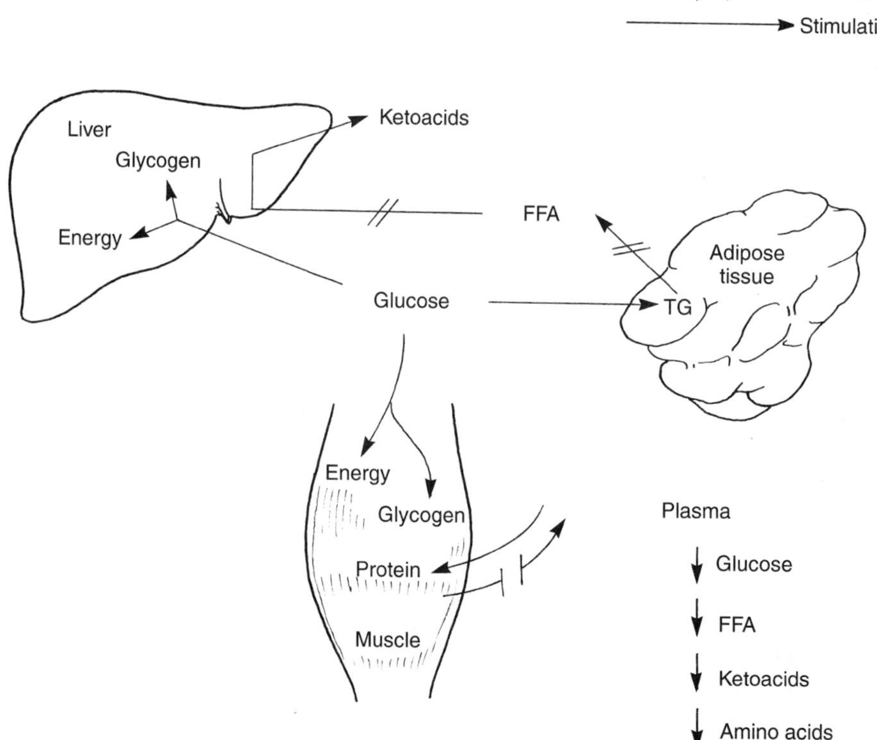

FIGURE **31-9**
The effect of insulin on the overall flow of metabolic substrates. Insulin promotes the uptake of glucose into insulin-responsive tissue to meet energy needs. In the liver and skeletal muscle, insulin promotes the storage of excess glucose as glycogen. In adipose tissue, excess glucose is stored as triglyceride. Insulin inhibits the breakdown of triglyceride into glycerol and free fatty acids. Amino acid uptake into muscle is increased for protein synthesis, and protein breakdown is inhibited.

be made available for local energy use or for delivery to the central nervous system.

Effects on Protein Metabolism. Insulin's actions on protein metabolism are also directed toward nutrient storage and growth (anabolism). Insulin stimulates the uptake of amino acids from the extracellular fluid to the cell, and once inside the cell it promotes the synthesis of specific proteins. Insulin also conserves amino acids in existing proteins by inhibiting the breakdown of protein stores. Because insulin is required for protein synthesis, it is firmly established as a hormone necessary for normal development and maintenance of healthy tissues.[44]

Effects on Fat Metabolism. The acute effects of insulin on fat metabolism are not as readily apparent as the effects on carbohydrate metabolism, but in the long run they are no less important.

Insulin favors fat storage. After a meal, carbohydrates not utilized for energy or stored as glycogen are converted, under the direction of insulin, to fatty acids and glycerol. These two substances combine in adipose tissue to form triglyceride, the storage form of fat. Insulin not only stimulates triglyceride storage in adipose tissue but also strongly inhibits the breakdown of stored triglyceride to free fatty acids and glycerol. Insulin blocks triglyceride hydrolysis and the liberation of free fatty acids into the circulating blood by suppressing the enzyme *hormone-sensitive lipase*. Under ordinary conditions, insulin continually exerts a "braking" effect on free fatty acid release. A major consequence of lower concentrations of circulating free fatty acids is the decreased use of fatty acids for fuel.[43] Insulin suppresses fatty acid mobilization in the fed state when glucose is readily available to meet energy needs.

In the fasted state, when insulin levels are low, free fatty acid release is promoted to provide metabolic fuel. The oxidation of fatty acids for energy during fasting spares glucose use.[43,44] Organic acids, called *ketoacids* or *ketone bodies*, are generated in the liver from fatty acid oxidation. Ketoacid production is increased in the fasted state, when insulin levels are low, and it is markedly reduced when insulin levels are high. Insulin is the body's major antiketogenic hormone.[44]

Effects on Ion Transport. Insulin stimulates the translocation of vital electrolytes from the extracellular compartment into cells. Potassium, phosphate, and magnesium uptake into cells is mediated by an insulin mechanism.[43] Exogenous insulin administration may appreciably lower serum potassium, phosphate, and magnesium levels. The precipitation of hypokalemia secondary to vigorous insulin treatment can be of great clinical significance.

Insulin's actions are complex and wide ranging. Overall, insulin promotes the formation of complex molecules for nutrient storage and growth and fosters glucose utilization, instead of fat or protein, for energy.

Control of Insulin Secretion. Insulin synthesis and secretion is stimulated by "feast" or energy abundance. Ingestion of a meal (fuel excess) increases the rate of insulin secretion fivefold to tenfold. Plasma insulin levels rise, reaching peak values 30 to 60 minutes after eating is initiated.[43] High insulin levels, in turn, direct nutrients to appropriate storage sites.

Between meals, insulin levels drift downward, the storage process is reversed, and metabolic substrates are mobilized in the form of glucose, free fatty acids, and amino acids. Plasma glucose is by far the most important stimulator of insulin release. Elevated plasma glucose levels directly activate β-cells of the pancreas, stimulating insulin synthesis and secretion. Low plasma glucose concentrations inhibit this response. A maximal insulin response occurs at blood glucose levels of 400 to 600 mg/dL.[44] Very little insulin is secreted at plasma glucose levels of 50 mg/dL and below.[43,46,47]

Amino acids also are potent stimulators of insulin release, although the β-cell response to amino acids is not as pronounced as the response to glucose. Fat has little if any stimulating effect on insulin release.[43]

Both adrenergic and cholinergic fibers of the autonomic nervous system innervate the islets. Parasympathetic vagal activity and β-adrenergic stimulation increase insulin release. A general sympathetic discharge has a suppressive effect on insulin release through α-adrenergic receptor stimulation.[14] Pancreatic insulin secretion, however, does not *require* intact autonomic innervation because appropriate secretion responses occur in the transplanted pancreas as well.

Gastrointestinal hormones that accompany the digestive process potentiate insulin secretion. Food ingestion seems to send an "anticipatory" signal to the pancreas to discharge insulin in preparation for the absorption of glucose and amino acids.[44] Box 31-3 lists some of the factors that influence insulin secretion.

Glucagon. Glucagon is a linear polypeptide hormone produced by the α-cells of the pancreatic islets as a biologic antagonist to insulin.[43,44] The most important role of glucagon is to enhance hepatic glucose output and increase plasma glucose. A decrease in blood glucose concentration below 90 mg/dL increases the plasma glucagon level by several times. Hyperglycemia, on the other hand, decreases glucagon release from the α-cells.

Insulin and glucagon have opposing biologic actions. Whereas insulin is considered a hormone of energy storage, glucagon is considered a hormone of energy release.[44] Between meals, when blood glucose levels are low, the concentration of glucagon increases relative to that of insulin to maintain fuel production at a level that meets the energy needs of the individual. Special priority for glucose delivery is given to the brain.

Glucagon works in concert with the counterregulatory hormones epinephrine, growth hormone, and cortisol. These hormones are strong defenders against hypoglycemia and are critical in restoring normal glucose levels during periods of hypoglycemic stress. They also are secreted in response to various other stresses, such as infection, toxemia, severe injury,

BOX **31-3**

Factors That Influence Insulin Release

Stimulators	Inhibitors
Glucose, mannose, fructose	Hypoglycemia
Glucagon, cortisol, growth hormone	Somatostatin
α-Adrenergic stimulation	
Amino acids	
Gastrointestinal hormones	
Acetylcholine (parasympathetic stimulation)	
β-Adrenergic stimulation	

and surgery.[43] Nondiabetic surgical patients may experience an increased plasma blood glucose, as much as 60 mg/dL above their preoperative levels, in response to surgical stress.[45]

Insulin Deficiency: Diabetes Mellitus. Diabetes mellitus (DM) is a complex metabolic derangement caused by relative or absolute insulin deficiency. Diabetes has been called "starvation in a sea of food." Glucose is present in abundance but, because of insulin lack, is unable to reach cells for energy provision. Recommended guidelines for diagnosing diabetes include a fasting plasma glucose (FPG) of 126 mg/dL or greater. This diagnostic level was reduced from a previous value of 140 mg/dL based on findings that patients with a FPG of 126 mg/dL are at risk for diabetes-related complications.[48]

The incidence of diabetes has increased by several times over the last 40 years. Today it affects nearly 17 million people in the United States; about 6% of our population.[49,50] The rise can be attributed to a combination of three factors: (1) an overweight population, (2) more sedentary lifestyles, and (3) a rise in the number of elderly.[51] As more of our population advances in age into the decades in which most cases of diabetes occur, the impact of the disease will become even more alarming. As outlined in Figure 31-10, many pathophysiologic features of diabetes mellitus are directly attributable to a lack of the normal effects of insulin on carbohydrate, fat, and protein metabolism.

Insulin-Dependent Diabetes Mellitus. About 10% of diabetics have *type 1* or *insulin-dependent diabetes mellitus (IDDM)*. This type of diabetes was formerly known as *juvenile-onset diabetes*. These patients have an absolute deficiency of insulin and are therefore entirely dependent on exogenous insulin therapy.[52] In the absence of sufficient exogenous insulin, the disease course may be complicated by periods of ketosis and acidosis.

Type 1 DM is believed to be caused by unusually vigorous autoimmune destruction of the β-cells of the pancreatic islets. Environmental exposure to infectious agents or other antigenic proteins is cited as a possible initiator of the immune assault.[53] A genetic predisposition for development of the disease also is involved.

Type 1 DM usually develops before the age of 40 years, but it can develop at any age. The classic symptoms of type 1 DM appear only when at least 90% of the β-cells are destroyed.[52] The remaining β-cells usually are eliminated inexorably over the next 2 or 3 years. In patients with type 1 DM, exogenous insulin therapy is essential for life. Some type 1 DM patients may be candidates for pancreatic transplant; the transplantation of isolated islets holds out promise for a future cure.

Non–Insulin-Dependent Diabetes Mellitus. About 90% to 95% of the patients with diabetes have *type 2* or *non–insulin-dependent diabetes mellitus (NIDDM)*, a disorder characterized by impaired insulin secretion or peripheral insulin resistance (a decreased number of insulin receptors or an insulin receptor or postreceptor defect), or by both. This form of diabetes was formerly known as *maturity-onset diabetes*.

Type 2 DM occurs in patients who have some degree of endogenous insulin production but who produce quantities insufficient for sustaining normal carbohydrate homeostasis.[52] Insulin levels may be low, normal, or even elevated, but a *relative* insulin deficiency exists. The ultimate expression is a hyperglycemic state.

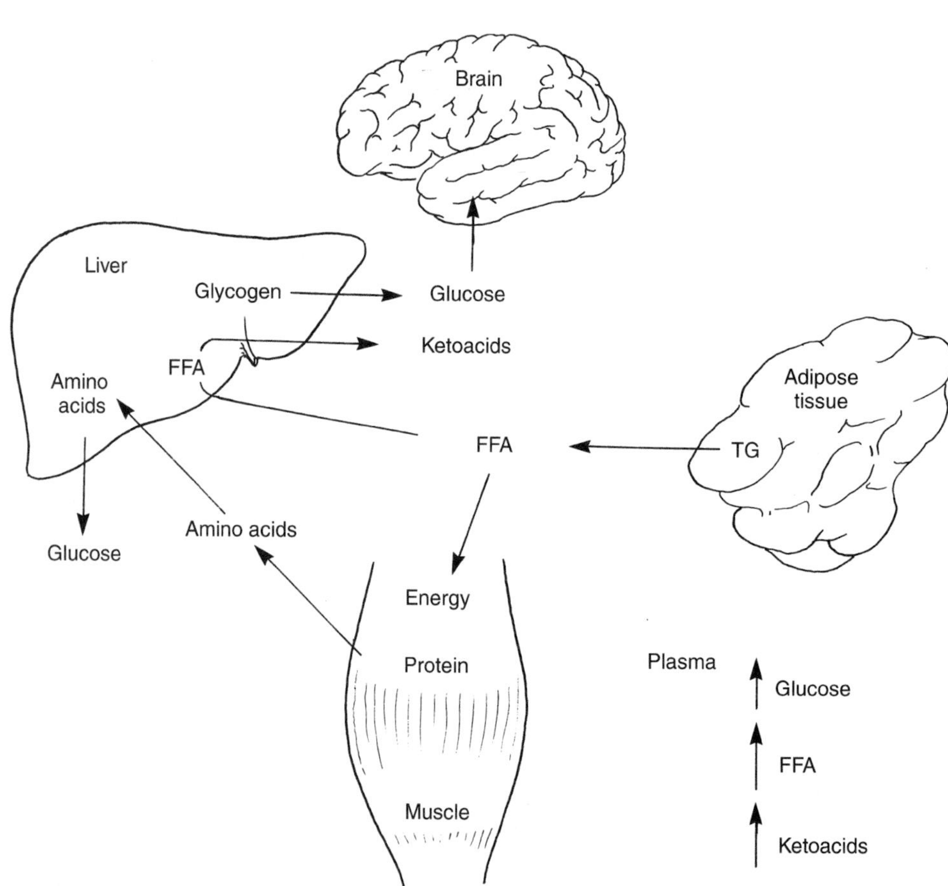

FIGURE **31-10**
The pattern of substrate flow in the diabetic state. Lack of insulin enhances hepatic glucose production because of increased gluconeogenesis and glycogenolysis. The diabetic state promotes protein breakdown, and the released amino acids are converted to glucose in the liver (gluconeogenesis). Lipolysis is augmented, and this increases free fatty acid supply to the liver, resulting in enhanced ketogenesis. Free fatty acids provide an energy source to muscle and other facultative tissue. Glucose uptake by the brain is sustained. *FFA*, free fatty acids; *TG*, triglyceride.

The distinction between *insulin-treated* diabetics and *insulin-dependent* diabetics is important. Some non-insulin-dependent diabetics may need exogenously administered insulin, especially during times of illness or stress. Insulin-dependent diabetics, on the other hand, require exogenous insulin daily to live.

Typically, type 2 DM occurs in patients who are older than 40 years of age, obese (80%), and with a family history of the disease.[52,54] Type 2 DM has an insidious onset, and it is estimated that one half of the people who have type 2 DM are not even aware of it. The disease course is rarely associated with ketosis or acidosis, but it may be complicated by a nonketotic, hyperosmolar, hyperglycemic state.

Treatment for this class of diabetes consists primarily of oral hypoglycemic agents and diet therapy. Weight reduction in the obese diabetic patient improves tissue responsiveness to endogenous insulin and often restores normoglycemia.

Diabetes Associated with Other Conditions. Diabetes may result from other conditions such as pancreatectomy, cystic fibrosis, or severe pancreatitis. Certain endocrine conditions, including Cushing's syndrome, glucagonoma, pheochromocytoma, and acromegaly, may also be associated with a diabetic condition. Steroid-induced diabetes may occur in the patient taking supraphysiologic doses of glucocorticoids. Gestational diabetes occurs with 2% to 5% of the pregnancies in the United States.

Effects of Insulin Deficiency on Carbohydrates. Insulin deficiency results in a decreased uptake and utilization of glucose by insulin-sensitive cells. Glycogen storage is decreased and gluconeogenesis is uninhibited with insulin lack, causing the liver to increase its glucose output. This produces an intracellular deficit and an extracellular surplus of glucose.[43]

The hyperglycemia produced by insulin lack has immediate adverse consequences. When the blood glucose concentration increases to a threshold level (about 180 to 200 mg/dL), the amount of glucose filtered at the kidney glomerulus cannot be totally reabsorbed. The excess filtered glucose spills into the urine (*glucosuria*) and acts as an osmotic diuretic, pulling water with it. The increased urine output (*polyuria*) contributes to extracellular dehydration and electrolyte depletion. Intracellular dehydration also occurs because of the osmotic transfer of water out of cells and into the hypertonic extracellular fluid. In an attempt to compensate for the hypovolemia, the diabetic patient may drink large quantities of water (*polydipsia*).[43,44]

Effects of Insulin Deficiency on Fat. As the diabetic state evolves, glucose-deprived cells meet their energy requirements by drawing on fat and protein reserves. Fat breakdown occurs normally between meals, when insulin levels are low, but it is enhanced greatly in diabetes. The lack of insulin activates hormone-sensitive lipase, which causes uninhibited lipolysis of stored triglycerides to free fatty acids and glycerol. This fat mobilization increases circulating lipids and may contribute to the atherosclerotic and angiopathic changes that complicate the disease course.[44]

Insulin deficiency produces a shift from carbohydrate to fat metabolism. Free fatty acids become the main energy substrate for essentially all tissues (the brain excluded). With uncontrolled diabetes, the excess free fatty acids are converted in the liver to ketone bodies (acetoacetic acid, β-hydroxybutyric acid, and acetone). This ultimately leads to greater circulating levels of ketoacids and an elevated hydrogen ion concentration in body fluids. The ketone body acetone is a volatile acid and is excreted via the lungs. Consequently, one can frequently identify ketonemia in uncontrolled diabetes by detecting on the patient a fruity "acetone breath."

Effects of Insulin Deficiency on Protein. The insulin deficiency of diabetes causes protein storage to halt and catabolism to ensue. When insulin levels are low or absent, the plasma amino acid concentration increases, and the excess circulating amino acids are converted in the liver to glucose (gluconeogenesis). The protein-wasting effects accompanying diabetes lead to loss of weight, weakness, and widespread organ dysfunction. The diabetic may attempt to compensate for the protein loss and caloric drain by increasing food intake (*polyphagia*).

Many proteins, including hemoglobin and structural tissue proteins, become glycosylated in the presence of high circulating blood glucose levels. Glucose adducts can alter protein function and may contribute to the organ damage and functional derangements observed in individuals with long-standing diabetes.[43]

Long-Term Diabetic Complications. Diabetics are subject to long-term complications that confer substantial morbidity and premature mortality. These complications include extensive arterial diseases, cataracts, peripheral neuropathies, and autonomic nervous system dysfunctions.

Arterial thrombotic lesions in the diabetic population are widely distributed in the extremities, kidneys, eyes, skeletal muscle, myocardium, and nervous system. As a result of these diffuse lesions, diabetes carries a serious risk for the development of nephropathy, atherosclerosis, stroke, retinopathy, and coronary artery disease.[55,56]

According to data from the Centers for Disease Control, the incidence of circulatory insufficiency to the legs and feet is fourfold to sevenfold greater in diabetic men and women compared with their nondiabetic counterparts. Gangrene is 17-fold more common in the diabetic than in the nondiabetic individual.[49,57] Not surprisingly, lower-extremity bypass grafting and amputations are common surgical procedures in the diabetic population. Heart disease is the leading cause of diabetes-related deaths. Adults with diabetes have heart disease death rates about 2 to 4 times higher than adults without diabetes. [49] Systolic dysfunction, decreased ejection fraction, and congestive heart failure may occur with severe and long-standing disease.

Further, 70% of diabetics have a medical history of hypertension, a rate of occurrence twofold to threefold that for nondiabetics.[57] In many of these patients the hypertension is uncontrolled. The risk of stroke is 2 to 4 times higher in people with diabetes, and the recovery rate for diabetics after a stroke is poor.[57]

The most frequent vascular complication of type 1 DM is diabetic retinopathy. The eyes are vulnerable to vascular disease because of the dense network of capillary vessels in the retina. This disorder is characterized by microaneurysm formation, swelling and narrowing of retinal blood vessels, and neovascularization. These vascular lesions may result in vitreous hemorrhage and retinal scarring or detachment. Loss of vision from diabetic retinopathy is the leading cause of new cases of blindness in people aged 20 to 74 years in the United States.[49]

Diabetic renal disease develops after 15 years in one third of patients with type 1 DM and in one fifth of patients with type 2 DM.[57] The nephropathy may be caused by inflammation and thickening of the glomerular capillary basement membrane (glomerulosclerosis). Renal insufficiency or chronic renal failure is often the end result.[58] Diabetics commonly are candidates for kidney transplantation.

The diabetic process also interferes with normal nerve function. Both the peripheral and autonomic nervous systems may be involved. Measurable defects of the autonomic nervous system affect as many as 40% of all diabetic patients.[49,59,60] Vagal denervation may occur early in the course of the disease. Dysfunction of the cardiac vagus nerve may be manifested as resting tachycardia, cardiac dysrhythmias, and the absence of heart rate variability with deep breathing. Postural hypotension may occur in the diabetic with autonomic neuropathy as a result of dysfunctional sympathetic nervous system vasoconstrictive processes. Manifestations of orthostatic hypotension may include postural syncope, dizziness, and lightheadedness.

Diabetic patients with autonomic neuropathy are at increased risk for developing painless myocardial ischemia. The possibility of a myocardial infarction should be considered in the presence of unexplained hypotension in these patients.[59,61]

Other signs of autonomic neuropathy in the diabetic include early satiety, lack of sweating, impotence, and nocturnal diarrhea.[14] The patient with diabetic autonomic neuropathy has impaired gastric emptying and is at risk for aspiration of stomach contents in the perioperative period.

There is a strong relationship between the hyperglycemia of diabetes and end-organ diseases. Sustained hyperglycemia seems to be prerequisite for significant nephropathy, retinopathy, and neuropathy to occur, at least in type 1 diabetes.[62] Other factors—genetic or environmental, or both—may also have roles in determining end-organ complications. The hemoglobin A1c or glycosylated hemoglobin level provides an estimate of the patient's overall plasma glucose control during the past 3 months. A value less than 7.5% suggests adequate blood glucose control.[9]

Anesthetic Management of the Diabetic Patient. Diabetes is the most common endocrine disorder encountered in surgical patients. Long-standing diabetes predisposes the patient to many diseases that require surgical intervention. Cataract extraction, kidney transplantation, ulcer debridement, and vascular repair are some of the operations frequently performed on diabetic patients. It is estimated that approximately 50% of diabetics have major surgery during their lifetimes.

Diabetic patients have higher morbidity and mortality in the perioperative period compared with nondiabetics of similar age. Increased complications are not because of the disease itself but primarily because of organ damage associated with long-term disease.[11,14] Ischemic heart disease is the most common cause of perioperative mortality in the diabetic patient.[9]

The diabetic surgical patient's operation should be scheduled early in the day if possible, to minimize disruptions in treatment and nutrition regimens. Day-stay for minor surgery may be utilized for patients with well-controlled diabetes who are knowledgeable about their disease and treatment and who have proper home support.[54]

Preoperative Considerations. The diabetic patient may come to the operating room with a spectrum of metabolic aberrations and end-organ complications that warrant careful preanesthetic assessment.

Cardiovascular complications account for most of the surgical deaths in diabetics.[63] The presence of hypertension, coronary artery disease, or autonomic nervous system dysfunctions can result in a labile cardiovascular course during anesthesia. It is essential that the cardiovascular and volume status of the patient be thoroughly evaluated before surgery. Preoperative electrocardiography is necessary for all adult diabetic patients because of the high incidence of cardiac disease.

Autonomic nervous system dysfunction may result in delayed gastric emptying. It is estimated that gastroparesis occurs in 20% to 30% of all diabetics.[9,64] These patients are prone to aspiration, nausea and vomiting, and abdominal distention. Routine preoperative aspiration prophylaxis with H_2-receptor blockers, metoclopramide, and/or preinduction antacids is recommended by many authorities for patients with diabetes.[11,14] Intubation during general anesthesia is a logical choice for the patient with gastroparesis.

Patients with significant autonomic neuropathy may have an impaired respiratory response to hypoxia. These patients are especially sensitive to the respiratory-depressant effects of sedatives and anesthetics and require particular vigilance in the perioperative period.[9,14,59]

Peripheral neuropathies (paresthesias, numbness in the hands and feet) should be adequately documented in the preanesthetic evaluation. Their presence may affect the decision to use regional anesthesia.

Glycosylation of tissue proteins may produce a stiff joint syndrome in diabetics. An estimated 30% to 40% of insulin-dependent diabetics demonstrate restricted joint mobility.[9] Limited motion of the atlantooccipital joint can make endotracheal intubation difficult.[55,65,66] Demonstration of the "prayer sign," an inability to approximate the palms of the hands and fingers, may help identify patients with tissue protein glycosylation and potentially difficult airways.[54]

Evidence of kidney disease should be sought, and basic tests of renal function (urinalysis, serum creatinine, blood urea nitrogen) performed preoperatively. The presence of renal impairment may influence the choice and dosage of anesthetic agents. The use of potentially nephrotoxic drugs should be avoided.

The anesthetist should examine the patient's history of glycemic control to ensure preoperative optimization of the patient's metabolic state. A recommended target blood glucose range for the perioperative period is 120 mg/dL to 180 mg/dL.[9] Glycosylated hemoglobin levels provide an "averaged" estimate of glucose control.

Sustained hyperglycemia, with attendant osmotic diuresis, should alert the anesthetist to possible fluid deficits and electrolyte depletion. Preoperative levels of electrolytes should be determined for all diabetic patients and adequate hydration and a good urine output should be maintained. Lactate-containing solutions are generally avoided as lactate conversion to glucose may contribute to hyperglycemia. An important part of the preoperative evaluation is a review of oral hypoglycemic and insulin regimens.

Oral Hypoglycemic Agents. Oral hypoglycemic agents are used as adjuncts to diet therapy for treating type 2 DM. Currently available oral hypoglycemic agents fall into the following classifications: (1) sulfonylureas, (2) α-glucosidase inhibitors, (3) thiazolidinediones, (4) biguanides, and (5) nonsulfonylurea

TABLE 31-3 Oral Drugs for Type 2 Diabetes

Drug	Usual Daily Dosage
Sulfonylurea: first generation	
Acetohexamide (Dymelor)	500 to 750 mg once or divided
Chlorpropamide (Diabinese)	250 to 375 mg once
Tolazamide (Tolinase)	250 to 500 mg once or divided
Tolbutamide (Orinase)	1000 to 2000 mg divided
Sulfonylurea: second generation	
Glimepiride (Amaryl)	1 to 4 mg once
Glipizide (Glucotrol)	10 to 20 mg once or divided
(Glucotrol XL sustained-release tablets)	5 to 20 mg once
Glyburide (DiaBeta, Micronase)	5 to 20 mg once or divided
(Glynase, micronized tablets,)	3 to 12 mg once or divided
α-Glucosidase inhibitors	
Acarbose (Precose)	50 to 100 mg tid with meals
Miglitol (Glyset)	50 to 100 mg tid with meals
Thiazolidinediones	
Rosiglitazone (Avandia)	4 to 8 mg once or divided
Pioglitazone (Actos)	15 to 45 mg once
Biguanides	
Metformin (Glucophage)	1500 to 2550 mg divided
(Glucophage XR)	1500 to 2000 mg once
Metformin/Glyburide (Glucovance)	500 mg/5 mg bid
Nonsulfonylurea secretagogues	
Repaglinide (Prandin)	1 to 4 mg tid before meals
Nateglinide (Starlix)	60 to 120 mg tid before meals

secretagogues. Table 31-3 lists commonly used medications used to treat type 2 diabetes.

Sulfonylureas increase the secretion of insulin from the pancreas, and improve tissue sensitivity to insulin. These agents require the presence of functioning β-cells and thus are not efficacious in patients with IDDM. Hypoglycemia is the most important adverse side effect of sulfonylureas.[14,52,54] Sulfonylurea therapy is also associated with a low incidence of cholestatic jaundice, rashes, and gastrointestinal symptoms. The syndrome of inappropriate ADH secretion and hyponatremia has been associated with chlorpropamide.

Acarbose (Precose) and miglital (Glyset) are *α-glucosidase inhibitors*. These medications block the intestinal enzymes that digest starches into absorbable monosaccharides, resulting in a slower and lower rise in plasma glucose.

Rosiglitazone (Avandia) and pioglitazone (Actos) are *thiazolidinedione derivatives*. Thiazolidinediones decrease hepatic glucose output and reduce insulin resistance in the type 2 DM patient by sensitizing the insulin receptor for glucose uptake.[52,67] Liver enzymes must be monitored closely with these agents. The thiazolidinedione *troglitazone* (Rezulin) was withdrawn from the market in March 2000 for serious liver complications associated with the drug.

Metformin, a *biguanide*, decreases hepatic glucose production and increases peripheral insulin sensitivity. Lactic acidosis, a rare but potentially fatal problem, has been reported with biguanides. Lactic acidosis is precipitated by drug accumulation; therefore, even mild renal impairment is a contraindication to metformin therapy.[54,68,69] Metformin is also not prescribed to patients with conditions that predispose to acidosis (e.g., liver failure, major surgery).

Newer oral hypoglycemic drugs such as the *meglitinides* (repaglinide) and *D-phenylalanine* (nateglinide) increase insulin production by pancreatic β-cells in a manner similar to the sulfonylureas.[67] Repaglinide and nateglinide must be taken before each meal, and if a meal is missed, the drug should be omitted.[67]

Insulin Preparations. Insulin preparations differ in onset and duration after subcutaneous administration.[67] In addition to subcutaneous injections, insulin delivery devices (implantable pumps, mechanical syringes) are used to facilitate exogenous administration. The greatest risk with all forms of insulin is hypoglycemia. Table 31-4 identifies three major classes of exogenous insulin: short-acting, intermediate-acting, and long-acting.

It is imperative to know the surgical patient's normal insulin dosage regimen and treatment compliance. Most diabetics are on a fixed regimen that consists of a mixture of rapid- and intermediate-acting insulins taken before breakfast

TABLE 31-4 Characteristics of Insulin Preparations

Insulin Type	Onset of Action	Peak Activity	Duration	Route
Short-acting				
Regular	30-60 min	1-2 h	5-12 h	IV, SC, IM
Rapid-acting				
Aspart (Novolog)	10-30 min	30-60 min	3-5 h	SC
Lispro (Humalog)	10-30 min	30-60 min	3-5 h	SC
Intermediate-acting				
NPH/Lente	1-2 h	4-8 h	10-20 h	SC
Long-acting				
Ultralente	2-4 h	8-20 h	16-24 h	SC
Glargine	1-2 h	No peak	24 hr	SC

IV, *intravenous;* SC, *subcutaneous;* IM, *intramuscular;* NPH, *neutral protamine Hagedorn. Time course is based on subcutaneous administration.*
Adapted from Treatment Guidelines from The Medical Letter, *vol 1, September 2002.*

and again at the evening meal.[9,47] Multiple injection regimens are designed to give tight control.[54] Insulin glargine (Lantus) is a recombinant DNA analog of human insulin taken once a day. It forms microprecipitates in subcutaneous tissue, which delay its absorption and prolong its effects. Unlike NPH and ultralente, it has no peak effect, but rather behaves like an insulin infusion.

The use of long-acting insulins (e.g., ultra-lente, glargine) is discouraged in the perioperative period because the dosage cannot be adjusted quickly for changes in blood glucose levels. Long-acting insulin regimens are often switched to intermediate- or short-acting insulin regimens for perioperative glucose control. Since glargine insulin maintains a stable level throughout the day, more experience with its use may demonstrate its safety as a basal insulin throughout the perioperative period.

Intraoperative Management. Surgery produces a catabolic stress response and elevates stress-induced counterregulatory hormones.[9,11] The hyperglycemic, ketogenic, and lipolytic effects of the counterregulatory hormones in the diabetic compound the state of insulin deficiency. For this reason, perioperative hyperglycemia and other metabolic aberrations are common in the surgical diabetic patient.

No specific anesthetic technique is superior overall for diabetic patients. Both general anesthesia and regional anesthesia have been used safely. General anesthesia, however, has been shown to induce hormonal changes that accentuate glycogenolysis and gluconeogenesis, compounding the diabetic patient's hyperglycemic state. Regional anesthesia may produce less deleterious changes in glucose homeostasis.[9,70,71]

The CRNA must be especially careful in positioning and padding the diabetic patient on the operating table. Decreased tissue perfusion and peripheral sympathetic neuropathy may contribute to the development of skin breakdown and ulceration.

Diabetic patients represent a heterogeneous group requiring individualized perioperative care. The specific approach to metabolic management depends on the type of diabetes (type 1 or type 2), the history of glycemic control, and the type of surgery being performed. Frequent blood sugar determinations should be an integral part of any diabetic management technique. A glucose meter or other accurate and rapid means of monitoring blood glucose levels should be available. Blood glucose should be routinely monitored in the preoperative and postoperative periods. An hourly intraoperative blood glucose measurement is the prudent course for the brittle diabetic patient, during a long surgical procedure, or for major surgery.

Persistent hyperglycemia has been shown to impair wound healing and wound strength.[72] In addition, reports suggest that postoperative infection is more prevalent in diabetic patients with uncontrolled blood sugar levels.[73,74] Studies also provide evidence that hyperglycemia worsens the neurologic outcome after ischemic brain injury.[75,76] Avoiding hyperglycemia is advisable, especially in the patient at risk for acute neurological insult (carotid endarterectomy, intracranial surgery, cardiopulmonary bypass).

Various regimens have been tendered on how to best manage the metabolic changes that occur in the surgical diabetic.[7,9,11,14,77-81] Experts differ on optimal protocols for case management. Current debate centers on the value of intensive or "tight" blood glucose control versus "nontight" control during surgery. The universal goal with all techniques is to avoid hypoglycemia and to minimize metabolic derangements. Patients under anesthesia are generally maintained with a mild transient hyperglycemia to avoid the potentially catastrophic effects of hypoglycemia. Frequent blood glucose determinations during surgery and in the immediate postoperative period are central to safe practice.

Three different approaches to the metabolic management of the surgical diabetic patient are described as follows; however, the reader should note that there are numerous variations.

Nontight Control of Blood Glucose Levels in the Perioperative Period. *Nontight control* of blood sugar levels refers to diabetic management techniques that involve less intensive control of plasma glucose but avoid marked hyperglycemia and dangerous hypoglycemia. This is a traditional method of managing the surgical diabetic patient and variations of this technique are used for stable diabetics undergoing elective operative procedures.[7,9,11,14]

Technique for nontight management of the diabetic patient:

1. On the morning of surgery, fasting blood sugar level is measured.
2. An intravenous (IV) infusion containing 5% dextrose is started at 125 mL/hr/70 kg body weight.
3. After the IV infusion is started, 30% to 50% of the patient's normal morning intermediate insulin (NPH or Lente) dose is administered subcutaneously.
4. The glucose-containing IV infusion is continued throughout surgery. Additional fluid requirements are met with the administration of a second, glucose-free infusate.
5. Blood glucose levels are checked every 1 to 2 hours during surgery.
6. If the blood glucose level exceeds an established maximum level, commonly 200 mg/dL, a bolus of regular insulin is administered intravenously, according to an established "sliding scale." Insulin sensitivity varies markedly from one patient to the next, but on the average, 1 unit of regular insulin can be expected to decrease the blood glucose level 40 to 50 mg/dL.[47]

This time-tested regimen is easy to implement, and it is usually successful in preventing significant hypoglycemia and the other metabolic extremes, diabetic ketoacidosis, and hyperosmolar states.[14,78,82,95]

The disadvantages of nontight control are as follows:

1. Absorption of preoperatively administered subcutaneous insulin is unpredictable and erratic in the surgical patient because of blood pressure, blood flow, and temperature variations that occur with anesthesia.
2. The onset and the peak effect of the preoperative intermediate-acting insulin may not correspond to the time of surgical stress, especially if the operation is delayed or prolonged.
3. The half-life of regular insulin is short and a "rollercoaster" glucose profile may occur. Plasma glucose levels will vary considerably.

Tight Control of Blood Glucose Levels in the Perioperative Period. *Tight control* of plasma glucose refers to diabetic management techniques in which the blood glucose concentration is maintained within relatively narrow boundaries—commonly 100 to 180 mg/dL. These regimens require the use of infusion pumps. Tighter control of blood glucose levels require more frequent blood glucose assays.[14,78] Intensive perioperative regulation of blood glucose prevents hyperglycemia, but it carries the risk of hypoglycemia.

Insulin infusion during surgery is advised for the type 1 diabetic having major surgery and for the patient with poorly controlled diabetes (type 1 or type 2).[54] A combined insulin/glucose infusion regimen is advised to prevent hypoglycemia caused by inadvertent blockage of a glucose infusion when separate glucose and insulin infusions are used.[31] An example of this regimen follows:

1. An infusion of 5% dextrose with 0.32 units regular insulin/g of dextrose (16 units per liter), with 20 mEq potassium/L is administered at 100 mL/hr.
2. The glucose/insulin containing IV infusion is started only when the patient's blood glucose level is 200 mg/dL or greater.
3. Blood glucose levels should be measured every hour during an insulin infusion, and potassium levels checked after the first hour of the infusion.
4. For patients with higher insulin needs, 1 to 2 units additional insulin can be added to the infusate bag.
5. Additional fluid requirements are met with the administration of a second, glucose-free infusate.

Blood glucose levels less than 80 mg/dL may be treated with $D_{50}W$ and remeasured in 30 minutes. In a 70-kg patient, 15 mL of $D_{50}W$ can be expected to raise the blood glucose concentration by about 30 mg/dL. Surgical patients undergoing renal transplantation or coronary artery bypass graft procedures, obese and septic patients, and patients on steroid therapy usually have higher insulin infusion requirements.[9,14,63,81,95]

The advantages of tight glucose management in the perioperative period are as follows:

1. The insulin infusion can be finely regulated to correspond to hourly variations in blood glucose levels.
2. Periods of hyperglycemia are less likely. Deleterious effects of hyperglycemia (hyperosmolarity, osmotic diuresis, impaired wound healing, infection) may be prevented.[78]
3. The insulin-glucose infusion can be continued into the postoperative period until the patient is ready to eat, at which time subcutaneous insulin or an oral hypoglycemic agent can be reinstated.

Type 2 Diabetes and Oral Hypoglycemic Agents. Patients treated with oral hypoglycemic agents demand the same individualized perioperative management as those with type 1 diabetes. The duration of action of the patient's oral agent must be noted. Discontinuing long-acting agents 2 to 3 days before surgery and converting to shorter-acting agents or insulin affords better perioperative glucose control.[7,80,83] Metformin should be discontinued 2 days or more before surgery because the surgical risks of hypotension and renal hypoperfusion place patients on this drug at increased risk for lactic acidosis.[7,9]

For the well-controlled surgical patient with type 2 diabetes who is scheduled for minor to moderate surgery, the patient's oral hypoglycemic agent may be continued until the evening before surgery. Glucose-containing fluids may be administered intraoperatively to protect against possible residual effects of oral hypoglycemic agents. Other experts adhere to a "no glucose, no insulin" technique for well controlled type II diabetics. Regardless of the technique chosen, plasma glucose should be measured regularly throughout the procedure and hyperglycemia treated with insulin on a "sliding scale."[83,84]

Acute Derangements in Glucose Homeostasis

Hypoglycemia. Hypoglycemia is encountered more frequently in the diabetic patient than in the healthy adult and it can develop insidiously during the perioperative period.

Medications (insulin, sulfonylureas, β-adrenergic receptor blocking agents) and toxins (ethanol) are common causes of hypoglycemia.[46] β-Adrenergic blockers reduce the hyperglycemic effects of epinephrine. Severe liver disease (impaired hepatic glucose output) or an insulin-secreting tumor of the islets of Langerhans (an insulinoma) are among the many other disorders that can cause hypoglycemia.

The blood glucose concentration at which signs and symptoms of hypoglycemia appear varies widely from one person to the next, but blood glucose levels in the range of 40 to 60 mg/dL commonly produce mild symptoms in the otherwise healthy patient.[44] Because the brain is the predominant organ of glucose consumption, it is most sensitive to glucose deprivation.[44,46] Manifestations of impaired cerebral function (confusion, dizziness, headache, weakness) are associated with glucose lack. As the blood sugar level declines to below 50 mg/dL, aberrant behavior, seizures, and loss of consciousness may occur.[44] Other signs of hypoglycemia (tachycardia, diaphoresis, anxiety, tremors, piloerection, pupillary dilation, and vasoconstriction) reflect sympathetic-adrenal hyperactivity.[44] Acute treatment for the hypoglycemic surgical patient is the intravenous administration of 25 mL of 50% glucose.[9] Unless prompt glucose therapy is provided, irreversible brain damage may result.

Hypoglycemia is potentially catastrophic during surgery because most of the neural indications of glucose lack are masked by general anesthesia. Signs of sympathetic adrenal discharge may also be blunted by general anesthesia or severe diabetic autonomic neuropathy, making the diagnosis of hypoglycemia extremely difficult. β-Adrenergic receptor blocking agents may further diminish the symptomatic warning signs of hypoglycemia.[46] Frequent blood glucose determinations, maintenance of mild hyperglycemia, and assiduous monitoring help to avoid this serious complication during anesthesia.

Diabetic Ketoacidosis. Diabetic ketoacidosis (DKA) is a medical emergency triggered by a hyperglycemic event, usually in an insulin-dependent diabetic. Treatment errors, critical illnesses (myocardial infarction, trauma, cerebral vascular accident, burns), and infections are common precipitants of DKA.[85,86,87] Gangrene and infection of an ischemic lower extremity are common surgical conditions associated with DKA.

Stressful events, such as an infection or a critical illness, stimulate the release of hyperglycemic counterregulatory hormones (glucagon, growth hormone, epinephrine, cortisol).[84,87] The insulin-dependent diabetic is unable to secrete insulin to counterbalance the serum elevations of glucose, free fatty acids, and ketone bodies produced by these stress-induced hormones. Unless exogenous insulin is provided, the glycemic event may progress to severe ketoacidosis, dehydration, and acute metabolic decompensation.

Major signs and symptoms of DKA include hyperglycemia (>250 mg/dL), volume depletion (average deficit of 3 to 8 L), tachycardia, metabolic acidosis (arterial pH <7.3) with ketonemia, electrolyte depletion, hyperosmolarity (>320 mOsm/L), nausea and vomiting, abdominal pain, and lethargy.[14,52,84,87] The blood levels of the organic acids, ketone bodies, are elevated and the patient's breath may have a fruity odor from the acetone. The respiratory center is typically stimulated by the low plasma pH, resulting in rapid, deep breathing (*Kussmaul's respiration*). Acidosis, hyperosmolarity, and dehydration may depress consciousness to the point of coma. Figure 31-11 outlines the pathophysiologic events leading to diabetic ketoacidosis.

Preoperative management of the surgical patient with DKA requires an aggressive approach to restore intravascular volume, correct electrolyte abnormalities, improve acid-base

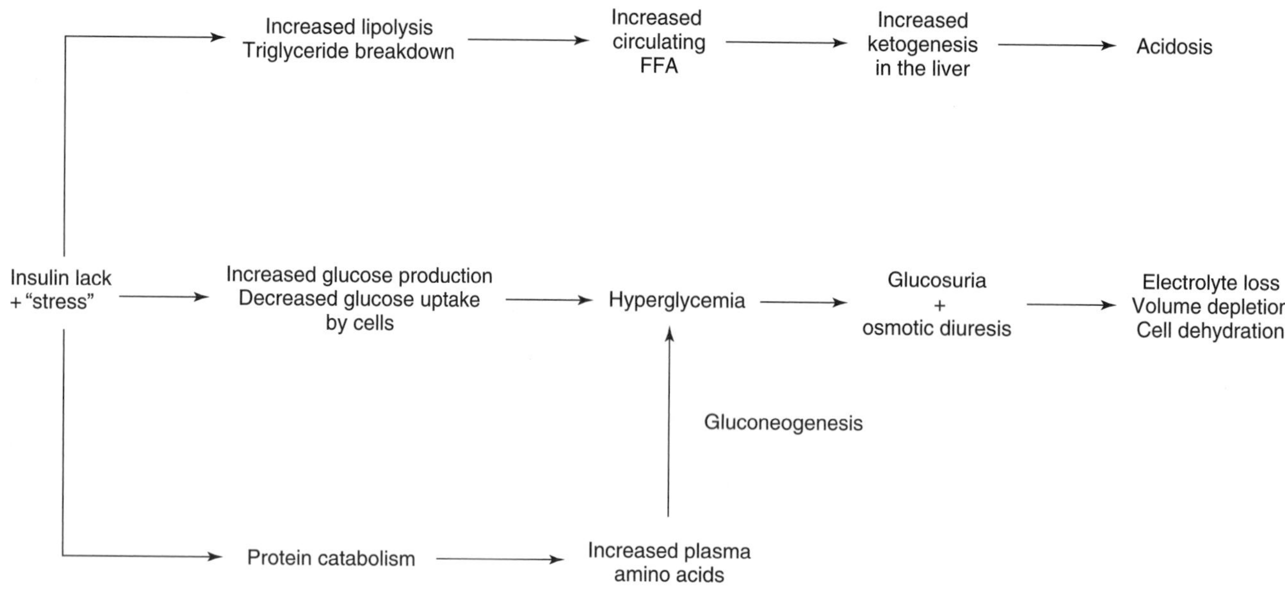

FIGURE **31-11**
Diabetic ketoacidosis

balance, and reduce blood glucose levels.[85] The airway must be protected in the obtunded patient. Emergency surgery should not be postponed in an attempt to correct DKA.[85] Once the surgical problem has resolved, medical management of DKA often is more effective.[52]

Hyperglycemic Hyperosmolar Nonketotic Syndrome. Hyperglycemic hyperosmolar nonketotic syndrome (HHNS) is a hyperosmolar state triggered by a hyperglycemic event. This syndrome commonly occurs in patients with type 2 DM, but it also develops in patients with no history of diabetes. Patients are typically middle aged or elderly; they generally have some endogenous insulin secretion, but the hyperglycemic episode overwhelms the pancreas and produces severe hyperglycemia and glucosuria. The amount of insulin secreted is usually sufficient to prevent lipolysis and ketone production. Therefore, unlike DKA, this syndrome usually is not associated with acidosis or significant ketogenesis. Table 31-5 compares common features of diabetic ketoacidosis and HHNS.

Common precipitating factors of HHNS include infection, steroid therapy, hyperalimentation and dextrose infusions, peritoneal dialysis, and myocardial infarction.

TABLE **31-5** Features of Diabetic Ketoacidosis and Hyperglycemic Hyperosmolar Nonketotic Syndrome

	DKA	HHNS
Plasma glucose	>250 mg/dL	>600 mg/dL
PH	<7.3	>7.3
Serum osmolarity	+	++
Ketonemia	++	Normal or slight+
Mental obtundation	Variable	Present
Hypovolemia	Present	Present

+ = increase; ++ = large increase.

A spectrum of symptoms is associated with HHNS, ranging from a small degree of hyperosmolarity with minimal central nervous system dysfunction to severe hyperosmolarity with coma. Laboratory evaluation may reveal the following biochemical profile: marked hyperglycemia (>600 mg/dL), a normal arterial pH, absent or minimal ketonemia and ketonuria, and hyperosmolarity (>330 mOsm/L).[14,52,86] Profound dehydration is always present.

The mortality rate for HHNS may be as high as 50%. The mortality figures for HHNS are higher than those for DKA, in part because this syndrome commonly affects an older population group.[9,52]

Treatment goals are similar to those for DKA and include judicious isotonic rehydration (average total body water deficit is 7 L), correction of hyperglycemia, and electrolyte replacement.[85] The hazards inherent in aggressive fluid administration in the elderly may be avoided by central hemodynamic monitoring.

ADRENAL GLANDS

The adrenal glands are located at the superior poles of each kidney. The glands consist of two distinct anatomical and physiological entities, the adrenal cortex and the adrenal medulla. The *adrenal medulla* comprises the central 20% of the adrenal gland and secretes the hormones epinephrine and norepinephrine. The *adrenal cortex* constitutes the outer part of the adrenal gland and secretes three main types of hormones: mineralocorticoids (aldosterone), glucocorticoids (cortisol), and androgenic hormones (dehydroepiandrosterone).

Adrenal Cortex

The adrenal cortex is composed of three layers, each having distinct properties. The *zona glomerulosa* is the outermost tissue of the cortex and it secretes mineralocorticoid hormones. The *zona fasciculata* is the middle layer and it secretes cortisol, other glucocorticoids, and androgenic hormones. The *zona reticularis* is the innermost layer of the adrenal cortex and it secretes adrenal androgenic hormones and glucocorticoids. (Fig. 31-12).

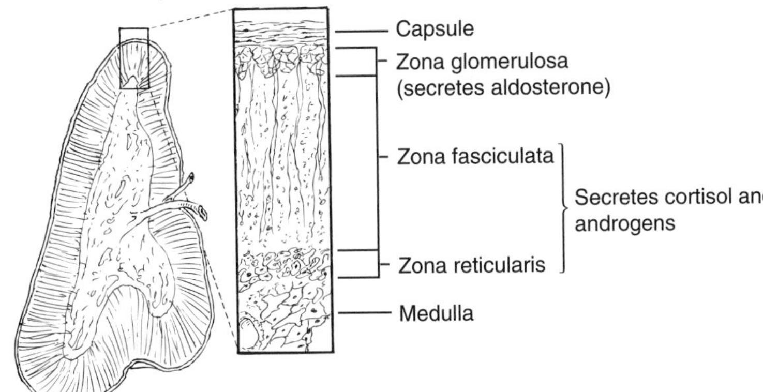

FIGURE **31-12**
Secretion of adrenocortical hormones by the different zones of the adrenal cortex. (From Guyton AC, Hall JE: *Textbook of Medical Physiology*, ed 10, Philadelphia, 2000, Saunders, p 870.)

Hormones Secreted from the Adrenal Cortex. All hormones secreted from the adrenal cortex have a steroidal structure and they share a common cholesterol backbone. As a group, these hormones are termed *corticosteroids*. Corticosteroids have similar chemical structures but widely diverse functions. Glucocorticoid and androgenic hormone production and release is controlled in large part by ACTH from the anterior pituitary gland. ACTH stimulates adrenocortical hormone synthesis by activating the enzyme desmolase. Desmolase causes the initial conversion of cholesterol to pregnenolone, the first step in corticosteroid hormone synthesis (Fig. 31-13).

The adrenal androgens, of which dehydroepiandrosterone is the most important, are secreted by the adrenal cortex. Androgenic hormones have effects similar to the male sex hormone testosterone, but display only weak effects in humans.[88] The glucocorticoids and mineralocorticoids are discussed in more detail in the following sections.

Glucocorticoids. The adrenal cortex synthesizes over 30 types of glucocorticoid hormones. Cortisol (hydrocortisone) is the prototypical glucocorticoid; it accounts for 95% of the glucocorticoids released from the adrenal cortex. *Corticosterone* exhibits a small but significant amount of glucocorticoid activity.

Cortisol secretion is almost entirely controlled by ACTH, and in turn, cortisol is the most potent regulator of ACTH. Cortisol has a direct negative feedback effect on the hypothalamus, inhibiting the release of CRH, and on the anterior lobe of the pituitary gland, decreasing ACTH release. When cortisol concentration is high, the feedback system reduces ACTH levels. Secretion rates of CRH, ACTH, and cortisol follow a circadian rhythm: they are high in the early morning and low in the late evening.[88] The daily cortisol production is 15 to 25 mg, and most of this is produced and released between 5 A.M. and 9 A.M.[101] Physical and mental stress increase the secretion of CRH, ACTH, and cortisol (Box 31-4). Stress can raise cortisol production levels to 250 mg/day.[101]

After release from the adrenal cortex, cortisol circulates in the blood bound to the proteins cortisol-binding globulin (transcortin), and albumin. Ninety-four percent of cortisol is transported in the bound form, and 6% is free. Cortisol becomes fixed in the target tissues within 1 to 2 hours after release. It is inactivated mainly in the liver and excreted in the urine as 17-hydroxycorticosteroids. The daily production of endogenous cortisol is approximately 20 mg, and the normal blood concentration averages 12 mcg/dL.[88]

Cortisol Actions. Glucocorticoids are necessary to maintain life. They are needed for the proper utilization of proteins, carbohydrates, and fats by the body and they are central to the body's response to physical and mental stress. Almost any stress, psychological or physical, causes an immediate and marked increase in ACTH and cortisol secretion. Important perioperative stressors may include trauma, infection, heat or cold, and surgery.

Glucocorticoids have weak mineralocorticoid and androgenic effects, which may become apparent with hormone excess.

Effect on Carbohydrate Metabolism. An important function of glucocorticoids is their ability to stimulate gluconeogenesis in the liver. The rate of gluconeogenesis increases six- to tenfold in the presence of cortisol. Further, cortisol mobilizes amino acids from extrahepatic tissues (mainly muscle), making them available for gluconeogenesis and glycogenesis in the liver. In extrahepatic tissues, cortisol moderately decreases the rate of glucose utilization. Cortisol is called "diabetogenic" because its overall effect increases blood glucose concentrations.

Effect on Protein Metabolism. Cortisol decreases protein synthesis and increases protein catabolism in essentially all body cells except those of the liver. Cortisol increases amino acid transport into liver cells. In the presence of sustained cortisol excess, the catabolic effects are marked. This is especially apparent in skeletal muscles, which become weak and atrophic.

Effect on Fat Metabolism. Plasma free fatty acids are mobilized from adipose tissue under cortisol's effect. Cortisol also enhances oxidation of fatty acids in the cells. These two effects help shift metabolic systems, in times of starvation or other stress, to the utilization of fatty acids instead of glucose for energy. With excess cortisol, a person can develop a distinctive obesity, with fat being deposited in the chest and head regions, leading to a buffalo-like torso and a "moon facies."

Effect on Inflammation and Immunity. Cortisol can diminish the inflammatory process by stabilizing lysosomal membranes and decreasing the amount of the proteolytic enzymes released by inflammatory mediators. Migration of white blood cells into the inflamed area is also decreased. These effects are the basis for the therapeutic use of corticosteroids to reduce the inflammatory responses associated with asthma, allergic reactions, and other inflammatory disorders.

Cortisol decreases the number of eosinophils and lymphocytes in the blood. T lymphocyte and antibody output are

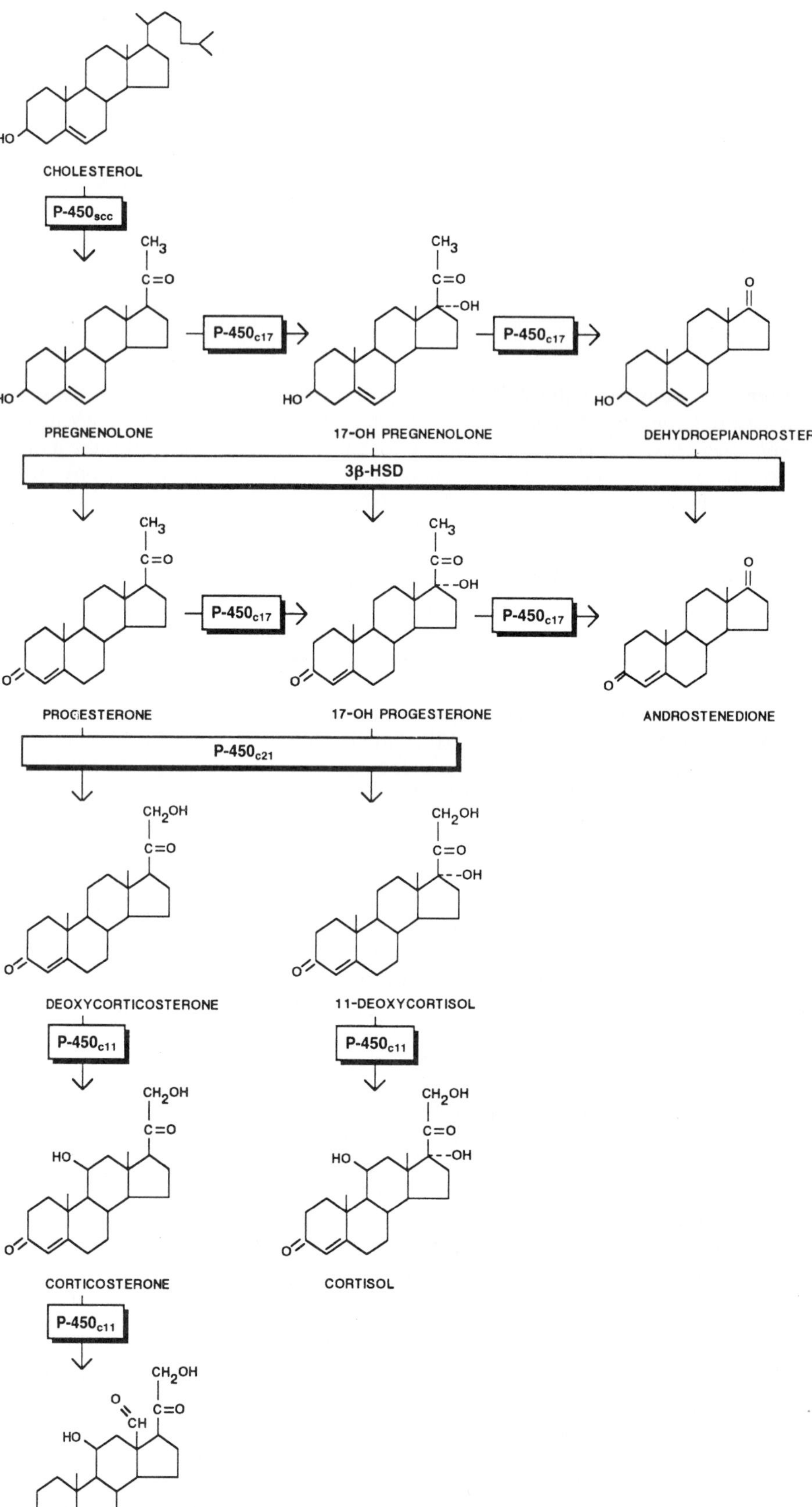

FIGURE **31-13**
Steroid biosynthetic pathways in the adrenal cortex. The branching pathways for glucocorticoids, mineralocorticoids, and adrenal androgens and the structures of these steroids and their biosynthetic precursors are shown. The biosynthetic enzymes are represented by the boxes. *3b-HSD*, 3-β-hydroxysteroid dehydrogenase. (From Wilson JD, Foster DW, Kronenberg HM, Larsen PR: *Williams Textbook of Endocrinology*, ed 9, Philadelphia, 1998, Saunders, p 523.)

BOX 31-4

Regulation of Adrenocorticotropic Hormone Secretion

Stimulation	Inhibition
Corticotropin-releasing hormone	
Cortisol decrease	
Stress	
Sleep-to-waking transition	
Hypoglycemia	
Sepsis	
Trauma	
α-Agonists	
β-Antagonists	ACTH
Cortisol increase	
Opioids	

From Stoelting RK: Pharmacology and Physiology in Anesthetic Practice, *ed 3, Philadelphia, 1999, Lippincott, p 711.*

decreased from the atrophy of lymphoid tissue. As a result, the level of immunity to almost all foreign invaders of the body is reduced. Fulminating infection and death may ensue from disease that would otherwise not be lethal. The ability of cortisol and other glucocorticoids to suppress immunity makes exogenous administration of these hormones useful in preventing the immunologic rejection of transplanted organs, and in treating several autoimmune disorders.

Mineralocorticoids. *Mineralocorticoids* are required for life. They play a major role in the regulation of extracellular sodium and potassium ion concentrations and total body fluid balance. *Aldosterone* is the body's principle mineralocorticoid. It is secreted from the zona glomerulosa, the thin zone of cells on the surface of the adrenal cortex, directly below the capsule. This zone functions mostly autonomous of the other two adrenal cortex zones. Most distinctly, control of aldosterone secretion from the zona glomerulosa is relatively independent of ACTH control. Adults secrete 50 to 250 mcg of aldosterone per day.[89] With a total loss of mineralocorticoid secretion, death ensues within days without treatment.[88,89]

Following secretion from the adrenal cortex, aldosterone circulates 50% bound to serum proteins. The hormone reaches its target sites within 30 minutes. It is degraded mainly in the liver and excreted in the bile, feces, and urine. The normal blood concentration of aldosterone is 6 nanograms/dL.

The four main physiologic stimulants of aldosterone release are, in order of importance, as follows:[88]

1. Hyperkalemia
2. Angiotensin II (activation of the renin-angiotensin system)
3. Hyponatremia
4. ACTH

Our body's most significant protector of volume status is the renin-angiotensin system. Renin is a proteolytic enzyme released from the juxtaglomerular cells of the kidney afferent arteriole in response to hypovolemia, sympathetic stimulation, hypotension, or hyponatremia.[88] Renin acts on the plasma protein angiotensinogen to form angiotensin I (a 10–amino acid peptide), which is acted on by *angiotensi-converting enzyme* (primarily in the lung) to form angiotensin II (an 8–amino acid peptide). Angiotensin II is an extremely powerful vasoconstrictor and a potent stimulus of aldosterone.

Mineralocorticoids—Aldosterone Functions. Aldosterone's primary target cells are *principal cells,* located in the kidney distal convoluted tubules and collecting tubules. Here, aldosterone causes the reabsorption of Na^+ from the tubular fluid and in exchange, secretion of K^+ into the tubular fluid for excretion. In addition to facilitating K^+ secretion, aldosterone works on kidney *intercalated cells* to cause secretion of H^+ into tubular fluid in exchange for Na^+ reabsorption. Aldosterone's effect on the extracellular sodium ion *concentration* is limited because simultaneous with the Na^+ absorption is absorption of nearly equivalent amounts of water. The resulting extracellular fluid volume increase expands circulating blood volume and elevates arterial blood pressure.

Aldosterone's effect on sweat and salivary glands is similar to the effect on renal tubules. The effect on sweat glands is important in hot environments, where body salt conservation is needed.

Disorders Associated with the Adrenal Cortex

Primary Aldosteronism. J. W. Conn described the first case of primary mineralocorticoid excess in 1954, 1 year after the biochemical composition of aldosterone was identified.[90] *Conn's syndrome*, the most common form of *primary aldosteronism*, represents hypersecretion of aldosterone from an adrenal adenoma independent of stimulus. Primary aldosteronism may also be caused by adrenocortical hyperplasia or rarely carcinoma.[91,92] An increase in the plasma concentration of aldosterone and an increase in the urinary excretion of potassium with coexisting hypokalemia is pathognomonic of hyperaldosteronism.

Manifestations of the syndrome reflect the exaggerated effects of aldosterone. Hypertension and hypernatremia are usually present. Aldosterone's action of promoting renal excretion of potassium (or H^+) in exchange for Na^+ results in a hypokalemic metabolic alkalosis. Hypertension associated with Conn's syndrome results from aldosterone-induced sodium retention and subsequent increase in extracellular fluid volume. Primary aldosteronism accounts for approximately 1% of all cases of hypertension. The hypertension is often recalcitrant to standard medical treatment.[91,92]

Primary aldosteronism is associated with low renin levels, a result of the elevated blood pressure's negative feedback to the juxtaglomerular cells. *Secondary hyperaldosteronism* is associated with an increase in circulating renin levels.

Treatment. Treatment of Conn's syndrome may involve surgical removal of the adenoma or medical management. Surgical intervention is more successful for primary aldosteronism caused by adrenocortical adenoma than for gland hyperplasia because adenomas are almost always unilateral. When the affected adrenal gland is removed, the patient is cured in most cases. For patients with hyperplasia, both glands are usually involved and unilateral gland resection is much less likely to be curative than bilateral adrenalectomy. For patients with adrenal hyperplasia, medical management has been used successfully to treat primary aldosteronism.[93,94]

Management of Anesthesia. Preoperative management of the patient with Conn's syndrome includes correcting electrolyte and blood glucose levels and managing hypertension.[7,9,11,14] Potassium should be replaced slowly to allow for equilibration of intracellular and extracellular potassium stores. Hypokalemia may alter nondepolarizing muscle relaxant responses, making peripheral nerve stimulation monitoring especially valuable. Plasma electrolyte concentrations and acid-base status should be checked often during the perioperative period. Inadvertent hyperventilation may further decrease plasma potassium concentration.[95]

Hypertension should be controlled prior to elective surgery with sodium restriction and potassium-sparing diuretics.[7,91,92] Spironolactone, 25 to 100 mg every 8 hours, is a potassium-sparing diuretic that slowly increases potassium levels by inhibiting the action of aldosterone on the distal convoluted tubule. Measurement of cardiac filling pressures may be needed to assess fluid volume status.[9] Patients with Conn's syndrome have a higher incidence of ischemic heart disease and cardiovascular complications.[96,97,98] Adrenalectomy may be associated with damage to anatomically adjacent structures, such as the parietal pleura.

Laparoscopic adrenalectomy is currently advocated as the operation of choice for surgically remediable mineralocorticoid excess. Compared to open laparotomy, patients who undergo laparoscopic adrenalectomy have fewer postoperative complications and similar improvement in blood pressure control and correction of hypokalemia.[99,100]

Glucocorticoid Excess (Cushing's Syndrome). *Cushing's syndrome* is a diverse complex of symptoms, signs, and biochemical abnormalities caused by excess glucocorticoid hormone.[101] Clinical features reflect cortisol excess, either from overproduction of the adrenal cortex or exogenously administered glucocorticoid. The clinical picture includes central obesity, hypertension, glucose intolerance, plethoric facies, purple striae, muscle weakness, bruising, and osteoporosis.[88,101] Mineralocorticoid effects include fluid retention and hypokalemic alkalosis. Women manifest a degree of masculinization (hirsutism, hair thinning, acne, oligomenorrhea, amenorrhea), and men manifest a degree of feminization (gynecomastia, impotence) due to androgenic effects of glucocorticoid excess. The catabolic effects of cortisol results in skin that is thin and atrophic and unable to withstand the stresses of normal activity. Patients with Cushing's syndrome typically gain weight and develop a characteristic redistribution of fat in a yokelike pattern over the clavicles, neck, trunk, abdomen, and cheeks.[88,101]

The most common cause of Cushing's syndrome today is the therapeutic administration of supraphysiologic doses of glucocorticoids for conditions such as arthritis, asthma, various autoimmune disorders, allergies, and a myriad of other diseases.[9,95,101]

Endogenous Cushing's syndrome is most often the result of one of three distinct pathogenic disorders: pituitary tumor (Cushing's disease), adrenal tumor, or ectopic hormone production.

Cushing's disease specifically denotes an anterior pituitary tumor cause of the syndrome. The pituitary tumor produces excessive amounts of ACTH and is associated with bilateral adrenal hyperplasia. Patients often develop skin pigmentation as a result of excess ACTH. Cushing's disease is the most common cause of endogenous Cushing's syndrome.[88]

Adrenal Cushing's syndrome is caused by autonomous cortisol production (ACTH-independent) by an adrenal tumor. This form of hyperadrenalism accounts for 20% to 25% of patients with Cushing's syndrome and is associated with suppressed plasma ACTH levels.[88] The tumors are usually unilateral. Adrenal tumors that are malignant are usually large by the time Cushing's syndrome becomes manifest.[101,102,103]

Ectopic Cushing's Syndrome results from autonomous ACTH production by extrapituitary malignancies, producing markedly elevated plasma levels of ACTH. Bronchogenic carcinoma accounts for most of these cases. Malignant tumors of the kidney and pancreas also can cause ectopic production of ACTH.[101]

Diagnosis. The most widely used test for the diagnosis of hyperadrenocorticism is measurement of the plasma cortisol concentration in the morning after a dose of dexamethasone. Dexamethasone suppresses plasma cortisol secretion in normal patients, but not in those with hyperadrenocorticism. Diagnosis of Cushing's syndrome is also based on elevations of plasma and urinary cortisol levels, and urinary 17-hydroxycorticosteroids.[7,9,101]

Treatment. Treatment for Cushing's syndrome depends on the cause.[104,105] Transsphenoidal hypophysectomy is a primary treatment option for Cushing's disease. Complications occur in about 5% of patients and include diabetes insipidus (usually transient), cerebrospinal fluid rhinorrhea, and hemorrhage.[105]

Adrenal Cushing's syndrome may be treated by surgical removal of the adrenal adenoma. Because the contralateral adrenal gland is preoperatively suppressed, glucocorticoid replacement may be necessary for several months until adrenal function returns. Bilateral adrenalectomy in the patient with Cushing's syndrome is associated with a high incidence of postoperative complications. Permanent glucocorticoid and mineralocorticoid deficiency results.[101,104,106]

The treatment of choice for an ectopic ACTH-secreting tumor is surgical removal, but this may not always be feasible because of the nature of the underlying process (e.g., metastatic carcinoma). Metyrapone, an 11β-hydroxylase inhibitor, and ketoconazole, an agent that blocks steroidogenesis at several levels, may be used to help normalize cortisol levels.

Management of Anesthesia. Perioperative considerations for the patient with Cushing's syndrome include normalizing blood pressure, blood glucose levels, intravascular fluid volume, and electrolyte concentrations.[7,9,11,14] Spironolactone is an effective diuretic for decreasing extracellular fluid volume and correcting hypokalemia.

Osteoporosis is a consideration in positioning the patient for the operative procedure. Special consideration must be given to the patient's skin, which can easily be abraded by tape or minor trauma. Glucocorticoids are lympholytic and immunosuppressive, placing the patient at increased risk for infection and mandating particular enforcement of aseptic techniques where indicated.

The choice of drugs for induction and maintenance of anesthesia is not specifically influenced by the presence of hyperadrenocorticism.[7,9,11] Muscle relaxants may have a more exaggerated effect in patients with preexisting muscle weakness; a conservative approach to muscle relaxant dosing is warranted when significant skeletal muscle weakness is present.

If unilateral or bilateral adrenal resection is planned, glucocorticoids can be administered at doses equivalent to adrenal output for maximum stress (hydrocortisone, 100 mg, IV, every 8 hours). This dose can be reduced over 3 to 6 days postoperatively until a maintenance dose is reached.

Thromboembolic phenomena occur more frequently in patients with Cushing's syndrome, with an 11% incidence of deep venous thrombosis, and a 2% to 3% incidence of pulmonary embolus postoperatively. The thromboembolic events are believed to be secondary to the prevalence of obesity, hypertension, elevated hematocrit, and increased factor VIII levels.[107,108]

Primary Adrenocortical Insufficiency (Addison's Disease). In 1855, an English physician, Dr. Thomas Addison, first described a clinical syndrome characterized by wasting and hyperpigmentation and identified its cause as destruction of the adrenal glands. Clinical manifestations of *primary adrenocortical insufficiency* (*Addison's disease*) become apparent when 90% of the gland is destroyed. Tuberculosis is a common cause of primary adrenocortical insufficiency worldwide. In the United States, approximately 70% to 80% of the cases of primary adrenocortical insufficiency are autoimmune mediated.[101,109] Autoimmune destruction of the adrenal glands may also be associated with other autoimmune disorders, such as type 1 diabetes and Hashimoto's thyroiditis.[101] Less commonly, primary adrenal insufficiency is congenital or caused by adrenal hemorrhage, malignancy, trauma, or infection.[110,111]

Clinical symptoms of Addison's disease reflect glucocorticoid and mineralocorticoid deficiency.[95,101,109,110] Weakness and fatigue are common clinical features. Reduced appetite with weight loss, vomiting, abdominal pain, and diarrhea are frequently reported. Hypoglycemia is often present.[101,109,110]

Volume depletion is a common feature of the disease and may be manifested by orthostatic hypotension. Hyponatremia and hyperkalemia are commonly revealed by laboratory screening.[101]

The adrenal-pituitary axis is intact in primary adrenal insufficiency. ACTH concentrations are elevated as a result of the reduced production of cortisol. Increased melanin formation in the skin and hyperpigmentation of the knuckles of the fingers, toes, knees, elbows, lips, and buccal mucosa may be evident. Women with adrenal insufficiency may experience oligomenorrhea or amenorrhea.

Treatment. Normal adults secrete 15 to 25 mg of cortisol (hydrocortisone) and 50 to 250 mcg of aldosterone per day (Table 31-6). Therapeutic replacement dosages of glucocorticoids are typically 50% greater than basal adrenal output so that the patient is covered for mild stress. A typical oral replacement dose may consist of prednisone, 5 mg in the morning and 2.5 mg in the evening, or hydrocortisone, 20 mg in the morning and 10 mg in the evening. Mineralocorticoid replacement may consist of 0.05 to 0.2 mg/d of fludrocortisone.[7,9,101] Standard glucocorticoid doses are increased during periods of increased stress (Table 31-7).

Secondary Adrenocortical Insufficiency. Secondary adrenocortical insufficiency has two primary causes: (1) hypothalamic-pituitary-adrenal axis suppression after exogenous glucocorticoid therapy, and (2) ACTH deficiency secondary to hypothalamic or pituitary gland dysfunction (tumor, infection, surgical or radiological ablation). Adrenal cortex suppression

TABLE 31-6 Physiologic Effects of Endogenous Corticosteroids (mg)

Corticosteroid	Daily Secretion	Sodium Retention*	Glucocorticoid Effect*	Antiinflammatory Effect*
Aldosterone	0.125	3000	0.3	Insignificant
Desoxycorticosterone		100	0	0
Cortisol	20	1	1	1
Corticosterone	Minimal	15	0.35	0.3
Cortisone	Minimal	0.8	0.8	0.8

**Relative to cortisol.*
From Stoelting RK: Pharmacology and Physiology in Anesthetic Practice, *ed 3, Philadelphia, 1999, Lippincott, p 714.*

TABLE 31-7 Comparative Pharmacology of Endogenous and Synthetic Corticosteroids

	Antiinflammatory Potency	Sodium Retaining Potency	Equivalent Dose (mg)	Elimination Half-Time (h)	Duration of Action (h)	Route of Administration
Cortisol	1	1	20	1.5-3	8-12	Oral, IV, IM, IA
Cortisone	0.8	0.8	25	0.5	8-36	Oral, IM
Prednisolone	4	0.8	5	2-4	12-36	Oral, IV, IM, IA
Prednisone	4	0.8	5	3-4	18-36	Oral
Methylprednisolone	5	0.5	4	2-4	12-36	Oral, IV, IM, IA
Betamethasone	25	0	0.75	5	36-54	Oral, IV, IM, IA
Dexamethasone	25	0	0.75	3.5-5	36-54	Oral, IV, IM, IA
Triamcinolone	5	0	4	3.5	12-36	Oral, IM, IA
Fludrocortisone	10	125	–	–	24	Oral

IV, *intravenous;* IM, *intramuscular;* IA, *intraarticular.*
Adapted from Nicholson G, Burrin, J, and Hall G: Perioperative steroid supplementation, Anaesthesia 53:1091, 1998; *Stoelting RK:* Pharmacology and Physiology in Anesthetic Practice, *ed 3, Philadelphia, 1999, Lippincott, p 416.*

due to glucocorticoid therapy is the leading cause of secondary adrenal insufficiency.[111] The longer the duration of glucocorticoid administration, the greater the likelihood of suppression, but the precise dose or duration of therapy that produces adrenal suppression is unknown. Sustained and clinically important adrenal suppression usually does not occur with treatment periods less than 14 days. Treatment periods long enough to provoke signs of Cushing's syndrome are usually associated with adrenal suppression of clinical importance.[7,112]

Manifestations of secondary adrenal insufficiency are less likely than primary insufficiency to be associated with severe hypovolemia, hyperkalemia, or hyponatremia because mineralocorticoid secretion is usually preserved.[9,101] Hyperpigmentation is absent. Cortisol levels are low with the secondary form of the disorder and patients demonstrate symptoms associated with cortisol deficiency.

Acute Adrenal Crisis. Acute adrenal crisis is a sudden exacerbation or onset of severe adrenal insufficiency. It is a rare event associated with high morbidity and mortality if allowed to progress unrecognized.[113,114] A patient with progressive chronic adrenal insufficiency may deteriorate rapidly into an acute insufficiency state as a result of some superimposed stress, such as infection, acute illness, or sepsis. The stress of surgery or trauma in the patient with inadequate adrenal reserves can precipitate acute adrenal crisis in the perioperative period.[14,111,113,114]

Symptoms of adrenal crisis reflect acute deficiency of corticosteroids and include severe weakness, nausea, hypotension, fever, and decreasing mental status. In the surgical setting, hemodynamic instability or cardiovascular collapse may herald adrenal crisis. The index of suspicion for adrenal crisis should be particularly high if the patient has hyperpigmentation, hyponatremia, and/or hyperkalemia; a history of autoimmune disease (hypothyroidism, diabetes); or recent prior use of exogenous steroids.[110,111,113,114] Etomidate transiently inhibits cortisol production and should be avoided in patients at risk for adrenal insufficiency.

Acute adrenal crisis is a medical emergency requiring aggressive treatment of the steroid insufficiency and associated hypoglycemia, electrolyte imbalance, and volume depletion. Early recognition and intervention are crucial steps in altering the course of acute adrenal insufficiency. Initial therapy begins with rapid intravenous administration of a glucose-containing isotonic crystalloid solution.[113,114] If the patient is hemodynamically unstable, advanced hemodynamic monitoring and inotropic support may be necessary. Steroid replacement therapy should begin with hydrocortisone, 100 mg IV, followed by hydrocortisone, 100-200 mg IV over 24 hours. If the patient is stable, hydrocortisone is tapered during recovery. An individualized replacement dose of mineralocorticoids is also initiated when primary adrenal insufficiency is diagnosed.

Perioperative Steroid Replacement. Case reports of perioperative cardiovascular collapse in surgical patients on supraphysiologic doses of glucocorticoids were first reported in 1952.[115] These reports and subsequent knowledge regarding the stress-response associated with surgery and the suppression of the hypothalamic-pituitary-adrenal cortex axis with supraphysiologic doses of corticosteroids, has led to the practice of administering perioperative glucocorticoids to patients who have taken steroids in the preceding year.

Several reports have suggested that clinically important suppression of the hypothalamic-pituitary-adrenal axis is extremely uncommon and that levels of glucocorticoids required for surgical stress are much lower than previously believed.[9,115,116,117] Debate exists regarding who should receive perioperative steroid coverage and what the appropriate dose should be.

Patients who have received pharmacologic doses of glucocorticoids (greater than 5 mg prednisone-equivalent per day) for more than 2 weeks during the 12 months before surgery may have adrenal-pituitary axis suppression.[11,101] Under these circumstances, inadequate perioperative replacement of corticosteroids can lead to adrenal crisis and death.[113,114] The benefits of perioperative steroid supplementation are tempered by the potentially negative effects of decreased glucose tolerance, immune system inhibition, and impaired wound healing, but because acute adrenal crisis is life threatening, most clinicians believe that the potential risks of short-term glucocorticoid administration are outweighed by the benefits.[7,9,14]

The adrenal glands secrete 116 to 185 mg of cortisol per day in the perioperative period in response to stress.[95] In general, major surgery of long duration produces a greater adrenal response than minor surgery of short duration. For the adult patient who has received supraphysiologic doses of glucocorticoids (oral, topical, or inhaled) during the year preceding surgery, supplemental intravenous administration of hydrocortisone is advocated to compensate for the amount the body manufactures in response to maximal stress.[7,95,115-117] A common perioperative protocol for major surgical stress is the administration of hydrocortisone, 100 mg IV at induction, followed by 100 mg IV for at least 24 hours. A more recently proposed "low-dose" regimen calls for hydrocortisone, 25 mg IV at induction, followed by hydrocortisone, 100 mg IV infusion over the next 24 hours.[9] If the surgical patient is undergoing treatment with glucocorticoids at the time of surgery, supplemental doses are administered in addition to the patient's daily maintenance dose. Therapeutic aims are to tailor the steroid dose considering the length and severity of surgical stress, while administering the minimal dose that will fully protect the patient.[112-119]

Adrenal Medulla

The adrenal medulla is a catecholamine-producing endocrine gland that is derived embryologically from neuroectodermal cells. It is enervated by preganglionic fibers of the sympathetic nervous system and can be thought of as analogous to a postganglionic neuron. Preganglionic fibers bypass the paravertebral ganglia and run directly from the spinal cord to the adrenal medulla. Epinephrine accounts for approximately 80% of the hormone secreted by the adrenal medulla, and norepinephrine accounts for 20%. The majority of norepinephrine synthesized in the adrenal medulla is converted to epinephrine by the enzyme *phenylethanolamine-N-methyltransferase*. The ability of the adrenal medulla to synthesize epinephrine is probably influenced by the flow of glucocorticoid-rich blood from the cortex through the medulla. High concentrations of glucocorticoids stimulate the enzyme phenylethanolamine-*N*-methyltransferase (Fig. 31-14, A through C). Catecholamines in the adrenal medulla are stored in chromaffin granules.[88,120]

Stimulation of the sympathetic nerves to the adrenal medulla causes large quantities of epinephrine and norepinephrine to be released into the circulation, which carries them to all tissues in the body. The effects of circulating epinephrine and norepinephrine are similar to the effects of direct sympathetic stimulation but last 5 to 10 times longer because of the slow removal of these hormones from the blood.

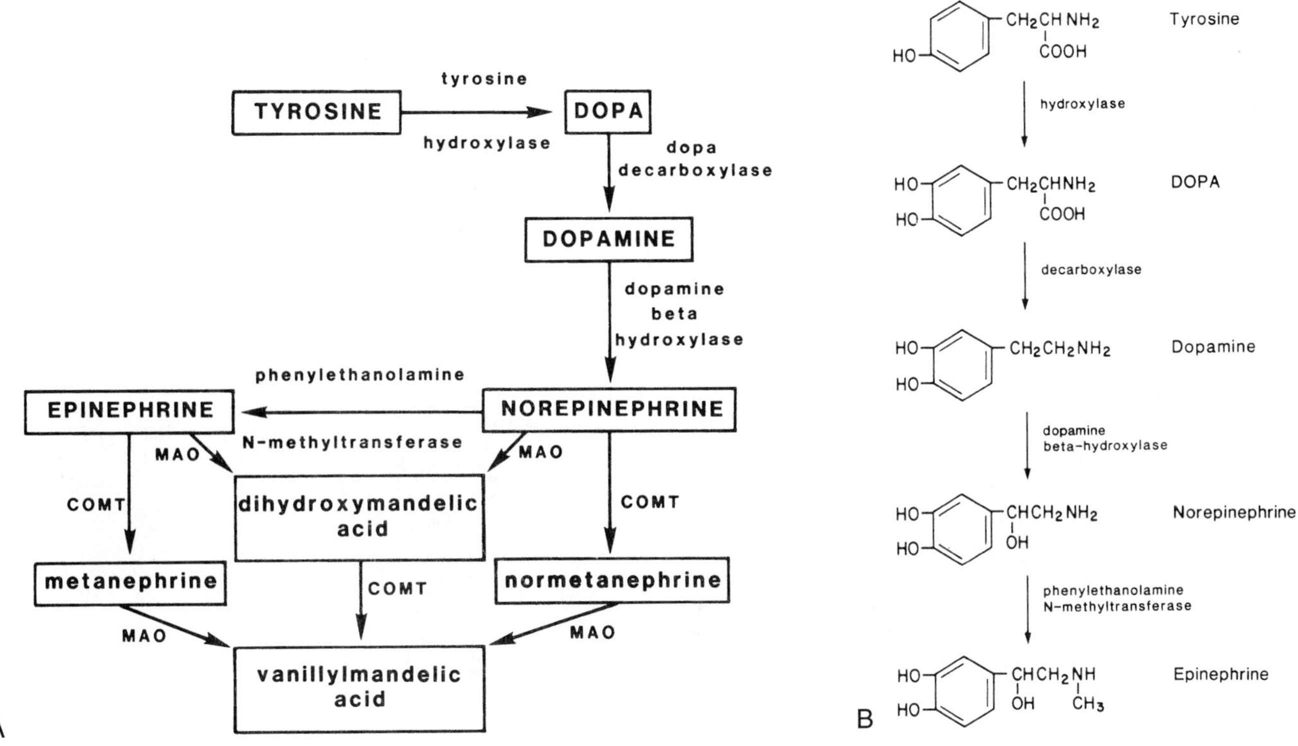

FIGURE **31-14**
A, The synthesis of endogenous catecholamines (dopamine, norepinephrine, and epinephrine) involves a series of enzyme-controlled steps, beginning with active transport of tyrosine from the circulation into postganglionic sympathetic nerve endings. The rate-limiting enzyme step is conversion of tyrosine to dopa by tyrosine hydroxylase. The inhibition of tyrosine hydroxylase by drugs or increased plasma concentrations of norepinephrine results in decreased synthesis or nonsynthesis of catecholamines. The metabolism of norepinephrine and epinephrine to normetanephrine, metanephrine, and vanillylmandelic acid is controlled by the enzymes monoamine oxidase (MAO) and catechol-O-methyltransferase (COMT). **B,** Steps in the enzymatic synthesis of endogenous catecholamines and neurotransmitters. **C,** Norepinephrine and epinephrine are initially deaminated by MAO or, alternatively, are first methylated by COMT. The resulting metabolites are then further metabolized by the other enzyme to form the principal end-metabolite, 3-methoxy-4-hydroxymandelic acid (vanillylmandelic acid, or VMA). (From Stoelting RK: *Pharmacology and Physiology in Anesthetic Practice*, ed 3, Philadelphia, 1999, Lippincott, p 623.)

Norepinephrine and epinephrine are metabolized in the liver and kidney by the enzyme *catechol-O-methyltransferase*. The by-products of metabolism, vanillylmandelic acid (VMA) and metanephrines, and free unchanged catecholamine are excreted in the urine.[7,120]

Norepinephrine stimulates α- and β-adrenergic receptors. It causes constriction of essentially all blood vessels of the body, increasing total peripheral resistance. High circulating norepinephrine levels increase the heart's activity, inhibit gastrointestinal function, and dilate the pupils. Epinephrine has a greater affinity for β-receptors. Its actions are seen primarily in the heart, producing chronotropic and inotropic effects. Epinephrine causes less constriction of blood vessels than does norepinephrine. Norepinephrine and epinephrine release from the adrenal medulla can increase the metabolic rate of the body by as much as 100% above normal.

Pheochromocytoma. In 1905, the term *pheochromocytoma* was first used to describe the appearance of a tumor that was noted during autopsy resection to be a dusky (*pheo*) color (*chromo*). Cesar Roux of Lausanne, Switzerland, and Charles Mayo in the United States were the first surgeons to successfully remove a pheochromocytoma (Fig. 31-15).

Pheochromocytomas are catecholamine-secreting tumors derived most commonly (90%) from adrenomedullary chromaffin cells or less commonly from extraadrenal chromaffin cells (Fig. 31-16). Pheochromocytomas involve both adrenal glands in 10% of adult patients with the tumor. Extraadrenal pheochromocytomas have been found anywhere from the pelvis to the skull base[121] (Table 31-8, 31-9) Malignant spread of pheochromocytomas occurs in approximately 10% of cases. These pheochromocytomas are more often extraadrenal and often secrete dopamine. Malignant pheochromocytomas usually proceed via venous and lymphatic channels to the liver.

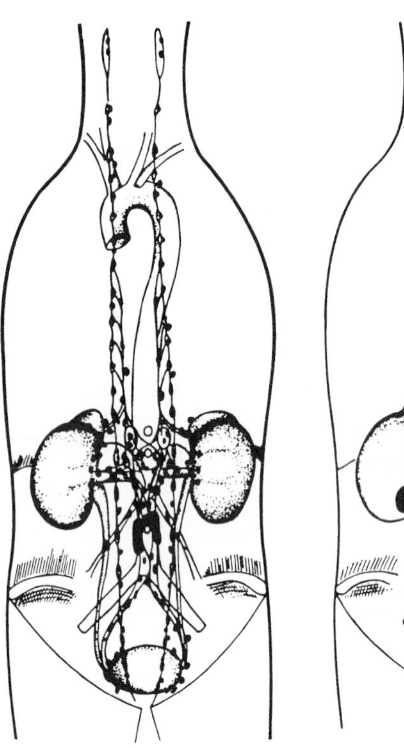

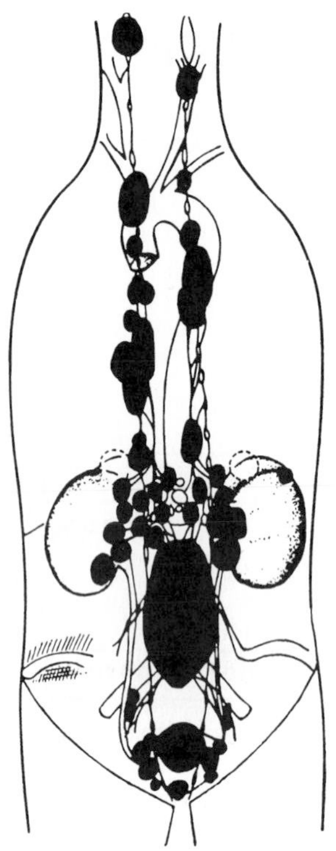

FIGURE **31-16**
Distribution of chromaffin tissue in the newborn compared with the distribution of extraadrenal pheochromocytomas. Extraadrenal pheochromocytomas (*right*) occur in sites containing chromaffin tissue in the newborn (*left*). (Modified from Coupland RE: *The natural history of the chromaffin cell*, London, 1965, Longmans, Green, p 192.)

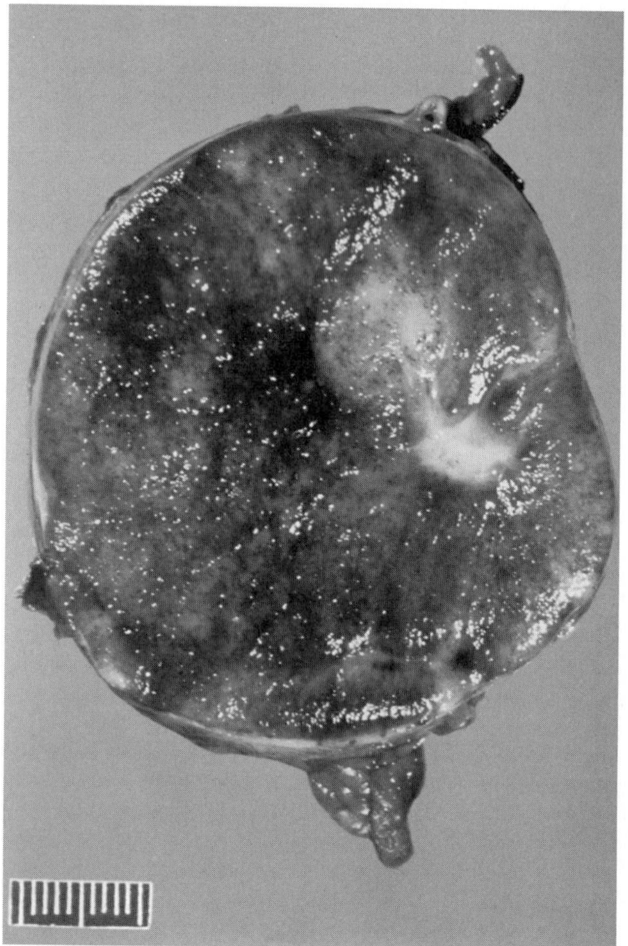

FIGURE **31-15**
Pheochromocytoma of the adrenal gland. (Courtesy of Dr. Terri L. Johnson, Department of Pathology, Henry Ford Hospital, Detroit, Michigan.)

TABLE **31-8** Location of Pheochromocytomas

Location	PERCENTAGE		
	Total*	Familial	Children
Solitary adrenal	80	<50	50
Extraadrenal	10	<10	25
Bilateral adrenal	10	>50	25

**95% of cases are sporadic and 5% familial; 10%-12% of all cases are in children.*
From Landsberg L, Young JB: Catecholamines and the adrenal medulla. In Wilson JD, Foster DW, editors: Williams Textbook of Endocrinology, *ed 9, Philadelphia, 1998, Saunders, p 707.*

TABLE **31-9** Location of Extraadrenal Pheochromocytomas*

Location	%
Cervical	2
Thoracic	10-20
Intraabdominal	70-80
Upper abdomen	40
Organ of Zuckerkandl	30
Bladder	15

**About 10% of all pheochromocytomas are extraadrenal.*
From Landsberg L, Young JB: Catecholamines and the adrenal medulla. In Wilson JD, Foster DW, editors: Williams Textbook of Endocrinology, *ed 9, Philadelphia, 1998, Saunders, p 707.*

TABLE 31-10 Values for Catecholamines and Catecholamine Metabolites

Hormone/Metabolite	Normal Value
Vanillylmandelic acid, urine	2.0-7.0 mg/24 hr
Metanephrines, urine	<1.3 mg/24 hr
Norepinephrine, urine	<100 mcg/24 hr
Norepinephrine, plasma	150-450 pg/mL
Epinephrine, plasma	<35 pg/mL
Catecholamines, free urinary	<110 mcg/24 hr

From Noble J, editor: Textbook of Primary Care Medicine, *ed 3, St Louis, 2001, Mosby.*

Diagnostic tests for determining the presence of a catecholamine tumor include measurements of urinary or plasma catecholamines or their metabolites, VMA, and metanephrines. Free norepinephrine measurement in a 24-hour urine sample is a sensitive index of pheochromocytoma (Table 31-10).

Incidence and Associated Diseases. Pheochromocytomas are rare, occurring in less than 0.5% of all hypertensive patients.[122,123] These tumors may be associated with neurocutaneous syndromes such as von Hippel-Lindau disease, tuberous sclerosis, Sturge-Weber syndrome, and as a component of multiple endocrine neoplasia (MEN) type 2A or 2B[124,125] (Table 31-11). Patients with a family history of MEN syndrome should be regularly screened for pheochromocytoma. Five to 10 percent of pheochromocytomas occur as part of an inherited autosomal dominant trait.[122] Five percent of patients with pheochromocytomas have neurofibromatosis, but only 1% of patients with neurofibromatosis have pheochromocytomas.

Pheochromocytomas can occur at any age, but usually occur within the third to the fifth decade of life. They occur with equal frequency in both sexes in adults.[7,9]

Pheochromocytomas produce, store, and secrete catecholamines, mostly norepinephrine and epinephrine. Unlike in a normal adrenal medulla, norepinephrine is the predominant catecholamine secreted by most of these tumors. In the majority of cases, however, it is impossible to predict the pattern of catecholamine secretion from the clinical features.

TABLE 31-11 Manifestations of Multiple Endocrine Neoplasia

Syndrome	Manifestations
MEN type 1 (Wermer's syndrome)	Hyperparathyroidism, pituitary adenomas, pancreatic islet cell tumors
MEN type 2A (Sipple's syndrome)	Medullary thyroid cancer, parathyroid adenoma, pheochromocytoma
MEN type 2B (mucosal neuroma syndrome)	Medullary thyroid tumor, pheochromocytoma, neuromas of the oral mucosa, marfanoid habitus

Multiple endocrine neoplasia (MEN) is a group of rare diseases caused by genetic defects that lead to hyperplasia and hyperfunction of two or more components of the endocrine system.
Adapted from Stoelting RK, Dierdorf SF: Endocrine disease. In Anesthesia and Co-existing Disease, *ed 4, New York, 2002, Churchill Livingstone, p 430.*

Clinical Manifestations. Manifestations of a pheochromocytoma reflect massive and sustained catecholamine release and include hypertension, diaphoresis, headache, tremulousness, palpitations, and weight loss. Symptoms may be paroxysmal or sustained. The combination of diaphoresis, tachycardia, and headache in the hypertensive patient is a frequently recognized and highly specific triad.[7,9,14,123]

A catecholamine-mediated paroxysm typically consists of a sudden and alarming increase in blood pressure, a severe throbbing headache, profuse sweating, palpitations with or without tachycardia, a sense of doom, anxiety, pallor (rarely flushing), nausea, abdominal pain, and orthostatic hypotension. Orthostatic hypotension is a result of plasma volume deficit.[7,9] Additionally, the postural reflexes that defend upright blood pressure may lose their tone with sustained excesses of catecholamines. Paroxysmal symptoms may last several minutes to days and are often followed by exhaustion. The frequencies of clinical symptoms associated with pheochromocytoma are outlined in Table 31-12.

TABLE 31-12 Frequency of Symptoms in 100 Patients with Pheochromocytoma

Symptom	%	Symptom	%	Symptom	%
Headache	80	Chest pain	19	Tinnitus	3
Excessive perspiration	71	Dyspnea	19	Dysarthria	3
Palpitation (with or without tachycardia)	64	Flushing or warmth	18	Gagging	3
Pallor	42	Numbness or paresthesia	11	Bradycardia	3
Nausea (with or without vomiting)	42	Blurring of vision	11	Back pain	3
Tremor or trembling	31	Tightness of throat	8	Coughing	1
Weakness or exhaustion	28	Dizziness or faintness	8	Yawning	1
Nervousness or anxiety	22	Convulsions	5	Syncope	1
Epigastric pain	22	Neck-shoulder pain	5	Unsteadiness	1
		Extremity pain	4	Hunger	1
		Flank pain	4		

From Landsberg L, Young JB: Catecholamines and the adrenal medulla. In Wilson JD, Foster DW, editors: Williams Textbook of Endocrinology, *ed 8, Philadelphia, 1998, Saunders, p 706.*

A paroxysm may be triggered by acute physical stress, abdominal palpation, defecation, hypotension, activation of the sympathetic nervous system, or micturition if pheochromocytoma is present in urinary bladder wall. In other patients, no clearly defined precipitating factor can be found. Mental or psychological stress does not usually initiate a crisis.

The symptoms associated with a pheochromocytoma reflect the usual predominance of α-adrenergic activity over β-adrenergic effects.[9] As a result of α-adrenergic inhibition of insulin, mild hyperglycemia may be present. The cardiac output and heart rate may be significantly increased. An overall increase in metabolism increases oxygen consumption and can cause hyperthermia. Vasoconstriction in the extremities may produce pain, paresthesias, intermittent claudication, or ischemia.

Hypertension is the most common symptom, occurring in over 90% of patients.[7,9] Paroxysmal hypertension is present in 40% to 50% of patients and is a distinctive manifestation of the disease.[7] Sustained hypertension is often resistant to conventional treatment. When pheochromocytomas are predominantly epinephrine secreting, hypertension can alternate with periods of hypotension associated with syncope. This may be due to the surges of epinephrine causing disproportionate β-adrenergic stimulation with vasodilation in the presence of a contracted vascular space.

A catecholamine-induced increase in myocardial oxygen consumption, hypertension, and possibly coronary artery spasm can precipitate myocardial infarction or congestive heart failure even in the absence of coronary artery disease.[9] ECG changes are common. Nonspecific ST-segment and T-wave changes and prominent U waves may be seen.[9] Sinus tachycardia, sinus bradycardia, supraventricular tachycardias, and premature ventricular contractions have been noted. Right and left bundle branch blocks and ventricular strain sometimes occur. Ventricular tachycardia has been reported. The ECG is abnormal in as many as 75% of patients with pheochromocytoma.[126,127,128]

Preoperative Management. The pharmacological effects of released catecholamines present major anesthetic challenges. Medical management, prior to tumor excision, aims to reverse the effects of excessive adrenergic stimulation. Preoperative antihypertensive therapy and volume replacement has helped to decrease the surgical mortality rate from 40%-60% to 1%-3%.[11] The preoperative use of α-adrenergic antagonists or calcium channel blockers and reexpansion of the intravascular fluid compartment greatly improve cardiovascular stability intraoperatively.[95,129,130] Myocardial infarction, congestive heart failure, cardiac dysrhythmias, and cerebral hemorrhage decrease in frequency when the patient has been treated preoperatively with α-adrenergic antagonists. Table 31-13 outlines drugs used in the management of pheochromocytoma.

α-Adrenergic Blockade. Phenoxybenzamine (Dibenzyline) is the drug of choice for preoperative α-adrenergic blockade and blood pressure stabilization.[11] It is a noncompetitive presynaptic (α-2) and postsynaptic (α-1) adrenergic receptor antagonist of long duration (24-48 hrs).[7] Most patients with pheochromocytoma require an oral dose of 60-250 mg/day.[14] Postural hypotension is a common side effect of this drug.

Typically, patients require 10 to 14 days of α-adrenergic antagonist therapy to stabilize blood pressure and decrease symptoms. Since pheochromocytomas spread slowly, little is lost by waiting until preoperative conditions are optimized by medical treatment.[7,9,14] Establishment of normotension facilitates reexpansion of the intravascular fluid volume. Satisfactory α-adrenergic blockade is implied if the hematocrit decreases by 5% during treatment.[9] One half to two thirds of the normal oral phenoxybenzamine dose may be given the morning of surgery.[14]

Prazocin (Minipress), a specific postsynaptic α-1 adrenergic antagonist, has also been used successfully to treat the hypertension of pheochromocytoma preoperatively. Labetalol (Trandate, Normodyne), a mixed α– and β– antagonist, has not been as effective as a first-line drug in controlling the blood pressure response, but it may be used as an adjunctive agent.[7,9,131]

β-Adrenergic Blockade. A β-adrenergic receptor antagonist is usually introduced in the preoperative period for control of tachycardia, hypertension, and catecholamine-induced supraventricular dysrhythmias. An important caveat is that β-adrenergic receptor antagonists should not be administered until after α-adrenergic blockade is established. Blocking β-receptor–mediated vasodilation in skeletal muscle without prior α-adrenergic blockade can increase the blood pressure even further in the patient with pheochromocytoma. In addition, β-adrenergic blockade prior to α-adrenergic blockade may depress the heart to the point that cardiac output suffers should unopposed α-mediated vasoconstriction occur from an abrupt catecholamine release.[7,9,14]

Other Treatment Regimens. Calcium channel blockers have been used with variable success as monotherapy for the perioperative management of pheochromocytoma.[11,132] Recommendations are that they be used in conjunction with adrenergic blocking drugs.[11]

α-Methyl tyrosine (Demser) is utilized for patients requiring long-term therapy—for instance, the patient for whom surgery is contraindicated.[130,133] The drug competitively inhibits catecholamine formation by blocking tyrosine hydroxylation, the rate-limiting step in catecholamine synthesis.

The following criteria may be used as end points for the patient awaiting surgery for pheochromocytoma resection:[95]

1. No in-hospital blood pressure reading higher than 165/90 mm Hg evident 48 hours prior to surgery.
2. Blood pressure on standing should not be lower than 80/45 mm Hg.
3. The ECG should have no ST-segment or T-wave abnormality prior to surgery that cannot be attributed to a permanent defect.
4. The patient should have no marked symptoms of catecholamine excess; no more than one premature ventricular contraction every 5 minutes.

Anesthetic Management. Effective anesthetic management is based on selecting drugs that do not stimulate catecholamine release, avoiding sympathetic nervous system activation, and implementing monitoring techniques that facilitate early and appropriate intervention when catecholamine-induced changes in the cardiovascular function occur.[7,95]

Most pheochromocytomas are excised by open laparotomy, but successful laparoscopic removal of pheochromocytoma has also been performed.[134-137] It is generally recommended that laparoscopic removal be reserved for small, solitary, and hormonally latent tumors.[136,137] During pneumoperitoneum, significant catecholamine release has been reported.[135]

A number of drugs and conditions can precipitate hypertension in the surgical patient with pheochromocytoma. Dopamine antagonists (metoclopramide, droperidol), radiographic contrast media, indirect acting amines (ephedrine), drugs that block neuronal catecholamine reuptake (tricyclic antidepressants, cocaine), histamine, glucagon, and pancuronium can trigger

TABLE 31-13 Drugs Used in the Management of Pheochromocytoma

Drug	Action	Pressor Crisis	Preoperative Blood Pressure Control	Comment
Phentolamine	α Blocker	iv 2-5 mg	—	Rapid onset, short-acting; give bolus every 5 min or infuse initially 1 mg·min^{-1}
Phenoxybenzamine	α Blocker	—	Oral 30 mg·day^{-1}, increasing daily dosage by 30 mg	Long half-life; may accumulate; give twice or three times daily
Prazosin	α Blocker	—	Oral 1.0 mg single dose, increasing to tid regimen	First-dose phenomenon; may cause syncope, so start with low dose before bedtime
Propanolol	β Blocker	iv 1.0 mg bolus to total of 10 mg	Oral 40 mg bid; increase to 480 mg·day^{-1}	Should never be given without first creating α blockade
Atenolol	β Blocker	—	Oral 50 mg·day^{-1} initially; may increase to 100 mg·day^{-1}	Long-acting, selective β_1 antagonist eliminated unchanged by kidney
Esmolol	β Blocker	iv 500 mcg·kg^{-1}·min^{-1} loading followed by maintenance infusion	—	Ultrashort-acting selective β_1 antagonist; may be used during anesthesia
Labetalol	α and β Blocker	iv 10 mg bolus to 150 mg	Oral 200 mg tid	A much weaker α blocker than β blocker; may cause pressor response in pheochromocytoma
Nitroprusside	Vasodilator	iv infusion initially 0.5-1.5 mcg·kg^{-1}·min^{-1}	—	Powerful vasodilator; short-acting; may be used during anesthesia
Magnesium sulfate	Vasodilator	iv 40-60 mg·kg^{-1} bolus followed by 2 g·h^{-1} and additional 20 mg·kg^{-1} boluses as needed	—	May potentiate neuromuscular blockade
Diltiazem	Calcium channel blocker	iv 3-10 mcg·kg^{-1}·min^{-1}	—	May also directly block release of catecholamines
Nicardipine	Calcium channel blocker	iv 2-6 mcg·kg^{-1}·min^{-1}	—	Better vasodilator than diltiazem
α-Methyl-tyrosine	Inhibitor of biosynthesis of cathecholamines	—	Oral 1-4 g·day^{-1}	Suitable for patients not amenable to surgery; may be nephrotoxic

iv = intravenous.
Adapted from Schwartz JJ, Rosenbaum S, Graf GJ: Anesthesia and the endocrine system. In Barash PG, Cullen BF, Stoelting RK, editors: Clinical Anesthesthia, *ed 4, Philadelphia, JB Lippincott, 2001, p 1132.*

catecholamine release from the tumor.[9,95,138,139] Hypoxia and hypercapnia can elicit a catecholamine response by stimulating the sympathetic nervous system.

Preoperative sedation is advised to decrease anxiety and prevent activation of the sympathetic nervous system. Benzodiazepines are especially useful.[9] Preoperative atropine should be avoided because of its potential for inducing tachydysrhythmias.

Large-bore intravenous lines and a peripheral arterial catheter should be established preoperatively. A central venous pressure or pulmonary artery catheter should be placed to help guide fluid management and intervention with inotropes or vasodilating drugs.[7,9] Arterial blood gases, electrolytes concentrations, and blood glucose levels should be assessed regularly during the anesthetic.

Critical intraoperative junctures are as follows: (1) during induction and intubation of the trachea, (2) during surgical manipulation of the tumor, and (3) after ligation of the tumor's venous drainage.

Induction can be accomplished with barbiturates, benzodiazepines, or propofol. Anesthetic depth can be enhanced by mask ventilation of the lungs with a volatile anesthetic and nitrous oxide prior to laryngoscopy and intubation of the trachea. Lidocaine (1-2 mg/kg, IV) administered 1 minute prior to intubation may attenuate the hemodynamic response to laryngoscopy. Rapid-acting vasodilating drugs such as nitroprusside and phentolamine should be readily available to treat persistent hypertension.[9] Short-acting opioids, such as fentanyl or sufentanil, administered prior to intubation may help attenuate blood pressure responses to intubation.[9] Morphine sulfate should be avoided due to its propensity for histamine release.

Selection of a volatile anesthetic should be based on its ability to decrease sympathetic nervous system activity and a low likelihood of sensitizing the myocardium to the dysrhythmic effects of catecholamines. Halothane is not recommended because of the potential for causing ventricular irritability in the presence of an increased catecholamine concentration. Sevoflurane and isoflurane provide cardiovascular stability and possess the ability to rapidly change anesthetic depth, attractive features in the anesthetic management of the patient with pheochromocytoma.[7,9,14] The tachycardia associated with desflurane makes it an undesirable choice for these cases.

The use of succinylcholine has been questioned, since compression of an abdominal tumor by drug-induced skeletal muscle fasciculations may provoke catecholamine release. However, a predictable adverse effect of succinylcholine has not been supported clinically when administered to patients with pheochromocytoma. Skeletal muscle paralysis with a nondepolarizing muscle relaxant devoid of vagolytic or histamine-releasing effects is desirable. Pancuronium should be avoided due to its known chronotropic effect.[7,9,14]

Particular efforts should be made to keep the rate of fluid replacement equal to the rate of loss. Hypotension generally responds to volume replacement. Adequate preparation should be in place for the hypertension and cardiac dysrhythmias that occur, especially during tumor manipulation. Hypertension can be treated with intravenous nitroprusside or phentolamine and high concentrations of inhaled anesthetic.[7,9,14,140] Propranolol, lidocaine, labetalol, or esmolol may be given intravenously to decrease tachydysrhythmias. β-Adrenergic antagonists must be used cautiously in patients with catecholamine-induced cardiomyopathy because even minimal β-adrenergic blockade can accentuate left ventricular dysfunction.[7,9] The short half-life of esmolol makes it an advantageous choice for β-adrenergic blockade. Dysrhythmias associated with hypertension may be resolved by simply lowering an abnormally high blood pressure. Norepinephrine or phenylephrine administration is usually satisfactory when a vasopressor is needed. Indirect-acting sympathomimetics have an unpredictable pressor effect in these patients and should be avoided.

Magnesium sulfate ($MgSO_4$) appears to be a useful addition to the armamentarium available for anesthetic management of patients with pheochromocytoma. Rationale for its use is based on its ability to inhibit catecholamine release from both the adrenal medulla and peripheral adrenergic nerve terminals, decrease the sensitivity of α-adrenergic receptors to catecholamines, and exert a direct vasodilator effect.[141]

After surgical ligation of the veins that drain a pheochromocytoma, the rapid decrease in circulating catecholamines and the associated downregulation of adrenergic receptors may precipitate a decrease in blood pressure. During this juncture, close communication with the surgical team is important. Decreasing the inhaled anesthetic agent concentration and increasing the administration of intravenous crystalloid or colloid solution should adequately increase blood pressure. Intravenous administration of phenylephrine or norepinephrine may be needed until the peripheral vasculature can adapt to the decreased level of endogenous α-stimulation.[9]

Hyperglycemia is common before excision of the pheochromocytoma. With tumor removal, the sudden withdraw of catecholamine stimulation can result in hypoglycemia.[142] Further, β-adrenergic blockade impairs both hepatic glucose production and the glucagon secretion mechanism. β-Adrenergic blockers may also mask hypoglycemic signs by preventing tachycardia and tremor. Blood glucose levels should be monitored at frequent intervals intraoperatively and postoperatively.

Regional anesthesia has been used successfully for the excision of pheochromocytomas. A specific disadvantage of this technique, for this procedure, is the blockade of sympathetic nervous system activity if hypotension accompanies vascular isolation of the pheochromocytoma. Additionally, spontaneous alveolar ventilation may be impaired during intra-abdominal manipulation and retraction.

Some pheochromocytomas may first present as a hypermetabolic state during anesthesia for unrelated surgery. The hypertension, tachycardia, hyperthermia, and respiratory acidosis of a pheochromocytoma may mimic light anesthesia, thyroid crisis, malignant hyperthermia, or sepsis.[143]

Postoperative Management. Fluid shifts, pain, hypoxia, hypercapnia, autonomic instability, urinary retention, or residual tumor are all potential causes of postoperative hypertension. Invasive monitoring is indicated during the initial postoperative period to keenly assess blood pressure changes and cardiac status.[7,9,95] Fifty percent of patients remain hypertensive during the postanesthesia recovery period despite removal of the pheochromocytoma.[9] Transient hypertension postoperatively usually reflects fluid shifts and autonomic instability. Postoperative catecholamine levels decrease to normal over several days. Normal blood pressure returns within about 10 days after surgery in 75% of patients.

Relief of postoperative pain can be accomplished with neuraxial opioids and may contribute to early tracheal extubation in otherwise healthy patients.

Thyroid Gland

The thyroid gland is an endocrine gland consisting of two lobes connected by an isthmus. It produces and secretes two important thyroid hormones: triiodothyronine (T3) and thyroxine (T4). The vascular supply to the gland is derived from the superior and inferior thyroid arteries. The blood flow is equivalent to about fivefold the weight of the gland, which is a blood supply as rich as almost any tissue in the body.

Microscopically, the thyroid is divided into lobules, each of which is composed of 20 to 40 follicles. The follicles are lined by epithelial cells that surround central deposits of the secretory substance *colloid.* The major constituent of the colloid is a large glycoprotein called *thyroglobulin,* which serves as the backbone for the synthesis and storage of thyroid hormones.[144,145]

Synthesis of Thyroid Hormones

Iodide Trapping. Approximately 1 mg of ingested iodine is required each week to form normal quantities of thyroid hormones. Dietary iodine is reduced in the gastrointestinal tract to *iodide.* Common table salt is iodized with one part sodium iodide for every 100,000 parts sodium chloride for the prevention of iodine deficiency.

The first stage of thyroid hormone formation is the transport of iodides from the extracellular fluid into the thyroid cells and follicles. About one fifth of the circulating iodide is removed from the blood by the thyroid cells and used for the synthesis of thyroid hormones. This process is dependent on the ability of the basal membrane of the thyroid gland cell to pump iodide actively to the interior of the cell, a process called *iodide trapping.* The iodide pump normally concentrates the iodide to about 30 times its concentration in the blood. Iodide trapping is the rate-limiting step in thyroid hormone synthesis and is under the control of TSH from the anterior pituitary. Once inside the thyroid gland, iodide ions are oxidized back to iodine.

Thyroid Hormone Formation. Thyroid hormones are formed in the follicles of the thyroid gland under the control of TSH. Thyroglobulin contains the amino acid tyrosine. Tyrosine combines with iodine to form various iodotyrosines, including the two major thyroid hormones. The binding of iodine to the tyrosine moieties of the thyroglobulin molecule is called *organification of thyroglobulin*. One iodine atom joined to tyrosine forms *monoiodotyrosine*; two iodine atoms joined to tyrosine forms *diiodotyrosine*.

Thyroid hormone synthesis progresses when two diiodotyrosine residues couple with each other to produce the molecule *thyroxine* (T_4). One molecule of monoiodotyrosine coupled with one molecule of diiodotyrosine forms *triiodothyronine* (T_3). The two newly formed hormones, thyroxine and triiodothyronine, remain part of the thyroglobulin molecule, stored as colloid within the thyroid follicle until release. Enough hormone is synthesized and stored under basal conditions to supply the body with its normal hormone requirements for 2 to 3 months.[144,145]

About three quarters of the iodinated tyrosine in the thyroglobulin is not converted to thyroid hormones but remains monoiodotyrosine or diiodotyrosine. Iodine from uncoupled monoiodotyrosine or diiodotyrosine is recycled within the gland for formation of additional thyroid hormones. An inactive stereoisomer of T_3 called *reverse* T_3 is formed at about the same rate as T_3.[144,145] Although iodine is required for hormone synthesis, excess iodine can inhibit gland production of thyroid hormone.

Release of Thyroxine and Triiodothyronine. During release from the thyroid gland, T_4 and T_3 are cleaved from the thyroglobulin molecule and secreted into the circulating blood. Thyroglobulin remains within the colloid. TSH controls release of hormones from the gland.

Under normal conditions, about 90% of the hormone released from the thyroid gland is T_4 and 10% T_3. The secretion of T_4 from the thyroid gland is 80 to 100 mcg/day and the circulating half-life is 6 to 7 days. When thyroid hormones reach their target tissues, most of the T_4 is deiodinated to T_3, T_4 serving mostly as a hormone precursor. Triiodothyronine is more potent and less protein bound than T_4 and it is the primary metabolically active hormone that stimulates target tissues. The circulating half-life of T_3 is 24 to 30 hours.[11,32] Figures 31-17 and 31-18 summarize the biosynthesis and chemical structure of thyroid hormones.

Transport of Thyroxine and Triiodothyronine to Tissues. Thyroid hormone exists in circulation in both free and bound forms. The amount of free hormone, which is the metabolically active fraction, is extremely small, less than 0.03% of total circulating T_4 and 0.3% of total circulating T_3. The majority of circulating hormone (99%) is bound to thyroid-binding proteins. Eighty percent of thyroid hormones bind to the circulating protein *thyroxine-binding globulin*, 10% to 15% to *thyroxine-binding prealbumin*, and the remainder to *albumin*. Thyroxine-binding globulin has a higher affinity for T_4 than for T_3.

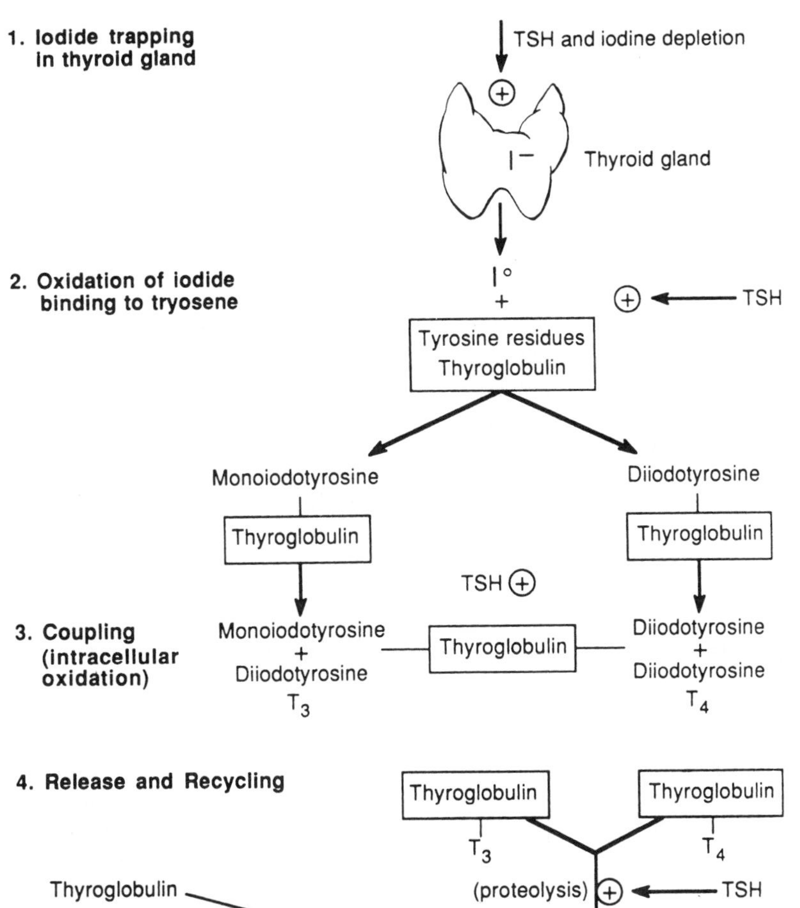

FIGURE **31-17**
Thyroid hormone biosynthesis consists of four stages: (1) iodide trapping, (2) oxidation, (3) coupling, and (4) release and recycling. *TSH*, thyroid-stimulating hormone. (From Schwartz JJ, Graf G, Rosenbaum S: Anesthesia and the endocrine system. In Barash PG, Cullen BF, Stoelting RK, editors: *Clinical Anesthesia*, ed 4, Philadelphia, 2001, Lippincott Williams & Wilkins, p 1120.)

FIGURE **31-18**
Thyroid gland hormones. (From Stoelting RK: *Pharmacology and Physiology in Anesthetic Practice*, ed 3, Philadelphia, 1999, Lippincott, 1999, p 410.)

Triiodothyronine (T_3)

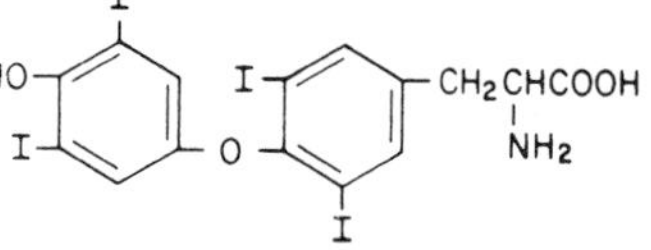

Thyroxine (tetraiodothyronine, T_4)

Various clinical situations can result in altered thyroxine-binding globulin levels. Estrogens, pregnancy, oral contraceptives, hepatitis, and porphyria can increase thyroxine-binding globulin levels, which can lead to a decline in circulating free T_4 concentration.[32] Androgens, cirrhosis, nephrosis, and genetic influences can decrease the level of thyroxine-binding globulin.

Because of the very high affinity of the plasma-binding proteins for thyroid hormones, the hormones are released to the tissue cells very slowly. The half-life of T_4 in the circulation is 6 to 7 days, and the half-life of T_3 is 24 to 30 hours.[10,12,144,145]

Functions of Thyroid Hormones

Increased Cellular Metabolic Activity. Thyroid hormones initiate widespread transcription and translation of large numbers of genes in virtually all cells of the body. Consequently, the level of enzymes, structural proteins, transport proteins, and other substances increases considerably under the direction of T_4 and especially T_3. The net result is a generalized increase in the metabolic activity, heat production, and oxygen consumption of all or almost all tissues in the body.[146] The basal metabolic rate can increase by as much as 60% to 100% above normal when large quantities of thyroid hormones are secreted. The utilization of energy substrates is greatly accelerated. Protein synthesis is increased; however, protein catabolism also is increased.

Effect of Thyroid Hormone on Growth. Thyroid hormone is necessary for normal growth in infants and children. In a hypothyroid state the rate of tissue growth is greatly reduced. Thyroid hormone is required for normal growth and development of the brain during fetal life and for the first few years of postnatal life.[144,145]

Effect of Thyroid Hormone on Specific Systems. Thyroid hormone probably has a direct effect on the excitability of the heart. The heart rate and the force of contraction are augmented with increasing thyroid hormone production. Thyroid hormones increase the number of β-adrenergic receptors.[147] The rate and depth of respiration increase due to the enhanced metabolic rate and increased oxygen utilization and carbon dioxide formation by cells. Thyroid hormones enhance the secretion of digestive juices and the motility of the gastrointestinal tract, in addition to increasing an individual's appetite and food intake. When the quantity of thyroid hormone is slightly increased, the muscles react with vigor; however, when the quantity is excessive, muscles become weakened from excess protein catabolism. Thyroid hormones enhance the rapidity of cerebration.

Thyroid hormones increase the rate of hormone secretion from most endocrine glands, especially the pancreas. The heightened cellular requirement for glucose mandates higher insulin secretion.

Regulation of Thyroid Hormone Secretion. Specific feedback mechanisms operate through the hypothalamus and anterior pituitary gland to precisely control the rate of thyroid secretion. Thyrotropin-releasing hormone (TRH) from the hypothalamus causes cells of the anterior pituitary lobe to produce and secrete TSH. TSH increases all known activities of thyroid gland cells, resulting in increased hormone synthesis and release. Circulating thyroid hormones inhibit the secretion of TSH and TRH through a negative feedback effect on the anterior pituitary lobe and hypothalamus.

Hyperthyroidism and Graves' Disease. Hyperthyroidism is thyroid gland hyperactivity that produces excess circulating thyroid hormone. The most common cause of hyperthyroidism in the United States is *Graves' disease*. Graves' disease is an autoimmune disease in which TSH receptor antibodies bind to and stimulate the thyroid gland, causing excessive production and secretion of T_4 and T_3.[148] The immunoglobulin G autoantibodies mimic the effect of TSH, but their effects are longer, lasting up to 12 hours compared to 1 hour for normal TSH.[148]

Graves' disease autoantibodies target the thyroid gland, extraocular muscles, and skin. There is a familial tendency and a higher incidence of other autoimmune disorders in patients with Graves' disease.[149] The disease occurs most often in women (female-to-male ratio is 5:1) and between 20 and 50 years of age.[10] Graves' disease has an unpredictable course, marked by relapses and exacerbations.

Hyperthyroidism can also be caused by benign follicular adenomas, which are not believed to have an autoimmune etiology. Exogenous iodine excess (radiocontrast agents or angiography dye) or the administration of thyroid hormones may induce iatrogenic thyrotoxicosis. Toxic multinodular goiter, subacute viral thyroiditis, postpartum thyroiditis, TSH-secreting pituitary tumors, and thyroid cancer are less common causes of hyperthyroidism. The antiarrhythmic agent amiodarone is iodine rich and may cause thyrotoxicosis.[32,150]

Signs and Symptoms. Clinical manifestations associated with thyrotoxicosis reflect the widespread hypermetabolic effects of excess thyroid hormones. Thyrotoxic patients complain of fatigue, thinning hair, fine muscle tremors, and anxiety. Sleep is often difficult. Menstrual cycles may become shorter, causing reversible infertility. Weight loss despite increased food consumption, muscle weakness, and heat intolerance are more specific indicators of thyrotoxicosis.

A goiter and proptosis ("thyroid stare") are highly specific findings of thyroid disease. The ophthalmopathy of Graves' disease may cause eye redness and a gritty sensation in early stages, with diplopia, ocular pain, and (rarely) loss of visual acuity in more advanced stages. Graves' ophthalmopathy results from antibody-mediated inflammation of the periorbital connective tissue and extraocular muscles.[151]

The blood volume increases slightly under the influence of excess thyroid hormone, a result of vasodilation. Mean arterial pressure usually remains unchanged, but the pulse pressure increases. The systolic pressure is typically elevated 10 to

15 mm Hg, and the diastolic pressure is reduced. Blood flow to the skin increases because of the increased need for heat elimination.

The effects of thyrotoxicosis on the heart are pronounced. Palpitations, tachycardia, and cardiac dysrhythmias affect most patients. The cardiac output increases, sometimes to 60% or more above normal. About 10% of thyrotoxic patients have atrial fibrillation. Mitral valve prolapse is more common in patients with Graves' disease than in the general population. With protracted high thyroid hormone levels, the heart muscle strength may become depressed as a result of protein catabolism. Diagnosis is more difficult in the elderly, as many of the hyperkinetic manifestations of hyperthyroidism are absent.[11] Elderly patients may present with myocardial failure.[9]

The hyperthyroid individual may feel a constant fatigue from the exhausting effect of thyroid hormone on the musculature and on the central nervous system.

Diagnosis. The diagnosis of primary disease is established in most cases by the combined findings of an abnormally high total or free serum T_4 assay and depressed TSH levels.[151] With Graves' disease, the diagnosis may be supported by the presence of stimulatory TSH receptor autoantibodies.[151,152] An elevated uptake of radioactive iodine (^{131}I) by the thyroid gland may be used to confirm gland hyperactivity. Serum alkaline phosphatase and calcium concentrations are mildly elevated in approximately 20% of patients with Graves' disease.[95,151] Mild normochromic normocytic anemia is sometimes present.[95,151]

Other autoimmune diseases such as myasthenia gravis, rheumatoid arthritis, systemic lupus erythematosus, and diabetes mellitus are more common in patients with Graves' disease. About 1% of patients with hyperthyroidism have myasthenia gravis.

Treatment of Graves' Disease. A variety of treatment options are available for patients with Graves' disease. The three primary treatment options for thyrotoxicosis are radioactive gland ablation, surgery, and antithyroid drug therapy.[149,153-156] β-Adrenergic receptor blockers are usually administered for controlling symptoms until the patient becomes euthyroid.[155]

Radioactive Iodine. A common therapy for Graves' disease is ablation of the thyroid gland with $Na^{131}I$. Two to 4 months is needed to reverse the hyperthyroidism, and hypothyroidism is common following $Na^{131}I$ treatment. Use of $Na^{131}I$ is contraindicated in pregnancy.[149,156]

Subtotal Thyroidectomy. Surgery for treatment of Graves' disease is usually performed only when radioactive iodine or antithyroid drugs are refused, for children or pregnant women who are allergic to antithyroid drugs, or if the thyroid goiter is exceptionally large. Patients should be treated preoperatively with antithyroid medication and rendered euthyroid prior to surgery. Complications associated with thyroid surgery occur in less than 1% of cases and include damage to the recurrent laryngeal nerve, hypoparathyroidism, and neck hematoma.[151]

Antithyroid Drugs and β-Adrenergic Receptor Blockade. Propylthiouracil (PTU) and methimazole (Tapazole) are thiourea derivatives that inhibit thyroid hormone synthesis and are used in the medical management of hyperthyroidism. These drugs inhibit the formation of thyroid hormone by interfering with the incorporation of iodine into tyrosine residues of thyroglobulin. PTU also inhibits conversion of T_4 to T_3. The usual dose for PTU is 50 to 200 mg/d in divided doses and a typical methimazole dose is 5 to 10 mg/d.[151] A euthyroid state is usually obtained in 6 to 7 weeks. Generally, the smaller the gland is, the shorter the amount of time necessary for achieving euthyroidism. Agranulocytosis is the most serious side effect of these drugs.[151] Figure 31-19 shows the chemical structure of antithyroid drugs.

β-Adrenergic receptor blockers are used to control tachycardia and reduce myocardial oxygen demand associated with hyperthyroidism. β-Adrenergic blockade does not affect goiter size or interfere with the synthesis of thyroid hormones.[149,155]

About 10 days before surgery, oral potassium iodide (Lugol's solution) may be added to the antithyroid regimen to decrease gland vascularity and to block hormone synthesis and release. The combination of propranolol and potassium iodide is frequently used preoperatively to reduce cardiovascular symptoms and decrease circulating T_4 and T_3 concentrations.[7,9,154,155] The combination of iodides and β-adrenergic receptor blockers may be used to blunt clinical symptoms and lower serum T_4 levels in a thyrotoxic patient being prepared for surgery if time is insufficient for administering PTU or methimazole.[95]

The optimal preoperative preparation usually requires 1 to 2 months of treatment with an antithyroid drug regimen.[7,11]

Preoperative Assessment—Hyperthyroidism. The key to successful preoperative preparation of the hyperthyroid surgical patient is a careful assessment of the extent of thyrotoxicosis and the severity of end-organ manifestations.[32] Severe disease is associated with increased operative risk.[11] Elective surgery should not proceed until the patient has been rendered euthyroid by medical management. Antithyroid medications should be continued through the morning of surgery.[7]

Hyperthyroid patients have increased blood volume, decreased peripheral resistance, and a wide pulse pressure. The cardiac output and systolic blood pressure may be increased. Appropriate corrections of the patient's fluid volume and electrolyte status should be accomplished before surgery. Hematocrit, hemoglobin, and total red cell count are usually normal, although 1% of patients with Graves' disease have pernicious anemia. Antithyroid medications can cause granulocytopenia.

A careful preoperative evaluation of the airway is mandatory in all hyperthyroid patients undergoing surgery. Thyroid gland enlargement can cause tracheal deviation and tracheoesophageal compression.[11,157] Assessment of the quality of voice should be documented. Hoarseness, coughing, or dyspnea suggests tracheal compression that can be caused by thyromegaly. A sore throat, the feeling of pressure in the neck, and dysphagia suggest tracheoesophageal compression. Chest and airway

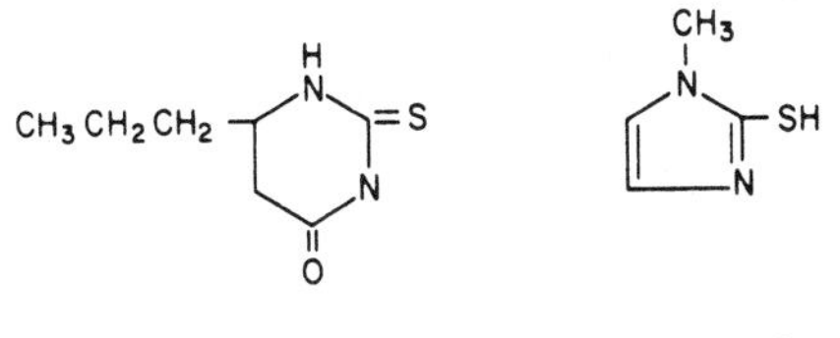

Propylthiouracil Methimazole

FIGURE **31-19**
Antithyroid drugs. (From Stoelting RK: *Pharmacology and Physiology in Anesthetic Practice*, ed 3, Philadelphia, 1999, Lippincott, p 410.)

radiographs and computerized tomography (CT) scans are useful to detect tracheal deviation and compression.[157]

A patient with a large goiter and an obstructed airway poses the same challenge as any other patient in whom airway management is problematic.[95] An awake fiberoptic intubation with topical anesthesia is of proven value under these conditions. Tracheomalacia weakens thyroid cartilage from chronic pressure and its presence may necessitate a more prolonged intubation after surgery.

Only life-threatening emergency surgery should be performed in an untreated symptomatic hyperthyroid patient.[7,9,95] In an emergency situation, the otherwise healthy patient can be expeditiously prepared for surgery with the oral administration of potassium iodide (3 to 5 drops every 6 hours) and intravenous administration of propranolol (1 to 10 mg) or esmolol (100 to 300 mcg/kg per minute).[11,95] Hyperthyroid patients who require emergency surgery and have rapid ventricular rates with congestive heart failure require central pressure monitoring to guide therapy.

Intraoperative Management. A major goal of the perioperative management of the hyperthyroid patient is prevention of sympathetic stimulation. This is accomplished by providing sufficient anesthetic depth and avoiding medications that stimulate the sympathetic nervous system.[7,9,14,95]

A preoperative anxiolytic medication is generally warranted. Atropine should be avoided as an antisialagogue because of its vagolytic effects and its ability to impair sweating.

Induction of anesthesia may be achieved with a number of intravenous medications. Thiopental is an attractive choice for induction because of its antithyroid activity, although significant antithyroid effect with an induction dose of this drug is unlikely.[9] Ketamine should be avoided because it can stimulate the sympathetic nervous system.[158]

If the airway is not compromised by an enlarged goiter, administration of a muscle relaxant can facilitate intubation of the trachea. Pancuronium should be avoided because it has the potential to increase the heart rate. Because of the increased incidence of myasthenia gravis and skeletal muscle weakness in the hyperthyroid patient, prudence dictates careful titration of muscle relaxant doses with use of a peripheral nerve stimulator.[7,9]

Hyperthyroid patients have been shown to metabolize more halothane and enflurane than euthyroid patients, as evidenced by higher plasma bromide and fluoride concentrations per hour of anesthesia at minimum alveolar concentration (MAC). Isoflurane or sevoflurane are attractive choices for inhalation anesthetics because of their ability to offset sympathetic nervous system responses to surgical stimulation and because they do not sensitize the myocardium to catecholamines.

Hyperthyroid patients do not generally require a higher MAC.[146] The increased cardiac output accompanying hyperthyroidism may accelerate the uptake of an inhaled anesthetic, resulting in the need to increase the delivered concentration, and this may be perceived clinically as an increased anesthetic requirement.[9,14,95]

Monitoring of the hyperthyroid patient should focus on early recognition of increased thyroid gland activity, suggesting the onset of thyroid storm. Core body temperature should be monitored closely. The ECG should be monitored for tachycardia or dysrhythmias.[159] Hypotension occurring during surgery is better treated with direct-acting vasopressors than with drugs that provoke the release of catecholamines.[7] Hypercarbia and hypoxia should be prevented because they stimulate the sympathoadrenal axis.

Meticulous care of the eyes is required. The patient with exophthalmos is at risk for corneal drying and ulceration, so special care should be taken to lubricate and protect the eyes perioperatively. Box 31-5 summarizes key anesthesia implications for patients with hyperthyroidism.

Thyroid Storm. A feared complication in the hyperthyroid patient is *thyroid storm*. Thyroid storm is a rare event that is caused by acute stress in the previously undiagnosed or incompletely treated hyperthyroid patient. Precipitating events may include trauma, surgery, the peripartum period, ^{131}I therapy, acute illness, and infection.[95,160,161]

Thyroid storm is a life-threatening medical emergency that represents a severe exacerbation of hyperthyroid signs and symptoms.[151] The clinical manifestations may include marked tachycardia, hyperthermia, hypertension, atrial fibrillation, sweating, tremor, vomiting, weakness, agitation, shock, and congestive heart failure.[151] Metabolic acidosis may be present secondary to increased lactate production from the overactive metabolism. Similarities exist between the clinical features of thyroid storm and those of pheochromocytoma, light anesthesia, and malignant hyperthermia.

Thyroid storm associated with surgery may occur intraoperatively but is more likely to occur 6 to 18 hours after surgery.[9] Treatment must be initiated as soon as the diagnosis is made to prevent substantial morbidity and mortality. Mortality rates have decreased from 20%-30% to less than 10% with early diagnosis and management.[11] The high mortality associated with thyroid storm underscores the importance of achieving a euthyroid state before surgery.

Management of perioperative thyroid storm includes identifying and treating the precipitating cause, administering antithyroid medications, and providing hemodynamic support. Carefully titrated β-adrenergic blockers, sodium iodide, and anthyroid drugs (PTU or methimazole) may be part of the treatment regimen.[162] Supplemental glucocorticoids should be administered as the turnover of endogenous steroids is accelerated by the hypermetabolism of thyrotoxicosis. Glucocorticoids also impair the peripheral conversion of T_4 to T_3.

Supportive measures include intravenous hydration with glucose-containing crystalloid solutions, correction of electrolyte and acid base imbalances, and management of hyperthermia.[151,161] Salicylates may displace T_4 from its carrier protein;

BOX 31-5

Anesthesia Implications for the Hyperthyroid Patient

Ensure a euthyroid state prior to surgery.
Determine the extent of thyrotoxicosis and end-organ complications.
Evaluate the airway closely.
Avoid sympathetic nervous system activation and sympathomimetic drugs.
Titrate muscle relaxants carefully, considering possible myopathy and myasthenia gravis.
Monitor closely for early signs of thyroid storm.
Pad and protect the eyes.

therefore, acetaminophen is the recommended antipyretic for lowering body temperature. Adequate oxygenation is of paramount importance during thyroid storm. Vasoactive medications and advanced hemodynamic monitoring may be necessary to help manage the labile cardiovascular course.

Hypothyroidism. *Hypothyroidism* is a state of thyroid gland hypofunction resulting in decreased circulating concentrations of T_3 and T_4. Circulating T_4 concentrations decrease and TSH levels increase in patients with primary hypothyroid disease.[11,151] The clinical spectrum of thyroid hormone deficiency can range from the asymptomatic patient with no overt physical findings to the classic myxedematous patient with profound symptoms.[151,163] Hypothyroidism is the most common disorder of thyroid function, occurring in 0.8% of the adult population.[9]

Primary hypothyroidism accounts for 95% of all cases of hypothyroidism. An autoimmune-mediated thyroiditis is the most common etiology in the United States.[151,164] This disorder, known as *Hashimoto's thyroiditis*, is characterized by a slow and progressive destruction of the thyroid gland. It is most common in females of middle age and is associated with other autoimmune disorders such as myasthenia gravis and adrenal insufficiency.[151]

Primary hypothyroidism may also be the result of severe iodine deficiency, previous thyroid surgery, neck irradiation, or treatment for hyperthyroidism (^{131}I therapy).[32,151,163] The antiarrhythmic agent amiodarone is associated with hyper- and hypothyroidism. Lithium inhibits the release of thyroid hormone and causes hypothyroidism in some patients.

Rarely, secondary hypothyroidism is the result of pituitary or hypothalamic disorder. Secondary hypothyroidism is associated with decreased concentrations of both thyroid hormones and TSH. Regardless of the etiology, the clinical manifestations of hypothyroidism are similar.[151]

Signs and Symptoms. Most cases of hypothyroidism are subclinical with no overt symptoms and the only finding an increased plasma TSH. Patients with more significant disease develop symptoms that reflect a slowed metabolism and impaired cellular functions. The thyroid gland usually is enlarged, nontender, firm, and indurated. Patients may have dry skin, cold intolerance, paresthesias, slow mental functioning, ataxia, puffy face, and constipation. Lack of thyroid hormones causes the muscles to become sluggish. Patients with severe hypothyroidism may be hypersomnolent with a decreased ventilatory response to hypoxia and hypercarbia. The hair and nails frequently are brittle. Modest weight gain may occur.[95,151,163-165]

The accumulation of proteinaceous fluid in serous body cavities is a well-recognized feature of hypothyroidism and may occur in mild cases. The most common sites of effusions associated with hypothyroidism are the pleural, pericardial, and peritoneal cavities.[166] Inappropriate ADH secretion and impaired free water clearance can lead to hyponatremia. Accumulation of mucopolysaccharides and fluid imparts the characteristic edematous appearance in these patients.[32]

Cardiovascular complications include sinus bradycardia, dysrhythmias, cardiomegaly, impaired contractility, congestive heart failure, and labile blood pressure.[95,151,163] Symptoms of low exercise tolerance and shortness of breath with exertion may be partially the result of decreased cardiac function. Bradycardia and decreased stroke volume are responsible for a reduction in cardiac output of up to 40%.[7] Chronic vasoconstriction produces diastolic hypertension and decreases the intravascular fluid volume.[32,167] The autonomic nervous system response is blunted and there is a decrease in the sensitivity and number of β-receptors.[167,168]

Overt hypothyroidism is associated with a number of abnormalities in lipid metabolism that may predispose patients to accelerated coronary artery disease. Hypothyroidism is associated with anemia and decreased erythrocyte production of 2,3-diphosphoglycerate, leading to a leftward shift of the oxyhemoglobin dissociation curve.

These "classic" clinical features of hypothyroidism are often lacking in the elderly hypothyroid patient. Thyroid status cannot always be predicted from clinical signs and symptoms in the elderly and diagnosing hypothyroidism is difficult based solely on clinical features.[169,170]

Treatment. Treatment of hypothyroidism requires replacement with thyroid hormone. The agent of choice is synthetic *levothyroxine sodium*, because of its long half-life (7 days) and its ability to attain physiologic levels of T_3.[151] The average replacement dosage in the United States is 112 mcg/day.[151]

Two areas of particular concern during thyroid hormone replacement are the effect on the cardiovascular system and the effect on bone. Initiation of thyroid hormone replacement in a patient with coexisting angina pectoris or underlying risk factors for coronary artery disease is potentially hazardous and requires careful monitoring of both cardiovascular and thyroid status. Myocardial oxygen consumption is augmented by thyroid hormone, and a hypothyroid patient with deficient coronary artery circulation may not tolerate full replacement doses.[171,172] Excessive L-thyroxine ingestion or thyrotoxicosis may lead to decreased bone density and predispose patients to osteoporosis.[165] The effects of T_4 on lipid measurements suggest that patients with subclinical hypothyroidism should receive replacement therapy.[173]

Anesthetic Management—Hypothyroidism. Patients with mild to moderate hypothyroid disease have an overall low risk of complications when undergoing anesthesia and surgery.[32] These patients should receive a careful preoperative evaluation and preoperative continuation of their levothyroxine therapy.[9,11] Patients with severe hypothyroidism are predisposed to multiple complications with anesthesia. Depression of myocardial function, abnormal baroreceptor function, and reductions in plasma volume may be present.[7,9,11,14,163] Slowed hepatic metabolism and renal clearance of injected drugs may prolong their effects, but MAC is not decreased significantly.[146] Elective surgical procedures should be postponed in the presence of severe symptomatic hypothyroidism.[11,95,172]

All patients with hypothyroidism should undergo careful preoperative evaluation of the airway. A large goiter may cause airway compromise in the form of tracheal deviation or compression. In some patients with severe hypothyroidism, adequate air exchange may be compromised by an enlarged tongue and myxedematous infiltration of the vocal cords.[174] Depression of the ventilatory responses to hypoxia and hypercarbia must be considered. Preoperative sedation should be avoided in the patient with macroglossia or preexisting hypoventilation. The risk of pulmonary aspiration is increased because of associated somatic obesity and delayed gastric emptying.[11,14]

Hypothyroid patients respond to opioids with increased central nervous system and respiratory depression and to volatile agents with increased hypotension and myocardial depression. Although ketamine has been proposed as the ideal induction agent, even ketamine can produce cardiovascular depression in the absence of an active sympathetic nervous system.[7,9] Thiopental has been used for induction of anesthesia in the hypothyroid patient without apparent excessive cardiovascular depression.[7,9]

Intubation of the trachea may be facilitated by the administration of succinylcholine or a nondepolarizing muscle relaxant; however, hypothyroid patients may be more sensitive to standard doses of nondepolarizing muscle relaxants because of coexisting muscle weakness, a propensity to develop hypothermia, and decreased hepatic metabolism and renal elimination of these drugs.[11,14] Acute severe hypothyroidism may interfere with both intraoperative monitoring of neuromuscular excitability and estimation of neuromuscular blockade.[175] Maintaining muscle paralysis with minimal doses of muscle relaxants is an appropriate goal.

Supplemental perioperative cortisol should be considered, as there exists a potential for adrenal insufficiency with stress.[7,165] In a severely hypothyroid, acutely ill patient with unstable vital signs, prescribing stress doses of glucocorticoids until the patient is stabilized is prudent.

In hypothyroidism, the number of β-receptors is diminished, possibly as a result of a reversible allosteric change from β-receptors to α–receptors, mediated by a lack of thyroid hormone.[168] Responses to inotropic drugs may be influenced by the accompanying alterations in the adrenergic receptor concentration. Inamrinone may be an appropriate inotrope for patients who may have an altered β-receptor pool.[167]

Body temperature should be monitored closely in hypothyroid patients, and mechanisms for warming the patient should be employed during surgery. The maintenance of body temperature may be facilitated by an increase in ambient air temperature, the warming and humidification of inhaled gases, covering of the patient's head, and the delivery of IV fluids through a blood-warming device. Box 31-6 summarizes the anesthesia implications of hypothyroidism.

Myxedema Coma. Myxedema coma is a rare syndrome that reflects the end stage of untreated, long-standing hypothyroidism. The presence of coma is a marker of the patient's clinical deterioration rather than a primary effect of hypothyroidism. A critical insult (infection, surgery, cerebrovascular accident, gastrointestinal bleeding, cold exposure) can precipitate myxedema coma in a patient with hypothyroidism.[32,151]

Generally, the patient has severe clinical features of hypothyroidism and is hypothermic, hypoventilating, and hyponatremic. The response to hypoxia and hypercapnia is measurably decreased and mechanical ventilation may be required. The patient is typically lethargic or stuporous. The skin often is pale as a result of cutaneous vasoconstriction.

Myxedema coma is a medical emergency with a mortality rate as high as 60%.[11,151] Vigorous therapeutic attention should be paid to hypothermia, shock, and ventilatory failure. Treatment consists of hemodynamic and ventilatory support, and the intravenous administration of levothyroxine with continuous ECG monitoring. Supplemental cortisol is appropriate since the myxedematous patient may have adrenal atrophy and decreased adrenal reserve. Because these patients may be vulnerable to water intoxication and hyponatremia, meticulous fluid replacement is important.[7] Only lifesaving surgery should proceed in a patient with myxedema coma.[9]

BOX **31-6**

Anesthesia Implications for the Hypothyroid Patient

Delay elective surgery for the patient with severe symptomatic disease.
Evaluate the airway closely.
Monitor for exaggerated central nervous system depression with anesthetic agents.
Titrate muscle relaxants carefully considering possible coexisting muscle weakness.
Consider decreased hepatic metabolism and renal elimination when dosing medications.
Maintain normothermia.
Monitor ventilation closely considering blunted ventilatory response to hypercarbia and hypoxia.

REFERENCES

1. Genuth SM: General principles of endocrine physiology. In Berne RM, Levy NM, editors: *Physiology*, St Louis, 1998, Mosby, p 779.
2. Lyons FM, Meeran K: The physiology of the endocrine system. In Desborough J, editor: *International Anesthesiology Clinics*, Philadelphia, 1997, Lippincott-Raven, p 1.
3. Guyton AC, Hall JE: Introduction to endocrinology. In Guyton AC, Hall JE, editors: *Textbook of Medical Physiology*, ed 10, Philadelphia, 2000, Saunders, p 836.
4. Wilson JD, Foster DW: Hormones and hormone action: introduction. In Melmed S, Larsen PR, Kroneneberg HM, Polonsky KS, editors: *Williams Textbook of Endocrinology*, ed 10, Philadelphia, 2002, Saunders, p 1.
5. Genuth SM: The hypothalamus and pituitary gland. In Berne RM, Levy NM, editors: *Physiology*, St Louis, 1998, Mosby, p 872.
6. Guyton AC, Hall JE: The pituitary hormones and their control by the hypothalamus. In *Textbook of Medical Physiology*, ed 10, Philadelphia, 2000, Saunders, p 846.
7. Schwartz JJ, Rosenbaum S, Graf G: Anesthesia and the endocrine system. In Barash PG, Cullen BF, Stoelting RK, editors: *Clinical Anesthesia*, Philadelphia, 2001, Lippincott Williams & Wilkins, p 1119.
8. Wicklund RA, Rosenbaum SH: Preoperative endocrine testing. In Fleisher LA, editor: *Problems in Anesthesia*, Philadelphia, 1997, Lippincott-Raven, p 182.
9. Stoelting RK, Dierdorf SF: Endocrine disease. In *Anesthesia and Co-existing Disease*, ed 4, New York, 2002, Churchill Livingstone, p 395.
10. Razis PA: Anesthesia for surgery of pituitary tumors. In Desborough J, editor: *International Anesthesiology Clinics*, Philadelphia, 1997, Lippincott-Raven, p 23.
11. Sieber FE: Evaluation of the patient with endocrine disease and diabetes mellitus. In Rogers MC, Tinker JH, Covino BG, Longnecker DE, editors: *Principles and Practice of Anesthesiology*, ed 3, St Louis, 1998, Mosby, p 303.
12. Klibanski A, Zervas NT: Diagnosis and management of hormone-secreting pituitary adenomas, *N Engl J Med* 324:822-831, 1991.
13. Black PM: Brain tumors, *N Engl J Med* 324:1555-1564, 1991.
14. Roizen MF: Diseases of the endocrine system. In Katz J, Benumof JL, Kadis LB, editors: *Anesthesia and Uncommon Diseases*, ed 4, Philadelphia, 1998, Saunders, p 223.
15. Salomon F, Cuneo RC, Hesp R, Sonksen PH: The effects of treatment with recombinant human growth hormone on body composition and metabolism in adults with growth hormone deficiency, *N Engl J Med* 321:1797-1804, 1989.

16. Molitch ME: Clinical manifestations of acromegaly, *Endocrinol Metab Clin North Am* 21:597-614, 1992.
17. Melmed S: Acromegaly, *N Engl J Med* 322:966-977, 1990.
18. Fahlbusch R, Honegger J, Buchfelder M: Surgical management of acromegaly, *Endocrinol Metab Clin North Am* 21:669-691, 1992.
19. Baxter MA: Acromegaly and transsphenoidal hypophysectomy: a case report, *AANA J* 62:182-185, 1994.
20. Hassan SZ, Matz GJ, Lawrence AM, Collins PA: Laryngeal stenosis in acromegaly: a possible cause of airway difficulties associated with anesthesia, *Anesth Analg* 55:57-60, 1976.
21. Muchler HC, Renz D, Ludecke DK: Anesthetic management of acromegaly. In Ludecke DK, Tolis G, editors: *Growth Hormone, Growth Factors, and Acromegaly*, New York, 1987, Raven Press, p 267.
22. Messick JM Jr, Cucchiara RF, Faust RJ: Airway management in patients with acromegaly (letter), *Anesthesiology* 56:157, 1982.
23. Buonocore CM, Robinson AG: The diagnosis and management of diabetes insipidus during medical emergencies, *Endocrinol Metab Clin North Am* 22:411-423, 1993.
24. Ayus JC, Arieff AI: Pathogenesis and prevention of hyponatremia encephalopathy, *Endocrinol Metab Clin North Am* 22: 425-446, 1993.
25. Sterns RH: Severe hyponatremia: the case for conservative management, *Crit Care Med* 20:534-539, 1992.
26. Berl T: Treating hyponatremia: what is all the controversy about? *Ann Intern Med* 113:417-419, 1990.
27. Guyton AC, Hall JE: Parathyroid hormone, calcitonin, calcium and phosphate metabolism, vitamin D, bone, and teeth. In *Textbook of Medical Physiology*, ed 10, Philadelphia, 2000, Saunders, p 899.
28. Genuth SM: Endocrine regulation of calcium and phosphate metabolism. In Berne RM, Levy NM, editors: *Physiology*, St Louis, 1998, Mosby, p 848.
29. Tohme JF, Bilezikian JP: Hypocalcemic emergencies, *Endocrinol Metab Clin North Am* 22:363-375, 1993.
30. Lyons FM, Meeran K: The physiology of the endocrine system. In Desborough J, editor: *International Anesthesiology Clinics*, Philadelphia, 1997, Lippincott-Raven, p 1.
31. Christopherson R, Parris WCV: Anesthesia for endocrine surgery. In Longnecker DE, Tinker JH, Morgan GE, editors: *Principles and Practice of Anesthesiology*, ed 2, St. Louis, 1998, Mosby, p 1948.
32. Edwards R: Thyroid and parathyroid disease. In Desborough J, editor: *International Anesthesiology Clinics*, Philadelphia, 1997, Lippincott-Raven, p 63.
33. DeRubertis FR: Recognition and reversal of hypocalcemia, *Hosp Med* 26:125-148, 1990.
34. Al-Zahrani, Levine MA: Primary hyperparathyroidism. *Lancet*. 349:1233, 1997.
35. Lufkin KG: Primary hyperparathyroidism, *Hosp Med* 27:98-116, 1991.
36. Irvin GL, 3rd, Carneiro DM, Solorzano CC: Progress in the operative management of sporadic primary hyperparathyroidism over 34 years, *Ann Surg* 239:704-711, 2004.
37. Pyrtek LJ, Belkin M, Bartus S, Schweizer R: Parathyroid gland exploration with local anesthesia in elderly and high-risk patient, *Arch Surg* 123:614-617, 1988.
38. Ditkoff BA, Chabot J, Feind C, Lo Gerfo P: Parathyroid surgery using monitored anesthesia care as an alternative to general anesthesia, *Am J Surg* 172:698-700, 1996.
39. Jossart GH, Clark OH: Thyroid and parathyroid procedures—surgical techniques, *Scientific American* 7:1-8, 1997.
40. Nussbaum SR: Pathophysiology and management of severe hypercalcemia, *Endocrinol Metab Clin North Am* 22:343-361, 1993.
41. Tominaga Y, Numano M, Tanaka Y, Uchida K, Takagi H: Surgical treatment of renal hyperparathyroidism, *Semin Surg Oncol* 13: 87-96, 1997.
42. Sonner JM, Hynson JM, Clark O, Katz JA: Nausea and vomiting following thyroid and parathyroid surgery, *J Clin Anesth* 9(5):398-402, 1997.
43. Genuth SM: Hormones of the pancreatic islets. In Berne RM, Levy NM, editors: *Physiology*, St. Louis, 1998, Mosby, p 822.
44. Guyton AC, Hall JE: Insulin, glucagon, and diabetes mellitus. In *Textbook of Medical Physiology*, ed 10, Philadelphia, 2000, Saunders, p 884.
45. Clarke RSJ: The hyperglycemic response to different types of surgery and anaesthesia. *Br J Anaesth* 42:45, 1970.
46. Comi RJ: Approach to acute hypoglycemia, *Endocrinol Metab Clin North Am* 22:247-262, 1993.
47. Nolte MS: Insulin therapy in insulin-dependent (type I) diabetes mellitus, *Endocrinol Metab Clin North Am* 21:281-303, 1992.
48. Report of the Expert Committee on the Diagnosis and Classification of Diabetes Mellitus, 20:1183-1197, 1997.
49. National Diabetes Fact Sheet—U.S. Department of Health and Human Services Centers for Disease Control and Prevention. Available at http://cdc.gov/diabetes. Accessed September 1, 2003.
50. National Institute of Diabetes and Digestive and Kidney Diseases of the National Institute of Health. Available at http://niddk.nih.gov. Accessed September 1, 2003.
51. Centers for Disease Control: *The Public Health of Diabetes in the United States: Surveillance Report 2002*, US Department of Health and Human Services. Available at http://www.cdc.gov/diabetes/statistics/. Accessed September 7, 2003.
52. Nathan DM: Diabetes mellitus, *Scientific American Medical* 9: 1-23, 1997.
53. MacLaren N, Atkinson M: Is insulin-dependent diabetes mellitus environmentally induced? *N Engl J Med* 327:348-349, 1992.
54. Milaszkiewicz RM: Diabetes mellitus and anesthesia: what is the problem? In Desborough J, editor: *International Anesthesiology Clinics*, Philadelphia, 1997, Lippincott-Raven, p 35.
55. Jorgensen BG, Holm HE: Anaesthetic implications of long-term diabetic complications, *Acta Anaesthesiol Scand* 39:560-562, 1995.
56. Lasker RD: The diabetes control and complications trial, *N Engl J Med* 329:1035-1036, 1993.
57. National Diabetes Data Group, editors. *Diabetes in America*, ed 2, Washington, DC, US Department of Health and Human Services, National Institutes of Health, National Institute of Diabetes and Digestive and Kidney Diseases, 1995. NIH publication no. 95-1468:339-48.
58. Reddi AS, Camerini-Davalos RA: Diabetic nephropathy, *Arch Intern Med* 150:3143, 1990.
59. Watkins PJ: Diabetic autonomic neuropathy, *N Engl J Med* 322:1078-1079, 1990.
60. Quasthoff S: The role of axonal ion conductances in diabetic neuropathy: a review, *Muscle Nerve* 21:1246-1255, 1998.
61. Mangano DT: Diabetic silent hearts and anesthesia: the duty to assess, *J Clin Anesth* 10:610-612, 1998.
62. Tamborlane WV, Ahern J: Implications and results of the diabetes control and complications trial, *Pediatr Clin North Am* 44:285-299, 1997.
63. Hirsch IB, McGill JB, Cryer PE, White PF: Perioperative management of surgical patients with diabetes mellitus, *Anesthesiology* 74:346-359, 1991.
64. Ishihara H, Singh H, Giesecke AH: Relationship between diabetic autonomic neuropathy and gastric contents, *Anesth Analg* 78:943, 1994.
65. Salzarulo HH, Taylor LA: Diabetic "stiff joint syndrome" as a cause of difficult endotracheal intubation, *Anesthesiology* 64:366-368, 1986.
66. Reissell E, Orko R, Maunuksela EL, Lindgren L: Predictability of difficult laryngoscopy in patients with long-term diabetes mellitus, *Anaesthesia* 45:1024, 1990.
67. Abramowicz M, editor: Drugs for diabetes, *The Medical Letter* 1:1, 2002.
68. DeFronzo RA, Goodman AM, and the Multicenter Metformin Study Group: Efficacy of metformin in patients with non-insulin-dependent diabetes mellitus, *N Engl J Med* 333:541-549, 1995.
69. DeFronzo RA: Pharmacologic therapy for type 2 diabetes mellitus. *Ann Intern Med* 131:281, 1999.

70. Weissamn C: The metabolic response to stress: an overview and update. *Anesthesiology* 73:308, 1990.
71. Engquist A, Brandt MR, Fernandes A, Kehlet H: The blocking effect of epidural analgesia on the adrenocortical and hyperglycemic responses to surgery. *Acta Anaesthesiol Scand* 21:330-335, 1977.
72. McMurry JF Jr: Wound healing with diabetes mellitus: better glucose control for better wound healing in diabetes, *Surg Clin North Am* 64:769-778, 1984.
73. Zerr KJ, Furnary AP, Grunkemeier GL, Bookin S, Kanhere V, Starr A: Glucose control lowers the risk of wound infection in diabetics after open heart operations, *Ann Thorac Surg* 63: 356-361, 1997.
74. Knight JW, Cordingley JJ, Palazzo MG: Epidural abscess following epidural steroid and local anaesthetic injection, *Anaesthesia* 52:576-578, 1997.
75. Longstretch WT, Invi TS: High blood glucose level on hospital admission and poor neurological recovery after cardiac arrest, *Ann Neurol* 15:59-63, 1984.
76. Pulsinelli WA, Levy DE, Sigsbee B, Scherer P, Plum F: Increased damage after ischemic stroke in patients with hyperglycemia with or without established diabetes mellitus, *Am J Med* 74: 540-544, 1983.
77. Maser RE, Ellers JM, DeCherney GS: Glucose monitoring of patients with diabetes mellitus receiving general anesthesia: A study of the practices of anesthesia providers in a large community hospital, *AANA J* 64:357-361, 1996.
78. Wiklund RA: Preoperative endocrine testing. In Fleisher LA, editor: *Problems in Anesthesia*, Philadelphia, 1997, Lippincott-Raven, p 182.
79. Eldridge AJ, Sear JW: Perioperative management of diabetic patients: Any changes for the better since 1985? *Anaesthesia* 51:45-51, 1996.
80. Kerner PA: Perioperative management of the diabetic patient, *Exp Clin Endocrinol Diabetes* 103:213-218, 1995.
81. Hirsch IB, Paauw DS: Diabetes management in special situations, *Endocrinol Metab Clin North Am* 26:631-645, 1997.
82. Raucoules-Aime M, Ichai C, Roussel LJ, et al: Comparison of two methods of i.v. insulin administration in the diabetic patient during the perioperative period, *Br J Anaesth* 72:5-10, 1994.
83. Raucoules-Aime M, Labib Y, Levraut J, Gastaud P, Dolisi C, Grimaud D: Use of i.v. insulin in well-controlled non-insulin-dependent diabetics undergoing major surgery, *Br J Anaesth* 76:198-202, 1996.
84. Hemmerling TM, Schmid MC, Schmidt J, Kern S, Jacobi KE: Comparison of a continuous glucose-insulin-potassium infusion versus intermittent bolus application of insulin on perioperative glucose control and hormone status in insulin-treated type 2 diabetics, *J Clin Anesth* 13:293-300, 2001.
85. Fleckman AM: Diabetic ketoacidosis, *Endocrinol Metab Clin North Am* 22:181-207, 1993.
86. Siperstein MD: Diabetic ketoacidosis and hyperosmolar coma, *Endocrinol Metab Clin North Am* 21:415-432, 1992.
87. Kitabchi AE, Wall BM: Diabetic ketoacidosis, *Med Clin North Am*. 79:9-37, 1995.
88. Guyton AC, Hall JE: The adrenocortical hormones. In Guyton AC, Hall JE, editors: *Textbook of Medical Physiology*, ed 10, Philadelphia, 2000, Saunders, p 869.
89. Genuth SM: The adrenal glands. In Berne RM, Levy MN, editors: *Physiology*, ed 4, St Louis, 1998, Mosby p 930.
90. Conn JW: Part I. Painting background. Part II. Primary aldosteronism, a new clinical syndrome, 1954. [historical article]. *J Lab Clin Med* 116:253-267, 1990.
91. Stewart PM: Mineralocorticoid hypertension, *Lancet* 17(9161): 1341, 1999.
92. Schamess A, Bernik T, Tenner S: Refractory hypertension due to Conn's syndrome, *Postgrad Med* 95(4):199-200, 203-206, 1994.
93. Bravo EL: Primary aldosteronism: Issues in diagnosis and management, *Endocrinol Metab Clin North Am* 23(2):271-283, 1994.
94. Favia G, Lumachi F, Scarpa V, D'Amico DF: Adrenalectomy in primary aldosteronism: a long-term follow-up study in 52 patients, *World J Surg* 16:680-684, 1992.
95. Roizen MF: Anesthetic implications of concurrent diseases. In Miller RD, editor: *Anesthesia*, New York, 2000, Churchill Livingstone, p 903.
96. Nishimura M, Uzu T, Fujii T, et al: Cardiovascular complications in patients with primary aldosteronism, *Am J Kidney Dis* 33(2):261-266, 1999.
97. Rossi GP, Sacchetto A, Visentin P, et al: Changes in left ventricular anatomy and function in hypertension and primary aldosteronism, *Hypertension* 27(5):1039-1045, 1996.
98. McLeod MK: Complications following adrenal surgery, *J Natl Med Assoc* 83:161-164, 1991.
99. Shen WT, Lim RC, Siperstein AE: Laparoscopic vs open adrenalectomy for the treatment of primary hyperaldosteronism, *Arch Surg* 134(6):628-631, 1999.
100. Puccini M, Iacconi P, Bernini G: Conn syndrome: 14 years' experience from two European centres, *Eur J Surg* 164(11):811-817, 1998.
101. Brunt MJ, Melby JC: Adrenal gland disorders. In Noble J, editor, *Textbook of Primary Care Medicine*, ed 3, Mosby, St Louis, 2001, p 863.
102. Hutter AM, Kayhoe DE: Adrenal cortical carcinoma: clinical features of 138 patients, *Am J Med* 41:572, 1966.
103. Goldfard DA: Contemporary evaluation and management of Cushing's syndrome, *World J Urol* 17(1):22-25, 1999.
104. Ernest I, Ekman H: Adrenalectomy in Cushing's disease: a long-term follow-up, *Acta Endocrinol Suppl* 160:3, 1972.
105. Tyrrell JB, Brooks RM, Fitzgerald PA, Cofoid PB, Forsham PH, Wilson CB: Cushing's disease: selected trans-sphenoidal resection of pituitary microadenomas, *N Engl J Med* 298:753, 1978.
106. Kemink L, Hermus A, Pieters G, Benraad T, Smals A, Kloppenborg P: Residual adrenocortical function after bilateral adrenalectomy for pituitary-dependent Cushing's syndrome, *J Clin Endocrinol Metab* 75:1211-1214, 1992.
107. Small M, Lowe GD, Forbes CD, Thomson JA: Thromboembolic complications in Cushing's syndrome, *Clin Endocrinol (Oxf)* 19:503-511, 1983.
108. Dal Bo Zanon R, Fornasiero L, Boscaro M, Cappellato G, Fabris F, Girolami A: Increased factor VIII associated activities in Cushing's syndrome: a probable hypercoagulable state, *Thromb Haemost* 47:116-117, 1982.
109. National Institute of Diabetes and Digestive and Kidney Diseases at the National Institute of Health. Available at http://www.niddk.nih.gov/. Accessed September 7, 2003.
110. Oelkers W: Adrenal insufficiency. *N Engl J Med* 335:1206, 1996.
111. Arit W, Allolia B: Adrenal insufficiency, *Lancet*. 361:1881, 2003.
112. Glowniak JV, Loriaux DL: A double-blind study of perioperative steroid requirements in secondary adrenal insufficiency, *Surgery* 121:123, 1997.
113. Werbel SS, Ober KP: Acute adrenal insufficiency, *Endocrinol Metab Clin North Am* 22:303-328, 1993.
114. Chin R: Adrenal crisis. *Crit Care Clin* 7:23, 1991.
115. Salem M, Tainsh RE Jr, Bromberg J, Loriaux DL, Chernow B: Perioperative glucocorticoid coverage. A reassessment 42 years after emergence of a problem, *Ann Surg* 219(4):416-425, 1994.
116. Udelsman R, Ramp J, Gallucci WT, et al: Adaptation during surgical stress: a re-evaluation of the role of glucocorticoids, *J Clin Invest* 77:1377-1381, 1986.
117. Henriques HF III, Lebovic D: Defining and focusing perioperative steroid supplementation, *Am Surg* 61(9):809-813, 1994.
118. Fallo F, Betterle C, Budano S, Lupia M, Boscaro M, Sonino N: Regression of cardiac abnormalities after replacement therapy in Addison's disease, *Eur J Endocrinol* 140(5):425-428, 1999.
119. Friedman RJ, Schiff CF, Bromberg JS: Use of supplemental steroids in patients having orthopaedic operations, *J Bone Joint Surg Am* 77(12):1801-1806, 1995.

120. Guyton AC, Hall JE: The autonomic nervous system; and the adrenal medulla. In Guyton AC, Hall JE editors: *Textbook of Medical Physiology*, ed 10, Philadelphia, 2000, Saunders, p 697.
121. Atiyeh BA, Barakat AJ, Abumrad NN: Extra-adrenal pheochromocytoma, *J Nephrol* 10(1):25-29, 1997.
122. Samaan NA, Hickey RC, Shutts PE: Diagnosis, localization, and management of pheochromocytoma: pitfalls and follow-up in 41 patients, *Cancer* 62:2451-2460, 1988.
123. Geoghegan JG, Emberton M, Bloom R, Lynn JA: Changing trends in the management of phaeochromocytoma, *Br J Surg.* 85:117, 1998.
124. Dougherty TB, Cronau LH Jr: Anesthetic implications for surgical patients with endocrine tumors, *Int Anesthesiol Clin* 36(3):31-44, 1998.
125. Neumann HP, Berger DP, Sigmund G, et al: Pheochromocytoma, multiple endocrine neoplasia type 2, and von Hippel-Lindau disease, *N Engl J Med* 329:1531-1538, 1993.
126. Cheng TO, Bashour TT: Striking cardiographic changes associated with pheochromocytoma masquerading as ischaemic heart disease, *Chest* 70:397, 1976.
127. Kaul U, Mohan JC, Rao PS, Mukhopadhyaya S, Singh SM, Bhatia ML: Pheochromocytoma presenting as recurrent syncope resulting from ventricular tachycardia: an annual presentation, *Indian Heart J* 36:118-120, 1984.
128. Shub C, Cueto-Garcia L, Sheps SG, Ilstrup DM, Tajik AJ: Echocardiographic findings in pheochromocytoma, *Am J Cardiol* 57:971-975, 1986.
129. Ulchaker JC, Goldfarb DA, Bravo EL, Novick AC: Successful outcomes in pheochromocytoma surgery in the modern era, *J Urol* 161(3):764-767, 1999.
130. Sand J, Salmi J, Saaristo J, Auvinen O: Preoperative treatment and survival of patients with pheochromocytomas, *Ann Chir Gynaecol* 86(3):230-232, 1997.
131. Briggs RSJ, Birtwell AJ, Pohl JEF: Hypertensive response to labetalol in pheochromocytoma, *Lancet* 1:1045-1046, 1978.
132. Colson P, Rychwaert F, Ribstein J, Mann C, Dareau S: Haemodynamic heterogeneity and treatment with the calcium channel blocker nicardipine during phaeochromocytoma surgery, *Acta Anaesthesiol Scand* 42(9): 1114-1119, 1998.
133. Perry RR, Keiser HR, Norton JA, et al: Surgical management of pheochromocytoma with the use of metyrosine, *Ann Surg* 212(5):621-628, 1990.
134. Pujol J, Viladrich M, Rafecas A, et al: Laparoscopic adrenalectomy: A review of 30 initial cases, *Surg Endosc* 13(5):488-492, 1999.
135. Joris JL, Hamoir EE, Hartstein GM, et al: Hemodynamic changes and catecholamine release during laparoscopic adrenalectomy for pheochromocytoma, *Anesth Analg* 88(1):16-21, 1999.
136. Col V, de Canniere L, Collard E, Michel L, Donckier J: Laparoscopic adrenalectomy for pheochromocytoma: endocrinological and surgical aspects of a new therapeutic approach, *Clin Endocrinol (Oxf)* 50(1):121-125, 1999.
137. Gagner M, Breton G, Pharand D, Pomp A: Is laparoscopic adrenalectomy indicated for pheochromocytoma? *Surgery* 120(6):1076-1079, 1996.
138. Fraley DS, Lemoncelli GL, Coleman A: Severe hypertension associated with pancuronium bromide, *Anesth Analg* 7:265-267, 1978.
139. Plouin PF, Menard J, Corvol P: Hypertensive crisis in patient with pheochromocytoma given metoclopramide, *Lancet* 2:1357, 1976.
140. Zakowski M, Kaufman B, Berguson P, Tissot M, Yarmush L, Turndorf H: Esmolol use during resection of pheochromocytoma: report of 3 cases, *Anesthesiology* 70:875-877, 1989.
141. James MF: Use of magnesium sulfate in the anaesthetic management of phaeochromocytoma: a review of 17 anaesthetics, *Br J Anaesth* 62:616-623, 1989.
142. Levin H, Heefetz M: Phaeochromocytoma and severe protracted postoperative hypoglycaemia, *Can J Anaesth* 37:477-478, 1990.
143. Allen GC, Rosenberg H: Pheochromocytoma presenting as acute malignant hyperthermia: a diagnostic challenge, *Can J Anaesth* 37:593-595, 1990.
144. Guyton AC, Hall JE: The thyroid metabolic hormones. In Guyton AC, Hall JE, editors: *Textbook of Medical Physiology*, Philadelphia, 2000, Saunders, ed 10, p 858.
145. Genuth SM: The thyroid glands. In Berne RM, Levy MN, editors: *Physiology*, ed 4, St Louis, 1998, Mosby, p 910.
146. Babad AA, Eger EI: The effects of hyperthyroidism and hypothyroidism on halothane and oxygen requirements in dogs, *Anesthesiology* 29:1087-1093, 1969.
147. Bilezikian J, Loeb JN: The influence of hyperthyroidism and hypothyroidism on alpha and beta adrenergic receptor systems and adrenergic responsiveness, *Endocr Rev* 4:378, 1983.
148. Smith BR, McLachlan SM, Furmaniak J: Autoantibodies to the thyrotropin receptor, *Endocr Rev* 9:106-120, 1988.
149. Caruso DR, Mazzaferri EL: Intervention in Graves' disease: choosing among imperfect but effective treatment options, *Postgrad Med* 92:117-134, 1992.
150. Surks MI, Sievert R: Drugs and thyroid function. *N Engl J Med.* 333:1688, 1995.
151. Farwell AP, Ebner SA: Thyroid Gland Disorders. In Noble J, editor: *Textbook of Primary Care Medicine*, ed 3, Mosby, St Louis, 2001, p 843.
152. Surks M, Chopra IJ, Mariash CN, Nicoloff JT, Solomon DH: American Thyroid Association Guidelines for the use of laboratory tests in thyroid disease, *JAMA* 263(11):1529-1532, 1990.
153. Gittoes NJL, Franklyn JA: Hyperthyroidism: Current treatment guidelines, *Drugs* 55:543, 1998.
154. Franklyn JA: The management of hyperthyroidism, *N Engl J Med*, 330:1731, 1994.
155. Geffner DL, Hershman JM: Beta-adrenergic blockade for the treatment of hyperthyroidism, *Am J Med* 93:61, 1992.
156. Tsuruta M, Nagayama Y, Yokoyama N, Izumi M, Nagataki S: Long-term follow-up studies on iodine-131 treatment of hyperthyroid Graves' disease based on the measurement of thyroid volume by ultrasonography, *Ann Nucl Med* 7:193-197, 1993.
157. Shaha AR: Surgery for benign thyroid disease causing tracheoesophageal compression, *Otolaryngol Clin North Am* 23:391-401, 1990.
158. Kaplan JA, Cooperman LH: Alarming reactions to Ketamine in patients taking thyroid medication: treatment with propranolol, *Anesthesiology* 35:229-230, 1971.
159. Valcavi R, Menozzi C, Roti E, et al: Sinus node function in hyperthyroid patients, *J Clin Endocrinol Metab* 75:239-242, 1992.
160. Robson NJ: Emergency surgery complicated by thyrotoxicosis and thyrotoxic periodic paralysis, *Anaesthesia* 40:27-31, 1985.
161. Bennett MH, Wainwright AP: Acute thyroid crisis on induction of anaesthesia, *Anaesthesia* 44:28-30, 1989.
162. Thorne AC, Bedford RF: Esmolol for perioperative management of thyrotoxic goiter, *Anesthesiology* 71:291-294, 1989.
163. Lindsay RS, Toft AD: Hypothyroidism, *Lancet* 349:413, 1997.
164. Toft AD: Subclinical hypothyroidism, *N Engl J Med* 345:512-516, 2001.
165. Mokshagundam S, Barzel SE: Thyroid disease in the elderly, *J Am Geriatr Soc* 41:1361-1369, 1993.
166. Kabadi VM, Kumar SP: Pericardial effusion in primary hypothyroidism, *Am Heart J* 120:1393-1395, 1990.
167. Whitten CW, Latson TW, Klein KW, Elmore J, Spencer R, Duggar P: Anesthetic management of a hypothyroid cardiac surgical patient (review), *J Cardiothorac Vasc Anesth* 5:156-159, 1991.
168. Kunos G, Vermes-Kunos I, Nickerson M: Effects of thyroid state on adrenoreceptor properties, *Nature* 250:779-781, 1974.

169. Bemben DA, Winn P, Hamm RM, Morgan L, Davis A, Barton E: Thyroid disease in the elderly: prevalence of undiagnosed hypothyroidism, *J Fam Pract* 38(6):577-582, 1994.
170. Bemben DA, Hamm RM, Morgan L, Winn P, Davis A, Barton E: Thyroid disease in the elderly: predictability of subclinical hypothyroidism, *J Fam Pract* 38(6):583-588, 1994.
171. Toft AD: Thyroxine therapy. *N Engl J Med.* 331:174, 1994.
172. Murkin JM: Anesthesia and hypothyroidism: a review of thyroxine physiology, pharmacology, and anesthetic implications, *Anesth Analg* 61(4): 371-383, 1982.
173. Franklyn JA, Daykin J, Betteridge J, et al: Thyroxine replacement therapy and circulating lipid concentrations, *Clin Endocrinol (Oxf)* 38(5):453-459, 1993.
174. Meares N, Braude S, Burgess K: Massive macroglossia as a presenting feature of hypothyroid-associated pericardial effusion, *Chest* 104:1632-1633, 1993.
175. Miller LR, Benumof JL, Alexander L, Miller CA, Stein D: Completely absent response to peripheral nerve stimulation in an acutely hypothyroid patient: case reports, *Anesthesiology* 7:779-781, 1989.

CHAPTER 32

Hematology and Anesthesia

Francis R. Gerbasi

HEMOSTASIS

Hemostasis is a process that stops bleeding and prevents the loss of blood from vessels. This process is complex and involves the combined activity of vascular, platelet, and plasma factors counterbalanced by regulatory mechanisms to limit the accumulation of platelets and fibrin in the area of injury. Hemostatic abnormalities can lead to excessive bleeding or thrombosis.[1]

Blood Vessel Wall

The blood vessel wall is composed of four layers: the endothelial lining, the subendothelial connective tissue layer, the muscular layer, and the adventitia. In the past, the *endothelial cell lining* was considered primarily a vascular barrier with a nonthrombogenic surface. It is now known that the endothelial cells have an important role in the modulation of hemostasis, thrombosis, and vascular permeability. The endothelial cell modulates hemostasis by synthesizing and secreting prostaglandins, especially prostacyclin, von Willebrand's factor, type IV procollagen, tissue plasminogen activator (t-PA), tissue plasminogen activator inhibitor (t-PAI), thrombomodulin, protein S, fibronectin, proteoglycans, and thromboplastin.

The diversity of the substances synthesized reflects the endothelial cell's ability to promote procoagulant as well as anticoagulant activity. The thromboresistance of the endothelial lining has been characterized as "nature's prototype for blood compatible surfaces."[2] The luminal surface of the endothelial cell has an endocapillary layer known as a *glycocalyx*. The glycocalyx is composed of intrinsic membrane glycoproteins, glycolipids, membrane-associated polysaccharides, and glycosaminoglycans. Among the glycosaminoglycans are sialic acid residues and heparan sulfate. Heparan sulfate is structurally similar to the anticoagulant heparin and, with antithrombin III, may serve to inhibit blood clotting. α_2-Macroglobulin also is found in the vascular lining. It is a potent antiprotease and may inactivate clotting factors.

The endothelial cell also inhibits platelet aggregation by several mechanisms. Primarily, the endothelial cell synthesizes prostacyclin (prostaglandin I_2 [PGI_2]), which is a potent antiaggregator and vasodilator. Endothelial cell injury and activation of the coagulation sequence stimulate the endothelial cell surrounding the injury to synthesize prostacyclin. In addition, the endothelial cell synthesizes plasminogen activators and inhibitors of blood coagulation, especially thrombomodulin and protein S. The plasminogen activators promote fibrinolytic activity in the blood, clear fibrin deposits from the endothelial surface, and dissolve intravascular thrombi.

In contrast, the endothelial cell can promote thrombosis through its secretory activities. The endothelial cell releases substances that activate either the coagulation sequence or platelets. Injury to the endothelium results in the release of tissue factor (thromboplastin), which activates the clotting system. The endothelial cell can also synthesize and secrete von Willebrand's factor. Von Willebrand's factor is a necessary cofactor for the adherence of platelets to subendothelial components.

The second layer of the vessel wall, the *subendothelial connective tissue*, consists of a basement membrane, elastin, and microfibrils. Collagen and fibronectin also are found throughout this layer. Collagen is a potent stimulus for platelet attachment, whereas fibronectin facilitates the anchoring of fibrin during the formation of a hemostatic plug. Damage to the endothelial cell barrier exposes a highly thrombogenic subendothelium, which activates hemostasis.

The flow of blood through a vessel is primarily determined by the degree of contraction of the third layer of the vessel wall, the *muscular layer*. Injury to a vessel causes acute vascular contraction, which decreases blood flow at the site of injury. Neurogenic mechanisms and vasoactive products released from platelets, such as epinephrine and serotonin, mediate vasoconstriction. A decrease in the diameter of the blood vessel retards blood loss and facilitates the formation of a primary hemostatic plug.

Platelets

Although the platelets are the smallest cellular elements in the blood (2 μm in diameter), they play a primary role in hemostasis. A platelet's plasma membrane serves as a physical barrier between the platelet's cytoplasm and the surrounding plasma. Located in the platelet membrane are receptors for substances such as thrombin, collagen, adenosine diphosphate (ADP), prostaglandins I_2 and D_2, prostacyclins, von Willebrand's factor, 5-hydroxytryptamine, fibrinogen, α-adrenergic agents, and endotoxins. Some of these substances (e.g., thrombin, collagen, ADP) activate platelets, whereas others such as prostacyclin (PGI_2) inhibit platelet activity. When activated, platelets exhibit a specific activation process that includes adhesion and morphologic transformation, secretion, and aggregation.

Damage to a blood vessel causes the rapid activation and attachment of platelets to the injured surface (Fig. 32-1). The adherence of platelets to the subendothelium involves the platelet membrane, substrate surface, and plasma cofactors. Three major glycoproteins (Ib, IIb, and IIIa) have been identified on the platelet membrane and appear to have a role in platelet adhesion. A defect in the group I glycoproteins causes

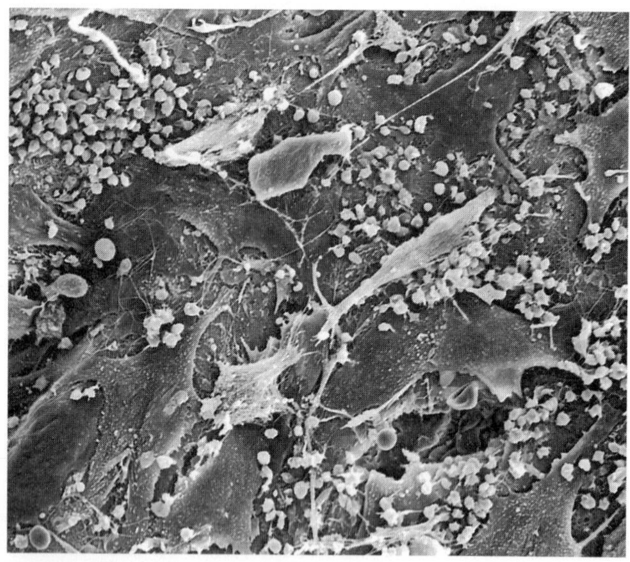

FIGURE **32-1**
Electron microscopic view of a damaged blood vessel showing platelet aggregation and attachment. (Photo courtesy of Marilyn L. Seymour HTL, William Beaumont Hospital, Royal Oak, Michigan.)

a reduction in platelet adhesion in patients with Bernard-Soulier disease. Other important plasma cofactors for platelet adhesion include von Willebrand's factor and calcium. Following adhesion, the attached platelets undergo a morphologic transformation that results in complete coverage of the damaged area. At this time, the platelets secrete the contents of their α-granules and dense bodies. The α-granules contain fibrinogen, fibronectin, platelet-derived growth factor, platelet factor 4, and β-thromboglobulin. It appears that fibronectin mediates platelet adhesion to collagen. The dense bodies contain ADP, ionized calcium, histamine, epinephrine, and serotonin. The secretion of these substances attracts additional platelets to the site of injury and activates the intrinsic coagulation pathway.

When platelets adhere and aggregate at a site of injury, they form the *first hemostatic plug*. This plug temporarily seals the site of injury; however, its structure is not sufficient for permanent repair. A more permanent plug results from the activation of the coagulation system. Thrombin produced concomitantly with ADP and thromboxane A_2 induces contraction of the primary platelet plug. Thrombin also produces fibrin at the site of injury. The fibrin, in conjunction with factor XIIIa, forms the stable *second hemostatic plug*. See Figure 32-2.

Blood Coagulation System

The blood coagulation system is complex. More than 20 substances with either procoagulant or anticoagulant activity participate in this process. The *coagulation cascade* represents the activation of blood zymogens by proteolytic enzymes, which convert these precursors into active enzymes that activate the next zymogens.

The coagulation cascade has been divided into two separate pathways (Fig. 32-3). The coagulation factors are listed in Table 32-1. The intrinsic pathway is initiated with the activation of factor XII. In vivo activation of the *intrinsic pathway* is normally initiated by changes in the endothelial cell surface or following the exposure of subendothelial components such as collagen. The *extrinsic pathway* is activated by the release of tissue thromboplastin, which occurs following damage to endothelial cells and other tissue. An important reaction for both pathways is the conversion of prothrombin to thrombin. Thrombin converts fibrinogen to fibrin; activates factor VIII, factor V, and factor XIII; and stimulates platelet aggregation. Thrombin's activity thus provides a positive feedback for the acceleration of clotting.

Activation of the intrinsic system results in the activation of three separate but interrelated systems. Activation of factor XII occurs whenever the factor "contacts" a nonendothelial surface (e.g., a negatively charged surface, injured endothelium, or collagen). In this process, factor XII changes its molecular configuration. This results in a biologic activity factor (factor XIIa). Factor XIIa interacts with high-molecular-weight kininogen and converts prekallikrein to kallikrein. High-molecular-weight kininogen is important in the optimal placement of the factor XII substrate on the contact area. Kallikrein converts more factor XII to XIIa, and both kallikrein and XIIa activate factor XI. Both enzymes also can convert plasminogen to plasmin, and plasmin can activate the complement system by cleaving C1, C2, C3, and C4 components. Kallikrein likewise converts high-molecular-weight kininogen to kinins, especially the vasoactive inflammatory and vasomediator bradykinin. Once factor XIa is formed, it converts factor IX to its active serine protease, factor IXa. However, this reaction and the remaining reactions of the cascade require the presence of calcium ions. Interaction of factor IXa with cofactor VIII, calcium ions, and a phospholipid surface (provided by activated platelets) yields the activation of factor X. Factor X also is converted to its active protease (factor Xa) by a complex composed of tissue thromboplastin, factor VIIa, and calcium ions. The latter activation represents the extrinsic pathway.

All necessary components for the extrinsic pathway are present in the plasma except tissue thromboplastin, which is released from injured tissues. Factor Xa in conjunction with cofactor V, calcium ions, and phospholipid surfaces converts prothrombin to thrombin.

The final phase of blood clotting is the interaction of thrombin with fibrinogen, which forms fibrin monomers. Fibrinogen is composed of a pair of alpha, beta, and gamma chains. During the first stage of this reaction, two fibrinopeptide A peptides are released from both alpha chains. This allows end-to-end association of the molecules. Following this, two fibrinopeptide B peptides are removed from the beta chains; this allows lateral association of the fibrin monomer molecules. Fibrin monomers combine and form fibrin polymers, which are cross-linked into an insoluble clot by factor XIIIa.

Fibrinolytic System

An intricate system of checks and balances maintains the blood in a fluid state and localizes clotting. The control mechanisms that ensure this balance include the inhibition of activated proteases, the depletion of clotting factors, and fibrinolysis. Normally, a number of protease inhibitors are present in the blood, keeping the hemostatic process localized by inactivating coagulation enzymes. Antithrombin III is the most important inhibitor of blood coagulation. Antithrombin has a wide spectrum of antiprotease activities and inhibits not only thrombin but also factors XIIa, XIa, IXa, Xa, and VIIa. In the presence of heparin, antithrombin's reaction with the clotting enzymes is enhanced several hundred–fold. Each molecule of antithrombin binds to one enzyme molecule. The rate of

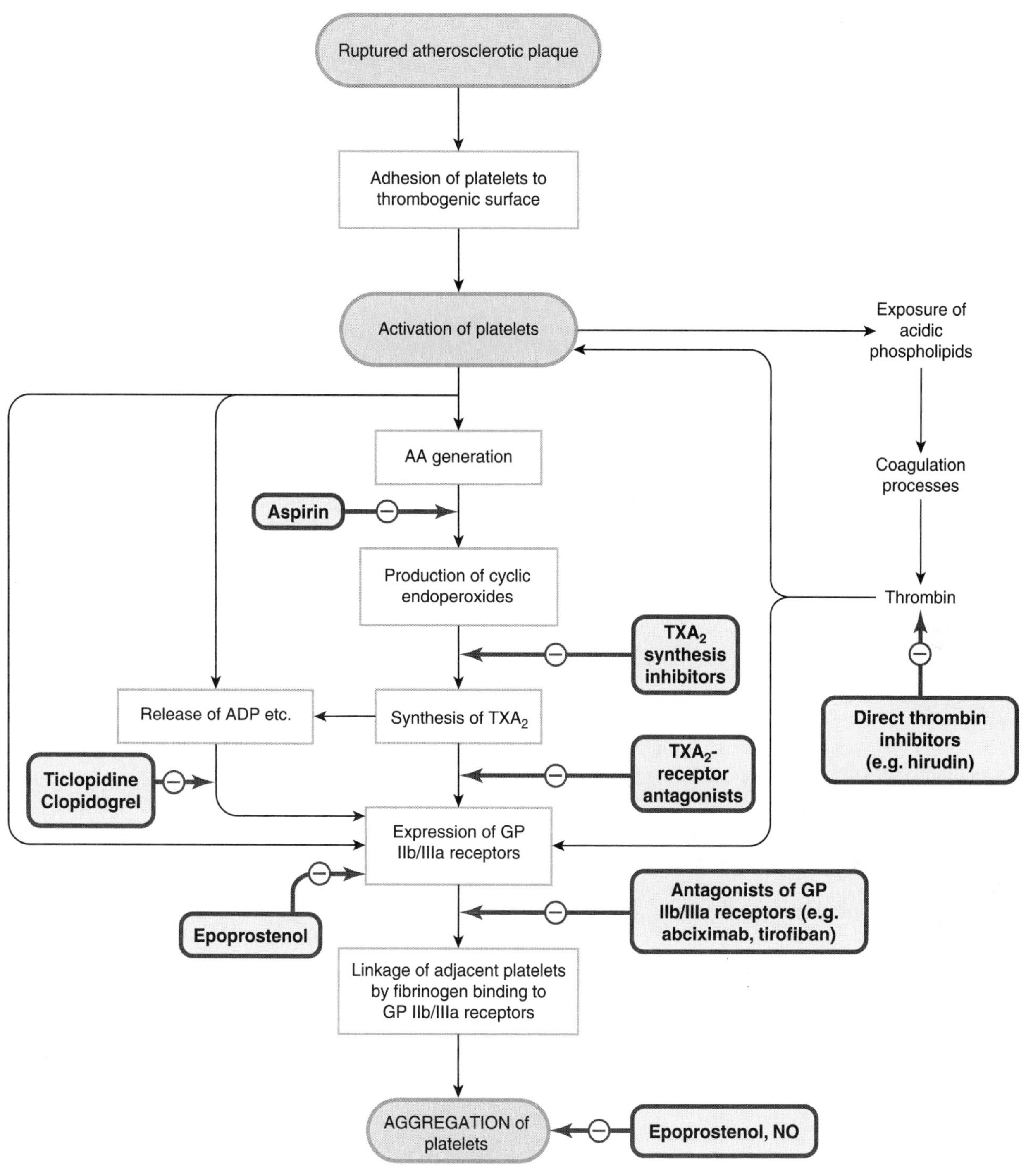

FIGURE **32-2**
Platelet activation. (From Rang HP, Dale MM, Ritter JM: *Pharmacology*, ed 5, Edinburgh, Scotland, 2003, Churchill Livingstone, p 324.)

complex formation with heparin is instantaneous. Heparin may dissociate from the thrombin-antithrombin complex and catalyze another round of thrombin-antithrombin interaction. The importance of antithrombin is apparent from numerous reports of families in which heterozygous antithrombin deficient members have a high incidence of recurrent venous thromboembolic disease (thrombophilia).

Other inhibitors of clotting include C1 inactivator protein, α_2-macroglobulin, α_1-antitrypsin, protein C, and protein S. In vivo, proteins C and S probably are the only ones with a significant regulatory function of clotting. Protein C is a vitamin K–dependent protein that circulates in the blood as a zymogen. It is converted to an active protease by thrombin in the presence of the endothelial cell–bound cofactor thrombomodulin. The activated form, protein Ca, is a powerful inhibitor of factors Va and VIIIa. It also stimulates fibrinolysis by proteolytically destroying plasminogen activator inhibitor. For these proteolytic actions, protein Ca requires protein S as a cofactor. Protein S, a vitamin K–dependent protein, also is an inhibitor of the membrane attack complex of human

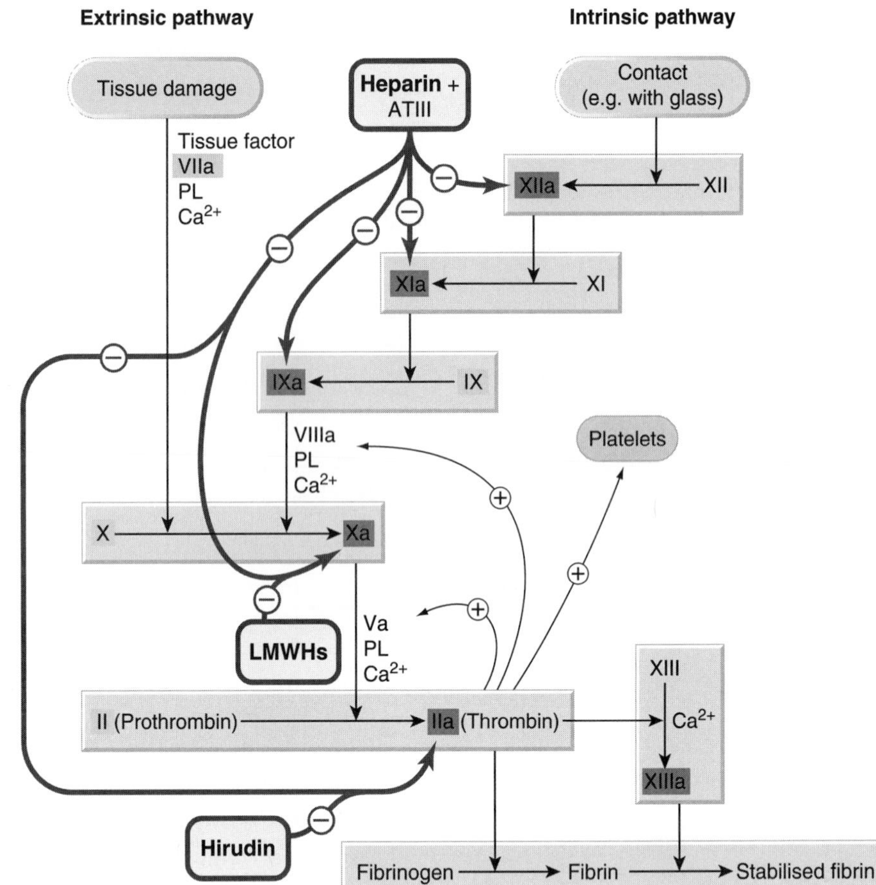

FIGURE **32-3**
The coagulation cascade: sites of action of anticoagulant drugs. (From Rang HP, Dale MM, Ritter JM: *Pharmacology*, ed 5, Edinburgh, Scotland, 2003, Churchill Livingstone, p 316.)

complement. Several families have been described in whom some members had protein C or protein S deficiency. These individuals suffered from recurrent thromboembolic events and were clinically indistinguishable from those with antithrombin deficiency.

Another important regulator mechanism of clotting is the removal of fibrin via enzymatic destruction by plasmin. Plasmin can be formed from plasminogen by factor XIIa, kallikrein, and other tissue activator substances (Fig. 32-4). Other nonphysiologic plasminogen activator substances include urokinase and streptokinase.

Tissue plasminogen activator has been obtained from various sources, including vascular perfusates, blood collected after exercise, and uterine tissue. Tissue plasminogen activator is

TABLE **32-1** Blood Coagulation Factors

Factor[a]	Synonym	Biologic Half-Life	Blood Product Source
I	Fibrinogen	100-150 h	Cryoprecipitate (200-300 mg/bag)
II	Prothrombin	50-80 h	FFP, PCC
V	Proaccelerin	24 h	FFP
VII	Proconvertin	6 h	Recombinant VIIa, FFP, PCC
VIII	Antihemophilic factor	12 h	FFP, PCC, factor concentrates, cryoprecipitate
IX	Christmas factor	24 h	FFP, PCC, factor concentrates
X	Stuart-Prower factor	25-60 h	FFP, PCC
XI	Plasma thromboplastin Antecedent	40-80 h	FFP
XII	Hageman factor	50-70 h	
XIII	Fibrin-stabilizing factor	150 h	FFP, cryoprecipitate

[a] *Coagulation factors are numbered with Roman numerals in order of their discovery. Factor III (tissue factor) and factor IV (calcium ions) have been omitted. There is no factor VI. PCC, prothrombin complex concentrate; FFP, fresh-frozen plasma.*
Adapted from Bickert B, Kwiatkowsy JL: Coagulation disorders. In DiPiro JT, Talbert RL, Yee GC, et al, editors: Pharmacotherapy: A Pathophysiologic Approach, *ed 5, New York, 2002, McGraw-Hill, p 1748.*

produced by endothelial cells and is released in response to various stimuli such as exercise, hypotension, and pharmacologic agents. The gene for human tissue plasminogen activator has been cloned and has made tissue plasminogen activator treatment possible in acute thromboembolic events.

Urokinase is a trypsinlike protease that activates plasminogen directly to form plasmin. Urokinase is secreted in an inactive form (prourokinase) that can be activated by plasmin. Streptokinase is a nonenzymatic protein not normally present in plasma but that is obtained from streptococcal cultures. Both streptokinase and urokinase are widely used as thrombolytic agents. Plasminogen activators cleave plasminogen peptide bonds to form plasmin, a two-chain enzyme. Plasmin cleaves fibrinogen and fibrin to yield fragments (fibrin[ogen] split products) that are no longer capable of forming a fibrin network. The fragments of fibrin produced as a result of plasmin degradation are designated X, Y, D, and E; the last two of these represent the major end products. The fibrin(ogen) split products act as anticoagulants by competitively inhibiting thrombin, by interfering with the polymerization of fibrin, and by interfering with platelet aggregation.

Another unique plasmin-derived cross-linked fibrin fragment, the D-dimer, is important in the clinical diagnosis of intravascular clotting processes, such as disseminated intravascular coagulation. The D-dimer represents a cross-linked chain remnant of fibrin and is composed of two cross-linked D-domains and one E-domain. The presence of D-dimer in plasma indicates that thrombin was there to form fibrin and that plasmin dissolved the fibrin.

The fibrinolytic system may be regulated at the level of plasmin or at the level of plasminogen activators (see Fig. 32-4). A specific rapid-acting inhibitor of tissue plasminogen activator has been identified. It is present in normal human plasma at low concentrations but at higher concentrations in some pathologic states. Higher levels have been noted in patients with severe liver disease, pancreatitis, malignancy, myocardial infarction, or deep vein thrombosis. Nilsson and Tengborn[3] first reported a family with defective fibrinolysis due to a five- to 50-fold greater tissue plasminogen activator inhibitor capacity. In addition, a number of patients with elevated tissue plasminogen activator inhibitor levels and thromboembolisms have been reported.

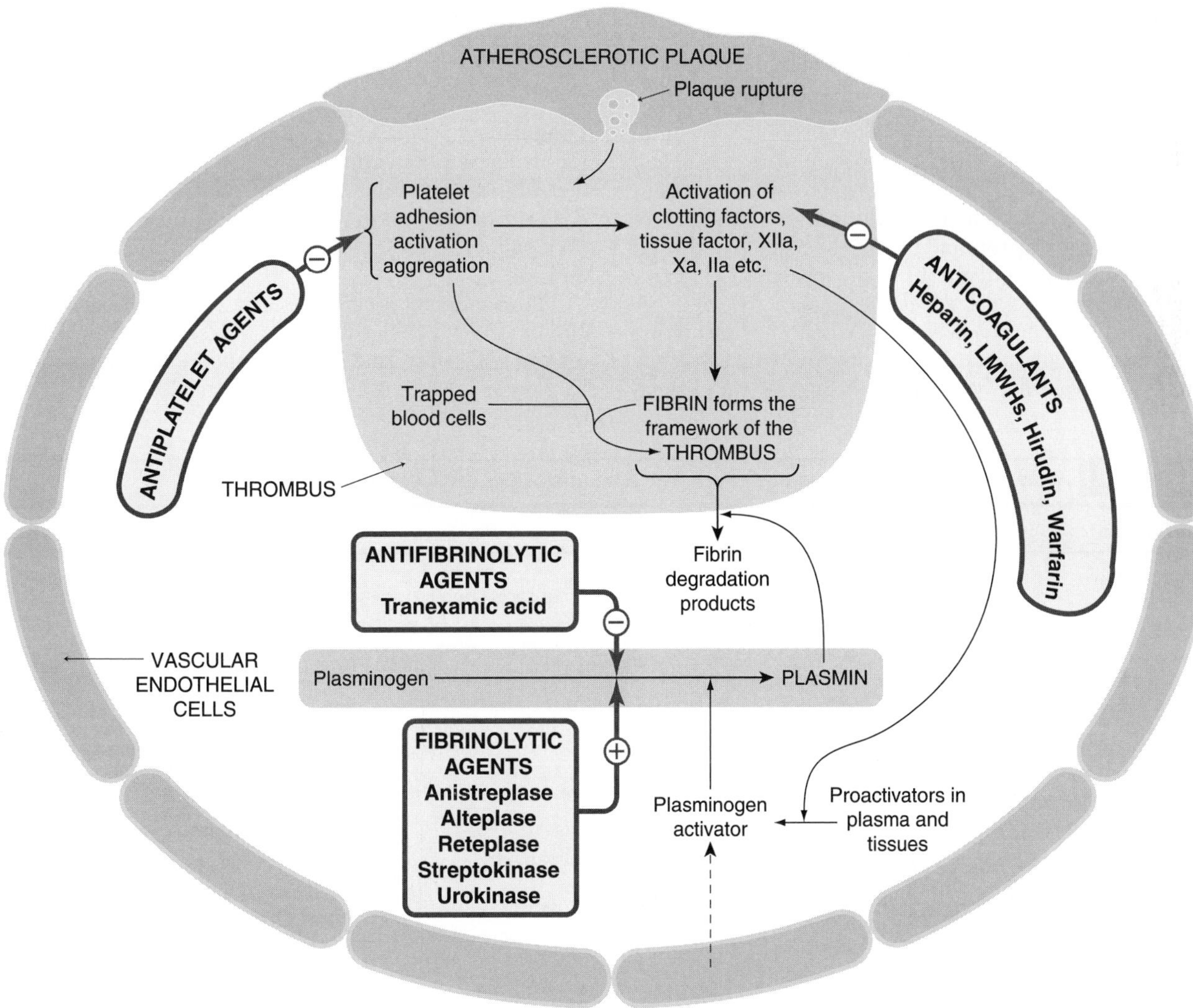

FIGURE **32-4**
Fibrinolytic system. (From Rang HP, Dale MM, Ritter JM: *Pharmacology*, ed 5, Edinburgh, Scotland, 2003, Churchill Livingstone, p 327.)

α_2-Antiplasmin is the plasma protein inhibitor of plasmin. The reaction of α_2-antiplasmin with plasmin results in the formation of an inactive complex. α_2-Antiplasmin also may be an important inhibitor of fibrin clot destruction by plasmin. Other inhibitors of plasmin are α_1-macroglobulin and α_1-antitrypsin. Fibrinolysis is regulated by the interaction of these components. Normally, very little plasminogen activation is noted in plasma. However, when fibrin is formed, plasminogen activators and plasminogen absorb to the fibrin, and plasmin is generated. The plasmin complex formed with fibrin is only slowly inactivated by α_2-antiplasmin, whereas the plasmin released into plasma is rapidly and irreversibly neutralized. The fibrinolytic process is normally triggered by and confined to fibrin. Thrombus formation may occur as the result of insufficient activation of the fibrinolytic system or the presence of excess inhibitors, whereas excessive activation of the fibrinolytic system or a deficiency of inhibitors might cause excessive plasmin formation and a tendency for bleeding.

The clearance of activated clotting factors is another important anticlotting mechanism. Activated factors are primarily cleared by the liver and the reticuloendothelial system. If venous stasis exists, activated factors remain in the vessel and may contribute to thrombosis.

A thrombus is likely to form when the vessel wall endothelium has been injured, when blood flow is decreased, or when alterations in the blood foster a state of hypercoagulability. Endothelial damage is seen in atherosclerosis and the hemodynamic stress of hypertension or when chemical agents (presented by cigarette smoke or hypercholesterolemia), bacterial toxins, or immunologic injuries are encountered. Stasis and sluggish venous drainage greatly contribute to the venous thrombosis. They prevent hepatic dilution and clearance of activated coagulation factors and permit the buildup of thrombin in the vessels. Also, alterations in the regulation of hemostasis may predispose to the development of a thrombus. A state of hypercoagulability may exist when the circulating blood requires a smaller quantity of clot-promoting substance to induce intravascular coagulation. Suggestive clinical evidence of a state of hypercoagulability includes thrombocytopenia; reduced levels of antithrombin III, protein C, and protein S; and decreased fibrinolytic activity.

In summary, the hemostasis system normally is in a state of dynamic equilibrium that maintains the vascular integrity and prevents pathologic thrombus formation. Alterations in the various components can predispose to bleeding or thrombosis. Hemostatic disorders can be caused by a variety of abnormal conditions (e.g., malignancy and sepsis) or by drugs. Disturbances in the hemostasis process may be shown clinically as bleeding, bruising, or a tendency for thrombosis. These disturbances can be acquired or inherited and encompass defects in the platelets, coagulation, and the fibrinolytic systems. A thorough history taking and physical examination identify most patients with bleeding or thrombotic tendencies. Several in vitro laboratory studies can be used for identifying the precise nature of the disorders.

Anesthetic Implications

The anesthetist should be familiar with the detection, evaluation, and treatment of hemostatic disorders. An undetected preoperative bleeding tendency can lead to life-threatening blood loss during surgery. Because it may be difficult for the anesthetist to acquire experience in detecting and managing bleeding disorders due to their relatively infrequent occurrence and complexity, the following section describes a practical approach to the detection and management of hemostatic disorders.

Coagulation Studies. Coagulation tests are primarily used for evaluating the ability of the hemostasis system to prevent bleeding and control traumatic hemorrhage. The platelets, coagulation, and fibrinolytic components can be screened with the commonly available coagulation tests shown in Table 32-2 and Table 32-3.

Platelet function can be evaluated on the basis of platelet counts (PCs) and bleeding times (BTs). PCs normally are performed with electronic instrumentation. Errors may occur due to platelet clumping or variations in platelet size, and large

TABLE 32-2 Commonly Used Hemostasis Values for Screening Specific Components

System/Function	Parameter	Values
Platelet function	BT	Normal: 2-9 min Abnormal: >12 min
	PC	Normal: 200,000450,000/mm³ Problem: <100,000/mm³ Surgical risk: <50,000/mm³ Spontaneous bleeding: <20,000/mm³
Coagulation system: intrinsic	APTT	Normal: 25-32 sec (reagent dependent) Abnormal: >35 sec
Coagulation system: extrinsic	PT	Normal: control Abnormal: >3 sec above control
Coagulation system: end stage	TT	Normal: 10-12 sec (reagent dependent) Abnormal: >15 sec
Fibrinolytic system	Fibrinogen	Normal: 200-350 mg/mL Abnormal: <100 mg/mL
	Fibrin(ogen) degradation products	Normal: <10 mcg/mL Questionable: 10-40 mcg/mL Abnormal: >40 mcg/mL

APTT, *Activated partial thromboplastin time;* BT, *bleeding time;* PC, *platelet count;* PT, *prothrombin time;* TT, *thrombin time.*

TABLE 32-3 Laboratory Procedures

Procedure	Identifies	Causes of Prolonged Value	Clinical Manifestations
Bleeding time	Platelet function: adhesion, aggregation, and release	Thrombocytopenia Inherited qualitative platelet defects von Willebrand's disease Uremia Collagen defects Antiplatelet drugs (i.e. aspirin) Factor V deficiency Afibrinogenemia	Bleeding from the gums Easy bruising Bleeding following surgery or tooth extraction Nosebleeds
Prothrombin time (PT)	Factors of common pathway: I, II, V, X Factors of extrinsic pathway: VII	Newborn Vitamin K deficiency Inherited factor deficiencies Warfarin Liver disease Lupus anticoagulant Afibrinogenemia	Bleeding: uterine surgery, childbirth, trauma Bleeding in newborn: umbilical cord, intracranial, gastrointestinal
Activated partial thromboplastin time (aPTT)	Factors of contact phase: HMWK, XII, prekallikrein Factors of intrinsic pathway: VIII, IX, XI	Inherited factor deficiencies Lupus anticoagulant Heparin therapy Liver disease	Increased incidence of thrombotic disease with lupus anticoagulant Joint and muscle bleeding factor deficiencies
	Factors of common Pathway: I, II, V, X	Afibrinogenemia von Willebrand's disease	Mucosal bleeding with von Willebrand's disease
Thrombin time (TT)	Fibrinogen Inhibitors of fibrin aggregation	Afibrinogenemia Heparin therapy	Life-long hemorrhagic disease

HMWK, *high-molecular-weight kininogen*
Adapted from Bickert B, Kwiatkowsy JL: Coagulation disorders. In DiPiro JT, Talbert RL, Yee GC, et al, editors: Pharmacotherapy: A Pahtophysiologic Approach, *ed 5, New York, 2002, McGraw-Hill, p 1749.*

platelets may be interpreted as red blood cells (RBCs). This results in falsely low PCs. Occasionally, platelets may aggregate when blood is collected in ethylenediaminetetraacetic acid (EDTA), resulting in "pseudothrombocytopenia." Collection in sodium citrate corrects the problem. Hemostasis is competent with counts greater than 100,000/mm^3, provided that the platelets are functioning. Preoperatively, PCs less than 100,000/mm^3 warrant further hematologic investigation, and counts less than 50,000/mm^3 place a patient at risk for increased operative bleeding. Spontaneous bleeding may occur when counts are less than 20,000/mm^3. A direct relationship between the severity of surgical bleeding and PC has been demonstrated.[4]

BTs provide a good measure of primary hemostasis; however, BTs may be inaccurate when obtained improperly or during surgery. BT is used for identifying both quantitative and qualitative platelet disorders. The currently used template procedure is more sensitive than older methods.[5] Prolonged BTs are seen when PCs are less than 100,000/mm^3, in qualitative (dysfunctional) platelet disorders, and in von Willebrand's disease (VWD). The most common causes of platelet abnormality are drugs, especially aspirin, which inhibits platelet function. Thrombocytopenia, disorders of platelet functions, and von Willebrand's disease may prolong the bleeding time. In the absence of drug ingestion, a prolonged BT suggests abnormal primary hemostasis and warrants further investigation.

The clotting system can be screened on the basis of activated partial thromboplastin time (APTT), prothrombin time (PT), and thrombin time (TT). These parameters, determined in vitro, reflect the ability of the blood to coagulate and can be used to screen a specific pathway of the coagulation cascade. Prolonged times suggest a potential tendency for bleeding.

The APTT is a modification of the old plasma recalcification time and reflects the activity of the intrinsic and common coagulation pathways. The APTT screens for abnormal blood coagulation reactions triggered by exposure of plasma to a negatively charged surface. In the United States, APTT determination is the most commonly used test for monitoring heparin therapy. It can be prolonged by deficiencies of 30% to 40%, abnormalities, or inhibition of any intrinsic (factors XII, XI, IX, VIII, prekallikrein, and high-molecular-weight kininogen) and common pathway (factors II, V, X, and fibrinogen) participants.[6] Only factors VII and XIII are not evaluated on the basis of APTT.

PT is a measure of the extrinsic activation of factor X by the tissue thromboplastin–factor VII complex. The test screens for abnormalities of factors V, VII, and X; prothrombin; and fibrinogen. The normal PT varies between 10 and 12 seconds, depending on the tissue factor reagent and technical details. A PT $\geq$2 seconds longer than a laboratory's normal control value should be considered abnormal and requires further investigation. The PT is valuable in screening for coagulation disorders in various acquired conditions (e.g., vitamin K deficiency, liver disease, disseminated intravascular coagulation [DIC]). The PT is the most commonly used test for monitoring oral anticoagulants, such as coumarin derivatives, which impair the proper production of factors II, VII, IX, and X. The therapeutic range of PT depends on the thromboplastin used in each laboratory. The international normalized ratio (INR normal = 0.9 to 1.1) has been introduced by the World Health Organization (WHO) to standardize control of anticoagulant therapy internationally. The INR is the ratio of patient PT to control PT raised to the power of the international sensitivity index (ISI).[7]

TT is a measure of the conversion of fibrinogen to fibrin by thrombin. It is a screening tool for assessing the end stage of the coagulation cascade. Like the APTT, TT may be used for monitoring heparin therapy. Prolonged TTs are seen in hypofibrinogenemia and dysfibrinogenemia, as well as in the presence of inhibitors, such as elevated levels of fibrin(ogen) degradation products (FDPs) and heparin. Also, the TT is useful in establishing whether a plasma sample contains heparin (residual heparin not neutralized after extracorporeal bypass or blood drawn from a line kept open with a heparin flush). In plasma that contains heparin, the thrombin time will be prolonged, but a repeat test will be normal if the reagent batroxobin (a snake venom enzyme insensitive to heparin that directly converts fibrinogen to fibrin) is substituted for thrombin.

The fibrinolytic system can be screened with measurement of fibrinogen, FDP, and D-dimer levels. The fibrinogen assay measures the quantity of fibrinogen present in plasma. A fibrinogen level lower than 100 mg/dL may be associated with bleeding. A latex agglutination test is used for detecting FDPs, and elevated levels are diagnostic for increased fibrinolytic activity. The D-dimer detects the D-D-E complex of factor XIIIa–stabilized fibrin. The presence of D-D-E complexes indicates clotting and fibrinolytic activity.

As a result of technologic advances, specific hematologic tests for clarifying abnormal screening tests are now available. Such studies include assays for platelet adhesion and aggregation, clot retraction, specific factors and inhibitors, D-dimer, and others. In vivo hemostasis activation can be determined by measuring the end products of clotting (e.g., fibrinopeptide A) and of platelet activation (e.g., β-thromboglobulin and platelet factor 4). Currently, tests for these parameters are not readily available in most hospital laboratories.

Preoperative Assessment. The greatest challenge to the hemostatic system frequently occurs during surgery. Therefore, a patient's hemostatic system should be in optimal condition before surgery.[8] To ensure this, one may use routine preoperative coagulation screening (see Table 32-2); however, such screening may be unnecessary in patients whose history and physical findings do not suggest a hemostatic disorder.[9]

The best method for identifying patients with bleeding or thrombosing tendencies is a *thorough* history taking and physical examination.[10] During history taking, the clinician may ask the patient to answer specific questions directed at identifying a problem with hemostasis. Physical findings such as mucous membrane hemorrhages, petechiae, epistaxis, and bruising suggest platelet or von Willebrand's disease. Coagulation tests may then be ordered based on the history and physical findings (Table 32-4). Despite a history or physical finding of bleeding, the results of coagulation screening tests may be normal. The APTT may be normal as long as factor levels are greater than 30% and in patients with mild von Willebrand's disease. Nevertheless, these patients are at risk of increased bleeding during surgery. Therefore a bleeding disorder should be diagnosed preoperatively.

TABLE 32-4 Indications for Preoperative Coagulation Studies*

Indication	PT/APTT	PC	BT
History			
Thrombocytopenia, splenectomy, prosthetic heart valves		X	
Chronic renal failure, splenic disease, platelet dysfunction, radiation therapy		X	X
Prolonged bleeding and easy bruising	X	X	X
Cirrhosis, jaundice, intestinal bypass for obesity	X	X	X
Metastatic carcinoma, thrombosis, family history of coagulopathy	X	X	X
Physical examination findings			
Hepatomegaly, nodular liver, ascites, jaundice	X	X	X
Petechiae, ecchymosis, splenomegaly	X	X	X
Medications			
Aspirin, dipyridamole (Persantine), antibiotics, antihistamines, sulfasalazine, nonsteroidal antiinflammatory drugs			X
Oral anticoagulants (coumarin derivatives)	X		
Heparin	X	X	
Laboratory results			
Decreased albumin, total protein	X		
Increased bilirubin, aspartate transaminase, alkaline phosphatase	X	X	X
Decreased hemoglobin	X	X	X

APTT, *Activated partial thromboplastin time;* BT, *bleeding time;* PC, *platelet count;* PT, *prothrombin time.*
**X designates suggested studies.*

The preoperative use of drugs, such as nonsteroidal antiinflammatory drugs, amitriptyline, cephalosporins, indomethacin, imipramine, and phenylbutazone, can be associated with a tendency for bleeding. Their ingestion may result in the prolongation of BT. A "safe" BT has not yet been established, but Barber and associates[11] found no excessive bleeding with BTs shorter than 12 minutes. To ensure primary hemostasis, one should withhold aspirin and other nonsteroidal antiinflammatory drugs 10 days to 2 weeks before surgery.[12] If platelet aggregation inhibition is needed, a patient may be placed on dipyridamole; its activity can be reversed within 12 hours when therapy with the drug is discontinued.

Patients with an inherited coagulation disorder (e.g., hemophilia A or B, von Willebrand's disease) must undergo an adequate preoperative coagulation workup in order to ensure surgical hemostasis. Consultation with a hematologist is strongly encouraged to aid in the preoperative preparation and to facilitate intraoperative and postoperative management. The majority of hemophiliacs are identified by the time they reach adulthood and wear a special identification band or tag. Hemophilia A and B are usually treated with factor VIII and IX concentrates, respectively. One unit of factor VIII per kilogram of body weight should increase the factor VIII concentration in plasma by 2%.[13] In the case of factor IX, the plasma concentration increases 1%. Preoperatively, factor levels should be close to

100% if an adequate level is to be maintained during surgery. Patients with von Willebrand's disease may be more difficult to diagnose. The PC and APTT are frequently normal. The only signs suggesting this hemostatic disorder may be a history of bleeding and a prolonged BT. Treatment that includes the administration of deamino-D-arginine vasopressin (DDAVP) and cryoprecipitate is used for increasing the level of factor VIII.

Any unexplained abnormal results of preoperative coagulation tests require thorough investigation and possibly hematologic consultation. Occasionally, despite the importance of knowing the cause of abnormal results, no further studies are undertaken. Causes of a prolonged APTT included poor sampling technique and the presence of "lupus anticoagulant" (anticardiolipin antibody). The patient with a lupus anticoagulant has an increased tendency for thrombosis. A hematologist should be consulted to assist in the management of this patient, who may require low-dose heparin therapy.

Planning anesthetic management in a patient with a known or suspected preoperative bleeding disorder requires special consideration. If general anesthesia is to be used, care must be taken to prevent soft tissue damage during laryngoscopy and endotracheal intubation. Also, uncontrolled bleeding may occur when a nasal endotracheal tube or nasal pharyngeal airway is placed.

Generally, hard and fast rules are impossible to establish for the use of regional anesthesia in patients with bleeding disorders or who are on anticoagulant therapy, but some precautions should be taken. The presence of a gross bleeding disorder, thrombocytopenia (PC less than 100,000/mm^3), or hemorrhage or the use of full-dose preoperative anticoagulant therapy is a relative contraindication to the use of most regional anesthetic techniques (e.g., spinal and epidural blocks). However, both spinal analgesia and epidural analgesia have been used successfully in patients receiving low-dose heparin, provided that the results of laboratory tests were within normal limits. Benzon and colleagues[14] performed epidural and spinal blocks in 100 patients receiving aspirin therapy without any signs or symptoms of hematoma formation. However, Locke and coworkers[15] described a case of epidural hematoma in a patient who received two doses of aspirin. Spinal and epidural analgesia also have been used successfully in patients receiving intraoperative anticoagulant therapy.[16] However, neurologic integrity should be monitored during the intraoperative and postoperative periods.

Anesthesia providers should also be aware of the potential effect of anesthetic agents and techniques on the hemostasis system. Most notably, regional anesthesia has been shown to decrease the incidence of thrombosis following orthopedic surgical procedures.[17]

Intraoperative Assessment. Abnormal intraoperative bleeding can be a life-threatening condition, requiring rapid patient assessment and therapy. Initial actions include the administration of blood components and the performance of coagulation studies. Suggested treatments for intraoperative hemostatic disorders identified on clinical assessment and laboratory results are presented in Table 32-5. The most common reason for intraoperative bleeding is loss of vascular integrity. This type of bleeding usually is localized and must be corrected by the surgeon.

Generalized intraoperative bleeding or oozing may be due to a dilutional coagulopathy, a consumptive coagulopathy (disseminated intravascular coagulation), or a transfusion reaction. Other known causes of intraoperative bleeding include liver disease, vitamin K deficiency, and congenital coagulation abnormalities that should have been identified and appropriately managed preoperatively. Intraoperative coagulation tests can aid in the differential diagnosis. These tests include PCs; measurement of fibrinogen and antithrombin III levels; determination of PT, APTT, FDPs, and D-dimers; and specific factor assays.

Intraoperative dilutional coagulopathy, especially thrombocytopenia (PC less than 100,000/mm^3), usually is the result of massive volume and blood replacement. Studies suggest that the use of packed RBCs for blood replacement is associated with significant decreases in the levels of platelets; fibrinogen; and factors V, VIII, and XI.[18] Also, whole blood stored for longer than 48 hours has no viable platelets. Its use may lead to thrombocytopathy (PC greater than 100,000/mm^3, BT greater than 15 minutes). Treatment may require the transfusion of fresh frozen plasma and platelet concentrates. Coagulation findings suggesting consumptive coagulopathy (disseminated intravascular coagulation) include decreased PCs and fibrinogen levels, prolonged PT or APTT, and increased FDP and D-dimer levels.[19,20]

TABLE 32-5 Possible Causes and Treatment of Hemostatic Disorders

	CLINICAL COAGULATION TESTS						
BL	**APTT**	**PT**	**BT**	**PC**	**Fib**	**Possible Cause**	**Treatment**
–	Abn	–	–	–	–	Factor VIII, heparin, "lupus anticoagulant," poor sample	No treatment
+	Abn	–	–	–	–	Factors XI, IX, VIII, heparin therapy	FFP, protamine
+	Abn	Abn	–	–	–	Factors V, X, II, dysfibrinogenemia, heparin, coumarin	FFP, cryoprecipitate, protamine
+	–	Abn	–	–	–	Factor VII	FFP
+	Abn	–	Abn	–	–	von Willebrand's disease	Desmopressin acetate, cryoprecipitate
+	Abn	Abn	Abn	–	Low	Hypofibrinogenemia	FFP, cryoprecipitate
+	–	–	Abn	Abn	–	Thrombocytopenia	Platelet concentrate (8-10 units)
+	–	–	Abn	–	–	Thrombocytopathy, aspirin, NSAIDs	Platelet concentrate
+	Abn	Abn	Abn	Abn	Abn	DIC, severe liver disease, dilutional coagulopathy	FFP, cryoprecipitate, platelet concentrate, whole blood

Abn, *Abnormal result;* BL, *bleeding;* DIC, *disseminated intravascular coagulation;* FFP, *fresh frozen plasma;* Fib, *fibrinogen;* NSAIDs, *nonsteroidal antiinflammatory drugs;* +, *increased clinical bleeding.*

Disseminated intravascular coagulation (DIC) is the result of systemic activation, and an imbalance in, the coagulation and fibrinolytic systems. It is characterized by a rapid and extensive depletion of coagulation factors and excessive fibrinolysis to compensate for microvascular clotting. Bleeding occurs due to the consumption of coagulation factors during clotting, platelet depletion or dysfunction, interference of fibrin formation, and lysis of clots by plasmin. Acute DIC occurs secondary to a variety of conditions.[21,22] Thirty percent to 50% of patients with gram-negative sepsis may develop DIC. Gram-positive, fungal, and viral infections may also be precipitators. Women in the late stages of pregnancy who present with placental abruption or placenta previa, a dead fetus, or amniotic fluid embolism have a greater than 50% incidence of acute DIC. It is also associated with prolonged surgery, burns, malignancies, certain vascular disorders, chronic liver disease, heatstroke, and acute promyelocytic leukemia. Optimal treatment remains controversial due to the differing mechanisms and clinical presentations. Treatment is primarily supportive and complex but may include administration of cryoprecipitate, fresh frozen plasma, platelets, whole blood, coagulation factors, aminocaproic acid, vitamin K, antibiotics, vasopressors, and anticoagulants.

Certain surgical procedures such as prostatectomy for prostatic carcinoma, liver transplantation, and coronary bypass surgery are frequently associated with intraoperative coagulation abnormalities. Intraoperative coagulation monitoring frequently is used during these types of surgery and in patients requiring intraoperative anticoagulation therapy. The activated coagulation time of whole blood has been used for monitoring heparin therapy during cardiopulmonary bypass (see Chapter 22, Cardiac Anesthesia) and for predicting the protamine dose for heparin neutralization. Studies suggest that the APTT may be a better indicator of heparin reversal. Also, a renewed interest in thromboelastography and Sonoclot coagulation analyzers has occurred. These instruments perform automated intraoperative measurement of clot formation.[23,24]

Postoperative Assessment. The postoperative patient must be monitored closely for signs and symptoms of bleeding or thrombosis. Factors that increase the likelihood of postoperative bleeding include abnormal preoperative clotting and elevated postoperative blood pressure. The most frequent cause of postoperative bleeding is a lack of hemostasis at either a suture line or surgically traumatized tissue. The use of postoperative antibiotics also can increase bleeding. If postoperative bleeding occurs, coagulation tests (see Table 32-2 and 32-3) may be used for screening hemostasis. If test results are normal, the bleeding may be related to a factor XIII deficiency or to a telangiopathy, such as Ehlers-Danlos syndrome. Two common reasons for abnormal postoperative APTT and PT are dilutional coagulopathy and consumption coagulopathy (disseminated intravascular coagulation). If multiple units of banked blood have been given, thrombocytopathy or factor V and VIII deficiencies (or both) may prevail.

Certain types of surgical procedures such as cardiopulmonary bypass surgery are associated with an increased risk of postoperative bleeding that may be due to thrombocytopathy, thrombocytopenia, or inadequate heparin reversal. Decreases in fibrinogen, antithrombin III, plasminogen, and α_2-antiplasmin are always noted (hemodilution) but may exceed the hemodilutional effect.[25] If bleeding is significant, administration of platelet concentrates, fresh frozen plasma, fresh whole blood, or protamine may be necessary.

Patients with an increased risk of thrombosis (e.g., those undergoing total hip replacement or knee replacement) may receive preoperative, intraoperative, and postoperative anticoagulant therapy. Caution must be exercised when epidural analgesia is used in conjunction with anticoagulant therapy. Postoperative care should include continued monitoring of anticoagulant activity and maintenance of normal arterial pressure.[16] Also, motor and sensory function must be evaluated for signs and symptoms of hematoma formation before each dose of local anesthetic is given.

Anesthetic care for the surgical patient with a hemostatic disorder is multifaceted. It requires a thorough preoperative history taking and physical examination; use of coagulation studies; and good communication between the surgeon, the anesthetist, and (if necessary) the hematologist. Hemostatic screening should include coagulation tests for identification of hemostatic defects and guiding treatment. The responsible use of coagulation tests can yield valuable information regarding a patient's hemostatic system and can help in identifying the best method of treatment.

HEMATOLOGIC DISORDERS

Anemia is characterized by a hemoglobin concentration that is less than normal for an individual's age and sex. It is a common hematologic disorder that decreases the oxygen-carrying capacity and reserve against tissue hypoxia. Causes of anemia include iron deficiency anemia, megaloblastic anemia, vitamin B_{12} and folate deficiency, hemolytic anemia, and sickle cell disease. Mild asymptomatic anemia is not considered the absolute contraindication to anesthesia and surgery that it was in the past. Recent practice surveys reveal that many clinicians do not consider transfusion for nonischemic, otherwise stable, patients whose hemoglobin is above 8 g/dL.[26]

Preoperatively, anemic patients must be evaluated for their ability to compensate by increasing their cardiac output, especially with acute blood loss. Signs and symptoms of lack of compensation include dyspnea, tachycardia, congestive heart failure, and angina. The decision to transfuse the patient must be individualized.

Anesthesia management should minimize drug-induced decreases in cardiac output or leftward shift of the oxygen dissociation curve. Symptoms of a blood loss greater than 20% of the blood volume include decreased central venous pressure, decreased blood pressure, and increased heart rate. Treatment for acute blood loss includes administration of blood products and crystalloid solutions.

Sickle cell disease is one of the more commonly encountered hemoglobinopathies. It is an inherited disease in which valine replaces glutamic acid at the sixth-position beta chain of hemoglobin. Desaturated hemoglobin S is 50% less solvent than desaturated hemoglobin A. The desaturated hemoglobin S forms long, rigid stacks that clump together.

Individuals may have either sickle cell trait or sickle cell disease. Sickle cell trait is a heterozygous disorder seen in 10% of black persons. Hemoglobin S levels are normally 30% to 50%, and sickling is seen with a PO_2 of 20 to 30 mm Hg. Sickle cell disease is a homozygous disorder seen in 0.5% to 1.0% of black persons. The majority of the hemoglobin is hemoglobin S, and sickling is seen with a PO_2 of 30 to 40 mm Hg. Sickle cell crisis may be caused by a decrease in oxygen saturation and temperature, infections, dehydration, stasis, and acidosis.

It has long been suggested that sickle cell disease is associated with increased surgical risk. There is no universal method of caring for these patients. A general guideline for preoperative preparation is a hemoglobin A level of at least 50% and a hematocrit of 35%.[27] The National Preoperative Study in Sickle Cell Disease concluded that a conservative transfusion regimen was as effective as an aggressive regimen in preventing perioperative complications.[28] In pediatric patients undergoing minor operations, no increase in complications was identified without preoperative transfusion.[29] In the majority of surgical procedures, there appears to be documented benefit of reducing preoperative hemoglobin S levels to 30% or 40%. However, there is a clear benefit of increasing hemoglobin levels to 10 to 12 g/dL preoperatively because lower levels are associated with higher complication rates.[30] Precipitating factors of an occlusive crisis include fever, infection, acidosis, hypoxia, stress, and hypothermia. Treatment is primarily supportive and includes hydration, analgesics, and possibly hydroxyurea.

Anesthetic management includes particular attention to maintenance of oxygenation, normal fluid and electrolyte status, and avoiding acidosis and hypothermia. Proper positioning is critical to avoid circulatory compromise.[31,32]

THROMBOEMBOLIC DISORDERS

Venous thromboembolism includes both deep vein thrombosis (DVT) and its most serious complication, pulmonary embolism (PE). It is estimated that there are approximately 600,000 cases of PE in the United States each year, with about 10% resulting in death. DVT is associated with numerous operations, especially orthopedic and major abdominal surgery. Thrombi that form in the larger leg veins are the most common source of pulmonary embolism.[33] A number of therapies are available for the prevention of DVT following anesthesia and surgery. These include minimal-dose heparin, coumadin, low-molecular-weight heparins, and occlusive stockings. Guidelines for prophylaxis for thromboembolism are listed in Table 24-22, Chapter 24. Some common anticoagulant agents used for the prophylaxis of DVT[34-40] are listed in Table 32-6.

Most surgical procedures require that the patient not be anticoagulated due to the risk of hemorrhage. However, some patients take anticoagulants, primarily coumadin, on a chronic basis if they have a history of atrial fibrillation or placement of a mechanical heart valve and other disorders. Most surgical procedures can be done if the patient's international normalized ratio (INR) is below 1.5. See Box 32-1 for a summary of drugs affecting blood coagulation.

TABLE 32-6 Drugs Used in Deep Vein Thrombosis Prophylaxis

Drug	Type	Dose	Comments
Enoxaprin (Lovenox, Clexane)	Low-molecular-weight heparin	30-40 mg SC bid	First dose given immediately after surgery and continued for 7-10 days
Dalteparin (Fragman)	Low-molecular-weight heparin	2500 anti-Xa units SC qd	First dose 1-2 hours preop and continued for 5 days (5000 anti-Xa units in high-risk patients)
Ardeparin (Normiflo)	Low-molecular-weight heparin	50 anti-Xa units/kg of actual weight SC bid	First dose in the evening of the day of surgery and continued for 14 days or until ambulatory
Heparin	Intravenous anticoagulant	Low-dose prophylaxis: 5000 units SC every 8-12 hours guided by coagulation tests	Pharmacokinetics highly variable; aPTT 1.5-2 × normal is considered adequate; first dose 2 hours preop then every 8-12 hours for 7 days guided by aPPT results; effects may be reversed with protamine
Warfarin (Coumadin)	Oral anticoagulant	2-5 mg/day adjusted to INR	Low-intensity therapy INR = 2.0-3.0; high-intensity therapy INR = 2.5-3.5; effects may be reversed with vitamin K
Danaparoid (Orgaran)	Subcutaneous anticoagulant	750 anti-Xa units SC bid	First dose given 1-4 hours preop and continued for 7-14 days or until ambulatory in patients undergoing total hip replacement
Desirudin (Iprivask)	Thrombin inhibitor	15 mg q 12 hrs Initial dose 5-15 min prior to surgery	Caution with neuraxial anesthesia
Anisindione (Miradon)	Prothrombin inhibitor	300 mg day 1, 200 mg day 2, 100 mg day 3, 25-250 maintenance	Prothrombin time of 2-2.5 times normal value is therapeutic goal
Tinzaparin (Innohep)	Low molecular weight heparin	175 anti-Xa IU/kg SC for 6 days	Caution with neuraxial anesthesia
Fondaparinux (Artrixa)	Factor Xa inhibitor	2.5 mg SC 6 hrs After surgery	Used following orthopedic surgery

INR, *international normalized ratio*; aPTT, *activated partial thromboplastin time*; SC, *subcutaneous*; qd, *once per day*; bid, *twice per day*.
Adapted from Mosby's Drug Consult, *St Louis*, 2004, *Mosby*.

BOX **32-1**

Drugs Affecting Blood coagulation

Clinical Uses of Anticoagulants

- Heparin or the low-molecular-weight heparins are used acutely for short-term action.
- Warfarin is used for long-term therapy.
- Anticoagulants are given to prevent perioperative deep vein thrombosis (DVT), extension of a DVT or recurrence of a pulmonary embolism, thrombosis and embolization in patients with atrial fibrillation, thrombosis on prosthetic heart valves, clotting during extracorporeal circulation such as dialysis or cardiopulmonary bypass, unstable angina.

Procoagulant Drugs (e.g., vitamin K)

- The reduced form of vitamin K is a cofactor in the posttranslational γ-carboxylation of a cluster of glutamic acid residues in each of factors II, VII, IX, and X; vitamin K is oxidized during the reaction. The γ-carboxylated glutamic acid residues are essential for the interaction of these factors with Ca^{2+} and negatively charged phospholipid.

Injectable Anticoagulants (e.g., heparin, low-molecular-weight heparins [LMWHs])

- These increase the rate of action of antithrombin III (AT III), a natural inhibitor that inactivates Xa and thrombin.
- They act both in vivo and in vitro.
- Anticoagulant activity results from a unique pentasaccharide sequence with high affinity for AT III.
- The effect of heparin is monitored by the APTT (activated partial thromboplastin time) and the dose is individualized.
- LMWHs have the same effect on factor X as heparin but less effect on thrombin; however, their anticoagulant effects are similar to heparin.
- LMWHs are given subcutaneously or intravenously and the onset of action is rapid. A standard dose (on a body weight basis) is given without the need for monitoring or individual dose adjustment. Patients can administer them at home.

Oral Anticoagulants (e.g., warfarin [Coumadin])

- These inhibit the reduction of vitamin K, thus inhibiting the γ-carboxylation of glutamic acid in II, VII, IX, and X.
- They act only in vivo and the effect is delayed.
- Many factors modify their action; drug interactions are especially important.
- There is wide variation in response; their effect is monitored by measuring the prothrombin time (PT) and INR (international normalized ratio) and the dose individualized accordingly.

Antiplatelet Drugs (e.g., aspirin)

- Aspirin, dipyridamole, and clopidogrel have different actions but their effects are additive.
- Their uses mainly relate to arterial thrombosis and include acute myocardial infarction, prevention of morbidity in post–myocardial infarction, angina, transient ischemic attacks and intermittent claudication, post–coronary bypass, post–angioplasty with stenting, transient cerebral ischemic attack (TIA), and atrial fibrillation.
- Their effects are monitored by measuring bleeding time.

From Rang HP, Dale MM, Ritter JM, Moore PK: Hemostasis and thrombosis. Human Pharmacology, *ed 5, Edinburgh, Scotland, 2003, Churchill Livingstone, pp 314-329.*

REFERENCES

1. Sere KM, Hackeng TM: Basic mechanisms of hemostasis, *Semin Vasc Med* 3:3-11, 2003.
2. Gimbrone MA: Endothelial dysfunction and the pathogenesis of atherosclerosis. In Gotto AM, Smith LC, Allen B, editors: *Atherosclerosis V: Proceedings of the Fifth International Symposium on Atherosclerosis*, New York, 1980, Springer-Verlag, pp 415-420.
3. Nilsson IM: A family with thrombosis associated with high level of tissue plasminogen activator inhibitor. *Hemostasis* 14:24, 1984 (abstract).
4. American Society of Anesthesiologists Task Force on Blood Component Therapy: Practice guidelines for blood component therapy, *Anesthesiology* 84:732-747, 1996.
5. Sirridge MS, Shannon R: *Laboratory evaluation of hemostasis and thrombosis*, ed 3, Philadelphia, 1983, Lea & Febiger.
6. Suchman AL, Grinder PF: Diagnostic uses of the activated partial thromboplastin time and prothrombin time. *Ann Intern Med* 104:810-816, 1986.
7. WHO Technical Report Series: Guidelines for thromboplastins and plasma used to control oral anticoagulant therapy. In WHO Expert Committee on Biological Standardization: *World Health Organization, Annex* 3 889:64-93, 1999.
8. Esler MD, Douglas MJ: Planning for hemorrhage: steps an anesthesiologist can take to limit and treat hemorrhage in the obstetric patient, *Anesthesiol Clin North Am* 21:127-144, 2003.
9. Rohrer MJ, Michelotti MC, Nahrnold DL: A prospective evaluation of the efficacy of preoperative coagulation testing, *Ann Surg* 208:554-557, 1988.
10. Cobas M: Preoperative assessment of coagulation disorders. In Hurford W, Gilbertson L, editors: *International Anesthesiology Clinics*, Philadelphia, 2001, Lippincott, pp 1-15.
11. Barber A, Green D, Galluzzo T, Ts'ao CH: The bleeding time as a preoperative screening test, *Am J Med* 78:761-764, 1985.
12. Russell MW, Jobes D: What should we do with aspirin, NSAIDs, and glycoprotein-receptor inhibitors? *Int Anesthesiol Clin* 40: 63-76, 2002.
13. Renck H: *Bleeding and Thrombotic Disorders in the Surgical Patient*, East Norwalk, CT, 1988, Appleton & Lange, p 26.
14. Benzon HT, Brunner EA, Vaisrub N: Bleeding time and nerve blocks after aspirin, *Reg Anesth* 9:86, 1984.
15. Locke GE, Giorgo AT, Biggers SL: Acute spinal epidural hematoma secondary to aspirin-induced prolonged bleeding, *Surg Neurol* 5:292, 1976.
16. Rao TLK, El-Etr AA: Anticoagulation following placement of epidural and subarachnoid catheters: an evaluation of neurologic sequelae, *Anesthesiology* 55:616-620, 1981.
17. Langenecker SAK: The effects of drugs used in anesthesia on platelet membrane receptors and on platelet function, *Current Drug Targets* 3:247-258, 2002.
18. Murray DJ, Olson J, Strauss R, Tinker JH: Coagulation changes during packed red cell replacement of major blood loss, *Anesthesiology* 69:839-845, 1988.

19. Toh CH: Laboratory testing in disseminated intravascular coagulation, *Semin Thromb Hemost* 27:664-665, 2001.
20. Horan JT, Francis CW: Fibrin degradation products, fibrin monomer and soluble fibrin in disseminated intravascular coagulation, *Semin Thromb Hemost* 27:657-665, 2001.
21. Hardaway R, Williams CH, Vasquez Y: Disseminated intravascular coagulation in sepsis, *Semin Thromb Hemost* 27:577-583, 2001.
22. Gando S: Disseminated intravascular coagulation in trauma patients, *Semin Thromb Hemost* 27:585-592, 2001.
23. Cammerer U, Dietrich W, Tobias R: The predictive value of modified computerized thromboelastography and platelet function analysis for postoperative blood loss in routine cardiac surgery, *Anesth Analg* 96:51-57, 2003.
24. Faraday N, Guallar E, Sera VA, et al: Utility of whole blood hemostatometry using the clot signature analyzer for assessment of hemostasis in cardiac surgery, *Anesthesiology* 96:1115-1122, 2002.
25. Mammen EF, Koets MH, Washington BC, et al: Hemostasis changes during cardiopulmonary bypass surgery, *Semin Thromb Hemost* 11:281-292, 1985.
26. Nuttall GA, Stehling LC, Beighley CM, Faust RJ, American Society of Anesthesiologists Committee on Transfusion Medicine: Current transfusion practices of members of the American Society of Anesthesiologists: a survey, *Anesthesiology* 99:1433-1443, 2003.
27. Schmalzer EA, Lee JO, Brown AK, Usami S, Chien S: Viscosity of mixtures of sickle and normal red cells at varying hematocrit levels: implications for transfusion, *Transfusion* 27:228-233, 1987.
28. Vichinsky EP, Haberkern CM, Neumayr L, et al: A comparison of conservative and aggressive transfusion regimens in the perioperative management of sickle cell disease: The Preoperative Transfusion in Sickle Cell Disease Study Group, *N Engl J Med* 333:206-213, 1995.
29. Griffin TC, Buchanan GR: Elective surgery in children with sickle cell disease without preoperative blood transfusion, *J Pediatr Surg* 28:681-685, 1993.
30. Koshy M, Weiner SJ, Miller ST, et al: Surgery and anesthesia in sickle cell disease: Cooperative study of sickle cell diseases, *Blood* 86:3676-3684, 1995.
31. Dix HM: New advances in the treatment of sickle cell disease: focus on perioperative significance. *AANA J* 69:281-286, 2001.
32. Marchant WA, Walker I: Anesthetic management of the child with sickle cell disease, *Paediatr Anaesth* 13:473-489, 2003.
33. Dunn AS, Turpie AG: Perioperative management of patients receiving oral anticoagulants: a systematic review, *Arch Intern Med* 163:901-908, 2003.
34. Geerts WH, Heit JA, Clagett GP, et al: Prevention of venous thromboembolism, *Chest* 121:2078-2079, 2002.
35. Whang PG, Leiberman JR: Low-molecular-weight heparin, *J Am Acad Orthop Surg* 10:299-302, 2002.
36. Hirsh J, Dalen JE, Anderson DR, et al. Oral anticoagulants: mechanism of action, clinical effectiveness, and optimal therapeutic range, *Chest* 119:8S-21S, 2001.
37. Wilde MI, Markham A: Danaparoid: a review of its pharmacology and clinical use in the management of heparin-induced thrombocytopenia, *Drugs* 54:903-924, 1997.
38. Hyers TM, Agnelli G, Hull RD, et al. Antithrombotic therapy for venous thromboembolic disease, *Chest* 119:176S-193S, 2001.
39. Jackson MR, Clagett GP: Antithrombotic therapy in peripheral arterial occlusive disease, *Chest* 119:283S-299S, 2001.
40. Hirsh J, Warkentin TE, Shaughnessy SG, et al: Heparin and low-molecular-weight heparin: mechanisms of action, pharmacokinetics, dosing, monitoring, efficacy, and safety, *Chest* 119: 64S-94S, 2001.

CHAPTER 33

THERMAL INJURY AND ANESTHESIA

JULIE ANN LOWERY

In the 1950s there were fewer than 10 recognized burn centers in the United States. This number now exceeds over 200, with established burn centers now located across the country, in virtually every major metropolitan area. Recent statistics reveal a decline in the national incidence of burn injury and medical care use during the past two decades.[1] This progress coincides with an increased national focus on burn prevention. Smoke detectors have come into widespread use, fire and burn prevention education has expanded, and regulation of consumer product and occupational safety has increased significantly.

In the United States more than 1.25 million people are treated annually for a burn injury, with 51,000 acute hospital admissions; approximately 5500 die from fire and burn injuries.[1] Roughly 35% of all burn victims are under 17 years of age, with more than 15,000 children requiring hospitalization as a result of their burn injuries. Scald injuries predominate among small children, with a progressive increase in the frequency of thermal-related burns in the elderly.[2] The major causes of death in burn patients are multiple organ failure and infection. Death following a burn injury is not related to the toxic biologic effect of thermally injured skin, but to the shock associated with metabolic and bacterial consequences of a large open wound, depletion of the patient's resistance to infection, inhalation injury, and extensive malnutrition, which set the stage for life-threatening bacterial infection originating from the burn wound.[3]

CLASSIFICATION OF BURN INJURY

Burn injuries, regardless of their etiology, are classified according to the depth and the extent of the skin and tissue destruction as well as the total body surface area (TBSA) involved. First-degree (superficial) burns are limited to the epidermis, which is the outermost layer of skin. The epidermis is primarily thin and avascular. First-degree burns heal spontaneously and do not usually require any medical intervention. Second-degree burns are also known as deep and superficial *partial-thickness burns*. They extend into the dermis, which lies below the epidermis. In contrast to the epidermis, the dermis is very vascular and contains numerous blood vessels and nerves. The severity of the type of burn varies, depending upon the amount and the depth of the dermal tissues involved. If the epithelial basement membrane of the dermis is intact, the skin will regenerate and grafting may not be required. Third-degree or *full-thickness burns* extend into the subcutaneous tissue lying below the dermis. The entire skin thickness is destroyed with third-degree burns.[4] Skin grafting is required for these types of burns, as the epithelium and the dermal appendages are destroyed. A fourth-degree burn classification is used by some institutions to describe structures burned below the dermis, such as muscle, fascia, and bone. See Table 33-1 for classification of burn depth with regard to the skin layers affected and Fig. 33-1 for description of the layers of burn injury.

TABLE 33-1 Degrees of Burn Injury

Classification	Tissue Level Involvement	Appearance
Superficial, first-degree burn	Epidermis destroyed	Skin, red tone (sunburn); painful with erythema and blisters; heals spontaneously with no scarring
Partial-thickness, second-degree burn		
Superficial dermal	Epidermis and some (upper) dermis destroyed	Red or pale ivory with a moist, shiny surface; painful, immediate blisters with minimal scarring
Deep dermal	Epidermis and deep dermis	Mottled with white, waxy, dry surface; blisters may or may not appear; significant scarring
Full-thickness, third-degree burn	All epidermis and dermis	White, cherry red, or black; dry, tissue-paper skin; grafting necessary; decreased scarring with early excision
Fourth-degree burn	Muscle, fascia, bone	Complete excision required; limited function

Modified from Faldmo L, Kravitz M: Management of acute burns and burn shock resuscitation, AACN Clin Issues Crit Care Nurs *4:351-366, 1993.*

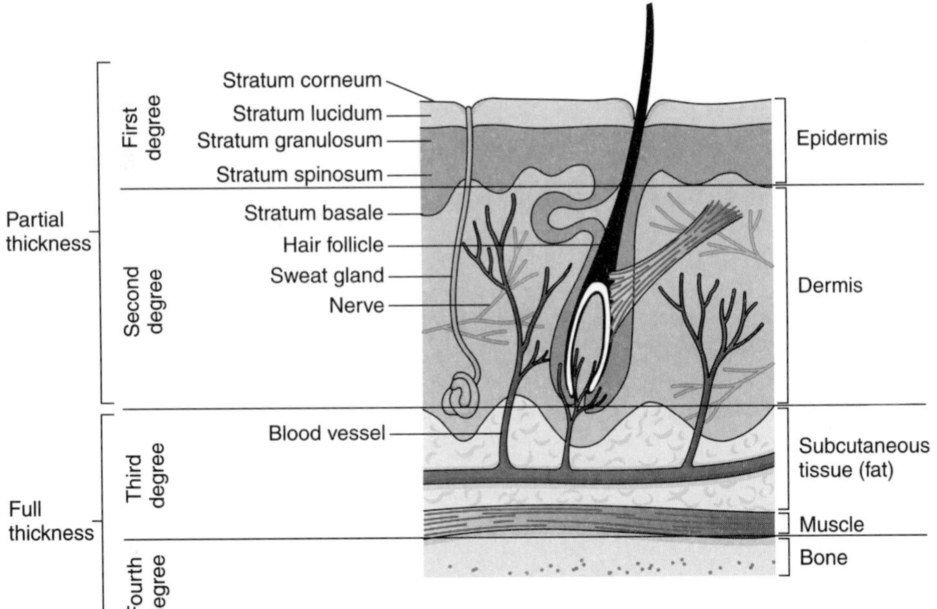

FIGURE **33-1**
Depth of a thermal injury determines whether a burn will heal without grafting. Superficial and partial-thickness burns do not destroy the dermal appendages and thus are able to heal readily. Full-thickness burns, particularly when they reach the muscle and bone, require skin grafting to prevent infection and promote healing. (From Beare PG, Myers JL: *Adult Health Nursing*, ed 3, St Louis, 1998, Mosby.)

It is necessary for the burn team to assess the extent of a burn and plan initial resuscitation efforts. Burn wounds can be readily quantified, but estimation of burn size remains subjective and assessor related. The most widely used estimation is the "rule of nines," which was first described by Lund and Browder (Fig. 33-2). The body is divided into regions that represent 9% or a multiple of 9% of the TBSA. Modifications are needed in children because the surface areas of their heads and trunks are proportionally larger than their extremities.[5] The rule of nines is a quick method to visually estimate a burn size; however, it is not definitive. The extensiveness of a burn injury can be more specifically quantified via use of the Lund and Browder chart. Figure 33-3 demonstrates the Lund and Browder method utilized at the University of North Carolina's burn center. Although more time consuming to utilize, deriving a burn victim's injury extent via this method is much more accurate, especially in the pediatric patient.

According to the American Burn Association's injury severity grading system, a major burn is a second-degree burn involving more than 10% of the TBSA in adults or 20% at extremes of age, a third-degree burn involving more than 10% of the TBSA in adults, and any electrical burn, or one complicated by smoke inhalation. A burn formula derived from the National Burn Registry estimating mortality is as follows: if the age of the patient + % TBSA of burn exceeds 115, the mortality is greater than 80%. Additionally, from clinical observations, it is estimated that the mortality of a burned victim is approximately doubled if there is an inhalation injury sustained in conjunction with a thermal burn.

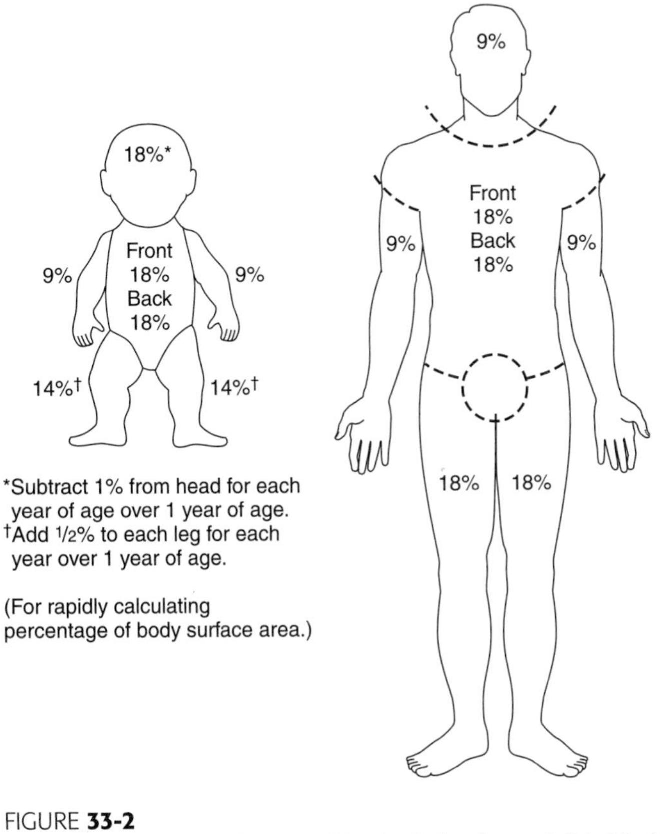

18%*
Front 18% Back 18%
9% 9%
14%† 14%†

9%
Front 18% Back 18%
9% 9%
18% 18%

*Subtract 1% from head for each year of age over 1 year of age.
†Add 1/2% to each leg for each year over 1 year of age.

(For rapidly calculating percentage of body surface area.)

FIGURE **33-2**
Total body surface area determined by the "rule of nines." (Modified from Berkow SG: A method of estimating the expansiveness of lesions based on surface area proportions, *Arch Surg* 8:138-148, 1924. Copyright 1924, American Medical Association.)

ETIOLOGIES OF BURN INJURIES

A burn is a burn is a burn . . . perhaps that is true for the treatment modalities sustained with a burn injury. However, it is vital for the burn team in a burn unit to ascertain the etiology of a burn victim's injury. Specific pathophysiological sequelae occur and are expected as a result of an electrical burn, or alternatively, a thermal burn. The global circumstances behind the burn injury must be examined. A good example is that of an individual burned in a contained space such as a house fire; such an individual should be highly suspected of having an inhalation injury as well.

There are four types of burn injuries: chemical, electrical, thermal/heat (also referred to as *flame* or *scald*), and inhalation. Chemical burns commonly occur in a laboratory setting or in an industrial environment. These types of burns occur when a

Date of admission: ______________

Date of burn: ______________

Age: __________ Sex: __________

Type of burn injury: (3)
Flame _______
Electrical _______
Scald _______
Chemical _______
Inhalation _______

Height (cm): _______

Weight (kg): _______

Body surface (m^2): _______

Date completed: ______________

Completed by: ______________
Name
____
ID# Required

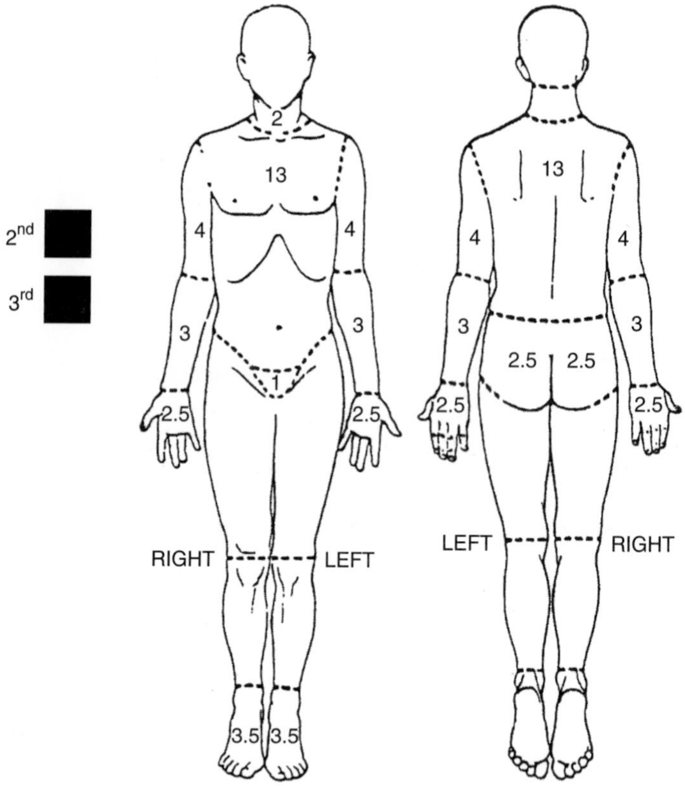

2nd ■
3rd ■

BURN ESTIMATE – AGE VS AREA

Area	Birth-1 year	1-4 years	5-9 years	10-14 years	15 years	Adult	2	3	TBS A%
Head	19	17	13	11	9	7			
Neck	2	2	2	2	2	2			
Anterior trunk	13	13	13	13	13	13			
Posterior trunk	13	13	13	13	13	13			
Right buttock	2.5	2.5	2.5	2.5	2.5	2.5			
Left buttock	2.5	2.5	2.5	2.5	2.5	2.5			
Genitalia	1	1	1	1	1	1			
Right upper arm	4	4	4	4	4	4			
Left upper arm	4	4	4	4	4	4			
Right lower arm	3	3	3	3	3	3			
Left lower arm	3	3	3	3	3	3			
Right hand	2.5	2.5	2.5	2.5	2.5	2.5			
Left hand	2.5	2.5	2.5	2.5	2.5	2.5			
Right thigh	5.5	6.5	8	8.5	9	9.5			
Left thigh	5.5	6.5	8	8.5	9	9.5			
Right leg	5	5	5.5	6	6.5	7			
Left leg	5	5	5.5	6	6.5	7			
Right foot	3.5	3.5	3.5	3.5	3.5	3.5			
Left foot	3.5	3.5	3.5	3.5	3.5	3.5			
						TOTAL			

FIGURE **33-3**
The Lund and Browder burn estimation chart. (Reprinted with permission from Jaycee Burn Center, University of North Carolina at Chapel Hill.)

noxious chemical substance comes in contact with the skin. Tissue damage and destruction result from the reaction of the chemical with the tissue proteins and cellular components. Skin disruption will continue until the chemical irritant is removed or neutralized. Initial treatment is with copious amounts of water or normal saline irrigation. Chemical burns are uncommon in children, although they can occur.

Electrical burns can be the most damaging to the skin and surrounding tissues. The extent of the burn depends on the amount of thermal energy conducted through the skin, based upon the voltage and the duration of contact with the electrical source. Significant tissue disruption can occur where the electrical current is the most concentrated—at the points of entry and exit, although two wounds are not always evident. Initially, the extensiveness of skin and underlying tissue involved may be hard to diagnose since surface damage may not reflect the extent of tissue damage and the entrance wounds may appear superficial. Electrical burns can cause severe damage to bones, blood vessels, muscle, and nerves. If the amount of muscle damaged from the conducted electrical current is significant, myoglobin can be released into the circulation, resulting in myoglobinemia. This places the electrical burn patient at great risk for developing renal failure secondary to myoglobinuria, affecting nephron and renal tubular function.

Thermal-related burns or burns sustained from any heat source commonly occur in and around the house. In children between 1 and 4 years of age, fires and burns are the second leading cause of accidental death. Scald burns in children remain one of the most common injuries resulting from abuse.[6]

Inhalation burn injuries often accompany thermal burns and should be suspected until aggressively ruled out.[7-9] Damage to the airway can vary, depending on whether or not the upper airway or lower airway is affected. Upper airway injuries result from inhalation of superheated air or steam and toxic compounds found in smoke.[10] Brief exposure of the epiglottis or larynx to either dry air at 300° C or steam at 100° C can lead to massive edema and rapid airway obstruction.[11] As mentioned earlier, the addition of an inhalation injury to a cutaneous burn of any size doubles the mortality rate[12] and is a stronger determinant of death (related to pneumonia) than is the size of the burn wound.[3] The inhalation of heated air can result in direct injury to the face, oropharynx, and upper trachea, with sparing of the lower airway. It is speculated that the heat entrained is readily dissipated in the upper airway and there is reflex closure of the vocal cords. These features are thought to protect the lower airways from heat-related injury. However, true thermal injury from exposure to live steam can occur in the lower respiratory tract because the heat-exchange mechanisms of the airway are unable to cool the gas sufficiently as it is inhaled. Lower airway injuries more commonly arise from the inhalation of soot particles and/or chemicals produced by a fire. Heat and excessive edema mainly obstruct the upper airway due to macroglossia and swelling of the pharyngeal soft tissue. In the lower airways, the inhaled toxins react with the airway mucosa, forming acidic and alkali substances. Capillary permeability is increased. Extensive alveolar and epithelial damage can occur, with the trachea and bronchi becoming necrotic. Warning signs of respiratory injury include hoarseness, sore throat, dysphagia, hemoptysis, tachypnea, the use of accessory muscles, wheezing, carbonaceous sputum production, and elevated carbon monoxide levels.[13]

Treatment of the burn patient involves three distinct phases: the resuscitative phase, debridement and grafting, and the reconstructive phase. Each phase has its own unique problems that the anesthesia provider must identify when developing an anesthetic plan.

RESUSCITATIVE PHASE

As for any trauma patient, the initial treatment of the burn patient should involve attention to the airway, breathing, and circulation and coexisting trauma. All burn patients must be considered at risk for pulmonary compromise, especially if the % TBSA involved is significant and signs of inhalation injury are present.

Diagnosis and Treatment: Airway Injury

It is necessary to aggressively rule out upper airway injury in patients at risk (e.g., involving a fire that occurred in a closed space or the development of unconsciousness or stupor that prevented the patient from protecting his or her airway). Diagnosis is made by history and physical examination. This is best achieved by direct visualization of the airway with a laryngoscope or fiberoptic bronchoscope[14] or xenon-133 lung scanning,[2] which detects ventilation/perfusion defects. The chest radiograph is usually normal in the early phase of inhalation injury unless aspiration of gastric or pharyngeal contents occurred during the accident, becoming abnormal after the injury when pulmonary edema or infiltration develops. Treatment of upper airway injury involves *early* endotracheal intubation, even if the burn patient is not yet demonstrating any signs of airway decompensation. It is important to add that even in the absence of an inhalation injury, the lungs are at risk for compromise if the burn is large.

Thermal damage to the soft tissues of the respiratory tract and trachea can make intubation an almost impossible task because of the malalignment of structures, swelling, and bleeding of the tissues involved. Intubation of the trachea is much easier to perform earlier than later, when there may be glottic or facial edema, which worsens after fluid resuscitation.[15] In the pediatric population, intubation should be performed with an uncuffed endotracheal tube, usually one size smaller than expected according to age and weight. Nasotracheal intubation in children is generally preferred, as it is better tolerated by the child and tube displacement with movement is less likely.[16,17]

In the absence of an airway abnormality, early tracheal intubation can usually be achieved using a rapid-sequence technique with an intravenous induction agent and a rapidly acting muscle relaxant. There is general agreement that succinylcholine administration to patients more than 24 hours after burn injury is unsafe,[18,19] although some authors extend this safe period to several days.[20] It is speculated that a denervation-like phenomenon occurs following a burn, with a proliferation of acetylcholine receptors throughout the muscle membrane. Succinylcholine is structurally similar to acetylcholine and can cause potassium (K^+) release from the entire muscle membrane rather than from discrete end plate junctions, leading to hyperkalemia and possibly cardiac arrest.[21] The magnitude of K^+ elevation appears to be related to the size of the burn. This process of receptor proliferation takes several days to develop, allowing an initial 24-hour window of safety. It is wise to avoid the use of succinylcholine in a burn patient more than 24 hours after injury[22] until complete wound closure has occurred and the patient is gaining weight.[23] Administering high doses of nondepolarizing muscle relaxants (e.g., rocuronium, vecuronium, or cisatracurium) is an alternative to succinylcholine.

Variations in acetylcholine receptors—specifically, an increased number of nicotinic acetylcholine receptors[24]—along with a change in volume and distribution associated with alterations in plasma protein binding, may account for a decreased sensitivity to nondepolarizing drugs. Both the dose administered and the serum concentrations required in the burn patient may be increased twofold to threefold if the desired paralysis with a nondepolarizer is to be achieved.[23]

With an abnormal airway or upper airway obstruction, the safest way to secure the airway is with the patient awake. Key actions include effective topical anesthesia, patient positioning, and supplemental oxygenation. Administration of sedatives may worsen airway obstruction and should be given cautiously. However, intravenous opioid administration may be appropriate for the alert patient in pain. Methods to secure the airway include flexible fiberoptic bronchoscopy, direct laryngoscopy, laryngeal mask airway, blind nasal intubation, and the Bullard laryngoscope. When the upper airway is badly damaged and endotracheal intubation is not possible, a direct surgical approach is indicated: needle cricothyroidotomy, surgical cricothyroidotomy, or tracheostomy. This should *only* be considered as a last resort.

For the most part, after airway management, the patient is taken to the intensive care unit and placed on ventilatory support.[25] The inspired gases should be humidified to aid clearing of tracheobronchial debris and prevent drying of secretions. The endotracheal tube must be kept in place until the surrounding laryngeal edema has subsided. A progressive air leak around the endotracheal tube, especially in uncuffed pediatric sizes, is an indication that edematous tissue is returning to normal.

Carbon Monoxide Poisoning. Any burn victim rescued from an enclosed space fire should be considered at high risk for carbon monoxide poisoning. It is estimated that 50%-60% of all fire victims die from carbon monoxide poisoning.[26] Symptoms depend on the carboxyhemoglobin level, although it is actually the tissue carbon monoxide level that determines the toxicity of carbon monoxide (Table 33-2).

TABLE **33-2** Clinical Manifestations of Carbon Monoxide Exposure

Carboxyhemoglobin Level (%)	Clinical Manifestations
0-5	None
5-10	Mild headache, confusion
11-20	Throbbing headache, blurred vision
21-40	Disorientation, nausea, vomiting, irritability, syncope
41-60	Tachycardia, tachypnea, agitation, combativeness, hallucination
>60	Death

Modified from Sharar SR, Heimbach DM, Hudson LD: Management of inhalation injury in patients with and without burns. In Haponik EF, Munster AM, editors: Respiratory Injury: Smoke Inhalation and Burns, *New York, 1990, McGraw-Hill.*

Carbon monoxide binds to the hemoglobin molecule with 200 times greater affinity than does oxygen.[27] Tissues are unable to extract oxygen, leading to the disruption of oxidative phosphorylation and metabolic acidosis at the cellular level. Analysis of blood gases reveals a normal arterial oxygen tension but a decreased total oxygen content, indicating that the hemoglobin oxygen saturation is markedly reduced.[23] Carbon monoxide increases the stability of the oxyhemoglobin molecule, decreasing the release of oxygen to the tissues—a leftward shift in the oxyhemoglobin curve (Fig. 33-4). Pulse oximeters do not detect CO Hgb and give falsely elevated readings for oxygen saturation in its presence. A co-oximeter, which measures the percentage of hemoglobin, oxyhemoglobin, carboxyhemoglobin, and methemoglobin, is needed to obtain an accurate oximetry saturation.[28]

The treatment is to displace the carbon monoxide molecule from the hemoglobin. Typical interventions include administering 100% oxygen via face mask or an endotracheal tube.

Oxygen displaces the carbon monoxide and shortens its half-life from roughly 4 hours to 40 minutes.[15,27] Hyperbaric oxygen treatments are an alternative therapy. The debate continues over the effectiveness of hyperbaric oxygen (HBO) to treat carbon monoxide poisoning. The major question is whether HBO reduces the incidence of delayed neurologic sequelae. Studies have been inconclusive.[14,29-31]

Hypovolemic Shock Associated with Thermal Injury

After the airway has been secured and other life-threatening injuries have been managed, the burn patient must be resuscitated with large volumes of fluid. Aggressive fluid administration and restoration of the blood volume are critical interventions for improving the patient's survival chances and preventing renal failure. Fluid losses are greatest in the first 12 hours after the burn and then begin to stabilize after 24 hours. Fluid losses occur secondary to direct transudation of plasma from the wound and from diffuse capillary leakage that shifts fluid from the intravascular space into the interstitium of unburned tissue. Capillary leak results from the loss of endothelial integrity and from reduction of intravascular

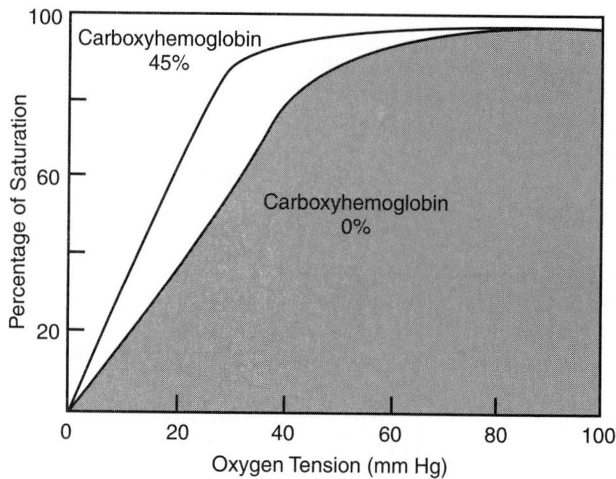

FIGURE **33-4**
Shift of the oxyhemoglobin dissociation curve to the left by 45% carboxyhemoglobin. (From Jackson DL, Menges H: Accidental carbon monoxide poisoning, *JAMA* 243:772, 1980. Copyright 1980, American Medical Association.)

oncotic pressure as plasma proteins are lost through the burn wound and incompetent capillary beds.[32] The end result of the changes in the microvasculature caused by thermal injury is disruption of normal capillary barriers separating intravascular and interstitial compartments, and rapid equilibrium of these compartments. This causes severe depletion of plasma volume with a marked increase in extracellular fluid, clinically manifested as hypovolemia and burn-induced edema.

Inflammatory mediators are released from burned tissues following the injury. These local mediators cause localized inflammation and burn wound edema. Localized mediators include oxygen radicals, arachadonic acid metabolites, histamine, prostaglandins, leukotrienes, products of platelet activation, and the complement cascade.[15,26,32] In minor burns, the inflammatory process seen remains sequestered in the wound itself. However, in major burn insults, this local injury signals the release of systemic circulatory mediators. This results in a systemic response to the burn.

Fluid Resuscitation

Within seconds after an acute burn injury, massive fluid shifts begin to occur. Therefore, fluid resuscitation and airway management are the hallmarks of initial therapy and should be instituted by the first response emergency medical providers. There are many formulas for calculating a burn patient's initial fluid resuscitation requirements. The current American Burn Association consensus formula for fluid resuscitation and urine output in burn patients is given in Table 33-3. Table 33-4 lists other commonly used fluid protocols. Common to all of these formulas is the need to know the patient's weight in kilograms and the percentage of TBSA involved. The American College of Surgeons Committee on Trauma has advocated that only crystalloid formulas be used for all burn resuscitation. Colloid solutions are not advocated in the first 24 hours, since capillary permeability remains enhanced and any colloids administered will not remain in the intravascular space. It is important to remember that the formulas for fluid guidelines are only that—guidelines. Individual factors must also be taken into account. It is crucial to resuscitate the patient with fluids according to patient response, hemodynamic variables, sensorium, and urinary output of 0.5 to 1.0 mL/kg/hr in adults and 1.0 mL/kg/hr in children under 60 pounds,[32] instead of by a fixed formula.[15,23] Because infants and small children have high volume–to–surface area ratios, formulas that base fluid requirements on surface area burned and weight may underestimate need.

Invasive hemodynamic monitoring (central venous pressure, pulmonary artery catheterization) is indicated in patients who do not respond to fluid resuscitation or who have preexisting cardiopulmonary disease. Catheters should be removed as quickly as possible to minimize the risk of local and systemic infection.

TABLE 33-3 Consensus Formula for Fluid Resuscitation and Urine Output in Burn Patients (American Burn Association)

Adults: Ringer's lactate 2-4 mL × kg body weight × percent BSA burned*

Children: Ringer's lactate 3-4 mL × kg body weight × percent BSA burned*†

*One half of the estimated volume of fluid should be administered in the first 8 hours after the burn. The remaining half should be administered over the subsequent 16 hours of the first postburn day.

†Infants and young children should receive fluid with 5% dextrose at a maintenance rate in addition to the resuscitation fluid noted above.

Minimum Urinary Output in Burn Patients

Adults: 0.5 mL/kg/hour

Children weighing less than 30 kg: 1 mL/kg/hour

Patients with high voltage electrical injuries: 1-1.5 mL/kg/hour

Source: *American Burn Association:* Advanced Burn Life Support Course Provider's Manual, *Chicago, 2001, American Burn Association, pp 33-39.*

TABLE 33-4 Fluid Resuscitation Formulas for Burn Patients

Formula	First 24 hr	Second 24 hr
Brooke		
Crystalloid	2 mL LR/% burn per kg	D_5W maintenance
1/2 in first 8 hr		
1/2 in next 16 hr		
Colloid	None	0.5 mL/% burn per kg
Parkland		
Crystalloid	4 mL LR/% burn per kg 1/2 in first 8 hr 1/2 in next 16 hr	D_5W maintenance
Colloid	None	0.5 mL/% burn per kg
MGH		
Crystalloid	1.5 mL LR/% burn per kg 1/2 in first 8 hr 1/2 in next 16 hr	Not specified
Colloid	0.5 mL LR/% burn per kg None in first 4 hr 1/2 in second 4 hr 1/2 in next 16 hr	Not specified
Evans		
Crystalloid	1.0 mL LR/% burn per kg 1/2 in first 8 hr 1/2 in next 16 hr	D_5W maintenance
Colloid	1.0 mL LR/% burn per kg 1/2 in first 8 hr 1/2 in next 16 hr	Not specified

D_5W, *5% dextrose in water;* LR, *lactated Ringer's solution;* MGH, *Massachusetts General Hospital.*

Hypermetabolic/Hyperhemodynamic Phase

Once a burn victim survives the initial 48 hours after the burn insult, a systemic inflammatory syndrome is noted: the hypermetabolic hyperhemodynamic phase. The hypermetabolic phase is associated with increased blood flow to the organs and tissues. The exact cause of the hypermetabolic phase remains unclear, but it may be related to heat loss from burn tissue and increased intrinsic sympathetic nervous system activity.[33] The state is manifested by hyperthermia, tachypnea, tachycardia, increased serum catecholamine levels, increased oxygen consumption, increased catabolism, and increased basal metabolic rate. The state persists for several weeks, gradually receding to normal when the wound healing is well underway.[23]

Pathophysiologic Changes

As with any disease entity, certain pathophysiological alterations occur after an acute burn injury. It is important for the anesthetist to understand the basis for these changes, as many of these changes must be managed intraoperatively. The anesthetic plan must reflect any changes present.

Cardiovascular System. The cardiovascular system is greatly affected in the burn patient. Almost immediately after an acute burn injury, intravascular fluid losses begin. Etiologies for this include the loss of vascular and endothelial integrity and the release of circulating mediators, as described earlier. There is also a loss of plasma proteins from within the intravascular compartment due to the disrupted endothelium. This persists for up to 36 hours after the initial burn injury. Hypovolemia results with subsequent hypotension and circulatory compromise. Indeed, the size and the extent of the burn determine the magnitude of this development. Hence, burn victims can develop "burn shock" within the first 24-36 hours following an acute burn injury. A reduction in cardiac output is a hallmark of burn shock and appears to occur within minutes after the injury. It is initially preserved via catecholamine responses—tachycardia and vasoconstriction. However, with the progressive loss of intravascular fluids and proteins, left ventricular filling declines, leading to a reduction in cardiac output. Additionally, cardiac output is thought to be depressed from the release, by burned tissues, of a myocardial depressant factor or proteins. The cardiovascular response to catecholamines is attenuated after a burn injury as a result of a reduction in adrenergic receptor affinity and decreased secondary messenger production. Coronary blood flow can be reduced as a result, further decreasing cardiac function. Systemic vascular resistance increases.

Aggressive fluid resuscitation administered over the first 24-36 hours aims to restore intravascular volume and cardiac function. What is seen is a systemic inflammatory response syndrome, characterized by increased cardiac output, tachycardia, and a reduction in systemic vascular resistance. The patient becomes hypermetabolic, with an increase in oxygen consumption and carbon dioxide production.

It is important to note that children with extensive burn injuries can become quite hypertensive weeks after their injury. A definite etiology is not clear but is speculated to be a result of increased catecholamine production, hypervolemia, and/or activation of the renin-angiotensin system during the postburn period. This occurs primarily within the first 2 weeks and can last for several weeks.[6]

Pulmonary System. The pulmonary system is greatly affected in burn patients, with resulting pathophysiologic changes (Table 33-5). Pulmonary function may decrease markedly, even in the absence of an inhalation injury. Functional residual capacity is reduced, and both lung and chest wall compliance decrease. The latter can be severely compromised if the chest is circumferentially burned. With progressive fluid shifts and interstitial edema formation in cases with eschar formation, the inability to adequately expand the lungs impairs ventilation. In some cases, escharotomies are necessary to alleviate the pressure in the tissues in order to improve oxygenation and ventilation. The oxygen gradient between alveoli and arterial blood increases as well. Ventilation can increase to as much as 40 L/min from a normal rate of 6 L/min.[23]

As stated, the lungs are still at risk for compromise without an inhalation injury. There are many mechanisms involved. A primary factor is the effect that released mediators have on the lung. Plasma oncotic pressure greatly decreases after a burn due to the loss of plasma proteins in both burned and nonburned tissues. Impaired vascular and capillary permeability, combined with the large amount of fluid resuscitation needed, sets the stage for pulmonary edema.[27]

Patients with varying degrees of hypoxemia and respiratory insufficiency require mechanical support and ventilation. High-frequency percussive ventilation may be superior to conventional, volume-controlled mechanical ventilation, presumably because barotrauma is minimized.[34,35] In severely burned patients, especially if there is an inhalation injury, prolonged endotracheal intubation and mechanical ventilation are likely. Despite this, early or routine tracheostomy placement in burned patients has not been shown to improve the overall outcome in this patient population.[36]

Immune System. Burn victims, regardless of age, are particularly susceptible to infection for various reasons. The protective barrier of the skin has been destroyed and the doorway to microbial invasion is wide open. Altered immune responses are also present and begin within hours after the burn injury occurs. Leukocyte activity is depressed, as well as humoral and cellular responses. Burn eschar is a prime medium for bacterial growth. Colonization of gram-negative bacteria increases mortality. These patients often become septic and subject to developing pneumonia, especially if prolonged endotracheal intubation is required. Strict asepsis is required. Of those patients who die after sustaining a burn, infection is the leading cause of death over the long term in nearly 100% of children and 75% of adults.

Renal System. The development of acute renal failure (ARF) after an acute burn injury is a serious complication, as mortality rates increase.[16] Decreases in renal blood flow can occur immediately after a burn injury, leading to alterations in glomerular filtration. Causes include the large intravascular depletion, hypovolemia, decreased cardiac output, and increased circulating plasma catecholamine levels. The renin-angiotensin-aldosterone system and the release of ADH are stimulated and act to conserve sodium and water.[37] Subsequently, alterations in electrolyte balance can take place. Electrical burns with massive muscle necrosis can result in myoglobinemia, which may damage renal tubules and impair renal function. Intravenous administration of sodium bicarbonate to alkalize the urine protects the kidneys by preventing the formation of myoglobin casts. With adequate fluid resuscitation, renal blood flow and glomerular filtration are preserved. Hourly urine output measurements remain the gold standard for assessing adequate fluid replacement and resuscitation. See Table 33-3.

TABLE 33-5 Pathophysiologic Effects of Major Burns

System	Considerations
Respiratory	
Upper airway	Thermal damage to soft tissue and respiratory tract requires early endotracheal intubation
Carbon monoxide poisoning	Considered in all victims of enclosed fires; treatment with 100% oxygen by mask or endotracheal tube
Cardiac	
Burn shock phase (0 to 48 hr)	Hypovolemia is a major concern; fluid resuscitation is mandatory; expect impaired cardiac contractility
Hypermetabolic phase (after 48 hr)	Increased blood flow to organs and tissues; manifested by hyperthermia, tachypnea, tachycardia, increased oxygen consumption, and increased catabolism
Renal	
Early	
Reduced renal blood flow	Secondary to hypovolemia and decreased cardiac output; adequate fluid resuscitation and diuresis prevents renal failure
Electrical burns and muscle necrosis damage renal tubules	Intravenous administration of sodium bicarbonate to alkalize the urine
Late	
Increased renal blood flow	Variable drug clearance
Nutrition	
Increased caloric requirements	Limited to no nothing-by-mouth (NPO) status required
Ileus and duodendal ulcers	Treatment with H_2-blockers and antacids
Pharmacokinetics	
Decreased albumin	Benzodiazepines, phenytoin, and salicylic acid have an increase in the free fraction and thus a larger volume of distribution
Increased α_1-acid glycoprotein	Lidocaine, meperidine, and propranolol have the opposite effect
Denervation phenomenon with spreading of acetylcholine receptors	Succinylcholine avoided 24 hours after injury.
Increased nicotinic acetylcholine receptors	Requires a twofold to threefold increased concentration of nondepolarizer for paralysis
Skin Integrity	
Vulnerable to nosocomial infections	Strict adherence to aseptic individual patient rooms; wound care, including topical antimicrobial agents and early excision/grafting of the burn wound

Acute renal failure can also occur 2-3 weeks after the burn injury. Associated causes include sepsis and delayed wound excision. Delayed renal failure in children is rare and usually not a problem.

Gastrointestinal System/Nutrition. Caloric requirements for a patient with a 40% thermal injury are estimated to be 132% higher than basal energy expenditure, compared with a 79% increase for sepsis and a 25% increase for major elective surgery.[38] The increased energy expenditure enhances a period of negative nitrogen balance and causes an erosion of lean body mass, requiring intensive nutritional support. This nutritional support is essential for the immune system function, wound healing, and the prevention of catabolism. In patients with large burns and a pronounced hypermetabolic response, carbohydrate is more effective than fat in maintaining body protein.[39] The burn patient has an injury-induced resistance to the action of insulin in the liver and skeletal muscle. Ongoing assessment of blood glucose with administration of exogenous insulin may be necessary.

The necessity for continued adequate caloric intake cannot be ignored during the preanesthetic evaluation. Because of the importance of nutrition, it is unwise to arbitrarily stop enteral feedings the night before surgery. This can result in an excessive loss of calories, especially if the patient must undergo multiple burn debridements in a short period. Preoperative nothing-by-mouth (NPO) status must be kept at a safe minimum to prevent the patient from reverting to a catabolic state. Tracheally intubated patients do not need the enteral feedings discontinued before surgery, and unintubated patients can remain on nutritional support as late as 4 hours before the scheduled surgical procedure.[40] This practice improves preoperative nutrition without increasing the risk for aspiration. On admission to the operating room, the nonintubated patient's nasogastric tube should be suctioned and induction tailored to ensure rapid protection of the airway.[33] If the patient is not receiving enteral feedings, but rather parenteral feedings via a central venous catheter, the hyperalimentation line should not be used for administration of fluids or drugs during anesthesia. Hyperalimentation and lipid infusions need not be discontinued intraoperatively.

Burn patients demonstrate a decrease in gastrointestinal function. If the % TBSA involved is greater than 20%, the development of an ileus is common.[41] Other gastrointestinal sequelae that burn patients can develop are acute ulcerations of the gastric and/or duodenal mucosa. These are known as *Curling's ulcers*. Treatment primarily entails the administration of H_2-blockers and antacids.[15] However, there has been an associated increased incidence of pulmonary infection with *Pseudomonas* in the intensive care unit patient treated with such medication. The clearance of cimetidine, but not ranitidine, is increased, so appropriate dosage adjustments are required.[24]

Pharmacokinetics. Burn injury causes considerable changes in plasma protein levels, with significant consequences for the protein binding of drugs. In general, patients with burns exhibit decreased albumin and increased α_1-acid glycoprotein (AAG) levels.[24,42,43] Because the pharmacologic effect is often related to the unbound fraction of a drug, alterations in protein binding can also affect the efficacy and tolerability of drug treatment in patients with burns. This alteration causes the plasma binding of predominantly albumin-bound drugs (e.g., benzodiazepines, phenytoin, salicylic acid) to be decreased, resulting in an increase in the free fraction and thus a larger volume of distribution for the drug. Drugs primarily bound to AAG (e.g., lidocaine, meperidine, propranolol) have the opposite effect.

Volume of distribution (V_d) may be increased or decreased in patients with burns. In general, two factors may cause alteration in V_d: changes in extracellular fluid volume and changes in protein binding.[24] Fluid loss to the burn wound and edema can decrease plasma concentrations of many drugs. After the initial resuscitation state, cardiac output increases as the hypermetabolic phase develops. This increases blood flow to the kidneys and liver with increased drug clearance. Dosage requirements may change if the drug has a small V_d and a narrow therapeutic range. Overall, there is significant patient variability based on fluid status and phase of recovery.

BURN MANAGEMENT: SURGICAL DEBRIDEMENT AND GRAFTING

Of all of the surgical procedures performed, the debridement and the grafting of burn wounds is one that an anesthetist must understand well. The course and dynamics of the surgical procedure can affect the anesthetic in many ways. Additionally, good communication is needed with the surgeon regarding the patient's hemodynamic tolerance.

A goal of burn therapy is to rapidly restore skin integrity after the burn. After thorough cleansing, the burn wound should be treated with antimicrobial agents as early as possible to limit bacterial proliferation on the wound surface and to avoid bacterial wound invasion. Wounds have been shown to reepithelialize more rapidly and with less pain and inflammation when occluded, and a thin layer of wound fluid is maintained in contact with the surface. The next treatment involves surgical procedures such as amputation, grafting, and multiple skin debridements.

There is varying opinion on the timing of burn wound excision, debridement, and grafting. Some surgeons favor early excision and grafting of the wound within the first 24 to 48 hours after injury. This point of view reflects the philosophy that the earlier the dead eschar is removed, the less time elapses for bacterial colonization to take place. Some authors suggest that this timeframe appears to decrease the mortality rate,[3,44,45] shorten the hospital stay,[44-46] improve cellular immunity, and provide a better cosmetic outcome.[3] Conversely, there is the opinion to defer surgical treatment of the burn wounds until at least 1 week to up to 3 weeks after the initial burn injury. With the latter option (i.e., to defer treatment), it is possible that some marginal burned sites may heal and/or tissue granulation will occur, promoting better skin graft adherence.[47,6]

Independent of the timing, a common shared approach involves an initial waiting period to stabilize and fluid resuscitate the patient, followed by excision and grafting of the wound. The primary plan is to control infection and remove sloughing burn eschar. It is suggested to limit an operation to approximately 20% of body surface;[15] however, larger areas may be excised depending on the patient's preoperative and perioperative hemodynamic stability and coagulation status. Additional surgery endpoints include a time of 2-3 hours, if the patient's core temperature decreases to 35° C or less, or if there has been a blood loss of 10 U packed red blood cells.[48] Usually, the patient will be brought to the operating room every 2-3 days until the burn wounds have been excised.

In patients with extensive burns and limited donor sites, biologic dressings provide temporary coverage for the excised wound. One effective biologic dressing is homograft skin, which derives a temporary blood supply from the underlying wound bed. New alternatives for the management of burns are being developed. Results with the use of recombinant human growth hormone have been encouraging, especially in children.[49] Artificial skin substitutes such as Integra provide an outer silicone layer for wound closure, while an inner layer establishes a vascular supply.[39,50] The outer layer is removed after 2 weeks and replaced with thin autologous skin grafts.

Anesthetic Implications

There are many anesthetic implications that accompany the burn patient—not only in the operating room, but beforehand as well. The anesthetist must be astute to the global picture of this patient, including the preoperative status, to facilitate the delivery of a safe and an effective anesthetic.

Preoperative Evaluation. The burn patient requires a thorough and complete preoperative assessment. A complete medical history, including laboratory studies, and a brief physical examination with lung auscultation, assessment of chest compliance, and inspection of the neck and oral cavity to evaluate for difficulties with intubation or reintubation should be implemented. There are specific data unique to the burn patient that the anesthesia provider should know, such as the underlying trauma, mechanism of burn (electrical, inhalation), percentage of TBSA burned, the location of the burn sites, the area and the amount that the surgeon intends to debride, and whether the patient will be grafted during the perioperative course. The assimilation of this information affects the anesthetic plan in terms of anesthetic agents selected, appropriate monitoring, positioning, vascular access, and blood product requirements. A review of prior anesthetic records can be helpful in determining the anesthetic plan. Quite often this is possible to do, since more often than not, these patients make several trips to the operating room.

The Set-Up and Preparation. A successful anesthetic for the excision and grafting of a burn wound requires planning and preparation of necessary equipment. There are specific anesthetic interventions that should be done for this patient before his or her arrival into the operating room. See Table 33-6 for suggested preparations.

Equipment and Monitoring. Burn patients require all of the standard monitors intraoperatively. It can be challenging at times to adapt the standard monitors to the burned patient. Electrocardiogram (ECG) leads are often difficult to place secondary to a lack of intact skin. It may be necessary to staple the leads or use needle electrodes on the patient to obtain an acceptable ECG tracing. Ideally, blood pressure cuffs should be placed on an unaffected limb or, at times, at a nonsurgical site. The placement of an arterial line for blood pressure monitoring may be warranted even in the healthy patient, if the planned amount of surgical debridement is extensive, or if manipulation of the patient's limbs intraoperatively limits the accuracy of noninvasive cuff readings. In large burns that are greater than 20%-30%, invasive blood pressure monitoring should be instituted after induction, if not in place preoperatively. Rapid blood losses, the potential for hemodynamic swings, and the need to check intraoperative laboratory values all validate this requirement. The standard sites for pulse oximetry placement may not be available. Alternative sites include the nose, the ear, and the cheek. Any preexisting invasive monitors such as arterial line, central venous, or pulmonary artery catheters should be continued in the operating room. Accurate temperature monitoring is essential, since burn patients can become very hypothermic intraoperatively. Temperature measurements should be obtained via an esophageal stethoscope. Skin temperature devices are highly inaccurate and there may not be a suitable place to place one.

Critically ill burn patients are usually transported by the anesthesia provider directly to the operating room from the burn intensive care unit and vice versa postoperatively. These patients are usually intubated, on continuous infusions of pharmacologic agents, and have invasive lines in place. Astute monitoring of the patient's vital signs during transport is mandatory. Care must be taken while transporting to not disrupt or dislodge any invasive lines or IVs. A portable oxygen delivery system is another component of required transport equipment. Careful handling and vigilant guarding of the airway is vital. The anesthetist must also consider the patient's comfort and privacy during transport. Amnestic and analgesic drugs should be administered as needed.

TABLE 33-6 Preoperative Anesthesia Planning for the Burn Patient

- Warm up the operating room ahead of time, well before the patient arrives.
- Check on the patient's blood status and order more if necessary, based on the patient's preoperative hemoglobin and hematocrit values, the size of the burn, and the extent of the planned debridement.
- Have the blood in the operating room and checked before surgical debridement is initiated. This is critical in the pediatric patient.
- Have at least one blood warmer primed, plugged in, and turned on. If the burn is large, have two.
- Make sure that you have adequate IV access before the surgeon begins debriding the burn.
- Have an adequate supply of narcotics.
- Know and plan ahead of time if invasive lines will need to be placed.
- Have a plan but be willing to modify it if needed.

Airway Management. Any acute airway problems that the patient may have had are usually handled upon admission to the burn unit. In the patient with a major burn or an inhalation injury, preoperative intubation is likely. In the nonintubated patient without an inhalation injury and whose airway is normal, induction and intubation of the airway can proceed as with any other anesthetic (except no succinylcholine). Preoperative airway evaluation is necessary as with any other patient. The anesthetist should exert good judgment in determining the degree of intubation difficulty. If the airway appears difficult, fiberoptic intubation should be considered or at least be readily available.

In the severely burned patient who is intubated preoperatively, vigilance is required to protect the airway from accidental extubation. Loss of the airway in this patient may be impossible to regain due to edema of the airway structures. Securing of such an airway can be problematic. Tape does not readily stick to burned skin. The use of soft beard straps to secure an endotracheal tube is a good option, especially if the plan is to extubate the patient at the end of the procedure. Cloth ties encircled around the head are frequently employed in the burn unit to secure endotracheal tubes and should not be disrupted.

Temperature Regulation. Depending upon the percentage TBSA affected by the burn, temperature regulation can be problematic in the burn patient. These patients are at high risk for hypothermia development due to the loss of the skin's insulating mechanisms, radiation and evaporative heat losses, and the large amount of body surface area exposure intraoperatively. The temperature in the operating room should be greater than 28° C.[23,26,38] Intravenous solutions and skin preparations should be warmed. All methods of heat conservation should be employed while the patient is in the operating room. The use of in-line humidivents or low gas flows reduces evaporative respiratory tract heat loss. Forced air warming blankets are very effective but their use can be limited. Over-body heating lamps can be utilized but need to be at a safe distance above the patient to prevent further skin burns. It can also be helpful to insulate any exposed body parts not being surgically operated on in plastic bags.

It is suggested that keeping a patient warm is more beneficial than rewarming. With hypothermia, vasoconstriction occurs, which may curtail any warming efforts later on. It has been shown that slow rewarming postoperatively in critically ill burn patients leads to an increase in mortality.[51] If the patient becomes hypothermic even despite the best effort put forth, the surgeon needs to be advised to stop the procedure.

Fluid and Blood Replacement. Surgical burn debridements may be extraordinarily bloody operations. Wound management involves removal of the burn eschar layer until brisk bleeding of the dermis is reached.[23] The surgical team may remove the eschar so rapidly that it becomes difficult to keep up with the massive blood loss, resulting in a suddenly hypovolemic patient. Some institutions stop the surgical procedure after 2 hours if more than two blood volumes have been lost or if the body temperature falls to 35° C or by greater than 1.5° C from baseline.

There are many formulas to approximate the amount of potential blood loss for a burn debridement. These vary from 200 to 400 mL of blood loss for each 1% of BSA excised and grafted[26] to as high as 4%-15% of the patient's blood volume for every percentage of skin debrided.[16] During and especially after the excision and debridement, gauzes soaked in a vasoconstrictor[15] (e.g., epinephrine, phenylephrine) are placed on the newly excised wound to control the bleeding. However, this may result in systemic absorption of vasoconstrictors, causing elevation of the patient's blood pressure, even in the face of hypovolemia. Thrombin-soaked sponges may be preferred for patients in whom systemic absorption of epinephrine may cause myocardial ischemia or arrhythmias.[26]

Adequate venous access is a must prior to the initiation of surgical debridement. The size and extent of the burn will mandate how much access is needed. It is optimal to have two large-bore peripheral IVs in place to ensure the quick administration of fluids and blood products. Critically ill patients will often have a central venous catheter in place, especially if the burn is extensive and access is difficult. Although a triple-lumen catheter is adequate in the intensive care unit setting, it is may not be ideal in the operating room when fluid and blood replacement is needed quickly.

The readiness of blood products should be ascertained before the patient is brought to the operating room. Ideally, the blood should be in the operating room, checked, and ready to go at the beginning of the surgical procedure. This is particularly necessary in pediatric patients. Some hospitals initiate blood transfusions before the beginning of the surgical debridement and apply compression dressings after excision and grafting.

Careful planning is necessary to manage the hemorrhage and potential complications associated with massive transfusion (citrate toxicity, loss of clotting factors) during the debridement. Visual estimation of the blood loss is subjective at best and prone to be miscalculated. Suction is not used during debridements. Sponges may be accidentally thrown away or covered up. Blood drips onto the floor, is covered up in the surgical drapes, or leaks under the patient. It is possible to be lulled into a false sense of security immediately after the eschar incision. Proper monitoring of the patient's urinary output, hematocrit, and hemodynamic status is necessary for keeping the patient within normal limits.

One intravenous catheter is adequate for the induction of anesthesia in most burned patients, but at least two large-bore intravenous catheters are necessary before beginning a major excision and grafting procedure. The use of central venous or pulmonary artery catheters is patient dependent. Risks of sepsis in the immunosuppressed patient must be weighed against the benefit of information gained.

The Anesthetic Agents

Induction. There is no single best anesthetic agent to administer to the burn patient. The anesthetic is individualized and should be based on the patient's preoperative status and medical history. The acute burn patient seldom comes to the operating room immediately after the injury. Patients are usually admitted and stabilized in the burn unit. If the patient requires surgery, the anesthetist must realize that the burn patient is quite "fragile" within the first 24 hours of the injury. Anesthetic agents can exert extreme depressant effects, especially if fluid resuscitation is not adequate or has not been fully completed. The loss of intravascular volume, coupled with the potential for a depressed myocardium, can result in a hemodynamically unstable patient under general anesthesia. Careful and slow titration of all anesthetic agents is vital. Premedicating stable patients with a benzodiazepine or a narcotic decreases anxiety and makes transfer to the OR tolerable. Anxiety, depression, and pain are interrelated in patients with burns.[52,53] To minimize patient discomfort, induction can be performed on the patient's ICU bed before moving the patient onto the OR table.

Regional anesthesia is sometimes considered for burn trauma limited to a small area or an extremity or for surgery during the reconstructive phase. One advantage of this technique is prolonged postoperative analgesia. Regional anesthesia is generally limited for a variety of reasons. The anesthesia provider must avoid performing any regional technique through burned tissue because of the potential for the spread of infection. There is an almost universal presence of hypotension (hypovolemia) and vasodilation with or without sepsis, which is a relative contraindication to the use of spinal or epidural routes for pain control until the burn wound is closed. Coagulopathy and cardiorespiratory instability are also reasons to avoid a regional anesthetic technique. The greatest limitation to the use of regional anesthesia is the extent of the surgical field. The anesthetized region must include both the area to be excised and the area to be harvested for donor skin.

In children, regional anesthesia blocks are sometimes a viable option for postoperative analgesia. A tried-and-true regional block to institute in children undergoing debridements in the lower extremities or skin harvesting from the buttocks or thighs is a single-shot caudal injection. This can be placed either after the induction of general anesthesia or at end of the case before emergence. Injection of 0.25% bupivacaine or 0.25% levobupivacaine with epinephrine 1:200,000 added are two options. The volume of local anesthetic injected into the caudal space is determined by the child's weight in kilograms and the analgesia level needed to be covered by the block. If the child is to be admitted postoperatively, the addition of morphine at 30-50 mcg/kg or Clonidine at 1-2 mcg/kg can be considered.

The standard induction drugs are all acceptable to use. Sodium thiopental is well tolerated, but it may require higher than normal dosages.[21] The use of this agent may produce hypotension on induction if the patient has not received adequate intravascular replacement.[54] Etomidate maintains hemodynamic stability during induction with less respiratory depression than barbiturates.[21] However, repeated doses may inhibit adrenocortical function. Propofol has greater negative inotropic effects than does either thiopental or etomidate, which may lead to hypotension after induction. The high lipid content of propofol may limit its use during initial resuscitation and in septic patients.[54] Another intravenous anesthetic is ketamine, a phencyclidine derivative that produces a dissociative anesthetic state of relatively short duration. Ketamine offers the advantage of stable hemodynamics and analgesia. Low doses produce adequate amnesia and analgesia for the debridement of superficial burns; higher doses may be administered for more extensive procedures, such as eschar excisions.[15,23,52] Hallucinogenic episodes can be minimized with the administration of benzodiazepines in small doses, and an anticholinergic prevents excessive pharyngeal and tracheobronchial secretions. In the pediatric burn patient, an inhalation induction with sevoflurane is certainly acceptable if the child does not have intravenous access prior to induction and if the airway appears normal.

Anesthesia should be maintained with opioid or inhalational agents as the hemodynamic status of the patient permits. Inhaled volatile agents have proven to be safe and effective, allowing rapid adjustment of anesthetic depth and the administration of high oxygen concentrations. The burn patient may be sensitive to the cardiovascular depressant effects of inhaled anesthetics, especially if acute fluid resuscitation is incomplete.[26] Inhaled agents do not provide analgesia during the postsurgical period. Intubated burn patients may require the continuance of specialized critical care ventilators (e.g., percussive ventilators) intraoperatively to maintain adequate oxygenation and ventilation. In this instance, a total intravenous anesthetic is indicated.

The main group of anesthetic agents that can exert altered effects in the burn patient are the muscle relaxants. Within the first 24 hours following the burn injury, the burn is considered stable. Succinylcholine is probably safe to use within this time frame. As stated previously, the postjunctional acetylcholine receptors begin to proliferate soon after a burn injury occurs. This phenomenon is thought to be fully complete by 7 days after the acute injury. Succinylcholine given after the initial 24-hour window has produced significant hyperkalemia as a result of this upregulation of receptors.

Nondepolarizing muscle relaxants are safe to use with the burn patient. The anesthetist should realize that the patient may demonstrate a resistance to their effects. Higher dosing or more frequent redosing may be necessary. The etiology of the phenomenon again is thought to result from the increase in postjunctional acetylcholine receptors. Since responses to the nondepolarizers can vary significantly, neuromuscular blockade monitoring should always be used .

Pain Management. There is an increased requirement for narcotics by the burn patient,[15,52,54] which may be accounted for by the activation of endogenous opioid pathways that occurs during stress-induced analgesia.[23,53] Pain sensations associated with a serious burn injury may start within a few minutes of trauma or may be delayed for several hours.[52-54] The intravenous route (patient-controlled analgesia) is preferred early in the course of burn care because the absorption from intramuscular sites may be erratic or too slow for rapid control of pain.[52]

Narcotics are a very important component in the anesthetic care of the burn patient. These are painful procedures. Pain from skin harvest sites frequently exceed that from burned debrided and grafted areas. Morphine, fentanyl, and sufentanil all provide intraoperative and postoperative analgesia and are acceptable choices. Remifentanil, a newer short-acting opioid, may be used in the burn population for dressing changes. Many times, burn patients will be on narcotic infusions preoperatively for pain control and/or sedation. As mentioned earlier, their narcotic requirements intraoperatively may be high. Narcotic-based anesthetics provide the advantage of minimal cardiac depression. In addition, postoperative analgesia must be a vital constituent incorporated into the anesthetic plan.

Nonsteroidal antiinflammatory agents can work peripherally to reduce pain through control of inflammation. However, these agents also inhibit the synthesis of thromboxane A, resulting in the failure of platelet aggregation, with potentially disastrous effects on hemostasis. This may cause problems during the surgical procedure, precluding their routine use to control peripheral pain.

Concern about possible addiction or the inability of burn patients to eliminate opioids has led to undermedication;[38,52,53,55] yet surveys have not indicated the prevalence of iatrogenic addiction. Painful procedures include multiple dressing changes, debridements, nursing care, hydrotherapy, physiotherapy, and surgical procedures. The very high level of pain associated with these treatments, and the fact that they are inflicted repeatedly (sometimes twice a day or more) over long periods of time, explains why patients require medication. Inadequate pain management is a problem in many burn units.[53]

Emergence from Anesthesia. The postoperative anesthetic course should be planned in advance and is frequently intuitive. Critically ill and intubated burn patients are kept intubated postoperatively and are directly transported to the burn unit. The anesthetist should safeguard the airway and be respectful of the patient's need for sedation and analgesia during this terminal phase of the anesthetic.

If the patient is to be extubated, emergence from anesthesia should be planned in advance as well, as with any other patient undergoing an anesthetic procedure. Neuromuscular blockade should be adequately reversed and, if possible, the patient allowed to begin spontaneously breathing at an appropriate time. Narcotics for postoperative analgesia should be titrated according to the patient's respiratory status. Keep in mind that these are painful procedures and the patient's narcotic requirements can be tremendous.

RECONSTRUCTIVE PHASE

It is important to address the ongoing effect a burn injury can have on an individual. After all skin grafting and surgery have been completed and some healing has taken place, there may remain the visible scars. Physical and occupational therapy is very important to assist these individuals in optimizing function and prevention of contractures and deformity. For months to years after hospital discharge, victims of major burns return for reconstructive procedures to remove or reduce scar tissue. These procedures improve cosmetic and functional outcomes. Patients may experience anxiety, stress, and depression from undergoing repeated procedures over a long period of time. The most important anesthetic concern is management of the airway, particularly if contractures of the face and neck are present. An awake fiberoptic technique is the safest method to intubate the patient.

The invisible scars may remain as well. Psychological issues must be explored as needed while the patient is in the hospital. This effort is especially important when dealing with children. Recreational therapists can help children reveal their feelings and fears. Once the child is at home and healed, burn camps are a great means to allow the child the freedom to be around other children who have experienced burn injuries, and to not be judged or feel ashamed of burn scars.

SUMMARY

The anesthetic implications with the burn patient are numerous and can be challenging. As burn centers continue to improve in their ability to extend life after a severe burn injury, the likelihood of an anesthesia provider being involved in the care of a burn patient increases. By understanding the pathophysiological changes that can occur, the anesthetic to these individuals. We must always remember that these patients are being challenged not only physically, but emotionally as well. As anesthesia providers and patient advocates, it is important to take into account each particular aspect of this patient's needs, so that delivery of anesthetic can be optimized.

REFERENCES

1. Brigham P, McLoughlin E: Burn incidence and medical care use in the United States: estimates, trends, and data sources, *J Burn Care Rehabil* 17:95-107, 1996.
2. Saffle J, Davis B, Williams P: Recent outcomes in the treatment of burn injury in the United States: a report from the American Burn Association patient registry, *J Burn Care Rehabil* 16: 219-231, 1995.
3. Donati P: Survival and therapy of burn patients at the threshold of the twenty first century: a review, *J Chemother* 7:475-502, 1995.
4. Kane A, Kumar V: Environmental and nutritional pathology. In Cotran R, Kumar V, Collins T, editors: *Robbins Pathologic Basis of Disease*, ed 6, Philadelphia, 1999, Saunders, pp 433-444.
5. Parks DH, Carvjal HF, Larson DL: Management of burns, *Surg Clin North Am* 57:875-894, 1977.
6. Clarke H, Chalain T: Burns and post-burn care: surgical considerations. In Bissonnette B, Dalens, B, editors: *Pediatric Anesthesia Principles and Practice*, New York, 2002, McGraw-Hill, pp 1414-1427.
7. Weiss Sm, Lakshminarayan S. Acute inhalation injury, *Clin Chest Med* 15(1):103-116, 1994.
8. Paus S, Bueno R. The burned trachea, *Chest Surg Clin North Am* 13(2):343-348, 2003.
9. Lee-Chiong TL Jr. Some inhalation injury, *Postgrad Med* 105(2):55-62, 1999.
10. Haponik EF, Summer W: Respiratory complications in burned patients, pathogenesis and spectrum of inhalation injury, *J Crit Care* 2:49-74, 1987.
11. Moritz AR, Henriques FC, McLean R: The effects of inhaled heat on the air passages and lungs: an experimental investigation, *Am J Pathol* 21:311, 1945.
12. Tredget EE, Shankowsky HA, Taerum TV, Moysa GL, Alton JD: The role of inhalation injury in burn trauma, *Ann Surg* 212: 720-727, 1990.
13. Haponik EF, Lykens MG: Acute upper airway obstruction in patients with burns, *Crit Care Report* 2:28-49, 1990.
14. Sharar S, Hudson DH: Toxic gas, fume, and smoke inhalation. In Parrillo JE, Bone RC, editors: *Critical Care Medicine: Principles of Diagnosis and Management*, St Louis, 1995, Mosby, pp 849-866.
15. MacLennan N, Heimbach D, Cullen B: Anesthesia for major thermal injury, *Anesthesiology* 89:749-770, 1998.
16. Berger M, Bernath M: Burns and post-burn care: anesthetic considerations and postoperative management. In Bissonnette B, Dalens B, editors: *Pediatric Anesthesia Principles and Practice*, New York, 2002, McGraw-Hill, pp 1428-1446.
17. Eckhauser FE, Billote J, Burke JF: Tracheostomy complicating massive burn injury: a plea for conservation, *Am J Surg* 127: 418-423, 1974.
18. Huggins RM, Kennedy WK, Melroy MJ, Tollerton DG: Cardiac arrest from succinylcholine-induced hyperkalemia, *Am J Health Syst Pharm* 60(7):694-697, 2003.
19. Maclennan N, Heimbach D, Cullen BF: Succinylcholine hyperkalemia after burns, *American Society of Anesthesiologists* 91(1): 320, 1999.
20. Gronert GA: Succinylcholine hyperkalemia after burns, *Anesthesiology* 91(1):320-322, 1999.
21. Martyn JA, Goudsouzian NG, Chang Y, Szyfelbein SK, Schwartz AE: Neuromuscular effects of mivacurium in 2- to 12-year old children with burn injury, *Anesthesiology* 92(1):31-37, 2000.
22. Diefenbach C, Busello W: Muscle relaxation in patients with neuromuscular disease *Dir Anaesthetist* 43:283-288, 1994.
23. Sartain-Spivak E: Anesthesia for the burn patient. In Nagelhout J, Zaglaniczny K, editors: *Nurse Anesthesia*, Philadelphia, 1997, Saunders, pp 988-995.
24. Jaehde U, Sorgel F: Clinical pharmacokinetics in patients with burns, *Clin Pharmacokinet* 29:15-28, 1995.
25. Clark WR: Smoke inhalation: diagnosis and treatment, *World J Surg* 16:24-29, 1992.
26. Creasman M, Bradshaw MJ: AANA journal course: update for nurse anesthetists—anesthetic considerations for the burn patient, *AANA J* 63:257-265, 1995.
27. Morgan EG, Mikhail M, Murry MJ: *Clinical Anesthesiology*, ed 3, New York, 2002, Lange Medical/McGraw-Hill, pp 974-975.
28. Vegfors M, Lennmarken C: Carboxyhemoglobinaemia and pulse oximetry, *Br J Anaesth* 66:625, 1991.
29. Weaver LK, Hopkins RO, Larson-Lohr V: Neuropsychologic and functional recovery from severe carbon monoxide poisoning without hyperbaric oxygen therapy, *Ann Emerg Med* 27:736-740, 1996.
30. Thom SR, Taber RL, Mendiguren II, Clark JM, Hardy KR, Fisher AB: Delayed neuropsychologic sequelae after carbon monoxide poisoning: prevention by treatment with hyperbaric oxygen, *Ann Emerg Med* 25:474-480, 1995.
31. Norkool DM: Treatment of acute carbon monoxide poisoning with hyperbaric oxygen: a review of 115 cases, *Ann Emerg Med* 14:1168-1171, 1985.
32. Carleton S, Tomasson A, Alexander J: The cardiovascular effects of environmental traumas, *Cardiol Clin* 13:257-262, 1995.
33. Funke D: The burn patient, *Nurse Anesthetist Forum* 1:4-12, 1997.
34. Monafo WW: Initial management of burns, *N Engl J Med* 335:1581-1586, 1996.
35. Rue LW, Cioffi WG, Mason AD, McManus WF, Pruitt BA Jr: Improved survival of burned patients with inhalational injury, *Arch Surg* 128:772-780, 1993.
36. Saffle J, Morris SE, Edelman L: Early tracheostomy does not improve outcome in burn patients, *J Burn Care Rehabil* 23: 431-438, 2002.
37. Aikawa N, Wakabayashi G, Ueda M, Shinozawa Y: Regulation of renal function in thermal injury, *J Trauma* 30:174-178, 1990.
38. Davis S, Kingsley C: Update on perioperative care of the burned patient. In Lake C, editor: *Advances in Anesthesia*, St Louis, 1996, Mosby, pp 149-191.
39. Shirani K, Vaughan GM, Mason AD Jr, Pruitt BA Jr: Update on current therapeutic approaches in burns, *Adv Burn Ther* 5:1-16, 1996.
40. Pearson KS, From RP, Symreng T, Kealey GP: Continuous enteral feeding and short fasting periods enhance perioperative nutrition in patients with burns, *J Burn Care Rehabil* 14:477-481, 1992.
41. Stoelting R, Dierdorf S: *Anesthesia and Co-existing Disease*, ed 4th, New York, NY, 2002, Churchill Livingstone, pp 725-735.
42. Zini R, Riant P, Barre J, Tillement JP: Disease-induced variations in plasma protein levels. Implications for drug dosage regimens, *Clin Pharmacokinet* 19:147-159, 1990.
43. Martyn JA, Abernethy DR, Greenblatt DJ: Plasma protein binding of drugs after severe burn injury, *Clin Pharmacol Ther* 35:539, 1984.
44. Heimbach DM: Early burn excision and grafting, *Surg Clin North Am* 67:93-107, 1987.
45. Deitch EA: A policy of early excision and grafting in elderly burn patients shortens hospital stay and improves survival, *Burns Including Thermal Injury* 12:109-114, 1985.
46. Still J Jr, Law EJ, Belcher K, Thiruvaiyarv D: Decreasing length of hospital stay by early excision and grafting of burns, *South Med J* 89:578-582, 1996.
47. Caldwell FT Jr, Wallace BH, Cone JB: Sequential excision and grafting of the burn injuries of 1507 patients treated between

1967 and 1986: End results and the determinants of death, *J Burn Care Rehabil* 17: 137-145, 1996.
48. Press BHJ, Solem LD, Giffard RG: Burn surgery. In Jaffe RA, Samuels SI, editors: *Anesthesiologist's Manual of Surgical Procedures*, Philadelphia, 1999, Lippincott Williams & Wilkins, pp 815-821.
49. Lal SO, Wolf SE, Herndon DN: Growth hormone, burns and tissue healing, *Growth Horm IGF Res* 10(suppl B):S39-43.
50. Heimbach D, Luterman A, Burke J, et al: Artificial dermis for major burns. A multi-center randomized clinical trial, *Ann Surg* 208:313-320, 1988.
51. Shiozaki T, Kishikawa M, Hiraide A, et al: Recovery from postoperative hypothermia predicts survival in extensively burned patients, *Am J Surg* 165: 326, 1993.
52. Ashburn M: Burn pain: the management of procedure-related pain, *J Burn Care Rehabil* 46:365-371, 1995.
53. Latarjet J, Choiner M: Pain in burn patients, *Burns* 71:344-348, 1995.
54. Beushausen T, Mucke K: Anesthesia and pain management in pediatric burn patients, *Pediatr Surg Int* 12:327-333, 1997.
55. Kealey GP: Pharmacologic management of background pain in burn victims, *J Burn Care Rehabil* 16:358-362, 1995.

CHAPTER 34

TRAUMA ANESTHESIA

CHARLES R. BARTON

Trauma is ubiquitous, a blight on humankind, and a source of pain and suffering through the ages.[1] Trauma and its final complication, death, pursue humankind relentlessly in this age of high-speed transportation, high-technology military incursions, civil disturbances, and terrorism. Additionally, the incidence of burns, sports-related injuries, industrial and farm accidents, falls, drownings, near-drownings, electrocutions, exposure to carbon monoxide and other toxic substances, and self-inflicted injuries are substantial causes of trauma. Trauma can be thought of as a "disease" that humankind has battled through the ages, especially during times of war. The pathophysiologic responses to injury are consistent enough to warrant use of the term *traumatic disease*.[2,3] It has been characterized as the neglected disease of modern society. Only recently has trauma been recognized as a specific disease entity and received the attention it deserves. The concept of the domestic emergency medical services system is primarily based on military field medicine. Overwhelming evidence indicates that the benefit of trauma care has extended to the civilian population as a direct result of military medicine's attempts to cope with injuries sustained in war. The Emergency Medical Services System Act of 1973, and as amended in 1976, is perhaps the most important factor affecting the development of emergency medical services systems in the United States. The term *trauma system* denotes an integrated approach to the care of the critically injured patient. The ideal system should include (1) triage and in-field treatment, (2) a communications network, (3) air and ground transportation, (4) patient treatment within the hospital, (5) education of paramedical personnel and the public on trauma care and accident prevention, and (6) evaluation of care.

Trauma is responsible for more than 160,000 deaths each year in the United States. Each year, approximately 340,000 individuals are disabled as a result of trauma. The rate of trauma death from all causes has increased by more than 1% each year since 1977.[4] Fatalities from motor vehicle accidents in 1999 numbered 41,345; in addition, 4695 pedestrians were killed in traffic accidents. An additional 3,200,000 persons suffered nonfatal injuries. Firearm injuries included 32,436 fatal and 64,207 nonfatal injuries. Trauma patients are hospitalized for 19 million days annually—more than the total days required for all heart patients and four times the days required for cancer patients. Because the increase in the incidence of trauma is projected to continue and because emergency medical care is improving dramatically, the number of severely injured trauma patients admitted to trauma facilities will continue to rise. According to the National Safety Council, accidents cost the nation approximately $107 billion a year in medical fees, hospital expenses, and lost productivity.[5]

Trauma is the leading cause of death in individuals younger than 37 years in the United States. It is the fourth leading cause of death, following heart disease, cancer, and cerebrovascular disease, when patients of all ages are included in the overall mortality rate. Unlike heart disease, cancer, and cerebrovascular disease, trauma strikes mainly between the ages of 1 and 37 years. Recognition of the tremendous loss of life in this age group prompted a group of concerned anesthesia professionals to form the International Trauma Anesthesia and Critical Care Society in 1988. The society has worked with several other groups of anesthesia and critical care providers who dedicate most or all of their professional attention to the care of trauma patients. This international society works to compile and share the collective knowledge and experience gained in trauma anesthesia and critical care management.

PATHOPHYSIOLOGIC CHANGES ARISING FROM TRAUMATIC INJURY

Cell injury can be defined as an alteration of normal homeostasis that leads to unfavorable consequences for the organism.[6] Depending on the severity of the cell injury, various morphologic and biochemical changes occur. After traumatic injury these changes may lead to eventual restoration of the cell or to ultimate death of the cell. When shock and hypoxia are involved, injured tissues that require high oxygen consumption are more vulnerable to injury and subsequent death. Metabolic rates, not tissue mass, are related to oxygen consumption. Consequently, tissues with the highest metabolic demand are likely to suffer damage and death. Therefore, the importance of early intervention, adequate ventilation, oxygenation, and perfusion in the treatment of the trauma patient is apparent.

The body's response to trauma and shock has been described as a complex series of neural and hormonal reflexes that are induced by injury. They result in an integrated attempt by the organism to preserve oxygen delivery, mobilize energy substrates, and reduce pain.[7] These reflexes intensify correspondingly with greater levels of traumatic injury. A point is eventually reached at which the reflexes can no longer compensate for the disturbances caused by the traumatic insult. This irreversible condition eventually leads to death.

Trauma causes the body to call on many physiologic defense mechanisms, including fever; immune system activation;

leukocytic and reticuloendothelial cell changes; metabolic effects; responses by the brain and autonomic nervous system; release of various hormones; and sometimes the activation of the coagulation, complement, and kinin systems.[8] These responses include a general acceleration of body metabolism, a catabolic degradation of skeletal muscle protein, the production of needed extra energy substrates from endogenous sources, and the production of new body cells and molecular products as needed for host defense and the healing process. Other responses include certain transient derangements in electrolyte and water metabolism; a redistribution of certain minerals and trace elements; a need for the elimination of toxic waste products and metabolites; and the direct participation of body cells in defensive mechanisms, such as inflammatory processes, immune responses, and tissue repair.

When trauma results in hemorrhagic blood loss or sequestration of extracellular fluid in the injured tissues, the loss of circulating volume triggers a response by low-pressure baroreceptors in the right atrium and by high-pressure baroreceptors in the carotid arteries and the aorta.[9,10] When the blood volume is reduced, the venous return and cardiac output are similarly diminished. This effect, in turn, results in a neuroendocrine response of increased secretion of adrenocorticotropic hormone (ACTH), vasopressin, and growth hormone through central pathways, and in the secretion of epinephrine, norepinephrine, renin, and glucagon via peripheral sympathetic pathways. In turn, some of these hormones stimulate a further hormonal response of inhibition of pancreatic secretion of insulin caused by the release of epinephrine or stimulation of adrenocortical secretion of aldosterone by ACTH and renin-angiotensin.[11] Pain, which is an almost universal finding after injury, stimulates a neuroendocrine response. Pain causes activation of nociceptive fibers, resulting in the release of endogenous opiates, vasopressin, ACTH, catecholamines, and other hormones.[12,13]

CHARACTERISTICS OF TRAUMA PATIENTS

Trauma patients often present to surgery and anesthesia with many unique characteristics. These differences are not always immediately apparent in a cursory evaluation. Frequently, trauma patients present in an obtunded state and are unable to supply information about past medical history, possible allergies, or previous response to anesthesia. The trauma patient frequently has a full stomach and is at high risk for developing aspiration pneumonitis. In dealing with trauma, medical personnel are frequently confronted with an acute disease process that is occurring in a previously healthy patient. Compensatory mechanisms often cannot be established as they can be in chronic disease processes; for example, if the popliteal artery is traumatically disrupted, collateral circulation cannot develop as it might develop in a chronic vascular disease state, such as coronary artery disease. Unlike elective surgery, anesthesia and surgery in the trauma patient generally cannot be postponed if an optimal outcome is to be achieved. The compensatory mechanisms, which evolve during the shock state, may eventually cause death. Injured tissues release factors or toxins that affect the metabolic and physiologic functioning of other organ systems. These factors include tissue thromboplastin, prostaglandin, myocardial toxic factor, and endotoxins released from dead gram-negative bacteria in the gut. In the past clinicians tended to look only at the injured organ when treating traumatic injuries. It is currently known that trauma often leads to depression of multiple organs and physiologic systems. Trauma has both direct and indirect effects on organs that are not directly involved with the trauma. For example, severe brain injury may lead to diabetes insipidus as a result of pituitary gland damage. Disseminated intravascular coagulation may occur as a result of tissue thromboplastin release. Neurogenic pulmonary edema may occur as a result of head injury. In addition, the trauma patient often presents with many conditions that may contraindicate the use of specific anesthetic agents (Box 34-1).

BOX **34-1**

Conditions Presented by Trauma Patients That Contraindicate the Use of Specific Anesthetic Agents

Shock

Most anesthetic agents cause dose-related cardiovascular depression. Intravenous induction agents are used cautiously in small incremental doses. Inhalation agents are added slowly as cardiovascular stability improves. Use of histamine-releasing muscle relaxants (e.g., atracurium, mivacurium) and narcotics (e.g., morphine, codeine) that aggravate shock are avoided.

Head Injury

Ketamine causes increases in ICP. N_2O causes increases in pneumocephalic tension. All inhalation agents tend to increase ICP as a result of increases in cerebral blood volume. The effects are attenuated by the hyperventilation of patients to $PaCO_2$ levels of 28-35 mm Hg. Succinylcholine causes rises in ICP that may be detrimental in certain situations of significant ICP elevations.

Burns, Spinal Cord Injury, and Crush Injuries

In these categories, succinylcholine can produce dangerous rises in potassium levels if it is administered approximately 24 h after the injury. This problem can occur indefinitely in patients with permanent spinal cord injuries (e.g., paraplegics, quadriplegics).

Pneumothorax, Pneumocephalus, and Pneumoperitoneum

N_2O causes a wide variety of problems in the trauma patient to the extent that it is not used in the acute anesthetic management of trauma patients. N_2O tends to accumulate in closed spaces, aggravating conditions such as pneumothorax, pneumocephalus, and distention of the bowel. N_2O exaggerates the effects of air embolisms.

Malignant Hyperthermia

All potent inhalation agents are absolutely contraindicated. Succinylcholine is known to trigger malignant hyperthermia and is absolutely contraindicated.

ICP, *intracranial pressure*; $PaCO_2$, *partial pressure of arterial carbon dioxide*; N_2O, *nitrous oxide*.

IDEAL TRAUMA CARE

In the ideal trauma center the anesthesia care providers consist of anesthesiologists and nurse anesthetists working together as a team to provide the best possible anesthesia care to the trauma patient.[14] As key members of the trauma team, these individuals bring a wealth of experience and expertise to the care of these patients. In few other anesthesia situations do the two specialties better complement one another. The role of the anesthetist in the care of trauma patients begins at the earliest possible moment when the patient is transported to the trauma facility. As a member of the admissions team, the anesthetist meets the patient immediately at the heliport or ambulance entrance. Radio transmissions from the field may give advance notice of the nature of the injuries so that the anesthetist and other trauma team members can be prepared to deal with the specific needs of the patient.

In a well-managed trauma center approach, assessment and treatment often have to be carried out in rapid succession. The anesthetist is primarily concerned with the management of the airway and ventilation during the initial resuscitation efforts. After these tasks are accomplished, highly skilled anesthesia practice is required for providing intraoperative critical care so that prompt surgical intervention can occur. Effects of anesthesia care delivery are manifested not only during the surgery but also long beyond the operative period. Therefore, proper anesthesia management in trauma patients must be conducted from the time of initial resuscitation and treatment through the completion of initial and follow-up surgical procedures and possible reconstructive procedures.

TRAUMA SYSTEMS AND LEVELS OF CARE

Trauma centers are classified into three levels, representing the best possible use of community resources. The organization of trauma services within the community or region must address the development of a good prehospital system. The practice of taking the severely injured patient to the nearest hospital is no longer acceptable.

Death resulting from trauma has a trimodal distribution.[15] The initial peak in deaths is within seconds or minutes of injury. Invariably, these deaths are the result of lacerations of the brain, brain stem, upper spinal cord, heart, or aorta or other large vessels. Few of these patients can be saved.

The second peak in deaths occurs within the first 2 hours after injury. Death is usually caused by subdural and epidural hematomas, hemopneumothorax, ruptured spleen, liver lacerations, fractured femur, or multiple injuries associated with significant blood loss. These patients, whose numbers are significant and who can usually be saved, benefit most from regionalized trauma care.

The third peak in deaths occurs days or weeks after the injury; these deaths usually result from sepsis and multiple organ failure. These patients can benefit also from a trauma center in which the concentration of the expertise of surgeons, anesthesia professionals, and other specialists allows for a rational therapeutic approach that positively affects patient outcomes.[16]

Level I and Level II Trauma Care

The goals of the Committee on Trauma of the American College of Surgeons are (1) improved care of the injured patient, (2) education for all personnel involved in trauma care, and (3) research in trauma. In keeping with these goals, the committee believes that the commitment to quality of patient care should be identical in level 1 and level II hospitals. Training and research programs are essential parts of level I and level II facilities. Invariably, in the planning for regional trauma needs, physicians, administrators, and health planners must decide how many hospitals should be so designated. Factors that they must consider include the maintenance of skills and experience, cost, population density, and geography.

Injuries can be divided into three general categories: severe, urgent, and nonurgent. *Severe injuries* are those that are immediately life threatening (Box 34-2). Although they represent only 5% of all injuries, they account for 50% of all trauma deaths. *Urgent injuries* are those that are not immediately life threatening but may become so or result in significant disability. Urgent injuries account for approximately 10% to 15% of all injuries, whereas *nonurgent injuries* account for 80% of all injuries. These injuries are not immediately life threatening, nor do they present a risk of permanent disability.

BOX 34-2

Common Problems in Trauma that Can Cause Life-Threatening Outcomes

- Undiagnosed and untreated pneumothorax
- Cardiac tamponade
- Cardiac contusion
- Cervical spine injury
- Open- and closed-head injuries
- Major blood vessel disruptions
- Airway disruptions

Level III Trauma Care

The level III hospital generally serves communities that do not have resources for a level I or level II institution. However, a level III hospital has a maximum commitment to trauma care, as reflected in its resources. Planning care for the injured in small community or suburban settings usually calls for transfer agreements and protocols for the most severely injured.

In the ideal system, the capability of the hospital and its personnel precisely matches the severity of the injury. Improved care for the seriously injured, with maximum efficiency and minimal costs in terms of life, disability, and dollars, depends on the appropriate use of trained personnel, specific trauma facilities, and equipment.

INITIAL RESUSCITATION AND STABILIZATION

At the scene of an accident, emergency medical technicians attempt to stabilize the patient. The major concern is ensuring a patent airway so that the patient can breathe adequately. At times, endotracheal intubation may be initiated before the patient is transported to the treatment facility. However, if the patient has adequate respiratory exchange, intubation should be performed at the trauma center, ideally after stabilization. Other advanced life support procedures that can be applied before the patient is transported include control of bleeding points, use of military antishock trousers (MAST), and initiation of intravenous fluid resuscitation.

The resuscitation efforts should occur within minutes of the team members' arrival at the scene. Speed is essential. Prompt, appropriate treatment provided during the first 60 minutes after a severe traumatic injury often determines whether a patient will survive. Not all trauma patients are in shock, but for patients who are in hemorrhagic shock, the time to adequate resuscitation is critical. If the effects of shock are not sufficiently corrected within the first 60 to 90 minutes, the mortality rate rises substantially. The term *golden hour* denotes the principles developed by R. Adams Cowley, M.D., founder of the University of Maryland Shock Trauma Center. This principle demonstrates that as more time elapses between the moment that a trauma patient develops hemorrhagic shock and the beginning of resuscitation, the rate of survival decreases.[17] The highest rate of mortality occurs at approximately 60 minutes. Awareness of the golden hour principle encourages trauma care providers to begin aggressive resuscitation efforts at the earliest possible moment.

Because trauma patients are susceptible to infection, vascular lines placed in the field under less-than-ideal conditions are replaced at the trauma center when possible. At the trauma center, arterial, central venous, and pulmonary artery catheters are inserted by use of an aseptic technique. Numerous factors are considered in the preparation of the trauma patient for surgery and anesthesia (Box 34-3). Fluid status is monitored, and appropriate fluid replacement is continued. Monitoring oxygenation allows early diagnosis of acute respiratory distress syndrome and a previously undiagnosed pneumothorax or other forms of pulmonary dysfunction.

AIRWAY MANAGEMENT AT THE TRAUMA CENTER

According to Scottish physiologist J. B. S. Haldane, hypoxia not only stops the machine, it also wrecks the machinery. It is beyond the scope of this chapter to provide a detailed description of specific techniques of airway management for all situations seen in the trauma patient (Boxes 34-4 and 34-5). General guidelines are given in this chapter that require the clinician's sound judgment for each trauma situation. All trauma cases require an individualized approach so that the airway can be properly assessed and secured.

Rapid control of the airway and ventilation with oxygen are critical for traumatic shock resuscitation (Box 34-6). Although in certain critical situations tracheal intubation must be accomplished immediately, intubation conditions are generally better after initial fluid resuscitation and general stabilization. If the patient can maintain adequate spontaneous respiration, the patient's cervical spine is radiographed before intubation for the evaluation of possible cervical spine injuries. Arterial blood gas values are obtained immediately after the patient arrives, and the results are used for guiding subsequent airway interventions. Placing the patient on a known fraction of inspired oxygen (FIO_2) before the arterial blood gases are measured is advantageous so that the adequacy of oxygen exchange can be evaluated.

With a cervical collar in place and the patient lying on a long spinal board, well-maintained axial stabilization of the head (in-line stabilization with the head in the neutral position) should be performed in all trauma patients with suspected or confirmed cervical spine injuries. Awake nasal intubation, although ideal in patients with cervical spine injuries, is often difficult to carry out in the inebriated, obtunded, frightened, or confused trauma patient. This unprepared emergency patient, who frequently has

BOX 34-3

Preoperative Anesthetic Considerations and Preparations for Trauma Patients

- Obtain initial radio or telephone report of patient's condition from field providers.
- Prepare anesthesia machine and ventilator and anticipated drugs, equipment, and supplies.
- Prepare for standard endotracheal intubation and alternative airway interventions.
- Have proper monitoring equipment and supplies, as well as equipment for rapid infusion of blood and fluids.
- Use gloves, gowns, proper eyewear protection, and universal precautions for contact with patient during placement of invasive lines, endotracheal intubation, and surgical procedures.
- Evaluate at the earliest feasible point after arrival of the patient to the trauma facility (e.g., at heliport or ambulance entrance).
- Elicit appropriate information from the patient at the earliest possible time to ascertain current and past history of trauma, surgeries, medical conditions, current medications, allergic reactions, previous anesthesia experiences, and current mechanism of injury.
- Evaluate airway and ventilation for adequacy of presenting status and need for immediate or delayed interventions.
- Evaluate airway to determine anticipated relative difficulty and plan for primary and possible secondary maneuvers for securing of the airway.
- Determine the Glasgow Coma Score and Trauma Severity Score at the time of arrival.
- Secure intravenous access with two or more large-bore catheters.
- Obtain venous and arterial blood samples for typing and cross-match, CBC, electrolyte levels, blood glucose levels, coagulation profile, toxicology screen, and blood gas analysis.
- Have appropriate crystalloids, colloids, and blood components available for use.
- Formulate the plan for use of anesthetic agents and techniques appropriate for the patient.
- Provide airway and anesthesia support as necessary for diagnostic procedures (e.g., CT, MRI, angiography, peritoneal lavage, examination during general anesthesia).
- Exercise care during transport of the trauma patient within the trauma facility in order to protect the spine, to ensure adequate ventilation, to maintain hemostasis, to maintain fluid infusion, and to maintain drug therapies.

CBC, *complete blood count;* CT, *computed tomography;* MRI, *magnetic resonance imaging.*

BOX 34-4

Factors Considered in the Securing of the Airway in the Trauma Patient

Severity of deterioration of ventilation and oxygenation
Need for rapid assessment and intervention in a limited time
Full stomach
Hemorrhagic shock and/or cardiovascular instability
Influence of alcohol and/or "street drugs"
Burns and/or inhalation injuries
Head injury and/or obtunded or combative patient
Maxillofacial injuries
Neck injuries and/or cervical spine injuries
Chest injuries to lungs, major airways, heart, great vessels
Penetrating eye injuries
Near-drowning
Anatomic distortion
Existing medical problems
Prior medication administration

BOX 34-5

Airway Evaluation and Interventions in the Trauma Patient

Administer oxygen immediately while the evaluation is being conducted.
Evaluate the patency of the natural airway and the adequacy of ventilation.
Evaluate the quality of gas exchange visually and with pulse oximetry and arterial blood gas analysis.
Obtain lateral cervical spine radiographs before airway manipulations are performed if the patient's oxygenation and general condition appear adequate.
Evaluate the neurologic status (e.g., level of consciousness, ability to follow commands, presence of head and spinal cord injury).
Evaluate blunt or penetrating facial and throat injuries that may complicate airway function or interventions.
Evaluate for evolving edema that may compromise the airway.
Evaluate complicated airway injuries with a surgeon who is prepared to establish an invasive primary or alternative "backup" airway (e.g., cricothyroidotomy, tracheostomy, or laryngeal mask airway) in the event that noninvasive attempts are ineffective.
Perform oral endotracheal intubation after induction of anesthesia and use an appropriate neuromuscular blocking agent with application of cricoid pressure and in-line axial immobilization of the cervical spine in most situations.
Awake oral or nasal intubation can be attempted in cooperative patients who are adequately oxygenated and hemodynamically stable; nasal intubation is contraindicated in head-injured patients who may have cribriform plate injuries because of the potential for the endotracheal tube to enter the brain vault.
Intubation over a flexible fiberoptic bronchoscope is useful in selected patients if no active bleeding exists that can obscure visualization.
Placement of chest tubes in the presence of a pneumothorax should be completed before, or simultaneously with, intubation in order to avoid acceleration of the size of the pneumothorax, with resultant mediastinal shift and hemodynamic compromise.

BOX 34-6

Recommended Equipment and Drugs for Emergency Airway Management

Face masks for adults and children
Oropharyngeal and nasopharyngeal airways
Long- and short-handled laryngoscope
Blades of several sizes and shapes
Endotracheal tubes with stylets sized appropriately for adults and children
Laryngeal mask airways appropriately sized for temporary airway rescue
Suction with large-bore openings connected to a vacuum source
Self-filling positive-pressure bag
Local and topical anesthetics for infiltration and spraying
Lubricant for endotracheal tubes
Drugs appropriate for sedation, analgesia, induction, and production of neuromuscular blockade

a full stomach, is often uncooperative and thrashes about during attempts at awake intubation. Local and topical anesthesia can obtund protective laryngeal reflexes and contribute to the possibility of pulmonary aspiration. Additionally, head-injured patients with suspected basilar skull fractures (e.g., those with raccoon eyes, Battle's sign, cerebrospinal fluid from the nose or ears) should have oral intubations in order to avoid penetration of the cribriform plate and subsequent entry of foreign material into the brain through the fracture site.

A laryngeal mask airway (LMA) may be useful as a temporary measure to oxygenate or assist intubation in patients who are in life-threatening situations and it is difficult to obtain a more secure airway. The concept that all trauma patients must be considered to have a "full stomach" precludes long-term use.

Awake nasal intubation may be ideal for patients who are about to undergo elective procedures; however, it is often not feasible in an emergency. Topical anesthesia and nerve blocks obtund the patient's cough reflex and potentially increase the chance of aspiration. Fiberoptic-guided nasal intubation should be attempted only in cooperative patients. A lighted wand may be helpful for guiding intubation of the trachea. This technique is based on transillumination of the soft tissues of the neck.

Nasal intubation has several disadvantages. It is time consuming, it depends on the patient's respiratory effort, and it commonly causes nosebleeds. Furthermore, foreign material may enter the brain through a basilar skull fracture. Muzzi and associates[18] published a case report involving a trauma patient with a basilar skull fracture in whom a nasopharyngeal airway was inserted into the cranial vault via a cribriform plate fracture. Additionally, the presence of an endotracheal tube in the nose can cause a sinus infection, and eventually late sepsis, because of prolonged obstruction of sinus drainage. These complications can be avoided with use of the oral intubation route.

Oral tubes also have disadvantages. They get in the way if surgery of the mouth is necessary, they make oral hygiene difficult, and they are not ideal for long-term use postoperatively. However, these disadvantages are minor; overall, oral intubation is usually preferable to nasal intubation in the trauma patient.

Many trauma patients have inadequate respiratory function and are hypoxic on arrival at the trauma center. Until the trachea can be intubated, these patients undergo continuous ventilation with a mask. Cricoid pressure is applied in order to occlude the esophagus when anesthesia is induced, thus preventing regurgitation of gastric or esophageal contents and preventing gastric distention. Maintaining continuous ventilation with cricoid pressure prevents further hypoxic insults that can otherwise occur during the apneic period between the administration of a neuromuscular blocking agent and completed intubation. If an intubation attempt fails, cricoid pressure is continued, and mask ventilation is resumed before the next attempt. It is often helpful to gently lift the mandible forward and bring the patient's face upward to meet the mask; otherwise, the pressure of the tongue against the posterior pharyngeal wall may obstruct the airway. Typically, until trauma patients can be intubated, they undergo continuous ventilation with a mask.

Lawes and colleagues[19] demonstrated the importance of applying sufficient pressure to the cricoid ring in order to press the esophagus firmly against the anterior vertebral bodies so that the esophagus is sealed against possible regurgitation. Delivering oxygen with mask-and-bag ventilation while applying cricoid pressure to protect the airway improves oxygenation before endotracheal intubation is performed. The feasibility of performing ventilation on a given patient is assessed ("testing the airway"); if the airway allows ventilation, muscle relaxants are used. Muscle relaxants should not be administered before the airway is opened and ventilation ensured by visible rising of the chest. This gives the anesthetist the knowledge that the patient can undergo adequate ventilation if attempts at intubation fail.[20]

Testing of the airway allows the anesthetist to assess his or her ability to support ventilation when intubation proves difficult or infeasible. It also ensures the ability to continue ventilation after failed intubation while the patient is prepared for emergency tracheostomy or cricothyroidotomy. All trauma patients should be considered to have full stomachs. Early intubation often prevents potential long-term problems, such as those caused by aspiration or hypoxic insult.

If endotracheal intubation is not possible because of severe facial injuries or other causes and if ventilatory effort is poor or absent because of partial or complete obstruction, an emergency cricothyroidotomy, tracheostomy, or percutaneous tracheal catheter should be placed in order to allow oxygenation. Emergency supplies and equipment must be readily available for this possibility. After intubation, general anesthesia may be required for further diagnostic workup with or without subsequent surgery.

Verification by end-tidal CO_2 concentration with normal waveform morphology is now considered the gold standard for ensuring proper placement of an endotracheal tube in the trachea. End-tidal CO_2 values also serve as a guide for adequate ventilation, in conjunction with arterial blood gas determinations. During cardiac arrest the endotracheal tube can be in the correct place, and yet no CO_2 is observed by the capnography unit. With no perfusion, CO_2 cannot be delivered to the lungs. As perfusion improves, CO_2 levels again begin to rise. Conversely, the endotracheal tube can be placed in the esophagus and CO_2 may be initially detected. This phenomenon can occur if the patient previously swallowed air or ingested a carbonated beverage. Generally, the waveform observed in this situation is flattened and is generally nonexistent after a few attempts at ventilation are completed.

MONITORING OF THE TRAUMA PATIENT

Initial noninvasive monitoring procedures should include continuous temperature measurements, pulse oximetry, continuous end-tidal CO_2 monitoring, end-tidal agent measurements, and automatic blood pressure cuff monitoring. An indwelling urinary catheter should also be inserted in this initial period.

Arterial, central venous, and pulmonary artery catheters are inserted, as indicated by use of an aseptic approach. Fluid status should be continuously assessed as appropriate fluid resuscitation is accomplished. Initially, volume replacement should be guided by monitoring of mean arterial pressure (MAP), pulse rate, central venous pressure (CVP), urinary output, and peripheral arterial oxygen saturation values. Measurements of cardiac output and derived hemodynamic variables help guide fluid and vasoactive drug management. Restoration of these values to normal ranges is a major goal of resuscitation. Sudden changes in any of the parameters being monitored are evaluated carefully because they may indicate the presence of significant clinical problems that need to be treated promptly (Box 34-7). A reasonable approximation of intravascular volume can be determined by observation of central venous and arterial pressure, pulse rate, external bleeding, chest tube drainage, and the rate and total volume of fluid infused. During the resuscitative efforts, venous and arterial lines should be evaluated for continued proper placement and function. The electrocardiogram should be monitored for heart rate, arrhythmias, and ST-T-segment abnormalities. The urinary output should be monitored for volume, concentration, and color.

Initial laboratory screening should include complete blood count, coagulation profile, electrolyte levels, blood glucose level, toxicology screen, blood alcohol level, serum osmolality, and arterial blood gas analysis. An upright chest radiograph should be obtained in order to screen for acute pathology, including pneumothorax, hemothorax, pulmonary contusion, and widening of the mediastinum that could suggest cardiac or major vascular injury.

TRAUMA-INDUCED SHOCK

The term *choc* was coined in 1743 by Le Dran,[21] a French physician, to note a sudden collapse in the clinical status of a patient after a serious traumatic episode. Later, E. A. Morris,[22] an English physician, used the term *shock* for the first time in a paper entitled "A Practical Treatise on Shock After Operations and Injuries." In *System of Surgery* (1850) S. P. Gross called it "a rude unhinging of the machinery of life." Shock is a generalized state of severe circulatory inadequacy that is caused by reduced perfusion and inadequate delivery of oxygen and nutrients to tissues. Shock results in a profound and sustained loss of effective circulating blood volume. It leads to hypoperfusion of peripheral tissues and to a deficit in transcapillary exchange function.[23] Traumatic shock that follows severe hemorrhage inevitably leads to depression of physiologic systems in multiple organs. The sooner emergency intervention begins, the greater the patient's chances for survival. Rapid control of the airway and ventilation with oxygen and appropriate fluid replacement is critical for traumatic shock resuscitation. Venous access must be rapidly established by use of several large-bore plastic cannulas. This measure facilitates volume restoration with appropriately selected fluids and provides a route for the administration of drugs. The rapid infusion of large volumes of fluid and blood can be optimized

BOX 34-7

Assessment and Interventions for Common Problems in Trauma

Hypotension

The most common cause of hypotension is generally hypovolemia. Fluid resuscitation should be undertaken and continued as the causes of the hypovolemia are investigated. Disruptions of major vessels in the chest, abdomen, and pelvis are the most common causes of hypovolemia. Cardiac tamponade must be considered as a cause of persistent hypotension. Inotropes and vasopressors are seldom indicated in the management of hypotension in the trauma patient. Exceptions may include the patient in spinal shock or the patient who has sustained myocardiac contusion.

Desaturation

Usually noted first by pulse oximetry measurements and/or arterial blood gas determination. Check for adequate FIO_2, adequate ventilation, adequate perfusion. Check breath sounds. Check for endobronchial intubation. Look for signs of pneumothorax (i.e., distended neck veins and increased resonance on affected side, and tracheal deviation). May be due to pulmonary contusion, which is often treated with increasing levels of PEEP in order to open atelectatic areas. Copious secretions and mucous plugs are considered as potential causes. A chest radiograph is helpful for ruling out many potential causes of desaturation. Aspiration of blood, stomach contents, or foreign bodies and postobstructive pulmonary edema are considered. Fiberoptic bronchoscopy can be both diagnostic and therapeutic. Consider the possibility of air embolism, especially in cases of penetrating injuries.

Hypertension

Trauma patients frequently become hyperdynamic after resuscitation; this problem is usually treated with adequate levels of anesthesia, including fairly large doses of potent narcotics, such as fentanyl or sufentanil. May need to consider use of antihypertensive agents

Tachyarrhythmias and Bradyarrhythmias

Hypoxemia and hypercarbia must be considered first. Myocardial injury is also considered. 12-lead ECG is obtained. Consider performing echocardiography to access cardiac motion and possible tamponade.

Sudden Cardiac Arrest

Check for obvious causes using ABCs (check for Airway patency, Breathing adequacy, and Circulatory adequacy). Sudden cardiac arrest is often a strong indication for open thoracotomy in order to inspect the heart for pericardiac tamponade or other injuries in addition to performing open-chest cardiac massage; abdominal incision may also be indicated in order to look for other sources of bleeding; rapid blood and fluid resuscitation need to be continued as indicated.

ECG, *electrocardiogram;* PEEP, *positive end-expiratory pressure;* FIO_2, *inspired concentration of oxygen.*

by pressurization of the fluid containers with an automated device. During cardiopulmonary resuscitation (CPR), placement of a 16-gauge or larger-sized catheter in the largest accessible peripheral vein is preferred. Ideally, the antecubital veins should be used for drug administration during CPR.[24] Insertion of a central line may hamper CPR. When possible after restoration of spontaneous circulation, a central venous catheter should be placed. Efforts at cannulating subclavian or internal jugular veins for central line placement are contraindicated during CPR because of the danger of inducing pneumothorax when these measures are attempted in the patient who is being bounced by cardiac compressions.[25] Additionally, attempts at inserting central lines during CPR interfere with ventilation, oxygenation, and cardiac compressions. It is advantageous to have at least one large-bore intravenous catheter above and below the diaphragm in patients with injuries to the abdomen or pelvis. If injuries to the superior or inferior vena cava are present, venous return is ineffective from catheters placed distal to vena caval disruptions. Use of lower-extremity veins is generally not suitable because these veins are often smaller and may be occluded from chronic venous stasis. In addition, MAST may impede venous drainage.

Three Phases of Shock

Stage I. Stage I of the three stages of shock is often called *nonprogressive shock* or *compensated shock.*[26] A negative-feedback control mechanism of the circulation tries to return the cardiac output and arterial pressure to normal levels. This phenomenon is mediated through the baroreceptor reflexes, central nervous system (CNS) ischemic responses, contraction of blood vessels, release of vasopressin (antidiuretic hormone), formation of angiotensin, and compensation mechanisms that tend to return the blood volume back toward normal by mobilization of fluids from other spaces of the body.

Stage II. Stage II of shock is also known as *progressive shock.* A positive-feedback mechanism comes into play with this phase of shock. When shock becomes severe enough, components of the cardiovascular system start to deteriorate. This deterioration is associated with cardiac depression caused by ischemia, vasomotor failure, thrombosis of small vessels, increased capillary permeability, release of endotoxins by ischemic tissues, and generalized cellular degeneration.

Stage III. Stage III of shock is also called *irreversible shock.* This stage occurs when adenosine triphosphate reserves are depleted. Death follows as the natural consequence of not successfully halting progressive shock.

Fluid Management and Resuscitation

The mortality rate for shock is approximately 50%, if treatment is initiated at 30 minutes from the onset; the rate rises to 90% if 1 hour elapses.[15,16] This high mortality rate associated with the delayed treatment of shock is the basis for the initiation of fluid resuscitation in the field. At the trauma center, red blood cells (RBCs) must be replaced in order to provide adequate oxygen-carrying capacity. Shed blood should be replaced with a 1:1 volume of packed RBCs and a 3:1 volume of crystalloids. Evaluation of the patient's fluid status is accomplished in part with CVP monitoring, pulmonary artery catheter monitoring, or both, and by observation of the clinical signs for a return of the heart rate and blood pressure to normal levels.

Serial electrolyte levels, hemoglobin and hematocrit levels, and arterial blood gas analysis should be obtained approximately every hour in severely injured, unstable patients in surgery until the patient is stable. Additionally, coagulation parameters should be observed closely in patients with signs of active bleeding. Colloids usually allow rapid restoration of intravascular volume but can contribute to a later episode of pulmonary edema in some patients. Balanced electrolyte solutions should be given in order to help maintain the CVP between 1 and 15 mm Hg (8 to 10 mm Hg in anesthetized patients). Up to 1500 mL of 5% plasma protein fraction (Plasmanate) or hetastarch (Hespan) can be used initially for restoration of intravascular volume in unstable patients. Fresh frozen plasma is indicated in single or multiple coagulation deficiencies. It should not be used for volume replacement or for any other nonspecific use.

Dextrose-containing solutions are generally undesirable for use in initial resuscitation fluid administration. Rapid determination of blood glucose levels is critical in patients with diabetes and in children. Traumatized infants and children in shock may rapidly consume their gluconeogenic substrate, allowing significant hypoglycemia to occur.[26] Although patients are more likely to become hyperglycemic than hypoglycemic after traumatic injury, hypoglycemia can occur. Significant hyperglycemia is associated with further neurologic injury.[27] Traumatically induced hyperglycemia is so common that it is often called *diabetes of injury*.[28] Withholding glucose or giving it in moderate amounts in order to maintain blood glucose levels at less than 150 mg/dL is advisable if brain ischemia occurs, because data have shown that hyperglycemia existing before an ischemic or a hypoxic event increases ischemic damage.[29]

Dilutional thrombocytopenia is the most common cause of coagulopathy in the trauma patient, followed by hypofibrinogenemia. These conditions should be treated with pooled platelets, fresh frozen plasma, or cryoprecipitate, as indicated. Cryoprecipitate is the most concentrated source of fibrinogen. Cryoprecipitate should also be given when fibrinogen or von Willebrand's factor is needed. Administration of supplemental platelets should be considered when the laboratory values for platelets are less than 50,000 or when the values are less than 70,000, if signs of unaccountable bleeding are present during surgical procedures. An autotransfusion device is an excellent alternative to homologous transfusions, considering the risks associated with banked blood (e.g., type and cross mismatches or transmission of infectious diseases). Autotransfusion blood has several advantages, including a higher oxygen-carrying capacity and elimination of incompatibilities and disease transmission. Use of Micropore blood filters should be considered. Standard blood administration sets have 170-m filters. Although these filters trap a notable share of cellular debris from blood transfusions, some of the materials bypass these standard pore-sized filters and become lodged in the lungs. Micropore filters, which have pore sizes of 20 to 40 m, retain a greater portion of cellular debris. Although the literature is inconsistent on this issue, if massive transfusions are given, use of Micropore filters probably provides some benefits.[30,31] An aseptic approach should be used for starting invasive lines because trauma patients are susceptible to infection. Meticulous preparing and draping while gloves are worn are imperative for the initiation of any vascular line.

Military antishock trousers (MAST) can be placed temporarily in order to improve cardiac and venous filling until fluid resuscitation is effective. Inflated MAST will compress the arterial inflow to the legs and effectively raise both the arterial resistance and the blood pressure, as measured in the arms. Complications observed with the use of MAST include ischemia of the skin and superficial tissues, acidosis, hyperkalemia, ventilatory embarrassment from pressure on the abdomen, muscle damage, increased capillary permeability, coagulopathy, and elevated levels of thrombolytic products. Initially, MAST was viewed as a panacea for hypovolemic trauma patients. Through decades of study, this view has not been substantiated. However, MAST seems to stabilize and decrease bleeding in pelvic and long-bone fractures of the lower extremities. It also appears useful in anaphylaxis and in nontraumatic intraabdominal hemorrhage. The suit has proven deleterious to trauma victims with moderate hypotension (systolic BP, 50-90 mm Hg) who face only a short ride to a hospital, especially those with thoracic injuries. Its role in patients with severe hypotension or long prehospital transport times remains unclear. In severely hypotensive patients, the improvement in BP and oxygenation to the heart and brain may override any negative effects of continued hemorrhage.[32]

MECHANISM OF INJURY

An understanding of the mechanism of injury is crucial because it determines the pattern of injuries that can be anticipated from a given type of traumatic insult. For proper resuscitation and anesthesia care for the trauma patient, the anesthetist must have a basic understanding of the various mechanisms of injury. Research and experience have demonstrated that certain types of injuries generally produce predictable pathophysiologic changes. A lack of understanding of these injury mechanisms can result in inadequate or inappropriate anesthesia care. At the earliest feasible time in the assessment and treatment of the trauma patient, a careful history of the sequence of physical events leading to the traumatic injury should be conducted.[33] This information may be obtained from many sources, including the patient (if he or she is conscious and coherent), paramedics, other rescue workers, and eyewitnesses. Blunt trauma is caused by high-velocity or low-velocity impact, generally from dull objects. Penetrating trauma usually results from the piercing of tissue by sharp objects, such as stab wounds produced by knives or bullet wounds produced by gunfire. Mixed blunt and penetrating injuries can be seen in impalement injuries. Falls from substantial heights can cause vertical high-velocity injuries. Burns are caused by thermal, electrical, or chemical exposure. Airway burns and smoke inhalation injuries are often associated with carbon monoxide poisoning. Chemical, biologic, and nuclear injuries are other forms of trauma that have a known basis. Environmental injuries can be caused by such events as poisonous insect bites, animal bites, or snake bites with venom.

Penetrating Injuries

With *neck penetration injuries*, large arteries and veins, nerves, and the vertebral column can be damaged from either direct impact or from the effects of cavitation. The airway can be damaged by either effect as well. With *penetrating head injuries*, cavitation within the brain from a high-velocity missile can cause massive damage, if not instant death. Transmitted energy from a tangential missile injury can cause skull fractures, brain contusions, or lacerations. Penetration of the chest cavity can cause severe injuries. A high-velocity missile can shatter the heart, causing instantaneous death. Low-velocity missiles may cause small holes in the heart that are usually repairable if tamponade or hemorrhage is not excessive. Major vessel penetration frequently causes death unless tamponade is sufficient to contain the hemorrhagic state. Isolated lung injuries can often be treated by placement of a chest tube. Significant major airway or blood vessel damage may require lobectomy. A high-velocity missile may rupture the diaphragm and cause damage to the upper abdominal organs from cavitation effect. A chest tube should be placed in patients with a pneumothorax before an endotracheal tube is placed or immediately after the intubation is completed. This measure helps prevent rapid progression of a tension pneumothorax accelerated by positive-pressure ventilation. The progression can lead to mediastinal shift, reduced venous return, reduced cardiac output, and cardiac arrest. Penetrating injuries to the abdomen by high-velocity bullets cause temporary cavity formation as they pulp the liver, spleen, and kidney. Low-velocity bullets usually produce less severe drill-hole injuries unless blood vessels are directly hit.

An injury from a high-velocity missile can produce trauma to the entire extremity. Low-velocity missiles cause drill-hole injuries through muscle, bone, and subcutaneous tissues. The presence or absence of a pulse distal to an injury is not a reliable indicator of vascular integrity.

Classification of Penetrating Trauma

Penetrating injuries can range from a simple pinprick to high-velocity projectile injury. Damage depends on three interactive factors:[34]

- The type of wounding instrument (e.g., knife, missile, fragment)
- The velocity of the missile at time of impact
- The characteristics of tissue through which it passes (e.g., bone, muscle, fat, blood vessels, nervous tissues, and organs)

The crush component of penetrating injuries causes destruction by fraying of the tissues as they are stretched to accommodate the wounding instrument (e.g., as occurs when a car falls onto the leg of an individual working under it). The blunter the penetrating instrument, the greater the crushing.

The science of ballistics classifies the types of penetrating wound missile injuries. The characteristics of ballistic injuries are studied in either animal models or artificial models, such as the "ordnance gelatin" model, while being photographed by high-speed cinematography. These types of injuries can be *penetrating*, in which only an entrance wound is present because the missile remains in the body. Conversely, they can be *perforating*, in which both entrance and exit wounds are present. High-velocity projectiles generally produce massive wounds, based on the following formula:

Equation 34-1

$$\text{Kinetic energy} = MV^2/2$$

As a result, doubling the mass (M) of a projectile doubles its energy, but doubling its velocity (V) quadruples its energy.

In perforating trauma, the energy deposited in the tissues equals the difference between the amount of energy that a missile had before it entered the body and the energy it retains after it leaves the body. In penetrating trauma, all the energy that the missile possesses at the time of impact is transferred to the body. Low-velocity and high-velocity bullets differ in the amount and the pattern of damage they create. Low-velocity bullets usually cut and crush tissues to form a drill hole, known as a *permanent cavity*, that approximates the same diameter as the missile. A high-velocity bullet creates a temporary cavity in addition to the permanent cavity. The temporary cavity forms in the wake of the high-velocity bullet, which creates a shock wave with a series of rapid tissue expansions, followed by collapse. This *cavitation effect* causes a stretching and tearing of tissues as far as 10 cm from the permanent cavity.

High-velocity bullets pulp less elastic organs, such as the liver, spleen, kidney, brain, or heart, as a result of the temporary cavity effect. More elastic tissues, such as the lung, bowel, skin, and muscle, tend to sustain less damage from high-velocity missiles.

Blunt Trauma

Direct impact, deceleration, continuous pressure, shearing, and rotary forces may all contribute to the resulting *blunt trauma*. These factors are associated with high levels of energy, such as may result from high-speed collisions and falls from heights. Newton's first law can explain most trauma: an object tends to remain in motion until it is affected by an outside force. Abrupt deceleration creates negative gravitational forces. As the human body decelerates, the internal organs continue forward at the original velocity. The organs that continue to move forward are torn from their attachments through rotary and shearing forces. These forces often cause disruption of connective tissue, blood vessels, and nerves.

Motor Vehicle Accident Trauma

The five types of *motor vehicle accidents* are classified as head-on, rear impact, side impact, rotational impact, and rollover. Because passengers are traveling in the same direction as the vehicle they are in, they often have injury locations that are similar to that of the vehicle. In addition, contralateral injuries can result. Depending on the passenger's position and the presence or absence of seat belts, various injuries can occur. "Down-and-under" injuries begin with the passenger slumping into the seat or dashboard with the knees moving forward. Forces can cause injuries to the knees, femurs, and acetabulum. The upper portion of the body may collide with the dashboard, steering wheel, or windshield, resulting in injuries of the head, neck, chest, abdomen, and upper extremities. Physical evidence of this down-and-under pattern includes imprints of the knees in the dashboard, starburst patterns in the windshield, and steering wheel imprints on the chest. Up-and-over injuries result as the body arcs forward so that the head has the first point of contact, usually with the windshield. The thorax impacts next, so that the cervical spine absorbs a large amount of energy. Resultant vertebral injuries are common as a result of hyperflexion, hyperextension, or direct compression. Direct impact to the trachea frequently produces laryngeal fractures (*padded dash syndrome*).

Understanding the concept of mechanisms of injuries is important in the management of trauma patients. A greater understanding of the many factors involved in a specific injury can enable the anesthetist to prepare an appropriate anesthesia care plan. A complete understanding of the factors involved in a particular traumatic injury can allow health care providers to see the complete picture instead of seeing only the second half of an otherwise "mysterious" picture.

Thoracic Trauma

Blunt *thoracic trauma* often results when drivers who are not wearing safety belts impact the steering wheel during a motor vehicle accident. Penetrating and blunt trauma to the chest may injure several structures and thus compromise optimal resuscitation. These structures include the chest wall, the lungs and airways, the heart and pericardium, and the great vessels of the thorax. Injuries to these structures also compromise anesthesia care by affecting gas exchange and cardiac output.

If the trauma patient is still in shock despite vigorous resuscitative measures, the differential diagnosis of traumatic shock must be reviewed again, other causes must be sought aggressively, and specific injuries may need to be treated immediately. Both blunt and penetrating chest injuries may be responsible for continued hemodynamic and ventilatory compromise. These problems can be caused by direct effects on the lungs and airways or by indirect effects—for example, pulmonary dysfunction resulting from cardiovascular pathology.[35]

Several life-threatening conditions require immediate interventions in patients with chest injuries. A *tension pneumothorax* develops when the pleural cavity is punctured, creating a one-way valve that controls the flow of air into this cavity. With each breath, more air becomes trapped in this space, increasing intrapleural pressure to the point that it eventually exceeds all other intrathoracic pressures. The enlarging pleural cavity then collapses the ipsilateral lung and shifts structures of the mediastinum (e.g., trachea, great vessels, heart) into the opposite hemithorax, thereby compressing the contralateral lung. The size of a pneumothorax rapidly increases during positive-pressure ventilation, especially if nitrous oxide is used in the field for analgesia or during anesthesia in the trauma facility. Patients with a pneumothorax often present with hypotension, subcutaneous emphysema of the neck or chest, unilateral decrease in breath sounds, diminished chest wall motion, hyperresonance to percussion of one hemithorax, distended neck veins, or tracheal shift. An upright expirational chest radiograph provides definite information if the problem is significant. However, if the trauma patient is unstable, a large-bore intravenous catheter should be inserted into the second superior portion of the intercostal space along the midclavicular line. A hissing sound may be created by the air's escaping under pressure. The catheter can then be attached to an intravenous line extension tube and placed under water seal by placing it in a bottle of sterile water that is kept beneath the level of the patient.

Many thoracic injuries can be life threatening. *Massive hemothorax,* which can be caused by bleeding from the heart and great vessels, must be treated immediately. Adequate fluid resuscitation should be accomplished before placement of chest tubes. Chest tubes allow drainage of blood from the pleural cavity but can lead to more extensive bleeding and hypotension. *Pericardial tamponade* that restricts filling of the cardiac chambers during diastole and produces a fixed low cardiac output is also a life-threatening emergency that requires immediate correction with pericardiocentesis. Patients with *cardiac rupture* without pericardial tamponade seldom survive because exsanguination is extremely rapid in this situation. *Traumatic aortic rupture,* if complete, is usually fatal, but with an intimal tear with a dissecting aneurysm, the patient can be saved if the diagnosis and repair are performed promptly during well-managed fluid resuscitation and anesthesia care. Management of these cases requires rapid and accurate assessment and appropriate surgical and anesthesia intervention. *Partial disruption of the trachea or major bronchi* can be handled in many cases through securing of the airway (by intubation or tracheostomy) and surgical correction. *Total disruption of the trachea* is commonly fatal unless rapid surgical retrieval of the distal disrupted airway segment is accomplished; this measure allows lifesaving mechanical ventilation.

Diagnosis of stable chest injuries is frequently enhanced by computed tomography (CT), magnetic resonance imaging (MRI), angiography, and other radiologic studies. Upright chest radiographs (in contrast to flat plate views) frequently reveal widening of the mediastinum in the patient who has mediastinal bleeding from any cause. Radiographs taken with the patient in an upright position generally display a narrow profile of the mediastinum because of the effects of gravity on the mediastinal contents. Widening of the mediastinum in an upright radiograph should cause the clinician to have a high index of suspicion for life-threatening conditions, such as disruption of a major vessel—for example, the aorta. Chest radiographs are also helpful in the diagnosis of hemothorax and pneumothorax. Arterial blood gas analysis can help in the assessment of ventilation and the treatment of acid-base disturbances. Serial evaluation of the hematocrit and coagulation profile helps guide fluid and blood component replacement.

Abdominal Trauma

Placement of a diagnostic peritoneal catheter for lavage and subsequent analysis of the obtained fluid can help prevent unnecessary exploratory laparotomy in patients with *abdominal trauma* (Box 34-8). The incidence of false-positive results from lavage is less than 2%.[36,37] This procedure can be performed with local anesthesia and intravenous analgesia as appropriate. Peritoneal washings are analyzed for the presence of RBCs, white blood cells, amylase, bacteria, feces, or bile. Peritoneal lavage is unreliable in patients with gunshot wounds of the

BOX 34-8

Diagnostic Peritoneal Lavage

- Diagnostic peritoneal lavage (DPL) is usually indicated when abdominal injury is suspected, because of the mechanism of injury (often blunt trauma). It is also indicated in cases of cardiovascular instability.
- DPL is used to screen patients with suspected hemoperitoneum.
- DPL can be performed by use of local anesthesia with supplemental sedation and analgesia. It may be performed during general anesthesia in the patient who has previously been intubated.
- The peritoneum is lavaged with a clear fluid that is subsequently examined for the presence of red blood cells (RBCs), bile, amylase, and white blood cells. In addition, a Gram stain can be performed.
- DPL can frequently prevent unnecessary exploratory laparotomy.
- Generally, a positive finding for bleeding that requires exploratory laparotomy would be a level greater than 100,000 RBCs/mL. Depending on other clinical conditions and laboratory findings, the surgeon may decide to explore the abdomen at a lower RBC level.
- The anesthesia team must be prepared to proceed immediately to an exploratory laparotomy after the DPL.
- Other diagnostic approaches to abdominal trauma include serial hematocrit value determinations, serial abdominal examinations, and CT or MRI of the abdomen.

lower chest and abdomen; in these patients, false-negative rates may reach 25%.[37,38] In stable trauma patients with abdominal injuries, CT, magnetic resonance imaging, or angiography may help in the diagnosis of specific injuries. Extremely unstable patients with abdominal trauma need immediate surgery.

Both blunt and penetrating injuries of the abdomen can cause serious bleeding or other damage that requires exploratory surgery. Retroperitoneal injuries can damage the abdominal aorta, inferior vena cava, kidneys, pancreas, and duodenum. Intraperitoneal injuries can occur to the spleen, liver, stomach, small bowel, colon, or rectum. Beyond peritoneal lavage, use of CT with contrast enhancement can help in the proper diagnosis of abdominal trauma. Knowing the mechanism of injury and performing a meticulous physical examination can yield valuable information regarding abdominal injuries.

Anesthetic problems in patients with abdominal trauma include hemorrhage, hypothermia, sepsis, and interference with ventilation. Major hemorrhage is associated with injuries to solid organs, liver, spleen, and kidney and with vascular injuries. The patient with significant abdominal trauma should have an indwelling arterial line in order to allow close monitoring of blood pressure and to provide a route for sampling blood for blood gas, hematologic, and chemistry analysis. Placement of a central line facilitates CVP measurements for volume assessment and provides a route for obtaining venous blood samples.

Hypothermia is a common complication of abdominal trauma surgery because of increased heat loss through the open mesentery and reduced heat production associated with shock and anesthesia. All intravenous fluids must be warmed with an efficient system, and factors that tend to encourage heat loss must be guarded against in all patients who have sustained major trauma (Box 34-9). Use of heat moisture exchangers in the airway circuit is beneficial in all trauma patients for preventing direct delivery of dry and cool gas to the lungs.

Orthopedic Trauma

Although most *orthopedic injuries* are not usually immediately life threatening and are considered in the secondary evaluation of the trauma patient, they can be associated with significant hemorrhage and other extensive systemic physiologic derangements, such as shock, fat emboli, and thromboembolic hypoxic respiratory failure. Major hemorrhage associated with fractures requires massive intraoperative fluid resuscitation, although rapid exsanguination from major fractures is unlikely. Modern intramedullary rodding devices often allow patients to ambulate within 24 hours of surgery, drastically reducing the incidence of thrombophlebitis and its subsequent morbidity.[39]

Because the ideal time to repair open fractures operatively is within the first few hours after injury, all patients brought to the operating room for emergency surgical repairs must be considered to have full stomachs and should be anesthetized by use of techniques that are aimed at reducing the risk of aspiration. Certain secondary vascular injuries commonly occur with specific fracture sites because the sharp edges of fractured bones are forced into blood vessels and nerves in proximity to the fracture site.[40] Massive hemorrhage can be associated with pelvic fractures. The displaced pelvic fragments can sever the arteries, veins, and nerves that exit the pelvis to the perineum and the lower extremities. This can result in major blood loss into the retroperitoneal space, with continued hemorrhage from movement of unstable fragments that shear away hemostatic elements that have formed in these ruptured blood vessels. Although blood loss from pelvic fractures involving the iliac artery is notorious, significant blood loss can also occur from fractures associated with disruption of the axillary, brachial, femoral, and popliteal arteries. Severe shock can result from major bleeding into fracture sites, particularly in pelvic and long-bone fractures. Close monitoring and replacement of initial and ongoing blood loss are needed during the anesthetic management of these cases.

Hypoxic respiratory failure is a common sequela of long-bone fractures. The hypoxia results from continuous seeding of marrow fat into the venous circulation. All patients with major fractures, especially fractures of the lower extremities and pelvis, should receive frequent monitoring of arterial blood gases. Endotracheal intubation and mechanical ventilation with large tidal volumes are recommended for the treatment of fracture-induced hypoxia and the prevention of further lung damage. If patients are extubated immediately after fracture fixation, despite evidence of poor oxygenation and a large pulmonary venous admixture, they develop acute respiratory distress syndrome and possibly fat emboli syndrome. These patients benefit from mechanical ventilation with large tidal volumes and positive end-expiratory pressure (PEEP) that is titrated for the reduction of intrapulmonary shunting.[41]

Head Injury

Patients with *head injury* may sustain initial damage from trauma that is beyond response to treatment. The goal of care is the prevention of secondary brain damage resulting from intracranial complications that are aggravated by intracranial bleeding, edema, and resultant increased intracranial pressure (ICP). Common extracranial causes of death in head-injured patients are hypoxia and shock. Anesthesia management of head-injured patients should include early control of the airway, establishment of cardiovascular stability, and avoidance of intracranial hypertension. Baseline evaluation of the patient's Glasgow Coma Scale score, pupillary reactivity, and motor function should be carefully documented before therapeutic maneuvers are initiated. Early oral endotracheal intubation with hyperventilation helps in the reduction of hypercarbia and hypoxemia and contributes to the reduction of intracranial pressure.

BOX **34-9**

Preventing and Treating Hypothermia in the Trauma Patient

- Remove all wet clothing and bedding, and dry skin as soon as possible at the time of admission.
- Warm the admission, surgery, and recovery areas.
- Use warming lights over the patient.
- Warm all fluids and blood products with an effective system (e.g., level I fluid warmer).
- Warm all irrigating fluids and topical cleansers.
- Use in-line heat-moisture exchangers in the breathing circuit.
- Use convection warming devices (e.g., Bair Hugger type of device).
- Use warm solution-circulating mattress devices (e.g., K-thermia unit).
- During rewarming, use neuromuscular blocking agents to prevent shivering—shivering may increase oxygen consumption by 200%-400% without improving oxygen delivery.

Judicious use of induction agents and neuromuscular blocking agents can facilitate a straightforward intubation. Attempts to perform an awake intubation in an obtunded, semicomatose, head-injured patient may promote coughing, bucking, and thrashing about, along with concomitant increases in the ICP that carry the risk of tentorial herniation. Nasal intubation may be problematic in the head-injured patient because of possible basilar skull fractures that can facilitate contamination and ultimate sepsis from nasal microorganisms introduced into the cranial vault. Late sepsis can also occur from a sinus infection caused by prolonged nasal tracheal intubation. Gastric tubes are placed orally in head-injured patients for these same reasons.[42]

Patients with a suspected open- or closed-head injury should be placed in a head-up position in order to help promote venous drainage and reduce ICP. Placement of an ICP measurement device may be indicated for the monitoring of changes in ICP. In addition, moderate hyperventilation to a $PaCO_2$ of 28 to 35 mm Hg helps reduce increased ICP. Prompt control of the airway with endotracheal intubation, diuretics, moderate hyperventilation, and possible cerebral spinal fluid drainage is necessary for the reduction of cerebral swelling and the prevention of further brain injury.

A judicious induction dose of thiopental, propofol, or etomidate is usually suitable in the preparation of the head-injured patient for intubation. Succinylcholine has traditionally been used for facilitating intubation in these patients, with the reminder however that succinylcholine may increase ICP, especially if the ICP is already elevated. Preceding succinylcholine administration with an induction agent and a pretreatment dose of a nondepolarizing muscle relaxant will minimize possible ICP increases. When contraindications to the use of succinylcholine exist, nondepolarizing neuromuscular blocking agents, which do not increase ICP, may be safely used.[43-45] Rocuronium exhibits the fastest onset among the nondepolarizing neuromuscular blocking agents. At a dose of 0.7 mg/kg, rocuronium can facilitate good-to-excellent intubation conditions in 60 seconds with a duration of approximately 60 to 90 minutes. Reasonably rapid recovery from neuromuscular blockade allows early neurologic evaluation of the head-injured patient.

Patients with significant head injury benefit from the placement of an arterial line in addition to the standard monitoring, which should include capnography and pulse oximetry. The placement of an ICP monitoring device facilitates the observation of changes in ICP dynamics that are influenced by drug administration and other manipulations. Intracranial hypertension exists when the ICP is at a sustained elevation of greater than 15 mm Hg.

An anesthetic technique in which fentanyl and a potent inhalation agent are administered after appropriate hyperventilation (to a $PaCO_2$ of 28 to 35 mm Hg) is performed with oxygen has been found to be satisfactory in head-injured patients. The safety of isoflurane, desflurane, and sevoflurane has been demonstrated. Avoidance of nitrous oxide is recommended at least until the full extent of injuries is known because it may aggravate potential pneumocephalus and pneumothorax in the traumatized patient. Ketamine should be avoided in the head-injured patient in order to avoid increasing the ICP; however, in the dying patient it may be the most appropriate alternative. Temporary reduction of ICP can often be accomplished by use of small incremental doses of thiopental or propofol, moderate hyperventilation, furosemide and/or mannitol for diuresis, and elevation of the patient's head in relation to the heart for a beneficial gravitational influence. Etomidate has been advocated for use in trauma patients due to its minimal hemodynamic effects. Etomidate may inhibit the adrenocortical response stress.[46] Although no significant clinical effects have been reported from single doses of etomidate, long-term use may be associated with increased mortality in multiple-trauma patients.[47]

Spinal Cord Injury. Approximately 10,000 *spinal cord injuries* (SCIs) occur each year in the United States. There are more than 250,000 spinal injury patients living in the United States. The leading cause of death in patients with SCI at the scene is aspiration pneumonia. Most injuries occur in young males in the second and third decades of life. The SCIs injuries are usually sustained from falls, motor vehicle accidents, diving injuries, penetrating missiles, and other sport injuries. Few severe injuries have as devastating physical and psychologic effects as those caused by spinal cord trauma. Eventual outcome after an acute SCI depends on three factors: (1) the severity of the acute injury; (2) the prevention of exacerbation of the injury during rescue, transport, and hospitalization; and (3) the avoidance of hypoxia and systemic hypotension, which can further compromise neural function.[48] See Table 34 -1 for the common mechanisms of spinal injuries.

TABLE **34-1** Classification of Spinal Injuries

Mechanisms of spinal injury	Stability
Flexion	
Wedge fraction	Stable
Flexion teardrop fracture	Extremely unstable
Clay shoveler's fracture	Stable
Subluxation	Potentially unstable
Bilateral facet dislocation	Always unstable
Atlantooccipital dislocation	Unstable
Anterior atlantoaxial dislocation with or without fracture	Unstable
Odontoid fracture with lateral displacement fracture	Unstable
Fracture of transverse process	Stable
Flexion-rotation	
Unilateral facet dislocation	Stable
Rotary atlantoaxial dislocation	Unstable
Extension	
Posterior neural arch fracture (CI)	Unstable
Hangman's fracture (C2)	Unstable
Extension teardrop fracture	Usually stable in flexion; unstable in extension
Posterior atlantoaxial dislocation with or without fracture	Unstable
Vertical compression	
Bursting fracture of vertebral body	Stable
Jefferson fracture (CI)	Extremely unstable
Isolated fractures of articular pillar and vertebral body	Stable

Hockberger RS, Kirshenbaum KJ: Spine. In Marx JA, Hockberger RS, Walls RM, editors: Rosen's Emergency Medicine, *ed 5, Mosby, St Louis, 2002, p 332.*

Spinal cord injury should be ruled out in any traumatized individual. The nature of the accident should help guide the diagnosis. The mechanism of injury usually helps in the diagnosis of possible SCI. If an individual has been thrown from an automobile, a 1 in 13 chance exists that a cervical fracture has been sustained. If the victim remains in the car, the chances of such an injury improve to 1 in 436. Cervical SCI should be assumed to be present in any patient who has sustained trauma to the head or face, in any unconscious trauma patient, and in any patient who complains of pain before or after careful palpation of the cervical spine. The anesthetist should be aware of the six conditions that are highly correlated with SCIs: paralysis, pain, position, paresthesias, ptosis, and priapism (Box 34-10). A comparison of cervical spine injuries and their acuity is noted in Table 34-1.

If SCI is suspected, care should be taken to prevent further extension of the injury. A properly fitted cervical collar should be carefully placed before the patient is moved or extricated.

Precautions should be taken for the prevention of further extension of actual or potential neurologic deficits. Spinal immobilization should be completed before the patient is moved. The head should be stabilized in neutral alignment with no extension, flexion, or rotation. Stabilization can be accomplished by placing a cervical collar on the patient, splinting, and/or sandbagging the head in neutral alignment. The patient should be placed on a long spinal back board before he or she is moved.[49]

All patients with suspected SCI must be assessed for adequacy of a patent airway. Care should be used to avoid extension, flexion, or rotation of the neck in the attempts to open the airway. A gentle "chin lift" maneuver may be adequate for securing a patent airway without disturbing the neutral neck position. Oxygen should be administered by mask immediately in the patient whose airway is secured at the scene. Hypoxia and hypercarbia can further accentuate the damage sustained with SCIs. These injuries at the C-1 or C-2 level result in complete respiratory paralysis. Death follows within a few minutes if artificial ventilation is not commenced rapidly. In such patients, an esophageal obturator airway or a Combi-tube may be placed in the patient at the scene by paramedics. Although these devices may be adequate initially for allowing transport to a medical facility, the esophageal obturator airway is associated with a high failure rate.[50] The esophageal obturator airway or Combi-tube should be replaced with an endotracheal tube as quickly as possible after the patient is admitted to a treatment facility. The head is maintained in a neutral position with in-line axial immobilization during the intubation. The anterior portion of the cervical collar should be removed before intubation so that movement of the mandible is facilitated for oral endotracheal tube placement. The esophageal obturator airway is removed only after the endotracheal tube is properly placed, its position verified, and the cuff inflated. If this procedure is not performed properly, a high risk of aspiration of stomach contents exists.

If the patient with an SCI is breathing spontaneously on arrival at the treatment facility, the anesthetist must evaluate the adequacy of ventilation. If the patient is not able to protect his or her airway (because he or she is unconscious or semiconscious; has an absent or diminished gag reflex or cough; or has intraoral or facial injuries with significant edema, or bleeding, or both), rapid intubation is needed. If ventilation appears to be reasonable, chest and cervical spine radiographic evaluation and neurologic examinations can be started while an arterial blood gas determination is completed. A lateral view of the cervical spine can be obtained quickly, and it reveals most unstable fractures. For a complete evaluation of the cervical spine, multiple films or CT scanning or MRI may be required. An adequate evaluation must include all seven cervical vertebrae; C-7 is the most common site of injury. In the stable, cooperative patient with an SCI, awake nasal intubation is the method of choice.[51] The nasal intubation can be accomplished blindly with the use of an Endotrol tube that has a trigger device that allows the tip of the endotracheal tube to be positioned with relative ease. The tube can also be guided by use of a direct fiberoptic laryngoscope. Sedation may be accomplished by use of small doses of midazolam and fentanyl. Topical anesthesia can be useful, but transtracheal injection should be avoided in patients with a possible full stomach because the possibility of pulmonary aspiration is increased in this situation. In children and uncooperative adults or in patients in whom awake intubation fails, a carefully selected dose of thiopental or propofol and a neuromuscular blocking agent is used for inducing general anesthesia for the intubation. Special care is given in the situation that requires oral intubation. SCI patients have the best chance of recovery if hypoxia, hypercarbia, and hypotension are avoided or rapidly corrected if encountered. Arterial blood gas values indicating that ventilation is suboptimal are corrected by intubation and mechanical ventilation. If there is a delay in establishing the airway, the patient is given ventilation by mask while cricoid pressure is maintained until the airway is secured. Severely traumatized patients who are hypoxic on arrival undergo ventilation by mask with application of cricoid pressure until the intubation is completed. This method prevents further hypoxic insults that can occur during the apneic period between the administration of a muscle relaxant and the completed intubation. Often, time does not allow the luxury of adequate preoxygenation in an already compromised hypoxic patient with respiratory inadequacy. In order to prevent further hypoxic insult and the resultant potential life-threatening

BOX **34-10**

Six Signs and Symptoms Correlated with Spinal Cord Injuries

Paralysis Inability to move the arms or legs should always raise suspicion of spinal cord injury.

Pain Conscious patient may complain of pain localized at the site of the spinal injury.

Position Patient holding the head upright or the neck with both hands may be indicating a Jefferson-type C-1 fracture; the "hold-up" position (arms and hands held over the head as in a robbery) can indicate a C-4, C-5 fracture; and the "prayer position," with the arms folded across the chest, indicates a possible C-5, C-6 fracture.

Paresthesias Complaints of numbness, a "pins-and-needles" sensation, a burning sensation (dysesthesia), a feeling of electric shock passing down the vertebral column or of water flowing down the back may indicate the presence of a spinal cord injury.

Ptosis Drooping eyelid and myotic pupil, which are signs of Horner's syndrome, may indicate a cervical spinal cord injury.

Priapism Penile erection occurs in about 3%-5% of spinal cord injuries. Its presence indicates that the sympathetic nervous system is involved.

dysrhythmias, these patients are continuously ventilated while cricoid pressure is applied. This measure helps maintain or improve oxygenation until laryngoscopy and intubation are completed.

Use of Muscle Relaxants in Patients with Spinal Cord Injury. *Succinylcholine* may precipitate cardiac arrest in patients with massive muscle injury or denervation, such as that seen in patients with SCIs, crush injuries of muscles, or burns.[45] The basis for this problem involves supersensitivity of the neuromuscular junction to the depolarizing effect of both acetylcholine and succinylcholine. This phenomenon results in the release of large quantities of potassium during muscle contraction. Normal depolarization results in a small potassium flux across the muscle cell membrane. If a muscle is crushed, burned, or denervated, acetylcholine receptors proliferate around the injured cell, so that when the muscle is depolarized, the flux of potassium is increased significantly. The problem is thought to develop in response to succinylcholine several days after the injury. Succinylcholine is not recommended for intubation of the patient with acute SCI because muscle fasciculation may exacerbate the SCI.[52] A conservative approach to caring for patients with SCI would be to avoid the use of succinylcholine by using nondepolarizing muscle relaxants or non-relaxant-assisted airway control techniques.

Spinal Shock. A triad of *hypotension*, *bradycardia*, and *hypothermia* frequently results from a relative sympathectomy in SCI patients. The *spinal shock* is progressively intensified the more cephalad the SCI. Patients with SCIs at the T-6 level or higher have severely impaired CNS function. Sympathetically mediated cardioaccelerator responses no longer oppose vagal innervation, allowing the heart rate to slow dramatically. Loss of sympathetic tone allows vasodilation, pooling of the peripheral circulation, and decreased venous return to the heart. This situation results in a decreased cardiac output and hypotension. The SCI also interrupts sympathetic pathways from the hypothalamus (temperature control center) to peripheral blood vessels. The patient in spinal shock is unable to constrict vessels or shiver in order to produce heat or to dilate vessels in order to dissipate heat. The patient's body temperature has a tendency to migrate toward the environmental level.

Treatment

Patients in spinal shock are hypotensive and bradycardiac with warm, pink extremities. In contrast, patients in hemorrhagic shock tend to be hypotensive and tachycardiac with cold, clammy skin. Use of invasive monitoring is critical for fluid resuscitation and appropriate intervention with vasoactive drugs. An indwelling arterial catheter is mandatory in the acute phase of spinal shock. Moment-to-moment control of arterial blood pressure is essential for the replacement of fluids and for the use of vasoactive drug therapy. In addition, arterial blood gas assessments are facilitated by an indwelling arterial catheter.

A pulmonary artery catheter may be helpful for managing fluid and drug therapy. It allows for measurement of the cardiac output and derived hemodynamic variables needed for proper therapy. SCI patients can readily develop pulmonary edema if their fluids and vasoactive drug therapy are not guided by the variables derived from use of a pulmonary artery catheter. A general principle in any therapeutic protocol is aimed at preventing the worsening of neurologic status after an acute SCI. In severe SCIs, electrical conduction through the injured cord segment ceases as a result of direct tissue disruption from the trauma and from the secondary concussion effect. Vasomotor reactivity of the injured cord is lost, leading to changes in the spinal cord flow. These local injury changes in the microcirculation may be compounded by cardiovascular instability secondary to the trauma itself. The resultant ischemia from these factors causes the accumulation of metabolic toxins and sets in motion a biochemical sequence of events that leads to further ischemia and irreversible damage. Because some of these secondary events are avoidable or reversible, recovery from SCI is limited but possible. Oxygen is supplemented by mask or endotracheal tube, with arterial blood gas values being used for determining the approximate FIO_2.

The SCI patient is frequently unable to maintain adequate cardiac filling pressures. However, over-aggressive fluid therapy can precipitate pulmonary edema. For the maintenance of adequate arterial blood pressure and cord perfusion, pressor therapy may be initiated.

Patients with a high cervical SCI who manifest cardiovascular instability are not be placed on a Stryker frame because of the rapid change in cardiovascular status that turning may cause. These patients are placed on a Roto-Rest bed or a regular bed after their spinal column has been stabilized.

Other Considerations. Patients with SCI are extubated as quickly as possible after spinal stabilization surgery. If the patient requires intubation because of associated pulmonary injuries or dysfunction, then a weaning program is started when it is tolerated by the patient. With frequent assessment of respiratory status, this weaning is usually begun within the first few days. Useful guidelines for assessing the adequacy of ventilation include measurement of the tidal volume (>5 mL/kg), negative inspiratory force (−20 to 25 cm H_2O pressure—needed for adequate cough), and vital capacity (>15 mg/kg). Patients with a high SCI often lose innervation of the intercostal and abdominal musculature.

For these reasons, continued assessment of adequate diaphragmatic innervation, a characteristic needed for the generation of adequate ventilation, is mandatory. Some patients require tracheostomies. Chest physiotherapy is initiated for all patients as soon as possible in order to reduce the risk of pulmonary congestion and infection. Oral or nasogastric tubes are placed for decompressing the stomach. This measure eases diaphragmatic excursion for improved ventilation and reduces the risk of aspiration. Peptic ulceration with loss of sympathetic innervation in the patient with a high SCI is a well-described complication, especially in patients receiving steroids.

Surgical Intervention and Anesthesia Approach. Although external immobilization devices, including a Halo vest, are sometimes used, many neurosurgeons believe that prolonged use of external fixation devices is contraindicated in patients with unsatisfactorily reduced spines. Frequently, spinal stabilization and/or decompression procedures are performed after initial resuscitation and diagnostic workup.

The neurosurgeon and anesthesia team document the current neurologic status and note any deficits before the start of anesthesia and intubation. In an awake intubation, the patient is assessed before and after endotracheal tube placement and after the patient is positioned for surgery.

Whether an anterior or a posterior surgical approach is used in cervical SCI depends on the nature of the injury. Internal fixation devices are commonly placed in the acute phase for stabilization of lower SCIs. At times, these procedures can be associated with significant surgical blood loss. Careful monitoring and replacement of blood loss are essential. Use of an autotransfusion device often saves considerable bank blood use in these procedures.

In patients deferred for elective spinal stabilization procedures, awake nasal intubations are performed. In controlled conditions, this measure allows the use of local, topical, and transtracheal anesthesia without the risk of pulmonary aspiration that is present in emergency procedures. In addition to moderate sedation, superior laryngeal nerve block and topical oral pharyngeal and transtracheal sprays are beneficial. Administration of oxymetazoline (Afrin) nasal spray before the patient arrives in surgery is helpful in reducing nasal congestion. Administration of topical 4% cocaine to both nares provides good topical anesthesia and helps constrict the nasal mucosa. Serial dilation of the nares with increasing sizes of soft nasal pharyngeal airways helps facilitate the passage of the endotracheal tube. Endotracheal tubes that have a trigger mechanism to help control the tube tip position are helpful. Most blind nasal intubations are readily accomplished. Some clinicians prefer fiberoptic placement of the endotracheal tube as the initial method of choice. Certainly, difficult intubations are often accomplished with the help of the fiberoptic bronchoscope.

Anesthetic techniques that avoid hypotension and provide good cardiovascular stability are recommended. Baseline analgesia is provided with opioids (generally fentanyl or sufentanil). Muscle relaxation is provided with a nondepolarizing neuromuscular blocking agent to promote cardiovascular stability. Succinylcholine is avoided during the patient's remaining lifetime following a spinal cord injury with permanent neuromuscular deficits. Nitrous oxide may be avoided because many SCI patients may have a head injury or possible pneumothorax. Following head injury, nitrous oxide can cause a pneumocephalus to develop, with a subsequent rise in the intracranial pressure. Following injury to the chest wall, use of nitrous oxide with positive pressure can cause rapid expansion of a subclinical pneumothorax into a rapidly increasing and life-threatening pneumothorax with mediastinal shift. Ketamine can be useful as an induction agent in unstable patients, but it is contraindicated if an associated head injury may be present, because it increases ICP.

Autonomic Hyperreflexia (Mass Reflex). Trauma centers frequently deal with acute trauma patients during the initial hospitalization and for future related surgery. In this setting, the anesthesia plan addresses the implications of *autonomic hyperreflexia*. Autonomic hyperreflexia is a sudden massive sympathetic discharge resulting from stimulation below the level of spinal cord transection. Hyperreflexia is seen in 85% of SCI patients with lesions above T-5. The incidence is progressively less if the lesion level is lower than T-5. Signs of this condition include paroxysmal hypertension, bradycardia, and cardiac dysrhythmias in response to stimuli below the level of transection (such as bladder catheterization). Hyperreflexia is not observed until after the spinal shock phase has passed. It is therefore usually seen when patients return to surgery for such procedures as cystoscopies, performed later in their recovery phase. The condition is caused by stimulation below the level of the lesion. It is typically caused by distention of the bladder or rectum that is caused by bladder distention, defecation, childbirth, and even cutaneous stimulation. It can occur intraoperatively with local, spinal, and nitrous oxide–opioid general anesthesia. No episodes have been reported with the use of potent inhalation anesthetics. Bradycardia is treated with atropine or glycopyrrolate.

Radiologic Studies. Diagnostic workup of suspected SCI patients consists of lateral cervical spinal radiographs and chest, pelvis, and skull radiographs performed in that sequence. Upright chest radiographs are taken until the cervical radiograph has been determined to be normal. Lumbar and thoracic spine radiographs are obtained if the workup suggests the presence of a lesion in these areas. If a question exists about pathologic findings in the cervical spine radiograph, the patient is accompanied by anesthesia personnel to CT for management of the airway, anesthesia, and vasoactive drug therapy.

Selection of Anesthetic Agents for the Trauma Patient

Trauma patients arriving in the admitting area are frequently unable to provide reliable information about their past medical history. The anesthetist may have no knowledge of the patient's possible allergies or previous response to anesthesia. Moreover, 30% to 50% of trauma patients are intoxicated, usually with ethyl alcohol and sometimes with illicit "street drugs." These substances may alter a patient's response to drugs administered during anesthesia; postoperative hallucinations or delayed recovery from anesthesia may occur. In shock trauma patients, maintenance of cardiovascular stability is the major criterion in the formulation of a safe plan for anesthesia management.

Because of the many problems that can occur if nitrous oxide is used, other techniques are preferable in acutely injured patients. Because of its affinity for diffusing into closed spaces, nitrous oxide is contraindicated if a pneumothorax, a closed-head injury with possible pneumocephalus, or a bowel injury has occurred. Isoflurane, desflurane, and sevoflurane may all be used successfully and anesthesia can be maintained with a mixture of oxygen and air to achieve an appropriate FiO_2 concentration. Vecuronium, rocuronium, and cisatracurium are very useful during the induction and maintenance of anesthesia in the trauma patient. They are not associated with histamine release that may cause bronchospasm and hypotension. Rocuronium has the fastest onset in intubating doses.

During the preoperative phase, midazolam in small doses helps provide consistent amnesia during the insertion of invasive monitoring lines. A narcotic such as fentanyl, sufentanil, or remifentanil can be used for supplementing the induction and maintenance of anesthesia.

Thiopental or propofol may be used as an induction agent in standard doses in stable patients and in reduced doses in unstable trauma patients. They are also useful in patients with brain injuries because they tend to reduce cerebral metabolic rate, ICP, and cerebral blood flow. Ketamine is not used in any patient with suspected head injury in order to avoid the risk of increased ICP. Propofol is a very useful agent for use in post–acute trauma patients who may undergo numerous follow-up corrective procedures following the primary surgical procedure that is done on admission to the trauma facility. Use of propofol in these patients allows for a rapid recovery with minimal residual drowsiness. This is in sharp contrast to the somnolence usually seen following use of thiopental. Nitrous oxide is contraindicated in cases of pneumothorax, closed-head injury, bowel injury, or possible air emboli. Because ruling out such conditions in acute trauma cases is often difficult, nitrous oxide should generally be avoided in acute trauma management.

Postoperative Analgesia. Shock trauma patients frequently experience severe postoperative pain. Intravenous narcotics, such as fentanyl and sufentanil, often help alleviate that pain. Patient-controlled analgesia systems can also maintain a stable level of pain relief. Alternatively, morphine can be continuously administered via epidural catheters. Continuous intercostal catheter techniques can be used for injecting local anesthetic agents in patients with chest injuries.

Operating Room Fires—Iatrogenically Induced Trauma

The days of ether and cyclopropane are gone, but fires in the OR are not. Fortunately, fires in the operating room are a relatively rare event. The most common ignition sources are electrosurgical equipment (68%) and lasers (13%). High-intensity light cords have also been reported to be a source of ignition. The most common locations of these fires are in the airway (34%), about the head or face (28%), and several other areas of or in the patient's body (38%).

On June 24, 2003, the Joint Commission on Accreditation of Healthcare Organizations (JACHO) issued a Sentinel Event Alert related to operating room (OR) fires.[53] The alert was issued due to an alarming number of surgical fires occurring in the United States each year. While anesthesia professionals may think that these fires are of greater concern to surgeons and surgical nurses, anesthesia providers appear to have had a major role in the occurrence of the majority of these fires. The classical fire triangle requires the presence of three elements for a fire to start: fuel, ignition source, and oxygen. In 74% of the approximately 100 surgical fires reported in the U.S. each year, an oxygen-enriched environment was a contributing factor. In essentially all cases that require anesthesia involvement (general, local-MAC, regional), the source of oxygen is under the direct control of the anesthetist. In virtually all OR fires, anesthesia professionals are shocked to discover that oxygen facilitated or significantly contributed to the fire that occurred. Of the approximately 100 surgical fires reported each year, approximately 20 cause major thermal injuries. One to two of the fires result in death.

Fuels commonly found in the OR consist of alcohol, solvents, sheets and drapes (cloth and disposable paper), and plastic or rubber materials (including endotracheal tubes). Oxygen is by far the most common oxidizing agent, although nitrous oxide will also support combustion. Materials that are only marginally combustible in air can produce a massive flame in the presence of high oxygen concentration. Lasers and electrocautery devices are the most common sources of ignition.

Recommendations

Surgeons, anesthesia personnel, and surgical nurses all have a part in reducing operating room fires. Surgeons generally control the ignition sources; anesthesia personnel generally control the air, oxygen, and nitrous oxide administration that constitutes the oxidizing agents; and the surgical nurses generally control flammable materials (flammable prep solutions and solvents, sheets, drapes) that become the fuel sources for fire production. The simultaneous presence of these three factors (ignition source, oxidizers, and fuel) is needed to initiate a fire. The absence of any one of these factors will prevent a fire from occurring.

Room air, oxygen, and nitrous oxide support combustion; as the enrichment of oxygen above 21% increases, the risk of ignition of combustible materials is progressively increased. Keep oxygen levels as low as can be safely done and keep leaks to the ambient air to a minimum. Be sure that oxygen and nitrous oxide leaks from the anesthesia mask are minimal. Attempt to reduce the oxygen concentration when a heat-producing device, such as a cautery unit or fiberoptic light source, is used. Although fiberoptic light is often called "cool light," heat is generated. Keep the total liter flow of oxygen as low as possible when using nasal cannulas or standard oxygen masks. Excessive oxygen can accumulate under the patient drape or about the operative site, creating an enriched oxygen environment. If a spark is created in these areas, a flash-fire can rapidly spread out of control.

Procedures performed near the head and neck are more likely to be associated with fires due to the frequent presence of enriched oxygen and nitrous oxide. Avoid petroleum-based ointments in the vicinity of surgery. This would include petroleum-based ophthalmic ointments when surgery is in the vicinity of the face.

Use the lowest possible concentration of oxygen when given by nasal cannula or oxygen mask. Keep the total liter per minute flow as low as possible consistent with the patient's status and response as monitored by standard physiological monitors, with special attention to the SaO_2 values as compared to the patient's baseline values. If the degree of sedation is minimal, consider using insufflation of medical-grade air with either a large face mask or a funnel that directs the high-flow of air across the patient's face. Don't try to make a patient with a baseline SaO_2 of 94% have a value of 100%. Don't oversedate the patient to the point of significantly depressed respirations. Stay in verbal contact with the patient so that the taking of deep breathes can be solicited on command. Despite many surgeons' belief to the contrary, the local-MAC technique, when properly conducted, is not a form of general anesthesia. During a well-conducted local-MAC technique, the patient is not necessarily totally pain-free and oblivious to his or her circumstances. This needs to be explained to the patient and surgeon in advance of the contemplated procedure.

Obtain and document the patient's baseline oxygen saturation value with pulse oximetry prior to the administration of opioids and sedation drugs; strive to maintain the oxygen saturation value during sedation at a similar value as the baseline value. If possible, administer higher values of inspired oxygen during the preparation and local anesthetic infiltration if needed, then reduce the inspired oxygen to the lowest possible level consistent with the patient's well-being during the use of electrosurgery, electrocautery, or laser units (drills, defibrillators, static electricity).

Under circumstances where surgical drapes are placed over the face (e.g., eye surgery) during local or local/MAC techniques, consider active evacuation of the ambient gases given off by nasal cannulas or face masks. This can be achieved by the placement of a funnel-like collection device that evacuates the gases by way of the hospital suction system. Consider giving an oxygen-air blend to the patient with a FiO_2 of .3 or less. This can be done by administering nasal O_2 via O_2 tubing connected with an approximately 5-mm endotracheal tube connector placed at the Y-connection outlet from the circle system anesthesia circuit. In this manner, a mixture of oxygen and medical-grade air can be blended from the anesthesia machine flowmeters while using the oxygen analyzer to regulate the O_2 level of (ideally) .3 or less.

The use of an incise drape (clear vinyl drape that is placed over the proposed surgical site so that the incision is made through the clear drape) has been recommended by some sources to keep the oxygen concentrated below the incision. This should not be considered a totally effective method of keeping the oxygen concentration low in the surgical field. Channeling of oxygen can occur through any small opening in the area between the incise drape and the skin. As well, if the oxygen is concentrated below the drape, any breach of the incise drape with an instrument or the electrosurgical cautery tip would have the potential of causing a catastrophic flash-fire below the drapes and directly on the skin. The hot tip of an electrocautery unit laid on a drape could cause ignition of the drapes. The cautery hand unit should always be placed in its holster when not in use. Activate heat sources only when the tip is in view and deactivate before the tip leaves the surgical site.

During surgical procedures in the head, neck, and upper chest areas, consider using blended supplemental oxygen/air by use of the anesthesia machine final gas outlet at the Y-piece of the anesthetic circuit; this allows for the monitoring of the FiO_2 by way of the machine's oxygen cell monitor.[54]

Communicate actively with the surgeon and other operating room personnel concerning the use of enriched oxygen during procedures about the head, neck, and upper chest. If possible, stop oxygen administration for a minimum of one minute prior to the use of electrosurgical units (cautery).

Consider avoiding the use of flammable solutions to prepare the skin in the operating room. If flammable solutions are used, allow them to dry completely before draping to prevent alcohol vapors from being trapped under the drapes. Do not allow flammable solutions to pool onto sheets or other absorptive materials that remain in contact with the patient or the operating room table. Prevent flammable solutions from getting into the patient's hair or beard. Place preoperative towels under both sides of the neck to absorb excess preoperative solution and remove towels before draping. If the solution accidentally gets into the hair, the drying time and release of flammable vapors will be prolonged. To shorten drying time, wipe hair with a towel. Check for pooled prep solutions in the umbilicus, skin folds, nape of the neck, and other potential areas of the skin and hair. Read and follow the manufacturer's recommendations for use of their particular prep solutions.

Arrange drapes to allow ready access to the patient's face and thus facilitate observation, maximal exchange of ambient room air, communications with the patient, and ready access for possible airway manipulations; this is generally achieved by placing the drapes in as near to a vertical position as possible. Remember that both oxygen and nitrous oxide are heavier than room air. This causes these gases to tend to drop down over the patient in a manner similar to that of water poured over a surface. Heavier-than-air gas tends to spread and become concentrated under the drapes. It also contributes to a phenomenon called *surface fiber flame propagation* (SFFP). When oxygen coats the fine fibers of a surface such as draping fabrics or even the fine facial (vellus) hair and other body hair surfaces, an enriched oxygen environment can cause the flames to rapidly spread by means of these fibers igniting rapidly in the presence of oxygen enrichment. Facial hair or any other hair should be coated with a water-soluble gel if it is in the area of surgery when cautery use is anticipated.

If a fire starts, immediately cut or tear off any burning drapes or other materials from the patient. Water should be readily available to extinguish fire, especially in the mouth or other open body cavities. Since many drapes (especially disposable ones) are liquid resistant, water will tend to bead up rather than soak the material to reduce flame propagation. Water mist extinguishers are also an option for extinguishing a surgical fire. Water mist canisters may decrease the risk of electrocution as the mist will not pool as readily as water spray. If tearing the material away is difficult or ineffective, use a CO_2 fire extinguisher. Fire blankets should be available to smother flames if they occur. However, if there is a concern that the fire started under a surgical drape due to an oxygen-enriched environment, a fire blanket may not be able to smother the fire and the fire could actually continue to thermally injury the patient.

Sponges, gauze, pledgets, and strings should be wet and kept moistened when in use in the area of surgery to help prevent airway fires. The anesthetist must be ever vigilant to prevent OR fires by treating oxygen and nitrous oxide as potentially dangerous elements in the fire triangle of fuel, ignition source, and oxidizing agent. Careful consideration of the use of such agents can help prevent the tragedy of the approximately 100 OR fires in the U.S. each year that result in approximately 20 serious burn injuries and one to two deaths. Be constantly on the lookout for ways to enhance patient safety by keeping the oxygen concentration as low as possible consistent with the patient's well-being. Work with OR personnel and surgeons to develop educational programs to provide periodic in-service on fire safety, prevention, and management for all surgical staff members that provide patient care. Display prevention reminders, posters, recommendations, guidelines, and information on fire safety where they are readily available for OR staff to read and review.[54]

SUMMARY

Trauma care is an important area in modern anesthesia practice. The organization of trauma care in the United States has substantially improved survival and quality of outcomes for traumatically injured patients. The anesthetist's involvement begins as soon as the patient reaches the trauma facility. The major concern is the evaluation of the patient's airway and the maintenance of ventilation until endotracheal intubation can be performed. The principles of successful management of the trauma patient are based on organization and preparation, assessment of the patient's injuries, proper priority for therapeutic interventions, achievement and maintenance of a patent airway, fluid resuscitation, application of appropriate continuous invasive and noninvasive monitoring, correction of acid-base and electrolyte disturbances, and careful titration of anesthetic and adjunctive agents. The degree of functional outcome of trauma patients is largely dependent on the early involvement of sound principles of anesthesia care in the resuscitation and overall anesthetic management during the perioperative period. In a well-managed team approach, assessment and treatment are carried out in rapid succession or even simultaneously.

REFERENCES

1. Barton CR, Beeson M, Campbell J: Anesthesia for the trauma patient, *Curr Rev Nurse Anesth* 20(24):241-252, 1998.
2. Booij LH: Pitfalls in anaesthesia for multiply injured patients, *Injury* 14:81, 1982.

3. Foex BA: Systemic responses to trauma, *Br Med Bull.* 55(4): 726-743, 1999.
4. Barker SJ: Anesthesia for trauma: a fresh look, In ASA: *Annual Refresher Course Lectures*, Parkridge, IL, 1999, ASA, p 244.
5. *Early Assessement of 2000 Crashes, Injuries, and Fatalities*. National Center for Statistics and Analysis Website, 2001. Available at:http://www-nrd.nhtsa.dot.gov/pdf/nrd-30/NCSA/Rpts/2001/Assess2K.pdf. Accessed Feb 15, 2004.
6. Lee CC, Marill KA, Carter WA, Crupi RS: A current concept of trauma-induced multiorgan failure, *Am Emerg Med.* 38(2):170-176, 2001.
7. Johnson D, Mayers I: Multiple organ dysfunction syndrome: a narrative review, *Can J Anaesth.* 48(5):502-509, 2001.
8. Beisel WR: Humoral mediators of cellular response and altered metabolism. In: Siegel JH, editor: *Trauma: Emergency Surgery and Critical Care*, New York, 1987, Churchill Livingstone, p 57.
9. Baertschi AJ, Ward DG, Gann DS: Role of atrial receptors in the control of ACTH, *Am J Physiol* 231:692, 1976.
10. Gann DS, Cryer GL, Pirkle JC: Physiological inhibition and facilitation of adrenocortical response to hemorrhage, *Am J Physiol* 232:R5, 1977.
11. Woolf PD: Hormonal responses to trauma, *Crit Care Med* 20(2):216-226, 1992.
12. Grundy PL, Harbuz MS, Jessop DS, Lightman SL, Sharples PM: The hypothalamo-pituitary-adrenal axis response to experimental traumatic brain injury, *J Neurotrauma* 18(12):1373-1381, 2001.
13. Pflug AE, Halter JB: Effect of spinal anesthesia on adrenergic tone and the neuroendocrine response to surgical stress in humans, *Anesthesiology* 55:120, 1981.
14. Biddle CJ, Barton CR: Trauma team. In Grande CM, editor: *Textbook of Trauma Anesthesia and Critical Care*, St Louis, 1993, Mosby, p 141.
15. Trunkey DD: Trauma centers and trauma systems, *JAMA* 289(12):1566-1567, 2003.
16. Trunkey DD: History and development of trauma care in the United States, *Clin Orthop* May(374):36-46, 2000.
17. Olson CJ, Brand D, Mullins RJ, Harrahill M, Trunkey DD: Time to death to hospitalized injured patients as a measure of quality of care, *J Trauma* 55(1):45-52, 2003.
18. Muzzi DA, Losasso TJ, Cucchiara RF: Complication from a nasal-pharyngeal airway in a patient with a basilar skull fracture, *Anesthesiology* 74:366-368, 1991.
19. Lawes EG, Campbell I, Mercer D: Inflation pressure, gastric insufflation and rapid sequence induction, *Br J Anaesth* 59:315-318, 1987.
20. Stene JK: Anesthesia for trauma. In Miller RD, editor: *Anesthesia*, ed 5, New York, 2000, Churchill Livingstone, p 2157.
21. Le Dran HF: A treatise, or reflections drawn from practice on gunshot wounds, London, 1743, Clark.
22. Morris EA: A practical treatise on shock after operations and injuries, London, 1867, Hardwicke.
23. Pinsky MR. Targets for resuscitation from shock. *Minerva Anestesiol* 69(4):237-244, 2003.
24. American Heart Association: Guidelines for cardiopulmonary resuscitation and emergency cardiac care: Adult advanced cardiac life support, *ACLS Provider Manual* 2001.
25. Babbs CF: Interposed abdominal compression CPR: a comprehensive evidence based review, *Resuscitation* 59(1):71-82, 2003.
26. Song EC, Chu K, Jeong SW, et al: Hyperglycemia exacerbates brain edema and perihematomal cell death after intracerebral hemorrhage, *Stroke* 34(9):2215-2220, 2003.
27. Nacht A, Kahn RC, Ramanathan S: Metabolic-endocrine response to trauma and nutritional support. In Capan LM, Miller SM, Turndorf H, editors: *Trauma Anesthesia and Intensive Care*, Philadelphia, 1991, Lippincott, 1991, p 665.
28. Sieber FE, Smith DS, Traystman RJ, Wollman H: Glucose: a reevaluation of its intraoperative use, *Anesthesiology* 67:72-81, 1987.
29. Coursin DB, Cicala RS: Perioperative care of the trauma patient. In Barash PG, editor: *Refresher Courses in Anesthesiology*, vol 20, Philadelphia, 1992, Lippincott, p 40.
30. Swank RL, Seaman GV: Microfiltration and microemboli: a history, *Transfusion* 40(1):114-119, 2000.
31. Joffe D, Silvay G: The use of microfiltration in cardiopulmonary bypass, *J Cardiothorac Vasc Anesth* 8(6):685-692, 1994.
32. Frank LR: Is MAST in the past? The pros and cons of MAST usage in the field, *J Emerg Med* 25(2):38-41, 44-45, 2000.
33. Colwell C, Murphy P, Bryan T: Detecting mechanism of injury, *Emerg Med Serv* 32(5):52-58, 2003.
34. Grande CM: Mechanisms and patterns of injury: the key to anticipation in trauma management, *Crit Care Clin* 6:25-35, 1990.
35. Liman ST, Kuzucu A, Tastepe AL, Ulasan GN, Topcu S: Chest injury due to blunt trauma, *Eur J Cardiothorac Surg* 23(3):374-378, 2003.
36. Demetriades D, Velmahos G: Technology-driven triage of abdominal trauma: the emerging era of nonoperative management, *Annu Rev Med* 54:1-15, 2003.
37. Chiquito PE: Blunt abdominal injuries: diagnostic peritoneal lavage, ultrasonography and computed tomography scanning, *Injury* 27(2):117-124, 1996.
38. Barton CR, Beeson M: Orthopedic anesthesia. In McIntosh LW, editor: *Essentials of Nurse Anesthesia*, New York, 1997, McGraw-Hill, p 439.
39. Litchtblau S: Hip fracture: surgical decisions that affect medical management, *Geriatrics* 55(5):50-52, 55-56, 2000.
40. Stene JK, Grande CM, Barton CR: Perioperative anesthetic management of the trauma patient: thoracoabdominal and orthopaedic injuries. In Stene JK, Grande CM, editors: *Trauma Anesthesia*, Baltimore, 1991, Williams & Wilkins, p 236.
41. Stene JK, Grande CM: Anesthesia for trauma. In Miller RD, editor: *Anesthesia*, ed 5, Philadelphia, 2000, Churchill Livingstone, pp 2157-2172.
42. Atkinson JLD, Faust R: Central nervous system trauma. In Cucchiara RF, Black S, Michenfelder JD, editors: *Clinical Neuroanesthesia*, ed 2, New York, 1998, Churchhill Livingstone, p 539-556.
43. Silber SH: Rapid sequence intubation in adults with elevated intracranial pressure: a survey of emergency medicine residency programs, *Am J Emerg Med* 15(3):263-267, 1997.
44. Li J, Murphy-Lavoie H, Bugas C, Martinez J, Preston C: Complications of emergency intubation with and without paralysis, *Am J Emerg Med* 17(2):141-143, 1999.
45. Orebaug SL: Succinylcholine: adverse effects and alternatives in emergency medicine, *Am J Emerg Med.* 17(7):715-721, 1999.
46. Absalom A, Pledger D, Kong A: Adrenocortical function in critically ill patients 24 h after a single dose of etomidate, *Anaesthesia* 54(9):861-867, 1999.
47. Ledingham I, McArthur A, Watt I: Influence of sedation on mortality in critically ill multiple trauma patients, *Lancet* 1:1270, 1983.
48. McKinley WO, Jackson AB, Cardenas DD, DeVivo MJ: Long term medical complications after traumatic spinal cord injury: a regional model systems analysis, *Arch Phys Med Rehabil* 80: 1402-1410, 1999.
49. Kopaniky DR: Pathophysiology and management of spinal cord trauma. In Frost E, editor: *Clinical Anesthesia in Neurosurgery*, ed 2, Boston, 1991, Butterworth-Heinemann, p 375.
50. Grande CM, Barton CR, Stene JK: Emergency airway management in trauma patients with a suspected cervical spine injury: in response, *Anesth Analg* 68:416-418, 1989.
51. Fuchs G, Schwartz G, Baumgarter A, et al: Fiberoptic intubation in 327 neurosurgical patients with lesions of the cervical spine, *J Neurosurg Anesthesiol* 11(1):11-16, 1999.
52. Vuksanj D, Fisher DM: Pharmokinetics of rocuronium in children aged 4-11 years, *Anesthesiology* 82:1104-1110, 1995.
53. Joint Commission on Accreditation of Healthcare Organizations: Preventing surgical fires, *Sentinel Event Alert*, Issue 29, June 24, 2003.
54. ECRI. A clinician's guide to surgical fires; how they occur, how to prevent them, how to put them out {guidance article}, *Health Devices* 32(1):5-24, 2003.

CHAPTER 35

Outpatient Anesthesia

Rex A. Marley

The concept of outpatient anesthesia is not unique to the past three decades. It was introduced in dentists' offices with the administration of nitrous oxide. Physicians' offices were next to offer this type of service for superficial procedures that required, at most, the administration of local anesthesia. In 1909 Nicoll[1] first reported on 8988 outpatient surgical procedures performed at the Glasgow Royal Hospital for Sick Children. In 1916 in Sioux City, Iowa, Waters[2] opened the first freestanding unit designed for outpatient surgery.

The evolution of and the demand for outpatient care have not slowed since first described by these pioneers. Ambulatory surgery is becoming increasingly popular as the needs of the patient and medical community are better met. More than 31 million ambulatory procedures were performed in the United States in 1996.[3] At present, more than 70% of all operations are performed on an outpatient basis.[4] The patient is expected to enter the outpatient surgical care facility, undergo the procedure, and then be released without needing an overnight stay. Outpatient surgery includes the "23-hour observation" patient, who may be admitted to the inpatient or overnight facility yet is discharged before staying in the hospital 24 hours. Surgical procedures requiring the expertise of an anesthesia provider in the office setting are becoming increasing popular. Office-based surgery can be performed more efficiently and at lower cost than in the hospital.[5] It is predicted that 24% of all elective surgeries will be office based by 2005, a total of almost 10 million operations per year.[6]

FEATURES OF OUTPATIENT SURGERY

Advantages

Financial. An advantage of ambulatory surgical settings has been the economic benefit for consumers, third-party payers, and medical facilities. Patients may benefit not only from reduced medical cost but also from minimized costs of outside child care and from resumption of normal living activities at an earlier time. Third-party payers concerned about cost containment are increasingly identifying procedures that may be performed only in the outpatient setting. Cost savings exceeding 50% have been reported for selected surgeries (e.g., laparoscopic cholecystectomy) performed on an outpatient basis.[7]

Medical. One medical advantage of ambulatory surgery is the increased availability of hospital beds for patients requiring hospital admission. For patients who are susceptible to infection (e.g., children, immunosuppressed patients, cancer patients, and transplant recipients), minimizing time in the hospital and contact with people in the hospital may decrease the risk of nosocomial infections.[8]

Social. Children benefit from outpatient surgery because it minimizes separation from parents and causes less disruption in the children's feeding schedule. The continued presence and care offered by the parents are beneficial for children with mental or physical impairments. Geriatric patients show better cognitive and physical capacity when separation from familiar surroundings and family is minimized.[9] The elderly are better able to maintain their normal living routines (e.g., diet, medication, and sleep pattern). Postoperative confusion is decreased in geriatric patients undergoing outpatient procedures because they receive less medication and are returned to a familiar environment sooner than their inpatient counterparts.

Staffing. The ambulatory surgery setting is more convenient than the inpatient surgery setting for the staff because it offers better use of time, uniform work schedules, and more predictable surgical outcomes.

Disadvantages

The outpatient setting may have several disadvantages, including the following:

1. The degree of patient privacy is less than that in the inpatient setting.
2. The patient must make multiple trips to the physician's office or the ambulatory setting for evaluation and screening.
3. Adequate home care must be ensured once the patient is discharged from the facility after surgery.
4. The lack of patient compliance with preoperative and postoperative instructions is a limitation that is minimized when the patient is admitted to the hospital before the surgery.
5. Because of the emphasis on efficiency, children are not allowed the time to adapt to the ambulatory setting, as they would as an inpatient.
6. The amount of observation time in which the patient is monitored for the occurrence of adverse events is less than that in the inpatient setting.

Demographic Considerations

Patient Age. Patients receiving outpatient anesthesia can be any age. Approximately 30% of outpatients are younger than 12 years of age,[10] and more than 10% are at least 60 years of age.[11]

Surgical Length. Earlier guidelines for the length of outpatient surgery recommended limiting the length to less than

1.5 to 2 hours.[12] A correlation between a greater duration of anesthesia and recovery time[13] and an increased incidence of hospital admission[14] has been suggested; yet this is not a consistent finding.[15] Other factors, such as the skill of the surgeon, the type of surgery performed, the patient's condition, and anesthetic technique used, must be considered. Arbitrarily limiting the length of surgery to less than 2 hours is not appropriate; procedures exceeding 4 hours are routinely performed without complications in ambulatory centers.

Suitable Procedures. The list of procedures suitable for the ambulatory setting is constantly evolving. Ophthalmologic procedures are now the most common type of outpatient procedure, and gynecologic surgery is the second.[16] The outpatient surgical procedure should not involve extensive blood loss or physiologic shifts of considerable fluid volumes, because these processes necessitate protracted patient observation and hydration. In the past, the potential for blood transfusion implied the need for the procedure to be conducted at an inpatient facility.[12] The increasing popularity of autologous blood donation for future transfusion has led to the application of transfusion during or after the outpatient surgery.[17]

Acceptable surgical procedures are expanding and routinely include such surgeries as laparoscopic cholecystectomy,[7] lumbar laminectomy,[18] thyroidectomy,[19] vaginal hysterectomy,[20] and tonsillectomy.[21] The tonsillectomy with or without adenoidectomy remains a controversial procedure when performed on an outpatient basis because of the potential for postoperative bleeding.[22] Chiang and coworkers[23] reported on 40,000 outpatient tonsillectomies in which no deaths occurred. The incidence of posttonsillectomy hemorrhage is 1.93% and is similar in outpatient and inpatient populations.[24] This review of 4662 patients over a 13-year period found that 46% of those with postoperative hemorrhage required return to the operating room for hemorrhage control. Interestingly, the age group at highest risk for hemorrhage was 21 to 30 years of age (3.61% incidence of hemorrhage). The minimum age for an ambulatory surgical facility to consider adenotonsillectomy is 3 years, and additionally the child must not have obstructive sleep apnea.[25,26] The 23-hour observation area, which is designed for extended patient inspection, is popular for outpatient tonsillectomy.

Procedures requiring prolonged immobilization are best conducted on an inpatient basis. For procedures associated with postoperative discomfort, arrangements for parenteral opioid therapy in the home may be made, provided that adequate pain relief can be achieved with safe doses of opioids.

PATIENT SELECTION

Proper patient selection minimizes the number of hospital admissions that follow outpatient surgery. The determination of which patients are appropriate for outpatient surgery and anesthesia requires consensus and cooperation between the surgical and the anesthesia staff. Factors to consider in the determination of the suitability of a patient for outpatient surgery include the following:

1. *The anticipated surgical procedure for the patient.* The proposed surgery should have an insignificant incidence of intraoperative and postoperative problems and should not require intense postoperative patient management.
2. *The physical and psychosocial health of the patient.* The patient is ideally in his or her usual good health, or if the patient is ill, the illness should be under proper control. The patient and family should be receptive to the outpatient philosophy and the perioperative adaptations that will be required of them.
3. *The surgeon's skills and cooperation.* Early referral to the anesthesia department for patients of questionable appropriateness helps streamline the outpatient process and helps minimize delays on the day of surgery.

Selection Criteria

Acute Substance Abuse. The patient with a history of substance abuse should be evaluated before the day of surgery. Counseling for such patients includes the warning that preoperative substance abuse will lead to the cancellation of the surgery. A distinction between long-term and acute substance abuse must be made. A urinary drug screen should be performed in patients suspected of substance abuse.[27] The patient with signs of acute substance intoxication is an inappropriate ambulatory surgery candidate because of the increased likelihood of impaired autonomic and cardiovascular responses.[28] The surgery should be rescheduled after the patient is detoxified and treated. Patient management strategies should emphasize methods of minimizing postoperative pain because substance abusers are typically intolerant to pain. Regional or local anesthetic techniques, if their use is suitable to the surgeon and appropriate for the type of operation being performed, may be used if the patient wishes to abstain from sedatives and opioids. Postoperatively, pain may be minimized by the use of local wound infiltration and the prophylactic use of nonsteroidal analgesics.

Age. Patient age, by itself, should not be the deciding factor for outpatient suitability. Meridy[15] retrospectively examined the charts of patients ranging in age from 9 months to 92 years and noted that most perioperative complications occurred in the 20-year to 49-year age group.

Premature Infant. The premature infant (gestational age of 37 weeks or less at birth) is an inappropriate candidate for outpatient surgery because of potential physiologic aberrations. The premature infant may do the following:

1. Exhibit anemia
2. Not have fully developed gag reflexes (and thus be more prone to aspiration of liquid or solid food)[29]
3. Have immature temperature control and be susceptible to the effects of hypothermia, thus contributing to postoperative apnea[30]
4. Demonstrate immature brain stem functioning, which predisposes the infant to pathologic respiratory conditions[10]

The infant with a hemoglobin value that is less than the predicted normal value for that age will require additional evaluation before surgery. Hemoglobin values in the premature infant may drop to between 7 and 8 g/100 mL 1 to 3 months after birth.[31] The presence of anemia (hematocrit value less than 30%) may increase the incidence of apnea in the newborn.[32] Some investigators have recommended delaying elective surgery until the hematocrit value is increased to greater than 30% through the supplementation of iron intake.[33]

In the perioperative period, the preterm infant is at greater risk for developing respiratory complications, including apnea, than is the full-term infant.[34] The preterm infant is susceptible to short apnea (6 to 15 seconds), prolonged apnea (greater than 15 seconds), or periodic breathing (three or more periods of apnea of 3 to 15 seconds separated by less than 20 seconds of normal respiration). Short or prolonged apnea and periodic breathing predispose the infant to hypoxemia and bradycardia. An obstructive component that leads to quicker oxyhemoglobin desaturation appears to be part of postoperative apnea in these infants.[35] These infants have developed prolonged apnea as late as 12 hours after surgery.[34]

The older the infant, the less likely that respiratory complications, such as apnea, will occur. In the decision regarding the suitability of the former preterm infant for outpatient surgery, conservative measures are best, and inpatient status should be assigned if significant concerns exist. These patients benefit from the intensive monitoring available in the inpatient setting. Much discussion has been held as to the postconceptual age (gestational age plus postnatal age) at which the former premature infant may safely undergo outpatient anesthesia. Healthy former premature infants whose postconceptual age is less than 50 to 60 weeks[36,37] should be admitted to the hospital for extended monitoring. Postoperative apnea has even been described in the full-term infant.[38] Our ability to exactly predict the susceptibility of an infant to postoperative apnea is lacking.[39] Patients should be evaluated individually for appropriateness for outpatient surgery, and consideration should be given to growth and development; feeding problems; upper respiratory tract infections (URTIs); apneic history; and disorders of metabolic, endocrine, neurologic, or cardiac systems.[29] All infants with a history of prematurity should be closely observed for signs of apnea and bradycardia, and if evidenced in the postanesthesia care unit, they should be admitted and observed. If the infant has a history of apnea or bradycardia, they need to be apnea free and without monitoring for at least 6 months to be considered for outpatient surgery.[40] Efforts should be made to schedule surgery for these patients as early in the day as possible to allow for extended observation time.

Attempts to minimize the likelihood of postoperative apnea in these susceptible infants, beyond simply delaying surgery, have been examined. Spinal anesthesia without sedation resulted in less prolonged apnea, oxyhemoglobin desaturation, and bradycardia than did general anesthesia[41] or spinal anesthesia with ketamine sedation.[42] However, apnea and delayed respiratory failure have been reported in children who have had spinal or caudal anesthesia.[43-46] Infants treated with endotracheal intubation or mechanical ventilation, or both, for respiratory distress syndrome at birth have been shown to have abnormal arterial blood gas values and abnormal pulmonary function results as late as 1 year after treatment.[47] Infants exhibiting signs of bronchopulmonary dysplasia should not be considered for outpatient surgery.[48] Patients with a history of bronchopulmonary dysplasia are at risk for sudden infant death.[49]

Infants with a history of apneic events or with siblings who developed sudden infant death syndrome (SIDS) are at risk for SIDS. The greatest at-risk age for the development of SIDS is between 1 month and 1 year of age.[50] In infants who have lost a sibling to SIDS, the risk of dying from the same syndrome is four to five times that of the general population.[51] Patients at risk for the development of SIDS should not be considered for outpatient surgical procedures until they are at least 6 months[52] to 1 year old.[53]

Full-Term Infant. Healthy, full-term infants (greater than 37 weeks' gestational age at birth) at least 2 weeks[54] to 4 weeks[17] of age can be considered for minor outpatient surgery. Full-term infants with histories of apneic episodes, failure to thrive, and feeding difficulties are not suitable candidates for outpatient surgery. Infants with a history of respiratory difficulties at birth are not suitable outpatient candidates unless they are free of respiratory symptoms at the time of surgery and at the time of discharge.[52]

Geriatric Patient. The decision whether ambulatory surgery should be performed in a geriatric patient (age 65 years or older) should be individualized and based on physiologic age rather than on chronologic age. Existing medical problems are a concern when considering the geriatric patient for outpatient surgery. There are more concomitant age-related diseases that should be optimally treated preoperatively in this group of patients. Patient age exceeding 85 years is a strong predictor of hospital admissions and death with 7 days of surgery.[55] Appropriate home care and transportation to and from the outpatient center with a responsible caregiver must be ensured.

Convulsive Disorders. Surgery for patients with seizure disorders should be scheduled early in the day so that the patients can be observed for 4 to 8 hours after the operation before they are discharged.[56] It is important to establish the patients' ability to maintain their schedule for anticonvulsant medications. Patients with uncontrolled seizure activity are not deemed appropriate for outpatient surgery by most institutions.

Cystic Fibrosis. The extent of pulmonary involvement is the primary determinant of appropriateness for ambulatory surgery in patients with cystic fibrosis. Such patients should be evaluated several days before the proposed surgery; patients with symptomatic respiratory distress are better treated in an inpatient setting, where appropriate respiratory care management and hydration can be administered.[57]

Malignant Hyperthermia Susceptibility. A malignant hyperthermia (MH)–susceptible patient is defined as having one or more of the following:[58]

1. A previous episode of MH
2. Masseter muscle rigidity with previous anesthesia
3. A first-degree relative with history of an MH episode or positive muscle biopsy

The MH-susceptible patient who has received a trigger-free anesthetic does not require overnight hospitalization based exclusively on being MH susceptible.[59] The ambulatory facility should have the requisite monitoring and resuscitation capabilities, including a minimum of 36 vials of dantrolene, for managing the MH patient.[59] The patient should be scheduled as early in the day as possible to allow for extended patient observation for at least 4 hours after surgery, and the lack of symptoms of MH should be ensured before discharge is considered.[60] Overnight monitoring of the patient has been advocated;[61] the role of the 23-hour ambulatory unit makes this a viable outpatient option.

Morbid Obesity. Morbidly obese patients who meet the criteria for American Society of Anesthesiologists (ASA) physical status classifications I and II are suitable candidates for ambulatory surgery. However, morbidly obese patients with preexisting cardiac, hepatic, pulmonary, or renal disease should be managed as inpatients.[61] The ability to sufficiently manage postoperative pain and address postoperative ambulation should be discussed preoperatively by the surgeon and anesthesia provider. The morbidly obese patient is at risk for persistent hypoxemia in the postanesthesia care unit (PACU),[62] which may necessitate overnight supplemental oxygen therapy.

Morbid obesity is associated with an increased risk of obstructive sleep apnea.[63] Preoperative airway evaluation (e.g., Mallampati classification, nuchal girth, redundant pharyngeal tissue) is important in the patient with obstructive sleep apnea. If continuous positive airway pressure (CPAP) is part of the patient's management of obstructive sleep apnea, it should be available for use in the immediate postoperative recovery phase. Consideration should be given to schedule the morbidly obese patient with obstructive sleep apnea early in the day to allow for prolonged observation.

Reactive Airway Disease. Before surgery is performed, the severity of the disease must be assessed, and optimal disease management should be achieved. A chest radiograph is indicated only if the patient is suspected of having an acute infiltrative process or if deterioration in the patient's physical condition has occurred.[64] Likewise, arterial blood gases are indicated when signs and symptoms of chronic respiratory insufficiency are suspected. The patient may be best managed as an inpatient if indications for a chest radiograph or arterial blood gases are met. Consultation with the patient's internist may help in formulating therapeutic modalities and in establishing baseline conditions for this patient. Patients receiving long-term medication therapy should continue to take their medications until the time of surgery. All parties involved must anticipate the possibility of admitting the patient to the hospital should the symptoms of the disease become exacerbated.

Sickle Cell Disease. The possibility of sickle cell hemoglobinopathy should be considered in every black American when obtaining the preoperative medical history. If individual or family history is suggestive of the disease, a Sickledex may be obtained in children 6 months of age and older to determine the presence of sickle-shaped red blood cells.[65] The patient with sickle cell disease is at risk for crisis development should acidosis, dehydration, or hypoxia occur. The patient diagnosed with only the sickle cell trait is an acceptable outpatient candidate, but this patient is not without risk. Sickling of the red blood cells may occur in the patient with sickle cell trait who is subjected to hypoxia.[66] The patient with sickle cell anemia would typically be cared for as an inpatient;[67] however, if this patient is to be cared for in the ambulatory setting, certain criteria must be satisfied:[68]

1. The patient should have no major organ disease as a result of the sickle cell disease.
2. The patient should have not had a sickle cell crisis for at least 1 year.
3. The patient should be compliant with the prescribed medical care.
4. On discharge, the patient should be within 15 minutes' travel time to a facility that is prepared to care for the patient.
5. The patient should receive close follow-up postoperative care.

The procedure should not be a prolonged surgery that is associated with blood loss. The patient should arrive earlier than normal so that he or she receives adequate intravenous hydration. The patient's surgery should be scheduled early in the day to allow for extended postoperative monitoring before the patient is discharged from the ambulatory center.

Social Considerations. Factors other than physical condition must be weighed in the consideration of a patient for outpatient surgery (Box 35-1). The lack of appropriate home conditions and care makes the outpatient option less desirable.

BOX 35-1

Social Considerations in Ambulatory Surgery

Patient compliance
Presence of responsible caregiver
Discharge accommodations
Access to assistance

Unacceptable Patient Conditions for Ambulatory Surgery

Certain situations make ambulatory surgery impractical. Each patient must be considered individually for acceptability as an outpatient surgical candidate. Adult patients believed to be unacceptable candidates[69] are those with any of the following:

- Unstable ASA physical status classification III or IV (e.g., cardiac, renal, endocrine, pulmonary, hepatic, or cancer diagnoses)
- Active substance/alcohol abuse
- Psychosocial difficulties (see Box 35-1)
- Poorly controlled seizures
- Previously unevaluated and managed obstructive sleep apnea
- Uncontrolled diabetes
- A current presentation of sepsis or infectious disease, which would necessitate separate isolation facilities
- Anticipated postoperative pain not expected to be controlled with oral analgesics

PATIENT EVALUATION AND PREPARATION

Preoperative evaluation is mandatory for all patients preparing to undergo outpatient anesthesia and surgery to assist in recognizing the anesthetic risk and the suitability of the patient to the planned procedure.[70-72] Organizing and accomplishing all of the necessary tests and evaluations while causing the least inconvenience to the patient and allowing for an expedient surgical process are challenges for the outpatient team. The preoperative interview permits the medical personnel to gather pertinent patient information, which helps them recognize risk factors that may affect the patient. Additionally, by obtaining a thorough current and past medical history, including a personal and family anesthetic history, the staff may determine what further patient workup is required before surgery. A formalized preanesthesia assessment clinic is the most comprehensive and cost-effective process for preoperative evaluation and preparation.[73] Preoperative screening also allows the staff to communicate what will be expected of the patient in the perioperative phases. Consultations, laboratory tests, and diagnostic procedures should be performed based on clinical findings rather than on a preestablished regimen of "standard" tests.[74] Without any discoveries from the medical history and physical examination, the probability of observing a significant abnormality is negligible in diagnostic procedures, including electrocardiogram,[75] chest radiograph,[75-77] and laboratory tests.[75,78,79] Abnormal tests results obtained from routine testing potentially alter patient care only 0.22% to 0.56% of the time.[75,79] Routine preoperative laboratory screening is neither cost-effective nor predictive of postoperative complications.[80,81]

Patient Interview

Patient screening should take place sufficiently in advance of the scheduled surgery to allow time for necessary risk assessment, preoperative testing, specialty consultations, and adjustments in patient care. Proper timing of the patient assessment, particularly for the patient with complex medical conditions, minimizes surgical delays and cancellations. The high-risk patient should be evaluated at least 1 week before the scheduled procedure. With respect to client convenience, the otherwise healthy individual who does not have the opportunity to visit the clinic can be evaluated on the day of surgery.[82] In this circumstance, there is a higher potential for surgical postponement or cancellation with last-minute discovery (e.g., inappropriate fasting, suspected difficult airway).

Patient Orientation

The preoperative interview allows the staff to convey, both verbally and in writing, what is expected of the patient and what the patient can expect perioperatively. Providing instructions to the patient both verbally and in writing results in improved patient compliance.[83] An information packet that is given to the patient at the interview and details specific instructions and concerns is beneficial (Box 35-2).

Orientation to Facility

At the time of the patient interview, or at a mutually agreeable time, patients and family members should have the opportunity to become acquainted with the ambulatory surgery facilities and the anticipated sequence of events. This would include orientation to the laboratory and procedure areas, changing areas, waiting room, play areas, and the short-stay area, where the patient remains after surgery until discharge. This orientation is designed to reduce patient and family fear by providing relevant perioperative information (e.g., directions, anticipated schedule, instructions for physiologic preparation of the child, expected postoperative course, and discharge instructions), offering reassurance, and enhancing coping skills through familiarity. A variety of techniques may be incorporated to prepare the child for the operative procedure. Children can be oriented to equipment that is commonly used in the perioperative setting (e.g., anesthetic mask, intravenous therapy equipment, the anesthesia machine and circuit, blood pressure cuff, thermometer, and postoperative oxygen therapy devices). Children can be told when and where they will be reunited with their parents after surgery.

History and Physical

A thorough medical history and physical examination performed by a member of the medical staff should be available in the patient's chart before the surgery is performed. A separate anesthesia history should be incorporated into a questionnaire that is specifically designed for preanesthetic evaluation; the anesthesia provider should review this history with the patient. Such a review may be accomplished in a written format and would include a general review of the major systems, history of

BOX 35-2

Preoperative Patient Instructions

Preoperative Instructions

Tell the patient when and where laboratory tests, consultations, and diagnostic procedures will be completed.
Clarify the appropriate time for the patient to be without food and drink.

Registration on the Day of Surgery

Tell the patient the time to report for surgery and mention that a wait can normally be expected.
Describe the location of the parking areas.
Tell the patient where to report for surgery.

Ambulatory Center Policies

Inform the patient about the expected conduct of the patient and the family.
Explain the ambulatory facility policies to the patient and family.
Describe the family waiting area and services (e.g., dining areas).
Review advance directive information as required by law in some states.
Review the patient's rights to privacy policies.
Outline the facility's cancellation policies: late arrival, nonadherence to fasting guidelines, inappropriate transportation home, lack of responsible person to help patient postoperatively, interim changes in patient's health status (e.g., upper respiratory tract infection [URTI]).

Personal Considerations

Tell patient to wear comfortable, loose-fitting clothing that may be easily stored.
Instruct patient to wear no jewelry or makeup (remove nail polish from at least one nail).
Instruct patient to bring personal toilet items (e.g., comb, brush, toothbrush) as required.
Caution patient to leave valuables at home.
Tell caregiver to bring child's favorite toy, comforter, or pacifier, or light reading material for the older patient.

Postoperative Considerations

Inform patient and family of the discharge time, including the time spent in the postanesthesia care unit and the customary length of stay until discharge.
Instruct patient in the manner of discharge, the appropriate transportation arrangements, and the necessity for the presence of a responsible caregiver.
Give the patient postoperative instructions: no driving, alcohol, or major decisions postoperatively for at least 24 to 48 hr after anesthesia (see Box 35-10 for additional information).
Inform the patient where, how, and to whom complications should be reported, including telephone numbers.
Indicate the possibility of hospital admission.

Considerations If the Patient's Physical Condition Changes

Tell the patient to contact the surgeon.
Tell the patient to contact the anesthetist.
Tell the patient to call regarding cancellations or physical condition changes (e.g., URTI).

allergies, current medicines, past and present medical problems, laboratory and diagnostic test results, and patient and family response to previous anesthetics. Prior anesthesia records should be examined for complications, response to anesthesia, and postoperative course. Patient evaluation should be conducted within 30 days of the scheduled surgery for medically stable patients and within 72 hours of the scheduled surgery for high-risk patients. The clinician should determine whether any changes might have occurred since the original history and physical examination were performed, and an update note should be made on the day of the procedure. A review of current vital signs, laboratory test results, diagnostic reports, and fasting status should be made.

Laboratory Evaluation

Each ambulatory center should have a consensus regarding the minimum testing requirement for surgery. These testing criteria depend on the proposed surgical procedure, the patient's medication history, and the patient's physical condition. Certain states and regions have established minimum testing requirements. However, conducting a battery of preoperative laboratory tests without specific indications has not been shown to reduce patient morbidity,[79] is not cost-effective, and may even place the patient at increased risk.[84] Discriminating laboratory testing, based on findings from the history and physical examination, designed to evaluate a patient's comorbidities and surgical risk, seems to be indicated.[85] Normal laboratory test and diagnostic procedure results are deemed current if the tests are performed within 60 days of surgery if the patient's physical condition remains stable.[86] Exceptions include serum potassium level determinations, which should be obtained within 7 days of surgery for patients receiving diuretics or digitalis, and blood glucose level determinations, which should be obtained on the same day of surgery for patients with diabetes that is controlled by medication.[87] Physical conditions and systemic illnesses in which preoperative laboratory testing is appropriate are listed in Box 35-3.

Pregnancy Testing

The medical facility should have established guidelines delineating when testing for pregnancy is appropriate. If the medical history and physical examination indicate that the patient may be pregnant, or if pregnancy might complicate the surgery, then pregnancy testing should be performed.[88] It is important that the patient be educated as to the potential risks of exposing a fetus to an anesthetic. Whenever possible, especially in the adolescent population, a female staff member should question the patient in the absence of family members.[89]

Urinalysis

The practice of routinely performing urinalysis before surgery on asymptomatic patients does not appear warranted except for specific procedures as indicated by the surgeon. An ambulatory study of preoperative laboratory evaluations noted that abnormal urinalysis findings were obtained in 39% of the subjects; yet these findings did not result in the postponement of the surgical procedure, nor was increased morbidity observed.[90,91] There appears to be no advantage to performing routine urinalysis rather than hematologic evaluation (e.g., glucose, blood urea nitrogen).[92]

Diagnostic Procedures

Chest Radiography. Performing routine preoperative chest radiography is not recommended without specific indications from the history and physical examination.[93] Its value as a screening tool has been questioned, and some contend that the history and physical examination are as efficient as chest radiography for screening for chronic lung pathology.[84] With asymptomatic individuals less than 75 years of age, the risk involved in obtaining a routine preoperative chest radiograph is greater than the benefit.[94] Box 35-4 cites indications for obtaining a preoperative chest radiograph or electrocardiogram.

Electrocardiography. Few data support the routine performance of 12-lead electrocardiographic screening before surgery because it has not been shown to be cost-effective,[91,95-97] is a poor predictor of perioperative complications,[98,99] and is of limited value in detecting ischemia[100] in asymptomatic individuals. The use of age as a criterion for obtaining baseline electrocardiograms has recently been questioned;[98,101] however, if a minimum age criterion is deemed appropriate, it has been argued that it should be raised to 60 years of age.[101-103] Acquiring a preoperative electrocardiogram routinely is not indicated in the elderly patient for ambulatory surgery.[104] Box 35-4 cites indications for obtaining a preoperative electrocardiogram.

Fasting Status and Aspiration Risk

Part of the preoperative evaluation process identifies patients who are at risk for aspirating gastric contents into the lungs and developing aspiration pneumonitis. Factors associated with an increased risk of pulmonary aspiration of gastric contents[105-115] are listed in Box 35-5.

Recent ingestion of food and liquid before surgery contributes to an increased risk of aspiration. Solid foods must be digested to a bolus diameter of less than 2 mm before the food can pass through the pylorus.[116] This process normally takes several hours for solids, whereas liquids pass through the pylorus in 1 to 2 hours. Historically, patients have been required to fast for extended periods in an attempt to ensure an empty stomach. However, sustained fasting does not ensure that the stomach will be empty at the time of surgery.[117] The traditional policy of fasting after midnight fails to address several variables that influence gastric emptying for surgery:

- The time of the scheduled surgery
- The time at which the patient retired for the night
- The variability of gastric emptying for solids and fluids across individuals

Several problems have been associated with prolonged fasting:

- Dehydration
- Hypoglycemia[118]
- Hypovolemia
- Increased irritability
- Enhanced preoperative anxiety[119]
- Reduced compliance with preoperative fasting orders
- Thirst and related discomfort (e.g., hunger, headache, unhappiness)

Data suggest that liquids (e.g., clear apple juice, clear broth, coffee, gelatin, popsicles, pulp-free orange juice, water, and weak tea) may be given to healthy, unpremedicated patients up to 2 hours[120-122] to 3 hours[123,124] before surgery without placing them at increased risk for aspiration; there is no increase in gastric volume, nor is there a decrease in gastric pH, at the time of elective surgery. The studies that allowed patients to consume clear liquids until 2 to 3 hours before surgery demonstrated that although the patients appeared to be at no greater risk of aspirating gastric contents, the pH of the stomach contents remained less than 2.5. In light of these findings, recommended fasting guidelines for the otherwise healthy individual have been liberalized (Table 35-1).[125]

BOX 35-3

Indications for Laboratory Testing

Complete Blood Count
Hematologic disorder
Vascular procedure
Chemotherapy
Unknown sickle cell syndrome status

Hemoglobin/Hematocrit
Age <6 months (<1 yr if born premature)
Hematologic malignancy
Recent radiation or chemotherapy
Renal disease
Anticoagulant therapy
Procedure with moderate to high blood loss potential
Coexisting systemic disorders (e.g., cystic fibrosis, prematurity, severe malnutrition, renal failure, liver disease, congenital heart disease)

White Blood Cell Count
Leukemia and lymphomas
Recent radiation or chemotherapy
Suspected infection that would lead to cancellation of surgery
Aplastic anemia
Hypersplenism
Autoimmune collagen vascular disease

Blood Glucose Level
Diabetes mellitus
Current corticosteroid use
History of hypoglycemia
Adrenal disease
Cystic fibrosis

Serum Chemistry
Renal disease
Adrenal or thyroid disease
Chemotherapy
Pituitary or hypothalamic disease
Body fluid loss or shifts (e.g., dehydration, bowel prep)
Central nervous system disease

Potassium
Digoxin therapy
Diuretic therapy

Creatinine and Blood Urea Nitrogen
Cardiovascular disease (e.g., hypertension)
Renal disease
Adrenal disease
Diabetes mellitus
Diuretic therapy
Digoxin therapy
Body fluid loss or shifts (e.g., dehydration, bowel prep)
Procedure requiring radiocontrast

Liver Function Tests
Hepatic disease
Exposure to hepatitis
Therapy with hepatotoxic agents

Coagulation Studies
Prothrombin Time and Partial Thromboplastin Time
Leukemia
Hepatic disease
Bleeding disorder
Anticoagulant therapy
Severe malnutrition or malabsorption
Platelet Count and Bleeding Time
Bleeding disorder
Abnormal hemorrhage, purpura, easy bruisability

Urinalysis
Not indicated as a routine screening test

Pregnancy
Possibility of pregnancy

Serum Medication Levels
Monitor for medications (e.g., theophylline, phenytoin, digoxin, carbamazepine) if the patient exhibits signs of ineffective therapy, potential drug side effects, or poor drug compliance or has recently changed medication therapy without documentation of the drug level

Modified from Marley RA: Preoperative preparation. In Zaglaniczny K, Aker J, editors: Clinical Guide to Pediatric Anesthesia, *Philadelphia, 1999, Saunders, pp 34-35.*

Special Considerations

Daily Medications. Patients should continue to take their prescribed cardiopulmonary medications on the morning of the surgery. The medications may be taken with a minimum of water (up to 150 mL in adults and up to 75 mL in children) up to 1 hour before anesthesia.[126]

Warfarin Sodium. An early decision of whether the administration of warfarin sodium should be continued must be made in consultation with the surgeon and the patient's internist. The question of whether the disadvantages of stopping the administration of this medication before surgery outweigh any advantage must be addressed. If the decision to withhold warfarin is made, the drug should be discontinued for 4 to 5 days before the scheduled surgery,[127] and a prothrombin time should be determined on the day of surgery.[128] Tinker and Tarhan[129] withheld oral anticoagulants preoperatively for 1 to 3 days, then reinstated the anticoagulant between 1 and 7 days after surgery; the investigators did not observe an increase in thromboembolic problems.

BOX 35-4

Indications for Diagnostic Procedures

Chest Radiograph

Previous abnormal results on chest radiography
A history of malignancy in which pulmonary metastasis might alter the surgical therapy
A history of tuberculosis or a positive skin test result for tuberculosis for which no treatment was given
A history suggestive of pulmonary infection (e.g., new or chronic productive cough or blood-tinged or purulent-appearing sputum)
Suspected intrathoracic pathologic condition (e.g., tumors, vascular ring)
History of congenital heart disease
History of prematurity associated with residual bronchopulmonary dysplasia
Severe obstructive sleep apnea (may have cardiomegaly)
Down syndrome (may have asymptomatic subluxation of the atlantoaxial junction)
Symptomatic or debilitating asthma, chronic obstructive pulmonary disease, or cardiovascular disease

Electrocardiogram

Patients at risk for cardiovascular disease (e.g., cocaine abuse, hypertension, renal disease, circulatory disease, thyroid disease, diabetes mellitus [age 40 years or older], significant pulmonary disease)
History of previously unevaluated pathologic-sounding murmur or palpitation
Family history reveals possibility of inherited prolonged QT syndrome
History of moderate to severe sleep apnea or those with chronic anatomic airway obstruction (e.g., Pierre Robin syndrome) may be at risk for right-sided heart strain

From Marley RA: Preoperative preparation. In Zaglaniczny K, Aker J, editors: Clinical Guide to Pediatric Anesthesia, *Philadelphia, 1999, Saunders, pp 29-45; and Cassidy J, Marley RA: Preoperative assessment of the ambulatory patient,* J Perianesth Nurs *11:334-343, 1996.*

Diabetes. The recommended care for the patient with diabetes who is undergoing ambulatory surgery is a subject of debate and lacks clear guidelines. The patient with diabetes should receive an early and thorough preoperative evaluation, including electrocardiography, history and physical examination, and laboratory analysis. The patient with insulin-dependent diabetes whose diabetes is not well controlled and whose serum glucose levels are prone to wide fluctuations may be best treated in the inpatient setting. Considerations for care of the patient with diabetes who is undergoing ambulatory surgery include the following:

1. Scheduling the diabetic patient early in the day
2. Instructing the patient to have nothing to eat or drink after midnight the night before surgery if the procedure is scheduled early in the day
3. Monitoring the patient's blood or serum glucose levels on arrival to the ambulatory center by use of a capillary test strip or laboratory analysis
4. Preventing hypoglycemia while maintaining blood glucose levels at less than 180 mg/dL[130]
5. Returning the patient to his or her preoperative activities of daily living (e.g., baseline activity status, nutrition habits) as soon as possible
6. Making the patient aware that admission to the hospital is likely if persistent nausea and vomiting prevent him or her from resuming normal dietary intake

BOX 35-5

Risk Factors for Pulmonary Aspiration

Age extremes (<1 yr or >70 yr)
Anxiety
Ascites
Collagen vascular disease (e.g., scleroderma)
Depression
Difficult airway management
Esophageal surgery
Exogenous medications (opioids or premedications [e.g., barbiturates] and anticholinergics)
Gastroesophageal junction dysfunction (e.g., hiatal hernia)
Inadequate anesthesia
Mechanical obstruction (e.g., pyloric stenosis, duodenal ulcer)
Metabolic disorders (e.g., hypothyroidism, chronic diabetes, hepatic failure, hyperglycemia, obesity, renal failure, and uremia)
Neurologic sequelae (e.g., those of developmental delays, head injury, hypotonia, and seizures)
Pain
Pregnancy
Prematurity with respiratory problems
Severe hypotension
Type and composition of gastric contents (e.g., solid foods and milk products)

TABLE 35-1 **Fasting Guidelines for Healthy Patients Undergoing Elective Procedures**

Ingested Material	Minimum Fasting Period (hr)—All Ages
Clear liquids*	2
Breast milk	4
Infant formula	6
Nonhuman milk†	6
Light meal‡	6

**Examples of clear liquids include water, fruit juices without pulp, carbonated beverages, clear tea, and black coffee.*
†Because nonhuman milk is similar to solids in gastric emptying time, the amount ingested must be considered when determining an appropriate fasting period.
‡A light meal typically consists of toast and clear liquids. Meals that include fried or fatty foods or meat may prolong gastric emptying time. Both the amount and type of foods ingested must be considered when determining an appropriate fasting period.
From Warner MA and others: Practice guidelines for preoperative fasting and the use of pharmacologic agents to reduce the risk of pulmonary aspiration: application to healthy patients undergoing elective procedures, Anesthesiology *90:896-905, 1999.*

Heart Murmur. The patient with a heart murmur who is undergoing surgery requires further workup if the condition was previously undetected. Heart murmurs are categorized as innocent or pathologic. Pathologic murmurs may be due to complex congenital malformations or heart disease and have accompanying physical dysfunction, whereas with innocent murmurs, the patient may be completely asymptomatic.[131] Whether the murmur is benign, functional, or caused by organic heart disease, cardiologic assessment should be obtained before the induction of anesthesia.[132]

Rhinorrhea. From 20% to 30% of all children display symptoms of rhinorrhea a good portion of the year.[29] Children younger than 2 years of age are prone to 5 to 10 viral respiratory infections annually.[133] Individual patient evaluation is required for the child undergoing ambulatory surgery who has a runny nose. The history and physical examination are beneficial in determining the cause of the runny nose. The differential diagnosis of rhinorrhea may include the following:

- Allergic (seasonal) rhinitis
- Bacterial infection (early stages)
- Flu syndrome
- URTI
- Vasomotor rhinitis
- Nothing found[54]

The clinician obtaining the patient history should try to ascertain the allergic and acute nature of the runny nose. The history taker must determine whether this runny nose is normal for the child or whether an illness has recently developed and worsened. Recently acquired (within 12 to 24 hours of surgery) rhinorrhea[54] or chronic rhinorrhea[134] in the otherwise fit child is not a contraindication to surgery. The differentiation between a noninfectious and an infectious runny nose might influence the decision of whether the procedure should be delayed (Box 35-6). Surgery might be delayed for only 1 to 2 weeks in the child with localized infectious rhinorrhea.[135]

BOX 35-6

Differential Diagnosis of Rhinorrhea

Noninfectious Runny Nose

Allergic rhinitis
- Seasonal
- Perennial

Vasomotor rhinitis
- Emotional (crying)
- Temperature

Infectious Runny Nose

Viral infections
- Nasopharyngitis (common cold)
- Contagious disease (e.g., chickenpox, measles)

Acute bacterial infections
- Streptococcal tonsillitis
- Meningitis

From Berry FA: Pre-existing medical conditions of pediatric patients, Semin Anesth *3:24-31, 1984.*

Considerations for Postponing Surgery

Lack of Drug Compliance. The patient with uncontrolled hypertension or diabetes who has wide swings in blood pressure or blood glucose levels may not be suitable for outpatient surgery; such conditions should be optimally managed before outpatient surgery and anesthesia are performed.

Fasting Status. For safety reasons, the patient not adhering to the fasting guidelines should not undergo surgery, and the rationale of not eating before surgery should be reinforced.

Suspicion of Pregnancy. If the patient responds that she may be pregnant or if clinical signs are indicative of pregnancy, the surgery should be delayed until the determination of whether or not the patient is pregnant can be made. A decision can then be made based on the test results as to whether the surgery should be performed and what type of anesthesia should be used.

Upper Respiratory Tract Infection. In patients with an acute infection, differentiating between a bacterial infection as causative of the URTI versus other causes—such as uncomplicated viral infection (afebrile, clear secretions) or allergic conditions—is important. Differentiating between a noninfectious process and an infectious process is paramount in the decision whether the procedure should be performed. This differentiation may be difficult to make early in the course of the disease. Symptoms of URTI include the following:

1. Elevated white blood cell count (greater than 12,000 to 15,000 with a left shift)[136]
2. Mucopurulent nasal secretions[136]
3. Inflamed and reddened mucosa (nasopharyngeal and oropharyngeal) (with allergic rhinitis, the nasal mucosa is ashen and boggy)[137]
4. Positive chest findings (e.g., congestion, rales)[138]
5. Temperature of 38° C or greater (usually associated with lower respiratory tract involvement)
6. Tonsillitis[29]
7. Viral ulcers in the oropharynx[29]

Other accompanying symptoms may include conjunctivitis, coughing (nonproductive), fatigue, itching, laryngitis, malaise, myalgias, sneezing, and sore throat.[138] Laboratory and diagnostic testing in children with suspected URTI includes nasal or throat cultures if signs of an infectious process are observed. A chest radiograph is not warranted, especially if chest sounds are clear.[139] Similarly, the value of obtaining a white blood cell count has been challenged because the results may be normal and typically do not influence whether to proceed with the surgery.[139]

Anesthetizing the patient who has a URTI has been shown to increase the incidence of respiratory-associated complications twofold to sevenfold.[140] The anesthetized patient with a URTI is more prone to experience breath holding, bronchospasm, coughing, hypoxemia, increased secretions, laryngospasm, pneumonia, atelectasis, croup, and stridor.[141,142] Risk factors for the development of perioperative adverse respiratory events in children with URTI include endotracheal intubation (<5 years of age), history of prematurity, history of reactive airway disease, paternal smoking, surgery involving the airway, the presence of copious secretions, and nasal congestion.[143] A minimum of 4 hours of postoperative observation is appropriate before the patient is considered for discharge from the ambulatory setting.[140]

Guidelines for the decision whether surgery should be performed in children with URTI[136] apply to both the symptomatic and the asymptomatic child. In the case of the symptomatic child (fever >38° C, mucopurulent sputum or secretions, wheezing, generally seems sick), the surgery should be canceled and rescheduled to at least 4 weeks later.[144] For the asymptomatic child (nonpurulent nasal secretions, unremarkable chest examination), anesthesia and surgery can be performed if the following conditions are met:

1. The child is older than 1 year.
2. The surgery is not of the thorax or the abdomen.
3. The child is otherwise healthy; no other illness that might complicate perioperative patient management exists.
4. Endotracheal intubation is not planned. The laryngeal mask airway has been found to contribute to fewer adverse respiratory events than the endotracheal tube.[145] Endotracheal intubation in a child increases the risk of adverse respiratory complications 11-fold.[140]

Each case has to be reviewed individually and consideration has to be given to the urgency of the surgery, the duration and complexity of the surgery, the number of times the procedure has been cancelled, and the wishes of the family and patient.

PREMEDICATION

Premedicating the ambulatory surgery patient with sedative agents remains controversial. The concern about giving anxiolytic and sedative medications is related to their potential to prolong the patient's stay. The use of premedication should not become routine; rather, the decision to administer these agents should be based on individual need and desired benefit. Common indications for preoperative medication include the following:

- To decrease patient anxiety and fear
- To facilitate smooth induction and emergence from anesthesia
- To supplement anesthesia and reduce the need for general anesthetic agents
- To reduce the volume and acidity of gastric contents
- To provide a more pleasant stay in the PACU[64]

Pulmonary Aspiration Prophylaxis

Patients at higher risk for aspirating gastric contents should be given medications before surgery to raise gastric pH and lower gastric volume with the hope of minimizing their risk for pulmonary aspiration. Pulmonary aspiration prophylaxis in the patient not at risk is not recommended.[115,125,146]

Antacids. The value of oral antacids lies in their ability to rapidly reduce gastric acidity; they are effective in raising pH in 15 to 20 minutes.[147] This characteristic is useful in emergency situations, but it is of limited application in the ambulatory setting. Although oral antacids raise gastric pH, they have the disadvantage of increasing gastric volume. Clear nonparticulate oral antacids (e.g., two tablets of Alka Seltzer Gold in 30 mL of water; 30 mL [0.4 mL/kg pediatric dose] of 0.3 M sodium citrate [Bicitra]) are preferred over particulate antacids, such as Maalox or Mylanta, because particulate antacids may produce pulmonary injury if they are aspirated.[148]

Gastrokinetics. Reducing the volume of gastric fluid with the gastrokinetic agent metoclopramide (Reglan) should help minimize the risk of aspiration. Metoclopramide has been demonstrated to decrease gastric fluid volume by reducing gastric emptying time without increasing pH in adults[149] and in children.[150] Metoclopramide may also reduce the risk of pulmonary aspiration by increasing lower esophageal sphincter tone[151]; it has been suggested to exert a central antiemetic effect (which is a dopaminergic receptor–blocking property of chemoreceptor trigger zone).[152] The antiemetic effect of metoclopramide has not been confirmed by other authors.[153] The combination of metoclopramide with a histamine$_2$ (H_2) receptor antagonist has been shown to be effective in raising gastric volume pH and decreasing gastric volume content.[154]

The intramuscular dose is 10 mg for adults (0.1 mg/kg for children[111]), given at least 45 minutes before surgery.[155] The intravenous dose is 10 to 20 mg (0.15 to 0.2 mg/kg) given over the course of 3 to 5 minutes[156] at least 30 minutes[157] to 45 minutes[155] before surgery. These regimens allow sufficient time for the desired results to be achieved. The oral dose, 10 mg for adults (0.1 mg/kg for children[111]), achieves peak plasma concentrations 40 to 120 minutes after administration.[158]

Histamine$_2$ Receptor Antagonists. Selective and competitive H_2 receptor antagonists, such as cimetidine (Tagamet), famotidine (Pepcid), and ranitidine (Zantac), block hydrogen ion release by gastric parietal cells.[159] These drugs do not alter the pH of gastric fluid already present in the stomach. These medications may be administered the night before surgery, on the day of surgery, or both, to reduce gastric acidity. Famotidine and ranitidine have longer durations of action,[160] are more potent,[161] and exhibit a lower potential for side effects than cimetidine.[162]

Cimetidine. In one study, the intravenous adult dose of 300 mg helped reduce the risk of pulmonary aspiration.[163] The oral dose is 300 mg (3 to 4 mg/kg) for adults[164] and 7.5 mg/kg for children,[165] given from 1.5 to 3 hours before surgery. This is effective in reducing the risk of chemical pneumonitis should pulmonary aspiration occur.

Famotidine. The intravenous dose is 20 mg for adults, given 15 to 30 minutes before surgery, and this is effective in increasing gastric pH.[166] When given electively, oral famotidine (40 mg) is given the night before surgery and on arising the morning of surgery. This results in a mean gastric pH of 6.2 and a gastric fluid volume of 7.8 mL at the time of the outpatient surgery.[162] When compared with ranitidine, famotidine was slower in raising the gastric pH to safe levels.[167]

Ranitidine. The intravenous dose is 50 to 100 mg[163] or 1.0 to 2.5 mg/kg.[168] This drug decreases the risk associated with pulmonary aspiration. The oral dose of 150 to 300 mg for adults (2.5 mg/kg for children[111]), given 1 to 3 hours before surgery, increases gastric pH, whereas gastric fluid volume may not be less than 25 mL.[169,170] Comparable results were noted when ranitidine (150 mg) was given at bedtime and again on arising on the morning of surgery[162] or when it was given orally 1 to 2 hours before surgery.[169]

Gastric Proton-Pump Inhibitor

Omeprazole. Omeprazole (Prilosec) causes dose-dependent intracellular inhibition of gastric acid secretion in humans without affecting gastric volume.[171] Omeprazole has a longer duration of effect than the H_2 receptor antagonist agents in suppressing gastric acid secretion[172] and appears to cause no significant side effects.[173]

The intravenous dose is 40 mg, administered after the induction of anesthesia. This is as effective as ranitidine in raising gastric pH above 2.5.[174]

The oral dose is 80 mg, given the evening before surgery. This has increased mean gastric pH to 4.56, compared with the pH of 2.05 that was achieved with the administration of a placebo.[171] Orally administered omeprazole, 40 mg, was not found to be as effective as either famotidine, 40 mg, or ranitidine, 300 mg, in protecting against pulmonary aspiration in parturients.[175]

Lansoprazole and Rabeprazole. Orally administered Lansoprazole (Prevacid), 30 mg, and rabeprazole (Aciphex), 20 mg, given the day prior to surgery and on the morning of surgery were not as effective in raising pH and lowering gastric volume as a single morning-of-surgery dose of ranitidine, 150 mg.[176]

Pantoprazole. Pantoprazole (Protonix) is marketed as an intravenous solution as well as tablets, which may prove useful for perioperative use. Intravenously administered pantoprazole, 40 mg, was comparable to ranitidine, 50 mg, in increasing pH and reducing gastric fluid volume.[177]

ANESTHETIC CONSIDERATIONS

Anesthetic techniques suitable for outpatient surgery include general anesthesia, regional anesthesia, and monitored anesthesia care. The goals for outpatient anesthesia, regardless of the type administered, are listed in Box 35-7, and factors influencing the choice of anesthesia are shown in Box 35-8. The ideal anesthetic agent for ambulatory anesthesia—whether it is administered via inhalational, intravenously, locally, or regionally—is one with the appropriate pharmacokinetic traits (i.e., rapid onset and offset, short beta-elimination half-lives, inert metabolites, and insignificant side effects).

General Anesthesia

General anesthesia is the most widely used anesthetic technique for ambulatory surgery. General anesthesia should be achieved with the less soluble inhalation agents or with the short-acting intravenous agents that have the capability of reversal if required. A combination of potent rapid-onset and -offset inhalation agents (e.g., desflurane, sevoflurane), along with intravenous agents (e.g., propofol, intravenous opioids, short-acting muscle relaxants, nonsteroidal antiinflammatory agents), comprise general anesthesia in contemporary practice.[178] The popularity of general anesthesia in the ambulatory setting is related to its acceptance by the patient, the anesthesia provider, and the surgeon, and to the consistent pace that can be maintained with regard to achieving a satisfactory state of anesthesia.

BOX 35-7

Goals of Outpatient Anesthesia

Minimize the physiologic changes associated with anesthesia
Provide a fast, smooth onset of anesthetic action
Promote intraoperative amnesia and analgesia
Afford suitable operating circumstances
Minimize perioperative anesthetic side effects
Allow rapid offset of anesthetic influence while maintaining patient comfort

BOX 35-8

Considerations for Choice of Anesthetic

Surgical requirements
Skill of the anesthesia provider
Patient choice
Patient age
American Society of Anesthesiologists physical status classification
Level of care available once the patient is discharged from the outpatient facility

Depth of Anesthesia Monitoring. Recent advances in depth-of-anesthesia monitoring technology have made their presence felt in ambulatory anesthesia. With appropriate application of depth-of-anesthesia monitoring principles, rapid emergence and recovery from ambulatory anesthesia may be optimized, thus promoting beneficial turnover and discharge times.[179] Bispectral index monitoring has been found to correlate well with levels of sedation and amnesia.[180] Some of the purported advantages of bispectral index monitoring in the outpatient setting include reducing the amount of anesthetic agent required,[181] faster emergence from anesthesia,[182,183] and a reduction in phase II vomiting.[184]

Airway Management. Issues regarding the use of general anesthesia with a face mask, a laryngeal mask airway, or an endotracheal tube in patients undergoing outpatient surgery are the same as those in patients undergoing inpatient surgery. The indications for intubating the trachea depend on the constraints of the surgery and the individual patient concerns (e.g., risk of regurgitation and aspiration, hypoventilation, access to the airway, use of muscle relaxants, and airway obstruction).

Drawbacks to endotracheal intubation specific to the outpatient setting must be considered. Resumption of dietary intake is prolonged in patients in whom the trachea was intubated for surgery.[185] More medications are administered to patients who require endotracheal intubation than to those who receive anesthesia through a mask.[186] The delayed oral intake and the increased total amount of medications required by endotracheal intubation may delay patient discharge. Irritation and trauma to the upper airway and trachea are a concern, especially in children. The development of postextubation croup is rare (0.1%),[187] but the potential for its occurrence must be considered in the plan for discharging the patient.[188] Careful attention paid to minimizing intubating trauma, ensuring that an air leak is present at less than 40 cm H_2O,[186] and avoiding large-diameter endotracheal tubes helps reduce the incidence of postextubation croup in children.

The laryngeal mask airway (LMA) has proven to be a popular and cost-effective airway management tool in the ambulatory setting.[189] Additional reported advantages of the LMA include less coughing, analgesic requirement, and sore throats following ambulatory surgery.[190,191]

Intravenous Fluid Therapy. Debate exists over whether all patients undergoing brief (less than 15 minutes) anesthesia require intravenous cannulation for uncomplicated surgery in which rapid recovery is expected. If an intravenous catheter is not inserted in children undergoing general anesthesia, the equipment and personnel trained in intravenous line placement should be immediately available in case they are needed. Keane and Murray[192] found quicker postoperative recovery (i.e., earlier discharge from the facility, earlier return to work) in fasting adult patients who received 2 L of intravenous fluid than in patients in whom fluids were withheld. Healthy adult outpatients undergoing laparoscopic surgery were found to have fewer problems after surgery if they received 20 mL/kg of lactated Ringer's solution (with or without dextrose) perioperatively.[193] These patients were less thirsty; reported a lower incidence of sore throat; and were not as prone to dizziness, drowsiness, and faintness on standing compared to patients for whom fluids were withheld perioperatively. Less thirst, dizziness, and drowsiness were observed in ambulatory patients undergoing short surgical procedures who were given 20 mL/kg of intravenous fluids when compared with patients who only received 2 mL/kg.[194]

Intravenous cannulation should be used and perioperative fluid should be administered in the following situations:

1. Procedures lasting longer than 30 minutes. Longer surgical times increase the risk of hypothermia, increase the amount of anesthetics delivered to the patient, and result in a delay of resumption of normal diet.[14]
2. Procedures with an increased incidence of postoperative nausea and vomiting. Intravenous access permits the administration of antiemetic medications and allows hydration.
3. Procedures associated with postoperative discomfort. If anticipated postoperative pain is unlikely to be controlled by nonintravenous means, an avenue should be established for the administration of intravenous analgesics.
4. Prolonged fasting before surgery. If the child has been fasting for more than 15 hours, intravenous hydration is desirable for the maintenance of fluid and glucose homeostasis.[118]
5. Procedures associated with intraoperative and postoperative bleeding.
6. Procedures associated with the use of perioperative antibiotics or patients who require the perioperative administration of antibiotics.

Regional Anesthesia

The use of regional anesthesia in the ambulatory setting is well established. Local wound infiltration, peripheral nerve block, intravenous regional anesthesia, ophthalmic blocks (e.g., retrobulbar or periorbital), brachial plexus anesthesia, spinal anesthesia, and epidural anesthesia are all successfully used for outpatient surgery. The proper application of outpatient regional anesthesia requires knowledge of the anticipated surgical procedure (e.g., anesthesia requirements, length of procedure), proper patient selection, and skillful anesthesia providers who are capable of providing the required block. The shortest-acting agent capable of providing satisfactory central neuraxial blockade should be used in the ambulatory setting if unreasonable delays in discharge are to be avoided. Peripheral nerve blockade with longer-acting local anesthetics can provide up to 24 hours of analgesia postoperatively. The advantages and disadvantages of the use of outpatient regional anesthesia are listed in Box 35-9.

Patients must understand and be willing to accept this type of anesthesia before it is used. Special consideration must be given to senile and mentally disabled patients. Preanesthesia patient education and appropriately administered sedation with continual reassurance and support promote patient acceptance, cooperation, and understanding regarding regional anesthesia.

BOX 35-9

Advantages and Disadvantages of Outpatient Regional Anesthesia

Advantages

Recovery times are shorter than those of general anesthesia.[15]
Unanticipated admission to the hospital is reduced.[14]
Provides excellent immediate postoperative pain relief.
Common side effects associated with general anesthesia (e.g., airway trauma, dizziness, "hangover," myalgia, nausea and vomiting, pharyngitis) are minimized.
The patient who fears general anesthesia or "loss of control" has a satisfactory alternative.

Disadvantages

Cooperation of the patient and the surgeon is required.
Regional anesthesia may require more time to provide than general anesthesia. In an ambulatory setting, where surgeries and patient stays tend to be of short duration, regional anesthesia may not be as well received. If a team approach is used, patient stays may be minimized by early placement of the proposed regional anesthetic, if appropriate.
Inherent problems associated with regional anesthesia, regardless of inpatient or outpatient status, include the sympathetic block associated with spinal and epidural anesthesia, which may complicate the discharge course if residual block results in orthostatic hypotension.

Patients' orientation to regional anesthesia can appropriately begin with support and an introductory dialogue with their surgeon.

The various types of regional anesthesia suitable for ambulatory surgery are reviewed in this chapter for their relevance to outpatient management.

Brachial Plexus Anesthesia. Brachial plexus anesthesia—involving the axillary, interscalene, and supraclavicular or infraclavicular approaches—is ideal for surgery on the arm or shoulder. A potential drawback for brachial plexus anesthesia is the length of time (longer than 15 minutes) required before complete anesthesia is achieved. This lengthy interval makes advance placement of the block in the preoperative area attractive. It does not appear that the addition of sodium bicarbonate to lidocaine[195] or bupivacaine[196] is beneficial in shortening the onset of the brachial plexus block; yet it appears to be of some benefit when mepivacaine is used as the anesthetic.[197,198] The shortest-acting agent for the surgical length should be used unless prolonged analgesia is desired. If discharge is considered before sensory and motor functions return, meticulous verbal and written instructions should be provided to the patient and the guardian, and the arm should be supported in a sling.[199] Approximately 85% of clinicians performing axillary or interscalene block with long-acting local anesthesia, routinely discharge patients home with a persistent block.[200]

For surgeries involving the forearm or hand, the axillary approach is the preferred method for use in outpatients and the least likely to create complications. Ideal for surgeries involving the arm, the supraclavicular approach is associated with a small likelihood of pneumothorax,[201] which may become apparent after the patient is discharged from the surgical facility.[202]

The risk of development of a pneumothorax is enhanced if the patient becomes quite active after these blocks are performed.[203] The interscalene approach, which is ideal for surgeries involving the shoulder, has a lower incidence of pneumothorax than the supraclavicular approach[199] and has been shown to promote earlier discharge and have fewer side effects (e.g., less pain and nausea) than general anesthesia.[204,205] However, the interscalene approach is associated with intradural injection of local anesthetic; vertebral artery puncture; and stellate ganglion, phrenic nerve, or recurrent laryngeal nerve block.[206]

Caudal Anesthesia. Although caudal anesthesia does not provide the same quality of block as that provided by spinal anesthesia, it is occasionally used in outpatients undergoing pelvic and perineal surgery[207] and in children requiring intraoperative and postoperative analgesia.[208,209] An advantage of caudal anesthesia in the geriatric patient is the absence of hypotension after the administration of this block.[10] Additionally, caudal analgesia has been shown to offer superior recovery features.[210] Caudal anesthesia appears to offer no advantage in preventing postoperative pain compared with treating the patient with intravenous ketorolac[211] or local anesthesia nerve block with wound infiltration.[212]

Epidural Anesthesia. Epidural anesthesia is successfully used in the ambulatory setting. The advantages of epidural anesthesia in this setting include a reduced incidence of nausea and vomiting and other problems that could delay discharge. With the epidural approach, the incidence of postdural puncture headache (PDPH) is lower, the control over level of block is greater, and the changes in blood pressure are fewer. Titration of a short- to intermediate-acting local anesthetic agent (e.g., 2-chloroprocaine, lidocaine, mepivacaine) through a continuous catheter technique is appropriate for outpatient surgery. Predictable surgical procedures, proper agent selection, and consideration for the addition of epinephrine may negate the necessity of catheter placement in favor of one-time injection. Disadvantages of outpatient epidural anesthesia include slower onset of anesthesia and a less reliable block than with spinal anesthesia.

Intravenous Regional Anesthesia. Intravenous regional anesthesia (Bier block) is suitable for some outpatient surgical procedures because it is simple to perform, it has a rapid onset with reliable results, and it has a rapid offset once the tourniquet is deflated. In the outpatient setting, it has been shown to cost less (approximately one half), be associated with fewer postoperative complications, and yield shorter discharge times when compared with general anesthesia.[213] The use of intravenous regional anesthesia need not be limited to adults. This type of block is successful in children undergoing outpatient surgery on an upper extremity.[214]

Nerve Blocks

Ankle. An ankle block is a simple, safe, and effective means of providing anesthesia and postoperative analgesia (12 to 24 hours with long-acting agents) for operations involving the foot. Limiting factors for an ankle block are the time it takes to block the nerves individually, and the delayed onset of anesthetic action. This makes early placement of the block desirable in the busy ambulatory setting. If the ankle and foot continue to be numb at the time of discharge, instructions on patient protection should be provided and emphasized.

Sciatic, Femoral, Lateral Femoral Cutaneous, and Obturator Nerves. Blocking these nerves singularly,[215] or, more commonly, in combination,[216-218] provides appropriate anesthesia and postoperative analgesia for procedures involving a lower extremity. The anesthesia given by this type of block may be extensive and is appropriate for longer procedures. When performed for complex knee surgeries, femoral or sciatic nerve blocks were associated with less postoperative pain in phase II recovery and fewer unplanned hospital admissions.[219] Discharge from the unit can be prolonged as a result of loss of coordination and loss of strength in the leg.[220] When proper preparation for home discharge with an insensate extremity is ensured, the likelihood of patient injury is minimal.[221]

Spinal Anesthesia. For the busy ambulatory surgery setting, a subarachnoid block may be preferable to epidural anesthesia because delays in the onset of block that result from epidural anesthesia may increase the time each patient spends in the preoperative holding room. The side effects of spinal anesthesia—such as orthostatic hypotension, PDPH, urinary retention, and transient neurologic sequelae following concentrated hyperbaric local anesthetic agents—are of particular concern for the patient who expects same-day discharge. The geriatric patient exhibits prolonged sympathetic block and thus is more prone to orthostatic hypotension and urinary retention than the younger patient.[222]

The choice of appropriate local anesthetic agents helps minimize the side effects associated with spinal anesthesia. Lidocaine and procaine are the preferred shorter-acting agents, whereas tetracaine and bupivacaine, because of their prolonged duration of effect, are best avoided.[199] If spinal anesthesia is deemed necessary for a procedure lasting longer than 1.5 to 2 hours, the use of bupivacaine or tetracaine may be required. In this instance, the surgery should be scheduled early in the day so that sufficient time is allowed for recovery. The use of lidocaine alone is appropriate for surgeries that are anticipated to last less than 1 hour. The addition of epinephrine (0.2 to 0.3 mg) or phenylephrine (1 to 5 mg) to lidocaine should prolong the anesthesia for procedures lasting between 1 and 2 hours. The addition of vasoconstrictive agents is not recommended for the longer-acting agents.[207] Should the surgical procedure last longer than anticipated, the surgeon may perform local wound infiltration with a longer-lasting local anesthetic agent in order to provide the anesthesia necessary for the completion of the surgery.

Efforts to optimize spinal anesthesia (i.e., minimize recovery time) in ambulatory surgery have placed increasing emphasis on maintaining patient comfort while reducing the total amount of the local anesthetic agent (lidocaine,[223-225] bupivacaine,[226-233] or ropivacaine[234]) administered plus the addition of intrathecal opioids to augment the sensory block.[223,224,230,231,235,236] Lidocaine remains the most useful local anesthetic for spinal anesthesia in the outpatient setting.[237]

Orthostatic Hypotension. Residual autonomic blockade, as manifested by such signs as dizziness or fainting, may be problematic when attempts are made to have the patient ambulate so that the patient can be discharged. These patients should be scheduled early in the day in order to allow recovery from the effects of sympathetic block. The use of the short-acting local anesthetics is preferred so that the duration of sympathetic block is minimized. The longer-lasting local anesthetic agents, which have a prolonged duration of action and recovery time, are not desirable for outpatient spinal anesthesia.

Postdural Puncture Headache. The likelihood of PDPH occurrence remains the major concern regarding the use of spinal anesthesia in the outpatient setting. With the employment of the smaller-gauge, noncutting spinal needles, the incidence of PDPH is very low.[238] The overall incidence of PDPH in the ambulatory population is 0% to 2%,[237] with less than 1% requiring management with an epidural blood patch.[239] Patient selection is important if spinal anesthesia is considered for ambulatory surgery. If the patient requires early resumption of normal activities without interference from the anesthesia, spinal anesthesia may not be the appropriate choice, because incapacitating headache may occur. The patient should be informed preoperatively that PDPH may occur and that treatment may be required. For this reason, patients receiving spinal anesthesia should remain within a convenient distance from the ambulatory surgery center for at least 72 hours in case treatment is required.[52]

Prior to discharge, the patient should be educated as to the typical presenting symptoms of a PDPH. Part of the patient's discharge instructions will include information on how to access assistance should a headache occur. If the patient complains of headache, conservative measures for mild symptoms (e.g., analgesics, bed rest, oral hydration, or oral caffeine) may be sufficient treatment. If an epidural blood patch is required, this may be easily performed on an outpatient basis.

Specific patient instructions should be reviewed before the patient is discharged from the ambulatory surgery center. Patients should be informed that lying flat is not required, because this measure does not affect the occurrence of PDPH.[240]

Transient Neurologic Symptoms. The term *transient neurologic symptoms* refers to a set of temporary pain or dysesthesia involving the back and legs after complete resolution of a spinal anesthetic.[241] The mechanism of this transient neural insult is believed to be a result of direct action on sensory neurons from a lidocaine-induced increase in intracellular calcium.[242] The symptoms appear between 1 and 24 hours following the spinal block resolution and usually resolve within 1 week. Risk factors for the development of transient neurologic symptoms include (1) certain types of surgeries (e.g., knee arthroscopy with the use of a tourniquet and urologic or gynecologic procedures performed in the lithotomy position), and (2) outpatient status (associated with early ambulation). Transient neurologic symptoms have been observed with local anesthetics other than lidocaine,[243-246] but lidocaine has the highest reported incidence (up to 12%) following ambulatory knee arthroscopy.[247] Clinical management typically involves the use of nonsteroidal antiinflammatory agents and the more potent analgesics that the patient might possess as a result of the surgery. See Chapter 9 for further discussion of transient neurologic symptoms.

Urinary Retention. Transient urinary retention secondary to sympathetic and parasympathetic block at the S2-S4 level of the nerves innervating the bladder, detrusor, and sphincter muscles results in loss of bladder tone and thus in loss of the reflex to void. This problem may require bladder catheterization and may prolong discharge or lead to hospital admission.[227] The incidence of urinary retention after regional anesthesia is affected by the type and the site of the surgery,[248] is higher in male patients,[199] and is influenced by the duration of the sympathetic block.[249] Strategies to reduce the incidence of urinary retention following spinal anesthesia include the following:

- Reduce the total amount of local anesthesia used for the spinal anesthetic.[250]
- Use the shorter-acting local anesthetic agent (e.g., lidocaine) as opposed to the longer-acting agents (e.g., tetracaine).[251,252]
- Add fentanyl to the local anesthesia agent. Reducing the total amount of lidocaine (from 50 mg to 20 mg) by adding fentanyl (10 mcg to 25 mcg) had a beneficial effect of reducing the time to patient voiding by approximately 30 minutes.[235]
- Omit the addition of epinephrine to the lidocaine because it prolongs the block and thus the time to micturition.[228,253]
- Careful attention to intravenous fluid administration and the avoidance of bladder distention.[254]

If these strategies are incorporated into the spinal anesthetic plan, and if the surgical procedure is not associated with a high incidence of urinary retention (high-risk surgeries include rectal and inguinal hernia operations), then the patient can be discharged without voiding.[255]

Concomitant Sedation. Comfort and safety are premier concerns in the care of patients undergoing regional or local anesthesia with monitored anesthesia care. Patients frequently verbalize their anticipated anxiety relating to discomfort and awareness during the time of the block and the procedure. The anesthesia provider's role during these procedures is to maximize patient comfort while ensuring patient protection. The anesthetist's continued presence, along with verbal reassurance and patient education, helps foster acceptance in the patient; even so, the use of agents that promote amnesia, analgesia, anxiolysis, and sedation is often required to create the ideal conditions for the patient and the surgical team. Several suitable techniques incorporating benzodiazepines, analgesics (opioid and nonopioid), and subhypnotic doses of intravenous anesthetic agents have been described that provide patient sedation during monitored anesthesia care for outpatient procedures. Alternate routes of drug administration (e.g., transmucosal) may have a place, but at present, the intravenous route remains the most popular means of administering these agents.

Some investigators have described the use of benzodiazepines (e.g., diazepam and midazolam) alone[256] or in combination with opioid analgesics, such as fentanyl;[257] nonopioid analgesics, such as ketorolac[258] and dezocine;[258] and hypnotics, such as propofol.[259] Because of its superior recovery profile, midazolam may be the preferred benzodiazepine in the ambulatory setting. It is now available in an easily administered oral formulation, as well as the traditional intravenous route. The use of other agents, such as opioid analgesics (e.g., remifentanil) and hypnotic agents (e.g., etomidate,[256] methohexital,[256] and propofol[260]), administered by bolus or continuous infusion, have been described for outpatient surgery. Propofol is associated with a more rapid recovery than that afforded by midazolam,[259] but the pain on injection and the short amnesia time it causes may contribute to diminished patient acceptance.[261] Opioid agents, when used in combination with benzodiazepines, have the advantage of promoting patient comfort. The shorter-acting opioid analgesics may be titrated until their therapeutic effect is demonstrated for procedures such as brachial plexus block, in which paresthesias are likely to be elicited. The patient should be comfortable, yet able to readily respond to a paresthesia. Patient-controlled analgesia may be desirable for some patients because it allows them additional control over their surgical experience.

POSTOPERATIVE CONSIDERATIONS

After the surgical procedure, care is provided in either the PACU (phase I) or the short-stay unit (phase II) until the patient is ready for discharge from the ambulatory setting. The location and the level of nursing care required vary according to the patient undergoing the procedure, the type of anesthesia used, and the surgical procedure. Properly addressing potential or realized complications in the most efficient manner possible expedites patient management and promotes a timely discharge process. Complications that might delay the patient's departure from the ambulatory facility include nausea, vomiting, and pain. Each outpatient facility has specific criteria for discharge that should be met before the patient is released from the facility.

Postanesthesia Care Unit

The care afforded to the recovering outpatient should be of the same quality as that afforded to comparable inpatients; patient monitoring capability and resuscitative equipment should be similar in both environments. These capabilities include methods of monitoring the patient's circulation, oxygenation, temperature, and ventilation. Respiratory care includes means of delivering supplemental oxygen therapy to the intubated and the nonintubated patient, as well as a method for evaluating the adequacy of such care. Mechanical ventilatory support should be available for the patient requiring postoperative ventilatory assistance.

An increasingly popular concept in ambulatory care relates to the bypassing of phase I recovery by taking select patients directly to the phase II recovery area.[262] This concept has seen increased popularity as a result of faster awakening times secondary to the rapid-offset anesthetic agents[263] and the ability to more accurately titrate the amount of anesthesia required by the patient as a result of intraoperative electroencephalogram monitoring.[264,265] "Fast-tracking" is designed to improve efficiency and reduce health-care expenses. A $50,000 to $160,000 per year savings was reported at institutions participating in the early evaluation of the fast-track concept.[266] A study in a community hospital–based ambulatory setting found 83% of their healthy outpatients could safely bypass phase I recovery.[267] Although this technique can significantly reduce the time patients spend in the PACU (variable cost savings), it is likely to have little effect on PACU productivity or labor costs (fixed costs).[268] An evaluation of lower extremity surgeries in a freestanding facility found successful bypass rates of 87% but noted that more nursing interventions were required of these patients in phase II than those patients who came to phase II after initially recovering in phase I recovery.[269] Phase I bypass eligibility criteria should be established to gauge the appropriateness of patients going directly to the phase II, and a less intensive monitoring, area (Table 35-2).[270]

TABLE 35-2 White's Fast-Tracking Scoring System

Criterion	Score*
Level of Consciousness	
Awake and oriented	2
Arousable with minimal stimulation	1
Responsive only to tactile stimulation	0
Physical Activity	
Able to move all extremities on command	2
Some weakness in movement of extremities	1
Unable to voluntarily move extremities	0
Hemodynamic Stability	
Blood pressure ± 15% of baseline	2
Blood pressure ± 30% of baseline	1
Blood pressure ± 50% of baseline	0
Respiratory Stability	
Able to breathe deeply	2
Tachypnea with good cough	1
Dyspnea with weak cough	0
Oxygen Saturation	
Maintains value >92% on room air	2
Requires supplemental oxygen	1
Saturation <92% with supplemental oxygen	0
Pain Assessment	
None or mild discomfort	2
Moderate to severe pain controlled with analgesics	1
Persistent severe pain	0
Emetic Symptoms	
None or mild nausea with no active vomiting	2
Transient vomiting or retching	1
Persistent moderate severe nausea and vomiting	0

**Total possible score is 14. A minimum score of 12 (with no score less than one in any category) would be required at the time the patient is transferred from the OR after general anesthesia.*

From Watkins AC, White PF: Fast-tracking after ambulatory surgery, J PeriAnesth Nurs *16:379-387, 2001.*

Postoperative Complications and Management

With today's standard of anesthesia care, major morbidity and mortality following ambulatory surgery is extremely rare. A review of ambulatory surgical care encompassing 45,090 patients during a 3-year period at a rural-based referral center found most major postoperative morbidities (myocardial infarction, stroke, pulmonary embolism, respiratory failure) to occur within the first 48 hours.[271] In a review of 17,638 patients who underwent ambulatory surgery, Chung and Mezei[272] reported on a variety of adverse postoperative events (Table 35-3), of which pain and vomiting occurred most frequently. Patel and Hannallah[273] described a 0.3% hospital admission rate from the short-stay unit for their pediatric population (Table 35-4). Recent publications have cited overall unanticipated hospital admissions following ambulatory surgery to range between 0.2% and 33%.[14,274-285] Certain procedures (laparoscopic sterilization; laparoscopic inguinal herniorrhaphy; head and neck; ear, nose, and throat; urologic; orthopedic) are associated with a higher incidence of hospital admissions;[276,279-281] otherwise, the hospital admission rate following ambulatory surgery approaches 0.5% to 1.5%.

Nausea and Vomiting. Persistent nausea and vomiting are responsible for delays in discharge and for increases in patient cost[286] and are a prominent factor in unanticipated hospital admission after outpatient surgery.[287] The reported incidence of postoperative nausea and vomiting ranges from 18% to 28% in adult patients[288,289] and 25% to 39% in children.[273,290,291] Nearly 50% of patients who experience vomiting in phase I or II

TABLE 35-3 Adverse Events Associated with Ambulatory Surgery

Adverse Event	Rate of Events (%)
Postanesthesia Care Unit	9.6
Excessive pain	4.7
Nausea, vomiting	2.2
Shivering/hypothermia	0.9
Drowsiness/sleepiness	0.4
Cardiovascular	0.6
Respiratory	0.4
Excessive bleeding	0.1
Ambulatory Surgical Unit	7.9
Nausea, vomiting	3.9
Excessive pain	1.9
Dizziness	1.3
Drowsiness	0.3
Cardiovascular	0.1
Excessive bleeding	0.1

From Chung F, Mezei G: Adverse outcomes in ambulatory anesthesia, Can J Anesth *46:R18-R26, 1999.*

TABLE 35-4 Reasons for Admission of Children to the Hospital from the Short-Stay Recovery Unit

Reason	Number of Patients (%) 1983-1986 (*n* = 10,000)	Number of Patients (%) 1988-1991 (*n* = 15,245)
Unexpected admissions rate	90 (0.9)	45 (0.3)
Protracted vomiting	30 (33)	17 (39)
Complicated surgery	15 (17)	4 (9)
Croup	8 (9)	5 (11)
Physician/parental request	6 (7)	2 (4)
Fever	6 (7)	0 (0)
Bleeding	3 (3)	4 (9)
Sleepiness	2 (2)	2 (4)
Pain	0 (0)	3 (7)
Respiratory monitoring	NA	2 (4)
Miscellaneous	20 (22)	6 (13)

From Patel RI, Hannallah RS: Complications following pediatric ambulatory surgery—less of the same? Anesthesiology *79:A223, 1993.*

recovery will continue to vomit once discharged.[292] Many anesthetic-related and non–anesthetic-related factors affect the susceptibility of patients to postoperative nausea and emesis.[293-295] Non–anesthetic-related factors contributing to increased episodes of emesis include the following:

1. *Age*. There is a higher incidence of postoperative vomiting in children,[296-298] particularly between 3 and 12 years of age.[290,299,300] A gradual decrease in the incidence of postoperative nausea and vomiting has been shown after 50 years of age.[301]
2. *Apprehension*. Preoperative anxiety may increase the likelihood of vomiting.[302] Proposed mechanisms by which apprehension contributes to vomiting include swallowed air[303] with resultant abdominal distention,[304] increased gastric volume,[305,306] and increased catecholamine levels.[307]
3. *Gastroparesis*[308] is associated with several pathologic conditions, such as ileus, bowel obstruction, diabetes mellitus, muscular dystrophies, collagen vascular disorders, uremia, raised intracranial pressure, and pregnancy.[293] The accompanying delayed gastric emptying means a greater gastric content and thus a greater chance of vomiting.[308,309]
4. *Gender*. Emesis occurs in adult females more than in males,[289,296,301,310,311] and differences are suggested to occur at various stages of the menstrual cycle (menses[312-314] or luteal phase[315]). Elevated preoperative estrogen levels may contribute to an increased incidence of emesis.[316] After 70 years of age, gender is no longer a distinction for developing postoperative nausea and vomiting.[297]
5. *Individual predisposition*. Patients relating a previous history of nausea and vomiting after anesthesia[297] or motion sickness[317,318] are at increased risk for nausea and vomiting after subsequent anesthetics.
6. *Food ingestion*. Recent ingestion of food before undergoing anesthesia increases the probability of vomiting,[319,320] as does vomiting during the induction of anesthesia.
7. *Obesity*. Increased patient weight correlates with an increased incidence of nausea and vomiting.[321] This relationship is thought to be caused by increased anesthetic requirements of the obese patient[298] or by increased residual gastric volume.[322] Not all studies have found a positive relationship between obesity and postoperative vomiting.[311]
8. *Nonsmoking status*. Cigarette smokers seem to experience less postoperative nausea and vomiting than nonsmokers.[323-325]
9. *Type of surgery*. Prolonged surgical times correspond to an increased risk of vomiting.[326] Certain surgical procedures[293]—for example, arthroscopy, laparoscopy,[327] lithotripsy, intestinal operations, ovum retrieval, orchiopexy, otoplasty, retinal detachment, tonsillectomy with or without adenoidectomy,[328] and strabismus[329]—are associated with an increased incidence of postoperative vomiting.

Anesthetic-related factors contributing to emesis include the following:

1. *Premedications*. Preoperatively administered opioid analgesics, primarily the longer-lasting agents,[330] can increase postoperative vomiting.[331,332] The proposed mechanisms for this to occur include opioid receptor site stimulation,[297] impaired gastric motility,[333] release of serotonin from the small intestine,[334] and vestibular system sensitization.[335]
2. *Induction of anesthesia*. Inhalation induction may result in gastric distention from positive pressure ventilation via the anesthesia face mask and is known to increase postoperative vomiting.[307] This coincides with increased vomiting in cases in which the anesthesia provider is relatively inexperienced and not familiar with proper mask ventilation technique.[336] For intravenous induction of anesthesia, propofol has been found to result in less postoperative vomiting than the other common hypnotic agents (e.g., etomidate, thiopental, ketamine, methohexital).[337-339]
3. *Maintenance of anesthesia*. Several variables are known to increase the incidence of postoperative vomiting:
   - Longer anesthesia times[289]
   - General anesthesia when compared with regional or local anesthetic techniques[340]
   - Older inhalation anesthetic agents (e.g., halothane, isoflurane) when compared with the newer volatile agents (e.g., desflurane,[341] sevoflurane[342])
   - Volatile inhalation anesthetics when compared with the intravenous hypnotic agents[333,343,344]
   - Intraoperative opioid administration[345,346]

- Nitrous oxide;[347-349] the proposed mechanisms leading to increased postoperative vomiting with nitrous oxide include increased middle ear pressure,[350,351] distention of the gut by nitrous oxide diffusing into the gastrointestinal tract,[326] interaction with opioid receptors,[352] and sympathetic nerve activation.[353]

Postanesthetic-related factors contributing to emesis include the following:

1. *Ambulation*. More commonly seen in phase II recovery when the patient is mobilized in preparation for discharge, especially in patients receiving opioid analgesics.[326]
2. *Postural hypotension*. Dizziness, syncope, and nausea may be a problem if there is a significant reduction in blood pressure on standing.[307]
3. *Uncontrolled pain*.[354] Etiologic factors may include increased catecholamine concentrations, increased level of consciousness, or peripheral sensitization after direct tissue injury with the resultant release of endogenous nociceptor activators (i.e., serotonin).[333]
4. *Postoperatively administered opioid analgesics*.[355]
5. *Oral intake* before discharge from phase II recovery results in approximately a 50% greater incidence of vomiting or prolonged phase II stay than in counterparts who only drank if they desired.[356-358] When oral fluids were held postoperatively for 4 to 6 hours, the incidence of postoperative nausea and vomiting was reduced in children from 56% to 38%.[359] In children receiving opioids, withholding of oral fluids saw a further reduction in vomiting by from 73% to 36%.
6. *Lower inspired oxygen concentrations*. Higher concentrations (50% to 80%) of intraoperative and postoperative supplemental oxygen therapy appear to reduce the incidence of vomiting for inpatients.[360-362] This appears to be of short-term benefit: once oxygen therapy is discontinued, the incidence approaches that of those breathing reduced concentrations of oxygen.[362] One study conducted in ambulatory patients found no benefit of supplemental oxygen in reducing the incidence of postoperative vomiting.[363]
7. *Reversal agents*. Opioid and benzodiazepine receptor antagonists and neuromuscular reversal agents may increase nausea and vomiting.[293] In regard to neuromuscular reversal, it appears that only the higher doses of neostigmine may demonstrate emetic tendencies.[364]

Suggested management of nausea and vomiting involves perioperatively administered pharmacologic interventions. However, evaluating the efficacy of these agents is difficult because the cause of nausea and vomiting is multifactorial. Oral fluids should be withheld and intravenous fluid hydration can be maintained with normal saline or lactated Ringer's solution until the emesis is controlled. Patients at high risk for postoperative nausea and vomiting will benefit from prophylactic antiemetic therapy. Prophylactic antiemetic therapy has been shown to be cost-effective in ambulatory surgery.[365] Circumstances that benefit from the perioperative administration of medications for the control of nausea and vomiting include the following:

- A history of protracted postoperative emesis
- Operations associated with a high incidence of nausea and vomiting
- Mandibular surgery when the jaws are wired shut
- Circumstances in which retching could jeopardize the surgical result (plastic or eye procedures)

Corticosteroids. Recent studies have found corticosteroids to be effective in reducing the incidence of postoperative nausea and vomiting. Betamethasone (12 mg) given intramuscularly 30 minutes before the start of surgery was more effective than placebo in preventing postoperative nausea.[366] Dexamethasone, 5 to 10 mg given to adults and up to 500 mcg/kg in children, given alone[367-378] or in combination with antiemetic agents,[379-385] was effective in reducing postoperative vomiting. Dexamethasone has been shown to be more effective the earlier it can be given to the patient.[386] The time until discharge from the phase II recovery area has been shortened following ambulatory surgery in patients receiving dexamethasone.[387,388] The incidence of vomiting in phase III is reduced if dexamethasone is administered during the surgery.[367] This beneficial effect could be secondary to its long duration of action. Adverse effects from a single dose of dexamethasone have not been reported.[389,390]

Dolasetron. Dolasetron (a selective serotonin type 3 receptor antagonist), 12.5 mg given intravenously, is effective in preventing[390] and treating[391] postoperative vomiting. Dolasetron should be administered within 15 minutes before the end of anesthesia.[392] A single oral dose of 100 mg of dolasetron given 1 to 2 hours before surgery is effective for the prevention of postoperative vomiting.[393] One comparative study found 50 mg of dolasetron given intravenously to be as effective as 4 mg of ondansetron for the prevention of postoperative nausea and vomiting.[394]

Droperidol. Droperidol (Inapsine, a butyrophenone/dopamine receptor antagonist), 10 to 20 mcg/kg given intravenously, has been effective in reducing vomiting.[395] Prophylactically administered droperidol, 20 mcg/kg given intravenously immediately after induction, was superior to metoclopramide, 5 or 10 mg orally, in reducing postoperative vomiting.[153] This dose appears to offer a compromise between the reduction of vomiting and the prolongation of the patient's stay that results from prolonged sedation.[396] Caution should be exercised with the use of larger doses of droperidol (50 to 75 mcg/kg) because the occurrence of side effects (anxiety, dizziness, drowsiness, extrapyramidal symptoms, hypotension) and the potential to delay discharge may be increased. In 2001 the Food and Drug Administration (FDA) placed a "black box" advisory on the packaging label regarding the use of droperidol and risk of fatal dysrhythmias. The FDA recommends 12-lead electrocardiographic monitoring of patients for 2 to 3 hours following drug administration, which creates concerns over time efficiency in the ambulatory setting.[397] The FDA has recently agreed to reassess this issue since the overwhelming consensus among anesthesiologists and nurse anesthetists is that droperidol is safe when used in small doses as an antiemetic.

Ephedrine. Ephedrine (an indirect-acting sympathomimetic agent), 0.5 mg/kg given intramuscularly at the end of surgery, was found to be as effective as droperidol, 40 mcg/kg given intramuscularly, in minimizing nausea and vomiting while producing less sedation.[398] Similarly, ephedrine 0.5 mg/kg, given at the end of abdominal surgery, reduced the incidence of nausea and vomiting during the first 3 hours postoperatively.[399] Ephedrine, 10 to 25 mg given intravenously, has been recommended for the treatment of nausea and vomiting associated with the postural hypotension of ambulation before the patient is discharged from the facility.[400]

Gastric Suctioning. Some investigators have suggested that intraoperatively inserting a gastric tube into the stomach and suctioning out the contents has a beneficial effect.[355]

However, other clinical evaluations have failed to show beneficial results with this maneuver,[401,402] and it may actually increase the incidence of emesis.[403]

Metoclopramide. Metoclopramide (a benzamide) exerts beneficial gastric effects by increasing lower esophageal sphincter tone, promoting gastric emptying by increasing gastric and small-bowel motility, and presumably by supposedly antidopaminergic and antiserotonin (at higher doses) receptor effect.[293,404] Conflicting reports have been published about the efficacy of metoclopramide as an antiemetic. A review of placebo controlled studies involving metoclopramide failed to find any clinically significant antinausea effect.[405] An advantage of metoclopramide is its lack of sedative traits; this quality reduces the potential for delayed discharge. The intravenous administration of 0.15 mg/kg of metoclopramide is recommended for the treatment of nausea and vomiting in patients in the PACU who appear sedated.[406] Metoclopramide is not without side effects; extrapyramidal symptoms have been associated with its use.[407]

Ondansetron. Ondansetron (a selective serotonin type 3 receptor antagonist), 0.15 mg/kg given intravenously over the course of 2 to 5 minutes, has been popular for the management of chemotherapy-induced nausea and vomiting, and recent studies have demonstrated its effectiveness in the treatment of anesthesia-related emesis. Ondansetron appears to be effective in the prevention of vomiting when it is administered preoperatively (intravenously[408] or orally[409]), intraoperatively, postoperatively, or in combination,[410] and it appears to be effective in the treatment of postoperative vomiting.[411] This drug is most effective at preventing postoperative nausea and vomiting when administered at the end of the surgical procedure.[412] In the adult patient, 4 mg of ondansetron appears to be as effective as 8 mg when it is administered intravenously in the PACU as a treatment for nausea and vomiting.[413,414] A repeat dose, given either intravenously or orally 8 hours later, has been employed as part of an antiemetic management regimen. Under select conditions, ondansetron was more effective in reducing the early (within the first 4 hours postoperatively) incidence of postoperative vomiting when compared with droperidol[408,414-417] and metoclopramide.[408,416,418]

Promethazine. Promethazine (a phenothiazine/dopamine receptor antagonist), in doses of 0.5 mg/kg given intravenously and 0.5 mg/kg given intramuscularly for strabismus repair before extraocular muscle manipulation, reduced the overall incidence of vomiting to 10%, compared with a 56% incidence for droperidol, in doses of 75 mcg/kg given intravenously.[419] The only difference in side effects between these agents was increased restlessness in the promethazine group. The potential for delays in recovery secondary to sedative and extrapyramidal effects must be taken into account when using promethazine.

Postoperative Pain. Appropriate postoperative pain management helps minimize the stress of surgery, thereby fostering a quicker convalescence. Uncontrolled postoperative pain causes a triggering of the stress response (i.e., elevated catecholamine release, increased oxygen consumption, increased cardiac work, tachycardia),[420] patient uneasiness, neurohumoral response (i.e., increased production of adrenocortical hormone, aldosterone, antidiuretic hormone, cortisol, follicle-stimulating hormone, growth hormone, luteinizing hormone, plasma renin activity, prolactin),[421] increased nausea and vomiting, psychologic distress,[422] discharge delays,[423] and unanticipated hospital admission.[15] Pain management should begin with the use of wound infiltration with local anesthesia, the use of peripheral or regional nerve block, and the administration of opioid and nonopioid (i.e., nonsteroidal antiinflammatory drugs) analgesics preoperatively or intraoperatively, particularly in procedures associated with discomfort after emergence from anesthesia. These practices decrease the analgesic requirements in the immediate recovery period.

The severity and the onset of postoperative discomfort are influenced by previously administered analgesics. Immediate control of pain in the PACU can be achieved by incremental titration of small intravenous doses of a short-acting opioid analgesic, such as fentanyl (12.5 to 75 mcg) or alfentanil (50 to 300 mcg), every 2 to 3 minutes until pain relief has been achieved.[424] Once patient discomfort has been controlled and the patient is tolerating oral fluids, early management of pain with oral analgesics (similar to those the patient will be taking after discharge) should be considered. This allows for the evaluation of the analgesic's effect on pain alleviation, the patient's mental condition, and the patient's respiratory drive. The outpatient's analgesic medication should be safe and easily managed by the patient or caregiver once the patient is discharged from the facility.

Discharge Criteria

Before the patient is discharged from the ambulatory facility, he or she must meet certain criteria of recovery from the effects of surgery and anesthesia. An organized approach to patient evaluation postoperatively allows for the most comprehensive and efficient means of judging the patient's readiness to be "weaned" from the immediate care of the anesthetist without compromising the patient's safety. A consistent method of evaluating the patient for discharge readiness offers the advantages of reproducibility, standardization, and objectivity; however, no universally accepted standard exists for determining discharge readiness. Several methods of patient evaluation have been proposed. Aldrete and Kroulik[425] were the first to describe a means of postoperative patient evaluation that was appropriate for all types of anesthesia; this method is based on physical signs that are frequently monitored. A minimum total Aldrete postanesthetic recovery (PAR) score of 8 is required before the patient is considered for discharge from phase I recovery.[426] More recently, Aldrete[427] has updated his original phase I PAR score to reflect the contemporary ability to monitor oxygenation in a more exact fashion with the use of pulse oximetry. The Aldrete phase I PAR scoring system is not meaningful for the phase II ambulatory population in regard to comprehensive "home-readiness." Newer, more discriminating models such as the postanesthesia discharge scoring system (PADS) for determining home-readiness[428] (Table 35-5) and Aldrete's phase II postanesthetic recovery score[427] (Table 35-6) address items specific to suitability for home discharge (i.e., ambulation, bleeding, comfort level, and nausea and vomiting). Although significant progress has been made in attempts to develop a meaningful discharge scoring system for the ambulatory surgical population, a definitive tool that is sensitive to the patient, surgical procedure, and anesthetic technique, as well as compatible with today's economic concerns, has yet to be finalized.[429]

For discharge to occur, the patient must be clinically stable and able to continue the recovery process at a remote recovery

TABLE 35-5 Postanesthesia Discharge Scoring System (PADS) for Determining Home-Readiness

Criterion	Score*
Vital Signs	
Vital signs must be stable and consistent with age and preoperative baseline.	
Blood pressure and pulse within 20% of preoperative baseline	2
Blood pressure and pulse 20%-40% of preoperative baseline	1
Blood pressure and pulse >40% of preoperative baseline	0
Activity Level	
Patient must be able to ambulate at preoperative level.	
Steady gait, no dizziness, or meets preoperative level	2
Requires assistance	1
Unable to ambulate	0
Nausea and Vomiting	
The patient should have minimal nausea and vomiting before discharge.	
Minimal: successfully treated with oral medication	2
Moderate: successfully treated with intramuscular medication	1
Severe: continues after repeated treatment	0
Pain	
The patient should have minimal or no pain before discharge.	
The level of pain that the patient has should be acceptable to the patient.	
Pain should be controllable by oral analgesics.	
The location, type, and intensity of pain should be consistent with anticipated postoperative discomfort.	
Acceptability:	
Yes	2
No	1
Surgical Bleeding	
Postoperative bleeding should be consistent with expected blood loss for the procedure.	
Minimal: does not require dressing change	2
Moderate: up to two dressing changes required	1
Severe: more than three dressing changes required	0

**Total possible score is 10. Patients who score 9 or 10 are considered fit for discharge.*

From Marshall S, Chung F: Assessment of "home readiness": discharge criteria and postdischarge complications, Curr Opin Anaesthesiol *10:445-450, 1997.*

TABLE 35-6 Aldrete's Phase II Postanesthetic Recovery Score

Patient Sign	Criterion	Score*
Activity	Able to move 4 extremities (voluntarily or on command)	2
	Able to move 2 extremities (voluntarily or on command)	1
	Able to move 0 extremities (voluntarily or on command)	0
Respiration	Able to breathe deeply and cough	2
	Dyspnea, limited breathing or tachypnea	1
	Apneic or on mechanical ventilator	0
Circulation	Blood pressure ± 20% of preanesthesia level	2
	Blood pressure ± 20%-49% of preanesthesia level	1
	Blood pressure ± 50% of preanesthesia level	0
Consciousness	Fully awake	2
	Arousable on calling	1
	Not responding	0
Oxygen saturation	SpO_2 >92% on room air	2
	Requires supplemental O_2 to maintain SpO_2 >90%	1
	SpO_2 <90% even with O_2 supplement	0
Dressing	Dry and clean	2
	Wet but stationary or marked	1
	Growing area of wetness	0
Pain	Pain free	2
	Mild pain handled by oral medications	1
	Severe pain requiring IV or IM medications	0
Ambulation	Can stand up and walk straight†	2
	Vertigo when erect	1
	Dizziness when supine	0
Fasting-feeding	Able to drink fluids	2
	Nauseated	1
	Nauseated and vomiting	0
Urine output	Has voided	2
	Unable to void but comfortable	1
	Unable to void and uncomfortable	0

**Total possible score is 20. A score of 18 or greater is required before patient discharge.*

†May be replaced by Romberg's test, or picking up 12 clips in one hand.

From Aldrete JA: Discharge criteria. In Thomson D, Frost E, editors: Baillieres Clinical Anaesthesiology—Postanaesthesia Care, *London, 1994, Bailliere Tindall, pp 763-773.*

location. The decision to discharge is best made on objective criteria outlined in the policies of each ambulatory surgical facility. Distinct objective discharge criteria must be addressed when assessing home-readiness of the patient. (*Note*: Before discharge from phase I, the patient's vital signs will be stable, there will be no respiratory impairment, protective reflexes of swallow and cough will be present, and the patient will be oriented to his or her preoperative level. It is assumed that the status of these parameters will not deteriorate during the patient's stay in phase I.) Individually, the following clinical markers should be evaluated in an organized, concise manner:[430]

1. Vital signs should be stable and age appropriate.
2. The patient should be oriented to person, place, and time or at a level appropriate for the patient's developmental and preoperative status.

3. Ambulation can be affected by the surgical procedure and the patient's developmental level. If assistance to ambulate is required, the home caregiver must be capable of meeting this need.
4. There should be no respiratory distress.
5. Swallowing and coughing protective airway reflexes must be present.
6. Bleeding should be minimal or appropriate for the surgical procedure.
7. Pain should be minimal or controlled with an appropriate analgesic regimen.
8. Nausea and vomiting should be minimal.
9. Oral intake prior to discharge is not necessary unless crucial to the patient's continued convalescence at home (e.g., diabetic patient, patient requiring oral analgesics).
10. Voiding is not mandatory before discharge except for patients at high risk for postoperative urinary retention (e.g., history of postoperative urinary retention, pelvic or urologic surgery, perioperative catheterization).[431,432]
11. A responsible caregiver should be available.

Discharge Considerations. During the preparatory phase, the availability of a responsible person who will oversee the patient's care once the patient is discharged should be ascertained before surgery. In some cases, inpatient admission may be necessary if a responsible individual cannot be located. Postoperative care may be required for up to 48 hours in such cases, especially in elderly patients.[433] The patient and responsible person should be provided with written instructions that are verbally reinforced before the patient is discharged. The information includes the physician's telephone numbers and steps that should be taken if questions or complications arise. Once the patient has satisfied the criteria for discharge from the outpatient facility, certain discharge instructions should be reviewed to expedite and streamline the discharge process (Box 35-10).

The period of patient recovery after discharge from the ambulatory facility until resumption of normal activities is termed *phase III*. This is an important and often forgotten aspect of postoperative ambulatory care as patient care issues

BOX **35-10**

Key Education Points for Discharge Instructions

Medications

Detail the name, purpose, and dosage schedule for each medication. Emphasize the importance of following the directions on the label.

The patient should resume medications taken before surgery per the physician's order.

If pain medication is not prescribed, nonprescription, nonaspirin analgesics (e.g., acetaminophen, ibuprofen) may be effective on mild aches and pains.

Additional pain medication may be ordered by the physician after surgery. The patient should take these medications as directed, preferably with food to prevent gastrointestinal upset.

Activity Restriction

Caution the patient to take it easy for the remainder of the day following surgery. Dizziness or drowsiness is not unusual after surgery and anesthesia.

For the next 24 hr, the patient should not drive a vehicle, operate machinery or power tools, consume alcohol (including beer), make important personal or business decisions, or sign important documents.

Activity level: in specific behavioral terms (e.g., do not lift objects greater than 20 lb), describe any limitation of activities.

Diet

Explain any dietary restrictions or instructions.

If no dietary restriction, instruct the patient to progress as tolerated to a regular diet.

Surgical and Anesthesia Side Effects

Anticipated sequelae of surgery, such as bleeding and pain, should be delineated.

Common side effects associated with anesthesia include dizziness, drowsiness, myalgia, nausea and vomiting, and sore throat.

Possible Complications and Symptoms

Instruct the patient and responsible caregiver in pertinent signs and symptoms that could be indicative of postoperative complications.

The patient should call his or her physician if any of the following develop:

- Fever >38.3° C (>101° F) orally
- Persistent, atypical pain
- Pain not relieved by pain medication
- Bleeding or unexpected drainage from the wound that does not stop
- Extreme redness/swelling around the incision or drainage of pus
- Urinary retention after 8 hr or otherwise instructed
- Continual nausea or vomiting

Treatment and Tests

Procedures that the patient or responsible caregiver are expected to perform, such as dressing changes or the application of warm moist compresses, should be described in detail.

A complete list of necessary supplies should be included.

If any postoperative tests are to be conducted, instructions as to the date, time, test location, and any previsit preparation should be listed.

Access to Postdischarge Care

The telephone number of the responsible and available physician.

The telephone number of the ambulatory center and the hours of operation.

The name, address, and telephone number of the appropriate emergency care facility.

Follow-Up Care

Identify the date, time, and location of the patient's scheduled return visit to the clinic or surgeon.

From Marley RA, Moline BM: Patient discharge issues. In Burden N, editor: Ambulatory Surgical Nursing, *ed 2, Philadelphia, 2000, Saunders.*

requiring attention continue to be important.[434] Up to 86% of all outpatients report minor complications following anesthesia and surgery.[435] Common postoperative complaints reported by outpatients after being discharged include drowsiness, pharyngitis, myalgia, vomiting (the most undesirable outcome),[436] pain, and headache. Greater than 60% of outpatients required 3 days of recuperation before they were able to resume their usual daily activities.[435] It is important to convey to patients that it will take several days before they begin to feel as they did before surgery.

SUMMARY

The numbers and types of surgeries performed on an ambulatory basis will continue to increase, as will facilities' ability to appropriately treat these patients. As anesthetic techniques and agents are refined, thereby increasing the safety and efficiency of patient care and discharge, new groups of patients will be evaluated for their appropriateness for outpatient surgery. These new groups will continue to challenge our resources for providing ambulatory anesthesia.

REFERENCES

1. Nicoll JH: The surgery of infancy, *BMJ* 2:753-754, 1909.
2. Waters RM: The down-town anesthesia clinic, *Am J Surg* 33(Anesth suppl):71-73, 1919.
3. Owings MF, Kozak LJ: Ambulatory and inpatient procedures in the United States, 1996: National Center for Health Statistics, *Vital Health Stat* 13:9, 1998.
4. Pregler JL, Kapur PA: The development of ambulatory anesthesia and future challenges, *Anesthesiol Clin North Am* 21:207-228, 2003.
5. Way JC, Culham BA: Establishment and cost analysis of an office surgical suite, *Can J Surg* 39:379-383, 1996.
6. SMG Marketing Group: SMG forecast of surgical volume in hospital/ambulatory settings: 1994-2001, Chicago, 1999.
7. Fleisher LA, Yee K, Lillemoe KD, et al: Is outpatient laparoscopic cholecystectomy safe and cost-effective? A model to study transition of care, *Anesthesiology* 90:1746-1755, 1999.
8. Herwaldt LA, Smith SD, Carter CD: Infection control in the outpatient setting, *Infect Control Hosp Epidemiol* 19:41-74, 1998.
9. Lichtiger M: Choice of anesthesia for the geriatric outpatient, *Curr Rev Nurse Anesthetists* 12:67-71, 1989.
10. Epstein BS, Hannallah RS: Outpatient anesthesia. In Gregory GA, editor: *Pediatric Anesthesia*, vol 2, ed 3, New York, 1994, Churchill Livingstone, pp 773-804.
11. FASA Special Study I, Alexandria, VA, 1986, Federated Ambulatory Surgery Association.
12. Epstein BS: Outpatient anesthesia. In Hershey SG, editor: *ASA Refresher Courses in Anesthesiology*, Philadelphia, 1984, Lippincott, pp 85-95.
13. Talamini MA, Stanfield CL, Chang DC, Wu AW: The surgical recovery index, *Surg Endosc* Mar 19, 2004.
14. Gold BS, Kitz DS, Lecky JH, Neuhaus JM: Unanticipated admission to the hospital following ambulatory surgery, *JAMA* 262:3008-3010, 1989.
15. Meridy HW: Criteria for selection of ambulatory surgical patients and guidelines for anesthetic management: a retrospective study of 1553 cases, *Anesth Analg* 61:921-926, 1982.
16. Henderson JA: Ambulatory surgery: past, present, and future. In Wetchler BV, editor: *Anesthesia for Ambulatory Surgery*, ed 2, Philadelphia, 1991, Lippincott, pp 1-27.
17. Conahan TJ, Young ML: Outpatient anesthesia. In Longnecker DE, Murphy FL, editors: *Dripps Eckenhoff Vandam Introduction to Anesthesia*, ed 9, Philadelphia, 1997, Saunders, pp 377-385.
18. Guthrie S: Laminectomy: an outpatient approach, *Nurs Case Manage* 1:31-34, 1996.
19. Lo Gerfo P: Local/regional anesthesia for thyroidectomy: evaluation as an outpatient procedure, *Surgery* 124:975-978, 1998.
20. Summitt RL Jr, Stovall TG, Lipscomb GH, Ling FW: Randomized comparison of laparoscopy-assisted vaginal hysterectomy with standard vaginal hysterectomy in an outpatient setting, *Obstet Gynecol* 80:895-901, 1992.
21. Pringle MB, Cosford E, Beasley P, Brightwell AP: Day-case tonsillectomy—is it appropriate? *Clin Otolaryngol* 21:504-511, 1996.
22. Rakover Y, Almog R, Rosen G: The risk of postoperative haemorrhage in tonsillectomy as an outpatient procedure in children, *Int J Pediatr Otorhinolaryngol* 41:29-36, 1997.
23. Chiang TM, Sukis AE, Ross DE: Tonsillectomy performed on an outpatient basis: report of a series of 40,000 cases performed without a death, *Arch Otolaryngol Head Neck Surg* 88:307-310, 1968.
24. Wei JL, Beatty CW, Gustafson RO: Evaluation of posttonsillectomy hemorrhage and risk factors, *Otolaryngol Head Neck Surg* 123:229-235, 2000.
25. Postma DS, Folsom F: The case for an outpatient "approach" for all pediatric tonsillectomies and/or adenoidectomies: a 4-year review of 1419 cases at a community hospital, *Otolaryngol Head Neck Surg* 127:101-108, 2002.
26. Ross AT, Kazahaya K, Tom LW: Revisiting outpatient tonsillectomy in young children, *Otolaryngol Head Neck Surg* 128: 326-331, 2003.
27. Cheng DCH: The drug addicted patient, *Can J Anaesth* 44:R101–R106, 1997.
28. Zahl K: Substance abuse. In Schmitter CR Jr, editor: Ambulatory surgery: is it for everyone? *Soc Ambulatory Anesth Newslett* 7:3, 1992.
29. Hannallah RS, Epstein BS: The pediatric patient. In Wetchler BV, editor: *Anesthesia for Ambulatory Surgery*, ed 2, Philadelphia, 1991, Lippincott, pp 131-195.
30. Van Vlymen JM, White PF: Outpatient anesthesia. In Miller RD, editor: *Anesthesia*, vol 2, ed 5, New York, 2000, Churchill Livingstone, pp 2213-2240.
31. Stockman JA III: Anemia of prematurity: current concepts in the issue of when to transfuse, *Pediatr Clin North Am* 33: 111-128, 1986.
32. Welborn LG, Hannallah RS, Luban NL, Fink R, Ruttimann UE: Anemia and postoperative apnea in former preterm infants. *Anesthesiology* 74:1003-1006, 1991.
33. Welborn LG, Greenspun JC: Anesthesia and apnea: perioperative considerations in the former preterm infant, *Pediatr Clin North Am* 41:181-198, 1994.
34. Kurth CD, Spitzer AR, Broennle AM, Downes JJ: Postoperative apnea in preterm infants, *Anesthesiology* 66:483-488, 1987.
35. Kurth CD, LeBard SE: Association of postoperative apnea, airway obstruction, and hypoxemia in former premature infants, *Anesthesiology* 75:22-26, 1991.
36. Malviya S, Swartz J, Lerman J: Are all preterm infants younger than 60 weeks postconceptual age at risk for postanesthetic apnea? *Anesthesiology* 78:1076-1081, 1993.
37. Cote CJ, Zaslavsky A, Downes JJ, et al: Postoperative apnea in former preterm infants after inguinal herniorrhaphy: a combined analysis, *Anesthesiology* 82:809-822, 1995.
38. Karayan J, LaCoste L, Fusciardi J: Postoperative apnea in a full-term infant, *Anesthesiology* 75:375, 1991.
39. Fisher DM: When is the ex-premature infant no longer at risk for apnea? *Anesthesiology* 82:807, 1995.
40. Stierer T, Fleisher LA: Challenging patients in an ambulatory setting, *Anesthesiol Clin North Am* 21:243-261, 2003.
41. Krane EJ, Haberkern CM, Jacobson LE: Postoperative apnea, bradycardia, and oxygen desaturation in formerly premature infants: prospective comparison of spinal and general anesthesia, *Anesth Analg* 80:7-13, 1995.

42. Welborn LG, Rice LJ, Hannallah RS, Broadman LM, Ruttimann UE, Fink R: Postoperative apnea in former preterm infants: prospective comparison of spinal and general anesthesia, *Anesthesiology* 72:838-842, 1990.
43. Watcha MF, Thach BT, Gunter JB: Postoperative apnea after caudal anesthesia in an ex-premature infant, *Anesthesiology* 71:613-615, 1989.
44. Cox RG, Goresky GV: Life-threatening apnea following spinal anesthesia in former premature infants, *Anesthesiology* 73: 345-347, 1990.
45. Tobias JD, Burd RS, Helikson MA: Apnea following spinal anaesthesia in two former pre-term infants, *Can J Anaesth* 45:985-989, 1998.
46. Kunst G, Linderkamp O, Holle R, Motsch J, Martin E: The proportion of high risk preterm infants with postoperative apnea and bradycardia is the same after general and spinal anesthesia, *Can J Anesth* 46:94-95, 1999.
47. Bryan MH, Hardie MJ, Reilly BJ, Swyer PR: Pulmonary function studies during the first year of life in infants recovering from the respiratory distress syndrome, *Pediatrics* 52:169-178, 1973.
48. Berry FA: Pre-existing medical conditions of pediatric patients, *Semin Anesth* 3:24-31, 1984.
49. Garg M, Kurzner SI, Bautista D, Keens TG: Hypoxic arousal responses in infants with bronchopulmonary dysplasia, *Pediatrics* 82:59-63, 1988.
50. Valdes-Dapena MA: Sudden infant death syndrome: a review of the medical literature 1974-1979, *Pediatrics* 66:597-614, 1980.
51. Guntheroth WG, Lohmann R, Spiers PS: Risk of sudden infant death syndrome in subsequent siblings, *J Pediatr* 116:520-524, 1990.
52. Wetchler BV: Outpatient anesthesia. In Barash PG, Cullen BF, Stoelting RK, editors: *Clinical Anesthesia*, ed 2, Philadelphia, 1992, Lippincott, pp 1389-1416.
53. Rockoff MA, McCann ME: Case report no 12. From Wong HC, Nkana CA: In the real world. In Wetchler BV, editor: *Anesthesia for Ambulatory Surgery*, ed 2, Philadelphia, 1991, Lippincott, pp 509-511.
54. Berry FA: Preoperative assessment of pediatric outpatients. In White PF, editor: *Outpatient Anesthesia*, New York, 1990, Churchill Livingstone, pp 147-162.
55. Stierer T, Fleisher LA: Challenging patients in an ambulatory setting, *Anesthesiol Clin North Am* 21:243-261, 2003.
56. Pasternak LR: Case report no 18. From Wong HC, Nkana CA: In the real world. In Wetchler BV, editor: *Anesthesia for Ambulatory Surgery*, ed 2, Philadelphia, 1991, Lippincott, pp 525-528.
57. Karlet MC: An update on cystic fibrosis and implications for anesthesia, *AANA J* 68:141-148, 2000.
58. McGoldrick K: Is malignant hyperthermia a contraindication for outpatient surgery? *Soc Ambulatory Anesth Newslett* 7:11, 1992.
59. Karlet MC: Malignant hyperthermia: considerations for ambulatory surgery, *J Perianesth Nurs* 13:304-312, 1998.
60. Malignant Hyperthermia Association of the United States: *Managing MH: Clinical Update*. Available at http://www.mhaus.org/index.cfm/fuseaction/OnlineBrochures.Display/BrochurePK/3FFCBC12-9479-49C3-8A9E0B304EF08746.cfm. Accessed October 28, 2003.
61. Apfelbaum JL: Outpatient anesthesia for adult patients. *ASA 1992 Annual Refresher Course Lecture*, Philadelphia, 1992, Lippincott, p 412.
62. Marley RA: Postoperative oxygen therapy, *J Perianesth Nurs* 13:394-412, 1998.
63. Siyam MA, Benhamou D: Difficult endotracheal intubation in patients with sleep apnea syndrome, *Anesth Analg* 95:1098-1102, 2002.
64. Marley RA: Preoperative preparation. In Zaglaniczny K, Aker J, editors: *Clinical Guide to Pediatric Anesthesia*, Philadelphia, 1999, Saunders, pp 29-45.
65. Aker J: Sickle cell disease: implications for perioperative care, *J Perianesth Nurs* 14(4):221-227, 1999.
66. McCormick F: Abnormal hemoglobins. II. The pathology of sickle cell trait, *Am J Med Sci* 92:329, 1961.
67. Kunichika ET, Graves SA: Case report no. 4. From Wong HC, Nkana CA: In the real world. In Wetchler BV, editor: *Anesthesia for Ambulatory Surgery*, ed 2, Philadelphia, 1991, Lippincott, pp 485-489.
68. Pasternak LR: Sickle cell disease. In Schmitter CR Jr, editor: Ambulatory surgery: is it for everyone? *Soc Ambulatory Anesth Newslett* 7:2, 1992.
69. Twersky RS: Ambulatory surgery update, *Can J Anaesth* 45(suppl):R76-R83, 1998
70. Accreditation Association for Ambulatory Health Care: Anesthesia services. In *1996/1997 Accreditation Handbook for Ambulatory Health Care*, Skokie, IL, AAAHC, 1996, p 39.
71. Joint Commission on Accreditation of Healthcare Organizations: Assessment of patients. In *1996 Comprehensive Accreditation Manual for Ambulatory Care*, Oakbrook Terrace, IL, AAAHC, 1995, pp 89-122.
72. American Association of Nurse Anesthetists: Documenting the standard of care: the anesthesia record. In *Professional Practice Manual for the Certified Registered Nurse Anesthetist*, Park Ridge, IL, AANA Press, 1991, p 1.
73. Conway JB, Goldberg J, Chung F: Preadmission anaesthesia consultation clinic, *Can J Anaesth* 39:1051-1057, 1992.
74. Cassidy J, Marley RA: Preoperative assessment of the ambulatory patient, *J Perianesth Nurs* 11:334-343, 1996.
75. Perez A, Planell J, Bacardaz C, et al: Value of routine preoperative tests: a multicentre study in four general hospitals, *Br J Anaesth* 74:250-256, 1995.
76. Archer C, Levy AR, McGregor M: Value of routine preoperative chest x-rays: a meta-analysis, *Can J Anaesth* 40:1022-1027, 1993.
77. Charpak Y, Blery C, Chastang C, Szatan M, Fourgeaux B: Prospective assessment of a protocol for selective ordering of preoperative chest x-rays, *Can J Anaesth* 35:259-264, 1988.
78. Narr BJ, Hansen TR, Warner MA: Preoperative laboratory screening in healthy Mayo patients: cost-effective elimination of tests and unchanged outcomes, *Mayo Clin Proc* 66:155-159, 1991.
79. Kaplan EB, Sheiner LB, Boeckmann AJ, et al: The usefulness of preoperative laboratory screening, *JAMA* 253:3576-3581, 1985.
80. Velanovich V: Preoperative laboratory screening based on age, gender, and concomitant medical diseases, *Surgery* 115:56-61, 1994.
81. Ransom SB, McNeeley SG, Hosseini RB: Cost-effectiveness of routine blood type and screen testing before elective laparoscopy, *Obstet Gynecol* 86:346-348, 1995.
82. Pollard JB, Olson L: Early outpatient preoperative anesthesia assessment: does it help to reduce operating room cancellations? *Anesth Analg* 89:502-505, 1999.
83. Malins AF: Do they do as they are instructed? A review of outpatient anaesthesia, *Anaesthesia* 33:832-835, 1978.
84. Roizen MF, Rupani G: Preoperative assessment of adult outpatients. In White PF, editor: *Outpatient Anesthesia*, New York, 1990, Churchill Livingstone, pp 181-200.
85. Dzankic S, Pastor D, Gonzalez C, Leung JM: The prevalence and predictive value of abnormal preoperative laboratory tests in elderly surgical patients, *Anesth Analg* 93:301-308, 2001.
86. Roizen MF, Fischer SP: Preoperative evaluation: adults and children. In White PF, editor: *Ambulatory Anesthesia and Surgery*, Philadelphia, 1997, Saunders, pp 155-172.
87. Health Care Standards Committee: *Ancillary Studies Screen for Ambulatory Surgery for Medicare Patients*, Aurora, CO, 1990, Colorado Foundation for Medical Care.
88. Pasternak LR: Preoperative screening for ambulatory patients, *Anesthesiol Clin North Am* 21:229-242, 2003.

89. Malviya S, D'Errico C, Reynolds P, Huntington J, Voepel-Lewis T, Pandit UA: Should pregnancy testing be routine in adolescent patients prior to surgery? *Anesth Analg* 83:854-858, 1996.
90. American Society of Anesthesiologists Task Force on Preanesthesia Evaluation: Practice advisory for preanesthesia evaluation, *Anesthesiology* 96:485-496, 2002.
91. Johnson H Jr, Knee-Ioli S, Butler TA, Munoz E, Wise L: Are routine preoperative laboratory screening tests necessary to evaluate ambulatory surgical patients? *Surgery* 104:639-645, 1988.
92. Stoelting RK, Miller RD: Outpatient surgery: hospital, Surgicenter or office based. In *Basics of Anesthesia*, ed 4, New York, 2000, Churchill Livingstone, pp 391-398.
93. *The Selection of Patients for X-Ray Examinations: Presurgical Chest X-Ray Screening Examinations*, HHS pub FDA-86-8265, Rockville, MD, 1986, US Department of Health and Human Services, Food and Drug Administration, Center for Devices and Radiological Health.
94. Roizen MF, Cohn S: Preoperative evaluation for elective surgery: what laboratory tests are needed? In Stoelting RK, editor: *Advances in Anesthesia*, St Louis, 1993, Mosby, pp 25-47.
95. Rabkin SW, Horne JM: Preoperative electrocardiography: its cost-effectiveness in detecting abnormalities when a previous tracing exists, *Can Med Assoc J* 121:301-306, 1979.
96. Gold BS, Young ML, Kinman JL, Kitz DS, Berlin J, Schwartz JS: The utility of preoperative electrocardiograms in the ambulatory surgical patient, *Arch Intern Med* 152:301-305, 1992.
97. Turnbull JM, Buck C: The value of preoperative screening investigations in otherwise healthy individuals, *Arch Intern Med* 147:1101-1105, 1987.
98. Tait AR, Parr HG, Tremper KK: Evaluation of the efficacy of routine preoperative electrocardiograms, *J Cardiothorac Vasc Anesth* 11:752-755, 1997.
99. Munro J, Booth A, Nicholl J: Routine preoperative testing: a systematic review of the evidence, *Health Technol Assess* 1:i-iv; 1-62, 1997
100. Orkin FK, Gold B: Selection. In Wetchler BV, editor: *Anesthesia for Ambulatory Surgery*, ed 2, Philadelphia, 1991, Lippincott, pp 81-129.
101. Callaghan LC, Edwards ND, Reilly CS: Utilisation of the preoperative ECG, *Anaesthesia* 50:488-490, 1995.
102. Wagner JD, Moore DL: Preoperative laboratory testing for the oral and maxillofacial surgery patient, *J Oral Maxillofac Surg* 49:177-182, 1991.
103. Haug RH, Reifeis RL: A prospective evaluation of the value of preoperative laboratory testing for office anesthesia and sedation, *J Oral Maxillofac Surg* 57:16-20, 1999.
104. Luirink MR, Pfaff A: Routine electrocardiography in elderly patients for ambulatory surgery, *Br J Anaesth* 82:6, 1999.
105. Cote CJ: Aspiration: an overrated risk in elective patients. In Stoelting RK, editor: *Advances in Anesthesia*, St Louis, 1992, Mosby, pp 1-26.
106. Yogendran S, Chung FF: How long should we fast our patients? *Soc Ambulatory Anesth Newslett* 7:10, 1992.
107. Simpson KH, Stakes AF: Effect of anxiety on gastric emptying in preoperative patients, *Br J Anaesth* 59:540-544, 1987.
108. Borland LM, Sereika SM, Woelfel SK, et al: Pulmonary aspiration in pediatric patients during general anesthesia: incidence and outcome, *J Clin Anesth* 10(2):95-102, 1998
109. Nimmo WS: Drugs, diseases and altered gastric emptying, *Clin Pharmacokinet* 1:189-203, 1976.
110. Morgan M: Anaesthetic contribution to maternal mortality, *Br J Anaesth* 59:842-855, 1987.
111. Morrison JE Jr, Lockhart CH: Preoperative fasting and medication in children, *Anesthesiol Clin North Am* 9:731-743, 1991.
112. Cote CJ: Changing concepts in preoperative medication and "NPO" status of the pediatric patient. In *ASA 1992 Annual Refresher Course Lecture*, Philadelphia, 1992, Lippincott, p 132.
113. Hinder RA, Kelly KA: Canine gastric emptying of solids and liquids, *Am J Physiol* 233:E335-E340, 1977.
114. Warner ME: Risks and outcomes of perioperative pulmonary aspiration, *J Perianesth Nurs* 12:352-357, 1997.
115. Nagelhout JJ: Aspiration prophylaxis: is it time for changes in our practice? *AANA J* 71:299-303, 2003.
116. Minami H, McCallum RW: The physiology and pathophysiology of gastric emptying in humans, *Gastroenterology* 86: 1592-1610, 1984.
117. Farrow-Gillespie A, Christensen S, Lerman J: Effect of the fasting interval on gastric fluid pH and volume in children, *Anesth Analg* 67:S59, 1988.
118. Dose VA, White PF: Effects of fluid therapy on serum glucose levels in fasted outpatients, *Anesthesiology* 66:223-226, 1987.
119. Sutherland AD, Stock JG, Davies JM: Effects of preoperative fasting on morbidity and gastric contents in patients undergoing day-stay surgery, *Br J Anaesth* 58:876-878, 1986.
120. Read MS, Vaughan RS: Allowing pre-operative patients to drink: effects on patients' safety and comfort of unlimited oral water until 2 hours before anaesthesia, *Acta Anaesthesiol Scand* 35:591-595, 1991.
121. Shevde K, Trivedi N: Effects of clear liquids on gastric volume and pH in healthy volunteers, *Anesth Analg* 72:528-531, 1991.
122. Splinter WM, Schaefer JD: Unlimited clear fluid ingestion two hours before surgery in children does not affect volume or pH of stomach contents, *Anaesth Intensive Care* 18:522-526, 1990.
123. Maltby JR, Lewis P, Martin A, Sutherland LR: Gastric fluid volume and pH in elective patients following unrestricted oral fluid until three hours before surgery, *Can J Anaesth* 38:425-429, 1991.
124. Splinter WM, Schaefer JD: Ingestion of clear fluids is safe for adolescents up to 3 h before anaesthesia, *Br J Anaesth* 66:48-52, 1991.
125. Practice guidelines for preoperative fasting and the use of pharmacologic agents to reduce the risk of pulmonary aspiration: application to healthy patients undergoing elective procedures, *Anesthesiology* 90:896-905, 1999.
126. Fasting S, Soreide E, Raeder JC: Changing preoperative fasting policies, *Acta Anaesthesiol Scand* 42:1188-1191, 1998.
127. Majerus PW, Tollesfen DM: Anticoagulant, thrombolytic, and antiplatelet drugs. In Hardman JG, Limbird LE, editors: *Goodman and Gilman's The Pharmacological Basis of Therapeutics*, ed 10, New York, 2001, McGraw-Hill, pp 1519-1538.
128. Long M: Ambulatory anesthesia. In Hurford WE, Bailin MT, Davison JK, Haspel KL, Rosow C, editors: *Clinical Anesthesia Procedures of the Massachusetts General Hospital*, ed 5, Philadelphia, 1998, Lippincott-Raven, pp 547-552.
129. Tinker JH, Tarhan S: Discontinuing anticoagulant therapy in surgical patients with cardiac valve prostheses: observations in 180 operations, *JAMA* 239:738-739, 1978.
130. Graham GW, Unger BP, Coursin DB: Perioperative management of selected endocrine disorders, *Int Anesthesiol Clin* 38: 31-67, 2000.
131. Saunders NR: Innocent heart murmurs in children: taking a diagnostic approach, *Can Fam Physician* 41:1507-1512, 1995.
132. McEwan AI, Birch M, Bingham R: The preoperative management of the child with a heart murmur, *Pediatr Anaesth* 5: 151-156, 1995.
133. Monto AS, Ullman BM: Acute respiratory illness in an American community: the Tecumseh study, *JAMA* 227:164-169, 1974.
134. Bailey AG, Valley RD: Myths in pediatric anesthesia. In Spielman FJ, editor: *Problems in Anesthesia: Myths in Anesthesiology*, Philadelphia, 1991, Lippincott, pp 483-496.
135. Hannallah RS: Selection of patients for paediatric ambulatory surgery, *Can J Anaesth* 38:887-890, 1991.
136. Cameron CB: The special patient: pediatrics. In Duncan PG, editor: *Problems in Anesthesia: Anesthetic Risk and Complications*, Philadelphia, 1992, Lippincott, pp 253-267.
137. Steward DJ: Preoperative evaluation and preparation for surgery. In Gregory GA, editor: *Pediatric Anesthesia*, vol 1, ed 3, New York, 1994, Churchill Livingstone, pp 179-198.

138. Tait AR, Knight PR: The effects of general anesthesia on upper respiratory tract infections in children, *Anesthesiology* 67: 930-935, 1987.
139. Tait AR, Malviya S: Anesthesia for the child with an upper respiratory tract infection, *Curr Rev Nurse Anesth* 21:170-175, 1999.
140. Cohen MM, Cameron CB: Should you cancel the operation when a child has an upper respiratory tract infection? *Anesth Analg* 72:282-288, 1991.
141. Rolf N, Cote CJ: Incidence of hypoxemic events during anesthesia in children with upper respiratory infection, *Anesthesiology* 73:A1124, 1990.
142. Malviya S, Voepel-Lewis T, Siewert M, Pandit UA, Riegger LQ, Tait AR: Risk factors for adverse postoperative outcomes in children presenting for cardiac surgery with upper respiratory tract infections, *Anesthesiology* 98:628-632, 2003.
143. Tait AR, Malviya S, Voepel-Lewis T, Munro HM, Seiwert M, Pandit UA: Risk factors for perioperative adverse respiratory events in children with upper respiratory tract infections, *Anesthesiology* 95:299-306, 2001.
144. Tait AR, Voepel-Lewis T, Malviya S: Perioperative considerations for the child with an upper respiratory tract infection, *J PeriAnesth Nurs* 15:392-396, 2000.
145. Tait AR, Pandit UA, Voepel-Lewis T, Munro HM, Malviya S: Use of the laryngeal mask airway in children with upper respiratory tract infections: a comparison with endotracheal intubation, *Anesth Analg* 86:706-711, 1998.
146. Ljungqvist O, Soreide E: Preoperative fasting, *Br J Surg* 90: 400-406, 2003.
147. Solanki DR, Nicholas DA, Williams KR: Comparative effects of oral sodium citrate and oral cimetidine on gastric pH in pediatric patients, *Anesth Analg* 65:S147, 1986.
148. Murrell GC, Rosen M: In vitro buffering capacity of Alka Seltzer Effervescent: a comparison with magnesium trisilicate mixture BP and sodium citrate 0.3 M, *Anaesthesia* 41:138-142, 1986.
149. Manchikanti L, Roush JR, Colliver JA: Effect of preanesthetic ranitidine and metoclopramide on gastric contents in morbidly obese patients, *Anesth Analg* 65:195-199, 1986.
150. Christensen S, Farrow-Gillespie A, Lerman J: Effects of ranitidine and metoclopramide on gastric fluid pH and volume in children, *Br J Anaesth* 65:456-460, 1990.
151. Brock-Utne JG, Dow TG, Welman S, Dimopoulos GE, Moshal MG: The effect of metoclopramide on the lower oesophageal sphincter in late pregnancy, *Anaesth Intensive Care* 6:26-29, 1978.
152. Diamond MJ, Keeri-Szanto M: Reduction of postoperative vomiting by preoperative administration of oral metoclopramide, *Can J Anaesth* 27:36-39, 1980.
153. Pandit SK, Kothary SP, Pandit UA, Randel G, Levy L: Dose-response study of droperidol and metoclopramide as antiemetics for outpatient anesthesia, *Anesth Analg* 68:798-802, 1989.
154. Dimich I, Katende R, Singh PP, Mikula S, Sonnenklar N: The effects of intravenous cimetidine and metoclopramide on gastric pH and volume in outpatients, *J Clin Anesth* 3:40-44, 1991.
155. Meyer PD: Preoperative interview and medication. In McGough EK, Monroe MC, editors: *Problems in Anesthesia: Preoperative Evaluation*, Philadelphia, 1991, Lippincott, pp 541-549.
156. Stoelting RK: Antacids and gastrointestinal prokinetics. In Stoelting RK, editor: *Pharmacology and Physiology in Anesthetic Practice*, ed 3, Philadelphia, 1999, Lippincott, pp 444-452.
157. Wyner J, Cohen SE: Gastric volume in early pregnancy: effect of metoclopramide, *Anesthesiology* 57:209-212, 1982.
158. Schulze-Delrieu K: Drug therapy: metoclopramide, *N Engl J Med* 305:28-33, 1981.
159. Stoelting RK: Histamine and histamine receptor antagonists. In Stoelting RK, editor: *Pharmacology and Physiology in Anesthetic Practice*, ed 3, Philadelphia, 1999, Lippincott, pp 385-397.
160. McCullough AJ: A multicenter, randomized, double-blinded study comparing famotidine and ranitidine in the treatment of active duodenal ulcer disease, *Am J Med* 81(suppl 4B):17-24, 1986.
161. Ostro MJ: Pharmacodynamics and pharmacokinetics of parenteral histamine (H_2)-receptor antagonists, *Am J Med* 83(suppl 6A): 15-22, 1987.
162. Dubin SA, Silverstein PI, Wakefield ML, Jense HG: Comparison of the effects of oral famotidine and ranitidine on gastric volume and pH, *Anesth Analg* 69:680-683, 1989.
163. Lam AM, Grace DM, Manninen PH, Diamond C: The effects of cimetidine and ranitidine with and without metoclopramide on gastric volume and pH in morbidly obese patients, *Can J Anaesth* 33:773-779, 1986.
164. Stoelting RK: Gastric fluid pH in patients receiving cimetidine, *Anesth Analg* 57:675-677, 1978.
165. Goudsouzian N, Cote CJ, Liu LM, Dedrick DF: The dose-response effects of oral cimetidine on gastric pH and volume in children, *Anesthesiology* 55:533-536, 1981.
166. Tatekawa S, Yukioka H, Fujimori M, et al: Comparison of effects of intravenous versus intramuscular famotidine on pH and volume of gastric juice, *Masui* 39:1619-1625, 1990.
167. Gardner JD, Ciociola AA, Robinson M, McIsaac RL: Determination of the time of onset of action of ranitidine and famotidine on intra-gastric acidity, *Aliment Pharmacol Ther* 16:1317-1326, 2002.
168. Manchikanti L, Colliver JA, Grow JB, et al: Dose-response effects of intravenous ranitidine on gastric pH and volume in outpatients, *Anesthesiology* 65:180-185, 1986.
169. Manchikanti L, Colliver JA, Marrero TC, Roush JR: Ranitidine and metoclopramide for prophylaxis of aspiration pneumonitis in elective surgery, *Anesth Analg* 63:903-910, 1984.
170. Escolano F, Sierra P, Ortiz JC, Cabrera JC, Castano J: The efficacy and optimum time of administration of ranitidine in the prevention of the acid aspiration syndrom, *Anaesthesia* 51: 182-184, 1996.
171. Haskins DA, Jahr JS, Texidor M, Ramadhyani U: Single-dose oral omeprazole for reduction of gastric residual acidity in adults for outpatient surgery, *Acta Anaesthesiol Scand* 36:513-515, 1992.
172. Gin T, Ewart MC, Yau G, Oh TE: Effect of oral omeprazole on intragastric pH and volume in women undergoing elective caesarean section, *Br J Anaesth* 65:616-619, 1990.
173. Ewart MC, Yau G, Gin T, Kotur CF, Oh TE: A comparison of the effects of omeprazole and ranitidine on gastric secretion in women undergoing elective caesarean section, *Anaesthesia* 45:527-530, 1990.
174. Atanassoff PG, Alon E, Pasch T: Effects of single-dose intravenous omeprazole and ranitidine on gastric pH during general anesthesia, *Anesth Analg* 75:95-98, 1992.
175. Escolano F, Castano J, Lopez R, Bisbe E, Alcon A: Effects of omeprazole, ranitidine, famotidine and placebo on gastric secretion in patients undergoing elective surgery, *Br J Anaesth* 69:404-406, 1992.
176. Nishina K, Mikawa K, Takao Y, Shiga M, Maekawa N, Obara H: A comparison of rabeprazole, lansoprazole, and ranitidine for improving preoperative gastric fluid property in adults undergoing elective surgery, *Anesth Analg* 90:717-721, 2000.
177. Memis D, Turan A, Karamanlioglu B, Saral P, Ture M, Pamukcu Z: The effect of intravenous pantoprazole and ranitidine for improving preoperative gastric fluid properties in adults undergoing elective surgery, *Anesth Analg* 97:1360-1363, 2003.
178. Nagelhout JJ, Boytim MJ: Pharmacologic rationale for anesthetic agents in ambulatory practice, *J Peri Anesth Nurs* 16: 371-378, 2001.
179. Chikungwa M, Smith I: Controversial issues in ambulatory anesthesia, *Anesthesiol Clin North Am* 21:313-327, 2003.
180. Liu J, Singh H, White PF: Electroencephalographic bispectral index correlates with intraoperative recall and depth of propofol-induced sedation, *Anesth Analg* 84:185-189, 1997.

181. Anez C, Papaceit J, Sala JM, Fuentes A, Rull M: The effect of encephalogram bispectral index monitoring during total intravenous anesthesia with propofol in outpatient surgery, *Rev Esp Anestesiol Reanim* 48:264-269, 2001.
182. Song D, Joshi GP, White PF: Titration of volatile anesthetics using bispectral index facilitates recovery after ambulatory anesthesia, *Anesthesiology* 87:842-848, 1997.
183. Pavlin DJ, Hong JY, Freund PR, Koerschgen ME, Bower JO, Bowdle TA: The effect of bispectral index monitoring on end-tidal gas concentration and recovery duration after outpatient anesthesia, *Anesth Analg* 93:613-619, 2001.
184. Nelskyla KA, Yli-Hankala AM, Puro PH, Korttila KT: Sevoflurane titration using bispectral index decreases postoperative vomiting in phase II recovery after ambulatory surgery, *Anesth Analg* 93:1165-1169, 2001.
185. Tomlin PJ, Howarth FH, Robinson JS: Postoperative atelectasis and laryngeal incompetence, *Lancet* 1:1402-1405, 1968.
186. Kurer FL, Welsh DB: Gynaecological laparoscopy: clinical experiences of two anaesthetic techniques, *Br J Anaesth* 56:1207-1212, 1984.
187. Litman RS, Keon TP: Postintubation croup in children, *Anesthesiology* 75:1122-1123, 1991.
188. Marley RA: Postextubation laryngeal edema: a review with consideration for home discharge, *J Perianesth Nurs* 13:39-53, 1998.
189. Macario A, Chang PC, Stempel DB, Brock-Utne JG: A cost analysis of the laryngeal mask airway for elective surgery in adult outpatients, *Anesthesiology* 83:250-257, 1995.
190. Cork RC, Depa RM, Standen JR: Prospective comparison of use of the laryngeal mask and endotracheal tube for ambulatory surgery, *Anesth Analg* 79:719-727, 1994.
191. Joshi GP, Inagaki Y, White PF, et al: Use of the laryngeal mask airway as an alternative to the tracheal tube during ambulatory anesthesia, *Anesth Analg* 85:573-577, 1997.
192. Keane PW, Murray PF: Intravenous fluids in minor surgery: their effect on recovery from anaesthesia, *Anaesthesia* 41:635-637, 1986.
193. Cook R, Anderson S, Riseborough M, Blogg CE: Intravenous fluid load and recovery: a double-blind comparison in gynaecological patients who had day-case laparoscopy, *Anaesthesia* 45:826-830, 1990.
194. Yogendran S, Asokumar B, Cheng DC, Chung F: A prospective randomized double-blinded study of the effect of intravenous fluid therapy on adverse outcomes on outpatient surgery, *Anesth Analg* 80:682-686, 1995.
195. Chow MY, Sia AT, Koay CK, Chan YW: Alkalinization of lidocaine does not hasten the onset of axillary brachial plexus block, *Anesth Analg* 86:566-8, 1998.
196. Candido KD, Winnie AP, Covino BG, et al: Addition of bicarbonate to plain bupivacaine does not significantly alter the onset or duration of plexus anesthesia, *Reg Anesth* 20:133-138, 1995.
197. Tetzlaff JE, Yoon HJ, O'Hara J, Reaney J, Stein D, Grimes-Rice M: Alkalinization of mepivacaine accelerates onset of interscalene block for shoulder surgery, *Reg Anesth* 15:242-244, 1990.
198. Quinlan JJ, Oleksey K, Murphy FL: Alkalinization of mepivacaine for axillary block, *Anesth Analg* 74:371-374, 1992.
199. Mulroy MF: Regional anesthesia for adult outpatients. In White PF, editor: *Outpatient Anesthesia*, New York, 1990, Churchill Livingstone, pp 293-311.
200. Klein S, Pietrobon R, Nielsen KC, et al: Peripheral nerve blockade with long-acting local anesthetics: a survey of The Society for Ambulatory Anesthesia, *Anesth Analg* 94:71-76, 2002.
201. Bridenbaugh LD, Mulroy MF: Neural blockade for outpatients. In Cousins MJ, Bridenbaugh PO, editors: *Neural Blockade in Clinical Anesthesia and Management of Pain*, ed 3, Philadelphia, 1998, Lippincott, pp 605-614.
202. Philip BK: Regional anaesthesia for ambulatory surgery, *Can J Anaesth* 39:R3-R6, 1992.
203. Allen GD: Outpatient anesthesia. In Waugaman WR, Foster SD, Rigor BM, editors: *Principles and Practice of Nurse Anesthesia*, ed 2, Norwalk, CT, 1992, Appleton & Lange, pp 591-600.
204. D'Alessio JG, Rosenblum M, Shea KP, Freitas DG: A retrospective comparison of interscalene block and general anesthesia for ambulatory surgery shoulder arthroscopy, *Reg Anesth* 20:62-68, 1995.
205. Brown AR, Weiss R, Greenberg C, Flatow EL, Bigliani LU: Interscalene block for shoulder arthroscopy: comparison with general anesthesia, *Arthroscopy* 9:295-300, 1993.
206. Davis WJ, Lennon RL, Wedel DJ: Brachial plexus anesthesia for outpatient surgical procedures on an upper extremity, *Mayo Clin Proc* 66:470-473, 1991.
207. Philip BK, Covino BG: Local and regional anesthesia. In Wetchler BV, editor: *Anesthesia for Ambulatory Surgery*, ed 2, Philadelphia, 1991, Lippincott, pp 309-374.
208. Wolf AR, Valley RD, Fear DW, Roy WL, Lerman J: Bupivacaine for caudal analgesia in infants and children: the optimal effective concentration, *Anesthesiology* 69:102-106, 1988.
209. Jamali S, Monin S, Gegon C, Dubousset AM, Ecoffey C: Clonidine in pediatric caudal anesthesia, *Anesth Analg* 78: 663-666, 1994.
210. May AE, Wandless J, James RH: Analgesia for circumcision in children: a comparison of caudal bupivacaine and intramuscular buprenorphine, *Acta Anaesthesiol Scand* 26:331-333, 1982.
211. Splinter WM, Reid CW, Roberts DJ, Bass J: Reducing pain after inguinal hernia repair in children, *Anesthesiology* 87:542-546, 1997.
212. Splinter WM, Bass J, Komocar L: Regional anaesthesia for hernia repair in children: local vs. caudal anaesthesia, *Can J Anaesth* 42:197-200, 1995.
213. Chilvers CR, Kinahan A, Vaghadia H, Merrick PM: Pharmacoeconomics of intravenous regional anaesthesia vs. general anaesthesia for outpatient hand surgery, *Can J Anaesth* 44:1152-1156, 1997.
214. Olney BW, Lugg PC, turner PL, Eyres RL, Cole WG: Outpatient treatment of upper extremity injuries in childhood using intravenous regional anaesthesia, *J Pediatr Orthop* 8:576-579, 1988.
215. Nakamura SJ, Conte-Hernandez A, Galloway MT: The efficacy of regional anesthesia for outpatient anterior cruciate ligament reconstruction, *Arthroscopy* 13:699-703, 1997.
216. Patel NJ, Flashburg MH, Paskin S, Grossman R: A regional anesthetic technique compared to general anesthesia for outpatient knee arthroscopy, *Anesth Analg* 65:185-187, 1986.
217. Goranson BD, Lang S, Cassidy JD, Dust WN, McKerrell J: A comparison of three regional anaesthesia techniques for outpatient knee arthroscopy, *Can J Anaesth* 44:371-376, 1997.
218. Vloka JD, Hadzic A, Mulcare R, Lesser JB, Kitain E, Thys DM: Femoral and genitofemoral nerve blocks versus spinal anesthesia for outpatients undergoing saphenous vein stripping surgery, *Anesth Analg* 84:749-752, 1997.
219. Williams BA, Kentor ML, Vogt MT, et al: Femoral-sciatic nerve blocks for complex outpatient knee surgery are associated with less postoperative pain before same-day discharge: a review of 1,200 consecutive cases from the period 1996-1999, *Anesthesiology* 98:1206-13, 2003.
220. Nakamura SJ, Conte-Hernandez A, Galloway MT: The efficacy of regional anesthesia for outpatient anterior cruciate ligament reconstruction, *Arthroscopy* 13:699-703, 1997.
221. Klein SM, Nielsen KC, Greengrass RA, Warner DS, Martin A, Steele SM: Ambulatory discharge after long-acting peripheral nerve blockade: 2382 blocks with ropivacaine, *Anesth Analg* 94:65-70, 2002.
222. Felts JA: Outpatient anesthesia in the geriatric patient, *Clin Anesthesiol* 4:1025-1034, 1986.
223. Vaghadia H, McLeod DH, Mitchell GW, Merrick PM, Chilvers CR: Small-dose hypobaric lidocaine-fentanyl spinal anesthesia for short duration outpatient laparoscopy. I. A randomized comparison with conventional dose hyperbaric lidocaine, *Anesth Analg* 84:59-64, 1997.
224. Chilvers CR, Vaghadia H, Mitchell GW, Merrick PM: Small-dose hypobaric lidocaine-fentanyl spinal anesthesia for short duration outpatient laparoscopy. II. Optimal fentanyl dose, *Anesth Analg* 84:65-70, 1997.

225. Pollock JE, Mulroy MF, Bent E, Polissar NL: A comparison of two regional anesthetic techniques for outpatient knee arthroscopy, *Anesth Analg* 97:397-401, 2003.
226. Kokki H, Tuovinen K, Hendolin H: Spinal anaesthesia for paediatric day-case surgery: a double-blind, randomized, parallel group, prospective comparison of isobaric and hyperbaric bupivacaine, *Br J Anaesth* 81:502-506, 1998.
227. Tarkkila P, Huhtala J, Tuominen M: Home-readiness after spinal anaesthesia with small doses of hyperbaric 0.5% bupivacaine, *Anaesthesia* 52:1157-1160, 1997.
228. Moore JM, Liu SS, Pollock JE, Neal JM, Knab JH: The effect of epinephrine on small-dose hyperbaric bupivacaine spinal anesthesia: clinical implications for ambulatory surgery, *Anesth Analg* 86:973-977, 1998.
229. Ben-David B, Solomon E, Levin H, Admoni H, Golkik Z: Spinal bupivacaine in ambulatory surgery: the effect of saline dilution, *Anesth Analg* 83:716-720, 1996.
230. Ben-David B, Solomon E, Levin H, Admoni H, Goldik Z: Intrathecal fentanyl with small-dose dilute bupivacaine: better anesthesia without prolonging recovery, *Anesth Analg* 85(3):560-565, 1997.
231. Liu SS: Optimizing spinal anesthesia for ambulatory surgery, *Reg Anesth* 22:500-510, 1997.
232. Korhonen AM, Valanne JV, Jokela RM, Ravaska P, Korttila K: Intrathecal hyperbaric bupivacaine 3 mg + fentanyl 10 microg for outpatient knee arthroscopy with tourniquet, *Acta Anaesthesiol Scand* 47:342-346, 2003.
233. Gupta A, Axelsson K, Thorn SE, et al: Low-dose bupivacaine plus fentanyl for spinal anesthesia during ambulatory inguinal herniorrhaphy: a comparison between 6 mg and 7. 5 mg of bupivacaine, *Acta Anaesthesiol Scand* 47:13-19, 2003.
234. Buckenmaier CC III, Nielsen KC, Pietrobon R, et al: Small-dose intrathecal lidocaine versus ropivacaine for anorectal surgery in an ambulatory setting, *Anesth Analg* 95:1253-1257, 2002.
235. Ben-David B, Maryanovsky M, Gurevitch A, et al: A comparison of minidose lidocaine-fentanyl and conventional-dose lidocaine spinal anesthesia, *Anesth Analg* 91:865-870, 2000.
236. Ben-David B, DeMeo PJ, Lucyk C, Solosko D: A comparison of minidose lidocaine-fentanyl spinal anesthesia and local anesthesia/propofol infusion for outpatient knee arthroscopy, *Anesth Analg* 93:319-325, 2001.
237. Urmey WF: Spinal anaesthesia for outpatient surgery, *Best Pract Res Clin Anaesthesiol* 17:335-346, 2003.
238. Vaghadia H: Spinal anaesthesia for outpatients: controversies and new techniques, *Can J Anaesth* 45:R64-R70, 1998.
239. Mulroy MF: Extending indications for spinal anesthesia, *Reg Anesth Pain Med* 23:380-383, 1998.
240. Carbaat PA, van Crevel H: Lumbar puncture headache: controlled study on the preventive effect of 24 hours' bed rest, *Lancet* 2:1133-1135, 1981.
241. Sime AC: Transient neurologic symptoms and spinal anesthesia, *AANA J* 68:163-168, 2000.
242. Gold MS, Reichling DB, Hampl KF, Drasner K, Levine JD: Lidocaine toxicity in primary afferent neurons from the rat, *J Pharmacol Exp Ther* 285:413-421, 1998.
243. Hampl KF, Keinzmann-Widmer S, Luginbuehl I, et al: Transient neurologic symptoms after spinal anesthesia: a lower incidence with prilocaine and bupivacaine than with lidocaine, *Anesthesiology* 88:629-633, 1998.
244. Freedman JM, Li DK, Drasner K, Jaskela MC, Larsen B, Wi S: Transient neurologic symptoms after spinal anesthesia: an epidemiologic study of 1,863 patients, *Anesthesiology* 89:633-641, 1998.
245. Liguori GA, Zayas VM, Chisholm MF: Transient neurologic symptoms after spinal anesthesia with mepivacaine and lidocaine, *Anesthesiology* 88:619-623, 1998.
246. Hodgson PS, Liu SS, Batra MS, Gras TW, Pollock JE, Neal JM: Procaine compared with lidocaine for incidence of transient neurologic symptoms, *Reg Anesth Pain Med* 25:218-222, 2000.
247. Mulroy MF, Larkin KL, Hodgson PS, Helman JD, Pollock JE, Liu SS: A comparison of spinal, epidural, and general anesthesia for outpatient knee arthroscopy, *Anesth Analg* 91:860-864, 2000.
248. Harris AP: Spinal anesthesia: it works, *Anesthesiol Rep* 3:56, 1990.
249. Bridenbaugh LD: Catheterization after long- and short-acting local anesthetics for continuous caudal block for vaginal delivery, *Anesthesiology* 46:357-359, 1977.
250. Ben-David B, Levin H, Solomon E, Admoni H, Vaida S: Spinal bupivacaine in ambulatory surgery: the effect of saline dilution, *Anesth Analg* 83:716-720, 1996.
251. Kamphuis ET, Ionescu TI, Kuipers PW, et al: Recovery of storage and emptying functions of the urinary bladder after spinal anesthesia with lidocaine and with bupivacaine in men, *Anesthesiology* 88:310-316, 1998.
252. Frey K, Holman S, Mikat-Stevens M, et al: The recovery profile of hyperbaric spinal anesthesia with lidocaine, tetracaine, and bupivacaine, *Reg Anesth Pain Med* 23:159-163, 1998.
253. Kito Km, Kato H, Shibata M, Adachi T, Nakao S, Mori K: The effect of varied doses of epinephrine on duration of lidocaine spinal anesthesia in the thoracic and lumbosacral dermatomes, *Anesth Analg* 86:1018-1022, 1998.
254. Breebaart MB, Vercauteren MP, Hoffmann VL, Adriaensen HA: Urinary bladder scanning after day-case arthroscopy under spinal anaesthesia: comparison between lidocaine, ropivacaine, and levobupivacaine, *Br J Anaesth* 90:309-313, 2003.
255. Mulroy MF, Salinas FV, Larkin KL, Polissar NL: Ambulatory surgery patients may be discharged before voiding after short-acting spinal and epidural anesthesia, *Anesthesiology* 97: 315-319, 2002.
256. Urquhart ML, White PF: Comparison of sedative infusions during regional anesthesia: methohexital, etomidate, and midazolam, *Anesth Analg* 68:249-254, 1989.
257. Tucker MR, Ochs MW, White RP: Arterial blood gas levels after midazolam or diazepam administered with or without fentanyl as an intravenous sedative for outpatient surgical procedures, *J Oral Maxillofac Surg* 44:688-692, 1986.
258. Ramirez-Ruiz M, Newson CD, White PF: Monitored anesthesia care: use of ketorolac, dezocine, and fentanyl, *Anesthesiology* 77:A27, 1992.
259. White PF, Negus JB: Sedative infusions during local and regional anesthesia: a comparison of midazolam and propofol, *J Clin Anesth* 3:32-39, 1991.
260. Church JA, Stanton PD, Kenny GN, Anderson JR: Propofol for sedation during endoscopy: assessment of a computer-controlled infusion system, *Gastrointest Endosc* 37:175-179, 1991.
261. Patterson KW, Casey PB, Murray JP, O'Boyle CA, Cunningham AJ: Propofol sedation for outpatient upper gastrointestinal endoscopy: comparison with midazolam, *Br J Anaesth* 67:108-111, 1991.
262. White PF: Ambulatory anesthesia—fast tracking concepts. IARS 1998 Review Course Lectures, *Anesth Analg* March(suppl): 153-156, 1998.
263. Song D, Joshi GP, White PF: Fast-track eligibility after ambulatory anesthesia: a comparison of desflurane, sevoflurane, and propofol, *Anesth Analg* 86:267-273, 1998.
264. Gan TJ, Glass PS, Windsor A, et al and the BIS Utility Study Group: Bispectral index monitoring allows faster emergence and improved recovery from propofol, alfentanil, and nitrous oxide anesthesia, *Anesthesiology* 87:808-815, 1997.
265. Song D, van Vlymen J, White PF: Is the bispectral index useful in predicting fast-track eligibility after ambulatory anesthesia with propofol and desflurane? *Anesth Analg* 87:1245-1248, 1998.
266. Apfelbaum JL: Bypassing PACU: a cost effective measure, *Can J Anaesth* 45:R91-R92, 1998.
267. Duncan PG, Shandro J, Bachand R, Ainsworth L: A pilot study of recovery room bypass ("fast-track protocol") in a community hospital, *Can J Anaesth* 48:630-636, 2001.

268. Macario A, Glenn D, Dexter F: What can the PACU manager do to decrease cost in the PACU? *J Perianesth Nurs* 14(5): 284-293, 1999.
269. Williams BA, Kentor ML, Williams JP, et al: PACU bypass after outpatient knee surgery is associated with fewer unplanned hospital admissions but more phase II nursing interventions, *Anesthesiology* 97:981-988, 2002.
270. Watkins AC, White PF: Fast-tracking after ambulatory surgery, *J PeriAnesth Nurs* 16:379-387, 2001.
271. Warner MA, Shields SE, Chute CG: Major morbidity and mortality within 1 month of ambulatory surgery and anesthesia, *JAMA* 270:1437-1441, 1993.
272. Chung F, Mezei G: Adverse outcomes in ambulatory anesthesia, *Can J Anesth* 46:R18-R26, 1999.
273. Patel RI, Hannallah RS: Complications following pediatric ambulatory surgery—less of the same? *Anesthesiology* 79:A223, 1993.
274. Osborne GA, Rudkin GE: Outcome after day-care surgery in a major teaching hospital, *Anaesth Intensive Care* 21:822-827, 1993.
275. Cardosa M, Rudkin GE, Osborne GA: Outcome from day-case knee arthroscopy in a major teaching hospital, *Arthroscopy* 10:624-629, 1994.
276. Cade L, Kakulas P: Ketorolac or pethidine for analgesia after elective laparoscopic sterilization, *Anaesth Intensive Care* 23:158-161, 1995.
277. Rudkin GE, Osborne GA, Doyle CE: Assessment and selection of patients for day surgery in a public hospital, *Med J Aust* 158:308-312, 1993.
278. Chung F: Recovery pattern and home-readiness after ambulatory surgery, *Anesth Analg* 80:896-902, 1995.
279. Brooks DC: A prospective comparison of laparoscopic and tension-free open herniorrhaphy, *Arch Surg* 129:361-366, 1994.
280. Helmus C, Grin M, Westfall R: Same-day-stay head and neck surgery, *Laryngoscope* 102:1331-1334, 1992.
281. Fortier J, Chung F, Su J: Unanticipated admission after ambulatory surgery—a prospective study, *Can J Anaesth* 45:612-619, 1998.
282. Fancourt-Smith PF, Hornstein J, Jenkins LC: Hospital admissions from the surgical day care centre of Vancouver General Hospital 1977-1987, *Can J Anaesth* 37:699-704, 1990.
283. Chye EP, Young IG, Osborne GA, Rudkin GE: Outcome after same-day oral surgery: a review of 1,180 cases at a major teaching hospital, *J Oral Maxillofac Surg* 51:846-849, 1993.
284. Biswas TK, Leary C: Postoperative hospital admission from a day surgery unit: a seven-year retrospective survey, *Anaesth Intensive Care* 20:147-150, 1992.
285. Meeks GR, Waller GA, Meydrech EF, Flautt FH Jr: Unscheduled hospital admission following ambulatory gynecologic surgery, *Obstet Gynecol* 80:446-450, 1992.
286. Green G, Jonsson L: Nausea: the most important factor determining length of stay after ambulatory anaesthesia: a comparative study of isoflurane and/or propofol techniques, *Acta Anaesthesiol Scand* 37:742-746, 1993.
287. Westman HR: Postoperative complications and unanticipated hospital admissions, *Semin Pediatr Surg* 8:23-29, 1999.
288. Forrest JB, Cahalan MK, Rehder K, et al: Multicenter study of general anesthesia. II. Results, *Anesthesiology* 72:262-268, 1990.
289. Larsson S, Lundberg D: A prospective survey of postoperative nausea and vomiting with special regard to incidence and relations to patient characteristics, anesthetic routines and surgical procedures, *Acta Anaesthesiol Scand* 39:539-545, 1995.
290. Karlsson E, Larsson LE, Nilsson K: Postanesthetic nausea in children, *Acta Anaesthesiol Scand* 34:515-518, 1990.
291. Cohen MM, Cameron CB, Duncan PG: Pediatric anesthesia morbidity and mortality in the perioperative period, *Anesth Analg* 70:160-167, 1990.
292. Kotiniemi LH, Ryhanen PT, Valanne J, Jokela R, Mustonen A, Poukkul E: Postoperative symptoms at home following day-case surgery in children: a multicentre survey of 551 children, *Anaesthesia* 52:963-969, 1997.
293. Marley RA: Postoperative nausea and vomiting: the outpatient enigma, *J Perianesth Nurs* 11:147-161, 1996.
294. Norred CL: Antiemetic prophylaxis: pharmacology and therapeutics, *AANA J* 71:133-140, 2003.
295. Cameron D, Gan FJ: Management of postoperative nausea and vomiting in ambulatory surgery, *Anesthesiol Clin North Am* 21:347-365, 2003.
296. Muir JJ, Warner MA, Offord KP, Buck CF, Harper JV, Kunkel SE: Role of nitrous oxide and other factors in postoperative nausea and vomiting: a randomized and blinded prospective study, *Anesthesiology* 66:513-518, 1987.
297. Purkis IE: Factors that influence postoperative vomiting, *Can Anaesth Soc J* 11:335-353, 1964.
298. Bellville JW, Bross IDJ, Howland WS: Postoperative nausea and vomiting IV: factors related to postoperative nausea and vomiting, *Anesthesiology* 21:186-193, 1960.
299. Lerman J: Surgical and patient factors involved in postoperative nausea and vomiting, *Br J Anaesth* 69(suppl):24S-32S, 1992.
300. Rowley MP, Brown TC: Postoperative vomiting in children, *Anaesth Intensive Care* 10:309-313, 1982.
301. Sinclair DR, Chung F, Mezei G: Can postoperative nausea and vomiting be predicted? *Anesthesiology* 91:109-118, 1999.
302. Quinn AC, Brown JH, Wallace PG, Asbury AJ: Studies in postoperative sequelae: Nausea and vomiting—still a problem, *Anaesthesia* 49:62-65, 1994.
303. Eger EI II: Nitrous oxide transfer to closed gas spaces. In *Anesthetic Uptake and Action*, Baltimore, MD, 1974, Williams & Wilkins, pp 171-183.
304. Foldes FF, Kepes ER, Ship AG: Severe gastrointestinal distention during nitrous oxide and oxygen anesthesia, *JAMA* 194:1146-1148, 1965.
305. Ong BY, Palahniuk RJ, Cumming M: Gastric volume and pH in out-patients, *Can Anaesth Soc J* 25:36-39, 1978.
306. White PF, Shafer A: Nausea and vomiting: causes and prophylaxis, *Semin Anesth* 6:300-308, 1987.
307. Watcha MF, White PF: Postoperative nausea and vomiting: its etiology, treatment, and prevention, *Anesthesiology* 77:162-184, 1992.
308. Read NW, Houghton LA: Physiology of gastric emptying and pathophysiology of gastroparesis, *Gastroenterol Clin North Am* 18:359-373, 1989.
309. Varis K: Diabetic gastroparesis, *Scand J Gastroenterol* 24:897-903, 1989.
310. Kovac AL, Scuderi PE, Boerner TF, et al and Dolasetron Mesylate PONV Treatment Study Group: Treatment of postoperative nausea and vomiting with single intravenous does of dolasetron mesylate: a multicenter trial, *Anesth Analg* 85: 546-552, 1997.
311. Cohen MM, Duncan PG, DeBoer DP, Tweed WA: The postoperative interview: assessing risk factors for nausea and vomiting, *Anesth Analg* 78:7-16, 1994.
312. Beattie WS, Lindblad T, Buckley DN, Forrest JB: The incidence of postoperative nausea and vomiting in women undergoing laparoscopy is influenced by the day of menstrual cycle, *Can J Anaesth* 38:298-302, 1991.
313. Fujii Y, Toyooka H, Tanaka H: Prevention of postoperative nausea and vomiting in female patients during menstruation: comparison of droperidol, metoclopramide and granisetron, *Br J Anaesth* 80:248-249, 1998.
314. Mollhoff T, Burgard G, Prien T: Propofol reduces the incidence of postoperative nausea and vomiting after gynecological laparoscopy, *Anesthesiology* 83:A37, 1995.
315. Honkavaara P, Lehtinen AM, Hovorka J, Korttila K: Nausea and vomiting after gynaecological laparoscopy depends upon the phase of the menstrual cycle, *Can J Anaesth* 38:876-879, 1991.
316. Beattie WS, Lindblad T, Buckley DN, Forrest JB: Menstruation increases the risk of nausea and vomiting after laparoscopy. A prospective randomized study, *Anesthesiology* 78:272-276, 1993.

317. Kamath B, Curran J, Hawkey C, et al: Anaesthesia, movement and emesis, *Br J Anaesth* 64:728-730, 1990.
318. Korttila K, Hovorka J, Erkola O: Nitrous oxide does not increase the incidence of nausea and vomiting after isoflurane anesthesia, *Anesth Analg* 66:761-765, 1987.
319. Bodman RI, Morton HJV, Thomas ET: Vomiting by outpatients after nitrous oxide anaesthesia, *BMJ* 30:1327-1330, 1960.
320. Riding JE: The prevention of postoperative vomiting, *Br J Anaesth* 35:180-188, 1963.
321. Jensen S, Wetchler BV: The obese patient: an acceptable candidate for outpatient anesthesia, *AANA J* 50:369-371, 1982.
322. Vaughan RW, Bauer S, Wise L: Volume and pH of gastric juice in obese patients, *Anesthesiology* 43:686-689, 1975.
323. Apfel CC, Roewer N: Risk factors for nausea and vomiting after general anesthesia: fictions and facts, *Anaesthesist* 49:629-642, 2000.
324. Chimbira W, Sweeney BP: The effect of smoking on postoperative nausea and vomiting, *Anaesthesia* 55:540-544, 2000.
325. Stadler M, Bardiau F, Seidel L, Albert A, Boogaerts JG: Difference in risk factors for postoperative nausea and vomiting, *Anesthesiology* 98:46-52, 2003.
326. Palazzo MGA, Strunin L: Anaesthesia and emesis. I. Etiology, *Can J Anaesth* 31:178-187, 1984.
327. Dering A, Dill-Russell P: Should all day-case anaesthesia patients be given prophylactic antiemetics? *Hosp Med* 65:125, 2004.
328. Ahlgren EW, Bennett EJ, Stephen CR: Outpatient pediatric anaesthesiology: a case series, *Anesth Analg* 50:402-408, 1971.
329. Hardy JF, Charest J, Girouard G, Lepage Y: Nausea and vomiting after strabismus surgery in preschool children, *Can J Anaesth* 33:57-62, 1986.
330. Pandit SK, Kothary SP: Intravenous narcotics for premedication in outpatient anaesthesia, *Acta Anaesthesiol Scand* 33:353-358, 1989.
331. Gerwels JW, Bezzant JL, Le Maire L, Pauley LF, Streisand JB: Oral transmucosal fentanyl citrate premedication in patients undergoing outpatient dermatologic procedures, *J Dermatol Surg Oncol* 20:823-826, 1994.
332. Shafer A, White PF, Urquhart ML, Doze VA: Outpatient premedication: use of midazolam and opioid analgesics, *Anesthesiology* 71:495-501, 1989.
333. Andrews PLR: Physiology of nausea and vomiting, *Br J Anaesth* 69(suppl):2S-19S, 1992.
334. Racke K, Schworer H: Regulation of serotonin release from the intestinal mucosa, *Pharmacol Res* 23:13-25, 1991.
335. Rubin A, Winston J: The role of the vestibular apparatus in the production of nausea and vomiting following the administration of morphine to man, *J Clin Invest* 29:1261-1266, 1950.
336. Hovorka J, Korttila K, Erkola O: The experience of the person ventilating the lungs does influence postoperative nausea and vomiting, *Acta Anaesthesiol Scand* 34:203-205, 1990.
337. de Grood PM, Harbers JB, van Egmond J, Crul JF: Anaesthesia for laparoscopy: a comparison of five techniques including propofol, etomidate, thiopentone and isoflurane, *Anaesthesia* 42:815-823, 1987.
338. Chittleborough MC, Osborne GA, Rudkin GE, Vickers D, Leppard PI, Barlow J: Double-blind comparison of patient recovery after induction with propofol or thiopentone for day-case relaxant general anaesthesia, *Anaesth Intensive Care* 20: 169-173, 1992.
339. Jobalia N, Mathieu A: A meta-analysis of published studies confirms decreased postoperative nausea/vomiting with propofol, *Anesthesiology* 81:A33, 1994 (abstract).
340. Cheng KP, Larson CE, Biglan AW, D'Antonio JA: A prospective, randomized, controlled comparison of retrobulbar and general anesthesia for strabismus surgery, *Ophthalmic Surg* 23:585-590, 1992.
341. Ghouri AF, Bodner M, White PF: Recovery profile after desflurane-nitrous oxide versus isoflurane-nitrous oxide in outpatients, *Anesthesiology* 74:419-424, 1991.
342. Johannesson GP, Floren M, Lindahl SGE: Sevoflurane for ENT-surgery in children: a comparison with halothane, *Acta Anaesthesiol Scand* 39:546-550, 1995.
343. Wrigley SR, Fairfield JE, Jones RM, Black AE: Induction and recovery characteristics of desflurane in day case patients: a comparison with propofol, *Anaesthesia* 46:615-622, 1991.
344. Fredman B, Nathanson MH, Smith I, Wang J, Klein K, White PF: Sevoflurane for outpatient anesthesia: a comparison with propofol, *Anesth Analg* 81:823-828, 1995.
345. Gaskey NJ, Ferriero L, Pournaras L, Seecof J: Use of fentanyl markedly increases nausea and vomiting in gynecological short stay patients, *AANA J* 54:309-311, 1986.
346. Zuurmond WWA, van Leeuwen L: Recovery from sufentanil anaesthesia for outpatient arthroscopy: a comparison with isoflurane, *Acta Anaesthesiol Scand* 31:154-156, 1987.
347. Divatia JV, Vaidya JS, Badwe RA, Hawaldar RW: Omission of nitrous oxide during anesthesia reduces the incidence of postoperative nausea and vomiting: a meta-analysis, *Anesthesiology* 85:1055-1062, 1996.
348. Tramer M, Moore A, McQuay H: Omitting nitrous oxide in general anaesthesia: meta-analysis of intraoperative awareness and postoperative emesis in randomized controlled trials, *Br J Anaesth* 76:186-193, 1996.
349. Tramer M, Moore A, McQuay H: Meta-analytic comparison of prophylactic antiemetic efficacy for postoperative nausea and vomiting: propofol anaesthesia vs omitting nitrous oxide vs total i.v. anaesthesia with propofol, *Br J Anaesth* 78:256-259, 1997.
350. Davis I, Moore JR, Lahiri SK: Nitrous oxide and the middle ear, *Anaesthesia* 34:147-151, 1979.
351. Perreault L, Normandin N, Plamondon L, et al: Middle ear pressure variations during nitrous oxide and oxygen anaesthesia, *Can Anaesth Soc J* 29:428-434, 1982.
352. Gillman MA: Possible mechanisms of action of nitrous oxide at the opioid receptor, *Med Hypotheses* 15:109-114, 1984.
353. Jenkins LC, Hahay D: Central mechanisms of vomiting related to catecholamine response: anaesthetic implications, *Can Anaesth Soc J* 18:434-441, 1971.
354. Andersen R, Krohg K: Pain as a major cause of postoperative nausea and vomiting, *Can J Anaesth* 23:366-369, 1976.
355. Rose DK, Cohen MM, Yee DA: Reducing postoperative nausea and vomiting: what works and what doesn't, *Anesth Analg* 80:S403, 1995 (abstract).
356. Byers GF, Doyle E, Best CJ, Morton NS: Postoperative nausea and vomiting in paediatric surgical inpatients, *Paediatr Anaesth* 5:253-256, 1995.
357. Schreiner MS, Nicolson SC, Martin T, Whitney L: Should children drink before discharge from day surgery? *Anesthesiology* 76:528-533, 1992.
358. Jin F, Norris A, chung F, Ganeshram T: Should adult patients drink fluids before discharge from ambulatory surgery? *Anesth Analg* 87:306-311, 1998.
359. Kearney R, Mack C, Entwistle L: Withholding oral fluids from children undergoing day surgery reduces vomiting, *Paediatr Anaesth* 8:331-336, 1998.
360. Greif R, Laciny S, Rapf B, Hickle RS, Sessler DI: Supplemental oxygen reduces the incidence of postoperative nausea and vomiting, *Anesthesiology* 91:1246-1252, 1999.
361. Goll V, Akca O, Greif R, et al: Ondansetron is no more effective than supplemental intraoperative oxygen for prevention of postoperative nausea and vomiting, *Anesth Analg* 92:112-117, 2001.
362. Purhonen S, Niskanen M, Wustefeld M, Mustonen P, Hynynen M: Supplemental oxygen for prevention of nausea and vomiting after breast surgery, *Br J Anaesth* 91:284-287, 2003.
363. Purhonen S, Turunen M, Ruohoaho UM, Niskanen M, Hynynen M: Supplemental oxygen does not reduce the incidence of postoperative nausea and vomiting after ambulatory gynecologic laparoscopy, *Anesth Analg* 96:91-96, 2003.

364. Fuchs-Buder T, Mencke T: Use of reversal agents in day care procedures (with special reference to postoperative nausea and vomiting), *Eur J Anaesthesiol Suppl* 23:53-59, 2001.
365. Frighetto L, Loewen PS, Dolman J, Marra CA: Cost-effectiveness of prophylactic dolasetron or droperidol vs rescue therapy in the prevention of PONV in ambulatory gynecologic surgery, *Can J Anesth* 46:536-543, 1999.
366. Aasboe V, Raeder JC, Groegaard B: Betamethasone reduces postoperative pain and nausea after ambulatory surgery, *Anesth Analg* 87:319-323, 1998.
367. Rothenberg DM, McCarthy RJ, Peng CC, Normoyle DA: Nausea and vomiting after dexamethasone versus droperidol following outpatient laparoscopy with a propofol-based general anesthetic, *Acta Anaesthesiol Scand* 42:637-642, 1998.
368. Splinter WM, Roberts DJ: Dexamethasone decreases vomiting by children after tonsillectomy, *Anesth Analg* 83:913-916, 1996.
369. Liu K, Hsu CC, Chia YY: Effect of dexamethasone on postoperative emesis and pain, *Br J Anaesth* 80:85-86, 1998.
370. Wang JJ, Ho ST, Lee SC, Liu YC, Liu YH, Liao YC: The prophylactic effect of dexamethasone on postoperative nausea and vomiting in women undergoing thyroidectomy: a comparison of droperidol with saline, *Anesth Analg* 89:200-203, 1999.
371. Thomas R, Jones N: Prospective randomized, double-blind comparative study of dexamethasone, ondansetron, and ondansetron plus dexamethasone as prophylactic antiemetic therapy in patients undergoing day-case gynaecological surgery, *Br J Anaesth* 87:588-592, 2001.
372. Lee Y, Lai HY, Lin PC, Huang SJ, Lin YS: Dexamethasone prevents postoperative nausea and vomiting more effectively in women with motion sickness, *Can J Anaesth* 50:232-237, 2003.
373. Elhakim M, Ali NM, Rashed I, Riad MK, Refat M: Dexamethasone reduces postoperative vomiting and pain after pediatric tonsillectomy, *Can J Anaesth* 50:392-397, 2003.
374. Wattwill M, Thorn WE, Lovqvist A, Wattwil L, Gupta A, Liljegren G: Dexamethasone is as effective as ondansetron for the prevention of postoperative nausea and vomiting following breast surgery, *Acta Anaesthesiol Scand* 47(7):823-827, 2003.
375. Wang JJ, Ho ST, Lee SC, Liu YC, Ho CM: The use of dexamethasone for preventing postoperative nausea and vomiting in females undergoing thyroidectomy: a dose-ranging study, *Anesth Analg* 91:1404-1407, 2000.
376. Huang JC, Shieh JP, Tang CS, Tzeng JI, Chu KS, Wang JJ: Low-dose dexamethasone effectively prevents postoperative nausea and vomiting after ambulatory laparoscopic surgery, *Can J Anaesth* 48:973-977, 2001.
377. Fujii Y, Uemura A: Dexamethasone for the prevention of nausea and vomiting after dilatation and curettage: a randomized controlled trial, *Obstet Gynecol* 99:58-62, 2002.
378. Wang JJ, Ho ST, Uen YH, et al: Small-dose dexamethasone reduces nausea and vomiting after laparoscopic cholecystectomy: a comparison of tropisetron with saline, *Anesth Analg* 95:229-232, 2002.
379. McKenzie R, Tantisira B, Karambelkar DJ, Riley TJ, Abdelhady H: Comparison of ondansetron with ondansetron plus dexamethasone in the prevention of postoperative nausea and vomiting, *Anesth Analg* 79:961-964, 1994.
380. Splinter WM, Rhine EJ: Low-dose ondansetron with dexamethasone more effectively decreases vomiting after strabismus surgery in children than does high-dose ondansetron, *Anesthesiology* 88:72-75, 1998.
381. Fujii Y, Tanaka H, Toyooka H: The effects of dexamethasone on antiemetics in female patients undergoing gynecologic surgery, *Anesth Analg* 85:913-917, 1997.
382. Elhakim M, Nafie M, Mahmoud K, Atef A: Dexamethasone 8 mg in combination with ondansetron 4 mg appears to be the optimal dose for the prevention of nausea and vomiting after laparoscopic cholecystectomy, *Can J Anaesth* 49:922-926, 2002.
383. Biswas BN, Rudra A: Comparison of granisetron and granisetron plus dexamethasone for the prevention of postoperative nausea and vomiting after laparoscopic cholecystectomy, *Acta Anaesthesiol Scand* 47:79-83, 2003.
384. Piper SN, Triem JG, Rohm KD, Kranke P, Maleck WH, Boldt J: Prevention of post-operative nausea and vomiting: randomised comparison of dolasetron versus dolasetron plus dexamethasone, *Anaesthesist* 52:120-126, 2003.
385. Fujii Y, Tanaka H: Granisetron versus granisetron/dexamethasone combination for treatment of nausea, retching, and vomiting after major gynecologic surgery: a randomized, double-blind study, *Clin Ther* 25:507-514, 2003.
386. Wang JJ, Ho ST, Tzeng JI, Tang CS: The effect of timing of dexamethasone administration on its efficacy as a prophylactic antiemetic for postoperative nausea and vomiting, *Anesth Analg* 91:136-139, 2000.
387. Coloma M, Duffy LL, White PF, Kendall Tongier W, Huber PJ Jr: Dexamethasone facilitates discharge after outpatient anorectal surgery, *Anesth Analg* 92:85-88, 2001.
388. Coloma M, White PF, Markowitz SD, et al: Dexamethasone in combination with dolasetron for prophylaxis in the ambulatory setting: effect on outcome after laparoscopic cholecystectomy, *Anesthesiology* 96:1346-1350, 2002.
389. Steward DL, Welge JA, Myer CM: Steroids for improving recovery following tonsillectomy in children, *Cochrane Database Syst Rev* 1:CD003997, 2003.
390. Graczyk SG, McKenzie R, Kallar S, et al: Intravenous dolasetron for the prevention of postoperative nausea and vomiting after outpatient laparoscopic gynecologic surgery, *Anesth Analg* 84:325-330, 1997.
391. Korttila K, Clergue F, Leeser J, et al: Intravenous dolasetron and ondansetron in prevention of postoperative nausea and vomiting: a multicenter, double-blind, placebo-controlled study, *Acta Anaesthesiol Scand* 41:914-922, 1997.
392. Philip BK, Pearman MH, Kovac AL, et al: Dolasetron for the prevention of postoperative nausea and vomiting following outpatient surgery with general anaesthesia: a randomized, placebo-controlled study. The Dolasetron PONV Prevention Study Group, *Eur J Anaesthesiol* 17(1):23-32, 2000.
393. Philip BK, McLeskey CH, Chelly JE, et al: Pooled analysis of three large clinical trials to determine the optimal dose of dolasetron mesylate needed to prevent postoperative nausea and vomiting. The Dolasetron Prophylaxis Study Group, *J Clin Anesth* 12(1):1-8, 2000.
394. Walker JB: Efficacy of single-dose intravenous dolasetron versus ondansetron in the prevention of postoperative nausea and vomiting, *Clin Ther* 23:932-938, 2001.
395. Valanne J, Korttila K: Effect of a small dose of droperidol on nausea, vomiting and recovery after outpatient enflurane anaesthesia, *Acta Anaesthesiol Scand* 29:359-362, 1985.
396. Lee Y, Lai HY, Lin PC, Lin YS, Huang SJ, Shyr MH: A dose ranging study of dexamethasone for preventing patient-controlled analgesia-related nausea and vomiting: a comparison of droperidol with saline, *Anesth Analg* 98:1066-1071, 2004.
397. Young D: FDA advisory panel discusses droperidol concerns, *Am J Health Syst Pharm* 61:219-220, 2004.
398. Rothenberg DM, Parnass SM, Litwack K, McCarthy RJ, Newman LM: Efficacy of ephedrine in the prevention of postoperative nausea and vomiting, *Anesth Analg* 72:58-61, 1991.
399. Hagemann E, Halvorsen A, Holgersen O, Tveit T, Raeder JC: Intramuscular ephedrine reduces emesis during the first three hours after abdominal hysterectomy, *Acta Anaesthesiol Scand* 44:107-111, 2000.
400. Wetchler BV: Management of nausea and vomiting in the ambulatory surgical patient, *Soc Ambulatory Anesth Newslett* 3:2-3, 1988.
401. Heyman HJ, Salem MR, Joseph NJ: Does gastric suction enhance the efficacy of droperidol prophylaxis of post-operative nausea and vomiting? *Anesthesiology* 73:A19, 1990.
402. Hovorka J, Korttila K, Erkola O: Gastric aspiration at the end of anaesthesia does not decrease postoperative nausea and vomiting, *Anaesth Intensive Care* 18:58-61, 1990.

403. Isabel L, Trepanier CA: Does gastric aspiration reduce postoperative nausea and vomiting in outpatients? *Can J Anaesth* 38:A42, 1991.
404. Albibi R, McCallum RW: Metoclopramide: pharmacology and clinical application, *Ann Intern Med* 98:86-95, 1983.
405. Henzi I, Walder B, Tramer MR: Metoclopramide in the prevention of postoperative nausea and vomiting: a qualitative systematic review of randomized placebo-controlled studies, *Br J Anaesth* 83:761-771, 1999.
406. Wetchler BV: Recovery room: the anesthesiologist's role as a problem solver in ambulatory surgery. In Barash PG, editor: *ASA Refresher Courses in Anesthesiology*, Philadelphia, 1991, Lippincott, pp 207-216.
407. Caldwell C, Rains G, McKiterick K: An unusual reaction to preoperative metoclopramide, *Anesthesiology* 67:854-855, 1987.
408. Alon E, Himmelseher S: Ondansetron in the treatment of postoperative vomiting: a randomized, double-blind comparison with droperidol and metoclopramide, *Anesth Analg* 75:561-565, 1992.
409. Leeser J, Lip H: Prevention of postoperative nausea and vomiting using ondansetron, a new, selective, 5-HT_3 receptor antagonist, *Anesth Analg* 72:751-755, 1991.
410. Monk TG, White PF, Lemon D: Ondansetron reduces nausea following outpatient lithotripsy, *Anesthesiology* 77:A19, 1992.
411. Larijani GE, Gratz I, Afshar M, Minassian S: Treatment of postoperative nausea and vomiting with ondansetron: a randomized, double-blind comparison with placebo, *Anesth Analg* 73:246-249, 1991.
412. Tang J, Wang B, White PF, Watcha MF, Qi J, Wender RH: The effect of timing of ondansetron administration on its efficacy, cost-effectiveness, and cost-benefit as a prophylactic antiemetic in the ambulatory setting, *Anesth Analg* 86:274-282, 1998.
413. Scuderi P, Wetchler B, Sung YF, et al: Treatment of postoperative nausea and vomiting after outpatient surgery with the 5-HT_3 antagonist ondansetron, *Anesthesiology* 78:15-20, 1993.
414. Kovac A, McKenzie R, O'Connor T, et al: Prophylactic intravenous ondansetron in female outpatients undergoing gynaecological surgery: a multicentre dose-comparison study, *Eur J Anaesthesiol* 9(suppl 6):37-47, 1992.
415. Davis PJ, McGowan FX Jr, Landsman I, Maloney K, Hoffmann P: Effect of antiemetic therapy on recovery and hospital discharge time: a double-blind assessment of ondansetron, droperidol, and placebo in pediatric patients undergoing ambulatory surgery, *Anesthesiology* 83:956-960, 1995.
416. Paxton LD, McKay AC, Mirakhur RK: Prevention of nausea and vomiting after day case gynaecological laparoscopy: A comparison of ondansetron, droperidol, metoclopramide and placebo, *Anaesthesia* 50:403-406, 1995.
417. Splinter WM, Rhine EJ, Roberts DW, et al: Ondansetron is a better prophylactic antiemetic than droperidol for tonsilectomy in children, *Can J Anaesth* 42:848-851, 1995.
418. Malins AF, Field JM, Nesling PM, Coooper GM: Nausea and vomiting after gynaecological laparoscopy: comparison of premedication with oral ondansetron, metoclopramide and placebo, *Br J Anaesth* 72:231-233, 1994.
419. Blanc VF, Ruest P, Milot J, Jacob JL, Tang A: Antiemetic prophylaxis with promethazine or droperidol in paediatric outpatient strabismus surgery, *Can J Anaesth* 38:54-60, 1991.
420. Tyler DC, Krane EJ: Postoperative pain management in children, *Anesthesiol Clin North Am* 7:155-170, 1989.
421. Collier CE: Pain management in the PACU. In Jacobsen WK, editor: *Manual of Postanesthesia Care*, Philadelphia, 1992, Saunders, pp 195-211.
422. Egan KJ: Psychological issues in postoperative pain, *Anesthesiol Clin North Am* 7:183-192, 1989.
423. Chung F, Ritchie E, Su J: Postoperative pain in ambulatory surgery, *Anesth Analg* 85:808-816, 1997.
424. Wetchler BV: What are the problems in the recovery room? *Can J Anaesth* 38:890-894, 1991.
425. Aldrete JA, Kroulik D: A postanesthetic recovery score, *Anesth Analg* 49:924-934, 1970.
426. Klepper ID: Paediatric patients. In Klepper ID, Sanders LD, Rosen M, editors: *Ambulatory Anaesthesia and Sedation: Impairment and Recovery*, Boston, 1991, Blackwell Scientific, pp 191-204.
427. Aldrete JA: Discharge criteria. In Thomson D, Frost E, editors: *Baillieres Clinical Anaesthesiology—Postanaesthesia Care*, London, 1994, Bailliere Tindall, pp 763-773.
428. Marshall S, Chung F: Assessment of "home readiness," *Curr Opin Anaesthesiol* 10:445-450, 1997.
429. Marley RA, Moline BM: Patient discharge from the ambulatory setting, *J Postanesth Nurs* 11:39-49, 1996.
430. Marley RA, Moline BM: Patient discharge issues. In Burden N, editor: *Ambulatory Surgical Nursing*, ed 2, Philadelphia, 2000, Saunders.
431. Mulroy MF, Salinas FV, Larkin KL, Polissar NL: Ambulatory surgery patients may be discharged before voiding after short-acting spinal and epidural anesthesia, *Anesthesiology* 97:315-319, 2002.
432. Pavlin DJ, Pavlin EG, Fitzgibbon DR, Koerschgen ME, Pitt TM: Management of bladder function after outpatient surgery, *Anesthesiology* 91:42-50, 1999.
433. Weintraub HD: Anesthetic management of the geriatric outpatient. In Barash PG, editor: *ASA Refresher Courses in Anesthesiology*, Philadelphia, 1986, Lippincott, pp 237-246.
434. Marley RA, Swanson J: Patient care after discharge from the ambulatory surgical center, *J PeriAnesth Nurs* 16:399-419, 2001.
435. Philip BK: Patient's assessment of ambulatory anesthesia and surgery, *J Clin Anesth* 4:355-358, 1992.
436. Macario A, Weigner M, Carney S, Kim A: Which clinical anesthesia outcomes are important to avoid? The perspective of patients, *Anesth Analg* 89:652-658, 1999.

CHAPTER 36

Anesthesia for Ear, Nose, Throat, and Maxillofacial Surgery

Gary D. Clark, Julie A. Stone

The practice of anesthesia for the ear, nose, throat (ENT) patient is challenging and rewarding. Decisions regarding difficult airway management are often necessary, as is the knowledge and skills to navigate abnormal and difficult anatomy. As a specialty, ENT presents specific concerns to the anesthetist for the preparation and management of surgical procedures (Box 36-1). There are several essential goals when providing anesthesia for ENT and maxillofacial (i.e., plastics and dental) surgical procedures. These essential goals of anesthesia should include the following:

1. Possessing a thorough knowledge of the airway anatomy and function
2. Selecting appropriate technique(s) and approach for airway management
3. Preventing and managing potential airway complications
4. Producing profound selective muscle relaxation during periods of extreme stimulation (e.g., suspension laryngoscopy)
5. Maintaining cardiovascular stability during periods of potent surgical stimulation
6. Omitting neuromuscular relaxation for surgical procedures that require isolation of nerves
7. Preventing and containing an endotracheal tube fire
8. Minimizing intraoperative and postoperative blood loss
9. Preventing adverse respiratory and cardiac responses resulting from manipulation of the carotid sinus and body
10. Taking the appropriate postoperative measures to prevent and treat postsurgical airway obstruction
11. Avoiding or limiting the use of nitrous oxide during tympanoplasty or other closed-space grafting

BOX 36-1

Special Considerations for ENT Procedures

Use of specialized ventilation techniques
- Insufflation
- Intermittent apnea
- Apneic oxygenation

Prevention of endotracheal tube fire
Shared airway
Surgical field avoidance
Restricted use of nitrous oxide
Restricted use of muscle relaxants
Use of specialized equipment
- Laser
- High-frequency jet ventilation (HFJV)

High percentage of pediatric patients
Minimizing blood loss

Surgical intervention for ENT procedures uses a variety of specialty equipment including the use of lasers, endoscopes, and specialized endotracheal tubes (e.g., laser and microlaryngeal tube), to name a few. The basis of many ENT and maxillofacial surgical procedures include endoscopic examination of the sinuses; tissue tumors of the head, neck, and oral cavity; abscesses; surgery to the middle ear; papillomas of the airway; hypertrophic tonsils and adenoids; acute epiglottitis; and traumatic or congenital facial deformities. The majority of these procedures involve the nose, facial and frontal sinuses, larynx, oropharynx, nasopharynx, tongue, trachea, mandible, and maxilla, as well as other supporting structures of the head and neck. These procedures necessitate sharing the airway with the surgeon and may lead to a tenuous airway and significant challenges for the anesthetist. Airway compromise in ENT patients may be subtle and can take several forms.

This chapter describes the pertinent anatomy and physiology of the head and neck for the anesthetist, reviews specialized anesthetic considerations, reviews surgical and anesthesia equipment used during ENT procedures, analyzes some of the common pharmacologic agents used for ENT procedures, and discusses principles of anesthesia for ENT.

FUNCTIONAL ANATOMY OF THE HEAD AND NECK

A fundamental knowledge of the anatomic and physiologic function of the structures of the head and neck is essential for dealing with the myriad decisions arising perioperatively during these procedures. Commonly, the ENT surgical procedure is being performed because the anatomic structures are abnormal, distorted, or deviated. Having a working knowledge of the structures and their relationships before subjecting the patient to respiratory changes produced by anesthesia is imperative.

The anatomic structures of the head and neck and their relationships are complex (Figure 36-1). The sensory and motor supply of the upper airway originates from cranial nerves and includes the trigeminal, glossopharyngeal, facial, and vagus nerves (Figure 36-2). Understanding the sensory supply allows the anesthetist to provide sufficient local and regional anesthesia. Likewise, motor function can be evaluated following

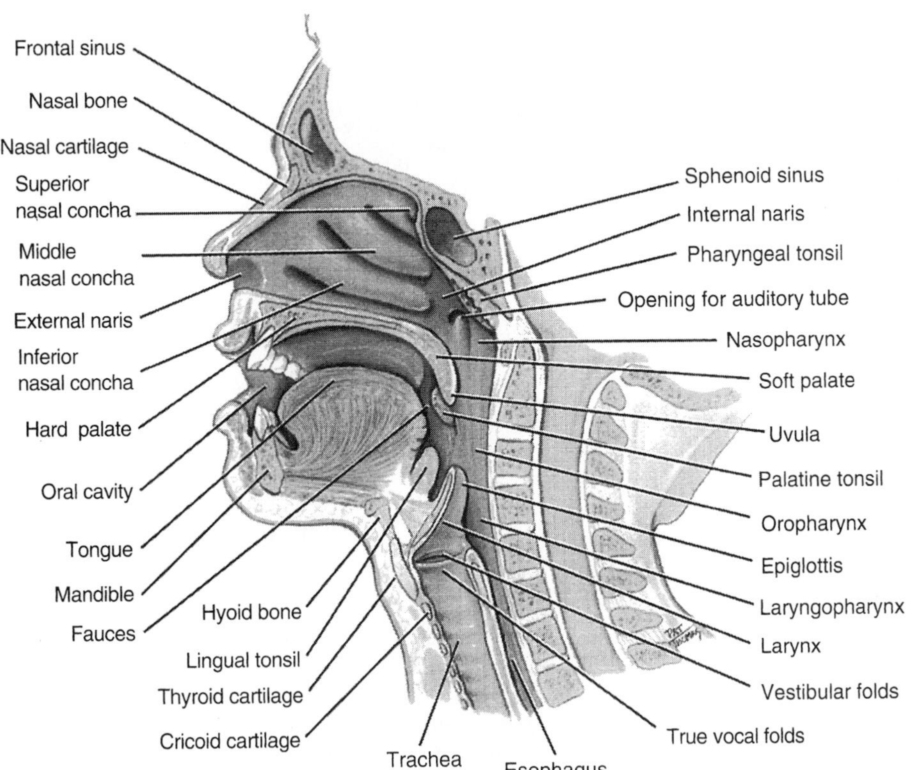

FIGURE **36-1**
Anatomic features of human head and neck. (From Applegate EJ: *The Anatomy and Physiology Learning System*, Philadelphia, 1995, Saunders, p 307.)

surgical procedures that may yield trauma or damage to muscles and the nerves controlling their function.

The relationships of the oropharynx; nasopharynx; nasal chambers; sinuses; esophagus; and lower airway structures such as the larynx, cricoid, thyroid, and vocal cords provide a basis for directing and providing care for the patient receiving ENT surgery. The nose is a major anatomic structure that is responsible for warming, filtering, and providing humidity to the air taken in during inspiration. The structures of the nose include the external nose; the nasal cavity; and frontal, maxillary, and ethmoid sinuses. The nares or nostrils are separated by the septum. The lateral margins of the nares are cartilaginous structures and extend posteriorly over the hard palate, leading to a confluence at the soft palate, oropharynx, and base of the tongue. The oropharynx rests superior to the epiglottis, vocal cords, larynx, and trachea.

The external nose is composed largely of cartilage that is supported primarily by soft connective tissue and delicate mucous membranes, as is the nasal septum. The nasal cavities are hollow structures formed by a floor, roof, lateral wall, and the septum. The lateral aspects of the nasal cavities contain concha or turbinates. The turbinates are highly vascular and are divided into three separate compartments: the superior, middle, and inferior. The turbinates greatly increase the surface area of the nasal cavities, aiding in the filtration and humidification of inspired gases. The extensive vascular supply of the turbinates may lead to severe bleeding if the endotracheal tube is not inserted along the superior margin of the hard palate. Congestion of the mucosal veins in the turbinates of the nose causes swelling of these tissues, reducing the size of the nasal cavity (most notably, the paranasal sinuses) and thus creating the feeling of "congestion" during respiration. These paired sinuses include the sphenoid, ethmoid, and frontal and the maxillary sinuses. They not only serve as resonators for the voice but also filter, humidify, and warm the air during inspiration. These hollow structures are formed of low-density bone and are lined with a thin layer of mucous membranes reducing the weight of the skull, making these bones more susceptible to fractures secondary to facial trauma.

The pharynx is composed of the terminal end of the nasopharynx, the oropharynx, and laryngopharynx or hypopharynx extending to sixth cervical vertebra. The medulla inhibits respiration with swallowing; the pharynx then serves as a muscular tube that constricts, allowing the passage of food. The pharynx allows the smooth passage of air and functions as a modulator for the voice. The nasopharynx is continuous with the internal nasal cavities and extends to the soft palate. The nasopharynx communicates with the oropharynx and forms the posterior aspect of the throat. Major structures of the oropharynx include the base of the tongue, soft palate, uvula, and lymphatic structures (tonsils). The tonsils are the most sensitive areas of the oropharynx and—beginning with the anterior margin and progressing bilateral and posterior—the oropharynx is defined by supporting structures including the soft palate, the base of the tongue, uvula, palatine tonsils, and adenoids, forming Waldeyer's ring.[1,2]

Hypertrophy of the palatine tonsils and adenoid tonsils (exaggerated many times by chronic infection) and of the soft palate and uvula can pose serious airway compromise, particularly in young children. The generous blood supply to the tonsils from branches of the external carotid, maxillary, and facial arteries and their close proximity to the facial and internal arteries are matters of concern regarding potential bleeding during "routine and simple" tonsillectomy. The laryngopharynx includes the epiglottis, which provides protection for the vocal cords, and is the region shared by the esophageal orifice and larynx.

The complexity of the neuromuscular system, which controls the epiglottis, allows the isolation of the trachea from the esophagus during swallowing.[1] Any interruption of this coordinated neuromuscular function of the epiglottis or of any

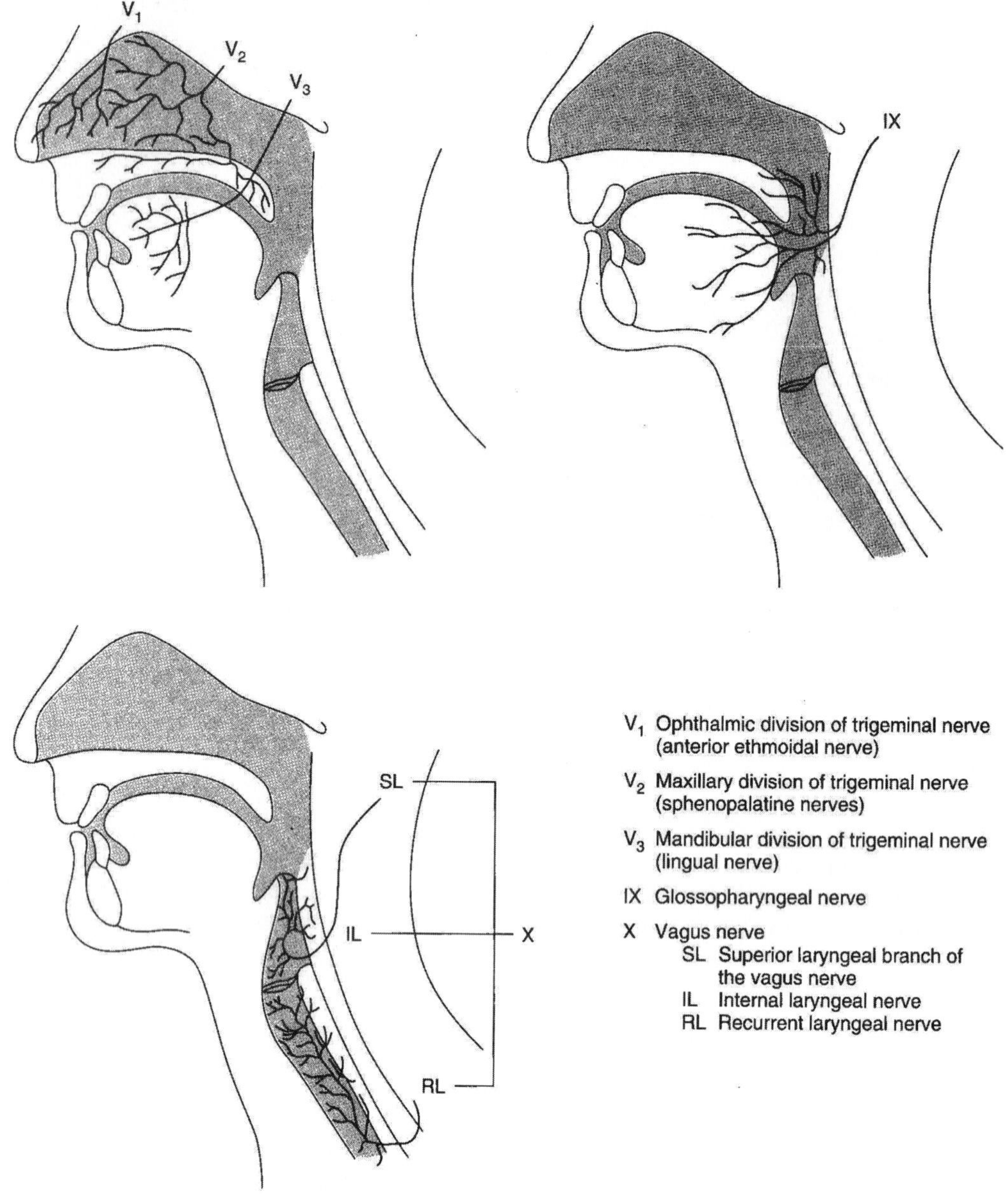

FIGURE **36-2**
Sensory nerve supply of the airway. (From Morgan GE, Mikhal HS, Murry MJ: *Clinical Anesthesiology*, ed 3, New York, 2002, McGraw-Hill, p 62.)

other protective reflexes can provide a potentially dangerous opportunity for the entrance of food or liquid into the larynx and lower airway. As food is squeezed posterior an automatic swallowing reflex is initiated. The larynx is pulled superior, allowing the epiglottis to cover and protect the opening of the larynx.[1] The epiglottis does not operate as a movable lidlike structure that falls to close the larynx during swallowing, as is often claimed. Passage of food into the trachea can occur if the muscles and protective elevation of the larynx become rigid or are changed due to nerve interruption. A series of reflex and involuntary processes mediated by the superior laryngeal, recurrent laryngeal, and glossopharyngeal nerves coordinates and regulates glottic closure during swallowing. Structures that provide both sensory and motor nerve innervation and functionality to the larynx are listed in Table 36-1.

The larynx is a rigid organ located distal to Waldeyer's ring and forms the connection between the oropharynx and the trachea. The larynx is composed of three cartilaginous structures (the epiglottis, thyroid, and cricoid cartilages) and is supported by the hyoid bone. This hollow structure forms a reservoir distal to Waldeyer's ring and provides the connection of the oropharynx to the trachea (Fig. 36-3). The primary functions of the larynx are vocalization and articulation; secondarily, it provides protection of the airway and allows respiration.[1] In the adult, the vocal cords or rima glottis is the narrowest portion of the larynx. In children, the cricoid ring is the narrowest portion of the airway until approximately 10 years of age. Cuffed tubes are then generally recommended for those older than 8 to 10 years of age to allow for a better seal of the airway, prevent subglottic edema, and reduce the incidence of postoperative airway compromise.[3]

Specific nervous structures of the head and neck are worthy of note because of their superficial location or proximity to operative sites. Surgeons may use audible or visual nerve-locating

TABLE 36-1 Structures and Innervation of the Larynx

Cartilages			
Paired			Unpaired
Arytenoid			Thyroid
Corniculate			Cricoid
Cuneiform			Epiglottis
Nerves			
Nerve	**Motor**	**Sensory**	**Innervation**
Internal laryngeal (vagus)		X	Laryngeal mucosa above vocal cords (inferior epiglottis)
Recurrent laryngeal		X	Laryngeal mucosa below vocal cords
Glossopharyngeal		X	Superior aspect of epiglottis and base of tongue
Recurrent laryngeal	X		All intrinsic muscles except cricothyroid
External laryngeal	X		Cricothyroid muscles

Muscles Controlling the Laryngeal Inlet	
Muscle	**Action**
Oblique arytenoids	Approximates aryepiglottic folds, narrows inlet
Aryepiglottic	Narrows inlet
Thyroepiglottic	Widens inlet by pulling aryepiglottic folds apart
Muscles Controlling Movements of Vocal Folds	
Muscle	**Action**
Cricothyroid	Tenses vocal cords; tilts cricoid and arytenoids posteriorly
Thyroarytenoid	Relaxes vocal cords; pulls arytenoids forward
Vocalis	
Lateral cricoarytenoid	Adducts vocal ligaments
Posterior cricoarytenoid	Abducts vocal ligaments
Transverse arytenoids	Closes posterior part of rima glottis

Modified from Snell RS, Katz J: Clinical Anatomy for Anesthesiologists, *Norwalk, CT, 1988, Appleton & Lange, pp 17, 25, 26.*

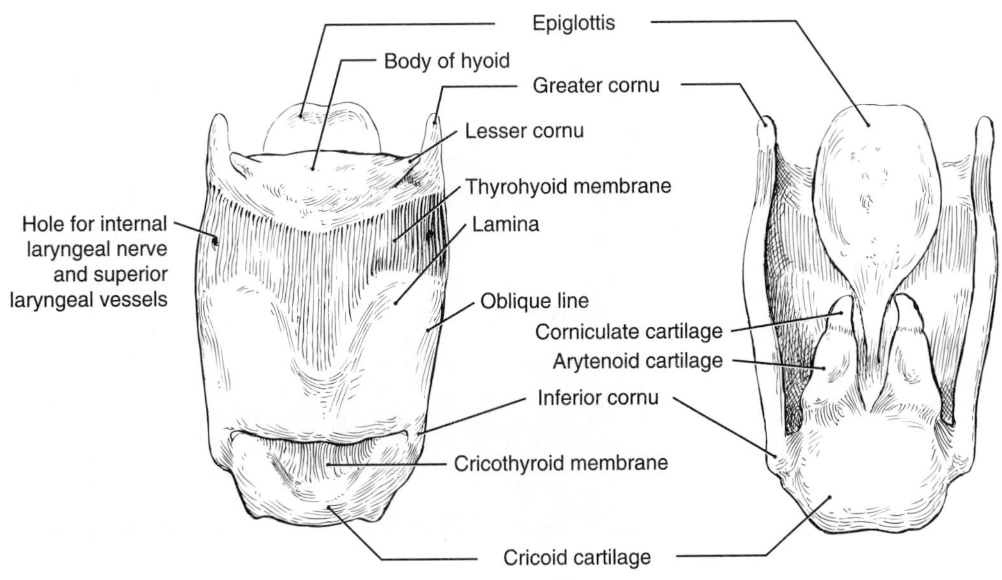

FIGURE **36-3** The larynx and its ligaments. **A,** Anterior view. **B,** Posterior view. (From Snell RS, Katz J: *Clinical Anatomy for Anesthesiologists,* Norwalk, CT, 1988, Appleton & Lange.)

devices to find these nerves and their appropriate branches. In order to accurately locate these nerves, neuromuscular blocking agents should be avoided during the maintenance of general anesthesia. The facial nerve (VII) has five branches: three anterior (temporal, zygomatic, buccal, and mandibular), one inferior (cervical), and one posterior (posterior auricular) branch. The facial nerve located at the tragus of the ear is the motor and sensory supply to the muscles for facial expressions. The zygomatic branch leaves the skull via the stylomastoid foramen and advances anteriorly over the maxilla. The corda tympani branch of the facial nerve conveys taste from the anterior two thirds of the tongue, and the more superficial tri-branched facial nerve controls facial expression. The trigeminal nerve begins at the Gasserian ganglion and divides into three branches; they are the ophthalmic (the first division, V_1), maxillary (the second division, V_2), and mandibular (the third division, V_3). All three divisions provide sensory and motor innervation to the nose, sinuses, palate, and tongue. They aid in the motor control of the face as well as mastication. The glossopharyngeal nerve provides motor and sensory innervation for the base of the tongue and nasopharynx and oropharynx. The glossopharyngeal is responsible for eliciting the gag reflex during instrumentation of the posterior pharynx and vallecula. The superior laryngeal and recurrent laryngeal are both branches of the vagus (X). The superior laryngeal descends to the hyoid bone and then branches into the internal laryngeal that passes through the thyrohyoid membrane and the exterior laryngeal nerve, which descends over the lateral thyroid cartilage to the distal trachea. The recurrent laryngeal nerve ascends from the vagus up the distal trachea, passing through the cricothyroid ligament into the proximal trachea and vocal cords. The recurrent laryngeal nerve lies between the trachea and esophagus and supplies sensory innervation to the trachea and vocal cords. This branch of the vagus nerve also affects vocal cord closure and sensory function up to the inferior aspect of the epiglottis. Stimulation of the epiglottis with the tip of a straight laryngoscope, blades, suction catheters, and placement of an endotracheal tube in the trachea can produce a vagal response.[3]

PREPARATION AND CONSIDERATIONS FOR EAR, NOSE, AND THROAT PROCEDURES

The Shared Airway and Considerations for Positioning

Operative procedures involving the airway, mouth, or bony structures of the face involve a true sharing of the airway between the surgeon and the anesthetist. Therefore, proper preparation requires planning and communication between the surgeon, surgical personnel, and the anesthetist prior to the surgical procedure. Sharing the airway with the surgeon also requires preparing and planning the use of the appropriate equipment. For example, during laryngoscopy the endotracheal tube may have to be smaller in diameter and moved to one side of the oropharynx to allow the surgeon to work around the tube and to facilitate the surgery. Many times the head of the table is rotated 90 to 180 degrees away from the anesthetist, resulting in a vulnerable airway to which the anesthetist may have little or no access. Of particular concern is the maintenance of adequate ventilation; patency of the anesthesia circuit and endotracheal tube; and prevention of extubation, disconnects, and leaks. Adequacy of ventilation is constantly assessed by observing chest movement, auscultation, pulse oximetry, end-tidal CO_2, and blood gas analysis.[4] A sudden loss of breath sounds, rising inspiratory pressures, or a reduction in end-tidal CO_2, particularly in the presence of a sharp reduction in inspiratory effort, may be due to a deflation of the endotracheal tube cuff, obstruction of the endotracheal tube, dislodgment of the endotracheal tube, a disconnection of the anesthesia circuit, or severing of the endotracheal tube during surgical dissection.[5] The precordial or esophageal stethoscopes are simple devices that when coupled with vigilance should not be overlooked in favor of more sophisticated mechanical devices.

Assessment of the airway prior to induction is critical in most ENT patients. While the induction of anesthesia and securing of the airway is performed in the usual manner, with the anesthetist at the head of the table, the management of the airway can become questionable and difficult while at a distance. Obtaining a thorough history and performing an extensive evaluation of the airway for the ENT patient is crucial. A good examination of the airway will (1) allow for a careful and deliberate approach to airway management, (2) aid in the determination of the need for additional equipment and assistance, and (3) include alternative approaches for the difficult airway should the initial plan not be successful. Once the induction is complete and the airway established, the anesthetist must be prepared to provide adequate ventilation, deliver necessary anesthetic and adjunct agents, place invasive lines, and safely monitor the patient, while remaining at a distance and isolated from the airway.

Orchestrating turning of the patient so that the patient's head is away from the anesthetist demands clear planning. The endotracheal tube should be secured with tape or suture to prevent removal. The breathing hoses, invasive line tubing, intravenous access lines, monitoring devices, and breathing circuit require added length to extend to the patient without creating tension at the site before induction. The patient's entire head is frequently draped and prepped into the surgical field, limiting access to the endotracheal tube and breathing circuit connections (Fig. 36-4). When

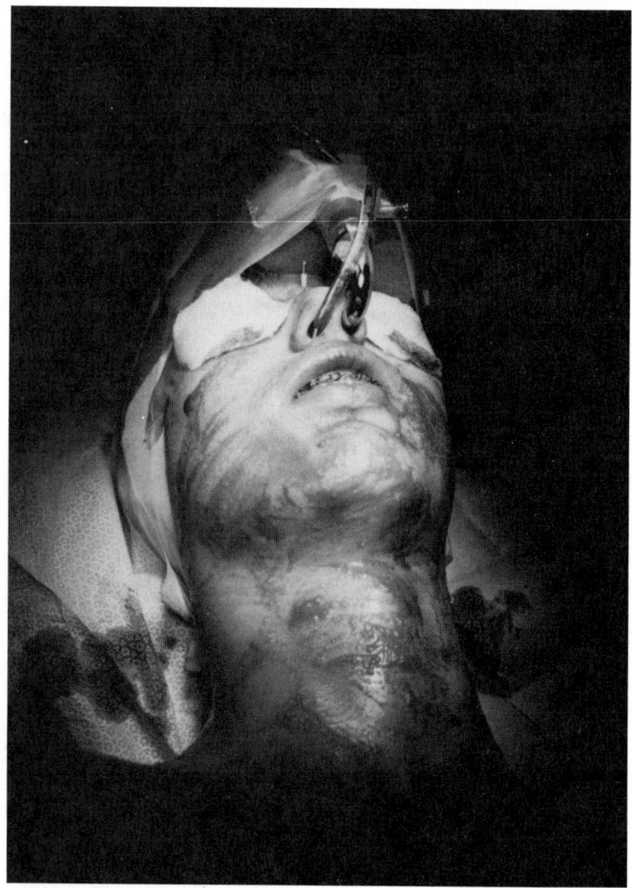

FIGURE **36-4**
Illustration of secured airway for a patient undergoing face, neck, or maxillofacial surgical procedures. Note that the tube is positioned to prevent pressure on the lip, nose, or forehead and secured with tape to prevent movement during surgery. The connection is covered by sterile surgical drapes and allows only limited access during the surgical procedure.

repositioning of the head is necessary, communication between the surgeon and anesthetist is important to reduce the possibility of extubation or position change of the endotracheal tube or occluding the endotracheal tube. Signs of air leaks around the endotracheal tube (bubbling, the sound of air escaping, or the smell of anesthetic agent from the patient's mouth) may well be more sensitive indicators than mechanical airway monitors. Occlusion of the endotracheal tube is best prevented but can be determined by good auscultation, watching chest wall motion, and monitoring inspiratory pressures. The surgeon must communicate and the anesthetist must be aware of any changes in the surgical field, such as changing the position of a suspended or fixed laryngoscope, dark blood, manipulation of carotid bodies, or the need for a change in the patient's head position.[6] Increased inspiratory pressures or a rapid loss of inspiratory pressure, decreased oxygen saturation, changes in end-tidal CO_2 measurements, or diminished breath sounds should in turn be communicated to the surgeon by the anesthetist so that inspection of the airway and anesthesia circuit may be undertaken. If unable to arrive at a cause, undraping the patient may become necessary for a thorough examination of tube placement and connections or to find a leak in the anesthesia circuit that could compromise patient ventilation.

Procedures of the head and neck typically require access to all planes of the head by several members of the surgical team. Because of the number of problems that can be encountered with the patient intubated during the surgical procedure, the surgeon may elect to perform a tracheostomy, then placing and suturing a flexible endotracheal tube in a fixed position during the procedure. The anesthetist should remain in a heightened state of vigilance for occlusions from mucous plugs or blood, disconnects, and other problems that may arise during the anesthetic. During some ENT procedures the surgical team may also need access to the chest and abdomen for securing grafts for the esophagus or oral cavity. Often, this requires the anesthetist to take residence at either the side of the patient or at the foot of the operating table (Fig. 36-5). Providing a smooth transition with protection of the established airway and prevention of hypoxia are the primary concerns during movement of an operating table with an anesthetized patient.

The anesthesia circuit and other monitors should be temporarily and briefly disconnected before the bed is turned. This will prevent undue tension on the circuit and other lines leading to a possible traumatic extubation or loss of access. While the average breathing circuit tubing is adequate for ventilation, the Bain non-rebreathing anesthesia circuit has certain advantages for procedures requiring circuit immobilization to the head of the patient. The Bain circuit has a single "tube within a tube" design that reduces breathing resistance and weight. One disadvantage of the Bain is that if the internal tube (which supplies the fresh gas flow for the circuit) becomes disconnected, it may be hard to detect and lead to extensive rebreathing.[7] The Bain should remain an option when choosing a circuit for ENT procedures. Ventilation of the patient with 100% oxygen and adequate tidal volumes for 3 to 5 minutes before disconnection will denitrogenate the functional residual volume and provides an extra reservoir of oxygen during the turn, preventing even a short period of hypoxia. However, the

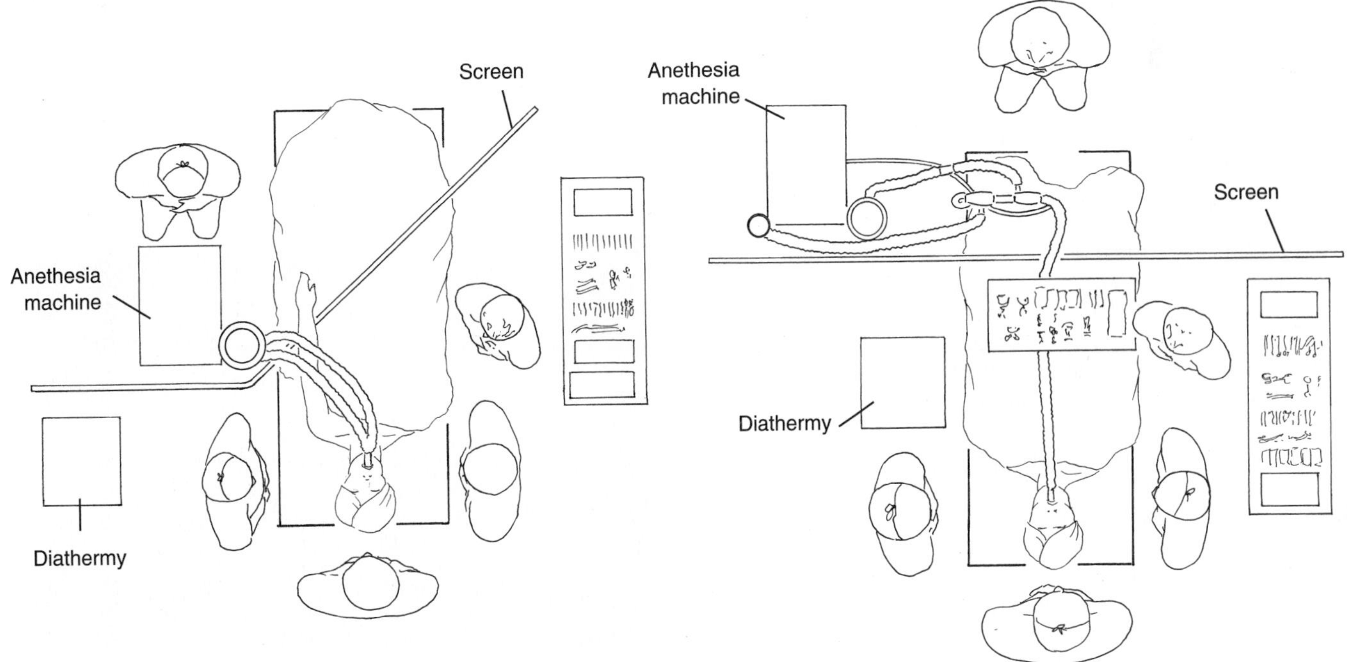

FIGURE **36-5**
Position of the anesthetist for surgery of the head and neck. *Left*, the anesthetist is positioned at the side of the table using a standard circle circuit; *Right*, the anesthetist is positioned at the foot of the bed using a coaxial (Bain) circuit. (From Brown CD: Anesthesia. In Cummings CW, Fredrickson JM, Harker LA, Krause CJ, Schuller DE, editors: *Otolaryngology: Head and Neck Surgery*, vol 1, ed 2, St Louis, 1993, Mosby, p 226.)

addition of intravenous anesthesia during this preoxygenation is necessary if volatile agent is the primary source of anesthesia to maintain an adequate level of anesthesia and/or amnesia during this period. A saturation of 100% is a reasonable goal before the disconnection and table movement.

The degree of table movement should be discussed with the surgeon before any interruption in the anesthesia or the breathing circuit. Turning of the operating table should be a well-organized procedure, understood by all members of the surgical team, that takes the minimum amount of time. Reconnection of the anesthesia circuit must be immediate once the turn is complete. Reevaluation and assessment of the tube placement, breath sounds, chest expansion, oxygen saturation, anesthetic level, line and intravenous access, and end-tidal CO_2 should be performed *before* prepping and draping is begun. Once adequate ventilation is established, the use of an "artificial nose" or airway humidifier will help in preserving heat and moisture during long periods of anesthesia.

Attention to simple practical points may prevent airway mishaps. At least one large-bore intravenous line, as well as arterial and central venous pressure lines, should be started on the nonoperative side and, if possible, the side of the patient that will be nearest to the anesthetist during the procedure. This will prevent obstruction of flow due to the surgical procedure, afford easier access for drug administration and blood sampling, facilitate the manipulation or maintenance of lines during surgery, and allow the surgeon easy access to the operative field. If such lines must be placed on extremities opposite the anesthetist or if the anesthetist is located a distance from the site, adequate Luer lock extensions should be placed before a change in position of the table to reduce the chance of lines being removed, infiltrating, or becoming disconnected during movement. The calf of the leg may be used for noninvasive blood pressure measurements to prevent dampening of intravenous fluid flows in the upper extremities. Monitoring of neuromuscular relaxation may be performed at locations other than the adductor pollicis. Stimulation of the tibial nerve produces flexion of the big toe and is similar to that of the adductor pollicis.[8] Recent investigations have indicated small differences in the response to train-of-four (TOF) nerve stimulation in the arm (adductor pollicis muscle) and the leg (flexor hallucis brevis muscle); these differences are probably of little clinical significance.[8,9] Since these procedures may take more than 2 hours and can require significant fluid administration, monitoring urinary output with a Foley catheter may be included in the plan.

Postoperative nausea and vomiting (PONV) are a common problem following ENT procedures with general anesthesia; proactive measures should be employed for control. Uncontrolled PONV can lead to delayed discharge, a compromised airway, bleeding, and poor patient satisfaction. The chemoreceptor trigger zone (CTZ), which is the central point responsible for vomiting, is stimulated by peripheral receptors such as the gastrointestinal (GI) tract, eye, and middle ear. Therefore, procedures that stimulate these peripheral sites are factors that increase the incidence of nausea and vomiting. There are several measures to reduce PONV, including adequate hydration and administration of drugs specific to these sites, such as the 5-HT_3 antagonists, metoclopramide, and propofol.[10] Other antiemetic therapies that may help reduce PONV are decompressing the stomach, avoiding nitrous oxide, controlling pain, and using nonsteroidal antiinflammatory agents for pain control.

SPECIALIZED EQUIPMENT FOR EAR, NOSE, AND THROAT PROCEDURES

Endotracheal Tubes

There are a number of endotracheal tubes to select from to secure an airway. Standard endotracheal tubes equipped with flexible or straight connectors are acceptable for many ENT procedures. The diameter and length of the endotracheal tube will affect ventilation and seal of the airway. Using a small-diameter endotracheal tube in a large adult airway will not only lead to less ventilation but will allow only a small portion of the cuff to contact the trachea. Using specialized tubes with small diameters (e.g., the microlaryngeal tube [Mallinckrodt MLT™]) allows more even distribution of the cuff over the trachea during inflation. Several of these specially designed endotracheal tubes have found wide acceptance in ENT anesthesia. A variety of designs are used by the anesthetist to limit encroachment of the endotracheal tube into the surgical field, prevent kinking of the endotracheal tube when severe angles are necessary, prevent fires in the airway during laser, and provide maximal patient ventilation and safety.

Preformed right-angled endotracheal (RAE) tubes, in cuffed and noncuffed types, are available for either oral or nasal intubation of adults or children (Fig. 36-6). The use of the oral RAE tubes is an excellent choice for cleft palate repair, tonsillectomy, uvulopalatopharyngoplasty, and procedures of the eye or upper face. Nasal RAE tubes are particularly well suited to maxillofacial surgery that does not allow for oral intubation. The nasal RAE can be used for cosmetic procedures of the face, surgical procedures of the oral cavity and mandible, or to correct malocclusion. However, while the preformed bend in the RAE tube prevents the endotracheal tube from kinking in many instances, the preformed bend may be too distal or proximal for an individual patient's airways. This then allows the tip of the endotracheal tube to rest well below or above the carina. A careful check of the breath sounds and inspiratory pressures is imperative following intubation with the RAE to ensure the proper positioning. Nasal intubation and placement of a nasogastric tube in the unconscious patient with facial trauma is best avoided to prevent possible penetration of the brain.[11]

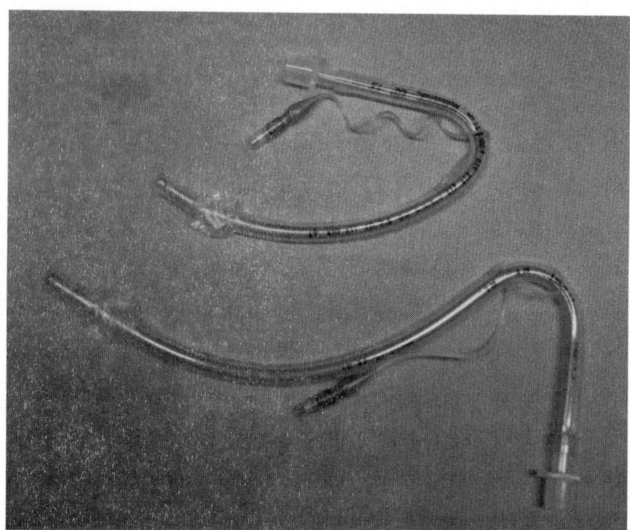

FIGURE **36-6**
Preformed RAE endotracheal tubes for procedures of the head, neck, and airway. *Top*, oral RAE; *Bottom*, nasal RAE.

Anode, armored, reinforced, and Kant Kink™ tubes all have an embedded coiled wire or plastic coil strand to produce a tube with greater flexibility and memory. Armored tubes, for oral or nasal intubations, resist kinking and retain their original integrity. They are useful when acute neck flexion or severe angles of the endotracheal tube are required, as in procedures involving the base of the skull or posterior aspect of the neck. Several varieties of metal-impregnated tubes are available for use with laser surgery and are designed to reduce the occurrence of an airway fire (Fig. 36-7). The cuff of the laser tube is usually filled with saline to dampen or prevent the ignition. Wrapping a standard endotracheal tube with reflective tape is not an adequate alternative to these commercially prepared tubes because the wrapped standard endotracheal tube will dry and lead to greater flammablility.[12,13]

The Carden tube, or the Xomed-Treace Mon-Jet Tube (Fig. 36-8), is a small-diameter, cuffed tube specifically designed to be used with high-flow jet ventilation for procedures of the larynx or subglottic area. A second method uses hand-controlled Venturi jet ventilation through needle tip. The needle fits into a side port of the laryngoscope or bronchoscope and entrains air for delivery as it exits at a high pressure. The jet ventilation system allows the intermittent delivery of oxygen and anesthetic gases during the procedure.

Although not classified as an endotracheal tube, the laryngeal mask (LMA) and intubating laryngeal mask airway (ILMA) may be used to facilitate intubations as well as diagnostic fiberoptic laryngoscopy and bronchoscopy.[14] The LMA is designed to be used for anesthesia when the patient is spontaneously breathing and is particularly well suited for visualization of the vocal cords or their function. The ILMAs or FastTrac LMAs have gained further popularity and acceptance in anesthesia as a means of establishing ventilation and intubation in patients with a difficult airway. With the use of a Portex™ connector that has a diaphragm port, a fiberoptic scope may be inserted into the lumen of the laryngeal mask airway without interrupting ventilation. The anesthetists must remember that the patient will be susceptible to laryngospasm if anesthesia is light or inadequate. The ILMA has a small flap that moves and is more conducive to placement of a laryngoscope or endotracheal tube. The LMA does not provide protection of the airway and is thus comparable to the endotracheal tube. The incidence of complications (e.g., aspiration of gastric contents, injury to the airway, dislodgment, failure of the device, and damage to the device) is reported to be related to the experience and expertise of the clinician.[15-18]

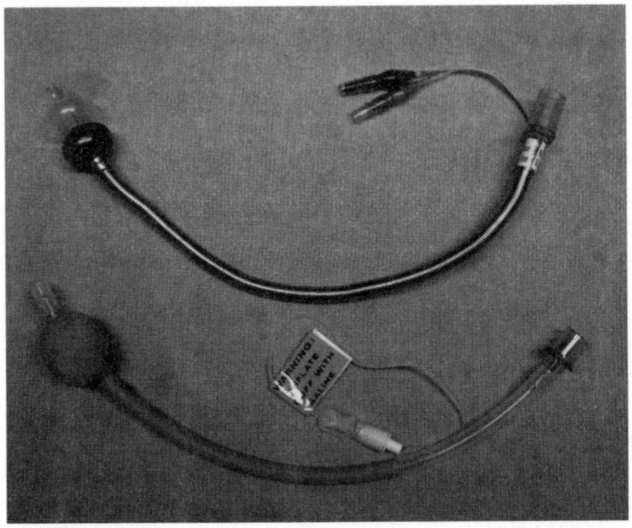

FIGURE **36-7**
Endotracheal tubes for laser surgery of the airway.

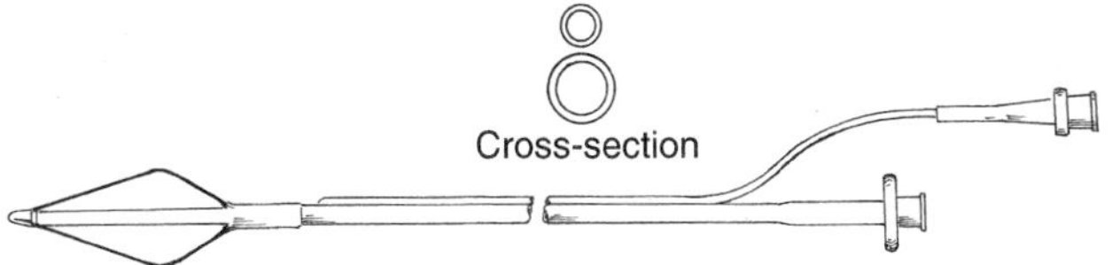

FIGURE **36-8**
Schematic drawing of the Xomed-Treace Mon-Jet Tube for jet ventilation.

Pharmacologic Considerations

The use of local anesthetics is particularly prevalent during nasal and sinus surgery. The most commonly used local anesthetics for ENT include the amide-based drugs. Many procedures are performed using topical and local anesthesia as the sole agent, in combination or supplemented with monitored anesthesia care, intravenous sedation, or general anesthesia. Local anesthetics are drugs that produce reversible conduction blockade of impulses along central and peripheral nerve pathways. The anesthetist using these agents or caring for patients receiving these drugs should be well versed in their pharmacology, duration of action, metabolism, toxicity, and effects on other anesthetics and dosages (Table 36-2). The anesthetist should also be familiar with physiologic changes such as acidosis, infection, and hyperthermia that will change or alter the effects of local anesthetic drugs. A practical point to remember is that the total dose based on patient weight must be determined prior to injection and must take into account all local anesthesia used during the case by the surgeon and the anesthetist. Additionally, multiple or large injection sites, hypercarbia, hypovolemia, and liver disease lower the toxic threshold of local anesthetics and are important considerations in calculating total dose. It has been suggested that mixing an ester and an amide may prevent the toxic effects of each and allow the better effects to prevail. For example, mixing 2-chloroprocaine (Nesacaine) with bupivacaine (Marcaine) allows a quick onset of action and an extended block. Mixing of agents may reduce the effectiveness of the block.[19]

Vasoactive Drugs

The duration of action of a local anesthetic is proportional to the time the drug is in contact with nerve fibers. For this reason, epinephrine in varying concentrations (1:200,000 or 5 mcg/mL; 1:100,000 or 10 mcg/mL; and 1:50,000 or 20 mcg/mL) may be added to local anesthetic solutions to produce vasoconstriction. Vasoconstriction limits systemic absorption and maintains a higher drug concentration in the vicinity of the nerve fibers to be anesthetized, thus extending the effects of the local anesthetic.[20,21] Addition of epinephrine to a lidocaine solution prolongs the duration of conduction blockade by approximately 50% and decreases systemic absorption and plasma concentrations of local anesthetics by approximately one third.[22,23] A generally accepted "safe" total dose of epinephrine is 200 micrograms, or 1.5 mcg/kg. The presence of volatile anesthetics may accentuate toxic reactions to epinephrine.[24,25] Caution must be

TABLE 36-2 Topical Anesthetic Drugs

Drug	Concentration	Dose	Notable Features
Cocaine	4%	3 mg/kg	Only local anesthetic with vasoconstrictive ability Blocks reuptake of norepinephrine and epinephrine at adrenergic nerve endings
Lidocaine	2% and 4% solution 2% viscous solution 10% aerosol 2.5% and 5% ointment 10%, 15%, 20%	4 mg/kg plain 7 mg/kg epinephrine 250-300 mg	Rapid onset Suitable for all areas of the tracheobronchial tree
Benzocaine	Cetacaine contains: 14% benzocaine, 2% butamben, and 2% tetracaine		Short duration of action (10 min) Can produce methemoglobinemia
Bupivacaine	0.25%, 0.5%, 0.75%	2.5 mg/kg plain	Slow hepatic clearance Long duration of action
Mepivacaine	1%, 2%	4 mg/kg	Intermediate potency with rapid onset
Dyclonine	0.5%, 1%	300 mg maximum	Topical spray or gargle Frequent use for laryngoscopy Absorbed through both skin and mucous membranes

exercised when using epinephrine in combination with volatile anesthesia agents. It has been reported that the dosages of epinephrine injected submucosally and necessary to produce ventricular dysrhythmias in 50% of patients anesthetized with 1.25 times the minimum alveolar concentration of halothane or isoflurane is 2.1or 6.7 mcg/kg, respectively.[26]

It is estimated that topical cocaine (4% to 10% solution) anesthesia is used in more than 50% of ENT procedures, specifically rhinolaryngologic procedures, performed annually in the United States.[27] Cocaine is a naturally occurring ester of benzoic acid that is hydrolyzed by plasma cholinesterase. Applied topically, it is an excellent local anesthetic and vasoconstrictor. The duration of action is approximately 45 minutes.[28] Cocaine produces vasoconstriction by blocking catecholamine reuptake into the adrenergic nerve ending, resulting in vasoconstriction and shrinking of the mucosa. Epinephrine is also injected for ENT procedures and is usually injected shortly after the application of cocaine. This combination of cocaine and epinephrine sets the stage for a significant interaction. Since cocaine that is absorbed into the plasma can block the uptake of epinephrine systemically, a toxic effect of epinephrine can result from the injection. This interaction can result in severe headaches, hypertension, tachycardia, and dysrhythmias.[29,30]

Anticholinergics

Anticholinergics were used liberally early in anesthesia predominately because of the excessive mucous production caused by early volatile inhalation agents. With the advent of newer anesthetic agents, mucous production is lower and the need for anticholinergics has been diminished. Premedication with anticholinergics helps reduce or diminish vagal tone, reduces secretions, and increases bronchodilation. The antisialagogue effects may be desired for intraoral procedures that require a dryer operative field. The addition of anticholinergics and the use of dry gases during anesthesia can increase the viscosity of secretions during long cases, limiting the evacuation of mucous or even creating a mucous plug in the bronchus or endotracheal tube. Anticholinergics can also precipitate closed angle glaucoma and should be avoided in the patients with a known history. It has also been recently suggested that the relaxation of the lower esophageal sphincter, produced by the current overuse of anticholinergics in the treatment of reflux, even in the short term may lead to adenocarcinoma.[31] However, when choosing an anticholinergic, glycopyrrolate may be a better choice than atropine. In comparison to atropine and scopolamine, glycopyrrolate does not readily cross the blood-brain barrier thus lacks sedative effects, and is less likely to raise intraocular pressure than atropine.

Corticosteroids

Glucocorticoids may be administered preoperatively and intraoperatively to decrease laryngeal edema formation, reduce nausea and vomiting, and prolong the analgesic effects of local anesthetics. They should be administered as early as possible in the perioperative period so as to reach their peak effect prior to initiating surgery. The use of steroids may reduce the nausea and vomiting experienced following surgery.[32,33] In a recent study, dexamethasone was also reported to prolong the analgesic effects of local anesthetics.[33] It has been asserted that prostaglandins, histamine, and other mediators increase the permeability of local vessels, changing the nociception at the site of trauma and leading to the sensation of pain. Steroids inhibit the production of prostaglandins and therefore reduce pain. While the use of steroids may be beneficial, they can also create sufficient immunosuppression so as to mask inflammation or infection.

Deliberate Controlled Hypotension

Extensive dissection is required for head and neck tumors with operative times extending to 12 or more hours. Considerable fluid replacement, blood loss, electrolyte imbalances, and cardiovascular and respiratory changes may occur during surgery. The surgeon may request deliberate controlled hypotension to reduce blood loss. Patients must be individually evaluated prior to controlled hypotension to determine a safe mean pressure. The effects of common intravenous controlled hypotensive techniques are compared in Table 36-3.[34-37] The practice of controlled hypotension focuses on reducing the mean arterial pressure to some predetermined level related to the limits of cerebral and systemic autoregulation. The mean pressure is not usually allowed to fall below 60 mm Hg, maintaining cerebral and renal autoregulation as well as adequate coronary artery blood flow. Patients with chronic hypertension may require a higher mean pressure to maintain adequate perfusion.[37] Regardless of the technique or medication chosen, it is imperative that urine output, mean arterial blood pressure, cerebral and cardiac perfusion pressure, and arterial blood gases be closely monitored and maintained. Due to the high acuity of this technique, the need for accurate blood pressure monitoring and frequent sampling for blood gases and electrolytes, an arterial line will provide the minute-to-minute access required during controlled hypotension.

PONV

All patients are at risk for postoperative nausea and vomiting (PONV). ENT procedures, particularly of the middle ear, are associated with a high incidence of PONV. Patients experiencing PONV are uncomfortable after surgery, their discharge may be delayed from the postanesthesia care unit (PACU), or they may have an unscheduled hospital admission. PONV delays recovery and reduces patient satisfaction.

The anesthetic drugs and the techniques used can affect both the central chemoreceptor trigger zone (CTZ) and peripheral receptors in the gastric area, eye, and middle ear that are thought to be responsible for PONV. Using a combination of drugs and treatments early in the preoperative period that attenuate both the central and peripheral effects may decrease the incidence of PONV. Since PONV is multifaceted it is not likely that one particular drug or treatment will prevent PONV in all paients. There are a number of factors attributed to the cause of PONV; these are listed in Table 36-4. A combination of drugs, fluid balance, and limiting exposure to anesthetics producing PONV may be beneficial. Highly selective serotonin receptor antagonists have been successful in treating PONV both preemptively and during emesis. Drugs such as metoclopramide increase lower esophageal sphincter tone, speed gastric emptying, lower gastric fluid volume, and may aid in the prevention of PONV.

Vigorous mask ventilation in the anesthetized patient may cause insufflation of air and irritating volatile agents into the stomach, creating PONV. Side effects from drugs such as opioids, nitrous oxide, edrophonium, and neostigmine can produce PONV. Decompressing the stomach after induction of general anesthesia empties the stomach of gas and fluid,

TABLE 36-3 Common Intravenous Agents for Hypotensive Techniques

Drug and Dosage	Advantages	Disadvantages
Sodium nitroprusside Variable age- and anesthetic-dependent effects; 1-5 mcg/kg/min young adults; 6-8 mcg/kg/min children	Potent; reliable; rapid onset and recover; cardiac output well preserved	Reflex tachycardia; rebound hypertension; pulmonary shunting; cyanide toxicity possible
Adenosine 0.06-0.35 mcg/kg/min	Reliable; rapid onset and recovery; increased coronary blood flow	Reflex tachycardia; possible inadequate cerebral perfusion when combined with hemodilution; greatly reduced urinary output
Esmolol 200 mcg/kg/min to achieve 15% reduction of mean arterial pressure	Particularly useful to control tachycardia	Potential for significant cardiac depression
Nitroglycerin 125-500 mcg/kg/min adults 10 mcg/kg/min children	Preserves myocardial blood flow; reduces preload; preserves tissue oxygenation	Increases intracranial pressure; highly variable dosage requirements
Fenoldopam 0.5-22 mcg/kg/min	Preserves renal blood flow	Reflex tachycardia; rebound hypertension; increased pulmonary shunting
Nicardipine* 5 mcg/kg/min	Ca++ channel blocker Preserves cerebral blood flow	
Remifentanil with propofol† Remi: 1 mcg/kg IV then continuous infusion 0.25-0.5 mcg/kg/min Prop: 2.5 mg/kg IV then infusion of 12o mcg/kg/min	Remifenanil reduces middle ear blood flow creating a dry surgical field for tympanoplasty Propofol may help reduce PONV	No analgesic effect once remifentanil infusion discontinued

*Tobias JD: *Controlled hypotension in children: A critical review of available agents*, Paediatr Drugs, 4(7):439-453, 2002.
†DeGoute CS, Ray MJ, Manchon M, Dubreuil C, Banssillon V: *Remifentanil and controlled hypotension; comparison with nitroprusside or esmolol during tympanoplasty*, Can J Anaesth, 48(1):20-27, 2001.
From McNulty SE: *Induced hypotension during head and neck surgery*, Otolaryngol Head Neck Surg 11:605, 1993; Kim KH, Moon IS, Park JS, Koh YB, Ahn H: *Nicardipine hypdrocloride injectable phase IV open label clinical tiral: Study on the antihypertensive effects and safety of nicardipine for acute aortic dissection*, J Int Med Rex, 3(30):337-345, 2002.

TABLE 36-4 Factors Related to Postoperative Nausea and Vomiting

Patient Considerations	Surgical Considerations	Anesthetic Agents and Techniques	Additional Considerations
Abdominal tumors	Operational site	Inhalation agents	Hypotension
Increased ICP	Duration of procedure	Intravenous agents	Hypoxia
Drug therapy		Opioids	Pain
Age		Gastric emptying	Hypercapnia
Obesity		Full stomach	Hypovolemia
Gender		Positioning	
Metabolic changes		Rapid position changes	

thereby diminishing gastric distention; this proceducre may decrease the likelihood of PONV. The accumulation of blood in the posterior oropharynx, which may drain into the stomach or be swallowed during the postoperative period, can lead to PONV. Packing the back of the throat with a surgical pack during the surgical procedure can prevent some drainage into the stomach. Care must be taken that the patient is awake, all surgical packs are removed, and suctioning of the airway precedes the extubation process, producing a clear airway and ensuring the control of protective airway reflexes.

Dehydration secondary to prolonged nothing by mouth (NPO) status or bleeding can contribute to PONV and electrolyte imbalance. Vigorous intravenous (IV) hydration and restoration with crystalloids, blood, and electrolytes during surgery to restore intravascular volume and electrolytes can offset PONV caused by the physiologic effects of hypovolemia. Certain anesthetic agents are known to increase nausea and vomiting, including etomidate, ketamine, opioids, nitrous oxide, and anticholinesterase agents.[38-41] Propofol possesses an antiemetic effect,[42] and isoflurane appears to be less emesis-provoking than halothane.[41,43] Ketorolac is a nonsteroidal antiinflammatory analgesic that is effective as a perioperative analgesic. It provides excellent postoperative analgesia and less emesis compared with equipotent doses of morphine.[44] A multimodal approach is advocated to attenuate PONV in ENT patients.[45]

Laser Surgery

Anesthesia and laser surgery is also discussed in Chapter 40. The term *laser* is an acronym for *l*ight *a*mplification by *s*timulated *e*mission of *r*adiation. Laser technology has been used in medicine for more than 25 years. The two most common lasers used in ENT surgery are the CO_2, Nd:YAG (neodymium-yttrium aluminum garnet), and recently the argon laser.[46] Laser light is different from standard light. Whereas standard light has a variety of wavelengths, lasers have only one wavelength (monochromatic); laser light oscillates in the same phase or all the photons are moving in the same direction (coherent), and its beam is parallel (collimated). The wavelength of the ND:YAG laser beam is shorter as it passes through the garnet than that of the CO_2 laser. The shorter wavelength allows less absorption by water and therefore less tissue penetration. For example, the shorter wavelength of the ND:YAG allows the laser light to pass through the cornea, whereas the longer wavelength of the CO_2 laser would burn the cornea. Laser light emits a small amount of radiation and can be infrared, visible, and ultraviolet in the spectrum. Lasers enable very precise excision, produce minimal edema and bleeding, and are favored by surgeons for resection of tumors and other obstructions of the airway. For operations in and around the larynx, the CO_2 laser is most often used because of its shallow depth of burn and extreme precision.[47] The CO_2 laser produces a beam with a relatively long wavelength that is absorbed almost entirely by the surface of these tissues, vaporizing cellular water. Intermittent bursts of the CO_2 laser produce intense, precisely directed energy that results in a clean cut through the target tissue with minimal amount of penetration of surrounding tissue. A low-energy helium-neon laser is commonly used to aim or direct CO_2 laser beams.

Compared with the CO_2 laser, the ND:YAG laser is poorly absorbed by water but easily absorbed by hemoglobin and pigmented tissues. The ND:YAG laser light is capable of producing deep tissue penetration that may not be apparent for hours or days after exposure to the laser. The ND:YAG allows debulking of larger tumors within body cavities. For this reason, the ND:YAG laser is best suited for resection of bronchial, esophageal, bladder, hepatic, and splenic tumors.[48]

Laser light beams are primarily used for their thermal effect and can be used to cut, coagulate, or vaporize tissues. The exact tissue interaction of a laser is dependent on several variables, including the types of tissues being irradiated, the wavelength of the emitted beam, and the power of the beam.

The use of laser technology mandates taking measures to ensure the safety of the patient and operating room personnel (Box 36-2). Specific concerns include eye protection with

BOX 36-2

General Safety Protocol for Surgical Lasers

1. Post warning signs outside any operating area: "WARNING: LASER IN USE."
2. Patient's eyes should be protected with appropriate colored glasses and/or wet gauze.
3. Matte-finish (black) surgical instruments reduce beam reflection and dispersion.
4. Use the lowest concentration of oxygen possible.
5. Avoid using N_2O since it supports combustion.
6. Lasers should be placed in STANDBY mode when not in use.
7. Use an endotracheal tube specifically prepared for use with lasers.
8. Inflate cuff of laser tube with normal saline.
9. All adjacent tissues should be shielded by wet gauze to prevent damage by reflected beams.
10. Plume should be suctioned and evacuated from the surgical field.

appropriate colored glasses, avoidance of the dispersion of noxious fumes, and fire prevention. Stray or reflected beams of the ND:YAG laser are capable of traversing the eye to the retina; therefore, green-lensed eye protection for all personnel is mandatory during its use. All persons in the operating room must wear goggles specifically designed to absorb ND:YAG laser beams. The required protective eye wear for CO_2 can be any clear glass or plastic that surrounds the face. Orange-red eye protection is required for the potassium-titanyl phosphate (KTP) laser and orange glasses for the argon laser.

When tissues are cut by a laser, the smoke and vapors that are formed are called laser "plume". This plume is an environmental concern and potentially toxic to operating room personnel. When the tissues vaporized by the laser are malignancies or viral papilloma, the concern arises as to whether these vapors are even more dangerous to operating room personnel if not removed from the environment. Because this issue remains under investigation, it is judicious to suction the laser plume and not allow it to circulate into the room.

The prevention of combustion within the airway is of primary concern to the anesthetist. Fire in the airway is relatively uncommon (0.4%) and it is usually due to penetration of the laser through the endotracheal tube, which exposes the beam to a rich oxygen supply. Nitrous oxide, although not flammable, also supports combustion and can propagate the flame.[49] Positive pressure ventilation in the presence of intraluminal combustion produces a blowtorch effect with serious damage to the respiratory tract of the unfortunate patient.[47,50] Steps to reduce the possibility of fire include using the lowest concentration of oxygen appropriate for a particular patient, avoiding paper surgical drapes, spraying the flame with a 60-ml syringe filled with normal saline, and using water-based rather than oil-based lubricants. Once a flame has been ignited, the endotracheal tube should be immediately removed and replaced with a new endotracheal tube large enough to allow the surgeon to assess the lungs with a bronchoscope.

The "perfect" endotracheal tube for use with lasers remains a major discussion (Table 36-5). The necessity of an inflatable cuff is a point of debate, although its ability to better ventilate the patient and keep the field free of combustible gases is an advantage. Cuff material must be made of thinner substance than the tube body, making it more susceptible to laser penetration. When filled with air, the cuff becomes a generous reservoir of combustion-supporting gas. If a cuffed tube is used, inflation with methylene blue–tinged normal saline is encouraged; then if a laser beam contacts the cuff, the colored liquid will absorb and disperse heat, alerting the surgeon and anesthetist to the penetration, and the liquid will reduce combustion.[51,52] Using high-flow jet ventilation (HFJV) can also be used but poses several problems. Many HFJV systems use oxygen only, which dries the tissues quickly and provides gases for ignition in the open airway.[53,54]

The American Society for Testing and Materials (ASTM) Subcommittee F29.02.10 of the Anesthesia Patient Safety Foundation developed guidelines for the provision of safe anesthesia during laser surgery for the upper airway. These guidelines compare and comment on the advantages and disadvantages of several anesthetic techniques and laser-resistant endotracheal tubes.[51-53]

Endoscopy

Endoscopic surgery includes panendoscopy, laryngoscopy, microlaryngoscopy (laryngoscopy aided by an operating microscope), esophagoscopy, and bronchoscopy. All of these procedures can be performed by using a rigid or flexible endoscope. If the rigid laryngoscope is used, the laryngoscope may be suspended from an arching support anchored to the patient's abdomen/chest or from a Mayo stand over the patient. One of the most common endoscopic procedures performed is the endoscopic sinus surgery. Endoscopic sinus surgery is often associated with multiple and seasonal allergies leading to polyps. Patients undergoing surgery are often also being

TABLE 36-5 Advantages and Disadvantages of Commonly Available Laser-Resistant Tracheal Tubes

Tube Type	Advantages	Disadvantages
Metal	Atraumatic external surface Double cuff maintains seal even if punctured by laser Kink resistant	Thick-walled nonflammable cuff reflects laser and transfers heat Cuff difficult to deflate if punctured Metal may reflect beam onto non-targeted tissue
Polyvinyl chloride (PVC)	Inexpensive Nonreflective Maintains shape well Double cuff maintains seal after proximal cuff puncture	Burns vigorously and yields pulmonary toxin (hydrogen chloride) Cuffed version contains flammable material
Red rubber	Wrapping protects flammable material, but dries tube Maintains structure Nonreflective	Red rubber itself is highly flammable Tubes are thick walled
Silicone rubber	Wrapping protects flammable material Methylene blue aids in detection of cuff perforation Nonreflective	Contains flammable material Turns to toxic ash Single cuff is vulnerable to laser damage

Modified from Pashayan A: Laser safety in the operating room, Current Rev Nur Anesth, *18:11-19, 1995; Sois MB: Which is the safest endotracheal tube for use with CO_2 laser: A comparative study,* J Clin Anesth *4:217, 1992; Sois M, Heller S: A comparison of five metallic tapes for endotracheal tube protection during CO_2 laser surgery,* Can J Anaesth *35:S63, 1988.*

evaluated for such pathology responsible for hoarseness, stridor, or hemoptysis. Other possible reasons for endoscopic examination include foreign-body aspiration, papillomas, trauma, tracheal stenosis, obstructing tumors, or vocal cord dysfunction. Several complications can arise with endoscopic surgery; eye trauma, epistaxis, laryngospasm, bronchospasm, and excessive plasma levels of local anesthesia and epinephrine have been reported.[55,56] Preoperatively, the patient should be examined for any signs of airway obstruction and proper measures taken to ensure safe and controlled airway management. Knowledge of the location and size of a mass is important and discussion with the surgeon about chest roentgenogram, magnetic resonance imaging (MRI), and computed tomography (CT) scan results can be invaluable.[55]

Light sedation is suggested for premedication since older children and adults may experience respiratory depression and worsening of airway obstruction. The airway must be protected from aspiration of gastric contents, especially during prolonged airway manipulation and deeper sedation. Premedication with an antisialagogue to dry secretions and a full regimen of acid aspiration prophylaxis in aspiration-prone patients may be indicated. An awake oral or nasal intubation with minimal sedation and topical anesthesia of the oral cavity, pharynx, larynx, and nasopharynx may be indicated. For shorter ENT procedures, anesthesia should be maintained with short-acting inhalation and intravenous agents to avoid patient movement and vocal cord movement, and to control sympathetic nervous system response to brief periods of extreme stimulation as in laryngoscopy.

Good muscle relaxation of the vocal cords is an essential part of anesthesia management for microsurgery of the larynx. A short-acting relaxant or infusion may be considered for brief cases. If the procedure is expected to last 30 minutes or more, use of an intermediate-duration neuromuscular blocking drug such as vecuronium, atracurium, cisatracurium, or rocuronium for the initial tracheal intubation allows the return of muscle strength and spontaneous respiration to meet extubation criteria at the end of the surgical procedure. Emergence should include adequate oropharyngeal suctioning, humidified oxygenation, and observation in the PACU for laryngeal spasm or postextubation croup.

One of the greatest management challenges during endoscopic procedures is to share the airway continuously with the surgeon. Several methods have been used to provide oxygenation and ventilation during the procedures. One method is to control the airway by using a small, cuffed endotracheal tube (5.0 to 6.0 mm for an adult). Since the 5.0-mm and 6.0-mm endotracheal tubes are designed for smaller patients, a better endotracheal tube selection might include the microlaryngeal endotracheal tube (MLT). The MLT in similar sizes (5.0 to 6.0 mm) has a cuff that is larger than the small standard endotracheal tubes (5.0 to 6.0 mm), allowing for a larger cuff distribution across the surface of the trachea, and creates a wider field of pressure on the tracheal surface. There are some distinct advantages of an endotracheal tube; these include a secure airway with easily controlled ventilation, a cuff to protect the lower airway from debris, monitoring of end-tidal CO_2, and the ability to administer inhalational anesthetics. Several drawbacks include the potential for extubation and loss of airway, complications during laser surgery, and interference with the operative field by the endotracheal tube.

Intermittent apnea is also used as a technique to ventilate patients in this shared space. The anesthetist or the surgeon repeatedly removes the endotracheal tube, operates during a brief period of apnea, and then allows the anesthesia provider to reintubate and ventilate the patient. One advantage of the technique is that no special equipment is needed to ventilate the patient. Many of the patients having these procedures have a long history of heavy smoking and alcohol use, which predisposes them to cardiovascular disease and labile vital signs. Some of the disadvantages of this approach include difficulty in reintubation of the patient and the time allotment between ventilations while preventing desaturations. The procedure must be interrupted frequently to ventilate the patient, and the airway is unprotected while the endotracheal tube is removed. During this technique the blood pressure and heart rate tend to fluctuate widely. The procedure resembles a series of stress-filled laryngoscopies and intubations, separated by varying periods of minimal surgical stimulation. Intravenous administration or topical application of agents such as lidocaine; small doses of alfentanil, remifentanil, sufentanil, or fentanyl; and/or a β-adrenergic receptor blocking drugs such as esmolol may help moderate the sympathetic response.

Jet Ventilation

Jet ventilation has been used extensively for laryngeal surgery. When the trachea is not intubated, a metal needle mounted in the operating laryngoscope or passed through the cords can be used for jet ventilation. Jet ventilation may be performed manually, using a simple hand valve attached to an appropriate oxygen source, or with the use of various mechanical devices that allow for adjustment of rate and oxygen concentration. Because oxygen can support combustion, the anesthetist should consider as low a concentration of oxygen as is possible. Many patients will tolerate an FiO_2 of 30% or less; however, oxygen requirements for each patient should be considered for their individual needs. Using lower levels of oxygen will be less likely to create a fire.

High-frequency jet ventilation (HFJV) was originally used as a technique to provide adequate oxygenation and alveolar ventilation for rigid bronchoscopy and laryngeal surgery. HFJV is typically ventilation at low tidal volumes with high respiratory rates. A needle connected to a high-pressure hose with a regulator to adjust rate and volume is used to deliver the ventilation. With the tip of the needle either above or below the glottis, the anesthetist directs a high-velocity jet stream of oxygen into the airway lumen. The lungs are ventilated as the mixture of oxygen forces air into the lumen. Introduction of high-pressure (up to 60 psi) jet-injected oxygen entrains room air into the lung, allowing the jet stream of gases into the airway for ventilation.[55,56] While inspiration is accomplished by HFJV pressurizing gas into the airway, the expiration is passive. Therefore, some pauses in ventilation may be necessary to provide adequate time for expiration, particularly in patients with severe respiratory disease.

If an airway mass lies above the level of delivery of the gas jet, it may be easy to force the gas down the trachea during inspiration. But the gases will be trapped during expiration. This air trapping can lead to increased airway pressure, subcutaneous emphysema, and pneumothorax particularly in patients with bullae. The anesthetist or surgeon may also find it difficult to aim the jet into the airway lumen, leading to hypoxia. If the jet is not accurately aimed, gastric distention, subcutaneous emphysema, or barotrauma may result. Patients with decreased pulmonary compliance or increased airway resistance from bronchospasm, obesity, or chronic obstructive pulmonary disease (COPD) are at high risk for hypoventilation with jet techniques. Jet ventilation is contraindicated in any situation in which an unprotected airway is a concern (e.g., full stomach, hiatal hernia, or trauma).[55]

Adequacy of ventilation is assessed by observing chest movement, auscultation with the precordial stethoscope, and a pulse oximeter. Total intravenous anesthesia (TIVA) is the primary anesthesia technique used with HFJV, since volatile agents cannot be delivered and environmental contamination is a concern. TIVA with short-acting agents such as propofol, mivacurium, alfentanil, fentanyl, and remifentanil provide an excellent anesthetic for these procedures.

Foreign Body Aspiration

Aspiration of foreign bodies is a common problem. There is a high morbidity and mortality, particularly in children, who aspirate foreign objects. Some common aspirants include peanuts, popcorn, jelly beans, coins, and bites of meat and hot dogs. The majority of aspirated items are food particles; however, beads, pins, and small toys are not unusual. A common site of foreign body aspiration is the right bronchus. If the patient is supine when the aspiration occurs, the object will most likely be found in the right upper lobe. If the patient is standing, the right lower lobe is most likely to be affected. Signs of aspiration include wheezing, choking, coughing, tachycardia, aphonia, and cyanosis. These signs indicate an obstructive severe irritation and swelling in the airway. As a result of the swelling, air may be trapped in the lungs, not allowing adequate expiration.

The anesthetic management depends on the location of the airway obstruction, the size and location of the object, and the severity of the obstruction. If it is located at the level of the larynx, a simple laryngoscopy with Magill forceps should allow for easy removal of the object. Care must be taken not to dislodge the object and allow the object to fall deeper in the airway. If the foreign body is located in the distal larynx or the trachea, the patient should have an inhalation induction performed in the operating room, maintaining spontaneous respiration. With the patient spontaneously breathing, the surgeon will most likely use a rigid bronchoscope for extraction of the foreign body. Usually, a gentle mask induction without cricoid pressure or positive pressure ventilation is the preferred induction technique.[57] The anesthetist should not assist with respirations because this may cause the object to move further into the airway and compromise ventilation with occlusion. Patients should be placed in the sitting position because it is known to produce the least adverse effect on airway symptoms. An antisialagogue, H_2 antagonist, and metoclopramide are often administered intravenously to decrease secretions and promote gastric emptying; the secretions may obscure the view through the bronchoscope. Patients with full stomachs who are induced with a rapid sequence must be prepared for complete occlusion of the airway.

Direct and sometimes rigid laryngoscopy is typically performed. A rigid bronchoscope is also used and passed through the vocal cords into the trachea. Ventilation is accomplished through a side port of the laryngoscope or bronchoscope that can be attached to the anesthesia circuit. If a foreign body is present, the telescope eyepiece within the bronchoscope is removed and optical forceps are inserted through the bronchoscope for retrieval of the item. While the telescopic eyepiece is being changed, a leak is present in the ventilation system and protracted periods can lead to hypoxia. When an anesthesia gas machine circuit is used, high fresh gas flow rates, large tidal volumes, and high concentrations of inspired volatile anesthetic agents are often necessary to compensate for leaks around the ventilating bronchoscope. Coughing, bucking, or straining during instrumentation with the rigid bronchoscope may cause difficulty for the surgeon and result in damage to the patient's airway; these must be avoided. The best anesthesia technique for rigid laryngoscopy and bronchoscopy is total intravenous anesthesia (TIVA), allowing greater control of cardiovascular stability and relaxation for short periods, as well as ventilation with 100% oxygen, allowing longer periods of hypoventilation without hypoxia.

A rigid bronchoscopy can lead to several complications including damage to dentition, gums, and upper lips and chipped or damaged teeth, all of which can be prevented to some degree with the use of a mouth guard and vigilance. Vagal stimulation may be noted from the extreme head extension, and tracheal tears can occur with the introduction of the bronchoscope. Inadequate ventilation manifests as hypoxemia, hypercarbia, barotrauma, and dysrhythmias. The surgeon must be prepared to perform an emergency tracheostomy or cricothyrotomy if partial obstruction suddenly becomes complete.

At the conclusion of the procedure, patients can be intubated to provide ventilation until returning to consciousness. Allow the patient to return to consciousness as quickly as possible with airway reflexes intact prior to extubation. Laryngeal and subglottic edema may occur for 24 hours after removal of a foreign body. To check for airway edema the cuff of the endotracheal tube can be deflated if not contraindicated, and the lumen of the endotracheal tube should be occluded for one or two breaths during inspiration and expiration while listening for air movement around the tube. If there is no air escaping around the endotracheal tube, postoperative sedation and ventilation might be considered. Close observation and use of humidified oxygen are suggested during the recovery period. Some additional supportive measures that can alleviate some of the postoperative complications that occur include racemic epinephrine, bronchodilators, and steroids.

Procedures of the Ear and Face

Some of the common surgical procedures for the ear and face include procedures such as myringotomy with insertion of tubes, mastoidectomy, acoustic neuroma, stapedectomy, and tympanoplasty. During ear surgery, the anesthetist must be concerned with four major issues: (1) nerve preservation (particularly cranial nerves VII, IX, X, XI, and XII), (2) the effect of nitrous oxide on the middle ear, (3) control of bleeding, and (4) PONV.

Nerve Preservation. Surgical procedures of the ear and face involve meticulous identification and preservation of the facial and other cranial nerves, especially during resection of a glomus tumor or an acoustic neuroma. The identification of these nerves requires the surgeon to isolate and verify function by means of an electrical stimulation. One method used for nerve isolation is the brain stem auditory evoked potential and electrocochleogram monitoring. It has been documented that the facial nerve is more sensitive to the train-of-four than is the ulnar nerve. Studies have also concluded that reliable intraoperative facial nerve monitoring may be performed despite significant neuromuscular blockade as monitored by conventional ulnar train-of-four monitoring.[58,59] However, profound skeletal muscle relaxation should be avoided and a volatile anesthetic drug, because of the muscle-relaxant properties, should be used judiciously as a primary anesthetic. If an opioid-relaxant technique is chosen, a minimum of 30% muscle response using the peripheral nerve stimulator should be preserved.[60] Selecting and using a combined or balanced technique may provide adequate anesthesia with minimal muscle relaxation, producing better outcomes. Opioids used with low-dose volatile agent may provide nerve integrity, allowing better assessment of function, and provide anesthesia adequate enough for the procedure.

Effect of Nitrous Oxide on the Middle Ear. Nitrous oxide is more soluble than nitrogen in blood. Therefore, nitrous oxide diffuses into air-containing cavities more rapidly than the bloodstream can absorb nitrogen. Normally, pressure increase in the middle ear is vented by the eustachian tube into the nasopharynx. Yawning and swallowing actively open the eustachian tubes, but these equalizing maneuvers cannot occur in anesthetized patients. Additionally, pressure may also be increased in the middle ear with positive pressure ventilation by forcing air into the compartment through the eustachian tubes.

During tympanoplasty, the middle ear is opened to the atmosphere and there is no pressure buildup. Once the surgeon has replaced a tympanic membrane graft, the middle ear becomes a closed space. If nitrous oxide is allowed to diffuse into this space, middle ear pressure will rise[61] and the graft may be displaced. Conversely, having administered nitrous oxide then discontinuing the gas after the graft has been placed will create a negative pressure in the middle ear that may last up to 6 weeks postoperatively. Either scenario may contribute to the development of serous otitis, disarticulation of the stapes, displacement of grafts, and impaired hearing.[62] There is no evidence that using N_2O 50% or less for general anesthesia for type 1 tympanoplasty interferes with the graft placement or changes the outcome of the surgical procedure.[63] If N_2O is used and in order to avoid complications, the anesthesia provider should discontinue the administration of N_2O at least 15 minutes before closure of the middle ear.

Control of Bleeding. During microscopic ear surgery, even a small drop of blood can make the procedure difficult. Injecting the ear with an epinephrine-containing solution, often in concentrations of 1:1000; 1:50,000; 1:100,000; and 1:200,000 is performed in the area of the tympanic vessels to produce vasoconstriction. Mild head elevation to decrease venous pressure, lowering of arterial pressure with volatile agents, and (although somewhat controversial) deliberate hypotensive techniques are other methods used to decrease blood loss during these procedures. At the completion of the surgical procedure, the patient's head is lifted, usually wrapped with a bandage; the anesthetist will want to avoid excessive coughing and bucking of the patient during this period. Provided there are no contraindications, a deep extubation might be considered.

Myringotomy and Tube Placement

Most often patients scheduled for myringotomy are young and healthy patients. A myringotomy allows the pressure to equalize between the middle ear and the atmosphere, reducing the pressure in the middle ear compartment. Simple tubes with a lumen are placed through the patient's tympanic membrane to alleviate the pressure created in the middle ear usually seen with chronic serous otitis media or recurrent otitis media. Chronic otitis media is manifested as fluid in the middle ear. Recurrent otitis media, a common pediatric disorder, is defined as six or more episodes of otitis media over the prior year. Untreated otitis media may lead to permanent middle ear damage and hearing loss; therefore, prompt treatment is necessary. Children with chronic otitis frequently have accompanying recurrent upper respiratory infections (URIs). Intervals between URIs may be brief, the patient is usually on a regimen of antibiotics, and scheduling surgery during these interludes is often impractical. Often the eradication of middle ear fluid and inflammation resolves the URI; therefore, surgery should not be delayed.

Bilateral myringotomies with tube insertions are typically very short operations. Sedative premedications may outlast the procedure and are usually not necessary. Mask or IV induction and maintenance using oxygen, nitrous oxide, and a volatile inhalation agent such as sevoflurane, desflurane, isoflurane, or halothane is routine. If IV access is established, it is usually after mask induction in children and may include fluid therapy or an injection cap for temporary access and administration of drugs. Nitrous oxide (N_2O) is often avoided in surgeries that involve the middle ear since it is 34 times more soluble in blood than nitrogen and can create pressure in the closed space.[63] Since the myringotomy surgical procedure is relatively short and a tube will be placed through tympanic membrane into the middle ear to relieve the pressure, the effects of nitrous oxide are often not relevant. For bilateral procedures, the inhalation anesthetic is discontinued during the second myringotomy to facilitate prompt emergence. Nitrous oxide is continued until the completion of the surgery. Intubation is performed only if airway difficulties are anticipated or encountered. However, the airway equipment is always prepared and available. The procedure is typically short and without much risk of bleeding.

The patient is supine with the head turned to expose the ear to the microscope. An ear speculum is inserted into the ear canal, cerumen is removed, and an incision is made in the tympanic membrane. Fluid is sometimes suctioned from the middle ear, and then a tympanostomy tube is inserted through the incision into the middle ear, straddling the tympanic membrane. Antibiotic and steroid eardrops frequently are inserted into the external auditory canal. The surgeon moves to the other side of the table, the microscope is repositioned, the head is turned, and the procedure is repeated in the other ear.

Tonsillectomy and Adenoidectomy

The lateral tonsils, tonsillar tissue at the base of the tongue, and adenoids form a tonsillar "ring" around the oropharynx that can lead to significant airway challenges following surgical intervention. An adenotonsillectomy, although often considered a simple procedure, requires a great degree of finesse by the anesthetist. Considerations of airway obstruction, shared airway, mechanical suspension of the airway, management of intubation and extubation, pain management, and the desire for a rapid awakening are all subtleties of anesthesia that challenge the anesthetist. In adult patients, a tonsillectomy may also accompany a uvulopalatopharyngoplasty (UPPP) for pickwickian syndrome or obstructive sleep apnea (OSA). OSA is typically seen with obesity and redundant pharyngeal tissue. OSA patients can also present with a history of right heart failure and congestive heart failure (CHF), which is not uncommon.[64-66]

The patient undergoing a tonsillectomy and/or adenoidectomy will probably have a higher incidence of airway obstruction because of the hypertrophied tissues. Chronic obstruction and infections of the tonsils can lead to potential systemic involvement, producing additional cardiac and respiratory anomalies. In the case of suspected airway obstruction, the clinician must choose wisely among routine intravenous induction, inhalation induction, awake intubation, or fiberoptic-assisted intubation before induction. Adult patients with severe obstructive sleep apnea may require a tracheostomy under local anesthesia in advance to secure the airway before the induction of general anesthesia. Such determination is based on the degree of obstruction, physical examination of the airway, and the clinical judgment of the anesthetist. Regardless of the induction technique chosen, the use of an antisialagogue is strongly encouraged.

In children, anesthesia is usually induced with a volatile drug, oxygen, and nitrous oxide by mask. Some institutions allow parental presence in the operating room during induction to prevent separation anxiety in the child. Tracheal intubation in children is best accomplished under deep inhalation anesthesia or aided by a short-acting nondepolarizing muscle relaxant. The airway generally is secured with an oral RAE or reinforced tube. A cuffed tube is recommended in those older than 8 to 10 years of age,[4] with continued attention to inflation pressures of the cuff. A properly sized pediatric endotracheal tube should allow a leak at 20 cm H_2O airway pressure, which reduces the likelihood of postoperative croup and edema. The tube must be secured midline. A simple yet effective method of securing the oral RAE tube is to apply a strip of tape directly to the chin, incorporating the endotracheal tube and another strip of tape over the tube. The first strip provides a secure base for the second strip, which actually holds the tube.

After the airway is secured, the mouth gag is inserted by the surgeon. An adequate depth of anesthesia is needed to facilitate gag insertion. The gag, designed to maintain an open mouth and tongue retraction, is equipped with a groove for the endotracheal tube to rest in (Fig. 36-9). The airway should be reevaluated at the time the gag is placed to ensure that the tube has not been moved from its original position and that occlusion of the endotracheal tube has not occurred as a result of compression from the gag. The table is frequently turned 45 to 90 degrees away from the anesthetist just prior to incision.

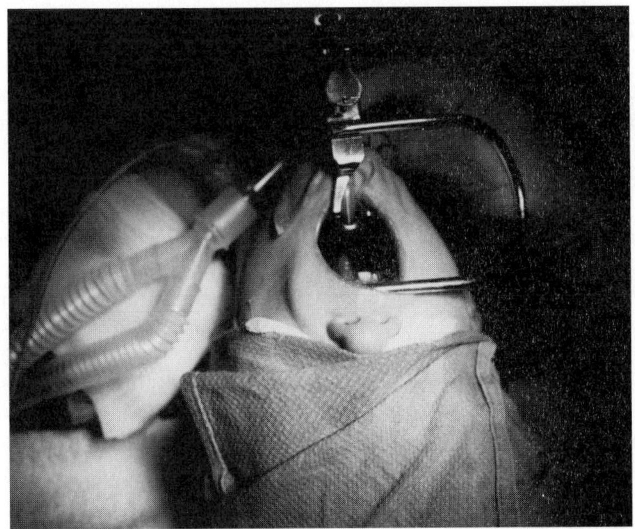

FIGURE **36-9**
Superior view of the suspension technique for tonsillectomy using the Crowe-Davis mouth gag. Note use of preformed RAE orotracheal tube.

The choice of techniques varies for the maintenance of anesthesia. There are four major goals to consider when choosing an anesthetic: (1) provide a depth of anesthesia adequate to blunt strong reflex activity elicited by the procedure, (2) a rapid return of protective reflexes, (3) good postoperative analgesia, and (4) reduced postoperative bleeding. The use of intermediate-acting muscle relaxants is acceptable, but their action must be completely reversed at the end of the case. Judicious narcotic supplementation will reduce the total amount of inhalation agent required and provide analgesia with minimal postoperative respiratory depression. Although postoperative bleeding has been a concern in the past regarding the use of ketorolac, it has been successfully used as an alternative to opioids, has not been found to accentuate bleeding, and has lead to shortened hospital stays following tonsillectomy.[67,68]

Blood loss during tonsillectomy is difficult to assess but has been estimated to average 4 mL/kg or 5% of blood volume.[7] Average blood loss during UPPP is slightly higher because the procedure frequently is performed in conjunction with adenotonsillectomy. Replacement for blood loss of less than 10% of the calculated volume may be accomplished with the administration of 3 mL of crystalloid per milliliter of blood loss. Although younger healthier patients can tolerate greater volumes of blood loss, transfusion should be considered if blood loss exceeds 10% of calculated preoperative blood volume.

At the end of the surgical procedure, the surgeon may release tension on the mouth gag to ensure that all bleeding has been controlled. The insertion of an orogastric tube and some irrigation may be used to remove blood and secretions from the stomach and oropharynx. This is thought to reduce the incidence of postoperative nausea and vomiting. Suctioning of the oropharynx and nares should be done very gently and briefly by avoiding the surgical beds and to prevent disruption of and prevent mucosal bleeding. Vigorous suctioning may also induce laryngospasm and bronchospasm.

During emergence from anesthesia after tonsillectomy or UPPP, the anesthetist should ensure that all protective reflexes have returned, the airway is free of blood and debris, and an adequate breathing pattern is present before the removal of the endotracheal tube. A topical spray of 2% lidocaine (maximum 3 mg/kg) on the glottic and supraglottic areas before intubation prevents postextubation stridor and laryngospasm following adenotonsillectomy. This approach has proved as effective as administering lidocaine, 1 mg/kg IV before extubation, but without higher sedation scores.[69]

The postoperative tonsillectomy patient should be transported to the recovery in the "tonsil position"—that is, on one side with the head slightly down. This allows blood or secretions to drain out of the mouth rather than flow back onto the vocal cords. Adults, however, frequently prefer a middle or high Fowler's position following UPPP. This position aids in ventilation and feeling of asphyxiation in the immediate postoperative period. The anesthetist must however make sure that the patient is awake enough to manage his/her own airway.

One hundred percent oxygen with a high-humidity mist is given by face mask or face tent to hydrate the airway. The pharynx should be rechecked directly for bleeding and edema before discharge from the recovery room.

Increasingly, tonsillectomies are being performed as an outpatient procedure. Although postoperative bleeding is the most serious complication, persistent vomiting and poor oral intake are the most common reasons for unscheduled overnight admission after ambulatory surgery. The incidence of postoperative nausea and vomiting can be as high as 70% during the first 24 hours after tonsillectomy.[70] As discussed previously, it is important to develop anesthetic techniques that incorporate the use of antiemetics in order to minimize episodes of nausea and vomiting.

Bleeding Tonsil

The incidence of posttonsillectomy bleeding that requires surgery is 0.3% to 0.6%. Approximately 75% of the postoperative tonsillar hemorrhages that occur are within 6 hours of the surgical procedure. The remaining 25% of the postoperative bleeds occur within the first 24 hours of surgery, although bleeding may be noted up until the sixth postoperative day.[71] Since the cautery is used for control of bleeding instead of ligatures a slow oozing of the tonsillar bed is far more common than profuse bleeding. One concern is that these patients may swallow large volumes of blood before bleeding is actually discovered. The patient may present with signs of hypovolemia, which are evidenced by tachycardia, hypotension, and agitation. If the blood is swallowed the patient may have nausea and vomiting. Appropriate laboratory tests (e.g., Hb and Hct) should be performed to determine replacement. If reoperation is deemed necessary, restoration of intravascular volume and/or blood based on the volume lost should precede induction. It is important to evaluate the adequacy of intravenous access (two lines may be appropriate), assess the coagulation variables, and be prepared to transfuse blood. All such patients should be assumed to have a significant amount of blood in the stomach, and an awake intubation of the trachea should be an initial consideration to maintain reflexes. At induction of anesthesia, an additional person should be available to provide suctioning of blood from the oropharynx. If an awake technique is not practical, a rapid-sequence induction with cricoid pressure should be implemented. The patient should be placed in a slight head-down position to protect the trachea and glottis from aspiration of blood. A nasogastric tube may be placed to removed stomach contents prior to induction and then removed after induction. The induction agent selected is based on the hemodynamics and condition of the patient.

Cleft Palate and Lip

Cleft Palate (Hard Palate and Soft Palate). Cleft palate repair is usually performed in stages, depending on the extent of the defect. For the more severe deformities, the initial operation repairs the lip and anterior portion of the hard palate. The soft palate and other deformities are usually corrected later, after 6 months of age. Infants with cleft lip deformities can have difficulty feeding and may be prone to malnutrition and congenital (heart) anomalies and disease.[72]

Intubation may sometimes be difficult if the laryngoscope blade slips into the cleft. However, packing the cleft with gauze may prevent this from occurring. An oral RAE tube or flexible connector is used and secured at the midline of the lower lip. A specialized mouth gag is used to hold the mouth open and the endotracheal tube in place during cleft palate surgery. All air bubbles should be carefully removed from IV lines to prevent an air embolus due to the incidence of associated cardiac anomalies, such as an atrial-ventricular defect (AVD), that may lead to air crossing from the venous to the arterial circulation. Congenital heart diseases may influence drugs that are selected for maintenance of anesthesia and for infiltration of the operative site, particularly if epinephrine is selected. Care must be implemented to protect the child's eyes since accidental damage may occur during the surgical procedure. Before emergence, a suture is often placed through the tip of the tongue and the suture is taped to the cheek. This suture eliminates the need for an oral airway and prevents damage to the palatal repair. If soft tissue obstruction occurs during emergence or recovery, traction on the suture can alleviate the problem. If edema occurs, a more aggressive and immediate airway management technique should be employed. Copious secretions and blood may cause laryngospasm after extubation, and therefore a clear airway is imperative.

Cleft Lip. Management of unilateral cleft lip repair consists of routine induction followed by oral intubation using an RAE tube or a flexible connector. Patients that have a documented common cold may have perioperative respiratory complications and should be postponed until the symptoms of the cold subside.[73] Secure the tube to the lower lip and midline via tape. To decrease tension on the surgical sutures at the end of the procedure, the surgeon may place a Logan bow across the upper lip of the patient.[74] When the Logan bow is placed, mask ventilation during emergence will become impaired or impossible. Extubation must be performed only with the patient fully awake and reflexes intact. The child's surgical site must also be protected from finger and hand manipulation. Some hospitals recommend the use of hand mittens or taping the extremities onto armboards during the postoperative period. Close monitoring or respiration should proceed into the postoperative period.

Dental Restoration

Dental restoration procedures are performed under general anesthesia for a multitude of reasons. These include rampant cavities, history of cerebral palsy or Down syndrome, and an uncooperative patient who would not be an appropriate candidate for local anesthetic and an office procedure.

Retarded patients develop a close personal relationship with either a family member or their long-term health care worker. It is often suggested that this individual accompany the patient to decrease anxiety and communicate a health history to the anesthesia provider. A thorough airway assessment should be performed before considering induction. Oral midazolam (0.5 mg/kg) or ketamine (3 to 4 mg/kg IM) is most effective in sedating retarded children in the preoperative arena. Since many patients requiring dental restoration have congenital anomalies, it is not uncommon to find patients with small oropharynx, enlarged tonsils, large tongues, and increased secretions. Atlantoaxial instability and congenital heart disease should also be considered in the preoperative preparation and anesthetic management.[72] Preparation and appropriate airway management must be planned and implemented for these patients. Patients who receive phenytoin to control seizures may have gingival hyperplasia. Because the gingiva is highly vascular, any surgical manipulation during restoration may lead to significant blood loss.

In patients with normal airways, a standard induction is appropriate and a nasal intubation usually facilitates the dental procedure. The application of a topical vasoconstrictive nasal spray during the preoperative period reduces or prevents bleeding during the insertion of the nasotracheal tube. Following loss of consciousness, lubricated intranasal trumpets may be inserted into the most patent nasal airway. Starting with a smaller nasal trumpet, several are placed in increasing sizes to dilate the airway. When full dilation of the nares has occurred, a well-lubricated endotracheal tube is passed through the nose into the trachea, either blindly or assisted by Magill forceps under direct laryngoscopy. The nasal endotracheal tube is preferably placed on the side opposite where the surgeon will be working. The endotracheal tube is often sewn to the nasal septum by the surgeon. Throat packs may be placed to prevent blood from entering the stomach and causing nausea and vomiting; monitoring their removal is essential to preventing respiratory obstruction following extubation.

Sinus and Nasal Procedures

Nasal and sinus procedures for drainage of chronic sinusitis, polyp removal, repair of deviated septum, or closed reduction of fractures generally involves the young and healthy patient population. Many of the patients having sinus and nasal surgery have chronic environmental and drug allergies; therefore, there is an increased incidence of reactive airway disease in these patients. The use of fiberoptics or functional endoscopic sinus surgery for nasal and sinus surgery has become a popular treatment for chronic sinusitis.

Nasal surgery may be successfully accomplished with local, monitored anesthesia care (MAC) or general anesthesia. All three methods of anesthesia require profound vasoconstriction. The mucous membranes of the sinuses and nose are highly vascular, and blood loss may be significant if vasoconstriction is not employed. The surgeon may select to control vasoconstriction with epinephrine or cocaine. The anesthetist may be asked to use a hypotensive technique or slight head elevation (10 to 20 degrees) during the procedure. Using general anesthesia has been associated with an increased blood loss even with the use of an epinephrine injection. This exaggerated blood loss may be related to the vasodilatory properties of the inhalation agents. Delivering general anesthesia for sinus surgery with propofol as well as other intravenous anesthetic techniques for the maintenance of anesthesia has been associated with less blood loss than occurs with the use of volatile agents for maintenance.[75] The placement of an oropharyngeal pack and light suctioning of the stomach at emergence may attenuate postoperative retching and vomiting. After all of the packing is removed, extubation should be performed on the awake patient who has regained control of protective reflexes.[76] The use of intravenous or topical lidocaine may reduce some of the coughing prior to extubation, leading to less bleeding in the postoperative period.

Trauma

Initial Assessment. Traumatic disruption of the bony, cartilaginous, and soft tissue components of the face and upper airway challenge the anesthesia provider to recognize the nature and extent of the injury and consequent anatomic alteration. It is imperative to create an anesthetic plan for securing the airway without promoting further damage or compromising ventilation. Possible mechanisms by which the upper or lower airway may become obstructed include edema; bleeding from the oral mucosa and palate; intraoral fracture sites; the presence of foreign bodies such as avulsed teeth, blood clots, or bony fragments; distortion of the nasal passages; injury of the pharynx and sinuses; and open lacerations.[77]

Initial management of the airway depends on the situation at hand. In the case of severe facial or neck trauma, alternative methods of tracheal intubation, such as fiberoptic laryngoscopy, retrograde wire placement, jet ventilation via a cricothyrotomy or emergent tracheostomy, may be necessary to secure the airway.

Injuries of the head and neck should alert the anesthetist to possible cervical spine injury. Although a complete evaluation of all cervical vertebrae is ideal, inspection of a lateral radiograph of the cervical spine is judicious to determine the presence or absence of dislocations and fractures. All seven cervical vertebrae must be visible in such studies. The seventh cervical vertebra is the most common site of traumatic fracture of the spine.[77] Vertebral artery injury must be suspect with a cervical injury since these fractures can lead to vertebral artery tear or occlusion.[78] If deteriorating respiratory function requires immediate airway management and intubation, the head should be maintained in a fixed position before any manipulation of the airway is performed. The use of manual in-line axial stabilization (MAIS) and/or a rigid cervical collar in place is recommended. The removal of the anterior segment of the collar can facilitate intubation and manipulation of the soft tissues of the neck.

Blunt trauma to the face or anterior neck may produce rapid airway occlusion, secondary to soft tissue edema, or hematoma formation, secondary to trauma of the vascular structures of the neck. The patient exhibiting smoke or blistering in the area of the mouth and nares or with a history of inhalation of toxic by-products of combustion should be intubated immediately. Edema of the face and glottis, which may lack symptoms in the early stages, has the potential to produce serious airway compromise several hours after injury. Securing the airway by either oral or nasal intubation is preferable to tracheostomy, which is associated with a higher incidence of complications.[79]

Maxillofacial Trauma and Orthognathic Surgery

Le Fort[80] determined the common fracture lines of the maxilla face by experimentation on cadavers in 1901. The fractures are divided into Le Fort I, II, and III.[81] Figure 36-10 shows the three classic patterns. The Le Fort I fracture is a horizontal fracture of the maxilla extending from the floor of the nose and hard palate, through the nasal septum, and through the pterygoid plates posteriorly. The palate, maxillary alveolar bone, lower pterygoid plate, and part of the palatine bone are all mobilized. The Le Fort II fracture is a triangular fracture running from the bridge of the nose, through the medial and inferior wall of the orbit, beneath the zygoma, and through the lateral wall of the maxilla and the pterygoid plates. The Le Fort III fracture totally separates the midfacial skeleton from the cranial base, traversing the root of the nose, the ethmoid bone, the eye orbits, and the sphenopalatine fossa.

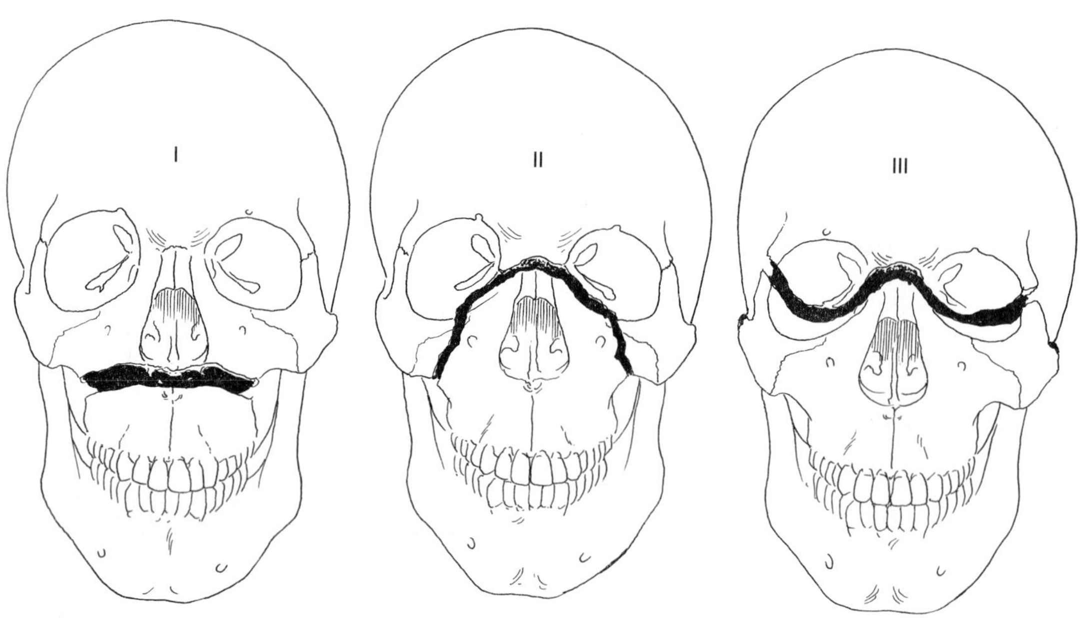

FIGURE **36-10**
Examples of the Le Fort I, II, and III facial fractures from left to right.

A Le Fort I fracture generally causes little difficulty for the anesthesia provider. Patients may be intubated orally or nasally and the airway secured without a problem. The Le Fort II and Le Fort III fractures are of particular concern to the anesthetist contemplating nasal intubation. In both of these fractures, disruption of the cribriform plate may occur, opening the underside of the cranial cavity. The presence of cerebral fluid in the nose, blood behind a tympanic membrane, periorbital edema, or "coon-eyes" hematoma are indications that attempts to pass an endotracheal tube or nasogastric tube through the nares could lead to inadvertent intracranial placement.[82] Although the insertion of a nasal tube may aid the surgeon, an attempted nasotracheal intubation of a patient with a basal skull fracture involves the very serious risk of introducing the tube into the skull, bringing contaminated material into the subarachnoid space and causing meningitis. The tube may also inflict damage to the brain itself.

The forces required to produce facial fractures are considerable and may be associated with other trauma. It is important that cervical spine injury, subdural hematoma, pneumothorax, and intraabdominal bleeding be investigated. Soft tissue injury to the airway and blood or debris in the oropharynx may make visualization impossible. If in doubt while in the emergency department, a tracheostomy under local anesthesia or an awake oral intubation with topical anesthesia should be considered. These patients should be treated with full stomach precautions.

As with any trauma victim, attention is first directed toward maintaining the ABCs: airway, breathing, and circulation. The repair of the facial fracture may be carried out at a later time. Once the patient arrives in the operating room for surgery (sometimes 24 to 48 hours after insult), it may be challenging to open the patient's mouth for intubation due to edema, pain, or trismus. It is necessary to differentiate the cause of the small mouth opening since it may be pain related or mechanical in nature. The administration of a short-acting narcotic or midazolam will sometimes assist the anesthesia provider in determining the cause of the restriction, which greatly influences the induction chosen. In mandibular or maxillary fractures, nasal intubation is usually best, because the patient's teeth are brought together via wires or rubber bands at the conclusion of surgery (intermaxillary fixation). Anesthesia is induced with an IV agent and maintained with narcotics, muscle relaxants, and inhalation agents. Blood loss from facial fractures can be extensive. The patient's blood should be typed and crossmatched so that blood is immediately available. The fixation process closes the teeth in proper occlusion and also prevents access to the oropharynx. Masking the patient at emergence requires that the patient be awake with intact reflexes at extubation. It also requires that wire cutters or scissors be available to cut the wire or rubber bands fixing the mandible to the maxilla in case an airway emergency occurs in the recovery area.

Orthopedic orthognathic procedures often require a sagittal splitting of the mandible to move the lower jaw either forward or back. A Le Fort I or Le Fort II osteotomy may be purposefully performed to move the maxilla in any direction to correct anomalies. Many of these patients have anomalies of the mandible and maxilla, small mouth openings, and appliances that make intubation difficult and airway management challenging. Since many of the malocclusions are treated orally, a nasal endotracheal tube is usually preferred over an oral intubation. Securing the nasotracheal tube away from the surgical field without causing necrotic injury of the nares is vital. Because blood loss during these procedures can be extensive, the patient is typed and crossmatched, and deliberate hypotensive anesthetic techniques are often employed. Rigid external or internal fixation devices are used to maintain stability in both the mandible and maxilla postoperatively; therefore the proper cutting tools should be at the patient's bedside for emergency airway issues. The anesthetist must also consider that edema will many times be extensive and progress over the first 24 hours following orthognathic surgery. To prevent postoperative respiratory problems the patient may remain intubated for several days. If extubation is necessary, it should only be done when the patient is awake and in full command of his or her reflexes.

Radical Neck Dissection

Radical neck dissection is required when cancerous tumors have invaded the musculature and other structures of the head and neck. Neoplastic growths can occur anywhere within the upper airway and may achieve significant size with little evidence of airway penetration or obstruction. These tumors are often friable and bleed readily. These patients are frequently heavy drinkers and smokers who have bronchitis, pulmonary emphysema, or cardiovascular disease. If the tumor interferes with eating then weight loss, malnutrition, anemia, dehydration, and electrolyte imbalance can be significant. Patients who have had radiation treatments of the neck and jaw prior to surgical intervention will have soft tissues that are less mobile, making intubation more difficult. Many of these patients are older. The number of complications in patients age 65 and older are nearly double those of younger patients.[82-84] Attempted tracheal intubation can induce significant hemorrhage and edema, causing severe compromise of the airway.

Consultation with a surgeon as to the nature, extent, and location of the tumor; therapy administered (radiation or chemotherapy); CT results; history and physical examination; and so on remains important in determining the appropriate techniques for airway management.

Head and neck reconstruction is an integral part of surgical removal of head and neck tumors. Traditional methods of reconstruction include regional pedicle flaps with microvascular reconstruction. These flaps include pectoralis major myocutaneous flap; trapezius flap; and local rotational flaps, such as forehead flap. Additionally, small bowel may be harvested to reconstruct the oropharynx and esophagus. The anesthesia team plays an important role in maximizing the overall success rate of a free flap and microvascular flow of the flap.[83] The anesthetist must communicate with the surgeon regarding the planned donor site, which will limit the available sites to place lines necessary for monitoring and venous access. Although the choice of monitoring is largely dependent on the general condition of the patient, the placement of a central venous pressure (CVP) line, a Foley catheter, and an arterial line (beat-to-beat and arterial blood gas trends) is suggested, particularly if deliberate hypotension during anesthesia is used. A pulmonary artery catheter may be useful if a history of cardiac problems is present. The internal jugular approach should be avoided because of proximity to the surgical site. Sites commonly used for the CVP and pulmonary catheter placement when the internal jugular is not accessible are the subclavian and femoral veins.

Maintenance of anesthesia is often performed with an inhalation agent and supplemental narcotics. The use of a nondepolarizing muscle relaxant must be discussed with the surgical team preoperatively because a nerve stimulator is frequently used (by the surgeon) to locate nerves distorted by the tumor during the procedure. Significant blood loss can be a problem; sometimes a controlled hypotension technique may be requested.[85] At least one and preferably two large-bore peripheral IV lines (16 to 14 gauge) should be in place. The patient's blood should be typed and crossmatched, with blood readily available. It is important to replace blood loss, but not to the point of overloading the patient. Monitoring estimated blood loss and measuring the hematocrit may provide some guidelines for replacement of blood. A positive fluid balance in the postoperative phase can result in edema and congestion of the flap, predisposing it to vascular compromise. Colloids may be used to help limit the amount of crystalloid required during the procedure. Patients undergoing a radical neck dissection are frequently hypovolemic and have electrolyte imbalances. This requires some fluid replacement and electrolyte balance intraoperatively to maintain cardiovascular stability.

In preparation for a tracheostomy or total laryngectomy to be performed during the surgical procedure, the patient should receive 100% oxygen. The trachea will be transected by the surgeon, which requires that the anesthesia provider suction the airway and remove the endotracheal tube only to a level above the tracheal incision. Once the tracheostomy tube has been placed by the surgeon and ventilation validated, the endotracheal tube can then be completely removed. A reinforced tube is usually placed in the distal airway by the surgeon and connected to the anesthesia machine. A reassessment of the ventilation should be performed including the entire procedure of listening to bilateral breath sounds, observing chest excursion, end-tidal CO_2, and positive inspiratory pressure (PIP) or negative inspiratory pressure (NIP). After the anesthesia provider has validated tube placement, the endotracheal tube is sutured to the chest wall for the entire surgical duration. At the end of surgery, the reinforced tube may be switched for a tracheostomy cannula.

During radical lymph node dissection of the neck for carcinoma, manipulation of the carotid sinus may elicit a vagal reflex, causing bradycardia, hypotension, or cardiac arrest. Small doses of local anesthetic injected near the carotid sinus or administration of an anticholinergic may block vagal reflexes. Due to the long duration of the surgery and interruption of venous flow, venous thrombus is commonly seen in patients who are undergoing radical neck dissection. Venous air embolism may also occur during radical neck dissection from the head-up position and open neck veins during surgery. Careful monitoring with precordial Doppler sonography or transesophageal echocardiography (TEE) provide the best detection of air embolism. Immediate removal of the air through the CVP is essential. Laryngeal edema and obstruction can also occur as a result of the venous stasis that follows major disruptions in venous flow during surgery. Further review of complications and treatments are necessary.[86]

Postoperative considerations consist of tracheostomy care; controlled ventilation; chest roentgenogram to rule out pneumothorax, hemothorax, and pulmonary edema; and monitoring for laryngeal edema induced by thrombosis. Postoperative characteristics of various surgical laryngectomy procedures are given in Table 36-6. It is suggested that these patients be admitted overnight in the intensive care unit because they have undergone major fluid and electrolyte shifts and altered ventilation/perfusion status and have spent an extensive time under the influence of anesthesia.

TABLE 36-6 Laryngectomy

Structures Removed	Structures Remaining	Postoperative Conditions
Total Laryngectomy		
Hyoid bone Entire larynx (Epiglottis, false cords, true cords) Cricoid cartilage Two or three rings of trachea	Tongue Pharyngeal wall Lower trachea	Loses voice; breathes through tracheostomy; no problem swallowing
Supraglottic or Horizontal Laryngectomy		
Hyoid bone Epiglottis False vocal cords	True vocal cords Cricoid cartilage Trachea	Normal voice; may aspirate occasionally, especially liquids; normal airway
Vertical (or HEMI-) Laryngectomy		
One true vocal cord False cord Arytenoid One half thyroid cartilage	Epiglottis One false cord One true vocal cord Cricoid	Hoarse but serviceable voice; normal airway; no problem swallowing
Laryngofissure and Partial Laryngectomy		
One vocal cord	All other structures	Hoarse but serviceable voice; occasionally almost normal voice; no airway problem; no swallowing problem
Endoscopic Removal of Early Carcinoma		
Part of one vocal cord	All other structures	May have a normal voice; no other problems

From Drain CB: Perianesthesia Nursing, *ed 4, Saunders, St. Louis, 2003, p 446.*

SUMMARY

The provision of anesthesia for ENT and maxillofacial procedures requires knowledge in basic and advanced anesthesia techniques. The anesthetist should not only subscribe to all the usual tenets of safe practice, but must apply these principles while remaining at a distant from the airway. Cooperation and communication between the surgeon and anesthetist is vital for all concerned, especially the patients in their charge.

REFERENCES

1. Guyton A, Hall J: *Textbook of Medical Physiology*, ed 10, Philadelphia, 2000, Saunders, p 487.
2. Marieb E: *Human Anatomy and Physiology*, ed 4, Benjamin/Cummings Science, Menlo Park, CA, 1998, p 804.
3. Murphy TM: Somatic blockade of the head and neck. In Cousins MJ, Bridenbaugh PO, editors : *Neural Blockade: In Clinical Anesthesia and Management of Pain*, ed. 3, Philadelphia, 1998, Lippencott-Raven, pp 493-505
4. Gronett B, Motoyama E: Induction of anesthesia and endotracheal intubation. In Motoyama E, Davis P, editors: *Smith's Anesthesia for Infants and Children*, ed 6, St Louis, 1996, Mosby, pp 33, 238.
5. Joseph M: Anesthesia for ear, nose and throat surgery. In Longnecker D, Tinker J, Morgan G, editors: *Principles and Practice of Anesthesiology*, ed 2, St Louis, 1998, Mosby, p 2202.
6. Philip J, Feinstein D, Raemer D: Monitoring anesthetic and respiratory gases. In Blitt C, Hines R, editors: *Monitoring in Anesthesia and Critical Care Medicine*, ed 3, New York, 1995, Churchill Livingstone, p 375.
7. Wetzel, RC, Maxwell, LG: Anesthesia for Children. In Longnecker, DE, Tinker, JH, Morgan, GE editors: *Principles and Practice of Anesthesiology*, ed 2, St Louis, 1998, Mosby Year Book, p 2081.
8. Sopher MJ, Sears DH, Walts LF: Neuromuscular monitoring comparing the flexor hallucis brevis and adductor pollicis muscles. *Anesthesiology* 69:129, 1988.
9. Brown ACD: Anesthesia. In Cummings CW, Fredrickson JM, Harker LA, Krause CJ, Schuller DE, editors: *Otolaryngology: Head and Neck Surgery*, vol 1, ed 2, Philadelphia, 1993, Mosby.
10. Gan TJ, Glass PSA, Howell ST, Howell ST, Canada AT, Grant AP, Ginsberg B. Determination of plasma concentrations of propofol associated with 50% reduction in postoperative nausea, *Anesthesiology*. 87:779, 1997.
11. Gregory JA, Tarter PT, Reynolds AF: A complication of nasogastric intubation: intracranial penetration, *J Trauma* 18:822, 1978.
12. Muzzi DA, Losasso TJ, Cucchiara RF: Complications from nasopharyngeal airway in a patient with a basilar skull fracture, *Anesthesiology* 74:366, 1991.
13. Patel KF, Hicks JN: Prevention of fire hazards associated with the use of carbon dioxide lasers, *Anesth Analg*. 60:885, 1981
14. Wat LI: The laryngeal mask airway for oral and maxillofacial surgery, *Int Anesthesiol Clin* 41(3):29-56, 2003.
15. Lopez-Gil M, Brimacombe J, Cebrian J, Arranz J: Laryngeal mask airway in pediatric practice: A prospective study of skill acquisition by anesthesia residents, *Anesthesiology* 84:807-811, 1996.
16. Hapberg C, Abramson D, Chilly J: A comparison of fiberoptic orotracheal intubations using two intubating conduits, *Anesthesiology* 83:A1220, 1995.
17. Frappier J, Guenoun T, Journois D, et al: Airway management using the intubating laryngeal mask airway for the morbidly obese patient, *Anesth Analg* 5:96, 2003.

18. Hagberg CA, Greger J, Chelly JE, Saad-Eddin HE: Instruction of airway management skills during anesthesiology residency, *J Clin Anesth* 2:15, 2003
19. de Jong RH, Bonin JD: Mixtures of local anesthetics are no more toxic than the parent drugs, *Anesthesiology* 54:177, 1981.
20. Catterall WA, Mackie K: Local anesthetics. In Hardman JG, Limbird LE, Gilman AG, editors: Goodman and Gilman's : *The Pharmacological Basis of Therapeutics*, ed 10, New York, 2001, McGraw-Hill, p 367-384.
21. Anderhuber W, Walch C, Nemeth E, Semmelrock HJ, Berghold A, Ranftl G, Stammberger H: Plasma adrenaline concentrations during functional endoscopic sinus surgery, *Laryngoscope* 109:204-207, 1999.
22. Stoelting R: *Pharmacology and Physiology in Anesthetic Practice*, ed 3, Philadelphia, 1999, Lippincott-Raven, p 163.
23. Catterall W, Mackie K: Local anesthetics. In Hardman JG, Limbird LE, Gilman AG, editors: Goodman and Gilman's: *The Pharmacological Basis of Therapeutics*, ed 10, New York, 2001, McGraw-Hill, p 377-384
24. Scott DB: Maximum recommended doses of local anaesthetic drugs, *Br J Anaesth* 63:373-374, 1989.
25. Bridenbaugh PO, Cruz ME, Helton LH: Anesthesia for otolaryngologic procedures. In Paperella MM, Shumrick DA, Paparella MM, Meyerhoff WL, editors: *Otolaryngology*, vol 1, ed 3, Philadelphia, 1991, Saunders.
26. Sumikawa K, Ishiazzka N, Suzaki M: Arrhythmogenic plasma levels of epinephrine during halothane, enflurane and pentobarbital anaesthesia in the dog, *Anesthesiology* 58:322, 1983.
27. Johnson RR, Eger IE, Wilson LC: A comparative interaction of epinephrine with enflurane, isoflurane and halothane in man, *Anesth Analg* 55:709, 1976.
28. Braid DP, Scott DB: The systemic absorption of local analgesic drugs, *Br J Anaesth* 37:394, 1965.
29. Myburgh JA, Upton RN, Grant C, Martinez A: The cerebrovascular effects of adrenaline, noradrenaline and dopamine infusions under propofol and isoflurane anaesthesia in sheep, *Anaesth Intensive Care* 30 (6):725-733, 2002.
30. Lange RA, Hillis LD: Cardiovascular complications of cocaine use, *N Engl J Med* 345:351-358, 2001.
31. Lagergren J, Bergstrom R, Adani HO, Nyren, O: Association between medications that relax the lower esophageal sphincter and risk for esophageal adenocarcinoma, *Annal Intern Med* 3(133):165-175, 2000.
32. Catlin FI, Grimes WJ: The effect of steroid therapy on recovery from tonsillectomy in children, *Arch Otolaryngol Head Neck Surgery* 6(117):649-652, 1991.
33. Holte K, Werner MS, Lacouture PG, Kehlet H: Dexamethasone prolongs local analgesia after subcutaneous infiltration of bupivacaine microcapsules in human volunteers, *Anesthesiology* 6(96): 1331-1325, 2002.
34. Goldberg ME, McNulty SE, Azad SS, et al: A comparison of labetalol and nitroprusside for inducing hypotension during major surgery, *Anesth Analg* 70:537-542, 1990.
35. Degoute CS, Ray MJ, Manchon M, Dubreuil C, Banssillon V: Remifentanil and controlled hypotension; comparison with nitroprusside or esmolol during tympanoplasty, *Can J Anaesth* 48(1), 20-27, 2001.
36. Kim KH, Moon IS, Park JS, Koh YB, Ahn H: Nicardipine hydrochloride injectable phase IV open label clinical trial: Study on the antihypertensive effects and safety of nicardipine for acute aortic dissection, *J Int Med Res* 3(30):337-345, 2002.
37. Tobias JD: Controlled hypotension in children: A critical review of available agents, *Paediatr Drugs* 4(7):439-453, 2002
38. Divatia JV, Vaidya JS, Badwe RA, Hawaldar RW: Omission of nitrous oxide during anesthesia reduces the incidence of postoperative nausea and vomiting: a meta-analysis, *Anesthesiology* 85:1055-1062, 1996.
39. Hartung J: Twenty-four of twenty-seven studies show a greater incidence of emesis associated with nitrous oxide than with alternative anesthetics, *Anesth Analg* 83:114-116, 1996.
40. Plazzo MGA, Scrunin L: Anesthesia and emesis: etiology, *Can Anaesth Soc J* 31:178-187, 1984.
41. White PF, Dworsky WA, Horai Y, Trevor AJ: Comparison of continuous infusion fentanyl or ketamine vs. thiopental: determining the mean effective serum concentrations for outpatients, *Anesthesiology* 59:564-569, 1983.
42. Borgeat A, Wilder-Smith OHG, Suter PM: The nonhypnotic therapeutic applications of propofol, *Anesthesiology* 80:642-656, 1994.
43. Frink EJ, Malan TP, Atlas M, et al: Clinical comparison of sevoflurane and isoflurane in healthy patients, *Anesth Analg* 74:241-245, 1992.
44. Souter AJ, Fredman B, White PF: Controversies in the perioperative use of nonsteroidal antiinflammatory drugs, *Anesth Analg* 79:1178-1190, 1994.
45. Krimmer H, Bullingham RE, Lloyd J, Bruch HP: Effects on biliary tract pressure in humans of intravenous ketorolac tromethamine compared with morphine and placebo, *Anesth Analg* 75:204-207, 1992.
46. Poe DS; Metson RB; Kujawski O: Laser eustachian tuboplasty: a preliminary report. *Laryngoscope* 113(4):583-591, 2003.
47. Pashayan A: Laser safety in the operating room, *Curr Rev Nurse Anesth* 18:11-19, 1995.
48. Evrards S, Mutter D, Marescaux J: Lasers in minimally invasive surgery. In Steichen FM, Welter R, editors: *Minimally Invasive Surgery and New Technology*, St Louis, 1994, Quality Medical, pp 85-90.
49. Neuman GG, Sidebotham G, Negoianu E, et al: Laparoscopy explosive hazards with nitrous oxide, *Anesthesiology* 78:875-879, 1993.
50. Munson ES: Transfer of nitrous oxide into body air cavities. *Br J Anaesth* 46:202, 1974.
51. Sois MB: Which is the safest endotracheal tube for use with CO_2 laser: A comparative study, *J Clin Anesth* 4:217, 1992.
52. Sois M, Heller S: A comparison of five metallic tapes for endotracheal tube protection during CO2 laser surgery. *Can J Anaesth* 35:S63, 1988.
53. Pashayan AG, Wolf G, Gottschalk A, et al: Anesthetic management guidelines for laser airway surgery: ASTM subcommittee, *Anesthesia Patient Safety Foundation Newsletter* 8:13, 1993.
54. Bourgain JL, Desruennes E, Fischler M, Ravussin P: Transtracheal high frequency jet ventilation for endoscopic airway surgery: a multicentre study, *Br J Anaesth* 87:870-875, 2001.
55. Brown M: ICU: critical care. In Barash P, Cullen B, Stoelting R, editors: *Clinical anesthesia*, ed 4, Philadelphia, 2001, Lippincott-Raven, p 1463-1484.
56. Chang JL, Meeuwis H, Bleyaert A, Babinski M, Petruscak J: Severe abdominal distention following jet ventilation during general anesthesia, *Anesthesiology* 49:216, 1978.
57. Kain ZN, O'Connor TZ, Berde CB: Management of tracheobronchial and esophageal foreign bodies in children, *J Clin Anesth* 6:28, 1994.
58. Caffrey RR, Warren ML, Becker KE: Neuromuscular blockade monitoring comparing the orbicularis oculi and adductor pollicis muscles, *Anesthesiology* 65:95, 1986.
59. Pathak D, Sokoll MD, Barcellos W, Kumar V: A comparison of the response of hand and facial muscles to non-depolarizing relaxants, *Anaesthesia* 43:747-748, 1988.
60. Levine RA, Ronner SF, Ojemann RG: Auditory evoked potential and other neurophysiologic monitoring techniques during tumor surgery in the cerebellopontine angle. In Loftus CM, Traynelis VC, editors: *Intraoperative Monitoring Techniques in Neurosurgery*, New York, 1994, McGraw-Hill, p 175.
61. Chinn K and others: Middle ear pressure variation: effects of nitrous oxide, *Laryngoscope* 107:357, 1997.

62. Stein SN, Canas LM, Zelman V: Complications rare and unusual, *Semin Anesth* 15:238, 1996.
63. Katayama M and others: Nitrous oxide and the middle ear, *Braz J Anesthesiol Int Issue* 3:1, 1992.
64. Strollo PJ, Rogers RM: Obstructive sleep apnea, *N Engl J Med* 334:99, 1996.
65. Sabers C; Plevak DJ; Schroeder DR; Warner DO: The diagnosis of obstructive sleep apnea as a risk factor for unanticipated admissions in outpatient surgery. *Anesth Analg* 96(5):1328-1335, 2003.
66. Benumof JL: Obstructive sleep apnea in the adult obese patient: implications for airway management. *Anesthesiol Clin North America* 20(4):789-811, 2002.
67. Agrawal A; Gerson CR; Seligman I; Dsida RM: Postoperative hemorrhage after tonsillectomy: use of ketorolac tromethamine. *Otolaryngol Head Neck Surg* 120(3):335-339, 1999.
68. Kokki H: Nonsteroidal anti-inflammatory drugs for postoperative pain: a focus on children. *Paediatr Drugs* 5(2):103-123, 2003.
69. Koc C, Kocaman F, Aygenc E, Ozdem C, Cekic A: The use of preoperative lidocaine to prevent stridor and laryngospasm after tonsillectomy and adenoidectomy, *Otolaryngol Head Neck Surg* 118:880, 1998.
70. Ferrari LR, Donlon JV: Metoclopramide reduces the incidence of vomiting after tonsillectomy in children, *Anesth Analg* 75:35, 1992.
71. Crysdale WD, Russel D: Complications of tonsillectomy and adenoidectomy in 9409 children observed overnight, *Can Med Assoc J* 135:1139, 1986.
72. Stoelting RK, Dierdorf SF: *Anesthesia and Co-existing Disease*, ed 4, New York, 2002, Churchill-Livingstone, p 708.
73. Takemura H; Yasumoto K; Toi T; Hosoyamada A: Correlation of cleft type with incidence of perioperative respiratory complications in infants with cleft lip and palate. *Paediatr Anaesth*, 12(7):585-588, 2002.
74. Gotta A, Ferrari L, Sullivan C: Otolaryngologic and maxillofacial surgery. In Kirby R, Gravenstein N, editors: *Clinical Anesthesia Practice*, ed 2, Philadelphia, 2002, Saunders, pp 1420-1441.
75. Blackwell K, Ross DA, Kapur P, Calcaterra TC: Propofol for endoscopic sinus surgery, *Am J Otolaryngol* 14:262-266, 1993.
76. Fedok FG; Ferraro RE; Kingsley CP; Fornadley JA: Operative times, postanesthesia recovery times, and complications during sinonasal surgery using general anesthesia and local anesthesia with sedation. *Otolaryngol Head Neck Surg* 2000, 4(122):560-566, 2000.
77. Phero JC, Weaver JM, Peskin RM: Anesthesia for maxillofacial/mandibular trauma, *Otolaryngol Head Neck Surg* 11:509-523, 1993.
78. Parks RE, Livoni JP: Detection of cervical spine injury in the multi-trauma patient. In Baisdell FW, Trunkey KK, editors: *Trauma Management III: Cervical Thoracic Trauma*, New York, 1986, Thieme Medical, p 56.
79. Eckhauser FE, Billote J, Burke JF: Tracheostomy complicating massive burn injury: a plea for conservation, *Am J Surg* 127:418, 1974.
80. Le Fort R: Experimental study of fractures of the upper jaw, *Plast Reconstr Surg* 30:6, 1963.
81. Gotta AW: Management of the traumatized airway, *ASA Refresher Course*, Park Ridge, IL, 1996, American Society of Anesthesiologists, p 121.
82. Tintinali JE, Claffey J: Complications of nasotracheal intubation, *Ann Emerg Med* 10:142, 1981.
83. van Aalst JA, McCurry T, Wagner J: Reconstructive considerations in the surgical management of melanoma, *Surg Clin North Am* 83:187-230, 2003.
84. Chick LR, Walton RL, Reus W, Colen L, Sasmor M: Free flaps in the elderly, *Plast Reconstr Surg* 90(1):87-94, 1992.
85. McNulty SE: Induced hypotension during head and neck surgery, *Otolaryngol Head Neck Surg* 11:604-605, 1993.
86. Veras LM, Pedraza-Gutierrez S, Castellanos J, Capellades J, Casamitjana J, Rovira-Canellas A: Vertebral artery occlusion after acute cervical spine trauma, *Spine* 25(9):1171-1177, 2000.

CHAPTER 37

Anesthesia for Ophthalmic Procedures

Donald Bell

Ophthalmic anesthesia is an exciting and growing segment of anesthetic practice. The specialty has grown tremendously since 1884, when the first retrobulbar block was performed with cocaine. The surgical technique of phacoemulsification has greatly simplified cataract surgery, resulting in a widespread shift from general to local anesthesia for these procedures.[1] Today, more than 1 million ocular blocks are performed annually for surgical procedures. This number will continue to increase as the population ages and undergoes the many ophthalmic procedures available. Ophthalmologists have recognized the value of ocular blocks and continue to request these services from anesthesia practitioners. Ocular regional blocks provide a satisfactory surgical environment for a variety of ophthalmic procedures that formerly required general anesthesia. Because our understanding of ocular blocks and the management of patients receiving them has continued to improve, nurse anesthetists throughout the United States who are performing regional ocular blocks have found eye anesthesia expertise to be a beneficial addition to their practice.

OPHTHALMIC ANATOMY

Extraocular Muscles

Six extraocular muscles exist (Figs. 37-1 through 37-4). The *superior rectus muscle* is located at the 12-o'clock position on the globe. This muscle moves the eye upward, or *supraducts* the eye. The *inferior rectus muscle* is located at the 6-o'clock position on the globe. This muscle moves the eye downward, or *infraducts* the eye. The *medial rectus muscle* is located 90° medially to the 12-o'clock position on the globe and moves the eyeball nasally, or *adducts* the eye. The *lateral rectus muscle* is located 90° laterally to the 12-o'clock position on the globe and moves the eyeball laterally, or *abducts* the eye. The *superior oblique muscle* is located on the superior aspect of the eye. This muscle rotates the eyeball on its horizontal axis toward the nose, or *intorts* the eye, and depresses the eyeball. The *inferior oblique muscle* is located on the inferior aspect of the globe. This muscle rotates the eyeball on its horizontal axis temporally, or *extorts* the eye, and elevates the eyeball (Table 37-1).

All the ocular muscles except the inferior oblique originate in the orbital apex around Zinn's annulus (Fig. 37-5), which is a fibrinous ring that encircles the optic foramen. The four rectus muscles move forward in a conal pattern that forms the muscle cone around the globe. These muscles, which are about 40 mm long, insert into the globe just anterior to its equator.[2] The superior oblique muscle arises just superior to Zinn's annulus and moves forward, becoming a tendon. This tendon passes through a cartilaginous ring called the *trochlea*, which is located on the medial supranasal orbital wall. After passing through the trochlea, the tendon is redirected in a posterolateral direction

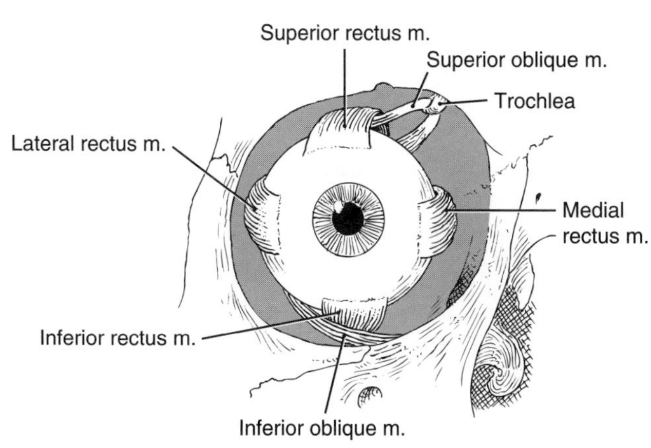

FIGURE **37-1**
Frontal view of the orbit. *m.*, muscle.

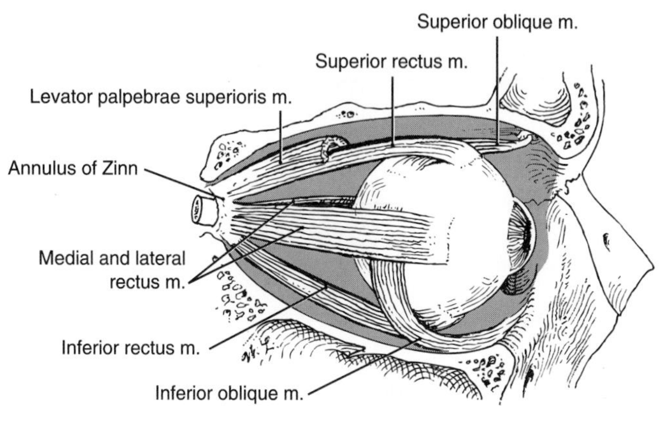

FIGURE **37-2**
Lateral view of the orbit.

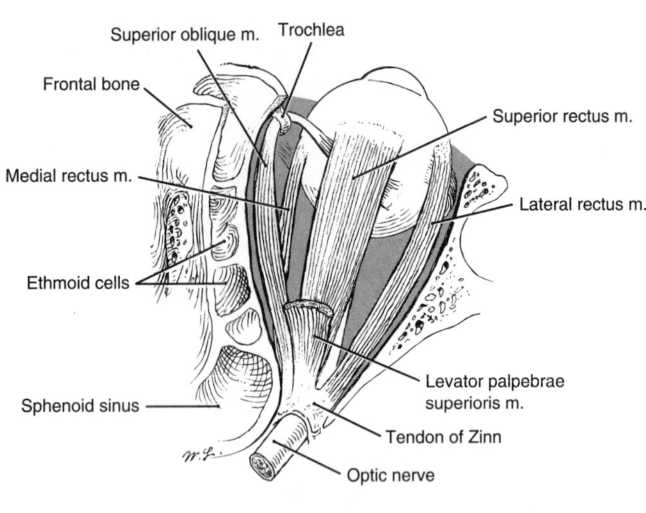

FIGURE **37-3**
Superior view of the orbit.

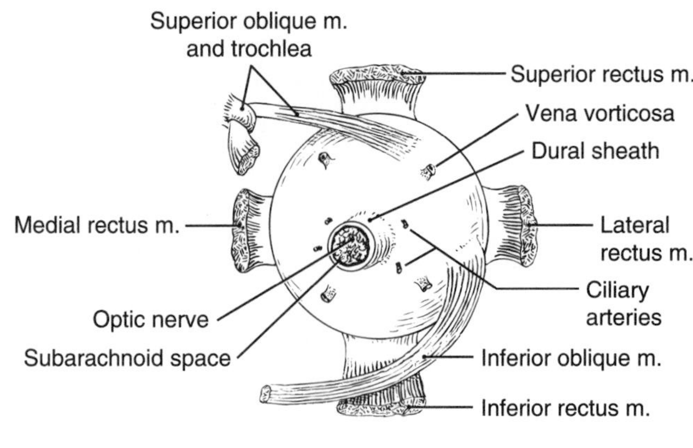

FIGURE **37-4**
Posterior view of the globe.

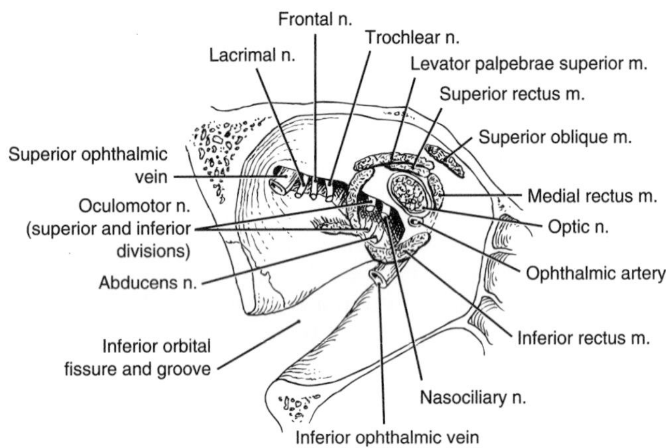

FIGURE **37-5**
View of the orbital apex. *n.*, nerve.

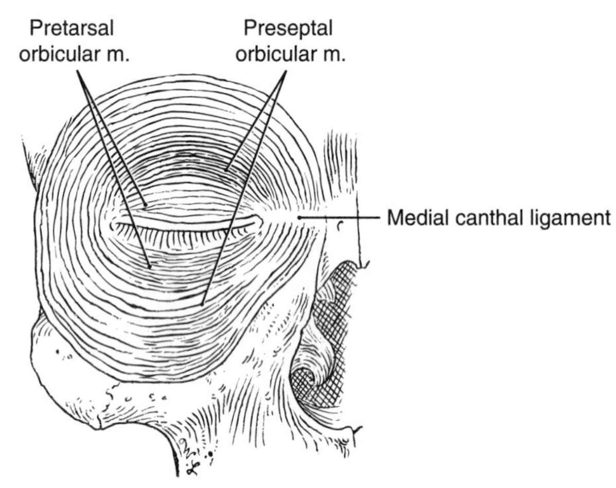

FIGURE **37-6**
Orbicularis oculi muscles.

TABLE 37-1 Orbital Muscles and Innervation

Muscle	Function	Cranial Nerve
Superior rectus	Supraduction	III
Inferior rectus	Infraduction	III
Medial rectus	Adduction	III
Lateral rectus	Abduction	VI
Superior oblique	Intorsion Depression	IV
Inferior oblique	Extorsion Elevation	III

and inserts on the superolateral aspect of the globe under the superior rectus muscle. The inferior oblique muscle originates from the anterior nasal orbit and moves in a posterolateral direction to the globe, inserting along the lateral aspect of the globe. The arching of both the inferior and the superior oblique muscles around the globe allows for the torsional movements of the eye.

Eyelid Muscles

The levator muscle of the upper eyelid is the primary muscle used for raising the upper eyelids. This muscle originates near Zinn's annulus (see Fig. 37-2). It moves forward just superior and slightly medial to the superior rectus muscle, inserting into the upper eyelid. Because the levator muscle only retracts and does not contract the eyelid, akinesia of this muscle is not necessary.

The *orbicular muscle* of the eye (Fig. 37-6) causes the eyelids to contract. This muscle has three divisions, *orbital*, *palpebral*, and *tarsal*, which are concentrically arranged around the eyelid. Akinesia of these muscles is generally desired for ocular procedures because if the muscles were allowed to contract around the globe, intraocular pressure would increase. However, the recent success of cataract and glaucoma procedures performed with the use of topical and subconjunctival anesthesia has demonstrated that akinesia of the orbicular muscle of the eye is not always mandatory.

Cranial Nerves

The orbital portion of the *optic nerve* (cranial nerve II) (Fig. 37-7) is from 25 to 30 mm long and travels posteriorly within the muscle cone from the globe into the cranial cavity.

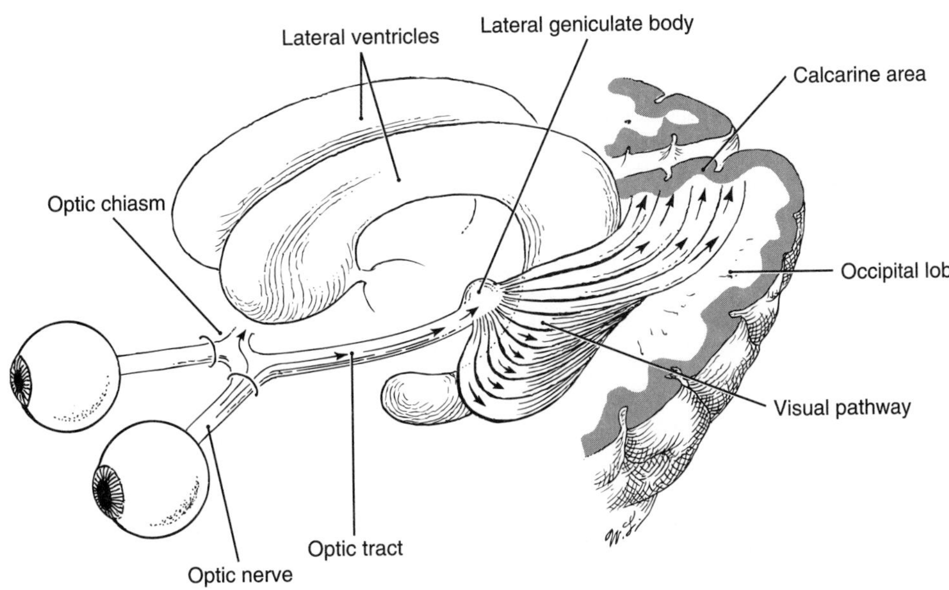

FIGURE **37-7**
Intraorbital and intracranial view of the optic nerve.

This distance is actually longer than that from the posterior portion of the globe to the orbital apex, giving the optic nerve an S-shaped configuration. This shape allows free movement of the nerve so that the many positions of the eye are accommodated. The optic nerve is myelinated and is about 4 mm in diameter.[2] The optic nerve extends through the *optic canal* and continues until it meets the *optic chiasm* intracranially. The optic chiasm is the junction of both optic nerve tracts. Here, suspended in and surrounded by cerebrospinal fluid, the optic nerve fibers partially decussate, sending visual fibers to the contralateral eye.

According to Wolff, the optic nerve is not a true cranial nerve but is actually an outgrowth of the brain.[2] As a result, the optic nerve is also covered by the *meninges*, the fibrous wrappings of the arachnoid, dura, and pia mater, which envelop the central nervous system (CNS).[3] Therefore, any anesthetic agent that is injected into the optic nerve sheath can find its way back to the midbrain through the cerebrospinal fluid and result in CNS depression and even lead to respiratory arrest. The optic nerve also carries the central retinal artery and vein into the globe. The central retinal artery and vein exit the optic nerve about 8 to 15 mm posterior to the globe.[4]

The *oculomotor nerve* (cranial nerve III) innervates the following muscles of the orbit: the superior rectus muscle, the inferior rectus muscle, the inferior oblique muscle, the medial rectus muscle, and the levator muscle of the upper eyelid. The oculomotor nerve is the primary motor nerve to the extraocular muscles of the orbit; this nerve branches superiorly and inferiorly (Fig. 37-8). The superior branch innervates the superior rectus muscle and the levator muscle of the upper eyelid. The inferior branch of the oculomotor nerve innervates the medial rectus muscle, the inferior rectus muscle, and the inferior oblique muscle. This nerve also sends parasympathetic fibers to the ciliary ganglion (Fig. 37-9), which is located adjacent to the optic nerve in the posterior portion of the orbit. The ciliary ganglion receives parasympathetic fibers from the oculomotor nerve and also sympathetic fibers from the carotid artery plexus and a sensory branch from the nasociliary nerve, a branch of the ophthalmic nerve. The parasympathetic fibers move from the ciliary ganglion forward to innervate the iris sphincter muscles, which cause constriction of the pupil. The sympathetic motor fibers move forward to control the radial muscle of the iris for pupillary dilation.

The *trochlear nerve* (cranial nerve IV) (see Fig. 37-8) provides the motor fibers for the superior oblique muscle. This nerve enters the orbit through the superior orbital fissure outside of the muscle cone. It is the only orbital cranial motor nerve that enters the orbit outside the muscle cone. Once inside the orbit, the nerve root moves in a medial direction to innervate the superior oblique muscle.

The *trigeminal nerve* (cranial nerve V) (see Fig. 37-9) has sensory and motor components. In ocular anesthesia, the sensory component is of primary importance. The intracranial portion of the nerve forms the trigeminal ganglion, which has three main divisions: the ophthalmic, the maxillary, and the mandibular nerves. The ophthalmic branch provides for the sensation of pain, touch, and temperature to the cornea, ciliary body, iris, lacrimal gland, conjunctiva, nasal mucosa, eyelid, eyebrow, forehead, and nose. The maxillary branch provides

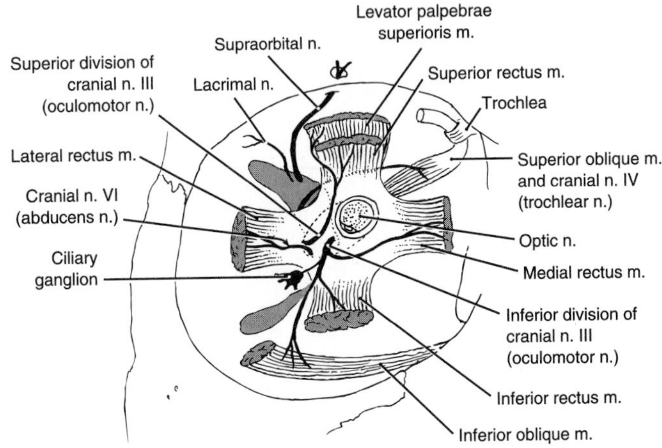

FIGURE **37-8**
Frontal view of the posterior orbit with its motor nerves and the extraocular muscles.

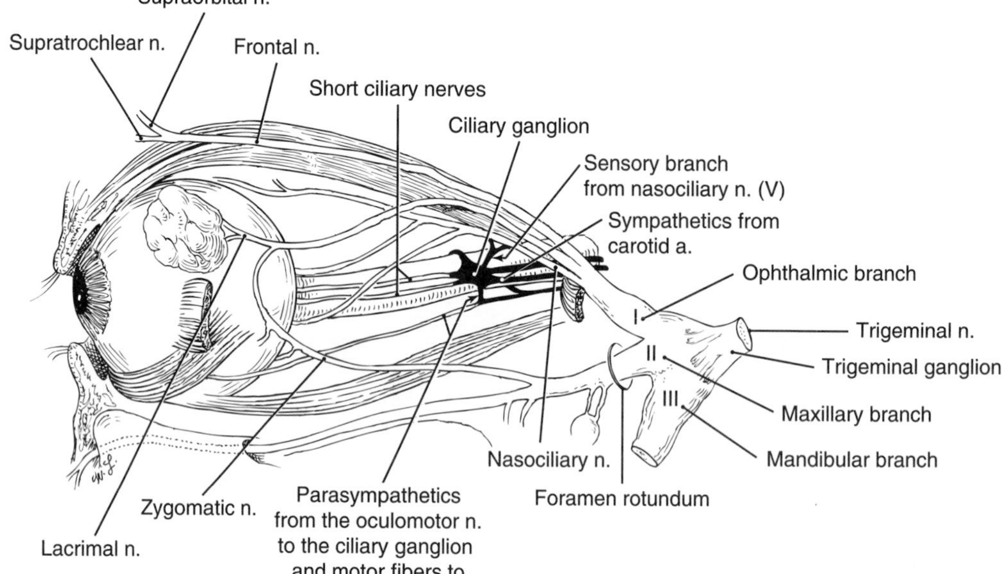

FIGURE **37-9**
Lateral orbital view of sensory nerves and ciliary ganglion. *a.*, artery.

for the sensation of pain, touch, and temperature to the upper lip, nasal mucosa, and scalp muscles.[5]

The *ophthalmic nerve* has three main branches: lacrimal, frontal, and nasociliary. The *lacrimal nerve branch* innervates the lacrimal gland in the superior lateral aspect of the orbit. The frontal branch is the largest branch of the ophthalmic nerve. This branch enters the orbit outside the muscle cone through the superior orbital fissure and travels anteriorly outside the muscle cone superior to the levator muscle. The frontal nerve itself splits into two branches. The larger, supraorbital branch continues forward into the orbit and exits the orbit through the supraorbital notch; this branch innervates the forehead. The smaller branch is the supratrochlear nerve, which moves in a medial direction, supplying nerve roots to the forehead and to the medial portion of the upper eyelid. The *nasociliary nerve branch* enters the orbit inside the muscle cone and crosses over the optic nerve, sending nerve fibers medially and to the ciliary ganglion. The fibers to the ciliary ganglion form the short ciliary nerves, which continue anteriorly, penetrating the posterior portion of the globe near the optic nerve. The nasociliary nerve also gives rise to the long ciliary nerves, which continue anteriorly and enter the posterior portion of the globe supplying the ciliary muscle, iris, and cornea. The long ciliary nerves also carry sympathetic fibers to the dilator muscle of the iris from the superior cervical ganglion. The nasociliary nerve continues along the medial aspect of the orbit just superior to the medial rectus muscle until it passes through the orbital septum to become the *infratrochlear nerve*. The infratrochlear nerve provides sensory input to the side of the nose, the medial aspect of the eyelids, the medial conjunctiva, the caruncle, and the lacrimal sac.

The *abducens nerve* (cranial nerve VI) (see Fig. 37-8) provides the motor function to the lateral rectus muscle. The nerve enters through the superior orbital fissure within the muscle cone and continues along the conal surface of the lateral rectus muscle, eventually inserting in the posterior one third of that muscle.

The *facial nerve* (cranial nerve VII) (Fig. 37-10) is predominantly a motor nerve for the muscles of the face. This nerve exits from the stylomastoid foramen. The facial nerve travels underneath the external auditory canal to the parotid gland, where it divides into an upper and a lower branch. Ocular anesthesia is more concerned with the upper branch of the facial nerve than with the lower. The upper branch further divides into the temporal and zygomatic branches, which innervate the orbicular muscle of the eye, the superficial facial muscles, and the scalp muscles.

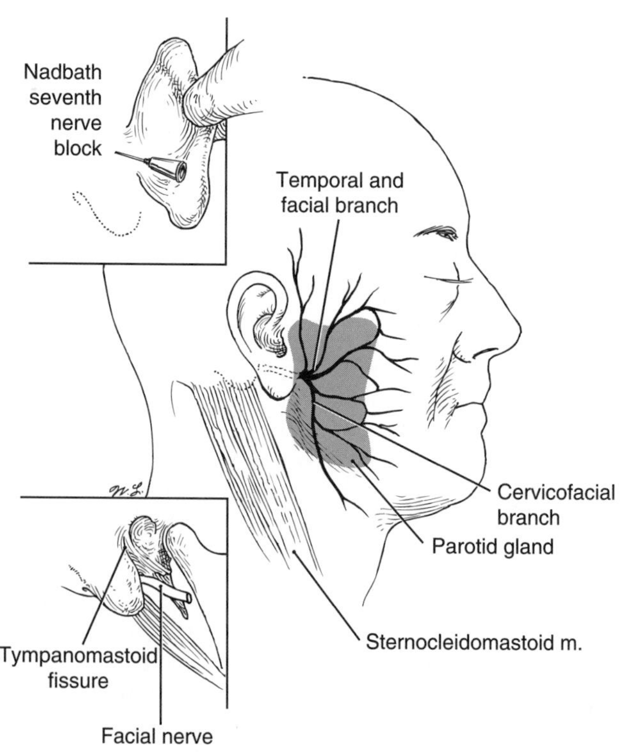

FIGURE **37-10**
The origin and branches of the facial nerve. *Upper inset,* Needle placement for the Nadbath seventh nerve block.

The *vagus nerve* (cranial nerve X) provides motor function to the intrinsic muscles in the larynx and the heart, and it provides major parasympathetic visceral innervation elsewhere. It is also the efferent pathway for the oculocardiac reflex, which can result in bradycardia and dysrhythmias.

Orbital Fossa

The *orbital fossa* has been described as pear shaped. The medial walls of the orbit extend almost straight back, whereas the lateral walls diverge medially at about a 90° angle to each other (Fig. 37-11). The *superior* and *inferior orbital fissures* are in the orbital apex, which is located in the posterior orbit. These fissures are the entry portals for the orbital nerves and vessels (Fig. 37-12). The *optic foramen* lies just medial to the superior orbital fissure and is the entry portal for the optic nerve and the ophthalmic artery from the intracranial to the intraorbital area. In the medial nasal aspect of the fossa, just behind the orbital rim, is the *lacrimal bone*, which is used as a landmark for the medial peribulbar block (Fig. 37-13). The *ethmoid bone* is just posterior to the lacrimal bone.

The *supraorbital nerve* exits the orbit in the supraorbital notch, which is in the superior nasal aspect of the orbital rim. The *infraorbital foramen*, where the infraorbital nerve and artery exit, is just below the infraorbital rim at about the 6-o'clock position. The *infraorbital nerve* is the sensory branch of the maxillary nerve. The *lacrimal*, *frontal*, and *trochlear nerves* all enter through the superior orbital fissure outside the muscle cone. The *oculomotor*, *abducens*, and *nasociliary nerves* all enter the orbit inside the muscle cone.

The *ophthalmic artery* (Fig. 37-14), which is the first branch of the internal carotid artery, passes into the orbit through the optic canal. The ophthalmic artery usually lies just inferolateral to the optic nerve. The artery extends along the optic nerve for a short distance, crossing over it in most cases, and continuing medially.[6] The first branch of the ophthalmic artery is usually the *central retinal artery*. The central retinal artery moves in an anterior direction underneath the optic nerve, usually entering the optic nerve on its inferomedial side 8 to 15 mm posterior to the globe.[4] The artery continues forward into the optic nerve head and branches into the retinal arteries. The ophthalmic artery gives rise to the long and short posterior ciliary arteries. The short posterior arteries move anteriorly and divide into many small

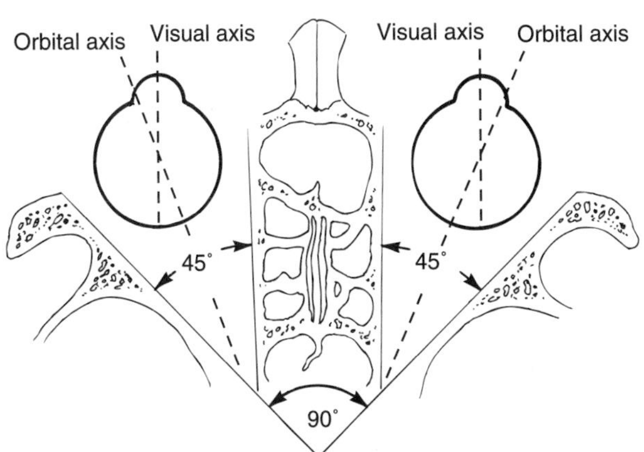

FIGURE **37-11**
Superior view of the bony orbit demonstrating the orbital and visual axes.

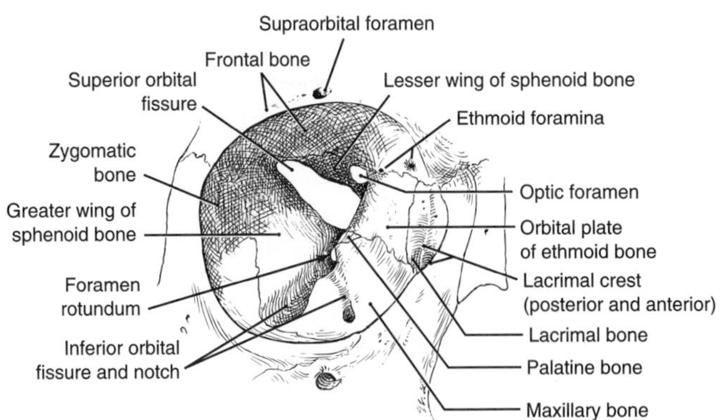

FIGURE **37-12**
Frontal view of the orbital bones.

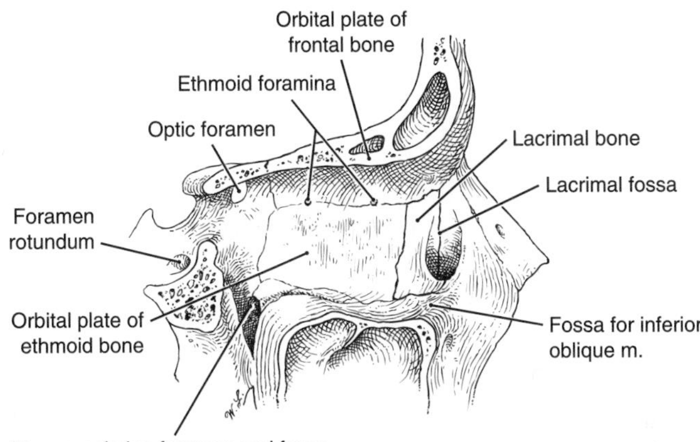

FIGURE **37-13**
Lateral view of the orbital bones.

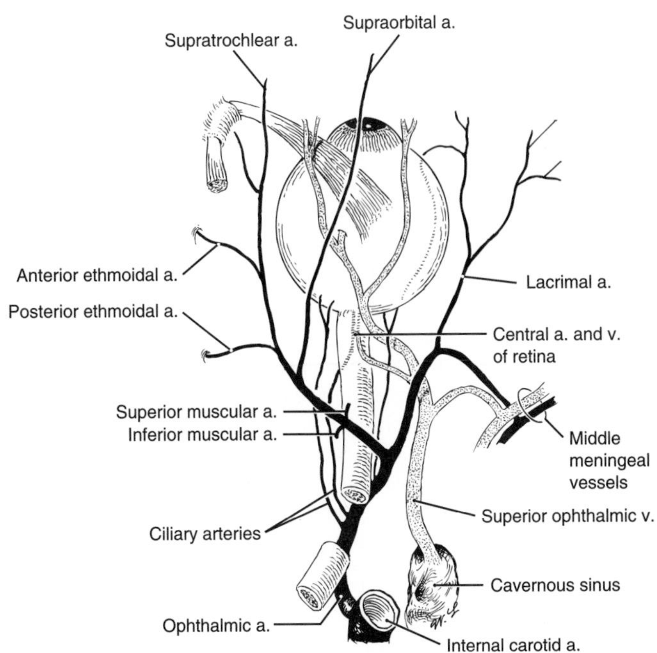

FIGURE **37-14**
Superior view of the orbital arteries and veins.

branches, which penetrate the globe close to the optic nerve and supply the choroid and the optic nerve head. The ophthalmic artery also provides branches to the optic nerve. The orbital branches of the ophthalmic artery include branches to the supraorbital arteries, the rectus muscles, and the lacrimal gland.

The *lacrimal artery* moves anteriorly along the superior aspect of the lateral rectus muscle to the lacrimal gland. The *supraorbital artery* branches from the ophthalmic artery as it crosses over the optic nerve and extends just medial to the superior rectus and levator muscles. It continues forward on a superior nasal route and exits through the *supraorbital notch* or *foramen*.

The *dorsal nasal artery* is one of the terminal branches of the ophthalmic artery. It exits the orbital septum above the medial canthal tendon and joins with the *angular artery*, thus establishing communication between the internal and external carotid arteries.[2] The *external carotid artery* gives branches to the facial artery (the external maxillary artery). The *facial artery* originates near the angle of the mandible, extends toward the stylohyoid muscles, and then proceeds forward to the lower border of the mandible. The artery then turns upward and moves toward the nose, where it joins with the dorsal nasal artery in the medial canthal area. The inferior orbital fissure is the entrance site for the *infraorbital artery*. This artery moves anteriorly through the infraorbital canal and exits to the face through the infraorbital foramen.

The venous drainage system (see Fig. 37-14) for the orbit includes the superior and inferior ophthalmic veins, which drain into the cavernous sinus that is located intracranially. Radiographic studies have demonstrated a unique characteristic of the orbital vascular system: the orbital veins are independent of the orbital arteries.[6] The venous system of the orbit is valveless, and blood flow in this area is determined by pressure gradients. The primary vein of the orbit is the *superior ophthalmic vein*. This vein travels posteriorly to the medial side of the superior rectus muscle, then beneath the superior rectus muscle inside a support hammock. The vein then emerges on the muscle's lateral aspect. The vein continues its posterior direction along the lateral aspect of the superior rectus, exiting the orbit through the superior orbital fissure, and terminating in the cavernous sinus.[7]

Several veins enter into the superior ophthalmic vein, such as the *ciliary veins*, the *lacrimal veins*, and the *superior vortex veins*, which are located on the posterior quadrants of the globe and drain the choroid, or second layer, of the globe. The *inferior ophthalmic vein* originates from a diffuse plexus on the floor of the orbit. This vein receives several branches, including the extraocular muscles and the inferior vortex veins located on the inferoposterior quadrants of the globe. The primary branch of the inferior ophthalmic vein also drains into the *superior ophthalmic vein* before the entrance of the superior ophthalmic vein into the cavernous sinus. The *central retinal vein* exits the globe inside the optic nerve. The central retinal vein then exits the optic nerve and enters the orbit between 8 and 15 mm posterior to the globe[4] and usually passes directly to the cavernous sinus.[2]

Orbit

An evaluation of the patient's orbit and globe size is important before ocular anesthesia is conducted. The usual volume of the orbit is 30 mL (Box 37-1). The volume of a typical globe (which has a diameter of about 25 mm) is 6.5 to 7 mL.[6] The balance of the orbital volume is approximately 23 mL and is composed of muscles, vessels, nerves, and fat. Katsev and associates[8] measured 120 orbits from 60 adult skulls and found an average orbital depth of 48 mm. The distance from the middle third and lateral third of the infraorbital rim to the superior aspect of the optic foramen was also measured and ranged from 42 to 52 mm. This distance should not be confused with the depth of the orbital floor. Because of the pear shape of the orbit, the orbital floor does not extend directly to the orbital apex. The orbital floor extends only to the posterior wall of the maxillary sinus, about two thirds of the depth of the orbital apex.

BOX 37-1

Orbital Measurements

Height of the orbit: 40 mm
Width of the orbit: 35 mm
Depth of the orbit: 42-52 mm
Approximate orbital volume: 30 mL
Approximate globe volume: 6.5-7.0 mL
Balance of orbital volume: 23 mL

Orbital fat is contained in both the extraconal and the intraconal areas. The orbital fat encircles and encapsulates all these areas of the orbit.

The *orbital septum* is a fibrinous tissue that defines the anatomic anterior boundary of the orbit and keeps the adipose tissue from protruding forward. The *visual axis* (also known as the *optic axis* or the *geometric axis*) is an imaginary line from the midpoint of the cornea (anterior pole) to the midpoint of the retina or macula (posterior pole) (Fig. 37-15). The horizontal (anteroposterior) diameter of the globe is an important consideration for ocular blocks. This measurement of the visual axis is referred to as the *axial length*. The axial length is measured preoperatively to determine the appropriate intraocular lens that should be placed in the eye after cataract removal. The axial length of the globe can be used *only* when measurements for intraocular lens implants are performed by the ophthalmologist. Normal axial lengths range from 23 to 23.5 mm. In the hyperopic (farsighted) eye, the globe is less than 22 mm long. This shorter eye length may allow a little more working area behind the eye during an ophthalmic block; however, this advantage may be offset by a smaller overall orbit.

The main concern regarding ophthalmic blocks involves the longer, myopic (nearsighted) eye, whose axial length is greater than 24 mm. As the globe stretches, it is believed that the fibrinous scleral layer thins, making the globe easier to penetrate by the needle. This increased posterior length of the globe also increases the chance of globe puncture. Therefore, because of a greater chance of contact in the posterior aspect of the orbit, the axial length of the eye, if this measurement is available, should be considered in the planning for the ocular block. If the axial length is unknown, which may be the case in glaucoma surgery, corneal transplants, retinal procedures, or muscle surgery, the practitioner's preoperative questions should include history of nearsightedness, previous retinal procedures, and general appearance of the eye.

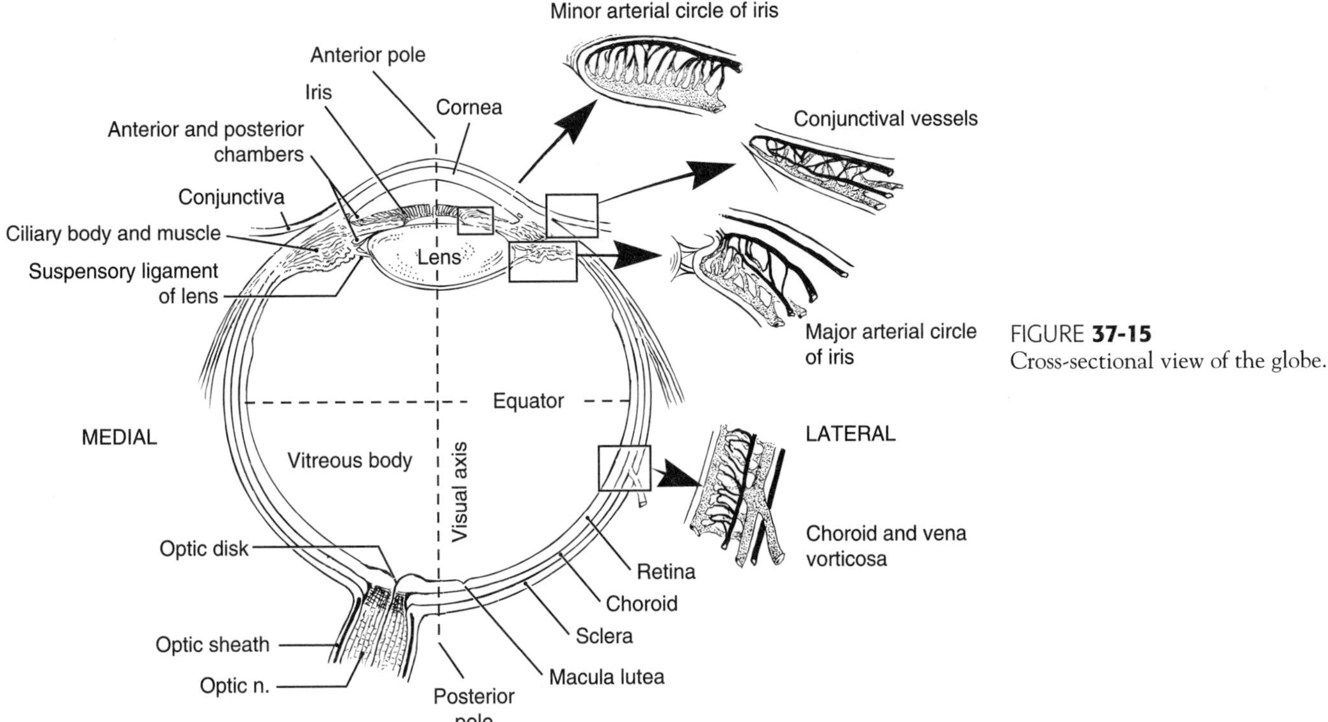

FIGURE **37-15**
Cross-sectional view of the globe.

The separate *coats*, or *tunics*, of the eyeball (see Fig. 37-15) start with the *sclera*, which is the outer, fibrinous protective layer. The sclera is white and opaque and lies just posterior to the cornea. The *cornea* is the outer, fibrinous protective layer located anteriorly, and it is transparent and colorless. The middle, or vascular, layer is called the *choroid*. The *retina* is the inner layer of the posterior half of the eye. The *limbal area* is defined as the area at the junction between the cornea and the sclera.[2] The *conjunctiva* is a thin, transparent mucous membrane that covers the posterior surface of the eyelids and the anterior surface of the sclera.

A *staphyloma* is a bulging of the uvea, which comprises the iris, the ciliary body, and the choroid, into a thin and stretched sclera. Staphylomas may occur in the anterior, equatorial, and posterior areas.[3]

Fascial Sheaths of the Orbit

Three connective tissue systems within the orbit have been defined by Koornneef.[6] They are Tenon's capsule, the orbital connective tissue, and the fascial sheaths of the extraocular muscles (Fig. 37-16).

Tenon's Capsule. *Tenon's capsule* (bulbar fascia) consists of fibrous connective tissue that covers the eyeball from near the corneal limbus, where it is fused to the conjunctiva, and extends behind the eye, with openings for the extraocular muscles and the optic nerve. Tenon's capsule serves primarily as a cavity in which the eye moves.

Orbital Connective Tissue. Koornneef demonstrated the presence of *connective tissue* attachments between both the globe and the periorbital area. The connective tissue begins at the orbital apex and continues anteriorly, becoming more complex and more clearly defined at the level of the globe. Koornneef[7] also noted that the tissue septa are in a 360° encapsulation of the globe (Fig. 37-17). These connective tissue septa encircle and support the globe within the bony orbit. Connective tissue septa were also noted between the superior and inferior oblique muscles, Tenon's capsule, the rectus muscles, and the ligaments stabilizing the globe within the orbit. This connective tissue septa meshwork limits displacement of the globe.

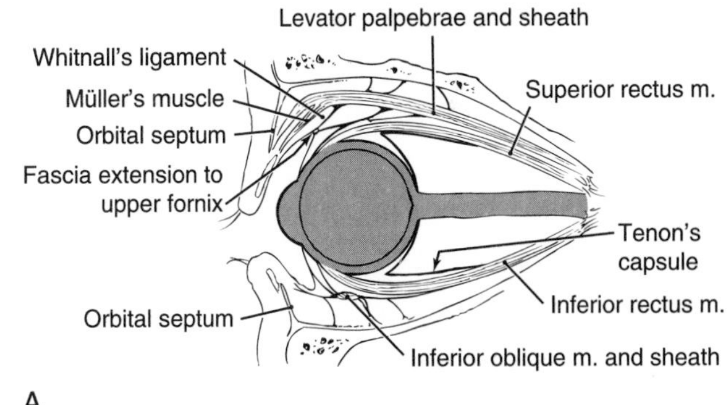

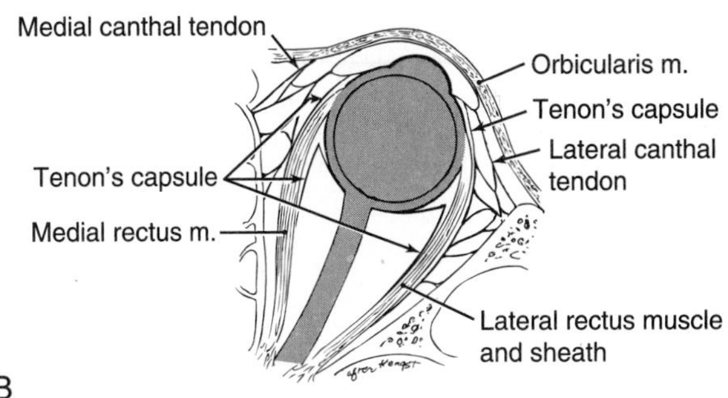

FIGURE **37-16**
A, Lateral view of the orbital connective tissue. **B,** Superior view of the orbital connective tissue.

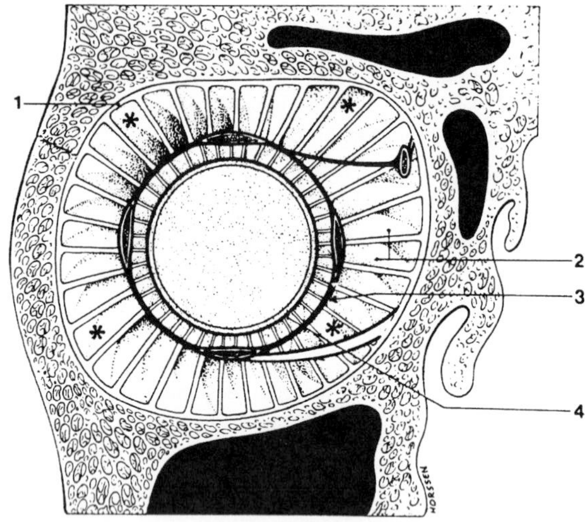

FIGURE **37-17**
Schematic representation of the anterior orbital connective tissue septa. *1*, periorbita; *2*, common muscle sheath around the eye; *3*, fibrous septa. (From Koornneef L: New insights in the human orbital connective tissue: results of a new anatomic approach, *Arch Ophthalmol* 95:1269, 1977. Copyright 1977, American Medical Association.)

Fascial Sheaths. The *intermuscular membrane* is a fibrous membrane that connects the four rectus muscle sheaths. Numerous extensions from these muscle sheaths form an intricate system of fibrinous attachments that interconnect the muscles into the orbit, support the globe, and check the ocular movements.

In the posterior orbit, the fascial sheaths of the extraocular muscles are not as well defined as they are immediately behind the globe.[9] Koornneef was not able to identify a common muscle cone throughout the orbit (Fig. 37-18). The muscle sheaths themselves contribute fibrinous septa to the periorbit; these septa serve as ligaments for the extraocular muscles. These fascial extensions promote the efficiency of the extraocular muscle functions.[7,9,10]

OCULAR DRUGS

Common ocular drugs are listed in Table 37-2

Mydriatic Agents

Mydriatic agents cause pupillary dilation by direct or indirect effect on the dilator muscle of the iris.

Phenylephrine. Phenylephrine (Neo-Synephrine) is a commonly used and effective mydriatic and vasoconstrictor that has no cycloplegic effects. The 2.5% concentration is generally safe for use in children and the elderly. The 10% solution may contain up to 5 mg per drop of phenylephrine. However, few adverse effects have been reported with 10% phenylephrine drops. The most common and generally transient responses are headache, tremors, hypertension, and tachycardia that may be accompanied by reflex bradycardia. More severe reactions include ventricular dysrhythmias and myocardial infarctions, including some that have been fatal. One case of acute hypertension secondary to concomitant use of 10% phenylephrine drops and systemic β-blockers resulted in the rupture of a congenital cerebral aneurysm. The vasopressor response may also

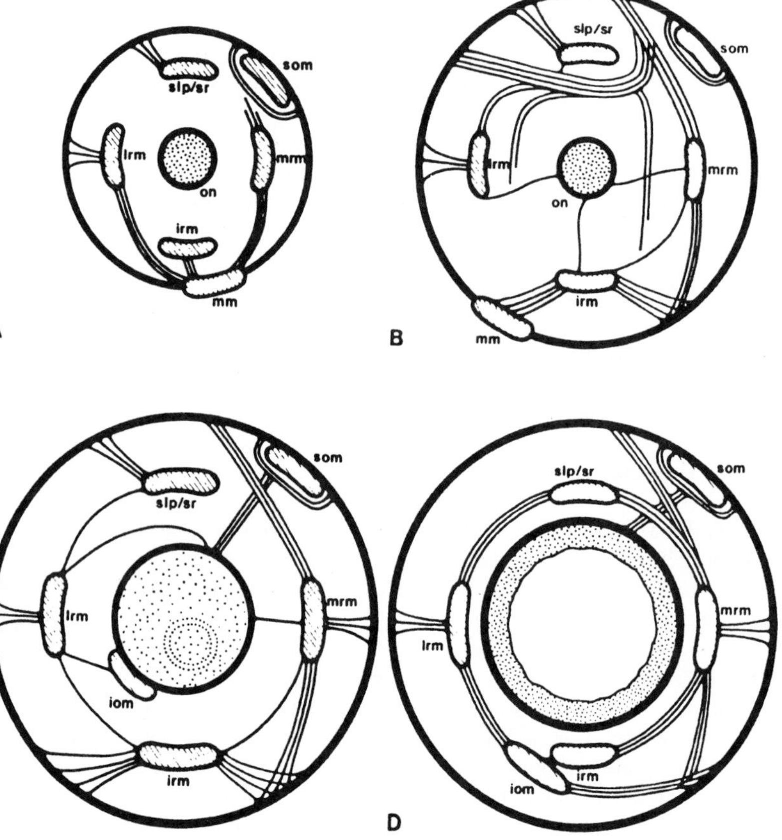

FIGURE **37-18**
Extraocular muscle connective tissue system. Highly schematic representation of the connective tissue system of the extraocular muscles. **A,** Coronal section near the orbital apex. **B,** Coronal section near the posterior portion of the globe. **C,** Coronal section lying just anterior to the posterior portion of the globe. **D,** Coronal section near the equator of the globe. *slp/sr*, levator palpebrae superioris–superior rectus complex; *lrm*, lateral rectus muscle; *iom*, inferior oblique muscle; *irm*, inferior rectus muscle; *m*, Müller's muscle; *mrm*, medial rectus muscle; *som*, superior oblique muscle; *on*, optic nerve. (From Koornneef L: Orbital septa: anatomy and function, *Ophthalmology* 86:876, 1979. Courtesy of *Ophthalmology*.)

TABLE 37-2 **Common Ocular Drugs**

Class	Generic name	Comments
β-Blockers	Timolol Levobunolol Betaxolol Carteolol Metipranolol	First-line therapy. Reduce production of aqueous humor. May produce systemic effect. Caution in patients with asthma, COPD, heart block, heart failure, and hypotension.
Carbonic anhydrase inhibitors	Acetazolamide Methazolamide Dorzolamide Brinzolamide	Reduce aqueous production. Usually used as second-line therapy for glaucoma.
Parasympathomimetic and anticholinesterase miotics	Carbachol Pilocarpine Physostigmine Echothiophate iodide	Promote aqueous outflow. Rarely used due to significant side effects and drug interactions.
Prostaglandins	Latanoprost Bimatoprost Travoprost Unoprostone	Promote aqueous outflow. Alternative to β-blockers in intolerant patients.
Sympathomimetics	Epinephrine Dipivefrin	Contraindicated in patients with narrow-angle glaucoma.
α_2-Agonists	Apraclonidine HCl Brimonidine	Reduce aqueous production. Contraindicated in patients on monoamine oxidase inhibitors.
Corticosteroids	Dexamethasone Fluorometholone Prednisolone Rimexolone	Antiinflammatory. May induce glaucoma with prolonged use.
Nonsteroidal antiinflammatory agents	Diclofenac Ketorolac	Antiinflammatory. Blocks cyclooxygenase pathway to inhibit prostaglandin and reduce inflammation.
Mydriatics and cycloplegics	Atropine Cyclopentolate Homatropine Phenylephrine Tropicamide	Used for eye exams. Phenylephrine and Tropicamide are mydriatic. The others produce mydriasis and cycloplegia.

be potentiated by reserpine, guanethidine, methyldopa, tricyclic antidepressants, monoamine oxidase inhibitors, and atropinelike drugs. If treatment becomes necessary, small doses of α-adrenergic blocking agents, such as phentolamine, chlorpromazine (Thorazine), or droperidol, have been suggested.[11]

Tropicamide. Tropicamide (Mydriacyl), which is available in strengths of 0.5% to 1%, is a synthetic antimuscarinic compound that provides good mydriatic activity but has weak cycloplegic effects.

Cycloplegic Agents

The *cycloplegic agents*, also referred to as *parasympatholytic compounds*, cause a temporary paralysis of the ciliary muscle and the muscles of accommodation.

Atropine. Topical atropine (1%) causes both mydriasis and cycloplegia, resulting in pupillary dilation. Intravenous atropine in doses of 0.4 to 0.6 mg has minimal ocular effects;[12,13] however, caution is advised in patients with narrow-angle glaucoma. Side effects of atropine include thirst, flushing, dry skin, tachycardia, irritability, and delirium.

Homatropine. Homatropine, which is available in strengths of 2% to 5%, is a topical cycloplegic with a rapid onset. Accommodation of the eye usually returns within 24 hours when the 2.5% concentration is used.

Cyclopentolate. Cyclopentolate (Cyclogyl), which is available in strengths of 0.5% to 2%, is a commonly used synthetic antimuscarinic agent that possesses potent mydriatic and cycloplegic properties. Reported toxic effects of cyclopentolate include speech impairment, disorientation, convulsions, and psychotic reactions.

Glaucoma Medications

β-Adrenergic Blockers. Several β-blockers are currently available and are the first line therapy for glaucoma. They work by reducing aqueous humor production. They have a long proven track record of effectiveness. Usually, β-blockers do not cause systemic problems, although the anesthetist must consider the patient's age, drug sensitivity, and underlying pulmonary and cardiovascular pathology before administering these drugs, since in some patients generalized systemic effects may occur. Contraindications for β-blockers are asthma, severe sinus bradycardia, heart block, burns more severe than first degree, hypotension, and severe heart failure.[14]

α_2-Agonists. These medications are slightly less effective than β–blockers; however, they may be used as first-line monotherapy for glaucoma in patients where β–blockers are not tolerated. They work by reducing aqueous production and possibly increasing uveoscleral outflow. Allergy and occasional headaches have been reported as side effects. Neuroprotective effects on retinal cell death have been observed in animals but not yet in humans with topical use.[14]

Echothiophate Iodide and Isoflurophate. Both echothiophate iodide (phospholine iodide), 0.03% to 0.25%, and isoflurophate (Floropryl), 0.025%, are indirect-acting organophosphorus anticholinesterase inhibitors. They differ from physostigmine primarily in their prolonged rate of degradation. These topical eye medications are absorbed into the system through the lacrimal apparatus. After covalently bonding with pseudocholinesterase, the drug begins to deactivate the enzyme within several days to a few weeks. The activity of the enzyme has been reported to take 3 to 6 weeks to return to normal after administration of the medication is discontinued. Therefore the anesthesia practitioner should anticipate prolonged apnea with the use of succinylcholine and delayed metabolism with the use of the local ester anesthetics.[12] Pilocarpine and Carbachol are rarely used in modern therapy.

Carbonic Anhydrase Inhibitors. Carbonic anhydrase inhibitors are relatively effective antiglaucoma medications that work by reducing the production of aqueous humor. Carbonic anhydrase isoenzyme 11 is the primary type found in the human ciliary body and its inhibition reduces the conversion of carbon dioxide and water to bicarbonate and hydrogen ion, additionally affecting sodium transport. Side effects are rare; however, fatigue and loss of appetite have been reported.[15]

Prostaglandins. These agents reduce intraocular pressure by reducing the resistance to aqueous uveoscleral outflow. They have been shown to be very effective and convenient. These agents are contraindicated in narrow-angle glaucoma.[16] Significant systemic effects have not been reported.[15]

Adrenergic Medications

Epinephrine Derivatives. Topical epinephrine eyedrops, such as Epitrate, Glaucon, Eppy/N or Epinal, and Propine, help reduce the production and increase the outflow of aqueous humor, thereby decreasing intraocular pressure. There is 0.5 to 1 mg of epinephrine per drop of a 2% solution. Side effects include headaches, nervousness, faintness, and palpitations. Other systemic side effects have been reported, including cardiac dysrhythmias, which are usually transient.

Intraocular Medications

Acetylcholine. Acetylcholine (Miochol) is an intraocular agent used to cause pupillary constriction, usually after lens extraction. Adverse effects of this cholinergic agent are uncommon, although bradycardia and bronchospasm have been reported. These symptoms respond well to intravenous atropine.

Sodium Hyaluronate. Sodium hyaluronate (Healon, Amvisc) is a physiologic viscoelastic substance that is distributed throughout the connective tissues in both animals and humans. It is used for maintaining a deep anterior chamber and for protecting the endothelial cells of the cornea from the surgical instrumentation and the intraocular lens in ocular surgery.

Epinephrine. For ocular procedures requiring continued mydriasis, such as cataract extraction, epinephrine is commonly placed in the intraocular irrigating solution. Fiore and Cinotti[17] studied the effects of epinephrine in intraocular irrigating solutions. They concluded that solutions containing low-dose epinephrine, specifically 0.5 mL of 1:1000 epinephrine in 500 mL of solution, were probably safe for maintaining surgical mydriasis and did not appear to cause systemic side effects. However, a sudden onset of epinephrine-induced side effects may warrant discontinuation of the solution.

Sulfur Hexafluoride and Perfluoropropane. Sulfur hexafluoride and perfluoropropane are gases that are used for the insufflation of the vitreous cavity and for the tamponade of a retinal detachment. For maintenance of the appropriate-sized bubble, it has been recommended that nitrous oxide be turned off 15 minutes before the gas is injected. The rest of the procedure should be performed with 100% oxygen and a small amount of volatile agent. Nitrous oxide should not be used for 10 days after the injection of sulfur hexafluoride or perfluoropropane.[13]

Osmotic Diuretic Agents

Mannitol. Mannitol (20% solution in water) is an effective agent for reducing intraocular pressure before surgery or in an acute glaucoma attack. The usual dosage is 1.5 to 2 g/kg, administered over a period of 30 to 60 minutes.[18] Maximum ocular hypotensive effects should be seen about 1 hour after the administration of the drug. This large dose must be carefully infused because rapid infusion can lead to electrolyte imbalance, hypertension or hypotension, pulmonary edema, congestive heart failure, and renal failure resulting from osmotic overload.[19]

Glycerin. Glycerin (Osmoglyn), an osmotic diuretic, is taken orally before ophthalmic procedures in dosages of 1 to 1.5 g/kg. This agent can increase the risk of aspiration with general anesthesia. The metabolism of glycerin may result in hyperglycemia and glycosuria. Common side effects of all osmotic diuretics include headache, nausea, and vomiting.

Topical Local Anesthetic Agents

Cocaine. Cocaine has limited use in ophthalmology today because of its many serious side effects. However, it still may be used in a nasal pack for dacryocystorhinostomy procedures. The maximum recommended dose for clinical use is 1.5 to 3 mg/kg. When used in conjunction with inhalation anesthetics, the dose should be cut in half. Intravenous labetalol has been recommended for the treatment of cocaine's cardiovascular side effects.[20,21]

Tetracaine. Tetracaine (Pontocaine), which is available in strengths of 0.5% to 1%, is an ester-linked local anesthetic. Each milliliter of the 0.5% solution contains 5 mg of tetracaine hydrochloride. As a topical agent, its onset is seen within 1 minute of administration, and its effects last about 30 minutes. Tetracaine tends to cause more stinging on instillation than proparacaine. Although very rare, topical dosages have been associated with systemic toxicity, usually seen as CNS stimulation followed by CNS and cardiovascular depression.

Proparacaine. Proparacaine hydrochloride (AK-Taine, Alcaine, Ophthaine) is a benzoate ester; however, it is chemically different from tetracaine and is much less irritating to the eye. The onset of action ranges from 13 to 20 seconds, and the duration of action is about 15 minutes.

Amide Anesthetic Agents

Bupivacaine, ropivacaine, levobupivacaine, lidocaine, and mepivacaine are common amide local anesthetics used in ophthalmic surgery. Bupivacaine (0.75%) may be used by itself or combined with lidocaine or mepivacaine as a means of decreasing its time of onset. In ophthalmic blocks, complete ocular analgesia usually precedes the onset of extraocular muscle akinesia. Therefore, the presence of akinesia determines the adequacy of the block, and analgesia must be assumed, yet not guaranteed. The use of long-acting bupivacaine in ocular anesthesia generally provides the patient with adequate postoperative pain relief.[21,22] Patients may also experience postoperative diplopia of 24 to 48 hours' duration with this agent. Postoperative diplopia after eye muscle surgery may be of concern; for this reason, a preoperative discussion with the ophthalmologist regarding the duration of action of the planned local anesthetic is in the patient's best interest.[23]

Although allergies to local anesthetics are rare, we have encountered four patients whose skin test results were positive for the preservative-free amides, and we have seen a few others whose results were positive for the preservative agents. For ocular anesthesia, local anesthesia may be used separately or in any combination in order to achieve the desired effect, as long as the total drug dosage does not exceed the recommended doses for the anesthetic administered.

Sodium Bicarbonate. Alkalization of local anesthesia with sodium bicarbonate may decrease the onset time and improve the quality of the neural blockade. The primary ocular anesthetic bupivacaine readily precipitates when alkalization dosages that are less than those recommended are used. The pH threshold for bupivacaine precipitation has been measured at between 6.7 and 6.9.[24] In clinical experience with properly placed modified retrobulbar anesthesia, lidocaine-bupivacaine results in an ocular block onset time of within 2 minutes with minimal to no patient discomfort from the anesthetic solution. However, a study performed in 1991 by Zahl and coworkers[25] on the effects of bicarbonate on peribulbar anesthetic mixtures demonstrated a measurable decrease in onset time of 2.9 to 4.5 minutes. Therefore, alkalization of ocular anesthetics may be of benefit, depending on the type of block used and its time of onset.

Hyaluronidase. Hyaluronidase (Wydase) is a protein enzyme that hydrolyzes hyaluronic acid, a cellular cement between connective tissue. This enzyme promotes the spread of local anesthesia. Clinical experience has demonstrated that hyaluronidase speeds up the onset of action of ocular anesthesia. It may also improve the quality of the block, especially the peribulbar type, by promoting a more uniform spread of anesthesia throughout the orbital fossa.[26] I use 3 U/mL for the modified retrobulbar block and 13 U/mL for the peribulbar block. Because in eyelid blocks the anesthetic agent should be concentrated in the orbicular muscle of the upper eyelid, the hyaluronidase should be omitted.

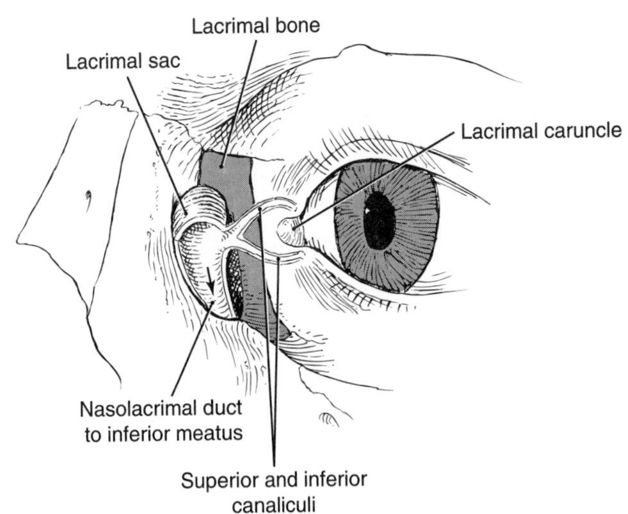

FIGURE **37-19**
Frontal view of the lacrimal drainage system.

Systemic Absorption of Eyedrops

The *lacrimal apparatus* includes the lacrimal gland, the puncta, the inferior and superior canaliculus, the common canaliculus, the lacrimal sac, and the nasolacrimal duct (Fig. 37-19). The lacrimal gland is located in a depression of the frontal bone in the superior temporal orbit.[27] Several ducts lead from the gland to the conjunctival surface of the upper eyelid. Tears pass from the lacrimal gland through the ducts, over the cornea and conjunctiva, keeping the eye moist. Near the medial canthus, the tears enter the puncta and travel through the canaliculus to the lacrimal sac, then drain into the nasolacrimal duct before entering the nasal mucosa.

Topical eye medications enter the bloodstream through the outer eye membrane and the lacrimal apparatus. If need be, the patient can take the following measures to reduce the amount of topical medications that enter the bloodstream:

1. Close the eyes for 60 seconds after drops are placed in order to encourage absorption by the eye and to minimize drainage to the nasal mucosa.
2. Avoid blinking, which rapidly moves the medication into the tear outflow canal and the systemic circulation.
3. Block the tear outflow canal by placing the index finger over the medial canthus after closing the eye.[3]

Patients may complain of a metallic taste after the administration of ocular anesthetics. This precursor to a toxic anesthetic level needs further evaluation. However, it is usually the result of the passing of local anesthesia into the nasal mucosa.

OCULAR REGIONAL ANESTHESIA

The term *ocular local anesthesia* has been used to refer to retrobulbar or peribulbar blocks. More correctly, local anesthesia should be defined as *superficial, topical,* or *cutaneous anesthesia,* used, for example, when skin laceration suturing is performed that poses minimal risks both to the body as a whole and to proximate vital organs. It is important to note that *topical anesthesia* is rapidly gaining popularity for use in a wide variety of outpatient ophthalmic surgical procedure. In fact, since 1998, topical anesthesia has been satisfactorily employed in greater than 37% of all cataract surgeries.[28] Its use continues to increase due to improved operating room management and safety.

Retrobulbar and peribulbar injections are categorized under regional anesthesia methods. These blocks are designed to anesthetize multiple cranial nerves (III, IV, V, VI, and VII). The optic nerve is a continuation of the brain. The dura mater divides at the entrance of the optic nerve into the orbit: the visceral layer of the dura covers the intraorbital part of the optic nerve, and the parietal layer blends into the periosteum of the orbit.[2] Therefore, by an anatomic definition, this procedure is performed in the orbital epidural space. As has been demonstrated in the anatomic reviews by Koornneef, no true muscle cone exists, especially in the posterior portion of the orbit.[7,9,10] Therefore, old anatomic concepts, such as the image of an intact muscle cone, must be set aside in favor of concepts that illustrate a communication throughout the orbit.

Techniques and Modifications

The original retrobulbar technique was described by Atkinson and is still performed today. The patient is instructed to look up and nasally (supranasal position). A 23-gauge retrobulbar (dull) needle is inserted, bevel up, through the skin in the inferotemporal area, just above the inferior orbital rim, and is advanced toward the orbital apex 35 mm (1.38 in) deep into the muscle cone (retrobulbar space). After negative aspiration, 2 to 4 mL of anesthetic solution is injected into the muscle cone. After the injection is completed, the eyelids are closed, and digital pressure is applied over the globe to the orbit. A few minutes later, the eyelids are opened, and the globe is inspected for akinesia.[29-31].

The reported complications from retrobulbar anesthesia include trauma to the optic nerve, the blood vessels, and the globe, all of which can lead to loss of vision. Respiratory arrest may result when anesthetic agents enter the cerebrospinal fluid of the optic nerve. Seizures may occur when even small amounts of local anesthetic are injected intravascularly. Complications have been occurring with greater frequency now that more than 1 million retrobulbar blocks are performed annually.

As a result of the increasing number of complications being reported, practitioners have begun to alter the Atkinson retrobulbar technique in an effort to increase the margin of safety for ocular anesthesia.[32,33] Three major problem areas in the Atkinson technique are identified in this chapter, and technique modifications are discussed (Fig. 37-20).

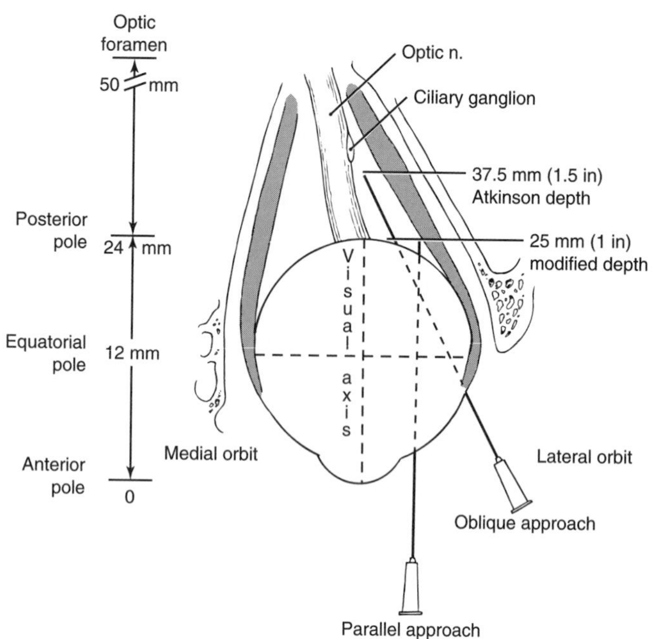

FIGURE **37-20**
Superior view of the parallel and oblique approach to retrobulbar anesthetic blocks.

Eye Position. The position of the eye during retrobulbar block anesthesia is an important consideration. When the patient looks upward and nasally, the optic nerve and blood vessels are placed in the path of the needle. Tension is created on the optic nerve and the surrounding vasculature, making the orbital structures more susceptible to trauma. In this position, the posterior pole of the globe also moves into the needle path. As a means of avoiding this problem, the following modification in technique has been recommended.

The primary gaze position, in which the patient is looking directly forward, allows the optic nerve to maintain its S-shaped curvature and also releases the tension on the blood vessels. The down-and-out gaze position allows the optic nerve and vessels to rotate toward the optic foramen and further away from the needle path. Both of these eye positions have the potential disadvantage of needle visualization by the patient. The upward-gaze position used in modified retrobulbar anesthesia should be used only as described by Gills and Lloyd.[32] Their technique allows the use of the upward-gaze position because the needle is placed lateral and parallel to both the optic nerve and the vessels.

Needle Depth. A second problem is the depth of the needle insertion. The vital structures in the ocular anatomy are more crowded in the posterior orbit. Therefore, the deeper the needle penetration in the orbit, the greater the likelihood of trauma to the optic nerve and vessels. If the depth of the needle insertion is decreased to approximately 25 mm (1 in), the needle would lie just posterior to the globe, thereby reducing the risk of puncture of the vital structures. Studies have demonstrated that because of the wide variation in orbital and globe sizes, a needle depth of 19 to 31 mm (0.75 to 1.25 in) is the safest.[8]

Needle Shape. A pertinent issue debated in the literature is the use of sharp versus dull needles for ocular blocks. Dull or flat-grind needles made specifically for retrobulbar anesthesia are touted by some clinicians as the only safe needles for use in ocular blocks. Currently, it is unclear whether needle choice reduces complications. Grizzard and colleagues[34] noted that it is not so much the type of needle, but where the needle is placed, that increases the risk. Dull retrobulbar needles may not be tolerated as well by awake patients because of the pressure pain they create on insertion. Other needles are available for ocular blocks, including a curved retrobulbar needle[35] and a dull pinhead needle, in which the injection port is proximal to the head of the needle.[36]

Needle Angle. The angle of the needle is a third area that may be considered for modification. The original modifications use an oblique approach; that is, the needle is inserted in the inferotemporal area just above the inferior orbital rim and is directed toward the orbital apex. The change in the eye position and the decrease in the depth of the needle are the significant primary changes to the original techniques that have significantly improved the degree of safety.

However, Gills and Lloyd[32] developed a technique that takes into consideration not only the aforementioned changes but also the length and the spherical shape of the globe. This technique changes the oblique approach to a parallel approach. The lateral limbic margin (corneoscleral junction) is identified, and the needle is inserted in the inferotemporal area transconjunctivally, just lateral and parallel to the lateral limbic margin. The needle is inserted to a depth of approximately 25 mm (1 in), entering the muscle cone just behind the globe. The advantages of this technique result from the needle position, which lies lateral and parallel to the optic nerve, the vasculature, and the posterior pole of the globe.

In summary, the original retrobulbar block technique described by Atkinson can be made safer by modification of the technique. Modifications that decrease the risk of adverse effects are as follows:

1. Position the globe to decrease the tension on the vital orbital structures and position them further away from the needle.
2. Use a depth of needle insertion of about 25 mm (1 in), which places the needle just behind the globe itself and avoids the structures deep in the orbit.
3. Consider using a more lateral to parallel approach to the orbit than was originally demonstrated by Atkinson.

In an effort to further improve the safety of ocular blocks, some investigators have advocated the use of peribulbar anesthesia.[37-39] With this technique, the needle is directed outside the muscle cone. The anesthetic is injected, creating a positive extraconal pressure that spreads the agent inside the muscle cone to anesthetize the cranial nerves. To accomplish this, the needle is inserted parallel to, or is angled away from, the visual axis of the globe in an effort to remain outside the muscle cone. Peribulbar injections may be performed in the superior, medial, and inferior orbital areas.[10] Peribulbar anesthesia requires larger volumes of anesthetic agents (8 to 12 mL).

Because of the many septal divisions of the orbit, which may divert the flow of anesthetic from its primary goal of diffusing into the inner muscle cone, true peribulbar blocks appear to have variable predictability. True peribulbar anesthetic injections may not consistently produce adequate akinesia and may necessitate repeat injections.[40]

Patients who may benefit from the peribulbar approach are those at increased risk for globe puncture, such as those with high myopia and resulting long axial length, significant enophthalmos, previous scleral buckling procedures, and staphylomas. However, peribulbar blocks have also been implemented in patients with globe punctures.[41]

The primary goal of peribulbar blocks is avoidance of the muscle cone and its vital structures. With a modified retrobulbar block, the goal is not only to avoid the vital structures but also to enter the muscle cone just posterior to the globe.

The least vascular areas in which ocular blocks can be performed were described by Koornneef and Kramer[10] (Fig. 37-21). The inferotemporal area can be used for both the modified retrobulbar and the peribulbar techniques. The superior orbital area just lateral to the 12-o'clock position through the skin and the medial orbital area may also be used. The medial orbital area may also be accessed through the caruncle conjunctiva.[33]

In conclusion, the most important considerations for ocular blocks are the position of the eye and the depth of the needle. Needle placement should avoid the optic nerve, the arteries and veins, the globe, and the extraocular muscles.

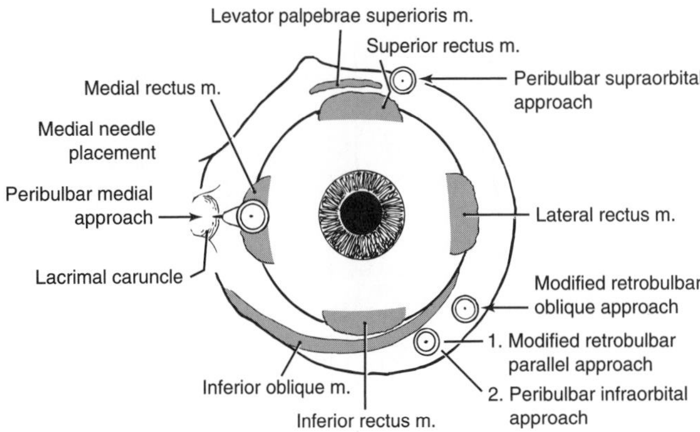

FIGURE **37-21**
Frontal view of needle placement for retrobulbar and peribulbar anesthetic blocks.

Anesthesia Techniques

Gills-Lloyd Modified Retrobulbar Technique

Equipment List

One 3-mL syringe
One 6-mL syringe
One 25- or 27-gauge needle
One 27- or 30-gauge needle
1-in paper tape
One 4 × 4 gauze pad

Description. Figures 37-22 through 37-27 and Box 37-2 present valuable reference aids for the Gills-Lloyd modified retrobulbar technique.

The patient should be in a comfortable, reclining position. Anesthetic drops are placed in the conjunctiva, the eyelids are closed, and the outer eyelids are cleansed. The patient is asked to look directly overhead and to stare at a finger or other object. The eye should not look inward but may look somewhat outward. Needle insertion through the skin is preferably avoided in this technique so that patient discomfort is minimized. The lateral limbic margin (corneoscleral junction) is identified. The lower eyelid is everted and controlled with a

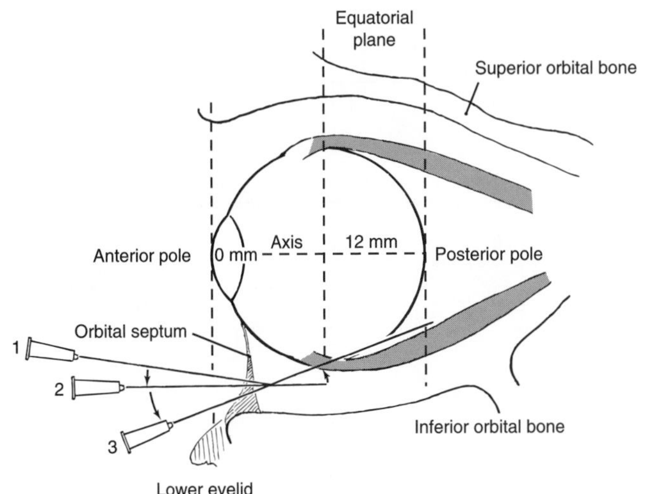

FIGURE **37-22**
Lateral view of needle angles for a modified retrobulbar block.

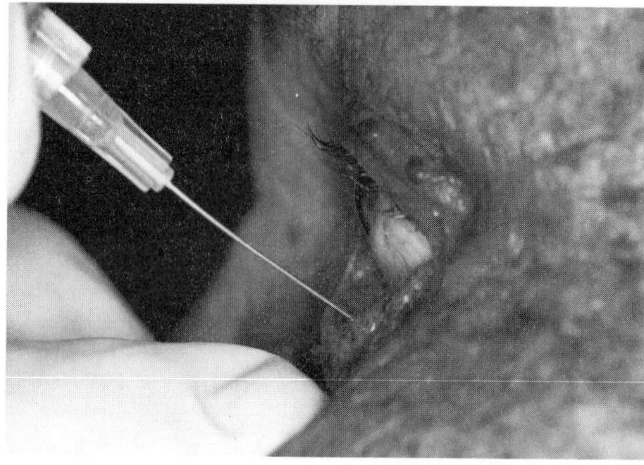

FIGURE **37-23**
In the Gills-Lloyd modified retrobulbar technique, the needle should be inserted transconjunctivally or transcutaneously, angled away from the visual axis of the globe toward the orbital floor until the orbital septum is penetrated.

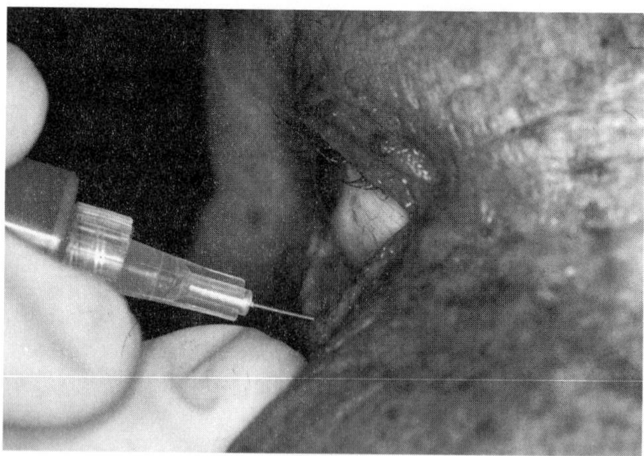

FIGURE **37-24**
The Gills-Lloyd modified retrobulbar technique. After penetrating the orbital septum, the needle should be redirected parallel to the visual axis to a depth of about 12 mm (0.5 in) to the equatorial plane of the globe.

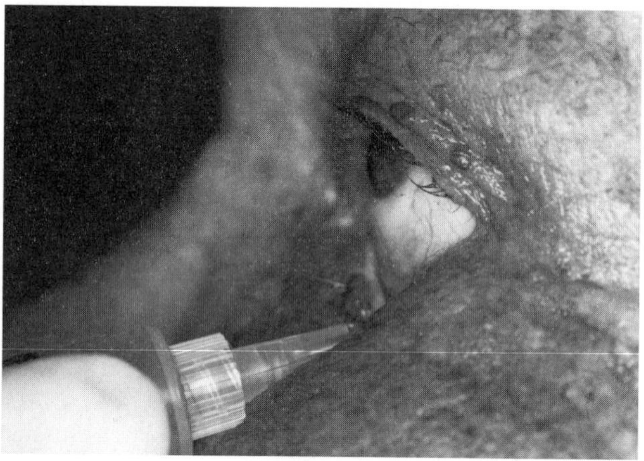

FIGURE **37-25**
The Gills-Lloyd modified retrobulbar technique. At the equatorial plane of the globe, the needle should be redirected toward the visual axis to a depth of about 25 mm (1 in). At this point, the needle enters the muscle cone, and the medication is injected.

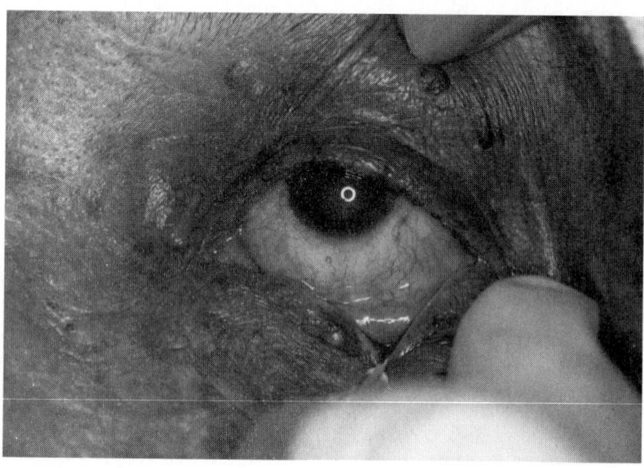

FIGURE **37-26**
Needle placement, which is lateral and parallel to the lateral limbic margin, is demonstrated for the Gills-Lloyd modified retrobulbar technique.

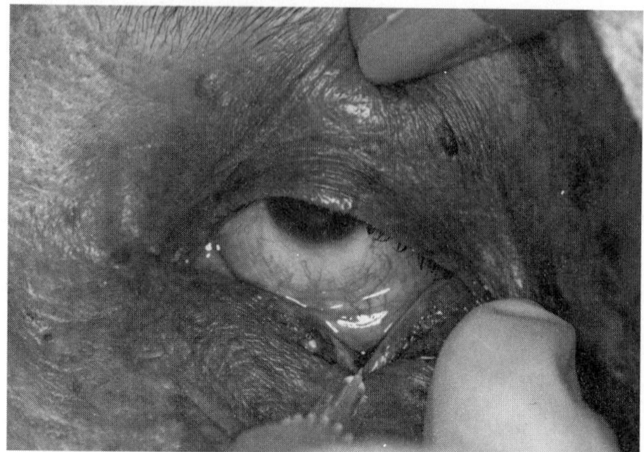

FIGURE **37-27**
Completion of the modified retrobulbar block. Some degree of globe proptosis and drooping of the upper eyelid should be expected.

BOX **37-2**

The Gills-Lloyd Modified Retrobulbar Technique: Parallel Approach

Insert the needle transconjunctivally or transcutaneously, angled away from the visual axis of the globe toward the orbital floor, until the orbital septum is penetrated (see Fig. 37-23).

After penetrating the orbital septum, redirect the needle parallel to the visual axis to a depth of about 12 mm (0.5 in) to the equatorial plane of the globe (see Fig. 37-24).

At the equatorial plane of the globe, redirect the needle toward the visual axis to a depth of about 25 mm (1 in), entering the muscle cone and injecting the medication (see Fig. 37-25).

finger. The needle is placed in the bevel-up position just above the inferior orbital rim, just lateral and parallel to the lateral limbic margin. The needle is then inserted through the conjunctiva and directed toward the orbital floor until the orbital septum is penetrated. The needle is then redirected parallel to the visual axis of the globe to a depth of 25 mm (1 in). At this time, 1 to 1.5 mL of lidocaine, 1% to 2%, is injected after negative aspiration is performed. This initial peribulbar technique is effective in reducing the potential discomfort from the needle and the anesthetic injection of the modified retrobulbar block in the awake patient.

The eye is closed briefly in preparation for the modified retrobulbar injection. The lower eyelid is again everted and controlled with a finger. The needle is placed bevel up, just above the inferior orbital rim, just lateral and parallel to the lateral limbic margin. The needle is then inserted through the conjunctiva and is directed toward the orbital floor until the orbital septum is penetrated. The needle is then redirected parallel to the visual axis of the globe to its equatorial plane, about 12 mm deep. At this point, the needle is rotated cephalad between the lateral and inferior rectus muscles. Resistance may or may not be felt as the needle penetrates the muscle cone. The needle should be inserted about 25 mm (1 in), depending on the size of the orbit and the globe (range, 19 to 31 mm). After negative aspiration, the anesthetic agent is injected slowly, 1 mL/10 sec, until the orbit is filled. Orbital size governs the total amount of anesthetic injected; however, 4 to 6 mL usually suffices. Once the orbit is full of anesthesia, as indicated by orbital tension, the needle is withdrawn. The eyelids are closed, a 4 × 4 gauze is placed over the eye, and positive digital pressure is applied. The pressure helps spread the anesthetic and detect any increasing orbital pressure, which might indicate a retrobulbar hemorrhage.

The fibrinous orbital septum may present considerable resistance to the needle, which, after penetration, may advance quickly into the periorbital space. Therefore, the initial needle insertion is directed away from the globe so that the risk of globe puncture is decreased. Resistance may or may not be felt as the needle enters the muscle cone, depending on the presence or absence of the fibrinous connective tissue in the area behind the globe, as described by Koornneef and Kramer.[10] The sharper the needle, the less resistance felt by the practitioner and the less discomfort felt by the patient. By comparison, use of a dull needle results in more resistance at the orbital septum and inner muscular membrane, potentially resulting in greater patient discomfort. Patients have described this resistance to the needle as pressure pain. Because a pop may or may not be felt as the needle enters the muscle cone, attention to needle depth is extremely important for the avoidance of deep penetration into the orbit.

During injection, the patient is told that if he or she experiences any discomfort, such as stinging or a mild headache, he or she should inform the practitioner, who will stop the injection to allow the agent to take effect. After the needle is placed, this pressure sensation appears to result from the local agent's spreading throughout the orbital area. The stinging is noticed more when the agent moves into the peripheral area along the upper and lower eyelids. This slow injection process is continued until the orbit is filled with the anesthetic agent. When the anesthetic is placed into the muscle cone, the effects are seen rapidly, and the block can be evaluated for akinesia after about 2 minutes. Generous traction must be applied to the lower eyelid because this technique is performed before the orbicular muscles of the eyelids are anesthetized (seventh nerve block). Seventh nerve blocks can be very painful and are not well tolerated by patients. An initial seventh nerve block may not be necessary because the anesthetic agent from the modified retrobulbar or peribulbar block spreads randomly throughout the orbit and eyelids, providing adequate akinesia of the eyelids.[42]

Peribulbar Techniques. Figures 37-28 through 37-30 and Box 37-3 serve as valuable reference aids for the peribulbar technique.

Peribulbar block may be performed by use of several different techniques. One is a supraorbital-only technique[39] of injecting a large volume (10 to 12 mL) of anesthetic agent, which should distribute throughout the orbit for completion of the block. An inferotemporal-only technique also involves injection of a large volume (10 to 12 mL) of anesthesia, which should distribute throughout the orbit and anesthetize the eye. The more common approach to peribulbar anesthesia is the use of both the inferior and the superior approaches. Each of these injections may be performed with a 6-mL syringe for a total volume of 10 to 12 mL. The combination technique generally

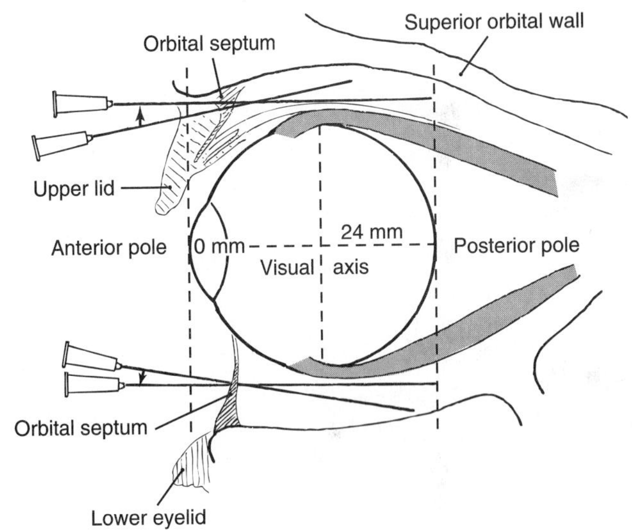

FIGURE **37-28**
Lateral view of needle angles for peribulbar block.

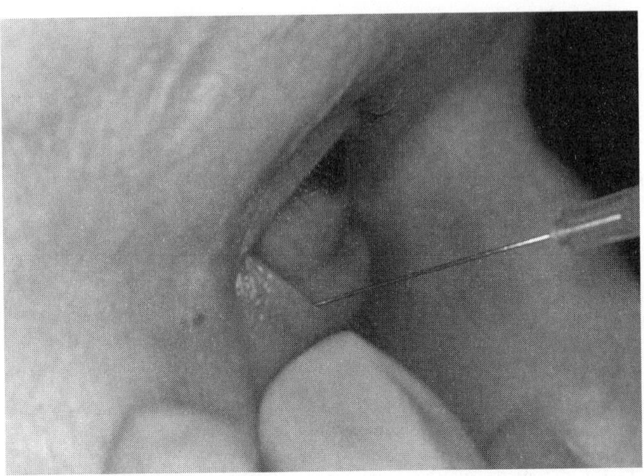

FIGURE **37-29**
In the infraorbital approach, the needle is inserted transconjunctivally or transcutaneously and angled away from the visual axis of the globe toward the orbital floor to a depth of about 25 mm (1 in), and the medications are injected.

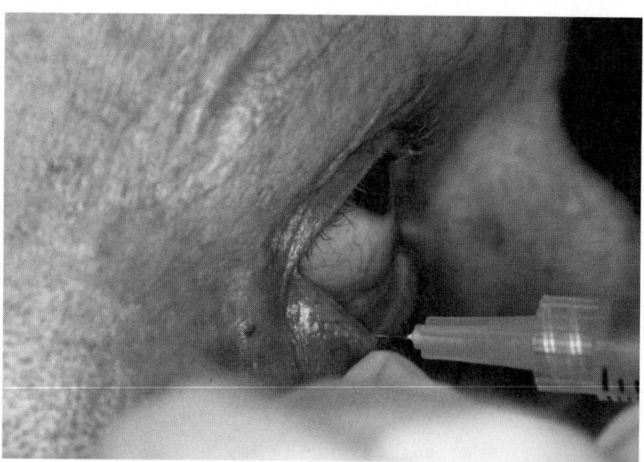

FIGURE **37-30**
In the infraorbital approach, after penetration of the orbital septum, as shown in Fig. 37-29, the needle is redirected parallel to the visual axis to a depth of about 25 mm (1 in), and the medications are injected.

BOX **37-3**

Peribulbar Techniques

Infraorbital Approach

Insert the needle transconjunctivally or transcutaneously, angled away from the visual axis of the globe toward the orbital floor, to a depth of about 25 mm (1 in) and inject the medications (see Fig. 37-29).

OR

After penetrating the orbital septum, as described in item 1, redirect the needle parallel to the visual axis to a depth of about 25 mm (1 in) and inject the medications (see Fig. 37-30).

Supraorbital Approach

Insert the needle *only transcutaneously*, angled away from the visual axis of the globe toward the orbital ceiling, to a depth of about 12 mm (0.5 in) and inject the medications.

OR

After penetrating the orbital septum, as described in item 3, redirect the needle parallel to the visual axis to a depth of about 25 mm (1 in) and inject the medications.

provides a more consistent result. It is usually easier to handle a 6-mL syringe rather than a 10-mL syringe around the eye.

Infraorbital Supraorbital Peribulbar Anesthesia

Equipment List

One 10-mL syringe or two 6-mL syringes
One or two 25- or 27-gauge needles
One 4 × 4 gauze pad
1-in paper tape
One alcohol or povidone-iodine (Betadine) wipe

Description. The patient is asked to look directly overhead. The lateral limbic margin is identified. The lower eyelid is everted and controlled with a finger. The needle is placed bevel up just above the inferior orbital rim, lateral and parallel to the lateral limbic margin. The needle is then inserted through the anesthetized conjunctiva and directed toward the orbital floor until the orbital septum is penetrated. The needle is then redirected parallel to, or angled away from, the visual axis of the globe to a depth of about 25 mm (1 in). After the syringe is secured and negative aspiration is performed, 6 mL of the anesthetic agent is slowly (1 mL/10 sec) injected. The rate of injection is determined by patient comfort. After the injection, the eyelids are closed, and positive pressure is applied for dispersal of the medication.

The supraorbital peribulbar injection is performed just inferior to the supraorbital rim and just lateral to the 12-o'clock position. The needle is inserted bevel down through the skin. This area is generally anesthetized from the original inferotemporal injection. The needle is inserted parallel to, or angled away from, the visual axis of the globe to a depth of about 25 mm (1 in). After negative aspiration is performed, the anesthetist must begin a slow injection of 4 to 6 mL of anesthetic solution until a tense orbital area is observed. A more tense orbit should be expected to result from the peribulbar technique because of the increased extraconal pressure necessary to move the anesthetic intraconally.

Once this technique is completed, the eyelids are closed and taped shut. A 4 × 4 gauze pad is placed over the closed eye. A positive pressure device is now placed over the eye to help distribute the agent throughout the orbit and achieve the desired analgesia and akinesia. The positive pressure device also decreases intraocular pressure to an acceptable surgical level. The eyelids must completely cover the eye in order to avoid a corneal abrasion. It may take up to 20 minutes for satisfactory surgical anesthesia to be established from a periorbital block. Should the periorbital block fail to attain adequate akinesia within 20 minutes, the appropriate muscles must be reblocked by use of the inferior technique for the inferior rectus, inferior oblique, and lateral rectus muscles. The superior technique is used for the superior rectus, superior oblique, and medial rectus muscles. The anesthetic volume of the second block should create an extraconal pressure that is adequate for reaching the inner conal area. The supraorbital approach should not be attempted through the conjunctiva, because of the potential for damage to the levator muscle of the upper eyelid; such damage may result in upper eyelid ptosis.

Medial Peribulbar Anesthesia

Equipment List

One 3-mL syringe
One 27- or 30-gauge needle

Description. Figures 37-31 and 37-32 and Box 37-4 serve as valuable reference aids for medial peribulbar anesthesia.

A medial peribulbar technique has been described in the literature.[33,34] In this technique, the anesthetic agent is placed in the periorbital space that exists between the medial wall of the bony orbit and the medial rectus muscle. This technique is very effective as a secondary block both for incomplete akinesia of the medial rectus muscle and the superior oblique muscle and as a primary block for the orbicular muscles of the eyelid.

The *medial peribulbar area* is a rather avascular fatty compartment that lies just medial to the medial rectus muscle. This area narrows significantly as it approaches the posterior surface of the globe, and the medial rectus muscle lies near the bony

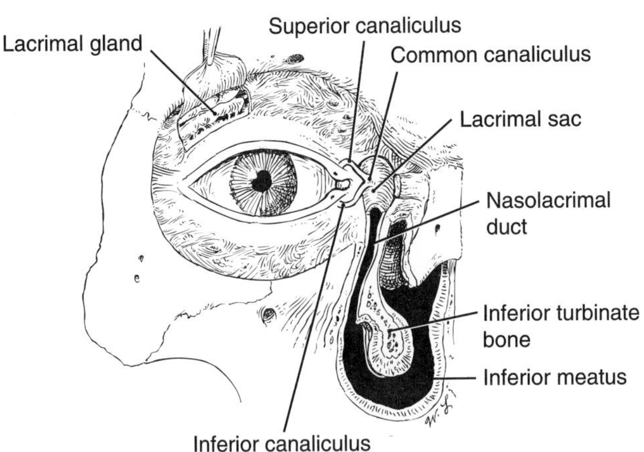

FIGURE **37-31**
Frontal view of the lacrimal drainage system.

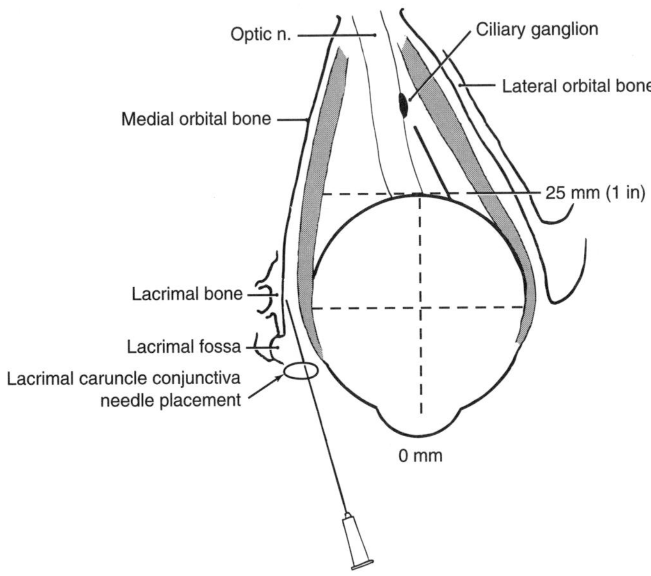

FIGURE **37-32**
Superior view of the needle angle for a medial peribulbar block.

orbit. Superior to the medial peribulbar area is the supranasal area. This area contains a portion of the superior ophthalmic vein and branches of the ophthalmic artery and should be avoided when ophthalmic blocks are performed.

The *caruncle*, a small mound at the inner canthus of the eye formed by a conjunctival fold at its junction with the skin, is the landmark for the medial peribulbar technique. The needle is inserted through the caruncle conjunctiva, tangential to the globe, and is directed medially and posteriorly toward the lacrimal bone, which is just posterior to the lacrimal sulcus. Great care must be taken to avoid trauma to the puncta, the lacrimal cuniculi, and the lacrimal sac. Once the needle is near or has made contact with the lacrimal bone, at a depth of about 12 mm (0.5 in), the anesthetic may be injected. If the bony orbit is contacted, the needle may be redirected more posteriorly. However, the anesthetist should maintain a slight angle away from the visual axis toward the bony orbit, and the insertion should not exceed the depth of the posterior surface of the globe, so that contact with the medial rectus muscle is

BOX **37-4**

Medial Peribulbar Technique

Penetrate the caruncle conjunctiva with the needle angled toward the lacrimal bone, to a depth of approximately 12 mm (0.5 in), and inject the medications.

OR

If bone is contacted, the needle may be redirected more posteriorly, with a slight angle maintained away from the visual axis and not exceeding the depth of the posterior surface of the globe.

avoided. After negative aspiration is performed, 2 mL or more of anesthetic agent may be injected for facilitation of the desired effect. After the block is completed, the eyelid should be closed and light pressure applied for reduction of the incidence of bleeding.

In the medial area are herniated orifices within the connective tissue that communicate anteriorly to the posterior surface of the orbicular muscle of the eye. Therefore, the anterior spread of the anesthetic agent also provides satisfactory akinesia of the eyelids for surgery. The medial peribulbar technique can also be used with minimal discomfort to provide eyelid akinesia before a modified retrobulbar is performed: in this sequence, proparacaine drops are applied to the caruncle before the block is administered.

Ocular Block Evaluation

After an ophthalmic block is performed, partial movement of one or more of the ocular muscles may occur. Residual movement should be assessed to determine which muscles are involved and whether additional anesthesia is required. Analgesia of the globe generally precedes akinesia of the eye muscles. Therefore, analgesia of the globe may be assumed, but not guaranteed, in the presence of an akinetic muscle. The effectiveness of a modified retrobulbar block may be evaluated 2 minutes after it is administered, and a peribulbar block 10 to 20 minutes after it is administered, by observing for eye movement in all four quadrants.

Eyelid Block

Once satisfactory akinesia of the globe is established, evaluation for movement of the eyelids is necessary. Partial-to-complete akinesia of the orbicular muscle is generally found after the ocular block, especially with the medial peribulbar block or techniques that require high anesthetic volumes. Should incomplete akinesia occur after an ocular block, an additional seventh nerve block may be required. Several seventh nerve blocks are described in the literature, including those by O'Brien, Nadbath, Van Lint, and Hustead.[29,33,43]

The Nadbath and O'Brien techniques block the seventh cranial nerve proximally, resulting in unilateral facial paralysis. The Nadbath technique is still used today; however, its popularity is decreasing as a result of its systemic side effects and the patient discomfort it causes. The Van Lint technique more appropriately addresses the need for eyelid akinesia, with less potential for adverse effects, by blocking the temporal and zygomatic branches of the facial nerve to the orbicular muscles. I have developed and used a variation of the Van Lint technique that I call an *orbicularis oculi block*. I believe that this technique is safer, less painful, and better accepted by the awake patient than the Van Lint block is. However, this technique still requires injections through the skin and has the potential for causing patient discomfort and eyelid ecchymosis. My preferred technique for eyelid akinesia remains the medial peribulbar block.

Orbicularis Oculi Block

Equipment List

One 6-mL syringe
One 30-gauge needle
One alcohol wipe

Description. Figure 37-33 and Box 37-5 serve as valuable reference aids for the orbicularis oculi block.

This technique is performed after a modified retrobulbar or peribulbar block in which residual eyelid movement remains. The inferotemporal area of the infraorbital rim is chosen. The needle is inserted bevel down, subcutaneously and tangentially to the eyelid. One to 2 mL of the anesthetic agent is injected just under the skin of the eyelid. After the needle is removed, the local anesthesia should be digitally spread to the medial and the lateral canthi; this measure avoids running the needle across the lower eyelid. The second injection is made supranasally in the upper eyelid. A finger should be placed over the closed eyelid, slightly depressing the globe. The needle is again inserted, bevel down, subcutaneously and tangentially to the eyelid. One to 2 mL of the agent is injected just under the skin of the eyelid. After the needle is removed, the local anesthetic is digitally spread to the medial and lateral canthi. After the anesthetic is spread throughout the eyelids, light to moderate pressure is applied over the eyelids for prevention or reduction of superficial bleeding.

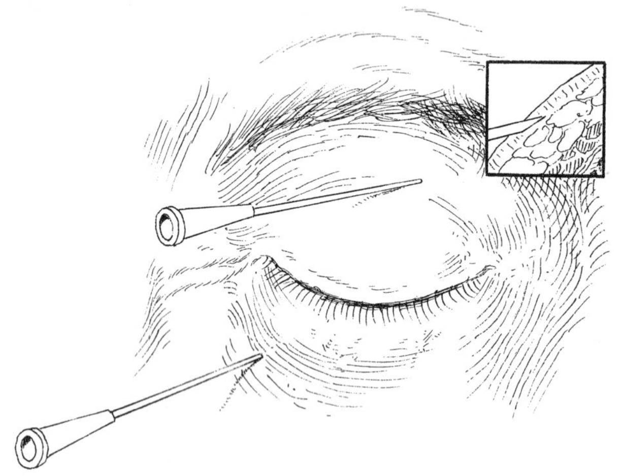

FIGURE **37-33**
Frontal view of the needle placement for an orbicularis oculi block.

BOX **37-5**

Orbicularis Oculi Block

Insert the needle subcutaneously, bevel down, and tangential to the lid in the infratemporal area and inject the medications.
While slightly depressing the globe, insert the needle subcutaneously, bevel down, and tangential to the lid in the supranasal area, and inject the medications.

Nadbath Technique

Equipment List

One 6-mL syringe
One 25- or 27-gauge needle
One 4 × 4 pad
One alcohol or povidone-iodine wipe

Description. Figure 37-10 provides valuable visual aids for the Nadbath technique.

The area immediately under the auricular cartilage is identified, just posterior to the ramus of the mandible. A 12.5-mm needle is inserted perpendicular to the skin in this location. The needle placement is in the area where the facial nerve exits the stylomastoid foramen. After negative aspiration is performed, 3 to 5 mL of anesthetic solution is injected. This block can be painful and has many side effects that are addressed later.

Van Lint Technique

Equipment List

One 6-mL syringe
One 25- or 27-gauge needle
One alcohol or povidone-iodine wipe
One 4 × 4 gauze pad

Description. A 37.5-mm (1.5-in) needle is inserted infratemporally into the subcutaneous tissue of the lateral canthus. The first injection of 1 to 2 mL of anesthetic agent is directed nasally along the lower margin of the orbit and then withdrawn back to its origination point. The second injection of 1 to 2 mL of anesthetic agent is directed upward along the supratemporal margin of the orbit. After the block is completed, light pressure is applied over the closed eyelids to disperse the medication and decrease ecchymosis.

Positive Orbital Pressure

The increased volume of local anesthetic required for both modified retrobulbar and peribulbar anesthetics causes an increase in orbital and intraocular pressures. The anesthetic agent not only tracks along and penetrates the fascial sheaths behind the globe, it also moves anteriorly underneath the conjunctiva, producing chemosis (subconjunctival edema) of the eye. These events make the surgical procedure more difficult to perform. The random dispersement of the orbital anesthetic that results in chemosis cannot be controlled. The agent merely tracks along the path of least resistance. Clinically, chemosis can begin with the injection of as little as 1 to 2 mL of anesthetic. In other instances, chemosis has not been seen even after the injection of as much as 12 mL of anesthetic agent.

Positive pressure devices are used to offset increased intraocular pressure and chemosis. Positive pressure devices are placed directly over the globe and orbit. They enhance the orbital spread of the anesthetic and reduce the intraocular pressure and chemosis, while returning the orbital anatomy to a more appropriate state for surgery. The deepened anterior chamber created by the reduction in the intraocular pressure allows greater room for surgical intervention.

Types of Positive Pressure Devices

Pinky Ball. The pinky ball, designed by Gills and Lloyd, is a commonly used positive pressure device. A head strap is placed behind the head, the eye is taped closed, and a 4 × 4 gauze pad is folded and placed over the eyelid. A rubber ball with an elastic strap running through it is placed over the center of the eye and secured to the head strap by the elastic straps. Light to moderate pressure is applied and maintained by adjustment of the elastic straps.

Honan Intraocular Pressure Device. With the Honan intraocular pressure device, a rubber head strap is placed behind the head. The eye is taped closed, and a folded 4 × 4 gauze pad is placed over the eye. The Honan cuff is placed over the gauze pad and secured with the Velcro head strap. The pressure gauge is inflated to 30 to 40 mm Hg, a value that is marked in yellow on the gauge.

Topical Anesthesia. For many years, it was believed that cataract and other ophthalmic surgical procedures required potent motor blockade to produce akinesia of the ocular structures. However, studies have now shown that excellent results may be achieved by employing topical anesthesia. The topical anesthesia technique includes eyedrop application of 0.5% tetracaine, sponge anesthesia utilizing intraocular lidocaine hydrochloride, and/or gel application of 2% lidocaine hydrochloride, with or without adjunctive sedation. Moreover, the topical anesthesia is gaining greater acceptance by nurse anesthetists because it provides the ophthalmic surgeon with optimal operating conditions, while avoiding the rare but serious complications associated with injected anesthetics, such as globe perforation, retrobulbar hemorrhage, and inadvertent dural or intravascular injection of local anesthetics.[44]

To control the discomfort of patients during cataract surgery using topical anesthesia, some practitioners employ an intracameral injection of local anesthetics.[1] The benefits derived from utilizing topical plus intracameral anesthesia as compared to pure topical application have been demonstrated in numerous studies.[45] Despite the many advantages of this technique, the variants in application have created a modicum of confusion as to the precise definition of "topical anesthesia" for ophthalmic surgical procedures.[44]

Sub-Tenon's Block. The sub-Tenon's (medial canthus episcleral) block has proven to be a safe and efficacious alternative to other regional anesthesia or injection techniques in high-risk cases, such as monocular patients, those with long eyes, and those on anticoagulants. The sub-Tenon's block, in which the local anesthetic is given with a blunt cannula underneath the Tenon's layer, utilizes a relatively high volume of approximately 10 mL. Under direct microscopic visualization, the ophthalmic surgeon utilizes scissors to make a small incision through the conjunctiva and sub-Tenon's capsule. A soft, curved cannula is inserted through the incision along the sclera approximate to the equator. The local anesthetic is then administered under the sub-Tenon's capsule under direct visualization and the sensory block occurs instantaneously. Since the technique does not use a sharp-tipped needle, it is considerably safer for the at-risk patient.[46]

As with other ocular blocks, some practitioners choose to supplement the injection with adjunctive medications, such as clonidine, midazolam, or propofol sedation. Studies in the extant literature comparing sub-Tenon injection to peribulbar or retrobulbar block have proven that it provides equivalent pain control, while avoiding most of the complications associated with needle injections.[46-48]

ANESTHESIA MANAGEMENT

Preoperative Preparation

Ophthalmic procedures are most commonly performed on young children and elderly persons. Each age group has a unique set of physical problems. For the young child, the questions regarding the patient's history should include any congenital, metabolic, and musculoskeletal abnormalities, such as malignant hyperthermia, that may affect anesthesia care. In the elderly patient, multisystem medical problems may be present, and drug interactions from multiple medication regimens may exist.[49] A thorough patient history is therefore paramount. Patients undergoing regional block, in which patients are awake for the procedure, must be evaluated for claustrophobia, severe arthritis, tremors, and any other physical derangements that may make it difficult for them to lie supine. Patients' mental status must also be evaluated so that their degree of cooperation and their ability to follow commands can be determined.

Elderly patients are often taking many medications and may not remember them; however, they are told to bring their medications to the surgery center the day of surgery. Patients are also seen by their primary medical physician and are evaluated as to their fitness for surgery.[50] However, the attending surgeon, in collaboration with the anesthesia practitioner, may allow patients to undergo surgery if they have no preexisting medical conditions or if the conditions are well controlled. An electrocardiogram (ECG) is also requested with the medical evaluation of such patients. This assessment furnishes a baseline so that the patient can be evaluated for any significant ECG changes that require further preoperative evaluation. Routine laboratory tests are not ordered unless they are medically necessary for patients receiving regional anesthesia.[51] *Appropriate laboratory data are necessary when general anesthesia is planned.*[52,53]

After a thorough patient history and physical examination are completed, the anesthetist must determine whether regional or general anesthesia is indicated (Box 37-6). Clearly, general anesthesia should be used for infants and young children. General anesthesia is also indicated in patients with severe claustrophobia; an inability to cooperate, communicate, or lie flat; or a history of uncontrolled acute anxiety attacks. It is also indicated for procedures of greater than 2 hours' duration. Most adults tolerate ophthalmic procedures well when

BOX **37-6**

Indications for General Anesthesia

Pediatric patient
Patient's lack of cooperation
Severe claustrophobia
Inability to communicate
Inability to lie flat
Open eye injuries
Procedures with durations greater than 2 hours

BOX 37-7

Disadvantages of General Anesthesia

Nausea/vomiting
Retching/bucking
Increased intraocular pressure
Aspiration
Complications secondary to other medical problems (e.g., cardiovascular disease)
Time and expense

regional anesthesia is used. Given the disadvantages associated with general anesthesia (Box 37-7), regional anesthesia should be considered the anesthetic of choice in these patients.

Regional Block with Minimal Sedation

Patients undergoing a regional block are requested to take their medications as usual on the day of surgery. An exception may be patients who complain of a frequent need to urinate after taking diuretic medications. Antiplatelet drugs (e.g., aspirin) and anticoagulants (e.g., warfarin [Coumadin]) are not mandatorily discontinued, because retrospective studies have shown no increase in hemorrhagic complications either operatively or postoperatively when these drugs were taken.[54,55] In addition, the risk of systemic complications, such as cardiovascular accidents and myocardial infarctions, is potentially greater if administration of these products is discontinued. Continuing anticoagulant administration, however, requires consultation and agreement between the anesthesia practitioner and the surgeon. If bleeding occurs, it may be more severe. Patients who are receiving or have previously been treated with chemotherapy may also have prolonged bleeding times.

Patients undergoing surgery in the morning may be instructed to eat a light breakfast the day of surgery, and those undergoing surgery in the afternoon may be told to eat a light lunch. They may also consume clear fluids until they are admitted to the facility.[56-58] We have followed this procedure since 1986 and have experienced improved compliance with medications, less nausea, and improved patient comfort without experiencing problems. Patients with diabetes are instructed to continue their regimen of medications and diet on the day of surgery.

Admissions on the Day of Surgery

Anesthesia practitioners must not forget how stressful a surgical procedure is for patients. A kind and professional attitude in those caring for these patients helps the patients to deal more effectively with their stress. The proper use of progressive relaxation and hypnotic techniques further helps alleviate anxiety. The establishment of a good patient-provider relationship works synergistically with pharmacologic agents in promoting the best possible surgical environment. On admission, the patient's mental and physical status, vital signs, and ECG should be reviewed, and any changes that may require postponement should be noted.

Regional Block Environment

Ocular blocks are commonly performed outside the operating room. This method facilitates a more efficient case flow and a more comfortable environment for the patient. The potentially life-threatening effects of orbital epidural blocks require that appropriate resuscitative equipment and trained personnel be available to monitor the patient. The area used for performing ocular blocks should have the following:

Oxygen
Bag-valve mask
Suction
Airways
ECG equipment
Blood pressure cuff
Oxygen saturation monitor
Intravenous access tubing
Canthotomy set
Ammonia capsules
Nitroglycerin tablets
Atropine
Glycopyrrolate tablets

Additional resuscitative equipment and medications as recommended by advanced cardiac life support guidelines should be available.

Sedation for Regional Blocks

Many techniques have been advocated for the relaxation of patients before ocular blocks are performed. Many of these techniques work well in the elderly patient. Sedation techniques should be designed to decrease anxiety (Box 37-8) and to reduce the discomfort of the block (Box 37-9). When the block is less painful, patients require less sedation for comfort. The surgeon's preference for an awake, relaxed, or sleeping patient during the procedure should be considered. Sleeping patients often snore or have sudden head movements on awakening.

The goal of sedation is to help patients gain and maintain control of themselves by reducing their heightened anxiety state.[58] If the patient will be asleep during the block, the patient should fast before the procedure, consistent with the facility's criteria for general anesthesia (Box 37-10). Methohexital (usually 0.5 to 1 mg/kg) has been a popular

BOX 37-8

Sedation Techniques

Good rapport between patient and clinician—no medications necessary
50% nitrous oxide and 50% oxygen inhalation
Intravenous benzodiazepine administration
Intravenous narcotic administration
Intravenous barbiturate or nonbarbiturate administration

BOX 37-9

Causes of Discomfort Resulting from Regional Blocks

Needle injection through the skin
Needle penetration of the orbital septum
Needle penetration of the intermuscular membrane
Rapid injection of anesthetic
Stinging from peripheral spread of anesthetic

BOX 37-10

Procedure for Patient Who Is Asleep During Regional Block

Tilt head to maintain patent airway.
Open patient's eye in primary gaze position.
Administer regional block.
Administer incremental sedation as required.

choice for this technique. It is slowly given intravenously until the patient's eyes close.[59] Thiopental has also been used;[60] however, its potential for causing prolonged sleeping during surgery can be disruptive to the surgeon. Propofol is an excellent choice for this technique because of its short duration of action.[61]

Monitoring for Regional Anesthesia

Communication is the cornerstone of dealing with the awake patient. Informing the patient of what to expect and what to do if he or she experiences any problems is mandatory. Questions and instructions must be clear and specific, especially if the patient is hearing impaired or if a language barrier exists.

The positioning of the patient is very important. Pillows may be used under the knees in order to decrease back strain. The patient with severe arthritis must be carefully padded and positioned. The patient's head and neck should be placed in a satisfactory surgical position. The practitioner should ensure that the patient is warm and is as comfortable as possible. Nasally administered oxygen is recommended. Monitoring equipment should consist of electrocardiograph, sphygmomanometer, and oxygen saturation monitor. Observing the surgical procedure on a television monitor is preferable to not seeing the surgery. This allows the anesthetist to follow the surgical progress and visualize critical points in the procedure in which patient movement would be most detrimental.

The surgical draping placed over the patient's face should be tented, and high-flow air may be used in order to decrease expired carbon dioxide. Claustrophobia can be a problem for awake patients, and some patients experience it for the first time during this procedure. Techniques for dealing with claustrophobia include taping the nonsurgical eye or adjusting the drape so that the patient can see the room with the nonsurgical eye. If a patient experiences a claustrophobic attack, the surgical drapes should be tented away from the face immediately, while the sterile field is maintained, and verbal control of the patient should be gained. At this point, the anesthetist must determine whether the patient can proceed with surgery with regional block.

Rarely, the patient may experience incomplete ocular analgesia, even in the presence of muscle akinesia. This problem responds well to tetracaine or proparacaine drops or subconjunctival anesthetic injection.

Acute increased intraocular pressure during the surgical procedure can be catastrophic and can cause loss of ocular contents. This problem can be created by coughing or a choroidal hemorrhage. The increased intrathoracic pressure created during coughing is reflected through the valveless orbital veins, resulting in an acutely increased intraocular pressure of 40 mm Hg or greater.[17] A choroidal hemorrhage occurs when a vessel in the vascular choroidal layer of the eye ruptures, bleeding into the closed cavity and creating an acute rise in intraocular pressure with potential expulsion of eye contents unless the eye is closed quickly. In the acute phase, medications that lower intraocular pressure may be of minimum benefit.

If the patient has a history of postnasal drip, vasoconstrictive nose drops may be given preoperatively. If the patient complains of a dry throat, small amounts of water may be given. These two remedies are helpful in reducing the incidence of coughing intraoperatively. The patient must also be instructed to give notice before he or she coughs. Instructing the patient to clear his or her throat effectively reduces the forcefulness of the cough. Quick, shallow breaths have been reported to help suppress the cough reflex.[62] Sedating the patient or using intravenous lidocaine to prevent further coughing can help but has minimal effect during an active coughing episode.[63]

After the surgery is completed, the patient walks or is transported from the operating room to the recovery room. Postoperative recovery time should be in accordance with the individual patient's physical and mental status and the amount of medication administered.

Postoperative nausea noted immediately after surgery may result from the sedative medications, increased intraocular pressure, or ocular pain.[64,65] On the afternoon or evening after their surgery, patients are generally called at home for evaluation of their status. A sudden onset of nausea at home after the procedure is more likely associated with increased intraocular pressure than anesthetic medications. Patients are usually examined the following day by the surgeon and are requested to fill out questionnaires regarding their experience on the day of surgery.

General Anesthesia

For general anesthesia, preoperative patient preparation should include the appropriate fasting guidelines for the patient's age and physical condition (e.g., diabetes). The patient should be reminded that the surgical eye will be patched when he or she awakens. Sedation should be administered as needed to help the patient relax. Benzodiazepines such as midazolam are effective in low doses. For reduction of the incidence of aspiration and postoperative nausea, the use of histamine$_2$ antagonists, metoclopramide, and other antiemetics should be considered. Induction of general anesthesia with any of the intravenous barbiturates is recommended because they all decrease intraocular pressure. In infants and children, inhalation induction also decreases intraocular pressure. Because of their emetic effect, narcotics should be used in low doses. Other than during examinations under anesthesia, endotracheal intubation is required for maintenance of the airway.

Depolarizing muscle relaxants, such as succinylcholine, cause a transient increase in intraocular pressure. However, they can be used safely for ocular procedures:

1. The sustained contracture of the extraocular muscles after succinylcholine could theoretically cause an expulsion of the intraocular contents. This assumption is theoretical. It is now felt that succinycholine may be safely used in eye surgery.
2. In eye muscle surgery, the sustained contraction may interfere with the forced duction test used by the surgeon in the planning of treatment.
3. Patients taking long-acting glaucoma medications, such as echothiophate, may have prolonged apnea.

The nondepolarizing muscle relaxants are also satisfactory for induction (Box 37-12) and have the advantage of decreasing intraocular pressure. Laryngoscopy, especially with light anesthesia, increases intraocular pressure. Intravenous lidocaine (1.5 to 2 mg/kg), given 1 to 1.5 minutes before laryngoscopy, helps attenuate this response. Inhalation anesthetics, which also decrease intraocular pressure, are commonly used for the maintenance of general anesthesia.

For intraocular procedures, the continued use of nondepolarizing muscle relaxants is recommended for the maintenance of an akinetic eye and a satisfactory intraocular pressure. The anesthetist must be aware of the potential adverse ECG changes that may result from the oculocardiac reflex, which may be elicited when traction is exerted on the extraocular muscles and orbital structures. Patients undergoing eye muscle surgery have an increased incidence of malignant hyperthermia and postoperative nausea. In retinal procedures in which sulfur hexafluoride or perfluoropropane is used as an intraocular gas, the use of nitrous oxide should be discontinued 15 minutes before injection.

When spontaneous ventilation returns, after neuromuscular blockade is reversed, the patient may be extubated while receiving deep anesthesia with 100% oxygen and may be placed in the lateral position until he or she awakens. In the patient with a difficult airway, full stomach, or incompetent esophageal sphincter, gastric suction and intravenous lidocaine (1.5 to 2 mg/kg) may be given before the patient is extubated awake. This method helps reduce the incidence of coughing and vomiting, along with their deleterious effects.

Postoperative care, with attention paid to alleviation of pain and control of nausea, helps maintain satisfactory intraocular pressure. For intraocular procedures, the ophthalmologist should be made aware of continued postoperative nausea because it may be the result of acute increased intraocular pressure.[64]

Open Eye Injury and the Full Stomach

Open eye injury in a patient with a full stomach is a difficult situation, at best, for the anesthesia practitioner. These injuries are commonly considered emergencies requiring general anesthesia. The clinician must protect the patient from aspiration and yet avoid increased intraocular pressure that could result in expulsion of intraocular contents. Authors are constantly debating the risks and advantages of using succinylcholine for this procedure.[17,66-68] Green and Lurenberg[69] and Coleman and Trokel[70] demonstrated that a normal eyelid blink increases intraocular pressure by 10 to 15 mm Hg, and a forceful eyelid closure increases intraocular pressure by more than 70 mm Hg. They concluded that a 10- to 12-mm Hg increase in intraocular pressure that is caused by succinylcholine administration was clinically insignificant and would not cause expulsion of intraocular contents.

This observation, coupled with the lack of any documented cases of extrusion of intraocular contents in open globes of humans when succinylcholine is used, causes us to question the traditional teaching that succinylcholine should be avoided in all cases when open globe is suspected or known.[68] Moreno and coworkers agreed with Libonati that, when indicated, succinylcholine should be considered in patients with suspected or known open globes.[71]

The location of the injury on the globe may place the eye at greater risk for intraocular expulsion.[72] The visual prognosis may also be poor because of the existing injury. If chances of repairing the eye to functional vision are minimal, it should be documented for legal reasons. Therefore, the ophthalmologist should be consulted preoperatively for documentation of the risks and advantages of the chosen induction technique.

OPHTHALMIC ANESTHESIA COMPLICATIONS

Anxiety coupled with underlying cardiovascular disease may promote marked hypertension, cardiac dysrhythmias, or angina in the patient before surgery. Vasovagal responses (e.g., fainting) secondary to anxiety are not unusual. Ammonia capsules are effective in preventing and treating fainting episodes.

Chronic coughing secondary to chronic obstructive pulmonary disease, asthma, or postnasal drip must be evaluated. Vasoconstrictive nose drops effectively decrease postnasal drip. Coughing and deep breathing before surgery helps clear the lungs of excess mucus in patients with chronic pulmonary disease. Proper evaluation and treatment help reduce undesired perioperative systemic and ocular sequelae.

Most complications of regional ocular anesthetics can be attributed to the direct traumatization of the orbital vessels, the globe, and the optic nerve. Trauma to these structures can result whenever a needle is placed near the eye. Frequently, the cause of complications during general anesthesia is patient movement.

Retrobulbar Hemorrhage

Retrobulbar hemorrhage results from trauma to an orbital vessel. The bleeding or proptosis moves the eye forward, and a subconjunctival hemorrhage is usually present. Venous hemorrhages are usually slow in onset. The arterial hemorrhage has a rapid onset and more pronounced proptosis and subconjunctival hemorrhage. Ecchymosis of the eyelids and orbit is usually present. The pressure caused by the bleeding in the bony orbital cavity produces an increased orbital pressure on the optic nerve, vessels, and globe. This positive orbital pressure usually resolves without problems. However, the increased intraorbital pressure may result in an occlusion or spasm of the central retinal artery or vein, resulting in partial to complete loss of vision.[73] One may detect a progressively increasing orbital pressure when digital pressure is applied over the eye after an ocular block. Continuous digital pressure may be all that is required for stopping a venous hemorrhage.[32] If the orbital pressure continues to increase in the presence of digital pressure, a lateral canthotomy should be performed immediately, and the ophthalmologist should be notified. *Canthotomy* is a procedure performed to increase the orbital space by cutting the lateral canthus. This procedure reduces the orbital pressure that results from a retrobulbar hemorrhage.

Any practitioner who performs ocular blocks should be instructed in how to perform a canthotomy, and a canthotomy set should be readily available (Box 37-11). The ophthalmologist should examine the central retinal artery and vein for patency. Occlusion of these vessels may warrant further surgical intervention for reduction of the elevated orbital pressure.

A localized scleral hemorrhage also causes subconjunctival bleeding. In this situation, however, no proptosis of the globe or increase in orbital pressure is noted. These episcleral vessels are the same ones the ophthalmologist cauterizes after a conjunctival incision. The vessels break as a result of the spread of local anesthesia through the subconjunctival area and are of no consequence. However, the ophthalmologist should be notified of their presence before the procedure begins.

Retrobulbar hemorrhage remains the most common sequela for ocular blocks (Box 37-12). Peribulbar injections can also

BOX **37-11**

Canthotomy Procedure

Equipment
1 straight hemostat
1 plastic scissors

Procedure
If possible, inject lidocaine along the lateral canthus.
Place the hemostat in a temporal direction along the lateral canthus 4-6 mm and clamp the hemostat.
Remove the hemostat.
Use the plastic scissors to incise *only* in the crush marks left by the hemostat.
Control local bleeding with the hemostat or with digital pressure.

BOX **37-12**

Measures for Preventing Retrobulbar Hemorrhage

Choose the least vascular areas for needle placement.
Avoid deep orbital injections.
Avoid supranasal position of gaze.
Use primary gaze position.
Use down-and-out gaze position.
Use upward-gaze position (Gills-Lloyd technique).
Insert needle slowly.

cause orbital hemorrhages.[41] Retrobulbar hemorrhages have been reported to occur in 1% to 3% of cases.[74]

Intravascular Injection

Grand mal seizures have been reported to occur after retrobulbar injections with lidocaine and lidocaine-bupivacaine combinations.[75,76] It is thought that a seizure may result from a less-than-toxic dose of local anesthesia by direct intraarterial injection, resulting in retrograde flow to the cerebral circulation (Box 37-13). In 1987 Mathers[77] surveyed 200 ophthalmologists. Sixty-six responded and reported three seizures occurring after retrobulbar injections. From these data, it appears that seizures after retrobulbar anesthesia may occur more frequently than reported in the literature. A reaction after an orbital vein injection has also been reported: the patient experienced uncontrolled shivering and rigor approximately 15 seconds after the retrobulbar injection. These symptoms resolved within 2 minutes of onset.[78]

Globe Puncture

Multiple reports have been published regarding globe perforations. Both sharp and dull needles have either penetrated or perforated the eye during retrobulbar and peribulbar injections. Although rare, globe punctures have occurred in the hands of experienced practitioners who have performed many thousands of ophthalmic blocks. The literature notes that patients may or may not exhibit signs and symptoms of a puncture immediately, and the diagnosis has been made anywhere from 1 to 14 days after the event.[34,79-84]

The myopic eye has an increased axial length of greater than 24 mm. Scleral thinning may result from this increased anteroposterior diameter of the myopic eye. The increased axial length brings the posterior pole of the globe near the retrobulbar needle. A previous scleral buckling procedure also increases the anteroposterior diameter of the eye. *Staphyloma*, a bulging of the sclera, may also predispose the patient to globe puncture. The risk of puncture increases when this abnormality is located inferoposteriorly on the globe. *Enophthalmos* is a recession of the eyeball into the orbit. This condition decreases the distance between the posterior pole of the globe and the posterior orbital wall. The supranasal gaze position rotates the posterior pole of the globe in line and closer to the retrobulbar needle. Multiple orbital injections have also been cited as a factor in globe punctures, along with unexpected patient movement (Box 37-14).

The choice of sharp versus dull retrobulbar needles is highly debated. The literature reviewed appears to draw conclusions based more on opinion than on fact. In 1991 Grizzard and colleagues[34] published a detailed review of the literature; this review confirmed a lack of safety with the use of blunt needles. The investigators quoted multiple authors who reported optic nerve penetration, ocular perforation, and CNS complications resulting from the use of blunt needles. The surgeon should be notified if a globe puncture is suspected (Box 37-15).

BOX **37-13**

Measures for Preventing Seizures Resulting from Intravascular Injection

Choose least vascular areas for needle placement.
Avoid deep orbital injections.
Avoid supranasal position of gaze.
Insert needle slowly.
Aspirate gently before injection; negative aspiration is no guarantee that you are not in a blood vessel.
Avoid injection against resistance.
Avoid forceful rapid injections.

BOX **37-14**

Measures for Preventing Globe Puncture

Use caution in patients with increased axial length.
Avoid supranasal position of gaze.
Direct needle away from the axis of the globe when inserting it through the orbital septum.
Observe globe movement with needle insertion.
Insert needle slowly.
Never forcefully inject anesthetic.
Use modified retrobulbar and peribulbar techniques (although globe punctures have also been reported with these).

BOX 37-15

Signs and Symptoms of Globe Puncture*

Increased resistance to injection
Immediate dilation and paralysis of the pupil
Rapid increase in intraocular pressure with edematous cornea
Subconjunctival hemorrhage
Pain and agitation
Hypotony of the globe
Intraocular hemorrhage

**Patient may or may not exhibit signs and symptoms of a puncture immediately.*

Optic Nerve Sheath Trauma

The *optic nerve sheaths* surround the optic nerve and are composed of the meninges of the brain. The outer sheath contains the *dura mater* and the inner sheath consists of the *arachnoid mater* and *pia mater*. The subarachnoid space contains cerebrospinal fluid and is continuous with the optic chiasma. The dura splits into two layers at the optic foramen. The outer dural layer becomes continuous with the orbital periosteum. The inner layer forms the dural covering of the optic nerve, creating the orbital epidural space.[2] Anesthetic agents injected into the subdural or subarachnoid space may track back to the optic chiasma. Here, the anesthetic can affect the contralateral eye by blocking cranial nerves II and III as they proceed through the subdural or subarachnoid space; this block can result in contralateral amaurosis.[85-87] This condition can be a precursor to the continued migration of the anesthetic to the respiratory centers of the midbrain, resulting in respiratory arrest.[75,88]

The anesthetist should observe the contralateral pupil before an ocular block is performed. The pupil may be dilated from accidental administration of preoperative eyedrops, a preoperative examination, or existing pathology. If the contralateral pupil is constricted before the ocular block and dilates after the ocular block (contralateral amaurosis), one must assume that subarachnoid or subdural injection has occurred and be prepared to treat a respiratory arrest.

The onset of respiratory arrest is usually within 2 to 5 minutes after injection; however, it may occur as late as 10 minutes after injection. Spontaneous ventilation usually returns in 15 to 20 minutes but may take up to 55 minutes for complete recovery. Treatment includes appropriate ventilatory and cardiovascular support, supplemental oxygen with oxygen saturation monitoring, ECG monitoring for cardiac dysrhythmias, and blood pressure monitoring. The surgeon should be notified immediately so that he or she can examine the eye for any optic nerve trauma that may require surgical intervention.

Retinal vascular occlusion or thrombosis has been reported after ocular blocks.[89,90] A retrobulbar hemorrhage resulting in increased extravascular pressure may result in occlusion of the central retinal artery or vein, or both. Also, direct trauma to the ophthalmic artery or the optic nerve by the retrobulbar needle may cause artery or vein occlusion without causing retrobulbar hemorrhage[91-93] (Box 37-16).

Optic nerve atrophy has been reported after intraocular surgery with either regional block or general anesthesia.[73] Direct trauma to the optic nerve may result in transient symptoms, such as contralateral amaurosis or respiratory arrest, or it may result in vascular occlusion or thrombosis, or both, with partial to complete loss of vision.

BOX 37-16

Measures for Preventing Optic Nerve Sheath Trauma

Avoid supranasal eye position.
Choose least vascular area for needle insertion.
Avoid deep orbital injection.
Insert needle slowly.
Avoid forceful injection of anesthetics.
Use modified retrobulbar or peribulbar techniques.

Extraocular Muscle Palsy and Ptosis

Inferior muscle palsy has been reported after retrobulbar anesthesia. Segmental inferior rectus muscle enlargement was noted posterior to the globe deep in the orbit.[94] This complication has not been reported to occur after general anesthesia.[95] The initial signs and symptoms of this problem manifest after surgery as persistent vertical diplopia. Surgical intervention is indicated for correction of this condition. Trauma to the superior oblique tendon–trochlea complex has also been reported to occur with peribulbar anesthesia[96] (Box 37-17).

In 1992 Carlson and coworkers[97] performed experiments on the rectus muscle of monkeys and humans; these investigators demonstrated minimal myotoxic damage to ocular muscles after retrobulbar administration of local anesthetics. Typically, after the injection of local anesthesia, the surface muscle fibers degenerate, then regenerate. However, direct injections of local anesthesia into the rectus muscle resulted in massive internal muscle lesions that were large enough to produce noticeable functional deficit. The myotoxicity of local anesthetics may also play a role in postoperative ptosis, especially in the elderly, because regeneration of their muscle fibers may not be as complete as that in younger patients.[97] However, ptosis is more commonly associated with the superior rectus stay suture and the eyelid speculum. Postoperative ptosis may take as long as 6 months to resolve.

Facial Nerve Blocks

Patients commonly experience discomfort as a result of seventh nerve blocks. Prolonged Bell's palsy has been seen after Nadbath and O'Brien blocks, probably secondary to direct nerve trauma.[98] Several authors have reported cases of dysphagia, hoarseness, coughing, and respiratory distress after Nadbath blocks (Box 37-18). They noted that these symptoms were consistent with paresis of the vagus, glossopharyngeal,

BOX 37-17

Measures for Preventing Extraocular Muscle Trauma

Avoid needle contact with extraocular muscles.
Avoid obliquely directing needles in the peribulbar space.
Avoid deep orbital penetration.
Avoid angling needle toward the visual axis of the globe when parallel to an extraocular muscle.

BOX 37-18

Prevention and Treatment of Complications from the Nadbath Block

Avoid using the Nadbath technique in patients weighing <45 kg.
Avoid using large volumes of anesthesia and hyaluronidase (Wydase).
Avoid using the Nadbath technique when patients have a preexisting unilateral vocal cord dysfunction.
Put patient in seated or lateral position in order to maintain a patent airway and patient comfort.
Intubate patient with an unsatisfactory airway.

and spinal accessory nerves. These nerves exit the skull about 10 mm medial to cranial nerve VII. Therefore, anesthesia injected for the seventh nerve block could also reach these nerves and result in unilateral vocal cord paralysis.[99-102]

Patients have also complained of jaw ache with movement for several weeks after the seventh nerve block. I am aware of one reported grand mal seizure when 3 mL of 2% lidocaine with epinephrine (1:200,000) was injected using the Nadbath technique.

Oculocardiac Reflex

The *oculocardiac reflex* is a trigeminal-vagal reflex that was first described in 1908 by Aschner. The stimulus for this reflex is generated by pressure on the globe, the orbital structures (e.g., the optic nerve), or the conjunctiva, or by traction on the extraocular muscles (particularly the medial rectus muscle). The afferent pathway for the stimulus is the trigeminal nerve via the ciliary ganglion. The efferent pathway consists of the vagus nerve to the cardioinhibitory center.

The reflex may be elicited during local infiltration anesthesia, retrobulbar blockade, and general anesthesia. However, ocular regional block (retrobulbar or peribulbar) may also inhibit the reflex. The occurrence of the reflex in ocular procedures is variable, but it is commonly seen in muscle procedures performed in children. The oculocardiac reflex reveals itself most often as an acute sinus bradycardia. However, it may also cause a wide variety of other cardiac dysrhythmias, such as nodal rhythms, atrioventricular block, ventricular ectopy, idioventricular rhythm, and asystole. Continuous ECG monitoring is essential for the diagnosis of dysrhythmias that result from the oculocardiac reflex. If cardiac dysrhythmias are observed, the surgeon must be instructed to immediately cease all pressure or traction on the orbit. Simultaneously, the patient should be assessed for adequate oxygenation and ventilation and for adequate anesthetic depth because one or more of these may be an underlying cause for the dysrhythmia. The aberrant rhythm usually resolves without intervention within a few seconds. However, if the aforementioned measures are taken and the dysrhythmia continues, thus threatening to cause hemodynamic instability, intravenous atropine should be administered. Two to 3 mg of atropine may be required for complete vagal blockade. Caution should be exercised with the administration of atropine, because atropine itself may induce cardiac dysrhythmias. The surgeon may proceed only after the dysrhythmia is resolved. If the reflex recurs, the aforementioned process should be repeated. The oculocardiac reflex, however, appears to fatigue with continued manipulations. The use of intravenous atropine or intravenous glycopyrrolate just before surgery may help reduce the incidence of the reflex, especially in children.[17,103,104]

Ocular Ischemia

While the risk has yet to be fully quantified, several studies of recent vintage have uncovered the possibility of ocular ischemia resulting from alterations in pulsatile ocular blood flow ostensibly caused by local anesthesia blockade.[105-108] Although intraocular pressure does not appear to rise significantly after the application of a retrobulbar or peribulbar blockade, there are indications that these blocks may induce a significant and sustained decrease in pulsatile ocular blood flow (POBF), which may have clinical implications in patients with preexisting compromised ocular circulation.[105-107] In response, some researchers have recommended monitoring of POBF in at-risk patients receiving retrobulbar or peribulbar blocks.[108]

General Anesthesia Complications

Corneal abrasion is the most common injury occurring after general anesthesia. It is believed to result from the drying of the exposed cornea or from direct trauma, such as an anesthesia mask injury. Ensuring that the eyelids are closed and secured with tape should provide satisfactory protection of the cornea. Movement during ocular surgery was identified as the single most common mechanism of injury. Movement was described as coughing and bucking, which resulted in poor visual outcome. In these reported cases, muscle relaxants were used less than 50% of the time and nerve stimulators were omitted. Chemical injury can result from the spilling of cleaning materials or preparatory solutions into the eye. In these cases, the eye should be flushed immediately with saline.[109]

Central retinal artery occlusion may result from prolonged pressure on the eye.[110] This type of injury may result with the patient in the prone position. Careful attention to padding and periodic checks of the eyes are necessary, especially for long procedures. Eye pads and gel donuts for the face may help prevent eye trauma. It is prudent to request an ophthalmic examination immediately after surgery if the patient complains of any eye problems or if the anesthesia provider suspects a problem.

REFERENCES

1. Venkatesan VG, Smith A: What's new in ophthalmic anaesthesia? *Curr Opin Anaesthesiol* 15:615-620, 2002.
2. Wolff E: *Anatomy of the Eye and Orbit*, ed 5, Philadelphia, 1966, Saunders.
3. Vaughn D, Asbury T: *General Ophthalmology*, ed 11, Norwalk, CT, 1986, Appleton-Century-Crofts.
4. Scheie H, Albert D: Anatomy of the human eye. In *Textbook of Ophthalmology*, ed 9, Philadelphia, 1977, Saunders, pp 45-78.
5. Netter F: *Nervous System*, vol 1, ed 11, Summit, NJ, 1972, Ciba Pharmaceutical.
6. Doxanas MT, Anderson, RL: *Clinical Orbital Anatomy*, Baltimore, 1984, Williams & Wilkins.
7. Ettl A, Koornneef L, Daxer A, Kramer J: High resolution magnetic resonance imaging of the orbital connective tissue system. *Ophtha Plas Reconstr Surg* 14(5):323-327, 1998.
8. Katsev D, Drews R, Rose B: An anatomic study of retrobulbar needle path length, *Ophthalmology* 96:1221-1224, 1989.

9. Meyer DR, Linberg JV, Wobig JL, McCormick SA: Anatomy of the orbital septum and associated eyelid connective tissues: Implications for ptosis surgery. *Ophthal Plas Reconstr Surg* 7(2): 104-113, 1991.
10. Koornneef L, Kramer N: *Anatomy and anesthesia*, Orbita Centrum, The Netherlands, 1988, University of Amsterdam (videotape).
11. McGoldrick K: Principles of ophthalmic anesthesia, *J Clin Anesth* 1:297-312, 1989.
12. Goodman LS, Gilman A, editors: *Goodman and Gilman's Pharmacological Basis of Therapeutics*, ed 10, New York, 2001, McGraw-Hill, p 1935.
13. McGoldrick K: Anesthesia and the eye. In Barash P, Cullen B, Stoelting R, editors: *Clinical Anesthesia*, ed 4, Philadelphia, 2001, Lippincott, pp 969-988.
14. Frishman WH, Kowalski M, Nagnur S, Warshafsky S, Sica D: Cardiovascular considerations in using topical, oral, and intravenous drugs for the treatment of glaucoma and ocular hypertension: focus on beta-adrenergic blockade, *Heart Dis* 3:386-397, 2001.
15. Hoyng PFJ, van Beek LM: Pharmacological therapy for glaucoma: a review, *Drugs* 59:411-434, 2000.
16. Alward WLM: Medical management of glaucoma, *N Engl J Med* 339:1298-1307, 1998.
17. Fiore P, Cinotti A: Systemic effects of intraocular epinephrine during cataract surgery, *Ann Ophthalmol* 20:23-25, 1988.
18. Mauger TF, Nye CN, Boyle KA. Intraocular pressure, anterior chamber depth and axial length following intravenous mannitol, *J Ocul Pharmacol Ther* 16(6):591-594, 2000.
19. Lichter P, Musch DC, Medzihradsky F, Standardi CL: Intraocular pressure effects of carbonic anhydrase inhibitors in primary open-angle glaucoma, *Am J Ophthalmol* 107:11-17, 1989.
20. McGoldrick K: Ocular drugs and anesthesia, *Int Anesthesiol Clin* 28:72-77, 1990.
21. Naor J, Slomovic AR: Anesthesia modalities for cataract surgery, *Curr Ophthalmol* 11(1):7-11, 2000.
22. Huha T, Ala-Kokko TI, Salomaki T, Alahuhta S: Clinical efficacy and pharmacokinetics of 1% ropivacaine and 0.75% bupivacaine in peribulbar anaesthesia for cataract surgery, *Anaesthesia* 54(2):137-141, 1999.
23. Nicholson G, Sutton B, Hall GM: Comparison of 1% ropivacaine with 0.75% bupivacaine and 2% lidocaine for peribulbar anaesthesia, *Br J Anaesth* 84(1):89-91, 2000.
24. Peterfreund R, Datta S, Ostheimer G: pH adjustment of local anesthetic solutions with sodium bicarbonate: laboratory evaluation of alkalinization and precipitation, *Reg Anesth* 14:74, 1989.
25. Zahl K, Jordan A, McGroarty J, Sorensen B, Gotta AW: Peribulbar anesthesia effect of bicarbonate on mixtures of lidocaine, bupivacaine, and hyaluronidase with or without epinephrine, *Ophthalmology* 98:239-242, 1991.
26. Kallio H, Paloheimo M, Maunuksela EL: Hyaluronidase as an adjuvant in bupivacaine-lidocaine mixture for retrobulbar/peribulbar block, *Anesth Analg* 91(4):934-937, 2000.
27. Paulsen F: The human nasolacrimal ducts, *Adv Anat Embryol Cell Biol* 170:iii-xi,1-106, 2003.
28. Leaming DV: Practice styles and preferences of ASCRS members: 1998 survey, *J Cataract Refract Surg* 25:851-859, 1999.
29. Aitkenhead AR, Rowbotham DJ, Smith G: Anesthesia for ophthalmic surgery. *Textbook of Anaesthesia*, ed 4, Edinburgh, Scotland, 2001, Churchill Livingstone, pp 594-605.
30. Hamilton RC, Gimbel HV, Strunin L: Regional anaesthesia for 12,000 cataract extraction and intraocular lens implantation procedures, *Can J Anaesth* 35(6):615-623, 1988.
31. Katz J: *Atlas of regional anesthesia*, ed 2, Norwalk, CT, 1993, Appleton-Century-Crofts, p 30.
32. Gills J, Lloyd T: A technique of retrobulbar block with paralysis of orbicularis oculi, *Am Intraocul Implant Soc J* 9:339-340, 1983.
33. Hustead RF, Hamilton RC, Loken RG: Periocular local anesthesia: medial orbital as an alternative to superior nasal injection, *J Cataract Refract Surg* 20:197-201, 1994.
34. Grizzard WS, Kirk NM, Pavan PR, et al: Perforating ocular injuries caused by anesthesia personnel, *Ophthalmology* 98: 1011-1016, 1991.
35. Straus J: A new retrobulbar needle and injection technique, *Ophthalmic Surg* 19:134-138, 1988.
36. Simonson D: Retrobulbar block: a review for the clinician, *AANA J* 58:456-461, 1990.
37. Bloomberg L: Anterior periocular anesthesia: five years' experience, *J Cataract Refract Surg* 17:508-511, 1991.
38. Davis D, Mandel M: Posterior peribulbar anesthesia: an alternative to retrobulbar anesthesia, *J Cataract Refract Surg* 12: 182-184, 1986.
39. Smith GB, Hamilton RC, Carr CA: *Ophthalmic Anaesthesia: A Practical Handbook*, ed 2, London, 1996, Arnold.
40. Wang H: Peribulbar anesthesia for ophthalmic procedures, *J Cataract Refract Surg* 14:441-443, 1988.
41. Shriver P, Sinha S, Galusha H: Prospective study of the effectiveness of retrobulbar and peribulbar anesthesia for anterior segment surgery, *J Cataract Refract Surg* 18:162-165, 1992.
42. Martin S, Baker S, Muenzler W: Retrobulbar anesthesia and orbicularis akinesia, *Ophthalmic Surg* 17:232-233, 1986.
43. Hustead RF: Techniques. In Gills J, Hustead RF, editors: *Ophthalmic Anesthesia*, Thorofare, NJ, 1993, Slack, pp 141-145.
44. Fichman RA: Use of topical anesthesia alone in cataract surgery, *J Refract Surg* 22:612-614, 1996.
45. Carino NS, Slomovic AR, Chung F, Marovich AL: Topical tetracaine versus topical tetracaine plus intracameral lidocaine for cataract surgery, *J Cataract Refract Surg* 24:1602-1608, 1998.
46. Guise PA: Single quadrant sub Tennon's block. Evaluation of a new local anaesthetic technique for eye surgery, *Anesth Intensive Care* 24:241-244, 1996.
47. Ripart J, Lefrant J-Y, Vivien B, Charavel P, Fabbro-Peray P, Jaussaud A, Dupeyron G, Eledjam J-J: Ophthalmic regional anesthesia: Medial canthus episcleral (sub-Tenon) anesthesia is more efficient than peribulbar anesthesia, *Anesthesiology* 92:1278-1285, 2000.
48. Stevens JD: A new local anaesthesia technique for cataract extraction by one quadrant sub-Tenons infiltration, *Br J Ophthalmol* 76:670-674, 1992.
49. Szmyd L, Schwartz B: Association of systemic hypertension and diabetes mellitus with cataract extraction, *Ophthalmology* 96:1248-1252, 1989.
50. Bartley G, Narr B: Preoperative medical examinations for patients undergoing ophthalmic surgery, *Am J Ophthalmol* 112:725-727, 1991.
51. Walters G, McKibbin M: The value of pre-operative investigations in local anaesthetic ophthalmic surgery, *Eye* 11(pt 6): 847-849, 1997.
52. Bellan L: Preoperative testing for cataract surgery, *Can J Ophthalmol* 29(3):111-114, 1994.
53. Schein OD, Katz J, Bass EB, Tielsch JM, Lubomski LH, Feldman MA, Petty BG, Steinberg EP: The value of routine preoperative medical testing before cataract surgery: Study of Medical Testing for Cataract Surgery, *N Engl J Med* 342(3):168-175, 2002.
54. Narendran N, Williamson TH: The effects of aspirin and warfarin therapy on haemorrhage in vitreoretinal surgery, *Acta Ophthalmol Scand* 81(1):38-40, 2003.
55. Alcalay, J: Cutaneous surgery in patients receiving warfarin therapy, *Dermatol Surg* 27(8):756-758, 2001.
56. Maltby J: Preoperative fasting guidelines undergo revision: Report on the Annual Meeting of the Society for Ambulatory Anesthesia, *Excerpta Medica* 21:3-14, 1991.
57. Daughtery J: Clear liquids before surgery offer ASC's more flexibility, *Same Day Surg* 15:105-107, 1991.
58. Practice guidelines for preoperative fasting and the use of pharmacologic agents to reduce the risk of pulmonary aspiration: application to healthy patients undergoing elective procedures: a report by the American Society of Anesthesiologist Task Force on Preoperative Fasting. *Anesthesiology*. 1999 Mar;90(3):896-905.

59. Sharvelle D: Brevital: a general anesthetic agent, *Ophthalmic Surg* 15:334, 1984 (letter).
60. Vindhya PK, Sheets JH, Tolia NH, Tomlinson LJ: Retrobulbar block using pentothal as a sedative for ambulatory surgery, *J Cataract Refract Surg* 13:321-322, 1987.
61. Habib NE, Balmer HG, Hocking G: Efficacy and safety of sedation with propofol in peribulbar anaesthesia, *Eye* 16(1):60-62, 2003.
62. Romano P: Coughing and the open eye, *Ophthalmic Surg* 14:1041-1042, 1983 (letter).
63. Stewart RH, Kimbrough RL, Engstrom PF, Cameron B: Lidocaine: an antitussive for ophthalmic surgery, *Ophthalmic Surg* 19:130-131, 1988.
64. Gross JG, Meyer DR, Robin AL, Filar AA, Kelley JS: Increased intraocular pressure in the immediate postoperative period after extracapsular cataract extraction, *Am J Ophthalmol* 150: 466-469, 1988.
65. Knopf H: Periocular anesthesia for relief of pain, *Ann Ophthalmol* 19:181, 1987.
66. Vinik HR: Intraocular pressure changes during rapid sequence induction and intubation: a comparison of rocuronium, atracurium, and succinylcholine, *J Clin Anesth* 11(2):95-100, 1999.
67. Poterack KA: How controversial are anesthetic controversies? *J Clin Anesth* 9(4):266-269, 1997.
68. Vachon CA, Warner DO, Bacon DR: Succinylcholine and the open globe. Tracing the teaching, *Anesthesiology* 99:220-223, 2003.
69. Green K, Lurenberg MN: Consequences of eyelid squeezing on intraocular pressure, *Am J Ophthalmol* 88:1072-1077, 1979.
70. Coleman DJ, Trokel S: Direct-recorded intraocular pressure variations in a human subject, *Arch Ophthalmol* 82:637-640, 1969.
71. Libonati MM, Leahy JJ, Ellison N: The use of succinylcholine in open eye surgery, *Anesthesiology* 62:637-640, 1985.
72. Morsman C: Succinylcholine in open eyes, *Ophthalmology* 98:1607-1608, 1991 (letter).
73. Ben-David, B: Complications of regional anesthesia: an overview, *Anesthesiol Clin North Am* 20(3):427-429, ix, 2002.
74. Mullins RM: Retrobulbar block. In Atlee JL, editor: *Complications in Anesthesia*, Philadelphia, 1999, Saunders, pp 782-784.
75. Gomez RS, Andrade LO, Costa JR: Brainstem anaesthesia after peribulbar anaesthesia. *Can J Anaesth* 44(7):732-734, 1997.
76. Rozentsveig V, Yagev R, Wecksler N, Gurman G, Lifshitz T: Respiratory arrest and convulsions after peribulbar anesthesia, *J Cataract Refract Surg* 27(6):960-962, 2001.
77. Mathers W: Occasional seizures that can follow retrobulbar anesthesia with bupicacaine 0.75%, *Ann Ophthalmol* 19:91 (letter).
78. Pearson PA, Solomon KD, Smith TJ, Epstein AD: Contralateral cavernous sinus syndrome after retrobulbar anesthetic injection, *Am J Ophthalmol* 111:773-774, 1991 (letter).
79. Gillow JT, Aggarwal RK, Kirkby GR: Ocular perforation during peribulbar anaesthesia, *Eye* 10(pt5):533-536, 1996.
80. Ahmad S, Ahmad A, Benzon HT: Clinical experience with the peribulbar block for ophthalmologic surgery, *Reg Anesth* 18(3):184-188, 1993.
81. Duker J: Inadvertent globe perforation during retrobulbar and peribulbar anesthesia, *Ophthalmology* 98:519-526, 1991.
82. Hay A, Flyn HW Jr, Hoffman JI, Rivera AH: Needle penetration of the globe during retrobulbar and peribulbar injections, *Ophthalmology* 98:1017-1024, 1991.
83. Rinkoff J, Doft B, Lobes L: Management of ocular penetration from injection of local anesthesia preceding cataract surgery, *Arch Ophthalmol* 190:1421-1425, 1991.
84. Joseph JP, McHugh JD, Franks WA, Chignell AH: Perforation of the globe—a complication of peribulbar anaesthesia, *Br J Ophthalmol* 75(8):504-505, 1991.
85. Friedberg H, Kline O: Contralateral amaurosis after retrobulbar injection, *Am J Ophthalmol* 101:688-690, 1986.
86. Follette J, LoCascio J: Bilateral amaurosis following unilateral retrobulbar block, *Anesthesiology* 63:237-238, 1985 (letter).
87. Antoszyk A, Buckley E: Contralateral decreased visual acuity and extraocular muscle palsies following retrobulbar anesthesia, *Ophthalmology* 93:462-465, 1986.
88. Loken RG, Kirker GE, Hamilton RC: Respiratory arrest following peribulbar anesthesia for cataract surgery: case report and review of the literature, *Can J Ophthalmol* 33(4):225-226, 1998.
89. Jindra L: Blindness following retrobulbar anesthesia for astigmatic keratotomy, *Ophthalmic Surg* 20:433-435, 1989.
90. Brod R: Transient central retinal artery occlusion and contralateral amaurosis after retrobulbar anesthetic injection, *Ophthalmic Surg* 20:643-646, 1989.
91. Paulter SE, Grizzard WS, Thompson LN, Wing GL: Blindness from retrobulbar injection into the optic nerve, *Ophthalmic Surg* 17:334-337, 1986.
92. Cowley M, Campochiaro PA, Newman SA, Fogle JA: Retinal vascular occlusion without retrobulbar or optic nerve sheath hemorrhage after retrobulbar injection of lidocaine, *Ophthalmic Surg* 19:859-861, 1988.
93. Hersch M, Baer G, Dieckert JP, Lambert HM, Shore JW: Optic nerve enlargement and central retinal artery occlusion secondary to retrobulbar anesthesia, *Ann Ophthalmol* 21:195-197, 1989.
94. Jan-Tjeerd H, de Faber N, von Noorden G: Inferior rectus muscle palsy after retrobulbar anesthesia for cataract surgery, *Am J Ophthalmol* 112:209-211, 1991 (letter).
95. Hamed L, Mancuso A: Inferior rectus muscle contracture syndrome after retrobulbar anesthesia, *Ophthalmology* 98: 1506-1512, 1991.
96. Erie JC: Acquired Brown's syndrome after peribulbar anesthesia, *Am J Ophthalmol* 109:349-350, 1990 (letter).
97. Carlson BM, Emerick S, Komorowski TE, Rainin EA, Shepard BM: Extraocular muscle regeneration in primates, *Ophthalmology* 99:582-589, 1992.
98. Spaeth G: Total facial nerve palsy following modified O'Brien facial nerve block, *Ophthalmic Surg* 18:518-519, 1987.
99. Koenig SB, Snyder RW, Kay J: Respiratory distress after a Nadbath block, *Ophthalmology* 95:1285-1287, 1988.
100. Birt CM, Dixon WS, Dionne CL: Vocal cord paralysis with Nadbath facial block, *Can J Ophthalmol* 29(5):231-233, 1994.
101. Rabinowitz L, Livingston M, Schneider H, Hall A: Respiratory obstruction following the Nadbath facial nerve block, *Arch Ophthalmol* 104:1115, 1986 (letter).
102. Shoch D: Complications of the Nadbath facial nerve block, *Arch Ophthalmol* 104:114, 1986 (letter).
103. Barnard NA, Bainton R: Bradycardia and the trigeminal nerve. *J Craniomaxfac Surg* 18:259-360, 1990.
104. Fayon M, Gauthier M, Blanc VF, Ahronheim GA, Michaud J: Intraoperative cardiac arrest due to the oculocardiac reflex and subsequent death in a child with occult Epstein Barr virus myocarditis, *Anesthesiology* 83:622-624, 1995.
105. Watkins R, Beigi B, Yates M, Chang B, Linardos E: Intraocular pressure and pulsatile ocular blood flow after retrobulbar and peribulbar anaesthesia, *Br J Ophthalmol* 85:796-798, 2001.
106. Chang B, Beigi B, Lum Hee W, Westlake W, West WR: Pulsatile ocular blood flow: peribulbar vs. subconjunctival local anesthesia, *Investigative Ophthalmology & Visual Science* 38(4), 1997.
107. Coupland SG, Deschenes MC, Hamilton RC: Intraocular pressure and pulsatile ocular blood flow during regional orbital anesthesia, *Can J Ophthalmol* 36:140-144, 2001.
108. Mori F, Konno S, Hikichi T, Yamaguchi Y, Ishiko S, Yoshida A: Factors affecting pulsatile ocular blood flow in normal subjects, *Br J Ophthalmol* 85:529-530, 2001.
109. Gild WM, Posner KL, Caplan RA, Cheney FW: Eye injuries associated with anesthesia: a closed claims analysis, *Anesthesiology* 76:204-208, 1992.
110. Locastro A, Novak K, Biglan A: Central retinal artery occlusion in a child after general anesthesia, *Am J Ophthalmol* 110:91-92, 1991 (letter).

CHAPTER 38

ANESTHESIA FOR ORTHOPEDICS AND PODIATRY

JOSEPH A. JOYCE

Historically, anesthesia has been closely associated with the field of orthopedic surgery from the first attempted anesthetic for rapid amputations using ethyl alcohol or laudanum. Most often this "anesthetic technique" was a futile effort that frequently resulted in a delirious patient and the surgeon or assistants being injured over the course of the surgical procedure.

Orthopedics is the branch of medicine that deals with maladies of the bones and joints, including congenital deformities, diseases, and injuries. The term *orthopedics* derives from the Greek words *orthos*, which means straight, and *paideia*, which means rearing of children; thus, a literal translation would be "straight rearing of children."[1] In fact, in its infancy, orthopedics dealt predominantly with children by attempting to correct maladies or deformities in children now known to have resulted from more nutritional and congenital abnormalities, for example, rickets. Over the past 20 to 30 years, this medical specialty has grown enormously. The development of metal prostheses for joint replacement and the refinement of the arthroscope have been the leading advances responsible for the tremendous growth in the field of orthopedics. Complete replacement of joints has allowed improvement in the quality of life for patients suffering from many forms of degenerative joint disease. The increasing interest in and refinement of arthroscopic procedures has reduced the invasive nature of many orthopedic procedures. The arthroscope allows the practitioner direct visualization of the affected area, such as the shoulder or knee, via comparatively small incisions. Patients undergoing arthroscopic procedures also benefit from greater mobility immediately postoperatively, reduced discomfort in the surgical area, and reduced length of hospitalization. Patients having arthroscopic procedures often receive treatment on an outpatient basis and may be discharged on the day of surgery or on the first postoperative day. Since the intense interest in arthroscopy was renewed in the 1970s, this subspecialty has continually expanded to include the foot, ankle, wrist, elbow, and shoulder in addition to the knee.

The choice of anesthetic technique to facilitate performance of the proposed orthopedic procedure mirrors that of other surgical specialties. General anesthesia, regional anesthesia, a combination of regional and general anesthesia, and monitored anesthesia care are possible.

The appropriate technique should take into consideration the following: the proposed procedure itself, the anticipated length of the procedure, the patient's position required to accomplish the procedure, the patient's state of health (including body habitus), and the patient's acceptance of the proposed anesthesia technique. There remain patients for whom no anesthetic is acceptable other than general anesthesia, despite the tremendous advances in regional anesthesia and reassurances given by the nurse anesthetist.

PNEUMATIC TOURNIQUET

One of the concerns when caring for the orthopedic surgical patient, as with any surgical procedure, is estimation of blood loss. A relatively bloodless surgical field is the desire of virtually any surgeon. The orthopedic surgeon can accomplish this desire by using a pneumatic tourniquet during many surgical procedures performed on the extremities. The pneumatic tourniquet consists of an inflatable cuff, similar to the sphygmomanometer, a pressurization source, connecting tubing, a pressure display, and a pressure regulator. The inflatable cuff differs from that of a sphygmomanometer in the following ways: first, it should provide at least 3 but no more than 6 inches of overlap. Second, the width of the cuff should cover approximately 50% of the target extremity, as opposed to two thirds for the sphygmomanometer. The area covered by the inflatable cuff must be padded using either stockinette or cotton wadding. The nurse anesthetist should take care to avoid wrinkling of the padding material because wrinkles may result in formation of bullous lesions while the cuff is pressurized.[2] The cuff should then be applied in such a manner that the cuff overlap is opposite the neurovascular bundle of the target extremity.[2] For example, for the upper extremity, when the cuff is applied to the humerus, the overlap should be situated on the lateral aspect of the humerus, which is 180 degrees away from the brachial plexus. After the cuff is properly and satisfactorily positioned, it is connected to the pressure source via the connecting tubing and the appropriate inflation pressure is determined. A guide to determining the appropriate inflation pressure is the initial systolic blood pressure measured before induction of anesthesia or administration of regional anesthesia. Adding 90 to 100 mm Hg of pressure to this initial systolic blood pressure has been demonstrated to effectively control hemostasis in lower extremities.[3] Inflation pressures for upper and lower extremities should not exceed 300 mm Hg and 500 mm Hg, respectively.[2] Before inflation of the pneumatic tourniquet, the operative extremity should be exsanguinated. Exsanguination is accomplished by very tightly wrapping the extremity with an Esmarch bandage, beginning with the digits and continuing proximally up to and including the distal edge of the inflatable cuff. While holding the Esmarch bandage in place, the cuff should be inflated to the predetermined pressure. The cuff should be palpated to ensure that inflation has occurred before the Esmarch bandage is removed. Additional checks of circulatory isolation can be accomplished by palpation of the arterial supply, such as the radial artery for the upper extremity or the popliteal artery for the lower extremity, or using the pulse oximeter to note its inability to obtain a reading. The use of the pneumatic tourniquet provides the advantages of dramatically reduced surgical blood loss and a virtually bloodless operative field, which helps reduce operative time, but it is not without potential problems and complications. Box 38-1 lists the physiologic changes that occur with pneumatic tourniquets.

Tourniquet Pain

Probably the best known problem encountered with the pneumatic tourniquet is the experience of tourniquet pain. When tourniquets were first used in surgery, and the potential complications were unknown, inflation pressures commonly exceeded 500 mm Hg. In 1944 Denny-Brown and Brenner[4] reported the first investigation into the cause of tourniquet discomfort. They listed characteristic anatomic changes associated with tourniquet ischemia that is caused by acute compression of the nerves under the inflated cuff. Compression of the intraneural blood vessels caused a secondary ischemia of the nerve fibers. The subjective discomfort occurred under the cuff and distal to the tourniquet. Similar reports of "tourniquet discomfort" or "aching" despite adequate spinal anesthesia prompted considerable attention toward discovering appropriate pressures required for hemostasis and minimizing subjective discomfort. Interestingly, from the first reports of tourniquet discomfort, the time to onset of subjective symptoms has been from 45 to 60 minutes. The first use of the term *tourniquet pain* was in 1952.[5]

Subsequent research into the cause of tourniquet pain, conducted between 1953 and 1979, resulted in the reduction of the effective pressures and accompanying reduction in the incidence of tourniquet pain. Not until 1979 and 1980, however, did reduction in tourniquet pressure become common practice. Patterson and Klenerman[6] reported histologic destruction of the ultrastructure of skeletal muscle under the tourniquet cuff in 1979. Based on this discovery and subsequent measurements of "occlusive pressure" in 1979, Klenerman and Hulands[7] suggested using tourniquet pressures of two times the patient's systolic blood pressure in order to minimize the subjective discomfort and destruction of tissues. Klenerman[8] modified this recommendation in 1980 to between 50 and 75 mm Hg more than the patient's systolic pressure.

The ischemic pain associated with tourniquet application is similar to that of thrombotic vascular occlusion and peripheral vascular disease.[9] At about 45 to 60 minutes after tourniquet pressurization, patients report various symptoms associated with dull aching that progress to burning and excruciating pain that may require general anesthesia. Once the pain begins, it is often resistant to analgesics and anesthetic agents, despite the anesthetic technique. Even with a well-controlled general anesthetic at the time of tourniquet inflation, ischemic pain may begin during this same time interval and may cause increasing heart rate and blood pressure that require pharmacologic intervention.[10]

Although specific neural and metabolic factors responsible for tourniquet pain are still unknown, several researchers have identified the nerve fibers responsible for the transmission of the impulses. The burning and aching pain corresponds to the activation of the small, slow-conducting, unmyelinated C fibers. The pinprick, tingling, and buzzing sensations that frequently accompany tourniquet application, often even after deflation, correspond to activation of the larger and faster myelinated A-delta fibers.

Activation of C fibers has been performed in the laboratory setting in which theorized metabolic effects of tourniquet ischemia were reproduced. In a study by MacIver and Tanelian[9] in 1992, hypoglycemia increased the activation of C fibers by more than 650% in as little as 15 minutes. Hypoxia increased the activation of C fibers by more than 200%, but when combined with hypoglycemia, it increased the activation of C fibers by more than 670%. Acidosis from pH 6.9 to 7.4 did not increase the activation of C fibers. Hypoxia and hypoglycemia, either alone or together, did not increase the activation of A-delta fibers.

Myelinated A-delta and unmyelinated C fibers differ in their sensitivity to local anesthetics. As the concentration of local anesthetic decreases, the activation of C fibers increases, but the A-delta fiber activation is still suppressed. This means that the C fibers may be more difficult to anesthetize than the A-delta fibers, and tourniquet pain therefore seems more consistent with pain sensation carried by C fibers.[9] Other research has shown that certain local anesthetics enhance the effect of

BOX 38-1

Physiologic Changes Caused by Limb Tourniquets

Neurologic Effects

Abolition of somatosensory evoked potentials and nerve conduction occurs within 30 minutes.
Application for more than 60 minutes causes tourniquet pain and hypertension.
Application for more than 2 hours may result in postoperative neuropraxia.
Evidence of nerve injury may occur at the skin level underlying the edge of the tourniquet.

Muscle Changes

Cellular hypoxia develops within 2 minutes.
Cellular creatinine value declines.
Progressive cellular acidosis occurs.
Endothelial capillary leak develops after 2 hours.

Systemic Effects of Tourniquet Inflation

Elevation in arterial and pulmonary artery pressures develops. This is usually slight to moderate if only one limb is occluded. The response is more severe in patients undergoing balanced anesthesia that does not include a potent anesthetic vapor.

Systemic Effects of Tourniquet Release

Transient fall in core temperature occurs.
Transient metabolic acidosis occurs.
Transient fall in central venous oxygen tension occurs but systemic hypoxemia is unusual.
Acid metabolites (e.g., thromboxane) are released into the central circulation.
Transient fall in pulmonary and systemic arterial pressures occurs.
Transient increase in end-tidal carbon dioxide occurs.

the blockade in the presence of increased stimulation of the isolated nerve fiber. For example, the potency of bupivacaine is enhanced by an increase in the rate of nerve stimulation and may offer an advantage by lowering the incidence of tourniquet pain.[11]

Some of these impulses travel with the sympathetic trunk and enter the spinal cord above the level of the sensory block with spinal or epidural anesthesia, but the incidence of tourniquet pain does not seem to be related to this level. It is apparent that a high-quality blockade of the sacral roots is more important than the thoracic sensory level in reducing the incidence of tourniquet pain because the intensity of pain may be due to ischemia of the entire leg, as well as under the cuff.[12] The addition of opioids to the local anesthesia solutions used for spinal and epidural anesthesia improves the quality of the block and may reduce the incidence of tourniquet pain.[13] If time permits, the superficial application of a eutectic mixture of local anesthetic (lidocaine-prilocaine [EMLA]) cream before tourniquet application may increase time before the onset of tourniquet pain.[14]

Postoperative Tourniquet Paresthesias

Properly placed tourniquets inflated to appropriate pressures rarely cause injury. The use of excessive tourniquet pressure for a prolonged time may cause postoperative paresthesias that are frustrating to treat and very painful for the patient. Excessive tourniquet pressure causes deformation of the underlying nerves—the myelin may be stretched on one side of the node and invaginated on the other. Nerve damage may be present because of rupture of the Schwann cell membrane. Use of proper padding, appropriate choice of tourniquet size, and adherence to recommendations of appropriate pressure and time minimize the incidence of this complication.

Tourniquet Inflation and Deflation

During the time of inflation, physiologic changes occur in the exsanguinated limb that are consistent with anaerobic metabolism. The nurse anesthetist must be aware of these changes (see Box 38-1) in order to anticipate the release of cold, acidotic metabolites into the patient's circulation when the tourniquet is released. Common effects of tourniquet release and reperfusion include serum potassium, bicarbonate, and carbon dioxide level increases and decreased pH, arterial oxygen partial pressure, and core temperature (0.6° C) for each hour of tourniquet time.[13]

The patient may experience lability in the blood pressure and heart rate as 300 to 500 mL of blood is acutely returned to systemic circulation on exsanguination and cuff inflation. Especially under general anesthesia, the inflation may cause increased vascular resistance and blood pressure, especially if the patient has preexisting cardiovascular disease. At the end of the procedure, sudden deflation of the tourniquet allows an acute reperfusion of the exsanguinated limb; this situation results in a decrease in the circulating blood volume by as much as 500 mL and washing out of the anaerobic metabolites. This change may cause transient hypotension and bradycardia, rapidly increased end-tidal carbon dioxide levels,[15] and dysrhythmias that may or may not require treatment.

Although the exsanguination of the extremity is an important part of the tourniquet application, several cases of fatal pulmonary embolism have been reported at tourniquet inflation.[16] The pathologic mechanism in these cases involved dislodgment of preexisting thrombi, either by the use of the Esmarch bandage or the inflation of the tourniquet.[17] Fat embolism syndrome is evident in 0.5% to 2% of patients with long-bone fractures, as evidenced by preoperative blood gas analysis.[18] Caution must be exercised in the use of tourniquets for patients with fractures, patients who are elderly, and patients with a history of risk factors for emboli formation, such as prolonged bed rest or immobilization.

Tourniquet Time

The research into complications associated with excessive tourniquet pressure also elucidated problems associated with excessive inflation time. Histologic and serum testing documented reversible changes that varied with changes in inflation duration. In 1977 Tountas and Bergman[19] reported that no significant changes relative to ischemia occurred in patients subjected to 2 hours of tourniquet time, but that permanent nerve damage sometimes occurred if tourniquet time was 4 hours. In 1980 Klenerman[8] measured biochemical changes in patients' blood that were associated with tourniquet ischemia during and serially after tourniquet deflation. He reported that serum parameters completely returned to normal in 20 minutes if the tourniquet was deflated at the end of 1 hour, but that parameters took 40 minutes to return to normal if the tourniquet was deflated at the end of 3 hours. Histologic changes, however, took 24 hours to return to normal if the tourniquet remained inflated for 3 hours. If the tourniquet was inflated for longer than 3 hours, muscle power in the extremity did not return to normal for 1 week. Klenerman recommended that the "safe" tourniquet time be no longer than 3 hours. Subsequent research has verified Klenerman's recommendations, and current "safe" tourniquet time should not exceed 2 hours routinely.[20] Safety measures for preventing or minimizing complications associated with the pneumatic tourniquet are listed in Box 38-2.

BOX 38-2

Safety Measures for Preventing Tourniquet Complications

- The tourniquet should be applied where the nerves are best protected in the underlying musculature.
- The nurse anesthetist must check proper availability and functioning of the equipment before it is operated.
- The tourniquet should be used for no longer than 2 hours.
- Only the minimally effective pressure should be used for occluding blood flow to the extremity. For the upper extremity, 70 to 90 mm Hg more than the patient's systolic blood pressure should be used. For the lower extremity, twice the patient's systolic pressure should be used. For Bier block anesthesia, a minimum standard tourniquet pressure of 300 mm Hg should be used unless the tourniquet is on the upper leg.[78] In this case, twice the patient's systolic pressure should be used unless this amount is less than 300 mm Hg.
- The pressure display must accurately reflect the pressure in the tourniquet bladder.
- The cuff must properly fit the extremity.
- The limb must be padded, and the cuff must be properly applied to the limb with care and attention.
- The tourniquet must be applied to the correct extremity.[20,79]

PATIENT POSITIONING

The discipline of orthopedic surgery is probably unique for the variety of patient positioning that may be used to facilitate a proposed surgical procedure. Patient positioning is a crucial component in the successful completion of an orthopedic procedure. Appropriate patient positioning must allow optimal exposure of the surgical site. Additionally, such positioning must afford adequate, appropriate monitoring throughout the procedure, provide good access to the patient's airway, provide comfort and warmth, minimize or prevent physiologic functioning compromise, protect all body systems, and maintain patient dignity.[21] Often surgery on one site (e.g., the elbow) may be accomplished using any one of the three main patient positions—that is, supine, lateral decubitus, or prone. The choice of patient position is dictated to a great extent by the nature of the surgery itself and to a somewhat lesser extent by the personal preference of the individual surgeon. For these reasons, good communication among the nurse anesthetist, operating room staff, and the surgeon is imperative.

The anesthetist is ultimately responsible for the proper positioning of the patient on the operating room table. Changes from the usual upright or erect position bring with them a multitude of potential injuries to the patient, as well as physiologic changes that the nurse anesthetist must be prepared to prevent or treat. Physical injury is deemed preventable, and the nurse anesthetist must be meticulous in ensuring maintenance of relatively normal anatomic positioning of the patient. Chapter 19 provides an excellent overview of the myriad potential injuries attributable to patient positioning. Physiologic changes are the areas about which the nurse anesthetist must demonstrate knowledge and understanding to adequately prepare for their occurrence and respond with appropriate measures to maintain homeostasis.

Human physiology has, over the millennia, adapted to being in an upright or erect position for the majority of the wakeful hours. For example, in the upright position there are three zones of ventilation/perfusion within the lungs: areas where alveolar pressure is greater than arterial pressure; areas of complex, variable pressure gradients between alveolar and arterial components; and areas where arterial pressure is greater than alveolar pressure (zones 1, 2, and 3, respectively)[22] (Fig. 38-1). Another example of the adaptations is the valves found in the dependent areas of the venous system, such as the extremities, as well as the absence of valves in nondependent areas, such as the cranium. Changes from the upright position produce physiologic changes.[21,23]

Supine Position

In the upright position, the majority of ventilation/perfusion distribution occurs in the variable, complex alveolar/arterial gradients known as zone 2 (Fig. 38-2).[21] The supine position redistributes the lung fields into predominately zone 3 ventilation/perfusion distribution.[24] The ventilation/perfusion distribution dynamics are further disturbed by an average 800 mL reduction in functional residual capacity (FRC) that accompanies being in the supine position;[25] if general anesthesia is used, the patient's FRC is further reduced by an average of 400 mL.[26-28] The initial FRC reduction is presumably the result of pressure being exerted on the diaphragm by the abdominal contents. The FRC reduction is further compounded by diaphragmatic relaxation brought about by general anesthesia. Furthermore, induction of general anesthesia results in almost immediate formation of areas of atelectasis, predominantly in

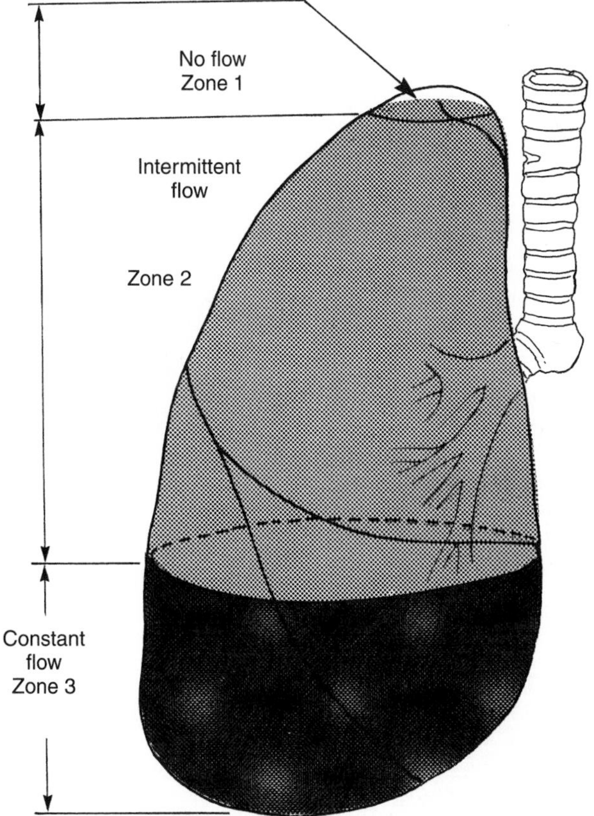

FIGURE **38-1**
Lung zones: the effect of gravity on ventilation/perfusion.

the dependent lung fields.[29] The areas of atelectasis are absolute or true shunting areas within the lung capillary—blood passes the capillary/alveolar interface without gas exchange occurring. However, with the change from upright posture to the supine position, the diaphragm demonstrates posterior displacement in a cephalad direction, which increases with unparalyzed general anesthesia and is further displaced with paralysis.[23] This diaphragmatic displacement produces greater muscle fiber stretch, which, in turn, improves the efficiency of muscle shortening. As a result of the greater efficiency of muscle fiber shortening, a greater portion of ventilation is directed to the dependent areas of the lung where gravity has already redistributed a larger portion of pulmonary blood flow; therefore, ventilation/perfusion is more closely matched than in the upright position.[23]

The central nervous system undergoes some dynamic changes when the patient is placed in the supine position. Both blood and cerebrospinal fluid drainage from the enclosed cranial vault are via valveless systems, which are gravity dependent. The directional forces of gravity within the cranial vault shift from parallel to the patient's position to perpendicular to that position when the supine position is assumed; these forces can be effectively reversed if the Trendelenburg variation of the supine position is used. These directional changes in the forces of gravity can increase the patient's intracranial pressure, which may, in turn, reduce the cerebral perfusion pressure (cerebral perfusion pressure equals mean arterial pressure minus intracranial pressure). Such changes in dynamics are of particular concern if the patient has or is suspected of having any form of closed head injury or pathology.

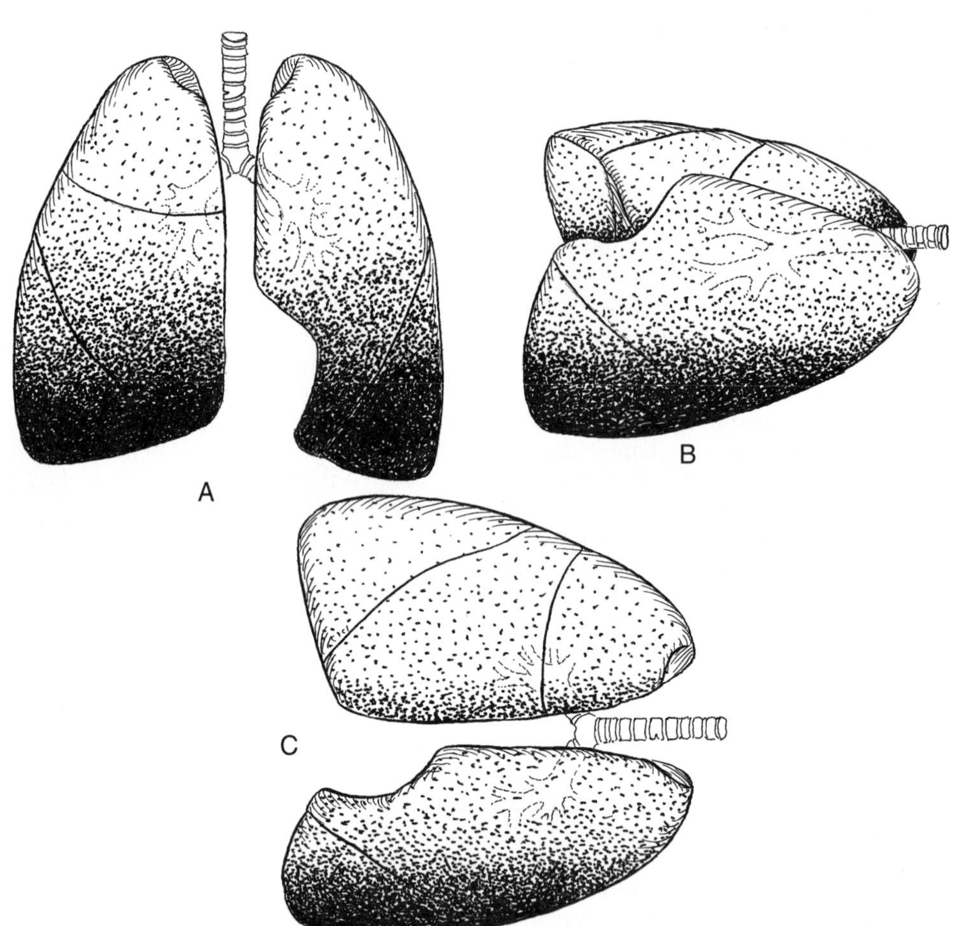

FIGURE **38-2**
Gravity dependence of ventilation and perfusion as noted by lungs depicted in the standing, supine, and lateral positions.

Lateral Decubitus Position

Placing the patient in a lateral decubitus position produces physiologic changes similar to those found in the supine patient. Although the majority of organ systems are unaffected, the physiologic alterations of most concern to the nurse anesthetist, once again, revolve around pulmonary and cardiovascular functioning.[30] Remember, in the upright position there are three zones of ventilation/perfusion distribution. Placing the patient in the lateral decubitus position results in a significantly greater proportion of the uppermost lung being classified as zone 1, where ventilation is more abundant than pulmonary blood flow, as well as a large portion of the dependent lung being classified as zone 3, where pulmonary blood flow exceeds alveolar ventilation[22] (see Fig. 38-2). In addition, the percentage of the zone 2 areas of the lung fields is reduced and split between the lungs, with the larger amount being in the dependent lung.

The alteration in ventilation/perfusion distribution is accompanied by reductions in vital capacity and tidal volume. On assuming the lateral decubitus position, healthy, conscious individuals experience about a 10% reduction in vital capacity[31] as a result of reduced anterior, as well as lateral, movement of the dependent rib cage along with restriction of the dependent hemidiaphragm.[32] Ventilation/perfusion distribution may be further altered as a result of the shift in the mediastinum toward the dependent side, which rotates the heart on its axis.[30] This cardiac rotation can impede venous return, thus reducing the cardiac output. The reduced cardiac output can produce hypotension, which must be judiciously treated with either fluid challenges or small doses of vasoactive medication.[30]

Prone Positioning

Physiologically and mechanically, the ventral surface of the thorax is not adapted to being a weight-bearing surface. Its structures are significantly more mobile than those of the dorsal surfaces.[33] However, placing a patient in the prone position puts just such requirements on the ventral structures. Maintaining normal cardiovascular function while in the prone position assumes the pressure of skeletal flexibility, normal muscle tone, cardiovascular reflexes that are intact, and sufficient energy reserves to increase ventilatory effort by lifting the torso.[33] Induction of general anesthesia or high levels of regional anesthesia nullifies most, and sometimes all, of those assumptions.

Cardiovascular functioning remains relatively normal when the patient is placed in the prone position, as long as occlusive pressure to the inferior vena cava and femoral veins is avoided.[33] If these routes of venous return become occluded, partially or completely, collateral routes must accomplish the task. However, the available collateral venous system has a greatly reduced capacity to accommodate the induced increase in flow rate,[34,35] and a reduction in venous return ensues, resulting in reduced cardiac output. In addition, placing a patient in the prone position produces significant increases in both systemic and pulmonary vascular resistance. These increases result in significant decreases in stroke volume and cardiac index.[36] It must be ensured that minimal pressure is exerted on the aforementioned vascular structures to maintain cardiac output as close to normal as possible.

Respiratory dynamics are greatly affected by placing the patient in the prone position. The three-zone model discussed earlier is rearranged. The proportion of zone 2 reduces, while that of zone 3 increases.[22] The spontaneously breathing patient must expend greater amounts of his or her energy reserves to elevate the weight of the thorax, as well as push the abdominal viscera back caudally, to inflate the lungs. This extra energy expenditure is of greatest concern to the nurse anesthetist when caring for patients with any type of limitations to their energy reserves, such as the elderly, the very young, and patients with moderate to severe chronic obstructive pulmonary disease or cardiac disease. The effort required to push the abdominal viscera back in a caudal direction during inspiration can be lessened by allowing the abdomen to rest free from pressure as much as possible; less pressure on the abdomen produces less intrusion of the viscera on the diaphragm. With general anesthesia, the patient's ventilatory effort is often abdicated to the nurse anesthetist, who assumes that role via positive pressure ventilation. The prone position necessitates higher airway pressures to achieve adequate ventilation. With the increased airway pressure in the prone position, the nurse anesthetist must be cognizant of the increased potential for barotrauma, particularly if the patient is not properly positioned.[33]

Finally, the prone position can alter central nervous system dynamics more than that of the supine position, which is of particular concern if head injury or closed head pathology is present or suspected. The anterior neck is particularly supple without considerable bony structural and protective support. In the spontaneously ventilating patient not under general anesthesia or unconscious, sensorium and protective reflexes remain largely intact. Such patients can assist the nurse anesthetist with positioning their head in a manner that is comfortable but does not alter blood flow via the carotid or vertebral arteries. With the unconscious patient or one under general anesthesia, head rotation during positioning must be done with great care. Should the patient's head be rotated 60 degrees, compression of the contralateral vertebral artery begins to constrain blood flow; if rotated 80 degrees, the contralateral vertebral artery becomes completely occluded.[37] The carotid artery and jugular vein on the upper side of the neck can become compressed by extreme degrees of head rotation, and those on the down side of the neck may become compressed by inappropriate head support.[33] Compression of the arterial supply to the brain can produce alterations in consciousness in the awake patient. Under general anesthesia, or with a patient whose level of consciousness is already altered, the alteration in arterial blood supply to the brain may not be easily recognized. Therefore, patients in whom any aberration in carotid blood flow is suspected or who have head injury should probably have the head maintained in a neutral anatomic alignment while in the prone position. In addition, even if no arterial or venous compression occurs, if the patient's head rests below the level of the heart, both blood and cerebrospinal fluid may accumulate within the closed cranial vault solely as a result of gravitational direction changes.[33] Such an accumulation can result in increased intracranial pressure and may reduce the cerebral perfusion pressure.

As previously stated, orthopedics has experienced virtually exponential growth in surgical procedures over the past 20 to 30 years. Three surgical areas are at the forefront of the growth in this field: arthroscopy, arthroplasty, and spinal/back surgery.

ARTHROSCOPY

Dorland's Pocket Medical Dictionary defines arthroscopy as "examination of the interior of a joint with an endoscope."[38] The concept of arthroscopy was first described and demonstrated by Takagi in 1918.[39,40] The concept was introduced into the United States in 1926.[41] However, without the availability of practical sources of illumination, arthroscopy languished. The development of fiberoptic light sources in the 1970s brought a resurgence of interest in the utilization of arthroscopy. Takagi's descriptions and demonstrations were predicated on using the techniques on the knee joint. Indeed, on the resurgence of interest in arthroscopy, the knee was the primary site for the procedure and currently remains the most common site for arthroscopy. Initially, arthroscopy was used to obtain definitive diagnosis of a patient's orthopedic malady so that a definitive, corrective surgical procedure could be performed. As interest in the procedure and technique increased, coupled with development of the necessary smaller surgical instrumentation, previously open surgical procedures on the knee, such as partial or complete meniscectomy, loose body removal, or cruciate ligament repair or reconstruction, were attempted and refined solely via the arthroscope.

Successful performance of arthroscopic procedures on the knee produced several benefits for the patient, including reduced blood loss, less postoperative discomfort, reduced length of hospitalization, and reduced length of rehabilitation. The success achieved with arthroscopic procedures on the knee led to application of the principles and techniques to other joints (e.g., the shoulder, elbow, wrist, hip, ankle, and phalangeal joints of the foot). Through the middle portion of the 1990s, application of arthroscopic procedures focused on the shoulder. Accordingly, shoulder arthroscopy utilization ranges from tendon debridement to rotator cuff repair.[40,41] The development and refinement of shoulder arthroscopic procedures mirrors that of knee arthroscopic procedures; that is, as more skill and comfort are obtained with initial procedures, more traditionally open surgical treatments are attempted solely via the arthroscope. Currently, arthroscopic techniques are being developed, refined, and expanded for the elbow, wrist, hip, and ankle.[40]

Anesthetic Management

Arthroscopic procedures may be anesthetically managed by almost any of the available anesthesia techniques (general anesthesia, regional anesthesia, combined regional and general anesthesia, local blockade, and sometimes monitored anesthesia care). Patient selection for a given anesthetic technique is crucial with arthroscopic procedures, as with all operative procedures. As previously mentioned, for some patients there is absolutely no substitute for receiving general anesthesia. Critical factors in the selection and presentation of the available anesthesia techniques appropriate for arthroscopic procedures are the patient positioning necessary to facilitate the proposed arthroscopic procedure and the overall state of health of the patient. For example, shoulder arthroscopy uses one of two positions to accomplish the surgery, either lateral decubitus or modified Fowler's ("beach chair") position.[41] The choice of position is determined, in part, by the nature and extent of the malady being surgically addressed. For some shoulder arthroscopy procedures, supplemental traction with weights and abduction may be necessary to provide optimum operative visualization (Fig. 38-3); for others, the modified

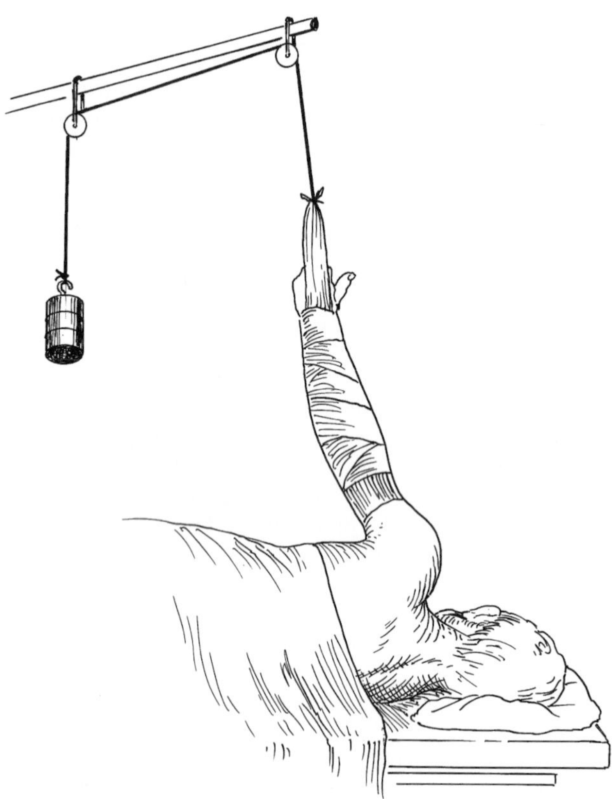

FIGURE **38-3**
Shoulder arthroscopy positioning.

Fowler's position may be used with the force of gravity or manual traction providing sufficient operative visibility. Reviewing the patient's chart and, most important, personally interviewing the patient, along with understanding the physiologic changes associated with various positions, will assist the nurse anesthetist in offering the best suggestion for anesthesia care for each patient. Box 38-3 lists important factors in this decision.

Patient positioning for arthroscopic procedures can encompass virtually the entire gamut of possible operative positions. Most often, arthroscopic procedures for lower extremity joints use the supine position, as do most arthroscopic procedures on the upper extremities. Arthroscopy on the knee requires the supine position with the foot of the operating room bed lowered (Fig. 38-4). The nonoperative leg should either be wrapped with an elastic bandage or have some form of antiembolic stocking in place to reduce pooling of blood and reduce the potential for thrombus formation. At times, patients undergoing elbow arthroscopy may be placed in the supine, lateral decubitus, or prone position; the position is dictated by operative necessity and surgeon preference (Figs. 38-5 and 38-6). The prone position is more advantageous primarily because of the better limb stability during the procedure.[42] Shoulder arthroscopy is usually accomplished via either the modified Fowler's position or the lateral decubitus position, based on optimal access to the injury and surgeon preference (see Fig. 38-3).[41] Hip arthroscopy is also typically accomplished via the lateral decubitus or the supine positions, with the patient on a fracture table[43] (Fig. 38-7). The fracture table is used to provide greater stability while traction is applied, using either weights and counterweights (lateral decubitus position) or mechanical traction attached to the leg-holding device of the fracture table (supine position).[43] Currently, wrist arthroscopy is seldom performed, but when used, the patient need only be in the supine position.

Complications from arthroscopic procedures represent a small percentage of the total number of procedures performed.[44-47]

BOX **38-3**

Anesthetic Selection in Orthopedics

What is the proposed surgical procedure?
How long is the procedure estimated to take?
What patient position will be necessary to accomplish the procedure?
Is this patient's overall health status sufficient to remain in the required position for an extended period of time without general anesthesia?
Is this patient receptive to an anesthesia technique (or techniques) other than general anesthesia?

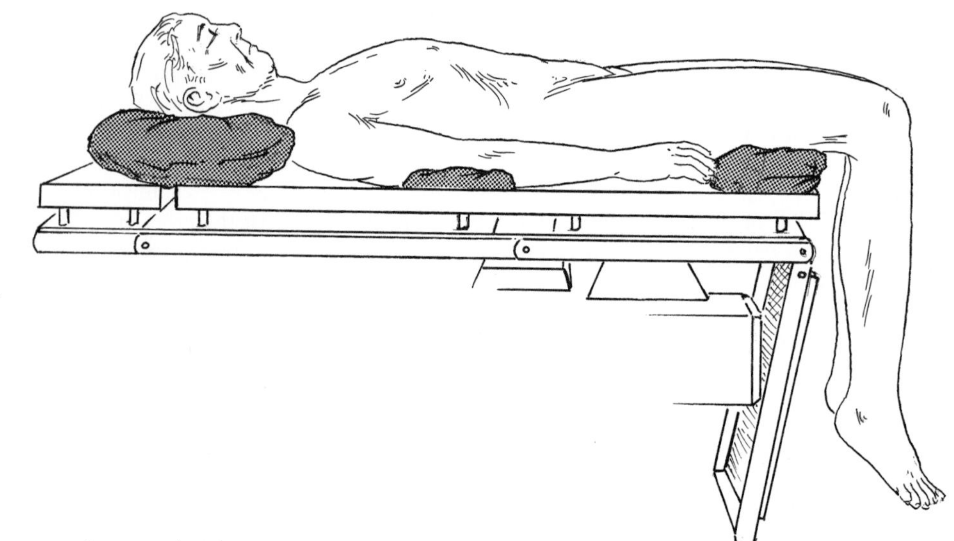

FIGURE **38-4**
Positioning for knee procedures.

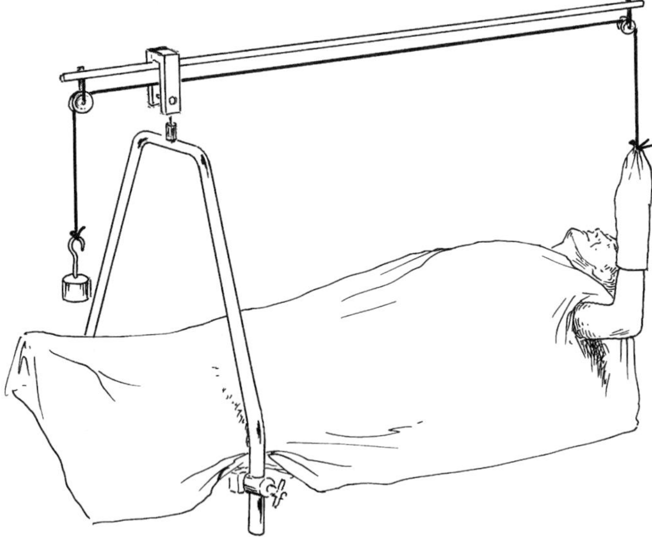

FIGURE **38-5**
Supine position for elbow surgery.

Accordingly, complications resulting from arthroscopic procedures that particularly concern the nurse anesthetist are relatively few. The full range of potential anesthetic complications associated with patient positioning apply (e.g., inadvertent extubation, eye/corneal injury, and nerve injury from improper patient positioning). Because of the less invasive nature of arthroscopic procedures, concerns over blood loss are typically minimal. However, sudden sustained hypotension is a cause for immediate investigation. With many arthroscopic procedures, the pneumatic tourniquet may be used to provide a clear, bloodless surgical field. Perforation of a major blood vessel may occur

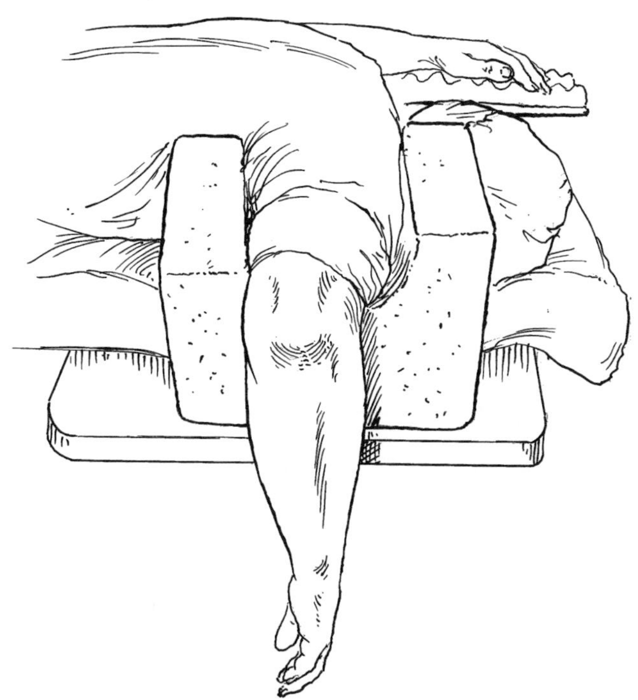

FIGURE **38-6**
Prone position for elbow surgery.

during trocar insertion and may not be detected until the tourniquet is deflated. Such vascular injury may result from pressure exerted by excess extravasated irrigation fluid during the procedure.[39] In the case of shoulder or hip arthroscopy, procedures in which pneumatic tourniquet use is not possible, any major vascular injury will be recognized significantly earlier than completion of the procedure.

In order to provide optimal visualization of joint structures during arthroscopic procedures, the irrigating fluid used to distend the operative joint is instilled under pressure. Pressurization of the irrigating solution is accomplished either by hanging the solution 3 to 4 feet higher than the operative joint or by using a mechanical pump device. Hanging the irrigation fluid 3 to 4 feet above the operative joint produces almost 90 mm Hg of fluid pressure entering the joint space.[39] Alternatively, mechanical pumps specifically designed for arthroscopic procedures are set to deliver fluid pressurized to between 60 and 80 mm Hg. As a result of the pressurization of the irrigating fluid, extravasation is not uncommon during arthroscopic procedures. The typical irrigation setup uses large bags of irrigating solution, 3 to 5 liters in volume. The nurse anesthetist should take note of any deficits of inflow versus outflow of irrigating solution throughout the procedure. Depending on the severity or complexity of the arthroscopic procedure, a large number of irrigation fluid bags may be required. Therefore, even small individual inflow/outflow deficits may result in significant fluid absorption by the patient over the course of an extended procedure. Fluid absorption is of particular concern to the nurse anesthetist for shoulder or hip arthroscopic procedures in which fluid absorption is not relatively limited by the use of the pneumatic tourniquet. Absorption of excessive extravasated fluid may lead to the development of signs and symptoms of congestive heart failure, pulmonary edema, volume overload, or hyponatremia (if a "salt-poor" fluid is used). Should the patient experience these symptoms, treatment with fluid restriction, supplemental oxygen, and diuresis should be instituted.

Although the mechanism of occurrence has not been delineated, subcutaneous emphysema, tension pneumothorax, and pneumomediastinum have been reported during shoulder arthroscopy, specifically subacromial decompression.[47] These complications appear to be associated, at least in part, with the use of mechanical irrigation pumps and power saver suction. The nurse anesthetist must be alert to the signs and symptoms of these complications in order to alert the surgeon to the need for immediate termination of the use of these arthroscopic adjunct devices and initiation of appropriate treatment measures. Box 38-4 lists the signs and symptoms of tension pneumothorax. Because tension pneumothorax is a potentially life-threatening event, early recognition and treatment are paramount. Ideally, placement of a chest tube is most desirable to relieve the pent-up intrathoracic pressure. However, an immediate, and very effective, treatment is needle decompression with a 14-gauge to 18-gauge intravenous stylet placed into either the second or third intercostal space, anteriorly, or the fourth or fifth intercostal space, laterally.[48,49] Successful decompression is accompanied by a sudden rush of air, as well as readjustment of physical symptoms and vital signs back toward the patient's normal parameters. After successful decompression, the intravenous catheter stylet should remain in place and be covered or capped to prevent air from being sucked back into the chest cavity until a chest tube can be properly inserted.

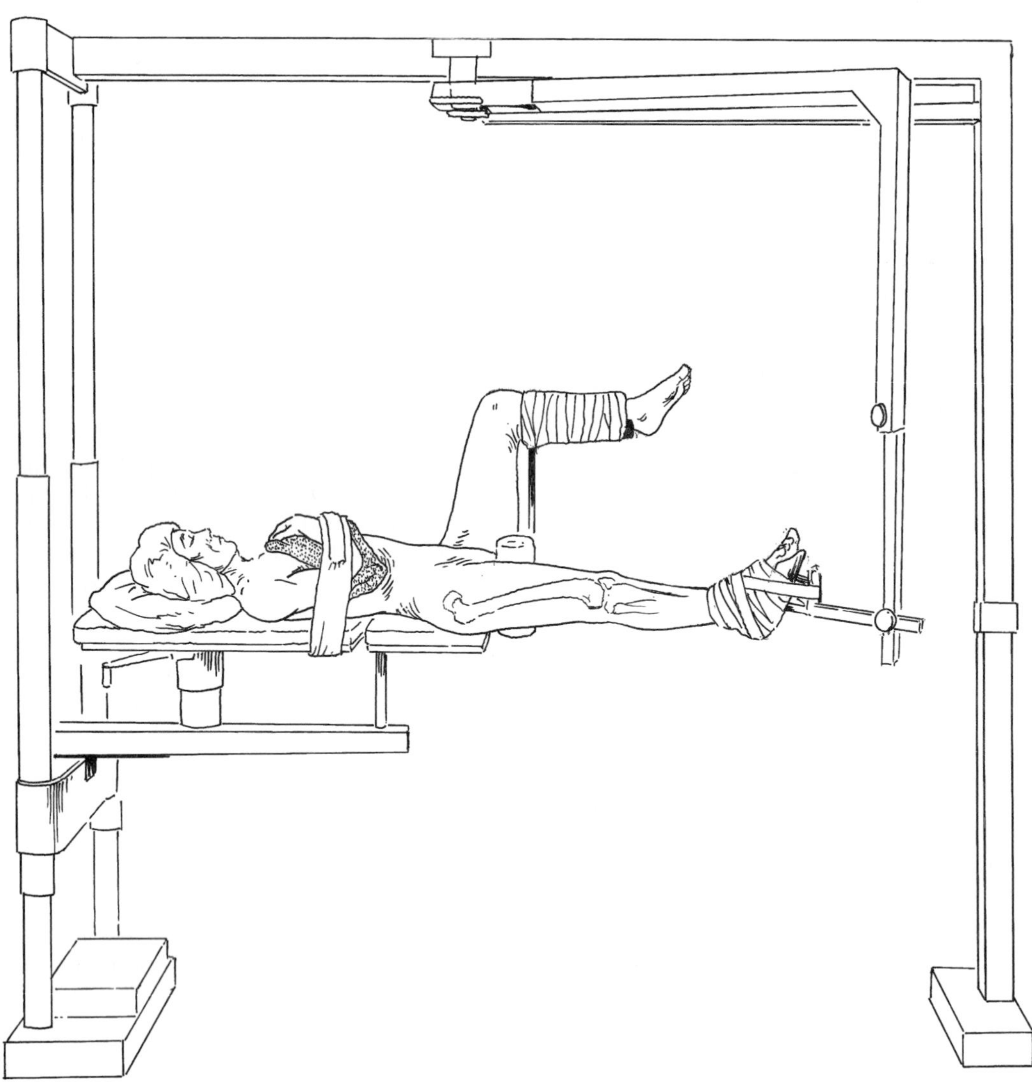

FIGURE **38-7**
Fracture table. Allows easy access for x-ray equipment.

BOX **38-4**

Signs and Symptoms of Tension Pneumothorax

Sudden, inexplicable hypoxemia
Elevated central venous pressure
Tachycardia
Absent breath sounds on the affected side
Tracheal shift
Agitation (may be observed in patients receiving regional anesthesia)
Hypotension
Jugular vein distention
Increased airway pressure
Asymmetric chest wall movement
Percussive hyperresonance over the affected side
Extreme anxiety (may be observed in patients receiving regional anesthesia)

ARTHROPLASTY

Arthroplasty is the surgical replacement of all (total arthroplasty) or part (hemiarthroplasty) of a joint to achieve a return of natural motion and function of the joint, as well as restoration of the controlling function of the surrounding soft tissues (i.e., the muscles, ligaments, and tendons). The goals of arthroplasty are: pain relief, stability of joint motion, and deformity correction.[50] The genesis of arthroplasty occurred in the mid-1800s, when surgeons of that era used simple resection to gain, for the short term, the aforementioned goals, but long-term results proved unsatisfactory. Orthopedic surgeons soon turned to interpositional grafting. For nearly 100 years, various autologous or exogenous substances were used in these grafting procedures. In the 1940s and 1950s, hemiarthroplasty was heavily investigated using molded metal alloy prosthetics as an alternative to interpositional grafting arthroplasty. Still, long-term results continued to be unsatisfactory. Finally, in the 1960s, Sir John Charnley developed a system for hip joint

$60 billion.[68,69] Virtually every industry now provides employees with education on body mechanics to attempt to reduce the number of back injuries.

In the past, laminectomies required large incisions to afford the surgeon optimal visualization of the affected area of the spinal column. The large incision resulted in large amounts of blood loss, prolonged wound healing, and lengthy hospitalization. Over the past decade, orthopedic surgeons have incorporated operative microscopes on an ever-increasing basis. Use of the operative microscope affords the surgeon better visualization while eliminating the need for the large incisions that were commonplace in the recent past, even for straightforward, "simple" lumbar laminectomies. In addition, the smaller incision results in reduced blood loss, faster wound healing, less trauma to surrounding soft tissues, shorter recovery, shorter length of hospitalization, and quicker return to a preinjury level of activity. In fact, often as a result of refined surgical technique, straightforward, "simple," single-level lumbar laminectomy patients are discharged from the hospital on the first postoperative day and, on occasion, may be discharged on the day of surgery.

The most common reasons for spinal surgery are intervertebral disk herniation and spinal stenosis. These maladies can potentially occur anywhere along the spinal column from C2–C3 through the L5–S1 vertebrae. Surgical intervention, via the posterior approach, consists of a midline incision and tissue dissection to expose the disk herniation or stenotic areas. The disk herniation is excised or the neuroforaminal space is enlarged to relieve compression of the nerve root. For the posterior approach, the patient is positioned prone. At times, other conditions exist that necessitate fusion of two vertebrae. Vertebral fusion is accomplished by a number of methods: bone grafting, either autologous or cadaveric; plate and screws; or the newest method, interbody cage devices. The goal is to prevent further degeneration and loss of the surgical correction achieved. Interbody cage devices facilitate fusion of the specific vertebral joint. They are designed to enhance the symptomatic relief that precipitated the fusion by restoring normal disk height, maintaining anatomically normal tension in the annular fibers, restoring lordosis in the affected segment, reducing subluxed facet joints, providing neuroforaminal space enlargement, and returning normal weight-bearing proportion through the anterior spinal column.[70] Interbody cage procedures, done by experienced surgeons, are more quickly accomplished than the previously standard bone-grafting procedure, are less costly, provide greater stability, and afford faster recovery and rehabilitation times.[69] Fusion within the cervical spine is most frequently accomplished by initial discectomy followed by a wedge of bone graft, often cadaveric, or by fusion of the joint with a plate and screws.

Scoliosis is lateral curvature of the spinal column. It is classified as either idiopathic, for which the cause is not known, or that of a known cause.[71] The majority (75% to 80%) of scoliosis cases are idiopathic. The remaining 20% to 25% can be identified as resulting from such conditions as congenital skeletal abnormalities (vertebral or extravertebral), neuromuscular disease, neurofibromatosis, arthrogryposis, trauma, and irritative phenomena resulting from nerve root compression or spinal cord tumor.[71] Untreated, scoliosis can lead to complex deformity in two planes (sagittal and coronal), chronic pain, neurologic and cardiopulmonary compromise, and cosmetic concerns.[72] Treatment pathways are determined by the severity and cause of the deformity and may be nonsurgical or surgical. Surgical intervention consists primarily of fusion of multiple joint spaces, with or without anterior release, and may include extensive instrumentation (e.g., Harrington rods and Dewer or Luque instrumentation). These surgical interventions may involve anterior or posterior approaches. Either approach is a major surgical intervention, but the anterior approach is more technically involved. The anterior approach to the thoracic spine requires performing a thoracotomy.

In conjunction with the development of "cage" technology, the principles of laparoscopy/endoscopy are being adapted and applied to spinal surgery. The first use of laparoscopy for lumbar discectomy was reported by Obenchain[73] in 1991. Laparoscopic techniques were first utilized by Mack and coworkers[74] for thoracic spinal surgery in 1993. Application of laparoscopic principles and techniques offers numerous advantages to anterior vertebral joint fusion (Box 38-5), not the least of which are dramatically reduced blood loss, improved ventilation (both intraoperatively and postoperatively), and reduced overall medical costs. The major disadvantage of the utilization of laparoscopic techniques in spinal surgery is acquisition of the technical skills necessary and level of comfort with the procedural requirements by the surgeon, which, in large part, is dependent on the frequency with which the newly acquired skills are used.

Not all patients should, at present, be considered for laparoscopic spinal surgery. For lumbar spinal surgery candidates, laparoscopy is currently contraindicated for patients with severe abdominal adhesions resulting from inflammatory processes, previous laparotomy, or severe abdominal trauma and patients with marked cardiac or pulmonary disease processes who may not be able to tolerate the hypercarbia that can result from abdominal insufflation of carbon dioxide, particularly during longer procedures.[75] For thoracic spinal surgery candidates, laparoscopy is currently contraindicated for patients unable to tolerate one-lung ventilation and those with severe or acute respiratory insufficiency, high positive airway pressures, and pleural symphysis. Patients who have required previous thoracotomy or chest tube placement must be more extensively evaluated preoperatively to determine if thorascopic spinal surgery will be employed. Also, at present, patients in need of internal fixation with extensive instrumentation of the anterior spine are not considered candidates for thorascopic spinal surgery.[75]

BOX **38-5**

Advantages of Laparoscopy for Anterior Spinal Surgery

Enhanced visualization
Decreased potential for infection
Reduced trauma to surrounding soft tissues
Shorter hospitalization
Shorter rehabilitation period
Decreased blood loss
Improved intraoperative and postoperative ventilation
Reduced intensive care unit time
Better cosmetic appearance
Reduced overall costs

Anesthetic Management

Almost all spinal surgery procedures are managed using general anesthesia because this technique affords a more secure airway along with the greatest degree of control over the patient's reflexive actions. Spinal anesthesia may be combined with general anesthesia when a lighter plane of anesthesia with a more secure airway would be better tolerated by the patient and produce a better postoperative course, as in a patient with severe chronic obstructive pulmonary disease.

A major anesthesia concern during spinal surgery centers on patient positioning. For spinal surgery involving the posterior approach, the patient will of necessity be placed in the prone position. While placing the patient in the prone position, the clinician must be vigilant in maintaining the security and integrity of the patient's airway so that inadvertent extubation, endobronchial intubation, or endotracheal tube kinking does not occur. The potential for eye or corneal injury is high in the prone position. It is important to avoid extremes in flexion or extension of the patient's neck, and ensure proper alignment and padding of the patient's upper extremities. When positioned prone, the patient's abdomen should not be compressed, because compression of the abdominal cavity will displace the organs and therefore the diaphragm cephalad, producing reduced functional residual capacity, reduced tidal volume, and increased airway pressures. Abdominal compression also contributes to engorgement of the epidural venous network and can be a contributing factor to a greater blood loss during the surgical procedure. To avoid abdominal compression, the abdomen must be elevated from the surface of the operating room bed.

Numerous methods and devices can be used to greatly reduce or eliminate abdominal compression. The simplest method is the use of "prone rolls," which are firm but compressible pads that extend from the shoulder to the iliac crest, bilaterally (Fig. 38-8). Other devices include the Wilson frame (Fig. 38-9), the Relton adjustable pedestal frame (Fig. 38-10), and the Andrews frame or spinal surgery table (Fig. 38-11). Each of these positioning devices is designed to allow the

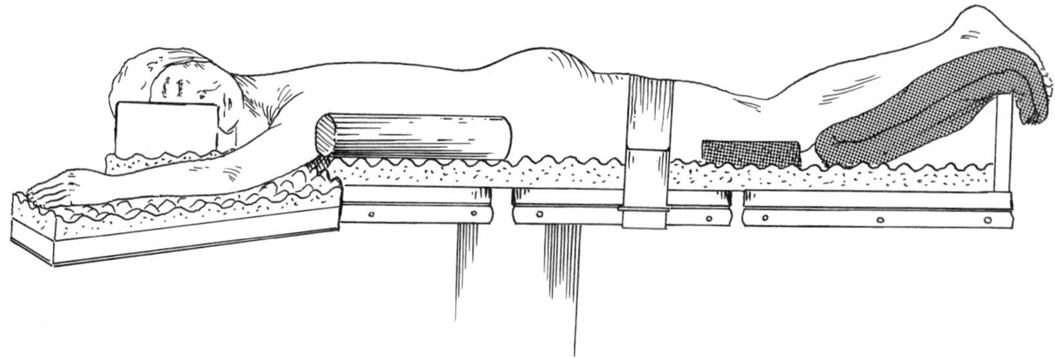

FIGURE **38-8**
Prone position using chest rolls.

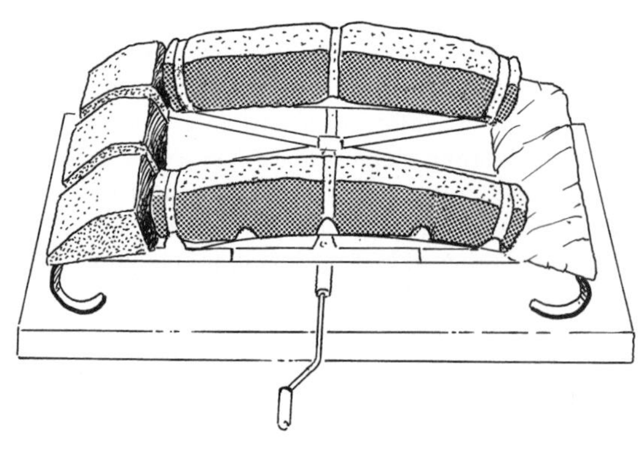

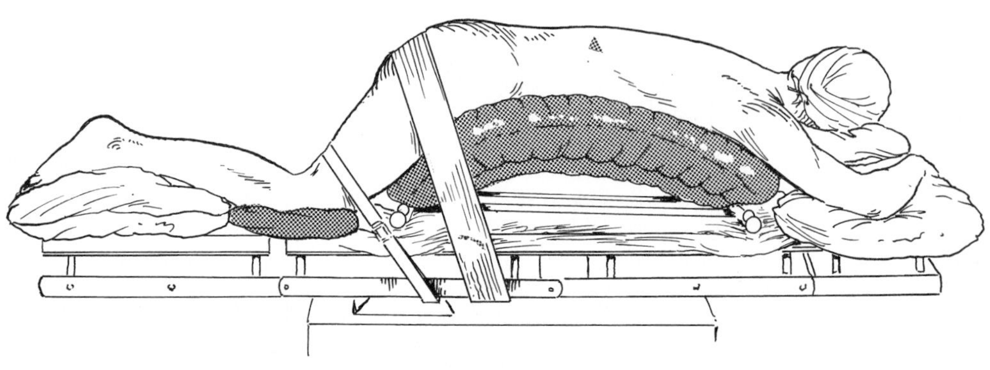

FIGURE **38-9**
Spinal operations using a convex saddle frame (Wilson frame).

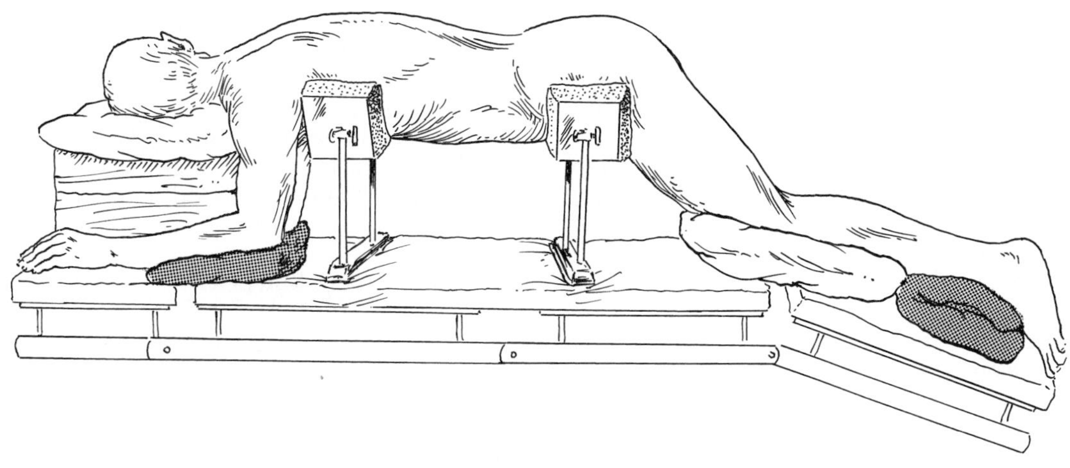

FIGURE **38-10**
The Relton adjustable pedestal frame.

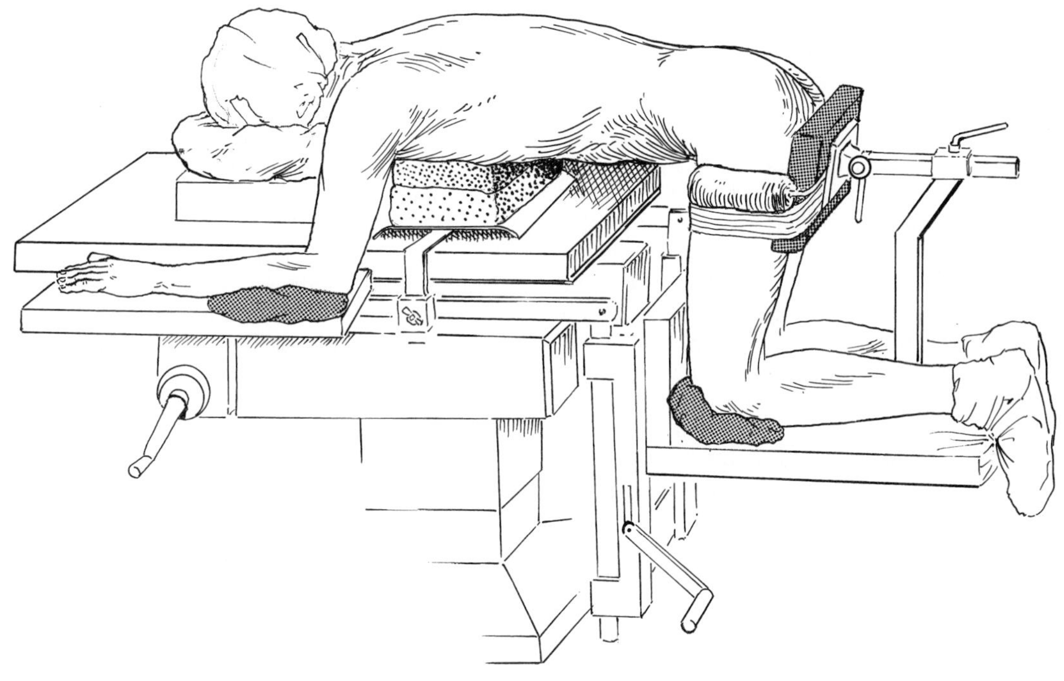

FIGURE **38-11**
The Andrews frame.

abdomen to "hang" freely and reduce the possibility of compressing major vascular structures.

The Andrews spinal surgery table is the most complex of the positioning devices. With the Andrews table, as with the other positioning devices, the patient is induced and intubated on the transportation stretcher, after which he or she is lifted onto the table. On initial positioning on the Andrews table, the patient lies flat with the legs resting perpendicular to the plane of the table. A buttock support is securely attached to the framework of the table, and the bony prominences of the hips and, particularly, the knees are adequately padded. The leg portion of the table is then lowered until the weight of the lower body rests on the knees, resulting in the patient's hips and knees being flexed at 90 degrees. This table produces a modified knee-chest position, allows the abdomen to "hang" freely, and greatly reduces the potential for compression of the major vascular structures of the lower abdomen and pelvic region (femoral arteries and veins). This position also maximizes the surgeon's visualization of the surgical site. Blood loss is decreased by using the Andrews spinal surgery table.[76] However, hypotension occurs frequently when using this table as a result of blood pooling in the dependent lower extremities. Antiembolic stockings may help counteract the tendency for blood to pool in the lower extremities, and any hypotensive event may be treated by judicious use of fluid challenges or small doses of vasoactive medications, such as ephedrine.

Scoliosis correction with large-scale instrumentation (e.g., Harrington instrumentation) is a major surgical intervention. The surgeon may choose a posterior, anterior, or thoracoabdominal approach to accomplish the procedure depending on the location and severity of the defect. The posterior approach requires the patient to be in the prone position. Scoliosis of the lower thoracic to upper lumbar spine may necessitate a thoracoabdominal incision and require the patient to be placed in a semilateral position. Scoliosis exclusively of the thoracic spine requires the patient to be placed in the lateral decubitus position.

Entry into the thoracic cavity will necessitate placement of a double-lumen endobronchial tube so that the ipsilateral lung can be deflated to facilitate visualization of the thoracic spine. Intubation may be difficult, at best, if the patient has a severe deformity. If the deformity has already produced significant cardiopulmonary compromise, the nurse anesthetist should carefully evaluate the anesthetic plan; specifically, because the patient's cardiopulmonary reserves may already be extremely poor to nonexistent, a more prudent course of action may be an awake, fiberoptic intubation. Endobronchial intubation can result in a host of untoward sequelae, including tracheal dissection and pneumomediastinum, right mainstem bronchus occlusion, and bronchial tree rupture or tear. For surgical correction of scoliosis by spinal fusion with anterior release, the patient is placed in the lateral decubitus position for the thoracotomy incision and requires endobronchial intubation. Depending on the direction of curvature of the thoracic spine, the heart may necessarily be manipulated, which may produce cardiac dysrhythmias.

With the large incision and complex dissection required for the multilevel spinal fusions and instrumentation needed to surgically correct the scoliosis, the nurse anesthetist should be prepared for a significant volume of blood loss. Blood transfusion is virtually ensured during the course of the procedure. Patient concerns about receiving a blood transfusion may be reduced by being encouraged to make an autologous blood donation of 1 to 2 units to the blood bank before the anticipated surgery date, assuming there are no conflicts with the patient's religious convictions. The nurse anesthetist can be instrumental in reducing the blood loss by maintaining the patient, as nearly as possible, at normothermic; employing deliberate hypotension; and using the cell saver to minimize the net blood loss incurred during the procedure.

As previously described, laparoscopic principles and techniques are beginning to be applied more frequently to spinal fusion surgery. Spinal fusion via laparoscopy provides the surgeon with enhanced visualization of the surgical site, reduces operative time once the surgeon and staff have acquired and are comfortable with the necessary skills, results in greatly reduced trauma to the surrounding soft tissues, produces dramatically less blood loss, reduces recovery and rehabilitation time, greatly reduces medical costs, contributes to an earlier return to preinjury level of activity, and is aesthetically more pleasing to the patient. It is important to compensate for any hypercarbia that may accompany insufflation of carbon dioxide, particularly during long procedures.

Sudden, dramatic, unanticipated, sustained hypotension requires rapid intervention and assessment of cause. The nurse surgeon should be informed and together a plan to rapidly determine the cause and initiate appropriate effective treatment measures may be instituted. Because of the close proximity to the spinal column, injury to the aorta can occur during surgery on the thoracic or lumbar spine. In addition to aortic injury, the inferior vena cava, iliac vessels, and common femoral vessels may be damaged as a result of traction during laparoscopic spinal procedures.[75] Injury to these vascular structures can be a truly emergent situation. If the patient is in the prone position, rapid closure of the surgical wound is imperative so the patient can be repositioned to facilitate repair to the damaged vessel. Large volumes of crystalloids, colloids, or blood transfusions may be required to maintain the patient's circulating blood volume and perfusion pressures while access to and repair of the injured vessel is achieved. If the patient has not been crossmatched, the worst-case scenario may involve transfusion of O-negative blood until crossmatched, banked blood becomes available.

FOOT AND ANKLE SURGERY

The feet and ankles are the basis of support on which the remainder of the body rests. Surgical correction of maladies and deformities of the feet and ankles falls under the scope of practice of two specialists: the orthopedic surgeon and the doctor of podiatric medicine (DPM), or podiatrist. Both of these specialists are highly skilled in the surgical correction of the multitude of maladies and deformities that occur with the feet and ankles.

The most commonly performed procedures on the ankle involve surgical repair of ankle fractures and fusion of the ankle joint. The Achilles tendon is also a frequent focus of surgery, particularly on the more physically active individuals. The most widely known surgical procedures on the feet are bunionectomy (with or without fusion), correction of hammertoe deformities (with or without fusion), and plantar fasciotomy (either open or endoscopic).

Open repair of ankle fractures is usually accomplished using plates and screws to hold the bone fragment in proper alignment until the fragments grow back together. Ankle fusion (arthrodesis) is performed for a multitude of medical reasons and may involve two or three bones being fused together to provide pain relief and greater joint stability. Incisions are usually made on both the medial and lateral aspects of the ankle joint to allow for optimal surgical access to the involved bones. The fracture is reduced, after which a plate is placed across the fracture site or sites. Holes are drilled with the plate acting as the template, and screws are placed into these holes. For ankle fusions, the incisions are typically made across the medial and lateral aspects of the joint and Kirschner wires or screws are used to fuse the appropriate bones in place. The incisions are closed and some type of inflexible stabilizing device is applied (e.g., cast or plaster splints or ambulatory boot) while under anesthesia. Pneumatic tourniquets are almost always employed to keep blood loss at a minimum and provide a clear surgical field.

Bunion deformity usually involves the first or great toe. Incision is made along the anterior surface from about midtoe across the metatarsophalangeal joint. The bony deformity is excised. Depending on the variation of the bunionectomy procedure chosen, excision of the bony deformity may be the totality of the procedure or the angular deformity may be corrected with a screw or Kirschner wire fusion.

Hammertoe deformity correction involves incision of the anterior surface of the malformed toe or toes. The incision crosses the joint containing the bony deformity. The surgeon dissects down to the joint and excises the bony deformity. Depending on the severity of the deformity, the interphalangeal joint may be fused by inserting a Kirschner wire.

Plantar fasciotomy is indicated for severe foot pain during or after ambulating, or on arising after sleep, resulting from chronic plantar fasciitis that has not responded to conservative therapy. Open fasciotomy is accomplished via a small incision along the posterior surface of the calcaneus. The plantar fascia is incised to relieve the tension across the plantar arch. Endoscopic plantar fasciotomy is accomplished via two "miniature" incisions, one medial and one lateral, at the beginning of the plantar arch. A small trocar is inserted through these incisions. The sheath of the trocar is slotted to allow visualization of the plantar fascia with the endoscope. The full thickness of the plantar fascia is incised, and the skin incisions are closed.

Anesthetic Management

Patients scheduled for foot or ankle surgery are excellent candidates for regional anesthesia. Most surgical procedures on the foot or ankle can be accomplished within a 2-hour time frame, often on an outpatient basis. Spinal anesthesia provides sufficient surgical anesthesia to allow completion of most procedures. However, the postanesthesia recovery phase may be unacceptably long and may require the patient to spend a night in the hospital or outpatient facility, which may be unacceptable to the patient.

Nerve blocks are especially effective for surgical procedures on the foot or ankle. Posterior tibial nerve block, Mayo blockade, and Bier block are examples of blocks that are effective for foot and ankle procedures. The nurse anesthetist can provide intravenous sedation by either continuous infusion or intermittent bolus to provide amnesia and minimize or eliminate any anxiety the patient may have. The surgeon can inject the surgical site with long-acting local anesthetic (e.g., bupivacaine) to maintain the patient's comfort immediately and for several hours postoperatively.

FOREARM AND HAND SURGERY

Surgical procedures on the hand or forearm may be precipitated by violent trauma resulting in complex or dislocated fractures to the bones of the forearm, hand, or fingers, or may be performed to alleviate numbness of the hand resulting from compression of the nerves of the forearm or wrist, as in carpal tunnel syndrome. Procedures on the fingers and hand are often relatively quick procedures requiring 1 hour or less to complete. Surgical correction of complex or dislocated fractures of the forearm may require considerable instrumentation and time to complete. For virtually all the surgical procedures of the hand and forearm, the pneumatic tourniquet is used.

Anesthetic Management

Patients scheduled for surgical procedures on the forearm or hand are excellent candidates for regional anesthesia. Axillary blockade and Bier block provide excellent surgical anesthesia for most surgical procedures of the forearm and hand that are anticipated to require 1 hour or less to accomplish.

For procedures precipitated by traumatic injury, such as complex, comminuted fractures or reconstruction of the vascular and nerve structures of the hand or forearm—procedures that may require considerable amounts of time to accomplish—the better anesthetic choice may be general anesthesia. Tourniquet pain becomes an issue with such longer procedures if regional anesthesia is chosen. Also, for the patient requiring surgery as the result of traumatic injury, the issue of the patient's nothing-by-mouth (NPO) status becomes important. Frequently, trauma patients have eaten or ingested liquids close to the time of the traumatic injury. Alcohol may be a precipitating factor in the traumatic injury as well. For these reasons, rapid-sequence induction of general anesthesia may be a more appropriate anesthetic course.

ARTHRITIC SYNDROMES

Of the many arthritic syndromes, two are especially disconcerting to the nurse anesthetist: rheumatoid arthritis (RA) and ankylosing spondylitis (AS). Both of these arthritic conditions extend beyond the primary affliction to the skeletal system and orthopedic medicine.

Rheumatoid arthritis is a chronic inflammatory process that primarily affects the synovial tissues. Even though RA has been investigated for decades, the etiology of the disease has yet to be delineated. Diagnosis of this malady is not made on the basis of a single biochemical, histologic, or immunologic entity; rather, it is confirmed as a result of a series of symptomatologic entities (Box 38-6).[77] Four of these criteria must be present, with symptoms A through D of Box 38-6, specifically, being present for a minimum of 6 weeks. One of the characteristics of RA is the spontaneous exacerbations and remissions. The chronic inflammatory processes at work destroy and remodel the articular surfaces, weaken surrounding soft tissues, and contribute to joint subluxation and muscle contractures.

Of particular concern are the effects of RA on the cervical spine, temporomandibular joint, larynx, and pulmonary system. Deposition of rheumatoid nodules causes inflammation of the intervertebral disks and dura, which is expressed as atlantoaxial joint subluxation. The synovium of the temporomandibular joint is also affected by RA and can result in severe limitation of joint range of motion. The cricoarytenoid joints are common sites for rheumatoid nodule deposition. The resultant chronic synovitis may cause fixation of the vocal cords in adduction and airway obstruction. Finally, RA is associated with nine forms of pulmonary disease, including pleural effusion, interstitial lung disease, obliterative bronchiolitis, and vasculitis (Box 38-7).

Ankylosing spondylitis is also a chronic inflammatory process. The primary target is the spinal column and surrounding soft tissues. The progressive nature of AS means the spine can be injured by seemingly inconsequential trauma. Patients with AS also experience cardiac valvular dysfunction, conduction delays, bundle branch blocks, and restrictive lung disease.

BOX **38-6**

American College of Rheumatology Criteria for Diagnosis of Rheumatoid Arthritis

A. One hour or more of morning stiffness around joints
B. Simultaneous swelling or presence of fluid at three or more joint areas, including the right and left proximal interphalangeal (PIP), metacarpophalangeal (MCP), wrist, elbow, knee, ankle, and metatarsophalangeal joints
C. Swelling or fluid in at least one wrist, MCP, or PIP joint area
D. Symmetric swelling or presence of fluid simultaneously at right and left target joint areas listed in criterion B
E. Subcutaneous rheumatoid nodules
F. The presence of serum rheumatoid factor determined by a laboratory test in which less than 5% of the normal control population is positive
G. Posteroanterior hand and wrist radiographs demonstrating erosions or unequivocal bony decalcifications

BOX 38-7

Classifications of Pulmonary Disease in Rheumatoid Arthritis Patients

Pleural effusion
Intrapulmonary nodules
Rheumatoid pneumoconiosis (Caplan's syndrome)
Interstitial lung disease
Vasculitis
Obliterative bronchiolitis
Upper lobe fibrosis
Pulmonary infections
Bronchogenic carcinoma

Anesthetic Management

The primary concern when caring for a patient with either RA or AS is the patient's airway. The mobility of the patient's cervical spine must be meticulously evaluated during the preoperative interview. Any neurologic symptoms that occur during movement of the cervical spine must be thoroughly documented at that time. As a result of RA or AS, cervical mobility may be severely restricted; therefore, the patient may prove to be extremely difficult to intubate. Because of the high risk to these patients from the cervical manipulation during direct laryngoscopy for tracheal intubation, awake fiberoptic intubation may be the safer course of action. The prudent anesthetic course may also include positioning the patient such that neurologic symptoms remain absent before induction of general anesthesia. The cervical spine must be neutrally positioned throughout any surgical procedure, during emergence, and during transfer to the postanesthesia care unit. Regional anesthesia is a safe approach to extremity surgery in these patients.[78,79]

SUMMARY

Orthopedic surgical procedures allow and require the nurse anesthetist to be proficient in more general and regional anesthetic techniques than in other specialty. The patient's health history and acceptability of various anesthetic techniques, the proposed surgery and its duration, the patient's intraoperative position, and the need for postoperative pain management are important considerations in the planning and preparation for a safe and comfortable outcome. The anesthetic plan must adapt to the needs of the patient and the proposed surgery rather than expect the patient to adapt to one anesthetic technique. As with any anesthetic, the nurse anesthetist must anticipate problems in order to avoid them, instead of treating them when they occur.

The innovations of orthopedic surgical procedures over the past 20 to 30 years have provided opportunities and challenges. Now, many procedures are performed with the aid of the arthroscope in same-day surgery, and anesthesia practice has adapted by introducing short-acting anesthetic agents with fewer residual side effects and by providing various regional anesthesia techniques. Trauma and high-profile surgeries corresponding to the increasing geriatric population have challenged nurse anesthetists to adapt techniques that reduce complications and provide postoperative pain management.

REFERENCES

1. Barnhart CL, Barnhart RK, editors: *The World Book Dictionary*, vol 2, Chicago, 1990, World Book, p 1468.
2. Aker J: Pneumatic tourniquet application in the perioperative period, *Curr Rev Nurse Anesth* 20:1-8, 1997.
3. Estersohn HS, Sourifman HA: The minimum effective mid-thigh tourniquet pressure, *J Foot Surg* 21:281-284, 1982.
4. Denny-Brown D, Brenner C: Paralysis of nerve induced by direct pressure and by tourniquet, *Arch Neurol Psychiatry* 51:1-26, 1944.
5. Cole F: Tourniquet pain, *Anesth Analg* 31:63-64, 1952.
6. Patterson S, Klenerman L: The effect of pneumatic tourniquets on the ultrastructure of skeletal muscle, *J Bone Joint Surg Br* 61:178-183, 1979.
7. Klenerman L, Hulands GH: Tourniquet pressures for the lower limbs, *J Bone Joint Surg Br* 61:124-127, 1979.
8. Klenerman L: Tourniquet time: how long? *Hand* 12:231-234, 1980.
9. MacIver MB, Tanelian DL: Activation of C fibers by metabolic perturbations associated with tourniquet ischemia, *Anesthesiology* 76:617-623, 1992.
10. Weidner WA: *A Comparison of the Tourniquet Pain Response Using One Versus Two Thigh Tourniquets During Orthopedic Procedures Under General Anesthesia*, (master's thesis), Richmond, VA, 1992, Virginia Commonwealth University, Medical College of Virginia.
11. Strichartz GR, Zimmerman M: An explanation for pain originating from tourniquets during regional anesthesia, *Reg Anesth* 94:44-48, 1984.
12. Bridenbaugh PO, Hagenouw RR, Gielen MJ, Edstrom HH: Addition of glucose to bupivacaine in spinal anesthesia increases incidences of tourniquet pain, *Anesth Analg* 65:1181-1185, 1986.
13. Bourke DL, Yates AJ Jr, Yates HM: Evaluation of the patient with musculoskeletal disease. In Longnecker DE, Tinker JH, Morgan GE Jr editors: *Principles and Practice of Anesthesiology*, ed 2, St Louis, 1998, Mosby, pp 287-302.
14. Lowire A, Jones MJ, Eastley RJ: Effect of a eutectic mixture of local anesthetic agents (EMLA) on tourniquet pain in volunteers, *Br J Anaesth* 63:751-753, 1989.
15. Bourke SL, Silberberg MS, Ortega R, Willock MM: Respiratory responses associated with release of intraoperative tourniquet, *Anesth Analg* 69:541-544, 1989.
16. Hofmann AA, Wyatt RWB: Fatal pulmonary embolism following tourniquet inflation: a case report, *J Bone Joint Surg Am* 67: 633-634, 1985.
17. Pollard BJ, Lovelock HA, Jones RM: Fatal pulmonary embolism secondary to limb exsanguination, *Anesthesiology* 58:373-374, 1983.
18. Concepcion M: Anesthesia for orthopedic surgery. In Longnecker DE, Tinker JH, Morgan GE Jr editors: *Principles and Practice of Anesthesiology*, ed 2, St Louis, 1998, Mosby, pp 2113-2137.
19. Tountas CP, Bergman RA: Tourniquet ischemia: ultrastructural and histochemical observations of ischemic human muscle and of monkey muscle and nerve, *J Hand Surg* 2:31-37, 1977.
20. Tourniquet Safety Home Study: *Use of Surgical Tourniquets, a Self-Instructional Program*, Dover, OH, 1993, Zimmer.
21. Hoshowsky VM: Surgical positioning, *Orthop Nurs* 17:55-65, 1998.
22. Shapiro BA, Harrison RA, Walton JR: *Clinical Application of Blood Gases*, ed 3, Chicago, 1982, Year Book Medical, pp 55-66.
23. O'Brien TJ, Ebert TJ: Physiologic changes associated with the supine position. In Martin JT, Warner MA, editors: *Positioning in Anesthesia and Surgery*, ed 3, Philadelphia, 1997, Saunders, pp 27-36.
24. West JB, Dollery GT, Naimark A: Distribution of blood flow in isolated lung: relation to vascular and alveolar pressures, *J Appl Physiol* 19:713, 1964.
25. Froese AB, Bryan CA: Effects of anesthesia and paralysis on diaphragmatic mechanics in man, *Anesthesiology* 41:242-255, 1974.

26. Fratacci MD, Kimball WR, Wain JC, Kacmarek RM, Polaner DM, Zapol WM: Diaphragmatic shortening after thoracic surgery in humans. Effects of mechanical ventilation and thoracic epidural anesthesia, *Anesthesiology* 79:654-655, 1993.
27. Rehder K, Sessler AD, Marsh HM: General anesthesia and the lung, *Am Rev Respir Dis* 112:541-563, 1975.
28. Vellody VP, Naaery M, Druz WS, Sharp JT: Effects of body position change on thoracoabdominal motion, *J Appl Physiol* 45:581-589, 1978.
29. Klingstedt C, Hedenstierna G, Lundquist H, Strandberg A, Tokics L, Brismar B: The influence of body position and differential ventilation on lung dimensions and atelectasis formation in anesthetized man, *Acta Anaesthesiol Scand* 34:315-322, 1990.
30. Lawson NW, Meyer DJ Jr: Lateral positions. In Martin JT, Warner MA, editors: *Positioning in Anesthesia and Surgery*, ed 3, Philadelphia, 1997, Saunders, pp 127-152.
31. Courington FW, Little DM Jr: The role of posture in anesthesia, *Clin Anesth* 3:23-54, 1968.
32. Campos JH: Lung isolation techniques, *Anesthesiol Clin North America* 19:455-474, 2001.
33. Martin JT: The ventral decubitus (prone) positions. In Martin JT, Warner MA, editors: *Positioning in Anesthesia and Surgery*, ed 3, Philadelphia, 1997, Saunders, pp 155-195.
34. Batson OV: Function of the vertebral veins and their role in the spread of metastases, *Ann Surg* 112:138, 1940.
35. McGregor AL: *Synopsis of Surgical Anatomy*, ed 7, Bristol, CT, 1950, Wright.
36. Backofen JE, Schauble JF: Hemodynamic changes with prone positioning during general anesthesia, *Anesth Analg* 64:194, 1985.
37. Toole JF: Effects of change of head, limb, and body position on cephalic circulation, *N Engl J Med* 279:307-311, 1968.
38. *Dorland's Pocket Medical Dictionary*, ed 22, Philadelphia, 1977, Saunders, p 75.
39. Phillips BB: General principles of arthroscopy. In Canala ST, editor: *Campbell's Operative Orthopaedics*, vol 3, ed 10, St Louis, 2003, Mosby, pp 2497-2514.
40. Miller GK: Operative arthroscopy into the next century, *Compr Ther* 24:383-387, 1998.
41. Long JS: Shoulder arthroscopy, *Orthop Nurs* 15:21-31, 1996.
42. Baker CL, Brooks AA: Arthroscopy of the elbow, *Clin Sports Med* 15:261-281, 1996.
43. Phillips BB: Arthroscopy of lower extremity. In Canala ST, editor: *Campbell's Operative Orthopaedics*, vol 3, ed 10, St Louis, 2003, Mosby, pp 2515-2612.
44. Small NC: Complications in arthroscopy: the knee and other joints. Committee on Complications of the Arthroscopy Association of North America, *Arthroscopy* 2:253-258, 1986.
45. Small NC: Complications in arthroscopic surgery performed by experienced arthroscopists, *Arthroscopy* 4:215-221, 1988.
46. Blumenthal S, Nadig M, Gerber C, Borgeat A: Severe airway obstruction during arthroscopic shoulder surgery, *Anesthesiology* 99:1455-1456, 2003.
47. Lee HC, Dewan N, Crosby L: Subcutaneous emphysema, pneumomediastinum, and potentially life threatening tension pneumothorax, *Chest* 101:1265-1267, 1992.
48. Hall S: Respiratory anatomy, physiology, and pathophysiology. In Nagelhout JJ, Zaglaniczny KL, editors: *Nurse Anesthesia*, ed 2, Philadelphia, 2001, Saunders, pp. 504-579.
49. Shapiro BA, Lichtenthal PR: Postoperative respiratory management. In Kaplan JA, editor: *Cardiac Anesthesia*, ed 4, Philadelphia, 1999, Saunders, pp 1215-1232.
50. Harkess JW and Daniels AU: Introduction and overview (arthroplasty). In Canala ST, editor: *Campbell's Operative Orthopaedics*, vol 1, ed 10, St Louis, 2003, Mosby, pp 223-242.
51. Sharrock NE, Savarese JJ: Anesthesia for orthopedic surgery. In Miller RD, editor: *Anesthesia*, ed 5, Philadelphia, 2000, Churchill-Livingstone, pp 2118-2139.
52. Scilco TP, Ranawat C: The use of spinal anesthesia for total hip replacement, *J Bone Joint Surg* 57:173-177, 1975.
53. Thornburn R, Louden JR, Vallance R: Spinal and general anesthesia in total hip replacement: frequency of deep vein thrombosis, *Br J Anaesth* 52:1117-1121, 1980.
54. Keith I: Anaesthesia and blood loss in total hip replacement, *Anaesthesia* 32:444-450, 1977.
55. Modig J, Borg T, Karlstrom G, Maripuu E, Sahlstedt B: Thromboembolism after total hip replacement: role of epidural and general anesthesia, *Anesth Analg* 62:174-180, 1983.
56. Modig J, Hjelmstedt A, Sahlstedt B, Maripuu E: Comparative influences of epidural and general anesthesia on deep vein thrombosis and pulmonary embolism after total hip replacement, *Acta Chir Scand* 147:125-130, 1981.
57. Fallon KM, Fuller JG, Morley-Forster P: Fat embolization and fatal cardiac arrest during hip arhtroplasty with methymethacrylate, *Can J Anaesth* 48:626-629, 2001.
58. Dandy DJ: Fat embolism following prosthetic replacement of the femoral head, *Injury* 3:85-88, 1971.
59. Sevitt S: Fat embolism in patients with fractured hips, *BMJ* 2:257-262, 1972.
60. Anderson KH: Air aspirated from the venous system during total hip replacement, *Anaesthesia* 38:1175-1178, 1983.
61. Evans RD, Palazzo GA, Ackers JWL: Air embolism during total hip replacement: comparison of two surgical techniques, *Br J Anaesth* 62:243-247, 1989.
62. Ngai SH, Stichfield FE, Triner LK: Air embolism during total hip arthroplasties, *Anesthesiology* 40:405-407, 1974.
63. Deuschle JA, Romeo AA: Understanding shoulder arthroplasty, *Orthop Nurs* 17:7-15, 1998.
64. Neer CS, Watson KC, Stanton FJ: Recent experience in total shoulder replacement, *J Bone Joint Surg* 64:319-337, 1982.
65. Gartsman GM, Russell JA, Gaenslen E: Modular shoulder arthroplasty, *J Shoulder Elbow Surg* 6:333-339, 1997.
66. Wilde AH: Shoulder arthroplasty: what is it good for and how good is it? In Matsen FAI, Fu FH, Hawkins RJ, editors: *The Shoulder: A Balance of Mobility and Stability*, Rosemont, IL, 1992, American Academy of Orthopedic Surgeons, pp 459-481.
67. Muntz JE: The risk of venous thromboembolism in non-large-joint surgeries, *Orthopedics* 26:s237-242, 2003.
68. Rucker S, Budge J, Bailes BK: Perioperative care of patients undergoing spinal stabilization with internal fixation, *Today's OR Nurse* 16:8-13, 1994.
69. Lestini WF: "Cage" technology revolutionizes approach to spinal fusion surgery, *N C Med J* 59:101-104, 1988.
70. Wener BK, Fraser RD: Spine update: lumbar interbody cages, *Spine* 23:634-640, 1998.
71. Freeman BL: Scoliosis and kyphosis. In Canala ST, editor: *Campbell's Operative Orthopaedics*, vol 2, ed 10, St Louis, 2003, Mosby, pp 1751-1954.
72. Hellman EW, Glassman SD, Dimar JR: Clinical outcome after fusion of the thoracic or lumbar spine in the adult patient, *Orthop Clin North Am* 29:859-869, 1998.
73. Obenchain TG: Laparoscopic lumbar discectomy, *J Laparoendosc Surg* 1:145-149, 1991.
74. Mack MJ, Regan JJ, Bobechko WP, Acuff TE: Application of thoracoscopy for diseases of the spine, *Ann Thorac Surg* 56:736-738, 1993.
75. Regan JJ, Guyer RD: Endoscopic techniques in spinal surgery, *Clin Orthop Relat Res* 335:122-139, 1997.
76. Bostman O, Hyrkas J, Hirvensalo E, Kallio E: Blood loss, operating time, and positioning of the patient in lumbar disc surgery, *Spine* 15:360-363, 1990.
77. Arnett FC, Edworthy SM, Bloch DA, et al: The American Rheumatism Association 1987 revised criteria for the classification of rheumatoid arthritis, *Arthritis Rheum* 31:315-324, 1988.
78. Brill S, Middleton W, Brill G, Fisher A: Bier's block; 100 years old and still going strong! *Acta Anaesthesiol Scan* 48:117-122, 2004.
79. Holmes C: Intravenous regional blockade. In Cousins MJ, Bridenbaugh PO, editors: *Neural Blockade in Clinical Anesthesia and Management of Pain*, ed 3, Philadelphia, 1998, Lippincott, pp 395-409.

CHAPTER 39

The Immune System and Anesthesia

BRENT SOMMER

The study of immunology has evolved as an appreciation and understanding of bodily response to invading pathogens and related diseases. More recent information regarding the immune system has resulted from the extensive study of infectious diseases, inflammatory processes, and related pathologic states. Protection from infection and disease is provided by two major components: the innate and adaptive (acquired) immune responses. This chapter highlights immune system function and pathology, including human immunodeficiency virus, with particular considerations appropriate to the practice of anesthesia.

IMMUNE SYSTEM OVERVIEW

A review of the cellular components of the immune system and their individual functions affords a thorough comprehension of their various interactions and overall clinical presentation. Table 39-1 lists the major components and the individual roles that they fulfill in contributing to immune system activity.[1] Cytokines associated with immune function are noted in Box 39-1.

Early Development

The human immune system begins to present and sustain competence at approximately the sixth week of gestational age. During this stage of embryogenesis, evidence of functional lymphocytes, the mainstay of cellular immunity, begins to appear. This early and somewhat rudimentary system eventually develops into a complex network that interacts with virtually every system within the body to support, protect, and vitalize functions and maintain homeostasis. Congenital immunodeficiencies such as graft-versus-host disease can present as early as the first month of life. Effective treatment for these more severe degrees of immunodeficiency may require bone marrow transplantation. The aging process is often associated with the attenuation of many immune system functions. The majority of humans who live to an advanced age express some degree of immunodeficiency or immunosenescence. While many theories exist, to date no singular explanation of the process responsible for these obvious and somewhat predictable changes has been confirmed.

Structure

Immune system function results from activities that occur within either the specific or the nonspecific components of the system. Specific responses result from the destruction of foreign materials and antigens that protect the body from insult and injury. The more refined areas of the specific immune system reactions belong to either the humoral or the cell-mediated systems. Specific and nonspecific pathways frequently intermingle and influence both function and response, resulting in overall immune system activity and a degree of stability.

TABLE 39-1 Cellular Components of the Nonspecific Human Immune System

Components	Functions
Mononuclear cells	Ingestion and destruction of damaged and neoplastic cells and bacteria
Polymorphonuclear cells	Ingestion or phagocytosis; killing of microorganisms; facilitation of bodily clearance of dead cells
Eosinophils	Phagocytosis, combating parasitic diseases; defense in allergic response
Neutrophils	Phagocytosis, cytokine release, secretion of hydrolytic enzymes, secretion of reactive oxygen species
Natural killer cells	Nonspecific tumor cell and antibody-dependent cytotoxicity
Basophils and mast cells	Sources of histamine and heparin, which combat insult by increasing vascular permeability, smooth muscle contractility, and inflammatory responses
Platelets	Facilitation of coagulation; influence of tissue reactivity to injury
B lymphocytes	Humoral immunity; transformation into plasma cells, which react to foreign substances by producing antibodies and immunoglobulins; active in the circulatory system, cytokine release
T lymphocytes	Recognition and reaction to foreign material inside fixed tissues and to harmful organisms such as neoplastic and tuberculosis cells; important in transplant rejection, cytokine release
Plasma cells	Active in protein synthesis for the formation of immunoglobulins

BOX 39-1

Cytokines

- Cytokines are peptides that, in immune and inflammatory reactions, are released from and regulate the action of inflammatory and immune system cells.
- The cytokine superfamily includes the interferons, numerous interleukins, tumour necrosis factor (TNF), various growth factors, the chemokines, and the colony-stimulating factors.
- They act in a complex interconnecting network on leukocytes, vascular endothelial cells, mast cells, fibroblasts, hemopoietic stem cells, and osteoclasts, controlling proliferation, differentiation, and/or activation through autocrine or paracrine mechanisms.
- Interleukin-1 and TNF-α are important primary inflammatory cytokines, inducing the formation of other cytokines.
- The interferons (IFNs) α and β have antiviral activity and IFN-α is used as an adjunct in the treatment of viral infections. IFN-γ has significant immunoregulatory function and is used in the treatment of multiple sclerosis.

Adapted from Rang HP, Dale MM, Ritter JM, Moore PK: Pharmacology, *ed 5, Edinburgh, Scotland, 2003, Churchill Livingstone, p 241, with permission.*

Specific Immune System. The body's ability to protect itself from damaging organisms and various toxins is characterized by two types of specific immunity. Innate immunity is a result of several general processes within the body that contain and destroy bacteria. Protective mechanisms such as phagocytosis facilitate the destruction of foreign toxins that are harmful to the body. The integument is another form of protection that prohibits bodily invasion by harmful organisms. Trace amounts of antibodies found throughout the body act to destroy more specific types of bacteria. Innate immunity serves as the primary line of defense against bacterial invasion.

Acquired (or adaptive) immunity is characterized by destruction of organisms and toxins by antibodies and specific lymphocytes. This system provides protection from invasive organisms to which the body has no innate or natural immunity. Specific resistance against such invasive agents is developed once they have entered the body.

The humoral branch of the immune system is composed of B lymphocytes, which originate from bone marrow and plasma cells and function primarily to combat bacterial infection. The cell-mediated portion consists of T lymphocytes, which are formed by the thymus to destroy microorganisms or antigenic materials in the prevention of viral infectivity.

Antigens are usually protein-based substances that interact with lymphocytes to formulate antibodies. This type of binding is responsible for many of the reactions elicited when drugs are administered. Antibodies are produced by B lymphocytes and are classified as immunoglobulins (Ig). These immunoglobulins (Table 39-2) provide support systems for fighting infection and defending against other potentially harmful insults to the body.

Nonspecific Immune System. The complement system contains a multitude of plasma proteins that contribute to the mechanism of inflammatory responses. Inflammatory responses and agents that affect the pathway are noted in Figure 39-1. This system also plays a major role in preventing infection. In a healthy individual, these detailed and complex networks function to stabilize and maintain vital functions of the immune system (see Table 39-1).

TABLE 39-2 Human Immunoglobulins

Type	Location	Function
IgA	Plasma, saliva, and tears	Topical defense
IgD	Plasma	Unknown/nonspecific
IgE	Plasma	Hypersensitivity/ anaphylaxis
IgG (gamma globulin)	Plasma, amniotic fluid	Defense against systemic infection
IgM	Plasma	Bacterial cell lysis

Vaccination is used to produce acquired immunity against specific diseases. Vaccination against bacterial diseases such as typhoid, diphtheria, and whooping cough is accomplished by administration of dead organisms that have retained their chemical antigens yet cannot cause an actual disease state. Other types of immunity against certain toxins such as tetanus and botulism can be prepared and have had their toxic components destroyed during such processes. Attenuated organisms that are grown or mutated contain specific antigens that protect against diseases such as poliomyelitis, measles, and smallpox.

Passive immunity occurs when antibodies, activated T cells, or some combination that provides protection from an invasive agent is administered. These substances are obtained from human or animal blood following immunization against the particular antigen. Such transfusions remain effective for a period ranging from a few hours to several weeks after their infusion.

SYSTEMIC RESPONSES

Allergic Reactions

Allergy and Hypersensitivity. Several types of allergy and hypersensitivity exist and vary in both magnitude and incidence of occurrence. Persons who have an increased allergic tendency are termed *atopic* and usually exhibit a genetic predisposition to such events while maintaining large quantities of circulating IgE antibodies.

The term *anaphylaxis* refers to a systemic immediate hypersensitivity reaction caused by the rapid, IgE-mediated immune release of potent mediators from tissue mast cells and peripheral blood basophils. The term *anaphylactoid* refers to those clinical events caused by mediator release from mast cells and basophils by non-IgE-mediated triggering events. These events are potentially life-threatening reactions, although some are self-limited without treatment. Clinically, the term *anaphylaxis* is most often used to describe rapidly developing generalized reactions that include pruritus; urticaria; angioedema (especially laryngeal edema); hypotension; wheezing and bronchospasm; nausea; vomiting; abdominal pain; diarrhea; uterine contractions; and/or direct cardiac effects, including arrhythmias. These clinical manifestations can occur singly or in various combinations and usually occur within moments of exposure. However, signs and symptoms may begin 30 to 60 minutes after exposure, and

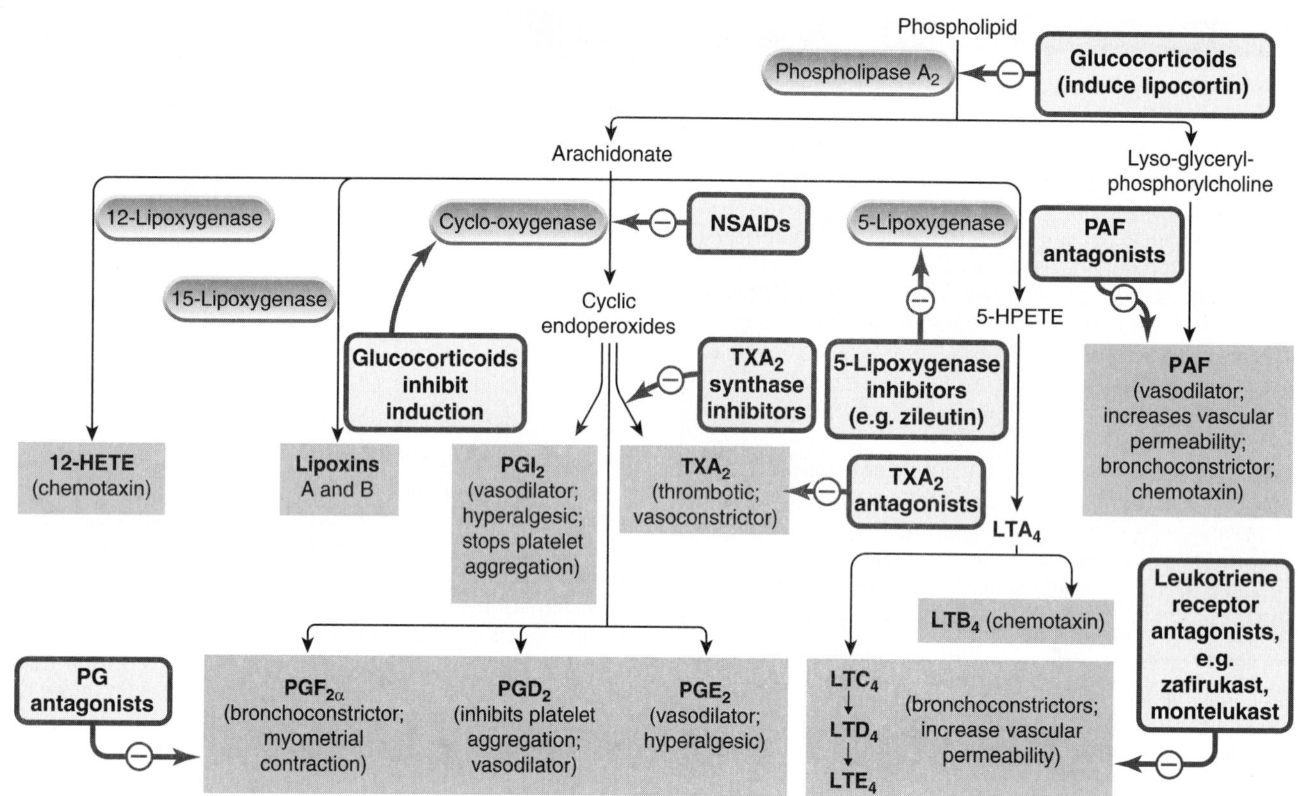

FIGURE **39-1**
Summary diagram of the inflammatory mediators derived from phospholipids with an outline of their actions and sites of action of antiinflammatory drugs. (From Rang HP, Dale MM, Ritter JM, Moore PK: *Pharmacology*, ed 5, Edinburgh, Scotland, 2003, Churchill Livingstone, p 232, with permission.)

in some cases onset may be delayed for longer than an hour. Signs and symptoms can be protracted and variably responsive to treatment. Biphasic anaphylaxis can also occur. In this situation, the early signs and symptoms clear (either spontaneously or after acute therapy) and reappear several hours later. Generally, the severity of an anaphylactic event will relate to the suddenness of its onset. Although the magnitude of the event also relates to the size of the challenge (i.e., the bigger the provocative dose, the more severe the reaction will be), severe reactions can occur after exposure to minute amounts of allergen in highly sensitive patients. Anaphylactoid reactions generally are dependent on systemic exposure to provoking agents and usually in amounts greater than would be expected to elicit anaphylaxis.

The sensitizing antibodies, or reagins, attach to mast cells or basophils and initiate changes within the cell membrane. As a result, histamines or similar substances that lead to abnormal tissue responses are released. A clinically apparent allergic reaction then results. Allergic reactions vary in presentation and magnitude and include urticaria, hay fever–like symptoms, asthma, and varying degrees of anaphylaxis.

Allergic reactions are usually the result of an antigen- or antibody-mediated response by the immune system, manifesting as varying degrees of anaphylaxis. Antigen-specific IgE antibodies are produced, sensitize the host, and elicit such reactions. Several factors often contribute a reaction to a specific agent. They include the underlying systemic condition present, the combination of agents administered, and adverse reactions on the system by each agent and its metabolites. Adverse reactions to anesthesia-related medications have long been appreciated and documented.[2]

Hypersensitivity reactions are classified into four types:

- Type I is a rapidly developing reaction that is IgE mediated and results in an anaphylactic response within minutes. This reaction is the result of an antigen combining with an antibody that is bound to basophils or mast cells in an individual who has been previously sensitized to the antigen. A shocklike state develops and usually elicits an initial response of vasodilation, vascular leakage, smooth muscle spasm, and increased glandular secretions. A delayed response may occur a few hours later and is characterized by allergic rhinitis and symptoms of bronchial asthma.
- Type II hypersensitivity occurs when antibodies specific to antigens attach to cell surfaces. These antibodies usually become bound to the cell surface antigens. Such a reaction is referred to as *cytotoxic*. An example of a type II immune disorder is an autoimmune hemolytic anemia.
- Type III response manifests as an immune complex disease, wherein humoral antibodies bind antigens that activate portions of complement to release neutrophilic enzymes that render tissue damage. Systemic lupus erythematosus, rheumatoid arthritis, and glomerulonephritis are examples.
- Type IV disorders are a delayed sensitivity such as contact dermatitis or graft rejection that occur as a cell-mediated response. Sensitized T lymphocytes release cytokines and are responsible for this classic delayed-type hypersensitivity.

Drug Reactions. Determining who will react adversely to a drug or combination of drugs is difficult. The incidence of an

BOX **39-2**

Classification of Adverse Reactions to Drugs

Reactions That May Occur in Any Patient

Drug overdose	Toxic reactions linked to excess dose or impaired excretion or both
Drug side effect	Undesirable pharmacologic effect at recommended doses
Drug interaction	Action of a drug on the effectiveness or toxicity of another drug

Reactions That Occur Only in Susceptible Patients

Drug intolerance	A low threshold to the normal pharmacologic action of a drug; hypersensitivity
Drug idiosyncrasy	A genetically determined, qualitatively abnormal reaction to a drug related to a metabolic change or enzyme deficiency
Drug allergy	An immunologically mediated reaction, characterized by specificity, transferability by antibodies or lymphocytes, and recurrence on re-exposure; involves anaphylaxis and immunoglobulin (IgE) release
Pseudoallergic reaction	A reaction with the same clinical manifestations as an allergic reaction, such as histamine release, but lacking immunological specificity; anaphylactoid

Adapted from Vervloet D, Durham S: ABCs of allergies: adverse reactions to drugs, BMJ *316:1511-1554, 1998.*

allergic drug reaction markedly increases with repeated dosing and relatively short periods of time between exposures. Of those reported reactions to medications from nearly 15% of the overall population, approximately 5% are thought to be an actual allergic response. Of these reported cases, approximately 0.1% are fatal.[3] Box 39-2 notes some definitions of adverse drug effects. Table 39-3 lists the drugs that commonly result in allergic responses in the perioperative period. Some of these are discussed in the following paragraphs.

Antibiotic preparations, for example, are responsible for a large number of documented medication allergies worldwide. Penicillin has been responsible for a significant portion of antibiotic-related anaphylaxis noted in the sixth report of a surveillance study in France, which has been ongoing since 1989.[4]

Cutaneous reactions to drugs are common (Box 39-3); however, life-threatening reactions to anesthetic drugs and adjuvants are unusual. These reactions occur approximately once in every 5,000 to 10,000 anesthetics. Over half of these serious reactions are immunologically mediated and the remainder are chemically mediated. Muscle relaxants are the primary etiologic agents of immunologically mediated reactions (58.2%). Rocuronium (43.1%) has surpassed succinylcholine (22.6%) as the drug most frequently implicated. This may reflect market share rather than a specific pharmacologic event. Reactions are more common in female subjects, which is thought to be due to common properties relaxants share with many cosmetics. This finding is consistent with the observation that many patients manifest an allergic reaction to muscle relaxants on first exposure. It can also be noted that drugs that do not elicit histamine release may still cause allergic reactions.[4,5]

TABLE **39-3** Agents Involved in Anaphylactic Reactions During Anesthesia

Causal Agent	Percentage
Neuromuscular blocking agents	***58.2 (total)***
Rocuronium	43.1
Succinylcholine	22.6
Atracurium	19.0
Vecuronium	8.5
Pancuronium	3.3
Mivacurium	2.6
Cisatracurium	0.6
Gallamine	0.3
Latex	***16.7***
Antibiotics	***15.1 (total)***
Penicillin	41.8
Cephalosporin	39.2
Vancomycin	11.4
Quinolone	5.1
Rifamycin	1.3
Aminoglycoside	1.3
Hypnotics	***3.4 (total)***
Propofol	66.7
Thiopental	16.7
Midazolam	16.6
Opioids	***1.3***
Nalbuphine	
Fentanyl	
Sufentanil	
Remifentanil	
Colloids	***4.0 (total)***
Gelatine	95.0
Hetastarch	5.0
Other agents	***1.3***
Protamine	
Ketoprofen	
Methylene blue	
Ethylene oxide	

From Mertes PM, Laxenaire MC, Alla F: Anaphylactic and anaphylactoid reactions occurring during anesthesia in France in 1999-2000, Anesthesiology *99(3):536-545, 2003.*

Tryptase is the marker of choice for mechanistic delineation. It is an enzyme that is released along with histamine, has a half-life of several hours, and is stable at room temperature, allowing for samples to be obtained after urgent clinical situations. It demonstrates a positive predictive value of 92.6% and a negative predictive value of 54.6% as an indication of an immunologically mediated event. The presence of a normal level does not exclude an immunologic reaction since elevated tryptase levels are not found in almost a third of anaphylactic cases. However, a significantly elevated tryptase level (>25 mcg/l) strongly suggests an allergic mechanism. The researchers caution that diagnosis of anaphylaxis should not rely on a single test. The high

BOX 39-3

Cutaneous Reactions to Drugs

Manifestation	Examples
Pruritis, urticaria or angio-oedema, maculopapular rash	Most drugs
Contact dermatitis	Antibiotics, ethylenediamine
Photodermatitis	Griseofulvin, sulphonamides
Fixed drug eruption	Metronidazole, penicillin
Toxic epidermal necrosis (potentially life threatening)	Sulphonamides, phenytoin, carbamazepine, barbiturates, allopurinol

Adapted from Vervloet D, Durham S: ABCs of allergies: adverse reactions to drugs, BMJ *316:1511-1554, 1998.*

BOX 39-4

Immediate Skin Testing for Diagnosing IgE-Dependent Allergy

Antibiotics
- Penicillin
- Cephalosporins

Anesthetic drugs
- Muscle relaxants
- Thiopental

Enzymes
- Chymopapain
- Streptokinase

Chemotherapeutic drugs
- Cisplatin

Others
- Insulin, latex

False-positive and false-negative reactions may occur with these skin tests. Adapted from Vervloet D, Durham S: ABCs of allergies: adverse reactions to drugs, BMJ *316:1511-1554, 1998.*

positive predictive value of tryptase, however, makes it useful both medicolegally and for subsequent patient management.[4,5]

Atopic patients frequently present with some history of hay fever, rhinitis, asthma, or food or drug allergy. There have been long-standing questions as to whether such patients are more likely to have an anaphylactic or anaphylactoid reaction during anesthesia. Such a correlation holds true for latex allergy. A history of generalized atopy or specific allergy to certain fruits, such as kiwi, avocado, or figs is recognized as a significant risk factor for latex reactions. However, other than for latex, a generalized history of allergy does not predispose a patient to anaphylactic and anaphylactoid reactions to anesthetics. There is, however, a significant cross-reactivity, as high as 80%, between anesthesia-related drugs such as muscle relaxants and a patient history of specific allergy to anesthetics. These patients merit a more thorough preoperative evaluation and possible referral to a clinical allergist for skin testing. If possible, a small test dose, administered intradermally, may help determine the likelihood of allergic response to drugs that do not elicit significant amounts of histamine (Box 39-4). Reliable, sophisticated, and more expensive methods for detecting the presence of specific IgE antibodies in sensitized plasma are available. The enzyme-linked immunosorbent assay (ELISA) and the radioallergosorbent test (RAST) are examples of these methods. In urgent circumstances, using an alternate anesthetic technique, such as regional anesthesia or avoidance of relaxants, may be the best clinical option.[4,5]

Most allergic reactions occur shortly after drug administration; however, delayed reactions can occur. Hallmark symptoms of cardiovascular and pulmonary responses usually occur within minutes following drug exposure and should warrant immediate response. Common allergic reactions frequently present as cutaneous lesions, edema, and urticaria, which may progress to anaphylactoid characteristics. Table 39-4 outlines the usual features of anaphylactoid reactions. The effect of histamine and its receptors is outlined in Box 39-5.

More than 10% of the general population exhibits some form of hypersensitivity when the immune response to some external antigen results in a significant reaction. Although these responses are usually far less intense than a full anaphylactoid reaction, the resultant hypersensitive state can be significant. This atopic state can be poorly differentiated and frequently is not completely understood or explained. An abnormal level of circulating IgE antibodies produces this hypersensitive state, with its wide range of presentations and varying degrees of severity.

A multitude of environmental components can cause these hypersensitivity reactions. Grass, pollen, dust, mites, molds, and animal dander cause an increase in circulating vasoactive substances, such as histamine, that can elicit a myriad of clinical symptoms. Usual allergic responses to these allergens include watery eyes, sneezing, runny nose, and occasional wheezing. The degree of this response is directly proportional to both the specific sensitization of the individual and the amount of allergen present in the immediate environment.

The unsuspected allergic response should always be anticipated and approached in as judicious a manner as possible. An appreciation of the magnitude and impact of a particular adverse reaction to a drug can best guide the appropriate response. Drug sensitivities particular to specific agents or techniques of anesthesia are varied and not particularly common. Pharmacologic agents that are capable of eliciting histamine release with detrimental results include basic compounds, hyperosmotic agents, and antibiotics. Muscle relaxants, opioids, and hypnotics are more likely to cause a nonimmunologic histamine release than are other agents. Although most drugs commonly used during anesthesia have at one time resulted in or contributed to allergic reactions, the incidence of life-threatening responses, as mentioned earlier, is rare. Considering the complexity, combinations, administration routes, and speed of injection of drugs employed in modern anesthesia practice, clinical complications are rare.

As discussed in detail in Chapter 9, local anesthetics from the ester group are more likely than amide agents to elicit an allergic response.[6] Solutions containing methylparaben and propylparaben as preservatives may also induce allergic responses in susceptible individuals. Metabolites such as para-amino benzoic acid (PABA) have been identified as responsible agents for this higher incidence of allergic response. A patient who reacts adversely to an amide local anesthetic agent can usually tolerate an ester group agent; the reverse can also be

TABLE 39-4 Anaphylactoid Responses

Presentation	Mechanism	Treatment
Cardiovascular		
Hypotension	Hypovolemia	Isotonic fluid, colloid administration
Tachycardia	Hypoxemia	Oxygen administration
Dysrhythmia		Standard antiarrhythmics
Pulmonary		
Bronchospasm	Histamine release	Epinephrine
Wheezing	Increase in oxygen demand	β_2-agonists
	Sensitization of tissues	Corticosteroids
	Stress	
Systemic		
Generalized edema	Increase in oxygen demand	Oxygen administration
	Angioedema	
Periorbital edema	Capillary permeability changes	
Laryngeal edema		Epinephrine, corticosteroids
Hypoxemia		
Local effects		
Flushing	Sensitization of tissues	Diphenhydramine
Urticaria	Local response	Corticosteroids

BOX 39-5

Histamine

- Histamine is a basic amine, stored in granules within mast cells and basophils and secreted when complement components C3a and C5a interact with specific membrane receptors, or when antigen interacts with cell-fixed IgE.
- It produces effects by acting on H_1-, H_2-, or H_3-receptors on target cells.
- The main actions in humans (with the receptors involved) are as follows:
  - –Stimulation of gastric secretion (H_2)
  - –Contraction of most smooth muscle other than that of blood vessels (H_1)
  - –Cardiac stimulation (H_2)
  - –Vasodilatation (H_1)
  - –Increased vascular permeability (H_1)
- Injected intradermally, histamine causes the "triple response": reddening from local vasodilatation, wheal by direct action on blood vessels and vasodilatation, and flare from an "axon" reflex in sensory nerves releasing a peptide mediator.
- The main pathophysiological roles of histamine are as follows:
  - –As a stimulant of gastric acid secretion (treated with H_2 receptor antagonists)
  - –As a mediator of type 1 hypersensitivity reaction such as urticaria and hay fever (treated with H_1-receptor antagonists)
- H_3-receptors occur at presynaptic sites and inhibit the release of a variety of neurotransmitters.

Adapted from Rang HP, Dale MM, Ritter JM, Moore PK: Pharmacology, *ed 5, Edinburgh, Scotland, 2003, Churchill Livingstone, p 231, with permission.*

true. Administration of preservative-free local anesthetics further ensures the lesser likelihood of an allergic response. Recent theories suggest that allergies to various antioxidants and certain sulfite components may be responsible for some degree of allergic reactions to local anesthetic agents. The application of histamine-1 and histamine-2 receptor antagonists preemptively has proved to be successful preventing reactions in many cases when a known or suspected sensitivity is present.

Avoiding known causal agents (particularly those that induce histamine release), combined with careful selection and application of additional drugs, further deters adverse reactions. A thorough history and discussion with the patient or the patient's guardian can usually reveal the potential for untoward effects and alert the anesthesia provider to avoid suspicious agents. The patient frequently mistakes a drug sensitivity or unpleasant response for an allergy. This is especially true with local anesthetic solutions containing epinephrine or with opiates. Careful investigation and cautious interviewing techniques are usually beneficial in clarifying these questionable areas. Reviewing past procedural notes and anesthesia records, and possible consultation with an allergist when appropriate, can further help in determining situational specifics and facilitate appropriate planning. Documentation of such findings is important to relate to future providers.

Treatment. Patients who do not appear to have life-threatening symptoms on initial presentation may progress to life-threatening anaphylaxis. Early administration of medications may be beneficial in halting this progression.

Standard therapy for non–life-threatening situations includes the following:

1. *Epinephrine*: The initial adult dose may range from 100 to 500 micrograms subcutaneously or intramuscularly. This may be repeated every 10 to 15 minutes as needed up to a maximum of 1 mg per dose. The dose in children is 10 mcg/kg up to a

maximum of 500 mcg per dose. This dose can be repeated every 15 minutes for two doses and then every 4 hours as needed. There is evidence that more rapid systemic absorption and higher peak plasma levels occur after intramuscular administration than occurs after subcutaneous administration.
2. *Diphenhydramine*: 1 to 2 mg/kg or 25 to 50 mg/dose (parenterally).
3. *Corticosteroids* may also be administered. However, the efficacy of corticosteroids in acute anaphylaxis or in reducing a late anaphylactic reaction has not been clearly established (Table 39-5).

Life-threatening anaphylaxis requires immediate administration of epinephrine and may require other immediate measures for support of cardiorespiratory status. Cardiopulmonary resuscitation (CPR) should be instituted if there is loss of circulation or respiration. Oxygen (100%) should be administered and the airway secured. Hypotension should be addressed by administration of vasopressors and infusions of large volumes of intravenous fluids and/or colloids to compensate for peripheral vasodilation and for intravascular fluid loss caused by third spacing. Bronchospasm should be treated with inhaled bronchodilators, theophylline, or both. For patients with life-threatening anaphylaxis who are poorly responsive to initial doses of epinephrine, more frequent or higher doses may be required. If the patient does not respond to subcutaneous epinephrine, intravenous administration of epinephrine must be initiated. Bolus doses of 50 to 100 micrograms should be titrated to effect. The infusion of epinephrine preparations should initially be titrated at 1 mcg/min, which can be increased to 2 to 10 mcg/min. For refractory cardiorespiratory arrest in children, the initial intravenous dose is 10 mcg/kg. Subsequent doses are 100 mcg/kg every 3 to 5 minutes, and if still refractory, the dose may be increased to 200 mcg/kg.

A good clinical response represents resolution of the reaction. If there is partial resolution or concern about biphasic anaphylaxis, continuous monitoring is suggested. Additional history might reveal previous episodes of anaphylaxis or asthma. Antihistamines may be useful in anaphylaxis particularly for urticaria, angioedema, or both. An H_2-receptor antagonist, used with an H_1 antihistamine, may be useful in reversing hypotension refractory to epinephrine and intravascular fluid replacement. Corticosteroids such as 200 mg intravenous hydrocortisone may reduce the risk of recurring or protracted anaphylaxis, although direct clinical evidence for this has not been clearly established.

Patients experiencing anaphylaxis may not always respond adequately to one injection of epinephrine. Epinephrine has a rapid onset but a short duration of action. At the same time, mediator release from effector cells (e.g., mast cells and basophils) may be prolonged, producing biphasic or protracted anaphylaxis. Therefore patients who receive epinephrine for the treatment of anaphylaxis may not improve sufficiently or may improve and then relapse. Additional doses of epinephrine may be necessary. Patients receiving β-adrenergic blocking agents may not respond to epinephrine and may require substantial fluid replacement. Patients receiving β-adrenergic blocking agents who do not respond to epinephrine and fluid replacement may respond to glucagon.

TABLE 39-5 Comparison of the Select Corticosteroid Agents

	APPROXIMATE RELATIVE POTENCY IN CLINICAL USE				
Compound	**Equivalent Dose in mg Oral and IV**	**Antiinflammatory**	**Sodium-Retaining**	**Duration of Action After Oral Dose***	**Comments**
Hydrocortisone (cortisol)	20	1	1	S	Drug of choice for replacement therapy
Cortisone	25	0.8	0.8	S	Inexpensive; inactive until converted to hydrocortisone; not used as antiinflammatory because of mineralocorticoid effects
Prednisolone	5	4	0.8	1	Drug of choice for systemic antiinflammatory and immunosuppressive effects
Prednisone	5	4	0.8	1	Inactive until converted to prednisolone
Methylprednisolone	4	5	0.5	I	Antiinflammatory and immunosuppressive
Triamcinolone	4	5	0	1	Relatively more toxic than others
Dexamethasone	0.75	25	0	L	Antiinflammatory and immunosuppressive, used especially where water retention is undesirable, e.g., cerebral edema; drug of, choice for suppression of ACTH production
Betamethasone	0.75	30	0	L	Antiinflammatory and immunosuppressive, used especially where water retention is undesirable
Fludrocortisone	Not used as glucocorticoid	10	125	I	Drug of choice for mineralocorticoid effects

Hydrocortisone is the standard for comparison.

**Duration of action (hours): S, short, 8-12; I, intermediate, 12-36; L, long , 36-72.*

Adapted from Chrousos GP, Margioris AN: Adrenocorticosteroids and adrenocortical antagonists. In Katzung BG, editor: Basic and Clinical Pharmacology, *ed 9, New York, 2004, McGraw-Hill; and Schimmer BP, Parker KL: Adrenocorticotropic hormone; adrenocortical steroids and their synthetic analogues; inhibitors of the synthesis and actions of adrenocortical hormones. In Hardman JG, Limbird LE, Gilman AG, editors:* Goodman and Gilman's The Pharmacological Basis of Therapeutics, *ed 10, New York, 2001, McGraw-Hill, p 1657.*

Transfusion Reactions

Because of advances in technological capabilities and quality control practices, blood transfusion reactions are, fortunately, not a common occurrence. The relative risk of an allergic transfusion reaction of mild severity (hives and pruritus) is calculated at a ratio of approximately 1:500, whereas a fatal hemolytic reaction can occur approximately 1:250,000 to 1:600,000 in those administered nationally. Mechanisms responsible for most transfusion reactions involve ABO compatibility, which is related to an individual's blood grouping and naturally occurring antibodies. In a transfusion resulting from inadvertent mismatching of blood types, recipient antibodies react to donor cells, causing their destruction with the potential for significant symptomology and consequences. Disseminated intravascular coagulation (DIC), renal failure, and death are not uncommon following this type of reaction. Reactions resulting from intravascular hemolysis can occur from excessive red cell warming and incompatibilities such as medications that may be concomitantly administered. Since the most common cause for a major hemolytic transfusion reaction is human error, it should never be assumed that another person is solely responsible for checking blood that you are preparing to administer to a patient.

Transfusion reactions are frequently masked, or at least delayed appreciably, during the administration of anesthetic agents. Hallmark symptoms of cardiovascular instability such as hypotension, fever, hemoglobinuria, and bleeding diathesis are indicative of an incompatibility and should be immediately treated.[7]

Latex Allergy

Allergies to latex-containing products continue to be the source of significant problems for specific populations. Health care workers and certain patients, particularly those with congenital neural tube deficits and those who have undergone multiple surgical procedures, have shown a particular sensitivity or allergy to latex-containing products.

Most estimates calculate that approximately 0.8% of the general population has some form of sensitivity to latex. Persons who are atopic react with skin dermatitis and are allergic to certain fruits (particularly kiwi and bananas) should be further evaluated for latex allergy. Health-care workers and patients who experience frequent exposure to devices and products that contain latex also exhibit such allergic reactions.[8] The incidence of health-care worker allergy to latex-containing products ranges between 8% and 25%. The most frequently clinically recognized reactions to latex include some form of contact dermatitis, type IV cell-mediated or delayed sensitivity, or type I IgE-mediated allergies wherein an immediate and potential anaphylaxis can occur. Box 39-6 lists such reactions in both awake and anesthetized patients.

BOX 39-6

Latex Reactions

Awake Patient	Anesthetized Patient
Itchy eyes	Tachycardia
Generalized pruritus	Hypertension
Shortness of breath	Wheezing
Feeling of faintness	Bronchospasm
Feeling of impending doom	Cardiorespiratory arrest
Nausea	Flushing
Vomiting	Facial edema
Abdominal cramping	Laryngeal edema
Diarrhea	Urticaria
Wheezing	

Preventive procedures and recommended protocols have been established for directing the management of latex allergies that can have significant anaphylactic consequences. Latex allergies have increased proportionately since medical glove usage has increased 10-fold to accommodate universal precautions and barrier protection during anesthesia, surgery, and obstetric care. Using gloves that do not contain latex can accommodate prevention of latex exposure. Gloves processed from polyvinyl or neoprene are appropriate for this application. While skin prick and patch testing and the radioallergosorbent (RAST) tests for latex allergy are available, all present various challenges in qualifying a diagnosis with conclusive results. The American Association of Nurse Anesthetists (AANA) Latex Protocol provides a detailed plan to avoid and treat latex allergic responses.[9]

IMMUNE SYSTEM PATHOLOGY

An intact immune system works to support and sustain routine physiologic functions while protecting the body from insult and injury. The healthy immune system accommodates changes and adverse insults that might otherwise alter or disrupt these vital functions. Pathophysiology affecting immune system function can involve a very complex network and can be responsible for significant impairment or even death.

Autoimmune Disease

Autoimmune diseases occur when an insufficient or limited response to antigens is superseded by a self-reactive state that is usually inadequate and dysfunctional. These pathologic states have a multitude of origins that range from genetic defects to environmental insults and acquired diseases. Breakdown of the usual sophisticated networking systems that maintain homeostasis leads to auto aggression and subsequent autoimmune disease states. The majority of autoimmune diseases affect women more often than men; in particular, they affect women of child-bearing and working age. There appears to be a specific genetic disposition to many autoimmune states.

Autoimmune disease results from alterations in the body's own response to cellular changes, tissue reaction, or immune responses to formerly latent antigens. In this state the immune system mistakenly attacks itself, targeting various cells, tissues, and organ systems throughout the body. A cross-reactive response may proliferate as another manifestation of autoimmune disease. An appreciable imbalance between suppressor and helper T lymphocytes that affects both humoral and cell-mediated responses occurs; as a result, several conditions, including anemias, arthritis, adrenal dysfunction, thyroid dysfunction, and platelet aberrations, can occur. Autoimmune lesions have also been traced to the administration of immune system antagonists, such as interleukin-2 and cyclosporine.[10] Cyclosporine has been used successfully for years for markedly combating allograft transplant rejection. In doing so, it concomitantly interferes with T-lymphocyte activation, thereby contributing to clinically significant autoimmune disease states.

Another well-documented disease process is cyclosporine-induced autoimmune syndrome, which is seen in bone marrow transplant recipients. In this situation, cyclosporine-induced autoimmune syndrome occurs following withdrawal from the drug.[11] Cyclosporine has been linked to the potentiation of both barbiturate anesthetics and narcotic analgesics. Cremophor, the solvent found in cyclosporine, has been found to potentiate muscle relaxants by significantly increasing neuromuscular blockade.[12,13]

Treatment of autoimmune disease consists of the induction of tolerance or suppression by means of system depletion, inactivation, and lymphocyte suppression. Self-tolerance can be restored through a usually prolonged and sophisticated networking of therapies[14] (Box 39-7).

Infection

Infection affects every organism in a unique manner, with a multitude of potential outcomes. These responses range from complete elimination of the microorganism, with resistance against recurrence, to incomplete elimination of antigens, with weakened immunity, sustained latency, or disease reactivation.

The stage and severity of infectivity from any source determine its impact on immune system stability, function, and future viability. The various effects that anesthetic agents have in contributing to infection have been studied extensively. Findings remain inconclusive as to what, if any, actual impact these agents have.[15]

Immunohematologic diseases resulting from blood transfusion and autoimmune reactions and drug-induced cytopenias can have significant impact on immune system function and subsequent viability. Thorough appreciation of these somewhat complex states and consequences may require substantial specialty consultation and multidisciplinary intervention. Early recognition and management of these situations is vital to both immediate and future outcomes.

Cancer

The immune system plays an extreme role in protecting the body from various malignancies by responding to cancer cells as antigens that it initially rejects and resists. Variables such as tumor cell type and growth influence immune system capability to respond effectively. An intact and healthy immune system can serve to combat cancers that do invade the body. The exact mechanism and role that all immune system components play in responding to various cancers is not completely understood.

Mixed activities—sometimes reflecting immune system protection and at other times supporting inhibition of neoplasms—are frequently observed during various cancer growth states. Immunotherapies are continuing to show promise in combating certain cancer types. Monoclonal antibodies are showing great potential in both the diagnosis and treatment of the side effects induced by various cytotoxic therapies (Box 39-8). Vaccination programs against breast and prostate cancers continue to show promise in combating cancers common to these areas.

BOX 39-7

Immunosuppressant Drugs

Most immunosuppressants act in the induction phase of the immunological response, reducing lymphocyte proliferation; some also inhibit aspects of the effector phase. The drugs used for immunosuppression can be roughly divided into agents that do the following:
- Inhibit interleukin-2 production or action e.g., cyclosporine, tacrolimus.
- Inhibit cytokine gene expression, e.g., the corticosteroids
- Inhibit purine or pyrimidine systhesis, e.g., azathioprine, myclophenolate mofetil
- Block the T cell surface molecules involved in signaling, e.g., monoclonal antibodies

Immunosuppressants are used for three main purposes:
- to suppress rejection of transplanted organs and tissues (kidneys, renal, bone marrow, heart, liver, etc)
- to suppress graft-versus-host disease (i.e., the response of lymphocytes in the graft to host antigens) in bone marrow transplants
- to treat a variety of conditions that, while not completely understood, are believed to have an important autoimmune component in their pathogenesis: idiopathic thrombocytopenic purpura, some forms of hemolytic anemia, some forms of glomerulonephritis, myasthenia gravis, systemic lupus erythematosus, rheumatoid arthritis, psoriasis, and ulcerative colitis

Therapy for this third category often involves a combination of glucocorticoid and cytotoxic agents.

For transplantation of organs or bone marrow, cyclosporine is usually combined with a glucocorticoid, a cytotoxic drug or an antilymphocyte immunoglobulin.

Adapted from Rang HP, Dale MM, Ritter JM, Moore PK: Pharmacology, *ed 5, Edinburgh, Scotland, 2003, Churchill Livingstone, p 257, with permission.*

DISEASE STATES

Although the human body has the innate capability of defending itself from insult and infection, a multitude of immunologic deficiencies can potentially prohibit or impair the usual course of immune system function from conception throughout adult life. More than four dozen primary immunodeficiency syndromes have been identified. An appreciation of the most common and significant of these processes is necessary for obtaining a complete understanding of immune system function.[16]

Presentation of Immunodeficiencies

Immunodeficiency results from an overwhelming insult to usual immune system function that is either inherent in a malformed system or develops over time. The presentation of specific immunodeficiencies reflects the functional portion of the system that is impaired. Bacterial infections result from malfunction within the humoral branch, whereas viral, fungal, protozoal, and mycobacterial insults are elicited by problems within the cell-mediated limb. These processes can occur in the presence of an intact immune system, but they tend to be more prominent and sustained in the presence of a preexisting immunodeficient state.

Preexisting conditions may make an immune system more vulnerable to insult. Some of these potentially compromising situations are listed in Table 39-6. These conditions result from concomitant systemic disease states, insufficient immune function due to significant illness, or pharmacologically induced immune depression from therapeutic measures.

Several clinically significant scenarios exist in conjunction with immune system impairment and dysfunction. A brief review serves to enhance a more thorough understanding of

BOX **39-8**

Monoclonal Antibodies

The monoclonal antibodies (mAbs) are genetically engineered immunoglobulins (IgGs) that react with specific molecular targets. They may be part mouse, part human (termed *humanized*, or *chimeric*), or fully human. In chimeric mAbs, the antigen-recognizing portion of a mouse antibody is joined to the framework of a human IgG molecule.

- **Abciximab** A chimeric mAb against the clotting receptor GpIIb/IIIa on platelets; used to prevent clotting in patients undergoing coronary angioplasty.
- **Adalimumab** A humanized mAb against the cytokine TNF-α used for rheumatoid arthritis.
- **Alemtuzumab** A humanized mAb against an antigen on T and B lymphocytes used to treat B-cell leukemia.
- **Basiliximab** A chimeric mAb against the receptor for the cytokine interleukin-2 on activated T cells; used in acute rejection of kidney transplants.
- **Daclizumab** A humanized mAb against the receptor for the cytokine interleukin-2 on activated T cells; used in acute refection of kidney transplants.
- **Gemtuzumab** A humanized mAb against an antigen on leukemia cells, used to treat relapsed acute myeloid leukemia.
- **Infliximab** A chimeric mAb against the cytokine TNF-α used for rheumatoid arthritis and Crohn's disease.
- **Muromonab** (Orthoclone OKT3) A murine mAb to the CD3 antigen of human T cells that functions as an immunosuppressant in heart, kidney and liver transplants.
- **Omalizumab** A humanized mAb against the binding of IgE to the high-affinity IgE receptor on the surface of mast cells and basophils for the treatment of asthma.
- **Palivizumab** A humanized mAb against a protein of respiratory syncytial virus (RSV); used to treat RSV infection in children.
- **Rituximab** A humanized mAb against the cytokine CD20 receptor on B cells; used in non-Hodgkin's lymphoma.
- **Satumomab** A conjugate produced from a murine mAb for imaging and diagnostics.
- **Trastuzumab** Herceptin is an mAb against HER2 used for breast cancer treatment.

Adapted from Mosby's Drug Consult, *St Louis, 2004, Mosby; Rang HP, Dale MM, Ritter JM, Moore PK:* Pharmacology, *ed 5, Edinburgh, Scotland, 2003, Churchill Livingstone, p 241, with permission.*

these pathophysiologic states and their applicability during the perioperative period.

Neutropenia occurs either secondary to cellular defects or in response to some overwhelming insult, such as immunosuppressive therapy. A myriad of organisms proliferate and contribute to secondary infections and further immune system disruption.

The immunocompromised patient may develop combined deficiencies that cause significant and often fatal outcomes. It is important to remember that organisms that are otherwise not pathogenic or routinely thought to be harmful can be the impetus for the demise of these patients. Meticulous technique in promoting infection control measures should be an initial focus in the care of these vulnerable patients throughout the perioperative period.

TABLE **39-6** Immune System Compromise States

Source	Cause	Presentation
Cancer	Neoplastic cells Immunotherapy Radiotherapy	Infection Exacerbation
Invasive	Intravenous cannulation Urinary catheterization	Infection Septicemia Infection Pyelonephritis
Pharmacologic	Side effects of therapeutic agents Chemotherapy Immunosuppressive agents (steroids, azathioprine)	Hematologic disorders Host infection and colonization
Systemic	Wounds Eczema Burns	Skin disruption Potential route Immunoglobulin defect Malabsorption syndrome Enteropathy
Viral	Human immunodeficiency virus	Multitudinal

Congenital Disease States

Congenital immunodeficiencies are classified according to the cellular level and immune system functions that are most specifically impacted. These include T- and B-cell defects, which affect cellular and humoral immunities respectively. Several immunodeficient states particular to the humoral system result in hypogammaglobulinemias. These processes are usually genetically determined and manifest at various stages of development. Those deficiency states that are treatable require intensive immune protective measures, antibiotics, and gamma-globulin replacement therapies. A thorough appreciation of genetic and formative history, past medical interventions, and surgical and anesthesia-related experience is vital to both the planning and implementation of further intervention for these patients.

Severe defects in cellular immunity frequently present within the first month of life and are often transmitted from maternal lymphocytes. Extensive and severe cellular immunodeficient states are often fatal, with bone marrow transplantation often providing the sole chance for survival. One instance of a defect in the cell-mediated branch of the immune system is the rare presentation of DiGeorge syndrome, a developmental aberrancy resulting in hypoplasia of the thymus and parathyroid glands. A multitude of connective tissue, skin and bone, and rare congenital diseases result as pathology of the immune system. A thorough appreciation for the particular presentation of these diseases and their anesthetic implications is essential in planning perioperative care. A secondary development frequently involves a hypocalcemic state and various vascular anomalies. Structural micrognathia frequently results during this syndrome, which can hinder laryngoscopy and related airway management efforts. It is necessary to monitor serum calcium level in these patients because inappropriate levels can interfere with the metabolism of neuromuscular blocking agents.

B-cell defects usually present as an IgG deficiency within the first year of life and can cause fatal respiratory compromise unless successfully treated, usually with gamma globulin. Phagocyte and hereditary complement deficiencies can also cause serious to fatal scenarios resulting from progressive infectious states that thrive secondary to such prevalent predispositions in these children.

ANESTHESIA AGENTS AND IMMUNE SYSTEM FUNCTION

General Effects

Immunocompetent patients without obvious or significant simultaneous disease processes can routinely metabolize and eliminate anesthesia-related agents with little or no appreciable consequence. Immune system insults caused by these drugs are usually negligible and of a transient nature. Individuals with organic disease frequently experience a more profound response to many agents and may experience a more direct and lasting effect on systemic functions. Efforts to elucidate more precisely the exact effects of anesthesia-related agents are ongoing.

Known effects on the human hematologic profile with or without concomitant diseases have been well documented.[17,18] Most studies completed to date that have examined immune system modification caused by anesthesia and surgery have failed to demonstrate a correlation between these alterations and significant adverse or persistent consequences.[19-22]

Specific Anesthetic Agents

Inhalation Agents. The effect of inhalation agents on immune system function and viability has been evaluated extensively and continues to remain controversial. No conclusive evidence has confirmed that general anesthetic agents have either significant or lasting immunosuppressant effects.[23,24] Nitrous oxide interacts with vitamin B_{12}, resulting in selective inhibition of methionine synthase, a key enzyme in methionine and folate metabolism. This effect of nitrous oxide may alter one-carbon and methyl-group transfer, which is important for DNA, purine, and thymidylate synthesis. Long-term exposure to high concentrations of nitrous oxide may cause megaloblastic bone-marrow depression and neurological symptoms. Exposure to high doses for less than 6 hours, as is common in clinical anesthesia, is considered harmless. Recent studies seem to suggest a correlation between nitrous oxide anesthesia and hyperhomocystinemia, which is an independent risk factor for coronary artery disease.[23] The ability of these agents to directly and substantially affect immune system function remains in most instances insignificant, yet present.[25-27]

Occupational exposure to inhalational anesthetics has often been associated with health hazards and reproductive toxicity, but the available evidence is weak and comes mostly from poorly designed epidemiological studies. Controlled studies generally showed no association between occupational exposure to anesthetic gases and reproductive effects. Animal studies also showed a lack of carcinogenicity, organ toxicity, and reproductive effects with trace concentrations found in modern operating rooms. The exception may be nitrous oxide, which in some (but not all) studies showed teratogenicity in rats chronically exposed to concentrations of 1000 ppm and higher, such as may occur in unscavenged operating rooms or dental settings without a proper ventilation system. At present, available data do not support the notion that exposure to trace amounts of nitrous oxide is associated with impaired fertility or an increased risk of developing cancer. It is good practice, however, to limit levels of exposure.[23,28,29]

The phenomenon of hepatotoxicity associated with halothane administration continues to be a subject of research, even though its use has all but ceased in the United States.

Hypnotics. At clinically appropriate dosages, thiopental has been associated with insignificant degrees of depression of immunoglobulin production.[30] Systemic responses to barbiturates and other intravenous sedative and hypnotic drugs have contributory effects that alter physiologic activities sufficiently to lead to interference with immunologic status. Delayed and decreased airway ciliary activity subjects the patient to potential insult and infection, and depressed respiratory efforts may contribute to pulmonary disease.

Propofol infusion syndrome, which has been recently reported, is a rare yet serious phenomenon that may have indirect immune consequences. This sometimes lethal syndrome of metabolic acidosis, acute cardiomyopathy, and skeletal myopathy is associated with infusions of propofol at rates of 5 mg/kg/hour for more than 48 hours. There is evidence to support the hypothesis that the syndrome is caused by the failure of free fatty acid metabolism due to inhibition of free fatty acid entry into the mitochondria and also specific sites in the mitochondrial respiratory chain. The syndrome mimics a mitochondrial myopathy.[31]

Opioids. Opioid preparations have been linked to specific changes in immune function, including organ atrophy, a lessening of cellular viability, and an increase in systemic stress.[32] Although several of these observations involved the consideration of marked levels of morphine and related drugs as clinically appropriate, dosages administered during routine anesthesia and postoperative recovery periods showed transient and reversible impact.[33,34] Cocaine, marijuana, and related drugs of abuse have all been implicated in the causation of proportional immune system insult and injury.

Regional Anesthesia. Regional anesthesia techniques have been implicated in transient and reversible effects on immune system function and reactivity.[35] Epidural block has been shown to cause a transient and significant alteration of lymphocyte and natural killer (NK)–cell activity regardless of pain status of the patient.[36] Controversies continue to exist regarding both the appropriateness and the impact of general and regional anesthesia techniques with regard to immune system function. It is important to weigh the potential insults against the possible benefits for each patient and to exercise proper judgment.

Additional Confounding Factors

More easily determined parameters such as age, degree of preexisting illness, systemic stress, and insults such as infection, cancer, and hematologic and metabolic disorders appear to have slightly greater predictive validity than other influential factors. The likelihood that anesthesia would cause more lasting and potentially harmful effects secondary to preexisting conditions may be greater under such circumstances.[37]

Overall, the majority of agents used in anesthesia, most of which have been evaluated extensively, show transient nonspecific immunosuppressant effects. The majority of effects noted were of short duration and of minimal, if any, final consequence. Most agents currently used, typically as combinations, provide valuable stress reduction during the perioperative period, which would prove to be beneficial under most circumstances. The benefits of this practice are believed to far exceed any potential adverse effects.

Viral infections that pose a threat to survival include various forms of hepatitis. Although an effective vaccine is available to combat hepatitis B, many people continue to succumb to this potentially lethal or chronic process. Hepatitis C has emerged as a far more detrimental disease state that can lie dormant for decades before total hepatic failure and related sequelae ensue. Prevention, surveillance, early detection, and appropriate therapeutic measures are key in controlling these significant factors for disability and death.

HUMAN IMMUNODEFICIENCY VIRUS

Human immunodeficiency virus (HIV) has escalated as a primary public health threat since the initial clinical presentation occurred over two decades ago. The magnitude and impact of this epidemic have been felt worldwide, and although a cure or potential preventive vaccine against this blood-borne pathogen does not currently exist, exhaustive studies have greatly broadened our understanding of immune system function.

Epidemiology

The epidemiologic basis for HIV begins with transmission through blood and certain body fluids. Box 39-9 lists the various sources of transmission of the virus, which can enter the body through blood contact, sexual transmission, and perinatal exposure. Since the disease was identified, approximately 50% of the cumulative number of reported victims have died. Although HIV infectivity has developed into a more chronic disease for the majority of those infected, it can progress to a fatal disease.[38] Early detection, evaluation, and pharmacologic intervention when indicated has proven to be extremely successful in controlling the disease while preserving immune system function and integrity.

BOX **39-9**

Routes of Transmission of Human Immunodeficiency Virus and Other Blood-Borne Pathogens

Absolute
Blood
Body fluids containing blood

Possible
Cerebrospinal fluid
Pericardial fluids
Amniotic fluids
Semen, vaginal secretions
Synovial fluid
Pleural fluid

Remote
Feces
Saliva
Sputum
Sweat
Tears
Urine
Wound drainage
Nasal secretions

Not Implicated in Health Care Settings
Human breast milk

Biology

HIV is a retrovirus that invades the cell-mediated branch of the immune system, resulting in an increased susceptibility to opportunistic disease and infections. Intracellular organisms such as viruses, fungi, and protozoa then proliferate, causing further damage, as reflected by the depletion of CD4 lymphocytes. These lymphocytes are normally responsible for initiating and sustaining immune responses.

The usual course of HIV is characterized by a decline in the number of helper T lymphocytes, which is indicative of dysfunction that is consistent with progressive disease. Early and initial stages of HIV disease progression were consistent with specific clinical signs and symptoms that correspond to decreases in T4 cell count (Table 39-7). More advanced stages of the disease that qualify due to clinical and hematologic parameters are classified as *acquired immune deficiency syndrome* (AIDS).

More recent progress in early detection and pharmacological intervention has literally redefined much of how the virus thrives and impacts the immune system. Childbearing women constitute a significant portion of recently reported cases of HIV and AIDS. Prophylactic cesarean section is frequently performed for the HIV-positive parturient according to current obstetrical practices and recommended guidelines in an attempt to control uteroplacental and fetal transmission of the virus by administering antiretroviral therapy during labor and delivery. Such practices have proven to diminish and in many cases eliminate fetal transmission of the virus.[39]

Treatment Modalities

Years of research and experience have produced several agents for combating HIV infection that are either currently used or under investigation. The International AIDS Society–USA Panel has published updated treatment guidelines for adult patients with HIV.[40]

Decisions regarding the appropriate timing and initiation of various agents to combat the virus and concomitant disease processes have been established. Regimen choices, monitoring parameters, appropriateness of adaptation and changes in

TABLE **39-7** **Stages of Human Immunodeficiency Virus–Related Disease**

Stage	Clinical Sign	T4 Cell Count
Acute	Mononucleosis-like illness	Normal
Early	Asymptomatic or persistent generalized lymphadenopathy Aseptic meningitis Dermatologic manifestations	>400
Middle	Asymptomatic or persistent generalized lymphadenopathy Thrush Hair leukoplakia Idiopathic thrombocytopenic purpura	200-400
Late	Opportunistic infections Malignancies Wasting Dementia	<200

therapeutic regimens, and alternative therapeutic approaches are more timely and individualized for each patient. Most current therapies involve a mixture or "cocktail" of drugs including protease inhibitors, nucleoside reverse transcriptase inhibitors (NRTIs), and nonnucleoside reverse transcriptase inhibitors (NNRTIs) retroviral agents. An example would be a three-drug regimen combining a protease inhibitor (e.g., indinavir, nelfinavir, saquinavir, amprenavir, or ritonavir) with two nucleoside reverse transcriptase inhibitors and some NNRTI preparation. Select combinations are recommended depending upon disease stage, clinical presentation, and general monitoring values[41-43] (Box 39-10). Most of these agents interrupt viral replication at various stages to protect cells that are not yet infected by the virus.

Agents commonly used to combat HIV infection usually work to combat receptor binding and subsequent entry of the virus into the cells. These agents act to inhibit viral reverse transcriptase, an enzyme that facilitates deoxyribonucleic acid proliferation and subsequent cellular infectivity. Pharmacologic intervention and treatment modalities for HIV-infected persons have experienced a rapid evolution and extreme complexity in recent years. Current recommendations suggest treatment for all persons who are experiencing acute HIV syndrome, those who have known seroconversion within the past 6 months, and those who are symptomatic. Treatment is currently offered in most cases to individuals whose laboratory values reflect fewer than 200 CD4 T cells/mm^3 or plasma HIV RNA levels (viral load) usually at or exceeding 50,000 copies/mL (DNA assay). Treatment for asymptomatic persons is addressed on an individual basis.

The immediate goal in administering antiretroviral therapy is to maximize viral suppression for as long a period as possible. Therapeutic approaches and treatment regimes are guided by individualized monitoring parameters, patient tolerance, and adherence patterns. Treatment objectives are to decrease HIV RNA levels significantly within 8 weeks of therapy initiation and eliminate detectable virus following 4 to 6 months of initial treatment. Therapeutic modalities may fail due to nonadherence, inadequacy of necessary potencies or suboptimal levels of antiretroviral agents, or resistance. Extensive options for combination therapy applications currently exist when initial recommended approaches fail. Management of HIV continues to evolve rapidly as experience and further research dictate. Treatment response continues to make remarkable progress. Further research continues to address resistance and investigate multiple strains of the virus that may not respond to current therapeutic modalities. Ultimate goals, of course, include prevention, isolation, and cure of HIV.

The first global clinical trials for HIV vaccine candidates were recently initiated in 18 cities around the world.[44] Vaccine safety, toleration, practicality, and response will be evaluated utilizing a vaccine that contains no live HIV in diverse populations around the globe.

It is important to understand the patient's status both in response and application of antiretroviral therapy and other treatments received when an operative procedure is planned. Appreciation of both recent and past therapeutic efforts and the patient's response is important in preparing the HIV-infected patient for anesthesia and related care. Consultation with and participation of the patient's primary care provider in the planning process can be beneficial (Table 39-8).

Zidovudine. One of the original antiretroviral agents available and approved by the Food and Drug Administration (FDA) for combating HIV disease is zidovudine (Retrovir), commonly referred to as AZT. This drug blocks HIV replication by means of competitive inhibition and interruption of the chemical bonding necessary for viral entry into the cell.[45,46] AZT was the first and only FDA-approved drug for the treatment of HIV infection for many years. A multitude of antiviral agents have more recently been approved for human use.

BOX 39-10

Treatment of HIV/AIDS

A consensus on the use of retroviral therapy in AIDS has emerged based on the following principles:

- Monitor plasma viral load and CD4+ cell count.
- Start treatment before immunodeficiency becomes evident.
- Aim to reduce plasma viral concentration as much as possible for as long as possible.
- Use combinations of at least three drugs (e.g., two reverse transcriptase inhibitors and one protease inhibitor).
- Change to a new regimen if plasma viral concentration increases.

Drugs for HIV Infection

- Reverse transcriptase inhibitors (RTIs).
- Nucleoside RTIs (NRTIs) are phosphorylated by host cells enzymes to give 5′-trisphosphate, which competes with the equivalent host cellular trisphosphates that are essential substrates for the formation of proviral DNA by viral reverse transcriptase. Examples are zidovudine and abacavir. They are used in combination with protease inhibitors. Unwanted effects with zidovudine (often serious) are blood dyscrasias, gastrointestinal disturbances, myopathy, CNS disturbances. Unwanted effects with abacavir are generalized hypersensitivity reactions (rare but serious).
- Nonnucleoside RTIs (NNRTIs) are chemically diverse compounds that bind to the reverse transcriptase near the catalytic site and denature it. An example is nevirapine. This can prevent mother-to-newborn transmission. Main unwanted effect is rash; Stevens-Johnson syndrome may occur. Drug interactions can be a hazard.
- Protease inhibitors inhibit cleavage of the translated inert protein into functional and structural proteins. They are used in combination with reverse transcriptase inhibitors. An example is saquinavir. All inhibit the liver P450 enzymes. Main unwanted effects are metabolic disorders, altered distribution of fat (some fat wasting, some fat accumulation).
- Combination therapy is essential (e.g., two NRTIs with either an NNRTI or one or two protease inhibitors).

Adapted from Rang HP, Dale MM, Ritter JM, Moore PK: Pharmacology, *ed 5, Edinburgh, Scotland, 2003, Churchill Livingstone, pp 661-662, with permission.*

TABLE 39-8 Centers for Disease Control HIV/AIDS Classification System

CD4+ T-Cell Categories	(A) Asymptomatic, Acute (Primary) HIV or PGL	Clinical Categories (B) Symptomatic (Not A or C) Conditions	(C) AIDS-Indicator Conditions
≥500/μl	A1	B1	C1
200-499/μl	A2	B2	C2
<200/μl	A3	B3	C3

Review of clinical categories

A. Patient must exhibit one or more of these documented conditions
   Asymptomatic HIV infection
   Persistent generalized lymphadenopathy
   Acute (primary) HIV infection or history of acute HIV infection
B. Conditions attributed to HIV or a defect in cell-mediated immunity, or conditions that are considered to have a clinical course or to require management that is complicated by HIV infection
   Candidiasis, oral and other
   Moderate-to-severe cervical dysplasia
   Fever of 38.5° C or diarrhea of 1 month's duration
C. Definitive diseases for AIDS diagnosis
   Cervical cancer
   Cytomegalovirus retinitis
   Mycobacteriosis
   Kaposi's sarcoma
   Pneumocystis carinii pneumonia
   Recurrent pneumonia
   Toxoplasmosis of the brain
   Primary tuberculosis

AIDS, *acquired immunodeficiency syndrome;* HIV, *human immunodeficiency virus;* PGL, *progressive general lymphadenopathy.*
Modified from Centers for Disease Control: 1993 revised classification system for HIV infection and expanded surveillance case definition for AIDS among adolescents and adults, MMWR Morb Mortal Wkly Rep *41/RR-17:1-19, 1992.*

Other studies have questioned the appropriateness of initiating AZT therapy before the actual presentation of clinical symptoms. The most significant side effect of AZT therapy is bone marrow suppression. Dose adjustments may limit the anemia and neutropenia associated with AZT administration. Other side effects such as headaches, malaise, and dizziness may subside with continued therapy or dose adjustment.

Other Pharmaceutical Agents. Additional antiviral agents—such as dideoxyinosine (didanosine, Videx), commonly referred to as DDI; D4T (Stavudine, Zerit); and 3TC (lamivudine)—have been approved by the FDA for use in patients who are unable to tolerate AZT or who demonstrate immunologic and clinical deterioration during single-agent therapy. Major side effects of these agents include pancytopenias, pancreatitis, hepatic toxicities, and peripheral neuropathies. It is critical that the anesthetist be aware of all medications that the patient is prescribed, know how well they have adhered to dosage regimes, and appreciate both the benefits and side effects that the patient has experienced in order to optimally accommodate this challenging disease throughout the perioperative period.

Planning for Procedures

Although several research studies are currently evaluating the effects of surgery and anesthesia on the HIV-infected patient, to date no conclusive evidence has been found to support any particular set of recommendations. Most alterations caused by various agents and techniques used for anesthesia are transient and have not been proved to contribute to any adverse outcome. The HIV-infected patient may require a variety of surgical interventions (Table 39-9).

When anesthesia care is planned, attention should be focused on end-organ and systemic impairment and resultant dysfunction. Several clinically significant alterations occur in most organ systems, particularly in the advanced disease states of HIV infection, when vigilant monitoring and, at times, intensive intervention may be necessary. The patient (or his or her legal representative or caregiver) should be included in the planning and evaluation of potential care options.

Clinical Presentation

A multitude of related clinical presentations have a potential to affect anesthesia for the person infected with HIV. A thorough preoperative assessment, including current physical examination, laboratory results, and radiographic examination, combined with other studies as indicated by patient presentation and current disease state, is critical before anesthesia care. Several clinical conditions may exist that have the ability to influence both anesthesia approach and patient outcomes.

Wasting syndrome results from disturbances in food absorption and metabolism and is defined as profound involuntary weight loss greater than 10% of baseline body weight. Chronic diarrhea frequently contributes to this scenario. Parenteral nutrition and appetite stimulation are usually required for this syndrome when persistent. Preoperative assessment should include extensive evaluation of volume status and related physiologic studies to plan appropriate management, intervention, and preparation.

TABLE 39-9 Common Abdominal Pathogens That May Necessitate Surgical Intervention

Pathogen	Effects
Virus	
Cytomegalovirus	Most common reason for surgery; potentially serious colitis, peritonitis, diarrhea, fever, hematochezia, gastrointestinal perforation, ulceration, ischemia resulting in small-bowel resection with diversion; acute cholecystitis
Tumors	
Kaposi's sarcoma	Gastrointestinal and biliary tree involvement results in hemorrhage, perforation; represents end stage of disease, so laparotomy for obstruction results in limited resection with reanastomosis
Lymphoma	Extranodal masses, usually distal to the esophagus; presents with abdominal pain, mass, bowel obstruction, hemorrhage, and peritonitis from perforation; most common presenting symptom is small-bowel obstruction resulting in emergency laparotomy
Bacteria	
Mycobacterium	Disseminated disease of the liver, spleen, lymph nodes, and small intestine; very poor prognosis with limited surgical intervention
Coexisting Gastrointestinal Pathogens	
Viruses	
Adenovirus	Colon involvement, chronic watery, nonbloody, nonmucoid diarrhea with weight loss
Herpes simplex	Chronic cutaneous ulcers; perianal lesions, proctitis; esophagitis
Protozoa	
Cryptosporidium	Debilitating, chronic, voluminous, watery diarrhea; severe dehydration; electrolyte imbalance and wasting; occasional biliary tract obstruction; malabsorption syndrome
Microsporida	Nonbloody, nonmucoid diarrhea, often requiring fluid and electrolyte replacement; patient retains good appetite
Bacteria	
Mycobacterium avium-intracellulare	Most common systemic bacterial infection
Salmonella	
Shigella	
Campylobacter	All bacterium-caused diarrhea requires rehydration and electrolyte supplementation as well as drugs to inhibit intestinal motility and secretion; occasional need for total parenteral nutrition; diarrhea recurs after withdrawal of antibiotics, but chronic suppressive regimens can result in resistant strains
Fungal	
Candida albicans	Invasive disease in oral cavity and esophagus

Modified from Smith PD, Quinn TC, Strober W, Janoff EN, Masur H: NIH conference. Gastrointestinal infections in AIDS, Ann Intern Med *116:63-77, 1992; Lowy AM, Barre PS:* Br J Surg *81:942-945, 1994.*

Neurologic evaluation is essential for the HIV-infected patient. Both the central and peripheral nervous systems can be impaired due to direct disease effects, concomitant opportunistic infections, or resultant side effects from therapeutic agents used to combat viral insult. AIDS-related dementia can influence both motor and cognitive states, particularly in advanced and late disease states.

Informed consent may be the responsibility of a legal guardian or durable power of attorney designee for the patient who may be mentally incompetent. It is critical that constant vigilance and attention to safety and orientation be directed toward these individuals.

Peripheral neuropathies may result in considerable discomfort or physical limitations. Autonomic effects may result in some degree of cardiovascular instability requiring immediate or continuous intervention. Anesthetic approach and planning should consider all factors that affect patient homeostasis during and after surgical intervention.

Hematologic abnormalities are not uncommon for the HIV patient. Platelet stability and functional activity are frequently impaired. Splenectomy may be indicated in an attempt to deter platelet-associated thrombocytopenias and cross-reactivities. Steroid therapy may precede these measures in an attempt to preserve platelet concentration and function.

Non-Hodgkin's lymphoma, manifesting as a space-occupying lesion within the central nervous system, may require surgical or chemotherapeutic intervention. Kaposi's sarcoma, a cancer that invades endothelial tissues, can attack both skin and internal organs. Women infected with HIV may develop cervical dysplasia and cancers.

Physical Complications of Human Immunodeficiency Virus Disease

As HIV disease progresses, advanced complexes of related diseases emerge that would otherwise be resisted in the immunocompetent host. These opportunistic disease processes increase in both manifestation and advancement as the immune system fails.

Opportunistic Infections

Bacterial Infection. Both acute and chronic infections tend to plague the HIV-infected person. *Mycobacterium avium-intracellulare* (MAI) infection is characterized by intractable diarrhea and resultant wasting states. Splenic and pulmonary infections with MAI lead to severe thrombocytopenia and tuberculosis. MAI attacks the immune-suppressed host easily and is transmittable.

Viral Infections. Several viral infections occur or recur from previously dormant states as HIV disease progresses. Herpes simplex and varicella infections can invade oral and esophageal tissues and the central nervous system. Cytomegalovirus can affect the gastrointestinal and pulmonary systems, resulting in colitis, pneumonia, or retinal invasion (possibly leading to marked visual disturbances and blindness). Ganciclovir is used to treat cytomegalovirus.

Protozoal Infections. *Pneumocystis carinii* pneumonia (PCP) is responsible for the majority of deaths in HIV-infected persons secondary to opportunistic infection. Fevers and impaired gas exchange frequently result in hypoxemia. Pneumothorax is not uncommon. Toxoplasmosis encephalitis can affect both central nervous system function and sensorium. Cryptosporidiosis can trigger considerable diarrhea. Significant dehydration and related electrolyte imbalance may exist as a result. Volume states must be judiciously evaluated and monitored.

Oxygenation, circulation, and most metabolic functions are frequently taxed and impaired during progressive HIV infection. Pulmonary infections and resultant insults frequently alter both gas exchange and perfusion. Dehydration and hypovolemia secondary to gastrointestinal disturbances can further complicate the patient's clinical course. This situation can present a significant challenge to both the surgeon and anesthetist when the additional stress of surgery and anesthesia becomes a factor. Thorough planning and preparedness usually contribute to the management of such scenarios and make it possible to avoid further complications. Thermoregulation and fluid management are often a considerable challenge for the anesthetist.

The pregnant patient with HIV presents a unique challenge for health maintenance. Anemia can be of great significance, frequently necessitating transfusion therapy, particularly in advanced states of HIV infection. Recent therapeutic advances and approaches to the HIV infected parturient, as referred to earlier, have markedly influenced and in many cases eliminated the incidence of HIV transmission from mother to fetus.

Perinatal transmission accounts for greater than 80% of all pediatric AIDS cases that have been reported in the United States.[39] Significant improvement continues in decreasing perinatal transmission with proactive antiretroviral therapy for antepartum care of the HIV-infected parturient.[47]

Because many physical manifestations of HIV-related illness involve neuromuscular disorders, pain management can be a difficult challenge during advanced HIV infection. Both routine and standardized modalities and agents combined with the use of various chemotherapies, nerve blocks, and complementary therapies have proven to be beneficial in treating acute postoperative and obstetrical pain in the HIV-infected patient.[48]

Patients with acute illness and injury who have histories of chemical dependency or who may currently be experiencing substance abuse states should be treated from a palliative perspective. Although recovery and abstinence are necessary for achievement of the ultimate goal of improved well-being, these patients are usually not candidates for aggressive recovery programs until acute situations are in check.

Managing HIV Infection

Fungal Infections. Fungal infectivity is responsible for histoplasmosis and aspergillosis pneumonia in the HIV patient. Such insults can frequently result in both febrile and hypoxic states of significant degrees, thereby impairing gas exchange and overall sensorium. Disseminated candidiasis infections are responsible for oropharyngeal and esophageal pathology that includes stomatitis, dysphagia, and esophagitis. Cryptococcal meningitis patients can experience increased intracranial pressure, and several therapeutic agents and antibiotics must be administered frequently to ensure their ultimate effectiveness.

The primary emphasis in managing HIV infection during anesthesia and all aspects of patient care is an effective prevention program. Because the routes of transmission of the virus are well known, an appropriate infection control program, with the consistent application of proven blood and body substance precautions, can prevent disease transmission. Universal precautions were developed after known modes of transmission of both HIV and hepatitis B virus (blood-borne pathogens) were clarified. More recent efforts to apply this practice throughout all patient care areas have resulted in the application of standard precautions consistently during patient care. The basic premise on which these guidelines are based is the prevention of parenteral, mucous membrane, and nonintact skin exposure to blood and certain body fluids from all patients. Guidelines include the following:

1. Gloves must be worn when contact with body substances is suspected or possible.
2. A plastic gown or apron must be worn when soiling with body substances is likely.
3. Protective masks and eyewear must be worn in the presence of airborne disease or for preventing splash or aerosolization of body substances to eyes or mucous membranes.
4. Hands must be thoroughly washed before and after body substances or articles possibly covered with body substances have been handled and after gloves have been removed at the completion of each task or procedure.
5. Uncapped needles and syringes must be discarded in puncture-resistant receptacles placed as close to their point of use as is practical.
6. Trash and linens must be discarded in impervious, sealed plastic bags that are labeled as infectious and transported according to standard precautions.

Optimal conformity to these guidelines requires a commitment by all involved parties to practice basic standard precautions in a diligent manner.

Occupational Safety

Human Immunodeficiency Virus Postexposure Prophylaxis. As of December 2001, the Centers for Disease Control and Prevention (CDC) had received voluntary reports of 57 documented cases of HIV seroconversion temporally associated with occupational exposure to HIV among U.S. health care personnel.[49,50] An additional 138 infections among health care personnel were considered possible cases of occupational HIV transmission. Since there is no cure or effective vaccine for AIDS, optimal postexposure care, including the administration of antiretroviral drugs to prevent HIV infection, remains a high priority for protecting health care personnel.[51]

Percutaneous injury, with a hollow-bore needle, is the most common mechanism of occupational HIV transmission. The CDC estimates that more than 380,000 needle-stick injuries occur in U.S. hospitals each year; approximately 61% of these injuries are caused by hollow-bore devices.[52] The proportion of injuries involving exposure to blood from HIV-infected sources is not known, but each exposure is an urgent health issue for the exposed person.

There are two main strategies for managing occupational exposure to blood. The first approach is to provide empirical treatment with two or more antiretroviral drugs unless additional information such as the results of an HIV test in the source patient or a detailed description of the exposure suggests that this treatment is not warranted. The second approach is to conduct a thorough assessment of the exposure (including an HIV test in the source patient if HIV infection has not already been diagnosed) and then initiate antiretroviral treatment only if the exposure poses a risk of HIV transmission.

A patient whose blood or other potentially infectious body fluid is involved in an occupational exposure should be evaluated to determine the likelihood of HIV infection, in accordance with relevant state regulations and local policies. The interval between the onset of viremia and the detection of HIV antibody, with the use of current enzyme immunoassays for HIV, is a few days at most.[53] If the result of a reliable HIV test in the source patient is negative, the risk of transmission is assumed to be zero, unless the patient has risk factors for infection and the clinical findings are compatible with acute HIV infection.

The use of a rapid HIV test can reduce the time needed to rule out HIV infection to a few hours or less. One test that is currently available, the Single Use Diagnostic System HIV-1 Test (Abbott-Murex Diagnostics), is highly sensitive, and a negative result is reliable evidence that infection is not present.[54] A positive test is presumptive evidence of HIV infection, but confirmatory tests should be performed, since false positive results do occur.

Pooled data from several prospective studies of health care personnel suggest that the average risk of HIV transmission is approximately 0.3% after a percutaneous exposure to HIV-infected blood and approximately 0.09% after a mucous-membrane exposure.[49] The average risk associated with exposure of nonintact skin and exposure to HIV-infected fluids and tissues other than blood or bloody fluids is too low to be estimated in prospective studies. In a retrospective study, the CDC found that the risk of transmission of HIV to health care workers was increased when the device causing the injury was visibly contaminated with blood, was used for insertion into a vein or artery, when a deep injury occurred , or when the source patient died within two months after the exposure.[55] A low plasma HIV RNA titer may indicate a lower inoculum but does not exclude the possibility of transmission, especially since this measurement does not account for cell-associated HIV. Transmission from source patients with undetectable HIV RNA has been documented.[49]

Suture needles have not been implicated as a source of infection in prospective studies, but occupational HIV infection has been reported among surgical personnel, and suture needles are one potential source of such infection. Exposure of intact skin to contaminated blood has not been identified as a risk for HIV transmission.

Chemoprophylactic Treatment. A convergence of indirect evidence suggests that treatment with antiretroviral drugs soon after occupational exposure to HIV decreases the risk of infection. The pathogenesis of the initial infection provides suggestive evidence that there is a window of opportunity in which antiretroviral treatment can prevent infection or abort it before irreversible systemic infection and HIV seroconversion occur (Tables 39-10 and 39-11).

In the CDC's retrospective case-control study of health care personnel, postexposure treatment with zidovudine was associated with an 81% reduction in the risk of HIV infection.[53] However, there are no data from randomized, controlled trials. Data from clinical trials of prophylaxis against perinatal HIV transmission consistently demonstrate that antiretroviral treatment can prevent HIV infection after exposure, even among neonates who are not treated until after birth.[56-61] The relevance of this clinical situation to occupational exposure is not known.

Although these data are encouraging, it is clear that, whatever benefit is afforded by postexposure treatment, the protection is not absolute. Twenty-one cases of HIV infection have been reported in health care personnel in the United States and elsewhere, despite postexposure antiretroviral treatment, which included two or more antiretroviral drugs in some cases.[49,62-67] A variety of factors may have contributed to the treatment failure, including an intrinsic lack of efficacy of prophylactic antiretroviral treatment and resistance to antiretroviral drugs.

It is unclear why 99.7% of occupational injuries involving percutaneous exposure to HIV do not transmit infection, and an assessment of the risk of transmission therefore remains imprecise. The most effective and safest antiretroviral regimen for exposed persons also remains uncertain. A combination of three or more antiretroviral agents is usually advised for the treatment of HIV infection, but there is no clinical evidence that such combinations are more effective in preventing infection after occupational exposure than is treatment with a single drug. In fact, of the five health care workers who are known to have acquired HIV infection despite prophylactic treatment with more than one antiretroviral drug, three received three or more drugs.[68]

The efficacy and safety of prophylactic treatment in pregnant and breastfeeding women has not been fully established, and there are few data on the effect of treatment on fertility, spermatogenesis, teratogenesis, and oncogenesis in otherwise healthy people.

HIV testing of exposed persons is recommended as soon as possible after exposure to establish that the infection was not already present and periodically during the first 6 months after the exposure to detect occupational transmission. Testing after 6 months is not usually indicated. An enzyme immunoassay for HIV antibody is the appropriate test for detecting new infections. The routine use of tests to detect plasma HIV RNA is not recommended. Since these tests are optimized to measure very low levels of HIV RNA, they have a relatively high rate of false-positive results and a low positive predictive value when used to detect occupational infection and can lead to unnecessary anxiety, unnecessary use of antiretroviral treatment, or both.[69,70]

Laboratory monitoring, including a complete blood count and tests of renal and hepatic function, is recommended at baseline and at 2 weeks. The use of additional tests depends on the specific regimen used and the medical condition of the source patient. The guidelines also recommend that persons who have acquired hepatitis C virus infection from the exposure be followed for 12 months, because anecdotal evidence indicates that they may be at risk for delayed HIV seroconversion.[49] All exposed persons, regardless of the postexposure treatment regimen, are advised to return for immediate evaluation if symptoms or signs that might be attributable to acute

TABLE 39-10 HIV Postexposure Prophylaxis (PEP) for Mucous Membrane Exposures and Nonintact Skin* Exposure

	INFECTION STATUS OF SOURCE				
Exposure type	HIV-Positive Class 1†	HIV-Positive Class 2†	Source of Unknown HIV Status§	Unknown Source¶	HIV-Negative
Small volume**	Consider basic 2-drug PEP††	Recommended basic 2-drug PEP	Generally, no PEP warranted; however, consider basic 2-drug PEP†† for source with HIV risk factors§§	Generally, no PEP warranted; however, consider basic 2-drug PEP†† in settings where exposure to HIV-infected persons is likely	No PEP warranted
Large volume¶¶	Recommended basic 2-drug PEP	Recommended expanded 3-drug PEP	Generally, no PEP warranted; however, consider basic 2-drug PEP†† for source with HIV Risk factors§§	Generally, no PEP warranted; however, consider basic 2-drug PEP†† in settings where exposure to HIV-infected persons is likely	No PEP warranted

*For skin exposures, follow-up is indicated only if there is evidence of compromised skin integrity (e.g., dermatitis, abrasion, or open would).
†HIV-positive, class 1, asymptomatic HIV infection or known low viral load (e.g., <1500 RNA copies/mL). HIV-positive, class 2, symptomatic HIV infection, AIDS, acute seroconversion, or known high viral load. If drug resistance is a concern, obtain expert consultation. Initiation of postexposure prophylaxis (PEP) should not be delayed pending expert consultation, and, because expert consultation alone cannot substitute for face-to-face counseling, resources should be available to provide immediate evaluation and follow-up care for all exposures.
§Source of unknown HIV status (e.g., deceased source person with no samples available for HIV testing).
¶Unknown source (e.g., splash from inappropriately disposed blood).
**Small volume (i.e., a few drops).
††The designation, "consider PEP," indicates that PEP is optional and should be based on an individualized decision between the exposed person and the treating clinician.
§§If PEP is offered and taken and the source is later determined to be HIV-negative, PEP should be discontinued.
¶¶Large volume (i.e., major blood splash).
From American Society of Health-System Pharmacists: ASHP therapeutic guidelines for nonsurgical antimicrobial prophylaxis, Am J Health-Syst Pharm 56:1201-1250, 1999.

HIV infection appear. Postexposure care must also address the risks of infection with hepatitis B virus and hepatitis C virus.

Body substance isolation techniques have been developed as a comprehensive system of barrier protection to be used during procedures in which the potential for personal contact with blood and body fluids exists. The major component of an adequate body substance isolation program is the readily available supply of effective protective barriers. Protective barriers appropriate during anesthesia care include gloves, masks, protective eyewear or face shields, gowns, and protective aprons and coverings that are worn when exposure is likely or anticipated. A major discrepancy exists in many practice settings in which such precautions are inappropriately applied. Failure to change gloves between successive contacts and tasks, for example, can further promote the spread of potential contaminants to otherwise clean objects or areas.

Respiratory isolation should be used when it is either known or suspected that airborne pathogens may be transmitted. Examples of such pathogens include the causative agents of tuberculosis (TB) and varicella. The immune system compromise resulting from HIV infection markedly increases the susceptibility to reactivation of TB. Recurrent or newly acquired TB is frequently the cause of death for persons infected with HIV. A striking clinical feature of TB in HIV-infected patients is a high incidence of extrapulmonary involvement, usually with concomitant pulmonary presentation.[71-73]

Intravenous and injectable administration apparatuses have a significant role in promoting universal precautions during anesthesia care. Needle-stick injuries account for the majority of workplace reports involving infection control and interventions. Protected needle devices and devices without needles are available and adaptable to all anesthesia delivery systems. The use of these devices should be promoted in all anesthesia care settings. Proactive efforts and compliance to manage these preventable incidents must be the foundation for all infection control programs.

Since most anesthetists are responsible for providing resuscitative care, it is important that they participate in the planning and preparation of resuscitation services at their workplace. Planning for and anticipation of practices and behaviors/procedures that carry risks of occupational exposure to blood-borne pathogens should be calculated and avoided by thoroughly preparing and planning, and by ongoing evaluation and risk determination. The appropriateness of disposable equipment and supplies, as well as their readiness and accessibility, should be addressed.

Although equipment preparedness is important for every patient to whom anesthesia is administered, it is of particular

TABLE 39-11 Recommendations for Prophylaxis against Human Immunodeficiency Virus (HIV) Infection After Percutaneous Injury, According to the Infection Status of the Source Person

	INFECTION STATUS OF SOURCE PERSON ±				
Risk Posed by Exposure†	**HIV-Positive, Class 1**	**HIV-Positive, Class 2**	**Unknown Status**	**Unknown Source Person**	**HIV-Negative**
Lower	Basic 2-drug prophylaxis is recommended	Expanded (3-drug) prophylaxis recommended	Generally, prophylaxis not warranted, but basic 2-drug prophylaxis can be considered if source person has risk factors for infection	Generally, prophylaxis not warranted, but basic 2-drug prophylaxis can be considered in settings where exposure to HIV-infected persons is likely	Prophylaxis not warranted
Higher	Expanded (3-drug) prophylaxis recommended	Expanded (3-drug) prophylaxis recommended	Generally, prophylaxis not warranted, but basic 2-drug prophylaxis can be considered if source person has risk factors for infection	Generally, prophylaxis not warranted, but basic 2-drug prophylaxis can be considered in settings where exposure to HIV-infected persons is likely	Prophylaxis not warranted

**The information is adapted from the recommendations issued in 2001 by the Public Health Service.*
†Injuries caused by solid needles and superficial injuries pose a lower risk of infection, and those involving a large-bore hollow needle, a deep puncture, a device visibly contaminated with blood, or a needle used in a patient's artery or vein pose a higher risk of infection.
±A class 1 positive status is defined by asymptomatic HIV infection or a lower viral load (e.g., <1500 RNA copies per millimeter): a class 2 positive status is defined as symptomatic HIV infection, the acquired immunodeficiency syndrome, acute seroconversion, or a high viral load. If drug resistance is a concern, an expert should be consulted. Initiation of prophylaxis should not be delayed pending such consultation. Resources should be available to provide immediate evaluation and follow-up care for all exposed persons.
If the source person has risk factors for HIV infection, prophylaxis is optional and should be based on an individualized decision made jointly by the exposed person and the treating clinician. If prophylaxis is administered and the source person is subsequently determined to be HIV negative, prophylaxis should be discontinued.
Gerberding, JL: Occupational exposure to HIV in health care settings, N Engl J Med. *348(9):826-833, 2003.*

significance to the immunocompromised patient. Meticulous attention to behaviors and adherence to strict aseptic technique in providing care to these most vulnerable patients is paramount to safe practice and quality patient care. The anesthesia machine and its multitude of components should be adequately maintained, cleaned, and disinfected, and appropriate sterile components should be changed between each use, in accordance with both approved infection control practices and manufacturers' recommendations. The AANA infection control guide details recommended practices for managing blood-borne pathogens during anesthesia care.[74] Several issues regarding the safety and well-being of anesthesia providers are relevant to the support of immune system viability and general health maintenance. Studies determining provider exposure risk to anesthetic agents and their effect on immune system function have shown minimal, reversible, or negligible effects during recommended practice and when standard protective mechanisms are in place. Although the particular measures for safeguarding against inadvertent and potentially harmful level of contaminants and exposure are known and can be readily implemented, all practitioners must be responsible for ensuring that these measures are judiciously maintained.

Appropriate and adequate infection control standards should be the foundation for every anesthesia practice setting. Immune system protection and preservation during anesthesia care is a primary responsibility of every provider. Careful planning and preparation provide for an environment free of or protected from known harmful agents. Situations that foster adverse conditions must be avoided.

Self-protection against HIV and all other infectious blood-borne pathogens such as hepatitis B and C viruses is an essential element of safe practice. Understanding the appropriate application of personal protective equipment in order to prevent exposures without hindering practice can be a challenge. The Occupational Safety and Health Administration (OSHA) Act, which became effective in 1992, mandates that employers minimize occupational exposure to all blood-borne pathogens in workplaces where a potential for such exposures exists. Known or suspected exposure to blood-borne pathogens should be responded to immediately with appropriate action, as recommended by OSHA and institutional infection control standards.

Every provider should know his or her hepatitis antibody status and seriously consider receiving the synthetically prepared hepatitis B vaccine, unless he or she is already sensitized. Anesthesia providers should be represented when committees and institutions are planning and implementing infection control programs for perioperative and obstetric areas. Management resources for occupational exposure to various pathogens are given in Box 39-11.

BOX 39-11

Occupational Exposure Management Resources

Resource	Contact
National Clinicians' Postexposure Prophylaxis Hotline (PEP-line) Run by University of California–San Francisco/San Francisco General Hospital staff; supported by the Health Resources and Services Administration Ryan White CARE Act, HIV/AIDS Bureau, AIDS Education and Training Centers, and CDC	Phone: (888) 448-4911 http://www.ucsf.edu/hivcntr
Needlestick! A website to help clinicians manage and document occupational blood and body fluid exposures. Developed and maintained by the University of California, Los Angeles (UCLA), Emergency Medicine Center, UCLA School of Medicine, and funded in party by CDC and the Agency for Healthcare Research and Quality.	http://www.needlestick.mednet.ucla.edu
Hepatitis Hotline	Phone: (888) 443-7232 http://www.cdc.gov/hepatitis
Reporting to CDC: Occupationally acquired HIV infections and failures of PEP	Phone: (800) 893-0485
HIV Antiretroviral Pregnancy Registry	Phone: (800) 258-4263 Fax: (800) 800-1052 1410 Commonwealth Drive, Suite 215 Wilmington, NC 28405 http://www.glaxowellcome.com/preg_reg/antiretrovial

From Updated U.S. Public Health Service guidelines for the management of occupational exposures to HBV, HCV, and HIV and recommendations for postexposure prophylaxis, MMWR Morb Mortal Wkly *50(RR-11):1-52, 2001.*

SUMMARY AND CONCLUSIONS

Sustaining a healthy immune system and ensuring proper functioning of all interrelated components can be extremely challenging to the health care provider who is faced with potential insults. Specific ways in which immune system functioning can be enhanced have been recognized and are continuing to be a major focus of current medical research.

Immunopathology continues to command the forefront of modern medical research and technological advancement. HIV-related disease has continued to challenge this branch of science, which hopes to conquer the fatal offender of immune system function. The hopes that a human trial to prevent the transmission of HIV disease brings new interest and hope to the world of research and epidemiology. More information regarding immune system components and their functions is continually being revealed. Through our committed efforts and dedication to knowledge and understanding, we will continue to appreciate this unique and highly complex network that virtually sustains the human body.

DEDICATION

I would like to dedicate this chapter to Mr. Charles Griffis, C.R.N.A., M.S., Ms. Marilyn Harrison, R.N., and Ms. Barbara Lamberto, R.N. (deceased), whose energy and commitment continues to make a difference for those who provide care for patients.

REFERENCES

1. Resistance of the body to infection, parts I and II. Guyton AC: *Textbook of Medical Physiology*, Philadelphia, 2000, ed 10, Saunders, pp 74-83.
2. Disease related to the immune system dysfunction. Stoelting R, Dierdorf S, McGammon R, editors: *Anesthesia and Coexisting Disease*, ed 4, New York, 2002, Churchill Livingstone, pp 611-628.
3. Vervloet D, Durham S: ABCs of allergies: adverse reactions to drugs, *BMJ* 316:1511, 1998.
4. Mertes PM, Laxenaire MC, Alla F: Anaphylactic and anaphylactoid reactions occurring during anesthesia in France in 1999-2000, *Anesthesiology* 99(3):536-545, 2003.
5. Moss J: Allergic to anesthetics, *Anesthesiology* 99(3):521-523, 2003.
6. Cox B, Durieux ME, Marcus MA: Toxicity of local anesthetics, *Best Pract Res Clin Anaesthesiol* 17(1):111-136, 2003.
7. Miller RD: Transfusion therapy. *Anesthesia*, ed 5, Philadelphia, 2000, Churchill Livingstone, pp 1628-1631.
8. Parisian S: Latex allergies causing more anesthesia problems, *Anesth Patient Safety Found News* 7:1-12, 1992.
9. American Association of Nurse Anesthetists: *Latex Protocol*, Park Ridge, IL, 1998, American Association of Nurse Anesthetists.
10. Kroemer G, Martinez C: The fail-safe paradigm of immunological self-tolerance, *Lancet* 338:1246-1249, 1991.
11. Jones RJ, Vogelsang GB, Hess AD: Induction of graft-versus-host disease following autologous bone marrow transplantation, *Lancet* 1:754-757, 1989.
12. Cirella VN, Pantuck CB, Lee YJ: Effects of cyclosporine on anesthetic action, *Anesth Analg* 66:703-706, 1987.
13. Gramstad L, Gjerlow JA, Hysing ES: Interaction of cyclosporine and its solvent Cremophor with atracurium and vecuronium, *Br J Anaesth* 58:1149, 1986.
14. Kutza J, Gratz I, Afshar M, Murasko DM: The effects of general anesthesia and surgery on basal and interferon stimulated natural killer cell activity of humans, *Anesth Analg* 85(4):918-923, 1997.
15. Khan FA, Kamal RS, Mithani CH, Khurshid M: Effect of general anesthesia and surgery on neutrophil function, *Anaesthesia* 50(9):769-775, 1995.
16. Overall JC: Viral infections of the fetus and neonate. In Feigin RD, Cherry JD, editors: *Textbook of Pediatric Infectious Diseases*, vol 1, ed 3, Philadelphia, 1992, Saunders, pp 924-959.

17. Bruce DL, Eide KA, Linde HW: Causes of death among anesthesiologists: a 20-year survey, *Anesthesiology* 29:565-569, 1968.
18. Waldron BA: Stabilization of the erythrocyte cell membrane by general anesthetics demonstrated by the autohemolysis test, *Br J Anaesth* 45:579-585, 1973.
19. Griffith CD, Rees RC, Platts A, Jermy A, Peel J, Rogers K: The nature of enhanced natural killer cell activity in patients with malignant disease of stomach and large bowel during intravenous anesthesia and surgery: preliminary report, *J Exp Clin Cancer Res* 4:339-402, 1983.
20. Tonnesen E, Mickley H, Grunnet N: Natural killer cell activity during premedication, anesthesia, and surgery, *Acta Anaesthesiol Scand* 27:238-241, 1983.
21. Kremer MJ: Surgery, pain, and immune function, *CRNA* 10:94-100, 1999.
22. Thompson DA: Anesthesia and the immune system, *J Burn Care Rehab* 8:483-487, 1987.
23. Mattila-Vuori A, Salo M, Iisalo E: Immune response in infants undergoing application of cast: comparison of halothane and balanced anesthesia. *Can J Anaesth* 46(11):1036-1042, 1999.
24. Weimann J: Toxicity of nitrous oxide, *Best Pract Res Clin Anaesthesiol* 17(1):47-61, 2003.
25. Van Achterbergh SM, Vorster BJ, Heyns AD: The effect of sepsis and short-term exposure to nitrous oxide on the bone marrow and the metabolism of vitamin B_{12} and folate, *S Afr Med J* 78:260, 1990.
26. Peric M, Vranes Z, Marusic M: Immunological disturbances in anaesthetic personnel chronically exposed to high occupational concentrations of nitrous oxide and halothane, *Anaesthesia* 46:531-537, 1991.
27. Bargellini A, Rovesti S, Barbieri A, et al: Effects of chronic exposure to anaesthetic gases on some immune parameters, *Sci Total Environ* 270(1-3):149-156, 2001.
28. Burm AG: Occupational hazards of inhalation anesthetics, *Best Pract Res Clin Anaesthesiol* 17(1):147-161, 2003.
29. Mazze RI, Fujinaga M, Rice SA, Harris SB, Baden JM: Reproductive and teratogenic effects of nitrous oxide, halothane, isoflurane, and enflurane in Sprague-Dawley rats, *Anesthesiology* 64:339-344, 1986.
30. Salo M: Effects of thiopentone on immunoglobulin production in vitro, *Br J Anaesth* 63:716-720, 1989.
31. Short TG, Young Y: Toxicity of intravenous anaesthestics, *Best Pract Res Clin Anaesthesiol* 17(1):77-89, 2003.
32. Donahoe RM, Falek A, Madden JJ: Neuro immunomodulation by opiates and other drugs of abuse: relationship to HIV infection and AIDS. In Bridge TP, Mirsdy AF, Goodwin FK, editors: *Psychological, Neuropsychiatric, and Substance Abuse Aspects of AIDS*, New York, 1988, Raven Press, pp 145-158.
33. Specter S, Lancz G: Effects of marijuana on human natural killer cell activity. In Friedman H, Specter S, Klein TW, editors: *Drugs of Abuse, Immunity, and Immunodeficiency*, New York, 1991, Plenum Press, p 47.
34. Donahoe RM, Falek A, Madden JJ: Effects of cocaine and other drugs of abuse on immune function, *Adv Exp Med Biol* 288:143-150, 1991.
35. Chen JE, Zheng ZX: Influence of operation under epidural anesthesia on peripheral T lymphocyte subsets, *Chin Med J (Engl)* 104:194-197, 1991.
36. Yokoyama M, Itano Y, Mizobuchi S, et al: The effects of epidural block on the distribution of lymphocytes subsets and natural-killer cell activity in patients with and without pain, *Anesth Analg* 92(2):463-469, 2001.
37. Thompson DA: Anesthesia and the immune system, *J Burn Care Rehabil* 8:483-487, 1987.
38. Statistics from the World Health Organization and the Centers for Disease Control (1988), *AIDS* 2:145-149, 1989.
39. Avidan M, Grovers P, Blott M, et al: Low complication rate associated with cesarean section under spinal anesthesia for HIV-1-infected women on antiretroviral therapy, *Anesthesiology* 97(2):320-324, 2002.
40. Yeni PG, Hammer SM, Carpenter CC, et al: Antiretroviral treatment for adult HIV infection in 2002: update recommendations of the International AIDS Society–USA Panel, *JAMA* 288(2):222-235, 2002.
41. Henkel J: Attacking AIDS with a "cocktail" therapy? *FDA Consum* 33:12-17, 1999.
42. King JR, Wynn H, Brundage R, Acosta EP: Pharmacokinetic enhancement of protease inhibitor therapy, *Clin Pharmacokinet* 43:291-310, 2004.
43. Carpenter CC, Cooper DA, Fischl MA, et al: Antiretroviral therapy in adults: updated recommendations of the International AIDS Society–USA Panel, *JAMA* 283:381-390, 2000.
44. Tramont EC, Johnston MI: Progress in the development of an HIV vaccine, *Expert Opin Emerg Drugs* 8(1):37-45, 2003.
45. Volberding PA, Lagakos SW, Koch MA: Zidovudine in asymptomatic human immunodeficiency virus infection: a controlled trial in persons with fewer than 500 CD4-positive cells per cubic millimeter, *N Engl J Med* 322:941-949, 1990.
46. Kuczkowski KM: Human immunodeficiency virus in the parturient, *J Clin Anesth* 15(3):224-233, 2003.
47. Visconti E, Celentano LP, Tamburrini E, Villa P, Oliva G, Fundaro C: Combination antiretroviral therapy in human immunodeficiency virus–infected pregnant women, *Obstet Gynecol* 95:636-637, 2000.
48. Newshan G: Pain management in HIV and AIDS, *GMHC Treatment Issues* 9(4):5,10-12, 1995.
49. Updated U.S. Public Health Service guidelines for the management of occupational exposures to HBV, HCV, and HIV and recommendations for postexposure prophylaxis, *MMWR Morb Mortal Wkly Rep* 50(RR-11):1-52, 2001.
50. Centers for Disease Control and Prevention: *HIV/AIDS Surveillance Report* 12(1):24, 2000, Atlanta, Centers for Disease Control and Prevention.
51. Gerberding, JL: Occupational exposure to HIV in health care settings, *N Engl J Med* 348(9):826-833, 2003.
52. *Occupational Safety: Selected Cost and Benefit Implications of Needlestick Prevention Devices for Hospitals*, Washington, DC, 2000, General Accounting Office (GAO-01-60R).
53. Busch M, Lee LL, Satten GA, et al: Time course of detection of viral and serologic markers preceding human immunodeficiency virus type 1 seroconversion: implications for screening of blood and tissue donors, *Transfusion* 35:91-97, 1995.
54. Salgado CD, Flanagan HL, Haverstick DM, Farr BM: Low rate of false-positive results with use of a rapid HIV test, *Infect Control Hosp Epidemiol* 23:335-337, 2002.
55. Cardo DM, Culver DH, Ciesielski CA, et al: A case-control study of HIV seroconversion in health care workers after percutaneous exposure, *N Engl J Med* 337:1485-1490, 1997.
56. Public Health Service Task Force recommendations for use of antiretroviral drugs in pregnant HIV-1-infected women for maternal health and interventions to reduce perinatal HIV-1 transmission in the United States (revised November 3, 2000), *HIV Clin Trials* 2:56-91, 2001.
57. Connor EM, Sperling RS, Gelber R, et al: Reduction of maternal-infant transmission of human immunodeficiency virus type 1 with zidovudine treatment, *N Engl J Med* 331:1173-1180, 1994.
58. Sperling RS, Shapiro DE, Coombs RW, et al: Maternal viral load, zidovudine treatment, and the risk of transmission of human immunodeficiency virus type 1 from mother to infant, *N Engl J Med* 335:1621-1629, 1996.
59. Wade NA, Birkhead GS, Warren BL, et al: Abbreviated regimens of zidovudine prophylaxis and perinatal transmission of the human immunodeficiency virus, *N Engl J Med* 339:1409-1414, 1998.
60. Musoke P, Guay LA, Bagenda D, et al: A phase I/II study of the safety and pharmacokinetics of nevirapine in HIV-1-infected pregnant Ugandan women and their neonates (HIVNET 006), *AIDS* 13:479-486, 1999.
61. Jackson JB, Musoke P, Fleming T, et al: Intrapartum and neonatal single-dose nevirapine compared with zidovudine for prevention of mother-to-child transmission of HIV-1 in Kampala,

Uganda: 18-month follow up of the HIVNET 012 randomized trial, *Obstet Gynecol Surv* 59:183-185, 2004.

62. Jochimsen EM: Failures of zidovudine postexposure prophylaxis, *Am J Med* 102(suppl 5B):52-55, 1997.
63. Pratt RD, Shapiro JF, McKinney N, Kwok S, Spector SA: Virologic characterization of primary human immunodeficiency virus type 1 infection in a health care worker following needlestick injury, *J Infect Dis* 172:851-854, 1995.
64. Lot F, Abiteboul D: Infections professionnelles par le VIH en France chez le personnel de sante: le point au 30 Juin 1995, *Bull Epidemiol Hebd* 44:193-194, 1995.
65. Weisburd G, Biglione J, Arbulu MM, Terrazzino JC, Pesiri A: HIV seroconversion after a workplace accident and treated with zidovudine. In *Abstracts of the XI International Conference on AIDS*, Vancouver, BC, July 7-12, 1996, p 460 (abstract).
66. Perdue B, Wolderufael D, Mellors J, Quinn T, Margolick J: HIV-1 transmission by a needlestick injury despite rapid initiation of four-drug postexposure prophylaxis. In *Program and Abstracts of the 6th Conference on Retroviruses and Opportunistic Infections*, Chicago, January 31-February 4, 1999. Chicago, 1999, Foundation for Retrovirology and Human Health, p 107 (abstract).
67. Beltrami EM, Luo C-C, Dela Torre N, Cardo DM: HIV transmission after an occupational exposure despite postexposure prophylaxis with a combination drug regimen. In *Program and Abstracts of the 4th Decennial International Conference on Nosocomial and Healthcare-Associated Infections: In Conjunction with the 10th Annual Meeting of SHEA*, Atlanta, March 5-9, 2000. Atlanta, 2000, Centers for Disease Control and Prevention, pp 125-126 (abstract).
68. Beltrami EM, Cheingsong R, Respess R, Cardo DM: Antiretroviral drug resistance in HIV-infected source patients for occupational exposures to healthcare workers. In *Program and Abstracts of the 4th Decennial International Conference on Nosocomial and Healthcare-Associated Infections: In Conjunction with the 10th Annual Meeting of SHEA*, Atlanta, March 5-9, 2000. Atlanta, 2000, Centers for Disease Control and Prevention, p 128 (abstract).
69. Rich JD, Merriman NA, Mylonakis E, et al: Misdiagnosis of HIV infection by HIV-1 plasma viral load testing: a case series, *Ann Intern Med* 130:37-39, 1999.
70. Roland ME, Martin JN, Grant RM, et al: Postexposure prophylaxis for human immunodeficiency virus infection after sexual or injection drug use exposure: identification and characterization of the source of exposure, *J Infect Dis* 184:1608-1612, 2001.
71. Barnes PF, Bloch AB, Davidson PT, Snider DE Jr: Tuberculosis in patients with human immunodeficiency virus infection, *N Engl J Med* 324:1644-1650, 1991.
72. Nicoll A, Godfrey-Faussett P: HIV and tuberculosis in the commonwealth, *BMJ* 319:1086, 1999.
73. Telenti A, Iseman M: Drug-resistant tuberculosis: what do we do now? *Drugs* 59:171-179, 2000.
74. *AANA Practice Manual*, Park Ridge, IL, 1996.

CHAPTER 40

Anesthesia and Laser Surgery

BERNADETTE T. ROCHE

The term *laser* is an acronym for *l*ight *a*mplification by the *s*timulated *e*mission of *r*adiation. In 1917 Albert Einstein described stimulated emission of radiation as a theoretic concept. Approximately 40 years later the laser was developed and patented by Arthur Schawlow and Charles Townes. The first laser (694-nm ruby laser) was built by Theodore Maiman in 1960.[1] A near-infrared laser (1060 nm) was developed soon after with glass rods doped with neodymium (Nd:Glass laser). In 1964 Townes won the Nobel Prize in physics for his work on masers and lasers. Lasers have widespread applications and are commonly used in industry, construction, medicine, communications, energy production, and entertainment.

The early lasers quickly found applications in medicine. In the mid sixties the ruby laser and the argon-ion laser were used successfully in retinal surgery. The neodymium:yttrium-aluminum-garnet (Nd:YAG) laser and the carbon dioxide (CO_2) laser, developed in 1964, were used as surgical instruments in otolaryngology and gynecology. By the early 1980s smaller and more powerful lasers were used in the new field of laparoscopic surgery. The first lasers were continuous wave (CW) and caused nonselective heat injury, which limited their use in medicine. After it was discovered that "pulsing" of the laser beam allowed selective destruction of abnormal tissue, the pulsed dye laser was introduced in the late 1980s for the treatment of pigmented skin lesions such as port-wine stains. Q-switched lasers were introduced soon afterward for removal of tattoos. In the early 1990s scanning devices were introduced, and computerized control of the laser beam became possible. Scanners had a significant impact on the use of surgical lasers, especially in cosmetic surgery.

Medical lasers are powerful instruments that make it possible to treat conditions that previously were untreatable. New, powerful lasers and delivery methods have made the surgical laser a standard in the operating room (OR). Lasers offer distinct advantages, such as precision and access, over traditional surgical techniques. They also present unique hazards to both patients and OR personnel. The anesthetist must have an understanding of the basic physics of lasers, indications for the laser treatment, hazards of the laser beam, and anesthetic implications of laser surgery.

BASIC PRINCIPLES OF LASERS

Light

Electromagnetic radiation is a broad spectrum of heat energy that can move through space. The electromagnetic spectrum is composed of radio waves, microwaves, infrared waves, visible light waves, ultraviolet waves, x-rays, and gamma rays (Figure 40-1). A wavelength is the distance between two successive points on a periodic wave that have the same phase. A progressive decease in wavelength and increase in frequency occur across the spectrum from radio waves to gamma waves. The optical portion of the electromagnetic spectrum has a wavelength range of 200 nm to 20 nm and contains ultraviolet, visible, and infrared waves. The visible light spectrum constitutes less than 0.1% of the electromagnetic spectrum of the optical spectrum. Visible light can be seen by the human eye and consists of red, orange, yellow, green, blue, indigo, and violet waves with a very narrow range of wavelengths—400 nm (violet) to 700 nm (red). Incandescent light is composed of several wavelengths; the observed white color is a mixture of the different wavelengths. The infrared portion of the optical spectrum is perceived as heat, whereas the ultraviolet waves cause a chemical reaction in human skin with little heat production. Both the infrared and the ultraviolet spectrums are invisible to the human eye.

Light can be thought of as both a wavelength and as a particle or quantum of energy, called a *photon*. The energy of an electromagnetic wave is inversely proportional to its wavelength and proportional to its frequency. The energy of a photon is defined by the energy emitted when an electron falls from an excited orbit to one of lower energy; the energy between the two orbits defines the wavelength of the emitted photon.[2] The relationship between the energy and the wavelength of light is expressed by the following equation:

Equation 40-1

$$E = hc/\lambda$$

where E = energy in joules, h = Planck's constant (6.63×10^{-34} J-s), c = the speed of light (2.998×10^{-8} m/s), and λ = wavelength in meters.

Spontaneous Absorption and Emission of Energy

Emission of light occurs as a result of two main processes: absorption of energy and spontaneous emission of energy. The electrons of an atom occupy shells, or orbits, and each orbit has a different energy. The higher the orbit, the greater the energy; ground state is an atom's lowest energy state. Electrons can move from one orbit or energy level to another by the spontaneous absorption or emission of energy. When an electron absorbs energy, it can jump to a higher energy (metastable) state; conversely, it emits energy if it falls to a lower orbit. Electrons have a tendency to return to the ground state spontaneously, releasing a photon of light energy in the process.

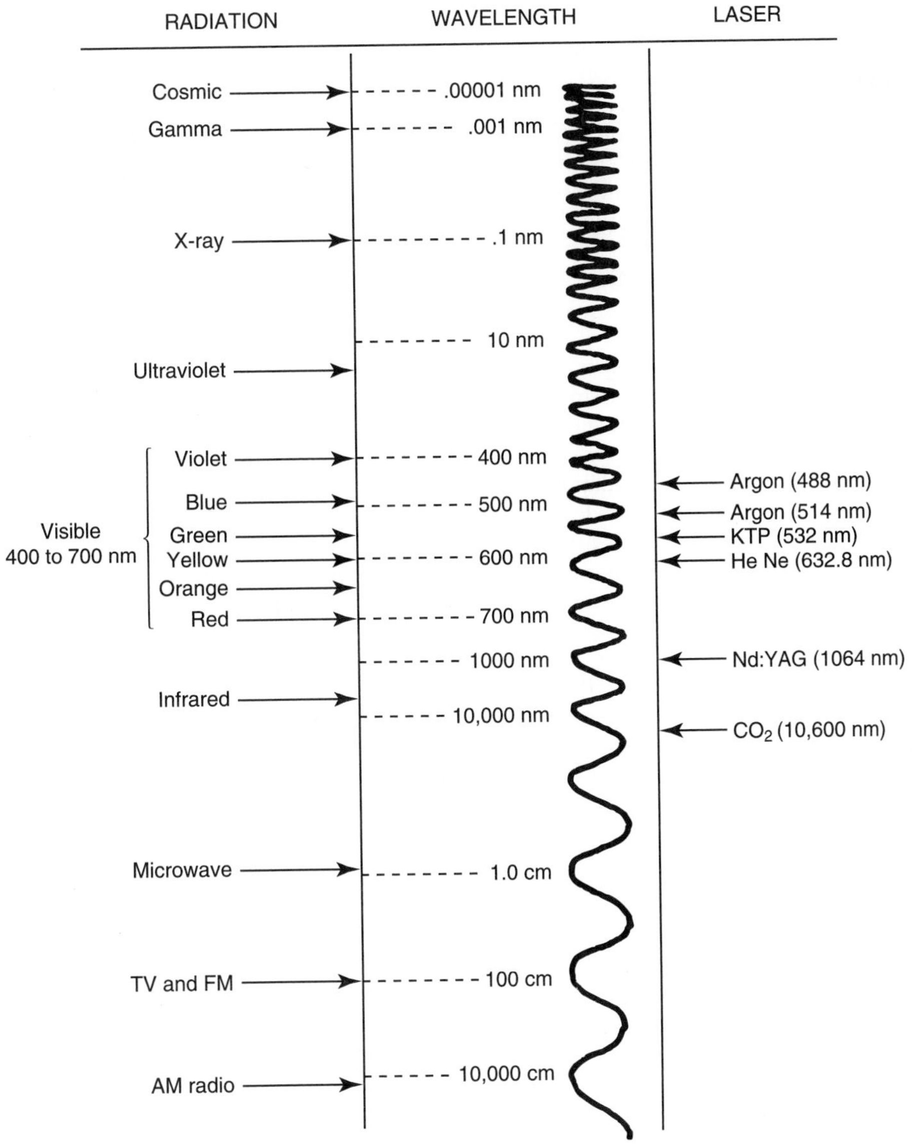

FIGURE **40-1**
Electromagnetic spectrum. (Modified from Arndt KA, Dover JS, Olbricht SM, eds. *Lasers in cutaneous and aesthetic surgery*. Philadelphia: Lippincott-Raven; 1997:4.)

This is called *spontaneous emission of radiation*. The energy of the photon and therefore its wavelength correspond to the energy levels between the two levels. Light produced by fluorescent lights or incandescent bulbs is a result of electrons that change orbits and return to ground state, releasing photons that radiate randomly in all directions. During emission the energy of the photon and the wavelength of the light are proportional to the energy difference between the excited state and the ground state of the atom. The light produced by spontaneous emission is composed of different wavelengths and frequencies; the photons oscillate randomly (noncoherence), and the light disperses as it travels.

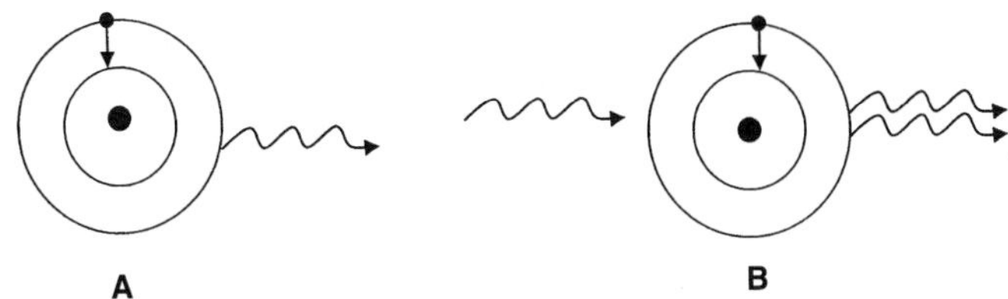

FIGURE **40-2**
A, Spontaneous emission of radiation. As an atom decays back to its ground state, it releases a photon of energy. **B,** Stimulated emission of radiation. When an exited atom is stimulated by a photon, it releases a photon of the same wavelength and frequency that travels in phase with and in the same direction as the stimulating photon.

Laser Radiation

Stimulated emission is crucial to the formation of laser light. When a photon strikes an atom in the excited state, the atom decays back to its ground state, emitting a second photon. If the energy of the photon is equal to the energy difference between the excited and ground states of the atom, the atom emits a photon of the same wavelength, energy, frequency, and direction and in phase with the stimulating photon. This process is known as *stimulated emission of radiation* (Figure 40-2). The two photons strike other excited atoms, stimulating further emission of photons. This process produces a sudden burst of coherent radiation as all the atoms return to ground state in a rapid chain reaction.

Properties of laser light include coherence, directionality, and monochromaticity. Unlike natural light, laser beam photons have the same wavelength and oscillate synchronously in identical phase with one another (coherence). Laser light displays

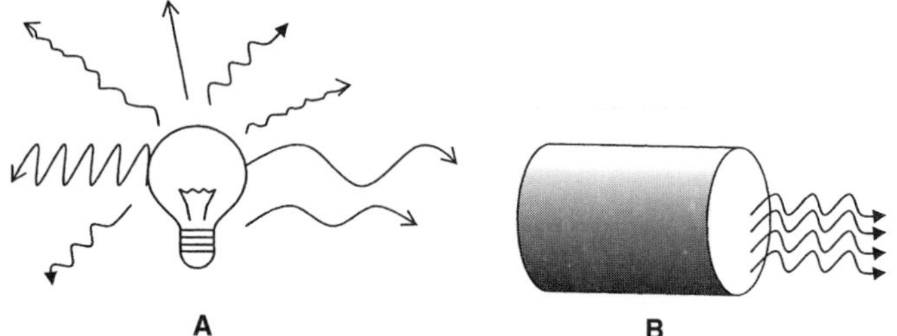

FIGURE **40-3**
Characteristics of laser light. In contrast to ordinary light **(A),** laser light **(B)** is coherent, collimated, and monochromatic.

minimal dispersion and moves in a parallel narrow beam (spatial coherence) over long distances. This spatial coherence, known as *collimation*, allows the laser to be focused on a very small area (Figure 40-3). Reflection of a laser beam reduces the collimation and increases the dispersion, especially if the reflecting surface has a matte or dull finish. Laser light is composed of specific and discrete wavelengths; consequently the light emitted is monochromatic and specific for each laser. A few lasers are tunable and can emit light at several different wavelengths. However, lasers can emit light of only one color at a time. A typical light bulb is more powerful than a laser, but its light is not collimated, and the dispersion of the light reduces its intensity. In contrast, the intensity of a 1-milliwatt (mW) laser can be six times that of a 100-watt (W) incandescent bulb. Although a typical laser emits only a few milliwatts of power, lasers can produce a highly intense beam of 1 to 2 mm.

Components of a Laser

Energy Source

A laser is a device that creates and amplifies a narrow, intense beam of coherent light. It consists of an energy source, an optical resonating cavity, and a lasing medium to create the laser light (Figure 40-4).[3] Lasers require an external energy source for excitation of the lasing medium. The external energy is used to transfer or pump up the energy of the laser medium. The electrons in the lasing medium absorb the energy and move to a higher energy state. Flash lamps, continuous light, high-voltage discharge, diodes, and, in some cases, another laser can be used as the energy source.

Optical Resonating Cavity

The optical resonating cavity is a tubelike structure that provides optimal amplification of the laser beam. It contains the lasing medium and one mirror at each of two ends of the tube. When the lasing medium is excited by the outside energy source (e.g., flash lamp, electric current), the atoms are "pumped" to a higher energy level, increasing the number of atoms in an excited state. Population inversion occurs when more atoms are in an unstable excited state than are in the resting state. Population inversion is necessary for stimulated emission of radiation. When one of the atoms spontaneously decays back to its ground state, it releases a photon that "stimulates" another excited molecule to decay back to its ground state, releasing another photon. The wavelength, frequency, phase, and direction of the second photon are identical to those of the first photon. The mirrors reflect the excited photons back into the resonant cavity, where they travel back and forth in a parallel fashion, stimulating the release of even more photons from other excited atoms. A cascade effect occurs, and the resultant light is amplified. One of the mirrors is partially transparent and allows a portion of the laser light (coherent, collimated, and monochromatic) to escape in a very thin beam that can be easily focused on a very small area.

Laser Medium

The laser medium is a substance that can be stimulated to a metastable state when pumped with an external energy source.

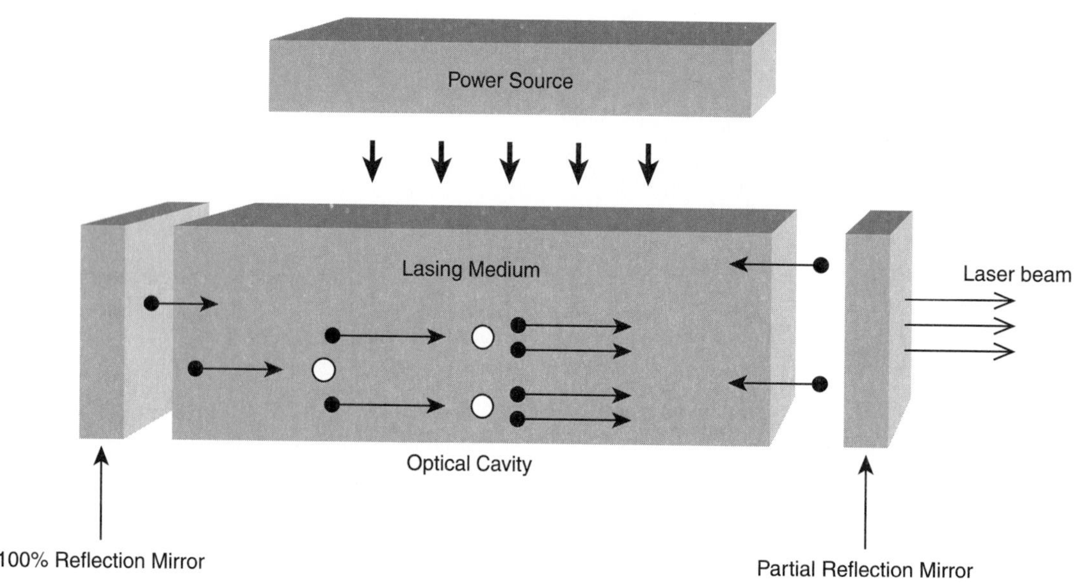

FIGURE **40-4**
Basic components of a laser. The power source (flash lamp, electric current, other laser) pumps up the electrons in the lasing medium to an excited state. The optical cavity contains the lasing medium (solid, liquid, gas) and two mirrors that reflect the photons back into the cavity, where they stimulate other excited atoms to emit identical photons that travel in the same direction within the medium. One mirror is partially transparent and allows the laser beam to exit the cavity.

The medium can be a solid, gas, liquid, or semiconductor. Lasers are commonly named after the laser medium, and the medium determines the wavelength output of the laser. Solid-state lasers such as the Nd:YAG laser use a solid matrix that is doped with a small amount of impurity (dopant). It is the impurity (Nd in this example) that provides the energy source for the laser. Solid-state lasers are more powerful than gas lasers and require optical pumping. Gas lasers use a variety of gases as lasing media, including argon, CO_2, helium, helium-neon, and krypton. An electrical source of energy is required for pumping. Complex liquid dyes, dissolved in a liquid such as alcohol, constitute the lasing media in liquid lasers. Optically pumped, liquid lasers are tunable over a broad range of wavelengths, mostly in the visible spectrum. Excimer lasers use electrical stimulation to produce a dimer of a halogen such as chlorine and fluorine and an inert gas such as argon, krypton, or xenon. The dimer is unstable and quickly breaks down into its constituent atoms, releasing energy in the form of light. Semiconductor lasers, also called *diode lasers*, are composed of semiconductor crystals that are pumped by a high-intensity current. They are commonly used in compact disc players, laser printers, and laser pointers. The gallium-arsenide laser is an example of a semiconductor laser.

Modes of Operation

Because most medical lasers deliver only one wavelength, laser selection is dependent on the targeted tissue and the desired effect. The wavelength or color of the laser light is dependent on the lasing medium, and the effect on tissue is dependent on the wavelength. In addition to selecting the appropriate wavelength, the surgeon must use the appropriate exposure time and energy density (power setting) to achieve the intended photothermolytic, photomechanical, or photochemical effect. The laser beam can be delivered in a CW mode, pulsed-wave mode, or Q-switched mode.

In the CW mode the laser emits a steady beam for as long as the laser medium is excited. The power output of a CW laser is measured in watts and can vary significantly among lasers; the power of the helium-neon laser is measured in milliwatts, whereas the output of the more powerful CO_2 laser is measured in kilowatts. Power density of the beam (irradiance or flux) varies from a few watts per square centimeter to hundreds of watts per square centimeter. Collateral tissue damage can be expected if the laser beam is held on tissue longer than the thermal relaxation time (the time it takes for 50% of the laser energy to be thermally conducted to surrounding tissue). Pulsing the laser beam or scanning a continuous beam limits the exposure time and minimizes thermal damage. Pulsing of the laser beam or electrical or mechanical interruption of a CW beam allows time for concentration of the energy. In the pulsed mode, the laser emit lights in individual pulses from femtoseconds (quadrillionths of a second) to seconds. The power of a pulsed laser is measured in joules, and energy intensity is expressed as joules per square centimeter. Scanners limit the duration of the laser beam by means of computerized scanning of the laser beam in a preset pattern before delivery of the beam to the tissue. In the Q-switched mode the laser emits high-energy, ultrashort pulses (approximately 10 to 250 nsec). A shutter is placed in the optical path to allow the buildup of a large population inversion. After release of the shutter the electrons fall rapidly to ground state, releasing a large amount of energy measured in megawatts. The effects of the laser on the tissue can be controlled by the mode of delivery. The Nd:YAG laser can be used in CW mode for coagulation of tumors, in the pulsed mode for hair removal, and in the Q-switched mode for tattoo removal. In the CW mode the CO_2 laser can be focused very tightly and used for incision, much like a scalpel. In contrast, the defocused CO_2 laser can vaporize a larger area. When delivered through a scanning device, the laser beam can remove a predetermined thickness of skin.

Fiberoptic cables are used for delivery of laser beams with visible and near-infrared wavelengths. Articulated arms with reflecting mirrors mounted in tubes are used to direct the beam of a far infrared laser (CO_2). Additional devices may be attached to the fiberoptic cables or articulated arms, including slit lamps (for use on the eye), operating microscopes, and insulated fibers (for use with endoscopes). Contact laser probes (sapphire) attached to the distal end of a fiberoptic bundle transform the light energy into heat for precise cutting and reduced penetration. Because of the high temperatures (>800° C) the probes require a compressed gas or liquid jet cooling system.

BIOLOGIC EFFECTS OF LASERS

Because it is monochromatic, laser light has very selective effects on biologic tissues. Depending on the tissue and the wavelength, the laser light undergoes transmission, scattering, reflection, or absorption. Light absorption is necessary for the laser to be effective. If the tissue transmits, reflects, or scatters the light, the laser will have little or no effect on the tissue. A specific wavelength may be absorbed by one type of tissue and transmitted by another. Biologic tissues can be thought of as an aqueous solution of light-absorbing molecules. Chromophores such as hemoglobin, melanin, and water are the main absorbing components, and they determine the reaction of the tissue to the light. To be effective the laser light must match the absorptive property of the tissue. When absorption occurs, the laser light is converted to heat. If the temperature reaches 100° C, vaporization or ablation of the tissue occurs. As the tissue is vaporized, the thermal energy of the laser beam cauterizes capillaries and provides immediate hemostasis. A lower temperature will produce tissue coagulation or denaturation rather than ablation.

A tissue's reaction to light absorption depends on the wavelength, intensity, and exposure time of the light. Powerful, short pulses of laser light cause an explosive tissue expansion (photomechanical reaction), whereas low-power, long pulses cause a rapid increase in temperature (photothermal reaction), resulting in tissue vaporization and coagulation. When applied for longer durations, low-power lasers can cause a chemical reaction or change in specific molecules (photochemical reaction). Laser light can also be used to activate a photosensitizing medication that is selectively absorbed by a specific tissue (photodynamic reaction). The effectiveness of nonthermal laser-assisted techniques is dependent on the ability of special drugs (photosynthesizers) to produce cytotoxicity in the presence of oxygen (O_2) after stimulation with light of an appropriate wavelength.

Tissue absorption is greatest with longer wavelengths such as the far-infrared wavelength of the CO_2 laser (10,600 nm). The CO_2 laser beam is completely absorbed by water in the first few cellular layers, resulting in explosive vaporization of the top layer but little or no damage to the underlying tissues. Excimer lasers (ultraviolet) are associated with an even more superficial effect because of their strong absorption by water. The light from lasers with visible wavelengths, such as the ruby, argon, and krypton lasers, is transmitted by water and absorbed by cells that contain dark pigment. It can penetrate the skin and the cornea to coagulate pigmented or vascular lesions. The light from near-infrared lasers, such as the Nd:YAG, is transmitted rather than absorbed by water. Because they have a greater tissue penetration, near-infrared lasers are better suited for deeper procedures such as tumor debulking.

MEDICAL LASERS

Lasers have a wide variety of uses in health care and treatment of disease. Because of their ability to cause rapid and precise vaporization or coagulation of tissues, lasers are commonly used in variety of unrelated diagnostic and therapeutic procedures. Advantages of lasers include precision, access to remote sites in the body, reduced blood loss, reduced damage to adjacent tissue, and improved patient satisfaction. A disadvantage of laser therapy may be delayed wound healing.[4,5]

Lasers were first used in ophthalmology. The excimer laser, a newer type of medical laser, is used for vision correction. Urology was another area of medicine in which laser therapy was used early, and such therapy continues to be a treatment option for a variety of urologic problems including strictures, genital condylomas, prostatic hypertrophy, urethral calculi, and interstitial cystitis.[6] Laser surgery of the upper and lower airways offers definite advantages over traditional surgery, including access, precision, anatomic preservation, and controlled hemostasis. Both fiberoptic and rigid bronchoscopes allow laser resection of endobronchial lesions.[7] Interstitial laser thermotherapy is used for destruction of both superficial and deep solid tumors.[5]

In orthopedics lasers are used in endoscopic laser-assisted disc surgery and arthroscopic procedures.[8-10] They also have several applications in cardiovascular surgery. During transmyocardial laser revascularization, laser-created channels in the myocardium allow the delivery of oxygenated blood to ischemic areas of the myocardium.[11-16] In addition to their use during percutaneous transluminal angioplasty, lasers have potential for use in ablation of cerebral thrombi.[17]

Lasers have revolutionized dermatology and plastic surgery and are indispensable in oral surgery and otolaryngology.[18-21] New applications for lasers in periodontal and general dentistry include gum reshaping, drilling, and whitening of teeth.[22,23] Laser stimulation of acupuncture point P6 is used as an alternative to antiemetics in surgical patients.[24] Low-power laser therapy appears to be useful in the management of chronic low back pain.[25]

TYPES OF MEDICAL LASERS

The major types of lasers used in medicine are far infrared (CO_2), mid infrared (erbium [Er]:YAG, holmium [Ho]:YAG, Nd:YAG), near infrared (alexandrite), visible (argon, krypton, ruby, diodes, copper and gold vapor), and ultraviolet (excimer). Commonly used surgical lasers are listed in Table 40-1.

TABLE 40-1 Common Surgical Lasers

Laser	Wavelength	Applications
Far Infrared		
CO_2	1700-1720 μm	Multiple uses: general surgery, orthopedics, gynecology, urology, otolaryngology, plastic surgery
Mid Infrared		
Nd:YAG	1064 nm	Multiple uses: GI, pulmonary, urology, ophthalmology, dermatology
Ho:YAG	2070 nm	Orthopedics, urology
Er:YAG	2940 nm	Dermatology
Near Infrared		
Diode	800-900 nm	Multiples uses: ophthalmology, otolaryngology, periodontics, cosmetic surgery, pain management
Visible		
Argon	488 and 514 nm	Multiple uses: ophthalmology, plastic surgery, dermatology, gynecology, otolaryngology
Krypton	476, 521, 568 nm	Dermatology
Copper bromide	511 and 577 nm	Dermatology, photosynthesizer
KTP	532 nm	Dermatology
Alexandrite	755 nm	Dermatology
Pulsed dye	577-585 nm	Dermatology
Ruby	694 nm	Dermatology
Ultraviolet (Excimer)		
Argon fluoride	193 nm	Ophthalmology, dermatology
Xenon fluoride	308 nm	Angioplasty

Er, *Erbium*; GI, *gastrointestinal*; HO, *holmium*; KTP, *potassium-titanyl-phosphate*; Nd, *neodymium*; YAG, *yttrium-aluminum-garnet*.

Carbon Dioxide Laser

The CO_2 laser is the most commonly used surgical laser. The infrared light produced by the CO_2 laser (10,600 nm) is invisible to the human eye, and a low-power helium-neon (He-Ne) laser (633 nm) is incorporated to provide a visible red beam for surgical aim. Because it emits light in the infrared region of the electromagnetic spectrum, the CO_2 laser is a powerful but dangerous laser. Infrared radiation is heat, and this laser basically melts through whatever its beam is focused on, including steel. The CO_2 laser beam is not transmitted by quartz, glass, or other transparent material and must be delivered as a free beam or through a rigid endoscope with a mirrored, articulated arm.

Light from the CO_2 laser is strongly absorbed by water, and vaporization of cells occurs within the first 100 to 200 μm of the irradiated surface. It can be used as both a CW and pulsed-wave laser. Blood loss is minimal during CO_2 laser procedures. Focused into a tight beam, the CO_2 laser is used for cutting. Defocusing the beam decreases the power density, and the tissue is vaporized or ablated. The CO_2 laser is used extensively in gynecology, otolaryngology, urology, orthopedics, and general surgery. When used with a scanning device, thin layers of the skin are ablated for skin resurfacing. Because of its high power the CO_2 laser is widely used in industry to drill, cut, and weld materials used in construction.

Argon Laser

The argon gas in an argon laser has one or more electrons removed, and the positive ions are excited by a large electrical discharge. The argon ion laser emits visible blue-green light with wavelengths of 488 nm and 514 nm simultaneously. The laser light is transmitted by water and absorbed by hemoglobin and melanin, where the main effect is photocoagulation. Penetration is approximately 1 to 2 mm, but this can vary depending on the degree of pigmentation. The beam passes through quartz optical fibers, and the laser can be used with a microscope or endoscope. The argon laser is used in ophthalmology, plastic surgery, dermatology, gynecology, and otolaryngology. A forced-air or water-cooling system is required to decrease heating.

Krypton Laser

The active medium is also a rare gas with one or more electrons removed, and the krypton ions are excited by an electrical discharge. The krypton laser produces visible green and blue light at 476, 521, and 568 nm. It is absorbed by hemoglobin and used for photocoagulation of vascular or pigmented lesions.

Yttrium-Aluminum-Garnet Lasers

The lasing medium for the YAG laser is a YAG crystal rod doped with atoms of rare earth minerals, which accounts for the different properties of the YAG lasers. The YAG lasers can be used in the CW, pulsed-wave, or Q-switched mode.

Neodymium:Yttrium-Aluminum-Garnet Laser

The active component is Nd. The Nd:YAG laser emits a near-infrared invisible light at 1064 nm and requires the addition of a visible aiming beam. It has a penetration of 5 to 7 mm and can be used to cut or coagulate tissue. In the Q-switched mode the laser removes black tattoo ink and hair. The Nd:YAG laser has important applications in internal debulking or destruction of lesions and is used to treat gastrointestinal and tracheal-bronchial tumors and genitourinary lesions. The pulsed and Q-switched Nd:YAG laser is used in ophthalmology. The energy of the Nd:YAG beam is more widely dispersed, and damage to adjacent tissues may not be evident for hours after the laser treatment.

Potassium-Titanyl-Phosphate Laser

The wavelength of the Nd:YAG laser is halved when it is passed through a potassium-titanyl-phosphate (KTP) crystal. A solid-state laser, the KTP laser is similar to the argon gas laser. The beam is transmitted by water and absorbed within 1 to 2 mm of vascular or pigmented tissue. A bright green light (532 nm) delivered through fiberoptics, scanners, or microscopes is used to cut tissue (CW mode) and to remove vascular lesions (pulsed mode) and red-orange and black tattoo ink (Q-switched mode). Although the power density of the KTP laser is sufficient to cut vascular tissue, it is insufficient to achieve effective hemostasis.

Erbium:Yttrium-Aluminum-Garnet Laser

When the YAG laser is doped with erbium (Er) it emits a mid-infrared beam at 2940 nm (peak absorption of water). Because the infrared beam is not transmitted by quartz or glass, the Er:YAG can be used only as a free beam or through a rigid endoscope. Because of its limited penetration and excellent precision, it is used extensively in laser resurfacing of the skin and vaporization of fibrous tissue, cartilage, and bone. Hemostasis is not possible because of limited penetration. The laser is also used as a dental drill.

Holmium:Yttrium-Aluminum-Garnet Laser

When doped with Ho, the YAG laser emits a mid-infrared beam at 2070 nm that is strongly absorbed by water. Output in the mid-infrared spectrum requires a coincident aiming beam. The Ho:YAG is used to vaporize, cut, coagulate, and sculpt avascular tissue with a minimal amount of thermal necrosis. Because of limited penetration (0.4 mm), the laser has a minimal effect on hemostasis. The primary applications of this new laser are in orthopedics (bone and cartilage ablation) and urology (stone removal and transurethral resection of the prostate [TURP]).

Ruby Laser

The first laser to be used in medicine, the ruby laser uses a synthetic ruby crystal of aluminum oxide doped with chromium. The laser emits a red light with a wavelength of 694 nm and a penetration >1 mm. The ruby laser light is absorbed by melanin and blue, green, and black pigment. Because the ruby laser has a low efficiency and requires a cooling system, its use has declined in favor of the use of newer and more powerful lasers. However, it is very effective for tattoo removal and treatment of pigmented lesions such as freckles, liver spots, and nevi (Q-switched mode). It is also used for hair removal.

Alexandrite Laser

The solid-state laser contains a rod of synthetic chrysoberyl (the alexandrite laser was named after Czar Alexander II) doped with chromium. It emits a deep red light at 755 nm, and frequency doubling of the alexandrite laser produces a tunable laser output of 360 to 400 nm. The beam is absorbed by blue and black pigments, with a lesser degree of absorption by melanin. Properties and uses are similar to those of the ruby laser.

Dye Lasers

Dye lasers use organic fluorescent materials dissolved in a solvent, such as methanol. The energy levels of the dyes are very close to one another and allow the lasers to release a wide range of wavelengths. Dye lasers are typically pumped with a flashlamp or another laser. The major advantage of the dye laser is the ability to tune the wavelength to maximize the laser-tissue interaction. CW and pulsed dye lasers have wavelengths of 400 to 1000 nm. They can produce extremely short pulses (measured in picoseconds). Dye lasers are used in dermatology for excision of vascular and pigmented lesions, in urology for treatment of urinary calculi, and in oncology for photodynamic therapy. The pulsed dye laser (PDL) uses a rhodamine dye to emit a yellow laser beam at 577 to 585 nm (peak absorption of hemoglobin). It is the laser of choice for treatment of port-wine stains in children and thick red scars. Because the laser ruptures the blood vessels (short pulse, high absorption), purpura is not uncommon after treatment.

Metal Vapor Lasers

The active medium is a neutral metal heated beyond its vapor point. A pulsed electrical discharge is used for excitation of the vapor. Vaporized copper bromide emits green light at 511 nm and yellow light at 577 nm and is used to treat vascular lesions as well as for facial resurfacing. The gold vapor laser (578 to 628 nm) is used in photodynamic therapy for cancer.

Excimer Lasers

Excimer lasers (derived from the terms *excited* and *dimers*) use a medium composed of a reactive noble gas (chlorine or fluorine) and an inert halogen gas (argon, krypton, or xenon). When the medium is electrically stimulated, an unstable pseudomolecule (dimer) is produced. As the dimer breaks down to its constituent atoms, it releases light in the ultraviolet range that is strongly absorbed by water. Excimer lasers have a photochemical effect on targeted tissues (pulsed mode) with a minimal thermal effect on the underlying tissue. The very short wavelength (ultraviolet) is capable of high resolution and has applications in microscopic surgery. Excimer lasers are currently used in ophthalmology for photorefractive keratectomy (PRK) and laser in situ keratomileusis (LASIK). They are also used for removal of arterial plaques. Examples of excimer lasers include argon-fluoride (193 nm), krypton-fluoride (249 nm), xenon-chloride (308 nm), and xenon-fluoride (351 nm) lasers.

Diode Lasers

Diode lasers are semiconductors that emit near-infrared light (800 to 900 nm) when pumped with a high-intensity electric current. Medical uses include otolaryngology, dermatology (hair removal), and periodontal surgery. Diode lasers are also used to "pump" other laser media such as YAG rods. They have multiple nonmedical applications and are used in laser printers, music recordings, and fiberoptic communication systems.

Cold Lasers

Cold lasers, also known as *low-level laser therapy (LLLT)* and *soft lasers*, use diodes to produce visible to infrared light. The laser beam can penetrate up to 2 inches without damaging tissues or producing a significant amount of heat. They work through biostimulation of cellular metabolism to increase healing of tissues. Currently they are used for treatment of carpal tunnel syndrome and other soft-tissues injuries.

HAZARDS OF LASERS

Lasers and laser systems are categorized in classes I to IV relative to their potential for causing biologic damage. Most medical lasers are class IV because they are high-power lasers that are hazardous if viewed under any condition (directly or diffusely scattered) and are a potential fire hazard because of their ability to ignite flammable objects. They also create hazardous airborne contaminants and require a high-voltage supply. Some of the dyes used in dye lasers can be toxic and hazardous to handle. The U.S. Food and Drug Administration (FDA) regulates the manufacturing and marketing of lasers used in medicine; however, it does not regulate laser safety. The Occupational Safety and Health Administration has identified the hazards associated with the use of medical lasers and has developed safety standards to protect patients and OR personnel.[26] The Association of Perioperative Registered Nurses has also developed recommendation for laser safety.[27] In addition, the American National Standards Institute (ANSI) has published specific laser safety standards; compliance with the ANSI guidelines is voluntary.[28]

The most common hazards of lasers are thermal trauma, eye injury, perforation of organs or vessels, gas embolization, pollution, and fire. The majority of laser-related accidents and injuries are attributable to inappropriate use or intentional use of malfunctioning equipment.[29] In addition to the risk of laser trauma incurred by patients, significant risks exist for OR personnel during laser procedures. Laser beams are transmitted through air and reflected by smooth metal surfaces. Misdirected beams are a potential source of trauma for patients and OR personnel.

Thermal Trauma

The most common cause of laser-induced tissue damage is thermal in nature. Tissue proteins are denatured after absorption of the laser energy.[30] Skin trauma is dependent on the energy and wavelength of the laser and can range from mild reddening to blistering and charring. Burns occur with exposure times greater than 10 μsec and wavelengths ranging from the near ultraviolet to the far infrared (0.315 μm to 103 μm). Ultraviolet radiation causes a photochemical reaction in the skin; aging and certain types of skin cancer are associated with chronic exposure to ultraviolet light. Exposure to visible and near-infrared lasers can cause photosensitive reactions and burns. The major skin damage associated with mid- and far-infrared lasers is burn. Lasers may also precipitate the development of or exaggerate existing skin lesions, including reactivation of viral infections[18,31,32] and delayed complications such as osteonecrosis.[33,34]

Patient protection should include saline-soaked towels applied to the skin surrounding the path of the laser beam. Skin protection for OR personnel can be provided by jackets and gloves for OR personnel. Topical application of a sunblock cream also protects against ultraviolet radiation in patients undergoing laser treatments.[26]

Eye Trauma

Incandescent and fluorescent lights are not harmful to the eye because the light is incoherent and only a small portion of the energy is spread out over the retina. The eye is extremely vulnerable to injury from the laser beam because laser radiation is coherent and all of its energy can be focused on a very small portion of the cornea or retina (Figure 40-5). Eye trauma is

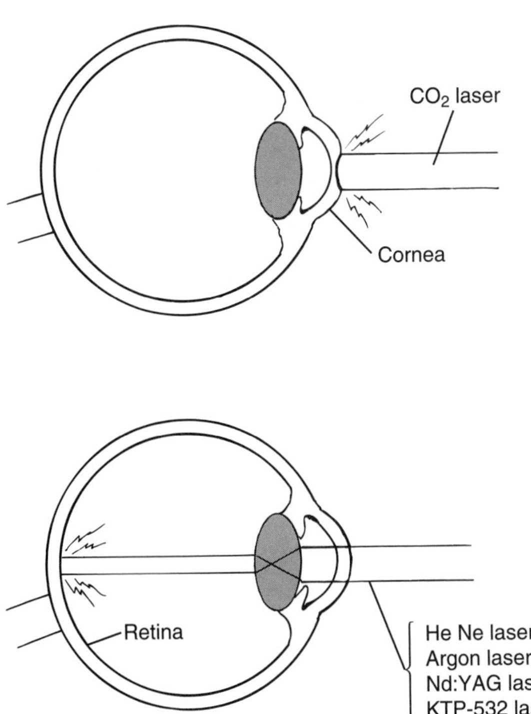

FIGURE **40-5**
Possible eye damage associated with various types of laser. (Modified from Boytim M. Anesthesia and laser surgery. In: Nagelhout JJ, Zaglaniczny KL, eds. *Nurse Anesthesia*. 2nd ed. Philadelphia: Saunders; 2001:963.)

dependent on the intensity and wavelength of the laser light and the exposed tissue.

Ultraviolet lasers (200 to 315 nm) may cause corneal photokeratitis and cataract formation. The cornea and the lens transmit lasers in the visible and near-infrared regions of the spectrum. Retinal damage is associated with visible and near-infrared (400 to 1400 nm) lasers such as the argon, KTP-YAG, Nd:YAG, and ruby lasers. The laser light is transmitted by the cornea and focused by the lens to produce an intense concentration of light energy on a small portion of the pigmented retina. The conversion of the light energy to heat can cause retinal burns, visual loss, or total blindness. Visible and near-infrared lasers can also increase the opacity of the lens, resulting in traumatic cataracts.[35] Laser light in the visible and near-infrared region (400 to 1400 nm) can create a hazardous concentration of laser energy. One milliwatt of visible laser radiation entering the eye deposits 100 W/cm^2 at the retina. Wavelengths less then 400 nm and greater than 1400 nm are not associated with retinal damage.

Rods make up the vast majority of the retina (over 95%) and are sensitive to light but not color. Cones make up less than 5% of the total retinal area (central retina, called the *fovea centralis*) and are responsible for color and fine detail. A visible laser beam produces a bright color flash of the emitted wavelength followed by an afterimage of its complementary color (e.g., a green, 532-nm laser light would produce a green flash followed immediately by a red afterimage). If an individual's cones are damaged, he or she may have difficulty discriminating blue and green colors. The Q-switched Nd:YAG laser beam (1064 nm) is especially hazardous to the eye because the beam is invisible and the retina lacks sensory innervation. Visual disorientation resulting from retinal damage may not be apparent until considerable thermal damage has occurred. No immediate signs of exposures to ultraviolet radiation occur, but severe eye pain and a sensation of sand in the eye may be present later.

Mid- and far-infrared wavelengths are absorbed by water; consequently, damage to the cornea and to a lesser extent the lens can occur if the unprotected eye is exposed to an aberrant laser beam from a mid- or far-infrared laser. Mid-infrared radiation (1400 to 3000 nm) can penetrate the lens, resulting in cataract formation. Far-infrared radiation (3000 to 10,000 nm) is absorbed by the cornea and can result in corneal burn and potential loss of vision. Inadvertent exposure to the invisible CO_2 laser beam (10,600 nm) causes burning pain of the cornea or sclera. After minor injury, regeneration of the epithelium occurs without any permanent abnormality, but corneal scarring and cataract formation may result with more extensive injury.

Eye Protection

Laser eye protection is required for class IV lasers and is advisable for class IIIB lasers. The aversion or blink response of 0.25 sec is triggered by bright visible light only, but it will not prevent the trauma of visible laser beams. The aversion response is absent or sluggish under general anesthesia, and in an OR that is darkened for video and microscope use the pupils of the eyes will be dilated, which increases the risk for laser exposure for OR personnel and the awake patient. The patient's eyes must be protected with laser safety lenses or covered with saline-moistened eye pads and metal shields. Petroleum-based eye ointments cannot be used during laser procedures, as they may cause severe burns.

Access to the laser area must be restricted to individuals wearing protective eyewear specific for the type of laser in use. Protective lenses must have the appropriate optical density (OD) and reflective properties based on the wavelengths of the beams encountered, the beam intensity, and the expected exposure conditions. *Optical density* refers to the attenuation or absorption of the laser light and transmission of sufficient ambient light for safe visibility. Historically, OR personnel have relied on the color of the lenses to indicate their use for specific lasers. However there is no current standard for protective lenses. For example, Nd:YAG laser protection can be provided with green lenses or specially coated clear lenses. OR personnel should not rely on the color of the lens to indicate use for specific lasers; they should check the OD and wavelength on the lenses relative to the laser in use. For example, protective eyewear for the Nd:YAG should be marked "OD5 or greater for 1,064 nm." Vision correction lenses may attenuate the effect of the CO_2 laser beam but do not completely protect the eye from direct or reflected laser beams. CO_2 lenses are usually clear and do not affect color perception, but tinted or colored lenses can affect color perception. Display lights and alarms of patient monitors should be set to maximum brightness or otherwise adjusted to compensate for the color restriction. The anesthetist should observe the monitors through the lenses before a case to ascertain the impact of the colored lenses.

Warning signs posted on the inside and outside of all entrances should include the type and wavelength of the laser in use as well as the wavelength and specific safety glasses required (Figure 40-6). Access should be restricted to authorized personnel. Entryway controls must be in place, such as a nondefeatable control on the door that cuts the beam off when the door is

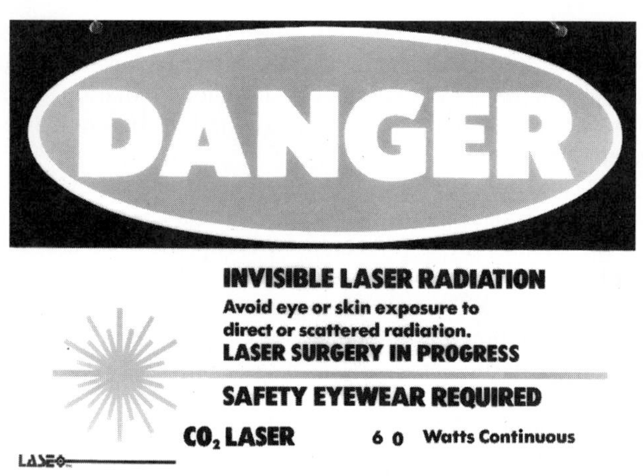

FIGURE **40-6**
Danger sign indicating laser procedure in progress. (From Boytim M. Anesthesia and laser surgery. In: Nagelhout JJ, Zaglaniczny KL, eds. *Nurse Anesthesia.* 2nd ed. Philadelphia: Saunders; 2001:962.)

opened. All other optical paths (windows) should be covered to reduce the transmitted intensity of the laser radiation.

Perforation

Perforation of a viscus or vessel can be attributed to operator error, such as a misdirected laser beam or failure to check for proper laser function before use.[36] Pneumothorax can be a life-threatening complication of a misdirected laser beam, especially during the administration of nitrous oxide (N_2O). Lasers cannot photocoagulate blood vessels larger than 5 mm; consequently, a beam misdirected at a vessel >5 mm can result in unexpected bleeding.[37] The Nd:YAG laser is associated with delayed tissue damage, as its beam is more widely disseminated and has greater penetration. The resultant perforation, bleeding, or edema may not be apparent for hours to days when necrosis and edema are maximal. Patients should be monitored for 24 to 48 hours after undergoing Nd:YAG laser surgery of the airway.[38]

Embolism

Venous gas embolism is a rare but potentially fatal hazard of laser procedures, and CO_2 emboli appear to be less damaging than air or nitrogen emboli. Several cases of coronary and cerebral embolism have been reported during endobronchial Nd:YAG therapy.[39] The emboli were attributed to the use of a gas coolant for the sapphire probe tip. Cerebral microembolization during transmyocardial laser revascularization has been confirmed.[40] Venous air embolism has also been reported with a diode laser.[41] During hysteroscopy, a procedure that carries risk for a venous air embolism, a liquid coolant will reduce the risk of air embolism but increase the risk of fluid overload.[37]

Pollution

According to the National Institute for Occupational Safety and Health (NIOSH), thermal destruction of tissue with a laser creates a smoke plume that can contain toxic gases and vapors including benzene, hydrogen cyanide, formaldehyde, bioaerosols, dead and live cellular material, and viruses.[42] The CO_2 laser produces the most smoke; the amount of smoke from 1 g of tissue is equivalent to 3 to 6 cigarettes.

High concentrations of smoke can cause ocular and upper respiratory irritation.[42] The smoke plume may contain fine particulates (0.3 μm) than can be deposited in the lower airways. Because lasers are commonly used to vaporize viral lesions and tumors, concern exists that the laser plume may contain infectious material. The laser plume may contain viral DNA and may transmit disease.[43]

As an addition to general room ventilation, NIOSH recommends the use of a local exhaust ventilation system such as a portable smoke evacuator as the most efficient method to control laser-generated smoke.[42] An in-line smoke filter attached to the wall suction can be used for laser procedures that produce a small smoke plume. A triple filtration smoke evacuator is indicated for evacuation of a large smoke plume. Smoke evacuators contain a either a high-efficiency particulate air filter (HEPA) that can filter 0.3-μm particulate matter or an ultra–low-penetration air filter (ULPA) that can filter particulate matter as small as 0.01 μm. The Filtresse Smoke Filtration System (Cortec Medical) and the SmartVac Smoke Evacuation System (Niche Medical) are three-stage disposable filter systems composed of a HEPA prefilter, a layer of activated charcoal for odor absorption, and a ULPA filter. The filtration system has an efficiency of >99.999% for 0.1-μm particles. To effectively capture airborne contaminants generated by surgical lasers, the smoke evacuator or room suction hose nozzle inlet must be kept within 2 inches of the surgical site. The smoke evacuator should be "on" (activated) at all times when airborne particles are produced during the laser procedure. The Laparoshield (Pall Medical) is a three-stage filter designed for use during laparoscopic procedures. High-filtration masks (0.3 μm) should be worn by OR personnel to filter out particulate matter and noxious odors. A close-fitting, surgical mask can filter particulate matter as small as 5 μm but is ineffective against particulate matter found in the smoke plumes.[44]

Fire

Historically the risk of fire in the OR was associated with the use of flammable anesthetics. The risk of an OR fire is still a very real hazard of modern surgery because of the use of surgical lasers and electrocautery units. Immediate recognition and management can limit patient injury, whereas delayed recognition and response can be fatal for the patient. For a fire to occur, a fuel, an ignition source, and an oxidizer must be present. Air, O_2, and N_2O are the oxidizers, and the laser is the source of ignition. Fuel sources include bowel gas, petroleum-based ointment, facial hair, surgical drapes, gloves, ointments, sponges, endotracheal tubes, Silastic stents, suction catheters, and tracheostomy tubes. Alcohol-based preparation solutions are very volatile; if adequate drying time is not achieved, the vapors can be ignited by the laser. This is more likely to occur in a confined space, as created by the use of tinted drapes, and in the presence of O_2.[45] The risk of fire is especially great during head and neck surgery, in which O_2 can build up under the surgical drapes, creating an oxidizer-enriched environment. Materials considered nonflammable may ignite easily and burn more quickly and at a higher temperature when exposed to an oxidizer-enriched environment. Even during monitored anesthesia care (MAC), the risk of fire is present if the patient is receiving supplemental O_2. It is imperative that all OR personnel be aware of the hazards of fire during laser procedures and know how to prevent and manage it.[46]

Laser-related fires are not confined to the airway, but airway fires can cause extensive damage.[29,45] The incidence of airway fires in the United States is estimated to be 0.5% to 1.5%.[47] It is also estimated that only 1 in 10 to 1 in 100 fires are reported, and serious patient injury occurrs in 20% of reported fires. Liability issues account for the underreporting of OR fires.[45] During airway surgery the laser beam is in close contact with the endotracheal tube. Fire can occur if the laser beam or the reflected laser light comes in direct contact with the endotracheal tube. Localized thermal trauma occurs if the fire is contained to the outside of the endotracheal tube. Rupture of the endotracheal tube cuff allows leakage of anesthetics gases into the path of the laser beam, increasing the risk of an ignition. If the fire burns through to the inner side of the tube, an intraluminal fire occurs, fed by both the anesthetics gases and the volatile products of combustion of the endotracheal tube wall. A blowtorch fire of the lower airway is possible and can cause extensive damage.

Anesthetic Gases

The gas mixture used during laser procedures of the airway should have the lowest potential for combustion. The volatile anesthetics currently used in clinical practice are nonflammable, but their use is not recommended during airway laser procedures because they may deteriorate to potentially toxic compounds in the presence of a fire.[28] N_2O readily supports combustion and should be avoided during laser procedures. Suitable gases include O_2 and air, O_2 and nitrogen, and O_2 and helium. Helium has a high thermal conductivity and is more resistant to ignition. In addition, its lower viscosity is beneficial for the increased resistance resulting from smaller internal diameter (ID) tubes or airway obstruction. O_2 concentration should be the lowest possible to support acceptable patient oxygenation and should be limited to 40%.

Endotracheal Tubes

Polyvinyl chloride (PVC) tubes ignite easily, producing toxic materials that can increase the amount of damage to the airway. PVC tubes appear to be more susceptible to damage by the CO_2 laser; however, the presence of blood on the tube makes a PVC tube susceptible to damage by the Nd:YAG laser. The radiopaque, barium sulfate strip found on most PVC tubes has a faster ignition rate than the PVC. Red rubber tubes appear to be more resistant to initial ignition, have a slower rate of burn, and produce less toxic smoke. However, red rubber tubes tend to melt and can produce carbon monoxide. Silicone tubes are also less combustible, but concern exists regarding the health hazards associated with inhalation of silica ash. Laser procedures of the airway require use of an endotracheal tube with a small ID. Increased resistance and tendency toward kinking are seen with smaller ID tubes.[48]

Several laser-resistant endotracheal tubes are available in the United States. The Laser-Flex Tracheal Tube (Nellcor) is a stainless steel, spiral wound tube with two PVC cuffs. In the event of a proximal cuff rupture the distal cuff maintains a tracheal seal and prevents anesthetic gases from leaking into the path of the laser beam. The Laser Flex is resistant to the CO_2 and KTP and Nd:YAG lasers. The Bivona Fome-Cuff (Portex) is a silicone and aluminum spiral tube designed for use with the CO_2 laser. It has a polyurethane self-inflating foam cuff covered with silicone that is designed to maintain a tracheal seal in the event of a cuff rupture. Inability to deflate the cuff before removal is a concern with the use of this tube. The Laser Shield II (Medtronic), a reflective aluminum-wrapped silicone tube covered with a smooth fluoroplastic, is specific for use with CO_2 and KTP lasers. The cuff is designed to be inflated with saline, and methylene blue is present in the inflation valve for immediate detection of cuff rupture. The Laser-Trach (Kendall/Sheridan) is a red rubber tube with an embossed copper foil for use with CO_2 and KTP lasers. The Lasertubus (Rüsch) is a soft white rubber tube, the lower 17 cm of which is covered with Merocel wrap. It has two high-volume cuffs, one inside the other.

Laser-Resistant Endotracheal Tube Wraps

Application of a metallic foil wrap (aluminum or copper) or a thin metal-coated plastic tape may protect the PVC and red rubber endotracheal tube during laser surgery of the airway with CO_2, KTP, and Nd:YAG lasers. Although the practice of using these foils is well supported in the medical literature, only the Merocel Laser-Guard Endotracheal Tube Wrap (Medtronic) has FDA approval for endotracheal tube protection. Meticulous application of the metallic tape is mandatory if it is to be to be effective in prevention of ignition of the endotracheal tube. Starting at the proximal edge of the cuff with a 60-degree angle cut, the practitioner should apply the tape in a spiral, overlapping manner (Figure 40-7). Leaving any area of the tube exposed to the laser beam negates the use of the metallic tape. A disadvantage of the metallic wrap tube is the need to use a smaller ID size, which increases airway resistance.

All endotracheal tubes carry the inherent risk of ignition. Use of a laser-resistant tube or a metallic-wrapped tube does not guarantee protection from the risk of a fire. When exposed to the CO_2 laser (CW) in room air, the silicone tube ignited in 0.3 seconds, the unwrapped PVC ignited in 0.8 seconds, and the Xomed laser tube ignited in 5 seconds. The Laser Flex and the aluminum-wrapped PVC did not ignite after 30 seconds.[49] The Nd:YAG laser (CW) will ignite clear PVC, red rubber,

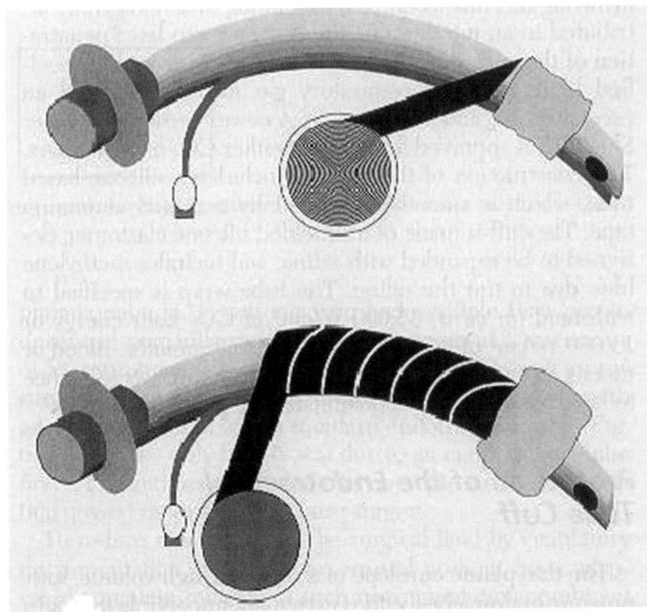

FIGURE **40-7**
Cuff-wrapping technique. The end of the tape, cut at a 60-degree angle, is aligned with the proximal end of the cuff, and wrapping is done is a spiral manner, allowing a 30% to 50% overlap between layers. Wrapping should include the inflation tube for the cuff and should be continued until just short of the pilot balloon. (Modified from Rampil IJ. Anesthesia for laser surgery. In: Miller RD, ed. *Anesthesia*. 5th ed. Philadelphia: Churchill Livingstone; 2000:2207.)

silicone, and laser resistant tubes, including the Bivona Fome Cuff and Laser Flex tubes. The clear PVC tube can withstand the pulsed Nd:YAG, but it is prone to ignition if blood is present on the tube or if the tube has radiopaque markings. Aluminum- and copper-wrapped red rubber tubes did not ignite with the Nd:YAG laser.[47] The potential for an airway fire still exists with the use of protective tapes.[50,51]

Endotracheal cuffs, including those on the laser-resistant tubes, are not laser resistant, and cuff rupture is often the prelude to an airway fire. The endotracheal tube cuff should be inflated with normal saline; the addition of methylene blue may alert the surgeon to cuff rupture. Saline-moistened cotton gauze should be placed proximal to the tube cuff; the gauze and the attached cotton strings should be constantly remoistened. The endotracheal cuff should be fully inflated and a stethoscope used to confirm the absence of a leak before the laser is used. At least 1 minute should elapse before a laser is used after reinflation of a cuff or repositioning of the tube for correction of a leak.

Laryngeal Mask Airway

The standard (silicone), intubating (silicone and steel), and disposable (PVC) laryngeal mask airways (LMAs) have been tested with the KTP and Nd:YAG lasers at two power densities common during airway surgery. The tube of the silicone mask was more resistant than the PVC tube, but the PVC cuff was more resistant than the silicone cuff. The intubating LMA was more sensitive to the KTP laser. The presence of blood increased the vulnerability of all the LMAs, especially with the KTP laser.[52] Additional precautions for use of the LMA during laser procedures include filling of the cuff with saline and methylene blue and covering of the cuff with moistened gauze.

Management of an Airway Fire

The OR team has approximately 6 seconds for recognition and removal of a tube that has ignited. Signs of an airway fire include darkening of the endotracheal tube or breathing circuit with soot, an orange or red glow to the endotracheal tube, and the presence of flames in or around the endotracheal tube. The endotracheal tube acts like a blowtorch, with high concentrations of O_2 adding to the intensity of the fire. Within seconds the flames can reach a height of 5 to 10 inches. Intraluminal fires will spread toward the proximal end of the tube—the source of the O_2. Severe thermal or chemical trauma is unlikely to occur if the flame is vented through the tube or oropharynx.[50,53] Downstream gases contain the products of oxidation and little O_2, but a free end fire can occur if the products of oxidation ignite in the O_2-rich alveoli.[54]

In rapid succession, ventilation should be discontinued, the breathing circuit disconnected, and the endotracheal tube removed and extinguished in a basin of water. The tube should be saved for later examination. A continuing airway fire should be extinguished with normal saline, and any residual smoldering material must be removed from the airway. The patient should be mask ventilated with air until all burning has stopped, at which time ventilation with 100% O_2 should be instituted.[50] Removal of the endotracheal tube is controversial, and the tube probably should not be removed if it is not burning or if concern exists regarding complete loss of the airway.[50,53,55] Cessation of gas flow will extinguish an intraluminal fire. If the tube is not removed, it should be lavaged with normal saline.[54] Leaving the patient intubated will allow acceptable ventilation, as the edematous airway provides a seal around the ruptured cuff. A tube exchanger or tracheostomy can be used to replace the damaged tube without the risk of losing the airway completely.[50,53] Recommendations for management of an airway fire are listed in Box 40-1.

Anesthesia should be continued to allow evaluation of the airway for direct thermal trauma, chemical inhalation injury, and smoke inhalation. Direct visualization of the tracheobronchial tree with a rigid bronchoscope is recommended for assessment of thermal injury and removal of foreign material. A flexible bronchoscope may be necessary for evaluation of distal airways, and tracheobronchial lavage with saline solution should be considered. After reintubation with a smaller tube, a chest x-ray examination and evaluation of arterial blood gases are indicated to guide postoperative management. Carboxyhemoglobulin levels are needed for assessment of smoke inhalation.

After an airway fire, 24-hour observation of the patient is indicated. For minor burns the patient should be monitored for development of laryngeal-tracheal edema, which often follows extubation. A patient with severe burns should remain intubated and receive humidified O_2 of 30% to 60%; a tracheostomy and mechanical ventilation with positive end-expiratory pressure (PEEP) should be considered. Corticosteroids have been recommended for the treatment of both smoke inhalation and the bronchospasm that may be precipitated in patients with irritable airways. Additional treatment is dependent on the extent of the injury and the response of the patient. Complications can be delayed, and tracheal stenosis has been documented 14 weeks after an airway fire.[56]

BOX **40-1**

Management of Airway Fire

- Discontinue use of laser.
- In rapid succession stop ventilation, turn off O_2, disconnect breathing circuit, and remove ETT.*
- If necessary, extinguish airway fire with normal saline.
- Assume mask ventilation with 100% O_2.
- Reintubate with a smaller ETT, and continue anesthetic.
- Examine airway and remove residual debris with rigid bronchoscope. Consider lavage with normal saline.
- Examine small and distal airways with flexible fiberoptic bronchoscope.
- Assess extent of thermal trauma with ABG and CXR.
- Consider administration of steroids.
- Postoperative intubation and administration of humidified O_2 should be performed if airway burn is present or suspect. Tracheostomy and mechanical ventilation should be considered.
- Extubation and administration of humidified O_2 by mask should be performed if airway damage is minimal and risk of laryngeal edema is low.
- Minimum 24 hours of ICU observation should be performed.

**Extubation may not be indicated if a risk of total loss of the airway is present.*
ABG, *Arterial blood gas*; CXR, *chest x-ray*; ETT, *endotracheal tube*; ICU, *intensive care unit*; O_2, *oxygen*.

LASER SAFETY

Laser equipment should be operated only by qualified personnel. An aiming beam should be used if the laser does not produce a visible light. When not in use, the laser should be disabled and stored in a secure location. When the laser is in use, appropriate laser warning signs should be posted inside and outside the laser area (see Figure 40-6). Safety controls should limit access to the laser area through the use of a safety interlock system that will prevent unexpected entry or shut-off of the laser if the door is unexpectedly opened. Doors should remain closed during laser operation, and windows should be covered to prevent the transmission of a misdirected laser beam. Eye-protective lenses must be worn when class IV lasers are used.

During any laser procedure, everyone in the OR must be alert to the possibility of a fire and be prepared to respond quickly. Personnel should be aware of the fire hazards in the laser area such as anesthetic gases, skin preparation solution, adhesive plastic tape, and surgical drapes. Oil-based lubricants should be avoided, and alcohol-based preparation solutions should be allowed adequate drying time before the patient is covered by drapes. Patients' eyes must be protected with laser-specific lenses or saline-moistened pads and metal eye guards. Fire resistant drapes are necessary, and saline-soaked towels should be placed on the skin surrounding the path of the laser beam. Application of a water-soluble surgical lubricant to a facial beard will reduce the chance of ignition.[57] Anodized, dull, nonreflective, or matte-finished equipment should be used when possible to decrease reflectivity of the beam. All OR personnel should know the location and be familiar with the use of fire extinguishers.

Additional precautions are required for the possibility of an airway fire. A basin of water or normal saline should be available during laser procedures to extinguish a burning endotracheal tube or other material. Two syringes filled with normal saline should be readily available to extinguish an endotracheal tube fire.[58] O_2 should be limited to the lowest concentration possible, and laser resistant tubes or metallic-wrapped endotracheal tubes should be used for laser procedures of the airway. Use of excessive tape to secure the endotracheal tube should be avoided to allow easier removal in the event of an airway fire. Emergency supplies, including a rigid bronchoscope and forceps, should be readily available. The use of 5 to 10 cm H_2O PEEP has been advocated during laser surgery of the airway to prevent the hot toxic gases from reaching the lower airways.[58]

Lasers require high power and carry the potential for electrical injury. In addition, liquid gases used for cooling of the laser medium, especially liquid nitrogen, are hazardous to the skin if accidentally spilled. Liquid nitrogen also decreases the O_2 concentration, and its use should be limited to well-ventilated spaces. Dyes used in the PDL have potential toxicity.

ANESTHETIC MANAGEMENT

Anesthesia is frequently required for laser procedures; the surgeon requires an immobile patient and an unrestricted view of the targeted tissue. Most anesthetic techniques are suitable for laser procedures. The anesthetist should realize that laser procedures have complications similar to those of traditional surgery.[59,60] The main anesthetic implications for laser surgery concern procedures in which the airway is shared between the anesthetist and the surgeon. Communication between the surgeon and the anesthetist is paramount to assure patient safety, maximize surgical access, and avoid complications. In addition to the shared airway, the proximity of the endotracheal tube and anesthetic gases to the laser beam creates a very real hazard of airway fire. During laser procedures of the airway, O_2 concentration should be limited to 40% and N_2O should be avoided as it supports combustion. Because of the hazards of room pollution, inhalation agents are best avoided if the patient is not intubated or during procedures with uncuffed endotracheal tubes.

Ventilation techniques during laser procedures of the airway depend on surgeon preference and the site of the laser application. For the patient receiving supplemental O_2 during MAC cases, good communication between the surgeon and anesthetist allows the discontinuation of the O_2 while the laser is in use, to reduce the risk of fire. To maximize surgical view and access, smaller-than-usual endotracheal tubes are necessary, and the anesthetist must be prepared to deal with increased resistance to ventilation. Some surgeons may prefer an apneic technique, in which case the airway is alternately shared between the surgeon and the anesthetist. After induction of general anesthesia and the administration of a muscle relaxant the patient is hyperventilated by mask after brief periods of laser application. The pulse oximeter must be monitored closely and ventilation immediately resumed if oxygenation decreases 2% to 3% below the patient's initial saturation or when 1.5 to 2 minutes have elapsed. A disadvantage of this technique is the potential aspiration of blood and resected tissue.

An alternative approach is the use of a jet ventilator to deliver O_2 through the operating laryngoscope.[61,62,63] Because the entrainment of room air during jet ventilation (Venturi effect) dilutes the final oxygenation concentration delivered to the patient, 100% O_2 should be used.

SUMMARY

Lasers are an integral part of modern surgery, and newer and more powerful lasers are in development. Their ability to cut, coagulate, vaporize, and selectively destroy abnormal tissue has numerous applications in medicine. Anesthetists are involved on a daily basis with patients undergoing laser procedures. Safe provision of anesthetic requires knowledge of laser physics, as well as the potential hazards associated with the use of lasers in the OR. The potential threat of fire, especially airway fires, requires prevention, reaction, and an appropriate management plan.

REFERENCES

1. Anderson RR. Dermatologic history of the ruby laser: the long story of short pulses. *Arch Dermatol.* 2003;139:70-74.
2. Davidovits P. *Physics in Biology and Medicine*. San Diego: Harcourt Academic; 2001.
3. Waynant RW, Merberg, GN. *Basics of Lasers*. In: Waynant RW, ed. *Lasers in Medicine*. Boca Raton, Fla: CRC; 2002.
4. Spector N, Spector J, Ellis DL, et al. Reduction in lateral thermal damage using heat-conducting templates: a comparison of continuous wave and pulse CO_2 lasers. *Lasers in Surgery and Medicine*. 2003;32:94-100.
5. Lippert BN, Teymoortash A, Folz BJ, Werner JA. Wound healing after laser treatment of oral and oropharyngeal cancer. *Lasers Med Sci.* 2003;18:36-42.

6. Rofeim O, Hom D, Fried RM, et al. Use of the neodymium:YAG laser for interstitial cystitis: a prospective study. *J Urol.* 2001; 166:134-136.
7. Duhamel DR. Laser bronchoscopy. *Chest Surg Clin North Am.* 2001;11:769-789.
8. Joseph TA, Williams JS, Brems JJ. Laser capsulorrhaphy for multidirectional instability of the shoulder. An outcomes study and proposed classification system. *Am J Sports Med.* 2003; 31:26-35.
9. Sherk HH, Vangsness CT, Thabit G, et al. Electromagnetic surgical devices in orthopaedics: lasers and radiofrequency. *J Bone Joint Surg.* 2002;84-A:675-681.
10. Takagi T, Koshino T, Okamoto R. Arthroscopic synovectomy for rheumatoid arthritis using a holmium:YAG laser. *J Rheumatol.* 2001;28:1518-1522.
11. Aaberge L, Rootwelt K, Blomhoff S, et al. Continued symptomatic improvement three to five years after transmyocardial revascularization with CO_2 laser: a late clinical follow-up of the Norwegian randomized trial with transmyocardial revascularization. *J Am Coll Cardiol.* 2002;39:1588-1593.
12. Bernheim MW. Transmyocardial laser vascularization. *AANA J.* 2001;69:195-197.
13. Burkhoff D, Schmidt S, Schulman S, et al. Transmyocardial laser revascularization compared with continued medical therapy for treatment of refractory angina pectoris: a prospective randomized trial. *Lancet.* 1999;354:885-890.
14. Clarke SC, Schofield PM. Percutaneous myocardial laser revascularization. *Heart.* 2000;83:253-254.
15. Huikeshoven M, van der Sloot JA, Tukkie R, et al. Transmyocardial laser revascularization and other treatment modalities for angina pectoris. *Lasers Med Sci.* 2003;18:2-11.
16. Nahrendorf M, Hiller KH, Theisen D, et al. Effects of transmyocardial laser revascularization on myocardial perfusion and left ventricular remodeling after myocardial infarction in rats. *Radiology.* 2002;225:487-493.
17. Bonn D. Laser thrombolysis: safe and rapid removal of clots? *Lancet.* 2000;355:1976.
18. Alster TS, Apfelberg DB, eds. *Cosmetic Laser Surgery.* New York: Wiley-Liss; 1999.
19. Biesman BS, Khan J. Laser incisional surgery. *Clin Plast Surg.* 2000;227:213-220.
20. Golz A, Goldenberg D, Westerman ST, et al. Laser partial epiglottidectomy as a treatment for obstructive sleep apnea and laryngomalacia. *Ann Otol Rhinol Laryngol.* 2000;109:1140-1145.
21. Newman J, Anand V. Applications of the diode laser in otolaryngology. *Ear, Nose and Throat Journal.* 2002;81:850-851.
22. Hoexter DL. Latest advances in laser systems and periodontal surgery. *Dent Clin North Am.* 2001;45:207-212.
23. Strauss RA. Lasers in oral and maxillofacial surgery. *Dent Clin North Am.* 2000;44:851-873.
24. Schlager A, Offer T, Baldissera I. Laser stimulation of acupuncture point P6 reduces postoperative vomiting in children undergoing strabismus surgery. *Br J Anaesth.* 1998;81:529-532.
25. Gur A, Karakoc M, Cevik R, et al. Efficacy of low power laser therapy and exercise on pain and function in chronic low back pain. *Lasers Surg Med.* 2003;32:233-238.
26. US Department of Labor Occupational Safety and Health Administration. Laser hazards. In: *OSHA Technical Manual* [Section II, Chapter 6]. Washington, DC: OSHA; 1999. Available at: http://www.osha.gov/pls/oshaweb/owadisp.show_document?p_table = DIRECTIVES&P_ID = 1705. Accessed May 22, 2003.
27. Recommended practices for laser safety in practice settings. *AORN J.* 1998;67:263-268.
28. American National Standards Institute. Pub No. Z136.3. *The Standard for the Safe Use of Lasers in Health Care Facilities.* Washington, DC: ANSI; 1996.
29. Barat K. Laser accidents: occurrence and response. *Health Phys.* 2003;84:593-595.
30. Grossman PH, Grossman AR. Treatment of thermal injuries from CO_2 laser resurfacing. *Plast Reconstr Surg.* 2002;109: 1435-1445.
31. Green JJ, Lawrence N, Heymann WR. Generalized ulcerative sarcoidosis induced by therapy with the flashlamp-pumped pulsed dye laser. *Arch Dermatol.* 2001;137:507-508.
32. Stratigos AJ, Tahan S, Dover J. Rapid development of non-melanoma skin cancer after CO_2 laser resurfacing. *Arch Dermatol.* 2002;138:696-698.
33. Cassatly MG, Rostock M, Gocke MW. Iatrogenic osteonecrosis of the maxilla caused by laser injury. *J Oral Maxillofac Surg.* 1999;57:184-186.
34. Janzen DL, Kosarek FJ, Helms CA, et al. Osteonecrosis after contact neodymium:yttrium-aluminum-garnet arthroscopic laser menisectomy. *Am J Roentgenol.* 1997;169:855-858.
35. Foroozan R, Buono LM, Savino PJ. Traumatic cataract after inadvertent laser discharge. *Arch Ophthalmol.* 2003;121:286-287.
36. Gueret G, Guischard F, Dumoulin JL, et al. Life-threatening bilateral pneumothorax caused by misconnection of the laser lens cooling system during gynecologic laparoscopy. *Anesthesiology.* 1999;91:1179.
37. Rampil IJ. Anesthesia for laser surgery. In: Miller R, ed. *Anesthesia.* 5th ed. Philadelphia: Churchill Livingstone; 2000.
38. Albelmalak B, Ryckman JV, Alhafddad S, et al. Respiratory arrest after successful neodymium: yttrium-aluminum-garnet laser treatment of subglottic tracheal stenosis. *Anesth Analg.* 2002;95: 485-486.
39. Tellides G, Ugurlu BS, Kim RW, et al. Pathogenesis of systemic air embolism during bronchoscopic Nd:YAG laser operations. *Ann Thorac Surg.* 1998;65:930-934.
40. von Knobelsdorff G, Brauer P, Tonner PH, et al. Transmyocardial laser revascularization induces cerebral microembolization. *Anesthesiology.* 1997;87:58-62.
41. Jacobson F, Gullaksen K, Johansen LV. Systemic air embolism as a possible cause of cardiac arrest during endoscopic treatment of pulmonary haemangioma using a diode laser. *Acta Anaesthesiol Scand.* 1998;42:742-744.
42. National Institute for Occupational Safety and Health. *Control of Smoke from Laser/Electric Surgical Procedures.* Washington, DC: NIOSH; 1998. Available at: http://www.cdc.gov/niosh/hc11.html. Accessed May 22, 2003.
43. Garden JM, O'Banion MK, Bakus AD, et al. Viral disease transmitted by laser-generated plume (aerosol). *Arch Dermatol.* 2002;138:1303-1307.
44. Ball K. The hazards of surgical smoke. *AANA J.* 2001;69: 125-132.
45. Barker SJ, Polson JS. Fire in the operating room: a case report and laboratory study. *Anesth Analg.* 2001;93:960-965.
46. Rogers ML, Nichalls RW, Brackenbury ET, et al. Airway fire during tracheostomy: prevention strategies for surgeons and anaesthetists. *Ann R Coll Surg Engl.* 2001;83:376-380.
47. Edwards BE, Barnes LK, Gibbs JB, Nguyen GB. Medical laser safety hazard evaluation. *Health Phys.* 2002;83:S36-S44.
48. Jacobs JS, Lewis M, DeSouza GJ, et al. Crimping of a laser tube resulting in hypoxemia. *Anesthesiology.* 1999;91:898.
49. Lai HC, Juang SE, Liu TJ, et al. Fires of endotracheal tubes of three different materials during carbon dioxide laser surgery. *Acta Anaesthesiol Sin.* 2002;40:47-51.
50. Benumof JL, Saidman LJ. *Anesthesia and Perioperative Complications.* 2nd ed. St Louis: Mosby; 1999.
51. Kuo CH, Tan PH, Chen JJ, et al. Endotracheal tube fires during carbon dioxide laser surgery on the larynx-a case report. *Acta Anaesthesiol Sin.* 2001;39:53-61.
52. Keller C, Brimacombe J, Coorey A, et al. Liability of laryngeal mask airway to thermal damages from KTP and Nd:YAG lasers. *Br J Anaesth.* 1999;82:29.
53. Chee WK, Benumof L. Airway fire during tracheostomy: extubation may be contraindicated. *Anesthesiology.* 1998;89: 1576-1580.

54. Wolf GL, Sidebotham GW. Endotracheal tube fires: comments on the advisability of not extubating. *Anesthesiology*. 1999;91: 888-889.
55. Ng J, Hartigan PM. Airway fire during tracheostomy: should we extubate? *Anesthesiology*. 2003;98:1303.
56. Ilgner J, Flater F, Westhofen M. Long-term follow up after laser-induced endotracheal fire. *J Laryngol Otol*. 2002;116: 213-215.
57. Massachusetts Department of Public Health. *Health Care Quality Safety Alert. Preventing Operating Room Fires during Surgery*. 2002. Available at: http:www.state.ma.us/dph/dhcq/pdfs/orfires.pdf. Accessed May 22, 2003.
58. Lierz P, Heinatz A, Gustorff B, et al. Management of intratracheal fires during laser surgery. *Anesth Analg*. 2002;95:502.
59. Kremer B, Schlondorff G. Late lethal secondary hemorrhage after laser supraglottic laryngectomy. *Arch Otolaryngol*. 2001;127: 203-205.
60. Matot I, Drenger B, Glantz L, et al. Coronary spasm during outpatient fiberoptic laser bronchoscopy. *Chest*. 1999;115:1744-1746.
61. Ihra G, Hieber C, Schabernig C, et al. Supralaryngeal tubeless combined high-frequency jet ventilation for laser surgery of the larynx and trachea. *Br J Anaesth*. 1999;83:940-942.
62. Medici G, Mallios C, Custers WT, van Meerbeek JP, Verhoeven GT, Hop WC. Anesthesia for endobronchial laser surgery: a modified technique. *Anesth Analg*. 1999;88:298-301.
63. Unzueta MC, Casas I, Merten A, Landeira JM. Endobronchial high-frequency jet ventilation for endobronchial laser surgery: an alternative approach. *Anesth Analg*. 2003;96:298-300.

CHAPTER 41

Obesity and Anesthesia Practice

Karen L. Zaglaniczny

OVERVIEW

Obesity is a complex, multifactorial, chronic disease that develops from an interaction between the genotype and the environment.[1-3] It is the second leading cause of preventable death in the United States.[1] The prevalence of overweight and obesity has increased significantly during the last three decades. Obesity is associated with an increased incidence of a wide spectrum of medical and surgical conditions and morbidity. As a result, anesthetists can expect to encounter overweight and obese patients frequently in their practices. These patients may provide the anesthetist with a considerable challenge. A thorough understanding of the pathophysiology, pharmacology, and specific anesthetic considerations associated with obesity will promote optimal anesthesia care.

Statistics

Obesity is a disease that affects one third of the adult U.S. population.[4-6] The number of overweight and obese adults has continued to increase over the past decade. It is estimated that 64.5% of U.S. adults (approximately 127 million) are either overweight or obese.[5] According to epidemiologic studies of the adult population aged 20 to 72 years, the estimated prevalence of obesity (body mass index [BMI] greater than or equal to 30) has doubled from approximately 15% to an estimated 31% since 1960.[6] Data from the National Health and Nutrition Examination Surveys (NHANES) reveal the significant growth in overweight and obesity from 1960 to 1994 (Figure 41-1). Demographically, obesity has dramatically increased among civilian, black, white, and Hispanic populations of both sexes and all ages. Obesity in children and adolescents has also increased significantly over the past decade. In the United

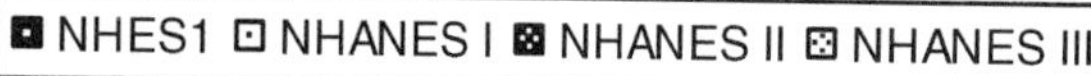

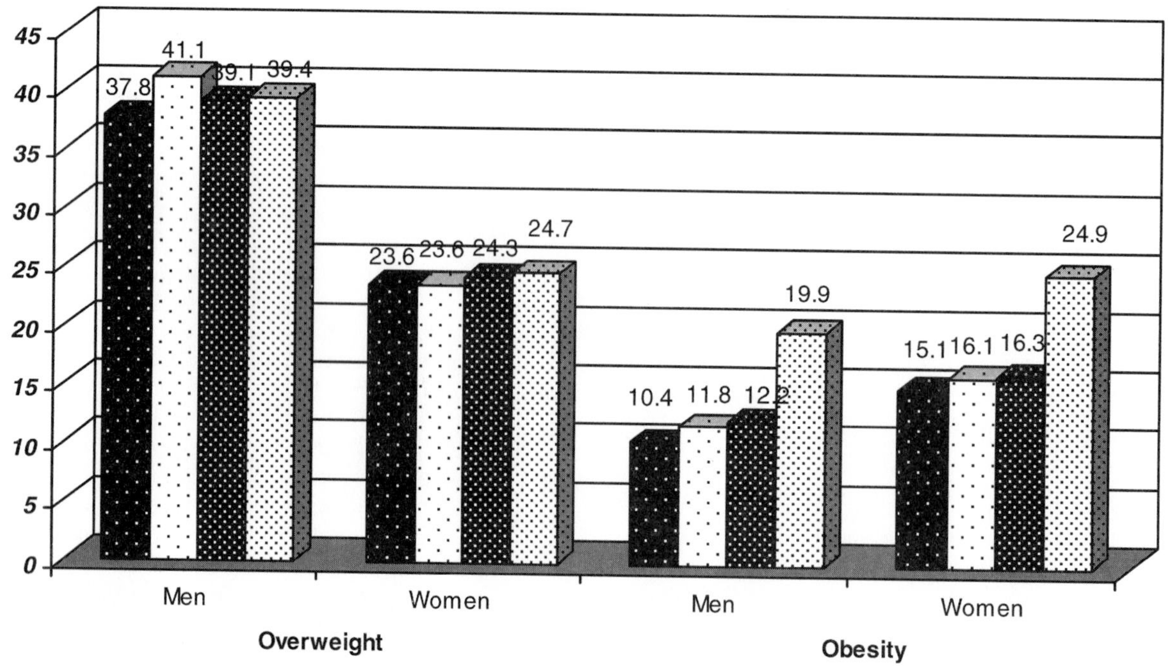

FIGURE **41-1**
Age-adjusted prevalence of overweight and obesity.

States, 30% of the members of this population are overweight, and 15% are obese.[1]

Definitions

BMI is the accepted measure of body habitus that normalizes adiposity for height.[1] BMI can be calculated according to the following formulas:

- BMI = Weight (in kilograms)/Height (in meters)^2
- BMI = (Body weight [in pounds]/Height [in inches]^2) × 703

Overweight is defined as a BMI of 25 to 29 kg/m^2, and obesity as a BMI of 30 kg/m^2.[1-3] The rationale for these definitions is based on epidemiologic data that reveal increasing mortality with BMIs over 25 kg/m^2.[6] For individuals with BMI >30 kg/m^2, mortality rates for a number of conditions, especially those associated with cardiovascular disease, are increased 50% to 100% above rates in individuals of normal weight. Guidelines for classification of weight status by BMI are summarized in Table 41-1.

Ideal body weight (IBW) is a term used interchangeably with the terms *normal weight*, *lean body weight*, and *desirable weight*.[1-3] IBW is a measurement of height and body mass that exhibits the lowest morbidity and mortality for a given population.[2] Determination of IBW is especially useful in the calculation of drug and intravenous infusion doses in morbidly obese patients. Certain drugs, if administered according to actual body weight, can produce toxicity, renal damage, or hemodynamic instability. Conversely, some drugs must be given according to actual body weight if therapeutic effects are to be achieved. The formula for IBW (in kilograms) is as follows:

- For men: IBW = Height (in centimeters) − 100
- For women: IBW = Height (in centimeters) − 105

Risk Factors

Obesity is associated with an increase in the incidence of more than 30 medical conditions (Table 41-2). The risk of cardiovascular disease, certain cancers, and diabetes and overall mortality are linearly related to weight gain.[1-3] Type 2 diabetes, coronary heart disease, hypertension, and hypercholesterolemia are prominent conditions in overweight and obese patients.[1-3] With increasing weight gain and increased adiposity, glucose tolerance deteriorates, blood pressure rises, and the lipid profile becomes more atherogenic.[2] Hormonal and nonhormonal mechanisms contribute to the greater risk of breast, gastrointestinal, endometrial, and renal cell cancers.[6] Psychologic health risks often stem from social ostracism, discrimination, and impaired ability to participate fully in activities of daily living. Coexistent feelings of worthlessness and low self-esteem can lead to depression that not only magnifies anesthetic morbidity, but also contributes to an increased incidence of suicide among morbidly obese persons.

TABLE 41-1 Classification of Overweight and Obesity by Body Mass Index

	Obesity Class	Body Mass Index (kg/m²)	Risk of Disease
Underweight	—	<18.5	Increased
Normal	—	18.5-24.9	Normal
Overweight	—	25-29.9	Increased
Obesity	I	30-34.9	High
	II	35-39.9	Very high
	III	>40	Extremely high

From National Institute of Health. Clinical Guidelines on the Identification, Evaluation, and Treatment of Overweight and Obesity in Adults: the Evidence Report. NIH publication no. 98-4083. Washington, DC: National Institute of Health; September, 1998; Klein S, Romijn J. Obesity. In: Larsen PR, Kroneberg HM, Mclmed S, Polonsky KS. Williams Textbook of Endocrinology. *10th ed. Philadelphia: Saunders; 2003:1619-1641; Flier JS. Obesity. In: Braunwald E, Fauci AS, Kasper DL, Hauser SL, Longo DL, Jameson JL, eds.* Harrison's Principles of Internal Medicine. *15th ed. New York: McGraw-Hill; 2001:479-486.*

TABLE 41-2 Conditions Associated with Obesity

Type 2 diabetes	Osteoarthritis
Coronary heart disease	Cancer: esophageal, gallbladder, colon, breast, uterine, cervical, prostate, renal
Hypertension	Chronic venous insufficiency
Dyslipidemia	Deep vein thrombosis
Cerebrovascular disease	Gallbladder disease
Thromboembolic disease	Urinary incontinence
Restrictive lung disease	Gastroesophageal reflux disease
Obesity hypoventilation syndrome	Pancreatitis
Obstructive sleep apnea	Nonalcoholic fatty liver disease: steatosis, cirrhosis, hepatomegaly
Gout	Low back pain
Infertility	Obstetric complications
Impaired immune response	Surgical infections
Wound infections	
Depression	

From National Institute of Health. Clinical Guidelines on the Identification, Evaluation, and Treatment of Overweight and Obesity in Adults: the Evidence Report. NIH publication no. 98-4083. Washington, DC: National Institute of Health; September, 1998; Klein S, Romijn J. Obesity. In: Larsen PR, Kroneberg HM, Mclmed S, Polonsky KS. Williams Textbook of Endocrinology. *10th ed. Philadelphia: Saunders; 2003:1619-1641; Flier JS. Obesity. In: Braunwald E, Fauci AS, Kasper DL, Hauser SL, Longo DL, Jameson JL, eds.* Harrison's Principles of Internal Medicine. *15th ed. New York: McGraw-Hill; 2001:479-486.*

ADIPOSE TISSUE

Adipose tissue has major integrative physiologic functions, secretes numerous proteins, and is considered an endocrine organ.[2] Its major functions as an organ are to provide a reservoir of readily convertible and usable energy and to maintain heat insulation.[2,3,7] Functions associated with liver fat metabolism include degradation of fatty acids into usable units of energy, synthesis of triglycerides from carbohydrates and proteins, and synthesis of other lipids from fatty acids, particularly cholesterol and phospholipids.[7] The ability of the liver to desaturate fatty acids is tremendously important, because all cells contain some unsaturated fats synthesized by the liver.

Body fat is also important in heat regulation and insulation. Fat cells, which arise from modified fibroblasts, enlarge and fill with liquid triglycerides to nearly 95% of their storage capacity.[7,8] During exposure of the skin to cold (several weeks), the fatty acid chains of the triglycerides shorten, or become more unsaturated.[3] This phenomenon lowers their melting point, which allows the fat in the fat cells to maintain a liquid state. Metabolically, this is significant. Only liquid fat can be hydrolyzed and transported from the cells to be used for energy.[3]

Body Fat Distribution

In early childhood, fat cell formation occurs very rapidly.[2] Overfeeding during this time accelerates fat storage and triggers hyperproliferation of fat cells. During adolescence the number of fat cells stabilizes and remains constant throughout adult life. Children become obese through an increase in fat cell numbers, whereas adults become obese through hypertrophy of existing fat cells.[2,3] The distribution of body fat, however, is a clearer indicator of increased health risk.[8]

Central, android, or abdominal visceral obesity ("apple" shape), with a waist/hip ratio greater than 0.85 in men and 0.92 in women, is perceived as a malignant form of fat accumulation[2,9] (Figure 41-2, *A*). Waist/hip ratio is calculated by dividing the narrowest waist measurement by the broadest hip measurement while the patient is standing.[2] Waist circumference is the newly established standard used as a marker for abdominal obesity. In men a waist circumference greater that 102 cm (40 inches) and in women a waist circumference of 88 cm (35 inches) denote increased risk for certain diseases and conditions.[2,7] These include ischemic heart disease, diabetes mellitus, hypertension, dyslipidemia, and death.[1-3]

Peripheral, gynecoid, or gluteal femoral obesity ("pear" shape) with a waist/hip ratio below 0.76 is associated with varicose vein development, joint disease, and reduced incidence of non–insulin-dependent diabetes mellitus (Figure 41-2, *B*). Medical risks accompanying gynecoid fat deposition are less perilous than those associated with the android pattern.[1,4]

Differences in morbidity between android and gynecoid fat distribution are caused by metabolic attributes of the adipose and tissues adjacent to it. Gynecoid repositories of fat, found primarily in women, are metabolically static and are proposed to function as energy depots for pregnancy and lactation.[3,4] Android fat distribution, typically seen in males, is metabolically active with regard to free fatty acid (FFA) release.[2] When elevated levels of FFAs are mobilized from adipose tissue, portal venous drainage delivers high concentrations of FFAs to the liver. Continual delivery of excessive FFAs stimulates hepatic synthesis of very–low-density lipoproteins (VLDLs) and circulation of low-density lipoproteins (LDLs).[2,3] Hepatic exposure to high concentrations of FFAs also increases gluconeogenesis and inhibition of insulin uptake, which induces non–insulin-dependent diabetes mellitus.[2,3] Although VLDLs, LDLs, and hyperglycemia are catalysts for the formation of associated cardiovascular and cerebrovascular disease, some studies support the possibility that hyperinsulinemia alone may cause hypertension.[2,3]

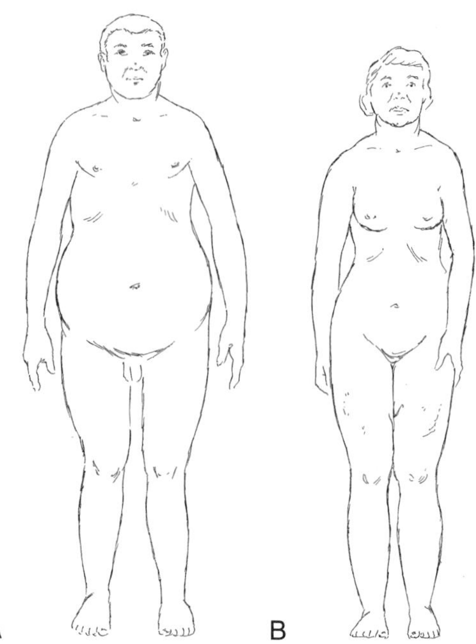

FIGURE **41-2**
Obesity. **A,** Central android, or abdominal visceral. **B,** Peripheral gynecoid, or gluteal.

CAUSES OF OBESITY

Body size is dependent on genetic and environmental factors. Genetic predisposition, believed to be a primary factor in the development of obesity, explains only 40% of the variance in body mass.[6] The significant increase in the prevalence of obesity has resulted from environmental factors that result in increased food intake and reduced physical activity.[6,7] Other factors such as socialization, age, sex, race, and economic status affect its progression. In the United States food consumption has risen as a result of the "super-sizing" of portions and the availability of high-fat fast food and snacks. Physical activity has been reduced as a result of modernization (television and computers) and sedentary lifestyle and work activities. Cultural and lifestyle variations play an important role in the development of obesity.[6] For example, some ethnic foods contain high levels of fats and carbohydrates, whereas others (e.g., Asian) focus on low-fat foods such as fish and vegetables.

Since the discovery of the adipose tissue protein leptin, advances have been made in understanding the molecular basis of body fat regulation. In 1994 the *ob* gene was identified in mice and was shown to control the production of the protein leptin.[10] Genetically obese *ob/ob* mice produce insufficient leptin and tend to overeat, which leads to obesity. Exogenous leptin reveres hyperphagia and induces weight loss. However, serum leptin levels increase exponentially with fat mass, suggesting that most obese patients are resistant or insensitive to weight regulation by exogenous leptin. Continued investigation into genetic-environmental interactions may provide further understanding and treatment of obesity.[4,9,10]

Public awareness of the problems that arise from obesity is corroborated by the $100 billion spent annually on medical treatment, weight reduction programs, exercise equipment, low-fat diet products, pharmacologic agents, advertising, and marketing.[11] Obesity is a major health concern, and obese patients admitted for surgery may exhibit one or more medical conditions in addition to the primary underlying problem.[12] Clearly, identification of obesity-related conditions is vital to the safe administration of an anesthetic.

PATHOPHYSIOLOGY OF OBESITY

A number of pathophysiologic changes occur as a result of overweight and obesity. These involve all of the major body organ systems, leading to an increase in morbidity and premature death. The risk of many of the medical conditions associated with obesity increases linearly with BMI.[2-4]

Cardiovascular Considerations

Cardiovascular considerations are predominantly a reflection of the progressive compensatory processes that evolve to meet the increased metabolic demands of the fat organ.[2-4,13]

Cardiovascular disease dominates the morbidity and mortality in obesity and manifests in the form of ischemic heart disease, hypertension, and cardiac failure.[12] Development and sustenance of the fat mass necessitates formation of extra blood vessels and increased circulatory, pulmonary, central, and peripheral blood volume.[2-4] For every 13.5 kg of fat gained, an estimated 25 miles of neovascularization occurs to provide blood flow at a rate of 2 to 3 ml/100 g of tissue per minute.[3] This represents an increased cardiac output of 0.1 L/min for each kilogram of fat acquired.[3] Expansion of blood volume, stimulated by hypoxia-induced, chronic respiratory insufficiency, is seen in severe obesity. Accelerated renin-angiotensin activity and the perfusion requirements of the fat organ further increase the vascular fluid compartment.[2-4,13]

Movement of the expanded blood volume through extensive vascular tissue, under compression by adipose tissue, places greater demand on the myocardium. Increased workload caused by elevation of the basal metabolic rate is reflected in increased cardiac output, increased oxygen (O_2) consumption, increased carbon dioxide production, and normal or slightly abnormal arteriovenous O_2 difference.[2,14] Chronically elevated cardiac output precedes increased left-sided heart pressures and left ventricular hypertrophy. Because heart rate usually remains the same, cardiac output must be augmented by an increase in stroke volume. Therefore cardiomegaly, atrial and biventricular dilation, and biventricular hypertrophy ensue. These contribute to the development of hypertension and eventual congestive heart failure[2-4,13] (Figure 41-3).

Hypertension is defined as a systolic pressure greater than 140 mm Hg, a diastolic pressure greater than 90 mm Hg, or both.[3] The prevalence rates of hypertension in obese patients are more than twice as high as those in lean men and women.[13,15] Blood pressure has been shown to increase 6.5 mm Hg for every 10% increase in body weight.[16] In the nonhypertensive remainder of the severely obese, decreased systemic vascular resistance may serve to facilitate forward blood flow through the doubled body habitus.[2,4] Hypertension is precipitated by increased blood viscosity, catecholamine kinetics, and possibly increased estrogen concentrations.[4] Hyperinsulinemia, elevated mineralocorticoids, and abnormal sodium reabsorption also are implicated as causes of hypertension.[4] Hypercholesterolemia (defined as a cholesterol level greater than 250 mg/dL) often coexists with hypertension, thereby predisposing obese patients to atherosclerosis and cerebrovascular accident.[14,15] Arrhythmias may occur as a result of hypoxemia, hypercapnia, electrolyte disorders, sleep apnea, ventricular hypertrophy, hypertension, and coronary artery disease.

Coronary artery disease in the obese is a frequently associated but independent risk factor. It appears with or without hypertension, hypercholesterolemia, diabetes mellitus, hyperlipidemia, or sedentary lifestyle.[2-4] Obesity coincident with coronary artery disease results in frequent angina, congestive heart failure, acute myocardial infarction, and sudden death.[12-14] Ischemic heart disease is more common in those obese individuals with a central distribution of fat.[13]

Respiratory Considerations

Compromise of respiratory function results from the compression of fat on abdominal, diaphragmatic, and thoracic structures. Over time, thoracic kyphosis and lumbar lordosis develop, resulting in impaired rib movement and fixation of the thorax in an inspiratory position.[1,3] As a result, chest wall, lung, parenchyma, and extrapulmonary compliance is reduced to 35% of predicted values.[17,18] Metabolic needs of the fat organ and the greater mechanical work of breathing stimulate increased myocardial O_2 consumption. Increases in carbon dioxide production and retention, coupled with decreased ventilation, coincide with reduced respiratory muscle efficiency.[2] Lung inflation is inhibited, which causes declinations in functional residual capacity (FRC) to less than closing capacity. Premature airway closure increases dead space and causes carbon dioxide retention, ventilation-perfusion mismatch, shunting, and hypoxemia[1,9] (Figure 41-4). Morbid obesity is associated with reductions in FRC, expiratory reserve volume (ERV), and total lung capacity.[17-19] FRC declines exponentially with increasing BMI.[2] Concomitant diminution of vital capacity, total lung capacity, ERV, and inspiratory capacity are demonstrated by rapid, shallow breathing. These ventilation patterns are characteristic of restrictive lung disease.[2,18,19] Eventual hypoventilation, hypercarbia, and acidosis result from depression of central nervous system responsiveness to chronic hypoxia.[3] Recurrent hypoxemia leads to secondary polycythemia and is associated with an increased risk of coronary artery disease and cerebrovascular disease.[8]

Obstructive Sleep Apnea

Approximately 5% of morbidly obese patients have obstructive sleep apnea (OSA). OSA is characterized by excessive episodes of apnea (10 seconds) and hypopnea during sleep that are caused by complete or partial upper airway obstruction.[20] Hypopnea is a 50% reduction in airflow or reduction sufficient to lead to a 4% decrease in arterial saturation.[8,18-20] Clinically significant episodes of five or more per hour or more than 30 per night result in hypoxia, hypercapnia, systemic and pulmonary hypertension, and cardiac arrhythmias. Daytime sleepiness and cardiopulmonary dysfunction result from interruption of sleep and arterial hypoxemia. Patients characterized with OSA have a BMI >30 kg/m^2, abdominal fat distribution, and a large neck girth (>17 inches in men and >16 inches in women).[2]

Obese Hypoventilation (Pickwickian) Syndrome

Of clinical significance during anesthetization of the morbidly obese patient is the presence of obesity-induced pulmonary syndromes. In conjunction with preexisting risk factors (e.g., history of smoking, emphysema, asthma, sleep apnea), more problems are encountered during the course of intraoperative management. Chaotic maintenance of oxygenation, ventilation, and anesthesia occurs because of alterations in neurologic and cardiopulmonary mechanisms.

Pickwickian syndrome is synonymous with obesity hypoventilation syndrome (OHS).[18-20] OHS, which occurs in 8% of the obese population, is clinically distinct from simple obesity.[19] With simple obesity the partial pressure of arterial carbon dioxide, pH, and pulmonary compliance are within normal ranges.[17] Hypoxia may be present, but no evidence of cardiac failure or arterioalveolar O_2 difference exists. In contrast, OHS is diagnosed when the morbidly obese patient exhibits inappropriate and sudden somnolence, sleep apnea, hypoxia, and hypercapnia.[3] Alveolar ventilation is reduced because of shallow and inefficient ventilation related to decreased tidal volume, inadequate inspiratory strength, and inadequate elevation of the diaphragm. Cardiac enlargement, cyanosis, polycythemia, and twitching also are evident on physical examination.[4] Activities of daily living are altered by the somnolent episodes. Operating machinery or driving a vehicle may cause injury or death.

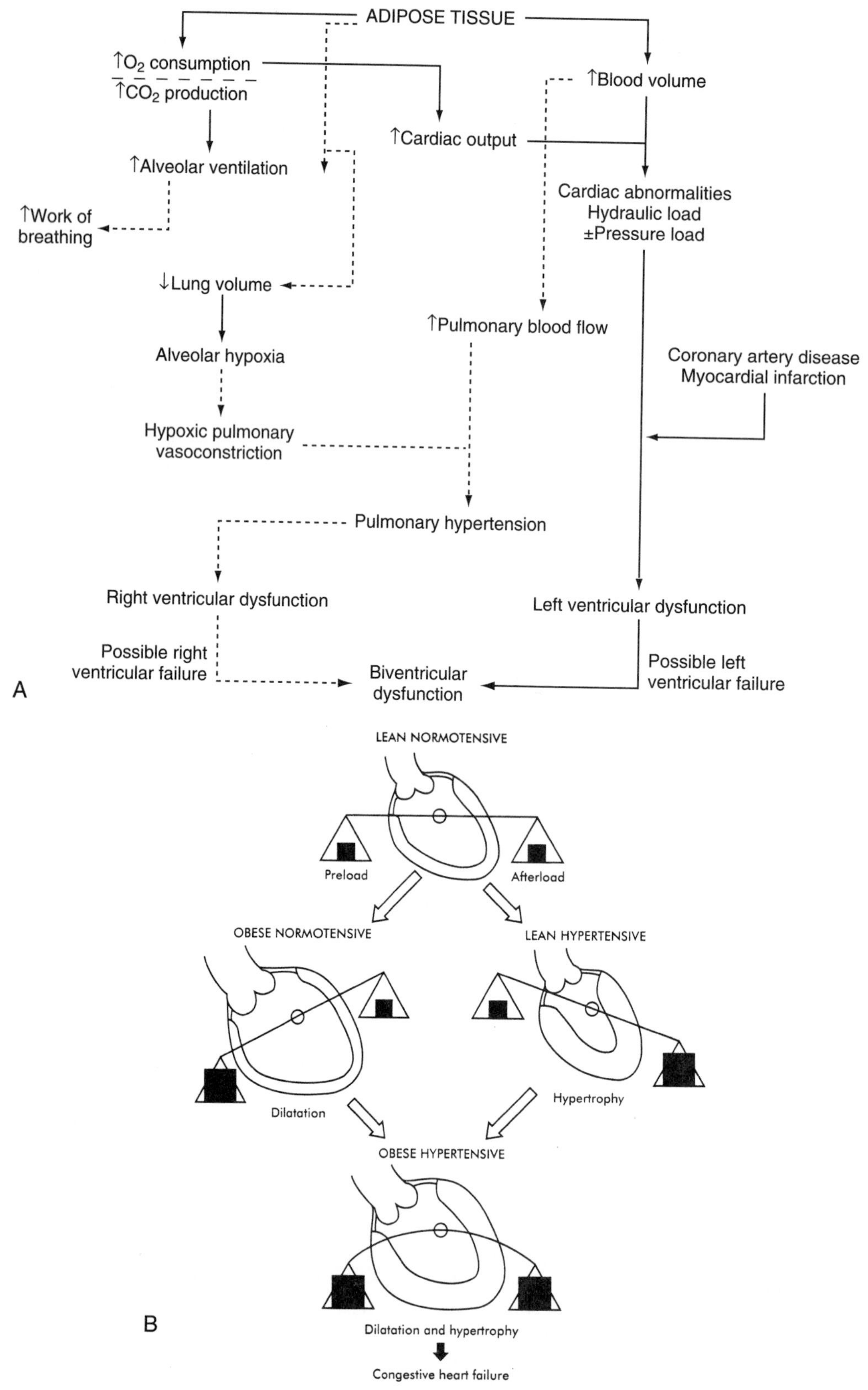

FIGURE **41-3**
A, Cardiovascular problems and morbid obesity. **B,** Adaptation of the heart to obesity, hypertension, and a combination of the two. Although hypertension produces concentric hypertrophy only, obesity plus hypertension produces hypertrophy and dilation (eccentric hypertrophy), associated with a high incidence of congestive heart failure. (**A,** Modified from Vaughan RW. Anesthetic management of the morbidly obese patient. In: *International Anesthesia Research Society 1987 Review Course Lectures*. New York: International Anesthesia Research Society; 1987:11-18. **B,** From Messerli FH. Cardiovascular effects of obesity and hypertension. *Lancet*. 1982;1:1165.)

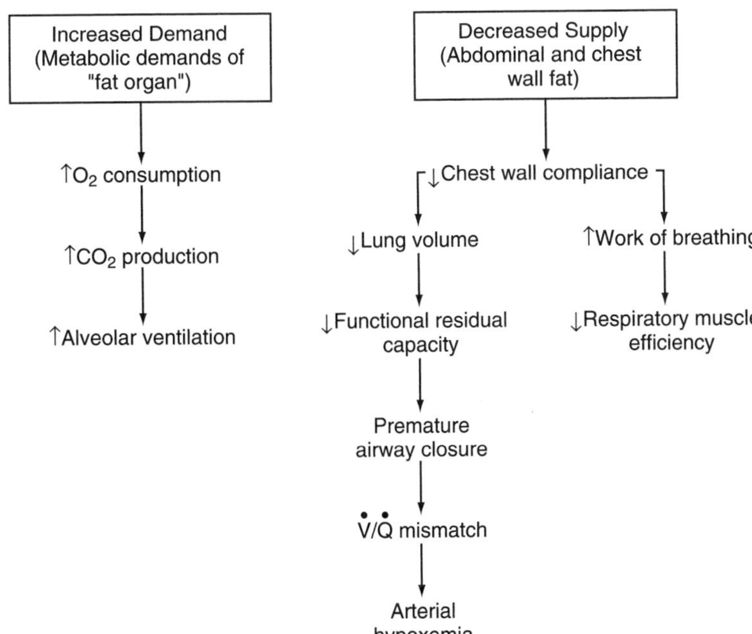

FIGURE **41-4**
Pulmonary problems and morbid obesity. (Modified from Vaughan RW. Pulmonary and cardiovascular derangements in the obese patient. In: Brown BR Jr, ed. *Anesthesia and the Obese Patient: Contemporary Anesthesia Practice*. Philadelphia: FA Davis; 1982:19-41.)

Gastrointestinal Disease

The incidence of gastroesophageal reflux disease, gallstones, and pancreatitis increases with obesity. Obesity is associated with a number of liver abnormalities referred to as *nonalcoholic fatty liver disease* (NAFLD).[21] NAFLD includes steatosis, steatohepatitis, fibrosis, cirrhosis, hepatomegaly, and abnormal liver biochemistry. Liver impairment in severely obese patients is caused by infiltration of hepatocytes with triglycerides. Continued deposition of lipid ruptures the cellular wall of the hepatocyte, causing extrusion of serum lactic dehydrogenase and aspartate aminotransferase.[3] Triglycerides block bile canaliculi and cause elevated serum alkaline phosphatase. Lipid-induced inflammation of the hepatic lobules degenerates to necrosis and intralobular collagen deposition.[4] Portal inflammation or fibrosis ensues in 29% of these patients, and 3% develop cirrhosis.[4] In obese patients the mortality rate from liver cirrhosis is 1.5 to 2.5 times higher than in nonobese persons.[8]

Gallstones

Gallstones are 30% more prevalent in obese than nonobese women, and this prevalence increases linearly with BMI.[4] Higher concentrations of cholesterol in the bile and an increased ratio of bile salts to lecithin are responsible for the development of gallstones.[22] Jaundice may also accompany bile duct obstruction. Laparoscopic and open cholecystectomies are commonly performed in this group of patients because of the increased incidence of gallbladder disease in the obese. Although technically more difficult for both surgical and anesthesia teams, the benefits of laparoscopic gallbladder removal (reduced postoperative pain, shorter hospitalization, earlier return to activities of daily living) may outweigh the risks.

Endocrine and Metabolic Disease

Obesity is seldom the result of primary endocrine dysfunction. Thyroid, adrenocortical, and pituitary function should be investigated with obesity that manifests atypical symptoms.[3] Menstrual problems such as oligomenorrhea, amenorrhea, menorrhagia, and the presence of hirsutism may herald hypothalamic-pituitary abnormalities.[4] Obese men may experience decreased libido or impotence indicative of hypogonadism. Low serum follicle-stimulating hormone and testosterone levels are evident.[4]

Within groups of individuals demonstrating non–insulin-dependent diabetes mellitus, 80% are obese.[2] The risk of type II diabetes increases linearly with BMI.[4] Hyperinsulinemia and impaired insulin receptor sensitivity lead to hyperglycemia and glycosuria.[2] A metabolic or insulin-resistant syndrome, or "syndrome X," has been described in patients with abdominal obesity.[2] It is characterized by insulin resistance, impaired glucose tolerance, type II diabetes, dyslipidemia, and hypertension.[2]

Orthopedic and Joint Disease

Obese persons often develop osteoarthritis from continued mechanical stress on weight-bearing joints. A linear relationship between degree of arthritis and weight exists.[2-4] Ankles, hips, knees, and lumbar spine are frequently burdened. Bone resorption secondary to limited physical activity may also reduce bone density and contribute to stress fractures. Reduction of weight can curb orthopedic injury and lessen the discomfort in the back and lower extremities.

TREATMENT OF OBESITY

A multimodal approach in the treatment of obesity includes dietary intervention, increased exercise, behavior modification, drug therapy, and surgery. Weight-loss programs are individualized to each patient based on the degree of obesity and coexisting conditions. Drug therapy is initiated in patients with a BMI >30 kg/m^2 or BMI between 27 and 29.9 kg/m^2 with a coexisting medical condition.[2-4] Pharmacologic management includes the administration of anorexiant drugs that affect the monoamine oxidase system. Through interactions with norepinephrine, dopamine, and serotonin, anorexiant agents affect satiation (level of fullness), satiety (level of hunger after eating), or both.[2] The most commonly used anorexiant drug is sibutramine hydrochloride (Meridia). Recently, gastrointestinal lipase inhibitors such as orlistat (Xenical) have been used to block the absorption of dietary fat. Overweight and obese patients may self-prescribe "natural" herbs and plant concoctions such as ma huang or diet teas that contain ephedra and unknown quantities of other stimulants.

Surgical Treatment

Besides common surgeries performed within the general population, obese persons undergo additional procedures to ameliorate obesity-related diseases (Box 41-1). Surgical approaches designed to treat obesity can be classified as malabsorptive or restrictive.[23-26] Malabsorptive procedures, which include jejunoileal bypass and biliopancreatic bypass, are rarely used at the present time. Restrictive procedures include the vertical banded gastroplasty (VBG) and gastric banding, including adjustable gastric banding (AGB). Roux-en-**Y** gastric bypass (RYGB) combines gastric restriction with a minimal degree of malabsorption.[23-26] VBG, AGB, and RYGB can all be performed laparoscopically. RYGB is the most commonly performed bariatric procedure in the United States, involves anastomosis of the proximal gastric pouch to a segment of the proximal jejunum, bypassing most of the stomach and the entire duodenum.[23-26] It is the most effective bariatric procedure for production of short-term and long-term weight loss in severely obese patients.[24] Advances in laparoscopic surgery have significantly improved surgical procedure times, morbidity, and mortality related to bariatric surgery.

BOX **41-1**

Obesity-Related Diseases Treated Surgically

Metabolic
Cholelithiasis
Thromboembolism
Peripheral vascular disease
Urolithiasis

Mechanical
Osteoarthritis
Varicose veins
Esophagitis
Hiatal hernia
Abdominal wall hernia

Neoplastic
Cancer (endometrial, breast, prostate, colorectal, renal)
Fibroadenoma of the breast

Gynecologic
Uterine fibroma
Ovarian cysts
Cesarean section
Stress urinary incontinence

From Kral JG. Obesity. In: Lubin MF, Walker HK, Smith RB III, eds. Medical Management of the Surgical Patient. *3rd ed. Philadelphia: Lippincott; 1995:415-423.*

Patients selected for weight-loss surgery are generally younger than 65 years of age and weigh 100 lb or more above IBW.[24] Previous attempts to lose weight must be documented.[23-26] A thorough examination must be performed to rule out underlying physiologic diseases or psychologic disorders.[25] Failure to assess appropriate candidates for surgical intervention and long-term follow-up care may lead to recidivism. Poor compliance with postoperative dietary and exercise regimens can negate any benefit derived from surgical intervention.

Postoperatively patients stay in close contact with multidisciplinary team members. Rehabilitation of previous lifestyle patterns is achieved through counseling and support provided by psychologists, dietitians, physical therapists, and internists.[24-26] Most patients, who are monitored for as long as 5 years postoperatively, achieve losses from their original weight of as much as 40% to 45% with gastric partitioning and 55% to 65% with gastric bypass.[3,24-26]

PHARMACOLOGIC CONSIDERATIONS

Obesity is associated with significant alterations in body composition and function that can alter the pharmacodynamics and pharmacokinetics of drugs.[27] Alterations in the volume of distribution are related to size of the fat organ, increased blood volume, increased cardiac output, decreased total body water, alterations in protein binding, and lipophilicity of the drug.[27] Highly lipophilic drugs have an increased volume of distribution in obese persons compared with normal-weight individuals.[23] The increased volume of distribution requires higher doses of lipophilic drugs to produce the required pharmacologic effect and prolongs the elimination of certain drugs such as Pentothal and benzodiazepines. Factors such as protein binding and end organ clearance affect volume of distribution.

No systemic relationship exists between the solubility and the distribution of some highly lipophilic drugs (digoxin, remifentanil, and procainamide) in obese patients.[23] Determination of dosage according to IBW is appropriate with these drugs. Dosages of drugs with weak or moderate lipophilicity are usually determined on the basis of IBW or lean body mass. Recommendations for determining the dosages of commonly used anesthetics are listed in Table 41-3.[23,27-31] Clinical judgment guides the determination of dosages for individual patients and the administration of pharmacologic agents in overweight and obese patients.

Elimination of drugs in obese individuals is normal or increased in phase I reactions (oxidation, reduction, hydrolysis) and increased in phase II reactions (metabolism). Renal clearance is increased because of augmented renal blood flow and glomerular filtration rate.[2]

Parenteral Drug Administration

The intravenous route allows dependable and precise drug administration in morbidly obese patients. Patient-controlled analgesia, commonly used in postoperative pain management, is an example of intravenous administration technology. Caution must be observed, however, when drugs are injected via the subcutaneous or intramuscular route. If the drug is deposited into adipose, absorption and efficacy of the drug is unpredictable because of reduced vascularization. As a result the patient may not receive adequate analgesia or maximum therapeutic drug response. Use of a longer needle inserted into the muscle with the least fat (deltoid) may be more reliable.

TABLE 41-3 Guidelines for Dosages of Intravenous Anesthetics in Obese Patients

Anesthetic Agent	Basis for Calculation of Dosage	Guidelines
Midazolam	TBW	Increase central V_D; increase initial dose to achieve therapeutic effect; prolonged sedation
Thiopental	TBW	Increase V_D; increase initial dose; prolonged time to awakening
Propofol	TBW (initial and infusion)	Increase V_D; increase initial dose; high affinity for fat; high hepatic extraction
Fentanyl	TBW	Increase V_D; increase elimination half-time
Sufentanil	TBW	Increase V_D; increase elimination half-time
Remifentanil	IBW	Consider age and lean body mass
cis-Atracurium	TBW	No difference from patients with normal weight
Vecuronium	IBW	Increase V_D; impaired hepatic clearance; prolonged duration of action
Rocuronium	IBW	Faster onset and similar duration of action than normal weight patient
Succinylcholine	TBW	Increase plasma pseudocholinesterase activity; increase dose

IBW, *Ideal body weight;* TBW, *total body weight;* V_D, *volume of distribution.*
From *Ogunnaike BO, Jones SB, Jones DB, et al. Anesthetic considerations for bariatric surgery.* Anesth Analg. 2002;95:1793-1805; *Hunter JD, Reid C, Noble D. Anesthetic management of the morbidly obese patient.* Hosp Med. 1998;59:481-483; *Song D, Whitten CW, White PF. Remifentanil infusion facilitates early recovery for obese outpatients undergoing laparoscopic cholecystectomy.* Anesth Analg. 2000;90:111-113; *Slepchenko G, Simon N, Goubaux B, Levron JC, Le Moing JP, Raucoules-Aime M. Performance of target-controlled sufentanil infusion in obese patients.* Anesthesiology. 2003;98:65-73; *Puhringer FK, Keller C, Kleinsaser A, et al. Pharmacokinetics of rocuronium bromide in obese female patients.* Eur J Anaesthesiol. 1999;16:507-510; *Salihoglu Z, Karaca S, Kose Y, Zengin K, Taskin M. Total intravenous anesthesia versus single breath technique and anesthesia maintenance with sevoflurane for bariatric operations.* Obes Surg. 2001;11:496-501.

Biotransformation of Inhaled Anesthetics

Intraoperative hepatic concerns stem from alterations in biotransformation and metabolism of drugs. Isoflurane, desflurane and sevoflurane have been used with minimal complications in overweight and obese patients.[32-34]

Sevoflurane is pleasant smelling and nonirritating to the airway. Sevoflurane causes increased levels of serum inorganic fluorides to be metabolized at a rate 100% faster in obese patients than in nonobese patients.[32-34] Its potential ability to enhance fluoride ion concentrations in obese patients with marginal renal function (creatinine greater than 1.5 mg/dL) and production of compound A (with low fresh gas flows less than 2 L/min) may necessitate the use of another inhalation agent.[32]

Sevoflurane and desflurane are the least soluble of all the potent inhalation anesthetics. Of the two, desflurane is the most resistant to hepatic degradation (less than 0.02% with desflurane versus 0.2% with sevoflurane). With its low solubility profile, rapid washout, absence of hepatic and renal toxicity, and support of blood pressure, desflurane may be the preferred inhalation agent in morbidly obese patients.[32-34]

ANESTHETIC MANAGEMENT: PREANESTHETIC EVALUATION

The goals of the preanesthetic evaluation are to obtain pertinent data regarding the patient's medical or surgical history, to optimize current physiologic functioning, and to determine an appropriate anesthetic plan (see Chapter 17). Of paramount importance is the need to establish a nonjudgmental and trusting relationship with the patient. Explanations of anticipated events during preoperative preparation (multiple venipunctures, central and arterial line insertions, awake intubation, pain management) and protection of the patient's privacy will allay anxiety.

Medications

Obese persons must be queried for concurrent use of weight-reducing substances, herbal supplements, and anorexiant drugs. Chronic use of noradrenergic and serotonergic therapy can produce hypertension, tachycardia, anxiety, psychosis, and catecholamine depletion.[27] Patients who take over-the-counter drugs including herbal medications often forget or are afraid to reveal that they are taking these preparations, which can have deleterious consequences on induction. Catecholamine depletion can summate in profound hypotension during induction and maintenance of anesthesia, which is refractory to indirect-acting vasopressors such as ephedrine. Phenylephrine hydrochloride (Neo-Synephrine) is usually effective in reversing low blood pressure. At least 2 weeks of abstinence from the drugs is recommended for adequate catecholamine levels to be recovered.[27]

Laboratory Tests

Given the current climate of cost-consciousness and cost-efficiency, only the laboratory tests appropriate in light of the patient's history, physical examination, and planned surgery should be ordered.[12] In morbidly obese patients baseline studies that may be directly affected by associated medical conditions are performed. Routine testing includes assessment of a complete blood count and electrolyte panel. Complete blood cell counts may reveal hematocrits as high as 65%, which can result from contracted blood volume or polycythemia associated with cardiopulmonary disease.[12,17] Leukocytosis (greater than 11,000 μL) is a strong predictor of risk for acute myocardial infarction independent of tobacco smoking.[7]

Arterial blood gas analysis that compares samples taken with the patient lying supine and sitting while breathing room air provides baseline values and can distinguish simple obesity from OHS. The renal panel may reflect abnormal glucose and potassium levels, which are indicators of insulin resistance and potentiation of myocardial irritability. Concomitant use of diuretics and certain cardiac medications can exacerbate electrolyte disturbances.[12] Blood urea nitrogen (BUN) and creatinine levels may be elevated in response to dehydration or renal dysfunction. Liver function tests are typically elevated in obese patients. This is generally not the result of hepatic disease but of infiltration of the hepatocytes with triglycerides (fatty liver, liver steatosis). The severity of fatty infiltration may alter pharmacologic effects of many anesthetic drugs, thereby requiring dose reductions.[27]

Coagulation studies are necessary if regional anesthesia is planned or if coagulopathy exists. Patients taking anticoagulants for treatment of deep vein thrombosis or atrial fibrillation may exhibit elevated prothrombin and partial thromboplastin times. Use of nonsteroidal antiinflammatory drugs may prolong bleeding times and affect surgical hemostasis.

In obese patients undergoing abdominal or thoracic surgery, pulmonary function tests are invaluable and essential for anesthetic planning; for selected procedures, the tests may be waived.[8] Chest radiography is necessary to determine the presence of cardiomegaly, pulmonary infiltrates, and evidence of chronic obstructive pulmonary disease.

Cardiac Assessment

Evaluation of cardiac function is essential in overweight and obese patients undergoing surgery. Investigation of prior myocardial infarction and the presence of hypertension, angina, or peripheral vascular disease is crucial. Limitations in exercise tolerance, history of orthopnea, and paroxysmal nocturnal dyspnea may indicate left ventricular dysfunction.[2-4] A careful elicitation of drug history is invaluable in garnering clues about the patient's coexistent diseases. When possible, cardiac medications should be continued up to and including the morning of surgery.

An electrocardiogram is essential for determination of resting rate, rhythm, and ventricular hypertrophy or strain. Ischemic changes or evidence of coronary artery disease must be investigated.[12,17] The electrocardiogram may be of low voltage because of the excess overlying tissue and therefore might result in underestimation of the severity of ventricular hypertrophy. Axis deviation and atrial tachyarrhythmias are relatively common.[4]

QT-interval prolongation, discovered retrospectively in severely obese patients who died from refractory dysrhythmias, is a marker for sudden cardiac arrest.[3] In cases of fatal and nonfatal dieting, prolonged QT intervals were also exhibited on patient electrocardiograms.[4] In addition, sudden cardiac death is more prevalent in morbidly obese patients with left ventricular hypertrophy and ventricular ectopy.[5]

Exercise testing may elicit valuable information about myocardial function in morbidly obese patients. Most are physically unable, however, to achieve adequate levels of exercise stress to make the studies worthwhile.[12] Alternative tests using dipyridamole-thallium are satisfactory for determining myocardial adequacy. In addition, echocardiography is useful for determining whether akinesis or wall motion abnormalities are present in the obese myocardium.

Cardiomegaly, pulmonary congestion, elevated diaphragm, and a tortuous aorta can be identified by use of chest radiography. Results of radiographic studies serve to guide preoperative pharmacologic and medical management (diuretics, β_1-agonists, antibiotics). Repeated radiographs may be required to obtain adequate penetration and visualization of all lung fields.[27] Unfortunately, standard stationary and portable x-ray machines cannot accommodate massively obese persons. As a result, diagnostic x-ray examinations or evaluation of central line placement may be impossible. Under these circumstances, clinical expertise and management of subtle symptoms is invaluable. If it is indicated, the patient should be referred to a cardiologist for further investigation and optimization of his or her condition (e.g., control of blood pressure, treatment of heart failure, or coronary angioplasty).[35]

Respiratory Evaluation

Careful preoperative evaluation of the patient's respiratory function identifies potential problems. A patient who becomes dyspneic and desaturates when recumbent experiences the same symptoms during induction in the supine position.[36] Questions must elicit information regarding the presence or absence of orthopnea, wheezing, sputum production, or smoking history. Recent upper respiratory infection, snoring, or sleep disturbances may indicate obstructive processes. Room air pulse oximetry saturations and blood gases obtained in supine and upright positions may reflect disturbances in cardiac compensation.[19]

Airway Evaluation

A thorough airway evaluation is warranted for determination of the optimal airway management technique in overweight and obese patients.[36] A variety of assessment criteria have been evaluated for prediction of difficult intubation in obese patients.[37-39] Most practitioners use evaluation of multiple patient physical characteristics to identify potential airway problems indicative of the unanticipated difficult airway. These include measurement of interincisor distance, thyromental distance, head and neck extension, Mallampati classification, body weight, and a history of difficult airway.[37-39] Inspection of the oropharynx is necessary to determine Mallampati classification for intubation difficulty (Figure 41-5). Evaluation of the length of upper incisors, visibility of the uvula, shape of the palate, compliance of the mandibular space, and length and thickness of the neck provides further criteria for assessment. Increasing neck circumference and Mallampati classification >3 have been identified as the two most important factors in morbidly obese patients.[37]

Anatomic aberrations of the upper airway induced by severe obesity include reduced temporomandibular and atlantooccipital joint movement. Unsatisfactory mouth opening, presence of neck or arm pain, or inability to place the head and neck into "sniffing position" (Figure 41-6) may indicate the need for awake fiberoptic intubation. Extreme airway narrowing, in conjunction with shortened mandibular-hyoid distance (less than three fingerbreadths) can complicate mask ventilation and intubation. Presence of a short, thick neck, pendulous breasts, hypertrophied tonsils and adenoids, or a beard can contribute to a difficult airway. Marginal room air pulse oximeter saturations, abnormal arterial blood gases, and history of complicated airway management also indicate a potentially difficult intubation.[37-39] (Refer to Chapter 20 for a full description of the assessment and management of a difficult airway.) Airway management techniques should be explained to the patient, with emphasis on awake intubation and the need for postoperative ventilation.[40,41]

Vascular Access

Venipuncture can be challenging in overweight and obese patients with excessive fat that obscures blood vessels from

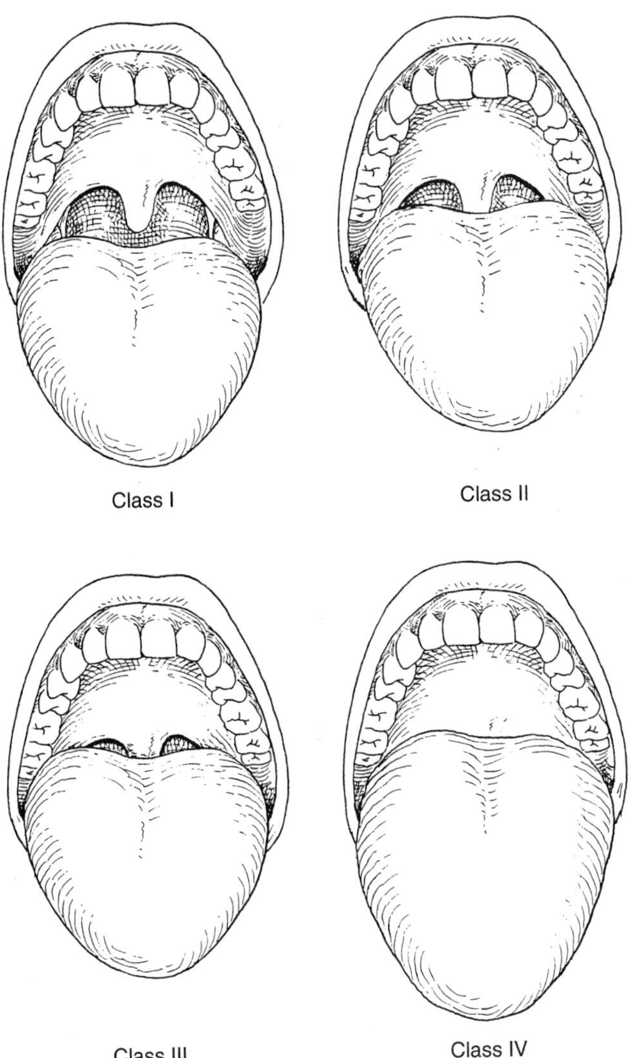

FIGURE **41-5**
Mallampati classification for intubation difficulty. (From Mallampati SR, Gatt SP, Gugino LD, et al. A clinical sign to predict difficult tracheal intubation: a prospective study. *Can Anaesth Soc J*. 1985;32:429-434.)

both visualization and palpation.[8] Central cannulation of vessels is impeded by distortions of the underlying anatomy by adipose tissue.[42] Hemorrhage, hypothermia, and trauma further reduce the likelihood of accessing vessels with ease. Use of a portable ultrasound machine may improve central venous catheter placement. As in all patients, iatrogenic pneumothorax must be avoided. Morbidly obese patients are less able than nonobese patients to tolerate the ensuing respiratory impairment.

ANESTHETIC MANAGEMENT: PREPARATION

Equipment

In preparation for emergent operating room procedures or nonemergent hospital admission, appropriate equipment must be readied. Newer model operating room tables can accommodate up to 600 pounds of weight. Older model standard operating room tables could hydraulically elevate 300 to 350 pounds of weight. In cases of extreme morbid obesity, "big boy" hydraulic beds are obtained and used in the operating room. Heavy-duty stirrups, extra-large retractors, elongated instruments, arm sleds, doubled arm boards, and extremity tourniquets must be obtained. Sometimes a sanitized engine crane or other hoisting device must be used to suspend the panniculus adiposus for optimal surgical exposure.

Extra-large thigh cuffs can be used on the upper arm or the lower leg (over the posterior tibial artery). A regular-size or large blood pressure cuff can be used on the forearm over the radial artery until arterial cannulation for blood pressure monitoring can be performed. Bed warming devices, fluid warmers, and warm airflow blankets should be employed to prevent hypothermia, which can occur rapidly when large areas of body surface are exposed.

Monitoring

Intraoperative monitoring, both basic and advanced, should address the specific needs of the patient.[27] Selection of electrocardiographic leads, when possible, should enhance detection of myocardial ischemia and pathology (leads II and V_5). Needle electrodes may be useful for obtaining a better tracing. Placement of an arterial catheter is appropriate for the monitoring of hemodynamic status and is advocated for all but the

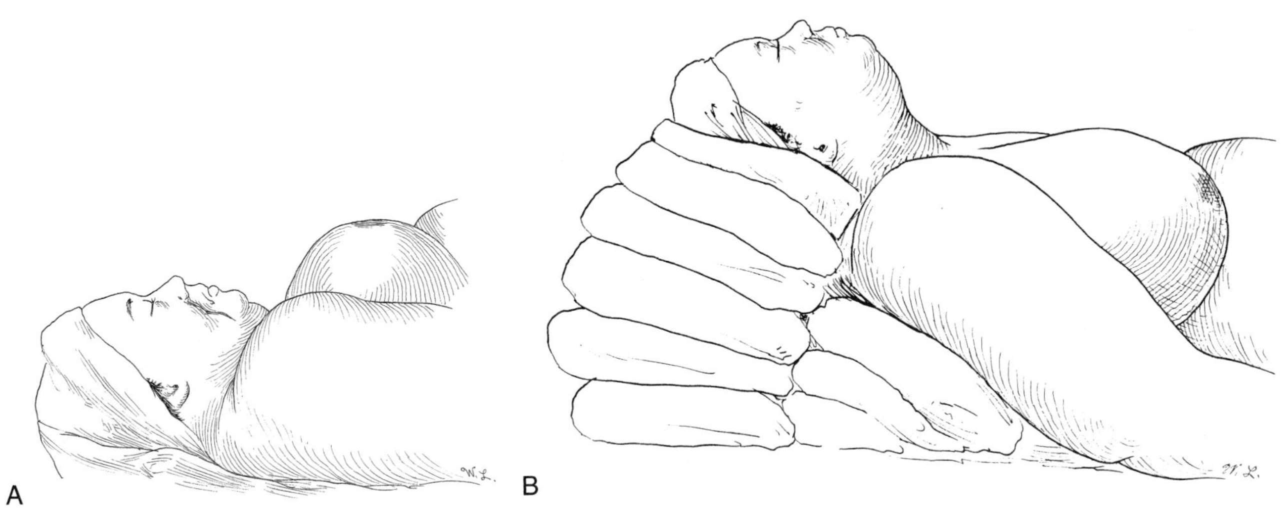

FIGURE **41-6**
A, Supine position. **B,** Sniffing position.

most minor procedures in the morbidly obese.[8] Use of central venous and pulmonary artery catheters should be considered in patients undergoing extensive surgery or those with serious cardiorespiratory disease.[27,42]

Aspiration Prophylaxis

Of further significance with the anesthetized obese airway is the increased risk of regurgitation (passive and active) and subsequent pulmonary aspiration.[43-45] Obese persons have greater volumes of and more acidic gastric fluid than persons of normal weight. Gastroesophageal reflux and hiatus hernia, which are more prevalent in the obese, also predispose them to esophagitis and pulmonary aspiration.[2] Other conditions that cause delayed gastric emptying, such as diabetes mellitus and traumatic injury, further increase the risk of aspiration. For these reasons the obese patient is considered to have a "full stomach," even if the prescribed nothing-by-mouth intake restriction has been followed. Debate and controversy exist regarding the relative risk of aspiration in obesity, with most practitioners using techniques to attenuate this complication.[45]

Timely preinduction administration of histamine-2 and dopamine receptor antagonists coupled with oral administration of nonparticulate antacids decreases morbidity resulting from pulmonary aspiration and Mendelson's syndrome.[8] Head-up positioning of the patient, with application of the Sellick maneuver during rapid-sequence induction, limits the volume of vomitus that enters the trachea if regurgitation occurs.[8] Nasogastric or orogastric suctioning before emergence further reduces the amount of fluid available for aspiration.

Airway Equipment

An equally important part of airway assessment is the preparation of equipment and personnel necessary to ventilate and intubate the morbidly obese patient. An assortment of blades, laryngoscopy handles, endotracheal tubes, masks, oral and nasopharyngeal airways, and stylets should be assembled. Laryngeal mask airways (LMAs), fiberoptic and bronchoscopic devices, Eschmann introducers, a jet ventilator (or Venturi apparatus), and emergency tracheotomy and cricothyrotomy kits must be available in the event that ventilation by mask or endotracheal tube is unsuccessful. Most departments have a difficult airway cart that has all of the available equipment that should be placed in the operating room.

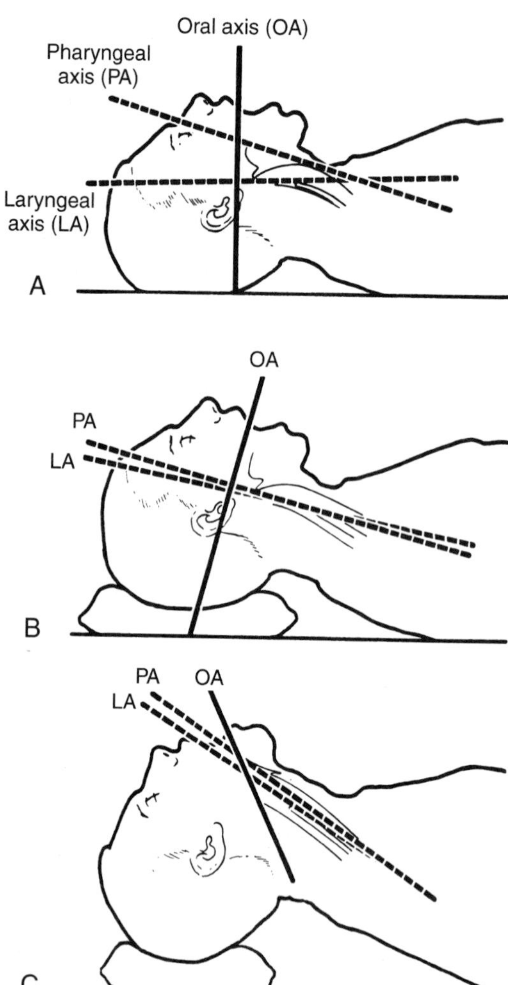

FIGURE **41-7**
Schematic diagram demonstrating head position for endotracheal intubation. **A,** Successful direct laryngoscopy for exposure of the glottic opening requires alignment of the oral, pharyngeal, and laryngeal axes. **B,** Elevation of the head approximately 10 cm with pads under the occiput with the shoulders remaining on the table aligns the laryngeal and pharyngeal axes. **C,** Subsequent head extension at the atlantooccipital joint serves to create the shortest distance and most nearly straight line from the incisor teeth to glottic opening. (From Stone DJ, Gal TJ. Airway management. In: Miller RD, ed. *Anesthesia.* 5th ed. New York: Churchill Livingstone; 2000:1419.)

ANESTHETIC MANAGEMENT: MAINTENANCE

Intubation

For airway management to be facilitated, the obese patient should be positioned with the head elevated (reverse Trendelenburg position) on the operating room table.[46] This position promotes patient comfort, reduces gastric reflux, provides easier mask ventilation, improves respiratory mechanics, and helps maintain FRC. The reduced FRC in obese patients contributes to the rapid desaturation that occurs with induction of general anesthesia.[46] To attenuate the desaturation and maximize O_2 content in the lungs, patients are preoxygenated with 100% mask O_2 for at least 3 to 5 minutes.[47] The patient's head, neck, and shoulders should be carefully moved into "sniffing position" by using pillows, "doughnuts," or foam head supports (see Figure 41-6, *B*). Without proper support and alignment of the oropharynx and trachea (Figure 41-7), ventilation may be obstructed and visualization of the laryngeal structures may be obscured.

Some practitioners advocate the use of an "awake look" to visualize the difficulty of the airway.[37-41] Careful administration of sedative drugs and application of topical anesthesia to the oropharyngeal structures, possibly including transtracheal and superior laryngeal nerve blocks, are performed. Nasal O_2 is used as a supplement during awake laryngoscopy. If the epiglottic and laryngeal architecture is easily visualized, successful asleep intubation can be done. If the airway structures cannot be visualized, an intubating LMA or awake fiberoptic intubation should be used.[40,48,49] The endotracheal tube must be safely secured to prevent movement during positioning and surgery.[50]

The surgeon and another skilled anesthesia provider must also be in attendance during the induction. Muscle hypotonus in the floor of the mouth, followed by rapid occurrence of soft tissue obstruction and hypoxia, requires one person to support the mask and airway while another person bag-ventilates the patient.[27] In the case of inability to ventilate or intubate, the American Society of Anesthesiologists' difficult airway algorithm should be followed (see Chapter 20). Intubation of the obese patient can be safely accomplished with careful assessment and planning and use of airway techniques familiar to the anesthetist.

Effects of General Anesthesia on Respiration

General anesthesia depresses respiration in normal subjects, so any preexisting pulmonary dysfunction is exaggerated by anesthesia.[8] The type of surgery, positioning, and underlying disease pathology further compound the undesirable respiratory responses caused by obesity and anesthesia.[51-56] General anesthesia causes a 50% reduction in FRC in the obese anesthetized patient, as compared with a 20% reduction in anesthetized nonobese patients.[50] FRC can be increased by ventilating with large tidal volumes (15 to 20 ml/kg), although this has been shown to improve arterial O_2 tension only minimally.[23,51] In contrast, the addition of positive end-expiratory pressure (PEEP) achieves an improvement in both FRC and arterial O_2 tension but only at the expense of cardiac output and O_2 delivery.[53,54] Current ventilation recommendations include using tidal volumes of 10 to 12 ml/kg to avoid barotrauma.[23] During laparoscopic surgeries the respiratory rate should be 12 to 14 breaths per minute.[23]

Prolonged (longer than 2 to 3 hours) and extensive procedures (those involving the abdomen, thorax, and spine) negatively influence respiratory function. Subdiaphragmatic packing, cephalad displacement of organs, and surgical retraction cause decreased alveolar ventilation, atelectasis, and pulmonary congestion.[51,52] Recumbent or Trendelenburg positioning further reduces diaphragmatic excursion, which is already impaired by the weight of the panniculus (which can be very large) (Figure 41-8). Trendelenburg positioning also causes elevated filling pressures, which then increase right ventricular preload. Subsequently, myocardial O_2 consumption, cardiac output, pulmonary artery occluding pressures, peak inspiratory pressures, and venous admixtures are increased above upright-sitting values.[53]

In a normal-weight person, cardiac output increases in response to supine posturing to maintain hemodynamic stability. By increasing left ventricular output the centrally located circulating volume is propelled forward, thereby minimizing pulmonary congestion and hypoxia. In a severely obese patient, positive-pressure ventilation (which impedes venous return) and inability to increase cardiac output may result in cardiopulmonary decompensation.[54,55] This is exhibited intraoperatively by hypoxia, rales, ventricular ectopy, congestive heart failure, and hypotension.[56] Bag ventilation by hand may be useful to attenuate hypotension resulting from positive pressure.

Use of ventilators powerful enough to inflate the morbidly obese thorax is critical to minimizing hypoxia. Pressure- or volume-controlled ventilators can be used to maintain adequate oxygenation and normocapnia. Avoidance of prolonged prone, Trendelenburg, or supine positioning also decreases ventilation-perfusion mismatch. Optimization of oxygenation by using no less than 50% flow of inspired O_2 is emphatically recommended.[8,19,23] Intermittent manual "sighs" of large volume can also augment the FRC.

Application of PEEP can reduce venous admixture and support adequate arterial oxygenation.[55] PEEP, however, can impair arterial oxygenation in some patients when it is superimposed on large tidal volumes.[55] For these reasons PEEP that exceeds 15 cm H_2O is not recommended.

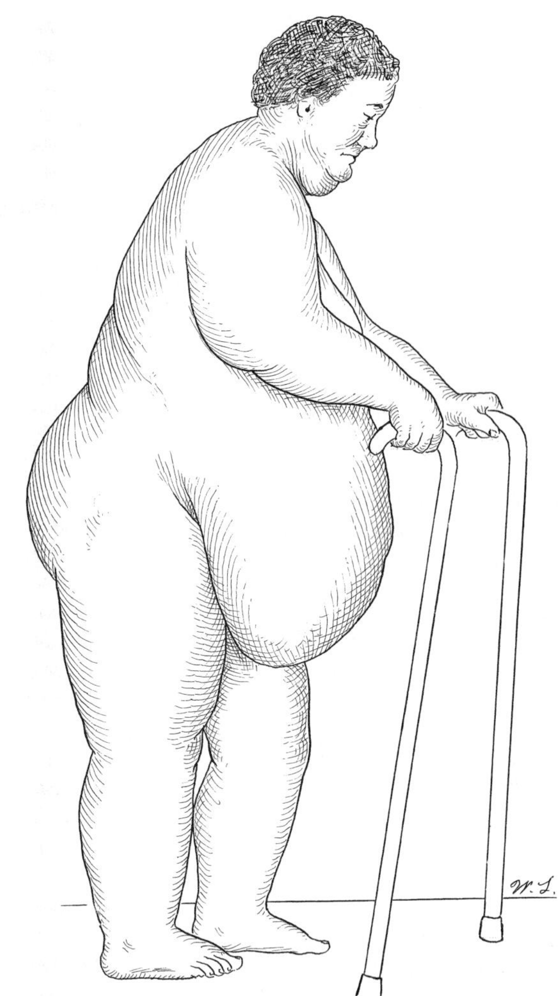

FIGURE **41-8**
Panniculus in a standing patient.

Other intraoperative events, such as hemorrhage or hypotension, further impair ventilatory homeostasis and result in hypoxemia that extends into the postoperative period.[18] A vertical abdominal incision, compared with a horizontal (transverse) incision, also prolongs postoperative hypoxia.[36] Pain causes further reductions in diaphragmatic excursion and vital capacity, leading to atelectasis and ventilation-perfusion mismatch.[8,23] For these reasons 24-hour postoperative admission to a monitored bed is prudent for severely obese patients, who already exhibit higher morbidity and mortality apart from anesthesia and surgery.

Choice of Anesthetic Technique

Selection of the anesthetic technique is dependent on the patient, coexisting history, planned surgical procedure, anesthetist skill and preference, and patient preference. Diverse anesthetic techniques have been described for use with obese patients undergoing surgical and diagnostic procedures.[57-61] Anesthetic management of obese patients can include local or monitored anesthesia; general (narcotic, inhalation) anesthesia; regional blocks; or a combination of techniques.

No demonstrable difference in emergence from inhalation versus narcotic technique has been discerned in the obese.[8,31,33,34] The use of short-acting water-soluble anesthetics facilitates smooth anesthetic induction, maintenance, and emergence from anesthesia.[31,33,34] Objectives for maintenance of anesthesia in the obese include strict maintenance of airway, adequate skeletal muscle relaxation, optimum oxygenation, avoidance of the residual effects of muscle relaxants, provision of appropriate intraoperative and postoperative tidal volume, and effective postoperative analgesia.[8,23] Depending on the patient's condition, these can be achieved by either general or regional anesthesia. An epidural anesthetic with concomitant "light" general anesthesia is frequently chosen. A light general anesthetic can facilitate management of the airway, ventilation, and the patient's level of consciousness, whereas the epidural provides surgical analgesia and anesthesia. The epidural catheter can be used for postoperative analgesic administration and will enhance earlier resumption of deep breathing and coughing maneuvers.

Volume Replacement

Despite the augmentation of circulatory fluid that accompanies morbid obesity, the estimated blood volume is actually diminished.[7] Fat, which contains only 8% to 10% water, contributes less fluid to total body water than equivalent amounts of muscle. The normal adult percentage of total body water is 60% to 65%.[8] In the severely obese it is reduced to 40%.[7] Therefore calculation of estimated blood volume should be 45 to 55 ml/kg of actual body weight rather than the 70 ml/kg apportioned in nonobese adults.[7] Use of reduced parameters for volume replacement and avoidance of rapid rehydration lessen cardiopulmonary compromise. Fluid management is guided by blood pressure, heart rate, and urine output measurements. Volume expanders, such as hetastarch (Hespan), should not be administered at greater than recommended volumes per kilogram of IBW (20 ml/kg). Dilutional coagulopathy, factor VIII inhibition, and decreased platelet aggregability can result from excessive administration. Albumin 5% and 25% should be used as indicated to support circulatory volume and oncotic pressure. When blood loss is replaced with crystalloid, the 3:1 ratio (3 ml of crystalloid to 1 ml of blood loss) is applicable in severely obese patients. Blood products, after careful identification, should be replaced according to the patient's laboratory values and hemodynamic or surgical need. No difference in the criteria between the administration of blood products in normal weight patients versus severely obese patients has been identified.

Intraoperative Positioning

Surgical positioning of morbidly obese patients necessitates extra precautions for the prevention of nerve, integumentary, and cardiorespiratory compromise. The type of surgery, combined with inordinate stretching or compression of nerve plexus, and prolonged immobility cause local tissue ischemia and damage, which begins at the cellular level.[62] Hypothermia, hypotension, table positioning, and the hydraulic pressure effect that the adipose places on orthopedic or cardiopulmonary structures potentiate impairment.[62]

Although many peripheral nerves are subjected to possible ischemia or necrosis, the lunar, brachial plexus, radial, personal, and sphenoid nerves are the most vulnerable to injury in any anesthetized patient.[62] In morbidly obese patients the incidence may be increased because of excessive weight on the anatomic structures.[62] Care is necessary when one is positioning obese extremities in slings, draping them on Mayo stands, or securing them in lithotomy stirrups. Excess weight and loose skin may "strangle" or macerate tissues on the dangling ankle or wrist. Cavalier draping of heavy upper extremities atop poorly secured Mayo stands can cause cuts, bruises, or abrasions of the arm, breast, or abdomen, as well as obscure early signs of skin breakdown or circulatory compromise.

Prolonged hyperextension, external rotation, or abduction greater than 90 degrees overstretches the brachial plexus and can cause postoperative muscle pain, nerve palsies, or paralysis. Often, obese patients do not have the range of motion that nonobese individuals possess. Therefore less flexion or abduction and rotation of hips, legs, and arms may be necessary. Frequent palpation of pulses, generous padding, correct alignment, and repeated inspection of extremities for color and temperature can help diminish the incidence of positioning-related injuries.[63]

Lower back pain can be aggravated by both spinal and general anesthesia because of ligamentous relaxation that results in loss of lumbar curvature. Surgical towels placed under the lumbar spine before induction will enhance lordosis and reduce postoperative discomfort.[62]

Treatment of the panniculus is often a major concern for both anesthetist and surgeon. Extra-long straps and wide adhesive tape can secure the panniculus and reduce shifting when the operating table is changed.[63] If Trendelenburg positioning is anticipated, some means to prevent its sliding cephalad must be devised. The head-down position, coupled with the crushing weight of the thorax and panniculus, compresses the brachial neurovascular bundle between the clavicle and first rib.[63] If the patient requires a fracture table, ensure that sufficient padding encircles the pole adjacent to the patient's vulva or penis.[63] Genital and pudendal nerve injury can be profound if adipose tissue surrounding the thigh is not carefully distracted to reveal proper placement of the padding.

Integumentary Concerns

Decubitus, skin infection, and wound dehiscence are exceedingly common in the severely obese. Decubitus arise from prolonged immobility and compression of the fat on bony prominences and vessels. Traction, external fixation devices, and straps may cause certain types of injury. Intertriginous creases of skin are subject to erosion and ulceration from sweat and constant friction of apposing skin surfaces. Inability to perform hygiene under the breasts, between neck folds, or beneath the abdominal pannus accommodates organismal proliferation. Concomitant diabetes, which interferes with leukocyte function, further accelerates the growth of bacterial or fungal infections.[2,3] As a result, wound dehiscence, particularly in the abdomen, can occur after suboptimal surgical closure in compromised skin. A poorly vascularized panniculus and torsion on the wound by the weight of the fat apron also contribute to malunion of the tissue.[63] Although atelectasis and hypoxia are less frequent with a horizontal laparotomy, a vertical laparotomy approach is often preferred by the surgical team. Compression of abdominal contents on superficial wound layers is lessened during ambulation and therefore may reduce the occurrence of dehiscence.[25]

Extubation

The risk of airway obstruction after extubation is increased in obese patients.[64] A decision to extubate depends on evaluation of the ease of mask ventilation and tracheal intubation, the length and type of surgery, and the presence of preexisting medical conditions, including OSA. Criteria for extubation include an awake state; tidal volume and respiratory rate at preoperative levels; ability to sustain head lift or leg lift for at least

5 seconds; strong, constant hand grip; effective cough; adequate vital capacity of at least 15 ml/kg; and inspiratory force of at least −25 to −30 cm H_2O. Patients must be placed with the head up or in a sitting position. If doubt exists regarding the ability of the patient to breathe adequately, the endotracheal tube is left in place Extubation over an airway exchange catheter or via a fiberoptic bronchoscope may be performed.[64]

Regional Anesthesia

Regional anesthesia can be used as the primary anesthetic in selected cases or as an accompaniment to postoperative pain and mobility management.[8,14,63] Difficulties are frequently encountered, though, in severely obese patients. Anatomic landmarks used to guide conduction blockade are not easily visualized or palpable. Brachial plexus anesthesia can be hampered by adipose tissue in the axillary region, inability to position the arm, and an undetectable pulse. Full-term pregnancy, obesity, and the coincident discomfort of active labor further inhibit the discernment of spinous processes and posterior iliac crests. Redundant rolls of fat, unsatisfactory ventilation, and inability of the patient to sustain optimal positioning make neuraxial anesthesia even more challenging (see Chapter 42).

For subarachnoid or epidural anesthesia it is recommended that the patient sit upright so that landmarks such as C7 or L3 to L4 can be more easily identified.[26] In addition, skin-fat folds will fall toward the operating table, and respiratory ventilation will be enhanced. A selection of longer needles (7 inches) should also be available before anesthetic administration is begun. Generous infiltration with local anesthetic will provide greater patient comfort during insertion of the "finder," Tuohy, or spinal needle. The importance of generous administration of local anesthetic cannot be overemphasized because repeated insertions and repositioning of the needle or introducer may be required before access to the epidural (or subarachnoid) space is achieved.

Another consideration regarding subarachnoid or epidural anesthesia in severely obese pregnant or surgical patients is the lack of predictability of spread of local anesthetic.[64] A significant correlation exists with increased body mass and rostral spread of epidural subarachnoid anesthetics when a patient is positioned supine.[64] Undesirable cephalad spread of local anesthetics can be obviated by reducing the volume and increasing the patient's upright sitting time.

ANESTHETIC MANAGEMENT: POSTOPERATIVE CARE

Pain Management

Optimal postoperative pain management is facilitated by the use of oral analgesics, nonsteroidal antiinflammatory agents, narcotics, patient-controlled analgesia, local infiltration of surgical site and epidural anesthesia. Obese patients are more sensitive to the respiratory depressant effects of opioid analgesics; therefore caution and close monitoring are warranted. Supplemental O_2 and pulse oximetry monitoring are mandated.[17]

Postoperative Complications

Morbidity and mortality rates are higher in obese patients than in normal-weight patients. Ventilation abnormalities are exacerbated in obese patients with OSA and OHS and may last for several days. The maximum decrease in partial pressure of arterial oxygen occurs 2 to 3 days postoperatively.[17] The risk of thromboembolism, wound infections, and atelectasis is amplified in patients with increased BMI.[17,65] Thromboembolism is facilitated by immobility (venous stasis), increased blood viscosity (polycythemia, hypovolemia), increased abdominal pressure, and abnormalities in serum procoagulants and anticoagulants.[6] Administration of minidose heparin (5000 units administered subcutaneously twice per day), low–molecular-weight heparin. Antiembolic stockings and correctly fitting pneumatic compression boots can lessen the occurrence of deep vein thrombosis in the early postoperative period. Early ambulation and maintenance of vascular volume further attenuate the likelihood that clots will develop. Wound infections and pulmonary embolism are 50% higher in obese patients than in normal-weight patients.

SUMMARY

Obesity is a complex and multifactorial disease, and its incidence is continuing to increase in the U.S. patient population. Through an understanding of the implications of associated conditions in obesity, the anesthetist can promote more favorable anesthetic outcomes. Consideration of the physiologic and pharmacologic changes and their implications for optimal anesthetic management guides clinical practice.

REFERENCES

1. National Institute of Health. Clinical Guidelines on the Identification, Evaluation, and Treatment of Overweight and Obesity in Adults: the Evidence Report. NIH publication no. 98-4083. Washington, DC: National Institute of Health; September, 1998.
2. Klein S, Romijn J. Obesity. In: Larsen PR, Kroneberg HM, Mclmed S, Polonsky KS. *Williams Textbook of Endocrinology*. 10th ed. Philadelphia: Saunders; 2003:1619-1641.
3. Flier JS. Obesity. In: Braunwald E, Fauci AS, Kasper DL, Hauser SL, Longo DL, Jameson JL, eds. *Harrison's Principles of Internal Medicine*. 15th ed. New York: McGraw-Hill; 1998:479-486.
4. *American Obesity Association Fact Sheet*. Available at: http://www.obesity.org/subs/fastfacts/obesity_US.shtml. Accessed May 13, 2004.
5. Flegal KM, Carroll MD, Ogden CL, et al. Prevalence and trends in obesity among US adults, 1999-2000. *JAMA*. 2002;288: 1723-1727.
6. Colditz GA. Epidemiology of obesity In: Gumbiner B. *Obesity*. Philadelphia: American College of Physicians–American Society of Internal Medicine; 2001:1-22.
7. Jensen M. Obesity. In: Goldman L, Ausiello D, eds. *Cecil Textbook of Medicine*. 22nd ed. Philadelphia: Saunders; 2004:1339-1347.
8. Adams JP, Murphy PG: Obesity in anaesthesia and intensive care. *Br J Anaesth*. 2000;85:91-108.
9. Woods SC, et al. Signals that regulate food intake and energy homeostasis. *Science*. 1998;280:1378-1386.
10. Comuzzie AG, Allison DB. The search for human obesity genes. *Science*. 1998;280:1374-1377.
11. Devlin MJ, Yanovski SZ, Wilson GT. Obesity: what mental health professionals need to know. *Am J Psychiatry*. 2000;157:854-866.
12. Roizen MF. Anesthetic implications of concurrent diseases. In: Miller RD, ed. *Anesthesia*. 5th ed. New York: Churchill Livingstone; 2000:903-1016.
13. Lean JM. Obesity and cardiovascular disease: the wasted years. *Br J Cardiol*. 1999;6:269-273.
14. Rosenbaum M, Leibel RL, Hirsch J. Obesity. *N Engl J Med*. 1997;337:396-407.
15. Brown CD, Higgins M, Donato KA, et al. Body mass index and the prevalence of hypertension and dyslipidemia. *Obes Res*. 2000;8:605-619.
16. Kannel W, Brand N, Skinner J, et al. The relationship of adiposity to blood pressure and development of hypertension. The Framingham Study. *Ann Intern Med*. 1967;67:48-59.

17. Stoelting RK, Dierdorf SF, McCammon RL. *Anesthesia and Co-existing Diseases*. 2nd ed. New York: Churchill Livingstone; 2002:441-451.
18. Benumof JL. Respiratory physiology and respiratory function during anesthesia. In: Miller RD, ed. *Anesthesia*. 5th ed. New York: Churchill Livingstone; 2000:578-618.
19. Biring MS, Lewis MI, Liu JI, Mohsenifar A. Pulmonary physiologic changes of morbid obesity. *Am J Med Sci*. 1999;318:293-297.
20. Benumof JL. Obstructive sleep apnea in the adult obese patient: implications for airway management. *J Clin Anesth*. 2001;13: 144-156.
21. Matteoni C, Younossi ZM, McCoullough A. Nonalcoholic fatty liver disease: a spectrum of clinical pathological severity. *Gastroenterology*. 1999;116:1413-1419.
22. Aria HE. Pitfalls in the diagnosis of gall bladder disease in clinically severe obesity. *Obes Surg*. 1998;8:444-451.
23. Ogunnaike BO, Jones SB, Jones DB, et al. Anesthetic considerations for bariatric surgery. *Anesth Analg*. 2002;95:1793-1805.
24. Provost DA, Jones DB. Minimally invasive surgery for the treatment of severe obesity. *Dallas Med J*. 1999;87:110-113.
25. Balsiger BM, Murr MM, Poggio J, et al:. Bariatric surgery: surgery for weight control in patients with morbid obesity. *Med Clin North Am*. 2000;84:477-489.
26. Scott DJ, Provost DA, Jones DB. Laparoscopic Roux-en-Y gastric bypass for morbid obesity. *Surg Rounds*. 2000;23:177-189.
27. Hunter JD, Reid C, Noble D. Anesthetic management of the morbidly obese patient. *Hosp Med*. 1998;59:481-483.
28. Song D, Whitten CW, White PF. Remifentanil infusion facilitates early recovery for obese outpatients undergoing laparoscopic cholecystectomy. *Anesth Analg*. 2000;90:111-113.
29. Slepchenko G, Simon N, Goubaux B, Levron JC, Le Moing JP, Raucoules-Aime M. Performance of target-controlled sufentanil infusion in obese patients. *Anesthesiology*. 2003;98:65-73.
30. Puhringer FK, Keller C, Kleinsaser A, et al. Pharmacokinetics of rocuronium bromide in obese female patients. *Eur J Anaesthesiol*. 1999;16:507-510.
31. Salihoglu Z, Karaca S, Kose Y, Zengin K, Taskin M. Total intravenous anesthesia versus single breath technique and anesthesia maintenance with sevoflurane for bariatric operations. *Obes Surg*. 2001;11:496-501.
32. Bedford RF, Ives HE. The renal safety of sevoflurane. *Anesth Analg*. 2000;90:505-508.
33. Torri G, Casati A, Albertin A, et al. Randomized comparison of isoflurane and sevoflurane for laparoscopic gastric banding in morbidly obese patients. *J Clin Anesth*. 2001;13:565-570.
34. Juvin P, Vadam C, Malek L, et al. Postoperative recovery after desflurane, propofol, or isoflurane anesthesia among morbidly obese patients: a prospective, randomized study. *Anesth Analg*. 1999;91:714-719.
35. Chung F, Mezei G, Tong D. Pre-existing medical conditions as predictors of adverse events in day-case surgery. *Br J Anesth*. 1999;83:262-270.
36. Dominguez-Cherit G, Gonzalez R, Borunda D, et al. Anesthesia for morbidly obese patients. *World J Surg*. 1998;22:1182.
37. Brodsky JB, Lemmens HJ, Brock-Utne JG, et al. Morbid obesity and tracheal intubation. *Anesth Analg*. 2002;94:732-736.
38. Siyam MA, Benhamou D. Intubation in morbidly obese patients. *Anesth Analg*. 2002;94:732-736.
39. Ezri T, Gewurtz G, Sessler D, et al. Prediction of difficult laryngoscopy in obese patients by ultrasound quantification of anterior neck soft tissue. *Anaesthesia*. 2003;58:1101-1118.
40. Frappier J, Guenoun T, Journois D, et al. Airway management using the intubating laryngeal mask airway for the morbidly obese patient. *Anesth Analg*. 2003;96:1510-1515.
41. Brodsky JB, Lemmens HJ, Brock-Utene JG, et al. Anesthetic considerations for bariatric surgery: proper positioning is important for laryngoscopy. *Anesth Analg*. 2002;95:1793-1805.
42. Jefferson P, Ball DR. Central venous access in morbidly obese patients. *Anesth Analg*. 2001;93:1363.
43. Mendelson CL. Aspiration of stomach contents into lungs during obstetric anesthesia. *Am J Obstet Gynecol*. 1946;53:196-205.
44. Sellick BA. Cricoid pressure to control regurgitation of stomach contents during induction of anesthesia. *Lancet*. 1961;2:404-406.
45. Juvin P, Fevre G, Merouche M, et al. Gastric residue is not more copious in obese patients. *Anesth Analg*. 2001;93:1621-1622.
46. Boyce JR, Ness T, Castroman P, et al. A preliminary study of the optimal anesthesia positioning for the morbidly obese patient. *Obes Surg*. 2003;13:4-9.
47. Cressey DM, Berthoud MC, Reilly CS. Effectiveness of continuous positive airway pressure to enhance pre-oxygenation in morbidly obese women. *Anesthesia*. 2001;56:680-684.
48. Keller C, Brimacombe J, Kleinsasser L. The laryngeal mask airway ProSeal as a temporary ventilatory device in grossly and morbidly obese patients before laryngoscope-guided tracheal intubation. *Anesth Analg*. 2002;94:737-740.
49. Natalini G, Franceschetti ME, Pantelidi MT, et al. A comparison of the standard laryngeal mask airway and the ProSeal laryngeal mask airway in obese patients. *Br J Anesth*. 2003;90:323-326.
50. Ezri T, Hazin V, Warters D, et al. The endotracheal tube moves more often in obese patients undergoing laparoscopy compared with open abdominal surgery. *Anesth Analg*. 2003;96:278-282.
51. Sprung J, Whalley DG, Falcone T, et al. The impact of morbid obesity, pneumoperitoneum, and posture on respiratory system mechanics and oxygenation during laparoscopy. *Anesth Analg*. 2002;94:1345-1350.
52. Sprung J, Whalley DG, Falcone T, et al. The effects of tidal volume and respiratory rate on oxygenation and respiratory mechanics during laparoscopy in morbidly obese patients. *Anesth Analg*. 2003;97:268-274.
53. Perilli V, Sollazzi L, Bozza P, et al. The effects of the reverse Trendelenburg position on respiratory mechanics and blood gases in morbidly obese patients during bariatric surgery. *Anesth Analg*. 2000;91:1520-1525.
54. Auler JO Jr, Miyoshi E, Fernandes CR, et al. The effects of abdominal opening on respiratory mechanics during general anesthesia in normal and morbidly obese patients: a comparative study. *Anesth Analg*. 2002;94:741-748.
55. Pelosi P, Ravagnan I, Giurati G, et al. Positive end-expiratory pressure improves respiratory function in obese but not in normal subjects during anesthesia and paralysis. *Anesthesiology*. 1999;91:1221-1231.
56. Tsueda K. Obesity supine death syndrome: report of two morbidly obese patients. *Anesth Analg*. 1979;58:345-347.
57. Coker LL. Continuous spinal anesthesia for cesarean section for a morbidly obese parturient patient: a case report. *AANA J*. 2002;70:189-192.
58. Kadar AG, Ing CH, White PF, et al. Anesthesia for electroconvulsive therapy in obese patients. *Anesth Analg*. 2002;94:360-361.
59. Ranucci M, Cazzaniga A, Soro G, et al. Obesity and coronary artery surgery. *J Cardiothorac Vasc Anesth*. 1999;13:280-284.
60. Michaloudis D, Fraidakas O, Petrou A, et al. Continuous spinal anesthesia/analgesia for perioperative management of morbidly obese patients undergoing laparotomy for gastroplastic surgery. *Obes Surg*. 2000;10:220-229.
61. Lippmann M, Rubin S, Ginsburg R, et al. An alternative anesthetic technique for the morbidly obese patient undergoing endovascular repair of an abdominal aortic aneurysm. *Anesth Analg*. 2003;97:981-983.
62. Martin JT. Patient positioning. In: Barash PG, Cullen BF, Stoelting RK, eds. *Clinical Anesthesia*. 3rd ed. Philadelphia: Lippincott; 1997:595-620.
63. Brodsky JB. Positioning the morbidly obese patient for anesthesia. *Obes Surg*. 2002;12:751-758.
64. Benumof JL. Airway exchange catheters: simple concept potentially great danger. *Anesthesiology*. 1999;91:342-344.
65. Eichenberger A, Proietti S, Wicky S, et al. Morbid obesity and postoperative pulmonary atelectasis: an underestimated problem. *Anesth Analg*. 2002;95:1788-1792.

CHAPTER 42

REGIONAL ANESTHESIA

JOE BURKARD, R. LEE OLSON, CHARLES A. VACCHIANO

Significant changes in anesthesia practice have occurred in the last decade, challenging the anesthesia provider to be proficient in regional anesthesia. The advantages of regional anesthesia include fewer recovery room admissions, decreased nausea and vomiting, decreased urinary retention, and improved postoperative analgesia. The introduction of long-acting local anesthetics has improved the ability to provide postoperative pain relief for up to 24 hours or longer. Clinical research has spawned new and more effective techniques for upper and lower extremity blocks. The development and continued use of catheter techniques will revolutionize regional anesthesia.

HISTORY OF REGIONAL ANESTHESIA

The contributions of many practitioners have brought regional anesthesia techniques to the state of the art that exists today. Much of the early motivation for the investigation of regional anesthesia came about because of the risks and mortality associated with general anesthesia. The early inhalation agents were difficult to administer, and toxicity was common.[1]

Without the contributions of LaFargue in 1836, Rynd in 1844, and Pravaz in 1851, regional anesthesia would not have advanced so quickly. Until that time opiates and other medications were applied to or rubbed into open wounds in order to provide analgesia. LaFargue devised a needle trocar for depositing morphine under the skin. Rynd invented the hollow needle, which was used for delivering hypodermic medications. Pravaz invented the hypodermic syringe, which was improved by Wood in 1854.[1,2]

Further investigation of local anesthetics began with the use of cocaine by Koller in 1884. Koller instilled cocaine drops into the eyes of patients, thereby providing anesthesia of the cornea and conjunctiva. However, concerns about toxicity and addiction led to the search for safer medications.

Halsted introduced the concept of nerve blocks for surgery in 1885. Both Halsted and Hall used a technique of injecting the nerve with cocaine to provide analgesia. The first nerve blocks were of the mandibular nerve. Before their addiction to cocaine, Hall and Halsted paved the way for the development of modern regional anesthesia and advanced the concepts of local anesthetic injections and nerve blocks.

Corning, a New York neurologist, experimented with the application of cocaine to the spinal nerves and the injection of cocaine solutions between the spinous processes of the inferior dorsal vertebrae. The technique and the development of analgesia after injection as he described them are similar to techniques and the development of modern epidural analgesia. However, not until Quincke demonstrated the usefulness and practicality of spinal puncture did its use increase. He described techniques used for entering the subarachnoid space and withdrawing cerebrospinal fluid (CSF) for diagnostic procedures.[1,2]

Bier is credited with the introduction of spinal anesthesia in 1898. He injected his assistant and then agreed to have the technique administered to him. He then used the technique during surgical procedures. When cocaine was introduced into the subarachnoid space, anesthesia lasted approximately an hour. With the development of newer and safer anesthetic drugs, needles, and techniques, regional anesthesia expanded to include many neural blocks for the enhancement of surgery and obstetrics and for the management of pain.[1,2]

Using the information described by Corning, Cathelin introduced caudal anesthesia in 1901. During the next decade most of the popular neural block techniques were described. Modern procedures have simplified, refined, and increased the safety and success of regional anesthesia techniques.[2]

SELECTION OF REGIONAL ANESTHESIA TECHNIQUES

When regional anesthesia is chosen for management of pain, the technique should be discussed with the patient before surgery. The patient is informed of all optional procedures available, their potential risks, and their potential complications before an anesthesia technique is selected. Once the patient is thus advised, the most appropriate anesthesia technique can be selected, and true informed consent can be obtained. Regional anesthesia is used extensively for surgical procedures involving the extremities or the lower abdomen, for the treatment of labor pain, for the management of obstetric procedures, and for the control of chronic pain syndromes. Frequently, regional anesthesia techniques are used in combination with other techniques to provide analgesia or anesthesia during surgical or obstetric procedures. Regional anesthesia may be the technique of choice when local anesthesia requires supplementation with heavy sedation. These techniques provide the patient with increased anesthesia options in the selection of an anesthetic for surgical or obstetric procedures.[3,4]

Before presenting the option of a regional anesthetic to the patient, the anesthesia practitioner should answer the following important questions about the procedure:

1. Would I be comfortable having this surgical procedure accomplished with the proposed regional anesthetic technique?
2. Can I remain in this position for the length of time required without difficulty?
3. What benefit will this technique provide for me that other anesthesia techniques would not provide?

The answers to these questions directly affect the choice of anesthetic techniques offered to the patient.

When the practitioner recommends any anesthetic technique to the patient, the practitioner has a responsibility to educate the patient, the patient's family, and other interested parties regarding the anesthesia procedure and the potential outcomes. The anesthesia practitioner must obtain an informed consent and the trust of the patient before performing any technique. Without this trust the best anesthetic technique may be a failure.

Patients who require anesthesia for some surgical or obstetric procedures are best cared for by use of regional anesthesia techniques. One primary example is the administration of an epidural anesthetic to the patient in labor. No other modality can provide the mother with relative relief from the most severe discomfort and still permit the baby to respond when delivered, all with minimal possibility of respiratory distress or depression.[4-6]

Urologic procedures may be accomplished with the use of regional anesthetics, whereas cystoscopies and transurethral resections can be performed with the use of spinal anesthesia. When awake and anesthetized to the level of the dome of the bladder (T10), the patient may respond to bladder distention, thereby helping the urologist minimize the potential for bladder rupture. In addition, patients who are awake are easier to monitor for developing conditions, such as hypervolemia, hyponatremia, and ammonium toxicity.[7]

Rectal procedures performed with the patient in the prone position can be accomplished with specialized spinal techniques. The spinal anesthetic technique is performed after the patient is positioned in the prone position. This technique restricts the spread of the local anesthetic medications, facilitates positioning, and provides the patient with postoperative analgesia.[8]

As a result of the introduction of spinal and epidural administration of narcotics in 1979, the anesthesia practitioner can provide the patient with extended analgesia through an epidural catheter or an intrathecal injection. The dose of the narcotic is reduced, permitting the patient to remain alert and to retain the ability to ambulate while experiencing analgesia.[4]

However, the administration of regional anesthesia to patients with a difficult airway or a full stomach presents both additional benefits and risks in selected patients. The use of regional anesthesia, when appropriate, permits the patient to retain upper airway and pharyngeal reflexes while being anesthetized in the area of the injury. Unless the sedation is reduced to a minimum, the airway may not be protected after the administration of the regional technique. Furthermore, block of the sympathetic nervous system theoretically results in increased gastric and intestinal motility, causing the stomach to empty sooner. However, this benefit may be negated by the perception of pain and anxiety that accompanies the injury. If hypotension develops, the patient may have increased nausea and vomiting. When an injury has occurred after the ingestion of alcohol, the pain caused by the injury may be the only stimulus for consciousness. When the block is instituted, the patient may lose consciousness as a result of the effects of the alcohol. At this point, airway support is required, and other problems may arise as well.[3,8]

Regional anesthesia should not become an alternative to securing of the airway. If the patient's airway cannot be secured in a safe manner in an emergent situation, use of a regional anesthetic should be avoided. The airway concerns must be addressed before the anesthetic technique is initiated so that the patient's ability to survive is maximized.[3,8]

Absolute Contraindications

Absolute contraindications to the selection of regional anesthesia techniques are few, and some remain controversial. Contraindications include patient refusal, uncorrected coagulation deficiencies, and infection at the site of the block. The most significant absolute contraindication to regional anesthesia is patient refusal. Each patient must be informed of the acceptable techniques that will provide analgesia or anesthesia, and each patient should be told of significant risks and potential benefits. The discussion must include the advantages and disadvantages of each proposed technique.[8] All of the patient's questions should be answered completely. This level of communication helps the practitioner uncover misconceptions while educating the patient about regional anesthesia.[8]

Another absolute contraindication is systemic anticoagulation in the patient. Certain drugs and systemic diseases can cause alterations in the coagulation profile. The long-term or extended use of aspirin products or nonsteroidal antiinflammatory drugs (NSAIDs) can prolong bleeding time without significantly altering other laboratory data. The patient's medical and pharmacologic history may provide information about increased bleeding time. Asking the patient about frequent bruising without injury may reveal the first indication of a problem. For instance, physical evaluation of the skin may show evidence of bruising or subcutaneous bleeding of which the patient may not recall the cause. If injury to a large epidural vessel were to occur during the performance of either a spinal or an epidural technique, major bleeding could develop in the epidural space. A similar injury to the axillary artery in the confined space of the axilla might result in a hematoma that would produce further complications. Injury to a large vessel in the neck during an interscalene technique could result in impairment of the airway.[8]

Insufficient data are available to quiet the controversy surrounding absolute laboratory values below which the practitioner should avoid using a regional anesthesia technique. Winnie suggested using arbitrary values for platelet counts of less than 100,000 and prothrombin time (PT), partial thromboplastin time (PTT), and bleeding times that are greater than two times normal values in the determination of whether a regional anesthetic technique should be avoided.[4,8] Severe bleeding with or without symptomatic hypovolemia or the potential for severe bleeding is a contraindication to the administration of a regional anesthetic. The contraindication can be considered either absolute or relative, depending on the clinical presentation of the patient. Trauma, along with physiologic or pathophysiologic conditions that cause contracted volume states and abruptio placentae, can result in the development of significant hypotension and tachycardia after the initiation of regional anesthesia, especially spinal or epidural anesthesia. A blockade of the sympathetic nervous system quickly develops, resulting in significant relaxation of the smooth muscles of the vascular bed. The extent of this block is dependent on the regional anesthesia technique, the dose of medication, and the volume of solution used when the procedure is performed.

When the patient demonstrates symptoms of hypovolemic shock on evaluation, his or her ability to safely tolerate the reduction in systemic vascular resistance and peripheral vasodilatation is reduced. The anesthetist's inability to compensate for falling blood pressure by increasing systemic vascular resistance places the patient at risk for potential hypoxic incidents in vital organs.

When an obstetric patient has abruptio placentae with or without fetal distress, the anesthesia practitioner must consider other anesthetic procedures. These alternatives should be considered so that hypotension and the compromise to fetal oxygen supply that results from decreased uterine blood flow can be minimized. Regional techniques require time in addition to the reduction in blood pressure that occurs with the establishment of the block. Uterine blood flow is dependent on arterial pressure and has few autoregulatory capabilities. However, when an epidural anesthetic is being used for labor, the time required for surgical anesthesia to be established may be less with epidural than with general anesthesia. The choice of anesthesia technique must focus on the possible effects of the sympathectomy, even if its development can be slowed or controlled. With the onset of the sympathetic blockade, the fall in blood pressure may be more than the mother and baby can tolerate. The anesthesia practitioner caring for the patient, in consultation with the patient's obstetrician, must decide whether administration of the regional anesthetic should be continued or whether another anesthesia procedure should be selected.[3-6,8]

If an active infectious process is present near the location at which regional anesthesia is to be performed, another anesthetic should be chosen. If active herpes lesions are present in the region in which the block procedure is to be performed, regional anesthesia should be avoided.[4]

Relative Contraindications and Precautions

One relative contraindication to regional anesthesia is patient age. In neonates with impairment in ventilatory regulation, regional anesthesia techniques are recommended when either surgery or pain management is required. The knowledge and the abilities of the practitioner are more important considerations, however.[4,7,8]

Small children tolerate the administration of a combination anesthetic for many surgical procedures, including hernia procedures, extremity procedures, and circumcision. A general anesthetic can be administered for the surgical procedure, and a regional technique can be used for postoperative pain management. Anatomic landmarks are easily identified in children, which permits implementation without extensive difficulty. Precautions must be taken when the patient is of short stature. This technique should be avoided in children who are unable to tolerate the loss of feeling and strength in the legs. As children begin to acquire independence through increased ambulation, the loss of feeling and movement in the legs may increase their fear. This phenomenon is especially common in children between the ages of 3 and 9 years.[7]

Interscalene and axillary blocks have been used to permit immobilization and analgesia of the upper extremity for extended periods of time. Bier's blocks (intravenous infusion blocks) have been used on small children, aged 8 to 12 years; in these cases reduced amounts of local anesthetic medication are used for the reduction of arm fractures.[9]

Patients who have difficulty understanding the procedures to be performed or who are unable to cooperate with the practitioner should undergo another type of anesthesia. Such patients may respond negatively to the presence of anyone behind them who may create confusion or cause discomfort; they could perceive this presence as an imminent threat and could respond inappropriately.

Patients with a history of headaches or backaches are at increased risk for experiencing these problems after spinal and epidural analgesia or anesthesia. Such patients should be evaluated and counseled regarding this potential before the administration of subarachnoid or epidural anesthesia. Postanesthesia symptoms of backache or headache become difficult to evaluate without information about the patient's previous pattern of headaches or backaches. Information about the position of the patient during the surgical or obstetric procedure assists in the evaluation of the patient.[4-6,10]

Patients with chronic neurologic disorders must be well informed of the potential effects of the regional anesthetic technique. The regional anesthetic may not cause an increase in the patient's symptoms; however, if symptoms of the disorder increase or deterioration results, the regional anesthetic technique may be identified as the cause of the problem.

Patients with a history of a documented local anesthetic allergy should undergo further evaluation in a controlled situation by an allergist. A true allergy to local anesthetic agents is rare. The problem may be caused by a preservative in the anesthetic solution or by a metabolic product of local anesthetic hydrolysis (para-aminobenzoic acid [PABA]). Skin testing is helpful but not always accurate. Patients may have negative results of the skin test and have a reaction when a concentration of the local anesthetic that is sufficient for the provision of anesthesia is administered. Alleged allergic reactions may be related to an intravenous injection of a local anesthetic solution that contains epinephrine.[11-13]

If a regional technique is used in a patient with an allergy, a local anesthetic that is unrelated to the suspected agent should be selected. For example, if the patient is allergic to an ester anesthetic, an amide anesthetic agent should be chosen. Before the anesthetic is administered, the patient should be medicated with histamine-1 and histamine-2 receptor blockers.

When the patient has a history of Mobitz type I, Mobitz type II, or third-degree heart block without a pacemaker, it may be advisable to choose another technique. In patients with increased plasma levels of local anesthetic after large-volume local anesthetic administration, stabilization of the cardiac cellular membrane may result in an increase in the degree of heart block.[3,8]

Patients with fixed-volume cardiac states are at risk for cardiovascular compromise after the initiation of a regional anesthetic. If the patient is unable to respond to changes in systemic vascular resistance by increasing stroke volume as a means of maintaining cardiac output, selected regional anesthesia techniques, including spinal and epidural anesthesia, should be reconsidered. As the heart rate increases to compensate for the falling pressure, the heart may fail, or ischemia may develop.[14]

COMPLICATIONS OF REGIONAL ANESTHESIA

Complications of regional anesthesia can be immediate or delayed. Cardiovascular problems are the most critical immediate complications. However, effects on the respiratory and gastrointestinal (GI) systems can have equally serious consequences. Delayed complications include problems involving the cardiovascular, musculoskeletal, genitourinary, and neurologic systems.

Immediate Complications

The initiation of a spinal or epidural technique causes anesthesia of the sympathetic nervous system. As this effect progresses, the potential for severe hypotension caused by a preganglionic sympathetic block increases. The blockade causes increased peripheral vasodilation and pooling of blood. This phenomenon results in a reduction in the reduced venous return. If the block is high enough, sympathetic nerve fibers that innervate the heart (T1 to T4) become anesthetized. These fibers are identified as the cardiac accelerators. This effect results in a slowing of the heart rate that is known as the *Bainbridge reflex*.[14] Rapid changes in position, changes in skeletal muscle tone caused by relaxation, decreased venous return, low preoperative volume status, reflex surgical stimulation, preoperative medications (especially narcotics and tranquilizers), and concurrent conditions, such as pulmonary embolism, pregnancy, and systemic reactions to medications, have all been implicated in increased severity of perioperative hypotension.[4,8,15-17]

Preventive management of hypotension includes the administration of nonglucose solutions before the regional technique is instituted. This initial infusion should include replacement of any fluid deficit caused by restricted oral intake. Initial treatment of hypotension includes the administration (in increments of 5 ml/kg of body weight) of balanced salt solutions that do not contain glucose.

Glucose-containing solutions can act as diuretics. The increased diuresis and the loss of circulating volume that occur decrease the blood volume. Continued treatment must be guided by the patient's presenting symptoms. The heart rate can be used for determination of pharmacologic intervention. If the heart rate is normal or elevated, an α-agonist, such as phenylephrine (Neo-Synephrine), causes increased systemic vascular resistance without further increasing the heart rate. In patients with symptomatic bradycardia the agent of choice is a mixed α-and β-agonist. Ephedrine causes an increase in peripheral vascular resistance and in heart rate. Severe hypotensive events should be treated vigorously with medication and fluids. Mortality increases when treatment is delayed.[8,15-17]

Although rare, hypertension may occur after the administration of a regional anesthesia technique. Several contributing factors, including anxiety, pain, prophylactic administration of vasopressors, and use of vasoconstrictors in the anesthetic mixture, are involved in the increase in systemic vascular resistance, the pulse rate, or both. The prophylactic or therapeutic use of vasopressors has been advocated for the prevention of hypotension. In patients receiving adequate hydration, medications should not be required. If the block fails, the action of the vasopressor is unopposed. Severe increases in blood pressure must be managed with vasodilators, narcotics, and anxiolytics.[8,15]

Hypoxia and hypercarbia can have severe systemic consequences, including death, if the problem is not recognized and treated immediately. As the level of the block moves cephalad, first the abdominal muscles and then the intercostal muscles become paralyzed. If the block is sufficiently high (C2 to C3), phrenic nerve paralysis, intercostal nerve paralysis, and loss of accessory muscles of ventilation increase the potential for hypoxia. With the loss of perception of intercostal and abdominal wall muscle movement as the sensory block reaches the level of T2 to T4, the patient may begin to feel dyspneic. Large doses of sedatives and narcotics further compound the problem by increasing hypoventilation. Ischemia of the respiratory center leads to hypoventilation and eventually respiratory arrest.[3,8,14,15]

When the abdominal muscles and the internal intercostal muscles are paralyzed, the patient is unable to cough effectively. Patients with this problem are unable to clear secretions or foreign materials from the airway. Once this occurs, patients are unable to protect the airway from potential aspiration.[3,8,15]

Total sympathetic blockade can theoretically result in acute pulmonary collapse and atelectasis. Total blockade is caused by the action of an unopposed parasympathetic system.

GI complications range from nausea to perforation of the bowel. Nausea and vomiting are the most common problems. However, GI causes of nausea and vomiting are not considered first in the evaluation of this problem. Nausea and vomiting should be considered to be signs of central hypoxia until proved otherwise. Use of high doses of vasopressors, obesity, ingestion of drugs and alcohol, and the prone position increase the potential for nonhypoxic nausea and vomiting in surgical and obstetric patients. Apprehension and fear can produce nausea and vomiting; this effect can occur even in patients who appear outwardly calm. Perforation of the bowel occurs very rarely and is caused by unopposed parasympathetic activity with increased peristalsis.[4,8]

The potential of an intravascular injection is increased when local anesthetics are injected into the tissues around nerves and blood vessels or in high volumes. If lidocaine is injected into the intravascular space, central nervous system toxicity can occur. The patient may first complain of tingling of the lips and a strange taste in the mouth and then visual disturbances. Seizures may also occur. In patients receiving an intravenous injection of 0.5% to 0.75% bupivacaine (Marcaine), the first symptom of intravascular injection must be a cardiac dysrhythmia. The most common dysrhythmias are of ventricular origin.[4,8,10-15]

Delayed Complications

The anesthesia practitioner must be prepared to manage complications that occur after the block has been established or during the postanesthesia recovery period. Some complications are less difficult to manage than are others.

Postdural puncture headache (PDPH) is one of the more commonly discussed and managed complications of subarachnoid block. It is caused by a decrease in the amount of available CSF in the subarachnoid space; this decrease causes the medulla and brain stem to drop into the foramen magnum. The subsequent stretching of the meninges and pulling on the tentorium caused by this movement may cause headache.[3,8,15-17] An additional complication of decreased CSF level is cranial nerve palsy. This condition causes stretching of the fibers of the nerve root, thereby decreasing the blood supply to the nerve.[8]

One theory proposes that loss of CSF is caused by a leak at the dural puncture site. The size and type of the needle, direction of the bevel, number of punctures that are made in the attempts to start the spinal anesthetic, dehydration, decreased intraabdominal pressure, patient position, and patient factors (e.g., age, sex, race, and history of headache) all influence the occurrence of headache. The patient's anticipation of untoward events must be considered during the evaluation of the headache.[8,15-17]

The incidence of headache is four times greater in 20-year-olds than in individuals aged 60 years and older. The incidence in female patients is two times greater than that in 20-year-old men. Headaches occur more frequently in white patients than in black patients of similar sex and age, and if the patient has a history of headaches, the incidence of headaches increases after the surgical procedure. Expectation of a headache increases the likelihood that a headache will occur.[8,16]

Spinal headaches usually occur within 1 week after the spinal anesthetic. The earlier the spinal headache occurs, the more severe it is. In addition, the headache is more severe in the upright position and is relieved by the supine position, and it occurs on both sides of the head in the occipital or frontal region, usually starting behind the eyes and radiating to the occiput, neck, or shoulders.[2] Occlusion of the jugular veins increases the severity of the headache, and occlusion of the carotid arteries reduces the headache's severity. Sore or stiff neck, backache, nausea and vomiting on standing, blurred vision, plugging of the ears, tinnitus, and vertigo can occur as well.[4,8]

Conservative treatment should be attempted before any invasive procedure is considered. Conservative management includes bed rest, rehydration, use of sedatives and opioids, and use of an abdominal binder before ambulation. Increasing fluids during the evaluation and early management period increases the central volume and increases the secretion of CSF from the choroid plexus. When appropriately applied, the abdominal binder increases intraabdominal pressure; this increase is transmitted directly to the subarachnoid space. The increased pressure in the subarachnoid space forces the brain stem and main stem to float above the foramen magnum in the remaining CSF. In addition, caffeine and niacin have been used to increase the production of CSF, with very limited results.[4,8,14,16]

Management of a PDPH includes the use of an epidural blood patch. The epidural space is identified, by use of either "loss-of-resistance" or "hanging-drop" technique (discussed later), at the level of the initial needle insertion. The availability of intravenous access is identified before the technique is begun. One of the most accessible routes is the antecubital fossa of one arm. Both the back of the patient and one arm are prepared and draped in a sterile manner. Venous blood (30 ml) is withdrawn from the vein in the arm by use of sterile procedures; the blood is then injected into the epidural space. The injection proceeds until the patient begins to feel pressure in the back. Bed rest should be maintained for 1 to 2 hours before the patient ambulates.

After bed rest the patient may ambulate slowly. When the blood patch is successfully accomplished, the patient experiences relief of the headache, often instantaneously. If the blood patch is attempted within 24 hours of the initial dural puncture, relief of symptoms may be less successful.[4,8,16,17]

The patient may develop a persistent backache after the administration of spinal or epidural anesthetic techniques. This problem may manifest as a continuous dull aching in the area of the block or as extensive pain that restricts movement. The most common cause of a backache is relaxation of the muscles of the back and flattening of the normal lordotic curve. As the muscles stretch, injury to tendons and ligaments can occur. The position of the patient might increase the severity of the problem. An exaggerated lithotomy position or a completely supine position can further increase tension on tendons, resulting in increased trauma to both the muscles and the tendons. Trauma from multiple punctures; hemorrhage; infections; use of large needles, retractors, and forceps; extremes of positions; preexisting diseases, such as arthritis and osteoporosis; use of chloroprocaine for epidural; and prolonged labor can contribute to backaches.[4,8,15-17] Management of this condition should include bed rest and direct application of heat to the area of injury. The use of antispasmodics may be required. The use of NSAIDs may reduce the discomfort, permitting ambulation and a more rapid recovery.[8,15,16]

Urinary retention commonly occurs after anesthesia and surgery because the spinal or epidural anesthetic blocks sympathetic fibers, thereby increasing the tone of the internal urethral sphincter. Further investigation can identify several contributing factors. The surgical procedure itself can cause the problem. Overdistention of the bladder caused by the administration of large volumes of intravenous fluids, trauma to the bladder, prolonged hypotension, incisional pain, prolonged labor, benign prostatic hypertrophy, use of narcotics intraoperatively, and position of the patient can all affect the patient's ability to urinate. An example of this problem is inability to urinate in the supine position. In such cases, invasive management may require the use of a catheter, but this method should be used only after noninvasive procedures, such as position change, have been attempted.[4,8,15]

When the practitioner does not maintain aseptic technique during the preparation or administration of the regional anesthesia, the potential for infection increases. Septic meningitis caused by bacterial contamination, and its consequences, can be devastating. Aseptic meningitis is caused by irritation of the meninges by a foreign substance. Hemorrhages into the subarachnoid or epidural space can be linked to aseptic meningitis. Other causes of aseptic meningitis include foreign bodies, local agent osmolarity, dextrose, indwelling catheters, detergents, antiseptics, coring of the epidermis as the needle is inserted, and previous myelography.[4,15]

If paraplegia develops, it is frequently thought to be caused by the anesthetic agent. However, the agent is usually not at fault. Blood can leak into the confined area of the epidural or subarachnoid space, causing compression of the cord. Undiagnosed neurologic disease, injection of the wrong drug, intraneural injections, intramedullary injections, and vascular syndromes can all lead to paralysis. In a study of 542 patients with neurologic symptoms, evaluation by electromyography revealed that only four patients' symptoms were related to the anesthetic.[4,8,15-17]

Inadequate or improper management of the physiologic effects of the regional technique results in hypotension, respiratory insufficiency, and hypoxia. These problems can result in central nervous system damage or death. A total spinal anesthetic can result in severe complications if the anesthesia practitioner does not maintain constant vigilance. Such complications can occur after an epidural technique in which the needle penetrates the dura. Large doses of medication are injected into the epidural space, and medication enters the subarachnoid space by way of the puncture in the dura. This situation can occur when inappropriate positions or hypobaric solutions are used, when the patient coughs or attempts to move and strain, when an exaggerated Trendelenburg position is used with a hyperbaric solution, or when large volumes of anesthetic solutions are administered. The problems occur because of brain stem ischemia that results from hypotension and total sympathetic block. These problems then cause apnea. Inattention is the cause of death.[4,8,15]

Technical Difficulties

Technical problems include difficulties with equipment and supplies. Broken needles, broken catheters, glass in the epidural and subarachnoid spaces, and injection of the wrong drugs are some of the problems that can be encountered.

Disposable needles are made in two parts: the hub and the barrel. The two parts are joined together and then fused to create a single unit. The weakest point on the needle is at the joint with the hub. Precautions should be taken so that the needle is not inserted into the hub. Also, the needle should not be bent. If extreme force is used while the needle is being inserted, the needle is stressed at the hub; this stress could cause the needle to break. If the needle is not inserted into the hub, some of the needle can be secured and removed, thus preventing its loss.[8,15,16]

Broken or sheared catheters are a concern in continuous regional anesthesia techniques. A visual inspection of the catheter should occur before it is inserted. The portion of the catheter that is inserted should have a radiopaque marker on the tip. Markings are placed at 1-cm divisions along the catheter, thereby providing an approximate measure for estimations of the length of the catheter that is inserted into the epidural or intrathecal space. When removed, the catheter should be inspected and its intactness verified. An epidural catheter should not be pulled back through the needle once the tip has passed beyond the bevel opening. The point where the two sides of the bevel join is the sharpest point of the entire needle. As the catheter is pulled back, it is forced against the joint and sheared off. If the catheter is sheared off, radiography can be used in order to locate the catheter, verify its position, and document the shearing. Catheters in use today have a radiopaque tip and are made of a material of low reactivity. Surgical procedures used in the search for a catheter can delay a patient's recovery. The patient should be told of the problem, where the catheter is located, the composition of the catheter, and any other information that might help reduce the patient's concerns about the catheter's location. Most catheters can remain in place without causing problems. However, when the remaining catheter is located in the subarachnoid space, it must be retrieved. The potential exists for the catheter to migrate cephalad, causing further problems once it reaches the level of the spinal cord or is directed through a foramen into a nerve root.[4,8,15,16]

Glass from broken ampules can be injected into the subarachnoid or epidural space or in the area of the nerve if care is not exercised during the preparation of the medication. Ampules should be broken away from the tray and enclosed within a sponge that is then discarded. A filter needle should be used during the withdrawal of all medications from ampules. The filter needle should then be discarded to prevent injection of the particles that had been filtered out. The glass particles may act as a foreign body, causing a local reaction and the development of a sterile abscess.[4,8]

TABLE 42-1 Classification of Nerve Fibers

Nerve Fiber	Myelination	CONDUCTION Diameter (μm)	Velocity (m/sec)	Function
A-α	Heavy	15-20	70-120	Motor
A-β	Moderate	5-12	30-70	Touch and pressure
A-γ	Moderate	5-10	30-70	Proprioception
A-δ	Light	2-5	12-30	Pain and temperature
B	Light	1-4	3-15	Preganglionic, autonomic
C	None	0.5-1	0.5-2	Pain and temperature

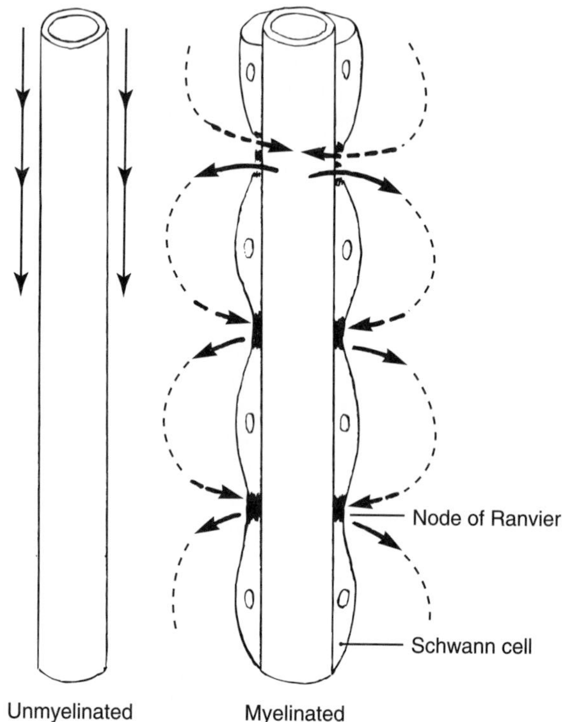

FIGURE **42-1**
Unmyelinated and myelinated nerve fibers. In myelinated fibers the stimulus is transmitted from one node of Ranvier to the next in a hopping fashion, resulting in saltatory conduction.

PHARMACOLOGY OF LOCAL ANESTHETICS

See Chapter 9 for a complete discussion of the pharmacology of local anesthetics. Local anesthetic agents temporarily block the transmission of a stimulus along the path of a nerve fiber through interference with the local ionic gradient across the cell membrane. Each nerve is composed of a cell and an axon. Many nerves are covered with a sheath that is made up of myelin. The sheath is produced by a Schwann cell and is interrupted in areas along the axon known as *nodes of Ranvier*. Electrical transmission along a myelinated fiber is different from that along an unmyelinated nerve fiber (Table 42-1). In a myelinated fiber the stimulus is transmitted from node of Ranvier to node of Ranvier in a hopping fashion (Figure 42-1). This phenomenon results in the more rapid transmission of the impulse; it is called *saltatory conduction*.[16] In an unmyelinated fiber the stimulus is transmitted along the fiber continuously.[11,17-20]

The cell membrane of the axon and nerve is important for the conduction of the stimulus. Several theories about the actual structure of the membrane have been proposed. A recent theory postulates that the cell membrane has two layers that are made up of lipid molecules with protein molecules interspersed throughout the space. Throughout the membrane are small openings, known as *pores* or *channels* that are the size of small ions and are controlled by gates. These gates restrict the movement of ions between the intracellular and extracellular spaces. The gates are influenced by changes in the electrical fields of the cell membrane.[18-20]

The primary function of most of the gates is to restrict the movement of sodium into the cell. Because the gates do not restrict the movement of potassium, it can freely move in and out of the cell for the maintenance of equilibrium. Several selective cells and conducting tissues have gates that regulate the flow of other ions, such as calcium and magnesium. One of the methods of action of the local anesthetics is the stabilization of the gate by maintaining it in the closed position. This action may be accomplished by the fixing of the local anesthetic with the intracellular calcium, which creates a large molecule and closes the gate. With the gate closed, sodium ion movement from the extracellular to the intracellular space is prevented. This prevents the change in the electrical potential of the axon and eliminates the transmission of the impulse and depolarization. The failure to change the resting potential results in interference with the action potential cycle of the cell.[11,19-21]

Current thoughts on the action of local anesthetic agents suggest that the following events occur:

1. Calcium ions are displaced from a receptor site at the cell membrane as a result of the local anesthetic moiety.
2. Reduction in cell permeability to sodium ions results.
3. The rate of depolarization of the membrane action potential is decreased.
4. The degree of depolarization of the cell is insufficient for reaching the threshold potential of the cell.
5. A propagated action potential does not occur.
6. Conduction blockade is the end result.

The synthetic local anesthetics are weakly basic amines that are not readily soluble in water. Because of this property the local anesthetic is usually made as a hydrochloride salt that is highly water soluble and stable. When in an aqueous solution, the anesthetic compound dissociates into a positively charged quaternary amine cation and an uncharged tertiary amine base.[12,13]

The direction of the reaction depends on the pH of the solution. Each anesthetic has a pK_a, which is the negative logarithm of the dissociation constant. When the pK_a equals the pH, 50% of the salt exists as a cation and 50% exists as an uncharged base. Because the pK_a for a specific compound is constant, the amount of free base or charged cation is dependent on the pH of the solution.[12,13]

As the pH of the solution decreases and the hydrogen ion concentration increases, the balance shifts, and more charged cation is present. The positively charged cation is responsible for the action of the local anesthetic drug. However, the positively charged cation is prevented from passing into the intracellular space. The free base ensures diffusion into the nerve cell or the axon. Once the anesthetic has crossed the cellular membrane, the ions dissociate. The positive cation acts to stabilize (close) the sodium channel gate, resulting in a blockage of movement of ions through the gate (Table 42-2).

Both forms of the local anesthetic are necessary for the action of the medication to occur. One of the hindrances to the administration of a local anesthetic drug is an acidic medium. When the tissues are acidotic, as is seen during an infection, the local anesthetic has difficulty both diffusing across the cellular membrane and having sufficient positively charged cations to cause membrane stabilization.[11,22]

Each local anesthetic has an aromatic lipophilic derivative of benzoic acid or alanine as well as a hydrophilic part. The hydrophilic portion is an amine derivative of ethyl alcohol or acetic acid. The two parts are linked by a hydrocarbon chain that is an ester or an amide. Changing a portion of the chain alters the activity of the compound. Within limits, lengthening the chain increases the potency of the compound. Surpassing this limit results in a decrease in the potency of the anesthetic. Chemical alterations to the compounds that change the protein binding change the duration of action of the local anesthetic (Table 42-3).[11,15,21]

Procaine, tetracaine, and 2-chloroprocaine are all ester-linked local anesthetics, which become hydrolyzed by plasma cholinesterases. This rapid chemical reaction results in the metabolism of the local anesthetic once it is absorbed into the vascular space. No plasma cholinesterases are in either the epidural space or the CSF. Lidocaine, bupivacaine, mepivacaine, etidocaine, levobupivacaine, and ropivacaine are amide-linked drugs. The amide-linked local anesthetics are

TABLE 42-2 Local Anesthetic Drugs

Local Anesthetic	pK_a	Nonionized Drug at pH 7.4 (%)	Mean Onset (min)	Mean Subarachnoid Block Onset (min)	Mean Epidural Onset (min)	Mean Brachial Plexus Duration (min)	Maximum Dose (mg) without Epinephrine
Esters							
Procaine	8.9	3	45-60	2-5	NA	NA	1000
Tetracaine	8.6	14	7-10	7-10	NA	60-180	100; 1-1.5 mg/kg
Chloroprocaine	9.8	2	6-12	5-12	5-12	30-45	800-1000
Amides							
Lidocaine	7	24	3-7	5-10	5-15	60-120	300-500; 3 mg/kg without epi; 7 mg/kg with epi
Mepivacaine	7.6	39	5-7	10-20	5-15	90-180	300-500; same as lidocaine
Bupivacaine	8.1	17	8-15	2-5	10-20	240-480	175-225
Chirocaine	8.1	17	8-15	2-5	10-20	240-480	175-225
Ropivacaine	8.1	17	5-13	2-5	11-26	3-8	300
Prilocaine	7.9	24	5-20	5-15	5-15	60-120	400-600; 8 mg/kg with epi

epi, *Epinephrine;* NA, *not applicable.*
Data from Mosby's Drug Consult. *St Louis:* Mosby; *2004.*

TABLE 42-3 Local Anesthetics Classified by Duration and Potency

Medication	Duration	Potency
Procaine	Short	Low
2-Chloroprocaine	Short	Moderate
Lidocaine	Moderate	Moderate
Prilocaine	Moderate	Moderate
Mepivacaine	Moderate	Moderate
Tetracaine	Long	High
Bupivacaine	Long	High
Ropivacaine	Long	High
Chirocaine	Long	High

metabolized by liver microsomes, and extended use of the medication in either repeated bolus doses or continuous infusions results in possible accumulation and toxicity. With the use of the short-acting, ester-linked local anesthetic 2-chloroprocaine, accumulation and eventual toxicity are unlikely to occur, because of its almost immediate hydrolysis.[11,22,23]

Etidocaine was developed by modification of the lidocaine molecule. A propyl group is substituted for an ethyl group at the amine end. One ethyl group is added to an alpha carbon in the intermediate chain. This medication is more soluble and more highly protein bound, and it has a greater potency and a longer duration of action than the parent compound. The affinity of etidocaine is higher for motor neurons when compared with sensory neurons. When a butyl group was added to the aromatic end of the procaine molecule, tetracaine was identified. Tetracaine has a greater potency, a longer duration of action, and a higher toxicity than procaine.

Changing the chemical structure of the compound results in changes in its intrinsic toxicity and duration of action. Tetracaine is hydrolyzed more slowly than procaine and has a greater potential for toxicity. 2-Chloroprocaine is rapidly hydrolyzed and is the least toxic of the ester-linked local anesthetics. Prilocaine is an amide-linked local anesthetic that is rapidly metabolized; it has a smaller potential for toxicity than any other agent in this group.[11-13,22-24]

The potential for allergic reaction is greatest in the ester-linked group of local anesthetics. Drugs in this group are derivatives of PABA. The ester-linked local anesthetics are hydrolyzed by plasma cholinesterases, resulting in the formation of PABA. This compound can produce an allergic reaction in some individuals.

The metabolism of amide-linked local anesthetics does not produce PABA. The documented incidence of allergic reactions to amide local anesthetics continues to be rare. Local anesthetics that are prepared for multiple-dose regimens contain a stabilizing agent that can be an allergen. Individuals who have allergic reactions to amide local anesthetics may have received an injection with either PABA in the solution or another antigen. Patients may believe that an intravenous injection of an epinephrine-containing solution causes an allergic reaction because of the symptoms that develop.[23]

The absorption and duration of action of local anesthetics are functionally dependent on the pharmacology of the agent, the dose administered, the anesthetic procedure performed, and the use of a vasopressor mixed with the solution. This may not be true of ropivacaine.[22]

In a 1990 study comparing solutions containing bupivacaine with those containing bupivacaine and epinephrine, no change in the duration of the anesthetic was observed when the epinephrine-containing solutions were used.[22] However, the actions of ropivacaine caused a reduction in the blood flow to the area of the injection, resulting in a reduction of the absorption of the medication when a vasopressor agent was not used concomitantly.

Pharmacologically, each drug's duration of action is related to the protein-binding characteristics of the local anesthetic compound, the direct action of the agent, the pH of the solution (as well as of the area surrounding the injection), the rate of metabolism, the excretion of the agent or metabolites, and the degree of vasodilatation in the area. The tissues being injected and the degree of vasodilatation in the area affect the duration of action.

Tetracaine, bupivacaine, levobupivacaine, and ropivacaine are highly protein bound; this quality results in a significantly higher duration of action than those of the medications that are less protein bound. Among the ester-linked anesthetics, tetracaine is 10 times more highly bound to protein than procaine and has a duration of action three to four times greater than that of procaine. Among the amide-linked local anesthetics, bupivacaine, ropivacaine, and levobupivacaine are highly bound to the protein molecule, whereas mepivacaine and lidocaine are less highly bound to protein. As a result the duration of action of bupivacaine, levobupivacaine, and ropivacaine is two to three times longer than that of lidocaine and mepivacaine.[25]

Vasodilatory activity and metabolic rate also influence the duration of action of the local anesthetic. When lidocaine and procaine are compared in vitro, they are very similar; however, when they are compared in vivo, the duration of procaine is much shorter than that of lidocaine because of the vasodilator effects of procaine. When 2-chloroprocaine is compared with procaine, it has a shorter duration of action because of its rapid rate of metabolism.

Most local anesthetic agents cause vasodilatation that is a result of direct smooth muscle relaxation. However, cocaine and ropivacaine cause vasoconstriction. Cocaine inhibits the uptake of norepinephrine, resulting in vasoconstriction. The mechanism that causes vasoconstriction with ropivacaine administration remains under investigation. Because of the potent vasodilator effects of tetracaine, epinephrine or another vasoconstrictor must be used when this medication is administered outside the subarachnoid or epidural space. Lidocaine is a more potent vasodilator than prilocaine. No significant difference occurs in the vasodilatation seen with either bupivacaine or etidocaine.[19]

Adding a vasoconstrictor such as epinephrine to the local anesthetic slows the uptake of the local anesthetic. Vasoconstriction decreases vascular absorption and removal of the local anesthetic from the local vicinity of the nerve, resulting in an increased intensity of the block and an increased duration of action (Table 42-4). The duration of action of levobupivacaine and bupivacaine is minimally affected by the addition of epinephrine. However, the absorption of the anesthetic solution is delayed, an effect that reduces the plasma levels of the medication. When epinephrine is added to the local anesthetic, fresh epinephrine solutions rather than prepared solutions should be used. Commonly used concentrations of epinephrine include 1:100,000, 1:150,000, and 1:200,000. The pH of the prepared solution is lower than that of the fresh solution, resulting in less available free cation per

TABLE 42-4 Duration of Action of Spinal Analgesia

Medication	Duration of Intraabdominal Analgesia (hr)	Duration of Perineal and Lower-Extremity Analgesia (hr)
Tetracaine	1.25-1.75	2-2.5
Tetracaine with 5 mg of phenylephrine	2.25-3.5	5-5.75
Tetracaine with 0.2 mg of epinephrine	1.75-2.5	2.5-3.75

milligram of the drug than if it were mixed when needed. Additionally, phenylephrine (100 mcg) can be used in place of epinephrine as a vasoconstrictor.[21]

Absorption of the local anesthetic determines its duration of action. The site of the injection directly affects the absorption of the agent, and injections into the intercostal area are the most rapidly absorbed. The slowest absorption results from cutaneous injections in areas of the body that have reduced blood supply. The rate of uptake changes the response to the medication. If the uptake is rapid, a less-than-toxic dose can cause toxic symptoms because of the rapid rise in the blood level of the medication.

As with other medications, local anesthetics are distributed throughout the body, following rules of diffusion and redistribution. The highest concentrations of local anesthetics are found in vessel-rich tissues, and the lowest concentrations are found in vessel-poor tissues. Bupivacaine affinity for cardiac muscle tissue may be one of the many factors that contribute to the increased toxicity of this drug, especially in cardiac tissue.

Placental transfer of the local anesthetics is dependent on the rate of diffusion and protein binding.[18] After epidural injection, bupivacaine and levobupivacaine appear to have the lowest concentrations in the umbilical vein, whereas lidocaine and mepivacaine have moderate concentrations. Agents that are highly protein bound in the mother, a quality that results in a low maternal plasma concentration, may have a higher concentration in the fetal circulation. Medication chosen for obstetric use should have reduced ability to cross the placenta.[10,26]

Excretion depends on metabolism of the drug. The metabolism of both groups of local anesthetics is dependent on liver function, either through direct degradation or through the production of pseudocholinesterases. The ester-linked local anesthetics are hydrolyzed by plasma pseudocholinesterase into PABA and diethyl amino-ethanol. The amide-linked local anesthetics undergo degradation in the liver. The rate of degradation or hydrolysis has a direct impact on toxicity. Prilocaine is the most rapidly metabolized and the least toxic of this group.

Although the metabolites of the amide-linked local anesthetics have been found, the complete mechanism of degradation has not yet been identified. Lidocaine oxidizes to become monoglycinexylidide. In normal patients, little concern exists regarding the toxic or pharmacologic effects of the residual metabolite. However, in patients with renal failure, this metabolite may accumulate and play a role in increased toxicity. Prilocaine is metabolized to *o*-toluidine, which can cause the development of methemoglobin, thus resulting in methemoglobinemia. This condition may develop when the dose of the local anesthetic exceeds 400 mg. Treatment of methemoglobinemia consists of administration of methylene blue, 1 to 5 mg/kg.

In addition, excretion of the local anesthetics is dependent on renal function. Less than 2% of procaine is excreted unchanged, whereas 100% of cocaine is excreted unchanged. An inverse relationship exists between renal clearance of the amide-linked local anesthetics and the degree of protein binding. Prilocaine is less protein bound than lidocaine, which results in more rapid renal clearance with prilocaine than with lidocaine.[11]

BRIEF HISTORICAL OVERVIEW OF SPINAL ANESTHESIA

Spinal anesthesia became popular after the discovery of the local anesthetic properties of cocaine, the invention of the hollow needle and syringe, and the written descriptions of the first lumbar puncture. The first clinical application of the technique was reportedly performed in the late 1890s.

Its prominence was short lived. The introduction of specific, reversible, neuromuscular blocking drugs and concurrent improvements in inhalation agents for general anesthesia soon displaced its popularity. Only recently has it regained popularity, in large part because of the introduction of newer agents, equipment, and techniques.

APPLIED ANATOMY AND PHYSIOLOGY OF THE NEURAXIS: REVIEW OF ANATOMY

Knowledge of anatomic landmarks and underlying structures aids the anesthetist in formation of a three-dimensional, "mind's-eye" picture. This picture, coordinated with the "feel" of the structures and tissues against the needle and a steady, sensitive hand, facilitates accurate placement of the needle tip and administration of appropriate medications. Although anatomy is the oldest of medical sciences, with detailed descriptions of the spinal column dating from the nineteenth century, modern imaging methods like computed tomography, magnetic resonance imagining, and endoscopic examination have permitted in vivo investigations that further our understanding of spinal anatomy. The following is therefore a current review of applied anatomy of the neuraxis.

The sequential interconnectivity of 33 bones called *vertebra* forms the spinal, or vertebral, column, which anesthetists use as a bony reference during the placement of various anesthetics or analgesics. This column is located in the posterior midline of the trunk and allows for truncal flexibility because movable joint surfaces and cartilaginous vertebral bodies exist between 24 of the 33 vertebrae (Figure 42-2). The vertebral column extends from the base of the skull and the foramen magnum to the tip of the coccyx. The vertebral bodies are stacked on top of one another, separated by a fibrocartilaginous intervertebral disc, to provide support for the cranium and trunk. The body is contiguous with two pedicles that stretch in a posterior and slightly lateral direction, joining to two lamina that stretch posteriorly and medially to complete an arch, creating an oval-triangular foramen. This foramen, known as the *vertebral foramen*, allows for the passage and protection of the spinal cord. Transverse processes on both sides of the pedicles allow for muscular attachments and the control of movement. A spinous process projects along the median plane from the union of the laminae in a posteroinferior direction. The spinous process is the long, slender, bony prominence that can

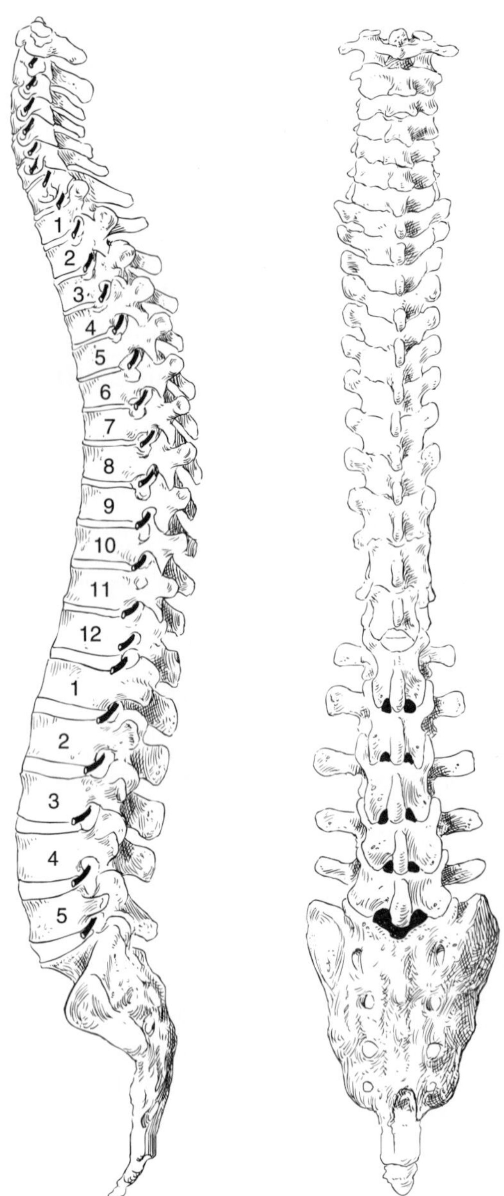

FIGURE **42-2**
The spinal, or vertebral, column with its 33 vertebrae.

often be seen and felt along the midline of the back. The spinous process also provides a place for muscular attachment and movement control. In addition, the inferior angle of the bone creates an overlap that further protects the spinal cord (Figure 42-3).[27] In general, each vertebra can be visualized as having two parts. The anterior, cylindric portion of the vertebra is solid and is called the *body*. This heavier portion of the vertebra forms the anterior portion of the vertebral arch.

The pedicles and processes of each vertebra have superior and inferior articular surfaces and have lateral notches. The superior notch is shallow when compared with the deeper inferior notch. When the vertebrae are stacked, the notches and the articulating surfaces, known as *zygapophyseal* or *facet joints*, form the intervertebral foramina. The intervertebral foramina provide safe passage for spinal nerves passing from the spinal cord to the rest of the body. The articular surfaces of the facet joints are covered with hyaline cartilage, which permits a gliding motion between the vertebrae. Because the facet joints are innervated by branches from closely associated spinal nerves, these joints often become clinically important. When the joint is injured, the associated spinal nerves may also be affected, leading to pain along associated dermatomes or muscle spasm along associated myotomes.[27]

The size and shape of vertebral lamina and spinous processes differ among the thoracic, lumbar, and sacral regions, and variation exists within each region. Knowledge of these variations is important in the practice of regional anesthesia in selection and administration of spinal and epidural anesthesia. For instance, cervical and thoracic vertebrae have spinous processes that angle acutely in a caudad direction such that the process of the superior vertebrae overlaps the inferior vertebrae and its process. This construction adds protection to the spinal cord when an individual stands erect but must also be allowed for when attempts are made to insert a needle into the cervical or thoracic regions.

In the lumbar region the vertebrae are larger and the spinous processes become shorter and broader and have a posterior orientation with less overlap than that in other vertebrae. Relatively large gaps, bridged by ligaments, exist between the spinous processes in the lumbar area. This provides the anesthesia practitioner easier access for needle placement, catheter passage, and the instillation of anesthetic into the epidural or subarachnoid space for surgical and obstetric procedures.

The sacrum is a triangle-shaped section of fused bodies of vertebrae. The broader portion is the base, which tapers as it approaches the coccyx. The sacrum is shaped so the weight of the body forces the base of the sacrum downward and forward. It is wedged tightly between the two iliac crests by the downward forces exerted on the spinal column. The lamina of the last sacral vertebra is incomplete and is bridged only by ligaments. This area is known as the *sacral hiatus* (Figure 42-4).[27] The coccyx is composed of four small segments of bone that become fused into two bones as an individual ages; by the age of 25 to 30 years, the fusion is complete. The bodies of the vertebrae can be identified with the transverse processes and articular processes. No pedicles or spinous processes are present. The last, or fourth, bone is small and is similar to a nodule. The changing size of the bone from the first to the fourth vertebra gives the coccyx the appearance of a triangle. The projections of the rudimentary articular processes are known as the *cornua*, and the superior pair is the most pronounced. These sacral cornua are the "horns" or bony protuberances that guard the area of the sacral hiatus.[27] Because they can be easily palpated in children and in most adults, they are important surface anatomic landmarks for the performance of a caudal anesthetic procedure.

Of the more than 35 pairs of muscles and ligaments in the back the supraspinous ligaments, the interspinous ligaments, and the ligamenta flava (yellow ligaments) are of special significance to the anesthesia practitioner. These three structures act as landmarks that help in identification of and access to the epidural and the subarachnoid spaces. The supraspinous ligament is a strong cordlike ligament that connects the apices of the spinous processes; it is thick and serves as the major ligament in the cervical and upper thoracic regions. The supraspinous ligament consists of three layers: the superficial layer extends over several vertebral spinous processes, the middle layer connects two or three spinous processes, and the inner layer connects only the neighboring spinous processes. The ligament blends at all levels with the thin interspinous ligaments that run between adjacent spinous processes. The

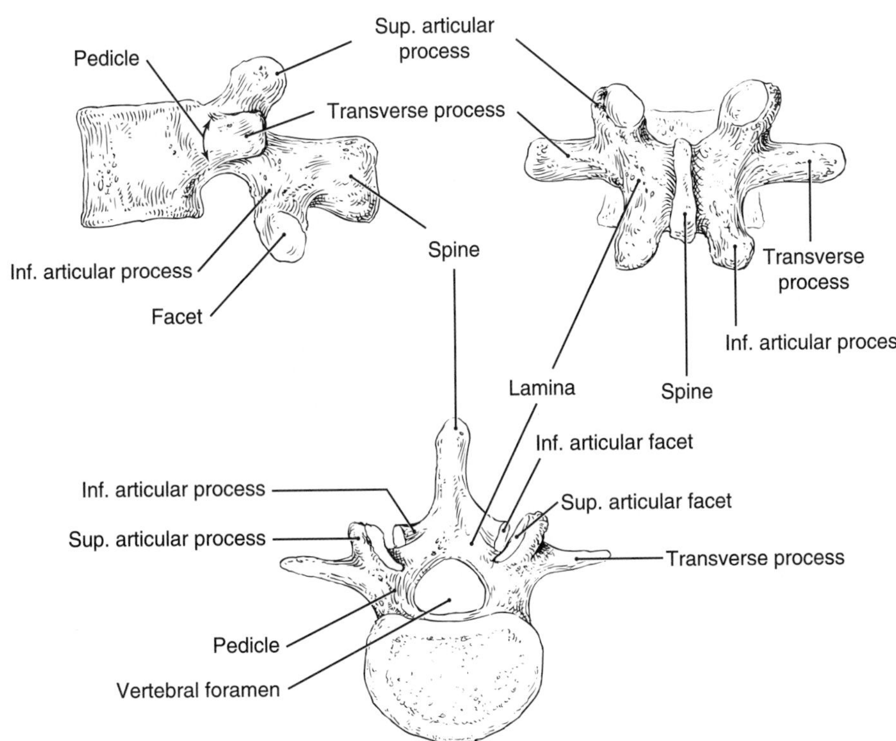

FIGURE **42-3**
Articular surfaces, transverse processes, and spinous process. *Inf*, Inferior; *Sup*, superior.

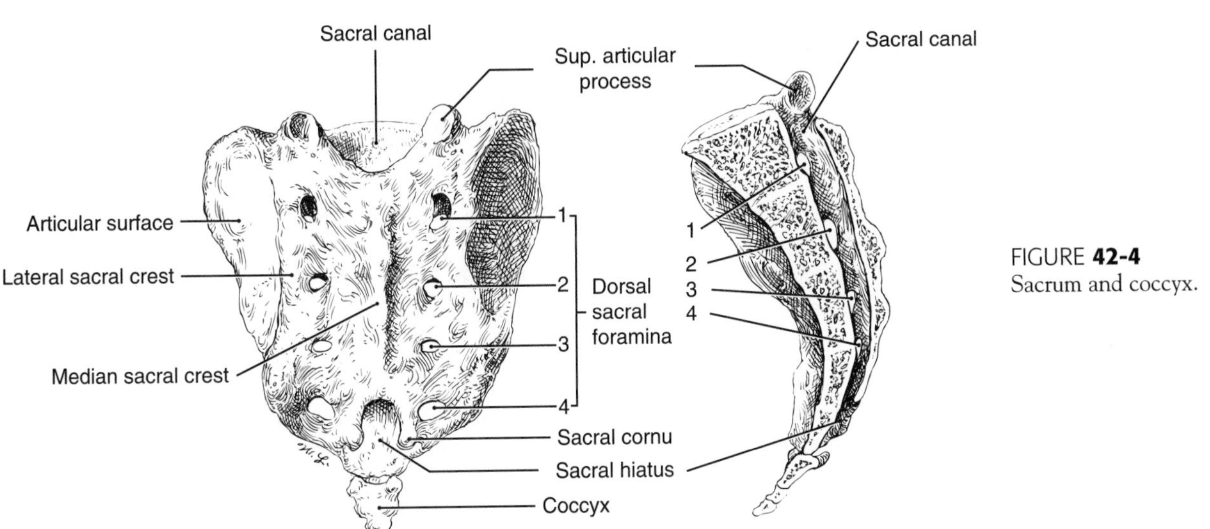

FIGURE **42-4**
Sacrum and coccyx.

interspinous ligaments are usually absent or of poor quality in the cervical region and can be exceptionally thin in the lumbar area, even in young people. The ligamenta flava are the strongest of the posterior ligaments. These broad elastic bands join the vertebral arches through vertical extensions from adjacent lamina. The ligamenta flava are paired flat ligaments that run caudad from the inferior border of one lamina to the upper border of the lower lamina on both sides of the midline. The two ligaments almost fill the space, leaving only a separation in the midline and thereby creating a **V** or wedge that points posteriorly to align with the interspinous and supraspinous ligaments. The **V** is thin on the lateral edge and thickest midline—in an adult approximately 3 to 5 mm at the L2-L3 interspace. The ligaments extend from each lamina with an overlapping of fibers that creates the appearance of a contiguous ligament from one vertebral body to the next. The ligament is thicker in the lumbar area than in the cervical area and is responsible for maintenance of upright posture. The ligaments' color comes from their high content of yellow elastic tissue.[28]

The spinal cord itself is a cylindric structure extending from the medulla oblongata through the spinal foramen to the level of the L2 vertebra in most adults and ranges from 42 to 45 cm in length (Figure 42-5). Because the vertebral column grows more rapidly than the spinal cord, the spinal cord in children extends initially to the level of the third lumbar vertebra. In approximately 1% of adults the spinal cord may extend below the second lumbar vertebra and rarely to the level of the L3 vertebra. The spinal cord tapers to the conus medullaris, and nerve pathways continue in a collection of rootlets, called the

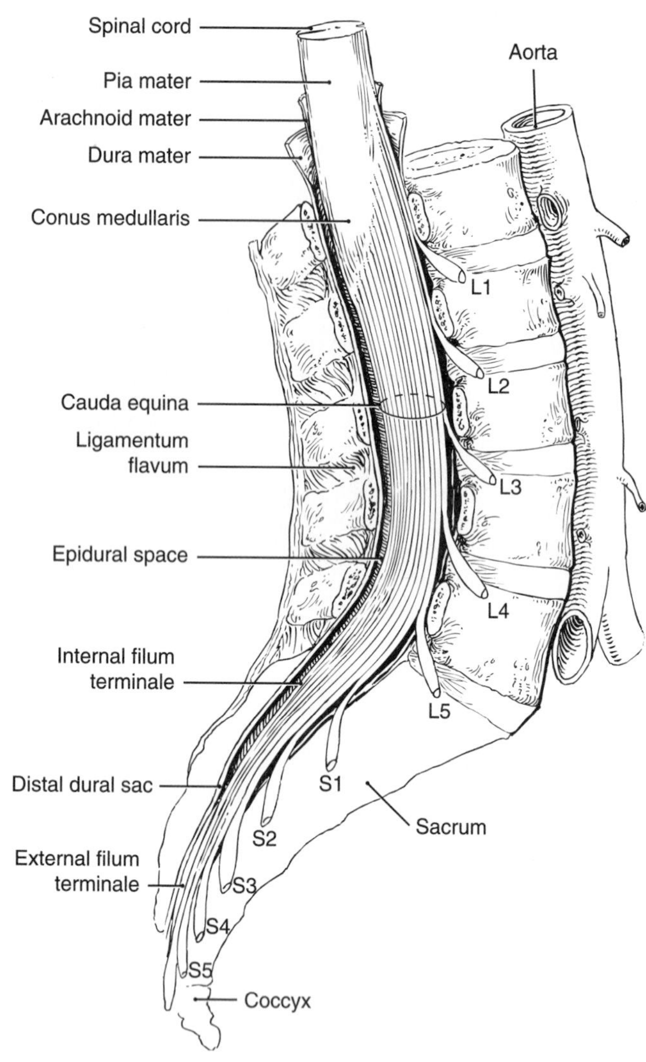

FIGURE **42-5**
Extension of the spinal cord to the second lumbar vertebra.

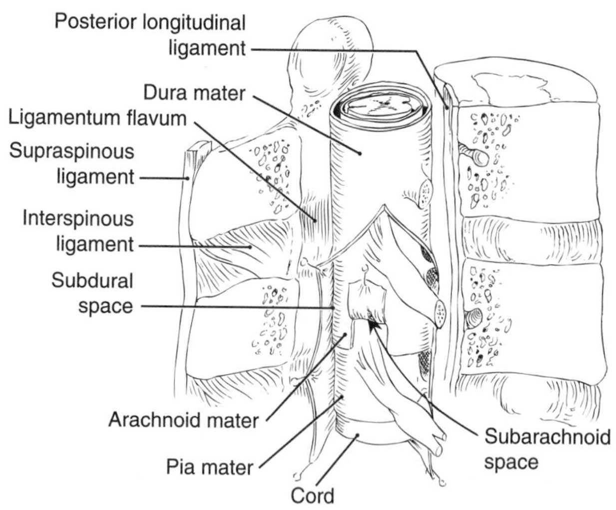

FIGURE **42-6**
The linings of the spinal cord and the posterior ligaments of the spinal column.

cauda equina or *horse's tail*, which extends from L1 to S5. The spinal cord is enlarged in two regions. The first, called the cervical enlargement, extends from the spinal segments C4 to T1. The ventral rami of the spinal nerves in this enlargement form the brachial plexus of nerves that innervates the upper limbs. The second enlargement stretches from the L2 to the S3 segment of the spinal cord. This lumbosacral enlargement contributes corresponding nerves to create the lumbar and sacral plexuses. It is important to note that the spinal cord levels do not directly correspond with vertebral levels. For example, in adults the lumbosacral enlargement (L2 to S3) usually extends from the body of the T11 vertebra to the level of the body of the L1 vertebra.[27]

The spinal cord is enveloped by the same three membranes that line the cranium, and they are collectively called the *meninges*. The meninges are nonnervous support tissues that provide a protective covering for the cord and nerve roots from the foramen magnum to the base of the cauda equina. The linings are identified as the dura mater, the arachnoid mater, and the pia mater. The dura mater is the outermost layer. It is a thick, tough membrane that provides most of the protection for the central cord structures. The nerve roots are covered with dura mater while inside the spinal canal. As the roots exit the canal via the intervertebral foramen, the dura blends into the root at a junction referred to as a *dural cuff* or *root sleeve*. The arachnoid mater is a thin, spider web–like covering that forms the middle layer. Beneath the arachnoid mater is a space that is continuous with the central canal of the cord and the ventricles. This space, which is filled with CSF, is known as the *subarachnoid space*. This mater and the fluid protect the spinal cord from shock injuries and are the medium for the interaction with local anesthetics and opioids that occurs during the administration of regional anesthesia. The innermost layer, the pia mater, is thin and is in direct contact with the outer surface of the spinal cord (Figure 42-6).[27]

The epidural space is a potential space outside the dural sac but inside the vertebral canal and is continuous from the base of the cranium to the base of the sacral sulcus. The epidural space contains epidural veins, fat, lymphatics, segmental arteries, and nerve roots. Fat in the epidural spaces is physiologically fluid, acting as a pad and lubricant for the movement of neural structures within the canal. The posterior epidural space, as it is approached by the anesthetist's advancing needle, is protected by the ligamenta flava, the lamina, and the spinous processes. It is easy but inaccurate to depict the epidural space as a uniform column surrounding an equally uniform and tapering spinal cord. A better mental picture is provided by a "look" along the longitudinal axes. The epidural space can be envisioned as a series of lateral, posterior, and anterior compartments existing among the vertebral body, lamina, and pedicles. The compartments, occupied mostly by fat but also by nerves and fibrous tissue, repeat at each segment in a metameric fashion. Of greatest interest to the anesthetist, the posterior epidural space is a series of fat-filled tripodal pads, shaped like a three-sided sand dune. The pad stretches and narrows in a caudad direction as it approaches the next inferior lamina. In areas of the vertebral canal surrounded by bone the dura actually contacts bone, leaving only a potential epidural space that physically separates the epidural fat-containing compartments. The posterior epidural space, therefore, is a discontinuous group of tapering fat pads that repeat throughout the length of the spinal canal and are separated by a potential space that allows the passage of fluids or small catheters.[28-31]

The distance from the skin to the epidural space and the depth of the epidural space, or the distance to the dura, is of interest to the anesthetist who wishes to avoid needle injury of neural and vascular tissues. The distance to the epidural space varies with vertebral level and is loosely correlated with patient weight. The distance from skin to the lumbar epidural space using a midline approach varies from 2.5 cm to 8 cm, with an average of 5 cm. Because the space itself is not a uniform shape, the depth of the epidural space from the ligamentum flavum to the dura varies considerably. Given the tripodal, dunelike shape of the epidural space, expect the space to narrow considerably when approaching laterally to the midline and in more caudad areas in the space. The depth of the epidural space is also relative to the vertebral level of approach and angle of needle entry; however, some clinical generalizations can be made. The epidural space is largest (posterior to anterior) in the midline of the midlumbar region, at 5 to 6 mm. The midline thoracic region epidural space may be 3 to 5 mm deep and is narrower there (lateral width). Caution is used when one approaches the lower cervical region, as the epidural space is very small (only 1.5 to 2 mm), which leaves little room for error.[29]

In addition to a larger epidural space, another anatomic reason to stay midline with an approaching anesthetic needle is the presence of the epidural veins. The epidural veins are valveless veins that form a plexus draining the blood from the spinal cord and the linings of the cord. The plexus is most prominent in the lateral portion of the epidural space, but in pregnant or obese patients the epidural veins become engorged and swollen as increased intraabdominal pressure results in venous congestion of the lumbar and sacral vessels. The potential for injury or accidental cannulation of these vessels is increased because of this compensatory physiologic change.[27,28,30]

A final anatomic consideration for neuraxial anesthesia is the existence of normal and abnormal curvatures of the spinal column. A median plane longitudinal view of the vertebral column reveals four curvatures in the normal adult. The thoracic and sacral curvatures have posterior curvatures (concave anteriorly), whereas the cervical and lumbar regions have anterior curvatures (concave posteriorly). In a supine patient the apex of the lumbar curve is usually at L3 to L4, and the trough of the thoracic curve is at T4.[32] Scoliosis, the most common abnormal curvature, is a lateral curvature of the spine, and kyphosis is an excessive posterior curvature or hump, usually of the thoracic region. Excessive lordosis or hollowing of the back may occur as a result of obesity as the body attempts to restore the center of gravity. A temporary lordosis may also occur during pregnancy. Changes in these anatomic curves will challenge the anesthesia provider during the performance of epidural or spinal anesthetic techniques.[27]

Consideration of patients' spinal curvatures is also important when anticipating the spread of local anesthetics in the subarachnoid space relative to the site of injection and patient position.

Neuroanatomic Mapping and Evaluation of Neuraxial Anesthesia

The goal of neuraxial anesthesia is to block pain transmission from areas of injury, disease, or surgical intervention. Therefore it is clinically useful to have knowledge of the innervations of body structures being operated on in relation to spinal nerve location within the vertebral column. Anatomic maps have been generated based on cutaneous sensation alone. These sensation maps are referred to as *dermatomal maps*, *charts*, or *levels*. A dermatome is defined as the area of cutaneous sensation supplied by a spinal nerve that is anatomically identified as it passes through an intervertebral foramen. For example, the umbilical area is directly anterior to the L3 vertebra but receives cutaneous innervations from T7 to T11 depending on the dermatomal map consulted.

For the practical clinician, use of accepted anatomic landmarks and test methods is perhaps the best method for documenting the sensory level achieved. The level of anesthetic can be evaluated in many ways, and tests can be used to evaluate several components of the neuraxial anesthetic. For motor function a straight leg raise or request to "step on the gas" works well as a clinical measure. Cutaneous sensation can be evaluated through use of multiple pinpricks with a blunted needle, pinwheels, and the stylet from the spinal or epidural needle, a peripheral nerve stimulator, or a portion of a broken wooden tongue blade. Such a "scratch" test is done using two surface anatomy points for comparison. Inform the patient that the sensation on a normal area, such as the skin surface of the shoulder, is scratchy or sharp. Next, scratch an area expected to be numb, such as the lateral thigh. Gradually work cephalad in two or three-inch bands until the patient notices a change in sensation. This approximates the upper level of sensory loss. Skin refrigerant, ice cubes, and alcohol pads can be used in a similar manner to identify changes in temperature sensation.

Physiology and Purported Mechanisms of Action

Despite over 90 years of research and experience with spinal and epidural anesthesia, much speculation remains regarding the exact cellular locations and molecular mechanisms involved when local anesthetics, opioids, and other pharmacologically active agents bind to produce spinal analgesia and anesthesia.[33,34] What is known and clinically important about spinal and epidural anesthesia is that the primary site of action for local anesthetics is on the nerve roots within the spinal cord. When a drug is injected directly into the CSF, the drug distributes through the subarachnoid space based on the physical and chemical properties of that injectant and the characteristics of the space in which it must spread. When the drug concentration reaches a minimal effective concentration, neuronal transmission is altered in a manner that clinically provides anesthesia. Neurons—some myelinated, others not; some relatively large, others smaller—differ in susceptibility to drugs such as local anesthetics, and these pharmacodynamic relationships are not easily explained (see Table 42-1). The processes involved at the cellular level are very complex, and *blockade* is perhaps a confusing term. Anesthetic drugs more accurately alter nerve transmission by affecting predominately sodium ion channels and affect the units of information that are transferred along the spinal cord. Complete blockade or a "chemical transection" of the cord is an oversimplification. For example, somatosensory evoked potentials have been recorded in individuals made functionally insensate from lidocaine epidural anesthesia. This suggests that neural transmissions are reaching the brain without causing sensory perceptions.[13,28]

When a local anesthetic interrupts nerve transmission of autonomic nerves, for example, but not sensory nerves or motor nerves because of a variation in susceptibility, then a "differential block" is said to have occurred. A differential block is seen in the more rostral spinal segments of a spinal anesthetic. As the spinal anesthetic spreads from the epicenter of injection, the distal reaches of drug distribution are presumably of lesser concentrations. A differential block is clinically important when sensory anesthesia is desired at a specific level; however, sympathetic blockade could be deleterious in a patient with coexisting disease. The level of sympathetic blockade could be as high as six or more dermatomal levels above the level of sensory blockade, therefore potentially contributing to hypotension and bradycardia.[34]

Drug injected into the epidural space is distributed to the same sites of action as a spinal anesthetic but in a slightly different manner. The drug must first distribute along the epidural space then diffuse through the meninges and dural cuffs to reach the nerve roots or reach the spinal cord through absorption into the radicular arteries.[17] Data exist to support the clinical impression that spinal anesthesia is generally more dense than epidural anesthesia. Epidural local anesthetics first act at sites, such as the dural cuffs, at which spinal nerves pass through the peridural spaces. This is consistent with the segmental onset often associated with epidural anesthesia. If the concentration and volume of the anesthetic agent is increased or if time is allowed for the drug to diffuse into the CSF or pass via radicular arteries into the spinal cord, then the epidural anesthetic can become more dense.[28,32]

Neuraxial Anesthesia: Indications and Contraindications

Spinal and epidural anesthesia (neuraxial anesthesia) can be used successfully for a variety of inpatient or ambulatory surgical procedures involving the lower extremities, perineum, and abdomen. In addition, spinal and epidural anesthesia or analgesia is used for the treatment of acute and chronic pain syndromes and for obstetric procedures and can be applied in patients at the extremes of age.[35] Spinal anesthesia techniques may also be used in combination with other techniques such as epidural catheter techniques, general or intravenous anesthetic techniques, and perhaps the use of a laryngeal mask airway to provide anesthesia during surgery. Such combinations or balanced techniques minimize the side effects of any one anesthetic technique and maximize the benefits.[36]

As with any anesthetic plan, proper preparation, patient selection, education, and collaboration with surgeons and nurses are the keys to success. Often the best time to obtain a truly informed consent is during the preoperative visit. It is important to establish rapport with patients, gaining their trust and cooperation. Patients eager to be involved in their own care often have the emotional maturity to understand the benefits of their anesthetic options and make rational choices. Anticipate patients' fears and anxieties; they are often easily dealt with through education and the reassurance provided by the calm voice of a confident and competent anesthetist.

Potential advantages of neuraxial anesthesia include less nausea, vomiting, and urinary retention; a reduced total opioid requirement; and greater mental alertness relative to patients who have received general anesthesia alone. After regional anesthesia, patients are quick to eat, void, and ambulate. Ambulatory surgical patients may or may not be discharged any sooner after spinal anesthesia when compared with those who have undergone general anesthesia, but they can avoid unnecessary overnight admissions resulting from complications of general anesthesia.[37] A growing body of evidence also supports improved outcomes for selected patients and situations. Spinal and epidural anesthesia blunt the body's stress response to surgery and may offer preemptive analgesia. In addition, studies have shown neuraxial anesthetics to decrease intraoperative blood loss, lower the incidence of postoperative thromboembolic events and postoperative ileus, increase patency of vascular grafts, improve respiratory function and cardiac stability, and improve outcome in high-risk surgical patients.

Patient safety may also be increased with spinal or epidural anesthesia. Urologic procedures such as cystoscopic examinations and transurethral resections of the prostate (TURP) are most often performed with the use of spinal anesthesia. When awake and anesthetized to the level of the dome of the bladder (T10), the patient may verbally respond to bladder overdistention, thereby helping the urologist minimize the potential for bladder rupture. In addition, the mental status of a responsive patient can easily be monitored and the development of conditions associated with the TURP syndrome such as hypervolemia, hyponatremia, and ammonium toxicity more readily detected.[38]

Safety is also an issue when the patient is placed in the prone or jackknifed position as for perianal procedures. A patient in such a position under general anesthesia is at risk for inadvertent extubation and positioning injury. A hypobaric spinal anesthesia technique offers several advantages. The anesthetic procedure can be performed after the patient is positioned and has verbalized that he or she is comfortably padded. With hypobaric spinal anesthesia the spread of the local anesthetic is controlled and spontaneous ventilation is maintained.

Patients often fear postoperative discomfort. Therefore another advantage of spinal anesthesia is the ability to administer long-acting spinal opioids or clonidine. Epidural catheter placement allows for opioids, low concentrations of local anesthetics, or mixtures containing both solutions to be continuously infused or administered by patient-controlled devices, thereby keeping patients comfortable well into the postoperative period. Because the total doses of opioids and local anesthetics are small, the patient remains alert and possibly ambulatory while experiencing analgesia with minimal side effects.[28,32] The patient's right to be fully informed also necessitates a discussion of the disadvantages of neuraxial anesthesia. Consider the patient's perspective and keep in mind that the disadvantages and risks inherent in any anesthetic plan are relative only to those of another anesthetic option. For example, patients with a history of headaches or backaches are at increased risk for experiencing these problems after spinal and epidural analgesia but may also experience exacerbations of these problems after a general anesthetic procedure. Such patients should be evaluated and counseled regarding this potential problem before the administration of any anesthetic. A thorough history of the patient's previous pattern of headaches or backaches is essential when faced with the challenge of evaluating similar symptoms in the postoperative period.

To many patients the risk of paralysis is the most important concern despite the extreme rarity of any neurologic sequela. The incidence rate of persistent paresthesia and sensory or motor dysfunction is less than 0.1%.[28,39-41] Common patient questions may also include the following:

- "Will the injections hurt?"
- "How long will I be numb?"
- "I am afraid of hearing (or smelling or feeling) the surgery. Can I be asleep?"

Patient perceptions can be corrected with thoughtful explanation and discussion of the clinician's expectations regarding the patient's case. Additional discussion should include the topic of intraoperative risks, such as the inability to obtain adequate anesthesia, paresthesia, hypotension, dyspnea, high or total spinal anesthesia, nausea and vomiting, use of additional sedation, and allergic reactions. Postoperative complications may include backache, PDPH, hearing loss, transient radicular irritation (TRI; transient neurologic symptoms), infection, and peridural abscess or hematoma formation.[15,29,39,42]

Before administration of any anesthetic a thorough preoperative history and physical examination must be conducted. During this part of the preoperative patient visit any concerns regarding administration of spinal anesthesia can be identified. Often the terms *absolute* and *relative contraindications* are used; the definition of these categories varies, and their use is therefore controversial. In my opinion it is more important to think of the anesthetic risks and associated complications relative to the possible benefits of the proposed anesthetic technique. An obvious example is patient refusal or lack of cooperation. Other preoperative concerns worthy of discussion during the preoperative patient visit include increased intracranial pressure; significant preexisting or therapeutic coagulopathy; skin infection at the site of injection; hypovolemia; spinal cord disease; patients with a fixed-volume cardiac state such as idiopathic hypertrophic subaortic stenosis or severe atrial stenosis; and an anticipated lengthy surgical time. Also, if a difficult airway is anticipated, it is discussed.

A dural puncture by a spinal needle or a larger epidural needle creates a rent in dural tissue that may or may not leak CSF. In patients with a preexisting increase in intracranial pressure the risk of brain herniation is increased. In the case of epidural catheter placement or epidural blood patch the addition of large volumes of fluid into the epidural or subarachnoid spaces would increase already elevated intracranial pressures. Other neurologic diseases are often listed as contraindications for neuraxial anesthesia. No evidence suggests that spinal or epidural anesthesia worsens or exacerbates conditions such as a gradually progressive diabetic neuropathy or the more fickle vacillations of multiple sclerosis; however, a legitimate medicolegal concern is that blame may be incorrectly placed on the anesthetic. If a neuraxial block is the appropriate anesthetic choice, then precise documentation of the patient's preexisting disease state and existing neurologic compromise is a mandatory precaution.[15,28,32,39]

The existence of a significant preexisting or therapeutic coagulopathy increases the risk of spinal or epidural hematoma. A spinal or epidural hematoma is a rare but devastating complication possibly resulting in permanent neurologic injury. Therefore, neuraxial anesthesia should be avoided in any patient with a coagulopathy. Substantial controversy has surrounded the use of spinal and epidural anesthesia when coagulopathy for thromboprophylaxis has been initiated or is planned. For example, patients routinely use aspirin or NSAIDs and are often preoperatively anticoagulated with heparin or warfarin. Also, with the increased use of natural and herbal medicines, anesthetists must be alert to the possibility of drug interactions when anticoagulation control becomes difficult and no other causes are apparent. However, if basic precautions are followed, some thromboprophylaxis therapies such as subcutaneous heparin and oral warfarin have had an extensive safety record when coadministered with neuraxial anesthetics. The usual recommendation is to place a needle or catheter at least 1 hour before administration of heparin. Anticoagulation should be monitored, PTT should be measured, and any catheters used should be pulled when heparin activity is at a minimal level, an hour before any subsequent dose. A similar approach is used with the oral anticoagulant warfarin. Coagulation should be closely monitored (via assessment of PT and international normalized ratio [INR]) because of considerable variability in patient response to this drug. Generally, the need for acute pain management exists within the first few days after surgery. If warfarin is started in the postoperative period, the epidural catheter is removed before warfarin has reached a therapeutic level. It is also important to remember that the tissue trauma and bleeding associated with needle placement and catheter insertion is as likely with catheter removal. Therefore, documentation of normal coagulation for catheter removal is a reasonable goal. This goal, however, may need to be weighed against the risks of ongoing trauma from an indwelling catheter and the need for ongoing coagulation.[41]

More recently, an increase has occurred in the use of low–molecular-weight heparins (LMWH). Since the introduction of these drugs, the incidence of spinal hematomas in the United States has increased from an estimated rate of approximately 1:200,000 to a rate between 1:1000 and 1:10,000 with neuraxial blocks.[41] New recommendations have been made based on successful use of these drugs in Europe, but because of the rarity of spinal hematomas this issue will be unresolved until more data and experience can be garnered. Based on the most current data and recommendations (such as the American Society of Regional Anesthesia consensus recommendations, 1998) our department has adopted the following recommendations:

1. The surgeon and anesthesia provider should consider the potential benefit versus risk before neuraxial intervention for patients who have been or will be anticoagulated for thromboprophylaxis.
2. Patients not receiving anticoagulant therapy and with no history or clinical signs of coagulopathy (easy bruising, bleeding gums, small cuts that bleed profusely) are routinely offered regional anesthetic options as appropriate.
3. Patients receiving antiplatelet medications alone may receive neuraxial anesthesia without regardless of when they received the last dose. It is preferred that aspirin be stopped 8 days before and NSAIDs 3 days before the procedure.
4. Subcutaneous or minidose heparin thromboprophylaxis does not preclude the use of neuraxial techniques. It is recommended that subsequent heparin doses be held for at least 1 hour after the placement of a neuraxial anesthetic and that catheters be placed and removed late in the interval between administration of heparin doses (10 hours after a dose or approximately 2 hours before the next anticipated dose).
5. Patients receiving chronic warfarin therapy should have this medication stopped at least 4 days before surgery.
6. If a patient receives more than one dose of warfarin within 24 hours of surgery, an INR should be checked immediately before the scheduled procedure. Neuraxial anesthesia can be administered if the preoperative INR is less than 1.4. The PT and INR values in patients with epidural catheters for continuous postoperative epidural analgesia should be evaluated daily. The catheter will not be pulled until the INR is less than 1.4.
7. Patients receiving fibrinolytic or thrombolytic drug therapy should not receive neuraxial anesthesia for 10 days. If the uses of such medications are anticipated in the postoperative period, these techniques should be avoided.
8. Patients receiving intravenous heparin therapy before surgery should not receive neuraxial anesthesia until a normal PTT can be documented.

9. Combinations of the previously listed medications place the patient at greater risk for the development of complications such as spinal or epidural hematoma formation and permanent neurologic injury. Therefore risks and benefits must be carefully weighed on an individual basis.
10. Patients may undergo single-dose and continuous catheter neuraxial techniques when LMWH thromboprophylaxis is anticipated. It is recommended that indwelling catheters be removed at least 2 hours before the initial dose of LMWH and that the first dose of LMWH be administered no earlier than 24 hours after surgery and only in the presence of adequate hemostasis.
11. Patients with medical indications for both an indwelling epidural catheter and the need for LMWH thromboprophylaxis should not receive any other medications that can potentially alter coagulation (aspirin, NSAIDs, dextrans, warfarin). Catheter removal should occur 8 to 12 hours after an administration of LMWH or 1 to 2 hours before the next dose.
12. Patients who have received a neuraxial anesthetic and who are on LMWH should be closely monitored for signs and symptoms of neurologic impairment. Any noted neurologic compromise is to be immediately reported, as emergent treatment is required.

The rarity of this event makes risk factor identification difficult, but case reports reveal a high incidence among elderly women with indwelling catheters undergoing orthopedic procedures. Most were receiving LMWH in addition to other antiplatelet therapy. Although a patient's status as a member of this high-risk group should raise one's index of suspicion, vigilant care must be maintained for all patients. Analysis of the known case reports found the median time to onset of neurologic dysfunction after initiation of LMWH therapy to be 3 days. The initial complaint was of new-onset weakness and sensory deficit, although bowel and bladder dysfunction and new-onset back pain can also occur. Emergent neurosurgical care is required; recovery is unlikely if surgical decompression of the hematoma is delayed more than 8 hours.[41,43]

The etiology of neuraxial infection is based on the theory that needle placement disrupts the body's physiologic protective mechanisms and deposits infectious or noxious agents beyond the skin, into underlying tissues and the peridural space and past the blood-brain barrier into subarachnoid spaces. Indeed, skin infection at the site of injection increases the risk of meningitis or epidural abscess formation. Although infectious complications of neuraxial anesthesia are exceedingly rare, the practitioner must maintain aseptic technique during the preparation and administration of any regional anesthetic to minimize the potential for infection. Septic meningitis or epidural abscess caused by bacterial contamination, and its consequences, can be devastating. Other factors that may theoretically increase the risk of infection include dermatologic conditions such as psoriasis that prevent aseptic skin preparation, underlying sepsis, diabetes, immunologic compromise (cancer, anorexia, chronic renal failure), steroid therapy, and the preexistence of chronic diseases such as infection with human immunodeficiency virus (HIV) or herpes simplex virus (HSV). Because meningitis after spinal or epidural anesthesia is so rare, it has been difficult to directly attribute causality to the anesthetic or to identify significant risk factors. In fact, based on the limited data available it would appear that regional anesthesia is safe in cases of secondary HSV infection and reasonable for patients in the early stages of HIV infection. Again, vigilance must be emphasized as patients are monitored for signs of meningeal irritation, fever, increasing back pain, neurologic changes, and local tenderness to injection sites. Epidural abscess, like epidural hematomas, with evidence of neurologic deficit can best be diagnosed by magnetic resonance imaging and requires early, aggressive surgical intervention and antibiotic administration.[28,39,44,45]

Arachnoiditis and aseptic meningitis are rare but can occur when foreign substances irritate the meninges. Precautions are taken to avoid introduction of glass or metal particles, highly concentrated local anesthetics or dextrose solutions, detergents or antiseptics, and the core of the epidermis as the needle is inserted. Indwelling catheters, previous myelography, and hemorrhages into the subarachnoid or epidural space have also been associated with meningeal irritation and scaring. Modern technology and techniques incorporate the use of disposable equipment; needles with matched stylets, filter needles, and improved pharmacologic agents have made this complication exceedingly rare.[27]

Shock and severe, uncorrected hypovolemia are contraindications to spinal or epidural anesthesia, because both techniques cause a sympathetic blockade. The resulting vasodilation prevents physiologic compensation and may worsen hypotension. In addition, management of shock and hypovolemia often requires aggressive fluid therapy and multisystem treatments that are often physiologically and psychologically uncomfortable for the aware patient.[28,32,39]

Disease involving the spinal cord precludes neuraxial anesthesia based on the presumption that abnormal tissues will not respond to pharmacologic agents in predictable ways. Because few objective data are available, use of neuraxial anesthesia in such patients becomes a medicolegal risk. However, musculoskeletal deformities such as severe kyphoscoliosis, arthritis, and fusion and scarring of the vertebrae are relative contraindications to neuraxial anesthesia. The location of the epidural or subarachnoid spaces by needle tip may be technically difficult, and spread of anesthetic agents may be limited by anatomic alterations.[39]

Patients with a fixed volume cardiac state such as idiopathic hypertrophic subaortic stenosis or severe atrial stenosis do not tolerate bradycardia, decreases in systemic vascular resistance, or decreases in venous return and left ventricular filling—all physiologic changes that can be anticipated with neuraxial block by local anesthetics. In these patients even transient episodes of hypotension can cause serious coronary hypoperfusion and cardiac arrest. Therefore spinal and usually epidural anesthesia are avoided; however, few things in anesthesia are truly absolute. For example, epidural administration of opioids has been used to provide obstetric analgesia and may provide cardiac benefit for these patients. Precautions in such a scenario might include close hemodynamic monitoring with an arterial line and pulmonary artery catheter, careful titration of the anesthetic, intervascular volume expansion, and use of ephedrine or phenylephrine to treat hypotension.[41]

Spinal anesthesia is typically a singular deposition of local anesthetic and therefore provides anesthesia for a fixed duration. If uncertainty exists about the anticipated length of surgery, then an epidural anesthetic is more appropriate, because catheter placement allows additional administration or continuous infusions of anesthetic agents. If the extent of the surgery is unknown, a neuraxial anesthetic may be initiated only to be converted at a later time to a general anesthetic when the surgeon exceeds the limits of the anesthetic block. This is rarely an ideal situation, as the patient may experience discomfort, albeit brief, and the anesthesia provider must contend with less-than-ideal intubating conditions. Despite the advantages of neuraxial anesthesia, many patients such as the elderly and those with arthritis or musculoskeletal limitations of the neck and upper extremities poorly tolerate prolonged immobility. The judicious use of conscious sedation can quickly evolve into a less-than-ideal "room air general," placing the patient at risk for hypoventilation, hypoxia, and hypercarbia. To avoid such circumstances, combined neuraxial and general anesthetic techniques have been advocated and may offer advantage by minimizing the total dose of general anesthetic used. Such techniques lower the risk of secondary effects of general anesthesia such as nausea and vomiting while gaining the advantages associated with neuraxial anesthesia such as attenuation of the stress hormone response and improved postoperative pain relief.[32]

The administration of spinal or any regional anesthesia to patients with a difficult airway or full stomach requires careful consideration. The use of spinal anesthesia permits the patient to retain upper airway and pharyngeal reflexes that block the sympathetic nervous system. This theoretically results in increased gastric and intestinal motility, causing the stomach to empty. However, such benefits may be negated by the perception of pain and anxiety that accompanies illness or injury. If sedation is used to counter such perceptions then the airway may again become compromised. Furthermore, if hypotension develops from the resulting sympathectomy, the patient may have increased nausea and vomiting. When an injury has occurred after the ingestion of alcohol or if the patient has been given opioid analgesics, the pain caused by the injury may be the only stimulus for consciousness. When spinal or other regional anesthesia is instituted, the reticular activating centers in the brain receive less input. This often results in somnolence in a normal patient but can result in unconsciousness in the overly sedated or inebriated patient. In addition, spinal or epidural anesthesia may reach an undesirably high level that is physically and psychologically intolerable for the patient and can even become a "total spinal." A total spinal is characterized by unresponsiveness accompanied by cardiac and respiratory compromise. With peripheral blocks local anesthetics can inadvertently enter the intravascular space, leading to toxicity and seizures. In such situations airway support is required, and the emergent management of any airway can severely compromise patient safety. Therefore any type of regional anesthesia is not an alternative for a secure airway. For patients identified as potentially difficult to intubate, equipment should be immediately available to secure the airway in a safe manner. Advances in airway management such as the laryngeal mask airway, improved fiberoptics and laryngoscopes, and light wands may tip the risk-benefit scale in favor of regional anesthesia.[3,32,34]

Spinal Anesthesia: Equipment and Techniques

Preparation for spinal anesthetic procedures, like that for any other regional technique, requires the immediate availability of emergency equipment and supplies should emergent resuscitation be required. Usually, spinal anesthetics are administered in the operating room where the minimal requirements—functional laryngoscopes, endotracheal tubes, induction agents, cardiovascular drugs including atropine and ephedrine or phenylephrine, suction, oxygen and ventilation equipment, a noninvasive blood pressure monitor, and pulse oximetry and electrocardiographic monitoring equipment—are readily available.

The original spinal technique, performed by August Bier in 1898, has been continuously examined and modified in hope of reducing the incidence of complications—primarily that of PDPH. The goal of needle design has been to create a needle that minimally rends, tears, or cuts dural tissues. As technology has improved, the use of sterile, disposable procedure trays containing needles, syringes, catheters, and drugs has virtually eliminated problems previously associated with dull needles or contaminated equipment and has allowed for the development of innovative needles. Currently two main types of needles are available for use in spinal anesthesia. The first type of needle, such as the Quincke-Babcock or Pitkin type needle, has a *cutting bevel tip*. These needles have matching stylets, which minimizes tissue coring, and the tip's cutting angle is more blunt than that of a standard needle. The newer noncutting-tip needles are either pencil-point shaped with lateral openings, such as the Sprotte, Whitacre, or Pencan type needles, or have the rounded bevel tip of the Greene type needle and an opening at the needle's end and also have matched stylets. These needles are marketed for spinal anesthesia use in sizes ranging from 22 to 29 gauge and in lengths of approximately 3.5 inches (88 mm) and 5 inches (120 mm). Most blocks are performed using 25- to 27-gauge, 3.5-inch (88-mm) needles.[39,46]

Recent data support the use of noncutting pencil-point needles over cutting needles for several reasons. Cadaver lumbar punctures performed with sharp cutting needles show piercing of the cauda equina roots without resistance appreciated by the anesthetist. This does not occur with pencil-point needles. The bevel of cutting tip needles encourages tip deviation on insertion, whereas symmetric noncutting needles stay midline, and the use of a beveled needle requires holding the bevel direction parallel to longitudinal dural tissue fibers to minimize the risk of PDPH. Noncutting needles may also drag less skin contaminants into subdermal tissue than cutting needles. Pencil-point needles pierce the dura with a clearly perceptible "click" or "pop" not as easily noticed with cutting needles. Newer, thin walled noncutting needles have improved CSF flow rates without compromise to strength. This allows for their use for CSF diagnostic procedures and helps simplify the identification of the intrathecal space by permitting quick return of CSF after stylet removal. Finally, unless prohibitively small cutting needles are used, the incidence of PDPH is clearly reduced with the use of noncutting needles. The newer, pencil-point needles are associated with less than a 1% risk of PDPH and a failure rate of approximately 5%.[32,39,46,47]

After the patient arrives in the surgical or obstetric preoperative area, the consents for surgery and anesthesia should be checked and any further patient questions or concerns should be addressed. Review of the anesthetic preoperative history and physical examination should include the addition of any last-minute changes in patient status and notation of recently obtained diagnostic results. Intravenous access is achieved, and a continuous crystalloid infusion is begun. Preoperatively, most patients benefit from low-dose anxiolysis. With the increased emphasis on same-day admission, surgery, and discharge, long-acting agents are avoided. A rapid-acting benzodiazepine with a relatively short duration, such as midazolam, is highly titratable in 0.5- to 1-mg increments given intravenously and minimally alters the patient's hemodynamic status when used in low doses, and the drug's effects can be reversed with flumazenil.

Monitors appropriate to the patient's physical status should be applied and minimally include blood pressure monitoring, a continuous electrocardiogram, and pulse oximetry. For the purpose of baseline comparisons, vital signs must be assessed with the patient in both the supine position and the position in which the block is being administered.

The surgical or obstetric procedure to be performed helps determine the patient's position for the administration of the block. For example, if vaginal or urologic surgery is planned, then a "saddle" block with the patient in a sitting position may be indicated. The prone position is useful for rectal surgery because the patient can be placed in position before the block is implemented. This reduces the time required for positioning by permitting the patient to move with minimal assistance and to personally verify comfort and adequacy of padding. A lateral position favors spinal drug spread for right- or left-sided extremity or abdominal procedures. When the patient is in the lateral position, a pillow placed under his or her head and perhaps shoulders helps maintain neutral alignment of the spinal column. Surgical table height or patient position may need to be adjusted to compensate for variations in anatomic structure or physiologic limitations and to maximize anesthetist ergonomics. To maximize the space between spinous processes the patient should arch the back (with assistance from the clinician) into the shape of a **C** or a "Halloween cat." Once the patient is positioned, anatomic surface landmarks are used to identify the lumbar region of the back to be used for dural puncture, a point below the end of the spinal cord (L2). The line formed between the tops of the iliac crests, called the intercristal line or Tuffier's line, crosses the vertebral column as high as the L3 to L4 disc or as low as the L5 to S1 disc (Figure 42-7). The accuracy of prediction of the precise level of needle insertion is at best 50%. This fact may account for variability in the spinal anesthesia level ultimately achieved, yet this landmark has been clinically useful since the advent of spinal anesthesia.[31] The skin overlying a prominent spinous process at this level is marked for easy identification after the skin is prepared and draped. A surgical skin marker or pen is useful for this purpose, with caution exercised to avoid scratching the skin surface and predisposing the patient to infection.

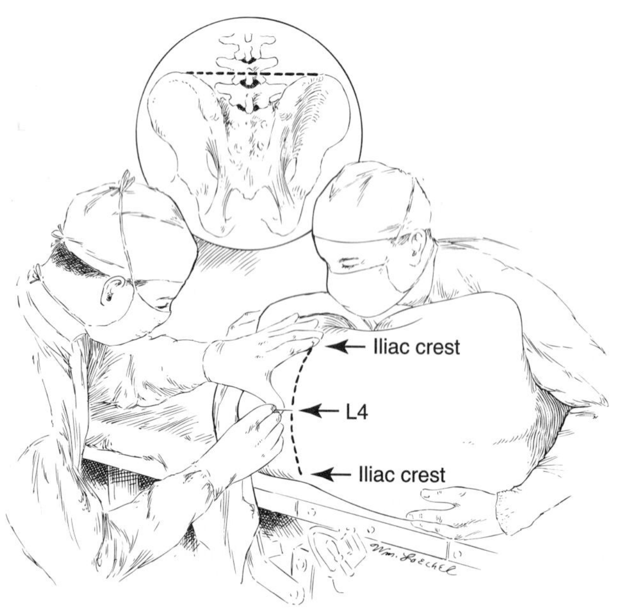

FIGURE **42-7**
Identification of landmarks in the lumbar region of the back.

Next, the spinal anesthesia tray is opened and sterile gloves are donned. The patient is prepared with an antiseptic solution, such as Betadine solution, which releases a concentration of 1% free iodine as it dries on a surface. The solution must remain in contact with the skin for at least 1 minute to be effective, and then the dry residue can be wiped away with sterile gauze to help prevent a chemical arachnoiditis. Do not use alcohol to remove antiseptic residue, because alcohol neutralizes the iodine solution and minimizes its antiseptic effect. Maintaining aseptic technique, apply the sterile drape to the back. Many spinal and epidural drapes have a circular window that is placed over the area of anticipated injection. Many drapes have adhesive strips to simplify application to the patient's back. Avoid touching the adhesive, because this has been shown to create small holes in gloves, increasing risk of infection in both patient and anesthesia provider.[48]

A rapid-acting local anesthetic such as 1% lidocaine is used for local infiltration of the area just caudad to the identified spinous process. Approach the skin of the back with the bevel of the needle facing away from the skin and at a 15- to 30-degree angle from the skin. Start injecting before the bevel of the needle is completely through the skin and raise a skin wheal to place local anesthetic into subdermal tissues most likely to contain nociceptors. Deep tissues, including the supraspinous ligament, can be anesthetized by spreading 3 to 5 ml of local anesthetic through the tissues in a fan pattern.[32,39]

Larger 22- to 25-gauge spinal needles and epidural needles (used for continuous spinal anesthetic techniques) have tensile strength that is sufficient to permit introduction of the needle without additional support. However, spinal needles smaller than 25 gauge often require an "introducer" needle to help stabilize the needle during insertion and to minimize infection in the surrounding dermis. The introducer is typically an 18- or 20-gauge needle with a "B" or blunt bevel. Introducer needles are approximately 3.8 cm long and matched to the spinal needles. The introducer is inserted through the skin and supraspinous ligament and into the interspinous ligament. Care must be taken, especially in thin individuals, not to enter the subarachnoid space with the introducer needle, as the dura may be only 2.5 cm beneath the skin. Depth to the epidural space and the nearby dura correlates with weight but typically averages approximately 4 to 5 cm and rarely exceeds 9 cm. An introducer needle placed into the subarachnoid space would be likely to cause a PDPH.[28,32,36,39]

Several common spinal anesthesia techniques can be used, including a straight midline approach. With this easy-to-learn technique the anesthesia practitioner inserts the needle directly midline between the spinous processes and toward the umbilicus perpendicularly to all planes or, at the lumbar level, with a slight cephalad angle (Figure 42-8). If bone is encountered early, the needle is withdrawn into the introducer, and subcutaneous tissue is then redirected in small angular increments in a cephalad direction. If bone is encountered when the needle is deeply inserted, the needle should be withdrawn and redirected caudad. As the tip of the spinal needle passes through the ligamentum flavum the sensation is similar to that felt when a needle is passed through a pencil eraser. As the needle tip passes through the dura the anesthesia provider may sense a "pop" or "click." The stylet is removed and several seconds are given for CSF to return through the small gauge needle. Once CSF return is confirmed, some authors recommend rotating the needle 360 degrees in 90-degree increments to ensure that the needle tip is seated well within the subarachnoid space (Figure 42-9).

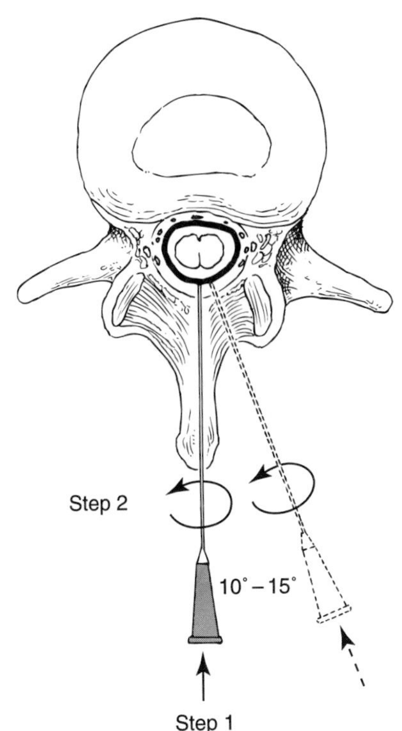

FIGURE **42-8**
Insertion of the needle between the spinous processes and toward the umbilicus.

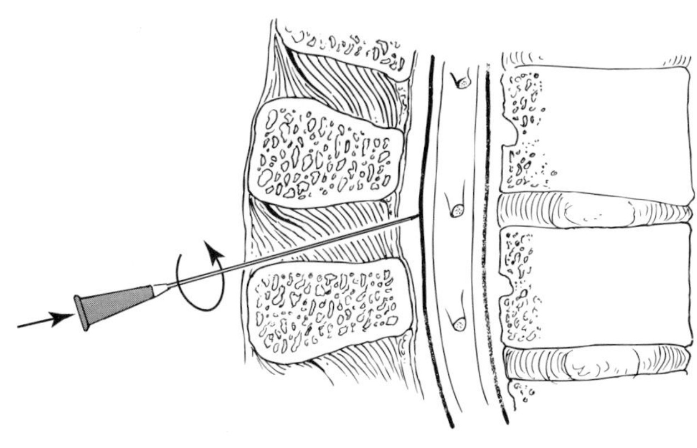

FIGURE **42-9**
The needle is rotated 360 degrees in order for its location in the subarachnoid space to be evaluated.

Other authors suggest that such needle manipulation risks a larger dural rent or needle dislodgment. Whichever method is used, secure needle handling is important. I recommend firmly placing the back of one's nondominant hand against the patient's skin and below the spinal needle. Grasp the needle hub with thumb and index finger. The patient's body then acts as a firm support for this needle-stabilizing hand and helps prevent advancement or withdrawal of the needle tip from the subarachnoid space when the syringe is applied to inject the anesthetic agent. A second technique is called the *paramedian approach*. With this technique the needle is inserted 1 cm or approximately one fingerbreadth lateral to the caudad aspect of the interspace. The needle is directed toward the spinal canal and angled slightly cephalad and then medially approximately 10 to 15 degrees. Elderly and arthritic patients may have decreased back flexibility and degenerating, calcified ligaments. For such patients this approach may be the only possible means of entering the subarachnoid space, as it aims for the largest area between processes and avoids calcified intraspinous ligaments. A third approach to the subarachnoid space known as the *Taylor approach* takes advantage of the L5 interspace, which is the largest interlaminar space. A point 1 cm medial and 1 cm caudad to the posterior superior iliac spine is located, and the needle is angled medially and cephalad at a 55-degree angle toward the fifth lumbar interspace. The Taylor approach is best used for pelvic and perineal surgical procedures.[28,31,32,36,39]

Intrathecal Drugs, Spread, and Block Levels

Once the anesthetic solution is delivered into the CSF, the distribution of its active molecules through the subarachnoid space is dependent on the chemical and physical characteristics of the solution in relation to the chemical and physical characteristics of the patient's CSF and the subarachnoid space. In adults approximately 500 ml of CSF is produced each day, predominately by the choroid plexuses of the cerebral ventricles. Much of the CSF is reabsorbed by arachnoid granulations along the sagittal sinus to regulate CSF pressure to 10 to 20 cm H_2O. At any given time a total of approximately 140 ml of CSF flows by bulk flow through the subarachnoid spaces, the central canal of the cord, and the ventricles of the brain. It is estimated that only 30 to 80 ml of the total CSF is present in the spinal canal. However, this quantity is difficult to measure, variable among individuals, and uncontrollable by the clinical anesthetist.

The density of a substance compared with the density of water is a ratio known as *specific gravity*. The specific gravity of CSF is 1.004 to 1.009 and can vary depending on variations in temperature and location of the fluid within the subarachnoid space. For example, the specific gravity of CSF sampled from the lumbar area is slightly greater than that of CSF from the ventricles. This difference is directly dependent on the protein in the CSF, as well as on the effects of gravity and the position of the patient. The specific gravity of CSF also tends to increase as patient age increases, correlating to increases in glucose and protein. Hyperglycemia and uremia increase specific gravity of CSF, whereas jaundice and related liver problems may decrease specific gravity. The change in specific gravity is related to the presence of bilirubin within the CSF. An increase in a solution's temperature decreases with its specific gravity. This change averages 0.001 points for each degree rise in Celsius temperature. Although all of these factors have been thought to influence the distribution of an anesthetic solution injected into the CSF, they are usually beyond the control of the anesthetist.[28,32,36,39,49]

A closely related concept, baricity, refers to the resting position of two fluids with differing specific gravities when the fluids are mixed in a single container, such as CSF and an anesthetic agent in the subarachnoid space. The baricity of the injected solution is compared with that of the CSF. Knowledge about the baricity of an injected solution provides the practitioner with information that helps determine the potential spread of the anesthetic mixture in the subarachnoid space. Therefore, when several medications are combined, the specific gravity of the combined solution at body temperature should be considered when the spread of the medication is anticipated. Unfortunately these bedside mixtures are rarely controlled or measured, and use becomes reliant on practical experience. When baricity (the ratio of specific gravity of local anesthetic to patient CSF) equals 1, the solution is referred to as being *isobaric*. Because the specific gravity of CSF is variable, it is not possible to prepare a solution that is precisely isobaric. Near-isobaric solutions remain and act in approximately the same location in which they are injected. A hyperbaric solution has a specific gravity that is greater than that of CSF. The solution would fall, or sink to the lowest anatomic point at which CSF is contained within the subarachnoid space in relation to gravity and the patient's position (presuming that, as previously mentioned, drug preparations are corrected for body temperature). Hypobaric solutions that are less dense than CSF rise or float to the highest anatomic position possible when injected into the subarachnoid space. Because the normal range for the specific gravity of CSF is variable, local anesthetics, opioids, or other solutions injected into the CSF must be predictably hypobaric or hyperbaric. By tradition, hypobaric solutions are defined as having a baricity of less than 0.999, and hyperbaric solutions have a baricity of greater than 1.0015. Clinically this is accomplished by dissolving the drug in either sterile water to create a hypobaric solution or 5% to 8% dextrose solutions to create a hyperbaric solution. If CSF or normal saline is added to the medications, then the specific gravity of the solution is similar to that of CSF and the drugs remain approximately where injected.[28,32,36,39,49]

Over 23 factors, including CSF density and local anesthetic baricity, have been thought to affect the spread of local anesthetics in CSF and therefore affect the level and quality of the anesthesia achieved. Less than half of these factors have been found to have clinical significance, and an even smaller number are controllable by the anesthetist performing the anesthetic procedure.[39] Clinically the most important factors are those that can be manipulated by the anesthesia provider. These are the total dose of the local anesthetic, the site of injection, the baricity of the drug (drug choice), and, when nonisobaric solutions are used, the position or posture of the patient during and after injection.[49]

The duration of a spinal anesthetic is based primarily on local anesthetic choice and total dose. Highly protein-bound drugs, such as tetracaine, bupivacaine, and ropivacaine, have long durations of action compared with less protein-bound drugs such as lidocaine and mepivacaine. Vasoconstrictors such as 0.2 mg of epinephrine are sometimes added to the local anesthetic solution to prolong the duration of action. Epinephrine is thought to prolong the duration of spinal anesthesia by causing vasoconstriction, thereby delaying normal uptake of local anesthetics, by direct antinociceptor action, or by a combination of these effects. The effect of added epinephrine on the prolongation of anesthesia is greatest with tetracaine, less with lidocaine, and minimal with bupivacaine. In addition, local anesthetic solutions may include opioids (10 to 25 mcg fentanyl, 10 mcg sufentanil, or 250 mcg morphine) or the α-agonist clonidine, 150 mcg, to prolong duration. These agents act at opioid and α_2-adrenergic receptors, respectively. The exact nature of the synergistic effect among opioids, α_2-agonists, and the local anesthetics is not clear, but the result is again prolonged spinal anesthesia. Volume, in the tested range of 1 to 14 ml, and therefore concentration minimally affect the duration of anesthesia or the final sensory level achieved. Increasing the total dose of a spinal local anesthetic will increase its duration of action and affect the sensory level achieved. Duration of sensory and motor blockade for local anesthetics, including spinal ropivacaine, has been shown to be predictable. For example, increasing the dose of hyperbaric bupivacaine from 10 mg to 15 mg prolongs the duration of sensory block by 50% and increases the maximum sensory level achieved. Based on these principles Table 42-5

TABLE 42-5 Choice of Medication for Spinal Anesthesia Used for Surgical Procedures

Procedure	Medication	Dosage	Duration without Epinephrine	Duration with Epinephrine
Vaginal delivery	Tetracaine	5 mg	1-1.5 hr	2.5-3 hr
	Bupivacaine	5-7 mg	1 hr	1.5 hr
	Lidocaine	25 mg	15-25 min	45 min-1 hr
Cesarean section	Tetracaine	8 mg	1-1.5 hr	2.5-3 hr
	Bupivacaine	10 mg	1-1.25 hr	1.5-2 hr
	Lidocaine	50-75 mg	30-45 min	1-1.25 hr
Anorectal surgery	Tetracaine (hyperbaric)	6 mg	1-1.5 hr	3 hr
	Tetracaine (hypobaric)	6 mg	1 hr	3 hr
	Bupivacaine	8 mg	1 hr	1.5-2 hr
	Lidocaine	25-50 mg	15-30 min	45 min
Genital or lower extremity procedure	Tetracaine	6-10 mg	1.5 hr	2-3 hr
	Bupivacaine	8-12 mg	1.5 hr	2 hr
	Lidocaine	75-100 mg	45-60 min	1.25-1.5 hr
Hernia, pelvic procedure	Tetracaine	10-12 mg	1.5 hr	2-3 hr
	Bupivacaine	12-15 mg	1.5 hr	2 hr
	Lidocaine	100 mg	45-60 min	1.25-1.5 hr
Intraabdominal surgery	Tetracaine	5 ft-5 ft 5 in = 12 mg 5 ft 6 in-6 ft = 15 mg >6 ft = 18 mg	1.5 hr	2-3 hr
	Bupivacaine	5 ft-5 ft 5 in = 15 mg 5 ft 6 in-6 ft = 18 mg >6 ft = 20 mg	1.5 hr	2 hr
Back and spine surgery	Tetracaine	10-15 mg	1-1.5 hr	2-2.5 hr
	Bupivacaine	15-20 mg	1-1.5 hr	1.5-2 hr

offers administration suggestions to achieve an approximate sensory level and duration of spinal anesthesia in a typical clinical setting.[49,50]

Selecting the precise site of injection, as already mentioned, is technically inaccurate at the clinical level.[31] The higher the site of injection, obviously, the higher the level of sensory block, but this is limited by the anatomy of the spinal cord and the anesthetist's desire to approach the subarachnoid space below the termination of the spinal cord. Theoretically, if a patient is administered a hyperbaric solution at the L3 level and placed supine, the local anesthetic would flow both cephalad and caudad from the relative peak of the lumbar lordosis to the troughs of the thoracic kyphosis and sacral regions. If a hyperbaric drug is placed below L3 with the patient in a sitting position and the patient is left sitting for 5 minutes, a lumbar and sacral root anesthetic known as a *saddle block* will occur. However, even under experimental conditions, using the second to fifth lumbar interspace, the data on the ability to control the maximum sensory block level achieved have been conflicting. Therefore, the site of injection can be a poor predictor of the final level of sensory anesthesia achieved.[49]

Several authors suggest that the level of the anesthetic can be adjusted or modified by use of position changes within the first few minutes after injection or until the medication becomes fixed on the nerve roots and the spinal cord. Some have even found that changes in position as late as 60 minutes after injection can alter the level of block achieved. For example, one of the suggested methods used to modify the level of the anesthetic is to raise a supine patient's legs 45 degrees. This position is thought to increase blood flow through the epidural venous plexus, indirectly altering CSF pressures. Such a position also flattens the lumbar lordosis, altering flow of hyperbaric local anesthetic within the subarachnoid space. The combined effects result in further cephalad spread of local anesthetic solutions. If one uses a similar line of thought, morbid obesity and third trimester pregnancy also are associated with epidural venous engorgement when the patient is supine, and a slightly higher level of spinal anesthesia is found when compared with controls. With traditional hyperbaric solutions, the block achieved may range from T3 to T6. Therefore the anesthetist's ability to precisely control the level of sensory anesthesia through baricity and changes in posture is associated with great variability and low predictability from patient to patient.[39,49] Once achieved, the final level of sensory blockade should be documented as discussed previously.

Continuous spinal anesthetics are administered using the same techniques used to establish a spinal or epidural anesthetic. A small epidural needle is used for the procedure, with the bevel turned parallel to dural fibers to help minimize the risk of PDPH. After the needle is inserted into the subarachnoid space, the bevel of the needle is turned either caudad or cephalad to facilitate passage of an epidural catheter into the subarachnoid space. The catheter is inserted only 2 to 3 cm into the subarachnoid space. Further insertion could result in advancement of the catheter along a nerve root or in curling of the catheter. The incidence of headache is minimal in elderly patients or when the catheter can remain in the subarachnoid space for at least 40 hours. In 1992 the Food and Drug Administration removed from the U.S. market small needles and microcatheters designed to further reduce the risk of PDPH because of reports of cauda equina syndrome. Cauda equina syndrome, or persistent paralysis of the nerves of the cauda equina, has subsequently been attributed to the deposition of neurotoxic concentrations of hyperbaric local anesthetics, particularly 5% lidocaine. This same solution in varying concentrations has been associated with *transient neurologic symptoms (TNS)*. These symptoms can include severe radicular back pain in up to 30% of patients and can require treatment with opioids; however, 90% of the cases resolve within 1 week. Some authors suggest that TNS is at the low end of the dose-effect curve that leads to cauda equina syndrome. However, not all studies support this theory, because changing concentrations of lidocaine does not seem to affect the incidence of transient symptoms. Other factors have been implicated as causing TNS and include knee and hip flexion, presumably stretching nerve roots, obesity, and ambulatory surgery. This complication has prompted many practitioners to modify their use of lidocaine by limiting the dose to a single, rapid, cephalad injection of less then 100 mg or to avoid its use altogether.[28,32,36,39,41,42,46,51]

Physiologic Alterations and Their Management

Spinal anesthesia causes several physiologic changes that are predictable and can usually be readily managed through anticipation and prevention or with minimal intervention. Physiologic changes include effects on the central nervous system, cardiovascular system, respiratory system, and GI system. In addition, physiologic alterations caused by central neural blockade affecting neuroendocrine, renal, and hepatic function are mentioned.

The obvious central nervous system effect of spinal anesthesia is the inhibition of nerve impulse conduction, resulting in spinal anesthesia. This occurs when the local anesthetic concentration exceeds the minimal blocking concentration of the particular nerve exposed to the drug. Neurons have different levels of susceptibility to local anesthetics, and this partially explains the differential block seen with spinal and epidural anesthesia. As a local anesthetic spreads from the epicenter of its injection site, the concentration of molecules decreases. As the local anesthetic spreads rostral and the concentration gradient lessens, only the most susceptible neurons will be blocked, and a differential block occurs. With spinal anesthesia, typically kinesthetic sense is inhibited at a dermatomal level higher than light touch or cold sensation, which in turn are inhibited at a more rostral dermatomal level than pinprick anesthesia. Therefore a differential blockade among the levels of sympathetic, somatic sensory, and somatic motor fibers can be identified. Attempts to demonstrate the numbers of segments between areas of differential blockade have found that sympathetic fibers are blocked a mean of six to seven segments higher than somatic sensory fibers.[33,34]

The reticular excitatory area in the brainstem is responsible for the brain's overall state of alertness or arousal. The primary determinant of the activity of the reticular excitatory area is the amount of sensory input from the body. Because spinal anesthesia greatly decreases the number of sensory impulses to the reticular excitatory area, normal patients often experience somnolence. Caution must be taken during administration of spinal anesthesia to a patient in pain and already under the influence of central depressants such as alcohol or opioids. The pain caused by the injury may be the only stimulus for consciousness, and when spinal or other regional anesthesia is instituted, unconsciousness may ensue.[34]

Spinal or epidural techniques using local anesthetics block sympathetic nerve transmission in addition to blocking sensory and motor fibers. Therefore the sum effect of neuraxial anesthesia on the cardiovascular system depends primarily on the overall degree of sympathetic blockade in terms of the rostral spread of the anesthetic and partially on the degree of patient sedation and central sympathetic inhibition. Blockade of the sympathetic nervous system causes arterial vasodilation, decreased systemic vascular resistance, venous pooling, and a reduction in venous return. These changes cause a redistribution of blood that often results in hypotension. If the block is high enough, the sympathetic nerve fibers that innervate the heart, known as the *cardiac accelerators* (T1 to T4) become anesthetized. An imbalance occurs between vagal fibers, and the heart rate often slows, further contributing to hypotension. Baroreceptor reflexes, volume receptor reflexes, and decreased central sympathetic outflow all contribute to the complexity of the cardiovascular response to neuraxial anesthesia. The overall result is loss of normal cardiovascular homeostatic reflexes and the ability to compensate for minor cardiovascular stresses.[14] Rapid changes in position; changes in skeletal muscle tone caused by relaxation; decreased venous return; low preoperative volume status; reflex surgical stimulation; preoperative medications (especially opioid and sedative-hypnotics); and concurrent conditions, such as pulmonary embolism, pregnancy, and systemic reactions to medications, have all been implicated in increased severity of perioperative hypotension.[34,52]

Hypotension is immediately relevant to the perfusion of critical organs like the heart and brain and is important to all organs in maintaining near homeostasis. Although normotensive patients have been shown to maintain cerebral blood flow despite a moderate decrease in blood pressure, hypertensive subjects may have altered cerebral blood flow autoregulation and are less tolerant of changes in mean arterial pressures.[34] A similar situation exists with elderly patients and patients with known coronary disease. With these caveats in mind, most clinicians allow a decrease in blood pressure of 20% from a patient's baseline before initiating treatment. Clinicians continue to debate the optimal treatment of spinal anesthesia–induced hypotension and bradycardia, and the treatment is often dependent on coexisting disease; however, some general recommendations can be made. Preventive management of hypotension includes the administration of non–glucose-containing crystalloid or colloid solutions in volumes of approximately 15 ml/kg 15 minutes before the start of the anesthetic procedure to maintain preload to the heart. This initial infusion should include replacement of any fluid deficit caused by restricted oral intake and has been shown to help prevent immediate cardiovascular side effects. Continuous infusions of α-adrenergic vasoconstrictors and sympathomimetic agents have been used to maintain volume preload by increasing central volume and have been shown to help reduce the incidence of cardiovascular side effects requiring treatment. Should the treatment of hypotension become necessary, the ongoing administration of intravenous solution is often the first response; however, excessive fluid therapy can lead to fluid overload and urinary retention, especially in the elderly.[52] Continued treatment is guided by the patient's presenting symptoms and coexisting disease. The heart rate can be used to help guide pharmacologic intervention. Ephedrine, a mixed α- and β-agonist in 5- to 10-mg intravenous boluses, is the agent of choice in patients with symptomatic bradycardia. Ephedrine's indirect effects cause an increase in peripheral vascular resistance and heart rate. If the heart rate is normal or elevated, an α-agonist, such as 50 to 100 mcg of intravenous phenylephrine, causes increased systemic vascular resistance without further increasing the heart rate. The use of phenylephrine may therefore be more efficacious in the elderly. Bradycardia is treated with intravenous atropine 0.4 to 0.8 mg. Severe hypotensive events should be treated vigorously with medication and fluids, because mortality from rare cardiac arrests increases when treatment is delayed.[28,34,36,52]

Most studies demonstrate that midthoracic levels of either spinal or epidural anesthesia have minimal effects on tidal volume, respiratory rate, minute ventilation, and arterial blood gas tensions in otherwise healthy individuals. The phrenic nerve is rarely paralyzed even when sensory levels reach the cervical dermatomes; however, the accessory abdominal and intercostal muscles for ventilation are impaired, and the ability to cough and clear secretions is inhibited. With the loss of perception of intercostal and abdominal wall muscle movement and the inability to cough, the patient may begin to feel dyspneic. Caution must be exercised if the accompanying anxiety is treated with large doses of sedatives or opioids. They may worsen ventilation and result in hypoxia. Although regional techniques have been shown to have minimal effects, adequate ventilatory ability during surgery is dependent on multiple factors, and improved pulmonary outcomes have not been clearly demonstrated. Some of the factors that affect ventilatory ability under spinal or epidural anesthesia include the presence of coexisting disease, depressant medications, patient position, type and location of the surgery and incision, and presence of hypotension and hemorrhage. The anesthetic plan must be adapted to the patient and the operation.[33,34]

The GI tract is regulated by the parasympathetic and sympathetic nervous systems. The parasympathetic innervation of the GI tract is primarily via the vagus nerves and is composed of both afferent and efferent fibers. Parasympathetic afferent nerves transmit sensations of satiety, distention, and nausea, whereas efferent outflow generally increases GI activities such as tonic contractions, sphincter relaxation, peristalsis, and secretion. Sympathetic innervation of the GI tract stems from the T5 to L2 spinal cord segments and via prevertebral ganglia. Sympathetic afferent nerves are responsible for transmitting pain information, whereas efferent nerves inhibit peristalsis and gastric secretion and cause sphincter contraction and vasoconstriction. When spinal and epidural anesthesia cause a sympathetic blockade, the result is unopposed or dominant parasympathetic activity. The neuraxial sympatholysis results in a generalized constriction of the bowel, normal to increased peristalsis, increased intraluminal pressure, and increased GI blood flow.[33,34,36] The combination of abdominal muscle relaxation and a contracted bowel offer improved operating conditions for intraabdominal procedures; however, because gastric motility can be increased, some clinicians have questioned the risk of wound disruption. Several studies have reported that the intraoperative and postoperative use of neuraxial anesthesia does not increase the risk of wound breakdown. Steinbrook and other researchers suggest that continued postoperative analgesia, especially with a thoracic epidural and local anesthetic infusion, has beneficial effects on the recovery of bowel function after major abdominal surgery.[33,34,53]

Nausea and vomiting are associated with neuraxial block in up to 20% of patients. Nausea and vomiting are primarily related to the GI hyperperistalsis of parasympathetic dominance, although other contributing factors may include hypoxemia, hypotension, systemic medications (opioids or rapidly infused antibiotics), and psychologic stimuli. A cardiac mechanism associated with spinal anesthesia, as proposed by some authors, may also lead to nausea and vomiting. Theoretically, cardiac vagal afferent nerves can be activated in response to a decrease in venous return via ventricular mechanoreceptors (Bezold-Jarish reflex), especially with high block levels. Therefore the vagolytic effect of atropine makes the drug an excellent antiemetic in the treatment of the nausea and vomiting associated with high spinal anesthesia.[34,36]

The neuroendocrine stress response is a combination of responses of the body to tissue trauma (like surgery) or critical illness. The response includes components of neural, immune, endocrine, metabolic, and inflammatory systems that are closely integrated through a complex mechanism of hormones, neurotransmitters, and receptors that affect cells throughout the body. These systems are activated in proportion to the level of critical illness or tissue injury experienced by the body.[34] The stress response is usually associated with increases in blood concentrations of adrenocorticotropins, cortisol, insulin, growth hormone, aldosterone, and glucose. Initially a protective response—the stress response—can lead to tachycardia, hypertension, catabolism, immunosuppression, and hypercoagulability.[33] Regional blocks, such as spinal and epidural techniques, moderate the stress response to surgery. Although spinal anesthesia blocks this response only for the duration of the anesthetic administration, the use of continuous epidural analgesia well into the postoperative period has the potential to improve perioperative outcome.

Renal blood flow and function are well preserved during spinal anesthesia when blood pressure is maintained. Hepatic blood flow is directly proportional to the mean arterial pressure and therefore depends on the treatment of any hypotension associated with the spinal or epidural anesthetic.[33] Spinal and epidural anesthetics block sympathetic fibers, thereby increasing the tone of the internal urethral sphincter; in addition, neuraxial opioids cause a decrease in detrusor contraction and an increase in bladder capacity. These changes in the genitourinary system can result in the rare complication of urinary retention.

Complications of Spinal Anesthesia

Postdural Puncture Headache

PDPH is perhaps the most commonly discussed and managed complication of neuraxial anesthesia, with a documented incidence that has varied over the years from 0.2% to 24%. Theoretically PDPH is caused by a decrease in the CSF available in the subarachnoid space through a leak created by the dural puncture with an intruding needle. The medulla and brainstem, having lost their hydraulic support, drop into the foramen magnum, stretching the meninges and pulling on the tentorium. This pulling, further irritated by movement and the upright position, causes a characteristic headache.[26,39,54] A contributing theory suggests that cerebrovasodilation may result from low CSF pressure. This theory is supported by the beneficial effects of vasoconstrictor drugs such as caffeine and theophylline.[54]

Several factors are known to increase the incidence of PDPH. The use of large, non–pencil-point needles or a cutting needle bevel direction that is perpendicular to the long axis of the body will make larger holes in the dural fibers, creating larger CSF leaks. Multiple punctures also increase CSF leak and the risk of headache. In addition, female patients are more likely than male patients to get a PDPH, and the young are more likely than the elderly to experience this complication. Most studies also demonstrate a higher incidence of PDPH in the pregnant population. Patients with a history of PDPHs are predisposed to another headache after a subsequent spinal anesthetic procedure. However, one should keep in mind that not all headaches that follow spinal anesthetic procedures are PDPHs. It is common for patients to experience headaches after surgery and even after general anesthetics. Factors that contribute to headaches may include anxiety, interrupted sleep, dehydration, hypoglycemia, and even simply the lack of normal morning caffeine intake. A differential diagnosis approach should be taken to identify serious complications such as subdural hematoma, subarachnoid hemorrhage, meningitis, sinusitis, or subarachnoid hemorrhage.[36,39,47,54]

Fortunately, PDPHs have several characteristic features that aid in diagnosis. Usually PDPHs occur within several hours to the first or second postoperative day. Historically, bed rest was thought to help prevent PDPH, but subsequent studies found that avoiding early ambulation simply postponed the onset of PDPH. The headache is typically described as a mild to incapacitating bilateral frontal headache that radiates from behind the eyes and across the head toward the occiput and often into the neck and shoulders. The headache is considered positional, because it completely subsides when the patient is lying down. The only other form of headache that has this positional component is caused by pneumocephalus. Other symptoms that may be associated with PDPH include nausea and vomiting, appetite loss, blurred vision or photophobia, a sensation of a plugging of the ears and loss of hearing acuity, tinnitus, vertigo, and depression.[32,39,54]

Although PDPHs are self-limiting, often resolving in less than 10 days, early identification and prompt treatment are essential if complications of immobility, depression, and patient dissatisfaction (a potential reason for litigation) are to be avoided. Conservative management includes a horizontal position, adequate hydration, oral analgesics, and the administration of 500 mg intravenous caffeine benzoate, 300 mg of oral caffeine, or theophylline. The horizontal position is impractical for most patients, especially mothers of newborns, and encourages further complications of immobility.[54] Abdominal binders, thought to increase epidural venous plexus blood flow and therefore CSF pressure, are also uncomfortable and often impractical. Increasing fluids during the evaluation and early management period was thought to increase the central volume and increase the secretion of CSF from the choroid plexus, but this has not been well supported in the literature. However, adequate hydration should be maintained in all patients.[39] Caffeine and theophylline are both methylxanthine derivatives that cause cerebral vasoconstriction and central nervous system stimulation. Caffeine therapy, both oral and parenteral, is the most commonly used pharmacologic treatment modality; however, theophylline and sumatriptan are potentially promising agents for the treatment of PDPH.[10,47] Caffeine has been shown to eliminate headache in up to 70% of patients, but this effect may be transient. Recently Panzer and co-workers have suggested that prophylactic intravenous caffeine administration may safely minimize PDPHs.[55]

An epidural blood patch is considered the definitive treatment for PDPH. Thought to work via clot formation that seals the dural rent and increases CSF pressure, the epidural blood patch is associated with a greater than 90% cure rate. Clinically an epidural blood patch is performed in a manner similar to that of placing an epidural catheter. First, the availability of intravenous access is identified, usually in the antecubital fossa, and informed consent is obtained. Both the patient's back and intravenous access site are prepared and draped in an aseptic manner. An insertion site at or below the level of the lowest initial needle insertion is chosen, because blood has been shown to spread in a predominately cephalad direction within the epidural space. The epidural space is identified by use of either loss-of-resistance or hanging-drop technique (discussed in the section on epidural anesthesia). Autologous venous blood (approximately 20 ml) is withdrawn from the vein and then slowly injected through the epidural needle into the epidural space. The injection proceeds until the patient senses pressure in the back, buttocks, or legs. Typically, this occurs at a volume of 12 to 15 ml, which is sufficient blood to patch most patients. A supine position should be maintained for $1/2$ to 1 hour before the patient ambulates. Relief of the headache is often instantaneous. In the rare case in which an epidural blood patch fails, a repeat blood patch may be attempted in 24 hours, with a similar success rate.[39,54]

The success rate and excellent safety record of the epidural blood patch encourages the use of this therapeutic option early in the treatment of PDPH. However, some risks, although minor or rare, are associated with this more invasive procedure. Backache, often associated with the administration of general, spinal, or epidural anesthetic techniques, occurs in up to 35% of patients after an epidural blood patch. Although rarely as debilitating as the headache itself, this risk should be explained to the patient. The most common cause of backache is relaxation of the muscles of the back and flattening of the normal lordotic curve. As the muscles stretch, injury to tendons and ligaments can occur. The position of the patient might increase the severity of the problem. An exaggerated lithotomy position or a completely supine position can further increase tension on tendons, resulting in increased trauma to both the muscles and the tendons. Trauma from multiple punctures, hemorrhage, infections, use of large needles, retractors, and forceps; extremes of positions; preexisting diseases such as arthritis and osteoporosis; and prolonged labor can contribute to backaches that may persist well into the postoperative period.

Management of backache includes the use of antispasmodics and NSAIDs to reduce discomfort, permit ambulation and promote a more rapid recovery. In addition, authors have reported a 5% incidence of transient (24- to 48-hour) temperature elevation, a 1% incidence of neck ache, radicular pain, nerve root irritation, cranial nerve palsy, and meningitis (although the cause was unproved).[39,54]

Several caveats regarding the treatment of PDPH are worth mentioning. Systemic infection, perhaps indicated by fever, presents a relative contraindication to epidural blood patch and warrants a trial of pharmacologic intervention. The risk of neurologic sequelae after epidural blood patch in the presence of HIV infection or sepsis is controversial, because few data are available, leading some authors to suggest alternative therapies such as epidural 0.9% sodium chloride or dextran.[36,44,54] Prophylactic epidural blood patch placement has not been proved consistently successful. In light of the relatively low incidence of PDPH and the effectiveness of the epidural blood patch, treatment should not begin until the problem exists. Finally, an alternative diagnosis should be sought if two epidural blood patches fail to resolve the patient's symptoms.[39,54]

Urinary Retention

Urinary retention can occur after anesthesia and surgery because spinal or epidural anesthetics block sympathetic fibers and increase the tone of the internal urethral sphincter. However, other factors are often contributory to the risk of urinary retention after surgery and anesthesia. These include the type of surgical procedure, bladder distention from the administration of large volumes of intravenous fluids, bladder trauma, prolonged hypotension, incisional pain, urethral edema caused by prolonged labor, benign prostatic hypertrophy, and the use of neuraxial or intraoperative opioids. Some authors suggest that spinal anesthesia may even carry a lower risk of urinary retention when compared with general anesthesia. In any case, urinary retention and subsequent catheterization can lead to complications such as urinary tract infections and urethral strictures. Attempts should first be made to allow the patient every opportunity to void in a natural position, saving urethral catheterization as a last resort.[37]

Neurologic Sequelae

Patients greatly fear the perceived risk of paraplegia resulting from neuraxial anesthetics, and the seriousness of such complications warrants our concern. However, several very large series have shown that the incidence of persistent motor paralysis is exceedingly rare (<1 per 10,000). Because neurologic sequelae are rare, the knowledge base of complications comes from case studies, and often cause is not proved but rather inferred by association. Direct needle or catheter nerve injury, drug-related neurotoxicity, anterior spinal artery syndrome, undiagnosed neurologic disease, intraneural or intramedullary injections, the presence of blood in the CSF, patient positioning, hematomas, and abscesses have all been associated with permanent neurologic deficits. Therefore good clinical practice depends on the use of appropriate anesthetic techniques that minimize risk and the conducting of postoperative assessments in a manner that promotes early detection, diagnosis, and treatment; especially as reversibility of complications is often time dependent.[36,39,41,56] Transient neurologic symptoms are discussed in Chapter 9.

Unexpected Cardiac Arrest

Hemodynamic collapse under neuraxial anesthesia, also a rare event, is often sudden and unexpected. Because unexpected cardiac arrest with spinal anesthesia has been reported in previously healthy patients, some authors consider this a physiologic response to neuraxial blocks. Some authors suggest a pattern of presentation with a gradual downward trend in heart rate followed by an abrupt onset of severe bradycardia or asystole.[34] Liguori and Sharrocks' review of 12 epidural anesthetic cases with arrest found that severe bradycardia or asystole could develop in seconds or minutes from a stable heart rate, a downward trend, or even increasing heart rate trends. Asystole or bradycardia may occur as late as 3 hours after epidural injection. It has been hypothesized that the Bezold-Jarisch reflex may be involved. This normally protective vasodepressor reflex has afferent and efferent pathways in the vagus, originating in mechanoreceptors in the left ventricle. With a rapid decrease in central venous return, as might occur with hemorrhage or the onset of spinal anesthesia, a paradoxic increase in parasympathetic tone and withdrawal of sympathetic tone results in severe bradycardia, further peripheral vasodilation, and hypotension. Other physiologic factors thought to be associated with arrest include hypoxemia and relative hypovolemia that leads to decreased ventricular filling pressures. Vigilance, awareness, and aggressive treatment are essential, because prophylaxis with volume loads, chronotropic support, or vagolysis is unproved. In addition to pacing and cardiopulmonary resuscitation, pharmacologic intervention might include fluids, atropine, or epinephrine.[34,57]

Auditory, Ocular, and Facial Complications

Unexpected complications or complications that a patient may not ascribe to anesthesia may be unreported or underreported, especially if they are transient in nature and not life-threatening. The complications of transient hypoacusis or hearing loss and retinal hemorrhage are thought to be caused by changes in CSF pressure, either from postdural puncture leaks or increases in pressure from the epidural administration of a large volume of solution. Epidural injection of 8 to 16 ml of fluid can increase CSF pressure by 85 cm H_2O for several minutes before compensation occurs. Horner's syndrome (ptosis, miosis, anhidrosis, and enophthalmos) and trigeminal nerve palsy probably result from a high spread of local anesthetic to the sympathetic fibers of the head and neck and to cranial nerve V, respectively. These problems are usually self-limiting; however, knowledge of their previous occurrence enables the compassionate anesthetist to provide council and reassurance to anxious patients.[42,58]

EPIDURAL ANESTHETIC TECHNIQUES

Indications

An epidural anesthetic technique is regional anesthesia produced by injection of local anesthetic solution into the peridural space. Local anesthetics or other analgesic solutions injected into the epidural space spread anatomically. Horizontal spread is to the region of the dural cuffs with diffusion into the CSF and leakage through the intravertebral foramen into paravertebral spaces. Longitudinal spread is preferentially cephalad in direction. Possible sites of anesthetic action include paravertebral nerve trunks, intradural spinal roots, dorsal and ventral spinal roots, the dorsal root ganglia, the spinal cord, and the brain. Initial blockade is probably a result of anesthetic blockade at the spinal roots within the dural sleeves. The dural cuffs or sleeves have a proliferation of arachnoid villi and granulations that effectively reduce the thickness of the dura mater, permitting rapid diffusion of anesthetics from the epidural space through the dura and into the CSF. Differences in physicochemical properties of anesthetics, such as lipid solubility, may account for the differences in diffusion rates across the dura, contributing to the variances seen in sensory, motor, and sympathetic blockade.[29] Because epidural anesthesia is diffusion dependent, relatively large volumes (20 ml) and higher concentrations of anesthetics must be used compared with spinal anesthesia (1 to 2 ml). In addition, because diffusion and spread take longer with an epidural anesthetic technique, spinal anesthesia has a faster onset. Given these caveats, any procedure that can be done with the patient under spinal anesthesia can also be done with epidural anesthesia.[28] However, epidural techniques allow for the placement of a continuous catheter, which is especially useful in cases of unpredictable duration, for prolonged postoperative analgesia, and for chronic pain control. In addition, labor epidural analgesia is the only method currently available that can relieve most of the discomfort of labor while minimally affecting maternal or fetal physiology. Labor epidural analgesia is highly satisfactory in these patients, because it permits their participation in a comfortable delivery and allows maternal-infant bonding after delivery. Labor analgesia also satisfies obstetricians and anesthesia providers, as its flexibility allows quick conversion from an analgesic technique to a surgical anesthetic technique for cesarean section.

Equipment and Techniques

Patient preparation and positioning and the availability of emergency equipment and monitors is similar to the preparation for a spinal anesthetic. With a spinal anesthetic the practitioner seeks CSF by piercing the dura, while the tip of the epidural needle seeks the fat-filled space deep to the ligamentum flavum and shallow to the dura. The epidural technique is performed most often with a 16-, 17-, or 18-gauge needle with a blunted tip designed to facilitate passage of the catheter into the epidural space. The most common designs available are the Tuohy, Hustead, and Crawford needles. The Tuohy needle has the most pronounced tip curve, to help control catheter direction within the epidural space. The Hustead needle has fewer curves than the Tuohy, and the Crawford needle tip is straight. Smaller, 20- to 22-gauge epidural needles, with correspondingly smaller catheters, are available for pediatrics and specialty use. Many needle designs incorporate wings near the base or hub. The wings provide a grip for the practitioner that permits distribution of pressure equally over the needle during insertion. Needles may also have clear hubs to allow detection of blood or CSF, plastic stylets, and 1-cm depth markings along the needle shaft.

Epidural catheters also come in a variety of materials and designs. Typically, catheter diameter is two gauges smaller than the needle. For example, a 20-gauge catheter would be used with an 18-gauge Tuohy needle. Catheters are constructed of physiologically inert materials designed to resist kinking, compression, and stretching and should be radiopaque. Generally, two catheter types are available: an open tip design and a closed tip design with multiple side ports. Catheters have markings that identify the tip of the catheter to help verify removal of the catheter and identify when the catheter is at the tip of the needle, with 1 cm markings to measure depth of catheter placement. An open tip catheter needs to be advanced 3 cm into the epidural space, whereas a multiple-orifice catheter should be advanced approximately 5 cm into the epidural space. It is always wise to refer to the manufacturer's recommendations, especially when using unfamiliar equipment.

Patient positioning (sitting or lateral), landmarks, aseptic preparation, draping, and localization are similar to those for a spinal anesthetic. The larger, more rigid epidural needle does not require the use of an introducer needle and offers better directional control than smaller spinal needles; however; needle-handling techniques must anticipate patient movement. Again, we recommend firmly placing the back of one's nondominant hand against the patient's skin and below the epidural needle. Grasp the needle and hub between the thumb and as much of the index finger and fist as possible. The patient's body then acts as a firm support for the needle-stabilizing hand. This firm grip, sometimes referred to as the *Bromage grip*, helps prevent advancement or withdrawal of the needle tip from its position if the patient moves, when the syringe is applied, and as the catheter is passed into the epidural space. The needle is placed bevel tip cephalad through the supraspinous ligament and seated in the interspinous ligament before the stylet is removed. After the stylet is removed, the needle is slowly advanced by use of either the hanging-drop technique or the loss-of-resistance technique.[29]

After the needle is seated in the interspinous ligament, the hanging-drop technique is accomplished by filling the hub of the needle with saline. The surface tension of the saline creates a droplet hanging on the needle hub. The needle is then advanced slowly. As the bevel of the needle enters the epidural space, the solution is drawn into the space because of negative pressure within the epidural space. Disadvantages to this technique are that a plug can form in the needle tip and that low or no negative pressure can exist in some epidural spaces.[29]

The more commonly used loss-of-resistance technique incorporates a syringe attached to the needle. The syringe is filled with 3 to 4 ml of air, normal saline, or a mixture of saline and air, thought by some to facilitate compression of the solution. To avoid dural puncture with the large epidural needle, pressure is applied to the plunger of the syringe filled with air or air and saline by "bouncing," or intermittently applying pressure to the plunger as the needle is slowly advanced. The needle is advanced toward the epidural space by application of pressure to the needle, not the syringe or syringe plunger. If normal saline is used, constant pressure may be applied to the syringe plunger. Contact with the needle or needle wings is maintained to control needle advancement. As the needle passes through the ligamentum flavum, resistance increases, and it is very difficult to inject either saline or air. Once the bevel of the needle completes the passage through the ligamentum flavum and enters the epidural space, an immediate loss of resistance occurs. The contents of the syringe then can be injected gently and without resistance. After the syringe is removed from the needle, an outward rush of a small amount of air or fluid may occur. Penetration of the dura with a large epidural needle usually results in profuse return of CSF, and the needle should be removed immediately to minimize CSF loss.

The loss of resistance experienced by a beginning practitioner, or the experienced practitioner with a patient with difficult anatomy, may not be easily discerned. Sometimes it may be necessary to further evaluate the needle tip's location. For example, several milliliters of air can be injected through the needle while the soft tissue lateral to the spinous process is palpated. If crepitus is felt, the needle is most likely located in the tissues adjacent and shallow to the spinous process. If fluid returns from either the needle or catheter, CSF can easily be distinguished from NS or local anesthetic. CSF is warm to the forearm, compared with recently administered room-temperature fluids. Glucose test paper will detect the glucose in CSF. Local anesthetics mixed with a similar volume of thiopental will immediately form a precipitate.

Once the practitioner is reassured of the needle tip's position, an epidural catheter is threaded through the needle and into the epidural space to a depth of 3 to 5 cm. As the catheter is passed into the epidural space, it is important to warn the patient that a "funny bone" sensation may be experienced down one or both legs. The catheter tip may brush a nerve root while passing from the bevel of the needle. The needle must be stabilized during catheter advancement, because the patient may move on such an unusual sensation. Limit catheter advancement to 3 to 5 cm to reduce the potential for complications related to catheter placement. The catheter is stabilized as the needle is withdrawn slowly over the catheter. The catheter must never be withdrawn through the needle because the needle tip can shear the catheter, leaving material imbedded in the patient's back. After the needle is removed, the catheter is taped securely. Avoid taping the catheter in the midline of the back to avoid pressure from the spinous processes.

The needle or catheter tip may be in the epidural space, in the subarachnoid space, in an intravascular space like an epidural vein, or simply in nearby tissues. Relatively safe administration of medications into the epidural space requires a series of logical steps to help ensure that medications will not be administered harmfully into the subarachnoid or vascular compartments. Once the needle is positioned or a catheter is inserted, return of CSF is sought by gravity flow. With the use of a catheter, aspiration is attempted to test for migration of the catheter tip into the subarachnoid space. Because tissue at the catheter tip may create a ball-valve effect, CSF or blood may not flow out; this test is therefore helpful only when fluid returns. A test dose must be injected for further evaluation of catheter tip placement. A test dose of 3 ml of a rapid-acting, low-toxicity local anesthetic agent, usually 1.5% lidocaine with 5 mcg/ml of epinephrine, is injected. If the needle or catheter tip is in the subarachnoid space, spinal anesthesia will occur within 3 minutes. A loss of sensory perception along the nerve root distribution in the area of injection occurs. If the test dose is injected into a blood vessel, the 15 mcg of epinephrine will result in a 20% rise in heart rate and systolic blood pressure within 30 seconds. The patient may also experience sensations from the intravascular lidocaine, describing symptoms such as tinnitus, a metallic taste, circumoral numbness, or a rushing sound in the ears. The duration is less than 5 minutes. After the test dose is injected, vital signs are reassessed. Additionally, 100 mcg of undiluted fentanyl can be injected. If the needle or catheter is intravascular, the patient will experience immediate dizziness and sleepiness from the opioid. Despite all efforts to avoid them, systemic toxic reactions can still occur. Be vigilant, be cautious, and be prepared to handle emergencies.[59,60]

Epidural Drugs, Spread, and Block Levels

As with any anesthetic technique, the clinical success of epidural anesthesia is often dependent on experience, as multiple factors must be managed and balanced to provide safe patient care. Two of these factors, dose and the site of injection, are the most important factors in determining the extent of dermatomal blockade. It should be remembered that the size of the segmental epidural spaces increases down the spinal cord as the spinal cord occupies less and less space. Very small volumes of local anesthetic will spread across more segments in the cervical region than in the thoracic region and even less segments in the lumbar and caudal regions. The suggested dose of local anesthetic is therefore dependent on the location of the catheter tip. Common clinical practice is to insert the epidural needle at a vertebral interspace such that the catheter tip falls near the middle of the spinal dermatomes of the proposed surgical incision. For example, an epidural catheter placed for labor or lower abdominal anesthesia would be placed at the L2 or L3 interspace; T8 to T10 for upper abdominal surgery; T4 to T5 for thoracic surgery; and C7 to T1 for chronic pain treatments or surgeries of the arms, shoulders, or upper chest. This has several advantages. The catheter tip, being the relative center of the spread of the local anesthetic, creates an area of high concentration at the spinal nerves specific to the site of the operation with the least amount of local anesthetic. This results in a rapid block onset and greater block density and often creates a differential blockade that can be controlled by dose. Dose is described as volume multiplied by concentration. The concentration of the local anesthetic generally affects the density of the block, whereas the volume, within limits, affects the spread from the needle or catheter tip throughout the epidural space. Successful analgesia can be achieved with relatively small volumes and high concentrations of local anesthetics. Clinically useful doses are based on volumes that permit an even filling of the anterior and posterior epidural spaces at the level of insertion. For example, the suggested volumes per segment at the cervical and thoracic levels are 0.7 to 1 ml per segment. The initial dose is usually less than 10 ml. At the lumbar level the spread of local anesthetic is approximately 1.25 to 1.5 ml per segment of block desired, with an initial total volume of 15 to 20 ml. Also, it should be remembered that spread of blockade tends to occur faster in the cephalad direction from the catheter tip, possibly because thoracic nerve roots are smaller in diameter than large lumbar and sacral nerve roots.[28,29,32]

Other factors thought to affect the level of blockade achieved with epidural anesthesia include height, weight, age, patient position during injection, pregnancy, and the speed or mode of injection. However, the clinical significance of these factors has been challenged. Correlations between patient height and weight and the spread of the epidural block are clinically insignificant except perhaps in the extremely tall or short or morbidly obese. Studies have examined patients in the sitting and lateral positions during administration of epidural anesthetics and found small differences in spread and onset that favor the dependent portion of the patient's body. Therefore provision of anesthesia to the sacral roots might be facilitated by having the patient sit up during the injection. In addition, leaving the patient on the operative side after the solution is injected may speed onset. However, these are clinically small differences and may not always be effective. Drugs should be injected slowly into the epidural space to avoid rapid increases in CSF pressure, headache, and increased intracranial pressure. A rapid speed of injection has not been shown to increase the spread of anesthetic. Also, incremental or bolus injection modes appear to have no influence on spread. The spread of epidural anesthetics may be three to four dermatomes greater in elderly patients, because age-related tissue changes create a less compliant and less leaky epidural space. Also, although conflicting data exist, some studies suggest that the epidural spread of anesthetics is greater in pregnant patients.[28,29,32] I therefore recommend that the volume of anesthetic solution administered to pregnant patients and elderly patients should initially be limited to 0.5 to 1 ml per segment (Table 42-6).

All solutions should be injected in increments of 3 to 5 ml every 3 minutes and titrated to the desired anesthetic level. With loading doses and intermittent injections, aspiration of the catheter should occur before any injection. This gradual administration of the medication slows the rate of onset of the anesthetic level and controls the development of the sympathetic blockade. After a loading dose is given, the anesthetic is maintained with either intermittent dosing or a continuous infusion technique. When a continuous infusion is used, block level should be monitored on a regular basis. Typical infusion rates range from as low as 2 ml/hr for concentrated hydrophilic opioid solutions such as preservative-free morphine up to 20 ml/hr for dilute solutions of local anesthesia (0.125% bupivacaine) used for postoperative or labor analgesia.

Management of Epidural Anesthesia

After epidural administration of local anesthetic the spread of the dermatomal block will continue and peak in an amount of time dependent on the factors previously mentioned and the local anesthetic solution used. Typically the time to maximal spread is between 10 and 25 minutes. The level of anesthesia should then be closely monitored for regression. When the block recedes one to two dermatomes, as detected by a simple scratch test, a second dose of 30% to 50% of the initial dose is given to maintain the initial level of anesthesia. Tachyphylaxis, or the need for an increase in the dosage required to maintain the level of blockade, may occur if the regression is allowed beyond two segments before the refill dose. Tachyphylaxis is also dependent on the number of injections administered. The phenomenon of tachyphylaxis is poorly understood but is more likely to occur with short-acting amides such as lidocaine or mepivacaine. Continuous infusions and the use of longer-acting agents such as bupivacaine and ropivacaine minimize this risk.

An inadequate block with "missed segments" or a one-sided block can make epidural catheter management frustrating. An initial attempt may be made to increase the spread of the anesthetic by administering half of the initial dose after 30 minutes. Placing the patient on his or her side with the unblocked side down may also help. Rarely an epidural catheter passes through dura without penetrating the arachnoid membrane. Spread of the injected anesthetic in this situation can be very

TABLE 42-6 Recommended Doses for Epidural Analgesia

Procedure	Position of Catheter	Dose (ml)
Chest	T12-L2	8-12
Upper Abdomen		
Cholecystectomy	L2	12-16
Gastric resection	L2	12-16
Incisional pain	L2	7-10
Lower Abdomen		
Colon resection	L2	12-16
Repair of aortic aneurysm	L2	12-16
Retropubic prostatectomy	L3	12-16
Herniorrhaphy	L3	8-12
Incisional pain	L3	8-12
Pancreatic pain	L3	5-7
Hysterectomy	L3	10-14
Lower Extremities		
Anesthesia	L4	10-14
Sympathetic block	L2	5-7
Perineum		
Transurethral resection of prostate	L4	8-12
Vaginal hysterectomy	L4	8-12
Back and Flank		
Nephrectomy	L2	10-14
Vaginal Delivery		
First-stage labor	L3	5-7
Second-, third-stage labor	L3	10-12

unpredictable. Anesthesia can range from a patchy, inadequate block to a rapid and high level of anesthesia requiring ventilatory support, similar to the total spinal anesthetic complication. Fortunately, subdural catheter placement is rare, and complications can be avoided by the careful use of test doses, maintained vigilance, and a high index of suspicion. Replacing the epidural catheter in a more cephalad interspace should be considered.[29,35]

Complications

As with spinal anesthesia, the hemodynamic changes seen with epidural anesthesia are attributed to sympathetic blockade and subsequent arterial and venous dilation. Use of plain local anesthetic solutions in the epidural space to create a high level of blockade will decrease the mean arterial pressure, cardiac output, stroke volume, heart rate, and peripheral vascular resistance. The addition of epinephrine (usually a 1:200,000 solution) to the epidural local anesthetic solution diminishes and slows systemic uptake, resulting in lower plasma levels of the local anesthetic and prolongation of its duration of action. However, the epinephrine is thought to be absorbed systemically in low levels, thereby causing β_2-adrenergic vasodilatation. The result is lower arterial pressure and peripheral resistance when compared with spinal anesthesia. Treatments of these hemodynamic alterations are very similar to those used for effects of spinal anesthesia. They include ephedrine 5 to 10 mg, phenylephrine 50 to 100 mcg, or a low- to moderate-rate infusion of dopamine, keeping in mind the caveats for use of these potent vasopressors. Atropine or glycopyrrolate are also useful for the treatment of bradycardia.[28,32]

Other complications associated with epidural catheters are similar to those associated with spinal anesthesia and have already been discussed in the sections covering neuraxial contraindications and spinal complications. For example, use of epidural needles, which are large in diameter compared with spinal needles, can inadvertently create a rather large dural rent. The overall risk of a postdural puncture headache is 1% to 2% with the placement of an epidural catheter. However, if a "wet tap" does occur with a 17-gauge Tuohy needle, the incidence of PDPH can be as high as 75% in young patients. Epidural catheters are also more likely to place a patient at risk for neuraxial anesthesia complications than the single passage of a smaller-gauge spinal needle, because the catheter acts as a foreign body remaining within the patient. The catheter causes mechanical tissue disruption, acts as a physical irritant, may provide a path for infection, and will cause tissue trauma on removal, perhaps as much trauma as is associated with catheter placement. Therefore, although complications are rare overall, patients must be followed closely in the postoperative period for signs and symptoms of neurologic compromise such as spinal ache, root pain, weakness, and bowel or bladder dysfunction.

COMBINED SPINAL AND EPIDURAL ANESTHESIA

Indications

First described in 1937, the combined spinal epidural anesthesia (CSE) technique has risen in popularity over the last 15 years and is currently being used successfully for orthopedic, urologic, and gynecologic surgeries and for providing postoperative pain relief. It has also gained favor in the obstetric suite for providing anesthesia and analgesia for labor and delivery and for cesarean section.[61,62]

CSE anesthesia and analgesia offers the advantages of each technique while reducing or eliminating disadvantages.[29,50] The CSE technique is appropriately employed in any setting in which the practitioner plans a spinal or epidural anesthetic and desires to exploit the advantages of each technique—usually the quicker onset of the spinal anesthetic combined with the flexibility of an epidural catheter.

History and Development

In 1937 Soresi described the sequential injection of local anesthetic, first into the epidural space then into the subarachnoid space, using the same small-gauge spinal needle. He used a needle without a stylet to identify the epidural space using the hanging-drop method and injected 7 to 8 ml of Novocain. He then advanced the needle through the dura into the subarachnoid space and injected 2 ml of Novocain, which provided anesthesia for 24 to 48 hours. His experience using this technique in more than 200 patients led him to report that "by combining the two methods many of the disadvantages of both methods are eliminated and their advantages are enhanced to an almost incredible degree."

In 1979 Curelaru provided CSE anesthesia to more than 150 patients using a two-puncture technique. He placed an epidural catheter first, and then performed the subarachnoid block one or two interspaces lower. Advantages of the technique included "the possibility of obtaining a high quality conduction anesthesia, virtually unlimited in time, the ability to extend over several anatomical regions the surgical field, minimal toxicity, the absence of postoperative pulmonary complications and the economy." Disadvantages included "the need for two vertebral punctures, the longer induction time of anesthesia and some difficulty in finding the subarachnoid space after catheterization of the epidural space."

In 1982 Coates, Mumtaz, and colleagues reported using a single space technique in which a long spinal needle was inserted through the epidural needle to provide the spinal component of the CSE technique.[63,64] Coates reported that the technique was "simple, reliable and quick to perform." He was, however, concerned that "the theoretical hazards of this technique include the possible passage of the epidural catheter through the hole in the dura mater and the possibility of subarachnoid effects from epidurally injected drugs by passage through the hole in the dura." Eldor and Brodsky reported finding metallic particles while using the needle-through-needle technique, supposedly formed by abrasion of the inner surface of the epidural needle by the passage of the spinal needle.[65] They were concerned that these particles might be introduced into the epidural space. In addition, they were concerned that distribution of the spinal local anesthetic would be uneven. They theorized that the delay inherent in introducing the epidural catheter after spinal puncture and injection into the subarachnoid space had occurred. These concerns led to the development of a combined spinal-epidural needle with two separate conduits to allow the epidural catheter to be placed first, followed by the spinal puncture. Because the needle had two conduits, it allowed both techniques to be performed with one puncture at one interspace. This innovation led to the development of several other needle types, each of which sought to improve on the others.

Equipment and Techniques: Two-Level Technique

This technique is unique in that each component is performed separately at two different interspaces. An epidural catheter is inserted first, followed by spinal anesthesia needle placed 1 to 2 interspaces lower. The primary advantage of this technique is the ability to insert and test the epidural catheter first, followed by placement of the spinal anesthetic needle. Once the spinal needle is placed, no delay occurs in positioning the patient, which may be an important factor when using a hyperbaric spinal anesthetic solution. Prior placement of the epidural catheter is not entirely benign. Potential problems include the inability to distinguish the epidural test dose from the spinal block; inability to differentiate the epidural test dose from CSF; epidural catheter laceration by the spinal needle; misdirection of the spinal needle by the catheter; inability to obtain CSF because of compression of the dural sac by the test dose; and an increased risk of dural puncture by the epidural catheter.[61] Other disadvantages include increased discomfort, tissue trauma and morbidity associated with multilevel interspinous space penetration, such as backache, epidural venous laceration, hematoma, infection, and technical difficulties.[66]

Single-Level Techniques: Needle through Needle

First described in 1982, the needle-through-needle technique involves insertion of an epidural needle at the appropriate interspace and then using the epidural needle as a guide for the spinal needle.[63,64] A small (25-, 27-, or 29-gauge) pencil-point spinal needle is inserted through the epidural needle into the subarachnoid space, and local anesthetic is injected. The spinal needle is removed and an epidural catheter is threaded into the epidural space. The epidural needle is removed and the catheter is secured. The main advantages are related to performance of a single interspace insertion (e.g., less tissue trauma, backache, and associated morbidity). Disadvantages include the possibility of inadequate spinal block if catheter placement is delayed; potential for increased nerve root trauma if paresthesias occur during catheter insertion; and the inability to reliably test the catheter with a preexisting spinal block. Inability to obtain CSF because of inadequate spinal needle length is a risk avoided by the use of the appropriate specialized needles.

Specialized Needles

Eldor was the first to develop and patent a combined spinal-epidural needle with two channels—one for the epidural catheter, the other for the spinal needle.[65] The needle is placed at the selected interspace, the epidural catheter is inserted through its designated conduit, and then the spinal needle is placed through its conduit. Once CSF is obtained, the chosen local anesthetic is injected and the needle is removed. The catheter is taped in place and the patient is positioned. Purported advantages and disadvantages are similar to those described for the single-level technique. Although the risk of metallic particle formation may be reduced, the risk of trauma to the interspinous ligaments is increased because of a larger needle diameter.

Several other needles have been developed, all seeking to minimize or eliminate potential problems.[65] In order to reduce external size, reduce needle abrasion, and allow for a direct angle of approach to the dura, a Tuohy needle was modified with a separate back eye at the bend of the needle, thereby permitting straight passage of the spinal needle. These needles are subject to their own limitations and failure rates as well. The spinal needle can miss the back-eye hole and exit the epidural needle through the main orifice, as occurs in the needle-through-needle technique.

Sequential Technique

Rawal described a single-level "sequential" technique that was developed in order to minimize the hypotensive effects of the spinal component of CSE anesthesia for cesarean section. An epidural needle is placed at the selected interspace and a low-dose (7.5 mg of hyperbaric bupivacaine) spinal anesthetic is placed using the needle-through-needle technique. The spinal needle is removed, the catheter is inserted and taped in place, and the patient is placed in the supine position with a left lateral tilt. After 15 minutes, the block is extended by titrating epidural local anesthetic until the desired level is achieved (1.5 to 2 ml for each unblocked segment). Although this technique takes longer to perform, it has been shown to decrease the frequency and severity of the hypotension seen with spinal anesthesia. This technique has also been applied in other types of surgery.[61]

Agents

As previously discussed, local anesthetic agents and their concentration are chosen depending on the effects desired. Appropriate anesthetics for the spinal component include isobaric or hyperbaric 5% lidocaine with or without epinephrine, hyperbaric 0.75% (spinal) bupivacaine, and isobaric or hyperbaric 1% tetracaine. Appropriate anesthetics for the epidural component include 2% lidocaine with or without epinephrine, 0.5% or 0.75% bupivacaine, 2% or 3% 2-chloroprocaine, and 1% ropivacaine. The concentration of these agents may be adjusted to provide postoperative analgesia in combination with opioids such as morphine and fentanyl. All agents should be preservative free in order to reduce or eliminate any potential neurotoxic effects.

Management

Although the CSE technique may be used in any type of surgical procedure in which a spinal or epidural would be acceptable, this technique may be particularly well suited to providing analgesia and anesthesia in obstetric patients. The CSE technique offers several potential advantages over conventional epidural anesthesia and analgesia[61]:

- Rapid onset of the intrathecal component for women who are in the later stages of labor and who are in significant pain and distress
- The use of intrathecal opioids (fentanyl, sufentanil, morphine, and meperidine) in early labor; the minimal to absent motor block associated with intrathecal opioids allows the patient to ambulate while in labor

The CSE technique for the laboring patient usually involves the placement of an epidural needle at the selected, usually lumbar, interspace, followed by the placement of the spinal needle using the needle-through-needle technique. Intrathecal opioids (5 to 15 mcg of sufentanil or 25 to 50 mcg of fentanyl) may be given alone or in combination with a small dose (2.5 mg of bupivacaine) of local anesthetic, saline, or both. The spinal needle is withdrawn, and the epidural catheter is inserted. The epidural needle is removed, and the catheter is taped in place. The catheter can be activated at any time should supplemental analgesia or anesthesia be required. Standard testing of the epidural catheter before use is always recommended.

The CSE technique can also be used to provide anesthesia for cesarean section if required. If the patient already has an epidural catheter in place, a test dose (3 ml 1.5% lidocaine with 1:200,000 epinephrine) is given to rule out intrathecal and intravascular placement. After a negative test dose, incremental administration of 2% lidocaine, 0.5% bupivacaine, or 3% 2-chloroprocaine can be used to establish a level of surgical anesthesia.

If a catheter has yet to be placed, and if time allows, proceed as with any new patient. After the spinal needle is placed, an intrathecal dose of local anesthetic (12 to 15 mg of 0.75% bupivacaine) with or without opioid (10 to 15 mcg of fentanyl, 0.2 to 0.3 mg of preservative-free morphine, or both) is given. The catheter is inserted and taped in place. The spinal anesthetic will set up quickly and allow for urgent (but maybe not emergent) delivery.

Despite the utility and flexibility of the CSE technique, several concerns related to its use exist. The first of these concerns is related to the use of intrathecal sufentanil and its associated hypotension.[67] Controversy exists with regard to whether intrathecal sufentanil causes clinically significant changes in blood pressure and fetal heart rate (fetal bradycardia). Purported mechanisms include pain relief, mild sympatholysis, and uterine hypertonus.[68-70] Studies show no differences in outcome between CSE using intrathecal sufentanil and epidural anesthesia.[71,72]

A second concern with CSE analgesia is the ability to ambulate after receiving intrathecal narcotics. The concern is related to possible motor weakness if low-dose local anesthetic is added and to effects on blood pressure.[73] Hypotension appears within the first 30 minutes after intrathecal fentanyl but remains stable through ambulation and follow-up doses of epidural local anesthetic. Studies demonstrate the safety of allowing ambulation with no apparent deleterious effects.[74]

A third concern with CSE technique in laboring patients is related to complications. Overall, the complications of itching and hypotension, although bothersome, do not appear to significantly affect outcome or patient satisfaction.[60] CSE anesthesia is associated with faster onset, denser motor block, lower anxiety, lower preoperative and intraoperative pain scores, and greater patient satisfaction preoperatively. There were no significant differences in the incidence or severity of hypotension or nausea, the need for supplemental analgesics, or the postoperative assessments of intraoperative pain, anxiety, and satisfaction.[75,76]

Complications

Spinal and epidural anesthesia both have their own associated complications as previously discussed. The CSE technique has the same complications and some additional unique complications. Therefore, as always, vigilance is prudent.

Failure to Obtain a Subarachnoid Block

The failure rate for subarachnoid block alone ranges from 3.1% to 17%.[77] With the single-level CSE technique for anesthesia the range is 0% to 24.5%, and for the two-level technique the range is 1.6% to 4%.[78-80] Failure with the single-level CSE technique may occur because the epidural needle is not in epidural space; the epidural needle is off midline; the spinal needle is too short (or dull) and does not penetrate the dura; or the angle of approach of the spinal needle is too oblique to puncture the dura.

One of the most important considerations is the length of the spinal needle, specifically, the length of needle that extends beyond the tip of the epidural needle.[66] Studies have shown an increased success rate when the tip of the spinal needle extends 7 to 15 mm beyond the tip of the epidural needle.[79,81] The angle at which the spinal needle approaches the dura may also be important. As the spinal needle exits a standard epidural needle tip, the angle caused by the epidural needle's curve may be 4 to 5 degrees or more.[82] This factor, combined with inadequate needle length, may result in failure to obtain CSF. This situation has led to the development of a modified Tuohy needle that has a separate back eye at the bend of the needle to allow for a straight-on approach to the dura. Pan determined that the success rate for the needles exiting the correct hole ranged from 50% to 67%.[83] The success rate can be improved to 81% to 94% by bending the spinal needle slightly in the direction of the epidural needle bevel and to 91% to 96% by orientating the epidural needle bevel upward.

Failure rates may also be directly related to level of experience with the technique and are not easily correctable. The problem of spinal needle displacement during connection of the syringe, aspiration, or injection of the local anesthetic has led to the development of "locking" devices that fix the spinal needle in the epidural needle once the dura has been punctured.[61] Their efficacy has not yet been confirmed.

Catheter Migration

Another potential problem with the needle-through-needle technique is the possibility of catheter migration through the dural puncture caused by the introduction of the spinal needle.[84] Studies that assessed the risk of catheter migration through a dural puncture site demonstrated little to no risk if the dural puncture was made with a 25-gauge or smaller spinal needle but an increased risk if the dural puncture was made by a larger (18-gauge) Tuohy needle.[62,85] Many factors may result in catheter placement in or migration into the subarachnoid space, including patient movement; undetected dural puncture with the epidural needle with subsequent catheter placement; and, least likely, diffusion of local anesthetic from the epidural space into the subarachnoid space through the dural puncture. The prudent practitioner is advised to adopt a conservative approach that includes a high index of suspicion and frequent aspiration and testing of the catheter.

However, even the question of when to test the epidural catheter can be problematic. The purpose of the epidural catheter test dose is to rule out inadvertent placement or migration of the catheter into the subarachnoid space or into an epidural vein. A preestablished subarachnoid block may preclude the ability to reliably test for subarachnoid catheter placement and mask intravascular placement. To date, no published studies have demonstrated reliable detection of inadvertent subarachnoid catheter placement in someone with a preexisting spinal block.

Increased Spinal Level after Epidural Administration

The CSE technique is known to cause an increased spread of spinal anesthesia after injection of solutions through the epidural catheter. Although controversial, several theories may help explain this phenomenon. The first—the "volume effect" theory—states that the volume of fluid injected into the epidural space compresses the subarachnoid space and the CSF within it, thereby increasing the spread of the intrathecal local anesthetic. This effect has been documented clinically and by the use of contrast media and radiography.[86,87] The second theory presupposes a "leak" or flow of local anesthetic from the epidural into the subarachnoid space through the dural puncture. This effect has also been demonstrated clinically and by radiography.[88,89] Other radiographic studies have been unable to confirm these results.[85,90]

Metallic Particles

Eldor and Levine noted the production of metallic particles when passing a spinal needle through a Tuohy epidural needle.[77] Subsequently Eldor has implied that scratches in the spinal needle and metallic particles may be associated with an increase in aseptic meningitis and cancer in patients who have received CSE anesthesia via the needle-through-needle technique.[91,92] No studies have been published to support these assertions, but several studies have examined the issue of metallic particle formation.[93] These studies used electron microscopy, atomic absorption spectrography, photomicrography, and microscopy; none were able to detect metallic particle formation.[85,94]

Postdural Puncture Headache

Conflicting evidence exists regarding whether or not a greater risk of PDPH is associated with the CSE technique compared with conventional epidural anesthesia and analgesia. Both techniques involve the placement of an epidural needle, with its attendant risk of dural puncture. In addition, the CSE technique involves a dural puncture, usually with a small-gauge, pencil-point spinal needle. Because this type of spinal needle is associated with an extremely low incidence of PDPH, one would expect an equally low incidence with the CSE technique. A review of the literature on the CSE technique shows a PDPH rate between 0% and 2.3% in laboring patients.[95] Theoretic reasons for a low incidence with the CSE technique include the following:

- The epidural needle serves as an introducer for the smaller-gauge spinal needles and allows for a straight approach at the dura.
- CSF leakage through the dural puncture is abated because of the presence of the epidural catheter and fluids, which increases pressure in the epidural space.
- The spinal needle penetrates the dura at a slight angle, which may help dural fibers seal the hole on withdrawal.

Studies suggest that the use of intrathecal opioids as part of the CSE technique may offer a protective effect from PDPH.[96,97] In addition, the success rate in obtaining CSF may be higher when the patient is in the sitting rather than the lateral position.[60] The sitting position allows for correct midline placement of the epidural needle and makes it more likely that CSF will be obtained with the spinal needle (higher hydrostatic pressure). Both of these factors contribute to minimization of the number of dural punctures and thereby decrease the risk of PDPH.

Infection

The incidence of infectious complications associated with epidural and spinal anesthesia has always been considered to be very low—in the range of 0% to 0.04%.[41,98,99] However, perhaps because of close monitoring of this newer technique, an increase has occurred in the number of case reports of patients who have developed complications that may be associated with the use of the CSE technique. Bouhemad and co-workers cite several recent cases (three since 1994) of bacterial meningitis associated with the use of CSE. The authors believe that potentially infectious skin matter was first introduced into the epidural space during the insertion of the epidural needle and was then introduced into the CSF by the passage of the spinal needle into the subarachnoid space.[100] Because the CSE technique requires invasion of both the epidural and subarachnoid spaces, strict aseptic technique should be practiced. As with other complications associated with the use of CSE, further study of this area is warranted.

Neurologic Injury

Neurologic injury associated with spinal and epidural anesthesia is also very low, ranging from 0.02% to 0.1%, and is usually transient in nature.[29] Although there does not appear to be any increased risk inherent in the CSE technique as compared with either spinal or epidural anesthesia alone, there have been several case reports of cauda equina syndrome in patients who underwent CSE anesthesia.[101,102] In none of these cases was the cause ever identified. Possible causes include preexisting spinal deformity (present in one case); use of lidocaine (present in one case); and an intrathecal catheter (never proved or disproved).

A final concern with the use of the CSE technique is paresthesia on epidural catheter insertion. A preexisting spinal block may mask a significant paresthesia on catheter insertion and result in neurologic injury. Paresthesias during epidural catheter placement range in frequency from 20% to 44%.[103] However, studies show no significant difference in the frequency of paresthesias reported for either technique.[79,103]

CAUDAL ANESTHESIA

Indications

Caudal anesthesia can be thought of as a distal approach to the epidural space. Therefore anesthetics administered or catheters placed via the caudal route will act as epidural administered anesthetics, but first on the sacral dermatomes. A caudal technique is therefore useful for perirectal surgery, urologic surgery, and orthopedic surgery of the lower extremity. Caudal techniques are especially useful in pediatrics but can also be used for labor and delivery and for chronic pain states. With the success of lumbar epidural catheters for labor and delivery, caudal anesthesia is rarely used in this population currently and is less likely to be used in the adult population in general. After the age of 12, sacral anatomy changes and bone growth makes identification of the epidural space by this approach difficult and the spread of anesthesia less reliable.[32] Therefore caudal anesthesia is most often used in combination with a light general anesthetic for postoperative analgesia in preadolescent pediatric patients.

Equipment and Techniques

The patient can be placed either prone or in a lateral position. The posterior iliac spines and the sacral hiatus are identified. Positioning the patient prone with the legs slightly apart, the heels rotated outward, and a pillow under the buttocks facilitates the palpation of the cornua of the sacral hiatus. In the lateral, Sims', or knee-chest position, identification of the cornua can be enhanced by adjusting the amount of hip flexion. Excess flexion can stretch the skin, making landmark identification difficult. An assistant is often useful when one is positioning patients who are anesthetized.

In pediatric patients general anesthesia is usually induced, the airway and intravenous access secured, and the patient turned prone or placed in a lateral decubitus position. After aseptic preparation is performed, the index and second finger of one hand are placed on the cornua of the sacrum with the hand cephalad and against the patient's back. A 22- to 25-gauge short needle attached to a 10-ml syringe filled with local anesthetic is inserted midline between the cornua at a steep angle to the skin into the sacral hiatus. Alternatively, a 20-gauge over-the-needle intravenous catheter is sufficiently long for the block, and the catheter can be passed into the epidural space while the needle is removed, allowing the anesthetist better control when administering the local anesthetic. The needle is inserted, with the bevel of the needle directed toward the sacrum. As the membranes are penetrated and the ventral canal of the sacrum is entered, a popping sensation can be felt. At this point the needle angle is lowered parallel to the sacrum and the spinal canal. The needle is advanced into the epidural space for a distance of 1 to 3 cm but no further than the second sacral interspace. The second sacral interspace lies 1 to 2 cm below a line drawn between the posterior iliac spines. The needle position is evaluated for entrance into the subarachnoid space or epidural veins via gentle aspiration and examination for CSF or blood return through the needle. Once the appropriate location of the needle is verified, the anesthetic is incrementally injected as with an epidural. During injection the skin area above the end of the needle is palpated. Bulging over the needle tip indicates subcutaneous or superficial injection rather than injection into the epidural space. If the needle is in the subperiosteal area, resistance to injection is felt and the needle must be repositioned.

Agents

In children 0.5 to 1 ml of solution per kilogram of body weight is injected to reliably achieve a level of analgesia to the umbilicus. Bupivacaine or ropivacaine, in concentrations of 0.125% to 0.5%, are usually administered with epinephrine 1:200,000, to a maximum dose of 2.5 mg/kg body weight. This provides analgesia or anesthesia for the lower extremities and the abdomen, urogenital surgery, inguinal hernia repair, or orthopedic procedures and lasts for 3 to 5 hours. Clonidine 1 mcg/kg of body weight added to the local anesthetic has been shown to be comparable to opioids that are added to enhance analgesia. Clonidine has fewer side effects than caudal opioids, such as delayed recovery, respiratory depression, and nausea. It should be remembered that some patients may be unable to tolerate the loss of lower extremity motor control. These patients should be identified before the anesthetic is administered and should be offered another technique. For example, infants too young to walk greatly benefit from caudal analgesia, but toddlers may be frightened by their inability to move their legs. Ropivacaine may have benefit over bupivacaine, because analgesia in the postoperative period is equivalent, but with shorter duration of motor blockade and less risk of cardiotoxicity.[32]

In adults the principles of epidural drug administration should be followed, with use of a 3-ml test dose and incremental injections and aspiration. Only 12 to 15 ml is necessary for sacral anesthesia, and up to 20 to 30 ml offers sufficient spread for lower extremity procedures to approximately the tenth thoracic dermatome. The spread of drug, duration of anesthesia, and desired level of anesthesia are less predictable than with epidural anesthesia because of the variability in the volume, content, and leakage of the caudal canal. The maximum recommended dose of lidocaine or mepivacaine is 10 mg/kg of body weight and 2.5 mg/kg of body weight for bupivacaine.[32] All agents injected into the epidural or subarachnoid spaces should be preservative free.

Management

Caudal anesthesia, like epidural anesthesia, is adaptable to a continuous catheter technique; however, the angle of the tip of a Tuohy needle must be kept in mind when one attempts to pass the catheter into the epidural space. Management is similar to that with an epidural catheter.

Complications

Caudal anesthesia has complications that are very similar to those of epidural anesthesia. The caudal canal has a sacral epidural venous plexus with vessels that can be unintentional recipients of a needle or catheter tip, with subsequent intravenous injection of local anesthetic. Dural puncture is also possible, although the dural sac usually ends in adults at the lower border of L2, and in infants the sac can extend to S4. High spinal punctures are less likely but have been reported. In addition, the anatomy of caudal anesthesia is variable enough, especially in adults, to cause a high (10% to 15%) failure rate as the needle is unintentionally inserted into false passages. The proximity of the caudal canal to the rectum makes infection a potential risk, although clinical infection is rarely reported.[32]

In 1899 Alice Magaw described the job of an anesthetist and best summarized the reality of the practice of regional anesthesia. She stated, "While one should be competent in the theoretical part of this important work, there is nothing so helpful to the anesthetist as the hard school of practical experience."[104]

UPPER EXTREMITY BLOCK

Frequent injury of the hand, arm, and shoulder combined with the accessibility of the nerves of the brachial plexus has encouraged the development of regional anesthesia techniques for surgical procedures of the upper extremity, as well as the diagnosis and control of pain.[105-110] The widespread use of upper extremity regional anesthesia is the result of numerous factors, including the availability of equipment to locate and deliver local anesthetics to the nerves of the plexus, the development of local anesthetics that can be applied alone and in combination to produce an appropriate duration of action for the procedure at hand, and the variety of techniques and approaches that can be used. The four primary approaches to block the brachial plexus are axillary, interscalene, supraclavicular, and infraclavicular. Because of the ease of performance, the relatively high success rate and low incidence of complications, and the ability to produce anesthesia of the forearm and hand, the most frequently used technique is the axillary approach. The requirement for anesthesia of the upper arm and shoulder is most often met through use of the interscalene approach. This is because of the potential complications associated with needle placement in close proximity to the apex of the lung necessary with supraclavicular and infraclavicular block. However, the decision to use one approach rather than another when both will produce satisfactory anesthesia of a specific region of the upper extremity is often driven by the training and experience of the anesthesia provider. Indeed, the decision to use regional anesthesia as opposed to general anesthesia, which may be viewed by the surgeon as failure-free and more expedient, for elective and emergency surgical procedures of the upper extremity requires a strong commitment to and expertise in the use of these techniques. Selection of brachial plexus block for the patient with upper extremity trauma who requires emergent surgery in the middle of the night by a practitioner who rarely uses these techniques during "normal" working hours does a disservice to both the patient and the surgical team. Moreover, the astute practitioner with experience and expertise in regional anesthesia does not lose sight of the fact that even in the best of hands upper extremity block is associated with a degree of failure. In this regard, one can never rule out the potential requirement for conversion to general anesthesia and therefore must be cognizant of elements of the patient's history and physical examination that would affect the ability to manage the airway and deliver general anesthesia safely.[105-110]

Despite the fact that existing patient pathology may suggest a regional anesthetic, it is unwise to base the decision to use an upper extremity block (or any regional technique) solely on the premise that general anesthesia should be avoided, because ultimately it may be unavoidable. The circumstances should dictate the degree to which "plan B" is considered and executed before administration of the block.[105-110]

Brachial Plexus Anesthesia

Approaches to Brachial Plexus Block

There are multiple approaches to local anesthetic block of the brachial plexus and various techniques applied with each approach. The choice of approach should be based on several factors including patient considerations, the location of the planned surgical intervention, and especially the skill and experience of the practitioner. Although surgical site and anesthesia practitioner preference often drive the decision as to which approach and technique are used, the patient's body habitus, comfort, and coexisting disease and the nature and location of the injury are as important, if not more so, than these other concerns. Patient-related considerations should be weighed in the context of the risk of potential complications associated with a given approach, technique and local anesthetic solution. The following discussion provides a practical approach to anesthesia of the brachial plexus with a focus on axillary and interscalene approaches.[105-110]

Applied Anatomy of the Brachial Plexus

An understanding of brachial plexus anatomy is mandatory if effective clinical application of regional block techniques of the upper extremity is to be achieved. This includes familiarity with muscle, facial, and vascular anatomy in relation to the origin and distribution of the brachial plexus. However, intimate knowledge of many of the anatomic details with regard to the evolution of nerve roots distributed to the brachial plexus and ultimately to peripheral nerves is not clinically essential for successful blockade. The brachial plexus is a large network of nerves that extend from the neck through the axilla and innervate the upper extremity (Figure 42-10). It is composed of ventral rami, trunks, divisions, cords, and their branches. The supraclavicular portion of the plexus, including the five primary ventral rami and the three nerve trunks and their six divisions, lies in the posterior triangle of the neck. The infraclavicular portion of the plexus, including the three cords and their four terminal branches, lies in the axilla. These nerves combine, divide, recombine, and divide again as they pass between the anterior and middle scalene muscles, through the posterior triangle of the neck, and into the axilla, where they end in the four terminal branches that supply the upper extremity. The resulting nerve pathway, when pictured and contemplated in two dimensions and without the associated bone, muscle, and vascular structures, often leads to difficulty in understanding and applying this anatomy in the clinical setting. Indeed, the value of augmenting written material when learning brachial plexus blockade with an apprenticeship at the hands of a master of the art cannot be overestimated.[105-110]

The archetypal brachial plexus is formed by the rami from the fifth (C5) to the eighth (C8) cervical nerves and the first thoracic (T1) nerve. In a small percentage of individuals the fourth cervical (C4) or the second thoracic (T2) nerve or a combination of the two contributes to the plexus. After the rami pass the lateral border of the scalene muscles, they reorganize into trunks. The rami from C5 and C6 combine to form the superior or upper trunk, and the ramus from C7 continues

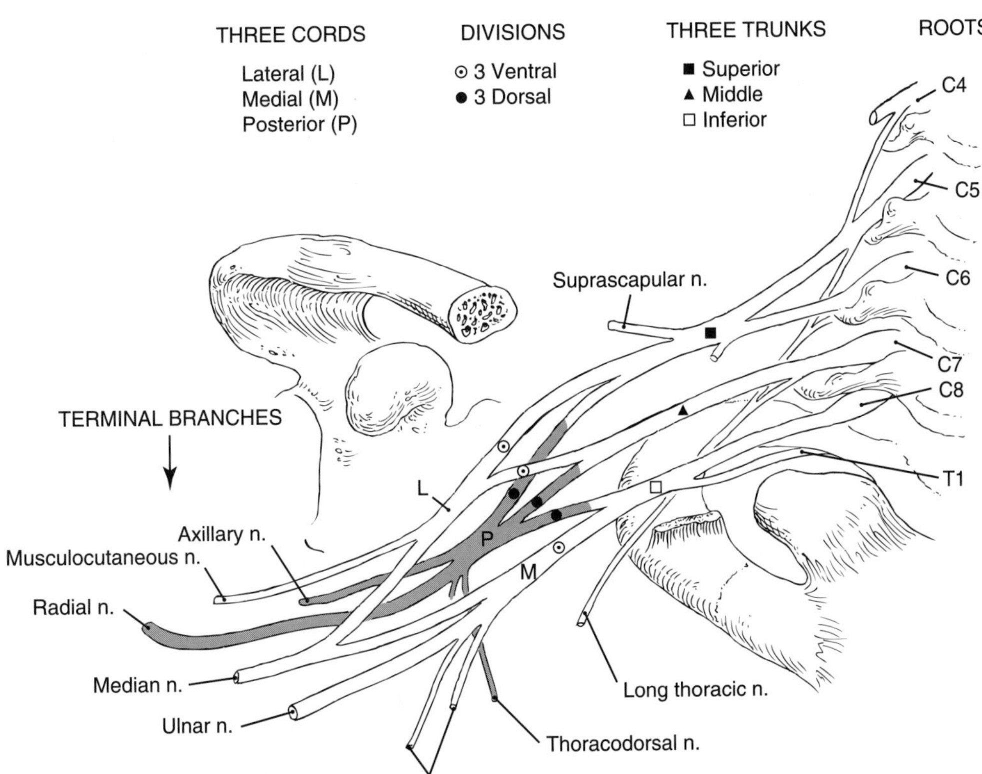

FIGURE **42-10** Derivation of the brachial plexus from the cervical spine. *n*, Nerve.

alone as the middle trunk. The rami from C8 and T1 combine to form the inferior or lower trunk, which lies on the first rib posterior to the subclavian artery. The nerve trunks are enveloped by a fascial "sheath," the origins of which are from the posterior fascia of the anterior scalene muscle and the anterior fascia of the middle scalene muscle. This forms a closed space known as the *interscalene space* at this level or more generally as the *sheath of the brachial plexus*. Cadaver studies have demonstrated the existence of extensive velamentous septa that can form compartments around the contents of this sheath. These septa appear to be incomplete and therefore may not function as mechanical barriers to the spread of local anesthetics. Indeed, a single injection of local anesthesia into this sheath commonly produces complete block of the upper extremity.[105-111] Nevertheless, anatomic variations do exist, and it is possible that in certain individuals septa occur that isolate nerves, resulting in so-called "patchy blocks" by preventing exposure to the injected local anesthetic. It has also been shown that injection even outside the sheath can produce neural blockade, albeit with a considerably greater latency period. The lesson to be learned with regard to clinical application of this information is that failure to allot a sufficient amount of time to perform an upper extremity block, and in particular to allow it to "set up," generally produces an unsatisfactory result.[105-111]

At the lateral border of the first rib and posterior to the clavicle each of the three trunks divides into ventral and dorsal divisions. These divisions are of significant clinical importance to application and evaluation of brachial plexus blockade, because the ventral divisions generally supply the ventral (flexor) portion of the upper extremity and the dorsal divisions generally supply the dorsal (extensor) portions. As these divisions enter the axilla, the three posterior divisions combine to form the posterior cord; the anterior divisions of the superior and middle trunks combine to form the lateral cord; and the anterior division of the inferior trunk continues to become the medial cord. At that point the cords are named according to their position in relation to the axillary artery. At the lateral border of the pectoralis minor muscle each of these cords divides into two branches, which reorganize to form the peripheral nerves of the upper extremity. The lateral cord divides and generates the musculocutaneous nerve and the lateral root of the median nerve. The medial cord divides and generates the ulnar nerve and the medial root of the median nerve. The posterior cord divides to generate the axillary and the radial nerves.

Understanding the anatomic relationships that result as the nerve cords give rise to the nerve branches and the areas of the upper extremity that these branches innervate is of paramount importance in the clinical application, evaluation, and supplementation of brachial plexus block. The branches of the lateral and medial cords (median, ulnar, and musculocutaneous nerves) predominately supply the ventral portions of the upper extremity, and the branches of the posterior cord (radial and axillary nerve) predominately supply the dorsal portions. However, in certain areas of the upper extremity, such as the posterior portion of the fingers and the hand, there exists considerable cutaneous representation of the "predominately ventral" median and ulnar nerves.[105-111]

The radial nerve (C5 to C8 and Tl) is the major nerve supply to the dorsal extensor muscles, such as the triceps, of the upper limb below the shoulder. It supplies sensory innervation to the extensor region of the arm, forearm, and hand. The musculocutaneous nerve (C5 to C7) supplies the flexor muscles, such as the biceps, brachialis, and coracobrachialis, of the ventral portion of the arm. It supplies sensory innervation to the lateral aspect of the forearm between the wrist and elbow as the lateral antebrachial cutaneous nerve. The median and ulnar nerves pass through the arm and provide sensory and motor innervation to the forearm and hand. The median nerve (C6 to Tl) is better represented than the ulnar nerve in the forearm, where it supplies most of the flexor and pronator muscles. It also supplies sensory innervation to the ventral portion of the thumb, the first and second fingers, the lateral half of the third finger, and the palm of the hand. The ulnar nerve (C8 and Tl) is better represented than the median nerve in the hand, where it supplies motor innervation to most of the small flexor muscles. It has no sensory innervation of the forearm but supplies sensation to the medial part of the third finger, the entire fourth finger, and the remaining portion of the palm of the hand.[105-111]

Interscalene Approach

With the patient in the supine position the anesthetist asks the patient to lower the shoulder on the side of the proposed anesthetic and surgery site to pull the shoulder away from the brachial plexus, intentionally trying to stretch the neck muscles and improve visualization and access. The patient's head can then either be turned so that the patient looks away from the area of the anesthetic or moved laterally away from the site, maintaining forward vision.

The cricoid cartilage ring is then palpated just below the thyroid cartilage. This anatomic landmark correlates to the vertebral body of C6 and the corresponding area of the transverse process called *Chassaignac's tubercle*. A straight line is drawn posteriorly to cross over the sternocleidomastoid (SCM) muscle, and the lateral border of the SCM is palpated. If this border is difficult to assess, the patient can be asked to raise the head against gentle resistance and then relax. Posterior to this border the anesthetist palpates for the groove between the anterior and middle scalene muscles with two fingers (Figure 42-11). This is the level of the trunks of the brachial plexus (Figure 42-12).

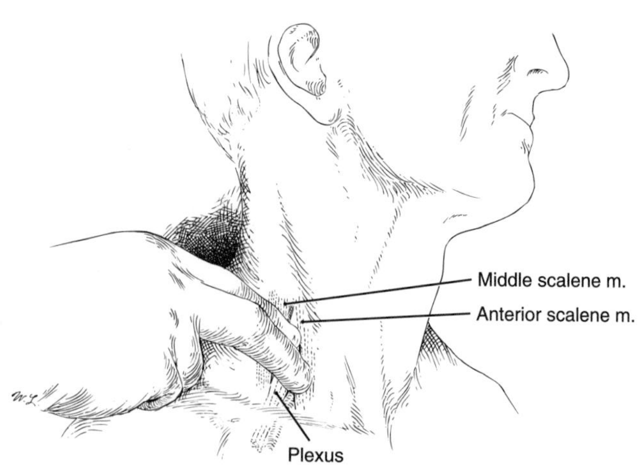

FIGURE **42-11**
Technique for identifying the anterior and middle scalene muscles and the major vessels so that the interscalene perivascular technique can be accomplished. *m*, Muscle.

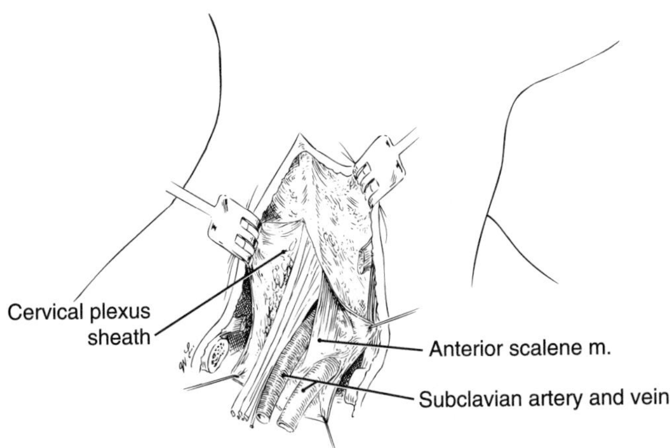

FIGURE **42-12**
Three trunks of the cervical plexus are revealed lying alongside the subclavian vessels. *m*, Muscle.

After cleansing of the patient's skin, an intradermal skin wheal of local anesthetic is made at this point on the groove. A 22-gauge insulated B-bevel needle usually $1^1/_2$ inches long is inserted gently through the skin wheal perpendicularly to the skin and then angled slightly caudad. The needle is attached to an intravenous extension tube with an anesthetic-filled syringe. The patient is told what to expect, and the needle is slowly advanced until a motor twitch response is elicited. The nerve stimulator current is lowered from 1 mA to 0.5 mA to minimize excessive current to the patient and to ensure proper needle position. After gentle aspiration is negative for blood or CSF, a test dose of 1 ml of local anesthetic solution is injected. A fade will be observed in the quality of the motor twitch experienced by the patient. This indicates that the needle is probably within the brachial plexus sheath. If no subjective symptoms of toxicity reaction are present, incremental injections of 3 to 5 ml of local anesthetic followed by aspiration to detect blood are administered until the intended volume is given. In adult patients the volume is usually 30 to 35 ml.[105-111]

Subclavian Approach

The patient is positioned and prepared as for the interscalene approach (Figure 42-13). In addition, some practitioners may place the patient's bed in a 30- to 45-degree head-up position or place a pillow under the patient's shoulder to accentuate the anatomy. The area above and including the clavicle on the surgical side is cleansed and draped.

The pulsations of the subclavian artery in the plexus are behind and below the clavicle, just above the superior surface of the first rib, and between the scalene muscles; the artery is palpated behind the midpoint of the clavicle. The anesthetist uses the nondominant hand to palpate for pulsations behind and 1 to 2 cm above the clavicle at this point and uses the dominant hand to place a skin wheal of local anesthetic immediately lateral to this site. Through the skin wheal, the 22-gauge insulated B-bevel needle, attached to a nerve stimulator, is advanced perpendicularly to the skin, inward, and caudad until a motor twitch is noted in the lower portion of the upper extremity (Figure 42-14). The nerve stimulator current is lowered from 1 mA to 0.5 mA to minimize excessive current to the patient and to ensure proper needle position. After gentle aspiration is negative for blood, a test dose of 1 ml of local anesthetic solution is injected. A fade will be observed in the quality of the motor twitch experienced by the patient. This indicates that the needle is probably within the brachial plexus sheath. If no subjective symptoms suggesting toxicity reactions are present, incremental injections of 3 to 5 ml of local anesthetic followed by aspiration to detect blood are administered

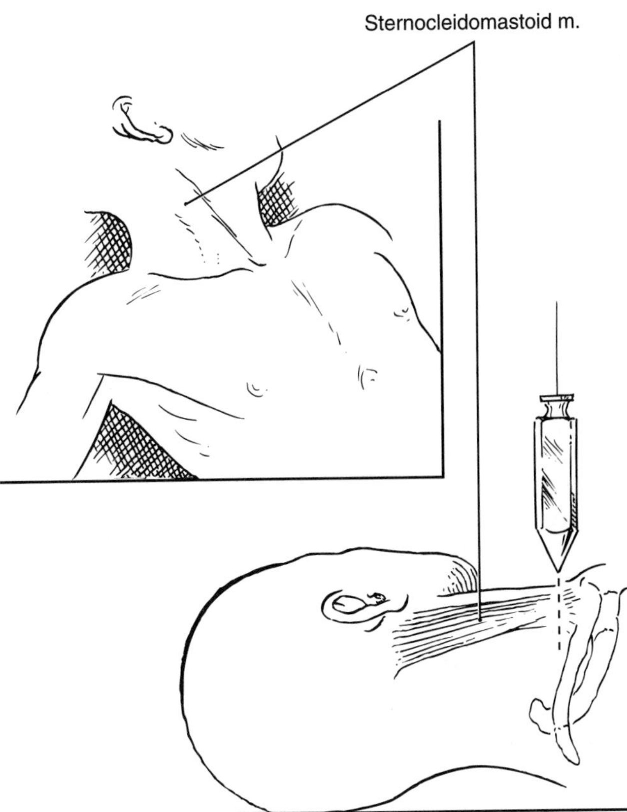

FIGURE **42-13**
The patient is placed in the supine position with the head supported and turned toward the opposite shoulder.

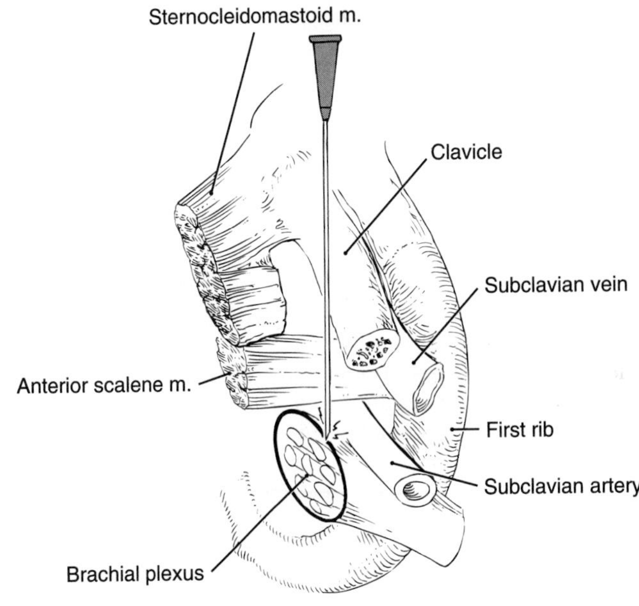

FIGURE **42-14**
The needle enters the sheath of the brachial plexus at the farthest possible distance from the subclavian artery. *m*, Muscle.

until the intended volume is given. In adult patients the volume is usually 30 to 35 ml.[105-111]

The anesthetist must watch for the onset of Horner's syndrome as a positive sign of a successful block. The most important complication of the supraclavicular approach is pneumothorax. The pleura of the lung is immediately inferior to the first rib, and careful needle placement as described previously is imperative. If landmarks are difficult to define, the patient is very thin, or the pleura of the lung is unusually high, the incidence of pneumothorax may increase. The increased incidence of pneumothorax with the supraclavicular approach and the high incidence of Horner's syndrome with the interscalene approach led to the development of a new approach to the brachial plexus called the *intersternocleidomastoid* (ISCM) *block* by Charles Pham Dang in 1997.[105-112]

Intersternocleidomastoid Block

The new supraclavicular approach to the brachial plexus is named the *intersternocleidomastoid block*, as the puncture site is situated between the heads of the SCM muscle. The novelty of the technique arises from many points: easy surface landmarks; minimized risk of pleural puncture; no risk of epidural, subarachnoid, or intravertebral artery injection; possible catheterization of perineural space.[105-112]

In the ISCM block, depending on the direction of the needle, the brachial plexus can be reached at the level of the trunks (i.e., superior, middle, and inferior). The needle passes successively between the heads of the SCM, behind the clavicular head, through the middle cervical fascia, next to the phrenic nerve, and through the anterior scalene muscle before arriving at the brachial plexus. The following nerves can be reached and stimulated depending on the direction of the needle, at a depth varying from 3 to 8 cm: suprascapular nerve, superior trunk, middle trunk, and the divisions and cord.[105-112]

The patient lies supine with the head turned away, arm at the side, and hand positioned on the abdomen. The anesthetist stands next to the patient's head, opposite the side on which the operation will be performed. The sternal and clavicular heads of the SCM, as well as the midclavicle, are marked. The puncture site is situated two fingerbreadths above the sternal notch, between the heads of the SCM, medial to the clavicular head. After disinfection and skin wheal infiltration the stimulating needle of appropriate length is introduced behind the posterior border of the clavicular head of the SCM. The needle, practically leaning on the sternal head, is advanced laterally, posteriorly, and caudally in the direction indicated by a point situated 1 cm lateral to the midclavicle. The needle makes an angle of 45 degrees to the table and 15 degrees to the clavicle. This initial orientation of the needle leads to the suprascapular nerve, the stimulation of which evokes glenohumeral coaptation and contraction of the supraspinatus and infraspinatus muscles. Stimulation of the superior trunk evokes contraction of the biceps brachi and deltoid muscles, elbow flexion, and abduction of the arm. Stimulation of the middle trunk evokes contraction of the triceps brachi muscle and elbow extension. Stimulation of the divisions and cord evokes flexion pronation of the hand and digit flexion in conjunction with pectoral contraction. Movements of the abdomen can be seen from stimulation of the phrenic nerve. They imply withdrawal and redirection of the needle. These motor responses are obtained at a depth of 2 to 8 cm depending on the collar size. The nerve stimulator current is lowered from 1 mA to 0.5 mA to minimize excessive current to the patient and to ensure proper needle position. After gentle aspiration is negative for blood, a test dose of 1 ml of local anesthetic solution is injected. A fade will be observed in the quality of the motor twitch experienced by the patient. This indicates that the needle is probably within the brachial plexus sheath. If no subjective symptoms suggesting toxicity reactions are present, incremental injections of 3 to 5 ml of local anesthetic followed by aspiration to detect blood are administered until the intended volume is given. In adult patients the volume is usually 30 to 35 ml.[105-112]

Axillary Approach

The axillary approach to anesthesia of the brachial plexus is best suited to surgical procedures at or below the elbow (hand and forearm). However, an injury to the hand or forearm, such as a fracture, which also limits the range of motion of the extremity because of patient discomfort, reduces the versatility of this approach. Under these conditions, patient comfort must be weighed against the need for profound anesthesia of the hand or forearm, often in the presence of a full stomach and the desire to avoid general anesthesia. In this instance, access to the axilla can generally be gained by the judicious use of intravenous opioids before slow, careful positioning and support of the extremity in preparation for placement of the block.[105-110]

The patient is placed in the supine position, with the arm to be blocked abducted 90 degrees from the body. The forearm is flexed to 90 degrees and rested parallel to the long axis of the body. The anesthetist uses the index and third fingers to identify the axillary artery, starting at the lateral margin of the pectoralis major muscle and tracing the artery into the mid to lower axilla (Figure 42-15). Needle insertion need not occur high in the axilla, as some authors suggest, for successful block. Insertion in the mid to lower axilla is just as effective; however, it reduces the chances that a local anesthetic will reach the point at which the musculocutaneous nerve leaves the sheath. A well-defined, localized pulsation of the axillary artery is more important to successful blockade than the point at which needle insertion occurs within the axilla. After appropriate preparation of the skin a local anesthetic intradermal skin wheal is raised just proximal and superior to the palpating index finger. During needle insertion moderate digital pressure should be applied to the artery in order to minimize the distance among the skin, subcutaneous tissue, and neurovascular bundle. An appropriate needle connected to a sterile extension tubing and syringe containing 50 ml of local anesthetic is inserted through the skin wheal. At this point the technique diverges depending on the endpoint used to determine when the needle tip lies within the sheath. These endpoints include loss of resistance to the advancing needle; penetration of the axillary artery; and elicitation of a paresthesia.[105-110]

Loss-of-Resistance Technique

The loss-of-resistance technique uses a distinct change in tissue resistance often described as a "pop" as the needle penetrates the fascia and enters the sheath. After the axillary artery is identified, a 22-gauge, 1-1/2-inch, short ("B") bevel needle is inserted medially at approximately a 20-degree angle to the skin and parallel to the longitudinal course of the artery (Figure 42-16). Use of a short bevel needle enhances the loss-of-resistance sensation on penetration of the sheath; however, the drag associated with the attachment of an extension tubing decreases this sensation. Some practitioners disconnect the

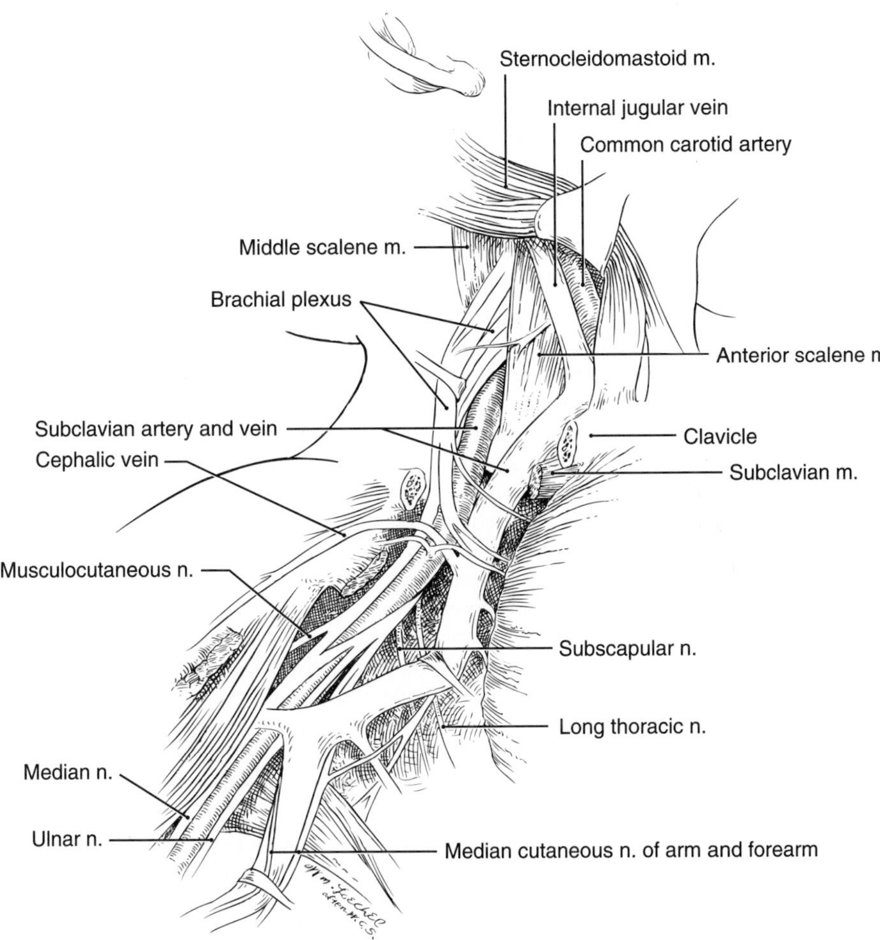

FIGURE **42-15**
The brachial plexus at the axilla. *m*, Muscle; *n*, Nerve.

extension tubing and observe the free needle for a pulsatile movement associated with the needle tip's close proximity to the axillary artery. This is considered a further indication of correct needle placement within the sheath, but it does not guarantee proper placement. The needle is then advanced medially an additional $^1/_2$ to 1 inch parallel to the axillary artery at an acute angle to the skin. Before local anesthesia is injected, the patient is instructed to immediately inform the anesthetist if symptoms indicative of rapid intravascular uptake or direct intravascular injection occur. These include dizziness, tinnitus, metallic taste in the mouth ("mouth full of nickels"), circumoral numbness or tingling, visual disturbances, and muscle twitching. If epinephrine has been added to the local anesthetic to reduce vascular absorption of the solution, the patient may also be instructed to report the sensation of having a "rapid" or "hard" heart beat. The needle is held fixed in position, and an assistant gently aspirates the syringe while the operator observes for blood in the extension tubing, which would indicate that the needle has entered the axillary artery or vein. In the absence of frank blood in the aspirate, a 5-ml test dose of the local anesthetic solution is injected and the patient observed and queried for the existence of any of the symptoms noted for a minimum of 1 minute. Barring an untoward event the remainder of the local anesthetic solution is injected in 5-ml increments, with each injection preceded by gentle aspiration and observation for blood in the extension tubing. Firm pressure should be applied to the area immediately behind the needle insertion site with several fingers during the injection to prevent retrograde flow of the anesthetic solution. Injection of each 5 ml of local anesthetic should be considered a "test dose," as unrecognized penetration of the artery or rapid uptake of the local anesthetic remains a possibility throughout the procedure. When 40 ml of the local anesthetic solution has been injected, the needle is withdrawn to the level of the skin in preparation for field block, if desired, of the musculocutaneous, medial brachial cutaneous, and intercostobrachial nerves (see Figure 42-16). These nerves may require individual blockade because they exit the sheath high in the axilla (musculocutaneous and medial brachial cutaneous) or lie outside the sheath altogether (intercostobrachial). If care is taken to apply continuous digital pressure immediately below the site of needle insertion during injection of a 40-ml bolus of local anesthetic solution, and the arm is adducted after injection, anesthesia of the musculocutaneous nerve and its terminal distribution, the lateral antebrachial nerve (sensory innervation to the lateral forearm from the elbow to the wrist), can be achieved. Before the needle is withdrawn from the skin, the musculocutaneous nerve can be independently blocked by injecting 3 to 5 ml of the remaining local anesthetic into the body of the coracobrachialis muscle. The coracobrachialis muscle is located immediately superior to the axillary artery and inferior to the biceps brachialis muscle. After block of the musculocutaneous nerve has been performed, the needle is again withdrawn to the level of the skin and redirected inferior and perpendicular to the artery into the subcutaneous tissue. The remaining 3 to 5 ml of local

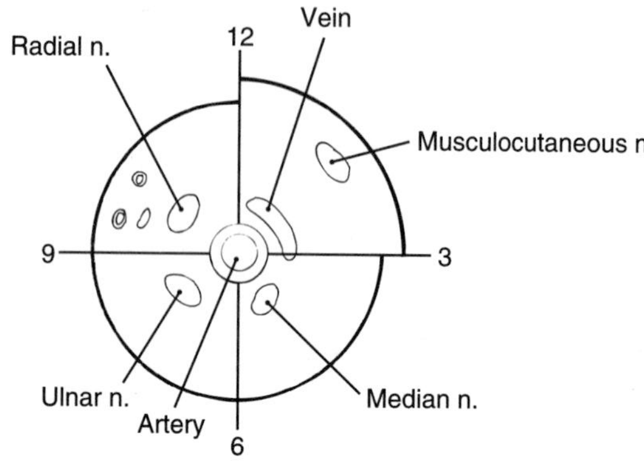

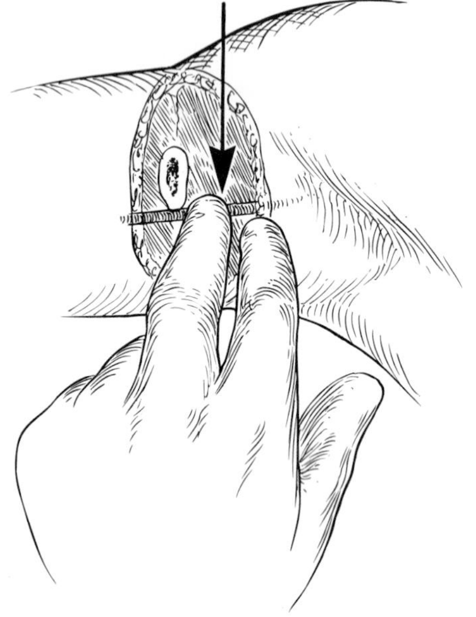

FIGURE **42-16**
Identification of the intercostobrachial and brachial cutaneous nerves after completion of the axillary block. *n*, Nerve.

anesthetic is injected into the subcutaneous tissue as the needle is advanced to the hub. This subcutaneous "bracelet" of local anesthetic produces conduction block of the medial brachial cutaneous and intercostobrachial nerves necessary to prevent discomfort if a tourniquet is to be used. After completion of the block the arm is immediately adducted and held close to the body to promote the cephalad spread of the local anesthetic solution, which can be obstructed by the abducted humeral head.[105-110]

Transarterial Technique

The transarterial technique uses intentional penetration of the axillary artery and aspiration of blood as the end point for determining that the needle is within the sheath. After the axillary artery is identified, a local anesthetic skin wheal is raised directly above the artery at the planned point of needle insertion (see Figure 42-16). A 21-gauge 1-1/2-inch needle is inserted perpendicularly to the skin and advanced slowly until blood is aspirated into the extension tubing by an assistant, who provides gentle aspiration of the syringe. The needle is then advanced along the same plane until blood can no longer be aspirated because the bevel has exited the posterior wall of the artery. Care must be taken to avoid advancing the needle through the posterior wall of the sheath after the artery is exited, which would result in deposition of the local anesthetic outside the sheath. Before local anesthetic is injected, the patient is instructed to immediately inform the anesthetist if symptoms indicative of rapid intravascular uptake or direct intravascular injection occur. The needle is held fixed in position, and an assistant gently aspirates the syringe while the operator observes for blood in the extension tubing, which would indicate that the needle has entered the axillary artery or vein. In the absence of frank blood in the aspirate a 5-ml test dose of the local anesthetic solution is injected, and the patient is observed for and queried regarding the existence of any of the symptoms previously noted for a minimum of 1 minute. Barring an untoward event the remainder of the local anesthetic solution is injected in 5-ml increments, with each injection preceded by gentle aspiration and observation for blood in the extension tubing. Firm pressure should be applied to the area immediately behind the needle insertion site with several fingers during the injection to prevent retrograde flow of the anesthetic solution. Injection of each 5 ml of local anesthetic should be considered a "test dose," as unrecognized penetration of the artery or rapid uptake of the local anesthetic remains a possibility throughout the procedure. When 40 ml of the local anesthetic solution has been injected, the needle is withdrawn to the level of the skin in preparation for field block, if desired, of the musculocutaneous, medial brachial cutaneous, and the intercostobrachial nerves. These nerves may require individual blockade because they exit the sheath high in the axilla (musculocutaneous and medial brachial cutaneous) or lie outside the sheath altogether (intercostobrachial). If care is taken to apply continuous digital pressure immediately below the site of needle insertion during injection of a 40-ml bolus of local anesthetic solution, and the arm is adducted after injection, anesthesia of the musculocutaneous nerve and its terminal distribution, the lateral antebrachial nerve (sensory innervation to the lateral forearm from the elbow to the wrist), can be achieved. Before the needle is withdrawn from the skin, the musculocutaneous nerve can be independently blocked by injecting 3 to 5 ml of the remaining local anesthetic into the body of the coracobrachialis muscle. The coracobrachialis muscle is located immediately superior to the axillary artery and inferior to the biceps brachialis muscle. After block of the musculocutaneous nerve has been performed, the needle is again withdrawn to the level of the skin and redirected inferiorly and perpendicularly to the artery into the subcutaneous tissue. The remaining 3 to 5 ml of local anesthetic is injected into the subcutaneous tissue as the needle is advanced to the hub. This subcutaneous "bracelet" of local anesthetic produces conduction block of the medial brachial cutaneous and intercostobrachial nerves necessary to prevent discomfort if a tourniquet is to be used. After completion of the block the arm is immediately adducted and held close to the body to promote cephalad spread of the local anesthetic solution, which can be obstructed by the abducted humeral head.[105-110]

Selective Blocks at the Elbow

Several other blocks in the arm can be of benefit and may become techniques of choice, especially in outpatients. Selective blocks at the elbow and wrist permit the surgeon to complete the procedure while minimizing the amount of anesthesia that is administered. The blocks at the elbow and the wrist are primarily sensory blocks. The patient retains the ability to move the hand during the procedure. Reduction of the area anesthetized, the amount of sedation administered, and the potential for complications minimizes the patient's stay in the outpatient center. The use of selective blocks avoids the use of a general anesthetic when the regional anesthetic technique is partially successful.[4,15,113]

Each nerve that supplies sensory branches into the arm can be blocked at the elbow and the wrist. Use of the nerve locator at the level of the elbow for the median and radial nerves and at the level of the wrist for the ulnar and median nerves can improve the success rate of the block.

When a tourniquet is used during the surgical procedure, the intercostobrachial nerve and the brachial cutaneous nerve should be blocked in the axilla. This blocking provides anesthesia sufficient to permit the patient to tolerate the pressure of tourniquet inflation. The coracobrachial muscle can also be blocked at the level of the shoulder in order to provide anesthesia so that the patient can better tolerate tourniquet inflation.

Ulnar Nerve Block at the Elbow

As the ulnar nerve traverses the ulnar sulcus of the humerus, it is tightly fixed in the groove. Performing a regional anesthetic technique in this location can increase the potential for nerve entrapment. The volume of the solution should be limited in order to reduce the amount of pressure exerted on the nerve and the potential ischemia that could develop from injection of a large volume (>3 ml).[4,15,113]

The technique should be performed 1 to 2 cm proximal to the sulcus. The patient's elbow is flexed 90 degrees, and the medial condyle of the humerus is identified. A finger is placed in the ulnar sulcus, extending approximately 1 cm proximal to the condyle (Figure 42-17). The insertion point for the needle is between the medial condyle of the humerus and the olecranon process of the ulna. The needle is inserted at a 45-degree angle to the skin and perpendicularly to a line drawn between the medial condyle and the olecranon process. If a paresthesia is elicited on introduction of the needle, the needle is withdrawn approximately 1 mm, and 2 to 3 ml of the solution is injected. If a paresthesia is not elicited, the volume of the solution can be increased. The total volume of the local anesthetic solution is 3 to 5 ml. The onset of action is determined by the local anesthetic used for the procedure. Epinephrine can be used at this level; however, this agent delays the onset.[4,15,113]

Median Nerve Block at the Elbow

For facilitation of forearm and hand anesthesia the median nerve block can be performed with the ulnar block as either a supplement to another technique or as the only anesthesia technique. The combination of a median nerve and an ulnar nerve block provides adequate anesthesia for procedures on the cutaneous portions of the lower forearm, the hand, and the second, third, and fourth fingers. The median block can be used to supplement partially successful brachial plexus blocks. The median nerve block should be avoided in patients with carpal tunnel syndrome. This block should be avoided if neuritis is present or if the artery is perforated. If anesthesia is administered to two of the three nerves in the foramen, limited function of the hand remains.[4,15,113]

The median nerve block is performed by positioning the patient's arm on a stable surface with the elbow slightly flexed. A line is drawn from the medial to the lateral condyles of the humerus on the anterior surface of the elbow. The brachial artery is then identified as it crosses this line (Figure 42-18). A short, B-bevel needle is inserted slightly medial to the brachial artery to a depth of 0.5 to 0.75 cm. Median nerve blocks at the

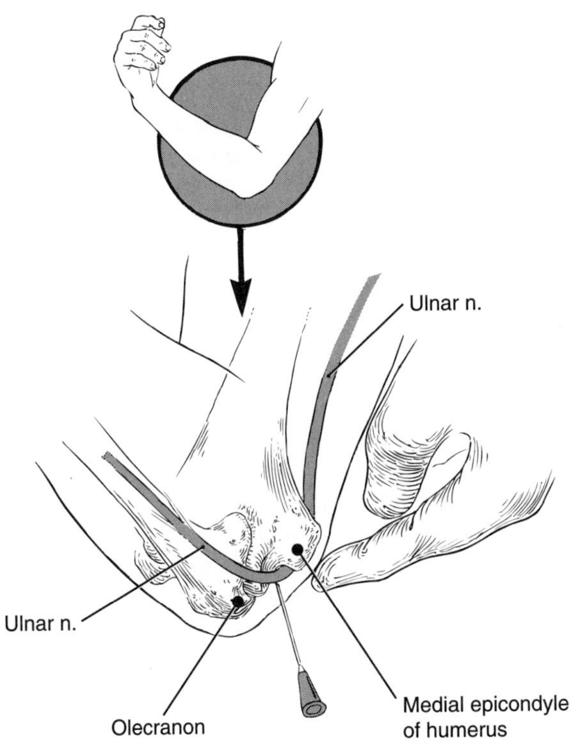

FIGURE **42-17**
Technique of ulnar block at the elbow. The patient's elbow is flexed 90 degrees, and the medial condyle of the humerus is identified. *n*, Nerve.

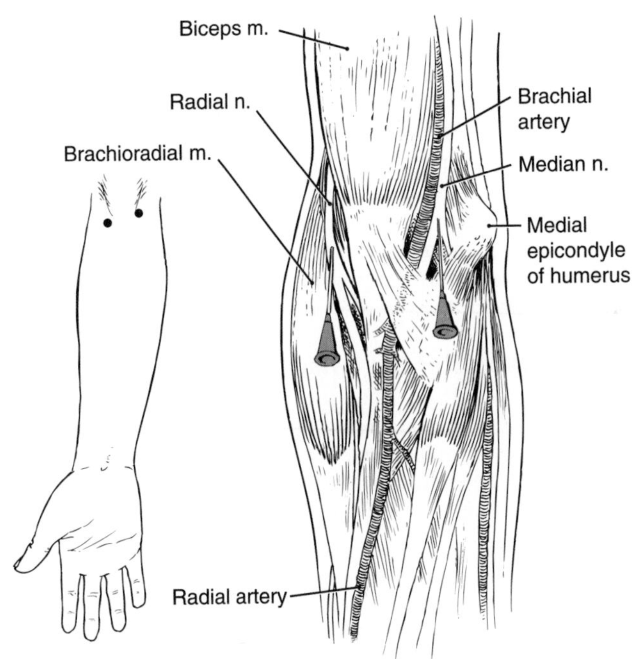

FIGURE **42-18**
Performance of median nerve block by positioning of the patient's arm on a stable surface with the elbow slightly flexed. After the brachial artery is identified, a short, B-bevel needle is inserted slightly medial to the brachial artery.

elbow can be facilitated with the nerve locator. When the nerve locator is used, a stimulus of low amplitude elicits a response along the path of the median nerve. If the nerve locator is not used, a paresthesia can be elicited by fan-wise movement of the needle. Identification of the median nerve is necessary for a successful anesthesia technique. Local anesthetic solution (3 to 5 ml) is injected after the nerve is located. As the needle is withdrawn through the fascia, an additional 1 to 2 ml of solution is injected in order to block cutaneous branches of the nerve.[4,15,113]

Radial Nerve Block at the Elbow

Blocking of the radial nerve can be used as an adjunct to axillary perivascular techniques. This block is also used successfully for surgery of the forearm and hand that is within the distribution of the radial nerve or in conjunction with other nerve blocks.

With the elbow extended and stabilized on a firm surface, the brachioradialis muscle and biceps tendon are identified. The radial nerve is located in the groove formed by the fascial border of the brachioradial muscle (see Figure 42-18) on the lateral edge, and the biceps tendon medially. A line is drawn between the medial and lateral condyles. A short, B-bevel needle is inserted along the medial border of the brachioradial muscle toward the lateral condyle at the point at which the line between the condyles crosses the facial groove. The needle is directed toward the anterior aspect of the lateral condyle so that gentle contact occurs. After contact with the condyle, the needle is withdrawn 2 mm. Local anesthetic solution (3 to 5 ml) is injected. This procedure is repeated two to three times while the needle is moved slightly more proximally for each injection. As the needle is withdrawn into the subcutaneous tissue, 3 to 5 ml of local anesthetic is injected.[4,15,113]

In an alternate approach to the radial nerve the lateral border of the brachioradial muscle is identified. Measuring 3 to 5 cm proximal from the lateral condyle along the border of the brachioradial muscle enables palpation of the radial nerve as it parallels the humerus. The nerve is adherent to the bone at this level and can be easily injured during trauma or during the performance of the regional anesthesia. By slight movement of the nerve, a paresthesia can be elicited. A short, B-bevel needle is inserted in a plane perpendicular to the humerus and is advanced to the proximity of the identified radial nerve. Because of its fixation against the humerus the needle must be slowly advanced, and the position must be evaluated in order to avoid injury to the nerve.[4,15,113]

Selective Blocks at the Wrist

Selective blocks of the ulnar, median, and radial nerves at the wrist can be used for supplying limited anesthesia for the outpatient or as a supplement to brachial plexus anesthesia. Procedures that require a motor block in addition to the sensory blockade should be accomplished by use of another anesthesia technique. Because of the nature of the small vessels of the wrist, hand, and fingers, epinephrine is not included in solutions used in nerve blocks below the elbow.[4,15,113]

Ulnar Block at the Wrist

With the wrist slightly flexed and stabilized on a firm surface, the ulnar flexor muscle of the wrist is identified (Figure 42-19). A line is then drawn across the forearm at the level of the styloid process of the ulna. A short, B-bevel needle is inserted perpendicularly to the skin on the radial side of the ulnar flexor muscle of the wrist, where it is crossed by the line. At this location the needle is slightly lateral to the ulnar artery, and a small deviation medially can place the needle over the artery. The ulnar artery can be palpated when the wrist is in moderately exaggerated extension. However, severe extension causes the artery to collapse. After the needle is inserted, 2 to 4 ml of local anesthetic solution is injected. An additional 2 ml is injected as the needle is withdrawn from the deep fascia. The dorsal branch of the ulnar nerve is blocked by injection of 3 to 5 ml of local anesthesia in a half-ring around the ulnar aspect of the wrist. The needle is placed subcutaneously at the radial margin of the ulnar flexor muscle of the wrist and is advanced to the midportion of the dorsal aspect of the wrist.[4,15,113]

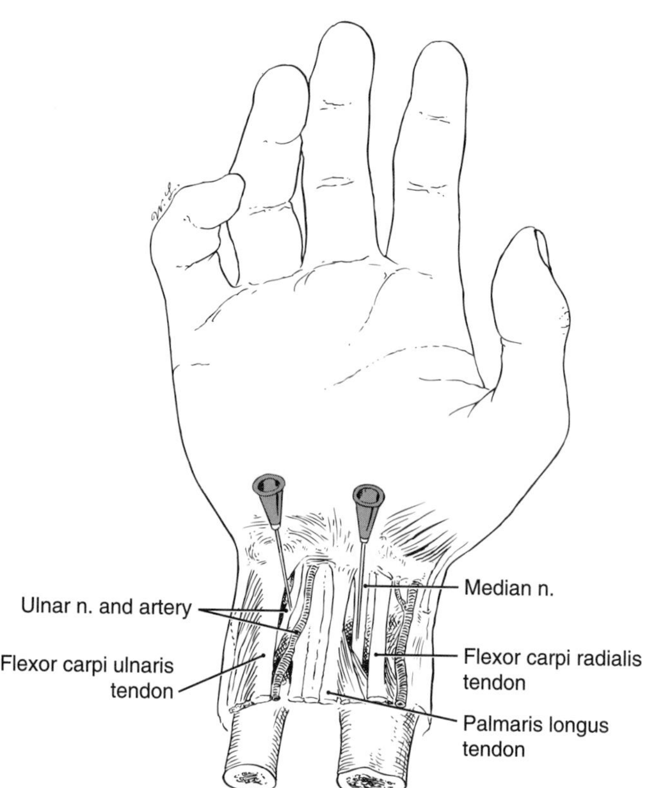

FIGURE **42-19**
With the patient's wrist slightly flexed and stabilized on a firm surface, the ulnar flexor muscle of the wrist is identified. A short, B-bevel needle is inserted perpendicularly to the skin on the radial side of the ulnar flexor muscle of the wrist. *n*, Nerve.

Median Block at the Wrist

The wrist is stabilized on a firm surface and is slightly flexed against resistance. When the wrist is flexed, the long palmar muscle and the radial flexor muscle of the wrist are easily identified (see Figure 42-19). A line is drawn across the wrist that parallels the proximal crease. A short, B-bevel needle is inserted perpendicularly to the skin between the two tendons for a distance of 0.5 to 1 cm. The carpal tunnel is a tightly confined space. The nerve is located in the superficial portion of the carpal tunnel. A paresthesia can be elicited during the performance of the procedure. If the sensation persists, the needle must be withdrawn and repositioned. Local anesthetic solution (2 to 5 ml) is injected within the carpal tunnel, and another 2 to 3 ml is injected after the needle is withdrawn from the fascia of the carpal tunnel.[4,15,113]

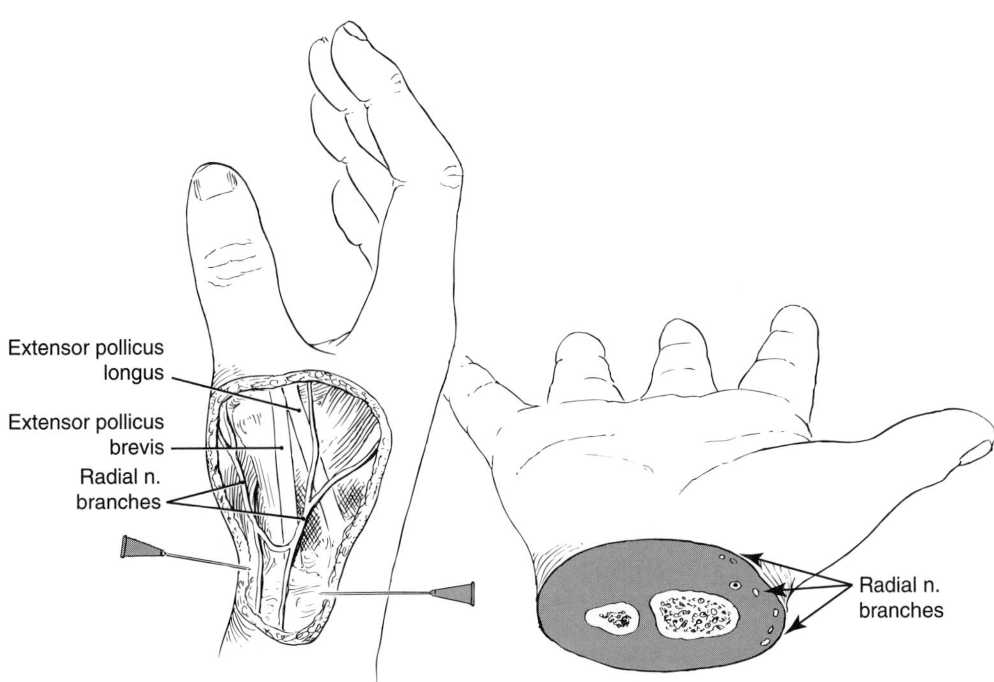

FIGURE **42-20**
Anesthesia of the radial fibers is achieved by injection of a subcutaneous ring of local anesthetic solution at the radial flexor muscle of the wrist and extending to the dorsal surface of the ulnar styloid.

Radial Block at the Wrist

The sensory fibers of the radial nerve to the hand are superficial branches at the wrist. Anesthesia of the radial fibers is achieved through the injection of a subcutaneous ring of local anesthetic solution beginning at the radial flexor muscle of the wrist and extending to the dorsal surface of the ulnar styloid (Figure 42-20). The anesthetist should avoid the formation of a continuous ring of local anesthetic around the wrist when this procedure is accomplished in conjunction with an ulnar block.

Another approach to anesthesia of the radial nerve is the identification of the brachioradial muscle proximal to the wrist. Approximately 6 to 8 cm proximal to the wrist, 5 to 7 ml of local anesthetic solution is injected under the brachioradial muscle. This technique is the least tolerated of all of the supplemental blocks and has limited success.[4,15,113]

INTRAVENOUS REGIONAL ANESTHESIA (BIER BLOCK)

Intravenous regional block is a technically simple, safe, and rapid means of producing surgical anesthesia of the extremity. The technique is best suited for upper extremity (hand and wrist) soft-tissue surgical procedures of 1 hour or less; however, it has also been used for lower extremity surgical procedures of the foot and ankle. The factor limiting the duration of anesthesia to approximately 1 hour is most commonly discomfort produced by the tourniquet required to initiate and maintain the block. Use of a dual tourniquet system and preoperative and or intraoperative administration of small doses of opioids may extend this time limit to 1-$^1/_2$ hours or longer. The greatest risk associated with intravenous regional anesthesia (IVRA) is the potential for rapid transfer of a large volume of local anesthetic from the extremity to the central circulation in the event of an improperly fitted or inflated tourniquet or tourniquet failure. Therefore it is important to have emergency equipment, medications, and monitors immediately available when this block is administered. Because of the rapid onset of the block and the limited duration, it is almost always performed in the operating area, where the emergency items needed are readily available. The necessity for intravenous access and manipulation of the affected extremity, the prerequisite for a tourniquet, and the density and duration of the block influence the clinical application of this technique.[105-107,114,115]

Intravenous Regional Anesthesia—Upper Extremity Block

A small-bore intravenous catheter is placed in a distal vein of the affected extremity and secured in place, and a heparin lock is attached and flushed with normal saline. The preferred location for access to the venous system of the upper extremity is the dorsum of the hand; however, forearm and antecubital fossa veins have been used. Evidence suggests that use of forearm or antecubital fossa veins increases the possibility of a partial or complete failure of the block when the hand or wrist is the surgical target. It is reasonable to assume that consideration should be given to the area on which surgery is to be performed with regard to access to the venous system, as attainment of surgical anesthesia is predicated on the adequate spread of the injected local anesthetic. The patient is placed supine, and several layers of a suitable padding material are wrapped around the arm in preparation for application of the tourniquet. Although a single tourniquet can be used, a dual tourniquet is recommended, as it provides a means to extend the length of the block after the initial onset of tourniquet pain. After application of the tourniquet the extremity is elevated and exsanguinated. Exsanguination is accomplished by wrapping an Esmarch bandage at close overlapping intervals tightly around the arm, starting at the fingertips and continuing until the bandage overlays the tourniquet itself. In cases in which application of an Esmarch bandage would cause undue discomfort; exsanguination by simple elevation of the extremity for a minimum of 5 minutes may be attempted. This method may or may not result in adequate block. In addition, an air-inflated splint may be used as an alternative to the Esmarch bandage. After exsanguination the proximal tourniquet is inflated to 250 mm Hg or 100 mm Hg above systolic blood pressure, and the Esmarch bandage is removed. A total of 50 ml of 0.5 % lidocaine is then injected via the intravenous catheter. The local anesthetic should be free of preservatives (methylparaben, metabisulfite) and contain no vasoconstrictor. The patient should be carefully monitored during the injection for signs of local anesthetic toxicity. An alternative technique employs the use of an additional "tourniquet" (Penrose drain) applied at mid forearm in the manner used to start an intravenous line after primary distal tourniquet inflation. Half of the 50-ml volume of local anesthetic is injected with the forearm tourniquet in place; the tourniquet is removed, and the remaining local anesthetic is injected. This technique results in a faster onset and a denser block. The addition of 15 to 30 mg of ketoralac to the local anesthetic solution can provide a degree of postoperative analgesia without increasing the risk of postoperative bleeding.[105-107,114,115]

Intravenous Regional Anesthesia—Lower Extremity Block

Indications for IVRA of the leg (lower extremity) include orthopedic surgery of short duration on the foot, removal of fixation plates and screws from the bones below the knee, and foreign body removal from the foot.

Two significant differences exist between IVRA of the arm and IVRA of the leg. First, the local anesthetic volume (and dose) in IVRA of the lower extremity has to be approximately double that used for the arm. This obviously may increase the risk of local anesthetic intoxication resulting from leakage under the inflated cuff and from release of a large bolus dose of local anesthetic when the cuff is deflated. Second, in order to occlude the arterial inflow at the thigh level (femoral artery), the tourniquet pressure must be higher than in the arm (usually 350 to 400 mm Hg), which increases the occurrence and intensity of tourniquet pain.

Two separate 9-cm-wide tourniquet cuffs (adult patient) are applied, and care must be taken that the pneumatic parts of the tourniquets surround the thigh by more than 1.5 turns. Otherwise, the technique is similar to that described for IVRA of the arm.

In short-lasting surgery of the foot or the ankle, the distal tourniquet cuff may be applied on the calf, clearly below the head of the fibula (away from the peroneal nerve), and the proximal cuff left on the thigh. The local anesthetic solution is injected with the distal tourniquet cuff inflated; therefore the volume and the dose can be the same as the arm of an adult, that is, 35 to 45 ml of 0.5% lidocaine. The proximal tourniquet is usually not inflated at all, but it is kept prepared as security in case the distal cuff fails.[105-107,114,115]

INTERCOSTAL NERVE BLOCKS

The use of the intercostal nerve block has increased in the past several years. The anatomic landmarks are easily identified, thereby facilitating the performance of the block. The procedure is not extremely painful, has a high rate of success, has a low incidence of complications, and provides the patient with significant analgesia on completion of the procedure. The most common complications are pneumothorax and toxicity from the local anesthetic. The patient who has been in pain with each breath is able to cough and breathe deeply with reduced discomfort. In the outpatient or ambulatory care setting, surgical procedures can be accomplished with the aid of this regional anesthesia technique.[116-118]

However, the use of multiple level intercostal blocks can lead to the highest plasma levels of local anesthetic of all regional techniques. The high vascularity of the area and large intercostal veins contribute to high plasma levels of local anesthetic. Because of the high plasma concentrations, toxic symptoms may develop with lower-than-toxic doses.

Intercostal blocks are used for supplementing balanced anesthesia techniques in order to increase tolerance of the surgical procedure. Sufficient analgesia can be provided to permit the performance of surgical procedures involving the abdominal wall without the need for supplemental blocks. For more involved procedures, additional anesthesia may be required.

The blocks can provide analgesia for postoperative pain control when epidural analgesia is not desired or possible. The procedure can provide analgesia during or after chest tube insertion to limit the patient's discomfort. The landmarks are easily identified in most patients. The procedure can be accomplished with the patient prone, in the lateral position, or sitting comfortably with the upper body supported over a table or a stand. Having obese patients sit up enables easier identification of landmarks. One advantage of using multiple-level intercostal blocks is the reduction in the amount of pain medication required and the work of breathing in the postoperative period. These factors result in a reduction in the potential development of respiratory depression related to the use of intravenous or intramuscular narcotics in obese patients; use of such agents may further compromise ventilation.

The intercostal nerve emerges from the intervertebral foramen and follows the rib in the costal groove. This groove is located on the anteroinferior aspect of the rib. The intercostal artery and vein accompany the nerve in the groove. Medial to the posterior angle of the rib, the neurovascular bundle lies between the pleura and the internal intercostal fascia. As the nerve passes the angle of the rib, it begins to run between the two layers of the internal intercostal muscle. At the midaxillary line the nerve branches send sensory fibers anteriorly and posteriorly to supply skin and subcutaneous tissue. Fibers also provide motor and sensory innervation to the bundles of the superior rectus muscle in the upper abdomen.

Positioning the patient may require modification in order to facilitate breathing during the procedure. The area of pain may have to be splinted, or other measures may need to be taken to reduce pain-induced movement during the procedure. Ideally the patient should be positioned in the prone position with the arms hanging down. This position pulls both scapulas away from the midline and permits the practitioner to perform the block as the nerve root begins to travel in the intercostal groove.

The block can be performed with the patient lying on the unaffected side with the arm extended over the head. This technique is helpful in obese patients and in patients experiencing severe pain, especially when such a patient is prone. When the patient is in the lateral position, preservation of circulation in the downward arm must be preserved.

In postoperative patients the supine position can be used with the anterior approach to the intercostal nerve. This position is less satisfactory and is associated with a higher incidence of complications.

The rib is palpated posterior to the midaxillary line in the prone patient so that the appropriate landmarks can be identified. In this position the rib becomes superficial to the muscle bodies. The lateral border of the sacrospinal muscle must be identified before the block is attempted. The sacrospinal muscle lies approximately 7 to 10 cm from the midline.

With a small-gauge (27- to 30-gauge) needle a skin wheal is raised over the point that is chosen for the injection. A 22-gauge B-bevel needle is then inserted perpendicularly to the rib through the skin wheal and is advanced until contact with the rib is made. The needle is slowly walked caudad off the rib. As the edge of the rib is cleared, the needle is advanced another 2 to 3 mm (Figure 42-21). The needle should be gently aspirated for verification of the needle placement. Use of a "free needle" as described in brachial plexus anesthesia can facilitate the maneuverability of the needle and increase control.

Once the needle is located in the appropriate location, 3 to 5 ml of the local anesthetic solution is injected. The procedure can be repeated for anesthesia at each dermatome level. If resistance is encountered during the injection, the injection should be terminated and the needle repositioned. If the patient begins to cough or move, the needle position should be re-evaluated before injection. Advancing the needle several millimeters can place the needle within the nerve itself, resulting in severe pain or direct injury to the nerve.

Procaine, bupivacaine, tetracaine, and lidocaine have all been used for blocking the intercostal nerves, with varying effects. Because the goal is to provide the patient with extended pain relief, a longer-acting agent is the most commonly used. An injection of 3 ml of bupivacaine (0.5%) into the tissues surrounding the intercostal nerve provides the patient with 3 to 9 hours of anesthesia and analgesia. Patient factors, such as temperature, presence of infection, and the response to local anesthetics, affect the duration of action. The addition of low–molecular-weight dextran added to the solution in a ratio of 1 ml of dextran to 3 ml of bupivacaine further extends the duration of action. Dextran slows the absorption of the local anesthetic, thereby reducing the plasma level of the anesthetic and permitting more of the concentrated local anesthetic solution to remain in close proximity to the neural tissue.[116-118]

Epinephrine 1:100,000 or 1:200,000 should be added to the local anesthetic solution. Bupivacaine's duration of action may be unchanged; however, the rise in the plasma concentration of the local anesthetic is slowed. The addition of epinephrine to tetracaine or lidocaine prevents the rapid absorption of the anesthetic and increases the duration of action. With the use of epinephrine, increased vasoconstriction occurs, an effect that reduces absorption of the local anesthetic. The increased contact time between the neural tissue and the local anesthetic increases the amount of local anesthetic present to be absorbed into the neural fibers.

In addition to the single-shot technique described previously, a continuous intercostal block can be used for providing additional pain relief. The technique was originally discussed in the mid 1960s. However, it did not gain popularity until 1983, when it was reintroduced as a new technique. The continuous technique permits the reinjection of the intercostal fibers without the need for additional invasive procedures. Narcotics have been injected in the intercostal nerve sheath with limited enhancement of the analgesia.

The continuous intercostal technique is performed by use of an epidural needle and a catheter in place of a single-shot needle technique. The intercostal groove is located by use of the technique described for the single-shot technique. When an epidural needle is used for the procedure, resistance is met as the needle passes through the sheath. The nerve can also be identified with a nerve locator or nerve stimulator. After the intercostal neural sheath is identified, the needle is adjusted so that the bevel of the needle directs the catheter toward the midline posteriorly. The epidural catheter is inserted slowly along the intercostal groove 2 to 3 cm. If severe pain or discomfort occurs during advancement of the catheter, the procedure is terminated, and the catheter is removed. Advancement of the catheter may produce electric-like shocks as the catheter

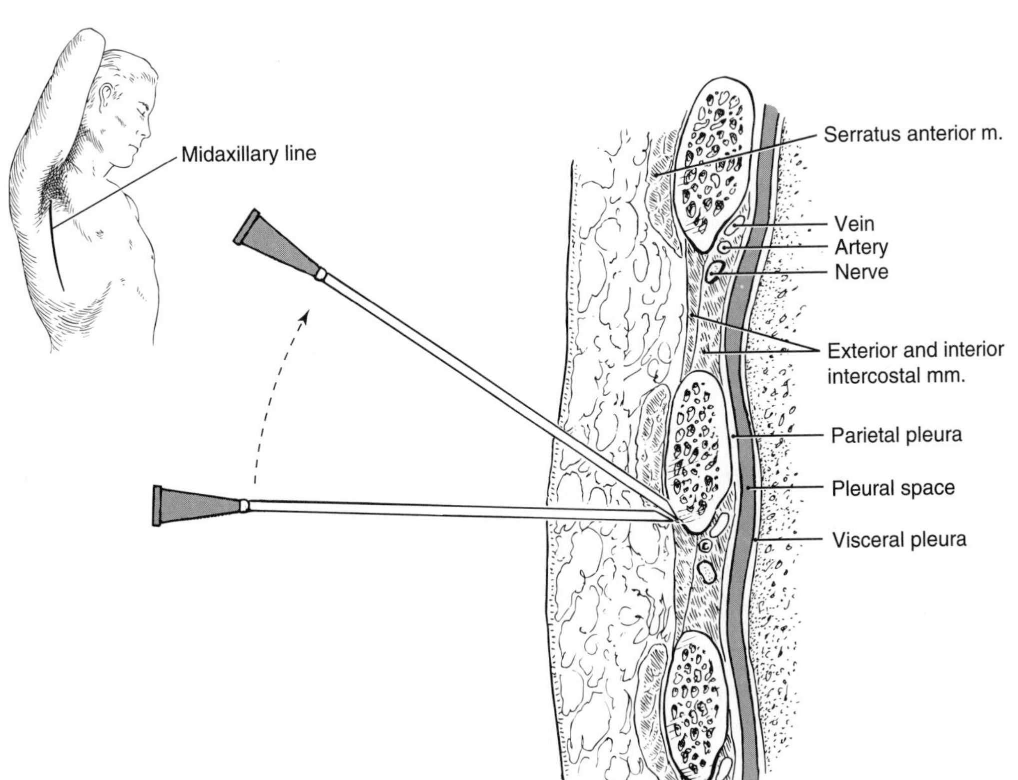

FIGURE **42-21**
A 22-gauge B-bevel needle is inserted perpendicularly to the rib and advanced until contact is made with the rib. The needle is slowly walked caudad off the rib.

brushes the nerve fibers. Severe pain should alert the practitioner of the possibility of an intraneural injection.[116-118]

As the medication is injected, a band of analgesia develops along the path of the catheter and spreads anteriorly and posteriorly. Other than the direct action of the local anesthetic on the neural fibers, the exact mechanisms of action are unknown. However, paravertebral or epidural distribution of the local anesthetic may facilitate and enhance the block. The medication is injected in 3-ml increments until the desired level and intensity of block are achieved. The onset of the extended block is slow; however, the onset of the block through direct actions of the anesthetic agent is rapid.

Tachyphylaxis develops with repeated injections of local anesthetic. Permitting resolution of the block before reinjection or using another local anesthetic allows the effect to be reduced. If an ester is used for the initial blockade, then an amide local anesthetic can be used when symptoms of tachyphylaxis develop.[116-118]

Injections of small doses of fentanyl and morphine have been accomplished with the use of the catheter. However, the uptake of medication into the vascular compartment is rapid, essentially negating the advantages of this route of administration. The use of narcotics in the intercostal space may increase the incidence of complications, including respiratory difficulties.

The likelihood of complications, such as pleural injection and pneumothorax, resulting from neural injection can be reduced by use of a short, B-bevel needle. In order to avoid an intraneural injection, the needle is directed cephalad as it passes over the ridge of the rib. A symptomatic pneumothorax can occur; however, use of a single 22-gauge short-beveled needle reduces the risk. A leak created by this needle can be minimal. When a larger or A-bevel needle is used, the risk of complications is increased.

In most patients a small leak of air does not cause a symptomatic pneumothorax. Most patients are able to compensate for any reduced ventilatory capacity, and the pneumothorax resolves without intervention. In a small percentage of patients intervention is needed for relief of the discomfort and dyspnea. Radiologic studies should be performed after the completion of the procedures so that the status or occurrence of a pneumothorax can be established. The studies can be used during follow-up evaluations and therapy if required.[116-118]

The use of intercostal blocks has enhanced the practice of anesthesia and pain control. This technique provides the patient with increased flexibility in the control of pain and reduces the need for narcotics. In the ambulatory surgery center this technique allows increased flexibility in the spectrum of techniques that can be offered to the patient who desires a regional anesthetic technique.[116-118]

BLOCKS OF THE LOWER EXTREMITY BLOCK

Lower extremity nerve blocks are well described and can provide high-quality anesthesia and analgesia for lower-extremity surgical procedures. Lower-extremity nerve blocks, although underused, have significant advantages compared with central neuraxial techniques, especially in the ambulatory setting.

Advantages of lower extremity blocks include reduced recovery room admissions, decreased nausea and vomiting and urinary retention, and improved postoperative analgesia. These benefits may translate into shortened hospital stays, decreased probability of hospital admission, and an overall reduction in hospital costs and patient charges.

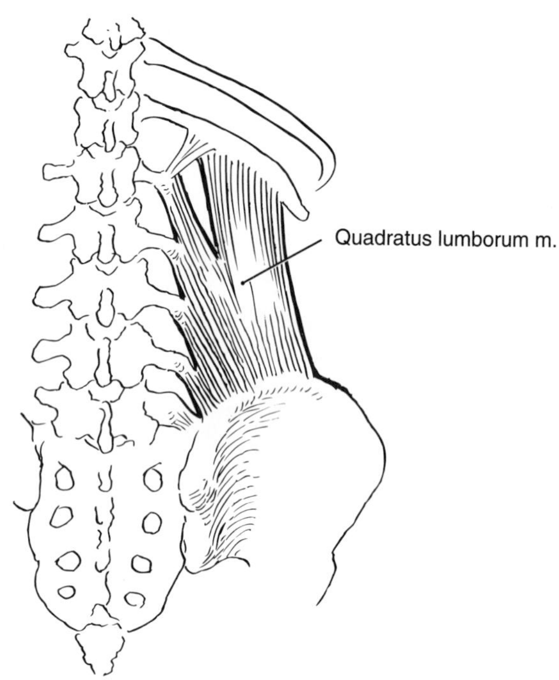

FIGURE **42-22**
Location of the lumbar plexus.

Anatomy of the Lumbar Plexus

The lumbar plexus is formed from the roots of the first, second, third, and fourth lumbar roots. Contributions to the plexus originate in the twelfth thoracic nerve. The plexus is formed in front of the quadratus lumborum muscle and behind the psoas major muscle (Figure 42-22). As the major branches from the plexus begin their descent into the leg, the muscle bodies and the connecting fascia tightly bind them. The lateral femoral cutaneous nerve is formed from the second and third lumbar nerves and is the first to leave the compartment. It emerges from the lateral border of the psoas major at its midpoint. The nerve then traverses the iliac muscle obliquely toward the anterior iliac spine. The lateral femoral cutaneous nerve passes under the lateral border of the inguinal ligament and then provides the sensory innervation to the lateral aspect of the thigh (Figure 42-23).

The obturator nerve arises from the second, third, and fourth lumbar nerves as an extension of the lumbar plexus. It emerges from the medial border of the psoas major at the level of the sacroiliac joint and is covered by the external iliac artery and vein. The nerve passes into the pelvis minor and runs anteroinferiorly to the obturator canal, which it traverses near the obturator vessels. Because of the proximity of the nerve to the external iliac artery, it can be injured during surgical procedures. This nerve is frequently injured when patients undergo extensive pelvic surgery. The obturator nerve is primarily a motor nerve that has some mixed sensory fibers to the hip, the medial aspect of the femur, and the skin and soft tissue of the lower portion of the thigh. The third nerve in the lumbar plexus is the femoral nerve, which is formed from the contributions of the second, third, and fourth lumbar nerve roots. This nerve forms and appears at the junction of the middle and lower third of the psoas major muscle. It remains within the groove of the psoas major and the iliac muscles and runs deep under the inguinal ligament, where it comes to lie anterior to

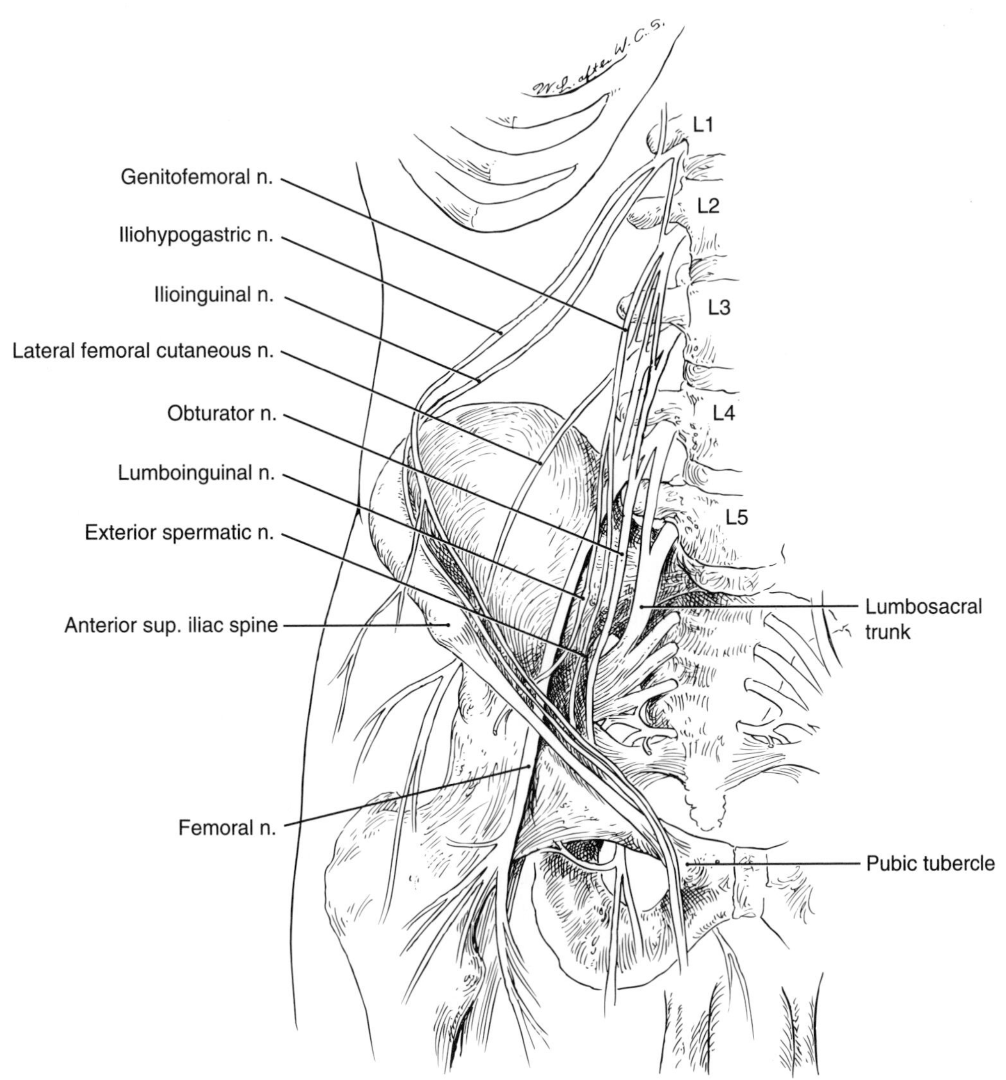

FIGURE **42-23**
Origin and position of the nerves of the lower extremity.

the iliopsoas muscle and lateral to the femoral artery. The femoral nerve forms two branches: the anterior and the posterior bundles. This formation usually occurs just after the nerve passes the inguinal ligament but may occur before it passes the inguinal ligament. The anterior branch provides the innervation to the anterior surface of the thigh and the sartorius muscle. The posterior branch provides the innervation to the quadriceps muscles, the knee joint, and its medial ligament and is the origin of the saphenous nerve. The femoral nerve is bound by several structures above and below the inguinal ligament. Above the inguinal ligament the iliac fascia encapsulates the femoral nerve laterally, the psoas fascia medially, and the transverse fascia anteriorly. The posterior border of this capsule or sheath is made up of the bony structure of the pelvis. As the femoral nerve joins the femoral artery to enter the leg, the iliopsoas fascia forms the posterolateral wall. The inguinal ligament and the fascia lata form the anterior wall, and the iliopectineal fascia forms the medial wall of the capsule. Winnie and associates suggested that the neural sheath originating with the femoral artery in conjunction with the fascial attachments form a structure similar to the neural sheath in the brachial plexus.[8] With this anatomic design, anesthesia can be provided for the lower extremity through techniques used in upper extremity anesthesia.

Psoas Compartment Block

Blockade of the lumbar plexus as a unit can be accomplished by injecting local anesthetic into the fascial sheath surrounding the plexus. This can be done at the level of the psoas compartment.[17,105,106]

Immediately after emerging from the intervertebral foramina, the nerve roots form the lumbar plexus. This approach attempts to block the plexus as it lies in the fascial plane bordered medially by the vertebral column, dorsally by the quadratus lumborum muscle, and ventrally by the psoas major muscle.

The patient is placed in either the lateral or sitting position. If placed in the lateral position, the patient should be in a relaxed but curled position similar to that used for spinal or epidural anesthesia, with the operative side uppermost (Figure 42-24).

From the spinous process of L4, a 3-cm line is drawn caudally in the interspinal line. From the end of this line, a 5-cm line is drawn perpendicularly and laterally toward the side to be blocked, usually ending at the medial edge of the iliac crest. This spot identifies the point of needle insertion. A 120-cm insulated block needle is used. A skin wheal is raised, and the needle is inserted perpendicularly to all planes and advanced until contact with bone is made, which identifies the transverse process of L5 and usually occurs at a depth of 5 to 10 cm.

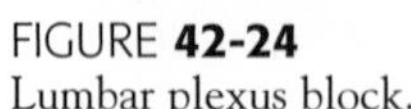

FIGURE **42-24**
Lumbar plexus block.

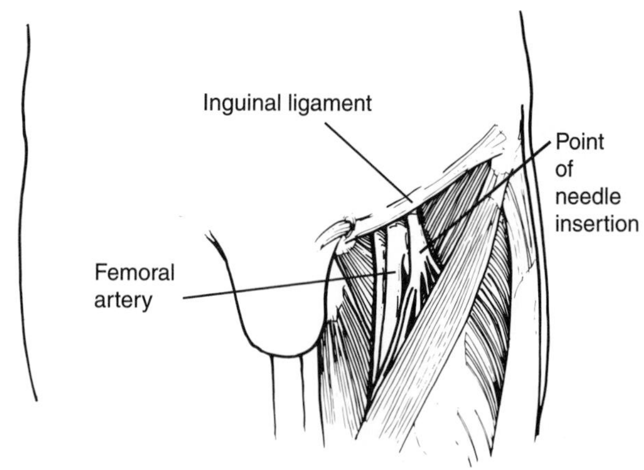

FIGURE **42-25**
Femoral nerve block.

The needle is then withdrawn, redirected slightly cephalad, and advanced until it slides over the transverse process of L5. Using the loss-of-resistance technique, the psoas compartment is usually encountered at the depth of 8 to 12 cm. The tip of the needle now lies in the psoas compartment. Needle placement can be confirmed with the aid of a nerve stimulator, by checking for stimulation of the quadriceps muscles, by eliciting paresthesias into the thigh, or by advancing the needle slightly into the psoas muscle and reconfirming a loss of resistance while withdrawing the needle slightly into the psoas compartment.

After the needle is properly placed, and after careful aspiration, 30 to 40 ml of local anesthetic is injected in 5-ml divided doses. It is often helpful to have the patient remain in the lateral position for a few minutes after injection to limit spread of the drug.[17,105,106]

Inguinal Perivascular Technique and Femoral Nerve Block

The inguinal perivascular technique, described by Winnie, is also known as the *three-in-one block* of the lower extremity. The lumber plexus is "sandwiched" among the psoas major, quadratus lumborum, and iliacus muscles and is enclosed by the fascia of these three muscles.[119,120]

After the patient is positioned supine, the groin is prepared and draped by use of aseptic technique. One possible complication is contamination of the deeper tissues. An immobile needle can be used for improved control of the needle.

The site of injection is 1 cm lateral to the femoral artery and 1 cm inferior to the inguinal ligament. The identified area is prepped with a Betadine solution and then infiltrated with 2 to 3 ml of 1% lidocaine solution subcutaneously. A 22-gauge, 4-cm insulated B-bevel needle is advanced perpendicularly to the skin just lateral to the artery until femoral nerve distribution is elicited with the aid of a peripheral nerve stimulator. With a stimulation frequency of 2 Hz, the intensity level is set at 1 mA until quadriceps extension is elicited, then decreased to less than 0.5 mA. Local anesthetic solution (20 to 30 ml) is injected in 5-ml increments with intermittent syringe aspiration. Digital pressure is applied firmly but gently distal to the needle. This action assists in limiting the distal spread of the anesthetic solution by forcing it proximal into the channel formed by the neural sheath and other structures. Digital pressure is continued after the injection for approximately 5 to 10 minutes. Winnie and associates indicated that the total volume of anesthetic solution required to maximize the block must exceed 20 ml. Volumes of less than 20 ml provide a spotty and unpredictable block. Increasing the volume of the solution to 30 ml increases the ability of the solution to contact all three nerves. Bupivacaine (0.5%), ropivacaine (0.5%), Levobupivacaine (0.5%), and lidocaine (1.5%) are commonly used for this procedure. Anesthesia to the sciatic distribution does not occur with this technique. If the surgical procedure requires anesthesia along the sciatic distribution, a separate procedure must be performed (Figure 42-25).[8,119,120]

Sciatic Nerve Block

Sciatic nerve blocks, in combination with lumbar plexus, femoral, or saphenous nerve blocks, provide complete anesthesia and postoperative analgesia for lower-extremity surgery. Contrary to common belief, sciatic nerve blocks are relatively easy to master and accomplish.[121] In a recent review of outpatients undergoing complex knee surgery, it was noted that among the patients who received a combination sciatic nerve block with a femoral nerve block, a lower incidence of nursing interventions for pain occurred in the step-down unit.[120] In addition, patients had fewer hospital admissions and were more satisfied with their surgical procedures.[119,120]

Anatomy of the Sciatic Nerve

The sciatic nerve is the continuation of the upper division of the sacral plexus and is the largest nerve trunk in the body. It supplies the muscles of the back of the thigh, the skin of the leg, and the muscles of the lower leg and foot. It passes out of the pelvis through the great sacrosciatic foramen, below the piriform muscle. It descends between the major trochanter and the tuberosity of the ischium to the lower third of the thigh, where it divides into the internal and external popliteal nerves.[24,27,119,120]

Technique of Sciatic Nerve Block

Although posterior and lateral popliteal approaches to the sciatic nerve are performed most commonly for ankle and foot surgery, and higher approaches to the sciatic nerve are performed more commonly for surgery below, above, and at the knee, it is important to recognize that no clinical evidence supports one particular sciatic approach over another. For any nerve the indications of a given approach are based on the specific surgical requirement (Figure 42-26).[119,120]

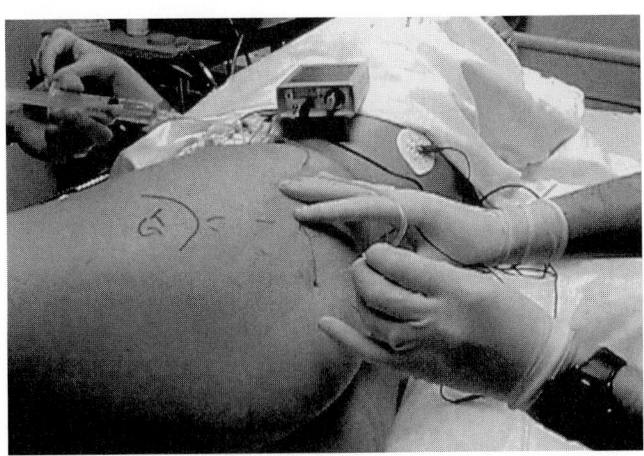

FIGURE **42-26**
Sciatic nerve block.

After standard monitors are placed, the patient is positioned in the Sims' position, with the operative leg positioned superiorly and flexed at the knee. A line is drawn from the posterior superior iliac spine to the greater trochanter of the femur. A second line is drawn from the sacral hiatus to the greater trochanter, and a third line is drawn perpendicular to and bisecting the first line. The intersection of the second and third lines is the point of needle entry. The identified area is prepared with a Betadine solution and then infiltrated with 2 to 3 ml of 1% lidocaine solution subcutaneously. A 22-gauge, 10-cm insulated B-bevel needle, aimed perpendicularly to the skin, is advanced until posterior tibial nerve distribution is elicited with the aid of a peripheral nerve stimulator. A stimulation frequency of 2 Hz and an intensity level of 1 mA is used until a plantar flexion motor response is elicited. The intensity level is decreased to less than 0.5 mA as long as motor response is still present. Local anesthetic solution (10 ml) is injected in 5-ml increments with intermittent syringe aspiration. The needle is redirected laterally and advanced until peroneal nerve distribution is elicited with the aid of a peripheral nerve stimulator. A stimulation frequency of 2 Hz and an intensity level of 1 mA is used until a dorsal flexion motor response is elicited. The intensity level is decreased to less than 0.5 mA as long as motor response is still present. Local anesthetic solution (10 ml) is injected in 5-ml increments with intermittent syringe aspiration. Bupivacaine (0.5%), ropivacaine (0.5%), Chirocaine (0.5%), and lidocaine (1.5%) are commonly used for this procedure.[119,120]

Popliteal Fossa Block

This approach is based on the use of the three anatomic landmarks that define the posterior popliteal fossa: the popliteal crease, the medial border of the femoris biceps muscle laterally, and the tendon of the semitendinous muscle medially.

A line is drawn joining the medial border of the femoris biceps muscle laterally and the lateral border of the semitendinous muscle medially at the level of the popliteal crease. From the middle of this line, a perpendicular line is extended 15 cm cephalad. The site of insertion of the needle is 1 cm laterally. A 100-mm, insulated needle connected to a nerve stimulator is introduced through a skin wheal of local anesthesia at a 45- to 60-degree anterior-superior angle. The sciatic nerve usually is located at a depth of 1 to 2 cm in an adult. After careful aspiration, 35 to 40 ml of a local anesthetic is injected (Figure 42-27).[119,120]

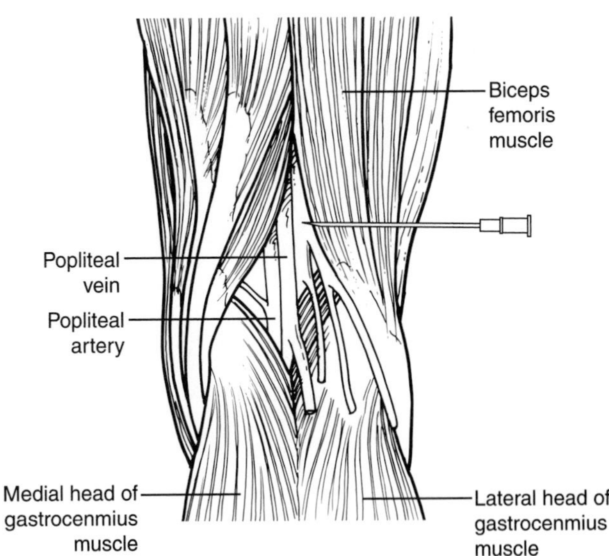

FIGURE **42-27**
Popliteal nerve block.

Ankle Blocks

The ability to administer anesthesia to patients who require surgery on the foot opens new and exciting vistas to anesthesia practitioners. Either a complete or a partial block of the foot can provide adequate anesthesia for many of the surgical procedures that are performed by podiatrists and orthopedic surgeons. The nerves are easy to locate, and the procedures can be rapidly accomplished. This tool can prove invaluable in the care of certain patients, such as those with gangrene of the foot or those with diabetes who have foot ulcers, in whom a local anesthetic procedure would be inadequate.[122-124]

Anatomy of the Ankle

The ankle block is performed by the blocking of five nerves at the level of the ankle: the tibial nerve, the sural nerve, the superficial peroneal nerve, the deep peroneal nerve, and the saphenous nerve.[122-124]

Tibial Nerve

The tibial nerve arises from the nerve roots of the fourth and fifth lumbar roots, along with the first, second, and third sacral roots. It is the largest of the two branches of the sciatic nerve. The path of this nerve lies on the medial side of the Achilles tendon. It passes into the ankle with the posterior tibial artery (Figure 42-28). At the level of the ankle this nerve lies behind the posterior tibial artery and between the tendons of the long flexor muscles of the toes and the long flexor muscles of the great toe. The nerve is covered by the flexor retinaculum. Several branches leave the neural bundle at the level of the medial malleolus. Two of the branches, the medial and the lateral plantar nerves, traverse the ankle, following under the cover of the abductor hallucis. They provide sensory innervation to the foot.[122-124]

Sural Nerve

The sural nerve is formed from the union of a branch of the tibial nerve and the common peroneal nerve. This nerve travels superficially with the short saphenous nerve behind the lateral malleolus into the ankle, where it provides the sensory innervation to the posterior portion of the sole of the foot, as well as to

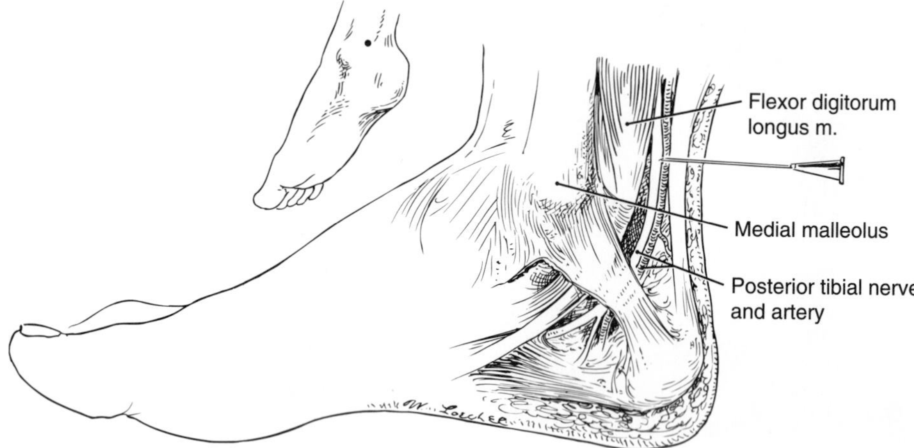

FIGURE **42-28**
Path of the posterior tibial nerve, with the posterior tibial artery past the Achilles tendon.

the posterior portion of the heel and the portion of the Achilles tendon immediately above the ankle (Figure 42-29).[122-124]

Superficial Peroneal Nerve

The superficial peroneal nerve arises from the roots of the fourth and fifth lumbar nerve roots, as well as the first and second sacral nerve roots. The nerve becomes superficial in the middle two thirds of the lower leg and remains subcutaneous as multiple branches proceed into the dorsum of the foot. Just above the ankle (Figure 42-30) the nerve begins to branch; for this reason a single injection site does not provide sufficient anesthesia.[122-124]

Deep Peroneal Nerve

The deep peroneal nerve arises from the same nerve roots as the superficial peroneal nerve. However, it remains within the protection of the anterior tibial muscle and the long extensor muscle of the great toe (Figure 42-30) as it traverses the leg and into the ankle. As it crosses the ankle, it is covered by the extensor retinaculum. The deep peroneal nerve provides innervation to the short extensors of the toes and provides sensory innervation to the skin on the lateral side of the hallux and on the medial side of the second digit. The nerve and the artery cross each other, so the nerve lies lateral to the anterior tibial artery and medial to the long extensor muscle of the great toe that is in the ankle. This nerve is frequently missed when anesthesia is administered to the ankle.[122-124]

Saphenous Nerve

The saphenous nerve is the terminal branch of the femoral nerve and travels subcutaneously from the lateral side of the knee joint. It follows the greater saphenous vein to the medial malleolus and provides sensory innervation to the medial side of the malleolus and the skin of the medial aspect of the lower leg (Figure 42-30). If the block of this nerve is inadequate, the patient is unable to tolerate a small tourniquet above the ankle.[122-124]

Ankle Block Technique

The approach to both the sural and the posterior tibial nerves can be enhanced by placing the patient in the prone position. However, this is not always the most comfortable position for the patient. Therefore the patient should be placed in the most comfortable position that permits sufficient mobility of the foot. Rotation of the foot from side to side can be facilitated by turning the patient onto either side or elevating the foot on towels or pillows. The posterior tibial artery is palpated at the level of the superior portion of the medial malleolus. After the artery is located, the needle is inserted lateral to the artery in a line drawn from the superior portion of the medial malleolus to the lateral malleolus across the Achilles tendon. If the artery is not palpated, the needle is inserted lateral to the Achilles tendon at the level of the superior portion of the medial malleolus. The needle is advanced toward the medial malleolus and lateral to the position of the posterior tibial artery. As the needle is

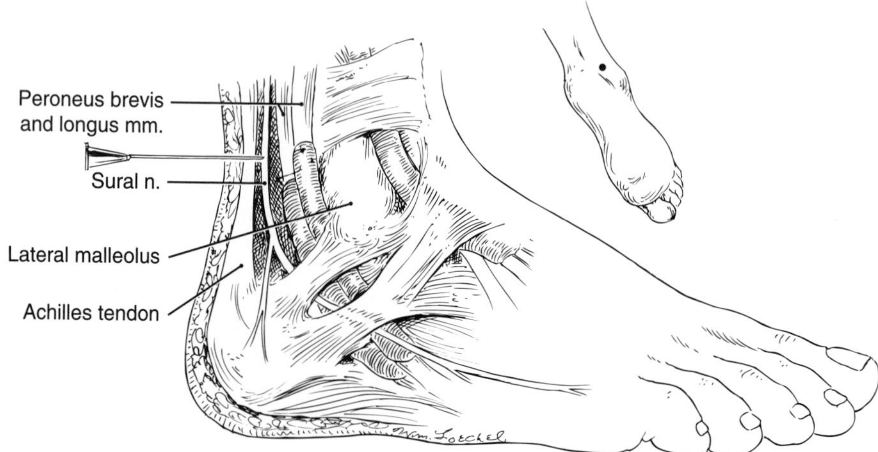

FIGURE **42-29**
Path of the sural nerve behind the lateral malleolus into the ankle.

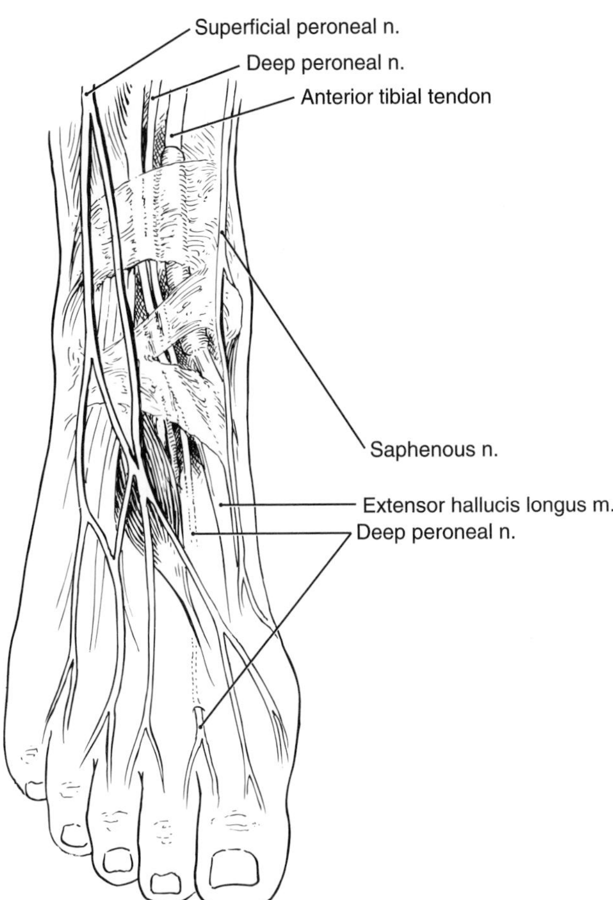

FIGURE **42-30**
The superficial peroneal nerve proceeds to the dorsum of the foot subcutaneously through multiple branches.

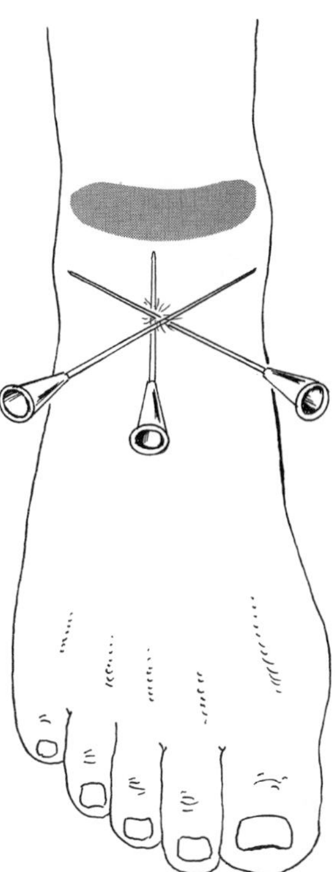

FIGURE **42-31**
Direction and redirection of the needle in the ankle block technique.

advanced toward the outer aspect of the medial malleolus, a paresthesia may be elicited. If this occurs, then 5 ml of the anesthetic solution is injected with the needle held in position, and an additional 3 ml is injected as the needle is withdrawn. If a paresthesia is not elicited, the medial malleolus is gently contacted with the needle tip and withdrawn 2 mm from the bone. The anesthetic solution is slowly injected at this position, and the location is gently massaged after the injection.[122-124]

With the patient in the same position the line from the medial malleolus across the Achilles tendon is identified on the lateral malleolus. The needle is inserted under the skin along the lateral border of the Achilles tendon in the plane with the line that is between the medial and lateral malleoli. The needle is advanced subcutaneously toward the superior edge of the lateral condyle. Five milliliters of solution is injected in the subcutaneous tissues as the needle is withdrawn. The solution must reach the superior edge of the lateral malleolus in order to anesthetize all of the fibers of the sural nerve.

The patient is then placed in the supine position, and the anterior ankle is prepared for the block. For blocking of the deep peroneal nerve a line is drawn from the superior edge of the medial malleolus to the superior border of the lateral malleolus across the anterior portion of the ankle. The tendons of the anterior tibial muscle and the long muscles of the great toe are identified by having the patient flex the foot against resistance. Where the line crosses the midpoint between the two tendons the needle is inserted toward the tibia (Figure 42-31). As the needle advances through the fascia, a paresthesia may be elicited. If the paresthesia is not obtained, the needle is slowly advanced until the needle gently contacts the tibia. As the needle is withdrawn from contact with the tibia, 5 ml of anesthetic solution is injected. The needle is then withdrawn through the fascia, and an additional 3 ml of solution is injected.[122-124]

With the needle remaining in the subcutaneous tissue the needle direction is changed. The needle is advanced toward the inferior border of the lateral malleolus. The superficial peroneal nerve is located in subcutaneous tissue at this level. While the needle is withdrawn, 5 ml of anesthetic solution is injected. A subcutaneous ring develops that should reach the lateral malleolus.[122-124]

The needle is withdrawn to the midpoint, and the needle direction is again changed. The needle is redirected to the inferior border of the medial malleolus. The saphenous nerve is in the subcutaneous tissue, superficial to the saphenous vein. If the needle is not superficial, the saphenous vein is entered. Five milliliters of solution is injected toward the medial malleolus. As the needle is withdrawn, 3 ml is injected.

The deep peroneal and the posterior tibial nerves are the only nerves of the ankle that are not in the subcutaneous tissue. The nerve locator can be used for facilitating the identification of the nerves and for improving the chances of success with the block. The technique of electrotranslocation of the nerves is similar to the technique employed with brachial plexus block.[3,122-124]

REGIONAL ANESTHESIA AND TRAUMA

Regional anesthesia techniques have become preferred for surgical procedures when the injury involves either the lower extremities or a single upper extremity. Postoperative pain management can be provided for the patient with an epidural catheter. Regional anesthesia to an extremity can provide muscle relaxation and sensory block while the patient remains awake in order to maintain his or her protective reflexes.[125]

When the patient is experiencing severe pain, technical difficulties may be encountered. Both the injury and the pain restrict movement of the extremities, making adjustments in position difficult or impossible. In patients who are experiencing pain, it is more difficult to optimize their position in order to facilitate the implementation of regional anesthesia.

Patel and associates[125] suggest that an epidural technique may be more advantageous than a subarachnoid block during the perioperative period. Many surgical procedures change once the full extent of the trauma is evaluated. These changes may require additional surgical and anesthesia time. With the gradual onset of a sympathetic block, management of changes in sympathetic tone and systemic vascular resistance can be more controlled.

The patient may be confused because of the effects of alcohol or drugs in addition to the effects of the trauma itself. Use of epidural narcotics in the postoperative period permits the surgeon and the anesthesia practitioner to evaluate the mental and physical status of the patient without having to be concerned about the cerebral effects of narcotics.

In the presence of alcohol, drugs, or other sedation the patient's ability to provide the anesthesia practitioner with an informed consent for the procedure must be evaluated. In this situation patient refusal may not be an indication of the patient's actual desires. However, a regional technique is significantly more difficult to manage in a noncooperative patient than in a cooperative one.

With trauma, sympathetic stimulation occurs and is continuously stressed during the initial evaluation and care of the patient. The patient's pulse and blood pressure may be maintained through this stimulation. Symptoms of hypovolemia and shock are masked by artificially induced hypertension that is mediated through the high circulating catecholamine level. When regional anesthesia is administered to such a patient, elimination of the stimulation to the sympathetic nervous system may precipitate hypotension. Decompensation can occur rapidly after the reduction of circulating catecholamines. The extent and rapidity of the decompensation are dependent on the type of regional technique used, the type of local anesthetics chosen, and the sedation administered to the patient when the block is instituted. When symptoms of hypovolemic shock are present, the patient is unable to compensate for the reduction in systemic vascular resistance.[125]

Winnie and colleagues state that initial alterations in blood pressure and heart rate occur during positioning. They suggest that the patient receive additional fluid boluses to compensate for this problem. Positioning the patient before administering the regional anesthetic minimizes this response. For example, hypobaric spinal anesthesia may be administered to a patient with a fractured femur. The patient is positioned for the surgical procedure, and the anesthetic is administered after the patient is stabilized.[8]

The administration of regional anesthesia to the patient with a full stomach must be a cause for concern to the practitioner. Regional techniques should provide anesthesia to the injured area while maintaining upper airway and pharyngeal reflexes. Theoretically a block of the sympathetic nervous system increases gastric and intestinal motility, causing the stomach to empty sooner. In practice this advantage is rarely seen. The development of hypotension after the administration of the anesthetic results in a higher incidence of nausea. If the patient's clinical situation is complicated by the ingestion of alcohol or the use of mind-altering substances, pain from the injury may be the only stimulus that causes the patient to maintain consciousness. After the regional anesthesia is administered, the patient may lose consciousness and require airway support.[4]

When the patient has a difficult airway to manage, regional anesthesia must not be selected, so that the airway need not be secured by other methods. When the patient has a difficult airway that prevents or limits the clinician's ability to secure it in an emergency, regional anesthesia should be avoided. The airway concerns must be addressed before the anesthesia is administered.[4]

Electrical Stimulators in Regional Anesthesia

Peripheral nerve stimulators have become an indispensable tool in the practice of regional anesthesia. Knowledge and in-depth understanding of how they function is required if their full potential in a clinical setting is to be realized.[126]

Electrical translocation devices provide a controlled stimulating pulse of variable amplitude that is administered through a conducting device (Figure 42-32). Location of neural fibers is improved without the need for eliciting repeated paresthesias. Specialized shielded needles have been designed to localize the distribution of the stimulating charge to the tip of the needle (Figure 42-33). This characteristic reduces confusion from wide-field stimulation of the area around the nerve, thereby enhancing the isolation of the appropriate nerve fibers. If specialized sheathed needles are not available, the alternative is preparation of a shielded needle through the use of an intravenous catheter and a short-beveled needle. The needle must be advanced slowly, and the amplitude of the unit must be adjusted as the needle approaches the nerve.

The electrical device must be equipped with an accurately adjustable amplitude from 0 to 5 mA. When a device is being selected for use with electrotranslocation techniques, it is advantageous to choose a device with a digital readout of the amplitude of the stimulus being delivered. The negative lead is attached to the skin with an electrocardiogram electrode, and

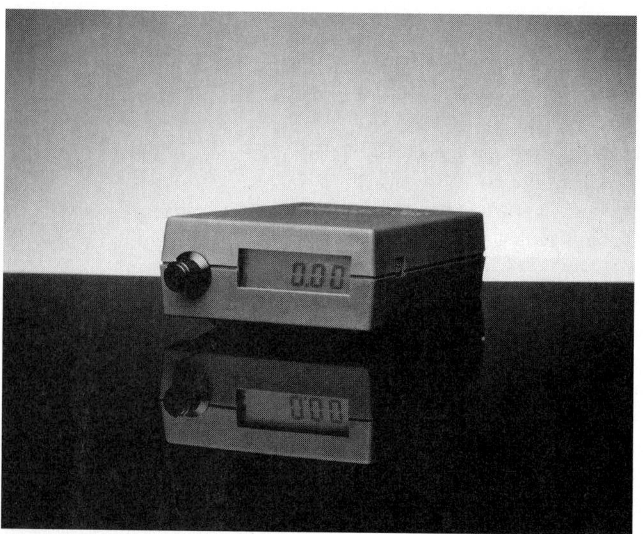

FIGURE **42-32**
Electrical translocation device, which provides a controlled stimulating pulse of variable amplitude. (Courtesy of Mercury Medical, Clearwater, Florida.)

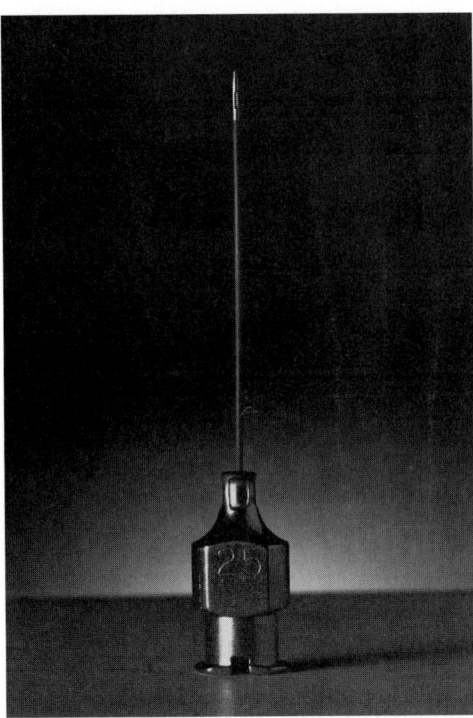

FIGURE **42-33**
Specialized shielded needle designed to localize the distribution of the stimulating charge to the tip of the needle. (Courtesy of Mercury Medical, Clearwater, Florida.)

the positive lead is attached to the needle. When this technique is used, the stimulator should not be turned on until the needle has entered the skin. This measure reduces the discomfort experienced by the patient during the initial advancement of the needle. The patient must be instructed to identify discomfort verbally and to not move during the advancement of the needle.[17,105,106,126]

Limiting the sedation helps the patient tolerate the procedure, maintain sufficient alertness to respond to the stimulus, and be cooperative. Use of an electrotranslocation device can assist the practitioner during the administration of nerve block anesthesia to patients with sensory perception difficulties or neural degeneration, such as that experienced during end-stage renal disease.

The stimulator is adjusted to deliver 2 mA after the needle has been introduced into the subcutaneous tissues. As the needle approaches the sheath, the amplitude is continuously reduced so that the muscle response to the stimulus is maintained. When the needle enters the sheath, the amplitude should be reduced to 0.5 mA. The muscle response to the stimulus continues to be the same as that obtained when the needle is outside of the sheath. The lower amplitude decreases the discomfort experienced by the patient while enhancing the anesthetist's ability to accurately identify the neurovascular bundle.

The use of an electrotranslocation device should not be restricted to brachial plexus techniques. Such a device can be used for enhancing any technique in which identification of specific nerve roots improves the success of the block and reduces the amount of medication required for anesthesia of the nerve root.

Electrotranslocation devices or a peripheral nerve stimulator can be used with continuous spinal and epidural techniques for monitoring of the level of the motor or sensory block. After the desired level of block is established, the nerve stimulator can be used for monitoring of the block. The stimulator leads are connected to the patient at the lowest level of motor block desired. When the patient responds to the stimulus at this level, local anesthetic can be administered in order to increase the level of the block. With the electrodes in place a stimulus is applied at an amplitude of 2.5 mA for 15 seconds at intervals of 10 to 15 minutes.

A peripheral nerve stimulator or an electrotranslocation device can be used for determining the level of the anesthetic with single-shot spinal and epidural techniques. If the patient is unable to interpret changes in temperature, single twitches or tetanus that results from lowered settings can provide information on the level of the block. This technique can minimize the patient's discomfort during the evaluation period. Patients may complain of aching or weakness along the path of the stimulated nerve after the regional anesthesia is terminated. This phenomenon is seen after the posterior tibial or the common peroneal nerves are stimulated. Severe or prolonged discomfort occurs when the stimulus is delivered over a long period or at a high current. Berger, Gravenstein, and Munson demonstrated the response to a stimulus with a lower amplitude. Placement of the negative electrode has been important in the enhancement of electrotranslocation of the nerve. If the path of the nerve fiber is located under the negative electrode, a lesser stimulus produces a significant response.[17,105,106,126]

SUMMARY

Regional anesthesia techniques can be primary tools for immediate and long-term pain relief. Although they can be highly effective in many settings, some contraindications to their use exist. These include patient refusal; systemic anticoagulation; platelet counts of less than 100,000; PT, PTT, and bleeding time greater than twice normal values; severe bleeding; hypovolemic shock; abruptio placentae; and active infection near the site of the regional technique. Patient age, ability to cooperate, history of headaches or backaches, chronic neurologic disorders, local anesthetic allergy, or heart block; and fixed volume cardiac states may all influence the decision to administer regional anesthesia.

Both immediate and delayed complications can result from regional anesthesia. One of the most common complications is the spinal headache. Technical problems include difficulties with equipment and supplies.

The pharmacology of local anesthetic agents indicates that they temporarily block the transmission of a stimulus along the path of a nerve fiber through interference with the local ionic gradient across the cell membrane. The action consists of displacement of calcium ions from a receptor site at the cell membrane, reduction in cell permeability to sodium ions, decrease in rate of depolarization, and inability of the cell to reach the threshold, resulting in lack of propagated action potential and subsequent conduction blockade.

Different methods of regional anesthesia include subarachnoid techniques, epidural anesthesia, caudal anesthesia, brachial plexus anesthesia, axillary perivascular techniques, selective blocks at the wrist, intravenous perfusion blocks, intercostal nerve blocks, blocks of the lower extremities, lumbar plexus blocks, sciatic nerve blocks, ankle blocks, and specialized trauma techniques, such as the use of electrical stimulators.

ACKNOWLEDGMENT

The authors of this chapter on regional anesthesia thanks Wayne Ellis for his initial contributions and framework.

REFERENCES

1. Orkin FK, Thomas SJ. Scope of modern anesthetic practice. In: Miller RD, ed. *Anesthesia.* 5th ed. New York: Churchill Livingstone; 2000:2577-2586.
2. Brown DL, Fink BR. History of neural blockade and pain management. In: Cousins MJ, Bridenbaugh P, eds. *Neural Blockade in Clinical Anesthesia and Management of Pain.* 3rd ed. Philadelphia: Lippincott; 1998:3-34.
3. Mulroy MF. Peripheral nerve blockade. In: Barash PG, Cullen BF, Stoelting RK, eds. *Clinical Anesthesia.* 4th ed. Philadelphia: Lippincott; 2001:715-742.
4. Winnie AP. Brachial plexus anesthesia. In: Winnie AP, ed. *Brachial Plexus Anesthesia.* Philadelphia: Saunders; 1987.
5. Ng K, Parsons J, Cyna A, Middleton P. Spinal versus epidural anaesthesia for caesarean section. *Cochrane Database Syst Rev.* 2004;2:CD003765.
6. Reynolds F. Epidural analgesia in obstetrics. *BMJ.* 1989;297: 751-752.
7. Monk TG, Weldon BC. The renal system and anesthesia for urologic surgery. In: Barash PG, Cullen BF, Stoelting RK, eds. *Clinical Anesthesia.* 4th ed. Philadelphia: Lippincott Williams & Wilkins; 2001:1005-1034.
8. Gogarten W. Spinal anaesthesia for obstetrics. *Best Pract Res Clin Anaesthesiol.* 2003;17:377-392.
9. Broadman LM, Rice LJ. Neural blockade for pediatric surgery. In: Cousins MJ, Bridgenbaugh P, eds. *Neural Blockade in Clinical Anesthesia and Management of Pain.* 3rd ed. Philadelphia: Lippincott; 1998:615-638.
10. Bromage P, Levinson G. Choice of local anesthetics in obstetrics. In: Wilkins W, ed. *Anesthesia for Obstetrics.* Baltimore: Williams & Wilkins; 1993:83-102.
11. Liu SS, Hodgson PS. Local anesthetics. In: Barash PG, Cullen BF, Stoelting RK, eds. *Clinical Anesthesia.* 4th ed. Philadelphia: Lippincott Williams & Wilkins; 2001:449-472.
12. Catterall WA, Mackie K. Local anesthetics. In: Hardman JG, Limbird LE, eds. *The Pharmacological Basis of Therapeutics.* New York: McGraw-Hill; 2001:331-348.
13. Berde CB, Strichartz GR. Pharmacology of local anesthetics. In: Miller RD, ed. *Anesthesia.* 5th ed. New York: Churchill Livingstone; 2000:491-522.
14. Guyton AC, Hall JE. Nervous regulation of the circulation. In: Guyton AC, Hall JE, eds. *Textbook of Medical Physiology.* Philadelphia: Saunders, 2002:184-193.
15. Veering BT, Burm AG, Feyen HM, Olieman W, M Souverign JH, Van Kleef JW. Pharmacokinetics of bupivacaine during postoperative epidural infusion: enantioselectivity and role of protein binding. *Anesthesiology.* 2002;96:1062-1069.
16. Turnbull DK, Shepherd DB. Post-dural puncture headache: pathogenesis, prevention and treatment. *Br J Anaesth.* 2003;91:718-729.
17. Harrington BE. Postdural puncture headache and the development of the epidural blood patch. *Reg Anesth Pain Med.* 2004;29:136-163.
18. Hawkins JM, Moore PA. Local anesthesia: advances in agents and techniques. *Dent Clin North Am.* 2002;46:719-732, ix.
19. Wood M. Local anesthetic agents. In: Wood M, Wood AJ, eds. *Drugs and Anesthesia: Pharmacology for Anesthesiologists.* Baltimore: Williams & Wilkins; 1990:319-346.
20. Butterworth JF 4th, Strichartz GR. Molecular mechanisms of local anesthesia: a review. *Anesthesiology.* 1990;72:711-734.
21. Nau C, Strichartz GR. Drug chirality in anesthesia. *Anesthesiology.* 2002;97:497-502.
22. Nagelhout J, Zaglaniczny K, Haglund V. *Handbook of Nurse Anesthesia.* 2nd ed. Philadelphia: Saunders; 2001.
23. Cox B, Durieux ME, Marcus MA. Toxicity of local anaesthetics. *Best Pract Res Clin Anaesthesiol.* 2003;17:111-136.
24. Hickey R, Blanchard J, Hoffman J. Plasma concentrations of ropivacaine given with or without epinephrine for brachial plexus block. *Can J Anaesth.* 1990;37:878-882.
25. Tetzlaff JE. *Clinical Pharmacology of Local Anesthetics.* Boston: Butterworth-Heinemann; 2000:47-54.
26. Arthur GR, Feldman HS, Covino BG. Comparative pharmacokinetics of bupivacaine and ropivacaine, a new amide local anesthetic. *Anesth Analg.* 1998;67:1053-1058.
27. Moore KL. The spinal cord. In: Moore KL, ed. *Clinically Oriented Anatomy.* Baltimore: Williams & Wilkins; 1992.
28. Bernards CM. Epidural and spinal anesthesia. In: Barash PG, Cullen BF, Stoelting RK, eds. *Clinical Anesthesia.* 4th ed. Philadelphia: Lippincott Williams & Wilkins; 2001:639-714.
29. Cousins MJ, Veering BT. Epidural neural blockade. In: Cousins MJ, Bridenbaugh P, eds. *Neural Blockade in Clinical Anesthesia and Management of Pain.* Philadelphia: Lippincott-Raven; 1998:243-321.
30. Portnoy D, Vadhera RB. Mechanisms and management of an incomplete epidural block for cesarean section. *Anesthesiol Clin North Am.* 2003;21:39-57.
31. Hogan Q. Anatomy of spinal anesthesia: some old and new findings. *Reg Anesth Pain Med.* 1998;23:340-343.
32. Stevens RA. Neuraxial blocks. In: Brown DL, ed. *Regional Anesthesia and Analgesia.* Philadelphia: Saunders; 1996:319-355.
33. Butterworth J. Physiology of spinal anesthesia: what are the implications for management? *Reg Anesth Pain Med.* 1998;23:370-373.
34. Mackey DC. Physiologic effects of regional blocks. In: Brown DL, ed. *Regional Anesthesia and Analgesia.* Philadelphia: Saunders; 1996:397-422.
35. Mulroy M. Extending indications for spinal anesthesia. *Reg Anesth Pain Med.* 1998;23:380-383.
36. Brown DL. Spinal, epidural and caudal anesthesia. In: Livingstone C, ed. *Anesthesia.* New York: Churchill Livingstone; 2000:1491-1519.
37. Greenberg CP. Practical, cost-effective regional anesthesia for ambulatory surgery. *J Clin Anesth.* 1995;7:614-621.
38. Monk TG, Weldon BC. The renal system and anesthesia for urologic surgery. In: Barash PG, Cullen BF, Stoelting RK, eds. *Clinical Anesthesia.* 3rd ed. Philadelphia: Lippincott-Raven; 1997:945-973.
39. Bridenbaugh PO, Greene NM, Brull SJ. Spinal (subarachnoid) neural blockade. In: Cousins MJ, Bridenbaugh PO, eds. *Neural Blockade in Clinical Anesthesia and Management of Pain.* 3rd ed. Philadelphia: Lippincott-Raven; 1998:203-241.
40. Liu SS, Stevens RA, Vasqez J. The efficacy of epinephrine test doses during spinal anesthesia in volunteers: Implications for combined spinal-epidural anesthesia. *Anesth Analg.* 1997;84:780-783.
41. Horlocker T, Wedel DL. Spinal and epidural blockade and perioperative low molecular weight heparin: smooth sailing on the Titanic. *Anesth Analg.* 1998;86:1153-1156.
42. Gielen M. Spinal anesthesia: hearing loss, failure, and transient radicular irritation (TRI). *Anaesthesia.* 1998;53:23-25.
43. Wulf H. Epidural anaesthesia and spinal haematoma. *Can J Anaesth.* 1996;43:1260-1271.
44. Royakkers AA, Willigers H, van der Ven A, Wilmink J, Durieux M, van Kleef M. Catheter-related epidural abscesses: don't wait for neurological deficits. *Acta Anaesthesiol Scand.* 2002;46:611-615.
45. Kindler CH, Seeberger MD, Staender SE. Epidural abscess complicating anesthesia and analgesia. *Acta Anaesthesiol Scand.* 1998;42:614-620.
46. Rosenberg PH. Novel technology: needles, microcatheters, and combined techniques. *Reg Anesth Pain Med.* 1998;23:363-369.
47. Spencer HC. Postdural puncture headache: what matters most in technique. *Reg Anesth Pain Med.* 1998;23:374-379.

48. Cork RC, Wood D, Evans B, deLanzac K, Naraghi M. Leak rate of latex gloves after tearing adhesive tape. *Am J Anesthesiol.* 1995;22:133-137.
49. Stienstra R, Veering BT. Intrathecal drug spread: is it controllable? *Reg Anesth Pain Med.* 1998;23:347-351.
50. Veering BT, Stienstra R. Duration of block: drug, dose, and additives. *Reg Anesth Pain Med.* 1998;23:352-356.
51. Liu SS. Drugs for spinal anesthesia: past, present, and future. *Reg Anesth Pain Med.* 1998;23:344-346.
52. Critchley LA. Hypotension, subarachnoid block and the elderly patient. *Anaesthesia.* 1996;51:1139-1143.
53. Steinbrook RA. Epidural anesthesia and gastrointestinal motility. *Anesth Analg.* 1998;86:837-844.
54. Weeks SK. Postpartum headache. In: Chestnut DH, ed. *Principles and Practice of Obstetric Anesthesia.* 3rd ed. Philadelphia: Mosby; 2004:562-578.
55. Panzer O, Ghazanfari N, Sessler DI, et al. Shivering and shivering-like tremor during labor with and without epidural analgesia. *Anesthesiology.* 1999;90:1609-1616.
56. Liu SS, Carpenter RL, Neal JM. Epidural anesthesia and analgesia. Their role in postoperative outcome. *Anesthesiology.* 1995;82:1474-1506.
57. Liguori GA, Sharrock NE. Asystole and severe bradycardia during epidural anesthesia in orthopedic patients. *Anesthesiology.* 1997;86:257-264.
58. Day CJ, Shutt LE. Auditory, ocular, and facial complications of central neural block. *Reg Analg.* 1996;21:197-201.
59. Mulroy M, Norris MC, Liu SS. Safety steps for epidural injection of local anesthetics: review of literature and recommendations. *Anesth Analg.* 1997;85:1346-1347.
60. Norris MC, Grieco W, Borkowski M. Complications of labor analgesia: epidural versus combined spinal epidural techniques. *Anesth Analg.* 1994;79:529-537.
61. Rawal N, Van Zundert A, Holmstrom B. Combined spinal-epidural technique. *Reg Analg.* 1997;22:406-423.
62. Holmstrom B, Rawal N, Axelsson K, Nydahl PA. Risk of catheter migration during combined spinal epidural block: Percutaneous epiduroscopy study. *Anesth Analg.* 1995;80:747-753.
63. Coates MB. Combined subarachnoid and epidural techniques: a single space technique for surgery of the hip and the lower limb. *Anesthesiology.* 1982;37:89-90.
64. Mumtaz MH, Daz M, Kuz M. Combined subarachnoid and epidural techniques: another single space technique for orthopaedic surgery. *Anaesthesia.* 1982;37:90.
65. Eldor J. The evolution of combined spinal-epidural anesthesia needles. *Reg Analg.* 1997;22:294-296.
66. Joshi G, McCaroll S. Evaluation of combined spinal-epidural anesthesia using two different techniques. *Reg Analg.* 1994;19:169-174.
67. D'Angelo R, Eisenach JC. Severe maternal hypotension and fetal bradycardia after a combined spinal epidural anesthetic. *Anesthesiology.* 1997;87:166-168.
68. Shnider S, Abboud TK, Artal R. Maternal catecholamines decrease during labor and after lumbar epidural anesthesia. *Am J Obstet Gynecol.* 1983;16:13-15.
69. Van de Velde M, Teunkens A, Hanssens M, Vandermeersch E, Verhaeghe J. Intrathecal sufentanil and fetal heart rate abnormalities: a double-blind, double placebo-controlled trial comparing two forms of combined spinal epidural analgesia with epidural analgesia in labor. *Anesth Analg.* 2004;98:1153-1159, table of contents.
70. Clarke V, Smiley R, Finster M. Uterine hyperactivity after intrathecal injection of fentanyl for analgesia during labor: a cause for fetal bradycardia? *Anesthesiology.* 1994;81:1083.
71. Albright GA, Forster RM. Does combined spinal-epidural analgesia with subarachnoid sufentanil increase the incidence of emergency cesarean delivery? *Reg Analg.* 1997;22:400-405.
72. Nielsen PE, Erickson JR, Abouleish EL. Fetal heart rate changes after intrathecal sufentanil or bupivacaine for labor analgesia: incidence and clinical significance. *Anesth Analg.* 1996;83:742-746.
73. Nageotte MP, Larson D, Rumney PJ, Sidhu M, Hollenbach K. Epidural analgesia compared with combined spinal-epidural analgesia during labor in nulliparous women. *N Engl J Med.* 1997;337:1715-1719.
74. Nageotte MP, Larson D, Rumney PJ. Epidural analgesia compared with combined spinal-epidural analgesia during labor in nulliparous women. *N Engl J Med.* 1997;337:1715-1719.
75. Davies SJ, Paech MJ, Welch H. Maternal experience during epidural or combined spinal-epidural anesthesia for cesarean section: a prospective, randomized trial. *Anesth Analg.* 1997;85:607-613.
76. Collis RE, Davies DW, Aveling W. Randomized comparison of combined spinal-epidural and standard epidural analgesia in labor. *Lancet.* 1995;345:1413-1416.
77. Eldor J, Levine S. Failed spinal anesthesia in combined spinal-epidural anesthesia. *Anaesth Intensive Care.* 1997;25:312-331.
78. Urmey WF, Stanton J, Peterson M. Combined spinal-epidural anesthesia for outpatient surgery: dose response characteristics of intrathecal isobaric lidocaine using a 27-gauge Whitacre spinal needle. *Anesthesiology.* 1995;83:528-534.
79. Casati A, D'Ambrosio A, De Negri P. A clinical comparison between needle-through-needle and double segment techniques for combined spinal and epidural anesthesia. *Reg Anesth Pain Med.* 1998;23:390-394.
80. Lyons G, MacDonald R, Mikl B. Combined epidural/spinal anesthesia for caesarian section. Through needle or in separate spaces? *Anaesthesia.* 1992;47:199-201.
81. Hoffman V, Vercauteren M, Buczkowski P. A new combined spinal-epidural apparatus: measurement of the distance to the epidural and subarachnoid spaces. *Anesthesiology.* 1997;52: 350-355.
82. Westbrook J, Donald F, Carrie L. An evaluation of a combined spinal/epidural needle set utilising a 26-gauge, pencil point spinal needle for caesarean section. *Anaesthesia.* 1992;47:990-992.
83. Pan P. Laboratory evaluation of single lumen, dual orifice combined spinal-epidural needles: effects of bevel orientation and modified technique. *J Clin Anesth.* 1998;10:286-290.
84. Robbins PM, Fernando R, Lim GH. Accidental intrathecal insertion of an extradural catheter during combined spinal-extradural anaesthesia for cesarean section. *Br J Anaesth.* 1995;75:355-357.
85. Holst D, Mollmann M, Schymroszcyk B. No risk of metal toxicity in combined spinal-epidural anesthesia. *Anesth Analg.* 1999;88:393-397.
86. Blumgart C, Ryall D, Dennison B. Mechanism of extension of spinal anesthesia by extradural injection of local anaesthetic. *Br J Anaesth.* 1992;69:457-460.
87. Takiguchi T, Okano T, Egawa H. The effect of epidural saline injection on analgesia level during combined spinal and epidural anesthesia assessed clinically and myelographically. *Anesth Analg.* 1997;85:1097-1100.
88. Stienstra R, Dahan A, Alhad BZ. Mechanism of action of an epidural top-up in combined spinal epidural anesthesia. *Anesth Analg.* 1996;83:382-386.
89. Leach A, Smith G. Subarachnoid spread of epidural local anesthetic following dural puncture. *Anaesthesia.* 1988;43:671-674.
90. Vartis A, Collier CB, Gatt SP. Potential intrathecal leakage of solutions injected into the epidural space following combined spinal epidural anesthesia. *Anaesth Intensive Care.* 1998;26: 256-261.
91. Eldor J. metallic particles in the spinal-epidural needle technique. *Reg Analg.* 1994;19:219-220.
92. Eldor J, Guedj P. Aseptic meningitis due to metallic particles in the needle-through-needle technique. *Reg Analg.* 1995;20:360.
93. Birnbach D, Danzer B. Comments on combined spinal-epidural anesthesia. *Reg Analg.* 1996;21:275.
94. Herman N, Molin J, Knape KG. No additional metal particle formation using the needle-through-needle combined epidural/spinal technique. *Acta Anaesthesiol Scand.* 1996;40: 227-231.

95. Mcloughlin L. Combined spinal-extradural analgesia in labour and post-dural puncture headache. *Br J Anaesth.* 1998;80: 123-124.
96. Boskovski N, Lewinski A. Epidural morphine for the prevention of headache following dural puncture. *Anaesthesia.* 1982;37: 217-218.
97. Johnson M, Herwig L, Vehring P. Intrathecal fentanyl may reduce the incidence of spinal headache (abstract). *Anesthesiology.* 1989;71:A911.
98. Scott D, Hibbard B. Serious non-fatal complications associated with extradural block in obstetric practice. *Br J Anaesth.* 1990;64:537-541.
99. Horlocker T, McGregor D, Matsushige D. A retrospective review of 4767 consecutive spinal anesthetics: central nervous system complications. *Anesth Analg.* 1997;84:578-584.
100. Bouhemad B, Dounas M, Mercier FJ. Bacterial meningitis following combined spinal-epidural analgesia for labor. *Anaesthesia.* 1998;53:292-295.
101. Kubina P, Gupta A, Oscarsson A. Two cases of cauda equina syndrome following spinal-epidural anesthesia. *Reg Analg.* 1997;22:447-450.
102. Paech MJ. Unexplained neurologic deficit after uneventful combined spinal and epidural anesthesia for cesarean delivery. *Reg Analg.* 1997;22:479-482.
103. Levin A, Segal S, Datta S. Does combined spinal-epidural analgesia alter the incidence of paresthesia during epidural catheter placement? *Anesth Analg.* 1998;86:448-449.
104. Koch E. Alice Magaw and the great secret of open drop anesthesia. *AANA J.* 1999;67:33-38.
105. Hahn MB, McQuillan PM, Sheplock GJ. *Regional Anesthesia: an Atlas of Anatomy and Techniques.* St Louis: Mosby; 1996.
106. Brown DL, ed. *Atlas of Regional Anesthesia.* Philadelphia: Saunders; 1999.
107. Pollock JE. Regional anesthesia for hand surgery. *Tech Reg Anesth Pain Manag.* 1999;3:79-84.
108. Panchal SJ. Upper extremity techniques for postoperative analgesia. *Tech Reg Anesth Pain Manag.* 2002;6:56-59.
109. Pham-Dang C, Gunst JP, Couin F, et al. A novel supraclavicular approach to brachial plexus block. *Anesth Analg.* 1997;85:111-116.
110. Narchi P, Bouaziz H, Antakly MC. A new approach to axillary brachial plexus block. Techniques in Regional Anesthesia and Pain Management 1997;1:178-180.
111. Urmey WF. New considerations in brachial plexus anesthesia. *Tech Reg Anesth Pain Manag.* 1997;1:185-193.
112. Pham Dang C. A novel supraclavicular approach to the brachial plexus. *Anesth Analg.* 1997;85:111-116.
113. Lofstrom B. Nerve block at the elbow. In: Eriksson E, ed. *Illustrated Handbook in Local Anesthesia.* Copenhagen, Denmark: Munksgaard; 1969.
114. Saga-Rumley SA. Intravenous regional anesthesia. *Curr Rev Nurse Anesth.* 1997;19:217-228.
115. Marchant AE, McConachie I. Intravenous regional anesthesia. *Curr Anaesth Crit Care.* 2003;14:32-37.
116. Covino BG, Lambert DH. Epidural and spinal anesthesia. In: Barash PG, Cullen BF, Stoelting RK, eds. *Clinical Anesthesia.* Philadelphia: Lippincott; 1992:809-840.
117. Lofstrom B. Intercostal nerve blocks. In: Eriksson E, ed. *Illustrated Handbook in Local Anesthesia.* Copenhagen, Denmark: Munksgaard; 1969:93-95.
118. Debreceni G, Molnar Z, Szelig L, Molnar TF. Continuous epidural or intercostal analgesia following thoracotomy: a prospective randomized double-blind clinical trial. *Acta Anaesthesiol Scand.* 2003;47:1091-1095.
119. Nielsen KC, Klien SM, Steele SM. Femoral nerve blocks. *Tech Reg Anesth Pain Manag.* 2003;7:8-17.
120. Williams BA, Kentor ML, Vogt MT, et al. Femoral-sciatic nerve blocks for complex outpatient knee surgery are associated with less postoperative pain before same-day discharge. *Anesthesiology.* 2003;98:1206-1213.
121. Chelly JE. Sciatic nerve block. *Tech Reg Anesth Pain Manag.* 2003;7:18-25.
122. Lofstrom B. Nerve block at the ankle. In: Eriksson E, ed. *Illustrated Handbook in Local Anesthesia.* Copenhagen, Denmark: Munksgaard; 1969:112-119.
123. Hadzic A, Vloka JD. Anesthesia for ankle and foot surgery. *Tech Reg Anesth Pain Manag.* 1999;3:113-119.
124. Kay J. Ankle block. *Tech Reg Anesth Pain Manag.* 1999;3:3-8.
125. Patel KP, Capan LM, Grant GJ, Miller mm. Musculoskeletal injuries. In: Capan L, Miller S, Turndorf H, eds. *Trauma: Anesthesia and Intensive Care.* Philadelphia: Lippincott; 1991: 511-546.
126. Visan A, Vloka JD, Koenigsamen J, Hadzic A. Peripheral nerve stimulators technology. *Tech Reg Anesth Pain Manag.* 2002;6: 155-157.

CHAPTER 43

Office-Based Anesthesia

Jeanne B. Learman

Office-based anesthesia now constitutes a significant portion of anesthesia practice. It is predicted that 24% of all elective surgeries will be office based by 2005, a total of almost 10 million operations per year.[1] Until 10 years ago office anesthesia received limited attention because of small numbers and a primarily private pay clientele. Office-based surgery is a practice setting distinct from hospital ambulatory surgery and ambulatory surgical centers.

A number of factors are driving this trend. Newer surgical techniques and safer anesthetics with faster recovery times and improved anesthesia monitors make it feasible to do many procedures in the office that only a few years ago would have been performed in the hospital or an ambulatory surgical facility. Advantages for patients include privacy and convenience, as well as lower overall costs when the procedure is self-pay. Surgeons enjoy the convenience and time efficiencies that office surgery affords, including control of the schedule and less driving time between sites. The surgeon realizes a financial gain when insurance pays a facility fee to the office.

PROBLEMS, STANDARDS, ACCREDITATION, STATE REGULATIONS

Problems and Adverse Events

Anesthesia sites in the office are less regulated than hospitals and ambulatory surgical centers. The reporting of anesthesia morbidity and mortality after office procedures is not mandatory in most states, so the incidence of adverse events cannot be calculated. Published studies are not consistent. A survey in the *Journal of Plastic and Reconstructive Surgery*[2] noted more than 400,000 surgical procedures performed in *accredited* offices had complications in fewer than 1% of cases. A report of 23,000 general anesthetic procedures in an office-based plastic surgical facility found no intraoperative or postoperative deaths and no significant complications.[3] A survey of the Massachusetts Society of Oral and Maxillofacial Surgeons, found no anesthesia deaths in 1,500,000 patients over a 5-year period.[4] In contrast to the apparent safety of office anesthesia suggested by these studies, Morell, reporting in the *Anesthesia Patient Safety Newsletter*[5] in 2000, highlighted some of the nationally publicized office deaths. This supports the view that in some settings the rapid growth of office-based procedures has occurred without appropriate consideration for safety. Examples include the following:

- No dantrolene was available in an office in which a 28-year-old woman received general anesthesia and developed malignant hyperthermia.
- No oxygen was available; oxygen tank was empty. Two deaths resulted.
- An unlicensed person left to oversee the recovery of a facelift patient injected narcotic pain medication (meperidine).
- Five California children died during dental procedures. Four received chloral hydrate.
- Respiratory arrest in a 50-year-old man during facial surgery resulted in death.
- A 25-year-old Florida woman and a 27-year-old Alabama woman died after returning home after breast augmentation.
- Five deaths in New York were associated with liposuction between 1993 and 1998.[6]

In many of these situations qualified anesthetists or anesthesiologists were not involved. In some situations surgeons have had minimal training in the surgical technique performed.

These problems were nationally publicized during the 1990s and came as a shock to many in the anesthesia community who have witnessed the significant reduction in anesthesia risk over the past 25 years as a result of improved monitoring, safer and shorter-acting anesthetic agents, and significant advancements in education of physicians and nurse anesthetists. Just when we had convinced ourselves that anesthesia had never been safer, the office problems were reported. Closer investigation reveals that the increased risk in the office setting is not usually a result of the anesthetic itself, which can be appropriately administered in the office. To control risk in the office, anesthetists must take control of the *entire process* of anesthesia administration, including credentialing practitioners; establishing emergency procedures; checking availability of equipment, drugs, and supplies; and training staff to handle emergencies. Significantly, anesthetists must embrace the concept of continuous quality improvement of all processes involved in patient care and realize that these processes involve much more than the anesthesia administration. This concept is difficult for many anesthetists and anesthesiologists who believe they alone control the anesthesia outcome. This chapter concentrates on the processes that, if followed, are likely to make an impact on risk reduction for patients who receive anesthesia in the office setting.

Office-Based Anesthesia Standards

Alarm over reported office anesthesia morbidity grew during the 1990s. Recognizing that appropriate support systems and protocols were lacking in some office settings, the American Association of Nurse Anesthetists (AANA) adopted the Office-Based Anesthesia Standards in March, 1999,[7] (Appendixes 43-A and 43-B), and the American Society of Anesthesiologists (ASA) adopted the ASA Guidelines for Office-Based Anesthesia in October, 1999.[8] Many groups made efforts to make office surgery safer (Box 43-1).

BOX 43-1

Measures for Improvement of Anesthesia Care in the Office Setting

- Adoption of standards for anesthesia monitoring (1980s)
- Accreditation of office-based surgical and anesthesia practices (rare until 1990s)
- AANA Office-Based Anesthesia Standards, March 1999
- ASA Guidelines for Office-Based Anesthesia, October 1999
- Adoption of state regulations or legislation for oversight of office surgical practices
- AMA and ACS Guidelines for Office-Based Facilities, May 2000
- Anesthesia Patient Safety Foundation devoted Spring, 2000 issue of newsletter to office anesthesia
- SOBA, 1996-2003, held meetings and developed a World Wide Web site to promote safety in office anesthesia

AANA, *American Association of Nurse Anesthetists;* ACS, *American College of Surgeons;* AMA, *American Medical Association;* ASA, *American Society of Anesthesiologists;* SOBA, *Society for Office Based Anesthesia.*

Before this time the major anesthesia associations and physicians' organizations felt that the adoption of "Standards for Anesthesia Monitoring" that had occurred during the 1980s was sufficient to protect patients who received intravenous (IV) sedation and regional and general anesthesia in all venues. Starting with the patient monitoring standards adopted by the Harvard Medical School Department of Anesthesia in 1985,[9] standards for patient monitoring during conscious sedation, deep sedation, and general anesthesia have been developed, publicized, and widely adopted by many groups, including the American Academy of Pediatric Dentistry, the American Academy of Pediatrics,[10] the ASA,[11] the AANA,[12] the American Dental Society of Anesthesiology,[13] and the American Society for Gastrointestinal Endoscopy.[14] The patient monitoring standards have been considered to be responsible for greater patient safety during conscious sedation and anesthesia.[15]

The AANA Office-Based Anesthesia Standards start with confirming the monitoring standards and then go further to provide guidance for setting up the anesthesia service in a setting that has little or no regulatory oversight. The use of AANA standards in the office setting emphasizes key safety concepts and reinforces the advocacy role of nurse anesthetists in patient care. The standards are completely reprinted in Appendix 43-A. Note the frequent references to documentation throughout the standards. It is emphasized that a complete anesthesia record is essential. In addition, in the office the nurse anesthetist may have the responsibility of ensuring documentation of narcotic use, equipment maintenance, provider credentials and staff training in emergency procedures (including cardiopulmonary resuscitation), malignant hyperthermia preparedness, and transfer protocols.

A checklist of minimum elements for providing anesthesia services in the office-based practice setting is reprinted in Appendix 43-B and is useful in setting up a new practice site or in evaluating an existing office-based practice. This checklist was developed as a supplement to the AANA Office-Based Anesthesia Standards and is especially useful for certified registered nurse anesthetists (CRNAs) who do not practice full time in the office setting and want a reliable tool to assess the readiness of a particular site.

Accreditation for Office-Based Surgery and Anesthesia

The American Association for Accreditation of Ambulatory Surgery Facilities (AAAASF),[16] formerly the American Association for Accreditation of Ambulatory Plastic Surgery Facilities (AAAAPSF), has been accrediting office surgical practices since 1980 for outpatient plastic surgical centers and since 1992 for other single-specialty and multispecialty ambulatory surgical facilities. Since July 2002 plastic surgeons must practice in an accredited facility to qualify for membership in the American Society of Plastic Surgeons (ASPS). The AAAASF program requires 100% compliance with all standards for a facility to be accredited. Key elements for accreditation include the requirement that all surgeons using the facility must be board certified or board eligible in an American Board of Medical Specialties (ABMS) surgical specialty. The director must be an ABMS board-certified surgeon or an anesthesiologist. Each surgeon must hold valid hospital privileges at an accredited or licensed hospital for those procedures that are performed within the facility. Multispecialty facilities must have a written transfer agreement with an accredited or licensed hospital in the community. AAAASF is the largest office-based accreditation program in the world, with approximately 900 facilities accredited in 2002. Facilities are reviewed according to differing levels of anesthesia capability. AAAASF has a 3-year accreditation cycle, and the cost for accreditation varies depending on the levels of anesthesia provided at the facility.

The Accreditation Association for Ambulatory Health Care (AAAHC)[17] has accredited office-based surgery practices since 1979 and currently accredits over 300 centers in the United States. The AAAHC reviews the office site for critical organizational structure including credentialing for anesthetists; policies and procedures; preanesthesia patient evaluation; informed consent; oxygen delivery; monitoring guidelines; discharge criteria; emergency equipment, supplies, medications, appropriately trained personnel, and emergency power for a safe patient environment. A transfer protocol and periodic resuscitation drills are required to demonstrate responsible anesthesia preparation. The AAAHC 2003 Anesthesia Standards allow the CRNA, designated as a "physician supervised qualified individual" approved by the governing board, to evaluate patients before surgery to evaluate the risks of anesthesia, develop a plan of anesthesia, and determine that the patient has met discharge criteria. The longest term of accreditation is 3 years. In a departure from the customary accreditation of surgical *sites*, the AAAHC also accredits anesthesiology *practices*.

The Joint Commission on Accreditation of Healthcare Organizations (JCAHO),[18] long involved in the accreditation of ambulatory surgical centers, approved Office-Based Surgery Standards in January 2001. They accredited their hundredth office in January 2003.[19,20] The length of accreditation is 3 years.

State Regulation of Office Surgery and Anesthesia

Surgical practice in physician offices has received increased scrutiny from the public, state legislators, and health regulators in the wake of publicity about injuries and deaths in the office setting (Table 43-1). The three ways that states have regulated

TABLE 43-1 Status of Office Anesthesia Laws, Regulations, Position or Policy Statements, and Guidelines among the States[a,b]

States with Laws	States with Regulations	States with Position or Policy Statement	States with Guidelines	States with Resolution to Study
California Connecticut Illinois Rhode Island Texas Virginia	Alabama (BOM)[c] California (BOM) Florida[h] (BOM) Illinois (DPR) Mississippi (BOM) New Jersey (BOM) Ohio (BOM) Rhode Island (DOH) Texas (BOM; BON) Virginia (BOM)	Colorado (BOM)[d] North Carolina[f] (BOM) Ohio (BOM)[i]	Massachusetts (BOM)[e] New York (DOH)[g] Colorado (BOM) North Carolina (BOM) Oklahoma (BOM) South Carolina (BOM)	Delaware
Total = 6	Total = 10	Total = 3	Total = 6	Total = 1

BOM, *Board of medicine or its generic equivalent;* BON, *board of nursing or its generic equivalent;* DPR, *department of professional regulation or its generic equivalent;* DOH, *department of health or its generic equivalent.*

[a]*Table identifies the states that have adopted laws, regulations, position or policy statements, or guidelines specifically concerning office anesthesia as of October 2003. Total of number of states that have taken an action in at least one of the categories noted above: 18 (Alabama, California, Colorado, Connecticut, Delaware, Florida, Illinois, Massachusetts, Mississippi, New Jersey, New York, North Carolina, Ohio, Oklahoma, Rhode Island, South Carolina, Texas, and Virginia).*

[b]*The laws, regulations, position or policy statements, and guidelines addressed in this table were enacted or adopted to apply specifically to physicians' office settings. Other laws, regulations, position or policy statements, or guidelines may also affect physicians' offices. For example, some ambulatory surgical center licensing statutes or regulations may be phrased in a way that includes or affects some physicians' offices.*

[c]*Alabama's regulations include so-called "general guidelines."*

[d]*The policy statement that the board of medicine adopted includes guidelines.*

[e]*Endorsed office-based surgery guidelines issued by the Massachusetts Medical Society.*

[f]*The position statement that the board of medicine adopted includes guidelines.*

[g]*Court decision declared guidelines null and unenforceable; defendant state has appealed.*

[h]*In Florida the adopted rules were originally effective in 1994. Subsequently, in 1998, the Florida Legislature enacted a law stating that the "board [of medicine] may establish by rule standards of practice and standards of care for particular practice settings, including, but not limited to, education and training, equipment and supplies, medications including anesthetics, assistance of and delegation to other personnel, transfer agreements, sterilization, records, performance of complex or multiple procedures, informed consent, and policy and procedure manuals." A Florida Court of Appeals decision has interpreted the phrase "practice settings" as giving the board of medicine authority to adopt rules concerning physicians' offices.*

[i]*The Ohio regulations appear to override the position statement.*

or provided oversight of office surgery and anesthesia are as follows:

1. Adoption of laws by state legislatures; sometimes these laws include provisions mandating that regulations be adopted and then identify which administrative entity, e.g. the state department of health or board of medicine, has the authority to adopt such regulations
2. Adoption of regulations or release of position statements or guidelines by boards of medicine
3. Adoption of regulations or guidelines by departments of health

As of 2003, six states have enacted laws: California, Connecticut, Illinois, Rhode Island, Texas, and Virginia. Ten states have adopted regulations: Alabama, California, Florida, Illinois, Mississippi, New Jersey, Ohio, Rhode Island, Texas, and Virginia (Table 43-1).

The content of these laws, regulations, position and policy statements, and guidelines varies from state to state. Some require accreditation of certain office surgical facilities, others recommend such accreditation, and some exempt certain office surgical facilities from further regulation or state licensure if the office surgical facilities are accredited. Many require a qualified anesthesia provider to administer general and major regional anesthesia; specify under what conditions a registered nurse or other health-care provider (such as a physician's assistant) can administer conscious sedation; and delineate the type of surgical qualifications or privileges a surgeon must have to perform surgical procedures in the office (e.g., board certification in the surgical specialty, hospital privileges, or alternative privileges granted by the medical board). Other types of provisions that may be found in state laws, regulations, position or policy statements, and guidelines include prohibitions or restrictions on overnight stays; lists of required equipment, supplies, and emergency medications; requirements for written transfer agreements; requirements that certain surgical or anesthesia personnel have current training in advanced cardiac life support (ACLS); requirements for written informed consent; limits on the duration of surgery; restrictions on the types of patients that can have surgery in the office setting (e.g., limiting surgery involving general or major regional anesthesia to class I and II patients); requirements for risk management programs or performance improvement programs; requirements for reporting adverse events; and infection control standards.

Practice Restrictions

Many of the laws, regulations, policy statements, and guidelines are reasonable and commendable in their efforts to establish equipment necessary for monitoring and emergencies, required medications, emergency power, and other provisions for safe care.

Unfortunately, in some cases anesthesiologists have also used the office anesthesia issue to seek unnecessary restrictions on CRNA practice. They have generally used two methods to do this: (1) advocating anesthesiologist supervision requirements for CRNAs in the laws or regulations (this has the practical effect of promoting the physician anesthesiologist as the provider because the patient and surgeon are not likely to pay two anesthesia providers); and (2) recommending extensive continuing medical education (CME) units or anesthesia training for the surgeon who works with or supervises the CRNA. This creates a disincentive for the surgeon to work with a CRNA.

Some states, influenced by the anesthesiologist's arguments, have imposed restrictions on CRNA practice that are not found in the nurse practice act and are not clinically justified. Examples of such restrictions include requiring surgeons who work with CRNAs to be physically present throughout the anesthetic procedure; requiring surgeons who work with CRNAs to perform or be available to perform anesthesia-related tasks; requiring supervision of CRNAs; and requiring surgeons who work with CRNAs to have detailed knowledge of anesthetic drugs. An example of a state anti-CRNA provision is the Florida Board of Medicine and Board of Osteopathic Medicine regulation that requires anesthesiologists to supervise CRNAs who provide general anesthesia, major conduction anesthesia, or deep sedation in the office. Another example is an Illinois regulation that requires surgeons who work with CRNAs in the office setting to obtain anesthesia-related CME.

OFFICE ANESTHETIC TECHNIQUES

A full range of anesthetic techniques from conscious sedation to general anesthesia, and from local anesthesia to major regional techniques, has been used in the office setting. All of these techniques are acceptable if the facility is equipped and staffed appropriately. Techniques that include a proactive approach to control postoperative pain, nausea, and vomiting *early* in the case favor quicker recovery, ambulation, and discharge and result in improved patient and surgeon satisfaction. The information learned from recent "fast-tracking" studies can be useful in the office setting. These techniques frequently use preemptive local analgesia and ketorolac or other nonsteroidal antiinflammatory drugs (NSAIDs) to reduce narcotic use and lower the incidence of nausea and vomiting.

Multimodal Analgesia

Pain relief is a basic tenet of anesthesia but has been poorly understood. New pain research is expanding our understanding of central sensitization to pain and late postsurgical pain. Mechanisms of pain production are complex. Tissue injury sends signals via afferent nerves into the spinal cord, and among other actions, initiates the cyclooxygenase (COX-2) pathway to release spinal prostaglandin, ultimately causing central sensitization to pain.[21] Blocking COX-2 preoperatively will reduce central sensitization to pain and reduce intensity and length of postoperative pain.[21] Reuben and colleagues reported that rofecoxib 50 mg given 1 hour before arthroscopic knee surgery reduced postoperative opioid use.[22] Activation of N-methyl-D-aspartate (NMDA) receptors leads to intracellular calcium flux and cell damage. NMDA receptor antagonists include ketamine, magnesium, and dextromethorphan[23] and can reduce the amount of postoperative analgesics required. Schumann[24] reported that preincision local anesthesia significantly reduced postoperative pain and believes that the development of local anesthetics such as levobupivacaine, which permits larger doses to be given without cardiac side effects, will extend opportunities for infiltration analgesia. NSAIDs such as ibuprofen and ketorolac have been instrumental in controlling pain, but NSAID-induced gastrointestinal (GI) toxicity is a common drug-related serious adverse event. It has been estimated that 100,000 patients are hospitalized and 16,500 die each year from NSAID-related GI events.[25] Because it is primarily COX-2 (and not COX-1) inhibition that decreases central sensitization to pain, and because the nonselective NSAIDs have several undesirable properties, much research has gone into development of COX-2–specific inhibitors. Celecoxib (Celebrex) was introduced in 1998, rofecoxib (Vioxx) in 1999, and valdecoxib (Bextra) in 2001. Paracoxib[26] is an injectable form of valdecoxib. Noor[25] reported on many studies, comparing the efficacy of the new COX-2 inhibitors with that of one another and that of ibuprofen. The results are not consistent. In one study rofecoxib 50 mg was equal to ibuprofen 400 mg. In another it took 800 mg of ibuprofen to achieve effects comparable with those of rofecoxib 50 mg or celecoxib 200 mg. A study by Recart and associates[27] verified the efficacy of celecoxib 400 mg premedication in reduction of postoperative pain after the dosage recommendation was increased from 200 mg to 400 mg. Clonidine, an α-agonist, is also useful for production of hypnosis and analgesia and reduction of anesthetic requirements.[28] Evidence continues to mount that use of multimodal analgesia preoperatively, intraoperatively, and postoperatively not only will manage perioperative pain, but also will reduce chronic pain after surgery[29-31] (Table 43-2).

Intravenous Sedation

An AANA survey of CRNAs involved in office practice revealed that sedation is the most common technique used in the office setting (88% of respondents).[7] Short-acting pharmacologic agents with increased potency, faster onset times, better amnesia-producing capabilities, and greater controllability contribute to the administration of IV sedation in a manner that optimizes patient safety and comfort and meets surgeons' needs. Deep IV sedation with propofol has increased significantly the types of surgical and diagnostic procedures that may be completed with sedation techniques with and without local or regional anesthesia.

The most important monitoring during deep sedation is respiratory monitoring. Carbon dioxide levels can rise to levels greater than 100 mm Hg in 15 to 20 minutes in the presence of serious hypoventilation. This can occur with relatively small decreases in oxygen saturation when supplemental oxygen is being administered. It is critical to remember that the monitoring of oxygenation and that of ventilation are two different requirements, and it is imperative to monitor respiratory rate and depth (or end-tidal carbon dioxide [$ETCO_2$]) in addition to arterial oxygen saturation (SaO_2).[32]

Remifentanil, introduced in 1996, is unique among the opioids because it does not accumulate with repeated or prolonged administration. It is important to note that its pharmacokinetics are not altered in disease states or in the elderly. The main advantage of remifentanil is that it rapidly equilibrates to meet the patient's need for varying levels of analgesia depending on the level of surgical stress. Hogue and co-workers[33] studied safety and efficacy of propofol-remifentanil regimens administered in a total IV technique (TIVA). Based on recovery, adverse events, and hemodynamic profiles, a combination of

TABLE 43-2 Multimodal Preemptive Analgesia*

Medication	Action	Dose	When Administered
Local anesthesia	Stops pain transmission by blocking sodium channels	Long-acting agents are preferable	Before incision
Narcotics	Blocks mu receptors in spinal cord, and stops pain signals in thalamus and cortex	Minimum effective dose should be used	Induction and 30 minutes before end of procedure
Ketamine	*N*-methyl-D-aspartate (NMDA)–receptor antagonist	0.1-0.2 mg/kg IV	Before incision
Dexamethasone	Inhibits prostaglandin synthesis	Children: 0.2 mg/kg up to 10-15 mg Adults: 6-10 mg	Start of surgery
Ketorolac	Inhibits prostaglandin synthesis in response to pain	30 mg IV or IM, or 15 mg in patients >65 yr old	
Rofecoxib	Block cyclooxygenase (COX-2)	50 mg PO	45-60 minutes before surgery
Clonidine	α-Agonist	1-2 mcg/kg orally	100 minutes before surgery

IM, *Intramuscular;* IV, *intravenous;* PO, *oral.*
**Polypharmacologic blockade of pain and pain processing at peripheral and nervous system sites for the purpose of preventing the central sensitization of pain pathways and reducing side effects of any one analgesic.*

propofol and remifentanil provided optimal TIVA conditions. Issues that have contributed to its limited use include the need to give other postoperative analgesics because of the fast offset of remifentanil and its relatively higher cost.

Ketamine can provide analgesia, sedation, and amnesia while maintaining respirations. This has made it the anesthetic of choice in many office operating suites, particularly for cosmetic surgery on the face, where the ability to avoid or minimize oxygen insufflation with laser surgery is critical. Unfortunately, awakening after ketamine anesthesia was often characterized by disagreeable dreams or visual disturbances until Vinnik[34] documented that the use of a benzodiazepine before ketamine decreases emergence reactions. In 1999 Friedberg[35] reported no hallucinations in 1264 cases in which propofol was substituted for a benzodiazepine. Ketamine is not indicated if the patient is hypertensive or if an increase in intraocular pressure could be detrimental.

Fire-safety techniques in the office must be kept in mind during procedures on the face in which supplemented oxygen and simultaneous electrocautery or laser techniques are used.[32] Use open draping techniques and administer oxygen through a small 10 French oxygen catheter placed deep in the nasopharynx. Reduce or turn oxygen off before cautery or use of laser. Flumazenil administration warrants a sufficient observation period postoperatively if used to reverse benzodiazepine sedation.[36]

Regional Anesthesia

Regional anesthesia should be considered whenever appropriate because it significantly reduces the possibility of problems with airway management, bronchospasm, prolonged sedation, malignant hyperthermia, nausea and vomiting, cardiac or respiratory depression, and drug interactions. Regional techniques may facilitate earlier fluid intake, ambulation, and discharge compared with general anesthesia. Knee arthroscopies are being performed with local anesthesia injections in the portal sites and intraarticular spaces. Patients have good postoperative anesthesia and early ambulation and appreciate the cost savings.[37,38] Regional facial blocks are now used for an increasing number of cutaneous laser procedures performed by dermatologists and plastic surgeons. Bing and colleagues[39] describe these techniques.

General Anesthesia

Desflurane and sevoflurane have made general anesthesia an acceptable choice in the office setting. The anesthetist, however, will be faced with a more complex preparation, including ensuring the availability of dantrolene and supplies for treatment of malignant hyperthermia, maintenance of the anesthesia machine, and availability of $ETCO_2$ monitoring, temperature monitoring, nerve stimulator, additional medications for muscle relaxation and reversal, and additional airway management devices. Use of the laryngeal mask airway (LMA) instead of the tracheal tube has been associated with a lower incidence of sore throat.[40] Use of the bispectral index (BIS) monitor may help to reduce the amount of general anesthesia or IV sedative to the minimum required.[41]

Trends

With new, minimally invasive techniques, surgeons are able to perform procedures with patients under local anesthesia and conscious sedation. Examples include minilaparoscopy,[42] tubal ligation, differential diagnosis of chronic pelvic pain, appendectomy, and saturation prostate biopsy with periprostatic block.[43]

Tumescent Anesthesia

A combination of IV fluid, dilute lidocaine 0.05% to 0.1%, and dilute epinephrine 1:1,000,000 is used to emulsify fat, provide anesthesia, and create hemostasis during liposuction. This combination has been used extensively since introduced in 1987 by Dr Jeffrey Kline,[44] a California dermatologist who reported good analgesia and almost no blood loss with the tumescent technique. Most significantly, he demonstrated that infiltration of up to 35 mg/kg of lidocaine in this dilute solution would bind to tissues and result in a slow release of lidocaine over 18 to 28 hours, which avoided the customary spike in serum lidocaine levels seen with injection of 1% and 2% lidocaine. Regardless of the recommended 7 mg/kg maximum, administration of lidocaine up to 50 mg/kg in tumescent solutions is used frequently (Box 43-2).

BOX 43-2

Office Liposuction Regulations and Recommendations by State and Date Enacted

California	If more than 5000 ml total aspirate, general anesthesia, or IV sedation, the liposuction must be performed in an acute care hospital (Medical Board of California Regulations, February 20, 2003).
Colorado	A maximum of 4500 ml of supernatant fat may be removed (1500 ml when combined with any other extensive procedure). A maximum of 55 mg/kg of lidocaine can be used in the tumescent technique, and the maximum for epinephrine should be 50 mcg/kg (Colorado Board of Medical Examiners, November 2001).
Florida	A maximum of 4000 ml of supernatant fat may be removed. A maximum of 50 mg/kg of lidocaine can be injected for tumescent liposuction. There is also an 8-hour limit on the time of combined procedures (Florida Board of Medicine Rules, 1999).
Mississippi	Recommendations were adopted for the amount of fat that can be removed within a range of weights and body mass indices (Mississippi Board of Medical Licensure, June 1, 2002).

IV, *Intravenous*.

The surgery and anesthesia community was surprised, then, when Grazer and de Jong,[45] after reviewing information in a 1999 census survey of aesthetic plastic surgeons, reported 95 deaths in nearly half a million liposuctions. This death rate of 19 in 100,000 is extreme when compared with the 3 in 100,000 death rate reported for elective hernia surgery. It was reported by de Jong[46] that pulmonary embolism is responsible for approximately 25% of the liposuction deaths, with causative factors including venous stasis, caval compression, and procedural fat mobilization. Other complications are more amenable to prevention: pulmonary edema caused by overzealous IV fluid administration, hemorrhage from perforation of a major blood vessel, or organ perforation from a misdirected cannula. Convulsions are extremely rare, but deJong hypothesizes that the deaths ascribed to "lidocaine toxicity" may have been caused by depression of cardiac conduction and contractility.

Although the census survey of aesthetic surgeons was alarming and appropriately focused attention on an entire range of concerns about surgery in the office, other reports verify low complication rates similar to those in the hospital setting. A study by the AAAHC reported a low 0.7% complication rate for tumescent liposuction.[47]

The anesthetist should monitor and chart the volume of injected fluid, lidocaine, and epinephrine. Using Klein's technique, cosmetic surgeons customarily administer no IV fluid. When IV fluids are administered as part of the IV sedation or general anesthesia along with the tumescent technique, caution is advised regarding volume. A urinary catheter may be the best guide when the liposuction will be in the 4000- to 5000-ml range. Abdominoplasty with the tumescent local technique and IV sedation allows the surgeon to perform a full abdominoplasty with suction-assisted lipectomy without general anesthesia.[48] Benefits include minimal blood loss, less postoperative pain, and less bruising.

BOX 43-3

Factors Associated with Postoperative Nausea and Vomiting

Surgical Procedures
Extraocular procedures
Ear procedures
Gynecologic surgery
Laparoscopy
Testicular traction
Abdominal procedures
Plastic and reconstructive procedures

Preexisting Conditions
Pregnancy
Menses
Obesity
Hiatal hernia

Patient Characteristics
Female
Young age
Anxiety
Gastroparesis
History of nausea, vomiting, or motion sickness

Drugs
Opiates
Nitrous oxide
Anticholinesterase agents
Etomidate
Ketamine

Perioperative Factors
Pain
Movement
Oral intake
Hypoglycemia
Swallowed blood
Dizziness
Hypotension
Gastric inflation from ventilation

Control of Nausea and Vomiting

Nausea and vomiting contribute to patient discomfort and dissatisfaction and delay patient discharge. Nausea and vomiting have been shown to be related to the type of surgical procedure, preexisting patient history, drugs, and other perioperative factors (Box 43-3).[49] Drug therapy for prevention and treatment of postoperative nausea and vomiting (PONV) is summarized in Table 43-3.[49]

Because not all patients will have a problem with nausea, treatment of all patients with the most expensive agents (the 5-HT_3–receptor antagonists) will not be considered cost

TABLE 43-3 Drugs for Treatment of Postoperative Nausea and Vomiting

Drug	Class	Dose	Comments
Ondansetron (Zofran)	Serotonin (5-HT_3) antagonist	2-8 mg IV 8-16 mg PO	Side effects minimal Occasional headache
Granisetron (Kytril)	Serotonin (5-HT_3) antagonist	1-3 mg IV 1-2 mg PO	Side effects minimal Occasional headache
Dolasetron (Anzemet)	Serotonin (5-HT_3) antagonist	12.5 mg IV 100 mg PO	Side effects minimal Occasional headache
Promethazine (Phenergan)	Antihistamine, sedative hypnotic	12.5-25 mg IV or IM 25 mg PO	Drowsiness, dry mouth
Hydroxyzine (Atarax, Vistaril)	Antihistamine, sedative hypnotic	10-25 mg IV	Drowsiness, dry mouth
Metoclopramide (Reglan)	Gastrokinetic	10 mg IV	Extrapyramidal, dystonic reaction
Meclizine	Antihistamine	25 mg PO	Minimal drowsiness
Prochlorperazine (Compazine)	Phenothiazine	2.5-10 mg IV 5-10 mg IM Oral: tablet 5-10 mg 3-4 times/day, capsule 5-10 mg q 12 h	Extrapyramidal, dystonic reaction Drowsiness, hypotension
Droperidol*	Butyrophenone	1.25-5 mg IV	Extrapyramidal, dystonic reaction; drowsiness, hypotension

IM, *Intramuscular;* IV, *intravenous;* OTC, *over the counter;* PO, *oral.*
**Reported ventricular arrhythmias in patients with prolonged QT syndrome.*

effective by most facilities. Formulation of a patient-specific plan is more cost effective and starts with identification of patients at higher risk for nausea and vomiting on the basis of a history of emetic symptoms or type of procedure. The plan should include patient input regarding known or perceived effective therapies, administration of selected antiemetics, good pain control, and careful choice of sedative and analgesic drugs. The incidence of PONV appears to be consistently reduced for patients who receive propofol as part of the anesthetic technique.[50] Dexamethasone has been shown to be very useful for prevention of "late" PONV, 6 to 24 hours after surgery.[51]

A multimodal approach for control of nausea and vomiting may include a combination of the following: (1) administration of meclizine, 25 mg orally (PO), 7 AM and 7 PM the day of surgery and the first postoperative day[52]; (2) use of propofol in the anesthesia technique; (3) dexamethasone 8 to 10 mg in adults early in the case[47]; (4) addition of an NSAID or COX-2 inhibitor before the end of surgery to decrease postoperative narcotic use; (5) encouragement of the surgeon to use a long-acting local anesthetic in the surgical area; (6) reduction of narcotics; and (7) administration of metoclopramide, 10 to 20 mg IV 30 minutes before the end of the surgery.[49] The use of ondansetron or dolasetron may be reserved for patients with a significant history of nausea and vomiting and for patients undergoing a procedure that is known to be associated with increased nausea and vomiting (e.g., long surgery, gynecologic surgery, rhinoplasty, breast augmentation). Eliminating neostigmine from the anesthesia technique by using the short-acting muscle relaxant mivacurium can also reduce the incidence of nausea and vomiting.[53] Droperidol is not as popular because of reports of ventricular arrhythmia in patents with a long QT interval and the manufacturer's recommendation of electrocardiographic (ECG) monitoring for 2 to 3 hours after administration. That is not practical for office anesthesia.[54]

Use of the "relief band," a battery-operated wrist band that stimulates the median nerve at the P-6 acupuncture point, showed a 60% reduction in nausea compared with placebo (about the same as antiemetic prophylaxis). It may produce a normalization of gastric motility.[55]

OFFICE ANESTHESIA: SAFETY AND GOOD BUSINESS PRACTICE

Anesthesia Policies Specific to the Office

Important questions related to provision of safe anesthesia in the office setting must not be overlooked. Who does the preoperative evaluation? Who trains the staff in emergency procedures? Where will the patient be transferred if there is a problem? Who is maintaining equipment and oxygen supplies? Who provides immediate recovery care? How will the extended recovery after long procedures be managed?

To set up appropriately for office-based anesthesia, the anesthetist must assume responsibility for quality, education, and infection control and ensure that maintenance functions are carried out. Discussion of these issues with surgeons and office staff will improve their understanding and cooperation. The best policies are brief, state the essentials clearly, and are readily available. Sample policies may be found in Appendix 43-C and include organization of anesthesia services, anesthesia safety guidelines, patient selection criteria for office anesthesia services, preanesthesia evaluation guidelines, intraoperative and postoperative anesthetic management recommendations, anesthesia infection control procedures, disposal guidelines for waste anesthetic gases, postanesthesia care, dispensation of and accounting for controlled substances, and local anesthesia guidelines.

Anesthesia Equipment and Supplies Checklist

It is accepted practice for CRNAs to check their equipment and supplies before starting each anesthetic procedure. In most instances an itemized checklist is not used, because the provider is familiar with the equipment and location of supplies. The office CRNA, however, will find the daily use of a checklist (Box 43-4) an important safety tool for the following reasons: (1) office CRNAs frequently practice at multiple office locations with different equipment and varied arrangements of supplies, and (2) it is essential that everything potentially needed be immediately available, because personnel, supplies, and equipment for backup in the office setting may be limited.

Clinical Privileges

Individual clinical privileges should be delineated regardless of the contractual or employment relationship that exists within the office practice. CRNAs are responsible for seeking clinical privileges that reflect their educational preparation, clinical experience, and level of professional competence.

Guidelines and forms for granting privileges to nurse anesthetists can be found in the *Professional Practice Manual for the Certified Registered Nurse Anesthetist.*[12] A credentialing file should be created at the office facility that includes professional licenses for physicians and RNs, as well as CRNAs.

BOX 43-4

Anesthesia Equipment and Supplies Checklist (to Be Kept in Log Book)

Date:_______ Checked out by:_______ Location:___________

- ☐ Oxygen pipeline pressure or primary source pounds per square inch (PSI)
- ☐ Oxygen tank pressure (second source) PSI
- ☐ Backup power
- ☐ Defibrillator and crash cart available
- ☐ Anesthesia cart supplies checked (e.g., intravenous [IV] equipment, anesthetics, stethoscope)
- ☐ Suction equipment tested
- ☐ Ambu bag tested
- ☐ Electrocardiogram operational
- ☐ Pulse oximeter operational
- ☐ Blood pressure (BP) monitor
- ☐ Backup BP cuff
- ☐ Atropine
- ☐ Epinephrine
- ☐ Ephedrine
- ☐ Lidocaine
- ☐ Other emergency medications as indicated
- ☐ Endotracheal equipment, airways

If general anesthesia is planned: anesthesia machine # ______.

- ☐ Leak test performed and other tests as indicated
- ☐ Oxygen analyzer ON
- ☐ Capnometer connected
- ☐ Temperature monitor available
- ☐ Emergency airways available (e.g., laryngeal mask airway [LMA], Combitube, or cricothyrotomy kit)
- ☐ Succinylcholine
- ☐ Dantrolene
- ☐ Other anesthesia medications as indicated

Note (if problem):______________________________

____

____

Follow-up (who; what):______________________________

____

____

Preanesthesia Evaluation

Medical providers are making every effort to reduce unnecessary preoperative tests. A complete medical history is the best tool for determining the necessity of further evaluation.[56] Asking questions about the patient's exercise tolerance elicits vital information regarding cardiovascular and respiratory function, which may have more value than a traditional ECG and chest x-ray examination. The American College of Cardiology/American Heart Association report entitled *Guidelines for Perioperative Cardiovascular Evaluation for Noncardiac Surgery*[57] provides help in determining which additional tests should be performed for patients with a history of cardiovascular disease and helps support decisions to forego cardiac testing when a patient is stable. If significant medical problems exist, consultation with the patient's primary physician will help optimize the patient for surgery. Physical assessment of heart sounds, lung sounds, and the airway should be performed immediately before anesthesia.

A reliable method of getting preoperative information to and from patients must be established. The AANA has developed a brochure that can help prepare patients for anesthetic choices and that has a preanesthesia questionnaire for patients to fill out and bring with them. The anesthesia group and surgical facility may prepare a customized brochure or letter. A sample preanesthesia testing policy may be found in Appendix 43-C, Policy 5. The office staff will need help to correctly inform patients regarding which medication to take or hold on the day of surgery. The preoperative medication guidelines in Appendix 43-D will help the surgeon and office nurse to pass on appropriate drug administration information.

Informed Consent

Informed consent is a legal principle that requires that the patient be knowledgeable about his or her choices for medical care and the possible consequences of that care before submitting to treatment. "Twenty-five thousand CRNAs administer more than 65% of the 26 million anesthetics given to patients in the United States each year. They are at greater risk for medical malpractice litigation if they are not well versed in the principle of informed consent."[58] In the office setting the same "production pressure" can exist as in the hospital setting, severely impinging on the CRNA's ability to achieve informed consent. Reviewing the nature of the anesthesia and the benefits and risks of anesthesia will be best achieved with a telephone call before the day of the procedure. The operating practitioner's agreement with the anesthesia plan should also be documented. In summary, the patient should be telephoned before anesthesia is administered, and the anesthesia plan should be discussed with the surgeon to improve patient and surgeon satisfaction.

Discharge Criteria

Newer anesthetics allow more rapid awakening and may reduce the time required to meet appropriate discharge criteria. In a review of discharge criteria and complications after ambulatory surgery, Marshall and Chung[59] have recommended that removing the drinking and voiding requirements from discharge criteria may help speed discharge. Requirements that the patient must drink fluids and void before discharge have been controversial. In a study of 998 children at the Children's Hospital of Philadelphia,[60] the children who were required to drink had a higher incidence of nausea and stayed longer in the ambulatory unit. The study concluded that drinking was not a mandatory discharge criterion.

Requiring patients to void can also delay discharge. Urinary retention is a known risk in patients having pelvic or urologic surgery or after spinal or epidural anesthesia. At least one study indicates that patients not at high risk of urinary retention can be discharged home before voiding.[61]

Recommended discharge criteria are listed in the postanesthesia care unit (PACU) policy—Policy 10 in Appendix 43-C.

Emergency Management

Office procedures may include high-risk patients and extensive procedures. Therefore medications and equipment must be available for the management of a wide range of physiologic changes that may occur, including respiratory depression, hypoxemia, hypertension, hypotension, bradycardia, tachycardia, allergic reactions, bronchospasm, arrhythmias, myocardial ischemia, and congestive heart failure. An LMA should be available for management of difficult airways.

Continuous Quality Improvement

An annual review of quality initiatives for the office anesthesia setting are listed in Box 43-5. CRNAs practicing in the office setting should be aware of new studies in anesthesia crisis resource management (CRM) training. As in aviation, in anesthesia it has been found that human error has a role in more than 70% of critical events. Joanne L Fletcher developed an AANA journal course to educate CRNAs in how to adapt the principles of CRM to their practice. CRM is based on the premise that we can provide the best patient care when we have a knowledgeable and fully coordinated health-care team. "Reluctance to call for help or accept help when it is offered is a dangerous attitude that endangers the patient," states Fletcher.[62] Because the "team" in office practice is smaller, it is essential to know how to use the resources of other members of the operating room team. Fletcher developed the acronym *ERR WATCH* to assist CRNAs in the use of the principles of CRM: *e*nvironment, *r*esources, *r*eevaluation, *w*orkload, *a*ttention, *t*eamwork, *c*ommunication, and *h*elp.

The High Reliability Organization (HRO) theory has been suggested by Dr David Gaba[63] to help improve anesthesia care through consistent systems, team training, prospective review of activities, and adoption of a "culture of safety."

BOX **43-5**

Annual Review for the Office-Based Surgical Facility: an Anesthesia Continuous Quality Improvement Form

- ☐ There is a credentialing file that includes current licensure for physicians, CRNAs, RNs, and LPNs.
- ☐ There is evidence that the anesthesia monitors, defibrillator, and anesthesia machine (if applicable) have been checked in the past year for electrical safety and function tested.
  Date checked:______________________________
- ☐ There are two oxygen sources with regulators attached.
- ☐ There is emergency backup power (e.g., generator or battery power) to operate monitors and lights for 2 hours.
  Date checked:______________________________
- ☐ Emergency phone numbers are posted with a protective cover near the operating room phone, including: Emergency Medical Response Team, usually 911 (or hospital code blue number if the office is physically attached to the hospital); Malignant Hyperthermia Hotline (1-800-MH-HYPER); emergency department number of the hospital with which you have a transfer agreement.
- ☐ Emergency protocols are readily available for advanced cardiac life support (ACLS), pediatric cardiac life support (if applicable), malignant hyperthermia, and management of the difficult airway.
- ☐ There is evidence of staff training during the past year in the areas of cardiopulmonary resuscitation (CPR), ACLS, and implementation of the emergency transfer protocol.
- ☐ Equipment includes at least the following: defibrillator, electrocardiograph, pulse oximeter, blood pressure monitor, positive pressure ventilation bag (e.g., Ambu bag), suction machine, temperature monitor oxygen analyzer, waste gas exhaust system, and oxygen fail-safe system.
- ☐ There is a mechanism for the ordering and stocking of anesthesia supplies and medications to ensure appropriate types and quantities for regular and emergency care.
- ☐ There is a system to check and replace outdated medications.
- ☐ There is a mechanism to lock DEA 222 forms and controlled substances and limit access to qualified individuals.
- ☐ Controlled pharmaceuticals are documented when used and tracked by a count at least weekly.
- ☐ Policies are reviewed annually for appropriateness for the types of procedures performed and the types of anesthesia administered in the facility.
  Date completed:______________________________
- ☐ There is evidence that anesthesia documentation is reviewed to determine the incidence of unusual, unexpected, or unplanned patient events during the perianesthesia period.
- ☐ There is evidence that appropriate actions were taken to improve care or correct identified problems.
  This review was completed by:______________________________
  Date:______________________________

CRNA, *Certified registered nurse anesthetist;* DEA, *Drug Enforcement Agency;* RN, *registered nurse;* LPN, *licensed practical nurse.*

Business Aspects

As office surgery suites increase, the anesthesia practice opportunities have also increased. These practice opportunities are not for every anesthetist. The administration of anesthesia can be a daunting task by itself. Many CRNAs and anesthesiologists do not want to deal with the logistics of facility setup and the business aspects of an anesthesia practice. If you do decide to pursue office opportunities, remember that (1) credibility with surgeons, (2) ability as an anesthesia consultant, and (3) willingness to provide the *entire* spectrum of anesthesia services are vital to creating an office-based anesthesia practice. Mannino[64] offers advice in her article "Setting up an Office Anesthesia Practice" and reports that trends appear to be moving toward the development of multispecialty office surgical facilities. Professional liability insurance is rarely provided by the surgeon or office facility. You and any subcontractors should purchase full- or part-time liability insurance from a qualified insurance carrier licensed to do business in your state. The problems you could create by purchasing from a nonadmitted insurance carrier are detailed in a 2003 article by John Fetcho.[65]

Spending time within the group to delineate responsibilities helps build long-term relationships. Issues such as scheduling, equipment, maintenance, drug and supply purchase must be addressed in order to establish an orderly and well-functioning practice. It is worth remembering that surgeons practicing in the office setting are running their own businesses, and a request for equipment and supplies will have an impact on their bottom line. The anesthetist will regularly need to make decisions about what is necessary for quality care. That is when it is more important than ever to adhere to standards and use them in discussions with the surgeons.

The CRNA as a Consultant for RN-Administered Conscious Sedation

RNs are increasingly providing conscious sedation in offices, many times in the same surgical office setting in which CRNAs are administering deep sedation or general anesthesia. The CRNA can play an important role in the development of policies for conscious sedation administered by RNs, emergency training, teach pharmacologic principles, and ensure that appropriate monitoring and safety precautions are followed.

Communication

Written communication is usually more effective than verbal communication. Useful forms and letters for office-based anesthesia include a sample patient letter with preanesthesia instructions and a form with common discharge instructions (see Appendix 43-E).

Controlled Substances

To purchase controlled substances, the physician will need to obtain Drug Enforcement Agency (DEA) 222 forms. Contact the DEA at 1-800-882-9539 for information on physician registration to acquire DEA 222 forms.

SUMMARY

Thousands of procedures have been safely performed in the office setting primarily with IV sedation, but also with regional and general anesthesia. In summary, elements key to the provision of quality care for office-based anesthesia include the following:

1. Appropriate patient selection
2. Preoperative communication with the patient
3. Emergency preparedness
4. Continuous intraoperative monitoring
5. Thorough knowledge of the pharmacokinetic profile of the medications used for producing sedation, analgesia, and general anesthesia
6. Adequate and early pain control with opiates, local anesthesia, and NSAIDs
7. Early planning for the prevention of nausea and vomiting
8. Appropriate monitoring of recovery care, with criteria-based discharge

REFFERENCES

1. *SMG Forecast of Surgical Volume in Hospital/Ambulatory Settings: 1994-2001*. Chicago: SMG Marketing Group; 1999.
2. Morello DC, Colon GA, Fredricks S, Iverson RE, Singer R. Patient safety in accredited office surgical facilities. *Plast Reconstr Surg*. 1997;99:1496-1500.
3. Hoefflin SM, Bornstein JB, Gordon M. General anesthesia in an office-based plastic surgical facility: a report on more than 23,000 consecutive office-based procedures under general anesthesia with no significant anesthetic complications. *Plast Reconstr Surg*. 2001;107:243-251.
4. D'eramo EM, Bookless SJ, Howard JB. Adverse events with outpatient anesthesia in Massachusetts. *J Oral Maxillofac Surg*. 2003;61:793-800.
5. Morell RC. OBA questions, problems just now being recognized, being defined. *APSF Newsletter*. 2000;15:2-4.
6. Rao RB, Ely SF, Hoffman RS. Deaths related to liposuction. *N Engl J Med*. 1999;340:1471-1475.
7. Tunajek SK. Office based anesthesia standards. *AANA J*. 1999;67:115-120.
8. American Society of Anesthesiologists. *ASA Guidelines for Office Based Anesthesia*, Park Ridge, Ill: American Society of Anesthesiologists; 1999.
9. Eichhorn JH, et al. Standards for patient monitoring during anesthesia: Harvard Medical School. *JAMA*. 1986;256: 1017-1020.
10. American Academy of Pediatrics, Committee on Drugs. Guidelines for monitoring and management of pediatric patients during and after sedation for diagnostic and therapeutic procedures. *Pediatrics*. 1992;89:1110-1115.
11. American Society of Anesthesiologists. *The American Society of Anesthesiologists Policy on Monitored Anesthesia Care*. Park Ridge, Ill: American Society of Anesthesiologists; 1986.
12. American Association of Nurse Anesthetists. *Patient Monitoring Standards: Professional Practice Manual for the Certified Registered Nurse Anesthetist*. Park Ridge, Ill: American Association of Nurse Anesthetists; 1996.
13. Rosenberg MB, Campbell RL. Guidelines for intraoperative monitoring of dental patients undergoing conscious sedation, deep sedation, and general anesthesia. *Oral Surg Oral Med Oral Pathol*. 1991;71:2-8.
14. Fleischer D. Monitoring the patient receiving conscious sedation for gastrointestinal endoscopy: issues and guidelines. *Gastrointest Endosc*. 1989;35:262-266.
15. ACS. *Guidelines for Office Based Facilities*. Chicago: American College of Surgeons; 2003.
16. American Association for Accreditation of Ambulatory Surgery Facilities. *American Association for Accreditation of Ambulatory Surgery Facilities*. Mundelein, Ill: American Association for Accreditation of Ambulatory Surgery Facilities; 2002.

17. Accreditation Association for Ambulatory Health Care. *AAAHC Guidebook for Office Based Surgery Accreditation*. Wilmette, Ill: Accreditation Association for Ambulatory Health Care; 2003.
18. Joint Commission on Accreditation of Healthcare Organizations: *Office Based Surgery Accreditation*. Oakbrook Terrace, Ill:; 2003. Website: http://www.jcaho.org/htba/office+based+surgery/index.htm. Accessed May 10, 2004.
19. *JACHO Ambulatory Care Advisor*. Website: http://www.jcaho.org/qualitycheck/directry/SearchResults.aspx. Accessed May 10, 2004. 1:2003.
20. Royer K. A case for office accreditation. *Outpatient Surg*. 2003;4:35-38.
21. Bertolini A, Ottani A, Sandrini M. Dual acting anti-inflammatory drugs: a reappraisal. *Pharmacol Res*. 2001;44:437-450.
22. Reuben SS, Bhopatkar S, Maciolek H, Joshi W, Sklar J. The preemptive analgesic effect of rofecoxib after ambulatory arthroscopic knee surgery. *Anesth Analg*. 2002;94:55-59.
23. Berry FA. Management of pain, nausea, and vomiting in pediatric patients. Eighth Annual Santa Fe Symposium, cosponsored by Scott and White Hospital and Clinic and Texas A&M University Health Science Center College of Medicine. *Audio Digest Anesthesiol*. 2003;45.
24. Schumann R, Shikora S, Weiss JM, Wurm H, Strassels S, Carr DB. A comparison of multimodal perioperative analgesia to epidural pain management after gastric bypass surgery. *Anesth Analg*. 2003;96:469-474.
25. Noor MG. Cyclooxygenase-2 inhibitors. *Anesth Analg*. 2003;96:1720-1738.
26. Tang J, Li S, White PF, et al. Effect of parecoxib, a novel intravenous cyclooxygenase type-2 inhibitor, on the postoperative opioid requirement and quality of pain control. *Anesthesiology*. 2002;96:1305-1309.
27. Recart A, Issioui T, White PF, et al. The efficacy of celecoxib premedication on postoperative pain and recovery time after ambulatory surgery: a dose ranging study. *Anesth Analg*. 2003;96: 1631-1635.
28. Hall JE, Uhrich TD, Ebert TJ. Sedative, analgesic and cognitive effects of clonidine infusion in humans. *Br Jr Anaesth*. 2001;86: 5-11.
29. Hartrick CT. Multimodal postoperative pain management. *Am J Health Syst Pharm*. 2004;Suppl 1:S4-S10.
30. DeKock M, et al. Balanced analgesia in the perioperative period: is there a place for ketamine? *Pain*. 2001;92:373.
31. Suzuki M, Tsueda K, Lansing PS, et al. Small-dose ketamine enhances morphine-induced analgesia after outpatient surgery. *Anesth Analg*. 1999;89:98-103.
32. Greco RI, et al. Potential dangers of oxygen supplementation during facial surgery. *Plast Reconstr Surg*. 1995;95:978.
33. Hogue CW, Jr, Bowdle TA, O'Leary C, et al. A multicenter evaluation of total intravenous anesthesia with remifentanil and propofol for elective inpatient surgery. *Anesth Analg*. 1996;83:279-285.
34. Vinnik CA. An intravenous. *Plast Reconstr Surg*. 1981;67: 100-105.
35. Friedberg BL. Propofol ketamine anesthesia for cosmetic surgery in the office suite. *Int Anesthesiol Clin*. 2003;41:39-50.
36. Nagelhout J, et al. The effect of flumazenil on patient recovery and discharge following ambulatory surgery. *AANA J*. 1999;67: 229-236.
37. Lintner S, et al. Local anesthesia in outpatient knee arthroscopy: a comparison of efficacy and cost. *Arthroscopy*. 1996;12:482-488.
38. Trieshmann HW Jr. Knee arthroscopy: a cost analysis of general and local anesthesia. *Arthroscopy*. 1996;12:60-63.
39. Bing J, et al. Regional anesthesia with monitored anesthesia care for dermatologic laser surgery. *Dermatol Clin*. 2002;20:123-134.
40. Joshi GP, et al. Use of laryngeal mask airway as an alternative to the tracheal tube during ambulatory surgery. *Anesth Analg*. 1997;85:573-577.
41. Friedberg BL, Sigl JC. Bispectral index (BIS) monitoring decreases propofol usage in propofol-ketamine office-based anesthesia. *Anesth Analg*. 1999;88:S54.
42. Palter SF. Office microlaparoscopy under local anesthesia. *Obstet Gynecol Clin North Am*. 1999;29:109-120.
43. Jones JS, Oder M, Zippe CD. Saturation prostate biopsy with periprostatic block can be performed in office. *J Urol*. 2002;168:2108-2110.
44. Klein JA. Tumescent techniques for regional anesthesia permits lidocaine doses of 35 mg/kg for liposuction. *J Dermatol Surg Oncol*. 1990;16:248-263.
45. Grazer FM, deJong RH. Fatal outcome from liposuction. Census survey of cosmetic surgeons. *Plast Reconstr Surg*. 2000;105:436-446.
46. de Jong RH. Lidocaine dosing duality in liposuction: "safe" only when highly diluted. *Plast Reconstr Surg*. 2004;113:1513-1514, author reply 1514-1515.
47. Accreditation Association for Ambulatory Health Care. *IQI study. Tumescent Liposuction*. Wilmette, Ill: Accreditation Association for Ambulatory Health Care; 2002.
48. Pravecek EJ, Worland RG. Tumescent abdominoplasty: full abdominoplasty under local anesthesia with IV sedation in an ambulatory surgical facility. *Plast Surg Nurs*. 1998;18:38-43.
49. Norred CL. Antiemetic prophylaxis: pharmacology and therapeutics. *AANA J*. 2003;71:133-140.
50. Sneyd JR, Carr A, Byrom WD, Bilski AJ. A meta-analysis of nausea and vomiting following maintenance of anaesthesia with propofol or inhalation agents. *Eur J Anaesthesiol*. 1998;15:433-445.
51. Henzi I, Walder B, Tramer MR. Dexamethasone for the prevention of postoperative nausea and vomiting: a quantitative systematic review. *Anesth Analg*. 2000;90:186-194.
52. Brown NJ, Roberts J. Histamine, bradykinin and their antagonists. In: Hardman JG, Limbird LE, eds. *Goodman & Gilman's the Pharmacological Basis of Therapeutics*. 10th ed. New York: Macmillan; 2001:645-668.
53. Ding Y, Friedman B, White PF. Use of mivacurium during laparoscopic surgery: effect of reversal drugs on postoperative recovery. *Anesth Analg*. 1994;78:450-454.
54. Dershwitz M. Droperidol: should the black box be light gray? *J Clin Anesth*. 2002;14:598-603.
55. Zarate E, Mingus M, White PF, et al. The use of transcutaneous acupoint electrical stimulation for preventing nausea and vomiting after laparoscopic surgery. *Anesth Analg*. 2001;92:629-635.
56. Huag RH, Reifeis RL. A prospective evaluation of the value of preoperative laboratory testing for office anesthesia and sedation. *J Oral Maxillofac Surg*. 1999;57:16-20.
57. Eagle KA, Berger PB, Calkins H, et al. ACC/AHA guideline update for perioperative cardiovascular evaluation for noncardiac surgery—executive summary. *Anesth Analg*. 2002;94:1052-1064.
58. Hartgerink BJ, McMullen P, McDonough JP, McCarthy EJ. A guide to understanding informed consent. *CRNA*. 1998;9:128-134.
59. Marshall SI, Chung F. Discharge criteria and complications after ambulatory surgery. *Anesth Analg*. 1999;88:508-517.
60. Schreiner MS, Nicolson SC, Martin T, Whitney L. Should children drink before discharge from day surgery? *Anesthesiology*. 1992;76:528-533.
61. Fritz WT, et al. Utilization of a home nursing protocol allows ambulatory surgery patients to be discharged prior to voiding. *Anesth Analg*. 1997;84:S6.
62. Fletcher JL. Update for nurse anesthetists—ERR WATCH: anesthesia crisis resource management from the nurse anesthetist's perspective. *AANA J*. 1998;66:595-602.
63. Gaba DM. Safety first: ensuing quality care in the intensely productive environment—the HRO model. *APSF Newsletter*. 2003; 18:1-16.
64. Mannino MJ. Setting up an office anesthesia practice. *CRNA*. 1999;10:54-58.
65. Fetcho J. Buyer beware: what you don't know about your professional liability insurance can hurt you. *AANA News Bull*. 2003;July/August:1-9.

APPENDIX CONTENTS

APPENDIX 43-A: AMERICAN ASSOCIATION OF NURSE ANESTHETISTS STANDARDS FOR OFFICE-BASED ANESTHESIA PRACTICE

Certified registered nurse anesthetists (CRNAs) have long been the predominant anesthesia practitioners and leaders in providing anesthesia services in physicians' offices. As the professional organization representing nurse anesthetists, the American Association of Nurse Anesthetists (AANA) advocates high-quality, appropriate standards of care for all patients in all settings, including the office-based practice setting. As they do in other settings, CRNAs provide anesthesia, working with physicians such as anesthesiologists, surgeons, and, where authorized, podiatrists, dentists, and other health-care professionals.

The AANA has been at the forefront in establishing clinical practice standards, including patient monitoring standards. The standards of care in the office-based setting are congruent with the AANA *Scope and Standards of Nurse Anesthesia Practice* and are intended to do the following:

1. Provide assistance to CRNAs and other practitioners by promoting a common base for the delivery of quality patient care in the office-based setting
2. Assist the public in understanding what to expect from the practitioner
3. Support the basic rights of patients

Although the standards are intended to promote high-quality patient care, they cannot ensure specific outcomes.

Anesthesia in the Office Setting

Some unique and specific responsibilities should be considered before administration of anesthesia in the office setting. When considering an office-based practice, anesthesia practitioners should determine if there are appropriate resources to manage the various levels of anesthesia for the planned surgical procedures and the patients' conditions. Most office-based practice settings are not regulated; therefore the CRNA should consider the benefit of uniform professional standards regarding practitioner qualifications, training, equipment, facilities, and policies that ensure the safety of the patient during operative and anesthesia procedures in the office setting. At a minimum the CRNA shall determine that there are policies to address all of the following:

1. Patient selection criteria
2. Monitoring equipment with a backup electrical source
3. Adequate numbers of well-trained personnel to support the planned surgery and anesthesia
4. Treatment of foreseeable complications
5. Patient transfer to other health-care facilities
6. Infection control practices, including Occupational Safety and Health Administration (OSHA) requirements
7. Minimal preoperative testing, including required consultations
8. Ancillary services (e.g., laboratory, pharmacy, consultation with outside specialists)
9. Equipment maintenance
10. Response to fire and other catastrophic events
11. Recovery and discharge of patients
12. Procedures for follow-up care

The CRNA shall comply with all applicable state and federal rules and regulations relating to licensure, certification, and accreditation of an office practice.

Standard 1

Perform a thorough and complete preanesthesia assessment

Interpretation. The responsibility for the care of the patient begins with the preanesthetic assessment. Except in emergency situations the CRNA has an obligation to complete a thorough evaluation and determine that relevant tests have been obtained and reviewed.

Application to Office Practice. Preanesthesia assessment of the patient undergoing office-based surgery should include documentation of at least the following:

1. Assigned physical status
2. Airway assessment
3. Anesthetic history
4. Allergies
5. Fasting status
6. History and physical examination

Standard 2

Obtain informed consent for the planned anesthetic intervention from the patient or legal guardian

Interpretation. The CRNA shall obtain or verify that an informed consent has been obtained by a qualified provider. Discuss anesthetic options and risks with the patient or legal guardian in language the patient or legal guardian can understand. Document in the patient's medical record that informed consent was obtained.

Application to Office Practice. The CRNA shall confirm that consent has been given for the planned surgical or diagnostic procedure and that the patient understands and accepts the plans and inherent risks for anesthesia in the office setting.

Standard 3

Formulate a patient-specific plan for anesthesia care

Interpretation. The plan of care developed by the CRNA is based on comprehensive patient assessment, problem analysis, anticipated surgical or therapeutic procedure, patient and surgeon preferences, and current anesthesia principles.

Application to Office Practice. A patient-specific plan of care is based on patient assessment and the anticipation of potential problems in the unique setting. The operating practitioner concurs that the patient is cleared for the planned anesthetic.

Standard 4

Implement and adjust the anesthesia care plan based on the patient's physiologic response

Interpretation. The CRNA shall induce and maintain anesthesia at required levels. The CRNA shall continuously assess the patient's response to the anesthetic and/or surgical intervention and intervene as required to maintain the patient in a satisfactory physiologic condition.

Application to Office Practice. The CRNA shall continuously assess and monitor the patient's response to the anesthetic. Before administration of anesthesia the CRNA shall verify a means to deliver positive pressure ventilation and to treat emergency situations, including the availability of necessary emergency equipment and drugs. If "triggering agents" associated with malignant hyperthermia are used, adequate dosages of dontrolene should be immediately accessible.

Standard 5
Monitor the patient's physiologic condition as appropriate for the type of anesthesia and specific patient needs

1. *Monitor ventilation continuously.* Verify intubation of the trachea by auscultation, chest excursion, and confirmation of carbon dioxide (CO_2) in the expired gas. Continuously monitor end-tidal CO_2 during controlled or assisted ventilation including any anesthesia or sedation technique requiring artificial airway support. Use spirometry and ventilatory pressure monitors as indicated.
2. *Monitor oxygenation continuously* by clinical observation, pulse oximetry, and, if indicated, arterial blood gas analysis.
3. *Monitor cardiovascular status continuously* via electrocardiogram (ECG) and heart sounds. Record blood pressure and heart rate at least every 5 minutes.
4. Monitor body temperature continuously in all pediatric patients receiving general anesthesia and when indicated in all other patients.
5. Monitor neuromuscular function and status when neuromuscular blocking agents are administered.
6. Monitor and assess patient positioning and protective measures at frequent intervals.

Interpretation. Continuous clinical observation and vigilance are the basis of safe anesthesia care. The standard applies to all patients receiving anesthesia care and may be exceeded at any time at the discretion of the CRNA. Unless otherwise stipulated in the standards, a means to monitor and evaluate the patient's status shall be immediately available for all patients. As new patient safety technologies evolve, integration into the current anesthesia practice shall be considered. The omission of any monitoring standards shall be documented, and the reason stated on the patient's anesthesia record. The CRNA shall be in constant attendance on the patient until the responsibility for care has been accepted by another qualified health-care provider.

Application to Office Practice. Minimum monitors in the office-based setting include pulse oximetry, ECG, blood pressure, an oxygen (O_2) analyzer and end-tidal CO_2 analyzer when administering general anesthesia, body temperature for the pediatric patient, an esophageal or precordial stethoscope, and peripheral nerve stimulator as indicated.

Standard 6
There shall be complete, accurate, and timely documentation of pertinent information on the patient's medical record

Interpretation. Document all anesthetic interventions and patient responses. Accurate documentation facilitates comprehensive patient care, provides information for retrospective review and research data, and establishes a medical-legal record.

Application to Office Practice. The CRNA confirms there is a plan for accurate record keeping and documentation of the following:

1. Informed consent
2. Preanesthesia and postanesthesia evaluations
3. Course of the anesthesia, including monitoring modalities and drug administration, doses, and wastage
4. Discharge follow-up

The CRNA shall confirm that there is a systematic mechanism for documentation of compliance with U.S. Drug Enforcement Agency rules, Board of Pharmacy regulations, Food and Drug Administration requirements, and U.S. Department of Transportation regulations for accountability and appropriate storage. Documentation of provider licensure and credentials, facility licensure, and continued competence is recommended.

Standard 7
Transfer the responsibility for care of the patient to other qualified providers in a manner that ensures continuity of care and patient safety

Interpretation. The CRNA shall assess the patient's status and determine when it is safe to transfer the responsibility of care to other qualified providers. The CRNA shall accurately report the patient's condition and all essential information to the provider assigned responsibility for the patient.

Application to Office Practice. Postanesthesia care is consistent with other practice settings in that there is a designated area staffed with appropriately trained personnel. At least one qualified provider—a surgeon, anesthesia practitioner, or advanced cardiac life support (ACLS)-certified registered nurse—remains in the facility until all patients are discharged. An accurate postanesthesia record is documented.

Standard 8
Adhere to appropriate safety precautions, as established within the institution, to minimize the risks of fire, explosion, electrical shock, and equipment malfunction. Document on the patient's medical record that the anesthesia machine and equipment have been checked

Interpretation. Before their use the CRNA shall inspect the anesthesia machine and monitors according to established guidelines. The CRNA shall check the readiness, availability, cleanliness, and working condition of all equipment to be used in the administration of the anesthesia care. When the patient is ventilated by an automatic mechanical ventilator, the CRNA will monitor the integrity of the breathing system with a device capable of detecting a disconnection by emitting an audible alarm. The CRNA will monitor oxygen concentration continuously with an oxygen supply failure alarm system.

Application to Office Practice. The CRNA confirms equipment is routinely maintained by appropriately trained professionals. Before use, equipment is inspected for risk of malfunction and electrical and fire hazards.

Standard 9
Precautions shall be taken to minimize the risk of infection to the patient, the CRNA, and other health-care providers

Interpretation Written policies and procedures for infection control shall be developed for personnel and equipment.

Application to Office Practice. The CRNA shall confirm that policies are in place and a process exists to document compliance with OSHA standards relating to blood-borne pathogens, medical waste, and hazardous materials, including personal protection devices, disposal of needles and syringes, and contaminated supplies.

Standard 10

Anesthesia care shall be assessed to ensure its quality and contribution to positive patient outcomes

Interpretation. The CRNA shall participate in the ongoing review and evaluation of the quality and appropriateness of anesthesia care. Evaluation shall be performed based on appropriate outcome criteria and reviewed on an ongoing basis. The CRNA shall participate in a continual process of self-evaluation and strive to incorporate new techniques and knowledge into practice.

Application to Office Practice. The CRNA shall participate in assessment and review of appropriateness of anesthesia care provided in the office setting. There should be a process to document patient satisfaction and outcomes.

Standard 11

The CRNA shall respect and maintain the basic rights of patients

Interpretation. The CRNA shall support and preserve the rights of patients to personal dignity and ethical norms of practice.

Application to Office Practice. The CRNA shall act as the patient advocate. The patient has the right to dignity, respect, and consideration of legitimate concerns in the office setting. Patients should be involved with all aspects of their care.

APPENDIX 43-B: MINIMUM ELEMENTS FOR PROVIDING ANESTHESIA SERVICES IN THE OFFICE-BASED PRACTICE SETTING–ASSESSMENT CHECKLIST*

Practitioners

Certified Registered Nurse Anesthetists

- ☐ Will the Board of Nursing and state laws allow the certified registered nurse anesthetist (CRNA) to work with this physician type?
- ☐ Will your liability insurance cover office anesthesia?
- ☐ Does the state have rules or regulations specific to the office-based anesthesia?
- ☐ What classes of patients, types of surgical procedures, and anesthesia will be performed?

Operating Physician

- ☐ Does the physician have liability coverage, current licensure, and DEA number?
- ☐ Does the physician have hospital privileges for procedures?
- ☐ Does the physician have admitting privileges at the nearest hospital?

Facility

- ☐ Is the facility licensed?
- ☐ By whom? Indicate name:______________________
- ☐ Is the facility accredited?
- ☐ By whom? Indicate name:______________________
- ☐ Operating room (OR)–size recovery room, preoperative area adequate for anesthesia and surgical procedures?
- ☐ Is there a transfer agreement?
- ☐ Does the facility have an emergency service agreement?
- ☐ Telephone numbers accessible and posted (e.g., emergency medical service, malignant hyperthermia hotline, hospital)?

Equipment

Local, Intravenous Sedation, Regional, and General Anesthesia

- ☐ Monitors include pulse oximeter, electrocardiograph, blood pressure monitor
- ☐ Oxygen supplies: a minimum of two oxygen sources must be available, with regulators attached
- ☐ Positive pressure ventilation sources including an Ambu bag and a mouth-to-mask unit
- ☐ Defibrillator (charged)
- ☐ Suction machine, tubing, suction catheters, and Yankauer suctions
- ☐ Anesthesia cart to provide for organization of supplies including endotracheal equipment, masks, airways, syringes, needles, intravenous catheters, intravenous fluids and tubing, alcohol, stethoscopes, and appropriate medications
- ☐ Emergency medication to include at a minimum, atropine, epinephrine, ephedrine, lidocaine, diphenhydramine, cortisone, and a bronchial dilator inhaler.

General Anesthesia

- ☐ An authorized factory technician or qualified service personnel has checked out anesthesia machine(s).

The following items are available as an integral part of the anesthesia machine:

- ☐ O_2 fail-safe system
- ☐ Waste gas exhaust system
- ☐ Vaporizers–calibration and exclusion system
- ☐ Pulse oximeter, electrocardiogram, blood pressure monitors
- ☐ Oxygen analyzer
- ☐ End-tidal carbon dioxide (CO_2) analyzer
- ☐ Alarm system

Emergencies

- ☐ Emergency equipment
  - ☐ Basic airway equipment (adult and pediatric)
    - ☐ Nasal and oral airway
    - ☐ Face mask (appropriate for patient)
    - ☐ Laryngoscopes, ET tubes (adult and pediatric)
    - ☐ Ambu bag
  - ☐ Difficult airway equipment (LMA, light wand, cricothyrotomy kit)
  - ☐ Supplemental oxygen (O_2)
  - ☐ Suction equipment (suction catheter, Yankauer type)
  - ☐ Defibrillator
  - ☐ Compression board
- ☐ Emergency drugs
- ☐ Drugs and equipment to treat malignant hyperthermia on site
- ☐ Backup power

Pharmaceutical Accountability

- ☐ Is there an appropriate mechanism for documenting and tracking use of pharmaceuticals, including controlled substances?
- ☐ Lock box
- ☐ Count sheets
- ☐ Expiration checklist or policy

*Part of the AANA *Standards for Office-Based Anesthesia Practice*.

- ☐ Drug Enforcement Agency (DEA) 222 forms
- ☐ Waste policy

Policies, Procedures, and Protocols

Are There Policies or Protocols Regarding the Following?

- ☐ Preoperative lab requirements
- ☐ Nothing-by-mouth (NPO) status
- ☐ Case cancellations
- ☐ Malignant hyperthermia
- ☐ Pediatric drug dosages
- ☐ Patient selection
- ☐ Discharge criteria
- ☐ Advanced cardiac life support (ACLS) algorithms
- ☐ Latex allergy protocols
- ☐ Emergency
  - ☐ Cardiopulmonary
  - ☐ Fire
  - ☐ Bomb threat
  - ☐ Chemical spill
  - ☐ Building evacuation
- ☐ Reporting adverse reactions
- ☐ Infection control in adherence to Occupational Safety and Health Administration (OSHA) rules for control of medical waste, disposal of sharps, and personal protection

Record Keeping

- ☐ Is there a system for record keeping for patients and providers?
  - ☐ Anesthesia record
  - ☐ Credentials
  - ☐ Patient satisfaction and follow-up
  - ☐ Purchasing agreements
  - ☐ Consent forms
  - ☐ Quality assurance mechanism
  - ☐ Preanesthesia equipment and supplies

Personnel

OR

☐ RN ☐ LPN ☐ OR tech

PACU

☐ RN ☐ LPN ☐ Anesthetist or Surgeon

ACLS Certified

☐ Surgeon ☐ Anesthetist ☐ RN

BCLS Certified

☐ RN ☐ LPN ☐ Others

APPENDIX 43-C: SAMPLE OFFICE ANESTHESIA POLICIES*

Policy 1—Organization of Anesthesia Services

Purpose. To establish the extent of anesthesia coverage, identify the mechanism of credentialing of anesthesia providers, and establish the responsibilities of the physician director of anesthesia services and the certified registered nurse anesthetist (CRNA) director of anesthesia services.

A. Anesthesia staff will be involved in the monitoring of all patients who undergo surgical, diagnostic, or other invasive procedures and receive general, spinal, or other major regional anesthesia and/or intravenous (IV), intramuscular (IM), or inhalation sedation or analgesia that, in the manner used, may result in the loss of the patient's protective reflexes.

B. Anesthesia staff will provide anesthesia services in the office surgical facility for scheduled procedures and during a reasonable recovery period after surgery.

C. CRNAs providing anesthesia care shall have the following on file: a current registered nurse (RN) license, nurse anesthetist specialty certification, certification or recertification by the Council on Certification of the American Association of Nurse Anesthetists; (AANA) a clinical privileges delineation form approved by the medical staff; and verification of professional liability insurance.

D. The CRNA director of anesthesia services in collaboration with the surgeon has responsibility for the following:
   1. Making recommendations regarding the clinical privileges of all anesthesia providers
   2. Participating with office staff to formulate mechanisms to provide a uniform quality of anesthesia services throughout the hospital, including
      a. Mechanisms designated to ensure that anesthesia services are consistent with patient needs and with current knowledge concerning anesthesia practice
      b. Recommendations concerning the type and amount of physical resources necessary for administering anesthesia and for providing any necessary resuscitative measures
      c. Approaches to effectively monitor and evaluate the quality of anesthesia care provided by all staff
      d. Guidelines for anesthesia safety
      e. Validation of continuing education for all individuals who provide anesthesia services

Policy 2—Anesthesia Safety Guidelines

Purpose. To provide mechanisms for the availability, maintenance, and use of devices and protocols designed to promote patient and staff safety during anesthesia.

A. Only nonflammable anesthetic gases will be used.

B. Anesthesia machines and attached monitors will be checked and preventive maintenance performed annually by qualified anesthesia maintenance persons.

C. When the anesthesia machine is used for general anesthesia, the following safety devices will be used:
   1. Oxygen analyzer
   2. Pressure and disconnect alarm
   3. Pin-index safety system
   4. Gas scavenging system
   5. Oxygen pressure interlock system

D. The CRNA will check the readiness, availability, cleanliness, and working condition of anesthesia equipment (before use) and document on the preanesthesia checklist. (The checklist will be kept for 2 years.) Any defects found in such testing that are not easily correctable should be reported to the Director of Anesthesia. Major repairs to anesthesia apparatus are to be done only by persons thoroughly familiar with such apparatus. If a patient is injured as a result of a machine malfunction, the involved equipment will be taken out of service and not reused until the malfunction is identified and repaired and the incident has been reported to the manufacturer and appropriate regulatory agencies.

*Developed by Donna J Smith, CRNA, MSA; Luanne Stencil, CRNA, MA; and Jeanne Learman, CRNA, MS for their office practices in Michigan.

E. Anesthesia machines, monitors, and supplies will be available to ensure the ability to monitor the patient according to the guidelines of the AANA and the American Society of Anesthesiologists (ASA).
F. Resuscitative equipment, supplies, and medications will be available to provide cardiopulmonary resuscitation (CPR) according to the guidelines of the American Heart Association, that is, advanced cardiac life support algorithms.
G. Resuscitative equipment, supplies, and medications will be available to treat malignant hyperthermia according to guidelines developed by the Malignant Hyperthermia Association of the United States. If triggering agents are used, a minimum of 12 vials of dantrolene will be available.

Policy 3—Patient Selection Criteria for Office Anesthesia Services

Patients will be considered for anesthesia care in the office if they are

1. Eighteen years of age or older. Patients who are 17 years of age or younger will be considered on an individual basis.
2. In good general health. Patients with mild to moderate medical problems will be considered on an individual basis if the condition is stable or the patient has received preoperative clearance by his or her regular physician, an internist, or other appropriate physician. Patients with significant medical problems may be cared for in the office setting with local or topical anesthesia and monitored anesthesia care (MAC) (e.g., cataract surgery).

Patients will *not* be considered for anesthesia services if they

1. Have uncontrolled hypertension, unstable diabetes, or angina.
2. Have a history of an unstable psychiatric disorder. *NOTE: Patients who are taking monoamine oxidase inhibitor (MAO) drugs must discontinue these drugs at least 2 weeks before surgery. This must be cleared in writing by the patient's psychiatrist. If discontinuance of MAO inhibitor is prohibited by the psychiatrist in the best interest of the patient, this patient will not be considered under any circumstance.*
3. Have undergone cardiac surgery within the last six months or continue to have unstable hypertension, angina, or dysrhythmia.
4. Have significantly abnormal liver function studies with diagnosed liver disease.
5. Have a known coagulopathy that is unstable or uncontrollable by medication.
6. Have a moderately to severely compromised pulmonary status.
7. Have an unstable or moderate to severe neuromuscular disorder (multiple sclerosis patients in remission will be considered on an individual basis).
8. Have a significant airway anatomic abnormality or a known history of difficult airway control or ventilation.
9. Are morbidly obese.

Policy 4—Preanesthesia Evaluation

Purpose. To determine the capacity of the patient to undergo anesthesia. To determine the overall condition of the patient through the patient's history, physical examination, and laboratory and other studies. To use this information to optimize the preparation of the patient for anesthesia. To select the most appropriate anesthetic based on the patient's condition, the surgical procedure to be performed, and the patient's preference.

A. Every patient will have a preanesthesia evaluation before administration of general, spinal, other major regional anesthesia or IV, IM, or inhalation sedation or analgesia that, in the manner used, may result in the loss of the patients' protective reflexes. This evaluation will include
   1. Current medications
   2. A review of complications of previous anesthetics and allergies
   3. A review of the patient's physical status with particular attention paid to anatomic abnormalities that could affect the administration of anesthesia: cardiac status, respiratory status, blood pressure, and airway anatomy
   4. A review of pertinent laboratory testing and other studies as indicated by the preanesthesia testing policy

Patients with significant cardiopulmonary disease or other systemic disease will obtain a clearance from their primary physician

A. Nothing by mouth (NPO) instructions:
   1. Routinely, patients scheduled for elective surgery and general, regional, or intravenous sedation anesthesia are instructed to be NPO after midnight the night before surgery.
   2. The following exceptions are appropriate:
      a. Patients may take necessary medications (e.g., antihypertensive medication) the morning of surgery with a sip of water.
      b. For children, for patients scheduled late in the day, and for those concerned about going without liquids, clear liquids (water, weak coffee, tea) may be consumed in small quantities up to 2 hours before surgery.
      c. For emergency surgeries when the patient has a "full stomach," a decision must be made jointly by the surgeon and the anesthetist regarding when to proceed with the anesthesia. The urgency of the surgery versus the risk of aspiration will be considered. If possible, the patient will be NPO for solid foods at least 6 hours and for liquids at least 2 hours before general anesthesia or major regional anesthesia.

B. Anesthesia plan:
   1. The anesthetist will discuss the anesthetic choices and probable risks with the patient and answer the patient's questions. Medications to be taken and held the morning of surgery will be discussed.
   2. The anesthetist will verify that the surgical and anesthesia consent form is signed.
   3. Immediately before anesthesia the patient is reevaluated and a determination is made that the patient is an appropriate candidate to undergo the planned anesthesia.
   4. The CRNA indicates the concurrence of the surgeon or physician with the anesthesia plan (i.e., general, regional, local, or IV sedation).

Policy 5—Preanesthesia Testing Policy

A. Patients who will have anesthesia services intraoperatively must have a preoperative hemoglobin test if they are menstruating females or are over age 60 (male or female) or if significant blood loss is anticipated. Those patients whose hemoglobin is below 10 will be considered on an individual basis.
B. The following tests should be considered when certain conditions exist:
   1. Age over 60 years: electrocardiogram (ECG), complete blood count (CBC)
   2. Diabetes, when patient is taking insulin: ECG, blood urea nitrogen (BUN), electrolytes, finger-stick glucose test immediately preoperatively and in postanesthesia care unit (PACU)

3. Hypertension: ECG, BUN, creatinine, electrolytes
4. Diuretic use: electrolytes
5. Heart disease: ECG, chest x-ray examination, CBC, BUN, creatinine, electrolytes; stress test or echocardiogram based on history
6. Pneumonia within last 6 months, emphysema, lung disease: chest x-ray examination, pulmonary function tests if indicated
7. Bleeding disorder, anticoagulant usage: coagulation studies
8. Reasonable possibility of pregnancy: pregnancy test
9. History of heavy alcohol use or other liver disease: liver function tests
10. History of renal disease: BUN, creatinine, electrolytes

C. Other tests may be required at the discretion of the CRNA.
D. Less testing may be required if procedure is minimally invasive and will be performed with local, topical, or minimal IV sedation (e.g., cataract surgery).

Policy 6–Intraoperative and Postoperative Anesthetic Management

Purpose. To provide guidelines for intraoperative anesthetic management, transfer to postanesthetic care, and postanesthetic follow-up.

A. The surgeon must be in the surgical facility before anesthesia may be induced.
B. The anesthesia care plan shall be skillfully implemented and the plan of care adjusted as needed to adapt to the patient's response to the anesthetic.
C. The patient's physiologic condition shall be monitored consistent with both the type of anesthesia care and specific patient needs. The patient will be monitored according to the AANA patient monitoring standards and the ASA monitoring standards.
D. There will be prompt, complete, and accurate documentation of pertinent information on the patient's record. Exhibit I from "Documenting the Standard of Care: the Anesthesia Record" (AANA, *Professional Practice Manual*) will be used as a guideline.
E. The responsibility for the care of the patient will be transferred to other qualified providers in a manner that ensures continuity of care and patient safety. The anesthetist will report all essential information to the personnel assuming responsibility for the care of the patient. Exhibit II F from "Documenting the Standard of Care: the Anesthesia Record" (AANA, *Professional Practice Manual*) will be used as a guideline.
F. A postanesthesia note that documents any adverse outcome related to anesthesia will be entered on the patient record within 48 hours.

Policy 7–Anesthesia Infection Control

Purpose. To define safety precautions to be taken to minimize the risk of infection for the patient, anesthetist, and other staff.

A. Universal blood and body fluid precautions will be used during anesthesia and related patient care activities.
B. The *Infection Control Guide* developed by the AANA will be used as a guideline for infection control practices related to anesthesia administration.
    1. Anesthesia machine components, ancillary instruments, medical devices, and accessory equipment that are in direct contact with a patient's blood or mucous membranes shall be cleaned, disinfected, and sterilized as recommended by the original manufacturer, before reuse. Items should be sterile if they enter a sterile area of the body. Items should be sterile or processed with a high-level disinfection technique if they make contact with mucous membranes. Items should be cleaned or processed with an intermediate or low-level disinfection technique if they come in contact with intact skin. Items that are soiled by blood or body fluids or exposed to blood-borne pathogens should be treated with high-level disinfection technique before reuse.
    2. A disposable bacterial filter with bacterial and viral removal efficiency greater than 99.999% will be positioned in the patient's breathing circuit at the Y-piece connection in such a manner as to efficiently entrap pathogenic particulate material from both the inspiratory and expiratory sides of the system and the sampling line of the respiratory gas monitor. The bacterial filter and mask will not be reused after the first patient exposure. The breathing circuit and breathing bag may be reused for subsequent patients so long as it is physically intact and passes the preanesthesia leak test.
    3. Disposal of regulated waste: disposable breathing circuits, rebreathing bags, airways, and any other accessory items contaminated during anesthesia shall be considered as regulated waste and placed in color-coded containers (in accordance with Occupational Safety and Health Administration [OSHA] standards) that are closeable and constructed to prevent leakage of fluids during handling, storage, transport, and shipping.

Policy 8–Waste Anesthetic Gases

Purpose. To minimize risk to operating room personnel of trace anesthetic gas exposure.

A. Waste gas scavenging systems shall be used for evacuating waste anesthetic gases from anesthetizing locations in which inhalation anesthetics are used.
B. Operation of the ventilation and air-conditioning system used in the surgical suite will be tested annually to ensure that complete room air exchanges occur at a rate of 15 times per hour or more.
C. Every effort will be made to minimize total exposure and keep waste anesthetics below recommended limits set forth by National Institute for Occupational Safety and Health (NIOSH): no more than 2 ppm over an 8-hour period of any halogenated agent, and no more than 25 ppm of nitrous oxide over an 8-hour period measured as a time-weighted average (TWA). Work practices to minimize exposure include the following:
    1. Avoid turning on nitrous oxide or any halogenated agent until the face mask is securely fitted to the patient's face.
    2. Avoid unnecessary disconnection of the breathing circuit. Empty the rebreathing bag into the waste gas scavenging system before disconnecting the breathing circuit from the patient.
    3. Administer 100% oxygen, when possible, before removing the mask or tracheal tube from patient.
    4. Conduct all leak tests using oxygen only.
    5. Avoid spilling anesthetic agent when filling calibrated vaporizers. Use key-filling mechanism if possible.
    6. Avoid sniffing the anesthetic agent. (The odor threshold for liquid anesthetic agents has been reported to be approximately 50 ppm.)

Policy 9—Anesthesia Continuous Quality Improvement

Purpose. To provide mechanisms to continuously review and improve the quality of anesthesia care and to provide a uniform quality of care throughout the office surgical facility.

A. Organization
   1. The director of anesthesia will coordinate functions for quality improvement (QI) for the anesthesia services.
   2. Data will be collected by each anesthetist for those cases in which he or she administers an anesthetic.
   3. Findings and actions concerning positive indicators will be reviewed and appropriate actions taken.

B. Comprehension
   The QI program will collect data on a broad range of anesthesia activities, including
   1. Preanesthesia evaluation and other preinduction activities
   2. Preexisting conditions
   3. Patient monitoring
   4. Anesthesia documentation
   5. Unusual, unexpected, or unplanned patient events during the perianesthesia period

C. QI activities
   1. Unusual, unexpected, or unplanned patient events (positive indicators) will be identified on the QI collection instrument and will require a narrative description of the event by the anesthetist involved.
   2. The postoperative note will include an assessment of patient status or outcome as it relates to the identified positive indicator.
   3. Thresholds for evaluation of positive indicators will be established by the anesthesia staff and based on internal statistics.
   4. Actions will be taken to improve care or to correct the identified problems.
   5. QI activities will be suggested by, implemented and evaluated by the anesthesia QI committee (QIC). All anesthesia staff members are members of the QIC.
   6. Checklist (see Box 43-5) will be completed annually to assess the capability of the surgical facility to provide safe and comprehensive care.

Policy 10—Postanesthesia Care

Purpose. To provide guidelines for postanesthesia care.

A. Patients undergoing operative, therapeutic, or invasive procedures under anesthesia shall be taken to the PACU before discharge. The PACU nurse will check readiness, availability, cleanliness, and working condition of equipment and supplies before arrival of the patient in the PACU.

B. In the absence of specific orders, routine PACU care shall be given to each patient:
   1. Begin initial assessment immediately on patient's arrival in PACU and include breath sounds, level of consciousness, oxygen saturation, blood pressure, pain level, dressings, drains, and condition of IV sites. Patients undergoing regional anesthesia will have motor and sensory levels monitored and documented.
   2. Monitor and document blood pressure, pulse, respirations, and pulse oximetry at least every 15 minutes until patient is discharged from PACU.
   3. Monitor electrocardiogram if
      a. The patient has a history of cardiac events
      b. The patient exhibits cardiac changes during the surgical procedure
      c. The best interest of the patient so indicates, at the discretion of the PACU RN
      d. The patient's condition deteriorates
      e. The attending physician or anesthetist requests monitoring
   4. Maintain an IV (except on order of responsible practitioner to discontinue IV). Add normal saline or lactated Ringer's solution as indicated.
   5. Suction secretions from oral and nasopharynx, nasogastric, and endotracheal tubes whenever indicated and after the removal of the tubes.
   6. Maintain normothermia to the extent possible: use active rewarming unit if necessary. Check the temperature of patients who receive general anesthesia, patients with an infection, and any patient who, in the RN's judgment, may be hyperthermic or hypothermic.
   7. Document any medications given, oxygen therapy, and changes from initial assessment.

C. The PACU nurse will be prepared to administer the following treatments/medications as indicated. These usually will be instituted in collaboration with the physician or anesthetist. If the urgency of a situation necessitates it, the treatment will be started while the physician or anesthetist is being notified.
   1. Oxygen therapy to maintain arterial oxygen saturation (SaO_2) greater than 94%: nasal cannula (2 to 6 L/min), mask (6 to 10 L/min), mouth-to-mask unit, or Ambu bag (15 L/min).
   2. Placement of an IV line or addition of fluids to existing intravenous line (5% dextrose in lactated Ringer's, lactated Ringer's, or normal saline).
   3. Administration of emergency medications as indicated, for example, atropine 0.4 to 1 mg IV when indicated for symptomatic bradycardia (e.g., bradycardia with hypotension or premature ventricular contractions [PVCs]), naloxone 0.1 to 1 mg IV when indicated to reverse respiratory depression from narcotics.
   4. CPR procedures when indicated. The PACU nurse must maintain current basic cardiac life support (BCLS) certification.

D. Criteria for discharge from PACU:
   1. Vital signs are stable, including temperature, pulse, respiration and blood pressure. Vital signs should remain stable (e.g., blood pressure ±20 mm Hg) for a period of not less than 30 minutes and be consistent with patient's age and preanesthesia levels.
   2. Patient has regained protective reflexes (e.g., can cough and swallow).
   3. Ability to ambulate: the patient demonstrates the ability to perform movement consistent with age and development level (sit, stand, walk).
   4. Bleeding is minimal or nonexistent.
   5. Nausea and vomiting are minimal.
   6. Alert and oriented: the patient is aware of surroundings and what has taken place and is interested in returning home, or level of consciousness has returned to preoperative level.
   7. Pain is controlled.
   8. Ability to void: *only* for patients who have received spinal or epidural anesthesia or have undergone pelvic or pelvic-related surgery.
   9. Oxygen saturation is 94% or greater in room air.
   10. Minimum of 30 minutes has elapsed since administration of IV analgesics or sedatives.

11. The patient will be discharged by both the anesthetist and the surgeon or their qualified designee.

E. The patient and his or her adult companion will be instructed in postoperative home care and will be given information on how to contact surgical center staff.

Policy 11—Dispensing and Accounting for Controlled Drugs

Purpose. To provide a standard for the accounting for and the administration of narcotic and federally controlled drugs.

A. In accordance with federal law, controlled drugs are locked in a designated and secured cabinet in the operating room. Each unit dose removed is immediately signed out on the controlled drug administration record.
B. Narcotic keys will be kept in the possession of an RN at all times.
C. Once per week the CRNA and RN will verify the physical count of controlled drugs and initial the audit record. Any discrepancies in the audit must be investigated immediately.
D. Any signs of tampering with the narcotics or narcotics box are immediately reported to the practice administrator or physician.

Policy 12—Guidelines for the use of Local Anesthetics

Listed below are local anesthetics used in the operating room, along with guidelines for determining safe, maximum doses over a relatively short duration. The dose in milligrams in a percentage is always the same, regardless of the drug (e.g., 1% always has 10 mg/ml). Examples of commonly used dose percentages used in the operating room are as follows:

- 0.25% = 2.5 mg/ml
- 0.5% = 5 mg/ml
- 1% = 10 mg/ml
- 2% = 20 mg/ml

Cocaine

Cocaine is used for topical application only, *not for injection*! Maximum is approximately 200 mg or 4 ml of 5%.

It is necessary to have twice the maximum dose of cocaine on the field because it is applied by applicators, packs, or NuGauze strips (tightly wrung out). It is estimated that less than half of the cocaine solution is absorbed from the packs. If any of the cocaine is unused it must be disposed of in front of two persons, one of whom is an RN.

- Symptoms of overdose: CNS stimulation, vasomotor collapse, restlessness, hyperactivity, and hallucinations
- Treatment of overdose: give IV tranquilizers (e.g., midazolam (Versed), diazepam (Valium), thiopental (Pentothal)

Lidocaine

Lidocaine is an amide local anesthetic. Maximum recommended dose with epinephrine equals approximately 7 mg/kg or 500 mg. Maximum recommended dose without epinephrine equals 4.5 mg/kg or 300 mg. When using the tumescent technique with dilute lidocaine 0.05% with epinephrine 1:1,000,000, doses up to 35 mg/kg have been used without lidocaine toxicity.[44]

Bupivacaine

Bupivacaine is an injectable local anesthetic that is approximately twice as toxic as lidocaine on a milligram per milligram basis. It is also an amide, as is lidocaine, and has an *additive* effect when used with lidocaine, rather than resulting in two separate maximum amounts (e.g., 115 mg of bupivacaine with 250 mg of lidocaine has approximately the same toxicity as 500 mg of lidocaine). The maximum dose is approximately 225 mg.

APPENDIX 43-D: PREOPERATIVE MEDICATION GUIDELINES (FOR USE BY SURGERY FACILITY STAFF)

Note: Patients should take medications as regularly scheduled with a small sip of water on the day of surgery as follows:

1. Acetaminophen (Tylenol): may be taken as needed.
2. Antibiotics: should be continued unless drug causes gastrointestinal upset; notify surgeon if withheld.
3. Anticoagulants (warfarin, heparin, dipyridamole, ticlopidine, aspirin): should be reviewed with primary care physician, because some should be held for several days before surgery, depending on the indication for use.
4. Anticonvulsants (phenytoin, carbamazepine, gabapentin): measurement of drug level needed within 30 days if patient has had a seizure in past year.
5. Antidepressants or antianxiety medications: should be taken, unless medication is a monoamine oxidase (MAO) inhibitor, which should be held for 14 days before surgery. Benzodiazepines such as diazepam, alprazolam, or lorazepam should be taken if customarily used regularly.
6. Antihistamines: may be taken as usual.
7. Antihypertensives: diuretics should be held, all others should be taken unless blood pressure <100 systolic.
8. Anti-Parkinson's medication: all can be taken, including selegiline (avoid meperidine with this medication).
9. Antipsychotics (e.g., haloperidol , risperidone, clozapine): may be taken.
10. Antacid or antireflux agents (e.g., ranitidine, famotidine, esomeprazole, omeprazole): should definitely be taken, but liquids such as Maalox or Mylanta should be avoided.
11. Bronchodilators (e.g., metered-dose inhalers, inhaled steroids): should definitely be taken the day of surgery.
12. Cardiac medications (i.e., digoxin, β-blockers, calcium channel blockers, and nitroglycerin [any form]): should be taken as usual.
13. Chemotherapy or immunosuppressants (methotrexate, azathioprine, cyclosporine): should be taken as usual unless they cause gastrointestinal upset.
14. Diabetes medications: oral hypoglycemic agents should not be taken the morning of surgery. May be taken postoperatively as eating resumes.
15. Eyedrops: if not undergoing eye surgery, patient may take per usual routine; if undergoing eye surgery, patient should follow ophthalmologist's orders.
16. Hormones and oral contraceptives: may be taken as usual.
17. Insulin: if patient has insulin-dependent diabetes, the anesthetist or surgeon should contact the patient's primary care physician to determine if patient is well controlled enough to have the surgery in an office setting and should get specific instructions about insulin administration. Patients should bring their own glucose meter and insulin.
18. Muscle relaxants: should be avoided if possible.
19. Narcotic analgesics: chronic maintenance dose should be continued; narcotics should be avoided unless absolutely necessary.
20. Nicotine patches: may be continued as usual.
21. Nose sprays: may be continued as usual.

22. Steroids: dose and whether to cover with stress dose steroids should be reviewed with primary care physician.
23. Vitamins, mineral supplements: should be held on day of surgery.
24. Herbals: should be stopped 7 days before surgery

NOTE This information sheet is not to be distributed to patients. If in doubt regarding type of medication or whether to hold, ask surgeon, anesthetist, or primary care physician.

APPENDIX 43-E: SAMPLE LETTERS AND FORMS

Sample Patient Letter with Preanesthesia Instructions

About Intravenous Sedation. . .

Dr. Jones has arranged with Office Anesthesia Associates to provide a service for selected patients to receive intravenous sedative medications before and during their surgical (or dental) procedure. This facilitates your surgical care by increasing your comfort during the procedure and allowing your surgeon to devote full attention to the details of your procedure.

You will be cared for by a Certified Registered Nurse Anesthetist (CRNA). Nurse anesthetists are specialists in providing anesthesia care and work closely with your physician to provide safe, high-quality anesthesia care.

Following is some pertinent information regarding the anesthesia for your procedure.

Before

1. The nurse anesthetist will call you 1 or 2 days before the procedure to review important health history information and the anesthesia care plan.
2. Make arrangements for a reliable adult to drive you home. *You will not be permitted to drive yourself home or take a cab by yourself.*
3. Do not eat solid food or drink milk during the 8 hours before your procedure. For late day surgeries, you may have small sips of water, black coffee, tea, or apple juice up to 3 hours before surgery. Morning medications or preoperative medications may be taken with a small sip of water. The CRNA may refuse to provide anesthesia services if these guidelines are not followed.
4. Do not smoke (including marijuana), drink alcohol, or use recreational drugs for 48 hours before your surgery.
5. Please take any medications as previously discussed with your physician and CRNA. If you have diabetes, your insulin dosage may be adjusted. Please bring your insulin and glucometer to the office with you on the day of your surgery.
6. Do not wear makeup, hair clips, jewelry, or a watch the day of your surgery. If you have nonremovable body jewelry, notify your CRNA. Please leave all valuables at home.
7. If you wear contact lenses, please leave them at home and wear your glasses.
8. Wear loose-fitting and comfortable clothing with tops that button or zip down the front. Warm socks are recommended. Women, please do not wear pantyhose or high-heeled shoes. Remove nail polish from left thumb or index finger and big toe nails to allow access for the blood oxygen sensor clip.
9. If you become ill between now and the time of your surgery, please contact your surgeon.

During

The nurse anesthetist will be in constant attendance. An intravenous line will be placed to give you fluids and medications. During your procedure the nurse anesthetist continually assesses your response to the sedation and will monitor blood pressure, heart rate, respirations, oxygen saturation, and electrocardiogram (commonly called an *ECG*). Only minimal changes in vital signs are expected during your procedure.

After

All procedures will require a recovery period. The length of time will vary depending on the nature of the procedure. Do not drive your car or any motorized vehicle the evening of your procedure. Although most of the sedative medication effects wear off quickly (within 1 to 2 hours), some minimal residual effects may impair your judgment or coordination. Therefore a responsible adult *must* drive you home.

Begin your food intake gradually. Start with sips of liquids and then soft foods. You may experience some discomfort after the procedure. Please follow the instructions carefully for pain medication. Using extra-strength Tylenol instead of the prescription pain medication will lessen your chances of postoperative nausea.

Sample Discharge Instructions

To be printed as a duplicate form: one copy to patient's chart. Please follow the instructions checked below.

1. General Anesthesia or Sedation

☐ Do not drive or operate machinery until instructed by doctor to do so. Do not consume alcohol, tranquilizers, sleeping medications, or any nonprescription medications for 24 hours. You will need to have an adult stay with you for the first night after surgery and drive you in for your follow-up appointment the next day.

2. Activity

☐ You are advised to go directly home. Restrict your activities and rest for a day. Do not engage in strenuous activity that may place stress on your incision.

☐ Special activity instructions:______________________________

3. Fluids and Diet

You'll feel better if you can eat and drink as soon as you are well enough.

☐ Begin with clear liquids, bouillon, dry toast, or soda crackers.

☐ If you are not nauseated, you may go to a regular diet. Greasy and spicy foods are not advised for 24 hours.

4. Medications

☐ Medications prescribed:______________________________

☐ When taking pain medications, you may experience dizziness or drowsiness. Do not drink alcohol or drive when you are taking these medications.

☐ You may take a nonprescription "headache remedy" type medication that does not contain aspirin or ibuprofen. Extra-strength Tylenol is suggested in place of prescription medication after 24 hours.

☐ You may resume your daily prescription medications.

5. Care of the Incision

☐ Do not change your dressing, but keep it clean and dry.

☐ Change your dressing when soiled or wet.

☐ You may shower and wash incision once dressing is removed.

☐ Apply ice bag or ☐ Swiss therapy______times per day for_____ minutes.

☐ Special instructions:______________________________

6. Tubes and Drains

☐ You are being discharged with a______________________________

☐ Empty the drain every________hours (see instruction sheet).

☐ Measure and record the drainage when you empty the drain. Bring these measurements to the doctor's office on your next visit along with used and unused drain tubes.

7. Compression Garment or Bra

☐ Wear the garment for________hours/day for________days.

☐ Special instructions:______________________________

8. Positioning

☐ Elevate________above the level of your heart to lessen swelling and discomfort.

☐ Keep arms elevated on pillow across chest

☐ Special instructions:______________________________

9. Complications

Call your surgeon if any of the following occur:

Fever over 100° F taken by mouth or 101° F taken rectally.
Pain not relieved by medication prescribed.
Blood-soaked dressing (small amounts of oozing may be normal).
Inability to urinate or completely empty your bladder.
Nausea and vomiting lasting longer than 24 hours.
Numbness, tingling, or cold fingers or toes.
Swelling around incision.
One side that becomes much larger than the other.
Increasing or continuous drainage from incision or examination site.
Increased redness, warmth, or hardness around incision area.

10. Follow-up Care

Within the first 24 to 48 hours after surgery, a representative may call you to check on your postoperative progress. Call your doctor's office for a follow-up appointment. Call your doctor if you have any questions or concerns.

11. Additional Instructions

____

____

If you need immediate attention, come to our emergency department or any hospital near your home.

I acknowledge receipt of the above discharge instructions:

____

Patient or Guardian Signature:____________________ Date:______

Registered Nurse Signature:____________________ Date:______

CHAPTER 44

Obstetric Anesthesia

Michael A. Fiedler

The anesthesia community has a long-standing history of valuable contributions to the care of pregnant patients. Approaches to pain relief during labor and delivery are continually being refined and updated in an effort to provide a comfortable and safe environment for the parturient. This chapter discusses the most current concepts in anesthesia care of the obstetric patient.

ANATOMY AND PHYSIOLOGY DURING NORMAL PREGNANCY

Physiologic changes in pregnancy fall into two categories: (1) those related to increased metabolic demands, that is, metabolic rate, oxygen (O_2) consumption, carbon dioxide (CO_2) production, cardiac output, and alveolar ventilation; and (2) anatomic changes.

Cardiovascular Changes

Myocardial Function

During pregnancy the heart enlarges and ventricular walls thicken. End-diastolic volume increases. By 24 to 32 weeks' gestation, cardiac output increases up to 50% above nonpregnant baseline. Considerable variability exists in baseline maternal cardiac output during the third trimester. Cardiac output increases even further immediately after delivery because of increases in heart rate (HR) and contractility. Cardiac output has been reported to be 0.76 ± 0.33 L/min (mean ± SD, $P = .027$) higher in nulliparous than in multiparous women.[1] Venous return (preload) increases because of an increase in plasma volume and, at delivery, because of an autotransfusion of blood from the contracting uterus. Pregnant women have greater baroreflex-mediated changes in HR at term than at 6 to 8 weeks postpartum.[2] This increase in baroreceptor responsiveness persists for even longer periods after delivery in some women.[3]

Maternal HR is increased at term compared with the nonpregnant state. In one study HR increased from 87 ± 2 beats per minute (bpm) (mean ± SD) at 10 to 18 weeks' gestation to 92 ± 1 bpm at 34 to 42 weeks' gestation (a 5.7% increase).[1] In another the increase was 17%, from 71 ± 10 bpm (nonpregnant) to 83 ± 10 bpm (term pregnant) (mean ± SD, $P < .05$).[4]

Several changes in heart sounds occur during pregnancy. Early closure of the mitral valve may cause a split first heart sound. A third heart sound can be heard in most women by 20 weeks' gestation. A benign grade I or grade II systolic murmur is also common. Diastolic murmurs are pathologic.

Blood Volume

Maternal blood volume increases to between 85 and 100 ml/kg at term. Increases occur in both plasma volume (50%) and red blood cell mass (up to 20%). Because the increase in plasma volume is greater than the increase in red blood cell volume, a relative (dilutional) anemia occurs. This results in reduced blood viscosity and in normal hemoglobin and hematocrit values of approximately 12 g and 35%, respectively.

Vasculature

Systemic vascular resistance (SVR) decreases as much as 21% by term pregnancy owing in large part to decreased resistance in the uteroplacental, pulmonary, renal, and cutaneous vascular beds.[1,4] Baseline central sympathetic outflow is twice as high in normal term pregnant women as in nonpregnant women.[5] The venous capacitance system loses tone, allowing pooling of the larger blood volume. Overall, systolic blood pressure changes little during normal pregnancy. A decrease in diastolic blood pressure of up to 15 mm Hg may occur, resulting in a decrease in mean pressure.

Renin

The pregnant woman is more dependent on the renin-angiotensin system for maintenance of blood pressure than her nonpregnant counterpart.[6] Plasma levels of renin and angiotensin II are increased during pregnancy[7] despite the increase in blood volume. Baseline plasma renin activity in the third trimester is 12 times greater than that in nonpregnant control women. Vascular sensitivity to angiotensin II is both clinically and statistically significantly reduced in third-trimester pregnant women,[8-10] whereas sensitivity to norepinephrine is unchanged. The magnitude of the reduction in sensitivity to angiotensin varies throughout the day in a diurnal pattern.[11]

Clearly, some dramatic changes occur in both vascular sensitivity to angiotensin II and plasma levels of renin and angiotensin II during pregnancy. What is not known is if a cause-and-effect relationship exists between these changes. Causes become exceedingly important when the effects of epidural anesthesia on renin release are considered. Because the renin-angiotensin system provides support for mean arterial pressure (MAP) in the absence of sympathetic nervous system–controlled vasoconstriction, understanding the cause of reduced vascular sensitivity to and increased plasma levels of angiotensin becomes important in the context of epidural anesthesia and maternal hypotension.

Vasopressin

The clearance of vasopressin at 36 to 38 weeks' gestation is three to four times greater than that observed before pregnancy ($P < .01$).[12] Vasopressinase levels increase by a factor of 50 between early and term pregnancy, likely accounting for the increased clearance rate observed. The vasopressin system is important because it is one of three systems with which the body defends against decreases in MAP.

Aortocaval Compression

In the early 1950s a syndrome of supine hypotension was identified in term or near-term pregnant women.[13,14] This syndrome of supine hypotension is caused by compression of the vena cava by the gravid uterus, which restricts venous return to the heart when the parturient lies in the supine position. Compression is more severe when the abdomen is tense or when the uterus is larger than normal, as in polyhydramnios or multiple gestation. Decreased venous return results in a significant reduction in stroke volume (SV) and cardiac output. Figure 44-1 depicts typical changes in vital signs during supine hypotension. The resultant hypotension can be severe enough to cause loss of consciousness in some women. Maximal decreases in blood pressure may require up to 10 minutes to develop; however, some women experience the decrease almost immediately. The normal physiologic responses to caval compression are tachycardia and vasoconstriction of the lower extremities. Despite this attempted compensation, uterine blood flow and therefore fetal oxygenation are reduced.[15] Figure 44-2 depicts changes in aortocaval compression with changes in position.

In addition to compressing the vena cava, the gravid uterus may compress the abdominal aorta. For this reason supine hypotensive syndrome is more correctly referred to as *aortocaval compression*. When the abdominal aorta is compressed, upper body blood pressure remains relatively normal while blood pressure distal to the L3 to L4 site of aortic compression (uterus and lower extremities) may be significantly reduced. It is by this mechanism that uterine blood flow and therefore fetal oxygenation may suffer, despite the presence of an apparently normal maternal systemic blood pressure.

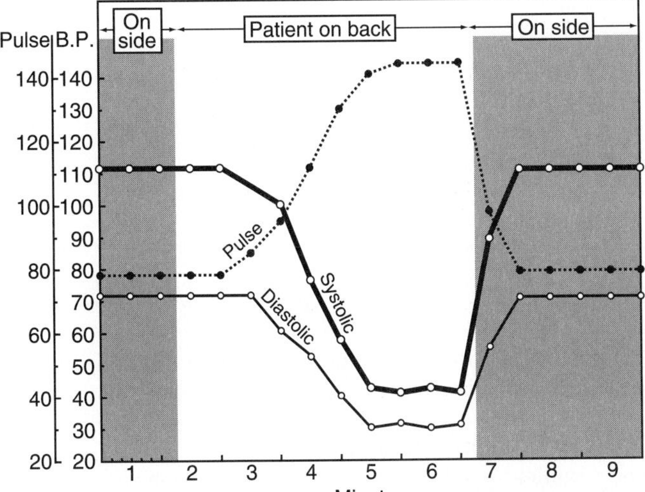

FIGURE **44-1**
Typical vital sign pattern in supine hypotensive syndrome. (From Howard BK, Goodson JH, Mengert WF. Supine hypotensive syndrome in late pregnancy. *Obstet Gynecol.* 1953;1:371-377.)

Compression of the aorta and vena cava can usually be relieved by shifting the uterus to the left (left uterine displacement) or, even more effectively, by lying on the side.[16] Left uterine displacement can be accomplished by rotation of the operating room table 15 degrees to the left or by placing a 15-cm-high wedge under the parturient's right hip and back, as shown in Figure 44-2. Care should be taken to ensure adequate left uterine displacement, as most anesthetists have been shown to underestimate the angle of tilt they have provided.[17] In women with an exceptionally large uterus, greater displacement may be necessary to be effective. In a small percentage of women, right uterine displacement may be more effective than left displacement, although in the majority of cases right uterine displacement results in SVs that are no better than those measured with the patient in the supine position.[16]

Left uterine displacement or the side-lying position is an essential component of obstetric care, especially when labor epidural analgesia (LEA) is administered. LEA defeats compensatory lower-extremity vasoconstriction by blocking the sympathetic nerves responsible for vasoconstriction, resulting in even greater hypotension.

Respiratory Changes

Capillary engorgement at term results in a variable amount of upper airway swelling. Swelling of the false vocal cords may cause narrowing of the glottis. Term pregnancy is accompanied by an increase in O_2 demand of up to 33% at baseline and 100% during the second stage of labor. At term, minute ventilation is increased by 50% because of an increase in both tidal volume (increased by 40%) and respiratory rate (increased by 15%). At term the normal arterial partial pressure of CO_2 ranges from 32 to 35 mm Hg, and the normal arterial partial pressure of O_2 is greater than 100 mm Hg. The functional residual capacity, expiratory reserve, and residual volume are decreased primarily as a result of upward pressure on the diaphragm, with results functionally similar to restrictive lung disease. The decrease in functional residual capacity, an important O_2 reserve, and the increase in O_2 consumption that occur in pregnancy commonly result in rapid arterial desaturation in the apneic pregnant patient, especially if she had been breathing room air before becoming apneic.[18] When the patient is supine, an increase in closing capacity occurs, often resulting in small airway closure before the tidal volume has been exhaled. This is evidenced clinically as wheezing and can result in hypoxia. This mechanism may explain the observation of reduced O_2 saturations in parturients during natural sleep. Compared with nonpregnant controls, whose average oxygen saturation as measured by pulse oximetry (SpO_2) during sleep was 98.5%, healthy near-term pregnant women averaged only 95.2%, with temporary desaturations below 90% being not uncommon.[19]

Coagulation Changes

In general the parturient is said to be "hypercoagulable." Levels of several clotting factors, including platelets and fibrinogen, are increased. The increased levels, when combined with periods of little to no physical activity, place the parturient at risk for deep venous thrombosis. In the nonpregnant state, fibrinogen levels average from 200 to 400 mg/dL. Late in pregnancy, fibrinogen levels are normally at least 400 mg/dL and may be as high as 650 mg/dL. Platelet counts are also elevated at term and may be as high as 400,000. Several pathologic conditions during pregnancy are associated with decreased levels of

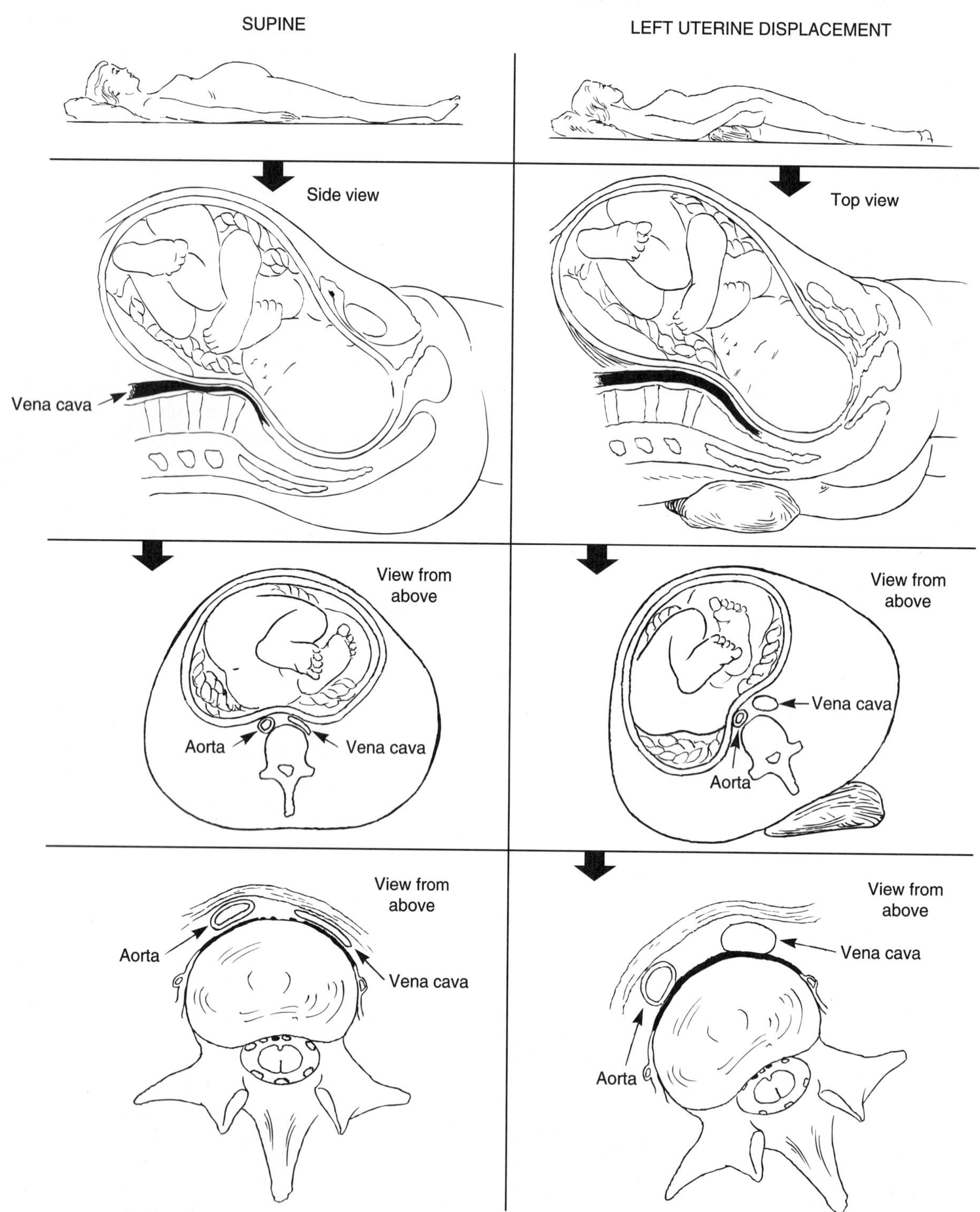

FIGURE **44-2**
Effects of left uterine displacement on the diameter of the abdominal aorta and vena cava.

fibrinogen, platelets, or both. In the parturient, platelet and fibrinogen levels that are within normal ranges for the nonpregnant state may actually represent a decrease from the parturient's baseline values; this has important implications if regional anesthesia is being considered.

Changes in the Nervous System

Animal studies have demonstrated a variable reduction in the minimum alveolar concentration (MAC) of inhalation agents necessary during pregnancy.[20,21] Both research and clinical experience have demonstrated an increase in the sensitivity of nerves to local anesthetic blockade during pregnancy.[22-24]

Gastrointestinal Changes

The parturient is at increased risk for regurgitation and aspiration of gastric contents because of anatomic and physiologic changes associated with pregnancy. A significant number of pregnant women and nonpregnant women immediately postpartum have gastric volumes in excess of 25 ml and gastric pH below 2.5. Ultrasound has demonstrated solid food in the stomach of almost two thirds of women in whom LEA had been instituted and in the stomach of more than 40% of laboring women who had not eaten in 12 to 24 hours.[25] Increased levels of gastrin during pregnancy result in greater gastric volume and lower pH. Upward displacement of the stomach by the gravid uterus may result in mechanical obstruction to outflow through the pylorus, delayed gastric emptying, and increased intragastric pressure. Elevated levels of progesterone, a smooth muscle relaxant, also decrease gastric motility and cause a reduction in lower esophageal sphincter tone. This explains the heartburn frequently experienced by pregnant women. Gastrointestinal changes do not completely normalize until several weeks postpartum.

Hepatic Changes

During pregnancy, levels of aspartate aminotransferase, alanine aminotransferase, lactate dehydrogenase, and alkaline phosphatase increase to the upper limits of nonpregnant normal levels. Serum albumin concentration decreases somewhat, and this decrease may result in increased free fractions of highly protein-bound drugs. Serum cholinesterase activity decreases by 30% or more during the first or second trimester; it recovers slightly by term, although it is still reduced compared with normal cholinesterase activity. Within a few days after delivery, cholinesterase levels dip again before returning to normal nonpregnant values over a few weeks. Despite decreases in cholinesterase activity, clinically relevant prolongation of the duration of action of drugs that depend on cholinesterase for elimination, such as succinylcholine and mivacurium, is uncommon in women with genotypically normal cholinesterase enzymes.

Renal Changes

During pregnancy both glomerular filtration rate and renal plasma flow increase. As a result the level of blood urea nitrogen decreases to approximately 8 mg/dL, and that of creatinine to approximately 0.5 mg/dL. Low levels of glucosuria and proteinuria commonly are present in the absence of disease. Mechanical obstruction of a ureter may occur if the gravid uterus is allowed to rest on it.

Uterine Changes

The uterus is altered tremendously during pregnancy. The uterus enlarges and its blood flow increases to meet both uterine and fetal metabolic demands. Uterine blood flow is supplied by two uterine arteries that are thought to be maximally dilated throughout pregnancy. Placental blood flow on the uterine side is supplied via the maternal arcuate, radial, and spiral arteries. The spiral arteries expel blood into the intervillous space. The maternal venous sinuses receive blood from the intervillous space and return it to the general circulation. Uterine blood flow increases to a maximum of 800 ml/min (approximately 10% of maternal cardiac output). Of this, approximately 150 ml/min supplies nutritive flow to the myometrium and 100 ml/min flows to the decidua (the lining of the uterus); the remainder flows to the intervillous space.

The fetus sends O_2-poor blood to the placenta via two umbilical arteries. These vessels perfuse capillary networks within placental villi that protrude into the pool of maternal blood. Placental villi are small, fingerlike projections, the purpose of which is to maximize the placental surface area in contact with maternal blood. Each villus contains a capillary network that exchanges respiratory gases, nutrients, and wastes with maternal blood (Figure 44-3). Both O_2 and CO_2 diffuse through placental tissue quickly. For clinical purposes diffusion does not limit the transfer of these gases. Both O_2 and CO_2 are said to be "perfusion limited," because their transfer to the fetus is limited only by the perfusion of the placenta, not by the

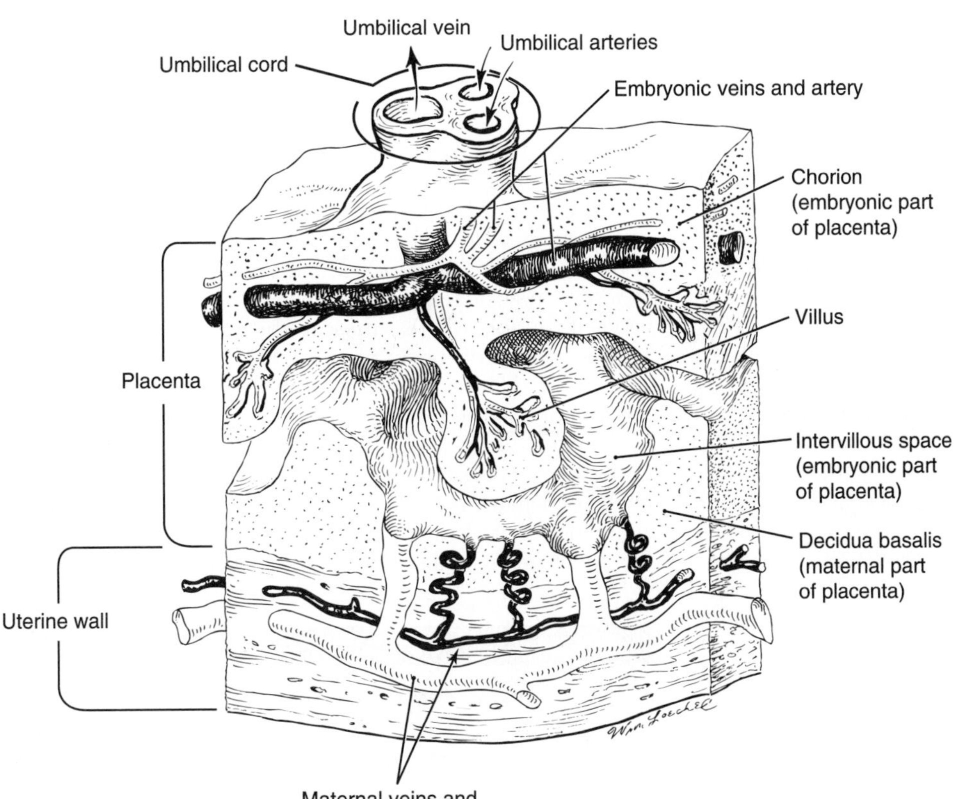

FIGURE **44-3**
Cross-section of the uteroplacental interface and the maternal and fetal blood supply.

rate of diffusion of the gases. Therefore decreases in maternal uterine artery blood flow or increases in placental vascular resistance will decrease fetal oxygenation.

Autoregulation of intervillous blood flow does not seem to occur. Spiral arteries, however, do constrict in response to α-agonists. Evidence of fetal embarrassment occurs if maternal systolic blood pressure drops below 100 mm Hg in awake, healthy patients during epidural anesthesia. Patients with preeclampsia (formerly called *pregnancy-induced hypertension* or PIH) can develop placental insufficiency at systolic pressures greater than 100 mm Hg. Unlike patients who receive LEA, patients receiving inhalation anesthesia seem to maintain adequate placental blood flow despite somewhat reduced blood pressure; this may be a function of altered uterine blood flow, altered fetal O_2 requirements, or both.

Placental Transfer and Fetal Effects of Drugs

Placental transfer of free (non–protein-bound) drug is dependent on the magnitude of the concentration gradient, molecular weight, lipid solubility, and drug ionization state. Drugs with molecular weights greater than 1000 daltons (d) cross the placenta poorly, whereas drugs with weights less than 500 d cross easily. Because cell membranes consist primarily of phospholipids, lipid solubility favors passage of drugs through cell membranes. Ionized molecules are polar and water soluble; therefore their diffusion through lipophilic cell membranes is inhibited.

After drugs have crossed the placenta, a variety of factors minimize their effects on the fetus. The chief factor responsible for minimizing these effects is dilution. Before reaching the fetus, a drug is diluted in intervillous blood, absorbed by the placenta, further diluted in placental blood, and circulated to the fetus. Once in the fetus, the drug is distributed within the fetal intravascular volume and redistributed to fetal tissues. Several other minor factors limit the effects of maternally administered drugs on a fetus. Some drugs, such as thiopental, are partially taken up by the fetal liver before gaining access to the general fetal circulation. Approximately one fifth of the fetal cardiac output returns directly to the placenta because of shunt flow through the foramen ovale and ductus arteriosus. This shunted blood does not circulate, and any drug it contains does not have a systemic fetal effect. For a full discussion of local anesthetics maternal-fetal ion trapping, see Chapter 9.

ANATOMY AND PHYSIOLOGY OF LABOR AND DELIVERY

The experience of pain is a highly personal phenomenon. During labor each woman's perception of pain is unique, because labor, the ability of the woman to modify the level of pain transmission, and tolerance to pain vary from one individual to the next. A few women are able to tolerate labor and delivery without significant discomfort; others experience pain in excess of their ability to cope. The combination of lack of control over the process in which the body is engaged, exhaustion, frustration, and seemingly unending pain can result in hyperventilation, screaming, cursing, and physical aggression. Effective labor analgesia not only makes the birth process more enjoyable but also provides women with more opportunity for control over their bodies and the environment, allowing them to maintain personal dignity.

In the absence of effective analgesia the onset of labor brings with it an intensification of many of the physiologic alterations of pregnancy. Serum catecholamine levels increase in response to pain, stress, and uterine activity. Whole body O_2 demand increases an additional 60% during painful contractions. Each uterine contraction expels blood from the uterus into the general circulation, acutely increasing venous return to the heart and therefore SV. Cardiac output in the first stage of labor increases 40% to 80% during contractions and returns to pregnant baseline between contractions.

Increases in minute ventilation of up to 300% may occur in response to pain and may occasionally cause maternal arterial partial pressure of CO_2 to drop below 15 mm Hg. Some evidence indicates that hyperventilation may cause a decrease in uterine blood flow. However, in animal studies this finding has usually been associated with stressful events, such as intubation and invasive procedures. In pregnant, laboring human volunteers, hyperventilation to an arterial partial pressure of CO_2 of 20 mm Hg does not seem to harm the fetus. Specifically, the fetus does not develop hypoxia or acidosis as determined by analysis of a scalp blood sample. A situation in which both hyperventilation and extreme stress are present is potentially detrimental to the fetus. When an anesthetized parturient is hyperventilated during stress, the neonate may be at risk of acidosis and hypoxia.

The onset of labor is accompanied by a further reduction in the rate of gastric emptying. If not contraindicated, administration of a histamine-2 (H_2) blocker and metoclopramide may benefit patients during anesthesia. The use of these drugs is advocated in the event that a general anesthetic or airway management becomes necessary. Ranitidine has been shown to reduce the acidity of gastric contents in the parturient within 30 minutes after an intravenous (IV) dose.[26] Unlike cimetidine, ranitidine does not inhibit the metabolism of amide local anesthetics. Metoclopramide and ranitidine are compatible with most IV solutions.

After delivery, cardiac output may increase further to as much as 180% above baseline because of the increase in fluid load from the now empty uterus and relief of aortocaval compression. This postpartum increase in cardiac output is the reason that pregnant cardiac patients are at greatest risk of dying after delivery. Cardiac output remains elevated for approximately 24 hours postpartum and returns to baseline 10 days later as HR and SV normalize.[27]

First Stage of Labor

During the late 1950s and early 1960s Bonica demonstrated that the pain of labor and delivery is mediated by T10 to L1 sympathetic nerve fibers and S1 to S4 somatic nerve fibers (Box 44-1 and Figure 44-4). The nerves at the T10 to L1 level were shown to be responsible for carrying pain sensation from cervical dilation, whereas those at the S1 to S4 level mediated vaginal and perineal pain perception.

Cervical dilation and possibly uterine muscle ischemia during contraction cause nonspecific nociceptor stimulation that is mediated by small, unmyelinated "C fibers." Pain transmission to the spinal cord occurs via nerves at the T10 to L1 level. Two modes of pain are perceived by laboring women: a nonlocalized cramping referred to the appropriate surface dermatomes on the abdomen from the level of the umbilicus to the inguinal

BOX 44-1

Pain Pathways during Labor

Uterus and cervix	T10 to L1-L2
Perineum	S2, S3, and S4

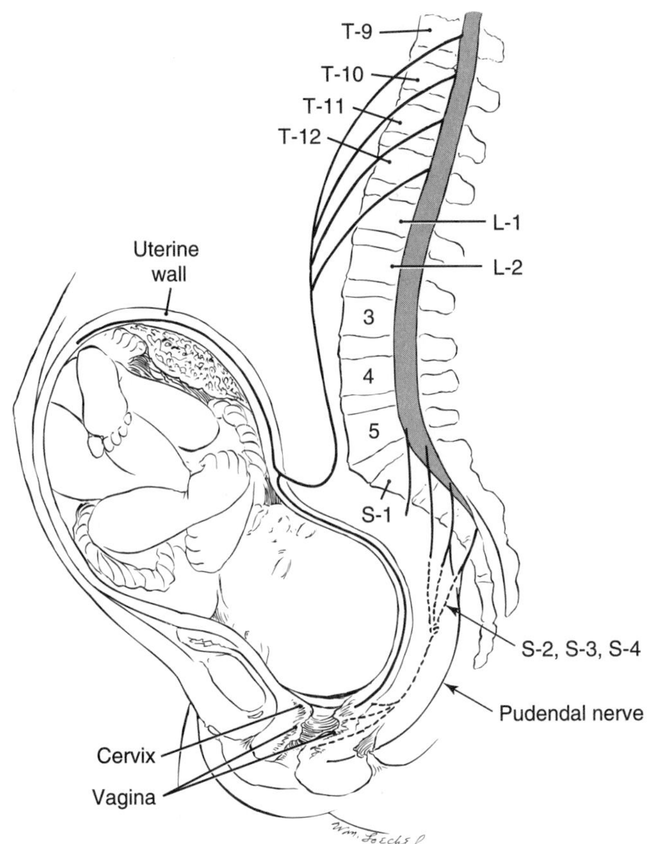

FIGURE **44-4**
Lower thoracic, lumbar, and sacral regions of the spine showing spinal cord, nerve roots, and sensory innervation to the uterus, cervix, and vagina.

ligament; and so-called "back labor," a sharp localized back pain that results from referred pain to dermatomes (cutaneous innervation) and sclerotomes (innervation of the bone and muscle). Sclerotomes are located several inches below the actual vertebral level of involvement, causing the pain to be felt over the L5 to S1 region. This pathway can be interrupted by a lumbar sympathetic block, a pericervical block, or an epidural sympathetic block with a local anesthetic level up to the T10 sensory dermatome.

Second Stage of Labor

As cervical dilation progresses and the fetal head descends into the pelvis, a second pain pathway becomes important. Compression and stretching of pelvic musculature and ligaments produce pain that is mediated by the sacral plexus. This pain can be eliminated with blockade of the pudendal nerve. In a normal laboring patient a lumbar epidural block effectively relieves the pain of uterine contraction and cervical dilation and under some circumstances also provides effective sacral analgesia. When sacral analgesia is not achieved with the epidural block, a pudendal block (usually placed by the obstetrician) provides nearly complete sacral relief.

Occasionally during labor, other sources of pain not mediated by these two pathways occur. They usually are mediated by lumbar somatic fibers and less frequently by sacral and thoracic somatic fibers. Such pain usually occurs in labors with abnormal presentations (e.g., occiput posterior presentation) or in cases of cephalopelvic disproportion.

Anesthetic Effects on the Progress of Labor

For years controversy has surrounded whether LEA prolongs labor or increases the need for assisted or operative delivery. The number of variables involved and the diversity of both patients and study methods make this a difficult topic about which to draw valid conclusions. It is generally accepted that LEA probably prolongs latent stage labor but if properly conducted has little effect on active labor. Even if LEA does prolong labor (and this "fact" is not universally accepted), most laboring women would agree that a slightly longer comfortable labor is preferable to a slightly shorter uncomfortable one.

An unnecessarily dense block does affect the progress of labor in many women. Complete sensory anesthesia eliminates a woman's signal to push and at best results in uncoordinated and less effective pushing during the second stage of labor. At worst it removes the urge to bear down; therefore some women will not participate in the second stage of labor. If the block is dense enough to include an effective motor block, even the most motivated, well-coached, and involved parturient may be unable to push. The goal of LEA is to provide analgesia for labor that does not remove maternal awareness of uterine contractions and that does not cause motor block. A minimally effective concentration of local anesthetic, perhaps in combination with an opioid, decreases the likelihood that LEA will interfere with the birth process.

FETAL HEART RATE MONITORING

Although the fetal heart rate (FHR) is not a specific predictor of fetal well-being, it is the most readily available method for the assessment of fetal well-being. From the FHR, information about the baseline status of a fetus can be obtained during a preanesthesia assessment. The FHR also reveals information about the fetal response to anesthetic intervention. This information is useful during LEA, anesthesia for assisted or operative delivery, and anesthesia for nondelivery surgery. Important information on which to build an anesthetic plan and evaluate its effects on both mother and fetus is available to the anesthetist knowledgeable in FHR monitoring.

The FHR is recorded on a graph running at 3 cm/min. Uterine tone, or pressure, is recorded concurrently on a second channel below the FHR tracing. In this way it is possible to relate FHR changes to uterine contractions. Two methods of detecting the FHR are used clinically. The first is noninvasive, using an abdominal ultrasound probe aimed at the fetal heart. Heart movement during each cardiac cycle is counted as a heartbeat, and the interval between beats is used to calculate the number of beats per minute. The FHR can also be measured invasively by inserting a spiral electrode approximately 2 mm into the fetal scalp. This method requires a ruptured amniotic sac and a partially dilated cervix through which the electrode is inserted.

Given a reasonable maternal O_2 saturation, fetal oxygenation is limited primarily by uteroplacental blood flow, not maternal oxygenation. Anything that decreases maternal blood pressure or uterine artery blood flow also decreases uteroplacental blood flow. This results in fetal hypoxia and eventually acidosis. Hypoxia results in FHR changes, and acidosis has been correlated with specific FHR responses.

The normal FHR in a term fetus is 120 to 160 bpm. An immature fetus has a higher HR. Fetal bradycardia down to 100 bpm is generally well tolerated if it lasts less than 2 minutes. Fetal bradycardia below 100 bpm is cause for concern, and bradycardia below 80 bpm is severe regardless of duration.

Changes in Fetal Heart Rate

Fetal tachycardia is defined as an HR above 160 bpm in a term fetus. In a few circumstances it may be the result of fetal hypoxia, but never when normal variability is present. More common causes of fetal tachycardia include fever, fetal arrhythmias, immaturity, and drugs such as terbutaline and atropine. Ephedrine, for example, can increase both FHR and variability if given to the parturient in large enough doses.[28]

Fetal bradycardia is present when the FHR is below 120 bpm. Transient decreases to as low as 100 bpm are generally not a cause for concern as long as FHR variability remains normal. Bradycardia can be caused by arrhythmias, drugs, and hypoxia or asphyxia. Prolonged bradycardia is the result of maternal hypoxemia or a sustained decrease in blood flow to the placenta.

Heart Rate Variability

Variability is a term used to describe small changes in the FHR. In general, baseline FHR variability increases with advancing gestational age. Short-term or beat-to-beat variability is the instantaneous change in rate that occurs between two consecutive heartbeats. The FHR monitor calculates HR based on the interval between two successive R waves on the fetal electrocardiogram. It records this rate on graph paper as a horizontal line. If each successive R wave–to–R wave interval is the same, then the HR is the same, and the line on the graph is flat. If successive R wave–to–R wave intervals are slightly different, then the resultant FHR calculation is different, and the line on the graph is irregular. This irregularity is the beat-to-beat variability. Indirect or external ultrasound monitoring of the FHR results in artifacts that can look very much like normal variability. For this reason, beat-to-beat variability can be accurately assessed only by direct FHR monitoring with a fetal scalp electrode.

Long-term variability, also called *reactivity*, is the acceleration of the FHR for short periods followed by a return to baseline HR. It often is associated with fetal movement. Long-term variability is described as "normal" when the baseline HR varies by 15 bpm for 15 seconds on a frequent and regular basis. Variability is decreased or absent when the baseline rate changes are less than this. During fetal sleep, beat-to-beat variability should continue, but long-term variability normally decreases for periods of up to 40 minutes. Examples of both normal beat-to-beat and long-term variability are shown in Figure 44-5.

FHR variability is the single best noninvasive clinical indicator of fetal well-being. In general, beat-to-beat variability and long-term variability are seen to occur together. They probably represent the presence of an intact central nervous system (CNS) regulatory mechanism. Changes in beat-to-beat variability are vagally mediated. Hypoxia causes CNS depression, which results in decreased variability. Other causes of decreased variability include fetal sleep, acidosis, anencephaly, drugs (CNS depressants or autonomic agents), and defects of the fetal cardiac conduction system. Administration of opioids to the mother, for example, decreases FHR variability for up to 30 minutes.[29-32] Maternal magnesium sulfate administration also may attenuate HR variability.[33]

FHR variability is indicative of fetal reserve. The presence of normal variability is a good sign that the fetus is either healthy or well compensated. Although nonpathologic causes of decreased FHR variability exist, decreased variability may be a sign that the fetus is beginning to decompensate. This is especially true when variability decreases in conjunction with variable or late FHR decelerations. Evidence shows that both beat-to-beat variability and long-term variability decrease when the fetal scalp pH is 7.2 or less. A fetus that is in trouble almost always loses variability

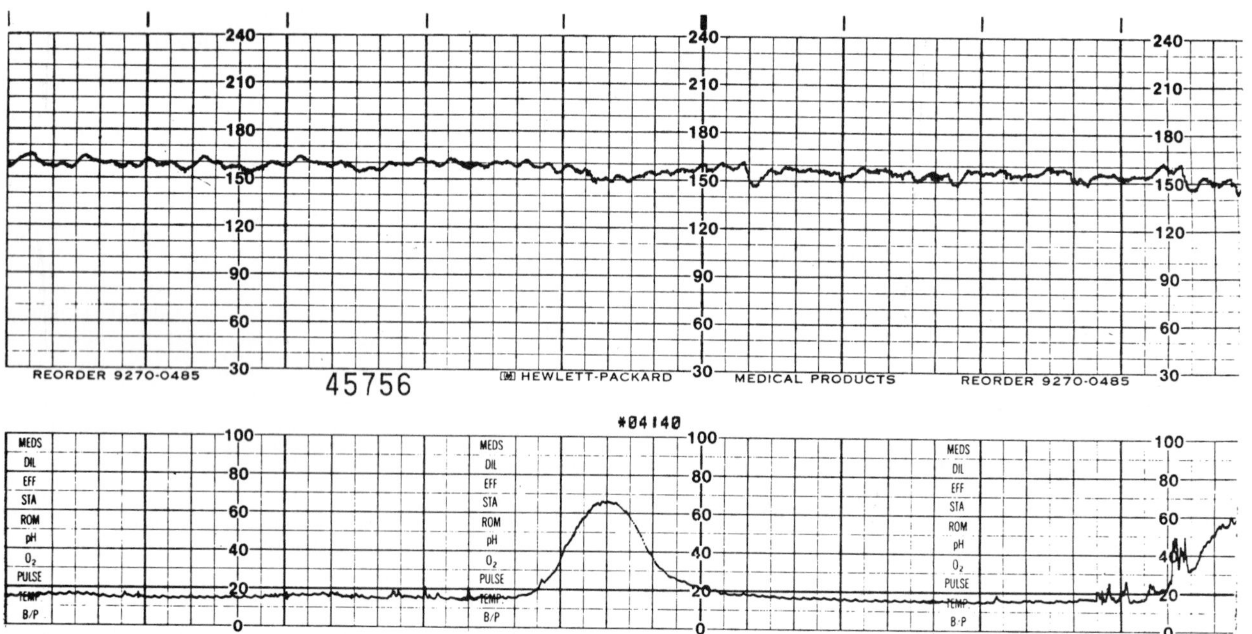

FIGURE **44-5**
Normal beat-to-beat and long-term variability with fetal heart rate (FHR) of 150 to 160 beats per minute (bpm). The distance between the heavy vertical lines represents 60 seconds. The lighter vertical lines are 10 seconds apart. The top graph is the FHR tracing; the bottom graph is intrauterine pressure. The rise in the bottom graph under the time stamp *04:40 represents a uterine contraction. Both FHR and uterine pressure are measured directly. (From Fiedler MA. An introduction to fetal heart rate monitoring. *AANA J*. 1989;57:257-264.)

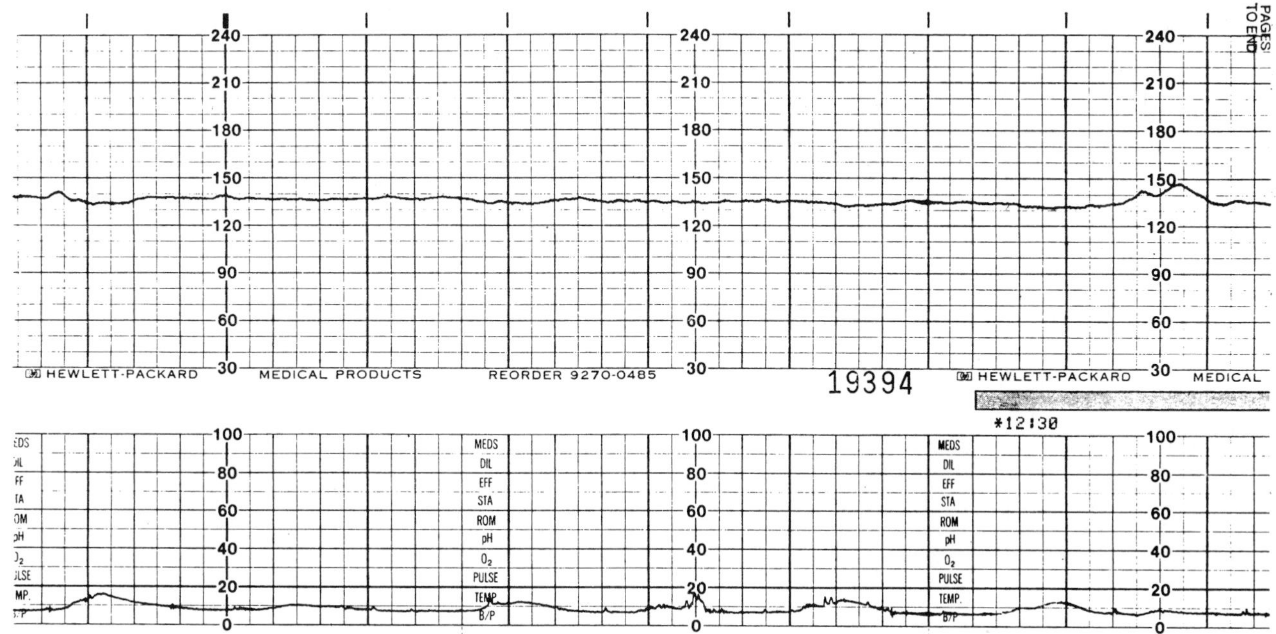

FIGURE **44-6**
Poor beat-to-beat and long-term variability. The fetal heart rate was measured with a scalp electrode. (From Fiedler MA. An introduction to fetal heart rate monitoring. *AANA J*. 1989;57:257-264.)

before death occurs. Figure 44-6 shows an example of poor beat-to-beat variability and almost no long-term variability.

Sinusoidal Fetal Heart Rate Pattern

An uncommon variant of FHR variability is the sinusoidal pattern (Figure 44-7). The cause of this variant is unknown in most circumstances but may be associated with fetal anemia. The sinusoidal FHR tracing is a pattern of consistent, repeating variability superimposed on a background of a normal FHR. It resembles a sine wave with a frequency of two to five cycles per minute and a wave amplitude of 5 to 10 bpm. The administration of as little as 0.5 mg of butorphanol (Stadol), an opioid agonist/antagonist commonly used for relief of obstetric pain, has been strongly associated with a sinusoidal FHR pattern.[34] The reported onset and duration of the sinusoidal pattern after butorphanol administration are highly variable, with the former ranging from 2 to 36 minutes and the latter from 10 to 92 minutes.

Early Decelerations

Early decelerations occur in concert with uterine contractions. The deceleration begins when the contraction begins, and it returns to baseline when the contraction ends. Early decelerations are smooth in appearance, and the change in HR is mild, usually no more than 20 bpm. An early deceleration occurs with each uterine contraction and has the same appearance from one contraction to the next. Compression of the fetal head as it passes through the birth canal is thought to be the cause of early decelerations via vagal stimulation. Early decelerations may be a sign that the parturient is pushing too early against a less-than-fully dilated cervix, or they may be a late sign of impending delivery. In either case early decelerations are physiologic unless they are seen with fetal tachycardia or loss of variability. Figure 44-8 shows early decelerations with poor baseline variability.

In summary, early decelerations have the following characteristics:

- Occur with each uterine contraction
- Start and end with the contraction
- Gradually decrease in rate and then end in a return to baseline
- Are uniform in appearance
- Are associated with a mild decrease in FHR (20 bpm or less)
- Are accompanied by a loss in beat-to-beat variability during the deceleration

Variable Decelerations

Variable decelerations occur with uterine contractions but usually not with every uterine contraction. The deceleration may begin when the contraction begins, or it may begin late. Also, a variable deceleration may end after the contraction ends, sometimes with a transient tachycardia. Variable decelerations are abrupt in both onset and recovery; at times the FHR plunges 60 bpm in only 1 or 2 seconds. Variable decelerations are variable in occurrence, onset, depth, duration, and appearance. Normally, beat-to-beat variability is still present during the decelerations. Variable decelerations are thought to be caused by a baroreflex-mediated response to umbilical cord compression. Variable decelerations are termed *severe* if the FHR decreases by 60 bpm from the baseline, if the FHR drops below 60 bpm, or if the decelerations are sustained for 60 seconds or longer. Less severe variable decelerations are still of concern if beat-to-beat variability is absent. If the fetus is compromised, then the recovery phase of the deceleration may be delayed. Figure 44-9 shows a variable deceleration on a baseline of good variability.

In summary, variable decelerations have the following characteristics:

- Vary in appearance, duration, depth, and shape
- Demonstrate abrupt onset and recovery
- Maintain beat-to-beat variability with the deceleration
- Are classified as severe if the FHR decreases by 60 bpm, if the FHR decreases to less than 60 bpm, or if the decelerations last 60 seconds or longer

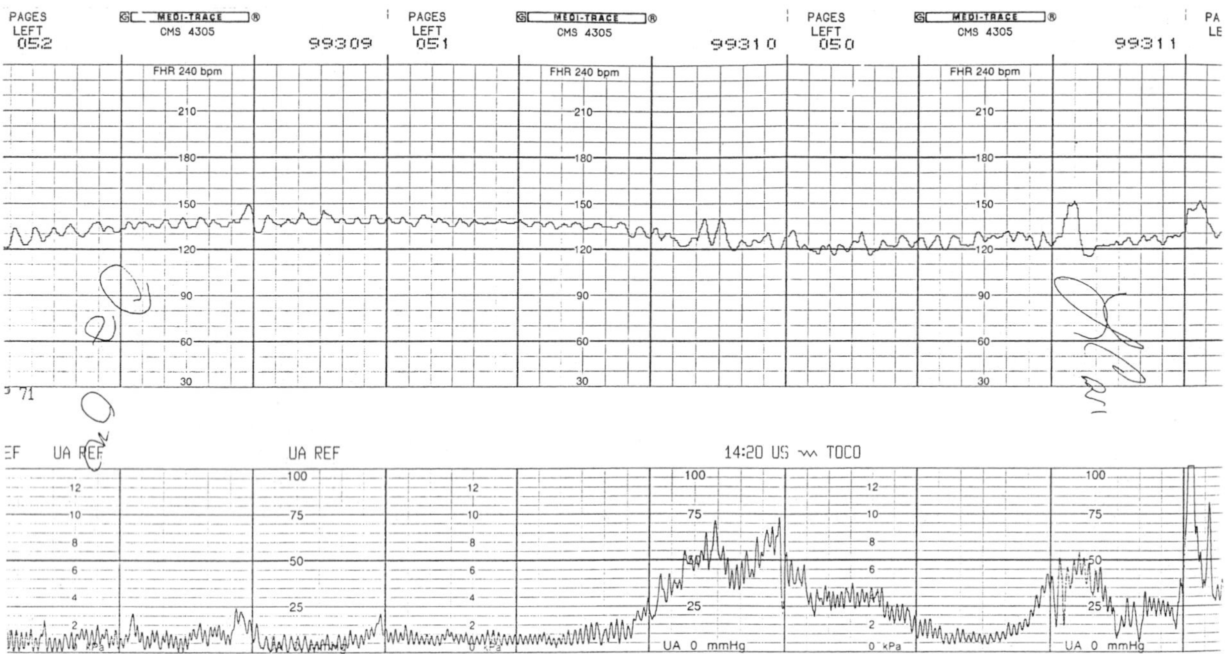

FIGURE **44-7**
Sinusoidal fetal heart rate pattern in a healthy 15-year-old primigravida who later delivered a healthy infant. Monitoring is external. (From Fiedler MA. An introduction to fetal heart rate monitoring. *AANA J.* 1989;57:257-264.)

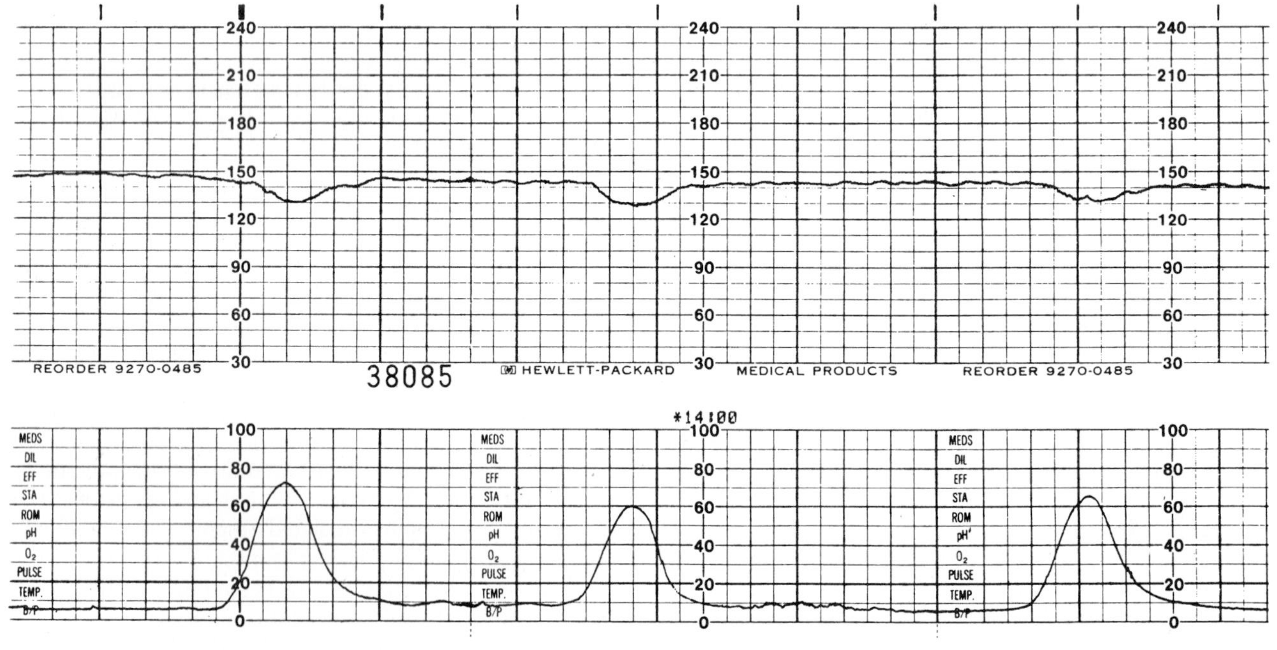

FIGURE **44-8**
Early decelerations with each of three uterine contractions and poor fetal heart rate variability. (From Fiedler MA. An introduction to fetal heart rate monitoring. *AANA J.* 1989;57:257-264.)

If variable decelerations continue to occur or are severe, the anesthetist should anticipate the possibility of obstetric intervention for which anesthesia will be required. Figure 44-10 shows two variable decelerations, the second of which is severe.

Late Decelerations

Late decelerations occur with a uterine contraction. In contrast to early decelerations, late decelerations begin between 10 and 30 seconds after the onset of the uterine contraction (Figure 44-11). Like early decelerations, they are smooth in both onset and recovery. Late decelerations are regular in occurrence. They occur with each uterine contraction, and they appear similar from one contraction to the next (however, as the fetus decompensates, recovery takes longer). Beat-to-beat variability may or may not be present during the deceleration, depending on the baseline level of fetal oxygenation. A fetus with late

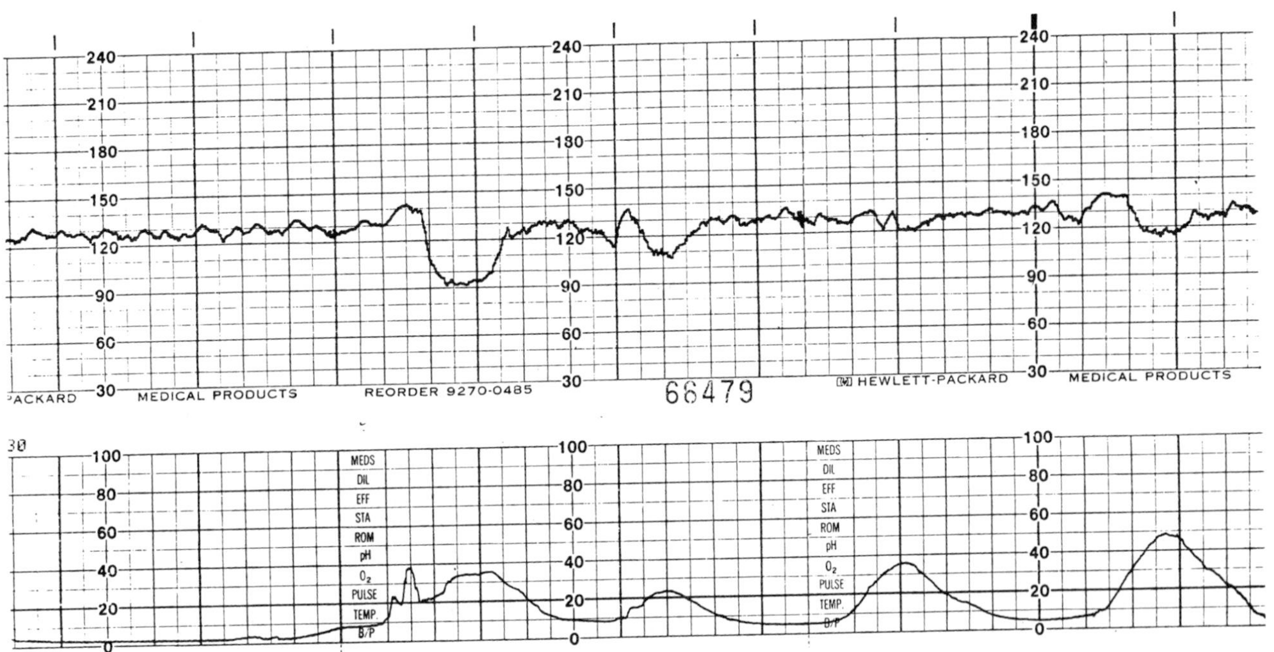

FIGURE **44-9**
Variable deceleration superimposed on a baseline of good variability. Note the quick descent and recovery characteristic of variable decelerations as well as the presence of beat-to-beat variability within the deceleration. The two peaks on the upslope of the uterine contraction are artifacts. (From Fiedler MA. An introduction to fetal heart rate monitoring. *AANA J.* 1989;57:257-264.)

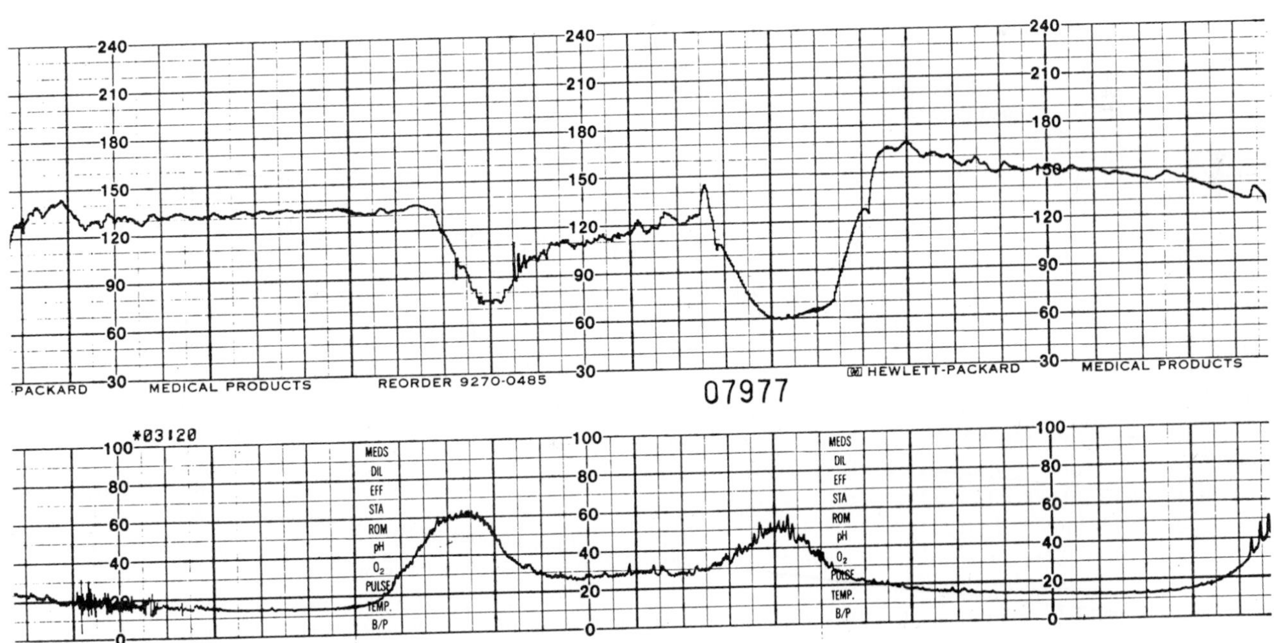

FIGURE **44-10**
Two variable decelerations on a baseline of poor long-term variability. The first deceleration recovers slowly, probably indicating fetal decompensation. Before recovery is complete, a second uterine contraction occurs, prompting another variable deceleration. The second deceleration meets the criteria for severity. The FHR drops by more than 60 bpm or to 60 bpm, and the deceleration persists for longer than 60 seconds. Note that the first uterine contraction did not relax to baseline before the second one began. The irregularity of the uterine pressure graph is artifact. (From Fiedler MA. An introduction to fetal heart rate monitoring. *AANA J.* 1989;57:257-264.)

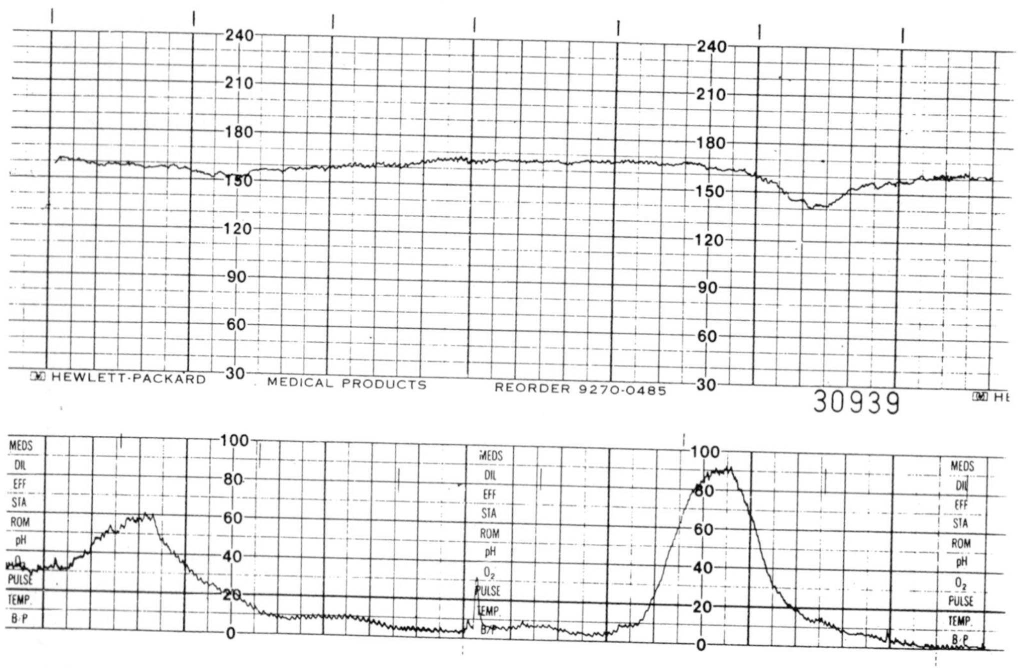

FIGURE **44-11**
Two late decelerations in a woman with a placental abruption. The first deceleration is significant, even though it is only 10 bpm in depth. Any late deceleration is a poor sign. Note the poor variability, which indicates that the fetus is already decompensated. (From Fiedler MA. An introduction to fetal heart rate monitoring. *AANA J.* 1989;57:257-264.)

decelerations and absent variability is much more likely to have metabolic acidosis than one in which variability is still present. When late decelerations are noted, it is important to evaluate beat-to-beat and long-term variability as well. The absence of variability in combination with late decelerations may indicate the presence of hypoxic myocardial depression.

In summary, late decelerations have the following characteristics:

- Occur with each uterine contraction
- Start between 10 and 30 seconds after the uterine contraction
- Gradually decrease in rate and end in a return to baseline
- Are uniform in appearance
- Vary in depth according to the strength of the uterine contraction
- May or may not be accompanied by beat-to-beat variability
- Are classified as severe if the FHR decreases by more than 45 bpm

Late decelerations are probably caused by a problem in the uteroplacental interface that results in fetal hypoxia and acidosis. Any late deceleration is a reason for concern. Even small, almost imperceptible late decelerations may represent severe fetal decompensation when they are combined with the absence of FHR variability. Intervention is needed to correct any cause of fetal hypoxia. If these efforts are not successful, the anesthetist should be prepared for emergency obstetric intervention for which anesthesia will be required.

Anesthetic Considerations

When presented with any FHR abnormality that may indicate hypoxia, the anesthetist must rule out anesthetic intervention as the cause. When related to anesthesia, such abnormality most commonly occurs in a parturient who has an epidural catheter in place for labor analgesia. Local anesthetics used to block labor pain also block sympathetic innervation to the vasculature; the resultant "chemical sympathectomy" allows peripheral vasodilation with pooling of blood, a reduction in venous return, and a decrease in cardiac output and therefore hypotension. Because fetal oxygenation is limited primarily by uteroplacental blood flow, maternal hypotension is sufficient to cause fetal hypoxia. If maternal hypotension is present, it should be treated. IV administration of fluid or ephedrine may be all that is necessary. Next, the sensory level of the epidural block should be assessed. If the level is higher than necessary for pain relief, it should be allowed to recede to a more appropriate level. This also decreases the amount of sympathetic blockade. In the majority of cases LEA is not essential for a safe delivery. If it is not possible to maintain a blood pressure adequate for fetal oxygenation, epidural analgesia should be discontinued.

If the FHR tracing made during the preanesthesia assessment suggests hypoxia, caution should be used in making the decision to proceed with epidural analgesia. Careful consideration must be given to the severity of the fetal hypoxia and to the possibility that it may be worsened by anesthetic intervention. Thoughtful consultation with the anesthesiologist or obstetrician involved is warranted.

When the obstetrician makes a decision that emergent operative delivery is warranted, the anesthetist must be prepared to move quickly. If the patient already has an epidural catheter in place, there are situations in which it can be used safely. When making the decision as to whether to use an epidural block for an emergent cesarean section, consider the following questions: Is the epidural block uniform or patchy? How likely is it that the patient will become hypotensive when additional local anesthetic is administered? How quickly can a sensory level sufficient for abdominal surgery be established? What are the chances that the block will fail?

If an epidural catheter is not already in place, general anesthesia is almost always preferable because it can be induced quickly and has a lower failure rate than regional anesthesia. An induction technique that minimizes the possibility of maternal hypotension (perhaps one that involves the use of ketamine) is chosen. Some clinicians would consider using a subarachnoid block; however, here again, hypotension is a risk.

Anesthesia care for a pregnant woman affects both the mother and the fetus. FHR monitoring provides useful information about how the fetus is tolerating the current circumstances. A basic understanding of the information contained in the FHR tracing allows the anesthetist to better plan for and assess anesthetic intervention in the pregnant patient.

PREPARATION FOR LIFE SUPPORT

Vascular Access

Because epidural anesthesia causes vasodilation and because childbirth sometimes results in an unexpectedly large loss of blood, generous venous access is recommended. Sites above the wrist are preferred, because wrist movement often causes fluid flow to be position dependent. When an IV infusion is started in the back of the hand, mechanical irritation of the vein by the end of the catheter results in perforation of the vein and in subcutaneous infiltration more often than it does when an IV catheter is placed in more proximal locations.

Drugs and Equipment

Emergency equipment and drugs for airway management, treatment of local anesthetic toxicity, maintenance of vital signs, and cardiopulmonary resuscitation (CPR) should always be immediately available wherever regional or general anesthesia is performed in the labor and delivery area. Carts containing epidural anesthesia trays, local anesthetics, tape, and other supplies are wheeled from room to room for epidural insertions. These carts also contain an Ambu bag, O_2 tubing, an anesthesia mask, oral and nasal airways, endotracheal tubes, two laryngoscope handles, and Miller and MacIntosh blades. Emergency drugs ready for use should include atropine, an induction drug (for terminating local anesthetic–induced seizure), succinylcholine, ephedrine, epinephrine, calcium chloride (for treating magnesium sulfate overdose), and sodium bicarbonate. A "crash cart" with a defibrillator must be available. Automatic blood pressure machines are required in each labor and delivery room, and pulse oximetry should be readily available. Operating rooms in the labor and delivery suite should be equipped exactly as main operating rooms and include up-to-date anesthesia machines, anesthesia gas analysis, pulse oximetry, and O_2 concentration monitoring. Although many institutions require that emergency drugs be discarded and replaced at 24-hour intervals because of infection control concerns, many emergency drugs (thiopental, succinylcholine, ephedrine, atropine, lidocaine, oxytocin) have been shown to remain sterile for up to 8 days in the obstetric anesthesia setting.[35] However, other reasons exist for replacement of emergency drugs. The concentration of atropine in a plastic syringe has been shown to decrease by 44% over 24 hours because of drug adsorption to the inner surface of the syringe.[36] Box 44-2 lists recommended equipment and drugs needed for neonatal resuscitation.

Personnel

In addition to proper drugs and equipment, knowledgeable assistants are needed for some anesthesia tasks. An additional anesthetist (either a physician or a certified registered nurse anesthetist) who can respond quickly to help with an emergency is desirable; a competent obstetric nurse is mandatory. An anesthetist cannot place an epidural catheter and at the same time steady a sitting parturient. If the patient becomes faint or apneic or has a seizure, a minimum of two professionals are needed to manage the situation. In the operating room an assistant who knows how to correctly apply cricoid pressure is essential. Circulating nurses can skillfully perform this maneuver after proper training. Some conditions associated with risk to newborns are given in Box 44-3. Some special circumstances in resuscitation of newborns is given in Table 44-1.

INTRAVENOUS ANALGESIA IN THE PARTURIENT

When LEA is unavailable, refused, or not indicated, IV opioids are still used for labor pain relief. From an anesthesia perspective the use of IV opioids presents several disadvantages. The pain relief they afford is often inadequate, and fetal CNS depression, maternal respiratory depression, nausea, vomiting, and decreased lower esophageal sphincter tone may all result. Nevertheless, IV analgesia can sometimes be a bridge to LEA or a necessary supplement to achieve complete anesthesia during cesarean section with the patient under regional anesthesia.

Opioids

Meperidine crosses the placenta easily and has been recovered from the fetus within 2 minutes of IV administration. Like all opioids, it is capable of causing neonatal respiratory depression, although less so than morphine or methadone. Because of differences in pH and protein binding, the level of meperidine in the fetus is likely to be higher than the maternal blood level. Normeperidine is an active metabolite of meperidine with an elimination half-life of 30 hours. Normeperidine remains in the neonate for several days after delivery and may lead to depression of neonatal behavioral assessment scores.[37]

Historically, larger doses of meperidine were used during labor than are used now, often in combination with other depressant drugs. With contemporary doses (generally $<$100 mg in total), neonatal depression is less of a problem. The interval from administration of the drug to delivery of the infant is important, however. A drug-to-delivery interval of 2 to 3 hours results in the greatest neonatal depression. Both meperidine and normeperidine can be antagonized by naloxone.

Butorphanol is an opioid agonist-antagonist. Two milligrams of butorphanol is equal to approximately 10 mg of morphine in analgesic potency and respiratory depression, although higher doses of butorphanol do not result in equally greater respiratory depression. The half-life of butorphanol is 3 hours. Unlike morphine, butorphanol increases pulmonary artery pressure and myocardial work. Butorphanol is a better sedative than are pure opioids.

Ketamine

In appropriate doses ketamine can be used advantageously in obstetric anesthesia without emergence reactions. In fact, many women report pleasant thoughts after receiving low doses of ketamine for sedation and analgesia.

Ketamine produces a centrally and peripherally mediated sympathomimetic effect. A dose-dependent increase in blood

BOX 44-2

Equipment and Drugs Needed for Neonatal Resuscitation

Suction Equipment
Bulb syringe
Mechanical suction and tubing
Suction catheters, 5-F or 6-F, 8-F, and 10-F or 12-F
8-F feeding tube and 20-mL syringe
Meconium aspiration device

Bag-and-Mask Equipment
Neonatal resuscitation bag with a pressure-release valve or pressure manometer (the bag must be capable of delivering 90% to 100% oxygen)
Face masks, newborn and preterm sizes (masks with cushioned rim preferred)
Oxygen with flowmeter (flow rate up to 10 L/min) and tubing (including portable oxygen cylinders)

Intubation Equipment
Laryngoscope with straight blades, No. 0 (preterm) and No. 1 (term)
Extra bulbs and batteries for laryngoscope
Tracheal tubes, 2.5, 3.0, 3.5, and 4.0 mm ID
Stylet (optional)
Scissors
Tape or securing device for tracheal tube
Alcohol sponges
CO_2 detector (optional)
Laryngeal mask airway (optional)

Medications
Epinephrine 1:10,000 (0.1 mg/mL): 3- or 10-mL ampules
Isotonic crystalloid (normal saline or Ringer's lactate) for volume expansion: 100 or 250 mL
Sodium bicarbonate 4.2% (5 mEq/10 mL): 10-mL ampules
Naloxone hydrochloride 0.4 mg/mL: 1-mL ampules (or 1.0 mg/mL: 2-mL ampules)
Normal saline, 30 mL
Dextrose 10%, 250 mL
Normal saline "fish" or "bullet" (optional)
Feeding tube, 5-F (optional)
Umbilical vessel catheterization supplies
- Sterile gloves
- Scalpel or scissors
- Povidone-iodine solution
- Umbilical tape
- Umbilical catheters, 3.5-F, 5-F
- Three-way stopcock

Syringes, 1, 3, 5, 10, 20, and 50 mL
Needles, 25-, 21-, and 18-gauge, or puncture device for needleless system

Miscellaneous
Gloves and appropriate personal protection
Radiant warmer or other heat source
Firm, padded resuscitation surface
Clock (timer optional)
Warmed linens
Stethoscope
Tape, ½- or ¾-inch
Cardiac monitor and electrodes and/or pulse oximeter with probe (optional for delivery room)
Oropharyngeal airways

From Niermeyer S (ed), Kattwinkel J, Van Reempts P, et al. International Guidelines for Neonatal Resuscitation: An excerpt from the Guidelines 2000 for Cardiopulmonary Resuscitation and Emergency Cardiovascular Care: International Consensus on Science, Pediatrics 2000;106:E29:1-16.

pressure is common after administration to awake patients. Ketamine is also a good bronchodilator and therefore may be helpful when pregnancy complicates asthma or other airway diseases. Although catecholamines may cause uterine vasoconstriction via an α-agonist effect, uterine arterial blood flow does not decrease after ketamine administration as it does with sympathomimetics; in fact, it may increase slightly.[38,39] Neonatal depression has not been demonstrated after maternal ketamine doses of up to 1 mg/kg. IV doses of 1 mg/kg or less are appropriate for induction of general anesthesia. Blood pressure will increase unless the sympathetics are already fully activated; if so, no additional sympathomimetic effect will be caused by ketamine. The temptation to exceed 1 mg/kg should be avoided. Because it has a high lipid solubility, ketamine crosses the placenta easily; larger doses result in neonatal depression and neonatal chest wall rigidity and may cause maternal dysphoric reactions on emergence.

Low-dose ketamine often preserves airway reflexes while causing somatic analgesia or anesthesia, sedation, increased blood pressure, and a dreamlike state. All these effects are dose dependent. Low IV doses of ketamine are within the range of 10 to 25 mg, up to a total of 1 mg/kg. Onset of drug action is within 1 minute, and its duration is dose dependent (usually 5 to 15 minutes at these doses).

REGIONAL ANALGESIA AND ANESTHESIA FOR LABOR AND VAGINAL DELIVERY

Obstetric Anesthesia History

The anesthetist should begin, as always, with an appropriate history-taking and physical examination. The taking of the history should include general questions about systemic disease that one would ask a nonpregnant patient. In a healthy parturient who desires labor analgesia a preanesthetic evaluation should include the following additional information: the extent of the patient's cervical dilation and percent effacement; the station of the fetal presenting part; the FHR and an assessment of FHR variability; whether the amniotic membrane is ruptured or intact; the gestational age of the fetus; and the parturient's gravity and parity. Some centers record the last of these using the designation $G_xP_xAb_x$, for gravity (the number of conceptions), *p*arity (the number of live

BOX 44-3

Risk Factors Suggesting an Increased Need for Neonatal Resuscitation

Antepartum risk factors:
- Maternal diabetes
- Pregnancy-induced hypertension
- Chronic hypertension
- Chronic maternal illness
  - Cardiovascular
  - Thyroid
  - Neurological
  - Pulmonary
  - Renal
- Anemia or isoimmunization
- Previous fetal or neonatal death
- Bleeding in second or third trimester
- Maternal infection
- Polyhydramnios
- Oligohydramnios
- Premature rupture of membranes
- Postterm gestation
- Multiple gestation
- Size-dates discrepancy
- Drug therapy, e.g.,
  - Lithium carbonates
  - Magnesium
  - Adrenergic-blocking drugs
- Maternal substance abuse
- Fetal malformation
- Diminished fetal activity
- No prenatal care
- Age <16 or >35 years

Intrapartum risk factors:
- Emergency cesarean section
- Forceps or vacuum-assisted delivery
- Breech or other abnormal presentation
- Premature labor
- Precipitous labor
- Chorioamnionitis
- Prolonged rupture of membranes (>18 hours before delivery)
- Prolonged labor (>24 hours)
- Prolonged second stage of labor (>2 hours)
- Fetal bradycardia
- Nonreassuring fetal heart rate patterns
- Use of general anesthesia
- Uterine tetany
- Narcotics administered to mother within 4 hours of delivery
- Meconium-stained amniotic fluid
- Prolapsed cord
- Abruptio placentae
- Placenta previa

From Niermeyer S (ed), Kattwinkel J, Van Reempts P, et al. International Guidelines for Neonatal Resuscitation: An excerpt from the Guidelines 2000 for Cardiopulmonary Resuscitation and Emergency Cardiovascular Care: International Consensus on Science, Pediatrics 2000;106:E29:1-16.

TABLE 44-1 Special Circumstances in Resuscitation of the Newly Born Infant

Condition	History/Clinical Signs	Actions
Mechanical blockage of the airway		
Meconium or mucus blockage	Meconium-stained amniotic fluid Poor chest wall movement	Intubation for suctioning/ventilation
Choanal atresia	Pink when crying, cyanotic when quiet	Oral airway Endotracheal intubation
Pharyngeal airway malformation	Persistent retractions, poor air entry	Prone positioning, posterior nasopharyngeal tube
Impaired lung function		
Pneumothorax	Asymmetrical breath sounds Persistent cyanosis/bradycardia	Needle thoracentesis
Pleural effusions/ascites	Diminished air movement Persistent cyanosis/bradycardia	Immediate intubation Needle thoracentesis, paracentesis Possible volume expansion
Congenital diaphragmatic hernia	Asymmetrical breath sounds Persistent cyanosis/bradycardia Scaphoid abdomen	Endotracheal intubation Placement of orogastric catheter
Pneumonia/sepsis	Diminished air movement Persistent cyanosis/bradycardia	Endotracheal intubation Possible volume expansion
Impaired cardiac function		
Congenital heart disease	Persistent cyanosis/bradycardia	Diagnostic evaluation
Fetal/maternal hemorrhage	Pallor; poor response to resuscitation	Volume expansion, possibly including red blood cells

From Niermeyer S (ed), Kattwinkel J, Van Reempts P, et al. International Guidelines for Neonatal Resuscitation: An excerpt from the Guidelines 2000 for Cardiopulmonary Resuscitation and Emergency Cardiovascular Care: International Consensus on Science, Pediatrics 2000;106:E29:1-16.

births), and *ab*ortus (the number of preterm dead births), with the subscript after each abbreviation representing the number of each. Other centers use the FPAL system (*f*ull-term, *p*remature, *a*bortus, and *l*iving children), documenting only the numbers for each category. Any previous analgesic interventions should be noted.

The parturient should be questioned about problems with previous pregnancies, deliveries, or anesthetics during pregnancy. Because a regional anesthetic is probably going to be considered, she should be asked specifically about bleeding or back problems. An assessment of her state of hydration is especially important, because obstetric patients are prone to increased fluid losses resulting from mouth-breathing and panting and may have taken nothing by mouth for an extended period. Oxygenation of the fetus is dependent on maintenance of an adequate maternal blood pressure, and epidural analgesia may produce significant hypotension in the presence of dehydration. Review of baseline laboratory values before the institution of LEA in healthy patients usually is not mandatory. In a 1995 survey of private practice anesthesiologists, however, 68% said they checked a complete blood cell count before administration of LEA, and 31% checked a platelet count.[40] If preeclampsia or other pathology with anesthetic implications is present, the performance of the anesthetic procedure should generally be delayed until appropriate laboratory results (e.g., coagulation studies) are available.

It is easier for a mother to cooperate during history-taking if she is not experiencing the pain of labor. Therefore it is helpful if the history is taken early in the labor and delivery process, often long before LEA is indicated. An added benefit of an early history-taking is that if anesthesia is needed emergently for fetal distress or maternal bleeding, much more is known about the patient than if history-taking had been postponed. For this reason, obtaining a history early is helpful in parturients in whom obstetricians suspect the possibility of problems.

At some point a general discussion of LEA that includes an explanation of both risks and benefits should be conducted with the parturient. In most circumstances the fact that epidural analgesia is not mandatory for labor or delivery and that other methods of pain relief are available should be addressed. Even the most insistent parturient normally should be told that any anesthetic procedure involves a small risk and that epidural analgesia is a type of anesthesia. Any problem for which the parturient is particularly at risk should be discussed. The risks of LEA should be discussed to the extent to which the parturient is comfortable and to her satisfaction.[41] It is not necessary to secure consent for the anesthesia accompanying a surgical procedure (e.g., cesarean section) at this time. If the potential for a problem does exist, the anesthetist may request consent for anesthesia in an emergency situation in which delay for a complete discussion would endanger the mother or her baby.

It is good to remember that LEA is optional. Babies are born safely without it. Although attempts should be made to prepare for the provision of pain relief as quickly as possible, rushing or pushing a patient into something or hurrying through the history-taking process to the point that injury to the patient may result is counterproductive. It is better to have a few women deliver without epidural analgesia than to cause injury to a mother or fetus because of inadequate preparation.

Local Anesthetics

For years the mainstay of LEA has been bupivacaine. Bupivacaine is not, however, the ideal obstetric local anesthetic. It tends to produce motor block, which is bothersome to many parturients, and can at times interfere with and prolong the second stage of labor. When excessive systemic absorption or intravascular injection occurs, bupivacaine also produces potent cardiac toxicity, which is worsened in pregnant women because of the increased level of progesterone. Although the incidence of cardiac toxicity is relatively low, given the risk of morbidity and mortality when it does occur in the parturient, consideration should be given to using a less cardiotoxic local anesthetic for LEA.

Ropivacaine is a pure S-isomer, rather than a racemic mixture of both isomers as is bupivacaine. The elimination half-life of ropivacaine in pregnant women is 5.2 hours, compared with 10.9 hours for bupivacaine.[42] This reduced elimination half-life makes it less likely that ropivacaine will accumulate to toxic levels over the course of a long labor epidural infusion. Ropivacaine produces approximately one third less motor block[43] and has a reduced potential to produce CNS and cardiac toxicity than does bupivacaine. A ropivacaine motor block develops more slowly, goes away more quickly, and is approximately one third less dense than that produced by bupivacaine.[43-46] Only slightly less potent than bupivacaine, ropivacaine is markedly less toxic,[47,48] and ropivacaine toxicity regresses more quickly once administration of the drug is terminated.[48] Whereas bupivacaine cardiac toxicity is enhanced in the parturient, that of ropivacaine is not.[49,50] Accidental intravascular injection of as little as 15 ml of 0.5% or 6.6 ml of 0.75% bupivacaine has resulted in maternal death,[51] while up to 20 ml of intravascular ropivacaine has resulted only in tinnitis.[52]

Epidural Insertion

Once the obstetrician approves and the parturient is in active labor, LEA may be begun. Active labor is generally present when cervical dilation is 4 cm in the primiparous patient or 3 cm in the multiparous patient. Earlier epidural analgesia can be initiated if the obstetrician is willing to use oxytocin to augment labor if necessary. The woman's pain perception should also be considered in the timing of LEA. If a woman with less cervical dilation perceives a significant amount of pain, and the obstetrician agrees, effective epidural analgesia is warranted, even if labor is temporarily slowed.

Before epidural block is administered, the room should be inspected for the presence of resuscitation supplies, an O_2 source, and ready-to-use suction. A large-bore IV catheter should be in place.

Epidural insertion should be preceded by skin surface disinfection using a newly opened container of povidone iodine (single-use container). Solution from single-use containers provides more effective skin disinfection than that from previously opened containers.[53] Of cultures taken after two applications of povidone iodine from previously opened containers, 40% grew bacterial colonies, fungal colonies, or both, and 70% of those grew multiple colonies. Only 5% of cultures taken after skin surface disinfection with solution from previously unopened containers grew any colonies at all, and when they did, they grew only one colony each. Although intuitively it would seem as though a container of povidone iodine should "self-sterilize," preventing growth of infectious organisms, this is not the case. Of cultures taken from the lid of previously opened povidone iodine bottles, 40% had a positive result, but there was no growth from any unopened container.

Baseline blood pressure should be measured, and blood pressure should be checked at regular intervals once the epidural anesthetic is begun. If the parturient is having difficulty cooperating because of her perception of pain, administration of 50 to 100 mcg of IV fentanyl (limit 1 mcg/kg) often provides significant relief while the epidural anesthetic is being administered. This dose has been shown to present little risk to the neonate,[54] especially when the fentanyl is given more than 2 hours before delivery. Although of shorter duration than meperidine, fentanyl results in fewer maternal side effects.[31,55]

Often the sitting position is easiest for the patient to maintain and usually offers the anesthetist the maximum interspace width. A knowledgeable obstetric nurse who helps to steady the parturient in the proper position while offering comfort is a great asset. If the patient is having a difficult time holding still during contractions, then placing her in the lateral position may help limit motion. A comforting attitude, patience, understanding, and complete explanation of what the anesthetist is doing often help minimize the parturient's fears.

When placing the epidural catheter, the anesthetist should take into consideration at what point in the labor and delivery process the patient is. If she is in the early stages of labor, she may need several hours of labor analgesia. In this case, introducing the catheter as high as safely possible (usually at the L2-3 interspace) and inserting it in a cephalad direction will be most likely to result in an optimal final catheter tip position of L1-2. From this position as little as 6 ml of local anesthetic volume may provide a truly segmental epidural block from T10 to L4, covering the nerves carrying pain from cervical dilation and uterine contractions (Figure 44-12). If the catheter is inserted at a point lower than L2-3, a greater volume of local anesthetic will be necessary in order to achieve a block up to the T10 dermatome. For optimal performance multiple side hole catheters (closed end) should be inserted 5 cm into the epidural space,[56] and single end hole catheters should be inserted 2 cm to 4 cm. Once inserted part of the way, the epidural catheter should not be pulled back through the needle or it may shear off in the patient. Rather, the needle and catheter should be withdrawn together and another attempt made.

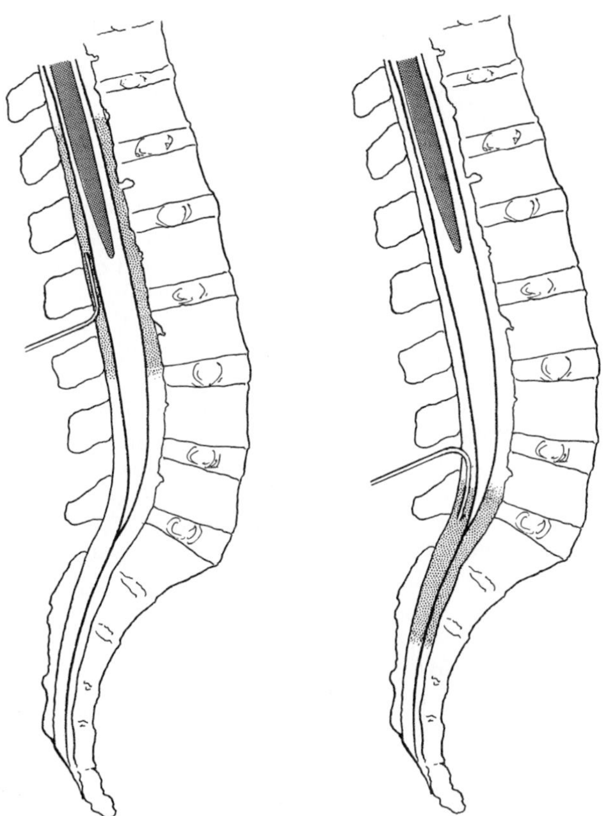

FIGURE **44-12**
Effect of epidural catheter position and direction on the spread of local anesthetic.

In the rare circumstance in which the epidural block is to be performed late in labor and analgesia is desired mainly for perineal pain caused by stretching and episiotomy, placing the catheter as low as possible (generally at L4-5) and directing it caudad results in a greater chance that a sacral block will be achieved. A sacral block can sometimes be difficult to achieve with epidural anesthesia and may require large volumes of local anesthetic. If epidural anesthesia has been established early in labor and a local anesthetic has been infusing for several hours, a sacral block is usually achieved before stage 2 (delivery of the fetus), when sacral analgesia is needed.

It has long been observed that the failure rate of epidural anesthetics is greater in the obese. It has been shown that the distance from the skin to the epidural space varies with changes in body position; and more so in the obese. The greatest increase in the distance from the skin to the epidural space is associated with a change from the sitting, flexed position to lying with the legs straight out. Because epidural catheters are usually secured to the back while the parturient is sitting up in a flexed position, when the parturient lies back down and the distance from the skin to the epidural space increases the catheter can actually be pulled out of the epidural space. The average increase in skin-to-epidural-space distance in those with a body mass index (BMI; equal to weight in kilograms divided by height in meters squared) between 25 and 30 is 0.75 cm, with a range of up to 2.72 cm. The average increase in distance in those with a BMI greater than 30 is 1.04 cm, with a range of up to 4.28 cm.[57] Withdrawing the epidural catheter a centimeter or more could certainly result in one or more of its openings exiting the epidural space. This problem can be avoided by having the patient lie on her side and straighten her legs before the epidural catheter is secured to the back, thereby allowing the catheter to be pulled in a bit as the distance to the epidural space increases. In obese patients the anesthetist can very often see the epidural catheter being "sucked in" during this position change.

The type of epidural catheter used has an influence on the effectiveness of the block. The incidence of unilateral or spotty epidural blocks is highest when a single-end hole catheter is used. Fewer unsatisfactory blocks occur when a closed-end catheter with several side holes is used.[58-60]

Test Doses

The test dose is designed to reveal subarachnoid or intravascular injection of local anesthetic without producing systemic toxicity or widespread subarachnoid block. The key is to think of the test dose as the amount of drug in milligrams required to produce a detectable effect either spinally or systemically. Unlike spread of local anesthetic within the epidural space, volume has little to do with the effectiveness of a test dose. It is generally agreed that 30 mg of lidocaine is an effective test dose for subarachnoid injection. Alternatively, 10 mg of bupivacaine has been shown to produce a noticeable increase in foot temperature and motor block at the ankle four minutes after subarachnoid but not epidural injection.[61] Disagreement exists regarding how best to test for intravascular injection. The most widely accepted test dose involves the administration of 15 mcg of epinephrine, which has been shown to reliably increase HR in nonpregnant patients when injected intravascularly. However, this test dose is not universally accepted for obstetric anesthesia. In the laboring parturient, increases in HR are a less specific indicator because of the changes in HR that occur during uterine contractions. Furthermore, concern exists that epinephrine may cause significant uterine artery constriction in a few patients,[62,63] resulting in a decrease in fetal O_2 delivery.

Minor CNS local anesthetic side effects are easily observed when they occur and, with the exception of those related to bupivacaine, carry little risk as long as administration is stopped when they become evident. Given this, an alternative test for intravascular injection is the slow administration of lidocaine or 2-chloroprocaine while the patient is observed for CNS side effects. For this technique to be successful, one must pay close attention and constantly stay in verbal communication with the patient. For example, CNS changes after the IV administration of 60 mg of 2-chloroprocaine often include ringing in the ears, auditory changes, or changes in mental functioning. Because of the rapid intravascular metabolism of 2-chloroprocaine, these changes are very transient and may be missed if the anesthetist is not observant. The transient nature of the changes is an advantage, however, as any problem that develops resolves quickly.

Given the limitations and occasional hazards of the epinephrine test dose in laboring patients an alternative method of detecting intravascular or subarachnoid placement would be desirable. Two nonpharmacologic methods have been described. Both rely on the detection of blood or cerebrospinal fluid (CSF) in the epidural catheter to indicate a positive test result.[64,65] Observing for blood or CSF while aspirating the epidural catheter had a 0% false-positive rate and a 0.2% false-negative rate in over 1000 women in whom 60 intravascular or subarachnoid catheter placements were performed.[65] Ideally, the administration of every dose should be observed as a test dose, with the anesthetist checking for signs of intravascular and subarachnoid injection with each dose administered. One of the most important factors in the safe administration of epidural analgesics is the physical presence of an observant anesthetist during administration and for a period of time after its completion.

Administration of the Epidural Anesthetic

The spread of analgesia when an epidural catheter is placed is primarily determined by the volume of local anesthetic solution injected. This is different from a subarachnoid block, in which the dose in milligrams, the baricity of the local anesthetic, and the patient's position are the chief determinants of the extent of the anesthesia. In a normal, healthy, term parturient in her late teens to twenties, an average of approximately 1 ml of local anesthetic is required for each dermatomal level of local anesthetic spread. This is an average volume per segment. Because the lumbar epidural space is larger than, for example, the thoracic epidural space, a larger volume of local anesthetic is required for the spread of analgesia across one level in the lumbar epidural space than in the thoracic epidural space. Therefore if the catheter is placed at L2, an average of 16 ml is required for spread up to T6 and down to S4.

Adequate analgesia must be balanced against loss of the sensation of labor, which is not desirable during the second stage, and motor block, which is bothersome to the mother during labor and prevents expulsive efforts during delivery. There are many ways to approach epidural administration. Following is a "cookbook" approach that can and should be developed further by the anesthetist as his or her knowledge of and experience with local anesthetics and obstetric regional anesthesia increases.

After the epidural catheter has been inserted and a test dose performed, 6 to 12 ml of either 0.1% to 0.2% ropivacaine or 0.125% to 0.25% bupivacaine may be injected incrementally through the catheter. Slow injection results in markedly lower peak plasma local anesthetic concentrations than rapid injection.[66] Alternatively, the bolus feature of an epidural pump can be used to inject the initial bolus slowly over several minutes, with monitoring performed by the anesthetist. The addition of small amounts of fentanyl to the initial local anesthetic dose speeds the onset, intensifies the analgesia provided, and allows the anesthetist to decrease the concentration of local anesthetic without reducing pain relief. Up to 100 mcg of fentanyl can be included in the epidural bolus dose without producing adverse fetal or neonatal effects,[67] but a smaller dose is frequently effective.

Occasionally the anesthetist encounters a woman in very early labor who perceives a great deal of pain. If her membranes have ruptured and the obstetrician intends that she remain hospitalized until delivery, the anesthetist might consider placing an epidural catheter, except for concerns of "stalling out" this early labor by administering local anesthetic via the epidural route. In this situation it may be appropriate to place the catheter and administer fentanyl until labor becomes active and local anesthetic can be used. The epidural catheter is placed in the usual fashion. The patient should receive 100 mcg of fentanyl in preservative-free, normal saline (as much as is needed to 10 ml). This dose commonly results in approximately 1 hour of good analgesia that is superior to what would have been obtained with IV opioids. Often, this hour gives the parturient time to develop active labor. Once active labor is present, the local anesthetic may be given in the usual fashion. If an additional dose of opioid is necessary in the interim, 50 to 75 mcg of fentanyl in a 10-ml volume can be used at hourly intervals without danger of depressing a healthy fetus.

Although the small amount of epinephrine present in an IV test dose should be safe for a healthy fetus, the larger amounts present in the volume of local anesthetic used to maintain LEA carry some risk of umbilical artery constriction in some parturients.[68] For this reason routine use of epinephrine-containing solutions may be unwise. Epinephrine-containing solutions are specifically indicated in a few circumstances and can be used safely in judicious amounts when the fetus is healthy.

After epidural analgesia has been instituted, the patient should be encouraged not to lie on her back, so that aortocaval syndrome can be avoided. The anesthetist should remain aware of cervical dilation and of the progress of labor after the epidural catheter has been placed. Communication with obstetric personnel is important to prevent use of a drug, dose, or concentration of local anesthetic that is inappropriate for the patient's circumstances. For example, readministration of 0.5% bupivacaine at the beginning of the second stage of labor is likely to result in a motor block that causes the patient to be unable to push or sense contractions.

Maintaining Epidural Analgesia for Labor and Delivery

Although it is possible to maintain LEA with intermittent bolus administration, less local anesthetic is administered and more effective analgesia achieved when analgesia is maintained with a continuous epidural infusion. Historically the most commonly chosen local anesthetic for epidural infusion has been bupivacaine, but ropivacaine produces less motor block and carries a lesser risk of life-threatening cardiotoxicity. During labor, the minimal effective concentration of local anesthetic should be used so that the risk of motor block is minimized. Ropivacaine or bupivacaine in concentrations of 0.0625% to 0.2% are commonly used. The lower concentration may be effective in mild to moderate labors as long as adequate spread is achieved. Maintaining an adequate sensory level usually necessitates an infusion rate of 10 to 15 ml/hr. In the majority of women, this dilute concentration is associated with minimal motor block, although block will become more dense the longer the infusion is maintained. A higher concentration may be needed as labor intensifies or in women who experience greater pain.

The addition of fentanyl to the local anesthetic speeds the onset, increases the density, and prolongs the duration of analgesia. In an epidural infusion this maximizes the pain relief while minimizing the concentration of local anesthetic needed. An epidural maintenance infusion of 0.1% or 0.15% ropivacaine or bupivacaine combined with 1 or 2 mcg/ml of fentanyl at a rate of 10 to 15 ml/hr produces better pain relief than higher concentrations of local anesthetic alone. However, even these low concentrations can result in motor block when they are infused for many hours. If the labor is prolonged, it may be necessary to decrease the concentration of local anesthetic over time.

If the onset of the second stage of labor occurs during a stable labor epidural block, and if the patient has good motor function, then the block may be maintained while the patient pushes. The ideal block provides analgesia for labor pain, dense analgesia of the perineum for delivery, and little motor block. If motor block hinders pushing or if sensory block prevents the parturient from sensing contractions and therefore knowing when to push, the epidural infusion should be turned off. If necessary, it can be restarted when the baby is beginning to crown or when perineal analgesia is needed. At that time perineal anesthesia, if lacking, can usually be achieved with the injection of 10 ml of 1.5% lidocaine with epinephrine, 2% 2-chloroprocaine, or 0.25% bupivacaine. If a more dense analgesia is needed, the addition of up to 100 mcg of fentanyl will produce very dense analgesia. If anesthesia is needed for a mid or high forceps delivery and the obstetrician does not need the parturient to push, the concentrations of bupivacaine, lidocaine, and 2-chloroprocaine are increased to 0.5%, 2%, and 3%, respectively, with or without fentanyl added.

Patient-Controlled Epidural Analgesia

Continuous infusion of local anesthetic solution into the epidural space is probably the most common method of maintaining analgesia during the first stage of labor. Several investigations of the efficacy of patient-controlled epidural analgesia (PCEA) have been conducted. PCEA may afford some advantages during labor, because it has been associated with a reduced need for top-up doses,[69,70] a high degree of patient satisfaction,[69-71] and a reduction in total doses of bupivacaine required.[69]

HYPOTENSION DURING REGIONAL ANESTHESIA IN THE OBSTETRIC PATIENT

The accepted cause of hypotension during regional anesthesia in obstetric patients has long been the fact that the block results in a sympathectomy that causes peripheral venous pooling, a reduction in venous return to the heart, reduced preload, reduced SV, and therefore reduced cardiac output and a fall in blood pressure. From this it followed that simply infusing additional volume would restore venous return to the heart and preserve cardiac output, thereby preventing hypotension. The most common measure undertaken to prevent maternal hypotension after epidural block has therefore been the infusion of IV fluid in an attempt to replace volume thought to pool because of sympatholytic-induced vasodilation. This hypothesis for the mechanism of maternal hypotension during regional anesthesia can now be seen to be lacking in a number of areas, which are enumerated in this section.

1. The proposed mechanism of maternal hypotension does not take into consideration differences in maternal physiology at term compared with the physiology of nonpregnant women. In addition, complete hemodynamic measurements in healthy pregnant women with which to consider these differences in the context of a regional block have been lacking.

Better understanding of the physiology of term-pregnant women has revealed considerable differences from that of nonpregnant women in terms of baseline peripheral sympathetic tone, concentrations of circulating vasoactive substances such as angiotensin II, and vascular reactivity to vasoactive substances. These differences were not taken into consideration when the mechanism of maternal hypotension after regional anesthesia was hypothesized. The proposed mechanism was based largely on a seminal work by Nicholas Greene,[72] but Green's conclusions were based on studies in nonpregnant individuals, most of whom were healthy volunteers.[73-77] Although studies have been reported in which SV, HR, SVR, and MAP were measured concurrently, these studies were in women with PIH or preeclampsia, not in healthy women.

2. Many studies spanning multiple years have failed to determine the volume of IV preload that prevents maternal hypotension after induction of regional anesthesia.

Numerous studies have reported the incidences and magnitude of hypotension after IV infusion of various solution types, volumes, and methods of administration. No study has identified a volume of intravascular fluid that comes close to eliminating hypotension in pregnant women undergoing regional anesthesia. Volume preload regimens have inconsistent efficacy and do not eliminate maternal hypotension.[78,79]

Crystalloid IV preloads with solutions such as lactated Ringer's of up to 30 ml/kg are commonly associated with an incidence of maternal hypotension of approximately 50%, often not statistically different from the incidence in controls who receive no preload at all.[80,81] One reason crystalloid preloads may be ineffective is that they remain in the circulation for a short period of time. Only 28%[82] of 1.5 L of lactated Ringer's solution infused over 30 minutes remains in the maternal circulation at the end of the 30-minute infusion period. Preloading with colloid solutions to prevent epidural anesthetic–induced hypotension nets a modest improvement in prevention of hypotension. Studies comparing preloads with hetastarch versus crystalloid solution often do show a significant difference between groups, but the incidence of hypotension remains high.[83] In addition, a study in which 1 L of 6% hetastarch was administered *in addition to* crystalloid solution as an IV preload still yielded 17% hypotension.[82] Clinically, colloid IV preloads are uncommonly used. They do not eliminate hypotension, and practitioners are often hesitant to use them because of their greater cost. In clinical practice, crystalloid solutions are used almost exclusively. The overall incidence of maternal hypotension is probably at least 38%, given the infrequent use of colloids.

3. A mechanism exists to suggest that aggressive crystalloid preloading may contribute to maternal hypotension during subarachnoid or epidural block.

Administering volume in excess of that needed to replace the deficit acquired during an overnight fast may play a role in maternal hypotension in the presence of subarachnoid or epidural block. The level of block necessary for effective anesthesia for cesarean section attenuates the ability of the sympathetic nervous system and the renin-angiotensin system to maintain normotension. The vasopressin system remains to support blood pressure. Vasopressin and antidiuretic hormone (ADH) are the same hormones, called by different names according to the context of the discussion. On the whole the body is more responsive to the antidiuretic role of ADH than it is to the vasoconstrictive role of vasopressin, with small reductions in plasma colloid osmotic pressure resulting in strong inhibition of ADH release. Vasopressin release in response to loss of intravascular volume, on the other hand, requires a fairly strong stimulus. Animal studies[84] have shown that infusion of 10 ml/kg of dextran 40 of in lactated Ringer's solution results in a 30% decrease in circulating vasopressin during mock operation, as opposed to a 250% increase during mock operation without dextran infusion. Three healthy nonpregnant women had vasopressin levels assayed before and after ingestion of 20 ml of water per kilogram.[12] Two hours after water ingestion vasopressin had decreased to unmeasureable levels. Therefore it is possible that the volumes of crystalloid IV preload commonly employed in an effort to prevent maternal hypotension may actually inhibit the body's efforts to support blood pressure by delaying or reducing the magnitude of the vasopressin response.

The Mechanism of Maternal Hypotension

In order to identify the mechanism of maternal hypotension during regional anesthesia, the factors directly responsible for controlling blood pressure (SV, HR, and SVR) must be observed during the onset of regional anesthesia. Such a study quantified the changes in maternal MAP during epidural anesthesia for cesarean section in a group of 60 healthy pregnant women[85] (Table 44-2). Changes in maternal MAP were closely tied to changes in SVR ($r = 0.8$). Neither SV ($r = -0.11$) nor HR ($r = 0.05$) had a significant total effect on MAP in comparison.

During epidural block setup, both MAP and SVR decreased, whereas SV and HR increased. Not only did SV not correlate with MAP during block set up, SV *increased* on average, whereas MAP declined. Because mean values for both SV and HR increased during the development of epidural block–induced hypotension, mean cardiac output increased and clearly was not the cause of maternal hypotension.

Because crystalloid intravascular fluid was infused in all patients in this study, the possibility remains that the primary cause of maternal hypotension during epidural anesthesia is indeed peripheral venous pooling and reduced venous return to the heart, resulting in a reduction in SV and cardiac output. This primary cause of maternal hypotension may simply have been masked by the infusion of fluid before the block. If this were so, one would expect that larger volumes of fluid preload would result in smaller reductions in maternal MAP. The opposite effect was observed. Intravascular fluid administered averaged 1956 ± 426 ml (1200 ml to 3000 ml). The correlation between intravascular fluid administered and change in MAP was −0.33 ($P < .01$). Though small, this statistically significant correlation indicates a greater reduction in MAP the larger the volume of intravascular fluid administered—opposite the expected effect. The volume of intravascular fluid administered did not correlate with changes in either SV or HR during block setup.

Regulation of MAP in healthy term pregnant women undergoing epidural anesthesia and cesarean section appears to be most strongly influenced by SVR. Although crystalloid IV fluid was administered before epidural anesthesia, when MAP fell SV did not. This indicates that reduced venous return to the heart did not cause the hypotension. Not only did crystalloid IV preloading fail to prevent hypotension, the correlation between IV fluid volume and MAP change indicated that greater fluid preloading may have increased the magnitude of hypotension. It appears, then, that effective prevention of maternal hypotension must include interventions to maintain maternal SVR (without increasing uterine arterial resistance), possibly in concert with administration of intravascular fluid that remains in the vascular space.

TABLE 44-2 Change in Maternal Hemodynamics during Induction of T4 Sensory Level Epidural Block*

	Mean	SD	Range
Δ MAP	−21.4%	1.7%	−55.2 – 9%
Δ SV	16.8%	11.9%	−18.6 – 30%
Δ HR	7.6%	16.8%	−25.2 – 40.9%
Δ SVR	−26.6%	19.5%	−58.7 – 24%
IV fluid	1956	426	1200 – 3000

Δ, *Change;* IV, *intravenous.*
**Calculated from data collected during block onset.*
From Fiedler MA. Maternal Hypotension and Epidural Anesthesia for Cesarean Section [dissertation]. Memphis, Tenn: University of Tennessee Center for the Health Sciences; 2002.

Prevention and Treatment of Maternal Hypotension during Regional Anesthesia

Hypotension is probably the most frequent complication in obstetric anesthesia. It can cause discomfort for the mother and result in dangerous decreases in fetal oxygenation by decreasing uteroplacental blood flow. Intervillous blood flow is dependent on maternal MAP.[86] Furthermore, in the presence of reasonable maternal arterial partial pressure of oxygen (PaO_2), fetal oxygenation is dependent on intervillous blood flow and maternal MAP. Maternal hypotension of sufficient magnitude and duration results in fetal hypoxia, which if allowed to progress results in fetal academia and death.[87-89] In a healthy pregnant woman the critical duration of hypotension is probably greater than 2 minutes.[88] The critical magnitude of hypotension is a systolic blood pressure below 100 mm Hg.[90] Because of pregnancy-related changes in vascular tone and cardiovascular dynamics the parturient is more dependent on vascular tone for maintenance of blood pressure than is a nonpregnant woman. In pregnant women receiving either subarachnoid or epidural block for cesarean section, which involves wide areas of chemical sympathectomy, hypotension is more likely than in nonpregnant patients who have received the same block.[91]

Ephedrine

Ephedrine is a synthetic, nonselective, noncatecholamine sympathomimetic drug. Doses of 5 to 25 mg intravenously are used to treat acute decreases in blood pressure. The duration of ephedrine's cardiovascular effects varies with the dose given. The effect of a 5- or 10-mg IV dose usually persists for 5 minutes.

Tachyphylaxis can occur with repeated administration of small doses, resulting in a noticeably reduced clinical effect after subsequent dosing. Ephedrine is metabolized in the liver, and up to 40% is excreted unchanged by the kidneys. It has an elimination half-life of 3 hours.

Ephedrine causes direct β stimulation and indirect α stimulation through the release of endogenous norepinephrine. It is the favorite vasoactive agent in obstetric anesthesia because it affects uterine artery blood flow less than other vasoactive drugs.[92] It does not constrict uterine arteries or compromise uteroplacental circulation when given as a bolus in clinically useful doses. The effect of ephedrine is similar to that of epinephrine, but ephedrine is much less potent (by a factor of 250) and has a longer duration. Ephedrine crosses the placenta. Fetal blood levels of the drug are directly related to maternal blood levels (the umbilical vein–to–maternal artery concentration ratio has been measured at 0.71).[93]

Given evidence that reduced SVR is the mechanism of maternal hypotension after regional anesthesia, and given the safety of ephedrine during pregnancy, an ephedrine infusion may currently be the most logical choice for treatment of maternal hypotension. Ephedrine infusion has been used during cesarean section with the patient under subarachnoid block anesthesia with or without a 1-L crystalloid preload without any evidence of fetal harm as assessed by Apgar score, umbilical arterial and venous pH, and neonatal adaptive capacity scoring.[94] Both groups required similar total ephedrine doses, and both had similar incidences of hypotension. Other studies employing an ephedrine infusion, with or without volume preloading, have shown a larger reduction in the incidence of hypotension after spinal or epidural anesthesia than that after large volumes of IV preload alone.[95-99]

Phenylephrine

In some situations ephedrine is ineffective or the increase in HR that it causes is undesirable. Though α-agonists were previously thought to cause fetal acidosis based on animal studies, phenylephrine has been shown to be safe for the treatment of maternal hypotension during regional anesthesia.[100] Neonatal blood gas values and Apgar scores remain within normal limits in all healthy subjects after the administration of 80-mcg[101] or 100-mcg[102] bolus doses of phenylephrine. Other investigators have also found reassuring results with the use of phenylephrine in healthy parturients.[102]

Nonpharmacologic Support of Blood Pressure

Another approach to maintenance of maternal SVR during regional anesthesia might be compression of the lower extremities much in the same way that the forearm is compressed in preparation for a Bier block. Though clinically uncommon, six investigations have reported the effects of leg compression either alone or in combination with IV preloading.

Elastic compression stockings appear to be of no benefit in prevention of maternal hypotension,[103] even in combination with a 500-ml IV preload of Hartmann's solution. Neither the incidence nor magnitude of hypotension was improved over controls.

Thromboembolic deterrent stockings are designed to aid venous return in the legs but are no more effective than regular elastic stockings[104] when applied after a 15-ml/kg IV preload of Hartmann's solution but before a bupivacaine subarachnoid block. These elastic stockings apply graduated pressure from 8 to 18 mm Hg to various parts of the legs when properly applied. No difference in the systolic blood pressure was present between the two groups after regional block.

In contrast to use of regular elastic or thromboembolic stockings, the wrapping of the legs with a tight rubber (Esmarch) bandage has been shown to reduce the incidence of maternal hypotension from 53% to 18% ($P = .004$)[105] in one study and from 83% to 17% ($P = 0.003$)[106] in another. Both groups in both studies also received a crystalloid IV preload.

Preliminary evidence suggests that applying sufficient pressure to the legs in the presence of left uterine displacement does reduce the incidence of maternal hypotension after regional block. Wrapping the legs with elastic compression stockings does not significantly reduce the incidence or severity of hypotension. Wrapping the legs with a rubber Esmarch bandage (a much tighter wrap) does so when left uterine displacement is also used. Compression stockings are designed only to compress veins and aid in venous return from the legs. Esmarch bandages are likely to compress not only veins, but, at least to some extent, arteries as well. The increased efficacy at preventing hypotension with the use of tight wraps compared with the use of elastic wraps may have been related to the difference between venous compression and arterial compression.

ANESTHESIA FOR CESAREAN SECTION

Aspiration Risk

From an anesthetic point of view, all obstetric patients have a full stomach. Routine measures to prevent aspiration pneumonitis in the obstetric patient are warranted. Unless contraindicated, a clear oral antacid, IV H_2 blocker, and IV metoclopramide are recommended for obstetric patients undergoing surgical procedures. Thirty milliliters of sodium citrate (Bicitra) or Alka-Seltzer Gold (defizzed) effectively raises the pH of gastric contents for up to an hour and is best administered near the time of the induction of anesthesia. The very sour taste of Bicitra is unpleasant, and it is better tolerated when gulped or given over crushed ice. Both agents are most effective when thoroughly mixed with gastric contents. The use of particulate antacids is best avoided, because animal studies have shown that they cause pulmonary damage when aspirated.

Ranitidine inhibits gastric acid secretion, thereby reducing future gastric volume. It can be given orally (150 or 300 mg) or intravenously (50 mg IV piggyback). A single oral or IV dose of ranitidine has been shown not to affect uterine contractions or neonatal neurobehavioral scores.[107] Unlike cimetidine, ranitidine does not inhibit the elimination of amide local anesthetics.[108] Metoclopramide (10 mg intravenously) increases gastric motility and increases sphincter tone between the esophagus and the stomach but should be administered slowly so that agitation and psychosis are avoided.[109] Metoclopramide inhibits the enzyme pseudocholinesterase (PCHE) and, to a lesser degree, acetylcholinesterase. By itself, this effect is unlikely to prolong the duration of succinylcholine or mivacurium to a clinically significant degree, but it does add to the depression of PCHE activity normally present at term pregnancy. Prolongation of neuromuscular block because of preeclampsia or magnesium administration could be intensified.

Positioning

During positioning of the parturient on the operative table, left uterine displacement should be provided as soon as possible; the table should be rolled to the left or a wedge placed under the right hip of the patient in order to shift the uterus off the inferior vena cava and abdominal aorta, thereby preserving fetal oxygenation. Fetuses delivered of mothers with left uterine displacement have a lower incidence of CNS depression and acidosis than those delivered of mothers in the supine position.[110]

Surgical Blood Loss

Blood loss during cesarean section is usually less when regional anesthesia is used than when general anesthesia is used. On average approximately 500 ml of blood is lost during cesarean section with regional anesthesia, and approximately 700 ml with general anesthesia. Despite this average the range of blood loss is great; in one study, from 164 to 1438 ml.[111] Many factors affect the volume of blood lost during cesarean section, including surgical time, surgical technique, blood pressure, fetal lie, fetal size, placental implantation, maternal coagulation status, and the ability of the uterus to contract after the placenta has been delivered. Statistically determined risk factors for excessive bleeding during cesarean section (with odds ratios) include general anesthesia (2.94), amnionitis (2.69), preeclampsia (2.18), protracted active phase of labor (2.4), second-stage arrest (1.9), and Hispanic ethnicity (1.82).[112]

General Anesthesia

Regional anesthesia is generally preferred for cesarean section. Properly conducted regional anesthesia may yield less neonatal depression (at least in the short term), and the mother is usually able to enjoy experiencing her newborn sooner.[113-116] Also, surgical blood loss is less when regional anesthesia rather than general anesthesia is used. A general anesthetic is indicated for cesarean section when the anesthetist is not knowledgeable in regional anesthetic techniques, when regional anesthesia is contraindicated, when the patient refuses regional anesthesia, or when anesthesia must be induced emergently.

Airway

When general anesthesia is chosen, use of a cuffed endotracheal tube is indicated, and rapid-sequence induction should be performed unless it is contraindicated. An airway evaluation is an important part of the preparation for anesthesia in any patient and even more so in the parturient. Airway problems tend to occur more frequently in obstetric patients than in other healthy patients; failure to intubate has been reported to occur as frequently as 1 in 250 obstetric patients.[117] This is true at least in part because of the soft-tissue edema often present in the hypopharynx. Breast enlargement and cephalad displacement of the thorax often make maneuvering the laryngoscope into the mouth difficult. Placement of a rolled towel lengthwise along the thoracic spine or widthwise under the shoulders helps to elevate the chest off the operating table. This makes it possible to flex the neck at the shoulders and extend the neck at the head more optimally, facilitating insertion of the laryngoscope blade and improving visualization of the glottis. Some anesthetists find short-handled laryngoscopes easier to use in these patients.

Induction

Induction of general anesthesia proceeds in the usual rapid-sequence manner, with cricoid pressure after denitrogenation and generous preoxygenation. Appropriate induction agents in the healthy parturient include thiopental, ketamine, etomidate, and propofol. Propofol produces no greater neonatal depression than thiopental and is rapidly cleared from the neonate.[118-120] It is cleared from the parturient more quickly than thiopental, resulting in more rapid emergence[119,120]; some studies have shown less variation in vital signs with the use of propofol than with thiopental.[121] Thiopental is usually used in doses of approximately 3 to 5 mg/kg. Ketamine, up to 1 mg/kg, is especially useful in patients who have airway disease or are hypotensive. It has also been associated with lower analgesic demands during the first 24 hours postoperatively compared with demands in women induced with thiopental.[122] The indirect sympathomimetic effect of ketamine helps support blood pressure until adequate volume can be replaced. The 1-mg/kg upper limit on ketamine should be observed to prevent depression of the neonate and maternal emergence reactions. Up to 0.3 mg/kg of etomidate can be used; the indications are the same in pregnant patients as they are in nonpregnant patients. All these lipid-soluble induction drugs cross the placenta rapidly, but neonatal depression is infrequently a problem when the cited doses are used.

Traditionally induction of anesthesia has been delayed until preparation for surgery is completed. Surgery starts immediately after verification of proper endotracheal tube placement. The reasoning behind this practice has been that the dose of depressant drugs to which the fetus is exposed before delivery should be minimized. An interesting study has called this practice into question because of concerns over maternal awareness during surgical incision. King and co-workers[123] have reported that as many as 96% of women given 3 mg of thiopental per kilogram, 50% nitrous oxide, and 0.5% halothane (the vaporizer setting, not the end-tidal concentration) with a 5-L fresh gas flow obeyed commands during skin incision; as many as 20% still responded 2 minutes after incision. They suggested that other means of providing anesthesia at skin incisions should be considered, such as the use of local infiltration or opioids. Perhaps ketamine should be used more often to induce anesthesia; ketamine is a good amnestic and, unlike thiopental, provides somatic analgesia.

Neonatal depression during routine cesarean section has not been observed despite anesthetic induction-to-delivery intervals of up to 10 minutes.[124] If this induction-to-delivery interval is safe, and if maternal awareness is a problem at the time of incision when traditional anesthetic techniques are used, then another alternative might simply be to delay incision until 3 minutes after anesthetic induction in healthy women.

Intubation

Succinylcholine remains the preferred muscle relaxant during induction of general anesthesia in the parturient. If the use of succinylcholine is contraindicated, a fast-acting nondepolarizer may be judiciously administered, or an awake intubation may be attempted. Although intubation can be accomplished quickly with a fast-onset nondepolarizing muscle relaxant, the duration of action will be longer than with succinylcholine.

Succinylcholine is metabolized by PCHE. PCHE activity is normally decreased approximately 30% in a healthy pregnant woman at term. If the parturient also has preeclampsia, PCHE levels may be decreased by 60%. Although a 30% decrease in PCHE has little clinical significance, a 60% decrease may prolong recovery time after succinylcholine neuromuscular blockade. Although magnesium sulfate seems to have no effect on PCHE activity, succinylcholine's duration of action is prolonged in patients receiving magnesium sulfate. Metoclopramide may also prolong the action of agents eliminated through ester hydrolysis.[125]

After adequate relaxation has been achieved, the trachea should be intubated expeditiously. Because the parturient's functional residual capacity is decreased by 25% and her whole-body O_2 demand is up to 30% greater than normal, desaturation occurs rapidly. Once apnea occurs, maternal O_2 partial pressure drops three times as quickly as it would in a nonpregnant woman.

The Difficult Airway. Airway problems resulting in a failure to oxygenate and ventilate the obstetric patient are still a significant anesthesia-related cause of maternal mortality. Although rapid-sequence induction is the technique most commonly employed to minimize the risk of gastric aspiration during induction of general anesthesia, it is *not* indicated if the laryngoscopist has doubts about his or her ability to intubate the patient. In such a case an alternative method, such as awake intubation, may be necessary. Blind nasal intubation should be performed cautiously, if at all, in the parturient, who commonly has swollen nasal mucosa that is prone to bleeding.

The anesthetist should be familiar with and able to perform the steps in an obstetric failed intubation algorithm. Such an algorithm is depicted in Figure 44-13. Those skilled with the laryngeal mask airway (LMA) would probably want to insert its use in the algorithm before cricothyrotomy. Pulse oximetry and capnography are essential monitors.

Maintenance of Anesthesia before Delivery

General anesthesia can be maintained by one of several methods. If propofol was used for induction, it can be used as an infusion for maintenance in the usual doses. Low doses of an inhalation agent also are appropriate. Up to two thirds MAC of an inhalation agent (0.75% isoflurane, 1.7% sevoflurane, 4.8% desflurane) has a long, safe history of use during cesarean section. However, all inhalation agents cause uterine relaxation, and the uterus must contract after delivery of the placenta to stop bleeding. Two thirds MAC inhalation agent depresses uterine contractility by approximately 25%,[126] and this amount of uterine relaxation usually can be overcome with clinically used doses of oxytocin.[127,128] If the woman has been laboring for an extended period, has received high doses of oxytocin before delivery, or has a uterus that has been stretched by multiple fetuses or hydramnios, her uterus will not contract well. In these circumstances, it is important to have as much of the inhalation agent as possible eliminated at the time of delivery. Under normal circumstances, low MAC levels of inhalation agent can be washed out quickly enough at delivery for undesirable uterine relaxation and bleeding to be avoided.

Disagreement exists regarding whether nitrous oxide should be used before delivery during cesarean section. If fetal distress is present or if maternal O_2 saturation is below 97%, high concentrations of O_2 should be used without nitrous oxide. Administering 100% O_2 does result in improved fetal oxygenation compared with 50% O_2,[129] but questions have been raised about the danger of free radical activity in neonates born to women administered greater than 50% O_2.[130] However, 50% nitrous oxide usually has been "allowable" during cesarean section in healthy women because it is believed that 50% O_2 is adequate if the fetus is healthy. Comparisons of Apgar scores, umbilical venous O_2 tension, time to breathing, and resuscitation efforts in neonates has revealed that infants born to women given 100% O_2 before delivery have a slightly better outcome.[131,132] Little benefit is associated with the discontinuation of nitrous oxide in order to deliver 100% O_2 only during the time from hysterotomy to delivery.[133]

After induction, if muscle relaxation is needed it can be accomplished with either a succinylcholine drip or a nondepolarizing agent. A succinylcholine drip is the classic technique for muscle relaxation during cesarean section but requires skill few anesthetists develop any longer. In inexperienced hands a succinylcholine drip may result in a phase 2 block that does not wear off quickly when the drip is discontinued. A phase 2 block may result either from too high a drip rate or from multiple boluses of succinylcholine. The duration of action of

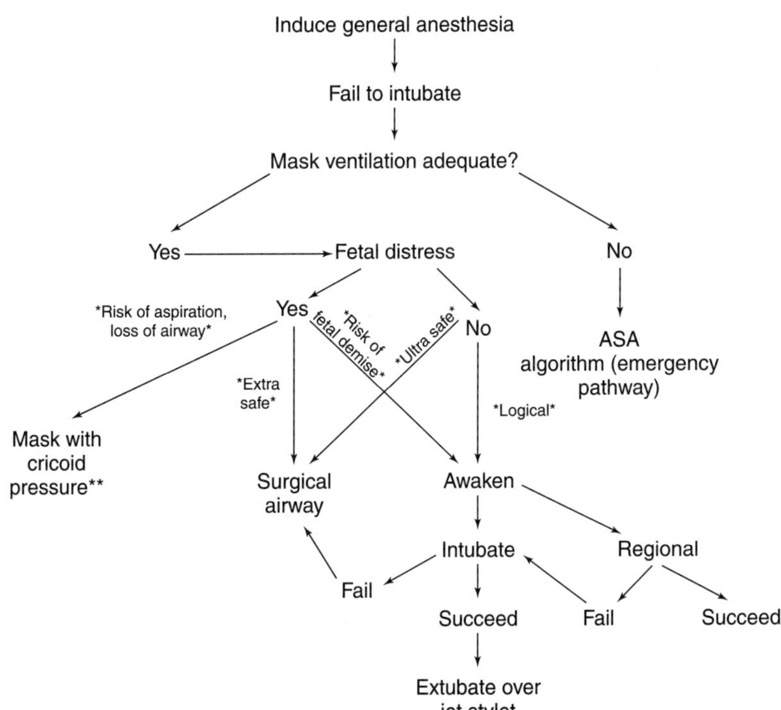

FIGURE **44-13**
Supplement to the difficult airway management algorithm, with special reference to the presence or absence of fetal distress. This algorithm includes options in the management of a recognized difficult airway in an uncooperative patient or in a cooperative patient with dire fetal distress. (From Chestnut DH. Obstetric anesthesia: principles and practice. 3rd ed. Philadelphia: Elsevier Mosby; 2004.)
*Denotes implications of this choice.
**Conventional face mask or laryngeal mask airway.

at least some nondepolarizers is slightly shorter than normal in a healthy term parturient.[134] If a tubal ligation is to be performed at the same time as the cesarean section, the surgery should easily last long enough to allow the use of a nondepolarizer. A final consideration should be whether a muscle relaxant is needed at all. Because a woman's skin and abdominal muscles are so stretched during pregnancy, the surgeon may not need additional muscle relaxation to perform the procedure if adequate anesthesia is provided.

Tasks at Delivery and Postdelivery Maintenance

The length of time from uterine incision to delivery has been shown to correlate with the degree of neonatal acidosis.[135] The interval should be recorded. An interval of 3 minutes seems to be the critical value[136]; neonates delivered later than 3 minutes after uterine incision are more likely to be depressed.

After the umbilical cord has been clamped, the anesthetist's options for anesthetic maintenance increase, because the administered drugs will no longer reach the baby. If adequate uterine contraction is achieved with oxytocin, there is no reason why the use of an inhalation anesthetic cannot be continued. A low-dose inhalation agent (up to 1 MAC), with or without nitrous oxide, and either fentanyl or sufentanil work well. The obstetrician also may want an antibiotic to be given. If uterine tone does not allow the use of an inhalation agent an opioid technique is useful. When opioids are used, nitrous oxide is usually needed. If nitrous oxide is not used, the anesthetist may consider giving a small dose of midazolam for amnesia. Opioid administration should be customized to the circumstances. One option is giving up to 5 mcg of fentanyl per kilogram or 0.5 mcg of sufentanil per kilogram, adjusting the dose according to the expected duration of the case and the patient's response. Another opioid choice is morphine 10 mg intravenously and 10 mg intramuscularly. One of these options should be selected, and nitrous oxide added. If midazolam is used, the dose of opioid should be reduced. If an inhalation agent is not used, paralysis must be maintained in order to prevent patient movement.

After the placenta has been delivered, oxytocin should be given immediately unless the obstetrician's plan for uterine contraction calls for the use of another agent. Pitocin is the clinically available synthetic equivalent of oxytocin, a naturally occurring hormone synthesized in the supraoptic and paraventricular nuclei of the hypothalamus. In the mature uterus of a pregnant woman, oxytocin causes an increase in the frequency and strength of uterine contractions. Endogenous oxytocin release occurs with stimulation of the cervix, vagina, and breasts.

The half-life of oxytocin varies from 4 to 17 minutes. It is metabolized by liver, kidney, and plasma enzyme pathways in the parturient. Commercially available preparations of oxytocin contain a preservative that causes systolic and especially diastolic hypotension, flushing, and tachycardia when infused at high doses.[137] The amount of oxytocin added to the IV solution should be tailored to the volume of solution remaining in the bag, the flow rate of the IV, and the patient's condition. If the IV bag is nearly empty or if IV solution is being administered rapidly, less oxytocin should be added to the bag. In general the obstetrician is likely to desire the administration of 30 to 40 units of oxytocin over the first hour postpartum. If an unusually large blood loss results in hypotension, and if fluid resuscitation is needed, it may be helpful to infuse the oxytocin at an appropriate rate and to start a second IV line for administering fluid volume at a rapid rate. If the solution with the added oxytocin is infused fast enough to replace volume, then it is likely that the high dose of oxytocin may cause further hypotension.

If oxytocin does not adequately stimulate uterine contraction, the next drug used is usually an ergot alkaloid (Methergine, Ergotrate). Because of their potent vascular effects, ergot alkaloids are not administered intravenously. Ergot alkaloids normally cause an increase in blood pressure, central venous pressure, and pulmonary capillary wedge pressure. IV administration may result in arterial and venous constriction, coronary artery constriction, severe hypertension, cerebral bleeding, headache, nausea, and vomiting. An intramuscular dose of 0.2 mg is commonly administered for stimulating uterine contractions. In some cases the obstetrician may choose to administer oxytocin or ergotamine directly into the uterine muscle to maximize effect. Ergot alkaloids are metabolized and eliminated chiefly by the liver. The plasma half-life is approximately 2 hours, but uterine effects last much longer.

Ergot alkaloids potentiate sympathomimetics, especially α-agonists (including ephedrine). Severe hypertension, cerebrovascular accidents, and retinal detachment have occurred when the two drugs were used simultaneously. These effects may persist even when the vasopressor is given well after the last dose of methylergonovine maleate.

When the uterus does not contract well despite the use of oxytocin and ergot alkaloids, prostaglandin F_{2a} (Prostin; 250 mcg) is administered either intramuscularly or directly into the uterine muscle. Prostaglandins are potent stimulators of uterine contractions. The contractions induced by prostaglandins are strong and painful. Nausea, vomiting, and diarrhea are frequent side effects. In addition to causing uterine contractions, prostaglandins may cause hypotension by relaxing vascular smooth muscle; however, cases of severe hypertension after prostaglandin administration have also been reported.[138-140] Prostaglandins may cause a recalcitrant uterus to contract and stop bleeding. If they do not, the surgeon is likely to extend the procedure and include hysterectomy, for which the anesthetist must be prepared.

Emergence from Anesthesia

Even when given drugs to empty the stomach, a parturient often has a large volume of gastric contents. Suctioning of the stomach with an orogastric tube while the patient is anesthetized decreases the incidence of vomiting after awake extubation. Before extubation the anesthetist should verify full recovery of neuromuscular function. Because cesarean section is usually a brief procedure involving fairly limited exposure to anesthetic, emergence is often quick. Advance preparation limits patient discomfort before extubation. A suggested method for providing general anesthesia for cesarean section is given in Box 44-4.

Epidural Block

Several local anesthetics are safe and effective for use in a cesarean section. Bupivacaine 0.5% provides good motor block and dense anesthesia but may require up to 30 minutes to take effect. The long time to onset is often considered a disadvantage. However, the sympathetic block also occurs more slowly; this means that there is more time to react to hemodynamic changes than when agents with a more rapid onset are used. Lidocaine 2% provides good motor block and dense anesthesia and has an onset time of approximately 10 minutes. If 1 mEq of sodium bicarbonate is added to each 10 ml of lidocaine

BOX **44-4**

General Anesthesia for Cesarean Section

Histamine$_2$-receptor antagonist or proton pump inhibitor and/or metroclopramide intravenously
Clear antacid orally
Left uterine displacement
Application of monitors
Denitrogenation (administration of 100% oxygen)
- Traditional 3-5 minutes versus four vital-capacity breaths

Cricoid pressure
Intravenous induction
- Thiobarbiturate, propofol, ketamine, or etomidate
- Succinylcholine (rocuronium or vecuronium if succinylcholine is contraindicated)

Intubation with a 6.0- to 7.0-mm cuffed endotracheal tube
Administration of 30% to 50% nitrous oxide in oxygen and a low concentration (e.g., 2/3 minimum alveolar concentration MAC) of a volatile halogenated agent.
After delivery
- Increased concentration of nitrous oxide, with or without a low concentration of a volatile inhalation agent
- Opioid titrated as needed
- Intravenous hypnotic agent (e.g., benzodiazepine, barbiturate, propofol), if needed
- Muscle relaxant (e.g., succinylcholine boluses or infusion, rocuronium, mivacurium, cisatracurium, vecuronium)

Extubation awake with intact airway reflexes

Modified from Kuczkowski KM, Reisner LS, Lim D. Anesthesia for Cesarean Section. In Obstetric Anesthesia, 3rd ed, Chestnut, DH (ed) Elsevier Mosby, Philadelphia, 2004, p 434.

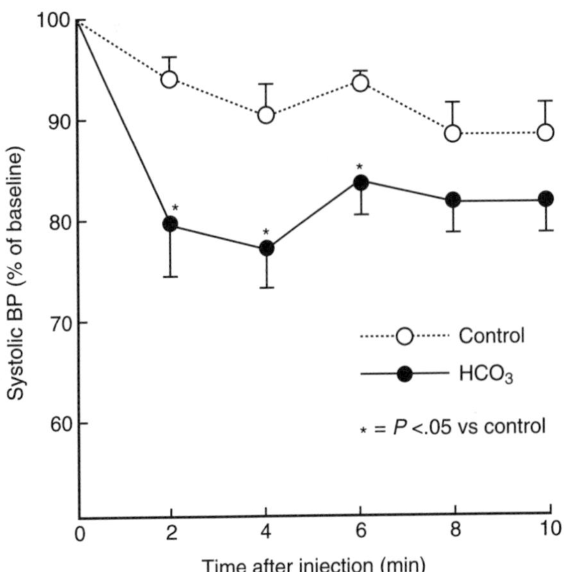

FIGURE **44-14**
Time course of average systolic blood pressure (*BP*) readings (mean SEM) expressed as a percentage of the baseline value after epidural injections of lidocaine alone or lidocaine with added sodium bicarbonate. (From Parnass SM, Curran MJA, Becker GL. Incidence of hypotension associated with epidural anesthesia using alkalinized and nonalkalinized lidocaine for cesarean section. *Anesth Analg.* 1987;66:1148-1150. Reprinted with permission from the International Anesthesia Research Society.)

solution, the onset time shortens to 5 minutes or less. Adding sodium bicarbonate increases the pH of the solution and shifts the equilibrium toward a greater percentage of nonionized local anesthetic base, thereby facilitating local anesthetic spread. Adding 1 mEq of sodium bicarbonate to each 10 ml of lidocaine solution results in faster onset of the block[141,142] and denser sensory[143] and motor[142] block. The density of motor block varies with the concentration of local anesthetic used but should be expected to be greater in the bicarbonate solution for any given concentration. A solution of lidocaine and sodium bicarbonate has a shelf life of at least 7 days and noticeably reduces stinging when it is injected in cutaneous and subcutaneous tissues.[144] Because bicarbonated lidocaine speeds the onset of sympathetic block, hypotension may develop quickly (Figure 44-14). No advantage is gained from the addition of sodium bicarbonate to bupivacaine; also, it is difficult to combine the two without causing precipitation. 2-Chloroprocaine 3% provides good motor block and dense anesthesia and has a very short time to onset, but bicarbonated lidocaine acts nearly as quickly. The use of 2-chloroprocaine 3% probably offers no clinical advantage other than its ester hydrolysis elimination pathway; also, its low pH results in a high incidence of backache.

Women not in labor, such as most of those undergoing elective cesarean sections, have been shown to have a greater incidence of hypotension after the institution of epidural anesthesia than women in labor.[87] This may be because of the lack of autologous transfusion provided to the woman in labor each time the uterus contracts and squeezes blood into the general circulation.

Although it may be tempting to administer epidural anesthesia for cesarean section through the Tuohy needle rather than an epidural catheter in order to save time, this administration technique has distinct disadvantages. If a complication related to the site of injection (e.g., intravascular injection) is going to occur, it will occur more quickly and be more severe when this technique is used. The incidence of hypotension after administration through the Tuohy needle is greater than it is when the dose is administered incrementally through the epidural catheter.[145]

The duration of action of bupivacaine and lidocaine, as well as the density of the block that they provide, can be increased by the addition of 5 mcg/ml or less of epinephrine.[146] Adding epinephrine to local anesthetics during cesarean section has been shown to be safe in healthy women with a healthy fetus.[147] An epidural anesthetic with added epinephrine may be preferable to spinal anesthesia with respect to the incidence of hypotension, umbilical artery Doppler pulsatility, FHR, and umbilical artery blood pH.[148]

In years past, women have almost universally complained of a diffuse, difficult-to-describe painful or noxious feeling during cesarean section despite "good," dense local anesthetic blocks. This uncomfortable feeling most commonly occurred during exteriorization of the uterus. Experience and scientific studies have verified that the use of local anesthetic solutions containing an opioid, both for epidural and subarachnoid blocks, significantly reduces this discomfort and results in greater patient satisfaction without danger of neonatal depression.[149-153] The addition of 100 mcg of fentanyl to the epidural local anesthetic

BOX 44-5

Epidural Anesthesia for Cesarean Section

- Metoclopramide 10 mg intravenously
- Clear antacid orally
- Intravascular volume replacement with Ringer's lactate or normal saline (15-20 ml/kg)
- Application of monitors
- Supplemental oxygen by face mask or nasal prongs
- Epidural catheter at L2-L3 or L3-L4
- Left uterine displacement
- Test dose
- Therapeutic dose
  - 5-mL boluses of 2% lidocaine + 1:400,000 epinephrine
    - Alternatively, 5-mL boluses of
      - 0.5% Bupivacaine,
      - 0.5% Ropivacaine,
      - or 3% 2-chloroprocaine (boluses of lidocaine or 2-chloroprocaine every 1-2 minutes, boluses of bupivacaine or ropivacaine every 2-5 minutes)
- Aggressive treatment of hypotension:
  - Exaggerated left uterine displacement
  - Intravenous fluids
  - Ephedrine and/or low-dose phenylephrine

Modified from Kuczkowski KM, Reisner LS, Lim D. Anesthesia for Cesarean Section. In Obstetric Anesthesia, 3rd ed, Chestnut, DH (ed) Elsevier Mosby, Philadelphia, 2004, p 431.

BOX 44-6

Spinal Anesthesia for Cesarean Section

- Metoclopramide 10 mg intravenously
- Clear antacid orally
- Intravascular volume
  Replacement with Ringer's lactate or normal saline (15-20 ml/kg)
- Application of monitors
- Supplemental oxygen by face mask or nasal prongs
- Prophylactic intramuscular ephedrine (25-50 mg) in patients with a baseline systolic blood pressure of less than 105 mm Hg
- Lumbar puncture at L3-L4
  - Right lateral or sitting position
  - 25- or 24-gauge Sprotte needle or 27- or 25-gauge Whitacre needle
  - Bupivacaine 12 mg in 8.25% dextrose
    - Morphine 0.1-0.25 mg for postoperative analgesia
  - Left uterine displacement
  - Aggressive treatment of hypotension
    - Exaggerated left uterine displacement
    - Intravenous fluids
    - Ephedrine and/or low-dose phenylephrine

Modified from Kuczkowski KM, Reisner LS, Lim D. Anesthesia for Cesarean Section. In Obstetric Anesthesia, 3rd ed, Chestnut, DH (ed) Elsevier Mosby, Philadelphia, 2004, p 429.

also results in less nausea and vomiting between delivery and the end of surgery.[154] A suggested method for epidural anesthesia for cesarean section is given in Box 44-5.

Subarachnoid Block

Both bupivacaine and lidocaine are good choices for cesarean section with subarachnoid block. Tetracaine 10 to 15 mg provides a block that lasts approximately 90 minutes within 15 minutes after administration. Bupivacaine, 10 to 15 mg, provides a solid anesthetic block and less motor blockade than tetracaine, and its duration of action is approximately 90 minutes. Bupivacaine sets up noticeably faster than tetracaine. A factor to consider when using bupivacaine is that in a patient placed in the lateral position for performance of the block the dose should be reduced compared with that in a patient in the sitting position. Failure to reduce the administered dose results in a noticeably higher spread of anesthetic block. Lidocaine, 75 to 100 mg, provides a block in 5 minutes or less, and the block lasts from 50 minutes to 1 hour. Transient neurologic symptoms appear not to be a concern in women undergoing cesarean section with lidocaine subarachnoid block.[155,156] Addition of fentanyl to either a subarachnoid or epidural block prolongs the block duration and increases its density, but without prolonging motor block or urinary retention as epinephrine does. A suggested method for spinal anesthesia for cesarean section is given in Box 44-6.

REGIONAL OPIOIDS

One of the chief advantages of combining local anesthetics and opioids in obstetric pain relief is that the use of opioids allows the concentration of local anesthetic to be decreased; this results in less motor blockade but equal relief. The onset of relief is also faster. Although opioids have centrally mediated effects, several areas in the spinal cord, including the substantia gelatinosa within the dorsal horn, are known to possess opioid receptors. These receptors can be stimulated by the application of opioids by the subarachnoid or epidural routes. Epidurally administered opioids are believed to be absorbed into the CSF, and ultimately the spinal cord, to exert their action on spinal opioid receptors.

Fentanyl

When used in combination with local anesthetics, fentanyl in epidural doses of 50 to 100 mcg and subarachnoid doses of 10 to 25 mcg produces good to excellent analgesia in 5 to 15 minutes. Administration of these doses, repeated as often as every 90 minutes in women in labor, has been shown not to affect neonatal Apgar scores, umbilical cord blood analysis, or neurobehavioral test results for up to 24 hours after delivery.[157-159] Epidural fentanyl, 100 mcg, is undetectable in breast milk.[160] Much higher doses of opioids are needed to provide labor analgesia if opioids are given alone, and even these higher doses are not entirely effective during the second stage of labor. When analgesia from fentanyl administration is at its peak, serum fentanyl levels are lower than those known to produce equivalent analgesia after IV administration. In fact, most women have undetectable plasma fentanyl levels after receiving 100 mcg of epidural fentanyl.[149]

Because fentanyl is so much more lipid soluble than morphine, it is absorbed into neural tissue faster, has a faster onset, and has a shorter duration of action than morphine. The dura-

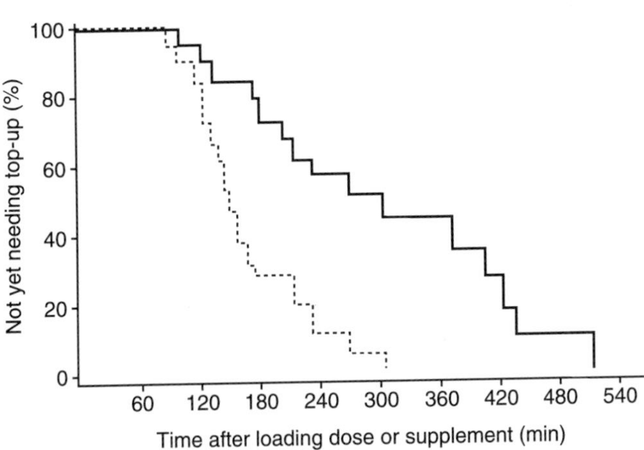

FIGURE **44-15**
Cumulative proportion of patients continuing epidural infusion and labor without the need for a top-up dose of local anesthetic. The dotted line represents group B (bupivacaine 0.08%). The solid line represents group F (bupivacaine 0.08% with fentanyl, 2.5 mg/ml). (From Jones G, Paul DL, Elton RA, McClure JH. Comparison of bupivacaine and bupivacaine with fentanyl in continuous extradural analgesia during labour. *Br J Anaesth*. 1989;63:254-259.)

tion of action is 3 to 4 hours. As a result the cephalad migration of fentanyl is much less than that of morphine; therefore fentanyl is associated with a significantly lower incidence of CNS side effects. This is probably why respiratory depression has rarely been reported after subarachnoid or epidural administration of fentanyl. In fact, subarachnoid doses of fentanyl up to 0.75 mcg/kg (much higher than the absolute limit of 25 mcg observed by most clinicians) result in a decrease in respiratory rate without undue respiratory depression.[150] An exceptionally high block with fentanyl, however, can result in respiratory depression. A young parturient who received 100 mcg of fentanyl and 0.5% bupivacaine in the epidural space for a cesarean section experienced a C4 block; this patient became apneic 100 minutes after the injection of the fentanyl. Spontaneous respirations resumed after the IV administration of naloxone.[161]

For continuous LEA, fentanyl concentrations up to 2.5 mcg/ml of local anesthetic can be used without adversely affecting neonatal respiration or neurobehavioral scores.[162] Bupivacaine (up to 0.125%) or ropivacaine (up to 0.2%) with 1 to 2 mcg/ml of fentanyl is a widely used combination. Figure 44-15 shows the percentage of women who did not need a repeat dose after epidural infusion of either plain bupivacaine (0.08%) (group B) or bupivacaine (0.08%) and fentanyl (2.5 mcg/ml) (group F). Both groups first received 6 ml of 0.5% bupivacaine, and the fentanyl group received 100 mcg of fentanyl with the loading dose. A 50- to 100-mcg dose of fentanyl may be used in the initial dose of local anesthetic in most situations.[163] The maintenance infusion rate was 15 ml/hr. Women who had fentanyl in their epidural solutions labored longer before they needed a repeat dose compared with women who had an equal concentration of bupivacaine without fentanyl in their epidural infusions.

For cesarean section, the addition of 50 to 100 mcg of fentanyl to the epidural local anesthetic of choice reduces the reported discomfort associated with some parts of the procedure[149]; however, doses as small as 25 mcg may be sufficient.[164] Mean pain scores were significantly lower and the number of parturients who reported no pain was greater when 100 mcg of fentanyl was added to 0.5% bupivacaine for cesarean section.[149] Adding fentanyl to solutions of 2-chloroprocaine may be an exception to this rule, as 2-chloroprocaine appears to have antagonistic properties at the mu opioid receptor[165,166] and therefore may antagonize the analgesic effect of the opioid.

Sufentanil

Sufentanil is highly lipid soluble, has a high receptor affinity, and is very potent. When injected into the epidural space, 98% of the dose is absorbed either by epidural fat or into epidural veins. Little sufentanil reaches the CSF. As a result, relatively higher plasma levels of sufentanil are achieved compared with those of fentanyl after the epidural injection of equipotent doses. When sufentanil is injected directly into the subarachnoid space, plasma levels of the drug are much lower than its CSF levels. One advantage of sufentanil is that it has a shorter plasma half-life than fentanyl; therefore accumulation should be even less likely to occur when it is used instead of fentanyl.

Sufentanil, 50 mcg, administered in the epidural space in combination with bupivacaine has been shown to decrease the slope of the CO_2 response curve by an average of approximately 40% (by <30% in patients who received 30 mcg). In a similar population of post–cesarean section women who received conventional subcutaneous morphine analgesia, the average decrease in the slope of the CO_2 response curve was 50%.[167,168]

Morphine

Morphine can be used in epidural doses of up to 5 mg to provide analgesia for 24 hours or longer. Subarachnoid administration of morphine, in doses of 0.1 to 1 mg, also may be used. With both epidural and subarachnoid blocks, a trend toward the use of lower doses is occurring in an effort to limit side effects. Morphine is lipid insoluble; therefore its onset of action after an epidural dose (approximately 1 hour) is longer than that of other opioids. Fentanyl has been added to the subarachnoid morphine infusion in healthy parturients in an effort to speed the onset of analgesia. Probably because of its limited lipid solubility, morphine continues to move cephalad long after injection into the subarachnoid or epidural space. It is thought that this mechanism accounts for respiratory depression, which can begin 12 hours or longer after epidural or subarachnoid morphine administration. Because of the long duration of action and absence of motor effects, epidural morphine is an excellent postoperative analgesic. Only preservative-free preparations should be used.

A series of 856 patients undergoing repeat cesarean section with subarachnoid block anesthesia[169] received hyperbaric 0.75% bupivacaine and 0.2 mg of preservative-free morphine in the subarachnoid space. Eighty-five percent of the patients were satisfied with the technique. Over half of the patients did not require any additional pain relief within the first 24 hours, and the average duration of pain relief for the group was in excess of 14 hours. The most common side effect was pruritus (42%), followed by vomiting (18%) and nausea (13%). Seventy percent of patients who had side effects were judged by the investigators not to require treatment. Fewer than 1% of these patients exhibited respiratory depression, which was defined as an SpO_2 of less than 85%. All the patients who had respiratory depression were obese and had a history of airway obstruction during sleep. Interestingly, none of the patients who experienced respiratory depression had a respiratory rate less than 10 breaths per minute. This suggests several conclusions:

- It may be unwise to use subarachnoid morphine in obese parturients.
- Respiratory rate alone may be an inadequate indicator of respiratory depression.
- Pulse oximetry may be a necessary postoperative monitor in parturients who have received subarachnoid morphine.

Side Effects of Regional Opioids

Side effects of epidural and subarachnoid opioid administration include respiratory depression, itching, urinary retention, nausea, and vomiting. These effects occur more commonly when the opioid is given by the subarachnoid than by the epidural route. IV doses of an opioid antagonist (naloxone) or agonist-antagonist (nalbuphine) are effective at reducing or eliminating the undesirable effects without antagonizing the analgesia and often are more effective against pruritus than an antihistamine.

The incidence and severity of pruritus after epidural morphine administration is greater in patients who have had epinephrine in their local anesthetic doses.[170] As little as 15 mcg of epinephrine in a test dose results in an increase in itching, even if the morphine is not given for up to 65 minutes after the epidural administration of epinephrine. Of interest, in some studies the incidence of shivering in parturients was decreased after administration of epidural fentanyl[171] or sufentanil,[172] but other investigations do not arrive at this conclusion.[148] As with other drugs, anaphylaxis is a rare risk of fentanyl administration. At least two cases of fentanyl-related anaphylaxis have been reported.

ANESTHETIC PROBLEMS

From 1987 to 1990 anesthesia complications accounted for 2.5% of all maternal deaths in the United States,[173] down from 3.3% for the 7 years preceding 1986.[174] Most anesthesia-related deaths were associated with general anesthesia for cesarean section.[175] Although the overall reduction in maternal deaths related to anesthesia is encouraging, complications of anesthesia resulted in maternal death six to seven times more frequently in black women than in white women.[173]

Nausea and Vomiting

Nausea and vomiting caused by anesthesia in the obstetric setting often are closely related to hypotension. The aggressive treatment of hypotension prevents much vomiting. Some clinicians believe that a sympathetic block results in unopposed gastrointestinal vagal stimulation, which predisposes the patient to nausea. The administration of an antimuscarinic agent (atropine, glycopyrrolate) before the institution of either an epidural or subarachnoid block may prevent nausea by this mechanism. Opioids administered in either the epidural or subarachnoid space may cause nausea. Scopolamine transdermal patches have been shown to significantly reduce the incidence of post–cesarean section nausea and vomiting resulting from regional opioids.[176] The transdermal scopolamine patch begins to be effective in 2 to 4 hours. Although this is longer than most drugs with which anesthetists are familiar, the duration of the scopolamine patch (48 hours or longer) makes up for the slow onset. The patch delivers a much smaller dose over time than did parenteral administration of scopolamine, and some women may experience side effects such as dry mouth or dizziness, which they judge to outweigh the benefits of scopolamine.

Postdural Puncture Headache

Postdural puncture headache (PDPH) results from a loss of CSF from within the dural and arachnoid membrane that surrounds the brain and spinal cord. The total volume of CSF present within this sac in an adult is approximately 150 ml. Approximately 500 ml of CSF is produced and reabsorbed each day.

PDPH occurs when CSF leaks out through a hole in the dura made during the performance of a subarachnoid block or accidentally during the attempted performance of an epidural block. Because the Tuohy needle used to place an epidural catheter has a large diameter, puncture of the dura with a Tuohy results in the loss of a significant volume of CSF. Diagnostic procedures that require dural punctures also result in PDPH, but these procedures are not commonly performed by an anesthetist. Loss of CSF is not the only cause of headache after regional anesthesia in the obstetric patient. Meningitis, although rare, can develop despite the adherence to aseptic technique, and this disease shares many of the signs and symptoms of PDPH (headache, nausea, and photophobia) in the initial stages.

Incidence

The incidence and severity of PDPH vary with factors thought to be related to the volume and rate of CSF leakage out of the subarachnoid space. PDPH is infrequent in the elderly and most frequent in young adults. Women seem to be slightly more susceptible than men. In general the use of large needles is more likely to be associated with PDPH than that of small ones. Even so, an 11% incidence of "mild and transient" headache was reported among 50 women undergoing cesarean section after dural puncture with a 30-gauge needle.[177] The configuration of the tip of the needle is also important. Other factors being equal, the use of beveled needles, like the Quincke needle, result in headache more frequently than the use of pencil-point or bullet-tip needles, like the Whitacre or Sprotte needle (Figure 44-16). No PDPH occurred in 38 patients after dural puncture with a 26-gauge pencil-point Portex needle.[178] Only one case of PDPH was reported in 50 parturients after dural puncture with a 26-gauge Becton

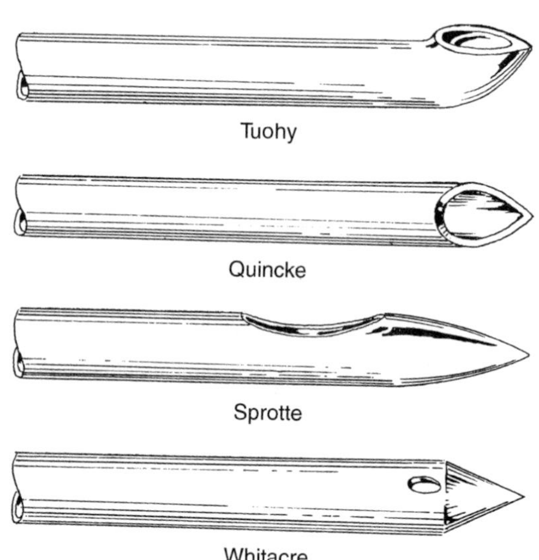

FIGURE **44-16**
Physical characteristics of four different types of spinal and epidural needles. Needle diameters are not to scale.

Dickinson needle,[179] and only one "slight" headache was reported in 271 parturients after dural puncture with a 24-gauge Sprotte needle.[180] In a retrospective study of 366 obstetric patients the incidence of PDPH after the use of a Sprotte needle was 1.5%, compared with 9% after the use of a beveled Quincke needle of similar gauge.[181] The orientation of the needle as it punctures the dural fibers also may be important. Spreading the fibers along their cephalad-to-caudad axis may result in less CSF leakage than cutting the fibers by inserting the bevel perpendicular to the axis of the dural fibers. In support of this theory, electron microscopy has confirmed that elastic fibers in the dura are arranged longitudinally.[182] Of course, this is true only with the use of beveled needles, not that of pencil-point or bullet-tip needles. The angle at which the needle approaches the dura may also modify the amount of CSF leakage and therefore the incidence of PDPH; however, the angle of approach most often is dictated by anatomy and therefore is difficult for the anesthetist to modify effectively.

Clinical Appearance

The hallmark of a PDPH is its postural nature. The headache is relieved by lying down and returns on sitting or standing up. It is commonly frontooccipital and sometimes is associated with neck and shoulder stiffness. Photophobia may be present in patients with severe headaches, whereas double vision occurs less frequently. Temporary deafness has occurred rarely. The onset of the headache is usually not immediate, but it may take 1 to 2 days to become bothersome. It may be mild or severe, and it often becomes worse if the patient feels sick and does not consume liquids.

Treatment

Patients should be given a choice of treatments ranging from the most conservative to the most aggressive. PDPH may be a mild irritation for a few days, or it may be debilitating. Patients with a mild PDPH may elect to rest in bed, as the horizontal position often provides complete relief from the headache, or to take over-the-counter analgesics if they are up and about. Adequate hydration should be encouraged. In hospitalized patients who are not taking fluids by mouth, IV hydration is warranted. Liberal hydration does not increase the production of CSF; however, it is important that the patient not be allowed to become dehydrated, because dehydration does decrease CSF production.

Caffeine is a cerebral vasoconstrictor and is effective in preventing or treating PDPH in some patients. In one trial 90% of patients with documented PDPH who were given 300 mg of caffeine showed significant improvement, compared with only 60% of patients who received a placebo.[183] For reference, Vivarin contains 200 mg of caffeine, NoDoz 200 mg, a cup of coffee approximately 100 mg, and soft drinks less. Like caffeine, serotonin also causes cerebral vasoconstriction. Case reports of serotonin type-1δ receptor agonists (sumatriptan) successfully relieving PDPH have also been published.[184]

The most effective treatment available for PDPH is an epidural blood patch. This treatment entails some risk because it is invasive; also, the headache is likely to become worse if another dural puncture is made in the course of placing the epidural (with a 17- or 18-gauge Tuohy needle). The usual contraindications to an epidural procedure also apply to this treatment.

To perform a blood patch the anesthetist places a Tuohy needle in the epidural space, preferably at the same interspace as the dural puncture or one interspace below. Once the Tuohy needle is in place, an assistant performs a peripheral venipuncture and draws 20 ml of the patient's own blood using strict aseptic technique. The blood is given to the anesthetist, who slowly injects it into the epidural space. The ideal volume for injection appears to be between 15 and 20 ml; the use of smaller volumes is associated with a significantly lower success rate, especially in the placement of prophylactic blood patches.[185,186] If discomfort develops in the back or neck, the injection is temporarily stopped. After the discomfort has passed, injection of the target volume of 15 to 20 ml may continue (unless discomfort returns). After the desired volume is injected, the Tuohy needle is withdrawn and the patient should lie quietly for at least 1 hour.[187] For the next several hours the patient should rest and not be overly active. This may need to be specifically discussed with the patient, because she may feel quite well for the first time in days and therefore may want to be more active. Excessive activity before complete clot consolidation may result in the clot being dislodged from the dural puncture site, allowing CSF leakage to resume.

The epidural blood patch is thought to plug the dural rent with a fibrin clot; the injected volume of blood applies pressure to the dura, in effect "autotransfusing" the cerebrum with CSF from around the spinal cord. An epidural blood patch is effective in more than 90% of patients when it is performed 24 hours after the dural puncture. A second patch is effective in approximately half of those who do not obtain relief from the first; this brings the total success rate to approximately 95%. Placing further patches does not increase the success rate significantly. Some authorities recommend earlier or prophylactic blood patches; however, the results obtained with them have been mixed. It is clear, however, that the success rate with early or prophylactic blood patches is not as high as that of blood patches performed 24 hours or more after the dural puncture. Still, only 21% of parturients who received a prophylactic blood patch after accidental dural puncture with a Tuohy needle experienced headache, compared with 80% of those who did not.[188] Likewise, in a study of 10 obstetric patients who received a prophylactic epidural blood patch after dural puncture with an 18-gauge Hustead needle, only one patient reported a "mild" headache; this patient's headache did not require further treatment.[189]

Accidental Intravascular Injection

Intravascular injection of local anesthetic may have CNS or cardiovascular consequences. CNS signs generally occur at lower plasma concentrations than does cardiovascular depression, although the effects of bupivacaine may be an exception to this rule at times. The first signs include ringing in the ears or other changes in hearing, confusion, inability to speak, a metallic taste in the mouth, or circumoral numbness. Higher blood levels eventually cause seizure and cardiovascular collapse. Obviously, the first step to be taken when any of these complications occurs is discontinuation of the injection of local anesthetic. If a seizure occurs, both mother and fetus are at risk of hypoxia. Quick action involving the administration of a barbiturate or benzodiazepine is necessary in order to end the seizure and to control the airway with an endotracheal tube. Thiopental, atropine, ephedrine, a self-inflating breathing bag, an anesthesia mask, laryngoscopes, oral and nasal airways, endotracheal tubes, and stylettes should all be on epidural insertion carts. Cardiovascular support is provided symptomatically, if needed. Positive-pressure ventilation through an endotracheal tube should be instituted as soon as possible. After this has been accomplished, maternal O_2 saturation, blood pressure, and pulse should be checked, and FHR and variability assessed.

Accidental Subarachnoid Injection

Subarachnoid injection results in a denser and more widespread block and one of more rapid onset than does epidural injection; therefore it may lead to the rapid onset of dyspnea, hypotension, or both. Treatment is directed at relief of symptoms. These complications may occur quickly after a bolus injection through a supposedly epidural catheter or insidiously after catheter migration in a patient receiving a continuous infusion of local anesthetic. The harmful effects of accidental subarachnoid injection can be greatly reduced if the anesthetic is administered through the catheter in increments no greater than 5 ml.

Accidental Subdural Injection

Occasionally the epidural catheter may be placed accidentally in the subdural space between the dura and the arachnoid membranes. After a negative intravascular and subarachnoid test dose, anesthetic is administered through the supposed epidural catheter in the normal fashion. After a delay of 10 to 25 minutes, a sudden excessive spread of the block is noted,[190] primarily in the cephalad direction.[191] The magnitude of the spread of the local anesthetic block is significantly greater than would be anticipated if the catheter were in the epidural space and very similar to what would be expected with a subarachnoid injection. Hypotension caused by extensive sympathetic block is usually the primary problem and is treated with ephedrine or other vasopressors as needed. If the block is sufficiently extensive to compromise respiration or airway maintenance, endotracheal intubation is necessary. This complication is uncommon and quite possibly unpreventable. The possibility of respiratory compromise emphasizes the necessity of being prepared to manage such a complication as well as the need for close monitoring after epidural administration.

Electrocardiographic Changes during Regional Anesthesia for Cesarean Section

In a series of 93 healthy parturients undergoing "routine" cesarean section, a 47% incidence of electrocardiographic (ECG) changes "characteristic" of myocardial ischemia was noted.[192] Although not all of the women with ECG changes had associated subjective complaints, 86% of the women with complaints of chest pain, pressure, nausea and vomiting, or dyspnea did have associated ECG changes. The investigators speculated that the superimposition of large fluid shifts involved with regional anesthesia on the already increased cardiac workload associated with term pregnancy may have resulted in myocardial ischemia. Further investigations of ECG changes during cesarean section have concluded that ST-segment changes are not caused by myocardial ischemia.[193] Observations of wall motion have shown no abnormality during ST changes, nor have myocardial-specific creatine kinase levels. Further studies indicate that few ST changes during regional anesthesia for cesarean section in healthy women are actually caused by myocardial ischemia.[194,195]

Cardiopulmonary Resuscitation in the Pregnant Patient

CPR has been accomplished successfully early in pregnancy, but use of the technique is problematic at best in the near-term parturient. The fetus does not tolerate decreases in maternal oxygenation and blood pressure well. The mother has a high O_2 demand and a small O_2 reservoir (residual volume). Perhaps most important, the term or near-term uterus obstructs central venous return in the supine parturient. It follows that left uterine displacement is important to the success of CPR in pregnant women. However, lateral tilt has been shown to decrease the force of cardiac compressions and, presumably, their effectiveness. Chest compressions done on a patient in 27-degree lateral tilt have only 80% of the force of compressions performed on a patient in the supine position.[196] As a result, a wedge that displaces the uterus while allowing closed-chest compressions has been developed. Presumably, any handy wedge that is positioned under the right hip would displace the uterus to the left while leaving the thorax fairly supine for effective chest compressions. In any case, when the near-term parturient does not respond to resuscitative efforts within 5 minutes, emergent cesarean section is often indicated. This makes possible direct oxygenation of the neonate and has resulted in substantially improved venous return in the mother,[197,198] ultimately allowing for successful resuscitation of her as well.

OBSTETRIC PROBLEMS

From 1982 to 1996 the maternal mortality rate in the United States was 7.5 per 100,000 live births.[199] Yet the range of mortality rates varied greatly by state and ethnicity (1987-1996), with a low of 2.7 for white women in Massachusetts to a high of 28.7 for black women in New York.[200] The most common causes of maternal death (from most to least) include hemorrhage, embolism, preeclampsia, infection, and cardiomyopathy.

Prematurity

Premature delivery is a leading cause of perinatal morbidity and mortality. Premature delivery is implicated in more than 50% of all perinatal deaths. Overall, up to 9% of the live births in the United States are of premature infants; in some segments of society the incidence of prematurity is even greater. Premature labor is an even more frequent occurrence.

Premature labor is defined as regular uterine contractions that occur between 20 and 37 weeks of gestation and that result in dilation or effacement of the cervix. When labor begins prematurely, the ability to halt it can allow the fetus additional time to mature. Stopping labor is termed *tocolysis* (from the Greek *tokos*, meaning "childbirth," and *lysis*, meaning "breaking up"). The cause of preterm labor is not well understood, but many associated risk factors exist, including race, weight, drug use, stress, parity, multiple gestation, extremes of maternal age, and the presence of obstetric complications.

Tocolysis

Historically, ethyl alcohol was used to stop premature labor. Ethanol depresses myometrial contractility and suppresses the release of oxytocin from the posterior pituitary. It was, however, the cause of many dangerous side effects, including increased gastric volume, depression or obliteration of airway reflexes, vomiting, lactic acidosis, and fluid and electrolyte abnormalities.

Magnesium Sulfate

Magnesium causes relaxation of vascular, bronchial, and uterine smooth muscle by altering calcium transport and availability. Motor end-plate sensitivity and muscle membrane excitability also are depressed.

The normal serum magnesium level during pregnancy is 1.8 to 3 mg/dL. A serum magnesium level of 4 to 8 mg/dL is therapeutic as a tocolytic, but even toxic levels do not always eliminate uterine contractility. At 10 to 12 mg/dL the patellar reflex is eliminated. Levels above 12 mg/dL cause respiratory depression; at approximately 18 mg/dL, respiratory depression progresses to apnea. The presence of higher levels (25 mg/dL) can cause cardiac arrest.

Side Effects. The side effects of magnesium sulfate administration are dose dependent. As magnesium levels increase, skeletal muscle weakness increases and CNS depression and vascular dilation occur. Magnesium sulfate infusion commonly results in a slight decrease in blood pressure during epidural anesthesia.[201] Magnesium antagonizes the vasoconstrictive effect of α-agonists, so ephedrine and phenylephrine are likely to less effectively increase maternal blood pressure when administered concomitantly with magnesium.[202] Cardiac muscle is not affected to a clinically evident degree when magnesium is administered at therapeutic levels, although magnesium can have profound myocardial effects during a gross overdose. Magnesium is eliminated unchanged by the kidneys. In a patient who is receiving a maintenance infusion of magnesium and who has decreasing urine output, blood levels of magnesium quickly increase, as do related side effects.

Side effects of magnesium sulfate include the following:

- Cutaneous vasodilation with flushing
- Headache and dizziness
- Nausea
- Skeletal muscle weakness
- Depression of deep tendon reflexes
- Respiratory depression
- ECG changes

Patients on magnesium sulfate therapy have partial, if subclinical, neuromuscular blockade. Both depolarizing and nondepolarizing[203,204] neuromuscular blocking drugs are potentiated by magnesium. Administration of priming or defasciculating doses of neuromuscular blocking drugs may cause significant paralysis when combined with magnesium therapy. The neuromuscular blocking effects of magnesium can be at least partially antagonized by calcium.

Magnesium sulfate overdose is treatable. In an excellent case report, a 23-year-old gravida received a 20-g bolus of magnesium sulfate superimposed on a therapeutic magnesium (Mg^{2+}) level. She attained a magnesium level of 38.7 mg/dL.[205] She had a respiratory arrest, became hypotensive and bradycardic, and developed a prolonged QRS complex. Resuscitation was successfully accomplished with discontinuation of the magnesium administration; endotracheal intubation and ventilation; IV administration of calcium chloride; and diuresis to facilitate the elimination of magnesium. Vital signs improved dramatically with ventilation and calcium administration, and the woman was extubated 8 hours later after her magnesium level had declined to a therapeutic level.

Neonatal side effects after maternal magnesium administration are rare. A few cases of hypotonia and respiratory depression in neonates after prolonged high-dose maternal magnesium administration have been reported; however, in general, magnesium administration is safe for the neonate. Magnesium is also used in the treatment of preeclampsia, a vasospastic disease of pregnancy that can result in severe hypertension, coagulopathy, and seizure. Magnesium sulfate causes relaxation of vascular smooth muscle, a decrease in SVR, and a decrease in blood pressure. At serum levels of 7 to 9.5 mg/dL, it is an anticonvulsant. It also decreases fibrin deposition, improving circulation to visceral organs that are vulnerable to vasospasm and failure.

β-Agonists

Stimulation of the β_2-receptor system causes smooth muscle relaxation, including relaxation of the uterus. The myometrium has β_2-receptors in cell membranes. Stimulation of these receptors triggers a cascade of biochemical effects, resulting in inhibition of myometrial contractility at the cellular level. β_2 stimulation also causes an increase in progesterone production. Progesterone, in turn, causes histologic changes in myometrial cells that limit the spread of contractile impulses.

The administration of β-agonists results in down regulation of β-receptors over time. This results in a decreased tocolytic effect during long-term β-agonist therapy that has been demonstrated in animals after as few as 24 hours of ritodrine administration.

Maternal Side Effects. All currently available β-agonists have both β_1 and β_2 effects, although some agents are fairly selective for one receptor subset over the other. The side effects of β-agonist therapy can be predicted on the basis of a knowledge of systemic β effects. Cardiovascular effects are generally the most clinically important and troublesome. β_1 Stimulation causes an increase in HR, myocardial contractility, and myocardial O_2 demand. Palpitations and premature ventricular contractions are not uncommon. β_2 stimulation causes vascular dilation, bronchial dilation, an increase in secretions, and various metabolic effects.

In one published case a young healthy parturient received an overdose of ritodrine (50 mg) in an IV bolus; the overdose resulted in flushing, tremor, tachycardia, and hypotension that lasted for 6 hours. She recovered with supportive treatment.

Maternal side effects of β-agonists include the following:

- Cerebral vasospasm
- Chest pain or tightness
- Glucose intolerance
- Hypokalemia
- Ileus
- Myocardial ischemia
- Nausea
- Palpitations
- Pulmonary edema
- Restlessness
- Tremor
- Ventricular arrhythmias

By the twenty-fourth week of gestation, maternal cardiac output is increased by up to 50% as a result of an increase in both HR and SV. β-Agonist therapy further increases the demand on the cardiovascular system. Complaints of palpitations and chest pain are not uncommon. ECG changes are sometimes seen, although myocardial ischemia is not always documented.

Both ritodrine and terbutaline can antagonize hypoxic pulmonary vasoconstriction through β_2-mediated vasodilation. Hypoxic pulmonary vasoconstriction causes pulmonary arteries that lead to areas of the lung with low O_2 tension to constrict and divert blood flow to well-oxygenated areas of lung. In patients with a significant degree of hypoxic pulmonary vasoconstriction, such as those with underlying pulmonary disease or pulmonary edema, dilation of constricted pulmonary arteries may result in a significant decrease in maternal O_2 tension.

Metabolic Effects. β stimulation increases blood glucose and insulin levels. When a β-agonist infusion is started, the blood glucose level increases within a few hours and returns to baseline within 72 hours without treatment. Potassium is redistributed from the extracellular to intracellular compartments. This results in a decrease in serum potassium level, sometimes to less than 3 mEq/L. As with glucose levels, serum potassium levels return to normal within 72 hours after initiation of β-agonist therapy.

Pulmonary Edema. There is a small but notable incidence of pulmonary edema among healthy parturients receiving β-agonists. The mechanism for the development of pulmonary edema in these patients is unclear. Fluid overload resulting from a physiologic increase in intravascular volume, antidiuresis, and IV fluid administration may have a role. Myocardial fatigue caused by tachycardia also has been suggested as a possible cause. Pulmonary artery pressures are not uniformly elevated, however, and sometimes they are low; this finding can be used to argue against both of these hypotheses. However, it is clear that the danger of pulmonary edema increases when parturients receiving β-agonists are preloaded for regional anesthesia.

Risk factors associated with pulmonary edema during β-agonist tocolysis include the following:

- Anemia
- Fluid overload
- Magnesium
- Multiple gestation
- Prolonged maternal tachycardia

Fetal and Neonatal Side Effects. Clinically used β-agonists cross the placenta and have fetal and neonatal effects. Fetal tachycardia (FHR >160 bpm) is common. Neonatal hypoglycemia may result, especially if maternal serum glucose is elevated at delivery. When maternal and therefore fetal blood glucose levels are elevated, the fetus increases insulin release in response. After delivery the neonate continues to release insulin at an increased rate, even though it is no longer receiving a glucose load from the mother. After the excess circulating glucose has been used up, continued release of insulin causes a rebound hypoglycemia. Because delivery of the infant during tocolysis is not the goal, these side effects are seldom a concern.

Ritodrine (Yutopar) is a selective β_2-agonist. Ritodrine therapy increases maternal HR by an average of 40 bpm. Systolic blood pressure commonly increases, and diastolic pressure decreases. The manufacturer's literature recommends that patients on ritodrine therapy receive no more than 2 L of IV fluid over 24 hours. Before spinal or epidural anesthesia for cesarean section is initiated, it is not uncommon for a 2-L IV preload to be given in less than 30 minutes. However, even smaller IV preloads are not recommended in patients receiving ritodrine until use of the drug has been discontinued for at least 1 hour. Ritodrine is eliminated by the kidneys and has an elimination half-life of approximately 30 minutes.

Terbutaline (Brethine, Bricanyl) is a synthetic, relatively β_2 receptor–selective, noncatecholamine sympathomimetic amine. When administered parenterally, terbutaline is less β_2 receptor–selective than ritodrine. Arrhythmias are more likely to occur with terbutaline use than during ritodrine administration, and tachycardia can be a problem. Terbutaline is approximately 50% eliminated by the kidneys and has a half-life of up to 16 hours. Like ritodrine, terbutaline has been associated with pulmonary edema when it is used for tocolysis.

Calcium channel blockers have been investigated for use as tocolytic agents but are not used clinically in the United States at present.

Anesthetic Considerations

When an anesthetic intervention is planned for a patient who is receiving a tocolytic agent, a knowledge of maternal and fetal physiology and of the pharmacology of the tocolytic agent must be integrated. β-Agonists may affect and mask indicators of volume status.

Regional Anesthesia

When tocolysis fails, preterm deliveries are often accomplished by cesarean section. In this situation 1- and 5-minute Apgar scores have been shown to be higher in neonates delivered with epidural anesthesia than in those delivered with general anesthesia.[206] Patients on magnesium therapy are often candidates for subarachnoid or epidural blocks as long as careful attention is devoted to volume status. Magnesium causes vasodilation, and maternal hemorrhage is tolerated poorly by both parturients on magnesium and their fetuses.[207,208] Subarachnoid block has the advantage of involving very small amounts of local anesthetic, and this reduces the chance for fetal local anesthetic toxicity. Epidural anesthesia can be used throughout labor for analgesia and can be induced slowly; this minimizes the risk of sudden hypotension caused by sympathetic block.

Even when volume status is accurately assessed, intravenous preloads before subarachnoid or epidural anesthesia are associated with an increased risk of pulmonary edema in parturients receiving β-agonist drugs. Use of ritodrine (and perhaps terbutaline) should almost always be discontinued, and enough time for the drug to be largely eliminated should be allowed to pass before regional anesthesia is induced. If time constraints do not permit the needed delay, induction of general anesthesia for an urgent or emergent procedure is almost always preferable. If the patient is already in pulmonary edema or has marginal to poor uterine artery blood flow because of vascular constriction, slowly induced epidural anesthesia may provide a beneficial vasodilation. Anesthesia-induced hypotension must be carefully avoided, however, because almost all therapies directed at restoration of blood pressure would be detrimental. Ephedrine could increase an already rapid HR, and IV fluid administration could precipitate or worsen pulmonary edema. A low dose of an α-agonist (e.g., 50 to 100 mcg of phenylephrine given intravenously) may be the least detrimental choice.

General Anesthesia. Succinylcholine is the muscle relaxant of choice during the rapid-sequence induction of an obstetric patient. In patients on magnesium therapy, defasciculation with a small dose of a nondepolarizing neuromuscular blocking agent is not recommended because significant paralysis may result, increasing the risk of aspiration of gastric contents. Magnesium potentiates depolarizing and, especially, nondepolarizing relaxants.[203,204] The amount of potentiation is variable, and a peripheral nerve stimulator is invaluable. The duration of paralysis after administration of a standard dose of succinylcholine may give a clue as to how much longer than normal the effect of a nondepolarizer will last.

Induction of general anesthesia in a patient receiving a β-agonist tocolytic can present a challenge. As with regional anesthesia, there are advantages to delaying induction of general anesthesia whenever possible until ritodrine has been largely eliminated (at least an hour).[209] Thiopental has a long, safe history of use in obstetric anesthesia, and its cardiovascular depression may offset some of the cardiac stimulation caused by the β-agonist. The use of a vagolytic, such as atropine, glycopyrrolate, or pancuronium bromide, is counterproductive.

Induction of general anesthesia should usually be delayed until the patient has been prepared and the operating surgeon and assistants are ready for incision. Preterm neonates have a significantly higher incidence of low Apgar scores at 1 minute. Reducing the interval from the induction of anesthesia to the delivery of the infant minimizes the depressant effects of the anesthetic that the neonate must overcome.

In nonpregnant patients, opioids such as the fentanyl analogues are often used to blunt the sympathetic response to laryngoscopy and intubation. In pregnant patients effective doses of fentanyl (5 to 8 mcg/kg) cross the placenta and result in significant neonatal depression. Fentanyl, 1 mcg/kg, administered before the induction of general anesthesia for cesarean section has been shown not to affect the Apgar score or neurobehavioral test results of neonates significantly.[210] By itself this dose is certainly not enough to blunt the sympathetic response to laryngoscopy and intubation but will contribute to the goal. Of course, as more depressants are added, the option to allow the parturient to awaken and breathe spontaneously if it is impossible to intubate or ventilate her is less conceivable.

Finally, because the tocolytic effect of a β-agonist is no longer needed, β-blockers may be used carefully before the induction of anesthesia and instrumentation of the airway. Labetalol, a selective α_1- and a nonselective β-receptor antagonist, has been used successfully to decrease maternal blood pressure while uteroplacental blood flow is maintained.[211,212] Neonatal side effects (hypotension, bradycardia) are apparently minimal.[213] In women with preeclampsia, labetalol has been administered before the induction of general anesthesia in order to decrease mean blood pressure at induction and during the first 10 minutes of anesthesia.[214]

Halothane is still used at some centers for maintenance of general anesthesia in obstetrics. However, it is well known that halothane sensitizes the myocardium to catecholamines and that its use should be avoided in patients receiving β-agonists. Terbutaline often precipitates premature ventricular contractions in a heart that is not sensitized and results in even more arrhythmias during halothane anesthesia.

Magnesium reduces the MAC of inhalation agents in rats to a clinically significant degree; ritodrine does not. Anesthetic depth has important implications for fetal oxygenation. Light anesthesia results in maternal catecholamine outflow in response to surgical stimulation, which, in turn, results in uterine artery constriction and a decrease in uterine artery blood flow. Anything that decreases uterine artery blood flow decreases uteroplacental blood flow and therefore results in fetal hypoxia.

Embolism

Thromboembolism

Thrombotic pulmonary embolism occurs in pregnant individuals fivefold more often than it does in nonpregnant individuals and is more likely to occur postpartum than antepartum. It is associated with prolonged inactivity, cesarean delivery, obesity, and increasing age and parity. The patient with pulmonary embolism may have a few minor complaints or a massive cardiovascular collapse. Pleuritic chest pain, dyspnea, hyperventilation, hypocapnia, coughing, hemoptysis, and distention of neck veins are associated with the disorder. Thromboembolism is a major cause of maternal mortality, but while the parturient is in the delivery area, it is less likely to occur than either amniotic fluid or air embolism.

Venous Air Embolism

Venous air embolism can occur during labor, spontaneous vaginal delivery, and operative delivery and is frequently associated with placenta previa. The overall incidence of subclinical venous air embolism in the parturient has been reported to be as high as 29%[215,216]; during general anesthesia, the incidence in the parturient may be as high as 97%.[217,218] Most venous air emboli are detected between delivery and uterine repair.[216,217] Air is entrained into open maternal venous sinuses in the uterine wall when the placenta separates or at the site of a surgical incision. Air returning to the heart may pass through a patent foramen ovale and form an embolism in any organ in the body. More often it passes through the right atrium and ventricle and lodges in the pulmonary arteries, impeding blood flow through the lungs. The resultant increase in pulmonary vascular resistance causes an increase in central venous pressure. A heavy, nonradiating, retrosternal chest pain may persist for 10 minutes after even a small venous air embolism. End-tidal CO_2 drops, because CO_2 cannot return to the lungs. A mill-wheel murmur may be heard over the precordium as a frothy air-blood mixture moves through the heart. This murmur is most pronounced when a large volume of air becomes trapped in the right ventricle. Dyspnea is common. If a sufficient number of pulmonary arteries are affected, cardiovascular collapse will occur.

The signs and symptoms of venous air embolism are as follows:

- Mill-wheel murmur detected over the precordium
- Chest pain
- Dyspnea
- Decreased end-tidal CO_2
- Elevated central venous pressure

Amniotic Fluid Embolism

Although rare, amniotic fluid embolism is almost uniformly fatal. It may occur during labor, vaginal delivery, or operative delivery and is associated with placental abruption. The pathogenesis is almost identical to that of venous air embolism except that patients who develop amniotic fluid embolism are prone to develop disseminated intravascular coagulation (DIC) if they survive the initial embolism. Signs and symptoms of amniotic fluid embolism include a chill, shivering, anxiety, cough, dyspnea, cyanosis, tachypnea, pulmonary edema, and cardiovascular collapse. O_2 saturation has been reported to decrease quickly.[218] This cascade often leads to death within a few minutes.

Anesthetic Implications

The incidence of postpartum thromboembolism can be affected by anesthetic interventions. Cesarean sections performed with general anesthesia are associated with accelerated maternal coagulation compared with those performed with regional anesthesia,[219] so the use of regional anesthesia may help reduce the incidence of postoperative thromboemboli. The anesthetist can help prevent prolonged inactivity in those who have had a cesarean section by providing analgesia sufficient to allow comfortable ambulation. Use of epidural opioid analgesia is often an appropriate solution to this problem. It may be specifically indicated in those at risk for thromboembolism, even if it must be administered after a general anesthetic has been given.

Because air embolism occurs when open veins are above the level of the heart, raising the head of the bed in order to position the uterus below the heart would seem to be useful for preventing embolization. However, a head-up tilt of between 5 and 10 degrees does not appear to decrease the incidence of venous air embolism during cesarean section and has increased the incidence of hypotension.[217,220] If embolism is suspected during spontaneous or operative delivery, the obstetrician should be informed immediately. The obstetrician can take steps to stop the entrainment of air or amniotic fluid, which include flooding the surgical field with saline, returning the uterus to within the abdomen, and stimulating uterine contractions.

One hundred percent O_2 should be administered by positive-pressure ventilation through a cuffed endotracheal tube. Nitrous oxide administration should be discontinued, as it rapidly expands the volume of an air embolus and prevents the delivery of 100% O_2. An arterial line may be needed for monitoring of oxygenation and blood pressure. IV fluids are administered as needed to bolster central venous pressure. A generous preload is necessary to enable the right side of the heart to pump volume forward against increased pulmonary vascular resistance. If the fetus has not been delivered, left uterine displacement improves uterine blood flow and facilitates venous return to the heart. Pharmacologic support of the cardiovascular system is likely to be needed.

Patient position has been suggested to hinder the movement of the foreign substance into the pulmonary arteries. A slight anti-Trendelenburg (head-up) position with left lateral tilt of at least 15 degrees is designed to trap air in the right atrium, from which it can be aspirated via a central venous catheter. Unfortunately, it often is difficult to place the patient in this position and insert a central line in time to prevent pulmonary artery embolization.

Blood Loss

Blood loss is difficult to estimate in the obstetric patient. Often, lost blood is hidden inside the women's body, soaked in laparotomy sponges, absorbed by drapes, or spilled onto the floor. In general, approximately 500 ml are lost during a spontaneous vaginal delivery and approximately 700 ml during a cesarean section with general anesthesia; 1500 ml or more are lost if a hysterectomy is performed during cesarean section. Because the term parturient has a 50% increase in blood volume, a great amount of blood can often be lost before the vital signs begin to change in response to the loss; 15% of the total blood volume may be lost without the occurrence of any compensatory tachycardia or vasoconstriction.[221] Hypotension may not occur until 30% of the total blood volume has been lost. Approximately 4% of all parturients who deliver vaginally experience excessive postpartum bleeding.[222]

Placenta Previa

When the placenta has implanted on the lower uterine segment and either partially or completely covers the opening of the cervix, placenta previa is present. Placenta previa has an incidence of up to 1%, and the mortality rate for those with it approaches 1%. Placenta previa is more common in women who have had it during a prior pregnancy. It most often results in painless vaginal bleeding before the onset of labor that may stop without intervention or hemodynamically significant blood loss. The potential exists, however, for *sudden* loss of large amounts of blood. The risk of bleeding increases if the placenta is disturbed by manual examination or cervical dilation. Postpartum bleeding is often increased as well, because the lower uterine segment, where the placenta previa was implanted, does not contract as well as the rest of the uterus.

Anesthetic Implications

The diagnosis of placenta previa normally indicates an operative delivery. The anesthetist should prepare for heavy blood loss. The anesthetist may choose either a general or regional anesthetic technique, taking into consideration the parturient's current volume status and the potential for blood loss. Regional techniques should be performed only by an anesthetist who is very experienced with regional anesthesia and only after careful assessment and preparation.

Placental Abruption

Abruption occurs when the placenta begins to separate from the uterus before delivery; this allows bleeding behind the placenta and jeopardizes the fetal blood supply. Placental abruption results in bleeding (often hidden), uterine irritability (often hypertonic), abdominal pain, and fetal distress or death. Open venous sinuses in the uterine wall may allow products of hemostasis and amniotic fluid to enter the maternal circulation; this results in an incidence of DIC of up to 50%. The reported incidence of abruption in the general population varies widely but is much higher in women with hypertension (up to 23% among women with preeclampsia). When fetal death occurs, maternal mortality can exceed 10%.

Anesthetic Implications

In cases of placental abruption without fetal distress, vaginal delivery may still be possible. Because fetal distress can occur without warning, the anesthetist should be prepared to administer anesthesia for an emergency cesarean section. Taking an anesthetic history as soon as the diagnosis of placental abruption becomes known and checking for adequate IV access is recommended. If the mother is unstable or if fetal distress is present, operative delivery is necessary. Regional anesthesia usually is not indicated because of the potential for coagulopathy and because of the uncertainty of uteroplacental blood flow and therefore of fetal oxygenation. Generous venous access should be established as soon as possible. Although placental abruption does not usually result in sudden blood loss, a large volume of blood may be lost. When abruption results in fetal death, the volume of lost maternal blood can be as great as 5 L, all of which may be concealed. Volume resuscitation should begin as soon as IV access has been secured. Large volumes of crystalloid and colloid solutions and of red blood cells may be needed.

General anesthesia can be induced with ketamine, up to 1 mg/kg. If the uterus is hypertonic, another drug should be chosen because the use of ketamine may further increase uterine tone, decreasing fetal O_2 supply. An alternate choice is etomidate, 0.3 mg/kg. If uterine tone is excessive, a volatile inhalation agent may be useful for maintenance of anesthesia and uterine relaxation. After the baby has been delivered, the uterus often becomes atonic; therefore the use of inhalation agents should normally be discontinued. IV or intramyometrial oxytocin and intramyometrial ergotamine may be used with uterine massage to facilitate uterine contraction and to halt bleeding.

Postpartum Bleeding

Postpartum bleeding in moderate amounts is a normal event. Excessive bleeding may occur because of uterine atony (which accounts for 80% of all postpartum bleeding), placental retention, abnormalities of the uterus, lacerations of the delivery channel, uterine inversion, and abnormalities of coagulation. Uterine atony is associated with multiparity, prolonged infusions of oxytocin before delivery, polyhydramnios, and multiple gestation. A retained placenta or retained placental fragments must be removed manually to stop the bleeding. In the past this has often required the administration of an inhalation agent for uterine relaxation. Nitroglycerin, a potent uterine relaxant with a relatively short duration of action, has been used successfully to provide uterine relaxation adequate for placental extraction. A dose of approximately 1 mcg/kg intravenously appears to be adequate.[223,224] Sublingual nitroglycerin spray has also been used effectively and offers the added benefits of long shelf life and a ready-to-use preparation.[225] Because nitroglycerin is a potent venodilator when given at low doses and is an arteriolar dilator when administered intravenously at a rate of 1 mcg/kg/min or higher, care should be taken to ensure that intravascular volume is adequate before this drug is administered. Analgesia for the procedure can be accomplished with a variety of methods, including the use of an already established epidural catheter or the administration of small IV doses of ketamine.

Anesthetic Implications

When postpartum bleeding is excessive, the anesthetist performs fluid resuscitation while simultaneously working with the obstetrician to eliminate the cause of the bleeding. Fundal massage, IV oxytocin, intramuscular methylergonovine maleate, or intramuscular prostaglandin often is all that is needed. In some cases anesthesia may be necessary for an additional procedure.

Uterine Rupture

Uterine rupture is most commonly associated with labor in the presence of a previous uterine incision (vaginal birth after cesarean, or VBAC) but may occur in an unscarred uterus.[226] The incidence of uterine rupture during attempted VBAC is approximately 0.6%.[227] Uterine rupture has also been associated with cocaine abuse during pregnancy.[228] The classic description of complete uterine rupture includes sudden, severe, tearing abdominal pain in a multiparous woman in hard labor. The pain may break through labor epidural anesthesia. Next, labor stops, and shock and fetal distress rapidly develop. Unfortunately, uterine rupture often does not present classically. For example, some ruptures occur during periods of mild labor.[229] The clinical finding most commonly associated with uterine rupture is an abnormal FHR tracing.[230,231] Whatever the presentation, bleeding is often severe. The uterus receives approximately 800 ml of blood per minute (approximately 10% of the cardiac output); therefore a tear in this organ holds the potential for rapid exsanguination. Mortality from uterine rupture accounts for half of the maternal deaths attributed to blood loss each year. Fetal mortality after uterine rupture is nearly 80%.

Anesthetic Implications

Uterine rupture requires surgery for hemostasis and, often, for delivery. Anesthetists should be prepared for heavy bleeding commensurate with any severe abdominal trauma. In the operating room, as much as 3500 ml of blood has been found in the abdomen at incision.

Abnormal Placental Implantation

The placenta normally implants into the endometrium. A placenta implanted on or in the myometrium, the underlying muscular layer of the uterus, is termed *placenta accreta* (on the myometrium), *placenta increta* (into the myometrium), or *placenta percreta* (completely through the myometrium). Any of these abnormal placental implantations means that separation of the placenta from the uterine wall will be difficult and that separation may be accompanied by severe bleeding. Placenta accreta, placenta increta, and placenta percreta are commonly associated with placenta previa and are more common in women who have had a previous cesarean section than in those who have not. The anesthetic implications are the same as those for other causes of increased blood loss.

Cesarean Hysterectomy

After delivery, when hemostasis is unobtainable despite the use of some combination of oxytocin, ergot alkaloids, and prostaglandin, the surgeon performs a hysterectomy to stop uterine bleeding. An atonic uterus, especially an incised uterus, can lose several liters of blood within a few minutes, outpacing the ability of even the most prepared anesthesia providers to replace intravascular volume. Anesthesia at this point becomes trauma anesthesia, the primary purpose of which is the maintenance of vital signs, vital organ perfusion, and oxygenation; maternal analgesia and amnesia are important but secondary concerns. Etomidate, ketamine, benzodiazepines, and opioids are useful because they cause minimal hemodynamic depression. If rapid blood loss begins during cesarean section with regional anesthesia, the anesthetist should consider the rapid induction of general anesthesia. It is difficult to manage volume resuscitation and to keep an awake patient both mentally and physically comfortable.

Disseminated Intravascular Coagulation

DIC is a generalized activation of the clotting system. It can occur when a large portion of the vascular system suffers damage or when thromboplastic material enters the general circulation. DIC is frequently associated with three obstetric problems: retention of a dead fetus, placental abruption, and amniotic fluid embolism. Circulatory shock, which often accompanies DIC, worsens the problem by decreasing peripheral and hepatic blood flow and causing further cell damage. Renal failure may result from the deposit of fibrin and cellular debris in the filtration system. Clinically the patient with DIC has uncontrolled bleeding because of the consumption of clotting factors. Laboratory studies show decreased levels of fibrinogen and platelets, increased prothrombin and partial thromboplastin times, and excessive amounts of fibrin degradation products.

Anesthetic Implications

The patient with DIC needs fluid resuscitation, and she almost always is hemorrhaging. Increasing intravascular volume dilutes activated clotting factors and slows the clotting process. Increased peripheral and hepatic perfusion limits cellular damage and improves clearance of activated clotting factors. Because the patient is bleeding and many clotting factors are depleted, it appears as if repletion of clotting factors is necessary; however, administration of clotting factors fuels an already out-of-control coagulation process. Definitive treatment of

DIC first requires elimination of the cause. Replacement of clotting factors in the obstetric patient should probably be postponed until the DIC has subsided.

Breech Presentation

Many obstetricians now choose to deliver fetuses in breech presentations by cesarean section. In this case, cesarean section usually is elective, and either a regional or a general anesthetic can be used. If the baby is to be delivered vaginally, an epidural anesthetic may be requested and, in fact, is considered strongly indicated at some centers. The muscle relaxation that it provides is helpful, and some sort of analgesia is required, at least for the forceps delivery of the fetal head. Breech deliveries often result in laceration of the birth canal and therefore cause more bleeding than head-first deliveries.

Multiple Gestation

Multiple-gestation pregnancies carry higher risk for both mother and fetuses than singleton pregnancies. Many of the risk factors affect anesthetic management. Multiple-gestation pregnancies, especially rare monoamniotic pregnancies, are associated with complications requiring emergent surgical intervention more often than singleton pregnancies. The anesthetist should constantly be prepared to provide anesthesia for an emergency cesarean section. The multiple fetuses are often small and premature. The large uterus compounds the problems of aortocaval compression; therefore left uterine displacement should be maintained at all times when the parturient is not lying on her side. If the fetuses are to be delivered vaginally, an epidural is valuable for maternal analgesia and neonatal safety. Because the neonate often is small and premature, a slow, controlled delivery through a well-relaxed birth canal makes birth trauma less likely. The epidural provides pelvic relaxation and reduces maternal discomfort, decreasing the likelihood that pain will induce a forceful reflexive expulsion of the fetus. Either regional or general anesthesia is appropriate for a cesarean section. After the babies have been delivered, the uterus may not contract well because it has been overstretched for many weeks. Larger-than-usual doses of oxytocin may be needed to induce the uterus to contract well and to stop bleeding. However, it is imperative that oxytocin administration not be started until after all the neonates have been delivered. Strong uterine contractions before the delivery of all neonates deprive any remaining fetuses of blood supply and oxygenation.

Prolapsed Umbilical Cord

A prolapsed umbilical cord is present when the cord protrudes through the cervix ahead of the fetus. Danger arises when compression of the cord against the wall of the cervix by the presenting part cuts off blood flow and oxygenation to the fetus. The obstetrician attempts either to restore blood flow in the umbilical cord by pushing the presenting part back into the uterus or to deliver the fetus abdominally before asphyxia causes permanent injury. In the first situation anesthesia is likely to be needed for uterine relaxation; in the second it is necessary for emergent cesarean section.

Preeclampsia

Description

Preeclampsia is a vasospastic disease of pregnancy that affects 2.6% to 6% of parturients. The incidence of preeclampsia is highest in primigravidas younger than 20 years or older than 35 years of age and in women who have had preeclampsia during a previous pregnancy. The exact cause of preeclampsia is unknown but probably involves an abnormality in the ratio of thromboxanes to prostacyclins. Thromboxanes are potent vasoconstrictors and platelet aggregators, whereas prostacyclins have the opposite effect. Thromboxane A_2 and prostacyclin levels normally increase during pregnancy. An imbalance of prostacyclins and thromboxanes, both of which are produced by the placenta, has been demonstrated in preeclampsia.[232-234]

Preeclampsia results in hypertension, 1+ to 2+ proteinuria, and edema after the twentieth week of gestation. Generally the diagnosis of preeclampsia is made when two of the three signs are present. Hypertension is defined as a blood pressure greater than 140/90, or more than 30 mm Hg above systolic baseline and more than 15 mm Hg above diastolic baseline.

Severe preeclampsia is said to exist when the following conditions are present: maternal blood pressure greater than 160/110, 3+ or 4+ proteinuria, urine output less than 20 ml/hr, CNS signs (blurred vision or changes in mentation), pulmonary edema, and epigastric pain. Blood pressure monitoring is a key indicator because it is technically easy to perform, and the severity of the hypertension frequently parallels the severity of the disease.

Preeclampsia results in maternal, fetal, and neonatal morbidity and mortality. The chief cause of maternal mortality is cerebral hemorrhage caused by hypertension. Pulmonary edema, renal failure, hepatic rupture, cerebral edema, and DIC also may cause maternal death. Brain edema results in CNS irritability, seizures (a significant percentage of which occur postpartum), and an increase in sensitivity to depressant drugs. Fetal death results primarily from placental abruption or infarct. Delivery of the fetus is curative.

Pathophysiology

No uniform agreement exists with regard to the pathophysiology of preeclampsia. One view is that preeclampsia is a hyperdynamic state involving an early increase in cardiac output and elevated SVR.[235,236] Another view is that preeclampsia is characterized by an increase in SVR and variable decrease in cardiac output.[237-240] In fact, SVRs of up to 4168 dyne • sec/cm^5 have been reported.[235] Thromboxane A_2 is found in increased levels during preeclampsia and has been correlated with disease severity.[241]

Increased vascular permeability results in extravasation of fluid and protein (proteinuria in the kidneys). Hypertension results in compensatory decreases in circulating blood volume and a loss of intravascular water and electrolytes via the kidney. Capillary injury stimulates platelet aggregation and fibrin deposition and may result in thrombocytopenia and, occasionally, DIC. It also results in multiple organ system dysfunction. Often, total body water is increased. Intravascular volume may decrease by as much as 40%. Marked peripheral and end-organ vasoconstriction is common, and it either causes or occurs in response to the decrease in vascular volume. An increased vascular sensitivity to vasopressin, angiotensin, and catecholamines has been demonstrated. Catecholamine levels often increase, and this results in decreased perfusion to the uterus, placenta, and fetus. Arteriolar constriction increases left ventricular work. When preeclampsia becomes severe, intravascular volume is either contracted or shifted centrally.

Central venous pressure may be low because of a contracted blood volume, or it may be relatively normal because of a redistribution of vascular volume into the central circulation. Pulmonary capillary occlusion pressure may be normal or high because of left-sided heart failure and often does not correlate well with the central venous pressure.

Uteroplacental insufficiency can result from a combination of decreased intravascular volume, vascular intimal deterioration, and increased vascular resistance. Placental perfusion in the preeclampsia patient may decrease by 70% compared with that in a healthy parturient. Decreased placental perfusion leads to intrauterine growth retardation and can cause fetal hypoxia and placental infarction.

Platelet aggregation and fibrin deposition increase in preeclampsia. Platelet counts may drop as the platelets are consumed; however, even in the presence of a normal platelet count, platelet function may be below normal.

Obstetric Management

Magnesium sulfate is almost always administered to women with preeclampsia in the United States. Although it is not curative, it has been shown to reduce the likelihood of eclampsia by 58% and the risk of maternal death by 45%.[242] Delivery presently is the only definitive way of ending the disease process of preeclampsia. When a fetus is at a gestational age of more than 37 weeks, obstetricians generally proceed with delivery. If the fetus is immature, delivery is delayed to allow the fetus time to mature. If preeclampsia is severe or fetal distress occurs, delivery is usually accomplished expeditiously. In any case, obstetric treatment is aimed at preventing eclampsia (seizures), avoiding decreases in uteroplacental blood flow, and maximizing organ perfusion. Magnesium sulfate, which is also used as a tocolytic, causes venodilation, mild CNS depression, a decrease in the rate of fibrin deposition, and a reduction in uterine activity, if present. Decreasing fibrin deposition prevents further decay in organ perfusion and often greatly decreases liver pain in parturients with hemolysis, elevated liver enzymes, and a low platelet count (HELLP syndrome). Magnesium therapy is continued after delivery for the suppression of seizures.

Regional Anesthesia and Preeclampsia

Epidural analgesia and anesthesia generally are preferred for both spontaneous vaginal delivery and cesarean section in the preeclampsia patient when they are not contraindicated. A carefully initiated epidural infusion helps control maternal hypertension and may improve organ blood flow. Characteristic changes in vital signs in women with preeclampsia before volume expansion, after volume expansion, and after institution of epidural analgesia are shown in Figure 44-17. Careful initiation of the block is necessary in women with preeclampsia, because their mean blood pressure tends to decrease more than that of healthy parturients (Figure 44-18). During a cesarean section, epidural anesthesia avoids stimulation of the airway, which can aggravate hypertension and possibly cause cerebral bleeding. During a vaginal delivery, epidural analgesia allows a slower, more controlled expulsion of the premature infant and decreases the likelihood of trauma to the fetal head. Even these advantages, however, must be weighed against the risks of regional anesthesia, primarily hypotension and bleeding.

Because thrombocytopenia and other coagulation problems are associated with preeclampsia, careful consideration should be given to the patient's coagulation status before regional anesthesia is begun. A careful history of bleeding should be taken

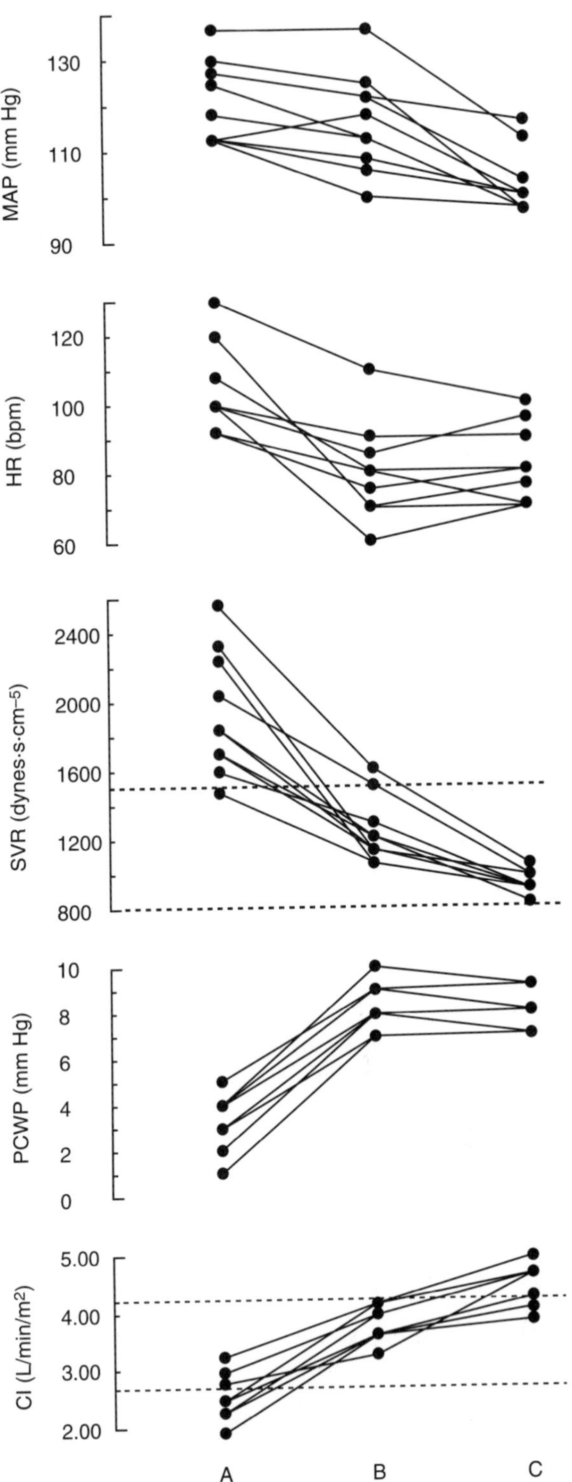

FIGURE **44-17**
Individual hemodynamic values before **(A)** and after **(B)** volume expansion and after vasodilation **(C)** in women with pregnancy-induced hypertension. The dotted lines represent the normal range for nonpregnant individuals. *CI*, Cardiac index; *HR*, heart rate; *MAP*, mean arterial pressure; *PCWP*, pulmonary capillary wedge pressure; *SVR*, systemic vascular resistance. (From Groenendijk R, Trimbos JB, Wallenburg HCS. Hemodynamic measurements in preeclampsia: preliminary observations. *Am J Obstet Gynecol*. 1984;150:232-236.)

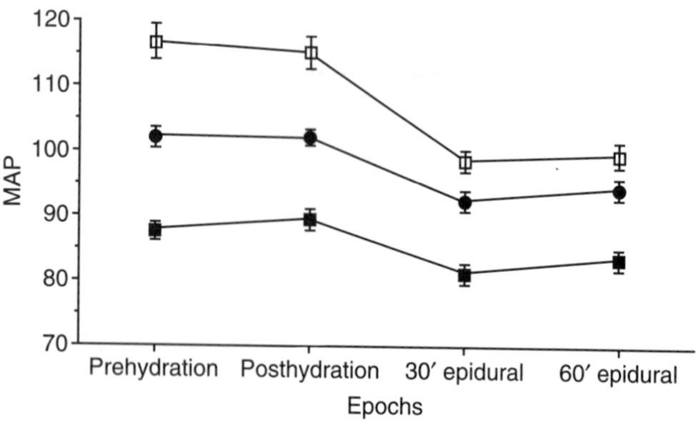

FIGURE **44-18**
Mean arterial pressure *(MAP)* of three study groups compared over four epochs. All values are expressed as group means; the bars represent standard errors. Maternal MAP decreased significantly in all groups after epidural blockade was established. *Closed circles*, Chronic hypertension; *closed squares*, normal; *open squares*, preeclampsia. (From Ramos-Santos E, Devoe LD, Wakefield ML, Sherline DM, Metheny WP. The effects of epidural anesthesia on the Doppler velocimetry of umbilical and uterine arteries in normal and hypertensive patients during active term labor. *Obstet Gynecol.* 1991;77:20-25. Reprinted with permission from The American College of Obstetricians and Gynecologists.)

and a platelet count evaluated before insertion of an epidural catheter in a patient with a diagnosis of preeclampsia. Coagulation problems are found almost exclusively in women with platelet counts below 100,000/mm^3.[243,244] Several studies indicate that significant decreases in platelet count occur almost exclusively in women with severe preeclampsia (diastolic blood pressure >110 mm Hg and urinary protein of at least 2+). Others do not believe that any correlation exists between the severity of preeclampsia and platelet count.[245] The normal bleeding time in healthy pregnant women appears to be approximately 5 minutes. When the platelet count was greater than 100,000/mm^3, 13% of women with mild preeclampsia and 34% of women with severe preeclampsia had prolonged bleeding times.[246] The platelet count correlated with prolongation of the bleeding time only when it was less than 100,000/mm^3.[245] When the platelet count falls below 100,000/mm^3, it is not likely to recover until several days after delivery.[247]

Some evidence indicates that epidural analgesia can improve uteroplacental perfusion, and therefore fetal oxygenation, by decreasing plasma catecholamines.[248,249] Epidural analgesia causes vascular dilation; this decreases blood pressure while maintaining—and, in some cases, improving—perfusion of the uterus and other organs, as long as hypotension is not allowed.[248-256] Uterine artery systolic/diastolic ratios in women with preeclampsia decrease after the initiation of epidural analgesia, suggesting that resistance to blood flow is lowered.[249] Diastolic blood pressure should not be reduced to less than 90 mm Hg in women with severe preeclampsia, because such a reduction will probably result in inadequate uteroplacental blood flow. Hypotension is a significant concern in the parturient with severe preeclampsia because of the sometimes constricted intravascular volume and the likelihood that the patient has already received an antihypertensive agent such as hydralazine or labetalol. When hypotension does occur, ephedrine and other vasopressors should be used cautiously, because they may produce an exaggerated response in the preeclampsia patient.

Epidural anesthesia can be accomplished safely in these patients if careful attention is devoted to volume status. Most but not all preeclampsia patients have a contracted blood volume.[255] IV preloading may be necessary because of the constricted intravascular volume; however, some patients have a normal central venous pressure or left ventricular dysfunction. Preloading in these patients can result in pulmonary edema. Placement of a central venous pressure line or pulmonary catheter may be indicated in severe preeclampsia when the patient is oliguric or hypoxic. Central line insertion probably is not indicated for anesthesia alone unless the line is needed for a general anesthetic and operative delivery. If so, the anesthetist must balance the benefits of infusing platelets and inserting a central line against the risks. The most useful platelet count is one of a continuous series and is as recent as possible, because the count may decrease precipitously as the disease progresses.

Bupivacaine is usually the local anesthetic of choice because of its long history of safe use in preeclampsia patients and because it has a slower onset than lidocaine and chloroprocaine. The slower onset allows time for the anesthetist to react to hemodynamic changes. Often, it is necessary to begin administering epidural anesthesia slowly with bupivacaine in these patients without any intravascular prehydration. Small incremental doses of bupivacaine can be administered and fluid given intravenously as needed when and if changes in blood pressure occur.

After epidural analgesia or anesthesia has been instituted, the sympathectomy should not be allowed to wear off abruptly, because the increased intravascular volume could precipitate a hypertensive crisis or pulmonary edema. Instead, the block should be allowed to recede slowly, when the body is able to eliminate the intravascular fluid load and adequate monitoring is available.

General Anesthesia

Coagulopathy or decay in maternal or fetal condition is the most common indication for general anesthesia in the patient with preeclampsia. The maternal brain is edematous and more sensitive to CNS-depressant drugs. Induction of general anesthesia is hazardous in persons with preeclampsia. Their exaggerated hypertensive response to laryngoscopy and endotracheal intubation is potentially lethal. Compounding the problem, upper airway swelling may make identification of landmarks and intubation more difficult. Swelling may preclude the insertion of an endotracheal tube of normal size. Difficulty in intubation increases the duration of airway stimulation and worsens hypertension. The challenge during induction of general anesthesia is prevention of a further increase in blood pressure, which may result in intracranial hemorrhage. Antihypertensives have long been used to control blood pressure during preeclampsia. Nevertheless, an average increase of 56 mm Hg in systolic blood pressure has been reported after induction of general anesthesia despite the use of β-blockers, trimethaphan, or both.[256] Comatose patients have even greater increases in systolic blood pressure (up to 70 mm Hg).[256] Control of blood pressure during induction of general anesthesia in these patients demands careful planning and skill in implementation.

Opioids to Control Blood Pressure

Opioids have long been known to attenuate the sympathetic response to laryngoscopy and intubation. Fentanyl, 5 to 8 mcg/kg, has been shown to be effective in nonpregnant

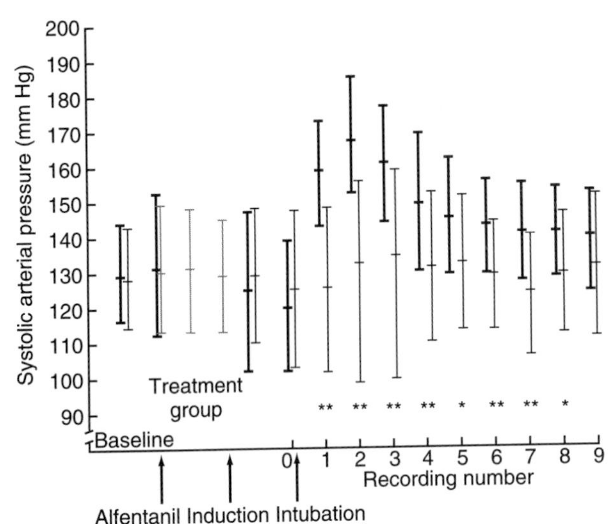

FIGURE **44-19**
Changes (1 SD) in systolic blood pressure before and after the induction of anesthesia, in the control group *(bold bars)* and the treatment group *(narrow bars)*. The shaded area represents the time from the administration of alfentanil to the administration of thiopental and therefore is of significance only for the treatment group. By *t*-test: **P*.05; ***P*.01; others not significant. (From Dann WL, Hutchinson A, Cartwright DP. Maternal and neonatal responses to alfentanil administered before induction of general anesthesia for cesarean section. *Br J Anaesth*. 1987;59:1392-1396.)

TABLE **44-3** Neonatal Results after Maternal Administration of Alfentanil, 10 mcg/kg 1 Minute before Induction of General Anesthesia

	Control (n = 16)	Alfentanil (n = 21)
Induction-to-delivery interval (min, mean [SD])	10.4 (2.6)	11.8 (2.5)
Weight (g, mean [SD])	3280 (690)	3240 (600)
Intubated	0	0
Received naloxone	0	0
Admitted to special baby unit	1	2
Apgar score at 1 min		
Median	9	9
Range	4-10	5-10
Apgar score at 10 min		
Median	10	10
Range	(All 10)	9-10

From Dann WL, Hutchinson A, Cartwright DP. Maternal and neonatal responses to alfentanil administered before induction of general anesthesia for cesarean section. Br J Anaesth. *1987;59:1392-1396.*

individuals, but this dose is infrequently used in obstetrics for fear of neonatal respiratory depression. For many years opioids were simply not used in obstetric anesthesia. However, studies have shown that small doses of fentanyl or alfentanil given before induction of general anesthesia helps attenuate the sympathetic response to laryngoscopy without causing neonatal respiratory depression.[257-260] Figure 44-19 shows the changes in systolic and diastolic blood pressure with and without the administration of 10 mcg of alfentanil per kilogram 1 minute before the induction of general anesthesia for cesarean section. The data in these figures were collected from healthy women undergoing cesarean section. Blood pressure changes in women with preeclampsia are likely to be more pronounced. Table 44-3 provides neonatal data for both control (no alfentanil before induction) and alfentanil induction groups. Using opioids to blunt blood pressure increases is not without risk. If the anesthetist is unable to manage the airway after a rapid-sequence induction, then the chance that the woman will reawaken and breathe in a reasonable amount of time is decreased.

Antihypertensives to Control Blood Pressure

Labetalol, a combined selective α_1- and nonselective β-antagonist, is widely used in obstetric anesthesia. Uteroplacental blood flow is maintained or increased when a total of up to 1 mg of labetalol per kilogram is used for treatment of preeclampsia.[211,212,214,261,262] Neonatal side effects (hypotension, bradycardia, hypoglycemia) are apparently minimal when this dose is used.[213,263-265] The fetal-to-maternal ratio of plasma levels for labetalol has been reported to be 0.5.[266] In women with preeclampsia, the administration of labetalol before induction of general anesthesia results in a lower mean blood pressure at induction and during the first 10 minutes of anesthesia.[214,267] Although the elimination half-life of labetalol is between 5 and 8 hours in nonpregnant adults, it is only 1.7 hours in pregnant adults.[266]

Hydralazine increases splanchnic, coronary, cerebral, uterine, and renal blood flow as long as hypotension is not allowed. Resistance vessels in these vascular beds are more affected than those of the skin and skeletal muscle. Hydralazine is favored in the preeclampsia patient because it may actually improve uteroplacental circulation. It is also a potent pulmonary arterial dilator. The long onset time (10 to 20 minutes) probably precludes use immediately before an emergent cesarean section.

IV nitroglycerin has a quick onset, but its antihypertensive effect is less predictable than that of other drugs. Nevertheless, it is widely used for this purpose. The fetal-to-maternal ratio of nitroglycerin blood levels in sheep is only 0.04.[268] If this is true in humans, it represents very low placental passage and could give nitroglycerin a significant advantage over other antihypertensives.

In one study, when a nitroglycerin infusion was begun before induction, the maximum MAP after intubation was 119 mm Hg in the nitroglycerin group and 155 mm Hg in the control group.[269] Nitroglycerin may, however, result in an increase in intracranial pressure in women with severe preeclampsia.

Nitroprusside has a fast onset and is easily titratable. Although at least theoretic concerns regarding neonatal cyanide toxicity exist, this should not be a problem if the drug is used briefly during the induction of anesthesia. Nitroprusside has been used for intracranial procedures during pregnancy without fetal toxicity. Probably to a greater degree than even nitroglycerin, nitroprusside may cause deleterious increases in maternal intracranial pressure.

Esmolol was initially thought to hold promise for attenuating the hypertension and tachycardia of laryngoscopy in preeclampsia patients, because early investigations reported the inability to measure any esmolol in fetal sheep 10 minutes after the discontinuation of an esmolol infusion, and because immature neonatal red blood cells hydrolyzed esmolol. A subsequent case report of a woman who was 22 weeks pregnant and underwent repair of a cerebellar arteriovenous malformation demonstrated only a mild effect on FHR both preoperatively and intraoperatively.[270] Unfortunately, more detailed studies have shown that, except at very low doses, esmolol does cross the placenta and may result in clinically significant fetal β-blockade.[271]

Whichever antihypertensive drug is used, it is wise to perform a test run before the induction of general anesthesia. This test indicates whether the agent will yield the desired result and also allows estimation of the proper dose.

Muscle Relaxants

Nondepolarizing relaxants are markedly potentiated in women with preeclampsia and therapeutic levels of magnesium. In these patients one half of an effective dose in 95% of the population dose produced 100% block for 35 minutes.[204] In healthy parturients not receiving magnesium sulfate, the same dose on average produced 42% blockade for approximately 9 minutes. Reduced doses of nondepolarizers can be used, if desired, but these drugs yield a longer-than-usual block.

HELLP Syndrome

HELLP syndrome consists of hemolysis, elevated liver enzymes, and a low platelet count. From 5% to 10% of the sickest women with preeclampsia develop HELLP syndrome. Clinical signs of HELLP syndrome include epigastric pain, upper abdominal tenderness, proteinuria, hypertension, jaundice, nausea, and vomiting. Rarely, HELLP syndrome may result in liver rupture. Some experts believe that a degree of compensated DIC is present in all patients with HELLP syndrome.

Anesthesia for the Pregnant Patient Undergoing a Nonobstetric Procedure

Occasionally anesthetists must provide anesthesia care for a pregnant woman having nonobstetric emergency procedures. Some key points are noted in Box 44-7.

BOX 44-7

Key Points for the Pregnant Patient Undergoing Nonobstetric Procedure

- A significant number of women undergo anesthesia and surgery during pregnancy for procedures unrelated to delivery.
- Maternal risks are associated with the anatomic and physiologic changes of pregnancy (e.g., difficult intubation, aspiration) and with the underlying maternal disease.
- The diagnosis of abdominal conditions often is delayed during pregnancy, which increases the risk of maternal and fetal morbidity.
- Maternal catastrophes involving severe hypoxia, hypotension, and acidosis pose the greatest acute risk to the fetus.
- Other fetal risks associated with surgery include increased fetal loss, increased incidence of preterm labor, growth restriction, and low birth weight. Clinical studies suggest that anesthesia and surgery during pregnancy do not increase the risk of congenital anomalies.
- It is unclear whether adverse fetal outcomes result from the anesthetic, the operation, or the underlying maternal disease.
- No anesthetic agent is a proven teratogen in humans, although some anesthetic agents, specifically nitrous oxide, are teratogenic in animals under certain conditions.
- Many anesthetic agents have been used for anesthesia during pregnancy, with no demonstrable differences in maternal or fetal outcome.
- The anesthesia management of the pregnant surgical patient should focus on the avoidance of hypoxemia, hypotension, acidosis, and hyperventilation.

From Naughton NN, Cohen SE. Nonobstetric Surgery During Pregnancy. In Obstetric Anesthesia, 3rd ed. Chestnut DH (ed). 3rd ed, Elsevier Mosby, Philadelphia, 2004, p 269.

REFERENCES

1. van Oppen AC, van der Tweel I, Alsbach GP, Heethaar RM, Bruinse HW. A longitudinal study of maternal hemodynamics during normal pregnancy. *Obstet Gynecol.* 1996;88:40-46.
2. Leduc L, Wasserstrum N, Spillman T, Cotton DB. Baroreflex function in normal pregnancy. *Am J Obstet Gynecol.* 1991;163:886-890.
3. Capeless EL, Clapp JF. When do cardiovascular parameters return to their preconception values? *Am J Obstet Gynecol.* 1991;163:883-886.
4. Clark SL, Cotton DB, Lee W, et al. Central hemodynamic assessment of normal term pregnancy. *Am J Obstet Gynecol.* 1989;161:1439-1442.
5. Greenwood JP, Scott EM, Stoker JB, Walker JJ, Mary DA. Sympathetic neural mechanisms in normal and hypertensive pregnancy in humans. *Circulation.* 2001;104:2200-2204.
6. August P, Mueller FB, Sealey JE, Edersheim TG. Role of renin-angiotensin system in blood pressure regulation in pregnancy. *Lancet.* 1995;345:896-897.
7. Schrier RW, Briner VA. Peripheral arterial vasodilation hypothesis of sodium and water retention in pregnancy: implications for pathogenesis of preeclampsia-eclampsia. *Obstet Gynecol.* 1991;77:632-639.
8. Magness RR, Cox K, Rosenfeld CR, Gant NF. Angiotensin II metabolic clearance rate and pressor responses in nonpregnant and pregnant women. *Am J Obstet Gynecol.* 1994;171: 668-679.
9. Lumbers ER. Peripheral vascular reactivity to angiotensin and noradrenaline in pregnant and non-pregnant women. *Aust J Exp Biol Med Sci.* 1970;48:493-500.
10. Chesley LC, Talledo E, Bohler CS, Zuspan FP. Vascular reactivity to angiotensin II and norepinephrine in pregnant and nonpregnant women. *Am J Obstet Gynecol.* 1965;91:837-842.
11. Delemarre FM, Didden MA, de Jong PA. Diurnal variation in angiotensin sensitivity in pregnancy. *Am J Obstet Gynecol.* 1996;174:259-261.
12. Davison JM, Sheills EA, Barron WM, Robinson AG, Lindheimer MD. Changes in the metabolic clearance of vasopressin and in plasma vasopressinase throughout human pregnancy. *J Clin Invest.* 1989;83:1313-1318.
13. Howard BK, Goodson JH, Mengert WF. Supine hypotensive syndrome in late pregnancy. *Obstet Gynecol.* 1953;1:371-377.
14. McRoberst WA Jr. Postural shock in pregnancy. *Am J Obstet Gynecol.* 1951;62:627.
15. Pirhonen JP, Erkkola RU. Uterine and umbilical flow velocity waveforms in the supine hypotensive syndrome. *Obstet Gynecol.* 1990;76:176-179.
16. Bamber JH, Dresner M. Aortocaval compression in pregnancy: the effect of changing the degree and direction of lateral tilt on maternal cardiac output. *Anesth Analg.* 2003;97: 256-258.
17. Jones SJ, Kinsella SM, Donald FA. Comparison of measured and estimated angles of table tilt at Caesarean section. *Br J Anaesth.* 2003;90:86-87.

18. Archer GW Jr, Marx GF. Arterial oxygen tension during apnea in parturient women. *Br J Anaesth*. 1974;46:358-360.
19. Bourne T, Ogilvy AJ, Vickers R, Williamson K. Nocturnal hypoxaemia in late pregnancy. *Br J Anaesth*. 1995;75:678-682.
20. Palahniuk RJ, Shnider SM, Eger EI II. Pregnancy decreases the requirements for inhaled anesthetic agents. *Anesthesiology*. 1974;41:82-83.
21. Datta S, Migliozzi RP, Flanagan HL, Krieger NR. Chronically administered progesterone decreases halothane requirements in rabbits. *Anesth Analg*. 1989;68:46-50.
22. Datta S, Lambert DH, Gregus J, Gissen AJ, Covino BG. Differential sensitivities of mammalian nerve fibers during pregnancy. *Anesth Analg*. 1983;62:1070-1072.
23. Flanagan HL, Datta S, Lambert DH, Gissen AJ, Covino B. Effect of pregnancy on bupivacaine-induced conduction blockade in the isolated rabbit vagus nerve. *Anesth Analg*. 1987;66:123-126.
24. Butterworth JF, Walker FO, Lyzak SZ. Pregnancy increases median nerve susceptibility to lidocaine. *Anesthesiology*. 1990;72:962-965.
25. Carp H, Jayaram A, Stoll M. Ultrasound examination of the stomach contents of parturients. *Anesth Analg*. 1992;74:683-687.
26. Rout CC, Rocke DA, Gouws E. Intravenous ranitidine reduces the risk of acid aspiration of gastric contents at emergency cesarean section. *Anesth Analg*. 1993;76:156-161.
27. Robson SC, Boys RJ, Hunter S, Dunlop W. Maternal hemodynamics after normal delivery and delivery complicated by postpartum hemorrhage. *Obstet Gynecol*. 1989;74:234-239.
28. Wright RG, Shnider SM, Levinson G, Rolbin SH, Parer JT. The effect of maternal administration of ephedrine on fetal heart rate and variability. *Am J Obstet Gynecol*. 1981;57:734-738.
29. Petrie RH, Yeh S, Murata Y, et al. The effect of drugs on fetal heart rate variability. *Am J Obstet Gynecol*. 1978;130:294-299.
30. Zimmer EZ, Divon MY, Vadasz A. Influence of meperidine on fetal movements and heart rate beat-to-beat variability in the active phase of labor. *Am J Perinatol*. 1988;5:197-200.
31. Rayburn WF, Smith CV, Parriott JE, Woods RE. Randomized comparison of meperidine and fentanyl during labor. *Obstet Gynecol*. 1989;74:604-606.
32. Alahuhta S, Räsänen J, Jouppila P, Jouppila R, Hollmén AI. Epidural sufentanil and bupivacaine for labor analgesia and Doppler velocimetry of the umbilical and uterine arteries. *Anesthesiology*. 1993;78:231-236.
33. Petrikovsky BM, Vintzileos AM. Magnesium sulfate and intrapartum fetal behavior. *Am J Perinatol*. 1990;7:154-156.
34. Hatjis CG, Meis PJ. Sinusoidal fetal heart rate pattern associated with butorphanol administration. *Obstet Gynecol*. 1986;67:377-380.
35. Driver RP Jr, Snyder IS, North FP, Fife TJ. Sterility of anesthetic and resuscitative drug syringes used in the obstetric operating room. *Anesth Analg*. 1998;86:994-997.
36. Lewis B, Jarvi E, Cady P. Atropine and ephedrine adsorption to syringe plastic. *AANA J*. 1994;62:257-260.
37. Kuhnert BR, Linn PL, Kennard MJ, Kuhnert PM. Effects of low doses of meperidine on neonatal behavior. *Anesth Analg*. 1985;64:335-342.
38. Craft JB Jr, Coaldrake LA, Yonekura JL, et al. Ketamine, catecholamines, and uterine tone in pregnant ewes. *Am J Obstet Gynecol*. 1983;146:429-434.
39. Levinson G, Shnider SM, Gildea JE, deLorimier AA. Maternal and foetal cardiovascular and acid-base changes during ketamine anaesthesia in pregnant ewes. *Br J Anaesth*. 1973;45:1111-1115.
40. Beilin Y, Bodian CA, Haddad EM, Leibowitz AB. Practice patterns of anesthesiologists regarding situations in obstetric anesthesia where clinical management is controversial. *Anesth Analg*. 1996;83:735-741.
41. Clarke S. Informed consent without bureaucracy. *J Clin Neurosci*. 2003;10:35-36.
42. Datta S, Camann W, Bader A, VanderBurgh L. Clinical effects and maternal and fetal plasma concentrations of epidural ropivacaine versus bupivacaine for cesarean section. *Anesthesiology*. 1995;82:1346-1352.
43. Lacassie HJ, Columb MO, Lacassie HP, Lantadilla RA. The relative motor blocking potencies of epidural bupivacaine and ropivacaine in labor. *Anesth Analg*. 2002;95:204-208.
44. Scott DA, Emanuelsson BM, Mooney PH, Cook RJ, Junestrand C. Pharmacokinetics and efficacy of long-term epidural ropivacaine infusion for postoperative analgesia. *Anesth Analg*. 1997;85:1322-1330.
45. Etches RC, Writer WD, Ansley D, et al. Continuous epidural ropivacaine 0.2% for analgesia after lower abdominal surgery. *Anesth Analg*. 1997;84:784-790.
46. Gautier P, De Kock M, Van Steenberge A, et al. A double-blind comparison of 0.125% ropivacaine with sufentanil and 0.125% bupivacaine with sufentanil for epidural labor analgesia. *Anesthesiology*. 1999;90:772-778.
47. Scott DB, Lee A, Fagan D, et al. Acute toxicity of ropivacaine compared with that of bupivacaine. *Anesth Analg*. 1989;69:563-569.
48. Knudsen K, Beckman Suurkula M, Blomberg S, Sjovall J, Edvardsson N. Central nervous and cardiovascular effects of IV infusions of ropivacaine, bupivacaine and placebo in volunteers. *Br J Anaesth*. 1997;78:507-514.
49. Moller RA, Covino BG. Effect of progesterone on the cardiac electrophysiologic alterations produced by ropivacaine and bupivacaine. *Anesthesiology*. 1992;77:735-741.
50. Moller RA, Datta S, Fox J, Johnson M, Covino BG. Effects of progesterone on the cardiac electrophysiologic action of bupivacaine and lidocaine. *Anesthesiology*. 1992;76:604-608.
51. Reiz S, Nath S. Cardiotoxicity of local anaesthetic agents. *Br J Anaesth*. 1986;58:736-746.
52. Morton CP, Bloomfield S, Magnusson A, Jozwiak H, McClure JH. Ropivacaine 0.75% for extradural anaesthesia in elective caesarean section: an open clinical and pharmacokinetic study in mother and neonate. *Br J Anaesth*. 1997;79:3-8.
53. Birnbach DJ, Stein DJ, Murray O, Thys DM, Sordillo EM. Povidone iodine and skin disinfection before initiation of epidural anesthesia. *Anesthesiology*. 1998;88:668-672.
54. Kleiman SJ, Wiesel S, Tessler MJ. Patient-controlled analgesia (PCA) using fentanyl in a parturient with a platelet function abnormality. *Can J Anaesth*. 1991;38:489-491.
55. Rayburn W, Rathke A, Leuschen P, Chleborad J, Weidner W. Fentanyl citrate analgesia during labor. *Am J Obstet Gynecol*. 1989;161:202-206.
56. Beilin Y, Bernstein HH, Zucker-Pinchoff B. The optimal distance that a multiorifice epidural catheter should be threaded into the epidural space. *Anesth Analg*. 1995;81:301-304.
57. Hamilton CL, Riley ET, Cohen SE. Changes in the position of epidural catheters associated with patient movement. *Anesthesiology*. 1997;86:778-784.
58. Michael S, Richmond MN, Birks RJS. A comparison between open-end (single hole) and closed-end (three lateral holes) epidural catheters. Complications and quality of sensory blockade. *Anaesthesia*. 1989;44:578-580.
59. D'Angelo R, Foss ML, Livesay CH. A comparison of multiport and uniport epidural catheters in laboring patients. *Anesth Analg*. 1997;84:1276-1279.
60. Dickson MAS, Moores C, McClure JH. Comparison of single, end-holed and multi-orifice extradural catheters when used for continuous infusion of local anaesthetic during labour. *Br J Anaesth*. 1997;79:297-300.
61. Dalal P, Gertenbach C, Harker H, O'Sullivan G. Assessing bupivacaine 10 mg/fentanyl 20 mcg as an intrathecal test dose. *Int J Obstet Anesth*. 2003;12:205-255.
62. Hood DD, Dewan DM, James FM. Maternal and fetal effects of epinephrine in gravid ewes. *Anesthesiology*. 1986;64:610-613.

63. Chestnut DH, Weiner CP, Herring JE, Wang J. Effect of intravenous epinephrine upon uterine blood flow velocity in the pregnant guinea pig. *Anesthesiology*. 1986;65:633-636.
64. Trojanowski A, Murray WB. A test to prevent subarachnoid and intravascular injections during epidural analgesia. *S Afr Med J*. 1995;85:531-534.
65. Norris MC, Fogel ST, Dalman H, et al. Labor epidural analgesia without an intravascular "test dose." *Anesthesiology*. 1998;88:1495-1501.
66. Jiang X, Wen X, Gao B, et al. The plasma concentrations of lidocaine after slow versus rapid administration of an initial dose of epidural anesthesia. *Anesth Analg*. 1997;84:570-573.
67. Viscomi CM, Hood DD, Melone PJ, Eisenach JC. Fetal heart rate variability after epidural fentanyl during labor. *Anesth Analg*. 1990;71:679-683.
68. Marx GF, Elstein ID, Schuss M, Anyaegbunam A, Fleischer A. Effects of epidural block with lignocaine and lignocaine-adrenaline on umbilical artery velocity wave ratios. *Br J Obstet Gynaecol*. 1990;97:517-520.
69. Purdie J, Reid J, Thorburn J, Asbury AJ. Continuous extradural analgesia: comparison of midwife top-ups, continuous infusions and patient controlled administration. *Br J Anaesth*. 1992;68:580-584.
70. Viscomi C, Eisenach JC. Patient-controlled epidural analgesia during labor. *Obstet Gynecol*. 1991;77:348-351.
71. Gambling DR, McMorland GH, Yu P, Laszlo C. Comparison of patient-controlled epidural analgesia and conventional intermittent "top-up" injections during labor. *Anesth Analg*. 1990;70:256-261.
72. Greene NM, Brull SJ. *Physiology of Spinal Anesthesia*. 4th ed. Baltimore: Williams & Wilkins; 1993.
73. Bonica JJ, Kennedy WF Jr, Ward RJ, Tolas AG. A comparison of the effects of high subarachnoid and epidural anesthesia. *Acta Anaesthesiol Scand Suppl*. 1966;23:429-437.
74. Sancetta SM, Lynn RB, Simeone FA, Heckman G, Janouskovec H. Studies of hemodynamic changes in humans following induction of spinal anesthesia. IV. Observations in low spinal anesthesia during surgery. *Surg Gynecol Obstet*. 1953;97:597-602.
75. Kennedy WF Jr, Everett GB, Cobb LA, Allen GD. Simultaneous systemic and hepatic hemodynamic measurements during high spinal anesthesia in normal man. *Anesth Analg*. 1970;49:1016-1024.
76. Sancetta SM, Lynn RB, Simeone FA, Scott RW. Studies of hemodynamic changes in humans following induction of low and high spinal anesthesia. *Circulation*. 1952;6:559-571.
77. Ward RJ, Bonica JJ, Freund FG, et al. Epidural and subarachnoid anesthesia. Cardiovascular and respiratory effects. *JAMA*. 1965;191:275-278.
78. Morgan PJ, Halpern SH, Tarshis J. The effects of an increase of central blood volume before spinal anesthesia for cesarean delivery: a qualitative systematic review. *Anesth Analg*. 2001;92:997-1005.
79. Kubli M, Shennan AH, Seed PT, O'Sullivan G. A randomised controlled trial of fluid pre-loading before low dose epidural analgesia for labour. *Int J Obstet Anesth*. 2003;12:256-260.
80. Park GE, Hauch MA, Curlin F, Datta S, Bader AM. The effects of varying volumes of crystalloid administration before cesarean delivery on maternal hemodynamics and colloid osmotic pressure. *Anesth Analg*. 1996;83:299-303.
81. Rout CC, Rocke DA, Levin J, Gouws E, Reddy D. A reevaluation of the role of crystalloid preload in the prevention of hypotension associated with spinal anesthesia for elective cesarean section. *Anesthesiology*. 1993;79:262-269.
82. Ueyama H, He YL, Tanigami H, Mashimo T, Yoshiya I. Effects of crystalloid and colloid preload on blood volume in the parturient undergoing spinal anesthesia for elective Cesarean section [see comments]. *Anesthesiology*. 1999;91:1571-1576.
83. Riley ET, Cohen SE, Rubenstein AJ, Flanagan B. Prevention of hypotension after spinal anesthesia for cesarean section: six percent hetastarch versus lactated Ringer's solution. *Anesth Analg*. 1995;81:838-842.
84. Shiraishi Y, Fujimura S, Handa M, et al. Vasopressin and atrial natriuretic peptide release in cardiopulmonary denervated dogs. *Am J Physiol*. 1990;258:R704-R710.
85. Fiedler MA. *Maternal Hypotension and Epidural Anesthesia for Cesarean Section* [dissertation]. Memphis, Tenn: University of Tennessee Center for the Health Sciences; 2002.
86. Jouppila R, Jouppila P, Kuikka J, Hollmen A. Placental blood flow during caesarean section under lumbar extradural analgesia. *Br J Anaesth*. 1978;50:275-279.
87. Brizgys RV, Dailey PA, Shnider SM, Kotelko DM, Levinson G. The incidence and neonatal effects of maternal hypotension during epidural anesthesia for cesarean section. *Anesthesiology*. 1987;67:782-786.
88. Corke BC, Datta S, Ostheimer GW, Weiss JB, Alper MH. Spinal anaesthesia for caesarean section: the influence of hypotension on neonatal outcome. *Anaesthesia*. 1982;37:658-662.
89. Antoine C, Young BK. Fetal lactic acidosis with epidural anesthesia. *Am J Obstet Gynecol*. 1982;142:55-59.
90. Hon EH, Reid BL, Hehre FW. The electronic evaluation of fetal heart rate. II. Changes with maternal hypotension. *Am J Obstet Gynecol*. 1960;79:209-215.
91. Goodlin RC. Venous reactivity and pregnancy abnormalities. *Acta Obstet Gynecol Scand*. 1986;65:345-348.
92. Ralston DH, Shnider SM, DeLorimer AA. Effect of equipotent ephedrine, metaraminol, mephentermine, and methoxamine on uterine blood flow in the pregnant ewe. *Anesthesiology*. 1974;40:354-370.
93. Hughes SC, Ward MG, Levinson G, et al. Placental transfer of ephedrine does not affect neonatal outcome. *Anesthesiology*. 1985;63:217-219.
94. Husaini S, Russell I. Volume preload: lack of effect in the prevention of spinal-induced hypotension at caesarean section. *Int J Obstet Anesth*. 1998;7:76-81.
95. Jackson R, Reid JA, Thorburn J. Volume preloading is not essential to prevent spinal-induced hypotension at caesarean section. *Br J Anaesth*. 1995;75:262-265.
96. Wennberg E, Frid I, Haljamäe H, Norén H. Colloid (3% dextran 70) with or without ephedrine infusion for cardiovascular stability during extradural caesarean section. *Br J Anaesth*. 1992;69:13-18.
97. Ramin SM, Ramin KD, Cox K, et al. Comparison of prophylactic angiotensin II versus ephedrine infusion for prevention of maternal hypotension during spinal anesthesia [see comments]. *Am J Obstet Gynecol*. 1994;171:734-739.
98. Gajraj NM, Victory RA, Pace NA, Van Elstraete AC, Wallace DH. Comparison of an ephedrine infusion with crystalloid administration for prevention of hypotension during spinal anesthesia. *Anesth Analg*. 1993;76:1023-1026.
99. Kang YG, Abouleish E, Caritis S. Prophylactic intravenous ephedrine infusion during spinal anesthesia for cesarean section. *Anesth Analg*. 1982;61:839-842.
100. Lee A, Ngan Kee WD, Gin T. A quantitative, systematic review of randomized controlled trials of ephedrine versus phenylephrine for the management of hypotension during spinal anesthesia for cesarean delivery. *Anesth Analg*. 2002;94:920-926.
101. Moran DH, Perillo M, LaPorta RF, Bader AM, Datta S. Phenylephrine in the prevention of hypotension following spinal anesthesia for cesarean delivery. *J Clin Anesth*. 1991;3:301-305.
102. Ramanathan S, Grant GJ. Vasopressor therapy for hypotension due to epidural anesthesia for cesarean section. *Acta Anaesthesiol Scand*. 1988;32:559-565.
103. Lee A, McKeown D, Wilson J. Evaluation of the efficacy of elastic compression stockings in prevention of hypotension during epidural anaesthesia for elective caesarean section. *Acta Anaesthesiol Scand*. 1987;31:193-195.
104. Sood PK, Cooper PJF, Michel MZ, Wee MYK, Pickering RM. Thromboembolic deterrent stockings fail to prevent hypotension associated with spinal anaesthesia for elective caesarean section. *Int J Obstet Anesth*. 1996;5:172-175.

105. Rout CC, Rocke DA, Gouws E. Leg elevation and wrapping in the prevention of hypotension following spinal anaesthesia for elective caesarean section. *Anaesthesia*. 1993;48:304-308.
106. Bhagwanjee S, Rocke JA, Rout CC, Koovarjee RV, Brijball R. Prevention of hypotension following spinal anaesthesia for elective caesarean section by wrapping the legs. *Br J Anaesth*. 1990;65:819-822.
107. McAuley DM, Moore J, McCaughey W, Donnelly BD, Dundee JW. Ranitidine as an antacid before elective caesarean section. *Anaesthesia*. 1983;38:108-114.
108. Brashear WT, Zuspan KJ, Lazenbnik N, Kuhnert BR, Mann LI. Effect of ranitidine on bupivacaine disposition. *Anesth Analg*. 1991;72:369-376.
109. Caldwell C, Rains G, McKiterick K. An unusual reaction to preoperative metoclopramide. *Anesthesiology*. 1987;67:854.
110. Crawford JS. Anesthesia for section: further refinements of a technique. *Br J Anaesth*. 1973;45:726-731.
111. Duthie SJ, Ghosh A, Ng A, Ho PC. Intra-operative blood loss during elective lower segment cesarean section. *Br J Obstet Gynaecol*. 1992;99:364-367.
112. Combs CA, Murphy EL, Laros RK Jr. Factors associated with hemorrhage in cesarean deliveries. *Obstet Gynecol*. 1991;77: 77-82.
113. Marx GF, Luykx WM, Cohen S. Foetal-neonatal status following caesarean section for foetal distress. *Br J Anaesth*. 1984;56:1009-1013.
114. Ong BY, Cohen MM, Palahniuk RJ. Anesthesia for cesarean section—effects on neonates. *Anesth Analg*. 1989;68:270-275.
115. Morgan BM, Magni V, Goroszenuik T. Anaesthesia for emergency caesarean section. *Br J Obstet Gynaecol*. 1990;97:420-424.
116. Evans CM, Murphy JF, Gray OP, Rosen M. Epidural versus general anaesthesia for elective caesarean section. Effect on Apgar score and acid-base status of the newborn. *Anaesthesia*. 1989;44:778-782.
117. Hawthorne L, Wilson R, Lyons G, Dresner M. Failed intubation revisited: 17-year experience in a teaching maternity unit. *Br J Anaesth*. 1996;76:680-684.
118. Dailland P, Cockshott ID, Lirzin JD, et al. Intravenous propofol during cesarean section: placental transfer, concentrations in breast milk, and neonatal effects. A preliminary study. *Anesthesiology*. 1989;71:827-834.
119. Gin T, Gregory MA, Chan K, Buckley T, Oh TE. Pharmacokinetics of propofol in women undergoing elective caesarean section. *Br J Anaesth*. 1990;64:148-153.
120. Valtonen M, Kanto J, Rosenberg P. Comparison of propofol and thiopentone for induction of anaesthesia for elective caesarean section. *Anaesthesia*. 1989;44:758-762.
121. Gin T, Gregory MA, Oh TE. The haemodynamic effects of propofol and thiopentone for induction of caesarean section. *Anaesth Intensive Care*. 1990;18:175-179.
122. Ngan Kee WD, Khaw KS, Ma ML, Mainland P-A, Gin T. Postoperative analgesic requirement after cesarean section: a comparison of anesthetic induction with ketamine or thiopental. *Anesth Analg*. 1997;85:1294-1298.
123. King HK, Ashley S, Brathwaite D, Decayette J, Wooten DJ. Adequacy of general anesthesia for cesarean section. *Anesth Analg*. 1993;77:84-88.
124. Bernstein K, Gisselsson SL, Jacobson L, Ohrlander S. Influence of two different anaesthetic agents on the newborn and the correlation between foetal oxygenation and induction delivery time in elective caesarean section. *Acta Anaesthesiol Scand*. 1985;29:157-160.
125. Kao YJ, Tellez J, Turner DR. Dose-dependent effect of metoclopramide on cholinesterase and suxamethonium metabolism. *Br J Anaesth*. 1990;65:220-224.
126. Munson ES, Embro WJ. Enflurane, isoflurane, and halothane and isolated human uterine muscle. *Anesthesiology*. 1977;46:11-14.
127. Marx GF, Kim YI, Lin CC, Halevy S, Schulman H. Postpartum uterine pressure under halothane or enflurane anesthesia. *Obstet Gynecol*. 1978;51:695-698.
128. Dogru K, Dalgic H, Yildiz K, Sezer Z, Madenoglu H. The direct depressant effects of desflurane and sevoflurane on spontaneous contractions of isolated gravid rat myometrium. *Int J Obstet Anesth*. 2003;12:74-78.
129. Ngan Kee WD, Khaw KS, Ma KC, Wong AS, Lee BB. Randomized, double-blind comparison of different inspired oxygen fractions during general anaesthesia for caesarean section. *Br J Anaesth*. 2002;89:556-561.
130. Khaw KS, Wang CC, Ngan Kee WD, Pang CP, Rogers MS. Effects of high inspired oxygen fraction during elective caesarean section under spinal anaesthesia on maternal and fetal oxygenation and lipid peroxidation. *Br J Anaesth*. 2002;88:18-23.
131. Piggott SE, Bogod DG, Rosen M, Rees GAD, Harmer M. Isoflurane with either 100% oxygen or 50% nitrous oxide in oxygen for caesarean section. *Br J Anaesth*. 1990;65:325-329.
132. Bogod DG, Rosen M, Rees GA. Maximum FIO_2 during caesarean section. *Br J Anaesth*. 1988;61:255-262.
133. Perrault C, Balise GA, Meloche R. Maternal inspired oxygen concentration and fetal oxygenation during cesarean section. *Can J Anaesth*. 1992;39:155-157.
134. Dailey PA, Fisher DM, Shnider SM, et al. Pharmacokinetics, placental transfer, and neonatal effects of vecuronium and pancuronium administered during cesarean section. *Anesthesiology*. 1984;60:569-574.
135. Bader AM, Datta S, Arthur GR, et al. Maternal and fetal catecholamines and uterine incision-to-delivery interval during elective cesarean. *Obstet Gynecol*. 1990;75:600-603.
136. Datta S, Ostheimer GW, Weiss JB, Brown WU, Alper MH. Neonatal effect of prolonged anesthetic induction for cesarean section. *Obstet Gynecol*. 1981;58:331-335.
137. Rosaeg OP, Cicutti NJ, Labow RS. The effect of oxytocin on the contractile force of human atrial trabeculae. *Anesth Analg*. 1998;86:40-44.
138. Veber B, Gauthé M, Michel-Cherqui M, Des Mesnards V, Fischler M. Severe hypertension during postpartum haemorrhage after IV administration of prostaglandin E_2. *Br J Anaesth*. 1992;68:623-624.
139. Silva D, Singh P, Bauman J, Miller R. Acute hypertensive response to prostaglandin F_2 alpha during anaesthesia administration. *J Reprod Med*. 1987;32:700-702.
140. Partridge BL, Key T, Reisner L. Life-threatening effects of intravascular absorption of PGF_2 alpha during therapeutic termination of pregnancy. *Anesth Analg*. 1988;67:1111-1113.
141. Parnass SM, Curran MJA, Becker GL. Incidence of hypotension associated with epidural anesthesia using alkalinized and nonalkalinized lidocaine for cesarean section. *Anesth Analg*. 1987;66:1148-1150.
142. Benzon HT, Toleikis JR, Dixit P, Goodman I, Hill JA. Onset, intensity of blockade and somatosensory evoked potential changes of the lumbosacral dermatomes after epidural anesthesia with alkalinized lidocaine. *Anesth Analg*. 1993;76:328-332.
143. Curatolo M, Petersen-Felix S, Arendt-Nielsen L, et al. Adding sodium bicarbonate to lidocaine enhances the depth of epidural blockade. *Anesth Analg*. 1998;86:341-347.
144. Bartfield JM, Homer PJ, Ford DT, Sternklar P. Buffered lidocaine as a local anesthetic: an investigation of shelf life. *Ann Emerg Med*. 1992;21:16-19.
145. Crochetière CT, Trépanier CA, Coté JJ. Epidural anaesthesia for caesarean section: comparison of two injection techniques. *Can J Anaesth*. 1989;36:133-136.
146. Ohno H, Watanabe M, Saitoh J, et al. Effect of epinephrine concentration on lidocaine disposition during epidural anesthesia. *Anesthesiology*. 1988;68:625-628.
147. Alahuhta S, Rasanen J, Jouppila R, Jouppila P, Hollmen AI. Effects of extradural bupivacaine with adrenaline for cesarean section on uteroplacental and fetal circulation. *Br J Anaesth*. 1991;67:678-682.
148. Robson SC, Boys RJ, Rodeck C, Morgan B. Maternal and fetal hemodynamic effects of spinal and extradural anesthesia for elective cesarean section. *Br J Anaesth*. 1992;68:54-59.

149. Paech MJ, Westmore MD, Speirs HM. A double-blind comparison of epidural bupivacaine and bupivacaine-fentanyl for caesarean section. *Anaesth Intensive Care*. 1990;18:22-30.
150. Ackerman WE, Colclough GC, Guiler JM, et al. Epidural fentanyl for the management of the pain caused by uterine manipulation during epidural anesthesia for elective cesarean section. *Anesthesiol Rev*. 1989;16:41-45.
151. Preston PG, Rosen MA, Hughes SC, et al. Epidural anesthesia with fentanyl and lidocaine for cesarean section: maternal effects and neonatal outcome. *Anesthesiology*. 1988;68:938-943.
152. Gaffud MP, Bansal P, Lawton C. Surgical analgesia for cesarean delivery and epidural bupivacaine and fentanyl. *Anesthesiology*. 1986;65:331-334.
153. Belzarena SD. Clinical effects of intrathecally administered fentanyl in patients undergoing cesarean section. *Anesth Analg*. 1992;74:653-657.
154. Vincent RD Jr, Chestnut DH, Choi WW, Ostman PL, Bates JN. Does epidural fentanyl decrease the efficacy of epidural morphine after cesarean delivery? *Anesth Analg*. 1992;74:658-663.
155. Aouad MT, Siddik SS, Jalbout MI, Baraka AS. Does pregnancy protect against intrathecal lidocaine-induced transient neurologic symptoms? *Anesth Analg*. 2001;92:401-404.
156. Philip J, Sharma SK, Gottumukkala VN, et al. Transient neurologic symptoms after spinal anesthesia with lidocaine in obstetric patients. *Anesth Analg*. 2001;92:405-409.
157. Celleno D, Capogna G. Epidural fentanyl plus bupivacaine 0.125% for labour analgesic effects. *Can J Anaesth*. 1988;35:375-378.
158. D'Athis F, Macheboeuf M, Thomas H, et al. Epidural analgesia with bupivacaine-fentanyl mixture in obstetrics: comparison of repeated injections and continuous infusion. *Can J Anaesth*. 1988;35:116-122.
159. Jones G, Paul DL, Elton RA, McClure JH. Comparison of bupivacaine and bupivacaine with fentanyl in continuous extradural analgesia during labour. *Br J Anaesth*. 1989;63:254-259.
160. Madej TH, Strunin L. Comparison of epidural fentanyl with sufentanil. *Anaesthesia*. 1987;42:1156-1161.
161. Brockway MS, Noble DW, Sharwood-Smith GH, McClure JH. Profound respiratory depression after extradural fentanyl. *Br J Anaesth*. 1990;64:243-245.
162. Porter J, Bonello E, Reynolds F. Effect of epidural fentanyl on neonatal respiration. *Anesthesiology*. 1998;89:79-85.
163. Yau G, Gregory MA, Gin T, Oh TE. Obstetric epidural analgesia with mixtures of bupivacaine, adrenaline, and fentanyl. *Anaesthesia*. 1990;45:1020-1023.
164. Yee I, Carstoniu J, Halpern S, Pittini R. A comparison of two doses of epidural fentanyl during caesarean section. *Can J Anaesth*. 1993;40:722-725.
165. Malinow AM, Mokurshi BLK, Wakefield ML. Does pH adjustment reverse Nesacaine antagonism of postcesarean epidural fentanyl analgesia? *Anesth Analg*. 1988;67(suppl):1376.
166. Camann WR, Hartigan PM, Gilbertson LI, Johnson MD, Datta S. Chloroprocaine antagonism of epidural opioid analgesia: a receptor-specific phenomenon? *Anesthesiology*. 1990;73:860-863.
167. Vertommen JD, Marcus MA, Van Aken H. The effects of intravenous and epidural sufentanil in the chronic maternal-fetal sheep preparation. *Anesth Analg*. 1995;80:71-75.
168. Abboud TK, Dror A, Mosaad P, et al. Mini-dose intrathecal morphine for the relief of post-cesarean section pain: safety, efficacy, and ventilatory responses to carbon dioxide. *Anesth Analg*. 1988;67:137-143.
169. Abouleish E, Rawal N, Rashad MN. The addition of 0.2 mg subarachnoid morphine to hyperbaric bupivacaine for cesarean delivery: a prospective study of 856 cases. *Reg Anesth*. 1991;16:137-140.
170. Douglas MJ, Kim JH, Ross PL, McMorland GH. The effect of epinephrine in local anaesthetic on epidural morphine-induced pruritus. *Can Anaesth Soc J*. 1986;33:737-740.
171. Shehabi Y, Gatt S, Buckman T, Isert P. Effect of adrenaline, fentanyl and warming of injectate on shivering following extradural analgesia in labor. *Anaesth Intensive Care*. 1990;18:31-37.
172. Sevarino FB, Johnson MD, Lema MJ, et al. The effect of epidural sufentanil on shivering and body temperature in the parturient. *Anesth Analg*. 1989;68:530-533.
173. Koonin LM, MacKay AP, Berg CJ, Atrash HK, Smith JC. Pregnancy-related mortality surveillance—United States, 1987-1990. *MMWR CDC Surveill Summ*. 1997;46:17-36.
174. Atrash HK, Koonin LM, Lawson HW, Franks AL, Smith JC. Maternal mortality in the United States, 1979-1986. *Obstet Gynecol*. 1990;76:1055-1060.
175. Hawkins JL, Koonin LM, Palmer SK, Gibbs CP. Anesthesia-related deaths during obstetric delivery in the United States, 1979-1990. *Anesthesiology*. 1997;86:277-284.
176. Kotelko DM, Rottman RL, Wright WC, et al. Transdermal scopolamine decreases nausea and vomiting following cesarean section in patients receiving epidural morphine. *Anesthesiology*. 1989;71:675-678.
177. Lesser P, Bembridge M, Lyons G, Macdonald R. An evaluation of a 30 gauge needle for spinal anaesthesia for cesarean section. *Anaesthesia*. 1990;45:767-768.
178. Carrie LES, Donald F. A 26-gauge pencil point needle for combined spinal-epidural anaesthesia for cesarean section. *Anaesthesia*. 1991;46:230-231.
179. Barker P. Are obstetric spinal headaches avoidable? *Anaesth Intensive Care*. 1990;18:553-554.
180. Cesarini M, Torrielli R, Lahaye F, Mene JM, Cabiro C. Sprotte needle for intrathecal anaesthesia for caesarean section: incidence of postdural puncture headache. *Anaesthesia*. 1990;45:656-658.
181. Ross BK, Chadwick HS, Mancuso JJ, Benedetti C. Sprotte needle for obstetric anesthesia: decreased incidence of post dural puncture headache. *Reg Anesth*. 1992;17:29-33.
182. Fink BR, Walker S. Orientation of fibers in human dorsal lumbar dura mater in relation to lumbar puncture. *Anesth Analg*. 1989;69:768-772.
183. Camann WR, Murray RS, Mushlin PS, Lambert DH. Effects of oral caffeine on postdural puncture headache A double-blind, placebo-controlled trial. *Anesth Analg*. 1990;70:181-184.
184. Carp H, Singh PJ, Vadhera R, Jayaram A. Effects of the serotonin-receptor agonist sumatriptan on postdural puncture headache: report of six cases. *Anesth Analg*. 1994;79:180-182.
185. Palahniuk RJ, Cumming M. Prophylactic blood patch does not prevent post lumbar puncture headache. *Can Anaesth Soc J*. 1979;26:132-133.
186. Loeser EA, Hill GE, Bennett GM, Sederberg JH. Time vs success rate for epidural blood patch. *Anesthesiology*. 1978;49:147-148.
187. Martin R, Jourdain S, Clairoux M, Tetrault JP. Duration of decubitus position after epidural blood patch. *Can J Anaesth*. 1994;41:23-25.
188. Colonna-Romano P, Shapira BE. Unintentional dural puncture and prophylactic epidural blood patch in obstetrics. *Anesth Analg*. 1989;69:522-523.
189. Cheek TG, Banner R, Sauter J. Prophylactic extradural blood patch is effective. *Br J Anaesth*. 1988;61:340-342.
190. Elliott DW, Voyvodic F, Brownridge P. Sudden onset of subarachnoid block after subdural catheterization: a case of arachnoid rupture? *Br J Anaesth*. 1996;76:322-324.
191. Mehta M, Maher R. Injection into the extra-arachnoid subdural space. Experience in the treatment of intractable cervical pain and in the conduct of extradural (epidural) analgesia. *Anaesthesia*. 1977;32:760-766.
192. Palmer CM, Norris MC, Giudici MC, Leighton BL, DeSimone CA. Incidence of electrocardiographic changes during cesarean delivery under regional anesthesia. *Anesth Analg*. 1990;70:36-43.
193. Zakowski MI, Ramanathan S, Baratta JB, et al. Electrocardiographic changes during cesarean section: a cause for concern? *Anesth Analg*. 1993;76:162-167.

194. Eisenach JC, Tuttle R, Stein A. Is ST segment depression of the electrocardiogram during cesarean section merely due to cardiac sympathetic block? *Anesth Analg*. 1994;78:287-292.
195. Burton A, Camann W. Electrocardiographic changes during cesarean section: a review. *Int J Obstet Anesth*. 1996;5:47-53.
196. Rees GA, Willis BA. Resuscitation in late pregnancy. *Anaesthesia*. 1988;43:347-349.
197. Lee RV, Rodgers BD, White LM, Harvey RC. Cardiopulmonary resuscitation of pregnant women. *Am J Med*. 1986;81:311-318.
198. Katz VL, Dotters DJ, Droegemueller W. Perimortem cesarean delivery. *Obstet Gynecol*. 1986;68:571-576.
199. Anonymous. Maternal mortality—United States, 1982-1996. *MMWR Morb Mortal Wkly Rep*. 1998;47:705-707.
200. State-specific maternal mortality among black and white women—United States, 1987-1996. *MMWR Morb Mortal Wkly Rep*. 1999;48:492-496.
201. Vincent RD Jr, Chestnut DH, Sipes SL, et al. Magnesium sulfate decreases maternal blood pressure but not uterine blood flow during epidural anesthesia in gravid ewes. *Anesthesiology*. 1991;74:77-82.
202. Sipes SL, Chestnut DH, Vincent RD Jr, et al. Does magnesium sulfate alter the maternal cardiovascular response to vasopressor agents in gravid ewes? *Anesthesiology*. 1991;75:1010-1018.
203. Kussman B, Shorten G, Uppington J, Comunale ME. Administration of magnesium sulphate before rocuronium: effects on speed of onset and duration of neuromuscular block. *Br J Anaesth*. 1997;79:122-124.
204. Baraka A, Yazigi A. Neuromuscular interaction of magnesium with succinylcholine-vecuronium sequence in the eclamptic parturient. *Anesthesiology*. 1987;67:806-808.
205. Bohman VR, Cotton DB. Supralethal magnesemia with patient survival. *Obstet Gynecol*. 1990;76:984-986.
206. Rolbin SH, Cohen MM, Levinton CM, Kelly EN, Farine D. The premature infant: anesthesia for cesarean delivery. *Anesth Analg*. 1994;78:912-917.
207. Chestnut DH, Thompson CS, McLaughlin GL, Weiner CP. Does the intravenous infusion of ritodrine or magnesium sulfate alter the hemodynamic response to hemorrhage in gravid ewes? *Am J Obstet Gynecol*. 1988;159:1467-1473.
208. Reynolds JD, Chestnut DH, Dexter F, McGrath J, Penning DH. Magnesium sulfate adversely affects fetal lamb survival and blocks fetal cerebral blood flow response during maternal hemorrhage. *Anesth Analg*. 1996;83:493-499.
209. Shin YK, Kim YD. Ventricular tachyarrhythmias during cesarean section after ritodrine therapy: interaction with anesthetics. *South Med J*. 1988;81:528-530.
210. Baraka A, Siddik S, Assaf B. Supplementation of general anaesthesia with tramadol or fentanyl in parturients undergoing elective caesarean section. *Can J Anaesth*. 1998;45:631-634.
211. Jouppila P, Kirkinen P, Koivula A, Ylikorkala O. Labetalol does not alter the placental and fetal blood flow or maternal prostanoids in pre-eclampsia. *Br J Obstet Gynaecol*. 1986;93:543-547.
212. Lubbe WF. Hypertension in pregnancy. Pathophysiology and management. *Drugs*. 1984;28:170-188.
213. Macpherson M, Pipkin FB, Rutter N. The effect of maternal labetalol on the newborn infant. *Br J Obstet Gynaecol*. 1986;93:539-542.
214. Ramanathan J, Sibai BM, Mabie WC, Chauhan D, Ruiz AG. The use of labetalol for attenuation of the hypertensive response to endotracheal intubation in preeclampsia. *Am J Obstet Gynecol*. 1988;159:650-654.
215. Malinow AM, Naulty JS, Hunt CO, Datta S, Ostheimer GW. Precordial ultrasonic monitoring during cesarean delivery. *Anesthesiology*. 1987;66:816-819.
216. Fong J, Gadalla F, Pierri MK, Druzin M. Are Doppler-detected venous emboli during cesarean section air emboli? *Anesth Analg*. 1990;71:254-257.
217. Lew TWK, Tay DHB, Thomas E. Venous air embolism during cesarean section: more common than previously thought. *Anesth Analg*. 1993;77:448-452.
218. Quance D. Amniotic fluid embolism: detection by pulse oximetry. *Anesthesiology*. 1988;68:951-952.
219. Sharma SK, Philip J. The effect of anesthetic techniques on blood coagulability in parturients as measured by thromboelastography. *Anesth Analg*. 1997;85:82-86.
220. Karuparthy VR, Downing JW, Husain FJ, et al. Incidence of venous air embolism during cesarean section is unchanged by the use of a 5 to 10 degree head-up tilt. *Anesth Analg*. 1989;69:620-623.
221. Breheny F, McCarthy J. Maternal mortality. A review of maternal deaths over twenty years at the National Maternity Hospital, Dublin. *Anaesthesia*. 1982;37:561-564.
222. Combs CA, Murphy EL, Laros RK Jr. Factors associated with postpartum hemorrhage with vaginal birth. *Obstet Gynecol*. 1991;77:69-76.
223. Abouleish AE, Corn SB. Intravenous nitroglycerin for intrapartum external version of the second twin. *Anesth Analg*. 1994;78:808-809.
224. Dayan SS, Schwalbe SS. The use of small-dose intravenous nitroglycerin in a case of uterine inversion. *Anesth Analg*. 1996;82:1091-1093.
225. Redick LF, Livingston E. A new preparation of nitroglycerin for uterine relaxation. *Int J Obstet Anesth*. 1995;4:14-16.
226. Schrinsky DC, Benson RC. Rupture of the pregnant uterus: a review. *Obstet Gynecol Surv*. 1978;33:217-232.
227. Chauhan SP, Martin JN Jr, Henrichs CE, Morrison JC, Magann EF. Maternal and perinatal complications with uterine rupture in 142,075 patients who attempted vaginal birth after cesarean delivery: a review of the literature. *Am J Obstet Gynecol*. 2003;189:408-417.
228. Gonsoulin W, Borge D, Moise KJ Jr. Rupture of unscarred uterus in primigravid woman in association with cocaine abuse. *Am J Obstet Gynecol*. 1990;163:526-527.
229. Chazotte C, Cohen WR. Catastrophic complications of previous cesarean section. *Am J Obstet Gynecol*. 1990;163:738-742.
230. Flamm BL, Newman LA, Thomas SJ, Fallon D, Yoshida MM. Vaginal birth after cesarean delivery: results of a 5-year multicenter collaborative study. *Obstet Gynecol*. 1990;76:750-754.
231. Johnson C, Oriol N. The role of epidural anesthesia in trial of labor. *Reg Anesth*. 1990;15:304-308.
232. Friedman SA. Preeclampsia: a review of the role of prostaglandins. *Obstet Gynecol*. 1988;71:122-137.
233. Walsh SW. Preeclampsia: an imbalance in placental prostacyclin and thromboxane production. *Am J Obstet Gynecol*. 1985;152:335-340.
234. Fitzgerald DJ, Entman SS, Mulloy K, FitzGerald GA. Decreased prostacyclin biosynthesis preceding the clinical manifestation of pregnancy-induced hypertension. *Circulation*. 1987;75:956-963.
235. Phelan JP, Yurth DA. Severe preeclampsia. I. Peripartum hemodynamic observations. *Am J Obstet Gynecol*. 1982;144:17-22.
236. Mabie WC, Ratts TE, Sibai BM. The central hemodynamics of severe preeclampsia. *Am J Obstet Gynecol*. 1989;161:1443-1448.
237. Zemel MB, Zemel PC, Berry S, et al. Altered platelet calcium metabolism as an early predictor of increased peripheral vascular resistance and preeclampsia in urban black women. *N Engl J Med*. 1990;323:434-438.
238. Groenendijk R, Trimbos JB, Wallenburg HC. Hemodynamic measurements in preeclampsia: preliminary observations. *Am J Obstet Gynecol*. 1984;150:232-236.
239. Belfort M, Uys P, Dommisse J, Davey DA. Haemodynamic changes in gestational proteinuric hypertension: the effects of rapid volume expansion and vasodilator therapy. *Br J Obstet Gynaecol*. 1989;96:634-641.
240. Gant NF, Daley GL, Chand S, Whalley PJ, MacDonald PC. A study of angiotensin II pressor response throughout primigravid pregnancy. *J Clin Invest*. 1973;52:2682-2689.

241. Fitzgerald DJ, Rocki W, Murray R, Mayo G, FitzGerald GA. Thromboxane A_2 synthesis in pregnancy-induced hypertension. *Lancet*. 1990;335:751-754.
242. Anonymous. Do women with pre-eclampsia, and their babies, benefit from magnesium sulphate? The Magpie Trial: a randomised placebo-controlled trial. *Lancet*. 2002;359:1877-1890.
243. Barker P, Callander CC. Coagulation screening before epidural analgesia in pre-eclampsia. *Anaesthesia*. 1991;46:64-67.
244. Leduc L, Wheeler JM, Kirshon B, Mitchell P, Cotton DB. Coagulation profile in severe preeclampsia. *Obstet Gynecol*. 1992;79:14-18.
245. Schindler M, Gatt S, Isert P, Morgans D, Cheung A. Thrombocytopenia and platelet functional defects in pre-eclampsia: implications for regional anaesthesia. *Anaesth Intensive Care*. 1990;18:169-174.
246. Ramanathan J, Sibai BM, Vu T, Chauhan D. Correlation between bleeding times and platelet counts in women with preeclampsia undergoing cesarean section. *Anesthesiology*. 1989;71:188-191.
247. Neiger R, Contag SA, Coustan DR. The resolution of preeclampsia-related thrombocytopenia. *Obstet Gynecol*. 1991;77:692-695.
248. Jouppila P, Jouppila R, Hollmen A, Koivula A. Lumbar epidural analgesia to improve intervillous blood flow during labor in severe preeclampsia. *Obstet Gynecol*. 1982;59:158-161.
249. Ramos-Santos E, Devoe LD, Wakefield ML, Sherline DM, Metheny WP. The effects of epidural anesthesia on the Doppler velocimetry of umbilical and uterine arteries in normal and hypertensive patients during active term labor. *Obstet Gynecol*. 1991;77:20-26.
250. Moore TR, Key TC, Reisner LS, Resnik R. Evaluation of the use of continuous lumbar epidural anesthesia for hypertensive pregnant women in labor. *Am J Obstet Gynecol*. 1985;152:404-412.
251. Jouppila R, Jouppila P, Hollmen A, Koivula A. Epidural analgesia and placental blood flow during labour in pregnancies complicated by hypertension. *Br J Obstet Gynaecol*. 1979;86: 969-972.
252. James FM, III, Davies P. Maternal and fetal effects of lumbar epidural analgesia for labor and delivery in patients with gestational hypertension. *Am J Obstet Gynecol*. 1976;126:195-201.
253. Giles WB, Lah FX, Trudinger BJ. The effect of epidural anaesthesia for caesarean section on maternal uterine and fetal umbilical artery blood flow velocity waveforms. *Br J Obstet Gynaecol*. 1987;94:55-59.
254. Hollmen AI, Jouppila R, Jouppila P, Koivula A, Vierola H. Effect of extradural analgesia using bupivacaine and 2-chloroprocaine on intervillous blood flow during normal labour. *Br J Anaesth*. 1982;54:837-842.
255. Clark SL, Greenspoon JS, Aldahl D, Phelan JP. Severe preeclampsia with persistent oliguria: management of hemodynamic subsets. *Am J Obstet Gynecol*. 1986;154:490-494.
256. Connell H, Dalgleish JG, Downing JW. General anaesthesia in mothers with severe pre-eclampsia/eclampsia. *Br J Anaesth*. 1987;59:1375-1380.
257. Cartwright DP, Dann WL, Huchinson A. Placental transfer of alfentanil at caesarean section. *Eur J Anaesthesiol*. 1989;6: 103-109.
258. Lawes EG, Downing JW, Duncan PW, et al. Fentanyl-droperidol supplementation of rapid sequence induction in the presence of severe pregnancy-induced and pregnancy-aggravated hypertension. *Br J Anaesth*. 1987;59:1381-1391.
259. Rout CC, Rocke DA. Effects of alfentanil and fentanyl on induction of anaesthesia in patients with severe pregnancy-induced hypertension. *Br J Anaesth*. 1990;65:468-474.
260. Dann WL, Hutchinson A, Cartwright DP. Maternal and neonatal responses to alfentanil administered before induction of general anaesthesia for caesarean section. *Br J Anaesth*. 1987;59: 1392-1396.
261. Eisenach JC, Mandell G, Dewan DM. Maternal and fetal effects of labetalol in pregnant ewes. *Anesthesiology*. 1991;74: 292-297.
262. Michael CA. The evaluation of labetalol in the treatment of hypertension complicating pregnancy. *Br J Clin Pharmacol*. 1982;13:127S-131S.
263. Mabie WC, Gonzalez AR, Sibai BM, Amon E. A comparative trial of labetalol and hydralazine in the acute management of severe hypertension complicating pregnancy. *Obstet Gynecol*. 1987;70:328-333.
264. Pickles CJ, Symonds EM, Pipkin FB. The fetal outcome in a randomized double-blind controlled trial of labetalol versus placebo in pregnancy-induced hypertension. *Br J Obstet Gynaecol*. 1989;96:38-43.
265. Plouin PF, Breart G, Maillard F, Papiernik E, Relier JP. Comparison of antihypertensive efficacy and perinatal safety of labetalol and methyldopa in the treatment of hypertension in pregnancy: a randomized controlled trial. *Br J Obstet Gynaecol*. 1988;95:868-876.
266. Rogers RC, Sibai BM, Whybrew WD. Labetalol pharmacokinetics in pregnancy-induced hypertension. *Am J Obstet Gynecol*. 1990;162:362-366.
267. Lavies NG, Meiklejohn BH, May AE, Achola KJ, Fell D. Hypertensive and catecholamine response to tracheal intubation in patients with pregnancy-induced hypertension. *Br J Anaesth*. 1989;63:429-434.
268. de Rosayro M, Nahrwold ML, Hill AB, et al. Plasma levels and cardiovascular effect of nitroglycerin in pregnant sheep. *Can Anaesth Soc J*. 1980;27:560-564.
269. Hood DD, Dewan DM, James FM, III, Floyd HM, Bogard TD. The use of nitroglycerin in preventing the hypertensive response to tracheal intubation in severe preeclampsia. *Anesthesiology*. 1985;63:329-332.
270. Losasso TJ, Muzzi DA, Cucchiara RF. Response of fetal heart rate to maternal administration of esmolol. *Anesthesiology*. 1991;74:782-784.
271. Eisenach JC, Castro MI. Maternally administered esmolol produces fetal beta-adrenergic blockade and hypoxemia in sheep. *Anesthesiology*. 1989;71:718-722.

CHAPTER 45

Pediatric Anesthesia

John Aker

The pediatric anesthetist must have a thorough understanding of normal pediatric growth and development, the anatomic and physiologic differences during various stages of maturation, and an understanding of how immature organ systems affect anesthetic pharmacokinetics and pharmacodynamics. Anesthetic management of the pediatric patient requires integration of this specialized knowledge, refinement of acquired technical skills, and the ability to apply this knowledge to the pediatric patient.

The adage that "children are simply small adults" represents a myopic view of the striking physiologic differences between infants and adults. However, by the time the newborn has matured to the age of 5 years, these physiologic differences are almost insignificant. Despite this, the anesthetist must consider the child's ongoing psychologic development, specifically the child's emotional, social, and physical needs.

Anesthetic morbidity and mortality are greater in pediatric patients than in adults. Accordingly, children require individualized and specialized anesthetic care. This chapter outlines the differences in the anesthetic care of the pediatric patient, providing an understanding of the differences in anesthetic morbidity and mortality. The focus of this chapter is to provide a clinical approach to the care of the pediatric patient rather than a comprehensive discussion of the specific anesthetic care of the child, reviewing growth and development, pharmacology, and perioperative anesthetic management. Recent developments in pediatric anesthesia, including the use of new volatile and intravenous anesthetic agents, the application of the laryngeal mask airway (LMA), and the emerging use of regional anesthetic techniques for postoperative analgesia, are discussed.

FETAL CIRCULATION

The fetal circulatory system relies on the placenta for delivery of oxygen and transport of carbon dioxide (CO_2) (Figure 45-1). The chorionic villus is the functional unit of the placenta. Normally, fetal blood is separated from the maternal blood in the placenta by a thin layer of cells known as *syncytial trophocytes*. Oxygen, CO_2, and small nonionized particles readily pass through this layer, whereas substances with a larger molecular weight are prevented from diffusing across the syncytial trophocytes.

Fetal circulation is characterized by high pulmonary vascular resistance (uninflated atelectatic lungs and hypoxic vasoconstriction) and low systemic circulatory resistance (high flow and low impedance of the placental vessels). Fetal deoxygenated blood travels down the aorta and through the internal iliac arteries, arriving in the placenta via paired umbilical arteries. The umbilical arteries divide, forming the arterioles, capillaries, and venules of the intervillous placental space. Oxygenated blood is delivered to the fetus from the placenta via a single umbilical vein. This oxygenated blood bypasses the lungs by flowing through extracardiac (ductus arteriosus, ductus venosus) and intracardiac (foramen ovale) shunts, forming a parallel circulation (see Figure 45-1). The ductus venosus routes oxygenated blood away from the sinusoids of the liver. The oxygenated blood in the inferior vena cava is directed by the eustachian valve toward the atrial septum and passes through the foramen ovale to enter the left side of the circulation. Oxygenated blood passes into the left ventricle and exits the aorta, supplying the coronary arteries. Blood entering the pulmonary artery from the right ventricle flows to the aorta via the ductus arteriosus. Only 5% to 10% of the combined ventricular output flows through the pulmonary circulation.

TRANSITIONAL CIRCULATION

The transitional circulation is established at the time of birth. With the cessation of placental blood flow aortic pressure increases. Clamping of the umbilical vein doubles systemic vascular resistance. Pulmonary vascular resistance falls with lung expansion, and increasing partial pressure of arterial oxygen (PaO_2) produces pulmonary vasodilation, resulting in further decreases in pulmonary resistance. These changes in systemic and pulmonary blood flow produce corresponding changes in intracardiac pressure. Decreases in right atrial pressure with accompanying increases in left atrial pressure change the direction of blood flow through the foramen ovale, resulting in the closure of the foramen ovale as left atrial pressure increases. The foramen ovale may reopen if right atrial pressure is greater than left atrial pressure (e.g., pulmonary hypertension), permitting venous blood to flow from right to left. Within a period of 2 to 3 months the foramen ovale will be permanently closed. Up to 25% of adult patients may demonstrate a probe patent foramen ovale at autopsy.[1]

Closure of the ductus arteriosus is precipitated in part by the increase in systemic vascular resistance and decrease in pulmonary vascular resistance. In utero prostaglandins maintain the patency of the ductus arteriosus. Within a few hours after birth the muscular wall of the ductus arteriosus constricts, preventing the retrograde flow of blood from the aorta into the pulmonary artery. This functional closure (thrombosis) occurs within 1 to 8 days. Anatomic closure (fibrosis of the ductus

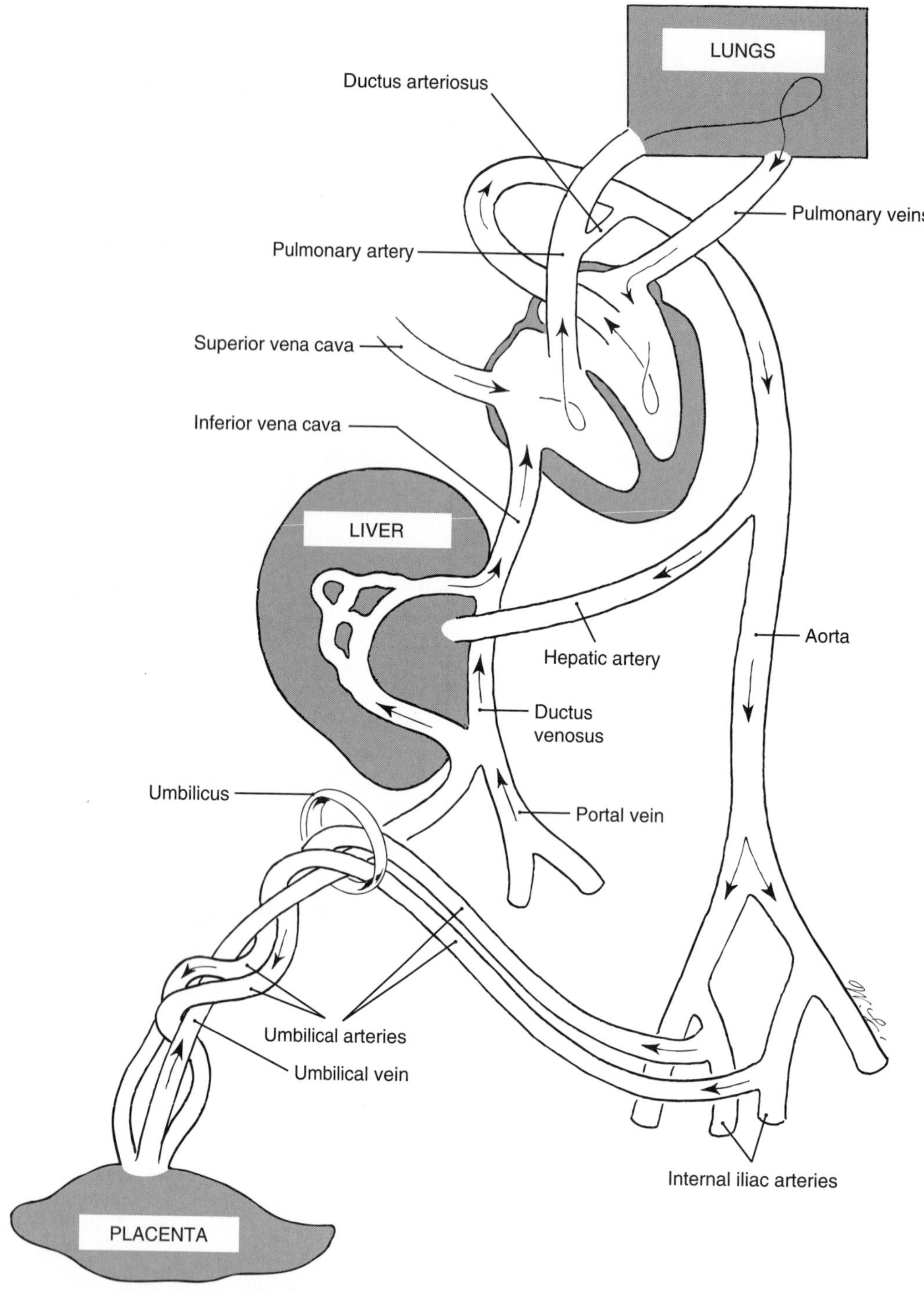

FIGURE **45-1**
Diagram of the circulatory system. Persistent fetal circulation in an infant can cause severe cyanosis secondary to high pulmonary vascular resistance. The high pulmonary vascular resistance causes right-to-left shunting across both the foramen ovale and the patent ductus arteriosus.

arteriosus) requires 1 to 4 months. Ductus closure may be influenced by elevations in the systemic PaO_2 that occur after birth.

The majority of portal blood flow continues to enter the ductus venosus after interruption of umbilical vein blood flow. While the cause of the initiating mechanisms of ductus venosus closure is unknown, the muscular wall of the ductus venosus begins to constrict 1 to 3 hours postnatally. Blood flow is directed into the liver, and portal venous pressure increases.

Persistent Pulmonary Hypertension of the Newborn

Before anatomic closure of the extracardiac and intracardiac shunts, fetal circulation may be reestablished and persist. Persistent pulmonary hypertension of the newborn (PPHN) (formerly persistent fetal circulation) is manifest by increases in pulmonary vascular resistance and accompanying pulmonary hypertension, which produces a right-to-left shunt across the foramen ovale and the ductus arteriosus, with resultant cyanosis. The presence of congenital cardiovascular or pulmonary disease inhibits functional and anatomic closure of these aforementioned fetal shunts. Persistent fetal circulation is common in preterm infants and infants with metabolic derangements (asphyxia, sepsis, meconium aspiration, congenital diaphragmatic hernia). Hypoxemia, acidosis, pneumonia, and hypothermia are primary precipitating factors of PPHN. Oxygenation, the avoidance of acidosis, and maintenance of normothermia will attenuate the increase in pulmonary vascular resistance. Continuous increases in pulmonary vascular pressure and resistance will precipitate the development of right ventricular hypertrophy (cor pulmonale). Although pulmonary vasodilators may have some utility in decreasing pulmonary vascular resistance, concurrent reductions in systemic vascular resistance can occur and may worsen the shunt. Nitric oxide (NO), a specific, short-acting pulmonary vasodilator, decreases pulmonary vascular resistance and produces antegrade flow through the ductus arteriosus while avoiding changes in systemic vascular resistance. Extracorporeal membrane oxygenation may be performed to maintain oxygenation in infants with PPHN and severe respiratory dysfunction.

GROWTH AND DEVELOPMENT

Cardiovascular System

A thorough understanding of the development of the pediatric cardiovascular system is essential when one is providing anesthetic care to every infant and child. The myocardium of the newborn is immature. The ventricles are of equal size and shape and possess a low contractile mass. Although the pediatric myocardium cannot mount the same stroke volume response as an adult's to maintain cardiac output, stroke volume changes do occur in pediatric patients. In the past, pediatric cardiac output was thought to be solely dependent on heart rate. Accordingly, atropine is often selected for the treatment of decreased cardiac output. More recent studies have shown that changes in contractility do have a role in maintaining cardiac output. Epinephrine, which increases both contractility and rate, is now used for the treatment of bradycardia and decreased cardiac output in pediatric patients.

Marked variation in the newborn heart rate and rhythm occur secondary to changes in autonomic tone. In utero autonomic control of heart rate occurs via the parasympathetic system; however, sympathetic control of heart rate takes control shortly after birth. The electrocardiogram (ECG) recording in the newborn reflects the immaturity of conduction and of the myocardium. The ECG axis is shifted to the right but shifts to the left with maturation and accompanying hypertrophy of the left ventricle. The P wave is evident; the PR is less than 0.12 seconds and increases until adolescence. T waves are upright in the recorded chest leads, reflecting the presence of right ventricular hypertrophy. The newborn heart rate averages 120 beats per minute during the first day of life, increasing to 160 beats per minute at 1 month of age, then steadily decreasing to an average of 75 beats during adolescents.

Blood pressure increases immediately after birth, rising to a mean of 70 to 75 mm Hg within the first 48 hours. Blood pressure is lower in the preterm infant. The heart rate will decrease as the infant develops, with a concurrent increase in blood pressure. Hypotension in an anesthetized newborn is defined as a systolic blood pressure of less than 60 mm Hg. In a 1-year-old, hypotension is defined as pressure less than 70 mm Hg. In the older child, it is approximately 70 mm Hg plus twice the child's age in years. Table 45-1 shows values for heart rate and blood pressure at different ages.

TABLE 45-1 Age-Related Changes in the Cardiovascular System

Age	Heart Rate	Systolic BP	Diastolic BP
Neonate	140	65	40
12 mo	120	95	65
3 yr	100	100	70
12 yr	80	110	60

BP, *Blood pressure*.

Fetal hemoglobin is the predominant hemoglobin species in the newborn. Fetal hemoglobin has a higher affinity for oxygen than does adult hemoglobin. In utero, this increased oxygen affinity of fetal hemoglobin facilitates oxygen uptake as fetal blood circulates through the placenta. This increases the binding of oxygen to fetal hemoglobin and allows the fetus to exist in a relatively low PaO_2 environment. After birth, oxygen delivery to the tissues is assured despite high levels of fetal hemoglobin because of increased concentrations of 2,3-diphosphoglycerate that shift the oxyhemoglobin dissociation curve to the right. Fetal hemoglobin is replaced by adult hemoglobin, which also produces a rightward shift of the oxyhemoglobin dissociation curve.

The newborn's blood volume is dependent on the time of cord clamping (transfusion from the placenta). Blood volume is approximately 80 to 90 ml/kg but may be as high as 100 ml/kg in the premature (Table 45-2). The intravascular volume decreases 25% in the immediate postnatal period with the loss of intravascular fluid. An elevated hemoglobin level (14 to 20 g/100 ml) inhibits erythropoiesis. Hemoglobin begins to fall shortly after birth. It is important to note that the premature infant may experience a dramatic fall in hemoglobin because of insufficient body stores of iron. A decrease in erythropoiesis and decreased lifespan of the newborn red blood cells (RBCs) produces a progressive decrease in hemoglobin, reaching a nadir by age 3 months. This "physiologic anemia" does not compromise the delivery of oxygen, because the oxyhemoglobin dissociation curve shifts to the right and RBC concentrations of 2,3-diphosphoglycerate increase (Figure 45-2).

Newborns should receive vitamin K prophylaxis, as the concentration of vitamin K–dependent clotting factors (II, VII, IX, and X) are 20% to 50% of adult levels. Premature infants generally have lower levels of vitamin K–dependent clotting factors. Maternally ingested drugs such as warfarin and isoniazid may precipitate the development of a coagulopathy.

TABLE 45-2 Estimated Blood Volumes by Age

Age Group	Volume (ml/kg)
Premature	90-100
Newborn (less than 1 mo of age)	80-90
Infants 3 mo–3 yr of age	75-80
Children older than 6 yr of age	65-70

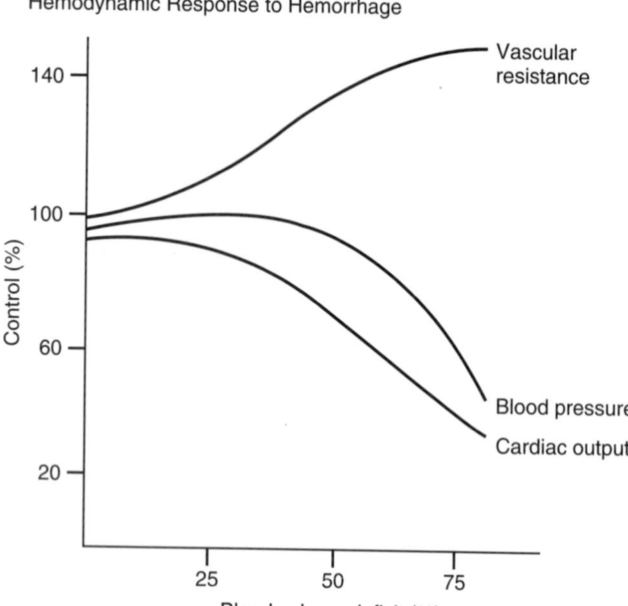

FIGURE **45-2**
Relationship of blood pressure to blood volume. (From Schwaitzberg SD, Bergman KS, Harris BH. Pediatric trauma model of continuous hemorrhage. *J Pediatr Surg.* 1988;23:605-609.)

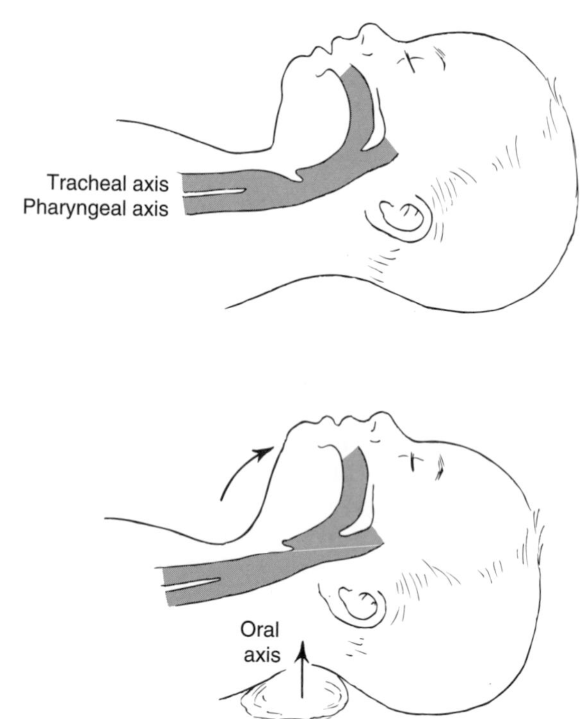

FIGURE **45-3**
Alignments of visual, oral, and laryngeal axes during laryngoscopy.

Respiratory System

The larynx is higher in the neck of a child than it is in an adult, extending from the second to the fourth cervical vertebrae (C2 to C4). The adult larynx lies between C3 and C6 and achieves this position by age 6. The epiglottis in a child is **U**-shaped and stiff, compared with the structure in an adult. The newborn tongue is large and difficult to manipulate because of the position of the hyoid. In addition, a smaller potential submental space is present in which to displace the tongue during laryngoscopy. The anterior position of the larynx and the large tongue make mask ventilation more difficult than in the adult. The newborn head is large (particularly the occiput). The placement of a rolled towel under the shoulders aids in the visual alignment of the oral, pharyngeal, and laryngeal axes during laryngoscopy (Figure 45-3 and Table 45-3).

TABLE **45-3** Differences between the Adult and the Pediatric Airway

	Pediatric	Adult
Laryngeal location	C2-C4	C3-C6
Narrowest location of airway	Cricoid	Glottis
Shape of epiglottis	Omega-shaped	**V**-shaped
Right mainstem bronchus	Less vertical	More vertical

The ring-shaped cricoid cartilage is the narrowest portion of the pediatric airway. Uncuffed endotracheal tubes are suitable to form a seal against the tracheal mucosa and to stop air leak, allowing delivery of positive-pressure ventilation. The prolonged use of cuffed endotracheal tubes may produce mucosal damage, leading to edema formation and airway obstruction. The use of uncuffed endotracheal tubes facilitates the selection of endotracheal tubes with a greater internal diameter. According to Poiseuille's law, increases in airway radius decrease the airway's resistance by a factor of four.

The newborn is an obligate nose breather. Infrequently, choanal atresia (failure of the development of the opening between the nasal cavity and the nasopharynx) produces airway obstruction. In the pediatric patient the mainstem bronchus branches from midline at a 55-degree angle. In the adult the right mainstem bronchus branches at a 25-degree angle, whereas the left mainstem bronchus is more horizontal, at an angle of 45 degrees. One possible consequence of this arrangement is an increase in the incidence of left mainstem intubations. Clinically, however, left mainstem intubation is rare in patients of both age groups.

Respiratory maturation is incomplete at birth. Surfactant production begins during the thirtieth week of gestation, reaching satisfactory levels at approximately 35 weeks. A postnatal increase occurs in the number of alveoli, as does vascularization. During maturation the pulmonary vasculature airway smooth muscle proliferates with extension to the alveoli. Prenatal lung development may be affected by congenital defects, such as congenital diaphragmatic hernia that produces a hypoplastic lung. Congenital heart lesions may also inhibit the maturation of the pulmonary vasculature and result in either a decrease or increase in pulmonary blood flow.

Airway resistance is greater in children, as airway caliber is smaller than in adults. According to Poiseuille's law, airway resistance is inversely proportional to the fourth power of the radius of the airway during laminar flow. Airway resistance changes with age. Although the larger airway resistance remains constant, airway resistance dramatically decreases in the small peripheral airways after the age of 5. Because of the increase in airway resistance, the infant and young child have an increased work of breathing. Small airway disease (e.g., pneumonia) produces additional increases in the work of breathing.

The newborn's chest wall is very pliable because it lacks developed musculature and because the skeletal structure is primarily composed of cartilage. The ribs are horizontal in orientation, providing minimal assistance in the expansion of the chest wall with inspiration. The premature infant has a more pliable chest wall, and paradoxic chest movement may occur with breathing during rest. To minimize the development of barotrauma, pressure-cycled ventilators are used in the neonatal intensive care unit. Pressure-cycled ventilators allow the peak airway pressure to be varied to optimize mechanical ventilation but limit the pressure, reducing the potential for trauma to the lungs. In normal newborns, the peak inspiratory pressure is set at approximately 24 to 25 cm H_2O. Although infants with diseased lungs may require higher pressures, an intermittent mandatory ventilation rate of 20 to 40 breaths per minute and a peak inspiratory pressure of 20 to 24 cm H_2O are typical ventilatory parameters for normal infants.

At birth, functional residual capacity is one half that of the adult. However, this difference rapidly disappears within the first few days of life. The infant's metabolic rate and oxygen consumption are approximately twice those of the adult. Table 45-4 illustrates the mean value for pulmonary function in the newborn and adult. The decreased reservoir for oxygen (decreased functional residual capacity), coupled with the increased demand for oxygen (increased metabolic rate), results in rapid desaturation when ventilation is interrupted. Airway closure produces a mismatching of ventilation and perfusion. The volume of these poorly ventilated alveoli that contribute to intrapulmonary shunting is greater in neonates than in adults. In addition, as previously discussed, increased pulmonary vascular resistance can produce a right-to-left shunt through the foramen ovale or a patent ductus arteriosus, resulting in the rapid development of cyanosis.

The control of ventilation is dependent on PaO_2 sensed via the peripheral chemoreceptors (carotid and aortic bodies), the partial pressure of arterial CO_2 ($PaCO_2$), and pH, which influence the central chemoreceptors within the respiratory control center of the medulla. High PaO_2 depresses respiration in the newborn, whereas low PaO_2 stimulates respiration. Although it initially stimulates an increase in ventilation, hypoxia ultimately produces ventilatory depression. This response is more profound in the premature infant than in the newborn. Increases in $PaCO_2$ produce corresponding increases in tidal volume and respiratory rate. The newborn may be noted to have periodic breathing or inspiratory pauses that last up to 10 seconds, followed by abrupt increases in ventilation. Periodic breathing is more common in the premature infant and occurs more often during REM sleep. Apnea is not uncommon in the premature infant. Apneic episodes produce arterial desaturation. Bradycardia and cardiac arrest may follow these apneic episodes. The suspected causes of apnea in premature infants include immature responses of the respiratory control center to hypercarbia or hypoxic stimuli and respiratory fatigue. Infants who have experienced apneic or bradycardic episodes are at risk for these episodes after general anesthesia. The anesthetic care of the premature infant with apnea or bradycardia is discussed later in this chapter.

TABLE 45-4 Mean Values for Normal Pulmonary Function in the Newborn and the Adult

	Newborn	Adult
Body weight (kg)	3	70
Tidal volume (ml/kg)	6	6
Respiratory rate (bpm)	35	15
Alveolar ventilation (ml/kg/min)	130	60
Oxygen consumption (ml/kg/min)	6.4	3.5
Total lung capacity (ml/kg)	63	86
Functional residual capacity (ml/kg)	30	34
Vital capacity (ml/kg)	35	70
Residual volume (ml/kg)	23	16
Closing capacity (ml/kg)	35	23
Arterial pH	7.38-7.41	7.35-7.45
$PaCO_2$	30-35	35-45
PaO_2	60-90	90-100
SaO_2 (%)	95-100	95-100

$PaCO_2$, *Partial pressure of arterial carbon dioxide;* PaO_2, *partial pressure of arterial oxygen;* SaO_2, *oxygen saturation.*

Nervous System

The central nervous system (CNS) is immature at birth. The primitive Moro response and grasp reflex are clinical demonstrations of this immaturity. Myelination of the nervous system is not complete until age 3. Because of the rapid maturation process of the CNS during infancy and childhood, proper nutrition is essential to ensure normal development. The infant cranial sutures are not fused, and therefore the cranium is pliable. The fullness of the fontanelle can be used as an indicator of fluid volume status. The spinal cord ends at approximately L3 in pediatric patients (it terminates at L1 in adults). This is an important consideration during lumbar puncture and spinal anesthesia.

The blood-brain barrier is incompletely developed in the newborn. Blood-brain barrier disruption follows traumatic head injury, subarachnoid or intracerebral hemorrhage, and cerebral ischemia. The cerebral vessels are very fragile in preterm and low–birth-weight infants. This fragility predisposes these patients to intracranial hemorrhage. Intracranial hemorrhage may be precipitated by hypoxia, hypercarbia, hyperglycemia, hypoglycemia, hypernatremia, and wide swings in arterial or venous pressure. The intravenous administration of hypertonic solutions may damage these fragile vessels. Therefore adult-strength sodium bicarbonate should not be administered to neonates.

Renal System

The kidneys become active in utero, and accompanying urine production contributes to the amniotic fluid volume. After birth the kidneys become responsible for excretion of metabolic by-products and acid-base balance. The newborn has the adult compliment of nephrons, although these nephrons are immature in function. For example, the GFR is only 15% to 30% that of GFR in adults. This function matures by the age of 6 to 12 months. The low GFR is the result of the lower systemic arterial pressure, increased renal vascular resistance, and decreased permeability of the glomerular capillaries. Infants are unable to tolerate fluid overload because of the lower GFR. By the end of the first month of life, renal function is approximately 70% of adult levels. By the end of the first year, renal function reaches adult levels. The ability of the kidneys' tubules to concentrate or dilute the urine does not mature until a child is 2 to 3 years of age. Infants are referred to as *obligate sodium excretors* because of their inability to conserve sodium, even in cases of severe sodium depletion. Although the renin-angiotensin-aldosterone system is functional, the renal tubules fail to respond. The renal tubules also have limited ability to reabsorb glucose. Increasing plasma glucose concentrations can produce an osmotic diuresis, depleting intravascular volume.

Hepatic System

Although active, hepatic function is immature at birth. The ability to metabolize protein and drugs is decreased at birth. The fetal liver is active in the synthesis of protein, specifically α-fetoprotein. Albumin, an essential protein that regulates colloidal osmotic pressure, is produced beginning at 3 to 4 months of gestation, reaching adult levels at the time of birth. As previously discussed, concentrations of clotting factors in the premature infant and the newborn are low; however, hepatic synthesis of essential clotting factors reaches adult levels during the first week after birth. In utero the liver is the organ responsible for hematopoiesis, but by 4 to 6 weeks after birth this function is assumed by the bone marrow. Glycogen storage capacity is greatly increased just before birth. Glycogen stores are not as large in preterm or small-for-gestational-age (SGA) infants. Therefore preterm and SGA infants should be monitored for the development of hypoglycemia.

Hyperbilirubinemia may develop in term infants within the first days of life. Bilirubin production is increased with the breakdown of RBCs. Enterohepatic circulation of bilirubin is increased because of the depressed activity of glucuronyl transferase that is required for hepatic conjugation. Bilirubin levels of 6 to 8 mg/100 ml are not uncommon in term infants. However, premature infants may have levels as high as 10 to 12 mg/ml on the third day of life. Phototherapy and, in rare cases, exchange transfusion are employed to avoid the development of encephalopathy (kernicterus). Infants with hyperbilirubinemia should be evaluated to rule out pathologic causes of jaundice.

Temperature Regulation

Core body temperature is controlled within a narrow range (37° C ± 0.4° C) by the hypothalamus via a negative feedback process. Afferent thermal input (warm and cold sensation) is relayed via the spinothalamic tracts to the hypothalamus from thermal sensors located in the skin, respiratory tract, gastrointestinal tract, and spinal cord. The hypothalamus compares these thermal inputs with the threshold temperature. When the temperature is either lower or higher than the threshold temperature, the hypothalamus activates effector organs (cutaneous circulation, sweat glands, respiration, skeletal muscle activity, and basal metabolism) to regulate heat loss or heat gain. Cutaneous blood vessels regulate conductive, convective, and radiant heat loss. Sweat glands are essential for evaporative heat loss from the skin. Heat loss is precipitated through an increase in both the rate and depth of respiration. Skeletal muscles contribute to heat production through shivering thermogenesis (infants and children), whereas the sympathetic stimulation of brown fat metabolism (nonshivering thermogenesis [NST]) increases heat production by 100% in neonates. Premature infants lack brown fat and have difficulty maintaining normothermia. Heat production follows an increase in the basal metabolic rate stimulated through the release of anterior pituitary hormones.

Afferent thermal input continues during general anesthesia, yet the previously mentioned effector organ responses are diminished. Core body temperature may decrease as much as 1° to 3° C. Heat loss occurs as a result of the internal redistribution of heat, reduced metabolism and heat production, increased heat loss to the environment, and the effects of anesthetic agents on thermoregulatory control. Heat loss occurs more rapidly in infants because of limited heat production (NST) and the larger body surface area. The infant skin (particularly the premature infant) is thinner and has less subcutaneous tissue, increasing the rate of evaporative heat loss. Shivering, an important mechanism for heat production, is impaired after the induction of general anesthesia and skeletal muscle paralysis.[2]

Perioperative hypothermia is common in pediatric patients and particularly problematic in premature infants because of the thin skin and limited body fat. Perioperative hypothermia has many contributing causes, including a cold operating room environment, anesthetic-induced vasodilation, the infusion of room-temperature intravenous fluids, evaporative heat loss from opened body cavities, use of cool irrigating solutions, and the inspiration of cool anesthetic gases.

NST is the infant's defense against hypothermia. NST is a metabolically derived method for heat production that does not involve muscular work. Brown fat stores are metabolically active tissue that contain a high density of mitochondria located in the scapulae, the axillae, and the mediastinum and surrounding the kidneys. Hypothermia stimulates the release of norepinephrine, which acts on brown fat to uncouple oxidative phosphorylation.[3]

Heat loss or gain occurs through the skin by radiation, conduction, convection, and evaporation. Radiant heat loss is responsible for the majority of heat loss.[4] Radiant heat loss is the transfer of heat from one object to another, the rate of which is dependent on the temperature gradient between the object losing heat and the objects near it. Placing an infant on a cold operating table results in heat transfer from the infant to the table, with a resultant drop in core body temperature. In this example, radiant heat loss may be minimized by wrapping the infant in a warm blanket, isolating the infant from the cold operating table, and decreasing the transfer of heat from the infant.

Radiant heat lamps may be used to maintain temperature during surgical positioning and preparation. Radiant heat lamps increase the temperature of the air between the infant and the lamps, thereby minimizing radiant heat loss. However, radiant heat lamps are ineffective when operating room personnel or large objects are placed between the lamp and the infant. In addition, the placement of a radiant heat lamp in close proximity to the infant may produce thermal injury (burn).

Conductive heat loss occurs with the transfer of heat to the environment and is dependent on the temperature differences between the child and the environment. Conductive heat loss is minimized with the use of warmed irrigating solutions, the use of warm blankets or heated forced-air blankets to cover the nonoperative areas of the child, and the prewarming of the operating room. Covering the child's head with a stockinette or reflective cap dramatically decreases conductive heat loss, as the infant's head may account for up to 60% of the total heat loss during the perioperative period.[5,6]

Convective heat loss is precipitated by moving air currents. The operating room air circulation is changed 6 to 12 times per hour and, in conjunction with cool ambient temperatures, increases heat loss. The air surrounding the body is warmed and subsequently rises, being replaced by the cooler ambient air. To minimize convective heat loss, the ambient air temperature must be increased. Prudent practice is to preheat the operating room to 26° C for premature and neonatal surgical patients. The premature infant or neonate arrives in the operating room in a heated isolette and is immediately covered with a warm blanket before being transferred to the operating table. Convective heat loss may be increased when wet cloth is in contact with the infant. Wet diapers and blankets soiled with preparation solutions must be replaced and not allowed to remain in contact with the skin.

Evaporative heat loss occurs through the vaporization of liquid from body cavities and the respiratory tract. Evaporative heat loss is either sensible loss (the evaporation of sweat) or insensible loss (the evaporation of water through the skin). The thin-skinned premature infant is particularly susceptible to insensible evaporative heat loss. Sensible evaporative heat loss may be prevented by removing wet clothing or blankets and thoroughly drying the infant. Insensible evaporative heat loss may be mitigated by increasing the relative humidity of the operating room, covering the child with a plastic barrier, and using warmed irrigating solutions. Insensible respiratory tract evaporative heat loss may be prevented with humidification of the inspired gases, which requires attentive temperature monitoring to avoid superheating of airway gases and subsequent airway burns. The addition of in-line humidifiers to the patient breathing circuit adds to the complexity and weight, perhaps increasing the likelihood of unintended tracheal extubation. These humidifiers may also contribute to unintended increases in core body temperature during lengthy surgical procedures. The use of a passive heat and moisture exchanger, added between the patient circuit and endotracheal tube, has been of questionable efficacy in pediatric patients.[7,8]

Although the previous discussion focuses on maintenance of core body temperature during the intraoperative period, iatrogenic increases in core body temperature also may occur. Attentiveness in covering the child may result in progressive increases in core temperature during prolonged surgical procedures. These steady increases in core temperature may be aggravated by the previous administration of atropine. Surgical procedures may also affect thermoregulation. An example may include hypothalamic manipulation during craniotomy. A recent report has noted core temperature increases in infants during video-assisted thoracoscopic ligation of patent ductus arteriosus, the cause of which was attributed to the heat generated by the light source and equipment.[8,9]

Pediatric Pharmacologic Considerations

The immaturity of organ systems is responsible for the noted pharmacologic differences among the premature, neonate, infant, and child. Physiologic characteristics that modify the pharmacokinetic (what the body does to the drug) and pharmacodynamic (what the drug does to the body) activity in the child include differences in total body water (TBW) composition; immaturity of metabolic degradation pathways; reduced protein binding; immaturity of the blood-brain barrier; greater proportion of blood flow to the brain, heart, liver and lungs; reduced glomerular filtration; smaller functional residual capacity; and increased minute ventilation.

Body water composition affects the volume of drug distribution. Water freely diffuses across cell membranes and is essential for the transport of cellular nutrients and substrates that support metabolic reactions. TBW, expressed in liters, is determined as a percentage of total body weight (1 L of water weighs 1 kg). TBW steadily decreases with increasing age and varies according to sex and body habitus. TBW is distributed into the intracellular fluid (ICF) compartment and the extracellular fluid (ECF) compartment. With maturation, there occurs an accompanying decrease of the relative fluid compartment volumes of TBW and ECF during the first year of life, followed by additional decreases in ECF later in childhood. Table 45-5 illustrates the changes in TBW, ICF, and ECF during stages of maturation.

TABLE 45-5 Fluid Compartment Volumes

	Premature	Infant	Child	Adult
Total Body Water (TBW)	80%-90%	75%	65%-70%	55%-60%
Extracellular Fluid (ECF)	50%-60%	40%	30%	20%
Intracellular Fluid (ICF)	60%	35%	40%	40%

From Aker J, O'Sullivan CT, Embrey JP. Pediatric fluid and blood therapy. In: Zaglaniczny K, Aker J, eds. Clinical Guide to Pediatric Anesthesia. *Philadelphia: Saunders; 1999:85.*

Alterations in fat content, muscle mass, and protein binding accompany the previously discussed age-related changes in TBW. Fat content is approximately 12% at birth, doubling by 6 months of age, and reaching 30% at 12 months of age.[10] A variety of drugs are bound to plasma proteins. Total protein is decreased in the neonate and infant and is equivalent in concentration to the adult level by childhood. Albumin is responsible for the binding of acidic compounds (benzodiazepines, barbiturates, acetylsalicylic acid), and α_1-acid glycoprotein (AAG) is responsible for the binding of basic drugs (local anesthetics, α-blockers, opioids, and skeletal muscle relaxants). Both albumin and AAG concentrations are diminished at birth but reach the adult equivalency by infancy.[10] Albumin concentrations decrease in chronic disease states, with parallel increases in AAG concentration.

Drugs are metabolized by the liver enzyme system (phase I reactions) known as P-450 (oxidation, reduction, and hydrolysis) or via conjugation (phase II reactions). Enzyme systems within the RBCs, plasma, and other extrahepatic tissues are capable of hydrolyzing a variety of pharmacologic agents such as local anesthetics, the nondepolarizing neuromuscular relaxant succinylcholine, and the depolarizing neuromuscular relaxants atracurium and *cis*-atracurium. Phase II reactions transform the metabolic product into a water-soluble compound, facilitating excretion within the bile or urine. Phase II reactions are inadequate at birth. Examples of conjugation reactions include glucuronidation, methylation, acetylation, and sulfation. The neonate lacks the capacity to efficiently conjugate bilirubin (decreased glucuronyl transferase activity), and metabolize acetaminophen, chloramphenicol, and sulfonamides.

Although the necessary enzyme systems are present at birth, enzyme activity is reduced, increasing drug elimination half-lives. Drugs that produce a prolonged plasma half-life in the newborn include bupivacaine (25 hours),[11] mepivacaine (8.5 hours),[12] diazepam (up to 100 hours),[13] indomethacin (15 to 20 hours),[14] meperidine (22 hours), and phenytoin (21 hours).[15]

Oral and Rectal Drug Administration

Oral and rectal drug administration is easy and convenient compared with parenteral drug administration. Drugs are usually formulated as liquids for oral administration in children. Midazolam may be administered orally for premedication, and the rectal route may be selected for the administration of acetaminophen, opioids, barbiturates (thiopental and methohexital), and benzodiazepines. Both routes rely on passive diffusion for drug absorption. The resulting plasma drug concentration is dependent on the molecular weight, degree of drug ionization, and lipid solubility.

The degree of ionization of orally administered drugs is dependent on gastric pH levels. Acidic drugs are non-ionized and are favorably absorbed in the low pH medium of the stomach. Basic drugs have more favorable absorption in the alkaline medium of the intestine. Orally administered drugs are generally reserved for older children, as gastric pH is elevated in the neonate at birth (pH 6 to 8), and although decreased to a pH level of 1 to 3 within 24 hours, adult gastric pH values are not consistent until age 2.[16,17,18] Gastric absorption is reduced after the oral administration of acidic drugs in neonates and infants. Gastric emptying time is also prolonged in the premature and in newborns but reaches adult values by 6 months of age. Although gastric emptying time does not affect drug absorption, peak drug concentration may be altered.

Rectal drug absorption is influenced by anatomic and physiologic factors, as well as by drug formulation. The superior (upper third of the rectum), middle, and inferior rectal veins carry blood away from the rectal mucosa. The superior rectal vein empties into the portal system, whereas the middle and inferior rectal veins empty into the systemic circulation by way of the inferior vena cava. For example, the administration of acetaminophen into the upper third of the rectum results in a lower plasma concentration because of first-pass metabolism.[13] Opioids, barbiturates, and midazolam undergo first-pass metabolism, and their administration in the upper third of the rectum should be avoided.

Acetaminophen, a metabolite of phenacetin, is a popular and safe analgesic and antipyretic commonly administered to children during the operative period. The inhibition of cyclooxygenase within the CNS is the proposed analgesic mechanism of action. This drug deserves some discussion because of its popularity as a supplemental intraoperative analgesic in pediatric patients.

The analgesic and antipyretic effects of acetaminophen are equivalent to those of aspirin when the drugs are administered in equipotent dosages. Acetaminophen is metabolized by the hepatic microsomal enzyme system, and approximately 80% of the parent drug is conjugated with glucuronic acid and sulfate (phase II metabolism). Animal data suggest that a small amount of the parent drug is metabolized by the cytochrome P-450 enzyme system (phase I metabolism), producing an intermediate metabolite that undergoes conjugation with glutathione and is excreted in the urine. High doses of acetaminophen may deplete glutathione, increasing the accumulation of this intermediate metabolite, which is thought to be responsible for acetaminophen-induced liver necrosis. Glutathione depletion may develop with continued administration of high doses of acetaminophen.[19]

Acetaminophen is frequently administered rectally to children after anesthetic induction to provide supplemental analgesia in the immediate postoperative period. It is my practice to administer the calculated dose into the distal rectum immediately after the induction of anesthesia, providing time for absorption. Suppositories should not be divided in an attempt to provide the exact calculated dose, because the suspended acetaminophen is distributed unevenly within the suppository. Recommended acetaminophen doses have been based on the age of the child, weight, body surface area calculations, and fractions of adult dosages. Doses calculated on patient weight are the most accurate for individual patients.[20] Currently recommended oral and rectal doses of acetaminophen range from 10 to 15 mg/kg every 4 hours.[21] Because of the variable absorption of acetaminophen suppositories, some practitioners have advocated the administration of larger rectal dosages during the perioperative period. Birmingham and colleagues examined the 24-hour pharmacokinetics of rectal acetaminophen, and based on the observed kinetics they recommend an initial dose of 40 mg/kg.[21] Analgesic efficacy was not studied, but rather the doses were based on resultant serum acetaminophen concentrations of 10 to 20 mcg/ml, which have been determined to be essential for antipyretic activity. Montgomery and colleagues administered 45 mg/kg of acetaminophen rectally to 10 pediatric patients who weighed between 13 and 15 kg.[22] Plasma sampling demonstrated a peak concentration that occurred 198 ± 70 minutes after administration. Resultant plasma concentrations were comparable to those after a 10- to 15-mg/kg oral dose, and no child attained plasma concentrations associated with acute toxicity. Although a number of studies have suggested an initial rectal dose of 40 to 45 mg/kg, I administer a rectal dose that does not exceed 25 to 30 mg/kg.

Parents are likely to continue to administer acetaminophen after outpatient anesthesia. The parents are informed as to the time of acetaminophen administration, and appropriate acetaminophen dosages (60 to 65 mg/kg/day) are discussed. Animal and human data are conflicting with regard to the impact of inhalation agents on the hepatic degradation of acetaminophen. Studies have suggested a decrease in acetaminophen conjugation,[23] an increase in acetaminophen metabolism via the oxidative metabolic pathway,[24] and an increase in hepatic metabolism on the first postoperative day.[25] Additional clinical studies are required to confirm the appropriate initial rectal dosages and the impact of inhalation anesthesia on serum acetaminophen concentrations and metabolism, as well as serum concentrations that provide optimum analgesia.

Transmucosal drug administration avoids first-pass metabolism. The vascular mucosa of the oral, nasal, and pulmonary passages is easily accessed. Sedation with nasally administered midazolam (0.2 mg/kg) may be achieved in as little as 10 to 20 minutes and is explained in part through drug absorption via the olfactory mucosa.[26,27] Nasal administration avoids first-pass metabolism. Oral fentanyl, although effective in producing significant sedation, has been plagued by significant side effects, including facial pruritus (up to 80%) and postoperative nausea and vomiting, seven times greater than when a child receives an oral meperidine, midazolam, or atropine premedicant.[28] Recall that water-soluble drugs (atropine, fentanyl, lidocaine, morphine) may be administered via inhalation; however, only 5% to 10% of the administered dose will reach the systemic circulation.

Inhalation Agents

Factors that affect inhalation anesthetic uptake include alveolar ventilation, the delivered inspired anesthetic concentration, the blood-gas partition coefficient, and the cardiac output. Pediatric patients have a greater minute ventilation

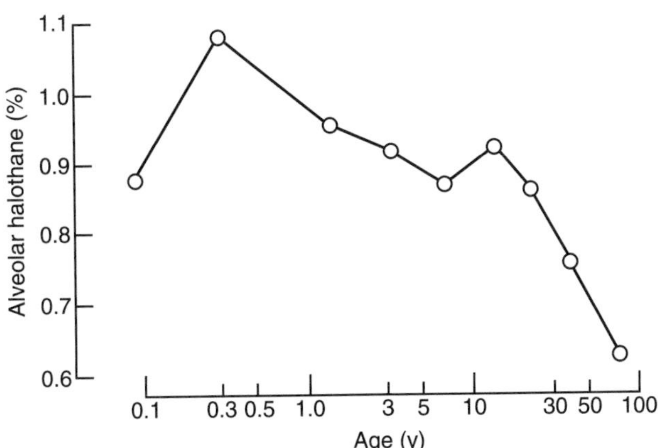

FIGURE **45-4**
Effects of age on maximum alveolar concentration. (Modified from Gregory GA, Eger E, Munson E. The relationship between age and halothane requirement in man. *Anesthesiology*. 1969;30:488-491; and Lerman J, Robinson S, Willis MM, Gregory GA. Anesthetic requirements for halothane in young children 0-1 month and 1-6 months of age. *Anesthesiology*. 1983;59:421-424.)

because of a smaller functional residual capacity and a higher cardiac output. In addition, their decreased distribution of adipose tissue and decreased muscle mass affect the rate of equilibration among the alveoli, blood, and brain. The percentage of blood flow to the vessel-rich organs (i.e., heart, brain, kidneys, and liver) is greater than in the adult, and the blood-gas partition coefficients are lower in infants and children.[29,30] Alveolar concentrations of inhaled agents increase more rapidly in both infants and children. Neonates have a somewhat lower minimum alveolar concentration (MAC), which peaks at around 30 days of age and decreases thereafter (Figure 45-4). The MAC is higher in infants from age 1 to 6 months of age; thereafter, MAC values are known to decrease with age.[31,32]

Myocardial depression may be exaggerated when inhalation anesthetics are administered to pediatric patients.[33,34] Higher anesthetic concentrations, a more rapid rise in the alveolar to inspired concentration ratio (F_A/F_I ratio), and the greater percentage of blood flow to the vessel-rich organs are central to the cause of myocardial depression. To summarize, inhalation induction is more rapid in pediatric patients and is accompanied by a higher incidence of myocardial depression than in adults.

Halothane. Halothane is less pungent than the ethers isoflurane and desflurane and is readily accepted for inhalation induction. Sevoflurane has emerged as a popular alternative to halothane for anesthetic induction. Children receiving halothane or sevoflurane have less airway-related incidents (bronchospasm, laryngospasm, breath-holding) compared with those induced with either isoflurane or desflurane.[35,36]

Halothane sensitizes the myocardium to the effects of endogenous and exogenous catecholamines. Ventricular dysrhythmias may occur with inadequate depths of anesthesia and in the presence of hypercarbia (stimulates the central release of catecholamines).[37] It has been suggested that epinephrine administration with local anesthetics should be limited to 10 mcg/kg body weight to minimize the potential of cardiac dysrhythmias.[38] Halothane produces a dose-dependent myocardial depression. The administration of high concentrations to neonates, infants, and children will decrease cardiac output, blood pressure, mean arterial pressure, and heart rate. Systolic blood pressure may decrease by as much as 30% at 1 MAC end-tidal concentrations. Myocardial contractility and left ventricular stroke work are depressed, whereas peripheral vascular resistance is minimally altered. Atropine administration increases both heart rate and blood pressure. The MAC of halothane in oxygen for neonates and infants is 0.87% and 1.2%, respectively.

Isoflurane. Inhalation induction with isoflurane produces more adverse respiratory events (breath-holding, coughing, and laryngospasm with copious secretions) than either halothane or sevoflurane. Administration of isoflurane to adults produces dose-dependent decreases in peripheral vascular resistance, although it increases heart rate, which acts to maintain blood pressure. This touted advantage (e.g., increase in heart rate to maintain blood pressure) does not occur in infants. Anesthetic induction in infants with isoflurane produces significant decreases in heart rate, blood pressure, and mean arterial pressure, which are not corrected with prior atropine administration.[39] The MAC of isoflurane in oxygen is 1.6% for neonates, infants, and children.

Desflurane. Desflurane has the lowest blood-gas partition coefficient of all the inhalation anesthetics, which facilitates a rapid induction, rapid alterations in anesthetic depth, and emergence. Like isoflurane, desflurane is pungent and is associated with more adverse respiratory events during inhalation induction. Dramatic increases in desflurane concentrations may produce tachycardia and hypertension.[40,41] The MAC of desflurane in oxygen is 9.2% for neonates, 9% for infants, and 6% to 10% for children.

Sevoflurane. Sevoflurane produces a more rapid induction and emergence than halothane because of its low blood-gas partition coefficient.[42] This clinical advantage is responsible for the increasing popularity of sevoflurane in pediatric anesthesia. Several clinical concerns have arisen as clinicians have gained experience in the administration of sevoflurane. During anesthetic induction, inspired concentrations in excess of 6% have been reported to produce seizure activity in an animal model. Seizure activity has been reported in two pediatric patients with epilepsy.[43,44] Severe postoperative agitation or delirium has also been reported after sevoflurane administration in children. Unpremedicated children experience a high incidence of emergence delirium.[45,46] Postoperative agitation is generally indicative of the need for postoperative analgesia, yet this postoperative agitation may continue despite the administration of opioids. Lapin and colleagues found that children undergoing myringotomy and tube placement who were premedicated with midazolam before receiving a sevoflurane anesthetic experienced less postoperative agitation and cried less than their unpremedicated counterparts. These children had longer recovery times but experienced less emergence delirium, although it was still greater than that witnessed in the halothane group.[47] Of the unpremedicated children receiving sevoflurane, 67% experienced some degree of postoperative agitation. A recent report of three children and one adult who were able to describe their emergence experiences after sevoflurane administration suggests that emergence delirium may be the result of a short-lived misperception of environmental stimuli or paranoia.[46]

Sevoflurane produces a greater depression of ventilation when compared with halothane. Both minute ventilation and respiratory rate are significantly lower after sevoflurane administration. With the introduction of high inspired concentrations, apnea is likely to occur.

Sevoflurane is unstable in CO_2 absorbents, producing fluoromethyl-2,2-difluoro-1-(trifluoromethyl) vinyl ether, known as *compound* A. Animal data suggest that compound A concentrations between 50 and 100 ppm may produce renal toxicity.[48,49] Compound A may be formed during high-flow, low-flow, and closed-circuit anesthesia.[50,51,52] A limited study of 19 children who received a 4-hour sevoflurane anesthetic using a 2-L total flow via a circle system produced compound A concentrations of up to 15 ppm. A 24-hour follow-up concluded that there was no renal or hepatic dysfunction.[53] However, reports have suggested that subtle renal abnormalities, including albuminemia and altered renal thresholds for glucose, occur in adults who volunteered to receive a sevoflurane anesthetic without surgical intervention.[54,55]

Sevoflurane metabolism may produce elevations in serum fluoride levels. These elevations are concentration-dependent and decline when sevoflurane is discontinued. However, it is important to note that sevoflurane has been administered to thousands of patients without evidence of fluoride-induced renal dysfunction.

Some clinicians, when performing longer procedures, use sevoflurane for anesthetic induction but introduce either desflurane or isoflurane for anesthetic maintenance. This clinical decision reduces patient cost and limits the sevoflurane exposure. Unlike halothane, sevoflurane does not sensitize the myocardium to the effects of endogenous and exogenous catecholamines. However, not unlike halothane, concentration-dependent myocardial depression may occur. The MAC of sevoflurane in oxygen is 2% to 3%.

Intravenous Anesthetics

As discussed previously, infants and children have a higher proportion of cardiac output delivered to vascular-rich tissues (i.e., heart, brain, kidneys, and liver). Intravenously administered drugs are readily taken up by these tissues and are subsequently redistributed to tissues less well perfused (muscle and fat). Intravenously administered drugs may have a prolonged duration of action in infants and children because of decreased percentages of muscle and fat. The CNS effects of opioids and barbiturates may also be prolonged because of the immaturity of the blood-brain barrier.[56] Although this evidence suggests that intravenously administered anesthetic doses should be reduced, one must also recall the effect of increased body water. Increased doses of thiopental, propofol, and ketamine are required, presumably because of a greater volume of distribution.[57,58]

Thiopental. Thiopental is supplied as a 2.5% solution. Intravenous induction dosages range from 4 to 6 mg/kg in children without significant cardiovascular disease.[59,60] Neonates have limited fat stores and may have an extended duration of action after thiopental administration. Thiopental, 25 to 30 mg/kg, may be administered rectally for anesthetic induction (see discussion of rectal induction).

Propofol. Propofol has a rapid onset and a short duration of action. Propofol may be delivered as a continuous infusion for short diagnostic and radiologic procedures. Its antiemetic properties may reduce the incidence of postoperative nausea and vomiting in children undergoing strabismus correction.[61] Infants require larger induction doses (2.5 to 3 mg/kg) than children (2 to 2.5 mg/kg).[62,63] These induction doses produce moderate decreases in systolic blood pressure.[64] The pain that accompanies intravenous administration may be reduced with the addition of as little as 0.2 mg/kg of lidocaine. Additional strategies have been advocated for decreasing the pain of injection, including the injection of propofol into a rapid-running intravenous line or the injection into larger intravenous catheters placed in the antecubital space.[65]

Methohexital. Methohexital, an oxybarbiturate, is supplied as a 1% solution that is suitable for intravenous and rectal administration (see discussion of rectal induction). Methohexital has a shorter elimination half-life than thiopental but may produce pain on injection, hiccups, coughing, and myoclonic movements. Methohexital may induce seizure activity in children with temporal lobe epilepsy.

Neuromuscular Blockers

Neuromuscular blocking drugs are highly ionized and have a low lipophilicity, which limits their ability to cross the blood-brain barrier. These pharmacologic properties restrict the distribution of neuromuscular blockers to the ECF compartment, which is larger in the neonate and infant than in the child and adult (see Table 45-5). Increases in ECF volume and the ongoing maturation of neonatal skeletal muscle and acetylcholine receptors affect the pharmacokinetics and pharmacodynamics of neuromuscular blockers. Table 45-6 references the effective doses of neuromuscular blocking drugs in various age groups.

The neuromuscular junction is incompletely developed at birth. The presynaptic release of acetylcholine is slowed at birth compared with that in the adult, which explains the decreased margin of safety for neuromuscular transmission in the neonate. The acetylcholine receptors of the newborn are anatomically different from the adult receptors, which may explain the sensitivity of the neonate to the nondepolarizing class of neuromuscular blockers.[66,67] This neuromuscular immaturity may be demonstrated with the appearance of fade after tetanic stimulation in the absence of neuromuscular blocking drugs.[68,69] Skeletal muscle, acetylcholine receptors, and biochemical processes essential in neuromuscular transmission mature during infancy into childhood, which accounts for the decreasing sensitivity and the child's development of resistance to neuromuscular blocking drugs.

TABLE 45-6 Effective Doses (ED_{95}) of Clinical Neuromuscular Blocking Drugs (mcg/kg)

	Neonate	Infant	Child	Adult
Succinylcholine*	620	729	423	290
Mivacurium	—	85	89-103	58-120
Atracurium	120	156-175	170-350	110-280
Vecuronium	47	42-47	56-80	27-56
Rocuronium	600	600	600	300
Pancuronium	—	55	55-81	50-70
Pipecuronium	46	48	49-79	42-59
Doxacurium	—	—	27-32	14-19

**Should be used for emergency airway stabilization in children younger than 12 years old. Not for routine intubation.*

Succinylcholine. Succinylcholine is composed of two acetylcholine molecules united by an ester bond. Succinylcholine is metabolized into the inactive metabolites succinylmonocholine, choline, and succinic acid by plasma (butyryl) cholinesterase. Succinylcholine has a number of well-defined side effects that can occur. These include increases in intragastric pressure, increases in intraocular and intracranial pressure, cardiac dysrhythmias, myalgia, and myoglobinemia.[70,71] Succinylcholine is also a known triggering agent for malignant hyperthermia (MH).

Because succinylcholine contains acetylcholine moieties, its intravenous administration will reproduce the effects of acetylcholine when it interacts with nicotinic and muscarinic receptors, provoking both sympathetic and parasympathetic cardiovascular responses. Stimulation of the parasympathetic ganglia or direct stimulation of cardiac muscarinic receptors will produce sinus bradycardia, junctional rhythms, unifocal premature ventricular contractions, and ventricular fibrillation.[72,73] The prior administration of 0.02 mg of atropine per kilogram will block cardiac muscarinic receptors and minimize the decreases in heart rate. Dysrhythmia is more common in children, particularly after repeated doses in the presence of hypoxia or concurrent electrolyte imbalance.

Myoglobinemia may occur in up to 20% of children who receive intravenous succinylcholine and in 40% of children who receive succinylcholine and halothane.[74] The prior administration of a small dose of a nondepolarizing neuromuscular blocking drug will modify the degree of myoglobinuria.[75]

Myalgia is common after succinylcholine administration. The cause of succinylcholine-induced myalgia has recently been hypothesized to follow the production of prostaglandins.[76] This hypothesis was successfully tested with the intravenous administration of acetylsalicylic acid (aspirin), which effectively reduced the incidence and intensity of postoperative myalgia.

Succinylcholine is known to be a triggering agent for the development of MH.[77] The North American and European estimates of the frequency of MH in children are approximately 1 in every 15,000 anesthetic procedures.[78] A resistance to mouth opening during endotracheal intubation has been described after succinylcholine administration. Increased masseter muscle tone, masseter muscle rigidity, or trismus occurs 0.2% of the time after the combination of halothane and succinylcholine.[78] Some clinical reports suggest that masseter spasm is a foreboding sign of MH and that as many as 50% of children with masseter muscle rigidity will develop MH.[79-82] This suggests that the incidence of MH is indeed higher than has been reported. It has been suggested that masseter muscle rigidity may occur as a result of inadequate succinylcholine intravenous doses in children.[81] A variety of opinions exist regarding the clinical management of the child with masseter muscle rigidity. Clearly, signs of MH should be sought in the child experiencing masseter rigidity. If the jaw can be forcefully opened to allow endotracheal intubation, the anesthetic procedure may proceed, with vigilance exercised for clinical signs of MH (rigidity of other skeletal muscle groups, increases in end-tidal CO_2 and core temperature). If the mouth cannot be forcefully opened, airway management may be difficult, necessitating the termination of the procedure. Such children should undergo laboratory serial determinations of creatinine kinase, electrolytes, and myoglobin.

Neonates are more resistant to the effects of succinylcholine than children and adults. This sensitivity is illustrated by the intravenous ED_{95} for neonates (620 mcg/kg), infants (729 mcg/kg), children (423 mcg/kg), and adults (290 mcg/kg) (see Table 45-6).[82] The increase in dose requirement is in part a result of the increased volume of distribution within the large extracellular compartment.[83] Plasma cholinesterase activity is reduced in neonates; however, the duration of action after a single dose is of expected duration (6 to 10 minutes). A longer duration of action after a single bolus dose suggests the presence of an inherited deficiency of plasma cholinesterase activity.

Historically, succinylcholine has been the only available neuromuscular blocker that can be administered intramuscularly to facilitate endotracheal intubation in the absence of intravenous access (see the discussion of rocuronium). Intramuscular succinylcholine may facilitate endotracheal intubation in children without suitable intravenous access. Because of the increased volume of distribution, a larger dose is required to achieve satisfactory relaxation. Although a dose of 3 mg/kg will produce satisfactory relaxation in 85% of patients, a dose of 4 mg/kg will provide skeletal muscle relaxation in all, with a duration of action of up to 21 minutes.[84,85] To attenuate the effects of succinylcholine at both the nicotinic and muscarinic receptors, atropine at a dose of 0.02 mg/kg may be combined in the same syringe with the calculated dose of succinylcholine or in an additional syringe, which is administered in a selected muscle group before succinylcholine administration.

Unexpected cardiac arrest has been reported after the routine administration of succinylcholine, and less than 40% of patients are successfully resuscitated. Boys younger than age 8 with undiagnosed Duchenne's muscular dystrophy may experience hyperkalemia and subsequent cardiac arrest after succinylcholine administration. In November 1993 the United States Food and Drug Administration (FDA) relabeled succinylcholine, restricting its use to emergency endotracheal intubation in children and adults.[86,87] After lengthy discussions between the FDA and clinicians, this was changed to a strong "warning" that noted that succinylcholine should not be routinely employed for airway management in children younger than 8 years of age.[87,88]

Nondepolarizing Neuromuscular Blocking Drugs. Neonates are sensitive, infants are less sensitive, and children are resistant to the effects of nondepolarizing neuromuscular blocking drugs (see ED_{95} doses, Table 45-6). This apparent sensitivity may be explained in part by the larger volume of drug distribution. The selection of a nondepolarizing neuromuscular blocker should take into consideration the desired degree and duration of skeletal muscle paralysis, the immaturity of organ systems, and the associated side effects of the selected relaxant. Interpatient variability in response to these drugs is greater than in adults, particularly in premature infants and neonates. Neuromuscular function monitoring must be employed to guide repeated administration of these drugs in all pediatric patients.

Mivacurium is a short-acting nondepolarizing neuromuscular blocker suitable for administration as a bolus or for continuous infusion. Mivacurium is metabolized by plasma cholinesterase at a rate that is 70% to 88% that of succinylcholine.[89] The ED_{95} for mivacurium during halothane administration is 85 mcg/kg in infants and 89 mcg/kg in children.[90] An intubating dose of 0.2 mg of mivacurium per kilogram will provide suitable intubating conditions in 2 to 3 minutes, with a duration of action approaching 20 minutes.[91] The time required for recovery to 25% of control twitch height is 6.3 minutes in infants and 10 minutes in children. Doses as high as 0.3 mg/kg do not prolong this recovery time.[92]

Although mivacurium is reported to produce flushing and mild hypotension in adults, doses as high as 0.3 mg/kg fail to produce these side effects in children. Continuous infusion doses range from 10 to 20 mcg/kg/min.

Atracurium is an intermediate-acting neuromuscular blocker that is metabolized by nonspecific esterases and spontaneous breakdown of the parent compound by Hofmann elimination. *cis*-Atracurium also uses Hofmann elimination and nonspecific ester hydrolysis for the metabolism of the parent compound. Unlike mivacurium, plasma cholinesterase deficiency does not affect the metabolism or elimination of atracurium or *cis*-atracurium. The ED_{95} for atracurium is higher in children, again reflecting the resistance in children to nondepolarizing neuromuscular blockers (see Table 45-6). Atracurium (intubating dose 0.5 mg/kg, maintenance dose 0.2 to 0.3 mg/kg) and *cis*-atracurium (intubating dose 0.1 mg/kg, maintenance dose 0.08 to 0.1 mg/kg) may be the drugs of choice in neonates and infants, because these drugs are not dependent on mature organ systems for elimination.

Vecuronium produces minimal alterations in cardiovascular function and stimulates the release of histamine. The ED_{95} are listed in Table 45-6. When administered in the newborn, vecuronium behaves as a long-acting relaxant, the duration of which approaches that of pancuronium.[93] Vecuronium may be administered as a continuous infusion at a rate of 0.8 to 1 mcg/kg/min. It is also important to note that prolonged infusions of vecuronium in the intensive care setting have been associated with prolonged paralysis.[94]

Rocuronium is an intermediate-acting neuromuscular blocker with a rapid-to-intermediate onset of 60 to 90 seconds after an intubating dose of 0.6 mg/kg. Unlike vecuronium, rocuronium in intubating doses may produce transient increases in heart rate.[95] Skeletal muscle relaxation can be maintained with repeat doses of 0.075 to 0.125 mg/kg. In clinical situations in which intravenous access is not available, rocuronium may be administered intramuscularly. Reynolds and colleagues found acceptable intubating conditions in lightly anesthetized infants 2.5 to 3 minutes after an intramuscular dose of 1000 mcg/kg and within 3 minutes after 1800 mcg/kg in children.[96] The onset of action approximates the onset of succinylcholine after intramuscular injection. Rocuronium injection into the deltoid provided a faster onset of twitch and ventilatory depression than did injection into the quadriceps muscle group. A disadvantage of this route of administration is the accompanying prolonged duration of relaxation—in excess of 60 minutes.[96] Whether intramuscular rocuronium is appropriate for the treatment of laryngospasm in children with contraindications to succinylcholine has not been studied. Rocuronium may also be administered by continuous infusion at doses of 0.004 to 0.016 mg/kg/min.

Reversal of Neuromuscular Blockade

The detection of residual neuromuscular blockade requires the integration of clinical criteria and the assessment of neuromuscular blockade via a peripheral nerve stimulator. Residual neuromuscular blockade places the pediatric patient at risk of hypoventilation and of the inability to independently and continuously maintain a patent airway. Conventional doses of the anticholinesterase inhibitors (0.4 to 0.7 mg of neostigmine per kilogram, 0.1 to 0.2 mg of pyridostigmine per kilogram, 0.5 mg of edrophonium per kilogram) combined with appropriate doses of atropine or glycopyrrolate are acceptable for the reversal of nondepolarizing neuromuscular blockade.

Clinical signs of adequate reversal of neuromuscular blockade in the adult patient include the ability to sustain a 5-second head lift, bilateral sustained grip strength, the ability to protrude the tongue, the absence of discoordinated movements, and a return to a normal train-of-four response as assessed by the peripheral nerve stimulator. The ability to generate a maximum inspiratory force (MIF) greater than -25 cm H_2O has been suggested to provide satisfactory inspiratory muscle function to maintain normal minute ventilation in adults.[97,98] Voluntary clinical tests are not applicable to the neonate and infant.

Clinical signs of the adequacy of neuromuscular function in the neonate and infant include spontaneous and sustained leg lift, spontaneous movement of the arms, and a return to a normal train-of-four response as assessed by the peripheral nerve stimulator. Neonates are capable of generating an MIF of -70 cm H_2O with the first few breaths after birth.[99] An MIF of at least -32 cm H_2O has been found to correspond with leg lift, which is indicative of the adequacy of ventilatory reserve required before tracheal extubation.[100]

Drug Preservatives

Premature neonates have a reduced ability to metabolize the preservatives benzoyl alcohol and sodium benzoate. These agents can produce severe CNS toxicity, seizures, and permanent brain damage. Use of preservative-free drugs and solutions is essential.

Pediatric Anesthesia Equipment

The child's age, weight, and proposed surgical procedure guide the selection of essential pediatric anesthesia equipment. The anesthesia workroom should be appropriately stocked with a variety of sizes of masks, airways, LMAs, laryngoscope blades, endotracheal tubes, endotracheal tube stylets, blood pressure cuffs, pulse oximeter probes, calibrated pediatric fluid sets, syringe pumps for the delivery of both fluids and drugs, an assortment of intravenous catheters, tape, and arm boards.

Airway Equipment

The pediatric face mask is designed to fit the smaller facial features of the child and eliminate mechanical dead space. Contemporary masks are manufactured from transparent plastics and have a soft inflatable cuff that sits on the face (Figure 45-5). The transparent feature allows continuous observation of skin color and the appearance of gastric contents should vomiting occur.

Oral and Nasal Airways

Appropriately sized oral airways must be readily available (Figure 45-6, A). The relatively large tongue of the infant predisposes to airway obstruction after the induction of general anesthesia. Oral airways that are too large may produce airway obstruction, inhibit venous and lymphatic drainage, and produce a subsequent macroglossia, producing further airway compromise. The oral airway should be inserted with the aid of a tongue blade, displacing the tongue toward the floor of the mouth to allow smooth insertion of the airway. The insertion and rotation of an oral airway should be avoided in children, as the rotation may dislodge deciduous or loose teeth.

Nasal airways are infrequently used in children less than 1 to 2 years of age. The internal diameter of the nasal airway may unnecessarily increase the work of breathing. Adenoid hypertrophy may make nasal airway placement difficult and produce

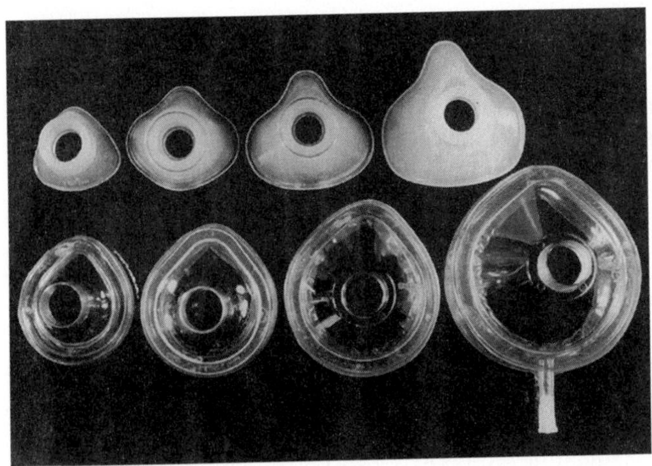

FIGURE **45-5**
Types of pediatric face masks. *Top row*, Rendell-Baker-Soucek masks, which have a low profile and the least amount of dead space. *Bottom row*, Transparent masks with pneumatic cushions, which have more dead space but with which provision of an effective seal for positive pressure ventilation is easier. Boytim M. Pediatric Equipment. (From Zaglaniczny K, Aker J, eds. *Clinical Guide to Pediatric Anesthesia*. Philadelphia: Saunders: 1999.)

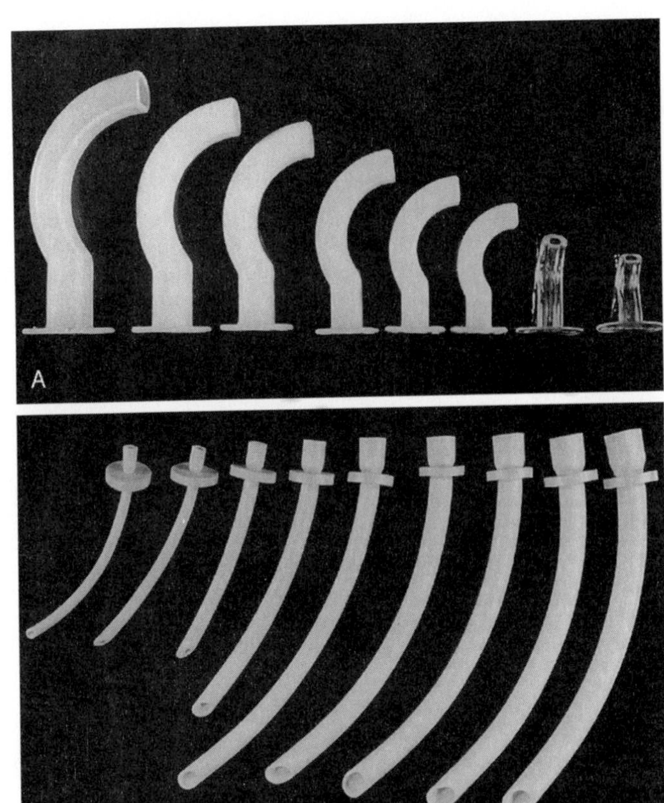

FIGURE **45-6**
A, Oral airways. Sizes range from neonate (*right*) to adolescent (*left*). **B,** Nasal airways. Sizes range from infant (*left*) to adolescent (*right*). Boytim M. Pediatric Equipment. (From Zaglaniczny K, Aker J, eds. *Clinical Guide to Pediatric Anesthesia*. Philadelphia: Saunders; 1999.)

severe epistaxis. If a nasal airway is required, a suitably sized, well-lubricated uncuffed endotracheal tube may be inserted through the nares (Figure 45-6, *B*).

Endotracheal Tubes. The cricoid is the narrowest portion of the pediatric airway. This anatomic fact allows the use of uncuffed endotracheal tubes in children up to 8 years of age. Many formulas exist for the selection of the correct size of endotracheal tube and depth of insertion. The approximate size of endotracheal tube for children 2 years of age and older may be determined by calculating as follows: age + 16 ÷ 4. The depth of endotracheal tube insertion from the dental alveoli may be estimated using the "1, 2, 3, 4/7, 8, 9, 10" rule—for example, the endotracheal tube should be inserted to a depth of 7 cm in a neonate weighing 1 kg and to a depth of 8 cm in a 2-kg neonate. Another approximate method is to insert the endotracheal tube to a depth in centimeters three times the internal diameter of the endotracheal tube in millimeters. For example, a 3-mm endotracheal tube should be inserted to a depth of 9 cm. Uncuffed endotracheal tubes are marked distally with a double black line that provides a visual indication of the depth of the endotracheal tube. During intubation the endotracheal tube should be passed until the double black line has reached the level of the vocal cords. This ensures that the distal tip of the tube is indeed cephalad to the carina. Table 45-7 provides approximate sizes of endotracheal tubes, suction catheters, and laryngoscope blades for preterm infants through 12-year-old children. To accommodate the variability in patient airway size, endotracheal tubes one-half size larger and one-half size smaller should be available at the bedside.

Proper endotracheal tube size is ultimately determined during endotracheal intubation. I select uncuffed endotracheal tubes for children younger than 8 years of age or until a size 6- to 6.5-mm tube is required. The endotracheal tube should be inserted below the level of the vocal cords without undue resistance. After proper placement is confirmed, the anesthetist should listen over the child's mouth while simultaneously squeezing the reservoir bag of the breathing circuit and noting the pressure at which an air leak is appreciated. Positive pressure ventilation will be ineffective when an air leak is detected at 8 to 10 cm H_2O. A large or tight-fitting endotracheal tube that does not permit a detectable air leak until

TABLE **45-7** Estimation of Endotracheal Tube Size by Age

	28-34 Wk	Newborn	6 Mo	1 Yr	2 Yr	4 Yr	6 Yr	8 Yr	10 Yr	12 Yr
Endotracheal tube size	2.5-3	3	4	4	4.5-5	5-5.5	5.5-6	6-6.5	6.5 cuffed	6.5-7 cuffed
Suction catheter (Fr)	6-8	8	10	10	10	14	14	14	14	14
Laryngo scope blade	0	0-1	1	1½	1½	2	2	2	2-3	2-3

30 to 40 cm H_2O may result in the development of postintubation laryngeal edema ("croup"). If the intended operative procedure is a lengthy one, I elected to reintubate with a smaller endotracheal tube. I am satisfied with the selected endotracheal tube size when an air leak is detected at 15 to 20 cm H_2O. The reader is referred to the comprehensive review by Marley of postextubation laryngeal edema.[101]

During the confirmation of proper endotracheal intubation, inadvertent endotracheal extubation may occur. Small endotracheal tubes are easily kinked and can be pulled from the mouth by the weight of the anesthesia breathing circuit. After intubation the endotracheal tube may be "pinned" against the palate at the desired depth of insertion with the index or middle finger of the left hand, freeing the right hand for stethoscope placement and the manual compression of the breathing bag. I secure the endotracheal tube with the application of an adhesive (tincture of benzoin) to both the face and the endotracheal tube before the application of cloth tape. The confirmation of breath sounds must be repeated after the application of tape and documented on the anesthesia record.

Specialized uncuffed and cuffed oral and nasal endotracheal tubes may be chosen for otolaryngologic, ophthalmologic, and dental procedures (Figure 45-7). The RAE (Mallinkrodt, Argyle, New York) endotracheal tube is premolded, with the acute angle of the tube designed to be positioned over the lower lip, and the nasal RAE is premolded with a 180-degree bend that directs the tube toward the top of the head. These tubes facilitate the routing of the breathing circuit away from the surgical field. RAE tubes are longer than straight endotracheal tubes and place the distal end of the tube in closer proximity to the carina, thereby minimizing the chance of inadvertent extubation with neck extension. The RAE tube is designed with not one, but two Murphy eyes located at the distal end of the tube, which may facilitate uninterrupted ventilation should the tube migrate in a caudad fashion. However, proper endotracheal tube placement must be ensured with confirmation of bilateral breath sounds, after intubation and the repositioning of the head. The use of a precordial stethoscope placed over the left anterior area of the chest will aid the detection of right bronchial migration of the RAE tube.

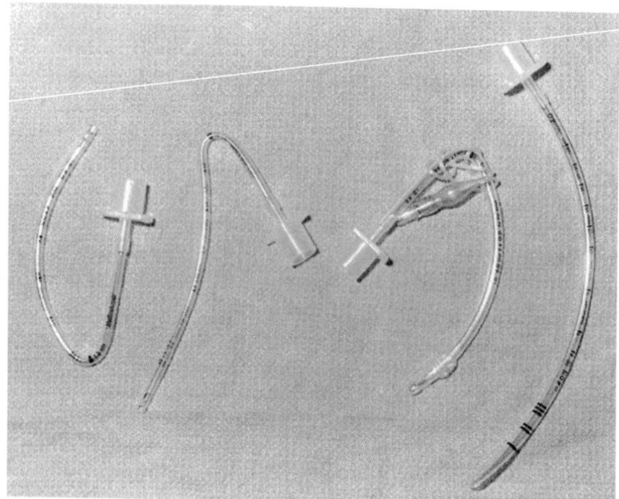

FIGURE **45-7**
Common pediatric endotracheal tubes. *From left,* Uncuffed oral RAE, uncuffed nasal RAE, cuffed oral RAE, and uncuffed straight endotracheal tube. Boytim M. Pediatric Equipment. (From Zaglaniczny K, Aker J, eds. *Clinical Guide to Pediatric Anesthesia.* Philadelphia: Saunders; 1999.)

The clinical application of laser technology (*l*ight *a*mplification by *s*timulated *e*mission of *r*adiation) for the treatment of airway pathology necessitates the use of a specialized endotracheal tube. Endotracheal tube ignition may occur in as many as 1.5% of patients during CO_2 laser laryngeal procedures.[102] Modern polyvinylchloride endotracheal tubes absorb infrared light and may be ignited with a direct hit from a CO_2 laser or as a result of burning material in close proximity to the tube. Laser-resistant or "laser-safe" endotracheal tubes are available from several manufacturers and marketed for specific laser applications (CO_2; neodymium:yttrium-aluminum-garnet [Nd:YAG]; and potassium titanyl phosphate [KTP]). An alternative is the wrapping of the external surface of a polyvinylchloride endotracheal tube with a metallic foil (Merocel Laser Guard, Merocel Corporation, Mystic, Connecticut) (see Chapter 40). A variety of straight and curved pediatric laryngoscope blades is available (Figure 45-8).

Laryngeal Mask Airway. The original LMA device was intended as an alternative to the anesthesia face mask rather than endotracheal intubation. The LMA is used for short surgical procedures that do not require endotracheal intubation (herniorrhaphy, peripheral extremity surgical procedures) and resuscitation situations. The LMA is available in sizes specific for the neonate, infant, child, and adolescent (Table 45-8). Many alternative designs are being introduced since "generic"

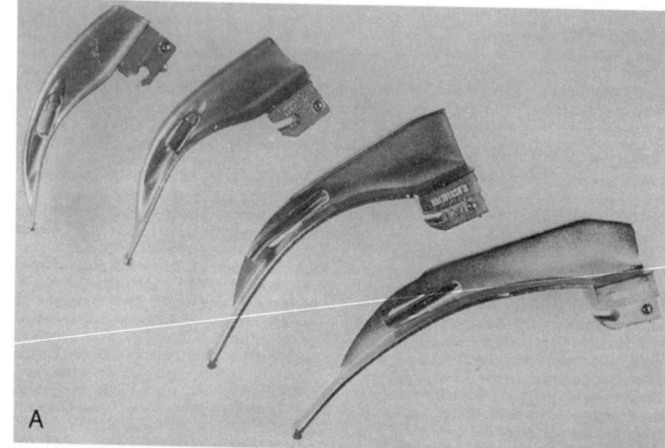

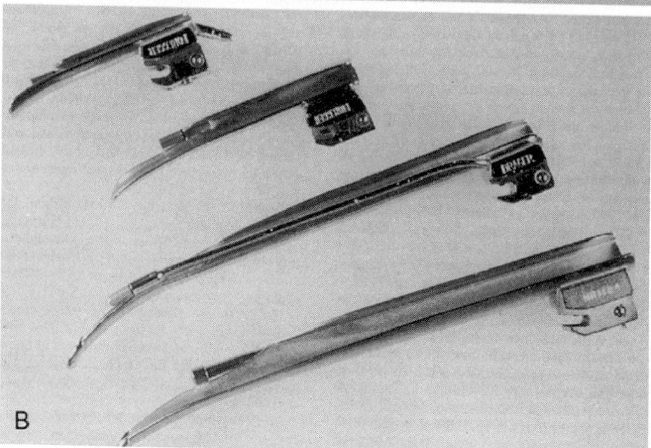

FIGURE **45-8**
Pediatric laryngoscope blades. **A,** Macintosh blades. **B,** Miller blades. Boytim M. Pediatric Equipment. (From Zaglaniczny K, Aker J, eds. *Clinical Guide to Pediatric Anesthesia.* Philadelphia: Saunders; 1999.)

TABLE 45-8 Laryngeal Airway Mask Sizes

Laryngeal Airway Mask Size	Suggested Inflation Volume
1	6 ml
1½	10 ml
2	15 ml
2½	21 ml
3	30 ml
4	45 ml
5	60 ml

From Brain AIJ, Denman WT, Goudsouzian NG. LMA-Classic and LMA-Flexible Instruction Manual. San Diego: LMA North America; 1998.

versions are now available. After inhalation or intravenous induction the LMA is inserted (after lubrication of its posterior surface) by pressing the cuff against the posterior pharyngeal wall. The distal end of the cuff rests in the inferior aspect of the hypopharynx superior to the esophageal sphincter; however, isolation of the esophageal sphincter is not guaranteed. Regurgitation, vomiting, and aspiration have all been reported with the use of the LMA. With a syringe the cuff is inflated with air to ensure a seal. Spontaneous respirations are allowed to resume after insertion. The device is removed on awakening, as is the custom when one removes an endotracheal tube.

The inflation of the pharyngeal cuff can produce undue pressure on pharyngeal structures. Like the adult endotracheal tube cuff, the LMA cuff may be expanded during the course of the anesthetic procedure with the administration of nitrous oxide. The initial volume of air injected into the laryngeal cuff may be regulated by identifying the amount of air and airway pressure that produces an audible leak. This pressure is generally between 15 and 25 cm H_2O. Algren and colleagues recommend that the LMA cuff be inspected before each use, that the volume of air required for cuff inflation should not exceed the manufacturer's recommendation, and that the LMA cuff should be periodically checked during the administration of nitrous oxide to prevent overinflation.[103]

Pediatric Breathing Circuits. Oxygen, nitrous oxide, air, and potent inhalation agents are mixed by the anesthesia machine and are delivered to the patient via the breathing circuit. The breathing circuit is essential for the removal of CO_2, the isolation of the anesthetic mixture from room air to prevent dilution of the desired anesthetic mixtures, and the maintenance of airway temperature and humidity. Spirometric and gas sampling connections to the breathing circuit allow the continuous monitoring of the end-tidal concentrations of oxygen, CO_2, nitrogen, and the potent inhalation agents. Additional accessories may be added to the breathing circuit, facilitating the pulmonary delivery of water-soluble and aerosol-derived pharmacologic agents.

The anesthesia machine should be equipped with an air flowmeter that allows the delivery of compressed air to the inspired mixture, drawn either from a central hospital supply or from an anesthesia machine–mounted cylinder. The blending of air with oxygen decreases the inspired concentration of oxygen, which is necessary for laser airway surgical procedures and for treatment of premature infants who are at risk for the development of retinopathy of prematurity. Nitrous oxide should be avoided in infants with acute intraabdominal disease (necrotizing enterocolitis), and the blending of air and oxygen permits the delivery of decreased inspired oxygen concentrations.

The circle system breathing circuit is popular for the delivery of anesthetic gases to adult patients. Advantages of the circle system include the conservation of potent inhalation agents, the ability to retain both heat and humidity, and the ease of collecting and scavenging waste gases. Components of the circle system include 1-m lengths of breathing tubing with a connected Y-piece through which inspiration and expiration take place, an elbowed or straight 15-mm connector that allows the attachment of the breathing circuit to a mask, an LMA or endotracheal tube, unidirectional respiratory valves that direct gas flow, a reservoir breathing bag, a CO_2 absorber, a port for the fresh-gas inflow, and the "pop-off" valve that directs exhaled gas to the scavenging system. The large dead space and high resistance produced by these components are ill-suited for spontaneous ventilation in anesthetized pediatric patients. Pediatric circle systems exist and are composed of smaller breathing tubing, smaller CO_2 canisters, and lower resistance valves. However, the newly designed circle systems compare in performance with the Mapleson F circuits that have comparable resistance and are acceptable for short periods of spontaneous ventilation in small infants.[104] Compliance of the circle system is greater than that of the Mapleson F circuit. The breathing tubing for the pediatric circle systems is of smaller diameter than the adult tubing and has a low compression volume, allowing accurate delivery of desired tidal volumes.

Although the adult circle system is satisfactory for the child and adolescent, the selection of the proper breathing circuit is more crucial for the neonate and infant. The ideal pediatric breathing circuit should be lightweight, minimize dead space, have a low resistance and a low compressible volume, be adaptable for both spontaneous and controlled ventilation, be capable of providing humidification and warming of inspired gases, and permit the collection and scavenging of exhaled anesthetic gases.

Contemporary pediatric breathing circuits include the traditional circle system, the Mapleson D and F circuits, and the Bain modification of the Mapleson breathing circuit. The Ayre's T-piece was first used for the delivery of anesthesia to infants undergoing cleft palate and cleft lip repair. This breathing circuit consists of a fresh-gas line that terminates in a **T** configuration. One limb of the **T** is directed toward the patient, while the opposite limb of the **T** is open to the atmosphere. Modifications of the Ayre's T-piece have been classified by Mapleson as A to E (Figure 45-9). The Mapleson D system contains an expiratory valve at the distal end of the expiratory limb. The Mapleson F system was modified by Jackson-Reese with the addition of a reservoir bag with an adjustable valve at the tail of the bag. The Mapleson F system has been described as the breathing circuit that nearly meets the ideal requirements for the pediatric patient.[105,106] Spontaneous ventilation is permitted with the opening of the adjustable valve, whereas closing the adjustable valve fills the reservoir bag, and repeated manual compression controls ventilation. With an expiratory pause of sufficient duration and sufficient fresh gas flows, exhaled CO_2 is washed from the reservoir tube, preventing the inhalation of exhaled CO_2 with subsequent inspiration. Fresh gas flows of two to three times the child's minute ventilation are required to prevent rebreathing of exhaled gases. Because of the required high fresh-gas flow rates, this circuit is not economical for children who weigh more than 20 kg.

The Bain circuit is a coaxial modification of the Mapleson D circuit. The inspiratory limb, which receives fresh gas from

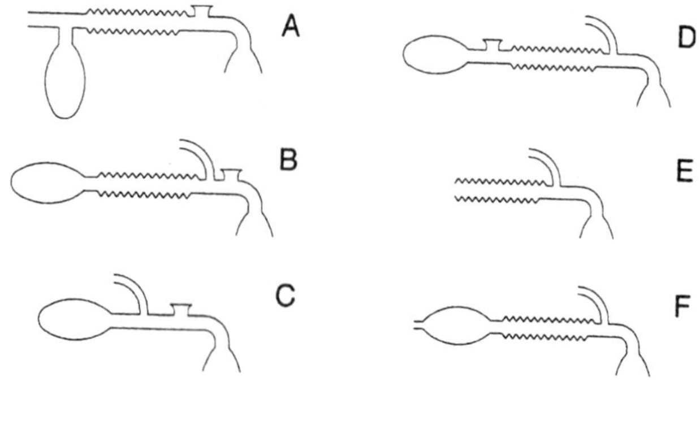

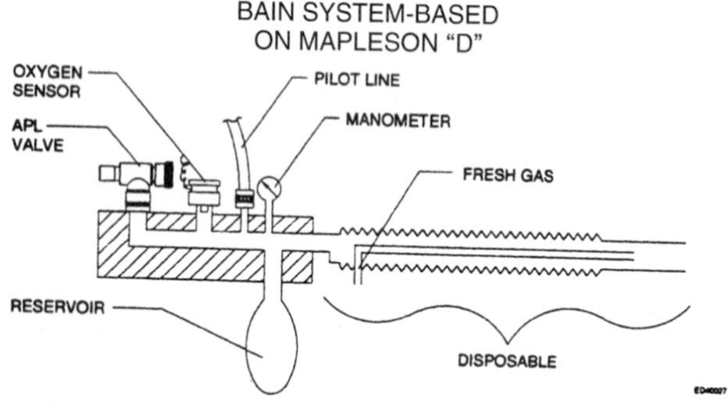

FIGURE **45-9**
Mapleson's classification of breathing systems. (From Zaglaniczny K, Aker J, eds. *Clinical Guide to Pediatric Anesthesia*. Philadelphia: Saunders; 1999.)

the anesthesia machine via a special adapter, is contained within the expiratory limb. The flow of expiratory gases over the inspiratory limb may aid in the warming of the inspired gas mixture and improve humidification. Recommended fresh gas flow rates producing normocarbia for spontaneous ventilation range from 200 to 300 $ml \cdot kg^{-1}$ and 70 to 100 $ml \cdot kg^{-1}$ for controlled ventilation. The circuit is lightweight and is adaptable for the collection and scavenging of exhaled anesthetic gases. Disadvantages of the Bain circuit include practitioner unfamiliarity, misconnection to the adapter mounted to the anesthetic machine, and kinking of the inner inspiratory limb. The integrity of the inner inspiratory limb must be ensured, otherwise inspired fresh gas will enter the expiratory limb, creating a large dead space.[106] Pethick's maneuver is used to test the integrity of the inspiratory limb.[107] The patient end of the inspiratory limb is occluded, and the reservoir bag is filled with the oxygen flush valve. The patient end is subsequently opened, and with continued high flow oxygen introduced from the oxygen flush, collapse of the reservoir bag (Venturi effect) should occur. If the inspiratory limb is fractured, the oxygen introduced via the oxygen flush will fill the reservoir bag.

The reservoir bag contains the anesthesia machine–delivered anesthetic mixture inspired by the patient and serves as a visual and tactile monitor of ventilation. Reservoir bags are shaped to allow compression with one hand and are constructed of rubber and latex, although latex-free bags are readily available. Reservoir bags range in size from 0.5 to 6 L. The selected reservoir bag must be appropriate for the patient's size, that is, capable of containing a volume in excess of the child's inspiratory capacity. The use of an inappropriately small reservoir bag may restrict respiratory efforts, and the use of a large reservoir bag inhibits the ability to use the reservoir bag as a monitor of ventilation.

We have briefly discussed the fresh gas flow requirements for spontaneous as well as controlled ventilation during the employment of the Mapleson F and Bain breathing circuits. The variables that must be considered to determine $PaCO_2$ during controlled ventilation when using these circuits include the ratio of dead space to tidal volume (V_D/V_T), the fresh gas flow rate, the child's CO_2 production, and the alveolar to arterial CO_2 difference. For children with decreased minute ventilation (recent opioid administration or high concentrations of potent inhalation agent), fresh gas flow rates may need to be increased or ventilation controlled.

Preoperative Preparation

The process of preoperative preparation has undergone extensive change with the move to outpatient day-care surgery. The preoperative evaluation may take place during a scheduled clinic visit days or weeks before, but typically is accomplished the morning of, and occasionally within minutes before, the scheduled operative procedure. The current time constraints of preoperative evaluation may disrupt the surgical schedule with cancellations for the medically unprepared or those who are acutely ill. Fortunately, the majority of pediatric surgical patients are in good health (American Society of Anesthesiologists [ASA] classes I and II). Accordingly, the preoperative evaluation is generally straightforward.[108]

Review of Systems

Appropriate anesthetic evaluation and management are dependent on a thorough understanding of the surgical and anesthetic requirements for the proposed procedure. All possible sources of medical information, including the patient chart, physical examination of the child, and the parental interview, are essential. The review of the chart should focus on the medical history (beginning with the gestational history), previous hospitalizations, previous medical or surgical experiences, the presence of chronic illness or infectious disease, and any family history of anesthetic complications (e.g., family history of atypical pseudocholinesterase). The child should also be evaluated for proper growth and development as determined by a review of norms and percentages for age and gender. Developmental delay may suggest a prenatal pathologic condition, the presence of a chronic illness, or the presence of a concurrent neurologic or neuromuscular disease. The examination of previous anesthetic records is invaluable in gleaning information regarding previous anesthetic encounters. Information obtained during the chart review is verified by the parent or guardian during the face-to-face interview and physical examination of the child.[109]

The physical examination allows the anesthetist to evaluate the child's general health. If not previously evaluated, the child's ears and nose should be examined. It is important to examine the throat for signs of redness when cough and rhinorrhea are present. This also provides the opportunity to evaluate the size of the pharyngeal tonsils, which may produce airway obstruction if hypertrophied. Airway obstruction secondary to adenotonsillar hypertrophy may be uncovered through a history of snoring with sleep. These children may also have obstructive sleep apnea and underlying pulmonary hypertension. Children between the ages of 5 and 9 should be examined for the presence of loose teeth, and these should be noted on the evaluation. A deciduous loose tooth that is in danger of being dislodged during airway management should be removed after anesthetic induction with the consent of a parent. Table 45-9 lists the anesthetic implications of the review of systems and history.

TABLE 45-9 Medical History and Review of Symptoms: Anesthetic Implications

System	History	Possible Anesthetic Implications
Central nervous and neuromuscular	Seizures	Medications: drug interactions, possible inadequate serum levels, valproate-induced hepatitis
	Head trauma	Elevated intracranial pressure
	Hydrocephalus	Possible elevated intracranial pressure
	CNS tumor	Possible elevated intracranial pressure, chemotherapeutic drugs and interactions
		Possible risk of malignant hypothermia
Cardiovascular	Heart murmur	Septal defect, avoid air bubbles in IV line
	Cyanosis	Right-to-left cardiac shunt
	History of squatting	Possible tetralogy of Fallot
	Diaphoresis with feedings	Congestive heart failure
	Hypertension	Possible coarctation of the aorta; renal disease; pheochromocytoma
	Transplant recipient	Fixed heart rate; insensitivity to anticholinergic drugs
Respiratory	Prematurity	Increased risk of postoperative apnea; possible lower respiratory tract illness
	Bronchopulmonary dysplasia	Lower airway obstruction; reactive airways; possible subglottic stenosis; possible postoperative hypoxia and apnea; pulmonary hypertension
	Lower respiratory infection, cough	Reactive airways; bronchospasm; medication history; drug interactions
	Croup	Possible subglottic stenosis or anomaly
	Snoring, sleep apnea	Perioperative airway obstruction; hypoxia
	Asthma	β-Agonist or theophylline drugs; pulmonary hypertension or cor pulmonale; steroid use; adrenal insufficiency; postoperative hypoxia
	Cystic fibrosis	Drug interactions; pulmonary toilet; pulmonary dysfunction; reactive airways
	Recent cold	Possible lower respiratory tract infection; reactive airways
Gastrointestinal and hepatic	Vomiting, diarrhea	Electrolyte abnormality; dehydration; full stomach
	Growth failure	Possible anemia
	Gastroesophageal reflux	Risk of aspiration; reactive airways; hypoxia
	Jaundice	Altered drug metabolism; risk of hypoglycemia
	Liver transplant recipient	Altered drug metabolism; immunosuppression
	Frequency, nocturia	Unrecognized diabetes, urinary tract infection
	Renal failure or dialysis	Electrolyte abnormality; hypervolemia or hypovolemia; anemia; medication history
	Renal transplant recipient	Immunosuppression
Endocrine and metabolic	Hypoglycemia	Hypoglycemia
	Diabetes	Insulin requirement; intraoperative hypoglycemia
	Steroid therapy	Adrenal insufficiency
	Pregnancy	Teratogenic effects of N_2O and other drugs; risk of spontaneous abortion
Hematologic	Anemia	Transfusion requirement
	Bruising, excessive bleeding	Coagulopathy
	Sickle cell disease	Anemia; transfusion; hydration; oxygenation; orthopedic tourniquet use
	AIDS	Susceptibility to infection; infectious risk to medical personnel
Allergies	Medication history	Drug reactions; drug interactions
Dental	Loose teeth	Dental trauma; aspiration of tooth

AIDS, *Acquired immunodeficiency syndrome;* CNS, *central nervous system;* IV, *intravenous;* N_2O, *nitrous oxide.*
Modified from Coté CJ, Ryan JF, Todres ID, Goudsouzian NG, eds. A Practice of Anesthesia for Infants and Children. *3rd ed. Philadelphia: Saunders: 1986:540.*

Preoperative Laboratory Testing. Preoperative laboratory tests should be ordered based on abnormal findings from the medical history and physical examination. Box 45-1 lists indications for preoperative laboratory testing. Preoperative hemoglobin determination has characteristically been obtained to provide an assessment of "anesthetic fitness." An "adequate" hemoglobin concentration is essential for oxygen delivery and has been arbitrarily defined as a hemoglobin of 10 g/dL or a hematocrit of 30%. No scientific studies support or refute this "acceptable" quantity. The determination of an acceptable value requires an understanding of the child's current medical history, the proposed surgical procedure, and an understanding of global oxygen transport and use. The value of a "routine" hemoglobin determination has been questioned for some time and has been found rarely to affect the anesthetic management of children.[108,109] The frequency of asymptomatic anemia in a prospective study of 2649 pediatric outpatients was found to be less than 1%, with 7 of 14 anemic patients younger than 1 year of age. However, the frequency of anemia may be as high as 12% in immigrant and indigent children.[110]

Children who benefit from preoperative hemoglobin determinations include premature infants less than 60 weeks' postconceptual age, children with concurrent cardiopulmonary disease, children with known hematologic dysfunction (sickle cell disease), and children in whom major blood loss is anticipated during the surgical procedure.

BOX **45-1**

Indications for Preoperative Laboratory Testing

Complete Blood Count
Hematologic disorder
Vascular procedure
Chemotherapy
Unknown sickle cell syndrome status

Hemoglobin and Hematocrit
<6 months of age (<1 year of age if born premature)
Hematologic malignancy
Recent radiation or chemotherapy
Renal disease
Anticoagulant therapy
Surgical procedures with potential for large blood loss
Coexisting systemic disorders (e.g., cystic fibrosis, prematurity, severe malnutrition, renal failure, hepatic disease, congenital heart disease)

White Blood Cell Count
Leukemia or lymphomas
Recent or concurrent radiation or chemotherapy
Suspected infectious process
Aplastic anemia
Hypersplenism
Autoimmune collagen vascular disease

Blood Glucose
Diabetes mellitus
Current corticosteroid use
History of hypoglycemia
Adrenal disease
Cystic fibrosis

Serum Chemistry
Renal disease
Adrenal or thyroid disease
Previous or concurrent hemotherapy
Pituitary or hypothalamic dysfunction
Body fluid loss or shifts (e.g., dehydration, bowel preparation)
Central nervous system disease

Potassium
Digoxin or diuretic therapy

Creatinine and Blood Urea Nitrogen
Hypertensive cardiovascular disease
Renal disease
Adrenal disease
Diabetes mellitus
Digoxin or diuretic therapy
Body fluid loss or shifts (e.g., dehydration, bowel preparation)
Administration of intravenous radiocontrast material

Liver Function Tests
Hepatic disease
Exposure to hepatotoxic agents

Coagulation Studies
Prothrombin Time
Activated partial thromboplastin time (aPTT)
Leukemia
Hepatic disease
Known coagulation disorder (e.g., hemophilia, Christmas disease)
Concurrent anticoagulant therapy
Severe malnutrition or malabsorption
Platelet Count or Bleeding Time
Known coagulation disorder (e.g., hemophilia, Christmas disease)
Purpura (increase in bruising)

Pregnancy Test
Serum human chorionic gonadotropin (HCG) in menstruating, sexually active patient

Electrocardiogram
Family history of prolonged QT interval
Congenital heart disease
History of sleep apnea or chronic airway obstruction (adenotonsillar hypertrophy)
Possible previously undiagnosed heart murmur

Chest Radiograph
Suspected intrathoracic pathology (e.g., tumors, vascular ring)
Congenital heart disease
History of prematurity with residual bronchopulmonary dysplasia
Obstructive sleep apnea with cardiomegaly

Cervical Spine Radiograph
Down's syndrome (rule out subluxation of atlantooccipital junction)

Modified from Cassidy J, Marley RA. Preoperative assessment of the ambulatory patient. J Perianesth Nurs. *1996;11:334-343.*

The time constraints of preoperative evaluation hinder the child's psychologic preparation, which has ostensibly become the responsibility of the parent or guardian and the surgeon. Children's exhibited behavior is age dependent and shaped by fears of parental separation, postoperative pain, the potential for disfigurement, and the loss of control. Children during the first 6 months of age readily accept strangers and can be separated from their parents, whereas children from 6 months to 5 years of age become distressed when separated from their parents.[111]

Parental preparation is important. The anesthetist will foster trust and confidence through a courteous and understandable explanation of the anesthetic experience. Parental anxiety may be driven by personal past anesthetic experiences, such as painful intravenous catheter placement, coerced mask induction, and postoperative pain, nausea, and vomiting.

Parents offer invaluable information regarding their child's past anesthetic experiences. When the child appears for a repeat surgical procedure, the parents may have important information relative to "what works" and may be helpful in detailing a successful approach. Parental presence during anesthetic induction in preschool-aged and young children may allay the fears of separation for both the parent and the child. The reader is referred to the excellent article by Azarnoff and Woody for additional information on psychologic preparation.[111]

Anesthetic Risk

The parent may inquire about the possibility of serious injury or death associated with the administration of anesthesia. I conduct this discussion with one or both parents out of the hearing of the child.

The anesthetic literature clearly suggests that pediatric patients have anesthetic experiences that are different from those of adults. Anesthetic morbidity and mortality is greater in pediatric patients.[112-117] The anesthetist must appreciate that, although multifactorial in origin, pediatric cardiac arrest is rarely a primary event, but follows the development of hypoxemia or acidosis that is either respiratory (failure to manage the airway) or circulatory (frank inhalation overdose) in origin. A 2000 review of the Pediatric Perioperative Cardiac Arrest Registry by the ASA Committee of the American Academy of Pediatrics Section on Anesthesiology has substantiated the cause of pediatric cardiac arrest to include excess inhalation agent administration, the intravascular injection of local anesthetic, and respiratory management problems. Intraoperative bradycardia is more frequent in infants. Because heart rate is an essential determinant of cardiac output in the infant, intraoperative bradycardia precipitated by high concentrations of inhalation agent or hypoxemia is associated with significant morbidity. Keenan and co-workers found the morbidity accompanying intraoperative bradycardia (heart rate <100 beats/min during the first year of life) to include hypotension, ventricular fibrillation, and death.[115]

A comparison of adult and pediatric closed claims reveals that respiratory complications are more frequent in the pediatric population, and associated outcome is significantly worse.[112] In addition, these respiratory events occur in healthy children of normal weight, as opposed to the adult populations with concurrent cardiopulmonary disease and obesity. Postoperative respiratory complications identified in the recovery room occur more frequently in pediatric patients (13 in 10,000) than in adults (5.9 in 10,000).[114] A reported European estimate of serious injury or death among pediatric patients during anesthesia found a threefold greater incidence in pediatric patients than in adults, and varied between 1 in 20,000 and 1 in 100,000.[113]

In a 6-year prospective examination of over 29,000 pediatric anesthetic procedures, Mooray and colleagues found that children less than 4 weeks of age have the greatest risk of experiencing adverse events during the perioperative period and the greatest risk of perioperative death.[114] These adverse events include hypotension, cardiac arrest, bronchospasm, laryngospasm, and apnea. The risk of complications requiring emergency surgical procedures is also increased in children.[114] Patients between the ages of 1 month and 12 years experience the fewest perioperative anesthetic complications.[114] Children between the ages of 1 and 5 and 6 and 10 have a greater incidence of intraoperative dysrhythmias than adults.[114]

Preoperative Fasting

Gastric regurgitation and pulmonary aspiration are known consequences of general anesthesia. Pathologic conditions that increase the risk of pulmonary aspiration include known difficult airway, impaired protective airway reflexes secondary to neurologic injury, gastroesophageal reflux, gastrointestinal obstruction, morbid obesity, chronic renal failure, and diabetes mellitus. Children undergoing emergency surgical intervention are also at risk. New guidelines for preoperative fasting have been published by the ASA; these guidelines are given in Table 45-10. A modified version is noted in Box 17-15.

The risk of pulmonary aspiration the pediatric patient is extremely low (1 in 10,000).[116] Accordingly, traditional fasting guidelines have become broader. Although the goal of preoperative fasting is to ensure an empty stomach at the time of anesthetic induction, consideration must be given to gastric volume and pH. The determination of risk is based on an experimentally derived case of gastric aspiration in Rhesus monkeys. These studies found that the development of Mendelson's syndrome required a gastric volume of 0.4 ml/kg and a gastric pH of less than 2.5.[117] This benchmark is frequently quoted, yet bears little resemblance to contemporary clinical practice. Gastric volume may be manipulated preoperatively with the administration of antacids (increases gastric pH) and metoclopramide 0.1 mg/kg (stimulates gastric emptying). Metoclopramide may be administered either intravascularly or intramuscularly. Antacids are generally refused by children preoperatively. Although the majority of children have a gastric pH of less than 2.5 and a gastric volume in excess of 0.4 ml/kg after an overnight fast, pulmonary aspiration remains an infrequent event.[118-120]

Prolonged fasting may produce irritability as a result of thirst and hunger. Prolonged fasting may also alter fluid balance, producing preinduction hypovolemia and hypoglycemia. Hypoglycemia is especially problematic in premature infants. Preoperative access to clear fluids (e.g., apple juice, water) 2 hours before anesthetic induction has been shown to have a minimal impact on the resultant gastric volume and pH.[121]

Several factors, including glucose content, osmolarity, and concentrations of proteins and lipids, affect the gastric emptying of infant formula and milk. Litman and colleagues found that fasting intervals of 2 hours after breast-feeding result in high residual gastric volumes (>1 ml/kg).[122]

The new guidelines are known loosely as the 2, 4, 6, 8 guidelines (Table 45-10). Many institutions have liberalized thin fasting guidelines to reflect local practice with no increase in morbidity.[121] Heavy meals and fatty foods require an 8-hour fasting time.

TABLE 45-10 Preoperative Fasting Recommendations

Ingested Materials	Minimum Fasting Period* (hr)
Clear liquids†	2
Breast milk	4
Infant formula	6
Non-human milk‡	6
Light meal§	6

These recommendations apply to healthy patients who are undergoing elective procedures. They are not intended for women in labor. Following the Guidelines does not guarantee complete gastric emptying.
**The fasting periods noted above apply to all ages.*
†Examples of clear liquids include water, fruit juices without pulp, carbonated beverages, clear tea, and black coffee.
‡Since non-human milk is similar to solids in gastric emptying time, the amount ingested must be considered when determining an appropriate fasting period.
§A light meal typically consists of toast and clear liquids. Meals that include fried or fatty foods or meat may prolong gastric emptying time. Both the amount and type of foods ingested must be considered when determining an appropriate fasting period.
Summary of Fasting Recommendations to Reduce the Risk of Pulmonary Aspiration. From Anesthesiology. *1999;90(3):896-905.*

Preoperative Controversies

Upper Respiratory Infection. Upper respiratory infections (URIs) are common in the pediatric age group, are seasonal in occurrence, and may be accompanied by cough, pharyngitis, tonsillitis, and croup. The child with an active or resolving URI has increased airway reactivity, a propensity for the development of atelectasis and mucous plugging of the airways, and the potential to experience postoperative arterial hypoxemia.[123] In addition, bronchial reactivity may persist for 6 to 8 weeks after a viral lower respiratory tract infection. The presence of chronic respiratory disease (asthma or bronchopulmonary dysplasia) requires a thorough assessment to ensure that the disease is well controlled and the child is not currently experiencing an exacerbation. The anesthetist must understand the child's routine pharmacologic management. A history of steroid use necessitates consideration of steroid supplementation throughout the perioperative period.

Healthy children who are scheduled for the placement of tympanostomy tubes frequently have rhinitis. In deciding whether to proceed with anesthesia, additional history must be obtained to differentiate between a chronic allergic or an acute infectious presentation and to determine whether involvement of the lower airway exists. The assessment of the color and the duration of nasal drainage will assist in deciding whether rhinorrhea is chronic or acute. Purulent nasal discharge associated with pharyngitis, cough, or fever is certainly indicative of a bacterial or viral URI. Additional information may be obtained by questioning the parents regarding their assessment of the child's current health. Does the child appear sick? Is the child eating, sleeping, and playing normally? Are siblings or anyone in the family currently ill? Children with chronic allergic rhinorrhea exhibited as clear nasal drainage without accompanying signs of illness (no cough, pharyngitis, wheezing, or associated fever) are probably in satisfactory condition for elective general anesthesia with no imposed increased risk.

Lower respiratory tract dysfunction typically accompanies viral or bacterial URI. This combination may be associated with a greater frequency of laryngospasm (fivefold greater incidence) and bronchospasm (tenfold greater incidence) during anesthetic management, particularly when endotracheal intubation is performed.[124] Although mild URI may be inconsequential during the intraoperative period, significant problems may develop in the immediate postoperative period. Studies have noted an increase in the incidence of postintubation croup, hypoxemia, and bronchospasm in patients with URIs compared with asymptomatic children.[124-126]

Multiple factors must be considered when one is deciding whether to cancel an elective procedure. Olsson and Hallen noted persistent spirometric changes indicative of bronchial hyperactivity for up to 7 weeks after URI and recommend postponing surgery for this period of time.[124] Postponement for 7 weeks may not be practical, because children experience multiple URIs (as many as 6 to 8 per year). Children with signs and symptoms of acute airway dysfunction should have further medical evaluation by a pediatrician. A white blood cell count of 12,000 to 15,000/mm^3 suggests the presence of infection, and the surgery should be canceled. Clearly, elective surgery should be postponed for children who have a cough and pharyngitis accompanied by fever and wheezing. Some recommendations based on a thorough review of the literature are shown in Box 45-2.

Heart Murmur. A history of a heart murmur may be relayed by the parent, or a murmur may be discovered during the physical examination. It is important that the significance of the heart murmur be understood before anesthesia. The murmur may not impose a functional limitation; however, this may change with the physiologic trespass of an anesthesia. For example, the child with aortic stenosis may function appropriately as long as the heart rate is capable of sustaining a normal cardiac output. Decreases in heart rate or acute hypotension after anesthetic induction with an inhaled agent will be poorly tolerated. For children with a previously diagnosed heart murmur, the parent may be able to provide information regarding the relevance of the murmur. Previous records may also contain information regarding its significance and whether additional testing was performed to assess its physiologic import. Children with "functional" murmurs are generally asymptomatic, without the presence of cyanosis, and are growing appropriately. An example of a functional murmur is the Still's vibratory systolic murmur, which is common in children between the ages of 2 and 6 years. It is important that previously undiagnosed murmurs be evaluated by a pediatrician or cardiologist before the induction of anesthesia. Auscultation of the chest and a detailed patient history may determine that the murmur is "functional" and that no additional studies are required. However, the consultant may wish to obtain additional information by means of an echocardiogram. The reader is directed to an excellent review by Pelech of the evaluation of the pediatric patient with a cardiac murmur.[127]

Bacterial Endocarditis Prophylaxis. Surgical procedures that involve invasion of mucosal surfaces may produce transient bacteremia in which bacteria may lodge on abnormal heart valves or within the endocardium. Accordingly, patients with abnormalities in cardiac structure require prophylaxis against the effects of these bacteremic periods. A great deal of confusion often surrounds the requirement of prophylaxis in particular patients. Box 45-3 lists the indications for which prophylaxis is indicated and not indicated as currently recommended by the American Heart Association's published guide-

BOX **45-2**

Recommendations for Patients With Upper Respiratory Tract Infections

These recommendations are neither clinical guidelines nor a consensus statement and should not replace clinical judgment, but they should serve as a guide to help make a rational decisions with parents, surgeons, and patients. The absence of a visit for preoperative evaluation does not eliminate the need for an exchange of information between families and the center, which should occur before the day of surgery. Efforts should make parents aware of the problems with respiratory tract infections and anesthesia, and parents should be encouraged to call before the day of surgery to discuss the symptoms and possible need for delay of surgery. There may be a role for pediatricians and other primary care practitioners to play in the process of perioperative evaluation and education.

- First, an emergency case mandates judicious airway management and logically must proceed regardless of the presence or absence of respiratory symptoms. In patients presenting for elective (nonurgent) surgery, initial consideration should be with respect to the severity of respiratory tract symptoms.
- Acute symptoms, such as runny nose and cough, must be differentiated from chronic symptoms related to underlying diseases such as allergic rhinitis (clear runny nose) and asthma (cough).
- Often careful questioning of parents can differentiate acute from chronic symptoms.
- Patients with severe symptoms such as fever (>38.4° C), malaise, productive cough, wheezing, or rhonchi should be considered for delay of elective surgery. A reasonable period of delay would be 4-6 weeks.
- If mild symptoms are present, such as nonproductive cough, sneezing, or mild nasal congestion, then surgery could proceed for those having regional or general anesthesia without endotracheal tube placement. However, those patients, especially children less than 1 year of age, who require endotracheal tube placement for anesthesia, should be considered carefully for other risk factors such as passive smoke exposure and underlying conditions (i.e., asthma, chronic lung disease, etc.) because they may benefit from a slight delay of 2-4 weeks.

Modified From Easley, RB, Maxwell LG. Should a Child with a Respiratory Tract Infection Undergo Elective Surgery? In: Fleisher LA, ed. Evidence-Based Practice of Anesthesiology, *WB Saunders, Philadelphia, 2004:424.*

lines. Tables 45-11 and 45-12 provide a schedule of the standard prophylactic regimen for pediatric patients at risk for subacute bacterial endocarditis who are undergoing dental, oral, esophageal, or respiratory procedures. For a detailed account of dosage regimens the reader is referred to the original reference by Dajani and colleagues.[128]

Dermatologic Eruptions. Skin rashes are common manifestations of a variety of infectious diseases in children. Children may appear for a preoperative evaluation and exhibit a skin rash after a recent illness. Common childhood diseases that have an accompanying rash may be viral (measles, rubella, fifth disease) or bacterial in origin (rheumatic fever, scarlet fever). An accurate

BOX **45-3**

Procedures for Which Prophylaxis against Bacterial Endocarditis Is Indicated and Not Indicated in Children

Prophylaxis Recommended

Dental procedures known to induce gingival or mucosal bleeding, including professional cleaning and scaling
Tonsillectomy or adenoidectomy
Surgery involving gastrointestinal or upper respiratory mucosa
Bronchoscopy with rigid bronchoscope
Sclerotherapy for esophageal varices
Gallbladder surgery
Cytoscopy, uretheral dilation
Urethral catheterization if urinary infection is present
Urinary tract surgery, including prostate surgery
Incision and drainage of infected tissue*
Vaginal hysterectomy
Vaginal delivery complicated by infection

Prophylaxis Not Recommended

Dental procedures not likely to cause bleeding, such as adjustment of orthodontic appliances and simple fillings above the gum line
Intraoral injection of local anesthetic
Shedding of primary teeth
Tympanostomy tube insertion
Endotracheal tube insertion
Bronchoscopy with flexible bronchoscope, with or without biopsy†
Cardiac catheterization
Gastrointestinal endoscopy, with or without biopsy
Cesarean section
In absence of infection: urethral catheterization, dilation and curettage, uncomplicated vaginal delivery, therapeutic abortion, insertion or removal of intrauterine device, sterilization procedures, laparoscopy

**In patients at highest risk, physicians may elect to use prophylaxis for these procedures.*
†Antibiotic prophylaxis should be directed against the most likely endocarditis-associated pathogen(s), often staphylococci.
Modified from Dajani AS, Bisno AL, Chung KJ, et al. Prevention of bacterial endocarditis: recommendations by the American Heart Association. JAMA. *1990;264:2919-2922.*

history of the course of illness and the identification of the morphology of the rash may provide clues to the cause. A pediatric or dermatologic consultation may be needed to determine the correct cause. The appearance of a skin rash may be delayed as a result of the long incubation period of the viral illness. Varicella (chicken pox) occurrence is most frequent between January and May. The incubation period of this viral illness is such that skin eruptions may not be apparent for up to 3 weeks after exposure. The taking of the medical history during the preoperative visit should therefore include questions about whether the child has been exposed to anyone with chicken pox or other infectious diseases. If an exposure has occurred within the 21-day incubation period and the child has failed to exhibit signs of the disease, it may be best to postpone elective surgery and await the development of the illness. Children who are

TABLE 45-11 Indications for Subacute Bacterial Endocarditis Prophylaxis

Endocarditis Prophylaxis Recommended
High-Risk Category
Prosthetic cardiac valves (bioprosthesis and homografts)
Previous bacterial endocarditis
Complex cyanotic congenital heart disease (e.g., single ventricle, transposition of great vessels, tetralogy of Fallot)
Surgically constructed systemic pulmonary artery shunts
Moderate-Risk Category
Congenital cardiac malformations (not noted above)
Acquired valvular dysfunction (e.g., rheumatic heart disease)
Hypertrophic cardiomyopathy
Mitral valve prolapse with valvular regurgitation or thickened leaflets
Endocarditis Prophylaxis Not Recommended
Negligible-Risk Category (No Greater than the General Population)
Isolated secundum atrial septal defect
Surgical repair of atrial septal defect, ventricular septal defect, or patent ductus arteriosis (without residua beyond 6 months)
Previous coronary artery bypass graft surgery
Mitral valve prolapse without valvular regurgitation
Physiologic, functional, or innocent heart murmurs
Previous Kawasaki disease without valvular dysfunction
Previous rheumatic fever without valvular dysfunction
Cardiac pacemakers (intravascular and epicardial) and implanted defibrillators

Modified from Dajani AS, Taubert KA, Wilson W, et al. Prevention of bacterial endocarditis: recommendations by the American Heart Association. JAMA. *1997;277:1794-1801.*

TABLE 45-12 Prophylactic Regimen for Dental, Oral, Esophageal, and Respiratory Tract Procedures in Children

Situation	Agent	Regimen
Standard prophylaxis	Amoxicillin	50 mg/kg orally 1 hr before procedure
Unable to take oral medication	Ampicillin	50 mg/kg IM, or IV within 30 min before procedure
Allergic to penicillin	Clindamycin	20 mg/kg orally 1 hr before procedure
	or	
	Cephalexin or cefadroxil	50 mg/kg orally 1 hr before procedure
	or	
	Azithromycin or clathromycin	15 mg/kg orally 1 hr before procedure
Unable to take penicillin or oral medication	Clindamycin	20 mg/kg IV within 30 min of procedure
	or	
	Cefazolin	25 mg/kg IM or IV within 30 min of procedure

IM, *Intramuscular;* IV, *intravenous.*
From Dajani AS, Taubert KA, Wilson W, et al. Prevention of bacterial endocarditis: recommendations by the American Heart Association. JAMA. *1997;277:1794-1801.*

exposed to an infectious agent may be infectious themselves before the development of the characteristic rash. Anesthetizing these children (in elective surgical cases) risks unnecessary exposure of additional individuals in the operating room and recovery room. Table 45-13 lists the typical skin eruptions, along with the characteristics of the accompanying disease and the recommended isolation and appropriate treatment.

The Premature Infant

Infants born before 37 weeks of gestation are considered premature. Advances in neonatal medicine have improved the survival of these infants. Accordingly, the premature infant is not an infrequent visitor to the operating room for either elective or emergent surgical intervention. Prematurity presents its own set of complications, which include anemia, aspiration with feeding, intraventricular hemorrhage, periodic apnea accompanied by bradycardia, and chronic respiratory dysfunction.

Premature infants are challenging to evaluate, and considerable controversy exists regarding the appropriateness of elective surgical intervention and proper postoperative care. Postconceptual age (gestational age + postnatal age) should be determined at the time of the anesthetic evaluation. Premature infants of less than 60 weeks postconceptual age have the greatest risk of experiencing postanesthetic complications; outpatient

TABLE 45-13 Dermatologic Eruptions and Clinical Characteristics

Pathogen	Lesion	Disease Course	Isolation	Treatment
Measles (rubeola) Spread by droplet (nasopharyngeal fluids, blood, urine, feces)	Generalized maculopapular or macular rash; enanthem (Koplik's spots) on oral mucosa	Infective 7-10 days until 5 days after appearance of rash; mild to moderate fever, worsening cough, conjunctivitis, photophobia	From onset until third day of rash; highly communicable; some quarantine, although it is of little value	Sedatives, antipyretics, bed rest, hydration
German measles (rubella) Spread by droplet and transplacentally	Generalized maculopapular or macular rash; facial exanthem that spreads rapidly, clearing on the third day; easily confused with rubeola	Incubation 14-21 days; infective 7 days before appearance of rash; tender posterior cervical lymph nodes	Avoid exposure throughout pregnancy	Symptomatic treatment
Scarlet fever Spread by droplet and food	Diffuse erythroderma (sandpaper rash on abdomen)	Derived from *Streptococcus aureus* infection; incubation 1-7 days; acute onset fever and chills, with development of rash in 12-36 hours; headache, pharyngitis with circumoral pallor; desquamation end of week 1		Penicillin and symptomatic treatment
Chicken pox (varicella) Spread by droplet and direct contact; peak age 5-9 yr	Vesicular, bulbous, pustular	Incubation 10-21 days; infective from 24 hours before rash appearance until all lesions crusted; fever, malaise, anorexia before rash; small red papules beginning on trunk, spreading to face, scalp with little involvement of extremities; vesicles scab but are easily broken because of accompanying pruritus	Isolated until all lesions have scabs	Topically applied antipruritics, perhaps topical or oral acyclovir
Erythema infectiosum (fifth disease) Mechanism of spread unknown	Maculopapular or macular "slapped-cheek" appearance with maculopapular rash on trunk, extremities, lasting up to 40 days	Incubation 7-28 days; low-grade or absent fever	Not required	None

From Aker J. *Preoperative preparation of the pediatric patient*. Nurse Anesth. 1996;1:1.

BOX 45-4

Factors Contributing to the Incidence of Apnea in the Premature Infant

Central Contributors
Inadequate development of respiratory center
Incomplete myelination of central nervous system

Metabolic Contributors
Hypothermia
Hypoglycemia
Hypocalcemia
Acidosis

Anesthetic Contributors
Residual inhalation anesthesia
Residual opioid plasma concentrations

From Aker J. Preoperative preparation of the pediatric patient: capsules and comments. Nurse Anesth. *1996;1:1.*

surgical care is not an acceptable venue for premature infants. The manifestations of prematurity are thought to occur as a result of inadequate development of respiratory drive and immature cardiovascular responses to hypoxia and hypercapnia. Therefore premature infants have a significant risk of postoperative apnea and bradycardia during the first 24 hours after general anesthesia.[129-131] Box 45-4 lists contributing factors that may influence the occurrence of apnea in premature infants.

Some generalities regarding the frequency of postoperative apnea can be made.[131-135] The incidence of apnea in the postoperative period is inversely related to postconceptual age and is most frequent in infants of less than 50 weeks postconceptual age. Apnea may still occur when regional anesthetic techniques have been substituted for general anesthesia.[133] Premature infants without a history of apnea or bradycardia may still experience postoperative apnea. Premature infants with histories of respiratory distress, concurrent respiratory disease, and periods of apnea are twice as likely to develop postoperative apnea.[132] Concurrent anemia (hematocrit <30%) places additional risk for the occurrence of postoperative apnea.[131]

Kurth and colleagues recommend the admittance of all premature infants of less than 60 weeks postconceptual age after general anesthesia, with continuous monitoring for apnea and bradycardia for at least the first 24 hours.[132] Such children should have a minimum of 12 apnea-free hours before dismissal.[132] Welborn recommends deferral of elective surgical procedures until 44 weeks postconceptual age. Infants younger than 44 weeks postconceptual age should be admitted postoperatively and monitored for at least 12 hours for the occurrence of apnea and bradycardia.[135] The care of these infants is further clouded by a recent report suggesting the need for oxygen monitoring in the postoperative period. Prolonged periods of hypoxemia may be unaccompanied by bradycardia or apnea in healthy premature infants.[136] The reader is encouraged to consult Welborn's comprehensive reviews of perioperative apnea in premature infants.[131,135]

Although the literature supports an increased risk for premature infants up to 60 weeks postconceptual age, debate continues as to when this risk decreases. Mestad and colleagues found that premature infants at 40 weeks postconceptual age without a history of apnea or bradycardia can be safely discharged after outpatient anesthesia.[134]

Premedication

The selection and administration of premedication for the pediatric patient requires an understanding of the desired goals, the planned surgical procedure (inpatient or outpatient procedure), the familiarity and previous experiences with the particular drug, and the availability of nursing staff to monitor the child after the drug's administration (Box 45-5). The ideal premedicant should be dependable, with a rapid and reliable onset and offset, and should be devoid of undesirable effects. The use of "cookbook" doses of premedicants is hazardous and may produce general anesthesia in some children while producing ineffective sedation in others. Table 45-14 lists commonly prescribed pediatric premedicants.

Premedication must be individualized to account for differences in maturation and development and the child's previous surgical experiences. The reliance on pharmacologic premedication in preparing the child for the surgical experience should not be routine; rather, it should be reserved for children who are extremely apprehensive. Anxiolytics and sedatives may prolong the time to discharge, thereby increasing patient care costs.[137-139] Children older than 1 year of age may benefit from anxiolytic premedication to decrease preoperative anxiety and modify behavioral changes after discharge.[140]

Midazolam has great utility as a premedicant in the pediatric patient. This short-acting, highly lipophilic benzodiazepine produces amnesia and anxiolysis and in sufficient dosages may also produce sleep (hypnosis). Serious respiratory events (respiratory depression, airway obstruction, apnea, and oxygen desaturation) may develop after the administration of midazolam. Resuscitative equipment must be immediately available.

Midazolam may be administered by a variety of routes, including parenteral (intravenous, intramuscular), transmucosal (intranasal, rectal), and oral. The parents should be instructed to hold the child or place the child on a cart, preventing ambulation. Appropriate monitoring is imperative after midazolam administration. A health-care provider should remain within

BOX 45-5

Goals for Premedication

Anxiolysis
Amnesia (insertion of invasive monitoring)
Analgesia (children in pain)
Antisialagogue (airway manipulation)
Increase gastric pH
Reduction of gastric volume
Reduce anesthetic requirements
Blunting of central nervous system reflex responses
Prophylaxis
Subacute bacterial endocarditis
  Allergic reactions (latex)
  Postoperative nausea and vomiting
  Infectious processes

Modified from Moline BM, Marley RA. Midazolam as a pediatric premedicant in the ambulatory setting. J Perianesth Nurs. *1997;12:42-47.*

TABLE 45-14 Commonly Prescribed Pediatric Premedicants—Premedicant Dose and Route of Administration

Anticholinergics	
Atropine	0.02 mg/kg PO, IV, IM
Glycopyrrolate	0.01 mg IV
Opioids	
Morphine sulfate	0.1-0.3 mg/kg IM
Meperidine	1.5-2 mg/kg PO 1-2 mg/kg IM
Benzodiazepines	
Diazepam	0.1-0.5 mg/kg PO
Midazolam	0.07-0.1 mg/kg IM 0.2 mg/kg nasally 0.025-0.05 mg/kg IV 0.25-0.5 mg/kg PO 0.5-1 mg/kg rectally
Barbiturates	
Methohexital (10%)	10 mg/kg IM 20-30 mg/kg rectally
Other	
Ketamine	3-6 mg/kg PO 3 mg/kg nasally 2-10 mg/kg IM

IM, *Intramuscular*; IV, *intravenous*; PO, *orally*.

eye contact of the child, and continuous oxygen saturation monitoring should be initiated by pulse oximetry.

The dose for intramuscular midazolam ranges from 0.07 to 0.1 mg/kg, with an onset time between 30 and 60 minutes. The intramuscular route is the least desirable because of the anxiety and the pain associated with parenteral injection, but this route may be necessary in children who refuse to swallow a liquid. The crying that accompanies intramuscular injection has been reported to produce oxygen desaturation in children with congenital heart disease.[141]

The intravenous route is rapid and reliable and allows for the titration of additional drug. An intravenous dose of 0.025 to 0.05 mg/kg produces on onset of action within 1 to 2 minutes. However, intravenous access is generally not established before the induction of anesthesia and is rarely indicated for the administration of a premedicant.

Intranasal administration of midazolam avoids first-pass metabolism and provides a rapid onset. A dose of 0.2 mg/kg produces effective sedation in 2 to 10 minutes. The calculated dose may be administered via a syringe, alternating nares, but parental assistance is required (the parent holds the child's head). Children frequently object to this route of administration, and this practice is falling out of favor. Midazolam administered intranasally may produce nasal burning and an unpleasant taste (the intravenous formulation contains benzyl alcohol). The intranasal route of drug administration may be disagreeable to parents and anesthesia providers, as it is commonly associated with the self-administration of recreational drugs.

Oral premedicants are generally accepted by children, particularly after an unexpected nothing-by-mouth (NPO) period. Rapid absorption occurs after the oral administration of midazolam. Oral administration is the least threatening but can also be the most challenging in uncooperative children. It may be difficult to determine the ingested dose, as children may swallow only a portion of the desired dose and refuse the remainder or may expectorate the dose after tasting the mixture (formulation with benzyl alcohol). Before the recent release of an oral formulation, intravenous midazolam was mixed with a variety of oral fluids, including apple juice, acetaminophen elixir, cherry and chocolate syrups, and flavored gelatins, in an attempt to disguise the unpleasant taste. A cherry-flavored midazolam syrup is now available (Roche Laboratories) and appears to be more palatable than the intravenous preparation.

Monitoring

As previously discussed, anesthetic morbidity and mortality are greater in pediatric patients, and intraoperative vigilance is imperative if poor anesthetic outcomes are to be averted. Patient blood pressure and heart rate are monitored for the assessment of the cardiovascular system. Pulse oximetry and capnography are used for the assessment of the adequacy of oxygenation and ventilation, a temperature probe for intermittent or continuous assessment of core body temperature, and a neuromuscular function monitor for the evaluation of the child's response to the administration of neuromuscular blocking drugs.[142] A precordial or esophageal stethoscope should be used for the continuous assessment of heart rate during anesthetic induction and throughout the perioperative period.

Pulse oximetry is essential for anesthetic induction. Artifactual alarms occur with excessive movement of the child, interference from environmental ultraviolet light and radiant lamps, and intermittent interference from electrocautery.[143] It may also be difficult to obtain an expired gas sample for accurate determination of end-tidal CO_2 when a nonrebreathing circuit is used. A more accurate determination may be obtained by sampling the expired gas as close as possible to the endotracheal tube or perhaps through aspiration from the endotracheal tube itself.[144,145] Thin sampling tubes are commercially available and may be inserted into the endotracheal tube for the sampling of expired gases.

Some circumstances require the application of arterial and central venous pressure monitoring. Fluid overload from the continuous heparinized flush is a real danger in the pediatric patient and may produce an iatrogenic coagulopathy. Small multilumen catheters are available for the pediatric patient. We find these catheters advantageous when large blood losses are expected (e.g., during burn débridement and skin grafting). However, these catheters have long thin lumens that may severely limit the rate at which intravenous fluid or blood may be administered. When rapid flow is advantageous, a peripheral intravenous line may be used for maintenance and deficit fluid replacement, and a single-lumen venous catheter placed within the femoral vein may be reserved for colloid and blood administration.

Anesthetic Induction

Mask Induction

Anesthetic induction may be accomplished in a variety of ways and is dependent on the child's current state of health, the age and level of anxiety, the proposed surgical procedure, and the parents' agreement with regard to the proposed anesthetic plan. Mask induction is the most popular and is easily accomplished in infants less than 8 months of age, as they are easily separated from their parents. The essential monitoring modalities for inhalation induction include a precordial stethoscope and a pulse oximeter. The remainder of the monitors are placed by an assistant during the induction period, after the patient has lost consciousness. Anesthetic induction is begun with a 70:30 mixture of nitrous oxide and oxygen via mask or a "cupped hand" that is placed on the infant's cheek with the anesthetic mixture directed toward the mouth and nose. The infant may suck a pacifier or the end of a finger, which quiets the infant. Either halothane or sevoflurane is added to the nitrous oxide–oxygen mixture beginning with a 0.5% concentration, with 0.5% incremental increases every four or five breaths. Breath-holding may occur if the inspired concentration is increased too quickly. The mask is then introduced as the inspired concentration is increased. The anesthetist should await the return of respiration and avoid the temptation to administer a breath, as this may produce coughing and laryngospasm. Unconsciousness is produced with inspired halothane concentrations of 3% to 4%, and 6% to 8% for sevoflurane. After the loss of consciousness, nitrous oxide is discontinued, with the continued administration of the selected inhalation agent in 100% oxygen. At this time the anesthetist should begin to assist respiration and promptly decrease the inspired anesthetic concentration of halothane to 1.5% to 2%, or of sevoflurane to 2% to 2.5%. Controlled ventilation with high inspired concentrations of inhalation agent aggravate myocardial depression, precipitating the development of sudden cardiac arrest.[112-115]

During assisted ventilation intravenous access should be established. The age of the child, proposed surgical procedure, and ease of airway management during induction are the determining factors for whether to proceed with intravenous access. It is my practice to establish intravenous access in all children before laryngoscopy and endotracheal intubation. For elective surgical procedures neonates may be managed with a 24-gauge catheter, infants with a 22-gauge catheter, and children with a 20-gauge catheter. Surgical procedures with expected large third-space fluid loss or blood loss require an additional intravenous catheter. Preferred sites for intravenous access include the nondominant upper extremity (dorsum of the hand, antecubital fossa) and the lower extremity (dorsum of the foot, the saphenous vein). Scalp veins are alternative sites in the premature or neonate. The scalp site should be reserved for fluid administration, as the injection of alkaline drugs (e.g., thiopental) into the scalp vein may produce necrosis and sloughing of the scalp. The deep saphenous vein is most easily accessed with a 20- or 22-gauge catheter. This vein can be identified by placing the thumb over the medial malleolus and moving it toward the anterior portion of the tibia. By extending the foot and piercing the skin parallel to the tibia and passing subcutaneously, the saphenous vein may be entered. Tincture of benzoin is applied to the intravenous site and adjacent skin, and the catheter is secured with a sterile clear dressing. The extremity is secured with a padded board, and the intravenous site is covered with a gauze dressing.

After the establishment of intravenous access, preparations are made for endotracheal intubation. Intubation may be accomplished using the inhaled anesthetic agent without muscle relaxation or after the administration of a nondepolarizing neuromuscular blocker. The administration of a neuromuscular blocker decreases the potential for the cardiovascular depression that accompanies the administration of high concentrations of inhalation agents that may be required to facilitate laryngoscopy and intubation (see the discussion of anesthetic risk). Endotracheal intubation in children ages 2 to 6 requires a 1.2% end-tidal concentration of halothane to provide acceptable conditions for laryngoscopy and intubation.[146] A recent survey of members of the Society of Pediatric Anesthesia found that inhalation agent administration without neuromuscular blockade was used to facilitate endotracheal intubation 38% of the time in infants (0 to 12 months) and 43.6% of the time in children (1 to 7 years old).[147] Whatever method is selected, I recommend that the inhalation agent be discontinued immediately before laryngoscopy. This practice minimizes the contamination of the operating room with free-flowing inhalation agent from the patient breathing circuit, and, more important, the delivery of high inspired anesthetic concentrations is avoided immediately after intubation during the confirmation of endotracheal tube placement. After confirmation of successful placement, the endotracheal tube is secured and the position of the tube at the alveolar ridge or lip is noted on the anesthetic record.

Older children (>1 year of age) may have difficulty with separation from their parents and may require premedication to ease their anxiety. To ease the anxiety of separation at my institution, one cooperative parent or guardian is invited to "dress up" and accompany the child to the operating room. Parental presence has been demonstrated to reduce anxiety and may obviate the need for premedication.[148,149] The child is placed in the lap of the parent, or the child may sit on the operating table while remaining in contact with the parent. Older children with previous anesthetic experiences may find mask induction unpleasant but generally prefer this method over a frightening attempt at intravenous access. Preoperatively the anesthetist may allow the child to select a scented mask or to choose a favorite scented oil, which is then coated inside the mask (Loran Oils, Lansing, Michigan). The child is persuaded to participate through conversation, and the parent or guardian is also encouraged to participate (to assist in holding the mask). The child may be fearful of the many "wires" and "tubes" of the various monitoring modalities. The child is introduced to the pulse oximeter, as this is the minimum monitoring for the initial induction of children who resist the application of a precordial stethoscope, ECG leads, and the noninvasive blood pressure cuff. Before induction an explanation is provided to the parent or guardian regarding the expected behavior of the child (excitement, spontaneous involuntary movements, snoring, floppy appearance with unconsciousness). Induction begins with the introduction of a 70:30 mixture of nitrous oxide and oxygen via a "cupped hand" or the selected mask, with the subsequent introduction of either halothane or sevoflurane as described previously. When the child becomes unconscious with a regular respiratory rate, he or she is carefully lifted from the lap of the parent or guardian and placed supine on the operating table (the parent is escorted out at this point). Subsequently the ECG and a noninvasive blood pressure cuff are applied, and intravenous access is established. Endotracheal intubation is accomplished as previously described.

Intravenous Induction

Intravenous induction is generally reserved for the child with an existing intravenous line. An intravenous induction may be clinically indicated when the child has a full stomach or a history of gastroesophageal reflux. Intravenous induction is quicker and more dependable, facilitating the rapid securing of the airway with endotracheal intubation. Venipuncture can be a frightening experience for the older child, particularly for the child who is afraid of needles. Oral premedication with midazolam before the child enters the operating room may be beneficial to decrease the child's anxiety and gain his or her cooperation. The following describes a successful technique I employ for venipuncture in nonemergent situations.

The child is brought to the operating room accompanied by two anesthesia providers and is encouraged to assume the supine position on the operating table. If the child is cooperative, we apply the essential monitors. One of the anesthetists is positioned on either side of the child and initiates a conversation. The pediatric breathing circuit is within easy reach of this anesthetist. The arm selected for venipuncture is positioned behind the hip of the anesthetist, minimizing the child's view of the preparations for venipuncture. During the casual conversation the anesthetist grasps and squeezes the upper arm, providing a tourniquet effect. This eliminates the application of a rubber tourniquet, which may increase the child's anxiety. The selected intravenous induction agent is drawn into a syringe and connected to the intravenous administration extension set through a stopcock. The venipuncture site is quickly prepared with alcohol, a subdermal injection of lidocaine is made with a 30-gauge needle, the selected intravenous catheter is inserted, the induction dose of thiopental is administered, and the intravenous catheter is secured with one strip of tape. I generally avoid the selection of propofol in this situation because of the discomfort associated with its injection immediately after intravenous catheter insertion.

The pain associated with preoperative intravenous access may be eased with the subcutaneous injection of local anesthetic via a 30-gauge needle. Additional analgesia may be provided by an anesthetist via the administration of a 70:30 mixture of nitrous oxide and oxygen during venipuncture. Cautious administration of nitrous oxide is warranted in children with gastroesophageal reflux or impaired swallowing, as nitrous oxide may blunt the protective airway reflexes, increasing the risk of aspiration. The timely application of EMLA cream, a eutectic mixture of local anesthetic, will also minimize the pain of venipuncture. Suitable intravenous sites are identified preoperatively and marked with an ink pen. EMLA is applied well in advance (30 to 60 minutes) to ensure effectiveness and covered with a Tegaderm dressing. Several over-the-counter preparations are now available, as described in Chapter 9. The child is then taken to the operating room and encouraged to lie on the operating table. At this time the essential monitors are applied. An operating room assistant is positioned next to and in full view of the child and initiates a conversation with the child and parent (if present). While the conversation is being conducted, the operating room assistant grasps the upper extremity selected for venipuncture, squeezing the arm to provide a tourniquet effect. The venipuncture site is quickly prepared with alcohol, and the selected intravenous catheter is inserted and secured with one piece of tape. The proper dose of intravenous induction agent is connected to the intravenous administration set via a stopcock, which facilitates its rapid administration and minimizes the time between venipuncture and unconsciousness.

Rectal Induction

Before parents were permitted to be present in the operating room or "induction" room, the rectal administration of thiopental or methohexital in the hospital room allowed the parent to remain with the child during anesthetic induction. The rectal administration of methohexital has been found to be safe and effective in children who are fearful of venipuncture or inhalation induction.[150-152] The absorption and bioavailability of rectal methohexital is influenced by the depth of catheter insertion in the rectum, drug absorption within the rectum, and the amount of drug absorbed by the upper rectum. Recall from the previous discussion that drug carried from the superior rectal vein (proximal rectum) into the portal system undergoes first-pass metabolism; drug absorbed by the middle and inferior rectal veins travels directly to the systemic circulation.

The rectal administration of methohexital is best suited for children between the ages of 1 and 3 years. Rectal methohexital is administered to children through a soft plastic catheter that is inserted no more than 3 cm into the rectum while the child is comforted by the parent. A dose of 25 to 30 mg/kg of a 2% solution produces higher plasma concentrations than a 10% solution and produces sleep (unconsciousness) within 15 minutes in 86% of children.[153,154] These large rectal doses of methohexital administered to healthy pediatric patients have been demonstrated to produce minimal hemodynamic alterations.[155]

Intramuscular Induction

On rare occasions an intramuscularly administered drug may be required in uncooperative children or in children who refuse alternative routes (oral, nasal, or rectal) for premedication. Ketamine, a derivative of phencyclidine, produces dose-dependent unconsciousness and analgesia via blockade of the excitatory neurotransmitter glutamic acid at the *N*-methyl-D-aspartate (NMDA) receptor. After administration the child may appear to be in a catatonic state. Parents who witness the administration of ketamine should be warned that their child may exhibit spontaneous involuntary movements and nystagmus. Ketamine is a cardiac stimulant that produces an increase in systemic blood pressure and heart rate. Additional undesirable effects include bronchodilation, increases in intraocular and intracranial pressure, disorientation, unpleasant dreaming, and hallucinations. The psychogenic effects may be decreased with the concomitant administration of a benzodiazepine. Intramuscular ketamine in a dose of 2 to 3 mg/kg facilitates inhalation induction in children who are reluctant to be subjected to inhalation induction or venipuncture.[156] Ketamine doses between 5 and 10 mg/kg are associated with a lengthy recovery period and the inability to accept oral fluids.[157] Ketamine may be injected in a small volume, as a variety of formulated concentrations exists. Ketamine is particularly advantageous in children with cardiovascular instability, as the cardiovascular system is stimulated via the CNS.

Intramuscular midazolam and methohexital may be used to induce sleep. Intramuscular midazolam (0.1 to 0.15 mg/kg) may also be used as a premedicant. The intramuscular administration of 6 mg/kg of methohexital produces sleep within 5 minutes in children between the ages of 1 and 3 years.[158] Intramuscular induction is less reliable and more uncomfortable for the child.

Intravenous Fluid and Blood Therapy

The maintenance of fluid homeostasis is essential in the comprehensive intraoperative care of the pediatric patient. The restoration and maintenance of the smaller pediatric intravascular volume is crucial if cardiac output is to be optimized and tissue oxygen delivery ensured.

Intravascular fluid balance is influenced by a number of preoperative and perioperative circumstances. Preoperative intravenous fluid administration minimizes the degree of dehydration that accompanies the NPO period. Unless there exists a compelling reason to place an intravenous catheter preoperatively, intravenous therapy is generally avoided in the pediatric patient until general anesthesia has been induced.

Perioperative fluid homeostasis is altered by a number of factors, including inhalation agent administration, the operating room environmental temperature, iatrogenic hyperventilation, and surgical stress. Inhalation agent administration produces peripheral vasodilation and some degree of myocardial depression, decreasing systemic blood pressure and end-organ blood flow. Dehydration after prolonged preoperative oral fluid abstinence aggravates these decreases in systemic blood pressure. The delivery of cold, dry anesthetic gases via an endotracheal tube bypasses normal anatomic humidification, increasing the loss of fluid from the respiratory tract. These insensible respiratory fluid losses can be minimized with the use of active or passive humidification systems during the intraoperative period. The operating room temperature also influences fluid balance. Basal caloric and water requirements are increased in a cold environment. Increases in core body temperature of 1° C may increase caloric expenditure by 12% to 14%.

General anesthesia modifies the neuroendocrine control of fluid balance. Surgical stress will increase plasma glucose levels. Hyperglycemia will act osmotically to increase renal losses of free water. Anesthetic agents themselves modify neuroendocrine regulation of fluids and electrolytes. Morphine as well as halothane have been demonstrated to increase the release of antidiuretic hormone (ADH) from the posterior pituitary.[159,160] ADH stimulates the release of aldosterone to conserve water through the renal reabsorption of sodium and water and the excretion of potassium. Decreased glomerular filtration, which parallels the decrease in renal perfusion, alters the kidneys' ability to handle administered fluid loads. Decreased renal perfusion stimulates the release of renin, which cleaves angiotensin I to form angiotensin II, a powerful vasoconstrictor that acts to increase systemic blood pressure. Renin stimulates the additional release of aldosterone.

Surgical trauma modifies fluid balance, the degree of which is dependent on the invasiveness of the surgical procedure. Intravenous fluids are used to replace intraoperative blood loss and fluid loss resulting from fluid shifts that develop from evaporative and third-space fluid losses. Physiologic parameters, such as heart rate, blood pressure, capillary refill time, urine output, and ongoing blood loss, are continually assessed. The rate of intraoperative fluid administration is continuously modified to maintain circulatory homeostasis. Peripheral surgical procedures (extremity procedures) have minimal evaporative or third-space fluid losses. However, intracavitary procedures (intraabdominal or intrathoracic procedures) are associated with greater blood loss, third-space fluid loss, and substantial evaporative fluid losses that approach 10 ml/kg of body weight per hour.

Pediatric Fluid Compartments

The growth of the newborn is accompanied by a decrease in the relative fluid compartment volumes of TBW and ECF volumes during the first year of life, followed by additional decreases in ECF later in childhood.[161] The TBW of the premature infant is as high as 80% of total body weight, whereas the TBW of the term infant is approximately 70% to 75% of total body weight. The adult value of TBW (55% to 60%) is reached between 6 months and 1 year of age. Knowledge of body fluid distribution is important when one is electing specific fluids and volumes for administration. Table 45-5 illustrates the differences in TBW as well as in the ICF and ECF compartments in the premature, infant, child, and adult.

Maintenance Fluid Calculation

The most direct and widely accepted method for determining intravenous fluid requirements is based on body weight. Holliday and Segar proposed a formula for the calculation of hourly maintenance fluids based on caloric expenditure studies in children. The hourly maintenance fluid level is determined by the "4-2-1" formula and is calculated as follows.[162] For the first 10 kg of body weight, 4 ml of crystalloid intravenous fluid (e.g., lactated Ringer's) is administered for each kilogram of body weight per hour. The hourly maintenance fluid requirement of a child who weighs 10 kg would be calculated as 10 kg × 4 ml/kg/hr = 40 ml/hr. Children weighing in excess of 10 kg but less than 20 kg would receive an additional 2 ml/kg/hr for body weight in excess of 10 kg. The child weighing 14 kg would receive 4 ml/kg/hr for the first 10 kg (40 ml) plus an additional 2 ml/kg/hr, for a total of 48 ml/hr. Children weighing in excess of 20 kg would receive an additional 1 ml/kg/hr in hourly fluid. This hourly maintenance fluid calculation serves as a basic guideline and does not take into account fluid deficits that develop during the NPO period and additional fluid losses (such as blood and third-space losses) that occur during the perioperative period. Table 45-15 summarizes the 4-2-1 formula and provides additional sample calculations.

Preoperative fluid deficits develop during the period of time in which the child has not received oral or intravenous maintenance fluids. The preoperative fluid deficit is calculated by determining the hourly maintenance fluid rate and multiplying this rate by the number of hours the child has been without intravenous or oral intake. The following calculations are used to determine the preoperative fluid deficit of an 8-kg child who has been NPO for 6 hours:

Equation 45-1

$$\begin{aligned}\text{Maintenance fluid} &= 8\ \text{kg} \times 4\ \text{ml/kg/hr} = 32\ \text{ml/hr}\\ \text{Deficit} &= \text{NPO hours} \times \text{maintenance fluid rate}\\ &= 6\ \text{hr} \times 32\ \text{ml/hr}\\ &= 192\ \text{ml}\end{aligned}$$

The calculated fluid deficit is replaced, following the guidelines of Furman and colleagues[163]: half of the fluid deficit is replaced during the first hour, with the remainder divided in half and replaced in the subsequent 2 hours. Using the calcu-

TABLE 45-15 Hourly Fluid Requirements: the "4-2-1" Formula

Weight (kg)	Fluid
0-10	4 ml/kg/hr for each kilogram of body weight
10-20	40 ml + 2 ml/kg/hr for each kg >10 kg
>20	60 ml + 1 ml/kg/hr for each kg >20 kg
Sample Calculated Fluid Requirements	***Maintenance Fluid per Hour***
4 kg	16 ml
9 kg	36 ml
15 kg	50 ml
30 kg	70 ml

TABLE 45-16 Fluid Replacement for Third-Space Fluid Losses

Expected Surgical Trauma	Administration Rate (ml/kg/hr)	Recommended Intravenous Fluid
Minimal	3-4	Lactated Ringer's 0.9% NS, Plasmalyte
Moderate	5-6	Lactated Ringer's 0.9% NS, Plasmalyte
Severe	7-10	Lactated Ringer's 0.9% NS, Plasmalyte

NS, *Normal saline*.

lations just presented, the following plan for intravenous fluids is developed.

Weight = 8 kg	Hour 1	Hour 2	Hour 3
Maintenance fluid (ml/hr)	32	32	32
Deficit (ml/hr)	96	48	48
Hourly total (ml)	128	80	80

In addition to the calculated maintenance and deficit fluids necessary to replace insensible fluid losses, additional intravenous fluid is required to replace third-space fluid losses that occur with surgical trauma. Lactated Ringer's solution, 0.9% normal saline, and Plasmalyte are acceptable for the replacement of insensible and third-space fluid losses at the rate of 1 to 2 ml/kg/hr. Expected third-space fluid losses can be categorized as minimal surgical trauma (an additional 3 to 4 ml/kg/hr), moderate surgical trauma (5 to 6 ml/kg/hr) and major surgical trauma (7 to 10 ml/kg/hr; Table 45-16).

Glucose-Containing Solutions

Glucose was previously administered during the perioperative period to prevent hypoglycemia, provide free-water to replace the insensible water lost during the NPO period, and conserve protein and prevent ketosis by preventing gluconeogenesis.[164] As previously discussed, surgical stress (e.g., surgical incision) elicits a neuroendocrine response, increasing plasma glucose levels. Despite extended periods of fasting, studies have noted that healthy pediatric patients infrequently become hypoglycemic.[165-167] However, very critically ill infants and those weighing less than 10 kg may develop hypoglycemia with prolonged periods of fasting.[168] Most anesthetists administer a glucose-free intravenous solution (lactated Ringer's) for maintenance fluid administration and to replace third-space and intraoperative blood loss. If the child has had an extended NPO period, a plasma glucose level may be determined after the induction of anesthesia at the time of intravenous catheter insertion.

Although the CNS is totally dependent on a continuous supply of exogenous glucose for the maintenance of cellular energy requirements, the continuous administration of glucose or elevated plasma glucose levels may worsen neurologic outcome in the event of an ischemic or hypoxic event. This association between hyperglycemia and worsened neurologic outcome has been noted in several reports.[169-171]

There exist clinical circumstances in which hypoglycemia is likely to develop. These occur in infants who are premature, infants of diabetic mothers, children with diabetes who have received a portion of daily insulin preoperatively, and children who receive glucose-based parenteral nutrition. A glucose-containing intravenous solution is administered in these patients as a controlled piggyback infusion, with frequent plasma glucose determinations performed to avoid hyperglycemia. Infants born of mothers with diabetes and infants of mothers who receive glucose-containing solutions during labor may require a continuation of these solutions for the prevention of rebound hypoglycemia. Premature infants have had less time to store glycogen in the liver than term infants and therefore are more susceptible to hypoglycemia. For this reason, premature infants routinely receive an infusion of 10% dextrose in 0.2% normal saline.

Crystalloid Intravenous Fluids

Crystalloid intravenous fluids contain water, various concentrations of electrolytes, and possibly varying amounts of glucose. These solutions move freely between the intravascular and interstitial fluid compartments. Crystalloid intravenous solutions are advantageous for perioperative administration, as they are the least expensive of the available intravenous solutions and are acceptable for the replacement of preoperative, intraoperative, and postoperative isotonic fluid deficits. Unlike colloid solutions, crystalloid solutions do not produce allergic reactions.

Crystalloid intravenous solutions can be further subdivided by their tonicity in relation to plasma (hypotonic, isotonic, or hypertonic). Tonicity is a measurement of the comparative osmolarity of solutions, which is determined by the sodium chloride content. For example, a hypotonic solution (e.g., 0.45% normal saline) has a lower sodium concentration (<130 mEq/L) and an osmolarity less than 280 mOsm/L; an isotonic solution (e.g., lactated Ringer's) has a sodium concentration between 130 and 155 mEq/L and an osmolarity between 280 and 310 mOsm/L; a hypertonic solution (e.g., 3% normal saline) has a sodium concentration greater than 155 mEq/L and an osmolarity in excess of 310 mOsm/L. These sodium-containing solutions move freely about the extracellular space, whereas the sodium-free intravenous solutions such as 5% dextrose in water (D_5W), will be distributed throughout all fluid compartments. Table 45-17 lists the physical constituents and the osmolarities of popular crystalloid solutions. An isotonic solution does not need to be equivalent to plasma in exact physical constituents (sodium, chloride, potassium) to be considered an isotonic solution, as it is the number of particles dissolved in solution (principally sodium) that determines the osmolarity.

Fluid Management of the Premature Infant

Proper fluid management of the premature infant requires an understanding of renal maturation. Renal tubular function develops after the thirty-fourth week of gestation, and nephrons mature by the thirty-sixth week.[172] In the term infant at birth the GFR is 15% to 30% of the adult value and reaches the adult value by the end of 1 year. The premature infant has a lower GFR and immature tubular function. The immature kidneys are unable to excrete sodium and excess fluid. The inability to concentrate urine secondary to the inability to reabsorb sodium leads to the excretion of large quantities of dilute urine. Therefore underestimation of fluid needs leads to more serious consequences than overestimation of fluid needs.[173] Healthy children over 6 months of age receive lactated Ringer's solution for maintenance, compensation for deficits, and third-space fluid replacement.

TABLE 45-17 Physical Characteristics of Popular Intravenous Crystalloid Solutions

	Na (mEq/L)	Cl (mEq/L)	K (mEq/L)	Ca (mg/ml)	Lactate (mg/ml)	Glucose (mg/dL)	mOsm/L
Hypotonic Solutions							
0.45% Normal saline	77	77					154
5% Dextrose in water						50	252
Isotonic Solutions							
0.9% Normal saline	154	154					308
Lactated Ringer's	130	109	4	3	28		273
Ringer's	130	109	4	3			309
Plasmalyte A	140	98	5				290
Hypertonic Solutions							
5% Sodium chloride	855	855					1700
7.5% Sodium chloride	1283	1283					2400

From Aker J. *The selection and administration of intravenous fluids*. Curr Rev Post-Anesth Care Nurses. *1995;17:63*.

Children younger than 6 months of age receive maintenance fluids of either 0.9% normal saline or 5% dextrose in 0.45% normal saline at the calculated ml/kg/hr rate. Preoperative dehydration may be corrected with the administration of 10 ml of crystalloid solution per kilogram of body weight. This fluid challenge is necessary to replace each 1% of dehydration.[174]

Estimation of Blood Volume

The goal of perioperative blood administration is the maintenance of acceptable oxygen-carrying capacity. Because pediatric patients have a relatively low intravascular volume compared with adults, vigilance and an accurate determination of intraoperative blood loss is fundamental to quality patient care.

The intravascular volume may be estimated by multiplying the child's weight by the estimated blood volume. The estimated blood volumes are as follows: premature infant, 90 to 100 ml/kg; full-term newborn, 80 to 90 ml/kg; infant age 3 months to 3 years, 75 to 80 ml/kg; and child older than 6 years of age, 65 to 70 ml/kg (see Table 45-2). For example, the estimated blood volume of a 6-month-old infant who weighs 7 kg is 525 ml (7 kg × 75 ml/kg = 525 ml).

The determination of intraoperative blood loss is difficult. Subjective estimates of blood loss are grossly inaccurate. Blood collected from the surgical field in suction canisters can be easily measured, but up to one half of blood lost during surgery can be contained in items such as surgical drapes, sponges, and towels and is difficult to measure. Accurate accounting of surgical blood loss related to these items requires weighing them. The weight of the dry item is subtracted from the weight of a blood-soaked item. Every 1 g of weight is equal to 1 ml of blood loss. Ongoing surgical blood loss requires frequent reassessment of the child's physiologic responses. Moderate to severe decreases in intravascular volume produce tachycardia, hypotension, narrowed pulse pressure, low urine output, decreased central venous pressure, pallor, and slow capillary refill. A sudden decrease in blood pressure in neonates and infants with rate-dependent cardiac output is indicative of significant intravascular volume depletion.

Permissible Blood Loss

What amount of blood loss may be permitted, while the patient still maintains adequate tissue oxygenation? No published studies are available to guide the anesthetist in determining the optimal and safe lower limits for hemoglobin concentration. Historically a hemoglobin of 10 g/L or a hematocrit of 30% triggered blood transfusion. This "transfusion trigger" has been redefined in light of the risks of blood-borne pathogen transmission. Permissible blood loss must be defined individually for each patient based on current medical condition, surgical procedure, and cardiovascular and respiratory function. Children with normal cardiovascular function may tolerate lower hematocrits and may compensate with an increased cardiac output if a higher inspired oxygen concentration is provided to improve oxygen delivery. An exception is the premature infant. As previously discussed, the incidence of apnea is higher in neonates and the premature with hematocrit levels below 30%. A target hematocrit level should be agreed on by the anesthetist, surgeon, and neonatologist, and this discussion should be documented in the medical record.

The permissible blood loss may be calculated by means of the following formula[175]:

Equation 45-2

$$ABL = EBV \times (H_O - H_L)/(H_A)$$

where ABL = allowable blood loss, EBV = estimated blood volume, H_O = the original hematocrit, H_L = the lowest acceptable hematocrit, and H_A = the average hematocrit, or $(H_O + H_L)/2$. For a 6-month-old infant who weighs 7 kg, with a starting hematocrit of 35% and the selection of the lowest acceptable hematocrit of 25%, we calculate the following:

Equation 45-3

$$ABL = 525 \times (35 - 25)/(25 + 35)/2 = 174 \text{ ml}$$

Blood loss may be replaced with suitable crystalloid solutions (0.9% normal saline, lactated Ringer's) by administering 3 ml for each ml of blood loss. Recall that the intravascular volume is one third of the ECF volume. Accordingly, one must administer 3 ml of an intravenous crystalloid solution to replace each ml of blood loss. A blood loss of 100 ml therefore requires replacement with 300 ml of crystalloid solution. Blood loss that is less than the calculated permissible blood loss may be replaced with colloid (1 ml for every 1 ml of blood loss).

When the blood loss equals or exceeds the calculated allowable loss, transfusion should be considered. Before transfusion is performed, a current hemoglobin and hematocrit should be obtained. The surgeon should be included in the decision process. These discussions and the resultant hemoglobin and hematocrit are recorded in the anesthetic record. The volume of packed RBCs to be infused may be determined by the following formula:

Equation 45-4

$$\text{Packed RBCs (ml)} = \frac{(\text{Blood loss} - \text{ABL}) \times \text{Desired hematocrit (30\%)}}{\text{Hematocrit of PRBCs (75\%)}}$$

Using the previous example of a 7-kg infant, with a total blood loss of 300 ml the volume of PRBCs would be $300 - 174 \times 30/75 = 50$ ml.

Blood Transfusion

Before blood component therapy is initiated, the proper equipment (filters, infusion devices, blood warming devices) should be obtained and tested. Standard blood transfusion sets contain a 170- to 200-μm filter. Microaggregate filters (20 to 40 μm) may be placed between the blood dispensing bag and the filtered infusion set, although no studies prove these filters to be of benefit over the standard 170- to 200-μm filter. Infusion pumps (syringe or piston driven) should be approved by the manufacturer for the infusion of blood and blood products. An excessive infusion rate can produce RBC lysis.

Blood is usually warmed before infusion. The American Association of Blood Banks has published standards for the use of blood-warming devices. Blood warmers must have a visible thermometer and an audible warning indicating excessive heating (>42° C). Warming devices for use in transfusions in adults (in-line water baths, counter-current heating with water through large-bore tubing) are cumbersome to use for the small volumes to be transfused in the pediatric patient. The selected blood component containers may be placed under the forced-air warming blanket, or the measured aliquot of blood that is drawn into a syringe may be warmed with the hand. Syringes should not be placed into water baths, as bacterial contamination may occur.

Blood administration need not be complicated. It is difficult to accurately determine the amount of blood administered when it is infused via adult-intended warming devices. Accurate accounting of the blood transfused is facilitated by drawing of the blood by syringe through the infusion tubing and delivery of the measured quantity to the child. A particularly suitable device is the Fenwal (Baxter Healthcare Corporation, Deerfield, Illinois) 80-μm blood component filter. This three-way infusion set is spiked into the blood component container, and the second limb of the set is placed into a stopcock, preferably located at the intravenous site. A syringe is attached to the remaining limb of the infusion set, allowing measured aliquots of blood to be drawn from the blood component container and then injected into the intravenous site.

The use of adult blood units is wasteful when a neonate or small infant undergoes transfusion. The blood bank can dispense small aliquots of blood into a calibrated syringe or provide 50- to 100-ml bags of blood, which are transferred from an assigned donor unit. Blood used for neonatal transfusion is preferably less than 1 week old, to preserve 2,3 diphosphoglycerate levels, and irradiated to prevent graft-versus-host disease. When packed RBCs are transfused, the blood should not be diluted before transfusion, as this may contribute to hypervolemia.

Considerations for Specialized Surgical Procedures

Laparoscopy. The application of laparoscopic procedures has been extended from adults to infants and children. Representative procedures in pediatric patients include appendectomy, cholecystectomy, and pyloromyotomy. The insufflation of CO_2 and the creation of a pneumoperitoneum produces significant cardiovascular and respiratory embarrassment. Increased intraabdominal pressure (IAP) may elicit bradycardia, limits ventilatory reserve, decreases cardiac output, decreases intraabdominal organ blood flow, and alters acid-base balance.[176]

The insufflation of CO_2 is accompanied by increased IAP, which increases peripheral vascular resistance, with accompanying decreases in venous return. Increased IAP impedes venous return from the lower extremities and decreases mesenteric, renal, and femoral arterial blood flow. Marked increases in IAP reduce preload and cardiac output, with subsequent cardiovascular collapse. This is of particular concern in infants, as decreases in preload may precipitate the return of fetal circulation. Therefore infants and children with congenital cardiopulmonary disease are not suitable candidates for laparoscopic surgical procedures. Bradycardia may occur with peritoneal and mesenteric stretching with insufflation. Bradycardia may be sudden and extreme, producing cardiac arrest. The administration of an anticholinergic (atropine 20 mcg/kg) before abdominal insufflation may be prudent.

The insufflation of CO_2 and the accompanying increases in IAP move the diaphragm cephalad, restricting lung expansion. The functional residual capacity is further reduced.[176] After insufflation, increases in $PaCO_2$ and end-tidal CO_2 occur secondary to CO_2 absorption from the peritoneal cavity, hypoventilation resulting from the restrictive defect created by the pneumoperitoneum, and decreased dead space ventilation, which accompanies the reduction in cardiac output. Additional respiratory embarrassment transpires after the child is placed in the Trendelenburg position.[177] The Trendelenburg position increases the required inspiratory pressures, producing further reductions in lung volume and increases in arteriovenous admixture. In addition, the Trendelenburg position may result in caudad migration of the endotracheal tube, creating a mainstem intubation, which will increase dead space ventilation.[178]

Marked increases in intracranial pressure may occur with excessive IAP. The neonate and infant are at risk for the development of intracerebral hemorrhage. The optimal IAP, which minimizes the risk of intracerebral bleeding, has not been studied. Vascular puncture with the introduction of the abdominal trocar may lead to gas embolization. This would be readily identified by a marked reduction in end-tidal CO_2. The absorption of CO_2 alters acid-base balance. The insufflated CO_2 combines with water contained within the peritoneal cavity to form H_2CO_3, which dissociates to form HCO_3^- and H^+. The pH will decrease over time during intraabdominal insufflation. Liem and colleagues used a swine model and noted a decrease in pH to 7.22 after 1 hour of CO_2 insufflation with a consistent IAP of 10 mm Hg.[178]

Intraoperative management for laparoscopy requires attention to detail. Endotracheal intubation is required to accomplish these procedures in order to effectively combat the accompanying respiratory embarrassment. Endotracheal tube placement must be reconfirmed after abdominal insufflation and with each change in the child's position (Trendelenburg or reverse Trendelenburg). Anesthetic maintenance may be accomplished with isoflurane or sevoflurane. Although halothane is suitable for anesthetic induction, its accompanying cardiovascular effects may further affect the physiologic alterations that accompany CO_2 insufflation. Alternatively, a balanced anesthetic technique using nitrous oxide and oxygen in combination with an opioid and a neuromuscular relaxant may be used. However, some surgeons request that nitrous oxide not be administered for fear of bowel distension. In such instances an inhalation technique for anesthetic maintenance is employed.

Before CO_2 insufflation the anesthetist should empty the stomach with a soft suction catheter to remove air that may have been delivered to the stomach during induction. Likewise, the surgeon should determine whether the urinary bladder should be catheterized and emptied. These considerations will prevent the inadvertent entry of the abdominal insufflating needle or trocars into these distended organs. The anesthetist must be vigilant and note peak airway pressures and the resulting end-tidal CO_2 after CO_2 insufflation and adjust ventilation accordingly. Finally, core body temperature should be monitored. Exposed body surface areas should be covered with warm blankets. Some degree of hypothermia is inevitable after the continuous insufflation of cold CO_2 into the abdominal cavity.

Pyloric Stenosis. Hypertrophic pyloric stenosis occurs more frequently in white male infants (4:1 male-to-female ratio) at a rate of 1 in every 1000 live births.[179] Pyloric stenosis is identified with the onset of vomiting between 2 to 4 weeks of age. The clinical history is classic and includes the onset of nonbilious projectile vomiting within 30 to 60 minutes of feeding. Affected children may be scheduled for "emergency" surgical procedures. The anesthetist should understand that pyloromyotomy is never an emergency. Disastrous outcomes may occur when the child's condition is treated as a surgical emergency without proper preoperative preparation.

The diagnosis of pyloric stenosis is made by history and physical examination. The clinical history of vomiting after feeding and the palpation of the diagnostic "olive" over the epigastric area confirm the diagnosis. Confirmation of pyloric stenosis when the clinical history or physical examination is suspicious may be facilitated with a gastric barium contrast roentgenogram. This complicates the subsequent anesthetic management, as a risk of barium regurgitation and aspiration exists with anesthetic induction. The use of an ultrasound examination may eliminate the need for barium examination.[180]

Sound preoperative evaluation and preparation are essential. The infant who has experienced prolonged vomiting may have severe dehydration. Electrolyte losses with prolonged vomiting create hypochloremic metabolic acidosis through the loss of H^+, Cl^-, Na^+, and K^+. ECF depletion stimulates aldosterone secretion, which increases the renal reabsorption of sodium. However, this increases the renal loss of K^+, and with the continued loss of Cl^- and HCO_3^-, the degree of alkalosis increases. This cycle can be interrupted only with the cessation of feeding to prevent vomiting and the deliberate administration of a balanced electrolyte solution (5% dextrose in lactated Ringer's). Before surgical intervention occurs, the infant should be euvolemic with a normal electrolyte balance.

The anesthetic plan must take consideration the diagnostic tests that were employed to make the diagnosis. Infants who received gastric barium should have their stomachs emptied with a large-bore catheter before anesthetic induction. However, this does not guarantee a barium-free stomach, nor does it decrease the potential for barium aspiration. Awake endotracheal intubation or a rapid-sequence induction may be preferred. Many argue that a rapid-sequence induction can quickly produce hypoxia in infants after intravenous induction agents. Hypoxia may also develop with repeated attempts to secure the airway in a vigorous infant. An alternative technique is to use an inhalation induction, applying cricoid pressure with the loss of consciousness and administering a nondepolarizing neuromuscular blocking drug before attempting endotracheal intubation. The ultimate selection of the induction technique is dependent on the anesthetist's experience with a given technique and the availability of skilled assistance.

Pediatric Regional Anesthesia. Pediatric regional anesthesia procedures are generally administered after general anesthesia for the management of postoperative pain. Recent studies highlight the advantages of combined regional anesthesia and general anesthesia in the pediatric patient.[181] Although the popularity of combined regional anesthetic techniques for adults has increased, the use of pediatric regional anesthesia has been more limited, because fewer anesthesia providers are properly trained in its administration. Additional concerns include the detection of intravascular injection, the ability to detect local anesthetic toxicity in preverbal infants and children, the consequences of accidental dural puncture, and the ethical and medical legal implications of regional anesthetic administration in anesthetized children.

The detection of intravascular injection in the child during the concurrent administration of inhalation agents has been the subject of several studies. Infants may have a greater risk of amide local anesthetic toxicity because of their decreased levels of AAG.[182] The routine administration of epinephrine-containing test doses of local anesthetics may be counterproductive during the concurrent administration of myocardial depressant drugs. Desparmet and colleagues found that the administration of halothane decreased the ability of epinephrine to produce tachycardia after intravascular injection.[183] Despite the intravascular injection of epinephrine, heart rate did not increase by greater than 10 beats per minute in 39% of the children studied. Desparmet and co-workers suggest that pretreatment with atropine increases the reliability of the detection of tachycardia after intravascular injection. In a recent study examining the reliability of an epidural test dose during sevoflurane administration, Tanaka and Nishikawa found that intravascular injection of epinephrine, when preceded by atropine administration, produced a heart rate increase exceeding 10 beats per minute and a systolic blood pressure increase of at least 15 mm Hg and concluded that an epinephrine test dose was a reliable indicator of intravascular injection.[184]

Fisher and colleagues have suggested that the ECG can be an effective marker of the intravascular injection of epinephrine.[185] They demonstrated that increased T-wave amplitude was a marker of intravascular injection, with the most prominent change in amplitude occurring within 15 to 45 seconds after intravascular injection.

The fear of neurologic injury in a combative child and the ethical considerations associated with the use of regional anesthetic techniques in preverbal children have led many to administer regional anesthesia after the induction of general anesthesia. The performance of a regional anesthetic procedure without general anesthesia requires that the child be sedated for the needed cooperation to be obtained. Perhaps the risk of neurologic injury is lower in the anesthetized child who is not resistant and combative during attempted epidural or caudal anesthesia. However, Bromage and Benumof report of a devastating neurologic injury in an adult after attempted epidural anesthesia.[186] These authors state that central neural axis techniques should not be attempted in patients who are under general anesthesia. A subsequent editorial in the same journal authored by a number of pediatric anesthesiologists experienced in pediatric regional anesthesia disagreed with this conclusion and proposed that the extrapolation of adult regional anesthetic experiences to children is inappropriate and may result in the denial of these beneficial procedures to children.[187] Regional anesthetic procedures in children should be performed only by anesthetists with previous training, demonstrated skill in adult regional anesthetic procedures, and knowledge of the appropriate applications of each technique.

REFERENCES

1. Konstadt SN, Louie EK, Black S, Rao TL, Scanlon P. Intraoperative detection of patent foramen ovale by transesophageal echocardiography. *Anesthesiology*. 1991;74:212-216.
2. Kranke P, Eberhart LH, Roewer N, Tramer MR. Postoperative shivering in children: a review on pharmacologic prevention and treatment. *Paediatr Drugs*. 2003;5:373-383.
3. Plattner O, Semstroth M, Sessler DI, Papousek A, Klasen C, Wagner O. Lack of nonshivering thermogenesis in infants anesthetized with fentanyl and propofol. *Anesthesiology*. 1997;86:772-777.
4. Jessen K. An assessment of human regulatory non-shivering thermogenesis. *Acta Anaesthesiol Scand*. 1980;24:138-143.
5. Dick W, Kreuscher H, Luhken D. Prevention of heat loss during anesthesia and operation in the newborn baby and small infant. *Acta Anaesthesiol Scand Suppl*. 1970;37:134.
6. Tempelman ML, Bell EF. Head insulation for premature infants in servocontrolled incubators, and radiant warmers. *Am J Dis Child*. 1986;140:940.
7. Arndt K. Inadvertent hypothermia in the OR. *AORN J*. 7i0(2):204-6, Aug 1999:208-214.
8. Bissonnette B, Sessler DI, LaFlamme P. Inspired gas humidification prevents intraoperative hypothermia in infants and children. *Anesth Analg*. 1989;68:528.
9. Sugi K, Katoh T, Gohra H, Hamano K, Fujimura Y, Esato K. Progressive hyperthermia during thoracoscopic procedures in infants and children. *Paediatric Anaesth*. 1998;8:211-214.
10. Mazoit JX, Dalens BJ. Pharmacokinetics of local anaesthetics in infants and children. *Clin Pharmacokinet*. 2004;43:17-32.
11. Caldwell J, Mofatt JR, Smith RL. Pharmacokinetics of bupivacaine administered epidurally during childbirth. *Br J Pharmacol*. 1976;3:956-957.
12. Gunter JB. Benefit and risks of local anesthetics in infants and children. *Paediatr Drugs*. 2002;4:649-672.
13. Morselli PL, Franco-Morselli R, Bossi L. Clinical pharmacokinetics in newborns and infants. *Clin Pharmacokinet*. 1980;5:485-527, 1980.
14. Jacqz-Aigrain E, Burtin P. Clinical pharmacokinetics of sedatives in neonates. *Clin Pharmacokinet*. 1996;31:423-443.
15. Battino D, Estienne M, Avanzini G. Clinical pharmacokinetics of antiepileptic drugs in paediatric patients. Part II. Phenytoin, carbamazepine, sulthiame, lamotrigine, vigabatrin, oxcarbazepine and felbamate. *Clin Pharmacokinet*. 1995;29:341-369.
16. Kearns GL, Reed MD. Clinical pharmacokinetics in infants and children: a reappraisal. *Clin Pharmacokinet*. 1989;17:29-67.
17. Milsap RL, Jusko WJ. Pharmacokinetics in the infant. *Environ Health Perspect*. 1994;102(Suppl 11):107-110.
18. Certana P, Maurelli M. Rectal administration of anesthetic agents. *Minerva Anesthesiol*. 1995;61:219-228.
19. Alcorn J, McNamara PJ. Pharmacokinetics in the newborn. *Adv Drug Deliv Rev*. 2003;55:667-686.
20. Temple AR. Pediatric dosing of acetaminophen. *Pediatr Pharmacol*. 1983;3:321.
21. Birmingham PK, Tobin MJ, Henthorn TK, et al. Twenty-four-hour pharmacokinetics of rectal acetaminophen in children: an old drug with new recommendations. *Anesthesiology*. 1997;87:244-252.
22. Montgomery CJ, McCormack JP, Reichert CC, Marsland CP. Plasma concentrations after high-dose (45 mg/kg) rectal acetaminophen in children. *Can J Anaesth*. 1995;42:982-986.
23. Bruun LS, Elkjaer S, Bitsch-Larsen D, Andersen O. Hepatic failure in a child after acetaminophen and sevoflurane exposure. *Anesth Analg*. 2001;92:1446-1448.
24. Berde CB, Sethna NF. Analgesics for the treatment of pain in children. *N Engl J Med*. 2002;347:1094-1103.
25. Ray K, Adithan C, Bapna JS, Kamatchi GL, Ray K, Mehta RB. Effect of halothane anesthesia on salivary elimination of paracetamol. *Eur J Clin Pharmacol*. 1986;30:371-373.
26. Geldner G, Hubmann M, Knoll R, Jacobi K. Comparison between three transmucosal routes of administration of midazolam in children. *Paediatr Anaesth*. 1997;7:103-109.
27. Weber F, Wulf H, el Saeidi G. Premedication with nasal s-ketamine and midazolam provides good conditions for induction of anesthesia in preschool children. *Can J Anaesth*. 2003;50:470-475.
28. Nelson PS, Streisand JB, Mulder SM, Pace NL, Stanley TH. Comparison of oral transmucosal fentanyl citrate and an oral solution of meperidine, diazepam, and atropine for premedication in children. *Anesthesiology*. 1989;70:616-621.
29. Eger EI 2nd, Bahlman SH, Munson ES. The effects of age on the rate of increase of alveolar anesthetic concentration. *Anesthesiology*. 1971;35:365-372.
30. Goldman LJ. Anesthetic uptake of sevoflurane and nitrous oxide during an inhaled induction in children. *Anesth Analg*. 2003;96:400-406.
31. Lerman J, Schmitt-Bantel BI, Gregory GA, Wilis MM, Eger EI, II. Effect of age on the solubility of volatile anesthetics in human tissues. *Anesthesiology*. 1986;65:307-311.
32. Lerman J, Robinson S, Willis MM, Gregory GA. Anesthetic requirements for halothane in young children 0-1 month and 1-6 months of age. *Anesthesiology*. 1983;59:421-424.
33. Copnstant I, Dubois MC, Pitat V, Moutard ML, McCue M, Murat I. Changes in electroencephalogram and autonomic cardiovascular activity during induction of anesthesia with sevoflurane compared with halothane in children. *Anesthesiology*. 1999;91:1604-1615.
34. Friesen RH, Lichtor JL. Cardiovascular depression during halothane anesthesia in infants: a study of three induction techniques. *Anesth Analg*. 1982;61:42-45.
35. Morimoto Y, Mayhew JF, Knox SL, Zornow MH. Rapid induction of anesthesia with high concentrations of halothane or sevoflurane in children. *J Clin Anesth*. 2000;12:184-188.
36. Fisher DM, Robinson S, Brett CM, Perin G, Gregory GA. Comparison of enflurane, halothane, and isoflurane for diagnostic and therapeutic procedures in children with malignancies. *Anesthesiology*. 1985;63:647-650.
37. Rolf N, Cote CJ. Persistent cardiac arrhythmias in pediatric patients: effects of age, expired carbon dioxide values, depth of anesthesia, and airway management. *Anesth Analg*. 1991;73:720.
38. Karl HW, Swedlow DB, Lee KW, Downes JJ. Epinephrine-halothane interactions in children. *Anesthesiology*. 1983;58:142-145.

39. Freisen RH, Lichtor JL. Cardiovascular effects of inhalation induction with isoflurane in infants. *Anesth Analg.* 1983;62:411-414.
40. Weiskopf RB, Moore MA, Eger EI 2nd, et al. Rapid increases in desflurane concentration is associated with greater transient cardiovascular stimulation than with rapid increase in isoflurane concentration in humans. *Anesthesiology.* 1994;80:1035-1045.
41. Marret E, Pruszkowski O, Deleuze A, Bonnet F. Accelerated idioventricular rhythm associated with desflurane administration. *Anesth Analg.* 2002;95:319-321, table of contents.
42. Moore EW, Pollard BJ, Elliott RE. Anaesthetic agents in paediatric day case surgery: do they affect outcome? *Eur J Anaesthesiol.* 2002;19:9-17.
43. Osawa M, Shingu K, Murakawa M, et al. Effects of sevoflurane on central nervous system electrical activity in cat. *Anesth Analg.* 1994;79:52-57.
44. Komatsu H, Taie S, Endo S, et al. Electrical seizures during sevoflurane anesthesia in two pediatric patients with epilepsy. *Anesthesiology.* 1994;81:1535-1537.
45. Kain ZN, Mayes LC, Wang SM, Hofstadter MB. Postoperative behavioral outcomes in children: effects of sedative premedication. *Anesthesiology.* 1999;90:758-765.
46. Wells LT, Rasch DK. Emergence "delirium" after sevoflurane anesthesia: a paranoid delusion? *Anesth Analg.* 1999;88:1308-1310.
47. Lapin SL, Auden SM, Goldsmith LJ, Reynolds AM. Effects of sevoflurane anaesthesia on recovery in children: a comparison with halothane. *Paediatr Anaesth.* 1999;9:299-304.
48. Baum JA, Woehlck HJ. Interaction of inhalational anaesthetics with CO_2 absorbents. *Best Pract Res Clin Anaesthesiol.* 2003;17:63-76.
49. Stabernack CR, Eger EI 2nd, Warnken UH, Forster H, Hanks DK, Ferrell LD. Sevoflurane degradation by carbon dioxide absorbents may produce more than one nephrotoxic compound in rats. *Can J Anaesth.* 2003;50:249-252.
50. Gentz BA, Malan TP, Jr. Renal toxicity with sevoflurane: a storm in a teacup? *Drugs.* 2001;61:2155-2162.
51. Conzen PF, Kharasch ED, Czerner SF, et al. Low-flow sevoflurane compared with low-flow isoflurane anesthesia in patients with stable renal insufficiency. *Anesthesiology.* 2002;97:578-584.
52. Versichelen LF, Bouche MP, Rolly G, et al. Only carbon dioxide absorbents free of both NaOH and KOH do not generate compound A during in vitro closed-system sevoflurane: evaluation of five absorbents. *Anesthesiology.* 2001;95:750-755.
53. Frink EJ, Jr, Green WB, Jr, Brown EA, et al. Compound A concentrations during sevoflurane anesthesia in children. *Anesthesiology.* 1996;84:566-571.
54. Eger EI 2nd, Koblin DD, Bowland T, et al. Nephrotoxicity of sevoflurane versus desflurane anesthesia in volunteers. *Anesth Analg.* 1997;84:160-168.
55. Iwasaka H, Itoh K, Miyakawa H, Kitano T, Taniguchi K, Honda N. Glucose intolerance during prolonged sevoflurane anesthesia. *Can J Anaesth.* 1996;43:1059-1061.
56. Raddle IC, McKerchner HG. Transport through membranes and the development of membrane transport. In: Macleod SM, Raddle IC, eds. *Textbook of Pediatric Clinical Pharmacology.* Littleton, Mass: PSG Publishing; 1985:1.
57. Cook DR. Neonatal anesthetic pharmacology: a review. *Anesth Analg.* 1974;53:544-548.
58. Lockhart CH, Nelson WL. The relationship of ketamine requirements to age in pediatric patients. *Anesthesiology.* 1974;40:507-508.
59. Brett CM, Fisher DM. Thiopental dose-response relations in unpremedicated infants, children and adults. *Anesth Analg.* 1987;66:1024.
60. Russo H, Bressolle F. Pharmacodynamics and pharmacokinetics of thiopental. *Clin Pharmacokinet.* 1998;35:95-134.
61. Olutoye O, Watcha MF. Management of postoperative vomiting in pediatric patients. *In Anesthesiol Clin.* 2003;41:99-117.
62. Hannallah RS, Baker SB, Casey W, McGill WA, Broadman LM, Norden JM. Propofol: effective dose and induction characteristics in unpremedicated children. *Anesthesiology.* 1991;74:217-219.
63. Aun CS, Short SM, Leung DH, Oh TE. Induction dose-response of propofol in unpremedicated children. *Br J Anaesth.* 1992;68:64-67.
64. Short SM, Aun CS. Hemodynamic effects of propofol in children. *Anaesthesia.* 1991;46:783.
65. Picard P, Tramer MR. Prevention of pain on injection with propofol: a quantitative systematic review. *Anesth Analg.* 2000;90:963-969.
66. Blount P, Merelis JP. Molecular basis of the two nonequivalent ligand-binding sites of the muscle nicotinic acetylcholine receptor. *Neuron.* 1989;3:349.
67. Guiton A. Contraction of skeletal muscle. In: *Textbook of Medical Physiology.* 10th ed. Philadelphia: Saunders; 2000:67-85.
68. Goudsouzian NG. Maturation of neuromuscular transmission in the infant. *Br J Anaesth.* 1980;52:205-213.
69. Goudsouzian NG, Standaert FG. The infant and the myoneural junction. *Anesth Analg.* 1986;65:1208-1217.
70. Sullivan M, Thompson WK, Hill GD. Succinylcholine-induced cardiac arrest in children with undiagnosed myopathy. *Can J Anaesth.* 1994;41:497-501.
71. Gronert GA. Cardiac arrest after succinylcholine: mortality greater with rhabdomyolysis than receptor upregulation. *Anesthesiology.* 2001;94:523-529.
72. Durant MM, Katz RI. Suxamethonium. *Br J Anaesth.* 1982;54:195-208.
73. Naguib M, Magboul MM. Adverse effects of neuromuscular blockers and their antagonists. *Drug Saf.* 1998;18:99-116.
74. Wong SF, Chung F. Succinylcholine-associated postoperative myalgia. *Anaesthesia.* 2000;55:144-152.
75. Cozanitis DA, Erkola O, Klemola UM, Makela V. Precurarisation in infants and children less than three years of age. *Can J Anaesth.* 1987;34:17-20.
76. Nagiub M, Farag H, Magbagbeola JAO. Effect of pretreatment with lysine acetyl salicylate on suxamethonium-induced myalgia. *Br J Anaesth.* 1995;59:606-610.
77. Blache JL. Anesthesia related malignant hyperthermia-clinical forms. In: Aubert M, et al, eds. *Malignant Hyperthermia.* Englewood, NJ: Normed Verlag; 1993:1.
78. Sambuughin N, Sei Y, Gallagher KL, et al. North American malignant hyperthermia population: screening of the ryanodine receptor gene and identification of novel mutations. *Anesthesiology.* 2001;95:594-599.
79. O'Flynn RP, Shutack JG, Rosenberg H, Fletcher JE. Masseter muscle rigidity and malignant hyperthermia susceptibility in pediatric patients: an update on management and diagnosis. *Anesthesiolgoy.* 1994;80:1228-1233.
80. Ellis FR, Halsall PJ. Suxamethonium spasm: a differential diagnosis conundrum. *Br J Anesth.* 1984;56:381-384.
81. Hannallah RS, Kaplan RF. Jaw relaxation after halothane/succinylcholine sequence in children. *Anesthesiology.* 1994;81:99.
82. Larach MG, Rosenberg H, Larach DR, Broennle AM. Prediction of malignant hyperthermia susceptibility by clinical signs. *Anesthesiology.* 1987;66:547-550.
83. Meakin G, McKiernan EP, Morris P, Baker RD. Dose-response curves for suxamethonium in neonates, infants and children. *Br J Anaesth.* 1989;62:655-658.
84. Cook DR, Fischer CG. Characteristics of succinylcholine in neonates. *Anesth Analg.* 1978;57:63-66.
85. Liu LM, DeCook TH, Goudsouzian NG, Ryan JF, Liu PL. Dose response to intramuscular succinylcholine in children. *Anesthesiology.* 1981;55:599-602.
86. Rosenberg H, Fletcher JE. Masseter muscle rigidity and malignant hyperthermia susceptibility. *Anesth Analg.* 1986;65:161.
87. Morell RC, Berman JM. Is succinylcholine safe for children? *Anesthesia Patient Saf Found Newsletter.* 1994;9:1-3.
88. Morell RC. Sux "contraindication" reduced to "warning." *Anesthesia Patient Saf Found Newsletter.* 1995;10:1-3.

89. Markakis DA, Lau M, Brown R, Luks AM, Sharma ML, Fisher DM. The pharmacokinetics and steady state pharmacodynamics of mivacurium in children. *Anesthesiology*. 1998;88: 978-983.
90. Gronert B, Woelfel S, Cook DR. Comparison of equipotent intubating doses of mivacurium and succinylcholine in infants 2-12 months old. *Anesthesiology*. 1993;79:A932.
91. Meakin GH. Muscle relaxants in paediatric day case surgery. *Eur J Anaesthesiol Suppl*. 2001;23:47-52.
92. Cook DR, Gronert BJ, Woelfel SK. Comparison of the neuromuscular effects of mivacurium and suxamethonium in infants and children. *Acta Anaesthesiol Scand Suppl*. 1995;106:35-40.
93. Meretoja OA, Wirtavuori K, Neuvonen PJ. Age-dependence of the dose-response curve of vecuronium in pediatric patients during balanced anesthesia. *Anesth Analg*. 1988;67:21.
94. Segredo V, Caldwell JE, Matthay MA, Sharma ML, Gruenke LD, Miller RD. Persistent paralysis in critically ill patients after long-term administration of vecuronium. *N Engl J Med*. 1992;327:524-528.
95. Eikermann M, Hunkemoller I, Peine L, et al. Optimal rocuronium dose for intubation during inhalation induction with sevoflurane in children. *Br J Anaesth*. 2002;89:277-281.
96. Reynolds LM, et al. Intramuscular rocuronium in infants and children. *Anesthesiology*. 1996;85:231-239.
97. Brandom BW. Neuromuscular blocking drugs in pediatric patients. *Anesth Analg*. 2000;90(suppl):S14-S18.
98. Bevan JC, Tousignant C, Stephenson C, et al. Dose responses for neostigmine and edrophonium as antagonists of mivacurium in adults and children. *Anesthesiology*. 1996;84:354-361.
99. Shoults D, Clarke TA, Benumof JL, Mannino FL. Maximum inspiratory force in predicting successful neonate tracheal extubation. *Crit Care Med*. 1979;7:485-486.
100. Brandom BW, Fine GF. Neuromuscular blocking drugs in pediatric anesthesia. *Anesthesiol Clin North Am*. 2002;20:45-58.
101. Marley RA. Postextubation laryngeal edema: a review with consideration for home discharge. *J Perianesth Nurs*. 1998;13:39-53.
102. Werkhaven JA. Microlaryngoscopy-airway management with anaesthetic techniques for CO_2 laser. *Paediatr Anaesth*. 2004;14:90-94.
103. Algren JT, Gursoy F, Johnson TD, Skjonsby BS. The effect of nitrous oxide diffusion on laryngeal mask airway cuff inflation in children. *Pediatr Anaesth*. 1998;8:31-36.
104. Conterato JP, Lindahl SG, Meyer DM, Bires JA. Assessment of spontaneous ventilation in anesthetized children with use of a pediatric circle or Jackson-Rees system. *Anesth Analg*. 1989;69:484-490.
105. Cote CJ. Pediatric equipment. In: Cote CJ, Todres ID, Goudsouzian NG, et al, (eds). *A Practice of Anesthesia for Infants and Children*. 3rd ed. Philadelphia: Saunders; 2001:715-738.
106. Bain JA. The Bain anesthesia circuit. *Int Anesthesiol Clin*. 1982;20:149-157.
107. Pethick SL. Letter to the editor. *Can Anaesth Soc J*. 1975;22:115.
108. Maxwell LG. Age-associated issues in preoperative evaluation, testing, and planning: pediatrics. *Anesthesiol Clin North Am*. 2004;22:27-43.
109. Hannallah RS. Preoperative investigations. *Paediatr Anaesth*. 1995;5:325-329.
110. Hackmann T, Steward DJ, Sheps SB. Anemia in pediatric day-surgery patients: prevalence and detection. *Anesthesiology*. 1991;75:27-31.
111. Azarnof P, Woody PD. Preparation of children for hospitalization in acute care hospitals in the United States. *Pediatrics*. 1981;68:361-368.
112. Morray JP, et al. A comparison of pediatric and adult anesthesia closed malpractice claims. *Anesthesiology*. 1993;78:461-467.
113. Morray JP. Anesthesia-related cardiac arrest in children: an update. *Anesthesiol Clin North Am*. 2002;20:1-28, v.
114. Morray JP, Geiduschek JM, Ramamoorthy C, et al. Anesthesia-related cardiac arrest in children: initial findings of the Pediatric Perioperative Cardiac Arrest (POCA) Registry. *Anesthesiology*. 2000;93:6-14.
115. Keenan RL, et al. Bradycardia during anesthesia in infants. *Anesthesiology*. 1994;80:976-982.
116. Warner MA, Warner ME, Warner DO, Warner LO, Warner EJ. Perioperative pulmonary aspiration in infants and children. *Anesthesiology*. 1999;90:66-71.
117. Roberts RB, Shirley MA. Reducing the risk of acid aspiration during cesarean section. *Anesth Analg*. 1974;53:859-868.
118. Olsson GL, Hallen B, Hambraeus-Jonzon K. Aspiration during anesthesia: a computer-aided study of 185,358 anaesthetics. *Acta Anaesthesiol Scand*. 1986;30:84-92.
119. Splinter WM, Schreiner MS. Preoperative fasting in children. *Anesth Analg*. 1999;89:80-89.
120. Ljungqvist, O, Soreide E. Preoperative fasting. *Br J Surg*. 2003;90:400-406.
121. Cook-Sather SD, Harris KA, Chiavacci R, Gallagher PR, Schreiner MS. A liberalized fasting guideline for formula-fed infants does not increase average gastric fluid volume before elective surgery. *Anesth Analg*. 2003;96:965-969, table of contents.
122. Litman RS, Wu CL, Quinlivan JK. Gastric volume and pH in infants fed clear fluids and breast milk prior to surgery. *Anesth Analg*. 1994;79:482-485.
123. Fishkin S, Litman RS. Current issues in pediatric ambulatory anesthesia. *Anesthesiol Clin North Am*. 2003;21:305-311, ix.
124. Tait AR, Voepel-Lewis T, Malviya S. Perioperative considerations for the child with an upper respiratory tract infection. *J Perianesth Nurs*. 2000;15:392-396.
125. Murat I, Constant I, Maud'huy H. Perioperative anaesthetic morbidity in children: a database of 24,165 anaesthetics over a 30-month period. *Paediatr Anaesth*. 2004;14:158-166.
126. Tait AR, Malviya S, Voepel-Lewis T, Munro HM, Seiwert M, Pandit UA. Risk factors for perioperative adverse respiratory events in children with upper respiratory tract infections. *Anesthesiology*. 2001;95:283-285.
127. Pelech A. Evaluation of the pediatric patient with a cardiac murmur. *Pediatr Clin North Am*. 1999;46:2.
128. Dajani AS, Taubert KA, Wilson W, et al. Prevention of bacterial endocarditis: recommendations by the American Heart Association. *JAMA*. 1997;277:1794-1801.
129. Fisher DM. When is the ex-premature infant no longer at risk for apnea? *Anesthesiology*. 1995;82:807-808.
130. Cote CJ, Zaslavsky A, Downes JJ, et al. Postoperative apnea in former preterm infants after inguinal herniorrhaphy: a combined analysis. *Anesthesiology*. 1995;82:809-822.
131. Welborn LG, Greenspun JC. Anesthesia and apnea: perioperative considerations in the former preterm infant. *Pediatr Clin North Am*. 1994;41:181-198.
132. Kurth CD, et al. Postoperative apnea in premature infants. *Anesthesiology*. 1987;66:483-487, 1987.
133. Cox RG, Goresky GV. Life-threatening apnea following spinal anesthesia in former premature infants. *Anesthesiology*. 73:345-347, 1997.
134. Mestad PH, Glenski JA, Binda BE. When is outpatient surgery safe in the preterm infant. *Anesthesiology*. 1988;69:A744.
135. Welborn LG. Preoperative apnea in the preterm infant. *Anesthesiol Clin North Am*. 1991;9:885-895.
136. Poets CF, et al. Prolonged episodes of hypoxemia in preterm infants undetectable by cardiopulmonary monitors. *Pediatrics*. 1995;95:860-863.
137. Tobias JD. Anaesthesia for minimally invasive surgery in children. *Best Pract Res Clin Anaesthesiol*. 2002;16:115-120.
138. Dawson B, Reed WA, Ogg TW. Use of anesthesia: implications of day-care surgery and anaesthesia. *BMJ*. 1980;281:212-214.
139. Stoelting RK, Miller RD. Pediatrics. In: *Basics of Anesthesia*. 4th ed. New York: Churchill Livingstone; 2000:364-375.
140. Eckhenhoff J. Relationship of anesthesia to postoperative personality changes in children. *Am J Dis Child*. 1953;86: 587-591.
141. Levine MF, et al. Oral midazolam premedication in children with congenital cyanotic heart disease undergoing

cardiac surgery: a comparative study. *Can J Anaesth*. 1993;40: 934-938.
142. *American Association of Nurse Anesthetist Patient Monitoring Standards*. Park Ridge, Ill: AANA; 1992.
143. Cote CJ, Rolf N, Liu LM, et al. A single-blind study of combined pulse oximetry and capnography in children. *Anesthesiology*. 1991;74:980-987.
144. Badgwell JM, McLeod ME, Lerman J, Creighton RE. End-tidal PCO_2 sampled at the distal and proximal ends of the endotracheal tube in infants and children. *Anesth Analg*. 1987;66:959-964.
145. Badgwell JM, Heavener JE. End-tidal carbon dioxide pressure in neonates and infants measured by aspiration and flow-through capnography. *J Clin Monit*. 1991;7:285.
146. Yakaitis RW, Blitt CD, Angiulo JP. End-tidal halothane concentration for endotracheal intubation. *Anesthesiology*. 1977;47: 386-388.
147. Politis GD, Tobin JR, Morell RC, James RL, Cantwell MF. Tracheal intubation of healthy pediatric patients without muscle relaxant: a survey of technique utilization and perceptions of safety. *Anesth Analg*. 1999;88:737-741.
148. Kain ZN, Caldwell-Andrews AA, Krivutza DM, Weinberg ME, Wang SM, Gaal D. Trends in the practice of parental presence during induction of anesthesia and the use of preoperative sedative premedication in the United States, 1995-2002: results of a follow-up national survey. *Anesth Analg*. 2004;98:1252-1259.
149. Kain ZN, Mayes LC, Want SM, Caramico LA, Hofstadter MB. Parental presence during induction of anesthesia versus sedative premedication: which intervention is more effective? *Anesthesiology*. 1998;89:1147-1156.
150. Audenaert SM, Montgomery CL, Thompson DE, Sutherland J. A prospective study of rectal methohexital; efficacy and side effects in 648 cases. *Anesth Analg*. 1995;81:957-961.
151. Pomeranz ES, Chudnofsky CR, Deegan TJ, et al. Rectal methohexital sedation for computed tomography imaging of stable pediatric emergency department patients. *Pediatrics*. 2000;105: 1110-1114.
152. Björkman S, et al. Pharmacokinetics of IV and rectal methohexitone in children. *Br J Anaesth*. 1987;59:1541-1547.
153. Forbes RB, Vandewalker GE. Comparison of two and ten percent rectal methohexitone for induction of anesthesia in children. *Can J Anaesth*. 1988;35:345-349.
154. Forbes RB, et al. Pharmacokinetics of two percent rectal methohexitone in children. *Can J Anaesth*. 1989;36:160-164.
155. Audenaert SM, Lock RL, Johnson GL, Pedigo NW Jr. Cardiovascular effects on rectal methohexital in children. *J Clin Anesth*. 1992;4:116-119.
156. Hannallah RS, Patel RI. Low dose intramuscular ketamine for anesthesia pre-induction in young children undergoing brief outpatient procedures. *Anesthesiology*. 1989;70:598.
157. Wyant GM. Intramuscular Ketalar in paediatric anaesthesia. *Can J Anaesth*. 1971;18:72-83.
158. Khazzam A, Karkas A. Intramuscular methohexital as a sole pediatric anesthetic-analgesic agent. *Anesth Analg*. 1972;51: 895-898.
159. Oyama T, Sato K, Kimura K. Plasma levels of antidiuretic hormone in man during halothane anesthesia and surgery. *Can Anaesth Soc J*. 1971;18:614.
160. Bozkurt P, Kaya G, Yeker Y, et al. Effects of systemic and epidural morphine on antidiuretic hormone levels in children. *Paediatr Anaesth*. 2003;13:508-514.
161. Friis-Hansen B. Body water compartments in children: changes during growth and related changes in body composition. *Pediatrics*. 1961;28:169-181.
162. Holliday MA, Segar WE. The maintenance need for water in parenteral fluid therapy. *Pediatrics*. 1957;19:823-832.
163. Furman EB, Roman DG, Lemmer LA, Hairabet J, Jasinska M, Laver MB. Specific therapy in water, electrolyte and blood-volume replacement during pediatric surgery. *Anesthesiology*. 1975;42:187-193.
164. Sieber FE, Smith DS, Traystman RJ, Wollman H. Glucose: a reevaluation of its intraoperative use. *Anesthesiology*. 1987;67: 72-81.
165. Aun CST, Panesar NS. Paediatric glucose homeostasis during anaesthesia. *Br J Anaesthesia*. 1990;64:413-418.
166. Van der Walt JH, Carter JA. The effect of different preoperative regimens on plasma glucose and gastric volume and pH in infancy. *Anaesth Intensive Care*. 1986;14:352-359.
167. Welborn LG, McGill WA, Hannallah RS, Nisselson CL, Ruttimann UE, Hicks JM. Perioperative blood glucose levels in pediatric outpatients [abstract]. *Anesthesiology*. 1986;65: 543-547.
168. Watson BG. Blood glucose levels in children during surgery. *Br J Anaesth*. 1972;44:712-715.
169. Ayers J, Graves SA. Perioperative management of total Parenteral nutrition, glucose containing solutions, and intraoperative glucose monitoring in paediatric patients: a survey of clinical practice. *Paediatr Anaesth*. 2001;11:41-44.
170. Lanier W, et al. The effect of glucose infusion and head position on neurologic outcome after complete cerebral ischemia in primates: examination of a model. *Anesthesiology*. 1987;66:39-48.
171. Pusinelli WA, et al. Moderate hyperglycemia augments ischemic brain damage. A neuropathological study in the rat. *Neurology*. 1982;32:1239-1246.
172. Dabbagh S, Ellis D, Gruskin AB. Regulation of fluids and electrolytes in infants and children. In: Motoyama EK, Davis PJ, eds. *Smith's Anesthesia for Infants and Children*. 6th ed. St Louis: Mosby; 1996:105.
173. Edelmann CM Jr, Barnett HL, Troupkou V. Renal concentrating mechanisms in newborn infants: effect of dietary protein and water content, role of urea, and responsiveness to antidiuretic hormone. *J Clin Invest*. 1960;39:1062-1069.
174. McManus ML. Pediatric fluid management. In: Cote CJ, Todres ID, Ryan JF, et al, eds. *A Practice of Anesthesia in Infants and Children*. 3rd ed. Philadelphia: Saunders; 2001:216-234.
175. Bennett EJ. Fluid balance in the newborn. *Anesthesiology*. 1975;43:210.
176. Manner T, Aantaa R, Alanen M. Lung compliance during laparoscopic surgery in pediatric patients. *Pediatr Anesth*. 1988;8:25-29.
177. Biddle C, Aker J. The cardiovascular and ventilatory effects of surgical positioning. *Curr Rev Nurse Anesth*. 1989;21:163.
178. Liem T, Applebaum H, Hertzberger B. Hemodynamic and ventilatory effects of abdominal CO_2 insufflation at various pressures in young swine. *J Pediatr Surg*. 1994;29:966-969.
179. Grant GA, McAleer JJA. Incidence of infantile hypertrophic pyloric stenosis, *Lancet* 1:1177, 1984.
180. Teele RL, Smith EH. Ultrasound in the diagnosis of idiopathic hypertrophic pyloric stenosis. *N Engl J Med*. 1977;296:1149-1150.
181. McNeely JK, Farber NE, Rusy LM, Hoffman GM. Epidural analgesia improves outcome following pediatric fundoplication: a retrospective analysis. *Reg Anesth*. 1997;22:16-23.
182. Booker PD, Taylor C, Saba G. Perioperative changes in alpha-1-acid glycoprotein concentrations in infants undergoing major surgery. *Br J Anaesth*. 1996;76:365-368.
183. Desparmet J, Mateo J, Ecoffey C, Mazoit X. Efficacy of an epidural test dose in children anesthetized with halothane. *Anesthesiology*. 1990;72:249-251.
184. Tanaka M, Nishikawa T. Simulation of an epidural test dose with intravenous epinephrine in sevoflurane-anesthetized children. *Anesth Analg*. 1998;86:952-957.
185. Fisher QA, Shaffner DH, Yaster M. Detection of intravascular injection of regional anaesthetics in children. *Can J Anaesth*. 1997;44:592-598.
186. Bromage PR, Benumof JL. Paraplegia following intracord injection during attempted epidural anesthesia under general anesthesia. *Reg Anesth Pain Med*. 1998;23:104-107.
187. Krane EJ, Dalens BJ, Murat I, Murrell D. The safety of epidurals placed during general anesthesia [editorial]. *Reg Anesth Pain Med*. 1998;23:433-438.

CHAPTER 46

GERIATRICS AND ANESTHESIA PRACTICE

DENISE MARTIN-SHERIDAN, SONJA MYERS

PERSPECTIVES ON AGING

The geriatric segment of the population is growing faster than any other age group (Figure 46-1). In the year 2000, as children of the "baby boom" entered their sixth decade, nearly 50 million Americans were older than 70 years of age and made up 13% of the general population (Figure 46-2). Providing anesthesia care to elderly individuals with diverse and variable age-induced physiologic changes constitutes a major part of modern adult anesthesia practice.

Although an absolute definition of who is elderly places an arbitrary marker on chronologic age, and because a concise definition has not been agreed on, individuals who are 65 years of age and older generally are considered to be part of the geriatric cohort. Over half of the members of this population will have at least one surgical procedure and anesthesia during their lifetime.[1] Despite the fact that conflicting data exist, the geriatric patient who undergoes anesthesia and surgery may be at increased risk for perioperative morbidity and mortality as a result of continuous physiologic aging processes and concomitant diseases. Anesthesia and surgery-related morbidity and mortality are likely to increase if the geriatric patient requires emergency surgery. When the nurse anesthetist plans the perioperative management for the geriatric patient, it is important to understand the influence that aging and disease processes have on patient outcome.

It should be noted that the extent to which systemic changes occur in the geriatric patient is not consistent across the population. For instance, individuals who maintain physical fitness may be less affected than patients who lead a sedentary lifestyle. The following sections discuss system changes that are predictable as functions of aging and of the decreased capacity for adaptation associated with it.

EXPECTED ANATOMIC AND PHYSIOLOGIC CHANGES

Aging is associated with structural changes of cells and organs. At the cellular level a genetically controlled number of cell divisions limits the number of human fibroblasts. After the maximum number of cell divisions has been reached, cells fail to grow and then die, despite apparent uniformity in the environment. The accumulation of random errors in the replication of deoxyribonucleic acid (DNA) and ribonucleic acid (RNA) and in protein synthesis is superimposed on the limitation of cellular division. When a sufficient number of cells fail to function, the organs eventually become unable to function effectively (Box 46-1).[2]

Human organ function shows a linear decline with age. The rate constant for this decline is slightly less than 1% per year of the functional capacity present at age 30 years. As a consequence, a 70-year-old geriatric patient may have a 40% decrease in the function of any specific organ compared with

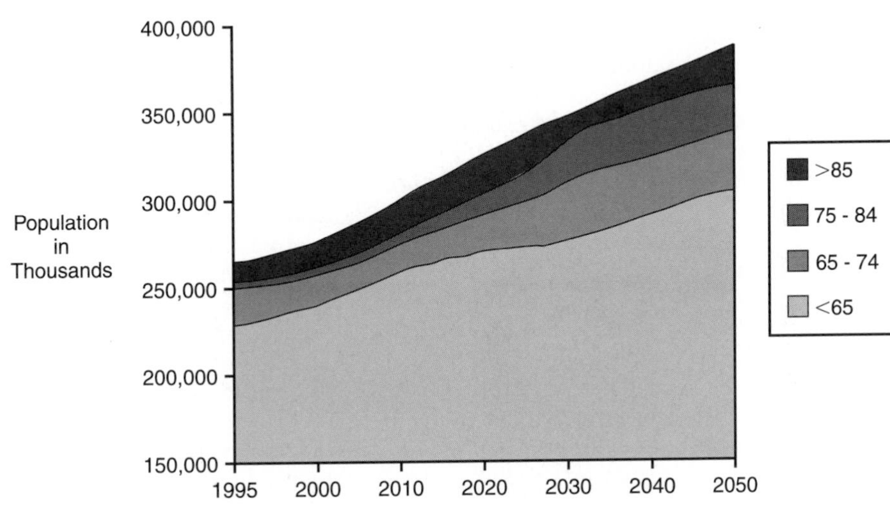

FIGURE **46-1**
Projected increase in the US population (in thousands) from 1995 to 2050, subdivided by age. (Data from United States Census Bureau, Population Division, Department of Commerce, Washington, DC. http://www.census.gov/population/www/socdemo/age.html#older.)

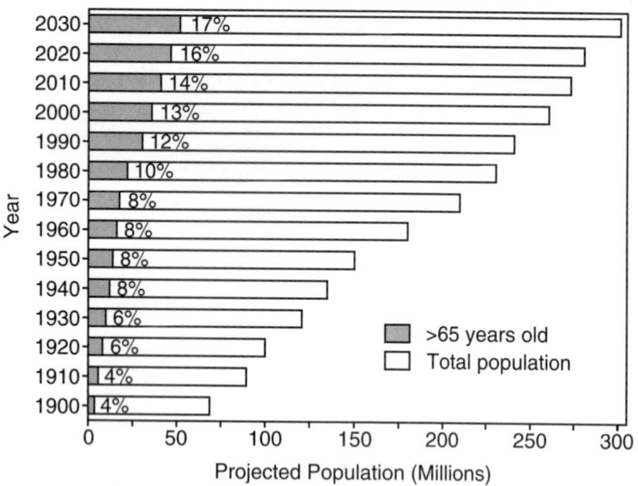

FIGURE **46-2**
The increasing population in the United States from 1900 to 1990, with projections to the year 2030. People who are now older than 65 years (*left portion of bars*) represent approximately 11% to 12% of the overall population. This proportion is expected to increase to 17% to 18% by the year 2030. (Data from United States Census Bureau, Population Division, Department of Commerce, Washington, DC. Available at: http://www.census.gov/population/www/socdemo/age.html#older. Accessed May 17, 2004.)

BOX **46-1**

Common Age-Related Anatomic and Physiologic Changes

- Decreased organ function
- Increased body fat
- Decreased blood volume
- Loss of protective reflexes
- Decreased ability to retain body heat
- Decreased lean body mass
- Decreased skin elasticity
- Collagen loss
- Decreased intracellular water

that present at the age of 30 years. Fortunately the healthy adult patient at age 30 years has 4 to 10 times the organ function required for maintenance of homeostasis.[3]

The degree of physiologic function that remains with increasing age varies. Changes in organ function manifest as decreased margins of reserve. Geriatric patients may be able to maintain homeostasis but become increasingly less able to restore it when they are subjected to trauma, disease, or drugs. For example, the response to a decrease in arterial oxygen tension or pH or to an increase in arterial carbon dioxide (CO_2) tension should be an increase in ventilation and heart rate. The response to hypoxemia and hypercarbia is blunted by aging and by residual anesthesia and narcotics. Postoperatively the geriatric patient may lack the reserve required to meet the added demands that residual anesthetics place on ventilatory capability. As a result the patient may be predisposed to hypoxemia and respiratory failure.

As a person ages, changes in body composition may have a significant impact on anesthetic patient care management. Overall a loss of skeletal muscle (lean body mass) and a 20% to 30% reduction in blood volume can be expected. The essentially contracted state of the vasculature may produce a higher than anticipated initial plasma concentration when anesthetic agents are administered. An increase in the amount of body fat also develops, with an increased availability of lipid storage sites and a greater reservoir for deposition of lipid-soluble anesthetic agents. As a consequence, it is likely that a greater than expected time period is required for lipid-soluble agents to be eliminated from storage sites, a prolonged effect may be seen, and hypotension can be anticipated.[4]

Geriatric patients are especially susceptible to decreases in temperature and may be unable to retain body heat when exposed to the cool environment of the operating room even for short periods of time. This characteristic is caused in part by the fact that basal metabolic rate declines with age and the fact that that the elderly become less able to adjust to a cold environment by means of autonomic peripheral vasoconstriction. Elderly patients in whom intraoperative normothermia is difficult to control have a greater incidence of shivering on arrival to the postanesthesia care unit and are prone to the development of significant postoperative protein catabolism.[5]

Protein catabolism may be compounded by nutritional deficiencies that occur in the elderly; these deficiencies are associated with a reduction in intracellular water and in potassium. The loss in total body water that renders the patient vulnerable to hypotension during anesthesia also makes it difficult for him or her to compensate for changes in position and posture.[6]

Great care must be taken to prevent trauma to skin and bony prominences when the geriatric patient is positioned for surgery on the operating table. Collagen loss and decreased elasticity of tissue make the skin more sensitive to damage from tape, monitoring devices, and contact with hard table surfaces. In addition, any invasive procedure—including insertion of intravenous, spinal, and epidural catheters—should be accomplished with the goal of protecting the integrity of the skin.

Waugaman and Rigor[6] point out that the airway of the geriatric patient may present several challenges to the anesthetist during patient care management. A progressive decrease in the reactivity of protective airway reflexes, such as coughing and swallowing, can be expected with age. Because the elderly often are edentulous, a sealed fit with the anesthetic face mask may be difficult. These factors may increase the likelihood of regurgitation of gastric contents, with aspiration of vomitus into the lungs. The changes that accompany cervical arthritis and osteoarthritis, limiting extension and flexion of the neck, often make endotracheal intubation difficult.

Cardiovascular System

Impaired myocardial pump function and reduced cardiac output in the elderly prolong circulation time and decrease the perfusion of such vital organs as the brain, heart, and liver. Prolonged circulation time may delay the onset of drug effects. This in turn may be reflected in delayed induction time and slow onset of drug action. Backlund noted no significant difference in cardiac output in response to exercise in elderly patients who were free of coronary artery disease and other complicating illnesses when compared with a population of younger patients.[7] Elderly patients, however, appear to be more dependent on an increase in end-diastolic volume than an increase in heart rate to produce an increase in cardiac output.[8] These factors make the geriatric patient more prone to

BOX **46-2**

Common Age-Related Cardiovascular Anatomic and Physiologic Changes

- Impaired pump function
- Prolonged circulation time
- Myocardial fiber atrophy
- Hypertension
- Impaired cardiac adrenergic receptor quality
- Increased peripheral vascular resistance
- Decreased cardiac output
- Decreased organ perfusion
- Left ventricular hypertrophy
- Coronary artery disease

congestive heart failure when large volumes of intravenous fluid are administered in the presence of anesthetic-induced myocardial depression and hypotension (Box 46-2).

Variable degrees of myocardial fiber atrophy occur as the fibers become replaced by connective tissue during the aging process. Loss of elasticity also is seen throughout the arterial vasculature, along with progressive loss of arterial distensibility. Left ventricular hypertrophy results from the related chronic increase in afterload to left ventricular ejection imposed by elevations in peripheral vascular resistance. Because increases in peripheral vascular resistance are greater than the decreases seen in cardiac output, and because blood vessels are poorly compliant, general systemic hypertension is common.

Replacement of elastic tissue by less resilient fibrous connective tissue also occurs in the coronary arteries. Coronary artery disease progressively increases in severity over the entire adult age span, but clinical symptoms may not be seen until a critical threshold is reached. The fact that coronary artery disease may be occult in many elderly patients should guide anesthetic patient care management in this population.

Cardiovascular function is altered with aging, even in the absence of arteriosclerotic, calcific, or hypertensive disease. The aging myocardium becomes thicker in both systole and diastole; an increase in the size and number of individual muscle fibers and in adipose tissue occurs. Atrial contraction, which normally produces 20% of the left ventricular end-diastolic volume, becomes even more important to the filling of these stiffer ventricles. Loss of the "atrial kick" in a nodal rhythm under anesthesia can cause a drop in systolic pressure.

Although the resting heart rate and heart response exercise loads in the elderly are similar to those seen in younger patients, the maximum heart rate that can be generated by an elderly patient is considerably lower. An age-related decrease in target organ responsiveness to the regulation of chronotropic and inotropic cardiac function results from impaired quality of adrenergic receptors in the heart. As a result, catecholamine effects that enhance calcium ion transport in the myocardium and improve calcium ion availability are less pronounced in the elderly.[8,9]

Pulmonary System

The effect of aging on the lung can be described as a generalized reduction of elasticity. The functional consequences of this are complex. In elderly patients, even in the absence of disease, emphysema-like decreases in lung compliance impair the matching of ventilation and perfusion. As a result, physiologic shunt is increased, and the efficiency of oxygen exchange is reduced at the alveolar level (Box 46-3).

BOX **46-3**

Common Age-Related Pulmonary Anatomic and Physiologic Changes

- Increased lung compliance
- Decreased forced expiratory volume
- Increased closing volume
- Decreased resting arterial oxygen tension
- Increased alveolar-arterial difference
- Ventilation-perfusion mismatch
- Decreased functional residual capacity
- Decreased total lung capacity

Functional efficiency also is impaired at the skeletal muscle level. A progressive decrease in forced expiratory volume in 1 second and forced vital capacity is caused by loss of elastic tissue around the alveoli and lung ducts. This loss of elasticity allows the alveoli to remain more distended at rest and less distensible at inspiration. The overall closing volume (i.e., the volume at which the small airways collapse) increases.[10] In the anesthetized elderly patient, closing capacity is much greater than functional residual capacity, more dependent airways are collapsed, and more of the tidal volume is distributed to areas of the lung that are less perfused.

Total lung capacity declines approximately 10% by 70 years of age, reflecting a loss of height because of deterioration of intervertebral disks. Increased stiffness of the thoracic cage and progressive dorsal kyphosis are accompanied by upward and anterior rotation of the ribs and sternum, which leads to an increase in the anterior-to-posterior diameter of the chest and in restricted chest expansion.[10]

Other major contributors to the decline in gas exchange efficiency include a reduction in the surface area of the alveoli, an increase in the alveolocapillary membrane thickness, and a reduction in pulmonary capillary blood volume. As a result, resting arterial oxygen tension (Pa_{O_2}) normally declines with age in accordance with the following equation:

Equation 46-1

$$Pa_{O_2} = 100 - (0.4 \text{ age [years] mm Hg})$$

The alveolar-arterial difference for oxygen increases from approximately 8 mm Hg at 20 years of age to more than 20 mm Hg at 70 years of age, and the Pa_{O_2} decreases 0.5 mm Hg per year after 20 years of age.[11,12] Because of the changes in pulmonary function that occur with age, elderly patients must be observed closely after surgery and anesthesia to ensure that they do not develop hypoxia and hypercarbia in the postoperative period. In addition, members of this population may require higher inspired intraoperative concentrations of oxygen because of their lower Pa_{O_2} values and reduced efficiency of gas exchange.

Nervous System

The extent to which central nervous system (CNS) function declines with age is debated in the literature. It has been thought that aging is associated with a progressive decline in

BOX **46-4**

Common Age-Related Central Nervous System Anatomic and Physiologic Changes

- Decreased activity
- Decreased oxygen consumption
- Reduced number of functioning receptors
- Reduced production of neurotransmitters
- Neuron loss
- Decreased cerebral blood flow

BOX **46-5**

Common Age-Related Renal Anatomic and Physiologic Changes

- Decreased renal blood flow
- Decreased urine-concentrating ability
- Decreased ability to conserve water
- Decreased elimination of drugs
- Decreased glomerular filtration rate

CNS activity and a loss of neurons, particularly in the cerebral cortex. The decreased CNS activity is related to a decrease in neuronal density, a decrease in cerebral metabolic oxygen consumption, a decrease in blood flow, a reduction in the number of receptor sites for neurotransmitter action, and a decrease in the rate of synthesis of neurotransmitters. Gradually the conduction velocity in peripheral nerves slows, and a reduction in the number of fibers in spinal cord tracts may occur (Box 46-4).[6,13]

However, the existence of an age-related decline in cerebral function does not appear to be conclusive. Much of the cognitive loss associated with aging may, in fact, be related to the degree to which the elderly exercise their mental functions and to nutritional changes that occur as people age rather than to the aging process itself. Cognitive loss may be preventable with better nutrition and stimulation of mental function in the elderly as a group.

Although the age-induced changes in CNS function remain controversial, the nervous system is the target organ for virtually every anesthetic agent administered to the patient. It is generally agreed that the geriatric patient has a reduced requirement for anesthetic agents. The variability of effect of the anesthetic agents may not be distinguishable in any given patient but has been observed between elderly patients and younger ones.[2,4]

Anesthetic requirements for the inhalation anesthetic agents decrease linearly with age as the minimum alveolar concentration (MAC) required falls. This applies not only to the inhalation agents but also to local anesthetics, opioids, barbiturates, benzodiazepines, and other intravenous agents. A comparable level of sedation at diazepam plasma concentrations significantly lower than that required for younger adults has been demonstrated in elderly patients.[14] Equivalent electroencephalographic suppression occurs at a lower plasma concentration of both fentanyl and alfentanil.[15]

Renal System

Aging has a profound effect on the renal vasculature and therefore exerts great influence on renal function. The glomerular filtration rate decreases approximately 6% to 8% per decade. Although the ability to concentrate urine and conserve water is progressively impaired, reduction in plasma flow is the primary source of loss of renal function with age. Renal blood flow decreases 1% to 2% each year after the age of 25 years and is decreased 40% to 50% by the age of 65 years.[16] Declines in renal blood flow are caused by decreases in cardiac output that accompany aging as well as to reductions in the size of the renal vascular bed (Box 46-5).

Renal function is sufficient for gross azotemia or uremia to be avoided, but the renal functional reserve needed to withstand water and electrolyte imbalance in elderly patients is minimal. The combination of decreased renal and reduced cardiac function makes geriatric patients prone to fluid overload. In addition, renal elimination of drugs may be impaired.

Hepatobiliary System

Hepatic blood flow decreases with age, paralleling reductions in cardiac output; nevertheless, hepatocellular function changes little. In normal individuals microsomal activity and nonmicrosomal activity appear well preserved, although some evidence suggests that plasma clearance of drugs known to be extensively metabolized in the liver is reduced (Box 46-6).[17]

The effect of an age-associated reduction of hepatic blood flow and a potential reduction in microsomal enzyme function impairs the liver's ability to metabolize anesthetics and nondepolarizing neuromuscular blocking agents. Reduced liver function, combined with the reduced filtration and excretory capacity of the aging kidney, results in a gradual decline in the plasma concentration of drugs and may contribute to a prolonged duration of drug effect.

Endocrine System

Pancreatic function declines during aging, and the incidence of diabetes mellitus increases as the ability to metabolize glucose load becomes impaired. Elderly patients have demonstrated an age-related increase in postprandial blood glucose levels. Mechanisms responsible for these alterations include a sluggish liberation of insulin in response to hyperglycemia and resistance to the effects of insulin at peripheral sites (Box 46-7).[18,19]

BOX **46-6**

Common Age-Related Hepatobiliary Anatomic and Physiologic Changes

- Decreased hepatic blood flow
- Decreased plasma drug clearance

BOX **46-7**

Common Age-Related Endocrine Anatomic and Physiologic Changes

- Decreased pancreatic function
- Increased incidence of diabetes
- Decreased tolerance to glucose load

Because insulin responsiveness varies from patient to patient, the anesthetist may be required to include the administration of exogenous insulin as part of perioperative patient care management. In addition, because intolerance to a glucose load is common, limitation of the administration of intravenous solutions that contain glucose also may be required for many surgical patients. Frequent intraoperative evaluation of blood glucose levels may be beneficial in the estimation of a patient's status.

PHARMACOKINETIC AND PHARMACODYNAMIC CONSIDERATIONS

The term *pharmacokinetics* of anesthetic agents employed during patient care management refers to the physiologic processes of drug absorption, tissue distribution, metabolism, and elimination. *Pharmacodynamics* refers to the relationship between drug quantity and drug effect. Physiologic changes occur during aging that affect the disposition and clearance of pharmacologic agents and the typical dose-response relationship produced. However, it is important to remember that the circumstances in which pharmacodynamics and pharmacokinetics interact reflect significant variability among patients.

Pharmacokinetics

The disposition and clearance of pharmacologic agents employed during anesthetic patient care management are characterized by age-related changes. However, the extent to which each process changes with age is debated in the literature.

Lee[20] points out that a reduction in plasma concentration in the elderly may produce clinically important changes in the amount of unbound drug in plasma after intravenous administration. The role that aging has in modifying the oral or parenteral uptake of drugs also is important. Changes in vascular volume, plasma protein binding, the percentage of body mass that is adipose or lean tissue, and the efficiency of metabolism and elimination of drugs are likely to affect an individual patient's response to anesthetic agents (Table 46-1).

As a result of a relatively contracted blood volume, higher-than-expected initial plasma drug levels occur in the elderly population after the administration of standard doses of drugs on the basis of calculated body weight. A reduced plasma protein binding capacity results in an increase in the amount of the free form of drug able to penetrate the blood-brain barrier. Significant increase in total body adipose tissue into which lipid-soluble drugs must be dispersed prolongs elimination, because the volume of drug that must be cleared is increased. Drug disposition also is altered as a result of reduced renal and hepatic function, slowing the elimination of drugs cleared through these pathways.

TABLE 46-1 Age-Related Changes and Pharmacokinetics

Change	Effect
Contracted vascular volume	High initial plasma concentration
Decreased protein binding	Increased availability of free drug
Increased total body lipid storage sites	Prolonged action of lipid-soluble drugs
Decreased renal and hepatic blood flow	Prolonged action of drugs dependent on kidney and liver elimination

Pharmacodynamics

Pharmacodynamic factors determine the relationship between the concentration of the drug at the site of action and the intensity of the effect produced. Although the exact mechanisms responsible have not been clearly described, a reduced need for anesthetic drugs, including reduced MAC requirements of the volatile anesthetic agents, is well established in the elderly. Possible responsible mechanisms elucidated are reductions in brain mass, absolute brain blood flow, and the number of neurons and axons in the CNS and peripheral nervous system. In addition, neurotransmitter activity and nervous system functional reserve also may be involved.

Clinically, the induction dose of barbiturates is reduced 30% to 40% in members of the geriatric population, compared with younger patients. The sensitivity may be explained on the basis of a higher plasma concentration after administration of barbiturates. Similarly, the dose of propofol required for induction is reduced. Significant hypotension may be seen if standard induction doses are administered.

The MAC of potent inhalation anesthetic agents decreases with age by approximately 4% for each decade of life after the age of 40 years. The age-related CNS changes discussed previously emphasize the pharmacodynamic correlation between cerebral metabolic function and anesthetic requirements for the potent inhalation anesthetic agents.[21] In addition, the contemporary inhalation anesthetic agents undergo little metabolism, have low solubility in blood, and produce less depression of myocardial contractility and left ventricular ejection fraction; these characteristics may make them well suited for use in elderly patients.

Overall reduction in hepatic clearance produces a prolonged half-life and duration of effect for the narcotics in general. Meperidine protein binding decreases with increasing age, thereby generating more unbound drug. Because nondepolarizing muscle relaxants are usually highly polarized, relatively fat insoluble, and dependent on urinary excretion for elimination (with the exception of atracurium and *cis*-atracurium), a reduction in clearance and increased elimination half-life are seen in elderly patients. No significant age-related changes have been found for atracurium and *cis*-atracurium. Succinylcholine may produce a longer effect in elderly men, because they appear to have a median effective dose that is significantly less than that in younger patients, as well as reduced levels of plasma cholinesterase.[22]

ANESTHETIC MANAGEMENT

Preparing a plan of anesthetic management for the geriatric patient requires that the anesthetist consider factors that may influence patient outcome. Those factors discussed previously include the anatomic and physiologic changes that occur with aging and the pharmacokinetic and pharmacodynamic processes that affect uptake, distribution, elimination, and the end-organ effect of pharmacologic agents employed during the anesthetic procedure. In addition, the anesthetist must tailor the anesthetic plan according to individual patient needs and predispositions, especially taking into account the impact of concomitant diseases.

History

Standard techniques used for accrual of anesthetic data are appropriate to the development of a plan of patient care management for the geriatric patient. Information relative to the history and status of the patient may be obtained directly from the patient, from the patient's family, and from others involved in caregiving.

An aspect that warrants consideration during patient assessment and evaluation is the importance of emotional and psychologic support in allaying patients' fears associated with surgery, anesthesia, and possible hospitalization. Although elderly patients may appear to have their emotions under control, the assumption that the geriatric patient is generally less intimidated by surgery and anesthesia may be incorrect. It is not uncommon to find patients who are reluctant to ask the anesthetist questions because of cultural predispositions or who are unable because of anxiety to understand questions asked of them. In addition, elderly patients may be unable to hear clearly the questions posed to them.

Patient Assessment

A thorough history-taking and physical examination of the elderly patient are essential, even when a minor procedure is planned. A baseline assessment of organ systems should be completed. In addition to changes that occur with aging, frequent coexisting diseases that may influence patient care management include hypertension, diabetes mellitus, coronary artery disease, chronic obstructive pulmonary disease, rheumatoid arthritis, and osteoarthritis. As discussed previously in this chapter, coexisting diseases and emergency surgery may increase the incidence of morbidity and mortality in this population.

It should be determined what prescription and over-the-counter medications the patient is currently receiving. It is likely that the geriatric patient is taking several different medications that have the potential to affect or interact with pharmacologic agents used during the anesthetic process. Nonopioid and nonsteroidal analgesics, as well as antiinflammatory drugs, may prolong bleeding time, produce renal and hepatic dysfunction, and precipitate allergic reactions. Sympathomimetics with β-adrenergic agonist effects as well as pancuronium may increase the likelihood of cardiac dysrhythmias in the presence of cardiac glycosides. Patients being treated with antihypertensive agents may display attenuated sympathetic activity and a modified response to sympathomimetic drugs and sedation.[21] It is important to ask about medication use during the review of systems; patients may fail to respond positively to a general question about what medications they use but may respond affirmatively, for example, to a direct question asking if they use eye drops.

Requests for specific laboratory data depend on the patient's overall state of health, nutritional status, and current drug regimen. The extent and duration of surgery and anesthesia also should be considered. Patients who have chronic diseases, such as diabetes mellitus and hypertension, may require electrolyte and glucose screening. In patients with chronic obstructive pulmonary disease and coronary artery disease, chest radiography and electrocardiography may be appropriate. Although not the overriding factor, a cost-benefit balance must be reached between "routine" laboratory screening tests and tests performed for recognizable indications. It is important to note that researchers continue to debate which screening tests are integral components of the assessment of the elderly patient and how they affect outcome.[23]

Perioperative Period

Premedication

Much controversy exists regarding the use of premedication in the geriatric population. After careful patient assessment has been performed, if a patient requires anxiety relief, administration of medication should be guided by the pharmacokinetic and pharmacodynamic concepts discussed previously in this chapter. Unwanted confusion, agitation, and prolonged duration of action may develop after administration of benzodiazepines because of their sedative-anxiolytic properties. The hepatic clearance of midazolam, for example, is decreased in the elderly, and the elimination half-life is 6 hours, compared with 2 hours in younger patients.[14]

Well-conducted studies investigating the effects of the opioids as premedication and patient outcome in the geriatric population have not been reported in the literature. It should be kept in mind that the use of sedatives and analgesics for premedication may be helpful in relieving anxiety without prolonging anesthetic recovery. Reduced dose requirements are necessary for preventing these centrally active sedatives and analgesics from producing a prolonged effect.[24] Many advocate the routine administration of oral antacids to all patients in whom general anesthesia is anticipated. Because elderly patients may be at increased risk for aspiration pneumonitis as a result of decreased reactivity of the protective airway reflexes, increased gastric residual volume, and dysfunction of the lower esophageal sphincter, the use of prophylactic oral antacids has been suggested. Others note that healthy geriatric patients are not at an increased aspiration risk and administration of multiple unnecessary drugs should be discouraged.[25]

Anesthetic Technique

As with the selection and administration of preoperative medication, the choice of anesthetic technique should be based on the changes in organ system function in the patient, the pharmacokinetic and pharmacodynamic effects anticipated, the surgical requirements, and the needs and predisposition of the patient. As a rule the geriatric patient is likely to be predisposed to hypotension as a result of reduced activity of the sympathetic nervous system and decreased intravascular volume. Decreased cardiac output and delayed drug clearance are likely to prolong the onset of drug effects and prolong the duration of action.

Regional, general, and MAC techniques are appropriate selections for the geriatric patient. Each technique has a cadre of supporters. No conclusive study has demonstrated the superiority of any one specific anesthetic technique. With regional and local techniques, maintenance of consciousness during the surgical procedure may be associated with less confusion during the postoperative period. However, general anesthesia with endotracheal intubation may be advantageous for promoting bronchopulmonary toilet and facilitating surgical conditions. It appears likely that the patient's preoperative health status and events during the course of the anesthesia that precipitate such physiologic changes as hypotension, hypoxia, hypercarbia, and hypertension do more to affect patient outcome than does anesthetic technique.[26,27]

Monitoring

Few clinicians would argue that all standard noninvasive monitors should be employed in the elderly surgical patient. Standard noninvasive monitors include electrocardiogram (ECG), pulse oximetry, temperature and blood pressure measurement, and end-tidal CO_2 determination. Some controversy exists regarding the application of invasive monitoring techniques, the extent to which they should be used in members of the geriatric population, and the benefit they may provide to improve a patient's outcome. Some clinicians believe that more intensive monitoring should be employed for the geriatric patient compared with the younger patient because of the limited physiologic reserves of the former. Studies report that invasive monitors may allow for earlier recognition and treatment of intraoperative problems and that they lower the incidence of morbidity and mortality. Other researchers question whether the use of invasive monitors has any effect on patient outcome overall, because definitive studies of patient outcome have not been conclusive.[28]

When decisions are made regarding the extent and intensity to which invasive monitors should be employed, it is important to consider that complications from the use of invasive monitors may be increased in the geriatric population. As with the selection of anesthetic agents and techniques, the geriatric patient must be viewed on an individual basis, according to the proposed surgical procedure, the status and age of the patient, and the value the monitor will likely have in enhancing the patient's outcome.[29]

Challenges in the Postanesthesia Care Unit

After operation, evaluation of hemodynamic and pulmonary status should be the focus in the elderly patient. Complications are often related to cardiac and pulmonary dysfunction and decreased reserves. Monitoring with a pulse oximeter may permit detection of the need for supplemental oxygenation or ventilation during the postoperative period, because ventilation-perfusion mismatch is common in geriatric patients. The elderly patient may be especially prone to regurgitation and aspiration from a reduction in airway reflexes. Responsiveness on the part of anesthesia and postanesthesia care unit staff to changes in patient status is especially important for the prevention of rapid deterioration.

In addition, renal and hepatic dysfunction may prolong the duration of action of pharmacologic agents administered to the patient. It is not uncommon to find ventilatory depression from the presence of residual anesthetic during the postoperative period. Postoperatively the patient may be less able to handle the fluid load administered during surgery and should be observed for signs of congestive failure.

The elderly patient also is prone to postoperative heat loss. In order to encourage rewarming and prevent problems associated with shivering, the patient should be placed in a warmed environment.

Finally, the geriatric patient may require special assistance in being oriented to time and place. Prolonged anesthetic effect may compound disorientation to an unfamiliar environment.

Development and implementation of a plan of anesthetic management for the geriatric patient must reflect an appreciation of the fact that the geriatric patient who undergoes surgery and anesthesia may be at increased risk for perioperative morbidity and mortality as a result of continuous physiologic aging processes and concomitant diseases. A thorough understanding of these changes, their impact on the anesthetic process, and variability among the cohort are essential components of continuous quality improvement directed toward decreasing morbidity and mortality in this ever-growing patient population.

REFERENCES

1. Beliveau MM, Multach M. Perioperative care for the elderly patient. *Med Clin North Am.* 2003;87:273-289.
2. Calabrese V, Scapagnini G, Giuffrida Stella AM, Bates TE, Clark JB. Mitochondrial involvement in brain function and dysfunction: relevance to aging, neurogenic disorders and longevity. *Neurochem Res.* 2001;26:739-764.
3. Muravchick S. Preoperative assessment of the elderly patient. *Anesthesiol Clin North Am.* 2000;18:71-89.
4. Kirkbride DA, Parker JL, Williams GD, Buggy DJ. Induction of anesthesia in the elderly ambulatory patient: a double-blinded comparison of propofol and sevoflurane. *Anesth Analg.* 2001; 93:1185-1187.
5. Nesher N, Insler SR, Sheinberg N, et al. A new thermoregulation system for maintaining perioperative normothermia and attenuating myocardial injury in off-pump coronary artery bypass surgery. *Heart Surg Forum.* 2002;5:373-380.
6. Waugaman W, Rigor B. Geriatrics in anesthesia. In: Waugaman WR, Foster SD, Rigor BM, eds. *Principles and Practice of Nurse Anesthesia.* 3rd ed. Norwalk, Conn: Appleton & Lange; 1999:283.
7. Backlund M, Lepantalo M, Toivonen L, et al. Factors associated with post-operative myocardial ischaemia in elderly patients undergoing major non-cardiac surgery. *Eur J Anaesthesiol.* 1999; 16:826-833.
8. Rooke GA. Autonomic and cardiovascular function in the geriatric patient. *Anesthesiol Clin North Am.* 2000;18:31-46.
9. Priebe HJ. The aged cardiovascular risk patient. *Br J Anaesth.* 2001;86:897-898.
10. Zaugg M, Lucchinetti E. Respiratory function in the elderly. *Anesthesiol Clin North Am.* 2000;18:47-58.
11. Raine J, Bishop M. Differences in O_2 tension and physiologic dead space in normal man. *J Appl Physiol.* 1963;18:284-288.
12. Kitamura H, Sawa T, Ikezono E. Postoperative hypoxemia: the contribution of age to the maldistribution of ventilation. *Anesthesiology.* 1972;36:244-252.
13. Rasmussen LS, Moller JT. Central nervous system dysfunction in the geriatric patient. *Anesthesiol Clin North Am.* 2000;18: 59-70.
14. Bjorkman S, Wada DR, Berling BM, Benoni G. Prediction of the disposition of midazolam in surgical patients by a physiologically based pharmacokinetic model. *J Pharm Sci.* 2001;90: 1226-1241.
15. Shafer SL. The pharmacology of anesthetic drugs in elderly patients. *Anesthesiol Clin North Am.* 2000;18:1-29.
16. Kumle B, Boldt J, Piper S, Schmidt C, Suttner S, Salopek S. The influence of different intravascular volume replacement regimens on renal function in the elderly. *Anesth Analg.* 1999;89: 1124-1130.
17. Suttner SW, Schmidt CC, Boldt J, Huttner I, Kumle B, Piper SN. Low-flow desflurane and sevoflurane anesthesia minimally affect hepatic integrity and function in elderly patients. *Anesth Analg.* 2000;91:206-212.
18. Bailes BK. Hypothyroidism in the elderly. *AORN J.* 1999; 69:1026-1030.
19. Bailes BK. Hyperthyroidism in the elderly. *AORN J.* 1999; 69:254-258.
20. Lee M. Drugs in the elderly: do you know the risks? *Am J Nurs.* 1996;96:25-31.
21. Stoelting R. *Pharmacology and Physiology in Anesthesia Practice.* 3rd ed. Philadelphia: Lippincott; 1999:302.
22. Jones AG, Hunter JM. Anaesthesia in the elderly, special considerations. *Drug Aging.* 1996;9:319-331.
23. Muravchick S. Preoperative assessment of the elderly patient. *Anesthesiol Clin North Am.* 2000;18:71-89, vi.
24. Rooke G, et al. Anesthesiology and geriatric medicine: mutual needs and opportunities. *Anesthesiology.* 2002;96:2-4.

25. Nagelhout JJ. Aspiration prophylaxis: is it time for changes in our practice? *AANA J.* 2003;71:299-303.
26. Gilbert TB, Hawkes WG, Hebel JR, et al. Spinal anesthesia versus general anesthesia for hip fracture repair: a longitudinal observation of 741 elderly patients during a 2-year follow-up. *Am J Orthop.* 2000;29:25-35.
27. Leung J, Dzankic S. Relative importance of preoperative health status versus intraoperative factors in predicting postoperative adverse outcomes in geriatric surgical patients. *J Am Geriatr Soc.* 2001;49:1080-1085.
28. O'Hara DA, Duff A, Berlin JA, et al. The effect of anesthetic technique on postoperative outcomes in hip fracture repair. *Anesthesiology.* 2000;92:947-957.
29. Mangano DT. Assessment of the patient with cardiac disease: an anesthesiologist's paradigm. *Anesthesiology.* 1999;91:1521-1526.

CHAPTER 47

POSTANESTHESIA RECOVERY

RICK BROWN

The term *perioperative patient care* implies a continuum of care, because the patient is moved from the preoperative holding or admitting area to the operating room (OR) and then to the postanesthesia care unit (PACU). *Postanesthetic recovery* refers to those activities undertaken to manage the patient after completion of a surgical or nonsurgical procedure in which anesthesia, analgesia, or sedation was administered. The focus of this chapter is on the perioperative management of patients,[1] with the goals of improving postanesthetic safety and quality of life, reducing postoperative adverse events, providing a uniform assessment of recovery, and streamlining postoperative care and discharge criteria.

POSTANESTHESIA CARE UNIT ADMISSION

Before the patient is transferred, PACU personnel should be notified not only to expect the transfer but also to have any necessary equipment (e.g., ventilator, nebulizer, invasive monitoring equipment, pharmacologic infusions) ready and waiting. Knowledge of the patient's acuity enables the PACU staff to best plan the patient's care and to assign that care to an appropriately experienced practitioner.

Both the anesthesia provider and the PACU nurse should collaborate in the patient's admission to the PACU. The immediate priority is evaluation of respiratory and circulatory adequacy. During this initial assessment any signs of inadequate oxygenation or ventilation are identified (Boxes 47-1 and 47-2). Although many of the signs of respiratory compromise could have multifactorial explanations, assessment of the adequacy of oxygenation and ventilation ensures that respiratory inadequacy is not contributory. Any evidence of respiratory compromise requires immediate correction.

Electrocardiographic (ECG) monitoring is initiated for determination of cardiac rate and rhythm. Any deviation from preoperative or intraoperative findings is noted and evaluated. Also, blood pressure is measured, and adequacy of organ perfusion is determined (Box 47-3). Any invasive monitoring, such as an arterial line, is initiated. Any evidence of cardiocirculatory compromise requires immediate correction.

The anesthesia provider should be active during the patient's transfer and stabilization in the PACU. Assistance in the initiation of oxygen therapy, the maintenance or verification of airway adequacy, and the assessment of circulatory status familiarizes PACU personnel with the patient and fosters a smooth transfer of care. After initially stabilizing the patient, the anesthesia provider can communicate relevant preoperative and intraoperative data to the PACU nurse.

BOX 47-1

Signs and Symptoms of Inadequate Oxygenation

Central Nervous System
Restlessness, agitation, confusion, coma
Muscular twitches or seizures

Cardiovascular System
Hypertension, tachycardia (sympathetic nervous system mediated)
Hypotension, bradycardia (direct hypoxic effect)
Dysrhythmias

Skin
Cyanosis (absent in severe anemia and vasoconstriction)
Poor capillary refill

Pulmonary System
Increased-to-absent respiratory efforts
Decreased Pao_2*
Oximetry saturation <90%

**Not standard practice to obtain during initial assessment.*
PaO_2, *Partial pressure of arterial oxygen.*
Modified from Litwack K. Immediate postoperative care: a problem-oriented approach. In: Vender J, Spiess B, eds. Post-Anesthesia Care. *Philadelphia: Saunders; 1992:2.*

ANESTHESIA REPORT

To ensure patient safety and continuity of care, the anesthesia provider must give a verbal report to the PACU nurse that specifies the details of the surgical and anesthetic course, the preoperative conditions that warrant or influence the surgical and anesthetic outcome, and the PACU treatment plan, including suggested interventions and end points. A coherent order for the presentation of this information is presented in Box 47-4.

The importance of the anesthesia report is reflected in the American Association of Nurse Anesthetists (AANA) guideline, from the *AANA Scope and Standards for Nurse Anesthesia Practice*[2]: "Standard VII: Transfer the responsibility for care of the patient to other qualified providers in a manner which assures continuity of care and patient safety."

BOX 47-2

Signs and Symptoms of Inadequate Ventilation

Spontaneous Ventilation
Increased or decreased respiratory frequency
Nasal flaring
Suprasternal or intercostal retractions
Decreased to absent movement of air at mouth, nares, or endotracheal tube
Abnormal airway sounds
Decreased to absent breath sounds
Diminished chest movement
Diaphragmatic breathing
Abnormal $ETCO_2$ or $PaCO_2$ values*
Signs of inadequate oxygenation (see Box 47-1)

Assisted or Controlled Ventilation
Increased frequency of respiratory efforts
Decreased chest expansion and contraction during ventilatory cycle
Abnormally high inflation pressures
Decreased to absent air movements in endotracheal tube
Decreased to absent breath sounds
Decreased air movement as assessed by monitors (apnea, capnography)
Abnormal $ETCO_2$ or $PaCO_2$ values*
Signs of inadequate oxygenation (see Box 47-1)

**Not standard practice to obtain during initial assessment.*
$ETCO_2$, *End-tidal carbon dioxide;* $PaCO_2$, *partial pressure of arterial carbon dioxide.*
Modified from Litwack K. Immediate postoperative care: a problem-oriented approach. In: Vender J, Spiess B, eds. Post-Anesthesia Care. *Philadelphia: Saunders; 1992:2.*

BOX 47-3

Signs of Adequate Organ Perfusion

Central Nervous System
Appropriate mentation
Intact sensation, motor function, reflexes
Electroencephalographic and evoked potential results appropriate for residual anesthetic exposure*

Cardiovascular System
Electrocardiography shows normal sinus rhythm without signs of ischemia
Cardiac output appropriate for preload and metabolic acuity*

Skin
Warm and dry with good color and capillary refill

Renal System
Urine production >0.5 ml/kg/hr (of appropriate specific gravity and composition)*
No evidence of osmotic diuresis
No evidence of postobstructive diuresis

Pulmonary System
Normal arterial blood gas results*
Normal intrapulmonary shunt activity*

**Not standard practice to obtain during initial assessment.*
Modified from Litwack K. Immediate postoperative care: a problem-oriented approach. In: Vender J, Spiess B, eds. Post-Anesthesia Care. *Philadelphia: Saunders; 1992:2.*

INITIAL POSTANESTHESIA CARE UNIT ASSESSMENT

Many postanesthesia assessment approaches (e.g., head-to-toe, major body systems assessments and scoring systems) are currently used in PACUs, and each approach has its benefits and limitations. The assessment approach should accomplish the following:

1. Determine the patient's physiologic status at the time of admission to the PACU
2. Allow the periodic reexamination of the patient so that physiologic trends become obvious
3. Establish the patient's baseline level so that the effect of previous medical conditions can be assessed and predicted as they affect current physiology
4. Assess the ongoing status of the surgical site and its effect on any preexisting conditions and recovery
5. Assess the patient's recovery from anesthesia and note residual effects
6. Allow the compilation and trend analysis of patient-specific characteristics that relate to discharge or transfer criteria[3]

Anesthesia personnel must manage the patient until PACU providers secure admission vital signs and attach appropriate monitors. To optimize safety the anesthesia provider cannot shift responsibility to PACU personnel until the patient's airway status, ventilation, and hemodynamics are appropriate.

Aldrete's Scoring System

The most commonly used assessment approach is a combination of the Aldrete scoring system[4] and the major body systems assessment. The Aldrete scoring system evaluates the patient's activity, respiration, circulation, consciousness, and color (Box 47-5). Patients receive a numeric score of 0, 1, or 2 in each area, with 2 representing the highest level of function. The Aldrete postanesthetic scoring system is the most widely used scoring system in PACUs, although its predictive value in determining recovery from anesthesia has not been studied prospectively.

Major Body Systems

The major body systems assessment systematically evaluates the body systems that are most affected by anesthesia and the surgical procedure. After the patient is admitted to the PACU, an assessment of cardiorespiratory stability and a more in-depth cardiac assessment are performed. The heart is auscultated, and the quality of heart sounds, the presence of any adventitious sounds, and any irregularities in rate or rhythm are noted. Unexpected findings are compared with preoperative data. Arterial pulses are evaluated for strength and equality. An ECG strip is obtained on admission to the PACU and compared with the preoperative ECG. In addition, body temperature and skin color and condition are assessed and the findings documented.

After respiratory and cardiac assessments are completed, the neurologic system is evaluated, with a focus on the level of

BOX **47-4**

Anesthesia Admission Report

General Information
Patient name
Patient age
Surgical procedure
Name of surgeon and anesthesia provider(s)

Intraoperative Management
Anesthetic agents, including dose
Time of last narcotic administration
Use of reversal agents
Intraoperative medications (antibiotics, antiemetics, vasopressors)
Estimated blood loss
Fluid and blood administration
Urine output

Intraoperative Course
Unexpected response to anesthetic administration
Unexpected surgical course
Laboratory results (arterial blood gas, glucose, hemoglobin)

Patient History
Acute (indication for surgery)
Chronic (medical history, medication use, allergies)

Postanesthesia Care Unit Plan
Potential and expected problems
Suggested interventions
Limits of acceptability of laboratory test
Discharge criteria
Responsible contact person

BOX **47-5**

Postanesthesia Recovery Score

Activity
0 = Unable to lift head or move extremities voluntarily or on command.
1 = Moves two extremities voluntarily or on command and can lift head.
2 = Able to move four extremities voluntarily or on command. Can lift head and has controlled movement. Exceptions: patients with a prolonged block such as with bupivacaine (Marcaine), who may not move an affected extremity for as long as 18 hours; patients who were immobile preoperatively.

Respiration
0 = Apneic; condition necessitates ventilator or assisted respiration.
1 = Labored or limited respirations. Breathes by self but has shallow, slow respirations. May have an oral airway.
2 = Can take a deep breath and cough well; has normal respiratory rate and depth.

Circulation
0 = Has abnormally high or low blood pressure; blood pressure within 50 mm Hg of preanesthetic level
1 = Blood pressure within 20-50 mm Hg of preanesthetic level
2 = Stable blood pressure and pulse. Blood pressure 2 mm Hg of preanesthetic level (minimum 90 mm Hg systolic). Exception: patient may be released by anesthesia provider after drug therapy.

Neurologic Status
0 = Not responding or responding only to painful stimuli.
1 = Responds to verbal stimuli but drifts to sleep easily.
2 = Awake and alert; oriented to time, place, and person.

O_2 Saturation
0 = O_2 saturation <90%, even with O_2 supplement
1 = Needs O_2 inhalation to maintain O_2 saturation >90%
2 = Able to maintain O_2 saturation >92% on room air

Modified from Aldrete J, Kroulik D. A post anesthetic recovery score. Anesth Analg. *1970;49:924-933; Aldrete JA. Discharge criteria.* Bailliere's Clin Anaesthesiol. *1994;8:763-773; and Odom J. Management and policy. In: Drain CB, ed.* Perianesthesia Nursing. *4th ed. Philadelphia: Saunders; 2003:38.*

consciousness, orientation, sensory and motor status, and pupil size, equality, and reactivity.

The renal system assessment focuses on fluid intake and output (blood, crystalloids, and colloids), as well as on volume and electrolyte status. The anesthesia provider gives intraoperative fluid totals in the verbal report, and the PACU nurse notes and documents all intravenous (IV) lines, irrigation solutions, and infusions that enter the patient. All output devices, including drains, catheters, and tubes, are inspected, and the color and consistency of any drainage are noted.

All data obtained in the admission assessment should be documented in a manner that facilitates data collection, trend analysis, and retrieval.

ONGOING ASSESSMENT

Perioperative and postanesthetic management of the patient includes periodic assessment and monitoring of the following[1]:

- Respiratory function (obstruction, hypoxemia, hypercarbia)
- Cardiovascular function (hypotension, hypertension, dysrhythmias)

- Neuromuscular function (inadequate reversal of neuromuscular blockade)
- Mental status (delayed awakening, emergence delirium)
- Pain
- Temperature (hypothermia)
- Nausea and vomiting
- Fluids
- Urine output and voiding

Respiratory Function

In postoperative patients, airway problems that interfere with oxygenation and ventilation are always related to an increase in the resistance to gas flow somewhere in the airways.[5]

Obstruction

In postanesthetic patients the tongue causes most upper airway obstructions. Obstruction occurs when the tongue falls back into a position that occludes the pharynx and blocks the flow of air into and out of the lungs. Signs and symptoms of an upper airway obstruction include snoring and activation of accessory muscles of ventilation. Intercostal and suprasternal retractions may be noted. However, patients are usually somnolent and may be difficult to arouse. Risk factors for an upper airway obstruction include anatomy (obesity, large neck, or short neck), poor muscle tone (secondary to narcotics, sedation, residual neuromuscular blockade, or neuromuscular disease), or swelling (secondary to surgical manipulation, edema, or anaphylaxis).

The goal for the relief of a tongue obstruction is a patent airway. Treatment consists of a series of interventions. The initial intervention may be as simple as stimulating the patient to take deep breaths, or it may require repositioning of the airway via a jaw thrust or a chin lift. Placement of an oral or a nasal airway may be required. The nasal airway is tolerated much better by patients emerging from general anesthesia, and unlike the oral airway, it is unlikely to cause gagging or vomiting. If the obstruction remains unrelieved, reintubation may be required, with or without adjunctive mechanical ventilation.

Laryngeal obstruction may occlude the airway as a result of partial or complete spasm of the intrinsic or extrinsic muscles of the larynx. Laryngospasm may be the result of a reflex closure of the glottis (intrinsic muscles) or of the larynx (extrinsic muscles).[5] Glottic closure usually manifests as intermittent obstruction; laryngeal closure manifests as complete obstruction. Airway irritation that predisposes a patient to laryngospasm may be the result of laryngoscopy, secretions, vomitus, blood, artificial airway placement, coughing, bronchospasm, or frequent suctioning. Symptoms that suggest laryngospasm include agitation, decreased oxygen saturation, absent breath sounds, and acute respiratory distress. Incomplete obstruction may manifest as a crowing sound or stridor.

Treatment of laryngospasm must be immediate. Positive-pressure ventilation with 100% oxygen is the initial intervention. If this intervention is ineffective, a subparalytic dose of IV succinylcholine (0.1 mg/kg) may be given. If succinylcholine is administered, assisted ventilation for 5 to 10 minutes is required, even if the obstruction has been relieved. Reintubation should be required only if severe airway edema is present or if the obstruction persists despite treatment interventions.

Steroids and topical or IV lidocaine have been included in the prevention and management of airway irritability. Other preventive strategies include obtaining meticulous hemostasis during surgery, suctioning the oropharynx before extubation to clear any retained blood or secretions, and extubating the patient when he or she is in either a very deep plane of anesthesia or the awake state.[5] When obstruction occurs, rapid intervention is imperative, because the arterial carbon dioxide pressure ($PaCO_2$) increases 6 mm Hg in the first minute of total obstruction and an additional 3 to 4 mm Hg each minute thereafter.[6]

Hypoxemia

Hypoxemia defined as low arterial oxygen pressure (PaO_2) (usually <60 mm Hg) is characterized by nonspecific signs and symptoms ranging from agitation to somnolence, hypertension to hypotension, and tachycardia to bradycardia. Pulse oximetry may confirm low oxygen saturation (<90%); arterial blood gas analysis may confirm a PaO_2 of less than 60 mm Hg. Hypoxemia, if untreated, can result in organ ischemia.

Hypoxemia can be the result of a delivered low concentration of oxygen, hypoventilation, impaired alveolar-capillary diffusion, ventilation-perfusion mismatches, or increased intrapulmonary shunting.[7] The most common causes of hypoxemia in the PACU include atelectasis, pulmonary edema, pulmonary embolism, aspiration, bronchospasm, and hypoventilation. A brief explanation of these pathologic states follows.

Atelectasis

Atelectasis is the most common cause of postoperative arterial hypoxemia and can lead to an increase in the right-to-left shunt. Atelectasis may be the result of bronchial obstruction caused by secretions or decreased lung volumes. Hypotension and low cardiac output conditions can also contribute to the development of decreased perfusion and atelectasis.[8] Treatment includes the use of humidified oxygen, coughing, deep breathing, postural drainage, and increased mobility. Incentive spirometry and intermittent positive-pressure ventilation may also be used.[8]

Pulmonary Edema. Pulmonary edema, which is caused by fluid accumulation within the alveoli, may be the result of an increase in hydrostatic pressure, a decrease in interstitial pressure, or an increase in capillary permeability.

An increase in hydrostatic pressure is usually the result of fluid overload, left ventricular failure (especially in the presence of systolic hypertension), mitral valve dysfunction, or ischemic heart disease. A decrease in interstitial pressure is often seen after prolonged airway obstruction. Increased capillary permeability may be the result of sepsis, aspiration, transfusion reaction, trauma, anaphylaxis, shock, or disseminated intravascular coagulation and is frequently referred to as *adult respiratory distress syndrome*.[5] Pulmonary edema is characterized by hypoxemia, rales on auscultation, decreased lung compliance, and pulmonary infiltrates seen on chest radiography.

Treatment of pulmonary edema is directed toward identification of the cause and toward reduction of hydrostatic pressure within the lungs. Oxygenation must be maintained, particularly in the presence of profound hypoxemia, via mask or, if necessary, intubation, mechanical ventilation, and the addition of positive end-expiratory pressure (PEEP) ventilation. Diuretics (most commonly furosemide) and fluid restriction are a part of treatment. Dialysis may be used if the fluid retention results from renal failure. Afterload reduction, which is achieved through the use of nitroglycerin or sodium nitroprusside, may be used in order to decrease myocardial work.[5]

Pulmonary Embolism

Pulmonary embolism is a leading cause of morbidity and mortality, accounting for 50,000 to 90,000 deaths annually in the United States. Most cases of pulmonary embolism are not fatal; however, two thirds of all deaths caused by a pulmonary embolism occur within 30 minutes of an acute event.[9]

Patients can be considered to be at risk for pulmonary embolism if three conditions, known as *Virchow's triad*, exist: venous stasis, hypercoagulability, and abnormalities of the blood vessel wall. These conditions are accentuated in the presence of obesity, varicose veins, immobility, malignancy, congestive heart failure, and increased age and after pelvic or long-bone surgery or injury. However, 90% of all pulmonary emboli arise from deep veins in the legs.[9-10]

A pulmonary embolism should be suspected in a patient who complains of or whose presenting signs include acute-onset tachypnea, dyspnea, and tachycardia, particularly when the patient is already receiving oxygen therapy. Signs and symptoms may also include chest pain, hypotension, hemoptysis, dysrhythmias, and congestive heart failure. Although the clinical symptomatology may be suggestive of a pulmonary embolism, confirmation requires pulmonary angiography. Pulmonary angiography is infrequently performed because of its high risk and associated mortality. A ventilation-perfusion scan may also prove useful.

Treatment of a pulmonary embolism is directed toward the correction of hypoxemia and support of hemodynamic stability. Preventive measures may include the use of antiembolic stockings or sequential compression devices. Subcutaneous heparin therapy may also be initiated. Once the occurrence of a pulmonary embolism has been confirmed, IV heparin therapy is started for the prevention of further clot formation. The goal of heparin therapy is an activated partial thromboplastin time that is 1.5 to 2 times the control value.

Aspiration

Aspiration is a potentially serious airway emergency that can compromise patient safety and stability on the induction of, or the emergence from, anesthesia. Aspiration may occur in the OR, in the PACU, or at any time during transfer. Patients may aspirate foreign matter (e.g., a tooth, food), blood, or gastric contents. Each type of material is associated with a characteristic clinical presentation.

Foreign matter aspiration may result in cough, airway obstruction, atelectasis, bronchospasm, and pneumonia. A profound reflex sympathetic nervous system (SNS) response might also cause hypertension, tachycardia, and dysrhythmias. In the absence of complete upper airway obstruction, complications are often localized and treated with supportive care once the foreign matter has been expelled or removed by bronchoscopy.[9]

Aspiration of blood may result from trauma or surgical manipulation and may also cause minor airway obstruction that is rapidly cleared by cough, resorption, and phagocytosis. Massive blood aspiration interferes with gas exchange through mechanical blockage of airways and leads to chronic fibrinous changes in air spaces or pulmonary hemochromatosis from iron accumulation in phagocytic cells. Aspiration of blood may result in infection, particularly if particles of soft tissue are aspirated along with the blood.[11] Treatment involves correction of hypoxemia, maintenance of airway patency, and initiation of antibiotic therapy, if indicated.

Aspiration of gastric contents is the most severe form of aspiration and may result in a chemical pneumonitis. Patients have diffuse bronchospasm (secondary to reflex airway closure), hypoxemia (compromised alveolar-capillary membrane), atelectasis (loss of surfactant), interstitial edema (loss of capillary integrity), hemorrhage, and adult respiratory distress syndrome. Gastric aspiration may also cause laryngospasm, infection, and pulmonary edema.

For this reason the prevention of gastric aspiration, rather than its treatment, is the goal. Patients who are at risk for gastric aspiration (e.g., obese or pregnant patients or those with a history of hiatal hernia, peptic ulcer, or trauma) may be given histamine-2 (H_2) blockers, gastrokinetic agents, nonparticulate antacids, or anticholinergics before anesthesia induction.[11] Rapid-sequence induction is likely used. Intraoperatively a nasogastric tube may be inserted and is usually then removed in order to decrease gastric volume and decompress the stomach. Postoperatively the patient should be left intubated until airway reflexes return.

Treatment of gastric aspiration is directed toward correction of hypoxemia and maintenance of hemodynamic stability. Antibiotics are indicated only if signs of infection (e.g., fever, leukocytosis, positive culture results) are present. Steroid use is controversial.[12] Clinicians who advocate the use of steroids cite their usefulness in decreasing inflammation, stabilizing the lysosomal membrane, and decreasing pulmonary cellular damage.[12] Clinicians who do not support the use of steroids argue that the agents have no therapeutic benefit, may mask infection, and do not improve long-term outcome.

If aspiration causes hypoxemia, increased airway resistance, atelectasis, or pulmonary edema, institution of support with supplemental oxygen, PEEP or continuous positive airway pressure, and mechanical ventilation is often necessary. Pulmonary edema is usually secondary to increased capillary permeability, so diuretics should not be used to decrease intravascular volume. Bacterial infection does not always occur, so prophylactic antibiotics might merely promote colonization by resistant organisms. If evidence of secondary bacterial infections appears, specific antibiotic therapy is instituted, based on sputum samples obtained for Gram stain and culture or on prevailing colonization experience within the institution.[11]

Bronchospasm

Bronchospasm results from an increase in bronchial smooth muscle tone with resultant closure of small airways. As a result of the strong increase in inspiratory force against these closed airways, airway edema develops, causing secretions to build up in the airway. Clinically, the patient demonstrates wheezing, dyspnea, use of accessory muscles, and tachypnea. Airway resistance is increased, and increased peak inspiratory pressures are noted if the patient is receiving mechanical ventilation.[5]

Bronchospasm may result from aspiration, pharyngeal or tracheal suctioning, endotracheal intubation, histamine release secondary to medications, or an allergic response and it may be seen in greater frequency in patients with a history of asthma or chronic obstructive pulmonary disease.

Treatment of bronchospasm requires confirmation and removal of the precipitating cause. Pharmacotherapy is instituted with the goals of decreasing airway irritability and promoting bronchodilation. Medications used in the management of bronchospasm include salmeterol (Serevent) and β_2-agonists such as albuterol (Proventil, Ventolin), salbutamol, and terbutaline and, if the condition is life threatening, IV epinephrine.[5] Cholinergics such as atropine sulfate and glycopyrrolate have been given via nebulization in order to decrease secretions.

Steroids have been used if the underlying cause is an inflammatory disease such as asthma.

Hypoventilation

Hypoventilation is a common, easily recognizable complication in the PACU. It is manifested clinically by a decrease in respiratory rate that results in an increase in $PaCO_2$ secondary to a decrease in alveolar ventilation.[6] This may occur because of a decrease in central respiratory drive, poor respiratory muscle function, or a combination of both.[8]

Depression of central respiratory drive can occur with both IV and inhalation anesthetics. Central respiratory depression is most profound on admission to the PACU, although the time and route of anesthetic administration may suggest otherwise. For example, an IV dose of fentanyl given just before the patient emerges from anesthesia may not peak until later in the PACU. An intramuscular dose of a narcotic takes substantially longer to peak than does an IV dose.[9]

Patients may also demonstrate a secondary stage of respiratory depression once certain stimuli are removed. For example, a patient may be admitted awake and breathing to the PACU with an endotracheal tube in place. After extubation, because of the loss of stimulation from the endotracheal tube, the patient may become hypercarbic secondary to residual narcotic effects and hypoventilation.[5]

Poor respiratory muscle function can result from many conditions. Some of the most common situations are inadequate reversal of neuromuscular blocking agents, surgery involving the upper abdomen, positioning, obesity, and diseases involving the neuromuscular system.

Inadequate reversal of neuromuscular blocking agents can result in hypoventilation secondary to respiratory muscle weakness. Factors that can adversely affect neuromuscular blockade and reversal include certain medications, hypokalemia, hypermagnesemia, hypothermia, and acidosis.[13]

Medications that have been associated with prolongation of blockade include the aminoglycoside antibiotics (gentamicin, clindamycin, and neomycin), as well as furosemide and propranolol.[14] Hypermagnesemia and hypothermia may potentiate neuromuscular blockade. Hypokalemia and respiratory acidosis inhibit reversal.[14]

Upper abdominal surgery can also affect respiratory muscle function. Hypoventilation occurs because of a reduced vital capacity secondary to poor diaphragmatic function.[15] A reduction in vital capacity of up to 60% has been noted on the first postoperative day.[15] Obesity, especially when combined with upper abdominal surgery, further contributes to hypoventilation because of the increased intraabdominal pressure in obese patients.

Diseases of the neuromuscular system can also affect ventilation. Patients with muscular dystrophy, myasthenia gravis, Eaton-Lambert syndrome, Guillain-Barré syndrome, or other muscle diseases can exhibit postoperative muscle weakness. Patients with severe scoliosis also exhibit poor respiratory muscle function. It is often in the best interest of the patients with these disorders that they remain intubated in the PACU until complete return of function occurs and any residual anesthetic effects are absent.

Cardiovascular Function

Hypotension

Classically, hypotension has been defined as a blood pressure of less than 20% of the baseline or preoperative blood pressure. However, the clinical signs of hypoperfusion, rather than numeric values, should be the indicators of compromise. Because the autonomic nervous system preferentially maintains blood flow to the brain, heart, and kidneys, signs of hypoperfusion to these organs (including disorientation, nausea, loss of consciousness, chest pain, oliguria, and anuria) reflect the failure of physiologic compensation. Hypoxia, which results from hypoperfusion, may cause lactic acidosis. Intervention must be implemented in a timely fashion so that cerebral ischemia, cerebrovascular accident (CVA), myocardial infarction or ischemia, renal ischemia, bowel infarction, and spinal cord damage do not develop.[16]

Hypotension in the PACU is most commonly caused by hypovolemia secondary to inadequate replacement of intraoperative fluid and blood loss. As a result initial treatment is directed toward the restoration of circulating volume. A 300- to 500-ml fluid bolus of physiologic saline or lactated Ringer's solution should be given. If no response is noted, myocardial dysfunction should be considered the cause of hypotension.

Primary cardiac dysfunction, as is the case with myocardial infarction, tamponade, or embolism, results in an acute fall in ventricular emptying and cardiac output. Secondary cardiac dysfunction occurs as a result of the negative chronotropic and negative inotropic effects of medications.

Low systemic vascular resistance (SVR) can also contribute to hypotension. Numerous anesthetic agents cause histamine release with subsequent vasodilation (e.g., barbiturates, morphine, atracurium, mivacurium), whereas others cause vasodilation by directly relaxing arterial smooth muscle (volatile inhalation anesthetics, local anesthetics used for producing spinal anesthesia). Sensitivity to vasodilators such as hydralazine, sodium nitroprusside, and nitroglycerin can also produce profound hypotension. Sepsis may be another cause of low SVR.

Arrhythmias that interfere with cardiac conduction and subsequently compromise cardiac output can also produce hypotension. Tachyarrhythmias prevent optimal ventricular filling and emptying. Conduction blocks compromise myocardial effectiveness, resulting in a lowered cardiac output and hypotension.

Intervention should always include supplemental oxygen therapy while the cause of the hypotension is investigated. Volume status should be evaluated, and preoperative and intraoperative fluid administration should be considered. Hypotension caused by artifact of the measurement system should also be considered, for example, a blood pressure cuff that is too large or too small or an inappropriate transducer height. The presence of hypotension secondary to myocardial dysfunction suggests the need for coronary vasodilators, inotropic therapy, and afterload reduction (e.g., through nitroglycerin therapy, dobutamine therapy, or both). Secondary myocardial dysfunction may require that administration of the causative medications be discontinued. Vasodilation resulting in lower SVR and symptomatic hypoperfusion can be treated with vasoconstrictive agents, either by IV bolus (ephedrine) or by infusion (dopamine or epinephrine).

Hypertension

Hypertension, defined as a 20% to 30% increase relative to the baseline blood pressure, is a common finding in the PACU and can be caused by stimulation of the SNS and pain, respiratory compromise, visceral distention, and significant increases in plasma catecholamine levels that produce vasoconstriction.

Pain remains the leading cause of hypertension and tachycardia in the PACU and results in stimulation of the somatic afferent nerves, producing a pressor response known as the *somatosympathetic reflex*.[16] The use of analgesics attenuates the sympathetic response, thereby normalizing blood pressure.

Hypoxemia and hypercarbia cause direct stimulation of the vasomotor area of the medulla, resulting in increased vasomotor tone, increased arteriolar constriction, and increased blood pressure.[16] Correction of the respiratory compromise should result in normalization of blood pressure.

Distention of the bladder, bowel, or stomach causes stimulation of afferent fibers of the SNS, producing an increase in plasma catecholamine levels. Catheterization of the bladder and decompression of the bowel or stomach remove the offending stimulus.

Hypertension may also develop as a sequela of hypothermia. Increased catecholamine secretion is an important endocrine response to cold.[16] As cooling occurs, blood vessels become more sensitive to catecholamines, resulting in arteriolar and venous constriction. Rewarming reverses the process. As vasodilation occurs, reperfusion of the extremities and skin decreases systemic elevations in pressure.

Preexisting hypertension exists in many of the patients who develop hypertension in the PACU. The degree of elevation in pressure is greater if preoperative antihypertensive medications are withdrawn suddenly. Ideally, patients receive their antihypertensive medications on the day of surgery.

Hypertension may also be seen after vascular or cardiac surgery, including carotid endarterectomy, secondary to revascularization and baroreceptor stimulation. Pharmacologic intervention is required for the protection of graft sites and the prevention of hemorrhage. Sodium nitroprusside and nitroglycerin are agents of choice for vasodilation.

Other agents that may be used for the reduction of blood pressure include hydralazine, labetalol hydrochloride, and nifedipine. Hydralazine relaxes vascular smooth muscle, preferentially favoring the arteriolar circulation. Labetalol is both an α- and a β-blocking agent, causing peripheral vasodilation and slowing of the heart rate. Nifedipine, a calcium channel blocker, relaxes coronary artery smooth muscle and dilates peripheral arteries.

Arrhythmias

Arrhythmias seen in the PACU most commonly have an identifiable cause that is not an actual myocardial injury. The major postanesthetic and surgical factors that lead to a relatively high incidence of perioperative arrhythmias include hypokalemia, hypoxia, hypercarbia, altered acid-base status, circulatory instability, and preexisting heart disease.

Arterial desaturation is a common postoperative complication that may result from obstruction or hypoventilation or less commonly from pulmonary embolism, pulmonary edema, or aspiration. A direct consequence of hypoxia is myocardial ischemia and depression of cardiac contractility. Signs of cardiac irritability may be manifested by atrial and ventricular arrhythmias, conduction delays, and heart block.

Hypercarbia caused by reduced alveolar ventilation results in elevation of the arterial carbon dioxide tension, which in turn stimulates the SNS and sensitizes the myocardium to the arrhythmic effects of endogenous catecholamines. Among the earliest signs of hypercarbia are tachycardia and hypertension, which may progress to ventricular arrhythmias.

Hypokalemia may occur secondary to hyperventilation, respiratory alkalosis, gastric suctioning, insulin administration, and diuretic use. The ECG may demonstrate widening of the QRS complex, U waves, and ST-segment abnormalities that may progress into premature ventricular complexes, ventricular tachycardia, and ventricular fibrillation.

Acid-base disturbances may occur as a result of alterations in ventilation, gastrointestinal losses, and lactic acid production during hypotension or shock. The cardiovascular effects include increased cardiac excitability and irritability.

Hypotension may result in impaired oxygen transport and compromised coronary circulation, leading to myocardial ischemia with associated conduction deficits. The use of vasoconstrictive medications designed to treat the hypotension may also contribute to the development of dysrhythmias.[17,18] Patients with preexisting heart disease, particularly those who have a history of myocardial infarction, are at continued risk for myocardial ischemia throughout the perioperative period.[19]

Hypothermia prolongs the refractory period, contributing to the development of sinus bradycardia and atrial fibrillation. Conduction deficits may progress to atrioventricular block and eventually to ventricular fibrillation.[20]

Vagal reflexes are usually transient and are produced by the Valsalva maneuver or direct eye, vagal nerve, or carotid sinus pressure. Severe sinus bradycardia with possible ventricular escape beats may occur. Vagotonic medications, such as neostigmine or pyridostigmine, can also produce these arrhythmias.[20]

The presence of residual anesthetics in both blood and tissue in patients admitted to the PACU may lower arrhythmia thresholds. Halothane sensitizes the myocardium to catecholamines and depresses sinoatrial and atrioventricular nodal function. Junctional rhythms and ventricular extrasystoles are most commonly seen. Ketamine may contribute to sympathetic stimulation, resulting in tachyarrhythmias and hypertension, as can vagolytic drugs such as atropine and glycopyrrolate.[21,22] Narcotics such as morphine, fentanyl, and sufentanil may result in the indirect development of dysrhythmias. Respiratory depression, a potential side effect of narcotics, may result in hypoxemia and hypercarbia, both of which are known to be arrhythmogenic. Narcotics, with the exception of meperidine, may also be direct myocardial depressants.[21] Succinylcholine has been associated with atrial, nodal, and ventricular arrhythmias.[21] Anticholinesterase agents may produce severe bradyarrhythmias or heart block.[21]

Surgical stress and pain can significantly increase plasma catecholamine levels. Although this sympathetic response may be mitigated by anesthetic administration, norepinephrine and epinephrine concentrations are consistently elevated in PACU patients who are in pain. Administration of analgesic medications may blunt this sympathetic response; however, cardiac irritability, tachycardia, and conduction dysrhythmias may occur.[18]

Neuromuscular Function

Reversal of Neuromuscular Blockade

Incomplete reversal of neuromuscular relaxation can lead to postoperative airway obstruction and hypoventilation. Residual paralysis compromises cough, airway patency, ability to overcome airway resistance, and airway protection. Intraoperative use of shorter-acting relaxants might decrease the incidence of residual paralysis but does not eliminate the problem.[23] Marginal reversal can be more dangerous than near total paralysis, because an agitated patient exhibiting uncoordinated movements and airway obstruction is more easily identified. A somnolent patient exhibiting mild stridor and shallow ventilation from marginal neuromuscular function might be overlooked. Insidious hypoventilation leading to respiratory acidemia or regurgitation with aspiration can occur later into recovery. Patients with coexisting neuromuscular abnormalities such as myasthenia gravis, Eaton-Lambert syndrome, or muscular dystrophies exhibit exaggerated or prolonged responses to muscle relaxants. Even without muscle relaxant administration, such patients can exhibit postoperative respiratory insufficiency from inadequate neuromuscular reserves.

Simple bedside tests help assess mechanical ability to ventilate. Forced vital capacity of 10 to 12 ml/kg and inspiratory pressure more negative than -25 cm H_2O imply that strength of ventilatory muscles is adequate to sustain ventilation. Sustained head elevation in a supine position, hand grip, and ability to bite down, swallow, and stick out the tongue are easily assessed parameters. These measures, along with tactile train-of-four and double-burst stimulation assessment, accurately predict a patient's ability to maintain sustained ventilation.

Mental Status

Emergence Delirium

Postoperatively, emergence delirium is the alteration in neurologic functioning that causes the most concern to the practitioner. *Delirium* is defined as a condition that is characterized by extreme disturbances of arousal, attention, orientation, perception, intellectual function, and affect and is most commonly accompanied by fear and agitation.[24] The incidence of postoperative delirium has been described to be 3% to 20%; with some procedures the incidence may be as high as 75%.[24] The causes of postoperative delirium have been classified into four categories: withdrawal psychosis, toxic psychosis, circulatory and respiratory origin, and functional psychosis.[24]

Withdrawal psychosis is caused by withdrawal of various substances, such as alcohol and illicit drugs. Alcohol withdrawal can be dangerous because it can cause delirium tremens. Clinical symptoms of delirium tremens may include hallucinations, extreme combativeness, and confusion.[24]

Amphetamine-induced delirium usually appears 1 hour after amphetamine use and disappears within 6 hours of use. Cocaine-induced delirium results from alteration of neurotransmitters. Management of withdrawal psychosis may include protection of patient safety and use of benzodiazepines or other sedatives.[24]

Toxic psychosis is caused by exposure to toxins, including toxic fumes that may occur in the OR, as from a malfunctioning laser. The Occupational Safety and Health Administration's regulations and its mandates on monitoring help to limit the occurrence of these events.[25]

Circulatory and respiratory causes of emergence delirium most commonly include hypoxemia and hypercarbia, which may be the result of central respiratory depression, airway obstruction, or perfusion deficits. The primary cause of postoperative emergence delirium is always considered to be hypoxemia until proved otherwise. As a result, sedation of the agitated patient should never be considered until hypoxemia has been ruled out as the cause of agitation.

Functional psychosis is defined as a brief reaction of paranoia and other changes not caused by an organic abnormality. This diagnosis is made by exclusion after known organic causes have been ruled out.[25]

Although this classification is useful, other, more frequently occurring causes of emergence delirium may be seen in the PACU. Confusion and agitation are common during recovery from inhalation anesthetics. Many drugs used during the perioperative period have been reported to contribute to postoperative delirium. Ketamine, a phencyclidine hydrochloride derivative, is associated with hallucinations, delirium, and unpleasant dreams, particularly in patients between 16 and 65 years of age.[26] Local anesthetics can cross the blood-brain barrier and may cause postoperative delirium. Nitrous oxide may cause acute mental status changes with prolonged exposure.[26] Other anesthetic adjuncts associated with delirium include butyrophenones (e.g., droperidol), naloxone, and muscle relaxants, which can cause dissociative reactions, heightened pain perception, and hypoxemia, respectively.[26] Delirium has also been reported as a side effect of antibiotic therapy (e.g., cefazolin, penicillin, streptomycin, chloramphenicol), antituberculosis drugs (e.g., isoniazid, cycloserine), antiviral agents (e.g., acyclovir), anticonvulsant medications (e.g., carbamazepine, phenytoin), and anti-Parkinson's agents (e.g., levodopa, bromocriptine).[26] Adverse reactions to medications that result in delirium have been reported with digitalis, antiarrhythmics (e.g., amiodarone, flecainide, lidocaine, mexiletine), β-blockers, calcium channel blockers, contrast dye, corticosteroids, chemotherapeutic agents, immunosuppressants, H_1 and H_2 blockers, antipsychotic medications, and clonidine.[26]

Premedicants, including anticholinergics, benzodiazepines, and opioids, may induce untoward reactions. Anticholinergics, specifically atropine and scopolamine, have been noted to cause central anticholinergic syndrome. These drugs cross the blood-brain barrier, altering the neurotransmitter balance and causing agitation, combativeness, and lack of cooperation. Central anticholinergic syndrome is reversible with physostigmine salicylate (Antilirium), which is the only anticholinesterase that crosses the blood-brain barrier. Benzodiazepines may contribute to postoperative delirium, especially in the elderly.[27] Flumazenil (Romazicon) remains the only benzodiazepine antagonist available to reverse the effects of benzodiazepine-induced delirium. Opioids, particularly morphine, have been cited as a contributing factor to postoperative delirium, secondary to respiratory depression and hypoxemia. In patients with renal failure, meperidine may cause excitation because of accumulation of normeperidine, a neuroexcitatory metabolic byproduct.

Metabolic disturbances associated with postoperative delirium include acidosis and alkalosis, electrolyte imbalance (magnesium, calcium, sodium), and porphyria. Treatment is directed at correction of the cause.[26]

Other causes of postoperative delirium include pain, visceral distention (bowel and bladder), anxiety (including separation anxiety in children), hyperthermia, and hypothermia.[26] Again, treatment is directed at correction of the cause.

Once hypoxemia has been eliminated as a cause of postoperative delirium and all known causes have been evaluated, sedation may prove useful in controlling the agitation and in providing for patient safety. Most events are time limited to the PACU and are resolved before discharge. Figure 47-1 summarizes the factors that contribute to postoperative delirium and treatment options.

Delayed Awakening

Delayed awakening is a common, often easily explained postoperative finding and can be defined as a clinician's expectation

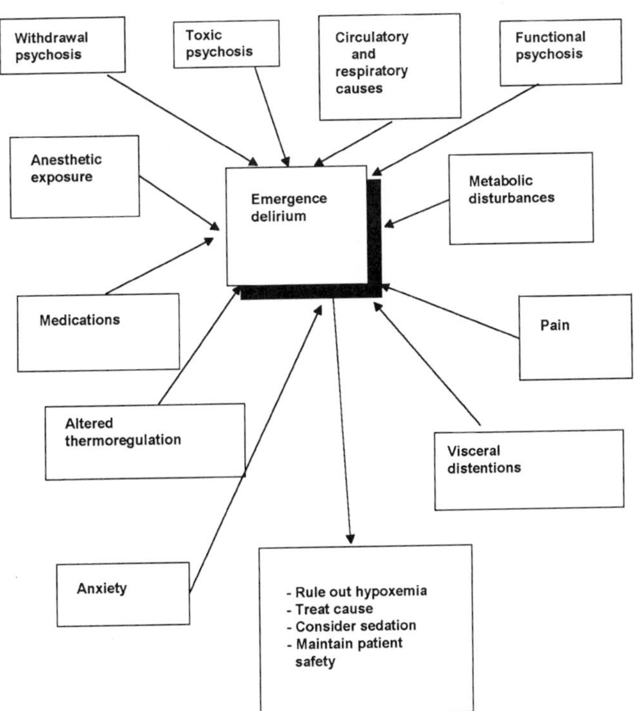

FIGURE **47-1**
Emergence delirium in the postanesthesia care unit: contributing factors and treatment.

in a specific circumstance that the patient "should be awake by now" but is not. Although delayed awakening may slow turnover of PACU beds and delay patient discharge from the PACU, the causes and consequences of delayed awakening are rarely serious. The most common causes of delayed awakening are the following:

1. Prolonged action of anesthetic drugs
2. Metabolic causes
3. Neurologic injury

Prolonged action of anesthetic drugs is the most common cause of delayed awakening. This may occur secondary to alterations in drug pharmacokinetics and pharmacodynamics. Pharmacokinetic alterations include changes in drug distribution secondary to mobilization of drugs from body tissue stores, redistribution, or decreased protein binding; changes in metabolism; and excretion secondary to renal or hepatic dysfunction. Pharmacodynamic alterations include increased patient sensitivity to drug effects because of extremes of age, hypothermia, or concomitant alcohol and drug use.[28]

Prolonged effects of inhalation anesthetics may be seen secondary to alterations in ventilation. Hypoventilation limits exhalation and prolongs elimination of inhalation agents.[29] Retention of carbon dioxide contributes to narcosis, particularly in the presence of inhalation agents, and compounds the problem.

The potentiating effects of combining inhalation agents with IV anesthetics and narcotics can also contribute to delayed awakening.[30] Premedications, particularly the long-acting benzodiazepines diazepam and lorazepam, may contribute to delayed awakening, especially in the elderly.[30] Prolonged effects of inhalation and IV agents may also occur secondary to accidental or intentional overdose and multiple drug interactions.

Metabolic causes of delayed awakening include hypoglycemia, hyperglycemia, and electrolyte disturbances. Diabetic patients have an increased risk of postoperative hypoglycemia. Taking the usual insulin dose (or half the dose) on the morning of surgery, the patient's nothing-by-mouth (NPO) status, and the stress of surgery all contribute to the development of hypoglycemia.[30] It is important to monitor serum glucose levels intraoperatively and postoperatively. Central nervous system changes may occur as blood glucose levels fall below 50 mg/dL.[31] It is good practice to obtain a baseline blood glucose level of all diabetic patients before they are admitted to surgery. Blood glucose levels of greater than 600 mg/dL can produce hyperosmolar, nonketotic, hyperglycemic coma. Approximately half of these patients have type 2 diabetes, but the syndrome can occur with severe dehydration (especially in the elderly), uremia, pancreatitis, sepsis, pneumonia, CVA, and large surface burns.[30]

Electrolyte disturbances, specifically alterations in sodium, calcium, and magnesium, can prolong awakening. Dilutional hyponatremia, occurring secondary to water intoxication, may develop after transurethral prostate resection surgery, producing sedation, coma, or even hemiparesis. Hypocalcemia, seen after parathyroidectomy and occasionally thyroidectomy, may delay awakening. Hypermagnesemia, which may occur after prolonged administration of magnesium sulfate to women with eclampsia or preeclampsia, may result in sedation and muscle weakness after general or regional anesthesia for cesarean section.[31]

Neurologic injury is a rare cause of delayed awakening of the nonneurosurgical patient. Potential causes of neurologic injury include CVA, intracranial hemorrhage, increased intracranial pressure, uncontrolled extreme hypertension (especially in the anticoagulated patient), air or fat emboli, and uncontrolled hypotension (especially in patients with hypertension or occlusive carotid disease.[31-35]

Evaluation of the patient who fails to awaken begins with an assessment of the patient's preoperative status and a review of intraoperative events. Oxygenation and gas exchange must be assessed and verified with pulse oximetry, physical assessment, and arterial blood gas analysis. When prolonged drug effects are suspected as the cause of delayed awakening, care must be taken to ensure the adequacy of ventilation and oxygenation through appropriate patient monitoring.

Residual drug effects should be considered. If possible and not contraindicated, reversal of medications should be attempted. Physostigmine reverses the anticholinergic drugs atropine and scopolamine. Flumazenil reverses benzodiazepines, and naloxone reverses the narcotics.

If other contributing factors are found, intervention should be initiated. Hypothermia necessitates rewarming, and electrolyte disturbances require correction. Hypoglycemia and hypocalcemia are treated with the IV administration of glucose and calcium, respectively. Hyperglycemia is treated with IV insulin to lower blood glucose levels and 0.5% normal saline to correct dehydration.

A neurologic cause of delayed awakening is usually either a diagnosis that is initially expected because of patient status or known intraoperative events or a diagnosis of exclusion (i.e., suspected after all other causes have been ruled out). At this point a neurologic consultation is warranted for a more in-depth evaluation.

Pain

Relief of surgical pain with minimal side effects is a primary goal of PACU care and a very high priority for both anesthesia provider and patient. Inadequate postoperative analgesia is a major source of preoperative fear and postoperative dissatisfaction in surgical patients. In addition to improving patient comfort, relief of pain reduces SNS response and helps avoid hypertension, tachycardia, and dysrhythmias. In hypovolemic patients who rely on SNS activity to maintain cardiovascular homeostasis, analgesics can precipitate hypotension. Eliminating pain may also precipitate hypoventilation by accentuating the depressant effects of previously administered opioids or residual anesthetics.[36]

Incisional pain may be effectively treated with careful titration of IV opioids with frequent cardiorespiratory assessments. Short-acting IV opioids are useful to expedite discharge and minimize nausea in ambulatory settings. Ketorolac is an effective analgesic with antiinflammatory characteristics that lowers opioid requirements, although the possibility of hemorrhage resulting from its antiplatelet properties must be taken into consideration.[37]

Other analgesic modalities provide effective pain relief beyond the PACU. IV opioid loading in the PACU is important for smooth transition to patient-controlled analgesia. Injection of opioids into the epidural or subarachnoid space during anesthesia or in the PACU often yields prolonged postoperative analgesia.[37] Epidural opioid analgesia is effective after thoracic and upper abdominal procedures and helps wean patients with obesity or chronic obstructive pulmonary disease from mechanical ventilation. Epidural analgesia may also improve surgical outcomes after orthopedic and urologic procedures. With epidural or intrathecal opioid administration, immediate and delayed ventilatory depression can occur, along with other side effects such as nausea and pruritus.

Placement of long-acting regional analgesic blocks reduces pain, controls SNS activity, and often improves ventilation. For example, interscalene block yields almost complete pain relief from shoulder or upper extremity procedures with only moderate inconvenience from motor impairment. Paralysis of the ipsilateral diaphragm can impair postoperative ventilation in patients with marginal respiratory reserve. Caudal analgesia is effective in children after inguinal or genital procedures, whereas infiltration of local anesthetic into joints, soft tissues, or incisions decreases the intensity of pain.

Opioid treatment for postoperative or chronic pain is frequently associated with adverse effects, the most common being dose-limiting and debilitating bowel dysfunction. Postoperative ileus, although attributable to surgical procedures, is often exacerbated by opioid use during and after surgery. Postoperative ileus is marked by increased inhibitory neural input, heightened inflammatory responses, decreased propulsive movements, and increased fluid absorption in the gastrointestinal tract. The current management of opioid-induced bowel dysfunction among patients receiving opioid analgesics consists primarily of nonspecific ameliorative measures. Recent clinical studies with the new agent alvimopan suggest that it may normalize bowel function without blocking systemic opioid analgesia in abdominal laparotomy patients with opioid-related postoperative ileus.[38]

Nonpharmacologic interventions may include verbal reassurance, touch, relaxation techniques, imagery, controlled breathing, and use of the patient's support system (e.g., parent or significant other), particularly in children.

Hypothermia

Hypothermia is a condition that is marked by an abnormally low internal body temperature, typically below 96° F (35.5° C), which occurs when systemic heat loss exceeds heat production.[39] Many patients are admitted into the PACU with hypothermia, which can prolong recovery, compromise physiologic stability, and contribute to postoperative morbidity.

The patient's interaction with the environment determines the degree of heat loss. Heat loss may occur via radiation, convection, conduction, or evaporation.

Radiant heat loss involves the loss of heat from a warm or hot surface (the body) to a cooler one (the environment); it does not require that the two surfaces be in direct contact with each other. Radiant heat loss accounts for 60% of heat loss to the environment. It is especially profound in the elderly, debilitated, and neonatal populations.

Convective heat loss depends on the existence of a temperature gradient between the body and the ambient air. This type of heat loss may occur in the OR, particularly in laminar flow rooms.

Conductive heat loss involves loss of heat from a warm surface that comes in contact with a cooler one. In the OR, patients lose heat to cooler OR tables, sheets, and drapes.

Evaporative heat loss involves transfer of heat during the change from a liquid to a gas. Evaporative heat loss occurs via perspiration and respiration.

Patients at high risk for the development of hypothermia can be identified. Elderly patients are at risk because of their decreased subcutaneous fat and alterations in their hypothalamic function.[40] Neonates are at risk because of their immature thermoregulatory center and their high surface-to-volume ratio.[40] Intoxicated individuals are at risk because of vasodilation and depression of their heat regulatory center. Patients taking vasodilators, nonsteroidal antiinflammatory agents, and phenothiazines have alterations in thermoregulation that are caused by either vasodilation or suppression of the thermoregulatory center.[40]

General anesthetics depress the thermoregulatory center. Narcotics and muscle relaxants depress voluntary shivering as a mechanism for the generation of heat. Any patient in whom a body cavity is entered may lose heat via convection and evaporation. Irrigation solutions used in genitourinary procedures or with cardioplegia in cardiac surgery cause internal cooling.[41]

Postoperative shivering consists of muscular tremor and rigidity. It is often associated with body heat loss, although hypothermia alone does not fully explain the occurrence of shivering. Shivering is self-limiting, never becomes chronic, and is rarely associated with major morbidity. However, it affects the comfort of patients and may sometimes lead to more serious complications.[42]

Physiologically, hypothermia results in decreased oxygen availability by shifting of the oxyhemoglobin dissociation curve to the left. Shivering may increase oxygen demand by 400% to 500%.[43] Metabolically dependent processes slow, thereby decreasing drug biotransformation. Renal transport processes are slowed, thereby decreasing glomerular filtration. Cardiac rate and rhythm disturbances, including bradyarrhythmias and premature ventricular contractions, may occur. Central nervous system depression may be profound.[43]

Treatment of hypothermia should ideally be focused on intraoperative prevention. As a result of positioning, operating time, and anesthetic exposure, therapeutic intervention most often begins in the PACU. Passive rewarming is designed to maximize basal heat production. Active rewarming consists of the use of external rewarming techniques and may include the use of heated blankets, heated water blankets, and radiant warmers. Forced-air rewarming systems are most effective for treating hypothermia.[1] Hypothermia is a common cause of shivering and should be treated with rewarming. However, when clinically indicated, meperidine can be effective in the treatment of shivering during emergence and recovery.[44]

Nausea and Vomiting

In 1914 the first journal devoted solely to the topic of anesthesia featured an original article entitled "Prophylaxis of Postanesthetic Vomiting."[45] More than 80 years later, postanesthetic vomiting is still one of the major problems faced in the PACU. Postoperative nausea and vomiting remain a leading cause of hospitalization of outpatients. These problems cause delays in recovery time, thereby increasing patient care costs, and are responsible for increased morbidity and mortality in postsurgical patients.[46] The increase in morbidity and mortality is the result of aspiration of gastric contents and the subsequent development of pneumonitis, wound disruption, atelectasis, pulmonary edema, and pneumonia.

Numerous risk factors have been associated with postoperative nausea and vomiting, including anesthetic techniques, anesthetic agents, narcotics, age, gender, weight, type of surgical procedure, pain, and history of nausea and vomiting or motion sickness.

Anesthetic technique, such as positive-pressure ventilation administered by mask, may affect the incidence of postoperative nausea and vomiting. This type of ventilation may force air into the stomach, causing gastric distention and subsequent postoperative nausea and vomiting. Positive-pressure ventilation may be especially problematic in the obese patient who is already difficult to ventilate. The length of anesthesia time (exposure time) has also been associated with an increase in postoperative nausea and vomiting.[47] Regional techniques also carry the risk of nausea and vomiting. Hypotension caused by sympathetic blockade in spinal anesthesia has been associated with medullary ischemia and resultant nausea and vomiting.[48]

The choice of anesthetic agent may influence the incidence of postoperative nausea and vomiting. Early vomiting in the PACU is usually the result of anesthetic agents.[49] Narcotic-based anesthesia increases the risk of postoperative nausea and vomiting by direct stimulation of the chemoreceptor trigger zone and, ultimately, of the medullary vomiting center. Narcotics also act peripherally to slow gastric motility and to prolong gastric emptying.

The use of nitrous oxide and its relationship to postoperative nausea and vomiting has been controversial.[50] Desflurane, isoflurane, and sevoflurane have not shown significant differences in the incidence of nausea and vomiting after their use. Propofol, used as an induction agent and IV anesthetic, is associated with a lower incidence of postoperative nausea and vomiting, whereas etomidate and ketamine may increase this adverse effect.[51]

Women are two to four times more likely to experience postoperative nausea and vomiting than men.[47] In addition, children and adolescents have an increased incidence of postoperative nausea and vomiting. Increased weight has also been associated with postoperative nausea and vomiting. Obese patients may sequester drugs in fat compartments, slowing metabolism and the elimination of anesthetics.[52] Pregnant women also have a high risk of nausea and vomiting as a result of delayed gastric emptying.

The type of surgical procedure has also been cited as a contributing factor in postoperative nausea and vomiting. In children, strabismus and orchiopexy surgery are associated with a higher incidence of postoperative nausea and vomiting.[53] Patients undergoing tonsillectomy and adenoidectomy have a high incidence of nausea and vomiting as a result of swallowed blood. In adults an increased incidence of nausea and vomiting has been noted in patients undergoing gastrointestinal procedures, diagnostic laparoscopy procedures, and otologic and ophthalmic procedures.[53]

Postoperative pain has also been shown to be a factor in postoperative nausea and vomiting. Thompson found that complete pain relief without simultaneous relief of nausea was unusual.[54] Narcotics used for pain relief may also cause nausea and vomiting.

Patients with a history of postoperative nausea and vomiting after previous surgeries and patients with a history of motion sickness have a significantly higher incidence of postoperative nausea and vomiting. A good preoperative history must be obtained, especially in ambulatory surgical patients. Figure 47-2 provides a schematic view of some of the stimuli that cause nausea and vomiting.

Management of nausea and vomiting should originate from a prophylactic rather than a therapeutic approach, particularly in patients identified as being at risk. The American Society of

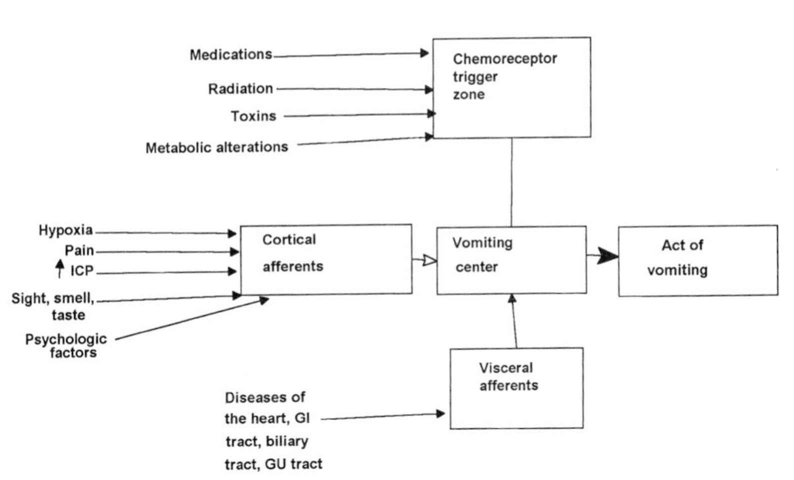

FIGURE **47-2**
Multiple pathways to the vomiting center. *GI*, Gastrointestinal; *GU*, genitourinary; *ICP*, intracranial pressure.

Anesthesiologists (ASA) Practice Guidelines[1] support the preoperative and intraoperative use of antiemetic agents (e.g., 5-HT_3 antagonists, droperidol, dexamethasone, and metoclopramide) for the prevention of nausea and vomiting. Side effects (e.g., agitation, restlessness, drowsiness) may be associated with the use of some antiemetics. Prophylaxis using a combination of antiemetic drugs has been suggested as an effective strategy for minimizing postoperative nausea and vomiting.[55] The use of diphenhydramine (Benadryl) may be effective for the prevention of vomiting. Pharmacologic prophylaxis of nausea and vomiting improves patient comfort and satisfaction, reduces time to discharge, and should be done selectively.[1] Ephedrine has also been used for the maintenance of systemic blood pressure, thereby minimizing cerebral ischemia and preventing postoperative nausea and vomiting.[48] It should be noted that in December, 2001, the U.S. Food and Drug Administration (FDA) specified changes to the droperidol labeling to include a "black box" warning, the most serious warning for an FDA-approved drug.[56] The new warning is intended to increase awareness of the potential for cardiac arrhythmias during drug administration and to encourage consideration of alternative medications for patients at high risk for cardiac arrhythmias. Droperidol currently carries a warning about cases of sudden death at high doses (greater than 25 mg) in patients at risk for cardiac arrhythmias. Recent research has shown QT prolongation (delayed recharging of the heart between beats) within minutes after injection of a dose of droperidol at the upper end of the labeled dose range. Prolonged QT is dangerous because it can cause a potentially fatal heart arrhythmia known as *torsades de pointes*. Historically the typical dose of droperidol given to adults with symptoms of postoperative nausea and vomiting has been 0.625 to 2.5 mg IV.[57]

In March 2003, a study was published comparing the use of inhaled 70% isopropyl alcohol and IV ondansetron for treatment of postoperative nausea and vomiting. For reasons unclear the inhalation of isopropyl alcohol vapors obtained from an alcohol wipe seemed to be effective for treatment of postoperative nausea and vomiting.[58]

Fluids

According to the ASA Practice Guidelines,[1] routine perioperative assessment of patients' hydration status and fluid management reduces adverse outcomes and improves patient comfort and satisfaction. On the patient's admission to the PACU, his or her intravascular volume is estimated, with consideration given to preoperative status, type and duration of surgery, estimated blood loss, fluid replacement, and hemostasis. Monitoring urine output as an index of intravascular volume can be misleading. Surgery and anesthesia impair renal tubular concentrating ability, and glycosuria causes osmotic diuresis, each falsely indicating that intravascular volume is adequate. Central venous, pulmonary arterial pressure, or transesophageal ultrasound monitoring can help to clarify volume status.

A reduction in circulating intravascular volume decreases ventricular filling and cardiac output. SNS-mediated tachycardia, increased SVR, and venoconstriction might compensate for a 15% to 20% loss of intravascular volume. Greater deficits can cause hypotension. Failure to replace preoperative fluid deficit and fluid or blood lost during surgery frequently causes hypovolemia. In the PACU, ongoing hemorrhage, sweating, and exudation of fluid into tissues (third-space losses) exacerbate hypovolemia. Blood loss is often occult, as with retroperitoneal bleeding, diffuse oozing related to coagulopathy, or hemorrhage into muscle after trauma or orthopedic procedures. Third-space losses can continue for up to 48 hours after surgery and can be massive during high permeability pulmonary edema or accumulation of ascites. In a hypothermic, venoconstricted patient, a low intravascular volume might maintain cardiac output on PACU admission but cause hypotension when venous capacity increases during rewarming.[20]

Urinary Output and Voiding

Monitoring kidney function during recovery reduces morbidity in patients with marginal cardiovascular or renal status. The ability to void should be assessed, because autonomic effects of regional anesthetics or opioids interfere with sphincter relaxation and promote urine retention.[59] Urinary retention is common after urologic, inguinal, and genital surgery and frequently delays discharge. It is reasonable to discharge inpatients to a surgical floor and selected ambulatory surgical patients from the facility before they void.[1] However, it is important to ensure that urine output is monitored after discharge from the PACU to avoid urinary retention. It is prudent to give ambulatory patients who are discharged without voiding a specific time interval in which to void (e.g., 10 to 12 hours after discharge). If retention persists, the patient should be instructed to contact a health-care facility. Patients with indwelling catheters should have urinary output recorded hourly.

Urine color is not useful for assessment of renal tubular function such as concentrating ability, but color can signal hematuria, hemoglobinuria, or pyuria. Urine osmolarity is a more reliable index of tubular function than is specific gravity, which is affected by molecular weight.

Oliguria ($<$0.5 ml/kg/hr) occurs frequently during recovery and usually reflects an appropriate renal response to hypovolemia or systemic hypotension. However, a decreased urine output might indicate abnormal renal function. The acceptable degree and duration of oliguria vary with underlying renal status, the surgical procedure, and the anticipated postoperative course. If events related to the surgical procedure could jeopardize renal function (e.g., aortic cross-clamping, severe hypotension, massive transfusion), oliguria must be aggressively evaluated. In patients without catheters, bladder volume and interval since last voiding should be checked to help differentiate between oliguria and inability to void. Urinary catheters should be checked for kinking and obstruction by blood clots or debris. Patient position might also place the catheter tip above the urinary level in the bladder.[20]

Polyuria, a state of profuse urine output, usually reflects generous intraoperative fluid administration. Osmotic diuresis caused by hyperglycemia and glycosuria is another cause, particularly if glucose-containing crystalloid solutions have been infused. Polyuria might also reflect intraoperative diuretic administration. Sustained polyuria (4 to 5 ml/kg/hr) can indicate abnormal regulation of water clearance, especially if urinary losses compromise intravascular volume and systemic blood pressure. Polyuria related to diabetes insipidus occurs secondarily to intracranial surgery, pituitary ablation, head trauma, increased intracranial pressure, and inadvertent omission of preoperative vasopressin. The diagnosis is made by comparing urine and serum electrolytes and osmolarity. High-output renal failure should also be considered as a cause.[60]

DISCHARGE FROM THE POSTANESTHESIA CARE UNIT

The patient leaving the PACU may be discharged to home, an ambulatory surgical unit, a surgical inpatient unit, or an intensive care unit. The choice of a discharge facility should depend on the patient's need and physical status and the availability of appropriate resources

When possible, before discharge, each patient should be sufficiently oriented to assess his or her physical condition and be able to summon assistance. Airway reflexes and motor function must be adequate to prevent aspiration. Ventilation and oxygenation should be acceptable and demonstrate sufficient reserve to safely cover minor deterioration in unmonitored settings. Oxygen saturation should be monitored for 15 minutes after discontinuation of supplemental oxygen in order to detect hypoxemia. Before discharge, patients should be observed for at least 15 minutes after the last IV opioid or sedative is administered to assess peak effects as well as side effects. Hemodynamic measurement and indexes of peripheral perfusion should be relatively constant for at least 15 minutes. Achievement of normal body temperature is not absolutely necessary for discharge, but resolution of shivering is important. Acceptable analgesia must be achieved, and vomiting appropriately controlled. Likely surgical complications must be assessed for (e.g., bleeding, vascular compromise, pneumothorax, complications of coexisting diseases such as coronary artery disease, diabetes, hypertension, or asthma). The results of postoperative diagnostic tests should be reviewed. The routine requirement for urination before discharge should not be part of a discharge protocol and may be necessary only for selected day-surgery patients.[1] Likewise, the requirement of drinking clear fluids should not be a part of a discharge protocol and may be necessary only for selected patients (e.g., diabetic patients) and determined on a case-by-case basis.[1]

The Joint Commission for Accreditation of Healthcare Organizations requires the use of outcome indicators as the basis for quality monitoring. Outcome indicators applied to discharge criteria should be written with a patient focus—for example, "before discharge the patient will maintain vital signs within the preoperative range." Examples of discharge criteria are found in Box 47-6. The patient's ability to meet these criteria clears him or her for discharge from the PACU but does not imply readiness for discharge to home. Two clinicians, Aldrete[61] and Chung,[62] have piloted scoring systems designed to evaluate the patients for outpatient discharge.

The Aldrete modified postanesthesia recovery (PAR) score for outpatient fitness is a modification of the original Aldrete score for PAR[3] (Table 47-1). Although it does address many areas unique to the ambulatory population, it has not so far been clinically validated to support its widespread use. A further modification of the Aldrete scoring system is given in Table 47-2.

Chung developed the Postanesthesia Discharge Scoring (PADS) system as a simple, objective tool to assess the readiness of patients to be discharged to home (Box 47-7). A score of 9 is needed for the patient to be discharged. Although studied retrospectively, the scoring system has yet to be tried as a predictive index in a widespread clinical trial. Regardless of the method

BOX 47-6

Postanesthesia Care Unit Discharge Criteria

- Regular respiratory pattern
- Respiratory rate appropriate for age
- Absence of restlessness and confusion
- Vital signs within preoperative range
- Pulse oximetry indicates 95% saturation or value equal to preoperative saturation
- Arterial blood gas values within normal limits*
- Ability to maintain patent airway
- Surgical stability of operative site or system

**Not routinely obtained before discharge.*

TABLE 47-1 Aldrete Postanesthesia Scoring System

			Admit	15 min	30 min	45 min	60 min
Activity	Able to move voluntarily on command	Four Extremities	2	2	2	2	2
		Two Extremities	1	1	1	1	1
		No Extremities	0	0	0	0	0
Respiration	Able to breathe deeply, cough freely		2	2	2	2	2
	Dyspnea or limited breathing		1	1	1	1	1
	Apnea		0	0	0	0	0
Circulation	BP + 20 mm Hg of preanesthesia level		2	2	2	2	2
	BP + 20-50 mm Hg of preanesthesia level		1	1	1	1	1
	BP + 50 mm Hg of preanesthesia level		0	0	0	0	0
Consciousness	Fully awake		2	2	2	2	2
	Arousable on calling		1	1	1	1	1
	Not responding		0	0	0	0	0
O_2 Saturation	Able to maintain O_2 saturation >90% on room air		2	2	2	2	2
	Needs O_2 inhalation to maintain O_2 saturation >90%		1	1	1	1	1
	O_2 saturation <90% even with O_2 supplementation		0	0	0	0	0

BP, *Blood pressure;* O_2, *oxygen.*
From Marshall S, Chung F. Assessment of 'home readiness' discharge criteria and postdischarge complications. Curr Opin Anesthesiol. *1997;10:445-480.*

TABLE 47-2 Modified Postanesthesia Recovery Score for Outpatients' Street Fitness

Activity	Able to move four extremities voluntarily on command	2
	Able to move two extremities voluntarily on command	1
	Able to move no extremities voluntarily on command	0
Respiration	Able to breathe deeply and cough freely	2
	Dyspnea or limited breathing	1
	Apneic	0
Circulation	BP + 20 mm Hg of preanesthetic level	2
	BP + 21-49 mm Hg of preanesthetic level	1
	BP + 50 mm Hg of preanesthetic level	0
Consciousness	Fully awake	2
	Arousable on calling	1
	Not responding	0
O_2 saturation	Able to maintain O_2 saturation >92% on room air	2
	Needs O_2 inhalation to maintain O_2 saturation >90%	1
	O_2 saturation <90% even with O_2 supplement	0
Dressing	Dry	2
	Wet but stationary	1
	Wet but growing	0
Pain	Pain free	2
	Mild pain handled by oral medications	1
	Pain requiring parenteral medications	0
Ambulation	Able to stand up and walk straight*	2
	Vertigo when erect	1
	Dizziness when supine	0
Fasting and feeding	Able to drink fluids	2
	Nauseated	1
	Nausea and vomiting	0
Urine output	Has voided	2
	Unable to void but comfortable*	1
	Unable to void and uncomfortable	0

**May be replaced by Romberg's test or the picking up of 12 clips in one hand.*
From Aldrete JA. The postanesthesia recovery score. Anesth News. *1995;7:89-91.*

BOX 47-7

Postanesthesia Discharge Scoring System

Vital Signs
2 = Within 20% of preoperative value
1 = 20%-40% of preoperative value
0 = >40% of preoperative value

Activity and Mental Status
2 = Oriented 3 separate times and a steady gait
1 = Oriented 3 separate times or a steady gait
0 = Neither

Pain, Nausea, Vomiting
2 = Minimal
1 = Moderate, requiring treatment
0 = Severe, requiring treatment

Surgical Bleeding
2 = Minimal
1 = Moderate
0 = Severe

Intake and Output
2 = Postoperative fluids and void
1 = Postoperative fluids or void
0 = Neither

From Chung F, Chan V, Ong D. A post-anesthetic discharge scoring system for home-readiness after ambulatory surgery. J Clin Anesth. *1995; 7:500-506.*

CHAPTER 48

Pain Management

Margaret Faut-Callahan, Walter R. Hand, Jr.

The nature and incidence of unrelieved pain are major concerns as we enter the twenty-first century. As providers of anesthesia care in the United States, certified registered nurse anesthetists (CRNAs) are integral to the study and management of acute, chronic, and cancer-related pain. CRNAs have often been removed from the decision-making processes related to pain management. Only recently have CRNAs been recognized as experts in the area of pain management, and their knowledge and skills are needed to address this major societal health-care problem. So important is the issue of unrelieved pain in the United States that the Agency for Health Care Policy and Research (AHCPR) (now the Agency for Healthcare Research and Quality [AHRQ]), a federally funded agency, chose pain as one of its initial health-care issues to address. Unrelieved pain associated with operative and medical procedures and trauma,[1] oncology,[2] and pediatric patients[3] has been thoroughly studied. Recommendations from the various study groups are being integrated throughout the health-care system. CRNAs must be fully aware of the issues that were addressed in these important studies.

Fundamentally the members of the study panels found that undermedication of patients in moderate to severe pain has been well documented in the literature for decades.[4-11] Many centers have tried to address this serious health issue through major interventional programs. Despite the implementation of various interventions, the problem of inadequately managed pain remains. Loeser and Egan,[12] experts in pain management, suggested a model of care that described the complexity of the phenomenon. Donovan and colleagues[13] modified this model to include an additional element, system response (Figure 48-1). The system response, or those of us in a position to intervene in a pain management situation, has been underemphasized. CRNAs must assume responsibility for being key members of the pain management team.

The role of health-care providers in the management of acute and chronic pain has become the focus of many professional and regulatory groups. The Joint Commission on Accreditation of Healthcare Organizations (JCAHO) has focused on the adequacy of pain management for a number of years. The JCAHO developed pain management standards and implemented them on January 1, 2001. The standards were developed through an effort of the JCAHO and the University of Wisconsin—Madison through a grant from the Robert Wood Johnson Foundation. The significance of this move by a regulatory agency is great and has had far-reaching effects. The JCAHO clearly outlined the responsibilities of hospitals, home-care agencies, nursing homes, behavioral health facilities, outpatient clinics, and health plans. The responsibilities are as follows:

- Recognize the right of patients to appropriate assessment and management of pain
- Assess the existence of pain and, if present, its nature and intensity in all patients
- Record the results of the assessment in a way that facilitates regular reassessment and follow-up
- Determine and assure staff competency in pain assessment and management, and address pain assessment and management in the orientation of all new staff
- Establish policies and procedures that support the appropriate prescription or ordering of effective pain medications
- Educate patients and their families about effective pain management
- Address patient needs for symptom management in the discharge-planning process [14]

Assessment of these standards includes review of policy and procedures, protocols, documentation, educational materials, and interviews with patients, families, and clinicians. The JCAHO has published three documents that explicitly define the agency's initiatives. *Pain: Current Understanding of Assessment, Management and Treatment* was published in December 2001.[15]

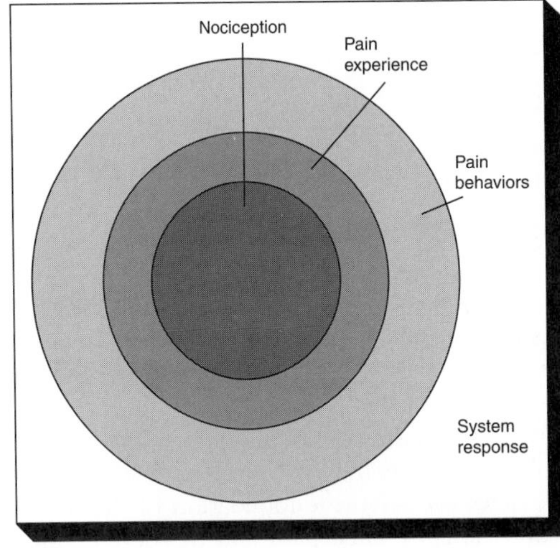

FIGURE **48-1**
Model for pain management. (Modified from Loeser J, Egan D. *Managing the Chronic Pain Patient. Theory and Practice at the University of Washington Multidisciplinary Pain Clinic.* New York: Raven; 1989:6.)

Improving the Quality of Pain Management through Measurement and Action was published in March 2003.[16] In 2003 the JCAHO published *Approaches to Pain Management: An Essential Guide for Clinical Leaders*.[17] This text provides advice regarding the development of a comprehensive pain management strategy for health-care organizations.

The American Pain Society (APS), a respected professional organization dedicated to the effective management of pain, developed standards for the relief of both acute and cancer-related pain. Key elements of the standards are as follows:

1. Recognize and treat pain promptly
   - Chart and display pain and relief (process)
   - Define pain and relief levels to trigger review (process)
   - Survey patient satisfaction (outcome)
2. Make information about analgesia readily available (process)
3. Promise patients attentive analgesic care (process)
4. Define explicit policies for use of advanced analgesic technologies (process)
5. Monitor adherence to standards (process)[18]

Further evidence of the importance now placed on effective management of pain is the introduction of a national strategy to alleviate pain in the United States. HR 1863, the National Pain Care Policy Act of 2003, was introduced. The purpose of the legislation is to provide resources for pain care research, education, and the establishment of treatment plans within federally funded health-care programs. This follows the declaration by the Congress that 2000 to 2010 is the Decade of Pain Control.

The complex issues related to effective pain management include an understanding of the physiologic, pathophysiologic, pharmacologic, and behavioral principles that occur. This chapter reviews the scientific foundation of the management of acute and cancer-related pain and the current methods of assessment, planning, implementation, and evaluation of a pain management plan.

DEFINING PAIN

The International Association for the Study of Pain and the APS developed a definition of pain. This was necessary because there existed a reluctance to look beyond the physiologic components of pain. Pain was defined as an unpleasant sensory and emotional experience associated with actual or potential tissue damage or described in terms of such damage.[19] This definition reminds us that pain is both a physiologic and a behavioral phenomenon.[20]

It is necessary to clarify terms associated with the understanding of pain. Nociception is the process of transduction, transmission, perception, and modulation of pain.[21] Two general categories of pain exist: nociceptive and neuropathic. Nociceptive pain is associated with the stimulation of specific nociceptors and can be either somatic or visceral. *Somatic pain* refers to pain that has an identifiable locus and follows the distribution of a somatic nerve. In addition, somatic pain is well localized, sharp in nature, and generally hurts at the point or area of stimulus. Conversely, visceral pain is diffuse, can be referred to another area, and is often described as dull and vague in nature. Visceral pain is often associated with the distention of an organ capsule or the obstruction of a hollow viscus. In contrast, neuropathic pain is caused by abnormal processing of painful stimuli. It is a dysfunction of the central nervous system (CNS) that allows for spontaneous excitation leading to severe pain. Neuropathic pain can be generated centrally or peripherally and is difficult to treat.[22] Patients describe their pain as burning, tingling, or shocklike.

PHYSIOLOGY OF PAIN

Pain is most commonly defined in terms of four processes: transduction, transmission, perception, and modulation. A noxious stimulus, be it chemical, mechanical, or thermal, is transformed into electrical energy during transduction. The electrical energy produces signals that are transmitted from the periphery to the CNS, and this process is called *transmission*. Perception occurs once the signal is recognized by the brain. Modulation occurs through descending mechanisms that modulate signal transmission in the spinal cord. Understanding of these distinct processes involved in the pain experience has allowed for the development of specific treatments to manage pain.

When peripheral tissues such as skin, bone, and viscera receive chemical, thermal, or mechanical stimuli or are traumatized by either surgery or injury, a series of biochemical events takes place. These events include the release of a number of endogenous chemicals (neurotransmitters) such as bradykinin, serotonin, and substance P. The most well known neurotransmitter as it relates to pain is substance P. As this process continues, the arachidonic acid cascade is activated. Collectively these substances generate an action potential that stimulates peripheral nerve receptors, causing nociceptive stimulation. This nociceptive stimulation results in a transduction of nociceptive impulses. Because the suspected chemical reactions have such far-reaching influence throughout the body, it is necessary to trace the effects (Figure 48-2).

The stimuli are then transmitted to the dorsal horn of the spinal cord, where a sympathetic reflex response is created. Afferent nerve fibers are classified as type A, B, or C. Type A fibers are further defined as alpha, beta, gamma, or delta. Types A and B fibers are known to be myelinated, whereas type C fibers are nonmyelinated.[23] In the spinal cord are several receptor systems that function as modulators in the neurotransmission of nociceptive impulses.[21,24] Information is transmitted via ascending tracts to the supraspinal sites, where it is then processed. Such sites include the cerebral cortex, hypothalamus, and periaqueductal gray matter. The neurochemical mechanisms of pain and nociception are complex. In recent years, several categories of pain receptors have been identified.

Both *N*-methyl-D-aspartate (NMDA) and α-amino-acid-3-hydroxyl-5-methyl-4-isoxazole propionic acid (AMPA) receptors are located throughout the brain and spinal cord.[25] However, their interaction in the transmission of pain is predominantly at the level of the dorsal horn. Both receptor subtypes are ionotropic glutamate receptors located postsynaptically on the second order neuron. When glutamate (excitatory neurotransmitter) is released from the depolarized primary afferent nerve terminals, it binds postsynaptically to these glutamate receptors to depolarize the second order neuron and continue transmission of the nociceptive impulse to the CNS. NMDA and AMPA antagonists are newer additions to pain management strategies.

Pathophysiology of Pain

Pathophysiologic alterations related to pain may complicate existing disease and alter outcome.[1] Inadequately relieved or unrelieved pain is a source of fear, anxiety, helplessness, depression, and demoralization. Pain management unfortunately is

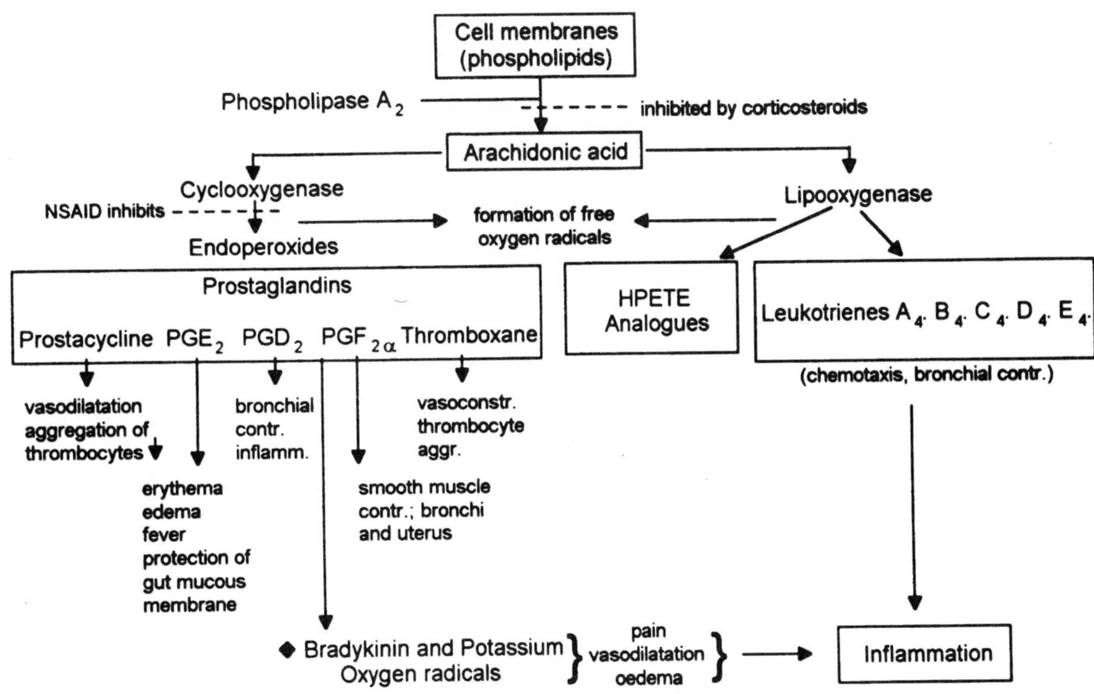

FIGURE **48-2**
Arachidonic acid cascade. (From Lundeberg T. Pain physiology and principles of treatment. *Scand J Rehabil Med Suppl.* 1995;32:13-42.)

still given a low priority and is associated with myths, misconceptions, and knowledge deficit among health-care providers.[22,24] We have learned a great deal about the effects of pain on the human body. In addition, factors such as the extent of the trauma or surgical field, the number of pain receptors involved in the particular area, bleeding, infection, anxiety, and physiologic stress accelerate the endocrine stress response to trauma (Figure 48-3).

Cardiovascular System

The stress of pain resulting from surgery or trauma causes many cardiovascular responses. The most significant of these is the activation of the sympathetic nervous system. Release of substances such as catecholamines, cortisol, and angiotensin II occurs. Common cardiovascular symptoms associated with unrelieved pain are increased heart rate, increased cardiac output, increased myocardial oxygen consumption, and increased vascular resistance (peripheral, systemic, and coronary). Hypertension, hypercoagulation, and deep vein thrombosis can be seen. These factors may negatively affect postoperative outcome. Aggressive pain management may reduce the postoperative incidence of cardiac complications.[24]

Respiratory System

The presence of pain can have a tremendous impact on the respiratory system. This impact is most pronounced in those patients having surgery or trauma in the area of the upper abdomen and thorax. Pain causes a measurable decrease in tidal volume because of limited thoracic and abdominal movement. Specifically, decreases in vital capacity, inspiratory capacity, and functional residual capacity, as well as a decreased physical ability to clear the airway, are the result of unrelieved pain. Muscle spasm below and above the site of injury caused by the noxious stimuli promotes limited movement of the respiratory muscles. Patients also voluntarily decrease the movement of the thorax and abdomen in an attempt to limit pain. Furthermore, patients are reluctant to breathe deeply and to cough, enhancing their respiratory compromise. As a result, atelectasis and pneumonia are common postoperative complications.[26] These alterations may be aggravated in those with preexisting pulmonary dysfunction (e.g., asthma, chronic obstructive pulmonary disease). Successful strategies to manage pain must include precautions against further respiratory compromise.

Gastrointestinal and Genitourinary System

Increased sympathetic activity results in a delay in gastric emptying and decreased intestinal motility. Intestinal secretions and smooth muscle sphincter tone increase.[26] Paralytic ileus with nausea and vomiting is a common problem related to postoperative pain. In addition to the physiologic consequences of pain, some commonly used analgesics also alter gastrointestinal functioning. Systemic opioids may cause delayed gastric emptying and may contribute to the development of paralytic ileus. In cases in which the speed of gastrointestinal recovery is of importance, local anesthetics have been shown to be beneficial.[26]

Pain can also result in hypomotility of the urethra and bladder, resulting in difficulty with urination. This increases the likelihood of having to catheterize the patient because of inability to void.[27]

Endocrine System

The neurohormonal response to pain is complex and involves an array of both anabolic and catabolic hormones. The endocrine response to pain is characterized by an increase in the secretion of hormones such as adrenocorticotropic hormone, cortisol, antidiuretic hormone, growth hormone, and

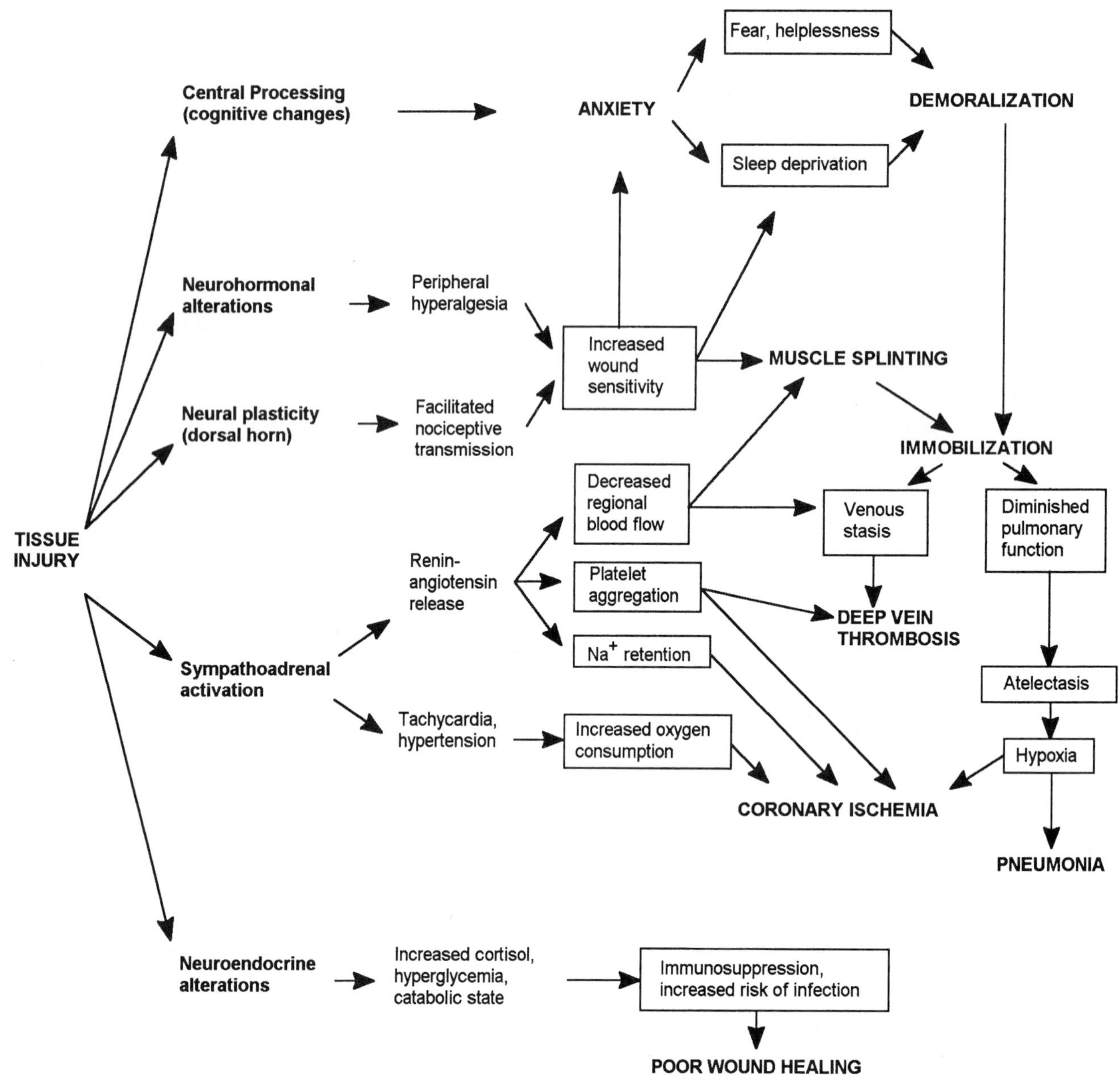

FIGURE **48-3**
Outline of pathophysiologic responses associated with surgical trauma and their impact on key target organs.

glucagon. Insulin and testosterone secretion is decreased.[24] In addition, hormones such as prolactin, vasopressin, and thyroxin are released as part of the endocrine response to pain.

Effective pain management decreases the neuroendocrine response to surgery or trauma. The timing of drug administration plays a major role in the blockade of the neuroendocrine response. In addition to the neuroendocrine response, a sympathoadrenal response and pathophysiologic change occur as a result of the increased release of norepinephrine from the sympathetic nerve endings (Figure 48-4).

Immune System

Pain, surgery, and trauma affect the competence of the immune system through neuroendocrine pathways. It is known that the degree of immunosuppression is closely linked to the magnitude of tissue damage.[28] Immunosuppression seen in the postoperative period may last as long as 1 to 2 weeks in healthy patients. Patients who are at higher risk for immunocompromise may experience more severe problems associated with immune dysfunction. Limiting pain and causes of surgical stress and infection is critical in these patients.

Psychologic Effects

The psychologic nature of pain must be recognized. The complex, subjective nature of pain is often difficult to comprehend.[29] The presence of pain can be a major source of fear and anxiety for the patient. An adversarial relationship may develop between the patient and doctors and nurses when pain is prolonged. This relationship may develop because the patient may perceive that the hospital staff is withholding pain relief, that the staff does not place a high priority on pain management, or that the staff believes that the patient's complaints of

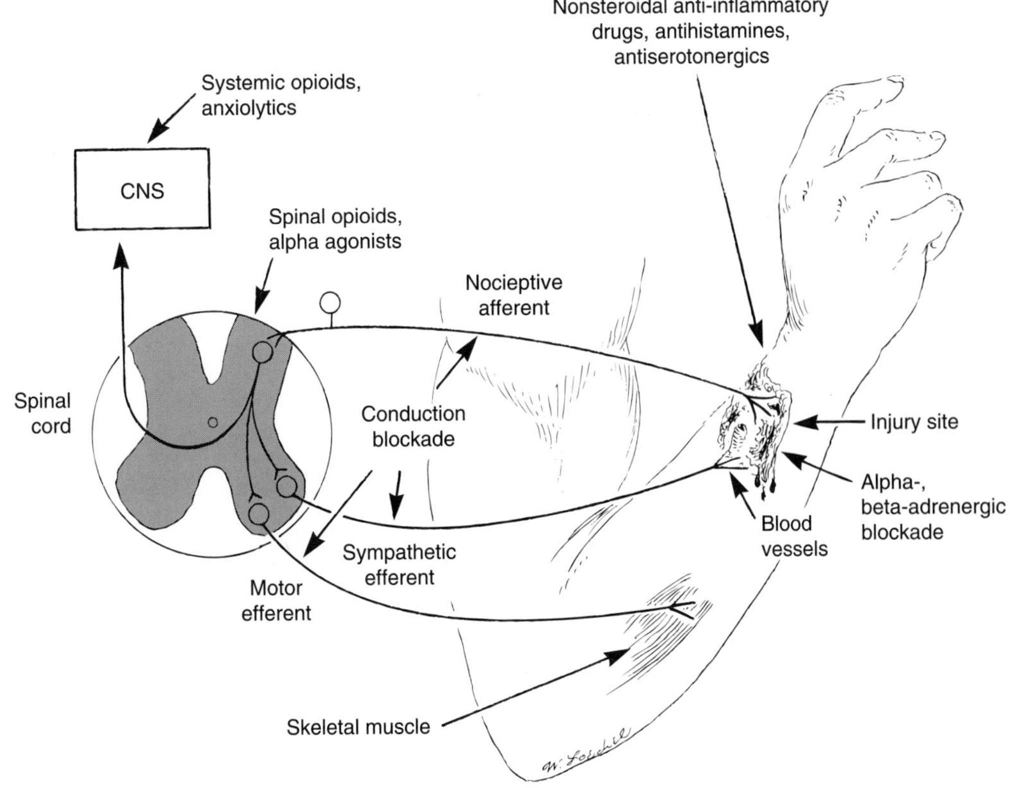

FIGURE **48-4**
Sympathoadrenal response occurring because of the increased release of norepinephrine from the sympathetic nerve endings.

pain are exaggerated or contrived. Every effort must be made to reassure the patient that his or her pain relief is important to the staff. The patient should know that his or her complaints of pain will be addressed in a timely and definitive manner.

GENERAL ASPECTS OF ACUTE PAIN MANAGEMENT

Preoperative planning should include a discussion of the patient's expectations of postoperative pain and its management. Goals for pain management should be set by both the patient and the care providers. The patient should be informed about the modalities available to him or her and should be given instructions on how to quantify pain intensity with instruments such as a verbal numeric scale, a visual analog scale, or another instrument appropriate to his or her cognitive skills. The patient should be encouraged to make use of simple nonpharmacologic techniques such as relaxation, simple imagery, and music.[1]

Regardless of the cause of the acute pain, a thorough patient interview, physical assessment, and review of the medical record (laboratory results, diagnostic studies, and so on) must be completed before the implementation of a plan to manage the patient's pain. The goal of the patient interview is to determine the existence of any history of pain, either malignant or nonmalignant (e.g., arthritis, chronic back pain). Patients should be asked if they have been taking any prescription or nonprescription medications to treat pain. A specific question regarding the use of any over-the-counter analgesics should be asked. In addition, CRNAs should know that there are a number of prescriptive adjunctive medications used to treat pain. It should not be assumed that a patient is being treated for a seizure disorder or depression because the patient is taking anticonvulsants or tricyclic antidepressants, both of which can effectively be used to treat different types of neuropathic pain. During the interview every effort should be made to try to determine what type of pain the patient is experiencing. Opioids are not as effective at alleviating neuropathic pain as they are in treating either somatic or visceral pain. Furthermore, the patient's perception, psychologic response, and behavioral and cognitive responses to the pain should be assessed. The perception should include location, description (qualitative), and intensity (via a verbally administered numeric rating scale), as well as factors that aggravate or relieve the pain (Figure 48-5).

Every assessment of a patient's pain should be accompanied by a physical assessment of the suspected locus of the pain. A visual inspection of the area may reveal signs and symptoms of infection, pressure, and so on. During the postoperative period it should not be assumed that the pain is related to the surgical procedure. The cause of the pain could be a burn from the electrocautery pad, an infiltrated intravenous (IV) line, angina, and so on.

Finally, a review of the medical record should be completed. A nursing summary or assessment completed when the admitting nurse interviews the patient or family can provide a wealth of information. This summary can be particularly useful when patients are poor historians or simply cannot remember information secondary to the presence of pain or the effects of medications. Laboratory and radiologic data can provide invaluable information regarding the cause of the pain (e.g., infection, tumor).

If optimal analgesic care is to be provided to the patient in pain, assessment and reassessment play a vital role. Assessment should be done at regular intervals and should be simple. Key

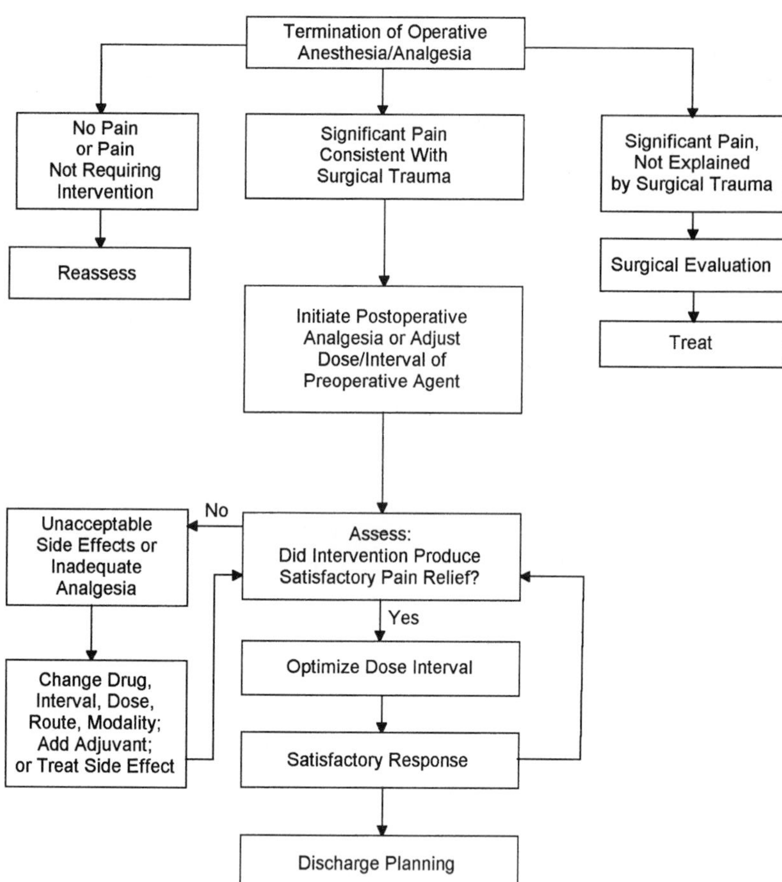

FIGURE **48-5**
Pain treatment flowchart, postoperative phase. (From Acute Pain Management Panel. *Acute Pain Management: Operative or Medical Procedures and Trauma. Clinical Practice Guidelines*. Rockville, Md: Agency for Health Care Policy and Research, Public Health Service, US Department of Health and Human Services; 1992:10. Publication 92-0032.)

to the success of a treatment plan are adequate documentation and communication among all care providers. Evidence suggests that the addition of a simple flowchart documenting the patient's pain increases successful management.[1]

PHARMACOLOGIC ASPECTS OF ACUTE PAIN MANAGEMENT

A clear understanding of the physiology of pain has led to the development of improved treatment modalities. Because pain is a complex phenomenon, the effective management of pain can be extremely difficult. Despite increasing knowledge in the area of pain physiology and pharmacology, many providers continue to treat the problem as if it is unidimensional. The use of multiple strategies to control pain is essential. Research in basic sciences and pharmacology suggests that the use of analgesic drugs in combination remains the most logical and efficient way to manage or decrease postoperative pain.[30] The optimal strategy for pharmacologic management of pain should include a combination of analgesics and nonpharmacologic strategies as determined through individual patient assessment.

PREEMPTIVE ANALGESIA

Preemptive analgesia is a concept first postulated approximately 100 years ago. It is postulated that pain perception can be decreased through the use of analgesics capable of inhibiting CNS sensitization before the painful stimulus occurs.[31,32]

After injury or surgery the tissue damage elicits peripheral sensitization and central sensitization. This causes a decrease in the pain threshold, hypersensitivity, and increased response to pain. Preemptive analgesia purports to prevent the sensitization of the CNS and may alter the overall pain response. The use of preemptive analgesia to limit central sensitization remains controversial, and some studies suggest that intraoperative administration of analgesics has little effect.

Although the use of preemptive analgesia has not been proved effective in decreasing central desensitization, research continues to evaluate the use of drugs that limit sensitization in the periphery. However, animal studies provide some evidence that this is an area for further study. Because many analgesics work in the periphery, it is postulated that they may be helpful in limiting peripheral sensitization. The use of nonsteroidal antiinflammatory drugs (NSAIDs), opioids, and local anesthetics is being studied. Reuben and Connelly found that preemptive use of cyclooxygenase (COX)-2 inhibitors decreased the use of morphine in a postoperative spinal fusion population.[33] Helmy and Bali found that the use of dextromethorphan (120 mg intramuscular [IM]) preincision decreased postoperative merperidine consumption.[34] The administration preoperatively of rofecoxib to arthroscopic knee surgery patients reduced postoperative pain.[35] Buvanendran and colleagues studied 70 randomized patients who underwent total knee replacement and found that preoperative administration of rofecoxib, followed by postoperative continuation, reduced opioid consumption and improved clinical outcomes.[36]

However, Kehlet reviewed 40 clinical studies and found little support for the use of preemptive analgesia.[30] Critics of this technique suggest that the use of NSAIDs in a surgical population, with limited evidence that preemptive analgesia is effective, does not warrant potential complications. Postoperative bleeding is a concern in a surgical population.

NONSTEROIDAL ANTIINFLAMMATORY DRUGS AND ACETAMINOPHEN

NSAIDs are best known for their use in the management of mild to moderate postoperative pain and pain related to inflammatory conditions. They represent a variety of chemical substances that inhibit the action of COX and thereby prevent conversion of arachidonic acid to prostaglandins; as a result the nociceptive response to endogenous mediators of inflammation is attenuated. Prostaglandins are responsible for sensitizing and amplifying peripheral nociceptors to the inflammatory mediators (substance P, bradykinin, serotonin) released when tissue is traumatized.

COX exists in two isoforms: COX-1 and COX-2. COX-1 is constitutive, widespread throughout the body, and necessary for homeostasis. It is located particularly in the kidneys, gastric mucosa, platelets, and endothelium. Conversely, COX-2 is normally present only in minute amounts, and synthesis is primarily induced in the presence of inflammation. Until recently, all of the NSAIDs were nonselective in their COX inhibition. As a result, in addition to the analgesia that results from the inhibition of the COX-2 isoform, inhibition of COX-1 leads to the detrimental side effects of gastric irritation, renal microvasculature constriction, and platelet inhibition. Presently there exist several selective COX-2–inhibiting NSAIDs. Although selective COX-2–inhibiting NSAIDs are not devoid of potential side effects, their introduction has greatly reduced the incidence of side effects associated with the use of nonselective NSAIDs, without sacrificing analgesic efficacy. Long used in the management of arthritis pain, the coxibs are now used for treatment of many other acute pain syndromes. Dysmenorrhea and dental pain have been shown to be successfully treated with coxibs. Chronic pain states, such as chronic back pain and cancer, are now being treated with these drugs. Postsurgical pain can now be successfully treated with the judicious use of coxibs because coxibs do not inhibit COX-1 platelet aggregation, which has been a limiting factor in the use of traditional NSAIDs in postsurgical patients. Buvanendran and colleagues did not find any bleeding complications in a postsurgical population.[36] In addition to the antiinflammatory properties of these drugs, recent research suggests that NSAIDs also work at the spinal and supraspinal levels.[37-40]

When an NSAID is used as a part of a postoperative pain regimen, nociception is diminished at the peripheral level. Evidence suggests that if an optimal dose of an NSAID is combined with an opioid, it produces an additive analgesic effect greater than that obtained by doubling the dose of either constituent.[41,42] The best time to initiate therapy is controversial. Research suggests that beginning NSAID therapy before activation of the inflammatory process and including NSAIDs as part of a preemptive analgesia regimen are effective.[30,42]

Some clinicians believe that the undesirable side effects of NSAIDs (gastrointestinal discomfort, the possibility of gastrointestinal bleeding, decreased platelet aggregation, potential renal insufficiency, and delayed wound healing) are sufficient grounds for avoiding their use in surgical patients, even for short periods. However, the short-term use of NSAIDs (<1 week) has not been shown to increase bleeding during surgery or to cause other major side effects.[42] NSAIDs are available primarily in oral form. Some are available as suppositories and can therefore be administered to patients denied oral intake. Ketorolac and indomethacin are available for parenteral administration. Ketorolac's analgesic potency is disproportionate to its antiinflammatory potency[43]; however, its side effect profile is similar to that of any other NSAID (Table 48-1).

Parecoxib is a new injectable COX-2 inhibitor. It is a prodrug of valdecoxib. Due to its ability to be given intravenously or intramuscularly, it is especially useful in the perioperative setting. Like other COX-2–inhibiting NSAIDs, it does not promote bleeding and is more useful than Ketorolac.

OPIOIDS

Opioids remain the drugs of choice for treatment of moderate to severe pain. Opioids are characterized on the basis of their specific affinity for the opioid receptors. Specific pharmacology is discussed in Chapter 10.

Adequate pain control may be hampered by fears of respiratory depression or hypotension. These misconceptions have little foundation provided that the dose, route of administration, and choice of drug are appropriate for the situation and that the pain management is based on thorough assessment and reassessment of the patient. Table 48-2 lists the opioids and opioid antagonists that are used for pain control.

The continued development of opioids indicates the focus the health-care industry has placed on the optimal management of pain. Many effective opioids are available, including meperidine, a commonly used opioid. It should be noted that meperidine has a neurotoxic metabolite, normeperidine, which has a half-life of 15 to 24 hours. The neurotoxic side effects of normeperidine (shakiness, tremor, twitches, multifocal myoclonus, and grand mal seizures[19,44-46]) are not reversible with naloxone. The recommendation for the use of meperidine in the AHCPR guidelines specifies that meperidine "should only be used for very brief courses, in otherwise healthy patients who have demonstrated an unusual reaction or allergic response during treatment with other opioids."[1] Meperidine should be used with caution in the elderly and in patients with compromised renal function.

A stigma is still associated with the prescription and administration of opioids because of the risk of habit formation or addiction. This phenomenon was referred to as "opiophobia" by Morgan,[47] who defined it as "undocumented fear that appropriate use of opioids causes addiction." Studies document that the risk of iatrogenic addiction is minimal.[48,49]

Misconceptions exist among both health professionals and patients about the principles of tolerance, pseudoaddiction, physiologic dependence, and psychologic dependence. Unfortunately, these misconceptions can result in the inappropriate labeling of patients as addicts.

Tolerance refers to a change in the dose-response relationship induced by exposure to the drug and manifested as a need for a higher dose to maintain an effect. The development of tolerance to an opioid is a normal physiologic response.

Pseudoaddiction is often confused with psychologic dependence because the behavior of the patients can be the same. That is, patients with both of these conditions exhibit what appears to be drug-seeking behavior. However, in the patient who is "pseudoaddicted," the origin of the behavior is inadequate analgesia. When these patients receive adequate analgesia, they no longer demonstrate drug-seeking behavior.

TABLE 48-1 Nonsteroidal Antiinflammatory Agents

Agent	Potency	Dose	Onset	Duration	Comments
Acetaminophen (Tylenol, Panadol, Phenaphen, Tempra; in Anacin-3, Excedrin, Vicodin, Tylox, Percocet, Darvon-N)	1	PO or rectal 325-650 mg (6-12 mg/kg) q4h	PO 5-30 min	PO 3-7 hr	Most commonly available analgesic. Does not produce gastric irritation, does not interfere with platelet function.
Aspirin (in Bufferin, Buffaprin, AlkaSeltzer, Anacin, Percodan, Talwin)	1	PO 325-650 mg (6-12 mg/kg) q4-8h	PO 5-30 min	PO 3-7 hr	Irreversibly inhibits platelet aggregation for the life of the platelet (7-10 days) and prolongs bleeding time. Enhances urinary excretion of uric acid and is useful for treatment of gout. May prevent arterial and possibly deep venous thrombosis. Increased risk of development of Reye's syndrome if used in children with influenza or chickenpox.
Celecoxib (Celebrex)	1-2	PO 100-200 mg bid	PO <45 min	PO 4-6 hr	NSAID that exerts its effect by selective inhibition of COX-2. GI effects and development of ulcers are reported to be less with this class of drugs. Avoid during pregnancy.
Choline salicylate (Arthropan)	1	PO 435-870 mg or 2.5-5 ml (8-16 mg/kg or 0.05-0.1 mg/kg) q4h	PO 5-30 min	PO 3-7 hr	Does not inhibit platelet aggregation. Useful in patients with GI intolerance to aspirin.
Diclofenac sodium (Voltaren)	15	PO 100-200 mg (2-4 mg/kg) daily in two to four divided doses	PO 15-30 min	PO 4-6 hr	Structurally related to mefenamic acid but more potent.
Diflunisal (Dolobid)	3.5-13	PO 1 g, then 500 mg q8-12h	PO <60 min	PO 3-7 hr	May be administered twice daily. In contrast to the prolonged effects of aspirin, platelet aggregation returns to normal within 24 hours.
Etodolac (Lodine)	3	PO 200-400 mg (4-8 mg/kg) q6-12h	PO 15-30 min	PO 4-6 hr	Better tolerated than indomethacin, naproxen, or ibuprofen; equipotent doses are associated with fewer gastric mucosal abnormalities.
Fenoprofen calcium (Nalfon)	3	PO 200 mg (4 mg/kg) q4-6h	PO 15-30 min	PO 4-6 hr	Better tolerated than aspirin; equipotent doses are associated with fewer gastric mucosal abnormalities.
Ibuprofen (Advil, Motrin)	1	PO 200-800 mg (8-16 mg/kg) q6h	PO 30 min	PO 6-8 hr	Better tolerated than aspirin or naproxen; equipotent doses are associated with fewer gastric mucosal abnormalities.
Indomethacin (Indocin)	20	PO 25-50 mg (0.5-1 mg/kg) q6-12h	PO 15-30 min	PO 4-6 hr	Potent NSAID. More effective than aspirin in relieving the pain of primary dysmenorrhea. Indomethacin has antiinflammatory effects comparable with those of colchicine in the treatment of gouty arthritis.
Ketoprofen (Orudis)	20	PO 25-50 mg (0.5-1 mg/kg) q6-8h	PO 15-30 min	PO 3-4 hr	Potent NSAID. Better GI tolerance than indomethacin or aspirin.
Ketorolac tromethamine (Toradol)	60 (PO)	Loading: IM or IV 30-60 mg (0.5-1 mg/kg) Maintenance: IM or IV 15-30 mg (0.25-0.5 mg/kg) PO 10 mg q4-6h	IV <1 min IM <10 min PO <1 hr	IV 3-7 hr IM 3-7 hr PO 3-7 hr	The only NSAID approved for parenteral administration for analgesia. To minimize serious adverse effects, duration of use should not exceed 5 days for parenteral and 14 days for oral administration.

TABLE 48-1 Nonsteroidal Antiinflammatory Agents—cont'd

Agent	Potency	Dose	Onset	Duration	Comments
Meclofenamate sodium (Meclomen)	3	PO 200-300 mg (4-6 mg/kg) daily in three or four divided doses	PO 30-60 min	PO 3-7 hr	Structurally related to mefenamic acid, but fewer incidences of hematologic abnormalities.
Mefenamic acid (Ponstel)	3	PO 500 mg (10 mg/kg), then 250 mg (5 mg/kg) daily q6h	PO 30-60 min	PO 3-7 hr	May be associated with hematologic abnormalities (e.g., decreased hematocrit, leukopenia, agranulocytosis, and pancytopenia).
Naproxen (Naprosyn, Aleve)	3	PO 500 mg (10 mg/kg), then 250 mg (5 mg/kg) q6-12h	P 30-60 min	PO 3-7 hr	Medium-potency NSAID. Better GI tolerance than aspirin. Available over the counter in the United States.
Oxphenbutazone (various)	20	Initial: PO 300-600 mg (6-12 mg/kg) daily in three or four divided doses Maintenance: PO 100-400 mg (2-8 mg/kg) daily in three or four doses	PO 15-30 min	PO 4-6 hr	Potent NSAID, may cause serious adverse effects. Should not be used as a simple analgesic or antipyretic. May compete with thyroxine for protein-binding sites and may reduce the uptake of iodine by the thyroid gland. May cause significant sodium retention.
Parecoxib (Dynastat)	10	IV or IM 20-40 mg	10-20 min	6-8h	COX-2 inhibitor for perioperative use. Allergic and anaphylactic responses have been reported.
Phenylbutazone (Butazolidin)	20	Initial: PO 300-600 mg (6-12 mg/kg) daily, in three or four divided doses Maintenance: PO 100-400 mg (2-8 mg/kg) daily in three or four doses	PO 15-30 min	PO 4-6 hr	Potent NSAID. May cause severe adverse effects; used only as a second-line agent. Has mild uricosuric activity and decreases tubular reabsorption of uric acid.
Piroxicam (Feldene)	3	PO 20-40 mg (0.4-0.8 mg/kg) daily, in one or two divided doses	PO 30-60 min	PO 48-72 hr	May be administered once daily. Structurally unrelated to other NSAIDs. Medium potency and long duration of action.
Rofecoxib (Vioxx)	8	PO 12.5-25 qd	PO <45 min	PO 12-24 hr	NSAID that exerts its effect by selective inhibition of COX-2. GI effects and development of ulcers are reported to be less with this class of drugs. Avoid during pregnancy.
Salsalate (Disalcid, Argesic)	1	PO 2-4 g (40-80 mg/kg) daily in two or three divided doses	PO 5-30 min	PO 3-7 hr	Useful in patients with GI intolerance to aspirin. Does not inhibit platelet aggregation. Increased risk of developing Reye's syndrome if used in children with influenza or chickenpox.
Sulindac (Clinoril)	20	PO 150-200 mg (3-4 mg/kg) bid	PO 15-30 min	PO 3-4 hr	Equipotent to indomethacin but associated with fewer gastric mucosal abnormalities.
Tolmetin sodium (Tolectin)	20	PO 400-600 mg (8-12 mg/kg) q8h	PO 15-30 min	PO 3-4 hr	Equipotent to indomethacin but associated with fewer gastric mucosal abnormalities
Valdecoxib (Bextra)	10	PO 10 mg qd to 20 mg bid	PO less than 45 min	PO 12-24 hr	COX-2 selective long-acting agent.

bid, *Twice daily*; COX, *cyclooxygenase*; GI, *gastrointestinal*; IM, *intramuscular*; IV, *intravenous*; NSAID, *nonsteroidal antiinflammatory drug*; PO, *by mouth*, qd, *once daily*.

Data from Mosby's Drug Consul. *St Louis: Mosby; 2004; Omoigui S:* The Pain Drugs Handbook. *St Louis: Mosby; 1995:495-499; Rofecoxib for osteoarthritis and pain.* Med Lett Drugs Ther. *1999;41:59-61; Boyce EG, Breen GA: Celecoxib: a COX-2 inhibitor for osteoarthritis and rheumatoid arthritis.* Formulary. *1999;34:405-417; Drugs for pain.* Med Lett Drugs Ther. *2000;42:73-78.*

TABLE 48-2 Opioids and Opioid Antagonists

Agent	Potency*	Dose	Onset	Duration	Comments
Buprenorphine HCl (PA) (Buprenex)	30	IV, IM, SL 0.3-0.6 mg (6-12 mcg/kg) q4-6h Epidural 50-60 mg (1 mg/kg)	IV <1 min IM 1 hr	IV, IM, SL 6 hr	Binds avidly to opioid receptors. Respiratory depression may not respond to naloxone; doxapram may be more suitable.
Butorphanol tartrate (Ag-An) (Stadol)	3.5-7	IV 0.5-2 mg (0.010.04 mg/kg) q3-4h IM 1-4 mg (0.02-0.08 mg/kg) q3-4h Nasal 1 mg Epidural 1-2 mg (20-40 mcg/kg)	IV 1-5 min IM 10 min Nasal <15 min	IV 2-4 hr IM 3-4 hr Nasal 4-5 hr Epidural 3-4 hr	May be administered by epidural route for acute and chronic pain.
Codeine phosphate or sulfate (Ag) (Tylenol with codeine, Phenaphen with codeine)	1/30-1/8	PO, IM, IV 15-60 mg (0.5 mg/kg) q4h	PO 15-30 min	PO 3-6 hr	May be used with acetaminophen or aspirin for mild to moderate pain. Has analgesic and antitussive properties.
Fentanyl citrate (Ag) (Sublimaze)	75-125	Oral (transmucosal) 200-400 mcg (5-15 mcg/kg) q4-6h IV, IM 25-100 mcg (0.7-2 mcg/kg) Epidural 50-100 mcg (1-2 mcg/kg) Spinal 5-20 mcg (0.1-0.4 mcg/kg) Transdermal 25-100 mcg/hr	Oral 5-15 min IV <30 sec IM <8 min Epidural 4-10 min Spinal 4-10 min Transdermal 12-18 hr	Oral 1-2 hr IV 30-60 min IM 1-2 hr Epidural 4-8 hr Spinal 4-8 hr Transdermal 3 days	Potent opioid. Related to meperidine. Transdermal and oral transmucosal forms useful in chronic pain.
Hydrocodone HCl (Ag) (Lortab, Lorcet, Co-Gesic, Vicodin)	1/30-1/8	PO 5-10 mg q4-6h	PO 15-30 min	PO 4-8 hr	Mild analgesic. Potency similar to codeine. Used in combination with aspirin or acetaminophen.
Hydromorphone HCl (Ag) (Dilaudid)	7	PO 2-4 mg q4-6h IM, SC 2-4 mg (0.04-0.08 mg/kg) Slow IV 0.5-2 mg (0.01-0.04 mg/kg) Epidural 1-2 mg (20-40 mcg/kg)	PO, IM, SC 15-30 min IV <30 sec Epidural 5 min	PO, IM, SC 4-6 hr IV 2-4 hr Epidural 10-16 hr	Potent, short-acting opioid. Used for breakthrough pain in conjunction with long-acting opioid (e.g., morphine). May be administered parenterally, rectally, or subcutaneously.
Levorphanol tartrate (Ag) (LevoDromoran)	5	PO, SC 2-4 mg q4-6h Slow IV 1 mg (0.02 mg/kg)	IV 10-15 min	SC 6-8 hr IV 6-8 hr	Highly concentrated. Useful for subcutaneous infusions requiring small volumes.
Meperidine HCl (Ag) (Demerol)	0.1	PO, IM. IV, SC 50-150 mg (1-3 mg/kg) Slow IV 25-100 mg (0.5-2 mg/kg) Epidural 50-100 mg (1-2 mg/kg) Spinal 0.2-1 mg (4-20 mcg/kg)	PO 10-45 min IM 1-5 min IV <1 min Epidural 2-12 min Spinal 2-12 min	IV, IM, PO 2-4 hr Epidural 1-8 hr Spinal 1-8 hr	Only opioid with local anesthetic properties and direct myocardial depressant effects.

TABLE 48-2 Opioids and Opioid Antagonists—cont'd

Agent	Potency*	Dose	Onset	Duration	Comments
Methadone HCl (Ag) (Dolophine)	1-3	PO, IM, SC 2.5-10 mg (0.05-0.1 mg/kg) q3-4h, then 5-20 mg/hr, q6-8h Epidural 1-5 mg (20-100 mcg/kg)	PO 30-60 min IV 1 min IM 1-5 min Epidural 5-10 min	IV, IM 4-6 hr PO 22-48 hr Epidural 6-10 hr	Long-acting opioid analgesic; accumulates with use, and administration frequency may be decreased.
Morphine sulfate (Ag) (Morphine, MS Contin, Duramorph, Astramorph)	1	PO 10-60 mg q4h PO (MS Contin) 15-100 mg q12h IM, SC 2.5-20 mg q4h Rectal 10-20 mg q4h IV 2.5-15 mg Epidural 2-5 mg (40-100 mcg/kg) Spinal 0.2-1 mg (4-20 mcg/kg)	PO $<$ 60 min IM 1-5 min IV 1 min Epidural 15-60 min Spinal 15-60 min	IV, IM, SC 2-7 hr Epidural 6-24 hr Spinal 6-24 hr	Principal alkaloid of opium. Prototype of the opiate agonists. Long-acting preparation used for chronic pain.
Nalbuphine HCl (Ag-An) (Nubain)	1	IV, IM, SC 5-10 mg (0.1-0.3 mcg/kg) q3-6h	IV 2-3 min IM, SC 15 min	IV, IM, SC 3-6 hr	Effective in reversing ventilatory depression of agonist opioids (e.g., morphine) while maintaining reasonable analgesia.
Nalmefene (Revex)	NA	IV 0.25 mcg/kg, repeat as necessary in 2- to 5-min intervals up to a total dose of 1 mcg/kg	IV 1-3 min	IV 6-8 hr	Reverses the side effects (e.g., respiratory depression and pruritus) of opioid agonists and the psychotomimetic and dysphoric effects of agonists-antagonists (e.g., pentazocine).
Naloxone HCl (Narcan)	NA	IV, IM, SC 0.1-2 mg (10-100 mcg/kg)	IV 1-2 min IM, SC 2-5 min	IV, IM, SC 1-4 hr	Reverses the side effects (e.g., respiratory depression and pruritus) of opioid agonists and the psychotomimetic and dysphoric effects of agonists-antagonists (e.g., pentazocine).
Naltrexone HCl (Ant) (Trexan)	NA	PO 12.5-50 mg daily	PO 15-30 min	PO 24-72 hr	May reverse the hypotension and cardiovascular instability secondary to endogenous endorphins (potent vasodilators) released in patients with septic or cardiogenic shock.
Oxycodone HCl (Ag) (Roxicodone; in Percocet, Percodan, Roxicet, Tylox)	2	PO 5-10 mg q4-6h	PO 10-15 min	PO 3-6 hr	Potency similar to morphine. Used often in combination with aspirin and acetaminophen.
Oxymorphone HCl (Ag) (Numorphan)	10	IV 0.5 mg q4-6h IM, SC 0.5-1.5 mg q4-6h Rectal 5 mg q4-6h	IV 5-10 min IM, SC 10-15 min	IV, IM 3-6 hr	Derivative of hydromorphone and with similar effects.
Pentazocine HCl (Ag-An) (Talwin)	1/3	PO 50-100 mg (1-2 mg/kg) q3-4h IM, SC 30-60 mg (0.5-1 mg/kg) q3-4h IV 15-30 mg (0.3-0.5 mg/kg) q3-4h	PO 15-30 min IM, SC 15-20 min IV 2-3 min	PO 3-6 hr IM 2 hr IV 1 hr	Oldest agonist-antagonist opioid. Like other agonist-antagonists, may be associated with psychotomimetic effects.

Continued

TABLE 48-2 Opioids and Opioid Antagonists—cont'd

Agent	Potency*	Dose	Onset	Duration	Comments
Propoxyphene HCl (Ag) (Darvon; in Genagesic, Wygesic)	1/50-1/25	PO 65 mg q4h	PO 15-60 min	PO 4-6 hr	Derivative of methadone. Weak analgesic. Used in combination with other analgesics (e.g., acetaminophen).
Sufentanil citrate (Ag) (Sufenta)	500-700	IV, IM 10-30 mcg (0.2-0.6 mcg/kg) Epidural 10-30 mcg (0.2-0.6 mcg/kg) Spinal 1-4 mcg (0.02-0.08 mcg/kg)	IV 1-3 min Epidural 4-10 min Spinal 4-10 min	IV 20-45 min IM 2-4 hr Epidural 2-4 hr Spinal 2-4 hr	Most potent opioid in clinical use, 700 times more potent than morphine. Administered via epidural or spinal route for chronic pain. Parenteral route used for general anesthesia.

Ag, *Agonist*; Ag-An, *agonist-antagonist*; An, *antagonist*; IM, *intramuscular*; IV, *intravenous*; NA, *not applicable*; PA, *partial agonist*; PO, *by mouth*; SC, *subcutaneous*; SL, *sublingual*.
**Compared with oral morphine sulfate.*
Data from Drugs for pain. Med Lett Drugs Ther. *2000;42:73-78;* Mosby's Drug Consult. *St Louis: Mosby; 2004; Valdecoxib (Bextra)—a New COX-2 Inhibitor.* Med Lett Drugs Ther. *2002;44:39-41.*

Physiologic dependence is a pharmacologic property of opioid drugs defined by the occurrence of an abstinence (withdrawal) syndrome after abrupt discontinuation of the drug or the administration of an opioid antagonist. Physiologic dependence should always be assumed to exist after repeated administration of an opioid for more than a few days.[50] Opioids should always be tapered before being discontinued in order to avoid this abstinence syndrome.

Psychologic dependence is characterized by the craving for an opioid drug to achieve a psychologic effect, resulting in the continual use of the drug despite harm to self or others. Iatrogenically induced psychologic dependence on opioids is rare when they are taken for medicinal reasons.[49]

ADJUVANTS

The use of adjuvant therapy can be beneficial for patients experiencing neuropathic pain. Anesthesia providers must be aware of this type of therapy, because patients may be on complex pharmacologic regimens that must be evaluated for effectiveness and maintained if appropriate. In addition, the anesthetist may need to add these agents to the armamentarium. It may be useful to use adjuvant drugs such as tricyclic antidepressants, anticonvulsants, corticosteroids, muscle relaxants, and local anesthetics.

The tricyclic antidepressants block the reuptake of serotonin and norepinephrine at the neuronal membrane. Although small doses (compared with the doses used for their primary indication) are effective, they produce anticholinergic effects, such as dry mouth; CNS effects, such as sedation and fatigue; and cardiovascular effects, such as orthostatic hypotension, arrhythmias, and tachycardia. The onset of the analgesic effect may not occur until 4 to 10 days after initiation of the treatment (Table 48-3).

Anticonvulsant drugs are used to alter the ion channels along the nerve fiber, thereby blocking pain stimuli by blocking the action potential. Carbamazepine, phenytoin, gabapentin, and clonazepam have been used. Common side effects include sedation and dizziness (Table 48-4).

Corticosteroids are used in the management of complex pain syndromes and work to reduce inflammation and swelling. Commonly used in the care of cancer patients, steroids may be indicated in other surgical and disease situations. Edema associated with tumors and the reduction of inflammatory mediators (e.g., prostaglandins and leukotrienes) is often associated with the use of corticosteroids (see Table 48-4).

The use of muscle relaxants in pain management is common. Some practitioners suggest that easing the tension of muscle spasm reduces various types of discomfort such as back pain, acute trauma, and surgical incision pain. Some clinicians do not believe that these drugs relieve muscle spasm but provide analgesia through a yet to be understood mechanism.[51]

NMDA receptor antagonists have been used for many years. Ketamine and dextromethorphan are common NMDA receptor antagonists. Ketamine has been used in the treatment of various neuropathic pain syndromes. Dextromethorphan has been used successfully in the treatment of diabetic neuralgia.[52]

Like clonidine, dexmedetomidine is an α2-adenoreceptor agonist. However, dexmedetomidine (Precedex) is a second-generation formulation of the medication. α_2-Receptors are located on or near the terminals of unmyelinated peripheral nerves and postsynaptically within the dorsal horn. Dexmedetomidine inhibits nociceptive neuron firing and the release of substance P centrally. Clinically, dexmedetomidine administered during the perioperative period has demonstrated anesthetic as well as opioid-sparing effects.[53,54] Patients undergoing off-pump coronary artery bypass[53] and bariatric surgery[54] have benefited from the administration of dexmedetomidine intraoperatively.

γ-Aminobutyric acid (GABA) is an inhibitory transmitter. Several GABA receptor agonists have been identified. The most commonly used drug is Baclofen, which acts in the spinal cord to prevent the release of excitatory neurotransmitters. Baclofen has been used in the treatment of trigeminal neuralgia.[55]

TABLE 48-3 Antidepressant Agents

Agent	Dose	Onset	Peak	Duration	Comments
Amitriptyline HCl (Elavil)	*Pain*: Initial PO 10-25 mg (0.2-0.5 mg/kg) daily hs Titrate up q3-4wk by 10-25 mg as necessary Maintenance: PO 10-150 mg (0.2-3 mg/kg) daily hs	Analgesic: PO 5 days			Classic tricyclic antidepressant. Like other tricyclics, may produce anticholinergic, antihistaminic, and sedating effects. Potentiates analgesic effects of opioids. May enhance ulcer healing (antihistaminic effect).
	Depression: Initial PO 75-100 mg (1.5-2 mg/kg) daily in one to four doses Maintenance: PO 25-150 mg/kg (0.5-3 mg/kg) daily in one to four doses IM 20-30 mg qid, then replace with oral Do not use intravenously	Antidepressant: PO 1-2 wk	PO 2-4 wk	PO variable	
Amoxapine HCl (Asendin)	*Pain*: Initial PO 50-150 mg (1-3 mg/kg) daily hs Titrate dose up q3-4wk by 25-50 mg as necessary Maintenance: PO 50-300 mg (1-6 mg/kg) daily hs	Analgesic: PO <5 days			Tricyclic antidepressant. Moderately sedating and has little anticholinergic effect. Rapid onset of activity. May be associated with the development of extrapyramidal symptoms. Toxic levels produce CNS manifestations rather than cardiovascular effects (as compared with other tricyclics).
	Depression: Initial PO 100-150 mg (2-3 mg/kg) daily in one to three doses Maintenance: PO 100-400 mg (2-8 mg/kg) daily in one to three doses Doses >300 mg should be administered in two to three doses	Antidepressant: PO 4-7 days	PO 2-4 wk	PO variable	
Citalopram (Celexa)	*Pain*: Initial PO 20 mg qd	Analgesic: PO 1 wk	PO 2-4 wk	PO variable	Selective serotonin reuptake inhibitor. Antidepressant activity is comparable with that of fluoxetine and superior to that of doxepin or trazadone with fewer adverse effects. Unlike the tricyclics, sedating, anticholinergic, and cardiovascular effects are minimal.
	Depression: PO 20-60 mg qd; dose increases are recommended at a rate of 20 mg/wk	Antidepressant: PO 1-2 wk	PO 2-4 wk	PO variable	

Continued

TABLE 48-3 Antidepressant Agents—cont'd

Agent	Dose	Onset	Peak	Duration	Comments
Desipramine HCl (Pertofrane)	*Pain*: Initial PO 50-100 mg (1-2 mg/kg) daily hs Titrate dose up q3-4wk by 25-50 mg as necessary Maintenance: PO 50-200 mg (1-4 mg/kg) daily hs	Analgesic: PO 5 days			Tricyclic antidepressant. Compared with the parent drug (imipramine), has fewer side effects (e.g., orthostatic hypotension, urinary retention). Used in patients who cannot tolerate the parent drug (imipramine).
	Depression: Initial PO 75-100 mg daily in one to four doses Maintenance: PO 50-300 mg in one to four doses Doses >200 mg not recommended for outpatients IM 100 mg daily in divided doses, then replace with oral	Antidepressant: PO 2-5 days	PO 2-3 wk	PO variable	
Fluoxetine (Prozac)	*Pain and depression*: Adults: 20 mg/day (two 10-mg capsules) in the morning; may increase after 4 wk in 10-20 mg/day increments; maximum: 80 mg/day; doses >20 mg should be divided into two daily doses. *Note*: Lower doses of 10 mg/day have been used for initial treatment.	PO 1-2 wk	PO 2-4 wk	PO variable	Selective serotonin reuptake inhibitor. Antidepressant-activity is comparable with that of paroxetine and superior to that of doxepin or trazadone with fewer adverse effects. Unlike the tricyclics, sedating, anticholinergic, and cardiovascular effects are minimal.
Nortriptyline HCl (Pamelor)	*Pain*: Initial PO 10-50 mg (0.5-1 mg/kg) daily hs Titrate dose up q3-4wk by 10-25 mg as necessary Maintenance: PO 10-150 mg (0.2-3 mg/kg) daily hs	Analgesic: PO 5 days			Compared with the parent drug (amitriptyline), nortriptyline has fewer side effects. The only tricyclic antidepressant with a therapeutic window for serum levels (50-150 ng/ml).
	Depression: Initial PO 50-100 mg (1.5-2 mg/kg) daily in one to four doses Maintenance: PO 50-150 mg (1-3 mg/kg) daily in one to four doses Monitor serum levels with doses >100 mg daily	Antidepressant: PO 1-2 wk	PO 2-4 wk	PO variable	
Paroxetine HCl (Paxil)	*Pain*: Initial PO 10-20 mg daily, preferably in the morning Titrate dose up qwk by 10 mg as necessary Maintenance: PO 10-50 mg daily in the morning	Analgesic: PO 5 days			Selective serotonin reuptake inhibitor. Antidepressant activity is comparable with that of fluoxetine and superior to doxepin or trazadone with fewer adverse effects. Unlike the tricyclics, sedating, anticholinergic, and cardiovascular effects are minimal.

TABLE 48-3 Antidepressant Agents—cont'd

Agent	Dose	Onset	Peak	Duration	Comments
	Depression: Initial PO 20 mg daily, preferably one dose in morning Titrate dose up by 10 mg/day by weekly intervals as necessary Maintenance: PO 20-50 mg daily in one dose in morning	Antidepressant: PO 1-2 wk	PO 3-4 wk	PO variable	
Protriptyline HCl (Vivactil)	*Pain*: Initial PO 5 mg (0.1 mg/kg) tid Maintenance: PO 5-10 mg (0.1-0.2 mg/kg) tid	Analgesic: PO 5 days			Tricyclic antidepressant. Protriptyline may have a more rapid onset of action than imipramine or amitriptyline. Like other secondary amines (e.g., amoxapine, nortriptyline, and desipramine), it is more effective in patients with low norepinephrine levels compared with serotonin-deficient patients.
	Depression: Initial PO 5 mg (0.1 mg/kg) tid Maintenance: PO 5-20 mg (0.1-0.4 mg/kg) tid	Antidepressant: PO 7 days	PO 2-4 wk	PO variable	
Sertraline (Zoloft)	*Pain and depression*: Initial PO 50 mg/day (half of a 100 mg tablet) as a single dose; dose may be increased at intervals of at least 1 wk to a maximum recommended dose of 200 mg/day	PO 1 week	PO 1-3 wk	PO variable	Selective serotonin reuptake inhibitor. Antidepressant activity is comparable with that of fluoxetine and superior to that of doxepin or trazadone with fewer adverse effects. Unlike the tricyclics, sedating, anticholinergic, and cardiovascular effects are minimal.
Trimipramine maleate (Surmontil)	*Pain*: Initial PO 25-100 mg (0.5-2 mg/kg) daily hs Titrate dose up q3-4wk by 25-50 mg as necessary Maintenance: PO 25-200 mg (0.5-4 mg/kg) daily hs	Analgesic: PO 5 days			Tricyclic antidepressant. Structurally related to imipramine.
	Depression: Initial PO 75-100 mg daily in one to four doses Maintenance: PO 50-300 mg daily in one to four doses Doses of >200 mg daily are not recommended for outpatients Do not administer intravenously	Antidepressant: PO 1-2 wk	PO 2-4 wk	PO variable	

CNS, *Central nervous system*; hs, *at bedtime*; IM, *intramuscular*; PO, *by mouth*; qd, *once daily*; qid, *four times a day*; tid, *three times a day*.
Data from Boyce EG, Breen GA: Celecoxib: a COX-2 inhibitor for osteoarthritis and rheumatoid arthritis. Formulary. *31:1999;4:405-417;* Med Lett Drugs Ther. *1998;40:113-114; and* Mosby's Drug Consult. *St Louis: Mosby; 2004.*

TABLE 48-4 Adjuvants Used in Pain Management

Drug Class	Indications	Drug and Routes	Starting Dose (mg/day)	Administration Schedule	Comments
Anticonvulsants	Multipurpose for chronic pain	Tizanidine PO (Zanaflex)	6	bid	
	First-line for paroxysmal or "shooting" pain; second-line for nonparoxysmal pain	Carbamazepine PO (Tegretol)	200	q6-8h	
		Clonazepam PO (Klonopin)	0.5	q8h	
		Divalproex sodium PO (Depakote)	500-1000	qd	
		Phenytoin PO (Dilantin)	300	qd	
		Phenytoin IV (Dilantin)	15-18 in divided doses	One to three doses	IV dose used for escalating neuropathic pain
		Valproate sodium IV (Depacon)	10-15 mg/kg/day	One to three doses	IV dose used for escalating neuropathic pain followed by PO doses
	Multipurpose for all types of neuropathic pain	Gabapentin PO (Neurontin)	900-1800	Three doses	May increase dose daily
Corticosteroids	Multipurpose analgesics	Dexamethasone PO (Decadron)	Low dose: 1-2	qd or bid	May also improve appetite, nausea, and malaise; used when pain persists after optimal opioid dose
			High dose: 100	qid	High doses used for acute episodic pain unresponsive to opioids; risk of serious toxicity increases with dose, duration of therapy, and NSAIDs
GABA-ergic	"Shooting" neuropathic pain	Baclofen PO (Lioresal)	15	q8h	
Local anesthetics	Neuropathic pain of any type	Mexiletine PO (Mexitil)	150	q8h	Mexiletine is safer than tocainide; plasma concentrations should be monitored
		Tocainide PO (Tonocard)	400	q8h	Analgesia occurs within 15-30 min
		Lidocaine IV	Brief infusion: 2-5 mg/kg over 20-30 min		
		Lidocaine SC, IV	Continuous infusion: 2.5 mg/kg/hr		

bid, *Twice daily;* GABA, *γ-aminobutyric acid;* IV, *intravenous;* NSAIDs, *nonsteroidal antiinflammatory drugs;* PO, *by mouth;* qd, *once daily.*
Modified from McCaffrey M, *Pasero* C. Pain: Clinical Manual. *St Louis: Mosby; 1999:342-344.*

MODE OF ADMINISTRATION

Previously, the most common approach to postoperative pain relief was IM injection of an opioid, administered as needed. However, this modality is painful and is associated with unpredictable absorption and with peaks and valleys in blood levels, creating inconsistent pain relief.[40] Today we know that pain medication should be administered around the clock via an IV or oral route in doses based on the assessment, dose response, and reassessment of the patient.[1,56]

The most reliable indicator of the existence and intensity of pain is the patient's own self-report. Opioids are often administered at fixed doses at arbitrary time intervals rather than on a dose-response basis. Correlation appears to be lacking between the opioid dose and subjective pain relief.

Of the less invasive modalities, the IV route is preferred for the administration of postoperative opioid therapy, with the sublingual or rectal route used as a secondary option.[1] Treatment of postoperative pain via subcutaneous (SC) or IM administration should not be considered as a primary choice.

Newer modalities, such as buccal or intranasal administration and perhaps the transdermal patch, may be considered when the traditional approaches fall short. The rationale behind this order of priority is to promote the titration of the opioid until pain relief is achieved and to avoid the unpredictability of absorption through the tissue.[1]

Patients should be switched to oral pain medication in equipotent doses as soon as the general condition permits or the patient is permitted to take food by mouth. When the oral route is chosen, the appropriate dose must be calculated on the basis of bioavailability and equipotency.[1] The importance of this point cannot be overstated. Too often patients are switched to oral medications too early or with little concern about required doses.

Patient-controlled analgesia was developed in the early 1970s with the advent of microprocessor technology. The administration technique has changed the face of pain management. It uses electronic devices programmed to inject set doses and incorporates lockout intervals, with or without basal infusions, and other built-in limitations to prevent peaks and valleys in analgesic blood levels. This technique makes the patient less dependent on the caregivers, within certain limits, for administration of the medication. The drugs most frequently used in these devices are morphine sulfate and hydromorphone. Meperidine use with patient-controlled analgesia is not recommended for the reasons cited earlier.

A new noninvasive patient-controlled analgesia delivery system is currently being evaluated and is demonstrating promise. The transdermal system was tolerated well by patients in this double-blind study.[57]

Local Anesthetics

Over the last few decades the use of local anesthetics administered as single injections or via continuous catheter techniques has gained popularity. Most peripheral nerve blocks consist of a bolus dose of local anesthetic injected to cause infiltration of an area or are applied at a peripheral nerve site. These techniques are primarily used for analgesia for minor surgical procedures, although they often provide pain relief in the immediate postoperative period as well.

The use of continuous local anesthetic techniques is becoming increasingly popular. These techniques may be applied where an anatomic structure allows the insertion of a temporary catheter adjacent to a nerve. The most commonly used technique is the brachial plexus block. Catheters can also be placed to provide nerve blocks in the intercostal, femoral, sciatic, and other major peripheral nerves.

Because nerve blocks only limit the path of nociceptive impulses, some clinicians favor adding an antiinflammatory agent to decrease inflammation at the peripheral (trauma) site. Several peripheral blocks are briefly discussed in this chapter.

Intercostal Blocks

Intercostal blocks have been used successfully as a means of pain relief for rib fractures. They are relatively easy to apply in the form of an injection but carry a potential risk of pneumothorax with repeated injections. Intercostal blocks may also be applied via a catheter after thoracic or upper-quadrant abdominal surgery or trauma. Intercostal local anesthetics can be administered as bolus injections as required.

Intrapleural Analgesia

Intrapleural analgesia is a modality that can be used for thoracic and upper abdominal surgery. A catheter can be placed in the intrapleural cavity for bolus injections or continuous infusion. This modality has the advantage of avoiding blockade of the sympathetic nervous system. It may not be as useful in thoracotomies with pleural drainage because of the unpredictable distribution and uptake of the local anesthetic agent. Cases of toxicity have been reported to result from systemic uptake. Other potential sequelae of continuous pleural analgesia include pneumothorax and ventilatory problems while the chest tube is clamped during equilibration in the pleural cavity.

Continuous Epidural Analgesia

A combination of a low-dose opioid and a low-concentration local anesthetic via an epidural route is an efficient treatment modality for postoperative pain. Continuous epidural analgesia was used in the late 1940s but lost popularity.[58] It regained popularity in the 1980s.[59,60]

Neuraxial blockade has been found to be useful in the management of postoperative pain; because it provides profound analgesia, some clinicians also use the epidural technique with light general anesthesia during the surgical procedure. At the end of the procedure, the epidural catheter is left in place for postoperative pain management. Drugs can then be administered as bolus injections or continuous infusion or via a patient-controlled device. The continuous epidural technique can be used for thoracic, abdominal, and lower extremity surgery, including trauma.

This technique is a powerful tool in the management of pain. Unfortunately, its implementation ideally requires that a pain management service be available for training the care providers and for coordination of pain management.

Analgesia is provided through the administration of a local anesthetic or an opioid alone or the combination of a diluted concentration of a local anesthetic and an opioid. The purpose of combining the two drugs is the use of the different sites of action and the provision of synergy.[61] If one of the agents is used alone, tachyphylaxis may develop. This is characterized by blockade of fewer dermatomes despite the injection of an increased amount of local anesthetic in identical concentration, as well as regression of a stable analgesic dermatomal level during continuous epidural infusion. Scott and coworkers[61] have reported evidence of a synergistic effect of the opioid–local anesthetic combination. Some clinicians advocate concomitant use of NSAIDs with the epidural modality to decrease inflammation at the peripheral site.

The analgesic solution can be administered either as a bolus or as a continuous infusion via a programmable pump. The placement of the epidural catheter and the initiation of treatment may vary. Some clinicians prefer to insert the catheter and start the treatment as part of the preoperative preparation; others insert it in the postoperative phase.

Individual preferences vary with regard to the level at which the epidural catheter should be placed. The following guideline is advocated by Lubenow[62]:

Procedure	Vertebral Range
Thoracic surgery	T2 through T8
Upper abdominal surgery	T4 through L1
Renal surgery	T6 through L1
Hip surgery	T12 through L3
Lower abdominal and gynecologic surgery	T10 through L3

The protocols used for monitoring patients with continuous epidural analgesia vary a great deal. Some institutions have the patients fully monitored in a critical care setting, whereas others have well-trained staff that care for these patients on regular floors. In many institutions with an acute pain management service, standard order sheets are used. The orders include drugs used, vital signs (including level of consciousness), and assessment of pain. Orders for treatment of respiratory depression, breakthrough pain, nausea, and itching should be available. It is important to instruct the nurses who provide bedside care to inspect the epidural catheter site when assessing for progressive loss of sensation or motor function and when evaluating for side effects of opioids.

Two commonly occurring side effects of epidural therapy are nausea, with or without vomiting, and pruritus. Nausea is related to the opioid level at the chemoreceptor zone in the medulla. Opioid-induced nausea can be reduced with commonly used antiemetics, such as phenothiazines. Also, intermittent low-dose naloxone (0.4 to 1 mg) may be administered intermittently via an IV route. If the nausea persists a continuous infusion of naloxone (1 mcg/kg/hr) may be used, with the dose increased until effective.

Although histamine plays a minimal role in pruritus caused by epidurally administered opioids, antihistamines such as diphenhydramine may be used to treat itching. For severe cases of itching, naloxone in doses similar to those used in the treatment of nausea may be administered.

Urinary retention is a well-recognized side effect of epidural pain management. The condition may be reversed with incremental doses of naloxone, although catheterization of the bladder often is the treatment of choice.

Local anesthetics in the epidural infusion, although diluted, may cause hypotension, as well as sensory and motor block.

The side effect of epidural opioids that causes the most concern is respiratory depression. This is caused by the rostral spread of the opioid and its subsequent effect on the respiratory control center in the brainstem. The poorer the opioid's lipid solubility, the greater the risk for delayed respiratory depression. When patients are treated with epidural opioids, equipment for airway management and assisted ventilation must be available. A patient who becomes apneic from epidural analgesia is treated with manual ventilation and incremental doses of naloxone. Alternatively, an infusion of naloxone (1 mcg/kg/hr) may be begun. The use of this modality may necessitate admission to a critical care or an intermediate care unit for observation.

Some controversy exists with regard to whether apnea or other monitors should be used as part of the protocol for the epidural treatment. This addition makes the modality extremely resource consuming. It is vital that nurses at the bedside be well trained in the observation of patients with epidural catheters. Lubenow states that the observation of vigilant nurses is paramount, and that it should be the complete responsibility of the pain management service to manage the analgesia and sedation.[62,63]

MANAGEMENT OF PAIN IN CHILDREN

The pediatric patient in pain poses numerous challenges. The anesthetist must keep in mind that both the patient and the family member responsible for the child should be included in the development of the pain management plan. Unfortunately, some health-care providers still believe that children do not have pain, and undermedication is more the rule than the exception. As with adult patients, several myths and misconceptions are related to the lack of adequate management of pediatric pain.[64-67]

One difficulty in providing adequate pain control in children is assessment and evaluation, owing to the child's cognitive development and individual emotions and reactions to pain. However, skilled pediatric nursing staff are still capable of providing adequate observation of the pediatric patient in discomfort or pain, as well as assessing the response to analgesics. Several scales are available for the quantification of pediatric pain and assessment of relief.

The modality and drugs of choice for the pediatric patient depend largely on the knowledge and skills of the staff involved in the care and the age of the child. The choices are the same as those available for the adult, with different dosages used because of the different pharmacokinetics (Table 48-5).

TABLE 48-5 Local Anesthetics for Pediatric Regional Anesthesia

Drug	Techniques	Concentration	Dose	Duration (min)
Bupivacaine (Marcaine)	Epidural or caudal	0.25%	2.5 mg/kg or 0.5-1 ml/kg	120-240
	Spinal*	Hyperbaric: 0.5% in 8% dextrose	<5 kg: 0.5 mg/kg 5-15 kg: 0.4 mg/kg >15 kg: 0.3 mg/kg	30-60
	Brachial plexus	0.25%	0.7 ml/kg up to 50 kg	150-360
Mepivacaine (Carbocaine)	Brachial plexus	0.5%-2%	5 mg/kg (maximum 8 mg)	60-90
	Caudal	0.5-1.5%	0.5 mg/kg	120-360
Lidocaine (Xylocaine)	Epidural or caudal	1%-2%	5 (7) mg/kg†	30-60
	Brachial plexus	0.5%-2%	5 (7) mg/kg†	45-160
	Spinal	5% with 7.5% dextrose	2 mg/kg	Variable
Tetracaine (Pontocaine)	Spinal*	0.5% in 10% dextrose	<5 kg: 0.4-0.8 mg/kg 5-15 kg: 0.4-0.8 mg/kg >15 kg: 0.3 mg/kg	60-90

**Indications: patient <60 wk postconceptional age, high risk for apnea and bradycardia.*
†*Without (with) epinephrine.*
From Kremer M, Faut-Callahan M. Regional anesthesia and pain management. In: Zaglaniczny K, Aker J, eds. Clinical Guide to Pediatric Anesthesia. *Philadelphia: Saunders; 1999:369.*

One goal of management of acute pain in children is minimizing the emotional trauma associated with treatment through a reliable method of administration. The pain experience of a pediatric patient largely influences the individual's future experiences with pain.

The fear of psychologic dependence in children is often a deterrent to adequate pain management. However, no evidence exists that children with moderate to severe postoperative pain, treated adequately, are likely to become drug dependent or craving.

The modality chosen should be as atraumatic as possible. Many children would rather suffer in silence than receive an IM injection. Because most children have IV access postoperatively, it is logical to give opioids intravenously. The technique depends on the age of the child. Older children may be able to use patient-controlled analgesia with or without a basal infusion. The determining factor for the implementation should be the cognitive development rather than the age. For younger children, an alternative is continuous infusion, which provides a uniform level of analgesia. Some may be reluctant to use this technique out of fear of side effects from the opioids, but the literature provides very little evidence of complications associated with this particular technique. In fact, one work advocates its superiority.[65]

Intermittent IV bolus injections are an alternative; however, they are associated with high peaks that are short lived, and they are just as labor intensive as IM injections. Respiratory depression may be more of a problem with this approach. If the patient still has the need for opioids when IV access is removed, oral medication should be strongly considered.

Postoperative pain relief should commence at the induction of the anesthesia, whenever applicable. Use of local anesthetics at the surgical site before incision has proven effective. The combination of regional analgesia and general anesthesia has also been promoted for management of pediatric postoperative pain.

Although limited by the lack of qualified providers, the use of regional analgesia in children is growing in popularity. Regional analgesia with the administration of local anesthetics or opioids modulates the transmission of afferent nociceptive impulses. Minimal side effects have been reported, and pain management is highly effective.[67]

It is unlikely that a child will tolerate the placement of a regional anesthetic. However, placement of a regional block may be done under sedation or once the child is anesthetized. A variety of peripheral nerve blocks can be used in the pediatric population. Wrist, ankle, femoral, and axillary blocks are common. Intercostal blocks have been used for thoracotomy and nephrectomy. Spinal, caudal, and epidural analgesia have also been used successfully. Local anesthetics can be used safely, provided close attention to dosage is maintained (see Table 48-5).

CANCER-RELATED PAIN

Cancer and cancer-related pathology are responsible for 20% of the deaths annually in the United States[68] and 10% of the deaths worldwide.[69] Presently more than 8 million Americans have cancer, and another 1 million are diagnosed yearly. Pain often accompanies the diagnosis and treatment of cancer. One third of cancer patients undergoing active therapy and two thirds of those with advanced disease experience pain. Studies have demonstrated that 70% to 90% of cancer-related pain can be effectively managed with pharmacotherapy alone. More sobering, however, is the fact that surveys suggest that 40% to 50% of patients experiencing cancer-related pain do not receive effective analgesia.[70] Numerous barriers prevent the achievement of this goal. All of the barriers can in some way be attributed to health professionals, the patients and family members, or the health-care system.[71] By obtaining the necessary knowledge and sharing this information with their colleagues, educating patients and families, and initiating or becoming involved in institutional pain management programs, CRNAs can have a significant impact on all three of these areas.

Untreated pain in patients with cancer can be psychologically devastating. Not only can pain cause unnecessary suffering, but many patients view the presence of pain as a constant reminder of the disease. In addition, patients who receive adequate analgesia are more likely to comply with potentially curative treatments and participate in activities of daily living.[72] Clearly, inadequate pain management affects patients' quality of life.

The AHCPR has established clinical practice guidelines for the management of cancer pain.[72] These guidelines provide a framework for CRNAs to accurately assess and effectively manage cancer-related pain. Despite the promulgation of these guidelines, CRNAs lack the assessment skills and pharmacologic knowledge base necessary to alleviate pain and suffering in patients with cancer. Although nurse anesthetists are proficient at the perioperative assessment of pain and opioid administration, they can no longer confine their practice to the perioperative period. As nurses in advanced practice, CRNAs should possess the knowledge to effectively assess and manage cancer-related pain during the preoperative and postoperative periods.

In a survey of 1777 cancer specialists, only 51% reported that patients in their treatment settings attained adequate relief.[72] Because the number of comprehensive cancer centers is small, CRNAs in smaller and rural hospitals must become involved in the pain management of these patients. This section provides the practicing CRNA with the rudimentary information necessary to effectively assess and pharmacologically manage patients with pain related to cancer. Other treatment modalities are mentioned for the sake of completeness, but the reader is cautioned that the information contained herein should be supplemented with additional reading and clinical exposure to affected patients.

Assessment of Cancer Pain

One of the greatest barriers to effective pain management is poor pain assessment.[73] The ability to complete a thorough assessment of pain in patients with cancer is an essential step. Initial assessment of the cancer pain must be comprehensive and completed in a stepwise fashion, beginning with data collection and finishing with a patient-oriented problem list and a strategy for pain management. The evaluation should be guided by the ability to conduct thorough physical and neurologic examinations. In addition, the CRNA should have knowledge of common pain syndromes, oncologic emergencies, and modalities available to treat a pain crisis.[71] Ultimately, the two main goals of the assessment are to gain an accurate characterization of the pain, including the pain syndrome and inferred pathophysiology, and to evaluate the impact of the pain and the role it plays in the overall suffering of the patient.[70]

Cancer-related pain can result from any of the following: (1) tumor invasion into bone, joint, muscle, or connective tissue; (2) diagnostic or therapeutic procedures (lumbar punctures, chemotherapy, radiation); and (3) unrelated pain (e.g., preexisting arthritis, infection). The overall incidence of pain in patients with cancer depends on the type and stage of the disease. When cancer is diagnosed at early and intermediate stages, 30% to 45% of patients experience pain, whereas nearly 75% of patients with advanced cancer have pain.[72]

The complete assessment of the patient with cancer-related pain has four facets[72]: (1) assessment of pain intensity and character, (2) psychosocial assessment, (3) physical and neurologic examinations, and (4) diagnostic evaluation. Evaluation of the intensity, quality, distribution, and temporal relationships of the pain can be beneficial in identification of cancer pain syndromes. Evaluating the intensity of the pain is critical, because it indicates the urgency with which pain relief is needed. Patient self-report should be the primary source of information regarding pain intensity. The use of validated and reliable tools, such as the numeric rating scale (0 through 10), the categoric scale (none, mild, moderate, severe, worst possible), or the Memorial Pain Assessment Scale,[74] enables the clinician to assess pain intensity as well as pain relief. Every effort should be made to assess the character of the pain, as well as the location; onset and duration; aggravating and relieving factors; past treatments, including what was effective or ineffective; and how the pain has affected the patient's physical and social function. In addition, assessment of pain intensity helps in determination of the analgesic drug to be used, the route of administration, and the rate at which the medication is titrated. Determination of pain intensity may also be beneficial in identifying the cause of the underlying syndrome. For example, nerve injury after radiation is rarely severe; however, severe pain in a previously irradiated region is suggestive of recurrent neoplasm.[70]

Assessing the quality of the patient's pain is crucial, because it can suggest the pathophysiology of the pain. Somatic pain is described as sharp, aching, throbbing, or pressure-like. Pain that is described as gnawing or cramping is most often visceral in nature secondary to obstruction of a hollow viscus. Visceral pain can be sharp or throbbing when it is associated with organ capsules or mesentery. Pain described as "burning," "tingling," or "shocklike," particularly when it is associated with subjective numbness, loss of sensation, and weakness, is likely to have a neuropathic origin.[72,75]

The distribution of the pain is particularly important when pain is experienced at a location with no evidence of pathology, when there is more than one site of pain, or when the patient complains of generalized pain. For example, patients can have referred pain in the iliac crest from a lesion at spinal cord level T12. Frequently, patients with advanced cancer experience pain at two or more sites. Complaints of diffuse, dull, aching pain can often indicate bone metastases.

Temporal relationships of pain refer to its acute or chronic nature. Acute cancer pain is generally related to therapeutic or diagnostic procedures. However, the patient can experience breakthrough pain—pain that is associated with incidental events such as coughing, movement, or defecation. *Chronic pain* is defined as pain that lasts for 3 months after the usual course of an acute illness, is associated with a chronic pathologic process, or recurs in a pattern over months or years.[73]

The psychosocial assessment encompasses the meaning of pain to the patient and his or her family, as well as how the individual and caregivers are coping with cancer and the pain that may be associated with the diagnosis. In addition, the patient's level of understanding with regard to expectations of treatment and opioid therapy must be addressed. Last, the nurse anesthetist must try to assess what provisions the patient and family have for dealing with the economic impact the disease will inevitably have on their lives.

The physical and neurologic examination should be focused and evaluate common referral of pain to other areas of the body. The diagnostic evaluation attempts to evaluate the recurrence or progression of disease or tissue injury related to cancer treatment. Appropriate radiologic studies and blood tests are performed, and their results correlated with the physical and neurologic examination. Every effort should be made to provide the patient with analgesia during the initial assessment and diagnostic evaluation. Patient comfort will improve compliance and will not result in an inadequate examination.[70]

The assessment of the patient's pain and the effectiveness of the treatment is an ongoing process. Results of evaluations should be continually documented, so that all people involved in the patient's care have access to the information. This ensures that all caregivers are aware of the current status of the patient's pain and efficacy of the present analgesic therapy. Patients are encouraged to report changes in pain patterns or new pain. These reports should trigger a diagnostic evaluation, because when patients have stable, controlled cancer pain, new complaints of pain are generally associated with progressive disease rather than opioid tolerance.[76,77]

The assessment of the patient is not complete without an attempt to quantify the impact of the entire cancer experience on the patient. This includes not only the physical pain that the patient may be experiencing, but also the amount of suffering that the pain and disease process have inflicted on the patient and the patient's family. *Suffering* is defined as "the state of severe distress associated with events that threaten the intactness of the person."[78] The CRNA must understand that pain and suffering are not synonymous. It is possible for a patient to experience suffering without pain. For example, the loss of a loved one can cause suffering without the perception of nociception (i.e., pain). The converse is also true. Determining whether a patient is suffering in addition to being in pain is important, because the presence of suffering undermines the patient's quality of life. However, determining whether a patient is suffering in addition to being in physical pain can be difficult. Establishing a relationship with the patient and family whereby they are comfortable discussing their financial concerns, their interactions with one another, and their fears can aid in this assessment. In addition, evaluation of the patient's appetite, sleep patterns, interactions with family, socioeconomic status, and so on is an integral part of this assessment.

Although the management of the patient's pain and suffering may seem like a daunting task, it is important to note that the comprehensive care of patients with cancer requires a multidisciplinary approach. The addition of pharmacists, physicians, clerics, psychologists, and social workers to the pain management team is invaluable.

Management of Cancer Pain

Comprehensive management of cancer pain incorporates primary therapy, pharmacologic therapy, and, if necessary, psychologic interventions and invasive therapies.[70] The initial management of the pain should never be delayed while diagnostic tests are being performed. Effective pain management during the initial stages of the diagnostic workup does not interfere with or lead to erroneous data from the tests. Tremendous benefit can be derived from primary therapy, but most patients eventually require some form of analgesic therapy. Pharmacologic therapy is the mainstay of analgesic therapy.

World Health Organization Analgesic Ladder

In 1990 the World Health Organization developed a three-step analgesic ladder to guide analgesic therapy for cancer patients (Figure 48-6).[79] This approach was adopted by the AHCPR (now the AHRQ) and has been shown to effectively relieve pain in 70% to 90% of patients with cancer pain. The first step of this approach uses an NSAID combined with an adjuvant drug to treat patients with mild pain. With persistent pain or an increase in pain from mild to moderate (step 2), an opioid conventionally used for this type of pain is added to the NSAID-adjuvant medication. Opioids used for this type of pain are codeine, hydrocodone, and oxycodone. When pain increases from moderate to severe (step 3), an opioid conventionally used for this type of pain is added to the NSAID-adjuvant medication. Opioids conventionally used for this type of pain are morphine, hdromorphone, oxycodone, methadone, levorphanol, and fentanyl.[80]

Nonopioid Analgesics

Nonopioid analgesics are useful in the treatment of mild pain or in combination with opioids or adjuvant drugs for the treatment of moderate to severe pain. Unlike opioid analgesics, these drugs have a "ceiling effect," whereby no additional analgesic effects can be derived from escalation of the dose past the recommended maximum daily amount. They also do not produce tolerance or physical dependence. Nonopioid analgesics are divided into numerous subclasses.[70] Aspirin and other NSAIDs exert their analgesic effect by inhibiting the enzyme COX. Inhibition of this enzyme blocks the synthesis of prostaglandins, inflammatory mediators known to sensitize peripheral nociceptors.[81] A central mechanism of action is also thought to contribute to NSAID analgesia and probably predominates with acetaminophen-induced analgesia.

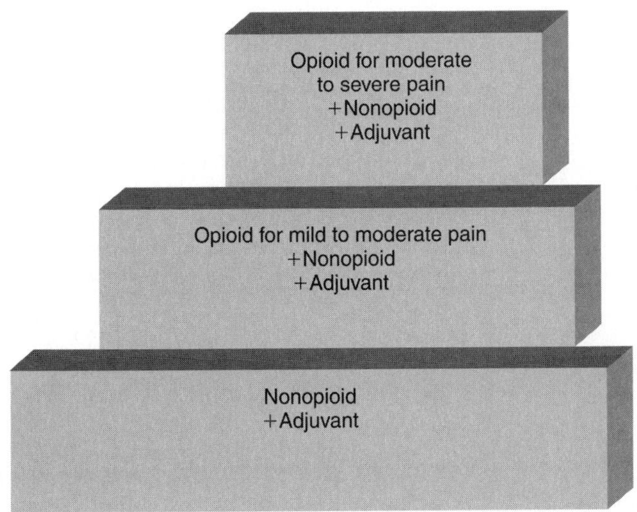

FIGURE **48-6**
Analgesic ladder. (From World Health Organization. *Cancer Pain Relief and Palliative Care*. Geneva: World Health Organization; 1990:9.)

In order to maximize the benefits of these drugs the CRNA must have a thorough understanding of their pharmacologic profiles, dosage guidelines, and potential adverse effects. Adverse effects secondary to nonselective NSAIDs include bleeding, renal failure, gastric ulceration, and hepatic dysfunction. Caution is required when administering these medications to patients at increased risk, including elderly patients; patients with blood clotting disorders, ulcer diathesis, or impaired renal function; and patients concurrently taking corticosteroids. Proton pump inhibitors have been shown to provide the greatest gastroprotection against nonselective NSAID-induced gastric mucosal damage. In addition, many of the potential adverse effects associated with nonselective NSAIDs can be avoided with the use of COX-2 selective drugs. Although no comparative studies demonstrate the analgesic efficacy of nonselective NSAIDs and COX-2 inhibitors in cancer patients, an initial trial of a COX-2 selective drug may be indicated in patients at risk for development of adverse reactions.[80]

The nonacetylated salicylates, choline magnesium trisalicylate and salsalate, have less effect on platelet function and do not affect bleeding times when administered at usual clinical doses. Acetaminophen doses in excess of 4000 mg/day can induce hepatic toxicity, particularly in patients with preexisting liver disease.

Opioid Analgesics

Expertise in opioid therapy is the single most important factor in the successful management of cancer-related pain.[82] This expertise should extend from the pharmacologic profiles of the opioids to the principles of tolerance, pseudoaddiction, physiologic dependence, and psychologic dependence. Opioids exert their analgesic effects through supraspinal, spinal, and possibly peripheral mechanisms by binding to the mu, delta, and kappa receptors.[83] For cancer pain management the pure opioid analgesic drugs are most commonly used. The use of mixed agonist-antagonist and partial agonist opioids is of limited value in this setting because of their ceiling effect for analgesia, ability to precipitate withdrawal symptoms in patients physiologically dependent on pure opioid drugs, and a higher incidence of psychomimetic side effects than pure opioids. Pure opioid analgesic drugs do not have a ceiling effect. Their ability to provide effective analgesia with escalating doses is limited only by the development of unmanageable or intolerable side effects.

Drug Selection

For young, healthy patients and patients without major organ system dysfunction, any of the opioid-agonist drugs can be used. Opioids with a short half-life (e.g., morphine, hydromorphone, oxycodone) are used to initiate therapy because they are easier to titrate than opioids with a longer half-life (e.g., methadone, levorphanol), which take longer to achieve a steady-state plasma concentration.

Particular caution must be used when initiating opioid therapy in patients with impaired renal function. These patients can accumulate the active metabolites of morphine sulfate (morphine-6-glucuronide), meperidine (normeperidine), and propoxyphene (norpropoxyphene). As discussed earlier, normeperidine has the most potentially detrimental side effects. This metabolite is twice as potent a convulsant as its parent compound. Accumulation of this metabolite can lead to CNS excitability manifested by irritability, myoclonus, and occasionally seizures. For these reasons the use of meperidine for the treatment of cancer pain must be discouraged.

Knowing how the patient has responded to previous trials of opioids is imperative. A particular opioid should be continued as long as effective analgesia can be maintained and unmanageable side effects are avoided. However, rotating to a different opioid should be considered when escalating doses become ineffective or when adverse effects become intolerable or unmanageable. Consequently, CRNAs must be familiar with several different opioids and possess the knowledge to initiate therapy with another opioid based on equianalgesic dosage data[19] and the incomplete cross-tolerance between opioids (Table 48-6).

Other medications that the patient is taking must be considered when one initiates opioid therapy. The metabolism and bioavailability of morphine can be altered by other medications. In addition, opioids are often indicted for causing excessive sedation when in fact it may be other centrally acting drugs or their interaction with the opioids.

Route of Administration

When considering which route of administration to use, the nurse anesthetist must determine the least invasive, most convenient, and most fiscally responsible method of providing effective analgesia. In the majority of cases this is the oral route. However, in patients in whom this route is precluded opioids can also be administered via the rectal, sublingual, transdermal, parenteral, and intraspinal routes.

The oral route is the most convenient and economic method of providing analgesia for cancer patients. In addition, most patients tolerate orally administered opioids throughout the course of the illness. Immediate-release preparations are available in both pill and syrup forms and have a peak onset of 45 to 60 minutes. Controlled-release opioids provide added convenience because of the 8-, 12-, or 24-hour doses and achieve their peak effectiveness within 3 to 5 hours for those medications administered every 8 to 12 hours and within 8 to 10 hours for those medications administered every 24 hours.

Rectal preparations of morphine, hydromorphone, and oxymorphone are available in the United States. Dosage of rectally administered opioids is approximately the same as that for oral medications.[84]

The sublingual route of administration, although not frequently used, provides an alternative route for those patients who lose their ability to take oral preparations for a short period of time. Bioavailability is limited with hydrophilic opioids (morphine), but lipophilic preparations (fentanyl and methadone) are well absorbed.[85]

Fentanyl is the only currently available opioid capable of being delivered via the transdermal route. Because interindividual pharmacokinetic variability is large, the administration interval can range from 48 to 72 hours. Transdermal fentanyl can be used only to treat stable pain, which necessitates that a short-acting opioid be provided to treat breakthrough pain.

The parenteral route encompasses IM, SC, and IV routes of administration. IM administration should be discouraged, because repetitive IM injections are painful and absorption is unreliable. Both the SC and IV routes can be used for bolus injections and continuous infusions. Bolus injections provide for rapid titration but can be associated with adverse effects at peak levels (excessive sedation) and trough levels (pain).

TABLE 48-6 Pharmacologic Management of Cancer Pain—Relative Potency, Half-Life, and Duration of Action of Commonly Used Opioid Drugs

Drug	Half-life (hr)	Equianalgesic Intramuscular Dose (mg)	Intramuscular or Oral Potency	Starting Oral Dose Range (mg)	Comments
Morphine	2-3	10	3 (Repeated dose)	15-30	Standard of comparison for opioid analgesics; multiple routes of administration; controlled release available; morphine-6-glucuronide accumulation in patients with renal failure; lower doses for the elderly
Hydromorphone	2-3	1.5	5	4-8	Useful alternative for morphine; no known active metabolite; multiple routes available
Methadone	15-190	10	2	5-10	May accumulate with repetitive administration
Levorphanol	12-15	2	2	2-4	May accumulate with repetitive administration
Meperidine	2-3	75	4	Not recommended	Central nervous system excitatory toxic metabolite, normeperidine; contraindicated for repetitive administration, for patients with renal failure, and for patients receiving monoamine oxidase inhibitors
Fentanyl	2	N/A	N/A	N/A	Short half-life; parenteral use by infusion; clinical experience suggests 2 mg MSO_4/hr = 100 mcg transdermal patch; patches available to deliver 25, 50, 75, 100 mcg/hr
Oxycodone	2-3	15	2	5-10	Available in liquid or tablet preparations; also in combination with a nonopioid
Codeine	2-3	130	1.5	30-60	Used orally for less severe pain; usually combined with a nonopioid

N/A, *Not applicable*; MSO_4, *morphine sulphate*.

Continuous infusions avoid bolus effects and can be administered via the SC or IV route. Opioids that are soluble, nonirritating, and well absorbed can be given subcutaneously via a needle that can remain in place for up to 1 week. Infusion rates should not exceed 5 ml/hr, and dosage is the same as IV. SC infusions are particularly beneficial in ambulatory patients and in patients in whom IV access is unavailable. IV infusions should be used when available and are recommended when large amounts of fluid are infused.

Intraspinal opioids can be administered in the intrathecal or epidural space. This route of administration is beneficial in a small number of cancer patients.

Dosage Schedule

Patients with continuous or frequently occurring pain should receive opioids "around the clock" (ATC). This type of administration provides the patient with opioids at a regular, fixed time. When immediate-release opioids are used, they should be administered should be every 3 to 4 hours. Controlled-release oral preparations (morphine, oxycodone, hydromorphone) are the most convenient form, because they reach peak serum levels in 3 to 5 hours and their analgesic half-life is 8 to 12 hours. Patients undergoing this regimen should also have access to an immediate-release form of the drug to treat breakthrough pain ("rescue dose"). Rescue doses are equivalent to 5% to 15% of the 24-hour baseline dose.[81] IV or SC rescue doses can be given every 15 to 30 minutes, and oral rescue doses can be offered every hour. "As needed" (prn) administration may be useful in opioid-naive patients beginning therapy or in those patients in whom rapid titration is necessary. This form of administration is not recommended in the routine management of continuous pain, because the patient can suffer needlessly if a time lag occurs between when the request is made and when the opioid is actually administered.

A patient in severe pain and beginning opioid therapy should receive a dose equivalent to 5 to 10 mg of IV morphine every 4 hours with rescue doses of 6 to 12 mg every hour (i.e., 15 to 30 mg every 4 hours with rescue doses of 18 to 36 mg every hour). If pain continues to be intolerable despite escalating doses or if adverse effects become unmanageable, rotation to another opioid should be considered. Equianalgesic dose charts are used to guide the conversion to the new drug. The starting dose of the new drug should be decreased by 50% to account for the incomplete cross-tolerance between opioids. If the new opioid is methadone, the dose should be decreased by 75% to account for the prolonged half-life of the drug.

Dose Titration

The severity of the pain should dictate the rate of dose titration. For patients with severe pain, parenteral administration of an opioid with a short half-life is the preferred method of dose titration. Doses can be administered intravenously every 15 to 30 min until adequate analgesia is obtained. Once analgesia is achieved the patient should receive a continuous infusion of the same opioid. During the titration process, doses can become quite high before adequate analgesia is obtained. CRNAs must understand that the total dose of opioid is immaterial as long as analgesia is obtained and adverse effects are not intolerable or unmanageable.

After effective analgesia is obtained, patients usually remain on a stable dose of opioid for pain control. Nurse anesthetists should not let their concern about tolerance deter the use of opioids early in the treatment of cancer pain. New complaints of pain and the need for continued dose escalation are seldom the result of analgesic tolerance. New pain or worsening pain should be aggressively pursued diagnostically, because once a stable dose of opioid has been achieved, worsening pain is often indicative of disease progression.[76,77]

Adverse Effects and Management

Successful cancer pain management mandates that the CRNA possess the skills necessary to assess and manage the adverse effects associated with opioid therapy. Clearly, the objective is for the analgesic effects of the opioid to outweigh the treatment-related adverse effects. The most common adverse effects of chronic opioid use are constipation, nausea, vomiting, sedation, and cognitive impairment. Also possible, but to varying degrees, are dysphoria, myoclonus, urinary retention, and respiratory depression.

The incidence of opioid-related constipation is extremely high, and tolerance to this side effect occurs very slowly, if at all. Patients who are dehydrated and immobile with advanced age or abdominal disease are particularly predisposed to this side effect. All patients receiving opioids should be on some type of bowel regimen. The aggressiveness of the regimen is dictated by the severity of the constipation, but patients should receive both a cathartic and a stool softener.

Nausea and vomiting are common adverse effects of opioid therapy, with an estimated incidence of between 10% and 40%. A treatment approach should be initiated based on the suspected cause. Opioid-induced nausea and vomiting can be mediated by the chemoreceptor trigger zone, vestibular sensitivity, and increased gastric tone.[86] Patients with nausea and vomiting secondary to enhanced vestibular sensitivity can be treated with scopolamine or meclizine. When nausea and vomiting are associated with increased gastric tone or delayed gastric emptying, prokinetic medications such as metoclopramide are indicated. Centrally induced nausea and vomiting can be treated with ondansetron, droperidol, haloperidol, benzodiazepines, metoclopramide, or chlorpromazine. Tolerance to opioid-induced nausea and vomiting generally develops very quickly.

Sedation generally occurs when opioid therapy is initiated, but patients become tolerant to this adverse effect rapidly. When sedation cannot be controlled by decreasing the dose of opioid and eliminating other centrally depressing drugs, psychostimulants such as methylphenidate, dextroamphetamine, or pemoline may be added. If sedation persists, administration of opioid-sparing drugs (NSAIDs or adjuvant) or rotation to a different opioid should be considered.

Respiratory depression is rare in cancer patients undergoing opioid therapy. If clinically significant respiratory depression is related to the opioid, other signs of CNS depression will be present (sedation and mental clouding). When respiratory depression is accompanied by tachypnea and anxiety, other causes must be sought (pneumonia or pulmonary embolism).[86]

Adjuvant Analgesics

The WHO recommends the use of adjuvant drugs with non-opioid and opioid medications at all levels of the analgesic ladder. Adjuvant analgesics are those drugs that have a primary indication other than the treatment of pain but have analgesic properties in certain painful conditions. Their use is indicated for specific painful conditions or when the adverse effects of opioid therapy become intolerable or unmanageable. The addition of an adjuvant may have an opioid-sparing effect and may allow the CRNA to decrease the total dose of opioid. Based on the indication for their use, adjuvant analgesics can be categorized broadly as follows: multipurpose adjuvants, adjuvants used to treat neuropathic pain, adjuvants used to treat bone pain, adjuvants used to treat sympathetically mediated pain, and adjuvants used to treat pain secondary to bowel obstruction. The interpatient response varies greatly with adjuvant medications, so numerous trials of several drugs may be necessary before any analgesia is appreciated. A list of the drugs, indications, and dosage regimens can be found in Table 48-4.[86]

Corticosteroids are the most common multipurpose adjuvants used to treat cancer pain. In addition to their ability to provide analgesia, corticosteroids have a beneficial effect on appetite, nausea, and mood. This class of drugs is most beneficial for pain secondary to metastatic bone disease, increased intracranial pressure, acute spinal cord compression, superior vena cava syndrome, neuropathic pain resulting from infiltration or compression by tumor, symptomatic lymphedema, and hepatic capsular distention.[86]

Much success has been enjoyed in the treatment of neuropathic pain. Although numerous drugs can provide analgesia for this type of pain, anticonvulsants and antidepressants are the mainstays of the therapy. In order to select the drug most likely to yield positive results, it is imperative for the CRNA to determine whether the neuropathic pain is continuous, lancinating, or sympathetically mediated.

The effective treatment of bone pain often requires a combination of opioid therapy and adjunctive therapies. The addition of NSAIDs or corticosteroids to opioid therapy can have tremendous benefits for patients suffering from bone pain. Bone pain that is localized to one area may respond to primary radiation therapy. However, if bone pain is multifocal and poorly controlled with opioids, bisphosphonates, calcitonin, or the radiopharmaceutical strontium 89 may be indicated.

Treatment of pain associated with bowel obstruction is aimed at decreasing intraluminal secretions and peristalsis.[82] For this purpose the anticholinergic drugs atropine and scopolamine are beneficial. In addition, the somatostatin analog octreotide has been used.

Anesthetic Implications

Providing an anesthetic to a patient receiving chronic opioid therapy for cancer-related pain presents numerous challenges for the nurse anesthetist. First, one may assume that patients on chronic opioid therapy are physiologically dependent on the medication. As a result patients scheduled for surgery should continue their opioids up to and including the morning of surgery with a sip of water. Failure to do so could result in the manifestation of an abstinence syndrome. In addition, these patients normally develop some degree of tolerance to opioids. This understanding may lead to the increased amount of opioids needed for opioid-based anesthetic procedures.

Extreme care should be taken when patients with bone metastases are positioned for surgery. Every effort to position the patient or manipulate the airway must be performed gently and with the least amount of trespass possible.

Succinylcholine should be used with extreme caution in patients with bone metastases and after prolonged immobility. In patients with advanced disease, succinylcholine-induced fasciculations in patients not precurarized can potentially cause pathologic fractures. Hyperkalemia after the use of succinylcholine after prolonged immobility is well documented and needs no further comment.

Comprehensive pain management for cancer patients can be both challenging and rewarding. With a select number of specialized cancer treatment hospitals available, CRNAs are in the ideal position to become actively involved with the management of pain in patients with cancer. Cancer pain management is much more than merely the management of symptoms. All management must begin with a thorough assessment of the patient. This involves assessment of the pain itself, a complete physical and neurologic examination, and evaluation of the diagnostic findings. Equally important is the psychosocial impact of the pain on the patient and his or her family.

In order to effectively achieve this goal, CRNAs must have an in-depth knowledge of the pharmacodynamics and pharmacokinetics of at least three different opioids, as well as adjuvant medications. In addition, the nurse anesthetist must know various routes of administration, equianalgesic dosages, and management of adverse effects of opioids.

CONCLUSION

As advanced practice nurses, CRNAs not only should learn how to effectively manage pain but should share this information with their anesthesia colleagues and primary care nurses. CRNAs are in a unique position to participate in the treatment of pain across the life span and across disease states. When patients receive effective analgesia, they are both inclined to participate in treatment protocols and empowered to participate in decisions that influence the plan of care.

REFERENCES

1. Acute Pain Management Panel. *Acute Pain Management: Operative or Medical Procedures and Trauma. Clinical Practice Guidelines.* Rockville, Md: Agency for Health Care Policy and Research, Public Health Service, US Department of Health and Human Services; 1992. Publication 92-0032.
2. Acute Pain Management Panel. *Acute Pain Management in Oncology.* Rockville, Md: Agency for Health Care Policy and Research, Public Health Service, US Department of Health and Human Services; 1994. Publication 94-0592.
3. Acute Pain Management Panel. *Acute Pain Management in Infants, Children and Adolescents: Operative and Medical Procedures.* Rockville, Md: Agency for Health Care Policy and Research, Public Health Service, US Department of Health and Human Services; 1992. Publication 92-0020.
4. Marks R, Sachar E. Under treatment of medical patients with narcotic analgesics. *Ann Intern Med.* 1973;78:173-181.
5. Cohen F. Postsurgical pain relief: patients' status and nurses' medication choices. *Pain.* 1980;9:265-274.
6. Mather L, Mackie J. The incidence of postoperative pain in children. *Pain.* 1981;15:271-282.
7. Sriwantanakul I, Weiss O, Alloza J. Analysis of narcotic usage in the treatment of postoperative pain. *JAMA.* 1983;250:926-929.
8. Donovan M, Dillon P, McGuire L. Incidence and characteristics of pain in a sample of medical surgical in-patients. *Pain.* 1987;30:69-78.
9. Faut M, Paice J, Mahon S. Factors associated with the adequacy of pain control in hospitalized surgical patients. In: *Proceedings of the Thirteenth Annual Midwest Nursing Research Society.* Oakbrook, Ill: Midwest Nursing Research Society; 1989:214.
10. Ballentyne J. Standards of treatment: American Pain Society quality assurance standards for relief of acute pain and cancer. In: *Massachusetts General Hospital Handbook of Pain Management.* Philadelphia: Lippincott Williams & Wilkins; 2001:539-541.

11. Ward S, Gordon D. Patient satisfaction and pain severity as outcomes in pain management: a longitudinal view of one setting's experience. *J Pain Symptom Manage.* 1996;11:242-251.
12. Loeser J, Egan D. *Managing the Chronic Pain Patient: Theory and Practice at the University of Washington Multidisciplinary Pain Center.* New York: Raven; 1989.
13. Donovan M, Slack J, Faut M. Factors associated with inadequate management of pain. In: *Proceedings of the Eighth Annual Scientific Meeting of the American Pain Society.* Glenville, Ill: American Pain Society; 1989.
14. *Joint Commission Focuses on Pain Management.* Oak Brook, Ill: JCAHO; August 3, 1999.
15. Joint Commission on Accreditation of Healthcare Organizations. *Pain: Current Understanding of Assessment, Management and Treatment* Oak Brook, Ill: JCAHO; 2001.
16. Joint Commission on Accreditation of Healthcare Organizations. *Improving the Quality of Pain Management through Measurement and Action.* Oak Brook, Ill: JCAHO; 2003.
17. Joint Commission on Accreditation of Healthcare Organizations. *Approaches to Pain Management: an Essential Guide for Clinical Leaders.* Oak Brook, Ill: JCAHO; 2003.
18. American Pain Society Quality of Care Committee. *Quality improvement guidelines for the treatment of acute pain and cancer pain.* JAMA. 1995;274:1874-1880.
19. American Pain Society. *Principles of Analgesic Use in the Treatment of Acute and Cancer Pain.* 5th ed. Glenview, Ill: APS; 2003.
20. Bonica J. Importance of effective pain control. *Acta Anaesthesiol Scand.* 1989;85:1-16.
21. Fields HL. *Pain: Mechanisms and Management.* New York: McGraw-Hill; 1987.
22. Greipp ME. Under medication for pain: an ethical model. *ANS Adv Nurs Sci.* 1992;15:44-53.
23. Heavener J. Pain mechanisms and pathways. In: Raj P, ed. *Pain Medicine: a Comprehensive Review.* 2nd ed. St Louis: Mosby; 2003.
24. McCaffery M, Pasero C. *Pain: Clinical Manual.* St Louis: Mosby; 1999.
25. Terman G, Bonica J. Spinal mechanisms and their modulation. In: *Bonica's Management of Pain.* 3rd ed. Hagerstown, Md: Lippincott, Williams & Wilkins; 2003.
26. Cousins M. Acute postoperative pain. In: Wall PD, Melzack R, eds. *Textbook of Pain.* 3rd ed. New York: Churchill Livingstone; 1994:357-385.
27. Ready LB. Acute perioperative pain. In: Miller RD, ed. *Anesthesia.* 5th ed. Philadelphia: Churchill Livingstone; 2000:2323-2350.
28. Kremer MJ. Surgery, pain, and immune function. *CRNA.* 1999;10:94-100.
29. Chapman CR, Turner J. Psychological aspects of pain. In: *Bonica's Management of Pain.* 3rd ed. Hagerstown, Md: Lippincott Williams & Wilkins; 2003:180-190.
30. Kehlet H, Dahl J. The value of "multimodal" or balanced analgesia in postoperative pain treatment. *Anesth Analg.* 1993;77:1048.
31. Gottschalk A, Smith DS, Jobes DR, et al. Preemptive epidural analgesia and recovery from radical prostatectomy: a randomized controlled trial. *JAMA.* 1998;279:1076-1082.
32. Gottschalk A, Wu CL, Ochroch EA. Current treatment options for acute pain. *Exp Opin Pharmacother.* 2002;3:1599-1611.
33. Reuben SS, Connelly NR. Postoperative analgesic effects of celecoxib or rofecoxib after spinal fusion surgery. *Anesth Analg.* 2000;91:1221-1225.
34. Helmy SA, Bali A. The effect of preemptive use of the NMDA receptor antagonist dextromethorphan on postoperative analgesic requirements. *Anesth Analg.* 2001;92:739-744.
35. Reuben SS, Bhopatker S, Maciolek H, Joshi W, Skar J. The preemptive analgesic effect of rofecoxib after ambulatory arthroscopic knee surgery. *Anesth Analg.* 2002;94:55-59.
36. Buvanendran A, Kroin JS, Tuman KJ, et al. Effects of perioperative administration of a selective cyclooxygenase 2 inhibitor on pain management and recovery of function after knee replacement: a randomized controlled trial. JAMA. 2003;290:2411-2418.
37. Ruoff G, Lema M. Strategies in pain management: new and potential indications for COX-2 specific inhibitors. *J Pain Symptom Manage.* 2003;25(suppl 2):S21-S31.
38. Yaksh T. Central sites and mechanisms of actions of NSAID drugs. In: *American Pain Society Twelfth Annual Scientific Meeting.* Palm Desert, Calif: Convention Cassettes; 1993.
39. Rowlingson JC, Rawal N. Postoperative pain guidelines: targeted to the site of surgery. *Reg Anesth Pain Med.* 2003;28:265-267.
40. Yaksh TL, Abram SE. Preemptive analgesia: a popular misnomer, but a clinically relevant truth? *APS J.* 1993;2:116-121.
41. Dahl JB, Kehlet H. Non-steroidal anti-inflammatory drugs: rationale for use in severe postoperative pain. *Br J Anaesth.* 1991;66: 703-712.
42. Dupuis R, et al. Preoperative flurbiprofen in oral surgery: a method of choice in controlling postoperative pain. *Pharmacotherapy.* 1988;8:193-200.
43. Denson DD, Katz JA. Nonsteroidal anti-inflammatory agents. In: Sinatra RS, et al, eds. *Acute Pain Mechanisms and Management.* St Louis: Mosby; 1992:112-123.
44. Miller RR, Jick J. Clinical effects of meperidine in hospitalized medical patients. *J Clin Pharmacol.* 1978;18:180-189.
45. Kaiko RF, Foley KM, Grabinski PY. Central nervous system excitatory effects of meperidine in cancer patients. *Ann Neurol.* 1983;13:180-185.
46. Marlowe KF, Chicella MF. Treatment of sickle cell pain. *Pharmacotherapy.* 2002;22:484-491.
47. Morgan JP. American opiophobia: customary underutilization of opioid analgesics. *Adv Alcohol Subst Abuse.* 1985/1986;5: 163-173.
48. Perry S, Heidrich G. Management of pain during débridement: a survey of US burn units. *Pain.* 1982;13:267-280.
49. Porter J, Jick H. Addiction rare in patients treated with narcotics. *N Engl J Med.* 1980;302:123.
50. McGuire DB, Yarbro CH, Ferrell BR. *Cancer Pain Management.* 2nd ed. Boston: Jones & Bartlett; 1995.
51. Portenoy R, McCaffery M. Adjuvant analgesics. In: McCaffery M, Pasero C, eds. *Pain: Clinical Manual.* 2nd ed. St Louis: Mosby; 1999:300-361.
52. Wall PD, Mexzack R. *Textbook of Pain.* 4 ed. New York: Churchill Livingstone.
53. Horswell JL, Mack MJ, Bachand DA, Michelsen L, Worley T. Use of dexmedetomidine as an adjunct to pain control following OPCAB: a randomized, double-blind study. *ASA Meeting Abstracts.* Philadelphia: Lippincott Williams & Wilkins; 2002.
54. Walker G, Donahue B, Costabile S. Dexmedetomidine in bariatric surgery patients. *ASA Meeting Abstracts.* Philadelphia: Lippincott Williams & Wilkins; 2002.
55. Fields HL, Baron R, Rowbotham MC. Peripheral Neuropathic pain: an approach to management. In: Melzcak R, Wall, PD, eds. *Handbook of Pain Management.* New York: Churchill Livingstone; 2003:598-620.
56. Austin KL, Stapleton JV, Mather LE. Multiple injections: a major source of variability in analgesic response to meperidine. *Pain.* 1980;8:47-62.
57. Viscusi ER, Reynolds L, Tait S, Melson T, Irani H. Evaluation of a non-invasive patient-controlled analgesia delivery system for the treatment of acute postoperative pain: a double-blind, multicenter, placebo-controlled trial incorporating JCAHO pain management standards. *ASA Meeting Abstracts.* Philadelphia: Lippincott Williams & Wilkins; 2003.
58. Cleland JG. Continuous peridural analgesia in surgery and early ambulation. *Northwest Med.* 1949;48:26.
59. El-Baz NM, Faber LP, Jensik RJ. Continuous epidural infusion of morphine for treatment of pain after thoracic surgery: a new technique. *Anesth Analg.* 1984;63:757-764.
60. Hjorts NC, et al. Epidural morphine improves pain relief and maintains sensory analgesia during continuous epidural bupivacaine after abdominal surgery. *Anesth Analg.* 1986;65: 1033-1036.

61. Scott NB, et al. Continuous thoracic extradural 0.05% bupivacaine with or without morphine: effect on quality of blockade, lung function and the surgical stress response. *Br J Anaesth.* 1989;62:253-257.
62. Lubenow T. Epidural analgesia: considerations and delivery methods. In: Sinatra RS, et al, eds. *Acute Pain Mechanisms and Management.* St Louis: Mosby; 1992:233-242.
63. Lubenow TR, Ivankovich AD, McCarthy RJ. Management of acute postoperative pain. In: Barash PG, Cullen BF, Stoelting RK, eds. *Clinical Anesthesia.* 4th ed. Philadelphia: Lippincott Williams & Wilkins; 2001:1305-1338.
64. Schecter NL. The under treatment of pain in children: an overview. *Pediatr Clin North Am.* 1989;36:781-794.
65. McIlvane MB. Overview of pediatric analgesia. In: Sinatra RS, et al, eds. *Acute Pain Mechanisms and Management.* St Louis: Mosby; 1992:445-452.
66. Schecter NL, Berde CB, Yaster M. *Pain in Infants, Children, and Adolescents.* Philadelphia: Lippincott Williams & Wilkins; 2003.
67. Kremer M, Faut-Callahan M. Regional anesthesia and pain management. In: Zaglaniczny K, Aker J, eds. *Clinical Guide to Pediatric Anesthesia.* Philadelphia: Saunders; 1999:359-382.
68. American Cancer Society. *Cancer Facts and Figures—1994.* Atlanta: American Cancer Society; 1994:1.
69. Stjernsward J, Teoh N. The scope of the cancer pain problem. In: Foley KM, Bonica JJ, Ventafridda V, eds. *Proceedings of the Second International Congress on Cancer Pain. Advances in Pain Research and Therapy.* Vol 16. New York: Raven; 1990:7-12.
70. Bruera ED, Portenoy RK. *Cancer Pain Management.* Cambridge, UK: Cambridge University Press; 2003.
71. Dahl J. Barriers to the management of cancer pain. In: *Innovations in Cancer Pain Management.* Titusville, NJ: Janssen Pharmaceutica; 1994.
72. Management of Cancer Pain Guideline Panel. *Management of Cancer Pain: Clinical Practice Guideline.* Rockville, Md: Agency for Health Care Policy and Research, Public Health Service, US Department of Health and Human Services; 1994. Publication 94-0592.
73. Von Roenn JH, et al. Physicians' attitudes and practice in cancer pain management: a survey from the Eastern Cooperative Oncology Group. *Ann Intern Med.* 1993;119:121-126.
74. Fishman B, et al. The Memorial Pain Assessment Card: a valid instrument for the evaluation of cancer pain. *Cancer.* 1987;60: 1151-1158.
75. Turk D, Okifugi A. Pain terms and taxonomy of pain. In: Bonica JJ, ed. *The Management of Pain.* 3rd ed. Philadelphia: Lippincott Williams & Wilkins; 2001:1725.
76. Coyle N, Adelhardt J, Foley KM. Disease progression and tolerance in the cancer pain patient. Second International Congress on Cancer Pain. *J Pain Symptom Manage.* 1988;3:S25.
77. Kanner RM, Foley KM. Patterns of narcotic drug use in a cancer pain clinic. *Ann N Y Acad Sci.* 1981;362:161-172.
78. Cassell EJ. The relationship between pain and suffering. In: Hill CS Jr, Fields WS, eds. *Drug Treatment of Cancer Pain in a Drug-Oriented Society. Advances in Pain Research and Therapy.* Vol 11. New York: Raven; 1989:61-70.
79. World Health Organization. *Cancer Pain Relief and Palliative Care. Report of a WHO Expert Committee. World Health Organization Technical Report Series 804.* Geneva: World Health Organization; 1990:1-75.
80. Viehlhaber A, Portenoy RK. Advances in cancer pain management. *Hematol Oncol Clin North Am.* 2002;16:527-541.
81. Caraceni A. Clinicopathologic correlates of common cancer pain syndromes. *Hematol Oncol Clin North Am.* 1996;10:57-78.
82. Portenoy RK. Management of cancer pain: opioid and adjuvant pharmacotherapy. In: Portenoy RK, ed. *Real Patients, Real Problems: Optimal Assessment and Management of Cancer Pain.* Glenview, Ill: American Pain Society; 1997 .
83. Gutstein HB, Akil H. Opioid analgesics. In: Gilman AG, Harman JG, Limbird LE, eds. *Gilman & Goodman's the Pharmacological Basis of Therapeutics.* 10th ed. New York: Pergamon; 2001:569-620.
84. Hanning CD. The rectal absorption of opioids. In: Benedette C, Chapman CR, Goron G, eds. *Opioid Analgesia. Advances in Pain Research and Therapy.* Vol 14. New York: Raven; 1990:259-269.
85. Weinberg DS, et al. Sublingual absorption of selected opioid analgesics. *Clin Pharmacol Ther.* 1988;44:335-342.
86. Cherny NI, Foley KM. Nonopioid and opioid analgesic pharmacotherapy of cancer pain. *Hematol Oncol Clin North Am.* 1996;10: 79-102.

CHAPTER 49

Anesthesia for Therapeutic and Diagnostic Procedures

Allan J. Schwartz

OVERVIEW

A common anesthesia dictum states, "There are cases of minor surgery, but there are no cases of minor anesthesia." Although most anesthetics were traditionally administered in the operating room, it is no longer unusual to provide services outside the operating suite in a variety of settings far from the traditional operating room, for different types of procedures. Box 49-1 provides a current and comprehensive list of procedures that could require anesthesia outside the operating room. Patients treated in these new settings deserve the same safe anesthetic administration and vigilant attention as those patients treated in the operating suite. Although certain therapeutic and diagnostic procedures are sometimes performed without anesthesia, the patient's condition or the requirements of the test or procedure may necessitate administration of an anesthetic. The anesthesia could range from local anesthetic infiltration to monitored anesthesia care or general anesthesia. Patients can range in age from pediatric, adolescent, or adult to geriatric. Patients treated in remote locations and who require anesthesia could be confused or disoriented, uncooperative, unwilling or unable to understand the requirements of the procedure, claustrophobic, anxious, or mentally disabled. The test or procedure might require the patient to lie still for an extended length of time or cause moments of painful stimulation to the patient, alternated with long periods of no stimulation.

Given the rapid advances in medical knowledge and technology, coupled with a strong societal impetus to reduce health-care costs, more therapeutic and diagnostic procedures will be performed in remote locations.[1]

Considerations for Remote Locations

The operating room provides an ideal environment for the administration of anesthesia and the performance of surgical procedures; the anesthesia setting in a remote location must possess the same level of safety and high standards. Modern anesthesia requires many pieces of equipment, utilities, supplies, and medications. Many considerations and plans must be made before a patient can safely receive anesthesia for a diagnostic or therapeutic procedure in a remote location. Box 49-2 provides a comprehensive checklist of the requisites for administration of anesthesia in remote locations that will facilitate planning and the gathering of needed equipment, supplies, and medications.

As part of the planning process before patient treatment, it is important that one familiarize oneself with the staff and the work area in the remote environment. The workplace allotted for anesthesia may be small, crowded, and different from the usual operating room setting. Some have advocated the use of total intravenous anesthesia (TIVA) in small workplaces in which the use of excessive equipment and supplies and an anesthesia machine with a ventilator, along with the handling of fresh and waste anesthetic gases, would be too costly or prohibitive.[2,3] No remote location should ever limit the ability to manage these anesthetic procedures or prevent equipment, medications, supplies, positive pressure ventilation, and suction from being readily available.

The American Association of Nurse Anesthetists (AANA)[4] and the American Society of Anesthesiologists (ASA)[5,6] have established written standards to provide for the basic rights and safety of patients, along with the safety of anesthesia providers and ancillary personnel. As technology advances, these standards are adapted.

Standards for the Delivery of Anesthesia in a Remote Location

A. Perform a complete preanesthesia assessment. The patient, parent, or legal guardian must be interviewed before the performance of an anesthetic procedure. During this assessment, information is obtained regarding the patient's medical history (prior allergy must be assessed), anesthesia history (noting any prior complications), surgical history, and medication history (including tobacco, alcohol, and any substance abuse). A complete physical assessment of the patient is made, along with inspection of the head, neck, mouth, and airway. Lung and heart sounds are auscultated. Review is made of objective diagnostic data such as patient laboratory values, radiographs, and electrocardiogram (ECG). Important findings are noted in the patient's anesthesia record. A physical status classification is then assigned the patient.

B. Obtain informed consent for the planned anesthetic intervention from the patient or legal guardian. The anesthesia provider should discuss the course of the anesthetic care and enumerate pertinent possible reactions or complications the patient might expect while receiving a typical anesthetic. It is far easier to discuss these points with the patient before the anesthetic procedure than to explain these points after the fact.

C. Formulate a patient-specific plan for anesthesia care. The art and science of anesthesia mandate that the safest and least invasive anesthetic technique be administered to the

BOX 49-1

Comprehensive List of Procedures That May Require Anesthesia Outside the Operating Room

Cardiologic Procedures
Angiography
Automatic implantable cardiac defibrillator insertion
Cardiac catheterization
Cardioversion
Pacemaker insertion
Radiofrequency catheter ablation

Emergency Room Procedures
Diagnostic peritoneal lavage
Central venous line insertion
Emergency endotracheal intubation
Insertion of intracranial pressure monitor
Orthopedic manipulations
Pericardiocentesis
Thoracocentesis
Tube thoracotomy
Vascular "cut down"

Gastroenterologic Procedures
Colonoscopy
Endoscopic retrograde cholangiopancreatography
Esophagogastroduodenoscopy
Liver biopsy
Percutaneous endoscopically placed gastrostomy
Upper endoscopy

Gynecologic Procedures
Assisted reproductive technologies
- In vitro fertilization
- Gamete intrafallopian transfer
- Peritoneal oocyte and sperm transfer
- Tubal embryo transfer
- Zygote intrafallopian transfer

Hematologic and Oncologic Procedures
Bone marrow aspiration and biopsy
Lumbar puncture
Removal of indwelling central venous catheters

Intensive Care Procedures
Bronchoscopy
Cardioversion
Central venous line insertion
Diagnostic peritoneal lavage
Endotracheal intubation
Percutaneous endoscopic gastrostomy
Percutaneous tracheostomy
Thoracocentesis
Thoracotomy and tube thoracotomy
Vascular "cut down"
Ventriculostomy

Office-Based Procedures
Neurophysiology Laboratory
Brain stem auditory evoked responses
Office-Based Surgeries
Dental surgery
- Pediatric dentistry
- Oral and maxillofacial surgery
- Periodontics
- Endodontics
- General dentistry
- Prosthodontics

Plastic Surgery
- Rhizotomy
- Removal of superficial skin lesions
- Liposuction

Ophthalmology suites
- Examination under anesthesia
- Retinoscopy and tonometry
- Electroretinography
- Selective eye surgeries

Orthopedic Procedures
Cast changes
Hardware removal
Joint aspiration

Psychiatric Procedures
Electroconvulsive therapy

Radiologic and Diagnostic Procedures
Brachytherapy
Computed tomography
Functional brain imaging
Interventional neuroradiology
Interventional radiology (vascular and nonvascular)
Intraoperative radiotherapy
Magnetic resonance imaging
Radiosurgery
Radiotherapy procedures
Teletherapy
Ultrasound-guided diagnostic and therapeutic procedures

Urologic Procedures
Cystoscopy procedures
Extracorporeal shock-wave lithotripsy

Other Procedures
Anesthesia in military bases and war fields
Veterinary anesthesia

Modified from Kotob F, Twersky RS. Anesthesia outside the operating room: general overview and monitoring standards. Int Anesthesiol Clin. *41: 1-15;2003.*

BOX **49-2**

Requisites for Administration of Anesthesia in Remote Locations

Utilities

Adequate work space
Adequate overhead lighting
Adequate numbers and current-carrying capacity of electrical outlets
Two-way communication devices—telephone, intercom
Backup power
(All building and safety codes and facility standards must be met.)

Equipment

Local Infiltration, Intravenous Sedation, Regional and General Anesthesia

Patient monitors
- Pulse oximeter
- Electrocardiograph
- Blood pressure monitor with a selection of adequate-sized cuffs
- Capnograph
- Body temperature monitor

Oxygen supplies
- Minimum of two oxygen sources must be available with regulators attached (compressed oxygen should be the equivalent of an E cylinder)

Positive pressure ventilation sources, including an Ambu bag and a mouth-to-mask unit
Defibrillator (charged)
Suction source or a suction machine, tubing, suction catheters, and Yankauer suctions
Anesthesia cart to permit organization of supplies, including endotracheal equipment, laryngeal mask airways, Combitubes, face masks, nasal cannulas, Connell airways, disposable face masks with oxygen tubing, oral and nasal airways, syringes (3 ml, 5 ml, 10 ml, 20 ml, 60 ml), needles, intravenous catheters, tourniquet, intravenous fluids and tubing, alcohol pads, adhesive tape, disposable gloves, face mask, stethoscopes, and appropriate anesthetic medications
Battery-powered flashlight
Syringe pump
Warm blankets or forced air warming devices and the appropriate blanket
Emergency medications to include, at a minimum, atropine, epinephrine, ephedrine, lidocaine, diphenhydramine, cortisone, and a bronchial dilator inhaler such as albuterol
Preoperative anesthesia evaluation forms
Anesthesia charts, black ink pens, indelible ink pens

Additional Requirements for General Anesthesia

Oxygen fail-safe system
Oxygen analyzer
Waste gas exhaust scavenging system
End-tidal carbon dioxide analyzer
Vaporizers—calibration and exclusion system
Alarm system
Anesthetic medications
In addition to the emergency medications listed above, consider the following:
- Induction drugs—propofol, etomidate, methohexital, thiopental
- Maintenance drugs—bottles of sevoflurane, isoflurane, desflurane, propofol
- Narcotics—midazolam, diazepam, fentanyl, alfentanil, sufentanil, remifentanil
- Muscle relaxants—succinylcholine, mivacurium, rocuronium, *cis*-atracurium, vecuronium
- Muscle relaxant reversal agents—edrophonium, neostigmine, atropine, glycopyrrolate
- Cardiovascular drugs—labetalol, esmolol, verapamil, hydralazine
- Narcotic reversal drugs—naloxone, flumazenil
- Antiemetic drugs—ondansetron, dolasetron, granisetron, droperidol

Emergency cart and equipment
- Basic airway equipment (adult and pediatric)
  - Nasal and oral airway
  - Face mask (appropriate for patient)
  - Laryngoscopes
  - Assortment of laryngoscope blades, endotracheal tubes (adult and pediatric), laryngeal mask airways
  - Combitube
  - Ambu bag
- Difficult airway equipment
  - Laryngeal mask airway
  - Light wand
  - Cricothyrotomy kit
- Defibrillator
- Supplemental oxygen and nitrous oxide tanks
- Emergency medications
- Succinylcholine
- Compression board
- Suction equipment (suction catheter, Yankauer type)
- Malignant hyperthermia drugs, equipment, and the phone number for the Malignant Hyperthermia Association of the United States (MHAUS) (United States and Canada, 1-800-MH HYPER or 1-800-644-9737; outside the United States and Canada, 0011 315 464-7079) for treatment of malignant hyperthermia on site

A policy must be developed that outlines the organization of emergency services for either in-hospital or office-based facilities. Office-based facilities should have a plan for emergency transportation to the nearest hospital emergency department.
Note: *An anesthesia machine and portable anesthesia cart with the listed equipment, supplies, and medications should be dedicated strictly for use in remote locations. This can save preparation time whenever a procedure is required in a remote location. It also decreases the risk of a mishap resulting from lack of necessary equipment and materials.*

patient to simplify delivery of the anesthetic and to avoid complications for the patient while in the remote location.

D. Implement and adjust the anesthesia care plan based on the patient's physiologic response. Immediately before implementation of anesthesia, reassess the patient and document a reassessment note in the anesthesia record. Also, make sure all anesthesia equipment, supplies, and medications are checked and immediately available in case the patient needs a change in the anesthetic plan.

E. Monitor the patient's physiologic condition as appropriate for the type of anesthesia and specific patient needs

1. *Monitor ventilation continuously*. Verify intubation of the trachea by auscultation, chest excursion, and confirmation of carbon dioxide in the expired gas. Continuously monitor end-tidal carbon dioxide ($ETCO_2$) during controlled, assisted, or spontaneous ventilation, including any anesthesia or sedation technique requiring artificial airway support. Use spirometry and ventilatory pressure monitors as indicated.
2. *Monitor oxygenation continuously* by clinical observation, pulse oximetry, and, if indicated, arterial blood gas analysis.
3. *Monitor cardiovascular status continuously* via electrocardiography and heart sounds. Record blood pressure and heart rate at least every 5 minutes.
4. *Monitor body temperature* continuously in all patients.
5. *Monitor neuromuscular function and status* when neuromuscular blocking agents are administered.
6. *Monitor and assess patient positioning and protective measures* at frequent intervals. Performance of a complete anesthesia equipment safety check must be made daily and documented on the patient medical record. An abbreviated check of all equipment is acceptable before each subsequent anesthetic is administered.

F. Precautions shall be taken to minimize the risk of infection to the patient, the operator, and ancillary personnel. Clean equipment and fresh medications and supplies should be used to ensure patient safety.

G. There shall be complete, accurate, and timely documentation of pertinent information on the patient's anesthesia record. Documentation must be made of all vital signs: heart rate, blood pressure, pulse oximeter readings, patient temperature, and the presence of $ETCO_2$. Also, documentation must be made of all fluids administered as well as the names and quantities of all drugs and agents administered. A narrative must be written concerning the technique(s) of anesthesia used and any unusual events that occurred during the anesthetic period.

H. After the anesthetic treatment for therapeutic or diagnostic procedures, transfer the responsibility for care of the patient to other qualified providers in a manner that assures continuity of care and patient safety. Anesthesia care does not end with the completion of the therapeutic or diagnostic procedure. The patient must be safely transported to a separate area for postanesthesia care. From there patient care can be transferred to another qualified health-care provider. Recovery from anesthesia can be divided into three phases. Phase I recovery encompasses the recovery from sedation, during which assessment is made of adequate patient oxygenation and respirations, cardiovascular function, neuromuscular function, mental status, body temperature, pain, nausea and vomiting, fluid status, urine output, the ability to void, and any bleeding or drainage, which must be noted and continuously observed for. Treatments may be administered as necessary for any adverse signs or symptoms elicited by the patient. Phase II recovery encompasses the adequate resumption of psychomotor functions such as the ability to communicate, ambulate, and consume fluids. Finally, before discharge from this area, a responsible individual must be present to escort the patient home. In phase III recovery the patient regains full preanesthetic psychologic and physical recovery. It is important to remember that phase III may occur several hours or days later, depending on the anesthetic technique and patient variables.

Post anesthesia recovery guidelines are discussed in Chapter 47.

I. Adhere to appropriate safety precautions as established with the institution, to minimize the risks of fire, explosion, electrical shock, and equipment malfunction. This standard is important for the patient, the anesthesia provider, and ancillary personnel. It is also important from a medicolegal standpoint.

Conclusion. The standards listed in this section describe the minimum requirements for treatment and monitoring of any patient who requires anesthesia care. The standards must be followed wherever and whenever anesthesia is given. Standards are considered essential in a malpractice case, and an anesthetic incident will be judged according to those standards.[7] The omission of any monitoring standard should be documented, and the reason stated on the patient's anesthesia record. Any anesthetic procedure, including those performed in a remote location, should not begin until the anesthetist feels sufficiently comfortable, safe, and well prepared to deliver the anesthetic treatment required for the patient.

Guidelines for Sedation

Many diagnostic and therapeutic procedures can be performed with various types of sedation. Sedation is possible with enteral, intravenous, and inhaled medications. It is important to remember that the depth of sedation in a patient is a continuum of progressive changes in cognition, respirations, and protective reflexes.[8] Sedation does not have strict boundaries.

The Joint Commission on Accreditation of Healthcare Organizations (JCAHO) is the organization whose mission is to continuously improve the safety and quality of care provided to the public. The JCAHO accredits health-care organizations and related service organizations and is recognized as one of the major authorities in the United States that supports performance improvement in health-care organizations. Many facilities that provide diagnostic and therapeutic procedures are accredited by the JCAHO (e.g., outpatient surgical facilities, group practices, and office-based surgical facilities such as plastic surgery centers). JCAHO recognition is a credible and important acknowledgment for the patient and for the accredited organization in the community.

The JCAHO publishes definitions for levels of sedation and anesthesia in their *Comprehensive Accreditation Manual for Hospitals: The Official Handbook*.[9] Box 49-3 lists the JCAHO definitions of the four levels of sedation and anesthesia. Figure 49-1 illustrates the continuum of sedation described by the JCAHO. From these definitions, standards are provided to practitioners for the administration of safe and high-quality care to patients. The JCAHO standards do not cover minimal sedation (anxiolysis), but patients undergoing moderate sedation and analgesia and deep sedation and analgesia.[9]

Standards for moderate sedation and analgesia and deep sedation and analgesia states the following:

1. The process from sedation to (general) anesthesia is a continuum, and individuals vary in their responses to medications.
2. Qualified individuals with appropriate credentials (nurses, certified registered nurse anesthetists [CRNAs], anesthesiologists) who are trained in professional standards and techniques do the following:

BOX **49-3**

The Four Levels of Sedation and Anesthesia

Minimal Sedation (Anxiolysis)

A drug-induced state during which patients respond normally to verbal commands. Although cognitive function and coordination may be impaired, ventilatory and cardiovascular functions are unaffected.

Moderate Sedation and Analgesia ("Conscious Sedation")

A drug-induced depression of consciousness during which patients respond purposefully to verbal commands, either alone or accompanied by light tactile stimulation. No interventions are required to maintain a patent airway, and spontaneous ventilation is adequate. Cardiovascular function is usually maintained. (*Note*: Reflexive withdrawal from a painful stimulus is not considered a purposeful response.)

Deep Sedation and Analgesia

A drug-induced depression of consciousness during which patients cannot be easily aroused but respond purposefully after repeated or painful stimulation. The ability to independently maintain ventilatory function may be impaired. Patients may require assistance in maintaining a patent airway, and spontaneous ventilation may be inadequate. Cardiovascular function is usually maintained.

Anesthesia

Consists of general anesthesia and spinal or major regional anesthesia. It does *not* include local anesthesia. General anesthesia is a drug-induced loss of consciousness during which patients are not arousable, even by painful stimulation. The ability to independently maintain ventilatory function is often impaired. Patients often require assistance in maintaining a patent airway, and positive pressure ventilation may be required because of depressed spontaneous ventilation or drug-induced depression of neuromuscular function. Cardiovascular function may be impaired.

Modified from Kaplan RF, Yang CI. Sedation and analgesia in pediatric patients for procedures outside the operating room. Anesthesiol Clin North Am. *2002;20:181-194*.

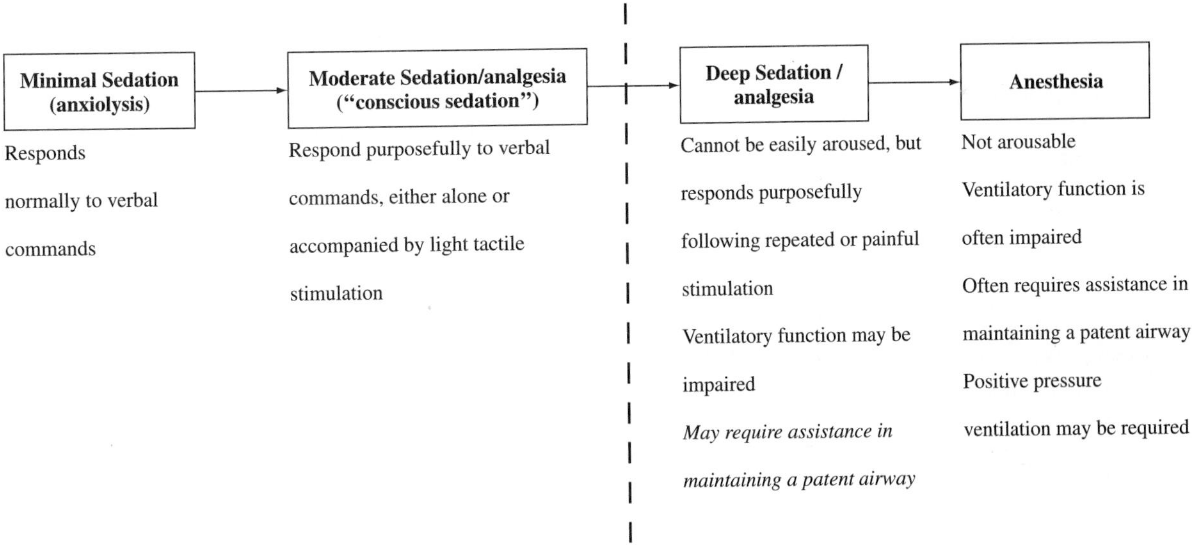

FIGURE **49-1**
The Joint Commission on Accreditation of Healthcare Organizations continuum of sedation and anesthesia. (From Kaplan RF, Yang CI. Sedation and analgesia in pediatric patients for procedures outside the operating room. *Anesthesiol Clin North Am* 2002;20:181-194.)

a. May administer pharmacologic agents to achieve a desired level of sedation.
b. Must monitor patients carefully in order to maintain the patient at the desired level of sedation. Appropriate equipment must be available for monitoring heart rate via ECG, respiratory rate and adequacy of pulmonary ventilation, oxygenation via pulse oximetry, and blood pressure measurement at regular intervals (at least every 5 minutes).
c. Must be competent to evaluate the patient before performing the moderate sedation and analgesia and deep sedation and analgesia.
d. Must be competent in the administration of moderate sedation and analgesia and deep sedation and analgesia.
e. Must be competent to rescue the patient who unavoidably or unintentionally slips into a deeper-than-desired level of sedation and analgesia. In the case of the CRNA,

competency is mandatory for all levels of the sedation continuum. This includes competency in management of a compromised airway and the provision of oxygenation. In addition, for patients undergoing deep sedation and analgesia, one must also have competency to manage an unstable cardiovascular system.
f. Must properly document the patient's response to care.
g. Must supervise recovery of the patient after the sedation in a postsedation area or a postanesthesia recovery area.
3. Adequate numbers of qualified personnel must be present during the performance of moderate sedation and analgesia, deep sedation and analgesia, and anesthesia (general).

It should be noted that the JCAHO has adopted a philosophy called, "Shared Visions, New Pathways." The new standards are more consistent across all areas of the accreditation process, more prescriptive in nature, and fewer.[10]

Anesthetic Considerations for the Pediatric Patient Receiving Anesthesia for a Therapeutic or Diagnostic Procedure in a Remote Location

The pediatric population can pose a challenge. Patients' behavior and degree of cooperation can range from very helpful to extremely anxious. Fortunately, several common anesthetic medications can help patients with slight to high levels of anxiety. Pediatric sedation and anesthesia increases the quality of care the patient receives by greatly reducing anxiety and by eliminating movement when necessary for therapeutic or diagnostic procedures.

The goals of pediatric anesthesia are listed in Box 49-4. First and foremost in the practice of nurse anesthesia are patient safety and guardianship of the welfare of patients. Important lessons can be learned from the literature regarding anesthesia in pediatric patients. Children ages 1 to 5 years seem to be at the greatest risk for adverse events, even with no underlying disease. Adverse events have been caused more commonly with the use of multiple drugs, especially sedative medications. The problems encountered most frequently are respiratory events: respiratory depression, respiratory obstruction, and apnea.[11,12]

Proper adherence to patient selection and a comprehensive preoperative assessment, proper dosage to minimize unexpected responses, proper monitoring, skilled administration of anesthesia, and proper recovery time can reduce adverse events. The anesthesia provider must plan to minimize the possibility of adverse reactions.[11,13] General patient selection criteria to help minimize the possibility of adverse events are seen with patients ≥6 months of age and applied during the preoperative assessment. It is during this time that the temperament of the child can be assessed.[14] Consideration must be made for the type of procedure to be performed. Will there be a great degree of patient stimulation, a large amount of blood loss, an inability to have close contact with the patient during the therapeutic or diagnostic procedure? It is found that adverse reactions are reduced with procedures that last less than 1 hour.[13] Clear communication with the technician and the medical practitioner is essential to clarify the requirements for the patient to be safe and properly anesthetized for the procedure.

BOX 49-4

Goals of Pediatric Anesthesia

1. Foremost, to provide safety and welfare to the patient.
2. To minimize physical discomfort or to provide more profound analgesia when necessary to the patient.
3. To minimize negative psychologic consequences of the therapeutic or diagnostic procedure. This can be accomplished by the provision of sedative medications, analgesics, and amnestic agents.
4. To control uncooperative or endangering behavior.
5. To provide the patient a safe discharge to the guardian and to home.
6. To minimize patient complications from applied therapeutic or diagnostic procedures and administered anesthetic medications.

Modified from Kaplan RF, Yang CI. Sedation and analgesia in pediatric patients for procedures outside the operating room. Anesthesiol Clin North Am. *2002;20:181-194.*

The pediatric patient and the parent or legal guardian must be properly prepared for the planned therapeutic or diagnostic procedure. Clear explanation of the entire anesthetic process to the parent or guardian is based on the developed treatment plan and is offered in age-appropriate terms for the pediatric patient.[14] "Inform before you perform."

Fasting times are constantly being reevaluated in clinical anesthesia and must be stringently adhered to. Fasting guidelines are discussed in Chapters 17 and 45.

Premedication with oral, intranasal, or rectal sedatives may be necessary. Common pediatric premedications and doses are listed in Table 49-1.

It is essential to have qualified personnel to assist in the safe care of pediatric patients receiving anesthesia in remote locations. An extra pair of trained hands enhances the ability for the patient to receive safer care throughout the entire procedure.

Anesthetic Considerations for the Geriatric Patient Receiving Anesthesia for a Therapeutic or Diagnostic Procedure in a Remote Location

As a result of a number of factors, including better nutrition, more physical activity, less tobacco and alcohol use, and improved medical care, more Americans are living longer lives.

The increasing population of the elderly is going to place many demands on the public health-care system. Medical technology is advancing, and therefore more procedures requiring anesthesia will be performed in elderly patients. Perioperative complications can increase with age. Special considerations related to the physiology of aging are necessary if anesthetic treatment is to be performed safely.[15]

The elderly have a greater prevalence of atherosclerosis, infections, autoimmune diseases, chronic disorders, and cancer. The immune system gradually and slowly diminishes in function with age. Therefore the ability to heal and fight foreign bacteria, viruses, and malignant cells diminishes. There are no fewer T cells than at a younger age, but T-cell function is decreased. Many of the body's cells begin to diminish in function or to function abnormally. Cells also may have increasing difficulty in membrane transfer of nutrients and waste.[15]

The normal aging process results in an increase in the ratio of adipose tissue to aqueous body tissues.[8,14,15] This means more lipid-soluble anesthetic drug is stored. Basal metabolic rate decreases with age.[16] Liver and kidney functions decrease with age. This results in a decrease in the rate of metabolism and excretion of anesthetic drugs. Nervous system function generally produces decreases in the perception of sight, hearing, touch,

TABLE 49-1 Common Pediatric Premedications and Doses

Medication	Dose	Route	Onset	Duration
Benzodiazepines				
Midazolam	0.1-0.15 mg/kg up to 10 mg	IM	5-10 min	0.5-2 h
	0.2 mg/kg	IN	10 min	0.5-2 h
	0.025-1 mg/kg	IV	1-3 min	0.5-2 h
	0.25-1 mg/kg up to 20 mg	PO	15-30 min	0.5-2 h
	0.3-1 mg/kg	PR	10-20 min	0.5-2 h
Diazepam	0.1-0.5 mg/kg	IM, PO, PR	60 min	>24 h
Narcotics				
Fentanyl	1-3 mcg/kg	IM	5-15 min	30-60 min
	0.5-1 mcg/kg	IV	1-3 min	30-60 min
	5 mcg/kg	OT	5-30 min	30-60 min
Sufentanil	1.5-4.5 mcg/kg	IN	7-10 min	30-60 min
Morphine sulfate	0.1-0.2 mg/kg	IM	30-45 min	4-5 h
	0.05-0.1 mg/kg	IV	3-10 min	
Dissociative Anesthetic				
Ketamine	1-2 mg/kg	IM	30s-2 min	12-25 min
	3 mg/kg	IN	20 min	
	0.2-1 mg/kg	IV	30s-1 min	
	6-10 mg/kg	PO	10-20 min	
	10 mg/kg	PR	10 min	
Reversal Agents				
Flumazenil	Adult 0.2 mg	IV	Over 15 seconds; wait 45 sec; if necessary give 0.2 mg; repeat at 60-sec intervals; maximum dose 3 mg/kg	
	Child 10 mcg	IV	Up to 1 mg cumulative dose	
Naloxone	Adult 0.4-2 mg	IV, SC, IM	Repeat in 2-3 min if needed	
	Child 0.5-2 mcg/kg	IV, SC, IM	Repeat in 1 min if needed	

IM, *Intramuscular;* IN, *intranasal;* IV, *intravenous;* OT, *oral transmucosal;* PO, *by mouth;* PR, *by rectum;* SC, *subcutaneous.*
From Mosby Drug Consult, *St Louis: Elsevier-Mosby, 2004.*

smell (taste), pain, and temperature sensations. Therefore the dose requirements for anesthetic drugs usually are decreased. Cardiovascular function is a function of the level of activity of the patient and generally decreases with age. Patients may be restricted in their activity because of arthritis or other debilitation. Circulation time is decreased. The ability of the cardiovascular system to respond to the effects of anesthetic drugs, fluid administration, and the stresses of therapeutic and diagnostic procedures can cause decreased cardiac function, resulting in hemodynamic instability and reduced circulation to vital organs.[8,14] Tissue oxygenation can decrease because of changes in ventilation ability and lung tissue. The ability to thermoregulate is also decreased.[8] Body metabolism is designed to function at 37° C. Changes in mental status or even delirium can occur more frequently in geriatric patients. All of these factors must be taken into consideration when one provides anesthesia to geriatric patients.

Significant variability exists in each of these vital functions among patients. Geriatric patients who are more physically fit have a decreased mortality, reduced incidence of cardiovascular disease, lower blood pressure, reduced blood cholesterol, and most important, better bodily reserves when they become surgically challenged or sick.[15] A thorough and comprehensive preanesthetic assessment is necessary, from which a plan of treatment can be deduced.

Complications related to anesthesia can be linked to poor preoperative planning and preparation of the patient. Agents with short half-lives are ideal for the elderly patient. Carefully consider the use of drugs that are synergistic or antagonistic in their effects. Such drugs as propofol, midazolam, fentanyl, alfentanil, remifentanil, and local anesthetics are ideal, and doses are calculated according to the patient's responses. The bispectral index (BIS) monitor is being evaluated as a tool for more precise titration of anesthetic medications to the patient's needs. Finally, care must be taken to ensure adequate body warmth, protection of skin both while moving the patient and during the procedure, and skin padding of bony prominences.[14]

ANESTHESIA FOR SPECIFIC THERAPEUTIC AND DIAGNOSTIC PROCEDURES IN REMOTE LOCATIONS

Cardiologic Procedures

Automatic Implantable Cardiac Defibrillator and Cardiac Pacemaker

Procedure Overviews. Patients who experience sudden cardiac death are usually approximately 60 years of age, and their most common underlying rhythm is pulseless ventricular tachycardia (VT) or ventricular fibrillation (VF).[17]

Ventricular defibrillation was first reported in the literature in 1947. Defibrillation is the application of a flow of electrical current through the appropriate chambers of the heart in order to restore a suitable heart rhythm to sustain life.[18] It has been proved that early defibrillation, along with cardiopulmonary resuscitation, can result in high long-term survival rates. The automatic implantable cardiac defibrillator (AICD) was conceived by Mirowski and co-workers to bypass the delay patients experienced before receiving defibrillation. The first AICD was implanted in a human by Mirowski, at Johns Hopkins University Medical Center in 1980. The AICD is composed of two basic parts: a pulse generator and a lead electrode for detection of arrhythmias, delivery of a defibrillating shock, cardiac pacing, telemetry, and provision of diagnostic data. The pulse generator is a hermetically sealed titanium can that contains a computer microprocessor, resistors, transformers, capacitors, and a battery. The battery is designed to deliver 120 shocks and usually lasts for 3 to 6 years. The computer is programmed with algorithms to detect VT and VF. If VF occurs, an electrical shock is administered within 10 to 15 seconds of detection (much of the time delay results from the charging of the capacitor). VT is treated with overdrive pacing called *antitachycardia pacing* (ATP). ATP is an extremely successful procedure. AICD implantation has been a crucial technique for prevention of sudden cardiac death.[18]

A cardiac pacemaker is used to treat bradycardia, atrioventricular block, sinus nodal dysfunction, and other arrhythmias. The pacemaker is used concurrently with other therapies for management of arrhythmia and hemodynamics. Pacemaker therapy was conceived in the 1950s and has been used since that time. The pacemaker consists of a pulse generator containing a computer and a battery that is designed to last 6 to 10 years. Attached to the pulse generator is a lead, which delivers the current used to depolarize the myocardium, and an anode, which completes the electrical circuit. Two different types of pacemaker leads are available. A unipolar pacemaker lead uses one lead as the cathode and the pulse generator as the anode. Unipolar leads are less likely to fail. A bipolar pacemaker lead uses two separate leads that are close together, the advantage of which is a sharper signal with less noise. The leads are inserted under fluoroscopic guidance via the cephalic vein or the subclavian vein into the cardiac chamber, usually the right ventricle in the case of an AICD and the right atrium and right ventricle for a cardiac pacemaker. The leads are then tunneled and connected to the pulse generator, which is then inserted into a subcutaneous pocket in the patient's pectoral region or into a subpectoral muscle pocket.[18] Figure 49-2 shows a postoperative radiograph of a pacemaker pulse generator, computer, and battery inserted into a patient. Figure 49-3 shows a postoperative radiograph of a unipolar pacemaker lead inserted into the right ventricle of a patient. Research and continual improvements allow more people to receive better and more reliable AICD and cardiac pacemaker therapy.

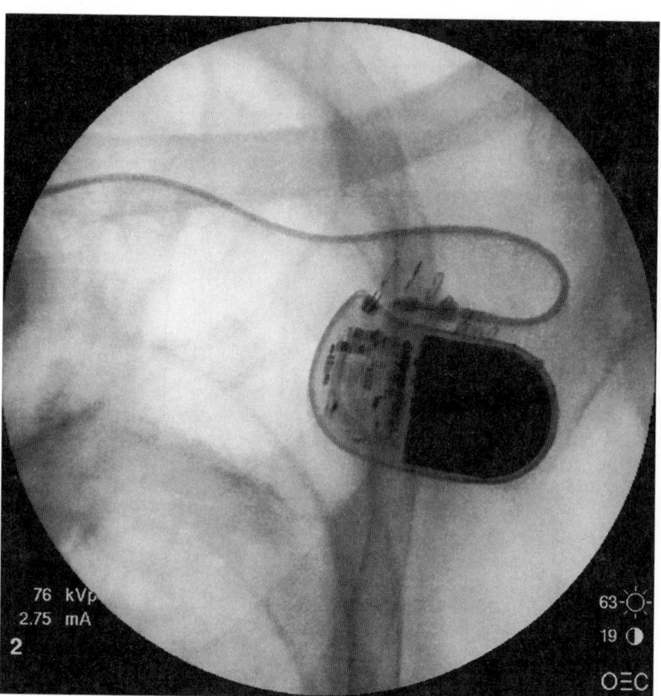

FIGURE **49-2**
Radiograph of a pacemaker pulse generator, computer, and battery inserted into a patient.

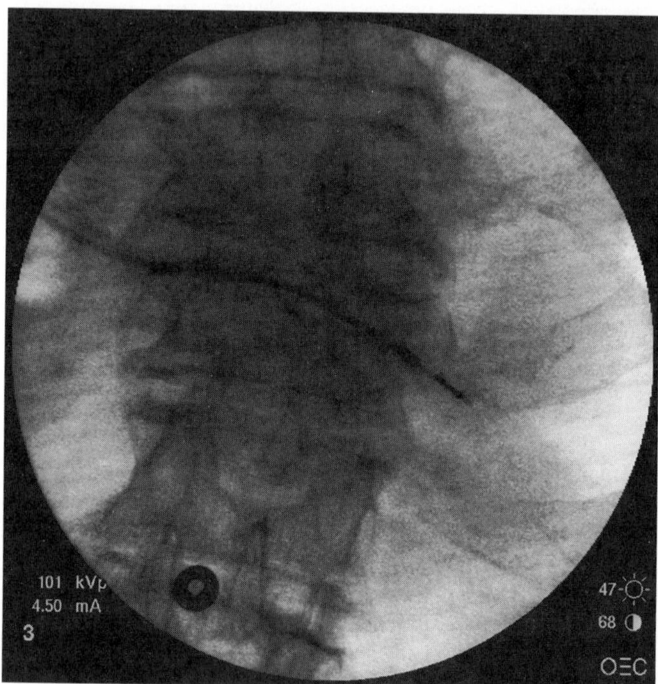

FIGURE **49-3**
Radiograph of a unipolar pacemaker lead inserted into the right ventricle of a patient.

Anesthetic Considerations. The AICD or cardiac pacemaker procedure may be performed in the operating room, in a special cardiac procedure room, or in the cardiac catheterization suite by a cardiologist or other physician.[19] Routine monitors are attached to the patient, with special attention paid to a properly functioning five-lead ECG. The ECG monitor screen must be available to the anesthesia team, the operating physician, and the AICD or pacemaker manufacturer's technical service representative, who is always present during insertion. The procedures are usually adequately performed with local anesthetic and moderate sedation or deep sedation, although some clinicians prefer a general anesthetic.[18]

AICD insertion requires purposeful triggering of VF in an attempt to test thresholds and functioning of the AICD. General anesthesia poses no significant difference to sedation in the amounts of energy needed to defibrillate.[20] As in all anesthetic procedures, endotracheal intubation may be required to secure the airway should a cardiac emergency arise.

After insertion of the cardiac pacemaker and before wound closure the device is threshold tested by the pacemaker manufacturer's technical service representative to ensure adequate contact between the leads and the myocardium.[18] After wound closure and dressing application, all computer function programming of either the AICD or the cardiac pacemaker can then be performed with a pacemaker programmer, which connects to a portable wand. The wand is placed within close proximity to the implanted pulse generator by the manufacturer's technical service representative and allows a telemetric connection to properly program or interrogate the AICD or cardiac pacemaker.

Postanesthesia Care. The patient is transported to the recovery room with oxygen when the procedure is completed, and the patient is observed during recovery from the anesthesia for any hemodynamic or cardiovascular ECG changes.

AICDs are generally well tolerated by patients. Some patients display anxiety or depression because of the possibility of sudden cardiac death, device failure, inappropriate shocks, and recalls of certain devices.[18] Shocks from the AICD are described as a sudden, heavy blow to the chest. Medical technology is ever improving, and the demand for AICDs and cardiac pacemakers increases annually. Better products with enhanced algorithms, along with better pharmacologic therapy, will minimize the risks associated with these devices and maximize their acceptability more quickly in a growing number of patients.

Cardioversion

Procedure Overview. Cardioversion is the synchronized discharge of electrical energy to convert hemodynamically unstable supraventricular rhythms, such as atrial flutter or atrial fibrillation, or hemodynamically stable VT.[18,21] These rhythms can be life threatening if left untreated. Atrial flutter and atrial fibrillation are associated with the development of congestive heart failure and with the formation of thromboemboli, which can lead to stroke.[18] The patient may also have symptoms of chronic fatigue.[21] Cardioversion usually is a scheduled and planned procedure. At times patient optimization is not possible because of the urgency for cardioversion as a result of hemodynamic instability. Much less electrical energy is required to cardiovert a patient when compared with defibrillation. Defibrillation is an unplanned and usually emergent application of unsynchronized electrical energy. Cardioversion is believed to be therapeutic because it closes an excitable gap in the myocardium, which causes currents to reenter and excite the electrical system of the heart.[18]

Anesthetic Considerations. Because cardioversion is usually a nonemergent and planned procedure, patient conditions usually can be optimized. Proper nothing-by-mouth (NPO) status must be observed unless the cardioversion is deemed urgent or emergent. Standard monitors are applied, with special attention paid to the ECG. The BIS monitor can be used to assess consciousness during cardioversion.[22,23] Intravenous access is necessary. The energy required for cardioversion is measured in joules (watt-seconds). The cardiologist or physician uses a cardioverter-defibrillator for the procedure. The operator applies cardioversion-defibrillator paddles with conduction gel or defibrillator patches to the patient. One paddle or patch is placed parasternally over the second and third intercostal space. The other paddle or patch is placed over the area of the apex of the heart. The cardioverter-defibrillator is set to the synchronous mode. Visual marks are placed by the cardioverter atop the tallest R waves of the ECG. Energy shocks are titrated progressively from 10 J up to 360 J as necessary, after observation after the synchronized shock.[18]

Midazolam may be administered as a sedative before cardioversion. The patient is then assisted in breathing oxygen via a face mask and Ambu bag with high-flow oxygen. Because of the intense and brief pain of cardioversion an ultra–short-acting general anesthetic such as propofol, thiopental, or methohexital is administered. After the loss of eyelash reflex occurs, an "all-clear" signal is given by the operator. Positive pressure respirations are temporarily suspended, with care taken not to touch any part of the patient or the patient's bed. Then the synchronized shock or shocks are administered.[21,23] Muscle relaxation is not necessary. As always, an assortment of oral airways, nasal airways, laryngeal mask airways (LMAs), endotracheal tubes, and laryngoscopes with blades and suction should be readily available in case complications occur. If cardioversion is required in a patient who has not fasted, general anesthesia with tracheal intubation is necessary to prevent aspiration of gastric contents.[23]

Postanesthesia Care. It is hoped that the patient's heart is now beating in a desirable cardiac rhythm and that the patient's blood pressure is stable. Spontaneous respirations return, along with swallowing and coughing if necessary. The patient is observed for any reactions to the anesthetic, and care is turned over to the nurse accompanying the patient.

Radiofrequency Catheter Ablation

Procedure Overview. Radiofrequency catheter ablation (RFCA) uses a catheter with an electrode at its tip, which is guided under fluoroscopy to an area of heart muscle that has demonstrated accessory electrical conductive pathways.[21] RFCA has all but replaced arrhythmia surgery and is now considered the foremost therapy for the treatment of many arrhythmias in pediatric and adult patients.[24,25] Supraventricular tachycardia is the most common tachyarrhythmia in children, and symptomatic supraventricular tachyarrhythmias are most often treated by RFCA.[26] Accessory electrical conductive pathways are distributed unevenly along the right and left atrioventricular valve annuli. Left-sided accessory pathways are most common, but both right- and left-sided accessory electrical pathways can be accessed and ablated.[24,26] Other treatments possible with RFCA are modification of the sinus node or AV node, ablation of atrial flutter and atrial tachycardia, and ablation of focal atrial fibrillation and VT foci.[18,21] Patients must undergo electrophysiologic studies to determine the origin and pathway of the arrhythmia, as well as the mechanism of action, before RFCA can be chosen as a therapy.

RFCA is an extremely safe and successful procedure, with success rates of 95% overall. Many patients no longer need their antiarrhythmic medications soon after therapy.[21]

Anesthetic Considerations. Electrophysiologic studies before RFCA are time-consuming procedures that may require moderate sedation in adults or general anesthesia in children. RFCA can be performed in the operating room, in a special cardiac procedure room, or in the cardiac catheterization suite, by a cardiologist. The electrode catheter is guided via the femoral artery and vein to the area of the accessory electrical pathway or an area of arrhythmogenic focus.[27,28] The internal jugular vein may also be used. The electrode is then energized with radiofrequency energy, and cells within the path of the electrode are painlessly obliterated.

RFCA is a short procedure. Patients must remain perfectly still, except for respiratory movement, during the procedure. Many adults can be anesthetized with moderate sedation and analgesia along with local anesthetic applied by the operator. Children may be best treated with general endotracheal anesthesia using either an LMA or endotracheal tube to secure the airway. Full monitors and an intravenous catheter are necessary. TIVA using propofol as the key medication has been used. Midazolam and thiopental, as well as a potent inhaled anesthetic gas such as isoflurane, have been used successfully for RFCA. TIVA with propofol and ondansetron has a much lower rate of nausea than does use of isoflurane and an antiemetic. Careful attention must be paid to the ECG, because the patient must stop taking any antiarrhythmic drugs before the electrophysiologic study and RFCA are performed.[28-30]

Postanesthesia Care. Patients must be monitored during recovery from administered anesthetics after RFCA. Patients must also be observed for possible RFCA procedural complications such as bleeding, ECG changes, cerebrovascular accidents, cardiac tamponade, or damage to the aortic valve.[18]

Gastroenterologic Procedures

Procedure Overview

Fiberoptic gastroscopy was first introduced in 1957. Endoscopy came into popular use in the early 1960s with the invention of a snare for collecting intestinal polyps for biopsy. Endoscopy for gastrointestinal procedures is the use of a flexible fiberoptic endoscope that transmits brilliant, coherent, high-resolution, magnified, direct visual images to the operator. The operator can then examine, biopsy, dilate, or cauterize portions of the gastrointestinal tract. The endoscopist may pass accessory devices down the endoscope such as biopsy forceps, dilation devices, cytology brushes, measuring devices, needles for injection, Doppler probes, ultrasound probes, and probes to measure electrical activity and pH. Even foreign bodies may be removed with the aid of a snare passed through an endoscope. Endoscopes are available in different diameters for use in pediatric to adult patients.[31]

An upper endoscopy, such as an esophagogastroduodenoscopy (EGD), is an accurate way for the operator to evaluate the mucosa of the esophagus, stomach, and duodenum. A colonoscopy allows total diagnostic visualization of the mucosa of the tortuous colon from the anus to the cecum. ERCP is used for the diagnosis of obstructive, neoplastic, or inflammatory pancreatobiliary structures. The use of ERCP is decreasing because of the availability of less-invasive and noninvasive techniques. Box 49-5 provides a brief list of indications for colonoscopy, EGD, and ERCP.[31]

Endoscopy for gastrointestinal procedures may be performed by a gastroenterologist, a general surgeon, a family practitioner, or a proctologist. The endoscope is passed into the gastrointestinal tract with the aid of lubricant. The endoscope has controls to change the direction of the flexible tip, allow flushing with water, apply suction, or insufflate air or carbon dioxide within the portion of the gastrointestinal tract being observed.

Anesthetic Considerations

Because of the expectations of patients, endoscopically caused discomfort, and the desirability of no patient movement, moderate sedation, deep sedation, and in some cases general endotracheal anesthesia are used. A proper preanesthetic assessment of the patient must be performed, focusing on the areas of age, ability to cooperate, level of anxiety, mental disability, allergies, fluid status, laboratory electrolyte values, cardiac history, hypertension, bleeding history, clotting status, respiratory status, obesity, drug and alcohol abuse, gastroesophageal reflux, and pregnancy.[8]

Endoscopy has been safely performed in pregnant patients.[31] Consideration should be given to any anesthetic

BOX **49-5**

Indications for Colonoscopy, Esophagogastroduodenoscopy, and Endoscopic Retrograde Cholangiopancreatography with Anesthetic Implications

Colonoscopy

Gastrointestinal bleeding and occult bleeding
Evaluation of an abnormality on barium enema
Polypectomy
Unexplained iron deficiency anemia
Significant diarrhea
Chronic inflammatory bowel disease
Malignancy
Dilation of stenotic lesions
Foreign body removal

Esophagogastroduodenoscopy

Persistent and recurrent dyspepsia (heartburn)
Persistent nausea or vomiting
Dysphagia (difficulty swallowing)
Chest pain with a negative cardiac evaluation
Iron deficiency anemia
Suspected small bowel malabsorption
Malignancy
Stomach or esophageal ulcer
Control of bleeding
Ligation or sclerosis of varices
Dilation of strictures
Percutaneous gastrostomy
Polypectomy
Removal of foreign body

Endoscopic Retrograde Cholangiopancreatography

Suspected biliary ductal disorder
Suspected pancreatic ductal disorder
Biliary drainage
Pancreatic drainage
Biopsy
Bile or pancreatic juice collection
Mapping of the pancreatic duct before intended surgery
Manometry of the sphincter of Oddi or other ductal mapping

Modified from. *Waye JD, Williams CB. Colonoscopy and Flexible Sigmoidoscopy.* *In* Textbook of Gastroenterology. *Yamada T, ed. Philadelphia: Lippincott Williams & Wilkins; 2003:2851-2865; Sherman S, Lehman GA. Endoscopic Retrograde Cholangiopancreatography, Endoscopic Sphincterotomy and Stone Removal, and Endoscopic Biliary and Pancreatic Drainage.* *In* Textbook of Gastroenterology. *Yamada T, ed. Philadelphia: Lippincott Williams & Wilkins; 2003:2866-2892.*

drugs administered to the parturient, because transfer can occur through the placenta to the fetus. Elective procedures should be reconsidered, although urgent procedures must be performed. None of the common sedative drugs such as propofol or the opioid fentanyl has been demonstrated to cause teratogenic changes in the fetus. Studies of the obstetric effect of anesthetic drugs are limited because of the infrequent requirements for surgery during pregnancy and the ethical difficulties associated with performing controlled trials. Regional anesthesia may expose the parturient to the fewest anesthetic drugs.[32]

Patients must adhere to proper NPO guidelines. Bacteremia is possible as a result of endoscopic procedures. Necessary medications may be given, such as cardiac medications, antihypertensives, and antibiotics.[31] Moderate sedation is usually accomplished with the short-acting midazolam and alfentanil, whereas deep sedation can be achieved with titration of propofol until effective.[8]

Colonoscopy requires thorough cleansing of the lumen of the colon of fecal material. The colon may be partly prepared with a cleansing enema. Full preparation of the colon is accomplished commonly with orally administered balanced electrolyte solutions in a volume of 4 L. Other types of solutions are available. Patients often find this the most distressing portion of the procedure. After the preparation can come abdominal cramping, diarrhea, weakness, and nausea. Patients who arrive for the procedure require reassessment and the insertion of an intravenous catheter with intravenous fluid, usually lactated Ringer's solution or normal saline. Patients are usually left reclining for the procedure in the transport cart. Conventional monitors, including pulse oximeter, noninvasive blood pressure monitor, and electrocardiograph, are attached. The patient is supplied with oxygen through a disposable nasal cannula or disposable face mask. The procedure is usually performed with the patient positioned in a lateral decubitus position, with the body flexed, the head and back bent downward toward the knees, and the legs bent upward toward the abdomen. Patient anxiety, distension because of insufflation, and acute discomfort during the maneuvering of the endoscope usually necessitates the administration of deep sedation or a general anesthetic in some cases.[33] The depth of sedation required may be titrated with the use of the BIS monitor.[34] Strong vagal nerve stimulation can occur as a result of distension of the colon. This may cause hypotension, bradydysrhythmia, and electrocardiographic changes.[31]

EGD requires a general patient assessment with special emphasis on any cardiac history, hypertension, bleeding disorders, nausea, dysphagia, and gastroesophageal reflux. The patient must be NPO according to guidelines. Most patients are able to have EGD performed with a spray or gargle of topical anesthetic such as cetacaine, benzocaine, or 4% lidocaine liquid.[35] Topical benzocaine can pose a small risk of methemoglobinemia if overused. Occasionally, patients require moderate sedation or deep sedation because topical anesthesia and even hypnosis have been found less effective.[36-38] An intravenous catheter is inserted, with fluids such as lactated Ringer's or normal saline attached. The patient is connected to standard monitors. Oxygen can be supplied through a disposable nasal cannula or a disposable face mask. EGD is generally performed with the patient positioned supine. After the patient is adequately sedated, the operator inserts a hollow oral airway gently into the patient's mouth, and the endoscope is advanced through this airway, allowing direct visualization of the larynx, hypopharynx, esophagus and stomach, and through the pylorus into the duodenal bulb.[31]

ERCP requires thorough assessment of the patient including a review of laboratory values of a complete blood count, serum liver chemistries and amylase or lipase levels to evaluate liver function, and clotting studies. Patients must also be evaluated for anticoagulant medications, bleeding history, and prosthetic heart valves.[31] Allergies must be evaluated, especially those to iodinated contrast media.[39] Patients who require ERCP are usually more ill than patients seen routinely for colonoscopy or EGD. The patient must be NPO according to guidelines. Intravenous access is obtained and fluid is administered. Standard monitors are applied, and oxygen is supplied to the patient via a disposable face mask. The procedure requires that the patient be in a prone or slightly left lateral decubitus position. Deep sedation is generally required, although painful or complex ERCP may require general anesthesia.[40,41]

Pediatric endoscopy has been performed with patients under deep intravenous sedation with agents such as propofol, midazolam, and alfentanil, when the patient will allow placement of the intravenous catheter, and under general endotracheal anesthesia.[42-45] Propofol has been found to provide anterograde amnesia during the procedure with no provided retrograde amnesia.[46] The use of a eutectic mixture of lidocaine and prilocaine local anesthetics (EMLA cream) facilitates the placement of the IV catheter. EMLA must be applied to undamaged skin, under an occlusive dressing for a period of 45-60 minutes, before the IV catheter is inserted.[47] The LidoSite Topical System (Vyteris, Inc.) is a delivery system indicated for use on normal intact skin to provide local topical anesthesia. The system is comprised of the LidoSite Patch (lidocaine HCl/epinephrine topical iontophoretic patch 10%/0.1%), and the LidoSite controller. The LidoSite System is intended for use in superficial dermatologic procedures such as venipuncture, intravenous cannulation, and laser ablation of superficial skin lesions. The prefilled LidoSite patch administers lidocaine medication through the skin via a mild electric current, regulated by the preprogrammed dose controller. It is intended to work in 10 minutes and may be used on patients aged 5 years and older. When general anesthesia is administered, a sturdily secured endotracheal tube should be considered because of relative inaccessibility to the airway, as in the patient position required for pediatric colonoscopy or for EGD in which the oral cavity will be shared with the operator.

These procedures can cause bowel rupture or duct rupture. One must be ready with immediate airway and hemodynamic support as necessary, along with monitored emergency transport to the operating room for surgical intervention.

Postanesthesia Care

Postprocedure morbidity differs with each of the described procedures. All patients must be monitored in a postanesthesia care area until they have recovered from the sedation or general anesthetic.

Colonoscopy patients have intestinal distension, which is relieved with encouragement to pass flatus. Rectal bleeding, nausea, hypotension, and vomiting may also be seen. Administration of a bolus of intravenous fluids along with an intravenous antiemetic agent, such as ondansetron, dolasetron, or granisetron is indicated.

EGD morbidity relates to bleeding, nausea, vomiting, aspiration, dysphagia, and hypotension. Treatments such as those used for colonoscopy may be indicated.

ERCP morbidity relates to possible reactions to iodinated contrast media. Patient reactions can be mild (such as nausea, vomiting, pruritus, diaphoresis, flushing, or mild urticaria), moderate (such as faintness, severe vomiting, profound urticaria, mild bronchospasm, mild hypotension, mild tachycardia, or bradycardia) or severe (hypotensive shock, angioedema, respiratory arrest, cardiac arrest, convulsions, or death).[39] Postprocedure bleeding, nausea, and vomiting are possible and can be treated as described previously.

Gynecologic Procedures

Procedure Overview

Assisted reproductive technologies (ART) refers to all techniques used to retrieve and fertilize the human oocyte. In vitro fertilization (IVF) is the most common technique used to artificially fertilize the human oocyte.[48,49] Research by reproductive endocrinologists has advanced technology since the first "test-tube baby" was born in 1978 and continues to result in new and more effective techniques.[8] The procedure is generally performed by a gynecologist who has had an advanced training fellowship in the ambulatory setting and takes approximately 20 to 30 minutes to complete.

The procedure is performed by initially stimulating maturation of the follicle with human chorionic gonadotropin (HCG). The oocyte is retrieved transvaginally with an ultrasonically guided probe 34 to 35 hours after HCG administration. Fertilization occurs in the IVF laboratory. The oocyte is identified and has minimal exposure to ambient room temperature, room air, and especially any chemical odors. Sperm are washed and centrifuged. Fresh media is added next to the centrifuged sperm, and those sperm that swim to the media, which can number 50,000 sperm, are placed with the oocyte. Fertilization then occurs, and the embryo, which has developed into 8 to 10 cells, is transferred into the uterus. Timing must be coordinated with proper maturation of the uterine endometrium.[48] ART is found to increase the risk of multiple gestations. Also, it has been reported that atypical implantations of the fertilized ovum or zygote, such as abdominal, cervical, ovarian, or tubal pregnancy, occur more frequently with ART.[50] Common ART techniques are listed in Box 49-6. IVF was first performed nearly 25 years ago and is accepted because of increased success rates, currently 25% for IVF.[48,50] Infertility affects approximately 20% of couples.[50]

Patients are assessed for antibodies to human immunodeficiency virus types 1 and 2 (HIV-1, HIV-2) and human T-cell lymphotropic virus type 1 (HTLV-1), hepatitis B antigen, and antibodies to hepatitis B and C. Patients are also tested for chlamydia, syphilis, gonorrhea, and cytomegalovirus. Smokers require twice as many attempts at successful IVF than nonsmokers, so smoking is extremely discouraged.[48]

BOX 49-6

Common Assisted Reproductive Technology Techniques

In vitro fertilization (IVF)	Oocytes are removed, fertilization occurs in the laboratory, and the embryo is placed transcervically into the uterus.
Gamete intrafallopian transfer (GIFT)	Oocytes and sperm are placed into the fallopian tube for fertilization.
Zygote intrafallopian transfer (ZIFT)	Fertilized oocytes are placed into the fallopian tube.
Tubal embryo transfer (TET)	Cleaving embryos are placed into the fallopian tube.
Peritoneal oocyte and sperm transfer (POST)	Oocytes and sperm are placed into the pelvic cavity.

Modified from Speroff L, Glass RH, Kase NG. Clinical Gynecologic Endocrinology and Infertility. *6th ed. Baltimore: Lippincott Williams & Wilkins; 1999:1133-1148.*

Anesthetic Considerations

IVF is generally performed on patients who are ASA class 1 or 2. Although IVF is a relatively simple procedure for the reproductive endocrinologist to perform, especially outside the operating room, IVF is an uncomfortable procedure and requires that patients do not move in order to for the probe to be guided for retrieval and later reimplantation. The vaginal wall must be pierced for the desired ovary to be accessed. Also, major blood vessels are present in the proximity of the ovaries, and their injury could lead to complications.[8]

Anesthesia requirements vary with the individual needs of the patient and the reproductive endocrinologist. Multiple ART procedures may need to be performed until one of them is successful, so safe yet inexpensive anesthetic techniques are desirable.[8] Minimal sedation (anxiolysis), moderate sedation and analgesia ("conscious sedation"), regional intrathecal anesthesia, paracervical block, or general anesthesia can be administered to assist in making the procedure as comfortable and successful as possible.[8,49,51-54] Moderate sedation with analgesia (conscious sedation) is usually sufficient for most patients. None of the anesthetic procedures caused differences in reproductive outcome.[49,52,53] Anesthetic medications described in the literature and their effects on ART are listed in Box 49-7. Consideration should be given to anesthetic techniques with quick onset and a short duration. It should be noted that propofol, lidocaine, and alfentanil have been shown

BOX 49-7

Anesthetic Medications Used for Assisted Reproductive Technologies

Intrathecal
Bupivacaine
Lidocaine
Fentanyl
Morphine

Paracervical Block
Bupivacaine
Lidocaine
Mepivacaine

Intravenous Sedation or Total Intravenous Anesthesia
Fentanyl
Midazolam
Propofol

Inhalational Agents
Nitrous oxide

to accumulate in the follicular fluid. Although no deleterious effects of any anesthetics have been identified, this area continues to be studied.[49,53] Morphine has been shown to adversely affect fertilization of sea urchin eggs in vitro and is not used because of the existence of safe alternatives such as fentanyl. The necessity for any medication given to the patient should be carefully considered, and the anesthetic technique should be kept simple and basic.

Postanesthesia Care

As in all cases of anesthetic administration, the patient is assessed in a postanesthetic recovery area. Vital signs and pulse oximetry are assessed and must be stable. If intrathecal anesthesia was used, the patient must have a recovery of sensorum, be able to ambulate, and be able to void. All patients must be free of nausea.

Office-Based Surgery

For further discussion of office-based surgery, see Chapter 43.

Procedure Overview

Anesthesia for dental surgery can present many challenges. The demand for dental care and visits from patients are increasing. The old mainstay was that 50% of the population never visited a dentist. This group used dentistry only for treatment of extreme pain or in an emergency. Demographic statistics show that this has changed. Overall, rates vary drastically across the U.S. population, with 43% of the population visiting a dentist at least once annually. More women see dentists annually than men, and as employment status, income, and educational levels increase, so do the number of annual visits to the dentist. Also, children aged 6 or younger and adults aged 65 or older are seeing dentists more frequently than in the past.[55,56]

Dental procedures may be performed in an operating room, a specially equipped hospital suite, or a dental office surgical area. Anesthesia may be required for dental procedures in the following areas of dentistry:

1. *Pediatric dentistry*—an age-defined specialty that provides primary and comprehensive preventive and therapeutic oral health care for infants and children through adolescence, including those with special health care needs.
2. *Oral and maxillofacial surgery*—the specialty that includes the diagnosis and surgical and nonsurgical treatment of diseases, injuries, and defects involving both the functional and esthetic aspects of the hard and soft tissues of the oral and maxillofacial region.
3. *Periodontics*—the specialty that encompasses the prevention, diagnosis, and treatment of diseases of the supporting and surrounding tissues of the teeth, or their substitutes, and the maintenance of the health, function, and esthetics of these structures and tissues.
4. *Endodontics*—the specialty that is concerned with the etiology, diagnosis, prevention, and treatment of diseases and injuries of the pulp and associated periradicular conditions.
5. *General dentistry and prosthodontics*—general dentistry encompasses the etiology, diagnosis, and treatment of conditions of oral, head, and neck tissues; the general dentist may perform procedures that encompass any or all of the dental specialty areas, depending on the training and abilities of the general dentist. Prosthodontics is a dental specialty that involves the more complicated restoration of missing teeth as well as oral and maxillofacial tissues, along with maintenance of oral functions, comfort, appearance, and patient health.

Anesthetic Considerations

Important considerations that must be part of the anesthesia treatment plan for the dental setting are outlined in Box 49-8. The patient may require minimal sedation (anxiolysis), moderate sedation and analgesia (conscious sedation), deep sedation and analgesia, or anesthesia (general anesthesia) for dental surgery. The anesthesia that is required depends on the patient-related factors of fear, anxiety, age, medical condition, level of cooperation and behavior, gagging, ineffective local anesthesia in the past, mental impairment, and physical disability. A thorough, documented patient assessment along with appropriate laboratory studies are necessary.[57-59] In pediatric dentistry a comprehensive and personalized discussion with the parent or guardian (with or without the patient present) of what the anesthetic procedure will entail, coupled with an opportunity for the parent or patient to engage in dialogue and ask questions, can alleviate the stress of the upcoming procedures for all parties.

The dental surgical area must be of adequate size, and the anesthetist must have full access to both the patient and all required equipment and supplies. Full monitors are necessary. Postoperative problems in dentistry generally are minimal but potentially can involve pain, swelling, bleeding, nausea and vomiting, the vasovagal response, airway problems, or hypoxemia as a result of anesthetic procedures other than local anesthesia administered.

Board-certified dental specialists are also trained to administer local anesthesia and are licensed by state dental boards to administer the continuum from minimal sedation to anesthesia (general anesthesia) while performing the dental surgery. The dental literature claims good success rates and safety, but caution is necessary.[60-65]

Each dental specialty has particular considerations, which are discussed in the following sections.

Pediatric Dentistry. Pediatric dentists usually require anesthesia (general anesthesia) for behaviorally uncooperative or mentally disabled patients or because of the necessity to perform all necessary dental surgery in one session. Anesthetic choices such as oral or intravenous ketamine; a mixture of oral chloral hydrate, meperidine, and hydroxyzine; intravenous diazepam; midazolam; and propofol have been used with success.[60,61,63,66,67] Premedication with oral, intranasal, or rectal midazolam can be used alone or given before general endotracheal anesthesia and has proved as effective as nitrous oxide for

BOX **49-8**

Considerations Related to Anesthesia in the Dental Setting

- Anesthesia may be administered in an unfamiliar area.
- The established airway may be shared with the dental surgeon.
- The potential exists for heavy bleeding because of the vast blood supply to the head and neck region.
- There exists the possibility of intense pain, transmitted primarily by the maxillary and mandibular divisions of the trigeminal nerve.
- Patients usually display a high level of anxiety, and adequate time must be incorporated into the schedule to allow for safe anesthetic treatment.

sedation.[67-70] Oral transmucosal fentanyl citrate has been used as an effective preoperative sedative.[71] After an inhaled mask or intravenous induction, nasal endotracheal intubation is usually performed to allow the pediatric dentist full access to the mouth. In one study 68% of children found induction to be an upsetting factor in their care.[72] Some dentists allow a secured oral endotracheal tube and are very cognizant of the importance of the airway during surgery. Typical pediatric dental procedures include restorative dentistry such as fillings and placement of stainless steel or polycarbonate crowns, pulpotomies, tooth extractions, and space maintainers. A study has shown that stainless steel crowns are more successful when the procedure is performed with the patient under general anesthesia.[73]

Oral and Maxillofacial Surgery. Procedures performed within the specialty of oral and maxillofacial surgery (OMS) are among the most invasive in dentistry. Oral surgeons perform uncovering of teeth for orthodontic treatment, extraction of impacted, severely carious, and multiple teeth, insertion of dental implants, treatment of infections of the head and neck, surgical remodeling of maxillary and mandibular alveolar bone, facial cosmetics, and removal of soft-tissue or bony tumors, as well as many other procedures. These procedures can produce both severe pain and heavy bleeding. Many OMS procedures are performed within the office setting. Oral and maxillofacial surgeons receive 6 years of postdoctoral training and become licensed by the state dental board to perform the continuum from minimal sedation to anesthesia (general anesthesia) care. Patients can have challenging physical and mental conditions; therefore a thorough preanesthetic assessment is necessary.[74] The patient's airway is shared with the oral surgeon; therefore nasal intubation may be necessary. It may be possible to perform some oral surgical procedures while carefully working around an unsecured tube or with a standard or reinforced LMA.[74-76] Local anesthesia in combination with intravenous sedation (propofol, midazolam), inhalation sedation (nitrous oxide), inhaled potent endotracheal anesthetics, and total intravenous general anesthesia are techniques available for office-based OMS.[74,77-79] Remifentanil has become a useful adjunct with the techniques listed, to counteract the intense stimulation of OMS.[80,81] The BIS monitor is also useful for careful anesthetic titration.[72,82]

Periodontics. Periodontic procedures can involve painful stimulation. Periodontists generally work in a particular quadrant of the patient's mouth and administer local anesthetic for the particular area of surgery. Periodontal treatment involves surgery of the teeth, gingiva, connective tissue, periodontal ligament, and alveolar bone, as well as insertion and maintenance of dental implants. Local anesthetics are administered with a normal epinephrine 1:100,000 concentration, unless contraindicated, along with greater than normal epinephrine concentrations (1:50,000) injected directly into the gingiva, because of its local anesthetic ability and for hemostasis. Periodontal surgery involves lengthy procedures and can be well managed with minimal sedation (both enteral or with inhalation sedation) or moderate sedation and analgesia (conscious sedation).[58] A full array of monitors is necessary. Midazolam with a propofol infusion helps achieve the goals of safety and comfort for periodontal surgical patients.[83]

Endodontics. Anesthesia for endodontic procedures is similar to that described for periodontal surgery. Local anesthesia provides adequate comfort, but in the presence of patient anxiety related to the length of endodontic procedures, minimal sedation (both enteral or with inhalation sedation) or moderate sedation and analgesia (conscious sedation) can make the procedure tolerable and less anxiety producing for the patient.

General Dentistry and Prosthodontics. General dentistry can encompass all procedures from all of the dental specialties, depending on the interest and training of the general dentist. Anesthesia can be delivered along the continuum of care to ensure safety for the patient and to fill the requirements of the particular dental procedure.[59,84,85]

Postanesthesia Care

Patients recover in a quiet, monitored environment. Intravenous access allows the titration of additional analgesia or antiemetics as necessary. Fortunately, patient morbidity from general anesthesia for dental procedures is low.[86] Patients who receive inhaled sedation are less stressed postoperatively than those who receive general anesthesia.[87]

Invasive dental procedures can be another source of distress in children, which can lead to crying, nausea, vomiting, and bleeding postoperatively.[88] The addition of the potent opioid morphine, ketorolac, or both greatly aids patient comfort in the postsurgical anesthesia recovery area. The use of oral minimal to moderate sedation in pediatric patients aged 2 to 34 months has been found to have no effect on behavior when the individual requires treatment later.[89] Adolescents who have undergone sedation for childhood dental therapy are found to possess a high level of anxiety regarding dentistry, when compared with adolescents without that history.[90]

Psychiatric Procedures

Procedure Overview

Electroconvulsive therapy (ECT) is the intentional inducement of a generalized seizure of the central nervous system for an adequate duration of time to treat patients with certain severe neuropsychiatric disorders.[91] In 2001 the American Psychiatric Association Committee on Electroconvulsive Therapy published a report approving ECT as a safe and effective treatment for severe and medication-resistant major depression, with response rates of 80% to 90% as a first-line treatment and 50% to 60% in patients unresponsive to adequate trials of antidepressant medications such as a combination of nortryptiline and lithium carbonate. Antidepressant medication administration, along with ECT, is well tolerated by patients, and both therapies can be beneficial to the patient. Major depressive disorder can occur at any age but typically begins to occur in the middle to late twenties and is ranked as the fourth leading burden of disease worldwide.[92] Symptoms develop over days to weeks and can be expressed as generalized anxiety, phobias, panic attacks, and depression.[93] Death from major depressive disorder occurs in 15% of patients, usually because of suicide.[20] Death from ECT itself is possible but is rare. ECT is also used in certain patients who experience mania, catatonia, vegetative dysregulation, inanition, suicidal drive, and schizophrenia with affective disorders.[91,92,94] Most patients receive three treatments per week and can undergo a total of 6 to 12 treatments overall.[92-94] Clinical improvement is seen within the first three to five treatments. ECT treatments exceed the total numbers of coronary revascularizations, herniorraphy, and appendectomy procedures performed in the United States.[94]

ECT is one of the most controversial and invasive treatments in medicine. The first documented use of ECT was in 1938. Early ECT was performed without anesthesia, with the occurrence of many adverse effects such as bitten tongues and broken bones and teeth. Treatment involves placement of electrodes with a conducting gel either right-sided unilaterally or bi-temporally bilaterally; an alternating current of electricity is passed through the electrodes.[91,92] Theories for the mechanism of ECT are related to profound changes in brain chemistry, such as enhancement of dopaminergic, serotonergic, and adrenergic neurotransmission. Another theory postulates the release of hypothalamic or pituitary hormones, which have antidepressant effects. Finally, ECT has anticonvulsant effects that raise the seizure threshold and decrease seizure duration, exerting a positive effect on the brain.[91]

Anesthetic Considerations

Anesthesia for ECT involves the administration of an ultrabrief general anesthetic to provide lack of consciousness to the patient for the procedure. Anesthetic medications and doses typically used are listed in Table 49-2.

A thorough preanesthetic assessment must be performed, with consideration given to the physiologic response generated by the induced seizure activity. Few absolute contraindications to ECT exist.[91] Patients with brain tumors, increased intracranial pressure, cerebral aneurysm, previous neurosurgery, skull fracture, stroke, myocardial infarction or cardiovascular disease, or neuroleptic malignant syndrome must be assessed, with the illness adequately documented to allow discussion with the treating psychiatrist.[91,94] Pheochromocytoma is an absolute contraindication to ECT. Patients may have results of laboratory studies, a pharmacologic regimen, and ECG readily available because of their psychiatric hospitalization. Informed consent is obtained whenever possible from the patient or legal guardian.

TABLE 49-2 Anesthetic Medications Used for Electroconvulsive Therapy

Drug	Dose
Anticholinergics	
Atropine	0.4-1 mg IV or IM
Glycopyrrolate	0.2-0.4 mg IV or IM
Anesthetics	
Alfentanil	0.2-0.3 mcg/kg IV
Etomidate	0.1-0.3 mg/kg IV
Ketamine	0.5-1 mg/kg IV
Methohexital	0.5-1 mg/kg IV
Propofol	0.75-1.5 mg/kg IV
Thiopental	1.5-2.5 mg/kg IV
Muscle Relaxants	
Depolarizing	
Succinylcholine	0.75-1.5 mg/kg IV
Nondepolarizing	
Atracurium	0.3-0.4 mg/kg IV (onset 6 minutes)
Mivacurium	0.1-0.2 mg/kg IV

IM, *Intramuscular;* IV, *intravenous.*
From Ding Z, White PF. Anesthesia for electroconvulsive therapy, Anesth Analg 2002;94:1351-1364.

An intravenous catheter is inserted in a peripheral vein. The patient is monitored with a pulse oximeter, ECG, noninvasive blood pressure monitor, temperature-monitoring device, and peripheral nerve stimulator. Use of $ETCO_2$ monitoring has been suggested, because hypercarbia and hypoxia shorten seizure duration. Suction, oxygen, a positive pressure Ambu bag and face mask, and rubber bite protectors must be present, as well as necessary airway and cardiovascular resuscitation equipment, medications, and supplies, as ECT is usually performed in a dedicated psychiatric suite or special treatment room.

The patient is preoxygenated before induction. Anticholinergics may be administered as an antisialagogue or to prevent asystole.[94] The induction agent is administered intravenously. Methohexital is the standard agent used for ECT. Methohexital produces rapid induction of general anesthesia, is associated with rapid recovery, and has convulsive properties because of its unique oxybarbiturate structure with a methyl radical.[95] Propofol, etomidate, thiopental, and ketamine have also been used.[96-98] Positive pressure ventilation is applied to the patient via the Ambu bag and a face mask, after loss of consciousness, and is continued until after treatment is completed and the patient is able to breathe spontaneously. The psychiatrist usually applies a tourniquet or a manual blood pressure cuff, inflated to slightly greater than the systolic blood pressure, above a lower extremity so that the muscle relaxant cannot reach the skeletal muscle in the extremity, in order to assess the duration of the induced convulsion. A rubber bite block is placed in the patient's mouth to prevent biting of the teeth, lips, and tongue, and a short-acting muscle relaxant such as succinylcholine or mivacurium is administered. Atracurium use has been described most often among the nondepolarizing relaxants.[94] A nerve stimulator must be used, and appropriate neuromuscular blockade reversal agents should be administered if necessary. The electrodes are applied, the proper waveform and current level are selected, and the electroconvulsive seizure is induced. The seizure lasts from 30 to 90 seconds; the motor seizure is shorter than the seizure duration as seen on an electroencephalogram (EEG). Use of the BIS monitor correlates with the EEG, and it can be a useful tool for the anesthetist and the psychiatrist.[99] The level of anesthesia displayed by the BIS monitor inconclusively correlates with seizure duration.[100,101] At the end of the seizure, spontaneous respirations resume, the patient is transferred to a recovery area, and vital signs are continually monitored until the patient is determined to be stable and able to be safely discharged.[91,102] Certain anesthetic medications and techniques such as hyperventilation can affect seizure duration. Box 49-9 summarizes typical anesthetic medications and techniques used in ECT and their effects on seizure duration.

Adult patients about to undergo ECT should follow fasting guidelines of at least 6 hours for solids and 2 hours for liquids.[91,94,102] Necessary bronchodilators may be taken.[102] Oral medications, such as antihypertensives, cardiac medications, anticoagulants, and thyroid medications, may be taken with a sip of water up to 1 hour before the procedure.[94,102] Rapid sequence induction of general anesthesia with applied cricoid pressure and endotracheal intubation can be performed. One must take into consideration the total number of ECT treatments to be received, weighed against the necessity for repeated intubations and the fact that most patients, even obese patients, have rarely been found to aspirate as a result of ECT.[103] The CRNA may perform a rapid-sequence induction and apply cricoid pressure until the protective reflexes return and the danger of aspiration is eliminated, rather than intubating the patient.

BOX 49-9

Common Medications and Their Effects on Seizure Duration

Medications That Can Prolong Seizure Duration
Alfentanil with methohexital or propofol
Aminophylline
Caffeine
Etomidate
Hyperventilation
Ketamine (is a proconvulsant)
Methohexital (some proconvulsant properties)
Remifentanil

Medications That Can Shorten Seizure Duration
Diltiazem
Fentanyl
Lidocaine
Lorazepam
Midazolam
Propofol
Thiamylal
Thiopental

Medications with No Apparent Effect on Seizure Duration
Clonidine
Dexmedetomidine
Esmolol (may shorten seizure duration)
Labetalol (may shorten seizure duration)
Nicardipine
Nifedipine
Nitroglycerin
Nitroprusside
Trimethaphan

Ding Z, White PF. Anesthesia for electroconvulsive therapy. Anesth Analg *2002;94:1351-1364.*

Postanesthesia Care

The intentional creation of central nervous system convulsions has profound effects on the patient's physiology. Patients usually experience temporary cognitive and memory impairment after ECT.

The first type of impairment that may be seen is postictal confusion, in which the patient is transiently restless, confused, and agitated immediately after the convulsive episode and for approximately 30 minutes. The agitation can be difficult to manage for the recovery nurse. Some patients require physical restraint or sedation with a benzodiazepine such as lorazepam or diazepam or an antipsychotic medication such as haloperidol. Researchers have recently hypothesized that high plasma lactate levels cause this agitation. The authors suggest that this is caused by inadequate neuromuscular blockade, and that increasing the dose of muscle relaxant is necessary.[94]

A second type of cognitive impairment that may be seen later is anterograde memory dysfunction, in which the patient may rapidly forget new information. The patient may not remember things that he or she does or is told in the days after ECT. Anterograde amnesia usually subsides within days or a few weeks. However, it can be frightening to the patient. A third cognitive dysfunction is retrograde memory dysfunction, which is the forgetting of memories from several weeks to several months before the ECT treatment. No evidence suggests that ECT causes any brain damage, nor does it impair the long-term ability for the patient to learn and retain new information. The cognitive effects described vary depending on the frequency and the number of ECT treatments the patient has received. The quantities of energy used to elicit the convulsions and the placement of the electrodes are also factors. Even the type of anesthetic drugs used is believed to be involved.[91-93,102]

Cardiovascular stimulation also occurs with ECT. The sympathetic and parasympathetic nervous systems are stimulated sequentially. Therefore the patient may experience an increase in heart rate and blood pressure, followed by a period of bradycardia or even asystole. This can lead to increases in myocardial oxygen demand, arrhythmias, and transient ischemic changes in susceptible individuals.[92,93] Transient cardiac changes can be managed before ECT with anticholinergics, intravenous local anesthetics such as lidocaine, or intravenous narcotics such as remifentanil.[94,105] Changes after ECT can be managed with β-blockers such as esmolol or labetalol, calcium channel blockers such as verapamil or nifedipine, or other antihypertensives such as nitroprusside or nitroglycerin.[91,94,106]

Finally, patients may also experience headache, muscle aches, or nausea. Symptoms of headache or muscle ache respond well to acetaminophen, aspirin, or nonsteroidal antiinflammatory agents such as intravenous or intramuscular ketorolac or oral ibuprofen.[93,120] Nausea can be caused by the stress and anxiety before the ECT treatment, the anesthetic agents used, the seizure itself, or air in the stomach from assisted ventilation. Nausea can be treated with agents such as ondansetron, dolasetron, granisetron, or metoclopramide.[92-94,102]

Radiologic and Diagnostic Procedures

Medical science has been able to use the sciences of physics, chemistry, and computers to produce remarkably accurate images of the internal structure and function of the body to aid medical diagnosis. Energy is transmitted to the patient and interacts with patient tissues. This energy is then detected, processed, and displayed on a computer console, which allows images to be selected for further investigation and diagnosis. These images can then be transferred to computer memory, e-mailed, printed onto paper, or printed onto x-ray or photographic film. Some medical images are created in real time and allow observation of flow or changes in tissue resulting from treatment.[107]

Procedure Overviews

Computed Tomography. The first computed tomography (CT) scanner was introduced in 1972. CT uses x-rays generated from a rotating anode x-ray generator. The patient is placed supine on a flat, wooden, wheeled platform and moved inside the scanning gantry. X-rays are then projected through the patient at different angles. The X-rays penetrate tissues differently according to the atomic numbers of the atoms within the tissue. Dense tissue such as bone attenuates (reduces the energy of) the x-ray beam more than less-dense tissue such as muscle. The patient images are then detected, and the computer acquires the image data. Finally, an image analyzer projects the analyzed data in the form of a tomogram or body section slice onto an operator console and a physician-viewing console. CT is excellent for imaging bone. The diagnostic quality of a CT scan is enhanced with the injection of intravenous contrast media (ICM).[108] Contrast media containing iodine may be administered to the patient enterally or parenterally to further attenuate the x-ray beam to enhance the images for CT vascular or gastrointestinal studies.[107,108]

Magnetic Resonance Imaging. Magnetic resonance imaging (MRI) uses the dipole moment (the ability of the atomic nucleus to behave as a magnet) of the hydrogen atom. Hydrogen is a simple atom that contains one proton and one electron. Hydrogen is selected because 70% to 85% of most cells of the human body contain water.[109] The patient is placed supine within the scanning gantry or bore of the magnet. The magnet used for MRI can be a permanent magnet or a powerful superconducting electromagnet cooled with liquid helium to 4° Kelvin. Magnetic strength is measured in tesla (T). 1 T is equivalent to 10,000 gauss or oersted. (The unit *gauss* has been renamed the *oersted*, so that 1 gauss is equal to 1 oersted.) MRI magnets generate field strengths of 0.3 to 4 T. The spin of the electron in hydrogen will align the hydrogen atoms parallel to this powerful magnetic field. The patient's water-containing tissues are then excited with variable radiofrequencies. After the proton in hydrogen receives this radiofrequency energy, it emits radiofrequency energy with three-dimensional–appearing spatial information. This information is then detected and analyzed by the computer and displayed on viewing consoles. MRI images can also be stored in computer memory, e-mailed, and printed onto x-ray or photographic film.[30,107] MRI technology now allows its use within the operating room with an open bore, portable, 0.12-T low-intensity magnet to assist the neurosurgeon with diagnostic decisions.[109] Contrast media are also used in MRI studies to enhance the patient's tissues and allow the scan to provide further diagnostic information. MRI contrast uses the element gadolinium bound as a chelated structure and administered primarily parenterally but rarely enterally.[110,111]

Interventional Radiology (Vascular and Nonvascular) and Radiotherapy or Radiosurgery. Interventional radiology (IR) involves minimally invasive procedures and therapies performed by radiologists, especially in patients at high medical risk.[12,112,113] Major IR therapies include angiography, the embolization of blood vessels such as arteriovenous malformations or for epistaxis, the delivery of chemical or physical vascular occlusive devices, the removal of thrombi, ablation of aneurysms, and angioplasty of blood vessels with stent placement.[12] See Chapter 23 for a discussion of interventional vascular surgery.

Radiation is a treatment itself for both benign tumors (low-grade astrocytoma, meningioma, pituitary adenoma, craniopharyngioma, schwannoma, pineocytoma, chemodectoma, low-grade papillary neoplasms) and aggressive tumors (germinoma, primitive neuroectodermal tumor, chorodoma, intermediate-grade pineal tumor, immature teratoma, undifferentiated sarcoma, anaplastic oligoastrocytoma, and metastatic tumors). Radiation surgery is the delivery of a single massive dose of radiation to the target tissue. Radiation therapy is the delivery of smaller doses of radiation over several sessions. Gamma radiation is used for radiotherapy and radiosurgery. The gamma radiation is produced by either a gamma knife, using beams from the radioactive decay of cobalt 60 or from gamma rays from a linear accelerator.

Interventional Neuroradiology. Interventional neuroradiology (INR) is the diagnosis and treatment of central nervous system diseases endovascularly to deliver therapeutic medications or devices.[112] INR was first used in the early 1980s, when digital subtraction angiography was developed.[114] Digital subtraction angiography first uses an original angiograph of the blood vessels to be studied. Then a contrast medium is injected into the same blood vessels, and opaque structures such as bone and tissues can be digitally subtracted or removed from the angiographic image, leaving a clear picture of the blood vessels.[107]

Improvements in vascular access techniques, new thin and flexible catheters and guide wires, and the development of innovative coils and therapeutic medications have made new treatments possible. Conditions that once required extensive surgery with accompanying patient morbidity and mortality can now be performed less invasively.[115] Some major procedures performed with INR are mechanical or chemical removal of emboli or thrombi that cause stroke, the physical occlusion of malformed vascular structures such as an arteriovenous malformations with chemicals or flow-directed balloons, dilation of stenotic blood vessels, and embolization (blocking blood flow) of cerebral vascular aneurysms using catheter-deployed coils.[115-118]

Box 49-10 lists some current uses for each of the above radiologic and diagnostic procedures. As technology advances, more uses will be seen in the future.

Anesthetic Considerations

Computed Tomography. CT scans require that the patient remain as motionless as possible for several minutes to an hour. Patient motion can produce artifacts in the diagnostic images to be read by the radiologist. Patients must lie on a flat, relatively hard wheeled platform, which is rolled into the short bore scanning gantry of the CT scanner. Although the majority of patients are able to cooperate and tolerate CT, others may not be able to cooperate because of extremes in age, concurrent medical conditions, or mental disability. The CT scan is neither physically invasive nor painful and is more rapidly performed than an MRI scan, especially if a spiral CT scanner is used.

The patient may require anesthesia anywhere along the continuum from minimal sedation (anxiolysis) to anesthesia (general anesthesia). Use of ferromagnetic anesthesia equipment and supplies around the CT scanner is not a concern. A standard anesthesia machine, laryngoscope and blades, and intravenous infusion pumps can be used as if in the operating room. An LMA is an appropriate alternative choice as a minimally invasive and secure airway in the patient without contraindications to its use. An LMA is contraindicated in patients with gastroesophageal reflux disease or a full stomach. Attention must be paid to securing the airway, and the anesthesia breathing circuit, the leads for the ECG, the noninvasive blood pressure cuff, the intravenous line, and the pulse oximeter must extend into the scanning gantry.

Sedation can be performed with a variety of agents, including midazolam, chloral hydrate, pentobarbital, diazepam, or propofol. General anesthesia can be performed with TIVA, such as with intravenous propofol, or with potent inhaled agents.

All personnel must be aware of the use of ionizing radiation during the CT scan and should take precautions to be shielded from any exposure to the radiation. Radiation exposure is

BOX 49-10

Some Indications for Radiologic and Diagnostic Procedures

Computed Tomography
Assessment of the airway with neck or thoracic tumors
Assessment of bony trauma especially the spine
Assessment of head trauma
Assessment of increased intracranial pressure
Assessment of neoplasms
Imaging of brain tumors
Imaging of intracerebral hemorrhage

Magnetic Resonance Imaging
Angiography
Central nervous system imaging
Imaging of the blood-brain barrier
Kidney imaging
Liver imaging
Urinary bladder imaging

Interventional Radiology (Vascular and Nonvascular), Radiotherapy, and Radiosurgery
Catheterization of ducts, vascular lesions, and tumors for: delivery of chemotherapy directly to tumors
Embolization or embolectomy or thrombofragmentation of vascular lesions and tumors (pulmonary thrombi or emboli)
Transluminal dilatation, angioplasty, and stent insertion for vascular stenosis or biliary stenosis
Radiotherapy
Radiosurgery

Interventional Neuroradiology
Intracranial aneurysm ablation
Brain arteriovenous malformation embolization
Dural arteriovenous malformation embolization
Carotid cavernous fistula and vertebral fistula treatment
Vein of Galen malformation treatment
Spinal cord lesion embolization
Carotid test occlusion
Therapeutic carotid occlusion
Balloon angioplasty of cerebral vasospasm
Sclerotherapy of venous angiomas
Angioplasty and stent placement for an atherosclerotic lesion
Thrombolysis of acute thromboembolic stroke
Embolization of highly vascularized intracranial tumors
Meningioma treatment
Juvenile nasopharyngeal angiofibroma treatment
Glomus tumor treatment

cumulative over a lifetime, and every precaution must be made to protect oneself from any unnecessary doses of radiation, which can cause genetic mutation and may lead to cancer.

ICM can cause an unexpected allergic reaction in some patients, varying from itching with hives to severe, life-threatening anaphylactoid and anaphylactic reactions that have lead to patient death.[108,119-122] ICM can also cause renal toxicity as well as local tissue damage if the ICM extravasates from the vein into the surrounding tissue.[119] ICM are water-soluble iodine-containing solutions of two available types: media that can dissociate into ions in solution and media that will remain in a neutral state in solution. ICM is also formulated as high-osmolar contrast media (HOCM), which contain few dissolved particles and iodine atoms, and low-osmolar contrast media (LOCM), which contain greater numbers of dissolved particles with iodine. An HOCM solution causes fluid shift from the cell to the vein with the ICM, whereas an LOCM solution is closely isoosmolar, inducing less fluid shift from the cell.[108] Nonionized LOCM is a more costly contrast medium for the patient. Some advocate that it should be the only contrast medium used for CT with dye studies.[119]

Reactions are possible with either type of ICM solution, although fewer reactions occur with LOCM.[119,123] Some reactions may present anywhere from one half hour to one week after the administration of the ICM. Reactions to ICM are theorized to be caused by the ICM molecule's serving as an antigen and affixing itself to either mast cells or basophils. This causes release of mediators such as histamine and tryptase, which can inhibit coagulation, dilate blood vessels, release complement, or even stimulate an IgE-modulated immune reaction.[108,120]

A thorough preanesthetic assessment for a patient about to undergo CT should include questions pertaining to asthma, allergies, and any previous reactions to any contrast media. Other patients at risk for reactions to ICM are patients with multiple medical problems, especially those with cardiac disease or with preexisting azotemia, patients of advanced age, and patients being treated with nephrotoxic agents such as the aminoglycoside antimicrobials gentamicin, tobramicin, streptomycin, amikacin, kanamycin, and neomycin or nonsteroidal antiinflammatory agents. ICM is contraindicated in pregnant patients.[95,119]

Clinicians may use preventive measures in patients who may be at risk for a reaction to ICM. The radiologist should use the smallest amount of contrast agent necessary. In order to safeguard against the possibility of renal failure, the patient should be adequately hydrated beginning 1 hour before the procedure and continuing for another 24 hours. Patients who are at risk for possible anaphylactoid reactions should be pretreated with corticosteroids such as methylprednisolone or prednisone administered by mouth or intravenously. In cases of moderate or severe previous ICM reactions a histamine-1 (H_1) blocker such as diphenhydramine and an H_2-blocker such as cimetidine or ranitidine should be given together either intravenously or by mouth.[108,119]

Extravasation of ICM into tissue can cause the sloughing of tissue and tissue necrosis, which are treated by elevation of the limb, along with the application of ice packs or a heating pad as necessary.

Anaphylactoid and anaphylactic reactions are rapidly life threatening and must be promptly recognized and treated. As little as 1 ml of ICM can initiate these reactions. Control of the airway is imperative. Treatments for anaphylactoid or anaphylactic reactions are listed in Box 49-11. The goals of treatment for anaphylactoid or anaphylactic reaction are to provide an airway, increase heart rate and contractility, and support blood pressure.[119,124]

Magnetic Resonance Imaging. MRI can take up to an hour. During this time the patient must remain extremely still in order to reduce motion artifacts. These artifacts can cause unfaithful representations of the tissues being studied. The

BOX **49-11**

Treatments for Anaphylactoid or Anaphylactic Reactions

Remember that this is a crisis situation and that immediate response is imperative.

Mild Allergic Reactions

Discontinue the causative agent
Administer diphenhydramine 50-100 mg IV

Moderate to Severe Reactions

Terminate administration of the causative agent
Administer 100% O_2 with ventilatory support
Discontinue all anesthetic medications
Administer a wide-open massive fluid bolus
Administer α-adrenergic agents as necessary to reverse severe hypotension:
- Epinephrine in 5- to 10-mcg boluses or as an intravenous drip of 0.05-0.1 mcg/kg/min titrated to effect an acceptable blood pressure
- Norepinephrine drip of 0.5-30 mcg/min IV for systolic BP <70 torr
- Dopamine 5-15 mcg/kg/min IV for systolic BP 70-100 torr with signs and symptoms of shock
- Dobutamine 2-20 mcg/kg/min IV for systolic BP 70-100 torr with no signs or symptoms of shock

Administer bronchodilators as necessary
- Aminophylline 5-6 mg/kg

Corticosteroids have been shown to have some positive effect in treatment of bronchospasm but have not been shown to be of help in an acute anaphylactoid or anaphylactic reaction

BP, *Blood pressure;* IV, *intravenous;* O_2, *oxygen.*

motions of breathing, the heart, blood flow, swallowing, and even cerebral spinal fluid flow produce artifacts in a highly sensitive MRI scan.

Patients must remain within the bore of the magnet for an MRI scan for longer periods of time than for a CT scan. During this time the MRI suite's ambient temperature is cold.

The patient is exposed to varying magnetic fields of up to 4 T, along with additional exposure to variable radiofrequency radiation. Blood flow is decreased by strong magnetic fields, and blood pressure compensates by rising. Patients also have reported symptoms of vertigo, nausea, headache, and visual sensations.[107]

The MRI machine produces loud vibratory and knocking noises as coils are switched on and off during the course of the study. The size of the MRI magnet bore may preclude the morbidly obese from MRI scanning, although a more open bore MRI is now available.

Most patients are content with an explanation of what to expect during the procedure and reassurance. Some patients need minimal or moderate sedation. Patients with claustrophobia or those who cannot or will not remain motionless during the study, as well as critically ill patients, may require deep sedation or general endotracheal anesthesia.[12,107,125-127] MRI is not painful, so opioids are not usually be required. Sedation has been performed with oral and intravenous midazolam, ketamine, pentobarbital, chloral hydrate, and propofol.[12,120,126,128,129] Minimal sedation requires full monitoring. Deep sedation or general anesthesia requires intravenous access and full monitoring. The LMA has served as an excellent, relatively noninvasive airway for MRI. Some anesthesia providers prefer general endotracheal intubation.[12] Manufacturers have developed an open-coil magnet for MRI, which has had a positive impact in those patients who could not tolerate MRI within the traditional closed bore magnet.[121] Children who cannot or will not cooperate experience better MRI scans with general endotracheal anesthesia in shorter periods of time, despite longer recovery times, when compared with sedation.[125-127]

Because of the intense magnetic field always present in the MRI suite, anesthesia providers must be aware of *every* item on their persons and every item that is to be used in conjunction with anesthesia administered to the patient. Ferromagnetic (iron-containing) substances are attracted at astonishing rates of speed into the bore of the magnet. Personal items such as pens, certain types of eyeglasses, jewelry, watches, pagers, personal computers, calculators, name badges, coins, audiotapes, videotapes, and credit cards are some of the items that should never enter the MRI suite, as well as any ferromagnetic anesthesia equipment, medication vials, and supplies. If a patient were present within the bore of the MRI, injury or death could be possible from the missile created.[130]

Certain patients may be prohibited from an MRI scan, such as those with cardiac pacemakers; AICDs; metallic aneurysm clips; cochlear implants; certain mechanical heart valves; internal plates, wires, or screws; shrapnel and metal fragments; permanent eyeliner; and certain metallic implants and prostheses.[107] Further investigation into the metal content of some of these may be necessary.

Manufacturers have developed a host of MRI-compatible anesthesia equipment and supplies, many of which are listed in Box 49-12. This host of equipment and supplies allows performance of the anesthetic procedure directly within the MRI

BOX **49-12**

List of Available MRI-Compatible Equipment and Supplies

- MRI-compatible anesthesia machine
- Pulse oximeter
- Intravenous bag pole
- Liquid crystal temperature monitoring strip
- Respiratory rate monitor
- Noninvasive blood pressure monitor
- Pulse oximeter
- Electrocardiograph
- Electrocardiograph patches
- Electrocardiograph cable
- Capnograph
- Laryngoscope with lithium batteries and aluminum spacers
- Laryngoscope blades
- Nerve stimulator
- Intravenous infusion pump
- Oxygen tanks
- Precordial stethoscope
- Esophageal stethoscope
- Patient carts
- Tables and trays

suite. Be aware that some equipment designated by the manufacturer as MRI compatible may not be compatible as magnet strengths increase.[130]

Facilities that cannot afford MRI-compatible equipment and supplies can provide anesthetic services to their patients by inducing anesthesia outside the MRI suite. With the aid of extra-long circuits, extension intravenous tubing, and properly insulated monitor cables, the anesthesia can be maintained with full monitors and a standard anesthetic machine outside the MRI suite. Attention should be paid to isolate any monitor leads or intravenous tubing from the skin of the patient. Any monitor leads and intravenous tubing should be kept in straight alignment, because the intense magnetic fields in the MRI suite can induce current flow and severely burn the patient. Flexible LMAs and endotracheal tubes that contain wire windings can also be sources of burns.

Consideration must be given to the MRI contrast media administered to patients. Fortunately, the dyes used for MRI contrast are nonionic gadolinium chelates and have extremely low allergy rates.[107,110,111] Nausea is a common side effect. Urticaria (hives) and anaphylactoid reactions occur in <1% of patients.[110] The risk of a reaction to MRI dye is increased in patients with a history of asthma or other allergies or drug sensitivities, especially to iodinated contrast dyes.[110,111] Proper equipment, medications, and supplies must be immediately available for management of a reaction if one occurs. Treatments for anaphylactoid and anaphylactic reactions are discussed in Box 49-11.

Although MRI does not use ionizing radiation, patients and personnel are exposed to constant levels of magnetic force while in the MRI suite. Acute exposure to magnetic fields <2.5 T have not been shown to have adverse effects in humans. All care providers must make their own determinations regarding how much magnetic exposure they will accept during a patient's MRI scan. Doses both to the patient and to all personnel should be minimized.[107] If the anesthesia provider is away from the patient during the procedure, it should be ensured that all airway circuitry, monitoring leads, and intravenous connections are secure and tight. A respiratory monitoring apparatus (RMA) built into the anesthesia circuit reservoir bag, will soon be available to monitor respiration with both visual and audible signals pertaining to movement of the RMA relative to the patient's respiratory rate and tidal volume.[131]

Interventional Radiology (Vascular and Nonvascular), Radiotherapy, Radiosurgery, Interventional Neuroradiology. As skills, techniques, and technology progress, more procedures will be performed with radiation or under radiologic guidance.[112-114] These procedures all require the absolute immobility of the patient, with periods of controlled apnea, which assist in the viewing or treatment of the targeted area of the patient, especially during whole-body therapeutic radiation treatment.[12,113,132] These procedures are also time consuming, taking up to several hours to complete. Procedures may be necessary in patients who are infants to those who are geriatric and in patients with more coexisting disease than those who undergo diagnostic scans only.[12,112] A thorough preanesthetic assessment is imperative.[112]

Procedures for INR are painful, are physically invasive to the patient, and may need to be accomplished over several treatment sessions. Patients may require anesthesia along the continuum from minimal or moderate sedation, with the trend moving toward anesthesia (general). Full monitors and intravenous access are required.[12,132] Additional catheterization and monitoring of arterial pressure and central venous pressure may be necessary.[12,112] Certain procedures require monitoring of the patient's neurophysiologic status for changes. The patient may also need to be assessed awake and then resedated at times during the procedure.[12,112,132] Anesthetics that can be used are midazolam, propofol, ketamine, isoflurane, and the other potent inhaled general anesthetics.[12,133]

It may be necessary to manipulate systemic or regional blood flow with deliberate hypertension or deliberate hypotension, manage anticoagulation, and manage unexpected procedural complications.[12,132]

Complications can occur rapidly and can be life threatening. Foremost is the possible complication of hemorrhage. A sedated patient experiencing hemorrhage may show sudden signs of headache, nausea and vomiting, and vascular pain. A patient under general anesthesia may experience sudden bradycardia. The airway must be secured first if necessary, followed by support of the cardiovascular system, discontinuation of heparin, and administration of protamine (1 mg/100 units of total heparin dose administered). Other possible complications are radiocontrast reactions, embolization of particles or tissue, perforation of an aneurysm, and obliteration of unintended physiologically necessary arteries.[12,132] Complications may necessitate the safe transfer of the patient to the operating room.

Postanesthesia Care

Physiologic stability is the goal in any patient undergoing a radiologic or diagnostic procedure. The patient must be observed for possible reactions to dyes administered by the radiologist. The patient must be relieved of pain. Cardiovascular status must be stable. Hospital admission may be necessary for observation after any complication experienced by the patient or suspected to have occurred. One should always err on the side of patient safety and patient welfare.

SUMMARY

New procedures and patient treatments are evolving and moving out of the traditional operating room. This demands evolution of anesthesia providers, anesthesia materiel, and techniques for the provision of anesthesia services to patients in need of such service. Those providing anesthesia for therapeutic and diagnostic procedures should adhere to the same standards of care in a remote location as they would in the operating room. An anesthetic procedure should be performed only when the provider is absolutely comfortable that all required equipment, medications, and supplies are available, as would be true in a typical, fully equipped operating room. It is easier and safer to prepare beforehand than to gather the items needed for safe anesthesia delivery later or go without them. Cases of minor surgery (patient interventions) exist, but cases of minor anesthesia do not.

Acknowledgments

I would like to acknowledge Anita Schwartz; David Brodsky; Jarad Schwartz; Colin Schwartz; Christina Sullivan at the Bernard Becker Medical Library of Washington University, St Louis, Missouri; Michael Campese and Sophie McCrary at the Medical Library; and St. Clair Anesthesia, Ltd, St Elizabeth's Hospital, Belleville, Illinois for their assistance in the preparation of this chapter.

REFERENCES

1. Kotob F, Twersky RF. Anesthesia outside the operating room: general overview and monitoring standards. *Int Anesthesiol Clin.* 2003;41:1-15.
2. Saissy JM. Simplified use of mixed propofol and alfentanil for anesthesia in remote locations. *Mil Med,* 2000;165:195-199.
3. Van de Velde M. Pediatric anesthesia and sedation in remote locations. *Acta Anaesthesiol Belg.* 2001;52:187-190.
4. Standards for office-based anesthesia practice. Available at American Association of Nurse Anesthetist website: http://www.aana.com/crna/prof/obstandards.asp Accessed May 20, 2004.
5. Guidelines for office-based anesthesia. Available at American Society of Anesthesiologist website: http://www.asahq.org/publicationsAndServices/standards/12.HTM. Accessed May 20, 2004.
6. American Society of Anesthesiologists Task Force on Postanesthetic Care. Practice guidelines for postanesthetic care. *Anesthesiology.* 2002;96:742-752.
7. Mannino MJ. Legal aspects of nurse anesthesia practice. *Nurs Clin North Am.* 1996;31:581-589.
8. Wiener-Kronish JP, Gropper MA. *Conscious Sedation.* Philadelphia: Hanley & Belfus; 2001:31-43, 45-57, 89-103, 105-115, 135-142.
9. Joint Commission on Accreditation of Healthcare Organizations. *2003 Comprehensive Accreditation Manual for Hospitals. The Official Handbook.* Oakbrook Terrace, Ill: JCAHO; 2003.
10. Tunajek SK. Matters of practice: JCAHO massive standards overhaul coming in 2004. *AANA News Bull.* 2003;June:11.
11. Kaplan RF, Yang CI. Sedation and analgesia in pediatric patients for procedures outside the operating room. *Anesthesiol Clin North Am.* 2002;20:181-194.
12. Osborn IP. Anesthesia for diagnostic and interventional radiology, *American Society of Anesthesiologists annual meeting refresher course lectures,* 145:pp 1-4, October 2002.
13. Kinder Ross A, Eck JB. Office-based anesthesia for children, *Anesthesiol Clin North America,* 2002;20:195-210.
14. Kirby RR, et al. *Clinical Anesthesia Practice.* 2nd ed. Philadelphia: Saunders; 2002:1-22.
15. Tonner PH, Kampen J, Scholz J. Pathophysiological changes in the elderly. *Best Pract Res Clin Anaesthesiol.* 2003;17:163-177.
16. Guyton AC, Hall JE. *Textbook of Medical Physiology.* 9th ed. Philadelphia: Saunders; 2000:815-821.
17. Goldberger JJ. Prevention of sudden cardiac death. *Heart Dis.* 2000 Jul-Aug;2(4):305-313.
18. Pinto DS, Josephson ME. Sudden Cardiac Death. In *Hurst's The Heart*: Fuster V, Alexander RW, O'Rourke RA, eds. 10th ed. New York: McGraw-Hill, 2004:1051-1078.
19. Bleasdale, RA, Ruskin JN, O'Callaghan PA. The Implantable Cardioverter Defibrillator. In *Hurst's The Heart*: Fuster V, Alexander RW, O'Rourke RA, eds. 11th ed. New York: McGraw-Hill, 2004:989-1002.
20. Knight BP, Pelosi F, Flemming M, Morady F, Strickberger SA. Effect of general anesthesia on the defibrillation energy requirement in patients undergoing defibrillator implantation. *J Interv Card Electrophysiol.* 1999;3:325-328.
21. Olgin JE, Zipes DP. Specific Arrythmia: Diagnosis and Treatment. In *Heart Disease: A Textbook of Cardiovascular Medicine.* Braunwald E, Zipes DP, Libby P, eds. 6th ed. Philadelphia: WB Saunders, 2001:815-889.
22. Baker GW, Sleigh JW, Smith P. Electroencephalographic indices related to hypnosis and amnesia during propofol anaesthesia for cardioversion. *Anaesth Intensive Care.* 2000;28: 386-391.
23. James S, Broome IJ. Anaesthesia for cardioversion. *Anaesthesia.* 2003;58:291-292.
24. Blaufox AD, Saul JP. Radiofrequency ablation of right-sided accessory pathways in pediatric patients. *Prog Pediatr Cardiol.* 2001;13:25-40.
25. Manolis AS, Vassilikos V, Maounis TN, Chiladakis J, Cokkinos DV. Radiofrequency ablation in pediatric and adult patients: comparative results. *J Interv Card Electrophysiol.* 2001;5:443-453.
26. Etheridge SP. Radiofrequency catheter ablation of left-sided accessory pathways in pediatric patients. *Prog Pediatr Cardiol.* 2001;13:11-24.
27. Kugler JD, Danford DA, Houston KA, Felix G. Pediatric radiofrequency catheter ablation registry success, fluoroscopy time, and complication rate for supraventricular tachycardia: comparison of early and recent eras. *J Cardiovasc Electrophysiol.* 2002;13:336-341.
28. Erb TO, Kanter RJ, Hall JM, Gan TJ, Kern FH, Schulman SR. Comparison of electrophysiologic effects of propofol and isoflurane-based anesthetics in children undergoing radiofrequency catheter ablation for supraventricular tachycardia. *Anesthesiology.* 2002;96:1386-1394.
29. Lai LP, Lin JL, Wu MH, et al. Usefulness of intravenous propofol anesthesia for radiofrequency catheter ablation in patients with tachyarrhythmias: infeasibility for pediatric patients with ectopic atrial tachycardia. *Pacing Clin Electrophysiol.* 1999;22:1358-1364.
30. Erb TO, Hall JM, Ing RJ, et al. Postoperative nausea and vomiting in children and adolescents undergoing radiofrequency catheter ablation: a randomized comparison of propofol- and isoflurane-based anesthetics. *Anesth Analg.* 2002;95:1577-1581.
31. Waye JD, Williams CB. Colonoscopy and Flexible Sigmoidoscopy. In *Textbook of Gastroenterology.* Yamada T, ed. Philadelphia: Lippincott Williams & Wilkins; 2003:2851-2865.
32. Naughton NN, Cohen SE. Nonobstetric Surgery During Pregnancy. In *Obstetric Anesthesia.* Chestnut DH, ed. 3rd ed: Philadelphia: Elsevier-Mosby, 2004:255-274.
33. Theodorou T, Hales P, Gillespie P, Robertson B. Total intravenous versus inhalational anaesthesia for colonoscopy: a prospective study of clinical recovery and psychomotor function. *Anaesth Intensive Care.* 2001;29:124-136.
34. Leslie K, Absalom, A, Kenny GN. Closed loop control of sedation for colonoscopy using the Bispectral Index. *Anaesthesia.* 2002;57:693-697.
35. Soma Y, Saito H, Kishibe T, Takahashi T, Tanaka H, Munakata A. Evaluation of topical pharyngeal anesthesia for upper endoscopy including factors associated with patient tolerance. *Gastrointest Endosc.* 2001;53:14-18.
36. Swaroop VS. Topical pharyngeal anesthesia for upper gastrointestinal endoscopy. *Am J Gastroenterol.* 2000;95:1360.
37. Davis DE, Jones MP, Kubik CM. Topical pharyngeal anesthesia does not improve upper gastrointestinal endoscopy in conscious sedated patients. *Am J Gastroenterol.* 1999;94:1853-1856.
38. Conlong P, Rees W. The use of hypnosis in gastroscopy: a comparison with intravenous sedation. *Postgrad Med J.* 1999;75:223-225.
39. Draganov P, Cotton PB. Iodinated contrast sensitivity in ERCP. *Am J Gastroenterol.* 2000;95:1398-1401.
40. Raymondos K, Panning B, Bachem I, Manns MP, piepenbrock S, Meier PN. Evaluation of endoscopic retrograde cholangiopancreatography under conscious sedation and general anesthesia. *Endoscopy.* 2002;34:721-726.
41. Cocking JB, Ferguson A, Mukherjee SK, Giancola G. Short-acting general anaesthesia facilitates therapeutic ERCP in frail elderly patients with benign extra-hepatic biliary disease. *Eur J Gastroenterol Hepatol.* 2000;12:451-454.
42. Kaddu R, Bhattacharya D, Metriyakool K, Thomas R, Tolia V. Propofol compared with general anesthesia for pediatric GI endoscopy: is propofol better? *Gastrointest Endosc.* 2002;55:27-32.
43. Sabra S, Kerner B, Latimer JS. Oxygen saturation during esophagogastroduodenoscopy in children: general anesthesia versus intravenous sedation. *J Pediatr Gastroenterol Nutr.* 1999;28:455.
44. Koh JL, Black DD, Leatherman IK, Harrison RD, Schmitz ML. Experience with an anesthesiologist interventional model for endoscopy in a pediatric hospital. *J Pediatr Gastroenterol Nutr.* 2001;33:314-318.

45. Hammer GB, Litalien C, Wellis V, Drover DR. Determination of the median effective concentration (EC50) of propofol during esophagogastroduodenoscopy in children. *Paediatr Anaesth.* 2001;11:549-553.
46. Rich JB, Yaster M, Brandt J. Anterograde and retrograde memory in children anesthetized with propofol. *J Clin Exp Neuropsychol.* 1999;21:535-546.
47. Bouchut JC. Deep sedation for upper gastrointestinal endoscopy in children. *J Pediatr Gastroenterol Nutr.* 2001;32:108.
48. Speroff L, Glass RH, Kase NG. *Clinical Gynecologic Endocrinology and Infertility.* 6th ed. Baltimore: Lippincott Williams & Wilkins; 1999:1133-1148.
49. Kim WO, Kil HK, Koh SO, Kim JI. Effects of general and locoregional anesthesia on reproductive outcome for in vitro fertilization: a meta-analysis. *J Korean Med Sci.* 2000;15:68-72.
50. Cunningham FG, Gan NF, Leveno KJ, Gilstrap LC, Hauth JC, Wenstrom KD. Ectopic Pregnancy. *Williams Obstetrics.* 21st ed. New York: McGraw-Hill; 2001:16, 771, 883-911.
51. Tsen LC, Schultz R, Martin R, Datta S, Bader AM. Intrathecal low-dose bupivacaine versus lidocaine for in vitro fertilization procedures. *Reg Anesth Pain Med.* 2001;26:52-56.
52. Pellicano M, Zullo F, Fiorentino A, Tommaselli GA, Palomba S, Nappi C. Conscious sedation versus general anaesthesia for mini laparoscopic gamete intra-Fallopian transfer: a prospective randomized study. *Hum Reprod.* 2001;16:2295-2297.
53. Martin R, Tsen LC, Tzeng G, Hornstein MD, Datta S. Anesthesia for in vitro fertilization: the addition of fentanyl to 1.5% lidocaine. *Anesth Analg.* 1999;88:523-526.
54. Eige S, Pritts EA, Palter SF, Olive DL. Anesthesia for office endoscopy. *Obstet Gynecol Clin North Am.* 1999;26:99-108.
55. Manski RJ, Moeller JF, Maas WR. Dental services: an analysis of utilization over 20 years. *J Am Dent Assoc.* 2001;132: 655-663.
56. Brown LJ, Lazar V. Dental care utilization: how saturated is the patient market? *J Am Dent Assoc.* 1999;130:573-580.
57. Haug RH, Reifeis RL. Prospective evaluation of the value of preoperative laboratory testing for office anesthesia and sedation. *J Oral Maxillofac Surg.* 1999;57:16-20.
58. Committee on Research, Science and Therapy, the American Academy of Periodontology. Guidelines: in-office use of conscious sedation in periodontics. *J Periodontol.* 2001;72: 968-975.
59. Ghezzi EM, Chavez EM, Ship JA. General anesthesia protocol for the dental patient: emphasis for older adults. *Spec Care Dentist.* 2000;20:81-92.
60. Manley MCG, Skelly, AM, Hamilton AG. Dental treatment for people with challenging behaviour: general anaesthesia or sedation. *Br Dent J.* 2000;188:358-360.
61. Leelataweedwud P, Vann WF. Adverse events and outcomes of conscious sedation for pediatric patients: study of an oral sedation regimen. *J Am Dent Assoc.* 2001;132:1531-1539.
62. Challen PD. Intra-venous sedation. *Br Dent J.* 1999;186:368.
63. Webb MD, Moore PA. Sedation for pediatric dental patients. *Dent Clin North Am.* 2002;46:803-814.
64. Cote CJ, Karl HW, Notterman DA, Weinberg JA, McCloskey C. Adverse sedation events in pediatrics: analysis of medications used for sedation. *Pediatrics.* 2000;106:633-644.
65. Cote CJ, Notterman DA, Karl HW, Weinberg JA, McCloskey C. Adverse sedation events in pediatrics: a critical incident analysis of contributing factors. *Pediatrics.* 2000;105:805-814.
66. Wilson S, Easton J, Lamb K, Orchardson R, Casamassimo P. A retrospective study of chloral hydrate, meperidine, hydroxyzine, and midazolam regimens used to sedate children for dental care. *Pediatr Dent.* 2000;22:107-112.
67. Bergman SA. Ketamine: review of its pharmacology and its use in pediatric anesthesia. *Anesth Prog.* 1999;46:10-20.
68. Wilson KE, Welbury RR, Girdler NM. A randomised, controlled, crossover trial of oral midazolam and nitrous oxide for paediatric dental sedation. *Anaesthesia.* 2002;57:860-867.
69. al-Rakaf H, Bello LL, Turkustani A, Adenubi JO. Intra-nasal midazolam in conscious sedation of young paediatric dental patients. *Int J Paediatr Dent.* 2001;11:33-40.
70. Jensen B, Matsson L. Oral versus rectal midazolam as a preanaesthetic sedative in children receiving dental treatment under general anaesthesia. *Acta Paediatr.* 2002;91:920-925.
71. Moore PA, Cuddy MA, Magera JA, Caputo AC, Chen AH, Wilkinson LA. Oral transmucosal fentanyl pretreatment for outpatient general anesthesia. *Anesth Prog.* 2000;47:29-34.
72. Vinckier F, Gizani S, Declerck D. Comprehensive dental care for children with rampant caries under general anaesthesia. *Int J Paediatr Dent.* 2001;11:25-32.
73. Al-Eheideb AA, Herman NG. Outcomes of dental procedures performed on children under general anesthesia. *J Clin Pediatr Dent.* 2003;27:181-183.
74. Ganzberg SI, Weaver JM. Anesthesia for office-based oral and maxillofacial surgery. *Dent Clin North Am.* 1999;43:547-562.
75. George JM, Sanders GM. The reinforced laryngeal mask in paediatric outpatient dental surgery. *Anaesthesia.* 1999;54:546-551.
76. Todd DW. A comparison of endotracheal intubation and use of the laryngeal mask airway for ambulatory oral surgery patients. *J Oral Maxillofac Surg.* 2002;60:2-4.
77. Cillo JE. Propofol anesthesia for outpatient oral and maxillofacial surgery. *Oral Surg Oral Med Oral Pathol Oral Radiol Endod.* 1999;87:530-538.
78. Fujii Y, Uemura A, Nakano M. Small dose of propofol for preventing nausea and vomiting after third molar extraction. *J Oral Maxillofac Surg.* 2002;60:1246-1249.
79. Leitch JA, Sutcliffe N, Kenny GN. Patient-maintained sedation for oral surgery using a target-controlled infusion of propofol—a pilot study. *Br Dent J.* 2003;194:43-45.
80. Ganzberg S, Pape RA, Beck FM. Remifentanil for use during conscious sedation in outpatient oral surgery. *J Oral Maxillofac Surg.* 2002;60:244-250.
81. Pendeville PE, Kabongo F, Veyckemans F. Use of remifentanil in combination with desflurane or propofol for ambulatory oral surgery. *Acta Anaesthesiol Belg.* 2001;52:181-186.
82. Sandler NA, Sparks BS. The use of bispectral analysis in patients undergoing intravenous sedation for third molar extractions. *J Oral Maxillofac Surg.* 2000;58:364-368.
83. Craig DC, Boyle CA, Fleming GJ, Palmer P. A sedation technique for implant and periodontal surgery. *J Clin Periodontol.* 2000;27:955-959.
84. Jackson DL, Johnson BS. Conscious sedation for dentistry: risk management and patient selection. *Dent Clin North Am.* 2002;46:767-780.
85. Jackson DL, Johnson BS. Inhalational and enteral conscious sedation for the adult dental patient. *Dent Clin North Am.* 2002;46:781-802.
86. Enever GR, Nunn JH, Sheehan JK. A comparison of postoperative morbidity following outpatient dental care under general anaesthesia in paediatric patients with and without disabilities. *Int J Paediatr Dent.* 2000;10:120-125.
87. Arch LM, Humphris GM, Lee GT. Children choosing between general anaesthesia or inhalation sedation for dental extractions: the effect on dental anxiety. *Int J Paediatr Dent.* 2001;11:41-48.
88. Bridgman CM, Ashby D, Holloway PJ. An investigation of the effects on children of tooth extraction under general anaesthesia in general dental practice. *Br Dent J.* 1999;186:245-247.
89. McComb M, Koenigsberg SR, Broder HL, Houpt M. The effects of oral conscious sedation on future behavior and anxiety in pediatric dental patients. *Pediatr Dent.* 2002;24:207-211.
90. Koroluk LD. Dental anxiety in adolescents with a history of childhood dental sedation. *ASDC J Dent Child.* 2000;67:200-205.
91. Sadock BJ, Sadock VA. *Comprehensive Textbook of Psychiatry.* 7th ed. Philadelphia: Lippincott Williams & Wilkins; 2000:2503-2515.
92. Glass RM. Electroconvulsive therapy time to bring it out of the shadows. *JAMA.* 2001;285:1346-1348.

93. Ebert M, Loosen PT, Nurcombe B. *Current Diagnosis and Treatment in Psychiatry*. New York: McGraw-Hill; 2000:304-307.
94. Ding Z, White PF. Anesthesia for electroconvulsive therapy. *Anesth Analg*. 2002;94:1351-1364.
95. Stoelting RK. *Pharmacology and Physiology in Anesthetic Practice*. 3rd ed. Philadelphia: Lippincott-Raven; 1999:113, 472-473.
96. Zaidi NA, Khan FA. Comparison of thiopentone sodium and propofol for electroconvulsive therapy (ECT). *J Pak Med Assoc*. 2000;50:60-63.
97. Sa Rego MM, Inagaki Y, White PF. The cost-effectiveness of methohexital versus propofol for sedation during monitored anesthesia care. *Anesth Analg*. 1999;88:723-728.
98. Kadoi Y, et al. The comparative effects of propofol versus thiopentone on left ventricular function during electroconvulsive therapy. *Anaesth Intensive Care*. 2003;31:172-175.
99. White PF, Rawal S, Recart A, Thornton L, Litle M, Stool L. Can the bispectral index be used to predict seizure time and awakening after electroconvulsive therapy? *Anesth Analg*. 2003;96: 1636-1639.
100. Lemmens HJ, Levi DC, Debattista C, Brock-Utne JG. The timing of electroconvulsive therapy and bispectral index after anesthesia induction using different drugs does not affect seizure duration. *J Clin Anesth*. 2003;15:29-32.
101. Nashihara F, Saito S. Preictal bispectral index has a positive correlation with seizure duration during electroconvulsive therapy. *Anesth Analg*. 2002;94:1249-1252.
102. Folk JW, et al. Anesthesia for electroconvulsive therapy: a review. *J ECT*. 2000;16:157-170.
103. Kadar AG, Ing CH, White PF, Wakefield C, Kramer BA, Clark K. Anesthesia for electroconvulsive therapy in obese patients. *Anesth Analg*. 2002;94:360-361.
104. Auriacombe M, et al. Post-ECT agitation and plasma lactate concentrations. *J ECT*. 2000;16:263-267.
105. Recart A, Rawal S, White PF, Byerly S, Thornton L. The effect of remifentanil on seizure duration and acute hemodynamic responses to electroconvulsive therapy. *Anesth Analg*. 2003;96: 1047-1050.
106. Wajima Z, Yoshikawa T, Ogura A, et al. Intravenous verapamil blunts hyperdynamic responses during electroconvulsive therapy without altering seizure activity. *Anesth Analg*. 2002;95: 400-402.
107. Hobbs G, Mahajan R. *Imaging in Anaesthesia and Critical Care*. London: Churchill Livingstone; 2000:1-10.
108. Howatson-Jones I. Adverse reactions to contrast media. *Prof Nurse*. 2000;15:771-774.
109. Berkenstadt H, Perel A, Ram Z, Feldman Z, Nahtomi-Shick O, Hadani M. Anesthesia for magnetic resonance guided neurosurgery: initial experience with a new open magnetic resonance imaging system. *J Neurosurg Anesthesiol*. 2001;13:158-162.
110. Runge VM. Safety of approved MR contrast media for intravenous injection. *J Magn Reson Imaging*. 2000;12:205-213.
111. Runge VM. Safety of magnetic resonance contrast media. *Top Magn Reson Imaging*. 2001;12:309-314.
112. Lai YC, Manninen PH. Anesthesia for cerebral aneurysms: a comparison between interventional neuroradiology and surgery. *Can J Anaesth*. 2001;48:391-395.
113. Watkinson AF, Francis IS, Torrie P, Platts AD. Commentary: the role of anaesthesia in interventional radiology. *Br J Radiol*. 2002;75:105-106.
114. Strother CM. Interventional neuroradiology. *AJNR Am J Neuroradiol*. 2000;21:19-24.
115. Nakstad PH. Interventional neuroradiology. *Acta Radiol*. 1999;40:344-359.
116. Wikholm G. Transarterial embolectomy in acute stroke. *AJNR Am J Neuroradiol*. 2003;24:892-894.
117. van der Schaaf IC, Brilstra EH, Buskens E, Rinkel GJ. Endovascular treatment of aneurysms in the cavernous sinus: a systematic review on balloon occlusion of the parent vessel and embolization with coils. *Stroke*. 2002;33:313-318.
118. Lusseveld E, Brilstra EH, Nijssen PC, et al. Endovascular coiling versus neurosurgical clipping in patients with a ruptured basilar tip aneurysm. *J Neurol Neurosurg Psychiatry*. 2002;73:591-593.
119. Maddox TG. Adverse reactions to contrast material: recognition, prevention, and treatment. *Am Fam Physician*. 2002;66: 1229-1234.
120. Laroche D, Namour F, Lefrancois C, et al. Anaphylactoid and anaphylactic reactions to iodinated contrast material. *Allergy*. 1999;54(suppl):13-16, 1999.
121. Hong SJ, Wong JT, Bloch KJ. Reactions to radiocontrast media. *Allergy Asthma Proc*. 2002;23:347-351.
122. Nakamura I, Hori S, Funabiki T, et al. Cardiopulmonary arrest induced by anaphylactoid reaction with contrast media. *Resuscitation*. 2002;53:223-226.
123. Webb JA, et al. Late adverse reactions to intravascular iodinated contrast media. *Eur Radiol*. 2003;13:181-184.
124. Hazinski MF, Cummins RO, Field JM. *2000 Handbook of Emergency Cardiovascular Care for Healthcare Providers*. Dallas: American Heart Association; 2000:21.
125. Sutherland P, Platt M. Sedation and general anaesthesia in children undergoing MRI and CT. *Br J Anaesth*. 2000;85:803-880.
126. Malviya S, Voepel-Lewis T, Eldevik OP, Rockwell DT, Wong JH, Tait AR. Sedation and general anaesthesia in children undergoing MRI and CT: adverse events and outcomes. *Br J Anaesth*. 2000;84:743-748.
127. Davis C, Razavi R, Baker EJ. Sedation versus general anesthesia for MRI scanning in children. *Arch Dis Child*. 2000;83:276.
128. Haeseler G, Zuzan O, Kohn G, Piepenbrock S, Leuwer M. Anaesthesia with midazolam and S-(+)-ketamine in spontaneously breathing paediatric patients during magnetic resonance imaging. *Paediatr Anaesth*. 2000;10:513-519.
129. Auden SM. This little piggy went to MRI: the tale of the toe test. *Anesth Analg*. 2001;93:241.
130. Farling P, McBrien ME, Winder RJ. Magnetic resonance compatible equipment: read the small print. *Anaesthesia*. 2003;58:86-87.
131. Schwartz AJ. Randall Pauley and the respiratory monitoring apparatus. *AANA Newsletter*. 2003;57:30.
132. Hashimoto T, Gupta DK, Young WL. Interventional neuroradiology—anesthetic considerations. *Anesthesiol Clin North America*. 2002;20:347-359.
133. Munte S, Munte TF, Kuche H, et al. General anesthesia for interventional neuroradiology: propofol versus isoflurane. *J Clin Anesth*. 2001;13:186-192.

Index